2000–2001 AHA Guide Code Chart

Hospital, Address, Telephone, Administrator, Approval, Facility, and Physician Codes, Health Care System, Network	Classi-fication Codes		Utilization Data					Expense (thousands) of dollars		
	Control	Service	Staffed Beds	Admissions	Census	Outpatient Visits	Births	Total	Payroll	Personnel
★ American Hospital Association (AHA) membership ☐ Joint Commission on Accreditation of Healthcare Organizations (JCAHO) accreditation + American Osteopathic Healthcare Association (AOHA) membership ○ American Osteopathic Association (AOA) accreditation △ Commission on Accreditation of Rehabilitation Facilities (CARF) accreditation Control codes 61, 63, 64, 71, 72 and 73 indicate hospitals listed by AOHA, but not registered by AHA. For definition of numerical codes, see page A4										
ANYTOWN—Universal County ★ COMMUNITY HOSPITAL, First Street and Main Avenue Zip 62835; tel 204/391–2345; Jane Doe, Administrator **A**1 2 3 4 6 9 10 **F**1 2 3 4 5 6 8 9 10 23 24 34; **P**1 2 3 4; **S** Acme HCS	23	10	346	10778	248	75953	1693	20695	9973	796

1 Approval Codes

Reported by the approving bodies specified, as of the dates noted.

1 Accreditation under the hospital program of the Joint Commission on Accreditation of Healthcare Organizations (March 2000).
2 Cancer program approved by American College of Surgeons (March 2000).
†3 Approval to participate in residency training, by the Accreditation Council for Graduate Medical Education (March 2000). As of June 30, 1975, internship (formerly code 4) was included under residency, code 3.
†5 Medical school affiliation, reported to the American Medical Association (March 2000).
6 Hospital–controlled professional nursing school, reported by National League for Nursing.
7 Accreditation by Commission on Accreditation of Rehabilitation Facilities (March 2000).
8 Member of Council of Teaching Hospitals of the Association of American Medical Colleges (January 2000).
9 Hospitals contracting or participating in a Plan, reported by the Blue Cross and Blue Shield Association (April 2000).
10 Certified for participation in the Health Insurance for the Aged (Medicare) Program by the U.S. Department of Health and Human Services (January 2000).
11 Accreditation by American Osteopathic Association (April 2000).
12 Internship approved by American Osteopathic Association (April 2000).
13 Residency approved by American Osteopathic Association (April 2000).
18 Critical Access Hospitals (January 2000).

Nonreporting indicates that the hospital was registered **after** the mailing of the 1999 Annual Survey, or, that the 1999 Annual Survey questionnaire for the hospital had not been received prior to publication.

2 Facility Codes

Provided directly by the hospital, its health care system, or network, or through a formal arrangement with another provider in the hospital's local community; for definitions, see page A6.

(Alphabetical/Numerical Order)

1 Adult day care program
2 Alcoholism–drug abuse or dependency inpatient unit
3 Alcoholism–drug abuse or dependency outpatient services
4 Angioplasty
5 Arthritis treatment center
6 Assisted living
7 Auxiliary organization
8 Birthing room–LDR room–LDRP room
9 Breast cancer screening/mammograms
10 Burn care services
11 Cardiac catheterization laboratory
12 Cardiac intensive care services
13 Case management
14 Children wellness program
15 Chiropractic services
16 Community health reporting
17 Community health status assessment
18 Community health status based service planning
19 Community outreach
20 Complementary medicine
21 Crisis prevention
22 CT scanner
23 Dental services
24 Diagnostic radioisotope facility
25 Emergency department
26 End of life care
27 Extracorporeal shock wave lithotripter (ESWL)
28 Fitness center
29 Freestanding outpatient care center
30 Geriatric services
31 Health facility transportation (to/from)
32 Health fair
33 Health information center
34 Health screenings
35 HIV–AIDS services
36 Home health services
37 Hospice
38 Hospital–based outpatient care center–services
39 Magnetic resonance imaging (MRI)
40 Meals on wheels
41 Medical surgical intensive care services
42 Neonatal intensive care services
43 Nutrition programs
44 Obstetrics services
45 Occupational health services
46 Oncology services
47 Open heart surgery
48 Outpatient surgery
49 Pain management services
50 Patient education center
51 Patient representative services
52 Pediatric intensive care services
53 Physical rehabilitation inpatient services
54 Physical rehabilitation outpatient services
55 Positron emission tomography scanner (PET)
56 Primary care department
57 Psychiatric acute inpatient services
58 Psychiatric child adolescent services
59 Psychiatric consultation–liaison services
60 Psychiatric education services
61 Psychiatric emergency services
62 Psychiatric geriatric services
63 Psychiatric outpatient services
64 Psychiatric partial hospitalization program
65 Radiation therapy
66 Reproductive health services
67 Retirement housing
68 Single photon emission computerized tomography (SPECT)
69 Skilled nursing or other long–term care services
70 Social work services
71 Sports medicine
72 Support groups
73 Teen outreach services
74 Transplant services
75 Trauma center (certified)
76 Ultrasound
77 Urgent care center
78 Volunteer services department
79 Women's health center/services

†Data from the Graduate Medical Education Database, Copyright 1999, American Medical Association, Chicago, Illinois.

Hospital, Address, Telephone, Administrator, Approval, Facility, and Physician Codes, Health Care System, Network	Classification Codes		Utilization Data					Expense (thousands) of dollars		
★ American Hospital Association (AHA) membership □ Joint Commission on Accreditation of Healthcare Organizations (JCAHO) accreditation + American Osteopathic Healthcare Association (AOHA) membership ○ American Osteopathic Association (AOA) accreditation △ Commission on Accreditation of Rehabilitation Facilities (CARF) accreditation Control codes 61, 63, 64, 71, 72 and 73 indicate hospitals listed by AOHA, but not registered by AHA. For definition of numerical codes, see page A4	Control	Service	Staffed Beds	Admissions	Census	Outpatient Visits	Births	Total	Payroll	Personnel
ANYTOWN—Universal County ★ COMMUNITY HOSPITAL, First Street and Main Avenue Zip 62835; tel 204/391–2345; Jane Doe, Administrator **A**1 2 3 4 6 9 10 **F**1 2 3 4 5 6 8 9 10 23 24 34; **P**1 2 3 4; **S** Acme HCS **N** ABC	23	10	346	10778	248	75953	1693	20695	9973	796

3 Physician Codes

Actually available within, and reported by the institution; for definitions, see page A9.

(Alphabetical/Numerical Order)
1. Closed physician–hospital organization (PHO)
2. Equity model
3. Foundation
4. Group practice without walls
5. Independent practice association (IPA)
6. Integrated salary model
7. Management service organization (MSO)
8. Open physician–hospital organization (PHO)

4 Health Care System Code and Name

A code number has been assigned to each health care system headquarters. The inclusion of one of these codes (1) indicates that the hospital belongs to a health care system and (2) identifies the specific system to which the hospital belongs.

6 Classification Codes

Control

Government, nonfederal
- 12 State
- 13 County
- 14 City
- 15 City–county
- 16 Hospital district or authority

Nongovernment not–for–profit
- 21 Church operated
- 23 Other

Investor–owned (for–profit)
- 31 Individual
- 32 Partnership
- 33 Corporation

Government, federal
- 41 Air Force
- 42 Army
- 43 Navy
- 44 Public Health Service other than 47
- 45 Veterans Affairs
- 46 Federal other than 41–45, 47–48
- 47 Public Health Service Indian Service
- 48 Department of Justice

Osteopathic
- 61 Church operated
- 63 Other not–for–profit
- 64 Other
- 71 Individual for–profit
- 72 Partnership for–profit
- 73 Corporation for–profit

Service
- 10 General medical and surgical
- 11 Hospital unit of an institution (prison hospital, college infirmary, etc.)
- 12 Hospital unit within an institution for the mentally retarded
- 22 Psychiatric
- 33 Tuberculosis and other respiratory diseases
- 44 Obstetrics and gynecology
- 45 Eye, ear, nose, and throat
- 46 Rehabilitation
- 47 Orthopedic
- 48 Chronic disease
- 49 Other specialty
- 50 Children's general
- 51 Children's hospital unit of an institution
- 52 Children's psychiatric
- 53 Children's tuberculosis and other respiratory diseases
- 55 Children's eye, ear, nose, and throat
- 56 Children's rehabilitation
- 57 Children's orthopedic
- 58 Children's chronic disease
- 59 Children's other specialty
- 62 Institution for mental retardation
- 82 Alcoholism and other chemical dependency

* Control codes 61, 63, 64, 71, 72 and 73 indicate hospitals listed by the AOHA but not registered by AHA.

When a hospital restricts its service to a specialty not defined by a specific code, it is coded 49 (59 if a children's hospital) and the specialty is indicated in parentheses following the name of the hospital.

7 Headings

Definitions are based on the American Hospital Association's Hospital Administration Terminology. In completing the survey, hospitals were requested to report data for a full year, in accord with their fiscal year, ending in 1999. Hospitals reporting for less than a 12–month period are so designated.

Utilization Data:

Beds–Number of beds, cribs, and pediatric bassinets regularly maintained (set up and staffed for use) for inpatients as of the close of the reporting period.

Admissions–Number of patients accepted for inpatient service during a 12–month period; does not include newborn.

Census–Average number of inpatients receiving care each day during the 12–month reporting period; does not include newborn.

Outpatient Visits–A visit by a patient who is not lodged in the hospital while receiving medical, dental, or other services. Each appearance of an outpatient in each unit constitutes one visit regardless of the number of diagnostic and/or therapeutic treatments that a patient receives.

Births–Number of infants born in the hospital and accepted for service in a newborn infant bassinet during a 12–month period; excludes stillbirths.

Expense: Expense for a 12–month period; both total expense and payroll components are shown. Payroll expenses include all salaries and wages.

Personnel: Represents personnel situations as they existed at the end of the reporting period; includes full-time equivalents of part–time personnel. Full-time equivalents were calculated on the basis that two part–time persons equal one full–time person.

AHA Guide™ to the Health Care Field

2000–2001 Edition

AHA Guide™ to the Health Care Field

AHA Institutional Members $180
Nonmembers $325
AHA Item Number 010000
Telephone ORDERS 1–800–AHA–2626

Online ORDERS www.ahaonlinestore.com

ISSN 0094–8969
ISBN 0–87258–757–6

Copyright © 1986–1996 American Hospital Association
Copyright © 1997–1998 Healthcare InfoSource, Inc., a subsidiary of the American Hospital Association
Copyright © 2000 Health Forum LLC, an affiliate of the American Hospital Association

All rights reserved. No portion of the AHA Guide may be duplicated or reproduced without prior written consent of Health Forum, LLC.
Printed in the U.S.A.

Contents

Section

	v	Acknowledgements and Advisements
	vi	Introduction
	viii	AHA Offices, Officers, and Historical Data

A — Hospitals Institutional and Associate Members

	A1	Contents of Section A
	2	Registration Requirements for Hospitals
	4	Explanation of Hospital Listings
	6	Annual Survey
	11	Hospitals in the United States, by State
	481	Hospitals in Areas Associated with the United States, by Area
	485	U.S. Government Hospitals Outside the United States, by Area
	486	Index of Hospitals
	521	Index of Health Care Professionals
	581	AHA Membership Categories
	582	Other Institutional Members
	588	Associate Members

B — Networks, Health Care Systems and Alliances

	B1	Contents of Section B
	2	Introduction
	3	Networks and their Hospitals
	49	Statistics for Multihospital Health Care Systems and their Hospitals
	50	Health Care Systems and their Hospitals
	156	Headquarters of Health Care Systems, Geographically
	163	Alliances

© 2000 AHA Guide

Section

C Lists of Health Organizations, Agencies and Providers

C1	Contents of Section C
2	Description of Lists
3	National Organizations
12	Healthfinder
29	International Organizations
31	U.S. Government Agencies
32	Blue Cross and Blue Shield Plans
34	Health Systems Agencies
35	Hospital Associations
37	Hospital Licensure Agencies
39	Medical and Nursing Licensure Agencies
42	Peer Review Organizations
43	State Health Planning and Development Agencies
44	State and Provincial Government Agencies
57	Health Maintenance Organizations
69	State Government Agencies for Health Maintenance Organizations
71	Freestanding Ambulatory Surgery Centers
98	State Government Agencies for Freestanding Ambulatory Surgery Centers
100	Freestanding Hospices
120	State Government Agencies for Freestanding Hospices
122	JCAHO Accredited Freestanding Long–Term Care Organizations†
146	JCAHO Accredited Freestanding Mental Health Care Organizations†
156	JCAHO Accredited Freestanding Substance Abuse Organizations†

D Indexes

D1	Abbreviations Used in the AHA Guide
2	Index

† List supplied by the Joint Commission on Accreditation of Healthcare Organizations

Acknowledgements and Advisements

Acknowledgements

The AHA Guide™ to the Health Care Field is published annually by Health Forum LLC, an affiliate of the American Hospital Association. Contributions made by Information Systems and Technology, Member Relations, Office of the President, Office of the Secretary, Printing Services Group and Resource Center.

Health Forum LLC acknowledges the cooperation given by many professional groups and government agencies in the health care field, particularly the following: American College of Surgeons; American Medical Association; American Osteopathic Healthcare Association; Blue Cross and Blue Shield Association; Council of Teaching Hospitals of the Association of American Medical Colleges; Joint Commission on Accreditation of Healthcare Organizations; Commission on Accreditation of Rehabilitation Facilities; American Osteopathic Association; Health Care Financing Administration; and various offices within the U.S. Department of Health and Human Services.

Advisements

The data published here should be used with the following advisements: The data are based on replies to an annual survey that seeks a variety of information, not all of which is published in this book. The information gathered by the survey includes specific services, but not all of each hospital's services. Therefore, the data do not reflect an exhaustive list of all services offered by all hospitals. For information on the availability of additional data, please contact Health Forum LLC at 800/821–2039.

Health Forum LLC does not assume responsibility for the accuracy of information voluntarily reported by the individual institutions surveyed. **The purpose of this publication is to provide basic data reflecting the delivery of health care in the United States and associated areas, and is not to serve as an official and all inclusive list of services offered by individual hospitals. The information reflected is based on data collected as of May 5, 2000.**

© 2000 AHA Guide

Introduction

Each of the three major sections of the AHA Guide begins with its own table of contents and pertinent definitions or explanatory information. Sections B, C and indices have bleed bar tabs for easy identification. The three major sections are:
- Hospitals
- Networks, Health Care Systems and Alliances
- Health Organizations, Agencies and other Health Care Providers

Please note that many area codes may have changed, check before you call.

Hospitals

This section lists:
- AHA–registered and osteopathic hospitals in the U.S. and associated areas, by state within city.
- U.S. government hospitals outside the United States.
- Index of hospitals alphabetically.
- Index of health care professionals.
- AHA Associate members.

AHA member hospitals are identified by a star (★). Hospitals accredited under one of the programs of the Joint Commission on Accreditation of Healthcare Organizations are identified by a hollow box (□). Preceding the list of hospitals is a statement of the formal requirements for registration by the AHA.

The lists provide a variety of information about each hospital, including the administrator's name; various approvals; selected facilities and services; relationship to a health care system; classification by control, service; physician arrangement relationships, and other selected statistical data from the 1999 AHA Annual Survey.

Also the *AHA Guide* includes state population data from the U.S. Bureau of the Census, *Statistical Abstract of the United States: 1999. (119th edition.) Washington, DC, 1999. They include the following:*
- Total resident population (in thousands)
- Percent of resident population in metro areas
- Birth rate per 1,000 population
- Percent of population 65 years and over
- Percent of persons without health insurance

Some of this information is coded. These include approval, facility and classification codes.

Approval codes refer to approvals held by a hospital; they represent information supplied by various national approving and reporting bodies. For example, code A–1 indicates accreditation under one of the programs of the Joint Commission on Accreditation of Healthcare Organizations – formal evidence that a hospital meets established standards for quality of patient care.

Physician codes refer to the different types of physician arrangements in which the hospital participates.

Health Care system names reference specific health care system headquarters. The presence of the system name indicates the hospital belongs to a health care system. Absence of a system name indicates that the hospital does not belong to a health care system.

Classification codes indicate the type of organization that controls or operates the hospital and type of service. Code numbers in the 10s denote nonfederal (states and local) government hospitals; in the 20s, nongovernment not–for–profit hospitals; in the 40s, federal government hospitals; and in the 60s and 70s, nonregistered osteopathic hospitals.

Among **service codes**, the most common code is 10, indicating a general hospital. Other numbers designate various special services. For example, code 22 indicates psychiatric hospitals and codes in the 50s indicate different types of children's hospitals.

Facility codes refer to facilities and services provided directly by the hospital, its health care system or network or through a formal arrangement with another provider.

(For easy reference, there is an alphabetical/numerical list for all of the codes on page A4).

Names of osteopathic hospitals, supplied by the American Osteopathic Healthcare Association are provided in the list of hospitals. Codes and symbols identifying these institutions are explained on page A4 and in the headnote at the top of each page of the list of hospitals. Also included in this section is an **index of hospitals** in alphabetical order by hospital name, followed by the city and state and the page reference to the hospital's listing in Section A. This section is designated by tabs along the side of the pages. Immediately following this section is an **index of health care professionals** in alphabetical order by name, followed by the hospital and/or health care system, the city and state and the page reference to the health care professional's listing in section A or B. This section is also designated by tabs along the side of the pages.

This section also lists **other AHA institutional members** not listed elsewhere in the AHA Guide and **AHA associate members.** The list of AHA institutional members includes Canadian hospitals, associated university programs in health administration, hospital schools of nursing, and nonhospital preacute and postacute care facilities. The list of associate members includes ambulatory centers and home care agencies, Blue Cross plans, health maintenance organizations/health care corporations, health system agencies, other inpatient care institutions, shared services organizations and other associate members.

Networks, Health Care Systems and Alliances

Networks
The *AHA Guide* lists the names and addresses of networks including network partners by state, alphabetically by name. **Please see page B2 for more information.**

Health Care Systems
This is an alphabetical listing of health care systems and their hospitals. Data on bed size for each hospital in the system is provided along with an indication of whether the hospital is owned, leased, sponsored, or contract–managed. Where available a health care system is assigned to one of five categories based on how much they differentiate and centralize their hospital services, physician arrangements, and provider-based insurance products.

Following this listing is an index for health care system headquarters listed geographically by state. **Please see page B2 for more information.**

Alliances
Alliances provide information on multistate alliances and their members. Alliances are listed alphabetically by name. Members are listed alphabetically by state, city and then by name. **Please see page B2 for more information.**

Health Organizations, Agencies and Other Health Care Providers

There are four major categories in this section.

First is an alphabetical listing of national, international, and regional organizations. Many voluntary organizations that are interested in, or of interest to, the health care field are included. Also included is the Healthfinder® listing.

© 2000 AHA Guide

The second category lists United States government agencies.

The third category presents a list of state and local organizations and government agencies. The list for states and provinces include Blue Cross and Blue Shield plans, health systems agencies, hospital associations and councils, hospital licensure agencies, medical and nursing licensure agencies, peer review organizations, state health planning and development agencies, and state and provincial government agencies.

The fourth category consists of lists of various health care providers including JCAHO accredited freestanding long-term care organizations, JCAHO accredited freestanding substance abuse organizations, and JCAHO accredited freestanding mental health care organizations, freestanding hospices, freestanding ambulatory surgery centers and health maintenance organizations (HMOs). **Please see page C2 for more information**.

These lists are provided for your information and are not exhaustive. Inclusion or omission of any organization's name indicates neither approval nor disapproval by Health Forum LLC.

We hope you find *AHA Guide* a valuable resource. If you have any questions or comments, please call Health Forum LLC, at 800/821–2039.

AHA Offices, Officers, and Historical Data

Chicago: One North Franklin, Chicago, IL 60606–3401; tel. 312/422–3000

Washington: 325 Seventh Street, N.W., Suite 700, Washington, DC 20004; tel. 202/638–1100

San Francisco: Health Forum, 425 Market Street, 34th Floor, San Francisco, CA 94105

Immediate Past Chairman of the Board of Trustees: Fred L. Brown, FACHE, BJC Health System, 120 S. Central, Suite 1200, St. Louis, MO 63105

Chairman of the Board of Trustees: Carolyn Boone Lewis, Washington Hospital Center, 2920 W Street, S.E., Washington, DC 20020

Chairman–Elect of the Board of Trustees: Gary A. Mecklenburg, Northwestern Memorial Hospital, Feinberg Inpatient Pavilion, Suite 3–708, 251 East Huron Street, Chicago, IL 60611

President: Richard J. Davidson, 325 Seventh Street, N.W., Suite 700, Washington, DC 20004

Senior Vice President and Secretary: Michael P. Guerin, One North Franklin, Chicago, IL 60606–3401

Treasurer: John Evans, One North Franklin, Chicago, IL 60606–3401

Past Presidents/Chairs†

Year	Name	Year	Name	Year	Name
1899	★James S. Knowles	1932	★Paul H. Fesler	1967	George E. Cartmill
1900	★James S. Knowles	1933	★George F. Stephens, M.D.	1968	★David B. Wilson, M.D.
1901	★Charles S. Howell	1934	★Nathaniel W. Faxon, M.D.	1969	★George William Graham, M.D.
1902	★J. T. Duryea	1935	★Robert Jolly	1970	★Mark Berke
1903	★John Fehrenbatch	1936	★Robin C. Buerki, M.D.	1971	★Jack A. L. Hahn
1904	★Daniel D. Test	1937	★Claude W. Munger, M.D.	1972	Stephen M. Morris
1905	★George H. M. Rowe, M.D.	1938	★Robert E. Neff	1973	★John W. Kauffman
1906	★George P. Ludlam	1939	★G. Harvey Agnew, M.D.	1974	★Horace M. Cardwell
1907	★Renwick R. Ross, M.D.	1940	★Fred G. Carter, M.D.	1975	Wade Mountz
1908	★Sigismund S. Goldwater, M.D.	1941	★B. W. Black, M.D.	1976	H. Robert Cathcart
1909	★John M. Peters, M.D.	1942	★Basil C. MacLean, M.D.	1977	John M. Stagl
1910	★H. B. Howard, M.D.	1943	★James A. Hamilton	1978	★Samuel J. Tibbitts
1911	★W. L. Babcock, M.D.	1944	★Frank J. Walter	1979	W. Daniel Barker
1912	★Henry M. Hurd, M.D.	1945	★Donald C. Smelzer, M.D.	1980	★Sister Irene Kraus
1913	★F. A. Washburn, M.D.	1946	★Peter D. Ward, M.D.	1981	Bernard J. Lachner
1914	★Thomas Howell, M.D.	1947	★John H. Hayes	1982	Stanley R. Nelson
1915	★William O. Mann, M.D.	1948	★Graham L. Davis	1983	Elbert E. Gilbertson
1916	★Winford H. Smith, M.D.	1949	★Joseph G. Norby	1984	Thomas R. Matherlee
1917	★Robert J. Wilson, M.D.	1950	★John H. Hatfield	1985	Jack A. Skarupa
1918	★A. B. Ancker, M.D.	1951	★Charles F. Wilinsky, M.D.	1986	Scott S. Parker
1919	★A. R. Warner, M.D.	1952	★Anthony J. J. Rourke, M.D.	1987	Donald C. Wegmiller
1920	★Joseph B. Howland, M.D.	1953	★Edwin L. Crosby, M.D.	1988	Eugene W. Arnett
1921	★Louis B. Baldwin, M.D.	1954	★Ritz E. Heerman	1989	Edward J. Connors
1922	★George O'Hanlon, M.D.	1955	★Frank R. Bradley	1990	David A. Reed
1923	★Asa S. Bacon	1956	★Ray E. Brown	1991	C. Thomas Smith
1924	★Malcolm T. MacEachern, M.D.	1957	★Albert W. Snoke, M.D.	1992	D. Kirk Oglesby, Jr.
1925	★E. S. Gilmore	1958	★Tol Terrell	1993	Larry L. Mathis
1926	★Arthur C. Bachmeyer, M.D.	1959	★Ray Amberg	1994	Carolyn C. Roberts
1927	★R. G. Brodrick, M.D.	1960	Russell A. Nelson, M.D.	1995	Gail L. Warden
1928	★Joseph C. Doane, M.D.	1961	★Frank S. Groner	1996	Gordon M. Sprenger
1929	★Louis H. Burlingham, M.D.	1962	★Jack Masur, M.D.	1997	Reginald M. Ballantyne III
1930	★Christopher G. Parnall, M.D.	1963	T. Stewart Hamilton, M.D.	1998	John G. King
1931	★Lewis A. Sexton, M.D.	1964	★Stanley A. Ferguson	1999	Fred L. Brown
		1965	Clarence E. Wonnacott		
		1966	★Philip D. Bonnet, M.D.		

Chief Executive Officers

Years	Name	Years	Name	Years	Name
1917–18	★William H. Walsh, M.D.	1943–54	★George Bugbee	1986–91	Carol M. McCarthy, Ph.D., J.D.
1919–24	★Andrew Robert Warner, M.D.	1954–72	★Edwin L. Crosby, M.D.	1991	Jack W. Owen (acting)
1925–27	★William H. Walsh, M.D.	1972	Madison B. Brown, M.D. (acting)	1991	Richard J. Davidson (current)
1928–42	★Bert W. Caldwell, M.D.	1972–86	J. Alexander McMahon		

Distinguished Service Award

Year	Name	Year	Name	Year	Name
1934	Matthew O. Foley	1959	Edwin L. Crosby, M.D.	1982	R. Zach Thomas, Jr.
1939	Malcolm T. MacEachern, M.D.	1960	Oliver G. Pratt	1983	H. Robert Cathcart
1940	Sigismund S. Goldwater, M.D.	1961	E. M. Bluestone, M.D.	1984	Matthew F. McNulty, Jr., Sc.D.
1941	Frederic A. Washburn, M.D.	1962	Mother Loretto Bernard, S.C., R.N.	1985	J. Alexander McMahon
1942	Winford H. Smith, M.D.	1963	Ray E. Brown	1986	Sister Irene Kraus
1943	Arthur C. Bachmeyer, M.D.	1964	Russell A. Nelson, M.D.	1987	W. Daniel Barker
1944	Rt. Rev. Msgr. Maurice F. Griffin, LL.D.	1965	Albert W. Snoke, M.D.	1988	Elbert E. Gilbertson
1945	Asa S. Bacon	1966	Frank S. Groner	1989	Donald G. Shropshire
1946	George F. Stephens, M.D.	1967	Rev. John J. Flanagan, S.J.	1990	John W. Colloton
1947	Robin C. Buerki, M.D.	1968	Stanley W. Martin	1991	Carol M. McCarthy, Ph.D., J.D.
1948	James A. Hamilton	1969	T. Stewart Hamilton, M.D.	1992	David H. Hitt
1949	Claude W. Munger, M.D.	1970	Charles Patteson Cladwell, Jr.	1993	Edward J. Connors
1950	Nathaniel W. Faxon, M.D.	1971	Mark Berke		Jack W. Owen
1951	Bert W. Caldwell, M.D.	1972	Stanley A. Ferguson	1994	George Adams
1952	Fred G. Carter, M.D.	1973	Jack A. L. Hahn	1995	Scott S. Parker
1953	Basil C. MacLean, M.D.	1974	George William Graham, M.D.	1996	John A. Russell
1954	George Bugbee	1975	George E. Cartmill	1997	D. Kirk Oglesby, Jr.
1955	Joseph G. Norby	1976	D. O. McClusky, Jr.	1998	Henry B. Betts, M.D.
1956	Charles F. Wilinsky, M.D.	1977	Boone Powell	1999	Mitchell T. Rabkin, M.D.
1957	John H. Hayes	1978	Richard J. Stull	2000	Gail L. Warden
1958	John N. Hatfield	1979	Horace M. Cardwell		
		1980	Donald W. Cordes		
		1981	Sister Mary Brigh Cassidy		

★Deceased

†On June 3, 1972, the House of Delegates changed the title of the chief elected officer to chairman of the Board of Trustees, and the title of president was conferred on the chief executive officer of the Association.

Award of Honor

1966	Senator Lister Hill	1992	Donald W. Dunn		Mothers Against Drunk Driving (MADD)
1967	Emory W. Morris, D.D.S.		Ira M. Lane, Jr.	1997	Paul B. Batalden, M.D.
1971	Special Committee on Provision of Health Services (staff also)	1993	Elliott C. Roberts, Sr. William A. Spencer, M.D.	1998	Habitat for Humanity International John E. Curley, Jr.
1982	Walter J. McNerney	1994	Robert A. Derzon		National Civic League
1989	Ruth M. Rothstein	1995	Russell G. Mawby, Ph.D.	1999	Joseph Cardinal Bernardin, Literacy
1990	Joyce C. Clifford, R.N.		John K. Springer		Volunteers of America
1991	Haynes Rice	1996	Stephen J. Hegarty	2000	Institute for Safe Medication Practices

Justin Ford Kimball Innovators Award

1958	E. A. van Steenwyk	1972	John R. Mannix	1988	Ernest W. Saward, M.D.
1959	George A. Newbury	1973	Herman M. Somers	1990	James A. Vohs
1960	C. Rufus Rorem, Ph.D.	1974	William H. Ford, Ph.D.	1993	John C. Lewin, M.D.
1961	James E. Stuart	1975	Earl H. Kammer	1994	Donald A. Brennan
1962	Frank Van Dyk	1976	J. Ed McConnell	1995	E. George Middleton, Jr.
1963	William S. McNary	1978	Edwin R. Werner		Glenn R. Mitchell
1964	Frank S. Groner	1979	Robert M. Cunningham, Jr.	1997	Harvey Pettry
1965	J. Douglas Colman	1981	Maurice J. Norby		D. David Sniff
1967	Walter J. McNerney	1982	Robert E. Rinehimer	1998	Montana Health Research and Education Foundation
1968	John W. Paynter	1983	John B. Morgan, Jr.		
1970	Edwin L. Crosby, M.D.	1984	Joseph F. Duplinsky	1999	Kenneth W. Kizer, M.D.
1971	H. Charles Abbott	1985	David W. Stewart		

Trustees Award

1959	Joseph V. Friel John H. Hayes	1974	James E. Hague Sister Marybelle	1987	Michael Lesparre
1960	Duncan D. Sutphen, Jr.	1975	Helen T. Yast	1988	Barbara A. Donaho, R.N.
1963	Eleanor C. Lambertsen, R.N., Ed.D.	1976	Boynton P. Livingston	1989	Walter H. MacDonald
1964	John R. Mannix		James Ludlam		Donald R. Newkirk
1965	Albert G. Hahn		Helen McGuire	1990	William T. Robinson
	Maurice J. Norby	1979	Newton J. Jacobson	1992	Jack C. Bills
1966	Madison B. Brown, M.D.		Edward W. Weimer		Anne Hall Davis
	Kenneth Williamson	1980	Robert B. Hunter, M.D.	1993	Theodore C. Eickhoff, M.D.
1967	Alanson W. Wilcox		Samuel J. Tibbitts		Stephen W. Gamble
1968	E. Dwight Barnett, M.D.	1981	Vernon A. Knutson		Yoshi Honkawa
1969	Vane M. Hoge, M.D.		John E. Sullivan	1994	Roger M. Busfield, Jr., Ph.D.
	Joseph H. McNinch, M.D.	1982	John Bigelow	1995	Stephen E. Dorn
1972	David F. Drake, Ph.D.		Robert W. O'Leary		William L. Yates
	Paul W. Earle		Jack W. Owen	1996	Leigh E. Morris
	Michael Lesparre	1984	Howard J. Berman		John Quigley
	Andrew Pattullo		O. Ray Hurst	1998	John D. Leech
1973	Tilden Cummings		James R. Neely	1999	Sister Carol Keehan
	Edmond J. Lanigan	1985	James E. Ferguson		C. Edward McCawley
			Cleveland Rodgers		Stephen Rogness
		1986	Rex N. Olsen	2000	Dennis May

Citation for Meritorious Service

1968	F. R. Knautz Sister Conrad Mary, R.N.		Susan Jenkins Gordon McLachlan	1982	Jorge Brull Nater
1971	Hospital Council of Southern California	1977	Theodore Cooper, M.D.	1983	David M. Kinzer
1972	College of Misericordia, Dallas, PA	1979	Norman D. Burkett	1984	Donald L. Custis, M.D.
1973	Madison B. Brown, M.D.		John L. Quigley	1985	John A. D. Cooper, M.D.
	Samuel J. Tibbitts		William M. Whelan		Imperial Council of the Ancient Arabic Order of the Nobles of the Mystic Shrine for North America
1975	Kenneth B. Babcock, M.D.	1980	Sister Grace Marie Hiltz		
	Sister Mary Maurita Sengelaube		Leo J. Gehrig, M.D.		
1976	Chaiker Abbis	1981	Richard Davi	1986	Howard F. Cook
			Pearl S. Fryar	1987	David H. Hitt Lucile Packard

This citation is no longer awarded

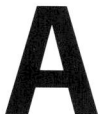

Hospitals, Institutional and Associate Members

A2	Registration Requirements for Hospitals
4	Explanation of Hospital Listings
6	Annual Survey
11	Hospitals in the United States, by State*
481	Hospitals in Areas Associated with the United States, by Area
485	U.S. Government Hospitals Outside the United States, by Area
486	Index of Hospitals
521	Index of Health Care Professionals
581	AHA Membership Categories
582	Other Institutional Members
582	*Types I–A Hospitals*
583	*Associated University Programs in Health Administration*
584	*Hospital Schools of Nursing*
585	*Nonhospital Preacute and Postacute Care Facilities*
587	*Provisional Hospitals*
588	Associate Members
588	*Ambulatory Centers and Home Care Agencies*
588	*Blue Cross Plans*
588	*Shared Services Organizations*
589	*Other Associate Members*

*AHA–registered hospitals in the United States and associated areas are approved for registration by the Executive Committee of the Board of Trustees of the American Hospital Association. This list of registered hospitals is complete as of April 2000. The list of osteopathic hospitals, integrated in this section is supplied by the American Osteopathic Healthcare Association.

Registration Requirements for Hospitals

This directory includes hospitals registered by the American Hospital Association and osteopathic hospitals listed by the American Osteopathic Association. Identification codes for both types of hospitals are explained fully on pages A4–5. For the reader's convenience, the codes for osteopathic hospitals are also summarized in the notes at the top of each page of this section. Beginning in November 1970, osteopathic hospitals became eligible to apply for registration with the American Hospital Association. Registered osteopathic hospitals carry the same codes as all other hospitals registered by the American Hospital Association.

The following requirements were approved by the Executive Committee of the Board of Trustees, May 13, 1986.

AHA–Registered Hospitals

Any institution that can be classified as a hospital according to the requirements may be registered if it so desires. Membership in the American Hospital Association is not a prerequisite.

The American Hospital Association may, at the sole discretion of the Executive Committee of the Board of Trustees, grant, deny, or withdraw the registration of an institution.

An institution may be registered by the American Hospital Association as a hospital if it is accredited as a hospital by the Joint Commission on Accreditation of Healthcare Organizations or is certified as a provider of acute services under Title 18 of the Social Security Act and has provided the Association with documents verifying the accreditation or certification.

In lieu of the preceding accreditation or certification, an institution licensed as a hospital by the appropriate state agency may be registered by AHA as a hospital by meeting the following alternative requirements:

Function: The primary function of the institution is to provide patient services, diagnostic and therapeutic, for particular or general medical conditions.

1. The institution shall maintain at least six inpatient beds, which shall be continuously available for the care of patients who are nonrelated and who stay on the average in excess of 24 hours per admission.
2. The institution shall be constructed, equipped, and maintained to ensure the health and safety of patients and to provide uncrowded, sanitary facilities for the treatment of patients.
3. There shall be an identifiable governing authority legally and morally responsible for the conduct of the hospital.
4. There shall be a chief executive to whom the governing authority delegates the continuous responsibility for the operation of the hospital in accordance with established policy.
5. There shall be an organized medical staff of fully licensed physicians* that may include other licensed individuals permitted by law and by the hospital to provide patient care services independently in the hospital. The medical staff shall be accountable to the governing authority for maintaining proper standards of medical care, and it shall be governed by bylaws adopted by said staff and approved by the governing authority.
6. Each patient shall be admitted on the authority of a member of the medical staff who has been granted the privilege to admit patients to inpatient services in accordance with state law and criteria for standards of medical care established by the individual medical staff. Each patient's general medical condition is the responsibility of a qualified physician member of the medical staff. When nonphysician members of the medical staff are granted privileges to admit patients, provision is made for prompt medical evaluation of these patients by a qualified physician. Any graduate of a foreign medical school who is permitted to assume responsibilities for patient care shall possess a valid license to practice medicine, or shall be certified by the Educational Commission for Foreign Medical Graduates, or shall have qualified for and have successfully completed an academic year of supervised clinical training under the direction of a medical school approved by the Liaison Committee onGAT Medical Education.
7. Registered nurse supervision and other nursing services are continuous.
8. A current and complete+ medical record shall be maintained by the institution for each patient and shall be available for reference.
9. Pharmacy service shall be maintained in the institution and shall be supervised by a registered pharmacist.
10. The institution shall provide patients with food service that meets their nutritional and therapeutic requirements; special diets shall also be available.

---

*Physician–Term used to describe an individual with an M.D. or D.O. degree who is fully licensed to practice medicine in all its phases.

‡The completed records in general shall contain at least the following: the patient's identifying data and consent forms, medical history, record of physical examination, physicians' progress notes, operative notes, nurses' notes, routine x–ray and laboratory reports, doctors' orders, and final diagnosis.

Types of Hospitals

In addition to meeting these 10 general registration requirements, hospitals are registered as one of four types of hospitals: general, special, rehabilitation and chronic disease, or psychiatric. The following definitions of function by type of hospital and special requirements for registration are employed:

General

The primary function of the institution is to provide patient services, diagnostic and therapeutic, for a variety of medical conditions. A general hospital also shall provide:
- diagnostic x-ray services with facilities and staff for a variety of procedures
- clinical laboratory service with facilities and staff for a variety of procedures and with anatomical pathology services regularly and conveniently available
- operating room service with facilities and staff.

Special

The primary function of the institution is to provide diagnostic and treatment services for patients who have specified medical conditions, both surgical and nonsurgical. A special hospital also shall provide:
- such diagnostic and treatment services as may be determined by the Executive Committee of the Board of Trustees of the American Hospital Association to be appropriate for the specified medical conditions for which medical services are provided shall be maintained in the institution with suitable facilities and staff. If such conditions do not normally require diagnostic x-ray service, laboratory service, or operating room service, and if any such services are therefore not maintained in the institution, there shall be written arrangements to make them available to patients requiring them.
- clinical laboratory services capable of providing tissue diagnosis when offering pregancy termination services.

Rehabilitation and Chronic Disease

The primary function of the institution is to provide diagnostic and treatment services to handicapped or disabled individuals requiring restorative and adjustive services. A rehabilitation and chronic disease hospital also shall provide:
- arrangements for diagnostic x-ray services, as required, on a regular and conveniently available basis
- arrangements for clinical laboratory service, as required on a regular and conveniently available basis
- arrangements for operating room service, as required, on a regular and conveniently available basis
- a physical therapy service with suitable facilities and staff in the institution
- an occupational therapy service with suitable facilities and staff in the institution
- arrangements for psychological and social work services on a regular and conveniently available basis
- arrangements for educational and vocational services on a regular and conveniently available basis
- written arrangements with a general hospital for the transfer of patients who require medical, obstetrical, or surgical services not available in the institution.

Psychiatric

The primary function of the institution is to provide diagnostic and treatment services for patients who have psychiatric-related illnesses. A psychiatric hospital also shall provide:
- arrangements for clinical laboratory service, as required, on a regular and conveniently available basis
- arrangements for diagnostic x-ray services, as required on a regular and conveniently available basis
- psychiatric, psychological, and social work service with facilities and staff in the institution
- arrangements for electroencephalograph services, as required, on a regular and conveniently available basis.
- written arrangements with a general hospital for the transfer of patients who require medical, obstetrical, or surgical services not available in the institution.

The American Hospital Association may, at the sole discretion of the Executive Committee of the Board of Trustees, grant, deny, or withdraw the registration of an institution.

AOHA-Listed Hospitals

The list of osteopathic hospitals includes both members and nonmembers of the American Osteopathic Healthcare Association.

---

*Physician–Term used to describe an individual with an M.D. or D.O. degree who is fully licensed to practice medicine in all its phases.

‡The completed records in general shall contain at least the following: the patient's identifying data and consent forms, medical history, record of physical examination, physicians' progress notes, operative notes, nurses' notes, routine x-ray and laboratory reports, doctors' orders, and final diagnosis.

Explanation of Hospital Listings

Hospital, Address, Telephone, Administrator, Approval, Facility, and Physician Codes, Health Care System, Network	Classification Codes		Utilization Data					Expense (thousands) of dollars		
★ American Hospital Association (AHA) membership □ Joint Commission on Accreditation of Healthcare Organizations (JCAHO) accreditation + American Osteopathic Healthcare Association (AOHA) membership ○ American Osteopathic Association (AOA) accreditation △ Commission on Accreditation of Rehabilitation Facilities (CARF) accreditation Control codes 61, 63, 64, 71, 72 and 73 indicate hospitals listed by AOHA, but not registered by AHA. For definition of numerical codes, see page A4	Control	Service	Staffed Beds	Admissions	Census	Outpatient Visits	Births	Total	Payroll	Personnel
ANYTOWN—Universal County ★ COMMUNITY HOSPITAL, First Street and Main Avenue Zip 62835; tel 204/391-2345; Jane Doe, Administrator **A**1 2 3 4 6 9 10 **F**1 2 3 4 5 6 8 9 10 23 24 34; **P**1 2 3 4; **S** Acme HCS	23	10	346	10778	248	75953	1693	20695	9973	796

1 Approval Codes

Reported by the approving bodies specified, as of the dates noted.

1. Accreditation under the hospital program of the Joint Commission on Accreditation of Healthcare Organizations (March 2000).
2. Cancer program approved by American College of Surgeons (March 2000).
†3. Approval to participate in residency training, by the Accreditation Council for Graduate Medical Education (March 2000). As of June 30, 1975, internship (formerly code 4) was included under residency, code 3.
†5. Medical school affiliation, reported to the American Medical Association (March 2000).
6. Hospital-controlled professional nursing school, reported by National League for Nursing.
7. Accreditation by Commission on Accreditation of Rehabilitation Facilities (March 2000).
8. Member of Council of Teaching Hospitals of the Association of American Medical Colleges (January 2000).
9. Hospitals contracting or participating in a Plan, reported by the Blue Cross and Blue Shield Association (April 2000).
10. Certified for participation in the Health Insurance for the Aged (Medicare) Program by the U.S. Department of Health and Human Services (January 2000).
11. Accreditation by American Osteopathic Association (April 2000).
12. Internship approved by American Osteopathic Association (April 2000).
13. Residency approved by American Osteopathic Association (April 2000).
18. Critical Access Hospitals (January 2000).

Nonreporting indicates that the hospital was registered **after** the mailing of the 1999 Annual Survey, or, that the 1999 Annual Survey questionnaire for the hospital had not been received prior to publication.

2 Facility Codes

Provided directly by the hospital, its health care system, or network, or through a formal arrangement with another provider in the hospital's local community; for definitions, see page A6.

(Alphabetical/Numerical Order)

1. Adult day care program
2. Alcoholism–drug abuse or dependency inpatient unit
3. Alcoholism–drug abuse or dependency outpatient services
4. Angioplasty
5. Arthritis treatment center
6. Assisted living
7. Auxiliary organization
8. Birthing room–LDR room–LDRP room
9. Breast cancer screening/mammograms
10. Burn care services
11. Cardiac catheterization laboratory
12. Cardiac intensive care services
13. Case management
14. Children wellness program
15. Chiropractic services
16. Community health reporting
17. Community health status assessment
18. Community health status based service planning
19. Community outreach
20. Complementary medicine
21. Crisis prevention
22. CT scanner
23. Dental services
24. Diagnostic radioisotope facility
25. Emergency department
26. End of life care
27. Extracorporeal shock wave lithotripter (ESWL)
28. Fitness center
29. Freestanding outpatient care center
30. Geriatric services
31. Health facility transportation (to/from)
32. Health fair
33. Health information center
34. Health screenings
35. HIV–AIDS services
36. Home health services
37. Hospice
38. Hospital-based outpatient care center–services
39. Magnetic resonance imaging (MRI)
40. Meals on wheels
41. Medical surgical intensive care services
42. Neonatal intensive care services
43. Nutrition programs
44. Obstetrics services
45. Occupational health services
46. Oncology services
47. Open heart surgery
48. Outpatient surgery
49. Pain management services
50. Patient education center
51. Patient representative services
52. Pediatric intensive care services
53. Physical rehabilitation inpatient services
54. Physical rehabilitation outpatient services
55. Positron emission tomography scanner (PET)
56. Primary care department
57. Psychiatric acute inpatient services
58. Psychiatric child adolescent services
59. Psychiatric consultation–liaison services
60. Psychiatric education services
61. Psychiatric emergency services
62. Psychiatric geriatric services
63. Psychiatric outpatient services
64. Psychiatric partial hospitalization program
65. Radiation therapy
66. Reproductive health services
67. Retirement housing
68. Single photon emission computerized tomography (SPECT)
69. Skilled nursing or other long-term care services
70. Social work services
71. Sports medicine
72. Support groups
73. Teen outreach services
74. Transplant services
75. Trauma center (certified)
76. Ultrasound
77. Urgent care center
78. Volunteer services department
79. Women's health center/services

---

†Data from the Graduate Medical Education Database, Copyright 1999, American Medical Association, Chicago, Illinois.

Explanation of Hospital Listings

Hospital, Address, Telephone, Administrator, Approval, Facility, and Physician Codes, Health Care System, Network	Classi-fication Codes		Utilization Data					Expense (thousands) of dollars		
★ American Hospital Association (AHA) membership ☐ Joint Commission on Accreditation of Healthcare Organizations (JCAHO) accreditation + American Osteopathic Healthcare Association (AOHA) membership ○ American Osteopathic Association (AOA) accreditation △ Commission on Accreditation of Rehabilitation Facilities (CARF) accreditation Control codes 61, 63, 64, 71, 72 and 73 indicate hospitals listed by AOHA, but not registered by AHA. For definition of numerical codes, see page A4	Control	Service	Staffed Beds	Admissions	Census	Outpatient Visits	Births	Total	Payroll	Personnel
ANYTOWN—Universal County ★ COMMUNITY HOSPITAL, First Street and Main Avenue Zip 62835; tel 204/391-2345; Jane Doe, Administrator **A**1 2 3 4 6 9 10 **F**1 2 3 4 5 6 8 9 10 23 24 34; **P**1 2 3 4; **S** Acme HCS **N** ABC	23	10	346	10778	248	75953	1693	20695	9973	796

4   6   7

3 Physician Codes

Actually available within, and reported by the institution; for definitions, see page A9.

(Alphabetical/Numerical Order)
1. Closed physician–hospital organization (PHO)
2. Equity model
3. Foundation
4. Group practice without walls
5. Independent practice association (IPA)
6. Integrated salary model
7. Management service organization (MSO)
8. Open physician–hospital organization (PHO)

4 Health Care System Code and Name

A code number has been assigned to each health care system headquarters. The inclusion of one of these codes (1) indicates that the hospital belongs to a health care system and (2) identifies the specific system to which the hospital belongs.

6 Classification Codes

Control

Government, nonfederal
12 State
13 County
14 City
15 City–county
16 Hospital district or authority

Nongovernment not–for–profit
21 Church operated
23 Other

Investor–owned (for–profit)
31 Individual
32 Partnership
33 Corporation

Government, federal
41 Air Force
42 Army
43 Navy
44 Public Health Service other than 47
45 Veterans Affairs
46 Federal other than 41–45, 47–48
47 Public Health Service Indian Service
48 Department of Justice

Osteopathic
61 Church operated
63 Other not–for–profit
64 Other
71 Individual for–profit
72 Partnership for–profit
73 Corporation for–profit

Service
10 General medical and surgical
11 Hospital unit of an institution (prison hospital, college infirmary, etc.)
12 Hospital unit within an institution for the mentally retarded
22 Psychiatric
33 Tuberculosis and other respiratory diseases
44 Obstetrics and gynecology
45 Eye, ear, nose, and throat
46 Rehabilitation
47 Orthopedic
48 Chronic disease
49 Other specialty
50 Children's general
51 Children's hospital unit of an institution
52 Children's psychiatric
53 Children's tuberculosis and other respiratory diseases
55 Children's eye, ear, nose, and throat
56 Children's rehabilitation
57 Children's orthopedic
58 Children's chronic disease
59 Children's other specialty
62 Institution for mental retardation
82 Alcoholism and other chemical dependency

* Control codes 61, 63, 64, 71, 72 and 73 indicate hospitals listed by the AOHA but not registered by AHA.
When a hospital restricts its service to a specialty not defined by a specific code, it is coded 49 (59 if a children's hospital) and the specialty is indicated in parentheses following the name of the hospital.

7 Headings

Definitions are based on the American Hospital Association's Hospital Administration Terminology. In completing the survey, hospitals were requested to report data for a full year, in accord with their fiscal year, ending in 1999. Hospitals reporting for less than a 12–month period are so designated.

Utilization Data:

Beds–Number of beds, cribs, and pediatric bassinets regularly maintained (set up and staffed for use) for inpatients as of the close of the reporting period.

Admissions–Number of patients accepted for inpatient service during a 12–month period; does not include newborn.

Census–Average number of inpatients receiving care each day during the 12–month reporting period; does not include newborn.

Outpatient Visits–A visit by a patient who is not lodged in the hospital while receiving medical, dental, or other services. Each appearance of an outpatient in each unit constitutes one visit regardless of the number of diagnostic and/or therapeutic treatments that a patient receives.

Births–Number of infants born in the hospital and accepted for service in a newborn infant bassinet during a 12–month period; excludes stillbirths.

Expense: Expense for a 12–month period; both total expense and payroll components are shown. Payroll expenses include all salaries and wages.

Personnel: Represents personnel situations as they existed at the end of the reporting period; includes full–time equivalents of part–time personnel. Full–time equivalents were calculated on the basis that two part–time persons equal one full–time person.

© 2000 AHA Guide

Annual Survey

Each year, an annual survey of hospitals is conducted by the American Hospital Association through its Health Forum affiliate.

The facilities and services found below are either provided by the hospital, its health care system, or network or through a formal arrangement with another provider in the local community of the hospital.

The AHA Guide to the Health Care Field does not include all data collected from the 1999 Annual Survey. Requests for purchasing other Annual Survey data should be directed to Health Forum LLC, an affiliate of the American Hospital Association, One North Franklin, Chicago, IL 60606–3401, 800/821–2039.

Definitions of Facility Codes

1. **Adult day care program** Program providing supervision, medical and psychological care, and social activities for older adults who live at home or in another family setting, but cannot be alone or prefer to be with others during the day. May include intake assessment, health monitoring, occupational therapy, personal care, noon meal, and transportation services.

2. **Alcoholism–drug abuse or dependency inpatient services** Provides, diagnosis and therapeutic services to patients with alcoholism or other drug dependencies. Includes care for inpatient/residential treatment for patients whose course of treatment involves more intensive care than provided in an outpatient setting or where patient requires supervised withdrawal.

3. **Alcoholism–drug abuse or dependency outpatient services** Organized hospital services that provide medical care and/or rehabilitative treatment services to outpatients for whom the primary diagnosis is alcoholism or other chemical dependency.

4. **Angioplasty** The reconstruction or restructuring of a blood vessel by operative means or by nonsurgical techniques such as balloon dilation or laser.

5. **Arthritis treatment center** Specifically equipped and staffed center for the diagnosis and treatment of arthritis and other joint disorders.

6. **Assisted living** A special combination of housing, supportive services, personalized assistance and health care designed to respond to the individual needs of those who need help in activities of daily living and instrumental activities of daily living. Supportive services are available, 24 hours a day, to meet scheduled and unscheduled needs, in a way that promotes maximum independence and dignity for each resident and encourages the involvement of a resident's family, neighbor and friends.

7. **Auxiliary Organization** A volunteer community organization formed to assist the hospital in carrying out its purpose and to serve as a link between the institution and the community.

8. **Birthing room–LDR room–LDRP room** A single room–type of maternity care with a more homelike setting for families than the traditional three–room unit (labor/delivery/recovery) with a separate postpartum area. A birthing room combines labor and delivery in one room. An LDR room accommodates three stages in the birthing process—labor, delivery, and recovery. An LDRP room accommodates all four stages of the birth process—labor, delivery, recovery and postpartum.

9. **Breast cancer screening/mammograms** Mammography screening–the use of breast x–ray to detect unsuspected breast cancer in asymptomatic women. Diagnostic mammography–the x–ray imaging of breast tissue in symptomatic women who are considered to have a substantial likelihood of having breast cancer already.

10. **Burn care services** Provides care to severely burned patients. Severely burned patients are those with any of the following: 1. Second–degree burns of more than 25% total body surface area for adults or 20% total body surface area for children; 2. Third–degree burns of more than 10% total body surface area; 3. Any severe burns of the hands, face, eyes, ears or feet or; 4. All inhalation injuries, electrical burns, complicated burn injuries involving fractures and other major traumas, and all other poor risk factors.

11. **Cardiac catheterization laboratory** Facilities offering special diagnostic procedures for cardiac patients. Available procedures must include, but need not be limited to, introduction of a catheter into the interior of the heart by way of a vein or artery or by direct needle puncture. Procedures must be performed in a laboratory or a special procedure room.

12. **Cardiac intensive care services** Provides patient care of a more specialized nature than the usual medical and surgical care, on the basis of physicians' orders and approved nursing care plans. The unit is staffed with specially trained nursing personnel and contains monitoring and specialized support or treatment equipment for patients who, because of heart seizure, open–heart surgery, or other life–threatening conditions, require intensified, comprehensive observation and care. May include myocardial infarction, pulmonary care, and heart transplant units.

13. **Case management** A system of assessment, treatment planning, referral and follow–up that ensures the provision of comprehensive and continuous services and the coordination of payment and reimbursement for care.

14. **Children wellness program** A program that encourages improved health status and a healthful lifestyle of children through health education, exercise, nutrition and health promotion.

15. **Chiropractic Services** An organized clinical service including spinal manipulation or adjustment and related diagnostic and therapeutic services.

16. **Community health reporting** Does your hospital either by itself or in conjunction with others disseminate reports to the community on the quality and costs of health care services?

17. **Community health status assessment** Does your hospital work with other providers, public agencies, or community representatives to conduct a health status assessment of the community?

18. **Community health status based service planning** Does your hospital use health status indicators (such as rates of health problems or surveys of self–reported health) for defined populations to design new services or modify existing services?

19. **Community outreach** A program that systematically interacts with the community to identify those in need of services, alerting persons and their families to the availability of services, locating needed services, and enabling persons to enter the service delivery system.

20. **Complementary Medicine** Organized hospital services or formal arrangements to providers that provide care or treatment not based solely on traditional western allopathic medical teachings as instructed in most U.S. medical schools. Includes any of the following; acupuncture, chiropractic, homeopathy, osteopathy, diet and lifestyle changes, herbal medicine, massage therapy, etc.

21. **Crisis prevention** Services provided in order to promote physical and mental well being and the early identification of disease and ill health prior to the onset and recognition of symptoms so as to permit early treatment.

22. **CT scanner** Computed tomographic scanner for head or whole body scans.

23. **Dental services** An organized dental service, not necessarily involving special facilities, that provides dental or oral services to inpatients or outpatients.

24. **Diagnostic radioisotope facility** The use of radioactive isotopes (Radiopharmaceutical) as tracers or indicators to detect an abnormal condition or disease.

25. **Emergency department** Hospital facilities for the provision of unscheduled outpatient services to patients whose conditions require immediate care. Must be staffed 24 hours a day.

26. **End of Life Care** An organized service providing care and/or consultative services to dying patients and their families based on formalized protocols and guidelines.

27. **Extracorporeal shock wave lithotripter (ESWL)** A medical device used for treating stones in the kidney or ureter. The device disintegrates kidney stones noninvasively through the transmission of acoustic shock waves directed at the stones.

28. **Fitness center** Provides exercise, testing, or evaluation programs and fitness activities to the community and hospital employees.

29. **Freestanding outpatient care center** A facility owned and operated by the hospital, but physically separate from the hospital, that provides various medical treatments on an outpatient basis only. In addition to treating minor illnesses or injuries, the center will stabilize seriously ill or injured patients before transporting them to a hospital. Laboratory and radiology services are usually available.

30. **Geriatric services** The branch of medicine dealing with the physiology of aging and the diagnosis and treatment of disease affecting the aged. Services could include: Adult day care program; Alzheimer's diagnostic–assessment services; Comprehensive geriatric assessment; Emergency response system; Geriatric acute care unit; and/or Geriatric clinics.

31. **Health facility transportation (to/from)** A long–term care support service designed to assist the mobility of the elderly. Some programs offer improved financial access by offering reduced rates and barrier–free buses or vans with ramps and lifts to assist the elderly or handicapped; others offer subsidies for public transport systems or operate mini–bus services exclusively for use by senior citizens.

32. **Health fair** Community health education events that focus on the prevention of disease and promotion of health through such activities as audiovisual exhibits and free diagnostic services.

33. **Health information center** Education which is directed at increasing the information of individuals and populations. It is intended to increase the ability to make informed personal, family and community health decisions by providing consumers with informed choices about health matters with the objective of improving health status.

34. **Health screenings** A preliminary procedure, such as a test or examination to detect the most characteristic sign or signs of a disorder that may require further investigation.

35. **HIV–AIDS services** Services may include one or more of the following: HIV–AIDS unit (special unit or team designated and equipped specifically for diagnosis, treatment, continuing care planning, and counseling services for HIV–AIDS patients and their families.) General inpatient care for HIV–AIDS (inpatient diagnosis and treatment for human immunodeficiency virus and acquired immunodeficiency syndrome patients, but dedicated unit is not available.) Specialized outpatient program for HIV–AIDS (special outpatient program providing diagnostic, treatment, continuing care planning, and counseling for HIV–AIDS patients and their families.)

36. **Home health services** Service providing nursing, therapy, and health–related homemaker or social services in the patient's home.

37. **Hospice** A program providing palliative care, chiefly medical relief of pain and supportive services, addressing the emotional, social, financial, and legal needs of terminally ill patients and their families. Care can be provided in a variety of settings, both inpatient and at home.

38. **Hospital–based outpatient care center–services** Organized hospital health care services offered by appointment on an ambulatory basis. Services may include outpatient surgery, examination, diagnosis, and treatment of a variety of medical conditions on a nonemergency basis, and laboratory and other diagnostic testing as ordered by staff or outside physician referral.

39. **Magnetic resonance imaging (MRI)** The use of a uniform magnetic field and radio frequencies to study tissue and structure of the body. This procedure enables the visualization of biochemical activity of the cell in vivo without the use of ionizing radiation, radioisotopic substances, or high–frequency sound.

40. **Meals on wheels** A hospital sponsored program which delivers meals to people, usually the elderly, who are unable to prepare their own meals. Low cost, nutritional meals are

delivered to individuals' homes on a regular basis.

41. **Medical surgical intensive care services** Provides patient care of a more intensive nature than the usual medical and surgical care, on the basis of physicians' orders and approved nursing care plans. These units are staffed with specially trained nursing personnel and contain monitoring and specialized support equipment of patients who, because of shock, trauma, or other life–threatening conditions, require intensified, comprehensive observation and care. Includes mixed intensive care units.

42. **Neonatal intensive care services** A unit that must be separate from the newborn nursery providing intensive care to all sick infants including those with the very lowest birth weights (less that 1500 grams). NICU has potential for providing mechanical ventilation, neonatal surgery, and special care for the sickest infants born in the hospital or transferred from another institution. A full–time neonatologist serves as director of the NICU.

43. **Nutrition programs** Those services within a health care facility which are designed to provide inexpensive, nutritionally sound meals to patients.

44. **Obstetrics services** Levels should be designated: (1) unit provides services for uncomplicated maternity and newborn cases; (2) unit provides services for uncomplicated cases, the majority of complicated problems, and special neonatal services; and (3) unit provides services for all serious illnesses and abnormalities and is supervised by a full–time maternal/fetal specialist.

45. **Occupational health services** Includes services designed to protect the safety of employees from hazards in the work environment.

46. **Oncology services** An organized program for the treatment of cancer by the use of drugs or chemicals.

47. **Open heart surgery** Heart surgery where the chest has been opened and the blood recirculated and oxygenated with the proper equipment and the necessary staff to perform the surgery.

48. **Outpatient surgery** Scheduled surgical services provided to patients who do not remain in the hospital overnight. The surgery may be performed in operating suites also used for inpatient surgery, specially designated surgical suites for outpatient surgery, or procedure rooms within an outpatient care facility.

49. **Pain Management Services** A hospital wide formalized program that includes staff education for the management of chronic and acute pain based on guidelines and protocols like those developed by the agency for Health Care Policy Research, etc.

50. **Patient education center** Written goals and objectives for the patient and/or family related to therapeutic regimens, medical procedures, and self care.

51. **Patient representative services** Organized hospital services providing personnel through whom patients and staff can seek solutions to institutional problems affecting the delivery of high–quality care and services.

52. **Pediatric intensive care services** Provides care to pediatric patients that is of a more intensive nature than that usually provided to pediatric patients. The unit is staffed with specially trained personnel and contains monitoring and specialized support equipment for treatment of patients who, because of shock, trauma, or other life–threatening conditions, require intensified, comprehensive observation and care.

53. **Physical rehabilitation inpatient services** Provides care encompassing a comprehensive array of restoration services for the disabled and all support services necessary to help patients attain their maximum functional capacity.

54. **Physical rehabilitation outpatient services** Outpatient program providing medical, health–related, therapy, social, and/or vocational services to help disabled persons attain or retain their maximum functional capacity.

55. **Positron emission tomography scanner (PET)** is a nuclear medicine imaging technology which uses radioactive (positron emitting) isotopes created in a cyclotron or generator and computers to produce composite pictures of the brain and heart at work. PET scanning produces sectional images depicting metabolic activity or blood flow rather than anatomy.

56. **Primary care department** A unit or clinic within the hospital that provides primary care services (e.g. general pediatric care, general internal medicine, family practice and gynecology) through hospital–salaried medical and or nursing staff, focusing on evaluating and diagnosing medical problems and providing medical treatment on an outpatient basis.

57. **Psychiatric acute inpatient services** Provides acute or long–term care to emotionally disturbed patients, including patients admitted for diagnosis and those admitted for treatment of psychiatric problems, on the basis of physicians' orders and approved nursing care plans. Long–term care may include intensive supervision to the chronically mentally ill, mentally disordered, or other mentally incompetent persons.

58. **Psychiatric child adolescent services** Provides care to emotionally disturbed children and adolescents, including those admitted for diagnosis and those admitted for treatment.

59. **Psychiatric consultation–liaison services** Provides organized psychiatric consultation/liaison services to nonpsychiatric hospital staff and/or department on psychological aspects of medical care that may be generic or specific to individual patients.

60. **Psychiatric education services** Provides psychiatric educational services to community agencies and workers such as schools, police, courts, public health nurses, welfare agencies, clergy and so forth. The purpose is to expand the mental health knowledge and competence of personnel not working in the mental health field and to promote good mental health through improved understanding, attitudes, and behavioral patterns.

61. **Psychiatric emergency services** Services or facilities available on a 24–hour basis to provide immediate unscheduled outpatient care, diagnosis, evaluation, crisis intervention, and assistance to persons suffering acute emotional or mental distress.

62. **Psychiatric geriatric services** Provides care to emotionally disturbed elderly patients, including those admitted for diagnosis and those admitted for treatment.

63. **Psychiatric outpatient services** Provides medical care, including diagnosis and treatment of psychiatric outpatients.

64. **Psychiatric partial hospitalization program** Organized hospital services of intensive day/evening outpatient services of three hours or more duration, distinguished from other outpatient visits of one hour.

65. **Radiation therapy** The branch of medicine concerned with radioactive substances and using various techniques of visualization, with the diagnosis and treatment of disease using any of the various sources of radiant energy. Services could include: megavoltage radiation therapy; radioactive implants; stereotactic radiosurgery; therapeutic radioisotope facility; X–ray radiation therapy.

66. **Reproductive health services** Services that include any or all of the following:

    Fertility counseling A service that counsels and educates on infertility problems and includes laboratory and surgical workup and management for individuals having problems conceiving children.

    In vitro fertilization Program providing for the induction of fertilization of a surgically removed ovum by donated sperm in a culture medium followed by a short incubation period. The embryo is then reimplanted in the womb.

67. **Retirement housing** A facility which provides social activities to senior citizens, usually retired persons, who do not require health care but some short–term skilled nursing care may be provided. A retirement center may furnish housing and may also have acute hospital and long–term care facilities, or it may arrange for acute and long term care through affiliated institutions.

68. **Single photon emission computerized tomography (SPECT)** is a nuclear medicine imaging technology that combines existing technology of gamma camera imaging with computed tomographic imaging technology to provide a more precise and clear image.

69. **Skilled nursing or other long–term care services** Provides non–acute medical and skilled nursing care services, therapy, and social services under the supervision of a licensed registered nurse on a 24–hour basis.

70. **Social work services** Services may include one or more of the following: Organized social work services (services that are properly directed and sufficiently staffed by qualified individuals who provide assistance and counseling to patients and their families in dealing with social, emotional, and environmental problems associated with illness or disability, often in the context of financial or discharge planning coordination.) Outpatient social work services (social work services provided in ambulatory care areas.) Emergency department social work services (social work services provided to emergency department patients by social workers dedicated to the emergency department or on call.)

71. **Sports medicine** Provision of diagnostic screening and assessment and clinical and rehabilitation services for the prevention and treatment of sports–related injuries.

72. **Support groups** A hospital sponsored program which allows a group of individuals with the same or similar problems who meet periodically to share experiences, problems, and solutions, in order to support each other.

73. **Teen outreach services** A program focusing on the teenager which encourages an improved health status and a healthful lifestyle including physical, emotional, mental, social, spiritual and economic health through education, exercise, nutrition and health promotion.

74. **Transplant services** The branch of medicine that transfers an organ or tissue from one person to another or from one body part to another to replace a diseased structure or to restore function or to change appearance. Services could includes: Bone marrow transplant program; kidney transplant; organ transplant (other than kidney); tissue transplant.

75. **Trauma center (certified)** A facility certified to provide emergency and specialized intensive care to critically ill and injured patients.

76. **Ultrasound** The use of acoustic waves above the range of 20,000 cycles per second to visualize internal body structures.

77. **Urgent care center** A facility that provides care and treatment for problems that are not life–threatening but require attention over the short term. These units function like emergency rooms but are separate from hospitals with which they may have backup affiliation arrangements.

78. **Volunteer services department** An organized hospital department responsible for coordinating the services of volunteers working within the institution.

79. **Women's health center/services** An area set aside for coordinated education and treatment services specifically for and promoted by women as provided by this special unit. Services may or may not include obstetrics but include a range of services other than OB.

Definitions of Physician Codes

1. **Closed physician–hospital organization (PHO)** A PHO that restricts physician membership to those practitioners who meet criteria for cost effectiveness and/or high quality.

2. **Equity model** Allows established practitioners to become shareholders in a professional corporation in exchange for tangible and intangible assets of their existing practices.

3. **Foundation** A corporation, organized either as a hospital affiliate or subsidiary, which purchases both the tangible and intangible assets of one or more medical group practices. Physicians remain in a separate corporate entity but sign a professional services agreement with the foundation.

4. **Group practice without walls** Hospital sponsors the formation of, or provides capital to physicians to establish, a 'quasi' group to share administrative expenses while remaining independent practitioners.

5. **Independent practice association (IPA)** An IPA is a legal entity that hold managed care contracts. The IPA then contracts with physicians, usually in solo practice, to provide care either on a fee–for–services or capitated basis. The purpose of an IPA is to assist solo physicians in obtaining managed care contracts.

6. **Integrated salary model** Physicians are salaried by the hospital or another entity of a health system to provide medical services for primary care and specialty care.

7. **Management services organization (MSO)** A corporation, owned by the hospital or a physician/hospital joint venture, that provides management

services to one or more medical group practices. The MSO purchases the tangible assets of the practices and leases them back as part of a full-service management agreement, under which the MSO employs all non-physician staff and provides all supplies/administrative systems for a fee.

8. **Open physician-hospital organization (PHO)** A joint venture between the hospital and all members of the medical staff who wish to participate. The PHO can act as a unified agent in managed care contracting, own a managed care plan, own and operate ambulatory care centers or ancillary services projects, or provide administrative services to physician members.

Hospitals in the United States, by State

ALABAMA

Resident Population 4,352 (in thousands)
Resident population in metro areas 67.7%
Birth rate per 1,000 population 14.1
65 years and over 13.1%
Percent of persons without health insurance 15.5%

Hospital, Address, Telephone, Administrator, Approval, Facility, and Physician Codes, Health Care System, Network	Classification Codes		Utilization Data					Expense (thousands) of dollars		
★ American Hospital Association (AHA) membership □ Joint Commission on Accreditation of Healthcare Organizations (JCAHO) accreditation + American Osteopathic Healthcare Association (AOHA) membership ○ American Osteopathic Association (AOA) accreditation △ Commission on Accreditation of Rehabilitation Facilities (CARF) accreditation Control codes 61, 63, 64, 71, 72 and 73 indicate hospitals listed by AOHA, but not registered by AHA. For definition of numerical codes, see page A4	Control	Service	Staffed Beds	Admissions	Census	Outpatient Visits	Births	Total	Payroll	Personnel
ALABASTER—Shelby County ✚ SHELBY BAPTIST MEDICAL CENTER, 1000 First Street North, Zip 35007-0488; tel. 205/620-8100; Charles C. Colvert, President (Total facility includes 18 beds in nursing home-type unit) (Nonreporting) **A**1 2 9 10 **S** Baptist Health System, Birmingham, AL Web address: www.bhsala.com	13	10	228	—	—	—	—	—	—	—
ALEXANDER CITY—Tallapoosa County ✚ RUSSELL MEDICAL CENTER, (Formerly Russell Hospital), U.S. 280 By-Pass, Zip 35010, Mailing Address: P.O. Box 939, Zip 35011-0939; tel. 256/329-7100; Frank W. Harris, President and Chief Executive Officer **A**1 9 10 **F**7 8 9 11 16 17 18 22 24 25 26 31 32 33 34 37 38 39 40 41 43 44 46 48 50 51 53 54 56 68 70 72 76 78 79 **P**7 Web address: www.russellmedcenter.com	23	10	81	4623	37	80273	411	26560	11681	435
ANDALUSIA—Covington County ✚ ANDALUSIA REGIONAL HOSPITAL, 849 South Three Notch Street, Zip 36420-5325, Mailing Address: P.O. Box 760, Zip 36420-0760; tel. 334/222-8466; Barry L. Keel, Chief Executive Officer (Nonreporting) **A**1 9 10 **S** LifePoint Hospitals, Inc., Brentwood, TN	33	10	101	—	—	—	—	—	—	—
ANNISTON—Calhoun County ✚ NORTHEAST ALABAMA REGIONAL MEDICAL CENTER, 400 East Tenth Street, Zip 36207-4716, Mailing Address: P.O. Box 2208, Zip 36202-2208; tel. 256/235-5121; Allen P. Fletcher, President and Chief Executive Officer **A**1 2 3 9 10 **F**8 9 11 16 17 18 19 22 24 25 32 33 34 35 36 38 39 41 44 45 46 48 50 51 54 57 59 60 61 62 63 64 65 70 71 72 75 76 78 Web address: www.rmccares.org	16	10	255	14746	175	116614	1703	90805	38954	1201
□ STRINGFELLOW MEMORIAL HOSPITAL, 301 East 18th Street, Zip 36207-0038, Mailing Address: P.O. Box 38, Zip 36207-0038; tel. 256/235-8900; Vincent T. Cherry, Jr, Administrator **A**1 9 10 **F**7 16 18 22 24 25 27 31 38 39 40 41 46 48 49 51 54 76 78 **S** Health Management Associates, Naples, FL	33	10	125	3317	37	33220	0	19402	8020	285
ASHLAND—Clay County ★ CLAY COUNTY HOSPITAL, 83825 Highway 9, Zip 36251, Mailing Address: P.O. Box 1270, Zip 36251-1277; tel. 256/354-2131; Linda U. Jordan, Administrator (Total facility includes 73 beds in nursing home-type unit) **A**9 10 **F**6 7 8 9 12 16 17 18 22 23 25 36 37 38 39 44 45 48 50 51 54 69 70 72 76 78	16	10	116	2657	98	19714	111	13971	6593	219
ATHENS—Limestone County ✚ ATHENS–LIMESTONE HOSPITAL, 700 West Market Street, Zip 35611-2457, Mailing Address: P.O. Box 999, Zip 35612-0999; tel. 256/233-9292; Philip E. Dotson, Chief Executive Officer **A**1 9 10 **F**7 8 9 13 17 18 22 24 25 28 30 32 33 34 36 41 43 44 45 48 50 54 70 76 77 **P**6 Web address: www.alhosp.com	16	10	101	4466	50	110364	410	35972	16347	521
ATMORE—Escambia County □ ATMORE COMMUNITY HOSPITAL, 401 Medical Park Drive, Zip 36502-3091; tel. 334/368-2500; Robert E. Gowing, Administrator (Nonreporting) **A**1 9 10 **S** Baptist Health Care Corporation, Pensacola, FL	13	10	51	—	—	—	—	—	—	—
BAY MINETTE—Baldwin County □ NORTH BALDWIN HOSPITAL, 1815 Hand Avenue, Zip 36507, Mailing Address: P.O. Box 1409, Zip 36507-1409; tel. 334/937-5521; Wilma D. Stuart, Administrator **A**1 9 10 **F**8 17 18 19 22 24 25 36 37 38 39 41 44 45 48 49 54 70 76 78	13	10	43	1287	11	18901	194	8708	4079	155
BESSEMER—Jefferson County ✚ BESSEMER CARRAWAY MEDICAL CENTER, 995 Ninth Avenue S.W., Zip 35022, Mailing Address: P.O. Box 847, Zip 35021-0847; tel. 205/481-7000; Dan M. Eagar, Jr, Administrator **A**1 2 9 10 **F**2 3 7 8 9 11 12 13 16 22 23 24 25 30 31 32 34 37 39 41 43 44 45 46 48 49 53 54 57 59 60 61 62 70 72 75 76 78 79 **P**4 6 7 Web address: www.bcmc.org	23	10	210	7045	105	65478	377	68989	25737	903
BIRMINGHAM—Jefferson County ✚ BROOKWOOD MEDICAL CENTER, 2010 Brookwood Medical Center Drive, Zip 35209; tel. 205/877-1000; John R. Nickens, II, Chief Executive Officer **A**1 2 9 10 **F**1 2 4 5 7 8 9 11 12 13 16 18 19 21 22 24 25 26 27 28 29 30 32 33 34 35 36 37 38 39 41 42 43 44 45 46 47 48 49 50 53 54 56 57 58 61 62 63 64 65 66 69 70 71 72 76 78 79 **P**6 **S** TENET Healthcare Corporation, Santa Barbara, CA Web address: www.brookwood–medical.com	33	10	497	20250	282	120564	3609	144545	46682	1205

Hospitals, U.S. / ALABAMA

Hospital, Address, Telephone, Administrator, Approval, Facility, and Physician Codes, Health Care System, Network	Classification Codes		Utilization Data					Expense (thousands) of dollars		
	Control	Service	Staffed Beds	Admissions	Census	Outpatient Visits	Births	Total	Payroll	Personnel

★ American Hospital Association (AHA) membership
☐ Joint Commission on Accreditation of Healthcare Organizations (JCAHO) accreditation
+ American Osteopathic Healthcare Association (AOHA) membership
○ American Osteopathic Association (AOA) accreditation
△ Commission on Accreditation of Rehabilitation Facilities (CARF) accreditation
Control codes 61, 63, 64, 71, 72 and 73 indicate hospitals listed by AOHA, but not registered by AHA. For definition of numerical codes, see page A4

Hospital	Control	Service	Staffed Beds	Admissions	Census	Outpatient Visits	Births	Total	Payroll	Personnel
☐ CALLAHAN EYE FOUNDATION HOSPITAL, (Formerly Eye Foundation Hospital), 1720 University Boulevard, Zip 35233–1816; tel. 205/325–8100; Steve C. Schultz, President **A**1 3 5 9 10 **F**17 18 19 22 25 33 34 39 45 48 76 78 **S** University of Alabama System, Birmingham, AL Web address: www.health.uab.edu/eyes	23	45	20	1037	4	14969	—	15714	5389	158
★ CARRAWAY METHODIST MEDICAL CENTER, 1600 Carraway Boulevard, Zip 35234–1990; tel. 205/502–6000; Cindy Williams, FACHE, Administrator **A**1 2 3 5 8 9 10 **F**2 4 8 9 11 12 13 16 17 18 19 22 24 25 28 29 30 32 34 35 37 38 39 41 43 44 45 46 47 48 49 50 51 53 54 56 57 58 59 60 61 62 63 65 68 70 72 75 76 78 79 **P**3 8 **S** Carraway Methodist Health System, Birmingham, AL Web address: www.carraway.org	23	10	383	14107	206	134347	459	143731	56349	1590
★ CHILDREN'S HOSPITAL OF ALABAMA, 1600 Seventh Avenue South, Zip 35233–1785; tel. 205/939–9100; Jim Dearth, M.D., Chief Executive Officer **A**1 3 5 9 10 **F**10 13 14 16 17 18 19 22 23 24 25 29 32 33 34 35 38 39 42 43 45 46 48 50 51 52 54 56 57 58 59 60 61 63 70 71 72 73 75 76 77 78 **P**7 Web address: www.chsys.org	23	50	211	11379	160	224472	0	150932	63218	2111
★ COOPER GREEN HOSPITAL, 1515 Sixth Avenue South, Zip 35233–1688; tel. 205/930–3200; Max Michael, M.D., Chief Executive Officer and Medical Director **A**1 3 5 9 10 **F**4 9 10 11 13 14 16 17 18 22 25 26 35 38 39 41 44 46 47 48 52 53 54 56 57 59 61 65 70 76 **P**5	13	10	141	5721	70	142390	1327	66918	28832	674
☐ HEALTHSOUTH LAKESHORE REHABILITATION HOSPITAL, 3800 Ridgeway Drive, Zip 35209–5599; tel. 205/868–2000; Terry Brown, Administrator and Chief Executive Officer **A**1 9 10 **F**16 17 18 22 23 24 25 29 31 34 38 39 45 46 48 49 51 53 54 56 70 71 72 76 **P**8 **S** HEALTHSOUTH Corporation, Birmingham, AL	33	46	100	2159	94	16229	0	—	—	236
★ HEALTHSOUTH MEDICAL CENTER, 1201 11th Avenue South, Zip 35205–5299; tel. 205/930–7000; Luke Standeffer, Administrator and Chief Executive Officer **A**1 10 **F**1 4 5 9 11 13 16 22 24 25 29 34 38 39 41 45 46 48 49 53 54 56 70 71 72 76 **S** HEALTHSOUTH Corporation, Birmingham, AL	33	10	169	6496	65	46160	0	73025	25272	704
☐ HILL CREST BEHAVIORAL HEALTH SERVICES, 6869 Fifth Avenue South, Zip 35212–1866; tel. 205/833–9000; Steve McCabe, Chief Executive Officer **A**1 9 10 **F**3 13 19 21 30 31 43 45 50 51 53 57 58 59 60 61 62 63 69 70 72 73 **P**5 **S** Ramsay Youth Services, Coral Gables, FL	33	22	119	1356	112	0	0	10034	6159	198
★ △ MEDICAL CENTER EAST, 50 Medical Park East Drive, Zip 35235–9987; tel. 205/838–3000; Gary R. Colberg, CHE, Chief Executive Officer **A**1 2 3 5 7 9 10 **F**1 4 6 7 8 9 11 12 13 16 17 19 22 24 25 28 30 31 32 33 34 35 36 37 38 39 41 42 43 44 45 46 47 48 50 51 53 54 56 61 65 67 69 70 72 75 76 77 78 79 **P**6 **S** Eastern Health System, Inc., Birmingham, AL Web address: www.ehs-inc.com	23	10	257	12284	145	123156	947	94576	33836	1088
★ MONTCLAIR BAPTIST MEDICAL CENTER, 800 Montclair Road, Zip 35213–1984; tel. 205/592–1000; John Shelton, President (Total facility includes 40 beds in nursing home–type unit) **A**1 2 3 5 8 9 10 **F**2 3 4 6 7 8 9 11 12 13 16 17 18 19 22 24 25 26 28 30 32 33 34 35 36 37 38 39 41 42 44 45 46 47 48 49 50 51 53 54 56 57 58 59 60 61 62 63 64 65 66 67 69 70 71 72 75 76 78 79 **P**5 **S** Baptist Health System, Birmingham, AL Web address: www.bhsala.com	21	10	463	19054	268	172346	966	156099	49851	1637
★ PRINCETON BAPTIST MEDICAL CENTER, 701 Princeton Avenue S.W., Zip 35211–1305; tel. 205/783–3000; Charlie Faulkner, President (Total facility includes 31 beds in nursing home–type unit) **A**1 2 3 5 8 9 10 **F**3 4 6 7 8 9 11 12 13 16 17 18 19 22 24 25 26 28 30 32 33 34 35 36 37 38 39 41 42 44 45 46 47 48 49 50 51 52 54 56 57 58 59 60 61 62 63 64 65 66 67 69 70 71 72 75 76 78 79 **P**5 **S** Baptist Health System, Birmingham, AL Web address: www.bhsala.com	21	10	320	12317	208	142058	472	131158	46531	1386
★ ST. VINCENT'S HOSPITAL, 810 St. Vincent's Drive, Zip 35205–1695, Mailing Address: P.O. Box 12407, Zip 35202–2407; tel. 205/939–7000; Curtis James, President and Chief Executive Officer **A**1 2 3 5 9 10 **F**4 7 8 9 11 12 13 17 18 22 24 25 26 31 32 34 36 37 38 39 41 42 43 44 45 46 47 48 49 51 54 65 70 71 72 76 78 79 **P**5 **S** Ascension Health, Saint Louis, MO Web address: www.stv.org	21	10	255	15554	198	133774	3021	133644	55990	1598
★ UNIVERSITY OF ALABAMA HOSPITAL, 619 South 19th Street, Zip 35233–6505; tel. 205/934–4011; Martin Nowak, Interim Executive Director (Total facility includes 39 beds in nursing home–type unit) **A**1 2 3 5 8 9 10 **F**2 3 4 5 7 8 9 10 11 12 13 16 17 18 19 22 23 24 25 26 28 29 30 31 32 33 34 35 36 37 38 39 41 42 43 44 45 46 47 48 49 51 53 54 55 56 57 58 59 60 61 62 63 65 66 68 69 70 71 72 73 74 75 76 77 78 79 **P**3 7 **S** University of Alabama System, Birmingham, AL Web address: www.uab.edu	12	10	870	41537	692	—	2888	507863	187854	5399
★ VETERANS AFFAIRS MEDICAL CENTER, 700 South 19th Street, Zip 35233–1927; tel. 205/933–8101; Y. C. Parris, Director **A**1 2 3 5 8 9 **F**1 2 3 4 5 9 11 12 13 16 17 18 22 23 24 25 29 30 31 32 33 34 35 36 37 38 39 41 43 45 46 47 48 49 50 51 53 54 55 56 57 59 61 63 65 68 69 70 72 74 77 78 79 **P**6 **S** Department of Veterans Affairs, Washington, DC Web address: www.va.gov	45	10	122	4282	100	280059	0	—	—	—

BOAZ—Marshall County

Hospital	Control	Service	Staffed Beds	Admissions	Census	Outpatient Visits	Births	Total	Payroll	Personnel
★ MARSHALL MEDICAL CENTER SOUTH, U.S. Highway 431 North, Zip 35957–0999, Mailing Address: P.O. Box 758, Zip 35957–0758; tel. 256/593–8310; J. Marlin Hanson, Administrator **A**1 9 10 **F**4 7 8 9 13 16 17 18 19 22 24 25 28 32 34 36 39 41 43 44 45 46 48 49 54 57 61 65 68 70 71 72 76 78 79 **S** Marshall County Health Care Authority, Guntersville, AL	13	10	102	5001	61	180839	667	46032	18592	533

Hospitals, U.S. / ALABAMA

Hospital, Address, Telephone, Administrator, Approval, Facility, and Physician Codes, Health Care System, Network	Classification Codes		Utilization Data					Expense (thousands) of dollars		
★ American Hospital Association (AHA) membership □ Joint Commission on Accreditation of Healthcare Organizations (JCAHO) accreditation + American Osteopathic Healthcare Association (AOHA) membership ○ American Osteopathic Association (AOA) accreditation △ Commission on Accreditation of Rehabilitation Facilities (CARF) accreditation Control codes 61, 63, 64, 71, 72 and 73 indicate hospitals listed by AOHA, but not registered by AHA. For definition of numerical codes, see page A4	Control	Service	Staffed Beds	Admissions	Census	Outpatient Visits	Births	Total	Payroll	Personnel
BREWTON—Escambia County										
□ D. W. MCMILLAN MEMORIAL HOSPITAL, 1301 Belleville Avenue, Zip 36426–1306, Mailing Address: P.O. Box 908, Zip 36427–0908; tel. 334/867–8061; Phillip L. Parker, Administrator **A**1 9 10 **F**8 9 16 17 18 22 24 25 31 32 34 36 38 39 41 43 44 46 48 50 54 70 72 76 78 **P**4 7 **S** Baptist Health Care Corporation, Pensacola, FL Web address: www.bhcpns.org	23	10	67	3036	32	36440	278	16269	7204	265
BRIDGEPORT—Jackson County										
□ NORTH JACKSON HOSPITAL, Mailing Address: 47005 U.S. Highway 72, Zip 35740; tel. 256/437–2101; Brad Hinton, Administrator (Total facility includes 90 beds in nursing home–type unit) **A**1 9 10 **F**8 10 19 22 23 25 44 45 48 54 68 69 78 79	16	10	129	1387	93	12007	24	—	5104	171
CAMDEN—Wilcox County										
J. PAUL JONES HOSPITAL, 317 McWilliams Avenue, Zip 36726–1610; tel. 334/682–4131; Arden Chesnut, Administrator **A**9 10 **F**9 22 25 36 69 70 76	15	10	32	462	3	9125	0	2019	898	45
CARROLLTON—Pickens County										
□ PICKENS COUNTY MEDICAL CENTER, Route 2, Zip 35447, Mailing Address: P.O. Box 478, Zip 35447–0478; tel. 205/367–8111; Tunisia Lavender, R.N., Chief Operating Officer (Nonreporting) **A**1 9 10	23	10	30							
CENTRE—Cherokee County										
★□ CHEROKEE BAPTIST MEDICAL CENTER, 400 Northwood Drive, Zip 35960–1023; tel. 256/927–5531; Barry S. Cochran, President **A**1 9 10 **F**7 9 13 16 17 18 19 22 24 25 28 32 34 36 37 39 41 48 49 54 67 71 75 76 78 **S** Baptist Health System, Birmingham, AL Web address: www.bhsala.com	23	10	45	1106	11	—	0	10474	3773	126
CENTREVILLE—Bibb County										
BIBB MEDICAL CENTER, 208 Pierson Avenue, Zip 35042–1199; tel. 205/926–4881; Terry J. Smith, Administrator (Total facility includes 113 beds in nursing home–type unit) **A**9 10 **F**8 22 25 36 48 54 67 69 70 76	13	10	138	783	106	13717	83	4023	3829	190
CHATOM—Washington County										
★ WASHINGTON COUNTY INFIRMARY AND NURSING HOME, St. Stephens Avenue, Zip 36518, Mailing Address: P.O. Box 597, Zip 36518–0597; tel. 334/847–2223; John S. Eads, Administrator (Total facility includes 73 beds in nursing home–type unit) **A**9 10 **F**16 17 18 25 32 34 37 38 56 69 70 76 **P**7 **S** Infirmary Health System, Inc., Mobile, AL	15	10	94	456	74	15773	0	4893	2684	124
CLANTON—Chilton County										
□ CHILTON MEDICAL CENTER, 1010 Lay Dam Road, Zip 35045; tel. 205/755–2500; Randy Smith, Chief Executive Officer (Nonreporting) **A**1 9 10 **S** NetCare Health Systems, Inc., Nashville, TN	33	10	45	—	—	—	—	—	—	—
CULLMAN—Cullman County										
★□ CULLMAN REGIONAL MEDICAL CENTER, 1912 Alabama Highway 157, Zip 35055, Mailing Address: P.O. Box 1108, Zip 35056–1108; tel. 256/737–2000; Jesse O. Weatherly, President **A**1 2 9 10 **F**4 7 8 9 11 13 16 17 18 19 22 24 25 28 32 33 34 36 37 38 39 41 44 45 46 48 49 50 51 54 65 70 71 72 76 78 79 **S** Baptist Health System, Birmingham, AL Web address: www.crmc–bhs.com	23	10	115	6918	67	320944	692	51839	19934	723
□ WOODLAND MEDICAL CENTER, 1910 Cherokee Avenue S.E., Zip 35055–5599; tel. 256/739–3500; Lowell S. Benton, Executive Director **A**1 9 10 **F**7 8 9 12 13 14 17 19 22 25 32 33 34 36 39 41 43 44 45 46 48 49 50 51 53 54 57 60 61 62 63 71 76 **S** Community Health Systems, Inc., Brentwood, TN Web address: www.woodlandmedicalcenter.com	33	10	100	2842	29	—	194	16826	6063	212
DADEVILLE—Tallapoosa County										
★ LAKESHORE COMMUNITY HOSPITAL, 201 Mariarden Road, Zip 36853, Mailing Address: P.O. Box 248, Zip 36853–0248; tel. 256/825–7821; Sue Boxx, Administrator **A**9 10 **F**7 22 25 36 38 48 76 **S** Healthcorp of Tennessee, Inc., Chattanooga, TN	23	10	28	1207	9	13320	0	5860	3322	149
DAPHNE—Baldwin County										
★□ MERCY MEDICAL, 101 Villa Drive, Zip 36526–4653, Mailing Address: P.O. Box 1090, Zip 36526–1090; tel. 334/626–2694; Sister Mary Eileen Wilhelm, President and Chief Executive Officer (Total facility includes 137 beds in nursing home–type unit) **A**1 10 **F**1 6 13 17 18 19 23 26 30 36 37 38 43 53 54 67 69 70 72 78 **P**7 **S** Catholic Health East, Newtown Square, PA Web address: www.mercymedical.com	21	46	162	1648	135	—	0	29935	15368	616
DECATUR—Morgan County										
★□ DECATUR GENERAL HOSPITAL, (Includes Decatur General Hospital, 1201 Seventh Street S.E., Mailing Address: P.O. Box 2239, Zip 35609–2239; tel. 256/341–2000; Robert L. Smith, President and Chief Executive Officer; Decatur General Hospital-West, 2205 Beltline Road S.W., Zip 35601–3687, Mailing Address: P.O. Box 2240, Zip 35609–2240; tel. 256/341–2000), 1201 Seventh Street S.E., Zip 35601, Mailing Address: P.O. Box 2239, Zip 35609–2239; tel. 256/341–2000; Robert L. Smith, President and Chief Executive Officer **A**1 2 9 10 **F**8 9 11 12 13 17 18 22 24 25 32 33 34 36 38 39 41 43 44 45 46 48 50 51 54 58 59 60 61 62 63 65 70 72 76 78 79 DECATUR GENERAL HOSPITAL–WEST See Decatur General Hospital	16	10	256	9946	125	147373	1539	74399	31391	1021
□ NORTH ALABAMA REGIONAL HOSPITAL, 4218 Highway 31 South, Zip 35609, Mailing Address: P.O. Box 2221, Zip 35609–2221; tel. 256/353–9433; Kay Greenwood, R.N., MS, Facility Director **A**1 10 **F**18 23 57 70 78 **P**6	12	22	74	515	68	0	0	7411	4736	155

© 2000 AHA Guide *Many Facility Codes have changed. Please refer to the AHA Guide Code Chart.*

Hospitals, U.S. / ALABAMA

Legend for Hospital, Address, Telephone, Administrator, Approval, Facility, and Physician Codes, Health Care System, Network:

- ★ American Hospital Association (AHA) membership
- ☐ Joint Commission on Accreditation of Healthcare Organizations (JCAHO) accreditation
- + American Osteopathic Healthcare Association (AOHA) membership
- ○ American Osteopathic Association (AOA) accreditation
- △ Commission on Accreditation of Rehabilitation Facilities (CARF) accreditation

Control codes 61, 63, 64, 71, 72 and 73 indicate hospitals listed by AOHA, but not registered by AHA. For definition of numerical codes, see page A4.

Hospital	Control	Service	Staffed Beds	Admissions	Census	Outpatient Visits	Births	Total	Payroll	Personnel
☐ PARKWAY MEDICAL CENTER HOSPITAL, 1874 Beltline Road S.W., Zip 35601–5509, Mailing Address: P.O. Box 2211, Zip 35609–2211; tel. 256/350–2211; Danny Crowe, Interim Chief Executive Officer (Nonreporting) **A**1 9 10 **S** Community Health Systems, Inc., Brentwood, TN	33	10	94	—	—	—	—	—	—	—
DEMOPOLIS—Marengo County										
★ BRYAN W. WHITFIELD MEMORIAL HOSPITAL, Highway 80 West, Zip 36732, Mailing Address: P.O. Box 890, Zip 36732–0890; tel. 334/289–4000; Charles E. Nabors, FACHE, Administrator and Chief Executive Officer **A**1 9 10 **F**1 7 9 13 14 16 17 18 22 24 25 28 29 34 36 37 39 41 43 44 46 48 50 51 56 65 68 70 72 73 76 78	16	10	99	3719	44	20841	458	20822	8880	339
DOTHAN—Houston County										
★ FLOWERS HOSPITAL, 4370 West Main Street, Zip 36305, Mailing Address: P.O. Box 6907, Zip 36302–6907; tel. 334/793–5000; Keith Granger, President and Chief Executive Officer (Nonreporting) **A**1 2 9 10 **S** Quorum Health Group, Brentwood, TN	33	10	215	—	—	—	—	—	—	—
☐ SOUTHEAST ALABAMA MEDICAL CENTER, 1108 Ross Clark Circle, Zip 36301–3024, Mailing Address: P.O. Box 6987, Zip 36302–6987; tel. 334/793–8111; Ronald S. Owen, Chief Executive Officer **A**1 2 9 10 **F**4 7 8 9 11 12 13 18 19 22 24 27 32 33 34 38 39 41 43 44 45 46 47 48 49 50 51 54 57 65 68 70 72 75 76 78 **P**6 7 Web address: www.samc.org	16	10	353	28364	217	274520	1187	141098	60276	2450
ELBA—Coffee County										
ELBA GENERAL HOSPITAL, 987 Drayton Street, Zip 36323–1494; tel. 334/897–2257; Ellen C. Briley, Administrator and Chief Executive Officer (Total facility includes 101 beds in nursing home–type unit) (Nonreporting) **A**9 10	16	10	121	—	—	—	—	—	—	—
ENTERPRISE—Coffee County										
★ MEDICAL CENTER ENTERPRISE, 400 North Edwards Street, Zip 36330–9981; tel. 334/347–0584; Keith Granger, President and Chief Executive Officer **A**1 9 10 **F**8 9 13 18 22 24 25 39 45 48 54 70 71 76 **S** Quorum Health Group, Brentwood, TN	33	10	117	4720	46	58824	933	23628	8879	307
EUFAULA—Barbour County										
☐ LAKEVIEW COMMUNITY HOSPITAL, 820 West Washington Street, Zip 36027–1899; tel. 334/687–5761; Carl A. Brown, Administrator (Nonreporting) **A**1 9 10 **S** Healthcorp of Tennessee, Inc., Chattanooga, TN	33	10	74	—	—	—	—	—	—	—
EUTAW—Greene County										
GREENE COUNTY HOSPITAL, 509 Wilson Avenue, Zip 35462–1099; tel. 205/372–3388; Robert J. Coker, Jr, Administrator (Nonreporting) **A**9 10	13	10	72	—	—	—	—	—	—	—
FAIRFIELD—Jefferson County										
★ HEALTHSOUTH METRO WEST HOSPITAL, (Formerly Lloyd Noland Hospital and Health System), 701 Richard M. Scrushy Parkway, Zip 35064; tel. 205/783–5121; Karen Davis, Chief Executive Officer **A**1 2 3 5 9 10 **F**2 3 9 11 13 16 17 18 19 22 24 25 29 30 31 32 34 36 38 39 41 45 46 48 49 50 57 58 61 62 63 72 76 78 **S** HEALTHSOUTH Corporation, Birmingham, AL	33	10	150	4043	71	165179	0	56315	21239	589
FAIRHOPE—Baldwin County										
★ THOMAS HOSPITAL, 750 Morphy Avenue, Zip 36532–1812, Mailing Address: P.O. Drawer 929, Zip 36533–0929; tel. 334/928–2375; G. Owen Bailey, Administrator (Nonreporting) **A**1 9 10 Web address: www.thomashosp.com	16	10	150	—	—	—	—	—	—	—
FAYETTE—Fayette County										
★ FAYETTE MEDICAL CENTER, 1653 Temple Avenue North, Zip 35555–1314, Mailing Address: P.O. Drawer 878, Zip 35555–0878; tel. 205/932–5966; Harold Reed, Administrator (Total facility includes 122 beds in nursing home–type unit) **A**1 9 10 **F**9 13 17 18 22 25 36 37 39 41 45 46 48 69 70 76 78 **S** DCH Health System, Tuscaloosa, AL	13	10	183	1699	142	45066	0	19968	8831	281
FLORALA—Covington County										
FLORALA MEMORIAL HOSPITAL, 515 East Fifth Avenue, Zip 36442–0189, Mailing Address: P.O. Box 189, Zip 36442–0189; tel. 334/858–3287; Blair W. Henson, Administrator (Nonreporting) **A**9 10 **S** United Hospital Corporation, Memphis, TN	33	10	23	—	—	—	—	—	—	—
FLORENCE—Lauderdale County										
★ ELIZA COFFEE MEMORIAL HOSPITAL, (Includes Mitchell–Hollingsworth Annex), 205 Marengo Street, Zip 35630–6033, Mailing Address: P.O. Box 818, Zip 35631–0818; tel. 256/768–9191; Richard H. Peck, President and Chief Executive Officer (Total facility includes 202 beds in nursing home–type unit) **A**1 9 10 **F**4 8 9 11 12 17 22 24 25 32 33 38 41 44 46 47 48 50 51 54 57 58 59 60 61 62 69 70 72 76 78 **S** Coffee Health Group, Florence, AL	16	10	455	13018	379	60313	1287	76672	39127	1520
FOLEY—Baldwin County										
★ SOUTH BALDWIN REGIONAL MEDICAL CENTER, 1613 North McKenzie Street, Zip 36535–2299; tel. 334/952–3400; Sandy D. McGill, Administrator (Nonreporting) **A**1 9 10 **S** Community Health Systems, Inc., Brentwood, TN Web address: www.southbaldwinrmc.com	16	10	82	—	—	—	—	—	—	—
FORT PAYNE—DeKalb County										
★ DEKALB BAPTIST MEDICAL CENTER, 200 Medical Center Drive, Zip 35968–3415, Mailing Address: P.O. Box 680778, Zip 35968–1608; tel. 256/845–3150; Barry S. Cochran, President **A**1 9 10 **F**7 8 9 13 16 17 18 22 24 25 26 28 30 32 34 35 36 37 38 39 41 44 45 48 49 51 54 67 70 71 72 73 75 76 78 79 **P**5 7 **S** Baptist Health System, Birmingham, AL Web address: www.bhsala.com	23	10	91	3541	35	50758	805	27002	9289	297

Hospitals, U.S. / ALABAMA

Hospital, Address, Telephone, Administrator, Approval, Facility, and Physician Codes, Health Care System, Network	Classification Codes		Utilization Data					Expense (thousands) of dollars		Personnel
	Control	Service	Staffed Beds	Admissions	Census	Outpatient Visits	Births	Total	Payroll	

★ American Hospital Association (AHA) membership
□ Joint Commission on Accreditation of Healthcare Organizations (JCAHO) accreditation
+ American Osteopathic Healthcare Association (AOHA) membership
○ American Osteopathic Association (AOA) accreditation
△ Commission on Accreditation of Rehabilitation Facilities (CARF) accreditation
Control codes 61, 63, 64, 71, 72 and 73 indicate hospitals listed by AOHA, but not registered by AHA. For definition of numerical codes, see page A4

Hospital	Control	Service	Staffed Beds	Admissions	Census	Outpatient Visits	Births	Total	Payroll	Personnel
FORT RUCKER—Dale County										
★ LYSTER U. S. ARMY COMMUNITY HOSPITAL, U.S. Army Aeromedical Center, Zip 36362–5333; tel. 334/255–7361; Lieutenant Colonel Donald Henderson, Jr, Deputy Commander for Administration **A**1 9 **F**3 9 13 14 16 17 18 19 21 22 32 33 34 35 38 43 45 48 49 51 54 56 59 63 70 72 76 78 79 **P**1 **S** Department of the Army, Office of the Surgeon General, Falls Church, VA	42	10	37	223	2	158796	0	27580	16754	479
GADSDEN—Etowah County										
★ GADSDEN REGIONAL MEDICAL CENTER, 1007 Goodyear Avenue, Zip 35903–1195; tel. 256/494–4000; James F. O'Loughlin, Chief Executive Officer **A**1 2 9 10 **F**41 44 57 **P**5 8 **S** Quorum Health Group, Brentwood, TN Web address: www.gadsdenregional.com	33	10	257	11547	145	109039	1122	83226	29125	1022
□ MOUNTAIN VIEW HOSPITAL, 3001 Scenic Highway, Zip 35901–9956, Mailing Address: P.O. Box 8406, Zip 35902–8406; tel. 256/546–9265; John A. Romano, Chief Executive Officer **A**1 9 10 **F**1 3 13 19 29 30 33 38 57 58 59 60 61 62 63 64 72 **P**5	33	22	68	1480	41	—	0	9196	4362	131
□ RIVERVIEW REGIONAL MEDICAL CENTER, 600 South Third Street, Zip 35901–5399, Mailing Address: P.O. Box 268, Zip 35999–0268; tel. 256/543–5200; J. David McCormack, Executive Director **A**1 9 10 **F**4 8 9 11 12 13 16 17 18 19 22 23 24 25 27 28 30 31 32 33 34 38 39 40 41 43 44 45 46 47 48 49 50 51 54 56 65 68 70 71 72 76 77 78 79 **S** Health Management Associates, Naples, FL	33	10	281	9036	122	161351	79	—	—	638
GENEVA—Geneva County										
★ WIREGRASS MEDICAL CENTER, (Formerly Wiregrass Hospital), 1200 West Maple Avenue, Zip 36340–1694; tel. 334/684–3655; John L. Robertson, Chief Executive Officer (Total facility includes 86 beds in nursing home–type unit) **A**1 9 10 **F**7 9 22 25 32 38 41 48 54 69 70 76	13	10	151	2829	115	23514	0	11882	4470	208
GEORGIANA—Butler County										
GEORGIANA HOSPITAL, (Formerly Georgiana Doctors Hospital), 515 Miranda Street, Zip 36033, Mailing Address: P.O. Box 548, Zip 36033–0548; tel. 334/376–2205; Harry Cole, Interim Administrator (Nonreporting) **A**9 10	33	10	22	—						
GREENSBORO—Hale County										
HALE COUNTY HOSPITAL, 508 Green Street, Zip 36744–0017, Mailing Address: P.O. Box 17, Zip 36744–0017; tel. 334/624–3024; Richard M. McGill, Administrator (Nonreporting) **A**9 10	13	10	30	—						
GREENVILLE—Butler County										
□ L. V. STABLER MEMORIAL HOSPITAL, 29 L. V. Stabler Drive, Zip 36037; tel. 334/382–2676; Tom R. McDougal, Jr, Chief Executive Officer (Nonreporting) **A**1 9 10 **S** Community Health Systems, Inc., Brentwood, TN	33	10	74	—						
GROVE HILL—Clarke County										
★ GROVE HILL MEMORIAL HOSPITAL, 295 South Jackson Street, Zip 36451–0935, Mailing Address: P.O. Box 935, Zip 36451–0935; tel. 334/275–3191; Hybard D. Sewell, Administrator **A**9 10 **F**7 8 9 13 17 18 19 21 22 23 25 26 34 38 40 43 44 45 48 51 54 59 62 69 70 **P**5 **S** Infirmary Health System, Inc., Mobile, AL	16	10	34	1165	10	18495	186	—	1443	79
GUNTERSVILLE—Marshall County										
★ MARSHALL MEDICAL CENTER NORTH, 8000 Alabama Highway 69, Zip 35976; tel. 256/753–8000; Gary R. Gore, Chief Executive Officer **A**1 9 10 **F**4 7 8 9 13 16 17 18 19 20 22 24 25 28 32 34 36 39 41 43 44 45 46 48 49 51 53 54 57 59 60 61 62 65 68 70 71 72 75 76 78 79 **P**8 **S** Marshall County Health Care Authority, Guntersville, AL Web address: www.mmcnorth.com	16	10	90	4300	47	—	604	31335	11381	384
HALEYVILLE—Winston County										
★ CARRAWAY BURDICK WEST MEDICAL CENTER, Highway 195 East, Zip 35565–9536, Mailing Address: P.O. Box 780, Zip 35565–0780; tel. 205/486–5213; Donald J. Jones, Administrator (Nonreporting) **A**1 9 10 **S** Carraway Methodist Health System, Birmingham, AL Web address: www.carraway.com	23	10	99	—						
HAMILTON—Marion County										
★ MARION BAPTIST MEDICAL CENTER, 1256 Military Street South, Zip 35570–5001; tel. 205/921–6200; Glenn C. Sisk, President (Total facility includes 69 beds in nursing home–type unit) **A**1 9 10 **F**9 13 16 17 18 22 24 25 28 30 32 34 36 37 38 39 41 46 48 51 54 56 68 69 70 71 76 78 79 **P**4 7 **S** Baptist Health System, Birmingham, AL Web address: www.bhsala.com	21	10	112	1754	88	20177	—	13995	5691	147
HARTSELLE—Morgan County										
□ HARTSELLE MEDICAL CENTER, 201 Pine Street N.W., Zip 35640–2309, Mailing Address: P.O. Box 969, Zip 35640–0969; tel. 256/773–6511; Mike H. McNair, Chief Executive Officer **A**1 9 10 **F**9 13 19 22 25 30 32 38 41 48 54 57 62 70 76 78 **S** Community Health Systems, Inc., Brentwood, TN	33	10	50	1747	22	22223	0	—	—	191
HUNTSVILLE—Madison County										
★ CRESTWOOD MEDICAL CENTER, One Hospital Drive, Zip 35801–3403; tel. 256/882–3100; Thomas M. Weiss, Chief Executive Officer (Nonreporting) **A**1 9 10 **S** Triad Hospitals, Inc., Dallas, TX	33	10	120	—						
□ HEALTHSOUTH REHABILITATION HOSPITAL OF NORTH ALABAMA, 107 Governors Drive S.W., Zip 35801–4329; tel. 256/535–2300; Rod Moss, Chief Executive Officer (Nonreporting) **A**9 10 **S** HEALTHSOUTH Corporation, Birmingham, AL	33	46	50	—						
★ HUNTSVILLE HOSPITAL, (Includes Huntsville Hospital East, 911 Big Cove Road S.E., Zip 35801–3784; tel. 256/517–8020), 101 Sivley Road, Zip 35801–4470; tel. 256/517–8020; L. Joe Austin, Chief Executive Officer **A**1 2 3 5 9 10 **F**4 7 8 9 11 12 13 16 17 18 19 22 24 25 28 29 32 33 34 36 38 39 41 42 43 44 45 46 47 48 49 50 51 52 54 57 60 61 62 63 64 65 70 76 77 78 79 **P**8 Web address: www.huntsvillehospital.org	16	10	702	35590	450	352270	4562	266165	124689	3500

© 2000 AHA Guide   *Many Facility Codes have changed. Please refer to the AHA Guide Code Chart.*

Hospitals, U.S. / ALABAMA

Hospital, Address, Telephone, Administrator, Approval, Facility, and Physician Codes, Health Care System, Network

★ American Hospital Association (AHA) membership
□ Joint Commission on Accreditation of Healthcare Organizations (JCAHO) accreditation
+ American Osteopathic Healthcare Association (AOHA) membership
○ American Osteopathic Association (AOA) accreditation
△ Commission on Accreditation of Rehabilitation Facilities (CARF) accreditation
Control codes 61, 63, 64, 71, 72 and 73 indicate hospitals listed by AOHA, but not registered by AHA. For definition of numerical codes, see page A4

Hospital	Control	Service	Staffed Beds	Admissions	Census	Outpatient Visits	Births	Total	Payroll	Personnel
JACKSON—Clarke County										
JACKSON MEDICAL CENTER, 220 Hospital Drive, Zip 36545-2459, Mailing Address: P.O. Box 428, Zip 36545-0428; tel. 334/246-9021; Teresa F. Grimes, Administrator **A**9 10 **F**7 8 9 13 22 25 32 36 48 76	33	10	21	1138	8	—	211	3869	1800	77
JACKSONVILLE—Calhoun County										
★ JACKSONVILLE HOSPITAL, 1701 Pelham Road South, Zip 36265-3399, Mailing Address: P.O. Box 999, Zip 36265-0999; tel. 256/435-4970; Charles Mitchener, Jr, Chief Executive Officer **A**1 9 10 **F**7 8 9 13 16 22 24 25 32 33 34 35 39 40 41 44 48 54 66 76 78 **P**1 7 **S** Quorum Health Group, Brentwood, TN **Web address:** www.jaxhosp.com	33	10	56	1891	16	32383	196	16073	5633	169
JASPER—Walker County										
★ WALKER BAPTIST MEDICAL CENTER, 3400 Highway 78 East, Zip 35501-8956, Mailing Address: P.O. Box 3547, Zip 35502-3547; tel. 205/387-4000; Evan S. Dillard, President **A**1 9 10 **F**1 7 8 9 11 13 16 17 18 19 22 24 25 32 34 36 37 39 41 44 45 46 48 50 54 57 59 60 62 70 75 76 78 **S** Baptist Health System, Birmingham, AL **Web address:** www.bhsala.com	23	10	157	7346	74	145573	695	46044	17375	569
LUVERNE—Crenshaw County										
CRENSHAW BAPTIST HOSPITAL, 101 Baptist Lane, Zip 36049; tel. 334/335-3374; Moultrie D. Plowden, CHE, Administrator **A**9 10 **F**2 7 8 16 17 18 19 22 25 29 32 36 38 45 48 50 54 57 61 62 70 71 76 78 **S** Baptist Health, Montgomery, AL	23	10	52	1071	18	21456	105	6601	3427	129
MADISON—Madison County										
BRADFORD HEALTH SERVICES AT HUNTSVILLE, 1600 Browns Ferry Road, Zip 35758-9769, Mailing Address: P.O. Box 176, Zip 35758-0176; tel. 256/461-7272; Bob Hinds, Executive Director (Nonreporting) **S** Bradford Health Services, Birmingham, AL	33	82	84	—	—	—	—	—	—	—
MOBILE—Mobile County										
★ △ MOBILE INFIRMARY MEDICAL CENTER, (Includes Rotary Rehabilitation Hospital), 5 Mobile Infirmary Drive North, Zip 36601, Mailing Address: P.O. Box 2144, Zip 36652-2144; tel. 334/435-2400; E. Chandler Bramlett, Jr, President and Chief Executive Officer **A**1 2 7 9 10 **F**4 5 6 7 8 9 11 12 13 14 16 17 19 22 24 25 28 29 31 32 33 35 36 37 38 39 41 43 44 45 46 47 48 49 50 51 52 54 56 57 58 59 60 62 63 64 65 66 67 68 69 70 71 72 76 77 78 79 **S** Infirmary Health System, Inc., Mobile, AL **Web address:** www.mimc.com	23	10	502	24091	346	241254	977	171242	67019	2178
★ PROVIDENCE HOSPITAL, 6801 Airport Boulevard, Zip 36608-3785, Mailing Address: P.O. Box 850429, Zip 36685-0429; tel. 334/633-1000; John R. Roeder, President and Chief Executive Officer **A**1 2 9 10 **F**4 7 8 9 11 12 13 17 18 19 22 24 25 27 28 34 35 36 37 38 39 40 41 44 46 47 48 49 50 51 54 65 70 71 72 76 78 **P**5 6 7 **S** Ascension Health, Saint Louis, MO **Web address:** www.providencehospital.org	21	10	349	16678	223	196648	1040	138821	50694	1630
ROTARY REHABILITATION HOSPITAL See Mobile Infirmary Medical Center										
□ SPRINGHILL MEMORIAL HOSPITAL, 3719 Dauphin Street, Zip 36608-1798, Mailing Address: P.O. Box 8246, Zip 36608-8246; tel. 334/344-9630; Bill A. Mason, President (Total facility includes 8 beds in nursing home-type unit) **A**1 9 10 **F**4 7 8 9 11 12 13 19 22 24 25 27 28 32 33 36 38 39 41 43 44 45 46 47 48 49 50 51 52 54 55 70 72 75 76 78 79 **Web address:** www.springhillmemorial.com	31	10	228	801040	27409	80008947	159	—	—	108
□ UNIVERSITY OF SOUTH ALABAMA KNOLLWOOD PARK HOSPITAL, 5600 Girby Road, Zip 36693-3398; tel. 334/660-5120; Thomas J. Gibson, Administrator (Nonreporting) **A**1 3 5 9 10 **S** University of South Alabama Hospitals, Mobile, AL	12	10	150	—	—	—	—	—	—	—
□ UNIVERSITY OF SOUTH ALABAMA MEDICAL CENTER, 2451 Fillingim Street, Zip 36617-2293; tel. 334/471-7000; Stephen H. Simmons, Administrator (Nonreporting) **A**1 2 3 5 8 9 10 **S** University of South Alabama Hospitals, Mobile, AL	12	10	316	—	—	—	—	—	—	—
□ USA CHILDREN'S AND WOMEN'S HOSPITAL, 1700 Center Street, Zip 36604-3391; tel. 334/415-1000; Stanley K. Hammack, Administrator **A**1 3 5 9 10 **F**4 7 8 9 10 11 12 13 14 19 22 24 25 35 36 39 41 42 43 44 45 46 47 48 50 51 52 53 54 56 59 63 65 66 68 69 70 71 72 74 75 76 77 78 79 **P**6 **S** University of South Alabama Hospitals, Mobile, AL	12	10	152	11350	137	25727	3700	69383	25432	—
MONROEVILLE—Monroe County										
□ MONROE COUNTY HOSPITAL, 1901 South Alabama Avenue, Zip 36460, Mailing Address: P.O. Box 886, Zip 36461-0886; tel. 334/575-3111; Joe Zager, Chief Executive Officer **A**1 9 10 **F**7 9 12 13 17 22 24 25 32 34 36 41 44 45 48 54 70 75 76 78 **S** Quorum Health Group, Brentwood, TN	13	10	59	2374	23	35766	264	13699	5827	202
MONTGOMERY—Montgomery County										
★ BAPTIST MEDICAL CENTER, 2105 East South Boulevard, Zip 36116-2498, Mailing Address: Box 11010, Zip 36111-0010; tel. 334/288-2100; Victor D. Butler, President and Chief Executive Officer (Nonreporting) **A**1 3 5 9 10 **S** Baptist Health, Montgomery, AL	23	10	454	—	—	—	—	—	—	—
★ BAPTIST MEDICAL CENTER EAST, 400 Taylor Road, Zip 36117-3512, Mailing Address: P.O. Box 241267, Zip 36124-1267; tel. 334/244-8178; John W. Melton, Administrator **A**1 9 10 **F**2 3 4 8 9 11 12 13 18 19 22 24 25 28 29 31 32 34 36 37 38 39 40 42 43 44 47 48 49 51 53 54 55 56 57 70 71 76 77 78 79 **S** Baptist Health, Montgomery, AL	23	10	130	6811	76	—	1192	30959	15026	545

Hospitals, U.S. / ALABAMA

Hospital, Address, Telephone, Administrator, Approval, Facility, and Physician Codes, Health Care System, Network	Classification Codes		Utilization Data					Expense (thousands) of dollars		
★ American Hospital Association (AHA) membership □ Joint Commission on Accreditation of Healthcare Organizations (JCAHO) accreditation + American Osteopathic Healthcare Association (AOHA) membership ○ American Osteopathic Association (AOA) accreditation △ Commission on Accreditation of Rehabilitation Facilities (CARF) accreditation Control codes 61, 63, 64, 71, 72 and 73 indicate hospitals listed by AOHA, but not registered by AHA. For definition of numerical codes, see page A4	Control	Service	Staffed Beds	Admissions	Census	Outpatient Visits	Births	Total	Payroll	Personnel
⊞ CENTRAL ALABAMA VETERAN AFFAIRS HEALTH CARE SYSTEM, (Includes Montgomery Division, 215 Perry Hill Road, tel. 334/272–4670; Veterans Affairs Health Care System–Tuskegee Division, 2400 Hospital Road, Tuskegee, Zip 36083–5001; tel. 334/727–0550), 215 Perry Hill Road, Zip 36109–3798; tel. 334/272–4670; Kenneth Rugle, Interim Director (Total facility includes 160 beds in nursing home–type unit) **A**1 5 **F**41 53 57 69 **S** Department of Veterans Affairs, Washington, DC Web address: www.va.gov/stations97/guide/home.asp?DIVISION=ALL	45	10	355	4020	293	200615	0	77021	61274	1569
□ HEALTHSOUTH REHABILITATION HOSPITAL OF MONTGOMERY, 4465 Narrow Lane Road, Zip 36116–2900; tel. 334/284–7700; Linda Wade, Administrator and Director of Operations **A**1 9 10 **F**5 13 16 17 18 29 30 31 32 34 38 43 45 49 50 53 54 70 71 72 78 **S** HEALTHSOUTH Corporation, Birmingham, AL	33	46	90	1399	78	7571	—	12819	7587	261
⊞ JACKSON HOSPITAL AND CLINIC, 1725 Pine Street, Zip 36106; tel. 334/293–8000; Donald M. Ball, President and Chief Executive Officer **A**1 2 9 10 **F**4 8 9 11 12 16 17 22 24 25 27 32 33 34 37 38 39 41 43 44 45 46 47 48 49 50 51 54 57 59 61 63 65 70 71 76 78 79 **P**6 Web address: www.jackson.org	23	10	280	14790	200	92325	1265	78522	43337	1472
★ LONG TERM CARE HOSPITAL AT JACKSON, (LONGTERM ACUTE CARE HOSPITAL), 1235 Forest Avenue, 5 North, Zip 36106, Mailing Address: P.O. Box 11649, Zip 36111; tel. 334/240–0532; Peter J. Miller, Administrator **F**13 22 24 26 30 39 46 49 50 65 70 76	23	49	25	169	12	0	0	3530	846	—
MOULTON—Lawrence County										
⊞ LAWRENCE BAPTIST MEDICAL CENTER, 202 Hospital Street, Zip 35650–0039, Mailing Address: P.O. Box 39, Zip 35650–0039; tel. 256/974–2200; Steven Honeycutt, Administrator (Nonreporting) **A**1 9 10 **S** Baptist Health System, Birmingham, AL Web address: www.bhsala.com	13	10	30	—	—	—	—	—	—	—
MOUNT VERNON—Mobile County										
□ SEARCY HOSPITAL, Mailing Address: P.O. Box 1001, Zip 36560–1001; tel. 334/829–9411; John T. Bartlett, Director (Total facility includes 142 beds in nursing home–type unit) **A**1 3 5 9 10 **F**16 17 18 51 57 60 62 69 70 **P**6	12	52	467	744	435	0	0	32600	19746	727
MUSCLE SHOALS—Colbert County										
⊞ SHOALS HOSPITAL, (Formerly Medical Center Shoals), 201 Avalon Avenue, Zip 35661–2805, Mailing Address: P.O. Box 3359, Zip 35662–3359; tel. 256/386–1600; Connie Hawthorne, Chief Executive Officer (Nonreporting) **A**1 9 10 **S** Coffee Health Group, Florence, AL	16	10	128	—	—	—	—	—	—	—
NORTHPORT—Tuscaloosa County										
⊞ NORTHPORT MEDICAL CENTER, (Formerly Northport Hospital–DCH), 2700 Hospital Drive, Zip 35476–1079, Mailing Address: P.O. Box 1079, Zip 35476–1079; tel. 205/333–4500; Charles L. Stewart, Administrator **A**1 9 10 **F**2 4 8 9 11 12 13 16 17 18 19 21 22 24 25 27 28 29 30 32 34 35 36 38 39 41 42 43 44 45 46 47 48 49 50 51 52 53 54 57 59 60 61 62 63 65 70 71 72 75 76 78 79 **P**7 8 **S** DCH Health System, Tuscaloosa, AL Web address: www.dchsystem.com	16	10	196	8015	144	60558	1217	49732	22126	621
ONEONTA—Blount County										
★ MEDICAL CENTER BLOUNT, (Formerly Blount Memorial Hospital), 150 Gilbreath, Zip 35121–2534, Mailing Address: P.O. Box 1000, Zip 35121–1000; tel. 205/274–3000; Jacki Jennings, Chief Executive Officer **A**9 10 **F**9 16 17 18 22 24 25 32 34 36 38 41 46 48 54 55 76 **S** Eastern Health System, Inc., Birmingham, AL	23	10	40	1839	20	46585	0	12993	4956	182
OPELIKA—Lee County										
⊞ EAST ALABAMA MEDICAL CENTER, 2000 Pepperell Parkway, Zip 36802–3201; tel. 334/749–3411; Terry W. Andrus, President (Total facility includes 28 beds in nursing home–type unit) **A**1 2 9 10 **F**1 4 6 7 8 9 11 12 13 16 17 18 19 22 24 25 28 30 35 36 37 38 39 41 43 44 46 47 48 49 50 54 57 58 61 62 65 69 70 75 76 78 **P**2 Web address: www.eamc.org	16	10	273	14709	193	84795	1468	105512	42894	1329
OPP—Covington County										
★ MIZELL MEMORIAL HOSPITAL, 702 Main Street, Zip 36467–1626, Mailing Address: P.O. Box 1010, Zip 36467–1010; tel. 334/493–3541; Allen Foster, Administrator **A**9 10 **F**7 8 9 12 13 17 18 19 22 24 25 32 35 36 37 39 44 46 48 49 51 54 68 70 76 78 79	23	10	57	1987	23	22251	125	7651	4349	226
OZARK—Dale County										
□ DALE MEDICAL CENTER, 100 Hospital Avenue, Zip 36360–2080; tel. 334/774–2601; Robert F. Bigley, Administrator **A**1 9 10 **F**7 9 11 13 15 19 20 22 24 27 28 29 32 34 36 38 39 41 44 45 48 54 70 71 75 76 77 78 **P**5	16	10	59	3095	30	37446	424	20863	9017	426
PELHAM—Shelby County										
BRADFORD HEALTH SERVICES AT OAK MOUNTAIN, (MENTAL HEALTH RTC), 2280 Highway 35, Zip 35124–6120; tel. 205/664–3480; William Weaver, Administrator **F**2 3 16 19 21 57 59 60 61 62 63 **S** Bradford Health Services, Birmingham, AL Web address: www.bradfordhealth.com	33	59	56	231	44	180	0	1905	1290	68
PELL CITY—St. Clair County										
★ ST. CLAIR REGIONAL HOSPITAL, 2805 Hospital Drive, Zip 35125–1499; tel. 205/338–3301 (Nonreporting) **A**9 10 **S** Eastern Health System, Inc., Birmingham, AL	13	10	51	—	—	—	—	—	—	—

© 2000 AHA Guide   *Many Facility Codes have changed. Please refer to the AHA Guide Code Chart.*

Hospitals, U.S. / ALABAMA

	Classification Codes		Utilization Data					Expense (thousands) of dollars		
Hospital, Address, Telephone, Administrator, Approval, Facility, and Physician Codes, Health Care System, Network	Control	Service	Staffed Beds	Admissions	Census	Outpatient Visits	Births	Total	Payroll	Personnel

★ American Hospital Association (AHA) membership
□ Joint Commission on Accreditation of Healthcare Organizations (JCAHO) accreditation
+ American Osteopathic Healthcare Association (AOHA) membership
○ American Osteopathic Association (AOA) accreditation
△ Commission on Accreditation of Rehabilitation Facilities (CARF) accreditation
Control codes 61, 63, 64, 71, 72 and 73 indicate hospitals listed by AOHA, but not registered by AHA. For definition of numerical codes, see page A4

PHENIX CITY—Russell County
★ PHENIX REGIONAL HOSPITAL, 1707 21st Avenue, Zip 36867–3753, Mailing Address: P.O. Box 190, Zip 36868–0190; tel. 334/291–8502; Lance B. Duke, FACHE, President and Chief Executive Officer **A**1 9 10 **F**2 3 7 8 9 11 13 17 18 19 21 22 24 25 28 30 32 33 34 35 36 38 39 41 42 44 45 46 48 49 50 51 52 53 54 56 57 59 60 61 65 68 69 70 72 73 75 76 77 78 79 **P**6 8 **S** Columbus Regional Health System, Columbus, GA — 23 10 114 3788 41 41442 529 21823 8710 308

PRATTVILLE—Autauga County
★ PRATTVILLE BAPTIST HOSPITAL, 124 South Memorial Drive, Zip 36067–3619, Mailing Address: P.O. Box 681630, Zip 36067–1638; tel. 334/365–0651; William E. Hines, Administrator **A**1 9 10 **F**3 4 6 7 8 9 11 13 14 16 17 18 19 22 24 25 27 28 29 30 31 32 33 34 35 36 37 38 39 41 43 45 46 47 48 49 50 51 54 56 58 59 60 61 62 63 64 65 66 67 70 71 72 73 75 76 77 78 79 **P**5 **S** Baptist Health, Montgomery, AL — 23 10 54 1591 15 27998 0 11630 4363 160

RED BAY—Franklin County
★ RED BAY HOSPITAL, 211 Hospital Road, Zip 35582–0490, Mailing Address: P.O. Box 490, Zip 35582–0490; tel. 256/386–4556; Ralph J. Wilson, Administrator **A**9 10 **F**9 22 25 34 36 38 45 48 54 69 76 — 16 10 25 934 11 21613 0 5959 2542 115

ROANOKE—Randolph County
★ RANDOLPH COUNTY HOSPITAL, 59928 Highway 22, Zip 36274, Mailing Address: P.O. Box 670, Zip 36274–0670; tel. 334/863–4111; Ronald L. Sparkman, Administrator (Nonreporting) **A**1 9 10 — 13 10 66 — — — — — — —

RUSSELLVILLE—Franklin County
★ RUSSELLVILLE HOSPITAL, (Formerly Russellville Medical Center), 15155 Highway 43, Zip 35653, Mailing Address: P.O. Box 1089, Zip 35653–1089; tel. 256/332–1611; Christine R. Stewart, President and Chief Executive Officer **A**1 9 10 **F**8 9 11 12 13 16 17 18 22 24 25 28 31 33 34 36 37 38 39 41 43 44 45 46 47 48 51 54 70 71 74 76 78 79 **S** Coffee Health Group, Florence, AL — 15 10 100 3864 43 22630 245 — — 396

SCOTTSBORO—Jackson County
□ JACKSON COUNTY HOSPITAL, 380 Woods Cove Road, Zip 35768–2428, Mailing Address: P.O. Box 1050, Zip 35768–1050; tel. 256/259–4444; Thomas O. Lackey, Chief Executive Officer (Total facility includes 50 beds in nursing home–type unit) **A**1 9 10 **F**8 12 16 17 18 22 25 36 39 44 48 69 71 76 78 — 13 10 142 3868 89 35931 318 27347 11736 390

SELMA—Dallas County
★ SELMA BAPTIST HOSPITAL, 1015 Medical Center Parkway, Zip 36701–6352; tel. 334/418–4100; Lee Ashbury, Chief Executive Officer **A**1 2 3 5 9 10 **F**4 7 8 9 11 13 16 17 18 22 25 30 32 33 34 41 43 44 45 46 48 54 57 62 64 70 71 72 75 76 78 **S** Baptist Health, Montgomery, AL — 23 10 130 5480 71 — 555 34530 11572 354

★ VAUGHAN REGIONAL MEDICAL CENTER, 1050 West Dallas Avenue, Zip 36701–6515, Mailing Address: P.O. Box 328, Zip 36702–0328; tel. 334/418–6000; Jerome H. Horn, President and Chief Executive Officer **A**1 3 5 9 10 **F**6 7 8 9 11 13 18 19 22 24 25 28 32 34 39 45 46 48 68 76 — 23 10 112 5078 61 31833 546 25033 9510 409

SHEFFIELD—Colbert County
★ HELEN KELLER HOSPITAL, 1300 South Montgomery Avenue, Zip 35660–6334, Mailing Address: P.O. Box 610, Zip 35660–0610; tel. 256/386–4196; William H. Anderson, President **A**1 9 10 **F**7 8 9 11 12 13 17 18 22 24 25 28 31 32 34 38 39 41 43 44 45 46 48 51 54 68 70 71 76 78 Web address: www.helenkeller.com — 16 10 151 6462 82 54478 737 42863 16524 625

SYLACAUGA—Talladega County
★ COOSA VALLEY BAPTIST MEDICAL CENTER, 315 West Hickory Street, Zip 35150–2996; tel. 256/249–5000; Steven M. Johnson, President (Total facility includes 75 beds in nursing home–type unit) (Nonreporting) **A**1 9 10 **S** Baptist Health System, Birmingham, AL Web address: www.bhsala.com — 21 10 176 — — — — — — —

TALLADEGA—Talladega County
★ CITIZENS BAPTIST MEDICAL CENTER, 604 Stone Avenue, Zip 35160–2217, Mailing Address: P.O. Box 978, Zip 35161–0978; tel. 256/362–8111; Steven M. Johnson, President (Nonreporting) **A**1 9 10 **S** Baptist Health System, Birmingham, AL Web address: www.bhsala.com — 23 10 97 — — — — — — —

TALLASSEE—Elmore County
★ COMMUNITY HOSPITAL, 805 Friendship Road, Zip 36078–1234, Mailing Address: P.O. Box 780700, Zip 36078–0700; tel. 334/283–6541; Jennie R. Rhinehart, Administrator and Chief Executive Officer (Nonreporting) **A**1 9 10 — 23 10 69 — — — — — — —

THOMASVILLE—Clarke County
THOMASVILLE INFIRMARY, 33700 Highway 43, Zip 36784; tel. 334/636–4431; Albert Ban, Jr, Administrator **A**9 10 **F**18 22 25 32 34 36 37 48 54 70 76 **P**5 **S** Infirmary Health System, Inc., Mobile, AL — 23 10 27 952 8 15055 — 5178 2029 87

TROY—Pike County
□ EDGE REGIONAL MEDICAL CENTER, 1330 Highway 231 South, Zip 36081–1224; tel. 334/670–5000; David E. Loving, Chief Executive Officer (Nonreporting) **A**1 9 10 **S** Community Health Systems, Inc., Brentwood, TN — 33 10 87 — — — — — — —

TUSCALOOSA—Tuscaloosa County
□ BRYCE HOSPITAL, 200 University Boulevard, Zip 35401–1294; tel. 205/759–0799; David E. Gay, Jr, Director (Total facility includes 354 beds in nursing home–type unit) **A**1 10 **F**18 23 43 50 51 57 58 59 69 70 78 **P**6 — 12 22 820 715 791 0 0 55897 33538 1202

Hospitals, U.S. / ALABAMA

Hospital, Address, Telephone, Administrator, Approval, Facility, and Physician Codes, Health Care System, Network	Classification Codes		Utilization Data					Expense (thousands) of dollars		
★ American Hospital Association (AHA) membership ☐ Joint Commission on Accreditation of Healthcare Organizations (JCAHO) accreditation + American Osteopathic Healthcare Association (AOHA) membership ○ American Osteopathic Association (AOA) accreditation △ Commission on Accreditation of Rehabilitation Facilities (CARF) accreditation Control codes 61, 63, 64, 71, 72 and 73 indicate hospitals listed by AOHA, but not registered by AHA. For definition of numerical codes, see page A4	Control	Service	Staffed Beds	Admissions	Census	Outpatient Visits	Births	Total	Payroll	Personnel
★ DCH REGIONAL MEDICAL CENTER, 809 University Boulevard East, Zip 35401–9961; tel. 205/759–7111; William H. Cassels, Administrator **A**1 2 3 5 9 10 **F**4 8 9 11 12 13 16 18 19 21 22 24 25 27 28 29 32 34 35 36 38 39 41 42 43 44 45 46 47 48 49 50 51 52 54 57 59 60 61 62 65 68 69 70 71 72 75 76 78 79 **P**7 **S** DCH Health System, Tuscaloosa, AL Web address: www.dchhealthcare.com	23	10	383	23173	344	257789	1772	190315	86509	2485
★ VETERANS AFFAIRS MEDICAL CENTER, 3701 Loop Road, Zip 35404–5015; tel. 205/554–2000; W. Kenneth Ruyle, Director (Total facility includes 195 beds in nursing home–type unit) (Nonreporting) **A**1 3 9 **S** Department of Veterans Affairs, Washington, DC Web address: www.va.gov/stations97/guide/home.asp?DIVISION=ALL	45	22	307	—	—	—	—	—	—	—
TUSKEGEE—Macon County VETERANS AFFAIRS HEALTH CARE SYSTEM–TUSKEGEE DIVISION See Central Alabama Veteran Affairs Health Care System, Montgomery										
UNION SPRINGS—Bullock County BULLOCK COUNTY HOSPITAL, 102 West Conecuh Avenue, Zip 36089–1303; tel. 334/738–2140; Jacques Jarry, Administrator (Nonreporting) **A**9 10	33	10	30	—	—	—	—	—	—	—
VALLEY—Chambers County ☐ LANIER HEALTH SERVICES, 4800 48th Street, Zip 36854–3666; tel. 334/756–3111; Robert J. Humphrey, Administrator (Total facility includes 93 beds in nursing home–type unit) (Nonreporting) **A**1 9 10 Web address: www.lanierhospital.com	23	10	175	—	—	—	—	—	—	—
WEDOWEE—Randolph County ★ WEDOWEE HOSPITAL, 209 North Main Street, Zip 36278–5138, Mailing Address: P.O. Box 307, Zip 36278–0307; tel. 256/357–2111; Kerlene Mitchell, Administrator (Nonreporting) **A**9 10	23	10	34	—	—	—	—	—	—	—
WETUMPKA—Elmore County ELMORE COMMUNITY HOSPITAL, 500 Hospital Drive, Zip 36092–1625, Mailing Address: P.O. Box 120, Zip 36092–0120; tel. 334/567–4311; Emily S. Mann, R.N., MSN, Acting Administrator (Nonreporting) **A**9 10	15	10	46	—	—	—	—	—	—	—
WINFIELD—Marion County ★ CARRAWAY NORTHWEST MEDICAL CENTER, Highway 78 West, Zip 35594, Mailing Address: P.O. Box 130, Zip 35594–0130; tel. 205/487–7000; Robert E. Henger, Administrator **A**1 9 10 **F**8 9 13 16 17 18 19 22 24 25 28 32 33 34 36 38 41 43 44 45 46 48 50 51 54 56 63 66 68 70 71 76 78 79 **P**1 5 **S** Carraway Methodist Health System, Birmingham, AL Web address: www.carraway.org	21	10	63	2835	29	89621	470	18846	7818	326

ALASKA

Resident Population 614 (in thousands)
Resident population in metro areas 41.3%
Birth rate per 1,000 population 16.3
65 years and over 5.5%
Percent of persons without health insurance 18.1%

Hospital, Address, Telephone, Administrator, Approval, Facility, and Physician Codes, Health Care System, Network	Classification Codes		Utilization Data					Expense (thousands) of dollars		
	Control	Service	Staffed Beds	Admissions	Census	Outpatient Visits	Births	Total	Payroll	Personnel

★ American Hospital Association (AHA) membership
□ Joint Commission on Accreditation of Healthcare Organizations (JCAHO) accreditation
+ American Osteopathic Healthcare Association (AOHA) membership
○ American Osteopathic Association (AOA) accreditation
△ Commission on Accreditation of Rehabilitation Facilities (CARF) accreditation
Control codes 61, 63, 64, 71, 72 and 73 indicate hospitals listed by AOHA, but not registered by AHA. For definition of numerical codes, see page A4

ANCHORAGE—2nd Judicial Division

Hospital	Control	Service	Staffed Beds	Admissions	Census	Outpatient Visits	Births	Total	Payroll	Personnel
✦ ALASKA NATIVE MEDICAL CENTER, (Formerly PHS Alaska Native Medical Center), 4315 Diplomacy Drive, Zip 99508; tel. 907/563-2662; Richard Mandsager, M.D., Administrator (Nonreporting) **A**1 9 10 **S** U. S. Public Health Service Indian Health Service, Rockville, MD	47	10	140	—	—	—	—	—	—	—
□ ALASKA PSYCHIATRIC INSTITUTE, 2900 Providence Drive, Zip 99508-4677; tel. 907/269-7100; Randall P. Burns, Chief Executive Officer (Nonreporting) **A**1 10	12	22	79	—	—	—	—	—	—	—
✦ △ ALASKA REGIONAL HOSPITAL, 2801 Debarr Road, Zip 99508, Mailing Address: P.O. Box 143889, Zip 99514-3889; tel. 907/276-1754; Edward H. Lamb, President and Chief Executive Officer (Total facility includes 16 beds in nursing home-type unit) **A**1 7 9 10 **F**3 4 7 8 9 11 12 13 14 17 18 22 24 25 26 27 28 29 31 32 33 34 38 39 41 42 44 45 46 47 48 49 50 51 53 54 58 59 60 61 63 64 65 68 69 70 72 76 78 79 **P**5 8 **S** HCA – The Healthcare Company, Nashville, TN	33	10	194	5177	76	85457	654	67099	29040	522
✦ CHARTER NORTH STAR BEHAVIORAL HEALTH SYSTEM, 1650 South Bragaw, Zip 99508-3467; tel. 907/258-7575; Kathleen Cronen, Chief Executive Officer (Nonreporting) **A**1 10 **S** Magellan Health Services, Atlanta, GA	33	22	34	—	—	—	—	—	—	—
✦ CHARTER NORTH STAR BEHAVIORAL HEALTH SYSTEM, 2530 DeBarr Road, Zip 99508; tel. 907/258-7575; Kathleen Cronen, Chief Executive Officer (Nonreporting) **A**1 10 **S** Magellan Health Services, Atlanta, GA Web address: www.charterbehavioral.com	33	22	80	—	—	—	—	—	—	—
✦ PROVIDENCE ALASKA MEDICAL CENTER, 3200 Providence Drive, Zip 99508, Mailing Address: P.O. Box 196604, Zip 99519-6604; tel. 907/562-2211; Gene L. O'Hara, Administrator **A**1 3 5 10 **F**3 4 6 7 8 9 11 12 13 17 18 22 24 25 32 34 36 38 39 41 42 43 44 46 47 48 50 51 52 53 54 55 57 58 59 61 62 63 64 65 68 69 72 76 78 **P**4 7 8 **S** Providence Health System, Seattle, WA Web address: www.providence.org	21	10	341	14451	210	359873	2663	203108	87956	1761

BARROW—4th Judicial Division

Hospital	Control	Service	Staffed Beds	Admissions	Census	Outpatient Visits	Births	Total	Payroll	Personnel
✦ SAMUEL SIMMONDS MEMORIAL HOSPITAL, (Formerly U. S. Public Health Service Alaska Native Hospital), 1296 Agvik Street, Zip 99723, Mailing Address: P.O. Box 29, Zip 99723; tel. 907/852-4611; Michael S. Herring, Administrator (Nonreporting) **A**1 10 **S** U. S. Public Health Service Indian Health Service, Rockville, MD	47	10	15	—	—	—	—	—	—	—

BETHEL—1st Judicial Division

Hospital	Control	Service	Staffed Beds	Admissions	Census	Outpatient Visits	Births	Total	Payroll	Personnel
✦ YUKON–KUSKOKWIM DELTA REGIONAL HOSPITAL, Mailing Address: P.O. Box 528, Zip 99559-3000; tel. 907/543-6300; Edwin L. Hansen, Vice President (Nonreporting) **A**1 10 **S** U. S. Public Health Service Indian Health Service, Rockville, MD	47	10	50	—	—	—	—	—	—	—

CORDOVA—2nd Judicial Division

Hospital	Control	Service	Staffed Beds	Admissions	Census	Outpatient Visits	Births	Total	Payroll	Personnel
★ CORDOVA COMMUNITY MEDICAL CENTER, 602 Chase Avenue, Zip 99574, Mailing Address: Box 160, Zip 99574; tel. 907/424-8000; Edward Zeine, Administrator and Chief Executive Officer (Total facility includes 13 beds in nursing home-type unit) (Nonreporting) **A**10	14	10	23	—	—	—	—	—	—	—

DILLINGHAM—1st Judicial Division

Hospital	Control	Service	Staffed Beds	Admissions	Census	Outpatient Visits	Births	Total	Payroll	Personnel
✦ KANAKANAK HOSPITAL, Mailing Address: P.O. Box 130, Zip 99576; tel. 907/842-5201; Darrel C. Richardson, Chief Operating Officer (Nonreporting) **A**1 10 **S** U. S. Public Health Service Indian Health Service, Rockville, MD	47	10	16	—	—	—	—	—	—	—

ELMENDORF AFB—2nd Judicial Division

Hospital	Control	Service	Staffed Beds	Admissions	Census	Outpatient Visits	Births	Total	Payroll	Personnel
✦ U. S. AIR FORCE REGIONAL HOSPITAL, 24800 Hospital Drive, Zip 99506-3700; tel. 907/552-4033 (Nonreporting) **A**1 **S** Department of the Air Force, Bowling AFB, DC	41	10	64	—	—	—	—	—	—	—

FAIRBANKS—1st Judicial Division

Hospital	Control	Service	Staffed Beds	Admissions	Census	Outpatient Visits	Births	Total	Payroll	Personnel
✦ FAIRBANKS MEMORIAL HOSPITAL, 1650 Cowles Street, Zip 99701; tel. 907/452-8181; Michael K. Powers, Administrator (Total facility includes 90 beds in nursing home-type unit) **A**1 2 9 10 **F**3 4 7 8 9 10 13 16 17 18 19 22 23 24 25 26 27 30 32 34 36 38 39 41 42 43 44 45 46 48 49 50 51 54 57 58 59 60 61 62 63 64 65 68 69 70 71 72 75 78 79 **S** Banner Health System, Fargo, ND Web address: www.lhsnet.org	23	10	209	5654	144	207643	1004	87313	36374	709

FORT WAINWRIGHT—1st Judicial Division

Hospital	Control	Service	Staffed Beds	Admissions	Census	Outpatient Visits	Births	Total	Payroll	Personnel
✦ BASSETT ARMY COMMUNITY HOSPITAL, 1060 Gaffney Road, Box 7400, Zip 99703-7400; tel. 907/353-5108; Lieutenant Colonel Dudley J. Schroeder, Deputy Commander (Nonreporting) **A**1 **S** Department of the Army, Office of the Surgeon General, Falls Church, VA	42	10	43	—	—	—	—	—	—	—

HOMER—3rd Judicial Division

Hospital	Control	Service	Staffed Beds	Admissions	Census	Outpatient Visits	Births	Total	Payroll	Personnel
★ SOUTH PENINSULA HOSPITAL, 4300 Bartlett Street, Zip 99603; tel. 907/235-8101; Charles C. Franz, Chief Executive Officer (Total facility includes 20 beds in nursing home-type unit) **A**9 10 **F**8 9 12 13 17 18 22 24 25 32 36 41 43 44 48 54 69 70 76 Web address: www.sphosp.com	16	10	40	1482	28	13547	128	14563	6578	189

Hospitals, U.S. / ALASKA

Hospital, Address, Telephone, Administrator, Approval, Facility, and Physician Codes, Health Care System, Network	Classification Codes		Utilization Data					Expense (thousands) of dollars		
★ American Hospital Association (AHA) membership ☐ Joint Commission on Accreditation of Healthcare Organizations (JCAHO) accreditation + American Osteopathic Healthcare Association (AOHA) membership ○ American Osteopathic Association (AOA) accreditation △ Commission on Accreditation of Rehabilitation Facilities (CARF) accreditation Control codes 61, 63, 64, 71, 72 and 73 indicate hospitals listed by AOHA, but not registered by AHA. For definition of numerical codes, see page A4	Control	Service	Staffed Beds	Admissions	Census	Outpatient Visits	Births	Total	Payroll	Personnel
JUNEAU—3rd Judicial Division										
★ BARTLETT REGIONAL HOSPITAL, 3260 Hospital Drive, Zip 99801; tel. 907/586–2611; Robert F. Valliant, Administrator (Nonreporting) **A**1 9 10 **S** Quorum Health Group, Brentwood, TN **Web address:** www.bartletthospital.org	15	10	64	—	—	—	—	—	—	—
KETCHIKAN—3rd Judicial Division										
★ KETCHIKAN GENERAL HOSPITAL, 3100 Tongass Avenue, Zip 99901–5746; tel. 907/225–5171; Edward F. Mahn, Chief Executive Officer (Total facility includes 29 beds in nursing home–type unit) **A**1 2 9 10 **F**9 16 17 22 25 33 36 44 45 46 48 54 63 69 70 78 **S** PeaceHealth, Bellevue, WA	23	10	65	2064	36	38237	282	27958	14085	304
KODIAK—2nd Judicial Division										
★ PROVIDENCE KODIAK ISLAND MEDICAL CENTER, 1915 East Rezanof Drive, Zip 99615; tel. 907/486–3281; Phillip E. Cline, Administrator (Total facility includes 19 beds in nursing home–type unit) **A**1 9 10 **F**8 9 16 17 18 22 25 32 34 35 36 41 43 44 45 48 53 57 59 60 61 63 69 70 76 78 **S** Providence Health System, Seattle, WA **Web address:** www.providence.org	21	10	44	849	26	11195	223	13883	6928	137
KOTZEBUE—2nd Judicial Division										
★ MANIILAQ HEALTH CENTER, Zip 99752–0043; tel. 907/442–3321; Tim J. Gilbert, Administrator (Nonreporting) **A**1 10 **S** U. S. Public Health Service Indian Health Service, Rockville, MD **Web address:** www.maniilaq.org	47	10	17	—	—	—	—	—	—	—
NOME—2nd Judicial Division										
★ NORTON SOUND REGIONAL HOSPITAL, Bering Straits, Zip 99762, Mailing Address: P.O. Box 966, Zip 99762–0966; tel. 907/443–3311; Charles Fagerstrom, Vice President (Total facility includes 15 beds in nursing home–type unit) (Nonreporting) **A**1 9 10 **S** U. S. Public Health Service Indian Health Service, Rockville, MD **Web address:** www.nshcorp.org	23	10	34	—	—	—	—	—	—	—
PALMER—2nd Judicial Division										
★ VALLEY HOSPITAL, 515 East Dahlia Street, Zip 99645, Mailing Address: P.O. Box 1687, Zip 99645; tel. 907/352–2860; Dave Pfeifer, Chief Executive Officer **A**1 9 10 **F**1 2 3 4 5 6 7 8 9 10 11 12 13 14 15 16 17 18 19 20 21 22 23 24 25 26 27 28 29 30 31 32 33 34 35 36 37 38 39 40 41 42 43 45 46 47 48 49 50 51 52 54 55 56 57 58 59 60 61 62 63 64 65 66 67 68 69 70 71 72 73 74 75 76 77 78 79 **Web address:** www.valley–hosp.com	23	10	36	2405	23	100131	375	34487	14241	384
PETERSBURG—3rd Judicial Division										
PETERSBURG MEDICAL CENTER, 103 Fram Street, Zip 99833, Mailing Address: Box 589, Zip 99833–0589; tel. 907/772–4291; John F. Bringhurst, Administrator (Total facility includes 15 beds in nursing home–type unit) **A**10 **F**1 2 8 9 12 16 17 18 19 25 32 34 35 36 44 46 48 56 57 61 66 69 70 72 76 77	14	10	27	183	17	12275	18	4958	2465	64
SEWARD—2nd Judicial Division										
★ PROVIDENCE SEWARD MEDICAL CENTER, 417 First Avenue, Zip 99664, Mailing Address: P.O. Box 365, Zip 99664–0365; tel. 907/224–5205; Judy Christine Rathje, Administrator **A**9 10 **F**8 14 16 17 18 25 32 36 43 56 72 76 **P**6 **S** Providence Health System, Seattle, WA **Web address:** www.providence.org	21	10	6	102	1	17431	1	4527	2481	49
SITKA—3rd Judicial Division										
★ SEARHC MT. EDGECUMBE HOSPITAL, 222 Tongass Drive, Zip 99835–9416; tel. 907/966–2411; Frank Sutton, Vice President Hospital Services **A**1 9 10 **F**8 9 13 16 17 18 22 23 25 28 31 32 38 43 44 48 57 58 59 61 62 63 70 72 73 76 79 **S** U. S. Public Health Service Indian Health Service, Rockville, MD **Web address:** www.searhc.org	23	10	60	1539	25	44112	69	—	—	278
★ SITKA COMMUNITY HOSPITAL, 209 Moller Avenue, Zip 99835–7145; tel. 907/747–3241; John H. Vowell, Interim Administrator **A**9 10 **F**16 17 18 22 24 36 48 49 70 76	14	10	24	556	5	—	78	—	—	—
SOLDOTNA—3rd Judicial Division										
★ CENTRAL PENINSULA GENERAL HOSPITAL, 250 Hospital Place, Zip 99669; tel. 907/262–4404; Martin I. Richman, Chief Executive Officer **A**1 9 10 **F**7 8 9 13 16 17 18 19 22 25 30 32 35 39 41 44 45 46 48 51 54 61 70 76 78 **P**5	23	10	46	2450	22	45783	407	24976	11342	242
VALDEZ—3rd Judicial Division										
★ VALDEZ COMMUNITY HOSPITAL, 911 Meals Avenue, Zip 99686–0550, Mailing Address: P.O. Box 550, Zip 99686–0550; tel. 907/835–2249; James R. Culley, Administrator **A**9 10 **F**3 7 8 16 17 19 21 25 32 48 59 63 70 72 76 **P**4 7 **Web address:** www.valdezrha.org	14	10	15	158	4	5570	33	3014	1439	35
WRANGELL—3rd Judicial Division										
★ WRANGELL MEDICAL CENTER, First Avenue and Bennett Street, Zip 99929, Mailing Address: P.O. Box 1081, Zip 99929; tel. 907/874–7000; Brian D. Gilbert, Chief Executive Officer (Total facility includes 14 beds in nursing home–type unit) **A**10 **F**7 8 9 23 25 32 36 38 48 69 70 76 **P**6 **Web address:** www.hisea.org/wgl.html	14	10	22	199	15	8647	14	4204	2502	65

Hospitals, U.S. / ARIZONA

ARIZONA

Resident Population 4,669 (in thousands)
Resident population in metro areas 87.6%
Birth rate per 1,000 population 16.6
65 years and over 13.2%
Percent of persons without health insurance 24.5%

★ American Hospital Association (AHA) membership
☐ Joint Commission on Accreditation of Healthcare Organizations (JCAHO) accreditation
+ American Osteopathic Healthcare Association (AOHA) membership
○ American Osteopathic Association (AOA) accreditation
△ Commission on Accreditation of Rehabilitation Facilities (CARF) accreditation
Control codes 61, 63, 64, 71, 72 and 73 indicate hospitals listed by AOHA, but not registered by AHA. For definition of numerical codes, see page A4

Hospital, Address, Telephone, Administrator, Approval, Facility, and Physician Codes, Health Care System, Network	Classification Codes		Utilization Data					Expense (thousands) of dollars		
	Control	Service	Staffed Beds	Admissions	Census	Outpatient Visits	Births	Total	Payroll	Personnel
BENSON—Cochise County ☐ BENSON HOSPITAL, 450 South Ocotillo Street, Zip 85602, Mailing Address: P.O. Box 2290, Zip 85602; tel. 520/586-2261; Ronald A. McKinnon, Chief Executive Officer (Nonreporting) **A**1 9 10 **Web address:** www.bensonhospital.theriver.com	16	10	22	—	—	—	—	—	—	—
BISBEE—Cochise County ☐ COPPER QUEEN COMMUNITY HOSPITAL, 101 Cole Avenue, Zip 85603-1399; tel. 520/432-5383; James J. Dickson, Administrator and Chief Executive Officer (Total facility includes 21 beds in nursing home–type unit) (Nonreporting) **A**1 9 10	23	10	49	—	—	—	—	—	—	—
BULLHEAD CITY—Mohave County ★ MOHAVE VALLEY HOSPITAL AND MEDICAL CENTER, 1225 East Hancock Road, Zip 86442-5941; tel. 520/758-3931; Ann Zimmerman, Acting Administrator (Nonreporting)	33	10	12	—	—	—	—	—	—	—
✯ WESTERN ARIZONA REGIONAL MEDICAL CENTER, 2735 Silver Creek Road, Zip 86442-8303; tel. 520/763-2273; James Sato, Senior Vice President and Chief Executive Officer (Total facility includes 120 beds in nursing home–type unit) (Nonreporting) **A**1 9 10 **S** Community Health Systems, Inc., Brentwood, TN **Web address:** www.baptisthealth.com	30	10	182	—	—	—	—	—	—	—
CASA GRANDE—Pinal County ✯ CASA GRANDE REGIONAL MEDICAL CENTER, 1800 East Florence Boulevard, Zip 85222-5399; tel. 520/426-6300; J. Marty Dernier, President and Chief Executive Officer (Total facility includes 128 beds in nursing home–type unit) **A**1 9 10 **F**8 9 11 13 22 25 28 32 39 41 44 48 49 54 69 70 76 78 **P**8 **S** Quorum Health Group, Brentwood, TN **Web address:** www.casagrandehospital.com	23	10	244	6202	163	52423	822	50385	17641	542
CHANDLER—Maricopa County ✯ CHANDLER REGIONAL HOSPITAL, 475 South Dobson Road, Zip 85224-4230; tel. 480/963-4561; David G. Covert, President and Chief Administrative Officer (Nonreporting) **A**1 9 10 **S** Catholic Healthcare West, San Francisco, CA **Web address:** www.evrhs.org	23	10	120	—	—	—	—	—	—	—
CHINLE—Apache County ✯ CHINLE COMPREHENSIVE HEALTH CARE FACILITY, Highway 191, Zip 86503, Mailing Address: P.O. Drawer PH, Zip 86503; tel. 520/674-7011; Ronald Tso, Chief Executive Officer **A**1 10 **F**8 9 13 14 17 18 20 23 25 29 31 34 41 44 48 51 54 56 58 60 61 63 64 66 70 76 79 **P**6 **S** U. S. Public Health Service Indian Health Service, Rockville, MD	47	10	46	3351	33	144786	636	—	—	517
COTTONWOOD—Yavapai County ✯ VERDE VALLEY MEDICAL CENTER, 269 South Candy Lane, Zip 86326; tel. 520/634-2251; Craig A. Owens, President and Chief Operating Officer (Nonreporting) **A**1 9 10	23	10	64	—	—	—	—	—	—	—
DAVIS–MONTHAN AFB—Pima County ★ U. S. AIR FORCE HOSPITAL, 4175 South Alamo Avenue, Zip 85707-4405; tel. 520/228-2930; Colonel James H. Young, Administrator (Nonreporting) **S** Department of the Air Force, Bowling AFB, DC	41	10	20	—	—	—	—	—	—	—
DOUGLAS—Cochise County ☐ SOUTHEAST ARIZONA MEDICAL CENTER, Route 1, Box 30, Zip 85607; tel. 520/364-7931; Thomas L. Haywood, Chief Executive Officer (Total facility includes 43 beds in nursing home–type unit) (Nonreporting) **A**1 9 10	23	10	75	—	—	—	—	—	—	—
FLAGSTAFF—Coconino County ✯ △ FLAGSTAFF MEDICAL CENTER, (Includes Aspen Hill Behavioral Health System, 305 West Forest Avenue, Zip 86001-1464; tel. 520/773-1060; Thor Kolle, Chief Executive Officer), 1200 North Beaver Street, Zip 86001-3198; tel. 520/779-3366; Stephen G. Carlson, President and Chief Operating Officer (Total facility includes 28 beds in nursing home–type unit) **A**1 7 9 10 **F**1 3 7 8 11 13 14 16 17 18 19 22 24 25 26 27 29 31 32 34 36 37 38 39 41 44 45 46 48 49 51 53 54 57 58 61 62 63 64 65 69 70 72 74 75 76 77 78 79 **P**5 8	23	10	174	9740	123	62230	1192	101809	21374	1128
FORT DEFIANCE—Apache County ✯ FORT DEFIANCE INDIAN HEALTH SERVICE HOSPITAL, Mailing Address: P.O. Box 649, Zip 86504-0649; tel. 520/729-5741; Franklin Freeland, Ed.D., Chief Executive Officer (Nonreporting) **A**1 10 **S** U. S. Public Health Service Indian Health Service, Rockville, MD	47	10	49	—	—	—	—	—	—	—
GANADO—Apache County ☐ SAGE MEMORIAL HOSPITAL, Highway 264, Zip 86505, Mailing Address: P.O. Box 457, Zip 86505-0457; tel. 520/755-4550; Elizabeth B. Johnson, Chief Executive Officer (Nonreporting) **A**1 9 10	23	33	25	—	—	—	—	—	—	—
GLENDALE—Maricopa County ✯ ARROWHEAD COMMUNITY HOSPITAL AND MEDICAL CENTER, 18701 North 67th Avenue, Zip 85308-5722; tel. 623/561-1000; Richard S. Alley, Executive Vice President and Chief Executive Officer **A**1 9 10 **F**1 4 7 8 9 11 12 13 16 17 19 22 25 32 33 34 36 37 38 39 41 43 44 45 46 47 48 54 67 69 70 72 76 78 **S** Vanguard Health System, Nashville, TN **Web address:** www.baptisthealth.com	23	10	115	6301	58	57297	1763	51415	18863	599

Many Facility Codes have changed. Please refer to the AHA Guide Code Chart.

© 2000 AHA Guide

Hospitals, U.S. / ARIZONA

Hospital, Address, Telephone, Administrator, Approval, Facility, and Physician Codes, Health Care System, Network	Classification Codes		Utilization Data					Expense (thousands) of dollars		
★ American Hospital Association (AHA) membership ☐ Joint Commission on Accreditation of Healthcare Organizations (JCAHO) accreditation + American Osteopathic Healthcare Association (AOHA) membership ○ American Osteopathic Association (AOA) accreditation △ Commission on Accreditation of Rehabilitation Facilities (CARF) accreditation Control codes 61, 63, 64, 71, 72 and 73 indicate hospitals listed by AOHA, but not registered by AHA. For definition of numerical codes, see page A4	Control	Service	Staffed Beds	Admissions	Census	Outpatient Visits	Births	Total	Payroll	Personnel
☐ HEALTHSOUTH VALLEY OF THE SUN REHABILITATION HOSPITAL, 13460 North 67th Avenue, Zip 85304–1042; tel. 602/878–8800; Michael J. Oliver, Administrator (Total facility includes 18 beds in nursing home–type unit) (Nonreporting) **A**1 10 **S** HEALTHSOUTH Corporation, Birmingham, AL	33	46	42	—	—	—	—	—	—	—
★ THUNDERBIRD SAMARITAN MEDICAL CENTER, (Includes Samaritan Behavioral Health Center–Thunderbird Samaritan Campus), 5555 West Thunderbird Road, Zip 85306–4696; tel. 602/588–5555; Robert H. Curry, Senior Vice President and Chief Executive Officer **A**1 9 10 **F**1 3 4 7 8 9 11 13 14 16 17 18 19 21 22 23 24 25 26 27 29 30 31 32 33 34 35 36 37 38 39 40 41 43 44 45 46 47 48 49 50 51 54 55 56 57 58 59 60 61 62 63 64 65 68 70 71 72 73 74 75 76 77 78 79 **P**5 7 **S** Banner Health System, Fargo, ND Web address: www.samaritan.edu	23	10	288	18779	184	99926	4057	127552	47107	1298
★ U. S. AIR FORCE HOSPITAL LUKE, Luke AFB, 7219 Litchfield Road, Zip 85309–1525; tel. 623/856–7501; Colonel Michael Lischak, MC, USAF, Commander (Nonreporting) **A**1 **S** Department of the Air Force, Bowling AFB, DC	41	10	23	—	—	—	—	—	—	—
GLOBE—Gila County										
★ COBRE VALLEY COMMUNITY HOSPITAL, 5880 South Hospital Drive, Zip 85501; tel. 520/425–3261; Charles E. Bill, CHE, Chief Executive Officer **A**1 9 10 **F**7 8 9 13 16 17 18 19 22 24 25 30 31 32 34 35 38 39 41 43 44 46 48 51 54 70 71 72 73 76 78 79 **S** Brim Healthcare, Inc., Brentwood, TN	23	10	49	2050	18	38898	390	18122	6810	222
KEAMS CANYON—Navajo County										
★ U. S. PUBLIC HEALTH SERVICES INDIAN HOSPITAL, Mailing Address: P.O. Box 98, Zip 86034–0098; tel. 520/738–2211; Anthony Marshall, Service Unit Director (Nonreporting) **A**1 10 **S** U. S. Public Health Service Indian Health Service, Rockville, MD	47	10	17	—	—	—	—	—	—	—
KINGMAN—Mohave County										
★ KINGMAN REGIONAL MEDICAL CENTER, 3269 Stockton Hill Road, Zip 86401–3691; tel. 520/757–2101; Brian Turney, Chief Executive Officer (Total facility includes 14 beds in nursing home–type unit) **A**1 9 10 **F**4 7 8 9 11 13 16 22 24 25 27 28 33 36 38 39 41 43 44 45 46 47 48 49 50 51 54 56 65 68 69 70 72 75 76 78 Web address: www.azkrmc.com	23	10	124	6826	81	64150	570	39913	18569	564
LAKE HAVASU CITY—Mohave County										
★ HAVASU REGIONAL MEDICAL CENTER, 101 Civic Center Lane, Zip 86403–5683; tel. 520/855–8185; Kevin P. Poorten, Chief Executive Officer (Total facility includes 20 beds in nursing home–type unit) (Nonreporting) **A**1 9 10 **S** Province Healthcare Corporation, Brentwood, TN	23	10	118	—	—	—	—	—	—	—
MESA—Maricopa County										
★ DESERT SAMARITAN MEDICAL CENTER, (Includes Samaritan Behavioral Health Center–Desert Samaritan Medical Center, 2225 West Southern Avenue, Zip 85202; tel. 602/464–4000), 1400 South Dobson Road, Zip 85202–9879; tel. 480/835–3000; Bruce E. Pearson, Senior Vice President and Chief Executive Officer (Total facility includes 166 beds in nursing home–type unit) **A**1 9 10 **F**1 3 4 7 8 9 11 13 14 16 17 18 19 21 22 23 24 25 26 27 29 30 31 32 33 34 35 36 37 38 39 40 41 43 44 45 46 47 48 49 50 51 54 55 56 58 59 60 61 62 63 64 65 66 68 70 71 72 74 75 76 77 78 79 **P**5 7 **S** Banner Health System, Fargo, ND Web address: www.samaritan.edu	23	10	551	28411	427	96561	6742	205189	72443	2093
★ ○ MESA GENERAL HOSPITAL MEDICAL CENTER, 515 North Mesa Drive, Zip 85201–5989; tel. 480/969–9111; Patrick T. Walz, Chief Executive Officer (Total facility includes 13 beds in nursing home–type unit) **A**1 9 10 11 12 13 **F**1 3 4 8 9 11 13 22 24 25 29 30 32 34 38 39 41 42 43 44 45 46 47 48 50 51 53 54 55 58 59 60 61 62 63 64 68 69 76 78 79 **P**5 7 8 **S** IASIS Healthcare, Nashville, TN	33	10	143	5331	62	63354	867	34053	17133	346
★ △ MESA LUTHERAN HOSPITAL, 525 West Brown Road, Zip 85201–3299; tel. 480/834–1211; James Gingerich, Senior Vice President and Chief Executive Officer (Total facility includes 60 beds in nursing home–type unit) (Nonreporting) **A**1 2 7 9 10 **S** Banner Health System, Fargo, ND	23	10	278	—	—	—	—	—	—	—
★ VALLEY LUTHERAN HOSPITAL, 6644 Baywood Avenue, Zip 85206–1797; tel. 480/981–2000; Robert A. Rundio, Executive Director of Hospital Operations (Nonreporting) **A**1 9 10 **S** Banner Health System, Fargo, ND	23	10	172	—	—	—	—	—	—	—
NOGALES—Santa Cruz County										
★ CARONDELET HOLY CROSS HOSPITAL, 1171 West Target Range Road, Zip 85621–2496; tel. 520/287–2771; Richard Polheber, Interim Vice President and Chief Executive Officer (Total facility includes 49 beds in nursing home–type unit) (Nonreporting) **A**1 9 10 **S** Carondelet Health System, Saint Louis, MO	21	10	80	—	—	—	—	—	—	—
PAGE—Coconino County										
★ PAGE HOSPITAL, 501 North Navajo Drive, Zip 86040, Mailing Address: P.O. Box 1447, Zip 86040–1447; tel. 520/645–2424; Richard Polheber, Chief Executive Officer **A**1 9 10 **F**8 9 13 16 17 18 22 25 32 34 35 36 38 39 44 45 46 48 51 54 70 76 **S** Banner Health System, Fargo, ND	23	10	25	493	4	11440	170	7463	3563	81
PARKER—La Paz County										
★ ○ LA PAZ REGIONAL HOSPITAL, 1200 Mohave Road, Zip 85344–6349; tel. 520/669–9201; William G. Coe, Executive Vice President and Chief Executive Officer (Nonreporting) **A**9 10 11	23	10	39	—	—	—	—	—	—	—
★ U. S. PUBLIC HEALTH SERVICE INDIAN HOSPITAL, Mailing Address: Route 1, Box 12, Zip 85344; tel. 520/669–2137; Gary Davis, Service Unit Director (Nonreporting) **A**1 10 **S** U. S. Public Health Service Indian Health Service, Rockville, MD	47	10	18	—	—	—	—	—	—	—

Hospitals, U.S. / ARIZONA

Hospital, Address, Telephone, Administrator, Approval, Facility, and Physician Codes, Health Care System, Network	Classification Codes		Utilization Data					Expense (thousands) of dollars		
★ American Hospital Association (AHA) membership ☐ Joint Commission on Accreditation of Healthcare Organizations (JCAHO) accreditation + American Osteopathic Healthcare Association (AOHA) membership ○ American Osteopathic Association (AOA) accreditation △ Commission on Accreditation of Rehabilitation Facilities (CARF) accreditation Control codes 61, 63, 64, 71, 72 and 73 indicate hospitals listed by AOHA, but not registered by AHA. For definition of numerical codes, see page A4	Control	Service	Staffed Beds	Admissions	Census	Outpatient Visits	Births	Total	Payroll	Personnel
PAYSON—Gila County										
☐ PAYSON REGIONAL MEDICAL CENTER, 807 South Ponderosa Street, Zip 85541–5599; tel. 520/474–3222; Russell V. Judd, Chief Executive Officer **A**1 9 10 **F**3 5 6 7 8 9 13 15 17 19 21 22 23 24 25 26 27 28 30 31 32 34 35 36 37 38 39 41 43 44 45 46 48 49 50 51 54 56 65 67 69 70 71 72 73 75 76 78 79 **P**6 7 **S** Community Health Systems, Inc., Brentwood, TN **Web address:** www.paysonhospital.com	33	10	66	2065	19	—	0	—	—	344
PHOENIX—Maricopa County										
☐ ARIZONA HEART HOSPITAL, 1930 East Thomas Road, Zip 85016; tel. 602/532–1000; John L. Harrington, Jr, FACHE, President (Nonreporting) **A**1 9 10 **S** MedCath, Inc., Charlotte, NC	33	49	56	—	—	—	—	—	—	—
☐ ARIZONA STATE HOSPITAL, 2500 East Van Buren Street, Zip 85008–6079; tel. 602/244–1331; Jack B. Silver, M.P.H., Chief Executive Officer (Nonreporting) **A**1	12	22	372	—	—	—	—	—	—	—
★ CARL T. HAYDEN VETERANS AFFAIRS MEDICAL CENTER, 650 East Indian School Road, Zip 85012–1892; tel. 602/277–5551; John R. Fears, Director (Total facility includes 104 beds in nursing home–type unit) **A**1 2 3 5 **F**1 3 4 9 11 13 16 17 18 19 21 22 23 24 25 26 27 28 29 30 31 32 33 34 35 36 37 38 39 41 43 45 46 47 48 49 50 51 54 55 56 57 59 61 62 63 65 68 69 70 72 74 76 77 78 79 **S** Department of Veterans Affairs, Washington, DC **Web address:** www.va.gov	45	10	285	8377	215	379380	0	172281	110623	1819
★ COMMUNITY HOSPITAL MEDICAL CENTER, 6501 North 19th Avenue, Zip 85015–1690; tel. 602/249–3434; Bryan D. Burklow, Chief Executive Officer (Nonreporting) **Web address:** www.tenethealth.com	33	10	59	—	—	—	—	—	—	—
★ △ GOOD SAMARITAN REGIONAL MEDICAL CENTER, 1111 East McDowell Road, Zip 85006–2666, Mailing Address: P.O. Box 2989, Zip 85062–2989; tel. 602/239–2000; Steven L. Seiler, Senior Vice President and Chief Executive Officer (Total facility includes 150 beds in nursing home–type unit) **A**1 2 3 5 7 8 9 10 **F**1 3 4 5 7 8 9 11 13 14 16 17 18 19 22 23 24 25 26 27 29 30 31 32 33 34 35 36 37 38 39 40 41 43 44 45 46 47 48 49 50 51 53 54 55 56 57 58 59 60 61 62 63 64 65 68 69 70 71 72 73 74 75 76 77 78 79 **S** Banner Health System, Fargo, ND **Web address:** www.samaritan.edu	23	10	687	30684	475	201380	7456	319080	112058	3422
★ ○ JOHN C LINCOLN HOSPITAL–DEER VALLEY, 19829 North 27th Avenue, Zip 85027–4002; tel. 623/879–6100; Tim Tracy, Executive Vice President and Chief Operating Officer (Total facility includes 23 beds in nursing home–type unit) **A**1 9 10 11 13 **F**1 4 8 9 11 12 13 14 17 18 19 21 22 23 25 30 31 32 33 34 36 37 38 39 40 41 44 45 46 47 48 49 50 54 55 59 65 69 70 71 74 75 76 77 78 79 **P**8 **S** John C Lincoln Health Network, Phoenix, AZ **Web address:** www.jcl.com	23	10	97	3927	48	37888	441	39431	14680	447
★ JOHN C. LINCOLN HOSPITAL – NORTH MOUNTAIN, (Formerly John C. Lincoln Health Network), 250 East Dunlap Avenue, Zip 85020–2446; tel. 602/943–2381; Dan C. Coleman, President and Chief Executive Officer **A**1 9 10 12 **F**1 4 6 7 8 9 11 12 13 14 16 17 18 19 22 24 25 28 29 32 33 34 36 37 38 39 40 41 43 44 45 46 47 48 50 53 54 59 65 67 68 69 70 71 72 73 75 76 78 79 **P**4 5 6 8 **S** John C Lincoln Health Network, Phoenix, AZ **Web address:** www.jcl.com	23	10	239	11295	126	70032	1156	100958	38685	1267
★ MARICOPA MEDICAL CENTER, 2601 East Roosevelt Street, Zip 85008–4956; tel. 602/344–5011; Mark Hillard, Chief Executive Officer (Nonreporting) **A**1 2 3 5 8 9 10 12 **S** Quorum Health Group, Brentwood, TN **Web address:** www.maricopa.gov/medcenter/mmc.html	13	10	481	—	—	—	—	—	—	—
★ MARYVALE HOSPITAL MEDICAL CENTER, 5102 West Campbell Avenue, Zip 85031–1799; tel. 623/848–5000; Art Layne, Chief Executive Officer **A**1 2 9 10 **F**8 9 11 13 14 17 18 19 22 24 25 27 31 32 33 34 38 39 41 44 45 46 48 51 53 54 65 70 72 75 76 77 78 79 **S** Vanguard Health System, Nashville, TN	33	10	171	11794	101	94758	3018	—	—	745
★ MAYO CLINIC HOSPITAL, 5777 East Mayo Boulevard, Zip 85054–4502; tel. 480/515–6296; Thomas C. Bour, Administrator (Total facility includes 24 beds in nursing home–type unit) **A**1 10 **F**4 9 11 13 18 22 24 25 27 38 39 41 45 46 47 48 51 53 54 69 70 74 76 77 78 **P**6 **S** Mayo Foundation, Rochester, MN	23	10	178	9555	120	—	0	117996	29210	1827
★ PARADISE VALLEY HOSPITAL, 3929 East Bell Road, Zip 85032–2196; tel. 602/867–1881; Rebecca C. Kuhn, Chief Executive Officer (Nonreporting) **A**1 2 9 10 **S** Triad Hospitals, Inc., Dallas, TX	33	10	140	—	—	—	—	—	—	—
★ PHOENIX BAPTIST HOSPITAL AND MEDICAL CENTER, 2000 West Bethany Home Road, Zip 85015–2110; tel. 602/249–0212; Jeffrey K. Norman, Executive Vice President and Chief Executive Officer **A**1 2 3 5 9 10 12 **F**1 4 7 8 9 11 12 13 17 18 19 22 24 27 29 32 33 34 36 37 38 39 41 43 45 46 47 48 49 50 51 54 56 65 67 69 70 72 76 78 79 **P**6 **S** Vanguard Health System, Nashville, TN **Web address:** www.baptisthealth.com	23	10	201	9073	97	106434	1813	93289	34655	906
★ PHOENIX CHILDREN'S HOSPITAL, 1111 East McDowell Road, Zip 85006–2666, Mailing Address: 1300 North 12th Street, Suite 404, Zip 85006–2896; tel. 602/239–5960; Burl E. Stamp, Chief Executive Officer (Nonreporting) **A**1 3 5 9 **Web address:** www.phxchildrens.com	23	50	205	—	—	—	—	—	—	—

Hospitals, U.S. / ARIZONA

Hospital, Address, Telephone, Administrator, Approval, Facility, and Physician Codes, Health Care System, Network

- ★ American Hospital Association (AHA) membership
- □ Joint Commission on Accreditation of Healthcare Organizations (JCAHO) accreditation
- + American Osteopathic Healthcare Association (AOHA) membership
- ○ American Osteopathic Association (AOA) accreditation
- △ Commission on Accreditation of Rehabilitation Facilities (CARF) accreditation

Control codes 61, 63, 64, 71, 72 and 73 indicate hospitals listed by AOHA, but not registered by AHA. For definition of numerical codes, see page A4

Hospital	Control	Service	Staffed Beds	Admissions	Census	Outpatient Visits	Births	Total	Payroll	Personnel
★ PHOENIX MEMORIAL HEALTH SYSTEM, (Formerly PMH Health Services Network), 1201 South Seventh Avenue, Zip 85007–3995; tel. 602/258–5111; Robert J. Conaway, Jr, Chief Executive Officer (Total facility includes 28 beds in nursing home–type unit) A1 2 9 10 12 13 F1 2 4 5 8 9 11 12 13 14 16 17 18 19 20 22 23 24 25 26 29 30 31 32 33 36 37 38 39 41 42 43 44 45 46 47 48 49 50 51 52 53 54 65 66 67 68 69 70 71 72 73 75 76 77 78 79 P5 8 S PMH Health Resources, Inc., Phoenix, AZ Web address: www.phzmemorialhospital.com	23	10	195	11643	114	175262	1379	167398	35880	834
★ △ ST. JOSEPH'S HOSPITAL AND MEDICAL CENTER, 350 West Thomas Road, Zip 85013–4496, Mailing Address: P.O. Box 2071, Zip 85001–2071; tel. 602/406–3000; Linda A. Hunt, President and Chief Administrative Officer (Nonreporting) A1 2 3 5 7 8 9 10 S Catholic Healthcare West, San Francisco, CA Web address: www.chw.edu	21	10	514	—	—	—	—	—	—	—
□ ST. LUKE'S BEHAVIORAL HEALTH CENTER, 1800 East Van Buren, Zip 85006–3742; tel. 602/251–8546; Patrick D. Waugh, Chief Executive Officer A1 9 10 F2 3 13 21 25 57 58 60 61 62 63 64 S IASIS Healthcare, Nashville, TN	33	22	70	3054	50	35203	0	10673	5670	138
★ ST. LUKE'S MEDICAL CENTER, 1800 East Van Buren Street, Zip 85006–3742; tel. 602/251–8100; Robert M. Luther, Chief Executive Officer (Total facility includes 39 beds in nursing home–type unit) A1 9 10 F4 9 11 12 13 17 18 19 22 24 25 26 27 30 32 34 37 38 39 41 43 45 46 47 48 49 50 51 53 54 55 57 62 65 68 69 70 71 72 76 78 P5 6 7 S IASIS Healthcare, Nashville, TN	33	10	282	7097	100	46114	0	64831	24295	764
★ U. S. PUBLIC HEALTH SERVICE PHOENIX INDIAN MEDICAL CENTER, 4212 North 16th Street, Zip 85016–5389; tel. 602/263–1200; Anna Albert, Chief Executive Officer (Nonreporting) A1 10 S U. S. Public Health Service Indian Health Service, Rockville, MD	44	10	137	—	—	—	—	—	—	—
□ VENCOR HOSPITAL–PHOENIX, 40 East Indianola Avenue, Zip 85012–2059; tel. 602/280–7000 A1 F13 18 22 24 30 31 37 39 41 43 45 46 51 55 59 65 68 70 76 S Vencor, Incorporated, Louisville, KY	33	10	58	424	43	0	0	14276	5923	148
WESTBRIDGE TREATMENT CENTER, 1830 East Roosevelt Street, Zip 85006–3641; tel. 602/254–0884; Mike Perry, Chief Executive Officer (Nonreporting) S Century Healthcare Development Corporation, Tulsa, OK	33	52	78	—	—	—	—	—	—	—
PRESCOTT—Yavapai County										
★ NORTHERN ARIZONA VA HEALTH CARE SYSTEM, (Formerly Veterans Affairs Medical Center), 500 Highway 89 North, Zip 86313–5000; tel. 520/445–4860; Patricia A. McKlem, Chief Executive Officer (Total facility includes 70 beds in nursing home–type unit) (Nonreporting) A1 S Department of Veterans Affairs, Washington, DC Web address: www.va.gov/stations97/guide/home.asp?DIVISION=ALL	45	10	287	—	—	—	—	—	—	—
★ YAVAPAI REGIONAL MEDICAL CENTER, 1003 Willow Creek Road, Zip 86301–1668; tel. 520/445–2700; Timothy Barnett, Chief Executive Officer A1 9 10 F8 9 11 12 16 17 18 19 22 24 25 28 29 32 34 36 37 38 39 44 45 46 48 49 50 51 53 54 61 68 70 72 76 78 P1 5 Web address: www.yrmc.org	23	10	95	7003	69	76121	—	55722	23307	605
SACATON—Pinal County										
★ HUHUKAM MEMORIAL HOSPITAL, Seed Farm and Skill Center Road, Zip 85247–0038, Mailing Address: P.O. Box 38, Zip 85247–0038; tel. 602/528–1200; Viola L. Johnson, M.P.H., Chief Executive Officer (Nonreporting) A1 9 10 S U. S. Public Health Service Indian Health Service, Rockville, MD	47	10	10	—	—	—	—	—	—	—
SAFFORD—Graham County										
★ MOUNT GRAHAM COMMUNITY HOSPITAL, 1600 20th Avenue, Zip 85546–4097; tel. 520/348–4000; Karl E. Johnson, Chief Executive Officer A1 9 10 F7 8 9 16 17 18 22 24 25 28 32 34 35 36 37 38 39 43 45 46 48 51 54 68 70 72 73 76 78 P8	16	10	44	3060	24	50118	552	20124	7871	257
SAN CARLOS—Gila County										
★ U. S. PUBLIC HEALTH SERVICE INDIAN HOSPITAL, Mailing Address: P.O. Box 208, Zip 85550–0208; tel. 520/475–2371; Nella Ben, Chief Executive Officer (Nonreporting) A1 10 S U. S. Public Health Service Indian Health Service, Rockville, MD	47	10	28	—	—	—	—	—	—	—
SCOTTSDALE—Maricopa County										
□ HEALTHSOUTH MERIDIAN POINT REHABILITATION HOSPITAL, 11250 North 92nd Street, Zip 85260–6148; tel. 480/860–0671; Elizabeth Lamkin, Administrator A1 10 F5 29 32 45 46 48 53 54 63 S HEALTHSOUTH Corporation, Birmingham, AL	33	46	40	628	27	5059	0	6320	3472	—
★ SAMARITAN BEHAVIORAL HEALTH CENTER–SCOTTSDALE, 7575 East Earll Drive, Zip 85251–6998; tel. 480/941–7500; Robert F. Meyer, M.D., Chief Executive Officer A1 10 F1 2 3 6 13 16 17 18 19 21 30 33 38 43 45 51 57 58 59 60 61 62 63 64 69 70 72 78 S Banner Health System, Fargo, ND	23	22	82	2197	57	5040	0	9750	6544	246
★ △ SCOTTSDALE HEALTHCARE–OSBORN, 7400 East Osborn Road, Zip 85251–6403; tel. 480/675–4000; Peggy Reiley, Senior Vice President and Chief Clinical Officer (Total facility includes 60 beds in nursing home–type unit) (Nonreporting) A1 2 3 5 7 9 10 S Scottsdale Healthcare, Scottsdale, AZ Web address: www.shc.org	23	10	258	—	—	—	—	—	—	—
★ SCOTTSDALE HEALTHCARE–SHEA, 9003 East Shea Boulevard, Zip 85260–6771; tel. 480/860–3000; Thomas J. Sadvary, FACHE, Senior Vice President and Chief Operating Officer A1 2 3 5 9 10 F1 2 3 4 5 6 7 8 9 10 11 12 13 14 16 17 18 19 21 22 23 24 25 26 27 28 29 30 31 32 33 34 35 40 41 42 43 44 45 46 47 48 49 50 51 52 53 54 55 56 57 61 65 66 68 69 70 72 73 74 75 76 77 78 79 P7 8 S Scottsdale Healthcare, Scottsdale, AZ Web address: www.shc.org	23	10	251	14161	144	79017	3040	127307	47138	1144

Hospitals, U.S. / ARIZONA

Hospital, Address, Telephone, Administrator, Approval, Facility, and Physician Codes, Health Care System, Network	Classification Codes		Utilization Data					Expense (thousands) of dollars		Personnel
★ American Hospital Association (AHA) membership □ Joint Commission on Accreditation of Healthcare Organizations (JCAHO) accreditation + American Osteopathic Healthcare Association (AOHA) membership ○ American Osteopathic Association (AOA) accreditation △ Commission on Accreditation of Rehabilitation Facilities (CARF) accreditation Control codes 61, 63, 64, 71, 72 and 73 indicate hospitals listed by AOHA, but not registered by AHA. For definition of numerical codes, see page A4	Control	Service	Staffed Beds	Admissions	Census	Outpatient Visits	Births	Total	Payroll	Personnel
SELLS—Pima County										
★ U. S. PUBLIC HEALTH SERVICE INDIAN HOSPITAL, Mailing Address: P.O. Box 548, Zip 85634-0548; tel. 520/383-7251; Darrell Rumley, Service Unit Director and Chief Executive Officer (Nonreporting) **A**1 10 **S** U. S. Public Health Service Indian Health Service, Rockville, MD	47	10	34	—	—	—	—	—	—	—
SHOW LOW—Navajo County										
★ NAVAPACHE REGIONAL MEDICAL CENTER, 2200 Show Low Lake Road, Zip 85901-7800; tel. 520/537-4375; Leigh Cox, Chief Executive Officer **A**1 9 10 **F**7 8 9 11 13 16 17 18 19 20 22 25 28 32 34 36 39 41 44 45 48 49 54 68 70 76 78 **S** Brim Healthcare, Inc., Brentwood, TN Web address: www.nrmc.org	23	10	54	4579	37	48402	779	30763	13095	408
SIERRA VISTA—Cochise County										
★ SIERRA VISTA REGIONAL HEALTH CENTER, 300 El Camino Real, Zip 85635-2899; tel. 520/458-4641; David R. Ressler, President and Chief Executive Officer **A**1 9 10 **F**7 8 9 22 24 25 27 29 32 33 34 36 37 38 39 41 44 46 48 54 68 70 75 76 Web address: www.svch.com	23	10	65	4326	32	154171	1044	32579	15189	451
SPRINGERVILLE—Apache County										
★ WHITE MOUNTAIN REGIONAL MEDICAL CENTER, 118 South Mountain Avenue, Zip 85938, Mailing Address: P.O. Box 880, Zip 85938-0880; tel. 520/333-4368; David Wanger, Chief Executive Officer (Total facility includes 64 beds in nursing home–type unit) (Nonreporting) **A**9 10	23	10	89	—	—	—	—	—	—	—
SUN CITY—Maricopa County										
★ WALTER O. BOSWELL MEMORIAL HOSPITAL, 10401 West Thunderbird Boulevard, Zip 85351-3092, Mailing Address: P.O. Box 1690, Zip 85372-1690; tel. 623/977-7211; George Perez, Executive Vice President and Chief Operating Officer (Total facility includes 40 beds in nursing home–type unit) **A**1 2 9 10 **F**3 4 6 7 9 11 12 13 17 18 19 22 24 25 26 27 28 30 31 32 33 34 36 37 39 40 41 43 45 46 47 48 49 50 51 53 54 56 59 60 61 62 63 64 65 67 69 70 71 72 76 77 78 79 **P**1 6 8 **S** Sun Health Corporation, Sun City, AZ Web address: www.sunhealth.org	23	10	313	16046	217	110164	0	120145	44605	1243
SUN CITY WEST—Maricopa County										
★ DEL E. WEBB MEMORIAL HOSPITAL, 14502 West Meeker Boulevard, Zip 85375-5299, Mailing Address: P.O. Box 5169, Sun City, Zip 85375-5169; tel. 623/214-4000; Thomas C. Dickson, Executive Vice President and Chief Operating Officer (Total facility includes 27 beds in nursing home–type unit) **A**1 9 10 **F**1 3 4 6 9 11 12 13 17 18 19 22 24 30 31 32 33 34 35 36 37 38 39 40 43 45 46 47 48 49 50 51 53 54 57 59 60 61 62 63 64 65 67 69 70 72 75 76 78 **P**1 5 **S** Sun Health Corporation, Sun City, AZ Web address: www.sunhealth.org	23	10	188	6974	120	85774	—	50187	21027	540
TEMPE—Maricopa County										
★ TEMPE ST. LUKE'S HOSPITAL, 1500 South Mill Avenue, Zip 85281-6699; tel. 480/784-5510; Joel F. Engles, Administrator (Nonreporting) **A**1 9 10 12 13 **S** IASIS Healthcare, Nashville, TN	33	10	110	—	—	—	—	—	—	—
TUBA CITY—Coconino County										
★ TUBA CITY INDIAN MEDICAL CENTER, 167 Main Street, Zip 86045-0611, Mailing Address: P.O. Box 600, Zip 86045-0600; tel. 520/283-2501; Susie John, M.D., Chief Executive Officer (Nonreporting) **A**1 10 **S** U. S. Public Health Service Indian Health Service, Rockville, MD	47	10	69	—	—	—	—	—	—	—
TUCSON—Pima County										
★ △ CARONDELET ST. JOSEPH'S HOSPITAL, 350 North Wilmot Road, Zip 85711-2678; tel. 520/296-3211; Wesley E. Colvin, Senior Vice President and Chief Executive Officer (Nonreporting) **A**1 7 9 10 **S** Carondelet Health System, Saint Louis, MO	21	10	287	—	—	—	—	—	—	—
★ △ CARONDELET ST. MARY'S HOSPITAL, 1601 West St. Mary's Road, Zip 85745-2682; tel. 520/622-5833 (Nonreporting) **A**1 7 9 10 **S** Carondelet Health System, Saint Louis, MO Web address: www.carondelet.org	21	10	345	—	—	—	—	—	—	—
★ EL DORADO HOSPITAL, 1400 North Wilmot Road, Zip 85712-4498, Mailing Address: P.O. Box 13070, Zip 85732-3070; tel. 520/886-6361; Rhonda Dean, Chief Executive Officer **A**1 9 10 **F**4 9 11 12 13 16 17 22 25 30 31 32 34 38 39 40 41 43 45 48 49 53 54 57 62 69 70 76 78 **P**6 **S** Triad Hospitals, Inc., Dallas, TX Web address: www.eldoradohospital.com	33	10	166	6096	84	41680	—	37413	16279	460
□ HEALTHSOUTH REHABILITATION INSTITUTE OF TUCSON, 2650 North Wyatt Drive, Zip 85712-6108; tel. 520/325-1300; Robbee Caseldine, Administrator **A**1 10 **F**5 13 16 17 18 19 20 29 30 31 33 34 38 43 45 46 49 53 54 72 78 **S** HEALTHSOUTH Corporation, Birmingham, AL	33	46	80	1513	57	10833	0	—	—	189
□ KINO COMMUNITY HOSPITAL, 2800 East Ajo Way, Zip 85713-6289; tel. 520/294-4471; Scott Floden, Administrator (Total facility includes 20 beds in nursing home–type unit) (Nonreporting) **A**1 3 5 9 10	13	10	155	—	—	—	—	—	—	—
★ NORTHWEST MEDICAL CENTER, 6200 North La Cholla Boulevard, Zip 85741-3599; tel. 520/742-9000; W. Jefferson Comer, FACHE, Chief Executive Officer **A**1 9 10 **F**4 7 8 9 11 13 17 18 19 22 24 25 30 32 33 34 38 39 40 41 43 44 45 46 47 48 49 50 51 55 65 68 70 72 77 78 79 **S** Triad Hospitals, Inc., Dallas, TX Web address: www.northwestmedicalcenter.com PALO VERDE MENTAL HEALTH SERVICES See Tucson Medical Center	33	10	134	11921	118	144617	1135	78208	33105	1092

Hospitals, U.S. / ARIZONA

Hospital, Address, Telephone, Administrator, Approval, Facility, and Physician Codes, Health Care System, Network	Classification Codes		Utilization Data					Expense (thousands) of dollars		
★ American Hospital Association (AHA) membership ☐ Joint Commission on Accreditation of Healthcare Organizations (JCAHO) accreditation + American Osteopathic Healthcare Association (AOHA) membership ○ American Osteopathic Association (AOA) accreditation △ Commission on Accreditation of Rehabilitation Facilities (CARF) accreditation Control codes 61, 63, 64, 71, 72 and 73 indicate hospitals listed by AOHA, but not registered by AHA. For definition of numerical codes, see page A4	Control	Service	Staffed Beds	Admissions	Census	Outpatient Visits	Births	Total	Payroll	Personnel
SIERRA TUCSON, 39580 South Lago Del Oro Parkway, Zip 85739–9637; tel. 520/624–4000; Terry A. Stephens, Executive Director **F**2 3 13 14 15 16 18 19 21 22 23 24 25 28 29 31 33 34 35 39 43 48 50 51 54 57 59 60 61 63 70 72 75 76 77 79 **P**1 **Web address:** www.sierratucson.com	33	82	77	883	57	0	0	11416	5896	147
★ △ SOUTHERN ARIZONA VETERANS AFFAIRS HEALTHCARE SYSTEM, (Formerly Veterans Affairs Medical Center), 3601 South 6th Avenue, Zip 85723–0002; tel. 520/792–1450; Jonathan H. Gardner, Chief Executive Officer (Total facility includes 84 beds in nursing home–type unit) **A**1 3 5 7 8 9 **F**1 2 3 4 5 6 9 11 13 16 17 18 19 22 23 24 25 26 29 30 31 32 33 34 35 36 37 38 39 41 43 45 46 47 48 49 50 51 53 54 55 56 57 59 60 61 62 63 64 65 66 68 69 70 72 76 77 78 79 **P**6 **S** Department of Veterans Affairs, Washington, DC **Web address:** www.va.gov/stations97/guide/home.asp?DIVISION=ALL	45	10	210	6379	185	294396	—	112402	57430	1301
★ ○ TUCSON GENERAL HOSPITAL, 3838 North Campbell Avenue, Zip 85719–1497; tel. 520/318–6300; Allan Harrington, Jr, Chief Executive Officer (Nonreporting) **A**1 9 10 11 13	33	10	80	—	—	—	—	—	—	—
★ TUCSON MEDICAL CENTER, (Includes Palo Verde Mental Health Services, 2695 North Craycroft, Zip 85712–2244; tel. 520/324–4340), 5301 East Grant Road, Zip 85712–2874; tel. 520/327–5461; Frank D. Alvarez, President and Chief Executive Officer (Total facility includes 30 beds in nursing home–type unit) **A**1 2 3 5 9 10 **F**4 7 8 9 11 12 13 17 18 22 24 25 28 30 31 33 37 38 39 41 42 43 44 45 46 47 48 49 50 51 52 53 54 57 58 59 60 61 62 63 64 65 69 70 75 76 77 78 79 **Web address:** www.home.tmcaz.com	23	10	457	29160	284	248994	4608	219818	102778	2858
★ UNIVERSITY MEDICAL CENTER, 1501 North Campbell Avenue, Zip 85724–5128; tel. 520/694–6148; Gregory A. Pivirotto, President and Chief Executive Officer **A**1 3 5 8 9 10 **F**4 5 8 9 11 12 13 19 20 22 24 25 26 27 28 29 30 32 33 34 35 36 37 38 39 41 42 44 46 47 48 49 50 51 52 54 55 57 58 59 60 61 62 63 64 65 68 70 72 74 75 76 77 78 79 **P**6	23	10	319	17172	229	303294	2450	233623	95905	2463
☐ VENCOR HOSPITAL – TUCSON, 355 North Wilmot Road, Zip 85711–2635; tel. 520/747–8200; Kevin Christiansen, Administrator (Nonreporting) **A**1 10 **S** Vencor, Incorporated, Louisville, KY	33	49	51	—	—	—	—	—	—	—
VETERANS AFFAIRS MEDICAL CENTER See Southern Arizona Veterans Affairs Healthcare System										
WHITERIVER—Navajo County										
★ U. S. PUBLIC HEALTH SERVICE INDIAN HOSPITAL, State Route 73, Box 860, Zip 85941–0860; tel. 520/338–4911; Carla Alchesay-Nachu, Service Unit Director (Nonreporting) **A**1 **S** U. S. Public Health Service Indian Health Service, Rockville, MD	47	10	45	—	—	—	—	—	—	—
WICKENBURG—Maricopa County										
★ WICKENBURG REGIONAL HOSPITAL, 520 Rose Lane, Zip 85390–1447; tel. 520/684–5421; David Garnas, Administrator (Total facility includes 57 beds in nursing home–type unit) (Nonreporting) **A**1 9 10 **S** Banner Health System, Fargo, ND	23	10	80	—	—	—	—	—	—	—
WILLCOX—Cochise County										
★ NORTHERN COCHISE COMMUNITY HOSPITAL, 901 West Rex Allen Drive, Zip 85643–1009; tel. 520/384–3541; Chris Cronberg, Chief Executive Officer (Total facility includes 24 beds in nursing home–type unit) **A**1 9 10 **F**7 9 13 16 17 18 22 25 29 32 33 38 43 48 50 51 56 69 70 76 78 **S** Brim Healthcare, Inc., Brentwood, TN	16	10	48	643	32	9432	4	6167	3050	114
WINSLOW—Navajo County										
★ WINSLOW MEMORIAL HOSPITAL, 1501 Williamson Avenue, Zip 86047–2797; tel. 520/289–4691; Anita Warboys, R.N., Administrator **A**9 10 **F**8 13 22 25 32 44 48 51 54	23	10	10	1228	10	15081	237	9083	4265	—
YUMA—Imperial County										
U. S. PUBLIC HEALTH SERVICE INDIAN HOSPITAL See Winterhaven, CA										
★ YUMA REGIONAL MEDICAL CENTER, 2400 South Avenue A, Zip 85364–7170; tel. 520/344–2000; Robert T. Olsen, CHE, President and Chief Executive Officer (Total facility includes 20 beds in nursing home–type unit) **A**1 9 10 **F**4 7 8 9 11 12 13 17 18 19 21 22 23 24 25 27 28 30 32 33 34 35 36 38 39 41 43 44 45 46 48 56 65 69 70 72 75 76 77 78 79 **Web address:** www.yumaregional.org	23	10	257	15237	169	98129	2890	99791	44199	1348

© 2000 AHA Guide   *Many Facility Codes have changed. Please refer to the AHA Guide Code Chart.*

ARKANSAS

Resident Population 2,538 (in thousands)
Resident population in metro areas 48.3%
Birth rate per 1,000 population 14.5
65 years and over 14.3%
Percent of persons without health insurance 24.4%

★ American Hospital Association (AHA) membership
☐ Joint Commission on Accreditation of Healthcare Organizations (JCAHO) accreditation
+ American Osteopathic Healthcare Association (AOHA) membership
○ American Osteopathic Association (AOA) accreditation
△ Commission on Accreditation of Rehabilitation Facilities (CARF) accreditation
Control codes 61, 63, 64, 71, 72 and 73 indicate hospitals listed by AOHA, but not registered by AHA. For definition of numerical codes, see page A4

Hospital, Address, Telephone, Administrator, Approval, Facility, and Physician Codes, Health Care System Network	Classification Codes		Utilization Data					Expense (thousands) of dollars		
	Control	Service	Staffed Beds	Admissions	Census	Outpatient Visits	Births	Total	Payroll	Personnel
ARKADELPHIA—Clark County										
★ BAPTIST HEALTH MEDICAL CENTER–ARKADELPHIA, (Formerly Baptist Medical Center Arkadelphia), 3050 Twin Rivers Drive, Zip 71923–4299; tel. 870/245-1100; Dan Gathright, Senior Vice President and Administrator **A**1 9 10 **F**7 8 9 13 17 18 22 24 25 31 34 35 36 37 39 40 41 44 46 48 54 70 75 76 78 **P**3 4 5 7 **S** Baptist Health, Little Rock, AR Web address: www.baptist-health.org	23	10	57	1583	19	20301	226	14118	6298	236
ASHDOWN—Little River County										
LITTLE RIVER MEMORIAL HOSPITAL, Fifth and Locke Streets, Zip 71822–0577, Mailing Address P.O. Box 577, Zip 71822–0577; tel. 870/898–5011; Judy Adams, Administrator and Chief Executive Officer **A**9 10 **F**9 12 17 18 22 25 36 45 48 54 68 76 **P**5	13	10	42	990	13	6129	0	4910	2371	119
BATESVILLE—Independence County										
★ △ WHITE RIVER MEDICAL CENTER, 1710 Harrison Street, Zip 72501–2197, Mailing Address P.O. Box 2197, Zip 72503–2197; tel. 870/793–1200; Gary Bebow, Administrator and Chief Executive Officer **A**1 7 9 10 **F**8 9 11 12 13 16 17 18 22 23 24 25 32 34 35 36 38 39 41 44 45 46 48 49 51 53 54 55 57 62 68 69 70 71 76 78 **P**3 8 Web address: www.wrmc.com	23	10	175	8478	99	73475	519	58214	24772	840
BENTON—Saline County										
☐ RIVENDELL BEHAVIORAL HEALTH SERVICES, 100 Rivendell Drive, Zip 72015–9100; tel. 501/316–1255; Mark E. Schneider, Chief Executive Officer (Nonreporting) **F**1 9 10 **S** Children's Comprehensive Services, Inc., Nashville, TN	33	52	77	—	—	—	—	—	—	—
★ SALINE MEMORIAL HOSPITAL, 1 Medical Park Drive, Zip 72015–3354; tel. 501/776–6000; Roger D. Feldt, FACHE, President and Chief Executive Officer (Total facility includes 4 beds in nursing home–type unit) **A**1 9 10 **F**7 8 9 11 13 15 16 19 22 24 25 28 32 34 36 37 39 41 44 45 46 48 49 51 53 54 57 58 59 60 61 62 63 69 70 76 78 **P**1 **S** Quorum Health Group, Brentwood, TN Web address: www.scmc.com	23	10	87	4721	64	41231	414	32381	13824	602
BERRYVILLE—Carroll County										
★ CARROLL REGIONAL MEDICAL CENTER, 214 Carter Street, Zip 72616–4303; tel. 870/423–3355; Rudy Darling, President and Chief Executive Officer **A**1 9 10 **F**8 9 13 17 19 22 24 25 26 27 28 32 33 34 35 36 37 41 44 45 46 48 49 50 54 70 71 72 76 78 **P**8 **S** Sisters of Mercy Health System–St. Louis, Saint Louis, MO Web address: www.carrollregional.com	23	10	31	1779	15	15846	225	10512	5439	182
BLYTHEVILLE—Mississippi County										
★ BAPTIST MEMORIAL HOSPITAL–BLYTHEVILLE, 1520 North Division Street, Zip 72315, Mailing Address: P.O. Box 108, Zip 72316–0108; tel. 870/838–7300; Brandt C. Wright, Administrator (Total facility includes 70 beds in nursing home–type unit) **A**1 9 10 **F**3 7 9 12 13 14 17 18 19 22 24 25 27 28 31 32 33 34 35 36 37 41 43 44 45 46 48 49 50 51 54 57 62 63 64 69 70 72 76 78 **P**7 8 **S** Baptist Memorial Health Care Corporation, Memphis, TN Web address: www.bmhcc.org	21	10	166	3528	99	36954	756	19733	7083	317
BOONEVILLE—Logan County										
★ BOONEVILLE COMMUNITY HOSPITAL, 880 West Main Street, Zip 72927–3420, Mailing Address: P.O. Box 290, Zip 72927–0290; tel. 501/675–2800; Robert R. Bash, Administrator **A**9 10 **F**7 9 13 16 17 18 22 25 30 32 34 36 38 48 54 70 76 **P**6 8	23	10	26	661	9	24690	0	3456	1882	79
CALICO ROCK—Izard County										
MEDICAL CENTER OF CALICO ROCK, 103 Grasse Street, Zip 72519, Mailing Address: P.O. Box 438, Zip 72519–0438; tel. 870/297–3726; Terry L. Amstutz, CHE, Chief Executive Officer and Administrator (Nonreporting) **A**9 10	23	10	26	—	—	—	—	—	—	—
CAMDEN—Ouachita County										
★ OUACHITA MEDICAL CENTER, 638 California Street, Zip 71701–4699, Mailing Address: P.O. Box 797, Zip 71701–0797; tel. 870/836–1000; C. C. McAllister, President and Chief Executive Officer (Nonreporting) **A**1 9 10 Web address: www.geocities.com/HotSprings/Spa/1295/	23	10	118	—	—	—	—	—	—	—
CHEROKEE VILLAGE—Sharp County										
★ EASTERN OZARKS REGIONAL HEALTH SYSTEM, 122 South Allegheny Drive, Zip 72529–7300; tel. 870/257–4101; Cindy Hall, Administrator (Nonreporting) **A**9 10	33	10	40	—	—	—	—	—	—	—
CLARKSVILLE—Johnson County										
JOHNSON REGIONAL MEDICAL CENTER, 1100 East Poplar Street, Zip 72830–4419, Mailing Address: P.O. Box 738, Zip 72830–0738; tel. 501/754-5454; Kenneth R. Wood, Administrator **A**9 10 **F**7 8 9 12 16 17 22 23 24 25 27 31 32 34 36 38 39 41 43 44 45 48 50 51 54 57 59 61 62 66 70 76 78 **P**1 3 Web address: www.jrmc.com	23	10	90	3101	32	29501	357	13258	6185	213

Hospitals, U.S. / ARKANSAS

Hospital, Address, Telephone, Administrator, Approval, Facility, and Physician Codes, Health Care System, Network	Classification Codes		Utilization Data					Expense (thousands) of dollars		
★ American Hospital Association (AHA) membership ☐ Joint Commission on Accreditation of Healthcare Organizations (JCAHO) accreditation + American Osteopathic Healthcare Association (AOHA) membership ○ American Osteopathic Association (AOA) accreditation △ Commission on Accreditation of Rehabilitation Facilities (CARF) accreditation Control codes 61, 63, 64, 71, 72 and 73 indicate hospitals listed by AOHA, but not registered by AHA. For definition of numerical codes, see page A4	Control	Service	Staffed Beds	Admissions	Census	Outpatient Visits	Births	Total	Payroll	Personnel
CLINTON—Van Buren County OZARK HEALTH MEDICAL CENTER, Highway 65 South, Zip 72031, Mailing Address: P.O. Box 206, Zip 72031-0206; tel. 501/745-7000; George S. Fray, Administrator (Total facility includes 120 beds in nursing home–type unit) (Nonreporting) **A**9 10 **S** United Hospital Corporation, Memphis, TN	23	10	144	—	—	—	—	—	—	—
CONWAY—Faulkner County ✠ CONWAY REGIONAL MEDICAL CENTER, 2302 College Avenue, Zip 72032-6297; tel. 501/329-3831; John N. Robbins, President and Chief Executive Officer **A**1 9 10 **F**7 8 9 11 12 13 16 17 18 22 24 25 27 28 32 36 37 39 41 44 45 46 48 49 51 54 57 62 65 69 70 71 76 78 **P**8 Web address: www.conwayregional.org	23	10	116	6564	72	59578	1278	54118	24035	816
CROSSETT—Ashley County ★ ASHLEY COUNTY MEDICAL CENTER, 1015 Unity Road, Zip 71635-2930, Mailing Address: P.O. Box 400, Zip 71635-0400; tel. 870/364-4111; Russ D. Sword, Administrator **A**9 10 **F**7 9 16 17 18 19 22 24 25 28 34 36 37 38 39 41 43 45 46 48 54 57 62 68 70 72 76	23	10	40	1228	12	22194	0	10351	4648	199
DANVILLE—Yell County CHAMBERS MEMORIAL HOSPITAL, Highway 10 at Detroit, Zip 72833, Mailing Address: P.O. Box 639, Zip 72833-0639; tel. 501/495-2241; Scott Peek, Administrator **A**9 10 **F**8 17 22 25 32 36 45 48 54 70 76 **P**5	23	10	41	1200	12	15515	61	7439	2909	130
DARDANELLE—Yell County DARDANELLE HOSPITAL, 200 North Third Street, Zip 72834-3802, Mailing Address: P.O. Box 578, Zip 72834-0578; tel. 501/229-4677; Shawn Cathey, Administrator **A**9 10 18 **F**9 18 22 24 25 30 32 34 36 48 54 56 57 62 76	13	10	44	776	7	7179	0	4639	1876	83
DE QUEEN—Sevier County ★ DE QUEEN REGIONAL MEDICAL CENTER, 1306 Collin Raye Drive, Zip 71832-2198; tel. 870/584-4111; Craig R. Cudworth, Chief Executive Officer (Nonreporting) **A**9 10 **S** Quorum Health Group, Brentwood, TN Web address: www.hcahealthcare.com	33	10	75	—	—	—	—	—	—	—
DE WITT—Arkansas County DEWITT CITY HOSPITAL, Highway 1 and Madison Street, Zip 72042, Mailing Address: P.O. Box 32, Zip 72042-0032; tel. 870/946-3571; Joe E. Smith, Administrator and Chief Executive Officer (Total facility includes 54 beds in nursing home–type unit) (Nonreporting) **A**9 10	14	10	88	—	—	—	—	—	—	—
DUMAS—Desha County ★ DELTA MEMORIAL HOSPITAL, 300 East Pickens Street, Zip 71639-2710, Mailing Address: P.O. Box 887, Zip 71639-0887; tel. 870/382-4303; Kurt Meyer, Administrator **A**9 10 **F**9 19 22 25 30 32 34 36 38 48 49 54 57 62 70 76 **P**6 8 **S** Quorum Health Group, Brentwood, TN	23	10	20	1463	13	12059	100	7222	3041	129
EL DORADO—Union County ✠ MEDICAL CENTER OF SOUTH ARKANSAS, (Includes Union Medical Center, 700 West Grove Street, Zip 71730, Warner Brown Hospital, 460 West Oak Street, Zip 71730; tel. 501/863-2000), 700 West Grove Street, Zip 71730-4416, Mailing Address: P.O. Box 1998, Zip 71731-1998; tel. 870/864-3200; Luther J. Lewis, Chief Executive Officer **A**1 3 5 9 10 **F**7 8 9 11 13 16 17 18 19 22 24 25 27 30 32 33 34 35 36 37 38 39 41 42 43 44 45 46 48 49 50 51 53 54 56 61 65 68 69 70 71 72 76 78 79 **P**7 8 **S** Triad Hospitals, Inc., Dallas, TX Web address: www.mcsaeldo.com	32	10	162	6190	85	56168	753	43073	18341	633
EUREKA SPRINGS—Carroll County ★ EUREKA SPRINGS HOSPITAL, 24 Norris Street, Zip 72632-3541; tel. 501/253-7400; Jack Morris, Administrator (Nonreporting) **A**9 10 18	23	10	16	—	—	—	—	—	—	—
FAYETTEVILLE—Washington County ☐ CHARTER BEHAVIORAL HEALTH SYSTEM OF NORTHWEST ARKANSAS, 4253 North Crossover Road, Zip 72703-4596; tel. 501/521-5731; Patrick Kelly, Chief Executive Officer (Nonreporting) **A**1 9 10 **S** Magellan Health Services, Atlanta, GA	33	22	49	—	—	—	—	—	—	—
☐ HEALTHSOUTH REHABILITATION HOSPITAL, 153 East Monte Painter Drive, Zip 72703-4002; tel. 501/444-2200; Dennis R. Shelby, Chief Executive Officer (Nonreporting) **A**1 9 10 **S** HEALTHSOUTH Corporation, Birmingham, AL Web address: www.healthsouth.com	33	46	60	—	—	—	—	—	—	—
✠ VETERANS AFFAIRS MEDICAL CENTER, 1100 North College Avenue, Zip 72703-6995; tel. 501/443-4301; Richard F. Robinson, Director **A**1 5 **F**3 9 22 23 26 31 33 34 35 37 38 41 43 45 46 48 50 51 54 56 57 63 66 70 72 76 77 78 79 **S** Department of Veterans Affairs, Washington, DC Web address: www.va.gov/stations97/guide/home.asp?DIVISION=ALL	45	10	51	2661	47	142858	—	—	—	541
✠ WASHINGTON REGIONAL MEDICAL CENTER, 1125 North College Avenue, Zip 72703-1994; tel. 501/713-1000; Jack C. Mitchell, Interim President and Chief Executive Officer **A**1 2 3 5 9 10 **F**4 6 7 8 11 12 13 14 16 17 18 19 22 24 25 27 28 29 30 31 32 33 34 36 37 39 41 42 43 44 45 46 47 48 50 51 54 57 62 69 70 72 75 76 78 79 **P**1 7 Web address: www.wregional.com	23	10	201	11288	136	78208	1998	89965	37150	1651
FORDYCE—Dallas County DALLAS COUNTY HOSPITAL, 201 Clifton Street, Zip 71742-3099; tel. 870/352-3155; Greg R. McNeil, Administrator (Nonreporting) **A**9 10 18 **S** Healthcorp of Tennessee, Inc., Chattanooga, TN	33	10	32	—	—	—	—	—	—	—
FORREST CITY—St. Francis County ✠ BAPTIST MEMORIAL HOSPITAL–FORREST CITY, 1601 Newcastle Road, Zip 72335, Mailing Address: P.O. Box 667, Zip 72336-0667; tel. 870/261-0000; Charles R. Daugherty, Administrator **A**1 9 10 **F**3 7 8 9 12 22 24 25 30 32 34 36 37 39 41 43 46 48 51 54 57 60 62 70 72 74 76 78 **S** Baptist Memorial Health Care Corporation, Memphis, TN Web address: www.bmhcc.org	23	10	86	2160	25	16460	577	11639	5332	182

© 2000 AHA Guide   *Many Facility Codes have changed. Please refer to the AHA Guide Code Chart.*

Hospitals, U.S. / ARKANSAS

Hospital, Address, Telephone, Administrator, Approval, Facility, and Physician Codes, Health Care System, Network	Classification Codes		Utilization Data					Expense (thousands) of dollars		Personnel
	Control	Service	Staffed Beds	Admissions	Census	Outpatient Visits	Births	Total	Payroll	

★ American Hospital Association (AHA) membership
☐ Joint Commission on Accreditation of Healthcare Organizations (JCAHO) accreditation
+ American Osteopathic Healthcare Association (AOHA) membership
○ American Osteopathic Association (AOA) accreditation
△ Commission on Accreditation of Rehabilitation Facilities (CARF) accreditation
Control codes 61, 63, 64, 71, 72 and 73 indicate hospitals listed by AOHA, but not registered by AHA. For definition of numerical codes, see page A4

FORT SMITH—Sebastian County

Hospital	Control	Service	Staffed Beds	Admissions	Census	Outpatient Visits	Births	Total	Payroll	Personnel
HARBOR VIEW MERCY HOSPITAL, 10301 Mayo Road, Zip 72903–1631, Mailing Address: P.O. Box 17000, Zip 72917–7000; tel. 501/484–5550; Richard Cameron, M.D., Administrator (Nonreporting) **A**9 10 **S** Sisters of Mercy Health System–St. Louis, Saint Louis, MO	21	22	80	—	—	—	—	—	—	—
☐ HEALTHSOUTH REHABILITATION HOSPITAL OF FORT SMITH, 1401 South J Street, Zip 72901–5155; tel. 501/785–3300; Raymond Lenz, Director Operations (Nonreporting) **A**1 9 10 **S** HEALTHSOUTH Corporation, Birmingham, AL Web address: www.healthsouth.com	33	46	80	—	—	—	—	—	—	—
★ SPARKS REGIONAL MEDICAL CENTER, 1311 South I Street, Zip 72901–4995, Mailing Address: P.O. Box 17006, Zip 72917–7006; tel. 501/441–4000; Michael D. Helm, President **A**1 2 3 5 9 10 **F**4 7 8 9 11 12 13 14 18 19 22 24 25 27 28 29 30 31 32 33 34 35 36 38 39 41 42 43 44 45 46 47 48 49 50 52 54 57 58 60 61 62 63 68 69 70 71 72 76 78 79 **P**1 3 Web address: www.sparks.org	23	10	370	17525	261	98774	1273	145792	67040	2736
★ △ ST. EDWARD MERCY MEDICAL CENTER, 7301 Rogers Avenue, Zip 72903–4189, Mailing Address: P.O. Box 17000, Zip 72917–7000; tel. 501/484–6000; Michael L. Morgan, President and Chief Executive Officer **A**1 2 5 7 9 10 **F**1 3 4 7 8 9 11 13 16 17 18 19 22 23 24 25 28 29 30 33 35 36 37 38 39 41 44 45 46 47 48 49 51 54 58 59 60 61 62 63 64 68 69 70 72 74 76 78 **P**8 **S** Sisters of Mercy Health System–St. Louis, Saint Louis, MO	21	10	343	15540	230	122829	2064	113053	42684	1479

GRAVETTE—Benton County

Hospital	Control	Service	Staffed Beds	Admissions	Census	Outpatient Visits	Births	Total	Payroll	Personnel
GRAVETTE MEDICAL CENTER HOSPITAL, 1101 Jackson Street S.W., Zip 72736–0450, Mailing Address: P.O. Box 450, Zip 72736–0450; tel. 501/787–5291; John F. Phillips, Administrator (Nonreporting) **A**9 10	23	10	58	—	—	—	—	—	—	—

HARRISON—Boone County

Hospital	Control	Service	Staffed Beds	Admissions	Census	Outpatient Visits	Births	Total	Payroll	Personnel
★ NORTH ARKANSAS REGIONAL MEDICAL CENTER, 620 North Willow Street, Zip 72601–2994; tel. 870/365–2000; Timothy E. Hill, Chief Executive Officer (Total facility includes 14 beds in nursing home–type unit) **A**9 10 **F**7 8 9 11 12 13 16 17 18 19 22 24 25 27 32 34 36 37 39 41 45 46 48 49 50 51 54 65 69 70 72 76 78 79 **P**8 Web address: www.narmc.com	23	10	125	5170	57	267094	480	34115	16301	617

HEBER SPRINGS—Cleburne County

Hospital	Control	Service	Staffed Beds	Admissions	Census	Outpatient Visits	Births	Total	Payroll	Personnel
★ BAPTIST HEALTH MEDICAL CENTER–HEBER SPRINGS, (Formerly Baptist Medical Center), 2319 Highway 110 West, Zip 72543; tel. 501/206–3000; Edward L. Lacy, Administrator **A**1 10 **F**7 9 16 17 18 22 25 32 34 36 38 39 48 76 **P**3 7 **S** Baptist Health, Little Rock, AR	23	10	24	519	5	8444	0	6991	3292	117

HELENA—Phillips County

Hospital	Control	Service	Staffed Beds	Admissions	Census	Outpatient Visits	Births	Total	Payroll	Personnel
★ HELENA REGIONAL MEDICAL CENTER, 1801 Martin Luther King Drive, Zip 72342, Mailing Address: P.O. Box 788, Zip 72342–0788; tel. 870/338–5800; Steve Reeder, Chief Executive Officer **A**1 9 10 **F**7 8 13 17 22 23 24 25 30 31 32 36 41 44 45 46 48 50 53 54 57 59 62 70 71 76 78 **P**8 **S** Quorum Health Group, Brentwood, TN	23	10	145	3205	34	31721	509	19089	8210	314

HOPE—Hempstead County

Hospital	Control	Service	Staffed Beds	Admissions	Census	Outpatient Visits	Births	Total	Payroll	Personnel
★ MEDICAL PARK HOSPITAL, 2001 South Main Street, Zip 71801–8194; tel. 870/777–2323; Jimmy Leopard, Chief Executive Officer **A**1 9 10 **F**9 13 19 22 24 25 32 38 39 41 42 48 49 51 54 57 62 68 69 70 76 78 79 **P**7 **S** Triad Hospitals, Inc., Dallas, TX	33	10	71	2998	34	27685	358	16231	7508	238

HOT SPRINGS—Garland County

Hospital	Control	Service	Staffed Beds	Admissions	Census	Outpatient Visits	Births	Total	Payroll	Personnel
★ △ NATIONAL PARK MEDICAL CENTER, 1910 Malvern Avenue, Zip 71901–7799; tel. 501/321–1000; Jerry D. Mabry, Executive Director **A**1 7 9 10 **F**4 7 8 9 11 13 18 22 24 25 27 31 32 33 36 38 39 41 43 44 45 46 47 48 49 50 51 53 54 57 60 61 62 68 69 70 72 76 78 79 **P**4 7 8 **S** TENET Healthcare Corporation, Santa Barbara, CA Web address: www.tenethealth.com	33	10	166	6361	114	78097	541	47405	15483	620

HOT SPRINGS NATIONAL PARK—Garland County

Hospital	Control	Service	Staffed Beds	Admissions	Census	Outpatient Visits	Births	Total	Payroll	Personnel
★ △ LEVI HOSPITAL, 300 Prospect Avenue, Zip 71901–4097; tel. 501/624–1281; Patrick McCabe, Jr, Executive Director **A**1 7 9 10 **F**1 5 17 18 22 24 30 31 32 33 34 36 37 38 39 54 57 58 59 61 62 63 64 70 71 72 76 78 Web address: www.levihospital.com	23	22	15	215	4	1842	0	5926	3989	156
★ ST. JOSEPH'S REGIONAL HEALTH CENTER, 300 Werner Street, Zip 71913–9937, Mailing Address: P.O. Box 29001, Zip 71913–9001; tel. 501/622–1000; Randall J. Fale, FACHE, President and Chief Executive Officer (Total facility includes 30 beds in nursing home–type unit) **A**1 2 9 10 **F**4 7 8 9 11 12 13 16 17 18 19 22 24 25 30 31 32 34 36 37 38 39 40 41 43 44 45 46 47 48 49 51 53 57 62 65 69 70 72 76 77 78 79 **P**7 **S** Sisters of Mercy Health System–St. Louis, Saint Louis, MO Web address: www.saintjosephs.com	21	10	248	11502	190	295928	879	103168	42099	1336

JACKSONVILLE—Pulaski County

Hospital	Control	Service	Staffed Beds	Admissions	Census	Outpatient Visits	Births	Total	Payroll	Personnel
★ △ REBSAMEN MEDICAL CENTER, 1400 West Braden Street, Zip 72076–3788; tel. 501/985–7000; Thomas R. Siemers, Chief Executive Officer **A**1 7 9 10 **F**7 8 9 11 12 13 22 24 25 27 30 32 33 34 36 38 39 41 44 48 49 51 53 54 57 62 68 70 71 72 76 78 79 **P**1 7 **S** Quorum Health Group, Brentwood, TN	23	10	113	4439	60	67353	516	37300	15281	442

JONESBORO—Craighead County

Hospital	Control	Service	Staffed Beds	Admissions	Census	Outpatient Visits	Births	Total	Payroll	Personnel
☐ HEALTHSOUTH REHABILITATION HOSPITAL OF JONESBORO, 1201 Fleming Avenue, Zip 72401–4311, Mailing Address: P.O. Box 1680, Zip 72403–1680; tel. 870/932–0440; Brenda Antwine, Administrator (Nonreporting) **A**1 9 10 **S** HEALTHSOUTH Corporation, Birmingham, AL Web address: www.healthsouth.com	33	46	60	—	—	—	—	—	—	—

Many Facility Codes have changed. Please refer to the AHA Guide Code Chart.

Hospitals, U.S. / ARKANSAS

Hospital, Address, Telephone, Administrator, Approval, Facility, and Physician Codes, Health Care System, Network	Classification Codes		Utilization Data					Expense (thousands) of dollars		
★ American Hospital Association (AHA) membership ☐ Joint Commission on Accreditation of Healthcare Organizations (JCAHO) accreditation + American Osteopathic Healthcare Association (AOHA) membership ○ American Osteopathic Association (AOA) accreditation △ Commission on Accreditation of Rehabilitation Facilities (CARF) accreditation Control codes 61, 63, 64, 71, 72 and 73 indicate hospitals listed by AOHA, but not registered by AHA. For definition of numerical codes, see page A4	Control	Service	Staffed Beds	Admissions	Census	Outpatient Visits	Births	Total	Payroll	Personnel
★ REGIONAL MEDICAL CENTER OF NORTHEAST ARKANSAS, (Formerly Methodist Hospital of Jonesboro), 3024 Stadium Boulevard, Zip 72401–7493; tel. 870/972–7000; Philip H. Walkley, Jr, Chief Executive Officer **A**1 5 9 10 **F**4 7 8 9 11 13 16 18 19 22 23 24 25 30 32 33 34 35 36 37 38 39 43 44 45 46 47 48 49 50 51 52 53 54 68 70 71 72 74 76 77 78 79 **P**8 **S** TENET Healthcare Corporation, Santa Barbara, CA Web address: www.tenethealth.com/jonesboro	33	10	104	4306	51	59469	704	30392	10227	331
☐ ST. BERNARD'S BEHAVIORAL HEALTH, 2712 East Johnson Avenue, Zip 72401–1874; tel. 870/932–2800; Andrew DeYoung, Administrator **A**1 9 10 **F**1 2 3 4 6 7 8 9 11 12 13 14 16 17 18 19 20 21 22 23 24 25 26 27 28 29 30 32 33 34 36 37 38 39 40 41 46 47 48 49 50 51 53 54 57 58 59 60 61 62 63 64 65 66 67 69 70 71 72 73 75 76 78 79 **P**3 8	21	22	60	793	26	2071	0	5824	2808	77
★ ST. BERNARDS REGIONAL MEDICAL CENTER, 224 East Matthews Street, Zip 72401–3156, Mailing Address: P.O. Box 9320, Zip 72403–9320; tel. 870/972–4100; Ben E. Owens, President (Total facility includes 27 beds in nursing home–type unit) **A**1 2 3 5 9 10 **F**6 7 8 9 11 12 13 14 15 16 17 18 19 21 22 24 25 26 27 28 29 30 31 32 33 34 35 36 37 38 39 40 41 43 44 45 46 47 48 49 50 54 58 59 60 61 62 63 65 66 67 69 70 71 72 74 76 77 78 79 **P**3 8 Web address: www.sbrmc.com	21	10	306	16417	212	61385	1483	122576	39271	1383

LAKE VILLAGE—Chicot County

★ CHICOT MEMORIAL HOSPITAL, 2729 Highway 65 and 82 South, Zip 71653, Mailing Address: P.O. Box 512, Zip 71653–0512; tel. 870/265–5351; Robert R. Reddish, Administrator and Chief Executive Officer **A**9 **F**7 8 9 12 13 16 22 25 32 34 36 37 38 41 48 49 54 58 61 70 72 73 76 **S** Quorum Health Group, Brentwood, TN	13	10	52	2476	24	16174	123	9215	4570	183

LITTLE ROCK—Pulaski County

★ △ ARKANSAS CHILDREN'S HOSPITAL, (PEDIATRIC), 800 Marshall Street, Zip 72202–3591; tel. 501/320–1100; Jonathan R. Bates, M.D., President and Chief Executive Officer **A**1 3 5 7 8 9 10 **F**3 4 5 7 10 11 12 13 14 18 19 22 23 24 25 26 28 31 32 34 35 38 39 42 43 45 46 47 48 50 51 52 53 54 56 59 61 63 65 66 68 70 71 72 74 76 78 **P**7 8 Web address: www.ach.uams.edu	23	59	248	10232	177	218671	0	105867	80283	2189
☐ ARKANSAS HEART HOSPITAL, (CARDIOVASCULAR), 1701 South Shackleford Road, Zip 72211; tel. 501/219–7000; David Blackburn, President **A**1 9 10 **F**4 11 12 13 19 22 23 24 25 32 34 38 39 41 45 47 48 50 53 70 72 76 **P**8 **S** MedCath, Inc., Charlotte, NC Web address: www.arheart.com	33	49	84	3850	55	—	0	46786	11460	250
★ ARKANSAS STATE HOSPITAL, 4313 West Markham Street, Zip 72205–4096; tel. 501/686–9000; Glenn R. Sago, Administrator (Nonreporting) **A**1 3 5 10 Web address: www.state.ar.us/dhs/dmhs	12	22	206	—	—	—	—	—	—	—
★ BAPTIST HEALTH MEDICAL CENTER–LITTLE ROCK, (Formerly Baptist Medical Center), 9601 Interstate 630, Exit 7, Zip 72205–7299; tel. 501/202–2000; Steven Douglas Weeks, Senior Vice President and Administrator **A**1 3 5 6 9 10 **F**2 3 4 6 7 8 9 11 12 13 14 16 17 18 19 20 21 22 23 24 25 27 28 29 30 31 32 33 34 35 36 37 38 39 41 42 43 44 45 46 47 48 49 50 51 53 54 55 57 58 59 60 61 62 63 64 65 66 67 68 69 70 71 72 73 74 75 76 77 78 79 **P**1 3 4 5 6 7 **S** Baptist Health, Little Rock, AR Web address: www.baptist-health.org	23	10	620	27557	452	—	2373	252073	97050	2871
★ △ BAPTIST HEALTH REHABILITATION INSTITUTE, (Formerly Baptist Rehabilitation Institute), 9601 Interstate 630, Exit 7, Zip 72205–7249; tel. 501/202–7000; Steven Douglas Weeks, Senior Vice President and Administrator **A**1 3 5 7 9 10 **F**2 3 4 6 7 8 9 11 12 13 14 16 17 18 19 21 22 23 24 25 27 28 29 30 31 32 33 34 35 36 37 38 39 40 41 42 43 44 45 46 47 48 49 50 51 53 54 55 57 58 59 60 61 62 63 64 65 66 67 68 69 70 71 72 74 75 76 77 78 79 **P**3 5 6 7 **S** Baptist Health, Little Rock, AR Web address: www.baptist-health.org	23	46	100	1742	69	58717	0	20345	9995	257
☐ BHC PINNACLE POINTE HOSPITAL, 11501 Financial Center Parkway, Zip 72211–3715; tel. 501/223–3322; Lucinda DeBruce, Chief Executive Officer **A**1 9 10 **F**3 13 57 58 59 60 61 62 63 64 70 72 **S** Behavioral Healthcare Corporation, Nashville, TN	33	22	102	1322	66	1089	0	—	—	158
★ CENTRAL ARKANSAS VETERANS AFFAIRS HEALTHCARE SYSTEM, (Includes North Little Rock Division, North Little Rock), 4300 West Seventh Street, Zip 72205–5484; tel. 501/257–1000; George H. Gray, Jr, Director (Total facility includes 152 beds in nursing home–type unit) **A**1 2 3 5 8 **F**1 3 4 5 11 12 13 18 19 21 22 23 24 25 28 30 32 34 35 36 38 39 41 43 45 46 48 50 51 53 54 56 57 59 60 61 62 63 64 66 68 69 70 72 76 78 79 **P**6 **S** Department of Veterans Affairs, Washington, DC Web address: www.visn16.med.va.gov	45	10	512	10691	483	436066	0	230548	114935	3058
☐ SOUTHWEST REGIONAL MEDICAL CENTER, 11401 Interstate 30, Zip 72209–7056; tel. 501/455–7100; Randall R. Cason, Chief Executive Officer **A**1 9 10 **F**7 8 9 11 13 22 24 25 32 38 39 40 41 45 48 49 54 57 62 70 76 78 **S** Health Management Associates, Naples, FL	33	10	76	1839	33	20853	106	—	—	223
★ ST. VINCENT DOCTORS HOSPITAL, 6101 West Capitol, Zip 72205–5331; tel. 501/661–4000; Larry Marr, Senior Vice President and Administrator (Nonreporting) **A**1 9 10 **S** Catholic Health Initiatives, Denver, CO	21	10	308	—	—	—	—	—	—	—

Hospitals, U.S. / ARKANSAS

	Classification Codes		Utilization Data					Expense (thousands) of dollars		
Hospital, Address, Telephone, Administrator, Approval, Facility, and Physician Codes, Health Care System, Network	Control	Service	Staffed Beds	Admissions	Census	Outpatient Visits	Births	Total	Payroll	Personnel

★ American Hospital Association (AHA) membership
☐ Joint Commission on Accreditation of Healthcare Organizations (JCAHO) accreditation
+ American Osteopathic Healthcare Association (AOHA) membership
○ American Osteopathic Association (AOA) accreditation
△ Commission on Accreditation of Rehabilitation Facilities (CARF) accreditation
Control codes 61, 63, 64, 71, 72 and 73 indicate hospitals listed by AOHA, but not registered by AHA. For definition of numerical codes, see page A4.

Hospital	Control	Service	Staffed Beds	Admissions	Census	Outpatient Visits	Births	Total	Payroll	Personnel
ST. VINCENT INFIRMARY MEDICAL CENTER, (Formerly St. Vincent Health System), Two St. Vincent Circle, Zip 72205–5499; tel. 501/660–3000; William A. McDonald, President and Chief Executive Officer A1 2 3 5 9 10 F3 4 5 6 7 8 9 11 12 13 16 17 18 19 20 21 22 23 24 25 26 27 28 30 31 32 33 34 35 36 37 38 39 41 42 43 44 45 46 47 48 49 50 51 53 54 55 56 57 59 60 61 62 63 64 65 68 69 70 73 75 76 78 79 P1 3 4 6 7 8 S Catholic Health Initiatives, Denver, CO Web address: www.stvincenthealth.org	21	10	605	25148	383	192144	2850	223926	87764	2876
UNIVERSITY HOSPITAL OF ARKANSAS, 4301 West Markham Street, Zip 72205–7102; tel. 501/686–7000; Richard Pierson, Executive Director, Clinical Programs A1 2 3 5 8 9 10 F4 5 7 8 9 11 12 13 16 17 18 22 23 24 25 30 32 33 34 35 36 38 39 41 42 43 44 45 46 47 48 49 50 51 54 55 56 58 59 60 61 62 63 65 66 68 69 70 71 72 74 76 77 78 79 P3 Web address: www.uams.edu/medcenter	12	10	285	14604	263	261990	2133	215411	85341	2670
MAGNOLIA—Columbia County										
MAGNOLIA HOSPITAL, 101 Hospital Drive, Zip 71753–2416, Mailing Address: Box 629, Zip 71753–0629; tel. 870/235–3000; Kirk Reamey, Chief Executive Officer A1 9 10 F7 8 9 12 19 22 24 25 32 34 36 43 44 45 48 50 51 53 54 69 70 72 76 78 S Christus Health, Irving, TX Web address: www.magnolia–net.com	14	10	62	2016	29	27586	170	13348	6697	281
MALVERN—Hot Spring County										
H.S.C. MEDICAL CENTER, 1001 Schneider Drive, Zip 72104–4828; tel. 501/337–4911; Jeff Curtis, President and Chief Executive Officer A9 10 F8 9 12 13 17 18 22 24 25 32 36 39 41 44 45 48 51 53 54 57 61 62 70 75 76 78 P8 S Sisters of Mercy Health System–St. Louis, Saint Louis, MO	23	10	92	2643	39	23549	76	14592	8108	315
MCGEHEE—Desha County										
MCGEHEE–DESHA COUNTY HOSPITAL, 900 South Third, Zip 71654–0351, Mailing Address: P.O. Box 351, Zip 71654–0351; tel. 870/222–5600; Barbara Wood, Administrator (Nonreporting) A9 10 Web address: www.menamedicaql.com	13	10	26	—	—	—	—	—	—	—
MENA—Polk County										
MENA MEDICAL CENTER, 311 North Morrow Street, Zip 71953–2516; tel. 501/394–6100; Travis W. Roderick, Administrator and Chief Executive Officer (Nonreporting) A9 10 S Quorum Health Group, Brentwood, TN	14	10	42	—	—	—	—	—	—	—
MONTICELLO—Drew County										
DREW MEMORIAL HOSPITAL, 778 Scogin Drive, Zip 71655–5728; tel. 870/367–2411; Darren Caldwell, Chief Executive Officer (Nonreporting) A9 10 Web address: www.drewmemorial.org	13	10	50	—	—	—	—	—	—	—
MORRILTON—Conway County										
ST. ANTHONY'S HEALTHCARE CENTER, 4 Hospital Drive, Zip 72110–4510; tel. 501/354–3512; Johnson L. Smith, Chief Executive Officer and Administrator A9 10 F1 8 9 12 13 18 19 22 24 25 30 31 36 37 39 41 44 45 48 51 54 57 61 62 64 70 71 72 76 78 P8	21	10	54	1790	28	13616	63	12442	5846	257
MOUNTAIN HOME—Baxter County										
△ BAXTER REGIONAL MEDICAL CENTER, (Formerly Baxter County Regional Hospital), 624 Hospital Drive, Zip 72653–2954; tel. 870/508–1000; Stephen M. Erixon, Chief Executive Officer (Total facility includes 26 beds in nursing home–type unit) A2 7 9 10 F4 7 8 9 11 13 17 18 22 24 25 27 32 34 36 37 38 39 41 44 45 46 47 48 49 53 54 65 69 70 72 76 78 79 P8 Web address: www.baxterregional.org	23	10	189	9799	125	70754	663	75311	34238	1114
MOUNTAIN VIEW—Stone County										
STONE COUNTY MEDICAL CENTER, Highway 14 East, Zip 72560, Mailing Address: P.O. Box 510, Zip 72560–0510; tel. 870/269–4361; Kaye Mallory, Administrator (Nonreporting) A9 10	33	10	48	—	—	—	—	—	—	—
MURFREESBORO—Pike County										
PIKE COUNTY MEMORIAL HOSPITAL, 315 East 13th Street, Zip 71958–9541; tel. 870/285–3182; Rosemary Fritts, Administrator A9 10 F25 36 69 76	13	10	32	608	5	4923	0	1791	975	51
NASHVILLE—Howard County										
HOWARD MEMORIAL HOSPITAL, 800 West Leslie Street, Zip 71852–0381, Mailing Address: Box 381, Zip 71852–0381; tel. 870/845–4400; Rex Jones, Chief Executive Officer A9 10 F9 13 18 22 24 25 30 32 33 34 36 41 48 51 54 57 62 69 70 72 76 78 P3 8 S Quorum Health Group, Brentwood, TN	23	10	50	846	12	19908	0	8690	3691	159
NEWPORT—Jackson County										
HARRIS HOSPITAL, 1205 McLain Street, Zip 72112–3533; tel. 870/523–8911; David W. Fuller, Chief Executive Officer (Nonreporting) A1 9 10 S Community Health Systems, Inc., Brentwood, TN	33	10	88	—	—	—	—	—	—	—
NEWPORT HOSPITAL AND CLINIC, 2000 McLain Street, Zip 72112–3697; tel. 870/523–6721; Eugene Zuber, Administrator A9 10 F9 11 12 19 22 24 25 32 34 35 36 38 39 44 46 48 54 76 78 Web address: www.biz.ipa.net/newporthospital	33	10	86	2576	31	16669	67	10659	4310	219
NORTH LITTLE ROCK—Pulaski County										
BAPTIST HEALTH BAPTIST MEMORIAL MEDICAL CENTER, (Formerly Baptist Memorial Medical Center), 3333 Springhill Drive, Zip 72117; tel. 501/202–3000; Harrison M. Dean, Senior Vice President and Administrator A1 9 10 F3 4 6 7 8 9 11 12 13 14 16 18 19 22 24 25 27 28 29 30 31 32 33 34 35 36 37 38 39 40 41 43 44 45 46 47 48 49 50 51 53 54 55 57 58 59 60 61 62 63 64 65 67 68 69 70 71 72 73 74 75 76 77 78 79 P1 3 5 7 S Baptist Health, Little Rock, AR Web address: www.baptist–health.org	23	10	200	8186	101	69487	638	70556	30020	913

Many Facility Codes have changed. Please refer to the AHA Guide Code Chart.

© 2000 AHA Guide

Hospitals, U.S. / ARKANSAS

Hospital, Address, Telephone, Administrator, Approval, Facility, and Physician Codes, Health Care System, Network	Classification Codes		Utilization Data					Expense (thousands) of dollars		
★ American Hospital Association (AHA) membership □ Joint Commission on Accreditation of Healthcare Organizations (JCAHO) accreditation + American Osteopathic Healthcare Association (AOHA) membership ○ American Osteopathic Association (AOA) accreditation △ Commission on Accreditation of Rehabilitation Facilities (CARF) accreditation Control codes 61, 63, 64, 71, 72 and 73 indicate hospitals listed by AOHA, but not registered by AHA. For definition of numerical codes, see page A4	Control	Service	Staffed Beds	Admissions	Census	Outpatient Visits	Births	Total	Payroll	Personnel
□ BRIDGEWAY, 21 Bridgeway Road, Zip 72113; tel. 501/771–1500; Barry Pipkin, Chief Executive Officer and Managing Director (Nonreporting) **A**1 9 10 **S** Universal Health Services, Inc., King of Prussia, PA NORTH LITTLE ROCK DIVISION See Central Arkansas Veterans Affairs Healthcare System, Little Rock	33	22	70	—	—	—	—	—	—	—
OSCEOLA—Mississippi County										
★ BAPTIST MEMORIAL HOSPITAL–OSCEOLA, 611 West Lee Avenue, Zip 72370–3001, Mailing Address: P.O. Box 607, Zip 72370–0607; tel. 870/563–7000; Joel E. North, Administrator **A**1 9 10 **F**13 16 17 18 22 25 32 34 36 37 41 48 51 58 61 70 76 **P**3 7 **S** Baptist Memorial Health Care Corporation, Memphis, TN **Web address:** www.bmhcc.org	21	10	59	2271	25	17157	0	8387	3668	—
OZARK—Franklin County										
★ MERCY HOSPITAL–TURNER MEMORIAL, 801 West River Street, Zip 72949–3000; tel. 501/667–4138; Jim L. Maddox, Regional Administrator (Nonreporting) **A**9 10 18 **S** Sisters of Mercy Health System–St. Louis, Saint Louis, MO	21	10	39	—	—	—	—	—	—	—
PARAGOULD—Greene County										
★ △ ARKANSAS METHODIST HOSPITAL, 900 West Kingshighway, Zip 72450–5942, Mailing Address: P.O. Box 339, Zip 72451–0339; tel. 870/239–7000; Ronald K. Rooney, President **A**1 7 9 10 **F**8 9 11 13 17 18 19 22 24 25 27 28 30 31 32 34 36 38 39 41 44 45 46 48 49 50 53 54 56 66 69 70 76 79 **P**5 8 **Web address:** www.amhparagould.com	23	10	129	4921	69	52499	388	28216	11407	488
PARIS—Logan County										
★ NORTH LOGAN MERCY HOSPITAL, 500 East Academy, Zip 72855–4099; tel. 501/963–6101 (Nonreporting) **A**9 10 18 **S** Sisters of Mercy Health System–St. Louis, Saint Louis, MO	21	10	16	—	—	—	—	—	—	—
PIGGOTT—Clay County										
★ PIGGOTT COMMUNITY HOSPITAL, 1206 Gordon Duckworth Drive, Zip 72454–1911; tel. 870/598–3881; James L. Magee, Executive Director (Nonreporting) **A**9 10	14	10	35	—	—	—	—	—	—	—
PINE BLUFF—Jefferson County										
★ JEFFERSON REGIONAL MEDICAL CENTER, 1515 West 42nd Avenue, Zip 71603–7089; tel. 870/541–7100; Robert P. Atkinson, President and Chief Executive Officer (Total facility includes 160 beds in nursing home–type unit) **A**1 2 3 5 6 9 10 **F**3 4 8 9 11 12 13 16 17 19 21 22 24 25 26 27 28 29 31 32 33 34 35 36 37 38 39 41 43 44 45 46 47 48 49 50 51 52 53 54 56 57 59 60 61 62 63 64 65 68 69 70 71 72 75 76 77 78 79 **Web address:** www.jrmc.org	23	10	516	13450	372	154057	1524	115127	46882	1869
POCAHONTAS—Randolph County										
RANDOLPH COUNTY MEDICAL CENTER, 2801 Medical Center Drive, Zip 72455–9497; tel. 870/892–6000; Michael G. Layfield, Chief Executive Officer **A**9 10 **F**9 13 17 18 22 24 25 30 32 34 36 39 41 44 53 54 57 62 68 70 75 76 78 **S** Community Health Systems, Inc., Brentwood, TN	33	10	50	1252	16	12846	0	9393	3163	110
ROGERS—Benton County										
★ ST. MARY–ROGERS MEMORIAL HOSPITAL, 1200 West Walnut Street, Zip 72756–3599; tel. 501/636–0200; Susan Barrett, President and Chief Executive Officer **A**1 2 9 10 **F**1 7 8 9 11 12 13 16 17 18 22 24 25 32 33 34 36 37 38 39 42 43 44 45 46 48 54 68 69 70 72 76 78 79 **P**6 **S** Sisters of Mercy Health System–St. Louis, Saint Louis, MO **Web address:** www.mercyhealthnwa.smhs.com	21	10	92	6059	58	51036	1205	46022	21276	719
RUSSELLVILLE—Pope County										
★ △ SAINT MARY'S REGIONAL MEDICAL CENTER, 1808 West Main Street, Zip 72801–2724; tel. 501/968–2841; Mike McCoy, Chief Executive Officer (Total facility includes 15 beds in nursing home–type unit) **A**1 7 9 10 **F**7 8 9 11 12 13 17 18 19 22 24 25 27 28 29 30 32 33 34 36 38 39 41 44 45 46 48 49 51 53 54 64 65 68 69 70 71 72 76 78 79 **P**8 **S** TENET Healthcare Corporation, Santa Barbara, CA **Web address:** www.tenethealth.com/saintmarys	33	10	150	5714	78	93018	989	36918	15034	437
SALEM—Fulton County										
FULTON COUNTY HOSPITAL, Highway 9, Zip 72576, Mailing Address: P.O. Box 517, Zip 72576–0517; tel. 870/895–2691; Franklin E. Wise, Administrator **A**9 10 **F**22 25 36 38 44 48 76	13	10	30	952	9	19483	29	3744	1938	104
SEARCY—White County										
★ △ CENTRAL ARKANSAS HOSPITAL, 1200 South Main Street, Zip 72143–7397; tel. 501/278–3131; David C. Laffoon, CHE, Chief Executive Officer **A**1 2 7 9 10 **F**4 7 8 9 11 13 18 22 23 24 25 27 28 31 32 34 36 38 39 41 45 46 47 48 49 53 57 61 62 63 64 65 70 72 76 79 **P**8 **S** TENET Healthcare Corporation, Santa Barbara, CA **Web address:** www.tenethealth.com	33	10	148	5046	78	82886	157	31112	13957	502
★ WHITE COUNTY MEDICAL CENTER, 3214 East Race, Zip 72143–4847; tel. 501/268–6121; Raymond W. Montgomery, II, President and Chief Executive Officer **A**1 2 9 10 **F**7 8 11 12 13 14 17 18 22 23 25 27 28 29 32 34 35 36 37 38 39 41 42 44 45 48 50 51 53 54 67 70 71 72 73 76 78 79 **Web address:** www.whitecmh.org	23	10	154	8004	81	38265	723	38489	16679	677
SHERWOOD—Pulaski County										
★ △ ST. VINCENT REHABILITATION HOSPITAL, 2201 Wildwood Avenue, Zip 72120–5074, Mailing Address: P.O. Box 6930, Zip 72124–6930; tel. 501/834–1800; C. Ronnie Sairls, Administrator **A**1 7 9 10 **F**13 16 17 18 30 31 49 50 53 54 70 72 78 **S** Catholic Health Initiatives, Denver, CO	32	46	60	933	44	12023	0	10657	5154	131

© 2000 AHA Guide   *Many Facility Codes have changed. Please refer to the AHA Guide Code Chart.*

Hospitals, U.S. / ARKANSAS

Hospital, Address, Telephone, Administrator, Approval, Facility, and Physician Codes, Health Care System, Network

★ American Hospital Association (AHA) membership
☐ Joint Commission on Accreditation of Healthcare Organizations (JCAHO) accreditation
+ American Osteopathic Healthcare Association (AOHA) membership
○ American Osteopathic Association (AOA) accreditation
△ Commission on Accreditation of Rehabilitation Facilities (CARF) accreditation
Control codes 61, 63, 64, 71, 72 and 73 indicate hospitals listed by AOHA, but not registered by AHA. For definition of numerical codes, see page A4.

Hospital	Control	Service	Staffed Beds	Admissions	Census	Outpatient Visits	Births	Total	Payroll	Personnel
SILOAM SPRINGS—Benton County ★ SILOAM SPRINGS MEMORIAL HOSPITAL, 205 East Jefferson Street, Zip 72761-3697; tel. 501/524-4141; Roy W. Wright, Chief Executive Officer (Nonreporting) **A**1 9 10 **S** Quorum Health Group, Brentwood, TN	14	10	52	—	—	—	—	—	—	—
SPRINGDALE—Washington County ★ NORTHWEST MEDICAL CENTER, 609 West Maple Avenue, Zip 72764-5394, Mailing Address: P.O. Box 47, Zip 72765-0047; tel. 501/751-5711 (Total facility includes 22 beds in nursing home-type unit) (Nonreporting) **A**1 2 9 10 **S** Quorum Health Group, Brentwood, TN **Web address:** www.northwesthealth.org	23	10	222	—	—	—	—	—	—	—
STUTTGART—Arkansas County ★ STUTTGART REGIONAL MEDICAL CENTER, North Buerkle Road, Zip 72160, Mailing Address: P.O. Box 1905, Zip 72160-1905; tel. 870/673-3511; John C. Neal, Chief Executive Officer (Nonreporting) **A**9 10	23	10	89	—	—	—	—	—	—	—
VAN BUREN—Crawford County ☐ CRAWFORD MEMORIAL HOSPITAL, East Main and South 20th Streets, Zip 72956, Mailing Address: P.O. Box 409, Zip 72957-0409; tel. 501/474-3401; Richard Boone, Executive Director **A**1 9 10 **F**8 9 12 13 17 18 19 22 24 25 27 30 31 32 33 34 36 37 38 39 41 43 44 45 48 49 51 54 70 71 72 76 78 79 **P**6 **S** Health Management Associates, Naples, FL **Web address:** www.noonanrusso.com	33	10	103	2864	30	24210	197	17403	7248	282
WALDRON—Scott County ★ MERCY HOSPITAL OF SCOTT COUNTY, Highways 71 and 80, Zip 72958-9984, Mailing Address: P.O. Box 2230, Zip 72958-2230; tel. 501/637-4135; Jim L. Maddox, Administrator (Total facility includes 105 beds in nursing home-type unit) (Nonreporting) **A**9 10 18 **S** Sisters of Mercy Health System—St. Louis, Saint Louis, MO	21	10	127	—	—	—	—	—	—	—
WALNUT RIDGE—Lawrence County LAWRENCE MEMORIAL HOSPITAL, (Includes Lawrence Hall Nursing Home), 1309 West Main, Zip 72476-1430, Mailing Address: P.O. Box 839, Zip 72476-0839; tel. 870/886-1200; Lee Gentry, President (Total facility includes 189 beds in nursing home-type unit) **A**9 10 **F**7 9 17 18 19 22 24 25 32 33 34 36 38 40 43 45 48 51 54 70 72 76	13	10	213	939	182	14546	0	7942	3320	248
WARREN—Bradley County ★ BRADLEY COUNTY MEDICAL CENTER, 404 South Bradley Street, Zip 71671; tel. 870/226-3731; Edward L. Nilles, President and Chief Executive Officer **A**9 10 **F**1 6 7 8 9 12 13 14 15 18 19 20 21 22 23 24 25 26 30 31 32 33 34 35 36 37 38 40 43 45 48 50 51 54 56 58 59 60 61 62 63 64 68 70 72 73 76 78 79 **P**1 3	23	10	56	1719	21	14705	167	10842	4914	199
WEST MEMPHIS—Crittenden County ☒ △ CRITTENDEN MEMORIAL HOSPITAL, 200 Tyler Avenue, Zip 72301-4223, Mailing Address: P.O. Box 2248, Zip 72303-2248; tel. 870/735-1500; Ross Hooper, Chief Executive Officer (Nonreporting) **A**1 7 9 10	23	10	95	—	—	—	—	—	—	—
WYNNE—Cross County ★ CROSSBRIDGE COMMUNITY HOSPITAL, (Formerly Cross County Hospital), 310 South Falls Boulevard, Zip 72396-3013, Mailing Address: P.O. Box 590, Zip 72396-0590; tel. 870/238-3300; Gary R. Sparks, Chief Executive Officer (Nonreporting) **A**9 10	13	10	53	—	—	—	—	—	—	—

CALIFORNIA

Resident Population 32,667 (in thousands)
Resident population in metro areas 96.6%
Birth rate per 1,000 population 16.3
65 years and over 11.1%
Percent of persons without health insurance 21.5%

Hospital, Address, Telephone, Administrator, Approval, Facility, and Physician Codes, Health Care System, Network	Classification Codes		Utilization Data					Expense (thousands) of dollars		
	Control	Service	Staffed Beds	Admissions	Census	Outpatient Visits	Births	Total	Payroll	Personnel

★ American Hospital Association (AHA) membership
□ Joint Commission on Accreditation of Healthcare Organizations (JCAHO) accreditation
+ American Osteopathic Healthcare Association (AOHA) membership
○ American Osteopathic Association (AOA) accreditation
△ Commission on Accreditation of Rehabilitation Facilities (CARF) accreditation
Control codes 61, 63, 64, 71, 72 and 73 indicate hospitals listed by AOHA, but not registered by AHA. For definition of numerical codes, see page A4

ALAMEDA—Alameda County

	Control	Service	Staffed Beds	Admissions	Census	Outpatient Visits	Births	Total	Payroll	Personnel
✣ ALAMEDA HOSPITAL, 2070 Clinton Avenue, Zip 94501; tel. 510/522–3700; William J. Dal Cielo, Chief Executive Officer (Total facility includes 23 beds in nursing home–type unit) **A**1 9 **F**8 9 17 18 22 24 25 32 33 36 37 38 43 45 46 48 50 54 68 76 78 **P**1 4 5 6 Web address: www.alamedahospital.org	23	10	123	3785	47	36225	370	35339	20814	329

ALHAMBRA—Los Angeles County

□ △ ALHAMBRA HOSPITAL MEDICAL CENTER, (Formerly Alhambra Hospital), 100 South Raymond Avenue, Zip 91801, Mailing Address: Box 510, Zip 91802–0510; tel. 626/570–1606; Lee Suyenaga, Chief Executive Officer (Total facility includes 42 beds in nursing home–type unit) (Nonreporting) **A**1 2 7 9 10	32	10	144	—	—	—	—	—	—	—

ALTURAS—Modoc County

MODOC MEDICAL CENTER, 228 McDowell Street, Zip 96101; tel. 530/233–5131; Teresa Jacques, Chief Executive Officer (Total facility includes 71 beds in nursing home–type unit) (Nonreporting) **A**9 10	13	10	87	—	—	—	—	—	—	—

ANAHEIM—Orange County

□ ANAHEIM GENERAL HOSPITAL, 3350 West Ball Road, Zip 92804–9998; tel. 714/827–6700; Michael F. Hunn, Chief Executive Officer **A**1 9 10 **F**8 9 13 16 17 18 19 22 24 25 31 32 33 38 39 41 44 45 48 49 54 56 57 59 62 64 66 69 70 76 78 79 **P**5 Web address: www.anaheimgeneral.com	32	10	101	3901	53	26328	854	33557	11985	327
✣ ANAHEIM MEMORIAL MEDICAL CENTER, (Includes Anaheim Memorial Outpatient Tower, 1830 West Romneya Drive, Zip 92801–1854; tel. 714/491–5200), 1111 West La Palma Avenue, Zip 92801; tel. 714/774–1450; Michael C. Carter, Chief Executive Officer (Nonreporting) **A**1 2 9 10 **S** Memorial Health Services, Long Beach, CA ANAHEIM MEMORIAL MEDICAL CENTER–WEST CAMPUS See Anaheim Memorial Medical Center ANAHEIM MEMORIAL OUTPATIENT TOWER See Anaheim Memorial Medical Center	23	10	375	—	—	—	—	—	—	—
✣ KAISER FOUNDATION HOSPITAL, 441 North Lakeview Avenue, Zip 92807; tel. 714/279–4100; Janice Head, Administrator **A**1 2 3 10 **F**2 3 4 7 8 9 11 12 13 14 16 17 19 21 22 23 24 25 27 31 32 33 34 35 36 37 39 41 42 43 44 45 46 47 48 50 51 52 54 56 57 58 59 60 62 63 64 65 66 68 69 70 71 72 73 74 76 77 78 **S** Kaiser Foundation Hospitals, Oakland, CA Web address: www.kaiserpermanente.org	23	10	150	9444	94	56326	3671	—	—	1444
✣ WEST ANAHEIM MEDICAL CENTER, 3033 West Orange Avenue, Zip 92804–3184; tel. 714/827–3000; David K. Culberson, Chief Executive Officer **A**1 2 9 10 **F**2 4 9 11 12 13 17 18 19 22 24 25 31 32 33 34 38 39 41 44 46 47 48 49 50 53 54 62 70 72 75 76 78 **S** Vanguard Health System, Nashville, TN	32	10	219	8179	104	22840	316	—	—	579
✣ WESTERN MEDICAL CENTER HOSPITAL ANAHEIM, 1025 South Anaheim Boulevard, Zip 92805; tel. 714/533–6220; Mark A. Meyers, President and Chief Executive Officer **A**1 9 10 **F**4 8 11 13 18 21 22 24 25 31 47 48 50 51 54 56 58 59 60 61 62 70 72 76 78 79 **P**5 **S** TENET Healthcare Corporation, Santa Barbara, CA Web address: www.tenethealth.com	33	10	183	6076	79	22860	1415	40615	17149	366

ANTIOCH—Contra Costa County

✣ SUTTER DELTA MEDICAL CENTER, 3901 Lone Tree Way, Zip 94509; tel. 925/779–7200; Linda Horn, Chief Executive Officer **A**1 9 10 **F**2 3 4 8 9 10 11 12 13 16 17 18 19 22 23 24 25 27 32 33 34 36 37 38 39 41 42 44 45 46 47 48 49 50 51 52 53 54 55 56 57 58 59 60 61 62 63 64 65 68 69 70 72 74 76 77 78 79 **P**3 5 7 **S** Sutter Health, Sacramento, CA Web address: www.sutterhealth.org	23	10	111	5280	57	66804	917	63069	22639	543

APPLE VALLEY—San Bernardino County

✣ SAINT MARY REGIONAL MEDICAL CENTER, 18300 Highway 18, Zip 92307–0725, Mailing Address: P.O. Box 7025, Zip 92307–0725; tel. 760/242–2311; Catherine M. Pelley, President and Chief Executive Officer (Nonreporting) **A**1 2 9 10 **S** St. Joseph Health System, Orange, CA	21	10	137	—	—	—	—	—	—	—

ARCADIA—Los Angeles County

✣ METHODIST HOSPITAL OF SOUTHERN CALIFORNIA, 300 West Huntington Drive, Zip 91007, Mailing Address: P.O. Box 60016, Zip 91066–6016; tel. 626/445–4441; Dennis M. Lee, President (Total facility includes 26 beds in nursing home–type unit) (Nonreporting) **A**1 2 9 10 **S** Southern California Healthcare Systems, Pasadena, CA	23	10	304	—	—	—	—	—	—	—

ARCATA—Humboldt County

□ MAD RIVER COMMUNITY HOSPITAL, 3800 Janes Road, Zip 95521, Mailing Address: P.O. Box 1115, Zip 95521–1115; tel. 707/822–3621; Douglas A. Shaw, Administrator (Nonreporting) **A**1 9 10	33	10	78	—	—	—	—	—	—	—

ARROYO GRANDE—San Luis Obispo County

□ ARROYO GRANDE COMMUNITY HOSPITAL, 345 South Halcyon Road, Zip 93420; tel. 805/489–4261; Gale E. Gascho, Chief Executive Officer (Nonreporting) **A**1 9 10	23	10	35	—	—	—	—	—	—	—

Hospitals, U.S. / CALIFORNIA

Hospital, Address, Telephone, Administrator, Approval, Facility, and Physician Codes, Health Care System, Network	Classification Codes		Utilization Data					Expense (thousands) of dollars		
★ American Hospital Association (AHA) membership ☐ Joint Commission on Accreditation of Healthcare Organizations (JCAHO) accreditation + American Osteopathic Healthcare Association (AOHA) membership ○ American Osteopathic Association (AOA) accreditation △ Commission on Accreditation of Rehabilitation Facilities (CARF) accreditation Control codes 61, 63, 64, 71, 72 and 73 indicate hospitals listed by AOHA, but not registered by AHA. For definition of numerical codes, see page A4	Control	Service	Staffed Beds	Admissions	Census	Outpatient Visits	Births	Total	Payroll	Personnel
ATASCADERO—San Luis Obispo County										
☐ ATASCADERO STATE HOSPITAL, 10333 El Camino Real, Zip 93422–7001, Mailing Address: P.O. Box 7001, Zip 93423–7001; tel. 805/461–2000; Jon Demorales, Executive Director **A**1 3 5 **F**17 23 35 45 50 51 57 70 78	12	22	1030	1128	1010	0	0	—	—	1717
AUBURN—Placer County										
★ SUTTER AUBURN FAITH COMMUNITY HOSPITAL, 11815 Education Street, Zip 95603; tel. 530/888–4500; Mitch Hanna, Chief Administrative Officer (Total facility includes 12 beds in nursing home–type unit) (Nonreporting) **A**1 9 10 **S** Sutter Health, Sacramento, CA **Web address:** www.sutterhealth.org	23	10	105	—	—	—	—	—	—	—
AVALON—Los Angeles County										
AVALON MUNICIPAL HOSPITAL AND CLINIC, 100 Falls Canyon Road, Zip 90704, Mailing Address: Box 1563, Zip 90704–1563; tel. 310/510–0700; Bonnie Hoh, R.N., MSN, Administrator (Total facility includes 4 beds in nursing home–type unit) (Nonreporting) **A**9 10	23	10	12	—	—	—	—	—	—	—
BAKERSFIELD—Kern County										
★ BAKERSFIELD MEMORIAL HOSPITAL, (Includes Memorial Center, 5201 White Lane, Zip 93309; tel. 805/398–1800), 420 34th Street, Zip 93301, Mailing Address: P.O. Box 1888, Zip 93303–1888; tel. 661/327–1792; C. Larry Carr, Regional Executive Vice President and President (Total facility includes 24 beds in nursing home–type unit) **A**1 2 9 10 **F**2 3 4 7 8 9 11 12 13 17 18 19 22 24 25 27 31 32 34 36 37 39 41 42 44 45 46 47 48 50 54 57 58 59 60 63 64 65 69 70 72 76 77 78 79 **P**1 4 5 7 **S** Catholic Healthcare West, San Francisco, CA **Web address:** www.chw.edu	23	10	299	11973	173	84712	1727	90003	34772	823
☐ GOOD SAMARITAN HOSPITAL, 901 Olive Drive, Zip 93308–4137; tel. 661/399–4461; David A. Huff, Administrator (Nonreporting) **A**1 9 10	33	10	64	—	—	—	—	—	—	—
☐ HEALTHSOUTH BAKERSFIELD REHABILITATION HOSPITAL, 5001 Commerce Drive, Zip 93309; tel. 661/323–5500; Robyn Field, Ph.D., Chief Operating Officer (Nonreporting) **A**1 9 10 **S** HEALTHSOUTH Corporation, Birmingham, AL	33	46	60	—	—	—	—	—	—	—
☐ KERN MEDICAL CENTER, 1830 Flower Street, Zip 93305–4197; tel. 661/326–2000; Peter K. Bryan, Chief Executive Officer **A**1 2 3 5 8 9 10 **F**1 3 4 8 9 11 12 13 16 17 18 19 21 22 24 25 29 30 32 33 34 35 36 38 39 40 41 42 43 44 45 46 47 48 50 51 54 56 57 58 59 61 65 66 70 76 77 78 **P**6 **Web address:** www.kernmedctr.com	13	10	171	11192	125	153108	2995	114781	50150	1268
MEMORIAL CENTER See Bakersfield Memorial Hospital										
★ MERCY HOSPITAL, (Includes Mercy Southwest Hospital, 400 Old River Road, Zip 93311; tel. 661/663–6000), 2215 Truxtun Avenue, Zip 93301, Mailing Address: P.O. Box 119, Zip 93302; tel. 661/632–5000; Bernard J. Herman, President and Chief Executive Officer (Total facility includes 50 beds in nursing home–type unit) **A**1 2 9 10 **F**7 8 9 12 13 17 18 19 22 24 25 27 32 33 36 39 41 42 43 44 45 46 48 51 54 65 69 70 72 76 77 78 **P**7 **S** Catholic Healthcare West, San Francisco, CA	21	10	422	12201	166	166978	2507	104823	39435	1223
★ SAN JOAQUIN COMMUNITY HOSPITAL, 2615 Eye Street, Zip 93301, Mailing Address: Box 2615, Zip 93303–2615; tel. 661/395–3000; Douglas L. Lafferty, President and Chief Executive Officer (Nonreporting) **A**1 9 10 **S** Adventist Health, Roseville, CA **Web address:** www.adventisthealth.org	23	10	178	—	—	—	—	—	—	—
BALDWIN PARK—Los Angeles County										
★ KAISER FOUNDATION HOSPITAL, 1011 Baldwin Park Boulevard, Zip 91706; tel. 626/851–1011; Gregory A. Adams, Senior Vice President and Service Area Manager **A**10 **F**8 9 13 17 18 22 25 29 33 34 36 39 41 42 43 44 45 48 49 50 51 54 56 59 63 70 76 78 **S** Kaiser Foundation Hospitals, Oakland, CA	23	10	158	8303	67	107997	2984	—	—	1121
BANNING—Riverside County										
★ SAN GORGONIO MEMORIAL HOSPITAL, 600 North Highland Springs Avenue, Zip 92220; tel. 909/845–1121; Donald N. Larkin, Chief Executive Officer (Total facility includes 16 beds in nursing home–type unit) **A**1 9 10 **F**7 9 13 14 17 18 19 22 25 32 41 44 48 54 62 63 68 69 70 72 76 77 78 **S** Brim Healthcare, Inc., Brentwood, TN **Web address:** www.sgmhf.org	23	10	68	3097	37	31990	291	17469	8291	227
BARSTOW—San Bernardino County										
☐ BARSTOW COMMUNITY HOSPITAL, 555 South Seventh Street, Zip 92311; tel. 760/256–1761; George F. Naylor, II, CHE, Chief Executive Officer **A**1 2 9 10 **F**7 8 9 12 13 17 22 24 25 30 32 33 34 39 43 44 48 49 76 78 **S** Community Health Systems, Inc., Brentwood, TN **Web address:** www.barstowhospital.com	33	10	56	2771	27	42364	335	—	—	211
BELLFLOWER—Los Angeles County										
☐ BELLFLOWER MEDICAL CENTER, 9542 East Artesia Boulevard, Zip 90706; tel. 562/925–8355; Stanley Otake, Administrator and Chief Executive Officer (Nonreporting) **A**1 9 10 **S** Pacific Health Corporation, Tustin, CA	33	10	145	—	—	—	—	—	—	—
☐ BELLWOOD GENERAL HOSPITAL, 10250 East Artesia Boulevard, Zip 90706; tel. 562/866–9028; Michael Kerr, Chief Executive Officer (Nonreporting) **A**1	33	10	65	—	—	—	—	—	—	—
★ KAISER FOUNDATION HOSPITAL–BELLFLOWER, 9400 East Rosecrans Avenue, Zip 90706–2246; tel. 562/461–3000; Karen K. Ringl, Director Hospital Operations **A**1 2 3 10 **F**2 3 4 8 9 10 11 13 14 15 16 17 18 19 20 21 22 23 24 25 26 27 29 30 32 33 34 35 36 37 38 39 41 42 43 44 45 46 47 48 49 50 51 52 53 54 55 56 57 58 59 60 61 62 63 64 65 66 68 69 70 72 73 74 76 77 78 79 **P**6 **S** Kaiser Foundation Hospitals, Oakland, CA **Web address:** www.ca.kaiserpermanente.org	23	10	282	17708	148	1518914	4275	—	—	1915

Hospitals, U.S. / CALIFORNIA

Hospital, Address, Telephone, Administrator, Approval, Facility, and Physician Codes, Health Care System, Network	Classification Codes		Utilization Data					Expense (thousands) of dollars		
★ American Hospital Association (AHA) membership ☐ Joint Commission on Accreditation of Healthcare Organizations (JCAHO) accreditation + American Osteopathic Healthcare Association (AOHA) membership ○ American Osteopathic Association (AOA) accreditation △ Commission on Accreditation of Rehabilitation Facilities (CARF) accreditation Control codes 61, 63, 64, 71, 72 and 73 indicate hospitals listed by AOHA, but not registered by AHA. For definition of numerical codes, see page A4	Control	Service	Staffed Beds	Admissions	Census	Outpatient Visits	Births	Total	Payroll	Personnel
BERKELEY—Alameda County										
★ △ ALTA BATES MEDICAL CENTER–ASHBY CAMPUS, (Includes Alta Bates Medical Center–Herrick Campus, 2001 Dwight Way, Zip 94704; tel. 510/204–4444), 2450 Ashby Avenue, Zip 94705; tel. 510/204–4444; Warren J. Kirk, President and Chief Administrative Officer (Total facility includes 81 beds in nursing home–type unit) (Nonreporting) **A**1 2 7 9 10 **S** Sutter Health, Sacramento, CA **Web address:** www.ahabates.com	23	10	468	—	—	—	—	—	—	—
BIG BEAR LAKE—San Bernardino County										
★ BEAR VALLEY COMMUNITY HOSPITAL, 41870 Garstin Road, Zip 92315, Mailing Address: P.O. Box 1649, Zip 92315–1649; tel. 909/866–6501; Mary Norman, Administrator and Chief Executive Officer (Total facility includes 15 beds in nursing home–type unit) (Nonreporting) **A**1 9 10	16	10	30	—	—	—	—	—	—	—
BISHOP—Inyo County										
★ NORTHERN INYO HOSPITAL, 150 Pioneer Lane, Zip 93514–2599; tel. 760/873–5811; Herman J. Spencer, Administrator **A**1 9 10 **F**7 8 9 22 25 37 38 39 41 44 48 54 70 76	16	10	30	1223	10	24121	283	20569	9294	249
BLYTHE—Riverside County										
☐ PALO VERDE HOSPITAL, 250 North First Street, Zip 92225; tel. 760/922–4115; M. Victoria Clark, Chief Executive Officer **A**1 9 10 **F**7 9 13 16 17 19 22 25 30 32 33 34 36 39 41 44 46 48 50 51 54 61 70 76 78 **S** Province Healthcare Corporation, Brentwood, TN	33	10	35	1808	15	19875	276	11266	4163	135
BRAWLEY—Imperial County										
★ PIONEERS MEMORIAL HEALTHCARE DISTRICT, 207 West Legion Road, Zip 92227–9699; tel. 760/351–3333; Claire Kuczkowski, Chief Executive Officer **A**1 9 10 **F**7 8 9 22 25 32 34 35 39 41 42 44 48 70 76 78 79 **P**5 **S** Brim Healthcare, Inc., Brentwood, TN **Web address:** www.pmhd.org	16	10	99	4175	38	48988	1059	35916	13695	363
BREA—Orange County										
☐ BREA COMMUNITY HOSPITAL, 380 West Central Avenue, Zip 92821; tel. 714/529–0211; Gaetano Zanfini, Chief Executive Officer (Nonreporting) **A**1 9 10 **S** Doctors Community Healthcare Corporation, Scottsdale, AZ	33	10	60	—	—	—	—	—	—	—
☐ VENCOR HOSPITAL–BREA, 875 North Brea Boulevard, Zip 92821; tel. 714/529–6842; Virgis Narbutas, Executive Director (Nonreporting) **A**1 10 **S** Vencor, Incorporated, Louisville, KY	33	10	48	—	—	—	—	—	—	—
BUENA PARK—Orange County										
ORANGE COUNTY COMMUNITY HOSPITAL OF BUENA PARK, 6850 Lincoln Avenue, Zip 90620–5703; tel. 714/827–1161; Michael Kerr, Chief Executive Officer (Nonreporting) **A**9 10 **S** Alta Healthcare System, Santa Monica, CA	33	22	55	—	—	—	—	—	—	—
BURBANK—Los Angeles County										
★ PROVIDENCE SAINT JOSEPH MEDICAL CENTER, 501 South Buena Vista Street, Zip 91505–4866; tel. 818/843–5111; Georgianne Jessen, Chief Executive Officer (Total facility includes 120 beds in nursing home–type unit) **A**1 2 9 10 **F**4 7 8 9 11 12 13 14 16 17 18 19 20 21 22 23 24 25 26 27 28 31 32 33 34 36 37 38 39 41 42 43 44 45 46 47 48 49 50 51 53 54 65 69 70 72 73 76 77 78 79 **P**5 **S** Providence Health System, Seattle, WA **Web address:** www.providence.org	21	10	448	20564	321	283911	2282	190247	83807	1937
BURLINGAME—San Mateo County										
★ MILLS–PENINSULA HEALTH SERVICES, (Includes Mills Hospital, 100 South San Mateo Drive, San Mateo, Zip 94401; tel. 415/696–4400; Peninsula Hospital, 1783 El Camino Real, tel. 415/696–5400), 1783 El Camino Real, Zip 94010–3205; tel. 650/696–5400; Robert W. Merwin, Chief Executive Officer (Total facility includes 75 beds in nursing home–type unit) **A**1 2 9 10 **F**1 2 3 4 5 7 8 9 11 12 13 16 17 18 19 20 21 22 23 24 25 27 28 30 31 32 33 34 35 36 38 39 41 44 45 46 47 48 49 50 51 53 54 57 58 59 60 61 62 63 64 65 68 70 72 76 77 78 79 **P**5 6 **S** Sutter Health, Sacramento, CA **Web address:** www.mphs.org	23	10	358	15353	238	402311	2174	186915	86007	1190
CAMARILLO—Ventura County										
★ ST. JOHN'S PLEASANT VALLEY HOSPITAL, 2309 Antonio Avenue, Zip 93010–1459; tel. 805/389–5800; William J. Clearwater, Vice President and Site Administrator **A**1 9 10 **F**8 9 16 17 18 19 22 24 25 27 32 33 34 35 39 41 44 48 50 51 54 68 69 70 72 76 78 **P**2 **S** Catholic Healthcare West, San Francisco, CA **Web address:** www.chw.edu	23	10	180	4043	109	43879	645	33186	16172	357
CAMP PENDLETON—San Diego County										
★ NAVAL HOSPITAL, Mailing Address: Box 555191, Zip 92055–5191; tel. 760/725–1288; Captain Thomas Burkhard, Commanding Officer (Nonreporting) **A**1 3 5 **S** Department of Navy, Washington, DC	43	10	209	—	—	—	—	—	—	—
CANOGA PARK—Los Angeles County, See Los Angeles										
CARMICHAEL—Sacramento County										
★ MERCY AMERICAN RIVER/MERCY SAN JUAN HOSPITAL, (Includes Mercy American River Hospital, 4747 Engle Road, tel. 916/484–2222; Mercy San Juan Hospital, 6501 Coyle Avenue), 6501 Coyle Avenue, Zip 95608, Mailing Address: P.O. Box 479, Zip 95608; tel. 916/537–5000; Michael H. Erne, President and Chief Executive Officer (Nonreporting) **A**1 2 9 10 **S** Catholic Healthcare West, San Francisco, CA	21	10	352	—	—	—	—	—	—	—

© 2000 AHA Guide   *Many Facility Codes have changed. Please refer to the AHA Guide Code Chart.*

Hospitals, U.S. / CALIFORNIA

Hospital, Address, Telephone, Administrator, Approval, Facility, and Physician Codes, Health Care System, Network	Classification Codes		Utilization Data					Expense (thousands) of dollars		
★ American Hospital Association (AHA) membership □ Joint Commission on Accreditation of Healthcare Organizations (JCAHO) accreditation + American Osteopathic Healthcare Association (AOHA) membership ○ American Osteopathic Association (AOA) accreditation △ Commission on Accreditation of Rehabilitation Facilities (CARF) accreditation Control codes 61, 63, 64, 71, 72 and 73 indicate hospitals listed by AOHA, but not registered by AHA. For definition of numerical codes, see page A4	Control	Service	Staffed Beds	Admissions	Census	Outpatient Visits	Births	Total	Payroll	Personnel
CASTRO VALLEY—Alameda County										
★ EDEN MEDICAL CENTER, 20103 Lake Chabot Road, Zip 94546; tel. 510/537-1234; George Bischalaney, President and Chief Executive Officer (Total facility includes 67 beds in nursing home–type unit) **A**1 9 10 **F**6 7 8 9 11 12 13 16 17 19 22 24 25 31 32 33 34 39 41 42 43 44 45 46 48 51 53 54 57 62 63 64 67 69 70 72 75 76 78 79 **P**5 **S** Sutter Health, Sacramento, CA **Web address:** www.edenmedcenter.org	23	10	258	9976	143	137860	1126	80403	36891	657
CEDARVILLE—Modoc County										
SURPRISE VALLEY COMMUNITY HOSPITAL, Main and Washington Streets, Zip 96104, Mailing Address: P.O. Box 246, Zip 96104–0246; tel. 530/279-6111; Joyce I. Gysin, Administrator (Total facility includes 22 beds in nursing home–type unit) **A**9 10 **F**16 17 18 23 25 30 32 34 36 38 40 43 48 69 76 78 **P**6	16	10	26	107	22	2844	5	2754	1687	67
CERRITOS—Los Angeles County										
□ COLLEGE HOSPITAL, 10802 College Place, Zip 90703–1579; tel. 562/924-9581; Stephen Witt, Chief Executive Officer **A**1 3 9 10 **F**17 57 58 61 62 64 72 **S** College Health Enterprises, Downey, CA	33	22	124	6014	90	15182	0	17507	7395	214
CHESTER—Plumas County										
SENECA DISTRICT HOSPITAL, 130 Brentwood Drive, Zip 96020, Mailing Address: Box 737, Zip 96020; tel. 530/258-2151; Bernard G. Hietpas, Chief Executive Officer (Total facility includes 16 beds in nursing home–type unit) **A**9 10 **F**8 9 16 25 32 35 37 38 44 48 69 70 76 77 78	16	10	26	417	20	25950	26	7990	3707	112
CHICO—Butte County										
★ ENLOE MEDICAL CENTER, (Includes Enloe Medical Center–Cohasset, 560 Cohasset Road, Zip 95926; tel. 530/332-7300; Dan Meister, Chief Operating Officer), 1531 Esplanade, Zip 95926–3386; tel. 530/891-7300; Philip R. Wolfe, President and Chief Executive Officer **A**1 2 9 10 **F**4 5 7 8 9 11 12 13 14 16 17 18 19 22 23 24 25 26 27 29 30 31 32 33 34 35 36 37 38 39 40 41 42 43 44 45 46 47 48 49 50 51 52 53 54 56 57 59 60 61 62 64 65 66 68 69 70 71 72 75 76 77 78 79 **P**5 7 **Web address:** www.enloehealth.com	23	10	291	13685	177	228394	1609	148998	61231	1683
CHINO—San Bernardino County										
□ CANYON RIDGE HOSPITAL, (Formerly BHC Canyon Ridge Hospital), 5353 G Street, Zip 91710; tel. 909/590-3700; Diana C. Hanyak, Chief Executive Officer **A**1 9 10 **F**3 18 19 21 30 31 57 58 59 60 61 62 63 64 70 72 **S** Behavioral Healthcare Corporation, Nashville, TN	32	22	59	670	38	999	0	1803	920	104
★ CHINO VALLEY MEDICAL CENTER, (Formerly Chino Valley Hospital), 5451 Walnut Avenue, Zip 91710; tel. 909/464-8600; Stephen E. Dixon, Chief Executive Officer (Total facility includes 14 beds in nursing home–type unit) (Nonreporting) **A**1 9 10 **S** HCA – The Healthcare Company, Nashville, TN **Web address:** www.cvmc.com	33	10	104	—	—	—	—	—	—	—
CHOWCHILLA—Madera County										
CHOWCHILLA DISTRICT MEMORIAL HOSPITAL, 1104 Ventura Avenue, Zip 93610, Mailing Address: Box 1027, Zip 93610; tel. 559/665-3781; Barbara Faller, Administrator (Nonreporting) **A**9 10	16	10	23	—	—	—	—	—	—	—
CHULA VISTA—San Diego County										
□ BAYVIEW HOSPITAL AND MENTAL HEALTH SYSTEM, 330 Moss Street, Zip 91911–2005; tel. 619/426-6310; Roy Rodriguez, Ph.D., Chief Executive Officer (Nonreporting) **A**1 9 10 **Web address:** www.bayviewhospital.com	33	22	64	—	—	—	—	—	—	—
★ SCRIPPS MEMORIAL HOSPITAL CHULA VISTA, (Formerly Scripps Hospital–Chula Vista), 435 H Street, Zip 91912, Mailing Address: P.O. Box 1537, Zip 91910–1537; tel. 619/691-7000; John Grah, Administrator **A**1 3 9 10 **F**7 8 13 16 17 18 19 22 24 25 31 32 33 36 39 40 41 44 46 48 51 54 68 70 72 76 78 79 **P**3 5 7 **S** Scripps Health, San Diego, CA **Web address:** www.scrippshealth.org	23	10	183	7527	99	67736	1649	50442	24267	490
★ SHARP CHULA VISTA MEDICAL CENTER, 751 Medical Center Court, Zip 91911, Mailing Address: Box 1297, Zip 91912; tel. 619/482-5800; JoAnne G. Schader, R.N., Interim Chief Executive Officer (Total facility includes 100 beds in nursing home–type unit) **A**1 2 3 9 10 **F**4 7 8 9 11 13 16 17 18 19 22 24 25 31 32 33 34 36 37 38 39 40 41 42 43 44 45 46 47 48 49 50 51 54 56 65 69 70 72 76 78 79 **S** Sharp Healthcare, San Diego, CA **Web address:** www.sharp.com	23	10	306	10412	221	52994	2087	74052	33275	751
CLEARLAKE—Lake County										
★ REDBUD COMMUNITY HOSPITAL, 18th Avenue and Highway 53, Zip 95422, Mailing Address: P.O. Box 6720, Zip 95422; tel. 707/994-6486; Richard D. Hathaway, Chief Operating Officer **A**1 10 **F**8 9 17 18 19 22 24 25 31 32 34 36 38 39 41 43 44 45 48 50 51 54 56 70 76 78 79 **S** Adventist Health, Roseville, CA **Web address:** www.adventisthealth.org	23	10	40	1466	15	—	174	21986	9326	261
CLOVIS—Fresno County										
★ COMMUNITY MEDICAL CENTER–CLOVIS, (Formerly Clovis Medical Center), 2755 Herndon Avenue, Zip 93611; tel. 559/324-4000; J. Philip Hinton, M.D., President and Chief Executive Officer (Nonreporting) **A**1 9 10 **S** Community Medical Centers, Fresno, CA **Web address:** www.communitymedical.org	23	10	143	—	—	—	—	—	—	—

Hospitals, U.S. / CALIFORNIA

Hospital, Address, Telephone, Administrator, Approval, Facility, and Physician Codes, Health Care System, Network

- ★ American Hospital Association (AHA) membership
- ☐ Joint Commission on Accreditation of Healthcare Organizations (JCAHO) accreditation
- + American Osteopathic Healthcare Association (AOHA) membership
- ○ American Osteopathic Association (AOA) accreditation
- △ Commission on Accreditation of Rehabilitation Facilities (CARF) accreditation
- Control codes 61, 63, 64, 71, 72 and 73 indicate hospitals listed by AOHA, but not registered by AHA. For definition of numerical codes, see page A4

Hospital	Classification Codes		Utilization Data					Expense (thousands of dollars)		
	Control	Service	Staffed Beds	Admissions	Census	Outpatient Visits	Births	Total	Payroll	Personnel
COALINGA—Fresno County										
COALINGA REGIONAL MEDICAL CENTER, 1191 Phelps Avenue, Zip 93210; tel. 559/935–6400; David P. Jacobsen, Administrator/Chief Executive Officer (Total facility includes 54 beds in nursing home–type unit) **A**9 10 **F**9 22 25 32 48 54 69 76 77 78	16	10	78	995	50	17191	45	8755	3442	121
COLTON—San Bernardino County										
★ ○ ARROWHEAD REGIONAL MEDICAL CENTER, (Formerly San Bernardino County Medical Center), 400 North Pepper Avenue, Zip 92324; tel. 909/580–1000; Mark H. Uffer, Chief Executive Officer **A**1 2 3 5 9 10 11 12 13 **F**4 8 9 10 11 13 16 17 18 19 20 22 23 24 25 26 29 30 31 32 33 34 35 36 38 39 41 42 43 44 45 46 48 49 50 51 54 56 57 58 59 60 61 62 63 66 68 70 72 74 75 76 77 78 79 **P**5	13	10	304	13096	210	235767	1343	180175	70356	2063
COLUSA—Colusa County										
☐ COLUSA COMMUNITY HOSPITAL, 199 East Webster Street, Zip 95932, Mailing Address: P.O. Box 331, Zip 95932–0331; tel. 530/458–5821; Woody J. Laughnan, Interim Chief Executive Officer **A**1 9 10 **F**7 8 9 13 22 25 30 36 41 43 44 45 48 54 69 70 72 76 78 **Web address:** www.communitymed.org	23	10	38	978	12	25241	166	9419	3373	107
CORCORAN—Kings County										
CORCORAN DISTRICT HOSPITAL, 1310 Hanna Avenue, Zip 93212, Mailing Address: Box 758, Zip 93212; tel. 559/992–5051; David R. Green, Chief Executive Officer **A**9 10 **F**22 25 32 36 38 48 54 56 70 76 78 **P**3 7 **S** Brim Healthcare, Inc., Brentwood, TN	16	10	32	857	10	12650	0	5227	2545	99
CORONA—Riverside County										
☐ CORONA REGIONAL MEDICAL CENTER, (Includes Corona Regional Medical Center–Rehabilitation, 730 Magnolia Avenue, Zip 91719; tel. 909/736–7200), 800 South Main Street, Zip 91720; tel. 909/737–4343; John A. Calderone, Ph.D., Chief Executive Officer **A**1 2 9 10 **F**4 6 8 9 11 13 14 16 17 18 19 22 25 32 33 34 36 37 38 39 41 43 44 45 46 47 48 49 50 51 53 54 57 62 63 64 65 69 70 72 74 76 77 78 79 **Web address:** www.coronaregional.com	23	10	210	8724	123	176754	1849	69520	24641	618
CORONADO—San Diego County										
★ SHARP CORONADO HOSPITAL, 250 Prospect Place, Zip 92118; tel. 619/522–3600; Marcia K. Hall, Chief Executive Officer (Total facility includes 149 beds in nursing home–type unit) (Nonreporting) **A**1 9 10 **S** Sharp Healthcare, San Diego, CA **Web address:** www.sharp.com	23	10	195	—	—	—	—	—	—	—
COSTA MESA—Orange County										
☐ COLLEGE HOSPITAL COSTA MESA, 301 Victoria Street, Zip 92627; tel. 949/574–3322; Dale A. Kirby, Chief Executive Officer (Nonreporting) **A**1 9 10 **S** College Health Enterprises, Downey, CA	33	22	119	—	—	—	—	—	—	—
COVINA—Los Angeles County										
☐ CHARTER BEHAVIORAL HEALTH SYSTEM OF SOUTHERN CALIFORNIA–CHARTER OAK, 1161 East Covina Boulevard, Zip 91724–1161; tel. 626/966–1632; Todd A. Smith, Chief Executive Officer (Nonreporting) **A**1 9 10	33	22	95	—	—	—	—	—	—	—
CITRUS VALLEY MEDICAL CENTER INTER–COMMUNITY CAMPUS, 210 West San Bernardino Road, Zip 91723–1901, Mailing Address: P.O. Box 6108, Zip 91722–5108; tel. 626/331–7331; Peter E. Makowski, President and Chief Executive Officer (Nonreporting) **A**2 9 10 **S** Citrus Valley Health Partners, Covina, CA	23	10	252	—	—	—	—	—	—	—
CRESCENT CITY—Del Norte County										
★ SUTTER COAST HOSPITAL, 800 East Washington Boulevard, Zip 95531; tel. 707/464–8511; John E. Menaugh, Chief Executive Officer **A**1 9 10 **F**7 8 9 17 18 22 25 27 31 34 36 37 39 41 44 48 76 77 **P**3 5 7 **S** Sutter Health, Sacramento, CA **Web address:** www.sutterhealth.org	23	10	59	2768	33	106293	297	31929	13594	335
CULVER CITY—Los Angeles County										
★ BROTMAN MEDICAL CENTER, 3828 Delmas Terrace, Zip 90231–2459, Mailing Address: Box 2459, Zip 90231–2459; tel. 310/836–7000; Sonja Hagel, Chief Executive Officer **A**1 9 10 **F**9 11 12 13 18 22 25 39 41 48 51 53 54 57 64 65 69 70 72 76 78 **S** TENET Healthcare Corporation, Santa Barbara, CA **Web address:** www.tenethealh.com	32	10	244	6902	150	28564	0	62642	34305	662
DALY CITY—San Mateo County										
★ SETON MEDICAL CENTER, 1900 Sullivan Avenue, Zip 94015; tel. 650/992–4000; Bernadette M. Smith, Chief Operating Officer (Total facility includes 91 beds in nursing home–type unit) **A**1 2 3 5 9 10 **F**1 2 3 4 7 8 9 10 11 12 13 14 16 17 18 19 22 24 25 27 29 30 31 32 33 34 36 38 39 41 42 43 44 45 46 47 48 49 51 52 53 54 57 58 61 62 63 64 65 69 70 71 72 76 77 78 79 **S** Catholic Healthcare West, San Francisco, CA **Web address:** www.chwwestbay.org	21	10	255	10833	226	—	1115	134848	55581	1071
DAVIS—Yolo County										
★ SUTTER DAVIS HOSPITAL, 2000 Sutter Place, Zip 95616, Mailing Address: P.O. Box 1617, Zip 95617; tel. 530/756–6440; Janet Wagner, Chief Administrative Officer (Nonreporting) **A**1 3 9 10 **S** Sutter Health, Sacramento, CA **Web address:** www.sutterhealth.org	23	10	48	—	—	—	—	—	—	—
DEER PARK—Napa County										
★ ST. HELENA HOSPITAL, 650 Sanitarium Road, Zip 94576, Mailing Address: P.O. Box 250, Zip 94576; tel. 707/963–3611; JoAline Olson, R.N., President and Chief Executive Officer (Total facility includes 23 beds in nursing home–type unit) (Nonreporting) **A**1 9 10 **S** Adventist Health, Roseville, CA **Web address:** www.sthelenahospital.org	21	10	168	—	—	—	—	—	—	—

Hospitals, U.S. / CALIFORNIA

Hospital, Address, Telephone, Administrator, Approval, Facility, and Physician Codes, Health Care System, Network	Classification Codes		Utilization Data					Expense (thousands) of dollars		
★ American Hospital Association (AHA) membership □ Joint Commission on Accreditation of Healthcare Organizations (JCAHO) accreditation + American Osteopathic Healthcare Association (AOHA) membership ○ American Osteopathic Association (AOA) accreditation △ Commission on Accreditation of Rehabilitation Facilities (CARF) accreditation Control codes 61, 63, 64, 71, 72 and 73 indicate hospitals listed by AOHA, but not registered by AHA. For definition of numerical codes, see page A4	Control	Service	Staffed Beds	Admissions	Census	Outpatient Visits	Births	Total	Payroll	Personnel

DELANO—Kern County

□ DELANO REGIONAL MEDICAL CENTER, 1401 Garces Highway, Zip 93215, Mailing Address: Box 460, Zip 93216; tel. 661/725–4800; Gerald A. Starr, Executive Officer (Total facility includes 45 beds in nursing home–type unit) (Nonreporting) **A**1 9 10
Web address: www.drmc.com

| 23 | 10 | 156 | — | — | — | — | — | — | — |

DINUBA—Tulare County

ALTA DISTRICT HOSPITAL, 500 Adelaide Way, Zip 93618–1698; tel. 559/591–4171; Russell Bloom, Chief Executive Officer (Total facility includes 18 beds in nursing home–type unit) (Nonreporting) **A**9 10

| 16 | 10 | 50 | — | — | — | — | — | — | — |

DOS PALOS—Merced County

DOS PALOS MEMORIAL HOSPITAL, 2118 Marguerite Street, Zip 93620; tel. 209/392–6106; Darryl E. Henley, Administrator (Nonreporting) **A**9 10

| 23 | 10 | 15 | — | — | — | — | — | — | — |

DOWNEY—Los Angeles County

□ DOWNEY REGIONAL MEDICAL CENTER, (Formerly Downey Community Hospital Foundation), (Includes Downey Community Hospital), 11500 Brookshire Avenue, Zip 90241–4990; tel. 562/904–5000; Donald H. Miller, Chief Operation Officer (Total facility includes 20 beds in nursing home–type unit) (Nonreporting) **A**1 9 10 12 13

| 23 | 10 | 222 | — | — | — | — | — | — | — |

★ △ LAC–RANCHO LOS AMIGOS NATIONAL REHABILITATION CENTER, 7601 East Imperial Highway, Zip 90242; tel. 562/401–7022; Consuelo C. Diaz, Chief Executive Officer **A**1 3 5 7 9 10 **F**1 4 5 6 8 9 11 13 14 16 17 19 22 23 24 25 27 29 30 31 32 33 34 35 38 39 41 43 44 45 46 47 48 49 50 51 53 54 55 56 58 59 60 61 62 63 64 65 66 68 70 71 73 74 75 76 77 78 79 **P**6 **S** Los Angeles County–Department of Health Services, Los Angeles, CA
Web address: www.rancho.org

| 13 | 10 | 207 | 3429 | 202 | 60970 | 0 | 185181 | 60101 | 1471 |

DUARTE—Los Angeles County

★ CITY OF HOPE NATIONAL MEDICAL CENTER, (ONCOLOGY), 1500 East Duarte Road, Zip 91010–3000; tel. 626/359–8111; Gil Schwartzberg, President and Chief Executive Officer **A**1 2 3 5 9 10 **F**9 13 17 19 22 23 24 26 32 33 34 35 36 38 39 41 46 48 49 50 51 52 54 65 68 70 72 74 76 77 78 **P**4 7
Web address: www.coh.org

| 23 | 49 | 137 | 3821 | 107 | 128222 | — | 203632 | 64606 | 2167 |

□ SANTA TERESITA HOSPITAL, 819 Buena Vista Street, Zip 91010–1703; tel. 626/359–3243; Robert G. Shell, Chief Executive Officer (Total facility includes 133 beds in nursing home–type unit) (Nonreporting) **A**1 2 9 10

| 21 | 10 | 283 | — | — | — | — | — | — | — |

EDWARDS AFB—Kern County

★ △ U. S. AIR FORCE HOSPITAL, 30 Hospital Road, Building 5500, Zip 93524–1730; tel. 661/277–2010; Lieutenant Colonel Thomas E. Yingst, USAF, MSC, Administrator (Nonreporting) **A**1 7 **S** Department of the Air Force, Bowling AFB, DC

| 41 | 10 | 10 | — | — | — | — | — | — | — |

EL CAJON—San Diego County

KAISER FOUNDATION HOSPITAL See Kaiser Foundation Hospital, San Diego

EL CENTRO—Imperial County

★ EL CENTRO REGIONAL MEDICAL CENTER, 1415 Ross Avenue, Zip 92243; tel. 760/339–7100; Ted Fox, Administrator and Chief Executive Officer **A**1 9 10 **F**7 8 9 17 19 22 24 25 27 31 32 33 34 38 39 41 43 44 45 48 50 51 54 56 68 70 72 74 76 77 78 79 **P**4 5 7

| 14 | 10 | 107 | 6433 | 69 | 107448 | 1250 | 47312 | 18075 | 479 |

ELDRIDGE—Sonoma County

SONOMA DEVELOPMENTAL CENTER, 15000 Arnold Drive, Zip 95431; tel. 707/938–6000; Timothy L. Meeker, Executive Director (Nonreporting) **A**9 10

| 12 | 62 | 996 | — | — | — | — | — | — | — |

ENCINITAS—San Diego County

□ BHC SAN LUIS REY HOSPITAL, 335 Saxony Road, Zip 92024–2723; tel. 760/753–1245; James S. Plummer, Chief Executive Officer (Nonreporting) **A**1 **S** Behavioral Healthcare Corporation, Nashville, TN

| 33 | 22 | 122 | — | — | — | — | — | — | — |

★ △ SCRIPPS MEMORIAL HOSPITAL–ENCINITAS, 354 Santa Fe Drive, Zip 92024, Mailing Address: P.O. Box 230817, Zip 92023; tel. 760/753–6501; Rebecca Ropchan, Administrator (Nonreporting) **A**1 2 7 9 10 **S** Scripps Health, San Diego, CA

| 23 | 10 | 145 | — | — | — | — | — | — | — |

ENCINO—Los Angeles County, See Los Angeles

ESCONDIDO—San Diego County

★ PALOMAR MEDICAL CENTER, 555 East Valley Parkway, Zip 92025–3084; tel. 760/739–3000; Gerald E. Bracht, Vice President and Administrator (Total facility includes 96 beds in nursing home–type unit) (Nonreporting) **A**1 2 9 10 **S** Palomar Pomerado Health System, San Diego, CA
Web address: www.pphs.org

| 16 | 10 | 395 | — | — | — | — | — | — | — |

EUREKA—Humboldt County

□ △ GENERAL HOSPITAL, 2200 Harrison Avenue, Zip 95501; tel. 707/445–5111; Martin Love, Chief Executive Officer (Nonreporting) **A**1 7 9 10 **S** Province Healthcare Corporation, Brentwood, TN

| 33 | 10 | 65 | — | — | — | — | — | — | — |

★ SAINT JOSEPH HOSPITAL, 2700 Dolbeer Street, Zip 95501; tel. 707/445–8121; Michael L. Purvis, President and Chief Executive Officer **A**1 2 9 10 **F**2 3 4 8 9 11 12 13 16 17 18 19 22 23 24 25 26 32 33 34 35 36 37 38 39 41 44 45 46 47 48 50 51 54 56 57 65 70 72 76 78 79 **P**3 6 **S** St. Joseph Health System, Orange, CA

| 21 | 10 | 96 | 4828 | 60 | 149972 | 421 | 60759 | 20573 | 611 |

EXETER—Tulare County

□ MEMORIAL HOSPITAL AT EXETER, 215 Crespi Avenue, Zip 93221–1399; tel. 559/592–2151; Thomas M. Johnson, Chief Executive Officer **A**1 9 10 **F**22 29 31 45 69 70 76

| 16 | 10 | 66 | 45 | 51 | 22393 | 0 | 7880 | 3827 | 143 |

Hospitals, U.S. / CALIFORNIA

Hospital, Address, Telephone, Administrator, Approval, Facility, and Physician Codes, Health Care System, Network	Classification Codes		Utilization Data					Expense (thousands) of dollars		
	Control	Service	Staffed Beds	Admissions	Census	Outpatient Visits	Births	Total	Payroll	Personnel

★ American Hospital Association (AHA) membership
☐ Joint Commission on Accreditation of Healthcare Organizations (JCAHO) accreditation
+ American Osteopathic Healthcare Association (AOHA) membership
○ American Osteopathic Association (AOA) accreditation
△ Commission on Accreditation of Rehabilitation Facilities (CARF) accreditation
Control codes 61, 63, 64, 71, 72 and 73 indicate hospitals listed by AOHA, but not registered by AHA. For definition of numerical codes, see page A4.

Hospital	Control	Service	Staffed Beds	Admissions	Census	Outpatient Visits	Births	Total	Payroll	Personnel
FAIRFIELD—Solano County										
★ NORTHBAY MEDICAL CENTER, 1200 B. Gale Wilson Boulevard, Zip 94533–3587; tel. 707/429–3600; Deborah Sugiyama, President (Total facility includes 11 beds in nursing home–type unit) A1 2 9 10 F1 6 8 9 11 13 14 16 17 18 19 22 24 25 27 32 34 36 37 39 40 41 43 44 45 46 48 54 65 69 70 72 76 78 P3 S NorthBay Healthcare System, Fairfield, CA Web address: www.northbay.org	23	10	121	5290	55	70624	1471	64106	26065	381
FALL RIVER MILLS—Shasta County										
MAYERS MEMORIAL HOSPITAL DISTRICT, Highway 299 East, Zip 96028, Mailing Address: Box 459, Zip 96028; tel. 530/336–5511; Judi Beck, Administrator and Chief Executive Officer (Total facility includes 50 beds in nursing home–type unit) (Nonreporting) A9 10 Web address: www.burneyfalls.com/mayers	16	10	72	—	—	—	—	—	—	—
FALLBROOK—San Diego County										
☐ FALLBROOK HOSPITAL DISTRICT, 624 East Elder Street, Zip 92028; tel. 760/728–1191; Corey A. Seale, Chief Executive Officer (Total facility includes 95 beds in nursing home–type unit) (Nonreporting) A1 9 10	16	10	142	—	—	—	—	—	—	—
FOLSOM—Sacramento County										
★ MERCY HOSPITAL OF FOLSOM, 1650 Creekside Drive, Zip 95630; tel. 916/983–7400; Donald C. Hudson, Vice President and Chief Operating Officer (Nonreporting) A1 9 10 S Catholic Healthcare West, San Francisco, CA Web address: www.mercysacramento.org	21	10	95	—	—	—	—	—	—	—
☐ VENCOR HOSPITAL–SACRAMENTO, 223 Fargo Way, Zip 95630; tel. 916/351–9151; Meredith Taylor, Administrator (Nonreporting) A1 9 10 S Vencor, Incorporated, Louisville, KY	33	10	32	—	—	—	—	—	—	—
FONTANA—San Bernardino County										
★ KAISER FOUNDATION HOSPITAL, 9961 Sierra Avenue, Zip 92335–6794; tel. 909/427–5000; Susan Caulk, Director Operations A1 2 3 5 10 F2 3 4 8 9 10 11 12 13 14 15 16 17 18 19 20 22 24 25 26 27 29 32 33 34 35 36 37 39 41 42 44 45 46 47 48 49 50 53 54 55 56 57 58 59 60 61 63 64 65 66 68 69 70 71 72 73 74 76 77 78 79 S Kaiser Foundation Hospitals, Oakland, CA Web address: www.kaiserpermanente.org	23	10	299	20795	206	88128	4067	—	—	3927
FORT BRAGG—Mendocino County										
☐ MENDOCINO COAST DISTRICT HOSPITAL, 700 River Drive, Zip 95437; tel. 707/961–1234; Bryan M. Ballard, Chief Executive Officer A1 9 10 F7 8 9 13 16 18 22 24 25 30 31 33 35 36 37 38 39 41 43 44 46 48 51 54 70 76 78 79 Web address: www.mcdh.net	16	10	54	1912	23	55519	216	21218	7853	222
FORT IRWIN—San Bernardino County										
★ WEED ARMY COMMUNITY HOSPITAL, Zip 92310–5065; tel. 760/380–3108; Colonel Michael McCaffrey, Commander (Nonreporting) A1 S Department of the Army, Office of the Surgeon General, Falls Church, VA	42	10	27	—	—	—	—	—	—	—
FORTUNA—Humboldt County										
★ REDWOOD MEMORIAL HOSPITAL, 3300 Renner Drive, Zip 95540; tel. 707/725–3361; Michael L. Purvis, President and Chief Executive Officer (Nonreporting) A1 2 9 10 S St. Joseph Health System, Orange, CA	21	10	35	—	—	—	—	—	—	—
FOUNTAIN VALLEY—Orange County										
★ FOUNTAIN VALLEY REGIONAL HOSPITAL AND MEDICAL CENTER, 17100 Euclid at Warner, Zip 92708; tel. 714/966–7200; Tim Smith, President and Chief Executive Officer A1 2 5 9 10 F1 4 8 9 11 12 13 14 16 17 18 19 22 24 25 27 30 31 32 33 34 35 38 39 41 42 43 44 45 46 47 48 49 50 51 52 54 57 62 64 66 68 69 70 71 72 76 77 78 79 P5 S TENET Healthcare Corporation, Santa Barbara, CA Web address: www.tenethealh.com	33	10	396	16596	218	62447	3862	115415	47524	1358
☐ ORANGE COAST MEMORIAL MEDICAL CENTER, 9920 Talbert Avenue, Zip 92708; tel. 714/378–7000; Barry S. Arbuckle, Ph.D., Chief Executive Officer A1 3 9 10 F2 3 4 7 8 9 10 11 13 14 15 16 17 18 19 20 22 24 25 26 27 28 29 30 31 32 33 34 36 37 38 39 41 42 43 44 45 46 47 48 49 50 51 52 53 54 55 56 57 58 59 60 61 62 63 64 65 66 68 69 70 71 72 73 74 75 76 77 78 79 P5 7 S Memorial Health Services, Long Beach, CA Web address: www.memorialcare.org	23	10	230	6346	66	26216	518	58729	19230	544
FREMONT—Alameda County										
☐ BHC FREMONT HOSPITAL, 39001 Sundale Drive, Zip 94538; tel. 510/796–1100; Edward Owen, Chief Executive Officer A1 9 10 F2 3 13 17 18 57 58 60 61 62 64 70 72 S Behavioral Healthcare Corporation, Nashville, TN Web address: www.fremonthospital.com	33	22	78	2250	43	4380	—	—	—	74
★ WASHINGTON TOWNSHIP HEALTH CARE DISTRICT, 2000 Mowry Avenue, Zip 94538–1716; tel. 510/797–1111; Nancy D. Farber, Chief Executive Officer A1 2 9 10 F4 7 8 9 11 12 13 16 17 18 19 21 22 24 25 32 33 34 38 39 41 43 45 46 47 48 51 54 57 59 61 65 70 72 76 77 78 P5 7 Web address: www.whhs.com	16	10	279	13984	165	117014	2520	134372	65326	1038
FRENCH CAMP—San Joaquin County										
△ SAN JOAQUIN GENERAL HOSPITAL, 500 West Hospital Road, Zip 95231, Mailing Address: P.O. Box 1020, Stockton, Zip 95201; tel. 209/468–6600; Michael N. Smith, Director Healthcare Services (Nonreporting) A3 5 7 9 10	13	10	195	—	—	—	—	—	—	—
FRESNO—Fresno County										
☐ BHC CEDAR VISTA HOSPITAL, 7171 North Cedar Avenue, Zip 93720; tel. 559/449–8000; Deborah Quinn, Administrator (Nonreporting) A1 9 10 S Behavioral Healthcare Corporation, Nashville, TN	33	22	61	—	—	—	—	—	—	—

Hospitals, U.S. / CALIFORNIA

Hospital, Address, Telephone, Administrator, Approval, Facility, and Physician Codes, Health Care System, Network

★ American Hospital Association (AHA) membership
☐ Joint Commission on Accreditation of Healthcare Organizations (JCAHO) accreditation
+ American Osteopathic Healthcare Association (AOHA) membership
○ American Osteopathic Association (AOA) accreditation
△ Commission on Accreditation of Rehabilitation Facilities (CARF) accreditation
Control codes 61, 63, 64, 71, 72 and 73 indicate hospitals listed by AOHA, but not registered by AHA. For definition of numerical codes, see page A4

Hospital	Classification Codes		Utilization Data					Expense (thousands) of dollars		Personnel
	Control	Service	Staffed Beds	Admissions	Census	Outpatient Visits	Births	Total	Payroll	
★ COMMUNITY MEDICAL CENTER–FRESNO, (Formerly Fresno Community Hospital and Medical Center), 2823 Fresno Street, Zip 93721, Mailing Address: P.O. Box 1232, Zip 93715–1232; tel. 559/459–6000; Marge Beekman, Facility Director (Nonreporting) **A**1 2 9 10 **S** Community Medical Centers, Fresno, CA Web address: www.communitymedical.org	23	10	375	—	—	—	—	—	—	—
FRESNO COMMUNITY HOSPITAL AND MEDICAL CENTER See Community Medical Center–Fresno										
FRESNO SURGERY CENTER–THE HOSPITAL FOR SURGERY, 6125 North Fresno Street, Zip 93710; tel. 559/431–8000; Toni Angle, Administrator **A**9 10 **F**17 38 46 48 Web address: www.fschealth.com	32	49	20	2019	11	3963	0	—	—	163
★ KAISER FOUNDATION HOSPITAL, 7300 North Fresno Street, Zip 93720; tel. 559/448–4555; Toni Flores, Director Operations **A**1 10 **F**2 3 4 7 8 9 10 11 12 13 17 18 19 22 24 25 26 27 28 30 33 34 35 36 37 39 41 42 44 46 47 48 51 52 53 54 57 65 69 70 75 76 78 **S** Kaiser Foundation Hospitals, Oakland, CA Web address: www.kaiserpermanente.org	23	10	121	11983	74	34148	2217	—	—	465
★ SAINT AGNES MEDICAL CENTER, 1303 East Herndon Avenue, Zip 93720–3309; tel. 559/449–3000; Sister Ruth Marie Nickerson, President and Chief Executive Officer **A**1 2 9 10 **F**1 2 3 4 7 8 9 10 11 12 13 14 15 16 17 18 19 21 22 23 24 25 26 27 30 31 32 33 34 35 36 37 38 39 41 42 43 44 45 46 47 48 49 50 51 52 53 54 55 57 58 59 60 61 62 63 64 65 68 69 70 71 72 75 76 77 78 79 **P**5 7 **S** Trinity Health, Novi, MI Web address: www.samc.com	21	10	326	21263	229	429068	2639	185753	92618	2157
☐ △ SAN JOAQUIN VALLEY REHABILITATION HOSPITAL, 7173 North Sharon Avenue, Zip 93720; tel. 559/436–3600; W. David Smiley, Chief Executive Officer (Nonreporting) **A**1 7 9 10	33	46	62	—	—	—	—	—	—	—
★ UNIVERSITY MEDICAL CENTER, 445 South Cedar Avenue, Zip 93702–2907; tel. 559/459–4000; Andres Fernandez, Director (Nonreporting) **A**1 8 9 **S** Community Medical Centers, Fresno, CA	13	10	334	—	—	—	—	—	—	—
★ VETERANS AFFAIRS MEDICAL CENTER, 2615 East Clinton Avenue, Zip 93703; tel. 559/225–6100; Alan S. Perry, Director (Total facility includes 60 beds in nursing home–type unit) **A**1 2 3 5 **F**2 3 16 18 22 24 25 26 28 30 31 32 33 34 35 36 37 38 39 41 43 45 46 48 49 50 51 54 56 57 59 61 62 63 70 72 76 78 79 **S** Department of Veterans Affairs, Washington, DC Web address: www.fresno.med.va.gov	45	10	145	3621	101	175066	0	67198	34591	796
FULLERTON—Orange County										
★ △ ST. JUDE MEDICAL CENTER, 101 East Valencia Mesa Drive, Zip 92835; tel. 714/992–3000; Robert J. Fraschetti, President and Chief Executive Officer (Nonreporting) **A**1 2 7 9 10 **S** St. Joseph Health System, Orange, CA Web address: www.mhrmc.com	21	10	347	—	—	—	—	—	—	—
GARBERVILLE—Humboldt County										
SOUTHERN HUMBOLDT COMMUNITY HEALTHCARE DISTRICT, 733 Cedar Street, Zip 95542–3292; tel. 707/923–3921; George Koortbojian, Interim Administrator (Total facility includes 8 beds in nursing home–type unit) (Nonreporting) **A**9 10 Web address: www.shchd.org	16	10	18	—	—	—	—	—	—	—
GARDEN GROVE—Orange County										
★ GARDEN GROVE HOSPITAL AND MEDICAL CENTER, 12601 Garden Grove Boulevard, Zip 92843–1959; tel. 714/537–5160; Mark A. Meyers, President and Chief Executive Officer (Total facility includes 12 beds in nursing home–type unit) (Nonreporting) **A**1 9 10 **S** TENET Healthcare Corporation, Santa Barbara, CA Web address: www.tenethealh.com	33	10	167	—	—	—	—	—	—	—
GARDENA—Los Angeles County										
☐ COMMUNITY HOSPITAL OF GARDENA, 1246 West 155th Street, Zip 90247–4062; tel. 310/323–5330; Raymond N. Smith, Chief Executive Officer (Total facility includes 20 beds in nursing home–type unit) (Nonreporting) **A**1 9 10	33	10	58	—	—	—	—	—	—	—
☐ MEMORIAL HOSPITAL OF GARDENA, 1145 West Redondo Beach Boulevard, Zip 90247; tel. 310/532–4200; Frank Katsuda, Administrator and Chief Executive Officer (Nonreporting) **A**1 9 10	33	10	107	—	—	—	—	—	—	—
GILROY—Santa Clara County										
★ ST. LOUISE REGIONAL HOSPITAL, (Formerly South Valley Hospital), 9400 No Name Uno, Zip 95020–2368; tel. 408/848–2000; Glenna L. Vaskelis, Interim Vice President and Chief Operating Officer (Total facility includes 21 beds in nursing home–type unit) (Nonreporting) **A**9 10	33	10	93	—	—	—	—	—	—	—
GLENDALE—Los Angeles County										
★ GLENDALE ADVENTIST MEDICAL CENTER, 1509 Wilson Terrace, Zip 91206–4007; tel. 818/409–8000; Fred M. Manchur, President and Chief Executive Officer (Nonreporting) **A**1 2 3 5 9 10 **S** Adventist Health, Roseville, CA Web address: www.glendaleadventist.com	21	10	396	—	—	—	—	—	—	—
★ GLENDALE MEMORIAL HOSPITAL AND HEALTH CENTER, 1420 South Central Avenue, Zip 91204–2594; tel. 818/502–1900; Arnold R. Schaffer, President and Chief Executive Officer **A**1 2 9 10 **F**3 4 5 7 8 9 10 11 12 13 14 16 17 18 19 22 24 25 30 31 32 33 34 35 36 37 38 39 41 42 43 44 45 46 47 48 49 50 53 54 57 59 60 61 62 63 64 65 68 69 70 72 73 74 76 77 78 79 **P**4 5 7 **S** Catholic Healthcare West, San Francisco, CA Web address: www.glendalememorial.com	23	10	290	15328	236	111867	1693	120944	52954	1409

Hospitals, U.S. / CALIFORNIA

Hospital, Address, Telephone, Administrator, Approval, Facility, and Physician Codes, Health Care System, Network	Classification Codes		Utilization Data					Expense (thousands) of dollars		
★ American Hospital Association (AHA) membership ☐ Joint Commission on Accreditation of Healthcare Organizations (JCAHO) accreditation + American Osteopathic Healthcare Association (AOHA) membership ○ American Osteopathic Association (AOA) accreditation △ Commission on Accreditation of Rehabilitation Facilities (CARF) accreditation Control codes 61, 63, 64, 71, 72 and 73 indicate hospitals listed by AOHA, but not registered by AHA. For definition of numerical codes, see page A4	Control	Service	Staffed Beds	Admissions	Census	Outpatient Visits	Births	Total	Payroll	Personnel
☐ VERDUGO HILLS HOSPITAL, 1812 Verdugo Boulevard, Zip 91208; tel. 818/790–7100; Bernard Glossy, President and Chief Executive Officer (Total facility includes 32 beds in nursing home–type unit) **A**1 9 10 **F**8 9 13 17 18 22 24 25 30 32 33 34 36 38 39 44 48 50 53 54 57 62 63 64 68 69 70 72 76 78 **P**5 **Web address:** www.verdugohillshospital.org	23	10	95	5565	88	85180	921	50084	18708	340
GLENDORA—Los Angeles County										
✣ FOOTHILL PRESBYTERIAN HOSPITAL–MORRIS L. JOHNSTON MEMORIAL, 250 South Grand Avenue, Zip 91741; tel. 626/963–8411; Larry S. Fetters, Administrator and Chief Operating Officer (Nonreporting) **A**1 2 9 10 **S** Citrus Valley Health Partners, Covina, CA	23	10	106	—	—	—	—	—	—	—
✣ HUNTINGTON EAST VALLEY HOSPITAL, 150 West Alosta Avenue, Zip 91740–4398; tel. 626/335–0231; James W. Maki, Chief Executive Officer (Nonreporting) **A**1 9 10 **S** Southern California Healthcare Systems, Pasadena, CA **Web address:** www.schs.com	23	10	128	—	—	—	—	—	—	—
GRANADA HILLS—Los Angeles County, See Los Angeles **GRASS VALLEY—Nevada County**										
✣ SIERRA NEVADA MEMORIAL HOSPITAL, 155 Glasson Way, Zip 95945, Mailing Address: P.O. Box 1029, Zip 95945–1029; tel. 530/274–6000; C. Thomas Collier, President and Chief Executive Officer (Total facility includes 13 beds in nursing home–type unit) **A**1 2 9 10 **F**7 8 9 11 12 13 16 17 18 22 25 27 31 36 37 38 39 41 44 46 48 50 54 65 69 70 76 77 **P**3 5 **S** Catholic Healthcare West, San Francisco, CA **Web address:** www.snmh.org	23	10	61	6049	61	128657	482	58795	25553	601
GREENBRAE—Marin County										
✣ MARIN GENERAL HOSPITAL, 250 Bon Air Road, Zip 94904, Mailing Address: Box 8010, San Rafael, Zip 94912–8010; tel. 415/925–7000; Henry J. Buhrmann, President and Chief Executive Officer **A**1 2 9 10 **F**4 7 8 9 11 12 13 16 17 18 19 21 22 24 25 26 27 31 32 33 34 35 36 38 39 41 42 44 45 46 47 48 50 51 57 58 59 60 61 62 63 64 65 69 70 72 76 78 79 **P**1 **S** Sutter Health, Sacramento, CA **Web address:** www.maringeneral.com	23	10	165	10398	112	91988	1828	119029	46247	841
GREENVILLE—Plumas County										
INDIAN VALLEY HOSPITAL DISTRICT, 184 Hot Springs Road, Zip 95947; tel. 530/284–7191; Lynn Seaberg, Administrator and Chief Executive Officer (Total facility includes 19 beds in nursing home–type unit) **A**9 10 **F**14 15 16 17 18 22 25 38 48 69 76 **P**6	16	10	26	311	22	17153	0	4539	2708	80
GRIDLEY—Butte County										
BIGGS–GRIDLEY MEMORIAL HOSPITAL, 240 Spruce Street, Zip 95948, Mailing Address: P.O. Box 97, Zip 95948; tel. 530/846–5671; Roger W. Cooper, Chief Executive Officer (Nonreporting) **A**9 10	23	10	55	—	—	—	—	—	—	—
HANFORD—Kings County										
✣ CENTRAL VALLEY GENERAL HOSPITAL, 1025 North Douty Street, Zip 93230, Mailing Address: Box 480, Zip 93232; tel. 559/583–2100; Kendall R. Fults, Chief Operating Officer (Nonreporting) **A**1 9 10 **S** Adventist Health, Roseville, CA **Web address:** www.hanfordhealth.com	33	10	40	—	—	—	—	—	—	—
✣ HANFORD COMMUNITY MEDICAL CENTER, 450 Greenfield Avenue, Zip 93230–0240, Mailing Address: Box 240, Zip 93232–0240; tel. 559/582–9000; Darwin R. Remboldt, President and Chief Executive Officer (Nonreporting) **A**1 9 10 **S** Adventist Health, Roseville, CA **Web address:** www.adventisthealth.org	21	10	59	—	—	—	—	—	—	—
HARBOR CITY—Los Angeles County, See Los Angeles **HAWTHORNE—Los Angeles County**										
HAWTHORNE HOSPITAL See Los Angeles Metropolitan Medical Center, Los Angeles										
✣ ROBERT F. KENNEDY MEDICAL CENTER, 4500 West 116th Street, Zip 90250; tel. 310/973–1711; Peter P. Aprato, President (Total facility includes 34 beds in nursing home–type unit) (Nonreporting) **A**1 9 10 **S** Catholic Healthcare West, San Francisco, CA **Web address:** www.chw.edu	23	10	195	—	—	—	—	—	—	—
HAYWARD—Alameda County										
✣ KAISER FOUNDATION HOSPITAL, 27400 Hesperian Boulevard, Zip 94545–4297; tel. 510/784–4313; Duayna Pucci, Director Operations **A**1 10 **F**3 4 8 9 11 12 13 16 17 18 22 24 25 27 29 30 31 33 34 35 36 37 39 41 42 43 44 45 46 47 48 49 50 51 54 56 58 59 60 61 62 63 64 65 66 70 71 72 73 74 75 76 77 78 79 **P**3 **S** Kaiser Foundation Hospitals, Oakland, CA **Web address:** www.kaiserpermanente.org	23	10	204	14800	142	652318	3160	—	—	—
☐ ST. ROSE HOSPITAL, 27200 Calaroga Avenue, Zip 94545–4383; tel. 510/264–4000; Michael P. Mahoney, President and Chief Executive Officer (Total facility includes 46 beds in nursing home–type unit) (Nonreporting) **A**1 2 9 10 **S** Via Christi Health System, Wichita, KS **Web address:** www.strosehospital.org	21	10	175	—	—	—	—	—	—	—
HEALDSBURG—Sonoma County										
☐ HEALDSBURG GENERAL HOSPITAL, 1375 University Avenue, Zip 95448; tel. 707/431–6500; Edward C. Bland, President and Chief Executive Officer (Nonreporting) **A**1 9 10 **Web address:** www.healdsburghospital.com	33	10	49	—	—	—	—	—	—	—

© 2000 AHA Guide *Many Facility Codes have changed. Please refer to the AHA Guide Code Chart.*

Hospitals, U.S. / CALIFORNIA

Hospital, Address, Telephone, Administrator, Approval, Facility, and Physician Codes, Health Care System, Network	Classification Codes		Utilization Data					Expense (thousands) of dollars		
★ American Hospital Association (AHA) membership □ Joint Commission on Accreditation of Healthcare Organizations (JCAHO) accreditation + American Osteopathic Healthcare Association (AOHA) membership ○ American Osteopathic Association (AOA) accreditation △ Commission on Accreditation of Rehabilitation Facilities (CARF) accreditation Control codes 61, 63, 64, 71, 72 and 73 indicate hospitals listed by AOHA, but not registered by AHA. For definition of numerical codes, see page A4	Control	Service	Staffed Beds	Admissions	Census	Outpatient Visits	Births	Total	Payroll	Personnel
HEMET—Riverside County ★ HEMET VALLEY MEDICAL CENTER, 1117 East Devonshire Avenue, Zip 92543; tel. 909/652–2811; Jack A. Burrows, Administrator (Nonreporting) **A**1 9 10 **S** Valley Health System, Hemet, CA	16	10	285	—	—	—	—	—	—	—
HOLLISTER—San Benito County ★ HAZEL HAWKINS MEMORIAL HOSPITAL, (Includes Hazel Hawkins Convalescent Hospital–Southside, 3110 Southside Road, Zip 95023; tel. 408/637–5711), 911 Sunset Drive, Zip 95023–5695; tel. 831/637–5711; Keith Mesmer, Chief Executive Officer (Total facility includes 52 beds in nursing home–type unit) **A**1 9 10 **F**7 8 9 12 16 17 18 19 22 23 25 29 30 32 33 34 35 36 38 39 41 44 45 46 48 49 50 51 54 56 62 63 69 70 71 72 76 78 **P**1 5 7 **S** Brim Healthcare, Inc., Brentwood, TN	16	10	72	2249	69	94381	563	26853	10589	242
HOLLYWOOD—Los Angeles County, See Los Angeles **HUNTINGTON BEACH—Orange County** ★ HUNTINGTON BEACH HOSPITAL, 17772 Beach Boulevard, Zip 92647–9932; tel. 714/842–1473; David K. Culberson, Chief Executive Officer (Total facility includes 14 beds in nursing home–type unit) **A**1 9 10 **F**4 7 9 11 13 16 18 22 24 25 31 32 34 38 39 41 48 49 51 57 59 60 61 62 63 64 69 70 76 78 **P**5 **S** Vanguard Health System, Nashville, TN	23	10	116	4151	65	52633	0	32442	14970	371
HUNTINGTON PARK—Los Angeles County ★ COMMUNITY HOSPITAL OF HUNTINGTON PARK, (Includes Mission Hospital of Huntington Park, 3111 East Florence Avenue, tel. 213/582–8261), 2623 East Slauson Avenue, Zip 90255; tel. 323/583–1931; Charles Martinez, Ph.D., Chief Executive Officer (Nonreporting) **A**1 9 10 **S** TENET Healthcare Corporation, Santa Barbara, CA Web address: www.tenethealh.com	33	10	226	—	—	—	—	—	—	—
INDIO—Riverside County ★ JOHN F. KENNEDY MEMORIAL HOSPITAL, 47–111 Monroe Street, Zip 92201, Mailing Address: P.O. Drawer LLLL, Zip 92202–2558; tel. 760/347–6191; Truman L. Gates, President and Chief Executive Officer **A**1 9 10 **F**1 4 7 8 9 11 12 13 14 16 17 18 19 22 24 25 27 29 32 33 34 35 36 37 38 39 40 41 42 43 44 45 46 47 48 51 52 54 56 57 59 60 61 62 63 64 65 69 70 72 75 76 77 78 79 **P**5 **S** TENET Healthcare Corporation, Santa Barbara, CA Web address: www.tenethealh.com	33	10	130	8521	83	63464	2048	42336	18080	503
INGLEWOOD—Los Angeles County ★ △ CENTINELA HOSPITAL MEDICAL CENTER, 555 East Hardy Street, Zip 90301–4073, Mailing Address: Box 720, Zip 90307–0720; tel. 310/673–4660; Michael A. Rembis, FACHE, Chief Executive Officer **A**1 2 3 7 9 10 **F**4 8 9 11 12 13 17 22 24 25 27 30 36 38 39 41 42 44 45 46 47 48 49 53 54 56 57 60 62 65 69 70 71 76 77 78 **P**5 **S** TENET Healthcare Corporation, Santa Barbara, CA Web address: www.tenethealh.com	33	10	377	12038	189	165957	2063	102554	41572	1206
★ △ DANIEL FREEMAN MEMORIAL HOSPITAL, 333 North Prairie Avenue, Zip 90301–4514; tel. 310/674–7050; Joseph W. Dunn, Ph.D., President and Chief Executive Officer (Total facility includes 29 beds in nursing home–type unit) **A**1 2 5 7 9 10 **F**1 2 3 4 7 8 9 11 12 13 17 18 19 20 21 22 24 25 27 28 29 31 34 36 38 39 40 41 42 43 44 45 46 47 48 49 50 51 53 54 57 58 60 61 62 63 64 65 68 69 70 76 78 79 **P**5 7 **S** Carondelet Health System, Saint Louis, MO Web address: www.danielfreeman.org	21	10	360	14250	213	93327	2921	139717	53883	1280
IRVINE—Orange County ★ IRVINE REGIONAL HOSPITAL AND MEDICAL CENTER, (Formerly Irvine Medical Center), 16200 Sand Canyon Avenue, Zip 92618–3714; tel. 949/753–2000; Dan F. Ausman, Chief Executive Officer (Total facility includes 35 beds in nursing home–type unit) **A**1 9 10 **F**4 7 8 9 11 13 16 17 18 19 22 24 25 31 32 33 34 38 39 41 42 44 45 46 48 49 50 51 54 57 61 62 65 69 70 72 76 78 79 **P**5 7 **S** TENET Healthcare Corporation, Santa Barbara, CA Web address: www.tenethealh.com	33	10	176	5605	67	64156	1271	38747	18343	377
JACKSON—Amador County ★ SUTTER AMADOR HOSPITAL, 200 Mission Boulevard, Zip 95642–2379; tel. 209/223–7500; Scott Stenberg, Chief Executive Officer (Total facility includes 44 beds in nursing home–type unit) (Nonreporting) **A**1 9 10 **S** Sutter Health, Sacramento, CA Web address: www.sutterhealth.org	23	10	85	—	—	—	—	—	—	—
JOSHUA TREE—San Bernardino County ★ HI–DESERT MEDICAL CENTER, 6601 White Feather Road, Zip 92252–6601; tel. 760/366–3711; John J. McCormick, Interim Chief Executive Officer (Total facility includes 86 beds in nursing home–type unit) **A**1 9 10 **F**7 9 13 16 18 19 22 23 24 25 29 30 31 32 34 35 36 37 38 39 41 43 45 48 50 51 54 64 69 70 72 76 78 **P**8 Web address: www.hdmc.org	16	10	128	2643	127	57140	0	33867	11355	394
KENTFIELD—Marin County ★ BHC ROSS HOSPITAL, 1111 Sir Francis Drake Boulevard, Zip 94904; tel. 415/258–6900; Judy G. House, Chief Executive Officer (Nonreporting) **S** Behavioral Healthcare Corporation, Nashville, TN	33	22	56	—	—	—	—	—	—	—
□ KENTFIELD REHABILITATION HOSPITAL, 1125 Sir Francis Drake Boulevard, Zip 94904; tel. 415/456–9680; David Smiley, Administrator and Chief Executive Officer (Total facility includes 12 beds in nursing home–type unit) (Nonreporting) **A**1 10	33	46	60	—	—	—	—	—	—	—

Hospitals, U.S. / CALIFORNIA

Hospital, Address, Telephone, Administrator, Approval, Facility, and Physician Codes, Health Care System, Network	Classification Codes		Utilization Data					Expense (thousands) of dollars		
★ American Hospital Association (AHA) membership ☐ Joint Commission on Accreditation of Healthcare Organizations (JCAHO) accreditation + American Osteopathic Healthcare Association (AOHA) membership ○ American Osteopathic Association (AOA) accreditation △ Commission on Accreditation of Rehabilitation Facilities (CARF) accreditation Control codes 61, 63, 64, 71, 72 and 73 indicate hospitals listed by AOHA, but not registered by AHA. For definition of numerical codes, see page A4	Control	Service	Staffed Beds	Admissions	Census	Outpatient Visits	Births	Total	Payroll	Personnel
KING CITY—Monterey County										
☐ GEORGE L. MEE MEMORIAL HOSPITAL, 300 Canal Street, Zip 93930–3410; tel. 831/385–6000; Walter G. Beck, Chief Executive Officer **A**1 9 10 **F**8 9 12 13 16 17 18 19 22 25 34 36 39 43 44 48 50 51 69 70 76 78 79	23	10	42	1345	22	28325	426	18993	8286	219
KINGSBURG—Fresno County										
KINGSBURG MEDICAL CENTER, (Formerly Kingsburg District Hospital), 1200 Smith Street, Zip 93631; tel. 559/897–5841; William J. Casey, Administrator (Total facility includes 20 beds in nursing home–type unit) (Nonreporting) **A**9 10	16	10	35	—	—	—	—	—	—	—
LA JOLLA—San Diego County										
★ SCRIPPS GREEN HOSPITAL, (Formerly Green Hospital of Scripps Clinic), 10666 North Torrey Pines Road, Zip 92037–1093; tel. 858/455–9100; Thomas C. Gagen, Senior Vice President and Regional Administrator (Nonreporting) **A**1 2 5 8 9 10 **S** Scripps Health, San Diego, CA Web address: www.chw.edu	23	10	165	—	—	—	—	—	—	—
★ △ SCRIPPS MEMORIAL HOSPITAL–LA JOLLA, 9888 Genesee Avenue, Zip 92037–1276, Mailing Address: P.O. Box 28, Zip 92038–0028; tel. 858/626–4123; Thomas C. Gagen, Senior Vice President and Regional Administrator (Total facility includes 29 beds in nursing home–type unit) (Nonreporting) **A**1 2 3 7 9 10 **S** Scripps Health, San Diego, CA	23	10	431	—	—	—	—	—	—	—
LA MESA—San Diego County										
★ △ GROSSMONT HOSPITAL, 5555 Grossmont Center Drive, Zip 91942, Mailing Address: Box 158, Zip 91944–0158; tel. 619/465–0711; Michele T. Tarbet, R.N., Chief Executive Officer (Total facility includes 30 beds in nursing home–type unit) **A**1 2 3 7 9 10 12 **F**3 4 7 8 9 11 12 13 17 18 19 22 23 24 25 26 29 30 31 34 35 36 37 38 39 40 41 42 43 44 45 46 47 48 49 51 53 54 56 57 58 59 60 61 62 63 64 65 66 68 69 70 71 72 74 75 76 77 78 79 **P**5 7 **S** Sharp Healthcare, San Diego, CA Web address: www.sharp.com	23	10	414	18089	233	209692	2425	145905	64769	1677
LA PALMA—Orange County										
★ △ LA PALMA INTERCOMMUNITY HOSPITAL, 7901 Walker Street, Zip 90623–5850, Mailing Address: P.O. Box 5850, Buena Park, Zip 90622; tel. 714/670–7400; David K. Culberson, Chief Executive Officer (Nonreporting) **A**1 2 7 9 10 **S** Vanguard Health System, Nashville, TN Web address: www.unihealth.org	23	10	139	—	—	—	—	—	—	—
LAGUNA HILLS—Orange County										
☐ SADDLEBACK MEMORIAL MEDICAL CENTER, 24451 Health Center Drive, Zip 92653; tel. 949/837–4500; Barry S. Arbuckle, Ph.D., Chief Executive Officer (Total facility includes 18 beds in nursing home–type unit) (Nonreporting) **A**1 2 9 10 **S** Memorial Health Services, Long Beach, CA Web address: www.memorialcare.org	23	10	220	—	—	—	—	—	—	—
LAKE ARROWHEAD—San Bernardino County										
☐ SAN BERNARDINO MOUNTAINS COMMUNITY HOSPITAL DISTRICT, 29101 Hospital Road, Zip 92352, Mailing Address: P.O. Box 70, Zip 92352; tel. 909/336–3651; James R. Hoss, Chief Executive Officer (Total facility includes 18 beds in nursing home–type unit) (Nonreporting) **A**1 9 10	16	10	36	—	—	—	—	—	—	—
LAKE ISABELLA—Kern County										
KERN VALLEY HEALTHCARE DISTRICT, (Formerly Kern Valley Hospital District), 6412 Laurel Avenue, Zip 93240, Mailing Address: P.O. Box 1628, Zip 93240; tel. 760/379–2681; Thomas D. Plantz, Interim Chief Executive Officer (Total facility includes 74 beds in nursing home–type unit) (Nonreporting) **A**9 10 Web address: www.kernvalleyhospdistrict.com	16	10	101	—	—	—	—	—	—	—
LAKEPORT—Lake County										
★ SUTTER LAKESIDE HOSPITAL, 5176 Hill Road East, Zip 95453–6111; tel. 707/262–5001; Gilbert Silbernagel, Chief Executive Officer (Nonreporting) **A**1 9 10 **S** Sutter Health, Sacramento, CA Web address: www.sutterlake.org	23	10	54	—	—	—	—	—	—	—
LAKEWOOD—Los Angeles County										
★ LAKEWOOD REGIONAL MEDICAL CENTER, 3700 East South Street, Zip 90712; tel. 562/531–2550; Kenneth I. Rivers, Chief Executive Officer (Nonreporting) **A**1 2 9 10 **S** TENET Healthcare Corporation, Santa Barbara, CA Web address: www.tenethealth.com	33	10	148	—	—	—	—	—	—	—
LANCASTER—Los Angeles County										
★ ANTELOPE VALLEY HOSPITAL, 1600 West Avenue J, Zip 93534–2894; tel. 661/949–5000; Mathew Abraham, Chief Executive Officer **A**1 9 10 **F**4 7 8 9 11 12 13 14 17 18 19 22 24 25 27 30 36 38 39 41 42 44 45 46 47 48 49 52 54 57 66 68 69 72 76 78 79 **P**7 Web address: www.avhospital.org	16	10	336	19941	241	133946	4752	144837	58679	1768
★ LAC–HIGH DESERT HOSPITAL, 44900 North 60th Street West, Zip 93536; tel. 661/945–8461; Mel Grussing, Administrator (Total facility includes 57 beds in nursing home–type unit) **A**1 9 10 **F**4 9 13 14 19 22 23 24 32 35 36 38 39 41 46 47 48 51 54 56 58 59 60 61 62 63 64 65 69 70 76 78 **P**6 **S** Los Angeles County–Department of Health Services, Los Angeles, CA	13	10	82	1799	84	48214	—	63745	18607	591
☐ LANCASTER COMMUNITY HOSPITAL, 43830 North Tenth Street West, Zip 93534; tel. 661/948–4781; Michael McAndrew, Chief Executive Officer (Total facility includes 22 beds in nursing home–type unit) (Nonreporting) **A**1 9 10 **S** Paracelsus Healthcare Corporation, Houston, TX	33	10	123	—	—	—	—	—	—	—

© 2000 AHA Guide *Many Facility Codes have changed. Please refer to the AHA Guide Code Chart.*

Hospitals, U.S. / CALIFORNIA

Hospital, Address, Telephone, Administrator, Approval, Facility, and Physician Codes, Health Care System, Network	Classification Codes		Utilization Data					Expense (thousands) of dollars		
★ American Hospital Association (AHA) membership ☐ Joint Commission on Accreditation of Healthcare Organizations (JCAHO) accreditation + American Osteopathic Healthcare Association (AOHA) membership ○ American Osteopathic Association (AOA) accreditation △ Commission on Accreditation of Rehabilitation Facilities (CARF) accreditation Control codes 61, 63, 64, 71, 72 and 73 indicate hospitals listed by AOHA, but not registered by AHA. For definition of numerical codes, see page A4	Control	Service	Staffed Beds	Admissions	Census	Outpatient Visits	Births	Total	Payroll	Personnel

LEMOORE—Kings County
★ NAVAL HOSPITAL, 930 Franklin Avenue, Zip 93246–5000; tel. 559/998–4201; Captain Christine M. Bruzek–Kohler, Commanding Officer (Nonreporting) **S** Department of Navy, Washington, DC
Web address: www.lenhfsa.med.navy.mil — 43 10 25 — — — — — — — —

LINDSAY—Tulare County
★ LINDSAY DISTRICT HOSPITAL, 740 North Sequoia Avenue, Zip 93247, Mailing Address: Box 40, Zip 93247; tel. 559/562–4955; Kelly C. Morgan, President and Chief Executive Officer (Total facility includes 53 beds in nursing home–type unit) **A**9 10 **F**8 9 17 22 25 26 30 32 34 38 41 44 45 48 54 70 76 **P**5 — 16 10 106 1842 56 35256 551 13133 5843 177

LIVERMORE—Alameda County
☐ VALLEYCARE MEMORIAL HOSPITAL, (Formerly Valley Memorial Hospital), 1111 East Stanley Boulevard, Zip 94550; tel. 925/447–7000; Marcy L. Feit, Chief Executive Officer (Total facility includes 14 beds in nursing home–type unit) (Nonreporting) **A**1 2 9 10 **S** ValleyCare Health System, Pleasanton, CA
Web address: www.valleycare.com — 23 10 110
VETERANS AFFAIRS PALO ALTO HEALTH CARE SYSTEM, LIVERMORE DIVISION See Veterans Affairs Palo Alto Health Care System, Palo Alto

LODI—San Joaquin County
⊕ LODI MEMORIAL HOSPITAL, (Includes Lodi Memorial Hospital West, 800 South Lower Sacramento Road, Zip 95242; tel. 209/333–0211), 975 South Fairmont Avenue, Zip 95240–5179, Mailing Address: P.O. Box 3004, Zip 95241–1908; tel. 209/334–3411; Joseph P. Harrington, Chief Executive Officer (Total facility includes 42 beds in nursing home–type unit) **A**1 9 10 **F**1 2 3 4 5 8 9 10 11 12 13 14 16 17 18 19 22 23 24 25 27 28 29 30 31 32 33 34 36 38 39 41 42 43 44 45 46 47 48 50 51 52 53 54 56 57 58 59 60 61 62 63 64 65 66 68 69 70 71 72 74 76 77 78 **P**6
Web address: www.lodihealth.org — 23 10 181 8201 111 154328 1287 61841 30518 762

LOMA LINDA—San Bernardino County
⊕ JERRY L. PETTIS MEMORIAL VETERANS MEDICAL CENTER, 11201 Benton Street, Zip 92357; tel. 909/825–7084; Dean R. Stordahl, Chief Executive Officer (Total facility includes 108 beds in nursing home–type unit) (Nonreporting) **A**1 3 5 8 **S** Department of Veterans Affairs, Washington, DC
Web address: www.desertpacific.med.va.gov — 45 10 315 — — — — — — — —

☐ △ LOMA LINDA UNIVERSITY MEDICAL CENTER, (Includes Loma Linda University Community Medical Center, 25333 Barton Road, Zip 92354–3053; tel. 909/558–6000), 11234 Anderson Street, Zip 92354–2870, Mailing Address: P.O. Box 2000, Zip 92354–0200; tel. 909/558–4000; B. Lyn Behrens, President and Chief Executive Officer (Nonreporting) **A**1 2 3 5 7 8 9 10 **S** Loma Linda University Health Sciences Center, Loma Linda, CA
Web address: www.llumc.edu — 21 10 653 — — — — — — — —

LOMPOC—Santa Barbara County
☐ LOMPOC HEALTHCARE DISTRICT, (Formerly Lompoc District Hospital), 508 East Hickory Street, Zip 93436, Mailing Address: Box 1058, Zip 93438; tel. 805/737–3300; James J. Raggio, Administrator (Total facility includes 110 beds in nursing home–type unit) **A**1 9 10 **F**9 13 17 18 22 25 27 29 39 40 41 44 46 48 54 69 70 75 76 — 16 10 170 3400 23 18000 600 — 13104 211

LONE PINE—Inyo County
SOUTHERN INYO COUNTY LOCAL HEALTH CARE DISTRICT, 501 East Locust Street, Zip 93545, Mailing Address: Box 1009, Zip 93545; tel. 760/876–5501; Donna M. Donald, Administrator (Total facility includes 33 beds in nursing home–type unit) **A**9 10 **F**7 19 22 25 30 31 32 37 38 43 54 56 69 76 77 78 **P**6 — 16 10 37 170 34 12472 — 4182 1928 57

LONG BEACH—Los Angeles County
⊕ LONG BEACH COMMUNITY MEDICAL CENTER, 1720 Termino Avenue, Zip 90804; tel. 562/498–1000; Thomas G. Hennessy, President and Chief Executive Officer **A**1 2 9 10 **F**1 4 7 8 9 11 12 13 14 15 17 18 19 22 25 26 27 29 30 31 32 33 34 35 39 41 43 44 45 46 47 48 49 51 54 57 59 60 61 62 63 64 65 68 69 70 72 75 76 77 78 79 **P**4 5 7 **S** Catholic Healthcare West, San Francisco, CA
Web address: www.lbcommunty.com — 21 10 278 7174 109 35520 1429 64622 21991 608

☐ △ LONG BEACH MEMORIAL MEDICAL CENTER, 2801 Atlantic Avenue, Zip 90806, Mailing Address: P.O. Box 1428, Zip 90801–1428; tel. 562/933–2000; Byron Schweigert, Chief Executive Officer (Total facility includes 62 beds in nursing home–type unit) (Nonreporting) **A**1 2 3 5 7 8 9 10 **S** Memorial Health Services, Long Beach, CA
Web address: www.memorialcare.org — 23 10 726 — — — — — — — —

☐ ○ PACIFIC HOSPITAL OF LONG BEACH, 2776 Pacific Avenue, Zip 90806–2699, Mailing Address: P.O. Box 1268, Zip 90801; tel. 562/595–1911; Michael D. Drobot, President and Chief Executive Officer (Total facility includes 27 beds in nursing home–type unit) **A**1 5 10 11 13 **F**9 12 13 17 18 22 23 24 30 34 35 36 37 38 39 41 44 45 46 49 54 56 57 60 61 62 66 70 71 72 73 74 **P**5 — 33 10 119 4639 97 — 543 53550 15307 446

REDGATE MEMORIAL HOSPITAL, 1775 Chestnut Avenue, Zip 90813; tel. 562/599–8444; Lawrence Gentile, Chief Executive Officer (Nonreporting) — 23 82 63 — — — — — — — —

⊕ ST. MARY MEDICAL CENTER, 1050 Linden Avenue, Zip 90801, Mailing Address: P.O. Box 887, Zip 90813–0887; tel. 562/491–9000; Thomas G. Hennessy, President and Chief Executive Officer (Total facility includes 80 beds in nursing home–type unit) (Nonreporting) **A**1 2 3 5 9 10 **S** Catholic Healthcare West, San Francisco, CA
Web address: www.sc.chw.edu — 23 10 479 — — — — — — — —

Hospitals, U.S. / CALIFORNIA

Hospital, Address, Telephone, Administrator, Approval, Facility, and Physician Codes, Health Care System, Network	Classification Codes		Utilization Data					Expense (thousands) of dollars		
★ American Hospital Association (AHA) membership □ Joint Commission on Accreditation of Healthcare Organizations (JCAHO) accreditation + American Osteopathic Healthcare Association (AOHA) membership ○ American Osteopathic Association (AOA) accreditation △ Commission on Accreditation of Rehabilitation Facilities (CARF) accreditation Control codes 61, 63, 64, 71, 72 and 73 indicate hospitals listed by AOHA, but not registered by AHA. For definition of numerical codes, see page A4	Control	Service	Staffed Beds	Admissions	Census	Outpatient Visits	Births	Total	Payroll	Personnel
★ VETERANS AFFAIRS MEDICAL CENTER, 5901 East Seventh Street, Zip 90822–5201; tel. 562/494–5400; Lawrence C. Stewart, Director (Total facility includes 110 beds in nursing home–type unit) **A**1 2 3 5 8 **F**1 2 3 4 5 6 7 9 11 13 16 17 18 19 21 22 23 24 29 30 31 32 33 34 35 36 37 38 39 41 43 45 46 48 49 50 51 53 54 55 56 57 59 60 61 62 63 64 65 70 71 72 74 76 77 78 79 **S** Department of Veterans Affairs, Washington, DC Web address: www.long–beach.va.gov	45	10	426	6351	294	402662	0	186343	—	2082
LOS ALAMITOS—Orange County										
★ LOS ALAMITOS MEDICAL CENTER, 3751 Katella Avenue, Zip 90720; tel. 562/598–1311; Michele Finney, Chief Executive Officer (Total facility includes 20 beds in nursing home–type unit) (Nonreporting) **A**1 2 9 10 **S** TENET Healthcare Corporation, Santa Barbara, CA Web address: www.tenethealth.com	33	10	173	—	—	—	—	—	—	—
LOS ANGELES—Los Angeles County (Mailing Addresses - Canoga Park, Encino, Granada Hills, Harbor City, Hollywood, Mission Hills, North Hollywood, Northridge, Panorama City, San Pedro, Sepulveda, Sherman Oaks, Sun Valley, Sylmar, Tarzana, Van Nuys, West Hills, West Los Angeles, Woodland Hills)										
★ BARLOW RESPIRATORY HOSPITAL, 2000 Stadium Way, Zip 90026–2696; tel. 213/250–4200; Margaret W. Crane, Chief Executive Officer **A**1 3 5 9 10 **F**17 18 22 38 39 70 72 76 **P**8 Web address: www.barlow2000.org	23	33	62	447	43	0	0	19289	8686	216
★ CALIFORNIA HOSPITAL MEDICAL CENTER, 1401 South Grand Avenue, Zip 90015–3063; tel. 213/748–2411; Melinda D. Beswick, President (Total facility includes 15 beds in nursing home–type unit) **A**1 2 3 5 9 10 **F**4 7 8 9 11 12 13 17 18 19 22 25 27 29 31 32 33 34 36 37 38 39 41 42 44 46 47 48 49 52 54 56 57 61 62 65 66 69 70 72 74 76 77 78 79 **P**5 **S** Catholic Healthcare West, San Francisco, CA Web address: www.chmcla.com	23	10	245	13396	164	142019	4449	108400	42677	1039
★ CEDARS–SINAI MEDICAL CENTER, 8700 Beverly Boulevard, Zip 90048–1865, Mailing Address: Box 48750, Zip 90048–0750; tel. 310/423–5000; Thomas M. Priselac, President and Chief Executive Officer **A**1 2 3 5 8 9 10 **F**3 4 5 8 9 11 12 13 14 16 17 18 19 20 21 22 23 24 25 26 27 30 32 33 34 35 36 37 38 39 40 41 42 43 44 45 46 47 48 49 50 51 52 53 54 55 56 57 58 59 60 61 62 63 64 65 66 68 69 70 71 72 73 74 75 76 78 79 **P**3 5 8 Web address: www.cedars–sinai.edu	23	10	849	43201	701	184264	6797	730437	314004	6450
★ CENTURY CITY HOSPITAL, 2070 Century Park East, Zip 90067; tel. 310/553–6211; Stephen M. Tullman, Chief Executive Officer (Nonreporting) **A**1 9 10 **S** TENET Healthcare Corporation, Santa Barbara, CA Web address: www.tenethealh.com	33	10	156	—	—	—	—	—	—	—
★ CHILDRENS HOSPITAL OF LOS ANGELES, 4650 Sunset Boulevard, Zip 90027–6089, Mailing Address: Box 54700, Zip 90054–0700; tel. 323/660–2450; Walter W. Noce, Jr, President and Chief Executive Officer **A**1 2 3 5 9 10 **F**4 7 11 12 13 14 17 18 19 22 23 24 25 26 31 32 35 39 42 46 47 48 49 50 51 52 53 55 56 65 68 70 71 72 73 74 75 76 77 78 **P**4 7 Web address: www.childrenshospitalla.org	23	50	286	11027	223	257822	0	256305	104967	2750
□ EAST LOS ANGELES DOCTORS HOSPITAL, 4060 Whittier Boulevard, Zip 90023–2596; tel. 323/268–5514; Frank Katsuda, Administrator and Chief Executive Officer (Total facility includes 25 beds in nursing home–type unit) (Nonreporting) **A**1 9 10	33	10	127	—	—	—	—	—	—	—
□ EDGEMONT HOSPITAL, 4841 Hollywood Boulevard, Zip 90027–5388; tel. 323/913–9000; Geri Beutler, Chief Executive Officer (Nonreporting) **A**1 9 10	33	22	61	—	—	—	—	—	—	—
★ ENCINO–TARZANA REGIONAL MEDICAL CENTER ENCINO CAMPUS, 16237 Ventura Boulevard, Encino, Zip 91436–2201; tel. 818/995–5000 **A**1 3 9 10 **F**10 12 17 18 22 24 25 31 32 33 34 36 38 39 41 43 48 50 51 53 54 57 62 65 69 71 73 74 76 78 **S** TENET Healthcare Corporation, Santa Barbara, CA	32	10	151	4403	37	16477	0	40600	16860	493
★ ENCINO–TARZANA REGIONAL MEDICAL CENTER TARZANA CAMPUS, 18321 Clark Street, Tarzana, Zip 91356; tel. 818/881–0800; Dale Surowitz, Chief Executive Officer **A**9 10 **F**2 4 8 9 10 11 12 13 17 18 20 22 24 25 30 31 32 33 34 36 38 39 41 42 43 44 46 47 48 50 51 52 53 54 57 62 65 66 69 70 71 72 73 74 76 77 78 79 **S** TENET Healthcare Corporation, Santa Barbara, CA Web address: www.tenethealh.com	32	10	232	12965	157	45566	3201	101237	42621	940
□ GATEWAYS HOSPITAL AND MENTAL HEALTH CENTER, 1891 Effie Street, Zip 90026–1711; tel. 323/644–2000; Saul Goldfarb, President and Chief Executive Officer **A**1 9 10 **F**3 17 57 58 59 60 62 63 64	23	22	55	634	30	5478	0	12951	8897	235
□ △ GOOD SAMARITAN HOSPITAL, 1225 Wilshire Boulevard, Zip 90017–2395; tel. 213/977–2121; Andrew B. Leeka, President and Chief Executive Officer **A**1 2 7 9 10 **F**4 7 8 9 11 13 17 18 19 22 24 25 27 28 31 32 34 36 38 39 42 44 45 46 47 48 49 51 53 54 65 66 68 69 70 71 72 75 76 78 79 Web address: www.goodsam.org	23	10	357	15328	234	92309	2694	167283	60998	1253
□ GRANADA HILLS COMMUNITY HOSPITAL, 10445 Balboa Boulevard, Granada Hills, Zip 91394–9400; tel. 818/360–1021; Thomas M. Wallace, President and Chief Executive Officer (Total facility includes 23 beds in nursing home–type unit) (Nonreporting) **A**1 9 10 Web address: www.ghch.com	23	10	139	—	—	—	—	—	—	—
HOLLYWOOD COMMUNITY HOSPITAL OF HOLLYWOOD, (Includes Hollywood Community Hospital of Van Nuys, 14433 Emelita Street, Zip 91401; tel. 818/787–1511), 6245 De Longpre Avenue, Zip 90028–9001; tel. 323/462–2271; Evan Rayner, Administrator (Nonreporting) **A**10 **S** Alta Healthcare System, Santa Monica, CA	33	10	160	—	—	—	—	—	—	—

Hospitals, U.S. / CALIFORNIA

★ American Hospital Association (AHA) membership
□ Joint Commission on Accreditation of Healthcare Organizations (JCAHO) accreditation
+ American Osteopathic Healthcare Association (AOHA) membership
○ American Osteopathic Association (AOA) accreditation
△ Commission on Accreditation of Rehabilitation Facilities (CARF) accreditation
Control codes 61, 63, 64, 71, 72 and 73 indicate hospitals listed by AOHA, but not registered by AHA. For definition of numerical codes, see page A4

Hospital, Address, Telephone, Administrator, Approval, Facility, and Physician Codes, Health Care System, Network	Classification Codes		Utilization Data					Expense (thousands) of dollars		
	Control	Service	Staffed Beds	Admissions	Census	Outpatient Visits	Births	Total	Payroll	Personnel
★ KAISER FOUNDATION HOSPITAL, (Includes Kaiser Foundation Mental Health Center, 765 West College Street, Zip 90012; tel. 213/580–7200), 4747 Sunset Boulevard, Zip 90027–6072; tel. 323/783–4011; Anthony A. Armada, Senior Vice President and Service Area Manager **A**2 3 5 10 **F**3 4 8 9 10 11 12 13 14 16 17 18 19 21 22 25 26 27 29 30 32 33 34 35 36 37 38 39 41 42 43 44 45 46 47 48 49 50 51 52 54 56 57 58 61 63 64 65 66 69 70 72 73 76 77 78 79 **P**1 **S** Kaiser Foundation Hospitals, Oakland, CA Web address: www.lac.usc.org	23	10	384	19906	256	23219	2826	—	—	1702
✠ KAISER FOUNDATION HOSPITAL, 25825 South Vermont Avenue, Harbor City, Zip 90710; tel. 310/325–5111; Carolyn Orlowski, Director Operations **A**1 2 10 **F**2 3 4 8 9 11 12 13 19 21 22 24 25 27 30 32 33 35 36 37 38 39 41 42 43 44 45 46 47 48 49 50 51 52 54 56 58 59 60 61 62 63 64 65 66 70 71 72 73 74 76 77 78 **S** Kaiser Foundation Hospitals, Oakland, CA Web address: www.kaiserpermanente.org	23	10	189	10063	96	82678	1886	—	—	1338
✠ KAISER FOUNDATION HOSPITAL, 13652 Cantara Street, Panorama City, Zip 91402; tel. 818/375–2000; Deborah M. Lee-Eddie, Administrator **A**1 5 10 **F**3 4 8 9 11 13 14 16 17 18 19 21 22 24 25 30 31 32 33 34 35 36 37 38 39 41 42 44 45 47 48 49 50 51 54 55 56 58 59 60 61 62 63 64 65 66 68 70 71 72 73 74 76 77 78 **S** Kaiser Foundation Hospitals, Oakland, CA Web address: www.kaiserpermanente.org	23	10	211	12062	108	105631	2074	—	—	1352
✠ KAISER FOUNDATION HOSPITAL, 5601 DeSoto Avenue, Woodland Hills, Zip 91365–4084; tel. 818/719–3808; Deborah M. Lee-Eddie, Administrator **A**1 3 5 10 **F**2 3 4 8 9 11 12 13 16 17 18 19 21 22 24 25 27 30 32 33 34 35 36 37 38 39 42 44 45 46 47 48 49 50 53 54 55 56 57 58 59 60 61 63 64 65 66 69 70 71 72 73 74 75 76 77 78 79 **S** Kaiser Foundation Hospitals, Oakland, CA Web address: www.kaiserpermanente.org	23	10	140	9975	102	88272	1971	—	—	929
✠ KAISER FOUNDATION HOSPITAL–WEST LOS ANGELES, 6041 Cadillac Avenue, Zip 90034; tel. 323/857–2201; Alice Isani, Acting Administrator **A**1 2 3 5 10 **F**2 3 4 8 9 10 11 13 16 17 18 19 22 23 24 25 27 29 30 31 32 33 34 35 36 37 38 39 41 42 43 44 45 46 47 48 49 50 51 52 53 54 55 56 57 58 59 60 61 62 63 64 65 66 68 69 70 71 72 73 74 75 76 77 78 79 **P**6 **S** Kaiser Foundation Hospitals, Oakland, CA Web address: www.kaiserpermanente.org KAISER FOUNDATION MENTAL HEALTH CENTER See Kaiser Foundation Hospital	23	10	180	11476	113	110854	1775	—	—	716
✠ LAC–KING–DREW MEDICAL CENTER, 12021 South Wilmington Avenue, Zip 90059 tel. 310/668–4321; Randall S. Foster, Administrator and Chief Executive Officer **A**1 2 3 5 8 9 10 **F**1 4 8 9 10 11 12 13 14 16 17 18 19 21 22 23 24 25 29 30 31 32 33 34 35 36 38 39 41 42 44 45 46 47 48 49 52 54 55 56 57 58 59 60 61 62 63 64 65 66 68 70 74 75 76 77 78 79 **P**8 **S** Los Angeles County–Department of Health Services, Los Angeles, CA	13	10	257	17551	243	260889	1547	450091	151394	3024
✠ LAC–OLIVE VIEW–UCLA MEDICAL CENTER, 14445 Olive View Drive, Sylmar, Zip 91342–1495; tel. 818/364–1555; Melinda Anderson, Administrator **A**1 3 5 9 10 **F**7 8 9 11 13 17 19 22 23 24 25 26 27 29 31 32 33 34 35 36 38 39 41 42 44 46 47 48 51 54 55 56 57 58 59 60 61 63 64 65 66 70 72 74 75 76 77 78 79 **P**6 **S** Los Angeles County–Department of Health Services, Los Angeles, CA	13	10	213	13052	187	172635	1574	288040	64179	1587
✠ LAC/UNIVERSITY OF SOUTHERN CALIFORNIA MEDICAL CENTER, (Includes General Hospital, 1200 North State Street, Zip 90033; Women's and Children's Hospital, 1240 North Mission Road, Zip 90033), 1200 North State Street, Zip 90033–1084; tel. 323/226–2622; Roberto Rodriguez, Executive Director and Chief Executive Officer **A**1 2 3 5 8 9 10 **F**1 3 4 5 6 7 8 9 10 11 12 13 14 16 17 18 19 20 21 22 23 24 25 27 29 30 31 32 33 34 35 36 38 39 41 42 43 44 45 46 47 48 49 50 51 52 54 56 57 58 59 60 61 62 63 64 65 66 68 70 71 72 73 74 75 76 77 78 79 **P**1 3 6 8 **S** Los Angeles County–Department of Health Services, Los Angeles, CA Web address: www.lacusc.org	13	10	756	47638	756	762233	2833	1027642	238744	6391
□ LINCOLN HOSPITAL MEDICAL CENTER, 443 South Soto Street, Zip 90033–4398; tel. 323/261–1181; Tim Kollars, Administrator and Chief Executive Officer (Nonreporting) **A**1 10	33	10	61	—	—	—	—	—	—	—
□ LOS ANGELES COMMUNITY HOSPITAL, (Includes Los Angeles Community Hospital of Norwalk, 13222 Bloomfield Avenue, Zip 90650; tel. 562/863–4763), 4081 East Olympic Boulevard, Zip 90023–3300; tel. 323/267–0477; Remy Hart, Chief Executive Officer (Nonreporting) **A**1 9 10 **S** Alta Healthcare System, Santa Monica, CA	33	10	186	—	—	—	—	—	—	—
LOS ANGELES COUNTY CENTRAL JAIL HOSPITAL, 441 Bauchet Street, Zip 90012–2994; tel. 213/473–6100; Tom Flaherty, Assistant Administrator (Nonreporting)	13	11	190	—	—	—	—	—	—	—
□ LOS ANGELES METROPOLITAN MEDICAL CENTER, (Includes Hawthorne Hospital, 13300 South Hawthorne Boulevard, Zip 90250; tel. 310/679–3321), 2231 South Western Avenue, Zip 90018–1399; tel. 323/730–7342; Marc A. Furstman, Chief Executive Officer (Nonreporting) **A**1 9 10 **S** Pacific Health Corporation, Tustin, CA	32	10	173	—	—	—	—	—	—	—
✠ MIDWAY HOSPITAL MEDICAL CENTER, 5925 San Vicente Boulevard, Zip 90019–6696; tel. 323/938–3161; Stephen M. Tullman, Chief Executive Officer (Total facility includes 21 beds in nursing home–type unit) (Nonreporting) **A**1 9 10 **S** TENET Healthcare Corporation, Santa Barbara, CA Web address: www.tenethealh.com MISSION COMMUNITY HOSPITAL–PANORAMA CITY CAMPUS See Mission Community Hospital–San Fernando Campus, San Fernando	33	10	150	—	—	—	—	—	—	—

Hospitals, U.S. / CALIFORNIA

Hospital, Address, Telephone, Administrator, Approval, Facility, and Physician Codes, Health Care System, Network	Classification Codes		Utilization Data					Expense (thousands) of dollars		
★ American Hospital Association (AHA) membership □ Joint Commission on Accreditation of Healthcare Organizations (JCAHO) accreditation + American Osteopathic Healthcare Association (AOHA) membership ○ American Osteopathic Association (AOA) accreditation △ Commission on Accreditation of Rehabilitation Facilities (CARF) accreditation Control codes 61, 63, 64, 71, 72 and 73 indicate hospitals listed by AOHA, but not registered by AHA. For definition of numerical codes, see page A4	Control	Service	Staffed Beds	Admissions	Census	Outpatient Visits	Births	Total	Payroll	Personnel
★ MOTION PICTURE AND TELEVISION FUND HOSPITAL AND RESIDENTIAL SERVICES, 23388 Mulholland Drive, Woodland Hills, Zip 91364–2792; tel. 818/876–1888; William F. Haug, FACHE, President and Chief Executive Officer (Total facility includes 165 beds in nursing home–type unit) (Nonreporting) **A**1 9 10 **Web address:** www.mptvfund.org	23	10	218	—	—	—	—	—	—	—
★ NORTHRIDGE HOSPITAL AND MEDICAL CENTER, SHERMAN WAY CAMPUS, 14500 Sherman Circle, Van Nuys, Zip 91405; tel. 818/997–0101; Richard D. Lyons, Senior Vice President and Chief Operating Officer (Total facility includes 38 beds in nursing home–type unit) (Nonreporting) **A**1 9 10 **S** Catholic Healthcare West, San Francisco, CA **Web address:** www.chw.edu	23	10	195	—	—	—	—	—	—	—
★ △ NORTHRIDGE HOSPITAL MEDICAL CENTER–ROSCOE BOULEVARD CAMPUS, 18300 Roscoe Boulevard, Northridge, Zip 91328; tel. 818/885–8500; Richard D. Lyons, Interim President and Chief Executive Officer (Total facility includes 31 beds in nursing home–type unit) **A**1 2 3 5 7 9 10 **F**1 3 4 7 8 9 11 12 13 17 18 19 21 22 23 24 25 28 30 34 35 36 37 38 39 41 42 43 44 45 46 47 48 49 50 51 52 53 54 55 57 58 59 60 61 62 63 64 65 68 69 70 72 73 75 76 77 78 79 **P**3 5 **S** Catholic Healthcare West, San Francisco, CA	23	10	413	14183	234	149561	2119	171457	58383	1485
□ ORTHOPAEDIC HOSPITAL, 2400 South Flower Street, Zip 90007–2697, Mailing Address: Box 60132, Terminal Annex, Zip 90060; tel. 213/742–1000; James V. Luck, Jr, M.D., Chief Executive Officer and Medical Director **A**1 2 3 5 9 10 **F**13 16 17 22 23 25 38 39 41 45 46 48 54 68 70 71 72 78 **P**4 7 **Web address:** www.orthohospital.org	23	47	73	1591	15	71918	0	33489	11511	264
□ PACIFIC ALLIANCE MEDICAL CENTER, 531 West College Street, Zip 90012–2385; tel. 213/624–8411; John R. Edwards, Administrator and Chief Executive Officer (Nonreporting) **A**1 9 10 **Web address:** www.pamc.net	32	10	89	—	—	—	—	—	—	—
□ PACIFICA HOSPITAL OF THE VALLEY, 9449 San Fernando Road, Sun Valley, Zip 91352; tel. 818/767–3310; Casey Fatch, Administrator and Chief Operating Officer **A**1 9 10 **F**4 8 11 12 13 14 16 17 18 19 21 22 25 31 32 39 43 44 45 48 57 60 61 63 65 70 76 78 **S** Doctors Community Healthcare Corporation, Scottsdale, AZ	33	10	204	4933	124	22367	600	47132	20102	500
□ PINE GROVE HOSPITAL, (Formerly ValueMark Pine Grove Health), 7011 Shoup Avenue, Canoga Park, Zip 91307; tel. 818/348–0500; Patty Lepe, Administrator **A**1 9 10 **F**1 3 13 19 21 30 31 43 57 58 59 60 61 62 63 65 70 72 **S** Doctors Community Healthcare Corporation, Scottsdale, AZ	12	22	80	1480	41	6938	0	7955	4271	—
★ PROVIDENCE HOLY CROSS MEDICAL CENTER, 15031 Rinaldi Street, Mission Hills, Zip 91345–1285; tel. 818/365–8051; Georgianne Jessen, Chief Executive Officer (Total facility includes 48 beds in nursing home–type unit) **A**1 9 10 **F**4 7 8 9 11 12 13 16 17 18 19 20 22 24 25 26 29 32 33 34 36 37 38 39 41 43 44 45 46 47 48 49 50 51 53 54 65 69 70 72 75 76 77 78 79 **P**5 **S** Providence Health System, Seattle, WA **Web address:** www.providence.org	21	10	255	10859	173	74823	1558	96238	38133	927
★ QUEEN OF ANGELS–HOLLYWOOD PRESBYTERIAN MEDICAL CENTER, 1300 North Vermont Avenue, Zip 90027–0069; tel. 323/413–3000; Lou Lazatin, Chief Executive Officer (Total facility includes 89 beds in nursing home–type unit) (Nonreporting) **A**1 2 9 10 **S** TENET Healthcare Corporation, Santa Barbara, CA **Web address:** www.tenethealh.com	33	10	409	—	—	—	—	—	—	—
□ △ SAN PEDRO PENINSULA HOSPITAL, 1300 West Seventh Street, San Pedro, Zip 90732; tel. 310/514–5233; John M. Wilson, President (Total facility includes 128 beds in nursing home–type unit) (Nonreporting) **A**1 2 7 9 10 **S** Little Company of Mary Sisters Healthcare System, Evergreen Park, IL **Web address:** www.lchms.org	23	10	309	—	—	—	—	—	—	—
□ SAN VICENTE HOSPITAL, 6000 San Vicente Boulevard, Zip 90036; tel. 323/937–2504; R. Wayne Ives, Administrator (Nonreporting) **A**1 10	33	44	17	—	—	—	—	—	—	—
★ SANTA MARTA HOSPITAL, 319 North Humphreys Avenue, Zip 90022–1499; tel. 323/266–6500; Harry E. Whitney, President and Chief Executive Officer **A**1 9 10 **F**4 13 17 19 22 25 29 31 36 38 41 43 44 45 48 50 51 54 70 76 78 79 **P**1 5 **S** Carondelet Health System, Saint Louis, MO **Web address:** www.santamarta.org	21	10	83	3273	45	17272	889	30611	12214	244
□ SHERMAN OAKS HOSPITAL AND HEALTH CENTER, 4929 Van Nuys Boulevard, Sherman Oaks, Zip 91403; tel. 818/981–7111; David Levinsonn, Chief Executive Officer **A**1 9 10 **F**1 9 10 12 13 17 22 24 25 30 31 32 34 35 38 39 41 43 45 46 48 49 50 51 54 57 62 64 68 69 70 71 72 76 78 **P**3 7 **Web address:** www.sohs.com	23	10	153	3497	59	11616	0	40154	17555	424
□ SHRINERS HOSPITALS FOR CHILDREN, LOS ANGELES, 3160 Geneva Street, Zip 90020–1199; tel. 213/388–3151; Frank LaBonte, FACHE, Administrator (Nonreporting) **A**1 3 5 **S** Shriners Hospitals for Children, Tampa, FL	23	57	50	—	—	—	—	—	—	—
★ ST. VINCENT MEDICAL CENTER, 2131 West Third Street, Zip 90057–0992, Mailing Address: P.O. Box 57992, Zip 90057; tel. 213/484–7111; William D. Parente, President (Total facility includes 27 beds in nursing home–type unit) (Nonreporting) **A**1 3 5 9 10 **S** Catholic Healthcare West, San Francisco, CA **Web address:** www.stvincentmedicalcenter.com	21	10	350	—	—	—	—	—	—	—
□ TEMPLE COMMUNITY HOSPITAL, 235 North Hoover Street, Zip 90004–3672; tel. 213/382–7252; Herbert G. Needman, Administrator and Chief Executive Officer (Total facility includes 11 beds in nursing home–type unit) (Nonreporting) **A**1 9 10	33	10	130	—	—	—	—	—	—	—

Hospitals, U.S. / CALIFORNIA

Hospital, Address, Telephone, Administrator, Approval, Facility, and Physician Codes, Health Care System, Network	Classification Codes		Utilization Data					Expense (thousands) of dollars		
★ American Hospital Association (AHA) membership □ Joint Commission on Accreditation of Healthcare Organizations (JCAHO) accreditation + American Osteopathic Healthcare Association (AOHA) membership ○ American Osteopathic Association (AOA) accreditation △ Commission on Accreditation of Rehabilitation Facilities (CARF) accreditation Control codes 61, 63, 64, 71, 72 and 73 indicate hospitals listed by AOHA, but not registered by AHA. For definition of numerical codes, see page A4	Control	Service	Staffed Beds	Admissions	Census	Outpatient Visits	Births	Total	Payroll	Personnel
✠ UNIVERSITY OF CALIFORNIA LOS ANGELES MEDICAL CENTER, 10833 Le Conte Avenue, Zip 90095–1730; tel. 310/825–9111; Michael Karpf, M.D., Vice Provost Hospital System and Director Medical Center **A**1 2 3 5 8 9 10 **F**4 5 7 8 9 11 12 13 14 17 19 22 23 24 25 26 27 28 29 30 31 32 33 34 35 36 38 39 40 41 42 43 44 45 46 47 48 49 50 51 52 53 54 55 56 65 66 68 70 71 72 74 75 76 77 78 79 **P**5 6 **S** University of California–Systemwide Administration, Oakland, CA **Web address:** www.medctr.ucla.edu	23	10	650	27194	438	720946	1618	588732	247467	6163
✠ UNIVERSITY OF CALIFORNIA LOS ANGELES NEUROPSYCHIATRIC HOSPITAL, 760 Westwood Plaza, Zip 90095; tel. 310/825–0511; Fawzy I. Fawzy, M.D., Medical Director (Nonreporting) **A**1 3 5 9 10 **S** University of California–Systemwide Administration, Oakland, CA **Web address:** www.npi.ucla.edu	12	22	117	—	—	—	—	—	—	—
✠ UNIVERSITY OF SOUTHERN CALIFORNIA–KENNETH NORRIS JR. CANCER HOSPITAL, 1441 Eastlake Avenue, Zip 90033–1085, Mailing Address: P.O. Box 33804, Zip 90033–3804; tel. 323/865–3000; Ted Schreck, Chief Executive Officer **A**1 2 3 5 9 10 **F**7 9 13 16 17 18 19 22 24 26 32 35 38 41 43 46 48 49 50 51 59 65 70 72 74 76 78 **P**5 6 **S** TENET Healthcare Corporation, Santa Barbara, CA **Web address:** www.uscnorris.com	23	10	60	2275	39	51820	0	52878	12031	391
✠ USC UNIVERSITY HOSPITAL, 1500 San Pablo Street, Zip 90033–4585; tel. 323/442–8500; Edward Schreck, Chief Executive Officer **A**1 3 5 8 9 10 **F**4 5 11 12 15 16 18 21 22 27 29 38 39 41 45 47 48 49 51 53 54 57 59 62 65 70 71 72 74 76 78 **P**7 **S** TENET Healthcare Corporation, Santa Barbara, CA **Web address:** www.uscuh.com	33	10	285	7619	168	55369	0	132175	50536	927
✠ VALLEY PRESBYTERIAN HOSPITAL, 15107 Vanowen Street, Van Nuys, Zip 91405; tel. 818/782–6600; Robert C. Bills, President and Vice Chairman (Total facility includes 32 beds in nursing home–type unit) (Nonreporting) **A**1 2 9 10 **Web address:** www.valleypres.org	23	10	347	—	—	—	—	—	—	—
□ VAN NUYS HOSPITAL, 15220 Vanowen Street, Van Nuys, Zip 91405; tel. 818/787–0123; Brent Lamb, Administrator (Nonreporting) **A**1 9 10	33	22	41	—	—	—	—	—	—	—
□ VENCOR HOSPITAL–LOS ANGELES, 5525 West Slauson Avenue, Zip 90056; tel. 310/642–0325; Judith McCurdy, Administrator and Chief Executive Officer **A**1 9 10 **F**4 11 12 13 16 18 22 27 38 39 41 46 47 48 65 70 76 **P**8 **S** Vencor, Incorporated, Louisville, KY	33	10	81	485	68	—	—	18044	8951	205
✠ △ VETERANS AFFAIRS MEDICAL CENTER–WEST LOS ANGELES, 11301 Wilshire Boulevard, Zip 90073–0275; tel. 310/268–3132; Philip P. Thomas, Chief Executive Officer (Total facility includes 240 beds in nursing home–type unit) (Nonreporting) **A**1 5 7 8 9 **S** Department of Veterans Affairs, Washington, DC **Web address:** www.va.gov/stations97/guide/home.asp?DIVISION=ALL	45	10	1327	—	—	—	—	—	—	—
✠ WEST HILLS HOSPITAL AND MEDICAL CENTER, (Formerly West Hills Medical Center), 7300 Medical Center Drive, West Hills, Zip 91307–9937, Mailing Address: P.O. Box 7937, Zip 91309–9937; tel. 818/676–4000; James F. Sherman, President and Chief Executive Officer (Total facility includes 24 beds in nursing home–type unit) **A**1 9 10 **F**4 7 8 9 11 13 16 17 18 19 22 24 25 28 29 30 32 33 34 38 39 41 42 43 44 45 46 47 48 49 50 51 54 65 68 70 71 72 76 77 78 79 **P**5 **S** HCA – The Healthcare Company, Nashville, TN **Web address:** www.westhillshospital.com	33	10	236	8179	104	57673	1435	77407	30447	765
✠ △ WHITE MEMORIAL MEDICAL CENTER, 1720 Cesar E Chavez Avenue, Zip 90033–2481; tel. 323/268–5000; Fred M. Manchur, President and Chief Executive Officer **A**1 2 3 5 7 9 10 **F**5 8 9 11 12 13 17 18 19 22 25 30 31 32 33 34 35 36 38 39 41 42 44 45 46 47 48 52 53 54 56 57 61 64 65 68 69 70 72 73 75 76 78 79 **P**3 5 **S** Adventist Health, Roseville, CA **Web address:** www.adventisthealth.org	21	10	344	13952	223	139945	0	126839	55287	1331
LOS GATOS—Santa Clara County										
✠ △ COMMUNITY HOSPITAL OF LOS GATOS, 815 Pollard Road, Zip 95030; tel. 408/378–6131; Daniel P. Doore, Chief Executive Officer (Nonreporting) **A**1 7 9 10 **S** TENET Healthcare Corporation, Santa Barbara, CA	33	10	153	—	—	—	—	—	—	—
LOYALTON—Sierra County										
SIERRA VALLEY DISTRICT HOSPITAL, 700 Third Street, Zip 96118, Mailing Address: Box 178, Zip 96118; tel. 530/993–1225; Chase Mearian, Administrator (Total facility includes 34 beds in nursing home–type unit) (Nonreporting) **A**9 10	16	10	40	—	—	—	—	—	—	—
LYNWOOD—Los Angeles County										
✠ ST. FRANCIS MEDICAL CENTER, 3630 East Imperial Highway, Zip 90262; tel. 310/603–6000; Gerald T. Kozai, President (Total facility includes 30 beds in nursing home–type unit) (Nonreporting) **A**1 6 9 10 **S** Catholic Healthcare West, San Francisco, CA	21	10	414	—	—	—	—	—	—	—
MADERA—Madera County										
□ MADERA COMMUNITY HOSPITAL, 1250 East Almond Avenue, Zip 93637–5606, Mailing Address: Box 1328, Zip 93639–1328; tel. 559/675–5501; Robert C. Kelley, President and Chief Executive Officer **A**1 9 10 **F**8 9 13 17 18 22 24 25 27 29 32 34 36 38 39 41 43 44 45 46 48 51 52 54 70 76 77 78 **P**5 **Web address:** www.maderahospital.org	23	10	100	5015	55	94265	1440	34666	16544	571
□ △ VALLEY CHILDREN'S HOSPITAL, 9300 Valley Children's Place, Zip 93638–8763; tel. 559/225–3000; William F. Haug, FACHE, President and Chief Executive Officer **A**1 3 5 7 9 10 **F**11 14 15 16 17 18 22 24 25 29 32 34 36 38 39 42 45 46 47 48 50 51 52 53 54 56 63 70 72 76 77 78 **P**1 5 **Web address:** www.valleychildrens.org	23	50	242	9145	152	148207	0	164784	66402	1881

Hospitals, U.S. / CALIFORNIA

Hospital, Address, Telephone, Administrator, Approval, Facility, and Physician Codes, Health Care System, Network	Classification Codes		Utilization Data					Expense (thousands) of dollars		
★ American Hospital Association (AHA) membership □ Joint Commission on Accreditation of Healthcare Organizations (JCAHO) accreditation + American Osteopathic Healthcare Association (AOHA) membership ○ American Osteopathic Association (AOA) accreditation △ Commission on Accreditation of Rehabilitation Facilities (CARF) accreditation Control codes 61, 63, 64, 71, 72 and 73 indicate hospitals listed by AOHA, but not registered by AHA. For definition of numerical codes, see page A4	Control	Service	Staffed Beds	Admissions	Census	Outpatient Visits	Births	Total	Payroll	Personnel

MAMMOTH LAKES—Mono County
□ MAMMOTH HOSPITAL, 85 Sierra Park Road, Zip 93546, Mailing Address: P.O. Box 660, Zip 93546; tel. 760/934–3111; Gary Myers, Administrator (Nonreporting) **A**1 9 10
Web address: www.mammothhospital.com | 23 | 10 | 15 | — | — | — | — | — | — | — |

MANTECA—San Joaquin County
★ DOCTORS HOSPITAL OF MANTECA, 1205 East North Street, Zip 95336; tel. 209/823–3111; Tim A. Joslin, Chief Executive Officer **A**1 9 10 **F**2 3 4 8 9 10 11 12 13 16 17 19 22 24 25 26 30 32 36 37 38 39 41 42 44 45 46 47 48 51 52 53 57 59 61 66 69 70 72 75 76 77 78 79 **P**3 7 **S** TENET Healthcare Corporation, Santa Barbara, CA | 33 | 10 | 73 | 2743 | 31 | 43585 | 411 | 22319 | 10202 | 249 |

★ ST. DOMINIC'S HOSPITAL, 1777 West Yosemite Avenue, Zip 95337; tel. 209/825–3500; Margaret Hepburn, Chief Administrative Officer and Chief Nurse Executive **A**1 9 10 **F**3 4 6 7 8 9 11 12 13 14 16 17 18 19 22 24 25 32 33 34 36 37 41 42 44 45 46 47 48 50 51 54 56 59 60 61 62 63 64 65 67 68 70 72 76 77 78 79 **P**7 **S** Catholic Healthcare West, San Francisco, CA
Web address: www.chw.edu | 21 | 10 | 77 | 1944 | 49 | 25446 | 471 | 20546 | 8002 | 264 |

MARIPOSA—Mariposa County
JOHN C. FREMONT HEALTHCARE DISTRICT, 5189 Hospital Road, Zip 95338, Mailing Address: P.O. Box 216, Zip 95338; tel. 209/966–3631; Elnora George, Administrator, Chief Executive Officer and Chief Financial Officer (Total facility includes 16 beds in nursing home–type unit) **A**9 10 **F**9 13 17 24 25 35 36 37 38 49 58 61 63 68 69 70 76 78 | 16 | 10 | 34 | 354 | 26 | 4216 | 0 | 7026 | 2934 | 106 |

MARTINEZ—Contra Costa County
□ CONTRA COSTA REGIONAL MEDICAL CENTER, 2500 Alhambra Avenue, Zip 94553; tel. 925/370–5000; Frank J. Puglisi, Jr, Executive Director **A**1 2 3 5 10 **F**1 3 4 7 8 9 11 13 14 15 17 18 19 20 21 22 23 24 25 27 30 31 32 33 34 35 36 38 39 40 41 42 43 44 45 46 47 48 50 51 54 56 57 58 59 60 61 62 63 64 65 66 70 72 73 74 75 76 78 **P**6 | 13 | 10 | 117 | 7830 | 117 | 337639 | 1379 | 183382 | 86759 | 1194 |

KAISER FOUNDATION HOSPITAL See Kaiser Foundation Hospital, Walnut Creek

MARYSVILLE—Yuba County
RIDEOUT MEMORIAL HOSPITAL, 726 Fourth Street, Zip 95901–2128, Mailing Address: 989 Plumas Street, Yuba City, Zip 95991; tel. 530/749–4300; Thomas P. Hayes, Chief Executive Officer (Total facility includes 11 beds in nursing home–type unit) **A**9 10 **F**8 9 11 16 17 18 22 24 25 29 30 34 35 36 37 38 39 41 45 48 49 54 65 69 70 76 **P**5 **S** Fremont–Rideout Health Group, Yuba City, CA
Web address: www.frhg.org | 23 | 10 | 89 | 5762 | 90 | 28047 | 0 | 56127 | 21981 | 797 |

MENLO PARK—San Mateo County
□ RECOVERY INN OF MENLO PARK, 570 Willow Road, Zip 94025; tel. 650/324–8500; Carole Wilson, MSN, CHE, Administrator (Nonreporting) **A**1 9 10 **S** Vencor, Incorporated, Louisville, KY | 33 | 10 | 16 | — | — | — | — | — | — | — |

MERCED—Merced County
★ MERCY HOSPITAL AND HEALTH SERVICES, 2740 M Street, Zip 95340–2880; tel. 209/384–6444; John Headding, Chief Administrative Officer (Nonreporting) **A**1 9 10 **S** Catholic Healthcare West, San Francisco, CA
Web address: www.chw.edu | 21 | 10 | 101 | — | — | — | — | — | — | — |

★ SUTTER MERCED MEDICAL CENTER, 301 East 13th Street, Zip 95340–6211; tel. 209/385–7000; Paul F. Dyer, Administrator (Nonreporting) **A**1 3 5 9 10 **S** Sutter Health, Sacramento, CA
Web address: www.sutterhealth.org | 23 | 10 | 158 | — | — | — | — | — | — | — |

MISSION HILLS—Los Angeles County, See Los Angeles

MISSION VIEJO—Orange County
★ △ MISSION HOSPITAL REGIONAL MEDICAL CENTER, 27700 Medical Center Road, Zip 92691; tel. 949/364–1400; Peter F. Bastone, President and Chief Executive Officer (Nonreporting) **A**1 2 5 7 9 10 **S** St. Joseph Health System, Orange, CA
Web address: www.mhrmc.com | 21 | 10 | 208 | — | — | — | — | — | — | — |

MODESTO—Stanislaus County
★ DOCTORS MEDICAL CENTER, 1441 Florida Avenue, Zip 95350–4418, Mailing Address: P.O. Box 4138, Zip 95352–4138; tel. 209/578–1211; Tim A. Joslin, Chief Executive Officer **A**1 2 3 5 9 10 **F**3 4 7 8 9 11 12 13 14 17 18 19 22 24 25 27 28 29 31 32 34 38 39 41 42 43 44 45 46 47 48 49 50 59 60 61 63 64 65 66 68 70 72 74 75 76 77 78 79 **P**5 **S** TENET Healthcare Corporation, Santa Barbara, CA | 33 | 10 | 392 | 19013 | 247 | 90056 | 3841 | 148697 | 64212 | 1584 |

★ MEMORIAL HOSPITALS ASSOCIATION, (Includes Memorial Hospital Los Banos, 520 West I Street, Los Banos, Zip 93635; tel. 209/826–0591; Memorial Medical Center, 1700 Coffee Road, Zip 95355), Mailing Address: P.O. Box 942, Zip 95353–0942; tel. 209/526–4500; David P. Benn, President and Chief Executive Officer **A**1 2 9 10 **F**4 7 8 9 11 13 17 22 24 25 36 39 41 42 43 44 45 46 47 48 50 51 65 69 70 75 76 78 79 **P**3 5 **S** Sutter Health, Sacramento, CA
Web address: www.sutterhealth.org | 23 | 10 | 296 | 16414 | 227 | 94340 | 2139 | 144736 | 59691 | — |

MONROVIA—Los Angeles County
□ MONROVIA COMMUNITY HOSPITAL, 323 South Heliotrope Avenue, Zip 91016, Mailing Address: P.O. Box 707, Zip 91017–0707; tel. 626/359–8341; Christopher A. Vito, Chief Executive Officer **A**1 9 10 **F**22 24 25 30 38 39 40 48 54 70 **S** Alta Healthcare System, Santa Monica, CA | 33 | 10 | 49 | 1856 | 25 | 2541 | — | 8882 | 3582 | 86 |

© 2000 AHA Guide   *Many Facility Codes have changed. Please refer to the AHA Guide Code Chart.*

Hospitals, U.S. / CALIFORNIA

Hospital, Address, Telephone, Administrator, Approval, Facility, and Physician Codes, Health Care System, Network	Classification Codes		Utilization Data					Expense (thousands) of dollars		
★ American Hospital Association (AHA) membership □ Joint Commission on Accreditation of Healthcare Organizations (JCAHO) accreditation + American Osteopathic Healthcare Association (AOHA) membership ○ American Osteopathic Association (AOA) accreditation △ Commission on Accreditation of Rehabilitation Facilities (CARF) accreditation Control codes 61, 63, 64, 71, 72 and 73 indicate hospitals listed by AOHA, but not registered by AHA. For definition of numerical codes, see page A4	Control	Service	Staffed Beds	Admissions	Census	Outpatient Visits	Births	Total	Payroll	Personnel
MONTCLAIR—San Bernardino County										
□ KPC GLOBAL MEDICAL CENTER, (Formerly U.S. FamilyCare Medical Center), 5000 San Bernardino Street, Zip 91763; tel. 909/625-5411; Ronald W. Porter, Chief Executive Officer (Nonreporting) **A**1 9 10 13	33	10	102	—	—	—	—	—	—	—
MONTEBELLO—Los Angeles County										
★ BEVERLY HOSPITAL, 309 West Beverly Boulevard, Zip 90640; tel. 323/726-1222; Matthew S. Gerlach, Chief Executive Officer and President **A**1 2 9 10 **F**4 8 9 11 12 13 16 17 18 19 22 24 25 27 31 32 34 36 39 41 42 43 44 45 46 47 48 51 54 72 73 76 78 79 **P**4 5 7 Web address: www.beverly.com	23	10	166	11126	129	75042	2433	67924	28977	730
MONTEREY—Monterey County										
★ COMMUNITY HOSPITAL OF THE MONTEREY PENINSULA, 23625 Holman Highway, Zip 93940, Mailing Address: Box 'HH', Zip 93942-1085; tel. 831/624-5311; Steven J. Packer, M.D., Chief Executive Officer **A**1 2 9 10 **F**1 3 7 8 9 13 16 17 18 19 22 24 25 26 27 29 32 34 35 36 37 38 39 41 44 45 46 48 54 57 58 59 60 61 62 63 64 65 68 69 70 72 76 78 **P**7 Web address: www.chomp.org	23	10	197	11537	131	252802	1721	172107	68472	1287
MONTEREY PARK—Los Angeles County										
★ △ GARFIELD MEDICAL CENTER, 525 North Garfield Avenue, Zip 91754; tel. 626/573-2222; Philip A. Cohen, Chief Executive Officer **A**1 2 7 9 10 **F**1 3 4 5 6 8 9 10 11 12 13 14 16 17 18 19 21 22 23 24 25 27 28 29 30 31 32 33 34 35 36 37 38 39 41 42 43 44 45 46 47 48 50 51 52 53 54 55 56 58 59 60 61 62 63 64 65 66 68 69 70 71 73 75 76 77 78 79 **P**5 7 **S** TENET Healthcare Corporation, Santa Barbara, CA Web address: www.tenethealh.com	33	10	211	11461	173	61214	3500	73863	34983	1204
★ MONTEREY PARK HOSPITAL, 900 South Atlantic Boulevard, Zip 91754; tel. 626/570-9000; Philip A. Cohen, Chief Executive Officer (Nonreporting) **A**1 2 9 10 **S** TENET Healthcare Corporation, Santa Barbara, CA Web address: www.tenethealh.com	33	10	95	—	—	—	—	—	—	—
MORENO VALLEY—Riverside County										
★ MORENO VALLEY COMMUNITY HOSPITAL, 27300 Iris Avenue, Zip 92555; tel. 909/243-0811; Janice Ziomek, Administrator (Nonreporting) **A**1 9 10 **S** Valley Health System, Hemet, CA	16	10	66	—	—	—	—	—	—	—
□ RIVERSIDE COUNTY REGIONAL MEDICAL CENTER, 26520 Cactus Avenue, Zip 92555; tel. 909/486-4000; Kenneth B. Cohen, Director (Nonreporting) **A**1 3 5 10 Web address: www.rivcohsa.org	13	10	239	—	—	—	—	—	—	—
MOSS BEACH—San Mateo County										
★ SETON MEDICAL CENTER COASTSIDE, 600 Marine Boulevard, Zip 94038; tel. 650/563-7100; John G. Williams, President and Chief Executive Officer (Total facility includes 116 beds in nursing home-type unit) **A**1 9 10 **F**1 2 3 4 5 6 7 8 9 10 11 12 13 16 17 18 19 22 24 25 26 29 30 31 32 33 34 35 36 37 38 39 40 41 42 43 44 45 46 47 48 49 50 51 52 53 54 56 57 58 59 60 61 62 63 64 65 66 68 69 70 71 72 73 76 77 78 79 **S** Catholic Healthcare West, San Francisco, CA Web address: www.chw.edu	21	48	121	137	111	6417	0	9044	4833	98
MOUNT SHASTA—Siskiyou County										
★ MERCY MEDICAL CENTER MOUNT SHASTA, 914 Pine Street, Zip 96067, Mailing Address: P.O. Box 239, Zip 96067-0239; tel. 530/926-6111; Richard J. Barnett, Executive Vice President and Chief Operating Officer (Total facility includes 47 beds in nursing home-type unit) **A**1 9 10 **F**8 9 17 19 22 25 28 29 30 31 32 35 37 39 41 43 44 45 48 61 69 70 71 75 76 78 **P**5 **S** Catholic Healthcare West, San Francisco, CA Web address: www.mercy.org	23	10	80	1697	48	52885	171	19612	8476	215
MOUNTAIN VIEW—Santa Clara County										
★ EL CAMINO HOSPITAL, 2500 Grant Road, Zip 94040, Mailing Address: P.O. Box 7025, Zip 94039; tel. 650/940-7000; Richard M. Warren, Chief Executive Officer (Total facility includes 22 beds in nursing home-type unit) **A**1 9 10 **F**3 4 7 8 9 11 13 17 19 21 22 24 25 29 31 32 33 34 38 39 41 42 44 45 46 47 48 54 57 59 60 61 62 63 64 65 69 70 72 73 76 78 79 Web address: www.sutterhealth.org	16	10	286	17324	249	217424	4160	172204	79313	2157
MURRIETA—Riverside County										
★ RANCHO SPRINGS MEDICAL CENTER, (Formerly Sharp Healthcare Murrieta), 25500 Medical Center Drive, Zip 92562-5966; tel. 909/696-6000; Harris Koenig, Chief Executive Officer (Total facility includes 50 beds in nursing home-type unit) **A**1 9 10 **F**7 8 9 11 13 16 18 19 22 24 25 27 29 31 34 39 41 43 44 46 48 51 54 69 70 76 78 **S** TENET Healthcare Corporation, Santa Barbara, CA Web address: www.tenethealh.com	33	10	99	4832	42	19770	505	—	—	333
NAPA—Napa County										
□ NAPA STATE HOSPITAL, 2100 Napa-Vallejo Highway, Zip 94558; tel. 707/253-5000; Dave Graziani, Acting Executive Director **A**1 3 9 10 **F**22 23 25 26 30 35 37 39 45 50 57 62 63 64 69 70 76 78	12	22	917	449	807	—	0	108259	69678	1887
★ QUEEN OF THE VALLEY HOSPITAL, 1000 Trancas Street, Zip 94558, Mailing Address: Box 2340, Zip 94558; tel. 707/252-4411; Dennis Sisto, President and Chief Executive Officer (Total facility includes 24 beds in nursing home-type unit) **A**1 9 10 **F**4 8 9 11 13 17 18 19 21 22 24 25 26 27 30 32 33 34 35 36 37 38 39 41 42 43 44 45 46 47 48 51 53 54 65 69 70 72 75 76 78 79 **S** St. Joseph Health System, Orange, CA Web address: www.thequeen.org	21	10	166	7605	110	200272	807	88570	36115	1014

Hospitals, U.S. / CALIFORNIA

Hospital, Address, Telephone, Administrator, Approval, Facility, and Physician Codes, Health Care System, Network	Classification Codes		Utilization Data					Expense (thousands) of dollars		
★ American Hospital Association (AHA) membership □ Joint Commission on Accreditation of Healthcare Organizations (JCAHO) accreditation + American Osteopathic Healthcare Association (AOHA) membership ○ American Osteopathic Association (AOA) accreditation △ Commission on Accreditation of Rehabilitation Facilities (CARF) accreditation Control codes 61, 63, 64, 71, 72 and 73 indicate hospitals listed by AOHA, but not registered by AHA. For definition of numerical codes, see page A4	Control	Service	Staffed Beds	Admissions	Census	Outpatient Visits	Births	Total	Payroll	Personnel
NATIONAL CITY—San Diego County										
★ △ PARADISE VALLEY HOSPITAL, 2400 East Fourth Street, Zip 91950; tel. 619/470–4321; David Butler, Chief Executive Officer (Total facility includes 12 beds in nursing home–type unit) (Nonreporting) **A**1 7 9 10 **S** Adventist Health, Roseville, CA Web address: www.adventisthealth.org	21	10	130	—	—	—	—	—	—	—
NEEDLES—San Bernardino County										
★ COLORADO RIVER MEDICAL CENTER, 1401 Bailey Avenue, Zip 92363; tel. 760/326–4531; James Arp, Chief Executive Officer **A**1 9 10 **F**7 9 13 16 17 19 22 25 29 30 32 34 36 38 39 40 41 43 44 45 48 49 51 53 54 66 70 71 72 76 78 79 **S** Province Healthcare Corporation, Brentwood, TN	33	10	49	1948	24	16779	119	14848	6424	186
NEWPORT BEACH—Orange County										
★ HOAG MEMORIAL HOSPITAL PRESBYTERIAN, One Hoag Drive, Zip 92663–4120, Mailing Address: Box 6100, Zip 92658–6100; tel. 949/645–8600; Michael D. Stephens, President and Chief Executive Officer **A**1 2 5 9 10 **F**1 2 3 4 7 8 9 11 12 13 16 17 18 19 22 25 27 29 31 32 33 34 35 36 38 39 40 41 42 43 44 45 46 47 48 49 50 51 54 55 65 66 70 72 74 76 77 78 79 **P**5 7 Web address: www.hoaghospital.org	23	10	350	22788	260	203665	4723	273986	96276	2379
NORTH HOLLYWOOD—Los Angeles County, See Los Angeles										
NORTHRIDGE—Los Angeles County, See Los Angeles										
NORWALK—Los Angeles County										
□ COAST PLAZA DOCTORS HOSPITAL, 13100 Studebaker Road, Zip 90650; tel. 562/868–3751; Gerald J. Garner, Chief Executive Officer **A**1 10 12 **F**8 18 22 25 31 39 44 48 55 63 68 69 70 75 76 78 **P**5	32	10	101	3700	49	—	1	28800	10700	—
LOS ANGELES COMMUNITY HOSPITAL OF NORWALK See Los Angeles Community Hospital, Los Angeles										
□ METROPOLITAN STATE HOSPITAL, 11400 Norwalk Boulevard, Zip 90650; tel. 562/863–7011; William G. Silva, Executive Director (Total facility includes 136 beds in nursing home–type unit) **A**1 5 9 10 **F**22 23 25 28 30 31 34 35 39 45 50 51 57 58 60 62 64 70 72 76 78	12	22	1096	1019	793	0	0	107036	67806	1653
NOVATO—Marin County										
★ NOVATO COMMUNITY HOSPITAL, 1625 Hill Road, Zip 94947, Mailing Address: P.O. Box 1108, Zip 94948; tel. 415/897–3111; Anne L. Hosfeld, Chief Administrative Officer (Total facility includes 11 beds in nursing home–type unit) **A**1 9 10 **F**4 7 8 9 12 13 16 17 18 19 21 22 24 25 26 27 32 33 34 35 36 38 39 41 42 44 45 46 47 48 50 51 54 57 58 59 60 61 62 63 64 65 69 70 76 78 79 **P**1 **S** Sutter Health, Sacramento, CA Web address: www.novatocommunity.com	23	10	33	2254	31	—	0	24396	9836	166
OAKDALE—Stanislaus County										
★ OAK VALLEY DISTRICT HOSPITAL, 350 South Oak Street, Zip 95361; tel. 209/847–3011; Dev Mahadevan, Chief Executive Officer (Total facility includes 115 beds in nursing home–type unit) **A**1 9 10 **F**8 9 13 14 17 18 19 22 23 24 25 30 32 33 34 38 39 41 44 45 48 49 50 51 54 69 70 76 77 78 **P**3 5 **S** Catholic Healthcare West, San Francisco, CA	16	10	148	2325	128	59670	348	26016	10093	368
OAKLAND—Alameda County										
ALAMEDA COUNTY MEDICAL CENTER–HIGHLAND CAMPUS, 1411 East 31st Street, Zip 94602; tel. 510/437–4800; Michael L. Walls, Chief Executive Officer **A**3 5 10 **F**1 3 9 13 14 17 18 19 22 23 24 25 29 31 32 33 34 35 36 38 39 41 43 44 45 46 48 50 51 52 54 56 58 59 60 61 62 63 64 69 70 72 73 75 76 77 78 79 **P**5 **S** Alameda County Health Care Services Agency, San Leandro, CA	13	10	269	13214	323	163994	1071	341403	103607	2475
□ CHILDREN'S HOSPITAL OAKLAND, 747 52nd Street, Zip 94609; tel. 510/428–3000; Antonie H. Paap, President and Chief Executive Officer **A**1 3 5 9 10 **F**4 11 13 14 16 17 18 19 22 23 24 25 29 31 32 33 34 35 38 43 45 46 47 48 49 50 54 56 58 59 60 61 63 70 72 73 74 75 76 77 78 **P**5 8 Web address: www.kidsfirst.org	23	50	204	10288	147	166131	0	173146	82998	1459
★ KAISER FOUNDATION HOSPITAL, 280 West MacArthur Boulevard, Zip 94611; tel. 510/987–1000; Bettie L. Coles, R.N., Administrator (Nonreporting) **A**1 3 5 10 **S** Kaiser Foundation Hospitals, Oakland, CA Web address: www.kaiserpermanente.org	23	10	264	—	—	—	—	—	—	—
□ SUMMIT MEDICAL CENTER, 350 Hawthorne Avenue, Zip 94609; tel. 510/655–4000; Irwin C. Hansen, President and Chief Executive Officer (Total facility includes 48 beds in nursing home–type unit) (Nonreporting) **A**1 2 9 10 **S** Sutter Health, Sacramento, CA	23	10	420	—	—	—	—	—	—	—
OCEANSIDE—San Diego County										
★ TRI–CITY MEDICAL CENTER, 4002 Vista Way, Zip 92056–4593; tel. 760/724–8411; Arthur A. Gonzalez, Dr.PH, President and Chief Executive Officer **A**1 2 9 10 **F**1 4 5 8 9 11 12 13 16 17 18 19 21 22 23 24 25 26 27 30 32 33 34 36 37 38 39 41 42 44 45 46 47 48 50 51 54 55 58 59 60 61 62 63 64 65 68 69 70 76 77 78 79 Web address: www.tri–citymed.com	16	10	397	17707	211	240791	2984	147286	55006	1685
OJAI—Ventura County										
□ OJAI VALLEY COMMUNITY HOSPITAL, 1306 Maricopa Highway, Zip 93023–3180; tel. 805/646–1401; Mark Turner, Chief Executive Officer (Total facility includes 66 beds in nursing home–type unit) **A**1 9 10 **F**8 9 13 17 22 25 38 39 41 43 44 48 54 69 70 76 **P**8 **S** Province Healthcare Corporation, Brentwood, TN	33	10	104	1532	75	37669	157	14113	6350	204

Hospitals, U.S. / CALIFORNIA

Hospital, Address, Telephone, Administrator, Approval, Facility, and Physician Codes, Health Care System, Network	Classification Codes		Utilization Data					Expense (thousands) of dollars		
	Control	Service	Staffed Beds	Admissions	Census	Outpatient Visits	Births	Total	Payroll	Personnel

★ American Hospital Association (AHA) membership
☐ Joint Commission on Accreditation of Healthcare Organizations (JCAHO) accreditation
+ American Osteopathic Healthcare Association (AOHA) membership
○ American Osteopathic Association (AOA) accreditation
△ Commission on Accreditation of Rehabilitation Facilities (CARF) accreditation
Control codes 61, 63, 64, 71, 72 and 73 indicate hospitals listed by AOHA, but not registered by AHA. For definition of numerical codes, see page A4

ONTARIO—San Bernardino County

☐ VENCOR HOSPITAL–ONTARIO, 550 North Monterey, Zip 91764; tel. 909/391–0333; Robert J. Trautman, Administrator (Nonreporting) **A**1 5 10 **S** Vencor, Incorporated, Louisville, KY — 33 10 100 — — — — — — —

ORANGE—Orange County

★ CHAPMAN MEDICAL CENTER, 2601 East Chapman Avenue, Zip 92869; tel. 714/633–0011; Maxine T. Cooper, Chief Executive Officer **A**1 9 10 **F**1 2 3 4 7 8 9 11 12 13 18 19 21 22 24 25 29 30 31 32 33 34 35 36 38 39 41 42 43 44 45 46 47 48 49 50 51 52 53 54 57 62 65 69 70 71 72 73 74 75 76 77 78 79 **P**5 7 **S** TENET Healthcare Corporation, Santa Barbara, CA
Web address: www.tenethealth.com — 33 10 40 2855 40 18996 492 — — 233

☐ CHILDREN'S HOSPITAL OF ORANGE COUNTY, 455 South Main Street, Zip 92868–3874; tel. 714/997–3000; Kimberly C. Cripe, Chief Executive Officer **A**1 2 3 5 9 10 **F**12 13 14 16 17 18 22 24 25 26 31 32 33 34 35 36 38 39 42 43 45 46 47 50 51 52 54 55 56 58 59 60 63 68 70 72 73 74 76 77 78 **P**1 4 5 7
Web address: www.choc.org — 23 50 192 6882 86 96194 0 107505 34823 869

★ ST. JOSEPH HOSPITAL, 1100 West Stewart Drive, Zip 92668, Mailing Address: P.O. Box 5600, Zip 92613–5600; tel. 714/633–9111; Larry K. Ainsworth, President and Chief Executive Officer (Total facility includes 34 beds in nursing home–type unit) **A**1 2 3 5 9 10 **F**2 3 4 6 7 8 9 10 11 12 13 16 17 18 19 20 22 23 24 25 26 27 32 33 34 36 37 38 39 41 42 43 44 45 46 47 48 49 50 51 52 53 54 57 61 62 63 64 65 69 70 72 74 76 78 79 **P**3 5 7 **S** St. Joseph Health System, Orange, CA
Web address: www.sjo.stjoe.org — 21 10 324 23411 266 229209 6154 284255 89520 2633

★ UNIVERSITY OF CALIFORNIA, IRVINE MEDICAL CENTER, 101 The City Drive, Zip 92868–3298; tel. 714/456–6011; Ralph Cygan, M.D., Interim Director **A**1 2 3 5 8 9 10 11 12 13 14 17 19 21 22 24 25 29 30 32 33 34 35 37 39 40 41 42 43 44 45 46 47 48 49 50 51 52 53 54 56 57 58 59 60 61 62 63 64 65 70 71 72 73 74 75 76 77 78 79 **P**6 **S** University of California–Systemwide Administration, Oakland, CA
Web address: www.ucihealth.com — 23 10 383 15043 246 452537 1100 211096 97836 2736

OROVILLE—Butte County

☐ OROVILLE HOSPITAL, 2767 Olive Highway, Zip 95966–6185; tel. 530/533–8500; Robert J. Wentz, President and Chief Executive Officer (Total facility includes 20 beds in nursing home–type unit) **A**1 9 10 **F**7 8 9 13 14 15 17 18 19 20 21 22 23 24 25 27 28 29 30 32 33 34 35 36 38 39 41 43 44 45 46 48 50 51 54 56 66 68 69 70 72 75 76 77 78 79 **P**8
Web address: www.orohealth.com — 23 10 120 5840 77 259894 555 63044 28699 952

OXNARD—Ventura County

★ ST. JOHN'S REGIONAL MEDICAL CENTER, 1600 North Rose Avenue, Zip 93030; tel. 805/988–2500; Charles E. Padilla, Administrator and Chief Operating Officer **A**1 9 10 **F**4 7 8 9 11 12 16 17 18 19 22 24 25 27 32 33 34 38 39 41 42 44 45 46 47 48 49 50 51 53 54 57 62 65 68 70 72 76 78 **P**2 **S** Catholic Healthcare West, San Francisco, CA
Web address: www.chw.edu — 23 10 230 12351 185 83083 2348 106348 44323 1100

PALM SPRINGS—Riverside County

★ DESERT REGIONAL MEDICAL CENTER, 1150 North Indian Canyon Drive, Zip 92262, Mailing Address: Box 2739, Zip 92263; tel. 760/323–6511; Truman L. Gates, President and Chief Executive Officer (Nonreporting) **A**1 2 9 10 **S** TENET Healthcare Corporation, Santa Barbara, CA
Web address: www.tenethealth.com — 33 10 348 — — — — — — —

PALO ALTO—Santa Clara County

★ LUCILE SALTER PACKARD CHILDREN'S HOSPITAL AT STANFORD, 725 Welch Road, Zip 94304; tel. 650/497–8000; Christopher G. Dawes, President **A**1 3 5 9 10 **F**4 7 8 9 11 12 13 14 16 17 18 19 20 21 22 23 24 25 26 27 28 29 30 31 32 33 34 35 36 37 38 39 41 42 43 44 45 46 47 48 49 50 51 52 53 54 55 56 57 58 59 60 63 64 65 66 68 69 70 71 72 73 74 75 76 77 78 79 **P**6 **S** Stanford Health Care, San Francisco, CA — 23 50 214 11156 163 82278 4419 187212 64714 1230

★ △ VETERANS AFFAIRS PALO ALTO HEALTH CARE SYSTEM, (Includes Palo Alto Division, 3801 Miranda Avenue, tel. 415/493–5000; Veterans Affairs Palo Alto Health Care System, Livermore Division, 4951 Arroyo Road, Livermore, Zip 94550; tel. 510/447–2560; Clarence H. Nixon, Director), 3801 Miranda Avenue, Zip 94304–1207; tel. 650/493–5000; James A. Goff, FACHE, Director (Total facility includes 393 beds in nursing home–type unit) **A**1 2 3 5 7 8 **F**1 2 3 4 5 6 9 11 12 13 14 15 16 17 18 19 21 22 23 24 25 26 27 28 29 30 31 32 33 34 35 36 37 38 39 41 43 44 45 46 47 48 49 50 51 53 54 55 56 57 59 60 61 62 63 64 65 66 68 69 70 72 73 76 77 78 79 **S** Department of Veterans Affairs, Washington, DC
Web address: www.icon.palo–alto.med.va.gov — 45 10 967 10063 816 437898 0 324079 162940 3178

PANORAMA CITY—Los Angeles County, See Los Angeles

PARADISE—Butte County

★ FEATHER RIVER HOSPITAL, 5974 Pentz Road, Zip 95969–5593; tel. 530/877–9361; Michael H. Schultz, Chief Executive Officer (Total facility includes 21 beds in nursing home–type unit) (Nonreporting) **A**1 9 10 **S** Adventist Health, Roseville, CA
Web address: www.adventisthealth.org — 21 10 122 — — — — — — —

Hospitals, U.S. / CALIFORNIA

Hospital, Address, Telephone, Administrator, Approval, Facility, and Physician Codes, Health Care System, Network	Classification Codes		Utilization Data					Expense (thousands) of dollars		
★ American Hospital Association (AHA) membership □ Joint Commission on Accreditation of Healthcare Organizations (JCAHO) accreditation + American Osteopathic Healthcare Association (AOHA) membership ○ American Osteopathic Association (AOA) accreditation △ Commission on Accreditation of Rehabilitation Facilities (CARF) accreditation Control codes 61, 63, 64, 71, 72 and 73 indicate hospitals listed by AOHA, but not registered by AHA. For definition of numerical codes, see page A4	Control	Service	Staffed Beds	Admissions	Census	Outpatient Visits	Births	Total	Payroll	Personnel

PARAMOUNT—Los Angeles County
★ SUBURBAN MEDICAL CENTER, 16453 South Colorado Avenue, Zip 90723; tel. 562/531–3110; Kenneth I. Rivers, Chief Executive Officer (Nonreporting) **A**1 9 10 **S** TENET Healthcare Corporation, Santa Barbara, CA
Web address: www.tenethealth.com/suburban
33	10	130	—	—	—	—	—	—	—

PASADENA—Los Angeles County
★ HUNTINGTON MEMORIAL HOSPITAL, 100 West California Boulevard, Zip 91105, Mailing Address: P.O. Box 7013, Zip 91109–7013; tel. 626/397–5000; Stephen A. Ralph, President and Chief Executive Officer (Total facility includes 75 beds in nursing home–type unit) **A**1 2 3 5 8 9 10 **F**4 8 9 11 12 13 17 18 19 22 24 25 27 30 32 33 34 35 36 38 39 41 42 43 44 45 46 47 48 50 52 53 54 56 57 59 60 61 62 63 64 65 70 72 75 76 77 78 79 **P**3 5 **S** Southern California Healthcare Systems, Pasadena, CA
Web address: www.schs.com
| 23 | 10 | 525 | 22737 | 320 | 186727 | 3964 | 224595 | 90911 | 2261 |

IMPACT DRUG AND ALCOHOL TREATMENT CENTER, 1680 North Fair Oaks Avenue, Zip 91103; tel. 323/681–2575; James M. Stillwell, Director (Nonreporting)
| 23 | 82 | 130 | — | — | — | — | — | — | — |

★ LAS ENCINAS HOSPITAL, 2900 East Del Mar Boulevard, Zip 91107–4375; tel. 626/795–9901; Roland Metivier, Chief Executive Officer **A**1 9 10 **F**2 3 16 17 18 57 58 59 60 61 62 63 64 **P**7 **S** HCA – The Healthcare Company, Nashville, TN
Web address: www.hcahealthcare.com
| 33 | 22 | 138 | 1575 | 62 | 8115 | 0 | 12288 | 6549 | 190 |

★ ST. LUKE MEDICAL CENTER, 2632 East Washington Boulevard, Zip 91107–1994; tel. 626/797–1141; Phyllis Bushart, R.N., Chief Executive Officer (Total facility includes 46 beds in nursing home–type unit) **A**1 2 9 10 **F**3 4 7 8 9 11 12 13 17 18 19 22 24 25 31 32 34 36 37 39 41 42 44 45 46 47 48 49 50 51 52 54 57 58 59 60 61 62 66 68 69 70 71 72 74 76 78 79 **S** TENET Healthcare Corporation, Santa Barbara, CA
Web address: www.tenethealh.com
| 33 | 10 | 148 | 4640 | 77 | 25058 | 646 | 38146 | 16694 | 418 |

PATTON—San Bernardino County
□ PATTON STATE HOSPITAL, 3102 East Highland Avenue, Zip 92369; tel. 909/425–7000; William L. Summers, Executive Director **A**1 9 **F**1 4 5 8 9 11 13 21 22 23 24 25 26 28 30 32 33 34 35 39 43 45 46 47 48 50 51 54 55 57 59 62 65 66 68 70 74 75 76 77 78 **P**6
| 12 | 22 | 1121 | 1085 | 1153 | — | — | 117659 | 77530 | 1885 |

PETALUMA—Sonoma County
★ PETALUMA VALLEY HOSPITAL, 400 North McDowell Boulevard, Zip 94954–2339; tel. 707/778–1111; Ramona Faith, R.N., MS, Site Administrator and Chief Nurse Executive **A**1 2 9 10 **F**4 7 8 9 10 11 12 13 17 19 20 22 23 24 25 26 27 30 31 32 34 35 36 37 38 39 40 41 42 43 44 45 46 47 49 50 51 52 53 54 55 57 59 61 62 63 64 65 66 68 69 70 72 73 74 75 76 77 78 **P**5 **S** St. Joseph Health System, Orange, CA
| 21 | 10 | 82 | 3963 | 47 | 271192 | 548 | 37958 | 18574 | 420 |

PINOLE—Contra Costa County
★ DOCTORS MEDICAL CENTER–PINOLE CAMPUS, 2151 Appian Way, Zip 94564; tel. 510/970–5000; Gary Sloan, Chief Executive Officer (Total facility includes 40 beds in nursing home–type unit) (Nonreporting) **A**1 9 10 **S** TENET Healthcare Corporation, Santa Barbara, CA
Web address: www.tenethealth.com
| 33 | 10 | 137 | — | — | — | — | — | — | — |

PLACENTIA—Orange County
★ PLACENTIA LINDA HOSPITAL, 1301 Rose Drive, Zip 92870; tel. 714/993–2000; Maxine T. Cooper, Chief Executive Officer **A**1 9 10 **F**7 8 9 12 13 16 17 18 19 21 22 24 25 30 31 32 33 34 35 36 38 39 41 43 44 45 46 48 49 51 54 66 68 70 71 72 76 78 **P**5 7 8 **S** TENET Healthcare Corporation, Santa Barbara, CA
Web address: www.tenethealth.com/placentialinda
| 33 | 10 | 114 | 3761 | 33 | 36633 | 639 | 23797 | 9411 | 282 |

PLACERVILLE—El Dorado County
★ MARSHALL HOSPITAL, 1100 Marshall Way, Zip 95667; tel. 530/622–1441; Frank Nachtman, Administrator **A**1 9 10 **F**7 8 9 13 16 17 18 19 22 24 25 28 32 33 34 35 36 38 39 41 43 44 45 46 48 49 50 51 56 65 68 69 70 72 76 78 **P**3 5 8
| 23 | 10 | 100 | 5448 | 56 | 322913 | 758 | 61993 | 23147 | 574 |

PLEASANTON—Alameda County
VALLEYCARE MEDICAL CENTER, 5555 West Positas Boulevard, Zip 94588, Mailing Address: 555 West Los Positas Boulevard, Zip 94588; tel. 925/847–3000; Marcy L. Feit, Chief Executive Officer (Nonreporting) **A**9 **S** ValleyCare Health System, Pleasanton, CA
| 23 | 10 | 68 | — | — | — | — | — | — | — |

POMONA—Los Angeles County
★ △ CASA COLINA HOSPITAL FOR REHABILITATIVE MEDICINE, 255 East Bonita Avenue, Zip 91767–9966, Mailing Address: P.O. Box 6001, Zip 91769–6001; tel. 909/593–7521; Felice Loverso, Ph.D., President and Chief Executive Officer (Total facility includes 11 beds in nursing home–type unit) (Nonreporting) **A**1 7 10
Web address: www.casacolina.org
| 23 | 46 | 38 | — | — | — | — | — | — | — |

LANTERMAN DEVELOPMENTAL CENTER, 3530 Pomona Boulevard, Zip 91768, Mailing Address: P.O. Box 100, Zip 91769; tel. 909/595–1221; Ruth Maples, Executive Director (Total facility includes 196 beds in nursing home–type unit) **A**9 10 **F**10 13 22 23 24 32 39 41 69 70
| 12 | 12 | 718 | 22 | 729 | 0 | 0 | — | — | 1422 |

★ POMONA VALLEY HOSPITAL MEDICAL CENTER, 1798 North Garey Avenue, Zip 91767–2918; tel. 909/865–9500; Richard E. Yochum, President and Chief Executive Officer (Total facility includes 38 beds in nursing home–type unit) **A**1 2 3 9 10 **F**4 7 8 9 11 12 13 14 16 17 18 19 22 23 24 25 28 29 32 33 34 38 39 40 41 42 43 44 45 46 47 48 49 50 51 52 54 56 65 68 69 70 71 72 76 77 78 79 **P**5
Web address: www.pvhmc.org
| 23 | 10 | 436 | 19731 | 249 | 744668 | 4780 | 205116 | 91560 | 1881 |

© 2000 AHA Guide   *Many Facility Codes have changed. Please refer to the AHA Guide Code Chart.*

Hospitals, U.S. / CALIFORNIA

★ American Hospital Association (AHA) membership
☐ Joint Commission on Accreditation of Healthcare Organizations (JCAHO) accreditation
+ American Osteopathic Healthcare Association (AOHA) membership
○ American Osteopathic Association (AOA) accreditation
△ Commission on Accreditation of Rehabilitation Facilities (CARF) accreditation
Control codes 61, 63, 64, 71, 72 and 73 indicate hospitals listed by AOHA, but not registered by AHA. For definition of numerical codes, see page A4

Hospital, Address, Telephone, Administrator, Approval, Facility, and Physician Codes, Health Care System, Network	Classification Codes		Utilization Data					Expense (thousands) of dollars		
	Control	Service	Staffed Beds	Admissions	Census	Outpatient Visits	Births	Total	Payroll	Personnel
PORT HUENEME—Ventura County										
☐ ANACAPA HOSPITAL, 307 East Clara Street, Zip 93041; tel. 805/488–3661; Shawn J. O'Connor, Chief Executive Officer **A**1 9 10 **F**13 19 21 31 38 45 50 57 58 60 61 63 64 70 72 73 **P**8	33	22	44	871	33	7569	0	6374	2657	106
PORTERVILLE—Tulare County										
PORTERVILLE DEVELOPMENTAL CENTER, 26501 Avenue 140, Zip 93257–9430, Mailing Address: Box 2000, Zip 93258–2000; tel. 559/782–2222; Norm Kramer, Executive Director **A**9 10 **F**4 16 18 19 21 22 23 24 30 32 33 39 43 45 48 50 51 55 58 59 62 65 69 70 72 78 **P**6	12	62	838	78	826	—	—	99536	62143	1885
SIERRA VIEW DISTRICT HOSPITAL, 465 West Putnam Avenue, Zip 93257–3320; tel. 559/784–1110; Kelly C. Morgan, President and Chief Executive Officer **A**9 10 **F**8 9 16 17 18 22 24 25 28 32 34 36 39 43 46 48 51 54 65 70 72 76 78 79 **P**5	16	10	120	6044	62	154973	1180	45616	16650	591
PORTOLA—Plumas County										
EASTERN PLUMAS DISTRICT HOSPITAL, 500 First Avenue, Zip 96122; tel. 530/832–4277; Charles R. Guenther, Administrator (Total facility includes 14 beds in nursing home–type unit) (Nonreporting) **A**9 10
Web address: www.ephc.org	16	10	24	—	—	—	—	—	—	—
POWAY—San Diego County										
★ POMERADO HOSPITAL, 15615 Pomerado Road, Zip 92064; tel. 858/485–6511; Marvin W. Levenson, M.D., Administrator and Chief Operating Officer (Total facility includes 149 beds in nursing home–type unit) (Nonreporting) **A**1 2 9 10
S Palomar Pomerado Health System, San Diego, CA
Web address: www.pphs.org	16	10	258	—	—	—	—	—	—	—
QUINCY—Plumas County										
☐ PLUMAS DISTRICT HOSPITAL, 1065 Bucks Lake Road, Zip 95971–9599; tel. 530/283–2121; R. Michael Barry, Administrator **A**1 9 10 **F**8 16 17 18 22 23 25 32 39 48 76 78 **P**6
Web address: www.pdh.org	16	10	18	404	4	108876	85	9557	4226	173
RANCHO MIRAGE—Riverside County										
★ EISENHOWER MEMORIAL HOSPITAL AND BETTY FORD CENTER AT EISENHOWER, 39000 Bob Hope Drive, Zip 92270; tel. 760/340–3911; Andrew W. Deems, President and Chief Executive Officer **A**1 2 5 9 10 **F**1 4 5 7 8 9 11 12 13 17 18 19 22 24 25 27 28 29 30 32 33 34 36 37 38 39 41 42 43 44 45 46 47 48 49 50 51 54 65 70 71 72 76 77 78 79 **P**7
Web address: www.emc.org	23	10	261	14812	162	292865	1617	169228	55627	1235
RED BLUFF—Tehama County										
★ ST. ELIZABETH COMMUNITY HOSPITAL, 2550 Sister Mary Columba Drive, Zip 96080–4397; tel. 530/529–8000; Thomas F. Grimes, II, Executive Vice President and Chief Operating Officer **A**1 9 10 **F**8 12 13 16 17 18 19 22 25 26 32 36 37 38 39 44 45 48 54 70 72 73 76 78 **P**3 **S** Catholic Healthcare West, San Francisco, CA
Web address: www.mercy.org	21	10	61	3445	33	57712	569	30765	13239	383
REDDING—Shasta County										
★ MERCY MEDICAL CENTER REDDING, 2175 Rosaline Avenue, Zip 96001, Mailing Address: P.O. Box 496009, Zip 96049–6009; tel. 530/225–6000; John Di Perry, Jr, Executive Vice President and Chief Operating Officer (Total facility includes 17 beds in nursing home–type unit) **A**1 2 3 5 9 10 **F**1 4 7 8 9 11 12 13 17 18 22 24 25 27 28 29 31 33 34 35 36 37 38 39 40 41 42 43 44 45 46 47 48 49 54 56 65 68 69 70 72 74 75 76 77 78 79 **P**3 5 **S** Catholic Healthcare West, San Francisco, CA
Web address: www.mercy.org	21	10	219	10463	122	156740	1595	123687	47737	1316
★ REDDING MEDICAL CENTER, 1100 Butte Street, Zip 96001–0853, Mailing Address: Box 496072, Zip 96049–6072; tel. 530/244–5454; Steve Schmidt, Chief Executive Officer **A**1 9 10 **F**4 7 8 9 11 12 13 18 19 21 22 25 27 28 29 30 31 32 33 34 36 38 41 42 43 44 45 46 47 48 49 50 51 54 56 65 70 71 72 76 77 78 79 **P**5 7 **S** TENET Healthcare Corporation, Santa Barbara, CA	33	10	188	8172	117	128451	372	—	—	1174
REDLANDS—San Bernardino County										
☐ LOMA LINDA UNIVERSITY BEHAVIORAL MEDICINE CENTER, 1710 Barton Road, Zip 92373; tel. 909/558–9200; Alan Soderblom, Administrator (Nonreporting) **A**1 5 9 10 **S** Loma Linda University Health Sciences Center, Loma Linda, CA	21	22	89	—	—	—	—	—	—	—
☐ REDLANDS COMMUNITY HOSPITAL, 350 Terracina Boulevard, Zip 92373, Mailing Address: Box 3391, Zip 92373–0742; tel. 909/335–5500; James R. Holmes, President and Chief Executive Officer (Nonreporting) **A**1 9 10
Web address: www.redlandshospital.com	23	10	194	—	—	—	—	—	—	—
REDWOOD CITY—San Mateo County										
★ KAISER FOUNDATION HOSPITAL, 1150 Veterans Boulevard, Zip 94063–2087; tel. 650/299–2000; Joanne Zimmerman, Administrator **A**1 3 5 10 **F**2 3 4 5 7 8 9 10 11 12 13 14 15 16 18 19 20 21 22 24 25 26 27 28 29 30 31 32 33 34 35 36 37 38 39 41 42 43 44 45 46 47 48 49 50 51 52 53 54 55 56 57 58 59 60 61 62 63 64 65 66 68 69 70 71 72 73 74 75 76 77 78 79 **P**3 **S** Kaiser Foundation Hospitals, Oakland, CA
Web address: www.kaiserpermanente.org	23	10	171	7226	83	618740	1458	—	—	583
★ SEQUOIA HOSPITAL, 170 Alameda De Las Pulgas, Zip 94062; tel. 650/369–5811; John Williams, Chief Executive Officer (Total facility includes 44 beds in nursing home–type unit) **A**9 10 **F**4 7 8 9 11 13 17 18 19 22 24 25 32 33 34 36 37 38 39 41 44 45 46 47 48 49 50 51 53 54 57 64 65 68 69 70 72 76 77 78 79 **P**3 **S** Catholic Healthcare West, San Francisco, CA
Web address: www.chwbay.org	23	10	245	10390	140	91076	1319	123998	51990	739

Hospitals, U.S. / CALIFORNIA

Hospital, Address, Telephone, Administrator, Approval, Facility, and Physician Codes, Health Care System, Network	Classification Codes		Utilization Data					Expense (thousands) of dollars		
★ American Hospital Association (AHA) membership □ Joint Commission on Accreditation of Healthcare Organizations (JCAHO) accreditation + American Osteopathic Healthcare Association (AOHA) membership ○ American Osteopathic Association (AOA) accreditation △ Commission on Accreditation of Rehabilitation Facilities (CARF) accreditation Control codes 61, 63, 64, 71, 72 and 73 indicate hospitals listed by AOHA, but not registered by AHA. For definition of numerical codes, see page A4	Control	Service	Staffed Beds	Admissions	Census	Outpatient Visits	Births	Total	Payroll	Personnel

REEDLEY—Fresno County

★ SIERRA–KINGS DISTRICT HOSPITAL, 372 West Cypress Avenue, Zip 93654; tel. 559/638–8155; Stan B. Berry, FACHE, Administrator **A** 1 9 10 **F** 8 9 13 16 17 18 19 22 25 28 32 34 38 43 44 48 50 54 70 76 78 79 **Web address:** www.skdh.org	16	44	39	1567	13	42285	712	11296	4731	163

RIDGECREST—Kern County

★ RIDGECREST REGIONAL HOSPITAL, 1081 North China Lake Boulevard, Zip 93555; tel. 760/446–3551; David A. Mechtenberg, Chief Executive Officer **A** 1 9 10 **F** 8 12 17 18 22 25 32 36 37 39 40 41 44 45 48 50 51 54 70 76 78 **Web address:** www.rrh.org	23	10	80	2547	23	23700	468	23569	10132	272

RIVERSIDE—Riverside County

★ KAISER FOUNDATION HOSPITAL–RIVERSIDE, 10800 Magnolia Avenue, Zip 92505–3000; tel. 909/353–4600; Gerald A. McCall, Chief Executive Officer **A** 1 2 3 10 **F** 3 4 8 9 11 13 16 17 18 24 25 35 36 37 39 41 44 45 46 47 50 51 58 59 60 61 63 68 70 74 76 77 78 79 **S** Kaiser Foundation Hospitals, Oakland, CA **Web address:** www.kaiserpermanente.org	23	10	188	12070	101	84984	2948	—	—	1850
□ PARKVIEW COMMUNITY HOSPITAL MEDICAL CENTER, 3865 Jackson Street, Zip 92503; tel. 909/688–2211; Norman Martin, President and Chief Executive Officer (Nonreporting) **A** 1 2 9 10 **Web address:** www.pchmc.org	23	10	193	—	—	—	—	—	—	—
★ RIVERSIDE COMMUNITY HOSPITAL, 4445 Magnolia Avenue, Zip 92501–1669, Mailing Address: P.O. Box 1669, Zip 92502–1669; tel. 909/788–3000; Bryan R. Rogers, President and Chief Executive Officer (Nonreporting) **A** 1 9 10 **S** HCA – The Healthcare Company, Nashville, TN **Web address:** www.pchmc.org	23	10	276	—	—	—	—	—	—	—

ROSEMEAD—Los Angeles County

□ BHC ALHAMBRA HOSPITAL, 4619 North Rosemead Boulevard, Zip 91770–1498, Mailing Address: P.O. Box 369, Zip 91770; tel. 626/286–1191; Peggy Minnick, R.N., Chief Executive Officer (Nonreporting) **A** 1 9 10 **S** Behavioral Healthcare Corporation, Nashville, TN	33	22	98	—	—	—	—	—	—	—

ROSEVILLE—Placer County

★ SUTTER ROSEVILLE MEDICAL CENTER, One Medical Plaza, Zip 95661–3477; tel. 916/781–1000; Patrick R. Brady, Chief Executive Officer (Total facility includes 14 beds in nursing home–type unit) (Nonreporting) **A** 1 2 9 10 **S** Sutter Health, Sacramento, CA **Web address:** www.sutterhealth.org	23	10	183	—	—	—	—	—	—	—

SACRAMENTO—Sacramento County

★ BHC HERITAGE OAKS HOSPITAL, 4250 Auburn Boulevard, Zip 95841; tel. 916/489–3336; Ingrid L. Whipple, Administrator and Chief Executive Officer (Nonreporting) **A** 1 9 10 **S** Behavioral Healthcare Corporation, Nashville, TN	33	22	76	—	—	—	—	—	—	—
□ BHC SIERRA VISTA HOSPITAL, 8001 Bruceville Road, Zip 95823; tel. 916/423–2000; Tom Pinizzotto, Administrator and Chief Executive Officer (Nonreporting) **A** 1 9 10 **S** Behavioral Healthcare Corporation, Nashville, TN	33	22	72	—	—	—	—	—	—	—
★ KAISER FOUNDATION HOSPITAL, 2025 Morse Avenue, Zip 95825–2115; tel. 916/973–5000; Edward S. Glavis, Administrator (Nonreporting) **A** 1 3 5 10 **S** Kaiser Foundation Hospitals, Oakland, CA **Web address:** www.kaiserpermanente.org	23	10	304	—	—	—	—	—	—	—
★ KAISER FOUNDATION HOSPITAL, 6600 Bruceville Road, Zip 95823; tel. 916/688–2430; Edward S. Glavis, Administrator (Nonreporting) **A** 1 3 10 **S** Kaiser Foundation Hospitals, Oakland, CA **Web address:** www.kaiserpermanente.org	23	10	221	—	—	—	—	—	—	—
★ MERCY GENERAL HOSPITAL, 4001 J Street, Zip 95819; tel. 916/851–2000; Thomas A. Petersen, Vice President and Chief Operating Officer (Total facility includes 95 beds in nursing home–type unit) **A** 1 2 9 10 **F** 4 8 9 11 12 13 17 19 21 22 24 25 26 27 29 30 32 33 34 36 37 38 39 41 42 43 44 45 46 47 48 51 53 54 55 58 59 60 61 62 63 65 66 69 70 71 72 75 76 77 78 79 **P** 3 5 **S** Catholic Healthcare West, San Francisco, CA **Web address:** www.mercysac.org	21	10	402	17077	240	109157	2298	202406	61866	1371
★ METHODIST HOSPITAL OF SACRAMENTO, 7500 Hospital Drive, Zip 95823; tel. 916/423–3000; Michael J. Finn, Acting Vice President and Chief Operating Officer (Total facility includes 171 beds in nursing home–type unit) **A** 1 3 9 10 **F** 4 8 9 11 12 16 17 18 19 22 23 24 25 27 28 29 30 31 32 33 34 35 38 39 41 42 43 44 45 46 47 48 49 51 53 54 55 56 58 59 60 61 62 63 64 65 68 69 70 71 72 74 76 77 78 79 **P** 3 5 **S** Catholic Healthcare West, San Francisco, CA **Web address:** www.mercysacto.org	23	10	325	7951	212	68837	1704	74964	30684	583
□ SHRINERS HOSPITALS FOR CHILDREN, NORTHERN CALIFORNIA, 2425 Stockton Boulevard, Zip 95817–2215; tel. 916/453–2000; Margaret Bryan, Administrator **A** 1 5 **F** 10 13 17 18 32 38 43 48 49 50 51 53 54 70 71 72 76 78 **P** 6 **S** Shriners Hospitals for Children, Tampa, FL **Web address:** www.shrinershq.org	23	57	50	1258	35	16675	—	—	—	385
★ SUTTER CENTER FOR PSYCHIATRY, 7700 Folsom Boulevard, Zip 95826–2608; tel. 916/386–3000; Diane Gail Stewart, Chief Administrative Officer **A** 9 10 **F** 3 4 7 8 9 11 12 14 15 17 19 20 22 24 25 30 31 32 33 34 35 36 37 38 39 41 42 43 44 45 46 47 48 49 50 51 52 53 54 55 56 57 58 59 60 61 62 63 64 65 66 67 68 69 70 71 72 73 74 76 77 78 79 **P** 5 **S** Sutter Health, Sacramento, CA **Web address:** www.sutterhealth.org	23	22	69	2283	41	3657	0	—	—	116

© 2000 AHA Guide   *Many Facility Codes have changed. Please refer to the AHA Guide Code Chart.*

Hospitals, U.S. / CALIFORNIA

Hospital, Address, Telephone, Administrator, Approval, Facility, and Physician Codes, Health Care System, Network	Classification Codes		Utilization Data					Expense (thousands) of dollars		
	Control	Service	Staffed Beds	Admissions	Census	Outpatient Visits	Births	Total	Payroll	Personnel

★ American Hospital Association (AHA) membership
☐ Joint Commission on Accreditation of Healthcare Organizations (JCAHO) accreditation
+ American Osteopathic Healthcare Association (AOHA) membership
○ American Osteopathic Association (AOA) accreditation
△ Commission on Accreditation of Rehabilitation Facilities (CARF) accreditation
Control codes 61, 63, 64, 71, 72 and 73 indicate hospitals listed by AOHA, but not registered by AHA. For definition of numerical codes, see page A4

Hospital	Control	Service	Beds	Admissions	Census	Outpatient	Births	Total	Payroll	Personnel
★ SUTTER MEDICAL CENTER, (Formerly Sutter Community Hospitals), (Includes Sutter General Hospital, 2801 L Street, Zip 95816; tel. 916/454-2222; Sutter Memorial Hospital, 5151 F Street, 5151 F Street, Zip 95819-3295; tel. 916/454-3333; Lawrence A. Maas, Chief Executive Officer (Total facility includes 186 beds in nursing home-type unit) **A**1 2 3 5 9 10 **F**1 2 3 4 5 6 7 8 9 11 12 13 16 17 18 19 20 21 22 23 24 25 27 29 30 31 32 33 34 35 36 37 38 39 40 41 42 43 44 45 46 47 48 49 50 51 52 54 55 57 58 59 60 61 62 63 64 65 66 68 69 70 72 73 74 75 76 77 78 79 **P**3 5 **S** Sutter Health, Sacramento, CA Web address: www.sutterhealth.org	23	10	469	27635	479	270623	4472	264393	111613	4077
★ UNIVERSITY OF CALIFORNIA, DAVIS MEDICAL CENTER, 2315 Stockton Boulevard, Zip 95817-2282; tel. 916/734-2011; Martha H. Marsh, Director **A**1 2 3 5 8 9 10 **F**4 5 7 8 9 10 11 12 13 14 16 17 18 19 21 22 23 24 25 27 28 29 30 31 32 33 34 35 36 37 38 39 41 42 43 44 45 46 47 48 49 50 51 52 54 55 56 65 68 70 71 72 74 75 76 77 78 79 **P**1 6 7 **S** University of California–Systemwide Administration, Oakland, CA	12	10	464	30491	374	961622	1406	582034	244424	7086
SALINAS—Monterey County										
★ NATIVIDAD MEDICAL CENTER, 1441 Constitution Boulevard, Zip 93906, Mailing Address: P.O. Box 81611, Zip 93912-1611; tel. 831/755-4111; Howard H. Classen, Chief Executive Officer (Total facility includes 52 beds in nursing home-type unit) (Nonreporting) **A**1 3 5 9 10 Web address: www.natividad.com	13	10	181	—	—	—	—	—	—	—
★ SALINAS VALLEY MEMORIAL HEALTHCARE SYSTEM, 450 East Romie Lane, Zip 93901-4098; tel. 831/757-4333; Samuel W. Downing, Chief Executive Officer (Nonreporting) **A**1 2 9 10 Web address: www.svmh.com	16	10	177	—	—	—	—	—	—	—
SAN ANDREAS—Calaveras County										
★ MARK TWAIN ST. JOSEPH'S HOSPITAL, 768 Mountain Ranch Road, Zip 95249-9710; tel. 209/754-2515; Michael P. Lawson, Administrator **A**1 9 10 **F**7 8 9 16 17 18 19 22 24 25 26 29 32 33 34 35 36 37 38 40 45 48 49 51 54 70 72 76 77 78 79 **P**5 **S** Catholic Healthcare West, San Francisco, CA Web address: www.chw.edu	23	10	30	1385	14	59949	29	18502	6674	223
SAN BERNARDINO—San Bernardino County										
★ COMMMUNITY HOSPITAL OF SAN BERNARDINO, 1805 Medical Center Drive, Zip 92411; tel. 909/887-6333; Bruce G. Satzger, President (Total facility includes 99 beds in nursing home-type unit) **A**1 9 10 **F**1 4 7 8 9 11 12 13 14 17 18 19 21 22 23 24 25 29 31 32 33 34 35 36 37 38 39 40 41 42 43 44 45 46 47 48 49 50 51 53 54 57 58 59 61 62 66 69 70 72 74 75 76 77 78 79 **P**5 **S** Catholic Healthcare West, San Francisco, CA Web address: www.chsb.org	23	10	373	10345	228	102799	2545	86253	35826	1225
★ ST. BERNARDINE MEDICAL CENTER, 2101 North Waterman Avenue, Zip 92404; tel. 909/883-8711; Steven R. Barron, President **A**1 2 9 10 **F**3 4 7 8 9 11 12 13 16 17 18 19 22 24 25 26 28 29 30 32 33 34 36 37 38 39 41 42 43 44 45 46 47 48 49 50 51 54 65 70 71 72 74 76 78 79 **P**4 5 6 7 **S** Catholic Healthcare West, San Francisco, CA	21	10	268	11555	170	92612	1414	108658	41967	1116
SAN CLEMENTE—Orange County										
☐ SAN CLEMENTE HOSPITAL AND MEDICAL CENTER, 654 Camino De Los Mares, Zip 92673; tel. 949/496-1122; Patricia L. Wolfram, R.N., Chief Executive Officer **A**1 9 10 **F**1 2 3 4 5 6 7 8 9 10 11 12 13 14 15 16 17 18 19 20 21 22 24 25 27 32 34 36 37 38 39 40 41 42 43 44 45 46 47 48 49 50 52 54 57 65 66 69 70 71 72 75 76 78 79 **P**1 2 3 4 5 6 7 8 **S** NetCare Health Systems, Inc., Nashville, TN Web address: www.sanclementehospital.com	33	10	71	2489	26	21403	279	17855	8518	253
SAN DIEGO—San Diego County										
★ ALVARADO HOSPITAL MEDICAL CENTER, 6655 Alvarado Road, Zip 92120-5298; tel. 619/287-3270; Barry G. Weinbaum, Chief Executive Officer (Nonreporting) **A**1 2 3 9 10 **S** TENET Healthcare Corporation, Santa Barbara, CA Web address: www.tenethealh.com	33	10	144	—	—	—	—	—	—	—
☐ CHARTER BEHAVIORAL HEALTH SYSTEM OF SAN DIEGO, 11878 Avenue of Industry, Zip 92128; tel. 619/487-3200; Robert A. Deney, Chief Executive Officer (Nonreporting) **A**1 9 10	33	22	80	—	—	—	—	—	—	—
☐ △ CHILDREN'S HOSPITAL AND HEALTH CENTER, 3020 Children's Way, Zip 92123-4282; tel. 858/576-1700; Blair L. Sadler, President and Chief Executive Officer (Total facility includes 59 beds in nursing home-type unit) (Nonreporting) **A**1 3 5 7 9 10 Web address: www.chsd.org	23	50	283	—	—	—	—	—	—	—
★ KAISER FOUNDATION HOSPITAL, (Includes Kaiser Foundation Hospital, 203 Travelodge Drive, El Cajon, Zip 92020; tel. 619/528-5000), 4647 Zion Avenue, Zip 92120; tel. 619/528-5000; Terry A. Belmont, Administrator **A**1 2 3 5 10 **F**2 3 4 8 9 11 13 14 16 17 18 19 21 22 24 25 27 29 30 32 33 34 35 36 37 39 41 42 43 44 45 46 47 48 49 50 51 56 57 58 61 63 66 68 69 70 72 76 77 78 79 **S** Kaiser Foundation Hospitals, Oakland, CA Web address: www.kaiserpermanente.org	23	10	310	24330	251	138775	5151	—	—	—
★ MISSION BAY HOSPITAL, (Formerly Mission Bay Memorial Hospital), 3030 Bunker Hill Street, Zip 92109-5780; tel. 619/274-7721; Deborah Brehe, Chief Executive Officer (Total facility includes 26 beds in nursing home-type unit) **A**1 9 10 **F**7 9 12 13 16 18 19 22 25 30 31 32 34 38 39 41 45 48 51 54 57 62 69 70 76 78 **S** Triad Hospitals, Inc., Dallas, TX Web address: www.mbhosp.com	33	10	91	3372	44	16021	—	23139	11560	243

Hospitals, U.S. / CALIFORNIA

Hospital, Address, Telephone, Administrator, Approval, Facility, and Physician Codes, Health Care System, Network	Classification Codes		Utilization Data					Expense (thousands) of dollars		
★ American Hospital Association (AHA) membership □ Joint Commission on Accreditation of Healthcare Organizations (JCAHO) accreditation + American Osteopathic Healthcare Association (AOHA) membership ○ American Osteopathic Association (AOA) accreditation △ Commission on Accreditation of Rehabilitation Facilities (CARF) accreditation Control codes 61, 63, 64, 71, 72 and 73 indicate hospitals listed by AOHA, but not registered by AHA. For definition of numerical codes, see page A4	Control	Service	Staffed Beds	Admissions	Census	Outpatient Visits	Births	Total	Payroll	Personnel
★ NAVAL MEDICAL CENTER, 34800 Bob Wilson Drive, Zip 92134–5000; tel. 619/532–6400; Rear Admiral Alberto Diaz, Jr, MC, USN, Commander **A**1 2 3 5 **F**3 4 5 8 9 11 12 13 14 18 21 22 23 24 25 27 28 29 32 33 34 38 39 41 42 43 44 45 46 47 48 49 50 51 52 54 56 57 58 59 61 63 65 66 68 70 71 72 74 76 78 **S** Department of Navy, Washington, DC	43	10	288	20697	176	1074746	3639	182871	41741	5496
□ SAN DIEGO COUNTY PSYCHIATRIC HOSPITAL, 3851 Rosecrans Street, Zip 92110, Mailing Address: P.O. Box 85524, Zip 92138–5524; tel. 619/692–8211; Karen C. Hogan, Administrator and Chief Executive Officer (Nonreporting) **A**1 10	13	22	109	—	—	—	—	—	—	—
★ SAN DIEGO HOSPICE, 4311 Third Avenue, Zip 92103; tel. 619/688–1600; Janet E. Cetti, President and Chief Executive Officer (Nonreporting) **A**10 **Web address:** www.sdhospice.com	23	49	24	—	—	—	—	—	—	—
★ SCRIPPS MERCY HOSPITAL, 4077 Fifth Avenue, Zip 92103–2180; tel. 619/294–8111; Thomas A. Gammiere, Senior Vice President and Regional Administrator **A**1 2 3 5 9 10 **F**2 3 4 7 9 11 12 13 16 17 18 19 21 22 24 25 26 28 30 31 32 33 34 38 39 41 42 43 44 45 46 47 48 50 51 52 53 54 56 57 58 59 60 61 62 63 64 65 69 70 71 72 74 75 76 77 78 79 **P**3 5 **S** Scripps Health, San Diego, CA	23	10	447	20746	262	105407	2830	149151	6086	1790
★ SHARP CABRILLO HOSPITAL, 3475 Kenyon Street, Zip 92110–5067; tel. 619/221–3400; Randi Larsson, Vice President (Total facility includes 79 beds in nursing home–type unit) (Nonreporting) **A**1 9 10 **S** Sharp Healthcare, San Diego, CA **Web address:** www.sharp.com	23	10	227	—	—	—	—	—	—	—
★ △ SHARP MEMORIAL HOSPITAL, 7901 Frost Street, Zip 92123–2788; tel. 858/541–3400; Dan Gross, Chief Executive Officer (Nonreporting) **A**1 2 3 7 9 10 **S** Sharp Healthcare, San Diego, CA **Web address:** www.sharp.com	23	10	488	—	—	—	—	—	—	—
★ SHARP MESA VISTA HOSPITAL, (Formerly Mesa Vista Hospital), 7850 Vista Hill Avenue, Zip 92123–2790; tel. 858/694–8300; Karenlee Robinson, Chief Operating Officer (Nonreporting) **S** Sharp Healthcare, San Diego, CA **Web address:** www.sharp.com	23	22	166	—	—	—	—	—	—	—
★ UNIVERSITY OF CALIFORNIA SAN DIEGO MEDICAL CENTER, 200 West Arbor Drive, Zip 92103–8970; tel. 619/543–6222; Sumiyo E. Kastelic, Director **A**1 2 3 5 8 9 10 **F**4 7 8 9 10 11 12 13 17 19 22 24 29 30 31 32 33 34 35 36 38 39 41 42 44 45 46 47 48 49 50 51 52 54 56 57 58 59 61 62 63 65 66 70 74 75 76 77 78 79 **P**1 5 **S** University of California–Systemwide Administration, Oakland, CA	12	10	468	20133	298	515448	1852	305886	111957	3400
□ VENCOR HOSPITAL–SAN DIEGO, 1940 El Cajon Boulevard, Zip 92104; tel. 619/543–4500; William Mitchell, Administrator (Nonreporting) **A**1 10 **S** Vencor, Incorporated, Louisville, KY	33	10	70	—	—	—	—	—	—	—
★ VETERANS AFFAIRS MEDICAL CENTER, 3350 LaJolla Village Drive, Zip 92161; tel. 858/552–8585; Gary J. Rossio, Director and Chief Executive Officer (Total facility includes 69 beds in nursing home–type unit) **A**1 2 3 5 8 9 **F**1 2 3 4 5 6 9 11 12 13 16 17 18 19 20 21 22 23 24 25 26 27 28 29 30 31 32 33 34 35 36 37 38 39 41 43 45 46 47 48 49 50 51 53 54 55 56 57 59 60 61 62 63 64 65 69 70 72 74 76 77 78 79 **P**6 **S** Department of Veterans Affairs, Washington, DC **Web address:** www.va.gov/stations97/guide/home.asp?DIVISION=ALL	45	10	232	6176	182	326671	0	185522	101975	1819
□ VILLAVIEW COMMUNITY HOSPITAL, 5550 University Avenue, Zip 92105, Mailing Address: P.O. Box 5587, Zip 92105; tel. 619/582–3516; Roy Rodriguez, Ph.D., Chief Executive Officer (Nonreporting) **A**1 9 10	23	10	100	—	—	—	—	—	—	—

SAN DIMAS—Los Angeles County

★ SAN DIMAS COMMUNITY HOSPITAL, 1350 West Covina Boulevard, Zip 91773–0308; tel. 909/599–6811; Garry M. Olney, R.N., Chief Executive Officer **A**1 2 9 10 **F**8 9 13 17 19 22 24 25 29 30 32 34 39 41 44 45 48 49 51 54 69 70 76 78 79 **P**5 **S** TENET Healthcare Corporation, Santa Barbara, CA **Web address:** www.tenethealth.com	33	10	93	3362	56	30378	816	—	—	292

SAN FERNANDO—Los Angeles County

□ MISSION COMMUNITY HOSPITAL–SAN FERNANDO CAMPUS, (Includes Mission Community Hospital–Panorama City Campus, 14850 Roscoe Boulevard, Panorama City, Zip 91402–4618; tel. 818/787–2222), 700 Chatsworth Drive, Zip 91340–4299; tel. 818/361–7331; William W. Daniel, Chief Executive Officer (Nonreporting) **A**1 9	23	10	152	—	—	—	—	—	—	—

SAN FRANCISCO—San Francisco County

★ △ CALIFORNIA PACIFIC MEDICAL CENTER, (Includes California Pacific Medical Center–Davies Campus, Castro and Duboce Streets, Zip 94114; tel. 415/565–6000), 2333 Buchanan Street, Zip 94115, Mailing Address: P.O. Box 7999, Zip 94120; tel. 415/563–4321; Martin Brotman, M.D., President and Chief Executive Officer (Total facility includes 95 beds in nursing home–type unit) (Nonreporting) **A**1 2 3 5 7 8 9 10 **S** Sutter Health, Sacramento, CA **Web address:** www.cpmc.org	23	10	520	—	—	—	—	—	—	—
★ CHINESE HOSPITAL, 845 Jackson Street, Zip 94133–4899; tel. 415/982–2400; Jan Robert Long, Chief Executive Officer **A**1 9 10 **F**4 7 8 9 10 11 12 13 16 17 18 19 22 24 25 29 31 32 33 34 36 37 39 41 42 44 45 46 47 48 50 51 52 53 55 57 65 68 69 70 72 74 75 76 78 **P**5 7	23	10	54	2010	30	45568	0	31500	9468	140
★ KAISER FOUNDATION HOSPITAL, 2425 Geary Boulevard, Zip 94115; tel. 415/202–2000; Julie A. Petrini, Administrator (Nonreporting) **A**1 3 5 10 **S** Kaiser Foundation Hospitals, Oakland, CA **Web address:** www.kaiserpermanente.org	23	10	210	—	—	—	—	—	—	—

Hospitals, U.S. / CALIFORNIA

Hospital, Address, Telephone, Administrator, Approval, Facility, and Physician Codes, Health Care System, Network

- ★ American Hospital Association (AHA) membership
- ☐ Joint Commission on Accreditation of Healthcare Organizations (JCAHO) accreditation
- + American Osteopathic Healthcare Association (AOHA) membership
- ○ American Osteopathic Association (AOA) accreditation
- △ Commission on Accreditation of Rehabilitation Facilities (CARF) accreditation

Control codes 61, 63, 64, 71, 72 and 73 indicate hospitals listed by AOHA, but not registered by AHA. For definition of numerical codes, see page A4.

Hospital	Control	Service	Staffed Beds	Admissions	Census	Outpatient Visits	Births	Total	Payroll	Personnel
★ LAGUNA HONDA HOSPITAL AND REHABILITATION CENTER, 375 Laguna Honda Boulevard, Zip 94116–1499; tel. 415/664–1580; Lawrence J. Funk, Executive Administrator (Total facility includes 1214 beds in nursing home–type unit) (Nonreporting) **A**10	15	48	1249	—	—	—	—	—	—	—
☐ PACIFIC COAST HOSPITAL, 1210 Scott Street, Zip 94115–4000; tel. 415/292–0554; Robert D. Roberts, President (Nonreporting) **A**1 9 10 Web address: www.ccpm.edu	23	49	28	—	—	—	—	—	—	—
★ △ SAINT FRANCIS MEMORIAL HOSPITAL, 900 Hyde Street, Zip 94109, Mailing Address: Box 7726, Zip 94120–7726; tel. 415/353–6000; Cheryl A. Fama, Administrator, Vice President and Chief Operating Officer **A**1 2 3 7 9 10 **F**1 4 8 9 10 11 12 13 16 17 18 19 20 21 22 24 25 26 27 28 29 31 32 33 34 35 36 37 38 39 41 42 44 45 46 47 48 49 50 51 52 53 54 56 57 58 59 60 61 62 63 64 65 66 67 69 70 71 72 73 74 75 76 77 78 79 **P**3 **S** Catholic Healthcare West, San Francisco, CA Web address: www.chw.edu	21	10	187	8777	130	144762	0	68241	35651	679
★ SAN FRANCISCO GENERAL HOSPITAL MEDICAL CENTER, 1001 Potrero Avenue, Zip 94110; tel. 415/206–8000; Gene O'Connell, Executive Administrator and Director Patient Care Services Community Health Network **A**1 2 3 5 8 10 **F**1 3 4 8 9 11 12 13 14 17 18 19 21 22 23 25 29 30 33 34 35 36 37 38 39 41 42 43 44 45 46 48 49 50 51 54 56 57 59 61 64 66 68 69 70 71 72 75 76 78 79 **P**1 Web address: www.sfgh.org	15	10	537	20603	437	503471	1471	314540	146201	3893
☐ ST. LUKE'S HOSPITAL, 3555 Cesar Chavez Street, Zip 94110; tel. 415/647–8600; Jack E. Fries, President (Total facility includes 33 beds in nursing home–type unit) (Nonreporting) **A**1 9 10 Web address: www.stlukes-sf.org	23	10	254	—	—	—	—	—	—	—
★ ST. MARY'S MEDICAL CENTER, 450 Stanyan Street, Zip 94117–1079; tel. 415/668–1000; Rosemary Fox, Vice President and Chief Operating Officer (Total facility includes 48 beds in nursing home–type unit) **A**1 2 3 5 8 9 10 **F**1 4 7 9 10 11 13 14 16 17 18 19 21 22 24 25 26 27 30 31 32 33 34 35 36 37 38 39 41 43 46 47 48 49 50 51 52 53 54 56 57 58 59 60 61 62 63 64 65 67 69 70 71 72 73 76 77 78 79 **P**5 **S** Catholic Healthcare West, San Francisco, CA	23	10	280	10075	201	112092	0	134590	61120	1053
★ UNIVERSITY OF CALIFORNIA SAN FRANCISCO MEDICAL CENTER, (Includes University of California–San Francisco Mount Zion Medical Center, 1600 Divisadero Street, Zip 94143–1601; tel. 415/567–6600), 500 Parnassus, Zip 94143–0296; tel. 415/476–1000; Mark R. Laret, Chief Executive Officer **A**1 2 3 5 8 9 10 **F**1 2 3 4 5 7 8 9 10 11 12 13 14 15 16 17 18 19 20 21 22 23 24 25 26 27 28 29 30 31 32 33 34 35 36 37 38 39 40 41 42 43 44 45 46 47 48 49 50 51 52 53 54 55 56 57 58 59 60 61 62 63 64 65 66 69 70 71 72 73 74 76 77 78 79 **P**5 6 **S** University of California–Systemwide Administration, Oakland, CA Web address: www.ucsfstanford.org	23	10	661	27296	478	564019	1727	789979	237674	4232
★ VETERANS AFFAIRS MEDICAL CENTER, 4150 Clement Street, Zip 94121–1598; tel. 415/221–4810; Sheila M. Cullen, Director (Total facility includes 112 beds in nursing home–type unit) **A**1 2 3 5 8 **F**1 3 4 7 11 12 18 19 22 23 24 25 26 28 29 30 31 32 33 34 35 36 37 38 39 41 43 45 46 47 48 49 50 51 54 56 57 59 61 62 63 64 68 69 70 72 74 76 78 79 **P**6 **S** Department of Veterans Affairs, Washington, DC Web address: www.va.gov/stations97/guide/home.asp?DIVISION=ALL	45	10	244	5073	204	316535	0	173395	84902	1797

SAN GABRIEL—Los Angeles County

Hospital	Control	Service	Staffed Beds	Admissions	Census	Outpatient Visits	Births	Total	Payroll	Personnel
★ SAN GABRIEL VALLEY MEDICAL CENTER, 438 West Las Tunas Drive, Zip 91776, Mailing Address: P.O. Box 1507, Zip 91778–1507; tel. 626/289–5454; Steven A. Fellows, President **A**1 9 10 **F**3 4 8 9 11 13 17 18 19 22 24 25 29 30 31 32 34 38 39 41 42 43 44 45 46 48 50 51 53 54 57 62 63 64 65 68 69 70 72 73 76 78 **P**4 5 7 **S** Catholic Healthcare West, San Francisco, CA Web address: www.sgvmc.org	23	10	274	7412	167	42556	1217	62092	25090	811

SAN JOSE—Santa Clara County

Hospital	Control	Service	Staffed Beds	Admissions	Census	Outpatient Visits	Births	Total	Payroll	Personnel
★ GOOD SAMARITAN HOSPITAL, 2425 Samaritan Drive, Zip 95124, Mailing Address: P.O. Box 240002, Zip 95154–2402; tel. 408/559–2011; William K. Piche, Chief Executive Officer **A**1 9 10 **F**3 4 7 8 9 11 12 13 18 22 25 28 34 39 41 42 44 45 46 47 48 54 57 59 63 64 65 70 76 78 79 **P**8 Web address: www.goodsamsj.org	33	10	332	18365	231	87380	4357	201831	81327	1289
★ O'CONNOR HOSPITAL, 2105 Forest Avenue, Zip 95128; tel. 408/947–2500; Joan A. Bero, Regional Vice President and Chief Operating Officer **A**1 2 9 10 **F**4 8 9 11 12 13 14 16 17 18 19 20 22 24 25 28 32 34 36 37 38 39 40 41 43 44 45 46 47 48 50 51 54 57 62 65 68 69 70 71 72 73 76 78 **P**5 7 **S** Catholic Healthcare West, San Francisco, CA Web address: www.chwbay.org	21	10	283	11393	147	97191	2546	111222	49622	799
★ REGIONAL MEDICAL CENTER OF SAN JOSE, 225 North Jackson Avenue, Zip 95116–1691; tel. 408/259–5000; Steven R. Barron, President and Chief Executive Officer (Nonreporting) **A**1 9 10 **S** HCA – The Healthcare Company, Nashville, TN	33	10	192	—	—	—	—	—	—	—
★ SAN JOSE MEDICAL CENTER, 675 East Santa Clara Street, Zip 95112, Mailing Address: P.O. Box 240003, Zip 95154–2403; tel. 408/998–3212; William L. Gilbert, Chief Executive Officer (Total facility includes 26 beds in nursing home–type unit) (Nonreporting) **A**1 2 3 5 9 10 **S** HCA – The Healthcare Company, Nashville, TN Web address: www.hcahealthcare.com	33	10	327	—	—	—	—	—	—	—

Many Facility Codes have changed. Please refer to the AHA Guide Code Chart.

Hospitals, U.S. / CALIFORNIA

Hospital, Address, Telephone, Administrator, Approval, Facility, and Physician Codes, Health Care System, Network	Classification Codes		Utilization Data					Expense (thousands) of dollars		
★ American Hospital Association (AHA) membership ☐ Joint Commission on Accreditation of Healthcare Organizations (JCAHO) accreditation + American Osteopathic Healthcare Association (AOHA) membership ○ American Osteopathic Association (AOA) accreditation △ Commission on Accreditation of Rehabilitation Facilities (CARF) accreditation Control codes 61, 63, 64, 71, 72 and 73 indicate hospitals listed by AOHA, but not registered by AHA. For definition of numerical codes, see page A4	Control	Service	Staffed Beds	Admissions	Census	Outpatient Visits	Births	Total	Payroll	Personnel
☐ SANTA CLARA VALLEY MEDICAL CENTER, (Formerly Santa Clara Valley Health and Hospital System), 751 South Bascom Avenue, Zip 95128; tel. 408/885–5000; Susan Murphy, Director (Nonreporting) **A**1 2 3 5 9 10 **Web address:** www.scvmea.org	13	10	377	—	—	—	—	—	—	—
✪ SANTA TERESA COMMUNITY MEDICAL CENTER, (Formerly Santa Teresa Community Hospital), 250 Hospital Parkway, Zip 95119; tel. 408/972–7000; Joann Zimmerman, Administrator (Nonreporting) **A**1 3 10 **S** Kaiser Foundation Hospitals, Oakland, CA	23	10	178	—	—	—	—	—	—	—
SAN LEANDRO—Alameda County										
☐ ALAMEDA COUNTY MEDICAL CENTER, 15400 Foothill Boulevard, Zip 94578–1091; tel. 510/437–4800; Michael L. Walls, Chief Executive Officer (Total facility includes 119 beds in nursing home–type unit) (Nonreporting) **A**1 **S** Alameda County Health Care Services Agency, San Leandro, CA	13	49	193	—	—	—	—	—	—	—
✪ SAN LEANDRO HOSPITAL, 13855 East 14th Street, Zip 94578–0398; tel. 510/357–6500; Carol B. Freeman, Interim Chief Executive Officer (Nonreporting) **A**1 9 10 **S** Triad Hospitals, Inc., Dallas, TX	33	10	136	—	—	—	—	—	—	—
☐ VENCOR HOSPITAL–SAN LEANDRO, 2800 Benedict Drive, Zip 94577; tel. 510/357–8300; Carole Wilson, MSN, CHE, Administrator and Chief Executive Officer (Nonreporting) **A**1 10 **S** Vencor, Incorporated, Louisville, KY	33	10	42	—	—	—	—	—	—	—
SAN LUIS OBISPO—San Luis Obispo County										
CALIFORNIA MENS COLONY HOSPITAL, Highway 1, Zip 93409–8101; Mailing Address: P.O. Box 8101, Zip 93409–8101; tel. 805/547–7913; Galen Kirn, Administrator (Nonreporting)	12	11	39	—	—	—	—	—	—	—
☐ FRENCH HOSPITAL MEDICAL CENTER, 1911 Johnson Avenue, Zip 93401; tel. 805/543–5353; Gale E. Gascho, Chief Executive Officer (Nonreporting) **A**1 9 10	33	10	124	—	—	—	—	—	—	—
☐ SAN LUIS OBISPO GENERAL HOSPITAL, 2180 Johnson Avenue, Zip 93401, Mailing Address: Box 8113, Zip 93403–8113; tel. 805/781–4800; Erich J. Wolters, Chief Executive Officer (Nonreporting) **A**1 9 10	13	10	46	—	—	—	—	—	—	—
✪ △ SIERRA VISTA REGIONAL MEDICAL CENTER, 1010 Murray Street, Zip 93405, Mailing Address: Box 1367, Zip 93406–1367; tel. 805/546–7600; Sean O'Neal, Administrator (Nonreporting) **A**1 7 9 10 **S** TENET Healthcare Corporation, Santa Barbara, CA **Web address:** www.tenethealth.com	33	10	117	—	—	—	—	—	—	—
SAN MATEO—San Mateo County										
MILLS HOSPITAL See Mills–Peninsula Health Services, Burlingame										
☐ SAN MATEO COUNTY GENERAL HOSPITAL AND CLINICS, 222 West 39th Avenue, Zip 94403–4398; tel. 650/573–2222; Timothy B. McMurdo, Chief Executive Officer (Total facility includes 94 beds in nursing home–type unit) **A**1 3 5 10 **F**4 8 9 11 12 13 16 17 18 19 22 23 24 25 27 29 31 34 35 37 38 39 40 41 42 43 46 47 48 52 54 56 57 59 61 65 66 69 70 73 75 76 78 79 **P**5 6	13	10	179	3570	158	182972	0	98431	40268	1123
SAN PABLO—Contra Costa County										
✪ DOCTORS MEDICAL CENTER–SAN PABLO CAMPUS, 2000 Vale Road, Zip 94806; tel. 510/970–5102; Gary Sloan, Chief Executive Officer (Total facility includes 106 beds in nursing home–type unit) (Nonreporting) **A**1 2 9 10 **S** TENET Healthcare Corporation, Santa Barbara, CA	33	10	286	—	—	—	—	—	—	—
SAN PEDRO—Los Angeles County, See Los Angeles										
SAN RAFAEL—Marin County										
✪ KAISER FOUNDATION HOSPITAL, 99 Montecillo Road, Zip 94903–3397; tel. 415/444–2000; Julie A. Petrini, Administrator **A**1 10 **F**4 9 11 13 14 16 17 19 22 24 25 29 33 34 35 36 38 39 41 43 45 46 47 48 50 51 54 56 63 65 68 70 72 76 77 78 79 **S** Kaiser Foundation Hospitals, Oakland, CA **Web address:** www.kaiserpermanente.org	23	10	119	4768	55	385384	0	—	—	143
SAN RAMON—Contra Costa County										
✪ △ SAN RAMON REGIONAL MEDICAL CENTER, 6001 Norris Canyon Road, Zip 94583; tel. 925/275–9200; Philip P. Gustafson, Administrator **A**1 7 9 10 **F**4 8 9 11 12 13 17 18 19 22 24 25 31 32 34 35 38 39 41 42 43 44 45 46 47 48 51 54 64 66 70 71 72 76 78 79 **P**4 5 7 **S** TENET Healthcare Corporation, Santa Barbara, CA **Web address:** www.sanramonmedctr.com	33	10	95	4374	45	50722	967	41167	19825	445
SANGER—Fresno County										
☐ SANGER GENERAL HOSPITAL, 2558 Jensen Avenue, Zip 93657–2296; tel. 559/875–6571; Jerry E. Gillman, Chief Executive Officer **A**1 9 10 **F**8 13 22 31 32 39 44 48 51 69 70 76 77	32	10	39	851	14	—	480	4786	2055	82
SANTA ANA—Orange County										
✪ COASTAL COMMUNITIES HOSPITAL, 2701 South Bristol Street, Zip 92704–9911; tel. 714/754–5454; Robert C. Caldwell, Chief Executive Officer (Total facility includes 46 beds in nursing home–type unit) **A**1 9 10 **F**7 9 13 17 18 22 23 24 25 31 38 39 41 43 44 45 48 51 56 57 62 65 68 69 70 76 79 **P**7 **S** TENET Healthcare Corporation, Santa Barbara, CA **Web address:** www.tenethealh.com	33	10	178	4040	88	21489	1743	—	—	398
✪ SANTA ANA HOSPITAL MEDICAL CENTER, 1901 North Fairview Street, Zip 92706; tel. 714/554–1653; Robert C. Caldwell, Chief Executive Officer **A**1 9 10 **F**2 3 4 7 8 9 10 11 12 13 18 19 21 22 24 25 27 29 30 31 32 33 34 36 37 38 39 41 42 43 44 45 46 47 48 49 50 51 52 53 54 57 62 65 66 70 71 72 75 76 77 78 79 **S** TENET Healthcare Corporation, Santa Barbara, CA **Web address:** www.tenethealth.com	33	10	90	3417	20	12999	2498	—	—	170

© 2000 AHA Guide   *Many Facility Codes have changed. Please refer to the AHA Guide Code Chart.*

Hospitals, U.S. / CALIFORNIA

Hospital, Address, Telephone, Administrator, Approval, Facility, and Physician Codes, Health Care System, Network	Classification Codes		Utilization Data					Expense (thousands) of dollars		
	Control	Service	Staffed Beds	Admissions	Census	Outpatient Visits	Births	Total	Payroll	Personnel

★ American Hospital Association (AHA) membership
☐ Joint Commission on Accreditation of Healthcare Organizations (JCAHO) accreditation
+ American Osteopathic Healthcare Association (AOHA) membership
○ American Osteopathic Association (AOA) accreditation
△ Commission on Accreditation of Rehabilitation Facilities (CARF) accreditation
Control codes 61, 63, 64, 71, 72 and 73 indicate hospitals listed by AOHA, but not registered by AHA. For definition of numerical codes, see page A4

Hospital	Control	Service	Staffed Beds	Admissions	Census	Outpatient Visits	Births	Total	Payroll	Personnel
SPECIALTY HOSPITAL OF SANTA ANA, 1901 North College Avenue, Zip 92706; tel. 714/564–7800; Richard Luna, Chief Executive Officer (Nonreporting) Web address: www.specialtyhealthcare.com	33	10	54	—	—	—	—	—	—	—
★ WESTERN MEDICAL CENTER–SANTA ANA, 1001 North Tustin Avenue, Zip 92705–3502; tel. 714/835–3555; Daniel Brothman, Chief Executive Officer (Total facility includes 14 beds in nursing home–type unit) A1 2 3 5 9 10 F1 4 7 8 9 11 12 13 17 18 19 20 22 24 25 27 31 32 34 36 39 40 41 42 44 45 46 47 48 49 51 52 54 57 58 59 61 62 64 65 69 70 72 73 75 76 77 78 P5 S TENET Healthcare Corporation, Santa Barbara, CA Web address: www.tenethealth.com/westermedical	33	10	296	11441	135	68002	2596	—	—	975

SANTA BARBARA—Santa Barbara County

Hospital	Control	Service	Staffed Beds	Admissions	Census	Outpatient Visits	Births	Total	Payroll	Personnel
☐ GOLETA VALLEY COTTAGE HOSPITAL, 351 South Patterson Avenue, Zip 93111, Mailing Address: Box 6306, Zip 93160; tel. 805/967–3411; James L. Ash, President and Chief Executive Officer (Nonreporting) A1 10 S Cottage Health System, Santa Barbara, CA Web address: www.sbch.org	23	10	79	—	—	—	—	—	—	—
☐ △ REHABILITATION INSTITUTE AT SANTA BARBARA, 427 Camino Del Remedio, Zip 93110; tel. 805/683–3788; Rusty Pollock, President and Chief Executive Officer (Nonreporting) A1 7 9 10	23	46	40	—	—	—	—	—	—	—
☐ SANTA BARBARA COTTAGE HOSPITAL, Pueblo at Bath Streets, Zip 93105, Mailing Address: Box 689, Zip 93102; tel. 805/682–7111; Ron Werft, President and Chief Executive Officer (Total facility includes 41 beds in nursing home–type unit) A1 2 3 5 9 10 F2 3 4 7 9 11 12 13 16 17 18 19 21 22 24 25 27 28 29 30 31 32 33 34 38 39 41 42 43 44 45 46 47 48 49 51 52 54 57 61 63 65 69 70 72 76 78 79 S Cottage Health System, Santa Barbara, CA Web address: www.cottagehealthsystem.org	23	10	336	17478	223	103017	2080	142723	56680	1859
★ ST. FRANCIS MEDICAL CENTER OF SANTA BARBARA, 601 East Micheltorena Street, Zip 93103; tel. 805/568–5705; Ron Biscaro, Administrator and Chief Operating Officer (Total facility includes 15 beds in nursing home–type unit) A1 9 10 F2 6 8 9 11 12 13 16 17 18 19 22 25 30 31 32 34 39 41 43 44 45 48 51 53 54 62 70 72 76 78 S Catholic Healthcare West, San Francisco, CA	21	10	85	3035	44	21364	336	27752	12244	265

SANTA CLARA—Santa Clara County

Hospital	Control	Service	Staffed Beds	Admissions	Census	Outpatient Visits	Births	Total	Payroll	Personnel
★ KAISER FOUNDATION HOSPITAL, 900 Kiely Boulevard, Zip 95051–5386; tel. 408/236–6400; Joann Zimmerman, Administrator (Nonreporting) A1 3 5 10 S Kaiser Foundation Hospitals, Oakland, CA Web address: www.kaiserpermanente.org	23	10	249	—	—	—	—	—	—	—

SANTA CRUZ—Santa Cruz County

Hospital	Control	Service	Staffed Beds	Admissions	Census	Outpatient Visits	Births	Total	Payroll	Personnel
★ DOMINICAN HOSPITAL, (Formerly Dominican Santa Cruz Hospital), 1555 Soquel Drive, Zip 95065; tel. 831/462–7700; Sister Julie Hyer, President and Chief Executive Officer (Total facility includes 41 beds in nursing home–type unit) A1 9 10 F4 6 7 8 9 11 13 14 16 17 19 22 25 29 34 36 38 39 41 44 45 46 47 48 49 50 51 53 54 57 59 61 64 65 67 69 70 71 72 73 74 76 77 78 79 P3 5 7 S Catholic Healthcare West, San Francisco, CA Web address: www.dominicanhospital.org	21	10	275	11914	158	124431	1159	112777	51017	969
★ SUTTER MATERNITY AND SURGERY CENTER OF SANTA CRUZ, 2900 Chanticleer Avenue, Zip 95065–1816; tel. 831/477–2200; David T. Hughes, FACHE, Chief Executive Officer A1 9 10 F8 16 17 18 19 20 27 32 33 36 38 44 48 49 70 77 78 P3 S Sutter Health, Sacramento, CA Web address: www.sutterhealth.org	23	10	30	1907	13	—	775	13835	3975	104

SANTA MARIA—Santa Barbara County

Hospital	Control	Service	Staffed Beds	Admissions	Census	Outpatient Visits	Births	Total	Payroll	Personnel
★ MARIAN MEDICAL CENTER, 1400 East Church Street, Zip 93454, Mailing Address: Box 1238, Zip 93456; tel. 805/739–3000; Charles J. Cova, Executive Vice President and Chief Operating Officer (Total facility includes 95 beds in nursing home–type unit) (Nonreporting) A1 2 9 10 S Catholic Healthcare West, San Francisco, CA Web address: www.chw.edu	21	10	225	—	—	—	—	—	—	—

SANTA MONICA—Los Angeles County

Hospital	Control	Service	Staffed Beds	Admissions	Census	Outpatient Visits	Births	Total	Payroll	Personnel
★ SAINT JOHN'S HOSPITAL AND HEALTH CENTER, 1328 22nd Street, Zip 90404–2032; tel. 310/829–5511; Bruce Lamoureux, Chief Executive Officer (Nonreporting) A1 2 9 10 S Sisters of Charity of Leavenworth Health Services Corporation, Leavenworth, KS Web address: www.stjohns.org	21	10	234	—	—	—	—	—	—	—
★ SANTA MONICA–UCLA MEDICAL CENTER, 1250 16th Street, Zip 90404–1200; tel. 310/319–4000; Ellen Pollack, R.N., Interim Chief Operating Officer and Director Nursing (Nonreporting) A1 2 3 5 9 10 S University of California–Systemwide Administration, Oakland, CA	12	10	221	—	—	—	—	—	—	—

SANTA PAULA—Ventura County

Hospital	Control	Service	Staffed Beds	Admissions	Census	Outpatient Visits	Births	Total	Payroll	Personnel
☐ SANTA PAULA MEMORIAL HOSPITAL, 825 North Tenth Street, Zip 93060–0270, Mailing Address: P.O. Box 270, Zip 93061–0270; tel. 805/525–7171; William M. Greene, FACHE, President and Chief Executive Officer A1 9 10 F7 8 9 16 17 18 19 22 24 25 29 34 38 39 41 43 44 46 48 54 70 76 78 P5 S Quorum Health Group, Brentwood, TN Web address: www.santapaulamemorial.org	23	10	34	1816	20	14195	271	14150	5838	197

SANTA ROSA—Sonoma County

Hospital	Control	Service	Staffed Beds	Admissions	Census	Outpatient Visits	Births	Total	Payroll	Personnel
★ KAISER FOUNDATION HOSPITAL, 401 Bicentennial Way, Zip 95403; tel. 707/571–4000; Julie A. Petrini, Administrator A1 10 F8 9 13 14 16 17 18 19 22 25 28 29 31 32 33 34 35 36 37 38 39 41 43 44 45 46 48 49 50 51 54 58 59 60 61 63 66 70 72 73 76 77 78 P6 S Kaiser Foundation Hospitals, Oakland, CA Web address: www.ca.kaiserpermanente.org	23	10	103	6670	58	608844	1412	—	—	1025

Many Facility Codes have changed. Please refer to the AHA Guide Code Chart.

© 2000 AHA Guide

Hospitals, U.S. / CALIFORNIA

Hospital, Address, Telephone, Administrator, Approval, Facility, and Physician Codes, Health Care System, Network	Classification Codes		Utilization Data					Expense (thousands) of dollars		
★ American Hospital Association (AHA) membership ☐ Joint Commission on Accreditation of Healthcare Organizations (JCAHO) accreditation + American Osteopathic Healthcare Association (AOHA) membership ○ American Osteopathic Association (AOA) accreditation △ Commission on Accreditation of Rehabilitation Facilities (CARF) accreditation Control codes 61, 63, 64, 71, 72 and 73 indicate hospitals listed by AOHA, but not registered by AHA. For definition of numerical codes, see page A4	Control	Service	Staffed Beds	Admissions	Census	Outpatient Visits	Births	Total	Payroll	Personnel
★ NORTH COAST HEALTH CARE CENTERS, (Formerly North Coast Hospital), 1287 Fulton Road, Zip 95401; tel. 707/543-2400; Jeffrey Flocken, Interim President and Chief Executive Officer (Nonreporting) **A**1 9 10 **S** St. Joseph Health System, Orange, CA	23	46	119	—	—	—	—	—	—	—
★ SANTA ROSA MEMORIAL HOSPITAL, 1165 Montgomery Drive, Zip 95405, Mailing Address: P.O. Box 522, Zip 95402; tel. 707/546-3210; David J. Ameen, President and Chief Executive Officer (Nonreporting) **A**1 2 9 10 **S** St. Joseph Health System, Orange, CA	21	10	225	—	—	—	—	—	—	—
★ SUTTER MEDICAL CENTER, SANTA ROSA, 3325 Chanate Road, Zip 95404; tel. 707/576-4000; Cliff Coates, Chief Executive Officer (Total facility includes 16 beds in nursing home-type unit) (Nonreporting) **A**1 3 5 9 10 **S** Sutter Health, Sacramento, CA **Web address:** www.sutterhealth.org	23	10	128	—	—	—	—	—	—	—
☐ WARRACK MEDICAL CENTER HOSPITAL, 2449 Summerfield Road, Zip 95405; tel. 707/542-9030; Dale E. Iversen, President and Chief Executive Officer (Nonreporting) **A**1 9 10 **Web address:** www.warrack.com	33	10	79	—	—	—	—	—	—	—
SEBASTOPOL—Sonoma County										
★ PALM DRIVE HOSPITAL, 501 Petaluma Avenue, Zip 95472; tel. 707/823-8511; Robert A. Schapper, Chief Executive Officer (Total facility includes 10 beds in nursing home-type unit) (Nonreporting) **A**1 9 **Web address:** www.palmdrivehospital.com	23	10	48	—	—	—	—	—	—	—
SELMA—Fresno County										
★ SELMA COMMUNITY HOSPITAL, 1141 Rose Avenue, Zip 93662-3293; tel. 559/891-2201; Richard L. Rawson, President (Total facility includes 14 beds in nursing home-type unit) (Nonreporting) **A**1 9 10 **S** Adventist Health, Roseville, CA **Web address:** www.adventisthealth.org	16	10	57	—	—	—	—	—	—	—
SEPULVEDA—Los Angeles County, See Los Angeles **SHERMAN OAKS—Los Angeles County, See Los Angeles** **SIMI VALLEY—Ventura County**										
★ SIMI VALLEY HOSPITAL AND HEALTH CARE SERVICES, (Includes Simi Valley Hospital and Health Care Services–South Campus, 1850 Heywood Street, Zip 93065; tel. 805/955-7000), 2975 North Sycamore Drive, Zip 93065-1277; tel. 805/955-6000; Alan J. Rice, President (Total facility includes 74 beds in nursing home-type unit) (Nonreporting) **A**1 2 9 10 **S** Adventist Health, Roseville, CA **Web address:** www.adventisthealth.org	21	10	225	—	—	—	—	—	—	—
SOLVANG—Santa Barbara County										
☐ SANTA YNEZ VALLEY COTTAGE HOSPITAL, 700 Alamo Pintado Road, Zip 93463; tel. 805/688-6431; Ron Werft, President and Chief Executive Officer (Nonreporting) **A**1 10 **S** Cottage Health System, Santa Barbara, CA **Web address:** www.cottagehealthsystem.org	23	10	20	—	—	—	—	—	—	—
SONOMA—Sonoma County										
☐ SONOMA VALLEY HOSPITAL, 347 Andrieux Street, Zip 95476-6811, Mailing Address: Box 600, Zip 95476-0600; tel. 707/935-5000; Barbara Bamberg, Chief Administrative Officer (Nonreporting) **A**1 9 10 **Web address:** www.svh.com	16	10	86	—	—	—	—	—	—	—
SONORA—Tuolumne County										
★ SONORA COMMUNITY HOSPITAL, 1 South Forest Road, Zip 95370; tel. 209/532-3161; Lary Davis, President (Total facility includes 68 beds in nursing home-type unit) **A**1 9 10 **F**7 8 9 12 13 17 18 19 20 22 24 25 29 30 31 32 33 34 36 38 39 41 43 44 45 46 48 49 50 51 54 56 69 70 71 72 76 77 78 **P**5 **S** Adventist Health, Roseville, CA **Web address:** www.sonoracom.com	21	10	118	3648	94	162760	551	50752	20610	594
☐ TUOLUMNE GENERAL HOSPITAL, 101 Hospital Road, Zip 95370; tel. 209/533-7100; Joseph K. Mitchell, Administrator (Total facility includes 36 beds in nursing home-type unit) **A**1 9 10 **F**1 7 9 12 13 16 17 19 21 22 25 26 27 29 30 32 33 34 35 36 37 38 39 41 43 45 46 48 49 50 51 54 56 57 58 59 60 61 63 66 69 70 72 76 78 **P**6 **Web address:** www.tghospital.com	13	10	80	1891	59	112291	0	21046	10350	310
SOUTH EL MONTE—Los Angeles County										
★ GREATER EL MONTE COMMUNITY HOSPITAL, 1701 South Santa Anita Avenue, Zip 91733-9918; tel. 626/579-7777; Deborah G. Webber, Chief Executive Officer (Total facility includes 13 beds in nursing home-type unit) **A**1 9 10 **F**2 4 5 6 7 8 9 10 11 12 14 15 17 18 19 21 22 23 24 25 26 27 30 31 32 33 34 35 36 37 38 39 40 41 42 43 44 45 46 47 48 49 50 51 52 53 54 55 56 57 58 59 60 61 62 63 64 65 66 68 69 70 71 73 74 75 76 77 78 79 **P**5 **S** TENET Healthcare Corporation, Santa Barbara, CA **Web address:** www.tenethealth.com	16	10	115	3887	49	23921	1107	21325	12043	276
SOUTH LAGUNA—Orange County										
★ SOUTH COAST MEDICAL CENTER, 31872 Coast Highway, Zip 92677; tel. 949/499-1311; T. Michael Murray, President (Total facility includes 29 beds in nursing home-type unit) **A**1 9 10 **F**2 3 7 8 9 12 13 16 17 19 22 24 25 29 31 32 33 34 35 36 38 39 40 41 43 44 45 46 48 50 51 54 57 61 62 63 64 65 69 70 72 76 78 79 **P**5 7 **S** Adventist Health, Roseville, CA **Web address:** www.southcoastmedcenter.com	21	10	155	4522	68	32504	396	43153	19817	361

© 2000 AHA Guide   *Many Facility Codes have changed. Please refer to the AHA Guide Code Chart.*

Hospitals, U.S. / CALIFORNIA

	Classification Codes		Utilization Data					Expense (thousands) of dollars		
Hospital, Address, Telephone, Administrator, Approval, Facility, and Physician Codes, Health Care System, Network	Control	Service	Staffed Beds	Admissions	Census	Outpatient Visits	Births	Total	Payroll	Personnel

★ American Hospital Association (AHA) membership
☐ Joint Commission on Accreditation of Healthcare Organizations (JCAHO) accreditation
+ American Osteopathic Healthcare Association (AOHA) membership
○ American Osteopathic Association (AOA) accreditation
△ Commission on Accreditation of Rehabilitation Facilities (CARF) accreditation
Control codes 61, 63, 64, 71, 72 and 73 indicate hospitals listed by AOHA, but not registered by AHA. For definition of numerical codes, see page A4

Hospital	Control	Service	Staffed Beds	Admissions	Census	Outpatient Visits	Births	Total	Payroll	Personnel
SOUTH LAKE TAHOE—El Dorado County ☐ BARTON MEMORIAL HOSPITAL, 2170 South Avenue, Zip 96158, Mailing Address: Box 9578, Zip 96158; tel. 530/541-3420; William G. Gordon, Chief Executive Officer (Nonreporting) A1 9 10	23	10	81	—	—	—	—	—	—	—
SOUTH SAN FRANCISCO—San Mateo County ✠ KAISER FOUNDATION HOSPITAL, 1200 El Camino Real, Zip 94080-3299; tel. 650/742-2401; Julie A. Petrini, Administrator (Nonreporting) A1 10 S Kaiser Foundation Hospitals, Oakland, CA	23	10	79	—	—	—	—	—	—	—
STANFORD—Santa Clara County ✠ STANFORD HOSPITAL AND CLINICS, 300 Pasteur Drive, Zip 94305-5584; tel. 650/723-4000; Malinda S. Mitchell, President and Chief Executive Officer A1 3 5 8 9 10 F4 9 11 12 13 16 17 18 19 20 22 24 25 26 30 31 33 34 35 36 37 38 39 41 43 46 47 48 49 50 51 53 54 56 57 59 60 61 62 63 64 65 66 69 70 71 72 74 75 76 77 78 79 P5 6 7 S Stanford Health Care, San Francisco, CA Web address: www.med.stanford.edu/sumc/	23	10	417	21479	307	576045	0	687971	213981	4314
STOCKTON—San Joaquin County ✠ DAMERON HOSPITAL, 525 West Acacia Street, Zip 95203; tel. 209/944-5550; Christopher Arismendi, M.D., Administrator (Nonreporting) A1 9 10 S Sutter Health, Sacramento, CA Web address: www.sutterhealth.org	23	10	211	—	—	—	—	—	—	—
✠ ST. JOSEPH'S BEHAVIORAL HEALTH CENTER, 2510 North California Street, Zip 95204-5568; tel. 209/948-2100; James Sondecker, Director A1 9 10 F3 4 6 8 9 11 12 13 14 16 17 19 21 22 23 24 25 26 27 29 30 31 32 33 34 35 36 37 38 39 41 44 45 47 48 49 50 51 54 57 58 59 60 61 62 63 64 65 67 69 70 71 72 73 74 76 77 78 79 P3 5 S Catholic Healthcare West, San Francisco, CA Web address: www.sjrhs.org	21	22	35	1097	21	3564	0	4037	2071	—
✠ ST. JOSEPH'S MEDICAL CENTER, 1800 North California Street, Zip 95204, Mailing Address: P.O. Box 213008, Zip 95213-3008; tel. 209/943-2000; Donald J. Wiley, Senior Vice President and Chief Operating Officer (Total facility includes 43 beds in nursing home-type unit) A1 2 9 10 F2 3 4 6 7 8 9 11 12 13 16 17 18 19 21 22 24 25 29 32 33 34 36 38 41 42 45 46 47 48 50 54 57 58 59 60 61 62 63 64 65 67 69 70 72 76 77 78 79 P3 5 7 S Catholic Healthcare West, San Francisco, CA Web address: www.sjrhs.org	21	10	291	16293	219	417455	1823	163977	64979	1727
SUN CITY—Riverside County ✠ MENIFEE VALLEY MEDICAL CENTER, 28400 McCall Boulevard, Zip 92585-9537; tel. 909/679-8888; Susan Ballard, Administrator (Nonreporting) A1 9 10 S Valley Health System, Hemet, CA	16	10	84	—	—	—	—	—	—	—
SUN VALLEY—Los Angeles County, See Los Angeles										
SUSANVILLE—Lassen County ✠ LASSEN COMMUNITY HOSPITAL, 560 Hospital Lane, Zip 96130-4809; tel. 530/257-5325; David S. Anderson, FACHE, Administrator (Total facility includes 31 beds in nursing home-type unit) A1 9 10 F7 8 9 13 17 18 22 25 32 34 36 37 39 41 44 48 69 70 76 78 S Banner Health System, Fargo, ND Web address: www.lshnet.org	23	10	59	1332	30	24671	269	12901	6132	140
SYLMAR—Los Angeles County, See Los Angeles										
TAFT—Kern County ★ MERCY WESTSIDE HOSPITAL, (Formerly Mercy West Side), 110 East North Street, Zip 93268; tel. 661/763-4211; Margo Arnold, Administrator (Total facility includes 63 beds in nursing home-type unit) A9 10 F2 3 4 7 8 9 11 12 13 17 18 19 22 24 25 31 32 34 36 37 38 39 41 42 45 46 47 48 49 50 51 54 57 58 59 60 63 64 65 69 70 72 76 77 78 79 P1 4 5 7 S Catholic Healthcare West, San Francisco, CA	21	10	84	363	63	13756	0	7539	3794	110
TARZANA—Los Angeles County, See Los Angeles										
TEHACHAPI—Kern County ★ TEHACHAPI VALLEY HEALTHCARE DISTRICT, (Formerly Tehachapi Hospital), 115 West E Street, Zip 93561, Mailing Address: P.O. Box 1900, Zip 93581; tel. 661/822-3241; Raymond T. Hino, Chief Executive Officer (Nonreporting) A9 10 S Brim Healthcare, Inc., Brentwood, TN	16	10	28	—	—	—	—	—	—	—
TEMPLETON—San Luis Obispo County ✠ TWIN CITIES COMMUNITY HOSPITAL, 1100 Las Tablas Road, Zip 93465; tel. 805/434-3500; Harold E. Chilton, Chief Executive Officer A1 9 10 F9 11 22 25 29 32 34 41 42 44 45 46 48 49 53 54 69 70 76 77 78 S TENET Healthcare Corporation, Santa Barbara, CA Web address: www.tenethealth.com	33	10	72	4321	48	64921	465	30558	13826	334
THOUSAND OAKS—Los Angeles County ✠ LOS ROBLES REGIONAL MEDICAL CENTER, 215 West Janss Road, Zip 91360-1899; tel. 805/497-2727; Robert C. Shaw, President and Chief Executive Officer (Total facility includes 42 beds in nursing home-type unit) A1 2 9 10 F4 7 8 11 12 13 16 17 18 19 22 24 25 30 32 33 34 35 38 39 40 41 42 43 44 45 46 47 48 50 51 53 54 57 59 62 65 68 69 70 72 76 77 78 79 S HCA - The Healthcare Company, Nashville, TN Web address: www.losrobleshospital.com	33	10	255	11669	177	86060	2054	113280	46352	847
TORRANCE—Los Angeles County ☐ DEL AMO HOSPITAL, 23700 Camino Del Sol, Zip 90505; tel. 310/530-1151; Lisa K. Montes, Administrator and Chief Executive Officer (Nonreporting) A1 9 10 S Universal Health Services, Inc., King of Prussia, PA	33	22	166	—	—	—	—	—	—	—

Hospitals, U.S. / CALIFORNIA

Hospital, Address, Telephone, Administrator, Approval, Facility, and Physician Codes, Health Care System, Network	Classification Codes		Utilization Data					Expense (thousands) of dollars		
★ American Hospital Association (AHA) membership ☐ Joint Commission on Accreditation of Healthcare Organizations (JCAHO) accreditation + American Osteopathic Healthcare Association (AOHA) membership ○ American Osteopathic Association (AOA) accreditation △ Commission on Accreditation of Rehabilitation Facilities (CARF) accreditation Control codes 61, 63, 64, 71, 72 and 73 indicate hospitals listed by AOHA, but not registered by AHA. For definition of numerical codes, see page A4	Control	Service	Staffed Beds	Admissions	Census	Outpatient Visits	Births	Total	Payroll	Personnel
★ LAC–HARBOR–UNIVERSITY OF CALIFORNIA AT LOS ANGELES MEDICAL CENTER, 1000 West Carson Street, Zip 90509; tel. 310/222-2101; Tecla A. Mickoseff, Administrator **A**1 2 3 5 9 10 **F**4 7 8 9 11 12 13 17 19 21 22 23 24 25 26 27 29 30 31 35 36 37 38 39 41 42 43 44 45 46 47 48 49 51 52 54 56 57 58 59 60 61 62 63 64 65 66 70 71 73 74 75 76 77 78 79 **P**6 **S** Los Angeles County–Department of Health Services, Los Angeles, CA	13	10	336	22843	326	330264	1386	450175	141815	2683
☐ LITTLE COMPANY OF MARY HEALTH SERVICES, (Formerly Little Company of Mary Hospital), 4101 Torrance Boulevard, Zip 90503-4698; tel. 310/540-7676; Blair Contratto, President and Chief Executive Officer (Total facility includes 121 beds in nursing home–type unit) (Nonreporting) **A**1 2 9 10 **S** Little Company of Mary Sisters Healthcare System, Evergreen Park, IL Web address: www.lcmhs.org	23	10	335	—	—	—	—	—	—	—
★ TORRANCE MEMORIAL MEDICAL CENTER, 3330 Lomita Boulevard, Zip 90505-5073; tel. 310/325-9110; George W. Graham, President and Chief Executive Officer **A**1 2 9 10 **F**3 4 7 8 9 11 13 17 18 19 22 24 25 27 29 30 31 32 33 34 35 36 37 38 39 43 45 46 47 48 49 50 51 54 56 59 60 61 62 63 64 65 70 72 76 77 78 79 **P**5 Web address: www.tmmc.com	23	10	360	22159	254	155830	4170	160164	62203	1635

TRACY—San Joaquin County

★ SUTTER TRACY COMMUNITY HOSPITAL, 1420 North Tracy Boulevard, Zip 95376-3497; tel. 209/835-1500; Gary D. Rapaport, Chief Executive Officer (Total facility includes 12 beds in nursing home–type unit) **A**1 9 10 **F**7 8 9 12 17 18 20 22 24 25 32 33 34 36 37 38 39 41 43 45 46 48 49 54 69 70 71 72 76 77 **P**3 4 5 6 7 **S** Sutter Health, Sacramento, CA Web address: www.suttertracy.org	23	10	71	2890	28	42293	464	27798	9941	302

TRAVIS AFB—Solano County

★ DAVID GRANT MEDICAL CENTER, 101 Bodin Circle, Zip 94535-1800; tel. 707/423-7300; Lieutenant Colonel David Costa, Administrator (Nonreporting) **A**1 2 3 5 **S** Department of the Air Force, Bowling AFB, DC	41	10	185	—	—	—	—	—	—	—

TRUCKEE—Nevada County

☐ TAHOE FOREST HOSPITAL DISTRICT, 10121 Pine Avenue, Zip 96161, Mailing Address: Box 759, Zip 96160; tel. 530/587-6011; Lawrence C. Long, Chief Executive Officer (Total facility includes 37 beds in nursing home–type unit) **A**1 9 10 **F**3 7 8 9 13 17 18 19 22 25 27 29 32 33 34 36 37 38 39 41 44 45 46 48 51 54 70 71 72 76 78 **P**5 Web address: www.tfhd.com	16	10	72	2468	55	99486	380	34423	12263	357

TULARE—Tulare County

★ TULARE LOCAL HEALTH CARE DISTRICT, (Formerly Tulare District Hospital), 869 Cherry Street, Zip 93274-2287; tel. 559/688-0821; Robert M. Montion, Chief Executive Officer (Nonreporting) **A**1 9 10	16	10	88	—	—	—	—	—	—	—

TURLOCK—Stanislaus County

★ EMANUEL MEDICAL CENTER, 825 Delbon Avenue, Zip 95382, Mailing Address: P.O. Box 819005, Zip 95381-9005; tel. 209/667-4200; Robert A. Moen, President and Chief Executive Officer (Total facility includes 145 beds in nursing home–type unit) **A**1 9 10 **F**6 7 8 9 12 13 16 17 18 19 22 23 24 25 26 27 29 30 31 32 33 34 36 37 38 39 40 41 43 45 46 48 54 67 69 70 72 76 77 79 **P**1 5 Web address: www.emanuelmed.org	21	10	270	7378	194	76645	1453	60570	23640	1058

TUSTIN—Orange County

☐ TUSTIN HOSPITAL AND MEDICAL CENTER, 14662 Newport Avenue, Zip 92680; tel. 714/838-9600; Jane Wingate, Chief Executive Officer (Total facility includes 24 beds in nursing home–type unit) (Nonreporting) **A**1 9	33	10	117	—	—	—	—	—	—	—
☐ TUSTIN REHABILITATION HOSPITAL, 14851 Yorba Street, Zip 92780; tel. 714/832-9200; Maureen Fakinos, Administrator (Nonreporting) **A**1 9 10	33	46	117	—	—	—	—	—	—	—

TWENTYNINE PALMS—San Bernardino County

★ NAVAL HOSPITAL, Mailing Address: Box 788250, MCAGCC, Zip 92278-8250; tel. 760/830-2190; Captain Joan M. Huber, Commanding Officer (Nonreporting) **A**1 **S** Department of Navy, Washington, DC Web address: www.nhtp.med.navy.mil/nhtp	43	10	29	—	—	—	—	—	—	—

UKIAH—Mendocino County

★ UKIAH VALLEY MEDICAL CENTER, (Includes Ukiah Valley Medical Center–Dora Street, 1120 South Dora Street; Ukiah Valley Medical Center–Hospital Drive), 275 Hospital Drive, Zip 95482; tel. 707/462-3111; Michael C. Wood, President and Chief Executive Officer **A**1 9 10 **F**8 9 11 13 16 17 18 22 24 25 27 34 36 39 41 42 44 45 46 48 50 51 54 69 70 76 77 78 79 **P**3 5 6 **S** Adventist Health, Roseville, CA Web address: www.adventisthealth.org	21	10	85	4053	40	30113	737	35927	15110	381

UPLAND—San Bernardino County

★ SAN ANTONIO COMMUNITY HOSPITAL, 999 San Bernardino Road, Zip 91786-4920, Mailing Address: Box 5001, Zip 91785; tel. 909/985-2811; George A. Kuykendall, President and Chief Executive Officer **A**1 2 9 10 **F**2 3 4 7 8 9 11 12 13 16 17 18 19 21 22 24 25 29 32 36 38 39 41 42 44 45 46 47 48 51 54 57 62 63 64 65 66 68 70 72 76 77 78 **P**7 Web address: www.sach.org	23	10	298	17597	185	261189	3479	142507	60184	1781

VACAVILLE—Solano County

CALIFORNIA MEDICAL FACILITY, 1600 California Drive, Zip 95696-2000; tel. 707/448-6841; Shelby Farrow, Administrator (Nonreporting)	12	11	215	—	—	—	—	—	—	—

Hospitals, U.S. / CALIFORNIA

Hospital, Address, Telephone, Administrator, Approval, Facility, and Physician Codes, Health Care System, Network	Classification Codes		Utilization Data					Expense (thousands) of dollars		Personnel
	Control	Service	Staffed Beds	Admissions	Census	Outpatient Visits	Births	Total	Payroll	

Key:
- ★ American Hospital Association (AHA) membership
- □ Joint Commission on Accreditation of Healthcare Organizations (JCAHO) accreditation
- + American Osteopathic Healthcare Association (AOHA) membership
- ○ American Osteopathic Association (AOA) accreditation
- △ Commission on Accreditation of Rehabilitation Facilities (CARF) accreditation

Control codes 61, 63, 64, 71, 72 and 73 indicate hospitals listed by AOHA, but not registered by AHA. For definition of numerical codes, see page A4.

Hospital	Control	Service	Staffed Beds	Admissions	Census	Outpatient Visits	Births	Total	Payroll	Personnel
★ VACAVALLEY HOSPITAL, 1000 Nut Tree Road, Zip 95687; tel. 707/446–4000; Deborah Sugiyama, President **A**9 10 **F**1 6 8 9 11 13 14 16 17 18 19 22 24 25 27 32 34 36 37 39 40 41 43 44 45 46 48 54 65 69 70 72 76 78 **P**3 **S** NorthBay Healthcare System, Fairfield, CA Web address: www.northbay.org	23	10	43	1978	19	22361	0	24242	9103	113

VALENCIA—Los Angeles County

Hospital	Control	Service	Staffed Beds	Admissions	Census	Outpatient Visits	Births	Total	Payroll	Personnel
□ △ HENRY MAYO NEWHALL MEMORIAL HOSPITAL, 23845 McBean Parkway, Zip 91355; tel. 661/253–8000; James T. Yoshioka, President and Chief Executive Officer (Total facility includes 62 beds in nursing home–type unit) (Nonreporting) **A**1 2 7 9 10	23	10	227	—	—	—	—	—	—	—

VALLEJO—Solano County

Hospital	Control	Service	Staffed Beds	Admissions	Census	Outpatient Visits	Births	Total	Payroll	Personnel
□ CALIFORNIA SPECIALTY HOSPITAL, 525 Oregon Street, Zip 94590; tel. 707/648–2200; JoAline Olson, R.N., President and Chief Executive Officer (Nonreporting) **A**1 9 10	33	22	61	—	—	—	—	—	—	—
★ KAISER FOUNDATION HOSPITAL AND REHABILITATION CENTER, 975 Sereno Drive, Zip 94589; tel. 707/651–1000; Sandra H. Small, Administrator (Nonreporting) **A**1 10 **S** Kaiser Foundation Hospitals, Oakland, CA Web address: www.kaiserpermanente.org	23	10	219	—	—	—	—	—	—	—
★ SUTTER SOLANO MEDICAL CENTER, 300 Hospital Drive, Zip 94589–2517, Mailing Address: P.O. Box 3189, Zip 94589; tel. 707/554–4444; Beverly Gilmore, Chief Executive Officer (Total facility includes 9 beds in nursing home–type unit) **A**1 9 10 **F**8 9 13 16 17 18 22 24 25 27 32 33 34 38 39 40 41 43 44 45 46 48 49 54 68 69 70 76 78 79 **S** Sutter Health, Sacramento, CA Web address: www.sutterhealth.org	23	10	111	4682	55	58999	759	43536	19491	486

VAN NUYS—Los Angeles County, See Los Angeles

VANDENBERG AFB—Santa Barbara County

Hospital	Control	Service	Staffed Beds	Admissions	Census	Outpatient Visits	Births	Total	Payroll	Personnel
★ U. S. AIR FORCE HOSPITAL, 338 South Dakota Street, Zip 93437–6307; tel. 805/606–1110; Colonel Alan D. Newton, Commander (Nonreporting) **A**1 **S** Department of the Air Force, Bowling AFB, DC	41	10	8	—	—	—	—	—	—	—

VENICE—Los Angeles County

Hospital	Control	Service	Staffed Beds	Admissions	Census	Outpatient Visits	Births	Total	Payroll	Personnel
★ DANIEL FREEMAN MARINA HOSPITAL, 4650 Lincoln Boulevard, Zip 90291–6360; tel. 310/823–8911; Joseph W. Dunn, Ph.D., Chief Executive Officer (Total facility includes 20 beds in nursing home–type unit) **A**1 9 10 **F**2 3 4 9 11 13 17 18 19 20 21 22 24 25 27 28 30 31 32 34 35 36 38 39 40 41 43 45 46 47 48 50 51 54 57 58 59 60 61 62 63 64 65 68 69 70 71 72 73 76 77 78 **P**5 **S** Carondelet Health System, Saint Louis, MO Web address: www.danielfreeman.org	21	10	138	5020	88	32850	0	36203	16850	327

VENTURA—Ventura County

Hospital	Control	Service	Staffed Beds	Admissions	Census	Outpatient Visits	Births	Total	Payroll	Personnel
□ BHC VISTA DEL MAR HOSPITAL, 801 Seneca Street, Zip 93001; tel. 805/653–6434; Diana L. Goulet, Administrator and Chief Executive Officer **A**1 9 10 **F**1 2 3 13 57 58 59 60 61 62 63 64 72 **S** Behavioral Healthcare Corporation, Nashville, TN	33	22	79	2104	47	5133	—	8071	4775	109
★ COMMUNITY MEMORIAL HOSPITAL OF SAN BUENAVENTURA, 147 North Brent Street, Zip 93003–2854; tel. 805/652–5011; Michael D. Bakst, Ph.D., Executive Director (Total facility includes 38 beds in nursing home–type unit) **A**1 9 10 **F**4 7 8 9 11 12 13 17 18 19 22 24 25 27 28 29 39 41 42 44 46 47 48 49 54 65 68 69 70 72 76 77 **P**5 7 Web address: www.cmhhospital.org	23	10	217	12956	154	112845	2696	92391	37418	1323
□ VENTURA COUNTY MEDICAL CENTER, 3291 Loma Vista Road, Zip 93003; tel. 805/652–6058; Samuel Edwards, Associate Administrator Hospital Services (Nonreporting) **A**1 3 5 9 10 Web address: www.ventura.org/hca/mc	13	10	162	—	—	—	—	—	—	—

VICTORVILLE—San Bernardino County

Hospital	Control	Service	Staffed Beds	Admissions	Census	Outpatient Visits	Births	Total	Payroll	Personnel
□ DESERT VALLEY HOSPITAL, 16850 Bear Valley Road, Zip 92392; tel. 760/241–8000; Ross Gassaway, Executive Director and Chief Executive Officer (Nonreporting) **A**1 9 10	31	10	83	—	—	—	—	—	—	—
□ VICTOR VALLEY COMMUNITY HOSPITAL, 15248 11th Street, Zip 92392; tel. 760/245–8691; Reggie Panis, Chief Executive Officer (Nonreporting) **A**1 2 9 10	23	10	119	—	—	—	—	—	—	—

VISALIA—Tulare County

Hospital	Control	Service	Staffed Beds	Admissions	Census	Outpatient Visits	Births	Total	Payroll	Personnel
★ KAWEAH DELTA HEALTH CARE DISTRICT, (Includes Community Health Center, 1633 South Court Street, Zip 93277, Mailing Address: Box 911, Zip 93277; tel. 209/824–2221; Lindsay K. Mann, Senior Vice President), 400 West Mineral King Avenue, Zip 93291; tel. 559/624–2000; Thomas M. Johnson, Chief Executive Officer (Total facility includes 52 beds in nursing home–type unit) **A**1 2 9 10 **F**1 3 4 7 8 9 11 13 16 17 18 19 22 24 25 27 28 30 31 32 33 34 36 38 39 41 43 44 45 46 47 48 49 50 51 53 54 57 62 63 64 65 69 70 72 73 76 77 78 79 Web address: www.kdhcd.org	16	10	258	16025	238	265909	3375	143714	65024	2034

WALNUT CREEK—Contra Costa County

Hospital	Control	Service	Staffed Beds	Admissions	Census	Outpatient Visits	Births	Total	Payroll	Personnel
□ BHC WALNUT CREEK HOSPITAL, 175 La Casa Via, Zip 94598; tel. 925/933–7990; Jay R. Kellison, Chief Executive Officer (Nonreporting) **A**1 **S** Behavioral Healthcare Corporation, Nashville, TN	33	22	108	—	—	—	—	—	—	—
★ JM/MD HEALTH SYSTEM, (Includes John Muir Medical Center, 1601 Ygnacio Valley Road, Zip 94598–3194; tel. 925/947–4433; Martin H. Diamond, President and Chief Administrative Officer; Mount Diablo Medical Center, 2540 East Street, Concord, Zip 94520, Mailing Address: P.O. Box 4110, Zip 94524–4110; tel. 925/674–2007; Thomas M. Harlan, President and Chief Administrative Officer), 1400 Treat Boulevard, Zip 94556; tel. 925/941–2100; J. Kendall Anderson, President and Chief Executive Officer (Total facility includes 501 beds in nursing home–type unit) (Nonreporting) **A**1 2 9	23	10	946	—	—	—	—	—	—	—

Hospitals, U.S. / CALIFORNIA

Hospital, Address, Telephone, Administrator, Approval, Facility, and Physician Codes, Health Care System, Network	Classification Codes		Utilization Data					Expense (thousands) of dollars		
★ American Hospital Association (AHA) membership ☐ Joint Commission on Accreditation of Healthcare Organizations (JCAHO) accreditation + American Osteopathic Healthcare Association (AOHA) membership ○ American Osteopathic Association (AOA) accreditation △ Commission on Accreditation of Rehabilitation Facilities (CARF) accreditation Control codes 61, 63, 64, 71, 72 and 73 indicate hospitals listed by AOHA, but not registered by AHA. For definition of numerical codes, see page A4	Control	Service	Staffed Beds	Admissions	Census	Outpatient Visits	Births	Total	Payroll	Personnel
★ KAISER FOUNDATION HOSPITAL, (Includes Kaiser Foundation Hospital, 200 Muir Road, Martinez, Zip 94553–4696; tel. 510/372-1000), 1425 South Main Street, Zip 94596; tel. 925/295–4000; Sandra H. Small, Administrator (Nonreporting) **A**1 10 **S** Kaiser Foundation Hospitals, Oakland, CA Web address: www.kaiserpermanente.org	23	10	210	—	—	—	—	—	—	—
WATSONVILLE—Santa Cruz County										
☐ WATSONVILLE COMMUNITY HOSPITAL, 75 Nielson Street, Zip 95076; tel. 831/724–4741; Barry S. Schneider, Chief Executive Officer (Total facility includes 13 beds in nursing home–type unit) (Nonreporting) **A**1 9 10 **S** Community Health Systems, Inc., Brentwood, TN Web address: www.watsonville.com\hospital	33	10	130	—	—	—	—	—	—	—
WEAVERVILLE—Trinity County										
TRINITY HOSPITAL, 410 North Taylor Street, Zip 96093, Mailing Address: P.O. Box 1229, Zip 96093–1229; tel. 916/623–5541; David L. Yarbrough, R.N., JD, Administrator (Total facility includes 26 beds in nursing home–type unit) **A**9 10 **F**7 8 9 13 16 17 18 19 22 25 26 30 31 32 33 34 35 36 43 44 48 50 69 70 72 73 76 78 79	13	10	65	755	32	23261	63	8421	3870	113
WEST COVINA—Los Angeles County										
☐ CITRUS VALLEY MEDICAL CENTER–QUEEN OF THE VALLEY CAMPUS, 1115 South Sunset Avenue, Zip 91790, Mailing Address: Box 1980, Zip 91793; tel. 626/962–4011; James T. Yoshioka, President (Nonreporting) **A**1 9 10 **S** Citrus Valley Health Partners, Covina, CA	23	10	263	—	—	—	—	—	—	—
☐ DOCTORS HOSPITAL OF WEST COVINA, 725 South Orange Avenue, Zip 91790–2614; tel. 626/338–8481; Gerald H. Wallman, Administrator (Total facility includes 24 beds in nursing home–type unit) **A**1 10 **F**22 39 41 44 45 48 54 63 64 69 70 76 **P**5	33	10	51	630	25	2179	245	—	—	—
SPECIALTY HOSPITAL, 845 North Lark Ellen Avenue, Zip 91791; tel. 626/339–5451; Nenda Estudillo, Administrator (Nonreporting) **A**9	32	10	76	—	—	—	—	—	—	—
WEST HILLS—Los Angeles County, See Los Angeles										
WEST LOS ANGELES—Los Angeles County, See Los Angeles										
WHITTIER—Los Angeles County										
☐ PRESBYTERIAN INTERCOMMUNITY HOSPITAL, 12401 Washington Boulevard, Zip 90602–1099; tel. 562/698–0811; Daniel F. Adams, President and Chief Executive Officer (Nonreporting) **A**1 2 3 5 9 10	23	10	312	—	—	—	—	—	—	—
★ WHITTIER HOSPITAL MEDICAL CENTER, 9080 Colima Road, Zip 90605; tel. 562/907–1541; Sandra M. Chester, Chief Executive Officer **A**1 9 10 **F**2 3 4 7 8 9 11 12 13 16 17 18 19 22 25 27 29 30 31 32 34 36 38 39 40 41 42 43 44 45 46 47 48 51 52 53 54 57 60 62 63 65 68 69 70 71 72 74 76 78 79 **P**5 7 **S** TENET Healthcare Corporation, Santa Barbara, CA Web address: www.tenethealth.com	33	10	181	10198	117	44170	2684	53740	2626	666
WILDOMAR—Riverside County										
☐ INLAND VALLEY REGIONAL MEDICAL CENTER, 36485 Inland Valley Drive, Zip 92595; tel. 909/677–1111; Christopher L. Boyd, Chief Executive Officer and Managing Director (Nonreporting) **A**1 9 10 **S** Universal Health Services, Inc., King of Prussia, PA	33	10	80	—	—	—	—	—	—	—
WILLITS—Mendocino County										
★ FRANK R. HOWARD MEMORIAL HOSPITAL, 1 Madrone Street, Zip 95490; tel. 707/459–6801; Kevin R. Erich, President (Nonreporting) **A**1 9 10 **S** Adventist Health, Roseville, CA Web address: www.adventisthealth.org	23	10	28	—	—	—	—	—	—	—
WILLOWS—Glenn County										
GLENN MEDICAL CENTER, 1133 West Sycamore Street, Zip 95988; tel. 530/934–1800; Bernard G. Hietpas, Chief Executive Officer (Nonreporting) **A**9 10	23	10	27	—	—	—	—	—	—	—
WINTERHAVEN—Imperial County										
★ U. S. PUBLIC HEALTH SERVICE INDIAN HOSPITAL, Mailing Address: P.O. Box 1368, Yuma, AZ, Zip 85366–1368; tel. 760/572–0217; Hortense Miguel, R.N., Service Unit Director (Nonreporting) **A**1 10 **S** U. S. Public Health Service Indian Health Service, Rockville, MD	47	10	34	—	—	—	—	—	—	—
WOODLAND—Yolo County										
★ WOODLAND HEALTHCARE, (Formerly Woodland Memorial Hospital), 1325 Cottonwood Street, Zip 95695–5199; tel. 530/662–3961; Margaret Cleary, Chief Executive Officer (Nonreporting) **A**1 9 10 **S** Catholic Healthcare West, San Francisco, CA Web address: www.chw.edu	23	10	103	—	—	—	—	—	—	—
WOODLAND HILLS—Los Angeles County, See Los Angeles										
YOUNTVILLE—Napa County										
VETERANS HOME OF CALIFORNIA, 100 California Drive, Zip 94599–1413; tel. 707/944–4500; Michael Madalao, Interim Administrator (Total facility includes 514 beds in nursing home–type unit) (Nonreporting) **A**10	12	10	540	—	—	—	—	—	—	—
YREKA—Siskiyou County										
☐ FAIRCHILD MEDICAL CENTER, 444 Bruce Street, Zip 96097; tel. 530/842–4121; Dwayne Jones, Chief Executive Officer **A**1 9 10 **F**7 8 9 17 18 19 22 24 25 32 36 39 44 48 54 68 76	23	10	20	1567	14	55638	154	17352	7188	243
YUBA CITY—Sutter County										
☐ FREMONT MEDICAL CENTER, 970 Plumas Street, Zip 95991; tel. 530/751–4000; Thomas P. Hayes, Chief Executive Officer **A**1 9 10 **F**2 3 6 8 9 11 16 17 18 22 24 25 29 30 36 37 38 39 41 42 44 45 48 49 54 65 70 76 78 79 **P**5 **S** Fremont–Rideout Health Group, Yuba City, CA Web address: www.frhg.org	23	10	90	7471	84	—	1970	44498	17627	500

© 2000 AHA Guide   *Many Facility Codes have changed. Please refer to the AHA Guide Code Chart.*

Hospitals, U.S. / COLORADO

COLORADO

Resident Population 3,971 (in thousands)
Resident population in metro areas 84.0%
Birth rate per 1,000 population 14.5
65 years and over 10.1%
Percent of persons without health insurance 15.1%

Hospital, Address, Telephone, Administrator, Approval, Facility, and Physician Codes, Health Care System, Network	Classification Codes		Utilization Data					Expense (thousands) of dollars		
	Control	Service	Staffed Beds	Admissions	Census	Outpatient Visits	Births	Total	Payroll	Personnel

★ American Hospital Association (AHA) membership
☐ Joint Commission on Accreditation of Healthcare Organizations (JCAHO) accreditation
+ American Osteopathic Healthcare Association (AOHA) membership
○ American Osteopathic Association (AOA) accreditation
△ Commission on Accreditation of Rehabilitation Facilities (CARF) accreditation
Control codes 61, 63, 64, 71, 72 and 73 indicate hospitals listed by AOHA, but not registered by AHA. For definition of numerical codes, see page A4

Hospital	Control	Service	Staffed Beds	Admissions	Census	Outpatient Visits	Births	Total	Payroll	Personnel
ALAMOSA—Alamosa County ★ SAN LUIS VALLEY REGIONAL MEDICAL CENTER, 106 Blanca Avenue, Zip 81101–2393; tel. 719/589–2511; Leslie K. Fleming, CPA, Co–Chief Executive Officer **A**1 9 10 **F**7 8 9 17 18 19 22 25 26 27 39 41 43 44 45 48 54 70 75 76 78 79 **Web address:** www.slvrmc.org	21	10	85	2815	22	35075	556	16796	7183	196
ASPEN—Pitkin County ☐ ASPEN VALLEY HOSPITAL DISTRICT, 401 Castle Creek Road, Zip 81611–1159; tel. 970/925–1120; Randy Middlebrook, Chief Executive Officer and Administrator (Nonreporting) **A**1 9 10 **Web address:** www.avhaspen.org	16	10	41	—	—	—	—	—	—	—
AURORA—Adams County ★ MEDICAL CENTER OF AURORA–SOUTH, (Formerly Aurora Regional Medical Center), (Includes Columbia Regional Medical Center–South Campus, 1501 South Potomac, Zip 80012; North Campus and Columbia Aurora Presbyterian Transitional Care Center, 700 Potomac Street, Zip 80011–6792; tel. 303/363–7200), 1501 South Potomac Street, Zip 80012–5499; tel. 303/695–2600; Sylvia Young, President and Chief Executive Officer (Nonreporting) **A**1 2 9 10 **S** HCA – The Healthcare Company, Nashville, TN **Web address:** www.hcahealthcare.com	33	10	334	—	—	—	—	—	—	—
★ △ SPALDING REHABILITATION HOSPITAL, 900 Potomac Street, Zip 80011–6716; tel. 303/367–1166 **A**1 5 7 10 **F**13 16 18 49 53 54 69 78 **S** HCA – The Healthcare Company, Nashville, TN	33	46	138	2203	69	11256	0	21906	11096	307
BOULDER—Boulder County ★ △ BOULDER COMMUNITY HOSPITAL, 1100 Balsam, Zip 80304–3496, Mailing Address: P.O. Box 9019, Zip 80301–9019; tel. 303/440–2273; David P. Gehant, President and Chief Executive Officer **A**1 2 7 9 10 **F**3 4 5 7 8 9 11 12 13 16 17 20 22 24 25 28 29 30 33 34 35 36 37 38 39 41 44 45 46 47 48 49 50 51 53 54 56 57 58 59 60 61 62 63 64 65 68 70 71 72 73 75 76 77 78 79 **P**6 7 **Web address:** www.bch.org	23	10	197	9361	113	206197	1596	119888	54514	1575
BRIGHTON—Adams County ★ PLATTE VALLEY MEDICAL CENTER, 1850 Egbert Street, Zip 80601–2404; tel. 303/659–1531; John R. Hicks, President and Chief Executive Officer **A**1 9 10 **F**8 9 13 16 17 18 19 22 24 25 28 31 32 34 36 38 39 43 44 45 46 48 51 54 56 69 70 71 72 76 78 **P**8 **Web address:** www.prmc.org	23	10	49	2506	19	33659	845	22410	9399	284
BRUSH—Morgan County ★ EAST MORGAN COUNTY HOSPITAL, 2400 West Edison Street, Zip 80723–1640; tel. 970/842–5151; Anne Platt, Administrator **A**9 10 18 **F**7 9 13 16 17 18 19 20 22 25 28 30 32 34 36 38 39 43 45 46 48 51 53 54 56 71 72 75 76 77 78 **P**6 8 **S** Banner Health System, Fargo, ND **Web address:** www.wphn.com	23	10	25	458	4	13910	0	7251	4002	92
BURLINGTON—Kit Carson County ★ KIT CARSON COUNTY MEMORIAL HOSPITAL, 286 16th Street, Zip 80807–1697; tel. 719/346–5311; James Jorden, Chief Executive Officer **A**9 10 **F**8 9 13 16 17 18 19 22 24 25 26 36 37 38 39 44 48 51 54 56 71 72 75 76	16	10	24	546	6	9952	76	4550	2221	97
CANON CITY—Fremont County ★ ST. THOMAS MORE HOSPITAL AND PROGRESSIVE CARE CENTER, 1338 Phay Avenue, Zip 81212–2221; tel. 719/269–2000; C. Ray Honaker, Chief Executive Officer (Total facility includes 163 beds in nursing home–type unit) (Nonreporting) **A**1 10 **S** Catholic Health Initiatives, Denver, CO **Web address:** www.centura.org	21	10	218	—	—	—	—	—	—	—
CHEYENNE WELLS—Cheyenne County ★ KEEFE MEMORIAL HOSPITAL, 602 North Sixth Street West, Zip 80810, Mailing Address: P.O. Box 578, Zip 80810–0578; tel. 719/767–5661; Curtis Hawkinson, Chief Executive Officer **A**9 10 **F**7 13 16 17 18 19 20 22 24 25 30 31 32 34 36 38 46 48 50 51 54 58 59 69 70 76 78 79 **P**6 **Web address:** www.yampa.com/npo/hprhn/keefe/keefe.htm	13	10	12	200	2	7685	0	2681	1498	53
COLORADO SPRINGS—El Paso County ☐ CEDAR SPRINGS BEHAVIORAL HEALTH SYSTEM, (Formerly Cedar Springs Psychiatric Hospital), 2135 Southgate Road, Zip 80906–2693; tel. 719/633–4114; Connie Mull, Chief Executive Officer **A**1 9 10 **F**1 2 3 13 17 23 30 51 57 58 59 60 61 62 63 64 70 72 **S** Brown Schools, Inc., Austin, TX **Web address:** www.brownschools.com	33	22	114	921	90	12142	0	—	—	129
★ MEMORIAL HOSPITAL, 1400 East Boulder Street, Zip 80909–5599, Mailing Address: Box 1326, Zip 80901–1326; tel. 719/365–5000; J. Robert Peters, Executive Director **A**1 2 9 10 **F**4 7 8 9 11 12 13 15 16 17 18 19 20 21 22 24 25 26 30 32 33 34 35 36 38 39 41 42 43 44 45 46 47 48 49 50 51 52 53 54 65 66 68 70 72 73 75 76 77 78 79 **P**5 7 8 **Web address:** www.memorialhospital.com	14	10	386	23114	287	317638	2794	217787	96071	2690

Hospitals, U.S. / COLORADO

Hospital, Address, Telephone, Administrator, Approval, Facility, and Physician Codes, Health Care System, Network	Classification Codes		Utilization Data					Expense (thousands) of dollars		
★ American Hospital Association (AHA) membership ☐ Joint Commission on Accreditation of Healthcare Organizations (JCAHO) accreditation + American Osteopathic Healthcare Association (AOHA) membership ○ American Osteopathic Association (AOA) accreditation △ Commission on Accreditation of Rehabilitation Facilities (CARF) accreditation Control codes 61, 63, 64, 71, 72 and 73 indicate hospitals listed by AOHA, but not registered by AHA. For definition of numerical codes, see page A4	Control	Service	Staffed Beds	Admissions	Census	Outpatient Visits	Births	Total	Payroll	Personnel
☒ △ PENROSE–ST. FRANCIS HEALTH SERVICES, (Includes Penrose Community Hospital, 3205 North Academy Boulevard, Zip 80917; tel. 719/776–3000; Penrose Hospital, 2215 North Cascade Avenue, Zip 80907; tel. 719/776–5000; St Francis Health Center, 825 East Pikes Peak Avenue, Zip 80903; tel. 719/776–8800), Rick O'Connell, President and Chief Executive Officer **A**1 2 3 5 7 9 10 **F**1 3 4 7 8 9 11 12 13 14 16 17 18 19 21 22 23 24 25 27 28 31 32 33 34 35 36 37 38 39 41 42 43 44 45 46 47 48 49 50 51 53 54 55 56 57 58 59 60 61 62 63 65 66 70 71 72 73 75 76 77 78 79 **P**8 **S** Catholic Health Initiatives, Denver, CO	21	10	384	20197	253	238831	2714	183342	69464	2505
CORTEZ—Montezuma County										
☒ SOUTHWEST MEMORIAL HOSPITAL, 1311 North Mildred Road, Zip 81321–2299; tel. 970/565–6666; Robert M. Peterson, President and Chief Executive Officer **A**1 9 10 **F**8 9 13 16 17 18 19 22 23 25 31 34 35 36 39 40 41 43 44 45 48 50 51 54 70 75 76 78 **P**3 8 **S** Quorum Health Group, Brentwood, TN	23	10	42	2381	17	—	243	19673	8265	250
CRAIG—Moffat County										
☒ MEMORIAL HOSPITAL, 785 Russell Street, Zip 81625–9906; tel. 970/824–9411; M. Randell Phelps, Administrator **A**1 9 10 **F**7 8 9 16 17 18 19 22 24 25 27 31 32 34 35 36 37 38 39 41 43 44 46 48 54 70 72 74 75 76 78 **P**8 **S** Quorum Health Group, Brentwood, TN	13	10	29	943	8	17057	101	10811	4431	104
DEL NORTE—Rio Grande County										
★ RIO GRANDE HOSPITAL, 1280 Grande Avenue, Zip 81132; tel. 719/657–2510; Rebecca Patterson, Administrator (Nonreporting) **A**18 **S** Brim Healthcare, Inc., Brentwood, TN	33	10	12	—	—	—	—	—	—	—
DELTA—Delta County										
☒ DELTA COUNTY MEMORIAL HOSPITAL, 100 Stafford Lane, Zip 81416–2297, Mailing Address: P.O. Box 10100, Zip 81416–5003; tel. 970/874–7681; Thomas Thomson, Administrator **A**1 9 10 **F**7 8 9 16 22 24 25 32 39 41 44 45 48 51 54 70 75 76 **P**5 8	16	10	44	2143	19	44595	233	12986	6016	235
DENVER—Denver, Adams and Arapahoe Counties										
☐ CENTURA SPECIAL CARE HOSPITAL, 1601 North Lowell Boulevard, Zip 80204–1597; tel. 303/899–5170; Silas M. Weir, Chief Executive Officer (Nonreporting) **A**1 Web address: www.centura.org	23	10	24	—	—	—	—	—	—	—
☒ CHILDREN'S HOSPITAL, 1056 East 19th Avenue, Zip 80218–1088; tel. 303/861–8888; Doris J. Biester, R.N., President and Chief Executive Officer **A**1 3 5 9 10 **F**7 10 11 13 14 16 17 18 19 20 22 23 25 26 29 32 33 34 35 36 37 38 39 42 43 44 45 46 47 48 49 50 51 52 54 55 56 57 58 59 60 61 63 64 66 68 70 71 72 73 74 75 76 77 78 **P**4 7 Web address: www.tehdeu.org.8000	23	50	198	7836	149	282562	0	188121	—	1978
☐ COLORADO MENTAL HEALTH INSTITUTE AT FORT LOGAN, 3520 West Oxford Avenue, Zip 80236–3197; tel. 303/761–0220; Garry A. Toenber, Ph.D., Director (Nonreporting) **A**1 9 10	12	22	315	—	—	—	—	—	—	—
☐ DENVER HEALTH MEDICAL CENTER, 777 Bannock Street, Zip 80204–4507; tel. 303/436–6000; Patricia A. Gabow, M.D., Chief Executive Officer and Medical Director **A**1 3 5 9 10 **F**2 3 4 7 8 9 11 12 13 14 16 17 18 19 22 23 24 25 29 30 31 33 34 35 36 38 39 41 42 43 44 46 47 48 51 52 53 54 55 56 57 58 59 61 63 64 65 66 68 70 71 72 73 74 75 76 77 78 79 **P**6	16	10	303	17167	205	583987	2873	247407	144178	3060
☒ EXEMPLA SAINT JOSEPH HOSPITAL, 1835 Franklin Street, Zip 80218–1191; tel. 303/837–7111; Jeffrey D. Selberg, President and Chief Executive Officer **A**1 2 3 9 10 **F**3 4 7 8 9 11 12 13 17 18 19 20 22 24 25 26 27 30 31 32 33 34 35 38 39 41 42 43 44 45 46 47 48 50 51 54 56 57 59 61 62 63 64 65 66 68 69 70 71 72 73 76 78 79 **P**6 **S** Exempla Healthcare, Inc., Denver, CO	23	10	480	25410	287	104421	5165	189785	96720	1997
☒ NATIONAL JEWISH MEDICAL AND RESEARCH CENTER, (ALLERGIC IMMUNOLOGICAL), 1400 Jackson Street, Zip 80206–2762; tel. 303/388–4461; Lynn M. Taussig, M.D., President and Chief Executive Officer **A**1 3 5 9 10 **F**13 16 19 22 24 31 34 38 45 50 51 54 70 76 77 78 **P**6 Web address: www.nationaljewish.org	23	49	24	305	7	15552	—	84775	26198	949
☒ PORTER ADVENTIST HOSPITAL, 2525 South Downing Street, Zip 80210–5876; tel. 303/778–1955; Ruthita J. Fike, Administrator (Total facility includes 35 beds in nursing home–type unit) **A**1 2 9 10 **F**3 4 6 7 8 9 11 12 13 19 20 22 24 25 26 28 29 30 32 33 34 35 36 39 41 42 43 44 45 46 47 48 50 51 53 54 56 57 59 60 61 62 63 64 65 66 67 68 69 70 71 72 73 74 75 76 77 78 79 Web address: www.centura.org	21	10	327	13932	189	97564	873	121192	51736	1179
☒ △ PRESBYTERIAN–ST. LUKE'S MEDICAL CENTER, (Includes Presbyterian–Denver Hospital, 1719 East 19th Avenue, Zip 80218–1124; tel. 303/839–6565), 1719 East 19th Avenue, Zip 80218–1281; tel. 303/839–6000; Madeleine Roberson, President and Chief Executive Officer (Nonreporting) **A**1 2 3 5 7 9 10 13 **S** HCA – The Healthcare Company, Nashville, TN	33	10	479	—	—	—	—	—	—	—
☒ △ ROSE MEDICAL CENTER, 4567 East Ninth Avenue, Zip 80220–3941; tel. 303/320–2121; Kenneth H. Feiler, President and Chief Executive Officer (Nonreporting) **A**1 2 3 5 7 9 10 **S** HCA – The Healthcare Company, Nashville, TN Web address: www.rosebabies.com	33	10	250	—	—	—	—	—	—	—
☒ ST. ANTHONY CENTRAL HOSPITAL, 4231 West 16th Avenue, Zip 80204–4098; tel. 303/629–3511; Matthew S. Fulton, Senior Vice President and Administrator **A**1 2 3 5 9 10 **F**1 4 6 7 8 9 10 11 12 14 16 17 18 19 22 24 25 28 29 30 31 32 34 36 37 38 39 41 44 45 47 48 49 51 53 54 56 57 62 63 65 69 70 72 74 75 76 77 78 79 **S** Catholic Health Initiatives, Denver, CO	21	10	417	18329	275	112238	1429	165983	66756	1558

Hospitals, U.S. / COLORADO

Hospital, Address, Telephone, Administrator, Approval, Facility, and Physician Codes, Health Care System, Network

- ★ American Hospital Association (AHA) membership
- ☐ Joint Commission on Accreditation of Healthcare Organizations (JCAHO) accreditation
- + American Osteopathic Healthcare Association (AOHA) membership
- ○ American Osteopathic Association (AOA) accreditation
- △ Commission on Accreditation of Rehabilitation Facilities (CARF) accreditation

Control codes 61, 63, 64, 71, 72 and 73 indicate hospitals listed by AOHA, but not registered by AHA. For definition of numerical codes, see page A4.

Hospital	Control	Service	Staffed Beds	Admissions	Census	Outpatient Visits	Births	Total	Payroll	Personnel
★ UNIVERSITY OF COLORADO HOSPITAL, 4200 East Ninth Avenue, Zip 80262; tel. 303/372-0000; Dennis C. Brimhall, President **A**1 2 3 5 8 9 10 **F**4 5 6 8 9 10 11 12 13 16 17 18 19 21 22 23 24 25 26 28 29 30 31 32 33 34 35 37 39 43 44 45 46 47 48 49 50 51 53 54 56 58 59 60 61 62 64 65 66 68 70 71 72 73 74 75 76 78 79 **P**4 Web address: www.uchsc.edu/uh/	16	10	332	14533	199	343185	1603	239622	91970	2554
★ △ VETERANS AFFAIRS MEDICAL CENTER, 1055 Clermont Street, Zip 80220-3877; tel. 303/399-8020; Ed Thorsland, Jr, Director (Total facility includes 60 beds in nursing home-type unit) (Nonreporting) **A**1 2 3 5 7 8 **S** Department of Veterans Affairs, Washington, DC Web address: www.va.gov/stations97/guide/home.asp?DIVISION=ALL	45	10	336	—	—	—	—	—	—	—
DURANGO—La Plata County										
★ MERCY MEDICAL CENTER, 375 East Park Avenue, Zip 81301; tel. 970/247-4311; Kirk Dignum, Ph.D., President and Chief Executive Officer (Total facility includes 10 beds in nursing home-type unit) **A**1 2 9 10 **F**4 7 8 9 11 12 13 16 17 19 22 23 24 25 26 27 28 32 36 37 38 39 40 41 42 43 44 45 46 48 51 52 53 54 56 65 69 70 71 72 75 76 77 78 79 **P**6 8 **S** Catholic Health Initiatives, Denver, CO Web address: www.mercydurango.org	21	10	81	3961	42	103871	605	55234	26382	532
EADS—Kiowa County										
★ WEISBROD MEMORIAL COUNTY HOSPITAL, 1208 Luther Street, Zip 81036, Mailing Address: P.O. Box 817, Zip 81036-0817; tel. 719/438-5401; Marvin O. Bishop, Chief Executive Officer and Administrator (Total facility includes 34 beds in nursing home-type unit) **A**9 10 **F**16 25 31 36 38 40 53 54 56 69 70 **P**6	16	10	42	102	24	16409	0	3025	1664	65
ENGLEWOOD—Arapahoe County										
★ CRAIG HOSPITAL, 3425 South Clarkson Street, Zip 80110-2899; tel. 303/789-8000; Dennis O'Malley, President **A**1 9 10 **F**13 16 17 18 19 22 23 24 25 27 28 38 39 43 45 48 50 51 53 54 55 65 68 70 72 75 76 78 Web address: www.craighospital.org	23	46	76	475	69	6453	—	35246	16016	448
★ SWEDISH MEDICAL CENTER, 501 East Hampden Avenue, Zip 80110-0101; tel. 303/788-5000; Mary M. White, President and Chief Executive Officer (Nonreporting) **A**1 2 3 5 9 10 **S** HCA – The Healthcare Company, Nashville, TN Web address: www.swedishhospital.com	33	10	368	—	—	—	—	—	—	—
ESTES PARK—Larimer County										
★ ESTES PARK MEDICAL CENTER, 555 Prospect Avenue, Zip 80517-2740, Mailing Address: P.O. Box 2740, Zip 80517-2740; tel. 970/586-2317; Andrew Wills, Chief Executive Officer (Total facility includes 60 beds in nursing home-type unit) **A**9 10 **F**8 9 25 32 36 37 38 44 48 54 67 69 76 **P**7	16	10	76	532	45	—	59	11430	5410	185
FORT CARSON—El Paso County										
★ EVANS U. S. ARMY COMMUNITY HOSPITAL, Zip 80913-5101; tel. 719/526-7200; Lieutenant Colonel Michael D. Wheeler, MSC, Deputy Commander, Administration **A**1 2 **F**2 8 9 10 11 12 13 14 15 17 18 19 21 22 23 24 25 26 28 29 32 33 34 35 36 37 38 39 41 42 43 44 45 46 47 48 49 50 51 52 53 56 57 63 66 69 70 71 72 74 75 76 77 78 79 **P**5 6 7 **S** Department of the Army, Office of the Surgeon General, Falls Church, VA	42	10	112	3434	26	397435	1167	57214	20843	1082
FORT COLLINS—Larimer County										
★ POUDRE VALLEY HOSPITAL, (Includes Mountain Crest Hospital, 4601 Corbett Drive, Zip 80525; tel. 970/225-9191), 1024 South Lemay Avenue, Zip 80524; tel. 970/495-7000; Rulon F. Stacey, President and Chief Executive Officer **A**1 2 3 9 10 **F**3 4 8 9 11 12 13 14 16 17 18 19 21 22 23 24 25 28 32 33 34 36 38 39 40 41 43 44 45 46 47 48 49 50 51 53 54 55 56 57 58 59 60 61 62 63 64 68 70 72 75 76 78 **P**1	23	10	254	14272	150	305715	2299	143169	59428	1581
FORT MORGAN—Morgan County										
★ COLORADO PLAINS MEDICAL CENTER, 1000 Lincoln Street, Zip 80701-3298; tel. 970/867-3391; Solon H. Boggus, Jr, Interim Chief Executive Officer **A**1 9 10 **F**8 9 13 16 17 18 19 22 23 24 25 30 31 32 33 34 35 36 38 39 40 41 44 45 46 48 49 50 51 53 54 56 70 72 73 75 76 78 79 **P**8 **S** Province Healthcare Corporation, Brentwood, TN	33	10	50	2300	25	31817	471	18314	6449	196
FRUITA—Mesa County										
FAMILY HEALTH WEST, 228 North Cherry Street, Zip 81521-2101, Mailing Address: P.O. Box 130, Zip 81521-0130; tel. 970/858-9871; Dennis E. Ficklin, Chief Executive Officer (Total facility includes 352 beds in nursing home-type unit) (Nonreporting) **A**9 10 18	23	10	358	—	—	—	—	—	—	—
GLENWOOD SPRINGS—Garfield County										
★ VALLEY VIEW HOSPITAL, 1906 Blake Avenue, Zip 81601-4259, Mailing Address: P.O. Box 1970, Zip 81602-1970; tel. 970/945-6535; Gary L. Brewer, Chief Executive Officer **A**1 9 10 **F**2 7 8 9 13 17 18 22 24 25 36 37 38 39 40 41 42 43 44 45 46 48 51 53 54 68 70 71 75 76 78 **P**5 **S** Quorum Health Group, Brentwood, TN Web address: www.vvh.com	23	10	63	2384	27	102880	521	33765	14288	404
GRAND JUNCTION—Mesa County										
☐ + ○ △ COMMUNITY HOSPITAL, 2021 North 12th Street, Zip 81501-2999; tel. 970/242-0920; Randall M. Phillips, President and Chief Executive Officer **A**1 7 9 10 11 **F**8 9 13 16 17 18 22 24 25 32 33 34 36 38 39 41 43 44 45 48 49 50 51 54 56 68 70 71 75 76 77 78 **P**8 Web address: www.gjhosp.org	23	10	58	1908	23	57786	270	21842	10143	325

Hospitals, U.S. / COLORADO

Hospital, Address, Telephone, Administrator, Approval, Facility, and Physician Codes, Health Care System, Network ★ American Hospital Association (AHA) membership □ Joint Commission on Accreditation of Healthcare Organizations (JCAHO) accreditation + American Osteopathic Healthcare Association (AOHA) membership ○ American Osteopathic Association (AOA) accreditation △ Commission on Accreditation of Rehabilitation Facilities (CARF) accreditation Control codes 61, 63, 64, 71, 72 and 73 indicate hospitals listed by AOHA, but not registered by AHA. For definition of numerical codes, see page A4	Classification Codes		Utilization Data					Expense (thousands) of dollars		
	Control	Service	Staffed Beds	Admissions	Census	Outpatient Visits	Births	Total	Payroll	Personnel
★ ST. MARY'S HOSPITAL AND MEDICAL CENTER, 2635 North 7th Street, Zip 81501–8204, Mailing Address: P.O. Box 1628, Zip 81502–1628; tel. 970/244–2273; Robert W. Ladenburger, President and Chief Executive Officer (Total facility includes 30 beds in nursing home–type unit) **A**1 2 3 9 10 **F**1 2 3 4 5 7 8 9 10 11 12 13 14 16 17 18 19 20 21 22 23 24 25 26 27 28 29 30 31 32 33 34 35 36 37 38 39 40 41 42 43 44 45 46 47 48 49 50 51 53 54 56 57 58 59 60 61 62 63 64 65 66 68 69 70 71 72 73 75 76 77 78 79 **P**3 6 **S** Sisters of Charity of Leavenworth Health Services Corporation, Leavenworth, KS	21	10	281	14097	186	338180	1433	135782	61667	1663
★ VETERANS AFFAIRS MEDICAL CENTER, 2121 North Avenue, Zip 81501–6499; tel. 970/242–0731; Kurt W. Schlegelmilch, M.D., CHE, Director (Total facility includes 30 beds in nursing home–type unit) **A**1 9 **F**3 4 6 9 10 11 12 13 16 17 18 19 22 23 24 25 26 27 28 29 30 31 32 33 34 35 36 37 38 39 41 43 45 46 47 48 49 50 51 54 56 57 59 61 62 63 64 65 69 70 72 74 76 78 79 **P**6 **S** Department of Veterans Affairs, Washington, DC Web address: www.va.gov/stations97/guide/home.asp?DIVISION=ALL	45	10	53	1346	48	74476	—	30586	14092	336
GREELEY—Weld County										
★ NORTH COLORADO MEDICAL CENTER, 1801 16th Street, Zip 80631–5199; tel. 970/352–4121; Jon Sewell, Administrator (Nonreporting) **A**1 2 3 9 10 **S** Banner Health System, Fargo, ND Web address: www.ncmcgreeley.com	23	10	262	—	—	—	—	—	—	—
GUNNISON—Gunnison County										
GUNNISON VALLEY HOSPITAL, 711 North Taylor Street, Zip 81230–2296; tel. 970/641–1456; Robert S. Austin, President **A**9 10 **F**7 8 9 10 13 15 16 17 18 19 22 23 24 25 32 33 36 38 39 41 44 45 48 51 54 71 75 76 Web address: www.montrose.net/gvh/	13	10	22	610	4	26186	114	7979	3310	108
HAXTUN—Phillips County										
★ HAXTUN HOSPITAL DISTRICT, 235 West Fletcher Street, Zip 80731–0308, Mailing Address: P.O. Box 308, Zip 80731–0308; tel. 970/774–6123; James E. Brundige, Administrator (Total facility includes 32 beds in nursing home–type unit) **A**9 10 **F**9 16 17 18 19 22 25 32 34 36 37 45 46 48 51 54 56 69 70 75 76 78 **P**6	16	10	48	349	31	13037	14	3519	1892	78
HOLYOKE—Phillips County										
★ MELISSA MEMORIAL HOSPITAL, 505 South Baxter Avenue, Zip 80734–1496; tel. 970/854–2241; George V. Larson, II, Administrator **A**9 10 **F**8 9 16 17 19 22 23 25 28 31 32 34 36 38 45 48 50 54 56 75 76 **P**3 6	16	10	18	407	4	11076	34	4697	2588	88
HUGO—Lincoln County										
★ LINCOLN COMMUNITY HOSPITAL AND NURSING HOME, 111 Sixth Street, Zip 80821–0248, Mailing Address: P.O. Box 248, Zip 80821–0248; tel. 719/743–2421; Herman Schreivogel, Administrator and Chief Executive Officer (Total facility includes 35 beds in nursing home–type unit) **A**9 10 **F**8 22 36 39 45 48 54 69 75 76	13	10	56	406	27	12930	37	2976	2404	119
JULESBURG—Sedgwick County										
SEDGWICK COUNTY HEALTH CENTER, 900 Cedar Street, Zip 80737–1199; tel. 970/474–3323; Bill Patten, Administrator (Total facility includes 32 beds in nursing home–type unit) (Nonreporting) **A**9 10	13	10	58	—	—	—	—	—	—	—
KREMMLING—Grand County										
KREMMLING MEMORIAL HOSPITAL, 214 South Grand Avenue, Zip 80459, Mailing Address: P.O. Box 399, Zip 80459–0399; tel. 970/724–3442; Thomas Andron, Administrator and Chief Executive Officer **A**9 10 **F**7 9 13 16 17 18 28 30 32 38 46 48 49 56 75 76 78 **P**6 Web address: www.centura.org	16	10	19	123	9	21944	0	3334	2008	73
LA JARA—Conejos County										
□ CONEJOS COUNTY HOSPITAL, 19021 U.S. Highway 285, Zip 81140–0639, Mailing Address: P.O. Box 639, Zip 81140–0639; tel. 719/274–5121; Richard Cormier, Ph.D., Chief Executive Officer (Total facility includes 34 beds in nursing home–type unit) **A**1 9 10 **F**3 4 5 7 8 9 10 11 12 13 14 15 17 18 19 20 22 25 26 29 31 32 33 34 36 37 38 41 42 43 44 45 46 47 48 49 50 51 52 54 56 58 59 60 61 62 63 64 69 70 71 72 75 76 **P**1 5	16	10	49	1050	9	9100	45	2588	—	144
LA JUNTA—Otero County										
★ ARKANSAS VALLEY REGIONAL MEDICAL CENTER, 1100 Carson Avenue, Zip 81050–2799; tel. 719/383–6000; Lynn Crowell, Chief Executive Officer (Total facility includes 115 beds in nursing home–type unit) **A**1 9 10 **F**7 8 9 13 17 19 22 25 27 29 32 34 36 37 38 39 41 43 44 45 46 48 51 54 69 70 72 75 76 **S** Quorum Health Group, Brentwood, TN	23	10	182	2807	135	62665	337	24047	11551	447
LAMAR—Prowers County										
★ PROWERS MEDICAL CENTER, 401 Kendall Drive, Zip 81052–3993; tel. 719/336–4343; Earl J. Steinhoff, Administrator and Chief Executive Officer **A**1 9 10 **F**1 2 3 4 5 7 8 9 10 11 12 16 17 18 19 22 23 24 25 27 29 30 31 32 33 34 36 37 38 39 40 41 42 43 44 45 46 47 48 50 51 52 53 54 55 56 57 58 59 60 61 62 63 64 65 66 68 69 70 71 72 74 75 76 78 79 **S** Quorum Health Group, Brentwood, TN Web address: www.pmchospital.org	16	10	40	1504	12	25362	262	14460	6888	221
LEADVILLE—Lake County										
ST. VINCENT GENERAL HOSPITAL, 822 West Fourth Street, Zip 80461–3897; tel. 719/486–0230; Phillip Lowe, Chief Executive Officer (Nonreporting) **A**9 10	16	10	38	—	—	—	—	—	—	—

Hospitals, U.S. / COLORADO

Hospital, Address, Telephone, Administrator, Approval, Facility, and Physician Codes, Health Care System, Network	Classification Codes		Utilization Data					Expense (thousands) of dollars		Personnel
★ American Hospital Association (AHA) membership ☐ Joint Commission on Accreditation of Healthcare Organizations (JCAHO) accreditation + American Osteopathic Healthcare Association (AOHA) membership ○ American Osteopathic Association (AOA) accreditation △ Commission on Accreditation of Rehabilitation Facilities (CARF) accreditation Control codes 61, 63, 64, 71, 72 and 73 indicate hospitals listed by AOHA, but not registered by AHA. For definition of numerical codes, see page A4	Control	Service	Staffed Beds	Admissions	Census	Outpatient Visits	Births	Total	Payroll	Personnel
LITTLETON—Arapahoe County ★ LITTLETON ADVENTIST HOSPITAL, 7700 South Broadway Street, Zip 80122–2628; tel. 303/730–8900; Ruthita J. Fike, Administrator **A**9 **F**3 4 6 7 8 9 11 13 19 22 24 25 26 28 29 30 32 33 34 35 36 37 38 39 41 42 43 44 45 46 47 48 50 51 54 56 59 60 61 62 63 64 65 66 67 68 70 71 72 73 74 75 76 77 78 79 **Web address:** www.centura.org	21	10	129	8396	77	98141	2119	58967	25743	571
LONGMONT—Boulder County ★ △ LONGMONT UNITED HOSPITAL, 1950 West Mountain View Avenue, Zip 80501–3162, Mailing Address: P.O. Box 1659, Zip 80502–1659; tel. 303/651–5111; Kenneth R. Huey, President and Chief Executive Officer (Total facility includes 15 beds in nursing home–type unit) **A**1 2 7 9 10 **F**1 3 7 8 9 11 13 16 17 18 19 20 22 23 24 25 28 29 30 31 32 33 34 35 36 37 38 39 41 43 44 45 46 48 50 51 53 54 57 58 59 60 61 62 63 64 65 69 70 71 72 74 75 76 78 **P**8 **Web address:** www.luhonline.org	23	10	122	6040	69	264507	1101	55486	24253	785
LOUISVILLE—Boulder County ★ AVISTA ADVENTIST HOSPITAL, 100 Health Park Drive, Zip 80027–9583; tel. 303/673–1000; John Sackett, Chief Executive Officer (Nonreporting) **A**1 3 9 10 **Web address:** www.centura.org	21	10	58	—	—	—	—	—	—	—
☐ CENTENNIAL PEAKS HEALTH, (Formerly Charter Centennial Peaks Health System), 2255 South 88th Street, Zip 80027–9716; tel. 303/673–9990; Richard Failla, Chief Executive Officer (Nonreporting) **A**1 9 10	33	22	72	—	—	—	—	—	—	—
LOVELAND—Larimer County ★ MCKEE MEDICAL CENTER, 2000 Boise Avenue, Zip 80538–4281, Mailing Address: P.O. Box 830, Zip 80539–0830; tel. 970/669–4640; Charles F. Harms, Administrator (Total facility includes 16 beds in nursing home–type unit) **A**1 9 10 **F**1 7 8 9 11 13 16 17 18 19 21 22 23 24 25 32 33 34 36 38 39 41 43 44 45 46 48 49 50 51 53 54 60 69 70 71 72 75 76 78 79 **P**1 6 7 **S** Banner Health System, Fargo, ND **Web address:** www.wphn.com	23	10	108	5531	59	63372	827	46683	22098	612
MEEKER—Rio Blanco County ★ PIONEERS HOSPITAL OF RIO BLANCO COUNTY, (Includes Walbridge Memorial Convalescent Wing), 345 Cleveland Street, Zip 81641–0000; tel. 970/878–5047; Thomas E. Lake, Administrator and Chief Executive Officer (Total facility includes 29 beds in nursing home–type unit) **A**9 10 **F**1 9 12 16 22 25 28 36 40 41 45 48 54 69 71 75 76 **P**1 **S** Quorum Health Group, Brentwood, TN	13	10	46	222	28	7309	0	5265	2398	96
MONTROSE—Montrose County ★ MONTROSE MEMORIAL HOSPITAL, 800 South Third Street, Zip 81401–4291; tel. 970/249–2211; Kenneth E. S. Platou, Chief Executive Officer **A**1 10 **F**2 3 7 8 9 12 13 16 17 18 19 21 22 23 24 25 26 27 28 30 32 33 34 37 38 39 41 43 44 45 46 48 50 51 52 53 54 57 58 59 60 61 62 63 64 65 69 64 70 71 72 73 75 76 77 78 79 **P**5 8 **S** Quorum Health Group, Brentwood, TN	13	10	62	2849	28	79410	439	30444	12675	382
PUEBLO—Pueblo County ☐ COLORADO MENTAL HEALTH INSTITUTE AT PUEBLO, 1600 West 24th Street, Zip 81003–1499; tel. 719/546–4000; Robert L. Hawkins, Superintendent **A**1 9 10 **F**2 5 8 9 10 11 12 17 18 22 24 25 39 41 42 43 44 47 48 49 52 53 55 57 58 62 65 66 68 70 75 76 78 **P**1	44	22	554	1984	523	1801	0	61489	35401	919
★ △ PARKVIEW MEDICAL CENTER, 400 West 16th Street, Zip 81003–2781; tel. 719/584–4000; C. W. Smith, President and Chief Executive Officer **A**1 7 9 10 **F**1 2 3 4 8 9 11 13 16 17 18 19 21 22 24 25 27 30 32 34 35 36 39 41 43 44 46 47 48 49 50 51 53 54 57 58 59 60 61 62 63 69 70 71 75 76 78 **P**8 **S** Quorum Health Group, Brentwood, TN **Web address:** www.parkviewmc.com	23	10	260	10794	146	118571	1157	89748	39979	1175
★ ST. MARY-CORWIN MEDICAL CENTER, 1008 Minnequa Avenue, Zip 81004–3798; tel. 719/560–4000; Thomas E. Anderson, Chief Executive Officer (Total facility includes 16 beds in nursing home–type unit) (Nonreporting) **A**1 2 3 9 10 **S** Catholic Health Initiatives, Denver, CO **Web address:** www.centura.org	21	10	261	—	—	—	—	—	—	—
RANGELY—Rio Blanco County ★ RANGELY DISTRICT HOSPITAL, 511 South White Avenue, Zip 81648–2104; tel. 970/675–5011; DeAnn K. Cure, Chief Executive Officer **A**9 10 **F**9 14 17 25 32 34 36 38 40 43 51 54 55 75 76 **P**6	16	10	25	65	10	16176	0	3392	1887	59
RIFLE—Garfield County ★ GRAND RIVER HOSPITAL DISTRICT, 701 East Fifth Street, Zip 81650–2970, Mailing Address: P.O. Box 912, Zip 81650–0912; tel. 970/625–1510; Patrick Howery, Chief Executive Officer (Total facility includes 57 beds in nursing home–type unit) (Nonreporting) **A**9 10	16	10	75	—	—	—	—	—	—	—
SALIDA—Chaffee County ★ HEART OF THE ROCKIES REGIONAL MEDICAL CENTER, 448 East First Street, Zip 81201–0429, Mailing Address: P.O. Box 429, Zip 81201–0429; tel. 719/539–6661; Howard D. Turner, Chief Executive Officer **A**9 10 **F**8 9 12 13 19 22 24 25 32 36 37 39 40 41 44 45 46 48 49 54 75 76 78 **P**5 **S** Quorum Health Group, Brentwood, TN **Web address:** www.hrrmc.com	16	10	33	1405	15	36152	139	13878	5690	200

Hospitals, U.S. / COLORADO

Hospital, Address, Telephone, Administrator, Approval, Facility, and Physician Codes, Health Care System, Network ★ American Hospital Association (AHA) membership ☐ Joint Commission on Accreditation of Healthcare Organizations (JCAHO) accreditation + American Osteopathic Healthcare Association (AOHA) membership ○ American Osteopathic Association (AOA) accreditation △ Commission on Accreditation of Rehabilitation Facilities (CARF) accreditation Control codes 61, 63, 64, 71, 72 and 73 indicate hospitals listed by AOHA, but not registered by AHA. For definition of numerical codes, see page A4	Classification Codes		Utilization Data					Expense (thousands) of dollars		
	Control	Service	Staffed Beds	Admissions	Census	Outpatient Visits	Births	Total	Payroll	Personnel
SPRINGFIELD—Baca County ★ SOUTHEAST COLORADO HOSPITAL AND LONG TERM CARE, 373 East Tenth Avenue, Zip 81073–1699; tel. 719/523–4501; Al Campbell, Chief Executive Officer (Total facility includes 56 beds in nursing home–type unit) **A**10 **F**7 9 15 16 18 19 22 25 29 31 32 36 37 38 39 40 41 48 54 69 70 76 79	16	10	81	404	57	26257	0	6382	3830	174
STEAMBOAT SPRINGS—Routt County ✣ YAMPA VALLEY MEDICAL CENTER, (Formerly Routt Memorial Hospital), 80 Park Avenue, Zip 80487–5010; tel. 970/879–1322; Margaret D. Sabin, Chief Executive Officer (Total facility includes 50 beds in nursing home–type unit) (Nonreporting) **A**1 10	23	10	74	—						
STERLING—Logan County ✣ STERLING REGIONAL MEDCENTER, 615 Fairhurst Street, Zip 80751–0500, Mailing Address: P.O. Box 3500, Zip 80751–0500; tel. 970/522–0122; Michael J. Gillen, Administrator **A**1 9 10 **F**7 8 9 13 14 16 18 19 22 24 25 26 27 28 30 32 33 34 35 36 37 38 39 40 41 43 44 45 46 48 49 50 51 52 53 54 56 69 70 71 72 75 76 78 79 **P**6 8 **S** Banner Health System, Fargo, ND Web address: www.lhsnet.org	23	10	36	1864	18	42399	255	25035	10778	259
THORNTON—Adams County ✣ NORTH SUBURBAN MEDICAL CENTER, 9191 Grant Street, Zip 80229–4341; tel. 303/451–7800; Margaret C. Cain, President and Chief Executive Officer (Total facility includes 15 beds in nursing home–type unit) (Nonreporting) **A**1 9 10 **S** HCA – The Healthcare Company, Nashville, TN Web address: www.hcahealthcare.com	33	10	125							
☐ SUNHEALTH SPECIALTY HOSPITAL FOR DENVER, (Formerly Mediplex Rehab–Denver), 8451 Pearl Street, Zip 80229–4804; tel. 303/288–3000; Walter Sackett, Chief Executive Officer **A**1 5 10 **F**3 17 18 22 24 30 31 38 39 49 53 54 55 57 62 68 70 76 78 Web address: www.sunh.com	33	46	92	839	61	279	0	15570	5776	209
TRINIDAD—Las Animas County ✣ MT. SAN RAFAEL HOSPITAL, 410 Benedicta Avenue, Zip 81082–2093; tel. 719/846–9213; Paul L. Herman, Chief Executive Officer **A**1 10 **F**7 8 9 16 17 18 19 22 24 25 32 33 34 35 36 39 41 43 44 48 51 54 70 72 75 76 **P**8 **S** Quorum Health Group, Brentwood, TN	23	10	31	1194	14	39451	152	9784	4287	155
USAF ACADEMY—El Paso County ✣ U. S. AIR FORCE ACADEMY HOSPITAL, 4102 Pinion Drive, Zip 80840–4000; tel. 719/333–5102; Colonel Jay D. Sprenger, USAF, Commander **A**1 9 **F**9 13 16 17 18 22 23 25 29 33 38 39 48 49 50 54 56 63 70 71 76 78 79 **S** Department of the Air Force, Bowling AFB, DC	41	10	30	1400	9	318596	0	—		
VAIL—Eagle County ✣ VAIL VALLEY MEDICAL CENTER, 181 West Meadow Drive, Zip 81657–5059; tel. 970/476–2451; Clifford M. Eldredge, President and Chief Executive Officer **A**1 3 9 10 **F**7 8 9 13 14 17 18 19 21 22 23 24 25 26 28 29 30 31 32 33 34 35 36 37 38 39 41 43 44 45 46 48 49 50 51 54 70 71 72 73 75 76 77 78 79 **P**5 Web address: www.vvmc.com	23	10	49	2298	18	43347	553	43347	14463	344
WALSENBURG—Huerfano County ★ HUERFANO MEDICAL CENTER, 23500 U.S. Highway 160, Zip 81089–9524; tel. 719/738–5100; Vonnie Maier, President and Chief Executive Officer **A**9 10 **F**3 5 9 17 18 19 22 23 25 30 31 32 33 34 35 36 37 38 39 43 46 48 50 51 54 69 70 71 76 78 79 Web address: www.huerfanomedicalcenter.org	16	10	24	756	11	21346	0	7130	3190	191
WESTMINSTER—Jefferson County CLEO WALLACE CENTERS HOSPITAL, 8405 Church Ranch Boulevard, Zip 80021; tel. 303/466–7391; Michael J. Montgomery, President and Chief Executive Officer (Nonreporting) **A**10	23	52	61	—						
★ ST. ANTHONY NORTH HOSPITAL, 2551 West 84th Avenue, Zip 80030–3887; tel. 303/426–2151; Peggy Gustafson, Administrator **A**10 **F**1 4 6 7 8 9 11 13 16 17 18 19 21 22 25 28 29 30 31 36 37 38 39 41 42 43 44 45 46 47 48 49 51 53 54 56 57 62 63 65 67 69 70 72 74 75 76 77 78 79 **S** Catholic Health Initiatives, Denver, CO Web address: www.centura.org	21	10	106	8054	74	71198	1209	52398	21426	545
WHEAT RIDGE—Jefferson County ✣ △ EXEMPLA LUTHERAN MEDICAL CENTER, (Includes Exempla West Pines, 3400 Lutheran Parkway, Zip 80033; tel. 303/467–4000), 8300 West 38th Avenue, Zip 80033–6005; tel. 303/425–4500; Jeffrey D. Selberg, President and Chief Executive Officer (Total facility includes 18 beds in nursing home–type unit) (Nonreporting) **A**1 2 7 9 10 **S** Exempla Healthcare, Inc., Denver, CO Web address: www.exempla.org	23	10	335	—						
WRAY—Yuma County ★ WRAY COMMUNITY DISTRICT HOSPITAL, 1017 West 7th Street, Zip 80758–1420; tel. 970/332–4811; Daniel Dennis, Administrator (Nonreporting) **A**3 9 10	16	10	25	—						
YUMA—Yuma County ★ YUMA DISTRICT HOSPITAL, 910 South Main Street, Zip 80759–3098, Mailing Address: P.O. Box 306, Zip 80759–0306; tel. 970/848–5405; Timothy F. Reardon, FACHE, Chief Executive Officer **A**10 **F**7 8 9 16 17 19 22 25 32 36 39 44 45 48 54 63 69 73 75 76 **P**2	16	10	11	271	2	19498	32	4567	2755	—

Hospitals, U.S. / CONNECTICUT

CONNECTICUT

Resident Population 3,274 (in thousands)
Resident population in metro areas 95.6%
Birth rate per 1,000 population 13.2
65 years and over 14.3%
Percent of persons without health insurance 12%

★ American Hospital Association (AHA) membership
□ Joint Commission on Accreditation of Healthcare Organizations (JCAHO) accreditation
+ American Osteopathic Healthcare Association (AOHA) membership
○ American Osteopathic Association (AOA) accreditation
△ Commission on Accreditation of Rehabilitation Facilities (CARF) accreditation
Control codes 61, 63, 64, 71, 72 and 73 indicate hospitals listed by AOHA, but not registered by AHA. For definition of numerical codes, see page A4

Hospital, Address, Telephone, Administrator, Approval, Facility, and Physician Codes, Health Care System, Network	Classification Codes		Utilization Data					Expense (thousands) of dollars		
	Control	Service	Staffed Beds	Admissions	Census	Outpatient Visits	Births	Total	Payroll	Personnel
BETHLEHEM—Litchfield County										
★ WELLSPRING FOUNDATION, 21 Arch Bridge Road, Zip 06751–0370, Mailing Address: P.O. Box 370, Zip 06751–0370; tel. 203/266–7235; Richard E. Beauvais, Ph.D., Chief Executive Officer **F**57 58 59 60 63 64
Web address: www.wellspring.org	23	22	36	73	21	1031	0	3375	2511	77
BRANFORD—New Haven County										
□ THE CONNECTICUT HOSPICE, (SPECIALTY SHORT–TERM HOSPITAL), 61 Burban Drive, Zip 06405–4096; tel. 203/481–6231; Rosemary Johnson Hurzeler, President and Chief Executive Officer **A**1 10 **F**13 16 17 18 19 20 23 26 31 33 35 36 37 38 49 59 70 72 78 **P**6
Web address: www.hospice.com	23	49	52	1447	40	93560	0	—	—	145
BRIDGEPORT—Fairfield County										
✠ BRIDGEPORT HOSPITAL, 267 Grant Street, Zip 06610–0120, Mailing Address: P.O. Box 5000, Zip 06610–5000; tel. 203/384–3000; Robert J. Trefry, President and Chief Executive Officer **A**1 2 3 5 6 8 9 10 **F**3 4 7 8 9 10 11 13 14 17 18 19 21 22 23 24 25 31 32 33 34 35 36 37 38 39 40 41 42 43 44 45 46 47 48 49 50 51 52 53 54 56 57 58 59 60 61 62 64 65 66 70 71 72 73 74 75 76 77 78 79 **P**1 **S** Yale New Haven Health System, New Haven, CT
Web address: www.bridgeporthospital.com	23	10	334	16684	233	147577	2542	190679	76903	1818
SOUTHWEST CONNECTICUT MENTAL HEALTH SYSTEM, (Formerly Greater Bridgeport Community Health Center), 1635 Central Avenue, Zip 06610–2700, Mailing Address: P.O. Box 5117, Zip 06610–5117; tel. 203/551–7444; James M. Pisciotta, Chief Executive Officer **A**10 **F**2 13 57 61 63 **S** Connecticut Department of Mental Health and Addiction Services, Hartford, CT	12	22	62	1878	57	131155	0	29234	23138	476
✠ ST. VINCENT'S MEDICAL CENTER, (Includes Hall–Brooke Hospital, A Division of Hall–Brooke Foundation, 47 Long Lots Road, Westport, Zip 06880–3800; tel. 203/227–1251; Seth Berman, President and Chief Executive Officer), 2800 Main Street, Zip 06606–4292; tel. 203/576–6000; William J. Riordan, President and Chief Executive Officer **A**1 2 3 5 8 9 10 **F**1 2 3 4 7 8 9 11 12 13 16 17 18 19 20 22 24 25 26 28 29 30 31 32 33 34 35 36 37 38 39 41 43 44 45 46 47 48 49 51 53 54 56 57 58 59 61 62 63 64 65 69 70 72 73 75 76 77 78 79 **P**1 5 7 8 **S** Ascension Health, Saint Louis, MO	21	10	291	16507	270	185797	1920	164064	78883	1612
BRISTOL—Hartford County										
✠ BRISTOL HOSPITAL, P.O. Box 977, Brewster Road, Zip 06011–0977; tel. 860/585–3000; Thomas D. Kennedy, II, President and Chief Executive Officer **A**1 2 9 10 **F**1 3 4 8 9 13 14 16 17 19 21 22 24 25 26 28 30 31 32 33 34 35 36 37 38 39 40 41 42 43 44 45 46 47 48 49 51 54 55 56 57 58 59 60 61 62 63 64 65 66 70 71 72 73 75 76 77 78 79 **P**5 7 8
Web address: www.bristolhospital.org	23	10	128	6315	76	181193	919	72387	33416	710
DANBURY—Fairfield County										
✠ DANBURY HOSPITAL, 24 Hospital Avenue, Zip 06810–6099; tel. 203/797–7000; Frank J. Kelly, President and Chief Executive Officer **A**1 2 3 5 8 9 10 **F**2 3 4 5 8 9 10 11 12 13 14 16 17 18 19 20 21 22 23 24 25 26 28 29 30 31 32 33 34 35 36 37 38 39 41 43 44 45 46 47 48 49 50 51 53 54 56 57 58 59 60 61 62 63 64 65 66 70 71 72 73 74 75 76 77 78 79 **P**1 6 7
Web address: www.danhosp.org	23	10	271	14168	171	224609	2457	194465	84855	1747
DERBY—New Haven County										
✠ GRIFFIN HOSPITAL, 130 Division Street, Zip 06418–1326; tel. 203/735–7421; Patrick Charmel, President and Chief Executive Officer **A**1 2 3 5 9 10 **F**3 8 9 16 17 18 20 22 24 25 32 33 34 38 39 41 44 45 46 48 49 50 51 54 56 57 61 62 63 64 66 76 77 78 79
Web address: www.lnvalley.org/griffin	23	10	160	5248	65	118508	614	62683	28139	649
FARMINGTON—Hartford County										
✠ UNIVERSITY OF CONNECTICUT HEALTH CENTER, JOHN DEMPSEY HOSPITAL, 263 Farmington Avenue, Zip 06030; tel. 860/679–2000; Gloria J. Opirhory, Ph.D., Director (Nonreporting) **A**1 2 3 5 8 9 10
Web address: www.uconnhealth.org	12	10	128	—	—	—	—	—	—	—
GREENWICH—Fairfield County										
✠ GREENWICH HOSPITAL, 5 Perryridge Road, Zip 06830–4697; tel. 203/863–3000; Frank A. Corvino, President and Chief Executive Officer **A**1 2 3 5 9 10 **F**2 3 7 8 9 11 12 13 14 15 16 17 18 19 20 21 22 23 24 25 26 28 30 32 33 34 35 36 37 38 39 41 42 43 44 45 46 48 49 50 51 54 56 58 59 60 61 62 63 65 66 69 70 71 72 73 75 76 78 79 **P**5 **S** Yale New Haven Health System, New Haven, CT
Web address: www.greenhosp.chime.org	23	10	160	7068	104	287266	1357	108010	54380	1155
HARTFORD—Hartford County										
✠ CONNECTICUT CHILDREN'S MEDICAL CENTER, 282 Washington Street, Zip 06106–3322; tel. 860/545–9000; Larry M. Gold, President and Chief Executive Officer **A**1 3 9 10 **F**7 11 14 16 19 22 24 25 33 34 35 36 38 39 42 43 45 46 47 48 50 52 54 56 58 59 61 65 70 71 72 74 75 76 78 **P**3
Web address: www.ccmckids.org	23	59	104	4410	73	99219	0	75553	27734	846

Hospitals, U.S. / CONNECTICUT

Hospital, Address, Telephone, Administrator, Approval, Facility, and Physician Codes, Health Care System, Network ★ American Hospital Association (AHA) membership ☐ Joint Commission on Accreditation of Healthcare Organizations (JCAHO) accreditation + American Osteopathic Healthcare Association (AOHA) membership ○ American Osteopathic Association (AOA) accreditation △ Commission on Accreditation of Rehabilitation Facilities (CARF) accreditation Control codes 61, 63, 64, 71, 72 and 73 indicate hospitals listed by AOHA, but not registered by AHA. For definition of numerical codes, see page A4	Classi-fication Codes		Utilization Data					Expense (thousands) of dollars		
	Control	Service	Staffed Beds	Admissions	Census	Outpatient Visits	Births	Total	Payroll	Personnel
★ △ HARTFORD HOSPITAL, (Includes Institute of Living, 400 Washington Street, Zip 06106–3392; tel. 860/545–7000), 80 Seymour Street, Zip 06102–5037, Mailing Address: P.O. Box 5037, Zip 06102–5037; tel. 860/545–5000; John J. Meehan, President and Chief Executive Officer (Total facility includes 104 beds in nursing home–type unit) A1 2 3 5 7 8 9 10 F1 3 4 7 8 9 11 12 15 16 17 18 19 20 22 23 24 25 28 29 30 32 33 34 35 36 37 38 39 40 41 42 43 44 45 46 47 48 49 50 51 52 53 54 55 56 57 58 59 60 61 62 63 64 65 66 68 69 70 71 72 74 75 76 77 78 79 P5 6 8 Web address: www.harthosp.org	23	10	874	31813	585	196902	4234	432523	206711	4127
★ SAINT FRANCIS HOSPITAL AND MEDICAL CENTER, 114 Woodland Street, Zip 06105–1200; tel. 860/714–4000; David D'Eramo, President and Chief Executive Officer A1 2 3 5 8 9 10 F3 4 7 8 9 11 12 13 14 16 17 18 19 20 22 23 24 25 28 30 34 35 36 37 38 39 40 41 42 44 45 46 47 48 49 50 51 54 55 56 57 58 59 60 61 62 63 64 65 66 68 70 71 72 73 75 76 77 78 79 P4 8 Web address: www.stfranciscare.org	21	10	545	25260	363	305563	3341	318151	141356	2576
MANCHESTER—Hartford County										
★ MANCHESTER MEMORIAL HOSPITAL, 71 Haynes Street, Zip 06040–4188; tel. 860/646–1222; Marc H. Lory, President and Chief Executive Officer A1 9 10 F1 3 7 8 9 12 13 14 16 17 18 19 21 22 24 25 27 30 32 33 34 35 36 37 38 39 40 41 43 44 46 48 49 50 51 54 56 57 58 59 60 61 62 63 64 65 68 69 70 71 72 73 76 77 78 P4 5 6 8 Web address: www.echn.org/ec01000.htm	23	10	161	7420	97	206669	933	100275	47709	1119
MANSFIELD CENTER—Tolland County										
☐ NATCHAUG HOSPITAL, 189 Storrs Road, Zip 06250–1638; tel. 860/456–1311; Stephen W. Larcen, Ph.D., Chief Executive Officer A1 9 10 F2 3 16 17 18 57 58 59 60 61 62 63 64 P1 6	23	22	58	1597	41	21840	0	14666	8496	220
MERIDEN—New Haven County										
★ MIDSTATE MEDICAL CENTER, (Includes East Campus, 883 Paddock Avenue, Zip 06450–7094), 435 Lewis Avenue, Zip 06451–2101; tel. 203/694–8200; Lucille A. Janatka, President and Chief Executive Officer A1 2 9 10 F1 3 7 8 9 13 17 18 19 21 22 24 25 26 27 28 29 30 33 34 35 36 37 38 39 41 43 44 46 48 49 50 51 57 58 59 60 61 62 63 64 65 68 70 72 73 76 77 78 P1 5 8 Web address: www.midstatemedical.org	23	10	94	7016	80	104669	1103	101961	33386	777
MIDDLETOWN—Middlesex County										
☐ CONNECTICUT VALLEY HOSPITAL, (Includes Whiting Forensic Division of Connecticut Valley Hospital, O'Brien Drive, Zip 06457, Mailing Address: Box 70, Zip 06457–3942; tel. 203/344–2541), Silver Street, Zip 06457–7023, Mailing Address: P.O. Box 351, Zip 06457–0351; tel. 860/262–5000; Garrell S. Mullaney, Chief Executive Officer (Nonreporting) A1 5 9 10 S Connecticut Department of Mental Health and Addiction Services, Hartford, CT	12	22	418	—	—	—	—	—	—	—
★ MIDDLESEX HOSPITAL, 28 Crescent Street, Zip 06457–3650; tel. 860/344–6000; Robert Gerard Kiely, President and Chief Executive Officer A1 2 3 5 9 10 F1 2 3 6 8 9 12 13 14 16 17 18 19 21 22 24 25 26 29 30 32 33 34 35 36 37 38 39 41 44 45 46 48 49 50 51 54 55 56 57 58 59 60 61 62 63 64 65 66 67 70 71 72 76 77 78 79 P5 8 Web address: www.midhosp.org	23	10	124	9123	98	870000	1182	130891	68090	1407
RIVERVIEW HOSPITAL FOR CHILDREN, 915 River Road, Zip 06457–3918, Mailing Address: P.O. Box 2792, Zip 06457–2792; tel. 860/704–4000; Robert Plant, Ph.D., Superintendent A3 F50 57 58 60 78	12	52	97	193	91	0	0	24222	16675	304
WHITING FORENSIC DIVISION OF CONNECTICUT VALLEY HOSPITAL See Connecticut Valley Hospital										
MILFORD—New Haven County										
★ MILFORD HOSPITAL, 300 Seaside Avenue, Zip 06460–4603; tel. 203/876–4000; Paul E. Moss, President A1 2 9 10 F7 8 9 13 16 17 18 19 22 24 25 32 34 36 38 39 40 41 43 44 46 48 49 51 61 68 70 72 73 76 77 78 P5 7 8 Web address: www.milfordhospital.org	23	10	51	3812	47	56648	471	43512	20305	515
NEW BRITAIN—Hartford County										
★ △ HOSPITAL FOR SPECIAL CARE, (CHRONIC DISEASE & REHAB), 2150 Corbin Avenue, Zip 06053–2263; tel. 860/827–4758; David Crandall, President and Chief Executive Officer A1 7 10 F13 16 17 18 23 28 30 38 43 45 53 54 59 70 71 72 78 P6 Web address: www.hfsc.org	23	49	199	569	180	18213	0	57066	32920	708
★ NEW BRITAIN GENERAL HOSPITAL, 100 Grand Street, Zip 06052–2017, Mailing Address: P.O. Box 100, Zip 06050–0100; tel. 860/224–5011; Laurence A. Tanner, President and Chief Executive Officer A1 2 3 5 8 9 10 F1 2 3 4 6 7 8 9 11 12 13 16 17 18 19 21 22 24 25 26 27 28 29 30 31 33 34 35 36 37 38 39 40 41 42 43 44 45 46 47 48 49 50 51 54 55 57 58 59 60 61 62 63 64 65 66 67 68 70 71 72 74 76 78 79 P8 Web address: www.nbgh.org	23	10	262	14072	170	245420	1945	169232	92319	1846
NEW CANAAN—Fairfield County										
★ SILVER HILL HOSPITAL, 208 Valley Road, Zip 06840–3899; tel. 203/966–3561; Richard J. Frances, M.D., President and Medical Director A1 9 10 F3 19 21 28 57 58 59 60 61 62 63 64 P6 Web address: www.silverhillhospital.com	23	22	64	1401	43	7615	0	14421	8504	156
NEW HAVEN—New Haven County										
☐ CONNECTICUT MENTAL HEALTH CENTER, 34 Park Street, Zip 06519–1187, Mailing Address: P.O. Box 1842, Zip 06508–1842; tel. 203/974–7144; Selby Jacobs, M.D., Director A1 3 5 9 10 F3 13 15 18 19 21 22 24 25 39 43 51 57 58 59 60 61 63 64 70 72 75 76 S Connecticut Department of Mental Health and Addiction Services, Hartford, CT	12	22	36	994	22	86276	—	—	—	513

© 2000 AHA Guide   *Many Facility Codes have changed. Please refer to the AHA Guide Code Chart.*   Hospitals   **A75**

Hospitals, U.S. / CONNECTICUT

Hospital, Address, Telephone, Administrator, Approval, Facility, and Physician Codes, Health Care System, Network

- ★ American Hospital Association (AHA) membership
- ☐ Joint Commission on Accreditation of Healthcare Organizations (JCAHO) accreditation
- + American Osteopathic Healthcare Association (AOHA) membership
- ○ American Osteopathic Association (AOA) accreditation
- △ Commission on Accreditation of Rehabilitation Facilities (CARF) accreditation

Control codes 61, 63, 64, 71, 72 and 73 indicate hospitals listed by AOHA, but not registered by AHA. For definition of numerical codes, see page A4

Hospital	Classification Codes - Control	Service	Staffed Beds	Admissions	Census	Outpatient Visits	Births	Expense Total	Payroll	Personnel
★ HOSPITAL OF SAINT RAPHAEL, 1450 Chapel Street, Zip 06511-1450; tel. 203/789-3000; David W. Benfer, FACHE, President and Chief Executive Officer **A**1 2 3 5 8 9 10 **F**1 3 4 7 8 9 11 12 13 14 16 17 18 19 21 22 23 24 25 26 30 31 32 33 34 35 36 38 39 41 43 44 45 46 47 48 50 51 53 54 56 57 58 59 60 61 62 63 64 65 66 68 69 70 72 73 75 76 77 78 79 **P**5 8 Web address: www.srhs.org	21	10	464	22220	347	217350	1236	276277	132447	2734
★ VETERANS AFFAIRS CONNECTICUT HEALTHCARE SYSTEM–WEST HAVEN DIVISION, (Includes West Haven Division, 950 Campbell Avenue, West Haven, Zip 06516-2700; tel. 203/932-5711), 950 Campbell Avenue, Zip 06516-2770; tel. 203/932-5711; Paul J. McCool, Director (Total facility includes 40 beds in nursing home–type unit) **A**1 2 3 5 8 9 **F**1 2 3 4 7 9 11 13 18 19 20 21 22 23 24 25 26 29 30 31 32 33 34 35 36 37 38 39 41 43 45 46 47 48 49 50 51 54 55 56 57 59 60 61 62 63 64 65 68 69 70 72 76 77 78 79 **P**6 **S** Department of Veterans Affairs, Washington, DC Web address: www.va.gov/stations97/guide/home.asp?DIVISION=ALL	45	10	200	4693	172	405603	0	180193	73890	1940
☐ YALE PSYCHIATRIC INSTITUTE, 184 Liberty Street, Zip 06520-8038, Mailing Address: P.O. Box 208038, Zip 06520-8038; tel. 203/785-7200; Thomas H. McGlashan, M.D., Director and Psychiatrist–in–Chief **A**1 3 5 9 10 **F**3 21 30 57 58 60 62 63 64 70 Web address: www.yale.edu	23	22	66	1914	55	—	0	—	—	—
★ YALE–NEW HAVEN HOSPITAL, 20 York Street, Zip 06504-3202; tel. 203/688-4242; Joseph A. Zaccagnino, President and Chief Executive Officer **A**1 2 3 5 8 9 10 **F**3 4 7 8 9 11 12 13 14 16 17 18 19 21 22 23 24 25 26 27 29 30 31 32 33 34 35 36 37 38 39 41 42 43 44 45 46 47 48 49 50 51 52 53 54 55 56 57 58 59 60 61 62 63 64 65 66 68 70 71 72 73 74 75 76 77 78 79 **P**4 5 7 8 **S** Yale New Haven Health System, New Haven, CT Web address: www.ynhh.org	23	10	722	34234	545	377663	4631	449552	208174	4658
NEW LONDON—New London County										
★ LAWRENCE & MEMORIAL HOSPITAL, 365 Montauk Avenue, Zip 06320-4769; tel. 860/442-0711; William T. Christopher, President and Chief Executive Officer **A**1 9 10 **F**7 8 9 11 12 13 14 16 17 18 19 22 24 25 29 34 35 37 38 39 41 42 43 44 45 46 48 49 50 51 53 54 57 58 59 60 61 62 63 64 65 66 70 71 72 76 77 78 79 **P**6	23	10	228	12282	181	114601	1769	145301	70575	1485
NEW MILFORD—Litchfield County										
★ NEW MILFORD HOSPITAL, 21 Elm Street, Zip 06776-2993; tel. 860/355-2611; Richard E. Pugh, President and Chief Executive Officer **A**1 9 10 **F**7 8 9 12 13 16 17 18 19 21 22 23 24 25 26 28 32 35 37 39 41 43 44 45 46 48 49 54 61 65 66 68 70 71 72 76 77 78 79 Web address: www.newmilfordhospital.org	23	10	62	3004	35	—	350	43491	19952	430
NEWINGTON—Hartford County										
☐ CEDARCREST HOSPITAL, 525 Russell Road, Zip 06111-1595; tel. 860/666-4613; Peter Mendelson, Superintendent **A**1 10 **F**2 3 7 16 17 18 31 33 35 50 51 57 59 60 61 62 63 64 70 72 78 **P**6 **S** Connecticut Department of Mental Health and Addiction Services, Hartford, CT	12	22	131	591	5	—	—	—	—	—
NORWALK—Fairfield County										
★ △ NORWALK HOSPITAL, 34 Maple Street, Zip 06856-5050; tel. 203/852-2000; David W. Osborne, President and Chief Executive Officer **A**1 2 3 5 7 9 10 **F**2 3 8 9 11 12 13 14 17 18 19 21 22 23 24 25 27 28 29 30 32 35 36 39 40 41 42 43 44 45 46 48 49 50 51 53 54 56 57 58 59 60 61 62 63 64 65 66 70 72 73 75 76 78 79 **P**5 7 Web address: www.norwalkhospital.org	23	10	286	13661	200	107725	2094	138507	74581	1746
NORWICH—New London County										
★ THE WILLIAM W. BACKUS HOSPITAL, 326 Washington Street, Zip 06360-2740; tel. 860/889-8331; Thomas P. Pipicelli, President and Chief Executive Officer **A**1 9 10 **F**4 7 8 9 11 13 16 17 18 19 22 24 25 26 27 29 32 33 34 35 36 37 38 39 41 42 43 44 45 46 48 49 50 54 56 57 59 60 61 62 63 64 65 68 70 72 73 75 76 77 78 Web address: www.backushospital.org	23	10	164	10215	127	646956	1137	104625	47855	—
PORTLAND—Middlesex County										
☐ SAINT FRANCIS CARE BEHAVIORAL HEALTH, (Formerly Elmcrest Behavioral Health Network), 25 Marlborough Street, Zip 06480-1829; tel. 860/342-0480; Richard Moed, President and Chief Executive Officer **A**1 9 10 **F**3 13 16 17 19 43 45 51 58 59 60 61 62 63 64 72 73 79 **P**6 Web address: www.stfranciscarebh.org	23	22	93	2953	80	69868	—	26942	16104	493
PUTNAM—Windham County										
★ DAY KIMBALL HOSPITAL, 320 Pomfret Street, Zip 06260-0901, Mailing Address: P.O. Box 6001, Zip 06260-6001; tel. 860/928-6541; Charles F. Schneider, President **A**1 9 10 **F**3 8 9 13 14 16 17 18 19 21 22 24 25 29 30 31 32 33 34 36 37 38 39 41 44 46 48 49 51 54 57 59 60 62 63 64 66 68 70 71 72 73 76 77 78 79 **P**8 Web address: www.hnne.org	23	10	101	4941	53	313036	575	58553	29727	547
ROCKY HILL—Hartford County										
☐ VETERANS HOME AND HOSPITAL, 287 West Street, Zip 06067-3501; tel. 860/529-2571; Joanne M. Blum, Administrator (Nonreporting) **A**1 10	12	48	296	—	—	—	—	—	—	—
SHARON—Litchfield County										
★ SHARON HOSPITAL, 50 Hospital Hill Road, Zip 06069-0789, Mailing Address: P.O. Box 789, Zip 06069-0789; tel. 860/364-4141; Michael R. Gallacher, President and Chief Executive Officer **A**1 2 9 10 **F**8 9 16 18 19 22 24 25 33 34 37 38 41 43 44 45 46 48 50 51 54 56 62 70 72 75 76 77 78 **P**5 7 Web address: www.sharon.org	23	10	85	2659	34	62703	328	31607	14295	323

Hospitals, U.S. / CONNECTICUT

Hospital, Address, Telephone, Administrator, Approval, Facility, and Physician Codes, Health Care System, Network ★ American Hospital Association (AHA) membership □ Joint Commission on Accreditation of Healthcare Organizations (JCAHO) accreditation + American Osteopathic Healthcare Association (AOHA) membership ○ American Osteopathic Association (AOA) accreditation △ Commission on Accreditation of Rehabilitation Facilities (CARF) accreditation Control codes 61, 63, 64, 71, 72 and 73 indicate hospitals listed by AOHA, but not registered by AHA. For definition of numerical codes, see page A4	Classification Codes		Utilization Data					Expense (thousands) of dollars		
	Control	Service	Staffed Beds	Admissions	Census	Outpatient Visits	Births	Total	Payroll	Personnel
SOMERS—Tolland County CONNECTICUT DEPARTMENT OF CORRECTION'S HOSPITAL, 100 Bilton Road, Zip 06071, Mailing Address: P.O. Box 100, Zip 06071-0100; tel. 860/749-8391; Edward A. Blanchette, M.D., Director (Nonreporting)	12	11	29	—	—	—	—	—	—	—
SOUTHINGTON—Hartford County ★ BRADLEY MEMORIAL HOSPITAL AND HEALTH CENTER, 81 Meriden Avenue, Zip 06489-3297; tel. 860/276-5000; Clarence J. Silvia, President and Chief Executive Officer **A**1 9 10 **F**7 9 12 13 17 19 22 24 25 27 30 32 33 34 37 38 39 41 43 45 46 48 50 54 59 60 61 63 68 70 72 76 78 79 **P**5 Web address: www.bradleymemorial.org	16	10	74	2530	33	83126	0	25749	12399	318
STAFFORD SPRINGS—Tolland County ★ JOHNSON MEMORIAL HOSPITAL, 201 Chestnut Hill Road, Zip 06076-0860, Mailing Address: P.O. Box 860, Zip 06076-0860; tel. 860/684-4251; Alfred A. Lerz, President and Chief Executive Officer **A**1 9 10 **F**3 8 9 13 14 16 17 18 19 21 22 24 25 28 29 30 32 33 34 35 36 37 38 39 41 43 44 45 46 48 50 51 54 56 57 58 59 60 61 62 63 64 68 70 72 73 76 78 79 **P**5 Web address: www.jmhosp.org	23	10	89	3722	42	67666	252	34622	17541	365
STAMFORD—Fairfield County ★ STAMFORD HEALTH SYSTEM, (Formerly Stamford Hospital), 6 Shelburne Road, Zip 06904-9317; tel. 203/325-7000; Philip D. Cusano, President and Chief Executive Officer **A**1 2 3 5 8 9 10 **F**1 3 6 8 9 11 12 13 16 17 18 19 22 23 24 25 26 28 29 30 31 32 33 34 35 36 37 38 39 41 42 43 44 45 46 48 49 50 51 53 54 56 57 58 59 60 61 62 63 64 65 66 68 69 70 72 74 75 76 77 78 79 **P**7 Web address: www.stamhealth.org	23	10	296	13800	199	155646	2798	150219	66694	1385
TORRINGTON—Litchfield County ★ CHARLOTTE HUNGERFORD HOSPITAL, 540 Litchfield Street, Zip 06790-0988, Mailing Address: P.O. Box 988, Zip 06790-0988; tel. 860/496-6666; Rosanne U. Griswold, President and Chief Executive Officer **A**1 2 9 10 **F**7 8 9 12 13 14 16 17 18 19 21 22 23 24 25 29 32 33 34 35 37 38 39 40 41 43 44 45 46 48 49 50 51 54 57 58 59 61 63 64 65 68 70 71 72 75 76 77 78 79 **P**6 8	23	10	102	5816	73	172579	596	71238	34099	778
VERNON ROCKVILLE—Hartford County ★ ROCKVILLE GENERAL HOSPITAL, 31 Union Street, Zip 06066-3160; tel. 860/872-0501; Marc H. Lory, President and Chief Executive Officer **A**1 9 10 **F**3 7 8 9 13 14 16 17 18 19 21 22 24 25 27 30 31 32 33 34 35 36 37 38 39 40 41 43 44 45 46 48 49 50 51 54 56 57 58 59 60 61 62 63 64 65 68 69 70 71 72 73 76 77 78 79 **P**4 5 6 8	23	10	50	3934	44	89384	590	44984	21483	485
WALLINGFORD—New Haven County □ △ GAYLORD HOSPITAL, Gaylord Farm Road, Zip 06492, Mailing Address: P.O. Box 400, Zip 06492; tel. 203/284-2800; Paul H. Johnson, President and Chief Executive Officer (Nonreporting) **A**1 5 7 10	23	46	88	—	—	—	—	—	—	—
★ MASONIC GERIATRIC HEALTHCARE CENTER, (LONG TERM CARE), 22 Masonic Avenue, Zip 06492-3048, Mailing Address: P.O. Box 70, Zip 06492-7002; tel. 203/284-3900; Arthur E. Santilli, President (Total facility includes 468 beds in nursing home-type unit) **A**1 10 **F**1 6 9 13 16 17 18 19 23 26 30 31 32 34 36 37 38 40 43 45 46 54 56 60 62 63 67 69 70 72 76 78 **P**4 7 Web address: www.masonicare.org	23	49	503	1294	435	14156	0	41157	20975	596
WATERBURY—New Haven County ★ ST. MARY'S HOSPITAL, 56 Franklin Street, Zip 06706-1201; tel. 203/574-6000; Sister Marguerite Waite, President and Chief Executive Officer **A**1 2 3 5 9 10 **F**3 5 7 8 9 11 12 13 14 16 17 18 19 21 22 23 24 25 29 30 32 33 34 35 37 38 39 41 43 44 45 46 48 50 51 54 56 57 59 60 61 63 64 65 68 70 72 75 76 77 78 **P**8 Web address: www.stmh.org	21	10	170	9296	118	193373	1344	135977	65883	1396
★ WATERBURY HOSPITAL, 64 Robbins Street, Zip 06708-2600, Mailing Address: P.O. Box 1589, Zip 06721-1589; tel. 203/573-6000; John H. Tobin, President and Chief Executive Officer **A**1 2 3 5 9 10 **F**3 5 7 8 9 11 12 13 16 17 18 19 21 22 23 24 25 27 28 31 32 33 34 35 36 38 39 41 42 43 44 45 46 48 50 51 54 56 57 58 59 60 61 62 68 69 70 71 72 74 75 76 77 78 79 **P**7 8 Web address: www.waterburyhospital.org	23	10	247	11410	160	123515	1335	134154	66410	1402
WEST HARTFORD—Hartford County ★ HEBREW HOME AND HOSPITAL, 1 Abrahms Boulevard, Zip 06117-1525; tel. 860/523-3800; Bonnie B. Gauthier, President and Chief Executive Officer (Total facility includes 293 beds in nursing home-type unit) (Nonreporting) **A**10 Web address: www.hebrew.home.hosp.org	23	49	334	—	—	—	—	—	—	—
WEST HAVEN—New Haven County VETERANS AFFAIRS CONNECTICUT HEALTHCARE SYSTEM, WEST HAVEN DIVISION, See New Haven										
WESTPORT—Fairfield County HALL-BROOKE HOSPITAL, See ST. VINCENT'S MEDICAL CENTER, Bridgeport										
WILLIMANTIC—Windham County ★ WINDHAM COMMUNITY MEMORIAL HOSPITAL, 112 Mansfield Avenue, Zip 06226-2040; tel. 860/456-9116; Richard A. Brvenik, President and Chief Executive Officer **A**1 9 10 **F**7 8 9 13 16 18 19 22 23 25 27 30 32 34 36 37 38 39 40 43 45 46 48 54 59 61 68 70 71 72 73 74 76 78 79 **P**8 Web address: www.windhamhospital.org	23	10	78	4811	52	109678	473	47356	20726	461

© 2000 AHA Guide *Many Facility Codes have changed. Please refer to the AHA Guide Code Chart.*

Hospitals, U.S. / DISTRICT OF COLUMBIA

DELAWARE

Resident Population 744 (in thousands)
Resident population in metro areas 81.9%
Birth rate per 1,000 population 14.0
65 years and over 13.0%
Percent of persons without health insurance 13.1%

★ American Hospital Association (AHA) membership
□ Joint Commission on Accreditation of Healthcare Organizations (JCAHO) accreditation
+ American Osteopathic Healthcare Association (AOHA) membership
○ American Osteopathic Association (AOA) accreditation
△ Commission on Accreditation of Rehabilitation Facilities (CARF) accreditation
Control codes 61, 63, 64, 71, 72 and 73 indicate hospitals listed by AOHA, but not registered by AHA. For definition of numerical codes, see page A4

Hospital, Address, Telephone, Administrator, Approval, Facility, and Physician Codes, Health Care System, Network	Classification Codes		Utilization Data					Expense (thousands) of dollars		
	Control	Service	Staffed Beds	Admissions	Census	Outpatient Visits	Births	Total	Payroll	Personnel
DOVER—Kent County										
★ BAYHEALTH MEDICAL CENTER, (Includes Bayhealth Medical Center at Kent General, 640 South State Street; Bayhealth Medical Center, Milford Memorial Hospital, 21 West Clarke Avenue, Milford, Zip 19963–1840; tel. 302/424–5613), 640 South State Street, Zip 19901–3597; tel. 302/674–4700; Dennis E. Klima, President and Chief Executive Officer **A**1 2 9 10 **F**3 8 9 11 12 13 14 17 18 19 22 24 25 27 28 29 31 32 33 34 35 36 38 39 41 42 43 44 45 46 48 50 51 53 54 55 56 57 58 59 60 61 62 64 65 66 68 70 71 72 75 76 77 78 79 **P**6 8 **Web address:** www.bayhealth.org	23	10	348	17095	230	329915	1841	147335	64103	1924
LEWES—Sussex County										
★ BEEBE MEDICAL CENTER, 424 Savannah Road, Zip 19958–0226; tel. 302/645–3300; Jeffrey M. Fried, FACHE, President and Chief Executive Officer **A**1 2 6 9 10 **F**1 3 7 8 9 11 13 14 15 16 17 18 19 20 21 22 24 25 27 29 30 31 32 33 34 35 36 38 39 41 43 44 45 46 48 49 50 51 54 56 68 69 70 72 75 76 77 78 79 **P**8 **Web address:** www.beebemed.org	23	10	212	8327	95	—	677	—	—	—
MILFORD—Sussex County										
BAYHEALTH MEDICAL CENTER, MILFORD MEMORIAL HOSPITAL See Bayhealth Medical Center, Dover										
NEW CASTLE—New Castle County										
□ DELAWARE PSYCHIATRIC CENTER, 1901 North Dupont Highway, Zip 19720–1199; tel. 302/577–4381; Jiro R. Shimono, Director (Total facility includes 83 beds in nursing home–type unit) **A**1 3 10 **F**13 16 19 21 22 23 24 26 30 33 39 43 45 49 50 51 54 55 57 61 62 63 68 70 72 76 78 **P**6	12	22	355	1236	329	0	0	36785	18974	724
□ MEADOW WOOD BEHAVIORAL HEALTH SYSTEM, 575 South Dupont Highway, Zip 19720–4600; tel. 302/328–3330; Joseph Pyle, Administrator **A**1 10 **F**16 17 18 57 58 62 63 64 **P**6	33	62	50	1644	41	5862	0	—	—	113
NEWARK—New Castle County										
★ △ CHRISTIANA HOSPITAL, (Includes Wilmington Hospital, 501 West 14th Street, Wilmington, Zip 19801, Mailing Address: Box 1668, Zip 19899; tel. 302/733–1000), 4755 Ogletown–Stanton Road, Zip 19718; tel. 302/733–1000; Charles M. Smith, M.D., President and Chief Executive Officer (Total facility includes 99 beds in nursing home–type unit) **A**1 2 3 5 7 8 9 12 **F**1 4 8 9 11 12 14 17 18 19 20 22 23 24 25 27 28 29 33 34 35 36 38 39 41 42 43 44 45 46 47 48 49 50 51 53 54 56 57 58 59 61 63 65 66 68 69 70 73 74 75 76 78 79 **S** Christiana Care Health System, Wilmington, DE **Web address:** www.christianacare.org	23	10	866	40931	670	496218	6481	531288	250300	5707
★ ROCKFORD CENTER, 100 Rockford Drive, Zip 19713–2121; tel. 302/996–5480; Barbara Neuse, Chief Executive Officer **A**1 10 **F**3 57 58 62 63 64	32	22	72	1933	44	—	0	—	—	—
SEAFORD—Sussex County										
★ NANTICOKE MEMORIAL HOSPITAL, 801 Middleford Road, Zip 19973–3698; tel. 302/629–6611; Edward H. Hancock, President (Total facility includes 90 beds in nursing home–type unit) **A**1 9 10 **F**2 3 4 7 8 9 11 13 16 17 18 19 22 25 28 32 34 39 41 43 44 45 46 48 49 50 51 53 54 61 62 63 64 69 70 71 72 76 78 79 **P**1 5 6	23	10	200	5971	152	54857	799	51314	25083	760
WILMINGTON—New Castle County										
★ △ ALFRED I. DUPONT HOSPITAL FOR CHILDREN, (Formerly duPont Hospital for Children), 1600 Rockland Road, Zip 19803–3616, Mailing Address: Box 269, Zip 19899–0269; tel. 302/651–4000; Thomas P. Ferry, Administrator and Chief Executive **A**1 3 5 7 9 10 **F**7 11 12 13 14 16 17 18 22 23 24 25 38 39 42 43 46 47 48 51 52 53 54 56 58 59 63 70 71 72 74 76 77 78 **P**3 **Web address:** www.kidshealth.org	23	50	152	6727	84	119643	0	59752	3734	—
★ ST. FRANCIS HOSPITAL, Seventh and Clayton Streets, Zip 19805–0500, Mailing Address: P.O. Box 2500, Zip 19805–0500; tel. 302/421–4100; M. Eileen Schmitt, M.D., President and Chief Executive Officer (Total facility includes 25 beds in nursing home–type unit) **A**1 2 3 5 9 10 **F**8 9 11 13 17 18 19 20 22 24 25 26 32 33 34 35 36 38 39 41 42 43 44 46 48 49 50 51 53 54 56 68 69 70 72 73 76 78 79 **S** Catholic Health Initiatives, Denver, CO	23	10	222	8149	117	204080	1098	123586	39303	913
★ VETERANS AFFAIRS MEDICAL CENTER, 1601 Kirkwood Highway, Zip 19805–4989; tel. 302/633–5201; Dexter D. Dix, Director (Total facility includes 60 beds in nursing home–type unit) **A**1 2 3 5 8 9 **F**1 3 4 5 7 8 9 11 13 16 17 18 19 22 23 24 25 26 27 28 29 30 31 32 33 34 35 36 37 38 39 41 43 45 46 47 48 49 50 51 54 56 59 63 65 68 69 70 72 74 76 78 79 **P**6 **S** Department of Veterans Affairs, Washington, DC **Web address:** www.va.gov/station WILMINGTON HOSPITAL See Christiana Hospital, Newark	45	10	118	2094	106	133911	0	50434	26894	540

Hospitals, U.S. / DISTRICT OF COLUMBIA

DISTRICT OF COLUMBIA

Resident Population 523 (in thousands)
Resident population in metro areas 100%
Birth rate per 1,000 population 15.0
65 years and over 13.9%
Percent of persons without health insurance 16.2%

★ American Hospital Association (AHA) membership
☐ Joint Commission on Accreditation of Healthcare Organizations (JCAHO) accreditation
+ American Osteopathic Healthcare Association (AOHA) membership
○ American Osteopathic Association (AOA) accreditation
△ Commission on Accreditation of Rehabilitation Facilities (CARF) accreditation
Control codes 61, 63, 64, 71, 72 and 73 indicate hospitals listed by AOHA, but not registered by AHA. For definition of numerical codes, see page A4

Hospital, Address, Telephone, Administrator, Approval, Facility, and Physician Codes, Health Care System, Network	Classification Codes		Utilization Data					Expense (thousands) of dollars		
	Control	Service	Staffed Beds	Admissions	Census	Outpatient Visits	Births	Total	Payroll	Personnel

WASHINGTON—District of Columbia County

★ CHILDREN'S NATIONAL MEDICAL CENTER, 111 Michigan Avenue N.W., Zip 20010–2970; tel. 202/884–5000; Edwin K. Zechman, Jr, President and Chief Executive Officer **A**1 3 5 8 9 10 **F**4 5 11 13 15 16 17 18 19 22 23 24 29 31 32 33 34 35 36 38 39 42 43 45 46 47 48 49 50 51 52 54 56 57 58 59 60 61 63 64 68 70 72 73 74 75 76 77 78 **P**6
Web address: www.cnmc.org | 23 | 50 | 188 | 8924 | 167 | 237553 | 0 | 198539 | 93864 | 2619

★ COLUMBIA HOSPITAL FOR WOMEN MEDICAL CENTER, 2425 L Street N.W., Zip 20037–1433; tel. 202/293–6500; Larry Wilson, President and Chief Executive Officer (Nonreporting) **A**1 9 10
Web address: www.chwmc.org | 23 | 44 | 75 | — | — | — | — | — | — | —

★ DISTRICT OF COLUMBIA GENERAL HOSPITAL, 1900 Massachusetts Avenue S.E., Zip 20003; tel. 202/675–5000; John A. Fairman, Chief Executive Officer (Nonreporting) **A**1 3 5 9 10 | 14 | 10 | 250 | — | — | — | — | — | — | —

★ GEORGE WASHINGTON UNIVERSITY HOSPITAL, 901 23rd Street N.W., Zip 20037–2377; tel. 202/715–4000; Phillip S. Schaengold, JD, Chief Executive Officer **A**1 2 3 5 8 9 10 **F**4 8 9 11 12 13 16 17 18 19 20 22 24 25 26 27 29 30 31 32 33 34 35 38 39 41 42 43 44 45 46 47 48 49 50 51 53 54 56 57 59 60 61 62 63 65 66 68 70 71 72 74 75 76 77 78 79 **S** Universal Health Services, Inc., King of Prussia, PA
Web address: www.gwumc.edu | 32 | 10 | 277 | 11596 | 171 | 154932 | 861 | 131168 | 58187 | 1370

★ GEORGETOWN UNIVERSITY HOSPITAL, 3800 Reservoir Road N.W., Zip 20007–2197; tel. 202/784–3000; Sharon Flynn Hollander, Chief Executive Officer **A**1 2 3 5 8 9 10 **F**3 4 5 8 9 11 13 14 16 19 21 22 24 25 27 29 30 31 32 33 34 35 36 38 39 41 42 43 44 45 46 47 48 49 50 51 52 54 55 56 57 58 59 60 61 62 63 64 65 66 68 70 71 72 73 74 75 76 78 79 **P**6
Web address: www.dml.georgetown.edu | 23 | 10 | 345 | 14314 | 245 | 187683 | 1440 | 225788 | 74996 | 1741

★ △ GREATER SOUTHEAST COMMUNITY HOSPITAL, 1310 Southern Avenue S.E., Zip 20032–4699; tel. 202/574–6000; Ana Raley, Chief Executive Officer (Total facility includes 24 beds in nursing home–type unit) (Nonreporting) **A**1 2 3 5 7 9 10 **S** Doctors Community Healthcare Corporation, Scottsdale, AZ | 33 | 10 | 305 | — | — | — | — | — | — | —

☐ HADLEY MEMORIAL HOSPITAL, 4601 Martin Luther King Jr. Avenue S.W., Zip 20032–1199; tel. 202/574–5700; Audrey Weston, Administrator (Total facility includes 39 beds in nursing home–type unit) (Nonreporting) **A**1 9 10 **S** Doctors Community Healthcare Corporation, Scottsdale, AZ
Web address: www.doctorscommunity.com | 33 | 10 | 109 | — | — | — | — | — | — | —

★ △ HOSPITAL FOR SICK CHILDREN, 1731 Bunker Hill Road N.E., Zip 20017–3096; tel. 202/832–4400; Thomas W. Chapman, President and Chief Executive Officer (Nonreporting) **A**1 7 9
Web address: www.hscsn.org | 23 | 56 | 114 | — | — | — | — | — | — | —

★ HOWARD UNIVERSITY HOSPITAL, 2041 Georgia Avenue N.W., Zip 20059–0002; tel. 202/865–6100; Sherman P. McCoy, Executive Director and Chief Executive Officer (Total facility includes 28 beds in nursing home–type unit) **A**1 2 3 5 8 9 10 **F**4 7 8 9 11 12 13 19 22 23 24 25 29 32 33 34 35 36 38 39 41 42 44 45 46 47 48 49 50 54 55 56 57 58 59 61 62 63 65 66 68 69 70 71 72 74 75 76 77 78 79
Web address: www.huhosp.org | 23 | 10 | 313 | 11924 | 240 | 112539 | 521 | 191247 | 94050 | 2142

★ MEDLINK HOSPITAL AND NURSING CENTER AT CAPITOL HILL, 700 Constitution Avenue N.E., Zip 20002; tel. 202/546–5700; Peter Shin, DPM, President and Chairman of the Board (Nonreporting) **A**10
Web address: www.medlink–dc.com | 23 | 49 | 35 | — | — | — | — | — | — | —

★ △ NATIONAL REHABILITATION HOSPITAL, 102 Irving Street N.W., Zip 20010–2949; tel. 202/877–1000; Edward A. Eckenhoff, President and Chief Executive Officer **A**1 3 5 7 9 10 **F**1 2 3 4 5 6 7 8 9 10 11 12 13 16 17 18 19 20 21 22 23 24 25 26 27 28 29 30 31 32 33 34 35 36 37 38 39 41 42 43 44 45 46 47 48 49 50 51 52 53 54 56 57 59 61 62 63 64 65 68 69 70 71 72 73 74 75 76 77 78 79 **P**1 5 6 7 **S** MedStar Health, Columbia, MD
Web address: www.nrhrehab.org/index.htm | 23 | 46 | 128 | 1683 | 97 | 58893 | 0 | 45434 | 23663 | 494

★ PROVIDENCE HOSPITAL, 1150 Varnum Street N.E., Zip 20017–2180; tel. 202/269–7000; Sister Carol Keehan, President and Chief Executive Officer (Total facility includes 240 beds in nursing home–type unit) **A**1 2 3 5 9 10 **F**1 2 3 4 5 6 7 8 9 10 11 12 13 14 15 16 17 18 19 20 21 22 23 25 26 27 28 29 30 31 32 33 34 35 36 37 38 39 40 41 42 43 44 45 46 47 48 50 52 53 54 56 57 59 60 61 62 63 64 66 69 70 72 75 76 77 78 79 **P**1 7 8 **S** Ascension Health, Saint Louis, MO
Web address: www.provhosp.org | 21 | 10 | 544 | 12456 | 445 | 98759 | 1452 | 133552 | 71490 | 1963

☐ PSYCHIATRIC INSTITUTE OF WASHINGTON, 4228 Wisconsin Avenue N.W., Zip 20016–2138; tel. 202/965–8550; Kenneth F. Courage, Chief Executive Officer and Chairman of the Board (Nonreporting) **A**1 5 9 10 | 33 | 22 | 99 | — | — | — | — | — | — | —

© 2000 AHA Guide   *Many Facility Codes have changed. Please refer to the AHA Guide Code Chart.*

Hospitals, U.S. / DISTRICT OF COLUMBIA

Hospital, Address, Telephone, Administrator, Approval, Facility, and Physician Codes, Health Care System, Network	Classification Codes		Utilization Data					Expense (thousands) of dollars		
	Control	Service	Staffed Beds	Admissions	Census	Outpatient Visits	Births	Total	Payroll	Personnel

★ American Hospital Association (AHA) membership
□ Joint Commission on Accreditation of Healthcare Organizations (JCAHO) accreditation
+ American Osteopathic Healthcare Association (AOHA) membership
○ American Osteopathic Association (AOA) accreditation
△ Commission on Accreditation of Rehabilitation Facilities (CARF) accreditation
Control codes 61, 63, 64, 71, 72 and 73 indicate hospitals listed by AOHA, but not registered by AHA. For definition of numerical codes, see page A4.

Hospital	Control	Service	Staffed Beds	Admissions	Census	Outpatient Visits	Births	Total	Payroll	Personnel
★ SIBLEY MEMORIAL HOSPITAL, 5255 Loughboro Road N.W., Zip 20016–2695; tel. 202/537-4000; Robert L. Sloan, Chief Executive Officer (Total facility includes 18 beds in nursing home–type unit) (Nonreporting) **A**1 2 3 5 9 10 **Web address:** www.sibley.org	23	10	252	—	—	—	—	—	—	—
★ ST. ELIZABETHS HOSPITAL, 2700 Martin Luther King Jr. Avenue S.E., Zip 20032–2698; tel. 202/373-7166; Saverio C. Fantasia, Chief Financial Officer (Nonreporting) **A**10	14	22	817	—	—	—	—	—	—	—
★ VETERANS AFFAIRS MEDICAL CENTER, 50 Irving Street N.W., Zip 20422–0002; tel. 202/745-8100; Sanford M. Garfunkel, Director (Total facility includes 120 beds in nursing home–type unit) **A**1 2 3 5 8 9 **F**1 3 4 9 11 13 18 19 22 23 24 25 26 29 30 31 32 33 34 35 36 37 38 39 41 43 45 46 47 48 49 50 51 54 56 57 59 60 61 62 63 64 65 66 70 72 76 78 79 **S** Department of Veterans Affairs, Washington, DC **Web address:** www.va.gov/station	45	10	287	6365	241	352282	0	162342	103851	1659
★ WALTER REED ARMY MEDICAL CENTER, 6900 Georgia Avenue N.W., Zip 20307–5001; tel. 202/782-3501; Colonel Michael A. Dunn, Commander (Nonreporting) **A**1 2 3 5 **S** Department of the Army, Office of the Surgeon General, Falls Church, VA	42	10	474	—	—	—	—	—	—	—
★ WASHINGTON HOSPITAL CENTER, 110 Irving Street N.W., Zip 20010–2975; tel. 202/877-7000; Michael H. Covert, FACHE, President **A**1 2 3 5 8 9 10 **F**3 4 5 7 8 9 10 11 12 13 16 17 18 19 20 21 22 23 24 25 26 28 29 30 31 32 33 34 35 36 37 38 39 41 42 43 44 45 46 47 48 49 50 51 53 54 56 57 59 61 62 63 64 65 68 69 70 71 72 73 74 75 76 77 78 **P**1 5 6 7 **S** MedStar Health, Columbia, MD **Web address:** www.whcenter.org	23	10	791	38301	623	286440	3812	552535	261903	5365

FLORIDA

Resident Population 14,916 (in thousands)
Resident population in metro areas 92.9%
Birth rate per 1,000 population 13.1
65 years and over 18.3%
Percent of persons without health insurance 19.6%

Hospital, Address, Telephone, Administrator, Approval, Facility, and Physician Codes, Health Care System, Network	Classification Codes		Utilization Data					Expense (thousands) of dollars		
★ American Hospital Association (AHA) membership ☐ Joint Commission on Accreditation of Healthcare Organizations (JCAHO) accreditation + American Osteopathic Healthcare Association (AOHA) membership ○ American Osteopathic Association (AOA) accreditation △ Commission on Accreditation of Rehabilitation Facilities (CARF) accreditation Control codes 61, 63, 64, 71, 72 and 73 indicate hospitals listed by AOHA, but not registered by AHA. For definition of numerical codes, see page A4	Control	Service	Staffed Beds	Admissions	Census	Outpatient Visits	Births	Total	Payroll	Personnel
ALTAMONTE SPRINGS—Seminole County										
FLORIDA HOSPITAL–ALTAMONTE See Florida Hospital, Orlando										
APALACHICOLA—Franklin County										
GEORGE E. WEEMS MEMORIAL HOSPITAL, 135 Avenue G., Zip 32320, Mailing Address: P.O. Box 580, Zip 32329–0580; tel. 850/653–8853; Susan Ficklen, Administrator and Chief Operating Officer (Nonreporting) **A**9 10	33	10	29	—	—	—	—	—	—	—
APOPKA—Orange County										
FLORIDA HOSPITAL–APOPKA See Florida Hospital, Orlando										
ARCADIA—De Soto County										
✣ DESOTO MEMORIAL HOSPITAL, 900 North Robert Avenue, Zip 34266–8765, Mailing Address: P.O. Box 2180, Zip 34265–2180; tel. 941/494–3535; Edward J. Hannon, President and Chief Executive Officer **A**1 9 10 **F**7 8 13 14 17 18 19 22 24 25 30 31 32 34 36 38 39 43 45 48 54 55 56 68 70 72 76 77 **P**6 **S** Quorum Health Group, Brentwood, TN	23	10	49	2381	21	34508	658	21331	10305	337
G. PIERCE WOOD MEMORIAL HOSPITAL, 5847 S.E. Highway 31, Zip 34266–9627; tel. 941/494–3323; Mike Murphy, Acting Administrator **A**5 10 **F**23 28 30 33 34 35 43 45 50 51 57 62 69 70 72 77 78	12	22	350	326	355	0	0	43808	26150	966
ATLANTIS—Palm Beach County										
✣ J. F. K. MEDICAL CENTER, 5301 South Congress Avenue, Zip 33462–1197; tel. 561/965–7300; Phillip D. Robinson, Chief Executive Officer (Total facility includes 20 beds in nursing home–type unit) (Nonreporting) **A**1 2 9 10 **S** HCA – The Healthcare Company, Nashville, TN Web address: www.hcahealthcare.com	33	10	363	—	—	—	—	—	—	—
AVON PARK—Highlands County										
FLORIDA CENTER FOR ADDICTIONS AND DUAL DISORDERS, 100 West College Drive, Zip 33825–9341; tel. 941/452–3858; Arthur J. Cox, Sr, Director (Nonreporting)	23	82	50	—	—	—	—	—	—	—
BARTOW—Polk County										
✣ BARTOW MEMORIAL HOSPITAL, 2200 Osprey Boulevard, Zip 33830, Mailing Address: P.O. Box 1050, Zip 33830–1050; tel. 941/533–8111; Brian P. Baumgardner, Administrator (Nonreporting) **A**1 9 10 **S** LifePoint Hospitals, Inc., Brentwood, TN Web address: www.koala.columbia.net	33	10	88	—	—	—	—	—	—	—
BAY PINES—Pinellas County										
✣ △ VETERANS AFFAIRS MEDICAL CENTER, Bay Pines & 100 Way, Zip 33744, Mailing Address: P.O. Box 5005, Zip 33744–5005; tel. 727/398–6661; Thomas H. Weaver, FACHE, Director (Total facility includes 142 beds in nursing home–type unit) **A**1 2 3 5 7 9 **F**1 2 3 4 5 6 9 10 11 13 15 18 19 21 22 23 24 25 26 27 28 29 30 31 32 33 34 35 36 37 38 39 41 45 46 47 48 49 50 51 53 54 55 56 57 59 60 62 63 64 65 66 69 70 72 74 75 76 77 78 79 **S** Department of Veterans Affairs, Washington, DC Web address: www.va.gov/stations97/guide/home.asp?DIVISION=ALL	45	10	453	7599	180	453568	0	158400	96108	2335
BELLE GLADE—Palm Beach County										
✣ GLADES GENERAL HOSPITAL, 1201 South Main Street, Zip 33430–4911; tel. 561/996–6571; James E. Purcell, II, Chief Executive Officer **A**1 9 10 **F**13 22 24 25 38 41 44 48 68 70 72 76 **S** Province Healthcare Corporation, Brentwood, TN	33	10	73	2642	30	31002	490	17156	6588	—
BLOUNTSTOWN—Calhoun County										
★ CALHOUN–LIBERTY HOSPITAL, 424 Burns Avenue, Zip 32424–1097, Mailing Address: P.O. Box 419, Zip 32424–0419; tel. 850/674–5411; Ben Burnham, Administrator (Nonreporting) **A**9 10	23	10	30	—	—	—	—	—	—	—
BOCA RATON—Palm Beach County										
✣ BOCA RATON COMMUNITY HOSPITAL, 800 Meadows Road, Zip 33486–2368; tel. 561/395–7100; Randolph J. Pierce, President and Chief Executive Officer (Nonreporting) **A**1 2 9 10 Web address: www.brch.com	23	10	331	—	—	—	—	—	—	—
✣ WEST BOCA MEDICAL CENTER, 21644 State Road 7, Zip 33428–1899; tel. 561/488–8000; Richard Gold, Chief Executive Officer (Nonreporting) **A**1 9 10 **S** TENET Healthcare Corporation, Santa Barbara, CA Web address: www.tenethealth.com	33	10	150	—	—	—	—	—	—	—
BONIFAY—Holmes County										
☐ DOCTORS MEMORIAL HOSPITAL, 401 East Byrd Avenue, Zip 32425–3007, Mailing Address: P.O. Box 188, Zip 32425–0188; tel. 850/547–1120; Dale Larson, Chief Executive Officer (Nonreporting) **A**1 9 10 **S** Community Health Systems, Inc., Brentwood, TN	33	10	34	—	—	—	—	—	—	—
BOYNTON BEACH—Palm Beach County										
✣ BETHESDA MEMORIAL HOSPITAL, 2815 South Seacrest Boulevard, Zip 33435–7995; tel. 561/737–7733; Robert B. Hill, President and Chief Executive Officer **A**1 2 9 10 **F**8 9 11 13 18 19 22 23 24 25 27 28 29 31 32 33 34 35 36 38 39 41 42 43 44 45 46 48 54 57 62 65 70 71 76 77 78 79 **P**5 7 Web address: bethesdaweb.com/	23	10	362	15616	207	129673	2351	126538	47461	1713

© 2000 AHA Guide   *Many Facility Codes have changed. Please refer to the AHA Guide Code Chart.*

Hospitals, U.S. / FLORIDA

Hospital, Address, Telephone, Administrator, Approval, Facility, and Physician Codes, Health Care System, Network	Classification Codes		Utilization Data					Expense (thousands) of dollars		
	Control	Service	Staffed Beds	Admissions	Census	Outpatient Visits	Births	Total	Payroll	Personnel

★ American Hospital Association (AHA) membership
☐ Joint Commission on Accreditation of Healthcare Organizations (JCAHO) accreditation
+ American Osteopathic Healthcare Association (AOHA) membership
○ American Osteopathic Association (AOA) accreditation
△ Commission on Accreditation of Rehabilitation Facilities (CARF) accreditation
Control codes 61, 63, 64, 71, 72 and 73 indicate hospitals listed by AOHA, but not registered by AHA. For definition of numerical codes, see page A4

Hospital	Control	Service	Staffed Beds	Admissions	Census	Outpatient Visits	Births	Total	Payroll	Personnel
BRADENTON—Manatee County										
★ △ BLAKE MEDICAL CENTER, 2020 59th Street West, Zip 34209–4669, Mailing Address: P.O. Box 25004, Zip 34206–5004; tel. 941/792–6611; Lindell W. Orr, Chief Executive Officer (Total facility includes 28 beds in nursing home–type unit) **A**1 2 7 9 10 **F**4 7 8 11 12 13 14 16 17 18 19 22 24 25 26 27 29 30 32 34 37 38 39 41 43 44 45 46 47 48 50 51 53 54 65 68 69 70 72 76 77 78 79 **S** HCA – The Healthcare Company, Nashville, TN **Web address:** www.hcahealthcare.com	33	10	284	13056	200	83458	471	76652	33742	941
☐ MANATEE MEMORIAL HOSPITAL, 206 Second Street East, Zip 34208–1000; tel. 941/746–5111; Michael Marquez, Chief Executive Officer (Total facility includes 10 beds in nursing home–type unit) **A**1 2 9 10 **F**2 3 4 8 9 11 12 13 16 17 18 19 22 24 25 28 29 32 34 36 38 41 42 44 45 46 47 48 50 51 57 58 63 64 69 70 72 76 77 78 79 **P**8 **S** Universal Health Services, Inc., King of Prussia, PA	32	10	512	16665	217	173236	1900	114694	47494	1311
BRANDON—Hillsborough County										
★ BRANDON REGIONAL HOSPITAL, 119 Oakfield Drive, Zip 33511–5799; tel. 813/681–5551; Michael M. Fencel, Chief Executive Officer (Nonreporting) **A**1 9 10 **S** HCA – The Healthcare Company, Nashville, TN **Web address:** www.brandonhospital.com	33	10	225	—	—	—	—	—	—	—
BROOKSVILLE—Hernando County										
☐ BROOKSVILLE REGIONAL HOSPITAL, 55 Ponce De Leon Boulevard, Zip 34601–0037, Mailing Address: P.O. Box 37, Zip 34605–0037; tel. 352/796–5111; Thomas D. Barb, Executive Director **A**1 9 10 **F**7 8 9 11 13 19 22 24 25 39 41 44 45 46 48 49 51 54 70 72 76 78 79 **S** Health Management Associates, Naples, FL	33	10	91	3893	113	—	0	—	—	616
☐ SPRINGBROOK HOSPITAL, (Formerly Greenbrier Hospital), 7007 Grove Road, Zip 34609–8610; tel. 352/596–4306; Susan L. Wright, Administrator (Nonreporting) **A**1 10	33	22	36	—	—	—	—	—	—	—
BUNNELL—Flagler County										
★ MEMORIAL HOSPITAL–FLAGLER, Moody Boulevard, Zip 32110, Mailing Address: HCR1, Box 2, Zip 32110; tel. 904/437–2211; Clark P. Christianson, Senior Vice President and Administrator (Total facility includes 8 beds in nursing home–type unit) **A**9 10 **F**7 9 13 17 18 19 22 23 24 25 29 30 32 33 34 35 36 37 38 41 43 45 46 48 49 50 51 54 69 70 71 72 76 77 78 79 **P**1 6 **S** Memorial Health Systems, Ormond Beach, FL **Web address:** www.memorialhealth.com	23	10	81	2385	29	30202	0	21024	9136	262
CAPE CORAL—Lee County										
CAPE CORAL HOSPITAL, 636 Del Prado Boulevard, Zip 33990–2695; tel. 941/574–2323; Earl Tamar, Chief Operating Officer **A**9 10 **F**1 3 4 5 6 7 8 9 11 12 13 15 19 20 21 22 23 24 25 26 27 28 29 30 31 32 33 34 35 36 37 38 39 40 41 42 43 44 45 46 47 48 49 50 51 52 53 54 55 56 58 59 60 61 62 63 64 68 69 70 71 72 75 76 77 78 79	23	10	212	10878	123	111968	962	66439	28158	708
CELEBRATION—Newton County										
FLORIDA HOSPITAL CELEBRATION See Florida Hospital, Orlando										
CHATTAHOOCHEE—Gadsden County										
FLORIDA STATE HOSPITAL, U.S. Highway 90 East, Zip 32324–1000, Mailing Address: P.O. Box 1000, Zip 32324–1000; tel. 850/663–7536; Diane R. James, Administrator **A**10 **F**4 9 11 12 13 19 22 23 24 25 27 30 32 33 34 35 39 41 43 44 45 46 47 50 51 57 59 60 62 65 68 70 72 75 76 78 79 **P**6	12	22	930	592	894	—	—	94454	58796	2329
CHIPLEY—Washington County										
★ NORTHWEST FLORIDA COMMUNITY HOSPITAL, 1360 Brickyard Road, Zip 32428–6303, Mailing Address: P.O. Box 889, Zip 32428–0889; tel. 850/638–1610; John E. Allen, Chief Executive Officer **A**1 9 10 **F**9 16 22 25 32 34 36 38 41 48 69 70 71 76 78	13	10	76	1309	47	26648	0	12530	5290	244
CLEARWATER—Pinellas County										
★ MORTON PLANT HOSPITAL, 323 Jeffords Street, Zip 33756, Mailing Address: P.O. Box 210, Zip 34657–0210; tel. 727/462–7000; Philip K. Beauchamp, FACHE, President and Chief Executive Officer (Total facility includes 126 beds in nursing home–type unit) (Nonreporting) **A**1 2 3 5 9 10 **S** Morton Plant Mease Health Care, Dunedin, FL	23	10	742	—	—	—	—	—	—	—
☐ WINDMOOR HEALTHCARE OF CLEARWATER, 11300 U.S. 19 North, Zip 33764; tel. 727/541–2646; C. William Brett, Ph.D., President and Chief Executive Officer **A**1 10 **F**2 3 16 17 18 19 34 35 57 60 61 70 72	33	22	163	1005	41	1594	0	7552	3770	137
CLERMONT—Lake County										
☐ SOUTH LAKE HOSPITAL, 1099 Citrus Tower Boulevard, Zip 34711; tel. 352/394–4071; Leslie Longacre, Executive Director and Chief Executive Officer **A**1 9 10 **F**7 9 13 17 18 22 25 28 32 36 39 41 43 45 46 48 49 54 68 72 76 78 **S** Orlando Regional Healthcare, Orlando, FL	23	10	68	2215	29	39059	0	17800	9889	222
CLEWISTON—Hendry County										
★ HENDRY REGIONAL MEDICAL CENTER, 500 West Sugarland Highway, Zip 33440–3094; tel. 941/983–9121; Joseph Gonzales, Chief Executive Officer **A**1 9 10 **F**1 7 12 13 22 25 32 34 36 37 38 39 43 45 54 64 76 **S** Quorum Health Group, Brentwood, TN	13	10	32	1315	12	—	0	13578	5944	168
COCOA BEACH—Brevard County										
★ HEALTH FIRST/CAPE CANAVERAL HOSPITAL, 701 West Cocoa Beach Causeway, Zip 32931–5595, Mailing Address: P.O. Box 320069, Zip 32932–0069; tel. 407/799–7111; Christopher S. Kennedy, President and Chief Operating Officer (Nonreporting) **A**1 9 10 **Web address:** www.health–first.org	23	10	128	—	—	—	—	—	—	—

Hospitals, U.S. / FLORIDA

Hospital, Address, Telephone, Administrator, Approval, Facility, and Physician Codes, Health Care System, Network	Classification Codes		Utilization Data					Expense (thousands) of dollars		
★ American Hospital Association (AHA) membership ☐ Joint Commission on Accreditation of Healthcare Organizations (JCAHO) accreditation + American Osteopathic Healthcare Association (AOHA) membership ○ American Osteopathic Association (AOA) accreditation △ Commission on Accreditation of Rehabilitation Facilities (CARF) accreditation Control codes 61, 63, 64, 71, 72 and 73 indicate hospitals listed by AOHA, but not registered by AHA. For definition of numerical codes, see page A4	Control	Service	Staffed Beds	Admissions	Census	Outpatient Visits	Births	Total	Payroll	Personnel
CORAL GABLES—Dade County										
★ CORAL GABLES HOSPITAL, 3100 Douglas Road, Zip 33134–6990; tel. 305/445–8461; Martha Garcia, Chief Executive Officer **A**1 9 10 **F**9 13 22 25 26 27 30 34 35 37 38 41 45 46 48 49 54 64 70 76 78 **P**1 5 7 **S** TENET Healthcare Corporation, Santa Barbara, CA **Web address:** www.tenethealth.com/coralgables	12	10	150	6273	95	27317	0	39632	18418	487
☐ HEALTHSOUTH DOCTORS' HOSPITAL, 5000 University Drive, Zip 33146–2094; tel. 305/666–2111; Lincoln S. Mendez, Chief Executive Officer (Total facility includes 29 beds in nursing home–type unit) (Nonreporting) **A**1 3 9 10 **S** HEALTHSOUTH Corporation, Birmingham, AL **Web address:** www.healthsouth.com	33	10	157	—	—	—	—	—	—	—
VENCOR HOSPITAL–CORAL GABLES, 5190 S.W. Eighth Street, Zip 33134–2495; tel. 305/445–1364; Jane Jackson, Chief Executive Officer (Nonreporting) **S** Vencor, Incorporated, Louisville, KY **Web address:** www.vencor.com	33	10	53	—	—	—	—	—	—	—
CORAL SPRINGS—Broward County										
★ CORAL SPRINGS MEDICAL CENTER, 3000 Coral Hills Drive, Zip 33065; tel. 954/344–3000; Deborah Mulvihill, Regional Vice President and Administrator **A**1 3 5 9 10 **F**3 4 5 6 7 8 9 11 12 13 14 16 17 18 19 20 21 22 23 24 25 26 27 28 29 30 31 32 33 34 35 36 37 38 39 41 42 43 44 45 46 47 48 49 50 51 52 54 55 56 58 59 60 61 62 63 64 65 66 68 70 71 72 73 74 75 76 77 78 79 **P**6 8 **S** North Broward Hospital District, Fort Lauderdale, FL	16	10	182	10285	112	96710	2028	69505	27789	798
CRESTVIEW—Okaloosa County										
☐ NORTH OKALOOSA MEDICAL CENTER, 151 Redstone Avenue S.E., Zip 32539–6026; tel. 850/689–8100; Roger L. Hall, Chief Executive Officer (Total facility includes 10 beds in nursing home–type unit) (Nonreporting) **A**1 9 10 **S** Community Health Systems, Inc., Brentwood, TN	33	10	91	—	—	—	—	—	—	—
CRYSTAL RIVER—Citrus County										
★ SEVEN RIVERS COMMUNITY HOSPITAL, 6201 North Suncoast Boulevard, Zip 34428–6712; tel. 352/795–6560; Donald McKenna, Chief Executive Officer (Nonreporting) **A**1 9 10 **S** TENET Healthcare Corporation, Santa Barbara, CA **Web address:** www.sevenrivershospital.com/	33	10	128	—	—	—	—	—	—	—
DADE CITY—Pasco County										
★ PASCO COMMUNITY HOSPITAL, 13100 Fort King Road, Zip 33525–5294; tel. 352/521–1100; William G. Buck, Chief Executive Officer **A**1 9 10 **F**4 7 8 9 11 13 16 17 18 19 22 24 25 30 32 33 34 38 43 44 48 49 50 51 54 68 70 72 75 76 78 79 **S** HCA – The Healthcare Company, Nashville, TN **Web address:** www.hcahealthcare.com	33	10	120	4083	41	31004	230	—	—	483
DAVENPORT—Polk County										
☐ HEART OF FLORIDA REGIONAL MEDICAL CENTER, 1615 U.S. Highway 27N, Zip 33837, Mailing Address: P.O. Box 67, Haines City, Zip 33844–0067; tel. 863/422–4971; Robert Mahaffey, Administrator (Nonreporting) **A**1 10 **S** Health Management Associates, Naples, FL	33	10	51	—	—	—	—	—	—	—
DAYTONA BEACH—Volusia County										
★ ATLANTIC MEDICAL CENTER, 400 North Clyde Morris Boulevard, Zip 32114–2770, Mailing Address: P.O. Box 9000, Zip 32120–9000; tel. 904/239–5000; Pam Corliss, Chief Executive Officer **A**1 9 10 **F**3 7 9 13 16 17 18 19 21 22 24 30 31 32 33 34 38 39 41 45 46 48 49 50 51 53 54 55 57 62 63 68 70 72 74 76 77 78 79 **P**2 **Web address:** www.hcahealthcare.com	12	10	214	2378	26	41380	—	21032	9079	266
★ HALIFAX MEDICAL CENTER, (Formerly Halifax Community Health System), (Includes Halifax Behavioral Services, 841 Jimmy Ann Drive, Zip 32117–4599; tel. 904/274–5333), 303 North Clyde Morris Boulevard, Zip 32114–2700; tel. 904/322–4785; Ron R. Rees, President and Chief Executive Officer **A**1 2 3 5 9 10 **F**1 3 4 8 9 11 12 13 14 15 16 17 18 19 21 22 23 24 25 26 27 28 29 30 31 32 33 34 35 36 37 38 39 41 42 43 44 45 46 47 48 49 50 51 52 54 56 57 58 59 60 61 62 63 64 65 66 68 69 70 71 72 73 74 75 76 77 78 79 **P**6 **Web address:** www.halifax.org	16	10	475	22609	300	362223	2017	227024	80789	2391
DE FUNIAK SPRINGS—Walton County										
HEALTHMARK REGIONAL MEDICAL CENTER, (Formerly Walton Regional Hospital), 4413 U.S. Highway 331 South, Zip 32433; tel. 850/892–5171; Jim Thompson, Ph.D., Chief Executive Officer **A**9 10 **F**7 9 13 22 25 30 36 38 39 41 48 49 50 51 54 71 76 78 **P**5	33	10	34	1206	12	15108	0	8000	3408	176
DE LAND—Union County										
★ MEMORIAL HOSPITAL–WEST VOLUSIA, 701 West Plymouth Avenue, Zip 32720–3291, Mailing Address: P.O. Box 6509, Zip 32721–6509; tel. 904/734–3320; Johnette L. Vodenicker, Administrator **A**1 9 10 **F**2 4 7 8 9 11 13 16 17 19 22 25 27 28 32 33 34 36 37 39 46 47 48 49 50 51 54 57 61 70 72 76 78 79 **P**6 **S** Memorial Health Systems, Ormond Beach, FL	23	10	156	7391	93	83048	1050	56500	19990	635
DELRAY BEACH—Palm Beach County										
★ DELRAY MEDICAL CENTER, (Includes Fair Oaks Hospital, 5440 Linton Boulevard, Zip 33484–6578; tel. 561/495–1000), 5352 Linton Boulevard, Zip 33484–6580; tel. 561/498–4440; Mitchell S. Feldman, Chief Executive Officer (Nonreporting) **A**1 9 10 **S** TENET Healthcare Corporation, Santa Barbara, CA FAIR OAKS HOSPITAL See Delray Medical Center	33	10	313	—	—	—	—	—	—	—

Hospitals, U.S. / FLORIDA

Hospital, Address, Telephone, Administrator, Approval, Facility, and Physician Codes, Health Care System, Network	Classification Codes		Utilization Data					Expense (thousands) of dollars		Personnel
	Control	Service	Staffed Beds	Admissions	Census	Outpatient Visits	Births	Total	Payroll	

Legend:
- ★ American Hospital Association (AHA) membership
- ☐ Joint Commission on Accreditation of Healthcare Organizations (JCAHO) accreditation
- + American Osteopathic Healthcare Association (AOHA) membership
- ○ American Osteopathic Association (AOA) accreditation
- △ Commission on Accreditation of Rehabilitation Facilities (CARF) accreditation

Control codes 61, 63, 64, 71, 72 and 73 indicate hospitals listed by AOHA, but not registered by AHA. For definition of numerical codes, see page A4

Hospital	Control	Service	Staffed Beds	Admissions	Census	Outpatient Visits	Births	Total	Payroll	Personnel
☐ △ PINECREST REHABILITATION HOSPITAL, 5360 Linton Boulevard, Zip 33484–6538; tel. 561/495–0400; Paul D. Echelard, Administrator (Nonreporting) **A**1 7 10 **S** TENET Healthcare Corporation, Santa Barbara, CA Web address: www.tenethealth.com	33	46	90	—	—	—	—	—	—	—
DUNEDIN—Pinellas County										
☐ MEASE HOSPITAL DUNEDIN, 601 Main Street, Zip 34698–5891, Mailing Address: P.O. Box 760, Zip 34697–0760; tel. 727/733–1111; James A. Pfeiffer, Chief Operating Officer (Total facility includes 20 beds in nursing home–type unit) (Nonreporting) **A**1 9 10 **S** Morton Plant Mease Health Care, Dunedin, FL	23	10	258	—	—	—	—	—	—	—
EGLIN AFB—Okaloosa County										
★ U. S. AIR FORCE REGIONAL HOSPITAL, 307 Boatner Road, Suite 114, Zip 32542–1282; tel. 850/883–8221; Colonel Monica A. Figun, MSC, USAF, Administrator (Nonreporting) **A**1 3 5 **S** Department of the Air Force, Bowling AFB, DC	41	10	85	—	—	—	—	—	—	—
ENGLEWOOD—Sarasota County										
★ ENGLEWOOD COMMUNITY HOSPITAL, 700 Medical Boulevard, Zip 34223–3978; tel. 941/475–6571; Robert C. Meade, Chief Executive Officer (Nonreporting) **A**1 9 10 **S** HCA – The Healthcare Company, Nashville, TN Web address: www.hcahealthcare.com	33	10	100	—	—	—	—	—	—	—
EUSTIS—Lake County										
★ FLORIDA HOSPITAL WATERMAN, 201 North Eustis Street, Zip 32726–3488, Mailing Address: P.O. Box B, Zip 32727–0377; tel. 352/589–3333; Kenneth R. Mattison, President and Chief Executive Officer (Total facility includes 49 beds in nursing home–type unit) **A**1 2 9 10 **F**7 8 9 11 13 16 17 18 19 22 24 25 28 29 31 32 34 36 37 38 39 41 43 44 46 48 49 50 51 54 60 62 63 64 68 69 70 71 72 73 76 78 79 **P**1 5 6 7 **S** Adventist Health System Sunbelt Health Care Corporation, Winter Park, FL Web address: www.fhwat.org	21	10	182	8135	135	123529	665	76619	36311	1049
FERNANDINA BEACH—Nassau County										
★ BAPTIST MEDICAL CENTER–NASSAU, (Formerly Baptist St. Vincent's Medical Center), 1250 South 18th Street, Zip 32034–3098; tel. 904/321–3501; Jim L. Mayo, Administrator **A**1 9 10 **F**7 8 9 12 13 19 22 24 25 26 39 41 44 48 53 54 76 78 **P**6 Web address: www.baptist-stvincents.com	23	10	32	2108	22	44859	390	17545	7074	265
FORT LAUDERDALE—Broward County										
☐ ATLANTIC SHORES HOSPITAL, 4545 North Federal Highway, Zip 33308–5274; tel. 954/771–2711; Edward J. Whitehouse, Chief Executive Office (Nonreporting) **A**1 10	31	22	86	—	—	—	—	—	—	—
BHC FORT LAUDERDALE HOSPITAL, 1601 East Las Olas Boulevard, Zip 33301–2393; tel. 954/463–4321; Andrew Fuhrman, Chief Executive Officer (Nonreporting) **A**10 **S** Behavioral Healthcare Corporation, Nashville, TN	33	22	100	—	—	—	—	—	—	—
★ BROWARD GENERAL MEDICAL CENTER, 1600 South Andrews Avenue, Zip 33316–2510; tel. 954/355–4400; Timothy P. Menton, Administrator (Total facility includes 20 beds in nursing home–type unit) **A**1 2 3 9 10 12 13 **F**4 7 8 9 11 12 13 14 16 17 18 19 21 22 23 25 27 28 29 31 32 33 34 35 36 37 38 39 41 42 43 44 45 46 47 48 49 50 51 52 53 54 56 57 59 61 62 63 64 65 68 69 70 71 72 75 76 77 78 79 **P**6 8 **S** North Broward Hospital District, Fort Lauderdale, FL	16	10	545	20795	353	157123	3184	184331	78628	1876
☐ CLEVELAND CLINIC HOSPITAL, 2835 North Ocean Boulevard, Zip 33308–7599; tel. 954/568–1000; Chantal Leconte, Administrator (Nonreporting) **A**1 3 9 10	23	10	120	—	—	—	—	—	—	—
★ FLORIDA MEDICAL CENTER, (Formerly Florida Medical Center Hospital), 5000 West Oakland Park Boulevard, Zip 33313–1585; tel. 954/735–6000; Joel Bergenfeld, Chief Executive Officer (Nonreporting) **A**1 9 10 **S** TENET Healthcare Corporation, Santa Barbara, CA Web address: www.tenethealth.com	32	10	459	—	—	—	—	—	—	—
☐ HEALTHSOUTH SUNRISE REHABILITATION HOSPITAL, 4399 Nob Hill Road, Zip 33351–5899; tel. 954/749–0300; Kevin R. Conn, Administrator **A**1 10 **F**1 3 5 13 16 17 18 19 22 28 29 30 31 32 34 38 39 43 45 46 49 51 53 54 70 71 72 76 78 79 **S** HEALTHSOUTH Corporation, Birmingham, AL Web address: www.healthsouth.com	33	46	116	1929	104	48911	0	24535	14480	373
★ △ HOLY CROSS HOSPITAL, 4725 North Federal Highway, Zip 33308–4668, Mailing Address: P.O. Box 23460, Zip 33307–3460; tel. 954/771–8000; John C. Johnson, Chief Executive Officer (Nonreporting) **A**1 2 7 9 10 **S** Catholic Health East, Newtown Square, PA Web address: www.holy-cross.com	21	10	437	—	—	—	—	—	—	—
★ IMPERIAL POINT MEDICAL CENTER, 6401 North Federal Highway, Zip 33308–1495; tel. 954/776–8500; Dorothy J. Mancini, R.N., Regional Vice President Administration **A**1 9 10 **F**4 5 8 9 11 13 16 17 18 19 20 22 25 27 28 30 32 34 35 36 37 38 39 41 43 45 46 47 48 49 54 56 57 61 62 63 64 65 70 71 75 76 78 **P**6 7 **S** North Broward Hospital District, Fort Lauderdale, FL	16	10	160	6316	109	73468	0	50875	21230	623
★ NORTH RIDGE MEDICAL CENTER, 5757 North Dixie Highway, Zip 33334–4182, Mailing Address: P.O. Box 23160, Zip 33307; tel. 954/776–6000; Clifford J. Bauer, Chief Executive Officer (Nonreporting) **A**1 9 10 **S** TENET Healthcare Corporation, Santa Barbara, CA Web address: www.tenethealth/northridge.com	33	10	391	—	—	—	—	—	—	—
☐ VENCOR HOSPITAL–FORT LAUDERDALE, 1516 East Las Olas Boulevard, Zip 33301–2399; tel. 954/764–8900; Lewis A. Ransdell, Administrator **A**1 10 **F**13 16 17 18 22 23 25 31 37 39 41 45 48 49 54 65 70 72 76 78 **S** Vencor, Incorporated, Louisville, KY Web address: www.vencor.com	33	10	64	528	55	0	0	—	—	223

Hospitals, U.S. / FLORIDA

Hospital, Address, Telephone, Administrator, Approval, Facility, and Physician Codes, Health Care System, Network	Classi-fication Codes		Utilization Data					Expense (thousands) of dollars		
★ American Hospital Association (AHA) membership □ Joint Commission on Accreditation of Healthcare Organizations (JCAHO) accreditation + American Osteopathic Healthcare Association (AOHA) membership ○ American Osteopathic Association (AOA) accreditation △ Commission on Accreditation of Rehabilitation Facilities (CARF) accreditation Control codes 61, 63, 64, 71, 72 and 73 indicate hospitals listed by AOHA, but not registered by AHA. For definition of numerical codes, see page A4	Control	Service	Staffed Beds	Admissions	Census	Outpatient Visits	Births	Total	Payroll	Personnel

FORT MYERS—Lee County

★ ○ GULF COAST HOSPITAL, 13681 Doctors Way, Zip 33912–4309; tel. 941/768–5000; Valerie A. Jackson, Chief Executive Officer (Nonreporting) **A**1 9 10 11 **S** HCA – The Healthcare Company, Nashville, TN — 33 10 120 — — — — — — —

★ △ LEE MEMORIAL HEALTH SYSTEM, 2776 Cleveland Avenue, Zip 33901–5855, Mailing Address: P.O. Box 2218, Zip 33902–2218; tel. 941/332–1111; James R. Nathan, Chief Executive Officer (Total facility includes 110 beds in nursing home–type unit) **A**1 2 7 9 10 **F**1 3 4 5 6 7 8 9 11 12 13 14 15 16 17 18 21 22 23 24 25 27 29 30 31 32 33 34 35 36 37 38 39 40 41 42 43 44 45 46 47 48 49 50 51 52 53 54 55 56 58 59 60 61 62 63 64 65 68 69 70 71 72 75 76 77 78 **P**6 8
Web address: www.leememorial.org — 16 10 757 28003 471 185328 2992 297906 146329 1149

★ SOUTHWEST FLORIDA REGIONAL MEDICAL CENTER, 2727 Winkler Avenue, Zip 33901–9396; tel. 941/939–1147; Stephen L. Royal, President and Chief Executive Officer (Nonreporting) **A**1 9 10 **S** HCA – The Healthcare Company, Nashville, TN
Web address: www.swfrmc.com — 33 10 400 — — — — — — —

FORT PIERCE—St. Lucie County

★ LAWNWOOD REGIONAL MEDICAL CENTER, (Includes Lawnwood Pavilion, 1860 North Lawnwood Circle, Zip 34950; tel. 361/466–1500), 1700 South 23rd Street, Zip 34950–0188; tel. 561/461–4000; Thomas R. Pentz, President and Executive Officer (Total facility includes 33 beds in nursing home–type unit) **A**1 9 10 **F**3 4 7 8 9 11 12 13 14 16 17 18 19 22 25 27 28 29 32 33 34 35 37 38 39 40 41 42 43 44 45 46 47 48 49 50 53 54 57 58 60 63 64 69 70 71 76 78 79 **S** HCA – The Healthcare Company, Nashville, TN
Web address: www.hcahealthcare.com — 33 10 375 13337 224 96160 1232 — — —

FORT WALTON BEACH—Okaloosa County

★ △ FORT WALTON BEACH MEDICAL CENTER, 1000 Mar–Walt Drive, Zip 32547–6795; tel. 850/862–1111; Wayne Campbell, Chief Executive Officer **A**1 7 9 10 **F**7 8 9 11 12 13 16 17 18 19 22 25 26 27 30 31 32 33 34 35 36 37 38 39 41 43 44 45 46 48 49 50 51 52 53 54 57 59 60 61 62 63 72 76 77 78 79 **S** HCA – The Healthcare Company, Nashville, TN
Web address: www.hcahealthcare.com — 33 10 247 10343 157 93273 940 56316 25012 708

GULF COAST TREATMENT CENTER, 1015 Mar–Walt Drive, Zip 32547–6612; tel. 850/863–4160; Raul D. Ruelas, M.D., Administrator (Nonreporting) **A**10 **S** Ramsay Youth Services, Coral Gables, FL — 33 52 79 — — — — — — —

GAINESVILLE—Alachua County

★ NORTH FLORIDA/SOUTH GEORGIA VETERANS HEALTH SYSTEM, (Formerly Malcom Randall Veterans Affairs Medical Center), 1601 S.W. Archer Roadl, Zip 32608–1197; tel. 352/376–1611; Elwood J. Headley, M.D., System Director (Total facility includes 253 beds in nursing home–type unit) **A**1 3 5 8 9 **F**1 2 3 4 9 11 13 16 17 18 19 21 22 23 24 29 30 31 32 33 34 35 36 38 39 41 43 45 46 47 48 49 51 54 56 57 59 60 61 62 63 64 65 66 68 69 70 72 76 78 79 **P**1 **S** Department of Veterans Affairs, Washington, DC
Web address: www.va.gov — 45 10 594 9156 418 563786 0 238193 107821 2569

★ NORTH FLORIDA REGIONAL MEDICAL CENTER, 6500 Newberry Road, Zip 32605–4392, Mailing Address: P.O. Box 147006, Zip 32614–7006; tel. 352/333–4000; Brian C. Robinson, Chief Executive Officer **A**1 2 9 10 **F**4 8 9 11 13 16 17 18 19 20 22 24 25 26 27 30 35 38 39 41 45 46 47 48 49 50 51 53 54 55 65 66 68 69 70 72 76 77 78 79 **P**5 **S** HCA – The Healthcare Company, Nashville, TN
Web address: www.hcahealthcare.com — 33 10 266 15492 200 108849 1736 — — 1135

★ SHANDS AT AGH, (Includes Shands at Vista, 8900 N.E. 39th Avenue, Zip 32606 904/338–0097), 801 S.W. Second Avenue, Zip 32601–6289; tel. 352/372–4321; Robert B. Williams, Administrator (Total facility includes 30 beds in nursing home–type unit) (Nonreporting) **A**1 2 3 5 9 10 **S** Shands HealthCare, Gainesville, FL
Web address: www.shands.org — 23 10 269 — — — — — — —

★ SHANDS AT THE UNIVERSITY OF FLORIDA, 1600 S.W. Archer Road, Zip 32610–0326, Mailing Address: P.O. Box 100326, Zip 32610–0326; tel. 352/395–0111; Jodi J. Mansfield, Executive Vice President and Chief Operating Officer **A**1 2 3 5 8 9 10 **F**1 2 3 4 7 8 9 10 11 12 13 14 15 17 18 19 20 21 22 23 24 25 27 29 30 32 34 35 36 38 39 40 41 42 43 44 45 46 47 48 49 50 51 52 53 54 55 56 57 58 59 60 61 62 63 64 65 66 69 70 71 72 73 74 75 76 78 79 **P**6 8 **S** Shands HealthCare, Gainesville, FL
Web address: www.shands.org — 23 10 558 25333 429 341875 2310 326628 133276 4473

★ △ SHANDS REHAB HOSPITAL, 8900 N.W. 39th Avenue, Zip 32606–5625; tel. 352/338–0091; Cynthia M. Toth, Administrator (Nonreporting) **A**7 9 10 **S** Shands HealthCare, Gainesville, FL
Web address: www.shands.org — 23 46 40 — — — — — — —

GRACEVILLE—Jackson County

CAMPBELLTON GRACEVILLE HOSPITAL, 5429 College Drive, Zip 32440; tel. 850/263–4431; Judy Schiros, Administrator **A**9 10 **F**13 16 17 18 19 22 25 26 32 33 34 37 38 43 50 51 56 70 75 76 78 — 16 10 40 584 7 5537 0 3551 1714 79

GREEN COVE SPRINGS—Clay County

□ VENCOR–NORTH FLORIDA, (LONG TERM ACUTE CARE HOSPITAL), 801 Oak Street, Zip 32043–4317; tel. 904/284–9230; Tim Simpson, Administrator **A**1 10 **F**16 17 18 22 25 41 49 70 76 **S** Vencor, Incorporated, Louisville, KY
Web address: www.vencor.com — 33 49 60 446 52 0 0 — — 185

Hospitals, U.S. / FLORIDA

★ American Hospital Association (AHA) membership
□ Joint Commission on Accreditation of Healthcare Organizations (JCAHO) accreditation
+ American Osteopathic Healthcare Association (AOHA) membership
○ American Osteopathic Association (AOA) accreditation
△ Commission on Accreditation of Rehabilitation Facilities (CARF) accreditation
Control codes 61, 63, 64, 71, 72 and 73 indicate hospitals listed by AOHA, but not registered by AHA. For definition of numerical codes, see page A4

Hospital, Address, Telephone, Administrator, Approval, Facility, and Physician Codes, Health Care System, Network	Classification Codes		Utilization Data					Expense (thousands) of dollars		
	Control	Service	Staffed Beds	Admissions	Census	Outpatient Visits	Births	Total	Payroll	Personnel
GULF BREEZE—Santa Rosa County										
GULF BREEZE HOSPITAL, 1110 Gulf Breeze Parkway, Zip 32561, Mailing Address: P.O. Box 159, Zip 32562; tel. 850/934–2000; Richard C. Fulford, Administrator (Nonreporting) **A**9 10 **S** Baptist Health Care Corporation, Pensacola, FL **Web address:** www.bhcpns.org	23	10	45	—	—	—	—	—	—	—
THE FRIARY OF BAPTIST HEALTH CENTER, 4400 Hickory Shores Boulevard, Zip 32561–9113; tel. 850/932–9375; Leo J. Donnelly, Executive Director (Nonreporting) **S** Baptist Health Care Corporation, Pensacola, FL	23	82	30	—	—	—	—	—	—	—
HIALEAH—Dade County										
★ HIALEAH HOSPITAL, 651 East 25th Street, Zip 33013–3878; tel. 305/693–6100; Aurelio Fernendez, Chief Executive Officer (Nonreporting) **A**1 9 10 **S** TENET Healthcare Corporation, Santa Barbara, CA **Web address:** www.tenethealth.com	33	10	411	—	—	—	—	—	—	—
□ PALM SPRINGS GENERAL HOSPITAL, 1475 West 49th Street, Zip 33012–3275, Mailing Address: Box 2804, Zip 33012–2804; tel. 305/558–2500; Carlos Milanes, Executive Vice President and Administrator **A**1 9 10 **F**7 9 19 22 25 30 31 34 38 39 41 48 49 54 70 72 76 78	33	10	190	8602	147	24818	—	—	—	650
★ PALMETTO GENERAL HOSPITAL, 2001 West 68th Street, Zip 33016–1898; tel. 305/823–5000; Ron Stern, Chief Executive Officer (Nonreporting) **A**1 9 10 12 13 **S** TENET Healthcare Corporation, Santa Barbara, CA **Web address:** www.tenethealth.com	33	10	360	—	—	—	—	—	—	—
□ ○ SOUTHERN WINDS HOSPITAL, 4225 West 20th Street, Zip 33012–5835; tel. 305/558–9700; Gilda Baldwin, Chief Executive Officer (Nonreporting) **A**1 10 11 13	33	22	60	—	—	—	—	—	—	—
HOLLYWOOD—Broward County										
★ △ HOLLYWOOD MEDICAL CENTER, 3600 Washington Street, Zip 33021–8216; tel. 954/966–4500; Steven MacLauchlan, Chief Executive Officer (Nonreporting) **A**1 7 9 10 **S** TENET Healthcare Corporation, Santa Barbara, CA **Web address:** www.tenethealth.com	33	10	238	—	—	—	—	—	—	—
□ HOLLYWOOD PAVILION, 1201 North 37th Avenue, Zip 33021–5498; tel. 954/962–1355; Karen Kallen–Zury, Chief Executive Officer (Nonreporting) **A**1 10	33	22	46	—	—	—	—	—	—	—
★ △ MEMORIAL REGIONAL HOSPITAL, (Includes Joe DiMaggio Children's Hospital), 3501 Johnson Street, Zip 33021–5421; tel. 954/987–2000; C. Kennon Hetlage, Administrator **A**1 2 3 7 9 10 **F**1 2 3 4 7 8 9 11 12 13 14 16 17 18 19 20 21 22 23 24 25 26 27 28 29 30 31 32 33 34 35 36 37 38 39 41 42 43 44 46 47 48 49 50 51 52 53 54 56 57 58 59 60 61 62 63 65 66 68 69 70 72 73 75 76 77 78 79 **P**5 8 **S** Memorial Healthcare System, Hollywood, FL **Web address:** www.mhs–net.com	16	10	672	29567	455	312843	3076	268816	110394	4950
HOMESTEAD—Dade County										
□ HOMESTEAD HOSPITAL, 160 N.W. 13th Street, Zip 33030–4299; tel. 305/248–3232; Bo Boulenger, Chief Executive Officer (Nonreporting) **A**1 9 10 **S** Baptist Health System of South Florida, Coral Gables, FL **Web address:** www.baptisthealth.net	23	10	100	—	—	—	—	—	—	—
HUDSON—Pasco County										
★ REGIONAL MEDICAL CENTER–BAYONET POINT, 14000 Fivay Road, Zip 34667–7199; tel. 727/863–2411; Don Griffin, Ph.D., President and Chief Executive Officer **A**9 10 **F**1 4 7 9 11 12 13 17 18 19 22 25 29 32 33 34 39 41 43 46 47 48 53 54 65 70 72 76 78 **P**1 **S** HCA – The Healthcare Company, Nashville, TN **Web address:** www.hcahealthcare.com	33	10	256	12749	171	50277	0	—	—	975
INVERNESS—Citrus County										
★ CITRUS MEMORIAL HOSPITAL, 502 West Highland Boulevard, Zip 34452–4754; tel. 352/344–6582; Charles A. Blasband, Chief Executive Officer **A**1 9 10 **F**7 8 9 11 13 17 22 24 25 29 32 36 38 39 40 43 48 54 56 70 72 76 77	23	10	171	8320	115	137334	425	68327	25971	814
JACKSONVILLE—Duval County										
★ BAPTIST MEDICAL CENTER, 800 Prudential Drive, Zip 32207–8203; tel. 904/202–2000; John F. Wilbanks, Administrator **A**1 2 3 5 9 10 **F**2 4 7 8 9 11 12 18 19 21 22 25 26 27 28 29 30 31 33 36 37 38 39 41 42 43 44 45 46 47 48 49 51 52 54 56 57 58 61 63 64 65 69 70 71 72 76 77 78 79 **P**6 7 **Web address:** www.baptist–stvincents.com	23	10	519	22292	296	378305	2691	248404	79900	2627
★ △ BROOKS REHABILITATION HOSPITAL, 3599 University Boulevard South, Zip 32216–4211, Mailing Address: P.O. Box 16406, Zip 32245–6406; tel. 904/858–7600; Charles A. Schauer, Ph.D., President and Chief Executive Officer (Nonreporting) **A**1 7 10 **Web address:** www.brookshealth.org	23	46	110	—	—	—	—	—	—	—
★ MEMORIAL HOSPITAL OF JACKSONVILLE, 3625 University Boulevard South, Zip 32216–4240, Mailing Address: P.O. Box 16325, Zip 32216–6325; tel. 904/399–6111; H. Rex Etheredge, President and Chief Executive Officer (Nonreporting) **A**1 2 9 10 **S** HCA – The Healthcare Company, Nashville, TN **Web address:** www.hcahealthcare.com	33	10	310	—	—	—	—	—	—	—
METHODIST MEDICAL CENTER See Shands Jacksonville Medical Center										
★ NAVAL HOSPITAL, 2080 Child Street, Zip 32214–5000; tel. 904/777–7300; Captain Barbara Vernoski, Commanding Officer (Nonreporting) **A**1 3 5 **S** Department of Navy, Washington, DC	43	10	84	—	—	—	—	—	—	—

Hospitals, U.S. / FLORIDA

Hospital, Address, Telephone, Administrator, Approval, Facility, and Physician Codes, Health Care System, Network	Classification Codes		Utilization Data					Expense (thousands) of dollars		
★ American Hospital Association (AHA) membership □ Joint Commission on Accreditation of Healthcare Organizations (JCAHO) accreditation + American Osteopathic Healthcare Association (AOHA) membership ○ American Osteopathic Association (AOA) accreditation △ Commission on Accreditation of Rehabilitation Facilities (CARF) accreditation Control codes 61, 63, 64, 71, 72 and 73 indicate hospitals listed by AOHA, but not registered by AHA. For definition of numerical codes, see page A4	Control	Service	Staffed Beds	Admissions	Census	Outpatient Visits	Births	Total	Payroll	Personnel
★ SHANDS JACKSONVILLE MEDICAL CENTER, (Includes Methodist Medical Center, 580 West Eighth Street, Zip 32209–6553; tel. 904/798–8000; Marcus E. Drewa, President and Chief Executive Officer), 655 West Eighth Street, Zip 32209–6595; tel. 904/549–5000; Robert G. Norton, President and Chief Executive Officer (Nonreporting) **A**1 2 3 5 8 9 10 **S** Shands HealthCare, Gainesville, FL	23	10	678	—	—	—	—	—	—	—
★ SPECIALTY HOSPITAL JACKSONVILLE, 4901 Richard Street, Zip 32207; tel. 904/737–3120; W. Raymond C. Ford, Chief Executive Officer **A**1 9 10 **F**3 4 8 9 10 11 12 13 19 22 24 25 27 28 29 30 32 33 34 35 36 38 39 41 43 44 46 47 48 49 50 51 53 54 55 56 59 60 61 62 63 64 66 70 71 72 76 78 79 **P**7 8 **S** HCA – The Healthcare Company, Nashville, TN Web address: www.heartofhealthcare.com	33	49	61	739	59	—	—	20845	8359	158
★ ST. LUKE'S HOSPITAL, 4201 Belfort Road, Zip 32216–5898; tel. 904/296–3700; Robert M. Walters, Administrator (Total facility includes 17 beds in nursing home–type unit) **A**1 2 3 5 8 9 10 **F**4 7 8 9 11 13 17 22 24 25 27 31 32 34 36 38 39 41 43 44 46 47 48 49 54 56 65 68 69 70 71 72 74 76 78 **P**3 6 **S** Mayo Foundation, Rochester, MN	23	10	240	11340	156	48960	1171	137061	51368	1474
★ ST. VINCENT'S MEDICAL CENTER, 1800 Barrs Street, Zip 32204–2982, Mailing Address: P.O. Box 2982, Zip 32203–2982; tel. 904/308–7300; John W. Logue, Executive Vice President and Chief Operating Officer (Total facility includes 240 beds in nursing home–type unit) (Nonreporting) **A**1 2 3 5 9 10 **S** Ascension Health, Saint Louis, MO Web address: www.baptist–stvincents.com	21	10	756	—	—	—	—	—	—	—
TEN BROECK HOSPITAL JACKSONVILLE, (Formerly St. Johns River Hospital), 6300 Beach Boulevard, Zip 32216–2782; tel. 904/724–9202; Patrick Hammer, Chief Executive Officer (Nonreporting) **A**10 **S** United Medical Corporation, Windermere, FL	33	22	60	—	—	—	—	—	—	—
JACKSONVILLE BEACH—Duval County										
★ BAPTIST MEDICAL CENTER–BEACHES, (Formerly Baptist St. Vincent's Beaches Medical Center), 1350 13th Avenue South, Zip 32250–3205; tel. 904/247–2900; Joseph Mitrick, Administrator **A**1 9 10 **F**4 7 8 9 11 12 13 19 22 24 25 27 28 31 32 34 36 39 41 42 44 45 46 47 48 50 51 52 54 55 56 57 58 59 60 61 62 64 65 68 69 70 71 75 76 77 78 79 **P**6 Web address: www.baptist–stvincents.com	23	10	82	4555	53	70976	748	34113	14400	433
JASPER—Hamilton County										
★ TRINITY COMMUNITY HOSPITAL, (Formerly Hamilton Medical Center), 506 N.W. Fourth Street, Zip 32052; tel. 904/792–7200; Kenneth E. Dykes, Sr, Administrator (Nonreporting) **A**9 10	33	10	42	—	—	—	—	—	—	—
JAY—Santa Rosa County										
JAY HOSPITAL, 221 South Alabama Street, Zip 32565–1070; tel. 850/675–8000; Mark Faulkner, Administrator (Total facility includes 24 beds in nursing home–type unit) **A**9 10 **F**2 3 4 6 7 8 9 11 12 13 16 17 18 19 20 21 22 24 25 26 27 28 29 30 31 32 33 34 35 36 37 38 39 41 43 44 45 46 47 48 49 50 51 54 56 57 58 59 60 61 62 63 64 65 66 67 68 69 70 71 72 73 75 76 77 78 79 **P**4 5 6 7 **S** Baptist Health Care Corporation, Pensacola, FL Web address: www.bhcpns.org	23	10	55	1741	26	18689	0	8273	3486	117
JUPITER—Palm Beach County										
★ JUPITER MEDICAL CENTER, 1210 South Old Dixie Highway, Zip 33458–7299; tel. 561/747–2234; R. Michael Barry, Chief Executive Officer (Total facility includes 120 beds in nursing home–type unit) **A**1 2 9 10 **F**7 9 12 13 14 18 19 20 22 24 25 28 31 32 34 36 38 39 43 46 48 49 54 65 68 69 70 72 76 79 **P**7 **S** Brim Healthcare, Inc., Brentwood, TN Web address: www.jupitermed.com	23	10	276	7717	195	82976	0	92870	38925	1019
KEY WEST—Monroe County										
□ LOWER KEYS MEDICAL CENTER, (Formerly Lower Florida Keys Health System), (Includes De Poo Hospital, 1200 Kennedy Drive, Zip 33041; tel. 305/294–4692; Florida Keys Memorial Hospital), 5900 College Road, Zip 33040–4396, Mailing Address: P.O. Box 9107, Zip 33041–9107; tel. 305/294–5531; Ronald L. Bierman, Chief Executive Officer (Nonreporting) **A**1 9 10 **S** Health Management Associates, Naples, FL	33	10	169	—	—	—	—	—	—	—
KISSIMMEE—Osceola County										
FLORIDA HOSPITAL KISSIMMEE See Florida Hospital, Orlando										
★ OSCEOLA REGIONAL MEDICAL CENTER, 700 West Oak Street, Zip 34741–4996, Mailing Address: P.O. Box 422589, Zip 34742–2589; tel. 407/846–2266; E. Tim Cook, Chief Executive Officer (Nonreporting) **A**1 9 10 **S** HCA – The Healthcare Company, Nashville, TN Web address: www.hcahealthcare.com	33	10	156	—	—	—	—	—	—	—
LAKE BUTLER—Union County										
NORTH FLORIDA RECEPTION CENTER HOSPITAL, State Road 231 South, Zip 32054, Mailing Address: P.O. Box 628, Zip 32054–0628; tel. 904/496–6111; Bob Torrescano, Administrator (Nonreporting)	12	11	153	—	—	—	—	—	—	—
LAKE CITY—Columbia County										
★ LAKE CITY MEDICAL CENTER, 1050 Commerce Boulevard North, Zip 32055–3718; tel. 904/719–9000; Todd Gallati, Chief Executive Officer (Total facility includes 5 beds in nursing home–type unit) **A**1 9 10 **F**7 9 11 13 16 18 19 22 24 25 27 28 30 32 34 35 37 38 39 41 43 45 46 48 49 50 51 54 57 59 60 61 62 63 64 69 70 76 78 **P**7 **S** HCA – The Healthcare Company, Nashville, TN Web address: www.lakecitymedical.com	33	10	75	3995	57	34211	—	20830	10206	315

Hospitals, U.S. / FLORIDA

Approval codes legend:
- ★ American Hospital Association (AHA) membership
- ☐ Joint Commission on Accreditation of Healthcare Organizations (JCAHO) accreditation
- + American Osteopathic Healthcare Association (AOHA) membership
- ○ American Osteopathic Association (AOA) accreditation
- △ Commission on Accreditation of Rehabilitation Facilities (CARF) accreditation

Control codes 61, 63, 64, 71, 72 and 73 indicate hospitals listed by AOHA, but not registered by AHA. For definition of numerical codes, see page A4.

Hospital, Address, Telephone, Administrator, Approval, Facility, and Physician Codes, Health Care System, Network	Classification Codes		Utilization Data					Expense (thousands) of dollars		
	Control	Service	Staffed Beds	Admissions	Census	Outpatient Visits	Births	Total	Payroll	Personnel
★ SHANDS AT LAKE SHORE, 560 East Franklin Street, Zip 32055–3047, Mailing Address: P.O. Box 1989, Zip 32056–1989; tel. 904/754–8000; Neil Whipkey, Administrator **A**1 9 10 **F**1 2 3 4 5 8 9 10 11 12 13 16 17 18 19 21 22 23 24 25 27 30 32 33 34 35 36 38 39 40 41 42 43 44 45 46 47 48 50 51 52 53 54 56 57 58 61 62 64 65 66 69 70 71 72 74 76 78 **S** Shands HealthCare, Gainesville, FL Web address: www.shands.org	23	10	83	4752	54	106283	601	26271	11923	339
★ VETERANS AFFAIRS MEDICAL CENTER, 801 South Marion Street, Zip 32025–5898; tel. 904/755–3016; Marlis Meyer, Division Director (Total facility includes 180 beds in nursing home–type unit) **A**3 5 9 **S** Department of Veterans Affairs, Washington, DC **(Data included with North Florida/South Georgia Veterans Health System, Gainesville)** Web address: www.va.gov/stations97/guide/home.asp?DIVISION=ALL										

LAKE WALES—Polk County
LAKE WALES MEDICAL CENTERS See Winter Haven Hospital, Winter Haven

LAKELAND—Polk County

Hospital	Control	Service	Staffed Beds	Admissions	Census	Outpatient Visits	Births	Total	Payroll	Personnel
☐ HEART OF FLORIDA BEHAVIORAL CENTER, 2510 North Florida Avenue, Zip 33805–2298; tel. 941/682–6105; David M. Polunas, Administrator and Chief Executive Officer (Nonreporting) **A**1 **S** Health Management Associates, Naples, FL	33	22	40	—	—	—	—	—	—	—
★ LAKELAND REGIONAL MEDICAL CENTER, 1324 Lakeland Hills Boulevard, Zip 33805–4543, Mailing Address: P.O. Box 95448, Zip 33804–5448; tel. 863/687–1100; Jack T. Stephens, Jr, President and Chief Executive Officer **A**1 2 5 9 10 **F**2 3 4 7 8 11 12 13 16 18 19 22 24 25 26 27 29 30 31 32 33 34 35 37 38 41 42 43 44 45 46 47 48 50 52 54 57 58 59 60 61 62 63 64 65 70 72 73 75 76 77 78 79 Web address: www.lrmc.com	23	10	615	30727	389	137674	2848	252754	101637	2692

LANTANA—Palm Beach County

Hospital	Control	Service	Staffed Beds	Admissions	Census	Outpatient Visits	Births	Total	Payroll	Personnel
A. G. HOLLEY STATE HOSPITAL, 1199 West Lantana Road, Zip 33462–1514, Mailing Address: P.O. Box 3084, Zip 33465–3084; tel. 561/540–3783; David Ashkin, M.D., Medical Executive Director **A**10 **F**3 13 16 17 19 23 26 28 30 32 33 35 38 50 51 64 70 78	12	33	50	93	43	8	0	9763	4787	174

LARGO—Pinellas County

Hospital	Control	Service	Staffed Beds	Admissions	Census	Outpatient Visits	Births	Total	Payroll	Personnel
☐ △ HEALTHSOUTH REHABILITATION HOSPITAL, 901 North Clearwater–Largo Road, Zip 33770; tel. 727/586–2999; Elaine D. Ebaugh, Chief Executive Officer (Nonreporting) **A**1 7 10 **S** HEALTHSOUTH Corporation, Birmingham, AL Web address: www.healthsouth.com	33	46	60	—	—	—	—	—	—	—
★ LARGO MEDICAL CENTER, 201 14th Street S.W., Zip 33770–3133, Mailing Address: P.O. Box 2905, Zip 33779–2905; tel. 727/588–5200; Thomas L. Herron, FACHE, President and Chief Executive Officer (Total facility includes 13 beds in nursing home–type unit) **A**1 2 9 10 **F**4 8 9 11 12 13 16 17 18 22 23 24 25 28 32 33 34 35 36 37 38 39 41 42 43 45 46 47 48 49 50 51 54 56 65 66 69 70 72 76 78 79 **S** HCA – The Healthcare Company, Nashville, TN Web address: www.largomedical.com	33	10	243	12064	135	61472	624	—	—	—
☐ + ○ SUN COAST HOSPITAL, 2025 Indian Rocks Road, Zip 33774, Mailing Address: P.O. Box 2025, Zip 33779–2025; tel. 727/581–9474; Jeffrey A. Collins, Chief Executive Officer (Total facility includes 14 beds in nursing home–type unit) (Nonreporting) **A**1 9 10 11 12 13 Web address: www.suncoasthealthcare.com	23	10	241	—	—	—	—	—	—	—

LEESBURG—Lake County

Hospital	Control	Service	Staffed Beds	Admissions	Census	Outpatient Visits	Births	Total	Payroll	Personnel
★ △ LEESBURG REGIONAL MEDICAL CENTER, 600 East Dixie Avenue, Zip 34748–5999; tel. 352/323–5000; Richard L. Wooten, President and Chief Executive Officer (Total facility includes 120 beds in nursing home–type unit) **A**1 7 9 10 **F**4 7 8 9 11 13 14 16 17 18 22 24 25 28 29 30 32 33 34 35 36 38 39 41 43 44 45 46 47 48 49 50 51 53 54 56 65 69 70 71 76 77 78 **S** Orlando Regional Healthcare, Orlando, FL Web address: www.Leesburgregional.org	23	10	414	14919	278	97442	1145	112368	42331	1382

LEHIGH ACRES—Lee County

Hospital	Control	Service	Staffed Beds	Admissions	Census	Outpatient Visits	Births	Total	Payroll	Personnel
★ EAST POINTE HOSPITAL, 1500 Lee Boulevard, Zip 33936–4897; tel. 941/369–2101; Valerie A. Jackson, Chief Executive Officer (Total facility includes 13 beds in nursing home–type unit) **A**1 9 10 **F**4 8 9 11 12 13 16 17 18 22 24 25 31 34 38 39 40 41 43 44 46 47 48 49 54 55 64 66 68 69 70 71 72 74 76 77 78 79 **P**8 **S** HCA – The Healthcare Company, Nashville, TN Web address: www.hcahealthcare.com	33	10	88	2678	33	34363	468	19006	8015	226

LIVE OAK—Suwannee County

Hospital	Control	Service	Staffed Beds	Admissions	Census	Outpatient Visits	Births	Total	Payroll	Personnel
★ SHANDS AT LIVE OAK, 1100 S.W. 11th Street, Zip 32060–3608, Mailing Address: P.O. Drawer X, Zip 32060; tel. 904/362–1413; Rhonda Sherrod, Administrator (Nonreporting) **A**1 9 10 **S** Shands HealthCare, Gainesville, FL Web address: www.shands.org	23	10	16	—	—	—	—	—	—	—

LONGWOOD—Seminole County

Hospital	Control	Service	Staffed Beds	Admissions	Census	Outpatient Visits	Births	Total	Payroll	Personnel
☐ ORLANDO REGIONAL SOUTH SEMINOLE HOSPITAL, (Formerly South Seminole Hospital), 555 West State Road 434, Zip 32750–4999; tel. 407/767–1200; Stephen M. Glazier, Executive Director (Nonreporting) **A**1 9 **S** Orlando Regional Healthcare, Orlando, FL	32	10	206	—	—	—	—	—	—	—

LOXAHATCHEE—Palm Beach County

Hospital	Control	Service	Staffed Beds	Admissions	Census	Outpatient Visits	Births	Total	Payroll	Personnel
★ PALMS WEST HOSPITAL, 13001 Southern Boulevard, Zip 33470–1150; tel. 561/798–3300; Heather J. Rohan, Chief Executive Officer (Nonreporting) **A**1 9 10 **S** HCA – The Healthcare Company, Nashville, TN Web address: www.hcahealthcare.com	33	10	117	—	—	—	—	—	—	—

Hospitals, U.S. / FLORIDA

Hospital, Address, Telephone, Administrator, Approval, Facility, and Physician Codes, Health Care System, Network	Classification Codes		Utilization Data					Expense (thousands) of dollars		
★ American Hospital Association (AHA) membership □ Joint Commission on Accreditation of Healthcare Organizations (JCAHO) accreditation + American Osteopathic Healthcare Association (AOHA) membership ○ American Osteopathic Association (AOA) accreditation △ Commission on Accreditation of Rehabilitation Facilities (CARF) accreditation Control codes 61, 63, 64, 71, 72 and 73 indicate hospitals listed by AOHA, but not registered by AHA. For definition of numerical codes, see page A4	Control	Service	Staffed Beds	Admissions	Census	Outpatient Visits	Births	Total	Payroll	Personnel
MACCLENNY—Baker County BAKER COMMUNITY HOSPITAL AND HEALTH CENTER, (Formerly Ed Fraser Memorial Hospital), 159 North Third Street, Zip 32063–0484, Mailing Address: P.O. Box 484, Zip 32063–0484; tel. 904/259–3151; Dennis R. Markos, Chief Executive Officer (Total facility includes 62 beds in nursing home–type unit) (Nonreporting) **A**9 10	23	10	68	—	—	—	—	—	—	—
MACDILL AFB—Hillsborough County ★ U. S. AIR FORCE HOSPITAL, 8415 Bayshore Boulevard, Zip 33621–1607; tel. 813/828–3258; Colonel Gregory C. Baggerly, MC, USAF, Commander (Nonreporting) **A**1 **S** Department of the Air Force, Bowling AFB, DC	41	10	50	—	—	—	—	—	—	—
MADISON—Madison County MADISON COUNTY MEMORIAL HOSPITAL, 201 East Marion Street, Zip 32340–2561; tel. 850/973–2271; Deena Hames, Administrator (Nonreporting) **A**9 10	23	10	26	—	—	—	—	—	—	—
MARATHON—Monroe County □ FISHERMEN'S HOSPITAL, 3301 Overseas Highway, Zip 33050–0068; tel. 305/743–5533; Alberto J. Aboud, Administrator (Nonreporting) **A**1 9 10 **S** Health Management Associates, Naples, FL	33	10	58	—	—	—	—	—	—	—
MARIANNA—Jackson County ★ JACKSON HOSPITAL, 4250 Hospital Drive, Zip 32446–1939, Mailing Address: P.O. Box 1608, Zip 32447–1608; tel. 850/526–2200; John West, Administrator (Nonreporting) **A**1 9 10 **S** Quorum Health Group, Brentwood, TN	16	10	84	—	—	—	—	—	—	—
MELBOURNE—Brevard County □ CIRCLES OF CARE, 400 East Sheridan Road, Zip 32901–3184; tel. 321/722–5200; James B. Whitaker, President (Nonreporting) **A**1 10 Web address: www.circlesofcare.org	23	22	72	—	—	—	—	—	—	—
DEVEREUX HOSPITAL AND CHILDREN'S CENTER OF FLORIDA, 8000 Devereux Drive, Zip 32940–7907; tel. 407/242–9100; Michael Becker, Executive Director **F**57 58 **P**6 **S** Devereux Foundation, Villanova, PA Web address: www.devereux.org	23	52	100	79	99	0	0	—	—	348
□ △ HEALTHSOUTH SEA PINES REHABILITATION HOSPITAL, 101 East Florida Avenue, Zip 32901–9966; tel. 321/984–4600; Denise B. McGrath, Chief Executive Officer (Nonreporting) **A**1 7 10 **S** HEALTHSOUTH Corporation, Birmingham, AL Web address: www.healthsouth.com	33	46	80	—	—	—	—	—	—	—
★ HOLMES REGIONAL MEDICAL CENTER, 1350 South Hickory Street, Zip 32901–3276; tel. 321/434–7000; Stephen P. Bunker, President **A**1 2 9 10 **F**4 6 7 8 9 11 12 13 14 16 17 18 19 22 24 25 26 27 28 29 31 32 33 34 36 37 38 39 41 42 44 45 46 47 48 49 51 54 58 59 60 61 62 63 64 65 69 70 72 75 76 78 79 **P**7 Web address: www.health–first.org	23	10	528	25050	326	178034	2084	226842	94831	2634
MIAMI—Dade County ★ AVENTURA HOSPITAL AND MEDICAL CENTER, 20900 Biscayne Boulevard, Zip 33180–1407; tel. 305/682–7100; Davide M. Carbone, Chief Executive Officer (Nonreporting) **A**1 9 10 **S** HCA – The Healthcare Company, Nashville, TN Web address: www.aventurahospital.com	33	10	407	—	—	—	—	—	—	—
★ △ BAPTIST HOSPITAL OF MIAMI, 8900 North Kendall Drive, Zip 33176–2197; tel. 305/596–1960; Lee S. Huntley, Chief Executive Officer (Nonreporting) **A**1 2 3 7 9 10 **S** Baptist Health System of South Florida, Coral Gables, FL Web address: www.baptisthealth.net	23	10	392	—	—	—	—	—	—	—
★ BASCOM PALMER EYE INSTITUTE–ANNE BATES LEACH EYE HOSPITAL, (EYE), 900 N.W. 17th Street, Zip 33136–1199, Mailing Address: Box 016880, Zip 33101–6880; tel. 305/326–6000; Richard C. Thomas, Administrator **A**1 3 5 9 10 **F**16 18 25 31 38 48 54 70 76 78 **P**4 7 **S** Quorum Health Group, Brentwood, TN Web address: www.bpei.med.miami.edu	23	45	35	682	4	146401	—	38171	16279	561
★ CEDARS MEDICAL CENTER, 1400 N.W. 12th Avenue, Zip 33136–1003; tel. 305/325–5511; Steven Sonenreich, Chief Executive Officer (Nonreporting) **A**1 2 3 5 9 10 **S** HCA – The Healthcare Company, Nashville, TN Web address: www.cedarsmed.com	33	10	500	—	—	—	—	—	—	—
★ DEERING HOSPITAL, 9333 S.W. 152nd Street, Zip 33157–1780; tel. 305/256–5100; Jude Torchia, Chief Executive Officer (Nonreporting) **A**1 9 10 **S** HCA – The Healthcare Company, Nashville, TN Web address: www.hcahealthcare.com	33	10	233	—	—	—	—	—	—	—
□ △ HEALTHSOUTH REHABILITATION HOSPITAL, 20601 Old Cutler Road, Zip 33189–2400; tel. 305/251–3800; Nelson Lazo, Chief Executive Officer **A**1 7 10 **F**13 29 31 45 49 53 54 70 **S** HEALTHSOUTH Corporation, Birmingham, AL Web address: www.healthsouth.com	33	46	45	632	43	—	0	—	—	—
★ △ JACKSON MEMORIAL HOSPITAL, (Includes Highland Park Hospital, 1660 N.W. Seventh Court, Zip 33136; tel. 305/324–8111; Stuart Podolnick, Administrator), 1611 N.W. 12th Avenue, Zip 33136–1094; tel. 305/585–6754; Ira C. Clark, President (Nonreporting) **A**1 2 3 5 7 8 9 10	13	10	1376	—	—	—	—	—	—	—
★ KENDALL MEDICAL CENTER, 11750 Bird Road, Zip 33175–3530; tel. 305/223–3000; Victor Maya, Chief Executive Officer **A**1 9 10 **F**1 2 3 4 5 8 9 11 12 13 16 17 18 22 23 24 25 27 30 31 32 34 35 36 37 38 39 41 43 44 45 46 47 48 49 50 51 53 54 57 58 59 60 61 62 63 64 65 68 70 72 73 74 76 77 78 79 **P**2 3 4 5 **S** HCA – The Healthcare Company, Nashville, TN Web address: www.kendallmed.com	32	10	316	12928	184	64963	1337	87921	34302	1199

© 2000 AHA Guide *Many Facility Codes have changed. Please refer to the AHA Guide Code Chart.*

Hospitals, U.S. / FLORIDA

Hospital, Address, Telephone, Administrator, Approval, Facility, and Physician Codes, Health Care System, Network	Classification Codes		Utilization Data					Expense (thousands) of dollars		
	Control	Service	Staffed Beds	Admissions	Census	Outpatient Visits	Births	Total	Payroll	Personnel

★ American Hospital Association (AHA) membership
☐ Joint Commission on Accreditation of Healthcare Organizations (JCAHO) accreditation
+ American Osteopathic Healthcare Association (AOHA) membership
○ American Osteopathic Association (AOA) accreditation
△ Commission on Accreditation of Rehabilitation Facilities (CARF) accreditation
Control codes 61, 63, 64, 71, 72 and 73 indicate hospitals listed by AOHA, but not registered by AHA. For definition of numerical codes, see page A4

Hospital	Control	Service	Staffed Beds	Admissions	Census	Outpatient Visits	Births	Total	Payroll	Personnel
★ △ MERCY HOSPITAL, 3663 South Miami Avenue, Zip 33133–4237; tel. 305/854–4400; Edward J. Rosasco, Jr, President and Chief Executive Officer A1 2 6 7 9 10 F4 7 8 9 11 12 13 18 19 20 22 24 25 26 27 29 31 34 35 36 37 38 39 41 42 43 44 45 46 47 48 53 54 56 57 60 61 63 64 65 68 70 72 76 77 78 79 P1 2 3 6 7 8 S Catholic Health East, Newtown Square, PA Web address: www.mercymiami.com	21	10	339	16702	251	78177	1757	164734	59233	1685
☐ MIAMI CHILDREN'S HOSPITAL, 3100 S.W. 62nd Avenue, Zip 33155–3009; tel. 305/666–6511; Thomas M. Rozek, President and Chief Executive Officer A1 3 5 9 10 12 13 F4 11 12 13 14 16 17 18 19 20 21 22 23 24 25 26 28 32 33 34 35 38 39 42 43 45 46 47 48 49 50 51 52 54 55 57 58 59 60 61 63 64 70 72 73 74 75 76 77 78 P1 7 Web address: www.mch.com	23	50	238	8682	135	182232	0	197862	89362	1745
★ MIAMI HEART INSTITUTE AND MEDICAL CENTER, 4701 North Meridian Avenue, Zip 33140–2910; tel. 305/674–3114; Ralph A. Aleman, Chief Executive Officer (Total facility includes 10 beds in nursing home–type unit) (Nonreporting) A1 9 10 12 13 S HCA – The Healthcare Company, Nashville, TN	32	10	278	—	—	—	—	—	—	—
★ MIAMI JEWISH HOME AND HOSPITAL FOR AGED, 5200 N.E. Second Avenue, Zip 33137–2706; tel. 305/751–8626; Terry Goodman, Chief Operating Officer (Nonreporting) A3 10 Web address: www.douglasgardens.com	23	10	32	—	—	—	—	—	—	—
★ NORTH SHORE MEDICAL CENTER, 1100 N.W. 95th Street, Zip 33150–2098; tel. 305/835–6000; Allan E. Atzrott, President and Chief Executive Officer (Nonreporting) A1 2 9 10 S TENET Healthcare Corporation, Santa Barbara, CA Web address: www.northshoremedical.com/	33	10	286	—	—	—	—	—	—	—
★ PAN AMERICAN HOSPITAL, 5959 N.W. Seventh Street, Zip 33126–3198; tel. 305/264–1000; Roberto Tejidor, Chief Executive Officer A1 9 10 F1 4 7 8 9 11 12 13 16 17 19 22 24 25 30 31 34 36 37 38 39 41 44 46 47 48 50 53 54 56 65 66 68 69 70 72 74 76 78 79 P8	23	10	146	7844	129	38980	0	69204	30574	944
☐ SOUTH FLORIDA EVALUATION AND TREATMENT CENTER, 2200 N.W. 7th Avenue, Zip 33127–4291; tel. 305/637–2500; Cheryl Y. Brantley, Administrator A1 F16 17 18 23 57 70	12	22	200	187	184	0	0	—	—	435
★ △ SOUTH MIAMI HOSPITAL, 6200 S.W. 73rd Street, Zip 33143–9990; tel. 305/661–4611; D. Wayne Brackin, Chief Executive Officer (Nonreporting) A1 7 9 10 S Baptist Health System of South Florida, Coral Gables, FL Web address: www.baptisthealth.net	23	10	397	—	—	—	—	—	—	—
★ UNIVERSITY OF MIAMI HOSPITAL AND CLINICS, 1475 N.W. 12th Avenue, Zip 33136–1002; tel. 305/243–6418; John Rossfeld, Administrator A1 2 3 5 9 10 F13 15 16 17 18 19 22 23 24 26 31 33 34 35 37 38 39 43 45 46 48 49 50 51 54 56 59 60 63 65 68 70 72 76 78 P1 S Quorum Health Group, Brentwood, TN	23	10	40	1009	20	151445	—	63797	19688	435
★ VETERANS AFFAIRS MEDICAL CENTER, 1201 N.W. 16th Street, Zip 33125–1624; tel. 305/324–4455; Thomas C. Doherty, Medical Director (Total facility includes 240 beds in nursing home–type unit) (Nonreporting) A1 3 5 8 9 S Department of Veterans Affairs, Washington, DC Web address: www.va.gov/stations97/guide/home.asp?DIVISION=ALL	45	10	669	—	—	—	—	—	—	—
+ ○ WESTCHESTER GENERAL HOSPITAL, 2500 S.W. 75th Avenue, Zip 33155–9947; tel. 305/264–5252; Gilda Baldwin, Chief Executive Officer A5 9 10 11 12 13 F5 9 13 16 17 22 25 29 30 41 45 48 57 58 59 61 62 64 70 76	33	10	160	3853	101	25724	0	29639	11932	521
☐ WINDMOOR HEALTHCARE OF MIAMI, 1861 N.W. South River Drive, Zip 33125–2787; tel. 305/642–3555; Audrey Delgado, Administrator (Nonreporting) A1 10	33	22	94	—	—	—	—	—	—	—
MIAMI BEACH—Dade County										
☐ △ MOUNT SINAI MEDICAL CENTER, 4300 Alton Road, Zip 33140–2800; tel. 305/674–2121; Bruce M. Perry, Chief Executive Officer (Total facility includes 150 beds in nursing home–type unit) A1 2 3 5 7 8 9 10 13 F2 3 4 5 8 9 11 12 13 16 17 18 19 22 23 24 25 29 30 31 32 33 34 35 36 37 38 39 41 42 43 44 45 46 47 48 49 50 51 53 54 56 57 59 60 61 62 63 64 65 66 68 69 70 71 72 76 78 79 P1 6 Web address: www.msmc.com	23	10	694	22602	511	206384	1659	327418	145452	2570
★ SOUTH SHORE HOSPITAL AND MEDICAL CENTER, 630 Alton Road, Zip 33139–5502; tel. 305/672–2100; William Zubkoff, Ph.D., Chief Executive Officer A1 9 10 F1 13 16 17 18 19 22 24 25 30 31 33 35 36 37 38 41 45 48 49 50 51 54 57 62 64 69 70 76 77 78 P5	23	10	155	4392	136	26323	0	41593	18178	631
MILTON—Santa Rosa County										
☐ SANTA ROSA MEDICAL CENTER, 1450 Berryhill Road, Zip 32570–4028, Mailing Address: P.O. Box 648, Zip 32572–0648; tel. 850/626–7762; M. P. Gandy, Jr, Chief Executive Officer (Total facility includes 10 beds in nursing home–type unit) (Nonreporting) A1 9 10 S Paracelsus Healthcare Corporation, Houston, TX	33	10	129	—	—	—	—	—	—	—
NAPLES—Collier County										
★ △ NAPLES COMMUNITY HOSPITAL, 350 Seventh Street North, Zip 34102–4746, Mailing Address: P.O. Box 413029, Zip 34101–3029; tel. 941/436–5000; William G. Crone, President and Chief Executive Officer (Total facility includes 24 beds in nursing home–type unit) A1 2 7 9 10 F2 3 4 7 8 9 10 11 12 13 14 16 17 18 19 22 24 25 26 27 28 29 30 31 32 33 34 35 36 37 38 39 40 41 42 43 44 45 46 47 48 49 50 51 52 53 54 56 57 61 62 63 64 65 69 70 71 72 75 76 77 78 79 P8 Web address: www.nchhcs.org	23	10	458	26000	342	—	2490	209689	83699	2493

Hospitals, U.S. / FLORIDA

Hospital, Address, Telephone, Administrator, Approval, Facility, and Physician Codes, Health Care System, Network	Classification Codes		Utilization Data					Expense (thousands) of dollars		
★ American Hospital Association (AHA) membership ☐ Joint Commission on Accreditation of Healthcare Organizations (JCAHO) accreditation + American Osteopathic Healthcare Association (AOHA) membership ○ American Osteopathic Association (AOA) accreditation △ Commission on Accreditation of Rehabilitation Facilities (CARF) accreditation Control codes 61, 63, 64, 71, 72 and 73 indicate hospitals listed by AOHA, but not registered by AHA. For definition of numerical codes, see page A4	Control	Service	Staffed Beds	Admissions	Census	Outpatient Visits	Births	Total	Payroll	Personnel
WILLOUGH HEALTHCARE SYSTEM, (Formerly Willough at Naples), 9001 Tamiami Trail East, Zip 34113–3316; tel. 941/775–4500; Patricia Perfetto, MSN, Executive Director (Nonreporting) **A**10	33	22	64	—	—	—	—	—	—	—
NEW PORT RICHEY—Pasco County										
✠ COMMUNITY HOSPITAL OF NEW PORT RICHEY, 5637 Marine Parkway, Zip 34652–4331, Mailing Address: P.O. Box 996, Zip 34656–0996; tel. 727/848–1733; Ernie Meier, Administrator (Nonreporting) **A**1 9 10 **S** HCA – The Healthcare Company, Nashville, TN	33	10	414	—	—	—	—	—	—	—
✠ △ MORTON PLANT MEASE–NORTH BAY HOSPITAL, (Formerly North Bay Hospital), 6600 Madison Street, Zip 34652–1900; tel. 727/842–8468; William M. Jennings, Administrator and Chief Operating Officer **A**1 7 9 10 **F**1 3 8 9 11 13 16 17 18 19 22 24 25 28 29 32 33 34 36 38 41 44 45 48 49 50 53 54 57 58 59 60 61 62 63 64 70 72 76 78 79 **P**1 6 **S** Catholic Health East, Newtown Square, PA	23	10	122	4442	59	30515	573	29760	12358	407
NEW SMYRNA BEACH—Volusia County										
✠ BERT FISH MEDICAL CENTER, 401 Palmetto Street, Zip 32168–7399; tel. 904/424–5000; James R. Foster, President (Nonreporting) **A**1 9 10 **Web address:** www.bertfish.com	16	10	82	—	—	—	—	—	—	—
NICEVILLE—Okaloosa County										
✠ TWIN CITIES HOSPITAL, 2190 Highway 85 North, Zip 32578–1045; tel. 850/678–4131; David Whalen, Chief Executive Officer (Nonreporting) **A**1 9 10 **S** HCA – The Healthcare Company, Nashville, TN **Web address:** www.hcahealthcare.com	33	10	60	—	—	—	—	—	—	—
NORTH MIAMI—Dade County										
☐ △ VILLA MARIA HOSPITAL, 1050 N.E. 125th Street, Zip 33161–5881; tel. 305/891–8850; Jack Rutenberg, Administrator (Total facility includes 212 beds in nursing home–type unit) (Nonreporting) **A**1 7 10	21	46	272	—	—	—	—	—	—	—
NORTH MIAMI BEACH—Dade County										
✠ △ PARKWAY REGIONAL MEDICAL CENTER, 160 N.W. 170th Street, Zip 33169–5576; tel. 305/654–5050; Peter A. Marmerstein, Chief Executive Officer (Nonreporting) **A**1 7 9 **S** TENET Healthcare Corporation, Santa Barbara, CA **Web address:** www.tenethealth.com	33	10	392	—	—	—	—	—	—	—
OCALA—Marion County										
☐ CHARTER SPRINGS HOSPITAL, 3130 S.W. 27th Avenue, Zip 34474–4485, Mailing Address: P.O. Box 3338, Zip 34478–3338; tel. 352/237–7293; Marina Cecchini, Chief Executive Officer (Nonreporting) **A**1 10 **S** Magellan Health Services, Atlanta, GA	33	22	92	—	—	—	—	—	—	—
✠ MUNROE REGIONAL MEDICAL CENTER, 131 S.W. 15th Street, Zip 34474–4059, Mailing Address: P.O. Box 6000, Zip 34478–6000; tel. 352/351–7200; Dyer T. Michell, President (Nonreporting) **A**1 5 9 10	23	10	319	—	—	—	—	—	—	—
✠ OCALA REGIONAL MEDICAL CENTER, 1431 S.W. First Avenue, Zip 34474–4058, Mailing Address: P.O. Box 2200, Zip 34478–2200; tel. 352/401–1000; Stephen Mahan, Chief Executive Officer **A**1 2 9 10 **F**4 7 8 9 11 12 13 16 22 24 25 34 36 37 39 41 43 44 45 46 47 48 49 54 65 68 70 71 76 78 79 **P**8 **S** HCA – The Healthcare Company, Nashville, TN	33	10	210	12659	157	72436	831	75188	31469	962
OCOEE—Orange County										
✠ HEALTH CENTRAL, 10000 West Colonial Drive, Zip 34761–3499; tel. 407/296–1000; Richard M. Irwin, Jr, President and Chief Executive Officer (Total facility includes 228 beds in nursing home–type unit) **A**1 9 10 **F**1 4 7 8 9 11 12 13 16 19 22 23 24 25 27 30 31 32 34 35 36 37 38 39 41 43 44 45 46 48 49 50 51 54 69 70 71 72 74 75 76 77 78 79 **Web address:** www.health–central.org	16	10	360	7191	280	82894	884	59930	24990	862
OKEECHOBEE—Okeechobee County										
✠ RAULERSON HOSPITAL, 1796 Highway 441 North, Zip 34972, Mailing Address: P.O. Box 1307, Zip 34973–1307; tel. 941/763–2151; Frank Irby, Chief Executive Officer **A**1 9 10 **F**7 9 12 13 17 18 19 22 25 27 29 32 34 37 38 39 41 43 45 46 48 49 51 54 76 78 **P**4 **S** HCA – The Healthcare Company, Nashville, TN	33	10	101	4509	70	50648	4	27037	13817	349
ORANGE PARK—Clay County										
✠ ORANGE PARK MEDICAL CENTER, 2001 Kingsley Avenue, Zip 32073–5156; tel. 904/276–8500; Robert M. Krieger, Chief Executive Officer (Nonreporting) **A**1 9 10 **S** HCA – The Healthcare Company, Nashville, TN	33	10	196	—	—	—	—	—	—	—
ORLANDO—Orange County										
✠ ○ △ FLORIDA HOSPITAL, (Includes Florida Hospital Celebration, 400 Clebration Place, Celebration, Zip 34747; tel. 407/303–4000; Florida Hospital East Orlando, 7727 Lake Underhill Drive, Zip 32822; tel. 407/277–8110; Florida Hospital Kissimmee, 200 Hilda Street, Kissimmee, Zip 34741–2301; tel. 407/846–4343; Florida Hospital–Altamonte, 601 East Altamonte Drive, Altamonte Springs, Zip 32701; tel. 407/830–4321; Florida Hospital–Apopka, 201 North Park Avenue, Apopka, Zip 32703; tel. 407/889–2566), 601 East Rollins Street, Zip 32803–1489; tel. 407/896–6611; Donald L. Jernigan, President (Total facility includes 37 beds in nursing home–type unit) **A**1 2 3 5 7 9 10 11 12 13 **F**3 4 6 7 8 9 10 11 12 13 14 16 17 18 19 20 21 22 23 24 25 26 27 28 29 30 32 33 34 35 36 37 38 39 40 41 42 43 44 45 46 47 48 49 50 51 52 53 54 56 57 58 59 60 61 62 63 64 65 66 67 68 69 70 71 72 73 74 75 76 77 78 79 **P**1 **S** Adventist Health System Sunbelt Health Care Corporation, Winter Park, FL **Web address:** www.flhosp.org	23	10	1389	65701	920	600623	7580	624403	298201	9311
LUCERNE MEDICAL CENTER See Orlando Regional–Lucerne										

Hospitals, U.S. / FLORIDA

Hospital, Address, Telephone, Administrator, Approval, Facility, and Physician Codes, Health Care System, Network	Classification Codes		Utilization Data					Expense (thousands) of dollars		
★ American Hospital Association (AHA) membership □ Joint Commission on Accreditation of Healthcare Organizations (JCAHO) accreditation + American Osteopathic Healthcare Association (AOHA) membership ○ American Osteopathic Association (AOA) accreditation △ Commission on Accreditation of Rehabilitation Facilities (CARF) accreditation Control codes 61, 63, 64, 71, 72 and 73 indicate hospitals listed by AOHA, but not registered by AHA. For definition of numerical codes, see page A4	Control	Service	Staffed Beds	Admissions	Census	Outpatient Visits	Births	Total	Payroll	Personnel
★ ORLANDO REGIONAL MEDICAL CENTER, (Includes Arnold Palmer Hospital for Children and Women; M. D. Anderson Cancer Center and Sand Lake Hospital), 1414 Kuhl Avenue, Zip 32806–2093; tel. 407/841–5111; Abe Lopman, Executive Director (Total facility includes 43 beds in nursing home–type unit) **A**1 2 3 5 8 9 10 **F**2 3 4 9 10 11 12 13 16 17 18 19 20 21 22 24 25 26 27 28 29 31 32 33 34 35 36 38 39 41 42 43 44 45 46 47 48 49 50 51 52 53 54 55 57 58 59 60 61 62 63 64 65 66 67 68 69 70 71 72 73 74 75 76 77 78 79 **S** Orlando Regional Healthcare, Orlando, FL **Web address:** www.orhs.org	23	10	1226	56155	757	547698	7609	555460	17428	8227
★ △ ORLANDO REGIONAL–LUCERNE, (Formerly Lucerne Medical Center), 818 Main Lane, Zip 32801; tel. 407/649–6111; James A. Shanks, Administrator (Total facility includes 20 beds in nursing home–type unit) (Nonreporting) **A**1 7 9 **S** Orlando Regional Healthcare, Orlando, FL **Web address:** www.cenflhealthcare.com	23	10	267	—	—	—	—	—	—	—
UNIVERSITY BEHAVIORAL CENTER, 2500 Discovery Drive, Zip 32826–3711; tel. 407/281–7000; David L. Beardsley, Administrator (Nonreporting) **A**10 **S** Health Management Associates, Naples, FL	33	22	100	—	—	—	—	—	—	—
ORMOND BEACH—Volusia County										
★ MEMORIAL HOSPITAL–ORMOND BEACH, 875 Sterthaus Avenue, Zip 32174–5197; tel. 904/676–6000; Clark P. Christianson, Senior Vice President and Administrator (Total facility includes 17 beds in nursing home–type unit) **A**1 9 10 **F**4 7 8 9 11 12 13 17 18 19 22 23 24 25 26 28 29 30 32 33 34 35 36 37 38 39 41 43 44 45 46 47 48 49 50 51 54 65 66 69 70 71 72 76 77 78 79 **P**1 6 **S** Memorial Health Systems, Ormond Beach, FL	23	10	205	9050	131	67065	715	83723	31461	—
★ ○ MEMORIAL HOSPITAL–PENINSULA, 264 South Atlantic Avenue, Zip 32176–8192; tel. 904/672–4161; Clark P. Christianson, Senior Vice President and Administrator (Nonreporting) **A**1 7 9 10 11 12 13 **S** Memorial Health Systems, Ormond Beach, FL	23	10	119	—	—	—	—	—	—	—
PALATKA—Putnam County										
★ PUTNAM COMMUNITY MEDICAL CENTER, Highway 20 West, Zip 32177, Mailing Address: P.O. Box 778, Zip 32178–0778; tel. 904/328–5711; Bland Eng, Interim Chief Executive Officer **A**1 9 10 **F**8 9 13 16 17 18 19 22 24 25 31 32 33 34 35 38 39 41 46 48 49 50 51 54 56 65 68 69 70 71 72 76 78 **S** HCA – The Healthcare Company, Nashville, TN **Web address:** www.hcahealthcare.com	33	10	141	6553	88	53177	484	—	—	440
PALM BEACH GARDENS—Palm Beach County										
★ PALM BEACH GARDENS MEDICAL CENTER, 3360 Burns Road, Zip 33410–4304; tel. 561/622–1411; Clint Matthews, Chief Executive Officer (Nonreporting) **A**1 9 10 **S** TENET Healthcare Corporation, Santa Barbara, CA **Web address:** www.tenethealth.com	33	10	204	—	—	—	—	—	—	—
PANAMA CITY—Bay County										
★ BAY MEDICAL CENTER, 615 North Bonita Avenue, Zip 32401–3600, Mailing Address: P.O. Box 59515, Zip 32402–2515; tel. 850/769–1511; Ronald V. Wolff, President and Chief Executive Officer **A**1 2 9 10 **F**4 7 8 9 11 12 13 17 18 19 22 24 25 28 29 31 32 33 34 35 36 37 38 39 41 43 44 45 46 47 48 49 51 53 54 57 61 64 65 68 69 70 71 76 77 78 79 **P**5 7 **Web address:** www.baymedical.org	16	10	315	12462	188	102422	638	129100	52879	1692
★ GULF COAST MEDICAL CENTER, 449 West 23rd Street, Zip 32405–4593, Mailing Address: P.O. Box 15309, Zip 32406–5309; tel. 850/769–8341; Brent A. Marsteller, Chief Executive Officer **A**1 2 9 10 **F**8 9 11 13 22 24 25 27 29 30 32 34 38 39 41 44 45 46 48 54 56 65 70 72 76 78 **S** HCA – The Healthcare Company, Nashville, TN **Web address:** www.hcahealthcare.com	33	10	165	8591	107	99915	1543	48289	19926	584
PEMBROKE PINES—Broward County										
★ MEMORIAL HOSPITAL PEMBROKE, 7800 Sheridan Street, Zip 33024; tel. 954/962–9650; J. E. Piriz, Administrator (Nonreporting) **A**1 9 10 **S** Memorial Healthcare System, Hollywood, FL **Web address:** www.mhs–net.com	16	10	301	—	—	—	—	—	—	—
★ MEMORIAL HOSPITAL WEST, 703 North Flamingo Road, Zip 33028; tel. 954/436–5000; Zeff Ross, Administrator **A**1 9 10 **F**1 2 3 4 8 9 11 12 13 14 16 17 18 19 21 22 23 24 25 26 27 28 29 30 31 32 33 34 35 36 37 38 39 41 42 43 44 46 47 48 49 51 52 53 54 56 57 58 59 60 61 62 63 64 65 66 67 68 69 70 71 72 73 75 76 77 78 79 **P**3 5 7 **S** Memorial Healthcare System, Hollywood, FL **Web address:** www.mhs–net.com	16	10	174	12687	130	185960	3451	80444	34978	925
□ SOUTH FLORIDA STATE HOSPITAL, 1000 S.W. 84th Avenue, Zip 33025; tel. 954/967–7000; Sal A. Barbera, FACHE, Administrator (Nonreporting) **A**1 10	12	22	355	—	—	—	—	—	—	—
PENSACOLA—Escambia County										
★ BAPTIST HOSPITAL, 1000 West Moreno, Zip 32501–2393, Mailing Address: P.O. Box 17500, Zip 32522–7500; tel. 850/469–2313; John R. Heer, Administrator (Total facility includes 57 beds in nursing home–type unit) **A**1 2 9 10 **F**2 3 4 6 7 8 9 11 12 13 16 17 18 19 20 21 22 24 25 26 27 28 29 30 31 32 33 34 35 36 37 38 39 41 43 44 45 46 47 48 49 50 51 54 56 57 58 59 60 61 62 63 64 65 66 69 70 71 72 73 75 76 77 78 79 **P**4 5 6 7 **S** Baptist Health Care Corporation, Pensacola, FL **Web address:** www.bhcpns.org	23	10	492	14176	232	229375	1095	123418	49669	1575

Hospitals, U.S. / FLORIDA

Hospital, Address, Telephone, Administrator, Approval, Facility, and Physician Codes, Health Care System, Network	Classification Codes		Utilization Data					Expense (thousands) of dollars		
★ American Hospital Association (AHA) membership □ Joint Commission on Accreditation of Healthcare Organizations (JCAHO) accreditation + American Osteopathic Healthcare Association (AOHA) membership ○ American Osteopathic Association (AOA) accreditation △ Commission on Accreditation of Rehabilitation Facilities (CARF) accreditation Control codes 61, 63, 64, 71, 72 and 73 indicate hospitals listed by AOHA, but not registered by AHA. For definition of numerical codes, see page A4	Control	Service	Staffed Beds	Admissions	Census	Outpatient Visits	Births	Total	Payroll	Personnel
★ NAVAL HOSPITAL, 6000 West Highway 98, Zip 32512-0003; tel. 850/505-6413; Mark F. Bernier, Director (Nonreporting) A1 3 5 **S** Department of Navy, Washington, DC REHABILITATION INSTITUTE OF WEST FLORIDA See West Florida Regional Medical Center	43	10	113	—	—	—	—	—	—	—
★ SACRED HEART HEALTH SYSTEM, (Formerly Sacred Heart Hospital of Pensacola), 5151 North Ninth Avenue, Zip 32504-8795, Mailing Address: P.O. Box 2700, Zip 32513-2700; tel. 850/416-7000; Patrick J. Madden, President and Chief Executive Officer (Total facility includes 89 beds in nursing home–type unit) A1 2 3 5 9 10 **F**4 7 8 9 11 12 13 14 17 18 19 22 23 24 25 27 28 29 30 32 33 34 35 36 37 38 39 41 42 43 44 45 46 47 48 49 50 51 52 54 56 61 65 66 68 69 70 71 72 75 76 77 78 79 **P**6 **S** Ascension Health, Saint Louis, MO Web address: www.sacred-heart.org	21	10	520	21456	355	246958	2853	154408	60678	2628
★ △ WEST FLORIDA REGIONAL MEDICAL CENTER, (Includes Rehabilitation Institute of West Florida, tel. 850/494-6000; The Pavilion, tel. 904/494-5000), 8383 North Davis Highway, Zip 32514-6088, Mailing Address: P.O. Box 18900, Zip 32523-8900; tel. 850/494-4000; Jerald F. Mitchell, President and Chief Executive Officer (Total facility includes 40 beds in nursing home–type unit) A1 7 9 10 **F**2 3 4 8 9 11 12 13 16 17 18 19 22 24 27 28 30 31 32 33 34 39 41 43 44 45 46 47 48 49 50 53 54 57 58 59 61 62 63 64 65 68 69 70 71 72 75 76 78 79 **S** HCA – The Healthcare Company, Nashville, TN Web address: www.hcahealthcare.com	33	10	531	13618	236	102386	694	95631	41266	1241
PERRY—Taylor County										
DOCTOR'S MEMORIAL HOSPITAL, 407 East Ash Street, Zip 32347-2104, Mailing Address: P.O. Box 1847, Zip 32348-1847; tel. 850/584-0800; James McKnight, Interim Chief Executive Officer (Nonreporting) A9 10	23	10	28	—	—	—	—	—	—	—
PLANT CITY—Hillsborough County										
★ SOUTH FLORIDA BAPTIST HOSPITAL, 301 North Alexander Street, Zip 33566-9058, Mailing Address: Drawer H, Zip 33564-9058; tel. 813/757-1200; William G. Ulbricht, Chief Operating Officer A1 9 10 **F**4 8 9 11 12 13 17 18 19 22 24 25 28 29 31 34 35 36 38 39 41 42 44 45 46 47 48 49 50 52 54 57 58 59 60 61 62 63 64 65 67 68 69 70 75 76 78 79 **P**1 **S** Catholic Health East, Newtown Square, PA	23	10	96	4155	48	—	547	27751	15128	609
PLANTATION—Broward County										
★ PLANTATION GENERAL HOSPITAL, 401 N.W. 42nd Avenue, Zip 33317-2882; tel. 954/587-5010; Anthony M. Degina, Jr, Chief Executive Officer (Nonreporting) A1 9 10 **S** HCA – The Healthcare Company, Nashville, TN Web address: www.hcahealthcare.com	33	10	264	—	—	—	—	—	—	—
★ WESTSIDE REGIONAL MEDICAL CENTER, 8201 West Broward Boulevard, Zip 33324-9937; tel. 954/473-6600; Michael G. Joseph, Chief Executive Officer A1 9 10 **F**2 3 4 5 8 9 11 13 14 17 18 19 22 23 24 25 26 27 29 30 31 32 33 34 35 37 38 39 41 43 45 46 48 49 50 51 53 54 56 58 59 60 61 62 63 65 66 69 70 71 72 73 74 76 77 78 79 **P**5 7 **S** HCA – The Healthcare Company, Nashville, TN Web address: www.hcahealthcare.com	33	10	204	11613	133	55652	0	62024	28089	662
POMPANO BEACH—Broward County										
★ △ NORTH BROWARD MEDICAL CENTER, 201 Sample Road, Zip 33064-3502; tel. 954/941-8300; James R. Chromik, Regional Vice President, Administration (Total facility includes 18 beds in nursing home–type unit) (Nonreporting) A1 2 7 9 10 **S** North Broward Hospital District, Fort Lauderdale, FL Web address: www.nbhd.org	16	10	334	—	—	—	—	—	—	—
★ NORTHWEST MEDICAL CENTER, 2801 North State Road 7, Zip 33063-5727, Mailing Address: P.O. Box 639002, Margate, Zip 33063-9002; tel. 954/978-4000; Gina Melby, Chief Executive Officer (Nonreporting) A1 9 10 **S** HCA – The Healthcare Company, Nashville, TN Web address: www.hcahealthcare.com	33	10	150	—	—	—	—	—	—	—
PORT CHARLOTTE—Charlotte County										
★ BON SECOURS–ST. JOSEPH HEALTHCARE GROUP, 2500 Harbor Boulevard, Zip 33952-5396; tel. 941/766-4122; Michael L. Harrington, Chief Executive Officer (Total facility includes 101 beds in nursing home–type unit) (Nonreporting) A1 5 9 10 **S** Bon Secours Health System, Inc., Marriottsville, MD	21	10	313	—	—	—	—	—	—	—
★ △ FAWCETT MEMORIAL HOSPITAL, 21298 Olean Boulevard, Zip 33952-6765, Mailing Address: P.O. Box 4028, Punta Gorda, Zip 33949-4028; tel. 941/629-1181; Thomas J. Rice, President and Chief Executive Officer (Total facility includes 25 beds in nursing home–type unit) A1 7 9 10 **F**5 9 11 13 16 17 18 22 24 25 29 30 31 32 33 34 38 39 43 45 46 48 49 50 51 53 54 61 64 69 70 71 72 75 76 78 **P**8 **S** HCA – The Healthcare Company, Nashville, TN Web address: www.hcahealthcare.com	33	10	241	7825	117	62953	0	56377	24923	587
PORT SAINT JOE—Gulf County										
GULF PINES HOSPITAL, 102 20th Street, Zip 32456-2356, Mailing Address: P.O. Box 70, Zip 32456-0070; tel. 850/227-1121; Hubert Steeley, Administrator (Nonreporting) A9 10	33	10	45	—	—	—	—	—	—	—
PORT ST. LUCIE—St. Lucie County										
□ SAVANNAS HOSPITAL, 2550 S.E. Walton Road, Zip 34952-7197; tel. 561/335-0400; Patricia W. Brown, Ph.D., Executive Director (Nonreporting) A1 10 **S** Liberty Management Group, Inc., Ramsey, NJ	33	22	70	—	—	—	—	—	—	—

© 2000 AHA Guide   *Many Facility Codes have changed. Please refer to the AHA Guide Code Chart.*

Hospitals, U.S. / FLORIDA

Hospital, Address, Telephone, Administrator, Approval, Facility, and Physician Codes, Health Care System, Network	Classification Codes		Utilization Data					Expense (thousands) of dollars		
	Control	Service	Staffed Beds	Admissions	Census	Outpatient Visits	Births	Total	Payroll	Personnel

Legend:
- ★ American Hospital Association (AHA) membership
- ☐ Joint Commission on Accreditation of Healthcare Organizations (JCAHO) accreditation
- + American Osteopathic Healthcare Association (AOHA) membership
- ○ American Osteopathic Association (AOA) accreditation
- △ Commission on Accreditation of Rehabilitation Facilities (CARF) accreditation

Control codes 61, 63, 64, 71, 72 and 73 indicate hospitals listed by AOHA, but not registered by AHA. For definition of numerical codes, see page A4

Hospital	Control	Service	Staffed Beds	Admissions	Census	Outpatient Visits	Births	Total	Payroll	Personnel
★ ST. LUCIE MEDICAL CENTER, 1800 S.E. Tiffany Avenue, Zip 34952–7580; tel. 561/335–4000; Gary Cantrell, President and Chief Executive Officer (Total facility includes 24 beds in nursing home–type unit) (Nonreporting) A1 9 10 S HCA – The Healthcare Company, Nashville, TN	33	10	150	—	—	—	—	—	—	—
PUNTA GORDA—Charlotte County										
☐ CHARLOTTE REGIONAL MEDICAL CENTER, 809 East Marion Avenue, Zip 33950–3898, Mailing Address: P.O. Box 51–1328, Zip 33951–1328; tel. 941/639–3131; Joshua S. Putter, Executive Director (Nonreporting) A1 9 10 S Health Management Associates, Naples, FL Web address: www.charlotteregional.com	33	10	148	—	—	—	—	—	—	—
QUINCY—Gadsden County										
GADSDEN COMMUNITY HOSPITAL, U.S. Highway 90 East, Zip 32353, Mailing Address: P.O. Box 1979, Zip 32353–1979; tel. 850/875–1100; Donald L. Bradford, Chief Executive Officer (Nonreporting) A9 10	23	10	51	—	—	—	—	—	—	—
ROCKLEDGE—Brevard County										
☐ WUESTHOFF HEALTH SYSTEM, (Formerly Wuesthoff Hospital), 110 Longwood Avenue, Zip 32955–2887, Mailing Address: P.O. Box 565002, Mail Stop 1, Zip 32956–5002; tel. 407/636–2211; Emil P. Miller, President and Chief Executive Officer (Nonreporting) A1 2 9 10	23	10	235	—	—	—	—	—	—	—
SAFETY HARBOR—Pinellas County										
MEASE COUNTRYSIDE HOSPITAL, 3231 McMullen–Booth Road, Zip 34695–1098, Mailing Address: P.O. 1098, Zip 34695–1098; tel. 727/725–6111; James A. Pfeiffer, Chief Operating Officer (Nonreporting) A9 10 S Morton Plant Mease Health Care, Dunedin, FL	23	10	100	—	—	—	—	—	—	—
SAINT AUGUSTINE—St. Johns County										
★ FLAGLER HOSPITAL, 400 Health Park Boulevard, Zip 32086–5779; tel. 904/829–5155; James D. Conzemius, President (Total facility includes 14 beds in nursing home–type unit) A1 9 10 F7 8 9 11 13 17 18 19 22 25 32 36 39 41 44 46 48 54 57 68 69 70 76 79	23	10	260	9988	162	99005	783	80323	33923	1096
SAINT CLOUD—Lowndes County										
ST. CLOUD HOSPITAL, A DIVISION OF ORLANDO REGIONAL HEALTHCARE SYSTEM, 2906 17th Street, Zip 34769–6099; tel. 407/892–2135; Jim A. Norris, Executive Director (Nonreporting) A9 10 S Orlando Regional Healthcare, Orlando, FL	23	10	68	—	—	—	—	—	—	—
SAINT PETERSBURG—Pinellas County										
☐ ALL CHILDREN'S HOSPITAL, 801 Sixth Street South, Zip 33701–4899; tel. 727/898–7451; J. Dennis Sexton, President (Nonreporting) A1 3 5 8 9 10 Web address: www.allkids.org	23	59	168	—	—	—	—	—	—	—
★ △ BAYFRONT MEDICAL CENTER, 701 Sixth Street South, Zip 33701–4891; tel. 727/823–1234; Sue G. Brody, President and Chief Executive Officer (Nonreporting) A1 2 3 5 7 9 10 S Catholic Health East, Newtown Square, PA Web address: www.bayfront.org	23	10	268	—	—	—	—	—	—	—
★ EDWARD WHITE HOSPITAL, 2323 Ninth Avenue North, Zip 33713–6898, Mailing Address: P.O. Box 12018, Zip 33733–2018; tel. 727/323–1111; Barry S. Stokes, President and Chief Executive Officer (Total facility includes 10 beds in nursing home–type unit) A1 9 10 F1 4 8 9 11 13 16 19 22 23 24 25 27 28 29 30 32 33 34 35 37 38 39 41 45 46 47 48 49 51 54 56 64 65 67 71 72 76 78 79 S HCA – The Healthcare Company, Nashville, TN Web address: www.hcahealthcare.com	33	10	134	3185	46	42503	0	23661	9670	275
★ ○ NORTHSIDE HOSPITAL AND HEART INSTITUTE, 6000 49th Street North, Zip 33709–2145; tel. 727/521–4411; Bradley K. Grover, Sr, Ph.D., FACHE, President and Chief Executive Officer A1 9 10 11 12 13 F2 4 8 9 10 11 12 13 14 17 18 22 23 24 25 26 27 28 29 30 31 32 33 34 35 36 37 38 39 40 41 42 43 44 45 46 47 48 49 50 51 52 53 54 55 56 57 58 59 60 61 62 63 64 65 66 67 68 69 70 71 72 73 74 75 76 77 78 79 S HCA – The Healthcare Company, Nashville, TN Web address: www.northsidehospital.com	12	10	288	8444	119	24946	—	—	—	—
★ PALMS OF PASADENA HOSPITAL, 1501 Pasadena Avenue South, Zip 33707–3798; tel. 727/381–1000; John D. Bartlett, Chief Executive Officer (Nonreporting) A1 2 9 10 S IASIS Healthcare, Nashville, TN Web address: www.tenethealth.com	33	10	267	—	—	—	—	—	—	—
★ ST. ANTHONY'S HOSPITAL, 1200 Seventh Avenue North, Zip 33705–1388, Mailing Address: P.O. Box 12588, Zip 33733–2588; tel. 727/825–1100; Sue G. Brody, President and Chief Executive Officer (Total facility includes 30 beds in nursing home–type unit) (Nonreporting) A1 2 9 10 S Catholic Health East, Newtown Square, PA Web address: www.stanthonys.org	23	10	329	—	—	—	—	—	—	—
★ ST. PETERSBURG GENERAL HOSPITAL, 6500 38th Avenue North, Zip 33710–1629; tel. 727/384–1414; Daniel J. Friedrich, II, President and Chief Executive Officer (Total facility includes 20 beds in nursing home–type unit) A1 9 10 F4 8 9 11 13 18 21 22 24 25 30 31 34 37 39 41 43 45 46 47 48 49 50 54 61 62 63 64 65 66 69 70 72 75 76 78 79 S HCA – The Healthcare Company, Nashville, TN Web address: www.stpetegeneralhospital.com	12	10	160	6310	79	—	994	44155	15837	477
VENCOR HOSPITAL–ST PETERSBURG, 3030 Sixth Street South, Zip 33705–3720; tel. 727/894–8719; Pamela M. Riter, R.N., Administrator (Nonreporting) S Vencor, Incorporated, Louisville, KY Web address: www.vencor.com	33	49	60	—	—	—	—	—	—	—

Many Facility Codes have changed. Please refer to the AHA Guide Code Chart.

Hospitals, U.S. / FLORIDA

Hospital, Address, Telephone, Administrator, Approval, Facility, and Physician Codes, Health Care System, Network	Classification Codes		Utilization Data					Expense (thousands) of dollars		
★ American Hospital Association (AHA) membership ☐ Joint Commission on Accreditation of Healthcare Organizations (JCAHO) accreditation + American Osteopathic Healthcare Association (AOHA) membership ○ American Osteopathic Association (AOA) accreditation △ Commission on Accreditation of Rehabilitation Facilities (CARF) accreditation Control codes 61, 63, 64, 71, 72 and 73 indicate hospitals listed by AOHA, but not registered by AHA. For definition of numerical codes, see page A4	Control	Service	Staffed Beds	Admissions	Census	Outpatient Visits	Births	Total	Payroll	Personnel
SANFORD—Seminole County ★ CENTRAL FLORIDA REGIONAL HOSPITAL, 1401 West Seminole Boulevard, Zip 32771–6764; tel. 407/321–4500; Rodney R. Smith, President and Chief Executive Officer (Nonreporting) **A**1 9 10 **S** HCA – The Healthcare Company, Nashville, TN **Web address:** www.hcahealthcare.com	33	10	226	—	—	—	—	—	—	—
SARASOTA—Sarasota County ★ DOCTORS HOSPITAL OF SARASOTA, 5731 Bee Ridge Road, Zip 34233–5056; tel. 941/342–1100; Charles F. Scott, President and Chief Executive Officer (Nonreporting) **A**1 2 9 10 **S** HCA – The Healthcare Company, Nashville, TN **Web address:** www.doctorsofsarasota.com	12	10	147	—	—	—	—	—	—	—
☐ △ HEALTHSOUTH REHABILITATION HOSPITAL OF SARASOTA, 3251 Proctor Road, Zip 34231–8538; tel. 941/921–8600; Jeff Garber, Administrator and Chief Executive Officer (Nonreporting) **A**1 7 10 **S** HEALTHSOUTH Corporation, Birmingham, AL **Web address:** www.healthsouth.com	33	46	60	—	—	—	—	—	—	—
★ △ SARASOTA MEMORIAL HOSPITAL, 1700 South Tamiami Trail, Zip 34239–3555; tel. 941/917–9000 **A**1 2 5 7 9 10 **F**2 3 4 7 8 9 11 12 13 16 17 18 19 22 24 25 26 27 29 30 32 33 34 35 36 37 38 39 41 42 43 44 46 47 48 49 50 51 53 54 56 57 58 59 60 61 62 63 65 68 69 70 71 72 76 77 78 79 **P**4 7 8 **Web address:** www.smh.com	16	10	568	26798	353	302421	2204	250133	86869	2605
SEBASTIAN—Indian River County ☐ SEBASTIAN RIVER MEDICAL CENTER, 13695 North U.S. Highway 1, Zip 32958–3230, Mailing Address: Box 780838, Zip 32978–0838; tel. 561/589–3186; Diane D. Torres, R.N., Executive Director (Nonreporting) **A**1 9 10 **S** Health Management Associates, Naples, FL **Web address:** www.srmcenter.com	33	10	133	—	—	—	—	—	—	—
SEBRING—Highlands County ★ FLORIDA HOSPITAL HEARTLAND DIVISION, 4200 Sun'n Lake Boulevard, Zip 33872, Mailing Address: P.O. Box 9400, Zip 33871–9400; tel. 863/314–4466; John R. Harding, President and Chief Executive Officer (Total facility includes 20 beds in nursing home–type unit) **A**1 9 10 **F**7 8 9 11 13 16 17 18 19 22 24 25 27 28 30 32 34 36 37 39 45 46 48 49 50 51 54 57 60 61 62 63 69 70 72 76 78 79 **P**6 7 8 **S** Adventist Health System Sunbelt Health Care Corporation, Winter Park, FL **Web address:** www.flhosp–heartland.org	21	10	195	9046	129	159502	621	64728	23152	874
☐ HIGHLANDS REGIONAL MEDICAL CENTER, 3600 South Highlands Avenue, Zip 33870–5495, Mailing Address: Drawer 2066, Zip 33871–2066; tel. 863/471–5800; Michael A. Callahan, Chief Executive Officer (Nonreporting) **A**1 9 10 **S** Health Management Associates, Naples, FL	33	10	126	—	—	—	—	—	—	—
SOUTH MIAMI—Dade County ☐ LARKIN COMMUNITY HOSPITAL, 7031 S.W. 62nd Avenue, Zip 33143–4781; tel. 305/284–7500; Jack Michel, M.D., Chief Executive Officer (Nonreporting) **A**1 9 10 **Web address:** www.larkinhospital.com	33	10	112	—	—	—	—	—	—	—
SPRING HILL—Hernando County ★ OAK HILL HOSPITAL, 11375 Cortez Boulevard, Zip 34611, Mailing Address: P.O. Box 5300, Zip 34611–5300; tel. 352/596–6632; Jaime A. Wesolowski, Chief Executive Officer **A**1 2 9 10 **F**4 8 9 11 12 13 17 18 19 22 23 24 25 29 32 33 34 38 39 41 43 44 45 46 48 51 54 68 70 76 78 **P**1 **S** HCA – The Healthcare Company, Nashville, TN **Web address:** www.hcahealthcare.com	33	10	204	10469	129	57935	540	54193	24069	708
SPRING HILL REGIONAL HOSPITAL, 10461 Quality Drive, Zip 34609; tel. 352/688–8200; Thomas Bard, Chief Executive Officer (Nonreporting) **A**9 10 **S** Health Management Associates, Naples, FL	33	10	75	—	—	—	—	—	—	—
STARKE—Bradford County ★ SHANDS AT STARKE, 922 East Call Street, Zip 32091–3699; tel. 904/368–2300; Jeannie Baker, Administrator **A**1 9 10 **F**7 9 16 17 18 19 22 25 32 34 36 37 38 43 45 48 53 54 56 72 76 78 **S** Shands HealthCare, Gainesville, FL **Web address:** www.shands.org	23	10	30	728	8	71025	0	9856	4583	140
STUART—Martin County ★ MARTIN MEMORIAL HEALTH SYSTEMS, (Includes Martin Memorial Hospital South, 2100 S.E. Salerno Road, Zip 34997; tel. 561/223–5945), 300 S.E. Hospital Drive, Zip 34995–9014, Mailing Address: P.O. Box 9010, Zip 34995–9010; tel. 561/223–5945; Richmond M. Harman, President and Chief Executive Officer **A**1 2 9 10 **F**4 5 7 8 9 11 13 14 16 17 18 19 20 22 24 25 27 28 29 30 31 32 33 34 35 36 37 38 39 40 41 43 44 45 46 48 49 50 51 54 56 59 62 63 64 65 68 70 72 76 77 78 79 **P**5 6 8 **Web address:** www.mmhs.com	23	10	324	18152	228	351421	1258	156079	68958	1946
SUN CITY CENTER—Hillsborough County ★ SOUTH BAY HOSPITAL, 4016 State Road 674, Zip 33573–5298; tel. 813/634–3301; Alan M. Levine, Chief Executive Officer (Nonreporting) **A**1 9 10 **S** HCA – The Healthcare Company, Nashville, TN **Web address:** www.hcahealthcare.com	33	10	112	—	—	—	—	—	—	—

Hospitals, U.S. / FLORIDA

Hospital, Address, Telephone, Administrator, Approval, Facility, and Physician Codes, Health Care System, Network	Classification Codes		Utilization Data					Expense (thousands) of dollars		
	Control	Service	Staffed Beds	Admissions	Census	Outpatient Visits	Births	Total	Payroll	Personnel

★ American Hospital Association (AHA) membership
☐ Joint Commission on Accreditation of Healthcare Organizations (JCAHO) accreditation
+ American Osteopathic Healthcare Association (AOHA) membership
○ American Osteopathic Association (AOA) accreditation
△ Commission on Accreditation of Rehabilitation Facilities (CARF) accreditation
Control codes 61, 63, 64, 71, 72 and 73 indicate hospitals listed by AOHA, but not registered by AHA. For definition of numerical codes, see page A4

SUNRISE—Broward County

Hospital	Control	Service	Staffed Beds	Admissions	Census	Outpatient Visits	Births	Total	Payroll	Personnel
☐ △ SUNRISE REGIONAL MEDICAL CENTER, (Formerly The Retreat), 555 S.W. 148th Avenue, Zip 33325–3072; tel. 954/370–0200; Humberto F. J. Munoz, Chief Executive Officer (Nonreporting) **A** 1 7 10 **S** Health Systems America, Sunrise, FL Web address: www.sunriseregional.com	33	22	100	—	—	—	—	—	—	—

TALLAHASSEE—Leon County

Hospital	Control	Service	Staffed Beds	Admissions	Census	Outpatient Visits	Births	Total	Payroll	Personnel
☐ △ HEALTHSOUTH REHABILITATION HOSPITAL OF TALLAHASSEE, 1675 Riggins Road, Zip 32308–5315; tel. 850/656–4800; Armando Colombo, Chief Executive Officer (Nonreporting) **A** 1 7 10 **S** HEALTHSOUTH Corporation, Birmingham, AL Web address: www.healthsouth.com	33	46	70	—	—	—	—	—	—	—
★ TALLAHASSEE COMMUNITY HOSPITAL, 2626 Capital Medical Boulevard, Zip 32308–4499; tel. 850/656–5000; Sharon L. Roush, Chief Executive Officer (Nonreporting) **A** 1 9 10 **S** HCA – The Healthcare Company, Nashville, TN Web address: www.hcahealthcare.com	33	10	180	—	—	—	—	—	—	—
★ TALLAHASSEE MEMORIAL HEALTHCARE, 1300 Miccosukee Road, Zip 32308–5093; tel. 850/431–1155; Duncan Moore, President and Chief Executive Officer (Total facility includes 102 beds in nursing home–type unit) **A** 1 2 3 5 9 10 **F** 3 4 7 8 9 11 12 16 17 18 19 22 24 25 26 27 28 29 30 31 32 33 34 35 36 38 39 41 42 43 44 45 46 47 48 49 50 51 52 54 56 57 58 59 60 61 62 63 64 65 66 68 69 70 71 72 74 76 78 79 **P** 6 Web address: www.tmrmc.com/	23	10	616	25638	431	248619	4068	226460	113470	3159

TAMARAC—Broward County

Hospital	Control	Service	Staffed Beds	Admissions	Census	Outpatient Visits	Births	Total	Payroll	Personnel
★ UNIVERSITY HOSPITAL AND MEDICAL CENTER, (Includes University Pavilion, 7425 North University Drive, Zip 33328; tel. 305/722–9933), 7201 North University Drive, Zip 33321–2996; tel. 954/721–2200; James A. Cruickshank, Chief Executive Officer (Nonreporting) **A** 1 9 10 **S** HCA – The Healthcare Company, Nashville, TN Web address: www.hcahealthcare.com	33	10	211	—	—	—	—	—	—	—

TAMPA—Hillsborough County

Hospital	Control	Service	Staffed Beds	Admissions	Census	Outpatient Visits	Births	Total	Payroll	Personnel
★ H. LEE MOFFITT CANCER CENTER AND RESEARCH INSTITUTE, (CANCER), 12902 Magnolia Drive, Zip 33612–9497; tel. 813/972–4673; John C. Ruckdeschel, M.D., Director and Chief Executive Officer **A** 1 2 3 5 8 9 10 **F** 7 9 13 16 17 18 19 20 22 23 24 26 30 31 32 33 34 35 36 37 38 39 41 43 46 48 49 50 51 54 55 59 60 63 65 66 73 74 76 77 78 79 Web address: www.moffitt.usf.edu	23	49	117	5299	83	113740	—	136251	50847	1365
★ △ JAMES A. HALEY VETERANS HOSPITAL, 13000 Bruce B. Downs Boulevard, Zip 33612–4798; tel. 813/972–2000; Richard A. Silver, Director (Total facility includes 209 beds in nursing home–type unit) (Nonreporting) **A** 1 3 5 7 8 9 **S** Department of Veterans Affairs, Washington, DC	45	10	640	—	—	—	—	—	—	—
★ MEMORIAL HOSPITAL OF TAMPA, 2901 Swann Avenue, Zip 33609–4057; tel. 813/873–6400; John Mainieri, Interim Chief Executive Officer **A** 1 5 9 10 **F** 1 3 4 9 11 12 13 18 19 21 22 24 25 28 30 32 33 34 35 36 37 39 41 42 43 45 46 48 49 50 52 54 57 58 61 62 63 64 68 69 70 71 75 76 78 79 **S** IASIS Healthcare, Nashville, TN Web address: www.tenethealth.com/tampa	33	10	140	4872	73	37779	—	36497	14760	394
☐ SHRINERS HOSPITALS FOR CHILDREN, TAMPA, 12502 North Pine Drive, Zip 33612–9499; tel. 813/972–2250; John Holtz, Administrator **A** 1 3 5 **F** 16 17 19 22 24 31 34 38 39 48 49 54 68 70 76 78 **S** Shriners Hospitals for Children, Tampa, FL	23	57	60	1144	29	10551	0	—	—	244
★ ST. JOSEPH'S HOSPITAL, (Includes Tampa Children's Hospital at St. Joseph's, St. Joseph's Women's Hospital – Tampa, 3030 West Dr. Martin L. King Boulevard, Zip 33607–6394; tel. 813/879–4730), 3001 West Martin Luther King Jr. Boulevard, Zip 33607–6387, Mailing Address: P.O. Box 4227, Zip 33677–4227; tel. 813/870–4000; Isaac Mallah, President and Chief Executive Officer **A** 1 2 5 9 10 **F** 4 6 8 9 11 12 13 17 18 19 22 24 25 28 29 31 33 34 35 36 38 39 41 42 44 45 46 47 48 49 50 52 54 57 58 59 60 61 62 63 64 65 67 68 69 70 72 75 76 78 79 **P** 1 7 **S** Catholic Health East, Newtown Square, PA	21	10	883	37164	538	—	6095	276080	114174	4366
★ △ TAMPA GENERAL HEALTHCARE, 2 Columbia Drive, Zip 33606, Mailing Address: P.O. Box 1289, Zip 33601–1289; tel. 813/251–7000; Ronald A. Hytoff, President and Chief Executive Officer (Total facility includes 31 beds in nursing home–type unit) **A** 1 3 5 7 8 9 10 **F** 4 7 8 9 10 11 12 13 14 16 17 18 19 22 24 25 27 28 29 31 33 34 35 38 39 41 42 43 44 45 46 47 48 49 50 51 52 53 54 56 57 61 65 66 69 70 71 74 75 76 77 78 79 Web address: www.tgh.org	23	10	722	22671	424	223964	3215	306393	106659	2838
★ TOWN AND COUNTRY HOSPITAL, 6001 Webb Road, Zip 33615–3291; tel. 813/885–6666; Phillip J. Mazzuca, Chief Executive Officer (Nonreporting) **A** 1 5 9 10 **S** IASIS Healthcare, Nashville, TN Web address: www.tenethealth.com	32	10	148	—	—	—	—	—	—	—
☐ UNIVERSITY COMMUNITY HOSPITAL, 3100 East Fletcher Avenue, Zip 33613–4688; tel. 813/971–6000; Norman V. Stein, President (Total facility includes 27 beds in nursing home–type unit) **A** 1 2 9 10 **F** 4 7 8 9 11 12 13 16 17 18 19 22 23 24 25 27 28 30 31 32 33 34 36 38 39 40 41 42 43 44 45 46 47 48 50 51 52 53 54 55 65 66 68 69 70 71 72 76 77 78 79 **P** 7 Web address: www.uch.org	23	10	384	19008	268	104547	2178	175541	76568	2656
○ UNIVERSITY COMMUNITY HOSPITAL–CARROLLWOOD, 7171 North Dale Mabry Highway, Zip 33614–2699; tel. 813/558–8001; Larry J. Archbell, Vice President Operations (Total facility includes 8 beds in nursing home–type unit) **A** 9 10 11 12 13 **F** 4 7 8 9 11 12 13 16 17 18 19 22 24 25 27 28 30 31 32 33 34 36 38 39 41 42 43 44 45 46 47 48 50 51 52 53 54 55 65 66 68 69 70 71 72 76 77 78 79 **P** 7 Web address: www.uch.org	23	10	120	4071	56	50387	0	29840	15057	500

Many Facility Codes have changed. Please refer to the AHA Guide Code Chart.

Hospitals, U.S. / FLORIDA

Hospital, Address, Telephone, Administrator, Approval, Facility, and Physician Codes, Health Care System, Network	Classification Codes		Utilization Data					Expense (thousands) of dollars		
★ American Hospital Association (AHA) membership ☐ Joint Commission on Accreditation of Healthcare Organizations (JCAHO) accreditation + American Osteopathic Healthcare Association (AOHA) membership ○ American Osteopathic Association (AOA) accreditation △ Commission on Accreditation of Rehabilitation Facilities (CARF) accreditation Control codes 61, 63, 64, 71, 72 and 73 indicate hospitals listed by AOHA, but not registered by AHA. For definition of numerical codes, see page A4	Control	Service	Staffed Beds	Admissions	Census	Outpatient Visits	Births	Total	Payroll	Personnel
☐ VENCOR HOSPITAL – CENTRAL TAMPA, (LONG TERM ACUTE CARE), 4801 North Howard Avenue, Zip 33603–1484; tel. 813/874–7575; Ken Stone, Administrator **A**1 5 9 10 **F**1 7 19 20 30 49 50 51 70 72 73 **S** Vencor, Incorporated, Louisville, KY **Web address:** www.vencor.com	33	49	73	362	49	0	0	—	—	—
☐ VENCOR HOSPITAL–TAMPA, 4555 South Manhattan Avenue, Zip 33611–2397; tel. 813/839–6341; Theresa Hunkins, Administrator (Nonreporting) **A**1 3 5 10 **S** Vencor, Incorporated, Louisville, KY **Web address:** www.vencor.com	33	49	73	—	—	—	—	—	—	—
TARPON SPRINGS—Pinellas County										
✳ HELEN ELLIS MEMORIAL HOSPITAL, 1395 South Pinellas Avenue, Zip 34689–3721, Mailing Address: P.O. Box 1487, Zip 34688–1487; tel. 727/942–5000; Joseph N. Kiefer, Administrator (Total facility includes 18 beds in nursing home–type unit) **A**1 9 10 **F**7 8 9 11 12 13 17 18 19 22 24 25 27 29 32 33 34 36 38 39 41 43 44 45 46 48 49 50 51 54 69 72 76 77 78 **P**8	23	10	127	7744	104	81377	697	61493	24767	745
TAVERNIER—Monroe County										
✳ MARINERS HOSPITAL, 91500 Overseas Highway, Zip 33070; tel. 305/853–1582; Robert H. Luse, Chief Executive Officer **A**1 9 10 **F**7 9 17 18 19 22 24 25 32 33 34 37 38 39 41 45 48 50 54 68 70 72 76 78 79 **P**1 **S** Baptist Health System of South Florida, Coral Gables, FL **Web address:** www.baptisthealth.net/	23	10	42	1415	16	18853	1	16055	6054	168
TEQUESTA—Martin County										
SANDYPINES, 11301 S.E. Tequesta Terrace, Zip 33469–8146; tel. 561/744–0211; Mary S. Bohne', Administrator (Nonreporting) **S** Health Management Associates, Naples, FL	33	52	60	—	—	—	—	—	—	—
TITUSVILLE—Brevard County										
☐ PARRISH MEDICAL CENTER, 951 North Washington Avenue, Zip 32796–2194; tel. 407/268–6111; Rod L. Baker, President and Chief Executive Officer **A**1 2 9 10 **F**1 3 5 7 8 9 11 12 13 16 17 18 19 22 23 24 25 27 28 29 31 32 33 34 35 36 37 38 39 41 43 44 46 48 49 50 51 54 61 65 68 70 71 72 74 76 77 78 79 **Web address:** www.parrishmed.com	16	10	210	9222	114	96437	593	65335	27420	746
TYNDALL AFB—Escambia County										
★ U. S. AIR FORCE HOSPITAL, 340 Magnolia Circle, Zip 32403–5612; tel. 850/283–7515; Colonel Michael J. Murphy, Commander (Nonreporting) **S** Department of the Air Force, Bowling AFB, DC	41	10	25	—	—	—	—	—	—	—
VENICE—Sarasota County										
✳ BON SECOURS–VENICE HOSPITAL, 540 The Rialto, Zip 34285–2900; tel. 941/485–7711; Michael G. Guley, Chief Executive Officer (Total facility includes 120 beds in nursing home–type unit) **A**1 2 9 10 **F**6 7 9 11 13 14 17 18 19 21 22 25 26 29 30 34 35 36 39 45 46 48 51 53 54 56 57 61 62 64 69 76 78 **P**5 7 **S** Bon Secours Health System, Inc., Marriottsville, MD **Web address:** www.bonsecours.org/florida/	21	10	281	9220	240	182943	0	77304	27084	1256
VERO BEACH—Indian River County										
☐ △ HEALTHSOUTH TREASURE COAST REHABILITATION HOSPITAL, 1600 37th Street, Zip 32960–6549; tel. 561/778–2100; Jason N. Roebuck, Chief Executive Officer **A**1 7 10 **F**5 13 16 17 18 29 33 34 38 39 48 49 50 53 54 71 72 78 **S** HEALTHSOUTH Corporation, Birmingham, AL **Web address:** www.healthsouth.com	33	46	90	1349	72	40583	—	16459	8323	256
✳ INDIAN RIVER MEMORIAL HOSPITAL, 1000 36th Street, Zip 32960–6592; tel. 561/567–4311; Jeffrey L. Susi, President and Chief Executive Officer (Nonreporting) **A**1 2 9 10 **Web address:** www.irmh.com	23	10	300	—	—	—	—	—	—	—
WEST PALM BEACH—Palm Beach County										
45TH STREET MENTAL HEALTH CENTER, 1041 45th Street, Zip 33407–2494; tel. 561/844–9741; Terry H. Allen, Executive Director (Nonreporting) **A**10	23	22	44	—	—	—	—	—	—	—
✳ ○ COLUMBIA HOSPITAL, 2201 45th Street, Zip 33407–2069; tel. 561/842–6141; Eric Goldman, Chief Operating Officer (Nonreporting) **A**1 9 10 11 12 **S** HCA – The Healthcare Company, Nashville, TN **Web address:** www.hcahealthcare.com	33	10	250	—	—	—	—	—	—	—
✳ GOOD SAMARITAN MEDICAL CENTER, Flagler Drive at Palm Beach Lakes Boulevard, Zip 33401–3499; tel. 561/655–5511; Steven R. Nathan, President and Chief Executive Officer **A**1 2 9 10 **F**2 3 4 7 8 9 11 12 13 14 16 17 18 19 21 22 24 25 26 27 28 29 30 32 33 34 35 36 37 38 39 40 41 42 43 44 45 46 47 48 49 50 51 52 53 54 55 57 58 59 61 62 63 64 65 66 68 70 71 72 74 75 76 78 79 **P**6 8 **S** Catholic Health East, Newtown Square, PA	23	10	341	11972	176	—	1742	113655	32892	884
HOSPICE OF PALM BEACH COUNTY, (HOSPICE), 5300 East Avenue, Zip 33401–2352; tel. 561/848–5200 **F**26 37 70 72 78	23	49	24	2645	24	—	0	13401	6443	217
★ △ ST. MARY'S HOSPITAL, 901 45th Street, Zip 33407–2495, Mailing Address: P.O. Box 24620, Zip 33416–4620; tel. 561/844–6300; Steven R. Nathan, President and Chief Executive Officer **A**7 9 10 **F**3 4 7 8 9 11 12 13 14 16 17 18 19 21 22 24 25 27 28 29 30 32 33 34 35 36 37 38 39 40 41 42 43 44 45 46 47 48 49 50 51 52 53 54 55 57 58 59 61 62 63 64 65 68 70 71 72 74 75 76 78 79 **P**6 8 **S** Catholic Health East, Newtown Square, PA	21	10	460	16318	269	114985	2493	162131	56289	1620

© 2000 AHA Guide   *Many Facility Codes have changed. Please refer to the AHA Guide Code Chart.*

Hospitals, U.S. / FLORIDA

Hospital, Address, Telephone, Administrator, Approval, Facility, and Physician Codes, Health Care System, Network	Classification Codes		Utilization Data					Expense (thousands) of dollars		
★ American Hospital Association (AHA) membership ☐ Joint Commission on Accreditation of Healthcare Organizations (JCAHO) accreditation + American Osteopathic Healthcare Association (AOHA) membership ○ American Osteopathic Association (AOA) accreditation △ Commission on Accreditation of Rehabilitation Facilities (CARF) accreditation Control codes 61, 63, 64, 71, 72 and 73 indicate hospitals listed by AOHA, but not registered by AHA. For definition of numerical codes, see page A4	Control	Service	Staffed Beds	Admissions	Census	Outpatient Visits	Births	Total	Payroll	Personnel
★ VETERANS AFFAIRS MEDICAL CENTER, 7305 North Military Trail, Zip 33410–6400; tel. 561/882–8262; Edward H. Seiler, Director (Total facility includes 98 beds in nursing home–type unit) **A**1 9 **F**1 3 5 9 13 22 23 24 29 31 34 35 38 39 41 43 45 46 48 49 50 51 54 56 57 61 62 63 66 69 70 72 76 77 78 79 **S** Department of Veterans Affairs, Washington, DC **Web address:** www.va.gov	45	10	192	3768	165	305816	0	112393	76445	1234
☐ ○ WELLINGTON REGIONAL MEDICAL CENTER, 10101 Forest Hill Boulevard, Zip 33414–6199; tel. 561/798–8500; Gregory E. Boyer, Chief Executive Officer (Nonreporting) **A**1 2 9 10 11 12 13 **S** Universal Health Services, Inc., King of Prussia, PA **Web address:** www.wrmhospital@icanect.net	33	10	93	—	—	—	—	—	—	—
WILLISTON—Levy County NATURE COAST REGIONAL HOSPITAL, (Formerly Nature Coast Regional Health Network), 125 S.W. Seventh Street, Zip 32696, Mailing Address: P.O. Drawer 550, Zip 32696–0550; tel. 352/528–2801; Steve Widener, Chief Executive Officer **A**9 10 **F**7 13 19 22 24 25 31 32 34 37 38 45 48 51 53 54 56 70 71 76 78 **P**4 7	33	10	40	826	11	15507	0	5830	2048	100
WINTER HAVEN—Polk County ★ △ WINTER HAVEN HOSPITAL, (Includes Lake Wales Medical Centers, 410 South 11th Street, Lake Wales, Zip 33853–4256, Mailing Address: P.O. Box 3460, Zip 33859–3460; tel. 941/676–1433; 200 Avenue F. N.E., Zip 33881–4193; tel. 941/297–1899; Lance W. Anastasio, President (Total facility includes 170 beds in nursing home–type unit) **A**1 7 9 10 **F**7 8 9 11 12 13 17 18 19 21 22 23 24 25 27 28 32 33 34 36 37 39 41 42 43 44 45 46 48 53 54 57 59 60 61 62 63 65 68 69 70 71 72 76 77 78 79 **P**6	23	10	676	20190	402	296058	2265	167225	82997	2781
WINTER PARK—Orange County ★ WINTER PARK MEMORIAL HOSPITAL, (Includes Winter Park Psychiatric Care Center, 1600 Dodd Road, Zip 32792; tel. 407/677–6842), 200 North Lakemont Avenue, Zip 32792–3273; tel. 407/646–7000; Douglas P. DeGraaf, Chief Executive Officer (Nonreporting) **A**1 2 9 10 **S** HCA – The Healthcare Company, Nashville, TN **Web address:** www.hcahealthcare.com	33	10	339	—	—	—	—	—	—	—
ZEPHYRHILLS—Pasco County ★ EAST PASCO MEDICAL CENTER, 7050 Gall Boulevard, Zip 33541–1399; tel. 813/788–0411; Paul Michael Norman, President (Total facility includes 12 beds in nursing home–type unit) **A**1 9 10 **F**7 8 9 11 13 16 17 18 19 22 25 28 29 33 36 38 39 41 44 45 48 49 51 54 56 65 69 70 72 76 78 79 **P**5 **S** Adventist Health System Sunbelt Health Care Corporation, Winter Park, FL	21	10	139	8879	95	65184	512	72769	30592	499

Hospitals, U.S. / GEORGIA

GEORGIA

Resident Population 7,642 (in thousands)
Resident population in metro areas 68.5%
Birth rate per 1,000 population 15.8
65 years and over 9.9%
Percent of persons without health insurance 17.6%

Hospital, Address, Telephone, Administrator, Approval, Facility, and Physician Codes, Health Care System, Network	Classification Codes		Utilization Data					Expense (thousands) of dollars		
★ American Hospital Association (AHA) membership □ Joint Commission on Accreditation of Healthcare Organizations (JCAHO) accreditation + American Osteopathic Healthcare Association (AOHA) membership ○ American Osteopathic Association (AOA) accreditation △ Commission on Accreditation of Rehabilitation Facilities (CARF) accreditation Control codes 61, 63, 64, 71, 72 and 73 indicate hospitals listed by AOHA, but not registered by AHA. For definition of numerical codes, see page A4	Control	Service	Staffed Beds	Admissions	Census	Outpatient Visits	Births	Total	Payroll	Personnel

ADEL—Cook County
★ MEMORIAL HOSPITAL OF ADEL, 706 North Parrish Avenue, Zip 31620–0677; Mailing Address: P.O. Box 677, Zip 31620–0677; tel. 912/896–2251; Greg Griffith, Chief Executive Officer (Total facility includes 95 beds in nursing home–type unit) (Nonreporting) **A**1 9 10 **S** New American Healthcare Corporation, Brentwood, TN — 33 10 155 — — — — — — —

ALBANY—Dougherty County
★ PALMYRA MEDICAL CENTERS, 2000 Palmyra Road, Zip 31702–1908, Mailing Address: P.O. Box 1908, Zip 31702–1908; tel. 912/434–2000; Allen Golson, Chief Executive Officer **A**1 9 10 **F**9 13 17 19 22 25 26 28 30 32 34 38 39 41 45 48 49 53 54 70 71 72 76 77 78 **P**5 **S** HCA – The Healthcare Company, Nashville, TN
Web address: www.palmyramedicalcenters.com — 33 10 163 4517 82 60103 0 41366 17998 477

★ PHOEBE PUTNEY MEMORIAL HOSPITAL, 417 Third Avenue, Zip 31701–1828, Mailing Address: P.O. Box 1828, Zip 31703–1828; tel. 912/883–1800; Joel Wernick, President and Chief Executive Officer (Nonreporting) **A**1 2 3 5 9 10
Web address: www.ppmh.org — 23 10 418 — — — — — — —

ALMA—Bacon County
□ BACON COUNTY HOSPITAL, 302 South Wayne Street, Zip 31510–2997, Mailing Address: P.O. Drawer 1987, Zip 31510–1987; tel. 912/632–8961; Oliver J. Booker, Chief Executive Officer (Total facility includes 88 beds in nursing home–type unit) (Nonreporting) **A**1 9 10
Web address: www.bchsi@almatel.net — 16 10 126 — — — — — — —

AMERICUS—Sumter County
★ SUMTER REGIONAL HOSPITAL, 100 Wheatley Drive, Zip 31709–3799; tel. 912/924–6011; Jerry W. Adams, President (Total facility includes 100 beds in nursing home–type unit) **A**1 9 10 **F**4 7 8 9 11 13 19 22 24 25 27 31 32 33 34 36 37 38 39 41 43 44 47 48 49 50 51 53 54 56 57 61 62 69 70 72 74 75 76 77 78 **P**8 — 15 10 232 4683 235 53256 903 40289 16493 555

ARLINGTON—Calhoun County
CALHOUN MEMORIAL HOSPITAL, 209 Academy & Carswell Streets, Zip 31713, Mailing Address: Drawer R, Zip 31713; tel. 912/725–4272; Peggy Pierce, Administrator (Nonreporting) **A**9 10 — 16 10 24 — — — — — — —

ATHENS—Clarke County
★ ATHENS REGIONAL MEDICAL CENTER, 1199 Prince Avenue, Zip 30606–2793; tel. 706/549–9977; John A. Drew, President and Chief Executive Officer **A**1 9 10 **F**3 4 8 9 11 12 13 16 17 18 19 22 24 25 27 29 34 35 38 39 41 42 44 45 46 47 48 54 57 62 64 65 66 70 71 72 76 78
Web address: www.armc.org — 16 10 315 15180 198 79864 1720 151839 61902 1908

★ ST. MARY'S HEALTH CARE SYSTEM, 1230 Baxter Street, Zip 30606–3791; tel. 706/548–7581; Thomas E. Fitz, Jr, FACHE, President and Chief Executive Officer (Total facility includes 120 beds in nursing home–type unit) **A**1 9 10 **F**6 7 8 9 11 13 17 18 19 22 23 24 25 28 30 31 32 33 34 35 36 37 38 39 41 42 43 44 45 46 48 49 50 51 54 67 69 70 71 72 76 78 79 **P**7 **S** Catholic Health East, Newtown Square, PA
Web address: www.stmarysathens.com — 23 10 292 7616 204 173205 1229 85561 40176 1089

ATLANTA—Fulton and De Kalb Counties County
★ △ ATLANTA MEDICAL CENTER, 303 Parkway Drive N.E., Zip 30312–1212; tel. 404/265–4000; Bruce F. Buchanan, FACHE, President and Chief Executive Officer (Total facility includes 72 beds in nursing home–type unit) (Nonreporting) **A**1 2 3 5 7 8 9 10 **S** TENET Healthcare Corporation, Santa Barbara, CA
Web address: www.atlantamedcenter.com — 33 10 450 — — — — — — —

□ CHARTER ANCHOR HOSPITAL, 5454 Yorktowne Drive, Zip 30349–5305; tel. 770/991–6044; Matthew Crouch, Chief Executive Officer (Nonreporting) **A**1 9 10 **S** Magellan Health Services, Atlanta, GA
Web address: www.talbottcampus.com — 33 82 84 — — — — — — —

□ CHARTER BEHAVIORAL HEALTH SYSTEM OF ATLANTA, 811 Juniper Street N.E., Zip 30308–1398; tel. 404/881–5800; John McKenna, Administrator (Nonreporting) **A**1 9 10 **S** Magellan Health Services, Atlanta, GA — 33 22 40 — — — — — — —

□ CHARTER BEHAVIORAL HEALTH SYSTEM OF ATLANTA AT PEACHFORD, 2151 Peachford Road, Zip 30338–6599; tel. 770/455–3200; Ron Fincher, Chief Executive Officer (Nonreporting) **A**1 9 10 **S** Magellan Health Services, Atlanta, GA — 33 22 224 — — — — — — —

□ CHILDREN'S HEALTHCARE OF ATLANTA AT EGLESTON, (Formerly Egleston Children's Hospital), (PEDIATRIC), 1405 Clifton Road N.E., Zip 30322–1101; tel. 404/325–6000; James E. Tally, Ph.D., President and Chief Executive Officer **A**1 3 5 8 9 10 **F**4 11 12 13 14 17 18 19 22 23 24 25 29 31 32 33 34 35 36 38 39 42 43 45 46 47 48 50 51 52 53 54 55 56 57 58 59 60 63 64 68 70 71 72 74 75 76 77 78 **P**8 **S** Children's Healthcare of Atlanta, Atlanta, GA — 23 59 206 12419 145 196937 0 143615 61140 1804

© 2000 AHA Guide   *Many Facility Codes have changed. Please refer to the AHA Guide Code Chart.*   Hospitals **A99**

Hospitals, U.S. / GEORGIA

Hospital, Address, Telephone, Administrator, Approval, Facility, and Physician Codes, Health Care System, Network	Classification Codes		Utilization Data					Expense (thousands) of dollars		
★ American Hospital Association (AHA) membership □ Joint Commission on Accreditation of Healthcare Organizations (JCAHO) accreditation + American Osteopathic Healthcare Association (AOHA) membership ○ American Osteopathic Association (AOA) accreditation △ Commission on Accreditation of Rehabilitation Facilities (CARF) accreditation Control codes 61, 63, 64, 71, 72 and 73 indicate hospitals listed by AOHA, but not registered by AHA. For definition of numerical codes, see page A4	Control	Service	Staffed Beds	Admissions	Census	Outpatient Visits	Births	Total	Payroll	Personnel
□ △ CHILDREN'S HEALTHCARE OF ATLANTA AT SCOTTISH RITE, (Formerly Scottish Rite Children's Center), (PEDIATRIC), 1001 Johnson Ferry Road N.E., Zip 30342–1600; tel. 404/256–5252; James E. Tally, Ph.D., President and Chief Executive Officer **A**1 3 5 7 9 10 **F**4 11 12 13 14 17 18 19 22 23 24 25 29 31 32 33 34 35 36 38 39 42 43 45 46 47 48 50 51 52 53 54 56 57 58 59 60 63 64 68 70 71 72 74 75 76 77 78 **P**8 **S** Children's Healthcare of Atlanta, Atlanta, GA **Web address:** www.srcmc.org	23	59	165	13786	129	220552	0	142605	70836	1889
★ CRAWFORD LONG HOSPITAL OF EMORY UNIVERSITY, 550 Peachtree Street N.E., Zip 30365–2225; tel. 404/686–4411; John Dunklin Henry, Sr, FACHE, Chief Executive Officer **A**1 2 3 5 8 9 10 **F**1 2 3 4 7 8 9 11 12 13 14 16 19 22 24 25 27 28 29 30 34 35 36 37 38 39 41 42 43 44 45 46 47 48 51 52 53 54 55 56 57 58 59 60 61 62 63 64 65 66 68 69 70 71 72 74 75 76 79 **Web address:** www.emory.org	23	10	397	19174	302	89594	2312	204734	78758	1868
★ EMORY DUNWOODY MEDICAL CENTER, 4575 North Shallowford Road, Zip 30338–6499; tel. 770/454–2000; Thomas D. Gilbert, President and Chief Executive Officer **A**1 9 10 **F**7 8 9 11 13 16 17 19 22 24 25 32 33 34 38 39 41 42 43 44 45 48 49 50 51 54 66 68 69 70 76 78 79 **S** HCA – The Healthcare Company, Nashville, TN **Web address:** www.hcahealthcare.com	33	10	140	3732	41	24234	1551	—	—	304
★ △ EMORY UNIVERSITY HOSPITAL, 1364 Clifton Road N.E., Zip 30322–1102; tel. 404/712–7021; John Dunklin Henry, Sr, FACHE, Chief Executive Officer **A**1 2 3 5 7 8 9 10 **F**1 2 3 4 6 8 9 11 12 13 16 18 19 21 22 23 24 25 26 27 28 29 30 31 32 33 34 35 36 37 38 39 40 41 43 44 45 46 47 48 49 50 51 53 54 55 56 57 59 60 61 62 63 64 65 66 67 68 69 70 71 72 74 76 77 78 79 **P**1 **Web address:** www.emory.org	23	10	473	21017	365	59408	0	301080	107403	2751
★ GRADY MEMORIAL HOSPITAL, 80 Butler Street S.E., Zip 30335–3801; Mailing Address: P.O. Box 26189, Zip 30335–3801; tel. 404/616–4252; Edward J. Renford, President and Chief Executive Officer (Total facility includes 354 beds in nursing home–type unit) **A**1 2 3 5 8 9 10 **F**3 4 5 7 8 9 10 11 12 13 14 16 17 18 19 22 23 24 25 26 29 30 31 32 33 34 35 36 37 38 39 41 42 43 44 45 46 47 48 49 50 51 52 54 56 57 58 59 60 61 62 63 64 65 66 69 70 72 73 75 76 77 78 79	16	10	1116	28071	533	737961	4349	475977	174826	4826
HILLSIDE HOSPITAL, 690 Courtney Drive N.E., Zip 30306–0206, Mailing Address: P.O. Box 8247, Zip 31106–0247; tel. 404/875–4551; Teresa Stoker, Chief Executive Officer **F**13 16 17 18 19 23 57 58 60 61 64	23	52	61	29	61	0	0	7618	4807	175
★ METROPOLITAN HOSPITAL, 3223 Howell Mill Road N.W., Zip 30327–4135; tel. 404/351–0500; Jean Calhoun, Administrator (Nonreporting) **A**1 9 10 **S** HCA – The Healthcare Company, Nashville, TN **Web address:** www.hcahealthcare.com	33	49	64	—	—	—	—	—	—	—
★ NORTHSIDE HOSPITAL, 1000 Johnson Ferry Road N.E., Zip 30342–1611; tel. 404/851–8000; Sidney Kirschner, President and Chief Executive Officer (Nonreporting) **A**1 2 9 10	23	44	352	—	—	—	—	—	—	—
★ △ PIEDMONT HOSPITAL, 1968 Peachtree Road N.W., Zip 30309–1231; tel. 404/605–5000; Richard B. Hubbard, II, President and Chief Executive Officer (Total facility includes 37 beds in nursing home–type unit) (Nonreporting) **A**1 2 3 5 7 9 10 **Web address:** www.piedmonthospital.org	23	10	444	—	—	—	—	—	—	—
★ SAINT JOSEPH'S HOSPITAL OF ATLANTA, 5665 Peachtree Dunwoody Road N.E., Zip 30342–1764; tel. 404/851–7001; Brue Chandler, President and Chief Executive Officer **A**1 2 9 10 **F**1 4 7 9 11 12 13 14 16 17 18 19 21 22 23 24 25 28 29 31 32 33 34 35 38 40 41 43 45 46 47 48 49 50 51 54 55 56 65 68 70 71 72 74 75 76 78 79 **P**1 **S** Catholic Health East, Newtown Square, PA **Web address:** www.stjosephsatlanta.org	23	10	346	17844	252	135133	0	216960	83788	2010
★ △ SHEPHERD CENTER, 2020 Peachtree Road N.W., Zip 30309–1465; tel. 404/352–2020; Gary R. Ulicny, Ph.D., President and Chief Executive Officer **A**1 7 10 **F**3 6 13 16 17 18 19 22 23 24 26 28 29 31 32 37 38 39 41 43 45 49 50 53 54 56 66 72 73 76 78 **P**1 6 **Web address:** www.shepherd.org	23	46	100	856	75	21199	0	45027	23405	671
□ SOUTHWEST HOSPITAL AND MEDICAL CENTER, 501 Fairburn Road S.W., Zip 30331–2099; tel. 404/699–1111; Marie Cameron, FACHE, President and Chief Executive Officer (Nonreporting) **A**1 3 5 9 10	23	10	80	—	—	—	—	—	—	—
□ VENCOR HOSPITAL–ATLANTA, 705 Juniper Street N.E., Zip 30365–2500; tel. 404/873–2871; Skip Wright, Administrator (Nonreporting) **A**1 10 **S** Vencor, Incorporated, Louisville, KY	33	49	66	—	—	—	—	—	—	—
★ WESLEY WOODS CENTER OF EMORY UNIVERSITY, (MULTI–DICIPLINARY ACUTE CARE), 1821 Clifton Road N.E., Zip 30329–5102; tel. 404/728–6200; William L. Minnix, Jr, President and Chief Executive Officer **A**1 3 5 9 10 **F**1 2 3 4 6 8 9 11 12 13 17 18 19 21 22 23 24 25 26 27 28 29 30 31 32 33 34 35 36 37 38 39 40 41 43 45 46 47 48 49 50 51 53 54 55 56 57 59 62 63 64 66 67 68 69 70 71 72 74 76 77 78 79 **P**6 **Web address:** www.emory.org	23	49	94	1821	64	32062	0	30438	12090	353

AUGUSTA—Richmond County

★ △ DOCTORS HOSPITAL, (Formerly Doctors Hospital of Augusta), 3651 Wheeler Road, Zip 30909–6426; tel. 706/651–3232; Michael K. Kerner, President and Chief Executive Officer **A**1 7 9 10 **F**7 8 9 10 11 13 18 19 22 23 25 27 29 30 32 34 36 38 39 41 43 44 45 46 48 49 53 54 65 70 71 72 76 78 79 **P**1 6 **S** HCA – The Healthcare Company, Nashville, TN **Web address:** www.doctors–hospital.net/	33	10	216	8234	125	93225	1111	72747	32197	872

Hospitals, U.S. / GEORGIA

Hospital, Address, Telephone, Administrator, Approval, Facility, and Physician Codes, Health Care System, Network	Classification Codes		Utilization Data					Expense (thousands) of dollars		
★ American Hospital Association (AHA) membership ☐ Joint Commission on Accreditation of Healthcare Organizations (JCAHO) accreditation + American Osteopathic Healthcare Association (AOHA) membership ○ American Osteopathic Association (AOA) accreditation △ Commission on Accreditation of Rehabilitation Facilities (CARF) accreditation Control codes 61, 63, 64, 71, 72 and 73 indicate hospitals listed by AOHA, but not registered by AHA. For definition of numerical codes, see page A4	Control	Service	Staffed Beds	Admissions	Census	Outpatient Visits	Births	Total	Payroll	Personnel
☐ GEORGIA REGIONAL HOSPITAL AT AUGUSTA, 3405 Mike Padgett Highway, Zip 30906–3897; tel. 706/792–7019; Benjamin H. Walker, Facility Administrator A1 3 9 10 F1 2 3 4 5 6 7 8 9 10 11 12 13 14 15 16 19 20 21 22 23 24 25 26 27 28 29 30 31 32 33 34 35 36 37 38 39 40 41 42 43 44 45 46 47 48 49 50 51 52 53 54 55 56 57 58 59 60 61 62 63 64 65 66 67 68 69 70 71 72 73 74 75 76 77 78 79 Web address: www.dhr.state.ga.us	12	22	172	1276	119	0	0	15797	9622	364
★ MEDICAL COLLEGE OF GEORGIA HOSPITAL AND CLINICS, 1120 15th Street, Zip 30912–5000; tel. 706/721–0211; Patricia Sodomka, FACHE, Executive Director A1 2 3 5 8 9 10 12 F4 8 9 11 12 13 14 17 18 19 22 23 24 25 30 31 32 33 34 35 38 39 41 42 43 44 45 46 47 48 49 51 52 54 56 57 58 59 60 61 62 63 64 65 66 68 70 71 72 74 75 78 79 P6 Web address: www.mcg.edu	12	10	461	14832	281	468450	1569	253168	125576	—
★ ST. JOSEPH HOSPITAL, 2260 Wrightsboro Road, Zip 30904–4726; tel. 706/481–7000; J. William Paugh, President and Chief Executive Officer A1 9 10 F8 9 11 13 16 17 18 19 22 25 26 27 29 30 32 33 34 36 37 38 39 41 42 43 44 46 48 50 54 56 70 72 76 78 79 P8 S Carondelet Health System, Saint Louis, MO Web address: www.stjoshosp.org	21	10	145	5582	72	—	1235	71241	31232	814
★ UNIVERSITY HEALTH CARE SYSTEM, 1350 Walton Way, Zip 30901–2629; tel. 706/722–9011; J. Larry Read, President and Chief Executive Officer (Nonreporting) A1 2 3 5 9 10 Web address: www.universityhealth.org	23	10	528	—	—	—	—	—	—	—
★ VETERANS AFFAIRS MEDICAL CENTER, 1 Freedom Way, Zip 30904–6285; tel. 706/733–0188; Ellen DeGeorge-Smith, FACHE, Director (Total facility includes 60 beds in nursing home–type unit) (Nonreporting) A1 2 3 5 8 9 S Department of Veterans Affairs, Washington, DC Web address: www.va.gov	45	10	587	—	—	—	—	—	—	—
★ △ WALTON REHABILITATION HOSPITAL, 1355 Independence Drive, Zip 30901–1037; tel. 706/724–7746; Dennis B. Skelley, President and Chief Executive Officer A1 7 10 F1 13 16 18 28 38 49 53 54 78 Web address: www.wrh.org	23	46	58	989	45	19898	0	16214	7925	181
AUSTELL—Cobb County										
★ △ WELLSTAR COBB HOSPITAL, 3950 Austell Road, Zip 30106–1121; tel. 770/732–4000; Thomas E. Hill, Chief Executive Officer (Nonreporting) A1 2 7 9 10 S WellStar Health System, Marietta, GA Web address: www.promina.org	23	10	311	—	—	—	—	—	—	—
BAINBRIDGE—Decatur County										
★ MEMORIAL HOSPITAL AND MANOR, 1500 East Shotwell Street, Zip 31717–4294; tel. 912/246–3500; James G. Peak, Chief Executive Officer (Total facility includes 131 beds in nursing home–type unit) A1 9 10 F6 7 8 9 13 18 19 22 23 24 25 27 32 34 37 39 41 43 44 48 49 50 51 54 69 70 71 72 74 76 78 79 P8	16	10	211	2947	146	44575	479	25513	11868	487
BAXLEY—Appling County										
☐ APPLING HEALTHCARE SYSTEM, 163 East Tollison Street, Zip 31513–2898; tel. 912/367–9841; Terry Stratton, Chief Executive Officer (Total facility includes 101 beds in nursing home–type unit) A1 9 10 F7 8 9 12 13 14 16 17 18 19 22 25 34 41 44 45 48 49 50 54 56 69 71 76 77 Web address: www.appling-hospital.org	16	10	140	1003	106	18498	95	12403	6374	254
BLAIRSVILLE—Union County										
★ UNION GENERAL HOSPITAL, 214 Hospital Drive, Zip 30512–6538; tel. 706/745–2111; Rebecca T. Dyer, Administrator (Total facility includes 147 beds in nursing home–type unit) A1 9 10 F7 8 9 16 17 18 22 23 24 25 31 32 34 39 44 46 48 49 69 70	13	10	192	1911	165	32535	247	16370	7846	305
BLAKELY—Early County										
☐ EARLY MEMORIAL HOSPITAL, 630 Columbia Street, Zip 31723–1798; tel. 912/723–4241; Kevin Taylor, Administrator (Total facility includes 127 beds in nursing home–type unit) A1 9 10 F9 13 16 17 18 22 25 32 36 37 38 48 54 69 P8 S Archbold Medical Center, Thomasville, GA	23	10	159	1044	136	8205	97	8104	4556	116
BLUE RIDGE—Fannin County										
☐ FANNIN REGIONAL HOSPITAL, 2855 Old Highway 5, Zip 30513; tel. 706/632–3711; Barry L. Mousa, Chief Executive Officer A1 9 10 F7 9 13 16 17 18 19 22 23 25 32 34 37 38 39 41 44 45 48 49 50 51 54 56 70 72 73 76 78 79 P6 S Community Health Systems, Inc., Brentwood, TN	33	10	32	1819	19	41470	134	11506	5523	161
BREMEN—Haralson County										
★ HIGGINS GENERAL HOSPITAL, 200 Allen Memorial Drive, Zip 30110–2012, Mailing Address: P.O. Box 655, Zip 30110–0655; tel. 770/537–5851; Robbie Smith, Administrator A1 9 10 F7 9 11 13 17 18 22 25 32 33 41 43 48 51 54 70 76 P6 7 S Quorum Health Group, Brentwood, TN	23	10	36	896	12	17544	0	8499	3563	123
BRUNSWICK—Glynn County										
★ SOUTHEAST GEORGIA REGIONAL MEDICAL CENTER, 3100 Kemble Avenue, Zip 31520–4252, Mailing Address: P.O. Box 1518, Zip 31521–1518; tel. 912/466–7000; E. Berton Whitaker, President and Chief Executive Officer (Total facility includes 16 beds in nursing home–type unit) A1 2 10 F7 8 9 11 12 13 16 17 18 22 24 25 27 29 32 33 34 35 37 38 39 41 44 45 46 48 49 51 54 57 61 65 69 70 72 76 77 78 P5 8 S Quorum Health Group, Brentwood, TN	15	10	316	11996	162	113403	2685	104109	42613	1221

Hospitals, U.S. / GEORGIA

Hospital, Address, Telephone, Administrator, Approval, Facility, and Physician Codes, Health Care System, Network	Classification Codes		Utilization Data					Expense (thousands) of dollars		
★ American Hospital Association (AHA) membership ☐ Joint Commission on Accreditation of Healthcare Organizations (JCAHO) accreditation + American Osteopathic Healthcare Association (AOHA) membership ○ American Osteopathic Association (AOA) accreditation △ Commission on Accreditation of Rehabilitation Facilities (CARF) accreditation Control codes 61, 63, 64, 71, 72 and 73 indicate hospitals listed by AOHA, but not registered by AHA. For definition of numerical codes, see page A4	Control	Service	Staffed Beds	Admissions	Census	Outpatient Visits	Births	Total	Payroll	Personnel
CAIRO—Grady County ☐ GRADY GENERAL HOSPITAL, 1155 Fifth Street S.E., Zip 31728–3142, Mailing Address: P.O. Box 360, Zip 31728–0360; tel. 912/377–1150; Glen C. Davis, Administrator **A**1 9 10 **F**7 8 9 13 16 17 18 19 22 23 25 31 32 33 34 36 37 38 39 41 43 44 45 48 50 51 54 70 76 78 **P**8 **S** Archbold Medical Center, Thomasville, GA Web address: www.archbold.org	23	10	49	1527	22	25066	257	11049	5137	171
CALHOUN—Gordon County ★ GORDON HOSPITAL, 1035 Red Bud Road, Zip 30701–2082, Mailing Address: P.O. Box 12938, Zip 30703–7013; tel. 706/629–2895; Carlene Jamerson, President and Chief Executive Officer **A**1 9 10 **F**7 8 9 11 13 17 19 22 24 25 30 32 34 38 39 41 44 46 48 49 50 54 55 62 68 70 76 77 78 79 **P**1 **S** Adventist Health System Sunbelt Health Care Corporation, Winter Park, FL	21	10	54	3112	30	126009	602	29204	13015	383
CAMILLA—Mitchell County ☐ MITCHELL COUNTY HOSPITAL, 90 Stephens Street, Zip 31730–1899, Mailing Address: P.O. Box 639, Zip 31730–0639; tel. 912/336–5284; Ronald M. Gilliard, FACHE, Administrator (Total facility includes 156 beds in nursing home–type unit) **A**1 9 10 **F**8 13 16 17 18 19 22 25 32 34 39 43 44 48 51 54 69 70 76 78 **P**6 **S** Archbold Medical Center, Thomasville, GA	23	10	179	760	167	13396	159	10934	6001	122
CANTON—Cherokee County ★ NORTHSIDE HOSPITAL – CHEROKEE, 201 Hospital Road, Zip 30114–2408, Mailing Address: P.O. Box 906, Zip 30114–0906; tel. 770/720–5100; Douglas M. Parker, Chief Executive Officer **A**1 9 10 **F**7 8 9 13 17 18 22 24 25 27 32 33 35 41 43 44 46 48 49 50 54 70 72 76 78 79	23	10	84	2884	29	41682	551	26632	9318	209
CARROLLTON—Carroll County ★ TANNER MEDICAL CENTER, 705 Dixie Street, Zip 30117–3818; tel. 770/836–9666; Loy M. Howard, Chief Executive Officer (Total facility includes 20 beds in nursing home–type unit) **A**1 9 10 **F**3 7 8 9 11 13 17 18 19 22 23 24 25 26 27 28 30 31 32 33 34 36 37 39 41 44 45 46 48 49 51 54 57 58 61 63 64 65 69 70 72 76 78 79 **P**7 8 **S** Quorum Health Group, Brentwood, TN Web address: www.tanner.org/	23	10	176	8329	115	159395	1147	64032	28325	958
CARTERSVILLE—Bartow County ★ EMORY CARTERSVILLE MEDICAL CENTER, (Formerly Columbia Cartersville Medical Center), 960 Joe Frank Harris Parkway, Zip 30120, Mailing Address: P.O. Box 200008, Zip 30120–9001; tel. 770/382–1530; Keith Sandlin, Chief Executive Officer (Nonreporting) **A**1 9 10 **S** HCA – The Healthcare Company, Nashville, TN	33	10	80	—	—	—	—	—	—	—
CEDARTOWN—Polk County ★ POLK MEDICAL CENTER, 424 North Main Street, Zip 30125–2698; tel. 770/748–2500; Mark Nichols, Chief Executive Officer **A**1 9 10 **F**16 17 18 22 24 25 32 34 39 48 51 68 70 76 78 **S** HCA – The Healthcare Company, Nashville, TN	33	10	40	771	8	25979	—	—	—	88
CHATSWORTH—Murray County ☐ MURRAY MEDICAL CENTER, 707 Old Ellijay Road, Zip 30705–2060, Mailing Address: P.O. Box 1406, Zip 30705–1406; tel. 706/695–4564; Mickey Rabuka, Administrator **A**1 9 10 **F**7 9 17 22 23 25 26 34 36 37 40 41 43 45 48 49 51 54 58 68 70 72	23	10	33	983	10	28394	1	11314	5001	164
CLAXTON—Evans County ☐ EVANS MEMORIAL HOSPITAL, 200 North River Street, Zip 30417–1659, Mailing Address: P.O. Box 518, Zip 30417–0518; tel. 912/739–5000; Eston Price, Jr, Administrator (Total facility includes 160 beds in nursing home–type unit) **A**1 9 10 **F**8 9 17 18 22 24 25 31 32 34 44 48 54 69 76 78	16	10	195	1880	172	30681	179	9398	4379	229
CLAYTON—Rabun County ★ RABUN COUNTY MEMORIAL HOSPITAL, 196 Ridgecrest Circle, Zip 30525, Mailing Address: P.O. Box 705, Zip 30525–0705; tel. 706/782–3100; Gerald E. Knepp, Chief Executive Officer (Nonreporting) **A**9 10 Web address: www.rabun.net	16	10	26	—	—	—	—	—	—	—
COCHRAN—Bleckley County BLECKLEY MEMORIAL HOSPITAL, 408 Peacock Street, Zip 31014–1559, Mailing Address: P.O. Box 536, Zip 31014–0536; tel. 912/934–6211; Cary Martin, Administrator **A**9 10 18 **F**14 16 17 19 22 25 36 38 48 54 66 70 71 72 76 78 79 **P**5 6 **S** Memorial Health Services, Adel, GA	16	10	25	520	4	4526	0	—	—	59
COLQUITT—Miller County MILLER COUNTY HOSPITAL, 209 North Cuthbert Street, Zip 31737–1015, Mailing Address: P.O. Box 7, Zip 31737–0007; tel. 912/758–3385; Harley Smith, Chief Executive Officer (Total facility includes 97 beds in nursing home–type unit) (Nonreporting) **A**10 18	16	10	135	—	—	—	—	—	—	—
COLUMBUS—Muscogee County BRADLEY CENTER OF ST. FRANCIS See St. Francis Hospital ★ DOCTORS HOSPITAL, 616 19th Street, Zip 31901–1528, Mailing Address: P.O. Box 2188, Zip 31902–2188; tel. 706/571–4262; Hugh D. Wilson, Chief Executive Officer **A**1 2 9 10 **F**3 8 9 11 13 18 22 24 25 30 31 32 33 34 38 41 43 44 46 48 50 51 57 62 63 64 66 70 72 73 75 76 78 79 **P**8 **S** HCA – The Healthcare Company, Nashville, TN Web address: www.hcahealthcare.com	33	10	171	5133	65	58164	1091	48226	16105	451
★ HUGHSTON SPORTS MEDICINE HOSPITAL, 100 First Court, Zip 31908–7188, Mailing Address: P.O. Box 7188, Zip 31908–7188; tel. 706/576–2101; Hugh C. Tappan, Chief Executive Officer **A**1 3 5 9 10 **F**2 3 4 8 9 11 12 13 17 18 19 22 24 25 30 32 33 38 39 41 44 47 48 50 51 53 54 57 65 70 71 76 78 79 **P**3 4 5 **S** HCA – The Healthcare Company, Nashville, TN Web address: www.hughstonsports.com	33	47	100	4247	38	6346	0	28297	8164	358

Many Facility Codes have changed. Please refer to the AHA Guide Code Chart.

Hospitals, U.S. / GEORGIA

Hospital, Address, Telephone, Administrator, Approval, Facility, and Physician Codes, Health Care System, Network	Classification Codes		Utilization Data					Expense (thousands) of dollars		
★ American Hospital Association (AHA) membership ☐ Joint Commission on Accreditation of Healthcare Organizations (JCAHO) accreditation + American Osteopathic Healthcare Association (AOHA) membership ○ American Osteopathic Association (AOA) accreditation △ Commission on Accreditation of Rehabilitation Facilities (CARF) accreditation Control codes 61, 63, 64, 71, 72 and 73 indicate hospitals listed by AOHA, but not registered by AHA. For definition of numerical codes, see page A4	Control	Service	Staffed Beds	Admissions	Census	Outpatient Visits	Births	Total	Payroll	Personnel
★ ST. FRANCIS HOSPITAL, (Includes Bradley Center of St. Francis, 2000 16th Avenue, Zip 31906–0308; tel. 706/320–3700), 2122 Manchester Expressway, Zip 31904–6878, Mailing Address: P.O. Box 7000, Zip 31908–7000; tel. 706/596–4000; Michael E. Garrigan, FACHE, President and Chief Executive Officer **A**1 9 10 **F**2 3 4 7 8 9 11 12 13 16 18 19 22 25 28 30 32 33 34 36 38 39 41 44 46 47 48 49 50 54 57 58 59 61 62 63 64 76 78 Web address: www.sfhga.com	23	10	217	7680	115	36226	0	75470	31921	1179
★ THE MEDICAL CENTER, 710 Center Street, Zip 31902, Mailing Address: P.O. Box 951, Zip 31902–0951; tel. 706/571–1000; Lance B. Duke, FACHE, President and Chief Executive Officer (Total facility includes 128 beds in nursing home–type unit) **A**1 2 3 5 9 10 12 **F**2 3 7 8 9 11 13 17 18 19 21 22 24 25 28 30 31 32 33 34 35 36 38 39 41 42 44 45 46 48 49 50 51 52 53 54 56 57 59 60 61 65 68 69 70 72 73 75 76 77 78 79 **P**6 8 **S** Columbus Regional Health System, Columbus, GA Web address: www.columbusregional.com	23	10	537	12908	310	126069	2637	129220	49617	1507
COMMERCE—Jackson County										
★ BJC MEDICAL CENTER, 70 Medical Center Drive, Zip 30529–9989; tel. 706/335–1000; J. David Lawrence, Jr, Chief Executive Officer (Total facility includes 167 beds in nursing home–type unit) **A**1 9 10 **F**7 9 12 17 18 22 24 25 32 34 37 43 44 48 50 51 54 69 70 72 76 78	16	10	233	1345	178	18735	65	8989	5275	211
CONYERS—Rockdale County										
★ ROCKDALE HOSPITAL AND HEALTH SYSTEM, 1412 Milstead Avenue N.E., Zip 30207–9990; tel. 770/918–3000; Nelson Toebbe, Chief Executive Officer **A**1 2 9 10 **F**7 8 9 12 13 17 18 19 22 25 27 32 33 34 36 38 39 41 43 44 46 48 50 51 54 65 70 71 72 76 77 78 79 **P**1 Web address: www.rockdale.org	23	10	107	6039	57	102282	1747	51103	20508	626
CORDELE—Crisp County										
★ CRISP REGIONAL HOSPITAL, 902 North Seventh Street, Zip 31015–5007; tel. 912/276–3100; D. Wayne Martin, President and Chief Executive Officer (Nonreporting) **A**1 9 10 Web address: www.crispregional.org	16	10	65	—	—	—	—	—	—	—
COVINGTON—Newton County										
★ NEWTON GENERAL HOSPITAL, 5126 Hospital Drive, Zip 30014; tel. 770/786–7053; James F. Weadick, Administrator and Chief Executive Officer **A**1 9 10 **F**7 8 9 17 19 22 25 27 32 33 34 36 37 38 39 41 44 45 48 49 50 61 68 70 72 74 76 78 **P**8	23	10	90	3869	40	108130	387	35987	16043	425
CUMMING—Forsyth County										
★ BAPTIST MEDICAL CENTER, (Formerly Baptist North Hospital), 1200 Baptist Medical Center Drive, Zip 30041; tel. 770/887–2355; Jim Litchford, Administrator **A**1 9 10 **F**7 9 16 17 18 19 22 24 25 28 32 34 36 37 38 39 41 46 48 49 51 54 58 59 60 61 63 70 72 76 78 **S** Georgia Baptist Health Care System, Atlanta, GA	21	10	41	2310	26	32671	0	23780	8783	286
CUTHBERT—Randolph County										
★ SOUTHWEST GEORGIA REGIONAL MEDICAL CENTER, 109 Randolph Street, Zip 31740–1338; tel. 912/732–2181; Keith J. Petersen, Chief Executive Officer (Total facility includes 80 beds in nursing home–type unit) **A**9 10 18 **F**7 16 17 18 22 25 37 54 69 76 **P**5	16	10	105	465	85	31196	5	7115	3540	146
DAHLONEGA—Lumpkin County										
☐ CHESTATEE REGIONAL HOSPITAL, 227 Mountain Drive, Zip 30533; tel. 706/864–6136; Charles T. Adams, Chief Executive Officer **A**1 9 10 **F**7 8 9 12 13 17 19 22 25 32 34 37 38 39 41 45 46 48 49 54 70 76 78 79 **P**1 **S** NetCare Health Systems, Inc., Nashville, TN	33	10	49	3081	11	22297	116	12225	5100	162
DALLAS—Paulding County										
★ WELLSTAR PAULDING HOSPITAL, 600 West Memorial Drive, Zip 30132–1335; tel. 770/445–4411; Thomas E. Hill, Chief Executive Officer (Total facility includes 169 beds in nursing home–type unit) (Nonreporting) **A**1 9 10 **S** WellStar Health System, Marietta, GA	23	10	208	—	—	—	—	—	—	—
DALTON—Whitfield County										
★ HAMILTON MEDICAL CENTER, 1200 Memorial Drive, Zip 30720–2529, Mailing Address: P.O. Box 1168, Zip 30722–1168; tel. 706/272–6000 **A**1 2 9 10 **F**1 2 3 6 8 9 11 13 14 17 18 19 21 22 24 25 27 28 29 31 32 34 35 36 37 38 39 41 43 44 45 46 48 49 50 51 54 57 58 59 60 61 62 63 64 65 67 70 71 72 75 76 78 **P**8	23	10	282	10201	119	204564	2329	103688	39954	1156
DECATUR—De Kalb County										
☐ DECATUR HOSPITAL, (LONG TERM ACUTE CARE), 450 North Candler Street, Zip 30030–2671; tel. 404/501–6700; Richard T. Schmidt, Executive Director **A**1 9 10 **F**5 7 8 9 11 12 14 16 17 18 22 24 25 28 29 30 32 33 34 35 37 38 39 41 42 43 44 45 46 48 49 50 51 53 54 56 57 65 69 70 71 76 77 78 79 **P**1	23	49	84	232	23	6585	0	11338	4410	—
★ △ DEKALB MEDICAL CENTER, 2701 North Decatur Road, Zip 30033–5995; tel. 404/501–1000; John R. Gerlach, Chief Executive Officer and Administrator (Total facility includes 47 beds in nursing home–type unit) **A**1 2 7 9 10 **F**2 3 5 7 8 9 11 12 13 17 18 19 20 22 24 25 26 27 28 29 30 31 32 33 34 35 36 37 38 39 41 42 43 44 45 46 48 49 50 51 53 54 56 57 59 60 61 62 63 64 65 66 68 69 70 71 72 73 75 76 77 78 79 **P**1 5 Web address: www.drhs.org	23	10	441	19784	326	243068	5251	210160	98594	2555

© 2000 AHA Guide   *Many Facility Codes have changed. Please refer to the AHA Guide Code Chart.*

Hospitals, U.S. / GEORGIA

- ★ American Hospital Association (AHA) membership
- ☐ Joint Commission on Accreditation of Healthcare Organizations (JCAHO) accreditation
- + American Osteopathic Healthcare Association (AOHA) membership
- ○ American Osteopathic Association (AOA) accreditation
- △ Commission on Accreditation of Rehabilitation Facilities (CARF) accreditation

Control codes 61, 63, 64, 71, 72 and 73 indicate hospitals listed by AOHA, but not registered by AHA. For definition of numerical codes, see page A4

Hospital, Address, Telephone, Administrator, Approval, Facility, and Physician Codes, Health Care System, Network	Classification Codes		Utilization Data					Expense (thousands) of dollars		Personnel
	Control	Service	Staffed Beds	Admissions	Census	Outpatient Visits	Births	Total	Payroll	
☐ GEORGIA REGIONAL HOSPITAL AT ATLANTA, 3073 Panthersville Road, Zip 30034–3828; tel. 404/243–2100; Ronald C. Hogan, Superintendent (Total facility includes 110 beds in nursing home–type unit) **A**1 3 5 9 10 **F**1 3 4 5 6 7 8 9 11 13 14 15 16 17 18 19 20 21 22 23 24 25 26 27 28 29 30 31 32 33 34 35 36 37 38 39 40 43 45 46 47 48 49 50 51 54 55 56 57 58 59 60 61 62 63 64 65 66 68 69 70 71 72 73 74 75 76 77 78 79 **P**6	12	22	366	5396	307	0	0	41423	24084	875
★ VETERANS AFFAIRS MEDICAL CENTER, 1670 Clairmont Road, Zip 30033–4004; tel. 404/321–6111; Robert A. Perreault, Director (Total facility includes 100 beds in nursing home–type unit) **A**1 3 5 8 9 **F**3 4 11 12 13 22 23 24 25 26 30 31 32 33 34 35 36 37 39 40 41 43 45 46 47 48 49 50 51 54 56 57 59 60 61 62 63 64 65 68 69 70 72 76 77 78 79 **S** Department of Veterans Affairs, Washington, DC **Web address:** www.va.gov/stations97/guide/home.asp?DIVISION=ALL	45	10	271	6954	242	353611	—	161638	92096	1859
DEMOREST—Habersham County										
★ HABERSHAM COUNTY MEDICAL CENTER, Highway 441, Zip 30535, Mailing Address: P.O. Box 37, Zip 30535–0037; tel. 706/754–2161; C. Richard Dwozan, President (Total facility includes 106 beds in nursing home–type unit) **A**1 9 10 **F**6 7 8 9 13 17 18 19 22 23 24 25 28 31 32 33 34 36 38 39 41 43 44 45 48 49 50 51 54 69 70 71 72 76 77 78 **P**7 **S** Quorum Health Group, Brentwood, TN	16	10	159	2654	132	36375	399	23400	9075	434
DONALSONVILLE—Seminole County										
☐ DONALSONVILLE HOSPITAL, Hospital Circle, Zip 31745, Mailing Address: P.O. Box 677, Zip 31745–0677; tel. 912/524–5217; Charles H. Orrick, Administrator (Total facility includes 75 beds in nursing home–type unit) **A**1 9 10 **F**16 17 18 22 24 25 39 48 54 69 76	23	10	140	2357	83	18123	0	12519	4997	235
DOUGLAS—Coffee County										
★ COFFEE REGIONAL MEDICAL CENTER, 1101 Ocilla Road, Zip 31533–3617, Mailing Address: P.O. Box 1287, Zip 31534–1287; tel. 912/384–1900; George L. Heck, II, President and Chief Executive Officer **A**1 9 10 **F**8 9 11 13 15 16 17 18 20 22 24 25 27 31 32 33 34 35 36 37 39 41 44 48 49 54 56 68 70 71 72 76 78 **P**5 **Web address:** www.coffeeregional.org	23	10	88	4661	41	79820	789	36416	16490	532
DOUGLASVILLE—Douglas County										
INNER HARBOUR HOSPITALS, 4685 Dorsett Shoals Road, Zip 30135–4999; tel. 770/942–2391; Maurice Jones, Administrator **A**9 **F**43 51 57 58 59 60 64 70 72 78 **P**6 **Web address:** www.innerharbour.org	23	52	165	319	136	0	0	16862	10337	404
★ WELLSTAR DOUGLAS HOSPITAL, 8954 Hospital Drive, Zip 30134–2282; tel. 770/949–1500; Thomas E. Hill, Chief Executive Officer (Nonreporting) **A**1 9 10 **S** WellStar Health System, Marietta, GA **Web address:** www.wellstar.org	23	10	98	—	—	—	—	—	—	—
DUBLIN—Laurens County										
★ FAIRVIEW PARK HOSPITAL, 200 Industrial Boulevard, Zip 31021–2997, Mailing Address: P.O. Box 1408, Zip 31040–1408; tel. 912/275–2000; James B. Wood, Chief Executive Officer **A**1 2 9 10 **F**8 9 12 13 16 17 18 19 22 24 25 27 28 29 30 32 34 36 37 38 39 41 43 44 45 46 48 49 50 53 54 65 68 70 71 76 78 79 **S** HCA – The Healthcare Company, Nashville, TN **Web address:** www.hcahealthcare.com	33	10	190	7590	88	61662	1045	37532	18060	617
★ VETERANS AFFAIRS MEDICAL CENTER, 1826 Veterans Boulevard, Zip 31021–3620; tel. 912/272–1210; James F. Trusley, II, Director (Total facility includes 112 beds in nursing home–type unit) (Nonreporting) **A**1 9 **S** Department of Veterans Affairs, Washington, DC **Web address:** www.va.gov/stations97/guide/home.asp?DIVISION=ALL	45	10	253	—	—	—	—	—	—	—
DULUTH—Gwinnett County										
JOAN GLANCY MEMORIAL HOSPITAL See Promina Gwinnett Hospital System, Lawrenceville										
EAST POINT—Fulton County										
★ SOUTH FULTON MEDICAL CENTER, 1170 Cleveland Avenue, Zip 30344; tel. 404/305–3500; H. Neil Copelan, President and Chief Executive Officer (Total facility includes 36 beds in nursing home–type unit) (Nonreporting) **A**1 2 9 10	23	10	369	—	—	—	—	—	—	—
EASTMAN—Dodge County										
☐ DODGE COUNTY HOSPITAL, 715 Griffin Street S.W., Zip 31023–2223, Mailing Address: P.O. Box 4309, Zip 31023–4309; tel. 912/374–4000; Meredith H. Smith, Administrator **A**1 9 10 **F**9 17 19 22 24 25 28 34 39 40 41 44 48 49 50 51 54 57 62 72 76 78	16	10	87	2917	36	25274	139	16724	8289	289
EATONTON—Putnam County										
☐ PUTNAM GENERAL HOSPITAL, Lake Oconee Parkway, Zip 31024–4330, Mailing Address: Box 4330, Zip 31024–4330; tel. 706/485–2711; Darrell M. Oglesby, Administrator **A**1 9 10 **F**7 17 22 25 32 38 41 48 49 76 **P**5	16	10	48	804	6	18139	0	5895	3138	118
ELBERTON—Elbert County										
★ ELBERT MEMORIAL HOSPITAL, 4 Medical Drive, Zip 30635–1897; tel. 706/283–3151; Mark LeNeave, Chief Executive Officer **A**1 9 10 **F**7 8 9 13 14 17 18 19 22 24 25 28 32 34 37 38 39 41 43 48 50 54 70 71 76 78 79 **P**5 **S** Quorum Health Group, Brentwood, TN	16	10	42	2163	26	10396	162	10563	4913	161
ELLIJAY—Gilmer County										
☐ NORTH GEORGIA MEDICAL CENTER, 1362 South Main Street, Zip 30540–0346, Mailing Address: P.O. Box 2239, Zip 30540–0346; tel. 706/276–4741; Jodi Beauregard, Chief Executive Officer (Total facility includes 100 beds in nursing home–type unit) (Nonreporting) **A**1 9 10 **S** NetCare Health Systems, Inc., Nashville, TN	33	10	150	—	—	—	—	—	—	—

Hospitals, U.S. / GEORGIA

Hospital, Address, Telephone, Administrator, Approval, Facility, and Physician Codes, Health Care System, Network	Classification Codes		Utilization Data					Expense (thousands) of dollars		
	Control	Service	Staffed Beds	Admissions	Census	Outpatient Visits	Births	Total	Payroll	Personnel

★ American Hospital Association (AHA) membership
☐ Joint Commission on Accreditation of Healthcare Organizations (JCAHO) accreditation
+ American Osteopathic Healthcare Association (AOHA) membership
○ American Osteopathic Association (AOA) accreditation
△ Commission on Accreditation of Rehabilitation Facilities (CARF) accreditation
Control codes 61, 63, 64, 71, 72 and 73 indicate hospitals listed by AOHA, but not registered by AHA. For definition of numerical codes, see page A4

Hospital	Control	Service	Staffed Beds	Admissions	Census	Outpatient Visits	Births	Total	Payroll	Personnel
FITZGERALD—Ben Hill County ☐ DORMINY MEDICAL CENTER, Perry House Road, Zip 31750, Mailing Address: Drawer 1447, Zip 31750–1447; tel. 912/424–7100; Steve Barber, Administrator **A**1 9 10 **F**16 22 24 34 37 39 41 44 47 54 55 68 70 76 78 Web address: www.dorminy-hosp.org	16	10	60	2159	26	25633	208	14696	7674	311
FOLKSTON—Charlton County ☐ CHARLTON MEMORIAL HOSPITAL, 1203 North Third Street, Zip 31537–1303, Mailing Address: P.O. Box 188, Zip 31537–0188; tel. 912/496–2531; John Lindsey, Administrator and Chief Executive Officer (Nonreporting) **A**1 9 10	16	10	35	—	—	—	—	—	—	—
FORSYTH—Monroe County ☐ MONROE COUNTY HOSPITAL, 88 Martin Luther King Jr. Drive, Zip 31029, Mailing Address: P.O. Box 1068, Zip 31029–1068; tel. 912/994–2521; Gale V. Tanner, Administrator **A**1 9 10 **F**7 9 17 18 22 25 35 38 39 48 53 70 76 78 **P**1	16	10	37	944	10	13763	0	6774	2915	109
FORT BENNING—Muscogee County ★ MARTIN ARMY COMMUNITY HOSPITAL, Mailing Address: P.O. Box 56100, Building 9200, Zip 31905–6100; tel. 706/544–2516; Lieutenant Colonel Joe W. Butler, Deputy Commander for Administration (Nonreporting) **A**1 2 3 **S** Department of the Army, Office of the Surgeon General, Falls Church, VA Web address: www.martin.amedd.army.mil	42	10	126	—	—	—	—	—	—	—
FORT GORDON—Richmond County ★ DWIGHT DAVID EISENHOWER ARMY MEDICAL CENTER, Hospital Drive, Building 300, Zip 30905–5650; tel. 706/787–8191; Lieutenant Colonel Julie Martin, Chief Operating Officer (Nonreporting) **A**1 2 3 5 **S** Department of the Army, Office of the Surgeon General, Falls Church, VA Web address: www.ddeamc.amedd.army.mil	42	10	313	—	—	—	—	—	—	—
FORT OGLETHORPE—Catoosa County ★ HUTCHESON MEDICAL CENTER, 100 Gross Crescent Circle, Zip 30742–3669; tel. 706/858–2000; Robert T. Jones, M.D., President and Chief Executive Officer (Total facility includes 109 beds in nursing home–type unit) **A**1 9 10 **F**1 7 8 9 11 12 13 16 17 18 22 24 25 29 32 33 34 36 37 39 41 42 44 45 46 48 49 50 51 54 58 59 60 61 62 63 64 69 70 71 72 75 76 77 78 79 Web address: www.hutcheson.org	16	10	288	7305	196	71464	1053	72495	32364	1203
FORT VALLEY—Peach County ☐ PEACH REGIONAL MEDICAL CENTER, 601 North Camellia Boulevard, Zip 31030–4599; tel. 912/825–8691; Nancy Peed, Administrator (Nonreporting) **A**1 9 10	16	10	41	—	—	—	—	—	—	—
GAINESVILLE—Hall County ★ LANIER PARK HOSPITAL, 675 White Sulphur Road, Zip 30505, Mailing Address: P.O. Box 1354, Zip 30503–1354; tel. 770/503–3000; Gerald N. Fulks, Chief Executive Officer (Total facility includes 10 beds in nursing home–type unit) **A**1 9 10 **F**4 9 11 13 16 17 18 19 22 24 25 27 32 33 34 36 38 39 41 43 45 46 48 50 54 68 69 70 72 76 78 79 **P**8 **S** HCA – The Healthcare Company, Nashville, TN Web address: www.lanierpark.com	33	10	119	3432	17	37900	0	29729	11992	304
★ △ NORTHEAST GEORGIA MEDICAL CENTER, 743 Spring Street N.E., Zip 30501–3899; tel. 770/535–3553; Henry Rigdon, Executive Vice President (Total facility includes 15 beds in nursing home–type unit) (Nonreporting) **A**1 2 7 9 10 Web address: www.nghs.com	23	10	338	—	—	—	—	—	—	—
GLENWOOD—Wheeler County WHEELER COUNTY HOSPITAL, 111 Third Street, Zip 30428, Mailing Address: P.O. Box 398, Zip 30428–0398; tel. 912/523–5113; Brenda Josey, Administrator **A**9 10 **F**13 16 17 18 22 25 32 39 48 51 70 76 **P**6 **S** Accord Health Care Corporation, Clearwater, FL	33	10	40	835	12	8057	0	4668	2431	81
GRACEWOOD—Richmond County GRACEWOOD STATE SCHOOL AND HOSPITAL, 100 Myrtle Boulevard, Zip 30812–1299; tel. 706/790–2030; Bruce D. Callander, Ed.D., Superintendent (Total facility includes 46 beds in nursing home–type unit) **A**9 10 **F**21 23 31 33 34 43 45 48 49 50 69 70 78 **P**6	12	12	582	94	588	0	0	52845	33604	1500
GREENSBORO—Greene County ★ MINNIE G. BOSWELL MEMORIAL HOSPITAL, 1201 Siloam Highway, Zip 30642–2811; tel. 706/453–7331; John M. Herron, Chief Executive Officer (Total facility includes 29 beds in nursing home–type unit) **A**1 9 10 **F**8 9 16 17 18 22 25 32 38 39 44 48 54 69 70 76 78 **S** Georgia Baptist Health Care System, Atlanta, GA	16	10	55	769	38	10927	101	7869	3352	112
GRIFFIN—Spalding County ★ SPALDING REGIONAL HOSPITAL, 601 South Eighth Street, Zip 30224–4294, Mailing Address: P.O. Drawer V, Zip 30224–1168; tel. 770/228–2721; Lex A. Guinn, Chief Executive Officer (Nonreporting) **A**1 2 9 10 **S** TENET Healthcare Corporation, Santa Barbara, CA	33	10	160	—	—	—	—	—	—	—
HAHIRA—Lowndes County SMITH HOSPITAL, 117 East Main Street, Zip 31632–1156, Mailing Address: P.O. Box 337, Zip 31632–0337; tel. 912/794–1912; Robert Bauer, Administrator **A**9 10 **F**9 13 16 17 18 19 22 26 29 30 32 34 38 39 43 44 48 54 59 62 70 72 76 77 78 **S** Memorial Health Services, Adel, GA	33	10	71	842	14	—	—	—	—	—
HARTWELL—Hart County ★ HART COUNTY HOSPITAL, Gibson and Cade Streets, Zip 30643–0280, Mailing Address: P.O. Box 280, Zip 30643–0280; tel. 706/856–6100; Jerry R. Wise, Administrator (Nonreporting) **A**1 9 10 Web address: www.tycobbhealthcare.org	13	10	65	—	—	—	—	—	—	—

Hospitals, U.S. / GEORGIA

Hospital, Address, Telephone, Administrator, Approval, Facility, and Physician Codes, Health Care System, Network	Classification Codes		Utilization Data					Expense (thousands) of dollars		Personnel
	Control	Service	Staffed Beds	Admissions	Census	Outpatient Visits	Births	Total	Payroll	

★ American Hospital Association (AHA) membership
☐ Joint Commission on Accreditation of Healthcare Organizations (JCAHO) accreditation
+ American Osteopathic Healthcare Association (AOHA) membership
○ American Osteopathic Association (AOA) accreditation
△ Commission on Accreditation of Rehabilitation Facilities (CARF) accreditation
Control codes 61, 63, 64, 71, 72 and 73 indicate hospitals listed by AOHA, but not registered by AHA. For definition of numerical codes, see page A4

Hospital	Control	Service	Staffed Beds	Admissions	Census	Outpatient Visits	Births	Total	Payroll	Personnel
HAWKINSVILLE—Pulaski County ☐ TAYLOR REGIONAL HOSPITAL, Macon Highway, Zip 31036, Mailing Address: P.O. Box 1297, Zip 31036–1297; tel. 912/783–0200; Dan S. Maddock, President **A**1 9 10 **F**7 9 11 13 17 18 22 24 25 32 36 39 43 46 48 49 54 76	23	10	55	2211	23	41412	333	—	—	320
HAZLEHURST—Jeff Davis County ☐ JEFF DAVIS HOSPITAL, 1215 South Tallahassee Street, Zip 31539–2921, Mailing Address: P.O. Box 1200, Zip 31539–1200; tel. 912/375–7781; Oreta Williams, Administrator **A**1 9 10 **F**7 8 9 17 22 25 32 39 41 48 76	16	10	50	893	8	18890	99	6547	5633	115
HIAWASSEE—Towns County ☐ CHATUGE REGIONAL HOSPITAL AND NURSING HOME, 110 Main Street, Zip 30546, Mailing Address: P.O. Box 509, Zip 30546–0509; tel. 706/896–2222; Lewis Kelley, Administrator (Total facility includes 76 beds in nursing home–type unit) (Nonreporting) **A**1 9 10	33	10	116	—	—	—	—	—	—	—
HINESVILLE—Liberty County ☐ LIBERTY REGIONAL MEDICAL CENTER, 462 East G. Parkway, Zip 31313, Mailing Address: P.O. Box 919, Zip 31313; tel. 912/369–9438; H. Scott Kroell, Jr, Chief Executive Officer **A**1 9 10 **F**8 9 16 17 18 21 22 25 34 39 44 45 48 50 53 54 76 78	16	10	28	1341	11	29475	294	13883	4813	219
✠ WINN ARMY COMMUNITY HOSPITAL, 1061 Harmon Avenue, Zip 31314–5611; tel. 912/370–6965; Colonel George V. Masi, Commander **A**1 **F**3 4 8 9 10 11 12 13 14 16 17 18 21 22 23 24 25 29 31 32 33 34 35 38 39 41 42 43 44 45 46 47 48 49 50 51 52 53 54 55 56 57 58 59 60 61 63 64 65 66 69 70 72 76 78 79 **P**1 **S** Department of the Army, Office of the Surgeon General, Falls Church, VA	42	10	93	4862	33	415075	1412	—	—	907
HOMERVILLE—Clinch County ★ CLINCH MEMORIAL HOSPITAL, 524 North Carswell Street, Zip 31634–1507, Mailing Address: P.O. Box 516, Zip 31634–0516; tel. 912/487–5211; Bruce Shepard, Administrator **A**9 10 **F**9 17 18 22 23 25 38 39 51 54 70 76 78	13	10	36	587	6	21272	0	4979	2152	74
JACKSON—Butts County ★ SYLVAN GROVE HOSPITAL, 1050 McDonough Road, Zip 30233–1599; tel. 770/775–7861; Jean Dodson, Administrator (Nonreporting) **A**9 10 **S** TENET Healthcare Corporation, Santa Barbara, CA Web address: www.tenethealth.com	33	10	28	—	—	—	—	—	—	—
JESUP—Wayne County ✠ WAYNE MEMORIAL HOSPITAL, 865 South First Street, Zip 31598, Mailing Address: P.O. Box 408, Zip 31598–0408; tel. 912/427–6811; Charles R. Morgan, Administrator **A**1 9 10 **F**7 8 9 13 16 17 22 25 32 33 34 38 39 41 43 44 45 48 50 51 54 70 76 78 **P**5 **S** Quorum Health Group, Brentwood, TN Web address: www.wmhweb.com	16	10	110	3639	47	35036	392	23275	10367	355
KENNESAW—Cobb County DEVEREUX GEORGIA TREATMENT NETWORK, 1291 Stanley Road N.W., Zip 30152–4359; tel. 770/422–2135; Elizabeth M. Chadwick, JD, Executive Director **F**16 17 18 25 57 58 60 **P**6 **S** Devereux Foundation, Villanova, PA Web address: www.devereux.org	23	52	125	106	98	0	0	12500	6417	199
LA GRANGE—Troup County ✠ WEST GEORGIA HEALTH SYSTEM, 1514 Vernon Road, Zip 30240–4199; tel. 706/882–1411; Charles L. Foster, Jr, FACHE, President and Chief Executive Officer (Total facility includes 278 beds in nursing home–type unit) **A**1 2 9 10 **F**1 3 6 7 8 9 11 13 14 16 17 18 19 20 21 22 24 25 27 30 31 32 33 34 36 37 38 39 41 42 43 44 45 46 48 49 50 51 54 55 56 57 58 59 60 62 63 64 65 68 69 70 72 73 75 76 78 79 **P**7 Web address: www.wghs.org	23	10	472	9410	381	293180	1098	79496	36006	1391
LAKELAND—Lanier County ★ LOUIS SMITH MEMORIAL HOSPITAL, 852 West Thigpen Avenue, Zip 31635–1099; tel. 912/482–3110; Randy Sauls, Administrator (Total facility includes 62 beds in nursing home–type unit) **A**9 10 **F**8 16 17 18 22 25 32 34 35 39 44 45 48 49 51 54 61 69 76 77 78 Web address: www.sgmc.org	23	10	102	628	66	7378	24	6394	2780	137
LAWRENCEVILLE—Gwinnett County ✠ PROMINA GWINNETT HOSPITAL SYSTEM, (Includes Gwinnett Medical Center, 1000 Medical Center Boulevard, Zip 30245; Joan Glancy Memorial Hospital, McClure Bridge Road, Duluth, Zip 30136; tel. 770/497–4800), Mailing Address: P.O. Box 348, Zip 30246–0348; tel. 770/995–4321; Franklin M. Rinker, President and Chief Executive Officer (Nonreporting) **A**1 2 9 10 Web address: www.promina.org	16	10	390	—	—	—	—	—	—	—
LITHIA SPRINGS—Douglas County ✠ EMORY PARKWAY MEDICAL CENTER, (Formerly Parkway Medical Center), 1000 Thornton Road, Zip 30122, Mailing Address: P.O. Box 570, Zip 30122–0570; tel. 770/732–7777; John D. Anderson, Chief Executive Officer **A**1 2 9 10 **F**2 3 7 8 9 11 13 16 17 18 19 21 22 24 25 30 32 35 38 39 41 43 44 45 46 48 51 53 54 57 59 60 61 63 64 65 68 70 72 76 78 79 **S** HCA – The Healthcare Company, Nashville, TN Web address: www.hcahealthcare.com/	33	10	182	3158	48	35181	1208	—	—	355
LOUISVILLE—Jefferson County ☐ JEFFERSON HOSPITAL, 1067 Peachtree Street, Zip 30434–1599; tel. 912/625–7000; Rita Culvern, Administrator (Nonreporting) **A**1 9 10	16	10	37	—	—	—	—	—	—	—

Hospitals, U.S. / GEORGIA

Hospital, Address, Telephone, Administrator, Approval, Facility, and Physician Codes, Health Care System, Network	Classification Codes		Utilization Data					Expense (thousands) of dollars		
★ American Hospital Association (AHA) membership □ Joint Commission on Accreditation of Healthcare Organizations (JCAHO) accreditation + American Osteopathic Healthcare Association (AOHA) membership ○ American Osteopathic Association (AOA) accreditation △ Commission on Accreditation of Rehabilitation Facilities (CARF) accreditation Control codes 61, 63, 64, 71, 72 and 73 indicate hospitals listed by AOHA, but not registered by AHA. For definition of numerical codes, see page A4	Control	Service	Staffed Beds	Admissions	Census	Outpatient Visits	Births	Total	Payroll	Personnel

MACON—Bibb County

Hospital	Control	Service	Staffed Beds	Admissions	Census	Outpatient Visits	Births	Total	Payroll	Personnel
★ COLISEUM MEDICAL CENTERS, 350 Hospital Drive, Zip 31213; tel. 912/765-7000; Timothy C. Tobin, Chief Executive Officer **A**1 9 10 **F**3 8 9 11 13 18 22 24 25 27 29 31 32 33 34 38 39 41 42 44 45 46 48 53 54 56 57 58 59 60 61 63 64 65 66 70 72 76 77 78 79 **P**7 **S** HCA – The Healthcare Company, Nashville, TN Web address: www.hcahealthcare.com	33	10	180	8786	120	92513	1456	—	—	877
★ COLISEUM PSYCHIATRIC CENTER, (Formerly Coliseum Psychiatric Hospital), 340 Hospital Drive, Zip 31217-8002; tel. 912/741-1355; Edward W. Ruffin, Administrator (Nonreporting) **A**1 9 10 **S** HCA – The Healthcare Company, Nashville, TN Web address: www.hcahealthcare.com	33	22	92	—	—	—	—	—	—	—
□ HEALTHSOUTH CENTRAL GEORGIA REHABILITATION HOSPITAL, 3351 Northside Drive, Zip 31210-2591; tel. 912/471-3536; Elbert T. McQueen, Chief Executive Officer **A**1 10 **F**1 2 3 4 5 6 7 8 9 10 11 12 13 14 15 16 17 18 19 20 21 22 23 24 25 26 27 28 29 30 31 32 33 34 35 36 37 38 39 40 41 42 43 44 45 46 47 48 49 50 51 52 53 54 55 56 57 58 59 60 61 62 63 64 65 66 67 68 69 70 71 72 73 74 75 76 77 78 79 **P**1 **S** HEALTHSOUTH Corporation, Birmingham, AL Web address: www.healthsouth.com	33	46	50	912	43	13636	0	10056	5129	153
★ MACON NORTHSIDE HOSPITAL, 400 Charter Boulevard, Zip 31210-4853, Mailing Address: P.O. Box 4627, Zip 31208-4627; tel. 912/757-8200; Bud Costello, Administrator and Chief Executive Officer **A**1 9 10 **F**2 3 8 9 11 13 16 17 18 19 22 24 25 27 30 32 34 38 39 41 42 44 46 48 51 53 54 57 58 59 60 61 62 63 64 65 68 72 77 78 79 **P**7 **S** HCA – The Healthcare Company, Nashville, TN Web address: www.hcahealthcare.com	33	10	103	2670	29	56646	286	28597	11363	301
★ MEDICAL CENTER OF CENTRAL GEORGIA, 777 Hemlock Street, Zip 31201-2155, Mailing Address: P.O. Box 6000, Zip 31208-6000; tel. 912/633-1000; A. Donald Faulk, FACHE, President **A**1 2 3 5 8 9 10 **F**4 7 8 9 10 11 12 13 16 17 18 19 22 25 28 29 30 32 33 34 35 36 37 38 39 41 42 43 44 45 46 47 49 50 51 54 56 57 60 61 62 63 65 66 70 71 72 75 76 77 78 79 **P**1 7 Web address: www.mccg.org	16	10	495	22323	305	—	2799	290473	15542	3542
★ MIDDLE GEORGIA HOSPITAL, 888 Pine Street, Zip 31201-2186, Mailing Address: P.O. Box 6278, Zip 31208-6278; tel. 912/751-1111; Richard L. McConahy, Chief Executive Officer (Nonreporting) **A**1 9 10 **S** HCA – The Healthcare Company, Nashville, TN Web address: www.hcahealthcare.com	33	10	119	—	—	—	—	—	—	—

MADISON—Morgan County

Hospital	Control	Service	Staffed Beds	Admissions	Census	Outpatient Visits	Births	Total	Payroll	Personnel
□ MORGAN MEMORIAL HOSPITAL, Canterbury Park, Zip 30650, Mailing Address: P.O. Box 860, Zip 30650-0860; tel. 706/342-1667; Patrick Green, Administrator (Total facility includes 21 beds in nursing home-type unit) **A**1 9 10 18 **F**7 9 13 16 17 18 22 23 25 31 32 38 39 43 45 48 51 53 54 69 70 71 75 76 78 Web address: www.mmh.org	13	10	41	481	12	10307	0	5231	2392	107

MARIETTA—Cobb County

Hospital	Control	Service	Staffed Beds	Admissions	Census	Outpatient Visits	Births	Total	Payroll	Personnel
★ △ WELLSTAR KENNESTONE HOSPITAL, 677 Church Street, Zip 30060-1148; tel. 770/793-5000; Thomas E. Hill, Chief Executive Officer (Nonreporting) **A**1 2 7 9 10 **S** WellStar Health System, Marietta, GA	23	10	439	—	—	—	—	—	—	—
★ WELLSTAR WINDY HILL HOSPITAL, 2540 Windy Hill Road, Zip 30067-8632; tel. 770/644-1000; Thomas E. Hill, Chief Executive Officer (Nonreporting) **A**1 10 **S** WellStar Health System, Marietta, GA	23	10	100	—	—	—	—	—	—	—

MCRAE—Telfair County

Hospital	Control	Service	Staffed Beds	Admissions	Census	Outpatient Visits	Births	Total	Payroll	Personnel
TELFAIR COUNTY HOSPITAL, U.S. 341 South, Zip 31055, Mailing Address: P.O. Box 150, Zip 31055-0150; tel. 912/868-5621; Gail Leggett, Administrator (Nonreporting) **A**9 10 18 **S** Memorial Health Services, Adel, GA	33	10	52	—	—	—	—	—	—	—

METTER—Candler County

Hospital	Control	Service	Staffed Beds	Admissions	Census	Outpatient Visits	Births	Total	Payroll	Personnel
□ CANDLER COUNTY HOSPITAL, Cedar Road, Zip 30439, Mailing Address: P.O. Box 597, Zip 30439-0597; tel. 912/685-5741; Michael Alexander, President and Chief Executive Officer **A**1 9 10 **F**9 17 22 25 39 41 48 54 72 76	16	10	42	1762	27	21430	0	10083	4400	178

MILLEDGEVILLE—Baldwin County

Hospital	Control	Service	Staffed Beds	Admissions	Census	Outpatient Visits	Births	Total	Payroll	Personnel
□ CENTRAL STATE HOSPITAL, Broad Street, Zip 31062; tel. 912/445-4128; Joseph T. Hodge, Jr, Facility Administrator (Total facility includes 1751 beds in nursing home-type unit) (Nonreporting) **A**1 3 9 10	12	49	1898	—	—	—	—	—	—	—
★ OCONEE REGIONAL MEDICAL CENTER, 821 North Cobb Street, Zip 31061-2351, Mailing Address: P.O. Box 690, Zip 31061-0690; tel. 912/454-3500; Brian L. Riddle, President and Chief Executive Officer **A**1 9 10 **F**4 7 8 9 13 16 17 18 19 22 24 25 27 28 31 32 34 37 39 40 41 43 44 46 48 50 51 54 65 69 70 71 72 75 76 77 78 79 **S** Quorum Health Group, Brentwood, TN	16	10	147	4382	59	74932	715	45916	18642	476

MILLEN—Jenkins County

Hospital	Control	Service	Staffed Beds	Admissions	Census	Outpatient Visits	Births	Total	Payroll	Personnel
★ JENKINS COUNTY HOSPITAL, 515 East Winthrope Avenue, Zip 30442-1600; tel. 912/982-4221; Pete Mills, Chief Executive Officer (Nonreporting) **A**9 10	16	10	35	—	—	—	—	—	—	—

MONROE—Walton County

Hospital	Control	Service	Staffed Beds	Admissions	Census	Outpatient Visits	Births	Total	Payroll	Personnel
★ WALTON MEDICAL CENTER, 330 Alcovy Street, Zip 30655-2140, Mailing Address: P.O. Box 1346, Zip 30655-1346; tel. 770/267-8461; Ronald L. Campbell, Chief Executive Officer (Total facility includes 58 beds in nursing home-type unit) **A**1 9 10 **F**7 8 9 18 22 23 24 25 28 32 34 38 39 41 44 46 48 54 69 70 72 75 76 78 79 **S** Quorum Health Group, Brentwood, TN	23	10	115	2058	80	60168	229	22551	10220	300

© 2000 AHA Guide *Many Facility Codes have changed. Please refer to the AHA Guide Code Chart.*

Hospitals, U.S. / GEORGIA

Legend:
- ★ American Hospital Association (AHA) membership
- ☐ Joint Commission on Accreditation of Healthcare Organizations (JCAHO) accreditation
- + American Osteopathic Healthcare Association (AOHA) membership
- ○ American Osteopathic Association (AOA) accreditation
- △ Commission on Accreditation of Rehabilitation Facilities (CARF) accreditation

Control codes 61, 63, 64, 71, 72 and 73 indicate hospitals listed by AOHA, but not registered by AHA. For definition of numerical codes, see page A4.

Hospital, Address, Telephone, Administrator, Approval, Facility, and Physician Codes, Health Care System, Network	Classification Codes		Utilization Data					Expense (thousands of dollars)		Personnel
	Control	Service	Staffed Beds	Admissions	Census	Outpatient Visits	Births	Total	Payroll	
MONTEZUMA—Macon County ★ FLINT RIVER COMMUNITY HOSPITAL, 509 Sumter Street, Zip 31063–0770, Mailing Address: P.O. Box 770, Zip 31063–0770; tel. 912/472–3100; Robert V. Deen, Interim Chief Executive Officer **A**1 9 10 **F**9 17 18 22 25 27 36 38 39 43 48 50 51 54 70 76 **S** Paracelsus Healthcare Corporation, Houston, TX	33	10	49	939	10	20438	0	9831	4746	158
MONTICELLO—Jasper County JASPER MEMORIAL HOSPITAL, 898 College Street, Zip 31064–1298; tel. 706/468–6411; Donna Holman, Administrator (Total facility includes 44 beds in nursing home–type unit) (Nonreporting) **A**9 10 18	16	10	72	—	—	—	—	—	—	—
MOULTRIE—Colquitt County ★ COLQUITT REGIONAL MEDICAL CENTER, 3131 South Main Street, Zip 31768–6701, Mailing Address: P.O. Box 40, Zip 31776–0040; tel. 912/985–3420; James R. Lowry, FACHE, Chief Executive Officer **A**1 9 10 **F**1 3 7 8 9 11 12 13 16 17 18 19 22 23 24 25 27 28 29 30 31 32 33 34 35 36 37 38 39 41 43 44 45 46 48 49 50 51 54 56 63 64 66 70 71 72 75 76 77 78 79 **P**1 2 5 Web address: www.colquittregional.com	16	10	84	3931	42	85926	646	40975	16293	653
TURNING POINT HOSPITAL, 319 East By–Pass, Zip 31768, Mailing Address: P.O. Box 1177, Zip 31776–1177; tel. 912/985–4815; Ben Marion, Chief Executive Officer (Nonreporting) **A**9 10 **S** Universal Health Services, Inc., King of Prussia, PA	33	82	59	—	—	—	—	—	—	—
NASHVILLE—Berrien County ☐ BERRIEN COUNTY HOSPITAL, 1221 East McPherson Street, Zip 31639–2326, Mailing Address: P.O. Box 665, Zip 31639–0665; tel. 912/686–7471; James L. Jarrett, Chief Executive Officer (Total facility includes 108 beds in nursing home–type unit) **A**1 9 10 **F**13 16 17 18 19 22 23 25 26 30 32 34 36 37 38 39 41 43 45 48 51 54 64 69 70 72 76 78 **S** Community Health Systems, Inc., Brentwood, TN	33	10	153	1144	114	15017	0	10282	5476	176
NEWNAN—Coweta County ★ EMORY PEACHTREE REGIONAL HOSPITAL, (Formerly Peachtree Regional Hospital), 60 Hospital Road, Zip 30264, Mailing Address: P.O. Box 2228, Zip 30264–2228; tel. 770/253–1912; Linda Jubinsky, Chief Executive Officer (Nonreporting) **A**1 9 10 **S** HCA – The Healthcare Company, Nashville, TN	33	10	144	—	—	—	—	—	—	—
★ NEWNAN HOSPITAL, 80 Jackson Street, Zip 30263–1941, Mailing Address: Box 997, Zip 30264–0997; tel. 770/253–2330; Glenn M. Flake, Executive Director (Total facility includes 143 beds in nursing home–type unit) **A**1 9 10 **F**7 9 11 13 17 18 22 24 25 27 28 34 39 41 43 45 46 48 49 51 54 65 69 70 76 78 Web address: www.newnanhospital.com	23	10	243	3848	187	49919	0	42892	16896	573
OCILLA—Irwin County ★ IRWIN COUNTY HOSPITAL, 710 North Irwin Avenue, Zip 31774–1098; tel. 912/468–3845; Sue Spivey, Administrator (Total facility includes 30 beds in nursing home–type unit) (Nonreporting) **A**1 9 10	16	10	64	—	—	—	—	—	—	—
PERRY—Houston County ★ PERRY HOSPITAL, 1120 Morningside Drive, Zip 31069–2906, Mailing Address: Drawer 1004, Zip 31069–1004; tel. 912/987–3600; Lora Davis, Administrator **A**1 9 10 **F**2 3 8 9 11 13 14 16 17 18 19 21 22 23 25 30 31 32 33 34 35 36 37 38 39 40 41 43 44 46 48 49 50 51 54 56 57 59 61 65 70 71 72 73 76 77 78 79 **P**7 Web address: www.hhc.org	16	10	45	1884	21	26724	266	14256	6450	231
QUITMAN—Brooks County ☐ BROOKS COUNTY HOSPITAL, 903 North Court Street, Zip 31643–1315, Mailing Address: P.O. Box 5000, Zip 31643–5000; tel. 912/263–4171; David Sanders, Administrator (Nonreporting) **A**1 9 10 **S** Archbold Medical Center, Thomasville, GA	23	10	35	—	—	—	—	—	—	—
REIDSVILLE—Tattnall County TATTNALL MEMORIAL HOSPITAL, Highway 121 South, Zip 30453, Mailing Address: Route 1, Box 261, Zip 30453; tel. 912/557–4731; Jim Riley, Administrator (Nonreporting) **A**10	16	10	40	—	—	—	—	—	—	—
RICHLAND—Stewart County STEWART–WEBSTER HOSPITAL, 300 Alston Street, Zip 31825–1406, Mailing Address: P.O. Box 190, Zip 31825–0190; tel. 912/887–3366; Stephen H. Noble, President (Nonreporting) **A**9 10 **S** Accord Health Care Corporation, Clearwater, FL	33	10	25	—	—	—	—	—	—	—
RIVERDALE—Clayton County ★ SOUTHERN REGIONAL MEDICAL CENTER, 11 Upper Riverdale Road S.W., Zip 30274–2600; tel. 770/991–8000; Eugene A. Leblond, FACHE, President and Chief Executive Officer (Nonreporting) **A**1 2 9 10 Web address: www.promina.org/healthsys/facilities.asp	23	10	324	—	—	—	—	—	—	—
ROBINS AFB—Houston County ★ U. S. AIR FORCE HOSPITAL ROBINS, 655 Seventh Street, Zip 31098–2227; tel. 912/327–7996; Colonel John A. Lee, USAF, MSC, Commander (Nonreporting) **S** Department of the Air Force, Bowling AFB, DC Web address: www.robins.af.mil/orgs/abw/78MEDGP/INEX/HTM	41	10	32	—	—	—	—	—	—	—
ROME—Floyd County ★ △ FLOYD MEDICAL CENTER, 304 Turner McCall Boulevard, Zip 30165–2734, Mailing Address: P.O. Box 233, Zip 30162–0233; tel. 706/802–2000; Kurt Stuenkel, FACHE, President and Chief Executive Officer **A**1 2 3 5 7 9 10 **F**3 4 5 7 8 9 11 12 13 14 16 17 18 19 20 21 22 23 24 25 26 27 28 29 30 31 32 33 34 35 36 37 38 39 41 42 43 44 45 46 48 49 50 51 52 53 54 56 59 60 61 62 63 64 66 68 70 71 72 73 75 76 77 78 79 **P**5 8 Web address: www.floydmed.org	23	10	216	10784	127	160418	2351	91502	37679	1542

Many Facility Codes have changed. Please refer to the AHA Guide Code Chart.

© 2000 AHA Guide

Hospitals, U.S. / GEORGIA

Hospital, Address, Telephone, Administrator, Approval, Facility, and Physician Codes, Health Care System, Network	Classification Codes		Utilization Data					Expense (thousands) of dollars		
★ American Hospital Association (AHA) membership ☐ Joint Commission on Accreditation of Healthcare Organizations (JCAHO) accreditation + American Osteopathic Healthcare Association (AOHA) membership ○ American Osteopathic Association (AOA) accreditation △ Commission on Accreditation of Rehabilitation Facilities (CARF) accreditation Control codes 61, 63, 64, 71, 72 and 73 indicate hospitals listed by AOHA, but not registered by AHA. For definition of numerical codes, see page A4	Control	Service	Staffed Beds	Admissions	Census	Outpatient Visits	Births	Total	Payroll	Personnel
☐ NORTHWEST GEORGIA REGIONAL HOSPITAL, 1305 Redmond Circle, Zip 30165-1393; tel. 706/295-6246; Thomas W. Muller, M.D., Superintendent (Nonreporting) A1 9 10	12	22	340	—	—	—	—	—	—	—
✠ REDMOND REGIONAL MEDICAL CENTER, 501 Redmond Road, Zip 30165-7001, Mailing Address: Box 107001, Zip 30164-7001; tel. 706/291-0291; James R. Thomas, Chief Executive Officer A1 2 9 10 F4 9 11 12 13 22 24 25 27 29 32 34 38 39 41 43 46 47 48 50 51 54 55 56 68 70 71 72 76 77 78 79 P4 7 S HCA – The Healthcare Company, Nashville, TN Web address: www.hcahealthcare.com/	33	10	199	10677	133	86692	0	88086	27503	810
ROSWELL—Fulton County										
✠ NORTH FULTON REGIONAL HOSPITAL, 3000 Hospital Boulevard, Zip 30076-9930; tel. 770/751-2500; John F. Holland, President A1 9 10 F7 8 9 22 24 25 29 32 33 34 38 39 42 43 44 45 46 48 49 51 53 54 70 71 72 75 78 79 P1 S TENET Healthcare Corporation, Santa Barbara, CA Web address: www.northfultonregional.com/	33	10	167	6401	84	64570	592	51010	21365	577
ROYSTON—Franklin County										
✠ COBB MEMORIAL HOSPITAL, (Includes Brown Memorial Convalescent Center, Cobb Health Care Center and Cobb Terrace Personal Care Center), 577 Franklin Springs Street, Zip 30662-3909, Mailing Address: P.O. Box 589, Zip 30662-0589; tel. 706/245-5071; Al Strickland, Administrator (Total facility includes 260 beds in nursing home–type unit) A1 9 10 F6 8 9 13 14 16 17 18 19 22 24 25 32 37 39 40 41 43 44 45 51 54 67 69 70 71 76 78 79 Web address: www.tycobbhealthcare.org	23	10	331	2265	298	38227	178	27303	13151	543
SAINT MARYS—Camden County										
★ CAMDEN MEDICAL CENTER, 2000 Dan Proctor Drive, Zip 31558; tel. 912/576-6200; Alan E. George, Administrator A9 10 F7 8 9 11 13 17 19 22 24 25 30 31 32 34 37 39 41 43 44 45 46 48 50 54 56 70 72 76 77 78 79 P8 S Quorum Health Group, Brentwood, TN	23	10	40	1940	14	31893	626	16992	6433	237
SAINT SIMONS ISLAND—Glynn County										
☐ CHARTER BY-THE-SEA BEHAVIORAL HEALTH SYSTEM, 2927 Demere Road, Zip 31522-1620; tel. 912/638-1999; Wes Robbins, Chief Executive Officer A1 9 10 F2 3 12 13 14 17 18 19 21 22 24 25 28 31 38 39 41 43 44 50 51 52 55 57 58 59 60 61 62 63 64 68 69 70 72 73 76 S Magellan Health Services, Atlanta, GA	33	22	98	1391	35	—	0	5963	3122	91
SANDERSVILLE—Washington County										
✠ WASHINGTON COUNTY REGIONAL MEDICAL CENTER, (Formerly Memorial Hospital of Washington County), 610 Sparta Highway, Zip 31082-1362, Mailing Address: P.O. Box 636, Zip 31082-0636; tel. 912/240-2000; Skip Wise, Chief Executive Officer (Total facility includes 60 beds in nursing home–type unit) A1 9 10 F8 17 18 19 22 24 25 28 30 32 34 37 38 39 41 43 44 45 46 48 54 58 59 60 61 62 63 69 70 71 75 76 78	16	10	116	2427	86	28271	211	21126	9451	331
SAVANNAH—Chatham County										
✠ CANDLER HOSPITAL, 5353 Reynolds Street, Zip 31405-6013; tel. 912/692-6000; Paul P. Hinchey, President and Chief Executive Officer A1 9 10 F1 4 5 7 8 9 11 13 16 17 18 19 22 24 25 27 28 30 31 32 33 34 35 36 38 39 41 43 44 45 46 48 49 50 51 53 54 56 65 68 69 70 71 72 76 78 79 P6	21	10	300	14271	214	133383	2684	125863	58207	1456
☐ CHARTER SAVANNAH BEHAVIORAL HEALTH SYSTEM, 1150 Cornell Avenue, Zip 31406-2797; tel. 912/354-3911; Jim Shaheer, Chief Executive Officer (Nonreporting) A1 9 10 S Magellan Health Services, Atlanta, GA	33	22	112	—	—	—	—	—	—	—
☐ GEORGIA REGIONAL HOSPITAL AT SAVANNAH, 1915 Eisenhower Drive, Zip 31406; tel. 912/356-2011; Gordon L. Ifill, M.D., Acting Facility Administrator A1 9 10 F57 58 61 62	12	22	140	1124	108	—	0	18487	11442	341
✠ △ MEMORIAL HEALTH, (Formerly Memorial Health System), 4700 Waters Avenue, Zip 31404-6283, Mailing Address: P.O. Box 23089, Zip 31403-3089; tel. 912/350-8000; Robert A. Colvin, President and Chief Executive Officer (Nonreporting) A1 2 3 5 7 8 9 10 S Quorum Health Group, Brentwood, TN Web address: www.memorialhealth.com	16	10	373	—	—	—	—	—	—	—
☐ △ ST. JOSEPH'S CANDLER HEALTH SYSTEM, (Formerly St. Joseph's Hospital), 11705 Mercy Boulevard, Zip 31419-1791; tel. 912/925-4100; Paul P. Hinchey, President and Chief Executive Officer A1 2 7 9 10 F4 11 12 13 16 17 18 22 24 25 31 39 41 43 45 46 47 48 49 50 51 53 54 68 69 70 71 72 76 78 P6 7 S Sisters of Mercy of the Americas–Regional Community of Baltimore, Baltimore, MD	21	10	216	8940	157	67829	—	106513	43692	1104
SMYRNA—Cobb County										
✠ EMORY-ADVENTIST HOSPITAL, 3949 South Cobb Drive S.E., Zip 30080-6300; tel. 770/434-0710; Dennis Kiley, President (Total facility includes 12 beds in nursing home–type unit) (Nonreporting) A1 9 10 S Adventist Health System Sunbelt Health Care Corporation, Winter Park, FL	23	10	54	—	—	—	—	—	—	—
✠ RIDGEVIEW INSTITUTE, 3995 South Cobb Drive S.E., Zip 30080-6397; tel. 770/434-4567; John E. Gronewald, Chief Operating Officer A1 3 5 9 10 F2 3 13 17 57 58 61 62 63 64 70 72 79 Web address: www.ridgeviewinstitute.com	23	22	56	2489	35	22095	0	13496	6713	212
SNELLVILLE—Gwinnett County										
✠ EMORY EASTSIDE MEDICAL CENTER, (Formerly Eastside Medical Center), 1700 Medical Way, Zip 30078, Mailing Address: P.O. Box 587, Zip 30078-0587; tel. 770/979-0200; Les Beard, Chief Executive Officer A1 9 10 F7 8 9 13 17 18 22 24 25 27 30 32 33 34 38 39 41 42 43 44 48 49 50 54 57 60 62 63 64 68 70 72 76 77 78 79 S HCA – The Healthcare Company, Nashville, TN	33	10	131	6517	87	91346	1658	49417	23079	718

© 2000 AHA Guide   *Many Facility Codes have changed. Please refer to the AHA Guide Code Chart.*

Hospitals, U.S. / GEORGIA

Hospital, Address, Telephone, Administrator, Approval, Facility, and Physician Codes, Health Care System, Network	Classification Codes		Utilization Data					Expense (thousands) of dollars		Personnel
	Control	Service	Staffed Beds	Admissions	Census	Outpatient Visits	Births	Total	Payroll	

★ American Hospital Association (AHA) membership
☐ Joint Commission on Accreditation of Healthcare Organizations (JCAHO) accreditation
+ American Osteopathic Healthcare Association (AOHA) membership
○ American Osteopathic Association (AOA) accreditation
△ Commission or Accreditation of Rehabilitation Facilities (CARF) accreditation
Control codes 51, 63, 64, 71, 72 and 73 indicate hospitals listed by AOHA, but not registered by AHA. For definition of numerical codes, see page A4.

SPARTA—Hancock County

★ HANCOCK MEMORIAL HOSPITAL, 453 Boland Street, Zip 31087–1105, Mailing Address: P.O. Box 490, Zip 31087–0490; tel. 706/444–7006; Henry T. Gibbs, Administrator and Chief Executive Officer (Nonreporting) **A**9 10	23	10	35	—	—	—	—	—	—	—

SPRINGFIELD—Effingham County

✠ EFFINGHAM HOSPITAL, 459 Highway 119 South, Zip 31329–3021, Mailing Address: P.O. Box 386, Zip 31329–0386; tel. 912/754–6451; Terrance R. Frech, Chief Executive Officer (Total facility includes 105 beds in nursing home–type unit) (Nonreporting) **A**1 9 10	16	10	146	—	—	—	—	—	—	—

STATESBORO—Bulloch County

☐ BULLOCH MEMORIAL HOSPITAL, 500 East Grady Street, Zip 30458–5105, Mailing Address: P.O. Box 1048, Zip 30459–1048; tel. 912/486–1000; C. Scott Campbell, Executive Director **A**1 2 9 10 **F**4 7 8 9 11 12 13 19 22 23 24 25 27 30 32 33 34 36 37 39 41 43 44 48 49 50 54 68 70 71 72 75 76 78 **S** Health Management Associates, Naples, FL	33	10	158	6325	75	71115	1148	32368	16698	505
WILLINGWAY HOSPITAL, 311 Jones Mill Road, Zip 30458–4765; tel. 912/764–6236; Jimmy Mooney, Chief Executive Officer (Nonreporting) **A**9 Web address: www.willingway.com	33	82	40	—	—	—	—	—	—	—

STOCKBRIDGE—Henry County

✠ HENRY MEDICAL CENTER, 1133 Eagle's Landing Parkway, Zip 30281–5099; tel. 770/389–2200; Joseph G. Brum, President and Chief Executive Officer **A**1 9 10 **F**8 9 11 16 17 18 19 22 24 25 32 33 34 38 39 42 43 44 45 48 49 50 65 70 72 73 75 76 77 78 79 **P**1 5 Web address: www.henrymedical.com	23	10	118	7007	85	59118	1641	62464	24645	709

SWAINSBORO—Emanuel County

✠ EMANUEL COUNTY HOSPITAL, 117 Kite Road, Zip 30401–3231, Mailing Address: P.O. Box 879, Zip 30401–0879; tel. 912/237–9911; Bob Via, Chief Executive Officer (Total facility includes 49 beds in nursing home-type unit) **A**1 9 10 **F**8 9 17 22 24 25 32 33 34 38 39 41 43 44 48 51 64 70 72 76 78 **P**6	16	10	91	1603	63	—	174	14236	6433	280

SYLVANIA—Screven County

★ SCREVEN COUNTY HOSPITAL, 215 Mims Road, Zip 30467–2097; tel. 912/564–7426; George H. St. George, Chief Executive Officer **A**9 10 **F**7 9 17 18 19 22 25 34 38 45 48 54 70 76	16	10	30	637	9	14669	1	4732	2137	81

SYLVESTER—Worth County

✠ BAPTIST HOSPITAL, WORTH COUNTY, (Formerly Worth County Hospital), 807 South Isabella Street, Zip 31791–0545, Mailing Address: Box 545, Zip 31791–0545; tel. 912/776–6961; Billy Hayes, Administrator **A**1 9 10 **F**8 9 17 18 19 22 25 32 39 41 44 48 51 54 76 78 **P**5 **S** Georgia Baptist Health Care System, Atlanta, GA	21	10	49	1039	11	28286	71	9482	4658	165

THOMASTON—Upson County

✠ UPSON REGIONAL MEDICAL CENTER, 801 West Gordon Street, Zip 30286–2831, Mailing Address: P.O. Box 1059, Zip 30286–1059; tel. 706/647–8111; Samuel S. Gregory, Administrator **A**1 9 10 **F**7 8 9 16 17 18 22 23 24 25 27 32 34 38 39 41 43 44 45 46 48 50 54 55 59 61 70 71 72 76 77 78 **S** Quorum Health Group, Brentwood, TN	23	10	115	5072	51	89932	789	37890	17124	592

THOMASVILLE—Thomas County

✠ JOHN D. ARCHBOLD MEMORIAL HOSPITAL, Gordon Avenue at Mimosa Drive, Zip 31792–6113, Mailing Address: P.O. Box 1018, Zip 31799–1018; tel. 912/228–2000; James L. Story, Jr, M.D., Acting President (Total facility includes 64 beds in nursing home–type unit) **A**1 2 9 10 **F**1 2 3 4 7 8 9 11 12 13 16 17 18 19 21 22 23 24 25 27 29 30 31 32 33 34 35 36 37 38 39 41 43 44 45 46 47 48 50 51 53 54 56 57 58 59 60 61 62 63 64 65 66 68 69 70 71 72 74 75 76 77 78 **P**8 **S** Archbold Medical Center, Thomasville, GA Web address: www.archbold.org	23	10	264	9543	149	163318	833	91834	39746	1175

THOMSON—McDuffie County

✠ MCDUFFIE REGIONAL MEDICAL CENTER, (Formerly McDuffie County Hospital), 521 Hill Street S.W., Zip 30824–2199; tel. 706/595–1411; Douglas C. Keir, Chief Executive Officer **A**1 9 10 **F**7 9 12 13 18 19 22 25 26 28 32 34 36 37 38 41 45 48 51 53 54 70 71 76 78 **S** Quorum Health Group, Brentwood, TN Web address: www.mcch.org	16	10	35	1641	18	27133	—	13126	5702	227

TIFTON—Tift County

✠ TIFT GENERAL HOSPITAL, 901 East 18th Street, Zip 31794–3648, Mailing Address: Drawer 747, Zip 31793–0747; tel. 912/382–7120; William T. Richardson, President and Chief Executive Officer (Total facility includes 15 beds in nursing home-type unit) **A**1 9 10 **F**7 8 9 11 13 16 17 18 19 22 24 25 27 31 32 37 39 41 44 46 48 50 51 53 54 65 69 70 72 76 77 78 79 **P**8 Web address: www.tiftgeneral.com	16	10	191	7303	82	86652	1059	67416	21531	833

TOCCOA—Stephens County

✠ STEPHENS COUNTY HOSPITAL, 2003 Falls Road, Zip 30577–9700; tel. 706/282–4200; Edward C. Gambrell, Jr, Administrator (Total facility includes 82 beds in nursing home–type unit) **A**1 9 10 **F**6 7 8 9 16 17 18 19 22 25 27 34 37 39 41 44 45 48 50 54 67 68 69 70 74 76 78 Web address: www.stephenscountyhospital.com	16	10	178	3649	109	35407	376	27439	13266	423

TUCKER—De Kalb County

✠ EMORY NORTHLAKE REGIONAL MEDICAL CENTER, (Formerly Northlake Regional Medical Center), 1455 Montreal Road, Zip 30084; tel. 770/270–3000; Thomas D. Gilbert, Chief Executive Officer **A**1 2 9 10 **F**8 9 13 16 19 22 23 24 25 32 35 39 41 42 43 44 45 46 48 53 54 70 76 78 **P**5 **S** HCA – The Healthcare Company, Nashville, TN	33	10	112	2298	36	29701	193	—	—	271

Hospitals, U.S. / GEORGIA

Hospital, Address, Telephone, Administrator, Approval, Facility, and Physician Codes, Health Care System, Network

- ★ American Hospital Association (AHA) membership
- □ Joint Commission on Accreditation of Healthcare Organizations (JCAHO) accreditation
- \+ American Osteopathic Healthcare Association (AOHA) membership
- ○ American Osteopathic Association (AOA) accreditation
- △ Commission on Accreditation of Rehabilitation Facilities (CARF) accreditation

Control codes 61, 63, 64, 71, 72 and 73 indicate hospitals listed by AOHA, but not registered by AHA. For definition of numerical codes, see page A4

Hospital	Control	Service	Staffed Beds	Admissions	Census	Outpatient Visits	Births	Total	Payroll	Personnel
VALDOSTA—Lowndes County										
GREENLEAF CENTER, 2209 Pineview Drive, Zip 31602–7316; tel. 912/247–4357; Michael Lane, Administrator and Chief Executive Officer (Nonreporting) **A**9	33	22	70	—	—	—	—	—	—	—
✠ △ SOUTH GEORGIA MEDICAL CENTER, 2501 North Patterson Street, Zip 31602–1735, Mailing Address: P.O. Box 1727, Zip 31603–1727; tel. 912/333–1000; James McGahee, Administrator and Chief Executive Officer **A**1 2 7 9 10 **F**1 3 6 7 8 9 11 12 13 14 16 17 18 19 21 22 23 24 26 27 29 30 31 32 33 34 35 36 37 38 39 41 42 43 44 45 46 47 48 49 50 51 53 54 56 57 58 59 60 61 62 63 64 65 67 68 70 71 72 74 75 76 77 78 79 **P**8 Web address: www.sgmc.org	16	10	335	13983	183	144879	1943	—	—	1838
VIDALIA—Toombs County										
□ MEADOWS REGIONAL MEDICAL CENTER, 1703 Meadows Lane, Zip 30474–8915, Mailing Address: P.O. Box 1048, Zip 30474–1048; tel. 912/537–8921; Alan Kent, Interim Chief Executive Officer (Total facility includes 35 beds in nursing home–type unit) **A**1 9 10 **F**7 8 9 15 16 17 18 22 24 25 26 27 29 32 34 35 37 38 39 43 44 45 48 49 50 51 54 68 69 70 71 72 76 77 78	23	10	108	3089	58	47133	530	23084	11134	353
VIENNA—Dooly County										
✠ DOOLY MEDICAL CENTER, 1300 Union Street, Zip 31092–7541, Mailing Address: P.O. Box 278, Zip 31092–0278; tel. 912/268–4141; Kenneth D. Rhudy, Chief Executive Officer (Nonreporting) **A**1 9 10	16	10	38	—	—	—	—	—	—	—
VILLA RICA—Carroll County										
✠ TANNER MEDICAL CENTER–VILLA RICA, 601 Dallas Road, Zip 30180–1202, Mailing Address: P.O. Box 638, Zip 30180–0638; tel. 770/456–3100; Larry N. Steed, Administrator **A**1 9 10 **F**7 8 9 13 17 18 19 20 22 24 25 31 32 34 36 39 41 44 45 48 54 68 70 76 78 79 **P**1 7 **S** Quorum Health Group, Brentwood, TN Web address: www.tanner.org	23	10	36	1081	8	19192	147	11673	4989	138
WARM SPRINGS—Meriwether County										
★ BAPTIST MERIWETHER HOSPITAL, 5995 Spring Street, Zip 31830, Mailing Address: P.O. Box 8, Zip 31830–0008; tel. 706/655–3331; Susan Milner, Administrator (Total facility includes 79 beds in nursing home–type unit) **A**9 10 **F**9 14 17 18 24 25 37 38 48 53 69 70 76 78 **S** Georgia Baptist Health Care System, Atlanta, GA Web address: www.gbhcs.org	23	10	117	659	87	9933	1	7070	3032	171
□ ROOSEVELT WARM SPRINGS INSTITUTE FOR REHABILITATION, Highway 27, Zip 31830, Mailing Address: P.O. Box 1000, Zip 31830–0268; tel. 706/655–5001; Frank C. Ruzycki, Executive Director (Nonreporting) **A**1 10 Web address: www.rooseveltrehab.org	12	46	78	—	—	—	—	—	—	—
WARNER ROBINS—Houston County										
✠ HOUSTON MEDICAL CENTER, 1601 Watson Boulevard, Zip 31093–3431, Mailing Address: Box 2886, Zip 31099–2886; tel. 912/922–4281; Arthur P. Christie, Administrator **A**1 9 10 **F**2 8 9 11 12 13 16 17 18 19 22 23 24 25 27 29 32 33 34 38 39 41 43 44 46 48 49 50 51 53 54 57 59 60 61 62 63 64 70 71 72 76 77 78 79 **P**7 Web address: www.hhc.org	16	10	186	8641	100	133793	1311	64226	28502	944
WASHINGTON—Wilkes County										
✠ WILLS MEMORIAL HOSPITAL, 120 Gordon Street, Zip 30673–1602, Mailing Address: P.O. Box 370, Zip 30673–0370; tel. 706/678–2151; Tim E. Merritt, Chief Executive Officer **A**1 9 10 **F**7 8 9 17 22 25 32 34 37 39 41 43 44 45 48 54 70 76 78	16	10	38	1309	17	9115	62	8489	3909	167
WAYCROSS—Ware County										
✠ SATILLA REGIONAL MEDICAL CENTER, 410 Darling Avenue, Zip 31501–5246, Mailing Address: P.O. Box 139, Zip 31502–0139; tel. 912/283–3030; Robert M. Trimm, President and Chief Executive Officer (Nonreporting) **A**1 9 10	23	10	116	—	—	—	—	—	—	—
WAYNESBORO—Burke County										
□ BURKE COUNTY HOSPITAL, 351 Liberty Street, Zip 30830–9686; tel. 706/554–4435; Michael A. Haddle, CPA, Chief Executive Officer and Chief Financial Officer **A**1 9 10 **F**7 16 17 18 22 25 48 76 78 Web address: www.burke.net	15	10	40	1707	18	17544	200	7663	3909	144
WILDWOOD—Dade County										
WILDWOOD LIFESTYLE CENTER AND HOSPITAL, Lifestyle Lane, Zip 30757, Mailing Address: P.O. Box 129, Zip 30757–0129; tel. 706/820–1493; Larry E. Clements, Administrator (Nonreporting) Web address: www.taquet.org/wildwood	23	10	13	—	—	—	—	—	—	—
WINDER—Barrow County										
✠ BARROW MEDICAL CENTER, (Formerly Columbia Barrow Medical Center), 316 North Broad Street, Zip 30680–2150, Mailing Address: P.O. Box 768, Zip 30680–0768; tel. 770/867–3400; Randy Mills, Chief Executive Officer **A**1 9 10 **F**7 8 9 13 17 18 19 22 24 25 32 33 34 38 39 41 43 44 48 49 50 65 70 75 76 78 79 **S** LifePoint Hospitals, Inc., Brentwood, TN Web address: www.barrowmedical.com	33	10	56	1272	11	34016	232	13281	5336	148

Hospitals, U.S. / HAWAII

HAWAII

Resident Population 1,193 (in thousands)
Resident population in metro areas 73.6%
Birth rate per 1,000 population 14.7
65 years and over 13.3%
Percent of persons without health insurance 7.5%

- ★ American Hospital Association (AHA) membership
- ☐ Joint Commission on Accreditation of Healthcare Organizations (JCAHO) accreditation
- + American Osteopathic Healthcare Association (AOHA) membership
- ○ American Osteopathic Association (AOA) accreditation
- △ Commission on Accreditation of Rehabilitation Facilities (CARF) accreditation
  Control codes 61, 63, 64, 71, 72 and 73 indicate hospitals listed by AOHA, but not registered by AHA. For definition of numerical codes, see page A4

Hospital, Address, Telephone, Administrator, Approval, Facility, and Physician Codes, Health Care System, Network	Classification Codes		Utilization Data					Expense (thousands) of dollars		
	Control	Service	Staffed Beds	Admissions	Census	Outpatient Visits	Births	Total	Payroll	Personnel
EWA BEACH—Honolulu County										
★ KAHI MOHALA, 91-2301 Fort Weaver Road, Zip 96706; tel. 808/671-8511; Margi Drue, Administrator **A**1 3 9 10 **F**3 16 18 29 31 38 57 58 59 63 64 70 **P**6 **S** Sutter Health, Sacramento, CA **Web address:** www.kahi.org	23	22	88	1211	67	29725	0	17456	10374	226
★ ST. FRANCIS MEDICAL CENTER–WEST, 91-2141 Fort Weaver Road, Zip 96706; tel. 808/678-7000; John V. Schleif, Administrator **A**1 10 **F**2 3 4 8 9 11 12 13 16 17 18 19 22 23 24 25 26 27 32 36 37 38 39 41 43 44 45 46 47 48 49 51 54 56 65 69 70 72 73 74 76 78 **P**8 **S** Sisters of the 3rd Franciscan Order, Syracuse, NY **Web address:** www.sfhs-hi.org	21	10	102	3890	84	106445	502	49049	18133	514
HILO—Hawaii County										
★ HILO MEDICAL CENTER, 1190 Waianuenue Avenue, Zip 96720-2095; tel. 808/974-4743; Ronald J. Schurra, Administrator (Total facility includes 108 beds in nursing home–type unit) **A**1 5 9 10 **F**8 9 12 16 17 18 22 23 24 25 29 30 33 35 36 37 39 41 44 45 46 48 49 54 57 59 60 61 62 64 65 69 70 76 78 **P**5 **S** Hawaii Health Systems Corporation, Honolulu, HI	12	10	164	7105	104	—	1085	53857	23318	700
HONOKAA—Hawaii County										
★ HALE HO'OLA HAMAKUA, 45-547 Plumeria Street, Zip 96727, Mailing Address: P.O. Box 237, Zip 96727-0237; tel. 808/775-7211; Romel Dela Cruz, Administrator (Total facility includes 48 beds in nursing home–type unit) **A**9 10 **F**17 18 24 30 69 70 72 78 **S** Hawaii Health Systems Corporation, Honolulu, HI	12	10	50	130	40	965	—	5172	2220	75
HONOLULU—Honolulu County										
★ KAISER FOUNDATION HOSPITAL, 3288 Moanalua Road, Zip 96819; tel. 808/834-5333; Robert Matsuwaka, Regional Administrator (Total facility includes 28 beds in nursing home–type unit) **A**1 2 3 5 9 10 **F**4 8 9 11 12 13 14 16 17 18 19 22 24 25 27 29 30 31 32 34 35 36 37 38 39 41 42 43 44 45 46 47 48 49 51 54 56 58 59 60 63 64 65 66 68 69 70 72 73 74 75 76 77 78 79 **P**3 **S** Kaiser Foundation Hospitals, Oakland, CA **Web address:** www.kaiserhawaii.com	23	10	190	10298	157	1134814	1874	—	—	1045
★ KAPIOLANI MEDICAL CENTER FOR WOMEN AND CHILDREN, 1319 Punahou Street, Zip 96826-1032; tel. 808/983-6000; Frances A. Hallonquist, Chief Executive Officer (Nonreporting) **A**1 3 5 9 10 **Web address:** www.kapiolani.org	23	44	276	—	—	—	—	—	—	—
★ KUAKINI MEDICAL CENTER, 347 North Kuakini Street, Zip 96817-2381; tel. 808/536-2236; Gary K. Kajiwara, President and Chief Executive Officer **A**1 2 3 5 9 10 **F**1 4 7 9 11 12 13 16 17 18 22 24 25 27 29 30 32 33 34 36 37 38 39 41 43 45 46 47 48 49 50 51 54 65 68 69 70 71 72 76 78 79 **P**8 **Web address:** www.kuakini.org	23	10	150	5704	123	38121	0	91480	45251	1091
★ LEAHI HOSPITAL, (SNF ICF TB), 3675 Kilauea Avenue, Zip 96816; tel. 808/733-8000; Jerry Walker, Administrator (Total facility includes 179 beds in nursing home–type unit) **A**3 5 9 10 **F**1 18 22 23 24 39 45 55 62 68 69 70 76 **S** Hawaii Health Systems Corporation, Honolulu, HI	12	49	192	107	170	—	0	16897	10390	293
★ QUEEN'S MEDICAL CENTER, 1301 Punchbowl Street, Zip 96813; tel. 808/538-9011; Arthur A. Ushijima, President and Chief Executive Officer (Total facility includes 28 beds in nursing home–type unit) **A**1 2 3 5 8 9 10 **F**3 4 7 8 9 11 12 13 14 16 17 18 21 22 23 24 25 27 29 30 32 33 34 35 36 37 38 39 40 41 43 44 45 46 47 48 49 50 51 54 55 56 57 58 59 60 61 62 63 64 65 68 69 70 74 75 76 77 78 **P**5 **S** Queen's Health Systems, Honolulu, HI **Web address:** www.queens.org	23	10	451	19241	377	198297	1538	313411	131198	2490
★ △ REHABILITATION HOSPITAL OF THE PACIFIC, 226 North Kuakini Street, Zip 96817-9881; tel. 808/531-3511; William D. O'Connor, President and Chief Executive Officer **A**1 7 9 10 **F**13 16 17 18 22 24 29 31 36 38 39 40 43 45 49 51 53 54 70 71 72 76 78 **P**2 **Web address:** www.rehabhospital.org	23	46	86	1558	66	72199	0	29151	14518	337
☐ SHRINERS HOSPITALS FOR CHILDREN, HONOLULU, 1310 Punahou Street, Zip 96826-1099; tel. 808/941-4466; Thomas J. Brotherton, Administrator **A**1 3 5 **F**5 17 24 38 53 54 70 76 78 **P**6 **S** Shriners Hospitals for Children, Tampa, FL **Web address:** www.shrinershq.org	23	50	40	442	25	4263	0	—	—	140
☐ ST. FRANCIS MEDICAL CENTER, 2230 Liliha Street, Zip 96817-9979, Mailing Address: P.O. Box 30100, Zip 96820-0100; tel. 808/547-6484; Cynthia Okinaka, Administrator (Total facility includes 46 beds in nursing home–type unit) **A**1 2 3 5 9 10 **F**2 3 4 8 9 11 17 18 19 22 23 24 25 30 32 34 36 37 38 39 41 43 44 45 46 47 48 49 50 51 54 56 59 60 61 63 65 68 69 70 72 73 74 76 78 **P**8 **S** Sisters of the 3rd Franciscan Order, Syracuse, NY **Web address:** www.stfrancishawaii.org	21	10	249	5145	204	358555	—	142013	48897	1471
☐ STRAUB CLINIC AND HOSPITAL, 888 South King Street, Zip 96813; tel. 808/522-4000; Jonathan D. Grimes, Chief Executive Officer (Nonreporting) **A**1 2 3 5 9 10 **Web address:** www.straubhealth.com	33	10	139	—	—	—	—	—	—	—

Hospitals, U.S. / HAWAII

Hospital, Address, Telephone, Administrator, Approval, Facility, and Physician Codes, Health Care System, Network	Classification Codes		Utilization Data					Expense (thousands) of dollars		
★ American Hospital Association (AHA) membership ☐ Joint Commission on Accreditation of Healthcare Organizations (JCAHO) accreditation + American Osteopathic Healthcare Association (AOHA) membership ○ American Osteopathic Association (AOA) accreditation △ Commission on Accreditation of Rehabilitation Facilities (CARF) accreditation Control codes 61, 63, 64, 71, 72 and 73 indicate hospitals listed by AOHA, but not registered by AHA. For definition of numerical codes, see page A4	Control	Service	Staffed Beds	Admissions	Census	Outpatient Visits	Births	Total	Payroll	Personnel
★ TRIPLER ARMY MEDICAL CENTER, Zip 96859–5000; tel. 808/433–6661; Major General Nancy R. Adams, Commander **A**1 2 3 5 **F**3 4 8 9 11 12 13 14 16 17 18 19 21 22 23 24 25 28 31 32 33 34 35 38 39 41 42 43 44 45 46 47 48 49 50 51 52 54 55 56 57 58 59 60 61 62 63 64 65 66 68 70 71 72 73 76 77 78 79 **P**6 **S** Department of the Army, Office of the Surgeon General, Falls Church, VA Web address: www.tamc.amedd.army.mil	42	10	256	11429	150	562444	2659	66255	45777	3193
KAHUKU—Honolulu County										
★ KAHUKU HOSPITAL, 56–117 Pualalea Street, Zip 96731–2052; tel. 808/293–9221; Wayne Fairchild, Chief Executive Officer (Nonreporting) **A**1 9 10	23	10	24	—	—	—	—	—	—	—
KAILUA—Honolulu County										
★ CASTLE MEDICAL CENTER, 640 Ulukahiki Street, Zip 96734–4498; tel. 808/263–5500; Robert J. Walker, President (Total facility includes 10 beds in nursing home–type unit) **A**1 9 10 **F**2 3 8 9 11 13 14 18 22 24 25 27 32 33 34 36 38 39 43 44 45 46 48 51 54 57 58 63 64 69 70 72 73 76 78 79 **S** Adventist Health, Roseville, CA Web address: www.cmc.ah.org	21	10	157	5846	86	94369	466	58456	27321	603
KANEOHE—Honolulu County										
☐ HAWAII STATE HOSPITAL, 45–710 Keaahala Road, Zip 96744–3597; tel. 808/236–8237; Wayne P. Law, Acting Administrator **A**1 3 5 **F**16 17 18 57 62	12	22	168	132	164	0	0	30000	—	545
KAPAA—Kauai County										
★ SAMUEL MAHELONA MEMORIAL HOSPITAL, 4800 Kawaihau Road, Zip 96746–1998; tel. 808/822–4961; Orianna A. Skomoroch, Regional Chief Executive Officer (Total facility includes 66 beds in nursing home–type unit) **A**9 10 **F**2 7 16 17 18 23 43 45 51 54 57 69 70 77 78 **P**6 **S** Hawaii Health Systems Corporation, Honolulu, HI Web address: www.mahelona.org	12	48	81	159	64	1219	—	7374	4067	137
KAUNAKAKAI—Maui County										
★ MOLOKAI GENERAL HOSPITAL, Mailing Address: P.O. Box 408, Zip 96748–0408; tel. 808/553–5331; Calvin M. Ichinose, Administrator (Total facility includes 14 beds in nursing home–type unit) **A**1 9 10 **F**2 3 4 8 9 10 11 12 16 17 18 19 22 23 24 25 26 27 28 32 33 34 35 37 39 40 41 42 43 44 45 46 47 48 49 51 52 53 54 55 57 65 66 68 69 70 71 72 73 75 76 77 79 **P**4 5 7 8 **S** Queen's Health Systems, Honolulu, HI Web address: www.queens.org	23	10	29	341	18	14227	42	7346	3271	79
KEALAKEKUA—Hawaii County										
★ KONA COMMUNITY HOSPITAL, Haukapila Street, Zip 96750, Mailing Address: P.O. Box 69, Zip 96750–0069; tel. 808/322–4429; Joseph C. Wall, Chief Executive Officer (Total facility includes 22 beds in nursing home–type unit) **A**1 9 10 **F**1 7 8 9 13 16 17 18 22 25 30 37 41 43 44 45 46 48 54 64 69 70 76 78 **S** Hawaii Health Systems Corporation, Honolulu, HI	12	10	75	3584	34	40483	474	26336	12264	295
KOHALA—Hawaii County										
★ KOHALA HOSPITAL, (RURAL ACUTE & LSC FACILITY), 54–383 Hospital Road, Zip 96755, Mailing Address: P.O. Box 10, Kapaau, Zip 96755–0010); tel. 808/889–6211; Herbert K. Yim, Administrator (Total facility includes 20 beds in nursing home–type unit) **A**9 10 **F**16 17 18 25 69 78 **S** Hawaii Health Systems Corporation, Honolulu, HI	12	49	26	47	23	1843	0	2612	1456	43
KULA—Maui County										
★ KULA HOSPITAL, 204 Kula Highway, Zip 96790–9499; tel. 808/878–1221; Alan G. Lee, Administrator (Total facility includes 103 beds in nursing home–type unit) (Nonreporting) **A**9 10 **S** Hawaii Health Systems Corporation, Honolulu, HI	12	49	105	—	—	—	—	—	—	—
LANAI CITY—Maui County										
★ LANAI COMMUNITY HOSPITAL, 628 Seventh Street, Zip 96763–0650, Mailing Address: P.O. Box 630650, Zip 96763–0650; tel. 808/565–6411; John Schaumburg, Administrator (Nonreporting) **A**9 10 **S** Hawaii Health Systems Corporation, Honolulu, HI	12	10	14	—	—	—	—	—	—	—
LIHUE—Kauai County										
★ WILCOX MEMORIAL HOSPITAL, 3420 Kuhio Highway, Zip 96766; tel. 808/245–1100; David W. Patton, Ph.D., President and Chief Executive Officer (Total facility includes 110 beds in nursing home–type unit) **A**1 2 9 10 **F**1 7 8 9 13 16 17 18 19 22 24 25 29 30 31 32 33 34 35 37 38 39 41 43 44 45 46 48 50 51 54 56 63 66 69 70 72 73 75 76 77 78 **P**5 6 Web address: www.wilcoxhealth.org	23	10	181	4991	148	69795	—	48009	23184	647
PAHALA—Hawaii County										
★ KAU HOSPITAL, 1 Kamani Street, Zip 96777, Mailing Address: P.O. Box 40, Zip 96777–0040; tel. 808/928–8331; Dawn S. Pung, Administrator (Total facility includes 19 beds in nursing home–type unit) (Nonreporting) **A**9 10 **S** Hawaii Health Systems Corporation, Honolulu, HI	12	10	21	—	—	—	—	—	—	—
WAHIAWA—Honolulu County										
★ WAHIAWA GENERAL HOSPITAL, 128 Lehua Street, Zip 96786; tel. 808/621–8411; Tyler A. Erickson, Chief Executive Officer (Total facility includes 93 beds in nursing home–type unit) **A**1 3 5 9 10 **F**7 8 9 11 19 22 23 25 26 30 32 34 36 38 39 44 45 46 48 51 54 56 69 70 71 72 73 76 78 **P**5 8 **S** Quorum Health Group, Brentwood, TN	23	10	162	2211	123	35275	291	25054	10376	322

Hospitals, U.S. / HAWAII

Hospital, Address, Telephone, Administrator, Approval, Facility, and Physician Codes, Health Care System, Network	Classification Codes		Utilization Data					Expense (thousands) of dollars		
★ American Hospital Association (AHA) membership ☐ Joint Commission on Accreditation of Healthcare Organizations (JCAHO) accreditation + American Osteopathic Healthcare Association (AOHA) membership ○ American Osteopathic Association (AOA) accreditation △ Commission on Accreditation of Rehabilitation Facilities (CARF) accreditation Control codes 61, 63, 64, 71, 72 and 73 indicate hospitals listed by AOHA, but not registered by AHA. For definition of numerical codes, see page A4	Control	Service	Staffed Beds	Admissions	Census	Outpatient Visits	Births	Total	Payroll	Personnel
WAILUKU—Maui County ★ MAUI MEMORIAL MEDICAL CENTER, 221 Mahalani Street, Zip 96793–2581; tel. 808/244–9056; William B. Kleefisch, Chief Executive Officer **A**1 2 9 10 **F**4 7 8 9 11 12 13 19 20 22 24 25 32 38 39 43 44 45 46 48 49 57 58 61 64 70 72 76 78 **S** Hawaii Health Systems Corporation, Honolulu, HI	12	10	194	9882	141	29826	1547	73982	29560	668
WAIMEA—Kauai County ★ KAUAI VETERANS MEMORIAL HOSPITAL, Waimea Canyon Road, Zip 96796, Mailing Address: P.O. Box 337, Zip 96796–0337; tel. 808/338–9431; Orianna A. Skomoroch, Regional Chief Executive Officer (Total facility includes 20 beds in nursing home–type unit) **A**1 9 10 **F**7 8 9 22 23 25 37 44 48 54 69 70 76 **S** Hawaii Health Systems Corporation, Honolulu, HI	12	10	49	806	28	10249	3	10797	6094	139

Hospitals, U.S. / IDAHO

IDAHO

Resident Population 1,229 (in thousands)
Resident population in metro areas 37.5%
Birth rate per 1,000 population 15.4
65 years and over 11.3%
Percent of persons without health insurance 17.7%

Hospital, Address, Telephone, Administrator, Approval, Facility, and Physician Codes, Health Care System, Network	Classification Codes		Utilization Data					Expense (thousands) of dollars		
★ American Hospital Association (AHA) membership □ Joint Commission on Accreditation of Healthcare Organizations (JCAHO) accreditation + American Osteopathic Healthcare Association (AOHA) membership ○ American Osteopathic Association (AOA) accreditation △ Commission on Accreditation of Rehabilitation Facilities (CARF) accreditation Control codes 61, 63, 64, 71, 72 and 73 indicate hospitals listed by AOHA, but not registered by AHA. For definition of numerical codes, see page A4	Control	Service	Staffed Beds	Admissions	Census	Outpatient Visits	Births	Total	Payroll	Personnel
AMERICAN FALLS—Power County										
★ HARMS MEMORIAL HOSPITAL DISTRICT, 510 Roosevelt Road, Zip 83211–0420, Mailing Address: P.O. Box 420, Zip 83211–0420; tel. 208/226–3200; Ronald O'Hallaron, Administrator (Total facility includes 31 beds in nursing home–type unit) **A**9 10 18 **F**17 25 29 32 56 69 70 77	16	10	41	117	26	10336	—	3509	1788	73
ARCO—Butte County										
★ LOST RIVERS DISTRICT HOSPITAL, 551 Highland Drive, Zip 83213–9771, Mailing Address: P.O. Box 145, Zip 83213–0145; tel. 208/527–8206; Harry Aubert, Chief Executive Officer (Total facility includes 33 beds in nursing home–type unit) (Nonreporting) **A**9 10 Web address: www.lrmc.net	16	10	41	—	—	—	—	—	—	—
BLACKFOOT—Bingham County										
⊞ BINGHAM MEMORIAL HOSPITAL, 98 Poplar Street, Zip 83221–1799; tel. 208/785–4100; Louis Kraml, Chief Executive Officer (Total facility includes 75 beds in nursing home–type unit) **A**1 9 10 **F**8 9 12 16 17 18 19 22 24 25 32 33 34 39 41 43 44 45 48 49 50 51 54 69 70 71 72 73 76 78 **P**8 **S** Quorum Health Group, Brentwood, TN Web address: www.binghammemorial.org	13	10	112	1947	71	21756	403	14690	6703	196
□ STATE HOSPITAL SOUTH, 700 East Alice Street, Zip 83221–0400, Mailing Address: Box 400, Zip 83221–0400; tel. 208/785–1200; Ray Laible, Administrative Director (Total facility includes 30 beds in nursing home–type unit) **A**1 9 10 **F**18 57 58 59 60 61 62 69 **P**6	12	22	136	345	110	—	—	14624	9231	259
BOISE—Ada County										
□ BHC INTERMOUNTAIN HOSPITAL, 303 North Allumbaugh Street, Zip 83704–9266; tel. 208/377–8400; Vernon G. Garrett, Chief Executive Officer **A**1 9 10 **F**3 16 57 58 59 61 63 64 70 **P**5 **S** Behavioral Healthcare Corporation, Nashville, TN	33	22	95	1610	63	8636	0	8767	4512	128
★ △ IDAHO ELKS REHABILITATION HOSPITAL, 600 North Robbins Road, Zip 83702–4597, Mailing Address: P.O. Box 1100, Zip 83701–1100; tel. 208/343–2583; Joseph P. Caroselli, Administrator (Total facility includes 12 beds in nursing home–type unit) **A**7 9 10 **F**7 13 18 28 31 32 45 49 53 54 69 70 71 72 78 Web address: www.ierh.org	23	46	64	1492	51	16900	0	13458	7513	300
⊞ △ SAINT ALPHONSUS REGIONAL MEDICAL CENTER, 1055 North Curtis Road, Zip 83706–1370; tel. 208/378–2121; Sandra B. Bruce, President and Chief Executive Officer **A**1 2 3 5 7 9 10 **F**3 4 7 8 9 11 12 13 14 16 17 18 19 20 21 22 24 25 29 30 32 33 34 35 36 38 39 41 43 44 45 46 47 48 49 50 51 53 54 56 57 58 59 60 61 62 63 65 69 70 71 72 73 74 75 76 77 78 79 **P**5 6 7 8 **S** Trinity Health, Novi, MI Web address: www.saintalphonsus.org	21	10	281	13711	183	356760	373	189092	74205	2014
⊞ ST. LUKE'S REGIONAL MEDICAL CENTER, 190 East Bannock Street, Zip 83712–6298; tel. 208/381–2222; Edwin E. Dahlberg, President (Nonreporting) **A**1 2 3 5 9 10 Web address: www.slrmc.org	23	10	312	—	—	—	—	—	—	—
⊞ VETERANS AFFAIRS MEDICAL CENTER, 500 West Fort Street, Zip 83702–4598; tel. 208/422–1100; Wayne C. Tippets, Director (Total facility includes 40 beds in nursing home–type unit) (Nonreporting) **A**1 3 5 9 **S** Department of Veterans Affairs, Washington, DC Web address: www.va.gov/stations97/guide/home.asp?DIVISION=ALL	45	10	176	—	—	—	—	—	—	—
BONNERS FERRY—Boundary County										
★ BOUNDARY COMMUNITY HOSPITAL, (Includes Boundary County Nursing Home), 6640 Kaniksu Street, Zip 83805–7532, Mailing Address: HCR 61, Box 61A, Zip 83805–9500; tel. 208/267–3141; William T. McClintock, FACHE, Chief Executive Officer (Total facility includes 52 beds in nursing home–type unit) **A**9 10 18 **F**7 9 13 16 17 18 19 25 30 31 32 34 36 38 43 45 48 54 56 61 69 70 72 73 77 78 79 **P**8 Web address: www.boundaryhospital.org	13	10	62	301	46	15266	0	5518	3783	155
BURLEY—Cassia County										
⊞ CASSIA REGIONAL MEDICAL CENTER, 1501 Hiland Avenue, Zip 83318–2648; tel. 208/678–4444; Michael R. Olson, Administrator (Total facility includes 34 beds in nursing home–type unit) (Nonreporting) **A**1 2 9 10 **S** Intermountain Health Care, Inc., Salt Lake City, UT Web address: www.ihc.com	23	10	87	—	—	—	—	—	—	—
CALDWELL—Canyon County										
⊞ WEST VALLEY MEDICAL CENTER, 1717 Arlington, Zip 83605–4864; tel. 208/459–4641; Mark Adams, Chief Executive Officer (Total facility includes 16 beds in nursing home–type unit) **A**1 9 10 **F**3 7 8 9 11 13 18 19 22 23 24 25 27 30 31 32 33 34 35 38 39 40 41 43 44 45 46 48 51 54 56 57 58 59 60 61 62 63 65 68 69 70 71 72 76 78 79 **S** HCA – The Healthcare Company, Nashville, TN Web address: www.westvalleymedctr.com	33	10	122	4809	49	47080	727	25518	12818	391

© 2000 AHA Guide   *Many Facility Codes have changed. Please refer to the AHA Guide Code Chart.*

Hospitals, U.S. / IDAHO

Hospital, Address, Telephone, Administrator, Approval, Facility, and Physician Codes, Health Care System, Network	Classification Codes		Utilization Data					Expense (thousands) of dollars		
★ American Hospital Association (AHA) membership ☐ Joint Commission on Accreditation of Healthcare Organizations (JCAHO) accreditation + American Osteopathic Healthcare Association (AOHA) membership ○ American Osteopathic Association (AOA) accreditation △ Commission on Accreditation of Rehabilitation Facilities (CARF) accreditation Control codes 61, 63, 64, 71, 72 and 73 indicate hospitals listed by AOHA, but not registered by AHA. For definition of numerical codes, see page A4	Control	Service	Staffed Beds	Admissions	Census	Outpatient Visits	Births	Total	Payroll	Personnel
CASCADE—Valley County										
★ CASCADE MEDICAL CENTER, 402 Old State Highway, Zip 83611, Mailing Address: P.O. Box 151, Zip 83611-0151; tel. 208/382-4242; Frank Clark, Chief Executive Officer (Nonreporting) **A**9 10 **S** Trinity Health, Novi, MI	13	10	10	—	—	—	—	—	—	—
COEUR D'ALENE—Kootenai County										
⊞ KOOTENAI MEDICAL CENTER, (Includes North Idaho Behavioral Health, Division of Kootenai Medical Center, 2301 North Ironwood Place, Zip 83814-2650; tel. 208/765-4800), 2003 Lincoln Way, Zip 83814-2677; tel. 208/666-2000; Joe Morris, Chief Executive Officer (Total facility includes 25 beds in nursing home-type unit) **A**1 2 9 10 **F**1 2 3 4 7 8 9 11 12 13 16 17 19 22 23 24 25 26 31 33 38 39 41 43 44 45 46 48 49 50 51 53 54 57 58 59 60 61 62 63 64 65 69 70 72 76 77 78 **P**4	16	10	250	12307	153	123125	1426	83425	36726	832
COTTONWOOD—Idaho County										
★ ST. MARY'S HOSPITAL, Lewiston and North Streets, Zip 83522, Mailing Address: P.O. Box 137, Zip 83522-0137; tel. 208/962-3251; Casey Uhling, Chief Executive Officer (Total facility includes 10 beds in nursing home-type unit) (Nonreporting) **A**9 10 **S** Benedictine Health System, Duluth, MN	21	10	28	—	—	—	—	—	—	—
COUNCIL—Adams County										
COUNCIL COMMUNITY HOSPITAL AND NURSING HOME, 205 North Berkley Street, Zip 83612; tel. 208/253-4242; Kay Garcia, Interim Administrator (Total facility includes 20 beds in nursing home-type unit) (Nonreporting) **A**9 10 18	13	10	26	—	—	—	—	—	—	—
DRIGGS—Teton County										
★ TETON VALLEY HOSPITAL, 120 East Howard Street, Zip 83422; tel. 208/354-2383; Susan Kunz, Administrator **A**9 10 **F**7 8 9 13 16 17 19 21 22 25 32 34 36 37 40 44 48 49 54 56 70 72 73 76 78 **P**3	13	10	13	410	3	11041	59	4384	2090	68
EMMETT—Gem County										
WALTER KNOX MEMORIAL HOSPITAL, 1202 East Locust Street, Zip 83617-2715; tel. 208/365-3561; Max Long, Chief Executive Officer **A**9 10 **F**7 8 9 19 22 25 32 36 38 39 44 48 49 50	13	10	17	496	3	14318	76	4008	1977	66
GOODING—Gooding County										
GOODING COUNTY MEMORIAL HOSPITAL, 1120 Montana Street, Zip 83330-1858; tel. 208/934-4433; Jim Henshaw, President and Chief Executive Officer **A**9 10 18 **F**7 9 14 15 16 17 18 19 20 21 23 25 29 32 34 36 38 43 45 48 51 54 67 70 76 77 **P**5	16	10	14	505	5	16342	0	4155	1905	68
GRANGEVILLE—Idaho County										
SYRINGA GENERAL HOSPITAL, 607 West Main Street, Zip 83530-1396; tel. 208/983-1700; Jess Hawley, Administrator **A**9 10 **F**7 8 9 13 22 25 32 34 36 37 38 44 48 54 60 72 76 78	16	10	16	450	4	6256	34	3833	1825	70
HAILEY—Blaine County										
BLAINE COUNTY MEDICAL CENTER See Wood River Medical Center, Sun Valley										
IDAHO FALLS—Bonneville County										
⊞ EASTERN IDAHO REGIONAL MEDICAL CENTER, 3100 Channing Way, Zip 83404-7533, Mailing Address: P.O. Box 2077, Zip 83403-2077; tel. 208/529-6111; Douglas Crabtree, Chief Executive Officer (Total facility includes 16 beds in nursing home-type unit) **A**1 10 **F**4 5 7 8 9 11 13 16 17 18 19 20 22 24 25 28 29 32 34 39 41 42 43 44 45 46 47 48 49 50 53 54 57 58 59 61 63 68 69 70 71 72 75 76 77 78 79 **P**8 **S** HCA – The Healthcare Company, Nashville, TN Web address: www.eirmc.org	33	10	289	13187	178	148343	1779	85181	35760	1118
★ IDAHO FALLS RECOVERY CENTER, (SURGICAL RECOVERY IV THERAPY), 1957 East 17th Street, Zip 83404-6429; tel. 208/529-5285; Jackie Street, President **A**9 10 **F**16 32 33 46 Web address: ifrc.ida.net	12	49	10	299	3	818	0	—	—	20
JEROME—Jerome County										
★ ST. BENEDICTS FAMILY MEDICAL CENTER, 709 North Lincoln Avenue, Zip 83338-1851, Mailing Address: P.O. Box 586, Zip 83338-0586; tel. 208/324-4301; Lynne M. Mattison, FACHE, Interim Administrator (Total facility includes 40 beds in nursing home-type unit) **A**9 10 **F**7 9 17 18 22 25 32 34 36 38 39 43 48 54 69 76 77 **S** Trinity Health, Novi, MI	23	10	60	921	34	21724	321	11262	4862	145
KELLOGG—Shoshone County										
⊞ SHOSHONE MEDICAL CENTER, 3 Jacobs Gulch, Zip 83837-2096; tel. 208/784-1221; Gary Moore, Chief Executive Officer **A**1 9 10 **F**2 3 8 9 12 16 17 22 25 28 30 34 36 38 39 44 45 48 54 70 76 77 **P**3 5 8 **S** Quorum Health Group, Brentwood, TN	16	10	26	986	11	20379	84	9538	4298	150
LEWISTON—Nez Perce County										
⊞ ST. JOSEPH REGIONAL MEDICAL CENTER, 415 Sixth Street, Zip 83501-0816; tel. 208/743-2511; Howard A. Hayes, President and Chief Executive Officer (Total facility includes 16 beds in nursing home-type unit) **A**1 2 9 10 **F**7 8 9 12 14 16 17 18 19 21 22 23 24 25 26 27 28 30 31 32 33 34 35 36 37 38 39 40 41 43 44 45 46 48 49 50 51 54 57 59 60 61 62 63 65 68 69 70 71 72 74 75 76 77 78 **P**5 **S** Carondelet Health System, Saint Louis, MO Web address: www.sjrmc.org	21	10	156	6586	80	109226	792	59385	25553	647
MALAD CITY—Oneida County										
ONEIDA COUNTY HOSPITAL, 150 North 200 West, Zip 83252-0126, Mailing Address: Box 126, Zip 83252-0126; tel. 208/766-2231; Todd Winder, Administrator (Total facility includes 41 beds in nursing home-type unit) (Nonreporting) **A**9 10 18	13	10	52	—	—	—	—	—	—	—

Hospitals, U.S. / IDAHO

Hospital, Address, Telephone, Administrator, Approval, Facility, and Physician Codes, Health Care System, Network	Classification Codes		Utilization Data					Expense (thousands) of dollars		
★ American Hospital Association (AHA) membership □ Joint Commission on Accreditation of Healthcare Organizations (JCAHO) accreditation + American Osteopathic Healthcare Association (AOHA) membership ○ American Osteopathic Association (AOA) accreditation △ Commission on Accreditation of Rehabilitation Facilities (CARF) accreditation Control codes 61, 63, 64, 71, 72 and 73 indicate hospitals listed by AOHA, but not registered by AHA. For definition of numerical codes, see page A4	Control	Service	Staffed Beds	Admissions	Census	Outpatient Visits	Births	Total	Payroll	Personnel
MCCALL—Valley County										
★ MCCALL MEMORIAL HOSPITAL, 1000 State Street, Zip 83638; tel. 208/634-2221; Karen J. Kellie, President **A**9 10 **F**8 9 16 17 22 25 32 39 41 43 44 45 48 50 54 70 76 78 **S** Trinity Health, Novi, MI	16	10	15	573	4	14831	73	5937	2048	66
MONTPELIER—Bear Lake County										
★ BEAR LAKE MEMORIAL HOSPITAL, 164 South Fifth Street, Zip 83254-1597; tel. 208/847-1630; Rod Jacobson, Administrator (Total facility includes 37 beds in nursing home-type unit) (Nonreporting) **A**9 10	13	10	58	—	—	—	—	—	—	—
MOSCOW—Latah County										
⊞ GRITMAN MEDICAL CENTER, 700 South Main Street, Zip 83843-3047; tel. 208/882-4511 (Nonreporting) **A**1 9 10 **S** Quorum Health Group, Brentwood, TN Web address: www.gritman.org	23	10	35	—	—	—	—	—	—	—
MOUNTAIN HOME—Elmore County										
★ ELMORE MEDICAL CENTER, 895 North Sixth East Street, Zip 83647, Mailing Address: P.O. Box 1270, Zip 83647-1270; tel. 208/587-8401; Gregory L. Maurer, Administrator (Total facility includes 55 beds in nursing home-type unit) (Nonreporting) **A**9 10 **S** Trinity Health, Novi, MI	16	10	78	—	—	—	—	—	—	—
MOUNTAIN HOME AFB—Elmore County										
⊞ U. S. AIR FORCE HOSPITAL MOUNTAIN HOME, 90 Hope Drive, Building 600, Zip 83648-5300; tel. 208/828-7600; Colonel Gwenda McClure, USAF, Commanding Officer (Nonreporting) **A**1 9 **S** Department of the Air Force, Bowling AFB, DC	41	10	29	—	—	—	—	—	—	—
NAMPA—Canyon County										
⊞ MERCY MEDICAL CENTER, 1512 12th Avenue Road, Zip 83686-6008; tel. 208/467-1171; Joseph Messmer, President and Chief Executive Officer (Total facility includes 17 beds in nursing home-type unit) **A**1 9 10 **F**2 3 4 8 9 11 16 17 18 22 24 25 29 31 36 37 39 40 41 44 48 54 69 70 76 78 **P**8 **S** Catholic Health Initiatives, Denver, CO	21	10	149	5944	75	124597	1243	46747	18989	583
OROFINO—Clearwater County										
★ CLEARWATER VALLEY HOSPITAL AND CLINICS, 301 Cedar, Zip 83544-9029; tel. 208/476-4555; Tim Zwickey, Administrator (Nonreporting) **A**9 10 **S** Benedictine Health System, Duluth, MN Web address: www.cvh-clrwater.com	13	10	23	—	—	—	—	—	—	—
STATE HOSPITAL NORTH, 300 Hospital Drive, Zip 83544-9034; tel. 208/476-4511; A. Jay Kessinger, Administrative Director **A**9 **F**2 16 18 43 57 59 70 72 **P**6	12	22	60	280	47	0	0	5532	3455	110
POCATELLO—Bannock County										
⊞ BANNOCK REGIONAL MEDICAL CENTER, 651 Memorial Drive, Zip 83201-4004; tel. 208/239-1000; Fred R. Eaton, Administrator (Total facility includes 118 beds in nursing home-type unit) **A**1 2 3 9 10 **F**4 7 8 9 11 12 13 14 17 19 22 23 24 25 26 27 29 30 32 33 34 35 36 38 39 41 42 43 44 45 46 47 48 49 50 51 52 54 56 65 66 68 69 70 71 72 74 75 76 77 78 79 **P**1 5 8 Web address: www.brmc.org	13	10	238	6019	149	134104	1355	56003	21374	719
⊞ △ POCATELLO REGIONAL MEDICAL CENTER, 777 Hospital Way, Zip 83201-2797; tel. 208/234-0777; Tracy J. Farnsworth, Administrator **A**1 3 7 9 10 **F**4 7 8 9 11 13 14 17 18 19 22 23 24 25 27 28 31 32 34 36 38 39 43 45 48 50 53 54 56 68 69 70 76 78 79 **P**6 **S** Intermountain Health Care, Inc., Salt Lake City, UT Web address: www.ihc.com	23	10	87	2352	30	32422	356	28677	13267	394
PRESTON—Franklin County										
★ FRANKLIN COUNTY MEDICAL CENTER, 44 North First East Street, Zip 83263-1399; tel. 208/852-0137; Michael G. Andrus, Administrator and Chief Executive Officer (Total facility includes 45 beds in nursing home-type unit) **A**9 10 **F**1 3 8 9 13 19 22 23 25 32 34 36 37 43 45 48 49 54 69 70 76 78 **P**1 Web address: www.fcmc.org	13	10	65	531	38	—	139	5482	2917	113
REXBURG—Madison County										
★ MADISON MEMORIAL HOSPITAL, 450 East Main Street, Zip 83440-2048, Mailing Address: P.O. Box 310, Zip 83440-0310; tel. 208/356-3691; Keith M. Steiner, Chief Executive Officer **A**9 10 **F**7 8 9 12 13 14 18 22 23 24 25 32 33 34 39 41 43 44 45 48 50 51 54 70 71 72 76 78 **P**8 Web address: www.rexburg.com/hospital	13	10	52	2766	19	31070	877	20518	7723	276
RUPERT—Minidoka County										
★ MINIDOKA MEMORIAL HOSPITAL AND EXTENDED CARE FACILITY, 1224 Eighth Street, Zip 83350-1599; tel. 208/436-0481; Carl Hanson, Administrator (Total facility includes 75 beds in nursing home-type unit) **A**9 10 **F**8 9 17 18 22 24 25 30 32 34 35 36 37 38 39 41 43 44 45 48 51 54 56 69 70 76 78	13	10	104	770	69	5055	178	11139	5358	178
SAINT MARIES—Benewah County										
★ BENEWAH COMMUNITY HOSPITAL, 229 South Seventh Street, Zip 83861-1894; tel. 208/245-5551; Camille Scott, Administrator **A**9 10 **F**7 8 9 13 16 17 18 19 20 22 25 32 34 38 39 41 43 44 45 46 48 54 56 66 70 71 76 78 79 **P**4 6 7	13	10	25	632	5	18001	83	9261	3282	107
SALMON—Lemhi County										
★ STEELE MEMORIAL HOSPITAL, Main and Daisy Streets, Zip 83467, Mailing Address: P.O. Box 700, Zip 83467-0700; tel. 208/756-4291; Roger Rife, Co-Administrator; Cecil Jackson, Co-Administrator (Nonreporting) **A**9 10 18	13	10	28	—	—	—	—	—	—	—
SANDPOINT—Bonner County										
⊞ BONNER GENERAL HOSPITAL, 520 North Third Avenue, Zip 83864-0877, Mailing Address: Box 1448, Zip 83864-0877; tel. 208/263-1441; Gene Tomt, FACHE, Chief Executive Officer **A**1 9 10 **F**7 8 9 12 13 19 22 25 32 34 35 36 37 38 43 44 48 50 54 61 70 71 76 78 **P**3 8 Web address: www.bonnergen.org	23	10	48	2277	17	36037	388	16929	8584	238

Hospitals, U.S. / IDAHO

	Hospital, Address, Telephone, Administrator, Approval, Facility, and Physician Codes, Health Care System, Network	Classification Codes		Utilization Data					Expense (thousands) of dollars		
		Control	Service	Staffed Beds	Admissions	Census	Outpatient Visits	Births	Total	Payroll	Personnel

Legend:
- ★ American Hospital Association (AHA) membership
- □ Joint Commission on Accreditation of Healthcare Organizations (JCAHO) accreditation
- + American Osteopathic Healthcare Association (AOHA) membership
- ○ American Osteopathic Association (AOA) accreditation
- △ Commission on Accreditation of Rehabilitation Facilities (CARF) accreditation

Control codes 61, 63, 64, 71, 72 and 73 indicate hospitals listed by AOHA, but not registered by AHA. For definition of numerical codes, see page A4.

SODA SPRINGS—Caribou County

★ CARIBOU MEMORIAL HOSPITAL AND LIVING CENTER, (Formerly Caribou Memorial Hospital and Nursing Home), 300 South Third West Street, Zip 83276–1598; tel. 208/547–3341; John L. Hoopes, Chief Executive Officer (Total facility includes 43 beds in nursing home–type unit) (Nonreporting) **A**9 10

Control	Service	Staffed Beds	Admissions	Census	Outpatient Visits	Births	Total	Payroll	Personnel
13	10	65	—	—	—	—	—	—	—

SUN VALLEY—Blaine County

★ WOOD RIVER MEDICAL CENTER, (Includes Blaine County Medical Center, 706 South Main Street, Hailey, Zip 83333, Mailing Address: Box 927, Zip 83333; tel. 208/788–2222; Moritz Community Hospital, Mailing Address: P.O. Box 86, Zip 83353; tel. 208/622–3333), Sun Valley Road, Zip 83353, Mailing Address: P.O. Box 86, Zip 83353–0086; tel. 208/622–3333; Jon Moses, Administrator (Total facility includes 25 beds in nursing home–type unit) (Nonreporting) **A**9 10
Web address: www.wrmc.org

| 15 | 10 | 64 | — | — | — | — | — | — | — |

TWIN FALLS—Twin Falls County

☒ MAGIC VALLEY REGIONAL MEDICAL CENTER, 650 Addison Avenue West, Zip 83301–5444, Mailing Address: P.O. Box 409, Zip 83303–0409; tel. 208/737–2000; Gerald L. Hart, Chief Executive Officer (Total facility includes 20 beds in nursing home–type unit) **A**1 2 9 10 **F**3 4 8 9 11 17 18 22 24 25 30 32 34 36 37 39 41 42 43 44 45 46 48 50 51 52 54 57 58 59 60 61 62 63 65 69 70 75 76 78
Web address: www.mvrmc.org

| 13 | 10 | 180 | 6714 | 79 | 114596 | 1246 | 54834 | 23206 | 789 |

TWIN FALLS CLINIC AND HOSPITAL, 666 Shoshone Street East, Zip 83301–6168, Mailing Address: P.O. Box 1233, Zip 83301–1233; tel. 208/733–3700; Michael Arehart, Chief Executive Officer **A**9 10 **F**9 17 18 19 20 22 24 25 27 28 32 34 39 41 45 46 48 51 56 71 72 76 77 79 **P**2

| 33 | 10 | 38 | 2018 | 22 | 7134 | 0 | 29528 | 13237 | 147 |

WEISER—Washington County

★ MEMORIAL HOSPITAL, 645 East Fifth Street, Zip 83672–2202; tel. 208/549–0370; Anne Oglevie, Administrator **A**9 10 **F**7 8 9 17 18 22 23 25 32 34 36 44 48 70 76 77 78 **P**6

| 16 | 10 | 25 | 454 | 3 | 7378 | 77 | 3894 | 2006 | 62 |

ILLINOIS

Resident Population 12,045 (in thousands)
Resident population in metro areas 84.1%
Birth rate per 1,000 population 15.2
65 years and over 12.4%
Percent of persons without health insurance 12.4%

Hospital, Address, Telephone, Administrator, Approval, Facility, and Physician Codes, Health Care System, Network	Classification Codes		Utilization Data					Expense (thousands) of dollars		
★ American Hospital Association (AHA) membership ☐ Joint Commission on Accreditation of Healthcare Organizations (JCAHO) accreditation + American Osteopathic Healthcare Association (AOHA) membership ○ American Osteopathic Association (AOA) accreditation △ Commission on Accreditation of Rehabilitation Facilities (CARF) accreditation Control codes 61, 63, 64, 71, 72 and 73 indicate hospitals listed by AOHA, but not registered by AHA. For definition of numerical codes, see page A4	Control	Service	Staffed Beds	Admissions	Census	Outpatient Visits	Births	Total	Payroll	Personnel

ALEDO—Mercer County
★ MERCER COUNTY HOSPITAL, 409 N.W. Ninth Avenue, Zip 61231-1296; tel. 309/582-5301; Bruce D. Peterson, Administrator (Total facility includes 18 beds in nursing home-type unit) **A**10 **F**7 9 17 18 19 22 25 26 32 34 36 37 38 40 41 43 44 48 49 54 56 66 69 70 71 72 76 78 **P**6 — 13 10 45 687 25 22921 41 8332 4289 216

ALTON—Madison County
✠ ALTON MEMORIAL HOSPITAL, One Memorial Drive, Zip 62002-6722; tel. 618/463-7311; Ronald B. McMullen, President (Total facility includes 64 beds in nursing home-type unit) **A**1 2 9 10 **F**7 8 9 11 13 17 18 19 22 23 24 25 32 34 36 37 38 39 40 41 43 44 46 48 49 51 54 65 68 69 70 72 76 78 **P**5 8 **S** BJC Health System, Saint Louis, MO
Web address: www.bjc.org — 23 10 202 5448 130 81779 694 56578 23242 663

☐ ALTON MENTAL HEALTH CENTER, 4500 College Avenue, Zip 62002-5099; tel. 618/474-3800; Karl Kruckeberg, Director and Network Manager (Nonreporting) **A**1 10 — 12 22 194 — — — — — — —

✠ △ SAINT ANTHONY'S HEALTH CENTER, (Includes Saint Clare's Hospital, 915 East Fifth Street, Zip 62002-6434; tel. 618/463-5151), 1 Saint Anthony's Way, Zip 62002-4579, Mailing Address: P.O. Box 340, Zip 62002-0340; tel. 618/465-2571; William E. Kessler, President (Total facility includes 42 beds in nursing home-type unit) **A**1 2 7 9 10 **F**1 2 3 4 5 8 9 11 13 14 16 17 18 19 21 22 23 24 25 26 27 30 32 33 34 35 36 37 38 39 40 41 43 44 45 46 48 50 53 54 56 57 59 60 61 62 63 64 65 66 68 69 70 72 76 77 78 79
Web address: www.sahc.org — 23 10 296 6714 93 134832 744 66840 27083 790

ANNA—Union County
☐ CHOATE MENTAL HEALTH CENTER, (Formerly Choate Mental Health and Development Center), 1000 North Main Street, Zip 62906-1699; tel. 618/833-5161; Paul M. Kaufmann, Ph.D., Chief Operating Officer (Nonreporting) **A**1 — 12 22 488 — — — — — — —

✠ UNION COUNTY HOSPITAL DISTRICT, 517 North Main Street, Zip 62906-1696; tel. 618/833-4511; Carol L. Goodman, Administrator and Chief Executive Officer (Total facility includes 22 beds in nursing home-type unit) **A**1 9 10 **F**7 9 13 16 17 18 19 22 24 25 28 30 32 34 36 37 38 43 48 50 51 54 56 69 70 75 76 77 78 — 16 10 58 848 33 44713 — 9829 5212 240

ARLINGTON HEIGHTS—Cook County
✠ NORTHWEST COMMUNITY HEALTHCARE, 800 West Central Road, Zip 60005-2392; tel. 847/618-1000; Bruce K. Crowther, President and Chief Executive Officer **A**1 2 9 10 **F**1 2 3 4 7 8 9 11 12 13 14 16 17 18 19 21 22 24 25 27 28 29 30 31 32 33 34 35 36 37 38 39 41 43 44 45 46 47 48 49 50 51 54 57 58 59 60 61 62 63 64 65 68 69 70 71 72 73 75 76 77 78 79 **P**8
Web address: www.nch.org — 23 10 395 19461 224 354534 2745 194902 89399 2279

AURORA—Du Page and Kane Counties County
✠ PROVENA MERCY CENTER, 1325 North Highland Avenue, Zip 60506; tel. 630/859-2222; John K. Barto, Jr, Interim President and Chief Executive Officer **A**1 2 9 10 **F**2 3 4 6 8 9 11 13 19 22 24 25 26 27 28 29 30 31 32 33 34 35 36 37 38 39 40 41 43 44 45 46 47 48 49 50 51 54 55 56 57 58 59 60 61 62 63 64 65 66 67 68 69 70 71 72 73 74 75 76 77 78 79 **S** Provena Health, Frankfort, IL
Web address: www.provenamercy.com — 21 10 180 11114 126 203764 1253 78846 31725 —

✠ △ RUSH–COPLEY MEDICAL CENTER, 2000 Ogden Avenue, Zip 60504-4206; tel. 630/978-6200; Martin Losoff, President and Chief Executive Officer (Total facility includes 10 beds in nursing home-type unit) **A**1 2 3 5 7 9 10 **F**1 3 4 5 6 8 9 11 12 13 14 15 16 17 18 19 20 21 22 23 24 25 26 27 28 29 30 31 32 33 34 35 36 37 38 39 41 42 43 44 45 46 47 48 49 50 51 53 54 55 56 58 59 60 61 62 63 64 65 66 67 68 69 70 71 72 73 74 75 76 77 78 79 **P**6 7 8 **S** Rush–Presbyterian–St. Luke's Medical Center, Chicago, IL
Web address: www.rushcopley.com — 23 10 142 8548 90 164424 1976 73680 28000 741

BARRINGTON—Lake County
✠ GOOD SHEPHERD HOSPITAL, 450 West Highway 22, Zip 60010-1901; tel. 847/381-9600; Alan Iftiniuk, Chief Executive **A**1 2 9 10 **F**7 8 9 13 17 18 19 21 22 24 25 27 36 38 39 40 41 44 54 56 57 65 68 70 71 72 75 76 78 **P**5 7 8 **S** Advocate Health Care, Oak Brook, IL
Web address: www.advocatehealth.com — 21 10 154 8122 85 99904 1929 80416 33196 909

BELLEVILLE—St. Clair County
✠ MEMORIAL HOSPITAL, 4500 Memorial Drive, Zip 62226-5399; tel. 618/233-7750; Harry R. Maier, President (Total facility includes 108 beds in nursing home-type unit) **A**1 2 9 10 **F**3 4 7 8 9 11 18 22 24 25 27 28 32 34 36 37 38 39 41 44 45 47 48 50 51 54 57 61 63 68 70 71 72 76 78 **P**8
Web address: www.memhosp.com — 23 10 449 15020 261 216245 1492 117410 51406 1722

© 2000 AHA Guide   *Many Facility Codes have changed. Please refer to the AHA Guide Code Chart.*

Hospitals, U.S. / ILLINOIS

Hospital, Address, Telephone, Administrator, Approval, Facility, and Physician Codes, Health Care System, Network	Classification Codes		Utilization Data					Expense (thousands) of dollars		
★ American Hospital Association (AHA) membership ☐ Joint Commission on Accreditation of Healthcare Organizations (JCAHO) accreditation + American Osteopathic Healthcare Association (AOHA) membership ○ American Osteopathic Association (AOA) accreditation △ Commission on Accreditation of Rehabilitation Facilities (CARF) accreditation Control codes 61, 63, 64, 71, 72 and 73 indicate hospitals listed by AOHA, but not registered by AHA. For definition of numerical codes, see page A4	Control	Service	Staffed Beds	Admissions	Census	Outpatient Visits	Births	Total	Payroll	Personnel
★ △ ST. ELIZABETH'S HOSPITAL, 211 South Third Street, Zip 62220–1998; tel. 618/234–2120; Gerald M. Harman, Executive Vice President and Administrator **A**1 2 3 7 9 10 **F**1 2 3 4 5 7 8 9 11 13 14 16 17 18 19 21 22 23 24 25 26 28 29 30 32 33 34 35 36 37 38 39 40 41 42 43 44 45 46 47 48 49 50 51 53 54 57 59 60 61 62 63 64 65 70 71 72 73 76 77 78 **P**8 **S** Hospital Sisters Health System, Springfield, IL Web address: www.steliz.org	21	10	289	12882	207	133684	699	111918	40365	1309
BELVIDERE—Boone County ☐ NORTHWEST SUBURBAN COMMUNITY HOSPITAL, 1625 South State Street, Zip 61008–5900; tel. 815/547–5441; Trevor J. Dyksterhouse, President and Chief Executive Officer (Nonreporting) **A**1 9 10	23	10	69	—	—	—	—	—	—	—
BENTON—Franklin County ★ FRANKLIN HOSPITAL AND SKILLED NURSING CARE UNIT, 201 Bailey Lane, Zip 62812–1999; tel. 618/439–3161; Becky Ashton, Administrator (Total facility includes 83 beds in nursing home–type unit) **A**1 9 10 **F**9 13 16 17 18 22 24 25 30 34 36 37 41 43 48 50 54 56 69 70 76 **P**7 **S** Southern Illinois Hospital Services, Carbondale, IL Web address: www.sih.net	16	10	117	1276	89	18311	—	10192	4524	197
BERWYN—Cook County ★ MACNEAL HOSPITAL, 3249 South Oak Park Avenue, Zip 60402–0715; tel. 708/783–9100; Brian J. Lemon, President (Total facility includes 40 beds in nursing home–type unit) **A**1 2 3 5 8 9 10 **F**2 3 4 8 9 11 12 13 16 17 18 19 21 22 23 24 25 26 29 30 31 32 33 34 35 36 37 38 39 40 43 45 46 48 49 50 51 54 55 56 57 58 59 60 61 62 63 64 65 66 68 69 70 71 72 73 75 76 78 79 **P**5 **S** Vanguard Health System, Nashville, TN Web address: www.macneal.com	23	10	315	18185	237	—	2191	150245	69445	1808
BLOOMINGTON—McLean County ★ OSF ST. JOSEPH MEDICAL CENTER, (Formerly St. Joseph Medical Center), 2200 East Washington Street, Zip 61701–4323; tel. 309/662–3311; Kenneth J. Natzke, Administrator (Total facility includes 13 beds in nursing home–type unit) **A**1 2 9 10 **F**4 7 8 9 11 13 16 17 18 22 24 25 27 29 32 33 34 35 36 37 38 39 41 43 44 45 46 47 48 49 50 51 54 56 65 69 70 71 72 75 76 77 78 **P**6 **S** OSF Healthcare System, Peoria, IL Web address: www.osfhealthcare.org	21	10	154	5688	73	104464	874	69423	28504	831
BLUE ISLAND—Cook County ★ SAINT FRANCIS HOSPITAL AND HEALTH CENTER, 12935 South Gregory Street, Zip 60406–2470; tel. 708/597–2000; Jay E. Kreuzer, FACHE, President **A**1 2 9 10 **F**4 8 9 11 13 16 18 19 22 23 24 25 28 29 33 34 35 36 37 38 40 41 43 44 45 46 47 48 54 59 65 68 70 72 76 77 78 79 **P**6 8 **S** SSM Health Care, Saint Louis, MO Web address: www.stfrancisblueisland.com	21	10	256	13069	153	81436	1113	120841	49777	1157
BREESE—Clinton County ★ ST. JOSEPH'S HOSPITAL, 9515 Holy Cross Lane, Zip 62230–0099; tel. 618/526–4511; Jacolyn M. Schlautman, Executive Vice President and Administrator **A**1 9 10 **F**8 9 16 17 18 22 24 25 32 34 36 37 39 41 44 46 48 54 70 76 78 **S** Hospital Sisters Health System, Springfield, IL	21	10	57	1920	17	48283	424	16674	7191	236
CANTON—Fulton County ★ GRAHAM HOSPITAL, 210 West Walnut Street, Zip 61520–2497; tel. 309/647–5240; D. Ray Slaubaugh, President (Total facility includes 54 beds in nursing home–type unit) **A**1 6 9 10 **F**1 7 8 9 13 16 17 18 19 22 24 25 32 34 36 37 39 41 44 46 48 51 69 70 72 76 78	23	10	124	2758	71	59520	265	26056	12125	—
CARBONDALE—Jackson County ★ MEMORIAL HOSPITAL OF CARBONDALE, 405 West Jackson Street, Zip 62901–1467, Mailing Address: P.O. Box 10000, Zip 62902–9000; tel. 618/549–0721; George Maroney, Senior Vice President and Administrator **A**1 2 3 5 9 10 **F**7 8 9 11 13 16 18 19 22 24 25 27 31 32 33 34 36 37 39 41 42 44 46 48 50 51 54 65 68 70 71 72 74 76 78 **P**7 **S** Southern Illinois Hospital Services, Carbondale, IL Web address: www.sih.net	23	10	132	8116	86	128502	2117	82474	28952	728
CARLINVILLE—Macoupin County ★ CARLINVILLE AREA HOSPITAL, 1001 East Morgan Street, Zip 62626–1499; tel. 217/854–3141; Robert W. Porteus, President and Chief Executive Officer **A**1 9 10 **F**7 9 13 18 22 25 28 30 36 37 38 39 45 48 54 71 76 Web address: www.cahcare.com	23	10	33	1211	14	24552	0	10940	4595	142
CARMI—White County ☐ WHITE COUNTY MEDICAL CENTER, 400 Plum Street, Zip 62821–1799; tel. 618/382–4171; Michael S. Thompson, Administrator (Total facility includes 98 beds in nursing home–type unit) (Nonreporting) **A**1 10	16	10	126	—	—	—	—	—	—	—
CARROLLTON—Greene County ★ THOMAS H. BOYD MEMORIAL HOSPITAL, (Includes Reisch Memorial Nursing Home), 800 School Street, Zip 62016–1498; tel. 217/942–6946; Deborah Campbell, Administrator (Total facility includes 38 beds in nursing home–type unit) (Nonreporting) **A**9 10 18	23	10	60	—	—	—	—	—	—	—
CARTHAGE—Hancock County ★ MEMORIAL HOSPITAL, South Adams Street, Zip 62321, Mailing Address: P.O. Box 160, Zip 62321–0160; tel. 217/357–3131; Keith E. Heuser, Chief Executive Officer **A**9 10 **F**7 8 9 13 17 22 24 25 32 33 37 38 39 40 44 46 48 49 54 63 70 72 76 78 79 **P**5 **S** Quorum Health Group, Brentwood, TN	23	10	59	1015	9	14958	98	8462	3754	127

Hospitals, U.S. / ILLINOIS

Hospital, Address, Telephone, Administrator, Approval, Facility, and Physician Codes, Health Care System, Network	Classification Codes		Utilization Data					Expense (thousands) of dollars		
★ American Hospital Association (AHA) membership ☐ Joint Commission on Accreditation of Healthcare Organizations (JCAHO) accreditation + American Osteopathic Healthcare Association (AOHA) membership ○ American Osteopathic Association (AOA) accreditation △ Commission on Accreditation of Rehabilitation Facilities (CARF) accreditation Control codes 61, 63, 64, 71, 72 and 73 indicate hospitals listed by AOHA, but not registered by AHA. For definition of numerical codes, see page A4	Control	Service	Staffed Beds	Admissions	Census	Outpatient Visits	Births	Total	Payroll	Personnel
CENTRALIA—Marion County										
★ ST. MARY'S HOSPITAL, 400 North Pleasant Avenue, Zip 62801–3091; tel. 618/532–6731; James W. McDowell, President **A**1 2 9 10 **F**1 2 3 7 8 9 11 13 16 17 18 19 21 22 23 25 26 30 31 34 35 36 37 38 39 41 43 44 45 46 48 50 51 54 56 57 58 59 60 61 62 63 64 65 68 70 71 72 74 76 78 79 **P**6 **S** SSM Health Care, Saint Louis, MO	21	10	276	7748	105	83184	537	64383	22900	795
CENTREVILLE—St. Clair County										
☐ TOUCHETTE REGIONAL HOSPITAL, 5900 Bond Avenue, Zip 62207; tel. 618/332–3060; Robert Klutts, Chief Executive Officer (Nonreporting) **A**1 9 10	23	10	104	—	—	—	—	—	—	—
CHAMPAIGN—Champaign County										
☐ THE PAVILION, 809 West Church Street, Zip 61820; tel. 217/373–1700; Nina W. Eisner, Chief Executive Officer (Nonreporting) **A**1 10 **S** Universal Health Services, Inc., King of Prussia, PA	33	22	46	—	—	—	—	—	—	—
CHESTER—Randolph County										
☐ CHESTER MENTAL HEALTH CENTER, Chester Road, Zip 62233–0031, Mailing Address: Box 31, Zip 62233–0031; tel. 618/826–4571; Stephen L. Hardy, Ph.D., Facility Director (Nonreporting) **A**1	12	22	314	—	—	—	—	—	—	—
★ MEMORIAL HOSPITAL, 1900 State Street, Zip 62233–0609, Mailing Address: P.O. Box 609, Zip 62233–0609; tel. 618/826–4581; Eric Freeburg, Administrator **A**1 9 10 **F**3 7 8 9 11 17 18 19 22 23 24 25 27 31 32 34 37 38 39 40 41 43 44 46 48 51 54 59 61 63 70 71 72 76	16	10	43	1181	18	42951	110	12365	5334	192
CHICAGO—Cook County										
BERNARD MITCHELL HOSPITAL See University of Chicago Hospitals										
★ BETHANY HOSPITAL, 3435 West Van Buren Street, Zip 60624–3399; tel. 773/265–7700; Lena Dobbs-Johnson, Chief Executive **A**1 9 10 **F**7 8 9 13 14 16 17 18 19 22 24 25 31 32 34 36 39 41 43 44 45 46 48 55 56 57 61 62 64 66 67 68 70 72 73 74 76 78 79 **P**6 8 **S** Advocate Health Care, Oak Brook, IL **Web address:** www.advocatehealth.com	23	10	102	5981	64	32622	947	44352	17862	384
★ CHICAGO LAKESHORE HOSPITAL, 4840 North Marine Drive, Zip 60640–4296; tel. 773/878–9700; Marcia S. Shapiro, Chief Executive Officer **A**1 3 5 10 **F**2 3 19 57 58 61 62 63 64 70 73	33	22	125	2702	77	15110	—	13013	6296	—
CHICAGO LYING–IN HOSPITAL See University of Chicago Hospitals										
☐ CHICAGO–READ MENTAL HEALTH CENTER, 4200 North Oak Park Avenue, Zip 60634–1457; tel. 773/794–4000; Thomas Simpatico, M.D., Facility Director and Network System Manager **A**1 10 **F**1 3 6 12 13 16 17 18 22 24 25 30 35 39 41 43 45 46 47 48 51 54 55 57 58 59 60 61 63 68 69 70 75 76 78	12	22	200	1599	184	0	0	34368	25685	518
CHILDREN'S HOSPITAL See University of Chicago Hospitals										
★ CHILDREN'S MEMORIAL HOSPITAL, 2300 Children's Plaza, Zip 60614–3394; tel. 773/880–4000; Patrick M. Magoon, President and Chief Executive Officer **A**1 2 3 5 8 9 10 **F**4 5 7 11 13 14 17 18 19 21 22 23 24 25 29 32 33 34 35 36 38 39 42 43 46 47 48 49 50 51 52 54 56 57 58 59 60 61 63 64 65 68 70 72 74 75 76 77 78 **P**8 **Web address:** www.childrensmemorial.org	23	50	218	8142	144	265785	0	220492	106522	—
★ COLUMBUS HOSPITAL, 2520 North Lakeview Avenue, Zip 60614–1895; tel. 773/388–7300; Arnold Kimmel, Interim President and Chief Executive Officer **A**1 3 5 9 10 **F**3 4 5 7 9 11 12 13 14 17 18 19 22 24 25 26 29 30 31 32 33 34 35 36 37 38 39 41 43 44 45 46 47 48 49 50 51 53 54 56 57 59 60 61 62 64 65 66 69 70 71 72 76 77 78 79 **P**6 8 **S** Catholic Health Partners, Chicago, IL **Web address:** www.cath–health.org	21	10	128	3304	72	24660	0	60971	21865	557
★ COOK COUNTY HOSPITAL, 1835 West Harrison, Zip 60612–3785; tel. 312/633–6000; Lacy Thomas, Director (Nonreporting) **A**1 2 3 5 8 9 10 12 **F**3 4 5 7 8 9 10 11 12 13 14 19 20 21 22 23 24 25 27 29 30 32 33 34 35 37 38 39 40 41 42 43 44 45 46 47 48 49 50 51 52 53 54 56 58 59 61 63 65 66 70 72 73 75 76 77 78 **S** Cook County Bureau of Health Services, Chicago, IL	13	10	593	24082	367	741111	1794	525926	301198	5026
★ EDGEWATER MEDICAL CENTER, 5700 North Ashland Avenue, Zip 60660–4086; tel. 773/878–6000; Joann A. Skvarek, Chief Executive Officer (Nonreporting) **A**1 2 10	23	10	215	—	—	—	—	—	—	—
★ △ GRANT HOSPITAL, 550 Webster Avenue, Zip 60614–9980; tel. 773/883–2000; Celeste L. Suchocki, Chief Executive Officer (Total facility includes 33 beds in nursing home–type unit) (Nonreporting) **A**1 7 9 10	23	10	213	—	—	—	—	—	—	—
☐ HARTGROVE HOSPITAL, 520 North Ridgeway Avenue, Zip 60624–1299; tel. 773/722–3113; Suzanne Barry, Administrator and Chief Operating Officer **A**1 10 **F**3 57 58 59 60 61 62 64 70 **S** Universal Health Services, Inc., King of Prussia, PA	33	22	128	2368	93	7123	0	—	—	254
★ HOLY CROSS HOSPITAL, 2701 West 68th Street, Zip 60629–1882; tel. 773/471–8000; Michael J. Peterson, Interim Chief Executive Officer (Total facility includes 37 beds in nursing home–type unit) **A**1 2 9 10 **F**7 8 9 11 12 13 14 17 18 19 22 24 25 31 33 34 36 37 38 39 41 43 44 45 46 48 50 51 53 54 61 69 70 72 76 78 79 **P**6 8	23	10	282	12784	169	156137	1340	111766	61244	1269
★ ILLINOIS MASONIC MEDICAL CENTER, 836 West Wellington Avenue, Zip 60657–5193; tel. 773/975–1600; Bruce C. Campbell, President and Chief Executive Officer (Total facility includes 224 beds in nursing home–type unit) **A**1 2 3 5 8 9 10 12 **F**1 3 4 5 6 7 8 9 11 13 14 16 17 18 19 20 21 22 23 24 25 26 29 30 31 32 33 34 35 36 37 38 39 43 45 46 47 48 49 50 51 54 56 58 59 60 61 62 63 64 65 66 68 70 71 72 73 74 75 76 77 78 79 **P**5 **Web address:** www.immc.org	23	10	550	19674	418	368240	3849	252301	134234	3019

Hospitals, U.S. / ILLINOIS

Hospital, Address, Telephone, Administrator, Approval, Facility, and Physician Codes, Health Care System, Network	Classification Codes		Utilization Data					Expense (thousands) of dollars		Personnel
★ American Hospital Association (AHA) membership ☐ Joint Commission on Accreditation of Healthcare Organizations (JCAHO) accreditation + American Osteopathic Healthcare Association (AOHA) membership ○ American Osteopathic Association (AOA) accreditation △ Commission on Accreditation of Rehabilitation Facilities (CARF) accreditation Control codes 61, 63, 64, 71, 72 and 73 indicate hospitals listed by AOHA, but not registered by AHA. For definition of numerical codes, see page A4	Control	Service	Staffed Beds	Admissions	Census	Outpatient Visits	Births	Total	Payroll	
☐ JACKSON PARK HOSPITAL AND MEDICAL CENTER, 7531 Stony Island Avenue, Zip 60649–3993; tel. 773/947–7500; Peter E. Friedell, M.D., President (Nonreporting) **A**1 2 3 9 10	23	10	254	—	—	—	—	—	—	—
JOHNSTON R. BOWMAN HEALTH CENTER See Rush–Presbyterian–St. Luke's Medical Center										
★ LARABIDA CHILDREN'S HOSPITAL AND RESEARCH CENTER, East 65th Street at Lake Michigan, Zip 60649–1395; tel. 773/363–6700; Paula Kienberger Jaudes, M.D., President and Chief Executive Officer **A**1 5 9 10 **F**13 14 19 22 23 24 25 31 32 38 39 50 54 55 56 68 70 72 75 76 77 78	23	58	62	1210	34	27342	0	26287	12657	381
☐ LORETTO HOSPITAL, 645 South Central Avenue, Zip 60644–9987; tel. 773/626–4300; Steve C. Drucker, President and Chief Executive Officer **A**1 10 **F**2 3 9 16 17 18 21 22 24 25 29 32 38 41 43 45 48 54 57 61 63 70 72 76 **P**5	23	10	223	5266	109	27970	0	32463	16606	461
★ LOUIS A. WEISS MEMORIAL HOSPITAL, 4646 North Marine Drive, Zip 60640–1501; tel. 773/564–5000; Edward A. Cucci, President (Nonreporting) **A**1 2 3 5 9 10 **S** The University of Chicago Hospitals and Health System, Chicago, IL **Web address:** www.weisshospital.org	23	10	200	—	—	—	—	—	—	—
★ MERCY HOSPITAL AND MEDICAL CENTER, 2525 South Michigan Avenue, Zip 60616–2477; tel. 312/567–2000; Dennis Patterson, Interim President and Chief Executive Officer (Total facility includes 28 beds in nursing home–type unit) **A**1 2 3 5 8 9 10 **F**2 3 4 5 8 9 11 12 13 14 17 18 19 20 21 22 23 24 25 26 29 30 31 32 34 35 36 37 38 39 41 43 44 46 47 48 49 50 51 53 54 56 57 58 59 63 64 65 66 68 69 72 73 76 78 **P**5 6 7 **Web address:** www.mercy-chicago.org	21	10	339	16504	207	107811	2643	165792	84958	2350
☐ METHODIST HOSPITAL OF CHICAGO, 5025 North Paulina Street, Zip 60640–2797; tel. 773/271–9040; Steven H. Friedman, Ph.D., Executive Vice President (Total facility includes 17 beds in nursing home–type unit) (Nonreporting) **A**1 2 10	23	10	189	—	—	—	—	—	—	—
★ △ MICHAEL REESE HOSPITAL AND MEDICAL CENTER, 2929 South Ellis Avenue, Zip 60616–3376; tel. 312/791–2000; Stephen M. Weinstein, President (Nonreporting) **A**1 2 3 5 7 8 9 10 **S** Doctors Community Healthcare Corporation, Scottsdale, AZ	33	10	523	—	—	—	—	—	—	—
★ MOUNT SINAI HOSPITAL MEDICAL CENTER OF CHICAGO, California Avenue and 15th Street, Zip 60608–1610; tel. 773/542–2000; Kenneth A. Richmond, President and Chief Executive Officer (Nonreporting) **A**1 2 3 5 8 9 10 **Web address:** www.sinai.org	23	10	315	—	—	—	—	—	—	—
★ NORTHWESTERN MEMORIAL HOSPITAL, (Includes Norman and Ida Stone Institute of Psychiatry, 320 East Huron Street; Prentice Women's Hospital, 333 East Superior Street), 251 East Huron Street, Zip 60611; tel. 312/926–2000; Gary A. Mecklenburg, President and Chief Executive Officer **A**1 2 3 5 8 9 10 **F**3 4 5 7 8 9 11 12 13 15 16 17 18 19 20 21 22 23 24 25 26 27 30 31 32 33 34 35 36 37 38 39 41 42 43 45 46 47 48 49 50 51 54 56 57 58 59 60 61 62 63 64 65 66 68 70 71 72 74 75 76 78 79 **P**5 6 8 **Web address:** www.nmh.org	23	10	642	30786	432	273572	6991	454385	203835	5197
☐ NORWEGIAN–AMERICAN HOSPITAL, Mailing Address: 1044 North Francisco Avenue, Zip 60622–2794; tel. 773/292–8200; Michael J. O'Grady, Jr, Interim President and Chief Executive Officer (Nonreporting) **A**1 9 10	23	10	230	—	—	—	—	—	—	—
★ OUR LADY OF THE RESURRECTION MEDICAL CENTER, 5645 West Addison Street, Zip 60634–4455; tel. 773/282–7000; Ronald E. Struxness, Executive Vice President and Chief Executive Officer (Total facility includes 66 beds in nursing home–type unit) **A**1 2 9 10 **F**1 2 3 4 6 7 8 9 10 11 12 13 17 18 19 20 21 22 23 24 25 28 29 30 31 32 33 34 35 36 37 38 39 40 41 42 43 44 45 46 47 48 49 50 51 52 53 54 55 57 58 59 60 61 62 63 64 65 66 67 68 69 70 72 74 76 77 78 79 **P**5 6 **S** Resurrection Health Care Corporation, Chicago, IL **Web address:** www.reshealthcare.org	21	10	282	11175	208	119520	0	83417	35694	1012
PRENTICE WOMEN'S HOSPITAL See Northwestern Memorial Hospital										
★ PROVIDENT HOSPITAL OF COOK COUNTY, 500 East 51st Street, Zip 60615–2494; tel. 312/572–2000; Stephanie Wright-Griggs, Chief Operating Officer **A**1 3 10 **F**2 3 4 5 8 9 10 11 12 13 14 16 17 18 19 21 22 23 24 25 27 29 30 32 33 34 35 38 39 41 42 44 45 46 47 48 50 51 52 54 57 65 68 69 70 71 72 73 74 75 76 77 78 79 **P**6 **S** Cook County Bureau of Health Services, Chicago, IL	13	10	113	5578	71	115084	895	91832	41247	806
★ △ RAVENSWOOD HOSPITAL MEDICAL CENTER, 4550 North Winchester Avenue, Zip 60640–5205; tel. 773/878–4300; John E. Blair, Chief Executive **A**1 2 3 5 6 7 9 10 **F**2 3 4 5 8 9 11 12 13 14 16 17 18 19 20 21 22 24 25 28 29 30 31 33 34 35 36 37 41 43 44 45 47 48 51 53 54 56 57 58 59 60 61 62 63 64 66 68 69 70 72 73 76 77 78 79 **P**1 **S** Advocate Health Care, Oak Brook, IL **Web address:** www.advocatehealth.com	23	10	324	12569	173	216628	1677	119297	55870	1506
★ △ REHABILITATION INSTITUTE OF CHICAGO, 345 East Superior Street, Zip 60611–4496; tel. 312/238–1000; Wayne M. Lerner, DPH, President and Chief Executive Officer **A**1 3 5 7 8 9 10 **F**5 13 16 17 18 22 24 30 33 34 38 39 45 49 50 53 54 55 68 70 71 76 78 79 **P**6 **Web address:** www.rehabchicago.org	23	46	155	2080	118	64920	0	56706	31246	808

Hospitals, U.S. / ILLINOIS

Hospital, Address, Telephone, Administrator, Approval, Facility, and Physician Codes, Health Care System, Network	Classification Codes		Utilization Data					Expense (thousands) of dollars		
★ American Hospital Association (AHA) membership ☐ Joint Commission on Accreditation of Healthcare Organizations (JCAHO) accreditation + American Osteopathic Healthcare Association (AOHA) membership ○ American Osteopathic Association (AOA) accreditation △ Commission on Accreditation of Rehabilitation Facilities (CARF) accreditation Control codes 61, 63, 64, 71, 72 and 73 indicate hospitals listed by AOHA, but not registered by AHA. For definition of numerical codes, see page A4	Control	Service	Staffed Beds	Admissions	Census	Outpatient Visits	Births	Total	Payroll	Personnel
★ △ RESURRECTION MEDICAL CENTER, 7435 West Talcott Avenue, Zip 60631–3746; tel. 773/774–8000; Sister Donna Marie, Executive Vice President and Chief Executive Officer (Total facility includes 298 beds in nursing home–type unit) **A**1 2 3 5 7 9 10 **F**3 4 7 8 9 11 17 18 19 22 24 25 28 33 35 36 38 39 41 42 44 45 46 47 48 49 50 51 53 54 58 59 60 61 62 63 64 65 69 70 71 72 76 78 79 **P**1 5 6 7 **S** Resurrection Health Care Corporation, Chicago, IL **Web address:** www.reshealthcare.org	21	10	667	19007	542	217305	1257	189960	77719	—
★ ROSELAND COMMUNITY HOSPITAL, 45 West 111th Street, Zip 60628–4294; tel. 773/995–3000; Oliver D. Krage, President and Chief Executive Officer **A**1 9 10 **F**7 9 13 16 18 19 22 24 25 29 30 31 32 34 35 37 38 41 43 44 46 48 50 51 54 56 59 61 70 72 76 77 78 **P**1	23	10	128	6399	70	58495	670	30476	14114	390
★ △ RUSH–PRESBYTERIAN–ST. LUKE'S MEDICAL CENTER, (Includes Johnston R. Bowman Health Center, 700 South Paulina, Zip 60612; tel. 312/942–7000; James T. Frankenbach, Senior Vice President, Corporate and Hospital Affairs), 1653 West Congress Parkway, Zip 60612–3833; tel. 312/942–5000; Leo M. Henikoff, M.D., President and Chief Executive Officer (Total facility includes 44 beds in nursing home–type unit) **A**1 2 3 5 7 8 9 10 **F**1 3 4 5 6 7 8 9 11 12 13 14 19 20 21 22 23 24 25 26 27 29 30 32 33 34 35 36 37 38 39 41 42 43 44 45 46 47 48 49 50 51 52 53 54 55 56 57 58 59 60 61 62 63 64 65 66 68 69 70 71 72 73 74 76 78 79 **P**6 7 8 **S** Rush–Presbyterian–St. Luke's Medical Center, Chicago, IL **Web address:** www.rush.edu	23	10	713	26493	492	185536	1852	530815	249609	7704
☐ SACRED HEART HOSPITAL, 3240 West Franklin Boulevard, Zip 60624–1599; tel. 773/722–3020; Edward Novak, President and Chief Executive Officer (Nonreporting) **A**1 10	33	10	96	—	—	—	—	—	—	—
★ SAINT ANTHONY HOSPITAL, 2875 West 19th Street, Zip 60623–3596; tel. 773/521–1710; Arnold Kimmel, Interim President and Chief Executive Officer **A**1 3 9 10 **F**3 4 5 8 9 11 12 13 14 17 18 19 22 24 25 29 31 32 33 34 35 36 37 38 39 41 42 43 44 45 46 47 48 49 50 51 53 54 57 59 60 61 62 63 64 65 66 68 69 70 71 72 76 77 78 79 **P**6 8 **S** Catholic Health Partners, Chicago, IL **Web address:** www.cath–health.org	21	10	163	7717	105	53972	2069	53261	25432	655
★ SAINT MARY OF NAZARETH HOSPITAL CENTER, 2233 West Division Street, Zip 60622–3086; tel. 312/770–2000; Sister Sally Marie Kiepura, President and Chief Executive Officer (Total facility includes 20 beds in nursing home–type unit) **A**1 2 3 9 10 **F**4 7 8 9 11 12 17 19 22 24 25 30 31 32 33 34 35 36 37 38 39 41 43 44 45 46 47 48 53 54 57 58 59 60 61 62 63 64 65 68 70 72 76 77 78 79 **P**5 6 8 **S** Sisters of the Holy Family of Nazareth–Sacred Heart Province, Des Plaines, IL **Web address:** www.stmaryofnazareth.org	23	10	325	14211	197	167273	1736	113012	54735	1369
★ △ SCHWAB REHABILITATION HOSPITAL AND CARE NETWORK, 1401 South California Boulevard, Zip 60608–1612; tel. 773/522–2010; Judith C. Waterston, President and Chief Executive Officer (Total facility includes 20 beds in nursing home–type unit) **A**1 3 7 8 9 10 **F**4 5 8 9 11 13 14 16 17 18 19 21 22 24 25 26 29 30 31 32 33 34 35 36 38 39 41 42 44 45 46 47 48 49 51 52 53 54 56 57 58 62 63 65 67 69 71 72 75 76 78 **P**6 **Web address:** www.schwabrehab.org	23	46	107	1416	90	114812	0	29801	17072	416
★ SHRINERS HOSPITALS FOR CHILDREN–CHICAGO, 2211 North Oak Park Avenue, Zip 60707; tel. 773/622–5400; A. James Spang, Administrator **A**1 3 5 **F**5 13 14 17 18 19 22 23 24 31 38 39 43 45 48 49 50 52 53 54 59 70 71 72 73 76 78 **P**6 **S** Shriners Hospitals for Children, Tampa, FL **Web address:** www.shrinerschicago.org	23	57	60	1684	25	17199	0	—	—	236
★ SOUTH SHORE HOSPITAL, 8012 South Crandon Avenue, Zip 60617–1199; tel. 773/768–0810; Jesus M. Ong, President **A**1 10 **F**2 9 13 19 22 24 25 32 35 37 41 48 50 51 54 70 76 78 **P**5 7 8	23	10	125	5033	72	—	—	28342	15761	—
☐ ST. BERNARD HOSPITAL AND HEALTH CARE CENTER, 326 West 64th Street, Zip 60621; tel. 773/962–3900; Sister Elizabeth Van Straten, President and Chief Executive Officer (Nonreporting) **A**1 10	21	10	194	—	—	—	—	—	—	—
★ ST. ELIZABETH'S HOSPITAL, 1431 North Claremont Avenue, Zip 60622–1791; tel. 773/278–2000; JoAnn Birdzell, President and Chief Executive Officer (Total facility includes 26 beds in nursing home–type unit) **A**1 2 3 9 10 **F**2 3 4 5 8 9 11 14 16 17 18 19 21 22 25 26 27 29 30 31 32 33 34 35 36 38 40 41 43 44 45 46 48 49 50 51 54 56 59 60 61 62 63 64 69 70 72 75 76 78 **P**3 6 7 8 **S** Ancilla Systems Inc., Hobart, IN **Web address:** www.ancilla.org	23	10	250	11112	160	84476	914	73161	34689	1001
★ ST. JOSEPH HOSPITAL, 2900 North Lake Shore Drive, Zip 60657–6274; tel. 773/665–3000; Arnold Kimmel, Interim President and Chief Executive Officer **A**1 2 3 5 9 10 **F**3 4 5 8 9 11 12 13 14 17 18 19 22 24 25 26 29 30 31 32 33 34 35 36 37 38 39 41 42 44 45 46 47 48 49 50 51 52 53 54 54 55 56 57 59 60 61 62 63 64 65 66 68 69 70 71 72 76 77 78 79 **P**6 8 **S** Catholic Health Partners, Chicago, IL **Web address:** www.cath–health.org	21	10	408	13342	227	75884	2169	134143	57206	1457
★ SWEDISH COVENANT HOSPITAL, 5145 North California Avenue, Zip 60625–3688; tel. 773/878–8200; Mark Newton, President and Chief Executive Officer (Nonreporting) **A**1 2 3 5 9 10	21	10	280	—	—	—	—	—	—	—

© 2000 AHA Guide *Many Facility Codes have changed. Please refer to the AHA Guide Code Chart.*

Hospitals, U.S. / ILLINOIS

Hospital, Address, Telephone, Administrator, Approval, Facility, and Physician Codes, Health Care System, Network	Classification Codes		Utilization Data					Expense (thousands) of dollars		
	Control	Service	Staffed Beds	Admissions	Census	Outpatient Visits	Births	Total	Payroll	Personnel

★ American Hospital Association (AHA) membership
☐ Joint Commission on Accreditation of Healthcare Organizations (JCAHO) accreditation
+ American Osteopathic Healthcare Association (AOHA) membership
○ American Osteopathic Association (AOA) accreditation
△ Commission on Accreditation of Rehabilitation Facilities (CARF) accreditation
Control codes 61, 63, 64, 71, 72 and 73 indicate hospitals listed by AOHA, but not registered by AHA. For definition of numerical codes, see page A4

Hospital	Control	Service	Staffed Beds	Admissions	Census	Outpatient Visits	Births	Total	Payroll	Personnel
★ THOREK HOSPITAL AND MEDICAL CENTER, 850 West Irving Park Road, Zip 60613–3099; tel. 773/525–6780; Frank A. Solare, President and Chief Executive Officer **A**1 9 10 **F**7 9 16 17 18 19 22 24 25 27 31 32 34 35 37 38 39 40 41 43 45 46 48 49 54 65 70 72 76 78 **P**8 **Web address:** www.thorek.org	23	10	137	4630	68	137540	0	43186	19737	456
★ TRINITY HOSPITAL, 2320 East 93rd Street, Zip 60617–9984; tel. 773/978–2000; John N. Schwartz, Chief Executive Officer **A**1 10 **F**2 3 4 7 8 9 11 13 14 17 18 19 22 23 24 25 26 28 31 32 33 34 36 38 39 41 43 44 45 46 48 49 50 51 54 56 59 63 64 66 67 70 72 73 76 77 78 79 **P**8 **S** Advocate Health Care, Oak Brook, IL **Web address:** www.advocatehealth.com	21	10	217	10480	129	96422	1710	80248	34406	809
★ UNIVERSITY OF CHICAGO HOSPITALS, (Includes Bernard Mitchell Hospital; Chicago Lying–in Hospital; Children's Hospital), 5841 South Maryland Avenue, Zip 60637–1470; tel. 773/702–1000; Ralph W. Muller, President and Chief Executive Officer **A**1 2 3 5 8 9 10 **F**4 5 8 9 10 11 12 13 14 17 18 19 22 23 24 25 27 29 30 31 32 34 35 37 38 39 41 42 43 44 46 47 48 49 50 51 52 53 54 55 56 58 59 60 61 62 63 64 65 66 68 70 71 72 74 75 76 78 79 **P**6 **S** The University of Chicago Hospitals and Health System, Chicago, IL	23	10	533	24487	411	443890	3184	472871	210345	5001
★ △ UNIVERSITY OF ILLINOIS AT CHICAGO MEDICAL CENTER, 1740 West Taylor Street, Zip 60612–7236; tel. 312/996–7000; John J. DeNardo, Executive Director **A**1 2 3 5 7 8 10 **F**3 4 5 8 9 11 12 13 16 17 18 19 21 22 23 24 25 27 29 30 31 32 33 34 35 38 39 41 42 43 44 45 46 47 48 49 50 51 52 53 54 56 57 58 59 60 61 62 63 64 65 66 70 71 72 73 74 75 76 78 79 **P**4 7 **Web address:** www.hospital.uic.edu	12	10	432	16871	295	417868	2390	309001	153091	2310
VENCOR HOSPITAL–CHICAGO CENTRAL, 4058 West Melrose Street, Zip 60641–4797; tel. 773/736–7000; Richard Cerceo, Administrator (Nonreporting) **A**10 **S** Vencor, Incorporated, Louisville, KY **Web address:** www.vencor.com	33	10	81	—	—	—	—	—	—	—
VENCOR HOSPITAL–CHICAGO NORTH, (LONG TERM ACUTE CARE), 2544 West Montrose Avenue, Zip 60618–1589; tel. 773/267–2622; Susan Legg, Administrator **F**22 23 25 26 31 39 41 49 50 51 57 70 **S** Vencor, Incorporated, Louisville, KY **Web address:** www.vencor.com	33	49	164	1519	136	0	0	35706	12794	378
★ VETERANS AFFAIRS CHICAGO HEALTH CARE SYSTEM, (Includes Veterans Affairs Chicago Health Care System, 333 East Huron Street, tel. 312/640–2100; Veterans Affairs Chicago Health Care System, 820 South Damon, Zip 60612–3776; tel. 312/943–6600), 333 East Huron Street, Zip 60611–3004; tel. 312/640–2100; Richard S. Citron, Director **A**1 2 3 5 8 **F**3 4 9 11 12 13 16 17 18 19 21 22 23 24 25 27 29 30 31 32 33 34 35 36 37 38 39 41 43 45 46 47 48 49 50 51 53 54 55 56 57 59 60 61 62 63 64 65 70 72 74 76 77 78 79 **S** Department of Veterans Affairs, Washington, DC	45	10	325	10722	267	489000	0	204783	124045	2091

CHICAGO HEIGHTS—Cook County

Hospital	Control	Service	Staffed Beds	Admissions	Census	Outpatient Visits	Births	Total	Payroll	Personnel
★ ST. JAMES HOSPITAL AND HEALTH CENTERS – CHICAGO HEIGHTS CAMPUS, 1423 Chicago Road, Zip 60411–3483; tel. 708/756–1000; Peter J. Murphy, President and Chief Executive Officer (Total facility includes 101 beds in nursing home–type unit) (Nonreporting) **A**1 2 9 10 **S** Sisters of St. Francis Health Services, Inc., Mishawaka, IN **Web address:** www.st jameshhc.org	21	10	332	—	—	—	—	—	—	—

CLINTON—Dewitt County

Hospital	Control	Service	Staffed Beds	Admissions	Census	Outpatient Visits	Births	Total	Payroll	Personnel
★ DR. JOHN WARNER HOSPITAL, 422 West White Street, Zip 61727–2199; tel. 217/935–9571; Hervey Davis, Administrator (Total facility includes 9 beds in nursing home–type unit) **A**9 10 18 **F**7 9 12 17 18 22 23 25 36 38 39 48 50 54 59 69 70 71 76	14	10	33	746	7	16416	0	9201	4152	215

DANVILLE—Vermilion County

Hospital	Control	Service	Staffed Beds	Admissions	Census	Outpatient Visits	Births	Total	Payroll	Personnel
★ PROVENA UNITED SAMARITANS MEDICAL CENTER, (Includes United Samaritans Medical Center, 600 Sager Avenue, Zip 61832; tel. 217/442–6300), 812 North Logan, Zip 61832–3788; tel. 217/443–5000; James W. Pope, President and Chief Executive Officer (Total facility includes 49 beds in nursing home–type unit) **A**1 2 9 10 **F**8 9 13 16 17 18 19 22 25 27 32 33 34 36 37 38 39 40 41 43 44 45 46 48 49 54 55 57 60 62 63 64 65 69 70 75 76 77 78 79 **P**3 5 7 8 **S** Provena Health, Frankfort, IL **Web address:** www.provenausmc.org	21	10	308	11042	156	232110	1024	85422	36942	—
★ VETERANS AFFAIRS MEDICAL CENTER, 1900 East Main Street, Zip 61832–5198; tel. 217/442–8000; Cathi Spivey-Paul, Acting Director (Total facility includes 175 beds in nursing home–type unit) **A**1 3 5 **F**1 3 6 9 13 16 17 18 19 21 22 23 24 25 26 28 29 30 31 32 33 34 35 36 38 43 45 48 49 50 51 54 56 59 60 62 63 64 68 70 72 74 76 78 79 **P**6 **S** Department of Veterans Affairs, Washington, DC **Web address:** www.va.gov/stations97/guide/home.asp?DIVISION=ALL	45	10	439	4216	431	195441	0	83344	47742	1129

DE KALB—De Kalb County

Hospital	Control	Service	Staffed Beds	Admissions	Census	Outpatient Visits	Births	Total	Payroll	Personnel
★ KISHWAUKEE COMMUNITY HOSPITAL, 626 Bethany Road, Zip 60115–4939, Mailing Address: P.O. Box 707, Zip 60115–0707; tel. 815/756–1521; Brad Copple, Administrator **A**1 2 9 10 **F**7 8 9 16 17 18 22 24 25 30 32 33 34 35 37 39 41 43 44 45 46 48 49 51 54 57 58 59 60 61 62 63 64 65 70 71 72 76 78 79 **P**1 **S** Kishwaukee Health System, De Kalb, IL **Web address:** www.kishhospital.org	23	10	114	4520	40	85386	839	44362	17235	641

DECATUR—Macon County

Hospital	Control	Service	Staffed Beds	Admissions	Census	Outpatient Visits	Births	Total	Payroll	Personnel
★ DECATUR MEMORIAL HOSPITAL, 2300 North Edward Street, Zip 62526–4192; tel. 217/876–8121; Kenneth L. Smithmier, President and Chief Executive Officer (Total facility includes 69 beds in nursing home–type unit) **A**1 2 3 5 9 10 **F**7 8 9 11 13 15 16 17 19 22 26 27 30 31 32 33 35 36 37 38 39 40 41 43 44 45 46 48 49 50 54 65 68 69 70 71 72 76 78 79 **P**6 8 **Web address:** www.dmhhs.org	23	10	243	10427	144	243623	1025	105091	46068	1531

Hospitals, U.S. / ILLINOIS

Hospital, Address, Telephone, Administrator, Approval, Facility, and Physician Codes, Health Care System, Network	Classification Codes		Utilization Data					Expense (thousands) of dollars		
★ American Hospital Association (AHA) membership □ Joint Commission on Accreditation of Healthcare Organizations (JCAHO) accreditation + American Osteopathic Healthcare Association (AOHA) membership ○ American Osteopathic Association (AOA) accreditation △ Commission on Accreditation of Rehabilitation Facilities (CARF) accreditation Control codes 61, 63, 64, 71, 72 and 73 indicate hospitals listed by AOHA, but not registered by AHA. For definition of numerical codes, see page A4	Control	Service	Staffed Beds	Admissions	Census	Outpatient Visits	Births	Total	Payroll	Personnel
✠ ST. MARY'S HOSPITAL, 1800 East Lake Shore Drive, Zip 62521–3883; tel. 217/464–2966; Anthony D. Pfitzer, Executive Vice President and Administrator (Total facility includes 45 beds in nursing home–type unit) **A**1 3 5 9 10 **F**1 3 8 9 13 16 17 18 19 21 22 24 25 27 30 31 32 33 34 36 37 38 39 40 41 43 44 45 46 48 49 50 52 54 57 58 59 60 61 62 63 64 65 69 70 72 76 78 **P**7 **S** Hospital Sisters Health System, Springfield, IL Web address: www.stmarys–hospital.com	21	10	176	9164	131	97768	716	69685	28587	967
DES PLAINES—Cook County										
□ HOLY FAMILY MEDICAL CENTER, 100 North River Road, Zip 60016–1255; tel. 847/297–1800; Sister Patricia Ann Koschalke, President and Chief Executive Officer (Nonreporting) **A**1 2 9 10 **S** Sisters of the Holy Family of Nazareth–Sacred Heart Province, Des Plaines, IL	23	10	183	—	—	—	—	—	—	—
DIXON—Lee County										
★ KATHERINE SHAW BETHEA HOSPITAL, 403 East First Street, Zip 61021–3187; tel. 815/288–5531; Darryl L. Vandervort, President and Chief Executive Officer (Total facility includes 15 beds in nursing home–type unit) **A**9 10 **F**1 3 7 8 9 12 13 16 17 18 19 20 22 23 25 28 30 31 32 33 34 35 37 38 39 40 41 43 44 45 46 48 50 51 54 56 57 58 59 60 61 62 63 64 65 67 68 69 70 71 72 76 78 **P**6 Web address: www.ksbhospital.com	23	10	100	3632	43	60710	324	39709	18377	485
DOWNERS GROVE—Du Page County										
✠ GOOD SAMARITAN HOSPITAL, 3815 Highland Avenue, Zip 60515–1590; tel. 630/275–5900; Jonathan R. Bruss, Chief Executive (Total facility includes 20 beds in nursing home–type unit) **A**1 2 9 10 **F**1 4 7 8 9 11 12 13 14 17 18 19 20 22 24 25 27 28 29 30 31 32 33 34 35 36 37 38 39 41 42 43 44 45 46 47 48 49 54 57 58 59 60 61 62 63 64 65 67 68 69 70 71 72 75 76 77 78 79 **P**7 8 **S** Advocate Health Care, Oak Brook, IL Web address: www.advocatehealth.com	21	10	258	15229	208	150935	2123	157157	62812	2750
DU QUOIN—Perry County										
✠ MARSHALL BROWNING HOSPITAL, 900 North Washington Street, Zip 62832–1230, Mailing Address: P.O. Box 192, Zip 62832–0192; tel. 618/542–2146; William J. Huff, Chief Executive Officer **A**1 9 10 **F**6 7 8 9 16 17 18 19 22 24 25 37 38 39 40 43 44 48 54 70 71 76	23	10	33	729	9	18852	33	8012	3267	121
EAST ST. LOUIS—St. Clair County										
✠ ST. MARY'S HOSPITAL OF EAST ST. LOUIS, 129 North Eighth Street, Zip 62201–2999; tel. 618/274–1900; Richard J. Mark, President and Chief Executive Officer **A**1 9 10 **F**2 3 9 13 14 16 17 18 19 21 22 23 25 31 32 33 34 35 36 37 38 41 43 48 49 50 51 54 57 58 59 60 63 64 70 72 75 76 78 79 **P**5 **S** Ancilla Systems Inc., Hobart, IN Web address: www.ancilla.org	23	10	119	4008	58	89067	0	33167	15992	531
EFFINGHAM—Effingham County										
✠ ST. ANTHONY'S MEMORIAL HOSPITAL, 503 North Maple Street, Zip 62401–2099; tel. 217/342–2121; Daniel J. Woods, Executive Vice President and Administrator (Total facility includes 13 beds in nursing home–type unit) **A**1 2 9 10 **F**7 8 9 16 17 18 22 24 25 27 32 36 37 38 39 40 41 44 46 48 54 65 68 69 70 72 76 78 **S** Hospital Sisters Health System, Springfield, IL Web address: www.stanthonyhospital.org	21	10	146	6431	78	175979	708	46375	17507	530
ELDORADO—Saline County										
★ FERRELL HOSPITAL, 1201 Pine Street, Zip 62930–1634; tel. 618/273–3361; William Hartley, Administrator **A**9 10 **F**7 13 22 25 34 38 48 54 70 76 **P**7 **S** Southern Illinois Hospital Services, Carbondale, IL Web address: www.sih.net	23	10	36	1294	18	7685	0	9400	3720	194
ELGIN—Kane County										
□ ELGIN MENTAL HEALTH CENTER, 750 South State Street, Zip 60123–7692; tel. 847/742–1040; Nancy Staples, Administrator **A**1 10 **F**9 12 17 23 25 41 44 46 50 51 57 70 75 78 **P**6	12	22	500	1409	530	0	0	64216	47924	1173
✠ △ PROVENA SAINT JOSEPH HOSPITAL, 77 North Airlite Street, Zip 60123–4912; tel. 847/695–3200; Larry Narum, President **A**1 2 7 9 10 **F**3 7 8 9 11 13 17 18 19 22 24 25 29 30 31 32 33 35 36 37 38 39 40 41 43 44 45 46 48 49 50 51 53 54 57 58 59 60 61 62 63 64 65 70 71 72 75 76 77 78 79 **P**5 **S** Provena Health, Frankfort, IL Web address: www.provenahealth.com	23	10	183	7019	106	243767	1129	73812	30084	894
✠ SHERMAN HOSPITAL, 934 Center Street, Zip 60120–2198; tel. 847/429–8000; John A. Graham, President and Chief Executive Officer **A**1 2 9 10 **F**4 7 8 9 11 12 13 14 16 17 18 19 22 24 25 27 29 30 31 32 33 34 35 36 37 38 39 40 41 43 44 45 46 47 48 49 50 54 56 60 61 68 69 70 71 72 73 75 76 77 78 79 **P**2 5 7 8 Web address: www.shermanhealth.com	23	10	238	10340	120	114537	1751	113840	43251	1454
ELK GROVE VILLAGE—Cook County										
✠ ALEXIAN BROTHERS MEDICAL CENTER, 800 Biesterfield Road, Zip 60007–3397; tel. 847/437–5500; Nancy R. Hellyer, President and Chief Executive Officer (Nonreporting) **A**1 2 9 10 **S** Alexian Brothers Health System, Inc., Elk Grove Village, IL Web address: www.alexian.org	21	10	391	—	—	—	—	—	—	—
ELMHURST—Du Page County										
✠ ELMHURST MEMORIAL HOSPITAL, 200 Berteau Avenue, Zip 60126–2989; tel. 630/833–1400; Leo F. Fronza, Jr, President and Chief Executive Officer (Total facility includes 38 beds in nursing home–type unit) **A**1 2 9 10 **F**3 4 5 7 8 9 11 12 15 17 18 22 24 25 27 28 29 31 33 34 36 37 38 39 40 41 42 43 44 45 46 47 48 49 50 51 54 57 58 59 60 61 62 63 65 66 68 69 70 72 75 76 78 79 **P**3 4 5 8 Web address: www.emhc.com	23	10	343	14758	232	305873	1908	172323	81787	2291

© 2000 AHA Guide *Many Facility Codes have changed. Please refer to the AHA Guide Code Chart.*

Hospitals, U.S. / ILLINOIS

Hospital, Address, Telephone, Administrator, Approval, Facility, and Physician Codes, Health Care System, Network	Classification Codes		Utilization Data					Expense (thousands) of dollars		
	Control	Service	Staffed Beds	Admissions	Census	Outpatient Visits	Births	Total	Payroll	Personnel

★ American Hospital Association (AHA) membership
□ Joint Commission on Accreditation of Healthcare Organizations (JCAHO) accreditation
+ American Osteopathic Healthcare Association (AOHA) membership
○ American Osteopathic Association (AOA) accreditation
△ Commission on Accreditation of Rehabilitation Facilities (CARF) accreditation
Control codes 61, 63, 64, 71, 72 and 73 indicate hospitals listed by AOHA, but not registered by AHA. For definition of numerical codes, see page A4

EUREKA—Woodford County
  EUREKA COMMUNITY HOSPITAL See BroMenn Healthcare, Normal

EVANSTON—Cook County

★ △ EVANSTON NORTHWESTERN HEALTHCARE CORPORATION, (Includes Evanston Northwestern Healthcare Corporation, 2650 Ridge Avenue, Zip 60201–1797; tel. 847/570–2000; Glenbrook Hospital, 2100 Pfingsten Road, Glenview, Zip 60025; tel. 847/657–5800; Highland Park Hospital, 718 Glenview Avenue, Highland Park, Zip 60035–2497; tel. 847/432–8000), 1301 Central Street, Zip 60201; tel. 847/570–2000; Mark R. Neaman, President and Chief Executive Officer (Total facility includes 56 beds in nursing home–type unit) **A**1 2 3 5 7 8 9 10 **F**1 2 3 4 5 7 8 9 10 11 12 13 15 16 17 18 19 20 21 22 23 24 25 27 28 29 30 31 32 33 34 35 36 37 38 39 40 41 42 43 44 45 46 47 48 49 50 51 53 54 56 57 58 59 60 61 62 63 64 65 66 68 69 70 71 72 73 74 75 76 77 78 79 **P**1 5 6 7 8
Web address: www.enh.org	23	10	618	39295	509	1050657	5787	436741	179894	5577
★ ST. FRANCIS HOSPITAL, 355 Ridge Avenue, Zip 60202–3399; tel. 847/316–4000; Kenneth W. Wood, Chief Executive Officer (Total facility includes 42 beds in nursing home–type unit) **A**1 2 3 5 9 10 **F**3 4 5 6 7 8 9 11 12 13 14 16 17 18 19 21 22 23 25 26 27 28 29 30 31 32 33 34 35 36 37 38 39 41 42 43 44 45 46 47 48 49 50 51 53 54 55 56 57 58 59 60 61 62 63 64 65 66 67 69 70 72 75 76 77 78 79 **P**5 6 7 8 **S** Resurrection Health Care Corporation, Chicago, IL	21	10	325	43765	201	144556	1129	120676	48370	1572

EVERGREEN PARK—Cook County

□ LITTLE COMPANY OF MARY HOSPITAL AND HEALTH CARE CENTERS, 2800 West 95th Street, Zip 60805–2795; tel. 708/422–6200; Sister Kathleen McIntyre, President **A**1 2 9 10 **F**1 3 7 8 9 11 12 13 14 17 18 19 21 22 24 25 26 29 30 32 33 34 35 36 37 38 39 41 42 43 44 45 46 48 50 51 52 54 56 57 58 59 60 61 62 63 64 65 68 70 72 76 77 78 79 **P**1 7 **S** Little Company of Mary Sisters Healthcare System, Evergreen Park, IL
Web address: www.lcmh.org	21	10	306	15587	192	184593	1618	128648	58651	1534

FAIRFIELD—Wayne County

★ FAIRFIELD MEMORIAL HOSPITAL, 303 N.W. 11th Street, Zip 62837–1203; tel. 618/842–2611 (Total facility includes 104 beds in nursing home–type unit) **A**1 9 10 **F**8 9 17 18 22 25 30 32 36 38 39 40 41 44 46 48 54 69 70 76 78 **S** Norton Healthcare, Louisville, KY	23	10	185	1127	123	17665	139	13156	5586	265

FLORA—Clay County

★ CLAY COUNTY HOSPITAL, 911 Stacy Burk Drive, Zip 62839–1823, Mailing Address: P.O. Box 280, Zip 62839–0280; tel. 618/662–2131; Tony Schwarm, President **A**1 9 10 **F**8 9 17 18 19 22 25 32 34 37 38 40 43 44 48 54 70 78 **S** BJC Health System, Saint Louis, MO
Web address: www.bjc.org	13	10	31	1444	14	23991	88	8150	3254	138

FOREST PARK—Cook County

★ RIVEREDGE HOSPITAL, 8311 West Roosevelt Road, Zip 60130–2500; tel. 708/771–7000; Mark R. Russell, Chief Executive Officer (Nonreporting) **A**1 10	33	22	120	—	—	—	—	—	—	—

FREEPORT—Stephenson County

★ FREEPORT MEMORIAL HOSPITAL, 1045 West Stephenson Street, Zip 61032–4899; tel. 815/599–6000; Dennis L. Hamilton, Chief Executive Officer (Total facility includes 43 beds in nursing home–type unit) **A**1 2 9 10 **F**8 9 11 12 13 17 18 19 21 22 23 24 25 26 27 28 32 34 36 37 39 40 44 45 46 48 49 50 54 58 59 60 61 62 63 65 69 70 71 75 76 77 78 **P**6
Web address: www.freeporthealthnet.com	23	10	191	6394	90	143206	590	49571	19457	728

GALENA—Jo Daviess County

★ GALENA–STAUSS HOSPITAL, 215 Summit Street, Zip 61036–1697; tel. 815/777–1340; Roger D. Hervey, Administrator (Total facility includes 57 beds in nursing home–type unit) **A**9 10 18 **F**1 9 17 25 28 32 43 45 54 69 70 76	16	10	82	381	59	18091	0	4440	2086	99

GALESBURG—Knox County

★ GALESBURG COTTAGE HOSPITAL, 695 North Kellogg Street, Zip 61401–2885; tel. 309/343–8131; Dennis J. Renander, President and Chief Executive Officer (Total facility includes 28 beds in nursing home–type unit) **A**1 10 **F**2 3 7 8 9 12 13 17 19 22 24 25 34 36 38 39 40 41 43 44 48 54 57 61 68 69 70 75 76 78 **P**6 8
Web address: www.cottagehospital.com	23	10	182	5559	86	63778	526	43491	19163	647
★ OSF ST. MARY MEDICAL CENTER, 3333 North Seminary Street, Zip 61401–1299; tel. 309/344–3161; Richard S. Kowalski, Administrator and Chief Executive Officer (Total facility includes 14 beds in nursing home–type unit) **A**1 2 9 10 **F**7 8 9 12 13 16 17 18 19 22 25 26 27 28 29 32 34 36 37 38 39 41 44 45 46 48 49 54 56 69 70 71 72 75 76 78 79 **P**6 **S** OSF Healthcare System, Peoria, IL
Web address: www.osfhealthcare.org	21	10	141	4425	60	61384	311	34225	15258	439

GENESEO—Henry County

★ HAMMOND–HENRY HOSPITAL, 210 West Elk Street, Zip 61254–1099; tel. 309/944–6431; Nathan C. Olson, President and Chief Executive Officer (Total facility includes 57 beds in nursing home–type unit) (Nonreporting) **A**1 9 10 **S** Brim Healthcare, Inc., Brentwood, TN	16	10	105	—	—	—	—	—	—	—

GENEVA—Kane County

★ DELNOR–COMMUNITY HOSPITAL, 300 Randall Road, Zip 60134–4200; tel. 630/208–3000; Craig A. Livermore, President and Chief Executive Officer **A**1 2 9 10 **F**6 7 8 9 10 12 15 17 18 19 22 23 24 25 28 31 32 33 34 36 37 39 41 43 44 45 46 48 49 50 51 54 58 68 70 71 72 75 76 78 79 **P**5 7
Web address: www.delnor.com	23	10	118	6892	70	89581	1545	64921	28147	778

Hospitals, U.S. / ILLINOIS

Hospital, Address, Telephone, Administrator, Approval, Facility, and Physician Codes, Health Care System, Network	Classification Codes		Utilization Data					Expense (thousands) of dollars		
★ American Hospital Association (AHA) membership □ Joint Commission on Accreditation of Healthcare Organizations (JCAHO) accreditation + American Osteopathic Healthcare Association (AOHA) membership ○ American Osteopathic Association (AOA) accreditation △ Commission on Accreditation of Rehabilitation Facilities (CARF) accreditation Control codes 61, 63, 64, 71, 72 and 73 indicate hospitals listed by AOHA, but not registered by AHA. For definition of numerical codes, see page A4	Control	Service	Staffed Beds	Admissions	Census	Outpatient Visits	Births	Total	Payroll	Personnel
GIBSON CITY—Ford County										
⊞ GIBSON AREA HOSPITAL AND HEALTH SERVICES, (Includes Gibson Community Hospital Nursing Home), 1120 North Melvin Street, Zip 60936–1066, Mailing Address: P.O. Box 429, Zip 60936–0429; tel. 217/784–4251; Craig A. Jesiolowski, Chief Executive Officer (Total facility includes 42 beds in nursing home–type unit) **A**1 9 10 **F**7 9 13 17 18 19 22 25 28 31 33 34 36 37 38 39 40 41 43 44 45 46 48 53 54 68 69 70 71 72 76 **P**1 7 **S** Quorum Health Group, Brentwood, TN	23	10	82	1124	51	40050	112	14454	5666	243
GLENDALE HEIGHTS—Du Page County										
⊞ GLENOAKS HOSPITAL, 701 Winthrop Avenue, Zip 60139–1403; tel. 630/545–8000; Brinsley Lewis, Senior Executive Officer **A**1 9 10 **F**3 7 8 9 12 13 14 16 17 19 21 22 24 25 26 32 33 34 35 36 37 38 41 42 43 44 45 46 48 49 54 56 58 59 60 61 62 63 64 70 71 72 73 75 76 78 **P**5 **S** Adventist Health System Sunbelt Health Care Corporation, Winter Park, FL Web address: www.glenoaks.org	21	10	116	3670	54	48940	535	36946	15497	366
GLENVIEW—Cook County										
GLENBROOK HOSPITAL See Evanston Northwestern Healthcare Corporation, Evanston										
GRANITE CITY—Madison County										
⊞ ST. ELIZABETH MEDICAL CENTER, 2100 Madison Avenue, Zip 62040–4799; tel. 618/798–3000; Ted Eilerman, President (Total facility includes 40 beds in nursing home–type unit) **A**1 9 10 **F**2 3 7 8 9 11 13 14 16 17 18 19 22 24 25 26 28 30 32 33 34 36 37 38 39 40 41 43 44 45 46 48 50 51 54 56 57 58 59 60 61 62 63 64 66 68 69 70 71 72 73 76 78 79 **P**4 7 Web address: www.sehs.com	21	10	236	6744	100	264209	373	60039	25454	881
GREAT LAKES—Lake County										
⊞ NAVAL HOSPITAL, 3001A Sixth Street, Zip 60088–5230; tel. 847/688–4560; Captain Elaine C. Holmes, MC, USN, Commanding Officer **A**1 2 **F**2 8 10 12 13 14 16 17 18 22 23 25 28 29 34 39 41 42 43 44 45 48 49 50 51 52 53 54 56 57 59 60 63 64 65 69 71 76 77 78 79 **S** Department of Navy, Washington, DC Web address: greatlakes.med.navy.mil	43	10	59	1602	24	457251	0	—	—	1317
GREENVILLE—Bond County										
⊞ EDWARD A. UTLAUT MEMORIAL HOSPITAL, (Includes Fair Oaks), 200 Health Care Drive, Zip 62246–1156; tel. 618/664–1230; Charles Bouis, President and Chief Executive Officer (Total facility includes 160 beds in nursing home–type unit) (Nonreporting) **A**1 9 10 Web address: www.utlaut.com	23	10	192	—	—	—	—	—	—	—
HARRISBURG—Saline County										
★ HARRISBURG MEDICAL CENTER, 100 Hospital Drive, Zip 62946–0017, Mailing Address: P.O. Box 428, Zip 62946–0428; tel. 618/253–7671; Claude Chatterton, Administrator **F**7 9 13 18 19 22 23 25 30 34 35 36 38 39 41 43 45 46 48 50 53 54 57 59 61 62 63 64 68 70 71 72 76 78 79 **P**6 **S** Ascension Health, Saint Louis, MO	23	10	80	2638	42	32133	0	17247	7609	316
HARVARD—McHenry County										
⊞ HARVARD MEMORIAL HOSPITAL, 901 Grant Street, Zip 60033–1898, Mailing Address: P.O. Box 850, Zip 60033–0850; tel. 815/943–5431; Dan Colby, President and Chief Executive Officer (Total facility includes 45 beds in nursing home–type unit) (Nonreporting) **A**1 9 10	16	10	81	—	—	—	—	—	—	—
HARVEY—Cook County										
⊞ △ INGALLS HOSPITAL, One Ingalls Drive, Zip 60426–3591; tel. 708/333–2300; Robert L. Harris, President and Chief Executive Officer **A**1 2 7 9 10 **F**2 3 4 7 8 9 11 12 16 18 19 20 21 22 23 24 25 28 29 30 31 32 33 34 35 36 37 38 39 41 42 43 44 45 46 47 48 49 50 51 53 54 55 56 57 59 60 61 62 63 64 65 66 69 70 71 72 75 76 77 78 79 **P**1 3 4 7 Web address: www.ingalls.org	23	10	409	19405	278	325301	1919	164325	75241	1964
HAVANA—Mason County										
⊞ MASON DISTRICT HOSPITAL, 615 North Promenade Street, Zip 62644–0530, Mailing Address: P.O. Box 530, Zip 62644–0530; tel. 309/543–4431; Harry Wolin, Administrator and Chief Executive Officer **A**1 9 10 **F**7 9 16 17 18 19 22 25 32 36 37 39 40 41 43 45 48 69 76 77 78 Web address: www.a2z.com/mdh	16	10	36	537	7	21923	0	8308	3954	152
HAZEL CREST—Cook County										
⊞ SOUTH SUBURBAN HOSPITAL, 17800 South Kedzie Avenue, Zip 60429–0989; tel. 708/799–8000; Patricia A. Martin, Chief Executive (Total facility includes 41 beds in nursing home–type unit) **A**1 2 9 10 **F**7 8 9 11 13 16 17 18 19 22 24 25 29 31 32 34 36 37 38 39 41 44 45 46 48 49 54 65 68 69 72 76 78 **P**1 7 **S** Advocate Health Care, Oak Brook, IL Web address: www.advocatehealth.com	23	10	235	12592	169	101757	1377	95857	43675	935
HERRIN—Williamson County										
⊞ HERRIN HOSPITAL, 201 South 14th Street, Zip 62948–3631; tel. 618/942–2171; Virgil Hannig, Senior Vice President and Administrator (Total facility includes 13 beds in nursing home–type unit) **A**1 9 10 **F**3 4 5 6 7 8 9 11 13 14 15 16 17 19 20 21 22 23 24 25 26 27 28 29 30 31 32 34 35 36 37 39 40 41 43 45 46 48 50 51 52 53 54 56 65 66 68 69 70 71 72 73 75 76 77 78 79 **P**7 **S** Southern Illinois Hospital Services, Carbondale, IL Web address: www.sih.net	23	10	92	2868	44	62821	0	30875	11841	367

Hospitals, U.S. / ILLINOIS

Hospital, Address, Telephone, Administrator, Approval, Facility, and Physician Codes, Health Care System, Network	Classi-fication Codes		Utilization Data					Expense (thousands) of dollars		
★ American Hospital Association (AHA) membership ☐ Joint Commission on Accreditation of Healthcare Organizations (JCAHO) accreditation + American Osteopathic Healthcare Association (AOHA) membership ○ American Osteopathic Association (AOA) accreditation △ Commission on Accreditation of Rehabilitation Facilities (CARF) accreditation Control codes 61, 63, 64, 71, 72 and 73 indicate hospitals listed by AOHA, but not registered by AHA. For definition of numerical codes, see page A4	Control	Service	Staffed Beds	Admissions	Census	Outpatient Visits	Births	Total	Payroll	Personnel
HIGHLAND—Madison County										
★ ST. JOSEPH'S HOSPITAL, 1515 Main Street, Zip 62249–1656; tel. 618/654–7421; Anthony G. Mastrangelo, Executive Vice President and Administrator (Total facility includes 30 beds in nursing home–type unit) **A**1 9 10 **F**7 9 13 19 22 24 25 31 32 33 34 35 36 38 39 41 43 45 46 48 51 54 59 68 69 70 71 72 76 78 79 **P**1 **S** Hospital Sisters Health System, Springfield, IL Web address: www.stjosephs–highland.org	21	10	106	1355	33	34904	0	14239	6575	211
HIGHLAND PARK—Lake County										
HIGHLAND PARK HOSPITAL See Evanston Northwestern Healthcare Corporation, Evanston										
HILLSBORO—Montgomery County										
☐ HILLSBORO AREA HOSPITAL, 1200 East Tremont Street, Zip 62049–1900; tel. 217/532–6111; Rex H. Brown, President (Total facility includes 40 beds in nursing home–type unit) **A**1 9 10 **F**8 9 16 17 18 22 25 38 39 44 48 54 69 70 76 78 **S** Brim Healthcare, Inc., Brentwood, TN	23	10	100	1443	35	28107	55	10191	4588	174
HINES—Cook County										
☐ JOHN J. MADDEN MENTAL HEALTH CENTER, 1200 South First Avenue, Zip 60141; tel. 708/338–7202; Ugo Formigoni, Metro–West Network Manager **A**1 10 **F**16 17	12	22	163	2269	164	—	0	24526	18258	386
★ △ VETERANS AFFAIRS EDWARD HINES, JR. HOSPITAL, Fifth Avenue & Roosevelt Road, Zip 60141–5000, Mailing Address: P.O. Box 5000, Zip 60141–5000; tel. 708/202–8387; John R. Fears, Acting Director **A**1 3 5 7 8 9 **F**1 2 4 11 12 19 22 23 24 25 26 30 35 36 37 38 39 41 43 46 47 48 50 51 53 54 57 59 62 63 64 65 68 69 70 76 78 **S** Department of Veterans Affairs, Washington, DC Web address: www.va.gov/stations97/guide/home.asp?DIVISION=ALL	45	10	385	8773	299	369121	0	227798	119164	2364
HINSDALE—Du Page County										
★ △ HINSDALE HOSPITAL, 120 North Oak Street, Zip 60521–3890; tel. 630/856–9000; Ernie W. Sadau, President and Chief Executive Officer **A**1 2 3 5 7 9 10 **F**2 3 4 5 7 8 9 11 12 13 14 16 17 18 19 21 22 23 24 25 26 29 30 32 33 34 35 36 37 38 39 41 43 44 45 46 47 48 49 50 51 52 53 54 56 57 58 60 61 62 63 64 65 66 68 70 71 72 74 75 76 77 78 79 **P**5 7 **S** Adventist Health System Sunbelt Health Care Corporation, Winter Park, FL Web address: www.keepingyouwell.com	21	10	331	14673	172	269440	3090	172411	68921	1924
☐ R. M. L. SPECIALTY HOSPITAL, 5601 South County Line Road, Zip 60521–8900; tel. 708/783–5800; James Richard Prister, President **A**1 9 10 **F**13 16 22 24 25 26 70 72 76 78 Web address: www.rmlspecialtyhospital.com	23	10	90	421	52	24	0	20252	8307	254
HOFFMAN ESTATES—Cook County										
★ ALEXIAN BROTHERS BEHAVIORAL HEALTH HOSPITAL, 1650 Moon Lake Boulevard, Zip 60194–5000; tel. 847/882–1600; Mark A. Frey, President and Chief Executive Officer (Nonreporting) **A**1 9 10 **S** Alexian Brothers Health System, Inc., Elk Grove Village, IL	21	22	94	—						
★ ST. ALEXIUS MEDICAL CENTER, 1555 Barrington Road, Zip 60194; tel. 847/843–2000; Edward M. Goldberg, President and Chief Executive Officer (Total facility includes 23 beds in nursing home–type unit) **A**1 2 9 10 **F**1 2 3 7 8 9 11 12 13 16 17 18 19 22 24 25 26 31 34 36 38 39 41 43 44 45 46 47 48 49 50 51 53 54 56 57 58 59 60 61 62 63 64 65 68 69 70 72 75 76 78 79 **P**6 7 **S** Alexian Brothers Health System, Inc., Elk Grove Village, IL Web address: www.stalexius.org	21	10	194	11681	135	94792	1945	—	—	611
HOOPESTON—Vermilion County										
★ HOOPESTON COMMUNITY MEMORIAL HOSPITAL, 701 East Orange Street, Zip 60942–1871; tel. 217/283–5531; Frank T. Caruso, Chief Executive Officer (Total facility includes 75 beds in nursing home–type unit) **A**1 9 10 **F**1 2 3 4 5 6 7 8 9 10 11 12 13 14 15 16 17 19 20 21 22 23 24 25 26 27 28 29 30 31 32 33 34 35 36 37 38 39 40 41 42 43 44 45 46 47 48 49 50 51 52 53 54 55 56 57 58 59 60 61 62 63 64 65 66 67 68 69 70 71 72 73 74 75 76 77 78 79 **P**6	23	10	100	341	77	14011	0	7408	3244	169
HOPEDALE—Tazewell County										
HOPEDALE MEDICAL COMPLEX, 107 Tremont Street, Zip 61747; tel. 309/449–3321; L. J. Rossi, M.D., Chief Executive Officer (Total facility includes 95 beds in nursing home–type unit) (Nonreporting) **A**9 10	23	10	119	—						
JACKSONVILLE—Morgan County										
★ PASSAVANT AREA HOSPITAL, 1600 West Walnut Street, Zip 62650–1136; tel. 217/245–9541; Chester A. Wynn, President and Chief Executive Officer (Total facility includes 15 beds in nursing home–type unit) **A**1 2 9 10 **F**4 7 8 9 17 18 19 20 22 24 30 32 33 34 37 39 40 41 43 44 45 46 48 50 51 54 56 58 62 64 65 68 70 71 72 75 78 Web address: www.passavanthospital.com	23	10	120	3999	55	35673	403	41399	17342	570
JERSEYVILLE—Jersey County										
☐ JERSEY COMMUNITY HOSPITAL, 400 Maple Summit Road, Zip 62052–2028, Mailing Address: P.O. Box 426, Zip 62052–0426; tel. 618/498–6402; Lawrence P. Bear, Administrator **A**1 9 10 **F**3 7 8 9 17 18 19 22 24 25 28 31 32 34 35 37 38 39 40 41 43 44 45 46 48 51 54 70 71 72 76 78 79 Web address: www.jch.org	16	10	67	2096	17	29211	220	14228	5940	235
JOLIET—Will County										
★ △ PROVENA SAINT JOSEPH MEDICAL CENTER, 333 North Madison Street, Zip 60435–6595; tel. 815/725–7133; Thomas A. Reitinger, Chief Executive Officer **A**1 2 7 9 10 **F**3 4 5 7 8 9 11 12 14 16 17 18 19 20 21 22 24 25 26 29 30 31 32 33 34 35 36 37 38 39 41 43 44 45 46 47 48 49 50 51 52 53 54 57 58 59 60 61 62 63 64 65 70 71 72 73 75 76 77 78 79 **P**1 6 7 **S** Provena Health, Frankfort, IL Web address: www.provena.org	21	10	369	18140	255	464853	2078	185814	80900	1914

Hospitals, U.S. / ILLINOIS

Legend for Hospital, Address, Telephone, Administrator, Approval, Facility, and Physician Codes, Health Care System, Network:

- ★ American Hospital Association (AHA) membership
- □ Joint Commission on Accreditation of Healthcare Organizations (JCAHO) accreditation
- + American Osteopathic Healthcare Association (AOHA) membership
- ○ American Osteopathic Association (AOA) accreditation
- △ Commission on Accreditation of Rehabilitation Facilities (CARF) accreditation

Control codes 61, 63, 64, 71, 72 and 73 indicate hospitals listed by AOHA, but not registered by AHA. For definition of numerical codes, see page A4.

Column headers: Classification Codes (Control, Service); Utilization Data (Staffed Beds, Admissions, Census, Outpatient Visits, Births); Expense (thousands) of dollars (Total, Payroll); Personnel.

Hospital	Control	Service	Staffed Beds	Admissions	Census	Outpatient Visits	Births	Total	Payroll	Personnel
★ SILVER CROSS HOSPITAL, 1200 Maple Road, Zip 60432–1497; tel. 815/740–1100; Paul Pawlak, President and Chief Executive Officer **A**1 2 9 10 **F**1 2 3 4 5 6 7 8 9 11 12 13 14 16 17 18 19 21 22 23 24 25 26 29 30 31 32 33 34 36 37 38 39 40 41 42 43 44 45 46 48 49 50 51 52 53 54 56 57 58 59 60 61 62 63 64 65 66 68 70 71 72 73 74 75 76 77 78 79 **P**5 6 7 8 Web address: www.silvercross.org	23	10	227	10024	111	148768	1210	93119	36325	820
KANKAKEE—Kankakee County										
★ PROVENA ST. MARY'S HOSPITAL, 500 West Court Street, Zip 60901–3661; tel. 815/937–2180; Paula Jacobi, President and Chief Executive Officer (Total facility includes 24 beds in nursing home–type unit) **A**1 2 10 **F**1 2 3 4 5 6 7 8 9 11 13 17 18 19 22 24 25 27 28 30 31 32 33 34 35 36 37 38 39 41 43 44 45 46 48 49 50 51 54 56 57 58 59 60 61 62 63 65 69 70 71 72 75 76 78 79 **P**8 **S** Provena Health, Frankfort, IL Web address: www.provena–stmarys.com	21	10	174	6778	89	163610	575	62115	24188	753
★ △ RIVERSIDE MEDICAL CENTER, 350 North Wall Street, Zip 60901–0749; tel. 815/933–1671; Dennis C. Millirons, President and Chief Executive Officer (Total facility includes 110 beds in nursing home–type unit) **A**1 2 7 9 10 **F**2 3 4 6 7 8 9 11 12 13 14 16 17 18 19 20 21 22 23 24 26 27 28 30 31 34 35 36 37 38 39 40 41 43 44 45 46 47 48 49 50 51 53 54 55 56 57 58 59 60 61 62 63 64 65 66 67 68 69 70 71 72 73 75 76 78 79 **P**1	23	10	388	9359	239	349409	1064	111219	46214	1358
KEWANEE—Henry County										
★ KEWANEE HOSPITAL, 719 Elliott Street, Zip 61443–2711, Mailing Address: P.O. Box 747, Zip 61443–0747; tel. 309/853–3361; William H. Thieben, Chief Executive Officer (Total facility includes 14 beds in nursing home–type unit) **A**1 9 10 **F**7 8 9 12 13 17 18 22 25 28 34 36 37 38 41 43 44 45 46 48 51 54 69 70 71 72 76 78 79 **P**6 Web address: www.kewaneehospital.com	23	10	63	2086	25	54014	178	26493	12824	422
LA GRANGE—Cook County										
★ LA GRANGE MEMORIAL HOSPITAL, 5101 South Willow Spring Road, Zip 60525–2680; tel. 708/352–1200; Todd S. Werner, Senior Executive Officer (Total facility includes 47 beds in nursing home–type unit) (Nonreporting) **A**1 2 3 5 9 10 **S** Adventist Health System Sunbelt Health Care Corporation, Winter Park, FL Web address: www.ahss.org	21	10	231	—	—	—	—	—	—	—
LAKE FOREST—Lake County										
★ △ LAKE FOREST HOSPITAL, 660 North Westmoreland Road, Zip 60045–1696; tel. 847/234–5600; William G. Ries, President (Total facility includes 88 beds in nursing home–type unit) **A**1 2 7 10 **F**1 3 5 7 8 9 13 15 17 19 20 22 24 25 26 28 29 30 32 34 35 36 38 39 40 41 43 44 45 46 48 49 50 51 54 56 59 61 63 65 66 68 69 70 71 72 75 76 78 79 **P**1 6 7 Web address: www.lakeforesthospital.com	23	10	214	8365	124	186954	2442	113667	50229	1197
LAWRENCEVILLE—Lawrence County										
★ LAWRENCE COUNTY MEMORIAL HOSPITAL, 2200 West State Street, Zip 62439–1853; tel. 618/943–1000; Gerald E. Waldroup, Administrator **A**9 10 **F**9 12 16 17 19 21 22 25 32 33 34 37 38 39 41 43 44 48 51 54 57 58 59 60 61 62 64 68 70 72 76 78	13	10	58	1509	20	30057	32	8311	3680	152
LEMONT—Cook County										
□ ROCK CREEK CENTER, 40 Timberline Drive, Zip 60439; tel. 630/257–3636; Wendy Mamoon, Chief Executive Officer (Nonreporting) **A**1 10 Web address: www.rockcreek–hosp.com	32	22	60	—	—	—	—	—	—	—
LIBERTYVILLE—Lake County										
★ CONDELL MEDICAL CENTER, 801 South Milwaukee Avenue on Condell Drive, Zip 60048–3199; tel. 847/362–2900; Eugene Pritchard, President **A**1 2 10 **F**1 3 7 8 9 11 13 17 18 19 21 22 24 25 28 29 30 32 33 34 35 36 37 38 39 41 43 44 45 46 48 49 50 51 54 57 59 60 61 62 64 70 71 75 76 77 78 79 **P**1 5 Web address: www.condell.org	23	10	183	10586	109	282100	1736	98492	43411	1038
LINCOLN—Logan County										
★ ABRAHAM LINCOLN MEMORIAL HOSPITAL, 315 8th Street, Zip 62656–2698; tel. 217/732–2161; Forrest G. Hester, President and Chief Executive Officer **A**1 9 10 **F**2 3 9 13 17 18 19 21 22 24 25 31 37 38 39 41 43 44 45 46 48 49 51 54 57 58 59 61 63 70 71 76 77 78 **P**3 5 **S** Memorial Health System, Springfield, IL Web address: www.almh.com	23	10	60	1841	20	44369	254	17737	7819	235
LINCOLN DEVELOPMENTAL CENTER, 861 South State Street, Zip 62656–2599; tel. 217/735–2361; Martin Downs, Facility Director (Nonreporting)	12	62	450	—	—	—	—	—	—	—
LITCHFIELD—Montgomery County										
★ ST. FRANCIS HOSPITAL, 1215 Franciscan Drive, Zip 62056, Mailing Address: P.O. Box 1215, Zip 62056–1215; tel. 217/324–2191; Michael Sipkoski, Executive Vice President and Administrator (Total facility includes 35 beds in nursing home–type unit) **A**1 9 10 **F**8 9 12 16 17 18 22 25 34 36 37 39 41 43 44 45 48 50 68 69 70 72 76 **S** Hospital Sisters Health System, Springfield, IL	21	10	97	2871	38	61368	—	20695	9410	304
MACOMB—McDonough County										
★ MCDONOUGH DISTRICT HOSPITAL, 525 East Grant Street, Zip 61455–3318; tel. 309/833–4101; Stephen R. Hopper, President and Chief Executive Officer (Total facility includes 16 beds in nursing home–type unit) **A**1 2 9 10 **F**1 3 7 8 9 13 16 17 18 19 22 24 25 27 28 30 32 33 34 36 37 39 41 43 44 45 46 48 49 50 51 54 58 62 63 69 70 71 72 76 78 79 **P**7 8 Web address: www.mdh.org	16	10	120	3724	44	43353	338	35326	16396	474

© 2000 AHA Guide — *Many Facility Codes have changed. Please refer to the AHA Guide Code Chart.*

Hospitals, U.S. / ILLINOIS

Hospital, Address, Telephone, Administrator, Approval, Facility, and Physician Codes, Health Care System, Network ★ American Hospital Association (AHA) membership ☐ Joint Commission on Accreditation of Healthcare Organizations (JCAHO) accreditation + American Osteopathic Healthcare Association (AOHA) membership ○ American Osteopathic Association (AOA) accreditation △ Commission on Accreditation of Rehabilitation Facilities (CARF) accreditation Control codes 61, 63, 64, 71, 72 and 73 indicate hospitals listed by AOHA, but not registered by AHA. For definition of numerical codes, see page A4	Classi-fication Codes		Utilization Data					Expense (thousands) of dollars		
	Control	Service	Staffed Beds	Admissions	Census	Outpatient Visits	Births	Total	Payroll	Personnel
MARION—Williamson County ☐ MARION MEMORIAL HOSPITAL, 917 West Main Street, Zip 62959-1836; tel. 618/997-5341; Ronald Seal, President and Chief Executive Officer **A**1 9 10 **F**7 8 9 12 13 16 17 18 22 24 25 32 39 40 44 45 46 48 49 50 51 54 68 76 **P**8 **S** Community Health Systems, Inc., Brentwood, TN	33	10	84	3709	36	74473	496	27105	10210	339
★ △ VETERANS AFFAIRS MEDICAL CENTER, 2401 West Main Street, Zip 62959-1194; tel. 618/997-5311; Earl F. Falast, Director (Total facility includes 60 beds in nursing home-type unit) **A**1 7 **F**3 9 11 13 18 19 22 23 24 25 26 29 30 31 32 34 35 36 37 38 39 41 43 45 46 48 49 51 54 56 57 59 61 62 63 65 68 69 70 72 74 76 78 79 **S** Department of Veterans Affairs, Washington, DC **Web address:** www.va.gov/stations97/guide/home.asp?DIVISION=ALL	45	10	99	2741	91	216932	0	51320	33534	678
MARYVILLE—Madison County ★ ANDERSON HOSPITAL, 6800 State Route 162, Zip 62062-8500, Mailing Address: P.C. Box 1000, Zip 62062-1000; tel. 618/288-5711; R. Coert Shepard, President **A**1 9 10 **F**4 7 8 9 11 13 16 17 18 19 22 24 25 28 30 32 33 34 35 36 37 38 39 40 41 43 44 46 48 49 50 51 54 61 68 69 70 71 72 75 76 78 79 **P**5	23	10	115	5957	67	82362	1083	40615	18729	638
MATTOON—Coles County ★ SARAH BUSH LINCOLN HEALTH CENTER, 1000 Health Center Drive, Zip 61938-0372, Mailing Address: P.O. Box 372, Zip 61938-0372; tel. 217/258-2525; Gary L. Barnett, President and Chief Executive Officer (Total facility includes 19 beds in nursing home-type unit) **A**1 2 9 10 **F**8 9 12 13 16 17 18 22 24 25 27 28 30 32 34 35 36 37 39 41 44 45 46 48 50 51 54 57 58 59 60 61 62 63 64 65 68 69 70 71 72 73 75 76 78 79 **P**5 6 **Web address:** www.sarahbush.org	23	10	152	7276	78	212733	927	87742	41231	1114
MAYWOOD—Cook County ☐ LOYOLA UNIVERSITY MEDICAL CENTER, 2160 South First Avenue, Zip 60153-5585; tel. 708/216-9000; Anthony L. Barbato, M.D., President and Chief Executive Officer (Nonreporting) **A**1 2 3 5 8 9 10 **Web address:** www.lumc.edu	23	10	536	—	—	—	—	—	—	—
MCHENRY—McHenry County ☐ △ NORTHERN ILLINOIS MEDICAL CENTER, 4201 Medical Center Drive, Zip 60050-9506; tel. 815/344-5000; Paul E. Laudick, President and Chief Executive Officer **A**1 2 7 9 10 **F**4 7 8 9 11 13 16 17 18 19 22 23 25 27 28 29 30 31 32 33 34 36 37 38 39 40 41 43 44 45 46 48 49 50 51 53 54 57 58 59 60 61 62 63 64 65 69 70 72 75 76 78 79 **P**6 **Web address:** www.centegra.org	23	10	133	8131	94	166661	894	82524	33866	706
MCLEANSBORO—Hamilton County ☐ HAMILTON MEMORIAL HOSPITAL DISTRICT, 611 South Marshall Avenue, Zip 62859-0429; tel. 618/643-2361; Randall W. Dauby, Chief Executive Officer (Total facility includes 60 beds in nursing home-type unit) **A**1 9 10 **F**17 18 22 24 25 32 34 36 38 39 48 50 51 54 69 70 76 **P**6 **Web address:** www.mcleansboro.com	16	10	91	1035	69	16590	0	7807	4064	115
MELROSE PARK—Cook County ★ GOTTLIEB MEMORIAL HOSPITAL, 701 West North Avenue, Zip 60160-1692; tel. 708/681-3200; John Morgan, President (Total facility includes 34 beds in nursing home-type unit) **A**1 5 9 10 **F**1 4 5 7 8 9 11 13 16 17 18 19 21 22 24 25 26 30 31 32 33 34 35 36 37 39 41 43 44 45 46 47 48 49 50 54 68 69 70 71 72 75 76 78 79 **P**6 8 **Web address:** www.gottliebhospital.org	23	10	210	9131	123	165371	1296	86931	—	1083
△ WESTLAKE HOSPITAL, (Formerly Westlake Community Hospital), 1225 Lake Street, Zip 60160-4000; tel. 708/681-3000; Patricia Shehorn, Chief Executive Officer (Total facility includes 17 beds in nursing home-type unit) **A**2 3 7 10 **F**1 3 4 8 9 11 12 13 18 22 24 25 28 29 32 33 34 36 37 38 39 41 42 43 44 45 46 47 48 53 54 57 59 62 63 65 67 68 69 70 72 76 77 78 **P**1 5 **S** Resurrection Health Care Corporation, Chicago, IL	21	10	247	8398	138	80035	661	75705	37882	912
MENDOTA—La Salle County ★ MENDOTA COMMUNITY HOSPITAL, 1315 Memorial Drive, Zip 61342-1496; tel. 815/539-7461; Susan Urso, Administrator (Total facility includes 14 beds in nursing home-type unit) **A**1 9 10 **F**3 7 8 9 13 16 17 18 19 22 24 25 32 33 34 36 37 40 43 45 46 48 49 50 51 54 56 69 70 72 76 78 **Web address:** www.mendotahospital.com	23	10	57	1572	21	71403	121	14229	7190	189
METROPOLIS—Massac County ★ MASSAC MEMORIAL HOSPITAL, 28 Chick Street, Zip 62960-2481, Mailing Address: P.C. Box 850, Zip 62960-0850; tel. 618/524-2176; Mark Edwards, Chief Executive Officer **A**1 9 10 **F**17 22 24 25 32 36 37 39 41 48 55 **S** Norton Healthcare, Louisville, KY	16	10	38	1410	15	18344	0	9150	4014	169
MOLINE—Rock Island County TRINITY MEDICAL CENTER-SEVENTH STREET CAMPUS See Trinity Medical Center-West Campus, Rock Island										
MONMOUTH—Warren County COMMUNITY MEDICAL CENTER AT WESTERN ILLINOIS, (Formerly Community Memorial Hospital), 1000 West Harlem Avenue, Zip 61462-1099; tel. 309/734-3141; Donald G. Brown, Chief Executive Officer (Total facility includes 35 beds in nursing home-type unit) **A**9 10 **F**7 9 13 16 17 18 19 21 22 23 24 29 30 32 34 36 37 43 45 48 49 50 51 54 56 68 69 70 72 75 76 78	23	10	66	1198	36	18332	0	7665	3515	153

Hospitals, U.S. / ILLINOIS

Hospital, Address, Telephone, Administrator, Approval, Facility, and Physician Codes, Health Care System, Network ★ American Hospital Association (AHA) membership ☐ Joint Commission on Accreditation of Healthcare Organizations (JCAHO) accreditation + American Osteopathic Healthcare Association (AOHA) membership ○ American Osteopathic Association (AOA) accreditation △ Commission on Accreditation of Rehabilitation Facilities (CARF) accreditation Control codes 61, 63, 64, 71, 72 and 73 indicate hospitals listed by AOHA, but not registered by AHA. For definition of numerical codes, see page A4	Classification Codes		Utilization Data					Expense (thousands) of dollars		
	Control	Service	Staffed Beds	Admissions	Census	Outpatient Visits	Births	Total	Payroll	Personnel
MONTICELLO—Piatt County ★ JOHN AND MARY KIRBY HOSPITAL, 1111 North State Street, Zip 61856–1116; tel. 217/762–2115; Thomas D. Dixon, Administrator **A**1 9 10 **F**7 9 16 17 18 25 32 33 34 36 37 38 45 48 50 51 56 61 72 74 75 76 77 78	23	10	16	360	5	25354	0	5392	2846	100
MORRIS—Grundy County ★ MORRIS HOSPITAL, 150 West High Street, Zip 60450–1497; tel. 815/942–2932; Clifford L. Corbett, President and Chief Executive Officer **A**1 2 9 10 **F**7 8 9 17 18 22 24 25 31 34 38 39 40 41 43 44 48 49 58 59 70 75 76 78 **Web address:** www.morrishospital.org	23	10	82	3326	33	97124	376	39731	18089	421
MORRISON—Whiteside County ★ MORRISON COMMUNITY HOSPITAL, 303 North Jackson Street, Zip 61270–3042; tel. 815/772–4003; Mark F. Fedyk, Administrator (Total facility includes 38 beds in nursing home–type unit) (Nonreporting) **A**9 10 **S** Trinity Health, Novi, MI	16	10	60	—	—	—	—	—	—	—
MOUNT CARMEL—Wabash County ★ WABASH GENERAL HOSPITAL DISTRICT, 1418 College Drive, Zip 62863–2638; tel. 618/262–8621; James R. Farris, CHE, Chief Executive Officer **A**1 9 10 **F**7 13 17 18 22 25 34 36 38 39 43 46 48 50 51 54 70 72 76 78 **S** Norton Healthcare, Louisville, KY	16	10	56	1001	12	28885	—	9451	3942	213
MOUNT VERNON—Jefferson County CROSSROADS COMMUNITY HOSPITAL, 8 Doctors Park Road, Zip 62864–6224; tel. 618/244–5500; Ruth McDaniel, Chief Executive Officer **A**9 10 **F**7 9 13 19 22 23 24 25 32 34 36 38 39 41 45 48 49 54 56 70 72 76 78 **S** Community Health Systems, Inc., Brentwood, TN	33	10	37	1897	23	39444	0	14208	6975	179
★ GOOD SAMARITAN REGIONAL HEALTH CENTER, 605 North 12th Street, Zip 62864–2899; tel. 618/242–4600; Leo F. Childers, Jr, FACHE, President (Total facility includes 14 beds in nursing home–type unit) **A**1 2 9 10 **F**4 7 8 9 11 13 16 17 18 19 21 22 23 24 25 27 28 29 32 33 34 35 36 37 38 39 41 43 44 45 46 48 49 50 51 53 54 56 65 69 70 72 76 78 79 **P**2 3 4 5 6 7 8 **S** SSM Health Care, Saint Louis, MO **Web address:** www.stmarys–goodsamaritan.com	21	10	141	5439	74	74571	635	64034	29052	864
MURPHYSBORO—Jackson County ★ ST. JOSEPH MEMORIAL HOSPITAL, 2 South Hospital Drive, Zip 62966–3333; tel. 618/687–3157; Betty Gaffney, Senior Vice President and Administrator **A**1 9 10 **F**8 9 13 17 18 19 22 25 27 34 35 37 38 44 48 51 54 61 70 72 73 76 78 79 **P**7 **S** Southern Illinois Hospital Services, Carbondale, IL **Web address:** www.sih.net	23	10	40	1923	26	21288	193	14287	6106	218
NAPERVILLE—Du Page County ★ EDWARD HOSPITAL, 801 South Washington Street, Zip 60566–7060; tel. 630/355–0450; Pamela Meyer Davis, President and Chief Executive Officer (Total facility includes 14 beds in nursing home–type unit) **A**1 2 9 10 **F**2 3 4 8 9 11 13 14 16 17 18 19 20 21 22 25 28 29 30 32 33 34 35 36 38 39 41 43 44 45 46 47 48 49 50 51 54 57 58 59 60 61 62 63 64 66 69 70 71 72 75 76 77 78 79 **P**5 6 7 8 **Web address:** www.edward.org	23	10	165	12192	140	227080	3024	139543	58340	2110
NASHVILLE—Washington County ★ WASHINGTON COUNTY HOSPITAL, 705 South Grand Avenue, Zip 62263; tel. 618/327–8236; Michael P. Ellermann, President and Chief Executive Officer (Total facility includes 32 beds in nursing home–type unit) **A**1 9 10 **F**3 4 5 7 8 9 10 11 12 13 14 16 19 21 22 24 25 29 31 33 34 35 36 37 38 39 41 42 43 44 45 46 47 48 50 52 53 54 55 57 58 59 60 61 62 63 64 65 66 68 69 70 71 72 74 75 76 77 78 79 **P**1 6 7	16	10	53	593	29	40408	50	7730	3535	149
NORMAL—McLean County ★ BROMENN HEALTHCARE, (Includes Bromenn Regional Medical Center, tel. 309/454–1400; Eureka Community Hospital, 101 South Major Street, Eureka, Zip 61530, Mailing Address: P.O. Box 203, Zip 61530; tel. 309/467–2371), Virginia and Franklin Streets, Zip 61761, Mailing Address: P.O. Box 2850, Bloomington, Zip 61702–2850; tel. 309/454–0700; Dale S. Strassheim, President **A**1 2 9 10 **F**1 2 3 7 8 9 11 13 14 17 18 19 22 24 25 26 28 29 30 31 32 33 34 36 37 38 39 41 43 44 45 46 48 49 50 51 53 54 56 57 58 59 60 61 62 63 64 65 69 70 72 74 75 76 77 78 **P**6 7 8 **Web address:** www.bromenn.org	21	10	242	7979	103	104890	1267	92781	39245	1365
NORTH CHICAGO—Lake County ★ VETERANS AFFAIRS MEDICAL CENTER, 3001 Green Bay Road, Zip 60064–3049; tel. 847/688–1900; Alfred S. Pate, Director (Total facility includes 373 beds in nursing home–type unit) (Nonreporting) **A**1 3 5 **S** Department of Veterans Affairs, Washington, DC **Web address:** www.va.gov/stations97/guide/home.asp?DIVISION=ALL	45	49	836	—	—	—	—	—	—	—
OAK FOREST—Cook County ★ △ OAK FOREST HOSPITAL OF COOK COUNTY, 15900 South Cicero Avenue, Zip 60452; tel. 708/687–7200; Cynthia T. Henderson, M.D., M.P.H., Director and Chief Operating Officer (Total facility includes 474 beds in nursing home–type unit) **A**1 3 5 7 10 **F**9 17 18 20 22 24 26 30 38 39 40 41 46 48 49 51 53 54 65 69 70 72 76 78 **P**6 **S** Cook County Bureau of Health Services, Chicago, IL	13	48	601	3254	561	60100	0	114948	69314	1669
OAK LAWN—Cook County ★ △ CHRIST HOSPITAL AND MEDICAL CENTER, (Includes Hope Children's Hospital), 4440 West 95th Street, Zip 60453–2699; tel. 708/425–8000; Carol Schneider, Chief Executive Officer **A**1 2 3 5 7 9 10 **F**1 2 3 4 7 8 9 11 12 13 14 17 18 19 21 22 24 25 28 29 30 31 32 33 34 35 36 37 38 39 40 41 42 43 44 45 46 47 48 49 51 52 53 54 55 57 58 59 60 62 63 64 65 66 67 69 70 71 72 73 75 76 78 79 **P**5 7 8 **S** Advocate Health Care, Oak Brook, IL **Web address:** www.advocatehealth.com	21	10	620	34271	498	293190	3730	373759	167129	3900

© 2000 AHA Guide *Many Facility Codes have changed. Please refer to the AHA Guide Code Chart.*

Hospitals, U.S. / ILLINOIS

Hospital, Address, Telephone, Administrator, Approval, Facility, and Physician Codes, Health Care System, Network	Classification Codes		Utilization Data					Expense (thousands) of dollars		
★ American Hospital Association (AHA) membership ☐ Joint Commission on Accreditation of Healthcare Organizations (JCAHO) accreditation + American Osteopathic Healthcare Association (AOHA) membership ○ American Osteopathic Association (AOA) accreditation △ Commission on Accreditation of Rehabilitation Facilities (CARF) accreditation Control codes 61, 63, 64, 71, 72 and 73 indicate hospitals listed by AOHA, but not registered by AHA. For definition of numerical codes, see page A4	Control	Service	Staffed Beds	Admissions	Census	Outpatient Visits	Births	Total	Payroll	Personnel
OAK PARK—Cook County										
★ △ OAK PARK HOSPITAL, 520 South Maple Avenue, Zip 60304–1097; tel. 708/383–9300; Bruce M. Elegant, President and Chief Executive Officer **A**1 2 5 7 9 10 **F**1 2 3 4 5 6 7 9 10 11 12 13 17 18 19 20 21 22 23 24 25 26 28 29 30 31 32 33 34 35 36 37 38 39 41 42 43 44 45 46 47 48 49 50 51 52 53 54 55 56 57 58 59 60 61 62 63 64 65 66 68 69 70 71 72 74 76 78 79 **P**1 6 7 **S** Wheaton Franciscan Services, Inc., Wheaton, IL	21	10	176	6462	119	74444	0	44894	22075	548
☐ WEST SUBURBAN HOSPITAL MEDICAL CENTER, 3 Erie Court, Zip 60302–2599; tel. 708/383–6200; Robert E. Landsman, Interim President and Chief Executive Officer (Total facility includes 59 beds in nursing home–type unit) **A**1 2 3 5 9 10 **F**4 5 7 8 9 11 13 14 15 17 18 19 20 21 22 23 24 25 29 30 31 32 33 34 35 36 37 38 39 41 43 44 45 46 47 48 49 50 51 54 56 59 61 65 66 68 69 70 71 72 73 75 76 77 78 79 **P**8 Web address: www.westsub.com	23	10	193	11844	120	205587	2098	160617	60697	1814
OLNEY—Richland County										
★ RICHLAND MEMORIAL HOSPITAL, 800 East Locust Street, Zip 62450–2598; tel. 618/395–2131; Harvey H. Pettry, President and Chief Executive Officer (Total facility includes 28 beds in nursing home–type unit) (Nonreporting) **A**1 2 9 10	13	10	97	—	—	—	—	—	—	—
OLYMPIA FIELDS—Cook County										
★ ○ ST. JAMES HOSPITALS AND HEALTH CENTERS – OLYMPIA FIELDS CAMPUS, (Formerly Olympia Fields Osteopathic Hospital and Medical Center), 20201 South Crawford Avenue, Zip 60461–1080; tel. 708/747–4000; David Scott Koenig, Chief Executive Officer **A**9 10 11 12 13 **F**3 4 5 8 9 11 12 13 14 16 17 18 19 21 22 24 25 26 27 29 30 31 32 33 34 36 37 38 39 41 43 44 45 46 47 48 49 50 51 53 54 55 57 58 59 60 61 62 64 65 66 68 70 72 73 74 75 76 77 78 79 **P**5 7 **S** Sisters of St. Francis Health Services, Inc., Mishawaka, IN	21	10	164	6088	8	117925	570	76043	27215	—
OTTAWA—La Salle County										
★ COMMUNITY HOSPITAL OF OTTAWA, 1100 East Norris Drive, Zip 61350–1687; tel. 815/433–3100; Robert Schmelter, President **A**1 9 10 **F**1 2 3 6 7 8 9 17 22 23 24 25 30 31 32 33 34 36 37 40 41 43 44 46 48 49 50 51 54 57 58 59 61 62 63 64 70 72 75 76 78 **P**8 Web address: www.community–hospital.org	23	10	113	3563	36	74569	377	33345	13931	410
PALOS HEIGHTS—Cook County										
★ PALOS COMMUNITY HOSPITAL, 12251 South 80th Avenue, Zip 60463–0930; tel. 708/923–4000; Sister Margaret Wright, President **A**1 2 9 10 **F**2 3 7 8 9 11 12 18 22 24 25 28 29 34 35 36 37 38 40 41 43 44 45 46 48 49 50 54 57 58 59 61 62 63 64 68 70 71 72 76 77 78	23	10	340	19674	233	217238	2273	180747	93457	1852
PANA—Christian County										
★ PANA COMMUNITY HOSPITAL, 101 East Ninth Street, Zip 62557–1785; tel. 217/562–2131; Vickie Holthaus, Interim Chief Executive Officer **A**1 9 10 **F**7 9 13 16 17 18 19 22 24 25 26 33 34 35 36 39 40 41 43 45 46 48 50 51 54 56 68 70 71 76 78	23	10	30	793	7	16696	0	6250	2859	95
PARIS—Edgar County										
★ PARIS COMMUNITY HOSPITAL, 721 East Court Street, Zip 61944–2420; tel. 217/465–4141; John D. Fajt, FACHE, President and Chief Operating Officer **A**1 9 10 **F**9 13 17 19 22 24 25 32 34 36 37 38 39 40 41 45 46 48 53 54 69 70 72 76 78 **P**6 **S** Norton Healthcare, Louisville, KY	23	10	49	940	22	28153	0	10882	4508	223
PARK RIDGE—Cook County										
★ △ LUTHERAN GENERAL HOSPITAL, 1775 Dempster Street, Zip 60068–1174; tel. 847/723–2210; Kenneth J. Rojek, Chief Executive **A**1 2 3 5 7 8 9 10 **F**1 3 4 5 6 7 8 9 10 11 12 13 14 15 16 17 18 19 20 22 24 25 26 28 29 30 31 32 33 34 35 36 38 39 40 41 42 43 44 45 46 47 48 49 50 51 52 53 54 55 56 57 58 59 60 61 62 63 64 65 66 67 68 70 71 72 73 75 76 77 78 79 **P**8 **S** Advocate Health Care, Oak Brook, IL Web address: www.advocatehealth.com	23	10	573	27315	385	241100	4256	327004	132334	3320
PEKIN—Tazewell County										
★ PEKIN HOSPITAL, 600 South 13th Street, Zip 61554–5098; tel. 309/347–1151; Robert J. Moore, CHE, Chief Executive Officer (Total facility includes 12 beds in nursing home–type unit) **A**1 9 10 **F**2 3 4 7 8 9 11 13 15 16 17 18 19 20 21 22 23 24 25 26 27 28 30 32 33 34 35 36 37 38 39 40 41 42 43 44 45 46 47 48 50 51 52 54 56 57 58 59 60 61 62 63 64 65 66 68 69 70 71 72 73 74 75 76 77 78 79 **P**1 Web address: www.pekin.net/hospital	23	10	109	4405	57	77810	453	37222	14863	654
PEORIA—Peoria County										
☐ GEORGE A. ZELLER MENTAL HEALTH CENTER, 5407 North University Street, Zip 61614–4785; tel. 309/693–5228; Robert W. Vyverberg, Ed.D., Director (Nonreporting) **A**1 10	12	22	154	—	—	—	—	—	—	—
★ △ METHODIST MEDICAL CENTER OF ILLINOIS, 221 N.E. Glen Oak Avenue, Zip 61636–4310; tel. 309/672–5522; W. Michael Bryant, President and Chief Executive Officer **A**1 2 3 5 6 7 10 **F**4 7 8 9 11 12 13 16 17 18 22 24 25 26 27 28 29 30 31 32 33 34 36 37 38 39 41 43 44 45 46 47 48 49 50 51 53 54 55 56 57 58 59 60 61 62 63 64 65 66 68 69 70 72 74 75 76 77 78 79 **P**1 7 Web address: www.mmci.org	23	10	300	14426	207	—	1674	186114	77947	1776
★ △ OSF SAINT FRANCIS MEDICAL CENTER, 530 N.E. Glen Oak Avenue, Zip 61637; tel. 309/655–2000; Keith E. Steffen, Administrator **A**1 2 3 5 7 9 10 **F**1 3 4 5 6 7 8 9 10 11 12 13 14 15 17 18 19 20 21 22 23 24 25 26 27 28 29 30 31 32 33 34 35 36 37 38 39 40 41 42 43 44 45 46 47 48 49 50 51 52 53 54 55 56 57 58 59 60 61 62 63 64 65 66 67 69 70 71 72 73 74 75 76 77 78 79 **P**4 5 8 **S** OSF Healthcare System, Peoria, IL Web address: www.osfhealthcare.org	21	10	532	23289	354	674782	2359	314339	138225	3541

Hospitals, U.S. / ILLINOIS

Hospital, Address, Telephone, Administrator, Approval, Facility, and Physician Codes, Health Care System, Network	Classification Codes		Utilization Data					Expense (thousands) of dollars		
★ American Hospital Association (AHA) membership □ Joint Commission on Accreditation of Healthcare Organizations (JCAHO) accreditation + American Osteopathic Healthcare Association (AOHA) membership ○ American Osteopathic Association (AOA) accreditation △ Commission on Accreditation of Rehabilitation Facilities (CARF) accreditation Control codes 61, 63, 64, 71, 72 and 73 indicate hospitals listed by AOHA, but not registered by AHA. For definition of numerical codes, see page A4	Control	Service	Staffed Beds	Admissions	Census	Outpatient Visits	Births	Total	Payroll	Personnel
☒ PROCTOR HOSPITAL, 5409 North Knoxville Avenue, Zip 61614–5094; tel. 309/691–1000; Norman H. LaConte, President and Chief Executive Officer (Total facility includes 40 beds in nursing home–type unit) **A**1 9 10 **F**2 3 4 7 8 9 11 13 14 16 17 18 22 24 25 28 29 32 33 34 36 38 39 40 41 43 44 45 47 48 50 51 54 56 68 69 70 75 76 77 78 **P**1 3 **Web address:** www.proctor.org **PERU—La Salle County**	23	10	169	7609	106	165312	581	65300	25625	882
☒ ILLINOIS VALLEY COMMUNITY HOSPITAL, 925 West Street, Zip 61354–2799; tel. 815/223–3300; Willis F. Fry, Administrator (Total facility includes 12 beds in nursing home–type unit) **A**1 9 10 **F**1 7 8 9 10 16 17 18 19 22 24 25 27 29 30 32 33 34 35 36 37 38 39 41 43 44 45 46 48 50 51 54 57 58 59 60 61 62 63 64 69 70 71 72 76 78 79 **P**8 **Web address:** www.ivch.org **PINCKNEYVILLE—Perry County**	23	10	100	3820	49	89769	551	32731	12737	459
★ PINCKNEYVILLE COMMUNITY HOSPITAL, 101 North Walnut Street, Zip 62274–1099; tel. 618/357–2187; Jerry L. Bolandis, CPA, Administrator and Chief Executive Officer (Total facility includes 50 beds in nursing home–type unit) **A**9 10 **F**17 18 22 24 25 28 36 37 39 46 48 54 69 70 76 **PITTSFIELD—Pike County**	16	10	61	959	41	37672	0	9806	5132	214
☒ ILLINI COMMUNITY HOSPITAL, 640 West Washington Street, Zip 62363–1397; tel. 217/285–2113; Connie L. Schroeder, Chief Executive Officer **A**1 9 10 **F**9 12 17 18 22 25 28 30 31 32 33 34 36 37 40 41 43 44 45 48 51 54 56 70 76 78 **P**6 **Web address:** www.ichcshealthcare.com **PONTIAC—Livingston County**	23	10	45	1208	10	35090	125	11375	5036	192
☒ OSF SAINT JAMES HOSPITAL, (Formerly Saint James Hospital), 610 East Water Street, Zip 61764–2194; tel. 815/842–2828; David T. Ochs, Administrator (Total facility includes 16 beds in nursing home–type unit) **A**1 9 10 **F**7 8 9 13 16 17 18 19 21 22 24 25 26 28 30 31 32 33 34 37 38 39 40 41 43 44 45 46 48 49 50 51 54 59 63 68 69 70 76 77 79 **P**6 7 **S** OSF Healthcare System, Peoria, IL **Web address:** www.osfhealthcare.org **PRINCETON—Bureau County**	21	10	81	2341	27	75171	342	20532	9354	226
☒ PERRY MEMORIAL HOSPITAL, 530 Park Avenue East, Zip 61356–2598; tel. 815/875–2811; Gregg Davis, Interim Chief Executive Officer (Total facility includes 15 beds in nursing home–type unit) **A**1 9 10 **F**7 8 9 13 17 19 22 24 25 28 29 30 32 33 34 38 39 40 41 43 44 45 46 48 50 54 69 70 72 76 78 **P**8 **Web address:** www.perry-memorial.org **QUINCY—Adams County**	14	10	87	2353	31	45127	165	22727	9735	304
☒ △ BLESSING HOSPITAL, (Includes Blessing Hospital, Broadway & 14th Street), Broadway at 11th Street, Zip 62301, Mailing Address: P.O. Box 7005, Zip 62305–7005; tel. 217/223–1200; Lawrence L. Swearingen, President and Chief Executive Officer (Total facility includes 40 beds in nursing home–type unit) **A**1 2 3 5 7 9 10 **F**1 2 7 8 9 11 13 14 16 17 18 19 22 23 24 25 27 28 30 32 33 34 35 36 37 38 39 40 41 43 44 45 46 48 49 50 51 53 54 57 58 59 61 62 63 64 65 68 69 70 72 75 76 77 78 79 **P**1 **Web address:** www.blessinghospital.org **RED BUD—Randolph County**	23	10	219	11938	199	260064	1181	98708	44184	1379
☒ ST. CLEMENT HEALTH SERVICES, (Formerly St. Clement Hospital), One St. Clement Boulevard, Zip 62278–1194; tel. 618/282–3831; Michael T. McManus, Administrator (Total facility includes 40 beds in nursing home–type unit) **A**1 9 10 **F**7 8 9 13 16 19 22 24 25 26 30 31 33 34 36 37 38 39 41 44 45 46 48 54 66 68 69 70 76 78 **P**5 6 7 8 **S** Sisters of Mercy Health System–St. Louis, Saint Louis, MO **ROBINSON—Crawford County**	21	10	75	1313	42	46817	145	16805	8621	245
☒ CRAWFORD MEMORIAL HOSPITAL, 1000 North Allen Street, Zip 62454; tel. 618/546–1234; Wallace R. Simmons, Chief Executive Officer (Total facility includes 48 beds in nursing home–type unit) **A**1 9 10 **F**7 8 9 14 16 17 18 21 22 25 28 30 31 32 34 36 37 38 39 40 41 43 44 45 46 48 49 51 54 56 69 70 71 72 76 78 **P**6 **S** Quorum Health Group, Brentwood, TN **ROCHELLE—Ogle County**	16	10	93	1718	54	29492	308	16626	6589	220
☒ ROCHELLE COMMUNITY HOSPITAL, 900 North Second Street, Zip 61068–0330; tel. 815/562–2181; Gregg Olson, Interim Chief Executive Officer **A**1 9 10 **F**7 9 13 16 17 18 19 20 22 24 25 26 28 32 33 34 35 36 37 38 39 41 43 44 45 46 48 50 51 54 56 61 70 71 72 76 78 **P**5 6 8 **Web address:** www.rcha.net **ROCK ISLAND—Rock Island County**	23	10	30	1032	11	—	41	9465	4498	151
☒ △ TRINITY MEDICAL CENTER–WEST CAMPUS, (Includes Trinity Medical Center–Seventh Street Campus, 500 John Deere Road, Moline, Zip 61265; tel. 309/779–5000), 2701 17th Street, Zip 61201–5393; tel. 309/779–5000; Eric Crowell, President and Chief Executive Officer (Total facility includes 29 beds in nursing home–type unit) **A**1 2 7 10 **F**2 3 4 7 8 9 11 13 16 17 18 19 20 22 24 25 26 27 28 29 30 31 32 33 34 35 36 37 38 39 41 42 43 44 45 46 47 48 49 50 51 53 54 56 57 58 59 60 61 62 63 64 65 66 69 70 71 72 73 75 76 77 78 79 **P**1 6 **S** Iowa Health System, Des Moines, IA **Web address:** www.trinityqc.com	23	10	338	17746	222	296012	1663	134123	59372	1560

© 2000 AHA Guide   *Many Facility Codes have changed. Please refer to the AHA Guide Code Chart.*   Hospitals **A133**

Hospitals, U.S. / ILLINOIS

Hospital, Address, Telephone, Administrator, Approval, Facility, and Physician Codes, Health Care System, Network	Classification Codes		Utilization Data					Expense (thousands) of dollars		
	Control	Service	Staffed Beds	Admissions	Census	Outpatient Visits	Births	Total	Payroll	Personnel

★ American Hospital Association (AHA) membership
□ Joint Commission on Accreditation of Healthcare Organizations (JCAHO) accreditation
+ American Osteopathic Healthcare Association (AOHA) membership
○ American Osteopathic Association (AOA) accreditation
△ Commission on Accreditation of Rehabilitation Facilities (CARF) accreditation
Control codes 61, 63, 64, 71, 72 and 73 indicate hospitals listed by AOHA, but not registered by AHA. For definition of numerical codes, see page A4

ROCKFORD—Winnebago County

□ H. DOUGLAS SINGER MENTAL HEALTH AND DEVELOPMENTAL CENTER, 4402 North Main Street, Zip 61103–1278; tel. 815/987–7096; Gail Tennant, Director (Nonreporting) **A**1 10 — 12 22 162 — — — — — — —

★ △ ROCKFORD MEMORIAL HOSPITAL, 2400 North Rockton Avenue, Zip 61103–3692; tel. 815/971–5000; Kate Wong, President and Chief Operating Officer **A**1 2 5 7 10 **F**2 3 4 5 7 8 9 11 12 13 14 17 18 19 21 22 24 25 32 33 34 35 36 37 38 39 40 41 42 43 44 45 46 47 48 49 50 51 52 53 54 56 57 58 59 60 61 62 63 64 65 66 68 70 71 72 75 76 77 78 79 **P**6
Web address: www.rhsnet.org — 23 10 344 14927 239 343036 2452 173719 72748 2148

★ SAINT ANTHONY MEDICAL CENTER, 5666 East State Street, Zip 61108–2472; tel. 815/226–2000; David A. Schertz, Administrator **A**1 2 5 9 10 **F**4 8 9 10 11 12 13 16 17 18 19 22 24 25 27 28 31 32 34 36 38 39 41 43 44 45 46 47 48 49 50 51 54 65 68 70 71 72 75 76 77 78 **P**6 **S** OSF Healthcare System, Peoria, IL
Web address: www.osfhealthcare.org — 21 10 221 9729 130 142781 871 134363 56472 1439

★ SWEDISHAMERICAN HEALTH SYSTEM, 1313 East State Street, Zip 61104; tel. 815/968–4400; Robert B. Klint, M.D., President and Chief Executive Officer **A**1 2 3 5 9 10 **F**2 3 4 8 9 11 12 13 14 16 17 18 19 20 21 22 23 24 25 26 27 28 30 31 32 33 34 35 36 37 38 39 41 43 44 45 46 47 48 49 50 51 52 53 54 56 57 58 59 60 61 62 63 64 65 68 69 70 72 75 76 77 78 79 **P**6 7 — 23 10 291 11749 155 140315 1772 120228 51824 1470

ROSICLARE—Hardin County

★ HARDIN COUNTY GENERAL HOSPITAL, Ferrell Road, Zip 62982; tel. 618/285–6634; Roby D. Williams, Administrator (Nonreporting) **A**1 9 10 — 23 10 48 — — — — — — —

RUSHVILLE—Schuyler County

★ SARAH D. CULBERTSON MEMORIAL HOSPITAL, 238 South Congress Street, Zip 62681–1472, Mailing Address: P.O. Box 440, Zip 62681–0440; tel. 217/322–4321; Michael C. O'Brien, Administrator (Total facility includes 30 beds in nursing home–type unit) **A**9 10 **F**7 8 9 16 22 25 34 37 38 40 44 48 54 67 69 76 77 78 **P**6
Web address: www.rushville.lib.il.us/community/culbertson/ — 16 10 58 820 34 22104 125 6821 2792 84

SALEM—Marion County

★ SALEM TOWNSHIP HOSPITAL, (Formerly Public Hospital of the Town of Salem), 1201 Ricker Drive, Zip 62881–6250; tel. 618/548–3194; James E. Robertson, Jr, President **A**1 9 10 **F**7 9 13 16 17 18 19 22 23 25 29 32 34 36 37 38 41 43 45 48 50 54 70 71 75 76 78 **S** BJC Health System, Saint Louis, MO — 14 10 31 1291 17 41199 0 12465 5285 205

SANDWICH—De Kalb County

★ VALLEY WEST COMMUNITY HOSPITAL, 11 East Pleasant Avenue, Zip 60548–0901; tel. 815/786–8484; Roger L. Holloway, Administrator **A**9 10 **F**7 8 9 17 22 24 25 32 34 38 39 41 43 44 45 48 50 54 70 76 78 **S** Kishwaukee Health System, De Kalb, IL
Web address: www.uwch.com — 23 10 35 780 11 10649 60 6869 2625 135

SCOTT AFB—St. Clair County

★ SCOTT MEDICAL CENTER, 310 West Losey Street, Zip 62225–5252; tel. 618/256–7456; Colonel Richard Weltzin, MSC, USAF, Administrator **A**1 3 5 9 **F**13 14 15 16 17 18 22 23 25 26 28 31 32 34 39 41 43 45 46 48 49 50 51 54 56 58 59 60 61 63 73 76 78 79 **P**6 **S** Department of the Air Force, Bowling AFB, DC
Web address: www.satx.disa.mil/mtf3751 — 41 10 25 2381 9 236522 379 36794 5420 183

SHELBYVILLE—Shelby County

★ SHELBY MEMORIAL HOSPITAL, 200 South Cedar Street, Zip 62565–1899; tel. 217/774–3961; John Bennett, President and Chief Executive Officer (Total facility includes 15 beds in nursing home–type unit) **A**1 9 10 **F**9 12 16 17 18 22 24 25 35 36 39 41 45 46 48 54 68 69 76 **P**5 — 23 10 52 2207 32 30195 — 9413 4262 169

SILVIS—Rock Island County

★ ILLINI HOSPITAL, 801 Hospital Road, Zip 61282–1893; tel. 309/792–9363; Gary E. Larson, Chief Executive Officer **A**1 10 **F**2 3 4 6 7 8 9 11 12 13 16 17 18 19 22 24 25 26 27 28 29 31 32 33 34 35 36 37 38 39 41 42 43 44 45 46 47 48 49 50 51 54 55 57 58 59 60 61 62 63 64 65 66 67 68 69 70 71 72 73 75 76 77 78 **P**6 8
Web address: www.genesishealth.com — 23 10 105 5398 53 108033 621 43086 18074 655

SKOKIE—Cook County

★ RUSH NORTH SHORE MEDICAL CENTER, 9600 Gross Point Road, Zip 60076–1257; tel. 847/677–9600; John S. Frigo, President (Total facility includes 13 beds in nursing home–type unit) **A**1 2 3 5 9 10 **F**4 8 9 11 13 17 18 19 22 24 25 26 27 30 32 34 38 39 40 41 43 44 46 47 48 50 54 57 63 64 65 68 69 70 75 76 78 79 **P**8 **S** Rush–Presbyterian–St. Luke's Medical Center, Chicago, IL
Web address: www.rush.edu — 23 10 226 10499 175 99664 632 107530 46993 1171

SPARTA—Randolph County

★ SPARTA COMMUNITY HOSPITAL, 818 East Broadway Street, Zip 62286–0297, Mailing Address: P.O. Box 297, Zip 62286–0297; tel. 618/443–2177; Joann Emge, Chief Executive Officer **A**1 9 10 **F**7 8 9 13 16 17 22 25 28 31 32 34 36 37 39 44 45 46 48 49 54 70 76 78 **P**5 — 16 10 35 1130 12 30210 135 10884 4991 184

SPRING VALLEY—Bureau County

★ ST. MARGARET'S HOSPITAL, 600 East First Street, Zip 61362–2034; tel. 815/664–5311; Tim Muntz, President (Total facility includes 33 beds in nursing home–type unit) **A**1 2 9 10 **F**8 9 16 17 18 22 24 25 28 31 32 33 34 35 36 37 41 43 44 45 46 48 50 51 53 54 67 69 70 71 72 76 78 79 **P**6 8 **S** Sisters of Mary of the Presentation Health Corporation, Fargo, ND
Web address: www.st.margarets.com — 21 10 123 3054 53 155778 248 33689 14914 361

Hospitals, U.S. / ILLINOIS

Hospital, Address, Telephone, Administrator, Approval, Facility, and Physician Codes, Health Care System, Network	Classification Codes		Utilization Data					Expense (thousands) of dollars		
★ American Hospital Association (AHA) membership ☐ Joint Commission on Accreditation of Healthcare Organizations (JCAHO) accreditation + American Osteopathic Healthcare Association (AOHA) membership ○ American Osteopathic Association (AOA) accreditation △ Commission on Accreditation of Rehabilitation Facilities (CARF) accreditation Control codes 61, 63, 64, 71, 72 and 73 indicate hospitals listed by AOHA, but not registered by AHA. For definition of numerical codes, see page A4	Control	Service	Staffed Beds	Admissions	Census	Outpatient Visits	Births	Total	Payroll	Personnel

SPRINGFIELD—Sangamon County

☐ ANDREW MCFARLAND MENTAL HEALTH CENTER, 901 Southwind Road, Zip 62703-5195; tel. 217/786-6994; Nieves Tan–Lachica, M.D., Superintendent (Nonreporting) **A**1 | 12 | 22 | 146 | — | — | — | — | — | — | — |

☐ DOCTORS HOSPITAL, 5230 South Sixth Street, Zip 62703-5194, Mailing Address: P.O. Box 19254, Zip 62794-9254; tel. 217/529-7151; Jim Bohl, President and Chief Executive Officer (Total facility includes 28 beds in nursing home–type unit) **A**1 9 10 **F**4 13 16 17 18 21 22 24 25 27 32 39 41 43 45 46 48 49 51 54 57 59 60 61 62 63 64 65 69 70 71 76 77 **P**2 | 32 | 10 | 96 | 2858 | 54 | 12116 | 0 | 27065 | 10785 | 438 |

★ △ MEMORIAL MEDICAL CENTER, 701 North First Street, Zip 62781-0001; tel. 217/788-3000; Robert T. Clarke, President and Chief Executive Officer **A**1 2 3 5 7 8 9 10 **F**3 4 7 8 9 10 11 12 13 16 17 18 19 21 22 23 24 25 26 27 29 30 31 32 33 34 35 36 37 38 39 40 41 43 44 45 46 47 48 49 50 51 53 54 56 57 58 59 60 61 62 63 64 65 66 70 71 72 73 74 75 76 77 78 79 **P**3 5 **S** Memorial Health System, Springfield, IL
Web address: www.memorialmedical.com | 23 | 10 | 453 | 18969 | 290 | 380430 | 1706 | 217319 | 90700 | 3634 |

★ ST. JOHN'S HOSPITAL, 800 East Carpenter Street, Zip 62769-0002; tel. 217/544-6464; Allison C. Laabs, Executive Vice President and Administrator (Total facility includes 43 beds in nursing home–type unit) **A**1 3 5 8 10 **F**1 3 4 7 8 9 11 13 14 16 17 18 20 22 25 30 32 34 36 37 39 41 42 43 44 46 47 48 49 51 52 54 55 57 62 64 65 69 70 71 73 75 76 78 79 **P**7 **S** Hospital Sisters Health System, Springfield, IL
Web address: www.st-johns.org | 21 | 10 | 568 | 21880 | 345 | 256387 | 1952 | 259453 | 104039 | 3167 |

STAUNTON—Macoupin County

★ COMMUNITY MEMORIAL HOSPITAL, 400 Caldwell Street, Zip 62088-1499; tel. 618/635-2200; Patrick B. Heise, Chief Executive Officer **A**1 9 10 **F**9 22 25 36 40 48 70 76 78 **S** Quorum Health Group, Brentwood, TN | 23 | 10 | 44 | 747 | 8 | 18516 | 0 | 8353 | 3837 | 141 |

STERLING—Whiteside County

★ CGH MEDICAL CENTER, 100 East LeFevre Road, Zip 61081-1279; tel. 815/625-0400; Edward Andersen, President and Chief Executive Officer **A**1 2 9 10 **F**7 8 9 13 16 17 18 19 22 23 24 25 27 31 32 33 36 37 39 43 46 48 49 51 54 65 68 70 72 76 78 **P**1 6
Web address: www.cghmc.com | 14 | 10 | 143 | 6277 | 62 | 63046 | 719 | 47086 | 19919 | 649 |

STREAMWOOD—Cook County

☐ BHC STREAMWOOD HOSPITAL, 1400 East Irving Park Road, Zip 60107-3203; tel. 630/837-9000; Jeff Bergren, Chief Executive Officer and Administrator **A**1 10 **F**10 12 41 42 44 45 52 57 58 59 60 61 62 63 64 70 **S** Behavioral Healthcare Corporation, Nashville, TN | 33 | 52 | 100 | 450 | 57 | 26041 | 0 | — | — | — |

STREATOR—La Salle County

★ ST. MARY'S HOSPITAL, 111 East Spring Street, Zip 61364-3399; tel. 815/673-2311; Thomas Whelan, Acting Administrator (Total facility includes 30 beds in nursing home–type unit) **A**1 2 10 **F**1 7 8 9 13 16 17 18 19 22 23 24 25 27 28 30 32 34 36 37 39 41 43 44 45 46 48 50 54 64 65 68 69 70 72 76 78 **P**8 **S** Hospital Sisters Health System, Springfield, IL
Web address: www.ortelco.com/~stmaryl | 21 | 10 | 170 | 4079 | 67 | 40355 | 289 | 30143 | 13505 | 418 |

SYCAMORE—De Kalb County

☐ VENCOR HOSPITAL–SYCAMORE, 225 Edward Street, Zip 60178-2197; tel. 815/895-2144; Laura S. Wills, R.N., Administrator (Nonreporting) **A**1 9 10 **S** Vencor, Incorporated, Louisville, KY
Web address: www.vencor.com | 33 | 10 | 50 | — | — | — | — | — | — | — |

TAYLORVILLE—Christian County

★ ST. VINCENT MEMORIAL HOSPITAL, 201 East Pleasant Street, Zip 62568-1597; tel. 217/824-3331; Daniel J. Raab, President and Chief Executive Officer (Total facility includes 50 beds in nursing home–type unit) **A**1 9 10 **F**7 9 13 14 16 17 18 20 22 24 25 30 32 33 34 35 36 37 38 39 40 41 44 45 46 48 50 51 54 56 68 69 70 72 76 78 79 **P**5 **S** Memorial Health System, Springfield, IL | 21 | 10 | 151 | 2150 | 64 | 39055 | 171 | 17619 | 8511 | 309 |

TINLEY PARK—Cook County

☐ TINLEY PARK MENTAL HEALTH CENTER, 7400 West 183rd Street, Zip 60477-3695; tel. 708/614-4000; Delores Newman, MS, Network Manager, Metro South Network (Nonreporting) **A**1 5 10 | 12 | 22 | 280 | — | — | — | — | — | — | — |

URBANA—Champaign County

★ △ CARLE FOUNDATION HOSPITAL, 611 West Park Street, Zip 61801-2595; tel. 217/383-3311; James Leonard, M.D., Interim Administrator (Total facility includes 240 beds in nursing home–type unit) **A**1 2 3 5 7 9 10 **F**4 6 7 8 9 11 12 13 14 16 17 18 19 22 25 27 29 30 31 32 33 34 35 36 37 38 39 41 42 43 44 45 46 47 48 49 50 51 53 54 56 65 66 67 69 70 71 72 75 76 77 78 79 **P**5
Web address: www.carle.com | 23 | 10 | 451 | 11498 | 289 | 56254 | 1811 | 120002 | 45404 | 1656 |

★ △ PROVENA COVENANT MEDICAL CENTER, 1400 West Park Street, Zip 61801-2396; tel. 217/337-2000; Diane Friedman, R.N., President and Chief Executive Officer (Total facility includes 12 beds in nursing home–type unit) **A**1 2 3 5 7 9 10 **F**4 8 11 13 17 18 19 22 24 25 30 34 37 38 39 41 42 43 44 46 47 48 50 51 53 54 57 59 60 61 63 68 69 70 72 76 78 **P**1 4 7 8 **S** Provena Health, Frankfort, IL
Web address: www.provenacovenant.org | 21 | 10 | 258 | 10942 | 121 | 142832 | 1297 | 89134 | 38825 | 1003 |

VANDALIA—Fayette County

★ FAYETTE COUNTY HOSPITAL, Seventh and Taylor Streets, Zip 62471-1296; tel. 618/283-1231; Daniel L. Gantz, President (Total facility includes 101 beds in nursing home–type unit) **A**1 9 10 **F**7 9 13 16 17 18 19 22 24 25 30 31 32 34 36 37 39 40 41 45 48 54 62 63 69 70 72 76 **P**7 **S** BJC Health System, Saint Louis, MO
Web address: www.provenamercy.com | 16 | 10 | 142 | 1600 | 101 | 28441 | — | 13161 | 5432 | 243 |

© 2000 AHA Guide   *Many Facility Codes have changed. Please refer to the AHA Guide Code Chart.*

Hospitals, U.S. / ILLINOIS

Hospital, Address, Telephone, Administrator, Approval, Facility, and Physician Codes, Health Care System, Network	Classification Codes		Utilization Data					Expense (thousands) of dollars		
★ American Hospital Association (AHA) membership □ Joint Commission on Accreditation of Healthcare Organizations (JCAHO) accreditation + American Osteopathic Healthcare Association (AOHA) membership ○ American Osteopathic Association (AOA) accreditation △ Commission on Accreditation of Rehabilitation Facilities (CARF) accreditation Control codes 61, 63, 64, 71, 72 and 73 indicate hospitals listed by AOHA, but not registered by AHA. For definition of numerical codes, see page A4	Control	Service	Staffed Beds	Admissions	Census	Outpatient Visits	Births	Total	Payroll	Personnel
WATSEKA—Iroquois County □ IROQUOIS MEMORIAL HOSPITAL AND RESIDENT HOME, 200 Fairman Avenue, Zip 60970–1644; tel. 815/432–5841; Rex D. Conger, President and Chief Executive Officer (Total facility includes 46 beds in nursing home–type unit) (Nonreporting) **A**1 9 10 Web address: www.iroquoismemorial.com	23	10	112	—	—	—	—	—	—	—
WAUKEGAN—Lake County ★ △ PROVENA SAINT THERESE MEDICAL CENTER, 2615 Washington Street, Zip 60085–4988; tel. 847/249–3900; Timothy P. Selz, President and Chief Executive Officer (Total facility includes 25 beds in nursing home–type unit) **A**1 7 9 10 **F**7 8 9 11 12 13 16 17 18 19 20 21 22 23 24 25 26 28 29 31 32 33 34 36 37 39 43 44 45 46 48 49 50 51 53 54 57 58 59 60 61 63 64 69 70 75 76 77 78 **P**3 7 8 **S** Provena Health, Frankfort, IL Web address: www.sainttherese.org	21	10	254	8498	117	226177	1379	67844	30452	862
★ VICTORY MEMORIAL HOSPITAL, 1324 North Sheridan Road, Zip 60085–2181; tel. 847/360–3000; Timothy Harrington, President **A**1 2 9 10 **F**4 6 8 9 11 13 16 17 18 22 24 25 27 29 30 32 33 34 37 38 39 40 41 43 44 46 48 49 50 51 54 57 59 60 61 62 63 64 65 67 68 69 70 72 76 78 **P**1 7	23	10	102	7367	85	65096	1133	55205	27349	707
WEST FRANKFORT—Franklin County ★ UNITED MINE WORKERS OF AMERICA UNION HOSPITAL, 507 West St. Louis Street, Zip 62896–1999; tel. 618/932–2155; Becky Ashton, Senior Vice President and Administrator **A**9 10 **F**16 17 18 22 25 36 37 76 78 **P**7 **S** Southern Illinois Hospital Services, Carbondale, IL Web address: www.sih.net	23	10	20	251	3	13337	0	4132	1828	54
WHEATON—Du Page County ★ △ MARIANJOY REHABILITATION HOSPITAL, (Formerly Marianjoy Rehabilitation Hospital and Clinics), 26 West 171 Roosevelt Road, Zip 60187–0795, Mailing Address: P.O. Box 795, Zip 60189–0795; tel. 630/462–4000; Kathleen C. Yosko, President and Chief Executive Officer **A**1 3 5 7 9 10 **F**5 7 13 17 18 19 20 23 25 30 31 32 33 34 38 43 45 49 50 53 54 72 78 **P**5 6 **S** Wheaton Franciscan Services, Inc., Wheaton, IL Web address: www.marianjoy.org	21	46	116	1584	85	30322	0	43049	19384	446
WINFIELD—Du Page County ★ CENTRAL DUPAGE HOSPITAL, (Includes Behavioral Health Center, 27 West 350 High Lake Road, tel. 630/653–4000), 25 North Winfield Road, Zip 60190; tel. 630/682–1600; David S. Fox, President **A**1 2 9 10 **F**2 3 4 6 7 8 9 11 12 13 16 17 18 19 22 23 24 25 27 28 29 32 33 34 35 37 38 39 41 42 44 45 46 47 48 49 50 51 52 54 56 57 58 59 61 62 63 64 67 69 70 72 75 76 77 78 **P**6	23	10	321	15173	173	281947	3277	179954	66654	1808
WOOD RIVER—Madison County ★ WOOD RIVER TOWNSHIP HOSPITAL, 101 East Edwardsville Road, Zip 62095–1332; tel. 618/251–7101; David G. Triebes, Chief Executive Officer **A**1 9 10 **F**3 7 8 9 14 16 17 18 19 22 24 25 26 30 37 39 40 41 44 45 48 53 54 57 70 76 78 **S** Brim Healthcare, Inc., Brentwood, TN Web address: www.ezl.com/~wrth101/	16	10	60	984	18	15886	168	14845	5611	173
WOODSTOCK—McHenry County ★ MEMORIAL MEDICAL CENTER, Highway 14 and Doty Road, Zip 60098–3797, Mailing Address: P.O. Box 1990, Zip 60098–1990; tel. 815/338–2500; Paul E. Laudick, President and Chief Executive Officer (Total facility includes 24 beds in nursing home–type unit) **A**1 2 9 10 **F**3 7 8 9 13 16 17 18 19 21 22 23 25 28 30 31 32 33 34 36 37 38 39 40 41 43 44 45 46 48 50 51 53 54 57 58 59 60 61 62 63 64 65 69 70 72 75 76 78 79 **P**6 Web address: www.centegra.org	23	10	122	5436	65	81421	577	51979	21792	459
ZION—Lake County □ MIDWESTERN REGIONAL MEDICAL CENTER, (ONCOLOGY), 2520 Elisha Avenue, Zip 60099–2587; tel. 847/872–4561; Roger C. Cary, President and Chief Executive Officer **A**1 2 10 **F**9 13 16 17 18 19 22 23 24 25 31 32 33 34 35 36 37 38 39 41 43 45 46 48 49 50 51 54 56 65 70 71 73 74 76 78 **S** Cancer Treatment Centers of America, Arlington Heights, IL Web address: www.pulbiconline.com/=mrmc	33	49	70	1860	29	22004	0	45281	15050	362

Hospitals, U.S. / INDIANA

INDIANA

Resident Population 5,899 (in thousands)
Resident population in metro areas 71.7%
Birth rate per 1,000 population 14.2
65 years and over 12.5%
Percent of persons without health insurance 11.4%

Hospital, Address, Telephone, Administrator, Approval, Facility, and Physician Codes, Health Care System, Network	Classification Codes		Utilization Data					Expense (thousands) of dollars		
★ American Hospital Association (AHA) membership ☐ Joint Commission on Accreditation of Healthcare Organizations (JCAHO) accreditation + American Osteopathic Healthcare Association (AOHA) membership ○ American Osteopathic Association (AOA) accreditation △ Commission on Accreditation of Rehabilitation Facilities (CARF) accreditation Control codes 61, 63, 64, 71, 72 and 73 indicate hospitals listed by AOHA, but not registered by AHA. For definition of numerical codes, see page A4	Control	Service	Staffed Beds	Admissions	Census	Outpatient Visits	Births	Total	Payroll	Personnel
ANDERSON—Madison County COMMUNITY HOSPITAL OF ANDERSON AND MADISON COUNTY See Community Hospitals Indianapolis, Indianapolis ✠ SAINT JOHN'S HEALTH SYSTEM, 2015 Jackson Street, Zip 46016-4339; tel. 765/649-2511; Jerry D. Brumitt, President and Chief Executive Officer (Total facility includes 29 beds in nursing home-type unit) **A**1 2 9 10 **F**2 3 7 8 9 11 13 14 16 17 18 19 21 22 23 24 25 26 27 29 31 32 33 34 35 36 37 38 39 41 43 44 45 46 48 49 50 53 54 57 58 63 64 65 69 70 71 72 73 76 77 78 79 **P**7 8 **S** Trinity Health, Novi, MI Web address: www.stjohnshealthsystem.org	21	10	205	7956	107	342057	604	95731	40702	1173
ANGOLA—Steuben County ★ CAMERON MEMORIAL COMMUNITY HOSPITAL, 416 East Maumee Street, Zip 46703-2015; tel. 219/665-2141; Dennis L. Knapp, President **A**9 10 **F**3 6 7 8 9 16 17 22 25 33 34 36 37 38 39 40 41 43 44 48 51 54 70 76 77 78 Web address: www.cameronhosp.com	23	10	30	1031	8	77184	300	16080	7593	258
AUBURN—De Kalb County ✠ DEKALB MEMORIAL HOSPITAL, 1316 East Seventh Street, Zip 46706-2515, Mailing Address: P.O. Box 542, Zip 46706-0542; tel. 219/925-4600; Jack M. Corey, President **A**1 9 10 **F**8 9 13 16 17 18 19 22 24 25 26 28 32 34 35 36 37 38 39 41 43 44 45 48 49 50 51 53 54 56 68 70 72 76 77 78 **P**6 7 8 Web address: www.dekalbmemorial.com	23	10	45	1892	14	66686	466	23862	10752	321
BATESVILLE—Franklin County ✠ MARGARET MARY COMMUNITY HOSPITAL, 321 Mitchell Avenue, Zip 47006-8953, Mailing Address: P.O. Box 226, Zip 47006-0226; tel. 812/934-6624; James L. Amos, President (Total facility includes 34 beds in nursing home-type unit) **A**1 9 10 **F**8 9 17 18 22 23 24 25 30 32 34 36 37 38 39 40 41 43 44 48 54 68 69 70 71 72 76 78 **P**6 Web address: www.mmch.org	23	10	81	2270	48	91792	403	22832	11089	304
BEDFORD—Lawrence County ✠ BEDFORD REGIONAL MEDICAL CENTER, 2900 West 16th Street, Zip 47421-3583; tel. 812/275-1200; Bradford W. Dykes, President and Chief Executive Officer **A**1 2 9 10 **F**7 8 9 13 16 17 18 19 20 22 23 24 25 29 31 32 33 34 36 37 38 39 43 44 45 46 48 49 50 51 54 56 59 63 68 70 72 76 77 78 79 **P**1 6 Web address: www.brmchealthcare.com	23	10	60	2528	25	177346	293	35790	14999	424
✠ DUNN MEMORIAL HOSPITAL, 1600 23rd Street, Zip 47421-4704; tel. 812/275-3331; Tony G. Sudduth, Chief Executive Officer (Nonreporting) **A**1 9 10 Web address: www.dunnmemorial.org	13	10	96	—	—	—	—	—	—	—
BEECH GROVE—Marion County ✠ ST. FRANCIS HOSPITAL AND HEALTH CENTERS – NORTH CAMPUS, (Includes St. Francis Hospital and Health Centers – South Campus, 8111 South Emerson Avenue, Indianapolis, Zip 46217), 1600 Albany Street, Zip 46107-1593; tel. 317/787-3311; Robert J. Brody, President and Chief Executive Officer (Total facility includes 41 beds in nursing home-type unit) **A**1 2 3 5 9 10 **F**3 4 8 9 11 12 13 16 17 18 19 21 22 24 25 30 32 33 34 36 37 38 39 41 42 43 44 45 46 47 48 49 51 54 57 58 59 60 61 62 63 64 65 68 69 70 71 72 73 76 77 78 79 **P**7 8 **S** Sisters of St. Francis Health Services, Inc., Mishawaka, IN Web address: www.stfrancis-indy.org	21	10	402	18651	238	187776	2721	215045	98346	3132
BLOOMINGTON—Monroe County ☐ BLOOMINGTON HOSPITAL, 601 West Second Street, Zip 47403-2317, Mailing Address: P.O. Box 1149, Zip 47402-1149; tel. 812/336-6821; Nancy S. Carlstedt, President and Chief Executive Officer (Total facility includes 750 beds in nursing home-type unit) **A**1 9 10 **F**1 2 3 4 6 7 8 9 11 12 13 16 17 18 19 21 22 24 25 26 27 28 29 30 31 32 33 34 35 36 37 38 39 40 41 42 43 44 45 46 47 48 50 51 54 57 58 59 60 61 62 63 64 65 67 69 70 71 72 75 76 77 78 79 **P**1 Web address: www.bhhs.org	23	10	1034	16177	669	338727	1935	168399	77755	2676
BLUFFTON—Wells County ✠ CAYLOR–NICKEL MEDICAL CENTER, One Caylor-Nickel Square, Zip 46714-2529; tel. 219/824-3500; William F. Brockmann, President and Chief Executive Officer (Total facility includes 19 beds in nursing home-type unit) **A**1 2 9 10 **F**3 5 8 9 12 13 16 17 18 19 22 23 24 25 28 29 30 34 36 37 39 41 43 44 45 46 48 49 50 51 54 56 57 58 59 61 62 63 64 65 69 70 72 76 78 **P**8 **S** Quorum Health Group, Brentwood, TN Web address: www.caylornickel.com	23	10	95	2840	35	107885	262	—	—	423
✠ WELLS COMMUNITY HOSPITAL, 1100 South Main Street, Zip 46714-3697; tel. 219/824-3210; Thomas A. Clark, Chief Executive Officer **A**1 9 10 **F**7 8 9 16 17 18 19 22 25 28 32 34 36 37 38 39 43 44 45 48 49 50 51 54 70 72 75 76 78 79 Web address: www.wellscommunityhospital.com	13	10	30	974	8	37436	171	12500	5487	159

© 2000 AHA Guide   *Many Facility Codes have changed. Please refer to the AHA Guide Code Chart.*   Hospitals **A137**

Hospitals, U.S. / INDIANA

Hospital, Address, Telephone, Administrator, Approval, Facility, and Physician Codes, Health Care System, Network	Classification Codes		Utilization Data					Expense (thousands) of dollars		
	Control	Service	Staffed Beds	Admissions	Census	Outpatient Visits	Births	Total	Payroll	Personnel

★ American Hospital Association (AHA) membership
☐ Joint Commission on Accreditation of Healthcare Organizations (JCAHO) accreditation
+ American Osteopathic Healthcare Association (AOHA) membership
○ American Osteopathic Association (AOA) accreditation
△ Commission on Accreditation of Rehabilitation Facilities (CARF) accreditation
Control codes 61, 63, 64, 71, 72 and 73 indicate hospitals listed by AOHA, but not registered by AHA. For definition of numerical codes, see page A4

BOONVILLE—Warrick County

☒ ST. ELIZABETH ANN SETON HOSPITAL, 1116 Millis Avenue, Zip 47601, Mailing Address: P.O. Box 290, Zip 47601–0290; tel. 812/897-7440; Reginald P. Gibson, FACHE, Executive Director (Nonreporting) **A**1 10 **S** Ascension Health, Saint Louis, MO — 23 10 25 — — — — — — —

☒ ST. MARY'S WARRICK, (Formerly St. Mary's Hospital Warrick), 1116 Millis Avenue, Zip 47601–0629, Mailing Address: Box 629, Zip 47601–0629; tel. 812/897–4800; James M. Hayes, Executive Vice President and Administrator **A**1 9 10 **F**9 16 17 18 19 22 23 25 32 34 35 36 41 45 48 53 54 70 76 78 **S** Ascension Health, Saint Louis, MO
Web address: www.stmarys.org — 23 10 28 864 10 13125 0 10994 5824 201

BRAZIL—Clay County

☒ CLAY COUNTY HOSPITAL, 1206 East National Avenue, Zip 47834–2797; tel. 812/448–2675; Jay P. Jolly, Administrator and Chief Executive Officer **A**1 9 10 **F**8 9 22 23 24 25 32 38 39 41 44 48 50 51 54 70 76 78 **P**8 — 13 10 36 1124 10 20950 97 7924 3199 134

BREMEN—Marshall County

★ COMMUNITY HOSPITAL OF BREMEN, 411 South Whitlock Street, Zip 46506, Mailing Address: P.O. Box 8, Zip 46506–0008; tel. 219/546–2211; Scott R. Graybill, Chief Executive Officer and Administrator **A**9 10 18 **F**7 9 13 17 19 22 25 26 30 31 32 34 36 37 38 43 44 45 48 49 54 56 58 59 60 61 62 63 64 70 71 76 78 **P**1 **S** Ancilla Systems Inc., Hobart, IN — 23 10 24 401 3 — 84 5201 2345 75

CARMEL—Hamilton County

ST. VINCENT CARMEL HOSPITAL See St. Vincent Hospitals and Health Services, Indianapolis

CHARLESTOWN—Clark County

☐ MEDICAL CENTER OF SOUTHERN INDIANA, 2200 Market Street, Zip 47111–0069, Mailing Address: P.O. Box 69, Zip 47111–0069; tel. 812/256–3301; Kevin J. Miller, FACHE, President and Chief Executive Officer (Nonreporting) **A**1 9 10
Web address: www.mcsin.org — 23 10 80 — — — — — — —

CLINTON—Vermillion County

☐ WEST CENTRAL COMMUNITY HOSPITAL, 801 South Main Street, Zip 47842–0349; tel. 765/832–2451; Marilyn J. Custer-Mitchell, Administrator **A**1 9 10 **F**8 9 16 17 18 22 25 28 29 32 38 41 43 44 46 48 51 54 70 76 78 **P**1 6 — 23 10 27 1406 15 42674 99 11916 4979 166

COLUMBIA CITY—Whitley County

☐ WHITLEY MEMORIAL HOSPITAL, 353 North Oak Street, Zip 46725–1623; tel. 219/244–6191; John M. Hatcher, President (Total facility includes 81 beds in nursing home–type unit) **A**1 9 10 **F**8 9 12 16 17 18 22 25 28 32 34 36 37 39 40 41 43 44 45 48 54 69 72 76 77 78 **P**6 7 8 **S** Parkview Health System, Fort Wayne, IN — 23 10 122 1786 92 40596 327 23389 10262 298

COLUMBUS—Bartholomew County

☐ BEHAVIORAL HEALTHCARE–COLUMBUS, 2223 Poshard Drive, Zip 47203–1844, Mailing Address: P.O. Box 1549, Zip 47203–1844; tel. 812/376–1711; Bryan W. Lett, Chief Executive Officer (Nonreporting) **A**1 9 10 **S** Behavioral Healthcare Corporation, Nashville, TN — 33 22 60 — — — — — — —

☒ COLUMBUS REGIONAL HOSPITAL, 2400 East 17th Street, Zip 47201–5360; tel. 812/379–4441; Douglas J. Leonard, Chief Executive Officer (Total facility includes 21 beds in nursing home–type unit) **A**1 2 9 10 **F**4 7 8 9 11 13 16 17 18 19 20 22 25 27 28 29 32 33 34 36 37 38 39 40 41 43 44 45 46 48 49 50 51 53 54 57 59 60 61 64 65 68 69 70 71 72 75 76 77 78 79 **P**3 5 8
Web address: www.crh.org — 13 10 218 10338 139 149772 1444 110698 48168 1438

CONNERSVILLE—Fayette County

☒ FAYETTE MEMORIAL HOSPITAL, 1941 Virginia Avenue, Zip 47331–9990; tel. 765/825–5131; David R. Brandon, Chief Executive Officer (Nonreporting) **A**1 9 10 — 23 10 111 — — — — — — —

CORYDON—Harrison County

☒ HARRISON COUNTY HOSPITAL, 245 Atwood Street, Zip 47112–1774; tel. 812/738–4251; Steven L. Taylor, Chief Executive Officer **A**1 9 10 **F**8 9 16 17 19 22 24 25 34 36 38 39 44 45 46 48 49 50 51 54 68 70 71 72 76 **P**2 7 **S** Norton Healthcare, Louisville, KY — 13 10 47 1277 14 37486 98 17514 7661 290

CRAWFORDSVILLE—Montgomery County

☒ ST. CLARE MEDICAL CENTER, (Formerly Culver Union Hospital), 1710 Lafayette Road, Zip 47933–1099; tel. 765/362–2800; Gregory D. Starnes, Chief Executive Officer (Total facility includes 17 beds in nursing home–type unit) **A**1 9 10 **F**8 9 13 16 17 18 22 25 26 32 34 36 37 38 39 40 41 43 44 45 48 53 54 57 59 61 62 69 70 71 72 76 78 79 **P**1 6 **S** Sisters of St. Francis Health Services, Inc., Mishawaka, IN — 21 10 89 3427 46 57924 287 26901 8969 329

CROWN POINT—Lake County

☒ ST. ANTHONY MEDICAL CENTER, 1201 South Main Street, Zip 46307–8483; tel. 219/738–2100; Stephen O. Leurck, President and Chief Executive Officer **A**1 2 6 9 10 **F**4 7 8 9 11 12 13 14 16 17 18 19 21 22 24 25 29 32 38 39 43 44 45 46 47 48 49 50 51 53 54 55 56 65 68 70 71 72 76 77 78 79 **P**6 7 8 **S** Sisters of St. Francis Health Services, Inc., Mishawaka, IN — 21 10 228 6180 92 86606 681 75093 29801 727

Hospitals, U.S. / INDIANA

Hospital, Address, Telephone, Administrator, Approval, Facility, and Physician Codes, Health Care System, Network	Classification Codes		Utilization Data					Expense (thousands) of dollars		
★ American Hospital Association (AHA) membership ☐ Joint Commission on Accreditation of Healthcare Organizations (JCAHO) accreditation + American Osteopathic Healthcare Association (AOHA) membership ○ American Osteopathic Association (AOA) accreditation △ Commission on Accreditation of Rehabilitation Facilities (CARF) accreditation Control codes 61, 63, 64, 71, 72 and 73 indicate hospitals listed by AOHA, but not registered by AHA. For definition of numerical codes, see page A4	Control	Service	Staffed Beds	Admissions	Census	Outpatient Visits	Births	Total	Payroll	Personnel
DANVILLE—Hendricks County ★ HENDRICKS COMMUNITY HOSPITAL, 1000 East Main Street, Zip 46122–0409, Mailing Address: P.O. Box 409, Zip 46122–0409; tel. 317/745–4451; Dennis W. Dawes, President **A**1 9 10 **F**2 7 8 9 13 16 17 18 22 23 24 25 28 32 33 34 35 36 38 39 40 41 43 44 45 46 48 50 54 56 57 59 60 61 62 63 65 70 71 72 76 77 78 79 **P**1 6 7 Web address: www.hendrickshospital.org	13	10	127	6323	67	206624	1008	60272	28421	740
DECATUR—Adams County ★ ADAMS COUNTY MEMORIAL HOSPITAL, 805 High Street, Zip 46733–2311, Mailing Address: P.O. Box 151, Zip 46733–0151; tel. 219/724–2145; Marvin L. Baird, Executive Director (Total facility includes 22 beds in nursing home–type unit) **A**1 9 10 **F**1 3 9 16 17 18 22 24 25 30 34 36 39 41 44 45 46 48 50 54 57 62 63 64 69 70 76	13	10	87	2569	42	55766	243	20042	8031	293
DYER—Lake County SAINT MARGARET MERCY HEALTHCARE CENTERS–SOUTH CAMPUS See Saint Margaret Mercy Healthcare Centers, Hammond										
EAST CHICAGO—Lake County ★ ST. CATHERINE HOSPITAL, 4321 Fir Street, Zip 46312–3097; tel. 219/392–7000; JoAnn Birdzell, President and Chief Executive Officer **A**1 9 10 **F**3 7 8 9 11 12 13 16 17 18 19 22 24 25 27 28 29 32 33 34 37 38 39 41 43 44 45 47 48 49 50 51 54 55 57 59 60 61 62 65 68 69 70 72 75 76 78 79 **P**1 **S** Ancilla Systems Inc., Hobart, IN	21	10	188	7914	119	78704	532	71747	27910	739
ELKHART—Elkhart County ★ △ ELKHART GENERAL HOSPITAL, 600 East Boulevard, Zip 46514–2499, Mailing Address: P.O. Box 1329, Zip 46515–1329; tel. 219/294–2621; Gregory W. Lintjer, President (Total facility includes 40 beds in nursing home–type unit) **A**1 7 9 10 **F**3 4 7 8 9 11 12 13 16 17 18 19 21 22 24 25 27 33 34 35 36 37 39 40 41 42 44 45 46 47 48 49 51 54 57 58 59 60 61 63 64 65 70 72 76 77 78 **P**5 8	23	10	309	13059	177	129502	1918	133091	55417	972
ELWOOD—Madison County ★ ST. VINCENT MERCY HOSPITAL, 1331 South A Street, Zip 46036–1942; tel. 765/552–4600; David Masterson, Administrator (Nonreporting) **A**1 9 10 **S** Ascension Health, Saint Louis, MO Web address: www.stvincent.org	21	10	40	—	—	—	—	—	—	—
EVANSVILLE—Vanderburgh County ★ DEACONESS HOSPITAL, 600 Mary Street, Zip 47747–0001; tel. 812/450–5000; Thomas H. Kramer, President and Chief Executive Officer (Total facility includes 48 beds in nursing home–type unit) **A**1 2 3 5 9 10 **F**3 4 7 8 9 11 12 13 16 17 18 19 20 21 22 24 25 26 27 28 29 30 31 32 33 34 35 36 37 38 39 40 41 43 44 45 46 47 48 51 52 54 56 58 59 60 61 62 63 65 66 67 68 69 70 72 75 76 77 78 79 **P**1 6 Web address: www.deaconess.com	23	10	335	15561	213	228615	1488	151689	66249	1965
☐ EVANSVILLE STATE HOSPITAL, 3400 Lincoln Avenue, Zip 47714–0146; tel. 812/473–2100; Ralph Nichols, Superintendent **A**1 13 **F**16 23 45 54 57 62 70 78	12	22	304	96	276	0	0	23743	12703	497
☐ △ HEALTHSOUTH TRI–STATE REHABILITATION HOSPITAL, 4100 Covert Avenue, Zip 47714–5567, Mailing Address: P.O. Box 5349, Zip 47716–5349; tel. 812/476–9983; Barbara Butler, Administrator and Chief Operating Officer (Nonreporting) **A**1 7 9 10 **S** HEALTHSOUTH Corporation, Birmingham, AL Web address: www.healthsouth.com	33	46	80	—	—	—	—	—	—	—
ST MARY'S HEALTH SERVICES–WELBORN CAMPUS See St. Mary's Medical Center ★ △ ST. MARY'S MEDICAL CENTER, (Includes St Mary's Health Services–Welborn Campus, 401 Southeast Sixth Street, Zip 47713–1299; tel. 812/426–8000; Richard C. Breon, Chief Executive Officer), 3700 Washington Avenue, Zip 47750–0002; tel. 812/485–4000; Jay D. Kasey, President (Total facility includes 137 beds in nursing home–type unit) **A**1 2 3 5 7 9 10 **F**1 2 3 4 6 7 8 9 11 12 13 14 15 16 17 18 19 20 22 24 25 26 27 28 29 30 32 33 34 36 37 38 39 41 42 43 44 45 46 47 49 51 52 53 54 56 57 58 59 60 61 62 63 64 65 66 69 70 71 72 73 76 77 78 79 **P**6 7 **S** Ascension Health, Saint Louis, MO	21	10	787	14418	381	243639	2191	168811	72745	2950
FORT WAYNE—Allen County ☐ CHARTER BEACON, 1720 Beacon Street, Zip 46805–4700; tel. 219/423–3651; Robert Hails, Chief Executive Officer (Nonreporting) **A**1 10 **S** Magellan Health Services, Atlanta, GA Web address: www.charterbeacon.com	33	22	97	—	—	—	—	—	—	—
★ LUTHERAN HOSPITAL OF INDIANA, 7950 West Jefferson Boulevard, Zip 46804–1677; tel. 219/435–7001; Thomas D. Miller, President and Chief Executive Officer **A**1 3 5 9 10 **F**3 4 8 9 11 12 13 16 17 18 19 22 24 25 27 29 30 31 32 33 34 35 38 39 40 41 42 43 44 45 46 47 48 50 52 54 57 59 60 61 62 63 64 65 69 70 72 74 76 77 78 79 **P**5 7 **S** Quorum Health Group, Brentwood, TN Web address: www.lutheran–hosp.com	33	10	377	17654	241	190811	2063	129222	53726	1620
★ △ PARKVIEW HOSPITAL, 2200 Randallia Drive, Zip 46805–4699; tel. 219/484–6636; Frank D. Byrne, M.D., President (Total facility includes 28 beds in nursing home–type unit) **A**1 3 5 7 9 10 **F**2 3 4 8 9 11 12 13 17 18 19 22 24 25 28 32 33 34 36 37 38 39 40 41 42 43 44 45 46 47 48 49 50 51 52 53 54 56 57 59 60 61 62 63 65 68 69 70 72 73 75 76 77 78 79 **P**6 7 8 **S** Parkview Health System, Fort Wayne, IN	23	10	505	24705	354	249556	3960	248417	114005	3003

© 2000 AHA Guide — *Many Facility Codes have changed. Please refer to the AHA Guide Code Chart.*

Hospitals, U.S. / INDIANA

Hospital, Address, Telephone, Administrator, Approval, Facility, and Physician Codes, Health Care System, Network	Classification Codes		Utilization Data					Expense (thousands) of dollars		
	Control	Service	Staffed Beds	Admissions	Census	Outpatient Visits	Births	Total	Payroll	Personnel

★ American Hospital Association (AHA) membership
□ Joint Commission on Accreditation of Healthcare Organizations (JCAHO) accreditation
+ American Osteopathic Healthcare Association (AOHA) membership
○ American Osteopathic Association (AOA) accreditation
△ Commission on Accreditation of Rehabilitation Facilities (CARF) accreditation
Control codes 61, 63, 64, 71, 72 and 73 indicate hospitals listed by AOHA, but not registered by AHA. For definition of numerical codes, see page A4

Hospital	Control	Service	Staffed Beds	Admissions	Census	Outpatient Visits	Births	Total	Payroll	Personnel
□ △ REHABILITATION HOSPITAL OF FORT WAYNE, 7970 West Jefferson Boulevard, Zip 46804–4140; tel. 219/436–2644; Norman F. Stephens, Chief Executive Officer **A**1 7 9 10 **F**3 4 5 7 8 9 11 13 14 16 20 22 24 25 26 27 28 30 31 33 35 36 37 38 39 45 46 47 48 49 50 51 53 54 56 58 59 60 61 62 63 64 70 71 72 74 76 77 78 79 **S** HEALTHSOUTH Corporation, Birmingham, AL	33	46	60	865	35	4313	0	8421	4547	114
★ △ ST. JOSEPH HOSPITAL, (Formerly St. Joseph Health System), 700 Broadway, Zip 46802–1493; tel. 219/425–3000; Michael H. Schatzlein, M.D., President and Chief Executive Officer (Nonreporting) **A**1 3 5 7 9 10 **S** Quorum Health Group, Brentwood, TN Web address: www.stjoehospital.com	33	10	194	—	—	—	—	—	—	—
★ VETERANS AFFAIRS NORTHERN INDIANA HEALTH CARE SYSTEM, (Includes Veterans Affairs Northern Indiana Health Care System–Marion Campus, 1700 East 38th Street, Marion, Zip 46953–4589; tel. 765/674–3321); 2121 Lake Avenue, Zip 46805–5347; tel. 219/460–1310; Michael W. Murphy, Ph.D., Director and Chief Executive Officer (Total facility includes 123 beds in nursing home–type unit) **A**1 **F**1 3 9 13 19 22 23 24 26 30 32 34 35 36 38 39 41 43 45 46 48 49 51 54 56 57 59 60 61 62 63 64 65 69 70 72 76 78 79 **P**1 **S** Department of Veterans Affairs, Washington, DC Web address: www.va.gov/stations97/guide/home.asp?DIVISION=ALL	45	10	423	2512	345	136198	—	78969	44059	1054

FRANKFORT—Clinton County

Hospital	Control	Service	Staffed Beds	Admissions	Census	Outpatient Visits	Births	Total	Payroll	Personnel
★ ST. VINCENT FRANKFORT HOSPITAL, (Formerly Clinton County Hospital), 1300 South Jackson Street, Zip 46041–3394, Mailing Address: P.O. Box 669, Zip 46041–0669; tel. 765/659–4731; Brian R. Zeh, Administrator **A**1 9 10 **F**3 7 8 9 13 22 23 24 25 30 32 33 34 38 39 41 43 44 45 46 48 49 50 54 59 60 63 68 70 72 76 78 79 **P**1 6 Web address: www.cchosp/accs.net	33	10	53	1320	12	39535	298	13680	5506	197

FRANKLIN—Johnson County

Hospital	Control	Service	Staffed Beds	Admissions	Census	Outpatient Visits	Births	Total	Payroll	Personnel
★ JOHNSON MEMORIAL HOSPITAL, 1125 West Jefferson Street, Zip 46131–2140, Mailing Address: P.O. Box 549, Zip 46131–0549; tel. 317/736–3300; Gregg A. Bechtold, President and Chief Executive Officer (Total facility includes 87 beds in nursing home–type unit) **A**1 9 10 **F**1 8 9 13 16 17 18 19 22 24 25 26 32 34 36 39 41 43 44 45 46 48 51 54 69 70 72 76 77 78 **P**6 8 Web address: www.johnsonmemorial.org	13	10	164	4302	110	105838	639	45446	17742	628

GARY—Lake County

Hospital	Control	Service	Staffed Beds	Admissions	Census	Outpatient Visits	Births	Total	Payroll	Personnel
★ △ METHODIST HOSPITALS, (Includes Northlake Campus; Southlake Campus, 8701 Broadway, Merrillville, Zip 46410; tel. 219/738–5500), 600 Grant Street, Zip 46402–6099; tel. 219/886–4000; John H. Betjemann, President (Total facility includes 62 beds in nursing home–type unit) **A**1 2 3 5 7 9 10 **F**2 3 4 7 8 9 11 13 14 15 17 18 19 20 21 22 24 25 27 29 32 33 34 35 38 39 41 42 43 44 45 46 47 48 49 50 51 53 54 56 57 58 59 63 65 66 68 69 70 71 72 74 75 76 77 78 79 **P**5 6 Web address: www.methodisthospitals.org	23	10	625	23466	369	210717	2160	222501	98627	2543

GOSHEN—Elkhart County

Hospital	Control	Service	Staffed Beds	Admissions	Census	Outpatient Visits	Births	Total	Payroll	Personnel
★ GOSHEN GENERAL HOSPITAL, 200 High Park Avenue, Zip 46526–4899, Mailing Address: P.O. Box 139, Zip 46527–0139; tel. 219/533–2141; James O. Dague, President and Chief Executive Officer **A**1 9 10 **F**1 2 3 4 6 7 8 9 11 13 14 16 17 18 19 22 23 24 25 26 27 28 30 31 32 33 34 35 36 37 38 39 40 41 43 44 45 46 48 49 50 51 54 56 57 58 59 60 61 62 63 64 66 67 69 70 71 72 73 75 76 77 78 79 **P**1 6	23	10	113	5392	62	99455	1216	48784	21969	592
OAKLAWN PSYCHIATRIC CENTER, INC., 330 Lakeview Drive, Zip 46528–9365, Mailing Address: P.O. Box 809, Zip 46527–0809; tel. 219/533–1234; Harold C. Loewen, President **A**10 **F**1 3 13 17 18 19 21 30 31 35 57 58 59 60 61 62 63 64 70 78 **P**1	21	22	16	974	15	153977	0	21397	10105	409

GREENCASTLE—Putnam County

Hospital	Control	Service	Staffed Beds	Admissions	Census	Outpatient Visits	Births	Total	Payroll	Personnel
★ PUTNAM COUNTY HOSPITAL, 1542 Bloomington Street, Zip 46135–2297; tel. 765/653–5121; Dennis Weatherford, Interim Administrator **A**1 2 9 10 **F**8 9 16 17 18 19 22 23 24 25 30 32 34 36 39 41 43 44 45 46 48 51 54 61 68 70 72 76 **P**8	13	10	85	1831	23	60517	217	16003	6763	267

GREENFIELD—Hancock County

Hospital	Control	Service	Staffed Beds	Admissions	Census	Outpatient Visits	Births	Total	Payroll	Personnel
★ HANCOCK MEMORIAL HOSPITAL AND HEALTH SERVICES, 801 North State Street, Zip 46140–1270, Mailing Address: P.O. Box 827, Zip 46140–0827; tel. 317/462–5544; Robert C. Keen, Ph.D., CHE, President and Chief Executive Officer (Total facility includes 21 beds in nursing home–type unit) **A**1 9 10 **F**1 3 7 8 9 11 12 13 16 17 18 19 20 21 22 25 26 27 28 30 32 34 35 36 37 38 39 41 43 44 46 48 49 50 51 54 57 62 63 64 66 70 71 72 73 76 77 78 79 **P**1 Web address: www.hmhhs.org	13	10	101	4416	60	162109	580	49469	22358	543

GREENSBURG—Decatur County

Hospital	Control	Service	Staffed Beds	Admissions	Census	Outpatient Visits	Births	Total	Payroll	Personnel
★ DECATUR COUNTY MEMORIAL HOSPITAL, 720 North Lincoln Street, Zip 47240–1398; tel. 812/663–4331; David V. Trexler, President **A**1 9 10 **F**1 7 8 9 22 24 25 27 32 34 36 39 44 45 46 48 49 53 54 56 68 70 71 72 76 79 **P**6 **S** Norton Healthcare, Louisville, KY	13	10	67	2184	29	67780	324	20474	9811	287

GREENWOOD—Johnson County

Hospital	Control	Service	Staffed Beds	Admissions	Census	Outpatient Visits	Births	Total	Payroll	Personnel
□ BHC VALLE VISTA HOSPITAL, 898 East Main Street, Zip 46143–1400; tel. 317/887–1348; Gordon L. Steinhauer, Chief Executive Officer (Nonreporting) **A**1 9 10 **S** Behavioral Healthcare Corporation, Nashville, TN	33	22	96	—	—	—	—	—	—	—

Hospitals, U.S. / INDIANA

Hospital, Address, Telephone, Administrator, Approval, Facility, and Physician Codes, Health Care System, Network	Classification Codes		Utilization Data					Expense (thousands) of dollars		Personnel
★ American Hospital Association (AHA) membership □ Joint Commission on Accreditation of Healthcare Organizations (JCAHO) accreditation + American Osteopathic Healthcare Association (AOHA) membership ○ American Osteopathic Association (AOA) accreditation △ Commission on Accreditation of Rehabilitation Facilities (CARF) accreditation Control codes 61, 63, 64, 71, 72 and 73 indicate hospitals listed by AOHA, but not registered by AHA. For definition of numerical codes, see page A4	Control	Service	Staffed Beds	Admissions	Census	Outpatient Visits	Births	Total	Payroll	
HAMMOND—Lake County ★ SAINT MARGARET MERCY HEALTHCARE CENTERS, (Includes Saint Margaret Mercy Healthcare Centers–North Campus, 5454 Hohman Avenue, Zip 46320; tel. 219/932-2300; Saint Margaret Mercy Healthcare Centers–South Campus, 24 Joliet Street, Dyer, Zip 46311-1799; tel. 219/865-2141), 5454 Hohman Avenue, Zip 46320-1999; tel. 219/933-2074; Eugene C. Diamond, President and Chief Executive Officer (Total facility includes 67 beds in nursing home–type unit) (Nonreporting) **A**1 2 9 10 **S** Sisters of St. Francis Health Services, Inc., Mishawaka, IN **Web address:** www.smmhc.com	21	10	624	—	—	—	—	—	—	—
HARTFORD CITY—Blackford County ★ BLACKFORD COUNTY HOSPITAL, 503 East Van Cleve Street, Zip 47348-1897; tel. 765/348-0300; Steven J. West, Chief Executive Officer **A**1 9 10 18 **F**7 8 9 13 17 18 22 23 25 32 34 36 39 44 48 70 72 76 78 **P**6 **S** Norton Healthcare, Louisville, KY	13	10	25	776	10	—	50	7983	2959	120
HOBART—Lake County ★ ST. MARY MEDICAL CENTER, 1500 South Lake Park Avenue, Zip 46342-6699; tel. 219/942-0551; Milton Triana, President and Chief Executive Officer **A**1 9 10 **F**1 2 3 4 5 6 7 8 9 10 11 12 13 14 15 16 17 18 19 20 21 22 23 24 25 26 27 28 29 30 31 32 33 34 35 36 37 38 39 40 41 42 43 44 45 46 47 48 49 50 51 52 53 54 55 56 57 58 59 60 61 62 63 64 65 66 67 68 69 70 71 72 73 74 75 76 77 78 79 **S** Ancilla Systems Inc., Hobart, IN **Web address:** www.stmary-hobart.com	21	10	146	7867	122	30862	414	70568	25547	667
HUNTINGBURG—Dubois County □ DEACONESS ST. JOSEPH'S HOSPITAL, (Formerly St. Joseph's Hospital), 1900 Medical Arts Drive, Zip 47542-9521; tel. 812/683-2121; John T. Graves, President and Chief Executive Officer **A**1 9 10 **F**7 8 9 13 21 22 25 26 32 33 34 35 36 37 41 43 44 45 48 50 51 53 54 57 59 60 61 70 72 73 76 78	23	10	60	1955	21	50197	219	15992	6993	267
HUNTINGTON—Huntington County ★ HUNTINGTON MEMORIAL HOSPITAL, 2001 Stults Road, Zip 46750-3696; tel. 219/356-3000; L. Kent McCoy, President **A**1 9 10 **F**3 4 5 6 8 9 11 13 14 16 17 18 19 20 21 22 24 25 28 29 30 31 32 33 34 35 36 37 38 39 40 43 44 47 48 49 50 51 54 55 56 58 59 60 61 62 63 64 65 66 67 70 71 72 73 74 75 76 77 78 79 **P**5 **S** Parkview Health System, Fort Wayne, IN	23	10	37	1634	12	38227	243	18377	8300	199
INDIANAPOLIS—Marion County ★ CLARIAN HEALTH PARTNERS, (Includes Indiana University Medical Center, 550 North University Boulevard, Zip 46202-5262; tel. 317/274-5000; Methodist Hospital of Indiana, 1701 North Senate Boulevard, Zip 46202, Mailing Address: I. 65 at 21st Street, P.O. Box 1367, Zip 46206-1367; tel. 317/929-2000; Riley Hospital for Children, 702 Barnhill Drive, Zip 46202-5225), I-65 at 21st Street, Zip 46206-5250, Mailing Address: P.O. Box 1367, Zip 46206-1367; tel. 317/274-5000; William J. Loveday, President and Chief Executive Officer (Total facility includes 45 beds in nursing home–type unit) **A**1 2 3 5 8 9 10 **F**2 3 4 5 7 8 9 10 11 12 13 14 16 17 18 19 20 21 22 23 24 25 26 27 29 30 32 33 34 35 36 37 38 39 40 41 42 43 44 45 46 47 48 49 50 51 52 53 54 55 56 57 58 59 60 61 62 63 64 65 66 68 69 70 71 72 73 74 75 76 77 78 79 **P**6 7	23	10	1245	51902	921	909142	4929	839241	358672	7861
□ △ COMMUNITY HOSPITALS INDIANAPOLIS, (Includes Community Hospital East, 1500 North Ritter Avenue, tel. 317/355-1411; Community Hospital North, 7150 Clearvista Drive, Zip 46256; tel. 317/849-6262; Community Hospital South, 1402 East County Line Road South, Zip 46227; tel. 317/887-7000; Community Hospital of Anderson and Madison County, 1515 North Madison Avenue, Anderson, Zip 46011-3453; tel. 765/642-8011), 1500 North Ritter Avenue, Zip 46219-3095; tel. 317/355-1411; William E. Corley, President (Total facility includes 30 beds in nursing home–type unit) (Nonreporting) **A**1 2 3 5 7 9 10 **Web address:** www.commhospindy.org	23	10	999	—	—	—	—	—	—	—
FAIRBANKS HOSPITAL, 8102 Clearvista Parkway, Zip 46256-4698; tel. 317/849-8222; Timothy J. Kelly, M.D., President **A**9 10 **F**2 3 17 18 19 21 23 57 58 61 70 **P**8 **Web address:** www.fairbankshospital.org INDIANA UNIVERSITY MEDICAL CENTER See Clarian Health Partners	23	82	70	2526	46	10832	0	6797	3519	108
□ LARUE D. CARTER MEMORIAL HOSPITAL, 2601 Cold Spring Road, Zip 46222-2273; tel. 317/941-4000; Diana Haugh, MS, Superintendent (Nonreporting) **A**1 3 5 10 METHODIST HOSPITAL OF INDIANA See Clarian Health Partners	12	22	146	—	—	—	—	—	—	—
□ △ REHABILITATION HOSPITAL OF INDIANA, 4141 Shore Drive, Zip 46254-2607; tel. 317/329-2000; Denny Armington, Chief Executive Officer (Nonreporting) **A**1 7 9 10 **Web address:** www.rehabhospind.org	23	46	80	—	—	—	—	—	—	—
★ △ RICHARD L. ROUDEBUSH VETERANS AFFAIRS MEDICAL CENTER, 1481 West Tenth Street, Zip 46202-2884; tel. 317/554-0000; Susan P. Bowers, Acting Director (Total facility includes 21 beds in nursing home–type unit) **A**1 2 3 5 7 8 **F**1 3 4 5 7 8 9 11 12 13 14 15 17 18 19 20 21 22 23 24 25 26 27 30 31 32 33 34 35 36 37 38 39 41 43 44 45 46 47 48 49 50 51 53 54 55 56 57 59 60 61 62 63 64 65 66 68 69 70 72 74 76 78 79 **P**6 **S** Department of Veterans Affairs, Washington, DC RILEY HOSPITAL FOR CHILDREN See Clarian Health Partners ST. FRANCIS HOSPITAL AND HEALTH CENTERS – SOUTH CAMPUS See St. Francis Hospital and Health Centers – North Campus, Beech Grove	45	10	139	8102	103	344817	0	144216	70552	1537

© 2000 AHA Guide   *Many Facility Codes have changed. Please refer to the AHA Guide Code Chart.*

Hospitals, U.S. / INDIANA

Hospital, Address, Telephone, Administrator, Approval, Facility, and Physician Codes, Health Care System, Network	Classification Codes		Utilization Data					Expense (thousands) of dollars		
	Control	Service	Staffed Beds	Admissions	Census	Outpatient Visits	Births	Total	Payroll	Personnel

- ★ American Hospital Association (AHA) membership
- □ Joint Commission on Accreditation of Healthcare Organizations (JCAHO) accreditation
- + American Osteopathic Healthcare Association (AOHA) membership
- ○ American Osteopathic Association (AOA) accreditation
- △ Commission on Accreditation of Rehabilitation Facilities (CARF) accreditation

Control codes 61, 63, 64, 71, 72 and 73 indicate hospitals listed by AOHA, but not registered by AHA. For definition of numerical codes, see page A4.

Hospital	Control	Service	Staffed Beds	Admissions	Census	Outpatient Visits	Births	Total	Payroll	Personnel
★ △ ST. VINCENT HOSPITALS AND HEALTH SERVICES, (Includes St. Vincent Carmel Hospital, 13500 North Meridian Street, Carmel, Zip 46032; tel. 317/582–7000; St. Vincent Stress Center, 8401 Harcourt Road, Zip 46260, Mailing Address: P.O. Box 80160, Zip 46280; tel. 317/338–4600; Paul Lefkovitz, Ph.D., Administrator), 2001 West 86th Street, Zip 46260–1991, Mailing Address: P.O. Box 40970, Zip 46240–0970; tel. 317/338–2345; Marsha N. Casey, President **A**1 2 3 5 7 8 9 10 **F**2 3 4 6 7 8 9 11 12 13 14 16 17 18 19 20 21 22 23 24 25 26 27 28 29 30 31 32 33 34 35 36 37 38 39 41 42 43 44 45 46 47 48 49 50 51 52 54 56 57 58 59 60 61 62 63 64 65 68 69 70 71 72 73 74 75 76 77 78 79 **P**6 8 **S** Ascension Health, Saint Louis, MO Web address: www.stvincent.org	21	10	752	34927	521	1024435	4527	492555	189756	5192
+ ○ WESTVIEW HOSPITAL, 3630 Guion Road, Zip 46222–1699; tel. 317/924–6661; David C. Dyar, Chief Executive Officer (Total facility includes 18 beds in nursing home–type unit) (Nonreporting) **A**9 10 11 12 13 Web address: www.westviewhospital.org	23	10	67	—	—	—	—	—	—	—
★ WINONA MEMORIAL HOSPITAL, 3232 North Meridian Street, Zip 46208–4693; tel. 317/924–3392; David L. Callecod, CHE, Chief Executive Officer **A**1 9 10 **F**2 3 4 9 11 12 13 16 17 18 19 22 24 25 30 31 32 33 34 36 38 39 41 43 45 46 48 49 50 51 53 54 57 59 60 61 62 63 70 72 76 78 79 **P**5 7 **S** TENET Healthcare Corporation, Santa Barbara, CA Web address: www.tenethealth.com	33	10	169	2930	47	48770	—	38159	15609	429
★ WISHARD HEALTH SERVICES, 1001 West 10th Street, Zip 46202–2879; tel. 317/630–7356; Randall L. Braddom, M.D., Chief Executive Officer and Medical Director (Total facility includes 240 beds in nursing home–type unit) (Nonreporting) **A**1 3 5 8 9 10	16	10	531	—	—	—	—	—	—	—
★ WOMEN'S HOSPITAL–INDIANAPOLIS, 8111 Township Line Road, Zip 46260–8043; tel. 317/875–5994; Steven B. Reed, President and Chief Executive Officer **A**1 9 10 **F**8 9 18 22 24 30 38 42 44 45 48 57 62 66 70 72 76 79 **S** HCA – The Healthcare Company, Nashville, TN Web address: www.womenshospital.org	33	44	102	3381	35	15638	2085	22773	11000	335

JASPER—Dubois County

Hospital	Control	Service	Staffed Beds	Admissions	Census	Outpatient Visits	Births	Total	Payroll	Personnel
★ MEMORIAL HOSPITAL AND HEALTH CARE CENTER, 800 West Ninth Street, Zip 47546–2516; tel. 812/482–2345; Raymond W. Snowden, President and Chief Executive Officer (Total facility includes 24 beds in nursing home–type unit) **A**1 2 9 10 **F**8 9 11 13 16 17 18 19 21 22 24 25 31 32 33 34 36 37 38 39 41 43 44 45 46 48 49 50 54 58 59 60 61 62 63 68 69 70 71 72 76 78 79 **S** Little Company of Mary Sisters Healthcare System, Evergreen Park, IL Web address: www.mhhcc.org	21	10	124	4866	62	98750	694	45666	22805	640

JEFFERSONVILLE—Clark County

Hospital	Control	Service	Staffed Beds	Admissions	Census	Outpatient Visits	Births	Total	Payroll	Personnel
★ CLARK MEMORIAL HOSPITAL, 1220 Missouri Avenue, Zip 47130–3743, Mailing Address: Box 69, Zip 47131–0069; tel. 812/282–6631; Merle E. Stepp, President and Chief Executive Officer (Total facility includes 66 beds in nursing home–type unit) **A**1 9 10 **F**3 4 7 8 9 11 13 16 17 19 21 22 24 25 28 29 32 33 34 36 37 38 39 41 43 44 45 46 47 48 50 51 54 56 57 58 59 60 61 62 63 65 70 71 72 74 76 78 79 **P**6 **S** Jewish Hospital HealthCare Services, Louisville, KY Web address: www.cmhl.com	13	10	243	8990	164	135484	1472	79515	39063	1221

KENDALLVILLE—Noble County

Hospital	Control	Service	Staffed Beds	Admissions	Census	Outpatient Visits	Births	Total	Payroll	Personnel
★ COMMUNITY HOSPITAL OF NOBLE COUNTY, (Formerly McCray Memorial Hospital), 951 East Hospital Drive, Zip 46755–2293, Mailing Address: P.O. Box 249, Zip 46755–0249; tel. 219/347–1100; John M. Hatcher, President (Nonreporting) **A**1 9 10 Web address: www.parkview.com	15	10	51	—	—	—	—	—	—	—

KNOX—Starke County

Hospital	Control	Service	Staffed Beds	Admissions	Census	Outpatient Visits	Births	Total	Payroll	Personnel
□ STARKE MEMORIAL HOSPITAL, 102 East Culver Road, Zip 46534–2299; tel. 219/772–6231; Kathryn J. Norem, Chief Executive Officer (Nonreporting) **A**1 9 10 **S** Province Healthcare Corporation, Brentwood, TN	13	10	35	—	—	—	—	—	—	—

KOKOMO—Howard County

Hospital	Control	Service	Staffed Beds	Admissions	Census	Outpatient Visits	Births	Total	Payroll	Personnel
□ HEALTHSOUTH REHABILITATION HOSPITAL OF KOKOMO, 829 North Dixon Road, Zip 46901–7709; tel. 765/452–6700; Allen Tyra, Administrator (Nonreporting) **A**1 9 10 **S** HEALTHSOUTH Corporation, Birmingham, AL Web address: www.healthsouth.com	33	46	60	—	—	—	—	—	—	—
★ HOWARD COMMUNITY HOSPITAL, 3500 South Lafountain Street, Zip 46904–9011; tel. 765/453–0702; James Alender, President and Chief Executive Officer (Total facility includes 18 beds in nursing home–type unit) **A**1 9 10 **F**3 4 8 9 11 12 13 16 17 18 21 22 24 25 27 28 30 32 33 34 36 39 41 42 43 44 45 46 48 50 54 57 58 59 60 61 62 63 64 65 69 70 72 75 76 78 79 **P**8	13	10	127	5425	71	173408	517	49298	21322	784
★ SCCI HOSPITAL OF KOKOMO, (LONG TERM ACUTE CARE), 1907 West Sycamore Street, Zip 46901; tel. 765/452–6730; Duane R. Vorseth, Chief Executive Officer **A**1 10 **F**16 17 18	33	49	19	166	12	0	0	4299	1979	44
★ ST. JOSEPH HOSPITAL & HEALTH CENTER, 1907 West Sycamore Street, Zip 46904–9010, Mailing Address: P.O. Box 9010, Zip 46904–9010; tel. 765/452–5611; Kathleen M. Korbelak, President (Total facility includes 13 beds in nursing home–type unit) **A**1 9 10 **F**2 3 7 8 9 11 13 16 17 18 19 22 23 24 25 26 27 28 29 30 32 34 36 37 38 39 40 41 43 44 45 46 48 49 51 54 57 58 59 60 61 62 63 64 65 68 69 70 72 73 76 77 78 79 **P**8 **S** Ascension Health, Saint Louis, MO Web address: www.stjhhc.org	21	10	167	5784	77	—	1022	58561	24138	763

Hospitals, U.S. / INDIANA

Hospital, Address, Telephone, Administrator, Approval, Facility, and Physician Codes, Health Care System, Network ★ American Hospital Association (AHA) membership □ Joint Commission on Accreditation of Healthcare Organizations (JCAHO) accreditation + American Osteopathic Healthcare Association (AOHA) membership ○ American Osteopathic Association (AOA) accreditation △ Commission on Accreditation of Rehabilitation Facilities (CARF) accreditation Control codes 61, 63, 64, 71, 72 and 73 indicate hospitals listed by AOHA, but not registered by AHA. For definition of numerical codes, see page A4	Classification Codes		Utilization Data					Expense (thousands) of dollars		
	Control	Service	Staffed Beds	Admissions	Census	Outpatient Visits	Births	Total	Payroll	Personnel
LA PORTE—La Porte County ★ △ LA PORTE REGIONAL HEALTH SYSTEM, (Formerly La Porte Hospital and Health Services), 1007 Lincolnway, Zip 46350, Mailing Address: P.O. Box 250, Zip 46352–0250; tel. 219/326–1234; Jonathan R. Goble, President and Chief Executive Officer (Total facility includes 55 beds in nursing home–type unit) **A**1 2 7 9 10 **F**3 6 7 8 9 11 13 16 17 18 19 20 21 22 23 24 25 27 28 29 31 32 33 34 35 36 37 38 39 40 41 43 44 45 46 48 50 54 55 56 57 58 59 60 61 62 63 65 66 68 69 70 71 72 76 77 78 79 **P**7 **Web address:** www.lph.org	23	10	227	5800	115	64019	689	74456	32772	818
LAFAYETTE—Tippecanoe County ★ △ GREATER LAFAYETTE HEALTH SERVICE, (Includes Lafayette Home Hospital, 2400 South Street, Zip 47904–3052, Mailing Address: P.O. Box 7518, Zip 47903–7518; St. Elizabeth Medical Center, 1501 Hartford Street, Zip 47904–2126, Mailing Address: Box 7501, Zip 47903–7501; tel. 765/423–6011), 2400 South Street, Zip 47904; tel. 765/447–6811; John R. Walling, President and Chief Executive Officer (Total facility includes 24 beds in nursing home–type unit) **A**1 2 6 7 9 10 **F**4 7 8 9 11 12 16 17 18 19 22 24 25 27 31 33 34 35 36 37 39 41 42 44 45 46 47 48 50 53 54 57 64 65 68 69 70 72 76 78 **Web address:** www.homehospital.com LAFAYETTE HOME HOSPITAL See Greater Lafayette Health Service ST. ELIZABETH MEDICAL CENTER See Greater Lafayette Health Service	23	10	418	16598	219	246151	85	130478	71625	2127
LAGRANGE—LaGrange County □ VENCOR HOSPITAL–LAGRANGE, 207 North Townline Road, Zip 46761–1325; tel. 219/463–2143; Shelleye Hicks, Administrator (Nonreporting) **A**1 9 10 **S** Vencor, Incorporated, Louisville, KY **Web address:** www.vencor.com	33	10	57	—	—	—	—	—	—	—
LAWRENCEBURG—Dearborn County ★ DEARBORN COUNTY HOSPITAL, 600 Wilson Creek Road, Zip 47025–1199; tel. 812/537–1010; Peter V. Resnick, Executive Director (Total facility includes 13 beds in nursing home–type unit) **A**1 9 10 **F**7 8 9 11 13 14 16 17 18 19 22 24 25 27 32 34 36 37 39 41 44 45 46 48 51 54 55 65 68 69 70 71 72 76 78 **P**6	13	10	87	3683	42	100064	422	34266	14909	462
LEBANON—Boone County □ WITHAM MEMORIAL HOSPITAL, 1124 North Lebanon Street, Zip 46052–1776, Mailing Address: P.O. Box 1200, Zip 46052–3005; tel. 765/482–2700; Raymond V. Ingham, President and Chief Executive Officer **A**1 9 10 **F**9 11 16 18 22 24 25 26 30 31 32 34 37 39 45 46 48 54 56 62 76 78 **Web address:** www.witham.org	13	10	49	1605	18	65692	0	23497	11380	339
LINTON—Greene County ★ GREENE COUNTY GENERAL HOSPITAL, Rural Route 1, Box 1000, Zip 47441–9457; tel. 812/847–2281; Jonas S. Uland, Executive Director **A**1 9 10 **F**8 9 16 17 18 22 23 25 32 33 34 36 38 41 44 46 48 54 59 61 76 78 **P**3 **Web address:** www.greenet.net/hospital	13	10	40	1483	17	—	79	15096	6940	238
LOGANSPORT—Cass County □ LOGANSPORT STATE HOSPITAL, 1098 South State Road 25, Zip 46947–9699; tel. 219/722–4141; Jeffrey H. Smith, Ph.D., Superintendent **A**1 **F**13 16 17 18 23 30 43 50 57 62 70 78	12	22	396	186	512	1227	—	34563	14136	709
★ MEMORIAL HOSPITAL, 1101 Michigan Avenue, Zip 46947–7013, Mailing Address: P.O. Box 7013, Zip 46947–7013; tel. 219/753–7541; Brian T. Shockney, President and Chief Executive Officer (Total facility includes 21 beds in nursing home–type unit) **A**1 9 10 **F**7 8 9 13 14 16 17 18 19 20 22 24 25 27 28 32 33 34 36 37 38 39 40 41 43 44 45 46 48 51 54 56 68 69 70 72 76 78 **P**8 **Web address:** www.mhlogan.org	13	10	104	2917	28	53790	570	28935	12840	480
MADISON—Jefferson County ★ KING'S DAUGHTERS' HOSPITAL AND HEALTH SERVICES, One King's Daughters' Drive, Zip 47250–3357, Mailing Address: P.O. Box 447, Zip 47250–0447; tel. 812/265–5211; Roger J. Allman, Chief Executive Officer (Total facility includes 29 beds in nursing home–type unit) **A**1 2 9 10 **F**8 9 11 16 17 18 22 24 25 27 29 32 34 36 37 38 39 43 46 48 49 54 65 69 70 71 72 76 78 79 **P**6	23	10	115	4886	70	129398	410	41077	18222	779
□ MADISON STATE HOSPITAL, 711 Green Road, Zip 47250–2199; tel. 812/265–2611; Nikki Morrell, Acting Superintendent **A**1 10 **F**17 18 23 58 62 70 78 **P**6	12	22	316	226	282	0	0	24752	14383	518
MARION—Grant County ★ MARION GENERAL HOSPITAL, 441 North Wabash Avenue, Zip 46952–2690; tel. 765/662–1441; Albert C. Knauss, President and Chief Executive Officer (Total facility includes 21 beds in nursing home–type unit) (Nonreporting) **A**1 9 10 **Web address:** www.mgh.net VETERANS AFFAIRS NORTHERN INDIANA HEALTH CARE SYSTEM–MARION CAMPUS See Veterans Affairs Northern Indiana Health Care System, Fort Wayne	23	10	191	—	—	—	—	—	—	—
MARTINSVILLE—Morgan County ★ MORGAN COUNTY MEMORIAL HOSPITAL, 2209 John R. Wooden Drive, Zip 46151–1840, Mailing Address: P.O. Box 1717, Zip 46151–1717; tel. 765/342–8441; John R. Whitcomb, Interim President and Chief Executive Officer **A**1 9 10 **F**8 9 13 16 17 18 22 25 32 33 34 36 38 39 40 41 43 44 45 46 48 50 56 70 71 76 78 **P**7 8 **Web address:** www.scican.net\hospital\mcmh.html	13	10	86	2295	25	80614	294	23377	10069	322

Hospitals, U.S. / INDIANA

Classification Codes / Utilization Data / Expense (thousands) of dollars

Legend:
- ★ American Hospital Association (AHA) membership
- □ Joint Commission on Accreditation of Healthcare Organizations (JCAHO) accreditation
- + American Osteopathic Healthcare Association (AOHA) membership
- ○ American Osteopathic Association (AOA) accreditation
- △ Commission on Accreditation of Rehabilitation Facilities (CARF) accreditation

Control codes 61, 63, 64, 71, 72 and 73 indicate hospitals listed by AOHA, but not registered by AHA. For definition of numerical codes, see page A4.

Hospital	Control	Service	Staffed Beds	Admissions	Census	Outpatient Visits	Births	Total	Payroll	Personnel

MERRILLVILLE—Lake County
SOUTHLAKE CAMPUS See Methodist Hospitals, Gary

MICHIGAN CITY—La Porte County
★ △ SAINT ANTHONY MEMORIAL HEALTH CENTERS, (Includes Memorial Hospital of Michigan City, 515 Pine Street, Zip 46360-3370; tel. 219/879-0202), 301 West Homer Street, Zip 46360-4358; tel. 219/879-8511; Bruce E. Rampage, President and Chief Executive Officer **A**1 7 9 10 **F**3 4 8 9 11 13 19 22 23 24 25 32 34 36 37 38 39 40 43 44 45 46 48 50 51 53 54 56 57 59 60 61 62 63 64 65 68 69 70 72 77 78 79 **S** Sisters of St. Francis Health Services, Inc., Mishawaka, IN
Web address: www.sahhc.org
— 21 | 10 | 207 | 8460 | 120 | 194846 | 723 | 66649 | 24979 | 673

MISHAWAKA—St. Joseph County
★ + ○ △ ST. JOSEPH COMMUNITY HOSPITAL, 215 West Fourth Street, Zip 46544-1999; tel. 219/259-2431; Mary Roos, President and Chief Executive Officer **A**1 7 9 10 11 12 13 **F**3 4 6 7 8 9 11 13 14 16 17 18 19 20 21 22 24 25 26 27 29 30 32 34 36 38 39 41 43 44 45 48 49 50 51 54 58 67 68 70 71 72 76 77 78 79 **P**6 7 8 **S** Ancilla Systems Inc., Hobart, IN
Web address: www.ancillahealthcare.org
— 21 | 10 | 100 | 4683 | 55 | 91627 | 1136 | 64375 | 27418 | 769

MONTICELLO—White County
□ WHITE COUNTY MEMORIAL HOSPITAL, 1101 O'Connor Boulevard, Zip 47960-1698; tel. 219/583-7111; John M. Avers, Chief Executive Officer (Nonreporting) **A**1 9 10
— 15 | 10 | 59 | — | — | — | — | — | — | —

MOORESVILLE—Morgan County
□ ST. FRANCIS HOSPITAL–MOORESVILLE, (Formerly Kendrick Memorial Hospital), 1201 Hadley Road N.W., Zip 46158-1789; tel. 317/831-1160; Charles D. Swisher, President (Nonreporting) **A**1 2 9 10 **S** Sisters of St. Francis Health Services, Inc., Mishawaka, IN
— 23 | 10 | 60 | — | — | — | — | — | — | —

MUNCIE—Delaware County
★ △ BALL MEMORIAL HOSPITAL, 2401 University Avenue, Zip 47303-3499; tel. 765/747-3111; Mitchell C. Carson, President (Total facility includes 39 beds in nursing home–type unit) **A**1 2 3 5 7 8 9 10 **F**2 3 4 7 8 9 11 12 13 14 16 17 18 19 22 23 24 25 26 27 28 29 30 32 33 34 35 36 37 38 39 40 41 42 43 44 45 46 47 48 49 50 51 53 54 56 57 61 62 65 66 68 69 70 71 72 76 77 78 79
Web address: www.cardinalhealthsystem.org
— 23 | 10 | 350 | 16198 | 220 | 157434 | 1781 | 164834 | 68446 | 1900

MUNSTER—Lake County
□ △ COMMUNITY HOSPITAL, 901 MacArthur Boulevard, Zip 46321-2959; tel. 219/836-1600; Edward P. Robinson, Administrator (Nonreporting) **A**1 2 7 9 10
— 23 | 10 | 292 | — | — | — | — | — | — | —

NEW ALBANY—Floyd County
★ FLOYD MEMORIAL HOSPITAL AND HEALTH SERVICES, 1850 State Street, Zip 47150-4997; tel. 812/949-5500; Bryant R. Hanson, President and Chief Executive Officer (Total facility includes 24 beds in nursing home–type unit) **A**1 2 9 10 **F**7 8 9 11 12 16 17 18 19 22 24 25 32 33 34 36 39 41 44 45 46 48 49 51 54 65 68 69 70 72 75 76 77 78 79 **P**1 6
Web address: www.floydmemorial.org
— 13 | 10 | 178 | 8607 | 101 | 195160 | 809 | 79238 | 34327 | 892

★ △ SOUTHERN INDIANA REHABILITATION HOSPITAL, 3104 Blackiston Boulevard, Zip 47150-9579; tel. 812/941-8300; Randy L. Napier, President and Chief Executive Officer **A**1 7 10 **F**4 7 8 10 11 12 13 17 18 19 22 23 24 25 28 29 30 31 32 33 34 36 38 39 41 44 45 46 47 48 49 50 51 53 54 55 56 57 65 69 70 71 72 74 76 77 78 79 **S** Jewish Hospital HealthCare Services, Louisville, KY
— 23 | 46 | 60 | 666 | 47 | 13865 | 0 | 11455 | 5470 | 155

NEW CASTLE—Henry County
★ HENRY COUNTY MEMORIAL HOSPITAL, 1000 North 16th Street, Zip 47362-4319, Mailing Address: P.O. Box 490, Zip 47362-0490; tel. 765/521-0890; Jack Basler, President **A**1 9 10 **F**7 8 9 16 17 18 19 22 24 25 36 37 38 39 45 46 48 49 51 54 56 65 70 71 72 76 78 79 **P**8
Web address: www.hcmhcares.org
— 13 | 10 | 107 | 3321 | 35 | 46359 | 469 | 34293 | 15194 | 580

NOBLESVILLE—Hamilton County
★ △ RIVERVIEW HOSPITAL, 395 Westfield Road, Zip 46060-1425, Mailing Address: P.O. Box 220, Zip 46061-0220; tel. 317/773-0760; Seward Horner, President (Total facility includes 25 beds in nursing home–type unit) **A**1 7 9 10 **F**4 7 8 9 11 12 13 16 17 18 21 22 25 28 32 34 36 37 38 39 40 41 43 44 45 46 48 49 51 53 54 65 68 69 70 71 72 76 77 78 79 **P**5 6 7 8
Web address: www.riverviewhospital.org
— 13 | 10 | 111 | 4442 | 58 | 167500 | 775 | 63501 | 26000 | 658

NORTH VERNON—Jennings County
★ ST. VINCENT JENNINGS HOSPITAL, (Formerly Jennings Community Hospital), 301 Henry Street, Zip 47265-1097; tel. 812/352-4200; Joseph Roche, Administrator (Nonreporting) **A**9 **S** Ascension Health, Saint Louis, MO
— 23 | 10 | 34 | — | — | — | — | — | — | —

OAKLAND CITY—Gibson County
★ WIRTH REGIONAL HOSPITAL, Highway 64 West, Zip 47660-9379, Mailing Address: Rural Route 3, Box 14A, Zip 47660-9379; tel. 812/749-6111; Jeff Probus, Interim Chief Executive Officer **A**9 10 **F**7 9 13 17 18 19 25 30 32 33 34 37 38 43 48 49 51 54 57 61 62 70 76 78 **S** Brim Healthcare, Inc., Brentwood, TN
— 23 | 10 | 20 | 220 | 2 | 10688 | 0 | 3662 | 1249 | 54

PAOLI—Orange County
□ BLOOMINGTON HOSPITAL OF ORANGE COUNTY, (Formerly Orange County Hospital), 642 West Hospital Road, Zip 47454-0499, Mailing Address: P.O. Box 499, Zip 47454-0499; tel. 812/723-2811; L. Gene Perry, Chief Executive Officer (Nonreporting) **A**1 9 10
— 13 | 10 | 37 | — | — | — | — | — | — | —

Many Facility Codes have changed. Please refer to the AHA Guide Code Chart.

© 2000 AHA Guide

Hospitals, U.S. / INDIANA

Hospital, Address, Telephone, Administrator, Approval, Facility, and Physician Codes, Health Care System, Network	Classification Codes		Utilization Data					Expense (thousands) of dollars		
★ American Hospital Association (AHA) membership ☐ Joint Commission on Accreditation of Healthcare Organizations (JCAHO) accreditation + American Osteopathic Healthcare Association (AOHA) membership ○ American Osteopathic Association (AOA) accreditation △ Commission on Accreditation of Rehabilitation Facilities (CARF) accreditation Control codes 61, 63, 64, 71, 72 and 73 indicate hospitals listed by AOHA, but not registered by AHA. For definition of numerical codes, see page A4	Control	Service	Staffed Beds	Admissions	Census	Outpatient Visits	Births	Total	Payroll	Personnel
PERU—Miami County ✠ DUKES MEMORIAL HOSPITAL, 275 West 12th Street, Zip 46970-1698; tel. 765/472-8000; R. Joe Johnston, President and Chief Executive Officer (Total facility includes 35 beds in nursing home-type unit) **A**1 9 10 **F**7 8 9 13 16 18 19 22 24 25 27 31 34 37 38 39 40 41 43 44 45 48 49 50 54 56 68 69 70 72 76 78 **P**6 Web address: www.dukeshospital.org	13	10	74	2931	40	93364	356	27654	11696	385
PLYMOUTH—Marshall County ☐ BEHAVIORAL HEALTHCARE OF NORTHERN INDIANA, 1800 North Oak Road, Zip 46563-3492; tel. 219/936-3784; Wayne T. Miller, Administrator **A**1 10 **F**2 3 17 18 57 58 59 60 61 62 63 64 **P**6 **S** Behavioral Healthcare Corporation, Nashville, TN	33	22	76	582	47	—	0	6265	3447	147
✠ SAINT JOSEPH'S REGIONAL MEDICAL CENTER–PLYMOUTH CAMPUS, 1915 Lake Avenue, Zip 46563-9905, Mailing Address: P.O. Box 670, Zip 46563-9905; tel. 219/936-3181; Brian E. Dietz, FACHE, Executive Vice President **A**1 9 10 **F**1 4 6 7 8 9 11 13 16 17 18 22 24 25 26 27 28 30 31 32 35 36 37 39 40 41 44 45 46 47 48 49 52 53 54 65 69 70 75 76 78 79 **P**8 **S** Trinity Health, Novi, MI Web address: www.sjmed.com	21	10	36	2212	21	97171	356	19309	7793	277
PORTLAND—Jay County ☐ JAY COUNTY HOSPITAL, 500 West Votaw Street, Zip 47371-1322; tel. 219/726-7131; Sheri Goforth, Chief Executive Officer (Nonreporting) **A**1 9 10	13	10	55	—	—	—	—	—	—	—
PRINCETON—Gibson County ✠ GIBSON GENERAL HOSPITAL, 1808 Sherman Drive, Zip 47670-1043; tel. 812/385-3401; Michael J. Budnick, FACHE, Administrator and Chief Executive Officer (Total facility includes 45 beds in nursing home-type unit) **A**1 9 10 **F**3 6 7 8 9 13 16 17 18 19 21 22 23 25 29 30 32 33 34 36 37 38 39 40 41 43 44 45 46 48 49 54 56 57 58 59 60 61 62 63 65 69 70 71 72 76 78 79 **S** Norton Healthcare, Louisville, KY Web address: www.gibsongeneral.org	23	10	109	1277	58	26264	159	14804	7332	249
RENSSELAER—Jasper County ★ JASPER COUNTY HOSPITAL, 1104 East Grace Street, Zip 47978-3296; tel. 219/866-5141; Timothy M. Schreeg, President and Chief Executive Officer (Total facility includes 21 beds in nursing home-type unit) **A**9 10 **F**8 9 12 17 19 22 25 27 28 32 34 36 37 38 39 40 41 44 45 46 48 54 69 70 71 72 76 78 **P**6	13	10	69	1457	34	45569	159	17483	8664	317
RICHMOND—Wayne County ✠ REID HOSPITAL AND HEALTH CARE SERVICES, 1401 Chester Boulevard, Zip 47374-1986; tel. 765/983-3000; Barry S. MacDowell, President (Total facility includes 17 beds in nursing home-type unit) **A**1 2 9 10 **F**3 7 8 9 11 12 13 16 17 18 19 22 24 25 26 27 31 34 37 38 39 41 44 45 46 48 49 50 51 54 57 61 65 69 70 72 75 76 78 **P**8 Web address: www.reidhosp.com	23	10	228	13111	166	123680	915	94757	40825	1339
☐ RICHMOND STATE HOSPITAL, 498 N.W. 18th Street, Zip 47374-2898; tel. 765/966-0511; Jeffrey Butler, Acting Superintendent (Nonreporting) **A**1 10	12	22	339	—	—	—	—	—	—	—
ROCHESTER—Fulton County ☐ WOODLAWN HOSPITAL, 1400 East Ninth Street, Zip 46975-8937; tel. 219/224-1173; James M. O'Keefe, President and Chief Executive Officer **A**1 9 10 **F**6 7 8 9 11 12 13 16 17 19 22 24 25 30 32 34 35 36 38 39 40 41 43 44 45 46 48 49 54 72 76 78 **P**6	13	10	35	1267	11	17627	255	14929	7401	194
RUSHVILLE—Rush County ★ RUSH MEMORIAL HOSPITAL, 1300 North Main Street, Zip 46173-1198; tel. 765/932-4111; J. Jay Purvis, Interim Chief Executive Officer **A**9 10 **F**9 12 17 18 19 22 25 30 32 33 34 36 38 39 43 46 48 50 51 54 56 70 71 76 78 **S** Norton Healthcare, Louisville, KY Web address: www.rushmemorial.com	13	10	46	973	24	26739	0	10597	4616	190
SALEM—Washington County ✠ WASHINGTON COUNTY MEMORIAL HOSPITAL, 911 North Shelby Street, Zip 47167; tel. 812/883-5881; Rodney M. Coats, President and Chief Executive Officer **A**1 9 10 **F**2 3 7 8 9 12 16 17 18 19 22 25 33 34 39 41 44 45 46 48 49 54 57 61 62 63 64 69 71 72 76 78 **P**6 **S** Jewish Hospital HealthCare Services, Louisville, KY	13	10	58	1263	19	30753	99	13635	5729	203
SCOTTSBURG—Scott County ✠ SCOTT MEMORIAL HOSPITAL, 1415 North Gardner Street, Zip 47170-0430, Mailing Address: Box 430, Zip 47170-0430; tel. 812/752-8500; Clifford D. Nay, Executive Director **A**1 9 10 **F**8 9 13 16 17 18 19 22 25 32 34 36 37 38 39 41 43 44 45 46 48 51 54 70 72 75 76 78 **S** Jewish Hospital HealthCare Services, Louisville, KY Web address: www.scottcounty.hsonline.com	13	10	45	1355	12	31701	120	12065	5437	150
SEYMOUR—Jackson County ✠ MEMORIAL HOSPITAL, 411 West Tipton Street, Zip 47274-5000, Mailing Address: P.O. Box 2349, Zip 47274-2349; tel. 812/522-2349; George H. James, Jr, President and Chief Executive Officer **A**1 2 9 10 **F**8 9 12 13 16 17 18 19 22 23 24 27 29 30 32 34 35 37 38 39 40 43 44 45 46 48 49 50 51 54 56 68 70 72 75 76 78 79	13	10	112	3869	41	95519	578	35233	16309	482
SHELBYVILLE—Shelby County ✠ MAJOR HOSPITAL, 150 West Washington Street, Zip 46176-1236; tel. 317/392-3211; Anthony B. Lennen, President and Chief Executive Officer **A**1 9 10 **F**8 9 13 16 17 18 19 22 25 32 33 34 36 38 39 40 41 43 44 45 46 48 49 50 51 54 56 59 61 63 68 70 71 72 76 78 79 **P**7 8 Web address: www.majorhospital.com	15	10	54	2773	27	92826	342	28224	12055	393

© 2000 AHA Guide   *Many Facility Codes have changed. Please refer to the AHA Guide Code Chart.*

Hospitals, U.S. / INDIANA

Hospital, Address, Telephone, Administrator, Approval, Facility, and Physician Codes, Health Care System, Network	Classification Codes		Utilization Data					Expense (thousands) of dollars		
★ American Hospital Association (AHA) membership □ Joint Commission on Accreditation of Healthcare Organizations (JCAHO) accreditation + American Osteopathic Healthcare Association (AOHA) membership ○ American Osteopathic Association (AOA) accreditation △ Commission on Accreditation of Rehabilitation Facilities (CARF) accreditation Control codes 61, 63, 64, 71, 72 and 73 indicate hospitals listed by AOHA, but not registered by AHA. For definition of numerical codes, see page A4	Control	Service	Staffed Beds	Admissions	Census	Outpatient Visits	Births	Total	Payroll	Personnel
SOUTH BEND—St. Joseph County										
★ △ MEMORIAL HOSPITAL OF SOUTH BEND, 615 North Michigan Street, Zip 46601-9986; tel. 219/234-9041; Philip A. Newbold, President and Chief Executive Officer **A**1 2 3 5 7 9 10 **F**1 2 3 4 5 7 8 9 11 12 13 14 16 17 18 19 21 22 23 24 25 28 29 30 31 32 33 34 35 36 38 39 41 42 43 44 45 46 47 48 49 51 52 53 54 55 56 57 58 59 60 61 62 63 64 65 66 68 69 70 71 72 73 75 76 77 78 79 **P**1 6 Web address: www.qualityoflife.org	23	10	405	14435	215	—	2439	170800	69199	1800
★ △ SAINT JOSEPH'S REGIONAL MEDICAL CENTER–SOUTH BEND CAMPUS, 801 East LaSalle, Zip 46617-2800; tel. 219/237-7111; Robert L. Beyer, President and Chief Executive Officer **A**1 2 3 5 7 9 10 **F**1 4 6 7 8 9 11 12 13 14 16 17 18 19 20 22 24 25 26 27 28 30 31 32 33 34 36 37 39 40 41 42 43 44 45 46 47 48 49 50 51 52 53 54 56 61 65 66 67 69 70 71 72 73 76 78 79 **P**6 8 **S** Trinity Health, Novi, MI Web address: www.sjmed.com	21	10	310	11749	167	112603	1335	146692	52672	1557
SULLIVAN—Sullivan County										
★ SULLIVAN COUNTY COMMUNITY HOSPITAL, (Formerly Mary Sherman Hospital), 2200 North Section Street, Zip 47882, Mailing Address: P.O. Box 10, Zip 47882-0010; tel. 812/268-4311; Thomas J. Hudgins, Administrator **A**1 9 10 **F**8 9 13 14 16 17 18 19 22 23 25 30 32 33 34 35 36 39 43 45 46 48 50 54 58 59 60 61 62 63 68 70 71 72 76 78 79 **S** Quorum Health Group, Brentwood, TN	13	10	37	1935	21	43259	187	11488	4547	178
TELL CITY—Perry County										
★ PERRY COUNTY MEMORIAL HOSPITAL, 1 Hospital Road, Zip 47586-0362; tel. 812/547-7011; Joseph A. Stuber, Chief Executive Officer **A**1 9 10 **F**7 8 9 13 17 18 19 21 22 23 24 25 30 32 33 34 36 37 38 39 41 43 44 45 46 48 50 51 54 60 61 63 68 69 70 72 76 78 **S** Norton Healthcare, Louisville, KY Web address: www.pchospital.org	13	10	38	1078	11	53648	55	11803	4565	173
TERRE HAUTE—Vigo County										
HAMILTON CENTER, 620 Eighth Avenue, Zip 47804-0323; tel. 812/231-8323; Galen Goode, Chief Executive Officer (Nonreporting) **A**9 10 Web address: www.hamiltoncenter.org	23	22	45	—	—	—	—	—	—	—
★ TERRE HAUTE REGIONAL HOSPITAL, 3901 South Seventh Street, Zip 47802-4299; tel. 812/232-0021; Jerry Dooley, Chief Executive Officer (Total facility includes 34 beds in nursing home–type unit) **A**1 9 10 **F**3 4 8 9 11 12 13 16 18 19 22 24 25 30 32 34 38 39 40 41 43 44 45 46 47 48 51 55 57 59 60 61 62 63 64 65 66 69 70 71 72 76 77 78 79 **P**5 7 8 **S** HCA – The Healthcare Company, Nashville, TN Web address: www.regionalhospital.com	33	10	238	8750	118	50005	733	45129	20100	879
★ △ UNION HOSPITAL, 1606 North Seventh Street, Zip 47804-2780; tel. 812/238-7000; David R. Doerr, Chief Executive Officer **A**1 2 3 5 7 9 10 **F**3 4 5 8 9 11 12 13 16 17 18 19 22 23 24 25 27 28 29 32 33 34 35 36 37 38 39 41 42 43 44 45 46 47 48 49 50 51 53 54 55 56 57 58 61 63 64 65 66 69 70 71 72 76 77 78 79 **P**1 5 6 Web address: www.uhhg.org	23	10	261	12853	183	377417	1549	150007	60808	1850
TIPTON—Tipton County										
★ TIPTON COUNTY MEMORIAL HOSPITAL, 1000 South Main Street, Zip 46072-9799; tel. 765/675-8500; Alfonso W. Gatmaitan, Chief Executive Officer (Total facility includes 50 beds in nursing home–type unit) **A**1 2 9 10 **F**6 7 8 9 13 19 22 32 33 34 36 39 40 41 43 44 45 46 48 50 51 54 68 69 70 71 76 78 79 **P**6 8 Web address: www.tiptonhospital.org	13	10	87	1792	55	52859	135	20796	9058	341
VALPARAISO—Porter County										
★ PORTER MEMORIAL HOSPITAL, 814 La Porte Avenue, Zip 46383-5898; tel. 219/465-4600; Wiley N. Carr, President and Chief Executive Officer (Total facility includes 25 beds in nursing home–type unit) **A**1 9 10 **F**2 3 4 8 9 11 16 17 18 19 21 22 24 25 27 29 31 32 34 36 37 38 39 40 41 42 43 44 45 46 47 48 49 50 54 66 68 69 70 71 73 75 76 77 78 79 **P**8 Web address: www.portermemorial.org	13	10	285	13255	184	352081	1295	125094	54454	1400
VINCENNES—Knox County										
★ GOOD SAMARITAN HOSPITAL, 520 South Seventh Street, Zip 47591-1098; tel. 812/882-5220; A. John Hidde, President and Chief Executive Officer (Total facility includes 49 beds in nursing home–type unit) **A**1 2 9 10 **F**3 4 7 8 9 11 12 13 14 16 17 18 21 22 23 24 25 26 27 28 32 33 34 36 37 38 39 41 43 44 45 46 47 48 49 50 51 54 57 58 59 60 61 62 63 64 65 68 69 70 72 76 77 78 79 **P**8 Web address: www.gshvin.org	13	10	289	9166	147	241287	474	93878	42811	1460
WABASH—Wabash County										
★ WABASH COUNTY HOSPITAL, 710 North East Street, Zip 46992-1924, Mailing Address: P.O. Box 548, Zip 46992-0548; tel. 219/563-3131; David C. Hunter, Chief Executive Officer (Total facility includes 25 beds in nursing home–type unit) **A**1 2 9 10 **F**7 8 9 13 14 17 18 19 22 23 24 25 28 32 33 34 36 37 38 39 40 43 44 45 46 48 49 50 51 54 69 70 71 72 76 78 Web address: www.wchospital.com	13	10	75	1653	31	43306	206	22093	9521	295
WARSAW—Kosciusko County										
★ KOSCIUSKO COMMUNITY HOSPITAL, 2101 East Dubois Drive, Zip 46580-3288; tel. 219/267-3200; Wayne Hendrix, Chief Executive Officer **A**1 9 10 **F**8 9 13 16 17 18 22 25 28 32 34 38 39 40 41 43 44 49 54 68 70 71 76 77 78 **P**6 **S** Quorum Health Group, Brentwood, TN Web address: www.kch.com	33	10	72	3257	26	187469	747	43043	17505	500

Hospitals, U.S. / INDIANA

Hospital, Address, Telephone, Administrator, Approval, Facility, and Physician Codes, Health Care System, Network	Classification Codes		Utilization Data					Expense (thousands) of dollars		
★ American Hospital Association (AHA) membership ☐ Joint Commission on Accreditation of Healthcare Organizations (JCAHO) accreditation + American Osteopathic Healthcare Association (AOHA) membership ○ American Osteopathic Association (AOA) accreditation △ Commission on Accreditation of Rehabilitation Facilities (CARF) accreditation Control codes 61, 63, 64, 71, 72 and 73 indicate hospitals listed by AOHA, but not registered by AHA. For definition of numerical codes, see page A4	Control	Service	Staffed Beds	Admissions	Census	Outpatient Visits	Births	Total	Payroll	Personnel
WASHINGTON—Daviess County										
✠ DAVIESS COUNTY HOSPITAL, 1314 East Walnut Street, Zip 47501-2198, Mailing Address: P.O. Box 760, Zip 47501-0760; tel. 812/254-2760; David G. Fuqua, R.N., Chief Executive Officer (Total facility includes 29 beds in nursing home-type unit) **A**1 9 10 **F**7 8 9 13 16 17 18 19 22 24 25 36 37 38 39 40 41 43 44 45 46 48 49 50 51 53 54 58 60 61 63 64 68 70 72 76 78 **P**3 7 8 **S** Quorum Health Group, Brentwood, TN Web address: www.dchosp.org	13	10	85	2660	40	87095	387	22514	10808	353
WEST LAFAYETTE—Tippecanoe County										
WABASH VALLEY HOSPITAL, 2900 North River Road, Zip 47906-3766; tel. 765/463-2555; R. Craig Lysinger, Administrator (Nonreporting) **A**10	23	22	70	—	—	—	—	—	—	—
WILLIAMSPORT—Warren County										
★ ST. VINCENT WILLIAMSPORT HOSPITAL, 412 North Monroe Street, Zip 47993-0215; tel. 765/762-4000; Jane Craigin, Chief Executive Officer (Nonreporting) **A**9 10 **S** Ascension Health, Saint Louis, MO Web address: www.stvincent.org	23	10	22	—	—	—	—	—	—	—
WINAMAC—Pulaski County										
✠ PULASKI MEMORIAL HOSPITAL, 616 East 13th Street, Zip 46996-1117; tel. 219/946-6131; Richard H. Mynark, Chief Executive Officer **A**1 9 10 **F**7 8 9 13 19 22 23 25 26 32 33 34 36 37 38 41 43 44 45 46 48 49 50 54 70 72 76 78 **P**8	13	10	19	997	10	33172	146	10999	5366	165
WINCHESTER—Randolph County										
✠ ST. VINCENT RANDOLPH HOSPITAL, (Formerly Randolph County Hospital and Health Services), 325 South Oak Street, Zip 47394-2235, Mailing Address: P.O. Box 407, Zip 47394-0407; tel. 765/584-9001; James M. Full, FACHE, Chief Executive Officer **A**1 9 10 18 **F**7 8 9 14 15 16 17 18 19 22 24 25 26 29 30 32 33 34 36 37 38 39 41 44 45 46 48 50 51 54 56 66 70 71 73 76 78 79 **S** Norton Healthcare, Louisville, KY	13	10	25	721	8	29823	145	10565	3228	188

© 2000 AHA Guide   *Many Facility Codes have changed. Please refer to the AHA Guide Code Chart.*   Hospitals **A147**

Hospitals, U.S. / IOWA

IOWA

Resident Population 2,862 (in thousands)
Resident population in metro areas 44.3%
Birth rate per 1,000 population 12.9
65 years and over 15.1%
Percent of persons without health insurance 12.0%

★ American Hospital Association (AHA) membership
☐ Joint Commission on Accreditation of Healthcare Organizations (JCAHO) accreditation
+ American Osteopathic Healthcare Association (AOHA) membership
○ American Osteopathic Association (AOA) accreditation
△ Commission on Accreditation of Rehabilitation Facilities (CARF) accreditation
Control codes 61, 63, 64, 71, 72 and 73 indicate hospitals listed by AOHA, but not registered by AHA. For definition of numerical codes, see page A4

Hospital, Address, Telephone, Administrator, Approval, Facility, and Physician Codes, Health Care System, Network	Classification Codes		Utilization Data					Expense (thousands) of dollars		
	Control	Service	Staffed Beds	Admissions	Census	Outpatient Visits	Births	Total	Payroll	Personnel
ALBIA—Monroe County MONROE COUNTY HOSPITAL, 6580 165th Street, Zip 52531; tel. 515/932-2134; Gregory A. Paris, Administrator **A**9 10 **F**7 9 13 17 18 22 24 25 32 34 36 37 39 40 45 48 54 72 76 **P**8	13	10	38	561	26	33101	0	6206	2268	110
ALGONA—Kossuth County ★ KOSSUTH REGIONAL HEALTH CENTER, 1515 South Phillips Street, Zip 50511-3649; tel. 515/295-2451; Scott Curtis, Administrator and Chief Executive Officer **A**9 10 **F**7 8 9 13 14 16 17 18 19 22 25 30 32 34 35 36 37 38 39 40 41 43 44 45 46 48 50 53 54 58 59 60 62 63 69 70 71 72 76 78 79 **P**1 **S** Trinity Health, Novi, MI	13	10	24	722	9	17556	85	9401	3165	120
AMES—Story County ✚ MARY GREELEY MEDICAL CENTER, 1111 Duff Avenue, Zip 50010-5792; tel. 515/239-2011; Kimberly A. Russel, President and Chief Executive Officer (Total facility includes 19 beds in nursing home-type unit) **A**1 2 9 10 **F**7 8 9 11 13 16 17 18 19 21 22 24 25 26 28 30 32 33 34 35 36 37 38 39 40 41 42 43 44 45 46 48 49 50 53 54 57 58 59 60 61 62 63 64 65 66 68 69 70 71 72 76 78 Web address: www.mgmc.com	14	10	196	9848	125	113533	1182	76635	32731	1041
ANAMOSA—Jones County ✚ JONES REGIONAL MEDICAL CENTER, (Formerly Anamosa Community Hospital), 104 Broadway Place, Zip 52205-1100; tel. 319/462-6131; Vickie Asbe, Administrator **A**1 9 10 **F**1 7 8 9 14 19 22 25 34 36 38 44 48 54 69 70 75 76 78 **P**1 **S** Iowa Health System, Des Moines, IA	23	10	17	534	6	23287	5	4641	1951	100
ATLANTIC—Cass County ★ CASS COUNTY MEMORIAL HOSPITAL, 1501 East Tenth Street, Zip 50022-1997; tel. 712/243-3250; Patricia Markham, Administrator **A**9 10 **F**1 7 8 9 13 17 18 22 24 25 32 34 36 37 38 39 40 41 43 44 45 46 48 54 57 58 60 61 62 63 64 68 70 72 76 **P**8	13	10	72	1867	28	42442	170	17225	7936	282
AUDUBON—Audubon County AUDUBON COUNTY MEMORIAL HOSPITAL, 515 Pacific Street, Zip 50025-1099; tel. 712/563-2611; Thomas G. Smith, Chief Executive Officer **A**9 10 **F**7 8 9 17 22 24 25 34 37 38 39 44 46 48 54 56 63 68 69 75 76 **P**1	13	10	29	472	5	14473	39	4430	1716	65
BELMOND—Wright County ★ BELMOND MEDICAL CENTER, (Formerly Belmond Community Hospital), 403 First Street S.E., Zip 50421-1201, Mailing Address: P.O. Box 326, Zip 50421-0326; tel. 515/444-3223; Kim Price, Administrator **A**9 10 18 **F**7 16 17 18 22 23 25 26 28 32 33 34 36 37 38 40 43 45 46 48 53 54 56 76 78 79 **P**8 **S** Trinity Health, Novi, MI	14	10	22	186	6	9962	0	2929	943	48
BLOOMFIELD—Davis County ★ DAVIS COUNTY HOSPITAL, 507 North Madison Street, Zip 52537-1299; tel. 515/664-2145; John E. Monnahan, Administrator (Total facility includes 32 beds in nursing home-type unit) **A**9 10 **F**8 9 14 16 17 18 22 23 25 34 35 36 37 38 39 40 41 43 44 46 48 50 54 56 69 76 78 **P**6	13	10	67	936	43	15662	59	9661	4584	175
BOONE—Boone County ✚ BOONE COUNTY HOSPITAL, 1015 Union Street, Zip 50036-4898; tel. 515/432-3140; Joseph S. Smith, Chief Executive Officer **A**1 9 10 **F**8 9 17 18 19 22 25 28 31 32 34 36 37 38 39 40 41 43 44 45 46 48 53 54 69 70 75 76 78 79 **P**6 **S** Quorum Health Group, Brentwood, TN Web address: www.boonehospital.com	13	10	57	1733	23	36000	113	14513	6246	241
BRITT—Hancock County ★ HANCOCK COUNTY MEMORIAL HOSPITAL, 532 First Street N.W., Zip 50423-0068, Mailing Address: P.O. Box 68, Zip 50423-0068; tel. 515/843-3801; Harriet A. Thompson, Administrator **A**9 10 **F**1 8 9 16 17 18 19 22 25 28 31 34 37 39 40 44 45 48 51 70 72 75 76 **P**1 **S** Trinity Health, Novi, MI	13	10	26	560	10	15637	0	5454	1800	72
CARROLL—Carroll County ✚ ST. ANTHONY REGIONAL HOSPITAL, 311 South Clark Street, Zip 51401, Mailing Address: P.O. Box 628, Zip 51401-0628; tel. 712/792-8231; Gary P. Riedmann, President and Chief Executive Officer (Total facility includes 79 beds in nursing home-type unit) **A**1 9 10 **F**1 7 8 9 13 16 17 18 19 22 23 24 25 30 32 33 34 35 36 37 38 39 40 43 44 45 46 48 49 50 51 54 56 57 58 59 60 61 62 63 64 65 67 68 69 70 71 72 73 76 78 **P**6 Web address: www.netins.net/showcase/sarh/	21	10	142	2404	104	62276	243	22335	10024	330
CEDAR FALLS—Black Hawk County ✚ SARTORI MEMORIAL HOSPITAL, 515 College Street, Zip 50613-2599; tel. 319/268-3000 (Total facility includes 16 beds in nursing home-type unit) **A**1 9 10 **F**3 7 9 13 19 22 23 25 28 34 36 38 39 40 41 43 45 46 48 54 56 69 70 71 72 76 78 **S** Wheaton Franciscan Services, Inc., Wheaton, IL	21	10	62	1633	21	66711	0	16596	7073	207

Hospitals, U.S. / IOWA

Hospital, Address, Telephone, Administrator, Approval, Facility, and Physician Codes, Health Care System, Network	Classification Codes		Utilization Data					Expense (thousands) of dollars		
★ American Hospital Association (AHA) membership □ Joint Commission on Accreditation of Healthcare Organizations (JCAHO) accreditation + American Osteopathic Healthcare Association (AOHA) membership ○ American Osteopathic Association (AOA) accreditation △ Commission on Accreditation of Rehabilitation Facilities (CARF) accreditation Control codes 61, 63, 64, 71, 72 and 73 indicate hospitals listed by AOHA, but not registered by AHA. For definition of numerical codes, see page A4	Control	Service	Staffed Beds	Admissions	Census	Outpatient Visits	Births	Total	Payroll	Personnel

CEDAR RAPIDS—Linn County

✠ △ MERCY MEDICAL CENTER, 701 Tenth Street S.E., Zip 52403-1292; tel. 319/398-6011; A. James Tinker, President and Chief Executive Officer (Total facility includes 84 beds in nursing home–type unit) **A**1 2 3 7 9 10 **F**2 3 4 7 8 9 11 13 16 17 18 22 24 25 28 30 32 33 34 35 36 37 38 39 41 42 44 45 46 48 49 50 51 52 54 55 57 59 60 61 62 63 64 65 68 69 70 72 74 75 76 78 79 **P**1 5 **Web address:** www.mercycare.org	21	10	364	10710	209	132602	1144	101029	46425	1404
✠ △ ST. LUKE'S HOSPITAL, 1026 A Avenue N.E., Zip 52402-3026, Mailing Address: P.O. Box 3026, Zip 52406-3026; tel. 319/369-7211; Stephen E. Vanourny, M.D., President and Chief Executive Officer (Total facility includes 28 beds in nursing home–type unit) **A**1 3 7 9 10 **F**3 4 8 9 11 12 13 16 17 18 19 22 23 24 25 27 28 29 30 31 32 33 34 35 36 37 38 39 40 41 42 43 44 45 46 47 48 50 51 52 53 54 55 56 57 58 59 60 61 62 63 64 66 68 69 70 71 72 73 75 76 77 78 79 **P**3 5 7 8 **S** Iowa Health System, Des Moines, IA	23	10	384	14471	210	282065	2237	134578	55935	1872

CENTERVILLE—Appanoose County

✠ MERCY MEDICAL CENTER–CENTERVILLE, (Formerly St. Joseph's Mercy Hospital), 1 St. Joseph's Drive, Zip 52544; tel. 515/437-4111; William C. Assell, President and Chief Executive Officer (Total facility includes 20 beds in nursing home–type unit) **A**1 9 10 **F**7 8 16 17 18 22 25 26 28 30 32 33 34 36 37 38 39 40 41 43 44 50 54 58 59 63 69 70 71 72 76 **S** Catholic Health Initiatives, Denver, CO	21	10	57	1237	41	31852	46	10223	4768	187

CHARITON—Lucas County

★ LUCAS COUNTY HEALTH CENTER, 1200 North Seventh Street, Zip 50049-1258; tel. 515/774-3000; Michael S. Wallace, Chief Executive Officer (Total facility includes 22 beds in nursing home–type unit) **A**9 10 **F**1 3 6 7 8 9 13 16 17 18 21 22 25 26 31 32 34 36 37 39 41 44 46 48 51 54 58 59 60 61 62 63 64 69 72 73 75 76 78 79	13	10	44	673	6	11986	88	8112	3549	143

CHARLES CITY—Floyd County

FLOYD COUNTY MEMORIAL HOSPITAL, 800 Eleventh Street, Zip 50616-3499; tel. 515/228-6830; Bill D. Faust, Administrator **A**9 10 **F**7 8 9 12 13 16 17 18 19 22 24 25 32 33 34 36 37 38 39 40 41 43 44 45 48 54 56 58 62 63 70 71 72 76 78 **S** Mayo Foundation, Rochester, MN **Web address:** www.willowtree.com/~fcmh/	13	10	31	1351	14	48585	97	9992	4121	151

CHEROKEE—Cherokee County

□ MENTAL HEALTH INSTITUTE, 1200 West Cedar Street, Zip 51012-1599; tel. 712/225-2594; Tom Deiker, Ph.D., Superintendent **A**1 10 **F**1 13 16 18 19 29 31 38 43 50 51 57 58 59 60 61 63 64 70 78 **P**6	12	22	110	921	67	478	0	13900	8276	227
★ SIOUX VALLEY MEMORIAL HOSPITAL, 300 Sioux Valley Drive, Zip 51012-1205; tel. 712/225-5101; John M. Comstock, Chief Executive Officer **A**9 10 **F**8 9 12 13 16 17 18 19 22 25 28 30 32 33 34 35 36 37 38 39 40 43 44 45 46 48 50 51 54 56 58 59 60 61 62 63 67 69 70 71 72 76 78 **P**4 6 7	23	10	40	1183	13	22714	113	8927	4157	165

CLARINDA—Page County

★ CLARINDA REGIONAL HEALTH CENTER, 17th and Wells Streets, Zip 51632, Mailing Address: P.O. Box 217, Zip 51632-0217; tel. 712/542-2176; Rudy Snedigar, Chief Executive Officer **A**9 10 **F**7 9 13 17 18 19 22 25 28 30 31 32 34 36 38 39 40 41 43 44 45 46 48 49 50 54 63 70 71 72 75 76 78 **P**3 **Web address:** www.clarindahealth.net	14	10	27	701	9	40703	73	8566	3824	154
MENTAL HEALTH INSTITUTE, Mailing Address: P.O. Box 338, Zip 51632-0338; tel. 712/542-2161; Mark Lund, Superintendent (Total facility includes 63 beds in nursing home–type unit) **F**16 17 18 23 28 30 41 45 53 57 60 62 69 70 78 **P**6	12	22	83	210	67	0	0	7058	5761	126

CLARION—Wright County

★ COMMUNITY MEMORIAL HOSPITAL, 1316 South Main Street, Zip 50525; tel. 515/532-2811; Steve J. Simonin, Chief Executive Officer **A**9 10 18 **F**1 7 8 9 22 23 25 28 34 36 37 38 39 40 41 43 44 45 46 48 54 67 69 70 76 78 **S** Iowa Health System, Des Moines, IA **Web address:** www.trcnet.net	14	10	33	626	14	25279	92	6538	2352	88

CLINTON—Clinton County

✠ MERCY MEDICAL CENTER–CLINTON, (Formerly Samaritan Health System), (Includes Mercy Services for Aging, 600 14th Avenue North, Zip 52732; tel. 319/244-3888), 1410 North Fourth Street, Zip 52732-2999; tel. 319/244-5555; Thomas J. Hesselmann, President and Chief Executive Officer (Total facility includes 212 beds in nursing home–type unit) **A**1 9 10 **F**7 8 9 11 12 13 17 18 19 20 21 22 23 24 25 26 27 28 29 30 32 33 34 35 36 37 38 39 43 44 46 48 49 51 54 56 57 58 59 60 61 62 64 65 69 70 72 76 78 **P**8 **S** Trinity Health, Novi, MI **Web address:** www.samhealth.com	21	10	364	7163	266	50782	662	49987	21927	755

CORNING—Adams County

★ ALEGENT HEALTH MERCY HOSPITAL, (Formerly Mercy Hospital), 703 Rosary Drive, Zip 50841, Mailing Address: P.O. Box 368, Zip 50841-0368; tel. 515/322-3121; James C. Ruppert, Administrator **A**10 **F**7 8 9 17 18 22 25 30 32 33 34 36 38 39 40 41 44 45 46 48 49 50 54 56 63 68 69 70 76 78 **P**6 **S** Catholic Health Initiatives, Denver, CO	21	10	22	436	6	—	—	5583	2348	108

CORYDON—Wayne County

★ WAYNE COUNTY HOSPITAL, 417 South East Street, Zip 50060-1860, Mailing Address: P.O. Box 305, Zip 50060-0305; tel. 515/872-2260; Bill D. Wilson, Administrator **A**9 10 **F**7 8 9 13 14 16 17 19 21 22 25 32 34 36 37 38 40 41 43 44 45 46 48 50 54 56 59 63 69 70 75 76 78	13	10	28	916	13	25922	92	6238	2703	122

© 2000 AHA Guide   *Many Facility Codes have changed. Please refer to the AHA Guide Code Chart.*   Hospitals **A149**

Hospitals, U.S. / IOWA

★	American Hospital Association (AHA) membership
□	Joint Commission on Accreditation of Healthcare Organizations (JCAHO) accreditation
+	American Osteopathic Healthcare Association (AOHA) membership
○	American Osteopathic Association (AOA) accreditation
△	Commission on Accreditation of Rehabilitation Facilities (CARF) accreditation

Control codes 61, 63, 64, 71, 72 and 73 indicate hospitals listed by AOHA, but not registered by AHA. For definition of numerical codes, see page A4.

Hospital, Address, Telephone, Administrator, Approval, Facility, and Physician Codes, Health Care System, Network	Classification Codes		Utilization Data					Expense (thousands) of dollars		
	Control	Service	Staffed Beds	Admissions	Census	Outpatient Visits	Births	Total	Payroll	Personnel

COUNCIL BLUFFS—Pottawattamie County

★ ALEGENT HEALTH MERCY HOSPITAL, (Formerly Mercy Hospital), 800 Mercy Drive, Zip 51503–3128, Mailing Address: P.O. Box 1C, Zip 51502–3001; tel. 712/328–5000; Charles J. Marr, Chief Executive Officer **A**1 9 10 **F**1 2 3 4 6 7 8 9 11 12 13 19 20 21 22 23 24 25 26 27 28 29 30 31 32 33 34 35 36 37 38 39 41 42 43 44 45 46 47 48 49 50 51 53 54 55 56 57 58 59 60 61 62 63 64 65 68 69 70 71 72 73 76 77 78 79 **P**6 8 **S** Catholic Health Initiatives, Denver, CO   21 10 189 5302 80 35374 470 41069 16481 640

★ JENNIE EDMUNDSON MEMORIAL HOSPITAL, 933 East Pierce Street, Zip 51503–4652, Mailing Address: P.O. Box 2C, Zip 51502–3002; tel. 712/328–6000; David M. Holcomb, President and Chief Executive Officer (Total facility includes 17 beds in nursing home–type unit) **A**1 2 5 9 10 **F**3 4 7 8 9 11 13 17 18 19 21 22 23 24 25 26 27 30 31 32 33 34 35 36 37 38 39 40 41 43 44 45 46 47 48 49 50 51 54 57 58 59 60 61 62 63 64 65 67 68 69 70 71 72 76 77 78 **P**6 8   23 10 112 6408 103 82878 615 55862 28301 679

CRESCO—Howard County

★ REGIONAL HEALTH SERVICES OF HOWARD COUNTY, 235 Eighth Avenue West, Zip 52136–1098; tel. 319/547–2101; Elizabeth A. Doty, President and Chief Executive Officer **A**9 10 **F**7 8 9 17 22 25 34 37 39 43 44 45 48 54 70 76 78 **P**4 5 8 **S** Trinity Health, Novi, MI
Web address: www.rhshc.com   13 10 32 400 4 17096 58 5779 2799 89

CRESTON—Union County

★ GREATER COMMUNITY HOSPITAL, 1700 West Townline, Zip 50801–1099; tel. 515/782–7091; Ronald D. Davis, Chief Executive Officer **A**9 10 **F**7 8 9 13 17 18 19 21 22 23 25 26 32 34 36 37 38 39 40 41 43 44 45 46 48 54 65 68 70 76 78 **P**6 **S** Iowa Health System, Des Moines, IA   13 10 49 1536 17 23561 172 11969 5416 187

DAVENPORT—Scott County

★ △ GENESIS MEDICAL CENTER, (Includes Genesis Medical Center–East Campus, 1227 East Rusholme Street, Zip 52803; tel. 319/421–1000; Genesis Medical Center–West Campus, 1401 West Central Park, Zip 52804–1769; tel. 319/421–1000), 1227 East Rusholme Street, Zip 52803–2498; tel. 319/421–1000; Leo A. Bressanelli, President and Chief Executive Officer (Total facility includes 40 beds in nursing home–type unit) **A**1 2 3 5 7 9 10 **F**2 3 4 6 7 8 9 11 13 16 17 18 19 21 22 23 25 27 31 32 33 34 35 36 37 38 39 41 42 43 44 45 46 47 48 49 50 51 53 54 55 57 58 59 60 61 62 63 65 66 68 69 70 72 73 75 76 77 78 **P**6 7 8
Web address: www.genesishealth.com   23 10 442 18805 329 181275 2323 203343 78504 2218

★ ○ TRINITY MEDICAL CENTER–NORTH CAMPUS, (Formerly Davenport Medical Center), 1111 West Kimberly Road, Zip 52806–5913; tel. 319/445–4020; Robert J. Lundin, II, Chief Executive Officer **A**1 9 10 11 12 13 **F**1 2 3 4 5 7 8 9 10 11 12 14 16 17 18 19 20 21 22 23 24 25 27 28 29 30 31 32 33 34 35 36 37 38 39 41 42 43 44 45 46 47 48 49 50 51 52 53 54 55 56 57 58 59 60 61 62 63 64 65 66 68 69 70 72 73 75 76 77 78 79 **P**1 **S** Iowa Health System, Des Moines, IA   23 10 105 1406 20 39792 138 16589 6750 224

DE WITT—Clinton County

★ DEWITT COMMUNITY HOSPITAL, 1118 11th Street, Zip 52742–1296; tel. 319/659–4200; Robert G. Senneff, Chief Executive Officer (Total facility includes 77 beds in nursing home–type unit) **A**1 9 10 **F**9 17 18 22 25 26 40 48 49 54 69 70 76   23 10 85 393 79 22290 0 6352 2816 126

DECORAH—Winneshiek County

★ WINNESHIEK COUNTY MEMORIAL HOSPITAL, 901 Montgomery Street, Zip 52101–2325; tel. 319/382–2911; Allan Atkinson, Chief Executive Officer **A**1 9 10 **F**7 8 9 12 13 16 17 19 22 24 25 32 34 35 36 37 38 39 40 41 43 44 45 46 48 50 54 70 71 76 78
Web address: www.winnhosp.org   13 10 83 1161 9 42574 292 12747 6060 213

DENISON—Crawford County

CRAWFORD COUNTY MEMORIAL HOSPITAL, 2020 First Avenue South, Zip 51442–2299; tel. 712/263–5021; Edwin A. Gast, Chief Executive Officer and Administrator **A**9 10 **F**7 8 9 16 18 19 22 23 24 25 30 31 32 33 34 35 38 39 41 43 44 46 48 54 56 70 71 72 76   13 10 28 849 9 25294 125 8460 4078 130

DES MOINES—Polk County

★ BROADLAWNS MEDICAL CENTER, 1801 Hickman Road, Zip 50314–1597; tel. 515/282–2200; Susan L. Hunsaker, CHE, Director and Chief Executive Officer **A**1 3 5 9 10 **F**1 3 7 8 9 13 14 16 17 18 19 21 22 23 24 25 30 31 35 37 38 39 41 43 44 45 46 48 49 51 54 56 57 58 59 60 61 63 64 65 70 72 75 76 77 78 79 **P**6
Web address: www.broadlawns.org
DES MOINES DIVISION See Veterans Affairs Central Iowa Health Care System   13 10 107 4815 55 198841 495 62284 29406 807

★ + ○ DES MOINES GENERAL HOSPITAL, 603 East 12th Street, Zip 50309–5515; tel. 515/263–4200; Stephen J. Harris, President and Chief Executive Officer (Total facility includes 15 beds in nursing home–type unit) **A**1 9 10 11 12 13 **F**2 3 4 7 8 9 10 11 12 13 15 16 18 19 22 24 25 26 28 29 30 32 33 35 37 38 39 41 42 43 44 45 46 47 48 49 50 51 52 53 54 55 57 59 60 61 62 63 64 68 69 70 72 75 76 78 79
Web address: www.dmgeneral.com   23 10 155 4126 92 29207 185 45695 18067 413

Hospitals, U.S. / IOWA

Hospital, Address, Telephone, Administrator, Approval, Facility, and Physician Codes, Health Care System, Network	Classification Codes		Utilization Data					Expense (thousands) of dollars		
★ American Hospital Association (AHA) membership □ Joint Commission on Accreditation of Healthcare Organizations (JCAHO) accreditation + American Osteopathic Healthcare Association (AOHA) membership ○ American Osteopathic Association (AOA) accreditation △ Commission on Accreditation of Rehabilitation Facilities (CARF) accreditation Control codes 61, 63, 64, 71, 72 and 73 indicate hospitals listed by AOHA, but not registered by AHA. For definition of numerical codes, see page A4	Control	Service	Staffed Beds	Admissions	Census	Outpatient Visits	Births	Total	Payroll	Personnel
☒ IOWA LUTHERAN HOSPITAL, 700 East University Avenue, Zip 50316–2392; tel. 515/263–5612; David Stark, Chief Operating Officer (Total facility includes 16 beds in nursing home–type unit) **A**1 3 5 9 10 **F**1 2 3 4 7 8 9 10 11 12 13 14 16 17 18 19 20 21 22 24 25 26 27 28 29 30 31 32 33 34 36 37 38 39 41 42 43 44 45 46 47 48 50 51 52 53 54 56 57 58 59 60 61 62 63 64 65 66 69 70 71 72 73 74 75 76 77 78 79 **P**1 3 6 7 **S** Iowa Health System, Des Moines, IA **Web address:** www.ihsdesmoines.org	23	10	232	9530	138	288898	1229	91828	44278	1387
☒ △ IOWA METHODIST MEDICAL CENTER, (Includes Powell Convalescent Center; Raymond Blank Memorial Hospital for Children; Younker Memorial Rehabilitation Center), 1200 Pleasant Street, Zip 50309–9976; tel. 515/241–6212; James H. Skogsbergh, President **A**1 2 3 5 6 7 9 10 **F**1 2 3 4 7 8 9 10 11 12 13 14 16 17 18 19 20 21 22 24 25 26 27 28 29 30 31 32 33 34 36 37 38 39 41 42 43 44 45 46 47 48 50 51 52 53 54 56 57 58 59 60 61 62 63 64 65 66 69 70 71 72 73 74 75 76 77 78 79 **P**1 3 6 7 **S** Iowa Health System, Des Moines, IA **Web address:** www.ihsdesmoines.org	23	10	464	20578	307	198435	2261	240103	98265	3077
☒ △ MERCY MEDICAL CENTER–DES MOINES, (Formerly Mercy Hospital Medical Center), (Includes Mercy Franklin Center, 1818 48th Street, Zip 50310; tel. 515/271–6000), 1111 6th Avenue, Zip 50314–2611; tel. 515/247–3121; David H. Vellinga, President and Chief Executive Officer (Total facility includes 35 beds in nursing home–type unit) **A**1 2 3 6 7 9 10 **F**1 3 4 5 6 7 8 9 11 12 13 16 17 18 19 20 22 23 24 25 26 27 28 29 30 32 33 34 35 36 37 38 39 41 42 43 44 45 46 47 48 49 50 51 52 53 54 55 56 57 58 59 60 61 62 63 64 65 67 68 69 70 71 72 73 74 75 76 77 78 79 **P**1 6 8 **S** Catholic Health Initiatives, Denver, CO **Web address:** www.mercydesmoines.org	21	10	591	28095	400	765403	3793	270747	113500	4270
☒ △ VETERANS AFFAIRS CENTRAL IOWA HEALTH CARE SYSTEM, (Includes Des Moines Division, 3600 30th Street; Knoxville Division, 1515 West Pleasant, Knoxville, Zip 50138–3399; tel. 515/842–3101), 3600 30th Street, Zip 50310–5774; tel. 515/699–5999; Donald C. Cooper, Director (Total facility includes 226 beds in nursing home–type unit) **A**1 2 3 5 7 **F**1 2 3 4 5 7 9 11 12 13 18 19 21 22 24 25 27 29 30 31 32 33 34 37 38 39 41 43 45 46 47 48 49 50 51 53 54 55 56 57 59 60 61 62 63 65 66 68 69 70 72 74 76 78 79 **S** Department of Veterans Affairs, Washington, DC **Web address:** www.va.gov/stations97/guide/home.asp?DIVISION=ALL	45	10	327	2968	288	192616	0	85142	51248	1213

DUBUQUE—Dubuque County

☒ FINLEY HOSPITAL, 350 North Grandview Avenue, Zip 52001–6392; tel. 319/582–1881; Kevin L. Rogols, President and Chief Executive Officer (Total facility includes 32 beds in nursing home–type unit) **A**1 2 9 10 **F**7 8 9 13 14 16 17 18 19 22 23 24 25 26 27 28 30 31 32 33 34 35 36 37 38 39 40 41 43 44 45 46 48 49 50 51 53 63 64 65 66 69 70 71 72 75 76 77 78 79 **P**1 5 **S** Iowa Health System, Des Moines, IA **Web address:** www.finleyhospital.org	23	10	139	5258	58	84380	609	49894	21538	760
☒ △ MERCY MEDICAL CENTER–DUBUQUE, (Formerly Mercy Health Center), (Includes Mercy Medical Center–Dyersville, 1111 Third Street S.W., Dyersville, Zip 52040; tel. 319/875–7101), 250 Mercy Drive, Zip 52001–7360; tel. 319/589–8000; Russell M. Knight, President and Chief Executive Officer (Total facility includes 69 beds in nursing home–type unit) **A**1 7 9 10 **F**1 2 3 4 7 8 9 11 12 13 14 17 18 19 21 22 23 24 25 26 27 28 30 31 32 33 34 35 36 37 38 39 41 42 43 44 45 46 47 49 50 53 54 55 56 57 58 59 60 61 62 63 64 65 69 70 71 72 73 75 76 77 78 79 **P**8 **S** Trinity Health, Novi, MI **Web address:** www.mercyhealth.com	21	10	385	9812	164	43745	935	85866	34218	1175

DYERSVILLE—Dubuque County

MERCY MEDICAL CENTER–DYERSVILLE See Mercy Medical Center–Dubuque, Dubuque

ELKADER—Clayton County

★ CENTRAL COMMUNITY HOSPITAL, 901 Davidson Street N.W., Zip 52043; tel. 319/245–7000; Fran Zichal, Chief Executive Officer **A**10 **F**7 9 12 17 18 19 22 25 28 30 32 33 34 36 37 41 43 48 50 54 56 69 70 72 76 **S** Trinity Health, Novi, MI	23	10	16	270	4	7941	0	2611	950	54

EMMETSBURG—Palo Alto County

★ PALO ALTO HEALTH SYSTEM, (Formerly Palo Alto County Hospital), 3201 First Street, Zip 50536–2599; tel. 712/852–5500; Darrell E. Vondrak, Administrator (Total facility includes 22 beds in nursing home–type unit) **A**9 10 **F**2 3 4 7 8 9 10 11 12 13 14 16 17 18 19 20 21 22 24 25 26 27 28 30 31 32 33 34 35 36 37 38 39 40 41 42 43 44 45 46 47 48 49 50 51 52 53 54 55 56 57 58 59 60 61 62 63 64 65 66 67 68 69 70 71 72 73 74 75 76 77 78 79 **P**1 **S** Trinity Health, Novi, MI **Web address:** www.northiowamercy.com	13	10	54	801	26	20443	73	8017	3344	124

ESTHERVILLE—Emmet County

☒ AVERA HOLY FAMILY HOSPITAL, (Formerly Avera Holy Family Health), 826 North Eighth Street, Zip 51334–1598; tel. 712/362–2631; William Bumgarner, Chief Executive Officer **A**1 9 10 **F**1 7 8 9 13 14 17 18 19 22 25 26 30 31 34 35 36 37 38 39 40 41 43 44 45 46 48 51 54 56 63 70 72 76 77 78 **P**3 5 **S** Avera Health, Yankton, SD	21	10	35	1063	13	28526	99	8582	3844	205

© 2000 AHA Guide *Many Facility Codes have changed. Please refer to the AHA Guide Code Chart.* Hospitals **A151**

Hospitals, U.S. / IOWA

Hospital, Address, Telephone, Administrator, Approval, Facility, and Physician Codes, Health Care System, Network	Classification Codes		Utilization Data					Expense (thousands) of dollars		
★ American Hospital Association (AHA) membership ☐ Joint Commission on Accreditation of Healthcare Organizations (JCAHO) accreditation + American Osteopathic Healthcare Association (AOHA) membership ○ American Osteopathic Association (AOA) accreditation △ Commission on Accreditation of Rehabilitation Facilities (CARF) accreditation Control codes 61, 63, 64, 71, 72 and 73 indicate hospitals listed by AOHA, but not registered by AHA. For definition of numerical codes, see page A4	Control	Service	Staffed Beds	Admissions	Census	Outpatient Visits	Births	Total	Payroll	Personnel
FAIRFIELD—Jefferson County										
★ JEFFERSON COUNTY HOSPITAL, 400 Highland Avenue, Zip 52556–3713, Mailing Address: P.O. Box 588, Zip 52556–0588; tel. 515/472–4111; Douglas Faus, Chief Executive Officer (Total facility includes 36 beds in nursing home–type unit) **A**10 **F**3 7 8 9 16 17 18 22 25 32 34 36 38 39 41 43 44 45 46 48 54 61 63 69 70 72 76 Web address: www.jchospital.org	13	10	67	1563	48	24717	96	11962	5010	193
FORT DODGE—Webster County										
✠ TRINITY REGIONAL HOSPITAL, 802 Kenyon Road, Zip 50501–5795; tel. 515/573–3101; Tom Tibbitts, President **A**1 9 10 **F**2 3 4 7 8 9 13 16 17 18 19 20 22 24 25 27 32 33 34 36 37 38 39 41 43 44 45 48 50 51 53 54 57 58 59 60 61 62 63 64 68 69 70 71 72 76 78 **P**6 **S** Iowa Health System, Des Moines, IA Web address: www.trh-fd.org	23	10	161	6905	80	141486	594	56571	24033	742
FORT MADISON—Lee County										
✠ FORT MADISON COMMUNITY HOSPITAL, 5445 Avenue O, Zip 52627–0174, Mailing Address: P.O. Box 174, Zip 52627–0174; tel. 319/372–6530; C. James Platt, Chief Executive Officer **A**1 9 10 **F**9 13 16 17 18 22 25 28 31 32 34 36 38 39 41 44 45 46 48 50 51 54 65 70 75 76 79 **S** Quorum Health Group, Brentwood, TN Web address: www.fmchcares.com	23	10	50	2483	28	39552	204	21333	9362	282
GLENWOOD—Mills County										
GLENWOOD STATE HOSPITAL SCHOOL, 711 South Vine, Zip 51534–1927; tel. 712/527–4811; William E. Campbell, Ph.D., Superintendent **F**17 18 23 40 58 63 70 **P**6	12	62	399	38	389	0	0	40586	27336	841
GREENFIELD—Adair County										
ADAIR COUNTY MEMORIAL HOSPITAL, 609 S.E. Kent Street, Zip 50849–9454; tel. 515/743–2123; Myrna Erb–Gundel, Administrator **A**9 10 **F**7 9 13 16 17 18 19 21 22 24 25 32 34 36 37 38 40 41 43 45 46 48 54 70 76 78	13	10	22	580	7	7062	14	4266	1935	86
GRINNELL—Poweshiek County										
✠ GRINNELL REGIONAL MEDICAL CENTER, 210 Fourth Avenue, Zip 50112–1833; tel. 515/236–7511; Todd C. Linden, President and Chief Executive Officer **A**1 9 10 **F**1 7 9 13 14 16 17 18 19 20 21 22 23 25 26 27 28 29 30 31 33 34 35 36 37 38 39 40 41 43 44 45 46 48 49 50 51 54 55 56 58 59 60 61 62 63 68 70 71 72 75 76 78 **P**7	23	10	46	2512	24	48324	185	23040	11112	335
GRUNDY CENTER—Grundy County										
★ GRUNDY COUNTY MEMORIAL HOSPITAL, 201 East J Avenue, Zip 50638–2096; tel. 319/824–5421; Janice McCart, Chief Executive Officer (Total facility includes 55 beds in nursing home–type unit) **A**9 10 **F**9 13 14 17 18 19 22 25 26 30 34 36 37 38 40 43 45 48 51 54 56 59 62 63 69 70 76 77 **P**5 **S** Iowa Health System, Des Moines, IA	13	10	71	271	59	14104	0	3530	1820	76
GUTHRIE CENTER—Guthrie County										
★ GUTHRIE COUNTY HOSPITAL, 710 North 12th Street, Zip 50115–1544; tel. 515/747–2201; Todd Hudspeth, Administrator and Chief Executive Officer **A**9 10 **F**7 9 12 13 17 18 19 20 22 23 25 28 32 34 37 38 39 40 43 46 48 54 56 63 70 71 75 76 **P**6 Web address: www.gcho.org	13	10	26	505	6	12040	0	3466	1444	66
GUTTENBERG—Clayton County										
★ GUTTENBERG MUNICIPAL HOSPITAL, Second and Main Street, Zip 52052–0550, Mailing Address: P.O. Box 550, Zip 52052–0550; tel. 319/252–1121; Kim Gau, Interim Chief Executive Officer **A**9 10 **F**7 8 9 12 22 25 26 28 34 36 37 38 39 40 41 43 44 45 46 48 51 54 70 75 76 **P**5 **S** Iowa Health System, Des Moines, IA	14	10	20	578	7	14611	43	4366	1755	79
HAMBURG—Fremont County										
GRAPE COMMUNITY HOSPITAL, 2959 U.S. Highway 275, Zip 51640; tel. 712/382–1515; Carolyn K. Hess, Administrator and Chief Executive Officer **A**9 10 **F**9 12 16 17 18 19 22 25 30 32 33 34 37 38 39 40 41 43 45 46 48 49 50 51 54 61 69 70 76	23	10	28	554	14	23916	8	5796	2748	88
HAMPTON—Franklin County										
★ FRANKLIN GENERAL HOSPITAL, 1720 Central Avenue East, Zip 50441–1859; tel. 515/456–5000; Scott Wells, Administrator (Total facility includes 52 beds in nursing home–type unit) **A**9 10 **F**3 4 5 7 8 9 11 12 13 16 17 18 21 22 23 25 26 27 30 31 33 34 35 36 37 38 39 41 43 46 47 48 49 50 54 56 58 59 60 61 62 63 64 65 67 69 70 71 72 75 76 77 78 79 **P**6 8 **S** Trinity Health, Novi, MI Web address: www.franklingeneral.com	13	10	82	405	58	16556	0	5605	2593	112
HARLAN—Shelby County										
★ SHELBY COUNTY MYRTUE MEMORIAL HOSPITAL, 1213 Garfield Avenue, Zip 51537–2057; tel. 712/755–5161; Stephen L. Goeser, Administrator **A**9 10 **F**7 8 9 13 14 17 18 19 21 22 24 25 26 28 32 34 36 37 38 39 40 43 44 45 46 48 49 54 56 58 59 63 71 72 73 76 78 **P**6 8 Web address: www.myrtue.org	13	10	52	1451	20	21648	84	10549	4198	176
HAWARDEN—Sioux County										
★ HAWARDEN COMMUNITY HOSPITAL, 1111 11th Street, Zip 51023–1999; tel. 712/551–3100; Stuart A. Katz, FACHE, Chief Executive Officer **A**9 10 **F**7 9 13 14 17 19 22 24 25 32 34 36 37 38 39 43 45 48 50 51 54 56 66 70 72 73 75 76 78 **P**7 **S** Trinity Health, Novi, MI Web address: www.acsnet.com/~commhosp/	14	10	17	218	6	14477	0	2762	1177	58

Hospitals, U.S. / IOWA

Hospital, Address, Telephone, Administrator, Approval, Facility, and Physician Codes, Health Care System, Network	Classi-fication Codes		Utilization Data					Expense (thousands) of dollars		
★ American Hospital Association (AHA) membership □ Joint Commission on Accreditation of Healthcare Organizations (JCAHO) accreditation + American Osteopathic Healthcare Association (AOHA) membership ○ American Osteopathic Association (AOA) accreditation △ Commission on Accreditation of Rehabilitation Facilities (CARF) accreditation Control codes 61, 63, 64, 71, 72 and 73 indicate hospitals listed by AOHA, but not registered by AHA. For definition of numerical codes, see page A4	Control	Service	Staffed Beds	Admissions	Census	Outpatient Visits	Births	Total	Payroll	Personnel
HUMBOLDT—Humboldt County										
★ HUMBOLDT COUNTY MEMORIAL HOSPITAL, 1000 North 15th Street, Zip 50548–1008; tel. 515/332–4200; Monte Neitzel, Administrator and Chief Executive Officer **A**9 10 **F**7 8 9 17 18 19 22 25 34 36 37 38 39 40 43 44 45 46 48 54 69 70 76 **S** Iowa Health System, Des Moines, IA Web address: trv1.trvnet.net/~hcmh/	13	10	49	374	32	45442	18	6300	3045	124
IDA GROVE—Ida County										
★ HORN MEMORIAL HOSPITAL, 701 East Second Street, Zip 51445–1699; tel. 712/364–3311; Dan Ellis, Administrator **A**9 10 **F**7 8 9 13 16 17 18 19 22 25 34 36 37 38 39 40 41 44 45 46 48 54 56 59 70 75 76	23	10	36	585	9	21805	61	4923	2436	72
INDEPENDENCE—Buchanan County										
□ MENTAL HEALTH INSTITUTE, 2277 Iowa Avenue, Zip 50644, Mailing Address: P.O. Box 111, Zip 50644; tel. 319/334–2583; Bhasker J. Dave, M.D., Superintendent **A**1 10 **F**16 17 18 23 25 31 57 58 59 60 61 70 72 78 **P**6	12	22	151	945	122	16	0	17963	12353	331
★ PEOPLE'S MEMORIAL HOSPITAL OF BUCHANAN COUNTY, 1600 First Street East, Zip 50644–3155; tel. 319/334–6071; Robert J. Richard, Administrator (Total facility includes 59 beds in nursing home–type unit) **A**9 10 **F**7 8 9 13 14 15 16 17 18 19 20 21 22 23 24 25 26 30 31 32 34 35 36 37 38 39 40 41 43 44 45 48 50 51 67 69 70 71 72 75 76	13	10	109	559	61	25334	44	7277	3616	159
IOWA CITY—Johnson County										
✪ MERCY HOSPITAL, 500 East Market Street, Zip 52245–2689; tel. 319/339–0300; Ronald R. Reed, President and Chief Executive Officer (Total facility includes 12 beds in nursing home–type unit) **A**1 2 3 5 9 10 **F**3 4 7 8 9 11 13 14 16 17 18 19 20 22 23 24 25 26 27 30 32 33 34 35 36 37 38 39 41 42 43 44 45 46 47 48 49 50 51 54 55 57 58 59 60 61 62 63 65 66 69 70 71 72 75 76 77 78 79 **P**1 Web address: www.mercyic.com STATE PSYCHIATRIC HOSPITAL See University of Iowa Hospitals and Clinics	21	10	240	8559	119	200474	1191	70474	32564	897
✪ UNIVERSITY OF IOWA HOSPITALS AND CLINICS, (Includes Chemical Dependency Center, tel. 319/384–8765; State Psychiatric Hospital, tel. 319/356–4658; University Hospital School, tel. 319/353–6456), 200 Hawkins Drive, Zip 52242–1009; tel. 319/356–1616; R. Edward Howell, Director and Chief Executive Officer **A**1 2 3 5 8 9 10 **F**2 3 4 5 7 8 9 10 11 12 13 14 16 17 18 19 20 21 22 23 24 25 26 27 29 30 31 32 33 34 35 36 37 38 39 41 42 43 44 45 46 47 48 49 50 51 52 53 54 55 56 57 58 59 60 61 62 63 64 65 66 68 70 71 72 74 75 76 77 78 79 **P**1 7 Web address: www.uihc.uiowa.edu	12	10	707	23399	471	711176	1199	440768	179705	5342
✪ VETERANS AFFAIRS MEDICAL CENTER, 601 Highway 6 West, Zip 52246–2208; tel. 319/338–0581; Gary L. Wilkinson, Director **A**1 3 5 8 **F**1 3 4 9 11 13 18 22 23 24 25 27 29 30 31 32 34 35 36 37 39 41 42 43 44 45 46 47 48 49 50 51 54 55 56 57 59 61 63 65 68 70 72 73 76 77 78 79 **S** Department of Veterans Affairs, Washington, DC Web address: www.va.gov/stations97/guide/home.asp?DIVISION=ALL	45	10	106	3654	65	180012	0	78160	44325	1147
IOWA FALLS—Hardin County										
✪ ELLSWORTH MUNICIPAL HOSPITAL, 110 Rocksylvania Avenue, Zip 50126–2431; tel. 515/648–4631; John O'Brien, Administrator **A**1 2 9 10 **F**3 7 8 9 13 19 20 22 24 25 26 28 29 32 33 34 36 37 38 39 41 43 44 45 48 50 51 54 57 58 59 60 61 63 64 68 70 72 76 78 **P**1 6 **S** Trinity Health, Novi, MI	14	10	40	1560	17	31243	123	8838	4240	182
JEFFERSON—Greene County										
✪ GREENE COUNTY MEDICAL CENTER, 1000 West Lincolnway, Zip 50129–1697; tel. 515/386–2114; Karen L. Bossard, Administrator and Chief Executive Officer (Total facility includes 74 beds in nursing home–type unit) **A**1 9 10 **F**7 8 9 12 13 14 16 17 18 19 21 22 24 25 30 32 33 34 35 36 37 38 39 41 43 44 45 46 48 50 54 67 69 70 72 73 76 78 **P**5 Web address: www.netins.net/showcase/gcmc/	13	10	127	776	83	23551	111	10518	5425	205
KEOKUK—Lee County										
✪ KEOKUK AREA HOSPITAL, 1600 Morgan Street, Zip 52632–3456; tel. 319/524–7150; Allan Zastrow, FACHE, Chief Executive Officer (Total facility includes 20 beds in nursing home–type unit) **A**1 10 **F**3 8 9 12 16 17 18 19 22 24 25 27 32 33 34 36 38 39 44 48 50 51 54 57 58 59 60 61 66 69 70 71 72 75 76 78 **P**7	23	10	113	3754	51	47283	227	21994	10583	378
KEOSAUQUA—Van Buren County										
★ VAN BUREN COUNTY HOSPITAL, Highway 1 North, Zip 52565, Mailing Address: P.O. Box 70, Zip 52565–0070; tel. 319/293–3171; Lisa Schnedler, Administrator **A**9 10 **F**3 4 5 7 8 9 11 13 14 15 17 18 19 22 24 25 27 31 32 33 34 35 36 38 39 43 45 46 47 49 50 51 54 55 56 58 59 60 61 62 63 64 65 66 68 69 70 71 72 74 75 76 78 79 **P**6 **S** Sisters of Mary of the Presentation Health Corporation, Fargo, ND Web address: www.netins.net/showcase/forhealth/	13	10	40	689	18	9802	31	6839	3391	147
KNOXVILLE—Marion County										
✪ KNOXVILLE AREA COMMUNITY HOSPITAL, 1002 South Lincoln Street, Zip 50138–3121; tel. 515/842–2151; Jim Murphy, Chief Executive Officer (Total facility includes 14 beds in nursing home–type unit) **A**1 9 10 **F**8 12 17 18 22 24 25 32 34 38 39 41 44 45 48 50 53 54 61 69 70 72 76 78 **P**8 **S** Quorum Health Group, Brentwood, TN KNOXVILLE DIVISION See Veterans Affairs Central Iowa Health Care System, Des Moines	23	10	52	1185	26	13944	93	8516	3274	141

© 2000 AHA Guide   *Many Facility Codes have changed. Please refer to the AHA Guide Code Chart.*

Hospitals, U.S. / IOWA

Hospital, Address, Telephone, Administrator, Approval, Facility, and Physician Codes, Health Care System, Network

- ★ American Hospital Association (AHA) membership
- ◻ Joint Commission on Accreditation of Healthcare Organizations (JCAHO) accreditation
- + American Osteopathic Healthcare Association (AOHA) membership
- ○ American Osteopathic Association (AOA) accreditation
- △ Commission on Accreditation of Rehabilitation Facilities (CARF) accreditation

Control codes 61, 63, 64, 71, 72 and 73 indicate hospitals listed by AOHA, but not registered by AHA. For definition of numerical codes, see page A4.

Hospital	Classification Codes		Utilization Data					Expense (thousands) of dollars		Personnel
	Control	Service	Staffed Beds	Admissions	Census	Outpatient Visits	Births	Total	Payroll	
LAKE CITY—Calhoun County										
★ STEWART MEMORIAL COMMUNITY HOSPITAL, 1301 West Main, Zip 51449–1585; tel. 712/464–3171; Kris Baumgart, Chief Executive Officer **A**9 10 **F**7 8 9 13 16 22 25 33 34 36 37 38 39 40 41 43 44 45 48 54 61 70 76 **P**5 6 Web address: www.smchospital.org	23	10	53	1780	26	37598	124	10366	5125	176
LE MARS—Plymouth County										
FLOYD VALLEY HOSPITAL/AVERA HEALTH, Highway 3 East, Zip 51031–0010, Mailing Address: P.O. Box 10, Zip 51031–0010; tel. 712/546–3398; Michael Donlin, Administrator **A**9 10 **F**6 7 8 9 14 17 18 19 22 24 25 28 32 33 34 36 37 38 39 40 43 44 45 46 48 49 50 51 54 61 69 72 75 76 78 **P**3 **S** Avera Health, Yankton, SD Web address: www.floydvalleyhospital.org	14	10	44	1364	17	36049	116	10373	3892	123
LEON—Decatur County										
◧ DECATUR COUNTY HOSPITAL, 1405 N.W. Church Street, Zip 50144–1299; tel. 515/446–4871; Roy E. White, Administrator **A**1 9 10 **F**7 8 9 16 17 18 22 25 36 38 39 44 45 46 48 51 54 58 59 60 61 62 63 64 70 72 76 **P**5	13	10	49	842	11	11265	56	5503	2517	120
MANCHESTER—Delaware County										
REGIONAL MEDICAL CENTER OF NORTHEAST IOWA AND DELAWARE COUNTY, (Formerly Delaware County Memorial Hospital), 709 West Main Street, Zip 52057–0359, Mailing Address: P.O. Box 359, Zip 52057–0359; tel. 319/927–3232; Lon D. Butikofer, R.N., Ph.D., Chief Executive Officer **A**9 10 **F**7 8 9 13 14 16 17 18 19 21 22 25 28 30 31 32 33 34 35 36 37 38 39 41 43 44 45 48 50 51 54 56 58 59 60 61 63 70 71 72 75 76 78 **P**5	13	10	35	825	9	52882	200	10879	5154	176
MANNING—Carroll County										
MANNING REGIONAL HEALTHCARE CENTER, 410 Main Street, Zip 51455–1093; tel. 712/653–2072; Michael S. Ketcham, Chief Executive Officer (Total facility includes 58 beds in nursing home–type unit) **A**9 10 **F**1 2 3 7 8 9 16 21 22 24 25 30 33 34 35 36 38 39 44 45 48 50 51 56 59 61 69 70 72 76 78 **P**5	23	10	87	449	58	12018	38	4357	2169	111
MAQUOKETA—Jackson County										
◧ JACKSON COUNTY PUBLIC HOSPITAL, 700 West Grove Street, Zip 52060–0910; tel. 319/652–2474; Curt Coleman, Chief Executive Officer (Total facility includes 18 beds in nursing home–type unit) **A**1 9 10 **F**7 8 9 17 18 22 24 25 28 34 36 38 40 41 43 44 48 50 51 68 69 70 76 78	13	10	61	809	25	19063	99	8415	4110	161
MARENGO—Iowa County										
MARENGO MEMORIAL HOSPITAL, 300 West May Street, Zip 52301–1261, Mailing Address: P.O. Box 228, Zip 52301–0228; tel. 319/642–5543; Michael D. Trachta, Administrator **A**9 10 **F**7 9 13 16 17 18 19 22 25 26 32 34 37 40 43 45 54 70 75 78	14	10	44	316	26	3724	0	3348	1551	76
MARSHALLTOWN—Marshall County										
◧ MARSHALLTOWN MEDICAL AND SURGICAL CENTER, 3 South Fourth Avenue, Zip 50158–2998; tel. 515/754–5151; Robert Cooper, Chief Executive Officer (Total facility includes 26 beds in nursing home–type unit) **A**1 9 10 **F**1 7 8 9 13 14 16 17 18 19 22 24 25 26 29 30 31 32 33 34 36 38 39 41 43 44 45 46 48 50 51 54 56 68 69 70 71 72 75 76 78 79 **P**6 7 Web address: www.mtnia.com/mmsc/INDEX.HTM	23	10	111	3845	48	154665	610	36616	16696	497
MASON CITY—Cerro Gordo County										
◧ MERCY MEDICAL CENTER – NORTH IOWA, (Formerly North Iowa Mercy Health Center), 1000 Fourth Street S.W., Zip 50401–2800; tel. 515/422–7000; James J. Sexton, President and Chief Executive Officer (Total facility includes 30 beds in nursing home–type unit) **A**1 2 3 5 9 10 **F**1 3 4 7 8 9 11 13 14 16 17 18 19 20 21 22 23 24 25 26 27 30 31 32 33 34 35 36 37 38 39 40 41 42 43 44 45 46 47 48 49 50 51 54 56 57 58 59 60 61 62 63 64 65 67 69 70 71 72 73 75 76 78 79 **P**1 6 **S** Trinity Health, Novi, MI Web address: www.mercynorthiowa.com	21	10	255	12077	135	769174	1201	148736	68388	1987
MISSOURI VALLEY—Harrison County										
★ ALEGENT HEALTH COMMUNITY MEMORIAL HOSPITAL, 631 North Eighth Street, Zip 51555–1199; tel. 712/642–2784; James A. Seymour, Regional Administrator **A**9 10 **F**7 9 13 17 18 22 25 29 32 33 34 36 37 38 43 45 46 48 54 56 58 59 61 63 70 72 76 **P**8	23	10	27	605	7	21251	0	6193	2953	136
MOUNT AYR—Ringgold County										
RINGGOLD COUNTY HOSPITAL, 211 Shellway Drive, Zip 50854–1299; tel. 515/464–3226; Gordon W. Winkler, Administrator **A**10 **F**2 3 7 9 22 25 32 34 37 38 43 48 54 56 70 76 **P**6	13	10	36	582	10	16682	0	6253	3154	93
MOUNT PLEASANT—Henry County										
★ HENRY COUNTY HEALTH CENTER, 407 South White Street, Zip 52641–2299; tel. 319/385–3141; Robert Miller, Chief Executive Officer (Total facility includes 49 beds in nursing home–type unit) **A**10 **F**7 8 9 13 14 16 17 18 19 22 24 25 30 32 33 34 36 37 38 39 41 44 45 46 48 49 50 54 56 61 69 70 71 72 75 76 77 78 **P**7 8 Web address: www.webtex.net/hchc	13	10	99	1406	65	23958	167	15814	6991	260
MENTAL HEALTH INSTITUTE, 1200 East Washington Street, Zip 52641–1898; tel. 319/385–7231; Ken Burger, Superintendent **A**10 **F**2 23 57 **P**5	12	82	89	880	60	105	0	6752	3316	79
MUSCATINE—Muscatine County										
◧ UNITY HOSPITAL, (Formerly Muscatine General Hospital), 1518 Mulberry Avenue, Zip 52761–3499; tel. 319/264–9100; Karmon T. Bjella, Chief Executive Officer (Total facility includes 8 beds in nursing home–type unit) **A**1 10 **F**3 7 8 9 17 18 19 22 25 30 32 34 39 40 41 43 44 46 48 54 69 70 76 Web address: www.mgh.edu	23	10	66	2627	29	38330	460	23136	9429	357

A154 Hospitals — *Many Facility Codes have changed. Please refer to the AHA Guide Code Chart.* © 2000 AHA Guide

Hospitals, U.S. / IOWA

Hospital, Address, Telephone, Administrator, Approval, Facility, and Physician Codes, Health Care System, Network	Classification Codes		Utilization Data					Expense (thousands) of dollars		
★ American Hospital Association (AHA) membership □ Joint Commission on Accreditation of Healthcare Organizations (JCAHO) accreditation + American Osteopathic Healthcare Association (AOHA) membership ○ American Osteopathic Association (AOA) accreditation △ Commission on Accreditation of Rehabilitation Facilities (CARF) accreditation Control codes 61, 63, 64, 71, 72 and 73 indicate hospitals listed by AOHA, but not registered by AHA. For definition of numerical codes, see page A4	Control	Service	Staffed Beds	Admissions	Census	Outpatient Visits	Births	Total	Payroll	Personnel
NEVADA—Story County ★ STORY COUNTY HOSPITAL AND LONG TERM CARE FACILITY, 630 Sixth Street, Zip 50201–2266; tel. 515/382–2111; Todd Willert, Administrator (Total facility includes 73 beds in nursing home–type unit) **A**9 10 **F**7 13 14 17 19 22 23 25 28 30 32 33 34 38 40 43 45 48 54 56 69 70 71 72 75 76 77 78 **P**8	13	10	91	341	77	22577	0	7531	3015	142
NEW HAMPTON—Chickasaw County ✠ MERCY MEDICAL CENTER–NEW HAMPTON, (Formerly Saint Joseph Community Hospital), 308 North Maple Avenue, Zip 50659–1142; tel. 515/394–4121; Carolyn Martin–Shaw, President (Total facility includes 35 beds in nursing home–type unit) **A**1 9 10 **F**7 8 9 13 16 17 18 19 21 22 24 25 30 32 34 36 38 43 44 45 48 54 63 69 70 71 72 76 78 **P**1 **S** Trinity Health, Novi, MI **Web address:** www.mercynewhampton.com	21	10	58	831	41	16907	61	6822	3111	100
NEWTON—Jasper County ✠ SKIFF MEDICAL CENTER, 204 North Fourth Avenue East, Zip 50208–3100, Mailing Address: P.O. Box 1006, Zip 50208–1006; tel. 515/792–1273; Eric L. Lothe, President and Chief Executive Officer **A**1 9 10 **F**7 8 9 14 17 18 22 25 36 37 38 39 41 43 44 45 48 54 68 70 71 72 76 **Web address:** www.skiffmed.com	14	10	52	2391	26	64672	170	18779	9423	268
OAKDALE—Johnson County IOWA MEDICAL AND CLASSIFICATION CENTER, Highway 965, Zip 52319, Mailing Address: IMCC, Box A, Zip 52319; tel. 319/626–2391; Russell E. Rogerson, Warden **F**2 4 5 8 9 10 11 12 22 23 24 26 27 31 33 34 35 39 41 43 44 46 47 48 49 50 51 53 55 56 57 59 60 61 62 63 65 68 69 70 72 74 75 76 77 79 **P**6	48	22	23	148	18	0	0	138697	115353	28
OELWEIN—Fayette County ✠ MERCY HOSPITAL OF FRANCISCAN SISTERS, 201 Eighth Avenue S.E., Zip 50662–2447; tel. 319/283–6000; Richard Schrupp, President and Chief Executive Officer (Total facility includes 39 beds in nursing home–type unit) **A**1 9 10 **F**3 7 8 9 11 17 22 24 25 30 31 32 33 34 36 37 38 39 40 41 43 44 45 46 48 50 51 56 68 69 70 71 72 75 76 78 **P**6 **S** Wheaton Franciscan Services, Inc., Wheaton, IL	21	10	64	1196	49	30264	29	9614	4616	167
ONAWA—Monona County ✠ BURGESS HEALTH CENTER, 1600 Diamond Street, Zip 51040–1548; tel. 712/423–2311; Francis Tramp, President **A**1 9 10 **F**7 8 9 16 17 18 19 22 25 28 32 34 36 37 38 39 43 44 46 48 49 54 56 63 70 71 76 78 **P**6	23	10	48	1297	18	43795	85	12182	5872	181
ORANGE CITY—Sioux County ★ ORANGE CITY HEALTH SYSTEM, (Formerly Orange City Hospital and Clinic), 400 Central Avenue N.W., Zip 51041–1398; tel. 712/737–4984; Martin W. Guthmiller, Administrator and Chief Executive Officer (Total facility includes 83 beds in nursing home–type unit) **A**9 10 **F**6 7 8 9 14 16 17 18 19 21 22 23 24 25 26 33 34 36 37 38 39 40 41 43 44 45 46 48 50 51 63 67 69 70 71 72 76 78 79 **P**6 **S** Sioux Valley Hospitals and Health System, Sioux Falls, SD	14	10	113	1097	99	51604	169	13486	5754	277
OSAGE—Mitchell County ★ MITCHELL COUNTY REGIONAL HEALTH CENTER, 616 North Eighth Street, Zip 50461–1498; tel. 515/732–6005; Kimberly J. Miller, CHE, Administrator and Chief Executive Officer **A**9 10 **F**7 8 9 12 16 17 18 21 22 25 26 32 33 34 36 37 38 39 43 44 45 46 48 54 70 72 75 76 78 **P**1 **S** Trinity Health, Novi, MI	13	10	28	777	7	53417	47	7966	2305	94
OSCEOLA—Clarke County ★ CLARKE COUNTY HOSPITAL, 800 South Fillmore Street, Zip 50213; tel. 515/342–2184; David M. Coates, Ph.D., Chief Executive Officer **A**9 10 **F**7 9 17 18 22 24 25 26 28 34 37 40 41 45 46 48 51 54 56 76 **S** Iowa Health System, Des Moines, IA **Web address:** www.clarkehosp.org	13	10	48	727	37	15074	0	5324	2221	109
OSKALOOSA—Mahaska County ✠ MAHASKA COUNTY HOSPITAL, 1229 C Avenue East, Zip 52577–4298; tel. 515/672–3100; Jay Christensen, Administrator **A**1 9 10 **F**3 7 8 9 12 13 14 16 17 18 19 22 24 25 26 29 30 32 33 34 35 36 37 38 39 40 41 43 44 45 46 48 49 50 51 54 56 58 59 60 61 62 63 64 69 70 71 72 73 76 77 78 79 **P**7	13	10	53	1495	17	64542	213	13051	5755	197
OTTUMWA—Wapello County ✠ OTTUMWA REGIONAL HEALTH CENTER, 1001 Pennsylvania Avenue, Zip 52501–2186; tel. 515/684–2300; Lynn W. Olson, President (Total facility includes 12 beds in nursing home–type unit) **A**1 2 9 10 **F**2 3 7 8 9 13 16 17 18 19 22 24 25 26 27 28 30 31 32 33 34 36 37 38 39 40 41 42 43 44 45 46 48 49 50 51 54 57 58 59 60 61 62 63 64 65 67 68 69 70 71 72 76 78 79 **P**6 8 **Web address:** www.orhc.com	23	10	87	5645	74	129157	763	48812	21653	743
PELLA—Marion County ✠ PELLA REGIONAL HEALTH CENTER, 404 Jefferson Street, Zip 50219–1257; tel. 515/628–3150; Robert D. Kroese, Chief Executive Officer (Total facility includes 109 beds in nursing home–type unit) **A**1 9 10 **F**1 8 9 12 16 17 18 22 25 27 33 34 36 37 38 39 43 45 46 48 49 50 51 54 68 69 70 71 72 76 78 **P**5 6	23	10	156	1943	136	100040	325	20669	9738	515
PERRY—Dallas County ★ DALLAS COUNTY HOSPITAL, 610 10th Street, Zip 50220–2221, Mailing Address: P.O. Box 608, Zip 50220–0608; tel. 515/465–3547; Kari L. Engholm, Administrator and Chief Executive Officer **A**9 10 **F**7 9 17 18 19 20 22 24 25 26 30 32 34 37 38 43 46 48 53 54 66 69 76 77 **P**6 **S** Iowa Health System, Des Moines, IA **Web address:** www.perryia.org/Healthcare/health.htm	13	10	33	582	10	15726	0	8074	2808	105

© 2000 AHA Guide *Many Facility Codes have changed. Please refer to the AHA Guide Code Chart.*

Hospitals, U.S. / IOWA

Hospital, Address, Telephone, Administrator, Approval, Facility, and Physician Codes, Health Care System, Network	Classification Codes		Utilization Data					Expense (thousands) of dollars		Personnel
★ American Hospital Association (AHA) membership □ Joint Commission on Accreditation of Healthcare Organizations (JCAHO) accreditation + American Osteopathic Healthcare Association (AOHA) membership ○ American Osteopathic Association (AOA) accreditation △ Commission on Accreditation of Rehabilitation Facilities (CARF) accreditation Control codes 61, 63, 64, 71, 72 and 73 indicate hospitals listed by AOHA, but not registered by AHA. For definition of numerical codes, see page A4	Control	Service	Staffed Beds	Admissions	Census	Outpatient Visits	Births	Total	Payroll	
POCAHONTAS—Pocahontas County ★ POCAHONTAS COMMUNITY HOSPITAL, 606 N.W. Seventh, Zip 50574–1099; tel. 712/335–3501 **A**9 10 **F**7 9 22 25 26 32 34 36 37 38 39 41 45 46 48 54 69 70 72 76 **S** Iowa Health System, Des Moines, IA	14	10	25	314	6	23070	0	3379	1534	68
PRIMGHAR—Obrien County ★ BAUM HARMON MERCY HOSPITAL, (Formerly Baum Harmon Memorial Hospital), 255 North Welch Avenue, Zip 51245–1034, Mailing Address: P.O. Box 528, Zip 51245–0528; tel. 712/757–2300; Trudy Pfeiffer, Administrator **A**9 10 18 **F**7 9 13 17 22 25 26 28 32 34 36 37 38 39 40 41 45 46 48 54 69 70 71 72 76 **P**6 8 **S** Trinity Health, Novi, MI	14	10	16	226	3	6923	0	2353	842	43
RED OAK—Montgomery County ★ MONTGOMERY COUNTY MEMORIAL HOSPITAL, 2301 Eastern Avenue, Zip 51566–1300, Mailing Address: P.O. Box 498, Zip 51566–0498; tel. 712/623–7000; Allen E. Pohren, Administrator **A**9 10 **F**7 8 9 13 16 17 19 22 25 27 28 32 33 34 36 37 38 39 40 41 43 44 45 46 48 51 54 63 68 70 75 76 78 79 **P**6 **Web address:** www.mcmh.org	13	10	40	1722	26	43999	96	15661	6901	222
ROCK RAPIDS—Lyon County ★ MERRILL PIONEER COMMUNITY HOSPITAL, 801 South Greene Street, Zip 51246–1998; tel. 712/472–2591; Gordon Smith, Administrator and Chief Executive Officer **A**9 10 **F**7 8 9 17 22 25 28 32 34 36 37 39 44 45 48 54 69 76 **P**6 **S** Sioux Valley Hospitals and Health System, Sioux Falls, SD	23	10	16	413	5	7929	37	2687	1160	49
ROCK VALLEY—Sioux County ★ HEGG MEMORIAL HEALTH CENTER/AVERA HEALTH, 1202 21st Avenue, Zip 51247–1497; tel. 712/476–8000; Vern Carda, Administrator (Total facility includes 95 beds in nursing home–type unit) **A**9 10 **F**7 8 9 16 17 18 19 22 25 26 28 30 32 33 34 36 37 38 39 40 41 43 44 45 46 48 50 54 64 67 69 70 71 72 76 78 **P**4 5 7 **S** Avera Health, Yankton, SD	23	10	123	368	90	22370	42	5311	2801	—
SAC CITY—Sac County ★ LORING HOSPITAL, 211 Highland Avenue, Zip 50583–0217, Mailing Address: P.O. Box 217, Zip 50583–0217; tel. 712/662–7105; Greg Miner, Administrator (Total facility includes 21 beds in nursing home–type unit) **A**9 10 **F**5 12 13 14 16 17 18 19 22 25 26 30 32 33 34 37 38 39 43 44 45 46 48 50 51 54 61 63 67 69 70 71 72 74 75 76 78 **P**7 **S** Iowa Health System, Des Moines, IA	23	10	54	845	28	10529	2	5342	2650	108
SHELDON—Obrien County ★ NORTHWEST IOWA HEALTH CENTER, 118 North Seventh Avenue, Zip 51201–1235, Mailing Address: P.O. Box 250, Zip 51201–0250; tel. 712/324–5041; Charles R. Miller, Chief Executive Officer (Total facility includes 103 beds in nursing home–type unit) **A**9 10 **F**9 13 16 17 18 19 22 25 28 30 32 34 36 37 38 39 40 43 45 46 48 50 51 54 69 70 71 72 76 78 **P**5 6 **S** Sioux Valley Hospitals and Health System, Sioux Falls, SD	23	10	127	918	79	19709	101	11434	5758	218
SHENANDOAH—Page County ★ SHENANDOAH MEDICAL CENTER, (Formerly Shenandoah Memorial Hospital), 300 Pershing Avenue, Zip 51601–2397; tel. 712/246–1230; Charles L. Millburg, CHE, Chief Executive Officer (Total facility includes 59 beds in nursing home–type unit) **A**9 10 **F**6 7 8 9 16 17 18 22 24 25 29 31 32 34 36 38 39 40 41 43 44 45 46 48 51 54 57 62 65 69 70 72 75 76 78 **P**1 7 **Web address:** www.shenandoahmedcenter.com	23	10	90	856	48	14247	90	11142	4836	203
SIBLEY—Osceola County ★ OSCEOLA COMMUNITY HOSPITAL, Ninth Avenue North, Zip 51249–0258, Mailing Address: P.O. Box 258, Zip 51249–0258; tel. 712/754–2574; Janet Dykstra, Administrator **A**9 10 **F**8 9 12 14 16 17 18 19 22 23 25 30 31 32 33 34 35 36 37 38 39 40 43 44 45 46 48 50 51 54 56 58 59 60 61 62 63 65 67 69 70 71 72 73 74 76 78 79 **P**5 **S** Avera Health, Yankton, SD	23	10	32	492	6	16777	87	4216	1752	75
SIGOURNEY—Keokuk County KEOKUK COUNTY HEALTH CENTER, 1312 South Stuart Street, Zip 52591–0286, Mailing Address: P.O. Box 286, Zip 52591–0286; tel. 515/622–2720; Michael D. Trachta, Chief Executive Officer **A**9 10 **F**16 18 24 25 26 37 38 45 50 51 54 70 76	13	10	25	114	6	6987	0	2110	1034	40
SIOUX CENTER—Sioux County SIOUX CENTER COMMUNITY HOSPITAL AND HEALTH CENTER/AVERA HEALTH, 605 South Main Avenue, Zip 51250–1398; tel. 712/722–1271; Marla Toering, Administrator (Total facility includes 69 beds in nursing home–type unit) **A**9 10 **F**6 7 8 9 12 13 14 16 17 19 22 25 26 30 33 34 36 37 38 39 43 44 45 48 49 50 51 54 63 67 69 70 71 72 76 78 79 **S** Avera Health, Yankton, SD	23	10	90	477	75	32633	196	9627	3823	185
SIOUX CITY—Woodbury County ★ △ MERCY MEDICAL CENTER–SIOUX CITY, (Formerly Marian Health Center), (Includes Mercy Behavioral Health Center, 4301 Sergeant Road, Zip 51106; tel. 712/279–2446), 801 Fifth Street, Zip 51102, Mailing Address: P.O. Box 3168, Zip 51102–3168; tel. 712/279–2010; Deborah VandenBroek, President and Chief Executive Officer (Total facility includes 20 beds in nursing home–type unit) **A**1 2 3 5 7 9 10 **F**3 4 6 7 8 9 11 12 13 14 16 17 18 19 22 24 25 27 30 31 32 33 34 35 36 37 38 39 40 41 43 45 46 47 48 49 50 51 53 54 56 57 58 59 60 61 62 63 64 65 68 69 70 72 75 76 77 78 **P**5 6 8 **S** Trinity Health, Novi, MI **Web address:** www.mercysiouxcity.com	21	10	284	11637	164	310313	773	140680	59964	1721

Hospitals, U.S. / IOWA

Hospital, Address, Telephone, Administrator, Approval, Facility, and Physician Codes, Health Care System, Network	Classification Codes		Utilization Data					Expense (thousands) of dollars		
★ American Hospital Association (AHA) membership □ Joint Commission on Accreditation of Healthcare Organizations (JCAHO) accreditation + American Osteopathic Healthcare Association (AOHA) membership ○ American Osteopathic Association (AOA) accreditation △ Commission on Accreditation of Rehabilitation Facilities (CARF) accreditation Control codes 61, 63, 64, 71, 72 and 73 indicate hospitals listed by AOHA, but not registered by AHA. For definition of numerical codes, see page A4	Control	Service	Staffed Beds	Admissions	Census	Outpatient Visits	Births	Total	Payroll	Personnel
✣ ST. LUKE'S REGIONAL MEDICAL CENTER, 2720 Stone Park Boulevard, Zip 51104–2000; tel. 712/279–3500; John D. Daniels, President and Chief Executive Officer **A**1 2 3 5 6 9 10 **F**4 6 7 8 9 10 11 13 14 16 17 18 19 22 23 24 25 27 31 32 33 34 36 37 39 40 41 42 43 44 45 46 48 50 52 54 56 57 61 64 66 67 69 70 72 74 76 77 78 79 **P**1 6 **S** Iowa Health System, Des Moines, IA **Web address:** www.siouxlan.com/stlukes	23	10	193	11049	133	102785	1813	84457	34946	1091
SPENCER—Clay County ★ SPENCER MUNICIPAL HOSPITAL, 1200 First Avenue East, Zip 51301–4321; tel. 712/264–6111; John Allen, President and Chief Executive Officer (Total facility includes 14 beds in nursing home–type unit) **A**9 10 **F**7 8 9 13 16 17 18 19 22 23 24 25 30 31 32 34 36 37 38 39 40 41 43 44 45 46 48 50 51 54 57 59 60 61 62 64 65 68 69 70 71 72 75 76 78 **S** Sioux Valley Hospitals and Health System, Sioux Falls, SD	14	10	85	2878	35	28554	244	24788	10930	379
SPIRIT LAKE—Dickinson County □ DICKINSON COUNTY MEMORIAL HOSPITAL, Highway 71 South, Zip 51360, Mailing Address: P.O. Box AB, Zip 51360; tel. 712/336–1230; Richard C. Kielman, President and Chief Executive Officer **A**1 9 10 **F**7 8 9 17 18 19 22 25 29 31 32 34 36 37 38 39 40 41 43 44 45 46 48 70 71 72 76 78	13	10	49	1554	18	32721	161	13153	5397	195
STORM LAKE—Buena Vista County ✣ BUENA VISTA COUNTY HOSPITAL, 1525 West Fifth Street, Zip 50588–0309, Mailing Address: P.O. Box 309, Zip 50588–0309; tel. 712/732–4030; James J. Sinek, Chief Executive Officer **A**1 9 10 **F**1 3 7 8 9 12 13 16 17 18 22 24 25 26 28 31 34 36 37 38 39 40 43 44 45 46 48 54 70 72 76 78 **S** Iowa Health System, Des Moines, IA	13	10	30	1585	17	60345	290	15332	6822	252
SUMNER—Bremer County COMMUNITY MEMORIAL HOSPITAL, 909 West First Street, Zip 50674–1203, Mailing Address: P.O. Box 148, Zip 50674–0148; tel. 319/578–3275; Mary Wells, Administrator **A**9 10 **F**3 8 9 16 17 18 22 25 34 36 37 38 39 40 43 45 48 54 70 76 78	23	10	13	492	5	13518	13	3826	1468	59
VINTON—Benton County ★ VIRGINIA GAY HOSPITAL, 502 North Ninth Avenue, Zip 52349–2299; tel. 319/472–6200; Michael J. Riege, Chief Executive Officer (Total facility includes 58 beds in nursing home–type unit) **A**9 10 **F**16 17 18 22 23 25 31 36 37 38 48 54 67 69 70 71 75 76 **P**6	23	10	87	521	64	58974	0	8025	3555	155
WASHINGTON—Washington County ★ WASHINGTON COUNTY HOSPITAL, 400 East Polk Street, Zip 52353–0909, Mailing Address: P.O. Box 909, Zip 52353–0909; tel. 319/653–5481; Donald E. Patterson, Chief Executive Officer (Total facility includes 43 beds in nursing home–type unit) **A**9 10 **F**8 9 14 22 25 32 34 36 37 39 40 41 44 45 48 50 54 69 70 76 78 **S** Quorum Health Group, Brentwood, TN **Web address:** www.wchc.org	13	10	91	1842	57	35426	111	10955	4776	179
WATERLOO—Black Hawk County ✣ ALLEN MEMORIAL HOSPITAL, 1825 Logan Avenue, Zip 50703–1916; tel. 319/235–3987; Richard A. Seidler, FACHE, Chief Executive Officer (Total facility includes 30 beds in nursing home–type unit) **A**1 3 5 6 9 10 **F**3 4 7 8 9 11 12 13 16 17 18 19 20 22 23 25 27 28 29 30 31 33 34 35 36 37 38 39 40 41 43 44 45 46 47 48 49 50 51 52 53 54 55 56 57 58 59 60 61 62 63 64 66 67 69 70 72 73 75 76 77 78 79 **P**1 3 6 **S** Iowa Health System, Des Moines, IA	23	10	202	9429	124	209440	870	84274	36483	1108
✣ △ COVENANT MEDICAL CENTER, (Includes Kimball–Ridge Center, 2101 Kimball Avenue, Zip 50702), 3421 West Ninth Street, Zip 50702–5499; tel. 319/272–8000; Raymond F. Burfeind, President (Total facility includes 44 beds in nursing home–type unit) **A**1 2 3 5 7 9 10 **F**2 3 4 6 7 8 9 11 13 17 18 19 20 21 22 23 24 25 27 28 31 32 33 34 35 36 37 38 39 41 42 43 44 45 46 48 49 50 53 54 56 57 58 59 60 61 62 63 64 65 68 69 70 71 72 73 75 76 77 78 79 **P**6 **S** Wheaton Franciscan Services, Inc., Wheaton, IL **Web address:** www.covhealth.com KIMBALL–RIDGE CENTER See Covenant Medical Center	21	10	283	11207	168	578055	1411	136291	68097	1852
WAUKON—Allamakee County VETERANS MEMORIAL HOSPITAL, 40 First Street S.E., Zip 52172–2099; tel. 319/568–3411; Michael D. Myers, Administrator **A**9 10 **F**3 7 8 9 16 17 18 19 22 25 28 32 33 34 36 37 38 39 43 44 45 46 48 54 63 70 71 72 73 76 77	14	10	25	724	7	36996	70	5327	2410	151
WAVERLY—Bremer County ✣ WAVERLY MUNICIPAL HOSPITAL, 312 Ninth Street S.W., Zip 50677–2999; tel. 319/352–4120; Arnold Flessner, Administrator **A**1 9 10 **F**7 8 9 16 17 18 22 25 28 32 34 36 38 39 43 45 48 54 69 70 72 76 78 **P**6	14	10	38	1039	10	23781	88	10406	4317	141
WEBSTER CITY—Hamilton County □ HAMILTON COUNTY PUBLIC HOSPITAL, 800 Ohio Street, Zip 50595–2824, Mailing Address: P.O. Box 430, Zip 50595–0430; tel. 515/832–9400; Roger W. Lenz, Administrator **A**1 9 10 **F**7 8 9 17 18 22 25 32 34 36 40 43 44 45 48 54 70 72 75 76 78 **Web address:** www.hamiltonhospital.com	13	10	40	2026	21	14086	153	11462	5256	189
WEST BURLINGTON—Monona County BURLINGTON MEDICAL CENTER See Great River Medical Center ✣ GREAT RIVER MEDICAL CENTER, (Formerly Burlington Medical Center), 1221 South Gear Avenue, Zip 52655; tel. 319/768–1000; Mark D. Richardson, President and Chief Executive Officer (Total facility includes 167 beds in nursing home–type unit) **A**1 9 10 **F**3 4 7 9 11 13 14 16 17 18 19 20 22 24 25 27 28 32 33 34 36 38 39 40 41 42 43 44 45 46 48 50 51 53 54 55 57 58 59 60 61 62 63 65 68 69 70 71 72 75 76 78	23	10	366	8393	247	192500	721	67076	28553	1031

© 2000 AHA Guide   *Many Facility Codes have changed. Please refer to the AHA Guide Code Chart.*

Hospitals, U.S. / IOWA

Hospital, Address, Telephone, Administrator, Approval, Facility, and Physician Codes, Health Care System, Network	Classification Codes		Utilization Data					Expense (thousands) of dollars		Personnel
	Control	Service	Staffed Beds	Admissions	Census	Outpatient Visits	Births	Total	Payroll	

★ American Hospital Association (AHA) membership
☐ Joint Commission on Accreditation of Healthcare Organizations (JCAHO) accreditation
+ American Osteopathic Healthcare Association (AOHA) membership
○ American Osteopathic Association (AOA) accreditation
△ Commission on Accreditation of Rehabilitation Facilities (CARF) accreditation
Control codes 61, 63, 64, 71, 72 and 73 indicate hospitals listed by AOHA, but not registered by AHA. For definition of numerical codes, see page A4

Hospital	Control	Service	Staffed Beds	Admissions	Census	Outpatient Visits	Births	Total	Payroll	Personnel
WEST UNION—Fayette County ★ PALMER LUTHERAN HEALTH CENTER, 112 Jefferson Street, Zip 52175-1022; tel. 319/422-3811; Debrah Chensvold, President **A**9 10 **F**2 8 9 10 12 18 19 22 25 30 32 33 34 35 36 37 38 39 41 42 44 45 46 48 52 53 54 57 62 63 69 70 71 72 76 77 78	23	10	30	814	11	63371	93	8281	3679	137
WINTERSET—Madison County MADISON COUNTY MEMORIAL HOSPITAL, 300 Hutchings Street, Zip 50273-2199; tel. 515/462-2373; Jill Kordick, Administrator **A**9 10 **F**3 9 13 17 18 19 22 25 30 34 35 36 37 38 39 41 43 46 48 49 50 54 56 58 59 60 61 62 63 64 70 71 72 73 76 78	13	10	31	736	12	32902	0	8928	3869	137
WOODWARD—Boone County WOODWARD STATE HOSPITAL-SCHOOL, Zip 50276-9999; tel. 515/438-2600; Michael J. Davis, Ph.D., Superintendent **F**4 5 9 10 11 12 22 23 24 25 27 35 39 41 46 47 48 52 55 57 58 59 60 61 62 63 65 68 75 76	12	62	287	21	278	0	0	30975	21065	685

Hospitals, U.S. / KANSAS

KANSAS

Resident Population 2,629 (in thousands)
Resident population in metro areas 55.4%
Birth rate per 1,000 population 14.4
65 years and over 13.5%
Percent of persons without health insurance 11.7%

Hospital, Address, Telephone, Administrator, Approval, Facility, and Physician Codes, Health Care System, Network	Classification Codes		Utilization Data					Expense (thousands) of dollars		
★ American Hospital Association (AHA) membership □ Joint Commission on Accreditation of Healthcare Organizations (JCAHO) accreditation + American Osteopathic Healthcare Association (AOHA) membership ○ American Osteopathic Association (AOA) accreditation △ Commission on Accreditation of Rehabilitation Facilities (CARF) accreditation Control codes 61, 63, 64, 71, 72 and 73 indicate hospitals listed by AOHA, but not registered by AHA. For definition of numerical codes, see page A4	Control	Service	Staffed Beds	Admissions	Census	Outpatient Visits	Births	Total	Payroll	Personnel
ABILENE—Dickinson County ★ MEMORIAL HOSPITAL, 511 N.E. Tenth Street, Zip 67410–2100, Mailing Address: P.O. Box 69, Zip 67410–0069; tel. 785/263–2100; Leon J. Boor, Chief Executive Officer and Administrator **A**9 10 **F**8 12 17 18 22 24 25 28 32 34 36 37 38 40 43 44 45 46 48 54 57 62 70 71 72 76 78 **P**8	16	10	57	1015	17	14692	65	7694	3733	164
ANTHONY—Harper County ★ HOSPITAL DISTRICT NUMBER SIX OF HARPER COUNTY, 1101 East Spring Street, Zip 67003–2122; tel. 316/842–5111; Cindy M. McCray, Administrator and Chief Executive Officer **A**9 10 **F**9 17 22 25 46 48 56 66 69 70 76 **P**6	16	10	30	253	20	19884	0	3551	1951	66
ARKANSAS CITY—Cowley County ★ SOUTH CENTRAL KANSAS REGIONAL MEDICAL CENTER, 216 West Birch Avenue, Zip 67005–1598, Mailing Address: P.O. Box 1107, Zip 67005–1107; tel. 316/442–2500; Webster T. Russell, Chief Executive Officer (Total facility includes 5 beds in nursing home–type unit) **A**9 10 **F**8 9 13 16 17 18 22 25 33 34 36 38 39 40 41 43 44 45 46 48 51 54 56 68 69 70 76 78 **P**8 Web address: www.sckrmc.com	14	10	50	1469	17	69331	168	9254	4058	144
ASHLAND—Clark County ★ ASHLAND HEALTH CENTER, 709 Oak Street, Zip 67831–0188, Mailing Address: P.O. Box 188, Zip 67831–0188; tel. 316/635–2241; Bryan Stacey, Administrator (Total facility includes 36 beds in nursing home–type unit) **A**9 10 18 **F**1 9 23 25 26 28 31 33 34 36 38 45 48 51 54 59 61 63 69 70 76 **S** Great Plains Health Alliance, Inc., Phillipsburg, KS Web address: www.phn.org	16	10	48	90	26	5259	0	2581	1235	60
ATCHISON—Atchison County ✠ ATCHISON HOSPITAL, 1301 North Second Street, Zip 66002–1297; tel. 913/367–2131; W. David Drew, President and Chief Executive Officer (Total facility includes 37 beds in nursing home–type unit) **A**1 9 10 **F**7 8 9 13 16 17 18 22 24 25 27 30 31 32 36 37 38 39 41 44 45 48 51 53 54 56 57 59 62 69 70 71 72 76 78 **P**6	23	10	77	1954	50	33423	188	17373	9345	275
ATWOOD—Rawlins County RAWLINS COUNTY HEALTH CENTER, 707 Grant Street, Zip 67730–4700, Mailing Address: P.O. Box 47, Zip 67730–4700; tel. 785/626–3211; Donald J. Kessen, Administrator and Chief Executive Officer **A**9 10 18 **F**3 9 16 17 18 19 21 22 25 30 31 34 38 39 43 46 48 54 67 68 70 76 78 **P**6 **S** Great Plains Health Alliance, Inc., Phillipsburg, KS Web address: www.gpha.com	13	10	24	343	3	7143	0	3131	1595	55
AUGUSTA—Butler County AUGUSTA MEDICAL COMPLEX, 2101 Dearborn Street, Zip 67010–0430, Mailing Address: P.O. Box 430, Zip 67010–0430; tel. 316/775–5421; Larry D. Wilkerson, Chief Executive Officer (Total facility includes 100 beds in nursing home–type unit) **A**9 10 **F**2 3 7 9 18 22 24 25 36 48 49 54 67 69 76	23	10	140	346	69	3777	0	6804	3555	146
BELLEVILLE—Republic County ✠ REPUBLIC COUNTY HOSPITAL, 2420 G Street, Zip 66935–2400; tel. 785/527–2254; Blaine K. Miller, Administrator (Total facility includes 38 beds in nursing home–type unit) **A**1 9 10 **F**8 9 13 16 17 19 22 23 24 25 30 32 37 38 43 45 46 48 50 51 54 69 70 71 76 **S** Great Plains Health Alliance, Inc., Phillipsburg, KS Web address: www.gpha.com	23	10	86	1171	51	9276	62	6826	3087	134
BELOIT—Mitchell County ★ MITCHELL COUNTY HOSPITAL, 400 West Eighth, Zip 67420–1605, Mailing Address: P.O. Box 399, Zip 67420–0399; tel. 785/738–2266; John M. Osse, Administrator (Total facility includes 40 beds in nursing home–type unit) **A**9 10 **F**7 8 9 13 19 22 23 25 30 36 37 38 39 40 45 46 48 50 54 69 70 72 76 **S** Great Plains Health Alliance, Inc., Phillipsburg, KS Web address: www.gpha.com	23	10	89	1678	59	13803	78	10175	4948	185
BURLINGTON—Coffey County ★ COFFEY COUNTY HOSPITAL, 801 North Fourth Street, Zip 66839–0189, Mailing Address: P.O. Box 189, Zip 66839–0189; tel. 316/364–2121; Dennis L. George, Chief Executive Officer (Total facility includes 42 beds in nursing home–type unit) **A**9 10 **F**8 9 12 17 22 25 29 32 34 36 38 39 41 43 44 45 48 54 67 69 70 76 78 **P**6	13	10	64	873	45	11620	47	10608	5388	183
CALDWELL—Sumner County SUMNER COUNTY HOSPITAL DISTRICT ONE, 601 South Osage Street, Zip 67022–1654; tel. 316/845–6492; Virgil Watson, Administrator **A**9 10 **F**9 17 22 25 32 34 36 37 39 46 48 56 69 70 76 78	16	10	27	223	3	7242	0	1938	947	41
CEDAR VALE—Chautauqua County CEDAR VALE COMMUNITY HOSPITAL, 501 Cedar Street, Zip 67024–0398, Mailing Address: P.O. Box 398, Zip 67024–0398; tel. 316/758–2266; William A. Lybarger, Ph.D., Administrator **A**9 10 18 **F**17 25 31 56 69 **P**5 Web address: www.gpha.com	23	10	25	247	20	4145	0	1167	1087	52

© 2000 AHA Guide   *Many Facility Codes have changed. Please refer to the AHA Guide Code Chart.*

Hospitals, U.S. / KANSAS

Hospital, Address, Telephone, Administrator, Approval, Facility, and Physician Codes, Health Care System, Network	Classification Codes		Utilization Data					Expense (thousands) of dollars		Personnel
	Control	Service	Staffed Beds	Admissions	Census	Outpatient Visits	Births	Total	Payroll	

★ American Hospital Association (AHA) membership
□ Joint Commission on Accreditation of Healthcare Organizations (JCAHO) accreditation
+ American Osteopathic Healthcare Association (AOHA) membership
○ American Osteopathic Association (AOA) accreditation
△ Commission on Accreditation of Rehabilitation Facilities (CARF) accreditation
Control codes 61, 63, 64, 71, 72 and 73 indicate hospitals listed by AOHA, but not registered by AHA. For definition of numerical codes, see page A4

Hospital	Control	Service	Staffed Beds	Admissions	Census	Outpatient Visits	Births	Total	Payroll	Personnel
CHANUTE—Neosho County ✠ NEOSHO MEMORIAL REGIONAL MEDICAL CENTER, 629 South Plummer, Zip 66720-0426, Mailing Address: P.O. Box 426, Zip 66720-0426; tel. 316/431-4000; Murray L. Brown, Administrator **A**1 9 10 **F**7 8 9 13 17 22 25 26 27 31 36 37 39 41 44 45 48 54 69 70 76 78 **P**8 **S** Quorum Health Group, Brentwood, TN	13	10	60	2471	26	16869	280	14664	6085	223
CLAY CENTER—Clay County ★ CLAY COUNTY MEDICAL CENTER, (Formerly Clay County Hospital), 617 Liberty Street, Zip 67432-0512, Mailing Address: P.O. Box 512, Zip 67432-0512; tel. 785/632-2144; Ronald Bender, Chief Executive Officer **A**9 10 **F**9 17 18 22 25 28 32 37 39 43 48 50 51 54 70 72 76 **P**8	13	10	32	787	11	24590	60	6614	3003	125
COFFEYVILLE—Montgomery County ✠ COFFEYVILLE REGIONAL MEDICAL CENTER, 1400 West Fourth, Zip 67337-0856; tel. 316/251-1200; Gerald J. Marquette, Jr, Chief Executive Officer (Total facility includes 29 beds in nursing home-type unit) **A**1 2 9 10 **F**7 8 9 16 17 22 24 25 30 31 32 34 36 39 41 44 45 46 48 54 57 58 62 65 69 70 76 78 79 **P**3 8 **S** Quorum Health Group, Brentwood, TN	23	10	116	3900	71	23780	250	24307	10637	379
COLBY—Thomas County CITIZENS MEDICAL CENTER, 100 East College Drive, Zip 67701-3799; tel. 785/462-7511; Michael E. Boyles, Chief Executive Officer (Total facility includes 80 beds in nursing home-type unit) **A**9 10 **F**7 8 9 12 16 17 22 24 25 33 36 38 39 40 41 44 45 46 48 50 51 54 56 69 70 72 76 78 Web address: www.nwkshealthcare.com	23	10	120	1270	78	11225	163	10657	4435	182
COLDWATER—Comanche County COMANCHE COUNTY HOSPITAL, Second and Frisco Streets, Zip 67029, Mailing Address: HC 65, Box 8A, Zip 67029; tel. 316/582-2144; Nancy Zimmerman, R.N., Administrator **A**9 10 18 **F**7 9 17 22 23 25 28 34 35 36 37 40 43 45 46 48 54 61 69 71 76 **P**6 **S** Great Plains Health Alliance, Inc., Phillipsburg, KS Web address: www.gpha.com	13	10	14	135	2	3684	0	1944	1008	39
COLUMBUS—Cherokee County ST. JOHN'S MAUDE NORTON MEMORIAL HOSPITAL, (Formerly Maude Norton Memorial City Hospital), 220 North Pennsylvania Street, Zip 66725-1110; tel. 316/429-2545; Cindy Neely, Administrator **A**9 10 18 **F**9 16 17 18 22 25 32 33 34 40 45 48 54 76 78	23	10	20	182	9	8946	0	1832	—	41
CONCORDIA—Cloud County CLOUD COUNTY HEALTH CENTER, 1100 Highland Drive, Zip 66901-3923; tel. 785/243-1234; Daniel R. Bartz, Chief Executive Officer (Total facility includes 9 beds in nursing home-type unit) **A**9 10 **F**7 8 9 17 19 22 24 25 27 30 31 32 37 38 39 40 41 43 44 45 48 49 50 51 54 56 58 59 60 61 62 63 69 70 72 75 76 78 **P**8	23	10	40	1254	16	19584	41	8687	3808	153
COUNCIL GROVE—Morris County MORRIS COUNTY HOSPITAL, 600 North Washington Street, Zip 66846-0275, Mailing Address: P.O. Box 275, Zip 66846-0275; tel. 316/767-6811; James H. Reagan, Jr, Ph.D., Chief Executive Officer **A**9 10 **F**7 8 9 16 17 18 19 22 25 29 32 34 36 37 38 39 41 43 44 45 46 48 51 54 70 72 76 78	13	10	28	876	11	13789	63	4545	2155	90
DIGHTON—Lane County ★ LANE COUNTY HOSPITAL, 243 South Second, Zip 67839-0969, Mailing Address: P.O. Box 969, Zip 67839-0969; tel. 316/397-5321; Donna McGowan, Administrator (Total facility includes 21 beds in nursing home-type unit) **A**9 10 18 **F**1 22 25 30 32 36 54 56 69 70 71 76 **P**6 **S** Great Plains Health Alliance, Inc., Phillipsburg, KS Web address: www.gpha.com	13	10	31	229	24	5342	0	2289	1260	47
DODGE CITY—Ford County ✠ WESTERN PLAINS MEDICAL COMPLEX, (Formerly Western Plains Regional Hospital), 3001 Avenue A, Zip 67801-6508, Mailing Address: P.O. Box 1478, Zip 67801-1478; tel. 316/225-8400; Ken Hutchenrider, President and Chief Executive Officer (Total facility includes 9 beds in nursing home-type unit) **A**1 9 10 **F**7 8 9 12 13 16 17 18 19 21 22 23 24 25 27 32 36 37 39 41 43 44 45 46 48 50 52 53 54 65 68 69 70 71 75 76 78 79 **S** LifePoint Hospitals, Inc., Brentwood, TN	33	10	99	3879	45	28394	781	—	—	261
EL DORADO—Butler County ✠ SUSAN B. ALLEN MEMORIAL HOSPITAL, 720 West Central Avenue, Zip 67042-2112; tel. 316/321-3300; Jim Wilson, President and Chief Executive Officer (Total facility includes 21 beds in nursing home-type unit) **A**1 9 10 **F**7 8 9 22 24 25 32 34 36 39 40 41 44 48 57 62 69 70 76 78 **P**8 Web address: www.sbamh.com	23	10	82	1964	33	46685	166	19418	9771	273
ELKHART—Morton County ★ MORTON COUNTY HEALTH SYSTEM, 445 Hilltop Street, Zip 67950-0937, Mailing Address: P.O. Box 937, Zip 67950-0937; tel. 316/697-2141; Bruce K. Birchell, Chief Executive Officer (Total facility includes 60 beds in nursing home-type unit) **A**9 10 **F**8 9 17 22 25 30 32 33 34 36 37 41 43 44 45 48 50 51 53 54 56 57 58 59 60 61 62 63 66 69 70 71 72 76 78 79 **P**5 6 Web address: www.phn.org	13	10	100	1149	76	9927	30	11421	6485	237
ELLINWOOD—Barton County ★ ELLINWOOD DISTRICT HOSPITAL, 605 North Main Street, Zip 67526-1440; tel. 316/564-2548; Marge Conell, Administrator **A**9 18 **F**7 9 22 23 25 38 39 40 45 54 69 70 74 76 **S** Great Plains Health Alliance, Inc., Phillipsburg, KS Web address: www.gpha.com	23	10	12	142	5	3924	0	1773	820	34

Hospitals, U.S. / KANSAS

Hospital, Address, Telephone, Administrator, Approval, Facility, and Physician Codes, Health Care System, Network	Classification Codes		Utilization Data					Expense (thousands) of dollars		Personnel
★ American Hospital Association (AHA) membership □ Joint Commission on Accreditation of Healthcare Organizations (JCAHO) accreditation + American Osteopathic Healthcare Association (AOHA) membership ○ American Osteopathic Association (AOA) accreditation △ Commission on Accreditation of Rehabilitation Facilities (CARF) accreditation Control codes 61, 63, 64, 71, 72 and 73 indicate hospitals listed by AOHA, but not registered by AHA. For definition of numerical codes, see page A4	Control	Service	Staffed Beds	Admissions	Census	Outpatient Visits	Births	Total	Payroll	
ELLSWORTH—Ellsworth County ELLSWORTH COUNTY MEDICAL CENTER, (Formerly Ellsworth County Hospital), 1604 Aylward Street, Zip 67439-0087, Mailing Address: P.O. Box 87, Zip 67439-0087; tel. 785/472-3111; Roger W. Pearson, Administrator **A**9 10 **F**7 13 22 24 25 32 45 50 51 54 69 70 76 78 **P**8 Web address: www.gpha.com	13	10	20	422	4	7447	0	3796	1550	65
EMPORIA—Lyon County ☒ NEWMAN MEMORIAL COUNTY HOSPITAL, 1201 West 12th Avenue, Zip 66801-2597; tel. 316/343-6800; Terry R. Lambert, CHE, Chief Executive Officer (Total facility includes 18 beds in nursing home–type unit) **A**1 9 10 **F**3 7 8 11 13 17 18 22 25 27 28 32 34 35 36 37 38 39 41 44 45 46 48 50 51 54 68 69 70 72 76 **S** Quorum Health Group, Brentwood, TN Web address: www.newmanhospital.org	13	10	110	3946	54	33625	568	29370	12458	425
EUREKA—Greenwood County ★ GREENWOOD COUNTY HOSPITAL, 100 West 16th Street, Zip 67045-1064; tel. 316/583-7451; Bruce K. Birchell, Administrator and Chief Executive Officer **A**9 10 **F**7 17 18 22 23 24 25 32 34 36 38 43 48 51 54 70 76	13	10	46	1032	17	7725	0	5775	2546	104
FORT RILEY—Geary County ☒ IRWIN ARMY COMMUNITY HOSPITAL, 600 Caisson Hill Road, Zip 66442-7037; tel. 785/239-7555; Colonel Dean R. Giulitto, Commander **A**1 2 **F**11 13 22 23 25 32 38 39 41 43 44 45 48 51 54 56 57 58 59 63 65 66 70 71 72 76 77 78 79 **P**1 **S** Department of the Army, Office of the Surgeon General, Falls Church, VA	42	10	44	3259	19	229747	847	—	—	650
FORT SCOTT—Bourbon County ☒ MERCY HEALTH SYSTEM OF KANSAS, (Formerly Mercy Hospital), 821 Burke Street, Zip 66701-2409; tel. 316/223-2200; Jerry L. Stevenson, President and Chief Executive Officer (Total facility includes 23 beds in nursing home–type unit) **A**1 9 10 **F**7 8 9 13 16 17 18 19 20 22 24 25 27 28 31 32 34 36 37 39 41 42 43 44 45 48 53 54 56 68 69 70 71 72 76 78 **P**6 **S** Sisters of Mercy Health System–St. Louis, Saint Louis, MO	21	10	94	3318	47	86038	209	22044	11667	380
FREDONIA—Wilson County ★ FREDONIA REGIONAL HOSPITAL, 1527 Madison Street, Zip 66736-1751, Mailing Address: P.O. Box 579, Zip 66736-0579; tel. 316/378-2121; Terry Deschaine, Chief Executive Officer (Total facility includes 9 beds in nursing home–type unit) **A**9 10 **F**7 16 17 22 25 36 39 48 54 57 62 67 69 70 76 **S** Great Plains Health Alliance, Inc., Phillipsburg, KS Web address: www.gpha.com	14	10	51	948	14	16104	0	5098	1954	79
GARDEN CITY—Finney County ☒ ST. CATHERINE HOSPITAL, 410 East Walnut, Zip 67846-5600; tel. 316/272-2222; Mark B. Steadham, President and Chief Executive Officer **A**1 9 10 **F**8 9 16 17 18 19 22 23 24 25 26 27 30 32 34 35 36 37 38 39 40 41 43 44 45 46 48 49 51 54 55 57 59 60 61 62 63 65 68 70 72 74 76 78 **S** Catholic Health Initiatives, Denver, CO Web address: www.phn.org	21	10	93	4831	54	61513	1038	38432	15503	536
GARDNER—Johnson County MEADOWBROOK REHABILITATION HOSPITAL, (Formerly Great Plains Rehabilitaion Hospital and Health Center), 427 West Main Street, Zip 66030-1183; tel. 913/856-8747; Susan Fitzpatrick, Administrator (Total facility includes 40 beds in nursing home–type unit) **A**10 **F**7 13 26 31 53 54 59 69 70 72 78	33	46	84	487	46	0	0	9909	3262	150
GARNETT—Anderson County ANDERSON COUNTY HOSPITAL, 421 South Maple, Zip 66032-1334, Mailing Address: P.O. Box 309, Zip 66032-0309; tel. 785/448-3131; Dennis A. Hachenberg, CHE, Chief Executive Officer (Total facility includes 32 beds in nursing home–type unit) **A**9 10 18 **F**7 9 17 22 25 30 32 34 36 37 38 39 43 46 48 54 69 70 76 77 **P**8 **S** Saint Luke's Shawnee Mission Health System, Kansas City, MO	23	10	57	715	37	25536	0	6262	3297	124
GIRARD—Crawford County ★ CRAWFORD COUNTY HOSPITAL DISTRICT ONE, 302 North Hospital Drive, Zip 66743-2000; tel. 316/724-8291; Dennis E. Nehls, Administrator and Chief Executive Officer **A**9 10 **F**3 6 7 8 9 12 20 22 23 24 25 31 32 34 36 37 38 39 40 41 43 44 49 54 56 61 62 67 68 69 71 76	16	10	38	1113	9	19552	107	8537	3985	138
GOODLAND—Sherman County GOODLAND REGIONAL MEDICAL CENTER, 220 West Second Street, Zip 67735-1602; tel. 785/899-3625; Jim Chaddic, Chief Executive Officer **A**9 10 **F**3 7 8 9 16 17 24 25 30 32 34 35 37 38 39 40 41 43 44 48 51 53 54 63 68 69 70 75 76 78	13	10	49	1072	13	30345	87	7429	3255	134
GREAT BEND—Barton County ☒ CENTRAL KANSAS MEDICAL CENTER, (Includes Central Kansas Medical Center–St. Joseph Campus, 923 Carroll Avenue, Larned, Zip 67550; tel. 316/285-3161), 3515 Broadway Street, Zip 67530-3633; tel. 316/792-2511; Thomas W. Sommers, President and Chief Executive Officer (Total facility includes 88 beds in nursing home–type unit) **A**1 9 10 **F**7 8 9 13 17 18 22 24 25 26 30 32 34 36 37 38 39 40 41 43 44 45 48 49 50 51 54 56 65 69 70 71 72 76 78 **P**8 **S** Catholic Health Initiatives, Denver, CO	21	10	184	3075	86	144047	454	33225	14474	491
GREENSBURG—Kiowa County KIOWA COUNTY MEMORIAL HOSPITAL, 501 South Walnut Street, Zip 67054-1951, Mailing Address: P.O. Box 616, Zip 67054-0616; tel. 316/723-3341; Cecilia Noll, Administrator (Total facility includes 8 beds in nursing home–type unit) **A**9 10 **F**9 17 25 28 32 34 36 38 40 43 48 54 57 69 70 76 **P**6 **S** Great Plains Health Alliance, Inc., Phillipsburg, KS Web address: www.gpha.com	13	10	46	495	22	—	0	4546	1784	68

Hospitals, U.S. / KANSAS

Hospital, Address, Telephone, Administrator, Approval, Facility, and Physician Codes, Health Care System, Network	Classification Codes		Utilization Data					Expense (thousands) of dollars		
	Control	Service	Staffed Beds	Admissions	Census	Outpatient Visits	Births	Total	Payroll	Personnel

★ American Hospital Association (AHA) membership
☐ Joint Commission on Accreditation of Healthcare Organizations (JCAHO) accreditation
+ American Osteopathic Healthcare Association (AOHA) membership
○ American Osteopathic Association (AOA) accreditation
△ Commission on Accreditation of Rehabilitation Facilities (CARF) accreditation
Control codes 61, 63, 64, 71, 72 and 73 indicate hospitals listed by AOHA, but not registered by AHA. For definition of numerical codes, see page A4

Hospital	Control	Service	Staffed Beds	Admissions	Census	Outpatient Visits	Births	Total	Payroll	Personnel
HALSTEAD—Harvey County ★ HALSTEAD HOSPITAL, 328 Poplar Street, Zip 67056-2014; tel. 316/835-4100; Daniel R. Kelly, President and Chief Executive Officer (Total facility includes 17 beds in nursing home–type unit) **A**1 9 10 **F**3 4 7 9 11 12 13 16 17 18 19 22 23 24 25 27 28 30 31 32 33 34 37 38 39 40 41 43 45 46 47 48 49 50 51 54 56 57 58 59 60 61 62 63 65 68 69 70 72 76 77 78 **P**5 Web address: www.halsteadhospital.com	33	10	137	2066	39	—	0	16559	7031	203
HANOVER—Washington County HANOVER HOSPITAL, 205 South Hanover, Zip 66945-8857, Mailing Address: P.O. Box 38, Zip 66945-0038; tel. 785/337-2214; Roger D. Warren, M.D., Administrator (Total facility includes 29 beds in nursing home–type unit) **A**9 10 **F**12 22 25 28 30 32 36 37 38 39 40 41 44 48 54 56 69 76	16	10	47	385	29	1663	16	2532	1281	60
HARPER—Harper County ★ HOSPITAL DISTRICT NUMBER FIVE OF HARPER COUNTY, 1204 Maple, Zip 67058-1438; tel. 316/896-7324; Richard P. O'Mara, Chief Executive Officer **A**9 10 **F**1 13 16 18 22 25 26 28 32 34 36 37 39 40 43 45 48 54 56 69 70 75 76 78	16	10	38	514	22	4122	1	3466	1778	86
HAYS—Ellis County ★ HAYS MEDICAL CENTER, (Includes Hadley Campus, 201 East Seventh Street, Zip 67601-4198; St. Anthony Campus, 2220 Canterbury Drive), 2220 Canterbury Drive, Zip 67601-2342, Mailing Address: P.O. Box 8100, Zip 67601-8100; tel. 785/623-5000; John H. Jeter, M.D., President and Chief Executive Officer (Total facility includes 20 beds in nursing home–type unit) **A**1 2 3 5 9 10 **F**4 7 8 9 11 12 13 14 16 17 18 19 21 22 24 25 30 31 32 33 34 35 36 37 38 39 40 41 42 43 44 45 46 47 48 49 50 53 54 56 57 58 59 60 61 63 65 68 69 70 72 76 78 79 **P**4 7 Web address: www.haysmed.com	23	10	191	6260	93	—	573	78514	34180	858
HERINGTON—Dickinson County HERINGTON MUNICIPAL HOSPITAL, 100 East Helen Street, Zip 67449-1606; tel. 785/258-2207; William D. Peterson, Administrator (Total facility includes 18 beds in nursing home–type unit) **A**9 **F**7 8 9 16 17 18 22 23 30 32 44 45 48 69 76	14	10	38	491	17	18666	27	3991	1845	92
HIAWATHA—Brown County ☐ HIAWATHA COMMUNITY HOSPITAL, 300 Utah Street, Zip 66434-2314; tel. 785/742-2131; John Moore, Administrator **A**1 9 10 **F**8 12 22 24 25 36 37 39 40 41 44 45 48 53 54 69 70 76 78 **P**6	23	10	43	883	11	33097	97	7269	3328	129
HILL CITY—Graham County ★ GRAHAM COUNTY HOSPITAL, 304 West Prout Street, Zip 67642-1435, Mailing Address: P.O. Box 339, Zip 67642-0339; tel. 785/421-2121; Fred J. Meis, Administrator and Chief Executive Officer **A**9 10 **F**1 9 17 18 22 25 28 32 36 37 38 39 40 43 48 54 76 Web address: www.ruraltel.net/gced/medical.htm	13	10	26	812	9	12267	0	4296	2083	81
HILLSBORO—Marion County HILLSBORO COMMUNITY MEDICAL CENTER, 701 South Main Street, Zip 67063-1595; tel. 316/947-3114; Tom Faulkner, Chief Executive Officer (Total facility includes 52 beds in nursing home–type unit) **A**9 10 **F**1 8 9 13 16 17 18 19 22 25 32 34 37 38 39 48 54 57 62 69 70 72 76 **P**5 Web address: www.hillsboromedicalcenter.org	23	10	78	580	50	8167	27	4864	2580	121
HOISINGTON—Barton County CLARA BARTON HOSPITAL, 250 West Ninth Street, Zip 67544-1706; tel. 316/653-2114; James Turnbull, Administrator and Chief Executive Officer (Total facility includes 12 beds in nursing home–type unit) **A**9 10 **F**8 17 22 25 38 39 40 41 44 45 48 54 69 76 78	23	10	40	537	10	17806	59	5049	2418	101
HOLTON—Jackson County ★ HOLTON COMMUNITY HOSPITAL, 1110 Columbine Drive, Zip 66436-1545; tel. 785/364-2116; Leonard Hernandez, Chief Executive Officer **A**9 10 18 **F**7 8 9 17 18 22 25 31 32 34 36 38 39 40 43 44 45 48 51 54 70 76 **P**4 7 Web address: www.aih.org	23	10	15	436	4	29733	16	3681	1873	73
HORTON—Brown County NORTHEAST KANSAS CENTER FOR HEALTH AND WELLNESS, (Formerly Horton Health Foundation), 240 West 18th Street, Zip 66439-1245; tel. 785/486-2642; Dale A. White, Chief Executive Officer **A**9 10 18 **F**7 9 13 16 17 18 22 32 34 36 38 39 40 43 46 48 70 76 **P**8 Web address: www.hhf-ks.org	23	10	35	376	4	—	0	4619	2466	90
HOXIE—Sheridan County SHERIDAN COUNTY HEALTH COMPLEX, (Formerly Sheridan County Hospital), 826 18th Street, Zip 67740-0167, Mailing Address: P.O. Box 167, Zip 67740-0167; tel. 785/675-3281; Brian Kirk, Chief Executive Officer (Total facility includes 48 beds in nursing home–type unit) **A**9 10 **F**1 6 9 16 17 18 22 25 26 32 36 37 40 43 44 48 63 68 69 70 72 76	13	10	66	244	48	6784	4	3548	1902	116
HUGOTON—Stevens County STEVENS COUNTY HOSPITAL, 1006 South Jackson Street, Zip 67951-2842, Mailing Address: P.O. Box 10, Zip 67951-0010; tel. 316/544-8511; Deryl E. Gulliford, Ph.D., Chief Executive Officer **A**9 10 **F**9 13 17 22 25 28 32 34 36 38 45 48 50 54 69 70 72 76 78 Web address: www.phn.org	13	10	17	481	6	12984	0	6121	3046	92

Hospitals, U.S. / KANSAS

Hospital, Address, Telephone, Administrator, Approval, Facility, and Physician Codes, Health Care System, Network	Classification Codes		Utilization Data					Expense (thousands) of dollars		
★ American Hospital Association (AHA) membership □ Joint Commission on Accreditation of Healthcare Organizations (JCAHO) accreditation + American Osteopathic Healthcare Association (AOHA) membership ○ American Osteopathic Association (AOA) accreditation △ Commission on Accreditation of Rehabilitation Facilities (CARF) accreditation Control codes 61, 63, 64, 71, 72 and 73 indicate hospitals listed by AOHA, but not registered by AHA. For definition of numerical codes, see page A4	Control	Service	Staffed Beds	Admissions	Census	Outpatient Visits	Births	Total	Payroll	Personnel
HUTCHINSON—Reno County										
★ HUTCHINSON HOSPITAL CORPORATION, 1701 East 23rd Avenue, Zip 67502–1191; tel. 316/665–2000; Gene E. Schmidt, President (Total facility includes 19 beds in nursing home–type unit) **A**9 10 **F**3 4 6 8 11 17 18 21 22 24 25 26 27 29 36 37 38 41 43 44 45 46 47 48 53 54 56 57 58 59 60 61 62 63 65 67 69 70 72 73 76 78	23	10	163	8100	130	98893	651	57911	23085	820
INDEPENDENCE—Montgomery County										
☒ MERCY HEALTH SYSTEM OF KANSAS, (Formerly Mercy Hospital), 800 West Myrtle Street, Zip 67301–9980, Mailing Address: P.O. Box 388, Zip 67301–0388; tel. 316/331–2200; Jerry L. Stevenson, President and Chief Executive Officer (Total facility includes 18 beds in nursing home–type unit) **A**1 9 10 **F**7 8 9 13 14 16 17 18 19 21 22 24 25 28 30 32 34 36 39 41 44 45 48 54 56 69 70 74 76 78 **P**6 **S** Sisters of Mercy Health System–St. Louis, Saint Louis, MO	21	10	58	1893	22	62280	210	14934	6350	216
IOLA—Allen County										
☒ ALLEN COUNTY HOSPITAL, 101 South First Street, Zip 66749–3505, Mailing Address: P.O. Box 540, Zip 66749–0540; tel. 316/365–1000; Bill May, Chief Executive Officer **A**1 9 10 **F**7 8 9 13 17 18 19 22 24 25 26 27 31 32 34 35 36 37 39 41 43 45 46 48 53 54 69 70 72 76 77 78 79 **S** Health Midwest, Kansas City, MO	23	10	49	1526	19	21204	124	10123	4049	149
JETMORE—Hodgeman County										
★ HODGEMAN COUNTY HEALTH CENTER, 809 Bramley Street, Zip 67854–9320, Mailing Address: P.O. Box 310, Zip 67854–0310; tel. 316/357–8361; Bill Lowrance, Administrator (Total facility includes 36 beds in nursing home–type unit) **A**9 10 **F**8 9 13 16 17 22 23 25 30 31 37 44 48 50 54 67 69 76 **Web address:** www.phn.org	13	10	52	386	37	3884	14	—	—	85
JOHNSON—Stanton County										
★ STANTON COUNTY HEALTH CARE FACILITY, 404 North Chestnut Street, Zip 67855–0779, Mailing Address: P.O. Box 779, Zip 67855–0779; tel. 316/492–6250; James E. Ferguson, Interim Administrator (Total facility includes 25 beds in nursing home–type unit) **A**9 10 **F**8 16 17 22 24 25 44 54 69 76 **Web address:** www.greenviewhospital.com	13	10	42	245	24	2589	62	2226	1273	57
JUNCTION CITY—Geary County										
☒ GEARY COMMUNITY HOSPITAL, 1102 St. Mary's Road, Zip 66441, Mailing Address: P.O. Box 490, Zip 66441–0490; tel. 785/238–4131; David K. Bradley, CHE, Chief Executive Officer **A**1 3 9 10 **F**7 8 9 13 14 17 18 19 22 24 25 30 35 36 37 38 39 41 43 44 46 48 50 51 52 53 54 56 62 70 72 76 79 **Web address:** www.gchks.org	13	10	69	1945	24	132538	260	16815	7968	189
KANSAS CITY—Wyandotte County										
☒ BETHANY MEDICAL CENTER, 51 North 12th Street, Zip 66102–5161; tel. 913/281–8400; Keith R. Poisson, President and Chief Executive Officer (Total facility includes 51 beds in nursing home–type unit) (Nonreporting) **A**1 2 3 5 9 10 **S** Sisters of Charity of Leavenworth Health Services Corporation, Leavenworth, KS	23	10	251	—	—	—	—	—	—	—
☒ PROVIDENCE MEDICAL CENTER, 8929 Parallel Parkway, Zip 66112–1636; tel. 913/596–4000; Francis V. Creeden, Jr, Senior Executive Officer (Total facility includes 40 beds in nursing home–type unit) **A**1 2 9 10 **F**4 8 9 11 13 17 18 19 21 22 23 24 25 30 31 32 33 34 35 36 37 38 39 41 43 44 45 46 47 48 49 50 51 54 57 65 68 69 70 71 72 73 76 78 79 **P**5 6 7 8 **S** Sisters of Charity of Leavenworth Health Services Corporation, Leavenworth, KS **Web address:** www.pmc–sjh.org	21	10	219	9713	135	59549	959	71884	31838	848
☒ △ UNIVERSITY OF KANSAS MEDICAL CENTER, 3901 Rainbow Boulevard, Zip 66160–7200; tel. 913/588–5000; Irene M. Cumming, Chief Executive Officer **A**1 2 3 5 7 8 9 10 **F**4 7 8 9 10 11 13 14 17 18 19 21 22 23 24 25 26 27 28 29 30 32 33 34 35 37 38 39 41 42 43 44 45 46 47 48 49 50 51 52 53 54 55 56 57 58 59 60 61 62 63 64 65 66 68 70 71 72 74 76 77 78 79 **P**1 6 **Web address:** www.kumc.edu	16	10	387	12665	216	404495	1014	187974	65807	1912
KINGMAN—Kingman County										
★ NINNESCAH VALLEY HEALTH SYSTEM, (Formerly Kingman Community Hospital), 750 Avenue D West, Zip 67068–0376, Mailing Address: P.O. Box 376, Zip 67068–0376; tel. 316/532–3147; Gary L. Tiller, Chief Executive Officer **A**9 10 **F**7 8 9 13 16 17 18 22 24 25 30 32 33 34 36 37 38 39 40 41 43 44 45 46 48 49 50 51 53 54 56 63 69 70 72 76 78 **P**3 6 7	23	10	45	676	10	19110	47	5908	2894	131
KIOWA—Barber County										
★ KIOWA DISTRICT HOSPITAL, 810 Drumm Street, Zip 67070–1626; tel. 316/825–4131; Paula Pickens, Interim Chief Executive Officer **A**9 10 **F**9 13 16 17 18 22 25 32 37 48 56 70 76 **P**6	16	10	24	316	3	3497	0	1965	1132	42
LA CROSSE—Rush County										
★ RUSH COUNTY MEMORIAL HOSPITAL, (Formerly Rush County Healthcare Center), 801 Locust Street, Zip 67548–9673, Mailing Address: P.O. Box 520, Zip 67548–0520; tel. 785/222–2545; Teresa L. Deuel, Administrator and Chief Executive Officer (Total facility includes 26 beds in nursing home–type unit) **A**9 10 **F**9 16 22 25 28 32 36 38 39 48 54 69 76 **P**5	13	10	50	380	31	1357	0	3033	1618	42
LAKIN—Kearny County										
★ KEARNY COUNTY HOSPITAL, 500 Thorpe Street, Zip 67860–0744; tel. 316/355–7111; Steven S. Reiner, Administrator (Total facility includes 52 beds in nursing home–type unit) **A**9 10 18 **F**1 6 8 9 14 16 17 18 19 22 23 25 26 28 30 32 34 36 37 38 40 41 44 48 54 56 67 69 70 72 76 79 **P**5 6 **Web address:** www.phn.org	13	10	77	267	19	10365	20	3792	2024	122

© 2000 AHA Guide   *Many Facility Codes have changed. Please refer to the AHA Guide Code Chart.*

Hospitals, U.S. / KANSAS

Hospital, Address, Telephone, Administrator, Approval, Facility, and Physician Codes, Health Care System, Network

★ American Hospital Association (AHA) membership
☐ Joint Commission on Accreditation of Healthcare Organizations (JCAHO) accreditation
+ American Osteopathic Healthcare Association (AOHA) membership
○ American Osteopathic Association (AOA) accreditation
△ Commission on Accreditation of Rehabilitation Facilities (CARF) accreditation
Control codes 61, 63, 64, 71, 72 and 73 indicate hospitals listed by AOHA, but not registered by AHA. For definition of numerical codes, see page A4

Hospital	Control	Service	Staffed Beds	Admissions	Census	Outpatient Visits	Births	Total	Payroll	Personnel
LARNED—Pawnee County										
CENTRAL KANSAS MEDICAL CENTER–ST. JOSEPH CAMPUS See Central Kansas Medical Center, Great Bend										
☐ LARNED STATE HOSPITAL, Mailing Address: Rural Route 3, P.O. Box 89, Zip 67550-9365; tel. 316/285-2131; Mani Lee, Ph.D., Superintendent A1 10 F2 8 9 12 22 24 27 35 39 41 43 44 45 46 48 50 51 52 57 58 61 62 65 70 72 76 77 78	12	22	342	1341	281	0	0	—	—	677
LAWRENCE—Douglas County										
☐ LAWRENCE MEMORIAL HOSPITAL, 325 Maine Street, Zip 66044-1389; tel. 785/749-6100; Eugene W. Meyer, President and Chief Executive Officer (Total facility includes 21 beds in nursing home-type unit) A1 5 9 10 F7 8 9 11 16 17 18 22 24 25 27 32 33 34 35 36 37 38 39 40 41 43 44 45 46 48 49 51 53 54 57 64 69 70 72 76 78 P6 Web address: www.lmh.org	14	10	154	6824	82	—	986	59807	27462	763
LEAVENWORTH—Leavenworth County										
☐ CUSHING MEMORIAL HOSPITAL, 711 Marshall Street, Zip 66048-3235; tel. 913/684-1100; Charles L. Rogers, President (Total facility includes 16 beds in nursing home-type unit) (Nonreporting) A1 9 10	23	10	74	—	—	—	—	—	—	—
DWIGHT D. EISENHOWER VETERANS AFFAIRS MEDICAL CENTER See Veterans Affairs Eastern Kansas Health Care System, Topeka										
✦ SAINT JOHN HOSPITAL, 3500 South Fourth Street, Zip 66048-5043; tel. 913/680-6000; Mark J. Jaeger, CHE, President and Chief Executive Officer (Total facility includes 6 beds in nursing home-type unit) A1 9 10 F7 8 9 17 18 19 22 25 27 30 32 34 35 36 37 38 41 44 45 46 48 54 68 69 70 72 76 78 79 P6 7 S Sisters of Charity of Leavenworth Health Services Corporation, Leavenworth, KS Web address: www.pmc–sjh.org	21	10	36	1879	22	45270	208	15935	7722	221
LEOTI—Wichita County										
★ WICHITA COUNTY HEALTH CENTER, (Formerly Wichita County Hospital), (Includes Wichita County Hospital Long Term Care), 211 East Earl Street, Zip 67861-0968, Mailing Address: Rural Route 2, Box 38, Zip 67861-0968; tel. 316/375-2233; Edward Finley, Administrator (Total facility includes 28 beds in nursing home-type unit) A9 10 18 F7 8 9 13 16 17 18 19 22 30 31 32 34 36 37 38 40 44 45 54 56 69 70 72 75 76 78 P6 Web address: www.phn.org	13	10	41	198	26	—	19	2692	1364	39
LIBERAL—Seward County										
✦ SOUTHWEST MEDICAL CENTER, 315 West 15th Street, Zip 67901-1340, Mailing Address: Box 1340, Zip 67905-1340; tel. 316/624-1651; Anthony A. Daigle, Administrator (Total facility includes 18 beds in nursing home-type unit) A1 9 10 F8 9 13 17 18 19 22 24 25 26 27 28 29 30 32 33 36 37 38 39 41 43 44 45 46 48 50 51 54 57 62 63 65 68 69 70 72 76 78 P6 Web address: www.phn.org	13	10	87	3620	47	32416	796	33669	12224	435
LINCOLN—Lincoln County										
LINCOLN COUNTY HOSPITAL, 624 North Second Street, Zip 67455-1738, Mailing Address: P.O. Box 406, Zip 67455-0406; tel. 785/524-4403; Jolene Yager, R.N., Administrator (Total facility includes 20 beds in nursing home-type unit) A9 10 F7 17 22 25 36 37 38 40 45 48 54 69 70 76 P6 S Great Plains Health Alliance, Inc., Phillipsburg, KS Web address: www.gpha.com	13	10	34	655	25	6623	0	4004	2233	86
LINDSBORG—McPherson County										
★ LINDSBORG COMMUNITY HOSPITAL, 605 West Lincoln Street, Zip 67456-2328; tel. 785/227-3308; Greg Lundstrom, Administrator and Chief Executive Officer A9 10 F9 17 25 28 34 36 38 40 48 69 70 76 P6	23	10	12	553	6	—	0	3271	1539	78
LYONS—Rice County										
★ RICE COUNTY HOSPITAL DISTRICT NUMBER ONE, 619 South Clark Street, Zip 67554-3003, Mailing Address: P.O. Box 828, Zip 67554-0828; tel. 316/257-5173; Robert L. Mullen, Chief Executive Officer A9 10 F6 7 9 16 17 18 19 22 23 30 36 40 43 44 48 54 67 70 76 Web address: www.rch-lyons.com	16	10	44	634	22	—	75	4752	2247	103
MANHATTAN—Riley County										
✦ MERCY HEALTH CENTER OF MANHATTAN, (Includes Memorial Hospital, 1105 Sunset Avenue, Zip 66502; tel. 913/776-3300; Saint Mary Hospital, 1823 College Avenue, Zip 66502), 1823 College Avenue, Zip 66502-3381, Mailing Address: P.O. Box 1289, Zip 66502-1289; tel. 785/776-3322; Richard L. Allen, President and Chief Executive Officer A1 9 10 F7 8 9 11 12 13 16 17 18 22 24 25 27 28 31 32 33 34 35 36 37 39 40 41 43 44 45 48 49 50 51 53 54 57 58 59 60 61 70 71 72 76 78 79 S Via Christi Health System, Wichita, KS	23	10	114	4582	53	75639	760	36780	16967	470
MANKATO—Jewell County										
JEWELL COUNTY HOSPITAL, 100 Crestvue Avenue, Zip 66956-2407, Mailing Address: P.O. Box 327, Zip 66956-0327; tel. 785/378-3137; Aloha Kier, Administrator (Total facility includes 40 beds in nursing home-type unit) A9 10 18 F1 6 7 9 13 14 16 17 18 19 22 23 25 26 30 31 32 33 34 35 37 38 43 50 51 54 59 61 62 69 72 76 78 P6 S Great Plains Health Alliance, Inc., Phillipsburg, KS	13	10	52	153	34	5829	0	2651	1362	62
MARION—Marion County										
★ ST. LUKE HOSPITAL AND LIVING CENTER, (Formerly St. Luke Hospital), 1014 East Melvin, Zip 66861-1299; tel. 316/382-2179; Craig Hanson, Administrator (Total facility includes 32 beds in nursing home-type unit) A9 10 F7 8 9 12 15 17 18 20 22 23 24 25 26 30 33 34 36 37 40 41 43 44 45 46 48 50 51 54 56 69 70 76 78 79 S Banner Health System, Fargo, ND Web address: www.lhsnet.com	23	10	54	432	36	16798	32	4436	2255	87

Hospitals, U.S. / KANSAS

Hospital, Address, Telephone, Administrator, Approval, Facility, and Physician Codes, Health Care System, Network	Classification Codes		Utilization Data					Expense (thousands) of dollars		
★ American Hospital Association (AHA) membership □ Joint Commission on Accreditation of Healthcare Organizations (JCAHO) accreditation + American Osteopathic Healthcare Association (AOHA) membership ○ American Osteopathic Association (AOA) accreditation △ Commission on Accreditation of Rehabilitation Facilities (CARF) accreditation Control codes 61, 63, 64, 71, 72 and 73 indicate hospitals listed by AOHA, but not registered by AHA. For definition of numerical codes, see page A4	Control	Service	Staffed Beds	Admissions	Census	Outpatient Visits	Births	Total	Payroll	Personnel
MARYSVILLE—Marshall County										
★ COMMUNITY MEMORIAL HEALTHCARE, 708 North 18th Street, Zip 66508–1338; tel. 785/562–2311; Jay M. Canter, Chief Executive Officer (Total facility includes 55 beds in nursing home–type unit) **A**9 10 **F**7 8 9 12 17 18 22 25 28 30 32 36 37 39 40 43 44 48 54 56 62 63 69 70 76 **P**3	23	10	104	1294	59	23830	78	10650	4711	219
MCPHERSON—McPherson County										
★ MEMORIAL HOSPITAL, 1000 Hospital Drive, Zip 67460–2321; tel. 316/241–2250; Stan Regehr, President and Chief Executive Officer **A**9 10 **F**7 8 9 16 17 18 19 22 24 25 28 32 35 36 37 39 40 41 43 44 45 46 48 49 50 51 54 70 76 78	23	10	41	1483	16	97358	186	14283	6306	185
MEADE—Meade County										
★ MEADE DISTRICT HOSPITAL, 510 East Carthage Street, Zip 67864–0680, Mailing Address: P.O. Box 680, Zip 67864–0680; tel. 316/873–2141; Michael P. Thomas, Administrator **A**9 10 **F**17 18 22 25 28 32 36 48 53 54 69 76 Web address: www.phn.org	16	10	20	532	6	—	1	3709	1747	72
MEDICINE LODGE—Barber County										
★ MEDICINE LODGE MEMORIAL HOSPITAL, 710 North Walnut Street, Zip 67104–1019, Mailing Address: P.O. Drawer C, Zip 67104; tel. 316/886–3771; Kevin A. White, CHE, Administrator **A**9 10 **F**7 9 17 18 22 25 28 30 38 48 54 76 **P**6 **S** Great Plains Health Alliance, Inc., Phillipsburg, KS Web address: www.gpha.com	16	10	42	584	18	7589	0	4862	2524	91
MINNEAPOLIS—Ottawa County										
★ OTTAWA COUNTY HEALTH CENTER, 215 East Eighth, Zip 67467–1999, Mailing Address: P.O. Box 290, Zip 67467–0290; tel. 785/392–2122; Joy Reed, R.N., Administrator (Total facility includes 23 beds in nursing home–type unit) **A**9 10 **F**6 16 17 18 19 23 24 25 28 30 31 36 38 40 50 54 63 69 70 76 **S** Great Plains Health Alliance, Inc., Phillipsburg, KS Web address: www.gpha.com	23	10	53	531	46	4261	0	3383	1828	79
MINNEOLA—Clark County										
★ MINNEOLA DISTRICT HOSPITAL, 212 Main Street, Zip 67865–8511, Mailing Address: P.O. Box 127, Zip 67865–0127; tel. 316/885–4264; Ronald D. Baker, Administrator **A**9 10 **F**9 18 25 32 37 38 48 54 61 67 69 70 76 **P**6 **S** Great Plains Health Alliance, Inc., Phillipsburg, KS Web address: www.gpha.com	16	10	15	486	7	5701	35	3057	1241	53
MOUNDRIDGE—McPherson County										
★ MERCY HOSPITAL, 218 East Pack Street, Zip 67107–0180, Mailing Address: P.O. Box 180, Zip 67107–0180; tel. 316/345–6391; Doyle K. Johnson, Administrator **A**9 10 **F**8 17 25 30 44 48	21	10	21	424	8	6141	37	1516	698	32
NEODESHA—Wilson County										
★ WILSON COUNTY HOSPITAL, 205 Mill Street, Zip 66757–1817, Mailing Address: P.O. Box 360, Zip 66757–0360; tel. 316/325–2611; Deanna Pittman, Administrator **A**9 10 **F**7 8 17 18 19 22 25 30 32 34 36 39 43 44 45 48 54 57 62 69 70 72 76 78	13	10	38	575	10	6125	51	4440	2238	95
NESS CITY—Ness County										
★ NESS COUNTY HOSPITAL, (Formerly Ness County Hospital District Two), 312 Custer Street, Zip 67560–1654; tel. 785/798–2291; Clyde T. McCracken, Administrator (Total facility includes 45 beds in nursing home–type unit) **A**9 10 **F**9 17 22 25 36 53 67 69 70 76 **P**6	16	10	65	320	37	4709	0	4152	2068	120
NEWTON—Harvey County										
✠ NEWTON MEDICAL CENTER, Mailing Address: P.O. Box 308, Zip 67114–0308; tel. 316/283–2700; Steven G. Kelly, President and Chief Executive Officer (Total facility includes 11 beds in nursing home–type unit) **A**1 9 10 **F**7 8 13 16 17 22 24 25 27 32 36 37 38 39 40 41 44 48 54 61 69 70 76 Web address: www.newtonmedicalcenter.com	23	10	66	2972	35	29709	455	20987	9282	288
□ PRAIRIE VIEW, 1901 East First Street, Zip 67114–5010, Mailing Address: P.O. Box 467, Zip 67114–0467; tel. 316/283–2400; Melvin Goering, Chief Executive Officer **A**1 9 10 **F**3 13 16 17 18 19 21 29 38 49 50 57 58 59 60 61 62 63 64 70 72 73 78 79 **P**6 Web address: www.pvi.org	23	22	38	1037	23	—	0	16645	10604	294
NORTON—Norton County										
★ NORTON COUNTY HOSPITAL, 102 East Holme, Zip 67654–0250, Mailing Address: P.O. Box 250, Zip 67654–0250; tel. 785/877–3351; Richard Miller, Administrator and Chief Executive Officer **A**9 10 **F**8 9 17 18 22 23 24 25 30 32 34 37 38 39 40 43 44 46 48 50 51 53 54 56 69 70 76 78 **P**4 7	13	10	24	728	15	15739	30	4576	2539	87
OAKLEY—Logan County										
★ LOGAN COUNTY HOSPITAL, 211 Cherry Street, Zip 67748–1201; tel. 785/672–3211; Rodney Bates, Administrator (Total facility includes 30 beds in nursing home–type unit) **A**9 10 **F**6 8 9 16 17 18 22 24 25 31 38 40 41 44 48 54 67 69 70 76	13	10	50	392	12	10835	23	2863	1597	59
OBERLIN—Decatur County										
★ DECATUR COUNTY HOSPITAL AND CEDAR LIVING CENTER, (Formerly Decatur County Hospital), 810 West Columbia Street, Zip 67749–2450, Mailing Address: P.O. Box 268, Zip 67749–0268; tel. 785/475–2208; Lynn Doeden, Administrator (Total facility includes 50 beds in nursing home–type unit) **A**9 10 **F**8 9 17 18 22 25 36 37 38 39 40 46 48 54 68 69 70 76 **S** Banner Health System, Fargo, ND Web address: www.lhsnet.com	23	10	74	737	52	13588	23	4220	2079	89

© 2000 AHA Guide *Many Facility Codes have changed. Please refer to the AHA Guide Code Chart.*

Hospitals, U.S. / KANSAS

Hospital, Address Telephone, Administrator, Approval, Facility, and Physician Codes, Health Care System, Network	Classification Codes		Utilization Data					Expense (thousands) of dollars		
	Control	Service	Staffed Beds	Admissions	Census	Outpatient Visits	Births	Total	Payroll	Personnel

★ American Hospital Association (AHA) membership
□ Joint Commission on Accreditation of Healthcare Organizations (JCAHO) accreditation
+ American Osteopathic Healthcare Association (AOHA) membership
○ American Osteopathic Association (AOA) accreditation
△ Commission on Accreditation of Rehabilitation Facilities (CARF) accreditation
Control codes 61, 63, 64, 71, 72 and 73 indicate hospitals listed by AOHA, but not registered by AHA. For definition of numerical codes, see page A4

Hospital	Control	Service	Staffed Beds	Admissions	Census	Outpatient Visits	Births	Total	Payroll	Personnel
OLATHE—Johnson County										
□ OLATHE MEDICAL CENTER, 20333 West 151st Street, Zip 66061-5350; tel. 913/791-4200; Frank H. Devocelle, President and Chief Executive Officer **A**1 2 9 10 **F**4 7 8 9 11 13 16 17 18 19 22 23 24 25 26 32 34 35 36 37 38 39 41 44 46 47 48 49 51 54 70 71 72 76 77 78 79 **P**3 8 Web address: www.ohsi.com	23	10	182	9485	98	90391	1474	66537	28878	801
ONAGA—Pottawatomie County										
★ COMMUNITY HOSPITAL ONAGA, 120 West Eighth Street, Zip 66521-0120; tel. 785/889-4272; Joseph T. Engelken, Chief Executive Officer (Total facility includes 173 beds in nursing home-type unit) **A**9 10 **F**1 2 3 6 7 8 9 12 13 14 16 17 18 19 20 22 23 25 28 30 31 32 33 34 35 36 37 38 39 40 41 43 44 45 46 48 49 50 51 53 54 56 57 58 59 60 61 62 63 66 67 69 70 71 72 73 75 76 77 78 79 **P**6	23	10	271	1473	150	35298	89	15587	9289	220
OSAWATOMIE—Miami County										
□ OSAWATOMIE STATE HOSPITAL, 500 State Hospital Drive, Zip 66064-0500, Mailing Address: P.O. Box 500, Zip 66064-0500; tel. 913/755-7000; Randy Proctor, Superintendent **A**1 10 **F**9 23 25 30 34 50 51 54 56 57 70 75 78 **P**6	12	22	289	830	177	0	0	—	12850	435
OSBORNE—Osborne County										
★ OSBORNE COUNTY MEMORIAL HOSPITAL, 424 West New Hampshire Street, Zip 67473-0070, Mailing Address: P.O. Box 70, Zip 67473-0070; tel. 785/346-2121; Patricia Bernard, R.N., Administrator **A**9 10 **F**7 8 9 22 23 25 37 38 40 48 69 76 **P**6 **S** Great Plains Health Alliance, Inc., Phillipsburg, KS Web address: www.gpha.com	13	10	29	431	5	5705	23	2848	1247	64
OTTAWA—Franklin County										
★ RANSOM MEMORIAL HOSPITAL, 1301 South Main Street, Zip 66067-3598; tel. 785/229-8200; Larry A. Felix, CHE, Administrator **A**1 9 10 **F**7 8 9 17 19 22 24 25 30 31 32 34 36 37 38 39 41 43 44 45 46 48 49 51 54 61 68 70 71 72 73 76 78 **P**8 Web address: www.ransom.org	13	10	46	1586	21	35408	157	14871	7300	205
OVERLAND PARK—Johnson County										
□ △ MID-AMERICA REHABILITATION HOSPITAL, 5701 West 110th Street, Zip 66211; tel. 913/491-2400; Mark J. Stepanik, Interim Chief Executive Officer **A**1 7 9 10 **F**13 16 17 18 22 23 24 29 31 38 39 45 46 51 53 54 65 70 71 72 76 78 **S** HEALTHSOUTH Corporation, Birmingham, AL	33	46	80	1099	63	27810	0	14651	6276	167
★ SAINT LUKE'S SOUTH HOSPITAL, 12300 Metcalf Avenue, Zip 66213; tel. 913/317-7000; William G. Robertson, Chief Executive Officer **A**1 **F**2 3 4 8 9 11 13 14 17 18 19 20 22 24 25 27 28 29 33 34 35 36 37 38 39 41 42 43 44 45 46 47 48 49 50 54 57 58 59 60 61 62 63 64 66 70 71 72 76 77 78 79 **P**4 5 6 7 8 **S** Saint Luke's Shawnee Mission Health System, Kansas City, MO	21	10	342	16641	196	190671	3150	157023	65858	1821
PAOLA—Miami County										
MIAMI COUNTY MEDICAL CENTER, 2100 Baptiste Drive, Zip 66071-0365, Mailing Address: P.C. Box 365, Zip 66071-0365; tel. 913/294-2327; Gerald Wiesner, Administrator **A**9 10 **F**7 9 18 22 24 25 28 34 35 36 38 43 45 46 48 51 54 56 61 70 71 76 78 **P**3 8	23	10	20	879	9	29995	0	10110	3913	125
PARSONS—Labette County										
★ LABETTE COUNTY MEDICAL CENTER, 1902 South U.S. Highway 59, Zip 67357-7404, Mailing Address: P.O. Box 956, Zip 67357-0956; tel. 316/421-4880; Robert E. Mac Devitt, Chief Executive Officer (Total facility includes 12 beds in nursing home-type unit) **A**1 9 10 **F**7 8 9 11 16 17 18 22 24 25 32 34 36 39 41 43 44 45 46 48 50 51 54 68 69 70 71 72 76 78 **P**4 7	13	10	70	2913	35	35893	280	29906	12276	416
PARSONS STATE HOSPITAL AND TRAINING CENTER, 2601 Gabriel Street, Zip 67357-0738, Mailing Address: P.O. Box 738, Zip 67357-0738; tel. 316/421-6550; Gary J. Daniels, Ph.D., Superintendent **F**9 19 22 23 24 25 32 39 41 46 48 53 57 69 70 76 78	12	62	223	29	198	0	0	20170	13314	218
PHILLIPSBURG—Phillips County										
★ PHILLIPS COUNTY HOSPITAL, 1150 State Street, Zip 67661-1799, Mailing Address: P.C. Box 607, Zip 67661-0607; tel. 785/543-5226; James Wahlmeier, Administrator (Total facility includes 33 beds in nursing home-type unit) **A**9 10 **F**1 7 9 17 22 23 25 37 38 39 46 48 49 51 54 69 70 76 78 **S** Great Plains Health Alliance, Inc., Phillipsburg, KS Web address: www.phillips.hpmin.com/	23	10	62	772	41	9934	30	7023	2969	111
PITTSBURG—Crawford County										
★ MOUNT CARMEL MEDICAL CENTER, 1102 East Centennial Drive, Zip 66762-6643; tel. 316/231-6100; John Daniel Lingor, President and Chief Executive Officer (Total facility includes 20 beds in nursing home-type unit) **A**1 2 9 10 **F**1 7 8 9 13 14 17 18 19 22 24 25 27 31 32 34 36 37 39 41 44 45 46 48 49 51 54 57 59 60 61 62 63 64 65 68 69 70 71 72 76 78 **P**3 6 7 8 **S** Via Christi Health System, Wichita, KS	21	10	126	4598	67	73968	338	36875	17226	580
PLAINVILLE—Rooks County										
PLAINVILLE RURAL HOSPITAL DISTRICT NUMBER ONE, 304 South Colorado Avenue, Zip 67663-0389; tel. 785/434-4553; Richard Q. Bergling, Administrator and Chief Executive Officer **A**9 10 18 **F**9 16 17 18 22 24 32 34 36 37 39 40 43 48 49 67 76 77 78	16	10	25	456	5	2497	5	2471	1178	43
PRATT—Pratt County										
★ PRATT REGIONAL MEDICAL CENTER, 200 Commodore Street, Zip 67124-2903; tel. 316/672-7451; Susan M. Page, President and Chief Executive Officer (Total facility includes 70 beds in nursing home-type unit) **A**9 10 **F**7 8 9 14 17 18 22 24 25 27 28 29 33 35 36 37 38 39 40 41 44 46 48 50 51 54 66 68 69 70 71 72 76 78 **P**6 7 Web address: www.prmc.org	23	10	139	1908	73	—	186	20711	9346	332

Hospitals, U.S. / KANSAS

Hospital, Address, Telephone, Administrator, Approval, Facility, and Physician Codes, Health Care System, Network ★ American Hospital Association (AHA) membership □ Joint Commission on Accreditation of Healthcare Organizations (JCAHO) accreditation + American Osteopathic Healthcare Association (AOHA) membership ○ American Osteopathic Association (AOA) accreditation △ Commission on Accreditation of Rehabilitation Facilities (CARF) accreditation Control codes 61, 63, 64, 71, 72 and 73 indicate hospitals listed by AOHA, but not registered by AHA. For definition of numerical codes, see page A4	Classification Codes		Utilization Data					Expense (thousands) of dollars		
	Control	Service	Staffed Beds	Admissions	Census	Outpatient Visits	Births	Total	Payroll	Personnel
QUINTER—Gove County GOVE COUNTY MEDICAL CENTER, 520 West Fifth Street, Zip 67752-0129, Mailing Address: P.O. Box 129, Zip 67752-0129; tel. 785/754-3341; Paul Davis, Administrator (Total facility includes 59 beds in nursing home–type unit) **A**9 10 **F**6 8 9 22 25 32 36 37 38 48 54 69 70 76 **P**5	13	10	80	968	63	24658	40	5431	2826	140
RANSOM—Ness County ★ GRISELL MEMORIAL HOSPITAL DISTRICT ONE, 210 South Vermont, Zip 67572-0268, Mailing Address: P.O. Box 268, Zip 67572-0268; tel. 785/731-2231; Kristine Ochs, R.N., Administrator (Total facility includes 34 beds in nursing home–type unit) **A**9 10 18 **F**9 22 23 25 30 36 37 40 45 48 54 56 61 69 70 76 **P**6 **S** Great Plains Health Alliance, Inc., Phillipsburg, KS Web address: www.gpha.com	16	10	46	210	35	3297	0	2818	1551	71
RUSSELL—Russell County ✠ RUSSELL REGIONAL HOSPITAL, 200 South Main Street, Zip 67665-2997; tel. 785/483-3131; Bruce Garrett, R.N., Administrator and Chief Executive Officer (Total facility includes 18 beds in nursing home–type unit) **A**1 9 10 **F**7 8 9 13 16 17 18 22 24 25 31 32 33 34 38 40 41 43 45 46 48 50 51 54 56 69 70 76 78 Web address: www.russellhospital.org	23	10	57	705	32	15757	8	7240	4149	164
SABETHA—Nemaha County ★ SABETHA COMMUNITY HOSPITAL, 14th and Oregon Streets, Zip 66534-0229, Mailing Address: P.O. Box 229, Zip 66534-0229; tel. 785/284-2121; Rita K. Buurman, Chief Executive Officer **A**9 10 **F**1 7 8 9 17 18 19 22 23 24 25 30 32 34 36 38 39 45 46 48 50 54 59 61 63 69 70 76 **P**6 **S** Great Plains Health Alliance, Inc., Phillipsburg, KS Web address: www.gpha.com	23	10	27	534	7	17919	52	4914	2601	75
SAINT FRANCIS—Cheyenne County ★ CHEYENNE COUNTY HOSPITAL, 210 West First Street, Zip 67756-0547, Mailing Address: P.O. Box 547, Zip 67756-0547; tel. 785/332-2104; Leslie Lacy, Administrator **A**9 10 18 **F**7 9 17 18 22 25 26 34 46 48 54 56 70 76 **P**6 **S** Great Plains Health Alliance, Inc., Phillipsburg, KS Web address: www.gpha.com	23	10	16	233	3	6589	1	3119	1483	57
SALINA—Saline County ✠ △ SALINA REGIONAL HEALTH CENTER, (Includes Salina Regional Health Center–Penn Campus, 139 North Penn Street, Zip 67401; Salina Regional Health Center–Santa Fe Campus, 400 South Santa Fe Avenue, Zip 67401), 400 South Santa Fe Avenue, Zip 67401-4198, Mailing Address: P.O. Box 5080, Zip 67401-5080; tel. 785/452-7000; Randy Peterson, President and Chief Executive Officer (Total facility includes 26 beds in nursing home–type unit) **A**1 2 3 7 9 10 **F**4 7 8 9 11 12 13 16 17 18 19 22 23 24 25 27 28 30 31 32 33 34 35 36 37 38 39 40 41 42 43 44 45 46 47 48 49 50 51 53 54 57 58 59 60 61 62 63 64 65 68 69 70 71 72 73 76 78 79 **P**8 Web address: www.srhc.com	23	10	241	9990	142	150442	1107	84335	37683	1204
★ ST. FRANCIS AT SALINA, 5097 West Cloud Street, Zip 67401-2348; tel. 785/825-0563; Father Phillip J. Rapp, President and Chief Executive Officer (Nonreporting) **A**9 Web address: www.st-francis.org	23	22	26	—	—	—	—	—	—	—
SATANTA—Haskell County ★ SATANTA DISTRICT HOSPITAL, 401 South Cheyenne Street, Zip 67870-0159, Mailing Address: P.O. Box 159, Zip 67870-0159; tel. 316/649-2761; T. G. Lee, Administrator (Total facility includes 32 beds in nursing home–type unit) **A**9 10 **F**7 8 9 15 17 19 22 25 26 36 38 39 43 45 48 49 51 69 70 76 **P**4 7 **S** Great Plains Health Alliance, Inc., Phillipsburg, KS Web address: www.gpha.com	16	10	45	259	29	4223	0	4938	2086	86
SCOTT CITY—Scott County ★ SCOTT COUNTY HOSPITAL, 310 East Third Street, Zip 67871-1203; tel. 316/872-5811; Greg Unruh, Chief Executive Officer **A**9 10 **F**7 8 9 16 19 22 25 32 34 38 39 40 43 44 45 46 48 54 69 70 72 76 78 79 Web address: www.phn.org	13	10	27	862	10	14315	63	5198	2658	144
SEDAN—Chautauqua County SEDAN CITY HOSPITAL, 300 North Street, Zip 67361-0427, Mailing Address: P.O. Box C, Zip 67361-0427; tel. 316/725-3115; Sheila Nettles, Administrator (Nonreporting) **A**9 10 18	14	10	30	—	—	—	—	—	—	—
SENECA—Nemaha County NEMAHA VALLEY COMMUNITY HOSPITAL, 1600 Community Drive, Zip 66538-9739; tel. 785/336-6181; Michael J. Ryan, Administrator **A**9 10 18 **F**7 8 9 17 18 22 23 25 30 32 34 36 38 39 43 44 45 48 54 70 72 75 76	23	10	24	667	7	11861	59	4431	1965	79
SHAWNEE MISSION—Johnson County ✠ MENORAH MEDICAL CENTER, 5721 West 119th Street, Zip 66209-3722; tel. 913/498-6000; Steven D. Wilkinson, President and Chief Executive Officer **A**1 2 10 **F**1 2 3 4 5 7 8 9 11 12 13 16 17 18 19 21 22 24 25 26 27 28 29 30 31 32 33 34 35 36 37 38 39 40 41 42 43 44 45 46 47 48 49 50 51 53 54 56 57 58 59 60 61 62 63 64 65 66 68 69 70 71 72 73 74 75 76 77 78 79 **P**1 5 **S** Health Midwest, Kansas City, MO Web address: www.healthmidwest.org MENORAH MEDICAL CENTER See	23	10	158	5736	76	51926	1159	63119	24830	649

© 2000 AHA Guide   *Many Facility Codes have changed. Please refer to the AHA Guide Code Chart.*   Hospitals **A167**

Hospitals, U.S. / KANSAS

★ American Hospital Association (AHA) membership
□ Joint Commission on Accreditation of Healthcare Organizations (JCAHO) accreditation
+ American Osteopathic Healthcare Association (AOHA) membership
○ American Osteopathic Association (AOA) accreditation
△ Commission on Accreditation of Rehabilitation Facilities (CARF) accreditation
Control codes 61, 63, 64, 71, 72 and 73 indicate hospitals listed by AOHA, but not registered by AHA. For definition of numerical codes, see page A4

Hospital, Address, Telephone, Administrator, Approval, Facility, and Physician Codes, Health Care System, Network	Classification Codes		Utilization Data					Expense (thousands) of dollars		
	Control	Service	Staffed Beds	Admissions	Census	Outpatient Visits	Births	Total	Payroll	Personnel
★ OVERLAND PARK REGIONAL MEDICAL CENTER, 10500 Quivira Road, Zip 66215–2306, Mailing Address: P.O. Box 15959, Zip 66215–5959; tel. 913/541–5000; Kevin J. Hicks, President and Chief Executive Officer (Total facility includes 17 beds in nursing home–type unit) **A**1 10 **F**1 3 4 9 11 12 13 14 17 18 19 21 22 23 24 25 26 28 29 30 31 32 33 34 35 36 37 38 39 41 42 43 44 45 46 47 48 49 50 51 54 55 56 57 62 65 66 69 70 72 74 75 76 77 78 79 **S** Health Midwest, Kansas City, MO **Web address:** www.healthmidwest.org	23	10	269	9031	126	84736	2221	83649	31614	738
★ SHAWNEE MISSION MEDICAL CENTER, 9100 West 74th Street, Zip 66204–4004, Mailing Address: Box 2923, Zip 66201–1323; tel. 913/676–2000; William G. Robertson, Chief Executive Officer (Nonreporting) **A**1 2 9 10 **S** Saint Luke's Shawnee Mission Health System, Kansas City, MO	21	10	333	—	—	—	—	—	—	—
SMITH CENTER—Smith County										
★ SMITH COUNTY MEMORIAL HOSPITAL, 614 South Main Street, Zip 66967–0349, Mailing Address: P.O. Box 349, Zip 66967–0349; tel. 785/282–6845; John Terrill, Administrator (Total facility includes 28 beds in nursing home–type unit) **A**9 10 **F**1 8 9 22 25 38 39 48 54 69 70 76 **P**6 **S** Great Plains Health Alliance, Inc., Phillipsburg, KS **Web address:** www.gpha.com	23	10	54	517	31	8702	35	3716	1863	88
STAFFORD—Stafford County										
★ STAFFORD DISTRICT HOSPITAL, 502 South Buckeye Street, Zip 67578–2035, Mailing Address: P.O. Box 190, Zip 67578–0190; tel. 316/234–5221; Vernon Minnis, Administrator and Chief Executive Officer **A**9 10 **F**25 32 36 69 70 76 **P**3	16	10	33	615	5	920	0	2010	1000	43
SYRACUSE—Hamilton County										
HAMILTON COUNTY HOSPITAL, East Avenue G and Huser Street, Zip 67878–0948, Mailing Address: P.O. Box 948, Zip 67878–0948; tel. 316/384–7461; Cynthia D. Akers, R.N., Administrator **A**9 10 18 **F**16 22 25 37 44 48 69 76 **Web address:** www.phn.org	13	10	68	210	3	6959	0	2129	1044	97
TOPEKA—Shawnee County										
□ C. F. MENNINGER MEMORIAL HOSPITAL, (Includes Child and Adolescent Services of the Menninger Clinic), 5800 West Sixth Avenue, Zip 66606–9699, Mailing Address: P.O. Box 829, Zip 66601–0829; tel. 785/350–5000; Efrain Bleiberg, M.D., President and Chief of Staff **A**1 3 9 10 **F**17 18 57 58 63 64 **P**1 **Web address:** www.menninger.edu	23	22	143	2238	125	92607	0	37220	19586	480
COLMERY–O'NEIL VETERANS AFFAIRS MEDICAL CENTER See Veterans Affairs Eastern Kansas Health Care System										
KANSAS NEUROLOGICAL INSTITUTE, 3107 West 21st Street, Zip 66604–3298; tel. 785/296–5301; Leon Owens, Superintendent **F**23 69 **P**1	12	12	214	9	203	0	0	24718	15859	668
□ △ KANSAS REHABILITATION HOSPITAL, 1504 S.W. Eighth Avenue, Zip 66606–1632; tel. 785/235–6600; Julie De Jean, Administrator and Chief Executive Officer **A**1 7 10 **F**13 16 28 31 45 49 51 53 54 63 70 71 72 78 79	33	46	79	924	41	—	0	8564	4409	182
★ △ ST. FRANCIS HOSPITAL AND MEDICAL CENTER, 1700 West Seventh Street, Zip 66606–1690; tel. 785/295–8000; Sister Loretto Marie Colwell, President and Chief Executive Officer **A**1 2 3 5 7 9 10 **F**3 4 7 8 9 11 13 17 18 19 22 23 24 25 27 28 31 32 34 35 36 37 38 39 41 43 44 45 46 47 48 49 50 51 53 54 55 56 61 65 68 70 72 76 78 **P**8 **S** Sisters of Charity of Leavenworth Health Services Corporation, Leavenworth, KS **Web address:** www.stfrancistopeka.org	21	10	269	10147	136	281841	1035	110343	51076	1366
★ STORMONT–VAIL HEALTHCARE, 1500 S.W. Tenth Avenue, Zip 66604–1301; tel. 785/354–6000; Maynard F. Oliverius, President and Chief Executive Officer **A**1 3 5 9 10 **F**4 7 8 9 11 12 13 16 17 18 19 22 24 25 27 28 30 31 32 33 34 35 36 37 38 39 40 41 42 43 44 45 46 47 48 49 50 51 52 54 57 60 61 62 63 65 70 71 72 76 78 79 **P**6 **Web address:** www.stormontvail.org	23	10	295	11859	160	111772	1933	171271	89343	2234
★ VETERANS AFFAIRS EASTERN KANSAS HEALTH CARE SYSTEM, (Includes Colmery–O'Neil Veterans Affairs Medical Center, 2200 Gage Boulevard, tel. 785/350–3111; Dwight D. Eisenhower Veterans Affairs Medical Center, 4101 South Fourth Street Trafficway, Leavenworth, Zip 66048–5055; tel. 913/682–2000), 2200 Gage Boulevard, Zip 66622–0002; tel. 785/350–3111; Edgar L. Tucker, Director (Total facility includes 388 beds in nursing home–type unit) **A**1 3 5 9 **F**3 4 5 6 9 11 13 16 17 18 19 21 22 23 24 25 26 27 28 29 30 31 32 33 34 35 36 37 38 39 41 43 44 45 46 47 48 49 50 51 53 54 56 57 59 60 61 62 63 64 65 66 68 69 70 72 75 76 77 78 79 **S** Department of Veterans Affairs, Washington, DC **Web address:** www.va.gov/stations97/guide/home.asp?DIVISION=ALL	45	10	588	5865	538	320798	0	127425	74323	1570
TRIBUNE—Greeley County										
★ GREELEY COUNTY HOSPITAL, 506 Third Street, Zip 67879–0338, Mailing Address: P.O. Box 338, Zip 67879–0338; tel. 316/376–4221; Jerrell J. Horton, Chief Executive Officer (Total facility includes 32 beds in nursing home–type unit) **A**9 10 **F**8 9 17 18 22 23 25 31 36 37 40 43 48 51 54 61 62 69 70 71 72 76 **P**6 **S** Great Plains Health Alliance, Inc., Phillipsburg, KS **Web address:** www.gpha.com	23	10	48	416	32	6580	44	3378	1691	105
ULYSSES—Grant County										
★ BOB WILSON MEMORIAL GRANT COUNTY HOSPITAL, 415 North Main Street, Zip 67880–2133; tel. 316/356–1266; Steven G. Daniel, Administrator **A**9 10 **F**8 9 18 22 25 32 36 37 39 41 44 48 54 59 70 76 **P**6 **S** Quorum Health Group, Brentwood, TN **Web address:** www.phn.org	13	10	30	795	7	13942	113	8088	3513	105

Hospitals, U.S. / KANSAS

Hospital, Address, Telephone, Administrator, Approval, Facility, and Physician Codes, Health Care System, Network	Classification Codes		Utilization Data					Expense (thousands) of dollars		
★ American Hospital Association (AHA) membership □ Joint Commission on Accreditation of Healthcare Organizations (JCAHO) accreditation + American Osteopathic Healthcare Association (AOHA) membership ○ American Osteopathic Association (AOA) accreditation △ Commission on Accreditation of Rehabilitation Facilities (CARF) accreditation Control codes 61, 63, 64, 71, 72 and 73 indicate hospitals listed by AOHA, but not registered by AHA. For definition of numerical codes, see page A4	Control	Service	Staffed Beds	Admissions	Census	Outpatient Visits	Births	Total	Payroll	Personnel
WAKEENEY—Trego County ★ TREGO COUNTY–LEMKE MEMORIAL HOSPITAL, 320 North 13th Street, Zip 67672–2099; tel. 785/743–2182; Lisa J. Freeborn, R.N., Administrator (Total facility includes 45 beds in nursing home–type unit) **A**9 10 **F**7 9 17 18 22 25 31 32 36 39 48 50 54 69 70 76 **S** Great Plains Health Alliance, Inc., Phillipsburg, KS Web address: www.gpha.com	13	10	73	769	52	4876	0	4755	2135	104
WAMEGO—Pottawatomie County ★ WAMEGO CITY HOSPITAL, 711 Genn Drive, Zip 66547–1179; tel. 785/456–2295; William K. Mahoney, Chief Executive Officer **A**9 10 **F**9 16 17 18 21 22 25 28 32 33 34 36 37 38 39 43 45 46 48 49 50 51 53 54 56 69 70 72 76 79 **P**6	14	10	24	534	6	10908	0	4341	2311	97
WASHINGTON—Washington County WASHINGTON COUNTY HOSPITAL, 304 East Third Street, Zip 66968–2033; tel. 785/325–2211; Everett Lutjemeier, Administrator **A**9 10 **F**1 8 9 10 16 17 18 22 25 28 32 36 39 40 41 44 48 54 56 69 70 76 **P**5	13	10	27	297	6	4172	7	1674	774	35
WELLINGTON—Sumner County ★ SUMNER REGIONAL MEDICAL CENTER, 1323 North A Street, Zip 67152–1323, Mailing Address: P.O. Box 509, Zip 67152–0509; tel. 316/326–7453; Raymond Williams, II, CHE, President and Chief Executive Officer (Total facility includes 13 beds in nursing home–type unit) **A**9 10 **F**7 8 9 16 17 18 22 24 25 34 36 38 39 40 44 45 46 48 51 54 57 62 69 76 **P**8	15	10	80	1305	22	29292	161	9465	4314	129
WICHITA—Sedgwick County + ○ RIVERSIDE HEALTH SYSTEM, 2622 West Central Avenue, Zip 67203–4902; tel. 316/946–5000; Robert Dixon, President and Chief Executive Officer (Total facility includes 22 beds in nursing home–type unit) **A**9 10 11 12 13 **F**7 8 9 12 13 14 16 17 18 19 20 22 23 24 25 26 30 32 33 34 35 36 38 39 42 43 45 46 48 49 50 51 54 59 61 66 69 70 71 72 76 77 78 **P**3 6 ST. JOSEPH CAMPUS See Via Christi Regional Medical Center	23	10	125	3685	49	35977	260	43030	21451	593
✠ VETERANS AFFAIRS MEDICAL AND REGIONAL OFFICE CENTER, 5500 East Kellogg, Zip 67218; tel. 316/685–2221; Kent D. Hill, Director **A**1 3 5 **F**1 2 3 4 9 11 12 13 16 17 18 19 20 22 23 24 25 26 30 31 32 34 35 36 37 39 41 43 45 46 47 48 49 50 51 53 54 56 57 59 60 61 62 63 64 65 69 70 72 76 77 78 79 **P**6 **S** Department of Veterans Affairs, Washington, DC Web address: www.va.gov/stations97/guide/home.asp?DIVISION=ALL	45	10	41	2062	38	129593	0	44025	26212	519
✠ △ VIA CHRISTI REGIONAL MEDICAL CENTER, (Includes St. Francis Campus, 929 North St. Francis Street, tel. 316/268–5000; St. Joseph Campus, 3600 East Harry Street, Zip 67218–3713; tel. 316/685–1111), 929 North St. Francis Street, Zip 67214–3882; tel. 316/268–5000; Randall G. Nyp, President and Chief Executive Officer **A**1 3 5 7 10 **F**2 4 5 6 7 8 9 10 11 12 13 14 17 18 19 20 21 22 24 25 27 28 29 30 31 32 33 34 35 36 38 39 41 42 43 44 45 46 47 48 49 50 51 52 54 55 56 57 59 60 61 62 63 64 65 66 68 69 70 71 72 73 74 75 76 77 78 79 **P**3 6 7 **S** Via Christi Health System, Wichita, KS Web address: www.via-christi.org	21	10	942	36037	552	291584	3642	357080	150571	4575
VIA CHRISTI REHABILITATION CENTER, 1151 North Rock Road, Zip 67206–1262; tel. 316/634–3400; Laurie Labarca, Chief Operating Officer (Total facility includes 20 beds in nursing home–type unit) **A**10 **F**1 2 3 4 6 7 8 9 10 11 12 13 14 16 17 18 19 20 21 22 23 24 25 26 27 28 29 30 31 32 33 34 35 36 37 38 39 41 42 43 44 46 47 48 49 50 51 52 53 54 55 57 58 59 60 61 62 63 64 65 67 68 69 70 71 72 73 75 76 77 78 79 **P**1 3 4 5 6 Web address: www.via-christi.org	21	46	60	735	35	49170	0	11757	6723	212
✠ WESLEY MEDICAL CENTER, 550 North Hillside Avenue, Zip 67214–4976; tel. 316/688–2000; Carl W. Fitch, Sr, President and Chief Executive Officer **A**1 2 3 5 9 10 **F**4 8 9 11 12 13 17 18 22 24 25 27 28 30 31 38 39 41 42 44 45 46 47 48 50 51 52 54 56 57 62 65 66 68 69 70 75 76 78 79 **P**6 **S** HCA – The Healthcare Company, Nashville, TN Web address: www.wesleymc.com	33	10	534	24473	344	247482	5022	233743	91298	2240
□ WESLEY REHABILITATION HOSPITAL, 8338 West 13th Street North, Zip 67212–2984; tel. 316/729–9999; Robyn Chadwick, Administrator **A**1 10 **F**16 17 18 38 49 53 54 71 **S** HEALTHSOUTH Corporation, Birmingham, AL	33	46	65	598	33	13028	0	7709	3457	139
WINCHESTER—Jefferson County JEFFERSON COUNTY MEMORIAL HOSPITAL, 408 Delaware Street, Zip 66097–4002, Mailing Address: Rural Route 1, Box 1, Zip 66097–0001; tel. 913/774–4340; Joye H. Huston, Acting Chief Executive Officer (Total facility includes 70 beds in nursing home–type unit) **A**9 18 **F**16 22 25 30 43 45 69 70 78	23	10	95	66	52	3133	0	3634	1953	66
WINFIELD—Cowley County ★ WILLIAM NEWTON MEMORIAL HOSPITAL, 1300 East Fifth Street, Zip 67156–2407; tel. 316/221–2300; Richard H. Vaught, Administrator (Total facility includes 14 beds in nursing home–type unit) **A**9 10 **F**7 8 9 14 15 17 18 22 24 25 31 32 34 36 39 40 41 43 44 45 46 48 49 50 51 54 57 63 69 70 71 72 76 78 **P**8 Web address: www.wnmh.org	14	10	63	1400	14	39555	284	14119	7574	258

© 2000 AHA Guide   *Many Facility Codes have changed. Please refer to the AHA Guide Code Chart.*

KENTUCKY

Resident Population 3,936 (in thousands)
Resident population in metro areas 48.2%
Birth rate per 1,000 population 13.6
65 years and over 12.5%
Percent of persons without health insurance 15.0%

★ American Hospital Association (AHA) membership
□ Joint Commission on Accreditation of Healthcare Organizations (JCAHO) accreditation
+ American Osteopathic Healthcare Association (AOHA) membership
○ American Osteopathic Association (AOA) accreditation
△ Commission on Accreditation of Rehabilitation Facilities (CARF) accreditation
Control codes 61, 63, 64, 71, 72 and 73 indicate hospitals listed by AOHA, but not registered by AHA. For definition of numerical codes, see page A4

Hospital, Address, Telephone, Administrator, Approval, Facility, and Physician Codes, Health Care System, Network	Classification Codes		Utilization Data					Expense (thousands) of dollars		
	Control	Service	Staffed Beds	Admissions	Census	Outpatient Visits	Births	Total	Payroll	Personnel
ALBANY—Clinton County CLINTON COUNTY HOSPITAL, 723 Burkesville Road, Zip 42602–1654; tel. 606/387–6421; Randel Flowers, Ph.D., Administrator **A**9 10 **F**7 9 17 18 22 25 38 41 54 70 76 78	23	10	42	1928	23	15191	—	6591	3140	122
ASHLAND—Boyd County ★ △ KING'S DAUGHTERS MEDICAL CENTER, 2201 Lexington Avenue, Zip 41101–2874, Mailing Address: P.O. Box 151, Zip 41105–0151; tel. 606/327–4000; Fred L. Jackson, Chief Executive Officer (Total facility includes 10 beds in nursing home–type unit) **A**1 2 7 9 10 **F**1 4 7 8 9 11 13 17 18 19 20 22 24 25 26 27 29 31 32 33 34 35 36 37 38 39 40 41 42 43 44 45 46 47 48 49 50 51 53 54 55 56 57 58 59 60 61 62 63 65 68 69 70 71 72 76 77 78 79 **P**8 Web address: www.kdmc.com	23	10	341	17650	252	146796	942	148568	60032	1645
□ OUR LADY OF BELLEFONTE HOSPITAL, St. Christopher Drive, Zip 41101, Mailing Address: P.O. Box 789, Zip 41105–0789; tel. 606/833–3333; Robert J. Maher, President (Nonreporting) **A**1 2 9 10 **S** Franciscan Health Partnership, Inc., Latham, NY Web address: www.olbh.com	21	10	194	—	—	—	—	—	—	—
BARBOURVILLE—Knox County ★ KNOX COUNTY HOSPITAL, 321 High Street, Zip 40906–1317, Mailing Address: P.O. Box 160, Zip 40906–0160; tel. 606/546–4175; Craig Morgan, Administrator (Total facility includes 16 beds in nursing home–type unit) (Nonreporting) **A**1 9 10 Web address: www.barbourville.com	13	10	58	—	—	—	—	—	—	—
BARDSTOWN—Nelson County ★ FLAGET MEMORIAL HOSPITAL, 201 Cathedral Manor, Zip 40004–1299; tel. 502/348–3923; Suzanne Reasbeck, President and Chief Executive Officer **A**1 9 10 **F**7 8 9 12 19 22 23 25 26 30 32 33 34 37 38 39 45 46 48 49 51 54 56 69 72 76 78 **S** Catholic Health Initiatives, Denver, CO Web address: www.flaget.com	23	10	52	2535	27	29431	345	20283	8870	386
BENTON—Marshall County ★ MARSHALL COUNTY HOSPITAL, 503 George McClain Drive, Zip 42025, Mailing Address: P.O. Box 630, Zip 42025–0630; tel. 270/527–4800; Kathy Long, Chief Executive Officer (Total facility includes 34 beds in nursing home–type unit) **A**1 9 10 **F**7 9 17 18 22 24 25 30 32 36 39 41 46 48 54 64 69 76 **P**6 **S** Quorum Health Group, Brentwood, TN Web address: www.healthcareonline.org	13	10	80	1051	51	18628	0	9393	4234	199
BEREA—Madison County ★ BEREA HOSPITAL, 305 Estill Street, Zip 40403–1909; tel. 859/986–3151; David E. Burgio, FACHE, President and Chief Executive Officer (Total facility includes 102 beds in nursing home–type unit) **A**1 9 10 **F**7 9 13 16 17 18 19 20 22 23 24 25 30 31 32 34 35 38 39 41 43 45 48 51 54 65 69 70 72 76 77 78 79 **P**6	23	10	150	2034	108	50495	0	22366	9186	422
BOWLING GREEN—Warren County ★ GREENVIEW REGIONAL HOSPITAL, 1801 Ashley Circle, Zip 42104–3384, Mailing Address: P.O. Box 90024, Zip 42102–9024; tel. 270/793–1000; Phillip A. Clendenin, Chief Executive Officer **A**1 9 10 **F**8 9 11 12 13 16 17 18 19 22 23 24 25 26 27 32 33 34 37 38 39 41 43 44 45 46 48 49 50 51 54 65 70 71 72 73 75 76 78 79 **P**7 8 **S** HCA – The Healthcare Company, Nashville, TN Web address: www.greenviewhospital.com	33	10	211	5535	81	54494	776	—	—	500
□ △ MEDIPLEX REHABILITATION HOSPITAL, 1300 Campbell Lane, Zip 42104–4162; tel. 270/782–6900; Shala S. Wilson, R.N., Chief Executive Officer **A**1 7 9 10 **F**13 16 53 70 72 **S** Sun Healthcare Group, Albuquerque, NM Web address: www.sunh.com	33	46	60	1093	57	0	0	15355	4102	166
★ THE MEDICAL CENTER AT BOWLING GREEN, (Includes Medical Center at Scottsville, 456 Burnley Road, Scottsville, Zip 42164–6355; tel. 502/622–2800; Sarah Moore, Vice President), 250 Park Street, Zip 42101–1795, Mailing Address: P.O. Box 90010, Zip 42102–9010; tel. 270/745–1000; Connie Smith, Chief Executive Officer (Total facility includes 105 beds in nursing home–type unit) **A**9 10 **F**1 4 8 9 11 12 13 19 20 21 22 23 24 25 28 29 30 31 32 33 34 35 36 38 39 41 42 43 44 45 46 47 48 49 50 51 54 55 56 57 59 60 61 62 63 64 65 69 70 72 75 76 77 78 79 **P**1	23	10	506	12406	305	50789	1217	—	—	1499
BURKESVILLE—Cumberland County ★ CUMBERLAND COUNTY HOSPITAL, Highway 90 West, Zip 42717–0280, Mailing Address: P.O. Box 280, Zip 42717–0280; tel. 270/864–2511; Edward J. Sanford, Chief Executive Officer **A**9 10 **F**9 17 22 24 25 32 33 38 54 70 76 **S** Quorum Health Group, Brentwood, TN	23	10	31	1530	18	17925	0	5685	2321	100
CADIZ—Trigg County ★ TRIGG COUNTY HOSPITAL, Highway 68 East, Zip 42211, Mailing Address: P.O. Box 312, Zip 42211–0312; tel. 270/522–3215; Richard Chapman, Administrator **A**9 10 **F**22 24 25 31 36 38 43 48 51 54 56 70 71 76 78	13	10	27	375	7	30196	—	4501	1976	87

Hospitals, U.S. / KENTUCKY

Hospital, Address, Telephone, Administrator, Approval, Facility, and Physician Codes, Health Care System, Network	Classification Codes		Utilization Data					Expense (thousands) of dollars		
★ American Hospital Association (AHA) membership □ Joint Commission on Accreditation of Healthcare Organizations (JCAHO) accreditation + American Osteopathic Healthcare Association (AOHA) membership ○ American Osteopathic Association (AOA) accreditation △ Commission on Accreditation of Rehabilitation Facilities (CARF) accreditation Control codes 61, 63, 64, 71, 72 and 73 indicate hospitals listed by AOHA, but not registered by AHA. For definition of numerical codes, see page A4	Control	Service	Staffed Beds	Admissions	Census	Outpatient Visits	Births	Total	Payroll	Personnel
CAMPBELLSVILLE—Taylor County										
✠ TAYLOR COUNTY HOSPITAL, 1700 Old Lebanon Road, Zip 42718-9600; tel. 270/465-3561; David R. Hayes, President **A**1 2 9 10 **F**7 8 9 11 16 17 20 22 24 25 26 27 31 32 33 34 36 37 39 41 43 44 46 48 49 50 51 54 55 68 75 76 78 **S** Jewish Hospital HealthCare Services, Louisville, KY	16	10	90	3332	41	43802	326	26572	9730	357
CARLISLE—Nicholas County										
✠ NICHOLAS COUNTY HOSPITAL, (Includes Johnson-Mathers Nursing Home), 2323 Concrete Road, Zip 40311-9721, Mailing Address: P.O. Box 232, Zip 40311-0232; tel. 606/289-7181; Doris Ecton, Administrator and Chief Executive Officer (Total facility includes 104 beds in nursing home-type unit) **A**1 9 10 **F**1 7 9 17 18 22 25 32 34 45 48 54 69 70 76 78	23	10	122	837	110	11883	0	6994	3621	156
CARROLLTON—Carroll County										
★ CARROLL COUNTY HOSPITAL, 309 11th Street, Zip 41008-1400; tel. 502/732-4321; Roger Williams, Chief Executive Officer (Nonreporting) **A**9 10 **S** Norton Healthcare, Louisville, KY **Web address:** www.nortonhealthcare.com	13	10	39	—	—	—	—	—	—	—
COLUMBIA—Adair County										
□ WESTLAKE REGIONAL HOSPITAL, Westlake Drive, Zip 42728-1149, Mailing Address: P.O. Box 468, Zip 42728-0468; tel. 270/384-4753; Rex A. Tungate, Administrator (Nonreporting) **A**1 9 10	16	10	80	—	—	—	—	—	—	—
CORBIN—Whitley County										
✠ BAPTIST REGIONAL MEDICAL CENTER, 1 Trillium Way, Zip 40701-8420; tel. 606/528-1212; John S. Henson, President (Total facility includes 23 beds in nursing home-type unit) **A**1 9 10 **F**2 3 7 8 9 11 12 13 17 18 19 21 22 24 25 28 32 34 38 39 41 44 48 50 53 54 57 58 59 60 61 62 63 64 68 69 70 72 76 78 79 **P**8 **S** Baptist Healthcare System, Louisville, KY **Web address:** www.bhsi.com	23	10	263	10623	159	66642	963	61435	25610	1085
COVINGTON—Kenton County										
HEALTHSOUTH NORTHERN KENTUCKY REHABILITATION HOSPITAL, 201 Medical Village Drive, Zip 41017-3407; tel. 606/341-2044; Timothy W. Mitchell, Chief Executive Officer **A**9 10 **F**13 19 22 24 30 31 33 38 39 43 45 46 50 53 54 70 71 72 76 78 79 **S** HEALTHSOUTH Corporation, Birmingham, AL	33	46	40	585	39	12433	0	6603	4250	120
NORTHKEY COMMUNITY CARE, (Formerly Children's Psychiatric Hospital), 502 Farrell Drive, Zip 41011-3799, Mailing Address: P.O. Box 2680, Zip 41012-2680; tel. 859/578-3200; Edward G. Muntel, Ph.D., President and Chief Executive Officer **A**9 10 **F**1 3 13 17 18 19 21 34 38 57 58 59 60 61 63 64 70 72 73 **P**5	23	52	51	438	17	0	0	3098	1387	54
ST. ELIZABETH MEDICAL CENTER-NORTH See St. Elizabeth Medical Center-South, Edgewood										
CYNTHIANA—Harrison County										
✠ HARRISON MEMORIAL HOSPITAL, Millersburg Road, Zip 41031-0250, Mailing Address: P.O. Box 250, Zip 41031-0250; tel. 859/234-2300; Darwin E. Root, Administrator (Total facility includes 38 beds in nursing home-type unit) **A**1 9 10 **F**7 8 9 16 22 24 25 28 30 32 34 36 37 38 39 41 43 44 46 48 54 68 69 70 72 76 78 **P**8	23	10	99	2069	55	40737	215	17326	7020	221
DANVILLE—Boyle County										
✠ EPHRAIM MCDOWELL REGIONAL MEDICAL CENTER, 217 South Third Street, Zip 40422-9983; tel. 606/239-1000; Thomas W. Smith, President and Chief Executive Officer (Total facility includes 25 beds in nursing home-type unit) (Nonreporting) **A**1 9 10 **Web address:** www.emrmc.com	23	10	177	—	—	—	—	—	—	—
EDGEWOOD—Kenton County										
□ ST. ELIZABETH MEDICAL CENTER-SOUTH, (Includes St. Elizabeth Medical Center-North, 401 East 20th Street, Covington, Zip 41014-1585; tel. 859/292-4000), One Medical Village Drive, Zip 41017; tel. 859/344-2000; Joseph W. Gross, President and Chief Executive Officer (Total facility includes 33 beds in nursing home-type unit) **A**1 2 3 9 10 **F**3 4 7 8 9 11 12 13 16 17 18 19 20 22 24 25 26 32 35 36 37 38 41 42 43 44 45 46 47 48 54 57 60 61 63 64 65 69 71 72 73 76 78 79 **P**6 **S** Catholic Healthcare Partners, Cincinnati, OH **Web address:** www.stelizabeth.com	21	10	397	21050	235	355175	2981	208244	96066	2528
ELIZABETHTOWN—Hardin County										
✠ HARDIN MEMORIAL HOSPITAL, 913 North Dixie Avenue, Zip 42701-2599; tel. 270/737-1212; David L. Gray, President (Total facility includes 15 beds in nursing home-type unit) **A**1 9 10 **F**4 7 8 9 11 12 13 17 18 22 23 24 25 27 32 33 34 36 38 39 41 43 44 45 46 47 48 49 50 51 54 57 61 63 65 68 69 70 72 76 77 78 79 **S** Baptist Healthcare System, Louisville, KY **Web address:** www.hmh.net	13	10	262	11402	169	130496	1335	88948	39369	1135
□ △ HEALTHSOUTH REHABILITATION HOSPITAL OF CENTRAL KENTUCKY, (Formerly Lakeview Rehabilitation Hospital), 134 Heartland Drive, Zip 42701-2778; tel. 270/769-3100; Mark K. Floro, Chief Operating Officer **A**1 7 9 10 **F**13 17 18 29 32 34 38 53 54 72 **S** HEALTHSOUTH Corporation, Birmingham, AL	33	46	40	728	35	9800	—	6848	3712	123
FLEMINGSBURG—Fleming County										
✠ FLEMING COUNTY HOSPITAL, 920 Elizaville Avenue, Zip 41041, Mailing Address: P.O. Box 388, Zip 41041-0388; tel. 606/849-5000; Luther E. Reeves, Chief Executive Officer **A**1 9 10 **F**7 9 13 22 25 32 37 39 41 45 46 48 54 70 76 **S** Quorum Health Group, Brentwood, TN	16	10	43	1464	17	27847	0	4692	4173	155

© 2000 AHA Guide   *Many Facility Codes have changed. Please refer to the AHA Guide Code Chart.*

Hospitals, U.S. / KENTUCKY

Hospital, Address, Telephone, Administrator, Approval, Facility, and Physician Codes, Health Care System, Network	Classification Codes		Utilization Data					Expense (thousands) of dollars		
★ American Hospital Association (AHA) membership ☐ Joint Commission on Accreditation of Healthcare Organizations (JCAHO) accreditation + American Osteopathic Healthcare Association (AOHA) membership ○ American Osteopathic Association (AOA) accreditation △ Commission on Accreditation of Rehabilitation Facilities (CARF) accreditation Control codes 61, 63, 64, 71, 72 and 73 indicate hospitals listed by AOHA, but not registered by AHA. For definition of numerical codes, see page A4	Control	Service	Staffed Beds	Admissions	Census	Outpatient Visits	Births	Total	Payroll	Personnel
FLORENCE—Boone County ★ ST. LUKE HOSPITAL WEST, 7380 Turfway Road, Zip 41042-1337; tel. 859/962-5200; Daniel M. Vinson, CPA, Senior Vice President (Total facility includes 24 beds in nursing home-type unit) **A**9 10 **F**2 3 4 5 7 8 9 10 11 12 13 14 15 16 17 18 19 20 21 22 23 24 25 26 27 28 29 30 31 32 33 34 35 36 37 38 39 40 41 42 43 44 45 46 47 48 49 50 51 53 54 55 56 57 58 59 60 61 62 63 64 65 66 68 69 70 71 72 73 74 75 76 77 78 79 **P**6 8 **S** Health Alliance of Greater Cincinnati, Cincinnati, OH **Web address:** www.health-alliance.com	23	10	168	8164	85	89695	879	55570	22210	612
FORT CAMPBELL—Christian County ☒ COLONEL FLORENCE A. BLANCHFIELD ARMY COMMUNITY HOSPITAL, 650 Joel Drive, Zip 42223-5349; tel. 270/798-8040; Colonel Virgil T. Deal, Commander (Nonreporting) **A**1 2 **S** Department of the Army, Office of the Surgeon General, Falls Church, VA **Web address:** 198.250.216.210/	42	10	107	—	—	—	—	—	—	—
FORT KNOX—Hardin County ☒ IRELAND ARMY COMMUNITY HOSPITAL, 851 Ireland Loop, Zip 40121-5520; tel. 502/624-9020; Lieutenant Colonel David Huddleston, Deputy Commander for Administration (Nonreporting) **A**1 5 **S** Department of the Army, Office of the Surgeon General, Falls Church, VA	42	10	76	—	—	—	—	—	—	—
FORT THOMAS—Campbell County ★ ST. LUKE HOSPITAL EAST, 85 North Grand Avenue, Zip 41075-1796; tel. 869/572-3100; Daniel M. Vinson, CPA, Senior Vice President (Total facility includes 26 beds in nursing home-type unit) **A**1 2 9 10 **F**2 3 4 5 7 8 9 10 11 12 13 14 15 16 17 18 19 20 21 22 23 24 25 26 27 28 29 30 31 32 33 34 35 36 37 38 39 40 41 42 43 44 45 46 47 48 49 50 51 53 54 55 56 57 58 59 60 61 62 63 64 65 66 68 69 70 71 72 73 74 75 76 77 78 79 **P**6 8 **S** Health Alliance of Greater Cincinnati, Cincinnati, OH **Web address:** www.health-alliance.com	23	10	211	8843	95	86172	855	61974	23449	801
FRANKFORT—Franklin County ☒ FRANKFORT REGIONAL MEDICAL CENTER, 299 King's Daughters Drive, Zip 40601-4186; tel. 502/875-5240; David P. Steitz, Chief Executive Officer **A**1 9 10 **F**2 7 8 9 11 12 13 16 17 19 22 23 24 25 32 33 36 37 38 39 41 43 44 45 46 48 50 51 54 56 57 59 63 65 68 70 71 72 76 78 79 **S** HCA - The Healthcare Company, Nashville, TN **Web address:** www.frankfortregional.com	33	10	146	4945	58	30354	549	29340	12875	510
FRANKLIN—Simpson County ★ THE MEDICAL CENTER AT FRANKLIN, (Formerly Franklin-Simpson Memorial Hospital), Brookhaven Road, Zip 42135-2929, Mailing Address: P.O. Box 2929, Zip 42135-2929; tel. 270/586-3253; Jeffrey L. Durham, Chief Executive Officer **A**9 10 **F**9 22 25 30 32 38 53 54 57 62 69 76	13	10	13	695	8	12197	0	5782	2266	79
FULTON—Fulton County ☐ PARKWAY REGIONAL HOSPITAL, 2000 Holiday Lane, Zip 42041; tel. 270/472-2522; Michael Patterson, Chief Executive Officer **A**1 9 10 **F**2 8 9 13 17 18 22 25 29 32 34 36 38 39 41 43 45 48 54 71 76 77 78 79 **S** Community Health Systems, Inc., Brentwood, TN	33	10	38	1436	15	14500	130	—	—	—
GEORGETOWN—Scott County ☒ GEORGETOWN COMMUNITY HOSPITAL, 1140 Lexington Road, Zip 40324-9362; tel. 502/868-1100; Jeffrey G. Seraphine, President and Chief Executive Officer **A**1 9 10 **F**8 9 13 17 18 22 24 25 32 39 40 41 44 45 48 54 68 69 70 71 76 78 **S** LifePoint Hospitals, Inc., Brentwood, TN	33	10	58	2022	20	28645	457	14302	6216	186
GLASGOW—Barren County ☒ T. J. SAMSON COMMUNITY HOSPITAL, 1301 North Race Street, Zip 42141-3483; tel. 270/651-4444; Dwayne Moss, Chief Executive Officer (Total facility includes 16 beds in nursing home-type unit) **A**1 3 9 10 **F**1 8 9 11 13 17 18 19 20 22 24 25 27 30 34 36 38 39 41 42 44 45 46 48 50 51 54 56 69 70 72 76 78 **P**5 8 **Web address:** www.glasgow.ky.com	23	10	186	7833	90	71744	952	48614	23337	891
GREENSBURG—Green County ★ JANE TODD CRAWFORD HOSPITAL, 202-206 Milby Street, Zip 42743-1100, Mailing Address: P.O. Box 220, Zip 42743-0220; tel. 270/932-4211; Eddy R. Stockton, Chief Executive Officer (Total facility includes 20 beds in nursing home-type unit) **A**9 10 **F**2 7 9 17 18 22 25 29 30 32 34 38 39 41 45 46 48 49 51 53 54 56 57 58 61 62 63 69 71 72 76	13	10	64	1392	36	27051	0	7830	3463	156
GREENVILLE—Muhlenberg County ☒ MUHLENBERG COMMUNITY HOSPITAL, 440 Hopkinsville Street, Zip 42345-1172, Mailing Address: P.O. Box 387, Zip 42345-0387; tel. 270/338-8000; Albert Pilkington, II, Chief Executive Officer (Total facility includes 45 beds in nursing home-type unit) (Nonreporting) **A**1 9 10 **S** Quorum Health Group, Brentwood, TN	23	10	135	—	—	—	—	—	—	—
HARDINSBURG—Breckinridge County ★ BRECKINRIDGE MEMORIAL HOSPITAL, 1011 Old Highway 60, Zip 40143-2597; tel. 270/756-7000; George Walz, CHE, Chief Executive Officer (Total facility includes 18 beds in nursing home-type unit) **A**9 10 **F**7 9 13 16 22 23 25 36 37 39 48 51 69 76 78 **P**5 **S** Norton Healthcare, Louisville, KY **Web address:** www.multiplan.com	23	10	45	1046	27	36796	0	6290	2825	133
HARLAN—Harlan County ☐ HARLAN ARH HOSPITAL, 81 Ball Park Road, Zip 40831-1792; tel. 606/573-8201; Daniel Fitzpatrick, Chief Executive Officer (Total facility includes 25 beds in nursing home-type unit) **A**1 9 10 **F**7 8 9 17 18 19 22 24 25 32 33 34 38 39 41 43 44 48 50 57 59 60 61 62 63 68 69 76 77 78 **S** Appalachian Regional Healthcare, Lexington, KY	23	10	130	5585	63	84177	288	35024	13369	477

Hospitals, U.S. / KENTUCKY

Hospital, Address, Telephone, Administrator, Approval, Facility, and Physician Codes, Health Care System, Network	Classification Codes		Utilization Data					Expense (thousands) of dollars		
★ American Hospital Association (AHA) membership □ Joint Commission on Accreditation of Healthcare Organizations (JCAHO) accreditation + American Osteopathic Healthcare Association (AOHA) membership ○ American Osteopathic Association (AOA) accreditation △ Commission on Accreditation of Rehabilitation Facilities (CARF) accreditation Control codes 61, 63, 64, 71, 72 and 73 indicate hospitals listed by AOHA, but not registered by AHA. For definition of numerical codes, see page A4	Control	Service	Staffed Beds	Admissions	Census	Outpatient Visits	Births	Total	Payroll	Personnel
HARRODSBURG—Mercer County ★ THE JAMES B. HAGGIN MEMORIAL HOSPITAL, 464 Linden Avenue, Zip 40330-1862; tel. 859/734-5441; Earl James Motzer, Ph.D., FACHE, Chief Executive Officer (Total facility includes 25 beds in nursing home–type unit) **A**9 10 **F**7 9 14 16 17 18 19 22 25 26 32 33 34 36 37 38 43 46 48 54 63 69 70 72 73 76 **S** Norton Healthcare, Louisville, KY	23	10	64	945	41	29326	0	9369	4072	153
HARTFORD—Ohio County ✠ OHIO COUNTY HOSPITAL, 1211 Main Street, Zip 42347-1619; tel. 270/298-7411; Blaine Pieper, Administrator **A**1 9 10 **F**7 8 9 12 13 17 19 20 21 22 23 25 26 28 32 34 37 38 41 45 46 48 49 50 51 54 69 70 76 **P**8 **S** Quorum Health Group, Brentwood, TN **Web address:** www.ohiocountyhospital.com	23	10	49	1353	13	25042	134	13520	5229	189
HAZARD—Perry County □ ARH REGIONAL MEDICAL CENTER, 100 Medical Center Drive, Zip 41701-1000; tel. 606/439-6833; Charles E. Housley, FACHE, Administrator **A**1 2 3 5 10 **F**8 9 11 13 16 17 18 19 22 23 24 25 27 29 33 36 37 39 41 43 44 46 48 49 50 53 54 57 59 60 61 62 65 70 72 76 78 **S** Appalachian Regional Healthcare, Lexington, KY **Web address:** www.arh.org	23	10	288	12308	117	106675	477	69715	27531	869
HENDERSON—Henderson County ✠ METHODIST HOSPITAL, (Formerly Community Methodist Hospital), 1305 North Elm Street, Zip 42420-2775, Mailing Address: P.O. Box 48, Zip 42420-0048; tel. 270/827-7700; Bruce D. Begley, Executive Director (Total facility includes 16 beds in nursing home–type unit) **A**1 9 10 **F**1 3 4 7 8 9 11 13 14 17 18 22 25 27 28 29 30 32 34 35 39 42 43 44 45 46 48 49 50 51 54 55 56 57 58 59 60 61 62 63 64 69 70 71 72 73 76 78 79 **P**8 **Web address:** www.methodisthospital.net	21	10	197	7485	123	172720	886	27140	26793	996
HOPKINSVILLE—Christian County □ CUMBERLAND HALL HOSPITAL, 210 West 17th Street, Zip 42240-1999; tel. 270/886-1919; William C. Heard, Administrator and Chief Executive Officer **A**1 9 10 **F**57 58 63 64 **P**5	33	52	48	939	48	3503	0	—	—	108
✠ JENNIE STUART MEDICAL CENTER, 320 West 18th Street, Zip 42241-2400, Mailing Address: P.O. Box 2400, Zip 42241-2400; tel. 270/887-0100; Lewis T. Peeples, Chief Executive Officer **A**1 2 9 10 **F**7 8 9 11 12 13 16 17 18 19 22 24 25 27 34 36 38 39 41 44 45 46 48 49 50 54 65 68 70 71 76 78 **S** Quorum Health Group, Brentwood, TN **Web address:** www.jsmc.org	23	10	139	6281	76	87058	615	50036	17168	558
□ WESTERN STATE HOSPITAL, Russellville Road, Zip 42241, Mailing Address: P.O. Box 2200, Zip 42241-2200; tel. 270/886-4431; Stephen P. Wiggins, Director (Total facility includes 144 beds in nursing home–type unit) **A**1 10 **F**23 31 43 45 50 51 57 60 61 62 69 70 72 78 **P**6	12	22	309	1310	278	0	0	19896	—	573
HORSE CAVE—Hart County ★ CAVERNA MEMORIAL HOSPITAL, 1501 South Dixie Street, Zip 42749-1477; tel. 270/786-2191; Alan B. Alexander, Administrator **A**9 10 **F**9 17 18 22 25 32 34 38 41 48 69 76 **S** Norton Healthcare, Louisville, KY	23	10	28	636	8	8403	24	1629	1550	73
HYDEN—Leslie County MARY BRECKINRIDGE HOSPITAL, 130 Kate Ireland Drive, Zip 41749-0000; tel. 606/672-2901; Mallie S. Noble, Administrator **A**9 10 **F**7 8 9 22 25 32 36 44 48 54 70 76 79	23	10	40	1692	16	45397	137	15576	7429	258
IRVINE—Estill County MARCUM AND WALLACE MEMORIAL HOSPITAL, 60 Mercy Court, Zip 40336-1331, Mailing Address: P.O. Box 928, Zip 40336-0928; tel. 606/723-2115; James F. Heitzenrater, President and Chief Executive Officer **A**9 10 **F**9 22 25 32 48 54 76 **P**8 **S** Catholic Healthcare Partners, Cincinnati, OH	21	10	25	584	6	45475	0	4971	2050	79
JACKSON—Breathitt County □ KENTUCKY RIVER MEDICAL CENTER, 540 Jett Drive, Zip 41339-9620; tel. 606/666-6305; O. David Bevins, Chief Executive Officer **A**1 9 10 **F**9 16 17 18 22 25 27 30 32 34 35 38 39 41 45 46 48 54 70 71 76 78 79 **P**7 **S** Community Health Systems, Inc., Brentwood, TN	33	10	49	3712	27	34599	2	22398	6952	199
JENKINS—Letcher County □ JENKINS COMMUNITY HOSPITAL, Main Street, Zip 41537-9614, Mailing Address: P.O. Box 472, Zip 41537-0472; tel. 606/832-2171; Sherrie Newcomb, Administrator **A**1 9 10 **F**13 17 22 25 28 32 36 38 41 48 76	31	10	60	608	4	100521	0	5987	3369	122
LA GRANGE—Oldham County ✠ TRI COUNTY BAPTIST HOSPITAL, 1025 New Moody Lane, Zip 40031-0559; tel. 502/222-5388; Dennis B. Johnson, Administrator (Total facility includes 30 beds in nursing home–type unit) **A**1 9 10 **F**7 8 9 13 17 18 22 24 25 32 34 38 41 43 44 45 46 48 49 51 54 59 61 63 69 70 72 76 78 79 **S** Baptist Healthcare System, Louisville, KY **Web address:** www.tri-countybaptist.com	23	10	105	3090	52	35313	362	21875	10112	269
LANCASTER—Garrard County GARRARD COUNTY MEMORIAL HOSPITAL, 308 West Maple Avenue, Zip 40444-1098; tel. 859/792-6844; John P. Rigsby, Administrator (Total facility includes 112 beds in nursing home–type unit) **A**9 10 **F**7 9 13 22 23 25 31 37 38 45 48 54 69 70 76 78 **P**5	13	10	131	677	102	11715	0	7753	3878	219

© 2000 AHA Guide   *Many Facility Codes have changed. Please refer to the AHA Guide Code Chart.*

Hospitals, U.S. / KENTUCKY

Hospital, Address, Telephone, Administrator, Approval, Facility, and Physician Codes, Health Care System, Network	Classification Codes		Utilization Data					Expense (thousands) of dollars		
★ American Hospital Association (AHA) membership ☐ Joint Commission on Accreditation of Healthcare Organizations (JCAHO) accreditation + American Osteopathic Healthcare Association (AOHA) membership ○ American Osteopathic Association (AOA) accreditation △ Commission on Accreditation of Rehabilitation Facilities (CARF) accreditation Control codes 61, 63, 64, 71, 72 and 73 indicate hospitals listed by AOHA, but not registered by AHA. For definition of numerical codes, see page A4	Control	Service	Staffed Beds	Admissions	Census	Outpatient Visits	Births	Total	Payroll	Personnel

LEBANON—Marion County

★ NORTON SPRING VIEW HOSPITAL, (Formerly Spring View Hospital), 320 Loretto Road, Zip 40033-0320; tel. 270/692-3161; Barry A. Papania, Chief Executive Officer (Total facility includes 38 beds in nursing home–type unit) **A**1 9 10 **F**3 4 5 7 8 9 11 12 13 14 16 17 18 19 21 22 23 25 26 27 28 30 32 33 34 35 36 37 38 39 41 42 43 44 45 46 47 48 49 50 51 52 54 57 58 59 60 61 62 63 64 65 66 68 69 70 71 72 73 74 75 76 77 78 79 **P**3 6 7 **S** Norton Healthcare, Louisville, KY
Web address: www.nortonhealthcare.com
23　10　85　2171　29　47564　353　15588　5057　195

LEITCHFIELD—Grayson County

★ TWIN LAKES REGIONAL MEDICAL CENTER, 910 Wallace Avenue, Zip 42754-1499; tel. 270/259-9400; Stephen L. Meredith, Chief Executive Officer **A**1 9 10 **F**9 13 18 22 25 28 36 41 44 48 50 51 54 67 70 71 76 78 **P**6 **S** Norton Healthcare, Louisville, KY
Web address: www.tlrmc.com
23　10　75　1881　26　45666　246　17670　7399　274

LEXINGTON—Fayette County

★ △ CARDINAL HILL REHABILITATION HOSPITAL, 2050 Versailles Road, Zip 40504-1499; tel. 859/254-5701; Kerry G. Gillihan, FACHE, President and Chief Executive Officer **A**3 5 7 9 10 **F**1 7 13 18 19 30 32 36 45 49 50 51 53 54 70 72 76 78 **P**6
Web address: www.cardinalhill.org
23　46　100　1636　74　32152　0　24902　13564　442

★ CENTRAL BAPTIST HOSPITAL, 1740 Nicholasville Road, Zip 40503; tel. 859/260-6100; William G. Sisson, President (Total facility includes 12 beds in nursing home–type unit) **A**1 2 3 5 9 10 **F**4 7 8 9 11 12 13 17 18 19 22 24 25 32 33 34 36 39 41 42 44 45 46 47 48 51 54 65 66 72 76 78 79 **S** Baptist Healthcare System, Louisville, KY
Web address: www.centralbap.com
21　10　355　19539　258　146030　3915　183494　70026　1912

☐ CHARTER RIDGE BEHAVIORAL HEALTH SYSTEM, (Formerly Charter Ridge Hospital), 3050 Rio Dosa Drive, Zip 40509-9990; tel. 606/269-2325; Barbara Kitchen, Chief Executive Officer **A**1 3 5 9 10 **F**2 3 22 23 25 39 57 58 60 63 64 70 72 76 **P**8 **S** Magellan Health Services, Atlanta, GA
33　22　110　2268　59　13721　0　—　—　117

☐ EASTERN STATE HOSPITAL, 627 West Fourth Street, Zip 40508-1294; tel. 606/246-7000; Joseph A. Toy, President and Chief Executive Officer (Nonreporting) **A**1 5 10
12　22　197　—　—　—　—　—　—　—

FEDERAL MEDICAL CENTER, 3301 Leestown Road, Zip 40511-8799; tel. 606/255-6812; Maryellen Thoms, Warden **F**18 29 37 45 49 50 51 70 72 **P**2
48　11　22　109　14　12000　—　—　—　102

★ SAINT JOSEPH HOSPITAL, One St. Joseph Drive, Zip 40504-3754; tel. 606/278-3436; Tom Matherlee, Interim Chief Executive Officer (Total facility includes 22 beds in nursing home–type unit) **A**1 2 3 5 9 10 **F**2 3 4 7 8 9 11 12 13 14 17 18 19 20 22 24 25 26 27 29 30 32 33 34 35 36 37 38 39 40 41 43 44 45 46 47 48 49 50 51 54 57 59 60 61 62 63 64 68 69 70 72 76 78 79 **P**1 3 **S** Catholic Health Initiatives, Denver, CO
Web address: www.sjhlex.org
21　10　361　14715　218　83203　0　148720　56251　1769

★ SAINT JOSEPH HOSPITAL EAST, (Formerly Jewish Hospital Lexington), 150 North Eagle Creek Drive, Zip 40509-1807; tel. 606/268-4800; Melinda Washburn, Chief Operating Officer (Total facility includes 8 beds in nursing home–type unit) **A**1 5 9 10 **F**3 4 7 8 9 11 12 13 14 17 18 19 20 22 24 25 26 27 29 30 32 33 34 35 36 37 38 39 40 41 43 44 45 46 47 48 49 50 51 54 59 60 61 62 63 64 68 69 70 72 76 78 79 **P**1 3 **S** Catholic Health Initiatives, Denver, CO
21　10　119　4419　65　25849　498　41580　15360　587

★ SAMARITAN HOSPITAL, 310 South Limestone Street, Zip 40508-3008; tel. 606/226-7151; Frank Beirne, Chief Executive Officer **A**1 9 10 **F**8 9 11 12 13 16 17 18 19 22 23 24 25 27 30 32 33 34 36 37 38 39 40 41 43 44 45 46 48 49 51 53 54 57 58 59 60 61 62 63 64 69 70 76 77 78 **P**6
Web address: www.samaritanhospital.com
33　10　173　4487　71　46642　0　—　—　490

☐ SHRINERS HOSPITALS FOR CHILDREN–LEXINGTON, 1900 Richmond Road, Zip 40502-1298; tel. 606/266-2101; Tony Lewgood, Administrator (Nonreporting) **A**1 3 5 **S** Shriners Hospitals for Children, Tampa, FL
23　57　50　—　—　—　—　—　—　—

★ UNIVERSITY OF KENTUCKY HOSPITAL, 800 Rose Street, Zip 40536-0084; tel. 859/323-5000; Frank Butler, Director **A**1 2 3 5 8 9 10 **F**4 8 9 10 11 12 13 14 16 17 18 19 21 22 24 25 27 30 32 33 34 35 36 37 39 41 42 43 44 45 46 47 48 49 50 51 52 54 55 56 57 59 60 61 62 63 65 66 68 70 71 72 73 74 75 76 77 78 79
Web address: www.ukhealthcare.uky.edu
12　10　396　20497　321　408048　2005　274723　92209　2430

★ VETERANS AFFAIRS MEDICAL CENTER–LEXINGTON, 2250 Leestown Pike, Zip 40511-1093; tel. 606/233-4511; Helen K. Cornish, Director (Total facility includes 215 beds in nursing home–type unit) **A**1 2 3 5 8 9 **F**1 3 4 8 9 11 12 13 18 19 22 23 24 25 26 28 30 31 32 33 34 35 37 38 39 41 43 45 46 47 48 49 50 51 53 54 56 57 59 61 62 63 65 68 69 70 72 76 78 79 **P**6 **S** Department of Veterans Affairs, Washington, DC
Web address: www.va.gov/stations97/guide/home.asp?DIVISION=ALL
45　10　413　6010　275　209628　0　125083　58299　1444

LONDON—Laurel County

★ MARYMOUNT MEDICAL CENTER, 310 East Ninth Street, Zip 40741-1299; tel. 606/877-3705; Lowell Jones, President and Chief Executive Officer (Total facility includes 24 beds in nursing home–type unit) **A**1 9 10 **F**7 8 11 12 13 16 17 18 22 23 24 25 32 36 37 39 43 44 46 47 48 49 50 51 54 69 70 72 76 77 78 79 **P**3 7 **S** Catholic Health Initiatives, Denver, CO
21　10　95　4638　51　151604　399　40033　19569　571

Hospitals, U.S. / KENTUCKY

Hospital, Address, Telephone, Administrator, Approval, Facility, and Physician Codes, Health Care System, Network	Classification Codes		Utilization Data					Expense (thousands) of dollars		
★ American Hospital Association (AHA) membership □ Joint Commission on Accreditation of Healthcare Organizations (JCAHO) accreditation + American Osteopathic Healthcare Association (AOHA) membership ○ American Osteopathic Association (AOA) accreditation △ Commission on Accreditation of Rehabilitation Facilities (CARF) accreditation Control codes 61, 63, 64, 71, 72 and 73 indicate hospitals listed by AOHA, but not registered by AHA. For definition of numerical codes, see page A4	Control	Service	Staffed Beds	Admissions	Census	Outpatient Visits	Births	Total	Payroll	Personnel
LOUISA—Lawrence County										
□ THREE RIVERS MEDICAL CENTER, Highway 644, Zip 41230, Mailing Address: P.O. Box 769, Zip 41230-0769; tel. 606/638-9451; Greg Kiser, Chief Executive Officer A1 9 10 F8 9 12 13 17 18 22 25 27 30 32 33 34 36 39 41 44 48 49 51 57 60 61 62 63 68 70 76 78 S Community Health Systems, Inc., Brentwood, TN Web address: www.trmc.net	33	10	90	3154	34	28184	113	—	—	231
LOUISVILLE—Jefferson County										
✠ △ BAPTIST HOSPITAL EAST, 4000 Kresge Way, Zip 40207-4676; tel. 502/897-8100; Susan Stout Tamme, President (Total facility includes 23 beds in nursing home-type unit) A1 2 7 9 10 F2 3 4 8 9 11 12 13 14 16 18 19 21 22 24 25 30 32 33 34 36 38 39 41 42 44 45 46 47 48 49 50 51 53 54 57 59 60 61 62 63 64 65 66 68 69 70 72 73 76 77 78 79 S Baptist Healthcare System, Louisville, KY Web address: www.baptisteast.com	23	10	407	22533	333	160768	2979	175891	78276	2120
✠ CARITAS MEDICAL CENTER, 1850 Bluegrass Avenue, Zip 40215-1199; tel. 502/361-6000; Peter J. Bernard, President and Chief Executive Officer (Total facility includes 33 beds in nursing home-type unit) A1 9 10 F1 2 3 6 7 9 11 12 13 16 17 18 22 24 25 26 32 36 38 39 40 41 42 43 45 48 49 51 54 56 57 58 59 60 61 62 63 64 65 69 70 71 72 73 76 78 P7 S Catholic Health Initiatives, Denver, CO Web address: www.chi-caritas.org	21	10	213	11541	172	118211	0	86170	38219	889
✠ CARITAS PEACE CENTER, 2020 Newburg Road, Zip 40205-1879; tel. 502/451-3330; Peter J. Bernard, President and Chief Executive Officer A1 9 10 F16 17 18 57 58 62 63 64 S Catholic Health Initiatives, Denver, CO	23	22	225	1856	158	19293	0	24727	11280	440
□ CENTRAL STATE HOSPITAL, 10510 LaGrange Road, Zip 40223-1228; tel. 502/253-7000; Paula Tamme Cooke, Chief Executive Officer A1 10 F58 59 60 61 62 63 64	12	22	192	944	139	—	—	—	—	—
★ △ FRAZIER REHABILITATION CENTER, 220 Abraham Flexner Way, Zip 40202-1887; tel. 502/582-7400; Barth A. Weinberg, Vice President, Inpatient Rehabilitation A3 5 7 9 F1 2 3 4 5 7 8 9 10 11 12 13 14 15 16 17 18 19 20 21 22 23 24 25 27 28 29 30 31 32 33 34 35 36 37 38 39 40 41 42 43 44 45 46 47 48 49 50 51 52 53 54 55 56 57 58 59 60 61 62 63 64 65 66 68 69 70 71 72 73 74 75 76 77 78 79 P6 S Jewish Hospital HealthCare Services, Louisville, KY Web address: www.jhhs.org	23	46	93	1789	76	68151	—	26749	12266	348
✠ JEWISH HOSPITAL, 217 East Chestnut Street, Zip 40202-1886; tel. 502/587-4011; Douglas E. Shaw, President A1 2 3 5 8 9 10 F2 3 4 7 8 9 10 11 12 13 16 17 18 19 22 24 25 27 28 29 30 32 33 34 35 36 38 39 41 42 43 44 46 47 48 49 50 51 52 53 54 55 56 57 58 59 60 61 62 63 64 65 66 68 69 70 71 72 73 74 75 76 77 78 79 P6 S Jewish Hospital HealthCare Services, Louisville, KY Web address: www.jhhs.org	23	10	435	21486	357	—	0	274919	84563	2335
KOSAIR CHILDREN'S HOSPITAL See Norton Hospital										
✠ NORTON AUDUBON HOSPITAL, One Audubon Plaza Drive, Zip 40217-1397, Mailing Address: P.O. Box 17550, Zip 40217-0550; tel. 502/636-7111; Thomas D. Kmetz, Chief Administrative Officer (Total facility includes 32 beds in nursing home-type unit) A1 2 5 9 10 F3 4 5 7 8 9 10 11 12 13 14 15 16 17 18 19 22 23 24 25 26 27 28 30 32 33 34 35 36 37 38 39 41 42 43 44 45 46 47 48 49 50 51 52 54 57 58 59 60 61 62 63 64 65 66 68 69 70 71 72 74 75 76 77 78 79 P3 6 7 S Norton Healthcare, Louisville, KY	23	10	235	11695	180	95130	15	92585	31210	847
✠ NORTON HEALTHCARE PAVILION, (Formerly Norton Medical Pavilion), 315 East Broadway, Zip 40202; tel. 502/629-2000; M. Michelle Hood, Chief Administrative Officer (Nonreporting) A1 2 3 9 10 S Norton Healthcare, Louisville, KY Web address: www.nortonhealthcare.com	23	10	178	—	—	—	—	—	—	—
✠ NORTON HOSPITAL, (Includes Kosair Children's Hospital, 231 East Chestnut Street, Zip 40202, Mailing Address: P.O. Box 35070, Zip 40232-5070; tel. 502/629-6000; Douglas J. Eighmey, Chief Administrative Officer), 200 East Chestnut Street, Zip 40202-1800, Mailing Address: P.O. Box 35070, Zip 40232-5070; tel. 502/629-8000; M. Michelle Hood, Chief Administrative Officer (Total facility includes 17 beds in nursing home-type unit) A1 2 3 5 9 10 F3 4 5 7 8 9 10 11 12 13 14 16 17 18 19 22 23 24 25 28 30 32 33 34 35 36 37 38 39 41 42 43 44 45 46 47 48 49 50 51 52 54 57 58 59 60 61 62 63 64 65 66 68 69 70 71 72 74 75 76 77 78 79 P3 6 7 S Norton Healthcare, Louisville, KY Web address: www.nortonhealthcare.com	23	10	687	28868	444	191813	5521	300535	100073	4065
✠ NORTON SOUTHWEST HOSPITAL, 9820 Third Street Road, Zip 40272-9984; tel. 502/933-8100; James W. Pope, Chief Executive Officer (Total facility includes 23 beds in nursing home-type unit) A1 9 10 F3 4 5 7 8 9 10 11 12 13 14 19 22 23 24 25 26 27 28 30 32 33 34 35 36 37 38 39 40 41 42 43 44 45 46 47 48 49 50 51 52 54 57 58 59 60 61 62 63 64 65 66 69 70 71 72 74 75 76 77 78 79 P3 6 7 S Norton Healthcare, Louisville, KY Web address: www.nortonhealthcare.com	23	10	108	3269	43	46285	0	27168	9994	250
✠ NORTON SUBURBAN HOSPITAL, 4001 Dutchmans Lane, Zip 40207-4799; tel. 502/893-1000; John D. Harryman, President and Chief Executive Officer A1 9 10 F3 4 5 7 8 9 10 11 12 13 14 16 17 18 19 21 22 23 24 25 26 27 28 30 32 33 34 35 36 37 38 39 41 42 43 44 45 46 47 48 49 50 51 52 54 57 58 59 60 61 62 63 64 65 66 68 69 70 71 72 74 75 76 77 78 79 P3 6 7 S Norton Healthcare, Louisville, KY Web address: www.nortonhealthcare.com	23	10	230	13628	181	99052	2847	92112	32358	893

Hospitals, U.S. / KENTUCKY

Hospital, Address, Telephone, Administrator, Approval, Facility, and Physician Codes, Health Care System, Network	Classification Codes		Utilization Data					Expense (thousands) of dollars		
	Control	Service	Staffed Beds	Admissions	Census	Outpatient Visits	Births	Total	Payroll	Personnel

★ American Hospital Association (AHA) membership
☐ Joint Commission on Accreditation of Healthcare Organizations (JCAHO) accreditation
+ American Osteopathic Healthcare Association (AOHA) membership
○ American Osteopathic Association (AOA) accreditation
△ Commission on Accreditation of Rehabilitation Facilities (CARF) accreditation
Control codes 61, 63, 64, 71, 72 and 73 indicate hospitals listed by AOHA, but not registered by AHA. For definition of numerical codes, see page A4

Hospital	Control	Service	Staffed Beds	Admissions	Census	Outpatient Visits	Births	Total	Payroll	Personnel
☐ TEN BROECK HOSPITAL, 8521 Old LaGrange Road, Zip 40242–3800; tel. 502/426–6380; Pat Hammer, Chief Executive Officer (Nonreporting) A1 9 10 S United Medical Corporation, Windermere, FL	33	22	94	—	—	—	—	—	—	—
★ UNIVERSITY OF LOUISVILLE HOSPITAL, 530 South Jackson Street, Zip 40202–3611; tel. 502/562–3000; James H. Taylor, President and Chief Executive Officer A1 2 3 5 8 9 10 F4 7 8 9 10 11 12 13 16 17 18 19 22 23 24 25 31 32 34 35 38 39 41 42 44 45 46 47 48 49 50 51 54 56 57 59 61 63 65 68 69 70 72 74 75 76 77 78 P4 7 S Jewish Hospital HealthCare Services, Louisville, KY Web address: www.ulh.org	23	10	271	13671	223	135140	1762	170723	56989	1650
☐ VENCOR HOSPITAL–LOUISVILLE, 1313 St. Anthony Place, Zip 40204–1765; tel. 502/587–7001; James H. Wesp, Administrator (Total facility includes 37 beds in nursing home–type unit) A1 9 10 F9 13 16 18 22 24 38 39 46 48 65 68 69 70 76 S Vencor, Incorporated, Louisville, KY Web address: www.vencor.com	32	10	156	457	111	83086	0	30705	14132	342
★ VETERANS AFFAIRS MEDICAL CENTER–LOUISVILLE, 800 Zorn Avenue, Zip 40206–1499; tel. 502/895–3401; Larry J. Sander, FACHE, Director A1 2 3 5 8 9 F3 4 9 11 12 16 18 19 22 23 25 26 28 29 30 31 32 33 34 35 36 37 38 39 41 43 45 46 47 48 49 50 51 54 56 57 59 61 63 65 69 70 72 74 76 78 79 P6 S Department of Veterans Affairs, Washington, DC Web address: www.va.gov/603louisville	45	10	110	5005	104	235181	0	107599	52879	1101
MADISONVILLE—Hopkins County ★ REGIONAL MEDICAL CENTER OF HOPKINS COUNTY, 900 Hospital Drive, Zip 42431–1694; tel. 270/825–5100; Bobby H. Dampier, Chief Executive Officer A1 2 3 5 9 10 F3 4 7 8 9 11 12 13 17 19 22 23 24 25 26 27 28 31 32 34 35 36 37 38 39 41 42 43 44 45 46 47 48 49 50 51 52 53 54 56 57 58 61 62 63 65 68 69 70 71 72 75 76 77 78 P6 Web address: www.troverfoundation.org	23	10	301	10326	139	—	781	79764	34041	1209
MANCHESTER—Clay County ★ MEMORIAL HOSPITAL, 401 Memorial Drive, Zip 40962–9156; tel. 606/598–5104; Jimm Bunch, President and Chief Executive Officer (Total facility includes 16 beds in nursing home–type unit) A1 9 10 F13 17 18 19 22 25 28 30 32 33 34 35 36 38 39 41 44 45 48 50 51 54 66 67 69 70 76 78 79 S Adventist Health System Sunbelt Health Care Corporation, Winter Park, FL	21	10	63	2694	35	50391	302	18707	7801	310
MARION—Crittenden County ★ CRITTENDEN COUNTY HOSPITAL, Highway 60 South, Zip 42064, Mailing Address: P.O. Box 386, Zip 42064–0386; tel. 270/965–5281; Greg Moore, Chief Executive Officer (Nonreporting) A1 9 10 S Quorum Health Group, Brentwood, TN Web address: www.crittenden–health.org	33	22	67	—	—	—	—	—	—	—
MARTIN—Floyd County ★ OUR LADY OF THE WAY HOSPITAL, 11022 Main Street, Zip 41649–0910; tel. 606/285–5181; Lowell Jones, Chief Executive Officer (Total facility includes 13 beds in nursing home–type unit) A1 9 10 F13 16 17 18 19 22 25 32 33 36 38 48 49 50 51 54 69 70 76 78 S Catholic Health Initiatives, Denver, CO Web address: www.olwh.org	23	10	39	1398	21	25711	0	13791	7005	163
MAYFIELD—Graves County ★ JACKSON PURCHASE MEDICAL CENTER, (Formerly Pinelake Regional Hospital), 1099 Medical Center Circle, Zip 42066–1179, Mailing Address: P.O. Box 1099, Zip 42066–1099; tel. 270/251–4100; Mary Jo Lewis, Chief Executive Officer (Total facility includes 14 beds in nursing home–type unit) A1 9 10 F8 9 11 13 16 17 18 22 24 25 27 32 33 34 38 39 41 43 44 45 46 48 50 54 59 68 69 70 71 72 75 76 78 79 P1 2 3 5 6 7 8 S LifePoint Hospitals, Inc., Brentwood, TN Web address: www.hcahealthcare.com	33	10	106	4482	54	67668	389	24066	9672	321
MAYSVILLE—Mason County ★ MEADOWVIEW REGIONAL MEDICAL CENTER, 989 Medical Park Drive, Zip 41056–8750; tel. 606/759–5311; Curtis B. Courtney, Chief Executive Officer (Total facility includes 10 beds in nursing home–type unit) A1 9 10 F8 9 11 13 16 17 18 19 22 25 26 32 34 39 41 44 45 46 48 49 51 54 65 69 70 72 76 78 S LifePoint Hospitals, Inc., Brentwood, TN	33	10	101	3800	38	37099	464	20288	8850	320
MCDOWELL—Floyd County ☐ MCDOWELL ARH HOSPITAL, Route 122, Zip 41647, Mailing Address: P.O. Box 247, Mc Dowell, Zip 41647–0247; tel. 606/377–3400; Dena C. Sparkman, Administrator A1 9 10 F2 3 4 7 8 9 12 13 16 17 22 24 25 29 30 32 33 34 36 39 41 42 43 44 45 46 48 51 52 53 54 56 57 58 59 60 61 62 63 64 69 70 71 72 76 78 79 S Appalachian Regional Healthcare, Lexington, KY Web address: www.arh.org	23	10	40	1421	13	—	0	13742	—	170
MIDDLESBORO—Bell County ☐ MIDDLESBORO APPALACHIAN REGIONAL HOSPITAL, 3600 West Cumberland Avenue, Zip 40965–2614, Mailing Address: P.O. Box 340, Zip 40965–0340; tel. 606/242–1101; Paul V. Miles, Administrator (Nonreporting) A1 9 10 S Appalachian Regional Healthcare, Lexington, KY	23	10	96	—	—	—	—	—	—	—
MONTICELLO—Wayne County ☐ WAYNE COUNTY HOSPITAL, 166 Hospital Street, Zip 42633–2416; tel. 606/348–9343; Patricia Brinson, Administrator A1 9 10 F8 22 24 25 30 38 48 54 70 76 78 Web address: www.users.kih.net/~wchospital/	23	10	30	1327	14	29760	0	—	—	128

Hospitals, U.S. / KENTUCKY

Hospital, Address, Telephone, Administrator, Approval, Facility, and Physician Codes, Health Care System, Network	Classification Codes		Utilization Data					Expense (thousands) of dollars		
★ American Hospital Association (AHA) membership □ Joint Commission on Accreditation of Healthcare Organizations (JCAHO) accreditation + American Osteopathic Healthcare Association (AOHA) membership ○ American Osteopathic Association (AOA) accreditation △ Commission on Accreditation of Rehabilitation Facilities (CARF) accreditation Control codes 61, 63, 64, 71, 72 and 73 indicate hospitals listed by AOHA, but not registered by AHA. For definition of numerical codes, see page A4	Control	Service	Staffed Beds	Admissions	Census	Outpatient Visits	Births	Total	Payroll	Personnel
MOREHEAD—Rowan County										
★ ST. CLAIRE MEDICAL CENTER, 222 Medical Circle, Zip 40351–1180; tel. 606/783–6500; Mark J. Neff, President and Chief Executive Officer **A**1 2 9 10 **F**3 7 8 9 11 16 17 18 19 21 22 23 24 25 26 29 30 32 33 34 35 36 37 38 39 41 43 44 45 46 48 49 51 54 56 57 58 59 60 61 62 63 65 68 70 72 76 78 79 **P**6 Web address: www.st–claire.com	21	10	133	5020	54	321166	478	56244	27400	908
MORGANFIELD—Union County										
□ METHODIST HOSPITAL UNION COUNTY, (Formerly Union County Methodist Hospital), 4604 Highway 60 West, Zip 42437–9570; tel. 270/389–3030; Patrick Donahue, Administrator (Total facility includes 16 beds in nursing home–type unit) **A**1 9 10 **F**9 13 17 18 22 23 25 30 32 34 36 37 39 41 43 45 48 54 58 61 62 63 64 69 70 76 78 Web address: www.methodisthospitaluc.net	21	10	53	582	21	18717	0	6304	2621	109
MOUNT STERLING—Montgomery County										
★ GATEWAY REGIONAL HEALTH SYSTEM, Sterling Avenue, Zip 40353–1158, Mailing Address: P.O. Box 7, Zip 40353–0007; tel. 859/497–6000; Patrick A. Romano, Interim Chief Executive Officer (Total facility includes 40 beds in nursing home–type unit) **A**1 9 10 **F**7 8 9 12 13 16 17 18 19 22 23 24 25 32 34 38 39 41 43 44 45 46 48 51 54 56 61 68 69 70 71 76 78 79 **P**6 7	23	10	103	2135	53	51348	667	21633	9382	358
MOUNT VERNON—Rockcastle County										
★ ROCKCASTLE HOSPITAL AND RESPIRATORY CARE CENTER, 145 Newcomb Avenue, Zip 40456–2733, Mailing Address: P.O. Box 1310, Zip 40456–1310; tel. 606/256–2195; Lee D. Keene, President and Chief Executive Officer (Total facility includes 60 beds in nursing home–type unit) **A**1 9 10 **F**9 16 17 18 22 24 25 38 54 69 76 **P**5 6	23	10	86	1063	70	24348	0	15625	8799	334
MURRAY—Calloway County										
★ MURRAY–CALLOWAY COUNTY HOSPITAL, 803 Poplar Street, Zip 42071–2432; tel. 270/762–1100; Isaac S. Coe, President (Total facility includes 214 beds in nursing home–type unit) **A**1 9 10 **F**1 7 8 9 11 13 17 18 19 22 23 24 25 26 30 32 33 34 36 37 38 39 41 43 44 45 46 48 51 54 59 60 61 62 63 65 68 69 70 71 72 75 76 78 79 **P**3	15	10	339	5419	271	165827	599	53579	22935	873
OWENSBORO—Daviess County										
★ △ OWENSBORO MERCY HEALTH SYSTEM, (Includes HealthPark, 1006 Ford Avenue, Zip 42301; tel. 502/686–6100), 811 East Parrish Avenue, Zip 42303–3268, Mailing Address: P.O. Box 20007, Zip 42303–0007; tel. 270/688–2000; Greg L. Carlson, President and Chief Executive Officer (Total facility includes 30 beds in nursing home–type unit) **A**1 2 7 9 10 **F**2 3 4 8 9 11 12 13 16 17 18 19 22 24 25 27 28 29 30 31 32 33 34 35 36 37 38 39 41 43 44 45 46 47 48 49 50 51 53 54 57 59 60 61 62 63 65 68 69 70 71 72 76 77 78 79 **P**7 8	23	10	347	17226	197	251519	1777	133063	54063	1913
RIVERVALLEY BEHAVIORAL HEALTH HOSPITAL, 1000 Industrial Drive, Zip 42301–8715; tel. 270/689–6500; Gayle DiCesare, President and Chief Officer **A**9 10 **F**16 17 18 57 58 61 63 **P**7 Web address: www.rvbh.com	23	52	69	636	75	0	0	5588	4706	170
OWENTON—Owen County										
OWEN COUNTY MEMORIAL HOSPITAL, 330 Roland Avenue, Zip 40359–1502; tel. 502/484–3441; Richard D. McLeod, Administrator (Total facility includes 20 beds in nursing home–type unit) (Nonreporting) **A**9 10	33	10	50	—	—	—	—	—	—	—
PADUCAH—McCracken County										
□ △ LOURDES HOSPITAL, 1530 Lone Oak Road, Zip 42003, Mailing Address: P.O. Box 7100, Zip 42002–7100; tel. 270/444–2444; Robert P. Goodwin, President and Chief Executive Officer (Total facility includes 30 beds in nursing home–type unit) (Nonreporting) **A**1 7 9 10 **S** Catholic Healthcare Partners, Cincinnati, OH Web address: www.lourdes–pad.org	21	10	290	—	—	—	—	—	—	—
★ WESTERN BAPTIST HOSPITAL, 2501 Kentucky Avenue, Zip 42003–3200; tel. 270/575–2100; Larry O. Barton, President (Total facility includes 24 beds in nursing home–type unit) **A**1 9 10 **F**2 3 4 7 8 9 10 11 12 13 17 18 19 22 24 25 28 31 32 33 34 36 38 39 41 43 44 45 46 47 48 49 50 53 54 56 57 58 59 60 61 62 63 64 65 69 70 72 76 77 78 79 **P**1 5 **S** Baptist Healthcare System, Louisville, KY Web address: www.bhsi.com	23	10	271	12521	161	122092	1105	104251	40384	1385
PAINTSVILLE—Johnson County										
□ PAUL B. HALL REGIONAL MEDICAL CENTER, 625 James S. Trimble Boulevard, Zip 41240–0000; tel. 606/789–3511; Deborah L. Trimble, Administrator (Nonreporting) **A**1 9 10 **S** Health Management Associates, Naples, FL	33	10	72	—	—	—	—	—	—	—
PARIS—Bourbon County										
★ BOURBON COMMUNITY HOSPITAL, 9 Linville Drive, Zip 40361–2196; tel. 606/987–3600; Rob Smart, Chief Executive Officer **A**1 9 10 **F**3 9 11 12 22 25 32 39 41 45 48 51 54 57 58 70 76 78 **S** LifePoint Hospitals, Inc., Brentwood, TN	33	10	58	1341	18	26135	0	10763	4847	156
PIKEVILLE—Pike County										
★ PIKEVILLE UNITED METHODIST HOSPITAL OF KENTUCKY, 911 South Bypass, Zip 41501–1595; tel. 606/437–3500; Walter E. May, Interim Administrator **A**1 2 9 10 **F**7 8 9 11 12 13 14 19 22 24 25 27 33 34 38 39 40 41 42 43 44 45 46 48 49 50 51 54 57 65 70 76 77 78	23	10	181	8390	108	115913	887	89447	36800	1096

© 2000 AHA Guide — Many Facility Codes have changed. Please refer to the AHA Guide Code Chart.

Hospitals, U.S. / KENTUCKY

★ American Hospital Association (AHA) membership
☐ Joint Commission on Accreditation of Healthcare Organizations (JCAHO) accreditation
+ American Osteopathic Healthcare Association (AOHA) membership
○ American Osteopathic Association (AOA) accreditation
△ Commission on Accreditation of Rehabilitation Facilities (CARF) accreditation
Control codes 61, 63, 64, 71, 72 and 73 indicate hospitals listed by AOHA, but not registered by AHA. For definition of numerical codes, see page A4

Hospital, Address, Telephone, Administrator, Approval, Facility, and Physician Codes, Health Care System, Network	Classification Codes		Utilization Data					Expense (thousands) of dollars		Personnel
	Control	Service	Staffed Beds	Admissions	Census	Outpatient Visits	Births	Total	Payroll	
PINEVILLE—Bell County										
★ PINEVILLE COMMUNITY HOSPITAL ASSOCIATION, 850 Riverview Avenue, Zip 40977–0850; tel. 606/337–3051; J. Milton Brooks, II, Administrator (Total facility includes 30 beds in nursing home–type unit) **A**1 9 10 **F**8 9 13 18 22 23 24 25 32 34 36 38 41 43 44 48 51 54 69 70 76 78	23	10	150	4444	87	23940	180	18602	8168	294
PRESTONSBURG—Floyd County										
★ HIGHLANDS REGIONAL MEDICAL CENTER, 5000 Kentucky Route 321, Zip 41653, Mailing Address: P.O. Box 668, Zip 41653–0668; tel. 606/886–8511; Harold C. Warman, Jr, President and Chief Executive Officer **A**1 2 9 10 **F**5 8 9 11 18 22 24 25 28 29 32 34 36 38 39 41 44 46 48 50 54 69 70 75 76 78 **P**7	23	10	148	6419	81	71616	647	46704	15829	442
PRINCETON—Caldwell County										
★ CALDWELL COUNTY HOSPITAL, 101 Hospital Drive, Zip 42445–0410, Mailing Address: Box 410, Zip 42445–0410; tel. 270/365–0300; William P. Macri, Chief Executive Officer **A**1 9 10 **F**7 9 13 16 17 18 22 23 24 25 32 33 34 36 38 40 41 43 48 50 51 54 68 70 71 76 78 **P**6 **S** Quorum Health Group, Brentwood, TN	23	10	38	985	11	—	0	9096	3085	131
RADCLIFF—Hardin County										
★ LINCOLN TRAIL BEHAVIORAL HEALTH SYSTEM, 3909 South Wilson Road, Zip 40160–9714, Mailing Address: P.O. Box 369, Zip 40159–0369; tel. 270/351–9444; Melvin E. Modderman, Administrator **A**1 9 10 **F**2 3 16 17 18 19 25 29 38 57 58 59 60 61 62 63 64 70 78	33	22	67	982	37	14269	0	6263	3577	107
RICHMOND—Madison County										
★ PATTIE A. CLAY HOSPITAL, EKU By–Pass, Zip 40475, Mailing Address: P.O. Box 1600, Zip 40476–2603; tel. 859/623–3131; Richard M. Thomas, President **A**1 9 10 **F**7 8 9 11 13 17 18 19 22 24 25 26 27 30 32 34 38 39 43 44 45 48 50 51 54 65 66 68 70 72 76 77 78 79 **S** Jewish Hospital HealthCare Services, Louisville, KY	23	10	105	3875	44	79114	882	30552	13859	465
RUSSELL SPRINGS—Russell County										
★ RUSSELL COUNTY HOSPITAL, Dowell Road, Zip 42642, Mailing Address: P.O. Box 1610, Zip 42642–1610; tel. 270/866–4141; Patricia Ekdahl, President and Chief Executive Officer **A**9 10 **F**7 9 16 17 18 22 23 24 25 32 34 37 40 41 48 53 54 70 72 76 78 **S** Norton Healthcare, Louisville, KY	13	10	45	912	11	15331	0	7585	3359	—
RUSSELLVILLE—Logan County										
★ LOGAN MEMORIAL HOSPITAL, 1625 South Nashville Road, Zip 42276–8834, Mailing Address: P.O. Box 10, Zip 42276–0010; tel. 270/726–4011; Michael Clark, Chief Executive Officer (Total facility includes 8 beds in nursing home–type unit) **A**1 9 10 **F**1 4 8 9 12 13 17 18 19 21 22 23 25 26 30 32 33 34 38 39 40 43 44 46 48 50 51 54 56 61 66 69 70 71 72 76 78 79 **S** LifePoint Hospitals, Inc., Brentwood, TN	33	10	63	1677	19	42757	158	15916	5690	178
SALEM—Livingston County										
★ LIVINGSTON HOSPITAL AND HEALTHCARE SERVICES, 131 Hospital Drive, Zip 42078; tel. 270/988–2299; Yvonne Maddux, Interim Chief Executive Officer **A**9 10 **F**9 16 17 18 19 22 32 34 36 37 39 46 48 51 53 54 76	23	10	26	1088	11	13533	0	8844	3466	127
SCOTTSVILLE—Allen County										
MEDICAL CENTER AT SCOTTSVILLE See The Medical Center at Bowling Green, Bowling Green										
SHELBYVILLE—Shelby County										
★ JEWISH HOSPITAL–SHELBYVILLE, 727 Hospital Drive, Zip 40065–1699; tel. 502/647–4000; Timothy L. Jarm, President (Total facility includes 8 beds in nursing home–type unit) **A**1 9 10 **F**2 4 8 9 10 11 12 13 14 16 17 18 19 21 22 24 25 27 28 29 30 31 32 33 34 35 36 37 38 39 41 43 44 45 46 47 48 49 50 51 53 54 55 57 58 59 60 61 62 63 64 65 67 68 69 70 71 72 74 75 76 78 79 **S** Jewish Hospital HealthCare Services, Louisville, KY Web address: www.jhhs.org	23	10	58	2788	37	37612	217	23437	10207	256
SOMERSET—Pulaski County										
★ △ LAKE CUMBERLAND REGIONAL HOSPITAL, 305 Langdon Street, Zip 42501, Mailing Address: P.O. Box 620, Zip 42502–2750; tel. 606/679–7441; Jon C. O'Shaughnessy, President and Chief Executive Officer (Nonreporting) **A**1 2 7 10 **S** LifePoint Hospitals, Inc., Brentwood, TN	33	10	227	—	—	—	—	—	—	—
SOUTH WILLIAMSON—Pike County										
☐ WILLIAMSON ARH HOSPITAL, 260 Hospital Drive, Zip 41503–4072; tel. 606/237–1710; Louis G. Roe, Jr, Administrator (Total facility includes 50 beds in nursing home–type unit) **A**1 9 10 **F**7 8 9 13 14 17 18 19 22 25 32 34 36 38 39 41 43 44 46 48 54 57 61 62 63 69 70 78 **P**1 **S** Appalachian Regional Healthcare, Lexington, KY Web address: www.arh.org	23	10	148	4424	111	52598	237	29960	13801	392
STANFORD—Lincoln County										
★ FORT LOGAN HOSPITAL, 124 Portman Avenue, Zip 40484–1200; tel. 606/365–2187; Terry C. Powers, Administrator (Total facility includes 30 beds in nursing home–type unit) **A**9 10 **F**7 8 9 16 22 23 25 30 34 35 44 48 54 69 70 76 78	23	10	73	1096	36	12600	163	7553	3466	155
TOMPKINSVILLE—Monroe County										
★ MONROE COUNTY MEDICAL CENTER, 529 Capp Harlan Road, Zip 42167–1840; tel. 270/487–9231; Mark E. Thompson, Chief Executive Officer **A**1 9 10 **F**9 17 18 22 25 31 36 38 48 50 54 75 76 **P**8 **S** Quorum Health Group, Brentwood, TN	23	10	49	2301	27	21714	0	11403	5227	214

Hospitals, U.S. / KENTUCKY

Hospital, Address, Telephone, Administrator, Approval, Facility, and Physician Codes, Health Care System, Network	Classification Codes		Utilization Data					Expense (thousands) of dollars		
★ American Hospital Association (AHA) membership ☐ Joint Commission on Accreditation of Healthcare Organizations (JCAHO) accreditation + American Osteopathic Healthcare Association (AOHA) membership ○ American Osteopathic Association (AOA) accreditation △ Commission on Accreditation of Rehabilitation Facilities (CARF) accreditation Control codes 61, 63, 64, 71, 72 and 73 indicate hospitals listed by AOHA, but not registered by AHA. For definition of numerical codes, see page A4.	Control	Service	Staffed Beds	Admissions	Census	Outpatient Visits	Births	Total	Payroll	Personnel
WEST LIBERTY—Morgan County ☐ MORGAN COUNTY APPALACHIAN REGIONAL HOSPITAL, 476 Liberty Road, Zip 41472-2049, Mailing Address: P.O. Box 579, Zip 41472-0579; tel. 606/743-3186; Dennis R. Chaney, Administrator (Total facility includes 25 beds in nursing home–type unit) **A**1 9 10 **F**7 9 13 17 18 19 22 25 29 32 33 34 36 37 38 44 50 51 54 56 69 70 76 78 **S** Appalachian Regional Healthcare, Lexington, KY **Web address:** www.2.arh.org	23	10	45	811	31	78005	1	10744	6058	161
WHITESBURG—Letcher County ☐ WHITESBURG APPALACHIAN REGIONAL HOSPITAL, 240 Hospital Road, Zip 41858-1254; tel. 606/633-3600; Donald Fields, Administrator **A**1 9 10 **F**7 8 9 11 13 16 17 18 19 22 24 25 33 34 36 37 38 39 41 44 46 48 51 54 58 59 60 61 63 65 68 70 76 78 **S** Appalachian Regional Healthcare, Lexington, KY	23	10	69	4379	44	76694	431	21089	8719	255
WILLIAMSTOWN—Grant County ST. ELIZABETH MEDICAL CENTER–GRANT COUNTY, 238 Barnes Road, Zip 41097-9460; tel. 606/824-2400; Chris Carle, Administrator (Nonreporting) **A**9 10 **S** Catholic Healthcare Partners, Cincinnati, OH	21	10	20	—	—	—	—	—	—	—
WINCHESTER—Clark County ✴ CLARK REGIONAL MEDICAL CENTER, West Lexington Avenue, Zip 40391, Mailing Address: P.O. Box 630, Zip 40392-0630; tel. 606/745-3500; Robert D. Fraraccio, Chief Executive Officer (Nonreporting) **A**1 9 10 **Web address:** www.clarkhospital.org	23	10	75	—	—	—	—	—	—	—

LOUISIANA

Resident Population 4,369 (in thousands)
Resident population in metro areas 75.2%
Birth rate per 1,000 population 15.2
65 years and over 11.5%
Percent of persons without health insurance 19.5%

Hospital, Address, Telephone, Administrator, Approval, Facility, and Physician Codes, Health Care System, Network

★ American Hospital Association (AHA) membership
☐ Joint Commission on Accreditation of Healthcare Organizations (JCAHO) accreditation
+ American Osteopathic Healthcare Association (AOHA) membership
○ American Osteopathic Association (AOA) accreditation
△ Commission on Accreditation of Rehabilitation Facilities (CARF) accreditation
Control codes 61, 63, 64, 71, 72 and 73 indicate hospitals listed by AOHA, but not registered by AHA. For definition of numerical codes, see page A4

Hospital	Classification Codes		Utilization Data					Expense (thousands) of dollars		Personnel
	Control	Service	Staffed Beds	Admissions	Census	Outpatient Visits	Births	Total	Payroll	
ABBEVILLE—Vermilion Parish										
☐ ABBEVILLE GENERAL HOSPITAL, 118 North Hospital Drive, Zip 70510–4077, Mailing Address: P.O. Box 580, Zip 70511–0580; tel. 318/893–5466; Ray A. Landry, Chief Executive Officer **A**1 9 10 **F**8 9 16 17 18 22 24 25 31 38 39 41 43 44 46 48 49 53 56 57 62 63 64 70 76 78	16	10	85	3858	60	51673	168	21334	10345	352
ALEXANDRIA—Rapides Parish										
★ △ CHRISTUS ST. FRANCES CABRINI HOSPITAL, 3330 Masonic Drive, Zip 71301–3899; tel. 318/487–1122; Stephen F. Wright, Chief Executive Officer (Total facility includes 19 beds in nursing home–type unit) (Nonreporting) **A**1 2 7 9 10 **S** Christus Health, Irving, TX	23	10	227	—	—	—	—	—	—	—
★ RAPIDES REGIONAL MEDICAL CENTER, 211 Fourth Street, Zip 71301–8421, Mailing Address: Box 30101, Zip 71301–8421; tel. 318/473–3000; A. C. Buchanan, President and Chief Executive Officer **A**1 2 3 5 10 **F**1 3 4 5 6 7 8 9 11 13 14 15 16 17 19 20 21 22 23 24 25 26 27 28 29 30 31 32 33 34 35 36 37 38 39 40 41 43 44 45 46 47 48 49 50 51 52 54 55 56 58 59 60 61 62 63 64 65 66 67 68 69 70 71 72 73 74 75 76 77 78 79 **P**8 **S** HCA – The Healthcare Company, Nashville, TN **Web address:** www.rapidesregional.com	32	10	320	14543	188	127095	1926	97257	40514	1540
★ VETERANS AFFAIRS MEDICAL CENTER, Shreveport Highway, Zip 71306–6002; tel. 318/473–0010; Allen J. Colston, Director (Total facility includes 149 beds in nursing home–type unit) **A**1 2 3 **F**1 3 7 9 13 19 21 22 23 24 25 26 27 29 30 31 32 34 35 36 37 38 39 41 46 48 50 51 54 56 57 59 60 61 62 63 65 66 69 70 72 74 76 78 79 **P**6 **S** Department of Veterans Affairs, Washington, DC **Web address:** www.va.gov/stations97/guide/home.asp?DIVISION=ALL	45	10	257	2884	249	122371	—	76274	48250	926
AMITE—Tangipahoa Parish										
★ HOOD MEMORIAL HOSPITAL, 301 West Walnut Street, Zip 70422–2098; tel. 504/748–9485; A. D. Richardson, Administrator (Nonreporting) **A**9 10	16	10	40	—	—	—	—	—	—	—
BARKSDALE AFB—Pierce Parish										
★ U. S. AIR FORCE HOSPITAL, 243 Curtiss Road, Suite 100, Zip 71110–5300; tel. 318/456–6004; Colonel Dennis Marquardt, USAF, Commander (Nonreporting) **S** Department of the Air Force, Bowling AFB, DC	41	10	25	—	—	—	—	—	—	—
BASTROP—Morehouse Parish										
★ MOREHOUSE GENERAL HOSPITAL, 323 West Walnut Street, Zip 71220–4521, Mailing Address: P.O. Box 1060, Zip 71221–1060; tel. 318/283–3600; William W. Bing, Administrator **A**1 9 10 **F**7 8 9 10 12 16 17 18 22 23 24 25 30 32 33 34 36 38 39 41 43 44 45 46 48 50 51 54 56 57 60 62 64 68 69 70 72 73 76 **Web address:** www.mghospital.com	16	10	95	3628	52	40970	458	28541	11390	403
BATON ROUGE—East Baton Rouge Parish										
★ BATON ROUGE GENERAL MEDICAL CENTER, (Includes Baton Rouge General Health Center, 8585 Picardy Avenue, Zip 70809–3679, Mailing Address: P.O. Box 84330, Zip 70884–4330; tel. 225/763–4500); 3600 Florida Street, Zip 70806–3889, Mailing Address: P.O. Box 2511, Zip 70821–2511; tel. 225/387–7000; Milton R. Siepman, Ph.D., President and Chief Executive Officer **A**1 2 3 5 6 8 9 10 **F**1 2 3 4 7 8 9 10 11 12 13 14 16 17 18 19 22 24 25 27 28 30 31 32 33 34 36 39 41 42 43 44 45 46 47 48 49 50 51 52 53 54 56 57 58 59 60 61 62 63 64 65 66 67 69 70 71 72 73 76 77 78 79 **S** General Health System, Baton Rouge, LA	23	10	423	15178	238	90091	775	159142	63791	—
☐ BHC MEADOW WOOD HOSPITAL, 9032 Perkins Road, Zip 70810–1507; tel. 225/766–8553; Ralph J. Waite, II, Chief Executive Officer (Nonreporting) **A**1 10 **S** Behavioral Healthcare Corporation, Nashville, TN	33	22	55	—	—	—	—	—	—	—
★ EARL K. LONG MEDICAL CENTER, 5825 Airline Highway, Zip 70805–2498; tel. 225/358–1000; Jonathan Roberts, Dr.PH, Administrator **A**1 3 5 10 **F**8 9 16 17 18 22 25 35 38 41 42 44 46 48 51 52 54 57 66 70 76 78 **P**1 **S** LSU Medical Center Health Care Services Division, Baton Rouge, LA	12	10	204	8346	133	198335	1603	75138	27937	1278
☐ HEALTHSOUTH REHABILITATION HOSPITAL OF BATON ROUGE, 8595 United Plaza Boulevard, Zip 70809–2251; tel. 225/927–0567; Michael D. Marshall, Chief Executive Officer (Nonreporting) **A**1 10 **S** HEALTHSOUTH Corporation, Birmingham, AL	33	46	80	—	—	—	—	—	—	—
★ △ OUR LADY OF THE LAKE REGIONAL MEDICAL CENTER, (Includes Our Lady of the Lake–Assumption, 135 Highway 402, Napoleonville, Zip 70390; tel. 504/369–3600), 5000 Hennessy Boulevard, Zip 70808–4350; tel. 225/765–6565; Robert C. Davidge, Chief Executive Officer **A**1 2 7 9 10 **F**1 2 3 4 6 7 9 11 12 13 14 17 18 19 20 21 22 23 24 25 27 28 29 30 31 32 33 34 35 36 37 38 39 41 43 45 46 47 48 49 50 51 52 53 54 55 56 57 58 59 60 61 62 63 64 65 67 68 69 70 71 72 73 74 76 77 78 79 **P**1 **S** Franciscan Missionaries of Our Lady Health System, Inc., Baton Rouge, LA **Web address:** www.ololrmc.com	21	10	668	28758	451	212908	0	261182	104107	3266

Hospitals, U.S. / LOUISIANA

Hospital, Address, Telephone, Administrator, Approval, Facility, and Physician Codes, Health Care System, Network	Classification Codes		Utilization Data					Expense (thousands) of dollars		
★ American Hospital Association (AHA) membership ☐ Joint Commission on Accreditation of Healthcare Organizations (JCAHO) accreditation + American Osteopathic Healthcare Association (AOHA) membership ○ American Osteopathic Association (AOA) accreditation △ Commission on Accreditation of Rehabilitation Facilities (CARF) accreditation Control codes 61, 63, 64, 71, 72 and 73 indicate hospitals listed by AOHA, but not registered by AHA. For definition of numerical codes, see page A4	Control	Service	Staffed Beds	Admissions	Census	Outpatient Visits	Births	Total	Payroll	Personnel
★ SUMMIT HOSPITAL, 17000 Medical Center Drive, Zip 70816-3224; tel. 225/755-4800; Steve Grimm, CHE, Chief Executive Officer (Total facility includes 24 beds in nursing home-type unit) (Nonreporting) **A**1 9 10 **S** Quorum Health Group, Brentwood, TN	33	10	183	—	—	—	—	—	—	—
★ WOMAN'S HOSPITAL, 9050 Airline Highway, Zip 70815-4192, Mailing Address: P.O. Box 95009, Zip 70895-9009; tel. 225/927-1300; Teri G. Fontenot, President and Chief Executive Officer **A**1 2 9 10 **F**7 8 9 13 16 17 18 19 21 22 24 28 29 32 33 34 36 38 41 42 43 44 45 46 47 48 50 51 54 66 70 72 73 76 78 79 **P**3 Web address: www.womans.com	23	44	220	11927	127	234069	7361	92609	46750	1188
BERNICE—Union Parish TRI-WARD GENERAL HOSPITAL, 409 First Street, Zip 71222-9709, Mailing Address: P.O. Box 697, Zip 71222-0697; tel. 318/285-9066; Charolette Thompson, Administrator (Nonreporting) **A**9 10	16	10	11	—	—	—	—	—	—	—
BOGALUSA—Washington Parish ★ BOGALUSA COMMUNITY MEDICAL CENTER, 433 Plaza Street, Zip 70427-3793; tel. 504/732-7122; William R. Hatton, Chief Executive Officer and Administrator **A**1 9 10 **F**7 12 13 22 24 25 34 36 39 43 45 48 50 53 54 70 72 76 78 **S** Quorum Health Group, Brentwood, TN	23	10	70	3033	46	—	51	18163	8352	269
★ WASHINGTON–ST. TAMMANY REGIONAL MEDICAL CENTER, 400 Memphis Street, Zip 70427-0040, Mailing Address: Box 40, Zip 70427-0040; tel. 504/735-1322; Larry R. King, Administrator **A**1 10 **F**22 25 35 45 48 50 51 57 64 70 76 **P**6 **S** LSU Medical Center Health Care Services Division, Baton Rouge, LA	12	10	50	1781	28	58220	0	13780	7259	200
BOSSIER CITY—Bossier Parish ★ △ CHRISTUS SCHUMPERT BOSSIER, (Formerly Christus Bossier Medical Center), 2105 Airline Drive, Zip 71111-3190; tel. 318/741-6000; Gary Kerr, Administrator (Total facility includes 20 beds in nursing home-type unit) (Nonreporting) **A**7 9 10 **S** Christus Health, Irving, TX	21	10	131	—	—	—	—	—	—	—
☐ SUMMIT HOSPITAL OF NORTHWEST LOUISIANA, 4900 Medical Drive, Zip 71112-4596; tel. 318/747-9500; Louise Wiggins, Chief Executive Officer and Administrator (Nonreporting) **A**1 10 **S** Specialty Hospital Group, Atlanta, GA	33	22	54	—	—	—	—	—	—	—
BREAUX BRIDGE—St. Martin Parish GARY MEMORIAL HOSPITAL, 210 Champagne Boulevard, Zip 70517-3852, Mailing Address: Box 357, Zip 70517-0357; tel. 318/332-2178; Burton Dupuis, Chief Executive Officer (Nonreporting) **A**9 10	16	10	12	—	—	—	—	—	—	—
BUNKIE—Avoyelles Parish ★ BUNKIE GENERAL HOSPITAL, 427 Evergreen Highway, Zip 71322, Mailing Address: P.O. Box 380, Zip 71322-0380; tel. 318/346-6681; Donald L. Kannady, Chief Executive Officer **A**9 10 **F**9 13 17 18 22 25 28 32 36 38 39 48 50 57 62 64 73 76	16	10	41	594	7	14314	0	7030	2349	102
CAMERON—Cameron Parish SOUTH CAMERON MEMORIAL HOSPITAL, 5360 West Creole Highway, Zip 70631-5127; tel. 337/542-4111; Michael J. Kornblatt, Chief Executive Officer (Nonreporting) **A**9 10	16	10	33	—	—	—	—	—	—	—
CHALMETTE—St. Bernard Parish ☐ CHALMETTE MEDICAL CENTER, (Includes Virtue Street Medical Pavilion, 801 Virtue Street, Zip 70043), 9001 Patricia Street, Zip 70043-1727; tel. 504/620-6000; Larry M. Graham, Chief Executive Officer (Nonreporting) **A**1 9 10 **S** Universal Health Services, Inc., King of Prussia, PA	33	10	196	—	—	—	—	—	—	—
CHURCH POINT—Acadia Parish ACADIA–ST. LANDRY HOSPITAL, 810 South Broadway Street, Zip 70525-4497; tel. 318/684-5435; Alcus Trahan, Administrator (Nonreporting) **A**9 10	23	10	39	—	—	—	—	—	—	—
COLUMBIA—Caldwell Parish CALDWELL MEMORIAL HOSPITAL, 411 Main Street, Zip 71418, Mailing Address: P.O. Box 899, Zip 71418-0899; tel. 318/649-6111; Faye Long, Administrator (Nonreporting) **A**10	33	10	31	—	—	—	—	—	—	—
COUSHATTA—Red River Parish ★ CHRISTUS COUSHATTA HEALTH CARE CENTER, (Formerly Coushatta Health Care Center), 1635 Marvel Street, Zip 71019-9022, Mailing Address: P.O. Box 589, Zip 71019-0589; tel. 318/932-2000; Sister Laureen Painter, Chief Executive Officer **A**9 10 **F**13 17 18 19 22 25 28 34 48 51 56 70 75 76 78 **P**7 **S** Christus Health, Irving, TX	23	10	49	1914	19	19944	0	7135	3393	131
COVINGTON—St. Tammany Parish ★ LAKEVIEW REGIONAL MEDICAL CENTER, 95 East Fairway Drive, Zip 70433-7507; tel. 504/867-3800; Max Lauderdale, Chief Executive Officer (Total facility includes 19 beds in nursing home-type unit) **A**1 10 **F**1 4 7 8 9 11 13 14 16 17 18 19 20 22 24 25 30 32 33 34 35 37 41 42 43 44 45 46 47 48 49 50 54 56 64 69 70 72 76 78 79 **S** HCA – The Healthcare Company, Nashville, TN	33	10	145	5143	64	60078	1152	42346	18153	479
★ ST. TAMMANY PARISH HOSPITAL, 1202 South Tyler Street, Zip 70433-2394; tel. 504/898-4000; Thomas J. Stone, Administrator and Chief Executive Officer (Total facility includes 24 beds in nursing home-type unit) **A**1 2 9 10 **F**4 8 9 11 13 16 17 19 22 24 25 27 28 29 30 34 35 36 37 38 39 40 41 42 43 44 45 46 47 48 50 51 54 56 68 69 70 76 77 78 79 **P**6 Web address: www.tamnet.com/dc/stphosp	16	10	157	9429	115	110820	1195	79077	36247	1021

© 2000 AHA Guide   *Many Facility Codes have changed. Please refer to the AHA Guide Code Chart.*

Hospitals, U.S. / LOUISIANA

Hospital, Address, Telephone, Administrator, Approval, Facility, and Physician Codes, Health Care System, Network	Classification Codes		Utilization Data					Expense (thousands) of dollars		Personnel
★ American Hospital Association (AHA) membership ☐ Joint Commission on Accreditation of Healthcare Organizations (JCAHO) accreditation + American Osteopathic Healthcare Association (AOHA) membership ○ American Osteopathic Association (AOA) accreditation △ Commission on Accreditation of Rehabilitation Facilities (CARF) accreditation Control codes 61, 63, 64, 71, 72 and 73 indicate hospitals listed by AOHA, but not registered by AHA. For definition of numerical codes, see page A4	Control	Service	Staffed Beds	Admissions	Census	Outpatient Visits	Births	Total	Payroll	Personnel
CROWLEY—Acadia Parish										
★ AMERICAN LEGION HOSPITAL, 1305 Crowley Rayne Highway, Zip 70526–9410; tel. 337/783–3222; Terry W. Osborne, Chief Executive Officer **A**9 10 **F**8 17 18 22 25 41 44 48 49 57 62 **P**2 Web address: www.alh.org	23	10	178	3813	36	34352	440	22862	9312	403
CUT OFF—Lafourche Parish										
✠ LADY OF THE SEA GENERAL HOSPITAL, 200 West 134th Place, Zip 70345–4145; tel. 504/632–6401; Lane M. Cheramie, Chief Executive Officer **A**1 9 10 **F**7 9 11 13 14 19 22 23 25 27 30 32 33 34 36 39 41 43 45 46 48 50 51 56 57 62 70 72 75 76 77 78 **S** Brim Healthcare, Inc., Brentwood, TN	16	10	55	1501	18	20445	0	15230	5092	195
DE RIDDER—Beauregard Parish										
✠ BEAUREGARD MEMORIAL HOSPITAL, 600 South Pine Street, Zip 70634–4998, Mailing Address: P.O. Box 730, Zip 70634–0730; tel. 318/462–7100; Theodore J. Badger, Jr, Chief Executive Officer **A**1 9 10 **F**9 11 17 18 22 23 24 25 27 28 32 34 36 37 38 39 41 43 46 48 54 68 69 70 76 78 **P**1 8 Web address: www.beauregard.org	16	10	93	4430	49	17377	581	22043	10412	398
DELHI—Richland Parish										
RICHLAND PARISH HOSPITAL–DELHI, 407 Cincinnati Street, Zip 71232–3009; tel. 318/878–5171; Michael W. Carroll, Administrator (Nonreporting) **A**9 10	16	10	42	—	—	—	—	—	—	—
DEQUINCY—Calcasieu Parish										
DEQUINCY MEMORIAL HOSPITAL, 110 West Fourth Street, Zip 70633–3508, Mailing Address: P.O. Box 1166, Zip 70633–1166; tel. 318/786–1200; John A. Matheson, Administrator (Nonreporting) **A**9 10 Web address: www.DeQuincym@aol.com	14	10	41	—	—	—	—	—	—	—
DONALDSONVILLE—Ascension Parish										
✠ PREVOST MEMORIAL HOSPITAL, 301 Memorial Drive, Zip 70346–4376, Mailing Address: P.O. Box 186, Zip 70346–0186; tel. 225/473–7931; Vince A. Cataldo, Administrator (Nonreporting) **A**1 9 10	16	10	35	—	—	—	—	—	—	—
EUNICE—St. Landry Parish										
✠ EUNICE COMMUNITY MEDICAL CENTER, (Formerly Moosa Memorial Hospital), 400 Moosa Boulevard, Zip 70535; tel. 318/457–5244; Larry D. Walker, Chief Executive Officer **A**1 9 10 **F**1 9 13 22 23 24 25 27 30 32 34 38 39 41 44 48 51 53 54 57 59 60 61 62 70 72 74 75 76 78 **S** Province Healthcare Corporation, Brentwood, TN Web address: www.eunicemedical.com/	16	10	62	1238	15	18345	1	10350	4165	149
FARMERVILLE—Union Parish										
UNION GENERAL HOSPITAL, 901 James Avenue, Zip 71241–2234, Mailing Address: P.O. Box 398, Zip 71241–0398; tel. 318/368–9751; Evalyn Ormond, Administrator **A**9 10 **F**9 14 19 22 25 30 32 34 36 38 39 40 43 48 53 54 57 60 61 62 63 70 72 76	23	10	27	653	7	24355	1	5300	2023	68
FERRIDAY—Concordia Parish										
PROFESSIONAL REHABILITATION HOSPITAL, 6818–A Highway 84, Zip 71334; tel. 318/757–7575; Chris Fox, Executive Director **A**10 **F**17 18 19 30 31 38 45 53 54 70 72 **P**6	33	46	40	365	20	8400	—	5791	2210	78
RIVERLAND MEDICAL CENTER, 1700 North E 'E' Wallace Boulevard, Zip 71334, Mailing Address: P.O. Box 111, Zip 71334–0111; tel. 318/757–6551; Vernon R. Stevens, Jr, Administrator (Nonreporting) **A**9 10	16	10	49	—	—	—	—	—	—	—
FORT POLK—Vernon Parish										
✠ BAYNE–JONES ARMY COMMUNITY HOSPITAL, 1585 Third Street, Zip 71459–5110; tel. 318/531–3928; Lieutenant Colonel Mark D. Moore, Deputy Commander and Administrator (Nonreporting) **A**1 **S** Department of the Army, Office of the Surgeon General, Falls Church, VA	42	10	58	—	—	—	—	—	—	—
FRANKLIN—St. Mary Parish										
✠ FRANKLIN FOUNDATION HOSPITAL, 1501 Hospital Avenue, Zip 70538–3724, Mailing Address: P.O. Box 577, Zip 70538–0577; tel. 318/828–0760; Patricia Luker, Chief Executive Officer (Nonreporting) **A**1 9 10 **S** Quorum Health Group, Brentwood, TN Web address: www.franklinfoundation.org	16	10	60	—	—	—	—	—	—	—
FRANKLINTON—Washington Parish										
✠ RIVERSIDE MEDICAL CENTER, 1900 Main Street, Zip 70438–3688; tel. 504/839–4431; Theodore M. Lewis, Chief Executive Officer **A**1 9 10 **F**9 13 22 24 25 32 34 36 38 39 41 45 48 70 78	16	10	48	1799	20	11566	0	11098	4741	163
GONZALES—Ascension Parish										
☐ ASCENSION HOSPITAL AND BEHAVIORAL HEALTH SERVICES, (LONG TERM ACUTE CARE), 615 East Worthy Road, Zip 70737–4240; tel. 225/647–2891; Michael J. Nolan, Chief Executive Officer **A**1 9 10 **F**13 16 17 18 22 24 32 33 34 38 41 45 48 51 54 57 64 70 76	16	49	87	300	27	8590	0	13079	5165	174
✠ RIVERVIEW MEDICAL CENTER, 1125 West Louisiana Highway 30, Zip 70737; tel. 225/647–5000; Kathy J. Bobbs, Chief Executive Officer (Total facility includes 15 beds in nursing home–type unit) (Nonreporting) **A**1 9 10 **S** LifePoint Hospitals, Inc., Brentwood, TN	33	10	104	—	—	—	—	—	—	—
GREENSBURG—St. Helena Parish										
ST. HELENA PARISH HOSPITAL, Highway 43 North, Zip 70441, Mailing Address: P.O. Box 337, Zip 70441–0337; tel. 225/222–6111; J. Scott Stafford, Chief Executive Officer and Administrator (Total facility includes 72 beds in nursing home–type unit) **A**9 10 18 **F**2 3 8 12 18 25 31 36 40 53 54 57 62 69 72 76 78 **P**5	16	10	97	509	74	7788	0	6552	3099	160

Many Facility Codes have changed. Please refer to the AHA Guide Code Chart.

Hospitals, U.S. / LOUISIANA

Hospital, Address, Telephone, Administrator, Approval, Facility, and Physician Codes, Health Care System, Network	Classification Codes		Utilization Data					Expense (thousands) of dollars		Personnel
★ American Hospital Association (AHA) membership □ Joint Commission on Accreditation of Healthcare Organizations (JCAHO) accreditation + American Osteopathic Healthcare Association (AOHA) membership ○ American Osteopathic Association (AOA) accreditation △ Commission on Accreditation of Rehabilitation Facilities (CARF) accreditation Control codes 61, 63, 64, 71, 72 and 73 indicate hospitals listed by AOHA, but not registered by AHA. For definition of numerical codes, see page A4	Control	Service	Staffed Beds	Admissions	Census	Outpatient Visits	Births	Total	Payroll	
GREENWELL SPRINGS—East Baton Rouge Parish										
EASTERN LOUISIANA MENTAL HEALTH SYSTEM/GREENWELL SPRING CAMPUS, (Formerly Greenwell Springs Hospital), 23260 Greenwell Springs Road, Zip 70739-0999, Mailing Address: P.O. Box 549, Zip 70739-0549; tel. 225/261-2730; Lauren Guttzeit, Acting Chief Executive Officer (Nonreporting) **S** Louisiana State Hospitals, New Orleans, LA	12	22	104	—	—	—	—	—	—	—
GRETNA—Jefferson Parish										
★ MEADOWCREST HOSPITAL, 2500 Belle Chase Highway, Zip 70056-7196; tel. 504/392-3131; Gerald L. Parton, Chief Executive Officer (Total facility includes 24 beds in nursing home-type unit) **A**1 3 9 10 **F**3 4 8 9 11 12 13 16 18 22 24 25 27 28 34 35 36 39 41 42 44 45 46 47 48 50 51 54 58 59 60 61 62 63 64 65 66 68 69 70 71 74 76 78 79 **P**1 5 7 **S** TENET Healthcare Corporation, Santa Barbara, CA Web address: www.tenethealth.com	33	10	181	7342	92	43187	1670	—	—	591
HAMMOND—Tangipahoa Parish										
★ △ NORTH OAKS MEDICAL CENTER, 15790 Medical Center Drive, Zip 70403-1436, Mailing Address: P.O. Box 2668, Zip 70404-2668; tel. 504/345-2700; James E. Cathey, Jr, Chief Executive Officer **A**1 7 9 10 **F**4 8 9 11 13 17 18 22 25 30 32 36 37 39 41 42 43 45 46 47 48 50 51 54 57 61 62 63 68 70 71 72 76 78 79 **P**6 **S** Quorum Health Group, Brentwood, TN Web address: www.northoaks.org	16	10	215	9877	133	192972	1551	94848	48406	1529
HOMER—Claiborne Parish										
HOMER MEMORIAL HOSPITAL, 620 East College Street, Zip 71040-3202; tel. 318/927-2024; James W. McClung, Acting Administrator **A**3 5 9 10 **F**8 9 17 18 22 25 26 30 31 32 34 36 37 38 41 44 45 48 51 57 61 62 63 70 72 76	14	10	60	2148	25	14647	114	—	—	451
HOUMA—Terrebonne Parish										
□ BAYOU OAKS BEHAVIORAL HEALTH SYSTEM, 8134 Main Street, Zip 70360-3404, Mailing Address: P.O. Box 4374, Zip 70361-4374; tel. 504/876-2020; Leonard W. Doucet, Interim Chief Executive Officer (Nonreporting) **A**1	16	22	70	—	—	—	—	—	—	—
★ LEONARD J. CHABERT MEDICAL CENTER, 1978 Industrial Boulevard, Zip 70363-7094; tel. 504/873-2200; Daniel M. Trahan, Administrator **A**1 3 10 **F**9 22 25 29 35 41 42 44 45 46 48 49 54 56 57 59 60 61 70 75 76 78 79 **S** LSU Medical Center Health Care Services Division, Baton Rouge, LA	12	10	123	6118	76	174487	1082	58509	24577	832
★ △ TERREBONNE GENERAL MEDICAL CENTER, 8166 Main Street, Zip 70360, Mailing Address: P.O. Box 6037, Zip 70361-6037; tel. 504/873-4141; Leonard W. Doucet, Interim Chief Executive Officer (Total facility includes 16 beds in nursing home-type unit) **A**1 7 9 10 **F**4 8 9 11 12 13 14 17 19 22 24 25 30 33 34 36 37 38 39 41 43 44 45 46 47 48 50 51 53 54 56 58 59 60 61 62 63 64 68 69 70 72 73 76 77 78 79 **P**6 7 Web address: www.tgmc.com	16	10	261	11763	144	102450	1254	106490	47371	1476
INDEPENDENCE—Tagipahoa Parish										
★ LALLIE KEMP MEDICAL CENTER, 52579 Highway 51 South, Zip 70443-2231; tel. 504/878-9421; LeVern S. Meades, Administrator **A**1 10 **F**9 13 14 17 18 20 22 23 25 29 31 32 34 35 36 38 41 43 45 46 48 49 50 51 54 56 65 68 69 70 72 75 76 77 78 79 **P**6 **S** LSU Medical Center Health Care Services Division, Baton Rouge, LA	12	10	68	1849	26	128463	0	28949	14207	481
JACKSON—East Feliciana Parish										
□ EAST LOUISIANA STATE HOSPITAL, Mailing Address: P.O. Box 498, Zip 70748-0498; tel. 225/634-0100; Warren T. Price, Jr, Chief Executive Officer (Nonreporting) **A**1 10 **S** Louisiana State Hospitals, New Orleans, LA	12	22	452	—	—	—	—	—	—	—
★ VILLA FELICIANA MEDICAL COMPLEX, 5002 Highway 10, Zip 70748-3627, Mailing Address: P.O. Box 438, Zip 70748-0438; tel. 225/634-4000; Hayden Ellis, Administrator (Total facility includes 253 beds in nursing home-type unit) **A**10 **F**23 30 31 59 62 69 70 78	12	48	275	95	246	0	0	16879	10377	426
JENA—La Salle Parish										
★ LASALLE GENERAL HOSPITAL, Highway 84 West, Zip 71342-2780, Mailing Address: P.O. Box 2780, Zip 71342-2780; tel. 318/992-9200; Mary B. Moffett, Administrator **A**9 10 **F**4 7 9 11 22 25 28 32 34 36 48 54 62 76	16	10	60	1747	36	12541	0	9947	4638	187
JENNINGS—Jefferson Davis Parish										
★ JENNINGS AMERICAN LEGION HOSPITAL, 1634 Elton Road, Zip 70546-3614; tel. 318/824-2490; Terry J. Terrebonne, Chief Executive Officer **A**1 9 10 **F**8 9 13 22 24 25 32 34 38 39 41 43 44 48 51 56 69 70 76 78 79 Web address: www.jalh.com	23	10	53	3318	30	34889	338	13569	4902	231
JONESBORO—Jackson Parish										
JACKSON PARISH HOSPITAL, 165 Beech Springs Road, Zip 71251-2059; tel. 318/259-4435; L. J. Pecot, Administrator (Nonreporting) **A**9 10	13	10	59	—	—	—	—	—	—	—
KAPLAN—Vermilion Parish										
ABROM KAPLAN MEMORIAL HOSPITAL, 1310 West Seventh Street, Zip 70548-2998; tel. 318/643-8300; Lyman Trahan, Chief Executive Officer **A**9 10 **F**9 19 22 24 25 32 34 36 37 45 48 57 62 76 78	16	10	40	694	6	—	0	6292	1892	75
KENNER—Jefferson Parish										
★ KENNER REGIONAL MEDICAL CENTER, 180 West Esplanade Avenue, Zip 70065-6001; tel. 504/468-8600; Deborah C. Keel, Chief Executive Officer (Nonreporting) **A**1 3 8 9 10 **S** TENET Healthcare Corporation, Santa Barbara, CA Web address: www.tenethealh.com	33	10	213	—	—	—	—	—	—	—

Hospitals, U.S. / LOUISIANA

Hospital, Address, Telephone, Administrator, Approval, Facility, and Physician Codes, Health Care System, Network	Classification Codes		Utilization Data					Expense (thousands) of dollars		
	Control	Service	Staffed Beds	Admissions	Census	Outpatient Visits	Births	Total	Payroll	Personnel

★ American Hospital Association (AHA) membership
□ Joint Commission on Accreditation of Healthcare Organizations (JCAHO) accreditation
+ American Osteopathic Healthcare Association (AOHA) membership
○ American Osteopathic Association (AOA) accreditation
△ Commission on Accreditation of Rehabilitation Facilities (CARF) accreditation
Control codes 61, 63, 64, 71, 72 and 73 indicate hospitals listed by AOHA, but not registered by AHA. For definition of numerical codes, see page A4

Hospital	Control	Service	Staffed Beds	Admissions	Census	Outpatient Visits	Births	Total	Payroll	Personnel
KINDER—Allen Parish ALLEN PARISH HOSPITAL, 108 North Sixth Avenue, Zip 70648–3519, Mailing Address: P.O. Box 1670, Zip 70648–1670; tel. 318/738–2527; William C. Jeanmard, Chief Executive Officer **A**9 10 **F**16 22 36 57 64 70 76 **P**5	16	49	24	751	13	3763	0	4203	1765	69
LA PLACE—St. John the Baptist Parish □ RIVER PARISHES HOSPITAL, 500 Rue De Sante, Zip 70068–5420; tel. 504/652–7000; B. Ann Kuss, Chief Executive Officer and Managing Director **A**1 9 10 **F**7 8 9 13 18 22 25 32 34 39 41 44 45 46 48 62 70 71 72 76 78 **P**8 **S** Universal Health Services, Inc., King of Prussia, PA	33	10	106	2626	26	79329	441	29465	11749	383
LAFAYETTE—Lafayette Parish ★ LAFAYETTE GENERAL MEDICAL CENTER, 1214 Coolidge Avenue, Zip 70503, Mailing Address: P.O. Box 52009 OCS, Zip 70505–2009; tel. 337/289–7991; James G. Thaw, President and Chief Executive Officer (Total facility includes 30 beds in nursing home–type unit) **A**1 2 6 9 10 **F**4 7 8 9 11 13 14 16 17 18 19 22 23 24 25 27 28 29 30 31 32 33 34 35 36 37 38 39 40 41 42 43 44 45 46 47 48 49 50 51 52 53 54 55 56 57 58 59 60 61 62 63 65 66 68 69 70 71 72 73 76 77 78 79 **P**7 8 Web address: www.lafayettegeneral.org	23	10	348	13991	194	55315	1324	120049	48783	1700
★ MEDICAL CENTER OF SOUTHWEST LOUISIANA, 2810 Ambassador Caffery Parkway, Zip 70506–5900; tel. 318/981–2949; Stephen K. Jones, Jr, Chief Executive Officer **A**1 9 10 **F**4 9 11 13 17 19 22 25 32 34 39 41 43 45 47 48 49 50 53 54 69 70 71 76 78 **P**8 **S** HCA – The Healthcare Company, Nashville, TN Web address: www.medicalcentersw.com	33	10	138	3489	55	44360	—	33455	12643	369
★ OUR LADY OF LOURDES REGIONAL MEDICAL CENTER, 611 St. Landry Street, Zip 70506–4697, Mailing Address: Box 4027, Zip 70502–4027; tel. 318/289–2000; Ronald W. Webb, Chief Executive Officer (Total facility includes 28 beds in nursing home–type unit) **A**1 2 9 10 **F**4 5 7 8 9 11 13 14 16 17 18 19 20 22 24 25 27 28 32 34 36 37 38 39 41 44 45 46 47 48 49 51 53 54 55 56 65 68 69 70 71 72 76 78 **P**6 8 **S** Franciscan Missionaries of Our Lady Health System, Inc., Baton Rouge, LA Web address: www.lourdes.net/	21	10	248	11079	180	86318	259	113276	45363	1367
★ UNIVERSITY MEDICAL CENTER, 2390 West Congress Street, Zip 70506–4298, Mailing Address: P.O. Box 69300, Zip 70596–9300; tel. 337/261–6001; Lawrence T. Dorsey, Administrator **A**1 2 3 5 10 **F**2 7 9 11 14 17 18 21 22 24 25 29 35 38 39 41 42 43 44 45 46 48 49 50 51 56 57 61 64 65 66 70 72 75 76 78 79 **P**6 **S** LSU Medical Center Health Care Services Division, Baton Rouge, LA Web address: www.umcip.lsums.edu	12	10	133	6309	102	129741	988	60278	25040	963
★ VERMILION HOSPITAL FOR PSYCHIATRIC AND ADDICTIVE MEDICINE, 2520 North University Avenue, Zip 70507–5306, Mailing Address: P.O. Box 91526, Zip 70509–1526; tel. 318/234–5614; William A. Ferry, Administrator (Nonreporting) **A**10 **S** General Health System, Baton Rouge, LA	23	22	54	—	—	—	—	—	—	—
★ WOMEN'S AND CHILDREN'S HOSPITAL, 4600 Ambassador Caffery Parkway, Zip 70508–6923, Mailing Address: P.O. Box 88030, Zip 70598–8030; tel. 337/981–9100; Susan Silverman, Chief Executive Officer **A**1 9 10 **F**8 9 13 16 17 18 19 22 32 33 34 38 42 43 44 45 48 54 66 70 72 76 77 78 79 **P**8 **S** HCA – The Healthcare Company, Nashville, TN	33	10	75	4690	54	50060	2668	—	—	—
LAKE CHARLES—Calcasieu Parish ★ CHRISTUS ST. PATRICK HOSPITAL, 524 South Ryan Street, Zip 70601–5799, Mailing Address: P.O. Box 3401, Zip 70602–3401; tel. 318/436–2511; James E. Gardner, Jr, Chief Executive Officer (Total facility includes 23 beds in nursing home–type unit) **A**1 2 7 9 10 **F**1 2 3 4 7 8 9 11 12 13 17 18 19 22 25 28 32 34 36 39 41 43 44 45 46 47 48 51 53 54 56 57 58 62 63 64 65 69 70 72 76 79 **P**7 8 **S** Christus Health, Irving, TX	21	10	359	9841	167	160567	257	89213	35412	1216
★ DUBUIS HOSPITAL FOR CONTINUING CARE, 524 South Ryan, 5th Floor, Zip 70601; tel. 318/491–7752; Tracey S. Richard, Administrator (Nonreporting) **A**1 9	21	48	20	—	—	—	—	—	—	—
□ △ LAKE CHARLES MEMORIAL HOSPITAL, 1701 Oak Park Boulevard, Zip 70601–8911, Mailing Address: P.O. Drawer M, Zip 70602; tel. 318/494–3000; Elton L. Williams, Jr, CPA, President **A**1 2 3 7 9 10 **F**1 2 3 4 8 9 11 13 14 17 18 19 21 22 23 24 25 27 28 29 32 33 34 36 37 38 39 41 43 44 45 46 47 48 49 51 52 53 54 57 58 61 62 63 65 69 70 71 72 73 75 76 77 78 **P**1 5 7 Web address: www.lcmh.com	23	10	301	12636	184	58672	1416	64819	32205	1892
★ WALTER OLIN MOSS REGIONAL MEDICAL CENTER, 1000 Walters Street, Zip 70605; tel. 318/475–8100; Clay Dunaway, Administrator **A**5 10 **F**7 9 13 14 22 25 32 35 38 39 41 46 48 50 51 54 56 57 70 76 78 **P**4 7 **S** LSU Medical Center Health Care Services Division, Baton Rouge, LA	12	10	74	2637	39	105056	0	28631	11152	406
★ WOMEN AND CHILDREN'S HOSPITAL–LAKE CHARLES, 4200 Nelson Road, Zip 70605–4118; tel. 318/474–6370; Bill Willis, Chief Executive Officer **A**1 9 10 **F**8 9 13 22 25 41 42 44 45 48 66 70 76 78 79 **S** Triad Hospitals, Inc., Dallas, TX Web address: www.women–childrens.com	33	10	80	2511	25	11476	1505	14516	7150	229
LAKE PROVIDENCE—East Carroll Parish EAST CARROLL PARISH HOSPITAL, 226 North Hood Street, Zip 71254–2194; tel. 318/559–2441; Ladonna Englerth, Administrator (Nonreporting) **A**9 10	16	10	29	—	—	—	—	—	—	—

Hospitals, U.S. / LOUISIANA

Hospital, Address, Telephone, Administrator, Approval, Facility, and Physician Codes, Health Care System, Network	Classification Codes		Utilization Data					Expense (thousands) of dollars		
★ American Hospital Association (AHA) membership □ Joint Commission on Accreditation of Healthcare Organizations (JCAHO) accreditation + American Osteopathic Healthcare Association (AOHA) membership ○ American Osteopathic Association (AOA) accreditation △ Commission on Accreditation of Rehabilitation Facilities (CARF) accreditation Control codes 61, 63, 64, 71, 72 and 73 indicate hospitals listed by AOHA, but not registered by AHA. For definition of numerical codes, see page A4	Control	Service	Staffed Beds	Admissions	Census	Outpatient Visits	Births	Total	Payroll	Personnel
LEESVILLE—Vernon Parish □ BYRD REGIONAL HOSPITAL, 1020 West Fertitta Boulevard, Zip 71446–4697; tel. 318/239–9041; Roger C. LeDoux, Chief Executive Officer (Nonreporting) **A**1 9 10 **S** Community Health Systems, Inc., Brentwood, TN	33	10	59	—	—	—	—	—	—	—
LULING—St. Charles Parish □ ST. CHARLES PARISH HOSPITAL, 1057 Paul Maillard Road, Zip 70070, Mailing Address: P.O. Box 87, Zip 70070–0087; tel. 504/785–6242; Fred Martinez, Jr, Chief Executive Officer **A**1 9 10 **F**9 13 16 17 22 30 32 33 34 38 39 41 45 46 48 49 50 54 57 59 60 61 62 70 71 72 76 78	16	10	56	1948	26	—	1	15613	8207	297
LUTCHER—St. James Parish ✠ ST. JAMES PARISH HOSPITAL, 2471 Louisiana Avenue, Zip 70071–5413; tel. 225/869–5512; Joan Z. Murray, R.N., Administrator and Chief Executive Officer **A**1 9 10 **F**9 17 18 19 22 25 26 30 32 33 34 36 38 40 43 45 48 50 51 54 57 60 62 70 72 76 78 79 Web address: www.stjamesparishhospital.com	16	10	26	350	5	15275	0	6530	2719	109
MAMOU—Evangeline Parish ✠ SAVOY MEDICAL CENTER, 801 Poinciana Avenue, Zip 70554–2298; tel. 318/468–5261; J. E. Richardson, Chief Executive Officer (Total facility includes 125 beds in nursing home–type unit) **A**1 10 **F**1 2 3 8 9 11 13 14 17 18 22 24 25 30 32 33 34 36 37 38 39 41 44 48 49 50 51 53 55 57 58 60 62 64 66 69 70 73 76 78 **P**1 **S** HCA – The Healthcare Company, Nashville, TN	33	10	330	5818	196	74796	550	33818	15720	601
MANDEVILLE—St. Tammany Parish □ SOUTHEAST LOUISIANA HOSPITAL, Mailing Address: P.O. Box 3850, Zip 70470–3850; tel. 504/626–6300; Joseph C. Vinturella, Chief Executive Officer **A**1 10 **F**17 18 57 58 59 61 62 63 64 78 **S** Louisiana State Hospitals, New Orleans, LA	12	22	231	618	199	0	0	28672	18325	603
MANSFIELD—De Soto Parish ★ DE SOTO REGIONAL HEALTH SYSTEM, 207 Jefferson Street, Zip 71052–2603, Mailing Address: P.O. Box 1636, Zip 71052–0672; tel. 318/871–3101; William F. Barrow, President and Chief Executive Officer **A**9 10 **F**9 13 14 16 17 22 28 29 31 32 34 36 38 39 43 45 46 48 51 54 57 59 62 63 64 70 72 76 79 **P**6	23	10	49	1438	20	17342	0	11626	4571	158
MANY—Sabine Parish □ SABINE MEDICAL CENTER, 240 Highland Drive, Zip 71449–3718; tel. 318/256–5691; Patrick W. Gandy, Chief Executive Officer **A**1 9 10 **F**13 17 18 22 23 25 32 33 34 39 41 48 51 54 68 76 **S** Community Health Systems, Inc., Brentwood, TN	33	10	48	1191	10	10822	0	5596	2539	85
MARKSVILLE—Avoyelles Parish ✠ AVOYELLES HOSPITAL, 4231 Highway 1192, Zip 71351, Mailing Address: P.O. Box 249, Zip 71351; tel. 318/253–8611; David M. Mitchel, Chief Executive Officer **A**1 9 10 **F**13 22 25 30 39 41 48 54 57 62 64 70 76 78 **P**1 7 **S** HCA – The Healthcare Company, Nashville, TN	32	10	47	1526	20	12979	0	9299	4181	156
MARRERO—Jefferson Parish ✠ △ WEST JEFFERSON MEDICAL CENTER, 1101 Medical Center Boulevard, Zip 70072–3191; tel. 504/347–5511; A. Gary Muller, FACHE, President and Chief Executive Officer **A**1 7 9 10 **F**2 3 4 7 8 9 11 12 13 14 19 22 23 24 25 27 28 29 33 34 36 38 39 41 42 44 45 46 47 48 49 50 51 52 53 54 57 61 65 68 69 70 71 72 75 76 78 79	16	10	309	13869	171	93801	1028	139707	53901	1691
METAIRIE—Jefferson Parish ✠ DOCTORS HOSPITAL OF JEFFERSON, 4320 Houma Boulevard, Zip 70006–2973; tel. 504/849–4000; John E. Walker, Chief Executive Officer (Total facility includes 10 beds in nursing home–type unit) **A**1 10 **F**1 2 3 4 5 6 8 9 10 11 13 14 16 17 18 19 21 22 23 24 25 27 28 29 30 31 32 33 34 35 36 37 38 39 40 41 42 43 44 45 46 47 48 49 50 51 52 53 54 56 57 58 59 60 61 62 63 64 65 66 67 68 69 70 71 72 74 75 76 77 78 79 **P**5 7 8 **S** TENET Healthcare Corporation, Santa Barbara, CA Web address: www.tenethealth.com	33	10	130	2404	36	17292	0	30631	8955	184
✠ △ EAST JEFFERSON GENERAL HOSPITAL, 4200 Houma Boulevard, Zip 70006–2996; tel. 504/454–4000; Peter J. Betts, President and Chief Executive Officer (Total facility includes 71 beds in nursing home–type unit) **A**1 2 3 5 7 9 10 **F**1 3 4 7 8 9 11 12 13 17 18 19 22 24 25 27 28 30 31 32 33 34 36 37 38 39 40 41 42 43 44 45 46 47 48 49 51 53 54 56 57 59 60 61 62 63 64 65 68 69 70 72 76 78 79 **P**6 7 Web address: www.eastjeffhospital.org/	16	10	460	20772	355	229704	2022	201642	88871	3004
✠ LAKESIDE HOSPITAL, 4700 I–10 Service Road, Zip 70001–1269; tel. 504/885–3342; Gerald A. Fornoff, Chief Executive Officer **A**1 9 10 **F**8 9 13 17 18 22 28 38 41 42 44 48 50 51 53 54 64 66 70 71 76 78 79 **P**5 7 8 **S** HCA – The Healthcare Company, Nashville, TN	33	10	75	2492	23	21962	1539	20405	8931	238
MINDEN—Webster Parish ✠ MINDEN MEDICAL CENTER, 1 Medical Plaza, Zip 71055–3330, Mailing Address: P.O. Box 5003, Zip 71058–5003; tel. 318/377–2321; George E. French, II, Chief Executive Officer **A**1 9 10 **F**8 9 13 16 17 18 19 22 25 30 32 33 34 36 37 39 41 44 45 46 48 51 54 62 64 70 76 78 79 Web address: www.mindenmedicalcenter.com	33	10	130	3451	32	38658	611	17633	10181	331
MONROE—Ouachita Parish ✠ E. A. CONWAY MEDICAL CENTER, 4864 Jackson Street, Zip 71202–6497, Mailing Address: P.O. Box 1881, Zip 71210–1881; tel. 318/330–7000; Aryon McGuire, Acting Administrator **A**1 3 5 10 **F**7 9 17 22 25 32 35 38 39 42 43 46 48 49 51 55 57 61 65 70 76 78 **P**1 **S** LSU Medical Center Health Care Services Division, Baton Rouge, LA	12	10	174	7890	122	162923	1638	58804	25002	1010

© 2000 AHA Guide *Many Facility Codes have changed. Please refer to the AHA Guide Code Chart.*

Hospitals, U.S. / LOUISIANA

Hospital, Address, Telephone, Administrator, Approval, Facility, and Physician Codes, Health Care System, Network	Classification Codes		Utilization Data					Expense (thousands) of dollars		
	Control	Service	Staffed Beds	Admissions	Census	Outpatient Visits	Births	Total	Payroll	Personnel

★ American Hospital Association (AHA) membership
□ Joint Commission on Accreditation of Healthcare Organizations (JCAHO) accreditation
+ American Osteopathic Healthcare Association (AOHA) membership
○ American Osteopathic Association (AOA) accreditation
△ Commission on Accreditation of Rehabilitation Facilities (CARF) accreditation
Control codes 61, 63, 64, 71, 72 and 73 indicate hospitals listed by AOHA, but not registered by AHA. For definition of numerical codes, see page A4

Hospital	Control	Service	Staffed Beds	Admissions	Census	Outpatient Visits	Births	Total	Payroll	Personnel
★ NORTH MONROE HOSPITAL, 3421 Medical Park Drive, Zip 71203–2399; tel. 318/388–1946; George E. Miller, Chief Executive Officer (Total facility includes 13 beds in nursing home–type unit) (Nonreporting) **A**1 9 10 **S** HCA – The Healthcare Company, Nashville, TN	33	10	210	—	—	—	—	—	—	—
★ ST. FRANCIS MEDICAL CENTER, 309 Jackson Street, Zip 71201–7498, Mailing Address: P.O. Box 1901, Zip 71210–1901; tel. 318/327–4000; H. Gerald Smith, President and Chief Executive Officer **A**1 2 9 10 **F**1 4 7 8 9 11 12 13 14 17 18 19 22 24 25 27 28 32 34 35 36 37 39 40 41 42 43 44 45 46 47 48 49 52 54 56 62 65 69 70 72 76 77 78 79 **P**6 8 **S** Franciscan Missionaries of Our Lady Health System, Inc., Baton Rouge, LA Web address: www.stfran.com	23	10	341	13405	214	96267	1271	141966	50573	1552
□ △ ST. FRANCIS SPECIALTY HOSPITAL, Mailing Address: P.O. Box 1532, Zip 71210–1210; tel. 318/327–4267; George W. Hightower, CHE, President and Chief Executive Officer **A**1 7 10 **F**1 4 7 8 9 11 13 17 18 19 22 25 26 27 28 29 30 31 32 33 34 35 36 37 39 45 46 47 48 49 50 53 54 56 62 64 65 70 72 73 74 75 76 77 78 79 Web address: www.stfran.com	23	46	50	402	29	0	—	12052	3804	139

MORGAN CITY—St. Mary Parish

	Control	Service	Staffed Beds	Admissions	Census	Outpatient Visits	Births	Total	Payroll	Personnel
★ LAKEWOOD MEDICAL CENTER, 1125 Marguerite Street, Zip 70380–1855, Mailing Address: Drawer 2308, Zip 70381–2308; tel. 504/384–2200; Clifford M. Broussard, Chief Executive Officer (Total facility includes 10 beds in nursing home–type unit) **A**1 9 10 **F**7 8 9 11 12 13 16 17 18 19 20 22 24 25 30 32 34 36 39 41 43 44 45 46 48 50 51 54 57 61 62 68 69 70 76 78 79	16	10	121	2781	29	38252	417	21222	9277	320

NAPOLEONVILLE—Assumption Parish

OUR LADY OF THE LAKE–ASSUMPTION See Our Lady of the Lake Regional Medical Center, Baton Rouge

NATCHITOCHES—Natchitoches Parish

	Control	Service	Staffed Beds	Admissions	Census	Outpatient Visits	Births	Total	Payroll	Personnel
★ NATCHITOCHES PARISH HOSPITAL, 501 Keyser Avenue, Zip 71457–6036, Mailing Address: P.O. Box 2009, Zip 71457–2009; tel. 318/214–4200; Mark E. Marley, Chief Executive Officer (Total facility includes 112 beds in nursing home–type unit) **A**1 9 10 **F**1 7 8 9 12 13 17 18 22 25 28 31 32 34 36 37 39 40 41 43 44 45 46 48 49 51 54 57 62 64 69 70 71 72 75 76 77 78 **P**5 **S** Christus Health, Irving, TX	16	10	166	3687	143	37940	646	21410	10216	398

NEW IBERIA—Iberia Parish

	Control	Service	Staffed Beds	Admissions	Census	Outpatient Visits	Births	Total	Payroll	Personnel
★ DAUTERIVE HOSPITAL, 600 North Lewis Street, Zip 70560, Mailing Address: P.O. Box 11210, Zip 70562–1210; tel. 318/365–7311; Kyle J. Viator, Chief Executive Officer **A**1 9 10 **F**8 9 11 16 18 22 25 30 33 44 48 49 50 54 57 62 63 64 69 70 71 76 78 79 **P**7 **S** HCA – The Healthcare Company, Nashville, TN	33	10	86	4301	52	39539	802	—	—	—
★ IBERIA MEDICAL CENTER, (Formerly Iberia General Hospital and Medical Center), 2315 East Main Street, Zip 70560–4031, Mailing Address: P.O. Box 13338, Zip 70562–3338; tel. 318/364–0441; James H. Youree, Interim Chief Executive Officer (Total facility includes 12 beds in nursing home–type unit) **A**1 9 10 **F**7 8 9 11 13 14 16 22 24 25 27 31 32 33 34 36 38 39 41 43 44 45 46 48 50 51 54 69 70 72 76 78 **S** Brim Healthcare, Inc., Brentwood, TN Web address: www.iberiamedicalcenter.com	16	10	90	3546	46	57596	345	30677	12686	382

NEW ORLEANS—Orleans Parish

	Control	Service	Staffed Beds	Admissions	Census	Outpatient Visits	Births	Total	Payroll	Personnel
BHC EAST LAKE HOSPITAL, 5650 Read Boulevard, Zip 70127–3145; tel. 504/241–0888; Darlene Brennan, Chief Executive Officer (Nonreporting) **S** Behavioral Healthcare Corporation, Nashville, TN	33	22	52	—	—	—	—	—	—	—
CHARITY CAMPUS See Medical Center of Louisiana at New Orleans										
□ △ CHILDREN'S HOSPITAL, 200 Henry Clay Avenue, Zip 70118–5799; tel. 504/899–9511; Steve Worley, President and Chief Executive Officer **A**1 2 3 5 7 9 10 **F**4 5 7 11 13 14 18 19 22 23 24 25 29 32 34 35 38 39 42 43 46 47 48 50 51 52 53 54 56 58 59 61 63 70 71 72 73 74 76 77 78 **P**8 Web address: www.chnola.org	23	50	175	7806	110	108069	0	—	—	1143
DEPAUL/TULANE BEHAVIORAL HEALTH CENTER See Tulane University Hospital and Clinic										
★ △ LAKELAND MEDICAL CENTER, 6000 Bullard Avenue, Zip 70128; tel. 504/241–6335; Tracy A. Rogers, Chief Executive Officer (Total facility includes 20 beds in nursing home–type unit) **A**1 7 9 10 **F**2 3 4 8 9 11 12 13 14 17 18 19 21 22 23 24 25 26 27 28 29 30 32 34 35 37 38 39 41 42 44 45 46 47 48 49 50 51 52 53 54 55 56 57 58 59 60 61 62 63 64 65 66 68 69 70 71 72 74 75 76 77 78 79 **P**7 8 **S** HCA – The Healthcare Company, Nashville, TN Web address: www.hcahealthcare.com	33	10	140	5279	84	33664	829	36574	16129	479
★ MEDICAL CENTER OF LOUISIANA AT NEW ORLEANS, (Includes Charity Campus, 1532 Tulane Avenue, Zip 70140; tel. 504/568–3201; University Campus, 2021 Perdido Street), 2021 Perdido Street, Zip 70112–1396; tel. 504/588–3000; John S. Berault, Chief Executive Officer **A**1 2 3 5 8 10 **F**4 8 9 11 13 17 18 19 21 22 23 24 25 26 27 32 34 35 36 37 38 39 41 42 43 44 45 46 47 48 51 52 53 54 56 57 59 63 64 65 68 70 71 72 73 74 75 76 78 **S** LSU Medical Center Health Care Services Division, Baton Rouge, LA	12	10	643	33400	548	571107	3579	394812	150780	4827
★ MEMORIAL MEDICAL CENTER, (Includes Memorial Medical Center–Baptist Campus, 2700 Napoleon Avenue, Zip 70115–6996; tel. 504/899–9311; Memorial Medical Center–Mercy Campus, 301 North Jefferson Davis Parkway, Zip 70119–5397; tel. 504/483–5000), Randall L. Hoover, Chief Executive Officer (Total facility includes 81 beds in nursing home–type unit) **A**1 2 3 5 8 9 10 **F**4 8 9 11 13 14 15 17 18 19 21 22 23 24 25 26 27 28 29 30 31 32 33 34 35 36 37 39 41 42 43 46 47 48 49 50 51 53 54 55 56 58 59 60 61 62 64 65 66 67 68 69 70 71 72 74 75 76 77 78 79 **P**5 7 8 **S** TENET Healthcare Corporation, Santa Barbara, CA	33	10	389	17490	287	281268	1808	163592	68559	1696

Hospitals, U.S. / LOUISIANA

Hospital, Address, Telephone, Administrator, Approval, Facility, and Physician Codes, Health Care System, Network	Classification Codes		Utilization Data					Expense (thousands) of dollars		
★ American Hospital Association (AHA) membership ☐ Joint Commission on Accreditation of Healthcare Organizations (JCAHO) accreditation + American Osteopathic Healthcare Association (AOHA) membership ○ American Osteopathic Association (AOA) accreditation △ Commission on Accreditation of Rehabilitation Facilities (CARF) accreditation Control codes 61, 63, 64, 71, 72 and 73 indicate hospitals listed by AOHA, but not registered by AHA. For definition of numerical codes, see page A4	Control	Service	Staffed Beds	Admissions	Census	Outpatient Visits	Births	Total	Payroll	Personnel
☐ METHODIST BEHAVIORAL RESOURCES, 5610 Read Boulevard, Zip 70127–3155; tel. 504/244-5661; Michael D. Moran, FACHE, Administrator (Nonreporting) **A**1 10 **Web address:** www.methodistpsych.com	32	22	36	—	—	—	—	—	—	—
☐ NEW ORLEANS ADOLESCENT HOSPITAL, 210 State Street, Zip 70118–5797; tel. 504/897-3400; William J. Malone, M.P.H., Acting Chief Executive Officer (Nonreporting) **A**1 3 10 **S** Louisiana State Hospitals, New Orleans, LA	12	52	95	—	—	—	—	—	—	—
★ △ OCHSNER FOUNDATION HOSPITAL, 1516 Jefferson Highway, Zip 70121–2484; tel. 504/842-3000; Eileen F. Skinner, Director (Total facility includes 34 beds in nursing home–type unit) **A**1 2 3 5 7 8 9 10 **F**3 4 5 8 9 11 12 13 14 17 18 19 20 21 22 23 24 25 26 27 28 29 31 33 34 35 36 38 39 41 42 43 44 45 46 47 48 49 50 51 52 53 54 56 57 58 59 60 61 62 63 64 65 66 68 69 70 71 72 74 76 77 78 79 **P**6 8	23	10	390	17191	264	1596324	1070	251419	91491	2893
★ PENDLETON MEMORIAL METHODIST HOSPITAL, 5620 Read Boulevard, Zip 70127–3154; tel. 504/244-5100; Frederick C. Young, Jr, President (Total facility includes 22 beds in nursing home–type unit) (Nonreporting) **A**1 9 10 **Web address:** www.pmmh.org	23	10	163	—	—	—	—	—	—	—
☐ PHYSICIANS HOSPITAL, 3125 Canal Street, Zip 70119–6285; tel. 504/822-8222; Steve E. Pallos, Administrator (Nonreporting) **A**1 10	33	10	40	—	—	—	—	—	—	—
☐ RIVER OAKS HOSPITAL, 1525 River Oaks Road West, Zip 70123–2199; tel. 504/734-1740; Daryl Sue White, Chief Executive Officer and Managing Director (Nonreporting) **A**1 10 **S** Universal Health Services, Inc., King of Prussia, PA **Web address:** www.riveroakshospital.com	33	22	94	—	—	—	—	—	—	—
★ ST. CHARLES GENERAL HOSPITAL, 3700 St. Charles Avenue, Zip 70115–4680; tel. 504/899-7441; L. Rene' Goux, Chief Executive Officer (Nonreporting) **A**1 9 10 **S** TENET Healthcare Corporation, Santa Barbara, CA **Web address:** www.tenethealth.com	33	10	137	—	—	—	—	—	—	—
ST. CLAUDE MEDICAL CENTER, 3419 St. Claude Avenue, Zip 70117–6198; tel. 504/948-8200; Gwendolyn M. McInnis, R.N., Chief Executive Officer (Nonreporting) **A**9 10 **S** United Medical Corporation, Windermere, FL	33	10	136	—	—	—	—	—	—	—
☐ △ TOURO INFIRMARY, 1401 Foucher Street, Zip 70115–3593; tel. 504/897-7011; Gary M. Stein, President and Chief Executive Officer (Total facility includes 53 beds in nursing home–type unit) **A**1 2 3 5 7 8 9 10 **F**1 4 6 7 8 9 11 13 18 19 20 21 22 24 27 28 29 30 32 33 34 36 38 39 41 42 43 44 45 46 47 48 49 50 51 53 54 56 57 59 60 61 62 63 64 65 66 67 68 69 70 71 72 75 76 77 78 79 **P**1 6 **Web address:** www.touro.com	23	10	336	9356	182	118503	1172	110902	51140	1424
★ TULANE UNIVERSITY HOSPITAL AND CLINIC, (Includes DePaul/Tulane Behavioral Health Center, 1040 Calhoun Street, Zip 70118–5999; tel. 504/899-8282), 1415 Tulane Avenue, Zip 70112–2632; tel. 504/588-5263; Shirley A. Stewart, President and Chief Executive Officer **A**1 2 3 5 8 9 10 **F**2 3 4 7 8 9 11 12 13 14 16 18 19 21 22 24 25 27 29 30 31 32 33 34 35 38 39 41 42 43 44 45 46 47 48 49 51 52 53 54 56 57 58 59 60 61 62 63 64 65 66 68 70 71 72 73 74 76 78 79 **P**1 **S** HCA – The Healthcare Company, Nashville, TN **Web address:** www.tuhc.com	32	10	336	11948	232	311253	583	190610	68224	1659
UNIVERSITY CAMPUS See Medical Center of Louisiana at New Orleans										
☐ VENCOR HOSPITAL – NEW ORLEANS, 3601 Coliseum Street, Zip 70115–3606; tel. 504/899-1555; Jan Turk, Chief Executive Officer (Nonreporting) **A**1 10 **S** Vencor, Incorporated, Louisville, KY	33	10	78	—	—	—	—	—	—	—
★ VETERANS AFFAIRS MEDICAL CENTER, 1601 Perdido Street, Zip 70112–1262; tel. 504/568-0811; John D. Church, Jr, Director (Total facility includes 60 beds in nursing home–type unit) **A**1 2 3 5 8 **F**3 4 6 7 9 11 13 16 17 18 19 20 21 22 23 24 25 26 29 30 31 32 33 34 35 36 37 38 39 41 43 45 46 47 48 49 50 51 54 55 56 57 60 61 62 63 64 65 68 69 70 72 75 76 77 78 79 **P**6 **S** Department of Veterans Affairs, Washington, DC **Web address:** www.va.gov/stations97/guide/home.asp?DIVISION=ALL	45	10	204	5029	144	309359	0	148857	71993	1981
NEW ROADS—Pointe Coupee Parish										
★ POINTE COUPEE GENERAL HOSPITAL, 2202 False River Drive, Zip 70760–2698; tel. 225/638-6331; Larry J. Ayres, Administrator and Chief Executive Officer **A**9 10 **F**7 9 17 18 22 25 36 41 45 48 76	16	10	27	1323	11	31752	0	9442	4238	166
OAK GROVE—West Carroll Parish										
WEST CARROLL MEMORIAL HOSPITAL, 706 Ross Street, Zip 71263, Mailing Address: P.O. Box 748, Zip 71263–0748; tel. 318/428-3237; R. Randall Morris, Administrator (Nonreporting) **A**9 10	23	10	21	—	—	—	—	—	—	—
OAKDALE—Allen Parish										
★ OAKDALE COMMUNITY HOSPITAL, 130 North Hospital Drive, Zip 71463–4004, Mailing Address: P.O. Box 629, Zip 71463–0629; tel. 318/335-3700; Kevin N. Fowler, Chief Executive Officer **A**1 10 **F**13 17 22 24 25 28 32 34 36 39 41 48 54 70 76 78 **P**8 **S** HCA – The Healthcare Company, Nashville, TN	32	10	54	2648	32	27632	0	12585	5143	184
OLLA—La Salle Parish										
HARDTNER MEDICAL CENTER, Highway 165 South, Zip 71465, Mailing Address: P.O. Box 1218, Zip 71465–1218; tel. 318/495-3131; David Hamner, Administrator **A**9 10 **F**7 9 13 17 22 25 27 30 48 50 54 57 62 70 76 **P**5	16	10	41	973	14	10569	—	5361	1850	76
OPELOUSAS—St. Landry Parish										
☐ DOCTORS' HOSPITAL OF OPELOUSAS, 3972 I-49 South Service Road, Zip 70570–8975; tel. 318/948-2100; Bethy W. Walker, Chief Executive Officer (Nonreporting) **A**1 9 10 **S** Province Healthcare Corporation, Brentwood, TN	32	10	105	—	—	—	—	—	—	—

© 2000 AHA Guide *Many Facility Codes have changed. Please refer to the AHA Guide Code Chart.*

Hospitals, U.S. / LOUISIANA

Hospital, Address, Telephone, Administrator, Approval, Facility, and Physician Codes, Health Care System, Network	Classification Codes		Utilization Data					Expense (thousands) of dollars		
★ American Hospital Association (AHA) membership □ Joint Commission on Accreditation of Healthcare Organizations (JCAHO) accreditation + American Osteopathic Healthcare Association (AOHA) membership ○ American Osteopathic Association (AOA) accreditation △ Commission on Accreditation of Rehabilitation Facilities (CARF) accreditation Control codes 61, 63, 64, 71, 72 and 73 indicate hospitals listed by AOHA, but not registered by AHA. For definition of numerical codes, see page A4	Control	Service	Staffed Beds	Admissions	Census	Outpatient Visits	Births	Total	Payroll	Personnel
⊞ OPELOUSAS GENERAL HOSPITAL, 539 East Prudhomme Street, Zip 70570; Mailing Address: P.O. Box 1208, Zip 70571–1208; tel. 318/948–3011; Daryl J. Doise, Administrator **A**1 2 9 10 **F**2 8 11 17 18 19 22 24 25 28 32 35 36 39 41 44 46 48 50 51 54 56 64 65 68 70 78 79 **P**7 8 **S** Quorum Health Group, Brentwood, TN Web address: www.opelousasgeneral.com	16	10	134	5727	68	80777	763	41883	16878	633
PINEVILLE—Rapides Parish										
□ CENTRAL LOUISIANA STATE HOSPITAL, 242 West Shamrock Avenue, Zip 71361–5031, Mailing Address: P.O. Box 5031, Zip 71361–5031; tel. 318/484–6200; Gary S. Grand, Chief Executive Officer **A**1 10 **F**16 23 57 58 60 70 78 **P**6 **S** Louisiana State Hospitals, New Orleans, LA	12	22	216	370	193	0	0	20264	12431	442
⊞ HUEY P. LONG MEDICAL CENTER, 352 Hospital Boulevard, Zip 71360, Mailing Address: P.O. Box 5352, Zip 71361–5352; tel. 318/448–0811; James E. Morgan, Administrator (Nonreporting) **A**1 3 5 10 **S** LSU Medical Center Health Care Services Division, Baton Rouge, LA	12	10	123	—	—	—	—	—	—	—
PLAQUEMINE—Iberville Parish										
□ RIVER WEST MEDICAL CENTER, 59355 River West Drive, Zip 70764–9543; tel. 225/687–9222; Mark Nosacka, Chief Executive Officer **A**1 9 10 **F**8 9 11 13 17 19 22 25 32 34 36 39 41 44 45 46 48 49 53 54 70 76 78 **S** Community Health Systems, Inc., Brentwood, TN	33	10	72	2854	29	24154	386	15709	5773	201
RACELAND—Lafourche Parish										
□ ST. ANNE GENERAL HOSPITAL, 4608 Highway 1, Zip 70394; tel. 504/537–6841; Milton D. Bourgeois, Jr, Administrator (Total facility includes 12 beds in nursing home–type unit) **A**1 9 10 **F**7 8 9 11 13 18 22 24 25 27 36 39 41 44 48 51 57 61 62 63 69 70 76	16	10	70	1829	16	19758	325	18115	7972	278
RAYVILLE—Richland Parish										
RICHARDSON MEDICAL CENTER, 254 Highway 3048, Christian Drive, Zip 71269–9985, Mailing Address: P.O. Box 388, Zip 71269–9985; tel. 318/728–4181; David D. Kervin, Administrator (Nonreporting) **A**9 10	16	10	60	—	—	—	—	—	—	—
RUSTON—Lincoln Parish										
□ HEALTHSOUTH NORTH LOUISIANA REHABILITATION HOSPITAL, 1401 Ezell Street, Zip 71270–7221, Mailing Address: P.O. Box 490, Zip 71273–0490; tel. 318/251–5354; Mark Rice, Chief Executive Officer (Nonreporting) **A**1 10 **S** HEALTHSOUTH Corporation, Birmingham, AL	33	46	90	—	—	—	—	—	—	—
⊞ LINCOLN GENERAL HOSPITAL, 401 East Vaughn Street, Zip 71270–5950, Mailing Address: P.O. Drawer 1368, Zip 71273–1368; tel. 318/254–2100; E. Allen Tuten, Administrator (Total facility includes 13 beds in nursing home–type unit) **A**1 9 10 **F**4 7 9 11 13 19 22 24 25 27 32 34 36 37 38 39 41 44 45 46 48 54 69 70 72 76 79	23	10	124	6428	79	35831	585	36859	15544	464
SAINT FRANCISVILLE—West Feliciana Parish										
⊞ WEST FELICIANA PARISH HOSPITAL, Mailing Address: P.O. Box 368, Zip 70775–0368; tel. 225/635–3811; John H. Green, Administrator (Nonreporting) **A**1 9 10	16	10	23	—	—	—	—	—	—	—
SHREVEPORT—Caddo Parish										
□ BRENTWOOD, A BEHAVIORAL HEALTH COMPANY, (Formerly Charter Brentwood Behavioral Health System), 1006 Highland Avenue, Zip 71101–4103; tel. 318/221–1436; Scott F. Blakley, Chief Executive Officer (Nonreporting) **A**1 3 9 10	33	22	200	—	—	—	—	—	—	—
⊞ CHRISTUS SCHUMPERT MEDICAL CENTER, One St. Mary Place, Zip 71101–4399, Mailing Address: P.O. Box 21976, Zip 71120–1076; tel. 318/681–4500; Wayne A. Sensor, Chief Executive Officer (Nonreporting) **A**1 2 3 5 9 10 **S** Christus Health, Irving, TX	21	10	486	—	—	—	—	—	—	—
□ △ DOCTORS' HOSPITAL OF SHREVEPORT, 1130 Louisiana Avenue, Zip 71101–3998, Mailing Address: P.O. Box 1526, Zip 71165–1526; tel. 318/227–1211; Charles E. Boyd, Chief Executive Officer and Managing Director (Nonreporting) **A**1 7 9 10 **S** Universal Health Services, Inc., King of Prussia, PA	33	10	118	—	—	—	—	—	—	—
★ HIGHLAND HOSPITAL, 1453 East Bert Kouns Industrial Loop, Zip 71105–6050; tel. 318/798–4300; Anthony S. Sala, Jr, Chief Executive Officer (Nonreporting) **A**9 **S** Christus Health, Irving, TX	33	10	121	—	—	—	—	—	—	—
⊞ LIFECARE HOSPITALS, (ACUTE LONG TERM CARE), 9320 Linwood Avenue, Zip 71106, tel. 318/688–8504; Robert A. Loepp, Jr, CHE, Administrator **A**1 10 **F**13 22 25 31 39 45 59 62 68 76 **S** LifeCare Management Services, Dallas, TX Web address: www.lifecare–hospitals.com	33	49	65	583	46	—	0	16877	5003	173
⊞ LSU MEDICAL CENTER–UNIVERSITY HOSPITAL, 1501 Kings Highway, Zip 71130–4299, Mailing Address: P.O. Box 33932, Zip 71130–3932; tel. 318/675–5000; Ingo Angermeier, FACHE, Administrator and Chief Executive Officer **A**1 2 3 5 8 10 **F**4 5 8 9 10 11 13 22 24 25 29 30 35 38 39 41 42 43 44 45 46 47 48 49 50 51 52 54 55 56 57 61 63 65 66 68 70 71 73 74 75 76 78 79 **P**1 Web address: www.lsumc.edu	12	10	413	18309	312	413351	2210	190746	115055	1969
⊞ OVERTON BROOKS VETERANS AFFAIRS MEDICAL CENTER, 510 East Stoner Avenue, Zip 71101–4295; tel. 318/221–8411; Billy M. Valentine, Director **A**1 2 3 5 8 **F**3 4 9 11 13 16 17 18 19 22 23 24 25 27 28 29 30 31 32 34 35 36 38 39 41 43 45 46 47 48 49 51 54 55 56 57 59 61 62 63 64 65 68 69 70 72 76 78 79 **P**6 **S** Department of Veterans Affairs, Washington, DC Web address: www.va.gov/stations97/guide/home.asp?DIVISION=ALL	45	10	100	4236	78	236976	0	90055	41080	1046

Hospitals, U.S. / LOUISIANA

Hospital, Address, Telephone, Administrator, Approval, Facility, and Physician Codes, Health Care System, Network	Classification Codes		Utilization Data					Expense (thousands) of dollars		
★ American Hospital Association (AHA) membership □ Joint Commission on Accreditation of Healthcare Organizations (JCAHO) accreditation + American Osteopathic Healthcare Association (AOHA) membership ○ American Osteopathic Association (AOA) accreditation △ Commission on Accreditation of Rehabilitation Facilities (CARF) accreditation Control codes 61, 63, 64, 71, 72 and 73 indicate hospitals listed by AOHA, but not registered by AHA. For definition of numerical codes, see page A4	Control	Service	Staffed Beds	Admissions	Census	Outpatient Visits	Births	Total	Payroll	Personnel
□ SHRINERS HOSPITALS FOR CHILDREN, SHREVEPORT, 3100 Samford Avenue, Zip 71103–4289; tel. 318/222–5704; Thomas R. Schneider, Administrator (Nonreporting) **A**1 3 5 **S** Shriners Hospitals for Children, Tampa, FL	23	57	45	—	—	—	—	—	—	—
✠ △ WILLIS–KNIGHTON MEDICAL CENTER, 2600 Greenwood Road, Zip 71103–2600, Mailing Address: P.O. Box 32600, Zip 71130–2600; tel. 318/632–4600; James K. Elrod, President and Chief Executive Officer (Nonreporting) **A**1 3 5 7 9 10 **Web address:** www.wkmc.com	23	10	426	—	—	—	—	—	—	—
SLIDELL—St. Tammany Parish										
□ NORTHSHORE PSYCHIATRIC HOSPITAL, 104 Medical Center Drive, Zip 70461–7838; tel. 504/646–5500; George H. Perry, Ph.D., Chief Executive Officer (Nonreporting) **A**1 9 10 **S** TENET Healthcare Corporation, Santa Barbara, CA **Web address:** www.tenethealth.com	33	22	58	—	—	—	—	—	—	—
✠ NORTHSHORE REGIONAL MEDICAL CENTER, 100 Medical Center Drive, Zip 70461–8572; tel. 504/649–7070; L. Rene' Goux, Chief Executive Officer (Total facility includes 13 beds in nursing home–type unit) (Nonreporting) **A**1 10 **S** TENET Healthcare Corporation, Santa Barbara, CA **Web address:** www.tenethealth.com	33	10	147	—	—	—	—	—	—	—
✠ △ SLIDELL MEMORIAL HOSPITAL AND MEDICAL CENTER, 1001 Gause Boulevard, Zip 70458–2987; tel. 504/643–2200; Monica P. Gates, FACHE, Chief Executive Officer (Total facility includes 18 beds in nursing home–type unit) **A**1 2 7 9 10 **F**4 8 9 11 13 16 17 18 19 22 25 28 30 32 33 34 36 37 38 39 41 42 43 44 45 46 47 48 49 50 51 53 54 56 68 69 70 71 72 73 76 78 79 **P**1 7 **Web address:** www.smhplus.org	16	10	173	8296	109	—	703	85878	35244	1006
SPRINGHILL—Webster Parish										
✠ SPRINGHILL MEDICAL CENTER, 2001 Doctors Drive, Zip 71075, Mailing Address: P.O. Box 920, Zip 71075–0920; tel. 318/539–1000; Kerry Wehmeyer, Chief Executive Officer (Nonreporting) **A**1 9 10 **S** LifePoint Hospitals, Inc., Brentwood, TN	33	10	86	—	—	—	—	—	—	—
STONEWALL—De Soto Parish										
★ STONEWALL MEDICAL CENTER, 960 Highway 171 South, Zip 71078, Mailing Address: P.O. Box 270, Zip 71078; tel. 318/925–5500; Suresh Donepudi, M.D., Chief Executive Officer (Nonreporting) **A**9	33	22	15	—	—	—	—	—	—	—
SULPHUR—Calcasieu Parish										
✠ WEST CALCASIEU CAMERON HOSPITAL, 701 East Cypress Street, Zip 70663–5000, Mailing Address: P.O. Box 2509, Zip 70664–2509; tel. 337/527–4240; Wayne A. Swiniarski, FACHE, Chief Executive Officer **A**1 9 10 **F**7 8 9 13 17 18 19 22 24 25 28 32 33 34 36 38 39 41 43 44 45 48 51 54 68 70 76 78 **P**5 **S** Specialty Hospital Group, Atlanta, GA	16	10	85	3685	33	40999	336	28556	13596	531
TALLULAH—Madison Parish										
MADISON PARISH HOSPITAL, 900 Johnson Street, Zip 71282–4537, Mailing Address: P.O. Box 1559, Zip 71284–1559; tel. 318/574–2374; Wendell Alford, Administrator (Nonreporting) **A**9 10	23	10	47	—	—	—	—	—	—	—
THIBODAUX—Lafourche Parish										
✠ △ THIBODAUX REGIONAL MEDICAL CENTER, 602 North Acadia Road, Zip 70301–4847, Mailing Address: P.O. Box 1118, Zip 70302–1118; tel. 504/447–5500; Greg K. Stock, Chief Executive Officer **A**1 7 9 10 **F**4 7 8 9 11 13 14 16 17 18 22 24 25 30 32 33 36 38 39 41 43 44 45 46 47 48 50 51 53 54 64 65 69 70 71 72 76 78 79 **S** Quorum Health Group, Brentwood, TN **Web address:** www.thibodaux.com	16	10	140	7525	75	87558	787	55627	22978	—
VILLE PLATTE—Evangeline Parish										
□ VILLE PLATTE MEDICAL CENTER, 800 East Main Street, Zip 70586–4618, Mailing Address: P.O. Box 349, Zip 70586–0349; tel. 337/363–5684; Linda F. Deville, Chief Executive Officer **A**1 9 10 **F**8 9 13 17 18 19 22 25 27 28 30 32 33 34 37 38 39 41 44 45 46 48 49 50 54 57 62 70 71 72 76 78 79 **P**8	23	10	80	3631	46	32681	—	17630	7668	272
VIVIAN—Caddo Parish										
NORTH CADDO MEDICAL CENTER, 1000 South Spruce Street, Zip 71082–3232, Mailing Address: P.O. Box 792, Zip 71082–0792; tel. 318/375–3235; Patricia S. Wilkins, Administrator **A**9 10 **F**8 17 18 22 23 25 34 36 37 43 48 49 50 54 76 **Web address:** www.l	16	10	35	724	22	2032	22	4380	2351	101
WEST MONROE—Ouachita Parish										
□ GLENWOOD REGIONAL MEDICAL CENTER, 503 McMillan Road, Zip 71291, Mailing Address: P.O. Box 35805, Zip 71294–5805; tel. 318/329–4200; Raymond L. Ford, President and Chief Executive Officer (Total facility includes 13 beds in nursing home–type unit) **A**1 2 9 10 **F**7 8 9 11 12 13 14 18 20 22 23 24 25 27 28 32 33 34 36 37 38 39 41 42 44 46 48 49 51 52 53 54 56 57 65 68 69 70 71 72 75 76 78 79 **P**8 **Web address:** www.grmc.com	23	10	189	9345	117	121765	388	70244	26874	868
WINNFIELD—Winn Parish										
✠ WINN PARISH MEDICAL CENTER, 301 West Boundary Street, Zip 71483–3427, Mailing Address: P.O. Box 152, Zip 71483–0152; tel. 318/628–2721; Bobby Jordan, Chief Executive Officer (Nonreporting) **A**1 10 **S** HCA – The Healthcare Company, Nashville, TN	33	10	103	—	—	—	—	—	—	—
WINNSBORO—Franklin Parish										
FRANKLIN MEDICAL CENTER, 2106 Loop Road, Zip 71295–3398; tel. 318/435–9411; Ann Netherland, Administrator **A**9 10 **F**7 13 16 17 19 22 24 27 30 31 32 36 41 46 48 57 62 70 75 76 78	16	10	47	2205	25	40868	0	11774	4381	180

© 2000 AHA Guide   *Many Facility Codes have changed. Please refer to the AHA Guide Code Chart.*

Hospitals, U.S. / LOUISIANA

Hospital, Address, Telephone, Administrator, Approval, Facility, and Physician Codes, Health Care System, Network	Classification Codes		Utilization Data					Expense (thousands) of dollars		Personnel
	Control	Service	Staffed Beds	Admissions	Census	Outpatient Visits	Births	Total	Payroll	

- ★ American Hospital Association (AHA) membership
- ☐ Joint Commission on Accreditation of Healthcare Organizations (JCAHO) accreditation
- + American Osteopathic Healthcare Association (AOHA) membership
- ○ American Osteopathic Association (AOA) accreditation
- △ Commission on Accreditation of Rehabilitation Facilities (CARF) accreditation

Control codes 61, 63, 64, 71, 72 and 73 indicate hospitals listed by AOHA, but not registered by AHA. For definition of numerical codes, see page A4

ZACHARY—East Baton Rouge Parish

Hospital	Control	Service	Staffed Beds	Admissions	Census	Outpatient Visits	Births	Total	Payroll	Personnel
★ LANE MEMORIAL HOSPITAL, 6300 Main Street, Zip 70791-9990; tel. 225/658-4000; Terry G. Whittington, Chief Executive Officer and Administrator (Total facility includes 50 beds in nursing home–type unit) **A** 1 9 10 **F** 7 8 9 13 19 22 23 24 25 30 32 33 34 35 36 38 41 43 45 48 51 54 69 70 76 78 **P** 6 7 **S** Quorum Health Group, Brentwood, TN Web address: www.lanehospital.org	16	10	137	4767	99	139469	465	34565	16768	485

A190 Hospitals — *Many Facility Codes have changed. Please refer to the AHA Guide Code Chart.* — © 2000 AHA Guide

Hospitals, U.S. / MAINE

MAINE

Resident Population 1,244 (in thousands)
Resident population in metro areas 35.8%
Birth rate per 1,000 population 11.0
65 years and over 14.1%
Percent of persons without health insurance 14.9%

Hospital, Address, Telephone, Administrator, Approval, Facility, and Physician Codes, Health Care System, Network	Classification Codes		Utilization Data					Expense (thousands) of dollars		
	Control	Service	Staffed Beds	Admissions	Census	Outpatient Visits	Births	Total	Payroll	Personnel

★ American Hospital Association (AHA) membership
□ Joint Commission on Accreditation of Healthcare Organizations (JCAHO) accreditation
+ American Osteopathic Healthcare Association (AOHA) membership
○ American Osteopathic Association (AOA) accreditation
△ Commission on Accreditation of Rehabilitation Facilities (CARF) accreditation
Control codes 61, 63, 64, 71, 72 and 73 indicate hospitals listed by AOHA, but not registered by AHA. For definition of numerical codes, see page A4

AUGUSTA—Kennebec County

□ AUGUSTA MENTAL HEALTH INSTITUTE, Arsenal Street, Zip 04330, Mailing Address: P.O. Box 724, Zip 04330-0724; tel. 207/287-7200; Rodney Bouffard, Superintendent (Nonreporting) **A**1 9 10 — 12 22 133 — — — — — — —

MAINEGENERAL MEDICAL CENTER–AUGUSTA CAMPUS See MaineGeneral Medical Center–Waterville Campus, Waterville

BANGOR—Penobscot County

★ ACADIA HOSPITAL, 268 Stillwater Avenue, Zip 04401-3945, Mailing Address: P.O. Box 422, Zip 04402-0422; tel. 207/973-6100; Ali A. Elhaj, President and Chief Executive Officer **A**1 9 10 **F**2 3 4 6 7 8 9 11 12 13 14 18 19 20 21 22 23 24 25 28 30 31 32 33 34 35 36 37 38 41 42 43 44 45 46 47 48 49 50 51 52 53 54 56 57 58 59 60 61 62 63 64 65 66 68 69 70 71 72 73 75 76 77 78 79 **P**5 6 7 8 **S** Eastern Maine Healthcare, Bangor, ME
Web address: www.emh.org — 23 22 91 1707 88 40731 0 24864 13242 385

□ BANGOR MENTAL HEALTH INSTITUTE, 656 State Street, Zip 04402-0926, Mailing Address: P.O. Box 926, Zip 04402-0926; tel. 207/941-4000; N. Lawrence Ventura, Superintendent (Nonreporting) **A**1 9 10 — 12 22 188 — — — — — — —

★ EASTERN MAINE MEDICAL CENTER, (Includes Ross Skilled Nursing Facility), 489 State Street, Zip 04401-6674, Mailing Address: P.O. Box 404, Zip 04402-0404; tel. 207/973-7000; Norman A. Ledwin, President and Chief Executive Officer (Total facility includes 15 beds in nursing home-type unit) **A**1 2 3 5 9 10 13 **F**2 3 4 6 7 8 9 11 12 13 16 18 19 20 21 22 23 24 25 28 30 31 32 33 34 35 36 37 39 41 42 43 44 45 46 47 48 49 50 51 52 53 54 56 57 58 59 60 61 62 63 64 65 66 68 69 70 71 72 73 75 76 77 78 79 **P**6 7 8 **S** Eastern Maine Healthcare, Bangor, ME
Web address: www.emh.org — 23 10 319 16499 247 285298 1640 212007 89632 2165

★ ST. JOSEPH HOSPITAL, 360 Broadway, Zip 04401-3897, Mailing Address: P.O. Box 403, Zip 04402-0403; tel. 207/262-1000; Sister Mary Norberta Malinowski, President **A**1 9 10 **F**7 9 13 17 18 19 22 24 25 26 27 30 32 36 37 38 39 41 43 45 46 48 49 50 51 54 70 71 72 76 78 79 — 21 10 84 3613 49 103793 0 42216 17694 481

BAR HARBOR—Hancock County

★ MOUNT DESERT ISLAND HOSPITAL, Wayman Lane, Zip 04609-0008, Mailing Address: P.O. Box 8, Zip 04609-0008; tel. 207/288-5081; Arthur Blank, Chief Executive Officer **A**1 9 10 **F**3 7 8 9 12 13 17 18 19 22 24 25 32 34 37 38 40 41 43 44 45 46 48 54 70 71 72 76 79 **P**6 7
Web address: www.mdihospital.org — 23 10 39 1442 16 27970 125 14278 6932 241

BATH—Sagadahoc County

BATH HEALTH CARE CENTER See Mid Coast Hospital

★ MID COAST HOSPITAL, (Includes Bath Health Care Center, Mailing Address: 1356 Washington Street, Zip 04530-2897; Mid Coast Hospital, 58 Baribeau Drive, Brunswick, Zip 04011-3286; tel. 207/729-0181), 1356 Washington Street, Zip 04530-2897; tel. 207/443-5524; Herbert Paris, President (Total facility includes 16 beds in nursing home-type unit) **A**1 9 10 **F**3 6 8 9 13 16 17 18 19 21 22 24 25 26 29 30 31 32 33 34 35 36 37 38 39 40 41 43 44 45 46 48 50 51 54 57 58 59 60 61 62 63 64 65 67 68 69 70 72 74 76 77 78 79 **P**6 — 23 10 88 4510 58 112364 421 33141 14868 442

BELFAST—Waldo County

□ WALDO COUNTY GENERAL HOSPITAL, Northport Avenue, Zip 04915, Mailing Address: P.O. Box 287, Zip 04915-0287; tel. 207/338-2500; Mark A. Biscone, Executive Director **A**1 9 10 **F**1 3 6 8 9 12 16 17 19 20 21 22 24 25 28 32 34 36 37 38 39 41 43 44 46 48 49 51 54 56 58 59 60 61 62 63 67 70 72 76 78
Web address: www.wchi.com — 23 10 45 1964 25 53636 206 19045 9841 346

BIDDEFORD—York County

★ SOUTHERN MAINE MEDICAL CENTER, One Medical Center Drive, Zip 04005-9496, Mailing Address: P.O. Box 626, Zip 04005-0626; tel. 207/283-7000; Edward J. McGeachey, President and Chief Executive Officer (Nonreporting) **A**1 2 9 10 13
Web address: www.smmctr.org — 23 10 112 — — — — — — —

BLUE HILL—Hancock County

★ BLUE HILL MEMORIAL HOSPITAL, Water Street, Zip 04614-0823, Mailing Address: P.O. Box 823, Zip 04614-0823; tel. 207/374-2836; Bruce D. Cummings, Chief Executive Officer **A**1 9 10 18 **F**6 7 8 9 13 16 17 18 19 22 25 26 32 33 36 37 38 41 43 44 45 46 48 50 54 56 63 67 70 72 76 77 78 79 **P**6
Web address: www.bhmh.org — 23 10 14 1378 11 28281 167 18217 10093 285

BOOTHBAY HARBOR—Lincoln County

★ ST. ANDREWS HOSPITAL AND HEALTHCARE CENTER, 3 St. Andrews Lane, Zip 04538-1732, Mailing Address: P.O. Box 417, Zip 04538-0417; tel. 207/633-2121; Margaret G. Pinkham, President and Chief Executive Officer (Total facility includes 30 beds in nursing home-type unit) **A**1 9 10 18 **F**7 9 13 14 16 17 18 19 25 32 36 38 45 48 54 56 69 70 71 72 76 **P**6 8
Web address: www.standrewshealthcare.org — 23 10 51 310 31 16912 0 7235 4226 142

© 2000 AHA Guide   *Many Facility Codes have changed. Please refer to the AHA Guide Code Chart.*   Hospitals **A191**

Hospitals, U.S. / MAINE

Hospital, Address, Telephone, Administrator, Approval, Facility, and Physician Codes, Health Care System, Network	Classification Codes		Utilization Data					Expense (thousands) of dollars		Personnel
★ American Hospital Association (AHA) membership ☐ Joint Commission on Accreditation of Healthcare Organizations (JCAHO) accreditation + American Osteopathic Healthcare Association (AOHA) membership ○ American Osteopathic Association (AOA) accreditation △ Commission on Accreditation of Rehabilitation Facilities (CARF) accreditation Control codes 61, 63, 64, 71, 72 and 73 indicate hospitals listed by AOHA, but not registered by AHA. For definition of numerical codes, see page A4	Control	Service	Staffed Beds	Admissions	Census	Outpatient Visits	Births	Total	Payroll	Personnel
BRIDGTON—Cumberland County ★ BRIDGTON HOSPITAL, (Formerly Northern Cumberland Memorial Hospital), South High Street, Zip 04009, Mailing Address: P.O. Box 230, Zip 04009-0230; tel. 207/647-8841; Laird P. Covey, President and Chief Executive Officer **A**1 9 10 **F**7 8 9 12 13 17 18 19 22 25 34 43 45 46 48 50 54 68 70 72 76 78 **P**5 6 8 Web address: www.ncmh.com	23	10	40	1012	9	15824	65	8217	3773	191
BRUNSWICK—Cumberland County ★ PARKVIEW HOSPITAL, 329 Maine Street, Zip 04011-3398; tel. 207/373-2000; Jon W. Gepford, President and Chief Executive Officer **A**1 9 10 **F**8 9 13 17 18 19 22 25 30 31 32 33 34 35 36 37 38 41 43 44 46 48 49 50 51 54 59 70 72 76 78 79 **P**8 Web address: www.parkviewhospital.com	21	10	48	2103	21	59677	485	18475	9585	272
CALAIS—Washington County ★ CALAIS REGIONAL HOSPITAL, 50 Franklin Street, Zip 04619-1398; tel. 207/454-7521; Ray H. Davis, Jr, Chief Executive Officer (Total facility includes 8 beds in nursing home-type unit) **A**1 9 10 **F**3 7 8 9 13 16 18 19 22 23 25 26 32 34 36 37 38 39 41 43 44 48 51 63 69 70 72 76 78 **S** Quorum Health Group, Brentwood, TN Web address: www.calaishospital.com	23	10	57	1237	18	32870	132	11702	5333	214
CARIBOU—Aroostook County ★ CARY MEDICAL CENTER, 163 Van Buren Road, Suite 1, Zip 04736-2599; tel. 207/498-3111; Kris Doody-Chabre, Chief Executive Officer (Total facility includes 9 beds in nursing home-type unit) **A**1 9 10 **F**4 7 8 9 11 12 13 14 16 17 18 19 21 22 23 24 25 26 28 29 30 31 32 33 34 35 36 37 38 39 40 41 43 44 45 46 48 49 50 51 53 54 55 56 58 59 60 61 62 63 64 65 66 68 70 71 72 74 75 76 77 78 79 **P**5 8 **S** Quorum Health Group, Brentwood, TN Web address: www.carymed.org	14	10	55	2152	26	—	112	26171	11268	419
DAMARISCOTTA—Lincoln County ★ MILES MEMORIAL HOSPITAL, Bristol Road, Zip 04543, Mailing Address: Rural Route 2, Box 4500, Zip 04543-9767; tel. 207/563-1234; Judith Tarr, Chief Executive Officer **A**1 9 10 **F**1 8 9 12 13 16 17 18 19 21 22 24 25 36 37 41 43 44 48 53 54 67 69 70 76 77 78 79 **P**2 Web address: www.mileshealthcare.org	23	10	32	1884	20	56375	193	19448	8723	326
DOVER-FOXCROFT—Piscataquis County ★ MAYO REGIONAL HOSPITAL, 75 West Main Street, Zip 04426-1099; tel. 207/564-8401; Ralph Gabarro, Chief Executive Officer **A**1 9 10 **F**1 7 8 9 16 17 18 19 22 25 32 34 39 41 44 45 46 48 56 59 61 70 76 78 **P**7 **S** Quorum Health Group, Brentwood, TN Web address: www.mayohospital.com	16	10	46	1612	15	41955	136	15143	6498	203
ELLSWORTH—Hancock County ★ MAINE COAST MEMORIAL HOSPITAL, 50 Union Street, Zip 04605-1599; tel. 207/667-5311; Douglas T. Jones, Chief Executive Officer **A**1 9 10 **F**8 9 13 17 18 19 21 22 24 25 28 29 30 32 33 34 35 37 38 39 41 43 44 45 46 48 50 51 54 56 61 68 70 71 72 76 77 78 79 **P**6 **S** Quorum Health Group, Brentwood, TN	23	10	48	2956	28	42185	199	33706	17196	461
FARMINGTON—Franklin County ★ FRANKLIN MEMORIAL HOSPITAL, 129 Hospital Drive, Zip 04938-9990; tel. 207/778-6031; Richard A. Batt, President and Chief Executive Officer **A**1 9 10 **F**3 8 9 13 14 16 17 18 19 22 23 25 28 30 31 32 33 34 35 36 37 38 39 41 43 44 45 46 48 49 50 54 58 59 60 61 62 63 64 67 70 71 72 73 76 78 79 **P**8 Web address: www.fchn.org	23	10	50	2500	27	28675	404	29272	13217	435
FORT FAIRFIELD—Aroostook County COMMUNITY GENERAL HEALTH CENTER See Aroostook Medical Center, Presque Isle										
FORT KENT—Aroostook County ★ NORTHERN MAINE MEDICAL CENTER, 143 East Main Street, Zip 04743-1497; tel. 207/834-3155; Martin B. Bernstein, Chief Executive Officer (Total facility includes 45 beds in nursing home-type unit) **A**1 9 10 **F**8 9 13 16 17 18 22 24 25 29 32 34 38 39 40 41 43 44 45 46 48 50 51 54 57 58 59 60 61 62 63 68 69 70 76 **P**6	23	10	97	1283	56	33848	97	15622	8466	282
GREENVILLE—Piscataquis County ★ CHARLES A. DEAN MEMORIAL HOSPITAL, Pritham Avenue, Zip 04441-1395, Mailing Address: P.O. Box 1129, Zip 04441-1129; tel. 207/695-2223; Philomena A. Marshall, R.N., President and Chief Executive Officer (Total facility includes 36 beds in nursing home-type unit) **A**9 10 18 **F**7 9 16 17 18 25 28 32 34 38 48 54 56 69 70 76 78 **S** Eastern Maine Healthcare, Bangor, ME Web address: www.moosehead.net/cadean	23	10	45	324	29	—	0	4643	2109	74
HOULTON—Aroostook County ★ HOULTON REGIONAL HOSPITAL, 20 Hartford Street, Zip 04730-9998; tel. 207/532-9471; Thomas J. Moakler, Chief Executive Officer (Total facility includes 26 beds in nursing home-type unit) **A**1 9 10 **F**3 7 8 9 13 16 17 18 19 22 23 24 25 28 32 33 34 36 37 38 39 40 41 43 44 45 46 48 49 50 51 54 59 61 62 69 70 72 73 76 78 **P**1 **S** Quorum Health Group, Brentwood, TN Web address: www.houlton.net/hrh	23	10	75	1929	39	47365	207	19940	9127	259

Hospitals, U.S. / MAINE

Hospital, Address, Telephone, Administrator, Approval, Facility, and Physician Codes, Health Care System, Network	Classification Codes		Utilization Data					Expense (thousands) of dollars		
★ American Hospital Association (AHA) membership ☐ Joint Commission on Accreditation of Healthcare Organizations (JCAHO) accreditation + American Osteopathic Healthcare Association (AOHA) membership ○ American Osteopathic Association (AOA) accreditation △ Commission on Accreditation of Rehabilitation Facilities (CARF) accreditation Control codes 61, 63, 64, 71, 72 and 73 indicate hospitals listed by AOHA, but not registered by AHA. For definition of numerical codes, see page A4	Control	Service	Staffed Beds	Admissions	Census	Outpatient Visits	Births	Total	Payroll	Personnel
LEWISTON—Androscoggin County										
★ CENTRAL MAINE MEDICAL CENTER, 300 Main Street, Zip 04240-0305; tel. 207/795-0111; Peter E. Chalke, President and Chief Executive Officer **A**1 2 3 5 9 10 **F**7 8 9 11 12 13 14 16 17 18 19 20 22 24 25 26 28 31 32 33 34 35 36 37 38 39 41 43 44 45 46 48 49 50 51 53 54 56 65 66 68 70 71 72 73 74 75 76 77 78 79 **P**5 6 8 Web address: www.cmmc.org	23	10	100	7576	100	184119	825	88286	37025	1041
★ ST. MARY'S REGIONAL MEDICAL CENTER, 45 Golder Street, Zip 04240-6033, Mailing Address: P.O. Box 291, Zip 04243-0291; tel. 207/777-8100; James E. Cassidy, President and Chief Executive Officer **A**1 2 9 10 **F**2 3 8 9 11 13 16 17 18 19 22 24 25 26 27 28 30 32 33 34 35 38 39 41 43 44 45 46 48 49 50 51 54 56 57 58 59 60 61 62 63 64 65 67 68 69 70 71 72 76 78 79 **P**6 **S** Covenant Health Systems, Inc., Lexington, MA Web address: www.stmarysmaine.com	23	10	187	6003	100	96000	408	54114	19549	552
LINCOLN—Penobscot County										
★ PENOBSCOT VALLEY HOSPITAL, Transalpine Road, Zip 04457-0368, Mailing Address: P.O. Box 368, Zip 04457-0368; tel. 207/794-3321; Ronald D. Victory, Administrator (Total facility includes 9 beds in nursing home-type unit) **A**1 9 10 **F**7 8 9 16 17 18 22 25 26 30 31 32 34 35 38 39 40 41 43 45 46 48 49 50 51 54 69 70 76 77 **P**6 8 **S** Quorum Health Group, Brentwood, TN	16	10	42	1181	17	41821	143	10702	5015	168
MACHIAS—Washington County										
★ DOWN EAST COMMUNITY HOSPITAL, Upper Court Street, Zip 04654, Mailing Address: Rural Route 1, Box 11, Zip 04654-9702; tel. 207/255-3356; Philo D. Hall, Chief Executive Officer **A**1 9 10 **F**7 8 9 16 17 18 19 22 24 25 32 34 38 39 41 44 46 48 54 68 70 72 76 78 **P**8 **S** Quorum Health Group, Brentwood, TN Web address: www.nemaine.com	23	10	36	1606	17	36565	108	16466	7033	213
MARS HILL—Aroostook County										
AROOSTOOK HEALTH CENTER See Aroostook Medical Center, Presque Isle										
MILLINOCKET—Penobscot County										
★ MILLINOCKET REGIONAL HOSPITAL, 200 Somerset Street, Zip 04462-1298; tel. 207/723-5161; Richard Waller, Chief Executive Officer **A**1 9 10 **F**1 7 13 22 25 26 28 34 38 39 41 43 46 48 53 54 61 68 69 70 71 76 79 **P**8 **S** Quorum Health Group, Brentwood, TN Web address: www.millinockethospital.com	23	10	20	912	12	23303	0	12211	5171	177
NORWAY—Oxford County										
★ STEPHENS MEMORIAL HOSPITAL, 181 Main Street, Zip 04268-1297; tel. 207/743-5933; Timothy A. Churchill, President **A**1 9 10 **F**3 6 7 8 9 16 17 18 19 22 32 33 36 37 41 44 45 46 48 50 54 59 61 69 70 76 78 **P**8 Web address: www.wmhcc.com	23	10	50	1843	21	102807	219	19435	9418	273
PITTSFIELD—Somerset County										
★ SEBASTICOOK VALLEY HOSPITAL, 99 Grove Street, Zip 04967-1199; tel. 207/487-5141; John C. May, Chief Executive Officer (Nonreporting) **A**9 10	23	10	28	—	—	—	—	—	—	—
PORTLAND—Cumberland County										
★ MAINE MEDICAL CENTER, (Includes Maine Medical Center, Brighton Campus, 335 Brighton Avenue, Zip 04102-9735; tel. 207/879-8000), 22 Bramhall Street, Zip 04102-3175; tel. 207/871-0111; Vincent S. Conti, President and Chief Executive Officer **A**1 2 3 5 8 9 10 **F**3 4 7 9 11 12 13 14 16 17 18 19 21 22 23 24 25 27 29 30 31 32 33 34 35 36 37 38 39 41 42 43 44 45 46 47 48 49 50 51 53 54 56 57 58 59 60 61 62 63 64 65 66 67 68 70 71 72 73 74 75 76 77 78 79 **P**4 6 7 8 Web address: www.mmc.org	23	10	560	28335	433	188918	2135	350951	154705	2779
★ MERCY HOSPITAL OF PORTLAND, (Includes Mercy Westbrook, 40 Park Road, Westbrook, Zip 04092-3158; tel. 207/854-8464; Charlene Wallace, Interim President), 144 State Street, Zip 04101-3795; tel. 207/879-3000; Howard R. Buckley, President **A**1 9 10 **F**2 3 7 8 9 14 17 19 20 22 24 25 29 30 31 32 33 34 35 36 37 38 39 41 43 44 46 48 49 54 56 59 61 63 70 72 76 77 78 79 **P**6 **S** Catholic Health East, Newtown Square, PA Web address: www.mercyhospital.com	21	10	166	9303	121	130986	1290	79840	34808	939
☐ NEW ENGLAND REHABILITATION HOSPITAL OF PORTLAND, 335 Brighton Avenue, Zip 04102; tel. 207/775-4000; Amy Morse, Chief Executive Officer (Nonreporting) **A**1 10 **S** HEALTHSOUTH Corporation, Birmingham, AL	33	46	76	—	—	—	—	—	—	—
PRESQUE ISLE—Aroostook County										
★ AROOSTOOK MEDICAL CENTER, (Includes Aroostook Health Center, 15 Highland Avenue, Mars Hill, Zip 04758; tel. 207/768-4900; Arthur R. Gould Memorial Hospital, 140 Academy Street, Zip 04769; tel. 207/768-4000; Community General Health Center, 3 Green Street, Fort Fairfield, Zip 04742; tel. 207/768-4700), 140 Academy Street, Zip 04769-3171, Mailing Address: P.O. Box 151, Zip 04769-0151; tel. 207/768-4000; David A. Peterson, President and Chief Executive Officer (Total facility includes 72 beds in nursing home-type unit) **A**1 9 10 **F**8 9 17 18 22 24 25 29 30 32 34 37 38 39 40 43 45 46 48 49 54 56 58 60 61 63 64 65 70 72 76 78 79 **P**2 6 **S** Eastern Maine Healthcare, Bangor, ME Web address: www.tamc.org	23	10	152	3338	90	74430	324	36347	16780	560
ROCKPORT—Knox County										
★ PENOBSCOT BAY MEDICAL CENTER, 6 Glen Cove Drive, Zip 04856-4241; tel. 207/596-8000; Roy A. Hitchings, Jr, FACHE, President and Chief Executive Officer (Total facility includes 62 beds in nursing home-type unit) **A**1 2 9 10 **F**2 3 8 9 12 17 18 22 24 25 31 32 33 36 37 39 41 43 44 45 46 48 51 53 54 57 59 61 62 68 69 70 72 76 78 79 **P**4 6 Web address: www.nehealth.org	23	10	147	4668	122	89768	376	44162	22482	587

© 2000 AHA Guide   *Many Facility Codes have changed. Please refer to the AHA Guide Code Chart.*

Hospitals, U.S. / MAINE

Hospital, Address, Telephone, Administrator, Approval, Facility, and Physician Codes, Health Care System, Network	Classi-fication Codes		Utilization Data					Expense (thousands) of dollars		
	Control	Service	Staffed Beds	Admissions	Census	Outpatient Visits	Births	Total	Payroll	Personnel

★ American Hospital Association (AHA) membership
☐ Joint Commission on Accreditation of Healthcare Organizations (JCAHO) accreditation
+ American Osteopathic Healthcare Association (AOHA) membership
○ American Osteopathic Association (AOA) accreditation
△ Commission on Accreditation of Rehabilitation Facilities (CARF) accreditation
Control codes 61, 63, 64, 71, 72 and 73 indicate hospitals listed by AOHA, but not registered by AHA. For definition of numerical codes, see page A4

RUMFORD—Oxford County
✸ RUMFORD HOSPITAL, (Formerly Rumford Community Hospital), 420 Franklin Street, Zip 04276–2145, Mailing Address: P.O. Box 619, Zip 04276–0619; tel. 207/364–4581; John H. Welsh, Chief Executive Officer **A**1 9 10 **F**3 7 8 9 12 13 16 17 18 19 22 23 24 25 28 32 34 44 48 54 70 72 76 78 **P**1
Web address: www.rumfordhospital.org
23 10 27 1206 13 30226 89 11584 5047 170

SANFORD—York County
✸ HENRIETTA D. GOODALL HOSPITAL, 25 June Street, Zip 04073–2645; tel. 207/324–4310; Peter G. Booth, President (Total facility includes 112 beds in nursing home–type unit) **A**1 9 10 **F**6 8 9 12 14 17 18 19 22 25 32 34 38 39 44 45 48 49 54 69 70 76 78 79
Web address: www.goodallhosp.org
23 10 161 2295 126 52224 289 26760 12612 423

SKOWHEGAN—Somerset County
✸ REDINGTON–FAIRVIEW GENERAL HOSPITAL, Fairview Avenue, Zip 04976, Mailing Address: P.O. Box 468, Zip 04976–0468; tel. 207/474–5121; Richard Willett, Chief Executive Officer **A**1 2 9 10 **F**8 9 13 17 18 19 22 24 25 28 32 34 36 37 39 41 44 45 46 48 54 59 63 68 70 71 72 76 78
23 10 65 2331 29 68696 223 23300 11393 328

SOUTH PORTLAND—Cumberland County
☐ SPRING HARBOR HOSPITAL, (Formerly Jackson Brook Institute), 175 Running Hill Road, Zip 04106; tel. 207/761–2200; Dennis King, President and Chief Executive Officer (Nonreporting) **A**1 10 **S** Community Care Systems, Inc.
Web address: www.springharbor.org
33 22 106 — — — — — — —

TOGUS—Kennebec County
✸ VETERANS AFFAIRS MEDICAL CENTER, 1 VA Center, Zip 04330; tel. 207/623–8411; John H. Sims, Jr, Director (Total facility includes 100 beds in nursing home–type unit) **A**1 2 3 5 9 **F**1 3 9 13 19 21 22 23 24 25 29 30 31 34 35 36 37 38 39 41 43 46 48 49 51 54 56 57 59 61 62 63 64 65 68 69 70 72 76 77 78 79 **P**6 **S** Department of Veterans Affairs, Washington, DC
Web address: www.visn1.med.va.gov
45 10 176 2565 161 181117 — 69607 34848 896

WATERVILLE—Kennebec County
★ + ○ INLAND HOSPITAL, 200 Kennedy Memorial Drive, Zip 04901–4595; tel. 207/861–3000; Wilfred J. Addison, President and Chief Executive Officer (Total facility includes 76 beds in nursing home–type unit) **A**9 10 11 **F**8 9 17 22 24 32 36 38 39 41 44 45 46 48 49 54 63 68 69 75 76 78 **S** Eastern Maine Healthcare, Bangor, ME
23 10 120 1900 88 73732 276 21164 10703 262

✸ MAINEGENERAL MEDICAL CENTER–WATERVILLE CAMPUS, (Includes MaineGeneral Medical Center–Augusta Campus, 6 East Chestnut Street, Augusta, Zip 04330–9988; tel. 207/626–1000), 149 North Street, Zip 04901–4974; tel. 207/872–1000; Scott B. Bullock, President (Total facility includes 29 beds in nursing home–type unit) **A**1 2 3 5 9 10 **F**1 2 3 7 8 9 12 13 14 17 18 19 22 24 25 26 27 30 34 35 36 37 38 39 41 43 44 45 46 48 51 53 54 56 57 58 59 61 63 64 65 68 69 70 71 72 75 76 77 78 79 **P**6 7 8
Web address: www.mainegeneral.org
23 10 323 13777 190 304168 1124 136536 62564 1927

WESTBROOK—Cumberland County
MERCY WESTBROOK See Mercy Hospital of Portland, Portland

YORK—York County
☐ YORK HOSPITAL, 15 Hospital Drive, Zip 03909–1099; tel. 207/351–2395; Jud Knox, President (Total facility includes 13 beds in nursing home–type unit) (Nonreporting) **A**1 9 10
Web address: www.yorkhospital.com
23 10 79 — — — — — — —

Hospitals, U.S. / MARYLAND

MARYLAND

Resident Population 5,135 (in thousands)
Resident population in metro areas 92.8%
Birth rate per 1,000 population 13.8
65 years and over 11.5%
Percent of persons without health insurance 13.4%

Hospital, Address, Telephone, Administrator, Approval, Facility, and Physician Codes, Health Care System, Network	Classification Codes		Utilization Data					Expense (thousands) of dollars		
	Control	Service	Staffed Beds	Admissions	Census	Outpatient Visits	Births	Total	Payroll	Personnel

★ American Hospital Association (AHA) membership
☐ Joint Commission on Accreditation of Healthcare Organizations (JCAHO) accreditation
+ American Osteopathic Healthcare Association (AOHA) membership
○ American Osteopathic Association (AOA) accreditation
△ Commission on Accreditation of Rehabilitation Facilities (CARF) accreditation
Control codes 61, 63, 64, 71, 72 and 73 indicate hospitals listed by AOHA, but not registered by AHA. For definition of numerical codes, see page A4

ANDREWS AFB—Prince George's County

★ MALCOLM GROW MEDICAL CENTER, 1050 West Perimeter, Zip 20762–6600, Mailing Address: 1050 West Perimeter, Suite A1–19, Zip 20762–6600; tel. 240/857-3000; Colonel Jeffrey L. Butler, Administrator **A**1 2 3 5 9 **F**2 3 8 9 10 12 13 14 16 17 18 19 22 23 25 28 29 32 33 34 35 38 39 41 42 43 44 45 46 48 49 50 51 52 53 54 56 57 58 63 64 66 70 71 72 74 75 76 78 79 **S** Department of the Air Force, Bowling AFB, DC	41	10	55	4472	44	348406	789	—	—	1515

ANNAPOLIS—Anne Arundel County

★ ANNE ARUNDEL MEDICAL CENTER, 64 Franklin Street, Zip 21401–2777; tel. 410/267-1000; Martin L. Doordan, President **A**1 2 9 10 **F**2 3 7 8 9 11 12 16 17 18 19 22 23 24 25 28 29 31 32 33 34 36 37 38 39 41 42 43 44 45 46 48 51 54 65 70 72 74 76 77 78 79 **P**6 7 Web address: www.aahcs.org	23	10	308	22589	195	185705	3785	136460	58642	2103

BALTIMORE—Baltimore City County

★ BON SECOURS BALTIMORE HEALTH SYSTEM, 2000 West Baltimore Street, Zip 21223–1597; tel. 410/362-3000; Percy Allen, II, FACHE, Chief Executive Officer (Total facility includes 32 beds in nursing home–type unit) (Nonreporting) **A**1 9 10 **S** Bon Secours Health System, Inc., Marriottsville, MD Web address: www.bonsecours.org	21	10	148	—	—	—	—	—	—	—
★ △ DEATON SPECIALTY HOSPITAL AND HOME, (SPECIALITY CHRONIC HOSP/NURSG), 601 South Charles Street, Zip 21230–3898; tel. 410/547-8500; James E. Ross, FACHE, Chief Executive Officer (Total facility includes 178 beds in nursing home–type unit) **A**1 7 9 10 **F**1 3 4 5 7 8 9 11 12 13 17 19 20 21 22 23 24 25 26 29 30 32 34 35 36 38 39 41 42 43 44 45 46 47 48 49 51 52 53 54 56 57 58 59 60 61 62 63 64 65 68 69 70 71 72 74 75 76 78 79 **S** University of Maryland Medical System, Baltimore, MD	23	49	277	992	277	0	0	29142	11859	351
★ FRANKLIN SQUARE HOSPITAL CENTER, 9000 Franklin Square Drive, Zip 21237–3998; tel. 410/682-7000; Carl J. Schindelar, President (Nonreporting) **A**1 2 3 5 8 9 10 **S** MedStar Health, Columbia, MD Web address: www.helix.org	23	10	405	—	—	—	—	—	—	—
★ △ GOOD SAMARITAN HOSPITAL OF MARYLAND, 5601 Loch Raven Boulevard, Zip 21239–2995; tel. 410/532-8000; Lawrence M. Beck, President and Chief Executive Officer (Total facility includes 23 beds in nursing home–type unit) **A**1 2 3 5 7 9 10 **F**1 3 4 5 6 7 8 9 10 11 12 13 16 17 18 19 21 22 23 24 25 26 27 28 29 30 31 32 33 34 35 36 37 38 39 40 41 42 43 44 45 46 47 48 49 50 51 53 54 56 57 58 59 60 61 62 63 64 65 66 67 68 69 70 71 72 73 74 76 77 78 79 **P**2 3 4 5 6 7 8 **S** MedStar Health, Columbia, MD Web address: www.helixhealth.com	23	10	254	11849	201	76352	0	111209	44875	1552
★ GREATER BALTIMORE MEDICAL CENTER, 6701 North Charles Street, Zip 21204–6892; tel. 410/828-2000; Laurence M. Merlis, President and Chief Executive Officer (Nonreporting) **A**1 2 3 5 8 9 10 Web address: www.gbmc.org	23	10	304	—	—	—	—	—	—	—
★ HARBOR HOSPITAL CENTER, 3001 South Hanover Street, Zip 21225–1290; tel. 410/350-3200; L. Barney Johnson, President and Chief Executive Officer (Total facility includes 26 beds in nursing home–type unit) **A**1 2 3 5 9 10 **F**1 7 8 9 11 13 14 17 18 19 22 24 25 28 29 30 31 32 33 34 35 37 38 39 41 44 46 48 50 51 54 56 59 61 62 63 66 69 70 72 73 76 78 79 **P**6 **S** MedStar Health, Columbia, MD Web address: www.helixhealth.com	23	10	182	11661	142	69411	1718	97068	45587	1154
★ △ JAMES LAWRENCE KERNAN HOSPITAL, (SPECIALITY ORTHO SURG & REHAB), 2200 Kernan Drive, Zip 21207–6697; tel. 410/448-2500; James E. Ross, FACHE, Chief Executive Officer (Total facility includes 30 beds in nursing home–type unit) **A**1 3 5 7 9 10 **F**2 3 4 5 7 8 9 11 12 13 19 20 21 22 23 24 25 26 28 29 30 32 34 35 36 38 39 41 42 43 44 46 47 48 49 51 52 53 54 56 57 58 59 60 61 62 63 64 65 66 69 70 71 72 74 75 76 78 79 **S** University of Maryland Medical System, Baltimore, MD	23	49	152	2718	100	38628	0	39675	17463	466
★ JOHNS HOPKINS BAYVIEW MEDICAL CENTER, 4940 Eastern Avenue, Zip 21224–2780; tel. 410/550-0100; Gregory F. Schaffer, President (Total facility includes 295 beds in nursing home–type unit) **A**1 3 5 8 9 10 **F**1 2 3 4 5 8 9 10 11 12 13 14 16 17 18 19 21 22 23 24 25 27 28 29 30 31 32 33 34 35 38 39 41 42 43 44 45 46 47 48 49 50 51 52 53 54 55 56 57 58 59 60 61 62 63 64 65 66 68 69 70 71 72 73 74 75 76 77 78 79 **P**5 6 **S** Johns Hopkins Health System, Baltimore, MD Web address: www.jhbmc.jhu.edu	23	10	658	20587	508	264146	1184	207883	77855	2593
★ △ JOHNS HOPKINS HOSPITAL, 600 North Wolfe Street, Zip 21287–2182; tel. 410/955-5000; Ronald R. Peterson, President **A**1 2 3 5 7 8 9 10 **F**1 2 3 4 5 7 9 10 11 12 13 14 16 17 18 19 21 22 23 24 25 26 27 28 29 30 31 32 33 34 35 36 37 38 39 41 42 43 44 45 46 47 48 49 50 51 52 53 54 55 56 57 58 59 60 61 62 63 64 65 66 68 69 70 71 72 73 74 75 76 77 78 79 **P**1 2 5 6 7 8 **S** Johns Hopkins Health System, Baltimore, MD Web address: www.med.jhu.edu	23	10	844	40339	704	283920	1879	601258	221185	6554

© 2000 AHA Guide *Many Facility Codes have changed. Please refer to the AHA Guide Code Chart.* Hospitals **A195**

Hospitals, U.S. / MARYLAND

Hospital, Address, Telephone, Administrator, Approval, Facility, and Physician Codes, Health Care System, Network	Classification Codes		Utilization Data					Expense (thousands) of dollars		
★ American Hospital Association (AHA) membership ☐ Joint Commission on Accreditation of Healthcare Organizations (JCAHO) accreditation + American Osteopathic Healthcare Association (AOHA) membership ○ American Osteopathic Association (AOA) accreditation △ Commission on Accreditation of Rehabilitation Facilities (CARF) accreditation Control codes 61, 63, 64, 71, 72 and 73 indicate hospitals listed by AOHA, but not registered by AHA. For definition of numerical codes, see page A4	Control	Service	Staffed Beds	Admissions	Census	Outpatient Visits	Births	Total	Payroll	Personnel
★ △ KENNEDY KRIEGER CHILDREN'S HOSPITAL, (CHILDRENS – OTHER SPECIALTY), 707 North Broadway, Zip 21205–1890; tel. 410/502–9000; Gary W. Goldstein, M.D., President **A**1 7 9 10 **F**13 16 17 18 19 22 24 38 39 43 50 51 53 54 55 58 59 60 63 68 70 72 76 78 **P**6 **Web address:** www.kennedykrieger.org	23	59	70	348	42	76161	0	47709	24140	1377
★ △ LEVINDALE HEBREW GERIATRIC CENTER AND HOSPITAL, 2434 West Belvedere Avenue, Zip 21215–5271; tel. 410/466–8700; Ronald Rothstein, President and Chief Executive Officer (Total facility includes 196 beds in nursing home–type unit) **A**7 9 10 **F**1 4 5 6 7 8 9 11 12 13 14 19 21 22 23 24 25 26 27 28 30 31 32 33 34 35 37 38 39 40 41 42 43 44 45 46 47 48 49 50 51 52 53 54 55 56 57 58 59 60 61 62 63 64 65 66 67 69 70 71 72 74 75 76 77 78 **P**1 3 5 8 **S** LifeBridge Health, Baltimore, MD **Web address:** www.sinai-balt.com	23	48	296	1204	99	0	0	32332	13959	451
★ MARYLAND GENERAL HOSPITAL, 827 Linden Avenue, Zip 21201–4681; tel. 410/225–8000; James R. Wood, Chairman and Chief Executive Officer (Total facility includes 24 beds in nursing home–type unit) **A**1 2 3 5 7 9 10 **F**3 5 7 8 9 11 12 13 16 17 18 19 21 22 24 25 29 30 31 32 33 34 35 36 38 39 41 43 44 45 46 48 50 51 53 54 56 57 59 60 61 62 63 64 65 66 68 69 70 72 73 75 76 77 78 79 **P**8 **S** University of Maryland Medical System, Baltimore, MD	23	10	225	8632	153	95288	758	87658	46702	1132
★ MERCY MEDICAL CENTER, 301 St. Paul Place, Zip 21202–2165; tel. 410/332–9000; Thomas R. Mullen, President and Chief Executive Officer **A**1 3 5 9 10 **F**2 3 7 8 9 11 12 13 16 17 18 19 22 23 24 25 26 29 32 33 34 37 39 41 42 43 44 45 46 48 50 51 53 54 65 70 72 73 76 78 79 **P**5 6 7 **S** Sisters of Mercy of the Americas–Regional Community of Baltimore, Baltimore, MD **Web address:** www.mercymed.com	21	10	200	13553	177	137086	2911	137253	49651	1454
★ △ MT. WASHINGTON PEDIATRIC HOSPITAL, (PEDIATRIC SPECIALTY), 1708 West Rogers Avenue, Zip 21209–4537; tel. 410/578–8600; Sheldon J. Stein, Chief Operating Officer **A**1 7 9 10 **F**13 17 26 29 36 38 53 54 58 63 64 70 72 **P**6 **Web address:** www.mwph.org	23	59	102	680	49	20000	0	24207	12786	290
☐ SHEPPARD AND ENOCH PRATT HOSPITAL, 6501 North Charles Street, Zip 21285–6815, Mailing Address: P.O. Box 6815, Zip 21285–6815; tel. 410/938–3000; Steven S. Sharfstein, M.D., President, Medical Director and Chief Executive Officer **A**1 3 5 9 10 **F**1 3 6 13 16 17 18 19 21 29 30 31 32 34 36 38 50 51 57 58 59 60 62 63 64 70 72 73 77 78 **P**4 **Web address:** www.sheppardpratt.org	23	22	188	5423	142	60837	0	65757	35298	1112
★ △ SINAI HOSPITAL OF BALTIMORE, (Includes Children's Hospital at Sinai), 2401 West Belvedere Avenue, Zip 21215–5271; tel. 410/601–9000; Neil M. Meltzer, President and Chief Operating Officer **A**1 2 3 5 7 8 9 10 **F**1 2 3 4 5 6 7 8 9 11 12 13 14 16 17 18 19 20 21 22 23 25 26 27 28 29 30 31 32 33 34 35 37 38 39 40 41 42 43 44 45 46 47 48 49 50 51 52 53 54 55 56 57 58 59 60 61 62 63 64 65 66 69 70 71 72 73 75 76 78 79 **P**1 6 **S** LifeBridge Health, Baltimore, MD **Web address:** www.lifebridgehealth.org	23	10	387	20939	288	179578	2023	250524	120650	2585
☐ SPRING GROVE HOSPITAL CENTER, 60 Wade Avenue, Zip 21228–4689; tel. 410/402–6000; Mark Pecevich, M.D., Superintendent (Total facility includes 70 beds in nursing home–type unit) (Nonreporting) **A**1 3 5 10 **Web address:** www.springgrove.com	12	22	360	—	—	—	—	—	—	—
★ ST. AGNES HEALTHCARE, 900 Caton Avenue, Zip 21229–5299; tel. 410/368–6000; Robert W. Adams, President and Chief Executive Officer (Total facility includes 24 beds in nursing home–type unit) (Nonreporting) **A**1 2 3 5 9 10 **S** Ascension Health, Saint Louis, MO **Web address:** www.stagnes.org	23	10	422	—	—	—	—	—	—	—
★ △ UNION MEMORIAL HOSPITAL, 201 East University Parkway, Zip 21218–2895; tel. 410/554–2000; Harrison J. Rider, II, President **A**1 2 3 5 7 9 10 **F**1 3 4 7 8 9 11 12 16 17 19 20 21 22 23 24 25 26 27 28 30 31 32 33 34 35 36 37 38 39 41 42 43 44 45 46 47 48 49 51 53 54 55 56 57 59 60 61 62 63 64 66 68 69 70 71 72 73 76 78 79 **S** MedStar Health, Columbia, MD **Web address:** www.medstarhealth.org	23	10	318	14746	183	87542	755	171620	67264	1611
★ UNIVERSITY OF MARYLAND MEDICAL CENTER, 22 South Greene Street, Zip 21201; tel. 410/328–8667; Stephen C. Schimpff, M.D., Chief Executive Officer **A**1 2 3 5 8 9 10 **F**1 3 4 5 7 8 9 11 12 13 14 16 17 18 19 20 21 22 23 24 25 27 28 29 30 31 32 33 34 35 36 37 38 39 41 42 43 44 45 46 47 48 49 50 51 52 53 54 55 57 58 59 60 61 62 63 64 65 66 68 69 70 71 72 73 74 75 76 77 78 79 **P**3 **S** University of Maryland Medical System, Baltimore, MD **Web address:** www.umm.edu	23	10	606	28972	490	203817	1007	455888	210158	4408
★ VETERANS AFFAIRS MARYLAND HEALTH CARE SYSTEM–BALTIMORE DIVISION, 10 North Greene Street, Zip 21201–1524; tel. 410/605–7001; Dennis H. Smith, Director (Total facility includes 140 beds in nursing home–type unit) (Nonreporting) **A**1 2 3 5 8 9 **S** Department of Veterans Affairs, Washington, DC	45	10	897	—	—	—	—	—	—	—
BERLIN—Worcester County										
★ ATLANTIC GENERAL HOSPITAL, 9733 Healthway Drive, Zip 21811–1155; tel. 410/641–1100; Barry G. Beeman, President and Chief Executive Officer (Total facility includes 24 beds in nursing home–type unit) **A**1 9 10 **F**1 2 3 4 6 7 9 11 13 14 16 17 18 19 21 22 23 24 25 29 30 31 32 33 34 35 36 37 38 39 40 41 44 45 46 47 48 49 50 51 55 58 59 60 61 62 63 64 65 66 67 69 70 71 72 73 74 75 76 77 78 79 **P**6 **Web address:** www.atlanticgeneral.org	23	10	86	2686	31	23711	—	17692	6812	289

Hospitals, U.S. / MARYLAND

Hospital, Address, Telephone, Administrator, Approval, Facility, and Physician Codes, Health Care System, Network	Classification Codes		Utilization Data					Expense (thousands) of dollars		
★ American Hospital Association (AHA) membership ☐ Joint Commission on Accreditation of Healthcare Organizations (JCAHO) accreditation + American Osteopathic Healthcare Association (AOHA) membership ○ American Osteopathic Association (AOA) accreditation △ Commission on Accreditation of Rehabilitation Facilities (CARF) accreditation Control codes 61, 63, 64, 71, 72 and 73 indicate hospitals listed by AOHA, but not registered by AHA. For definition of numerical codes, see page A4	Control	Service	Staffed Beds	Admissions	Census	Outpatient Visits	Births	Total	Payroll	Personnel
BETHESDA—Montgomery County										
★ NATIONAL NAVAL MEDICAL CENTER, 8901 Wisconsin Avenue, Zip 20889–5600; tel. 301/295–5800; Rear Admiral Bonnie B. Potter, Commander **A**1 2 3 5 9 **F**4 8 9 12 13 14 15 16 17 18 22 23 25 28 32 33 34 35 39 41 42 43 44 45 46 47 49 50 51 54 55 56 57 58 59 60 61 62 63 65 66 68 70 71 72 76 77 78 79 **P**6 **S** Department of Navy, Washington, DC	43	10	135	10291	109	590116	1918	257398	232304	3559
★ SUBURBAN HOSPITAL, 8600 Old Georgetown Road, Zip 20814–1497; tel. 301/896–3100; Brian G. Grissler, President and Chief Executive Officer (Total facility includes 31 beds in nursing home–type unit) **A**1 2 3 5 9 10 **F**2 3 4 6 7 9 11 12 13 16 17 18 19 20 21 22 24 25 30 31 32 33 34 36 38 39 41 45 46 48 49 50 51 54 57 59 60 61 62 63 64 65 66 67 68 69 70 72 73 75 76 77 78 79 **P**4 7 8 **Web address:** www.suburbanhospital.org	23	10	228	11657	181	64267	0	116373	50854	1232
★ WARREN G. MAGNUSON CLINICAL CENTER, NATIONAL INSTITUTES OF HEALTH, (BIOMEDICAL RESEARCH), 9000 Rockville Pike, Zip 20892–1504; tel. 301/496–4114; John I. Gallin, M.D., Director **A**1 3 5 8 **F**3 4 9 11 22 23 24 28 30 31 33 35 38 39 41 43 46 48 51 54 55 57 58 59 60 62 63 64 65 68 70 72 76 78 **S** U. S. Public Health Service Indian Health Service, Rockville, MD **Web address:** www.cc.nih.gov	44	49	290	6069	139	72798	0	219728	100552	1911
CAMBRIDGE—Dorchester County										
★ DORCHESTER GENERAL HOSPITAL, 300 Byrn Street, Zip 21613–1908; tel. 410/228–5511; Joseph P. Ross, President and Chief Executive Officer **A**1 2 9 10 **F**7 9 13 17 18 21 22 24 25 32 33 34 35 36 41 43 45 46 48 54 56 57 58 59 61 62 63 64 70 71 76 78 79 **P**3 7	23	10	60	3618	45	70026	0	23850	10301	304
☐ EASTERN SHORE HOSPITAL CENTER, Route 50, State Route 479, Zip 21613, Mailing Address: P.O. Box 800, Zip 21613–0800; tel. 410/221–2525; Mary Kay Noren, Superintendent **A**1 10 **F**16 17 18 41 50 51 53 57 59 60 62 63 70 78 **P**6	12	22	61	105	45	0	0	11970	7786	202
CHESTERTOWN—Kent County										
★ KENT & QUEEN ANNE'S HOSPITAL, 100 Brown Street, Zip 21620–1499; tel. 410/778–3300; William R. Kirk, Jr, President and Chief Executive Officer **A**1 9 10 **F**4 7 8 9 12 13 16 17 18 19 22 23 24 25 27 28 34 36 37 39 41 43 44 46 48 49 51 54 61 68 69 70 72 74 76 78	23	10	64	2830	33	42043	218	21869	9728	269
☐ UPPER SHORE COMMUNITY MENTAL HEALTH CENTER, Scheeler Road, Zip 21620, Mailing Address: P.O. Box 229, Zip 21620–0229; tel. 410/778–6800; Mary Kay Noren, Chief Executive Officer **A**1 10 **F** 16 17 57 59 60 61 70 72 78	12	22	64	208	35	0	0	—	—	102
CHEVERLY—Prince George's County										
GLADYS SPELLMAN SPECIALTY HOSPITAL AND NURSING CENTER, 2900 Mercy Lane, Zip 20785–1157; tel. 301/618–2010; Stewart R. Seitz, Chief Executive Officer (Nonreporting)	33	48	30	—	—	—	—	—	—	—
★ PRINCE GEORGE'S HOSPITAL CENTER, 3001 Hospital Drive, Zip 20785–1189; tel. 301/618–2000; Phyllis Wingate-Jones, President **A**1 3 5 9 10 **F**3 4 6 7 8 9 11 12 13 16 17 18 19 21 22 23 24 25 27 28 29 30 31 32 33 34 35 38 39 40 41 42 43 44 46 47 48 49 50 51 53 54 56 57 58 59 61 63 64 65 67 68 69 70 72 73 75 76 77 78 79 **P**7 8 **S** Dimensions Health Corporation, Largo, MD **Web address:** www.princegeorgeshospital.org	23	10	370	14857	230	110078	2529	143091	65690	1386
CLINTON—Prince George's County										
★ SOUTHERN MARYLAND HOSPITAL, 7503 Surratts Road, Zip 20735–3397; tel. 301/868–8000; Francis P. Chiaramonte, M.D., Chief Executive Officer (Total facility includes 20 beds in nursing home–type unit) **A**1 2 9 10 **F**4 8 9 11 12 13 16 17 19 22 24 25 27 28 29 31 32 33 34 36 39 41 44 48 51 54 55 56 57 58 60 61 62 63 64 65 68 69 70 72 76 77 78 79 **P**6	33	10	350	12180	148	70286	1548	92146	34149	1069
COLUMBIA—Howard County										
★ HOWARD COUNTY GENERAL HOSPITAL, 5755 Cedar Lane, Zip 21044–2912; tel. 410/740–7710; Victor A. Broccolino, President and Chief Executive Officer **A**1 2 5 9 10 **F**8 9 11 12 13 14 17 18 19 21 22 24 25 29 30 32 33 34 36 37 38 39 42 43 44 45 46 48 50 51 54 57 58 59 60 61 63 64 65 66 68 70 72 76 77 78 79 **S** Johns Hopkins Health System, Baltimore, MD **Web address:** www.hcgh.org	23	10	163	11531	110	62188	2950	85218	32075	1064
CRISFIELD—Somerset County										
☐ EDWARD W. MCCREADY MEMORIAL HOSPITAL, 201 Hall Highway, Zip 21817–1299; tel. 410/968–1200; J. Allan Bickling, Chief Executive Officer **A**1 9 10 **F**9 14 16 17 19 20 21 22 24 25 27 28 29 30 31 33 34 35 36 38 39 43 45 46 48 49 50 54 57 58 59 60 61 62 63 70 76 **P**5 6	23	10	45	1107	11	16087	0	11480	5143	261
CROWNSVILLE—Anne Arundel County										
☐ CROWNSVILLE HOSPITAL CENTER, 1520 Crownsville Road, Zip 21032–2306; tel. 410/729–6000; Ronald Hendler, Chief Executive Officer (Nonreporting) **A**1 10	12	22	248	—	—	—	—	—	—	—
CUMBERLAND—Allegany County										
★ △ MEMORIAL HOSPITAL AND MEDICAL CENTER OF CUMBERLAND, 600 Memorial Avenue, Zip 21502–3797; tel. 301/723–4000; Thomas C. Dowdell, Executive Director and Senior Vice President **A**1 2 7 9 10 **F**1 7 8 9 11 13 16 17 18 19 22 24 25 26 30 32 34 35 36 37 38 39 40 41 43 44 46 48 49 50 51 53 54 57 61 65 68 70 71 72 75 76 77 78 **S** Ascension Health, Saint Louis, MO **Web address:** www.wmhs.com	23	10	187	8142	108	81042	519	66347	30682	937

Hospitals, U.S. / MARYLAND

Hospital, Address, Telephone, Administrator, Approval, Facility, and Physician Codes, Health Care System, Network	Classification Codes		Utilization Data					Expense (thousands) of dollars		
	Control	Service	Staffed Beds	Admissions	Census	Outpatient Visits	Births	Total	Payroll	Personnel

★ American Hospital Association (AHA) membership
□ Joint Commission on Accreditation of Healthcare Organizations (JCAHO) accreditation
+ American Osteopathic Healthcare Association (AOHA) membership
○ American Osteopathic Association (AOA) accreditation
△ Commission on Accreditation of Rehabilitation Facilities (CARF) accreditation
Control codes 61, 63, 64, 71, 72 and 73 indicate hospitals listed by AOHA, but not registered by AHA. For definition of numerical codes, see page A4

Hospital	Control	Service	Staffed Beds	Admissions	Census	Outpatient Visits	Births	Total	Payroll	Personnel
★ SACRED HEART HOSPITAL, 900 Seton Drive, Zip 21502–1874; tel. 301/759–4200; Francis A. Pommett, Jr, Executive Director and Senior Vice President (Total facility includes 88 beds in nursing home–type unit) **A**1 2 9 10 **F**1 3 7 8 9 11 12 13 16 17 18 22 25 27 32 34 36 37 39 40 41 44 45 46 48 53 54 57 61 63 65 69 70 71 75 76 78 **S** Ascension Health, Saint Louis, MO Web address: www.wmhs.com	23	10	287	8383	190	63608	566	66435	30920	833
□ THOMAS B. FINAN CENTER, 10102 Country Club Road S.E., Zip 21501, Mailing Address: P.O. Box 1722, Zip 21501–1722; tel. 301/777–2240; Archie T. Wallace, Chief Executive Officer **A**1 10 **F**16 17 18 57 58 59 60 62 63 **P**6	12	22	114	363	88	19	0	—	—	225
EAST NEW MARKET—Dorchester County										
WARWICK MANOR BEHAVIORAL HEALTH, (Formerly Charter Behavioral Health System at Warwick Manor), 3680 Warwick Road, Zip 21631–1420; tel. 410/943–8108; Marie McBee, Chief Executive Officer (Nonreporting)	33	82	42	—	—	—	—	—	—	—
EASTON—Talbot County										
★ MEMORIAL HOSPITAL AT EASTON MARYLAND, 219 South Washington Street, Zip 21601–2996; tel. 410/822–1000; Joseph P. Ross, President and Chief Executive Officer (Total facility includes 31 beds in nursing home–type unit) **A**1 2 6 9 10 **F**3 7 8 9 11 17 18 19 20 22 23 24 25 29 30 32 33 34 35 36 37 38 39 41 43 44 45 46 48 49 50 51 54 59 61 65 68 69 70 72 76 77 78 79 **P**5 6 7 Web address: www.shorehealth.org	23	10	164	9519	117	433942	976	75234	27826	943
ELKTON—Cecil County										
★ UNION HOSPITAL, 106 Bow Street, Zip 21921–5596; tel. 410/398–4000; Michael V. Sack, President and Chief Executive Officer (Nonreporting) **A**1 9 10 Web address: www.uhcc.com	23	10	105	—	—	—	—	—	—	—
ELLICOTT CITY—Howard County										
□ TAYLOR MANOR HOSPITAL, 4100 College Avenue, Zip 21043–5506, Mailing Address: P.O. Box 396, Zip 21041–0396; tel. 410/465–3322; Morris L. Scherr, Executive Vice President and Chief Operating Officer **A**1 9 10 **F**16 17 18 22 24 39 51 55 57 58 60 62 63 64 68 70 76 **P**7	33	22	146	1824	108	6852	—	14673	9374	285
EMMITSBURG—Frederick County										
MOUNTAIN MANOR TREATMENT CENTER, Route 15, Zip 21727, Mailing Address: Box E, Zip 21727; tel. 301/447–2361; William J. Roby, Executive Vice President (Nonreporting)	33	82	140	—	—	—	—	—	—	—
FALLSTON—Harford County										
★ FALLSTON GENERAL HOSPITAL, 200 Milton Avenue, Zip 21047–2777; tel. 410/877–3700; Lyle Ernest Sheldon, President and Chief Executive Officer **A**1 9 10 **F**8 9 13 17 18 19 22 24 25 27 32 34 36 37 38 39 41 45 48 51 54 61 68 70 72 76 78 **S** Upper Chesapeake Health System, Fallston, MD	23	10	113	7320	81	51408	—	45776	19126	564
FORT HOWARD—Baltimore County										
★ VETERANS AFFAIRS MARYLAND HEALTH CARE SYSTEM–FORT HOWARD DIVISION, 9600 North Point Road, Zip 21052–9989; tel. 410/477–1800; Dennis H. Smith, Director (Total facility includes 47 beds in nursing home–type unit) (Nonreporting) **A**5 9 **S** Department of Veterans Affairs, Washington, DC	45	49	245	—	—	—	—	—	—	—
FORT WASHINGTON—Prince George's County										
★ FORT WASHINGTON HOSPITAL, 11711 Livingston Road, Zip 20744–5164; tel. 301/292–7000; Judith Burk, Administrator (Nonreporting) **A**1 9 10	23	50	35	—	—	—	—	—	—	—
FREDERICK—Frederick County										
★ FREDERICK MEMORIAL HOSPITAL, 400 West Seventh Street, Zip 21701–4593; tel. 301/698–3300; James K. Kluttz, President and Chief Executive Officer (Total facility includes 16 beds in nursing home–type unit) **A**1 2 9 10 **F**7 8 9 11 13 14 16 17 18 19 21 22 23 24 25 26 27 28 29 32 33 34 35 36 37 38 39 41 43 44 45 46 48 49 50 51 54 57 59 60 61 62 63 64 68 69 70 71 72 76 77 78 79 **P**6 Web address: www.fmh.org	23	10	171	14143	176	322843	1925	117140	60710	1542
GLEN BURNIE—Anne Arundel County										
★ NORTH ARUNDEL HOSPITAL, 301 Hospital Drive, Zip 21061–5899; tel. 410/787–4000; James R. Walker, FACHE, President and Chief Executive Officer (Total facility includes 17 beds in nursing home–type unit) **A**1 9 10 **F**6 7 9 11 12 13 14 17 18 19 22 24 25 29 30 31 32 34 36 38 41 42 46 48 52 53 54 57 58 59 61 62 64 69 70 76 77 78 **P**2 6 Web address: www.northarundel.org.	23	10	224	13837	162	122405	12	102379	51578	1631
HAGERSTOWN—Washington County										
□ BROOK LANE HEALTH SERVICES, (Formerly Brook Lane Psychiatric Center), 13218 Brook Lane Drive, Zip 21742–1945, Mailing Address: P.O. Box 1945, Zip 21742–1945; tel. 301/733–0330; R. Lynn Rushing, Chief Executive Officer **A**1 9 10 **F**3 16 17 22 24 29 30 34 38 39 43 50 51 57 58 59 60 61 62 63 64 70 72 **P**1 6 Web address: www.brooklane.org	23	22	39	1128	25	18690	—	8535	5310	172
★ △ WASHINGTON COUNTY HEALTH SYSTEM, 251 East Antietam Street, Zip 21740–5771; tel. 301/790–8000; Horace W. Murphy, President (Total facility includes 47 beds in nursing home–type unit) **A**1 2 7 9 10 **F**3 4 6 7 8 9 11 12 13 14 16 17 18 19 21 22 23 24 25 27 29 30 32 33 34 35 36 37 38 39 40 41 43 44 45 46 48 49 50 51 53 54 56 57 58 59 60 61 62 63 64 65 66 68 69 70 71 72 73 75 76 78 79 **P**6 8 Web address: www.wchsys.org	23	10	334	14837	192	174020	1699	121788	61005	1507

Hospitals, U.S. / MARYLAND

Hospital, Address, Telephone, Administrator, Approval, Facility, and Physician Codes, Health Care System, Network	Classification Codes		Utilization Data					Expense (thousands) of dollars		
★ American Hospital Association (AHA) membership □ Joint Commission on Accreditation of Healthcare Organizations (JCAHO) accreditation + American Osteopathic Healthcare Association (AOHA) membership ○ American Osteopathic Association (AOA) accreditation △ Commission on Accreditation of Rehabilitation Facilities (CARF) accreditation Control codes 61, 63, 64, 71, 72 and 73 indicate hospitals listed by AOHA, but not registered by AHA. For definition of numerical codes, see page A4	Control	Service	Staffed Beds	Admissions	Census	Outpatient Visits	Births	Total	Payroll	Personnel
□ WESTERN MARYLAND CENTER, 1500 Pennsylvania Avenue, Zip 21742–3194; tel. 301/791–4400; Cynthia Miller Pellegrino, Director and Chief Executive Officer (Total facility includes 60 beds in nursing home–type unit) (Nonreporting) **A**1 10	12	48	120	—	—	—	—	—	—	—
HAVRE DE GRACE—Harford County										
★ HARFORD MEMORIAL HOSPITAL, 501 South Union Avenue, Zip 21078–3493; tel. 410/939–2400; Lyle Ernest Sheldon, President and Chief Executive Officer (Total facility includes 17 beds in nursing home–type unit) **A**1 9 10 **F**6 8 13 17 18 19 22 24 25 27 32 34 36 37 38 39 41 44 45 46 48 51 54 57 61 68 69 70 72 76 78 **S** Upper Chesapeake Health System, Fallston, MD	23	10	157	7314	87	55142	678	45056	20300	613
JESSUP—Anne Arundel County										
□ CLIFTON T. PERKINS HOSPITAL CENTER, 8450 Dorsey Run Road, Zip 20794–9486, Mailing Address: P.O. Box 1000, Zip 20794–1000; tel. 410/724–3000; M. Richard Fragala, M.D., Superintendent **A**1 3 **F**57	12	22	250	120	210	—	0	—	—	400
LA PLATA—Charles County										
★ CIVISTA HEALTH, 701 East Charles Street, Zip 20646–1070, Mailing Address: P.O. Box 1070, Zip 20646–1070; tel. 301/609–4000; Christine M. Stefanides, R.N., CHE, President and Chief Executive Officer (Total facility includes 10 beds in nursing home–type unit) **A**1 2 9 10 **F**8 9 13 16 17 18 19 22 25 29 36 38 39 41 43 44 48 49 54 61 70 72 76 78 79 Web address: www.civista.org	23	10	131	5825	65	50305	850	46950	19972	420
LANHAM—Prince George's County										
★ DOCTORS COMMUNITY HOSPITAL, 8118 Good Luck Road, Zip 20706–3596; tel. 301/552–8118; Philip B. Down, President **A**1 9 10 **F**4 9 11 12 13 16 18 19 22 24 25 27 32 33 34 36 37 38 39 41 43 45 46 48 50 54 65 68 70 72 76 78 Web address: www.doctors–community.com	23	10	198	7708	113	47671	—	75281	32646	802
LAUREL—Prince George's County										
★ △ LAUREL REGIONAL HOSPITAL, 7300 Van Dusen Road, Zip 20707–9266; tel. 301/725–4300; Patrick F. Mutch, President **A**1 7 9 10 **F**2 3 4 6 7 8 9 11 12 13 17 19 21 22 23 24 25 29 30 32 33 34 35 36 37 38 39 40 41 42 43 44 45 46 47 49 50 51 52 53 54 56 57 58 59 60 61 62 63 64 69 70 72 73 74 75 76 77 78 **P**1 6 7 **S** Dimensions Health Corporation, Largo, MD Web address: www.laurelregionalhospital.org	23	10	133	6928	102	37937	857	57168	27144	566
LEONARDTOWN—St. Marys County										
★ ST. MARY'S HOSPITAL, 25500 Point Lookout Road, Zip 20650–9999, Mailing Address: P.O. Box 527, Zip 20650–0527; tel. 301/475–6001; Christine R. Wray, Chief Executive Officer **A**1 2 9 10 **F**7 8 9 13 14 17 18 19 20 21 22 23 24 25 27 30 32 33 34 35 36 37 38 39 41 43 44 45 46 48 49 50 51 54 57 58 59 60 61 62 63 64 68 70 72 76 77 78 79 **P**1 5 Web address: www.smhwecare.com	23	10	100	5654	60	116184	790	40368	18557	566
OAKLAND—Garrett County										
★ GARRETT COUNTY MEMORIAL HOSPITAL, 251 North Fourth Street, Zip 21550–1398; tel. 301/533–4000; Donald P. Battista, President and Chief Executive Officer (Total facility includes 10 beds in nursing home–type unit) **A**1 9 10 **F**1 3 6 7 8 9 11 13 14 16 17 18 21 22 23 24 25 26 28 31 32 33 34 36 37 41 43 44 45 46 48 68 69 70 71 72 75 76 78 79 **P**8 Web address: www.gcmh.com	23	10	86	2825	27	57716	281	19438	8592	258
OLNEY—Montgomery County										
★ MONTGOMERY GENERAL HOSPITAL, 18101 Prince Philip Drive, Zip 20832–1512; tel. 301/774–8882; Peter W. Monge, President and Chief Executive Officer (Total facility includes 21 beds in nursing home–type unit) **A**1 2 9 10 **F**1 2 3 7 8 9 11 12 13 18 19 21 22 24 25 30 32 33 36 39 41 43 44 45 46 48 54 57 58 61 62 63 64 68 69 70 72 73 76 78 **P**8 Web address: www.montgomerygeneral.com	23	10	174	8666	121	48497	859	65229	31236	665
PERRY POINT—Cecil County										
★ VETERANS AFFAIRS MARYLAND HEALTH CARE SYSTEM–PERRY POINT DIVISION, Circle Drive, Zip 21902; tel. 410/642–2411; Dennis H. Smith, Director (Total facility includes 80 beds in nursing home–type unit) (Nonreporting) **A**5 9 **S** Department of Veterans Affairs, Washington, DC	45	22	526	—	—	—	—	—	—	—
PRINCE FREDERICK—Calvert County										
★ CALVERT MEMORIAL HOSPITAL, 100 Hospital Road, Zip 20678–9675; tel. 410/535–4000; James J. Xinis, President and Chief Executive Officer (Total facility includes 16 beds in nursing home–type unit) **A**1 2 9 10 **F**7 8 9 13 16 17 18 19 20 22 25 26 27 28 29 32 33 34 37 38 39 40 41 43 44 45 46 48 49 50 51 54 57 58 59 61 64 65 70 71 72 73 76 77 78 79 **P**7 8	23	10	125	6458	74	67178	804	40451	19114	494
RANDALLSTOWN—Baltimore County										
★ NORTHWEST HOSPITAL CENTER, 5401 Old Court Road, Zip 21133–5185; tel. 410/521–2200; Robert W. Fischer, President (Total facility includes 17 beds in nursing home–type unit) **A**1 2 9 10 **F**1 4 7 8 9 11 13 17 19 22 24 25 28 31 32 33 34 37 38 39 40 41 43 44 46 47 48 49 50 51 54 55 58 59 61 65 66 68 69 70 75 76 77 78 79 **P**1 7 **S** LifeBridge Health, Baltimore, MD	23	10	160	9905	127	72906	0	83575	38604	1021
ROCKVILLE—Montgomery County										
CHARTER BEHAVIORAL HEALTH SYSTEM See Potomac Ridge										
★ CHESTNUT LODGE HOSPITAL, 500 West Montgomery Avenue, Zip 20850–3894; tel. 301/424–8300; Steven Goldstein, Ph.D., President and Chief Executive Officer (Nonreporting) **A**1 9 10 Web address: www.chestnutlodge.com	33	22	50	—	—	—	—	—	—	—

© 2000 AHA Guide *Many Facility Codes have changed. Please refer to the AHA Guide Code Chart.*

Hospitals, U.S. / MARYLAND

Hospital, Address, Telephone, Administrator, Approval, Facility, and Physician Codes, Health Care System, Network	Classification Codes		Utilization Data					Expense (thousands) of dollars		
	Control	Service	Staffed Beds	Admissions	Census	Outpatient Visits	Births	Total	Payroll	Personnel

Membership/Accreditation key:
- ★ American Hospital Association (AHA) membership
- ☐ Joint Commission on Accreditation of Healthcare Organizations (JCAHO) accreditation
- + American Osteopathic Healthcare Association (AOHA) membership
- ○ American Osteopathic Association (AOA) accreditation
- △ Commission on Accreditation of Rehabilitation Facilities (CARF) accreditation

Control codes 61, 63, 64, 71, 72 and 73 indicate hospitals listed by AOHA, but not registered by AHA. For definition of numerical codes, see page A4.

Hospital	Control	Service	Staffed Beds	Admissions	Census	Outpatient Visits	Births	Total	Payroll	Personnel
☐ POTOMAC RIDGE, (Formerly Charter Behavioral Health System), 14901 Broschart Road, Zip 20850–3321; tel. 301/251–4500; Craig S. Juengling, Chief Executive Officer (Nonreporting) **A**1 9 10	33	22	140	—	—	—	—	—	—	—
☐ SHADY GROVE ADVENTIST HOSPITAL, 9901 Medical Center Drive, Zip 20850–3395; tel. 301/279–6000; Cory Chambers, President and Chief Executive Officer **A**1 2 9 10 **F**1 3 4 6 8 9 11 13 14 16 17 18 22 24 25 27 28 31 32 33 34 35 36 37 39 40 41 43 44 45 46 48 49 50 51 54 56 58 59 60 61 62 63 64 65 66 68 70 72 76 78 79 **P**1 **S** Adventist Healthcare, Rockville, MD Web address: www.adventisthealthcare.com	21	10	253	16507	201	117594	4793	131245	47235	1380
SALISBURY—Wicomico County										
☐ DEER'S HEAD CENTER, (LONG TERM CARE), 351 Deer's Head Hospital Road, Zip 21802, Mailing Address: P.O. Box 2018, Zip 21802–2018; tel. 410/543–4000; Dorothy A. Bradshaw, Director (Total facility includes 65 beds in nursing home–type unit) **A**1 10 **F**4 7 9 11 12 15 16 17 18 22 23 24 25 26 30 32 33 34 35 37 39 41 43 46 48 50 51 53 54 57 58 59 60 61 62 63 65 69 70 72 74 76 78 **P**6	12	49	75	82	71	24102	0	16021	8281	261
☐ △ HEALTHSOUTH CHESAPEAKE REHABILITATION HOSPITAL, 220 Tilghman Road, Zip 21804–1921; tel. 410/546–4600; William Roth, Chief Executive Officer (Nonreporting) **A**1 7 9 10 **S** HEALTHSOUTH Corporation, Birmingham, AL	33	46	42	—	—	—	—	—	—	—
★ PENINSULA REGIONAL HEALTH SYSTEM, (Formerly Peninsula Regional Medical Center), 100 East Carroll Street, Zip 21801–5422; tel. 410/546–6400; R. Alan Newberry, President and Chief Executive Officer (Total facility includes 30 beds in nursing home–type unit) **A**1 2 9 10 **F**4 7 8 9 11 12 13 14 16 17 18 19 22 23 24 25 26 27 28 29 30 32 33 34 35 36 37 39 41 43 44 45 46 47 48 50 51 54 56 57 59 61 62 63 65 69 70 72 75 76 77 78 79 **P**5 6 7 8 Web address: www.peninsula.org	23	10	330	17783	233	434675	1942	152710	65865	1990
SILVER SPRING—Montgomery County										
★ HOLY CROSS HOSPITAL OF SILVER SPRING, 1500 Forest Glen Road, Zip 20910–1484; tel. 301/754–7000; Kevin J. Sexton, President and Chief Executive Officer (Total facility includes 90 beds in nursing home–type unit) **A**1 3 5 8 9 10 **F**1 4 8 9 11 12 13 17 18 19 20 21 22 24 25 26 29 30 31 32 33 34 35 36 37 38 39 40 41 42 43 44 45 46 48 49 50 51 54 56 59 61 65 69 70 71 72 74 76 78 79 **P**1 5 6 **S** Trinity Health, Novi, MI	21	10	460	23049	367	226116	5751	193371	82478	1524
SAINT LUKE INSTITUTE, 8901 New Hampshire Avenue, Zip 20903–3611; tel. 301/445–7970; Father Stephen J. Rossetti, Ph.D., President and Chief Executive Officer (Nonreporting)	23	22	24	—	—	—	—	—	—	—
SYKESVILLE—Carroll County										
☐ SPRINGFIELD HOSPITAL CENTER, 6655 Sykesville Road, Zip 21784–7966; tel. 410/795–2100; Paula A. Langmead, Chief Executive Officer (Nonreporting) **A**1 10	12	22	360	—	—	—	—	—	—	—
TAKOMA PARK—Montgomery County										
☐ WASHINGTON ADVENTIST HOSPITAL, 7600 Carroll Avenue, Zip 20912–6392; tel. 301/891–7600; Kiltie Leach, Chief Operating Officer (Nonreporting) **A**1 9 10 **S** Adventist Healthcare, Rockville, MD Web address: www.adventisthealthcare.com	21	10	300	—	—	—	—	—	—	—
TOWSON—Baltimore County										
★ ST. JOSEPH MEDICAL CENTER, 7601 York Road, Zip 21204–7582; tel. 410/337–1000; James J. Cullen, President and Chief Executive Officer (Total facility includes 26 beds in nursing home–type unit) **A**1 9 10 **F**4 7 8 9 11 12 13 16 17 18 19 20 22 24 25 26 27 28 30 32 33 34 36 37 38 39 41 42 43 44 45 46 47 48 49 50 51 53 54 56 57 58 59 60 61 62 63 64 65 66 68 69 70 71 72 73 75 76 77 78 79 **P**2 5 7 **S** Catholic Health Initiatives, Denver, CO Web address: www.sjmcmd.org	21	10	381	21756	265	231875	2315	168905	67641	2250
WESTMINSTER—Carroll County										
★ CARROLL COUNTY GENERAL HOSPITAL, 200 Memorial Avenue, Zip 21157–5799; tel. 410/871–6900; John M. Sernulka, President and Chief Executive Officer **A**1 9 10 **F**8 9 11 13 16 19 21 22 25 27 29 30 32 34 36 37 39 41 43 44 45 46 48 49 51 54 57 58 59 60 61 62 63 64 70 72 76 78 79 **P**3 7 Web address: www.ccgh.com	23	10	168	10201	117	107708	1114	67148	30605	862

Hospitals, U.S. / MASSACHUSETTS

MASSACHUSETTS

Resident Population 6,157 (in thousands)
Resident population in metro areas 96.1%
Birth rate per 1,000 population 13.1
65 years and over 14.0%
Percent of persons without health insurance 12.6%

Hospital, Address, Telephone, Administrator, Approval, Facility, and Physician Codes, Health Care System, Network	Classification Codes		Utilization Data					Expense (thousands) of dollars		
★ American Hospital Association (AHA) membership ☐ Joint Commission on Accreditation of Healthcare Organizations (JCAHO) accreditation + American Osteopathic Healthcare Association (AOHA) membership ○ American Osteopathic Association (AOA) accreditation △ Commission on Accreditation of Rehabilitation Facilities (CARF) accreditation Control codes 61, 63, 64, 71, 72 and 73 indicate hospitals listed by AOHA, but not registered by AHA. For definition of numerical codes, see page A4	Control	Service	Staffed Beds	Admissions	Census	Outpatient Visits	Births	Total	Payroll	Personnel

AMHERST—Hampshire County
UNIVERSITY HEALTH SERVICES, University of Massachusetts, Box 34310, Zip 01003–4310; tel. 413/577–5000; Bernette A. Melby, Executive Director (Nonreporting) **A**3 10
| 12 | 11 | 6 | — | — | — | — | — | — | — |

ANDOVER—Essex County
ISHAM HEALTH CENTER, 180 Main Street, Zip 01810–4161; tel. 978/749–4455; Nneka Anaebonam, Administrator (Nonreporting)
| 23 | 59 | 20 | — | — | — | — | — | — | — |

ATHOL—Worcester County
☐ ATHOL MEMORIAL HOSPITAL, 2033 Main Street, Zip 01331–3598; tel. 978/249–3511; Donna Ditch, Interim President and Chief Executive Officer **A**1 9 10 **F**1 2 3 4 5 6 7 8 9 10 11 12 13 14 15 17 19 20 21 22 23 24 25 26 27 28 29 30 31 32 33 34 35 36 37 38 39 40 41 42 43 44 45 46 47 48 49 50 51 52 53 55 56 57 58 59 60 61 62 63 64 65 66 67 68 69 70 71 72 73 74 75 76 77 78 79 **P**5
Web address: www.atholhospital.org
| 23 | 10 | 30 | 1131 | 12 | 28851 | 0 | 13651 | 6326 | 130 |

ATTLEBORO—Bristol County
☐ ARBOUR–FULLER HOSPITAL, (Formerly Fuller Memorial Hospital), 200 May Street, Zip 02703–5515; tel. 508/761–8500; Gary M. Gilberti, Chief Executive Officer (Nonreporting) **A**1 10 **S** Universal Health Services, Inc., King of Prussia, PA
| 33 | 22 | 46 | — | — | — | — | — | — | — |

FULLER MEMORIAL HOSPITAL See Arbour–Fuller Hospital
★ STURDY MEMORIAL HOSPITAL, 211 Park Street, Zip 02703–3137, Mailing Address: P.O. Box 2963, Zip 02703–2963; tel. 508/222–5200; Linda Shyavitz, President and Chief Executive Officer **A**1 2 9 10 **F**7 8 9 13 14 16 17 18 19 20 21 22 23 24 25 27 29 30 32 33 34 35 37 38 39 41 43 44 45 46 48 49 50 51 54 56 59 66 68 70 72 73 76 77 78 79
| 23 | 10 | 124 | 5532 | 63 | 159779 | 999 | 63113 | 32372 | 833 |

AYER—Middlesex County
★ DEACONESS–NASHOBA HOSPITAL, 200 Groton Road, Zip 01432–3300; tel. 978/784–9000; Jeffrey R. Kelly, President and Chief Executive Officer **A**1 9 10 **F**1 4 5 6 7 8 9 11 12 13 14 17 18 19 20 22 24 25 27 28 29 30 32 33 34 35 36 37 39 43 45 46 47 48 49 50 51 54 56 70 72 76 78 79 **P**5 8 **S** CareGroup, Boston, MA
| 23 | 10 | 41 | 2071 | 21 | 94019 | 0 | 24140 | 11507 | 283 |

BEDFORD—Middlesex County
★ EDITH NOURSE ROGERS MEMORIAL VETERANS HOSPITAL, 200 Springs Road, Zip 01730–1198; tel. 781/687–2000; William A. Conte, Director (Total facility includes 204 beds in nursing home–type unit) **A**1 3 5 9 **F**1 3 4 8 9 11 13 22 23 24 25 26 27 30 31 32 34 35 36 37 38 39 43 46 47 48 49 51 54 55 56 57 59 61 62 63 64 65 66 68 69 70 74 76 78 79 **P**1 **S** Department of Veterans Affairs, Washington, DC
Web address: www.va.gov/stations97/guide/home.asp?DIVISION=ALL
| 45 | 22 | 411 | 1633 | 418 | 188000 | 0 | 67870 | 41434 | 936 |

BELMONT—Middlesex County
★ MCLEAN HOSPITAL, 115 Mill Street, Zip 02478–9106; tel. 617/855–2000; Bruce M. Cohen, M.D., Ph.D., President and Psychiatrist–in–Chief **A**1 3 5 9 10 **F**2 3 4 5 6 7 8 9 10 11 12 13 14 15 19 20 21 22 23 24 25 27 28 30 32 33 34 35 36 37 38 39 40 41 42 43 44 45 46 47 48 49 50 51 52 53 54 55 56 57 58 59 60 61 62 63 65 66 68 69 70 71 72 74 75 76 78 79 **P**1 3 4 5 6 7 8 **S** Partners HealthCare System, Inc., Boston, MA
Web address: www.mcleanhospital.org
| 23 | 22 | 150 | 3118 | 130 | 39257 | 0 | 77098 | 31046 | 852 |

BEVERLY—Essex County
★ BEVERLY HOSPITAL, (Includes Addison Gilbert Hospital, 298 Washington Street, Gloucester, Zip 01930–4887; tel. 978/283–4000; Kathleen Allen Bliss, President), 85 Herrrick Street, Zip 01915–1777; tel. 978/922–3000; Robert R. Fanning, Jr, President and Chief Executive Officer **A**2 3 9 10 **F**1 3 5 6 8 9 11 13 16 17 18 19 21 22 25 26 27 30 32 33 34 35 37 38 39 40 41 43 44 45 46 48 49 50 51 54 56 57 58 59 60 61 62 63 64 65 66 67 69 70 71 72 73 74 76 78 79 **P**1 6
Web address: www.nhs–healthlink.org
| 23 | 10 | 339 | 17702 | 222 | 101491 | 2634 | 134743 | 66651 | 1715 |

BOSTON—Suffolk County
☐ ARBOUR HOSPITAL, 49 Robinwood Avenue, Zip 02130–2156, Mailing Address: P.O. Box 9, Zip 02130; tel. 617/522–4400; Roy A. Ettlinger, Chief Executive Officer (Nonreporting) **A**1 9 10 **S** Universal Health Services, Inc., King of Prussia, PA
| 33 | 22 | 118 | — | — | — | — | — | — | — |

★ BETH ISRAEL DEACONESS MEDICAL CENTER, 330 Brookline Avenue, Zip 02215–5491; tel. 617/667–2203; James Reinertsen, M.D., Chief Executive Officer (Total facility includes 48 beds in nursing home–type unit) **A**1 2 5 8 9 10 **F**1 3 4 5 7 8 9 11 12 13 14 16 17 18 19 20 21 22 23 24 25 26 27 28 29 30 31 32 33 34 35 36 37 38 39 40 41 42 43 44 45 46 47 48 49 50 51 52 54 56 57 58 59 60 61 62 63 64 65 66 68 69 70 71 72 73 74 75 76 77 78 79 **P**2 3 4 5 6 7 8 **S** CareGroup, Boston, MA
Web address: www.bidmc.harvard.edu
| 23 | 10 | 589 | 32818 | 460 | — | 4902 | 748014 | 273185 | 6482 |

© 2000 AHA Guide   *Many Facility Codes have changed. Please refer to the AHA Guide Code Chart.*   Hospitals **A201**

Hospitals, U.S. / MASSACHUSETTS

Hospital, Address, Telephone, Administrator, Approval, Facility, and Physician Codes, Health Care System, Network	Classification Codes		Utilization Data					Expense (thousands) of dollars		
	Control	Service	Staffed Beds	Admissions	Census	Outpatient Visits	Births	Total	Payroll	Personnel

★ American Hospital Association (AHA) membership
□ Joint Commission on Accreditation of Healthcare Organizations (JCAHO) accreditation
+ American Osteopathic Healthcare Association (AOHA) membership
○ American Osteopathic Association (AOA) accreditation
△ Commission on Accreditation of Rehabilitation Facilities (CARF) accreditation
Control codes 61, 63, 64, 71, 72 and 73 indicate hospitals listed by AOHA, but not registered by AHA. For definition of numerical codes, see page A4

Hospital	Control	Service	Staffed Beds	Admissions	Census	Outpatient Visits	Births	Total	Payroll	Personnel
★ BOSTON MEDICAL CENTER, One Boston Medical Center Place, Zip 02118–2393; tel. 617/638–8000; Elaine S. Ullian, President and Chief Executive Officer (Total facility includes 17 beds in nursing home–type unit) **A**1 2 3 5 8 9 10 **F**4 5 8 9 11 12 13 14 16 17 18 19 20 21 22 23 24 25 26 30 31 32 33 34 35 38 39 41 42 43 44 45 46 47 48 49 50 51 52 53 54 56 58 59 60 61 62 63 65 66 69 70 71 72 74 75 76 77 78 79 **P**7 **Web address:** www.bmc.org	23	10	354	22337	332	451318	1809	466488	172355	4821
★ BRIGHAM AND WOMEN'S HOSPITAL, 75 Francis Street, Zip 02115–6195; tel. 617/732–5500; Jeffrey Otten, President **A**1 2 3 5 8 9 10 **F**3 4 5 7 8 9 10 11 12 13 14 15 16 17 18 19 20 21 22 23 24 25 26 27 28 29 30 31 32 33 34 35 36 37 38 39 41 42 43 44 45 46 47 48 49 50 51 54 55 56 58 59 60 61 62 63 64 65 66 68 70 71 72 73 74 75 76 77 78 79 **P**1 3 8 **S** Partners HealthCare System, Inc., Boston, MA **Web address:** www.partners.org	23	10	694	39848	572	744066	9718	853098	290298	7624
★ CHILDREN'S HOSPITAL, 300 Longwood Avenue, Zip 02115–5737; tel. 617/355–6000; David S. Weiner, Chief Executive Officer **A**1 3 5 8 9 10 **F**4 11 12 13 14 16 17 18 19 20 21 22 23 24 25 26 29 31 34 35 36 39 42 43 45 46 47 48 49 50 51 52 54 55 56 57 58 59 60 61 63 65 66 68 70 71 72 73 74 75 76 77 78 **P**3 5 **Web address:** www.childrenshospital.org/	23	50	324	17530	240	302274	0	359966	154937	4491
★ DANA–FARBER CANCER INSTITUTE, (COMPREHENSIVE CANCER CENTER), 44 Binney Street, Zip 02115–6084; tel. 617/632–3000; David G. Nathan, M.D., President and Chief Executive Officer **A**1 3 5 9 10 **F**7 9 13 17 18 19 20 22 24 25 26 32 33 34 35 36 37 38 39 41 43 45 46 48 49 50 51 52 54 55 58 59 60 61 62 63 65 68 70 72 74 75 76 78 79 **P**6 **Web address:** www.dfci.harvard.edu	23	49	30	957	21	103896	0	242968	87122	2440
★ FAULKNER HOSPITAL, Mailing Address: 1153 Centre Sreet, Zip 02130–3400; tel. 617/983–7000; David J. Trull, President and Chief Executive Officer **A**1 2 3 5 8 9 10 **F**1 3 4 7 9 11 13 16 17 18 19 21 22 24 25 29 31 33 34 35 38 39 41 43 45 46 47 48 49 50 51 54 56 57 59 60 61 62 63 64 65 70 71 72 76 77 78 79 **P**5 **S** Partners HealthCare System, Inc., Boston, MA **Web address:** www.faulknerhospital.org	23	10	125	6010	83	146682	0	66982	34866	749
□ △ FRANCISCAN CHILDREN'S HOSPITAL AND REHABILITATION CENTER, Mailing Address: 30 Warren Street, Zip 02135–3680; tel. 617/254–3800; Paul J. Dellarocco, President and Chief Executive Officer **A**1 5 7 10 **F**1 13 17 18 19 23 26 34 36 37 38 43 48 53 54 56 57 58 63 64 70 72 76 77 78 **P**6 **Web address:** www.fch.com/	23	56	60	571	50	33203	0	33049	19077	496
★ HEBREW REHABILITATION CENTER FOR AGED, (CHRONIC DISEASE HOSP LONG–TERM), Mailing Address: 1200 Centre Street, Zip 02131–1097; tel. 617/325–8000; Maurice I. May, President and Chief Executive Officer **A**10 **F**1 6 7 17 18 19 23 26 28 30 31 32 34 36 37 38 40 43 45 51 54 56 59 62 63 67 69 70 72 78 **P**6 **Web address:** www.hebrewrehab.org	23	49	725	181	695	620	0	58442	32674	822
★ JEWISH MEMORIAL HOSPITAL AND REHABILITATION CENTER, 59 Townsend Street, Zip 02119–9918; tel. 617/442–8760; Paul J. Dellarocco, President and Chief Executive Officer (Nonreporting) **A**1 3 5 10 **Web address:** www.jmhrc.org	23	49	110	—	—	—	—	—	—	—
★ LEMUEL SHATTUCK HOSPITAL, 170 Morton Street, Jamaica Plain, Zip 02130–3787; tel. 617/522–8110; Robert D. Wakefield, Jr, Chief Executive Officer (Nonreporting) **A**1 3 5 6 10	12	10	230	—	—	—	—	—	—	—
□ MASSACHUSETTS EYE AND EAR INFIRMARY, 243 Charles Street, Zip 02114–3096; tel. 617/523–7900; F. Curtis Smith, President **A**1 3 5 9 10 **F**13 14 16 17 18 19 22 24 25 29 31 32 34 38 39 43 45 46 48 49 50 51 54 55 65 70 72 75 76 77 78 **P**8 **Web address:** www.meei.harvard.edu	23	45	42	2037	20	225792	0	82877	26391	1169
★ MASSACHUSETTS GENERAL HOSPITAL, 55 Fruit Street, Zip 02114–2696; tel. 617/726–2000; James J. Mongan, M.D., President **A**1 2 3 5 8 9 10 **F**1 3 4 5 6 7 8 9 10 11 12 13 14 16 17 18 19 20 21 22 23 24 25 26 27 29 30 31 32 33 34 35 36 37 38 39 41 42 43 44 45 46 47 48 49 50 51 52 53 54 55 56 57 58 59 60 61 62 63 64 65 66 67 68 69 70 71 72 73 74 75 76 77 78 79 **P**5 7 8 **S** Partners HealthCare System, Inc., Boston, MA **Web address:** www.mgh.harvard.edu/	23	10	853	37569	633	767141	2702	995155	333650	11665
★ NEW ENGLAND BAPTIST HOSPITAL, 125 Parker Hill Avenue, Zip 02120–3297; tel. 617/754–5800; Alan H. Robbins, M.D., President (Total facility includes 32 beds in nursing home–type unit) **A**1 3 5 6 9 10 **F**9 11 13 16 17 18 19 22 23 24 27 28 29 30 32 33 34 38 39 41 43 45 46 48 49 51 54 59 69 70 71 76 77 78 **P**8 **S** CareGroup, Boston, MA **Web address:** www.nebh.org	23	10	162	6274	96	94091	0	88368	37480	889
★ NEW ENGLAND MEDICAL CENTER, 750 Washington Street, Zip 02111–1845; tel. 617/636–5000; Thomas F. O'Donnell, Jr, M.D., FACS, President and Chief Executive Officer **A**1 2 3 5 8 9 10 **F**3 4 5 8 9 11 12 13 14 16 17 18 19 21 22 23 24 25 26 27 29 30 31 32 33 34 35 38 39 41 42 43 44 45 46 47 48 49 50 52 54 56 57 58 59 60 61 62 63 64 65 66 68 70 71 72 73 74 75 76 77 78 79 **P**3 5 7 **S** Lifespan Corporation, Providence, RI **Web address:** www.nemc.org/home/	23	10	323	15399	274	366515	1491	369431	176647	3767
□ SHRINERS HOSPITALS FOR CHILDREN, SHRINERS BURNS HOSPITAL–BOSTON, (PEDIATRIC BURNS), 51 Blossom Street, Zip 02114–2699; tel. 617/722–3000; Robert F. Bories, Jr, FACHE, Administrator **A**1 3 **F**18 22 24 25 39 50 54 58 70 72 76 78 **S** Shriners Hospitals for Children, Tampa, FL **Web address:** www.shrinershq.org	23	59	30	731	19	3919	0	—	—	243

Hospitals, U.S. / MASSACHUSETTS

Hospital, Address, Telephone, Administrator, Approval, Facility, and Physician Codes, Health Care System, Network	Classification Codes		Utilization Data					Expense (thousands) of dollars		
★ American Hospital Association (AHA) membership □ Joint Commission on Accreditation of Healthcare Organizations (JCAHO) accreditation + American Osteopathic Healthcare Association (AOHA) membership ○ American Osteopathic Association (AOA) accreditation △ Commission on Accreditation of Rehabilitation Facilities (CARF) accreditation Control codes 61, 63, 64, 71, 72 and 73 indicate hospitals listed by AOHA, but not registered by AHA. For definition of numerical codes, see page A4	Control	Service	Staffed Beds	Admissions	Census	Outpatient Visits	Births	Total	Payroll	Personnel
★ △ SPAULDING REHABILITATION HOSPITAL, 125 Nashua Street, Zip 02114–1198; tel. 617/573–7000; John E. Cupples, President (Total facility includes 37 beds in nursing home–type unit) **A**1 3 7 10 **F**2 3 4 5 6 7 8 9 10 11 12 13 16 17 18 19 20 21 22 23 24 25 26 27 30 31 32 34 35 36 38 39 41 42 43 44 45 46 47 48 49 51 52 53 54 55 56 57 58 59 60 61 62 63 64 65 66 67 68 69 70 71 72 73 74 75 76 77 78 79 **P**1 3 5 6 **S** Partners HealthCare System, Inc., Boston, MA **Web address:** www.spauldingrehab.org	23	46	333	4941	299	85254	0	102019	55542	1443
□ VENCOR HOSPITAL–BOSTON, 1515 Commonwealth Avenue, Zip 02135–3696; tel. 617/254–1100; Donald E. Schwarz, Administrator (Nonreporting) **A**1 10 **S** Vencor, Incorporated, Louisville, KY **Web address:** www.vencor.com	33	49	59	—	—	—	—	—	—	—
★ VETERANS AFFAIRS BOSTON HEALTHCARE SYSTEM, (Formerly Veterans Affairs Medical Center), Mailing Address: 150 South Huntington Avenue, Jamaica Plain Station, Zip 02130–4820; tel. 617/232–9500; Michael E. Lawson, Director **A**1 2 3 5 8 **F**1 3 4 5 7 9 11 12 13 17 19 20 21 22 23 24 25 26 28 29 30 31 32 33 34 35 37 38 39 41 43 45 46 48 49 50 51 53 54 55 56 57 59 60 61 62 63 64 65 66 68 69 70 71 72 74 75 76 77 78 79 **S** Department of Veterans Affairs, Washington, DC **Web address:** www.va.gov/stations97/guide/home.asp?DIVISION=ALL	45	10	188	6874	193	369006	0	97456	79232	3424
BRAINTREE—Norfolk County										
□ HEALTHSOUTH BRAINTREE REHABILITATION HOSPITAL, 250 Pond Street, Zip 02185–9020; tel. 781/848–5353; Anne M. MacRitchie, Chief Executive Officer **A**1 3 10 **F**5 13 22 31 39 45 46 51 53 54 55 70 71 72 76 78 **P**5 6 **S** HEALTHSOUTH Corporation, Birmingham, AL	33	46	187	2511	156	199047	0	43182	27543	919
□ MASSACHUSETTS RESPIRATORY HOSPITAL, 2001 Washington Street, Zip 02184–8664; tel. 781/848–2600; M. Lynne Francis, Chief Executive Officer (Nonreporting) **A**1	13	48	110	—	—	—	—	—	—	—
BRIDGEWATER—Plymouth County										
BRIDGEWATER STATE HOSPITAL, 20 Administration Road, Zip 02324–3201; tel. 508/279–4521; Kenneth W. Nelson, Superintendent (Nonreporting)	12	22	350	—	—	—	—	—	—	—
BRIGHTON—Suffolk County										
★ ST. ELIZABETH'S MEDICAL CENTER OF BOSTON, 736 Cambridge Street, Zip 02135–2997; tel. 617/789–3000; Michael F. Collins, M.D., President (Total facility includes 22 beds in nursing home–type unit) **A**1 2 3 5 6 8 9 10 **F**1 2 3 4 7 8 9 11 12 13 16 17 18 19 20 21 22 23 24 25 27 29 30 32 33 34 35 36 37 38 39 41 43 44 45 46 47 48 49 50 51 54 56 57 59 60 61 62 63 64 65 66 68 69 70 71 72 75 76 77 78 79 **P**3 5 **S** Caritas Christi Health Care, Boston, MA **Web address:** www.semc.org	21	10	247	14832	239	114206	1602	204371	85576	2570
BROCKTON—Plymouth County										
★ BROCKTON HOSPITAL, 680 Centre Street, Zip 02302–3395; tel. 508/941–7000; Norman B. Goodman, President and Chief Executive Officer (Total facility includes 26 beds in nursing home–type unit) **A**1 2 3 5 6 9 10 **F**3 4 7 8 9 11 12 13 14 16 17 18 19 20 21 22 23 24 25 27 30 31 32 33 36 38 39 41 43 44 45 46 48 49 51 54 56 57 58 59 60 61 62 63 64 65 68 69 70 71 72 73 76 77 78 79 **P**6 8 **Web address:** www.brocktonhospital.com	23	10	232	11086	142	193139	1132	93316	55275	1195
★ BROCKTON VETERANS AFFAIRS MEDICAL CENTER, 940 Belmont Street, Zip 02401–5596; tel. 508/583–4500; Roland E. Moore, Director (Total facility includes 120 beds in nursing home–type unit) **A**1 3 5 8 **F**1 2 3 9 11 19 21 22 23 24 25 29 30 31 32 34 35 38 41 43 45 46 47 48 51 53 54 56 57 59 60 61 62 63 64 69 70 72 76 77 78 79 **S** Department of Veterans Affairs, Washington, DC **Web address:** www.va.gov/stations97/guide/home.asp?DIVISION=ALL	45	10	495	1771	463	297356	0	—	—	—
★ CARITAS GOOD SAMARITAN MEDICAL CENTER, (Formerly Good Samaritan Medical Center), (Includes Good Samaritan Medical Center – Cushing Campus), 235 North Pearl Street, Zip 02401–1794; tel. 508/427–3000; Peter J. Holden, President **A**1 2 3 5 9 10 **F**8 9 12 13 16 17 18 19 22 23 24 25 27 30 32 34 37 39 41 43 44 45 46 48 49 51 54 70 72 76 77 78 79 **P**5 **S** Caritas Christi Health Care, Boston, MA **Web address:** www.caritaschristi.org/locations.html	23	10	193	10987	132	141681	1262	89658	43298	939
BROOKLINE—Norfolk County										
□ ARBOUR H. R. I. HOSPITAL, 227 Babcock Street, Zip 02146; tel. 617/731–3200; Roy A. Ettlinger, Chief Executive Officer (Nonreporting) **A**1 5 10 **S** Universal Health Services, Inc., King of Prussia, PA **Web address:** www.arbourhealth.com	33	22	51	—	—	—	—	—	—	—
□ BOURNEWOOD HOSPITAL, 300 South Street, Zip 02467–3694; tel. 617/469–0300; Nasir A. Khan, M.D., Director (Nonreporting) **A**1 9 10 **Web address:** www.bournewood.com	33	22	76	—	—	—	—	—	—	—
BURLINGTON—Middlesex County										
★ LAHEY CLINIC HOSPITAL, 41 Mall Road, Zip 01805; tel. 781/744–8500; David M. Barrett, M.D., Chief Executive Officer **A**1 2 3 5 8 9 10 **F**4 5 7 9 11 12 13 14 16 17 18 19 21 22 24 25 27 29 30 31 32 33 34 35 36 38 39 41 43 45 46 47 48 49 50 51 53 54 56 58 59 60 61 62 63 65 66 68 70 71 72 74 75 76 77 78 79 **P**6 **Web address:** www.lahey.org	23	10	234	15999	201	689358	—	275601	120370	3360

© 2000 AHA Guide   *Many Facility Codes have changed. Please refer to the AHA Guide Code Chart.*

Hospitals, U.S. / MASSACHUSETTS

Hospital, Address, Telephone, Administrator, Approval, Facility, and Physician Codes, Health Care System, Network	Classification Codes		Utilization Data					Expense (thousands) of dollars		
★ American Hospital Association (AHA) membership ☐ Joint Commission on Accreditation of Healthcare Organizations (JCAHO) accreditation + American Osteopathic Healthcare Association (AOHA) membership ○ American Osteopathic Association (AOA) accreditation △ Commission on Accreditation of Rehabilitation Facilities (CARF) accreditation Control codes 61, 63, 64, 71, 72 and 73 indicate hospitals listed by AOHA, but not registered by AHA. For definition of numerical codes, see page A4	Control	Service	Staffed Beds	Admissions	Census	Outpatient Visits	Births	Total	Payroll	Personnel

CAMBRIDGE—Middlesex County

★ CAMBRIDGE HEALTH ALLIANCE, (Includes Cambridge Hospital, 1493 Cambridge Street; Somerville Hospital, 230 Highland Avenue, Somerville, Zip 02143; tel. 617/666–4400), 1493 Cambridge Street, Zip 02139–1099; tel. 617/498–1000; John G. O'Brien, Chief Executive Officer **A**1 3 5 6 9 10 **F**1 2 3 4 7 8 9 11 13 14 16 17 18 19 21 22 23 24 25 29 30 31 32 33 34 35 36 37 38 39 40 41 43 44 45 46 48 50 51 54 56 57 58 59 60 61 62 63 64 66 69 70 71 72 73 76 78 79 **P**6
Web address: www.challiance.org — 16 10 269 8261 163 461329 643 179993 94440 1853

☐ M. I. T. MEDICAL DEPARTMENT, 77 Massachusetts Avenue, Zip 02139–4307; tel. 617/253–4481; Arnold N. Weinberg, M.D., Director (Nonreporting) **A**1 — 23 11 18 — — — — — — —

★ MOUNT AUBURN HOSPITAL, 330 Mount Auburn Street, Zip 02138; tel. 617/499–5700; Jeanette G. Clough, President and Chief Executive Officer **A**1 2 3 5 8 9 10 **F**3 4 7 8 9 11 12 13 16 17 18 19 22 24 25 27 30 32 33 34 35 36 38 40 41 43 44 45 46 47 48 49 50 51 54 56 57 59 60 61 62 63 64 65 66 68 70 71 72 76 77 78 79 **P**5 6 7 **S** CareGroup, Boston, MA
Web address: www.mtauburn.caregroup.org/ — 23 10 172 9998 122 208211 1209 120841 56434 1516

☐ STILLMAN INFIRMARY, HARVARD UNIVERSITY HEALTH SERVICES, 75 Mount Auburn Street, Zip 02138–4960; tel. 617/495–2010; David S. Rosenthal, M.D., Director (Nonreporting) **A**1 10 — 23 11 18 — — — — — — —

☐ △ YOUVILLE LIFECARE, 1575 Cambridge Street, Zip 02138–4398; tel. 617/876–4344; Daniel P. Leahey, President and Chief Executive Officer (Total facility includes 140 beds in nursing home–type unit) (Nonreporting) **A**1 6 7 10 **S** Covenant Health Systems, Inc., Lexington, MA — 21 46 286 — — — — — — —

CANTON—Norfolk County

★ MASSACHUSETTS HOSPITAL SCHOOL, (CHRONIC PEDIATRIC), 3 Randolph Street, Zip 02021–2397; tel. 781/828–2440; John H. Britt, Executive Director **A**1 5 10 **F**17 18 19 23 38 49 54 57 70 76 — 12 59 98 19 51 1700 0 — — 240

CHELSEA—Suffolk County

★ LAWRENCE F. QUIGLEY MEMORIAL HOSPITAL, 91 Crest Avenue, Zip 02150–2199; tel. 617/884–5660; Michael Resca, Chief Executive Officer (Total facility includes 88 beds in nursing home–type unit) (Nonreporting) **A**1 9 10 — 12 49 159 — — — — — — —

CLINTON—Worcester County

☐ CLINTON HOSPITAL, 201 Highland Street, Zip 01510–1096; tel. 978/368–3000; Thomas Devins, President (Nonreporting) **A**1 5 9 10 — 23 10 46 — — — — — — —

CONCORD—Middlesex County

★ EMERSON HOSPITAL, 133 Old Road to Nine Acre Corner, Zip 01742–9120; tel. 978/369–1400; Geoffrey F. Cole, President and Chief Executive Officer (Nonreporting) **A**1 2 5 9 10
Web address: www.emersonhosp.org — 23 10 165 — — — — — — —

DORCHESTER—Suffolk County

★ CARNEY HOSPITAL, 2100 Dorchester Avenue, Zip 02124–5666; tel. 617/296–4000; Joyce A. Murphy, President (Total facility includes 27 beds in nursing home–type unit) **A**1 2 5 9 10 **F**9 11 16 17 18 19 22 25 28 29 32 33 34 35 38 39 41 43 45 46 48 50 51 54 56 57 59 60 61 63 64 67 70 73 76 78 79 **P**5 6 7 **S** Caritas Christi Health Care, Boston, MA
Web address: www.caritaschristi.org/locations.html — 21 10 174 8301 135 90703 0 85184 48156 1032

EVERETT—Middlesex County

WHIDDEN MEMORIAL HOSPITAL See Hallmark Health System, Malden

FALL RIVER—Bristol County

CHARLTON MEMORIAL HOSPITAL See Southcoast Hospitals Group

★ SAINT ANNE'S HOSPITAL, 795 Middle Street, Zip 02721–1798; tel. 508/674–5741; Michael W. Metzler, President (Total facility includes 16 beds in nursing home–type unit) **A**1 2 9 10 **F**1 3 9 13 14 16 17 18 19 20 22 24 25 32 34 35 36 37 38 39 41 43 45 46 48 49 51 54 58 59 61 62 63 64 65 68 69 70 72 76 78 **P**5 7 **S** Caritas Christi Health Care, Boston, MA — 21 10 155 5020 89 104429 0 66200 27562 609

★ SOUTHCOAST HOSPITALS GROUP, (Includes Charlton Memorial Hospital, 363 Highland Avenue, Zip 02720–3794; tel. 508/679–3131; St. Luke's Hospital of New Bedford, 101 Page Street, New Bedford, Zip 02740, Mailing Address: P.O. Box H–3000, Zip 02741–3000; tel. 508/997–1515; Tobey Hospital, 43 High Street, Wareham, Zip 02571–0880), 363 Highland Avenue, Zip 02720–3703; tel. 508/679–7555; Ronald B. Goodspeed, M.D., M.P.H., President **A**1 2 9 10 **F**3 4 6 7 8 9 11 12 14 15 17 18 19 20 21 22 23 24 25 26 28 29 30 31 32 33 34 35 36 37 38 39 41 43 44 45 46 48 49 50 51 53 54 56 57 58 59 60 61 62 63 64 65 66 68 69 70 71 72 73 76 77 78 79 **P**4 5 6 7 8
Web address: www.southcoasthealth.org — 23 10 790 34446 578 815326 3568 305603 152791 3718

FALMOUTH—Barnstable County

★ FALMOUTH HOSPITAL, 100 Ter Heun Drive, Zip 02540–2599; tel. 508/548–5300; Robert A. Gunderson, Executive Vice President **A**1 9 10 **F**1 4 6 8 9 11 12 13 16 17 18 19 20 21 22 24 25 26 29 30 31 32 33 34 35 36 37 38 39 41 44 45 46 48 49 50 51 53 54 57 58 60 61 62 63 64 65 69 70 71 72 76 77 78 79 **P**5 **S** Cape Cod Healthcare, Inc., Hyannis, MA — 23 10 83 5346 56 66457 584 58846 24339 388

FITCHBURG—Worcester County

HEALTH ALLIANCE–BURBANK HOSPITAL See Health Alliance Hospitals, Leominster

Hospitals, U.S. / MASSACHUSETTS

Hospital, Address, Telephone, Administrator, Approval, Facility, and Physician Codes, Health Care System, Network	Classification Codes		Utilization Data					Expense (thousands) of dollars		
	Control	Service	Staffed Beds	Admissions	Census	Outpatient Visits	Births	Total	Payroll	Personnel

★ American Hospital Association (AHA) membership
□ Joint Commission on Accreditation of Healthcare Organizations (JCAHO) accreditation
+ American Osteopathic Healthcare Association (AOHA) membership
○ American Osteopathic Association (AOA) accreditation
△ Commission on Accreditation of Rehabilitation Facilities (CARF) accreditation
Control codes 61, 63, 64, 71, 72 and 73 indicate hospitals listed by AOHA, but not registered by AHA. For definition of numerical codes, see page A4

FRAMINGHAM—Middlesex County

| ★ METROWEST MEDICAL CENTER, (Includes Framingham Union Hospital, 115 Lincoln Street, tel. 508/383-1000; Leonard Morse Hospital, 67 Union Street, Natick, Zip 01760; tel. 508/650-7000), 115 Lincoln Street, Zip 01702; tel. 508/383-1000; Mary Jo Gregory, Chief Executive Officer (Nonreporting) **A**1 2 3 5 6 9 10 **S** TENET Healthcare Corporation, Santa Barbara, CA
Web address: www.mwmc.com | 33 | 10 | 398 | — | — | — | — | — | — | — |

GARDNER—Worcester County

| □ HEYWOOD HOSPITAL, 242 Green Street, Zip 01440-1373; tel. 978/632-3420; Daniel P. Moen, President and Chief Executive Officer **A**1 9 10 **F**5 7 8 9 13 17 18 19 22 23 24 25 26 30 32 34 37 38 39 41 43 44 45 46 48 54 57 58 62 66 68 70 71 72 76 78 79 **P**5 8 | 23 | 10 | 126 | 4438 | 70 | 115386 | 519 | 39471 | 20479 | 532 |

GLOUCESTER—Essex County

ADDISON GILBERT HOSPITAL See Beverly Hospital, Beverly

GREAT BARRINGTON—Berkshire County

| ★ FAIRVIEW HOSPITAL, 29 Lewis Avenue, Zip 01230-1713; tel. 413/528-0790; Eugene A. Dellea, Interim President (Total facility includes 21 beds in nursing home–type unit) **A**1 9 10 **F**2 3 6 7 8 9 11 12 13 14 17 18 19 20 21 22 23 24 25 26 27 30 31 32 33 34 36 37 38 39 41 44 45 46 48 49 51 53 54 56 57 59 60 61 63 64 65 69 70 71 72 73 75 76 77 78 **P**6 **S** Berkshire Health Systems, Inc., Pittsfield, MA
Web address: www.bhs1.org/fairviewhospital.htm | 23 | 10 | 46 | 1536 | 32 | 43144 | 168 | 16877 | 6595 | 143 |

GREENFIELD—Franklin County

| ★ FRANKLIN MEDICAL CENTER, 164 High Street, Zip 01301-2613; tel. 413/773-0211; Harlan J. Smith, President and Chief Executive Officer **A**1 2 9 10 **F**1 3 7 8 9 13 17 18 19 22 24 25 26 30 31 33 34 35 36 37 38 39 41 43 44 45 46 48 49 50 53 54 56 57 58 59 60 61 62 63 64 70 72 76 78 **P**3 5 6 7 8 **S** Baystate Health System, Inc., Springfield, MA
Web address: www.baystatehealth.com | 23 | 10 | 85 | 4572 | 54 | — | 537 | 54258 | 26575 | 644 |

HAVERHILL—Essex County

BALDPATE HOSPITAL, 83 Baldpate Road, Zip 01833-2399; tel. 978/352-2131; Lucille M. Batal, Administrator (Nonreporting) **A**9 10	33	22	59	—	—	—	—	—	—	—
★ HALE HOSPITAL, 140 Lincoln Avenue, Zip 01830-6798; tel. 978/374-2000; Robert J. Ingala, Chief Executive Officer (Total facility includes 21 beds in nursing home–type unit) **A**1 9 10 **F**7 8 9 11 12 16 17 18 22 23 25 32 33 34 37 39 43 44 45 46 48 49 50 51 54 59 61 66 68 69 70 72 73 76 78 79 **S** Quorum Health Group, Brentwood, TN	14	10	129	4499	69	53535	370	41403	19884	549
★ △ WHITTIER REHABILITATION HOSPITAL, 76 Summer Street, Zip 01830-5896; tel. 978/372-8000; Alfred J. Arcidi, M.D., Senior Vice President (Nonreporting) **A**1 7 10	33	46	60	—	—	—	—	—	—	—

HOLYOKE—Hampden County

| ★ HOLYOKE HOSPITAL, 575 Beech Street, Zip 01040-2296; tel. 413/534-2500; Hank J. Porten, President and Chief Executive Officer (Total facility includes 14 beds in nursing home–type unit) **A**1 2 9 10 **F**3 5 7 8 9 12 13 16 17 18 19 21 22 24 25 26 29 30 31 32 33 34 35 36 37 38 39 41 43 44 45 46 48 49 50 51 54 55 56 57 58 59 60 61 62 63 64 65 66 68 69 70 72 73 76 78 79 **P**8
Web address: www.holyokehealth.com | 23 | 10 | 117 | 7627 | 117 | 204549 | 480 | 65892 | 33406 | 827 |
| ★ SOLDIERS' HOME IN HOLYOKE, 110 Cherry Street, Zip 01040-7002; tel. 413/532-9475; Paul A. Morin, Superintendent (Total facility includes 260 beds in nursing home–type unit) **A**1 10 **F**17 18 23 32 34 43 54 69 78 **P**6 | 12 | 10 | 287 | 328 | 268 | — | 0 | 17905 | 11142 | 327 |

HYANNIS—Barnstable County

| ★ CAPE COD HOSPITAL, 27 Park Street, Zip 02601; tel. 508/771-1800; Gail M. Frieswick, Ed.D., Executive Vice President **A**1 2 9 10 **F**4 5 6 8 9 11 12 13 17 18 19 22 25 27 30 31 32 33 34 35 36 38 39 41 43 44 46 48 49 50 51 54 56 57 58 59 60 61 62 63 64 65 66 70 71 72 76 77 78 **P**4 5 6 7 **S** Cape Cod Healthcare, Inc., Hyannis, MA | 23 | 10 | 214 | 14073 | 173 | 253223 | 974 | 156641 | 65480 | 1187 |

LAWRENCE—Essex County

| □ LAWRENCE GENERAL HOSPITAL, 1 General Street, Zip 01842-0389, Mailing Address: P.O. Box 189, Zip 01842-0389; tel. 978/683-4000; Joseph S. McManus, President and Chief Executive Officer **A**1 2 3 9 10 **F**7 8 9 11 12 17 18 19 22 24 25 27 29 32 33 34 35 38 39 41 43 44 45 48 49 51 65 66 68 70 76 77 78 79 **P**4 5 7
Web address: www.lawrencegeneral.org | 23 | 10 | 189 | 8492 | 118 | 168479 | 1400 | 84560 | 40971 | 948 |

LEEDS—Hampshire County

| ★ VETERANS AFFAIRS MEDICAL CENTER, 421 North Main Street, Zip 01053-9764; tel. 413/584-4040; Bruce A. Gordon, Director (Total facility includes 55 beds in nursing home–type unit) **A**1 **F**1 3 16 18 19 22 23 25 26 28 29 30 31 32 33 34 35 36 37 38 43 45 48 49 50 51 54 56 57 59 61 63 69 64 69 70 72 76 78 79 **S** Department of Veterans Affairs, Washington, DC
Web address: www.va.gov/stations97/guide/home.asp?DIVISION=ALL | 45 | 22 | 197 | 1570 | 176 | 140687 | 0 | 55446 | 27093 | 625 |

LEOMINSTER—Worcester County

| ★ HEALTH ALLIANCE HOSPITALS, (Includes Health Alliance–Burbank Hospital, 275 Nichols Road, Fitchburg, Zip 01420-8209; tel. 978/343-5000), 60 Hospital Road, Zip 01453-8004; tel. 978/466-2000; Jonathan H. Robbins, M.D., President and Chief Executive Officer **A**1 3 5 9 10 **F**1 3 8 9 11 13 19 21 22 24 25 30 32 34 35 36 37 38 40 41 43 44 45 46 48 51 53 54 57 58 59 60 61 62 63 64 66 69 70 72 73 75 76 77 78 **P**5
Web address: www.healthalliance.com | 23 | 10 | 173 | 7385 | 97 | 194520 | 1426 | 72590 | 35283 | 959 |

Hospitals, U.S. / MASSACHUSETTS

Hospital, Address, Telephone, Administrator, Approval, Facility, and Physician Codes, Health Care System, Network	Classification Codes		Utilization Data					Expense (thousands) of dollars		
	Control	Service	Staffed Beds	Admissions	Census	Outpatient Visits	Births	Total	Payroll	Personnel

★ American Hospital Association (AHA) membership
☐ Joint Commission on Accreditation of Healthcare Organizations (JCAHO) accreditation
+ American Osteopathic Healthcare Association (AOHA) membership
○ American Osteopathic Association (AOA) accreditation
△ Commission on Accreditation of Rehabilitation Facilities (CARF) accreditation
Control codes 61, 63, 64, 71, 72 and 73 indicate hospitals listed by AOHA, but not registered by AHA. For definition of numerical codes, see page A4

Hospital	Control	Service	Staffed Beds	Admissions	Census	Outpatient Visits	Births	Total	Payroll	Personnel
LOWELL—Middlesex County										
★ LOWELL GENERAL HOSPITAL, 295 Varnum Avenue, Zip 01854-2195; tel. 978/937-6000; Robert A. Donovan, President and Chief Executive Officer (Total facility includes 21 beds in nursing home-type unit) **A**1 2 9 10 **F**1 3 7 8 9 11 13 16 17 18 19 20 22 24 25 26 30 33 34 35 36 37 38 41 43 44 45 46 48 49 50 51 54 57 59 60 61 62 63 64 65 69 70 71 72 75 76 78 79 **P**8 Web address: www.lowellgeneral.org	23	10	231	9586	127	180832	2071	83821	41646	1101
★ SAINTS MEMORIAL MEDICAL CENTER, One Hospital Drive, Zip 01852-1389; tel. 978/458-1411; Thomas Clark, President and Chief Executive Officer **A**1 2 9 10 **F**7 8 9 11 13 17 18 19 22 24 25 26 27 32 33 34 35 37 38 39 40 41 43 44 45 46 48 49 50 51 54 56 58 59 60 61 63 64 68 70 72 73 76 78 79 **P**5 Web address: www.saints-memorial.org	23	10	150	6822	89	250868	662	77104	35292	974
LUDLOW—Hampden County										
★ HEALTHSOUTH REHABILITATION HOSPITAL OF WESTERN MASSACHUSETTS, 14 Chestnut Place, Zip 01056-3460; tel. 413/589-7581; R. David Richer, Administrator (Nonreporting) **A**1 10 **S** HEALTHSOUTH Corporation, Birmingham, AL	33	46	40	—	—	—	—	—	—	—
LYNN—Essex County										
★ THE UNION HOSPITAL, (Formerly Atlanticare Medical Center), 500 Lynnfield Street, Zip 01904-1487; tel. 781/581-9200; Judith Ritchie, President and Chief Executive Officer (Total facility includes 24 beds in nursing home-type unit) (Nonreporting) **A**1 2 9 10 **S** Partners HealthCare System, Inc., Boston, MA	23	10	189	—	—	—	—	—	—	—
MALDEN—Middlesex County										
★ HALLMARK HEALTH SYSTEM, (Includes Lawrence Memorial Hospital of Medford, 170 Governors Avenue, Medford, Zip 02155-1643; tel. 781/306-6000; Malden Medical Center, 100 Hospital Road, tel. 781/338-7100; Melrose-Wakefield Hospital, 585 Lebanon Street, Melrose, Zip 02176; Whidden Memorial Hospital, 103 Garland Street, Everett, Zip 02149-5095; tel. 617/389-6270), 100 Hospital Road, Zip 02148-3591; tel. 781/338-7100; Richard S. Quinlan, President and Chief Executive Officer (Total facility includes 73 beds in nursing home-type unit) **A**1 2 6 9 **F**1 3 7 8 9 11 13 14 16 17 18 19 20 21 22 24 25 27 29 30 32 33 34 35 36 37 38 39 41 43 44 45 46 48 49 50 54 56 57 59 60 62 63 64 65 68 69 70 71 72 73 76 77 78 79 **P**1 5 7 Web address: www.hallmarkhealth.org	23	10	460	24183	355	730648	2083	234898	105306	2797
MARLBOROUGH—Middlesex County										
★ UMASS MARLBOROUGH HOSPITAL, 57 Union Street, Zip 01752-1297; tel. 508/481-5000; Annette B. Leahy, President and Chief Executive Officer **A**1 5 9 10 **F**3 7 9 13 14 17 19 21 22 23 25 26 30 32 33 34 36 37 38 40 41 43 45 46 48 50 51 54 56 57 58 59 61 63 64 68 70 71 72 75 76 77 78 79 **P**5 8	23	10	66	3360	40	69967	0	29312	13978	339
MEDFIELD—Norfolk County										
☐ MEDFIELD STATE HOSPITAL, 45 Hospital Road, Zip 02052-1099; tel. 508/359-7312; Margaret E. LaMontagne, R.N., Chief Operating Officer **A**1 10 **F**4 5 7 9 11 12 16 21 22 23 24 25 28 31 32 33 34 35 39 41 43 45 46 47 48 50 51 55 57 65 68 69 70 72 76 78 79 **S** Massachusetts Department of Mental Health, Boston, MA	12	22	147	141	141	0	0	—	—	386
MEDFORD—Middlesex County										
LAWRENCE MEMORIAL HOSPITAL OF MEDFORD See Hallmark Health System, Malden										
MELROSE—Middlesex County										
MELROSE-WAKEFIELD HOSPITAL See Hallmark Health System, Malden										
METHUEN—Essex County										
★ HOLY FAMILY HOSPITAL AND MEDICAL CENTER, 70 East Street, Zip 01844-4597; tel. 978/687-0151; William L. Lane, President (Total facility includes 21 beds in nursing home-type unit) **A**1 2 9 10 **F**1 3 7 8 9 11 12 13 14 16 17 18 19 21 22 23 24 25 26 27 29 30 32 33 34 35 36 37 38 39 41 42 43 44 45 46 48 49 50 51 54 55 56 57 58 59 60 61 62 63 64 65 68 69 70 71 72 73 74 76 77 78 79 **P**5 7 **S** Caritas Christi Health Care, Boston, MA Web address: www.holyfamilyhosp.org	21	10	249	10015	163	81702	1360	78074	37371	1094
MILFORD—Worcester County										
★ MILFORD-WHITINSVILLE REGIONAL HOSPITAL, (Includes Whitinsville Medical Center, 18 Granite Street, Whitinsville, Zip 01588; tel. 508/234-6311), 14 Prospect Street, Zip 01757-3090; tel. 508/473-1190; Francis M. Saba, President and Chief Executive Officer **A**1 2 5 9 10 **F**7 8 9 13 16 17 18 19 22 24 25 32 33 34 36 38 39 41 43 44 45 46 48 49 50 51 54 63 68 70 72 76 77 78 79 **P**4 5 7 8 Web address: www.mwrh.com	23	10	108	5691	63	174668	580	62848	31898	817
MILTON—Norfolk County										
★ MILTON HOSPITAL, 92 Highland Street, Zip 02186-3807; tel. 617/696-4600; George A. Geary, President (Total facility includes 32 beds in nursing home-type unit) **A**1 9 10 **F**9 12 13 16 17 18 19 22 24 25 32 33 34 38 39 40 41 43 45 46 48 49 51 54 59 68 69 70 71 76 78 79 **P**6 Web address: www.miltonhospital.org	23	10	120	5334	85	78588	0	40232	19238	516
NANTUCKET—Nantucket County										
★ NANTUCKET COTTAGE HOSPITAL, 57 Prospect Street, Zip 02554-2799; tel. 508/228-1200; Lucille C. Giddings, R.N., CHE, President and Chief Executive Officer **A**1 9 10 **F**1 3 8 9 16 17 18 19 22 25 32 34 35 36 37 39 41 43 44 45 46 48 49 54 70 72 76 Web address: www.nantuckethospital.org	23	10	19	547	5	31101	87	11612	5851	115

Hospitals, U.S. / MASSACHUSETTS

Hospital, Address, Telephone, Administrator, Approval, Facility, and Physician Codes, Health Care System, Network	Classification Codes		Utilization Data					Expense (thousands) of dollars		
★ American Hospital Association (AHA) membership ☐ Joint Commission on Accreditation of Healthcare Organizations (JCAHO) accreditation + American Osteopathic Healthcare Association (AOHA) membership ○ American Osteopathic Association (AOA) accreditation △ Commission on Accreditation of Rehabilitation Facilities (CARF) accreditation Control codes 61, 63, 64, 71, 72 and 73 indicate hospitals listed by AOHA, but not registered by AHA. For definition of numerical codes, see page A4	Control	Service	Staffed Beds	Admissions	Census	Outpatient Visits	Births	Total	Payroll	Personnel

NATICK—Middlesex County
  LEONARD MORSE HOSPITAL See MetroWest Medical Center, Framingham
NEEDHAM—Norfolk County

| ★ DEACONESS–GLOVER HOSPITAL CORPORATION, 148 Chestnut Street, Zip 02192–2483; tel. 781/453–3000; John Dalton, President and Chief Executive Officer **A**1 2 9 10 **F**7 9 13 16 17 18 19 22 24 25 30 32 33 34 36 37 38 40 41 43 45 46 48 49 54 70 76 78 **P**7 8 **S** CareGroup, Boston, MA
Web address: www.glover.caregroup.org/ | 23 | 10 | 41 | 2014 | 25 | 75008 | 0 | 22020 | 9953 | 263 |

NEW BEDFORD—Bristol County
  ST. LUKE'S HOSPITAL OF NEW BEDFORD See Southcoast Hospitals Group, Fall River
NEWBURYPORT—Essex County

| ★ ANNA JAQUES HOSPITAL, 25 Highland Avenue, Zip 01950–3894; tel. 978/463–1000; Scott W. Goodspeed, FACHE, President and Chief Executive Officer (Total facility includes 20 beds in nursing home–type unit) **A**1 9 10 **F**7 8 9 11 13 14 17 18 19 21 22 24 25 27 32 33 34 35 36 37 38 39 40 41 43 44 45 46 48 49 50 51 54 57 58 59 60 61 63 64 68 70 71 72 76 78 79 **P**4 5 7
Web address: www.ajh.org | 23 | 10 | 156 | 6749 | 100 | 110085 | 985 | 58039 | 27563 | 709 |

NEWTON LOWER FALLS—Middlesex County

| ★ NEWTON–WELLESLEY HOSPITAL, 2014 Washington Street, Zip 02462–1699; tel. 617/243–6000; John P. Bihldorff, President and Chief Executive Officer **A**1 2 3 5 9 10 **F**4 5 8 9 13 14 16 17 18 19 21 22 24 25 27 29 30 31 32 33 34 35 36 38 39 41 42 43 44 45 46 48 49 50 51 54 56 57 58 59 60 61 62 63 64 66 70 71 72 73 75 76 77 78 79 **P**1 2 3 6 7 8 **S** Partners HealthCare System, Inc., Boston, MA
Web address: www.nwh.org | 23 | 10 | 228 | 12541 | 149 | 74078 | 3615 | 137139 | 69856 | 1459 |

NORTH ADAMS—Berkshire County

| ★ NORTH ADAMS REGIONAL HOSPITAL, 71 Hospital Avenue, Zip 01247–2584; tel. 413/663–3701; John C. J. Cronin, President and Chief Executive Officer (Total facility includes 20 beds in nursing home–type unit) **A**1 2 9 10 **F**2 9 12 13 17 18 19 22 25 26 30 32 33 34 35 36 37 38 40 43 44 45 46 48 50 53 54 57 58 59 61 62 63 64 65 67 69 70 72 76 78 **P**6 | 23 | 10 | 89 | 4035 | 59 | 78960 | 336 | 32044 | 16502 | 335 |

NORTHAMPTON—Hampshire County

| ★ COOLEY DICKINSON HOSPITAL, 30 Locust Street, Zip 01061–5001, Mailing Address: P.O. Box 5001, Zip 01061–5001; tel. 413/582–2000; Craig N. Melin, President and Chief Executive Officer **A**1 2 9 10 **F**3 7 8 9 13 16 17 18 19 20 21 22 23 24 25 26 29 30 32 33 34 35 36 37 38 39 41 43 44 45 46 48 49 50 51 54 57 59 60 61 62 63 64 65 68 70 71 72 73 75 76 78 **P**8
Web address: www.hitchcock.org/pages/tha/cdh.html | 23 | 10 | 125 | 7563 | 85 | 167624 | 919 | 61942 | 29932 | 636 |

  VETERANS AFFAIRS MEDICAL CENTER See Leeds
NORWOOD—Norfolk County

| ★ CARITAS NORWOOD HOSPITAL, 800 Washington Street, Zip 02062–3487; tel. 781/278–6001; Delia O'Connor, President (Total facility includes 40 beds in nursing home–type unit) **A**1 2 5 9 10 **F**2 3 4 7 8 9 11 12 13 16 17 18 19 22 24 25 27 31 39 43 44 46 48 49 54 57 62 63 64 65 68 69 70 72 76 77 78 **P**5 7 **S** Caritas Christi Health Care, Boston, MA | 21 | 10 | 329 | 10460 | 141 | — | 778 | — | — | — |

OAK BLUFFS—Dukes County

| ★ MARTHA'S VINEYARD HOSPITAL, One Hospital Road, Zip 02557, Mailing Address: P.O. Box 1477, Zip 02557–1477; tel. 508/693–0410; Kevin R. Burchill, Chief Executive Officer **A**1 9 10 **F**3 6 8 9 13 16 17 18 19 21 22 25 26 30 34 35 38 40 41 43 44 45 46 48 54 56 58 61 62 67 70 72 76 77 78 79 **P**5
Web address: www.vineyard.net | 23 | 10 | 21 | 1009 | 9 | — | 124 | 18647 | 9160 | 171 |

PALMER—Hampden County

| ★ WING MEMORIAL HOSPITAL AND MEDICAL CENTERS, 40 Wright Street, Zip 01069–1138; tel. 413/283–7651; Charles E. Cavagnaro, M.D., President and Chief Executive Officer (Nonreporting) **A**1 5 9 10
Web address: www.winghealth.org | 23 | 10 | 46 | — | — | — | — | — | — | — |

PEABODY—Essex County

| ☐ VENCOR HOSPITAL NORTH SHORE, 15 King Street, Zip 01960–4268; tel. 978/531–2900; Steven E. Levitsky, Administrator **A**1 10 **F**16 17 18 41 62 70 78 **S** Vencor, Incorporated, Louisville, KY
Web address: www.vencor.com | 33 | 10 | 50 | 377 | 45 | — | 0 | — | — | 163 |

PEMBROKE—Plymouth County

| PEMBROKE HOSPITAL, 199 Oak Street, Zip 02359–1953; tel. 781/826–8161; Kenneth A. Davis, Chief Executive Officer **A**9 **F**17 18 57 58 61 62 63 **P**6 **S** Magellan Health Services, Atlanta, GA | 33 | 22 | 80 | 2358 | 65 | 2761 | 0 | 10594 | 5960 | 183 |

PITTSFIELD—Berkshire County

| ★ △ BERKSHIRE MEDICAL CENTER, (Includes Hillcrest Hospital, 165 Tor Court, Zip 01201–3099, Mailing Address: Box 1155, Zip 01202–1155; tel. 413/443–4761; Eugene A. Dellea, President), 725 North Street, Zip 01201–4124; tel. 413/447–2000; Ruth P. Blodgett, Chief Operating Officer (Total facility includes 20 beds in nursing home–type unit) **A**1 2 3 5 7 8 9 10 12 13 **F**2 3 4 6 8 9 11 13 14 17 18 19 21 22 23 24 25 30 32 34 35 36 38 39 41 43 44 45 46 48 49 50 51 53 54 56 57 58 59 60 61 62 63 64 65 69 70 71 75 76 77 78 79 **S** Berkshire Health Systems, Inc., Pittsfield, MA
Web address: www.bhs1.org | 23 | 10 | 310 | 12425 | 221 | 75218 | 835 | 142833 | 69266 | 1647 |

© 2000 AHA Guide   *Many Facility Codes have changed. Please refer to the AHA Guide Code Chart.*   Hospitals **A207**

Hospitals, U.S. / MASSACHUSETTS

Hospital, Address, Telephone, Administrator, Approval, Facility, and Physician Codes, Health Care System, Network	Classification Codes		Utilization Data					Expense (thousands) of dollars		
	Control	Service	Staffed Beds	Admissions	Census	Outpatient Visits	Births	Total	Payroll	Personnel

★ American Hospital Association (AHA) membership
☐ Joint Commission on Accreditation of Healthcare Organizations (JCAHO) accreditation
+ American Osteopathic Healthcare Association (AOHA) membership
○ American Osteopathic Association (AOA) accreditation
△ Commission on Accreditation of Rehabilitation Facilities (CARF) accreditation
Control codes 61, 63, 64, 71, 72 and 73 indicate hospitals listed by AOHA, but not registered by AHA. For definition of numerical codes, see page A4

PLYMOUTH—Plymouth County

★ JORDAN HOSPITAL, 275 Sandwich Street, Zip 02360–2196; tel. 508/746–2001; Alan D. Knight, President and Chief Executive Officer (Total facility includes 25 beds in nursing home–type unit) **A**1 2 9 10 **F**1 2 3 4 8 9 12 13 16 17 18 19 20 22 24 25 27 28 31 32 33 34 35 36 37 39 41 43 44 45 46 47 48 49 50 51 54 57 59 61 65 70 71 72 73 76 78 79 **P**4 5 6 7 **Web address:** www.jordan.org	23	10	119	7799	110	232123	786	70641	33197	597

POCASSET—Barnstable County

BARNSTABLE COUNTY HOSPITAL, 870 County Road, Zip 02559–2199; tel. 508/563–5941; Edward B. Leary, President (Nonreporting) **A**10	13	46	39	—	—	—	—	—	—	—

QUINCY—Norfolk County

★ QUINCY MEDICAL CENTER, (Formerly Quincy Hospital), 114 Whitwell Street, Zip 02169–1899; tel. 617/773–6100; Christine C. Schuster, Chief Executive Officer (Total facility includes 38 beds in nursing home–type unit) **A**1 9 10 **F**7 9 11 13 17 18 19 22 24 25 30 31 32 34 36 37 38 39 40 41 43 45 46 48 49 50 51 54 57 59 60 61 62 63 64 65 66 69 70 72 76 77 78 79 **Web address:** www.quincyhospital.com/	14	10	172	6935	125	120750	33	77070	35836	707

SALEM—Essex County

★ SALEM HOSPITAL, (Includes North Shore Children's Hospital, tel. 978/745–2100), 81 Highland Avenue, Zip 01970–2768; tel. 978/741–1200; Judith Ritchie, President and Chief Executive Officer (Nonreporting) **A**1 2 3 5 9 10 **S** Partners HealthCare System, Inc., Boston, MA **Web address:** www.nsmc.partners.org	23	10	291	—	—	—	—	—	—	—
★ △ SHAUGHNESSY-KAPLAN REHABILITATION HOSPITAL, Dove Avenue, Zip 01970–2999; tel. 978/745–9000; Anthony Sciola, President and Chief Executive Officer (Total facility includes 40 beds in nursing home–type unit) **A**1 7 10 **F**2 3 8 9 11 12 13 16 18 19 20 21 22 24 25 26 28 31 32 33 34 35 36 37 38 41 42 43 44 45 46 48 49 50 51 53 54 56 57 58 59 60 61 62 63 64 65 66 68 70 71 72 73 76 77 78 79 **P**6 **S** Partners HealthCare System, Inc., Boston, MA **Web address:** www.nsmc.partners.org	23	46	160	2208	118	38744	0	24657	12564	329

SOMERVILLE—Middlesex County

SOMERVILLE HOSPITAL See Cambridge Health Alliance, Cambridge

SOUTH WEYMOUTH—Norfolk County

★ SOUTH SHORE HOSPITAL, 55 Fogg Road, Zip 02190–2455; tel. 781/340–8000; David T. Hannan, President and Chief Executive Officer (Total facility includes 25 beds in nursing home–type unit) **A**1 2 9 10 **F**7 8 9 11 12 13 16 17 18 19 22 24 25 27 31 32 34 36 37 38 39 41 43 44 45 46 48 49 51 54 65 66 69 70 71 72 76 77 78 79 **P**8 **Web address:** www.sshosp.org	23	10	298	15318	156	228679	3872	169120	87864	2200

SOUTHBRIDGE—Worcester County

★ HARRINGTON MEMORIAL HOSPITAL, 100 South Street, Zip 01550–4045; tel. 508/765–9771; Richard M. Mangion, President and Chief Executive Officer **A**1 5 9 10 **F**3 7 8 9 12 16 17 19 21 22 25 30 32 33 34 36 37 38 39 41 43 44 45 46 48 49 50 51 54 56 57 58 59 60 61 62 63 64 65 66 70 72 76 78 **P**1 **Web address:** www.harringtonhospital.org/	23	10	113	3068	44	171806	431	38734	22874	491

SPRINGFIELD—Hampden County

★ BAYSTATE MEDICAL CENTER, 759 Chestnut Street, Zip 01199–0001; tel. 413/794–0000; Mark R. Tolosky, Chief Executive Officer **A**1 2 3 5 6 8 9 10 **F**2 3 4 8 9 11 12 13 14 16 17 18 19 20 21 22 24 25 26 27 28 29 30 31 32 33 34 35 36 37 39 41 42 43 44 45 46 47 48 49 50 51 52 54 56 57 58 59 61 62 63 64 65 66 68 69 70 72 74 75 76 77 78 79 **P**1 5 **S** Baystate Health System, Inc., Springfield, MA **Web address:** www.baystatehealth.com	23	10	564	28345	400	369937	5295	408049	160208	3853
★ △ MERCY HOSPITAL, 271 Carew Street, Zip 01104–2398, Mailing Address: P.O. Box 9012, Zip 01102–9012; tel. 413/748–9000; Vincent J. McCorkle, President **A**1 2 7 9 10 **F**1 2 3 7 8 9 11 12 13 16 17 18 19 21 22 24 25 26 27 30 31 32 34 35 36 39 41 44 45 46 48 49 50 51 53 54 55 57 58 59 60 61 62 64 65 68 69 70 72 73 76 78 79 **P**6 7 **S** Catholic Health East, Newtown Square, PA	21	10	311	13063	242	342648	803	122609	51347	1308
☐ OLYMPUS SPECIALTY HOSPITAL–SPRINGFIELD, 1400 State Street, Zip 01109–2589; tel. 413/787–6700; Linda K. Rahm, Chief Executive Officer (Total facility includes 220 beds in nursing home–type unit) (Nonreporting) **A**1 5 10	14	49	394	—	—	—	—	—	—	—
☐ SHRINERS HOSPITALS FOR CHILDREN, SPRINGFIELD, 516 Carew Street, Zip 01104–2396; tel. 413/787–2000; Mark L. Niederpruem, Administrator (Nonreporting) **A**1 3 5 **S** Shriners Hospitals for Children, Tampa, FL **Web address:** www.shrinerspfld.org	23	57	40	—	—	—	—	—	—	—

STOCKBRIDGE—Berkshire County

★ AUSTEN RIGGS CENTER, 25 Main Street, Zip 01262–0962, Mailing Address: P.O. Box 962, Zip 01262–0962; tel. 413/298–5511; Edward R. Shapiro, M.D., Medical Director and Chief Executive Officer **A**1 3 **F**17 19 57 64 **P**7 **Web address:** www.austenriggs.org	23	22	47	70	6	0	0	7530	4327	95

STOUGHTON—Plymouth County

GOOD SAMARITAN MEDICAL CENTER See Caritas Good Samaritan Medical Center, Brockton

Hospitals, U.S. / MASSACHUSETTS

Hospital, Address, Telephone, Administrator, Approval, Facility, and Physician Codes, Health Care System, Network	Classification Codes		Utilization Data					Expense (thousands) of dollars		
★ American Hospital Association (AHA) membership ☐ Joint Commission on Accreditation of Healthcare Organizations (JCAHO) accreditation + American Osteopathic Healthcare Association (AOHA) membership ○ American Osteopathic Association (AOA) accreditation △ Commission on Accreditation of Rehabilitation Facilities (CARF) accreditation Control codes 61, 63, 64, 71, 72 and 73 indicate hospitals listed by AOHA, but not registered by AHA. For definition of numerical codes, see page A4	Control	Service	Staffed Beds	Admissions	Census	Outpatient Visits	Births	Total	Payroll	Personnel
★ △ NEW ENGLAND SINAI HOSPITAL AND REHABILITATION CENTER, (REHABILITATION/LONG TERM CARE), 150 York Street, Zip 02072–1881; tel. 617/364–4850; Donald H. Goldberg, President (Total facility includes 21 beds in nursing home–type unit) **A**1 3 7 10 **F**1 5 7 13 17 18 19 22 23 30 32 37 38 39 43 46 53 54 59 65 69 70 71 72 76 78 **Web address:** www.newenglandsinai.org	23	49	212	2098	174	—	0	48365	26235	581
TAUNTON—Bristol County										
★ MORTON HOSPITAL AND MEDICAL CENTER, 88 Washington Street, Zip 02780–2499; tel. 508/828–7000; Thomas C. Porter, President (Total facility includes 21 beds in nursing home–type unit) **A**1 2 9 10 **F**3 7 8 9 11 13 16 17 18 19 22 24 25 28 29 30 32 33 34 36 38 39 41 43 44 45 46 48 49 51 54 56 57 58 59 61 62 66 69 70 71 72 76 77 78 **P**4 5 7	23	10	152	6580	101	69669	635	78420	36521	836
☐ TAUNTON STATE HOSPITAL, 60 Hodges Avenue Extension, Zip 02780–3034, Mailing Address: P.O. Box 4007, Zip 02780–4007; tel. 508/977–3000; Katherine Chmiel, R.N., MS, Administrator and Chief Operating Officer **A**1 10 **F**1 13 17 18 19 21 23 43 57 58 61 62 63 64 70 78 **P**1 **S** Massachusetts Department of Mental Health, Boston, MA	12	22	185	310	172	0	0	31121	14275	—
TEWKSBURY—Middlesex County										
★ TEWKSBURY HOSPITAL, 365 East Street, Zip 01876–1998; tel. 978/851–7321; Raymond D. Sanzone, Executive Director **A**1 6 10 **F**1 2 3 17 18 22 23 26 27 30 31 32 34 35 37 38 39 45 46 51 54 57 58 59 60 61 62 64 65 70 72 78 **P**6 **Web address:** www.state.ma.us/dph/hosp/th.htm	12	48	720	1990	596	0	0	40643	27332	735
WALTHAM—Middlesex County										
★ DEACONESS WALTHAM HOSPITAL, Hope Avenue, Zip 02453; tel. 781/647–6000; Dana W. Ramish, FACHE, President and Chief Executive Officer **A**1 2 5 9 10 **F**1 2 3 4 5 8 9 11 13 14 16 17 18 19 21 22 23 24 25 27 28 29 30 31 32 33 34 35 37 38 39 40 41 43 44 45 46 47 48 50 51 54 56 57 58 59 60 61 62 63 65 66 68 69 70 71 72 73 74 75 76 77 78 79 **P**5 6 8 **S** CareGroup, Boston, MA	23	10	199	6955	106	87722	395	63565	32637	806
☐ OLYMPUS SPECIALTY HOSPITAL, 775 Trapelo Road, Zip 02254, Mailing Address: P.O. Box 9151, Zip 02254–9151; tel. 781/895–7000; William J. DiFederico, Chief Executive Officer **A**1 10 **F**13 16 18 26 37 45 53 57 59 70	33	48	60	540	55	0	0	12758	6225	67
WARE—Hampshire County										
★ MARY LANE HOSPITAL, 85 South Street, Zip 01082–1697; tel. 413/967–6211; Christine Shirtcliff, Executive Vice President **A**1 9 10 **F**1 3 8 9 13 17 18 19 22 24 25 31 32 33 34 36 37 38 41 43 44 45 46 48 49 50 51 54 59 63 66 70 72 73 76 77 78 79 **P**1 5 8 **S** Baystate Health System, Inc., Springfield, MA **Web address:** www.baystatehealth.com	23	10	31	1326	13	77794	237	16488	8603	212
WAREHAM—Plymouth County										
TOBEY HOSPITAL See Southcoast Hospitals Group, Fall River										
WEBSTER—Worcester County										
★ HUBBARD REGIONAL HOSPITAL, 340 Thompson Road, Zip 01570–0608; tel. 508/943–2600; Gerald J. Barbini, Administrator and Chief Executive Officer (Total facility includes 21 beds in nursing home–type unit) **A**1 9 10 **F**9 17 18 22 24 25 31 34 38 41 43 45 46 48 50 51 54 62 63 69 70 76 77 78 79 **P**3 7 **S** Quorum Health Group, Brentwood, TN **Web address:** www.hubbard–hospital.org	23	10	47	1760	27	55169	0	17334	8012	238
WELLESLEY—Norfolk County										
☐ CHARLES RIVER HOSPITAL, 203 Grove Street, Zip 02482–7413; tel. 781/416–5300; Frederick J. Thacher, President and Chief Executive Officer (Nonreporting) **A**1 9 10	33	22	62	—	—	—	—	—	—	—
SIMPSON INFIRMARY, WELLESLEY COLLEGE, 106 Central Street, Zip 02481–8203; tel. 781/283–2810; Charlotte K. Sanner, M.D., Director Health Service **F**16 17 18 32 33 43 50 56 66 79	23	11	11	55	0	7691	0	—	—	15
WESTBOROUGH—Worcester County										
☐ WESTBOROUGH STATE HOSPITAL, Lyman Street, Zip 01581–0288, Mailing Address: P.O. Box 288, Zip 01581–0288; tel. 508/366–4401; Theodore E. Kirousis, Area Director (Nonreporting) **A**1 10 **S** Massachusetts Department of Mental Health, Boston, MA	12	22	220							
WESTFIELD—Hampden County										
★ NOBLE HOSPITAL, 115 West Silver Street, Zip 01086–1634; tel. 413/568–2811; George J. Koller, President and Chief Executive Officer **A**1 2 5 9 10 **F**3 6 7 9 13 16 17 18 19 21 22 25 26 29 31 32 33 34 36 37 38 39 41 43 45 46 48 49 50 51 53 54 56 57 58 59 60 62 63 64 67 70 71 72 76 77 78 79 **P**5 6 7 8 **Web address:** www.noblehealth.org	23	10	97	3251	60	88607	0	31188	16089	387
WESTWOOD—Norfolk County										
WESTWOOD LODGE HOSPITAL, 45 Clapboardtree Street, Zip 02090–2930; tel. 781/762–7764; Kenneth A. Davis, Chief Executive Officer **A**10 **F**17 18 57 58 61 63 64 **P**6	33	22	80	2398	86	4261	0	13998	7920	236
WHITINSVILLE—Worcester County										
WHITINSVILLE MEDICAL CENTER See Milford–Whitinsville Regional Hospital, Milford										
WINCHESTER—Middlesex County										
★ WINCHESTER HOSPITAL, 41 Highland Avenue, Zip 01890–9920; tel. 781/729–9000; Dale M. Lodge, President and Chief Executive Officer (Total facility includes 21 beds in nursing home–type unit) **A**1 2 5 9 10 **F**8 9 13 16 17 18 22 23 24 25 29 30 31 32 33 34 36 37 38 39 40 41 43 44 45 46 48 49 50 51 54 56 66 69 70 72 73 76 77 78 79 **P**3 5 7 **Web address:** www.winchesterhospital.org	23	10	182	9857	117	398100	2326	106419	49634	1160

© 2000 AHA Guide   *Many Facility Codes have changed. Please refer to the AHA Guide Code Chart.*

Hospitals, U.S. / MASSACHUSETTS

★ American Hospital Association (AHA) membership
☐ Joint Commission on Accreditation of Healthcare Organizations (JCAHO) accreditation
+ American Osteopathic Healthcare Association (AOHA) membership
○ American Osteopathic Association (AOA) accreditation
△ Commission on Accreditation of Rehabilitation Facilities (CARF) accreditation
Control codes 61, 63, 64, 71, 72 and 73 indicate hospitals listed by AOHA, but not registered by AHA. For definition of numerical codes, see page A4

Hospital, Address, Telephone, Administrator, Approval, Facility, and Physician Codes, Health Care System, Network	Classification Codes		Utilization Data					Expense (thousands) of dollars		
	Control	Service	Staffed Beds	Admissions	Census	Outpatient Visits	Births	Total	Payroll	Personnel
WOBURN—Middlesex County										
☐ △ HEALTHSOUTH NEW ENGLAND REHABILITATION HOSPITAL, Two Rehabilitation Way, Zip 01801–6098; tel. 781/935–5050; Mary Moscato, Chief Executive Officer (Total facility includes 75 beds in nursing home–type unit) **A**1 7 10 **F**13 16 18 19 20 38 53 54 59 69 70 71 72 78 **S** HEALTHSOUTH Corporation, Birmingham, AL	33	46	273	2709	168	126051	0	37344	22295	786
WORCESTER—Worcester County										
ADCARE HOSPITAL OF WORCESTER, 107 Lincoln Street, Zip 01605–2499; tel. 508/799–9000; David W. Hillis, President and Chief Executive Officer **A**9 10 **F**2 3 13 **P**8 **Web address:** www.adcare.com	33	82	114	4219	66	0	0	—	—	146
☐ △ FAIRLAWN REHABILITATION HOSPITAL, 189 May Street, Zip 01602–4399; tel. 508/791–6351; Peter M. Mantegazza, President and Chief Executive Officer (Nonreporting) **A**1 5 7 9 10 **S** HEALTHSOUTH Corporation, Birmingham, AL	33	46	110	—	—	—	—	—	—	—
★ SAINT VINCENT HOSPITAL, 25 Winthrop Street, Zip 01604–4593; tel. 508/798–1234; Robert E. Maher, Jr, President and Chief Executive Officer (Nonreporting) **A**1 2 3 5 8 9 10 12 **S** TENET Healthcare Corporation, Santa Barbara, CA **Web address:** www.svh–worc.com	33	10	369	—	—	—	—	—	—	—
★ UMASS MEMORIAL HEALTH CARE, (Includes Hahnemann Campus, 281 Lincoln Street, Zip 01605; tel. 508/334–1000; Memorial Campus, 119 Belmont Street, Zip 01605; tel. 508/334–1000; University Campus, 55 Lake Avenue North, Zip 01655–0002; tel. 508/334–1000), 119 Belmont Street, Zip 01605–2982; tel. 508/334–1000; Peter H. Levine, M.D., President and Chief Executive Officer **A**1 2 3 5 8 9 10 12 **F**3 4 8 9 10 11 12 13 14 16 17 18 19 20 21 22 23 24 25 26 28 29 30 31 32 33 34 35 36 37 38 39 40 41 42 43 44 45 46 47 48 50 51 52 54 55 56 57 58 59 60 61 62 63 64 65 66 68 70 71 72 73 74 75 76 77 78 79 **P**1 6 **Web address:** www.umassmemorial.org	23	10	634	36159	510	788866	3940	580791	212873	5050
☐ WORCESTER STATE HOSPITAL, 305 Belmont Street, Zip 01604–1695; tel. 508/368–3300; Raymond Robinson, Chief Operating Officer (Nonreporting) **A**1 5 10 **S** Massachusetts Department of Mental Health, Boston, MA	12	22	176	—	—	—	—	—	—	—

Hospitals, U.S. / MICHIGAN

MICHIGAN

Resident Population 9,817 (in thousands)
Resident population in metro areas 82.4%
Birth rate per 1,000 population 13.7
65 years and over 12.5%
Percent of persons without health insurance 11.6%

★ American Hospital Association (AHA) membership
□ Joint Commission on Accreditation of Healthcare Organizations (JCAHO) accreditation
+ American Osteopathic Healthcare Association (AOHA) membership
○ American Osteopathic Association (AOA) accreditation
△ Commission on Accreditation of Rehabilitation Facilities (CARF) accreditation
Control codes 61, 63, 64, 71, 72 and 73 indicate hospitals listed by AOHA, but not registered by AHA. For definition of numerical codes, see page A4

Hospital, Address, Telephone, Administrator, Approval, Facility, and Physician Codes, Health Care System, Network	Classification Codes		Utilization Data					Expense (thousands) of dollars		
	Control	Service	Staffed Beds	Admissions	Census	Outpatient Visits	Births	Total	Payroll	Personnel
ADDISON—Lenawee County										
□ ADDISON COMMUNITY HOSPITAL, 421 North Steer Street, Zip 49220-9409; tel. 517/547-6151; Robert A. Brown, Senior Vice President and Chief Operating Officer (Nonreporting) **A**1 9 10	16	10	24	—	—	—	—	—	—	—
ADRIAN—Lenawee County										
★ BIXBY MEDICAL CENTER, LENAWEE HEALTH ALLIANCE, 818 Riverside Avenue, Zip 49221-1496; tel. 517/265-0900; John R. Robertstad, President and Chief Executive Officer **A**1 2 9 10 **F**3 6 7 8 9 12 13 16 17 19 22 24 25 28 29 30 34 36 37 38 39 41 43 44 45 46 48 49 50 51 54 57 59 60 61 62 63 64 65 66 67 69 70 71 72 73 75 76 77 78 79 **P**1 7 8 **S** ProMedica Health System, Toledo, OH **Web address:** www.lhanet.org	23	10	77	3792	37	143030	766	48774	19733	781
ALBION—Calhoun County										
□ TRILLIUM HOSPITAL, 809 West Erie Street, Zip 49224-1556; tel. 517/629-2191; Michael G. Boff, President **A**1 9 10 **F**9 13 16 17 18 19 22 23 24 25 30 31 32 33 34 36 39 41 43 45 48 53 54 56 70 76 77 78 **Web address:** www.trillum.org	23	10	56	1311	15	23186	0	16053	6978	175
ALLEGAN—Allegan County										
★ ALLEGAN GENERAL HOSPITAL, 555 Linn Street, Zip 49010-1594; tel. 616/673-8424; James A. Klun, President **A**1 9 10 **F**7 8 9 12 13 16 17 18 19 21 22 24 25 31 32 34 36 38 39 41 43 44 45 46 48 50 51 54 56 57 59 60 61 63 70 71 72 76 77 78 **S** Quorum Health Group, Brentwood, TN **Web address:** www.aghosp.org	23	10	63	1804	18	77176	216	20229	8279	250
ALMA—Gratiot County										
★ △ GRATIOT COMMUNITY HOSPITAL, 300 East Warwick Drive, Zip 48801-1096; tel. 517/463-1101; Bob M. Baker, President and Chief Executive Officer (Nonreporting) **A**1 7 9 10	23	10	127	—	—	—	—	—	—	—
ALPENA—Alpena County										
★ ALPENA GENERAL HOSPITAL, 1501 West Chisholm Street, Zip 49707-1498; tel. 517/356-7390; John A. McVeety, Chief Executive Officer **A**1 2 9 10 **F**2 3 4 7 8 9 11 13 17 18 19 22 24 25 31 32 33 34 35 36 37 38 39 40 41 44 45 46 48 49 50 51 54 57 58 59 60 61 62 63 68 70 71 72 75 76 78 79 **Web address:** www.agh.org	13	10	121	6053	72	67427	520	59292	28679	782
ANN ARBOR—Washtenaw County										
★ △ SAINT JOSEPH MERCY HEALTH SYSTEM, (Includes St. Joseph Mercy Hospital), 5301 East Huron River Drive, Zip 48106, Mailing Address: P.O. Box 995, Zip 48106-0995; tel. 734/712-3456; Garry C. Faja, President and Chief Executive Officer **A**1 2 3 5 7 8 9 10 **F**1 3 4 5 7 8 9 11 12 13 14 16 17 18 19 20 21 22 23 24 25 26 29 30 31 32 33 34 35 36 37 38 39 41 43 44 45 46 47 48 49 50 51 53 54 56 57 58 59 60 61 62 68 70 71 72 73 75 76 77 78 79 **P**1 5 **S** Trinity Health, Novi, MI **Web address:** www.sjmh.com	21	10	467	26865	362	646926	3850	367768	149104	3533
□ UNIVERSITY OF MICHIGAN HOSPITALS AND HEALTH CENTERS, 300 North Ingalls, Zip 48109-0477, Mailing Address: 300 North Ingalls, N14A04, Zip 48109-0477; tel. 734/764-1505; Larry Warren, Executive Director **A**1 2 3 5 8 9 10 **F**2 3 4 5 8 9 10 11 12 13 14 16 17 18 19 21 22 23 24 25 27 28 29 30 32 33 34 35 36 38 39 40 41 42 44 45 46 47 48 49 50 51 52 53 54 55 56 57 58 59 60 61 62 63 64 65 66 68 70 71 72 73 74 75 76 77 78 79 **Web address:** www.med.umich.edu	23	10	726	36971	580	1231216	2522	728256	263069	8179
★ VETERANS AFFAIRS MEDICAL CENTER, 2215 Fuller Road, Zip 48105-2399; tel. 734/769-7100; James W. Roseborough, CHE, Director (Total facility includes 36 beds in nursing home–type unit) **A**1 2 3 5 8 9 **F**3 4 9 10 11 12 13 16 18 22 23 24 25 26 27 29 30 31 32 34 35 36 37 38 39 41 43 44 45 46 47 48 49 50 51 54 55 56 57 59 60 61 62 63 64 65 68 69 70 72 74 76 77 78 79 **S** Department of Veterans Affairs, Washington, DC **Web address:** www.va.gov/stations97/guide/home.asp?DIVISION=ALL	45	10	162	4235	89	201821	0	110424	64079	1417
AUBURN HILLS—Oakland County										
□ HAVENWYCK HOSPITAL, 1525 University Drive, Zip 48326-2675; tel. 248/373-9200; Robert A. Kercorian, Chief Executive Officer **A**1 9 10 **F**13 18 21 34 43 51 57 58 59 60 61 62 63 64 70 72 **S** Ramsay Youth Services, Coral Gables, FL	33	22	150	2857	116	4011	0	11670	8260	232
BAD AXE—Huron County										
★ HURON MEMORIAL HOSPITAL, 1100 South Van Dyke Road, Zip 48413-9799; tel. 517/269-8933; Larry R. Davis, President and Chief Executive Officer **A**1 9 10 **F**7 8 9 17 22 24 25 31 32 34 36 37 38 39 41 43 44 45 46 48 54 68 70 72 76 **P**6	23	10	64	1967	20	51008	358	20471	9253	242

Hospitals, U.S. / MICHIGAN

Hospital, Address, Telephone, Administrator, Approval, Facility, and Physician Codes, Health Care System, Network	Classification Codes		Utilization Data					Expense (thousands) of dollars		
	Control	Service	Staffed Beds	Admissions	Census	Outpatient Visits	Births	Total	Payroll	Personnel

★ American Hospital Association (AHA) membership
☐ Joint Commission on Accreditation of Healthcare Organizations (JCAHO) accreditation
+ American Osteopathic Healthcare Association (AOHA) membership
○ American Osteopathic Association (AOA) accreditation
△ Commission on Accreditation of Rehabilitation Facilities (CARF) accreditation
Control codes 61, 63, 64, 71, 72 and 73 indicate hospitals listed by AOHA, but not registered by AHA. For definition of numerical codes, see page A4

BATTLE CREEK—Calhoun County

★ BATTLE CREEK HEALTH SYSTEM, (Includes Community Hospital, 183 West Street, Zip 49016; Fieldstone Center, 165 North Washington Avenue, Zip 49016; tel. 616/964-7121; Leila Hospital, 300 North Avenue, Zip 49016), 300 North Avenue, Zip 49016-3396; tel. 616/966-8000; Patrick R. Garrett, Chief Executive Officer (Total facility includes 122 beds in nursing home-type unit) **A**1 2 9 10 **F**3 6 7 8 9 11 13 16 17 18 19 22 24 25 29 32 33 36 37 39 41 44 48 49 51 54 55 56 57 58 62 63 64 65 69 70 72 76 78 79 **P**1 **S** Trinity Health, Novi, MI Web address: www.bchealth.com	21	10	378	11431	248	136041	1255	126597	48765	1442
★ △ SOUTHWEST REHABILITATION HOSPITAL, 183 West Street, Zip 49017-3424; tel. 616/965-3206; Diane D. Giannunzio, President **A**1 7 9 10 **F**13 17 18 19 30 34 38 53 54 70	23	46	30	533	15	37814	0	6197	2063	84
★ VETERANS AFFAIRS MEDICAL CENTER, 5500 Armstrong Road, Zip 49016; tel. 616/966-5600; Michael K. Wheeler, Director (Total facility includes 124 beds in nursing home-type unit) **A**1 5 9 **F**2 3 6 9 13 17 18 19 22 29 31 32 34 35 36 37 38 45 51 54 57 59 60 69 70 72 76 78 79 **S** Department of Veterans Affairs, Washington, DC Web address: www.va.gov/stations97/guide/home.asp?DIVISION=ALL	45	22	376	3531	343	—	0	95826	49705	1144

BAY CITY—Bay County

★ △ BAY MEDICAL CENTER, (Includes Bay Medical Center–West Campus, 3250 East Midland Road, Zip 48706; tel. 517/667-6750; Samaritan Health Center, 713 Ninth Street, Zip 48708; tel. 517/894-3799), 1900 Columbus Avenue, Zip 48708-6880; tel. 517/894-3000; Robert N. Wright, President and Chief Operating Officer **A**1 2 7 9 10 12 13 **F**2 3 4 7 8 9 11 12 13 15 16 17 18 19 22 25 27 30 31 32 33 34 36 37 38 39 40 41 42 44 45 46 47 48 49 51 53 54 56 57 59 60 61 62 63 64 65 66 68 70 71 72 73 76 77 78 79 **P**8	23	10	332	14269	188	241563	1008	128767	56261	1448
BAY SPECIAL CARE, 3250 East Midland Road, Zip 48706-2835, Mailing Address: 3250 East Midland Road, Suite 1, Zip 48706-2835; tel. 517/667-6802; Cheryl A. Burzynski, President **A**10 **F**2 3 4 7 8 9 11 12 13 14 16 17 19 22 24 25 30 31 32 33 34 36 37 39 40 41 43 44 45 46 47 48 49 51 53 54 56 57 58 59 61 62 63 64 65 68 70 71 72 76 77 78 79 **P**8	23	49	21	261	19	0	0	4611	2304	94

BERRIEN CENTER—Berrien County

LAKELAND MEDICAL CENTER, BERRIEN CENTER See Lakeland Medical Center–St. Joseph, Saint Joseph

BIG RAPIDS—Mecosta County

★ △ MECOSTA COUNTY GENERAL HOSPITAL, 405 Winter Avenue, Zip 49307-2099; tel. 231/796-8691; Thomas E. Daugherty, Administrator **A**1 7 9 10 **F**7 8 9 11 17 18 22 35 36 37 38 40 44 45 48 49 50 53 54 68 70 76 77 **P**7 8 **S** Quorum Health Group, Brentwood, TN Web address: www.mecoscountygeneral.com	13	10	50	2464	26	86280	683	21756	9188	262

BRIGHTON—Livingston County

★ BRIGHTON HOSPITAL, 12851 East Grand River Avenue, Zip 48116-8596; tel. 810/227-1211; Frank P. Iacobell, Interim President **A**10 **F**2 3 16 17 18 43 Web address: www.brightonhospital.org	23	82	83	1612	39	11222	0	8357	4223	132

CADILLAC—Wexford County

★ MERCY HOSPITAL, (Formerly Mercy Health Services–North), 400 Hobart Street, Zip 49601-9596; tel. 231/876-7131; John L. MacLeod, Chief Executive Officer **A**1 9 10 **F**7 9 11 13 16 22 24 25 34 36 37 39 41 43 44 48 54 56 57 68 70 76 78 **P**5 8 **S** Trinity Health, Novi, MI Web address: www.mercyhealth.com	21	10	89	5513	45	76654	545	40317	14876	508

CARO—Tuscola County

☐ CARO CENTER, 2000 Chambers Road, Zip 48723-9240; tel. 517/673-3191; Rose Laskowski, R.N., Hospital Director **A**1 10 **F**3 4 5 8 9 10 11 12 13 16 17 18 21 22 23 24 25 27 30 34 35 37 39 41 43 44 46 47 48 50 51 54 57 58 59 60 61 62 63 64 65 66 70 72 74 75 76 79	12	22	214	277	196	0	0	28438	—	538
★ CARO COMMUNITY HOSPITAL, 401 North Hooper Street, Zip 48723-1476, Mailing Address: P.O. Box 71, Zip 48723-0071; tel. 517/673-3141; William P. Miller, President and Chief Executive Officer **A**9 10 **F**7 9 17 18 22 24 25 32 36 37 39 43 46 48 51 54 70 76 **P**6	23	10	18	713	6	51610	0	7305	3442	128

CARSON CITY—Montcalm County

+ ○ CARSON CITY HOSPITAL, 406 East Elm Street, Zip 48811-0879, Mailing Address: P.O. Box 879, Zip 48811-0879; tel. 517/584-0053; Bruce L. Traverse, President **A**9 10 11 12 13 **F**7 8 16 17 18 19 22 23 25 32 34 36 37 38 39 41 44 45 46 48 49 51 63 70 72 76 78 79 **P**6 Web address: www.carsoncityhospital.com	23	10	63	2247	25	50277	355	21696	10594	393

CASS CITY—Tuscola County

★ HILLS AND DALES GENERAL HOSPITAL, 4675 Hill Street, Zip 48726-1099; tel. 517/872-2121; Dee McKrow, Chief Executive Officer **A**1 9 10 **F**9 13 16 17 18 19 21 22 24 25 28 32 33 34 35 36 37 38 39 43 45 46 48 49 50 51 54 56 59 63 66 68 70 71 72 76 77 78 79 **P**5	23	10	47	897	10	37393	0	11103	5634	185

CHARLEVOIX—Charlevoix County

★ CHARLEVOIX AREA HOSPITAL, 14700 Lake Shore Drive, Zip 49720-1931; tel. 231/547-4024; William Jackson, President **A**1 9 10 **F**7 8 9 16 17 18 22 23 25 32 34 41 44 45 48 70 71 76 78 Web address: www.cah.org	23	10	33	1527	15	25054	243	14766	7048	212

CHARLOTTE—Eaton County

★ HAYES–GREEN–BEACH MEMORIAL HOSPITAL, 321 East Harris Street, Zip 48813-1697; tel. 517/543-1050; Matthew Rush, President **A**1 9 10 **F**8 9 14 16 17 18 22 24 25 28 29 30 32 34 36 38 39 43 44 45 46 48 51 54 56 69 70 71 72 76 77 78 79 **P**6 **S** Quorum Health Group, Brentwood, TN Web address: www.hgbadmin@voyager.net	23	10	35	1500	13	26193	221	17489	9857	331

Hospitals, U.S. / MICHIGAN

Hospital, Address, Telephone, Administrator, Approval, Facility, and Physician Codes, Health Care System, Network	Classification Codes		Utilization Data					Expense (thousands) of dollars		Personnel
★ American Hospital Association (AHA) membership ☐ Joint Commission on Accreditation of Healthcare Organizations (JCAHO) accreditation + American Osteopathic Healthcare Association (AOHA) membership ○ American Osteopathic Association (AOA) accreditation △ Commission on Accreditation of Rehabilitation Facilities (CARF) accreditation Control codes 61, 63, 64, 71, 72 and 73 indicate hospitals listed by AOHA, but not registered by AHA. For definition of numerical codes, see page A4	Control	Service	Staffed Beds	Admissions	Census	Outpatient Visits	Births	Total	Payroll	
CHEBOYGAN—Cheboygan County ★ COMMUNITY MEMORIAL HOSPITAL, 748 South Main Street, Zip 49721-2299, Mailing Address: P.O. Box 419, Zip 49721-0419; tel. 231/627-5601; Howard J. Purcell, Jr, President (Total facility includes 50 beds in nursing home–type unit) **A**1 9 10 **F**7 9 12 16 17 18 22 23 24 25 26 28 29 36 37 41 43 44 46 48 54 68 69 72 76 78 **P**8	23	10	92	2264	71	98967	226	23860	12366	356
CHELSEA—Washtenaw County ☐ △ CHELSEA COMMUNITY HOSPITAL, 775 South Main Street, Zip 48118-1399; tel. 734/475-1311; Kathleen S. Griffiths, President and Chief Executive Officer **A**1 3 5 7 9 10 **F**3 7 9 16 17 18 19 20 22 24 25 26 28 29 30 32 33 34 36 38 41 43 45 46 48 49 50 51 53 54 57 58 59 60 62 63 64 66 70 72 76 78 79 **Web address:** www.cch.org	23	10	97	3061	59	140279	0	43800	20980	608
CLARE—Clare County ★ ○ MIDMICHIGAN MEDICAL CENTER–CLARE, 104 West Sixth Street, Zip 48617-1409; tel. 517/386-9951; Lawrence F. Barco, President **A**1 9 10 11 **F**8 9 17 19 22 24 25 32 34 36 37 38 39 44 45 46 48 49 54 68 72 76 77 78 79 **P**8 **S** MidMichigan Health, Midland, MI	23	10	64	2566	26	59370	270	18287	7762	275
CLINTON TOWNSHIP—Macomb County ST. JOSEPH'S MERCY HOSPITAL–WEST See St. Joseph's Mercy Hospitals and Health Services ★ ST. JOSEPH'S MERCY HOSPITALS AND HEALTH SERVICES, (Includes St. Joseph's Mercy Hospital–East, 215 North Avenue, Mount Clemens, Zip 48043; tel. 810/466-9300; St. Joseph's Mercy Hospital–West, 15855 19 Mile Road, Zip 48038; tel. 810/263-2300; St. Joseph's Mercy–North, 80650 North Van Dyke, Romeo, Zip 48065; tel. 810/798-3551), Jack Weiner, President and Chief Executive Officer **A**1 9 10 **F**2 3 6 8 9 11 13 17 18 19 20 21 22 24 25 26 29 30 31 32 33 34 35 36 37 38 39 40 41 42 43 44 45 46 48 50 51 54 57 58 59 60 61 62 63 64 65 67 68 69 70 72 73 76 77 78 79 **P**6 8 **S** Trinity Health, Novi, MI **Web address:** www.stjoe-macomb.com	23	10	462	16203	258	101315	1651	—	—	1495
COLDWATER—Branch County ★ + ○ COMMUNITY HEALTH CENTER OF BRANCH COUNTY, 274 East Chicago Street, Zip 49036-2088; tel. 517/279-5400; Randy DeGroot, Chief Executive Officer **A**1 9 10 11 12 13 **F**3 7 8 9 11 16 18 22 24 25 32 33 34 35 36 37 39 41 44 45 46 48 49 54 56 57 59 60 61 62 63 64 68 70 72 75 76 77 78 **P**6 8 **S** Quorum Health Group, Brentwood, TN **Web address:** www.chcbc.com	13	10	88	3668	38	99644	393	34645	16382	469
COMMERCE TOWNSHIP—Oakland County ★ HURON VALLEY–SINAI HOSPITAL, 1 William Carls Drive, Zip 48382-2201; tel. 248/937-3300; Robert J. Yellan, President **A**1 5 9 10 **F**7 8 9 11 16 17 22 24 25 31 32 34 35 37 41 43 44 45 46 48 49 50 51 54 59 65 66 70 72 76 78 **P**4 6 **S** Detroit Medical Center, Detroit, MI	23	10	136	8797	98	74046	2108	89896	29136	940
DEARBORN—Wayne County ★ OAKWOOD HOSPITAL AND MEDICAL CENTER–DEARBORN, 18101 Oakwood Boulevard, Zip 48124-4093, Mailing Address: P.O. Box 2500, Zip 48123-2500; tel. 313/593-7000; Joseph Tasse, Administrator **A**1 2 3 5 8 9 10 **F**1 3 4 6 7 8 9 11 12 13 14 16 17 19 20 21 22 23 24 25 26 27 29 30 31 32 34 35 36 37 38 39 42 43 44 45 46 47 48 49 51 54 56 57 58 59 60 61 62 63 64 65 66 67 68 70 71 72 73 74 76 77 78 79 **P**5 **S** Oakwood Healthcare, Inc., Dearborn, MI **Web address:** www.oakwood.org	23	10	585	29318	441	518309	5327	276782	130056	2984
DECKERVILLE—Sanilac County ★ DECKERVILLE COMMUNITY HOSPITAL, 3559 Pine Street, Zip 48427-0126, Mailing Address: P.O. Box 126, Zip 48427-0126; tel. 810/376-2835; Edward L. Gamache, Administrator **A**1 9 10 **F**7 9 16 17 18 22 25 32 33 34 38 43 46 48 50 51 72 76 **S** Trinity Health, Novi, MI	23	10	17	251	2	14842	0	4163	4266	70
DETROIT—Wayne County ★ △ CHILDREN'S HOSPITAL OF MICHIGAN, 3901 Beaubien Street, Zip 48201-9985; tel. 313/745-0073; Larry Fleischmann, M.D., President **A**1 3 5 7 8 9 10 **F**10 11 13 14 17 19 21 22 24 25 26 29 31 32 33 34 35 36 37 38 39 41 42 43 46 47 48 50 52 53 54 55 56 58 59 61 63 65 70 72 73 74 75 76 77 78 79 **S** Detroit Medical Center, Detroit, MI **Web address:** www.dmc.org/chm	23	50	218	12895	151	180138	0	168565	59855	1530
★ DETROIT RECEIVING HOSPITAL AND UNIVERSITY HEALTH CENTER, 4201 St. Antoine Boulevard, Zip 48201-2194; tel. 313/745-3603; Leslie C. Bowman, Senior Vice President Operations **A**1 3 5 8 9 10 **F**1 2 3 4 8 9 10 11 12 13 14 16 17 18 19 21 22 23 24 25 26 27 28 29 30 31 32 33 34 35 36 37 38 39 41 42 43 44 45 46 47 48 49 50 51 52 53 54 55 56 57 59 61 62 63 65 66 70 72 74 76 77 78 **S** Detroit Medical Center, Detroit, MI **Web address:** www.dmc.org	23	10	258	12694	216	127955	0	172926	56395	1214
★ HARPER HOSPITAL, 3990 John R, Zip 48201-9027; tel. 313/745-8040; Jeff Dankins, Vice President Operations **A**1 2 3 5 8 9 10 **F**3 4 7 8 9 11 12 13 17 18 19 22 23 24 25 26 27 30 31 32 33 34 37 38 39 40 41 42 43 44 45 46 47 48 49 50 51 54 57 61 62 64 65 66 70 74 76 77 78 79 **S** Detroit Medical Center, Detroit, MI	23	10	542	28001	447	298399	5300	466801	148469	—
★ HENRY FORD HOSPITAL, 2799 West Grand Boulevard, Zip 48202-2689; tel. 313/916-2600; Stephen H. Velick, Chief Executive Officer **A**1 2 3 5 8 9 10 **F**1 2 3 4 5 6 7 8 9 11 12 13 14 15 16 17 18 19 20 21 22 23 24 25 26 27 28 29 30 31 32 33 34 35 36 37 38 39 40 41 42 43 44 45 46 47 48 49 50 51 52 53 54 55 56 57 58 59 60 61 62 63 65 66 69 70 71 72 73 74 75 76 77 78 79 **P**1 5 6 **S** Henry Ford Health System, Detroit, MI **Web address:** www.henryfordhealth.org	23	10	668	37421	545	—	2392	386210	178557	6632

© 2000 AHA Guide *Many Facility Codes have changed. Please refer to the AHA Guide Code Chart.*

Hospitals, U.S. / MICHIGAN

Hospital, Address, Telephone, Administrator, Approval, Facility, and Physician Codes, Health Care System, Network	Classification Codes		Utilization Data					Expense (thousands) of dollars		
★ American Hospital Association (AHA) membership ☐ Joint Commission on Accreditation of Healthcare Organizations (JCAHO) accreditation + American Osteopathic Healthcare Association (AOHA) membership ○ American Osteopathic Association (AOA) accreditation △ Commission on Accreditation of Rehabilitation Facilities (CARF) accreditation Control codes 61, 63, 64, 71, 72 and 73 indicate hospitals listed by AOHA, but not registered by AHA. For definition of numerical codes, see page A4	Control	Service	Staffed Beds	Admissions	Census	Outpatient Visits	Births	Total	Payroll	Personnel
★ HUTZEL HOSPITAL, 4707 St. Antoine Boulevard, Zip 48201–0154; tel. 313/745–7555; Mark McNash, Vice President Operations (Nonreporting) **A**1 3 5 8 9 **S** Detroit Medical Center, Detroit, MI **(Data included with Harper Hospital)**										
★ JOHN D. DINGELL VETERANS AFFAIRS MEDICAL CENTER, 4646 John R Street, Zip 48201–1932; tel. 313/576–1000; Carlos B. Lott, Jr, Director (Total facility includes 84 beds in nursing home–type unit) **A**1 2 5 8 9 **F**2 3 4 5 6 7 9 11 12 13 16 17 18 19 21 22 23 24 25 26 27 30 31 32 33 34 35 36 37 38 39 41 43 45 46 47 48 49 50 51 54 55 56 57 59 60 61 63 64 65 66 68 69 70 72 74 75 76 77 78 79 **P**6 **S** Department of Veterans Affairs, Washington, DC Web address: www.va.gov/stations97/guide/home.asp?DIVISION=ALL	45	10	218	4904	196	265427	—	132289	70046	1445
★ △ REHABILITATION INSTITUTE OF MICHIGAN, 261 Mack Boulevard, Zip 48201–2495; tel. 313/745–1203; Paul Thompson, Jr, Interim Senior Vice President **A**1 3 5 7 9 10 **F**3 4 5 7 8 9 10 11 12 13 16 17 18 19 22 23 24 25 26 27 28 29 30 31 32 33 34 35 36 37 38 39 41 42 43 44 46 47 48 49 50 51 52 54 55 56 57 58 59 60 61 62 63 64 65 66 68 69 70 71 72 74 75 76 77 78 79 **P**4 5 6 7 8 **S** Detroit Medical Center, Detroit, MI Web address: www.mdc.org	23	46	94	1630	68	95830	—	42416	23349	527
★ ○ △ SINAI/GRACE HOSPITAL, (Formerly Grace Hospital), 6071 West Outer Drive, Zip 48235–2679; tel. 313/966–3300; Anne M. Regling, Senior Vice President (Nonreporting) **A**1 3 5 7 8 9 10 11 **S** Detroit Medical Center, Detroit, MI Web address: www.dmc.org	23	10	821	—	—	—	—	—	—	—
★ ○ ST. JOHN DETROIT RIVERVIEW HOSPITAL, 7733 East Jefferson Avenue, Zip 48214–2598; tel. 313/499–4000; Richard T. Young, President (Nonreporting) **A**1 9 10 11 12 13 **S** Ascension Health, Saint Louis, MO	23	10	230	—	—	—	—	—	—	—
★ ST. JOHN HOSPITAL AND MEDICAL CENTER, (Includes St. John Hospital–Macomb Center, 26755 Ballard Road, Harrison Township, Zip 48045–2458; tel. 810/465–5501; David Sessions, President), 22101 Moross Road, Zip 48236–2172; tel. 313/343–4000; Timothy J. Grajewski, President and Chief Executive Officer **A**1 2 3 5 8 9 10 **F**1 2 3 4 5 6 7 8 9 11 12 13 14 15 17 18 19 20 21 22 23 24 25 26 27 28 29 30 31 32 33 34 35 36 37 38 39 40 41 42 43 44 45 46 47 48 49 50 51 52 53 54 55 56 57 58 59 60 61 62 63 64 65 66 67 68 69 70 71 72 73 74 75 76 77 78 79 **P**3 5 6 8 **S** Ascension Health, Saint Louis, MO	21	10	656	30073	432	—	3496	368099	184547	4203
★ ST. JOHN NORTHEAST COMMUNITY HOSPITAL, (Formerly Holy Cross Saratoga Hospital), 4777 East Outer Drive, Zip 48234–0401; tel. 313/369–9100; Michael F. Breen, President **A**1 9 10 **F**1 3 9 11 13 16 17 19 21 22 24 25 30 31 32 33 34 37 41 43 45 48 49 50 51 53 54 56 57 59 60 62 63 64 68 70 72 75 76 78 **P**8 **S** Ascension Health, Saint Louis, MO Web address: www.stjohn.org	23	10	222	7449	168	66915	0	68952	34858	932
☐ VENCOR HOSPITAL–METRO DETROIT, 2700 Martin Luther King Boulevard, Zip 48208; tel. 313/361–8000; Daniel A. Eppley, FACHE, Executive Director (Nonreporting) **A**1 9 10 **S** Vencor, Incorporated, Louisville, KY Web address: www.vencor.com	33	10	112	—	—	—	—	—	—	—
DOWAGIAC—Cass County										
★ LEE MEMORIAL HOSPITAL, 420 West High Street, Zip 49047–1907; tel. 616/782–8681; Fritz Fahrenbacher, President and Chief Executive Officer **A**1 9 10 **F**3 7 9 12 16 17 18 19 22 24 25 29 32 33 34 37 39 40 43 45 46 48 49 50 51 54 58 59 60 61 62 63 64 70 71 72 73 76 77 78 79 **P**6 8 **S** Ascension Health, Saint Louis, MO	21	10	40	1953	22	38959	0	16044	6844	230
EAST CHINA—St. Clair County										
★ ST. JOHN RIVER DISTRICT HOSPITAL, 4100 River Road, Zip 48054; tel. 810/329–7111; Frank W. Poma, President **A**1 9 10 **F**3 7 8 9 13 17 18 19 22 25 30 32 34 41 44 45 46 48 49 50 51 54 56 58 59 61 63 70 72 76 78 79 **P**6 8 **S** Ascension Health, Saint Louis, MO	21	10	68	2809	27	115488	608	26023	13523	347
EATON RAPIDS—Eaton County										
☐ EATON RAPIDS MEDICAL CENTER, (Formerly Eaton Rapids Community Hospital), 1500 South Main Street, Zip 48827–0130; Mailing Address: P.O. Box 130, Zip 48827–0130; tel. 517/663–2671; Jack L. Denton, President **A**1 9 10 **F**7 9 13 16 22 25 32 34 38 39 40 43 45 46 48 49 51 54 61 70 72 76 77 78	23	10	21	584	6	29391	0	7495	3385	137
ESCANABA—Delta County										
★ ST. FRANCIS HOSPITAL, 3401 Ludington Street, Zip 49829–1377; tel. 906/786–3311; Roger M. Burgess, Administrator **A**1 9 10 **F**7 8 9 16 17 18 19 22 25 28 30 32 34 36 37 39 41 43 44 45 46 48 50 54 56 70 71 72 73 76 77 79 **S** OSF Healthcare System, Peoria, IL Web address: www.osfhealthcare.com	21	10	66	3511	36	71733	452	31229	13906	370
FARMINGTON HILLS—Oakland County										
★ + ○ △ BOTSFORD GENERAL HOSPITAL, 28050 Grand River Avenue, Zip 48336–5933; tel. 248/471–8000; Gerson I. Cooper, President **A**7 9 10 11 12 13 **F**1 3 6 8 9 11 12 13 14 16 17 18 19 20 22 24 25 28 30 31 32 33 34 35 37 38 39 41 44 45 46 48 49 50 51 53 54 56 57 59 62 64 67 69 70 71 72 76 77 78 **P**5 6 7 Web address: www.botsfordsystem.org	23	10	325	12893	217	403121	964	180518	85986	2242
FERNDALE—Oakland County										
★ HENRY FORD KINGSWOOD HOSPITAL, (Formerly Kingswood Hospital), 10300 West Eight Mile Road, Zip 48220–2198; tel. 248/398–3200; Glenn Black, Associate Vice President and Chief Operating Officer **A**3 9 10 **F**18 30 31 57 58 59 60 62 63 64 70 72 **S** Henry Ford Health System, Detroit, MI	23	22	64	1796	56	—	0	9976	5746	164

Many Facility Codes have changed. Please refer to the AHA Guide Code Chart.   © 2000 AHA Guide

Hospitals, U.S. / MICHIGAN

Hospital, Address, Telephone, Administrator, Approval, Facility, and Physician Codes, Health Care System, Network	Classification Codes		Utilization Data					Expense (thousands) of dollars		
★ American Hospital Association (AHA) membership □ Joint Commission on Accreditation of Healthcare Organizations (JCAHO) accreditation + American Osteopathic Healthcare Association (AOHA) membership ○ American Osteopathic Association (AOA) accreditation △ Commission on Accreditation of Rehabilitation Facilities (CARF) accreditation Control codes 61, 63, 64, 71, 72 and 73 indicate hospitals listed by AOHA, but not registered by AHA. For definition of numerical codes, see page A4	Control	Service	Staffed Beds	Admissions	Census	Outpatient Visits	Births	Total	Payroll	Personnel
FLINT—Genesee County										
★ △ HURLEY MEDICAL CENTER, One Hurley Plaza, Zip 48503–5993; tel. 810/257–9000; Glenn A. Fosdick, President and Chief Executive Officer **A**1 2 3 5 7 8 9 10 **F**7 8 9 10 11 12 13 14 16 17 18 19 21 22 23 24 25 28 29 30 31 32 33 34 35 36 37 38 41 42 43 44 45 46 47 48 49 50 51 52 53 54 56 57 58 59 60 61 62 63 65 66 68 69 70 71 72 74 75 76 77 78 79 **P**8 Web address: www.hurleymc.com	14	10	463	19810	311	472727	3046	246735	111400	2596
★ △ MCLAREN REGIONAL MEDICAL CENTER, 401 South Ballenger Highway, Zip 48532–3685; tel. 810/342–2000; Gregory L. Beckman, President and Chief Executive Officer (Total facility includes 23 beds in nursing home–type unit) **A**1 2 3 5 7 8 9 10 **F**2 3 4 7 8 9 11 12 13 14 16 17 18 19 20 21 22 23 24 25 26 28 29 30 31 32 33 34 35 36 37 38 39 41 42 43 44 45 46 47 48 49 50 51 52 53 54 56 57 58 59 60 61 62 63 64 65 66 68 69 70 71 72 74 75 76 77 78 79 **P**6 7 Web address: www.mclaren.org	23	10	459	17265	247	363768	939	189949	84094	1881
FRANKFORT—Benzie County										
★ PAUL OLIVER MEMORIAL HOSPITAL, 224 Park Avenue, Zip 49635; tel. 231/352–9621; James D. Austin, CHE, Administrator (Total facility includes 40 beds in nursing home–type unit) **A**9 10 18 **F**1 3 7 9 16 17 18 19 21 22 23 24 25 26 28 30 31 33 34 35 36 37 38 40 43 46 48 49 50 54 56 58 59 60 61 62 63 64 66 67 69 70 71 76 78 79 **P**1 3 5 7 **S** Munson Healthcare, Traverse City, MI Web address: www.benzie.com	23	10	48	299	40	26981	0	6663	2503	58
FREMONT—Newaygo County										
★ GERBER MEMORIAL HEALTH SERVICES, (Formerly Gerber Memorial Hospital), 212 South Sullivan Street, Zip 49412–1596; tel. 231/924–3300; Ned B. Hughes, Jr, President **A**1 9 10 **F**8 9 16 17 18 19 21 22 24 25 30 34 36 38 39 41 43 44 45 46 48 49 50 51 54 55 56 63 65 70 71 72 76 78 79 **P**6 Web address: www.gmhs.org	23	10	73	2487	30	73645	376	27146	12854	382
GARDEN CITY—Wayne County										
+ ○ △ GARDEN CITY HOSPITAL, 6245 North Inkster Road, Zip 48135–4001; tel. 734/421–3300; Gary R. Ley, President and Chief Executive Officer **A**7 9 10 11 12 13 **F**2 3 7 8 9 11 12 13 16 17 18 19 20 22 25 31 32 33 35 36 37 38 39 41 43 44 45 46 48 51 53 54 56 63 65 70 71 72 75 76 77 78 **P**5 6 8 Web address: www.gchosp.org	23	10	270	10237	171	96388	704	101318	48512	1154
GAYLORD—Otsego County										
★ OTSEGO MEMORIAL HOSPITAL, (Includes McReynolds Hall), 825 North Center Street, Zip 49735–1560; tel. 517/731–2100; Thomas R. Lemon, Chief Executive Officer (Total facility includes 34 beds in nursing home–type unit) **A**1 9 10 **F**3 7 8 9 11 13 14 16 17 18 21 22 23 25 28 29 31 32 33 34 36 37 38 39 40 41 43 44 45 46 48 49 50 51 53 54 56 58 59 60 61 62 63 64 65 67 68 69 70 71 72 73 74 75 76 77 78 79 **P**6 8 Web address: www.gaylordhospital.org	23	10	87	1752	46	—	250	23010	10701	346
GLADWIN—Gladwin County										
★ MIDMICHIGAN MEDICAL CENTER–GLADWIN, 515 South Quarter Street, Zip 48624–1918; tel. 517/426–9286; Mark E. Bush, Executive Vice President **A**1 9 10 **F**7 9 14 17 18 19 22 25 32 34 36 37 43 45 48 50 54 56 59 63 69 72 73 76 77 **S** MidMichigan Health, Midland, MI	23	10	42	1457	16	41776	—	10617	4200	176
GRAND BLANC—Genesee County										
★ + ○ △ GENESYS REGIONAL MEDICAL CENTER, One Genesys Parkway, Zip 48439–8066; tel. 810/606–5000; Elliot T. Joseph, President and Chief Executive Officer **A**1 2 3 5 7 9 10 11 12 13 **F**1 3 4 7 8 9 11 12 13 16 17 18 19 20 21 22 24 25 26 27 29 30 31 32 34 35 36 37 38 39 41 43 44 45 46 47 48 49 50 51 53 54 56 58 59 61 62 63 65 68 69 70 72 73 75 76 77 78 79 **P**1 2 5 6 **S** Ascension Health, Saint Louis, MO Web address: www.genesys.org	21	10	379	24058	296	319561	3034	237260	113216	2490
GRAND HAVEN—Ottawa County										
★ NORTH OTTAWA COMMUNITY HOSPITAL, 1309 Sheldon Road, Zip 49417–2488; tel. 616/842–3600; Michael J. Funk, Chief Executive Officer **A**1 9 10 **F**7 8 9 13 16 17 18 22 24 25 30 32 34 35 36 37 38 39 40 41 43 44 45 46 48 49 51 54 70 71 72 76 77 78 79	23	10	81	2493	24	145560	595	32168	12655	340
GRAND RAPIDS—Kent County										
□ FOREST VIEW HOSPITAL, 1055 Medical Park Drive S.E., Zip 49546–3671; tel. 616/942–9610; John F. Kuhn, Chief Executive Officer (Nonreporting) **A**1 9 10 **S** Universal Health Services, Inc., King of Prussia, PA Web address: www.forestview.com	33	22	62	—	—	—	—	—	—	—
★ △ MARY FREE BED HOSPITAL AND REHABILITATION CENTER, 235 Wealthy S.E., Zip 49503–5299; tel. 616/242–0300; William H. Blessing, President **A**1 7 9 10 **F**16 17 22 24 36 39 45 53 54 71 76 Web address: www.mfbrc.com	23	46	66	1091	50	27431	0	22276	13306	493
+ ○ △ METROPOLITAN HOSPITAL, 1919 Boston Street S.E., Zip 49506–4199, Mailing Address: P.O. Box 158, Zip 49501–0158; tel. 616/252–7200; Michael D. Faas, President and Chief Executive Officer **A**7 9 10 11 12 13 **F**4 8 9 11 13 16 17 19 22 24 30 34 35 36 38 39 41 43 44 45 48 49 50 51 53 54 56 58 59 60 61 62 63 66 68 70 71 72 75 76 78 79 **P**6 7 8 Web address: www.metrohealth.net	23	10	214	8294	116	204374	1394	96290	48726	1006

© 2000 AHA Guide   *Many Facility Codes have changed. Please refer to the AHA Guide Code Chart.*

Hospitals, U.S. / MICHIGAN

Hospital, Address, Telephone, Administrator, Approval, Facility, and Physician Codes, Health Care System, Network	Classification Codes		Utilization Data					Expense (thousands) of dollars		
★ American Hospital Association (AHA) membership □ Joint Commission on Accreditation of Healthcare Organizations (JCAHO) accreditation + American Osteopathic Healthcare Association (AOHA) membership ○ American Osteopathic Association (AOA) accreditation △ Commission on Accreditation of Rehabilitation Facilities (CARF) accreditation Control codes 61, 63, 64, 71, 72 and 73 indicate hospitals listed by AOHA, but not registered by AHA. For definition of numerical codes, see page A4	Control	Service	Staffed Beds	Admissions	Census	Outpatient Visits	Births	Total	Payroll	Personnel
★ PINE REST CHRISTIAN MENTAL HEALTH SERVICES, 300 68th Street S.E., Zip 49501-0165, Mailing Address: P.O. Box 165, Zip 49501-0165; tel. 616/455-5000; Daniel L. Holwerda, President and Chief Executive Officer (Nonreporting) A1 3 5 9 10 Web address: www.pinerest.org	23	22	106	—	—	—	—	—	—	—
★ SAINT MARY'S MERCY MEDICAL CENTER, (Formerly Saint Mary's Health Services), 200 Jefferson Avenue S.E., Zip 49503-4598; tel. 616/752-6090; Joyce A. Helms, Interim President and Chief Executive Officer (Nonreporting) A1 2 3 5 9 10 S Trinity Health, Novi, MI Web address: www.trinity-health.org/	21	10	287	—	—	—	—	—	—	—
★ SPECTRUM HEALTH, (Includes Ferguson Campus, 72 Sheldon Boulevard S.E., Zip 49503-4294; tel. 616/356-4000; Spectrum Health-Downtown Campus, 100 Michigan Street N.E., Zip 49503-2551; tel. 616/391-1774), 1840 Wealthy Street S.E., Zip 49506-2921; tel. 616/774-7444; Terrence M. O'Rourke, President A1 2 3 5 8 9 10 F4 5 8 9 10 11 12 13 14 16 17 18 19 22 24 25 27 29 30 33 34 36 37 38 39 41 42 43 44 45 46 47 48 49 50 51 52 54 56 65 66 68 70 71 72 74 75 76 77 78 79 P1 6 S Spectrum Health, Grand Rapids, MI Web address: www.spectrum-health.org	23	10	857	44766	580	—	8285	502785	246579	6471
□ SPECTRUM HEALTH-KENT COMMUNITY CAMPUS, (Formerly Kent Community Hospital), (CHEMICAL DEPENDENCY LONG TERM), 750 Fuller Avenue N.E., Zip 49503-1995; tel. 616/336-3300; Lori Portfleet, Chief Executive Officer (Total facility includes 314 beds in nursing home-type unit) A1 9 10 F2 3 4 5 8 9 10 11 12 13 14 16 17 18 19 22 23 24 25 27 29 30 33 34 36 37 38 39 41 42 43 44 45 46 47 48 49 50 51 52 54 55 65 66 68 69 70 71 72 73 74 75 76 77 78 79 S Spectrum Health, Grand Rapids, MI	23	49	356	578	250	0	0	5752	2582	309
GRAYLING—Crawford County ★ MERCY HEALTH SERVICES NORTH-GRAYLING, 1100 East Michigan Avenue, Zip 49738-1398; tel. 517/348-5461; Stephanie J. Riemer-Matuzak, Chief Executive Officer (Total facility includes 40 beds in nursing home-type unit) A1 9 10 F7 8 9 11 12 13 17 18 20 21 22 24 25 33 34 37 38 39 43 44 45 48 54 69 70 72 76 78 P6 8 S Trinity Health, Novi, MI Web address: www.mercyhealth.com/north	21	10	74	3217	66	31182	279	26571	10837	386
GREENVILLE—Montcalm County ★ UNITED MEMORIAL HEALTH CENTER, (Formerly United Memorial Hospital Association), (Includes Kelsey Memorial Hospital, 418 Washington Avenue, Lakeview, Zip 48850; tel. 517/352-7211; James Cliborne, Chief Operating Officer), 615 South Bower Street, Zip 48838-2628; tel. 616/754-4691; Lorne J. Archer, Chief Executive Officer (Total facility includes 82 beds in nursing home-type unit) A1 9 10 F7 8 9 14 17 18 19 22 25 28 29 31 32 34 36 37 38 39 41 43 44 45 49 51 53 54 56 69 70 72 73 76 77 78 79 P3 6 7 8	23	10	171	2744	99	154198	301	35827	14503	505
GROSSE POINTE—Wayne County ★ BON SECOURS COTTAGE HEALTH SERVICES-BON SECOURS HOSPITAL, (Formerly Bon Secours Hospital), 468 Cadieux Road, Zip 48230-1592; tel. 313/343-1000; Richard Van Lith, Chief Executive Officer A1 3 5 9 10 F3 8 9 11 17 18 19 21 22 24 25 28 29 30 31 32 33 34 35 36 37 40 41 43 44 46 48 50 51 54 56 68 70 72 76 78 79 P5 S Bon Secours Health System, Inc., Marriottsville, MD Web address: www.bonsecoursmi.com	21	10	237	12074	160	131204	1558	113187	58446	1429
GROSSE POINTE FARMS—Wayne County ★ BON SECOURS COTTAGE HEALTH SERVICES-COTTAGE HOSPITAL, (Formerly Cottage Hosptal), 159 Kercheval Avenue, Zip 48236-3692; tel. 313/640-1000; Richard Van Lith, Chief Executive Officer A1 3 9 10 F1 8 9 16 17 18 21 22 24 25 31 32 33 34 35 36 37 38 48 50 51 53 54 57 59 60 61 62 63 64 68 70 71 72 76 77 78 79 S Bon Secours Health System, Inc., Marriottsville, MD	21	10	65	2812	57	—	89	40052	22151	580
HANCOCK—Houghton County ★ PORTAGE HEALTH SYSTEM, 500 Campus Drive, Zip 49930-1569; tel. 906/483-1000; James Bogan, Chief Executive Officer (Total facility includes 30 beds in nursing home-type unit) A1 9 10 F1 7 8 9 13 14 15 16 17 18 19 22 23 25 28 30 33 34 36 37 38 39 40 41 43 44 45 48 49 50 54 56 61 66 68 69 70 71 72 76 77 78 79 P6 Web address: www.phsys.org	23	10	74	1752	49	67683	393	24429	13678	357
HARBOR BEACH—Huron County ★ HARBOR BEACH COMMUNITY HOSPITAL, 210 South First Street, Zip 48441-1236, Mailing Address: P.O. Box 40, Zip 48441-0040; tel. 517/479-3201; Pauline Siemen-Messing, R.N., President and Chief Executive Officer (Total facility includes 40 beds in nursing home-type unit) A9 10 F7 9 18 22 25 30 34 38 48 54 56 69 70 72 76 P6 Web address: www.hbch.com	23	10	61	442	41	16903	0	6659	3440	100
HARRISON TOWNSHIP—Macomb County ST. JOHN HOSPITAL-MACOMB CENTER See St. John Hospital and Medical Center, Detroit										
HASTINGS—Barry County □ PENNOCK HOSPITAL, 1009 West Green Street, Zip 49058-1790; tel. 616/945-3451; Daniel Hamilton, Chief Executive Officer A1 9 10 F7 8 9 12 13 16 17 18 22 25 28 29 33 34 36 37 38 39 43 44 46 48 49 50 51 54 56 61 67 68 70 71 72 76 77 78	23	10	88	2998	37	137686	393	29928	13345	411

Hospitals, U.S. / MICHIGAN

Hospital, Address, Telephone, Administrator, Approval, Facility, and Physician Codes, Health Care System, Network	Classification Codes		Utilization Data					Expense (thousands) of dollars		
★ American Hospital Association (AHA) membership □ Joint Commission on Accreditation of Healthcare Organizations (JCAHO) accreditation + American Osteopathic Healthcare Association (AOHA) membership ○ American Osteopathic Association (AOA) accreditation △ Commission on Accreditation of Rehabilitation Facilities (CARF) accreditation Control codes 61, 63, 64, 71, 72 and 73 indicate hospitals listed by AOHA, but not registered by AHA. For definition of numerical codes, see page A4	Control	Service	Staffed Beds	Admissions	Census	Outpatient Visits	Births	Total	Payroll	Personnel

HILLSDALE—Hillsdale County ★ HILLSDALE COMMUNITY HEALTH CENTER, 168 South Howell Street, Zip 49242-2081; tel. 517/437-4451; Charles A. Bianchi, President (Total facility includes 21 beds in nursing home–type unit) **A**1 9 10 **F**3 7 8 9 12 13 16 17 18 19 22 24 25 32 34 35 36 38 39 40 41 43 44 45 46 48 49 51 54 58 59 60 61 62 63 66 68 69 70 71 72 75 76 77 78 **P**8	23	10	73	2927	49	96661	369	23967	9599	296
HOLLAND—Ottawa County ★ △ HOLLAND COMMUNITY HOSPITAL, 602 Michigan Avenue, Zip 49423-4999; tel. 616/392-5141; Judeth Newham, R.N., President and Chief Executive Officer **A**1 7 9 10 **F**3 7 8 11 13 16 17 18 19 22 23 24 25 32 33 34 35 36 38 39 40 41 43 44 45 46 48 49 50 54 57 58 59 60 61 62 63 68 70 72 75 76 77 78 **P**8 Web address: www.hoho.org	23	10	155	7615	66	200255	1961	65948	30032	852
HOWELL—Livingston County ★ MCPHERSON HOSPITAL, 620 Byron Road, Zip 48843-1093; tel. 517/545-6000; Patricia Claffey, Executive Director **A**1 9 10 **F**1 2 3 4 5 7 8 9 11 12 13 14 16 17 18 19 20 21 22 23 24 25 26 29 30 31 32 33 34 35 36 37 38 39 41 43 44 45 46 47 48 49 50 51 53 54 56 57 58 59 60 61 62 63 64 65 70 71 72 73 75 76 77 78 79 **P**1 5 **S** Trinity Health, Novi, MI Web address: www.sjmh.com	21	10	45	3264	31	280813	769	43280	19626	502
IONIA—Ionia County ★ IONIA COUNTY MEMORIAL HOSPITAL, 479 Lafayette Street, Zip 48846-1834, Mailing Address: Box 1001, Zip 48846-1899; tel. 616/527-4200; Evonne G. Ulmer, JD, Chief Executive Officer **A**1 9 10 **F**7 8 9 14 16 17 18 22 25 26 30 32 33 34 36 37 38 39 41 43 44 45 46 48 49 51 54 56 70 71 72 76 77 78 79 **P**6 Web address: www.ioniahospital.org	23	10	51	1193	12	—	137	12941	5982	195
IRON MOUNTAIN—Dickinson County ★ DICKINSON COUNTY HEALTHCARE SYSTEM, 1721 South Stephenson Avenue, Zip 49801-3637; tel. 906/774-1313; John Schon, Administrator and Chief Executive Officer **A**1 9 10 **F**1 2 3 4 6 8 9 10 11 12 13 15 16 17 18 19 21 22 23 24 25 28 29 30 32 33 34 35 36 37 38 39 40 42 43 44 45 46 47 48 49 50 51 52 54 55 57 58 59 61 63 65 66 68 69 70 71 72 75 76 77 78 **P**6 Web address: www.dchs.org	13	10	96	4609	53	138961	558	42289	20311	521
★ VETERANS AFFAIRS MEDICAL CENTER, 325 East H Street, Zip 49801-4792; tel. 906/774-3300; Deborah A. Thompson, Director (Total facility includes 40 beds in nursing home–type unit) **A**1 5 9 **F**3 9 13 19 22 23 24 25 26 30 31 34 35 37 38 41 43 46 47 50 51 54 56 59 60 61 62 63 64 69 70 76 77 78 79 **P**6 **S** Department of Veterans Affairs, Washington, DC Web address: www.va.gov/stations97/guide/home.asp?DIVISION=ALL	45	10	74	1569	55	80423	0	—	—	369
IRON RIVER—Iron County ★ IRON COUNTY COMMUNITY HOSPITAL, 1400 West Ice Lake Road, Zip 49935-9594; tel. 906/265-6121; David L. Hoff, Chief Executive Officer (Total facility includes 54 beds in nursing home–type unit) **A**1 9 10 **F**8 9 12 13 14 16 17 18 19 22 24 25 28 30 32 34 36 38 41 43 44 45 46 48 49 50 51 54 56 66 69 70 71 72 76 78 79 Web address: www.icch.org	23	10	72	1516	72	38563	26	18270	8843	241
IRONWOOD—Gogebic County ★ GRAND VIEW HOSPITAL, N10561 Grand View Lane, Zip 49938-9359; tel. 906/932-2525; Frederick Geissler, Chief Executive Officer **A**1 9 10 **F**8 9 12 13 16 17 19 22 25 26 29 32 34 36 37 38 41 43 44 45 46 48 49 54 56 66 70 71 72 75 76 78 79 **P**6 Web address: www.gvhs.org	23	10	54	1824	19	48291	155	16690	7160	203
ISHPEMING—Marquette County □ BELL MEMORIAL HOSPITAL, 101 South Fourth Street, Zip 49849-2151; tel. 906/486-4431; Kevin P. Calhoun, President and Chief Executive Officer (Nonreporting) **A**1 9 10 Web address: www.bellmemorial.org	23	10	30	—	—	—	—	—	—	—
JACKSON—Jackson County ★ + ○ DOCTORS HOSPITAL OF JACKSON, 110 North Elm Avenue, Zip 49202-3595; tel. 517/787-1440; Michael J. Falatko, President and Chief Executive Officer **A**9 10 11 **F**9 13 17 18 19 22 24 25 26 27 34 38 39 45 46 48 51 54 68 70 71 76 77 78 **P**1 Web address: www.doctorshospital.org	21	10	65	1274	21	29271	0	14907	6071	255
□ DUANE L. WATERS HOSPITAL, 3857 Cooper Street, Zip 49201-7521; tel. 517/780-5600; Gerald De Voss, Acting Administrator (Nonreporting) **A**1	12	11	86	—	—	—	—	—	—	—
□ W. A. FOOTE MEMORIAL HOSPITAL, 205 North East Avenue, Zip 49201-1789; tel. 517/788-4800; Georgia R. Fojtasek, President and Chief Executive Officer **A**1 9 10 **F**2 3 7 8 9 11 12 13 16 17 18 19 20 21 22 24 25 28 29 30 31 32 33 34 36 37 38 39 40 41 43 44 45 46 48 49 50 51 54 56 57 58 59 60 61 62 63 64 65 68 70 71 72 76 77 78 79 **P**6 Web address: www.foote.com	23	10	422	15484	194	261563	1772	146709	69747	1931
KALAMAZOO—Kalamazoo County ★ △ BORGESS MEDICAL CENTER, (Includes Borgess–Pipp Health Center, Plainwell), 1521 Gull Road, Zip 49001-1640; tel. 616/226-4800; Randall Stasik, President and Chief Executive Officer **A**1 2 3 5 7 9 10 **F**3 4 5 7 8 9 11 13 16 17 18 19 21 22 23 24 25 26 27 28 29 30 32 33 34 35 36 37 38 39 43 45 46 47 48 49 50 51 54 55 56 58 59 60 61 62 63 65 68 70 71 72 74 75 76 77 78 79 **P**3 6 8 **S** Ascension Health, Saint Louis, MO Web address: www.borgess.com	21	10	383	17722	231	450358	1812	246322	97755	2050

Hospitals, U.S. / MICHIGAN

Hospital, Address, Telephone, Administrator, Approval, Facility, and Physician Codes, Health Care System, Network

★ American Hospital Association (AHA) membership
□ Joint Commission on Accreditation of Healthcare Organizations (JCAHO) accreditation
+ American Osteopathic Healthcare Association (AOHA) membership
○ American Osteopathic Association (AOA) accreditation
△ Commission on Accreditation of Rehabilitation Facilities (CARF) accreditation
Control codes 61, 63, 64, 71, 72 and 73 indicate hospitals listed by AOHA, but not registered by AHA. For definition of numerical codes, see page A4

Hospital	Control	Service	Staffed Beds	Admissions	Census	Outpatient Visits	Births	Total	Payroll	Personnel
★ △ BRONSON METHODIST HOSPITAL, 252 East Lovell Street, Zip 49007-5345; tel. 616/341-6000; Frank J. Sardone, President and Chief Executive Officer **A**1 2 3 5 7 9 10 **F**2 3 4 6 8 9 10 11 12 13 14 16 17 18 19 20 21 22 23 24 26 27 29 30 31 32 33 34 35 36 37 38 39 41 42 43 44 45 46 47 48 50 51 52 53 54 56 57 58 59 60 61 62 63 64 65 66 68 70 71 72 73 75 76 77 78 79 **P**5 6 7 **S** Bronson Healthcare Group, Inc., Kalamazoo, MI Web address: www.bronsonhealth.com	23	10	307	15083	206	321343	2915	190637	74314	1843
□ KALAMAZOO REGIONAL PSYCHIATRIC HOSPITAL, 1312 Oakland Drive, Zip 49008-1205; tel. 616/337-3000; James Coleman, Director **A**1 9 10 **F**4 5 9 11 16 18 20 22 23 24 25 26 28 31 33 34 35 37 46 47 48 49 50 51 56 58 59 60 61 62 65 68 70 75 76 77 78 79	12	22	163	263	122	0	0	32069	15922	370
KALKASKA—Kalkaska County										
★ KALKASKA MEMORIAL HEALTH CENTER, 419 South Coral Street, Zip 49646; tel. 231/258-7500; James D. Austin, CHE, Administrator (Total facility includes 68 beds in nursing home–type unit) **A**9 10 18 **F**16 17 18 22 25 32 38 54 69 70 72 76 77 78 79 **S** Munson Healthcare, Traverse City, MI	16	10	81	260	68	31747	0	8809	4448	100
L'ANSE—Baraga County										
□ BARAGA COUNTY MEMORIAL HOSPITAL, 770 North Main Street, Zip 49946-1195; tel. 906/524-3300; John P. Tembreull, Administrator (Total facility includes 28 beds in nursing home–type unit) **A**1 9 10 **F**9 17 18 22 24 25 34 36 37 48 54 68 69 70 72 76 Web address: www.bcmh.org	13	10	52	884	35	19475	0	10183	4892	145
LAKEVIEW—Montcalm County KELSEY MEMORIAL HOSPITAL See United Memorial Health Center, Greenville										
LANSING—Ingham County										
★ ○ △ INGHAM REGIONAL MEDICAL CENTER, (Includes Ingham Regional Medical Center, Greenlawn Campus, 401 West Greenlawn Avenue; Ingham Regional Medical Center, Pennsylvania Campus, 2727 South Pennsylvania Avenue, Zip 48910; tel. 517/372-8220), 401 West Greenlawn Avenue, Zip 48910-2819; tel. 517/334-2121; Dennis M. Litos, President and Chief Executive Officer (Total facility includes 50 beds in nursing home–type unit) **A**1 5 7 8 9 10 11 12 13 **F**4 7 8 9 11 12 13 14 16 17 18 19 22 24 25 26 29 30 32 33 34 35 36 38 39 41 43 44 45 46 47 48 49 51 53 54 56 57 59 62 65 69 70 71 72 75 76 78 79 **P**1 6 Web address: www.irmc.org	23	10	382	16388	259	226612	1268	194513	95323	1958
★ ○ △ SPARROW HEALTH SYSTEM, (Includes St. Lawrence Hospital and Healthcare Services, 1210 West Saginaw Street, Zip 48915-1999; tel. 517/372-3610), 1215 East Michigan Avenue, Zip 48912-1811, Mailing Address: P.O. Box 30480, Zip 48909-7980; tel. 517/483-2700; Joseph F. Damore, President and Chief Executive Officer (Total facility includes 193 beds in nursing home–type unit) **A**1 2 3 5 7 9 10 11 12 **F**2 3 4 5 6 7 8 9 10 11 12 13 16 17 18 19 21 22 24 25 26 27 28 29 30 31 32 33 34 35 36 37 38 39 40 41 42 43 44 45 46 47 48 49 50 51 52 53 54 56 57 58 59 60 61 62 63 64 65 66 68 69 70 71 72 75 76 77 78 79 **P**1 6 Web address: www.sparrow.com ST. LAWRENCE HOSPITAL AND HEALTHCARE SERVICES See Sparrow Health System	23	10	706	23932	549	599964	4285	345441	164914	4431
LAPEER—Lapeer County										
□ △ LAPEER REGIONAL HOSPITAL, 1375 North Main Street, Zip 48446; tel. 810/667-5500; Donald C. Kooy, President and Chief Executive Officer (Total facility includes 19 beds in nursing home–type unit) **A**1 7 9 10 **F**2 3 4 7 8 9 10 11 12 13 14 16 17 18 19 20 21 22 23 24 25 26 28 29 30 31 32 33 34 35 36 37 38 39 41 42 43 44 45 46 47 48 49 50 51 52 54 55 57 58 59 60 61 62 63 65 66 68 69 70 71 72 75 76 77 78 79 **P**6 7	23	10	163	6003	89	74396	777	48313	21851	626
LAURIUM—Houghton County										
★ KEWEENAW MEMORIAL MEDICAL CENTER, 205 Osceola Street, Zip 49913-2199; tel. 906/337-6500; Rick Wright, FACHE, CPA, President and Chief Executive Officer **A**1 9 10 **F**7 8 9 12 13 18 19 22 24 25 28 32 34 35 36 39 41 44 48 51 54 66 70 71 72 76 78 79 **P**6 Web address: www.kmmc.org	23	10	49	1592	19	33046	121	17254	9287	283
LIVONIA—Wayne County										
★ ST. MARY HOSPITAL, 36475 West Five Mile Road, Zip 48154-1988; tel. 734/655-4800; Sister Mary Renetta Rumpz, FACHE, President and Chief Executive Officer **A**1 9 10 **F**2 3 4 6 8 9 11 12 13 14 16 17 18 19 22 23 24 25 26 30 31 32 33 34 35 36 37 38 39 41 43 44 46 47 48 49 50 51 54 57 59 60 61 62 63 64 70 72 74 75 76 77 78 79 Web address: www.stmaryhospital.org	21	10	263	11875	162	132654	1484	100301	50357	1149
LUDINGTON—Mason County										
MEMORIAL MEDICAL CENTER OF WEST MICHIGAN, One Atkinson Drive, Zip 49431-1999; tel. 231/843-2591; Robert C. Marquardt, FACHE, President and Chief Executive Officer **A**9 10 **F**7 8 9 16 17 18 19 22 24 25 34 36 38 39 43 44 45 46 48 49 54 56 57 61 68 70 72 76 78 79 **P**8 Web address: www.mmcwm.com	23	10	85	2955	38	74613	370	28506	12486	286
MADISON HEIGHTS—Oakland County										
★ MADISON COMMUNITY HOSPITAL, 30671 Stephenson Highway, Zip 48071-1678; tel. 248/588-8000; Ram Gunabalan, M.D., Chief Executive Officer (Nonreporting) **A**1 9 10	23	10	56	—	—	—	—	—	—	—

Hospitals, U.S. / MICHIGAN

Hospital, Address, Telephone, Administrator, Approval, Facility, and Physician Codes, Health Care System, Network	Classification Codes		Utilization Data					Expense (thousands) of dollars		Personnel
★ American Hospital Association (AHA) membership □ Joint Commission on Accreditation of Healthcare Organizations (JCAHO) accreditation + American Osteopathic Healthcare Association (AOHA) membership ○ American Osteopathic Association (AOA) accreditation △ Commission on Accreditation of Rehabilitation Facilities (CARF) accreditation Control codes 61, 63, 64, 71, 72 and 73 indicate hospitals listed by AOHA, but not registered by AHA. For definition of numerical codes, see page A4	Control	Service	Staffed Beds	Admissions	Census	Outpatient Visits	Births	Total	Payroll	
□ + ○ ST. JOHN OAKLAND HOSPITAL, 27351 Dequindre, Zip 48071-3499; tel. 248/967-7000; Robert Deputat, President **A**1 9 10 11 12 13 **F**1 2 3 4 5 6 7 8 9 10 11 12 13 14 15 16 17 18 19 20 21 22 23 24 25 26 27 28 29 30 31 32 33 34 35 36 37 38 39 40 41 42 43 44 45 46 47 48 49 50 51 52 53 54 55 56 57 58 59 60 61 62 63 64 65 66 67 68 69 70 71 72 73 74 75 76 77 78 79 **P**4 5 7 8 **S** Ascension Health, Saint Louis, MO	21	10	196	6545	113	63119	0	61428	30234	820
MANISTEE—Manistee County										
WEST SHORE MEDICAL CENTER, (Formerly West Shore Hospital), 1465 East Parkdale Avenue, Zip 49660-9785; tel. 231/398-1000; Burton O. Parks, II, President **A**9 10 **F**4 7 8 9 12 13 16 17 18 19 21 22 23 24 25 28 30 32 33 34 36 37 38 39 43 44 45 46 48 50 51 54 68 70 72 76 78 **P**3 8	13	10	54	1846	21	49340	168	20036	8865	253
MANISTIQUE—Schoolcraft County										
✠ SCHOOLCRAFT MEMORIAL HOSPITAL, 500 Main Street, Zip 49854-0000; tel. 906/341-3200; David B. Jahn, Administrator and Chief Financial Officer **A**1 9 10 18 **F**2 3 4 7 8 9 10 11 12 16 17 18 19 20 21 22 23 24 25 27 28 30 31 32 33 34 35 36 37 38 39 40 41 42 43 44 45 46 47 48 49 50 51 52 53 54 56 57 58 59 60 61 62 63 64 65 68 69 70 71 72 75 76 77 78 79 **P**4 7 Web address: www.scmh.org	13	10	20	675	5	33854	98	10227	5623	130
MARLETTE—Sanilac County										
✠ △ MARLETTE COMMUNITY HOSPITAL, 2770 Main Street, Zip 48453-0307, Mailing Address: P.O. Box 307, Zip 48453-0307; tel. 517/635-4000; David S. McEwen, Chief Executive Officer (Total facility includes 43 beds in nursing home–type unit) **A**1 7 9 10 **F**7 9 14 16 17 18 19 21 22 23 24 25 26 30 32 33 34 37 38 39 40 43 48 51 53 54 67 69 70 71 72 73 76 78 **P**6 **S** Quorum Health Group, Brentwood, TN	23	10	91	1413	58	35102	0	19143	9336	355
MARQUETTE—Marquette County										
✠ △ MARQUETTE GENERAL HEALTH SYSTEM, 580 West College Avenue, Zip 49855-2794; tel. 906/228-9440; William Nemacheck, Chief Executive Officer **A**1 2 3 5 7 9 10 **F**2 3 4 6 7 8 9 11 12 13 14 15 16 17 18 19 21 22 23 24 25 27 30 31 32 33 34 35 36 37 38 39 41 42 43 44 45 46 47 48 49 50 51 53 54 55 57 58 59 60 61 62 63 65 66 69 70 71 72 75 76 77 78 79 **P**6 Web address: www.mgh.org	23	10	282	10433	160	313516	594	156531	78191	1808
MARSHALL—Calhoun County										
✠ OAKLAWN HOSPITAL, 200 North Madison Street, Zip 49068-1199; tel. 616/781-4271; Rob Covert, President and Chief Executive Officer **A**1 9 10 **F**3 5 8 9 13 16 17 18 19 21 22 24 25 28 32 33 34 36 37 38 39 40 41 43 44 45 46 48 49 50 51 54 56 57 59 60 61 62 63 64 65 67 70 71 72 76 78	23	10	94	2451	25	71693	556	30045	14881	394
MIDLAND—Midland County										
✠ △ MIDMICHIGAN MEDICAL CENTER–MIDLAND, 4005 Orchard Drive, Zip 48670; tel. 517/839-3000; David A. Reece, President **A**1 2 3 5 7 9 10 **F**4 6 7 8 9 11 12 13 17 18 19 22 23 24 25 27 28 30 31 32 33 34 35 36 37 38 39 40 41 43 44 45 46 48 49 50 51 53 54 56 57 58 59 60 62 63 64 65 68 69 70 71 72 76 77 78 79 **P**7 8 **S** MidMichigan Health, Midland, MI Web address: www.midmichigan.org	23	10	250	10713	133	238926	1257	134463	54611	1380
MONROE—Monroe County										
✠ MERCY MEMORIAL HOSPITAL, 740 North Macomb Street, Zip 48161-9974, Mailing Address: P.O. Box 67, Zip 48161-0067; tel. 734/241-1700; Richard S. Hiltz, President and Chief Executive Officer (Total facility includes 70 beds in nursing home–type unit) **A**1 9 10 **F**1 2 3 4 5 6 7 8 9 10 11 12 13 14 15 16 17 18 19 20 21 22 23 24 25 26 27 28 29 30 31 32 33 34 35 36 37 38 39 40 41 42 43 44 45 46 47 48 49 50 51 52 53 54 55 56 57 58 59 60 61 62 63 64 65 66 67 68 69 70 71 72 73 74 75 77 78 79 Web address: www.mercymemorial.org	23	10	243	8871	155	136336	932	70032	36270	934
MOUNT CLEMENS—Macomb County										
★ MOUNT CLEMENS GENERAL HOSPITAL, 1000 Harrington Boulevard, Zip 48043-2992; tel. 810/493-8000; Robert Milewski, President and Chief Executive Officer **A**9 10 11 12 13 **F**4 7 8 9 11 13 14 16 17 18 19 20 21 22 23 24 25 26 28 29 30 31 32 33 34 35 36 37 38 39 40 41 43 44 45 46 47 48 49 50 51 54 56 66 68 70 71 72 75 76 77 78 79 **P**8 Web address: www.mcgh.org	23	10	242	12460	156	559695	1549	175121	79464	1803
MOUNT PLEASANT—Isabella County										
✠ + ○ CENTRAL MICHIGAN COMMUNITY HOSPITAL, 1221 South Drive, Zip 48858-3234; tel. 517/772-6700; Stephen C. Lada, President **A**1 9 10 11 **F**7 8 9 16 17 18 22 25 28 32 33 34 35 36 38 39 43 45 48 50 54 58 59 60 61 62 63 68 70 71 72 76 77 78 79 **P**8 Web address: www.cmch.org	23	10	118	3673	35	99516	576	34877	13972	414
MUNISING—Alger County										
□ MUNISING MEMORIAL HOSPITAL, 1500 Sand Point Road, Zip 49862-1406; tel. 906/387-4110; Carl J. Velte, Chief Executive Officer (Nonreporting) **A**1 9 10	23	10	40	—	—	—	—	—	—	—
MUSKEGON—Muskegon County										
□ HACKLEY HEALTH, 1700 Clinton Street, Zip 49443-3302, Mailing Address: P.O. Box 3302, Zip 49443-3302; tel. 231/726-3511; Gordon A. Mudler, President and Chief Executive Officer **A**1 2 9 10 **F**3 7 8 9 11 13 16 17 18 19 20 22 23 24 25 26 28 30 31 33 34 35 36 39 41 43 44 45 46 48 49 50 51 53 54 56 57 58 59 60 61 63 64 65 68 70 71 72 73 76 77 78 **P**5 6 7 Web address: www.hackley.org	23	10	181	9190	121	292195	1152	103943	48662	849

© 2000 AHA Guide   *Many Facility Codes have changed. Please refer to the AHA Guide Code Chart.*

Hospitals, U.S. / MICHIGAN

Hospital, Address, Telephone, Administrator, Approval, Facility, and Physician Codes, Health Care System, Network	Classification Codes		Utilization Data					Expense (thousands) of dollars		
	Control	Service	Staffed Beds	Admissions	Census	Outpatient Visits	Births	Total	Payroll	Personnel

★ American Hospital Association (AHA) membership
☐ Joint Commission on Accreditation of Healthcare Organizations (JCAHO) accreditation
+ American Osteopathic Healthcare Association (AOHA) membership
○ American Osteopathic Association (AOA) accreditation
△ Commission on Accreditation of Rehabilitation Facilities (CARF) accreditation
Control codes 61, 63, 64, 71, 72 and 73 indicate hospitals listed by AOHA, but not registered by AHA. For definition of numerical codes, see page A4

Hospital	Control	Service	Staffed Beds	Admissions	Census	Outpatient Visits	Births	Total	Payroll	Personnel
★ + ○ MERCY GENERAL HEALTH PARTNERS, (Includes Mercy General Health Partners–Oak Avenue Campus, 1700 Oak Avenue, Zip 49442–2407; tel. 616/773–3311; Mercy General Health Partners–Sherman Boulevard Campus, 1500 East Sherman Boulevard), 1500 East Sherman Boulevard, Zip 49443; tel. 231/739–9341; Roger Spoelman, President and Chief Executive Officer **A**1 9 10 11 12 13 **F**4 7 8 9 11 13 16 17 18 19 20 22 23 24 25 28 30 32 33 34 36 38 39 41 43 44 45 46 47 48 49 50 51 53 54 56 63 66 68 70 71 72 76 77 78 79 **P**6 8 **S** Trinity Health, Novi, MI	23	10	191	9787	127	197229	1168	141446	61091	1516
NEW BALTIMORE—Macomb County										
☐ HARBOR OAKS HOSPITAL, 35031 23 Mile Road, Zip 48047–2097; tel. 810/725–5777; Judi Schiop, Administrator **A**1 9 10 **F**16 17 18 57 58 59 60 61 62 63 64 70 **P**1 6 **S** Pioneer Behavioral Health, Peabody, MA	33	22	64	1292	24	0	—	—	—	88
NEWBERRY—Luce County										
★ HELEN NEWBERRY JOY HOSPITAL, (Includes Helen Newberry Joy Hospital Annex), 502 West Harrie Street, Zip 49868–0070; tel. 906/293–9200; Wayne P. Hellerstedt, Chief Executive Officer (Total facility includes 48 beds in nursing home–type unit) (Nonreporting) **A**1 9 10 18 Web address: www.hnjh.org	13	10	86	—	—	—	—	—	—	—
NILES—Berrien County										
LAKELAND MEDICAL CENTER–NILES See Lakeland Medical Center–St. Joseph, Saint Joseph										
NORTHPORT—Leelanau County										
★ LEELANAU MEMORIAL HEALTH CENTER, 215 South High Street, Zip 49670, Mailing Address: P.O. Box 217, Zip 49670–0217; tel. 231/386–0000; Jayne R. Bull, Administrator (Total facility includes 72 beds in nursing home–type unit) **A**1 9 10 18 **F**7 9 13 16 17 18 19 20 25 28 31 32 33 35 36 37 38 40 43 45 48 50 51 54 56 69 70 72 76 77 78 **P**1 7 **S** Munson Healthcare, Traverse City, MI	23	10	85	161	64	21650	0	6353	3131	138
NORTHVILLE—Wayne County										
☐ HAWTHORN CENTER, 18471 Haggerty Road, Zip 48167–9575; tel. 248/735–6790; Neil H. Wasserman, Chief Executive Officer **A**1 3 5 9 **F**57 58	12	52	118	170	111	0	0	21825	14246	331
☐ NORTHVILLE PSYCHIATRIC HOSPITAL, 41001 West Seven Mile Road, Zip 48167–2698; tel. 248/349–1800; Shobhana Joshi, M.D., Director **A**1 9 10 **F**4 9 10 11 12 22 23 24 25 39 41 44 46 47 53 55 57 62 65 68 75 76	12	22	425	428	379	0	0	57839	34631	826
ONTONAGON—Ontonagon County										
ONTONAGON MEMORIAL HOSPITAL, 601 Seventh Street, Zip 49953–1496; tel. 906/884–4134; Fred Nelson, Administrator (Total facility includes 46 beds in nursing home–type unit) **A**9 10 **F**9 16 19 22 23 24 25 29 30 32 33 34 40 43 45 48 54 56 69 70 71 76 **P**2 Web address: www.uphcn.org/uphcn/omh.html	14	10	72	772	52	15304	0	6561	3368	143
OWOSSO—Shiawassee County										
★ MEMORIAL HEALTHCARE CENTER, 826 West King Street, Zip 48867–2198; tel. 517/723–5211; Margaret S. Gulick, President and Chief Executive Officer (Total facility includes 16 beds in nursing home–type unit) **A**1 2 9 10 **F**3 7 8 9 13 16 17 18 19 21 22 24 25 26 29 31 32 33 34 36 37 39 40 41 43 44 45 46 48 51 53 54 57 58 59 60 61 62 63 64 69 70 71 72 73 76 77 78 79 **P**1 6 Web address: www.healthcare.org	23	10	130	5859	75	278659	611	54174	30306	852
PAW PAW—Van Buren County										
★ LAKEVIEW COMMUNITY HOSPITAL, 408 Hazen Street, Zip 49079–1019; tel. 616/657–3141; Sue E. Johnson–Phillippe, Chief Executive Officer (Total facility includes 120 beds in nursing home–type unit) **A**1 9 10 **F**8 9 13 16 17 18 19 22 23 25 30 34 36 38 41 43 44 45 48 49 50 54 57 59 60 62 66 69 70 72 76 77 78 79 **S** Quorum Health Group, Brentwood, TN	16	10	168	1588	140	63301	0	27969	13260	341
PETOSKEY—Emmet County										
★ NORTHERN MICHIGAN REGIONAL HEALTH SYSTEM, (Formerly Northern Michigan Hospital), 416 Connable Avenue, Zip 49770–2297; tel. 231/487–4000; Jeffrey T. Wendling, President and Chief Executive Officer **A**1 2 9 10 **F**1 2 3 4 6 7 8 9 11 12 13 14 15 16 17 18 19 20 21 22 23 24 25 26 27 28 30 31 32 33 34 35 36 37 38 39 40 41 42 43 44 45 46 47 48 49 50 52 54 57 58 59 61 63 64 65 66 67 68 69 70 71 72 73 76 77 78 79 **P**5 7 Web address: www.healthshare.org	23	10	204	8238	105	125331	817	100721	7015	1448
PIGEON—Huron County										
★ SCHEURER HOSPITAL, 170 North Caseville Road, Zip 48755–9704; tel. 517/453–3223; Dwight Gascho, President and Chief Executive Officer (Total facility includes 19 beds in nursing home–type unit) **A**1 9 10 **F**7 9 13 16 17 18 19 22 24 25 31 32 33 34 36 37 38 39 40 43 44 46 48 51 54 56 59 67 68 69 70 72 76 78 **P**6	23	10	42	630	25	35560	0	13843	6921	219
PLAINWELL—Allegan County										
BORGESS–PIPP HEALTH CENTER See Borgess Medical Center, Kalamazoo										
PONTIAC—Oakland County										
★ △ NORTH OAKLAND MEDICAL CENTERS, 461 West Huron Street, Zip 48341–1651; tel. 248/857–7200; Robert L. Davis, President and Chief Executive Officer **A**1 3 5 7 9 10 **F**4 7 8 9 11 13 16 17 18 19 20 21 22 23 24 25 29 30 32 33 34 35 36 37 38 41 42 43 44 45 46 48 49 50 51 53 54 56 57 59 60 61 62 63 64 65 66 68 70 72 73 76 77 78 79	23	10	220	8442	115	180778	1544	104186	47618	1145
+ ○ POH MEDICAL CENTER, 50 North Perry Street, Zip 48342–2253; tel. 248/338–5000; Patrick Lamberti, Chief Executive Officer (Total facility includes 120 beds in nursing home–type unit) **A**9 10 11 12 13 **F**3 7 9 11 13 16 17 18 19 20 22 26 29 33 34 36 39 41 43 45 48 49 50 54 68 69 70 71 72 75 76 77 78 **P**8 Web address: www.pohmedical.org	23	10	250	6769	201	95560	—	82766	39984	1064

A220 Hospitals — *Many Facility Codes have changed. Please refer to the AHA Guide Code Chart.* — © 2000 AHA Guide

Hospitals, U.S. / MICHIGAN

Hospital, Address, Telephone, Administrator, Approval, Facility, and Physician Codes, Health Care System, Network	Classification Codes		Utilization Data					Expense (thousands) of dollars		
★ American Hospital Association (AHA) membership ☐ Joint Commission on Accreditation of Healthcare Organizations (JCAHO) accreditation + American Osteopathic Healthcare Association (AOHA) membership ○ American Osteopathic Association (AOA) accreditation △ Commission on Accreditation of Rehabilitation Facilities (CARF) accreditation Control codes 61, 63, 64, 71, 72 and 73 indicate hospitals listed by AOHA, but not registered by AHA. For definition of numerical codes, see page A4	Control	Service	Staffed Beds	Admissions	Census	Outpatient Visits	Births	Total	Payroll	Personnel
★ ST. JOSEPH MERCY OAKLAND, 900 Woodward Avenue, Zip 48341–2985; tel. 248/858–3000; Thomas L. Feurig, President and Chief Executive Officer **A**1 3 5 9 10 **F**2 3 4 6 7 8 9 11 12 13 14 16 17 18 19 20 21 22 24 25 26 28 29 30 31 33 34 35 36 37 38 39 40 41 42 43 44 45 46 47 48 49 51 52 53 54 56 57 58 59 60 61 62 63 64 65 66 67 69 70 71 72 73 75 76 77 78 79 **P**1 **S** Trinity Health, Novi, MI **Web address:** www.mercyhealth.com/oakland	21	10	428	19437	269	703630	2615	211828	89833	2037
PORT HURON—St. Clair County										
★ △ MERCY HOSPITAL, 2601 Electric Avenue, Zip 48060; tel. 810/985–1510; Mary R. Trimmer, President and Chief Executive Officer **A**1 2 7 9 10 **F**4 7 9 11 13 16 17 18 19 22 24 25 28 32 34 35 36 37 38 39 41 43 45 46 47 48 49 50 51 53 54 65 68 70 71 72 75 76 78 79 **P**8 **S** Trinity Health, Novi, MI **Web address:** www.mercyporthuron.com	21	10	119	4891	69	113668	0	55459	21759	671
★ PORT HURON HOSPITAL, 1221 Pine Grove Avenue, Zip 48061–5011; tel. 810/987–5000; Donald C. Fletcher, President and Chief Executive Officer **A**1 2 9 10 **F**3 4 7 8 9 11 12 13 16 17 18 19 20 22 23 24 25 30 32 33 34 35 38 39 41 44 45 46 47 48 49 50 51 54 57 59 60 61 62 63 64 68 70 71 72 76 78 79 **P**8 **S** Blue Water Health Services Corporation, Port Huron, MI **Web address:** www.porthuronhosp.org	23	10	173	8361	105	188693	1274	76405	33502	850
REED CITY—Osceola County										
★ SPECTRUM HEALTH–REED CITY CAMPUS, (Formerly Reed City Hospital), 300 North Patterson Road, Zip 49677–0075; tel. 231/832–3271; Gary L. Petersen, President and Chief Executive Officer (Total facility includes 54 beds in nursing home–type unit) **A**1 9 10 **F**7 9 11 17 18 19 21 22 24 25 26 28 30 32 34 36 38 41 45 46 48 53 54 65 69 70 71 76 77 78 79 **S** Spectrum Health, Grand Rapids, MI	23	10	85	1421	63	45200	0	16451	6051	193
ROCHESTER—Oakland County										
☐ △ CRITTENTON HOSPITAL, 1101 West University Drive, Zip 48307–1831; tel. 248/652–5000; Joseph W. Ferguson, Vice President of Administration (Nonreporting) **A**1 2 7 9 10	23	10	224	—	—	—	—	—	—	—
ROGERS CITY—Presque Isle County										
☐ △ ROGERS CITY REHABILITATION HOSPITAL, 555 North Bradley Highway, Zip 49779–1599; tel. 517/734–7545; Nancy Dextrom, Executive Director (Nonreporting) **A**1 7 9 10	33	46	17	—	—	—	—	—	—	—
ROMEO—Macomb County										
ST. JOSEPH'S MERCY–NORTH See St. Joseph's Mercy Hospitals and Health Services, Clinton Township										
ROYAL OAK—Oakland County										
★ WILLIAM BEAUMONT HOSPITAL–ROYAL OAK, 3601 West Thirteen Mile Road, Zip 48073–6769; tel. 248/551–5000; John D. Labriola, Senior Vice President and Hospital Director **A**1 2 3 5 8 9 10 **F**1 3 4 6 8 9 11 12 13 16 17 18 19 20 22 23 24 25 26 27 28 29 30 31 32 33 34 35 36 37 38 39 41 42 43 44 46 47 48 49 50 51 52 53 54 55 56 57 59 60 61 62 63 64 65 66 68 69 70 71 72 74 75 76 77 78 79 **P**6 8 **S** William Beaumont Hospital Corporation, Royal Oak, MI **Web address:** www.beaumont.edu	23	10	899	51359	788	863692	6475	649553	287796	7939
SAGINAW—Saginaw County										
★ ALEDA E. LUTZ VETERANS AFFAIRS MEDICAL CENTER, 1500 Weiss Street, Zip 48602–5298; tel. 517/497–2500; Robert H. Sabin, Director (Total facility includes 81 beds in nursing home–type unit) **A**1 5 9 **F**2 3 4 5 7 9 10 11 12 13 17 18 19 22 24 25 26 27 28 29 30 31 32 34 35 36 37 38 39 41 43 44 45 46 47 48 49 50 51 54 55 56 57 59 63 65 68 69 70 72 74 76 77 78 79 **P**6 **S** Department of Veterans Affairs, Washington, DC	45	10	114	1648	100	78033	—	—	—	457
★ △ COVENANT HEALTHCARE, (Includes Covenant Medical Center–Cooper, 700 Cooper Avenue, Zip 48602–5399; tel. 517/583–0000; Covenant Medical Center–Harrison, 1447 North Harrison Street, tel. 517/583–0000), 1447 North Harrison, Zip 48602–4785; tel. 517/583–0000; Spencer Maidlow, President **A**1 3 5 7 9 10 **F**4 7 8 9 11 12 13 17 18 19 22 24 25 29 30 31 32 34 35 36 37 38 39 41 42 43 44 45 46 47 48 49 50 51 52 53 54 56 57 66 69 70 71 72 75 76 77 78 79 **P**1 **Web address:** www.covenanthealthcare.com	23	10	504	25087	366	319322	3394	259216	117675	3335
☐ △ HEALTHSOURCE SAGINAW, (LONG TERM CARE REHAB PSYCH), 3340 Hospital Road, Zip 48603–9623, Mailing Address: P.O. Box 6280, Zip 48608–6280; tel. 517/790–7700; Lester Heyboer, Jr, President and Chief Executive Officer (Total facility includes 213 beds in nursing home–type unit) **A**1 7 9 10 **F**2 3 23 30 43 45 50 51 53 54 57 58 59 60 62 63 69 70 72 **P**6	13	49	319	1807	204	11098	0	20153	9595	360
★ ST. MARY'S MEDICAL CENTER, 800 South Washington Avenue, Zip 48601–2594; tel. 517/776–8000; Frederic L. Fraizer, President and Chief Executive Officer **A**1 2 3 5 9 10 **F**4 7 9 10 11 12 16 17 18 19 22 24 25 26 27 29 31 32 33 34 37 38 39 41 43 46 47 48 49 50 51 54 56 59 61 65 68 70 72 75 76 78 **P**6 8 **S** Ascension Health, Saint Louis, MO **Web address:** www.saintmarys–saginaw.org	21	10	268	13225	197	224899	0	155162	62994	1597
SAINT IGNACE—Mackinac County										
MACKINAC STRAITS HOSPITAL AND HEALTH CENTER, 220 Burdette Street, Zip 49781–1792; tel. 906/643–8585; Rodney M. Nelson, President and Chief Executive Officer (Total facility includes 99 beds in nursing home–type unit) **A**9 10 **F**6 7 17 18 25 32 43 45 51 54 56 61 69 72	16	10	107	88	99	13345	0	8662	4999	180

© 2000 AHA Guide   *Many Facility Codes have changed. Please refer to the AHA Guide Code Chart.*   Hospitals **A221**

Hospitals, U.S. / MICHIGAN

Hospital, Address, Telephone, Administrator, Approval, Facility, and Physician Codes, Health Care System, Network	Control	Service	Staffed Beds	Admissions	Census	Outpatient Visits	Births	Total	Payroll	Personnel
SAINT JOHNS—Clinton County										
✦ CLINTON MEMORIAL HOSPITAL, 805 South Oakland Street, Zip 48879–0260; tel. 517/224–6881; Kathryn A. Bangs, President and Chief Executive Officer **A**1 9 10 **F**7 8 9 14 16 17 18 19 22 25 26 28 30 32 33 34 36 37 38 39 40 43 45 46 48 54 56 70 71 72 76 77 78 **P**1 Web address: www.sparrow.com	23	10	28	1046	9	38546	116	19270	5433	188
RIVENDELL OF MICHIGAN, 101 West Townsend Road, Zip 48879–9200; tel. 517/224–1177; Roger Rohall, Chief Executive Officer **A**9 **F**16 17 57 58 59 60 61 70 **S** Children's Comprehensive Services, Inc., Nashville, TN	33	22	31	422	10	0	0	1758	975	73
SAINT JOSEPH—Berrien County										
☐ △ LAKELAND MEDICAL CENTER–ST. JOSEPH, (Includes Lakeland Medical Center, Berrien Center, 6418 Dean's Hill Road, Berrien Center, Zip 49102–9704; tel. 616/471–7761; Lakeland Medical Center–Niles, 31 North St. Joseph Avenue, Niles, Zip 49120–2287; tel. 616/683–5510), 1234 Napier Avenue, Zip 49085–2112; tel. 616/983–8300; Joseph A. Wasserman, President and Chief Executive Officer (Total facility includes 193 beds in nursing home–type unit) **A**1 2 7 9 10 **F**4 6 7 8 9 11 13 14 16 17 18 19 22 24 25 32 33 34 35 36 39 41 43 44 45 46 47 48 49 53 54 57 61 65 70 71 72 76 78 **P**1 7	23	10	360	14662	282	306053	1941	158411	68540	2082
SALINE—Washtenaw County										
✦ SALINE COMMUNITY HOSPITAL, 400 West Russell Street, Zip 48176–1101; tel. 734/429–1500; Garry C. Faja, President and Chief Executive Officer **A**1 9 10 **F**1 2 3 4 5 7 8 9 11 12 13 14 16 17 19 20 21 22 23 24 25 26 29 30 31 32 33 34 35 36 37 38 39 41 43 44 45 46 47 48 49 50 51 53 54 56 57 58 59 60 61 62 63 64 65 68 70 71 72 73 75 76 77 78 79 **P**1 5 **S** Trinity Health, Novi, MI Web address: www.sjmh.com	21	10	39	1453	15	159074	0	21154	9535	215
SANDUSKY—Sanilac County										
★ MCKENZIE MEMORIAL HOSPITAL, 120 Delaware Street, Zip 48471–1087; tel. 810/648–3770; Joseph W. Weiler, President **A**9 10 **F**3 9 13 17 18 22 24 25 30 32 37 38 39 41 44 45 46 48 50 51 54 59 61 68 70 74 76 78 **P**6	23	10	25	824	7	19604	73	10741	5596	137
SAULT STE. MARIE—Chippewa County										
✦ CHIPPEWA COUNTY WAR MEMORIAL HOSPITAL, 500 Osborn Boulevard, Zip 49783–4467; tel. 906/635–4460; Daniel Wakeman, Chief Executive Officer (Total facility includes 51 beds in nursing home–type unit) **A**1 9 10 **F**3 7 8 9 13 16 17 19 20 22 23 24 25 28 32 34 35 36 41 44 45 46 48 50 51 53 54 68 69 70 72 73 76 77 78 79 **P**5 6 8	23	10	86	2401	75	94855	413	29916	13224	394
SHELBY—Oceana County										
☐ LAKESHORE COMMUNITY HOSPITAL, 72 South State Street, Zip 49455–1299; tel. 231/861–2156; Jay Bryan, Chief Executive Officer **A**1 9 10 **F**1 2 3 4 6 7 8 9 11 12 13 16 17 19 22 24 25 31 34 35 36 37 39 40 41 42 43 44 45 47 48 49 50 52 53 54 56 57 59 61 65 68 69 70 72 75 76 78 **P**3 4	23	10	24	817	6	28026	133	5554	2518	89
SHERIDAN—Montcalm County										
+ ○ SHERIDAN COMMUNITY HOSPITAL, 301 North Main Street, Zip 48884–9220, Mailing Address: P.O. Box 279, Zip 48884–0279; tel. 517/291–3261; Christopher Noland, Chief Executive Officer **A**9 10 11 **F**7 9 16 17 18 19 22 25 32 34 38 45 46 48 50 51 54 56 72 76 77 78	23	10	18	322	3	24101	1	7353	3981	124
SOUTH HAVEN—Van Buren County										
✦ SOUTH HAVEN COMMUNITY HOSPITAL, 955 South Bailey Avenue, Zip 49090; tel. 616/637–5271; Craig J. Marks, President and Chief Executive Officer (Nonreporting) **A**1 9 10 Web address: www.shch.org	16	10	52	—	—	—	—	—	—	—
SOUTHFIELD—Oakland County										
○ △ GREAT LAKES REHABILITATION HOSPITAL, 22401 Foster Winter Drive, Zip 48075–3708; tel. 248/483–5545; William H. Restum, Ph.D., President and Chief Executive Officer (Total facility includes 26 beds in nursing home–type unit) **A**7 9 10 11 **F**18 31 49 51 53 54 69 70 **P**5	33	46	52	999	43	4544	0	10150	6295	117
✦ PROVIDENCE HOSPITAL AND MEDICAL CENTERS, 16001 West Nine Mile Road, Zip 48075–4854, Mailing Address: Box 2043, Zip 48037–2043; tel. 248/424–3000; Robert F. Casalou, President **A**1 2 3 5 8 9 10 **F**1 4 6 7 8 9 11 13 14 16 17 18 19 20 22 24 25 26 29 30 31 32 33 34 35 36 37 38 39 43 45 46 47 48 49 50 51 54 56 59 60 61 62 63 64 65 68 70 71 72 76 78 79 **P**1 6 **S** Ascension Health, Saint Louis, MO Web address: www.providence–hospital.org	21	10	379	21492	301	549183	3636	356837	162684	3695
✦ STRAITH HOSPITAL FOR SPECIAL SURGERY, 23901 Lahser Road, Zip 48034–3296; tel. 248/357–3360; Gregory R. Hoose, Chief Executive Officer **A**1 9 10 **F**13 16 17 48 70	23	10	23	1019	13	4640	0	9277	4310	128
STANDISH—Arenac County										
☐ STANDISH COMMUNITY HOSPITAL, 805 West Cedar Street, Zip 48658–9526, Mailing Address: P.O. Box 579, Zip 48658–0579; tel. 517/846–3400; John L. Stindt, Chief Executive Officer (Total facility includes 44 beds in nursing home–type unit) (Nonreporting) **A**1 9 10 18	23	10	72	—	—	—	—	—	—	—
STURGIS—St. Joseph County										
✦ STURGIS HOSPITAL, 916 Myrtle, Zip 49091–2001; tel. 616/651–7824; James N. Browne, Interim Chief Executive Officer **A**1 9 10 **F**7 8 9 12 13 16 17 19 21 22 24 25 26 28 31 32 33 34 36 37 38 39 43 44 45 46 48 49 50 51 54 56 68 70 72 76 77 78 **P**5 6 **S** Quorum Health Group, Brentwood, TN	14	10	67	2400	21	107573	395	28022	12840	349

Hospitals, U.S. / MICHIGAN

Hospital, Address, Telephone, Administrator, Approval, Facility, and Physician Codes, Health Care System, Network	Classification Codes		Utilization Data					Expense (thousands) of dollars		Personnel
★ American Hospital Association (AHA) membership ☐ Joint Commission on Accreditation of Healthcare Organizations (JCAHO) accreditation + American Osteopathic Healthcare Association (AOHA) membership ○ American Osteopathic Association (AOA) accreditation △ Commission on Accreditation of Rehabilitation Facilities (CARF) accreditation Control codes 61, 63, 64, 71, 72 and 73 indicate hospitals listed by AOHA, but not registered by AHA. For definition of numerical codes, see page A4	Control	Service	Staffed Beds	Admissions	Census	Outpatient Visits	Births	Total	Payroll	

	Control	Service	Staffed Beds	Admissions	Census	Outpatient Visits	Births	Total	Payroll	Personnel
TAWAS CITY—Iosco County ✠ ST. JOSEPH HEALTH SYSTEM, (Formerly Tawas St. Joseph Hospital), 200 Hemlock Street, Zip 48763, Mailing Address: P.O. Box 659, Zip 48764–0659; tel. 517/362–3411; Patrick Murtha, President and Chief Executive Officer **A**1 9 10 **F**7 8 9 12 13 14 16 17 18 19 22 25 26 29 31 32 33 34 36 37 38 39 41 43 44 46 48 49 51 54 56 68 70 72 76 77 78 **P**8 **S** Ascension Health, Saint Louis, MO	21	10	49	2221	24	121465	305	33961	15317	445
TAYLOR—Wayne County ✠ OAKWOOD HERITAGE HOSPITAL, (Formerly Oakwood Hospital–Heritage Center), 10000 Telegraph Road, Zip 48180–3349; tel. 313/295–5000; Edward E. Freysinger, Administrator **A**1 9 10 **F**7 9 13 16 17 18 19 21 22 23 24 25 31 32 34 37 38 39 41 43 48 49 51 53 54 57 59 60 61 62 64 68 70 72 76 78 **P**5 7 **S** Oakwood Healthcare, Inc., Dearborn, MI	23	10	257	7552	174	55605	0	52786	27347	616
TECUMSEH—Lenawee County ✠ HERRICK MEMORIAL HOSPITAL, LENAWEE HEALTH ALLIANCE, 500 East Pottawatamie Street, Zip 49286–2097; tel. 517/424–3000; John R. Robertstad, President and Chief Executive Officer (Total facility includes 25 beds in nursing home–type unit) **A**1 9 10 **F**3 7 8 9 12 16 17 19 22 24 25 27 28 30 32 33 34 36 37 39 43 46 48 49 50 51 53 54 57 58 59 60 61 62 63 64 65 66 67 69 70 71 73 76 77 78 79 **P**1 7 8 **S** ProMedica Health System, Toledo, OH Web address: www.lhanet.org	23	10	88	2454	45	54036	174	22663	8528	218
THREE RIVERS—St. Joseph County ✠ △ THREE RIVERS AREA HOSPITAL, 1111 West Broadway, Zip 49093–9362; tel. 616/278–1145; Matthew Chambers, Chief Executive Officer **A**1 7 9 10 **F**8 9 13 17 18 19 22 24 25 28 32 34 35 36 37 38 39 41 43 44 45 46 48 50 51 53 54 59 66 70 72 76 77 78 79 **P**6 8 **S** Quorum Health Group, Brentwood, TN Web address: www.trah.org	16	10	60	1619	23	—	148	23473	9285	329
TRAVERSE CITY—Grand Traverse County ✠ △ MUNSON MEDICAL CENTER, 1105 Sixth Street, Zip 49684–2386; tel. 231/935–5000; Ralph J. Cerny, President and Chief Executive Officer **A**1 2 3 7 9 10 12 13 **F**3 4 7 8 9 11 13 14 16 17 18 19 20 21 22 23 24 25 27 28 29 30 31 32 33 34 35 36 37 39 40 41 42 43 45 46 47 48 49 50 51 52 53 54 56 59 60 61 62 63 64 65 66 70 71 72 73 74 76 77 78 79 **P**6 8 **S** Munson Healthcare, Traverse City, MI Web address: www.mhc.net	23	10	368	16969	224	373548	1873	179101	78487	2264
TRENTON—Wayne County ✠ OAKWOOD SEAWAY HOSPITAL, (Formerly Oakwood Hospital Seaway Center), 5450 Fort Street, Zip 48183–4625; tel. 734/671–3800; Brian Peltz, Administrator **A**1 9 10 **F**1 2 3 4 6 7 8 9 11 12 13 14 16 17 18 19 20 21 22 24 25 26 27 28 29 30 31 32 33 34 37 38 39 40 41 42 43 44 45 46 47 48 49 50 51 53 54 55 56 57 58 59 60 61 62 63 64 65 66 67 68 69 70 71 72 73 76 77 78 79 **P**1 2 5 6 7 **S** Oakwood Healthcare, Inc., Dearborn, MI Web address: www.oakwood.org	23	10	82	3141	33	50422	190	27164	14216	301
★ + ○ RIVERSIDE OSTEOPATHIC HOSPITAL, 150 Truax Street, Zip 48183–2151; tel. 734/676–4200; Dennis R. Lemanski, D.O., Vice President and Chief Executive Officer **A**9 10 11 12 13 **F**8 9 11 13 16 17 18 19 21 22 24 25 28 30 32 33 34 36 37 38 39 40 41 43 44 45 46 48 50 51 54 57 59 60 61 62 65 66 68 70 71 72 75 76 78 79 **S** Henry Ford Health System, Detroit, MI Web address: www.henryfordhealth.org	23	10	138	5712	72	86172	803	59683	26495	593
TROY—Oakland County ✠ WILLIAM BEAUMONT HOSPITAL–TROY, 44201 Dequindre Road, Zip 48098–1198; tel. 248/828–5100; Eugene F. Michalski, Senior Vice President and Director **A**1 2 3 9 10 **F**1 3 4 6 9 11 12 13 15 17 18 19 20 21 22 23 24 25 26 27 28 29 30 31 32 33 34 35 36 37 38 39 40 41 42 43 44 47 48 49 50 51 52 53 54 55 56 57 59 60 61 62 63 64 65 66 68 69 70 71 72 74 75 76 77 78 79 **P**6 8 **S** William Beaumont Hospital Corporation, Royal Oak, MI Web address: www.beaumont.edu	23	10	189	13336	165	349584	1797	146811	67440	1912
VICKSBURG—Kalamazoo County ✠ △ BRONSON VICKSBURG HOSPITAL, 13326 North Boulevard, Zip 49097–1099; tel. 616/649–2321; Frank J. Sardone, President **A**1 7 9 10 **F**4 8 9 11 13 14 16 19 22 24 25 27 29 30 32 33 34 35 36 38 39 41 42 44 45 46 47 48 49 50 51 54 59 65 66 70 75 76 77 78 79 **S** Bronson Healthcare Group, Inc., Kalamazoo, MI Web address: www.bronsonhealth.com	23	46	41	524	16	34829	0	8416	3526	99
WARREN—Macomb County ☐ ARBORVIEW HOSPITAL, 6902 Chicago Road, Zip 48092–4784; tel. 810/264–8875; Donald L. Warner, Chief Executive Officer **A**1 9 10 **F**16 17 57 59 60 61 63 64 **P**5	32	22	43	645	24	3540	0	5101	2531	80
★ + ○ △ BI–COUNTY COMMUNITY HOSPITAL, 13355 East Ten Mile Road, Zip 48089–2065; tel. 810/759–7300; Gary W. Popiel, Executive Vice President and Chief Executive Officer **A**7 9 10 11 12 13 **F**3 8 9 11 13 14 16 17 18 19 22 24 25 28 31 32 34 35 36 37 38 39 40 41 44 45 46 48 50 51 53 54 56 58 59 60 61 65 66 68 70 71 76 78 79 **P**1 6 **S** Henry Ford Health System, Detroit, MI	23	10	164	5650	87	117477	402	72740	33299	782

Hospitals, U.S. / MICHIGAN

Hospital, Address, Telephone, Administrator, Approval, Facility, and Physician Codes, Health Care System, Network	Classification Codes		Utilization Data					Expense (thousands) of dollars		
	Control	Service	Staffed Beds	Admissions	Census	Outpatient Visits	Births	Total	Payroll	Personnel

★ American Hospital Association (AHA) membership
☐ Joint Commission on Accreditation of Healthcare Organizations (JCAHO) accreditation
+ American Osteopathic Healthcare Association (AOHA) membership
○ American Osteopathic Association (AOA) accreditation
△ Commission on Accreditation of Rehabilitation Facilities (CARF) accreditation
Control codes 61, 63, 64, 71, 72 and 73 indicate hospitals listed by AOHA, but not registered by AHA. For definition of numerical codes, see page A4

Hospital	Control	Service	Staffed Beds	Admissions	Census	Outpatient Visits	Births	Total	Payroll	Personnel
☐ KERN HOSPITAL AND MEDICAL CENTER, 21230 Dequindre, Zip 48091–2287; tel. 810/427-1000; Manoj K. Prasad, M.D., President and Chief Executive Officer **A**1 9 10 **F**14 15 23 30 31 32 34 36 38 45 48 49 53 54 56 59 66 70 76 77 79	33	10	13	95	1	14352	0	—	—	93
★ △ ST. JOHN MACOMB HOSPITAL, 11800 East Twelve Mile Road, Zip 48093–3494; tel. 810/573-5000; John E. Knox, President **A**1 2 7 9 10 **F**2 3 4 7 8 9 11 12 14 16 17 18 19 20 21 22 23 24 25 27 29 30 31 32 33 34 35 36 37 38 39 41 42 43 44 45 46 47 48 49 50 51 53 54 56 57 58 59 60 61 62 63 64 65 66 68 70 71 72 73 74 75 76 77 78 79 **P**8 **S** Ascension Health, Saint Louis, MO **Web address:** www.stjohn.org	21	10	274	12185	206	—	1432	115551	61253	1195
WATERVLIET—Berrien County										
★ △ COMMUNITY HOSPITAL, Medical Park Drive, Zip 49098–0158, Mailing Address: P.O. Box 158, Zip 49098–0158; tel. 616/463-3111; David L. McMann, Chief Executive Officer **A**1 7 9 10 **F**7 8 9 13 17 18 22 25 30 32 33 34 36 37 38 39 41 44 48 50 51 53 54 68 70 72 76 77 78 **P**1 **S** Quorum Health Group, Brentwood, TN	23	10	56	1822	25	44557	174	18407	8980	265
WAYNE—Wayne County										
★ OAKWOOD ANNAPOLIS HOSPITAL, (Formerly Oakwood Hospital Annapolis Center), (Includes Oakwood Hospital Merriman Center–Westland, 2345 Merriman Road, Westland, Zip 48185; tel. 313/467-2300), 33155 Annapolis Road, Zip 48184–2493; tel. 734/467-4000; Thomas Kochis, Chief Administrative Officer **A**1 9 10 **F**1 2 3 4 6 7 8 9 11 12 13 14 16 17 18 19 20 21 22 23 24 25 26 27 29 30 31 32 34 35 36 37 38 39 41 42 43 44 45 46 47 48 49 51 53 54 56 57 58 59 60 61 62 63 64 65 66 67 68 69 70 71 72 73 74 76 77 78 79 **P**5 7 **S** Oakwood Healthcare, Inc., Dearborn, MI **Web address:** www.oakwood.org	23	10	183	7888	100	84752	874	52677	25424	557
WEST BRANCH—Ogemaw County										
★ WEST BRANCH REGIONAL MEDICAL CENTER, (Formerly Tolfree Memorial Hospital), 2463 South M–30, Zip 48661–1199; tel. 517/345-3660; Douglas E. Pattullo, Chief Executive Officer **A**1 9 10 **F**7 8 9 11 12 17 18 19 22 25 32 36 37 38 43 44 45 46 48 54 68 70 76 **Web address:** www.wbrmc.com	14	10	88	3460	42	56736	347	19642	8453	302
WESTLAND—Wayne County										
OAKWOOD HOSPITAL MERRIMAN CENTER–WESTLAND See Oakwood Annapolis Hospital, Wayne										
☐ WALTER P. REUTHER PSYCHIATRIC HOSPITAL, 30901 Palmer Road, Zip 48185–5389; tel. 734/722-4500; Norma C. Josef, M.D., Director **A**1 9 10 **F**16 22 23 24 30 39 53 55 57 59 61 62 68 70 78 **P**5	12	22	230	299	211	0	0	29910	17444	403
WYANDOTTE—Wayne County										
★ △ HENRY FORD WYANDOTTE HOSPITAL, 2333 Biddle Avenue, Zip 48192–4693; tel. 734/246-6000; William R. Alvin, President **A**1 7 9 10 **F**1 2 3 4 6 7 8 9 11 12 13 14 16 17 18 19 20 21 22 23 24 25 26 27 28 29 30 31 32 33 34 35 36 37 38 39 40 41 42 43 44 45 46 47 48 49 50 51 52 53 54 55 56 57 58 59 60 61 62 63 64 65 66 67 68 69 70 71 72 73 74 75 76 77 78 **P**6 **S** Henry Ford Health System, Detroit, MI **Web address:** www.henryfordhealth.org	23	10	355	14410	221	—	1007	123979	65285	1584
ZEELAND—Ottawa County										
★ ZEELAND COMMUNITY HOSPITAL, 100 South Pine Street, Zip 49464–1619; tel. 616/772-4644; Henry A. Veenstra, President **A**1 9 10 **F**8 9 12 13 16 17 18 19 22 25 32 34 37 40 43 44 45 46 48 49 50 53 54 65 70 76 77 78 79 **P**4 7 8	23	10	57	2105	22	54203	298	19944	9249	286

MINNESOTA

Resident Population 4,725 (in thousands)
Resident population in metro areas 69.7%
Birth rate per 1,000 population 13.8
65 years and over 12.3%
Percent of persons without health insurance 9.2%

Hospital, Address, Telephone, Administrator, Approval, Facility, and Physician Codes, Health Care System, Network	Classi-fication Codes		Utilization Data					Expense (thousands) of dollars		
★ American Hospital Association (AHA) membership ☐ Joint Commission on Accreditation of Healthcare Organizations (JCAHO) accreditation + American Osteopathic Healthcare Association (AOHA) membership ○ American Osteopathic Association (AOA) accreditation △ Commission on Accreditation of Rehabilitation Facilities (CARF) accreditation Control codes 61, 63, 64, 71, 72 and 73 indicate hospitals listed by AOHA, but not registered by AHA. For definition of numerical codes, see page A4	Control	Service	Staffed Beds	Admissions	Census	Outpatient Visits	Births	Total	Payroll	Personnel
ADA—Norman County ★ BRIDGES MEDICAL SERVICES, 201 9th Street West, Zip 56510–0233, Mailing Address: P.O. Box 233, Zip 56510–0233; tel. 218/784–5000; Kyle Rasmussen, Administrator **A**9 10 **F**15 17 20 22 23 25 34 36 38 43 45 48 54 56 69 70 76 79 **P**6	14	10	8	440	3	8062	—	3210	1699	50
ADRIAN—Nobles County ★ ARNOLD MEMORIAL HEALTH CARE CENTER, 601 Louisiana Avenue, Zip 56110–0279, Mailing Address: P.O. Box 279, Zip 56110–0279; tel. 507/483–2668; Gerald E. Carl, Administrator (Total facility includes 41 beds in nursing home–type unit) (Nonreporting) **A**9 10 **S** Sioux Valley Hospitals and Health System, Sioux Falls, SD Web address: www.siouxvalley.org	15	10	50	—	—	—	—	—	—	—
AITKIN—Aitkin County ★ RIVERWOOD HEALTHCARE CENTER, 301 Minnesota Avenue South, Zip 56431–1697; tel. 218/927–2121; Debra Boardman, Chief Executive Officer (Total facility includes 48 beds in nursing home–type unit) **A**9 10 **F**1 8 9 12 17 18 19 22 25 30 31 32 36 37 41 44 45 46 48 54 69 70 71 72 75 76 **P**6 Web address: www.riverwoodhealthcarectr.com	23	10	70	1095	55	25297	54	13319	7004	200
ALBANY—Stearns County ★ ALBANY AREA HOSPITAL AND MEDICAL CENTER, 300 Third Avenue, Zip 56307–9363; tel. 320/845–2121; Ben Koppelman, Administrator **A**9 10 **F**7 8 9 17 18 19 22 25 34 36 37 38 44 45 48 54 70 72 76 **P**6 **S** Catholic Health Initiatives, Denver, CO	21	10	15	406	3	9644	62	4499	2098	79
ALBERT LEA—Freeborn County ✠ △ ALBERT LEA MEDICAL CENTER, 404 West Fountain Street, Zip 56007–2473; tel. 507/373–2384; Ronald A. Harmon, M.D., Chief Executive Officer (Total facility includes 61 beds in nursing home–type unit) (Nonreporting) **A**1 7 9 10 **S** Mayo Foundation, Rochester, MN	23	10	129	—	—	—	—	—	—	—
ALEXANDRIA—Douglas County ✠ DOUGLAS COUNTY HOSPITAL, 111 17th Avenue East, Zip 56308–3798; tel. 320/762–1511; William G. Flaig, Administrator **A**1 9 10 **F**3 7 8 9 16 17 20 22 24 25 27 32 33 35 36 37 38 39 40 41 44 45 46 48 50 54 59 60 61 63 64 70 71 72 75 76 78 Web address: www.dchospital.com	13	10	99	4577	50	49919	537	36296	16364	349
ANOKA—Anoka County ☐ ANOKA–METROPOLITAN REGIONAL TREATMENT CENTER, 3300 Fourth Avenue North, Zip 55303–1119; tel. 612/712–4000; Judith Krohn, Ph.D., Chief Executive Officer (Nonreporting) **A**1 10	12	22	247	—	—	—	—	—	—	—
APPLETON—Swift County APPLETON MUNICIPAL HOSPITAL AND NURSING HOME, 30 South Behl Street, Zip 56208–1699; tel. 320/289–2422; Mark E. Paulson, Administrator (Total facility includes 84 beds in nursing home–type unit) **A**9 10 **F**8 16 19 22 25 36 37 38 40 43 45 48 50 54 63 67 68 69 70 76 78 **P**7	14	10	104	375	83	5010	7	6117	2971	108
ARLINGTON—Sibley County ARLINGTON MUNICIPAL HOSPITAL, 601 West Chandler Street, Zip 55307; tel. 507/964–2271; Michael Schramm, Administrator **A**9 10 **F**1 17 22 25 32 36 39 40 48 54 56 70 76	14	10	17	341	4	4615	0	2935	1330	37
AURORA—St. Louis County ★ WHITE COMMUNITY HOSPITAL, 5211 Highway 110, Zip 55705–1599; tel. 218/229–2211; Larry Ravenberg, Administrator (Total facility includes 69 beds in nursing home–type unit) (Nonreporting) **A**9 10 Web address: www.whitech.org	23	10	85	—	—	—	—	—	—	—
AUSTIN—Mower County ☐ AUSTIN MEDICAL CENTER, 1000 First Drive N.W., Zip 55912–2904; tel. 507/437–4551; Timothy Johnson, M.D., President (Nonreporting) **A**1	23	10	108	—	—	—	—	—	—	—
BAGLEY—Clearwater County ★ CLEARWATER HEALTH SERVICES, 203 Fourth Street N.W., Zip 56621–8307, Mailing Address: Rural Route 3, Box 46, Zip 56621–0046; tel. 218/694–6501; Larry Laudon, Administrator (Total facility includes 70 beds in nursing home–type unit) (Nonreporting) **A**9 10 Web address: www.clearwaterhs.com	13	10	92	—	—	—	—	—	—	—
BAUDETTE—Lake of the Woods County ★ LAKEWOOD HEALTH CENTER, 600 Main Avenue South, Zip 56623; tel. 218/634–2120; SharRay Palm, President and Chief Executive Officer (Total facility includes 52 beds in nursing home–type unit) **A**9 10 **F**6 7 8 9 14 16 17 18 19 22 25 31 32 36 37 39 44 48 55 68 69 70 76 **S** Catholic Health Initiatives, Denver, CO	21	10	64	351	52	9836	32	6018	2867	111

Hospitals, U.S. / MINNESOTA

Hospital, Address, Telephone, Administrator, Approval, Facility, and Physician Codes, Health Care System, Network	Classification Codes		Utilization Data					Expense (thousands) of dollars		Personnel
	Control	Service	Staffed Beds	Admissions	Census	Outpatient Visits	Births	Total	Payroll	

★ American Hospital Association (AHA) membership
□ Joint Commission on Accreditation of Healthcare Organizations (JCAHO) accreditation
+ American Osteopathic Healthcare Association (AOHA) membership
○ American Osteopathic Association (AOA) accreditation
△ Commission on Accreditation of Rehabilitation Facilities (CARF) accreditation
Control codes 61, 63, 64, 71, 72 and 73 indicate hospitals listed by AOHA, but not registered by AHA. For definition of numerical codes, see page A4

BEMIDJI—Beltrami County
★ NORTH COUNTRY REGIONAL HOSPITAL, 1100 West 38th Street, Zip 56601–9972; tel. 218/751–5430; James F. Hanko, President and Chief Executive Officer (Total facility includes 78 beds in nursing home–type unit) **A**1 9 10 **F**6 7 8 9 13 16 17 18 19 22 24 25 26 27 29 32 33 34 36 37 39 41 43 44 45 48 50 51 53 54 67 69 70 72 76 78 **P**6
Web address: www.nchs.com
| | 23 | 10 | 163 | 5407 | 126 | 46692 | 827 | 42715 | 19218 | 520 |

BENSON—Swift County
★ SWIFT COUNTY–BENSON HOSPITAL, 1815 Wisconsin Avenue, Zip 56215–1653; tel. 320/843–4232; Frank Lawatsch, Chief Executive Officer **A**9 10 **F**7 8 9 19 22 25 31 32 34 36 37 38 39 40 41 43 44 45 46 48 53 54 57 63 67 72 76 77 **P**6
| | 16 | 10 | 17 | 477 | 5 | — | 18 | 3978 | 1716 | 62 |

BIGFORK—Itasca County
★ NORTHERN ITASCA HEALTH CARE CENTER, 258 Pine Tree Drive, Zip 56628, Mailing Address: P.O. Box 258, Zip 56628–0258; tel. 218/743–3177; Richard M. Ash, Chief Executive Officer (Total facility includes 40 beds in nursing home–type unit) (Nonreporting) **A**9 10
Web address: www.nihcc.com
| | 16 | 10 | 56 | — | — | — | — | — | — | — |

BLUE EARTH—Faribault County
★ UNITED HOSPITAL DISTRICT, 515 South Moore Street, Zip 56013–2158, Mailing Address: P.O. Box 160, Zip 56013–0160; tel. 507/526–3273; Chad Cooper, Administrator (Nonreporting) **A**1 9 10 **S** Allina Health System, Minneapolis, MN
Web address: www.uhd.org
| | 16 | 10 | 43 | — | — | — | — | — | — | — |

BRAINERD—Crow Wing County
□ BRAINERD REGIONAL HUMAN SERVICES CENTER, 1777 Highway 18 East, Zip 56401–7389; tel. 218/828–2201; Harvey G. Caldwell, Administrator and Chief Executive Officer (Nonreporting) **A**1 10
| | 12 | 22 | 288 | — | — | — | — | — | — | — |

□ ST. JOSEPH'S MEDICAL CENTER, 523 North Third Street, Zip 56401–3098; tel. 218/829–2861; Thomas K. Prusak, President **A**1 9 10 **F**2 3 7 8 9 12 13 17 18 22 24 25 32 33 34 35 36 37 38 39 43 44 45 46 48 51 53 54 57 58 59 60 61 63 64 65 70 71 72 76 78 **S** Benedictine Health System, Duluth, MN
Web address: www.stjosephsmedicalctr.com
| | 21 | 10 | 152 | 6420 | 78 | 108278 | 643 | 51176 | 22247 | 535 |

BRECKENRIDGE—Wilkin County
★ ST. FRANCIS MEDICAL CENTER, 415 Oak Street, Zip 56520–1298; tel. 218/643–3000; David A. Nelson, President and Chief Executive Officer (Total facility includes 124 beds in nursing home–type unit) (Nonreporting) **A**1 9 10 **S** Catholic Health Initiatives, Denver, CO
| | 21 | 10 | 171 | — | — | — | — | — | — | — |

BUFFALO—Wright County
★ BUFFALO HOSPITAL, 303 Catlin Street, Zip 55313–1947; tel. 612/682–7180; Mary Ellen Wells, Administrator **A**1 9 10 **F**2 4 7 8 9 10 11 12 13 14 16 17 18 19 22 25 26 29 30 34 36 37 39 41 42 44 45 46 48 49 51 52 53 54 57 58 59 60 61 62 63 64 65 71 72 75 76 77 78 **P**5 6 **S** Allina Health System, Minneapolis, MN
Web address: www.allina.com
| | 23 | 10 | 30 | 2074 | 16 | 37163 | 482 | 18480 | 9077 | 200 |

BURNSVILLE—Dakota County
★ FAIRVIEW RIDGES HOSPITAL, 201 East Nicollet Boulevard, Zip 55337–5799; tel. 612/892–2000; Mark M. Enger, Senior Vice President and Administrator **A**1 9 10 **F**3 7 8 9 16 17 19 22 24 25 26 33 37 38 39 41 42 43 44 45 46 48 50 51 54 70 71 72 76 78 **P**1 6 **S** Fairview Health Services, Minneapolis, MN
Web address: www.fairview.org
| | 23 | 10 | 127 | 10805 | 89 | 74024 | 3148 | 52936 | 27413 | 536 |

CAMBRIDGE—Isanti County
★ CAMBRIDGE MEDICAL CENTER, 701 South Dellwood Street, Zip 55008–1920; tel. 763/689–7700; Dennis J. Doran, Administrator **A**1 9 10 **F**2 3 7 8 9 12 13 17 18 19 22 23 24 25 26 30 34 35 36 37 38 39 40 43 44 45 46 48 49 50 51 54 56 57 59 60 61 62 63 65 67 70 71 72 75 76 77 78 **P**8 **S** Allina Health System, Minneapolis, MN
| | 23 | 10 | 81 | 3682 | 44 | 244259 | 461 | 53856 | 27466 | 567 |

CANBY—Yellow Medicine County
★ SIOUX VALLEY CANBY CAMPUS, (Includes Senior Haven Convalescent Nursing Center), 112 St. Olaf Avenue South, Zip 56220–1433; tel. 507/223–7277; Robert J. Salmon, Chief Executive Officer (Total facility includes 75 beds in nursing home–type unit) **A**9 10 **F**7 8 9 17 18 19 22 23 25 28 30 31 32 34 36 37 39 41 43 44 46 54 67 68 69 70 76 77 78 **P**6 **S** Sioux Valley Hospitals and Health System, Sioux Falls, SD
Web address: www.siouxvalley.org
| | 23 | 10 | 94 | 560 | 79 | 7071 | 26 | 8213 | 4362 | 185 |

CANNON FALLS—Goodhue County
★ COMMUNITY HOSPITAL, 1116 West Mill Street, Zip 55009–1898; tel. 507/263–4221; Randy Ulseth, Administrator **A**9 10 **F**7 9 13 17 18 19 20 22 25 26 28 30 31 33 34 36 37 38 43 45 48 53 54 69 71 76 77
| | 16 | 10 | 14 | 430 | 4 | 4621 | 0 | 4312 | 2036 | 63 |

CASS LAKE—Cass County
★ U. S. PUBLIC HEALTH SERVICE INDIAN HOSPITAL, 7th Street and Grant Utley Avenue N.W., Zip 56633, Mailing Address: Rural Route 3, Box 211, Zip 56633; tel. 218/335–2293; Luella Brown, Service Unit Director (Nonreporting) **A**1 10 **S** U. S. Public Health Service Indian Health Service, Rockville, MD
| | 47 | 10 | 13 | — | — | — | — | — | — | — |

CLOQUET—Carlton County
★ CLOQUET COMMUNITY MEMORIAL HOSPITAL, 512 Skyline Boulevard, Zip 55720–1199; tel. 218/879–4641; James J. Carroll, Administrator (Total facility includes 88 beds in nursing home–type unit) **A**9 10 **F**8 9 13 22 25 32 34 36 38 39 40 41 43 44 45 46 48 50 51 54 69 70 72 76 77 78 **P**3 8
| | 23 | 10 | 124 | 1223 | 96 | 25915 | 112 | 14399 | 7409 | 227 |

Hospitals, U.S. / MINNESOTA

Hospital, Address, Telephone, Administrator, Approval, Facility, and Physician Codes, Health Care System, Network

★ American Hospital Association (AHA) membership
□ Joint Commission on Accreditation of Healthcare Organizations (JCAHO) accreditation
+ American Osteopathic Healthcare Association (AOHA) membership
○ American Osteopathic Association (AOA) accreditation
△ Commission on Accreditation of Rehabilitation Facilities (CARF) accreditation
Control codes 61, 63, 64, 71, 72 and 73 indicate hospitals listed by AOHA, but not registered by AHA. For definition of numerical codes, see page A4

Hospital	Control	Service	Staffed Beds	Admissions	Census	Outpatient Visits	Births	Total	Payroll	Personnel
COOK—St. Louis County COOK HOSPITAL AND CONVALESCENT NURSING CARE UNIT, 10 Fifth Street S.E., Zip 55723–9745; tel. 218/666–5945; Allen J. Vogt, Administrator (Total facility includes 41 beds in nursing home–type unit) A9 10 F1 7 9 16 17 18 19 25 28 30 37 38 45 54 58 59 60 63 69 70 71 76 78 P5	16	10	55	385	46	11854	0	4649	2451	86
COON RAPIDS—Anoka County ★ MERCY HOSPITAL, 4050 Coon Rapids Boulevard, Zip 55433–2586; tel. 763/421–8888; Marvin L. Dehne, Executive Officer A1 9 10 F2 3 4 7 8 9 11 12 13 17 18 19 20 22 24 25 26 27 28 31 33 34 36 37 39 40 41 43 44 45 46 47 48 49 51 53 54 56 57 58 61 63 64 66 69 70 72 73 74 75 76 77 78 79 S Allina Health System, Minneapolis, MN Web address: www.allina.com	23	10	198	12817	127	118403	2259	137250	59463	1475
CROOKSTON—Polk County ★ RIVERVIEW HEALTHCARE ASSOCIATION, 323 South Minnesota Street, Zip 56716–1600; tel. 218/281–9200; Thomas C. Lenertz, President and Chief Executive Officer (Total facility includes 162 beds in nursing home–type unit) A1 9 10 F1 2 3 6 7 8 9 15 17 18 22 23 33 34 36 37 39 40 41 44 45 46 48 51 54 61 69 70 71 72 75 76 78 P5 Web address: www.riverviewhealth.org	23	10	234	1801	168	22894	136	17956	9823	347
CROSBY—Crow Wing County ★ CUYUNA REGIONAL MEDICAL CENTER, 320 East Main Street, Zip 56441–1690; tel. 218/546–7000; Thomas F. Reek, Chief Executive Officer (Total facility includes 130 beds in nursing home–type unit) A9 10 F6 8 9 17 18 22 25 30 32 34 35 36 37 38 39 41 44 45 46 48 69 70 71 76 78 P8	16	10	160	1499	136	53110	165	20105	9931	308
DAWSON—Lac Qui Parle County JOHNSON MEMORIAL HEALTH SERVICES, 1282 Walnut Street, Zip 56232–2333; tel. 320/769–4323; Vern Silvernale, Administrator (Total facility includes 70 beds in nursing home–type unit) (Nonreporting) A9 10	16	10	94	—	—	—	—	—	—	—
DEER RIVER—Itasca County ★ DEER RIVER HEALTHCARE CENTER, 1002 Comstock Drive, Zip 56636–9700; tel. 218/246–2900; Jeffry Stampohar, Chief Executive Officer (Total facility includes 50 beds in nursing home–type unit) A9 10 F1 6 7 8 9 11 12 17 18 19 20 22 26 30 31 32 34 36 37 38 44 45 48 49 53 54 67 69 70 75 76 78 P6	23	10	70	548	4	3025	45	4128	—	146
DETROIT LAKES—Becker County ★ ST. MARY'S REGIONAL HEALTH CENTER, 1027 Washington Avenue, Zip 56501–3598; tel. 218/847–5611; Thomas R. Thompson, Chief Executive Officer (Total facility includes 100 beds in nursing home–type unit) A1 9 10 F7 8 11 13 17 18 19 22 24 25 30 31 32 34 36 37 38 39 41 43 44 45 46 48 51 54 65 67 69 70 71 72 74 76 78 79 S Benedictine Health System, Duluth, MN Web address: www.stmaryshealthcenter.com	21	10	163	2228	109	11681	365	15683	7098	236
DULUTH—St. Louis County ★ △ MILLER DWAN MEDICAL CENTER, 502 East Second Street, Zip 55805–1982; tel. 218/727–8762; William H. Palmer, President A1 2 7 9 10 F2 3 6 10 16 17 18 19 21 22 27 29 30 32 35 38 39 41 43 45 46 48 49 51 53 54 57 58 60 61 62 63 64 65 70 72 76 78 P5 Web address: www.miller-dwan.com	23	10	152	3570	76	83444	0	53708	26411	680
★ △ ST. LUKE'S HOSPITAL, 915 East First Street, Zip 55805–2193; tel. 218/726–5555; John Strange, President and Chief Executive Officer A1 2 3 5 7 9 10 F3 4 8 9 11 12 16 17 19 20 21 22 23 24 25 26 27 32 34 36 37 38 39 41 44 45 46 47 48 49 51 53 54 57 58 61 62 64 66 68 70 72 74 75 76 77 78 P1 Web address: www.slhduluth.com	23	10	242	8140	108	66638	824	95901	42696	1327
★ ST. MARY'S MEDICAL CENTER, 407 East Third Street, Zip 55805–1984; tel. 218/786–4000; Sister Kathleen Hofer, President A1 2 3 5 9 10 F2 3 4 5 6 7 8 9 10 11 12 16 17 18 19 21 22 23 24 25 26 27 28 31 32 33 34 35 36 37 38 39 40 41 42 43 44 46 47 48 49 50 52 53 54 56 57 58 59 60 61 62 63 64 65 66 67 68 69 70 71 72 75 76 77 78 P6 S Benedictine Health System, Duluth, MN Web address: www.smdc.org	23	10	288	16190	202	83047	1483	155948	68009	1939
ELBOW LAKE—Grant County ★ GRANT COUNTY HEALTH CENTER, 930 First Street N.E., Zip 56531–4699; tel. 218/685–4461; Larry Rapp, M.D., Chief Medical and Executive Officer (Nonreporting) A9 10	23	10	15	—	—	—	—	—	—	—
ELY—St. Louis County ★ ELY–BLOOMENSON COMMUNITY HOSPITAL, 328 West Conan Street, Zip 55731–1198; tel. 218/365–3271; John Fossum, Administrator (Total facility includes 99 beds in nursing home–type unit) A9 10 F1 7 8 9 12 15 17 19 20 22 23 24 25 36 37 38 39 40 44 48 54 69 70 72 76 77 78 P6	23	10	125	738	107	7284	37	10216	5600	183
FAIRMONT—Martin County ★ FAIRMONT COMMUNITY HOSPITAL, (Includes Lutz Wing Convalescent and Nursing Care Unit), 835 Johnson Street, Zip 56031, Mailing Address: P.O. Box 835, Zip 56031–0835; tel. 507/238–8100; Gerry Gilbertson, Administrator (Total facility includes 40 beds in nursing home–type unit) A1 9 10 F6 7 8 9 16 17 18 19 21 23 24 32 33 36 37 38 39 41 44 45 46 48 49 50 51 54 58 59 61 62 63 65 66 68 69 70 71 72 76 77 78	23	10	92	2033	58	36209	263	19672	9132	279
FARIBAULT—Rice County ★ DISTRICT ONE HOSPITAL, 631 S.E. First Street, Zip 55021–6345; tel. 507/334–6451; James N. Wolf, Chief Executive Officer A1 9 10 F7 8 9 17 19 22 24 25 26 32 34 37 38 39 40 41 43 44 45 46 48 53 54 70 71 72 76 77 78 79	16	10	52	2169	21	37711	437	19838	8057	212

Hospitals, U.S. / MINNESOTA

Hospital, Address, Telephone, Administrator, Approval, Facility, and Physician Codes, Health Care System, Network	Classification Codes		Utilization Data					Expense (thousands) of dollars		
	Control	Service	Staffed Beds	Admissions	Census	Outpatient Visits	Births	Total	Payroll	Personnel

★ American Hospital Association (AHA) membership
☐ Joint Commission on Accreditation of Healthcare Organizations (JCAHO) accreditation
+ American Osteopathic Healthcare Association (AOHA) membership
○ American Osteopathic Association (AOA) accreditation
△ Commission on Accreditation of Rehabilitation Facilities (CARF) accreditation
Control codes 61, 63, 64, 71, 72 and 73 indicate hospitals listed by AOHA, but not registered by AHA. For definition of numerical codes, see page A4

Hospital	Control	Service	Staffed Beds	Admissions	Census	Outpatient Visits	Births	Total	Payroll	Personnel
☐ WILSON CENTER PSYCHIATRIC FACILITY FOR CHILDREN AND ADOLESCENTS, 1800 14th Street N.E., Zip 55021, Mailing Address: P.O. Box 917, Zip 55021–0917; tel. 507/334–5561; Janine Sahagian, Administrator and Chief Executive Officer (Nonreporting) **A**1	33	22	50	—	—	—	—	—	—	—
FARMINGTON—Dakota County										
✠ TRINITY HOSPITAL, 3410–213th Street West, Zip 55024–1197; tel. 651/463–7825; David A. Grundstrom, Chief Executive Officer (Total facility includes 65 beds in nursing home–type unit) **A**1 9 10 **F**6 7 8 9 17 18 22 25 26 30 32 33 36 37 38 44 45 46 48 50 51 54 56 67 69 70 72 76 77 78 **P**6 **S** Benedictine Health System, Duluth, MN	23	10	85	328	67	2836	16	9614	4103	121
FERGUS FALLS—Otter Tail County										
☐ FERGUS FALLS REGIONAL TREATMENT CENTER, 1400 North Union Avenue, Zip 56537–1200; tel. 218/739–7200; Cynthia Skorick, Chief Executive Officer (Nonreporting) **A**1 10	12	22	281	—	—	—	—	—	—	—
✠ LAKE REGION HEALTHCARE CORPORATION, 712 South Cascade Street, Zip 56537–2900, Mailing Address: P.O. Box 728, Zip 56538–0728; tel. 218/736–8000; Edward J. Mehl, Chief Executive Officer (Total facility includes 44 beds in nursing home–type unit) **A**1 9 10 **F**8 17 22 24 25 36 38 39 41 44 45 48 54 57 58 59 60 61 62 69 70 71 72 76 78 Web address: www.lrhc.org	23	10	136	3550	79	34536	345	29828	15004	417
FOSSTON—Polk County										
★ FIRST CARE MEDICAL SERVICES, 900 South Hilligoss Boulevard East, Zip 56542–1599; tel. 218/435–1133; Patricia Wangler, Chief Executive Officer (Total facility includes 50 beds in nursing home–type unit) **A**9 10 **F**8 9 16 18 22 25 26 28 31 34 36 37 38 39 40 44 45 48 54 69 70 72 76 Web address: www.firstcare.org	23	10	72	525	53	45110	33	8145	3700	160
FRIDLEY—Anoka County										
★ UNITY HOSPITAL, 550 Osborne Road N.E., Zip 55432–2799; tel. 763/421–2222 **A**2 9 **F**2 3 4 7 8 9 11 12 13 17 18 19 20 22 24 25 26 27 28 31 33 34 36 37 38 39 40 41 43 44 45 46 47 48 49 51 53 54 56 57 58 61 63 64 66 69 70 72 74 75 76 77 78 79 **S** Allina Health System, Minneapolis, MN Web address: www.allina.com	23	10	201	11632	118	72326	1832	105634	46423	1046
GLENCOE—McLeod County										
★ GLENCOE REGIONAL HEALTH SERVICES, (Formerly Glencoe Area Health Center), 705 East 18th Street, Zip 55336–1499; tel. 320/864–3121; Jon D. Braband, President and Chief Executive Officer (Total facility includes 110 beds in nursing home–type unit) **A**9 10 **F**1 6 7 8 9 12 17 18 19 22 24 25 30 31 32 34 36 37 38 39 41 44 45 46 48 49 54 67 69 70 72 76 78 **P**5 **S** HealthSystem Minnesota, Saint Louis Park, MN Web address: www.glencoeregionalhealth.org	14	10	149	1418	120	15310	136	16944	7872	278
GLENWOOD—Pope County										
★ GLACIAL RIDGE HOSPITAL AND HEALTHCARE SERVICES, 10 Fourth Avenue S.E., Zip 56334–1898; tel. 320/634–4521; Douglas J. Reker, Administrator and Chief Executive Officer **A**9 10 **F**7 8 9 16 17 19 22 24 25 28 32 33 34 36 37 38 39 41 44 45 46 48 54 70 72 75 76 78 **P**6 Web address: www.runestone.net/~grh	16	10	19	561	6	9708	36	4348	2167	103
GOLDEN VALLEY—Hennepin County										
✠ VENCOR HOSPITAL–MINNEAPOLIS, 4101 Golden Valley Road, Zip 55422; tel. 612/588–2750; Thomas N. Theroult, Administrator (Nonreporting) **A**1 9 10 **S** Vencor, Incorporated, Louisville, KY	33	10	111	—	—	—	—	—	—	—
GRACEVILLE—Big Stone County										
GRACEVILLE HEALTH CENTER, 115 West Second Street, Zip 56240–0157, Mailing Address: P.O. Box 157, Zip 56240–0157; tel. 320/748–7223; Helen Jorve, Chief Executive Officer (Total facility includes 60 beds in nursing home–type unit) (Nonreporting) **A**9 10 **S** Missionary Benedictine Sisters American Province, Norfolk, NE	23	10	92	—	—	—	—	—	—	—
GRAND MARAIS—Cook County										
COOK COUNTY NORTH SHORE HOSPITAL, Gunflint Trail, Zip 55604, Mailing Address: P.O. Box 10, Zip 55604–0010; tel. 218/387–3040; Diane Pearson, Administrator (Total facility includes 47 beds in nursing home–type unit) **A**9 10 **F**8 9 12 22 24 25 31 36 41 44 53 54 69 70 76 **P**8	16	10	59	349	47	—	28	5874	3096	94
GRAND RAPIDS—Itasca County										
✠ ITASCA MEDICAL CENTER, 126 First Avenue S.E., Zip 55744–3698; tel. 218/326–3401; Gary Kenner, President and Chief Executive Officer (Total facility includes 35 beds in nursing home–type unit) **A**1 9 10 **F**1 7 8 9 12 17 19 22 24 25 30 36 38 39 41 43 44 45 46 48 51 54 61 68 69 70 71 72 76 78 79 **S** Benedictine Health System, Duluth, MN	23	10	84	2520	56	28644	340	22193	10491	281
GRANITE FALLS—Yellow Medicine County										
✠ GRANITE FALLS MUNICIPAL HOSPITAL AND MANOR, 345 Tenth Avenue, Zip 56241–1499; tel. 320/564–3111; George Gerlach, Administrator (Total facility includes 64 beds in nursing home–type unit) (Nonreporting) **A**1 9 10 **S** Allina Health System, Minneapolis, MN	14	10	87	—	—	—	—	—	—	—
HALLOCK—Kittson County										
★ KITTSON MEMORIAL HEALTHCARE CENTER, 1010 South Birch Street, Zip 56728, Mailing Address: P.O. Box 700, Zip 56728–0700; tel. 218/843–3612; Richard J. Failing, Chief Executive Officer (Total facility includes 88 beds in nursing home–type unit) **A**9 10 **F**9 12 22 24 25 30 36 37 39 41 44 48 53 54 69 76 **P**1	23	10	109	271	81	6641	19	5661	2932	141

Hospitals, U.S. / MINNESOTA

Hospital, Address, Telephone, Administrator, Approval, Facility, and Physician Codes, Health Care System, Network	Classification Codes		Utilization Data					Expense (thousands) of dollars		
★ American Hospital Association (AHA) membership ☐ Joint Commission on Accreditation of Healthcare Organizations (JCAHO) accreditation + American Osteopathic Healthcare Association (AOHA) membership ○ American Osteopathic Association (AOA) accreditation △ Commission on Accreditation of Rehabilitation Facilities (CARF) accreditation Control codes 61, 63, 64, 71, 72 and 73 indicate hospitals listed by AOHA, but not registered by AHA. For definition of numerical codes, see page A4	Control	Service	Staffed Beds	Admissions	Census	Outpatient Visits	Births	Total	Payroll	Personnel
HASTINGS—Dakota County ☐ REGINA MEDICAL CENTER, 1175 Nininger Road, Zip 55033–1098; tel. 651/480–4100; Stewart Laird, Interim Chief Executive Officer (Total facility includes 61 beds in nursing home–type unit) (Nonreporting) **A**1 9 10 **Web address:** www.reginamedical.com	23	10	118	—	—	—	—	—	—	—
HENDRICKS—Lincoln County ★ HENDRICKS COMMUNITY HOSPITAL, 503 East Lincoln Street, Zip 56136–0106; tel. 507/275–3134; Kirk Stensrud, Administrator (Total facility includes 70 beds in nursing home–type unit) **A**9 10 **F**1 6 8 9 12 13 17 18 19 22 23 25 26 28 32 35 36 37 38 39 41 44 45 46 48 53 54 67 68 69 70 76 78 **P**5	23	10	84	389	70	6453	27	4789	2461	111
HIBBING—St. Louis County ✠ UNIVERSITY MEDICAL CENTER-MESABI, 750 East 34th Street, Zip 55746–4600; tel. 218/262–4881; Richard W. Dinter, M.D., Chief Operating Officer (Nonreporting) **A**1 9 10 **S** Fairview Health Services, Minneapolis, MN	23	10	132	—	—	—	—	—	—	—
HUTCHINSON—McLeod County ✠ HUTCHINSON AREA HEALTH CARE, 1095 Highway 15 South, Zip 55350–3182; tel. 320/234–5000; Philip G. Graves, Administrator (Total facility includes 127 beds in nursing home–type unit) (Nonreporting) **A**1 9 10 **S** Allina Health System, Minneapolis, MN	14	10	187	—	—	—	—	—	—	—
INTERNATIONAL FALLS—Koochiching County ✠ FALLS MEMORIAL HOSPITAL, 1400 Highway 71, Zip 56649–2189; tel. 218/283–4481; Mary Klimp, Administrator and Chief Executive Officer **A**1 9 10 **F**7 8 9 12 13 16 17 18 19 22 25 32 34 39 41 44 45 48 51 53 54 61 69 76 77 78 **S** Quorum Health Group, Brentwood, TN	23	10	35	960	8	23626	126	7741	3146	92
IVANHOE—Lincoln County ★ DIVINE PROVIDENCE HEALTH CENTER/AVERA HEALTH, 312 East George Street, Zip 56142–0136, Mailing Address: P.O. Box 136, Zip 56142–0136; tel. 507/694–1414; Patrick Branco, Administrator (Total facility includes 51 beds in nursing home–type unit) (Nonreporting) **A**9 10 **S** Avera Health, Yankton, SD	23	10	79	—	—	—	—	—	—	—
JACKSON—Jackson County ★ JACKSON MEDICAL CENTER, 1430 North Highway, Zip 56143–1098; tel. 507/847–2420; Charlotte Heitkamp, Chief Executive Officer (Total facility includes 21 beds in nursing home–type unit) **A**9 10 **F**1 7 22 25 37 48 63 69 76 **P**6 **S** Sioux Valley Hospitals and Health System, Sioux Falls, SD	23	10	41	448	24	10044	0	3093	1620	69
LAKE CITY—Wabasha County ✠ LAKE CITY MEDICAL CENTER, 904 South Lakeshore Drive, Zip 55041–1899; tel. 651/345–3321; Mark Rinehardt, Administrator (Total facility includes 97 beds in nursing home–type unit) **A**1 9 10 **F**3 7 8 9 17 18 19 22 24 25 26 30 36 37 40 44 48 51 54 69 70 76 78	23	10	115	610	102	6365	57	9162	4762	175
LE SUEUR—Le Sueur County MINNESOTA VALLEY HEALTH CENTER, (Includes Gardenview Nursing Home), 621 South Fourth Street, Zip 56058–2298; tel. 507/665–3375; Jerry Boerboom, Chief Executive Officer (Total facility includes 85 beds in nursing home–type unit) **A**9 10 **F**1 7 8 9 12 17 18 19 22 25 26 33 34 37 38 39 40 44 45 46 48 54 69 70 72 76 78 **P**3	23	10	102	170	82	12433	16	5317	2834	134
LITCHFIELD—Meeker County ★ MEEKER COUNTY MEMORIAL HOSPITAL, 612 South Sibley Avenue, Zip 55355–3398; tel. 320/693–3242; Ronald E. Johnson, Administrator **A**9 10 **F**7 8 9 17 18 22 24 25 30 32 33 34 38 39 41 44 46 48 50 54 68 70 72 76	13	10	38	1378	14	17987	192	8836	3962	112
LITTLE FALLS—Morrison County ✠ ST. GABRIEL'S HOSPITAL, 815 Second Street S.E., Zip 56345–3596; tel. 320/632–5441; Larry A. Schulz, President and Chief Executive Officer (Total facility includes 150 beds in nursing home–type unit) **A**1 9 10 **F**1 3 6 7 8 9 13 17 18 19 22 24 25 26 30 31 32 34 35 36 37 38 39 41 43 44 45 46 48 49 50 51 54 58 59 60 62 63 64 67 68 69 70 71 72 76 77 78 **S** Catholic Health Initiatives, Denver, CO **Web address:** www.stgabriels.com	21	10	199	1904	160	55000	243	27221	12325	425
LONG PRAIRIE—Todd County ✠ LONG PRAIRIE MEMORIAL HOSPITAL AND HOME, 20 Ninth Street S.E., Zip 56347–1404; tel. 320/732–2141; Clayton R. Peterson, President (Total facility includes 105 beds in nursing home–type unit) **A**9 10 **F**1 8 9 12 16 17 18 22 25 31 32 36 37 38 39 40 44 45 48 54 69 70 78 **P**3 **S** CentraCare, Long Prairie, MN	23	10	117	671	106	—	90	8989	4264	152
LUVERNE—Rock County ★ LUVERNE COMMUNITY HOSPITAL, 305 East Luverne Street, Zip 56156–2519, Mailing Address: P.O. Box 1019, Zip 56156–1019; tel. 507/283–2321; Gerald E. Carl, Administrator (Nonreporting) **A**9 10 **S** Sioux Valley Hospitals and Health System, Sioux Falls, SD **Web address:** www.siouxvalley.org	14	10	38	—	—	—	—	—	—	—
MADELIA—Watonwan County ✠ MADELIA COMMUNITY HOSPITAL, 121 Drew Avenue S.E., Zip 56062–1899; tel. 507/642–3255; Candace Fenske, Administrator **A**1 9 10 **F**7 8 9 16 17 18 19 22 23 25 32 36 37 38 39 40 44 45 48 50 54 70 76 **P**5	23	10	25	509	6	4396	42	2998	1437	51
MADISON—Lac Qui Parle County MADISON HOSPITAL, 820 Third Avenue, Zip 56256–1014, Mailing Address: P.O. Box 184, Zip 56256–0184; tel. 320/598–7556; Thomas Richter, Chief Executive Officer **A**9 10 **F**8 9 22 25 32 34 35 37 38 39 40 44 48 54 70 76	23	10	13	345	3	—	8	1971	795	30

Hospitals, U.S. / MINNESOTA

Hospital, Address, Telephone, Administrator, Approval, Facility, and Physician Codes, Health Care System, Network	Classification Codes		Utilization Data					Expense (thousands) of dollars		
★ American Hospital Association (AHA) membership ☐ Joint Commission on Accreditation of Healthcare Organizations (JCAHO) accreditation + American Osteopathic Healthcare Association (AOHA) membership ○ American Osteopathic Association (AOA) accreditation △ Commission on Accreditation of Rehabilitation Facilities (CARF) accreditation Control codes 61, 63, 64, 71, 72 and 73 indicate hospitals listed by AOHA, but not registered by AHA. For definition of numerical codes, see page A4	Control	Service	Staffed Beds	Admissions	Census	Outpatient Visits	Births	Total	Payroll	Personnel

MAHNOMEN—Mahnomen County

MAHNOMEN HEALTH CENTER, 414 Jefferson Avenue, Zip 56557, Mailing Address: P.O. Box 396, Zip 56557–0396; tel. 218/935–2511; Charlotte Whittey, Chief Executive Officer (Total facility includes 48 beds in nursing home–type unit) (Nonreporting) **A**9 10 18	23	10	66	—	—	—	—	—	—	—

MANKATO—Blue Earth County

★ IMMANUEL ST. JOSEPH'S–MAYO HEALTH SYSTEM, 1025 Marsh Street, Zip 56002–4700, Mailing Address: P.O. Box 8673, Zip 56002–8673; tel. 507/625–4031; W. Neath Folger, M.D., President and Chief Executive Officer **A**1 2 3 5 9 10 **F**2 3 4 7 8 9 11 13 17 18 19 22 23 24 25 26 27 32 33 34 35 36 37 38 39 41 43 44 45 46 48 49 50 54 57 58 59 60 61 62 63 64 65 68 70 72 76 78 79 **P**6 8 **S** Mayo Foundation, Rochester, MN
Web address: www.isj-mhs.net/isjmhs.html
— 23 10 147 7891 91 73659 1203 67932 33994 839

MAPLEWOOD—Ramsey County

★ ST. JOHN'S HOSPITAL, (Formerly HealthEast St. John's Hospital), 1575 Beam Avenue, Zip 55109; tel. 651/232–7000; Douglas P. Cropper, Vice President and Administrator (Nonreporting) **A**3 5 9 10 **S** HealthEast, Saint Paul, MN
Web address: www.healtheast.org
— 23 10 150 — — — — — — —

MARSHALL—Lyon County

★ WEINER MEMORIAL MEDICAL CENTER, 300 South Bruce Street, Zip 56258–3900; tel. 507/532–9661; Richard G. Slieter, Jr, Administrator (Total facility includes 76 beds in nursing home–type unit) **A**1 9 10 **F**1 6 7 8 9 12 13 16 17 18 19 22 24 25 26 28 30 31 32 33 35 36 37 38 39 41 43 44 45 46 48 50 51 53 54 55 61 62 63 69 70 72 76 78
Web address: www.wmmc.org
— 14 10 125 1788 91 18209 412 18350 9198 246

MELROSE—Stearns County

MELROSE AREA HOSPITAL, 11 North Fifth Avenue West, Zip 56352–1098; tel. 320/256–4231; Joan Jackson, Administrator (Total facility includes 75 beds in nursing home–type unit) **A**9 10 **F**1 8 9 16 17 18 19 22 23 25 26 30 31 36 37 38 39 40 41 43 44 45 48 54 56 62 63 67 69 70 71 72 76 **P**5 **S** CentraCare, Long Prairie, MN
— 23 10 87 559 78 9372 60 3522 1858 57

MINNEAPOLIS—Hennepin County

★ △ ABBOTT NORTHWESTERN HOSPITAL, (Includes Sister Kenny Institute), 800 East 28th Street, Zip 55407–3799; tel. 612/863–4000; Mark Dixon, Administrator **A**1 2 3 5 7 9 10 **F**3 4 5 7 8 9 11 12 13 15 17 18 19 20 22 24 25 26 27 28 29 30 31 32 33 34 35 36 37 38 39 41 43 44 45 46 47 48 49 50 51 54 55 56 57 58 59 60 61 62 63 64 65 66 68 69 70 71 72 73 74 76 77 78 79 **P**5 8 **S** Allina Health System, Minneapolis, MN
Web address: www.allina.com
— 23 10 642 33739 465 — 3225 417762 176955 3536

☐ CHILDREN'S HOSPITALS AND CLINICS, MINNEAPOLIS, (PEDIATRIC), 2525 Chicago Avenue South, Zip 55404–9976; tel. 612/813–6100; Brock D. Nelson, Chief Executive Officer **A**1 2 3 9 10 **F**4 11 13 14 17 18 19 22 23 24 25 26 27 29 31 33 34 35 36 37 38 39 42 43 45 46 47 48 49 50 51 52 53 54 55 56 58 59 60 61 63 65 68 70 72 73 75 76 78 **P**1
Web address: www.childrenshc.org
— 23 59 163 6971 126 68166 0 137875 69315 —

FAIRVIEW RIVERSIDE HOSPITAL See Fairview–University Medical Center

★ FAIRVIEW SOUTHDALE HOSPITAL, 6401 France Avenue South, Zip 55435–2199; tel. 612/924–5000; Mark M. Enger, Senior Vice President and Administrator **A**1 9 10 **F**1 2 3 4 8 12 13 16 17 18 19 22 24 25 27 30 31 32 33 34 36 37 38 39 40 41 42 43 44 45 46 47 48 49 50 51 54 55 57 58 62 63 64 65 67 69 70 71 72 74 75 76 77 78 79 **P**1 6 **S** Fairview Health Services, Minneapolis, MN
Web address: www.fairview.org
— 23 10 348 21080 232 105561 3507 146086 73902 1645

★ FAIRVIEW–UNIVERSITY MEDICAL CENTER, (Includes Fairview Riverside Hospital, 2312 South Sixth Street, Zip 55454; St. Mary's Hospital and Rehabilitation Center, 2414 South Seventh Street, Zip 55454; tel. 612/338–2229; University of Minnesota Hospital and Clinic, 420 S.E. Delaware Street, Box 502, Zip 55455–0392; tel. 612/626–3000), 2450 Riverside Avenue, Zip 55454–1400; tel. 612/672–6000; Gordon L. Alexander, M.D., Senior Vice President and Chief Executive Officer (Total facility includes 80 beds in nursing home–type unit) **A**1 2 5 6 8 9 10 **F**1 2 3 4 6 7 8 9 10 11 12 13 15 16 17 18 19 20 21 22 23 24 25 26 27 30 31 32 33 34 35 36 37 38 39 40 41 42 43 44 45 46 47 48 49 50 51 52 53 54 55 57 58 59 60 62 63 64 65 67 69 70 71 72 73 74 75 76 77 78 79 **S** Fairview Health Services, Minneapolis, MN
Web address: www.fairview.org
— 23 10 1028 35311 609 404180 4349 504279 192376 6457

★ △ HENNEPIN COUNTY MEDICAL CENTER, 701 Park Avenue South, Zip 55415–1829; tel. 612/347–2121; Jeff Spartz, Administrator **A**1 2 3 5 7 8 9 10 **F**3 4 7 8 9 10 11 12 13 14 15 16 17 19 20 21 22 23 24 25 26 27 29 30 31 32 33 34 35 36 37 38 39 41 42 43 44 45 46 47 48 49 50 51 52 53 54 55 56 57 58 59 60 61 62 63 64 65 66 70 71 72 75 76 77 78 79 **P**6
— 13 10 360 21494 298 413903 2425 319505 172219 3285

★ PHILLIPS EYE INSTITUTE, (EYE SPECIALTY HOSPITAL), 2215 Park Avenue, Zip 55404–3756; tel. 612/336–6000; Shari E. Levy, Administrator **A**1 9 10 **F**1 3 4 5 6 7 8 9 11 13 14 15 16 17 18 19 20 21 22 23 24 25 26 27 28 29 30 31 32 33 34 35 36 37 39 40 43 45 46 47 48 51 54 55 56 58 59 60 61 62 63 64 65 66 67 68 70 71 72 73 74 75 76 77 78 79 **P**1 4 **S** Allina Health System, Minneapolis, MN
Web address: www.allina.com
— 23 49 10 653 2 16844 0 18521 6091 110

Hospitals, U.S. / MINNESOTA

Hospital, Address, Telephone, Administrator, Approval, Facility, and Physician Codes, Health Care System, Network	Classification Codes		Utilization Data					Expense (thousands) of dollars		
★ American Hospital Association (AHA) membership □ Joint Commission on Accreditation of Healthcare Organizations (JCAHO) accreditation + American Osteopathic Healthcare Association (AOHA) membership ○ American Osteopathic Association (AOA) accreditation △ Commission on Accreditation of Rehabilitation Facilities (CARF) accreditation Control codes 61, 63, 64, 71, 72 and 73 indicate hospitals listed by AOHA, but not registered by AHA. For definition of numerical codes, see page A4	Control	Service	Staffed Beds	Admissions	Census	Outpatient Visits	Births	Total	Payroll	Personnel
□ SHRINERS HOSPITALS FOR CHILDREN, TWIN CITIES, 2025 East River Parkway, Zip 55414-3696; tel. 612/596-6100; Laurence E. Johnson, Administrator **A**1 3 5 **F**7 17 19 22 34 38 39 48 50 51 54 58 70 72 76 78 **P**6 **S** Shriners Hospitals for Children, Tampa, FL **Web address:** www.shrinershq.org ST. MARY'S HOSPITAL AND REHABILITATION CENTER See Fairview–University Medical Center UNIVERSITY OF MINNESOTA HOSPITAL AND CLINIC See Fairview–University Medical Center	23	57	40	749	13	8910	0	—	—	141
★ △ VETERANS AFFAIRS MEDICAL CENTER, One Veterans Drive, Zip 55417-2399; tel. 612/725-2000; Steven Kleinglass, Acting Director (Total facility includes 104 beds in nursing home–type unit) **A**1 2 3 5 7 8 **F**1 3 4 9 11 12 13 17 18 19 21 22 23 24 25 28 30 31 32 33 34 35 36 38 39 41 43 45 46 47 48 49 50 51 53 54 55 56 57 59 61 62 63 64 65 70 72 74 76 77 78 79 **S** Department of Veterans Affairs, Washington, DC	45	10	361	9750	258	403481	0	244738	117759	1751
MONTEVIDEO—Chippewa County CHIPPEWA COUNTY MONTEVIDEO HOSPITAL, 824 North 11th Street, Zip 56265-1683; tel. 320/269-8877; Fred Knutson, Administrator (Nonreporting) **A**9 10	15	10	29	—	—	—	—	—	—	—
MONTICELLO—Wright County ★ MONTICELLO BIG LAKE HOSPITAL, 1013 Hart Boulevard, Zip 55362-8230; tel. 763/295-2945; Barbara Schwientek, Executive Director (Total facility includes 91 beds in nursing home–type unit) **A**1 9 10 **F**1 3 7 8 9 16 17 21 22 25 37 38 39 46 48 49 63 69 70 76 77 78 **Web address:** www.mblch.com	16	10	103	1343	100	32296	365	18601	9176	485
MOOSE LAKE—Carlton County ★ MERCY HOSPITAL AND HEALTH CARE CENTER, 710 South Kenwood Avenue, Zip 55767-9405; tel. 218/485-4481; Dianne Mandernach, Chief Executive Officer (Total facility includes 94 beds in nursing home–type unit) (Nonreporting) **A**9 10	16	10	119	—	—	—	—	—	—	—
MORA—Kanabec County ★ KANABEC HOSPITAL, 300 Clark Street, Zip 55051-1590; tel. 320/679-1212; Thomas D. Kaufman, Administrator **A**1 9 10 **F**7 8 9 13 17 18 19 22 25 26 27 37 39 41 43 44 45 46 48 54 68 70 72 76 78	13	10	35	1152	11	15675	168	10688	4869	145
MORRIS—Stevens County ★ STEVENS COMMUNITY MEDICAL CENTER, 400 East First Street, Zip 56267-1407, Mailing Address: P.O. Box 660, Zip 56267-0660; tel. 320/589-1313; John Rau, Administrator **A**1 9 10 **F**3 6 7 8 9 16 17 18 19 21 22 23 25 26 31 32 34 35 36 37 38 39 41 43 44 45 46 48 50 51 54 56 58 59 60 61 62 63 70 72 76 **P**6 **S** Allina Health System, Minneapolis, MN	23	10	39	1456	16	3821	116	13187	6489	203
NEW PRAGUE—Le Sueur County ★ QUEEN OF PEACE HOSPITAL, 301 Second Street N.E., Zip 56071-1799; tel. 612/758-4431; Sister Jean Juenemann, Chief Executive Officer **A**1 9 10 **F**7 8 9 12 22 23 24 25 28 34 36 38 39 43 44 45 46 48 49 50 51 54 56 67 72 76 77 78	23	10	31	1440	11	80699	164	14461	6693	193
NEW ULM—Brown County ★ NEW ULM MEDICAL CENTER, 1324 Fifth Street North, Zip 56073-1553, Mailing Address: P.O. Box 577, Zip 56073-0577; tel. 507/354-2111; Brian Kief, Administrator **A**1 9 10 **F**2 3 8 9 12 13 17 18 19 20 22 25 26 28 31 34 36 37 38 40 41 43 44 45 46 48 50 51 54 56 57 58 59 61 62 63 64 66 70 71 72 76 77 78 **P**2 **S** Allina Health System, Minneapolis, MN	23	10	47	2223	—	59448	402	—	10737	—
NORTHFIELD—Rice County ★ NORTHFIELD HOSPITAL, (Includes H. O. DILLEY SKILLED NURSING FACILITY), 801 West First Street, Zip 55057-1697; tel. 507/645-6661; Kendall C. Bank, Administrator (Total facility includes 40 beds in nursing home–type unit) **A**1 9 10 **F**8 9 12 17 18 22 23 25 26 32 34 36 37 38 39 40 43 44 45 46 48 50 51 54 56 69 70 71 72 76 78 **S** Allina Health System, Minneapolis, MN **Web address:** www.allina.com	14	10	67	1842	52	21389	334	17581	8803	236
OLIVIA—Renville County RENVILLE COUNTY HOSPITAL, 611 East Fairview Avenue, Zip 56277-1397; tel. 320/523-1261; Dean G. Slagter, Administrator (Nonreporting) **A**9 10	13	10	30	—	—	—	—	—	—	—
ONAMIA—Mille Lacs County ★ MILLE LACS HEALTH SYSTEM, 200 North Elm Street, Zip 56359-7978; tel. 320/532-3154; Randall A. Farrow, Administrator (Total facility includes 80 beds in nursing home–type unit) (Nonreporting) **A**1 9 10 **S** Allina Health System, Minneapolis, MN	23	10	98	—	—	—	—	—	—	—
ORTONVILLE—Big Stone County ★ ORTONVILLE AREA HEALTH SERVICES, 750 Eastvold Avenue, Zip 56278-1133; tel. 320/839-2502; Kenneth W. Archer, Administrator (Total facility includes 74 beds in nursing home–type unit) (Nonreporting) **A**9 10 **S** Sioux Valley Hospitals and Health System, Sioux Falls, SD	14	10	105	—	—	—	—	—	—	—
OWATONNA—Steele County ★ OWATONNA HOSPITAL, 903 Oak Street South, Zip 55060-3234; tel. 507/451-3850; Daniel J. Werner, Administrator **A**1 9 10 **F**7 8 9 13 17 18 19 20 22 25 26 28 32 34 36 37 39 40 41 43 44 45 48 54 57 58 61 62 64 71 72 76 77 78 **P**6 **S** Allina Health System, Minneapolis, MN **Web address:** www.allina.com	23	10	44	2177	21	10604	487	17447	7224	215

© 2000 AHA Guide   *Many Facility Codes have changed. Please refer to the AHA Guide Code Chart.*

Hospitals, U.S. / MINNESOTA

Hospital, Address, Telephone, Administrator, Approval, Facility, and Physician Codes, Health Care System, Network	Classification Codes		Utilization Data					Expense (thousands) of dollars		
	Control	Service	Staffed Beds	Admissions	Census	Outpatient Visits	Births	Total	Payroll	Personnel

★ American Hospital Association (AHA) membership
☐ Joint Commission on Accreditation of Healthcare Organizations (JCAHO) accreditation
+ American Osteopathic Healthcare Association (AOHA) membership
○ American Osteopathic Association (AOA) accreditation
△ Commission on Accreditation of Rehabilitation Facilities (CARF) accreditation
Control codes 61, 63, 64, 71, 72 and 73 indicate hospitals listed by AOHA, but not registered by AHA. For definition of numerical codes, see page A4

Hospital	Control	Service	Staffed Beds	Admissions	Census	Outpatient Visits	Births	Total	Payroll	Personnel
PARK RAPIDS—Hubbard County										
ST. JOSEPH'S AREA HEALTH SERVICES, 600 Pleasant Avenue, Zip 56470–1432; tel. 218/732–3311; Peter Jacobson, President and Chief Executive Officer **A**1 9 10 **F**7 8 9 13 14 17 18 19 22 24 25 26 32 33 34 36 37 38 39 41 43 44 48 49 50 51 54 68 70 72 76 78 **S** Catholic Health Initiatives, Denver, CO	23	10	39	1750	21	25929	146	16325	7248	205
PAYNESVILLE—Stearns County										
★ PAYNESVILLE AREA HEALTH CARE SYSTEM, 200 First Street West, Zip 56362–1496; tel. 320/243–3767; William M. LaCroix, Administrator **A**9 10 **F**1 7 8 9 12 17 18 22 24 25 28 30 31 36 37 38 39 40 43 44 46 48 57 63 67 69 70 72 76 **P**8 Web address: www.pahcs.com	16	10	94	745	65	19314	98	12163	5327	117
PERHAM—Otter Tail County										
PERHAM MEMORIAL HOSPITAL AND HOME, 665 Third Street S.W., Zip 56573–1199; tel. 218/346–4500; Chuck Hofius, Administrator (Total facility includes 102 beds in nursing home–type unit) (Nonreporting) **A**1 9 10 Web address: www.pmhh.com	16	10	123	—	—	—	—	—	—	—
PIPESTONE—Pipestone County										
PIPESTONE COUNTY MEDICAL CENTER/AVERA HEALTH, 911 Fifth Avenue S.W., Zip 56164–0370, Mailing Address: P.O. Box 370, Zip 56164–0370; tel. 507/825–6125; Carl P. Vaagenes, Administrator (Total facility includes 43 beds in nursing home–type unit) (Nonreporting) **A**9 10 **S** Avera Health, Yankton, SD	13	10	76	—	—	—	—	—	—	—
PRINCETON—Sherburne County										
FAIRVIEW NORTHLAND REGIONAL HEALTH CARE, 911 Northland Drive, Zip 55371–2173; tel. 612/389–6300; Jeanne Lally, Senior Vice President and Administrator (Nonreporting) **A**1 9 10 **S** Fairview Health Services, Minneapolis, MN Web address: www.fairview.org	23	10	41	—	—	—	—	—	—	—
RED WING—Goodhue County										
FAIRVIEW RED WING HOSPITAL, 1407 West Fourth Street, Zip 55066–2198; tel. 651/388–6721; Scott Wordelman, President and Chief Executive Officer **A**1 9 10 **F**2 3 7 8 9 12 17 18 19 22 25 26 30 32 33 34 35 36 37 38 39 40 41 43 44 45 46 48 49 50 51 54 56 58 59 60 63 67 68 69 70 71 72 75 76 77 78 **P**6 **S** Fairview Health Services, Minneapolis, MN Web address: www.fairview.org	23	10	70	2307	28	16537	328	25564	10913	366
REDLAKE—Beltrami County										
U.S. PUBLIC HEALTH SERVICE INDIAN HOSPITAL, Highway 1, Zip 56671; tel. 218/679–3912; Essimae Stevens, Service Unit Director (Nonreporting) **A**1 10 **S** U. S. Public Health Service Indian Health Service, Rockville, MD	47	10	23	—	—	—	—	—	—	—
REDWOOD FALLS—Redwood County										
★ REDWOOD FALLS MUNICIPAL HOSPITAL, 100 Fallwood Road, Zip 56283–1828; tel. 507/637–4500; James E. Schulte, Administrator (Nonreporting) **A**9 10	14	10	35	—	—	—	—	—	—	—
ROBBINSDALE—Hennepin County										
△ NORTH MEMORIAL HEALTH CARE, 3300 Oakdale Avenue North, Zip 55422–2900; tel. 612/520–5200; Scott R. Anderson, President and Chief Executive Officer **A**1 2 3 5 7 9 10 **F**4 7 8 9 11 12 13 16 17 18 19 21 22 24 25 26 30 31 36 37 38 39 40 41 42 43 44 45 46 47 48 49 50 51 52 53 54 56 57 59 61 66 70 71 72 75 76 77 78 79 **P**1 5 6 Web address: www.northmemorial.com	23	10	376	23878	267	206483	3180	279936	142236	3147
ROCHESTER—Olmsted County										
OLMSTED MEDICAL CENTER, 1650 Fourth Street S.E., Zip 55904, Mailing Address: 210 Ninth Street S.E., Zip 55904; tel. 507/288–3443; Noel Peterson, M.D., President and Chief Executive Officer **A**1 9 10 **F**8 9 17 18 22 25 39 40 41 43 44 45 48 51 56 58 63 76 Web address: www.olmmed.org	23	10	63	2372	16	—	882	52951	30592	640
ROCHESTER METHODIST HOSPITAL, 201 West Center Street, Zip 55902–3084; tel. 507/266–7890; John M. Panicek, Administrator (Nonreporting) **A**1 3 5 9 10 **S** Mayo Foundation, Rochester, MN	23	10	335	—	—	—	—	—	—	—
△ SAINT MARYS HOSPITAL, 1216 Second Street S.W., Zip 55902–1970; tel. 507/255–5123; John M. Panicek, Administrator (Nonreporting) **A**1 3 5 7 8 9 10 **S** Mayo Foundation, Rochester, MN	23	10	797	—	—	—	—	—	—	—
ROSEAU—Roseau County										
ROSEAU AREA HOSPITAL AND HOMES, 715 Delmore Avenue, Zip 56751–1599; tel. 218/463–2500; David F. Hagen, President and Chief Executive Officer (Total facility includes 124 beds in nursing home–type unit) **A**1 9 10 **F**8 9 11 12 13 14 16 17 18 22 24 25 26 31 32 34 36 37 38 39 43 45 46 48 49 50 54 63 65 68 69 70 72 76 78 **P**5	23	10	161	1080	130	22691	193	14422	7979	256
SAINT CLOUD—Stearns County										
ST. CLOUD HOSPITAL, 1406 Sixth Avenue North, Zip 56303–0016; tel. 320/251–2700; John Frobenius, President and Chief Executive Officer (Total facility includes 291 beds in nursing home–type unit) **A**1 2 3 9 10 **F**1 2 3 4 6 7 8 9 11 12 13 14 16 17 18 19 21 22 24 25 26 27 30 32 33 34 35 36 37 38 39 40 41 42 43 44 45 46 47 48 49 50 51 53 54 56 57 58 59 60 61 62 63 64 65 66 67 68 69 70 72 75 76 77 78 79 **P**6 **S** CentraCare, Long Prairie, MN Web address: www.stcloudhospital.com	21	10	697	18607	444	241171	2374	190152	90384	2419
VETERANS AFFAIRS MEDICAL CENTER, 4801 Eighth Street North, Zip 56303–2099; tel. 320/252–1670; Barry I. Bahl, Director (Total facility includes 220 beds in nursing home–type unit) **A**1 **F**1 2 3 9 13 16 18 19 22 23 26 28 29 30 32 33 34 35 36 37 38 39 43 45 48 51 54 56 57 59 62 63 64 69 70 72 76 77 78 79 **P**6 **S** Department of Veterans Affairs, Washington, DC	45	22	382	2727	350	138424	0	53795	41955	815

Hospitals, U.S. / MINNESOTA

Hospital, Address, Telephone, Administrator, Approval, Facility, and Physician Codes, Health Care System, Network	Classification Codes		Utilization Data					Expense (thousands) of dollars		
★ American Hospital Association (AHA) membership □ Joint Commission on Accreditation of Healthcare Organizations (JCAHO) accreditation + American Osteopathic Healthcare Association (AOHA) membership ○ American Osteopathic Association (AOA) accreditation △ Commission on Accreditation of Rehabilitation Facilities (CARF) accreditation Control codes 61, 63, 64, 71, 72 and 73 indicate hospitals listed by AOHA, but not registered by AHA. For definition of numerical codes, see page A4	Control	Service	Staffed Beds	Admissions	Census	Outpatient Visits	Births	Total	Payroll	Personnel
SAINT JAMES—Watonwan County										
ST. JAMES HEALTH SERVICES, 1207 Sixth Avenue South, Zip 56081–2415, Mailing Address: P.O. Box 460, Zip 56081–0460; tel. 507/375-3261; Lee Holter, Chief Executive Officer (Nonreporting) **A**9 10	23	10	24	—	—	—	—	—	—	—
SAINT LOUIS PARK—Hennepin County										
△ METHODIST HOSPITAL HEALTHSYSTEM MINNESOTA, 6500 Excelsior Boulevard, Zip 55426–4702, Mailing Address: P.O. Box 650, Minneapolis, Zip 55440–0650; tel. 952/993-5000; Mark Skubic, Vice President (Total facility includes 35 beds in nursing home–type unit) (Nonreporting) **A**2 3 5 7 9 10 **S** HealthSystem Minnesota, Saint Louis Park, MN Web address: www.healthsystemminnesota.com	23	10	376	—	—	—	—	—	—	—
SAINT PAUL—Ramsey County										
✠ △ BETHESDA REHABILITATION HOSPITAL, (Formerly HealthEast Bethesda Rehabilitation Hospital), 559 Capitol Boulevard, Zip 55103–2101; tel. 651/232-2000; Scott Batulis, Vice President and Administrator (Nonreporting) **A**1 7 9 10 **S** HealthEast, Saint Paul, MN Web address: www.healtheast.org	23	48	127	—	—	—	—	—	—	—
★ CHILDREN'S HOSPITAL AND CLINICS, 345 North Smith Avenue, Zip 55102–2392; tel. 651/220-6000; Brock D. Nelson, Chief Executive Officer **A**3 5 9 10 **F**2 3 4 8 11 13 14 16 17 18 19 20 22 23 24 25 26 27 28 31 35 36 37 38 39 42 43 45 46 47 48 49 50 51 52 53 54 56 57 58 59 60 61 63 64 65 66 70 71 72 73 75 76 78 **P**1 Web address: www.childrenshc.org	23	50	105	5297	81	68807	0	86571	44422	739
□ △ GILLETTE CHILDREN'S SPECIALTY HEALTHCARE, 200 University Avenue East, Zip 55101–2598; tel. 651/291-2848; Margaret Perryman, Chief Executive Officer (Nonreporting) **A**1 3 5 7 9 10 Web address: www.gillettechildrens.org	23	59	43	—	—	—	—	—	—	—
✠ △ REGIONS HOSPITAL, 640 Jackson Street, Zip 55101–2595; tel. 651/221-3456; Terry S. Finzen, President (Nonreporting) **A**1 2 3 5 7 8 9 10 Web address: www.healthpartners.com	23	10	409	—	—	—	—	—	—	—
✠ ST. JOSEPH'S HOSPITAL, (Formerly HealthEast St. Joseph's Hospital), 69 West Exchange Street, Zip 55102–1053; tel. 651/232-3000; Douglas P. Cropper, Vice President and Administrator (Nonreporting) **A**1 2 3 5 9 10 **S** HealthEast, Saint Paul, MN Web address: www.healtheast.org	23	10	292	—	—	—	—	—	—	—
✠ UNITED HOSPITAL, 333 North Smith Street, Zip 55102–2389; tel. 651/220-8000; M. Barbara Balik, MSN, Ed.D., Administrator **A**1 2 3 5 9 10 **F**3 4 8 9 11 13 16 17 18 19 20 22 24 25 27 28 31 33 35 36 38 39 41 43 44 45 46 47 48 49 50 51 53 54 55 56 57 58 59 60 63 64 65 66 68 70 71 72 74 76 78 79 **S** Allina Health System, Minneapolis, MN Web address: www.allina.com	23	10	483	25237	321	148295	4570	241537	105935	2222
SAINT PETER—Nicollet County										
★ COMMUNITY HOSPITAL AND HEALTH CARE CENTER, 618 West Broadway Avenue, Zip 56082–1327; tel. 507/931-2200; Colleen A. Spike, Administrator (Total facility includes 85 beds in nursing home–type unit) (Nonreporting) **A**10 **S** Allina Health System, Minneapolis, MN	14	10	118	—	—	—	—	—	—	—
MINNESOTA SECURITY HOSPITAL See St. Peter Regional Treatment Center										
□ ST. PETER REGIONAL TREATMENT CENTER, (Includes Minnesota Security Hospital, Sheppard Drive, Zip 56082; tel. 507/931-7100), 100 Freeman Drive, Zip 56082–1599; tel. 507/931-7100; William L. Pedersen, Chief Executive Officer (Nonreporting) **A**1 9 10	12	22	560	—	—	—	—	—	—	—
SANDSTONE—Pine County										
★ PINE MEDICAL CENTER, 109 Court Avenue South, Zip 55072–5120; tel. 320/245-2212; Michael D. Hedrix, Administrator (Total facility includes 86 beds in nursing home–type unit) **A**9 10 **F**7 9 13 17 18 19 22 24 25 34 45 48 54 69 70 76 **P**6 **S** Benedictine Health System, Duluth, MN	23	10	106	246	84	5817	1	6765	3162	125
SAUK CENTRE—Stearns County										
★ ST. MICHAEL'S HOSPITAL, 425 North Elm Street, Zip 56378–1010; tel. 320/352-2221; Delano Christianson, Administrator (Nonreporting) **A**9 10	14	10	78	—	—	—	—	—	—	—
SHAKOPEE—Scott County										
✠ ST. FRANCIS REGIONAL MEDICAL CENTER, 1455 St. Francis Avenue, Zip 55379–3380; tel. 952/403-3000; Venetia Kudrle, Administrator (Nonreporting) **A**1 2 9 10 **S** Allina Health System, Minneapolis, MN	21	10	63	—	—	—	—	—	—	—
SLAYTON—Murray County										
★ MURRAY COUNTY MEMORIAL HOSPITAL, 2042 Juniper Avenue, Zip 56172–1016; tel. 507/836-6111; Jerry Bobeldyk, Administrator **A**9 10 **F**9 17 22 25 39 48 76 **S** Sioux Valley Hospitals and Health System, Sioux Falls, SD	13	10	25	558	5	9995	0	3431	1458	56
SLEEPY EYE—Brown County										
SLEEPY EYE MUNICIPAL HOSPITAL, 400 Fourth Avenue N.W., Zip 56085–1109; tel. 507/794-3571; David Hartberg, Administrator (Nonreporting) **A**9 10	14	10	20	—	—	—	—	—	—	—
SPRING GROVE—Houston County										
TWEETEN HEALTH SERVICES, (Formerly Tweeten Lutheran Health Care Center), 125 Fifth Avenue S.E., Zip 55974–1309; tel. 507/498-3211; Penny Solberg, Administrator (Total facility includes 70 beds in nursing home–type unit) **A**9 10 **F**16 17 18 19 23 30 31 32 33 34 43 45 50 53 54 69 70 78 79 **P**6	23	10	80	176	64	5257	0	3270	1838	91
SPRINGFIELD—Brown County										
□ SPRINGFIELD MEDICAL CENTER–MAYO HEALTH SYSTEM, 625 North Jackson Avenue, Zip 56087–1714, Mailing Address: P.O. Box 146, Zip 56087–0146; tel. 507/723-6201; Scott Thoreson, Administrator **A**1 9 10 **F**8 9 17 18 22 25 32 34 36 39 48 54 69 70 76	23	10	23	607	5	12964	36	3362	1365	60

Hospitals, U.S. / MINNESOTA

Hospital, Address, Telephone, Administrator, Approval, Facility, and Physician Codes, Health Care System, Network

- ★ American Hospital Association (AHA) membership
- □ Joint Commission on Accreditation of Healthcare Organizations (JCAHO) accreditation
- + American Osteopathic Healthcare Association (AOHA) membership
- ○ American Osteopathic Association (AOA) accreditation
- △ Commission on Accreditation of Rehabilitation Facilities (CARF) accreditation

Control codes 61, 63, 64, 71, 72 and 73 indicate hospitals listed by AOHA, but not registered by AHA. For definition of numerical codes, see page A4

Hospital	Classification Codes		Utilization Data					Expense (thousands) of dollars		Personnel
	Control	Service	Staffed Beds	Admissions	Census	Outpatient Visits	Births	Total	Payroll	
STAPLES—Wadena County LAKEWOOD HEALTH SYSTEM, 401 East Prairie Avenue, Zip 56479–3201; tel. 218/894–0300; Tim Rice, President **A**9 10 **F**7 8 9 13 17 18 20 22 24 25 30 31 32 33 34 36 37 38 39 43 44 45 46 48 50 51 54 70 71 72 76 **P**7 Web address: www.lakewoodsystem.com	23	10	40	849	7	22270	117	8592	3955	239
STARBUCK—Pope County ★ MINNEWASKA DISTRICT HOSPITAL, 610 West Sixth Street, Zip 56381, Mailing Address: P.O. Box 160, Zip 56381–0160; tel. 320/239–2201; Roxann A. Wellman, Chief Executive Officer **A**9 10 **F**1 7 8 9 15 16 17 18 19 20 22 25 30 31 32 36 37 38 39 40 41 43 44 46 48 67 69 70 76	16	10	19	447	6	2726	7	2634	1193	35
STILLWATER—Washington County ⊞ LAKEVIEW HOSPITAL, 927 West Churchill Street, Zip 55082–5930; tel. 651/439–5330; Jeffrey J. Robertson, Chief Executive Officer **A**1 6 9 10 **F**6 7 8 9 12 16 17 18 19 20 22 24 25 28 32 36 37 38 39 41 44 45 46 48 49 50 51 54 67 70 71 72 73 76 78 79 **P**5 Web address: www.lakeview.org	23	10	62	3449	26	32060	693	34604	13944	392
THIEF RIVER FALLS—Pennington County ⊞ NORTHWEST MEDICAL CENTER, 120 LaBree Avenue South, Zip 56701–2819; tel. 218/681–4240; Richard A. Spyhalski, Chief Executive Officer (Total facility includes 90 beds in nursing home–type unit) **A**1 9 10 **F**7 8 9 16 17 18 19 21 22 24 25 27 32 33 34 38 39 40 41 43 44 46 48 50 54 57 58 59 60 61 62 63 65 69 70 71 72 76 78 79 Web address: www.nwmc.org	23	10	130	2373	112	14249	225	20097	11039	324
TRACY—Lyon County ★ TRACY AREA MEDICAL SERVICES, 251 Fifth Street East, Zip 56175–1536; tel. 507/629–3200; Dan Reiner, Administrator and Chief Executive Officer **A**9 10 **F**7 9 12 16 17 18 19 22 25 30 32 33 34 35 36 37 38 39 41 43 44 45 46 48 50 53 54 56 59 63 67 69 70 71 76 79 **P**6 **S** Sioux Valley Hospitals and Health System, Sioux Falls, SD	23	10	27	563	5	16949	5	3371	1742	68
TWO HARBORS—Lake County LAKE VIEW MEMORIAL HOSPITAL, 325 11th Avenue, Zip 55616–1360; tel. 218/834–7300; Brian J. Carlson, FACHE, President and Chief Executive Officer (Total facility includes 50 beds in nursing home–type unit) **A**9 10 **F**3 7 8 17 18 19 24 25 26 32 34 40 43 44 45 48 51 54 59 69 70 76 77 78 **P**5	23	10	66	383	52	10522	36	5584	2969	104
TYLER—Lincoln County ★ TYLER HEALTHCARE CENTER/AVERA HEALTH, 240 Willow Street, Zip 56178–0280, Mailing Address: P.O. Box 280, Zip 56178–0280; tel. 507/247–5521; Douglas P. Schweikhart, Administrator (Total facility includes 43 beds in nursing home–type unit) (Nonreporting) **A**9 10 **S** Avera Health, Yankton, SD	23	10	63	—	—	—	—	—	—	—
VIRGINIA—St. Louis County ⊞ △ VIRGINIA REGIONAL MEDICAL CENTER, 901 Ninth Street North, Zip 55792–2398; tel. 218/741–3340; Kyle Hopstad, Administrator (Total facility includes 116 beds in nursing home–type unit) **A**1 7 9 10 **F**4 7 8 9 16 17 18 22 24 25 27 30 32 34 38 39 40 41 44 46 48 49 53 54 69 70 72 76 78 **S** Quorum Health Group, Brentwood, TN Web address: www.vrmc-mn.com	14	10	199	3581	151	30461	313	32399	14027	411
WABASHA—Wabasha County ⊞ ST. ELIZABETH HOSPITAL, 1200 Fifth Grand Boulevard West, Zip 55981–1098; tel. 651/565–4531; Thomas Crowley, President (Total facility includes 130 beds in nursing home–type unit) **A**1 9 10 **F**1 3 4 6 7 8 9 11 13 16 17 18 19 22 23 25 26 28 30 31 32 34 35 36 37 38 39 40 44 45 46 48 49 54 61 62 63 64 67 69 70 72 75 76 77 78 79 **P**1 3 6 **S** Marian Health System, Tulsa, OK Web address: www.ministryhealthcare.org	21	10	155	762	117	21841	61	11494	5866	248
WACONIA—Carver County ⊞ RIDGEVIEW MEDICAL CENTER, 500 South Maple Street, Zip 55387–1791; tel. 952/442–2191; Robert Stevens, President and Chief Executive Officer **A**1 9 10 **F**7 8 9 12 16 17 19 21 22 23 24 25 26 29 32 33 34 36 37 38 39 41 43 44 45 46 48 49 50 51 54 57 62 65 66 68 70 71 72 76 77 78 79 Web address: www.ridgeviewmedical.org	14	10	102	5601	51	75267	1012	51681	26402	633
WADENA—Wadena County ⊞ TRI-COUNTY HOSPITAL, 415 Jefferson Street North, Zip 56482–1297; tel. 218/631–3510; Dennis C. Miley, Administrator **A**1 9 10 **F**7 8 9 12 16 17 18 19 22 24 30 32 34 36 37 38 39 40 41 43 44 45 46 48 54 58 59 63 70 71 72 76 78 Web address: www.tricountyhospital.org	23	10	30	1544	17	13539	143	14119	6496	174
WARREN—Marshall County ★ NORTH VALLEY HEALTH CENTER, 109 South Minnesota Street, Zip 56762–1499; tel. 218/745–4211; Jon Linnell, Administrator (Nonreporting) **A**9 10	23	10	18	—	—	—	—	—	—	—
WASECA—Waseca County ⊞ WASECA MEDICAL CENTER, 501 North State Street, Zip 56093; tel. 507/835–1210; Michael Milbrath, Administrator **A**1 9 10 **F**3 7 8 9 12 17 18 19 22 25 28 32 34 36 37 39 40 44 45 48 50 53 54 58 60 61 62 63 70 71 72 76 77 78 **P**6	23	10	26	587	4	13392	64	7747	3548	123
WESTBROOK—Cottonwood County ★ WESTBROOK HEALTH CENTER, 920 Bell Avenue, Zip 56183–0188, Mailing Address: P.O. Box 188, Zip 56183–0188; tel. 507/274–6121; Dan Reiner, Administrator and Chief Executive Officer (Nonreporting) **A**9 10 **S** Sioux Valley Hospitals and Health System, Sioux Falls, SD	23	10	8	—	—	—	—	—	—	—

Hospitals, U.S. / MINNESOTA

Hospital, Address, Telephone, Administrator, Approval, Facility, and Physician Codes, Health Care System, Network	Classification Codes		Utilization Data					Expense (thousands) of dollars		
★ American Hospital Association (AHA) membership ☐ Joint Commission on Accreditation of Healthcare Organizations (JCAHO) accreditation + American Osteopathic Healthcare Association (AOHA) membership ○ American Osteopathic Association (AOA) accreditation △ Commission on Accreditation of Rehabilitation Facilities (CARF) accreditation Control codes 61, 63, 64, 71, 72 and 73 indicate hospitals listed by AOHA, but not registered by AHA. For definition of numerical codes, see page A4	Control	Service	Staffed Beds	Admissions	Census	Outpatient Visits	Births	Total	Payroll	Personnel
WHEATON—Traverse County WHEATON COMMUNITY HOSPITAL, 401 12th Street North, Zip 56296-1099; tel. 320/563-8226; James J. Talley, Administrator **A**9 10 **F**7 8 9 12 14 16 17 18 19 22 23 24 25 28 32 33 34 36 37 38 39 43 44 46 48 50 54 55 58 59 60 61 62 63 65 68 72 76 78 **P**5	14	10	25	849	8	9221	11	3349	1428	54
WILLMAR—Kandiyohi County ✴ RICE MEMORIAL HOSPITAL, 301 Becker Avenue S.W., Zip 56201-3395; tel. 320/235-4543; Lawrence J. Massa, Chief Executive Officer (Total facility includes 80 beds in nursing home-type unit) **A**1 2 9 10 **F**7 8 9 17 22 24 25 27 34 36 37 38 39 41 44 45 46 48 50 54 57 59 60 61 62 63 65 68 69 70 72 76 78 **Web address:** www.ricehospital.com	14	10	198	4931	129	31366	746	52819	25515	520
☐ WILLMAR REGIONAL TREATMENT CENTER, North Highway 71, Zip 56201-1128, Mailing Address: Box 1128, Zip 56201-1128; tel. 320/231-5905; Gregory G. Spartz, Chief Executive Officer **A**1 10 **F**1 2 3 6 13 16 17 18 19 21 22 23 24 25 29 30 31 33 36 38 39 45 48 50 51 57 58 59 60 61 62 63 64 70 72 78 **P**6	12	22	182	1051	147	122	0	30147	20398	452
WINDOM—Cottonwood County ★ WINDOM AREA HOSPITAL, Highways 60 and 71 North, Zip 56101, Mailing Address: P.O. Box 339, Zip 56101-0339; tel. 507/831-2400 **A**9 10 **F**7 8 9 18 19 22 25 32 34 37 38 39 43 44 46 48 53 54 69 70 72 76 **P**6 **S** Sioux Valley Hospitals and Health System, Sioux Falls, SD	14	10	35	844	8	14565	160	5732	2522	76
WINONA—Winona County ✴ WINONA COMMUNITY MEMORIAL HOSPITAL, 855 Mankato Avenue, Zip 55987-4894, Mailing Address: P.O. Box 5600, Zip 55987-0600; tel. 507/454-3650; Patrick M. Booth, President (Total facility includes 104 beds in nursing home-type unit) **A**1 9 10 **F**1 2 6 7 8 9 11 17 18 19 22 24 25 27 28 30 33 34 36 37 39 41 43 44 45 48 50 51 54 56 57 58 59 60 61 62 68 69 70 72 76 78 **P**8 **Web address:** www.winonahealth.org	23	10	180	3107	127	—	403	27744	14563	402
WORTHINGTON—Nobles County ✴ WORTHINGTON REGIONAL HOSPITAL, 1018 Sixth Avenue, Zip 56187-2202, Mailing Address: P.O. Box 997, Zip 56187-0997; tel. 507/372-2941; Melvin J. Platt, Administrator **A**1 10 **F**7 8 16 17 19 22 24 25 31 34 36 37 39 40 41 43 44 45 48 49 50 54 57 60 70 71 76 78 **S** Sioux Valley Hospitals and Health System, Sioux Falls, SD	14	10	66	2514	28	34193	319	15607	7403	199
WYOMING—Chisago County ✴ FAIRVIEW LAKES REGIONAL MEDICAL CENTER, 5200 Fairview Boulevard, Zip 55092-8013; tel. 651/982-7000; Daniel K. Anderson, Senior Vice President and Administrator (Total facility includes 40 beds in nursing home-type unit) **A**1 9 10 **F**3 4 6 7 8 9 11 13 14 16 17 18 19 20 21 22 24 25 26 27 28 29 30 31 32 33 34 35 36 37 38 39 41 44 45 46 48 49 50 51 54 55 56 58 59 60 61 62 63 64 65 66 68 69 70 71 72 73 76 77 78 79 **P**1 6 **S** Fairview Health Services, Minneapolis, MN **Web address:** www.fairview.org	23	10	78	3139	55	282026	621	56474	30399	718
ZUMBROTA—Goodhue County ✴ ZUMBROTA HEALTH CARE, 383 West Fifth Street, Zip 55992-1699; tel. 507/732-5131; Daniel Will, Administrator (Total facility includes 70 beds in nursing home-type unit) (Nonreporting) **A**1 9 10	23	10	94	—	—	—	—	—	—	—

© 2000 AHA Guide   *Many Facility Codes have changed. Please refer to the AHA Guide Code Chart.*

MISSISSIPPI

Resident Population 2,752 (in thousands)
Resident population in metro areas 35.3%
Birth rate per 1,000 population 15.2
65 years and over 12.2%
Percent of persons without health insurance 20.1%

Hospital, Address, Telephone, Administrator, Approval, Facility, and Physician Codes, Health Care System, Network

★ American Hospital Association (AHA) membership
☐ Joint Commission on Accreditation of Healthcare Organizations (JCAHO) accreditation
+ American Osteopathic Healthcare Association (AOHA) membership
○ American Osteopathic Association (AOA) accreditation
△ Commission on Accreditation of Rehabilitation Facilities (CARF) accreditation
Control codes 61, 63, 64, 71, 72 and 73 indicate hospitals listed by AOHA, but not registered by AHA. For definition of numerical codes, see page A4

	Classification Codes		Utilization Data					Expense (thousands) of dollars		
	Control	Service	Staffed Beds	Admissions	Census	Outpatient Visits	Births	Total	Payroll	Personnel

ABERDEEN—Monroe County
ABERDEEN–MONROE COUNTY HOSPITAL, 400 South Chestnut Street, Zip 39730–3335, Mailing Address: P.O. Box 747, Zip 39730–0747; tel. 601/369–2455; Frank Harrington, Administrator **A**9 10 **F**9 17 18 19 22 25 54 62 69 70 76 78 **P**5 6 | 15 | 10 | 37 | 633 | 13 | 13538 | 0 | 6102 | 2967 | 90

ACKERMAN—Choctaw County
CHOCTAW COUNTY MEDICAL CENTER, 148 West Cherry Street, Zip 39735–0417, Mailing Address: P.O. Box 417, Zip 39735–0417; tel. 601/285–6235; Berry Gilbert, Administrator (Total facility includes 68 beds in nursing home–type unit) **A**9 10 **F**17 18 22 25 69 76 **P**6 | 33 | 10 | 81 | 280 | 78 | 3914 | 0 | — | — | 72

AMORY—Monroe County
★ GILMORE MEMORIAL HOSPITAL, 1105 Earl Frye Boulevard, Zip 38821–0459, Mailing Address: P.O. Box 459, Zip 38821–0459; tel. 662/256–7111; Robert F. Letson, President and Chief Executive Officer **A**1 9 10 **F**8 9 12 13 16 17 18 22 25 27 28 39 41 42 43 44 45 48 52 53 54 69 70 76 78 79 **P**8 | 23 | 10 | 95 | 3330 | 45 | 42765 | 758 | — | — | 461

BATESVILLE—Panola County
SOUTH PANOLA COMMUNITY HOSPITAL, 155 Keating Road, Zip 38606, Mailing Address: P.O. Box 433, Zip 38606–0433; tel. 601/563–5611; Richard W. Manning, Administrator **A**9 10 **F**8 22 24 25 44 45 48 70 76 78 **P**3 8 | 13 | 10 | 70 | 1961 | 33 | 17738 | 188 | 10088 | 4382 | 177

BAY SAINT LOUIS—Hancock County
★ HANCOCK MEDICAL CENTER, 149 Drinkwater Boulevard, Zip 39521–2790, Mailing Address: P.O. Box 2790, Zip 39521–2790; tel. 228/467–8600; Hal W. Leftwich, FACHE, Administrator **A**1 9 10 **F**8 9 12 13 16 17 18 19 22 24 25 27 39 41 43 44 48 50 51 53 54 56 70 76 78 79 **S** Quorum Health Group, Brentwood, TN
Web address: www.hmc.org | 13 | 10 | 104 | 4081 | 51 | 43526 | 389 | 30459 | 12745 | 394

BAY SPRINGS—Jasper County
JASPER GENERAL HOSPITAL, (Includes Jasper County Nursing Home), 15 A South Sixth Street, Zip 39422–9738, Mailing Address: P.O. Box 527, Zip 39422–0527; tel. 601/764–2101; M. Kenneth Posey, FACHE, Administrator (Total facility includes 104 beds in nursing home–type unit) **A**9 10 **F**9 17 36 69 70 76 | 13 | 10 | 124 | 164 | 109 | 0 | 0 | — | — | 141

BELZONI—Humphreys County
★ HUMPHREYS COUNTY MEMORIAL HOSPITAL, 500 CCC Road, Zip 39038–3806, Mailing Address: P.O. Box 510, Zip 39038–0510; tel. 662/247–3831; Debra L. Griffin, Administrator **A**9 10 **F**8 16 17 18 22 25 28 31 48 78 | 13 | 10 | 28 | 1091 | 14 | 4535 | 1 | — | — | 97

BILOXI—Harrison County
☐ BILOXI REGIONAL MEDICAL CENTER, 150 Reynoir Street, Zip 39530–4199, Mailing Address: P.O. Box 128, Zip 39533–0128; tel. 228/432–1571; Keith G. Leblanc, Chief Executive Officer **A**1 2 9 10 **F**1 2 8 9 10 12 13 16 17 18 19 22 23 24 25 28 30 31 35 36 37 39 40 41 42 43 44 45 46 48 50 51 52 53 54 56 57 66 68 70 71 72 73 75 76 77 78 79 **P**5 8 **S** Health Management Associates, Naples, FL | 33 | 10 | 153 | 6616 | 83 | 55033 | 711 | — | — | 453

★ GULF COAST MEDICAL CENTER, (Includes Gulf Oaks Hospital, 180–C Debuys Road, Zip 39531; tel. 601/388–0600), 180–A Debuys Road, Zip 39531–4405; tel. 228/388–6711; Gary L. Stokes, Chief Executive Officer **A**1 9 10 **F**2 3 8 9 12 13 17 18 19 22 24 25 35 36 37 39 41 43 44 45 46 48 51 57 58 60 61 62 63 69 70 72 74 76 77 78 **P**1 2 4 5 6 8 **S** TENET Healthcare Corporation, Santa Barbara, CA | 33 | 10 | 189 | 4140 | 69 | 34091 | 312 | 34347 | 16490 | 565

★ VA GULF COAST VETERANS HEALTH CARE SYSTEM, (Formerly Veterans Affairs Medical Center), (Includes Veterans Affairs Medical Center, Gulfport Division, East Beach, Gulfport, Zip 39501; tel. 228/563–2500), 400 Veterans Avenue, Zip 39531–2410; tel. 228/523–5000; Julie A. Catellier, Director (Total facility includes 320 beds in nursing home–type unit) (Nonreporting) **A**1 2 3 5 9 **S** Department of Veterans Affairs, Washington, DC | 45 | 10 | 510 | — | — | — | — | — | — | —

BOONEVILLE—Prentiss County
★ BAPTIST MEMORIAL HOSPITAL–BOONEVILLE, 100 Hospital Street, Zip 38829–3359; tel. 662/720–5000; Al Sypniewski, Administrator **A**1 9 10 **F**8 9 12 16 17 18 19 22 23 24 25 28 39 41 43 44 48 50 51 56 57 59 62 70 72 76 78 **P**1 3 7 **S** Baptist Memorial Health Care Corporation, Memphis, TN | 21 | 10 | 99 | 2322 | 34 | 21785 | 174 | 14398 | 4596 | 218

BRANDON—Rankin County
☐ RANKIN MEDICAL CENTER, 350 Crossgates Boulevard, Zip 39042–2698; tel. 601/825–2811; Robert L. Hammond, Jr, Executive Director **A**1 2 9 10 **F**9 12 13 17 18 19 22 23 24 25 28 31 36 39 41 43 45 46 49 50 51 52 53 54 56 57 59 60 62 68 70 72 73 76 78 **P**1 4 5 6 7 **S** Health Management Associates, Naples, FL | 33 | 10 | 90 | 3887 | 58 | 46751 | 0 | — | — | 398

BROOKHAVEN—Lincoln County
★ KING'S DAUGHTERS MEDICAL CENTER, (Formerly King's Daughters Hospital), 427 Highway 51 North, Zip 39601–2600, Mailing Address: P.O. Box 948, Zip 39602–0948; tel. 662/833–6011; Phillip L. Grady, Chief Executive Officer **A**1 9 10 **F**2 8 9 10 11 12 13 17 18 19 22 23 24 25 27 28 31 35 36 37 39 40 41 43 44 45 46 47 48 50 52 53 54 57 65 66 68 69 70 71 72 73 74 75 76 77 78 79 **P**3 **S** Quorum Health Group, Brentwood, TN
Web address: www.kdmc.org | 23 | 10 | 109 | 3829 | 50 | 45214 | 583 | — | — | 433

Many Facility Codes have changed. Please refer to the AHA Guide Code Chart.

© 2000 AHA Guide

Hospitals, U.S. / MISSISSIPPI

Hospital, Address, Telephone, Administrator, Approval, Facility, and Physician Codes, Health Care System, Network	Classification Codes		Utilization Data					Expense (thousands) of dollars		
★ American Hospital Association (AHA) membership ☐ Joint Commission on Accreditation of Healthcare Organizations (JCAHO) accreditation + American Osteopathic Healthcare Association (AOHA) membership ○ American Osteopathic Association (AOA) accreditation △ Commission on Accreditation of Rehabilitation Facilities (CARF) accreditation Control codes 61, 63, 64, 71, 72 and 73 indicate hospitals listed by AOHA, but not registered by AHA. For definition of numerical codes, see page A4	Control	Service	Staffed Beds	Admissions	Census	Outpatient Visits	Births	Total	Payroll	Personnel
CALHOUN CITY—Calhoun County HILLCREST HOSPITAL, 140 Burke–Calhoun City Road, Zip 38916–9690; tel. 601/628–6611; James P. Franklin, Administrator **A**9 10 **F**17 22 25 48 51 57 62 70 76	14	10	30	803	12	6143	0	3317	1160	66
CANTON—Madison County MADISON COUNTY MEDICAL CENTER, Highway 16 East, Zip 39046, Mailing Address: P.O. Box 1607, Zip 39046–1607; tel. 601/859–1331; G. Wayne Schuler, Executive Director (Total facility includes 60 beds in nursing home–type unit) **A**9 10 **F**1 2 3 9 18 19 22 23 25 30 35 36 37 41 44 48 56 57 59 61 62 63 64 70 76 **P**6	13	10	127	1827	113	24084	360	—	—	204
CARTHAGE—Leake County LEAKE MEMORIAL HOSPITAL, 300 Ellis Street, Zip 39051–0557, Mailing Address: P.O. Box 557, Zip 39051–0557; tel. 601/267–4511; Cindy Tadlock, Interim Administrator (Total facility includes 44 beds in nursing home–type unit) **A**9 10 **F**16 17 18 22 25 30 48 51 57 61 62 69 70 76 78 **P**6	33	10	76	925	62	17388	0	—	—	110
CENTREVILLE—Wilkinson County ★ FIELD MEMORIAL COMMUNITY HOSPITAL, 270 West Main Street, Zip 39631, Mailing Address: P.O. Box 639, Zip 39631–0639; tel. 601/645–5221; Brock A. Slabach, Administrator **A**1 9 10 **F**8 9 13 18 19 22 23 25 35 36 43 44 45 48 50 53 54 66 69 70 72 76 **S** Quorum Health Group, Brentwood, TN	13	10	66	1368	16	13666	86	7677	3064	98
CHARLESTON—Tallahatchie County TALLAHATCHIE GENERAL HOSPITAL, 201 South Market, Zip 38921–2236, Mailing Address: P.O. Box 230, Zip 38921–0230; tel. 662/647–5535; F. W. Ergle, Jr, Administrator (Total facility includes 61 beds in nursing home–type unit) **A**9 10 **F**1 2 3 8 9 10 11 12 13 19 22 23 24 25 27 28 30 31 35 36 37 39 40 41 42 43 44 45 46 47 48 50 51 52 53 54 55 56 57 58 59 60 61 62 63 64 65 66 68 69 70 71 72 73 74 76 77 78 79 **P**8	13	10	77	383	67	2201	0	—	—	102
CLARKSDALE—Coahoma County ☐ NORTHWEST MISSISSIPPI REGIONAL MEDICAL CENTER, 1970 Hospital Drive, Zip 38614–7204, Mailing Address: P.O. Box 1218, Zip 38614–1218; tel. 601/627–3410; John M. Faulkner, Executive Director (Total facility includes 20 beds in nursing home–type unit) **A**1 5 9 10 **F**8 9 11 12 13 16 17 18 19 22 24 25 35 39 41 44 45 46 48 50 54 68 69 70 71 76 78 **S** Health Management Associates, Naples, FL	33	10	195	8034	121	24682	1024	—	—	534
CLEVELAND—Bolivar County ★ BOLIVAR MEDICAL CENTER, 901 Highway 8 East, Zip 38732–9722, Mailing Address: P.O. Box 1380, Zip 38732–1380; tel. 662/846–0061; Robert L. Hawley, Jr, Chief Executive Officer (Total facility includes 35 beds in nursing home–type unit) **A**1 9 10 **F**8 9 12 13 18 19 22 23 24 25 28 31 37 41 42 44 45 48 50 51 52 54 56 68 69 70 71 72 73 76 78 **P**2 8 **S** Province Healthcare Corporation, Brentwood, TN	13	10	148	4653	94	15712	668	27486	12494	432
COLLINS—Covington County ☐ COVINGTON COUNTY HOSPITAL, Sixth and Holly Streets, Zip 39428, Mailing Address: P.O. Box 1149, Zip 39428–1149; tel. 601/765–6711; Irving Hitt, Administrator **A**1 9 10 **F**8 9 12 13 16 17 19 22 23 25 30 36 41 44 48 50 51 53 54 57 62 69 70 76 78	13	10	82	1618	31	19203	188	8715	4508	165
COLUMBIA—Marion County MARION GENERAL HOSPITAL, 1560 Sumrall Road, Zip 39429–2654, Mailing Address: P.O. Box 630, Zip 39429–0630; tel. 601/736–6303; Jerry M. Howell, Chief Operating Officer **A**9 10 **F**1 2 8 9 10 11 12 13 17 19 22 23 24 25 27 28 31 35 36 37 39 40 41 42 44 45 47 48 51 52 53 54 56 57 65 66 70 71 74 76 77 78	13	10	79	1834	33	28620	0	—	—	229
COLUMBUS—Lowndes County ★ BAPTIST MEMORIAL HOSPITAL–GOLDEN TRIANGLE, 2520 Fifth Street North, Zip 39703–2095, Mailing Address: P.O. Box 1307, Zip 39701–1307; tel. 662/244–1000; Dean A. Griffin, Chief Executive Officer **A**1 9 10 **F**1 2 3 8 9 10 11 12 13 17 18 19 22 23 24 25 27 28 30 31 35 36 37 39 40 41 42 43 44 45 46 47 48 50 51 52 53 54 56 57 58 59 60 61 62 63 64 66 70 71 72 73 76 77 78 79 **P**3 5 **S** Baptist Memorial Health Care Corporation, Memphis, TN **Web address:** www.bmhcc.org	23	10	328	8733	125	92230	988	62367	24963	919
★ U. S. AIR FORCE HOSPITAL, 201 Independence, Suite 235, Zip 39701–5300; tel. 662/434–2297; Lieutenant Colonel Mark L. Allen, MSC, USAF, Administrator (Nonreporting) **S** Department of the Air Force, Bowling AFB, DC	41	10	7	—	—	—	—	—	—	—
CORINTH—Alcorn County ★ MAGNOLIA REGIONAL HEALTH CENTER, 611 Alcorn Drive, Zip 38834–9368; tel. 662/293–1000; Douglas Garner, Chief Executive Officer **A**1 9 10 **F**8 9 11 12 13 16 17 18 19 22 23 24 25 27 28 31 36 37 39 41 43 44 45 46 47 48 50 51 52 53 54 57 60 61 63 64 65 70 71 72 76 78 **P**8 **S** Quorum Health Group, Brentwood, TN	15	10	163	6614	101	83459	492	48404	19084	722
DURANT—Holmes County UNIVERSITY HOSPITALS AND CLINICS OF HOLMES COUNTY–DURANT, 713 Northwest Avenue, Zip 39063–3007; tel. 662/653–3081; Thomas G. Honaker, II, FACHE, Administrator **A**10 **F**16 17 18 23 25 51 70 76 78 **P**6	12	10	29	319	6	10846	0	—	—	89
EUPORA—Webster County ☐ WEBSTER HEALTH SERVICES, 500 Highway 9 South, Zip 39744; tel. 601/258–6221; Harold H. Whitaker, Administrator (Total facility includes 33 beds in nursing home–type unit) **A**1 9 10 **F**9 16 17 18 19 22 24 25 28 35 36 37 50 51 53 65 69 70 72 76 **P**4 **S** North Mississippi Health Services, Inc., Tupelo, MS	23	10	76	1958	56	10376	0	7954	3781	146

© 2000 AHA Guide — *Many Facility Codes have changed. Please refer to the AHA Guide Code Chart.*

Hospitals, U.S. / MISSISSIPPI

Hospital, Address, Telephone, Administrator, Approval, Facility, and Physician Codes, Health Care System, Network

★ American Hospital Association (AHA) membership
☐ Joint Commission on Accreditation of Healthcare Organizations (JCAHO) accreditation
+ American Osteopathic Healthcare Association (AOHA) membership
○ American Osteopathic Association (AOA) accreditation
△ Commission on Accreditation of Rehabilitation Facilities (CARF) accreditation
Control codes 61, 63, 64, 71, 72 and 73 indicate hospitals listed by AOHA, but not registered by AHA. For definition of numerical codes, see page A4

Hospital	Classification Codes		Utilization Data					Expense (thousands) of dollars		Personnel
	Control	Service	Staffed Beds	Admissions	Census	Outpatient Visits	Births	Total	Payroll	
FAYETTE—Jefferson County										
JEFFERSON COUNTY HOSPITAL, 809 South Main Street, Zip 39069, Mailing Address: P.O. Box 577, Zip 39069-0577; tel. 601/786-3401; Jerry Kennedy, Administrator **A**9 10 **F**17 18 25 50	13	10	27	560	9	2954	0	—	—	51
FOREST—Scott County										
LACKEY MEMORIAL HOSPITAL, 330 Broad Street, Zip 39074-0428, Mailing Address: P.O. Box 428, Zip 39074-0428; tel. 601/469-4151; Donna Riser, Administrator (Total facility includes 30 beds in nursing home-type unit) **A**9 10 **F**9 13 16 17 18 19 22 24 25 30 48 50 59 62 63 64 69 70 71 76 78 **P**5	23	10	74	1330	47	6285	0	—	—	126
GREENVILLE—Washington County										
✠ DELTA REGIONAL MEDICAL CENTER, 1400 East Union Street, Zip 38703-3246, Mailing Address: P.O. Box 5247, Zip 38704-5247; tel. 662/378-3783; Barton A. Hove, Chief Executive Officer **A**1 9 10 **F**2 3 8 9 10 11 12 13 18 19 22 23 24 25 27 31 36 37 39 41 43 44 46 47 48 54 55 57 61 68 70 72 76 78 **P**8 **S** Quorum Health Group, Brentwood, TN	13	10	160	6327	115	34471	600	51169	22108	741
☐ KING'S DAUGHTERS HOSPITAL, 300 Washington Avenue, Zip 38701-3614, Mailing Address: P.O. Box 1857, Zip 38702-1857; tel. 601/378-2020; Donald Joe Fisher, Administrator **A**1 9 10 **F**8 9 10 11 12 13 16 17 19 22 23 24 25 31 41 43 44 45 48 50 51 53 54 68 70 72 76 78 79 **S** Community Health Systems, Inc., Brentwood, TN	33	10	103	2665	37	49957	600	20858	10058	323
GREENWOOD—Leflore County										
✠ GREENWOOD LEFLORE HOSPITAL, 1401 River Road, Zip 38930-4030, Mailing Address: Drawer 1410, Zip 38935-1410; tel. 662/459-7000; Terrell M. Cobb, Executive Director **A**1 9 10 **F**8 9 11 12 16 18 19 22 23 24 25 27 28 30 31 35 39 41 43 44 46 48 50 51 54 57 68 70 72 73 76 78 79 **P**6 8	15	10	204	8097	127	123846	765	—	—	974
GRENADA—Grenada County										
✠ GRENADA LAKE MEDICAL CENTER, 960 Avent Drive, Zip 38901-5094; tel. 662/227-7101; Linda J. Gholston, Chief Executive Officer **A**1 9 10 **F**2 8 9 11 12 13 16 17 18 19 22 24 25 28 35 36 37 39 40 41 42 43 44 45 46 48 51 52 53 54 59 61 68 70 72 76 78 **P**8	13	10	114	6217	93	37850	657	31972	14704	489
GULFPORT—Harrison County										
✠ COLUMBIA GARDEN PARK HOSPITAL, 1520 Broad Avenue, Zip 39501, Mailing Address: P.O. Box 1240, Zip 39502-1240; tel. 228/864-4210; William E. Peaks, Chief Executive Officer **A**1 9 10 **F**2 8 9 12 13 16 17 18 19 22 23 24 25 28 30 31 37 39 41 44 45 46 48 51 53 54 56 57 66 69 70 71 72 76 77 78 79 **P**5 6 7 8 **S** HCA – The Healthcare Company, Nashville, TN	33	10	97	2937	41	21192	420	22235	9341	321
MEMORIAL BEHAVIORAL HEALTH, (Formerly BHC Sand Hill Behavioral Healthcare), 11150 Highway 49 North, Zip 39503-4110; tel. 228/831-1700; Michael A. Zieman, Administrator (Nonreporting) **A**9 10 **S** Behavioral Healthcare Corporation, Nashville, TN	33	22	60	—	—	—	—	—	—	—
✠ △ MEMORIAL HOSPITAL AT GULFPORT, 4500 13th Street, Zip 39501-2569, Mailing Address: P.O. Box 1810, Zip 39502-1810; tel. 228/867-4000; W. R. Burton, Administrator **A**1 2 7 9 10 **F**2 3 8 9 11 12 13 17 18 19 22 24 25 27 28 30 35 37 39 41 42 44 45 46 47 48 51 52 53 54 56 57 58 60 61 62 63 64 66 68 70 71 72 76 77 78 79 **P**3 8 Web address: www.mhg.com	15	10	335	14975	250	264928	1156	161097	66224	2135
VETERANS AFFAIRS MEDICAL CENTER, GULFPORT DIVISION See VA Gulf Coast Veterans Health Care System, Biloxi										
HATTIESBURG—Forrest County										
✠ FORREST GENERAL HOSPITAL, 6051 U.S. Highway 49, Zip 39401-7243, Mailing Address: P.O. Box 16389, Zip 39404-6389; tel. 601/288-7000; William C. Oliver, President **A**1 2 9 10 **F**2 3 8 9 11 12 13 16 17 18 19 22 23 24 25 27 36 37 39 41 42 43 44 45 46 47 48 50 51 53 54 57 58 59 60 61 63 64 65 68 69 70 71 72 74 76 78 79 **P**8	13	10	537	27374	374	126953	2896	184865	75495	2700
✠ WESLEY MEDICAL CENTER, 5001 Hardy Street, Zip 39402, Mailing Address: P.O. Box 16509, Zip 39404-6509; tel. 601/268-8000; Dan H. Akin, Interim Chief Executive Officer **A**1 9 10 **F**8 9 11 12 13 16 17 18 19 22 23 24 25 27 28 30 35 36 39 41 42 43 44 45 46 48 50 51 53 54 56 70 71 72 76 78 79 **P**8 **S** Quorum Health Group, Brentwood, TN Web address: www.wesley.com	32	10	211	8173	118	77868	660	—	—	808
HAZLEHURST—Copiah County										
★ HARDY WILSON MEMORIAL HOSPITAL, 233 Magnolia Street, Zip 39083-2229, Mailing Address: P.O. Box 889, Zip 39083-0889; tel. 601/894-4541; L. Pat Moreland, Administrator **A**9 10 **F**9 22 25 31 44 48 54 57 62 70 76	13	10	49	1474	26	32944	207	—	—	137
HOLLY SPRINGS—Marshall County										
ALLIANCE HEALTHCARE SYSTEM, (Formerly Marshall County Medical Center), 1430 East Salem, Zip 38635, Mailing Address: P.O. Box 6000, Zip 38634-6000; tel. 602/252-1212; Perry E. Williams, Administrator **A**9 10 **F**13 17 18 19 22 25 30 31 37 43 48 51 56 57 62 63 64 70 72 76 78	33	10	40	811	11	18106	0	6100	2600	94
HOUSTON—Chickasaw County										
☐ TRACE REGIONAL HOSPITAL, Highway 8 East, Zip 38851, Mailing Address: P.O. Box 626, Zip 38851-0626; tel. 662/456-3700; Charles Nasem, Chief Executive Officer **A**1 9 10 **F**9 12 18 22 24 25 35 41 43 48 57 62 64 70 76 **P**6 **S** NetCare Health Systems, Inc., Nashville, TN Web address: www.traceregional.com	33	10	84	1679	22	13785	0	—	—	156
INDIANOLA—Sunflower County										
✠ SOUTH SUNFLOWER COUNTY HOSPITAL, 121 East Baker Street, Zip 38751-2498; tel. 662/887-5235; H. J. Blessitt, Administrator **A**1 9 10 **F**8 12 22 25 41 44 48 70 76 **P**1	13	10	69	2292	25	12254	398	10469	4527	151

Many Facility Codes have changed. Please refer to the AHA Guide Code Chart.

© 2000 AHA Guide

Hospitals, U.S. / MISSISSIPPI

Hospital, Address, Telephone, Administrator, Approval, Facility, and Physician Codes, Health Care System, Network	Classification Codes		Utilization Data					Expense (thousands) of dollars		
★ American Hospital Association (AHA) membership ☐ Joint Commission on Accreditation of Healthcare Organizations (JCAHO) accreditation + American Osteopathic Healthcare Association (AOHA) membership ○ American Osteopathic Association (AOA) accreditation △ Commission on Accreditation of Rehabilitation Facilities (CARF) accreditation Control codes 61, 63, 64, 71, 72 and 73 indicate hospitals listed by AOHA, but not registered by AHA. For definition of numerical codes, see page A4	Control	Service	Staffed Beds	Admissions	Census	Outpatient Visits	Births	Total	Payroll	Personnel

IUKA—Tishomingo County

☐ IUKA HOSPITAL, 1777 Curtis Drive, Zip 38852-1001, Mailing Address: P.O. Box 860, Zip 38852-0860; tel. 662/423-6051; Daniel Perryman, Administrator **A**1 9 10 **F**9 12 13 16 17 18 19 22 24 25 28 31 36 37 41 43 45 48 50 51 54 70 72 73 76 78 **P**3 5 6 **S** North Mississippi Health Services, Inc., Tupelo, MS	23	10	48	1995	27	8473	0	8305	3771	128

JACKSON—Hinds and Rankin County

☐ CENTRAL MISSISSIPPI MEDICAL CENTER, 1850 Chadwick Drive, Zip 39204-3479, Mailing Address: P.O. Box 59001, Zip 39204-9001; tel. 601/376-1000; John R. Finnegan, Chief Executive Officer **A**1 2 5 9 10 **F**8 9 11 12 13 16 17 18 19 22 24 25 27 35 36 39 41 42 43 44 46 47 48 50 51 52 53 54 56 57 59 61 68 69 70 72 76 78 79 **P**8 **S** Health Management Associates, Naples, FL	33	10	317	10472	185	64077	1353	88566	36935	1149
★ G.V. MONTGOMERY VETERANS AFFAIRS MEDICAL CENTER, 1500 East Woodrow Wilson Drive, Zip 39216-5199; tel. 601/364-1201; Richard F. Miller, Director (Total facility includes 120 beds in nursing home-type unit) (Nonreporting) **A**1 2 3 5 8 **S** Department of Veterans Affairs, Washington, DC Web address: www.visn16.med.va.gov	45	10	443	—	—	—	—	—	—	—
★ MISSISSIPPI BAPTIST HEALTH SYSTEMS, (Includes Baptist Behavioral Health, 5354 I-55 South Frontage Road, Zip 39212; tel. 601/372-9788; D. Preston Smith, Jr, Administrator), 1225 North State Street, Zip 39202-2002; tel. 601/968-1000; Kurt W. Metzner, President and Chief Executive Officer **A**1 2 3 5 9 10 **F**1 2 3 8 9 11 12 13 16 17 18 19 22 24 25 27 28 30 31 35 36 37 39 41 42 43 44 45 46 47 48 50 52 53 54 57 59 62 63 68 69 70 72 76 77 78 79 **P**1	23	10	639	17806	291	92197	878	179811	72925	2467
★ MISSISSIPPI HOSPITAL RESTORATIVE CARE, 1225 North State Street, Zip 39202-2097, Mailing Address: P.O. Box 23695, Zip 39225-3695; tel. 601/968-1000; Sallye M. Wilcox, R.N., Ph.D., Executive Director **A**1 **F**1 2 3 8 9 11 12 16 17 18 19 22 24 25 27 28 30 31 35 36 37 39 41 42 43 44 45 46 47 48 50 52 53 54 57 59 62 63 68 69 70 72 74 76 77 78 79 **P**1	23	49	25	244	19	0	0	7472	2422	62
★ MISSISSIPPI METHODIST HOSPITAL AND REHABILITATION CENTER, 1350 Woodrow Wilson Drive, Zip 39216-5198; tel. 601/981-2611; Mark A. Adams, President and Chief Executive Officer **A**1 5 9 10 **F**13 19 22 31 36 39 43 45 48 50 51 53 54 70 72 76 78 Web address: www.mmhcrehab.org	23	46	124	1653	80	—	0	36915	16377	615
★ RIVER OAKS HOSPITAL, 1030 River Oaks Drive, Zip 39208-9729, Mailing Address: P.O. Box 5100, Zip 39296-5100; tel. 601/932-1030; John J. Cleary, President and Chief Executive Officer **A**1 10 **F**8 9 12 13 16 17 18 22 23 24 25 31 37 41 42 43 44 46 48 50 51 52 57 68 70 76 78 79 **S** Health Management Associates, Naples, FL	33	10	109	6012	68	—	1283	48732	17058	542
★ ST. DOMINIC-JACKSON MEMORIAL HOSPITAL, 969 Lakeland Drive, Zip 39216-4699; tel. 601/982-0121; Claude W. Harbarger, President **A**1 2 3 5 9 10 **F**2 3 9 11 12 13 18 19 22 23 24 25 27 28 35 37 39 41 43 46 47 48 50 53 54 56 57 58 59 60 61 62 63 64 68 70 72 76 77 78 **P**8 Web address: www.stdom.com	23	10	571	15003	330	56889	0	126351	53724	2041
★ UNIVERSITY HOSPITALS AND CLINICS, UNIVERSITY OF MISSISSIPPI MEDICAL CENTER, 2500 North State Street, Zip 39216-4505; tel. 601/984-1000; Frederick Woodrell, Director **A**1 2 3 5 8 9 10 **F**1 9 10 11 12 13 17 18 22 23 24 25 27 35 39 41 42 43 44 45 46 47 48 50 51 52 53 54 56 57 59 60 62 63 66 68 69 70 71 72 73 74 75 76 77 78 **P**6 **S** Quorum Health Group, Brentwood, TN	12	10	613	23238	442	199890	3141	249950	107481	3212
☐ WOMAN'S HOSPITAL AT RIVER OAKS, (Formerly River Oaks East), 1026 North Flowood Drive, Zip 39208-9599, Mailing Address: P.O. Box 4546, Zip 39296-4546; tel. 601/932-1000; Sherry J. Smith, Executive Director **A**1 9 10 **F**8 9 12 13 16 17 18 19 22 23 24 25 31 41 42 44 45 46 48 50 51 52 53 56 57 69 70 78 79 **S** Health Management Associates, Naples, FL	33	10	76	2726	29	7842	1353	17414	7355	218

KEESLER AFB—Harrison County

★ U. S. AIR FORCE MEDICAL CENTER KEESLER, 301 Fisher Street, Suite 1A132, Zip 39534-2519; tel. 228/377-6510; Colonel Randall W. Hartley, Administrator (Nonreporting) **A**1 2 3 5 **S** Department of the Air Force, Bowling AFB, DC Web address: www.81mdg06.keesler.af.mil/index.cgi	41	10	185	—	—	—	—	—	—	—

KILMICHAEL—Montgomery County

KILMICHAEL HOSPITAL, 301 Lamar Avenue, Zip 39747-0188, Mailing Address: P.O. Box 188, Zip 39747-0188; tel. 601/262-4311; Calvin D. Johnson, Chief Executive Officer **A**9 10 **F**1 9 11 12 17 18 19 22 24 27 28 30 31 39 41 42 44 46 47 48 50 52 62 65 70 71 76 **P**8	13	10	19	544	9	3148	0	—	—	36

KOSCIUSKO—Attala County

MONTFORT JONES MEMORIAL HOSPITAL, Highway 12 West, Zip 39090-3209, Mailing Address: Box 677, Zip 39090-0677; tel. 601/289-4311; Thomas Bland, Administrator **A**9 10 **F**2 8 9 12 17 22 23 24 25 30 37 41 44 48 52 53 54 57 62 70 76	13	10	72	1950	35	19594	182	5763	4318	155

LAUREL—Jones County

★ SOUTH CENTRAL REGIONAL MEDICAL CENTER, (Includes South Central Extended Care, Ivy Street, Ellisville, Zip 39437; tel. 601/477-9159), 1220 Jefferson Street, Zip 39440-4374, Mailing Address: P.O. Box 607, Zip 39441-0607; tel. 601/426-4000; G. Douglas Higginbotham, Executive Director (Total facility includes 60 beds in nursing home-type unit) **A**1 9 10 **F**2 8 9 11 12 16 17 18 19 22 23 24 25 27 28 30 31 36 37 39 41 43 44 45 46 48 50 51 53 54 57 62 68 69 70 72 75 76 78 79 **P**3 4 7	13	10	261	9609	199	80713	1055	56405	25390	1103

© 2000 AHA Guide   *Many Facility Codes have changed. Please refer to the AHA Guide Code Chart.*

Hospitals, U.S. / MISSISSIPPI

Hospital, Address, Telephone, Administrator, Approval, Facility, and Physician Codes, Health Care System, Network	Classification Codes		Utilization Data					Expense (thousands) of dollars		
★ American Hospital Association (AHA) membership □ Joint Commission on Accreditation of Healthcare Organizations (JCAHO) accreditation + American Osteopathic Healthcare Association (AOHA) membership ○ American Osteopathic Association (AOA) accreditation △ Commission on Accreditation of Rehabilitation Facilities (CARF) accreditation Control codes 61, 63, 64, 71, 72 and 73 indicate hospitals listed by AOHA, but not registered by AHA. For definition of numerical codes, see page A4	Control	Service	Staffed Beds	Admissions	Census	Outpatient Visits	Births	Total	Payroll	Personnel
LEXINGTON—Holmes County ✠ UNIVERSITY HOSPITALS AND CLINICS – HOLMES COUNTY, (Formerly Methodist Healthcare of Middle Mississippi), 239 Bowling Green Road, Zip 39095–9332; tel. 662/834–1321; Thomas Honacker, Interim Chief Executive Officer **A**1 10 **F**9 16 22 24 25 31 48 70 75 76	23	10	80	2330	38	16596	84	—	—	144
LOUISVILLE—Winston County WINSTON MEDICAL CENTER, 562 East Main Street, Zip 39339–2742, Mailing Address: P.O. Box 967, Zip 39339–0967; tel. 601/773–6211; W. Dale Saulters, Administrator (Total facility includes 120 beds in nursing home–type unit) **A**9 10 **F**9 12 22 25 36 41 48 62 69 70 76 78	23	10	185	993	135	22343	0	—	—	133
LUCEDALE—George County GEORGE COUNTY HOSPITAL, 859 Winter Street, Zip 39452–6603, Mailing Address: P.O. Box 607, Zip 39452–0607; tel. 601/947–3161; Paul A. Gardner, CPA, Administrator **A**9 10 **F**1 2 8 9 10 12 13 16 17 18 19 22 24 25 28 30 31 36 37 39 40 41 42 43 44 45 46 48 50 51 52 53 54 56 57 66 69 70 71 72 73 75 76 77 78 79 **P**8	13	10	47	2611	25	34809	140	—	—	295
MACON—Noxubee County ★ NOXUBEE GENERAL HOSPITAL, 606 North Jefferson Street, Zip 39341–2236, Mailing Address: P.O. Box 480, Zip 39341–0480; tel. 662/726–4231; Arthur Nester, Jr, Administrator (Total facility includes 60 beds in nursing home–type unit) **A**9 10 **F**2 9 10 12 17 23 25 30 35 41 42 44 52 53 57 62 69 70 75 78	13	10	109	1044	75	7376	0	6546	3267	96
MAGEE—Simpson County MAGEE GENERAL HOSPITAL, 300 S.E. Third Avenue, Zip 39111–3698; tel. 601/849–5070; Althea H. Crumpton, Administrator **A**9 10 **F**22 24 25 48 54 57 62 68 70 76 78	23	10	64	2260	33	28405	0	—	—	175
MAGNOLIA—Pike County BEACHAM MEMORIAL HOSPITAL, 205 North Cherry Street, Zip 39652–2819, Mailing Address: P.O. Box 351, Zip 39652–0351; tel. 601/783–2351; Marilyn Speed, Administrator **A**9 10 **F**16 18 23 69 70 76	23	10	37	975	21	4001	0	3396	1650	69
MARKS—Quitman County QUITMAN COUNTY HOSPITAL AND NURSING HOME, 340 Getwell Drive, Zip 38646–9785; tel. 601/326–8031; Richard E. Waller, M.D., Interim Administrator (Total facility includes 60 beds in nursing home–type unit) **A**9 10 **F**2 8 10 12 16 17 18 22 25 30 37 40 41 42 44 48 50 51 52 53 54 57 62 69 70 76 78	33	10	96	970	78	12489	0	—	—	102
MCCOMB—Pike County ✠ SOUTHWEST MISSISSIPPI REGIONAL MEDICAL CENTER, 215 Marion Avenue, Zip 39648–2798, Mailing Address: P.O. Box 1307, Zip 39648–1307; tel. 601/249–5500; Norman M. Price, FACHE, Administrator **A**1 9 10 **F**8 9 11 12 13 17 18 19 22 23 24 25 27 31 35 39 41 43 44 46 48 50 51 53 54 68 70 72 74 76 78 79 **P**6 Web address: www.smrmc.com	15	10	120	7068	92	74136	947	56569	26256	855
MEADVILLE—Franklin County FRANKLIN COUNTY MEMORIAL HOSPITAL, Hospital Road, Zip 39653, Mailing Address: P.O. Box 636, Zip 39653–0636; tel. 601/384–5801; Semmes Ross, Jr, Administrator **A**9 10 **F**2 13 16 17 19 22 25 30 31 48 50 53 54 57 62 64 70 72 76	13	10	43	1083	20	3191	0	6664	3069	96
MENDENHALL—Simpson County SIMPSON GENERAL HOSPITAL, 1842 Simpson Highway 149, Zip 39114–3592; tel. 601/847–2221; Wayne Harris, Administrator **A**9 10 **F**17 18 19 22 24 25 28 30 35 48 50 51 53 54 62 70 72 76 78 **P**5	13	10	49	1191	23	9282	1	—	—	131
MERIDIAN—Lauderdale County EAST MISSISSIPPI STATE HOSPITAL, 4555 Highland Park Drive, Zip 39307–5498, Mailing Address: Box 4128, West Station, Zip 39304–4128; tel. 601/482–6186; Ramiro J. Martinez, M.D., Director (Total facility includes 226 beds in nursing home–type unit) **F**2 13 16 17 18 23 30 51 57 58 62 69 70 78 **S** Mississippi State Department of Mental Health, Jackson, MS	12	22	633	1330	591	0	0	43772	26046	1158
✠ JEFF ANDERSON REGIONAL MEDICAL CENTER, 2124 14th Street, Zip 39301–4093; tel. 601/553–6000; Mark D. McPhail, Chief Executive Officer **A**1 9 10 **F**8 9 11 12 13 16 17 18 19 22 24 25 27 28 35 39 41 42 44 45 46 47 48 50 51 52 53 54 57 65 68 70 71 72 74 76 78 **P**7 8	23	10	260	9464	136	40661	811	—	—	797
□ LAUREL WOOD CENTER, 5000 Highway 39 North, Zip 39303–1021; tel. 601/483–6211; Gregory Z. Cantrell, Chief Executive Officer **A**1 10 **F**2 3 13 19 40 50 51 57 58 59 60 62 64 70 72	33	22	79	533	15	0	0	—	—	85
□ RILEY MEMORIAL HOSPITAL, 1102 21st Avenue, Zip 39301–4096, Mailing Address: P.O. Box 1810, Zip 39301–1810; tel. 601/693–2511; Carl J. Etter, Chief Executive Officer **A**1 9 10 **F**2 8 9 10 12 18 19 22 24 25 28 36 39 41 43 44 45 46 48 50 51 52 53 54 57 68 70 71 72 76 78 79 **P**7 8 **S** Health Management Associates, Naples, FL	33	10	180	6333	86	52745	580	—	—	542
✠ RUSH FOUNDATION HOSPITAL, 1314 19th Avenue, Zip 39301–4195; tel. 601/483–0011; Dan M. Harrison, Executive Vice President and Administrator **A**1 9 10 **F**1 2 8 9 10 11 12 13 17 18 19 22 23 24 25 27 30 31 35 36 37 40 41 42 43 44 45 46 47 48 50 51 52 53 54 56 57 65 66 68 69 70 71 72 73 74 76 77 78 79 **P**3 5 6 8 **S** Rush Health Systems, Meridian, MS	23	10	195	8525	124	23161	1122	—	—	901
★ SPECIALTY HOSPITAL OF MERIDIAN, 1314 19th Avenue, Zip 39301; tel. 601/486–4211; Annette V. Drennan, R.N., President **A**10 **F**9 11 13 22 24 27 39 43 45 46 51 53 69 70 76 77 **S** Rush Health Systems, Meridian, MS	23	49	40	362	28	0	0	8895	2810	188

Hospitals, U.S. / MISSISSIPPI

Hospital, Address, Telephone, Administrator, Approval, Facility, and Physician Codes, Health Care System, Network	Classification Codes		Utilization Data					Expense (thousands) of dollars		Personnel
	Control	Service	Staffed Beds	Admissions	Census	Outpatient Visits	Births	Total	Payroll	

★ American Hospital Association (AHA) membership
☐ Joint Commission on Accreditation of Healthcare Organizations (JCAHO) accreditation
+ American Osteopathic Healthcare Association (AOHA) membership
○ American Osteopathic Association (AOA) accreditation
△ Commission on Accreditation of Rehabilitation Facilities (CARF) accreditation
Control codes 61, 63, 64, 71, 72 and 73 indicate hospitals listed by AOHA, but not registered by AHA. For definition of numerical codes, see page A4

Hospital	Control	Service	Staffed Beds	Admissions	Census	Outpatient Visits	Births	Total	Payroll	Personnel
MONTICELLO—Lawrence County										
LAWRENCE COUNTY HOSPITAL, Highway 84 East, Zip 39654-0788, Mailing Address: P.O. Box 788, Zip 39654-0788; tel. 601/587-4051; Deborah Roberts, Administrator A9 10 F2 10 12 19 23 24 25 36 41 42 50 51 62 70 76	13	10	53	1248	24	6738	0	4715	2522	125
NATCHEZ—Adams County										
☐ NATCHEZ COMMUNITY HOSPITAL, 129 Jefferson Davis Boulevard, Zip 39120-5100, Mailing Address: P.O. Box 1203, Zip 39121-1203; tel. 601/445-6200; Raymond Bane, Executive Director A1 9 10 F8 9 12 16 18 22 24 25 27 35 39 41 44 46 48 51 70 76 78 P1 6 8 S Health Management Associates, Naples, FL	33	10	101	3534	46	28123	499	20005	7947	243
★ NATCHEZ REGIONAL MEDICAL CENTER, Seargent S Prentiss Drive, Zip 39120, Mailing Address: P.O. Box 1488, Zip 39121-1488; tel. 601/443-2100; Karen A. Fiducia, Interim Chief Executive Officer A1 9 10 F8 9 12 13 16 17 18 19 22 24 25 39 41 43 44 46 48 50 51 53 54 56 68 70 71 72 76 77 78 79 S Quorum Health Group, Brentwood, TN	13	10	112	4232	57	32496	535	28533	12390	357
NEW ALBANY—Union County										
★ BAPTIST MEMORIAL HOSPITAL-UNION COUNTY, 200 Highway 30 West, Zip 38652-3197; tel. 601/538-7631; John Tompkins, Administrator A1 9 10 F8 9 12 13 17 19 22 23 24 25 30 34 39 41 43 44 48 50 51 53 54 68 69 70 72 76 78 79 S Baptist Memorial Health Care Corporation, Memphis, TN	21	10	153	5152	54	33021	932	22754	8495	327
OCEAN SPRINGS—Jackson County										
☐ OCEAN SPRINGS HOSPITAL, 3109 Bienville Boulevard, Zip 39564-4361; tel. 228/818-1111; Dwight Rimes, Administrator A1 F2 3 8 9 11 12 13 16 17 18 19 22 23 24 25 27 31 35 36 37 39 41 43 44 45 46 47 48 52 53 57 59 60 61 62 68 69 70 72 76 P3 4 S Singing River Hospital System, Gautier, MS	13	10	108	5150	73	83608	373	49238	20180	515
OKOLONA—Chickasaw County										
★ OKOLONA COMMUNITY HOSPITAL, (Includes SHEARER-RICHARDSON MEMORIAL NURSING HOME), Rockwell Drive, Zip 38860-0420, Mailing Address: P.O. Box 420, Zip 38860-0420; tel. 662/447-3311; Brenda Wise, Administrator (Total facility includes 66 beds in nursing home-type unit) A9 10 F23 27 35 36 37 39 53 65 69 70 76 78	23	10	76	94	68	0	0	2584	1358	63
OLIVE BRANCH—De Soto County										
☐ PARKWOOD BEHAVIORAL HEALTH SYSTEM, (Formerly Charter Parkwood Health System), 8135 Goodman Road, Zip 38654-2199; tel. 662/895-4900; M. Andrew Mayo, Chief Executive Officer A1 10 F2 3 9 12 13 17 18 19 25 28 31 37 39 41 43 46 48 52 55 57 58 59 60 61 63 64 68 69 70 72 76 77 S Magellan Health Services, Atlanta, GA	33	22	66	1357	42	0	0	—	—	73
OXFORD—Lafayette County										
★ BAPTIST MEMORIAL HOSPITAL-NORTH MISSISSIPPI, 2301 South Lamar Boulevard, Zip 38655, Mailing Address: P.O. Box 946, Zip 38655-0946; tel. 662/232-8100; James Hahn, Administrator A1 9 10 F8 9 11 12 13 16 17 18 19 22 23 24 25 27 28 36 37 39 41 44 45 46 47 48 50 51 52 53 57 63 69 70 71 72 76 78 79 P3 4 5 7 S Baptist Memorial Health Care Corporation, Memphis, TN Web address: www.bmhcc.org	23	10	204	9866	138	61204	756	—	—	823
PASCAGOULA—Jackson County										
★ SINGING RIVER HOSPITAL, 2809 Denny Avenue, Zip 39581-5301; tel. 228/809-5000; Lynn Truelove, Administrator A1 2 9 10 F2 3 8 9 11 12 13 16 17 18 19 22 23 24 25 27 31 35 36 37 39 41 43 44 45 46 47 48 52 53 57 59 60 61 62 68 69 70 72 74 76 P3 8 S Singing River Hospital System, Gautier, MS Web address: www.srhshealth.com	13	10	273	11827	187	200346	942	104602	50470	1483
PHILADELPHIA—Neshoba County										
★ CHOCTAW HEALTH CENTER, Highway 16 West, Zip 39350, Mailing Address: Route 7, Box R-50, Zip 39350; tel. 601/656-2211; James D. Wallace, Executive Director (Nonreporting) A1 10 S U. S. Public Health Service Indian Health Service, Rockville, MD	47	10	35	—	—	—	—	—	—	—
★ NESHOBA COUNTY GENERAL HOSPITAL, 1001 Holland Avenue, Zip 39350-2161, Mailing Address: P.O. Box 648, Zip 39350-0648; tel. 601/663-1200; Lawrence Graeber, Administrator (Total facility includes 118 beds in nursing home-type unit) A9 10 F9 22 24 25 30 31 35 37 39 48 53 62 69 70 76 78 S Quorum Health Group, Brentwood, TN	13	10	166	1629	141	30465	4	—	—	165
PICAYUNE—Pearl River County										
★ CROSBY MEMORIAL HOSPITAL, 801 Goodyear Boulevard, Zip 39466-3221, Mailing Address: P.O. Box 909, Zip 39466-0909; tel. 601/798-4711; Harry Albis, Interim Chief Executive Officer A9 10 F2 8 9 12 16 17 18 19 22 23 24 25 28 30 31 35 36 37 39 40 41 43 44 45 46 48 50 53 54 57 60 62 68 70 71 72 73 74 76 78 79 S New American Healthcare Corporation, Brentwood, TN Web address: www.crosbyhospital.com	33	10	71	2488	35	37286	369	17319	7288	252
PONTOTOC—Pontotoc County										
PONTOTOC HOSPITAL AND EXTENDED CARE FACILITY, 176 South Main Street, Zip 38863-3311, Mailing Address: P.O. Box 790, Zip 38863-0790; tel. 662/488-7640; Fred B. Hood, Administrator (Total facility includes 44 beds in nursing home-type unit) A9 10 F9 17 18 19 25 31 36 37 40 43 50 51 53 64 69 70 72 74 76 78 P3 8 S North Mississippi Health Services, Inc., Tupelo, MS	23	10	71	675	61	12520	0	7637	3246	89
POPLARVILLE—Pearl River County										
PEARL RIVER COUNTY HOSPITAL, 305 West Moody Street, Zip 39470-7242, Mailing Address: P.O. Box 392, Zip 39470-0392; tel. 601/795-4543; Dorothy C. Bilbo, Administrator (Total facility includes 66 beds in nursing home-type unit) A9 10 F16 17 18 51 53 54 69 70 76 78	13	10	90	663	72	0	0	—	—	86

© 2000 AHA Guide   *Many Facility Codes have changed. Please refer to the AHA Guide Code Chart.*

Hospitals, U.S. / MISSISSIPPI

Hospital, Address, Telephone, Administrator, Approval, Facility, and Physician Codes, Health Care System, Network	Classification Codes		Utilization Data					Expense (thousands) of dollars		
	Control	Service	Staffed Beds	Admissions	Census	Outpatient Visits	Births	Total	Payroll	Personnel

★ American Hospital Association (AHA) membership
☐ Joint Commission on Accreditation of Healthcare Organizations (JCAHO) accreditation
+ American Osteopathic Healthcare Association (AOHA) membership
○ American Osteopathic Association (AOA) accreditation
△ Commission on Accreditation of Rehabilitation Facilities (CARF) accreditation
Control codes 61, 63, 64, 71, 72 and 73 indicate hospitals listed by AOHA, but not registered by AHA. For definition of numerical codes, see page A4

PORT GIBSON—Claiborne County
★ CLAIBORNE COUNTY HOSPITAL, 123 McComb Avenue, Zip 39150–2915, Mailing Address: P.O. Box 1004, Zip 39150–1004; tel. 601/437–5141; Wanda C. Fleming, Administrator and Chief Executive Officer **A**9 10 **F**18 19 22 25 44 48 50 51 54 57 62 69 70 76 78 — 13 10 32 552 10 4075 1 — — 68

PRENTISS—Jefferson Davis County
PRENTISS REGIONAL HOSPITAL AND EXTENDED CARE FACILITIES, 1102 Rose Street, Zip 39474; tel. 601/792–4276; Mike Boleware, Administrator (Total facility includes 60 beds in nursing home–type unit) **A**9 10 **F**16 17 18 19 22 25 50 51 54 57 62 70 76 — 23 10 101 1070 76 18143 0 — — 124

QUITMAN—Clarke County
★ H. C. WATKINS MEMORIAL HOSPITAL, 605 South Archusa Avenue, Zip 39355–2398; tel. 601/776–6925; Lawrence H. McAvoy, Interim President and Chief Executive Officer (Total facility includes 13 beds in nursing home–type unit) **A**9 10 **F**2 9 12 22 24 25 39 41 48 53 54 57 69 70 76 78 **S** Quorum Health Group, Brentwood, TN — 23 10 45 1230 37 7004 0 — — 116

RICHTON—Perry County
★ PERRY COUNTY GENERAL HOSPITAL, 206 Bay Avenue, Zip 39476, Mailing Address: P.O. Drawer Y, Zip 39476; tel. 601/788–6316; Bobby Welborn, Administrator (Total facility includes 73 beds in nursing home–type unit) **A**9 10 **F**9 17 19 23 25 36 48 53 54 69 70 76 — 13 10 95 452 72 3094 0 — — 85

RIPLEY—Tippah County
⊞ TIPPAH COUNTY HOSPITAL, 1005 City Avenue North, Zip 38663–0499; tel. 601/837–9221; Jerry Green, Administrator (Total facility includes 40 beds in nursing home–type unit) **A**1 9 10 **F**9 12 17 18 22 24 25 35 37 41 48 52 69 70 76 **S** Baptist Memorial Health Care Corporation, Memphis, TN — 13 10 110 1346 56 22074 0 8786 4570 169

RULEVILLE—Sunflower County
NORTH SUNFLOWER COUNTY HOSPITAL, 840 North Oak Avenue, Zip 38771–0369, Mailing Address: P.O. Box 369, Zip 38771–0369; tel. 601/756–2711; Joseph Hammond, CHE, Administrator (Total facility includes 47 beds in nursing home–type unit) **A**9 10 **F**2 3 17 18 25 31 36 44 48 54 59 62 63 69 70 75 76 **P**8 — 13 10 91 1080 71 5093 9 — — 163

SENATOBIA—Tate County
☐ NORTH OAK REGIONAL MEDICAL CENTER, (Formerly Senatobia Community Hospital), 401 Getwell Drive, Zip 38668–2213, Mailing Address: P.O. Box 648, Zip 38668–0648; tel. 601/562–3100; James D. Tesar, Chief Executive Officer **A**1 10 **F**8 9 13 17 18 22 23 25 30 35 37 44 48 50 51 53 57 62 70 76 78 **S** Associates Capital Group, LLC, Birmingham, AL — 33 10 52 1068 13 16829 26 — — 110

SOUTHAVEN—De Soto County
⊞ △ BAPTIST MEMORIAL HOSPITAL–DESOTO, 7601 Southcrest Parkway, Zip 38671–4742; tel. 662/349–4000; Melvin E. Walker, Administrator (Total facility includes 120 beds in nursing home–type unit) **A**1 7 9 10 **F**2 8 9 11 12 13 16 17 18 19 22 23 24 25 27 28 30 31 35 36 37 39 41 42 43 44 45 46 47 48 50 51 53 54 56 57 65 68 69 70 71 72 74 76 77 78 79 **P**1 3 8 **S** Baptist Memorial Health Care Corporation, Memphis, TN
Web address: www.bmhcc.org — 23 10 260 7410 192 57687 1148 24068 16704 640

STARKVILLE—Oktibbeha County
⊞ OKTIBBEHA COUNTY HOSPITAL, 400 Hospital Road, Zip 39759–2163, Mailing Address: Drawer 1506, Zip 39760–1506; tel. 662/323–4320; Arthur C. Kelly, Administrator and Chief Executive Officer **A**1 9 10 **F**8 9 12 13 16 17 18 19 22 23 24 25 28 35 37 39 41 44 45 48 51 52 53 54 57 68 70 71 72 74 76 78 — 13 10 96 4038 49 63093 1134 26366 13061 458

TUPELO—Lee County
☐ △ NORTH MISSISSIPPI MEDICAL CENTER, 830 South Gloster Street, Zip 38801–4934; tel. 601/841–3000; Jeffrey B. Barber, Dr.PH, President and Chief Executive Officer (Total facility includes 100 beds in nursing home–type unit) **A**1 2 5 7 9 10 **F**2 3 8 9 11 12 13 16 17 18 19 20 22 24 25 27 28 30 36 37 39 40 41 42 43 44 45 46 47 48 50 51 52 53 54 56 57 58 60 62 63 64 65 68 69 70 71 72 76 77 78 79 **P**4 **S** North Mississippi Health Services, Inc., Tupelo, MS
Web address: www.nmhs.net — 23 10 724 27312 515 150900 2393 249693 101133 3211

TYLERTOWN—Walthall County
WALTHALL COUNTY GENERAL HOSPITAL, 100 Hospital Drive, Zip 39667–2099; tel. 601/876–2122; Jimmy Graves, Administrator **A**9 10 **F**9 17 22 23 25 30 36 48 51 54 57 62 70 76 78 — 13 10 49 1798 26 17240 0 7138 3001 147

UNION—Newton County
LAIRD HOSPITAL, 25117 Highway 15, Zip 39365–9099; tel. 601/774–8214; Georgia Buchanan, President **A**9 10 **F**9 22 24 25 36 41 48 51 54 70 76 78 — 33 10 50 1708 25 12216 0 7072 3911 229

VICKSBURG—Warren County
★ PARKVIEW REGIONAL MEDICAL CENTER, 100 McAuley Drive, Zip 39180–2897, Mailing Address: P.O. Box 590, Zip 39181–0590; tel. 601/631–2131; R. Allan Daugherty, Chief Executive Officer (Total facility includes 14 beds in nursing home–type unit) (Nonreporting) **A**2 10 **S** Quorum Health Group, Brentwood, TN
(Data included with Vicksburg Medical Center)
★ VICKSBURG MEDICAL CENTER, 1111 North Frontage Road, Zip 39180; tel. 601/619–3800; Rob Followell, Chief Operating Officer and Administrator (Total facility includes 17 beds in nursing home–type unit) **A**9 10 **F**2 3 8 9 10 11 12 13 18 22 24 25 27 30 36 37 39 40 41 42 43 44 46 48 50 51 54 57 62 69 70 75 76 78 79 **P**1 2 **S** Quorum Health Group, Brentwood, TN — 33 10 365 9667 169 — 1252 70297 25209 1121

Hospitals, U.S. / MISSISSIPPI

	Hospital, Address, Telephone, Administrator, Approval, Facility, and Physician Codes, Health Care System, Network	Classification Codes		Utilization Data					Expense (thousands) of dollars		
		Control	Service	Staffed Beds	Admissions	Census	Outpatient Visits	Births	Total	Payroll	Personnel

★ American Hospital Association (AHA) membership
□ Joint Commission on Accreditation of Healthcare Organizations (JCAHO) accreditation
+ American Osteopathic Healthcare Association (AOHA) membership
○ American Osteopathic Association (AOA) accreditation
△ Commission on Accreditation of Rehabilitation Facilities (CARF) accreditation
Control codes 61, 63, 64, 71, 72 and 73 indicate hospitals listed by AOHA, but not registered by AHA. For definition of numerical codes, see page A4

Hospital	Control	Service	Staffed Beds	Admissions	Census	Outpatient Visits	Births	Total	Payroll	Personnel
WATER VALLEY—Yalobusha County YALOBUSHA GENERAL HOSPITAL, Highway 7 South, Zip 38965, Mailing Address: P.O. Box 728, Zip 38965-0728; tel. 601/473-1411; John R. Jones, Administrator (Total facility includes 65 beds in nursing home-type unit) **A**9 10 **F**13 22 23 43 45 53 69 70 76 78 **P**4 7	13	10	91	578	78	3936	0	—	—	100
WAYNESBORO—Wayne County WAYNE GENERAL HOSPITAL, 950 Matthew Drive, Zip 39367-2590, Mailing Address: P.O. Box 1249, Zip 39367-1249; tel. 601/735-5151; Donald Hemeter, Administrator **A**9 10 **F**8 9 17 19 23 24 25 28 35 36 37 41 43 44 48 50 52 53 54 68 70 76 78	13	10	80	3591	45	33207	327	—	—	313
WEST POINT—Clay County □ CLAY COUNTY MEDICAL CENTER, 835 Medical Center Drive, Zip 39773-9320; tel. 601/495-2300; David M. Reid, Administrator **A**1 9 10 **F**8 9 12 16 17 18 19 22 23 24 25 28 37 41 43 44 45 46 48 50 51 53 54 56 66 68 70 71 72 76 78 79 **S** North Mississippi Health Services, Inc., Tupelo, MS	23	10	60	3823	38	38517	449	15164	7086	227
WHITFIELD—Rankin County ★ MISSISSIPPI STATE HOSPITAL, (Includes Whitfield Medical Surgical Hospital, Oak Circle, Zip 39193; tel. 601/351-8023), Zip 39193-0157; tel. 601/351-8000; James G. Chastain, Director (Total facility includes 479 beds in nursing home-type unit) **A**1 **F**2 8 9 10 11 12 13 17 19 22 23 24 25 27 31 35 39 41 42 43 44 45 46 47 48 50 51 52 53 54 57 58 59 60 61 62 63 64 65 66 69 70 71 73 74 76 78 79 **P**8 **S** Mississippi State Department of Mental Health, Jackson, MS	12	22	1297	2022	1246	4581	0	89809	55171	2250
WINONA—Montgomery County TYLER HOLMES MEMORIAL HOSPITAL, 409 Tyler Holmes Drive, Zip 38967-1599; tel. 601/283-4114; Gregory S. Mullen, Administrator **A**9 10 **F**17 18 19 22 24 25 30 36 40 44 48 51 57 62 66 70 76 **P**8	13	10	49	1178	24	12161	37	6531	2861	142
YAZOO CITY—Yazoo County KING'S DAUGHTERS HOSPITAL, 823 Grand Avenue, Zip 39194-3233; tel. 601/746-2261; Noel W. Hart, Administrator **A**9 10 **F**9 12 16 18 22 23 24 25 28 30 35 40 41 48 51 57 70 76 78	23	10	54	1586	25	33960	0	10763	3953	172

Hospitals, U.S. / MISSOURI

MISSOURI

Resident Population 5,439 (in thousands)
Resident population in metro areas 68.0%
Birth rate per 1,000 population 13.7
65 years and over 13.7%
Percent of persons without health insurance 12.6%

Hospital, Address, Telephone, Administrator, Approval, Facility, and Physician Codes, Health Care System, Network	Classification Codes		Utilization Data					Expense (thousands) of dollars		
	Control	Service	Staffed Beds	Admissions	Census	Outpatient Visits	Births	Total	Payroll	Personnel

★ American Hospital Association (AHA) membership
☐ Joint Commission on Accreditation of Healthcare Organizations (JCAHO) accreditation
+ American Osteopathic Healthcare Association (AOHA) membership
○ American Osteopathic Association (AOA) accreditation
△ Commission on Accreditation of Rehabilitation Facilities (CARF) accreditation
Control codes 61, 63, 64, 71, 72 and 73 indicate hospitals listed by AOHA, but not registered by AHA. For definition of numerical codes, see page A4

ALBANY—Gentry County
★ GENTRY COUNTY MEMORIAL HOSPITAL, 705 North College Street, Zip 64402–1499; tel. 660/726–3941; John W. Richmond, President and Chief Executive Officer (Total facility includes 10 beds in nursing home–type unit) **A**9 10 **F**7 9 13 15 16 17 18 19 22 23 24 25 30 32 33 34 35 36 37 38 39 41 45 46 48 50 51 54 56 60 66 68 70 71 72 76 78 79 **P**6
Web address: www.gcmh.org
— 23 10 35 1060 18 35921 0 6476 3142 112

APPLETON CITY—St. Clair County
ELLETT MEMORIAL HOSPITAL, 610 North Ohio Avenue, Zip 64724–1609; tel. 660/476–2111; Joseph Moss, Administrator **A**9 10 18 **F**17 22 25 33 39 45 48 54 70 76
— 16 10 25 409 4 2038 0 1877 878 44

AURORA—Lawrence County
AURORA COMMUNITY HOSPITAL, 500 Porter Street, Zip 65605–2399; tel. 417/678–2122; Don Buchanan, Chief Operating Officer **A**10 **F**7 8 9 12 13 17 19 22 24 25 28 31 32 33 34 36 38 40 41 43 44 45 48 50 51 54 56 70 72 76 78 **P**6
— 14 10 27 1832 12 33428 281 10041 5170 172

BELTON—Cass County
★ RESEARCH BELTON HOSPITAL, 17065 South 71 Highway, Zip 64012–2165; tel. 816/348–1200; Daniel F. Sheehan, Administrator (Total facility includes 7 beds in nursing home–type unit) **A**9 **F**1 2 3 4 5 6 7 8 9 10 11 12 13 14 15 16 17 18 19 21 22 23 24 25 26 28 30 32 33 34 35 36 37 38 39 41 42 43 44 45 46 47 48 49 51 52 53 54 57 58 59 60 61 62 63 64 65 66 68 70 74 75 76 78 79 **P**4 6 7 8 **S** Health Midwest, Kansas City, MO
Web address: www.healthmidwest.org
— 23 10 47 1615 19 24489 1 14545 6134 152

BETHANY—Harrison County
HARRISON COUNTY COMMUNITY HOSPITAL, 2600 Miller Street, Zip 64424, Mailing Address: P.O. Box 428, Zip 64424–0428; tel. 660/425–2211; Dan P. Broyles, CHE, Administrator **A**9 10 **F**2 6 7 9 14 15 16 17 18 19 22 23 24 25 26 28 30 31 32 33 34 35 36 37 38 40 41 43 45 46 48 49 50 51 53 54 56 58 59 60 61 62 63 64 65 67 68 70 71 72 73 74 76 78 79 **P**5
— 16 10 21 695 8 33382 0 5892 2721 94

BLUE SPRINGS—Jackson County
✠ ST. MARY'S HOSPITAL OF BLUE SPRINGS, 201 West R. D. Mize Road, Zip 64014; tel. 816/228–5900; Gordon Docking, Chief Executive Officer **A**1 9 10 **F**4 6 7 8 9 11 12 13 17 18 19 22 23 24 25 26 28 29 30 32 33 34 35 36 37 38 39 41 42 43 44 45 46 47 48 49 50 51 53 54 65 68 70 71 72 76 77 78 **P**1 6 **S** Carondelet Health System, Saint Louis, MO
— 23 10 115 4729 61 73228 984 40707 16273 349

BOLIVAR—Polk County
✠ CITIZENS MEMORIAL HOSPITAL, 1500 North Oakland Avenue, Zip 65613–3099; tel. 417/326–6000; Donald J. Babb, Chief Executive Officer **A**1 9 10 **F**7 8 9 16 17 18 19 22 24 25 30 31 32 33 34 35 36 37 38 39 41 43 44 45 46 48 49 50 51 54 56 57 60 61 62 63 70 71 72 75 76 78 79 **P**6
Web address: www.citizensmemorial.com
— 16 10 74 2929 35 139749 374 33337 13927 449

BONNE TERRE—St. Francois County
PARKLAND HEALTH CENTER–BONNE TERRE See Parkland Health Center, Farmington

BOONVILLE—Cooper County
✠ COOPER COUNTY MEMORIAL HOSPITAL, 17651 B Highway, Zip 65233–2839, Mailing Address: P.O. Box 88, Zip 65233–0088; tel. 660/882–7461; Wilbert E. Meyer, Administrator and Chief Executive Officer (Total facility includes 24 beds in nursing home–type unit) **A**1 9 10 **F**7 9 13 16 17 18 19 22 25 32 33 34 36 38 39 43 45 46 48 54 59 60 69 70 72 76 78
— 13 10 49 695 28 29097 0 — 3497 161

BRANSON—Taney County
✠ SKAGGS COMMUNITY HEALTH CENTER, Business Highway 65 and Skaggs Road, Zip 65616–2035, Mailing Address: P.O. Box 650, Zip 65615–0650; tel. 417/335–7000; Bob D. Phillips, Administrator (Total facility includes 23 beds in nursing home–type unit) **A**1 9 10 **F**7 8 9 11 16 17 18 19 21 22 24 25 26 27 30 31 32 33 34 35 36 37 38 39 41 43 44 45 46 48 49 50 51 54 56 59 60 70 72 75 76 78 **P**8
— 23 10 99 5208 59 290241 445 46507 20596 708

BRIDGETON—St. Louis County
☐ ALL SAINTS SPECIAL CARE HOSPITAL, (LONG TERM ACUTE), 12303 De Paul Drive, 2nd Floor, Zip 63044–2588; tel. 314/344–7838; Maureen E. Hanneken, Chief Executive Officer **A**1 10 **F**13 16 18 22 24 26 31 33 39 45 46 48 49 51 55 59 60 62 65 68 70 74 76
— 23 49 20 194 16 0 0 1615 542 59
ST. VINCENT'S PSYCHIATRIC DIVISION See DePaul Health Center, Saint Louis

BROOKFIELD—Linn County
GENERAL JOHN J. PERSHING MEMORIAL HOSPITAL, 130 East Lockling Avenue, Zip 64628–0130, Mailing Address: P.O. Box 408, Zip 64628–0408; tel. 660/258–2222; Phil Hamilton, R.N., Chief Executive Officer **A**10 **F**7 9 13 16 17 18 19 20 22 25 28 29 32 33 34 35 36 37 38 45 46 48 51 54 56 60 70 76 78 **P**6
— 23 10 29 930 8 52360 0 9678 4672 113

A244 Hospitals *Many Facility Codes have changed. Please refer to the AHA Guide Code Chart.* © 2000 AHA Guide

Hospitals, U.S. / MISSOURI

Hospital, Address, Telephone, Administrator, Approval, Facility, and Physician Codes, Health Care System, Network	Classification Codes		Utilization Data					Expense (thousands) of dollars		
★ American Hospital Association (AHA) membership □ Joint Commission on Accreditation of Healthcare Organizations (JCAHO) accreditation + American Osteopathic Healthcare Association (AOHA) membership ○ American Osteopathic Association (AOA) accreditation △ Commission on Accreditation of Rehabilitation Facilities (CARF) accreditation Control codes 61, 63, 64, 71, 72 and 73 indicate hospitals listed by AOHA, but not registered by AHA. For definition of numerical codes, see page A4	Control	Service	Staffed Beds	Admissions	Census	Outpatient Visits	Births	Total	Payroll	Personnel
BUTLER—Bates County										
BATES COUNTY MEMORIAL HOSPITAL, 615 West Nursery Street, Zip 64730–0370; tel. 660/679–4135; Bob S. Edwards, Jr, Chief Executive Officer (Total facility includes 12 beds in nursing home–type unit) **A**9 10 **F**7 8 9 13 16 18 22 24 25 26 28 32 33 34 36 37 38 39 41 43 44 45 46 48 50 51 54 60 70 76 78 **Web address:** www.bcmhospital.com	13	10	52	1966	30	38956	26	12970	5418	198
CAMERON—Clinton County										
CAMERON COMMUNITY HOSPITAL, 1015 West Fourth Street, Zip 64429–1498; tel. 816/632–2101; Joseph F. Abrutz, Jr, Administrator **A**9 10 **F**7 9 12 13 16 17 18 19 20 22 23 24 25 26 28 30 31 32 33 34 35 36 37 38 39 41 43 45 46 48 49 51 54 57 59 62 63 70 71 72 76 78 **P**6	23	10	48	2006	32	98358	0	16841	8458	308
CAPE GIRARDEAU—Cape Girardeau County										
☒ SAINT FRANCIS MEDICAL CENTER, 211 St. Francis Drive, Zip 63703–8399; tel. 573/331–3000; Steven C. Bjelich, President and Chief Executive Officer (Total facility includes 26 beds in nursing home–type unit) **A**1 2 10 **F**4 5 7 9 11 12 13 14 17 18 19 20 21 22 23 24 25 27 28 31 32 34 35 36 38 39 41 43 45 46 47 48 49 50 51 52 53 54 60 68 70 71 72 76 77 78 79 **Web address:** www.showme.net/sfmc/	23	10	264	8056	131	83176	0	96775	37308	1125
☒ SOUTHEAST MISSOURI HOSPITAL, 1701 Lacey Street, Zip 63701–5299; tel. 573/334–4822; James W. Wente, CPA, CHE, Administrator (Total facility includes 20 beds in nursing home–type unit) **A**1 2 10 **F**4 7 8 9 11 12 14 17 18 19 21 22 23 24 25 26 27 28 33 34 35 36 37 38 39 40 41 42 43 44 45 46 47 48 49 50 51 52 54 57 60 61 62 65 68 70 72 73 76 78 **Web address:** www.sehosp.org	23	10	240	9455	129	137931	1603	100828	37445	1306
CARROLLTON—Carroll County										
CARROLL COUNTY MEMORIAL HOSPITAL, 1502 North Jefferson Street, Zip 64633–1999; tel. 660/542–1695; Jerry Dover, Chief Executive Officer **A**9 10 **F**1 9 17 18 22 23 25 30 32 33 34 35 36 37 38 43 45 46 48 51 54 70 76 78 **P**6	23	10	50	581	37	19792	0	4038	1993	83
CARTHAGE—Jasper County										
★ MCCUNE–BROOKS HOSPITAL, 627 West Centennial Avenue, Zip 64836–0677; tel. 417/358–8121; Robert Y. Copeland, Jr, Chief Executive Officer (Total facility includes 7 beds in nursing home–type unit) **A**10 **F**7 9 17 19 22 25 30 32 33 34 36 39 40 41 43 45 48 57 62 70 71 72 76 **P**8 **Web address:** www.mccune–brooks.org	14	10	54	1900	32	36179	0	17221	7074	288
CASSVILLE—Barry County										
SOUTH BARRY COUNTY MEMORIAL HOSPITAL, 94 Main Street, Zip 65625–1610; tel. 417/847–4115; Deborah Stubbs, Chief Executive Officer **A**10 **F**9 16 17 22 25 28 32 33 34 35 37 45 48 54 56 76 **P**6	16	10	18	675	7	16732	0	4019	2729	104
CHESTERFIELD—St. Louis County										
☒ ST. LUKE'S HOSPITAL, 232 South Woods Mill Road, Zip 63017–3480; tel. 314/434–1500; Gary R. Olson, President **A**1 2 3 5 9 10 **F**1 2 3 4 5 6 7 8 9 10 11 12 13 14 16 17 18 19 20 21 22 23 24 25 26 27 28 29 30 31 32 33 34 35 36 37 38 39 40 41 42 43 44 45 46 47 48 49 50 51 52 53 54 56 57 58 59 60 61 62 63 64 65 66 67 68 70 71 72 73 74 75 76 77 78 79 **P**1 **S** Sisters of Mercy Health System–St. Louis, Saint Louis, MO	21	10	369	16150	198	211845	2561	183336	81523	2045
CHILLICOTHE—Livingston County										
☒ HEDRICK MEDICAL CENTER, 100 Central Avenue, Zip 64601–1599; tel. 660/646–1480; James K. Johnson, Chief Executive Officer **A**1 9 10 **F**7 8 13 16 17 18 19 20 21 22 25 26 32 33 34 36 37 38 39 40 41 43 44 45 46 48 49 50 51 54 60 63 70 72 76 78 **S** Health Midwest, Kansas City, MO **Web address:** www.healthmidwest.org	23	10	80	1396	18	100029	334	14167	6089	240
CLINTON—Henry County										
☒ GOLDEN VALLEY MEMORIAL HOSPITAL, 1600 North Second Street, Zip 64735–1197; tel. 660/885–5511; Randy S. Wertz, Administrator (Total facility includes 12 beds in nursing home–type unit) **A**1 9 10 **F**7 8 9 16 17 18 19 22 24 25 26 32 33 34 35 36 37 39 41 43 44 45 46 48 49 54 57 58 59 60 61 62 63 64 68 70 71 72 76 78 79	16	10	106	3857	54	25562	329	26347	12400	420
COLUMBIA—Boone County										
☒ BOONE HOSPITAL CENTER, 1600 East Broadway, Zip 65201–5897; tel. 573/815–8000; Michael B. Shirk, President and Senior Executive Officer (Total facility includes 19 beds in nursing home–type unit) **A**1 2 3 5 10 **F**4 7 8 9 11 13 16 17 18 19 20 22 24 25 26 28 29 30 32 34 35 36 37 38 39 41 42 43 44 45 46 47 48 49 50 51 53 54 57 58 59 60 61 62 63 64 65 66 68 70 72 73 74 76 77 78 79 **P**5 8 **S** BJC Health System, Saint Louis, MO **Web address:** www.boone.org	23	10	335	14354	214	204613	1736	133979	47595	1527
☒ △ COLUMBIA REGIONAL HOSPITAL, 404 Keene Street, Zip 65201–6698; tel. 573/875–9000; James C. Poehling, Director **A**1 2 5 7 10 **F**4 7 8 9 11 13 16 17 18 19 21 22 23 24 25 27 30 32 34 35 36 38 39 41 43 44 45 46 48 50 51 53 54 57 58 62 68 70 71 72 76 78 79 **P**8 **Web address:** www.tenethealth.com	33	10	265	4448	71	58155	179	60229	17564	556
ELLIS FISCHEL CANCER CENTER See University Hospitals and Clinics										
☒ HARRY S. TRUMAN MEMORIAL VETERANS HOSPITAL, 800 Hospital Drive, Zip 65201–5297; tel. 573/814–6300; Gary L. Campbell, Director (Total facility includes 38 beds in nursing home–type unit) **A**1 3 5 8 **F**3 4 9 11 12 13 16 18 19 22 23 25 26 30 31 33 34 37 38 39 40 41 43 45 46 47 48 49 50 51 53 54 56 57 58 59 60 61 62 63 64 65 66 68 70 72 73 74 76 77 78 79 **P**6 **S** Department of Veterans Affairs, Washington, DC	45	10	104	3724	90	312565	0	78166	38968	852

© 2000 AHA Guide   *Many Facility Codes have changed. Please refer to the AHA Guide Code Chart.*

Hospitals, U.S. / MISSOURI

Hospital, Address, Telephone, Administrator, Approval, Facility, and Physician Codes, Health Care System, Network

- ★ American Hospital Association (AHA) membership
- ☐ Joint Commission on Accreditation of Healthcare Organizations (JCAHO) accreditation
- + American Osteopathic Healthcare Association (AOHA) membership
- ○ American Osteopathic Association (AOA) accreditation
- △ Commission on Accreditation of Rehabilitation Facilities (CARF) accreditation

Control codes 61, 63, 64, 71, 72 and 73 indicate hospitals listed by AOHA, but not registered by AHA. For definition of numerical codes, see page A4

Hospital	Control	Service	Staffed Beds	Admissions	Census	Outpatient Visits	Births	Total	Payroll	Personnel
☐ MID MISSOURI MENTAL HEALTH CENTER, 3 Hospital Drive, Zip 65201–5296; tel. 573/884–1300; Dennis R. Canote, Chief Executive Officer **A**1 3 5 10 **F**17 18 33 57 58 59 60 61 62 63 64	12	22	69	1562	55	5971	0	12347	7956	248
☐ △ UNIVERSITY HOSPITALS AND CLINICS, (Includes Ellis Fischel Cancer Center, 115 Business Loop 70 West, Zip 65203; tel. 573/882–5460), One Hospital Drive, Zip 65212–0001; tel. 573/882–4141; Keith J. Weinhold, Interim Director **A**1 2 3 5 7 8 10 **F**2 3 4 5 7 8 9 10 11 12 14 17 18 19 20 21 22 23 24 25 26 27 28 30 31 32 33 34 35 36 37 38 39 41 42 43 44 45 46 47 48 49 50 51 52 53 54 55 56 57 58 59 60 61 62 63 64 65 66 68 70 71 72 73 74 75 76 77 78 79 **P**1 Web address: www.hsc.missouri.edu/~2000	12	10	378	11727	188	514519	1221	260122	103799	3410
CREVE COEUR—St. Louis County BARNES–JEWISH WEST COUNTY HOSPITAL See Saint Louis										
CRYSTAL CITY—Jefferson County ☐ JEFFERSON MEMORIAL HOSPITAL, Highway 61 South, Zip 63019, Mailing Address: P.O. Box 350, Zip 63019–0350; tel. 314/933–1000; Mark S. Brodeur, Chief Executive Officer (Total facility includes 187 beds in nursing home–type unit) **A**1 9 10 **F**2 3 4 6 7 8 9 11 13 17 18 19 22 24 25 26 27 28 29 31 32 33 34 36 37 38 39 41 43 44 45 46 47 48 49 51 53 54 56 57 58 59 60 61 62 63 64 65 68 70 71 72 76 77 78 **P**8 Web address: www.jeffersonmemorialhospital.org	23	10	395	8376	267	88119	782	73260	34455	1033
DEXTER—Stoddard County DEXTER MEMORIAL HOSPITAL, 1200 North One Mile Road, Zip 63841–1099; tel. 573/624–5566; Randal Tennison, Chief Executive Officer **A**9 10 **F**9 12 13 17 22 23 25 29 30 32 33 34 35 36 37 38 40 41 43 48 50 53 54 56 68 70 72 76 77 78 **S** NetCare Health Systems, Inc., Nashville, TN	33	10	48	972	12	67176	0	10973	5118	159
DONIPHAN—Ripley County RIPLEY COUNTY MEMORIAL HOSPITAL, 109 Plum Street, Zip 63935–1299; tel. 573/996–2141; Charles Ray Freeman, Administrator **A**9 10 **F**9 17 19 22 25 32 33 34 36 38 45 48 50 51 54 56 76	13	10	26	577	8	29318	0	4344	1647	107
EL DORADO SPRINGS—Cedar County CEDAR COUNTY MEMORIAL HOSPITAL, 1401 South Park Street, Zip 64744–2096; tel. 417/876–2511; Jackie Boyles, Administrator **A**10 **F**7 8 9 17 18 19 22 25 28 32 33 34 35 36 38 40 43 44 48 51 54 70 73 76 78 79 **P**6	13	10	34	925	7	36550	99	5734	3082	117
EXCELSIOR SPRINGS—Clay County ☐ EXCELSIOR SPRINGS MEDICAL CENTER, 1700 Rainbow Boulevard, Zip 64024–1190; tel. 816/630–6081; Sally S. Nance, Chief Executive Officer (Total facility includes 80 beds in nursing home–type unit) **A**1 9 **F**6 7 9 13 16 17 18 19 22 23 25 26 30 31 32 33 34 36 37 38 39 41 43 45 46 48 49 50 51 54 70 72 76 78	14	10	104	977	85	27440	0	11712	5507	146
FAIRFAX—Atchison County COMMUNITY HOSPITAL ASSOCIATION, Highway 59, Zip 64446–0107; tel. 660/686–2211; Larry S. Goodloe, Administrator **A**9 10 **F**7 8 9 22 23 25 33 34 36 37 38 39 41 43 44 45 48 51 54 63 70 76	23	10	41	764	17	25393	54	6122	2774	94
FARMINGTON—St. Francois County + ○ MINERAL AREA REGIONAL MEDICAL CENTER, 1212 Weber Road, Zip 63640–3309; tel. 573/701–7304; Stephen L. Crain, Chief Executive Officer (Total facility includes 10 beds in nursing home–type unit) **A**9 10 11 12 13 **F**2 3 7 8 9 13 17 19 20 21 22 23 24 25 31 32 33 34 35 36 37 38 39 41 44 46 48 50 51 54 56 58 59 60 61 62 63 70 71 72 75 76 77 78 **P**1 Web address: www.marmc.org	23	10	120	4158	53	109812	376	33489	16219	548
★ PARKLAND HEALTH CENTER, (Includes Parkland Health Center–Bonne Terre, 7245 Vo–Tech Road, Bonne Terre, Zip 63628; tel. 573/358–1400), 1101 West Liberty Street, Zip 63640–1997; tel. 573/756–6451; Richard L. Conklin, President **A**1 10 **F**3 4 7 8 9 13 16 17 18 19 20 21 22 23 24 25 26 28 29 32 33 34 35 36 37 38 39 40 41 43 44 45 46 48 49 50 51 54 56 58 59 60 61 62 63 68 70 71 72 76 78 **P**5 6 7 **S** BJC Health System, Saint Louis, MO Web address: www.bjc.org/phc.html	23	10	94	3264	32	89626	458	29934	11819	503
☐ SOUTHEAST MISSOURI MENTAL HEALTH CENTER, 1010 West Columbia, Zip 63640–2997; tel. 573/218–6792; Donald L. Barton, Superintendent **A**1 10 **F**16 17 18 19 25 28 32 33 34 45 50 57 60 61 62 64 78	12	22	221	1728	170	0	0	24673	16198	624
FLORISSANT—St. Louis County CHRISTIAN HOSPITAL NORTHWEST See Christian Hospital Northeast–Northwest, Saint Louis										
FORT LEONARD WOOD—Pulaski County ★ GENERAL LEONARD WOOD ARMY COMMUNITY HOSPITAL, 126 Missouri Avenue, Zip 65473–8952; tel. 573/596–0414; Lieutenant Colonel Mark A. Miller, Deputy Commander for Administration **A**1 2 **F**1 2 3 4 5 6 7 8 9 10 11 12 13 14 15 16 17 18 19 20 21 22 23 24 25 26 27 28 29 30 31 32 33 34 35 36 37 38 39 41 42 43 44 45 46 47 48 49 50 51 52 53 54 55 56 57 58 59 60 61 62 63 64 65 66 67 68 70 71 72 73 74 75 76 77 78 79 **S** Department of the Army, Office of the Surgeon General, Falls Church, VA Web address: glwach.leonardwood.amedd.army.mil	42	10	97	1861	17	295655	344	53837	23032	885
FREDERICKTOWN—Madison County MADISON MEDICAL CENTER, 611 West Main, Zip 63645, Mailing Address: P.O. Box 431, Zip 63645–0431; tel. 573/783–3341; Floyd D. Bounds, Administrator (Total facility includes 123 beds in nursing home–type unit) **A**9 10 **F**7 9 16 17 18 19 22 25 33 34 36 38 39 41 43 44 45 48 51 54 56 70 76	13	10	143	480	116	36477	54	10798	4490	228

Many Facility Codes have changed. Please refer to the AHA Guide Code Chart.

© 2000 AHA Guide

Hospitals, U.S. / MISSOURI

Hospital, Address, Telephone, Administrator, Approval, Facility, and Physician Codes, Health Care System, Network	Classification Codes		Utilization Data					Expense (thousands) of dollars		
	Control	Service	Staffed Beds	Admissions	Census	Outpatient Visits	Births	Total	Payroll	Personnel

★ American Hospital Association (AHA) membership
☐ Joint Commission on Accreditation of Healthcare Organizations (JCAHO) accreditation
+ American Osteopathic Healthcare Association (AOHA) membership
○ American Osteopathic Association (AOA) accreditation
△ Commission on Accreditation of Rehabilitation Facilities (CARF) accreditation
Control codes 61, 63, 64, 71, 72 and 73 indicate hospitals listed by AOHA, but not registered by AHA. For definition of numerical codes, see page A4

FULTON—Callaway County

☐ CALLAWAY COMMUNITY HOSPITAL, 10 South Hospital Drive, Zip 65251-2513; tel. 573/642-3376; Gerald M. Torba, Chief Executive Officer **A** 9 10 **F** 7 8 9 14 16 17 18 19 22 25 28 29 32 33 34 36 38 39 41 43 44 45 46 48 51 54 70 72 76 78   23   10   31   1175   10   59064   155   —   10973   142

☐ FULTON STATE HOSPITAL, 600 East Fifth Street, Zip 65251-1798; tel. 573/592-4100; Felix T. Vincenz, Ph.D., Chief Executive Officer (Total facility includes 24 beds in nursing home–type unit) **A**1 10 **F**2 13 21 23 26 30 31 32 33 34 37 38 43 50 51 56 57 58 59 60 62 64 70 72 78 **P**6
Web address: www.modmh.state.mo.us/fulton/   12   22   510   504   428   0   0   59868   34738   1387

HANNIBAL—Marion County

★ HANNIBAL REGIONAL HOSPITAL, Highway 36 West, Zip 63401, Mailing Address: P.O. Box 551, Zip 63401-0551; tel. 573/248-1300; John C. Grossmeier, President and Chief Executive Officer **A**1 2 9 10 **F**7 8 9 11 16 17 18 19 21 22 23 24 25 26 27 32 33 34 35 36 38 39 41 43 44 45 46 48 49 50 51 54 57 59 60 61 62 63 64 66 68 70 71 72 76 77 78 79 **P**1 6
Web address: www.hrhonline.org   23   10   105   5097   67   119837   578   45087   18622   623

HARRISONVILLE—Cass County

★ CASS MEDICAL CENTER, 1800 East Mechanic Street, Zip 64701-2099; tel. 816/380-3474; Alan O. Freeman, Chief Executive Officer **A**1 9 10 **F**7 9 13 16 17 18 22 23 24 25 32 33 34 37 38 39 41 43 45 46 48 49 50 51 54 56 57 58 59 60 61 62 63 68 70 71 72 76 78 **P**6 **S** Health Midwest, Kansas City, MO
Web address: www.healthmidwest.org   13   10   37   1061   19   71754   1   17469   6380   210

HAYTI—Pemiscot County

PEMISCOT MEMORIAL HEALTH SYSTEM, Highway 61 and Reed, Zip 63851, Mailing Address: P.O. Box 489, Zip 63851-0489; tel. 573/359-1372; Darrell Jean, Administrator and Chief Executive Officer (Total facility includes 120 beds in nursing home–type unit) **A**10 **F**2 7 8 9 10 12 13 17 22 24 25 29 30 31 32 33 34 35 36 38 39 40 41 42 43 44 45 46 48 49 51 52 54 55 56 58 59 61 62 63 64 70 74 76 77 78 79 **P**6 8   13   10   229   3367   178   89018   259   23233   12690   440

HERMANN—Gasconade County

HERMANN AREA DISTRICT HOSPITAL, Mailing Address: P.O. Box 470, Zip 65041-0470; tel. 573/486-2191; Dan McKinney, Administrator **A**10 **F**7 9 13 17 18 19 22 24 25 32 33 34 36 38 39 40 43 45 46 48 51 54 70 76 78 **P**6   16   10   41   373   26   26898   0   5225   2596   112

HOUSTON—Texas County

TEXAS COUNTY MEMORIAL HOSPITAL, 1333 Sam Houston Boulevard, Zip 65483-2046; tel. 417/967-3311; William L. Sword, President and Chief Executive Officer **A**10 **F**7 8 9 13 15 18 22 23 25 28 29 31 32 33 34 35 36 37 38 40 41 43 44 45 48 50 51 54 56 60 70 76 78 **P**6   13   10   66   2455   26   68526   279   13663   6491   243

INDEPENDENCE—Jackson County

★ INDEPENDENCE REGIONAL HEALTH CENTER, 1509 West Truman Road, Zip 64050-3498; tel. 816/836-8100; Michael W. Chappelow, President and Chief Executive Officer (Total facility includes 70 beds in nursing home–type unit) **A**1 2 9 10 **F**1 2 3 4 5 6 7 8 9 10 11 12 13 14 16 17 18 19 21 22 23 24 25 26 27 28 29 30 31 32 33 34 35 36 37 38 39 40 41 42 43 44 45 46 47 48 49 50 51 52 53 54 56 57 58 59 60 61 62 63 64 65 66 68 70 71 72 73 74 75 76 78 79 **P**5 **S** Health Midwest, Kansas City, MO
Web address: www.healthmidwest.org   23   10   329   9060   166   104756   0   74013   33178   930

★ MEDICAL CENTER OF INDEPENDENCE, 17203 East 23rd Street, Zip 64057-1899; tel. 816/478-5000; J. Kent Howard, President and Chief Executive Officer **A**1 9 10 13 **F**1 2 3 4 5 7 8 9 10 11 12 13 14 16 17 18 19 21 22 23 24 25 28 29 30 31 32 33 34 35 36 37 38 39 40 41 42 43 44 45 46 47 48 49 50 51 52 53 54 56 57 58 59 60 61 62 63 64 65 66 68 70 71 72 73 74 75 76 78 79 **P**5 8 **S** Health Midwest, Kansas City, MO
Web address: www.healthmidwest.org   23   10   99   4652   49   46061   1088   34254   15331   419

JEFFERSON CITY—Cole County

☐ + ○ △ CAPITAL REGION MEDICAL CENTER, 1125 Madison Street, Zip 65101-1128, Mailing Address: P.O. Box 1128, Zip 65102-1128; tel. 573/632-5002; Edward F. Farnsworth, President (Total facility includes 20 beds in nursing home–type unit) **A**1 7 10 11 12 13 **F**1 3 4 7 8 9 11 12 13 14 16 17 18 19 20 21 22 24 25 26 27 28 29 30 32 33 34 35 36 37 38 39 40 41 42 43 44 45 46 47 48 49 50 51 53 54 59 60 61 62 63 64 65 66 70 71 72 75 76 77 78 79 **P**8
Web address: www.crmc.org   23   10   134   6712   97   264754   463   85744   36877   1037

★ ST. MARYS HEALTH CENTER, 100 St. Marys Medical Plaza, Zip 65101-1601; tel. 573/761-7000; Mark R. Taylor, President (Total facility includes 10 beds in nursing home–type unit) **A**1 2 9 10 **F**4 7 8 9 11 13 16 17 18 19 21 22 23 24 25 27 28 32 33 34 35 36 37 38 39 41 43 44 45 46 47 48 49 50 51 53 54 56 57 58 59 60 61 62 63 64 65 68 70 72 75 76 77 78 79 **P**1 4 7 **S** SSM Health Care, Saint Louis, MO
Web address: www.stmarys-jeffcity.com/internet/home/stmaryjeff.nsf   23   10   167   8847   109   356214   1178   88603   34732   1029

JOPLIN—Newton County

★ + ○ △ FREEMAN HEALTH SYSTEM, (Includes Freeman Hospital East, 932 East 34th Street, Zip 64804-3999; Freeman Hospital West, 1102 West 32nd Street), 1102 West 32nd Street, Zip 64804-3599; tel. 417/623-2801; Gary D. Duncan, President and Chief Executive Officer (Total facility includes 32 beds in nursing home–type unit) **A**2 10 11 12 13 **F**2 3 4 5 7 8 9 11 12 13 14 16 17 18 19 20 21 22 23 24 25 26 27 30 31 32 33 34 35 36 37 38 39 41 43 44 45 46 47 48 50 51 54 55 56 57 58 59 60 61 62 63 64 65 66 70 71 72 75 76 77 78 79 **P**1 6
Web address: www.freemanhospitals.org   23   10   269   12455   165   506387   2606   160526   78054   1917

© 2000 AHA Guide   *Many Facility Codes have changed. Please refer to the AHA Guide Code Chart.*

Hospitals, U.S. / MISSOURI

Hospital, Address, Telephone, Administrator, Approval, Facility, and Physician Codes, Health Care System, Network

- ★ American Hospital Association (AHA) membership
- ☐ Joint Commission on Accreditation of Healthcare Organizations (JCAHO) accreditation
- + American Osteopathic Healthcare Association (AOHA) membership
- ○ American Osteopathic Association (AOA) accreditation
- △ Commission on Accreditation of Rehabilitation Facilities (CARF) accreditation

Control codes 61, 63, 64, 71, 72 and 73 indicate hospitals listed by AOHA, but not registered by AHA. For definition of numerical codes, see page A4.

Hospital	Classification Codes		Utilization Data					Expense (thousands of dollars)		Personnel
	Control	Service	Staffed Beds	Admissions	Census	Outpatient Visits	Births	Total	Payroll	
★ △ ST. JOHN'S REGIONAL MEDICAL CENTER, 2727 McClelland Boulevard, Zip 64804–1694; tel. 417/781–2727; Gary L. Rowe, President and Chief Executive Officer (Total facility includes 10 beds in nursing home–type unit) **A**1 2 7 10 **F**4 7 8 9 11 12 13 16 17 18 19 21 22 23 24 25 26 27 29 31 32 33 34 35 36 37 38 39 40 41 43 44 45 46 47 48 49 50 51 53 54 56 57 58 59 60 61 62 63 64 65 70 71 72 73 75 76 77 78 79 **P**1 6 **S** Catholic Health Initiatives, Denver, CO Web address: www.stj.com	23	10	367	13573	208	262907	627	160248	55932	1724
KANSAS CITY—Jackson County										
★ BAPTIST MEDICAL CENTER, 6601 Rockhill Road, Zip 64131–1197; tel. 816/276–7000; Darrell W. Moore, President and Chief Executive Officer (Total facility includes 23 beds in nursing home–type unit) **A**1 2 3 5 9 10 **F**1 2 3 4 5 7 8 9 11 12 13 14 16 17 18 19 20 21 22 23 24 25 26 27 28 29 30 31 32 33 34 35 36 37 38 39 40 41 42 43 44 45 46 47 48 49 50 51 53 54 56 57 58 59 60 61 62 63 64 65 66 68 70 71 72 73 74 75 76 77 78 79 **P**1 5 **S** Health Midwest, Kansas City, MO Web address: www.healthmidwest.org	23	10	265	10200	154	148944	1459	93359	39713	1058
★ CHILDREN'S MERCY HOSPITAL, (Includes Children's Mercy South, 5808 West 110th Street, Kansas, Zip 66211), 2401 Gillham Road, Zip 64108–9898; tel. 816/234–3000; Randall L. O'Donnell, Ph.D., President and Chief Executive Officer **A**1 2 3 5 8 9 10 **F**4 5 7 10 11 12 13 14 17 18 19 20 22 23 24 25 29 32 33 35 36 38 39 41 42 43 45 46 47 48 49 50 51 52 54 56 59 63 65 70 72 73 74 75 76 78 **P**4 5 6 7 8 Web address: www.childrens–mercy.org	23	50	177	8945	132	224814	0	181310	93753	2640
☐ CRITTENTON, 10918 Elm Avenue, Zip 64134–4199; tel. 816/765–6600; Gary L. Watson, FACHE, Senior Executive Officer **A**1 10 **F**2 3 12 13 16 17 18 19 21 33 34 38 41 43 44 50 51 53 57 58 59 60 61 63 64 70 72 78 **P**8 **S** Saint Luke's Shawnee Mission Health System, Kansas City, MO Web address: www.saint–lukes.org	23	52	127	1423	102	29857	0	13735	8756	297
☐ HALLMARK YOUTHCARE OF KANSAS CITY, (Formerly ValueMark Behavioral Healthcare System of Kansas City), 4800 N.W. 88th Street, Zip 64154–2757; tel. 816/436–3900; James R. Laws, Chief Executive Officer **A**1 10 **F**2 13 16 17 18 21 25 31 32 33 34 43 45 50 51 56 57 58 59 60 61 63 64 70 72 **S** ValueMark Healthcare Systems, Inc., Atlanta, GA	33	22	97	358	31	0	0	—	—	118
★ △ REHABILITATION INSTITUTE, 3011 Baltimore, Zip 64108–3465; tel. 816/751–7900; Ronald L. Herrick, President **A**7 9 10 **F**1 2 3 4 5 6 7 8 9 10 11 12 13 14 15 16 17 18 19 20 21 22 23 25 26 27 28 29 30 32 33 35 36 37 38 40 41 42 43 44 45 46 47 48 49 50 51 52 53 54 56 57 58 59 60 61 62 63 64 65 66 70 71 72 73 74 75 76 77 78 79 **P**5 8 **S** Health Midwest, Kansas City, MO Web address: www.healthmidwest.org	23	46	32	249	13	12479	0	12979	7652	215
★ RESEARCH MEDICAL CENTER, 2316 East Meyer Boulevard, Zip 64132–1199; tel. 816/276–4000; Steven R. Newton, President and Chief Executive Officer (Total facility includes 35 beds in nursing home–type unit) **A**1 2 3 5 9 10 **F**1 2 3 4 5 7 8 9 10 11 12 13 14 16 17 18 19 21 22 23 24 25 26 27 28 29 30 31 32 33 34 35 36 37 38 39 40 41 42 43 44 45 46 47 48 49 50 51 52 53 54 56 57 58 59 60 61 62 63 64 65 66 68 70 71 72 73 74 75 76 77 78 79 **P**1 7 8 **S** Health Midwest, Kansas City, MO Web address: www.healthmidwest.org	23	10	483	14972	252	298008	1689	183870	76652	2150
★ RESEARCH PSYCHIATRIC CENTER, 2323 East 63rd Street, Zip 64130–3495; tel. 816/444–8161; Todd Krass, Administrator and Chief Executive Officer **A**1 10 **F**1 2 3 4 5 6 7 8 9 10 11 12 13 14 15 17 18 19 20 21 22 23 25 26 27 28 29 30 31 32 33 34 35 36 37 38 39 40 41 42 43 44 45 46 47 48 49 50 51 52 53 54 55 56 57 58 59 60 61 62 63 64 65 66 67 68 70 71 72 73 74 75 76 77 78 79 **P**5 **S** Health Midwest, Kansas City, MO Web address: www.healthmidwest.org	23	22	100	1828	41	—	0	8911	4630	129
★ SAINT JOSEPH HEALTH CENTER, 1000 Carondelet Drive, Zip 64114–4673; tel. 816/942–4400; Michele Schaefer, Chief Executive Officer **A**1 2 5 9 10 **F**4 7 8 9 11 13 14 17 18 19 22 24 25 26 28 32 33 34 35 36 37 38 39 41 42 43 44 45 46 47 48 49 50 51 53 54 65 68 70 71 72 75 76 77 78 **P**1 6 **S** Carondelet Health System, Saint Louis, MO	23	10	267	11628	181	127128	1766	121087	41146	1023
★ SAINT LUKE'S HOSPITAL, 4401 Wornall Road, Zip 64111–3238; tel. 816/932–2000; G. Richard Hastings, President and Chief Executive Officer (Total facility includes 30 beds in nursing home–type unit) **A**1 2 3 8 9 10 **F**2 3 4 5 7 8 9 11 12 13 14 16 17 18 19 21 22 23 24 25 26 28 32 33 34 35 36 37 38 39 41 42 43 44 45 46 47 48 49 50 51 53 54 55 56 57 58 59 60 61 62 63 64 65 66 70 71 72 73 74 75 76 77 78 79 **P**6 8 **S** Saint Luke's Shawnee Mission Health System, Kansas City, MO Web address: www.saint–lukes.org	23	10	510	20407	329	212052	2597	272848	98029	2514
☐ SAINT LUKE'S NORTHLAND HOSPITAL, 5830 N.W. Barry Road, Zip 64154; tel. 816/891–6000; N. Gary Wages, President and Chief Executive Officer **A**1 **F**2 3 4 5 6 7 8 9 11 12 13 14 16 17 18 19 20 21 22 23 24 25 26 28 29 30 31 32 33 34 35 36 37 38 39 40 41 42 43 44 45 46 47 48 49 50 51 52 53 54 55 56 57 58 59 60 61 62 63 64 65 66 68 70 71 72 74 75 76 77 78 79 **P**6 8 **S** Saint Luke's Shawnee Mission Health System, Kansas City, MO Web address: www.saint–lukes.org	23	10	63	3677	37	43604	1028	34314	13566	347

ST. MARY'S HOSPITAL See Trinity Lutheran Hospital

Hospitals, U.S. / MISSOURI

Hospital, Address, Telephone, Administrator, Approval, Facility, and Physician Codes, Health Care System, Network	Classification Codes		Utilization Data					Expense (thousands) of dollars		
★ American Hospital Association (AHA) membership □ Joint Commission on Accreditation of Healthcare Organizations (JCAHO) accreditation + American Osteopathic Healthcare Association (AOHA) membership ○ American Osteopathic Association (AOA) accreditation △ Commission on Accreditation of Rehabilitation Facilities (CARF) accreditation Control codes 61, 63, 64, 71, 72 and 73 indicate hospitals listed by AOHA, but not registered by AHA. For definition of numerical codes, see page A4	Control	Service	Staffed Beds	Admissions	Census	Outpatient Visits	Births	Total	Payroll	Personnel
★ TRINITY LUTHERAN HOSPITAL, (Includes St. Mary's Hospital, 101 Memorial Drive, Zip 64108; tel. 816/751–4600), 3030 Baltimore Avenue, Zip 64108–3404; tel. 816/751–4600; Ronald A. Ommen, President and Chief Executive Officer (Total facility includes 30 beds in nursing home–type unit) **A**1 2 3 5 9 10 **F**1 3 4 5 7 8 9 11 12 13 17 18 19 20 21 22 24 25 26 27 28 29 30 31 32 33 34 35 36 37 38 40 41 42 43 44 45 46 47 48 49 50 51 54 56 57 58 59 60 61 62 63 64 65 66 69 70 71 72 73 74 75 76 77 78 79 **P**1 5 6 **S** Health Midwest, Kansas City, MO **Web address:** www.healthmidwest.org	21	10	334	6934	114	106076	0	—	—	—
★ △ TRUMAN MEDICAL CENTER–EAST, 7900 Lee's Summit Road, Zip 64139–1241; tel. 816/373–4415; James R. Kelly, Chief Operating Officer (Total facility includes 212 beds in nursing home–type unit) **A**3 5 7 9 10 **F**3 7 8 9 11 12 13 14 16 17 18 19 20 21 22 23 24 25 29 30 31 33 34 35 36 38 39 41 42 43 44 45 46 48 50 51 53 54 56 57 58 59 60 61 62 63 64 66 70 71 75 76 77 78 79 **S** Truman Health System, Kansas City, MO	23	10	302	4166	245	186738	850	50040	23922	752
★ TRUMAN MEDICAL CENTER–HOSPITAL HILL, (Formerly Truman Medical Center–West), 2301 Holmes Street, Zip 64108–2677; tel. 816/556–3000; Catherine D. Disch, Chief Operating Officer (Total facility includes 12 beds in nursing home–type unit) **A**1 2 3 5 8 9 10 **F**2 3 7 8 9 11 12 13 14 16 17 18 19 20 21 22 23 24 25 29 30 31 32 33 35 36 38 39 41 42 43 44 45 46 48 49 50 51 53 54 56 57 58 59 60 61 62 63 64 65 66 68 70 71 72 73 75 76 77 78 79 **P**5 **S** Truman Health System, Kansas City, MO	23	10	227	10980	156	307749	1948	128426	64665	1280
□ TWO RIVERS PSYCHIATRIC HOSPITAL, 5121 Raytown Road, Zip 64133–2141; tel. 816/356–5688; Linda Berridge, Chief Executive Officer **A**1 10 **F**16 18 19 21 30 31 33 43 45 50 51 57 58 59 60 61 62 64 70 72 **S** Universal Health Services, Inc., King of Prussia, PA **Web address:** www.tworivershospital.com	33	22	80	1240	38	0	0	8346	3749	125
□ VENCOR HOSPITAL–KANSAS CITY, 8701 Troost Avenue, Zip 64131–3495; tel. 816/995–2000; E. Bradley Strecker, Chief Executive Officer (Total facility includes 16 beds in nursing home–type unit) (Nonreporting) **A**1 10 **S** Vencor, Incorporated, Louisville, KY	33	49	100	—	—	—	—	—	—	—
★ VETERANS AFFAIRS MEDICAL CENTER, 4801 Linwood Boulevard, Zip 64128–2295; tel. 816/861–4700; Hugh F. Doran, Director **A**1 2 3 5 8 **F**1 2 3 4 6 9 11 12 14 19 20 21 22 23 24 25 26 27 28 30 31 32 33 34 35 36 37 38 39 41 43 44 45 46 47 48 49 50 51 53 54 56 57 59 60 61 62 63 64 65 66 68 70 72 76 77 78 79 **S** Department of Veterans Affairs, Washington, DC	45	10	126	5484	106	223606	0	101064	50533	1226
□ WESTERN MISSOURI MENTAL HEALTH CENTER, 600 East 22nd Street, Zip 64108–2675; tel. 816/512–4000; Gloria Joseph, Superintendent **A**1 3 5 10 **F**2 3 6 7 13 17 18 19 20 21 22 24 25 28 31 32 33 34 39 43 45 50 51 57 58 59 60 61 62 63 68 70 72 76 77 78 **P**6	12	22	110	2562	98	45279	0	26756	17973	652

KENNETT—Dunklin County
★ TWIN RIVERS REGIONAL MEDICAL CENTER, 1301 First Street, Zip 63857–2508; tel. 573/888–4522; Dale R. Mulder, Chief Executive Officer **A**1 10 **F**8 9 12 13 16 17 18 22 24 25 28 31 32 33 34 36 38 39 41 43 44 46 48 51 53 54 57 58 60 70 76 78 **P**7 8 **S** TENET Healthcare Corporation, Santa Barbara, CA **Web address:** www.tenethealth.com	33	10	116	3418	37	77523	263	22927	10207	373

KIRKSVILLE—Adair County
□ + ○ △ NORTHEAST REGIONAL MEDICAL CENTER–JEFFERSON CAMPUS, (Includes Northeast Regional Medical Center–Patterson Campus, 112 East Patterson Avenue, tel. 660/785–1000), 315 South Osteopathy, Zip 63501–8599, Mailing Address: P.O. Box C8502, Zip 63501–8599; tel. 660/785–1100; Charles M. Boughton, Chief Executive Officer (Total facility includes 14 beds in nursing home–type unit) **A**1 7 10 11 12 13 **F**4 5 7 8 9 11 13 15 16 17 18 19 20 21 22 23 24 25 28 32 33 34 35 36 38 39 41 43 44 45 46 48 49 50 51 54 60 65 68 70 71 72 75 76 78	33	10	164	5697	66	103642	598	52246	23073	676

LAKE SAINT LOUIS—St. Charles County
★ ST. JOSEPH HOSPITAL WEST, 100 Medical Plaza, Zip 63367–1395; tel. 314/625–5200; Kevin F. Kast, President, Chief Executive Officer and Market Executive (Total facility includes 11 beds in nursing home–type unit) **A**10 **F**2 3 4 5 6 7 8 9 11 12 13 14 16 17 18 19 20 21 22 23 24 25 26 27 28 29 30 31 32 33 34 35 36 37 38 39 41 42 43 44 45 46 47 48 49 50 51 52 53 54 56 57 58 59 60 61 62 63 64 65 66 67 68 70 71 72 73 74 76 77 78 79 **P**6 8 **S** SSM Health Care, Saint Louis, MO	23	10	58	3295	30	70668	661	24720	11858	251

LAMAR—Barton County
★ BARTON COUNTY MEMORIAL HOSPITAL, Second and Gulf Streets, Zip 64759–0626; tel. 417/682–6081; R. Mark Frye, Chief Executive Officer **A**10 **F**7 8 9 12 17 18 22 23 24 25 32 33 34 36 37 38 41 43 44 45 48 51 53 54 70 71 72 76 77 **Web address:** www.freemanhospitals.org/barton.htm	13	10	42	1146	15	43639	103	8256	3732	126

LEBANON—Laclede County
★ BREECH REGIONAL MEDICAL CENTER, 100 Hospital Drive, Zip 65536–2317; tel. 417/533–6100; Gary W. Pulsipher, President **A**1 10 **F**7 8 9 19 22 24 25 26 32 33 34 36 37 38 39 41 43 44 45 48 49 51 54 56 60 70 71 76 **P**6 **S** Sisters of Mercy Health System–St. Louis, Saint Louis, MO	23	10	41	1690	15	33610	268	14557	6913	219

LEES SUMMIT—Jackson County
★ LEE'S SUMMIT HOSPITAL, 530 North Murray Road, Zip 64081–1497; tel. 816/969–6000; John L. Jacobson, President and Chief Executive Officer **A**1 9 10 **F**2 3 4 5 7 8 9 10 11 12 13 16 17 19 20 21 22 24 25 26 27 28 29 30 31 32 33 34 36 37 38 39 40 41 42 43 44 45 46 47 48 49 50 51 52 53 54 57 58 59 60 61 62 63 64 65 66 70 71 72 74 76 77 78 79 **P**4 7 8 **S** Health Midwest, Kansas City, MO **Web address:** www.healthmidwest.org	23	10	83	3168	38	62833	0	26424	11730	278

© 2000 AHA Guide   *Many Facility Codes have changed. Please refer to the AHA Guide Code Chart.*   Hospitals **A249**

Hospitals, U.S. / MISSOURI

Hospital, Address, Telephone, Administrator, Approval, Facility, and Physician Codes, Health Care System, Network	Classification Codes		Utilization Data					Expense (thousands) of dollars		
	Control	Service	Staffed Beds	Admissions	Census	Outpatient Visits	Births	Total	Payroll	Personnel

★ American Hospital Association (AHA) membership
☐ Joint Commission on Accreditation of Healthcare Organizations (JCAHO) accreditation
+ American Osteopathic Healthcare Association (AOHA) membership
○ American Osteopathic Association (AOA) accreditation
△ Commission on Accreditation of Rehabilitation Facilities (CARF) accreditation
Control codes 61, 63, 64, 71, 72 and 73 indicate hospitals listed by AOHA, but not registered by AHA. For definition of numerical codes, see page A4

Hospital	Control	Service	Staffed Beds	Admissions	Census	Outpatient Visits	Births	Total	Payroll	Personnel
LEXINGTON—Lafayette County ✣ LAFAYETTE REGIONAL HEALTH CENTER, 1500 State Street, Zip 64067–1199; tel. 660/259–2203; Jeffrey S. Tarrant, Administrator **A**1 9 10 **F**7 8 13 17 18 22 25 33 34 35 37 38 39 41 43 44 45 46 48 49 50 51 54 56 60 70 76 78 **P**1 5 7 **S** Health Midwest, Kansas City, MO Web address: www.healthmidwest.org	23	10	37	1478	17	27824	2	10061	4007	124
LIBERTY—Clay County ✣ LIBERTY HOSPITAL, 2525 Glenn Hendren Drive, Zip 64069–1002, Mailing Address: P.O. Box 1002, Zip 64069–1002; tel. 816/781–7200; Joseph W. Crossett, Administrator (Total facility includes 12 beds in nursing home–type unit) **A**1 9 10 **F**4 5 7 8 9 11 17 18 19 22 24 25 26 27 30 31 32 33 34 36 37 38 39 40 41 42 43 44 45 46 48 49 54 65 70 72 75 76 78 **P**5 Web address: www.Libertyhospital.org	16	10	180	7764	113	89561	726	66989	29633	878
LOUISIANA—Pike County ✣ PIKE COUNTY MEMORIAL HOSPITAL, 2305 West Georgia Street, Zip 63353–0020; tel. 573/754–5531; Gregory C. Reed, Administrator **A**1 9 10 **F**7 9 13 16 17 18 22 25 31 32 33 34 38 39 43 48 54 60 70 72 76 78 **P**8 **S** SSM Health Care, Saint Louis, MO	13	10	31	889	7	24354	0	7011	3536	121
MACON—Macon County SAMARITAN MEMORIAL HOSPITAL, 1205 North Missouri Street, Zip 63552; tel. 660/385–3151; Bernard A. Orman, Jr, Administrator **A**10 **F**3 7 8 9 13 16 17 18 19 20 21 22 25 26 27 28 30 31 32 33 34 35 36 37 38 39 43 44 45 46 48 50 54 56 57 59 62 70 71 72 74 76 78 79 **P**3	13	10	28	1054	15	40132	94	—	—	157
MARSHALL—Saline County ★ FITZGIBBON HOSPITAL, 2305 South 65 Highway, Zip 65340–0250, Mailing Address: P.O. Box 250, Zip 65340–0250; tel. 660/886–7431; Ronald A. Ott, Chief Executive Officer (Total facility includes 13 beds in nursing home–type unit) **A**9 10 **F**7 8 9 17 18 19 22 24 25 28 32 33 34 36 37 38 39 41 43 44 45 48 49 51 54 68 70 71 72 76 79 **P**6	23	10	56	2412	32	86935	361	24636	10863	388
MARYVILLE—Nodaway County ✣ ST. FRANCIS HOSPITAL AND HEALTH SERVICES, 2016 South Main Street, Zip 64468–2693; tel. 660/562–2600; Michael Baumgartner, President **A**1 9 10 **F**7 8 9 11 13 16 17 18 21 22 23 24 25 32 33 34 36 37 38 39 43 44 48 54 57 59 60 61 62 63 64 70 72 76 78 **P**5 6 8 **S** SSM Health Care, Saint Louis, MO	21	10	53	2008	21	53860	264	17998	8724	322
MEMPHIS—Scotland County ○ SCOTLAND COUNTY MEMORIAL HOSPITAL, Sigler Avenue, Zip 63555, Mailing Address: Route 1, Box 53, Zip 63555; tel. 660/465–8511; Marcia R. Dial, Administrator **A**9 10 11 **F**5 7 8 9 13 14 16 17 18 19 21 22 23 25 30 32 33 34 36 37 38 40 41 43 44 45 46 48 50 51 53 54 56 59 70 71 72 76 **P**6	16	10	32	598	7	24009	36	4565	1967	130
MEXICO—Audrain County ✣ AUDRAIN MEDICAL CENTER, 620 East Monroe Street, Zip 65265–0858; tel. 573/582–5000; Douglas R. Trembath, President and Chief Executive Officer (Total facility includes 40 beds in nursing home–type unit) **A**1 9 10 **F**3 4 7 8 9 11 13 14 16 17 18 19 20 21 22 23 24 25 26 27 29 30 31 32 33 34 36 37 38 39 41 43 44 45 46 48 49 50 51 54 56 57 58 59 60 61 62 63 64 70 71 72 73 76 78 79 **P**6 Web address: www.amc–healthcare.org	23	10	154	4816	82	199026	268	54243	22824	700
MILAN—Sullivan County ★ ○ SULLIVAN COUNTY MEMORIAL HOSPITAL, 630 West Third Street, Zip 63556–1098; tel. 660/265–4212; Martha Gragg, Chief Executive Officer (Total facility includes 12 beds in nursing home–type unit) **A**10 11 **F**13 14 16 17 18 19 22 23 25 28 32 33 34 37 38 43 45 48 50 51 54 56 70 76	13	10	38	168	25	15106	0	2759	1425	62
MOBERLY—Randolph County ☐ MOBERLY REGIONAL MEDICAL CENTER, 1515 Union Avenue, Zip 65270–9449, Mailing Address: P.O. Box 3000, Zip 65270–3000; tel. 660/263–8400; Cathryn A. Hibbs, Chief Executive Officer **A**1 9 10 **F**8 9 11 12 13 17 18 19 21 22 23 24 25 28 30 32 33 34 36 37 38 41 43 44 45 48 50 51 54 56 57 60 62 64 68 70 71 72 73 75 76 77 78 79 **S** Community Health Systems, Inc., Brentwood, TN	33	10	92	3090	41	45704	296	24885	8295	315
MONETT—Barry County COX MONETT HOSPITAL, 801 Lincoln Avenue, Zip 65708–1698; tel. 417/354–1400; Gregory D. Johnson, Administrator **A**9 10 **F**3 7 9 17 18 19 21 22 23 24 25 29 30 31 32 33 34 36 37 38 41 43 45 46 48 50 51 54 56 58 59 60 61 62 63 68 70 71 72 76 77 78 **P**1 8 **S** Cox Health System, Springfield, MO Web address: www.coxnet.org/whoarewe/hospital_seche.cfm	23	10	53	806	9	52610	0	9569	5045	226
MOUNT VERNON—Lawrence County ☐ △ MISSOURI REHABILITATION CENTER, 600 North Main, Zip 65712–1099; tel. 417/465–3711; Dennis Stambaugh, Director **A**1 7 10 **F**3 6 7 13 22 24 26 30 31 33 34 35 37 38 41 43 45 46 51 53 54 56 63 70 72 76 78 **P**6 Web address: www.hsc.missouri.edu/~rehab/	12	10	135	476	69	35215	0	21740	12377	440
MOUNTAIN VIEW—Howell County ✣ ST. FRANCIS HOSPITAL, Highway 60, Zip 65548, Mailing Address: P.O. Box 82, Zip 65548–0082; tel. 417/934–2246; Gary W. Jordan, President and Chief Executive Officer **A**1 9 10 **F**7 9 16 17 22 23 25 32 33 36 37 38 43 44 54 60 70 75 76 77 **P**6 **S** Sisters of Mercy Health System–St. Louis, Saint Louis, MO Web address: www.stfran@socket.net	23	10	17	516	6	18423	0	4090	1685	90

A250 Hospitals   *Many Facility Codes have changed. Please refer to the AHA Guide Code Chart.*   © 2000 AHA Guide

Hospitals, U.S. / MISSOURI

Hospital, Address, Telephone, Administrator, Approval, Facility, and Physician Codes, Health Care System, Network	Classification Codes		Utilization Data					Expense (thousands) of dollars		
★ American Hospital Association (AHA) membership □ Joint Commission on Accreditation of Healthcare Organizations (JCAHO) accreditation + American Osteopathic Healthcare Association (AOHA) membership ○ American Osteopathic Association (AOA) accreditation △ Commission on Accreditation of Rehabilitation Facilities (CARF) accreditation Control codes 61, 63, 64, 71, 72 and 73 indicate hospitals listed by AOHA, but not registered by AHA. For definition of numerical codes, see page A4	Control	Service	Staffed Beds	Admissions	Census	Outpatient Visits	Births	Total	Payroll	Personnel
NEOSHO—Newton County FREEMAN NEOSHO HOSPITAL, 113 West Hickory Street, Zip 64850–1799; tel. 417/455–4352; Phil Willcoxon, Chief Executive Officer **A**9 10 **F**2 3 4 5 7 8 9 10 11 12 13 17 18 19 21 22 23 24 25 26 30 32 33 34 35 36 37 38 41 42 43 44 45 46 47 48 50 51 52 53 54 56 57 58 59 60 61 62 63 64 68 70 71 72 76 77 78 **P**1 4 Web address: www.freemanhospitals.org	23	10	54	2253	30	97390	0	18245	6603	242
NEVADA—Vernon County □ HEARTLAND BEHAVIORAL HEALTH SERVICES, 1500 West Ashland Street, Zip 64772–1710; tel. 417/667–2666; David Morrison, Chief Executive Officer **A**1 10 **F**16 30 33 57 58 59 60 61 62 70 **S** Ramsay Youth Services, Coral Gables, FL Web address: www.hardtoplacekids.com	33	22	30	472	17	0	0	—	—	54
★ NEVADA REGIONAL MEDICAL CENTER, 800 South Ash Street, Zip 64772–3223; tel. 417/667–3355; Robert B. Ohlen, President and Chief Executive Officer (Total facility includes 14 beds in nursing home–type unit) **A**1 9 10 **F**7 8 9 14 16 17 18 19 22 23 25 27 29 31 32 33 34 35 36 37 38 39 40 41 43 44 45 46 48 49 51 54 70 71 76 78 **S** Quorum Health Group, Brentwood, TN Web address: www.nrmchealth.com	14	10	85	2135	26	45175	292	18660	7449	309
NORTH KANSAS CITY—Clay County ★ NORTH KANSAS CITY HOSPITAL, 2800 Clay Edwards Drive, Zip 64116–3281; tel. 816/691–2000; David R. Carpenter, FACHE, President and Chief Executive Officer (Total facility includes 39 beds in nursing home–type unit) **A**1 9 10 **F**4 7 8 9 10 11 12 13 17 18 19 22 23 24 25 26 27 32 33 34 35 36 37 38 39 40 41 42 43 44 45 46 47 48 49 51 52 53 54 57 59 60 61 62 64 65 68 70 72 75 76 78 **P**6	14	10	350	16017	243	141393	1724	148446	57676	1549
OSAGE BEACH—Camden County ★ LAKE REGIONAL HEALTH SYSTEM, (Formerly Lake Regional Hospital), 54 Hospital Drive, Zip 65065–9699; tel. 573/348–8000; Michael E. Henze, Chief Executive Officer (Total facility includes 10 beds in nursing home–type unit) **A**1 9 10 **F**4 7 8 9 11 12 13 16 17 18 19 22 23 24 25 27 32 33 34 36 37 38 39 41 43 44 45 46 47 48 49 50 51 54 60 68 70 71 72 75 76 78 **P**6 Web address: www.lakeregional.com	23	10	94	4370	57	129967	625	59306	20834	611
OSCEOLA—St. Clair County ★ SAC–OSAGE HOSPITAL, Junction Highways 13 & Business 13, Zip 64776, Mailing Address: P.O. Box 426, Zip 64776–0426; tel. 417/646–8181; Terry E. Erwine, Administrator **A**1 9 10 **F**7 8 9 17 18 22 25 32 33 34 35 38 41 43 44 45 46 48 50 51 54 70 72 76 78 Web address: www.sac–osagehospital.com	16	10	47	1294	19	6691	43	5877	3197	115
PERRYVILLE—Perry County □ PERRY COUNTY MEMORIAL HOSPITAL, 434 North West Street, Zip 63775–1398; tel. 573/547–2536; Ralph Paulding, President and Chief Executive Officer **A**1 9 10 **F**1 7 8 9 13 17 18 19 22 25 27 28 29 30 31 32 33 34 36 38 39 43 44 45 48 49 50 54 58 60 63 68 70 71 72 74 76 77 78 79 Web address: www.pchmo.org	23	10	47	823	11	40816	157	13784	5681	204
POPLAR BLUFF—Butler County □ △ DOCTORS REGIONAL MEDICAL CENTER, 621 Pine Boulevard, Zip 63901; tel. 573/686–4111; Timothy F. Brady, FACHE, Chief Executive Officer (Total facility includes 15 beds in nursing home–type unit) **A**1 2 7 9 10 **F**2 3 7 8 9 11 13 17 18 19 21 22 23 24 25 26 27 28 29 30 32 33 34 35 36 37 38 39 41 43 44 45 46 48 49 50 51 53 54 56 57 58 59 60 61 62 63 70 71 72 76 77 78 79	33	10	170	6387	81	119673	375	37287	14814	596
★ JOHN J. PERSHING VETERANS AFFAIRS MEDICAL CENTER, 1500 North Westwood Boulevard, Zip 63901–3318; tel. 573/686–4151; Nancy Arnold, Director (Total facility includes 40 beds in nursing home–type unit) **A**1 **F**1 2 3 7 9 16 17 22 23 24 25 29 30 31 32 33 34 36 38 39 41 43 45 46 48 51 54 56 57 59 60 63 64 70 76 78 79 **P**6 **S** Department of Veterans Affairs, Washington, DC	45	10	56	1515	37	87510	0	30374	14639	322
★ LUCY LEE HOSPITAL, 2620 North Westwood Boulevard, Zip 63901–2341, Mailing Address: P.O. Box 88, Zip 63901–2341; tel. 573/785–7721; Timothy F. Brady, FACHE, Chief Executive Officer (Total facility includes 24 beds in nursing home–type unit) **A**1 2 10 **F**4 7 8 9 11 12 13 17 19 22 23 24 25 27 28 30 32 33 34 35 36 38 39 41 43 44 45 46 48 49 50 51 53 54 65 68 70 71 72 76 77 78 79 **P**1 7 **S** TENET Healthcare Corporation, Santa Barbara, CA Web address: www.tenethealth.com	33	10	173	7509	100	283952	1163	66672	24073	604
POTOSI—Washington County WASHINGTON COUNTY MEMORIAL HOSPITAL, 300 Health Way, Zip 63664–1499; tel. 573/438–5451; Clarence E. Lay, Administrator **A**9 10 **F**7 9 16 17 18 19 22 25 29 30 32 33 34 36 38 39 41 45 48 51 54 60 70 72 76 77 78 79 Web address: www.wcmhosp.org	13	10	42	788	9	44877	0	8519	3531	166
RICHMOND—Ray County RAY COUNTY MEMORIAL HOSPITAL, 904 Wollard Boulevard, Zip 64085–2243; tel. 816/470–5432; Tommy L. Hicks, Administrator (Total facility includes 11 beds in nursing home–type unit) **A**9 10 **F**7 9 17 22 25 26 33 36 37 38 39 41 43 45 46 48 49 51 54 60 70 76 78	13	10	50	1149	17	16382	0	10650	4622	187

Hospitals, U.S. / MISSOURI

	Classification Codes		Utilization Data					Expense (thousands) of dollars		
Hospital, Address, Telephone, Administrator, Approval, Facility, and Physician Codes, Health Care System, Network	Control	Service	Staffed Beds	Admissions	Census	Outpatient Visits	Births	Total	Payroll	Personnel

★ American Hospital Association (AHA) membership
☐ Joint Commission on Accreditation of Healthcare Organizations (JCAHO) accreditation
+ American Osteopathic Healthcare Association (AOHA) membership
○ American Osteopathic Association (AOA) accreditation
△ Commission on Accreditation of Rehabilitation Facilities (CARF) accreditation
Control codes 61, 63, 64, 71, 72 and 73 indicate hospitals listed by AOHA, but not registered by AHA. For definition of numerical codes, see page A4

ROLLA—Phelps County

★ ○ △ PHELPS COUNTY REGIONAL MEDICAL CENTER, 1000 West Tenth Street, Zip 65401–2905; tel. 573/364–3100; David Ross, Chief Executive Officer (Total facility includes 26 beds in nursing home–type unit) **A**1 7 9 10 11 12 **F**2 3 7 8 9 11 13 15 17 18 19 20 21 22 23 24 25 26 27 31 32 33 34 36 37 38 39 41 43 44 45 46 48 49 50 51 53 54 57 60 61 63 64 65 68 70 71 72 75 76 77 78 79
Web address: www.rollanet.org/~pcrmc/ — 13 10 202 8481 119 135550 894 62306 27108 883

SAINT CHARLES—St. Charles County

☐ BHC SPIRIT OF ST. LOUIS HOSPITAL, 5931 Highway 94 South, Zip 63304–5601; tel. 314/441–7300; Susan Young, Chief Executive Officer **A**1 9 10 **F**1 2 3 13 21 33 38 57 58 59 60 61 63 64 70 72 **S** Behavioral Healthcare Corporation, Nashville, TN — 33 22 104 465 52 0 0 — — —

★ ST. JOSEPH HEALTH CENTER, 300 First Capitol Drive, Zip 63301–2835; tel. 636/947–5000; Kevin F. Kast, President, Chief Executive Officer and Market Executive (Total facility includes 24 beds in nursing home–type unit) **A**1 2 9 10 **F**2 3 4 5 7 8 9 11 12 13 14 16 17 18 19 21 22 23 24 25 26 27 28 29 30 32 33 34 35 36 37 38 39 41 42 43 44 45 46 47 48 49 50 51 52 53 54 56 57 58 59 60 61 62 63 64 65 66 67 70 71 72 73 74 75 76 77 78 79 **P**4 6 7 **S** SSM Health Care, Saint Louis, MO — 23 10 273 11918 138 112060 731 91141 39004 936

SAINT JOSEPH—Buchanan County

★ △ HEARTLAND REGIONAL MEDICAL CENTER, (Includes Heartland Hospital East, 5325 Faraon Street, Zip 64506; Heartland Hospital West, 801 Faraon Street, Zip 64501; tel. 816/271–7111), 5325 Faraon Street, Zip 64506–3398; tel. 816/271–6000; Lowell C. Kruse, Chief Executive Officer **A**1 2 5 7 9 10 **F**4 5 7 8 9 11 12 13 14 16 17 18 19 22 24 25 29 30 32 33 34 35 36 37 38 39 41 42 44 45 47 48 49 50 51 53 54 55 56 57 59 60 61 62 65 68 70 71 75 77 78 **P**6 — 23 10 522 15149 176 336920 1600 174819 80028 2073

☐ NORTHWEST MISSOURI PSYCHIATRIC REHABILITATION CENTER, (Includes Woodson Childrens Psychiatric Hospital, 3510 Frederick, Zip 64506–2913; tel. 816/387–2320), 3505 Frederick Avenue, Zip 64506; tel. 816/378–2300; Laurent D. Javois, Superintendent **A**1 10 **F**17 33 57 58 59 60 61 62 78 WOODSON CHILDRENS PSYCHIATRIC HOSPITAL See Northwest Missouri Psychiatric Rehabilitation Center — 12 22 120 169 113 0 0 24043 8581 459

SAINT LOUIS—St. Louis County

★ ALEXIAN BROTHERS HOSPITAL, 3933 South Broadway, Zip 63118–9984; tel. 314/865–3333; Patricia F. Cook, R.N., Vice President Operations (Total facility includes 40 beds in nursing home–type unit) **A**1 9 10 **F**2 3 4 5 7 8 9 10 11 12 13 14 16 17 18 19 21 22 23 25 26 29 30 31 32 33 34 35 36 37 38 39 40 41 42 43 44 45 46 47 48 49 50 51 52 53 54 56 57 58 59 60 61 62 63 64 65 66 70 71 75 76 77 78 79 **P**5 6 7 8 — 23 10 203 5075 85 53629 0 43178 17573 533

★ △ BARNES–JEWISH HOSPITAL, One Barnes–Jewish Hospital Plaza, Zip 63110–1094; tel. 314/747–3000; Ronald G. Evens, M.D., President **A**1 2 3 5 7 8 9 10 **F**1 2 3 4 5 6 7 8 9 10 11 12 13 14 15 16 17 18 19 20 21 22 23 24 25 26 27 28 29 30 31 32 33 34 35 36 37 38 39 40 41 42 43 44 45 46 47 48 49 50 51 52 53 54 55 56 57 58 59 60 61 62 63 64 65 66 67 68 70 71 72 73 74 75 76 77 78 79 **P**1 4 5 6 7 **S** BJC Health System, Saint Louis, MO
Web address: www.bjc.org/bjh.html — 23 10 941 45826 758 249754 3934 725828 266787 7821

★ BARNES–JEWISH WEST COUNTY HOSPITAL, 12634 Olive Boulevard, Zip 63141–6354; tel. 314/996–8000; Ronald G. Evens, M.D., Interim President and Senior Executive Officer (Total facility includes 10 beds in nursing home–type unit) **A**1 9 10 **F**1 2 3 4 5 6 7 8 9 10 11 12 13 14 15 19 20 21 22 23 24 25 26 27 28 29 30 31 32 33 34 35 36 37 38 39 40 41 42 43 44 45 46 47 48 49 50 51 52 53 54 55 56 57 58 59 60 61 62 63 64 65 66 67 68 70 71 72 73 74 75 76 77 78 79 **P**1 7 **S** BJC Health System, Saint Louis, MO
Web address: www.bjc.org/chnenw.html — 23 10 91 2823 37 44673 0 40666 11358 306

★ CARDINAL GLENNON CHILDREN'S HOSPITAL, 1465 South Grand Boulevard, Zip 63104–1095; tel. 314/577–5600; Douglas A. Ries, President **A**1 3 5 9 **F**2 3 4 5 6 7 10 11 13 14 16 17 18 19 20 21 22 23 24 25 26 27 28 29 31 32 33 34 35 36 37 38 39 42 43 45 46 47 48 49 50 51 52 53 54 55 56 57 58 59 60 61 63 64 65 68 70 71 72 73 74 75 76 77 78 79 **P**7 8 **S** SSM Health Care, Saint Louis, MO
Web address: www.cardinalglennon.com/internet/net10hom.nsf/?Open — 23 50 172 7922 118 174024 0 101119 41100 1179

★ △ CHRISTIAN HOSPITAL NORTHEAST–NORTHWEST, (Includes Christian Hospital Northwest, 1225 Graham Road, Florissant, Zip 63031; tel. 314/953–6000), 11133 Dunn Road, Zip 63136–6192; tel. 314/653–5000; Mark A. Eustis, President (Total facility includes 36 beds in nursing home–type unit) **A**1 2 7 9 10 **F**1 2 3 4 5 6 7 8 9 10 11 12 13 14 15 16 17 18 19 20 21 22 23 24 25 26 27 28 30 31 32 33 34 35 36 37 38 39 40 41 42 43 44 45 46 47 48 49 50 51 52 53 54 55 57 58 59 60 61 62 63 64 65 66 67 68 69 70 71 72 73 74 75 76 77 78 79 **P**5 7 8 **S** BJC Health System, Saint Louis, MO
Web address: www.bjc.org — 23 10 546 22004 341 192615 1488 — — —

★ △ COMPTON HEIGHTS HOSPITAL, 3545 Lafayette Avenue, Zip 63104–9984; tel. 314/865–6500; Leona D. Stoll, Chief Executive Officer (Total facility includes 56 beds in nursing home–type unit) **A**1 7 9 10 **F**2 3 4 5 8 9 12 13 15 16 17 18 19 20 21 22 25 27 29 30 31 32 33 34 35 36 37 38 39 40 41 43 44 45 46 47 48 49 50 51 53 54 55 56 57 58 59 60 61 62 63 64 65 66 67 68 70 71 72 74 75 76 77 78 79 **P**8 **S** TENET Healthcare Corporation, Santa Barbara, CA
Web address: www.tenethealth.com — 33 10 192 4693 107 81487 0 38543 19433 412

Hospitals, U.S. / MISSOURI

Hospital, Address, Telephone, Administrator, Approval, Facility, and Physician Codes, Health Care System, Network	Classification Codes		Utilization Data					Expense (thousands) of dollars		
★ American Hospital Association (AHA) membership ☐ Joint Commission on Accreditation of Healthcare Organizations (JCAHO) accreditation + American Osteopathic Healthcare Association (AOHA) membership ○ American Osteopathic Association (AOA) accreditation △ Commission on Accreditation of Rehabilitation Facilities (CARF) accreditation Control codes 61, 63, 64, 71, 72 and 73 indicate hospitals listed by AOHA, but not registered by AHA. For definition of numerical codes, see page A4	Control	Service	Staffed Beds	Admissions	Census	Outpatient Visits	Births	Total	Payroll	Personnel
★ DEPAUL HEALTH CENTER, (Includes ST, ANNE'S SKILLED NURSING DIVISION; DePaul Hospital, Bridgeton; St. Vincent's Psychiatric Division, Bridgeton), 12303 DePaul Drive, Zip 63044-2588; tel. 314/344-6000; Robert G. Porter, President (Total facility includes 84 beds in nursing home-type unit) **A**1 2 9 10 **F**2 3 4 7 8 9 10 11 12 13 14 16 17 18 19 21 22 23 24 25 26 27 28 30 31 32 33 34 35 36 37 38 39 40 41 42 43 44 45 46 47 48 49 50 51 52 53 54 56 57 58 59 60 61 62 63 64 65 68 70 71 72 73 74 75 76 78 79 **P**6 8 **S** SSM Health Care, Saint Louis, MO	21	10	375	13331	264	147108	856	111083	42976	1192
★ + ○ △ DES PERES HOSPITAL, (Includes Metropolitan Medical Center-West), 2345 Dougherty Ferry Road, Zip 63122-3313; tel. 314/768-3000; Michele C. Meyer, Chief Executive Officer **A**7 9 10 11 12 13 **F**2 3 4 5 8 9 10 11 12 13 15 18 19 21 22 24 25 27 29 30 31 32 33 35 36 37 38 39 40 41 43 44 45 46 47 48 49 50 51 53 54 55 56 57 58 59 60 61 62 63 64 65 66 68 70 71 72 74 75 76 77 78 79 **S** TENET Healthcare Corporation, Santa Barbara, CA Web address: www.tenethealth.com	33	10	93	3448	48	24080	0	34916	14646	443
★ △ FOREST PARK HOSPITAL, 6150 Oakland Avenue, Zip 63139-3297; tel. 314/768-3000; John W. Sanders, Chief Executive Officer (Total facility includes 20 beds in nursing home-type unit) **A**1 2 3 5 7 9 10 12 **F**1 2 3 4 7 8 9 11 12 13 16 17 18 19 22 24 26 29 30 31 33 34 36 37 38 39 40 41 44 45 46 47 48 49 53 54 56 57 59 60 61 62 63 64 65 67 68 70 71 72 75 76 77 78 79 **P**6 **S** TENET Healthcare Corporation, Santa Barbara, CA Web address: www.tenethealth.com	33	10	288	12389	192	180437	1481	125250	53367	1317
METROPOLITAN MEDICAL CENTER-WEST See Des Peres Hospital										
☐ METROPOLITAN ST. LOUIS PSYCHIATRIC CENTER, 5351 Delmar, Zip 63112-3198; tel. 314/877-0500; Bonnie DiFranco, Chief Executive Officer **A**1 3 5 10 **F**2 6 7 13 16 19 22 25 33 39 43 45 50 51 57 59 60 61 62 63 64 70 72 78	12	22	104	1698	95	5289	0	11218	10895	379
MISSOURI BAPTIST MEDICAL CENTER See Town and Country										
★ SAINT LOUIS UNIVERSITY HOSPITAL, 3635 Vista at Grand Boulevard, Zip 63110-0250, Mailing Address: P.O. Box 15250, Zip 63110-0250); tel. 314/577-8000; Lee D. Stoll, Chief Executive Officer **A**1 3 5 8 9 10 **F**2 3 4 5 7 8 9 11 12 13 15 16 17 18 19 20 21 22 23 24 25 27 29 30 31 32 33 34 35 36 37 38 39 40 41 42 43 44 46 47 48 49 50 51 53 54 55 56 57 58 59 60 61 62 63 64 65 66 67 68 70 71 72 74 75 76 77 78 79 **P**1 6 **S** TENET Healthcare Corporation, Santa Barbara, CA Web address: www.stlucare.edu	33	10	303	12341	205	217256	0	194301	58397	2161
☐ SHRINERS HOSPITALS FOR CHILDREN, ST. LOUIS, 2001 South Lindbergh Boulevard, Zip 63131-3597; tel. 314/432-3600; Carolyn P. Golden, Administrator **A**1 3 5 **F**13 16 17 22 31 32 33 34 38 39 45 49 50 51 54 56 68 70 71 72 78 **S** Shriners Hospitals for Children, Tampa, FL	23	57	80	1931	30	12378	0	—	—	240
★ △ SOUTHPOINTE HOSPITAL, 2639 Miami Street, Zip 63118-3999; tel. 314/772-1456; Doug Doris, Chief Executive Officer (Total facility includes 30 beds in nursing home-type unit) **A**1 6 7 9 10 **F**1 2 3 4 5 7 8 9 11 13 15 16 17 18 19 21 22 25 26 29 30 31 32 33 35 36 37 38 39 41 43 44 45 46 47 48 49 50 51 53 54 55 56 57 58 59 60 61 62 63 64 65 66 68 70 71 72 74 75 76 77 78 79 **P**6 **S** TENET Healthcare Corporation, Santa Barbara, CA Web address: www.tenethealth.com	33	10	249	5991	134	72243	216	41148	21037	554
★ △ SSM REHAB, 6420 Clayton Road, Suite 600, Zip 63117-1861; tel. 314/768-5300; Melinda Clark, President (Total facility includes 20 beds in nursing home-type unit) (Nonreporting) **A**1 7 9 10 **S** SSM Health Care, Saint Louis, MO	21	46	78	—	—	—	—	—	—	—
★ ST. ANTHONY'S MEDICAL CENTER, 10010 Kennerly Road, Zip 63128-2185; tel. 314/525-1000; David P. Seifert, President and Chief Executive Officer (Total facility includes 96 beds in nursing home-type unit) **A**1 9 10 **F**1 2 3 4 5 7 8 9 10 11 12 13 14 16 17 18 19 21 22 23 24 25 26 27 28 29 30 31 32 33 34 35 36 37 38 39 40 41 42 43 44 45 46 47 48 49 50 51 52 53 54 56 57 58 59 60 61 62 63 64 65 66 68 70 71 72 73 74 75 76 77 78 79 **P**1 2 3 4 5 6 7 8	23	10	684	24542	388	241039	1549	217420	88742	2573
★ △ ST. JOHN'S MERCY MEDICAL CENTER, (Includes St. John's Mercy Hospital, 200 Madison Avenue, Washington, Zip 63090; tel. 314/239-8000), 615 South New Ballas Road, Zip 63141-8277; tel. 314/569-6000; Mark Weber, FACHE, President (Total facility includes 22 beds in nursing home-type unit) **A**1 2 3 5 7 8 9 10 **F**1 2 3 4 5 6 7 8 9 10 11 12 13 14 15 16 17 18 19 20 21 22 23 24 25 26 27 28 29 30 31 32 33 34 35 36 37 38 39 40 41 42 43 44 45 46 47 48 49 50 51 52 53 54 55 56 57 58 59 60 61 62 63 64 65 66 67 68 69 70 71 72 73 74 75 76 77 78 79 **P**1 5 6 7 8 **S** Sisters of Mercy Health System-St. Louis, Saint Louis, MO	21	10	898	34631	476	510315	7746	—	—	2967
★ ST. JOSEPH HOSPITAL OF KIRKWOOD, 525 Couch Avenue, Zip 63122-5594; tel. 314/966-1500; Carla S. Baum, President (Total facility includes 44 beds in nursing home-type unit) **A**1 2 9 10 **F**2 3 4 5 7 8 9 10 11 12 13 14 16 17 19 20 21 22 23 25 26 27 28 29 30 31 32 33 35 36 37 38 39 40 41 42 43 44 45 46 47 48 49 50 51 52 53 54 57 58 59 60 61 62 63 64 65 66 70 71 72 73 74 75 76 77 78 79 **P**6 8 **S** SSM Health Care, Saint Louis, MO Web address: www.stjosephkirkwood.com/internet/home/stjokirk.nsf	23	10	213	7285	98	134452	869	61454	27648	810
★ △ ST. LOUIS CHILDREN'S HOSPITAL, One Children's Place, Zip 63110-1077; tel. 314/454-6000; Ted W. Frey, President and Senior Executive Officer **A**1 3 5 7 8 9 10 **F**2 3 5 7 8 11 12 13 14 15 16 17 19 21 22 23 24 25 26 27 28 29 30 31 32 34 35 36 37 38 39 40 41 42 43 44 45 47 48 49 50 51 52 53 54 55 56 57 58 59 60 61 62 63 64 65 66 67 68 69 70 71 72 73 74 75 76 77 78 79 **P**6 **S** BJC Health System, Saint Louis, MO Web address: www.STLOUISCHILDRENS.ORG	23	50	235	10947	163	112516	0	175840	67634	1963

© 2000 AHA Guide   *Many Facility Codes have changed. Please refer to the AHA Guide Code Chart.*

Hospitals, U.S. / MISSOURI

Hospital, Address, Telephone, Administrator, Approval, Facility, and Physician Codes, Health Care System, Network	Classification Codes		Utilization Data					Expense (thousands) of dollars		
	Control	Service	Staffed Beds	Admissions	Census	Outpatient Visits	Births	Total	Payroll	Personnel

★ American Hospital Association (AHA) membership
□ Joint Commission on Accreditation of Healthcare Organizations (JCAHO) accreditation
+ American Osteopathic Healthcare Association (AOHA) membership
○ American Osteopathic Association (AOA) accreditation
△ Commission on Accreditation of Rehabilitation Facilities (CARF) accreditation
Control codes 61, 63, 64, 71, 72 and 73 indicate hospitals listed by AOHA, but not registered by AHA. For definition of numerical codes, see page A4

Hospital	Control	Service	Staffed Beds	Admissions	Census	Outpatient Visits	Births	Total	Payroll	Personnel
□ ST. LOUIS PSYCHIATRIC REHABILITATION CENTER, 5300 Arsenal Street, Zip 63139–1494; tel. 314/644–8000; Roberta Gardine, Chief Executive Officer **A**1 10 **F**7 13 23 28 33 34 43 57 59 60 78 **P**6	12	22	212	52	207	0	0	29814	17216	610
★ ST. MARY'S HEALTH CENTER, 6420 Clayton Road, Zip 63117–1811; tel. 314/768–8000; James B. Rigby, Interim President (Total facility includes 50 beds in nursing home–type unit) **A**1 2 3 5 8 9 10 **F**3 4 5 7 8 9 11 12 13 14 16 17 18 19 21 22 23 24 25 26 27 28 29 30 32 33 34 35 36 37 38 39 40 41 42 43 44 45 46 47 48 49 50 51 52 53 54 56 57 58 59 60 61 62 63 64 65 66 68 70 71 72 73 74 76 77 78 79 **P**6 8 **S** SSM Health Care, Saint Louis, MO	23	10	460	21161	284	184316	2409	138969	57249	1394
★ △ VETERANS AFFAIRS MEDICAL CENTER, 1 Jefferson Barracks Drive, Zip 63125–4199; tel. 314/652–4100; Linda Kurz, CHE, Director (Total facility includes 114 beds in nursing home–type unit) **A**1 2 3 5 7 **F**3 4 5 9 11 13 18 19 21 22 23 24 25 26 27 28 29 30 31 33 34 35 36 37 38 39 41 43 45 46 47 48 49 50 51 54 55 56 57 59 60 61 62 63 64 65 70 72 74 76 78 79 **S** Department of Veterans Affairs, Washington, DC	45	10	355	7583	300	311401	0	171190	102125	1960

SAINT PETERS—St. Charles County

Hospital	Control	Service	Staffed Beds	Admissions	Census	Outpatient Visits	Births	Total	Payroll	Personnel
★ BARNES–JEWISH ST. PETERS HOSPITAL, 10 Hospital Drive, Zip 63376–1659; tel. 636/916–9000; Carmelo J. Moceri, President (Total facility includes 8 beds in nursing home–type unit) **A**1 9 10 **F**7 8 9 11 13 16 17 19 22 24 25 30 32 33 34 35 36 37 38 39 41 43 44 45 46 48 49 50 54 68 70 71 72 76 77 78 79 **P**2 5 8 **S** BJC Health System, Saint Louis, MO Web address: www.bjc.org/bjsph.html	23	10	84	4745	48	96810	973	41595	17421	453

SALEM—Dent County

Hospital	Control	Service	Staffed Beds	Admissions	Census	Outpatient Visits	Births	Total	Payroll	Personnel
SALEM MEMORIAL DISTRICT HOSPITAL, Highway 72 North, Zip 65560, Mailing Address: P.O. Box 774, Zip 65560; tel. 573/729–6626; Dennis P. Pryor, Administrator (Total facility includes 18 beds in nursing home–type unit) **A**9 10 **F**7 8 9 13 17 18 22 25 27 31 32 33 34 36 37 38 43 44 45 48 50 51 54 70 71 76 78	16	10	51	1345	33	24106	97	8272	3768	162

SEDALIA—Pettis County

Hospital	Control	Service	Staffed Beds	Admissions	Census	Outpatient Visits	Births	Total	Payroll	Personnel
★ BOTHWELL REGIONAL HEALTH CENTER, 601 East 14th Street, Zip 65301–1706, Mailing Address: P.O. Box 1706, Zip 65302–1706; tel. 660/826–8833; James T. Rank, Administrator **A**1 9 10 **F**4 7 8 9 11 12 15 17 18 22 23 24 25 27 32 33 34 36 37 38 39 41 44 46 48 49 50 51 53 54 57 60 62 65 70 71 72 76 77 Web address: www.brhc.org	14	10	167	5694	77	75741	687	46104	21294	745

SIKESTON—Scott County

Hospital	Control	Service	Staffed Beds	Admissions	Census	Outpatient Visits	Births	Total	Payroll	Personnel
□ MISSOURI DELTA MEDICAL CENTER, 1008 North Main Street, Zip 63801–5099; tel. 573/471–1600; Charles D. Ancell, President (Total facility includes 14 beds in nursing home–type unit) **A**1 9 10 **F**3 4 5 6 7 8 9 11 13 15 16 17 18 19 21 22 23 24 25 26 27 28 29 30 31 32 33 34 35 36 37 38 39 40 41 43 44 45 46 47 48 49 50 51 54 56 57 59 60 61 62 63 64 65 67 68 70 71 72 74 76 77 78 79	23	10	154	4605	69	71915	529	38088	16767	574

SMITHVILLE—Clay County

Hospital	Control	Service	Staffed Beds	Admissions	Census	Outpatient Visits	Births	Total	Payroll	Personnel
★ SAINT LUKE'S NORTHLAND HOSPITAL–SMITHVILLE CAMPUS, 601 South 169 Highway, Zip 64089–9334; tel. 816/532–3700; Don Sipes, Chief Executive Officer (Total facility includes 16 beds in nursing home–type unit) **A**1 9 10 **F**2 3 4 5 6 7 8 9 11 12 13 14 16 17 18 19 20 21 22 23 24 25 26 27 28 29 30 31 32 33 34 35 36 37 38 39 40 41 42 43 44 45 46 47 48 49 50 51 53 54 55 56 57 58 59 60 61 62 63 64 65 66 68 70 71 72 73 74 75 76 77 78 79 **P**6 8 **S** Saint Luke's Shawnee Mission Health System, Kansas City, MO Web address: www.saint-lukes.org	23	10	59	1060	22	18949	0	10665	5044	116

SPRINGFIELD—Greene County

Hospital	Control	Service	Staffed Beds	Admissions	Census	Outpatient Visits	Births	Total	Payroll	Personnel
DOCTORS HOSPITAL OF SPRINGFIELD, 2828 North National, Zip 65803; tel. 417/837–4000; John Moran, Chief Executive Officer (Nonreporting) **A**10	32	10	45	—	—	—	—	—	—	—
□ LAKELAND REGIONAL HOSPITAL, 440 South Market Street, Zip 65806–2090; tel. 417/865–5581; John William Thompson, Ph.D., President and Chief Executive Officer **A**1 10 **F**16 17 18 21 22 25 29 33 38 39 43 51 57 58 59 60 61 63 64 70 76 **P**6 **S** Youth and Family Centered Services, Austin, TX	33	22	78	1922	78	9808	0	11526	6365	203
★ △ LESTER E. COX MEDICAL CENTERS, (Formerly Cox Medical Center), (Includes Lester E. Cox Medical Center North, 1423 North Jefferson Avenue, Zip 65802; tel. 417/269–3000; Lester E. Cox Medical Center South, 3801 South National Avenue, Zip 65807; tel. 417/269–6000), 1423 North Jefferson Street, Zip 65802–1988; tel. 417/269–3000; Larry D. Wallis, President and Chief Executive Officer (Total facility includes 36 beds in nursing home–type unit) (Nonreporting) **A**1 2 3 6 7 9 10 **S** Cox Health System, Springfield, MO Web address: www.coxnet.org/whoarewe/coxsystem.cfm	23	10	676	—	—	—	—	—	—	—
★ △ ST. JOHN'S REGIONAL HEALTH CENTER, 1235 East Cherokee Street, Zip 65804–2263; tel. 417/885–2000; Robert T. Brodhead, President (Total facility includes 62 beds in nursing home–type unit) **A**1 2 6 7 10 **F**3 4 5 7 8 9 10 11 12 13 14 15 16 17 18 19 20 21 22 23 24 25 26 27 28 31 32 33 34 36 37 38 39 40 41 42 43 44 45 46 47 48 49 50 51 52 53 54 56 57 58 59 60 61 62 63 64 65 68 70 71 72 73 75 76 77 78 79 **P**6 **S** Sisters of Mercy Health System–St. Louis, Saint Louis, MO	23	10	743	28414	391	289026	2478	251310	119842	3555
□ U. S. MEDICAL CENTER FOR FEDERAL PRISONERS, 1900 West Sunshine Street, Zip 65807–2240, Mailing Address: P.O. Box 4000, Zip 65808–4000; tel. 417/862–7041; R. H. Rison, Warden (Nonreporting) **A**1	48	10	587	—	—	—	—	—	—	—

Hospitals, U.S. / MISSOURI

Hospital, Address, Telephone, Administrator, Approval, Facility, and Physician Codes, Health Care System, Network	Classification Codes		Utilization Data					Expense (thousands) of dollars		
★ American Hospital Association (AHA) membership ☐ Joint Commission on Accreditation of Healthcare Organizations (JCAHO) accreditation + American Osteopathic Healthcare Association (AOHA) membership ○ American Osteopathic Association (AOA) accreditation △ Commission on Accreditation of Rehabilitation Facilities (CARF) accreditation Control codes 61, 63, 64, 71, 72 and 73 indicate hospitals listed by AOHA, but not registered by AHA. For definition of numerical codes, see page A4	Control	Service	Staffed Beds	Admissions	Census	Outpatient Visits	Births	Total	Payroll	Personnel
STE. GENEVIEVE—Ste. Genevieve County STE. GENEVIEVE COUNTY MEMORIAL HOSPITAL, Highways 61 and 32, Zip 63670–0468; tel. 573/883–2751; Michael J. Laird, FACHE, Chief Executive Officer **A**9 10 **F**7 8 9 13 17 18 19 20 21 22 23 24 25 27 30 32 33 34 36 37 38 39 41 43 44 45 46 48 50 51 54 70 71 72 76 78 79 **P**6 **Web address:** www.stgenevievehospital.org	13	10	34	1722	21	92638	63	15236	7398	207
SULLIVAN—Crawford County ★ MISSOURI BAPTIST HOSPITAL OF SULLIVAN, 751 Sappington Bridge Road, Zip 63080–2354, Mailing Address: P.O. Box 190, Zip 63080–0190; tel. 573/468–4186; Davis D. Skinner, President (Total facility includes 6 beds in nursing home-type unit) **A**9 10 **F**7 8 9 13 16 17 18 19 21 22 23 24 25 27 30 31 32 33 34 35 36 37 38 39 41 43 44 45 46 48 49 50 51 54 56 70 76 78 **P**6 **S** BJC Health System, Saint Louis, MO **Web address:** www.bjc.org/mbhs.html	23	10	46	1494	17	70617	150	21946	7176	266
TOWN AND COUNTRY—St. Louis County ⊞ MISSOURI BAPTIST MEDICAL CENTER, 3015 North Ballas Road, Zip 63131–2374; tel. 314/996–5000; Mark A. Eustis, President and Senior Executive Officer **A**1 2 6 9 10 **F**1 3 4 5 6 7 8 9 11 12 13 14 15 17 18 19 20 21 22 23 24 25 26 27 28 29 30 31 32 33 34 35 36 37 38 39 40 41 42 43 44 45 46 47 48 49 50 51 53 54 55 56 57 58 59 60 61 62 63 64 65 66 67 68 70 71 72 73 74 75 76 77 78 79 **P**1 **S** BJC Health System, Saint Louis, MO	23	10	370	18445	240	280699	3282	189438	70858	2192
TRENTON—Grundy County ☐ WRIGHT MEMORIAL HOSPITAL, 701 East First Street, Zip 64683–0648, Mailing Address: P.O. Box 628, Zip 64683–0628; tel. 660/359–5621; Ralph G. Goodrich, Chief Executive Officer **A**1 9 10 **F**7 8 9 12 16 17 18 19 22 25 30 31 32 33 34 36 37 38 40 43 44 48 54 56 66 70 71 76 78 **P**8 **S** Saint Luke's Shawnee Mission Health System, Kansas City, MO **Web address:** www.saint-lukes.org	23	10	34	774	8	44675	157	8125	4200	137
TROY—Lincoln County ☐ LINCOLN COUNTY MEMORIAL HOSPITAL, 1000 East Cherry Street, Zip 63379–1599; tel. 314/528–8551; Floyd B. Dowell, Jr, Administrator (Total facility includes 8 beds in nursing home-type unit) **A**1 9 10 **F**7 9 12 13 16 17 18 19 22 23 25 27 29 32 33 34 36 38 39 41 43 45 48 50 51 54 60 70 71 72 76 **P**1	13	10	28	1374	17	63661	0	—	—	203
UNIONVILLE—Putnam County PUTNAM COUNTY MEMORIAL HOSPITAL, 1926 Oak Street, Zip 63565–1100; tel. 660/947–2411; Ray Magers, Administrator (Total facility includes 10 beds in nursing home-type unit) **A**10 **F**7 9 17 25 33 34 38 48 54 60 68 76	13	10	26	292	13	7399	0	2504	1376	72
WARRENSBURG—Johnson County ☐ WESTERN MISSOURI MEDICAL CENTER, 403 Burkarth Road, Zip 64093–3101; tel. 660/747–2500; Gregory B. Vinardi, President and Chief Executive Officer (Total facility includes 11 beds in nursing home-type unit) **A**1 9 10 **F**7 8 9 13 14 16 17 18 22 23 24 25 27 32 33 34 35 36 37 38 39 40 41 43 44 45 46 48 49 50 51 54 66 70 71 72 73 75 76 78 79 **P**6 **Web address:** www.wmmconline.org	13	10	67	2504	28	49299	572	21887	10577	325
WASHINGTON—Franklin County ST. JOHN'S MERCY HOSPITAL See St. John's Mercy Medical Center, Saint Louis										
WENTZVILLE—St. Charles County ☐ DOCTORS HOSPITAL, 500 Medical Drive, Zip 63385–0711; tel. 314/327–1000; Joan Phillips, R.N., Interim Chief Executive Officer (Total facility includes 27 beds in nursing home-type unit) **A**1 9 10 **F**7 8 9 13 17 18 22 24 25 27 30 33 34 36 37 38 39 41 43 44 45 46 48 49 51 54 57 60 61 62 68 70 72 75 76 77 78 79 **S** New American Healthcare Corporation, Brentwood, TN **Web address:** www.healthmidwest.org	33	10	94	2087	25	32840	123	—	—	215
WEST PLAINS—Howell County ⊞ OZARKS MEDICAL CENTER, 1100 Kentucky Avenue, Zip 65775–2029, Mailing Address: P.O. Box 1100, Zip 65775–1100; tel. 417/256–9111; Graham J. O'Neal, Interim Chief Executive Officer (Total facility includes 16 beds in nursing home-type unit) **A**1 9 10 **F**3 6 7 8 9 11 13 16 17 18 21 22 24 25 27 31 32 33 34 35 36 37 38 39 41 43 44 45 46 48 49 50 51 54 57 58 59 60 61 62 63 65 68 70 71 72 75 76 77 78 79 **P**8 **Web address:** www.ozarksmedicalcenter.com	23	10	120	5977	71	242102	699	56202	26501	870

MONTANA

Resident Population 880 (in thousands)
Resident population in metro areas 33.7%
Birth rate per 1,000 population 12.3
65 years and over 13.3%
Percent of persons without health insurance 19.5%

- ★ American Hospital Association (AHA) membership
- ☐ Joint Commission on Accreditation of Healthcare Organizations (JCAHO) accreditation
- + American Osteopathic Healthcare Association (AOHA) membership
- ○ American Osteopathic Association (AOA) accreditation
- △ Commission on Accreditation of Rehabilitation Facilities (CARF) accreditation

Control codes 61, 63, 64, 71, 72 and 73 indicate hospitals listed by AOHA, but not registered by AHA. For definition of numerical codes, see page A4

Hospital, Address, Telephone, Administrator, Approval, Facility, and Physician Codes, Health Care System, Network	Classification Codes		Utilization Data					Expense (thousands) of dollars		Personnel
	Control	Service	Staffed Beds	Admissions	Census	Outpatient Visits	Births	Total	Payroll	
ANACONDA—Deer Lodge County ★ COMMUNITY HOSPITAL OF ANACONDA, 401 West Pennsylvania Street, Zip 59711–1999; tel. 406/563–8500; Sam J. Allen, Chief Executive Officer (Total facility includes 67 beds in nursing home–type unit) **A**9 10 **F**7 8 9 13 17 18 22 25 31 37 39 43 44 48 54 69 70 76 **P**4 **S** Quorum Health Group, Brentwood, TN	23	10	92	1106	69	140493	35	10521	4851	191
BAKER—Fallon County FALLON MEDICAL COMPLEX, 202 South 4th Street West, Zip 59313–0820, Mailing Address: P.O. Box 820, Zip 59313–0820; tel. 406/778–3331; David Espeland, Chief Executive Officer (Total facility includes 40 beds in nursing home–type unit) **A**9 10 **F**7 8 9 12 14 16 17 18 22 23 25 30 32 35 36 38 39 40 43 44 46 48 56 67 69 70 71 **P**1 6	23	10	52	261	41	19082	13	5027	2601	100
BIG SANDY—Chouteau County ★ BIG SANDY MEDICAL CENTER, Mailing Address: P.O. Box 530, Zip 59520–0530; tel. 406/378–2188; Harry Bold, Administrator (Total facility includes 22 beds in nursing home–type unit) **A**10 18 **F**17 18 25 36 38 69	23	10	30	39	22	5425	0	1458	784	24
BIG TIMBER—Sweet Grass County PIONEER MEDICAL CENTER, 301 West Seventh Avenue, Zip 59011, Mailing Address: P.O. Box 1228, Zip 59011–1228; tel. 406/932–4603; Cody Langbehn, Administrator (Total facility includes 52 beds in nursing home–type unit) **A**10 18 **F**1 16 24 25 30 31 34 37 38 40 43 48 54 56 69 70 72 76	13	10	60	130	49	8053	0	2731	1116	71
BILLINGS—Yellowstone County ⊞ DEACONESS BILLINGS CLINIC, 2800 10th Avenue North, Zip 59101–0799, Mailing Address: P.O. Box 37000, Zip 59107–7000; tel. 406/657–4000; Nicholas J. Wolter, M.D., Chief Executive Officer (Total facility includes 90 beds in nursing home–type unit) **A**1 3 9 10 **F**3 4 6 7 9 11 12 13 16 17 18 19 21 22 24 25 27 30 31 32 33 34 35 37 41 43 45 46 47 48 50 51 54 55 56 57 58 59 60 61 62 63 64 65 66 69 70 71 72 75 76 77 78 79 **P**1 3 Web address: www.billingsclinic.org	23	10	306	11015	257	631377	0	175617	81570	1724
⊞ △ SAINT VINCENT HOSPITAL AND HEALTH CENTER, 1233 North 30th Street, Zip 59101–0165, Mailing Address: P.O. Box 35200, Zip 59107–5200; tel. 406/237–7000; Patrick M. Hermanson, Senior Executive Officer (Total facility includes 28 beds in nursing home–type unit) **A**1 7 9 10 **F**4 6 7 8 9 11 13 14 16 17 18 19 20 21 22 24 25 26 27 30 32 33 34 35 37 38 39 41 42 43 44 45 46 47 48 49 50 51 53 54 56 65 66 69 70 71 72 73 75 76 77 78 79 **P**6 8 **S** Sisters of Charity of Leavenworth Health Services Corporation, Leavenworth, KS Web address: www.svhhc.org	21	10	249	13065	151	340954	1939	125598	54606	1465
BOZEMAN—Gallatin County ★ BOZEMAN DEACONESS HOSPITAL, 915 Highland Boulevard, Zip 59715–6999; tel. 406/585–5000; John A. Nordwick, President and Chief Executive Officer (Nonreporting) **A**9 10	23	10	70	—	—	—	—	—	—	—
BROWNING—Glacier County ⊞ U. S. PUBLIC HEALTH SERVICE BLACKFEET COMMUNITY HOSPITAL, Mailing Address: P.O. Box 760, Zip 59417–0760; tel. 406/338–6100; Reis Fisher, Service Unit Director (Nonreporting) **A**1 10 **S** U. S. Public Health Service Indian Health Service, Rockville, MD	47	10	25	—	—	—	—	—	—	—
BUTTE—Silver Bow County ⊞ ST. JAMES COMMUNITY HOSPITAL, 400 South Clark Street, Zip 59701–2328, Mailing Address: P.O. Box 3300, Zip 59702–3300; tel. 406/723–2500; Robert Rodgers, Administrator and Senior Executive Officer **A**1 9 10 **F**7 8 11 13 17 19 22 24 25 26 27 30 32 38 39 41 43 44 45 46 48 49 50 51 54 65 68 69 70 71 72 75 76 **P**8 **S** Sisters of Charity of Leavenworth Health Services Corporation, Leavenworth, KS Web address: www.svhhc.org	23	10	100	4599	65	39072	505	41610	16325	448
CHESTER—Liberty County LIBERTY COUNTY HOSPITAL AND NURSING HOME, Mailing Address: P.O. Box 705, Zip 59522–0705; tel. 406/759–5181; Douglas Faus, Chief Executive Officer (Total facility includes 53 beds in nursing home–type unit) **A**9 10 **F**1 6 9 25 36 38 48 69 76	23	10	64	366	53	5928	16	3664	1695	84
CHOTEAU—Teton County TETON MEDICAL CENTER, 915 Fourth Street N.W., Zip 59422–9123; tel. 406/466–5763; Lorin C. MacKay, Administrator (Total facility includes 42 beds in nursing home–type unit) **A**10 18 **F**1 7 9 18 19 25 26 28 32 35 37 45 48 54 69	16	10	47	105	29	5742	0	2254	1046	52
CIRCLE—McCone County MCCONE COUNTY MEDICAL ASSISTANCE FACILITY, Mailing Address: P.O. Box 48, Zip 59215–0048; tel. 406/485–3381; Mack N. Simpson, Administrator (Total facility includes 30 beds in nursing home–type unit) **A**10 18 **F**1 14 16 19 23 24 25 30 31 36 40 43 69 70 78	23	10	38	69	23	2440	0	1320	756	34

Many Facility Codes have changed. Please refer to the AHA Guide Code Chart.

Hospitals, U.S. / MONTANA

Hospital, Address, Telephone, Administrator, Approval, Facility, and Physician Codes, Health Care System, Network	Classification Codes		Utilization Data					Expense (thousands) of dollars		
★ American Hospital Association (AHA) membership ☐ Joint Commission on Accreditation of Healthcare Organizations (JCAHO) accreditation + American Osteopathic Healthcare Association (AOHA) membership ○ American Osteopathic Association (AOA) accreditation △ Commission on Accreditation of Rehabilitation Facilities (CARF) accreditation Control codes 61, 63, 64, 71, 72 and 73 indicate hospitals listed by AOHA, but not registered by AHA. For definition of numerical codes, see page A4	Control	Service	Staffed Beds	Admissions	Census	Outpatient Visits	Births	Total	Payroll	Personnel

COLUMBUS—Stillwater County
  STILLWATER COMMUNITY HOSPITAL, 44 West Fourth Avenue North, Zip 59019, Mailing Address: P.O. Box 959, Zip 59019–0959; tel. 406/322–5316; Tim Russell, Administrator (Total facility includes 10 beds in nursing home–type unit) **A**9 10 **F**8 9 11 13 14 17 19 22 24 25 30 32 34 36 43 44 48 54 67 69 70 72 76 | 23 | 10 | 23 | 229 | 13 | 4563 | 31 | 2219 | 1184 | 31

CONRAD—Pondera County
★ PONDERA MEDICAL CENTER, 805 Sunset Boulevard, Zip 59425–1721, Mailing Address: P.O. Box 757, Zip 59425–0757; tel. 406/278–3211; Vicky Newmiller, Interim Chief Executive Officer (Total facility includes 59 beds in nursing home–type unit) **A**9 10 **F**1 7 8 9 13 18 19 22 24 25 36 45 48 51 54 56 65 68 69 70 78 | 23 | 10 | 79 | 776 | 62 | 7365 | 18 | 6590 | 3505 | 107

CROW AGENCY—Big Horn County
⚕ U. S. PUBLIC HEALTH SERVICE INDIAN HOSPITAL, Mailing Address: P.O. Box 9, Zip 59022–0009; tel. 406/638–2626; Tennyson Doney, Service Unit Director **A**1 9 10 **F**3 8 9 14 16 17 18 21 23 25 32 34 35 38 48 54 61 63 70 76 77 79 **P**6 **S** U. S. Public Health Service Indian Health Service, Rockville, MD | 47 | 10 | 24 | 1464 | 11 | 99149 | 238 | 23430 | 9906 | 269

CULBERTSON—Roosevelt County
★ ROOSEVELT MEMORIAL MEDICAL CENTER, 818 Second Avenue East, Zip 59218, Mailing Address: P.O. Box 419, Zip 59218–0419; tel. 406/787–6281; Audrey Stromberg, Administrator (Total facility includes 44 beds in nursing home–type unit) **A**10 18 **F**14 17 19 25 30 31 32 34 36 38 40 43 51 54 56 69 70 78 **P**6 | 23 | 10 | 54 | 278 | 41 | 8093 | 0 | 3056 | 1827 | 73

CUT BANK—Glacier County
★ GLACIER COUNTY MEDICAL CENTER, 802 Second Street S.E., Zip 59427–3331; tel. 406/873–2251; Dale E. Polla, Chief Executive Officer (Total facility includes 39 beds in nursing home–type unit) (Nonreporting) **A**9 10 **S** Quorum Health Group, Brentwood, TN | 13 | 10 | 59 | — | — | — | — | — | — | —

DEER LODGE—Powell County
★ POWELL COUNTY MEMORIAL HOSPITAL, 1101 Texas Avenue, Zip 59722–1828; tel. 406/846–2212; Tony Pfaff, Chief Executive Officer (Total facility includes 16 beds in nursing home–type unit) **A**9 10 18 **F**8 17 18 22 25 36 40 41 43 44 45 48 69 76 | 23 | 10 | 35 | 254 | 12 | 4992 | 26 | 4279 | 1967 | 51

DILLON—Beaverhead County
★ BARRETT MEMORIAL HOSPITAL, 1260 South Atlantic Street, Zip 59725–3597; tel. 406/683–3000; John M. Mootry, Chief Executive Officer **A**9 10 **F**8 9 12 16 17 18 22 24 25 32 33 34 36 37 39 41 43 44 45 46 48 66 68 69 70 71 72 76 78 **P**8 **S** Brim Healthcare, Inc., Brentwood, TN
  Web address: www.barretthospital.org | 13 | 10 | 23 | 864 | 7 | 21365 | 85 | 9594 | 4117 | 120

ENNIS—Madison County
  MADISON VALLEY HOSPITAL, 217 North Main Street, Zip 59729–0397, Mailing Address: P.O. Box 397, Zip 59729–0397; tel. 406/682–4222; Pete Brekhus, Chief Executive Officer **A**9 10 **F**7 25 32 34 41 48 54 76 **P**5 | 23 | 10 | 9 | 142 | 2 | 13038 | 0 | 1526 | 846 | 31

FORSYTH—Rosebud County
★ ROSEBUD HEALTH CARE CENTER, 383 North 17th Avenue, Zip 59327; tel. 406/356–2161; John M. Chioutsis, Chief Executive Officer (Total facility includes 55 beds in nursing home–type unit) **A**9 10 **F**9 12 30 32 34 36 48 69 72 76 78 **P**6 | 23 | 10 | 75 | 385 | 49 | 8071 | 0 | 4168 | 2094 | 93

FORT BENTON—Chouteau County
  MISSOURI RIVER MEDICAL CENTER, 1501 St. Charles Street, Zip 59442–0249, Mailing Address: P.O. Box 249, Zip 59442–0249; tel. 406/622–3331; Jay Pottenger, Administrator (Total facility includes 45 beds in nursing home–type unit) **A**10 18 **F**1 6 9 25 30 32 36 37 38 54 69 **P**6 | 16 | 10 | 52 | 125 | 39 | — | 0 | 3109 | 1806 | 77

FORT HARRISON—Lewis and Clark County
⚕ VETERANS AFFAIRS MONTANA HEALTHCARE SYSTEM, (Formerly Veterans Affairs Hospital), Highway 12 and William Street, Zip 59636; tel. 406/442–6410; Joseph Underkofler, Director (Total facility includes 30 beds in nursing home–type unit) **A**1 9 **F**3 4 9 11 12 16 17 18 22 23 24 25 26 28 30 33 34 35 36 37 38 39 40 41 43 45 46 48 49 50 51 54 56 57 59 61 62 63 65 69 70 72 76 78 **P**6 **S** Department of Veterans Affairs, Washington, DC
  Web address: www.va.gov/stations97/guide/home.asp?DIVISION=ALL | 45 | 10 | 45 | 2225 | 38 | 136637 | 0 | 52263 | 24685 | 447

GLASGOW—Valley County
☐ FRANCES MAHON DEACONESS HOSPITAL, 621 Third Street South, Zip 59230–2699; tel. 406/228–3500; Randall G. Holom, Chief Executive Officer **A**1 3 9 10 **F**9 12 17 22 24 25 30 32 35 36 38 39 46 48 55 59 68 70 76 | 23 | 10 | 32 | 1090 | 10 | 24634 | 98 | 12265 | 4987 | 163

GLENDIVE—Dawson County
⚕ GLENDIVE MEDICAL CENTER, 202 Prospect Drive, Zip 59330–1999; tel. 406/345–3306 (Total facility includes 75 beds in nursing home–type unit) **A**1 9 10 **F**6 7 9 16 17 19 21 22 24 25 30 32 34 35 36 37 38 39 40 41 43 44 45 46 48 51 54 69 70 72 75 76 78 **P**7 8
  Web address: www.gmc.org | 23 | 10 | 101 | 953 | 79 | 24946 | 88 | 10330 | 4926 | 198

GREAT FALLS—Cascade County
⚕ △ BENEFIS HEALTHCARE, (Includes Benefis Health Care–East Campus, 1101 26th Street; Benefis Health Care–West Campus, 500 15th Avenue South), 1101 26th Street South, Zip 59405; tel. 406/455–5000; Lloyd V. Smith, President and Chief Executive Officer (Total facility includes 140 beds in nursing home–type unit) **A**1 2 7 9 10 **F**2 16 17 18 22 39 41 42 44 48 50 51 53 54 57 58 59 60 61 62 63 64 65 68 69 70 71 72 76 77 78 79 **P**5 8 **S** Providence Services, Spokane, WA
  Web address: www.benefis.org | 21 | 10 | 470 | 12177 | 325 | 140014 | 1371 | 132174 | 63107 | 1545

© 2000 AHA Guide   *Many Facility Codes have changed. Please refer to the AHA Guide Code Chart.*

Hospitals, U.S. / MONTANA

Hospital, Address, Telephone, Administrator, Approval, Facility, and Physician Codes, Health Care System, Network

- ★ American Hospital Association (AHA) membership
- ☐ Joint Commission on Accreditation of Healthcare Organizations (JCAHO) accreditation
- + American Osteopathic Healthcare Association (AOHA) membership
- ○ American Osteopathic Association (AOA) accreditation
- △ Commission on Accreditation of Rehabilitation Facilities (CARF) accreditation

Control codes 61, 63, 64, 71, 72 and 73 indicate hospitals listed by AOHA, but not registered by AHA. For definition of numerical codes, see page A4

Hospital	Control	Service	Staffed Beds	Admissions	Census	Outpatient Visits	Births	Total	Payroll	Personnel
HAMILTON—Ravalli County										
★ MARCUS DALY MEMORIAL HOSPITAL, 1200 Westwood Drive, Zip 59840–2395; tel. 406/363–2211; John M. Bartos, Administrator **A**9 10 **F**7 8 9 16 17 18 19 22 25 26 32 33 34 36 37 39 45 46 48 50 53 54 70 72 76 77 79 **P**8	23	10	48	1729	18	31835	182	18564	9928	319
HARDIN—Big Horn County										
★ BIG HORN COUNTY MEMORIAL HOSPITAL, 17 North Miles Avenue, Zip 59034–0430, Mailing Address: P.O. Box 430, Zip 59034–0430; tel. 406/665–2310; Robert G. Notarianni, Chief Executive Officer (Total facility includes 37 beds in nursing home–type unit) **A**9 10 **F**6 7 8 17 18 25 32 36 37 45 48 54 67 69 70 74 76 **S** Brim Healthcare, Inc., Brentwood, TN Web address: www.mcn.net/~medlab/	23	10	53	490	36	6075	37	4179	2147	89
HARLEM—Blaine County										
★ U. S. PUBLIC HEALTH SERVICE INDIAN HOSPITAL, Rural Route 1, Box 67, Zip 59526; tel. 406/353–3100; Charles D. Plumage, Director (Nonreporting) **A**9 10 **S** U. S. Public Health Service Indian Health Service, Rockville, MD	47	10	12	—	—	—	—	—	—	—
HARLOWTON—Wheatland County										
★ WHEATLAND MEMORIAL HOSPITAL, 530 Third Street North, Zip 59036, Mailing Address: P.O. Box 287, Zip 59036–0287; tel. 406/632–4351; Craig E. Aasved, Administrator (Total facility includes 36 beds in nursing home–type unit) **A**9 10 **F**1 3 4 5 6 7 8 9 11 12 13 14 15 16 17 18 19 20 21 22 23 24 25 26 27 28 29 30 31 32 33 34 35 36 37 38 39 40 41 43 46 47 48 49 50 51 54 55 56 58 59 60 61 62 63 64 65 66 67 68 69 70 71 72 73 74 75 76 77 78 79 **S** Quorum Health Group, Brentwood, TN	13	10	54	173	37	4601	0	3042	1578	68
HAVRE—Hill County										
✭ NORTHERN MONTANA HOSPITAL, 30 13th Street, Zip 59501–5222, Mailing Address: P.O. Box 1231, Zip 59501–1231; tel. 406/265–2211; David Henry, Chief Executive Officer (Total facility includes 167 beds in nursing home–type unit) **A**1 9 10 **F**2 3 6 7 8 9 17 18 22 24 25 32 34 36 37 39 41 44 45 48 54 57 58 60 61 62 63 64 69 70 71 72 75 76 78 **P**6 **S** Brim Healthcare, Inc., Brentwood, TN	23	10	259	3323	157	82607	394	35092	19012	612
HELENA—Lewis and Clark County										
✭ SHODAIR CHILDREN'S HOSPITAL, 2755 Colonial Drive, Zip 59601, Mailing Address: P.O. Box 5539, Zip 59604–5539; tel. 406/444–7500; Jack Casey, Administrator **A**1 10 **F**17 18 57 58 60 61 63 64 66 69 70	23	52	44	300	32	6102	0	6305	3512	136
✭ ST. PETER'S HOSPITAL, 2475 Broadway, Zip 59601; tel. 406/442–2480; John H. Solheim, President and Chief Executive Officer (Total facility includes 8 beds in nursing home–type unit) **A**1 9 10 **F**8 9 11 13 16 17 18 19 22 24 32 33 34 35 36 37 38 39 41 42 43 44 45 46 48 49 50 51 54 57 59 60 61 62 63 64 65 68 69 70 72 75 76 78 **P**8 Web address: www.stpetes.org	23	10	63	4764	45	79939	723	48787	21202	657
KALISPELL—Flathead County										
✭ △ KALISPELL REGIONAL MEDICAL CENTER, (Includes Pathways Treatment Center, 200 Heritage Way, Zip 59901; tel. 406/756–3950), 310 Sunnyview Lane, Zip 59901–3199; tel. 406/752–5111; Velinda Stevens, President and Chief Executive Officer (Total facility includes 100 beds in nursing home–type unit) **A**1 7 9 10 **F**1 2 3 4 8 9 11 13 17 18 19 21 22 23 24 25 28 30 31 32 34 35 36 37 38 39 41 43 44 45 46 48 50 51 53 54 56 57 58 59 60 61 62 63 64 65 68 69 70 71 72 76 78 **P**5 6 8 Web address: www.krmc.org	23	10	250	6641	153	93185	753	55689	23321	722
LEWISTOWN—Fergus County										
★ CENTRAL MONTANA MEDICAL CENTER, 408 Wendell Avenue, Zip 59457–2261; tel. 406/538–7711; David M. Faulkner, Chief Executive Officer (Total facility includes 85 beds in nursing home–type unit) **A**9 10 **F**1 7 8 9 13 16 17 22 24 25 28 30 32 34 36 37 38 39 41 43 44 46 48 54 68 69 70 71 72 75 76 78 **S** Quorum Health Group, Brentwood, TN	23	10	124	1341	101	30761	113	14434	7117	260
LIBBY—Lincoln County										
★ ST. JOHN'S LUTHERAN HOSPITAL, 350 Louisiana Avenue, Zip 59923–2198; tel. 406/293–0100; Richard L. Palagi, Chief Executive Officer **A**9 10 **F**6 7 8 16 19 22 25 30 32 34 36 38 43 45 46 48 49 54 76 77 Web address: www.sjlh.com	23	10	26	1034	11	26509	102	8319	4039	127
LIVINGSTON—Park County										
★ LIVINGSTON MEMORIAL HOSPITAL, 504 South 13th Street, Zip 59047–3798; tel. 406/222–3541; Richard V. Brown, Chief Executive Officer **A**9 10 **F**8 9 13 14 16 17 18 19 22 24 25 28 32 33 34 35 36 37 38 41 43 44 45 46 48 50 54 68 70 76 79 **P**6	23	10	32	1083	10	21840	131	12411	6668	202
MALTA—Phillips County										
PHILLIPS COUNTY MEDICAL CENTER, 417 South Fourth East, Zip 59538, Mailing Address: P.O. Box 640, Zip 59538–0640; tel. 406/654–1100; Larry E. Putnam, Administrator **A**10 18 **F**16 17 18 25 31 32 36 43 46 48 54 71 76 78 79	23	10	14	124	1	5412	1	2369	1020	62
MILES CITY—Custer County										
✭ HOLY ROSARY HEALTH CENTER, 2600 Wilson Street, Zip 59301–5094; tel. 406/233–2600 (Total facility includes 107 beds in nursing home–type unit) **A**1 9 10 **F**3 8 9 12 13 14 16 17 18 19 22 24 25 26 28 31 32 34 36 37 39 40 41 43 44 46 48 53 54 57 58 59 60 61 62 68 69 70 72 76 78 **S** Sisters of Charity of Leavenworth Health Services Corporation, Leavenworth, KS Web address: www.svhhc.org	21	10	151	1835	88	—	212	18297	7433	263

Many Facility Codes have changed. Please refer to the AHA Guide Code Chart.

Hospitals, U.S. / MONTANA

Hospital, Address, Telephone, Administrator, Approval, Facility, and Physician Codes, Health Care System, Network	Classification Codes		Utilization Data					Expense (thousands) of dollars		
★ American Hospital Association (AHA) membership □ Joint Commission on Accreditation of Healthcare Organizations (JCAHO) accreditation + American Osteopathic Healthcare Association (AOHA) membership ○ American Osteopathic Association (AOA) accreditation △ Commission on Accreditation of Rehabilitation Facilities (CARF) accreditation Control codes 61, 63, 64, 71, 72 and 73 indicate hospitals listed by AOHA, but not registered by AHA. For definition of numerical codes, see page A4	Control	Service	Staffed Beds	Admissions	Census	Outpatient Visits	Births	Total	Payroll	Personnel
MISSOULA—Missoula County										
★ △ COMMUNITY MEDICAL CENTER, 2827 Fort Missoula Road, Zip 59804; tel. 406/728–4100; Grant M. Winn, President **A**1 7 9 10 **F**8 9 13 16 17 18 19 22 24 25 26 27 32 34 36 37 38 39 41 42 43 44 45 46 48 49 51 52 53 54 56 69 70 71 72 76 77 78 79 **P**1 6	23	10	117	5223	74	196117	1519	55312	28547	593
★ ST. PATRICK HOSPITAL, 500 West Broadway, Zip 59802–4096, Mailing Address: Box 4587, Zip 59806–4587; tel. 406/543–7271; Lawrence L. White, Jr, President (Total facility includes 18 beds in nursing home–type unit) **A**1 2 9 10 **F**2 3 4 11 13 16 17 18 19 22 24 25 26 27 28 31 33 34 36 37 38 39 40 41 43 45 46 47 48 49 50 54 57 58 59 60 61 62 63 64 65 68 69 70 71 72 73 74 76 78 **P**7 **S** Providence Services, Spokane, WA **Web address:** www.saintpatrick.org	21	10	195	8289	109	101969	0	95610	35257	1065
PHILIPSBURG—Granite County										
GRANITE COUNTY MEMORIAL HOSPITAL AND NURSING HOME, Mailing Address: P.O. Box 729, Zip 59858–0729; tel. 406/859–3271; Jodi M. Martz, Administrator (Total facility includes 32 beds in nursing home–type unit) **A**10 18 **F**1 17 23 25 32 36 37 38 54 56 69 70 76 **P**5	13	10	35	43	24	2328	0	1367	780	34
PLAINS—Sanders County										
★ CLARK FORK VALLEY HOSPITAL, Mailing Address: P.O. Box 768, Zip 59859–0768; tel. 406/826–3601; John Serle, Administrator (Total facility includes 28 beds in nursing home–type unit) **A**9 10 **F**9 22 25 32 36 38 41 44 48 54 69 76 **P**6	23	10	44	657	33	35856	59	7115	3559	111
PLENTYWOOD—Sheridan County										
SHERIDAN MEMORIAL HOSPITAL, 440 West Laurel Avenue, Zip 59254–1596; tel. 406/765–1420; Ella Gutzke, Administrator (Total facility includes 78 beds in nursing home–type unit) (Nonreporting) **A**9 10	23	10	97	—	—	—	—	—	—	—
POLSON—Lake County										
★ ST. JOSEPH HOSPITAL, Skyline Drive and 14th Avenue, Zip 59860, Mailing Address: P.O. Box 1010, Zip 59860–1010; tel. 406/883–5377; John W. Glueckert, President **A**1 9 10 **F**7 8 9 11 15 19 22 25 36 38 48 54 70 71 76 78 79 **S** Providence Services, Spokane, WA	21	10	22	713	5	20012	104	5877	2555	98
POPLAR—Roosevelt County										
POPLAR COMMUNITY HOSPITAL See Northeast Montana Health Services, Wolf Point										
RED LODGE—Carbon County										
★ BEARTOOTH HOSPITAL AND HEALTH CENTER, 600 West 20th Street, Zip 59068, Mailing Address: P.O. Box 590, Zip 59068–0590; tel. 406/446–2345; Kelley Evans, Administrator (Total facility includes 30 beds in nursing home–type unit) **A**9 10 **F**16 17 18	23	10	52	377	32	1862	31	4055	2120	101
RONAN—Lake County										
★ ST. LUKE COMMUNITY HOSPITAL, 107 Sixth Avenue S.W., Zip 59864–2634; tel. 406/676–4441; Shane Roberts, Administrator (Total facility includes 75 beds in nursing home–type unit) **A**9 10 **F**1 8 9 16 17 18 25 32 34 35 36 37 38 45 48 71 76 **P**6	23	10	99	733	68	56538	98	12519	6798	187
ROUNDUP—Musselshell County										
★ ROUNDUP MEMORIAL HOSPITAL, 1202 Third Street West, Zip 59072–1816, Mailing Address: P.O. Box 40, Zip 59072–0040; tel. 406/323–2302; Dave McIvor, Administrator (Total facility includes 37 beds in nursing home–type unit) **A**9 10 **F**1 7 17 25 36 69 76 **P**6 **S** Brim Healthcare, Inc., Brentwood, TN	23	10	48	361	36	4584	0	3566	1815	82
SCOBEY—Daniels County										
DANIELS MEMORIAL HOSPITAL, 105 Fifth Avenue East, Zip 59263, Mailing Address: P.O. Box 400, Zip 59263–0400; tel. 406/487–2296; Glenn Haugo, Administrator (Total facility includes 48 beds in nursing home–type unit) **A**9 10 **F**1 7 8 9 13 14 16 19 22 23 25 34 36 38 39 40 43 45 48 54 56 58 59 63 65 69 76 78 **P**6	16	10	54	181	27	412	0	2496	1343	57
SHELBY—Toole County										
MARIAS MEDICAL CENTER, 640 Park Drive, Zip 59474–1663, Mailing Address: P.O. Box 915, Zip 59474–0915; tel. 406/434–3200; Jerry Morasko, Administrator (Total facility includes 68 beds in nursing home–type unit) **A**9 10 **F**6 7 8 9 12 16 22 24 25 31 34 36 38 39 41 43 44 45 46 48 49 50 51 54 69 70 72 76 78 **P**6 **Web address:** www.mariasmedicalcenter.org	13	10	84	1059	67	9980	61	8622	3405	82
SHERIDAN—Madison County										
RUBY VALLEY HOSPITAL, 220 East Crofoot Street, Zip 59749, Mailing Address: P.O. Box 336, Zip 59749–0336; tel. 406/842–5453; Steve Lang, Administrator **A**9 10 **F**25 36 54	16	10	8	193	2	7021	0	1239	697	31
SIDNEY—Richland County										
SIDNEY HEALTH CENTER, 216 14th Avenue S.W., Zip 59270–3586; tel. 406/488–2100; Donald J. Rush, Chief Executive Officer (Total facility includes 93 beds in nursing home–type unit) **A**9 10 **F**1 8 9 12 13 22 24 28 32 34 36 37 39 40 44 46 48 49 54 69 70 71 72 76 78 **P**8 **Web address:** www.sidneyhealth.com	23	10	135	1425	97	39244	126	17960	7767	339
SUPERIOR—Mineral County										
★ MINERAL COMMUNITY HOSPITAL, Roosevelt and Brooklyn, Zip 59872, Mailing Address: P.O. Box 66, Zip 59872–0066; tel. 406/822–4841; Steven Smoot, Chief Executive Officer (Total facility includes 20 beds in nursing home–type unit) (Nonreporting) **A**9 10 **S** Brim Healthcare, Inc., Brentwood, TN	23	10	30	—	—	—	—	—	—	—

Hospitals, U.S. / MONTANA

Hospital, Address, Telephone, Administrator, Approval, Facility, and Physician Codes, Health Care System, Network	Classification Codes		Utilization Data					Expense (thousands) of dollars		
★ American Hospital Association (AHA) membership □ Joint Commission on Accreditation of Healthcare Organizations (JCAHO) accreditation + American Osteopathic Healthcare Association (AOHA) membership ○ American Osteopathic Association (AOA) accreditation △ Commission on Accreditation of Rehabilitation Facilities (CARF) accreditation Control codes 61, 63, 64, 71, 72 and 73 indicate hospitals listed by AOHA, but not registered by AHA. For definition of numerical codes, see page A4	Control	Service	Staffed Beds	Admissions	Census	Outpatient Visits	Births	Total	Payroll	Personnel
TERRY—Prairie County ★ PRAIRIE COMMUNITY MEDICAL ASSISTANCE FACILITY, 312 South Adams Avenue, Zip 59349–0156, Mailing Address: P.O. Box 156, Zip 59349–0156; tel. 406/635–5511; James R. Mantz, Administrator (Total facility includes 19 beds in nursing home–type unit) **A**10 18 **F**7 9 14 17 25 30 32 40 56 69	16	10	21	34	18	1448	0	1104	667	33
TOWNSEND—Broadwater County BROADWATER HEALTH CENTER, 110 North Oak Street, Zip 59644–2399; tel. 406/266–3186; Nancy Taylor, Chief Executive Officer (Total facility includes 32 beds in nursing home–type unit) (Nonreporting) **A**9 10	23	10	44	—	—	—	—	—	—	—
WARM SPRINGS—Deer Lodge County MONTANA STATE HOSPITAL, Zip 59756; tel. 406/693–7000; Carl Keener, M.D., Medical Director (Nonreporting)	12	10	32	—	—	—	—	—	—	—
WHITE SULPHUR SPRINGS—Meagher County ★ MOUNTAINVIEW MEDICAL CENTER, 16 West Main Street, Zip 59645, Mailing Address: P.O. Box Q, Zip 59645; tel. 406/547–3321; Katharine Ann Campbell, Administrator (Total facility includes 31 beds in nursing home–type unit) **A**10 18 **F**7 14 19 25 30 31 32 34 36 40 43 50 54 56 69 70 76 78 **P**6	23	10	37	125	26	—	0	1981	1086	42
WHITEFISH—Flathead County ★ NORTH VALLEY HOSPITAL, 6575 Highway 93 South, Zip 59937; tel. 406/863–3500; Craig E. Aasved, Chief Executive Officer (Total facility includes 56 beds in nursing home–type unit) **A**9 10 **F**1 7 8 9 19 22 25 30 32 34 36 38 41 44 45 48 51 54 69 70 71 72 76 77 78 **P**5 **S** Quorum Health Group, Brentwood, TN **Web address:** www.nvhosp.org	23	10	99	1158	65	41191	181	14112	6389	195
WOLF POINT—Roosevelt County NORTHEAST MONTANA HEALTH SERVICES, (Includes Poplar Community Hospital, H and Court Avenue, Poplar, Zip 59255, Mailing Address: P.O. Box 38, Zip 59255; tel. 406/768–3452; Trinity Hospital, 315 Knapp Street, Zip 59201; tel. 406/653–2100), 315 Knapp Street, Zip 59201–1898; tel. 406/653–2110; Margaret Norgaard, Administrator (Total facility includes 82 beds in nursing home–type unit) **A**9 **F**1 8 16 17 18 22 25 30 31 32 34 36 40 41 44 46 48 50 51 67 69 70 76 **P**6	23	10	117	1111	82	16088	165	8339	4545	235

NEBRASKA

Resident Population 1,663 (in thousands)
Resident population in metro areas 51.3%
Birth rate per 1,000 population 14.1
65 years and over 13.8%
Percent of persons without health insurance 10.8%

Hospital, Address, Telephone, Administrator, Approval, Facility, and Physician Codes, Health Care System, Network	Classification Codes		Utilization Data					Expense (thousands) of dollars		
★ American Hospital Association (AHA) membership □ Joint Commission on Accreditation of Healthcare Organizations (JCAHO) accreditation + American Osteopathic Healthcare Association (AOHA) membership ○ American Osteopathic Association (AOA) accreditation △ Commission on Accreditation of Rehabilitation Facilities (CARF) accreditation Control codes 61, 63, 64, 71, 72 and 73 indicate hospitals listed by AOHA, but not registered by AHA. For definition of numerical codes, see page A4	Control	Service	Staffed Beds	Admissions	Census	Outpatient Visits	Births	Total	Payroll	Personnel
AINSWORTH—Brown County BROWN COUNTY HOSPITAL, 945 East Zero Street, Zip 69210–1547; tel. 402/387–2800; Victor Lee, FACHE, Interim Administrator **A**9 10 **F**8 9 16 18 22 25 36 38 45 48 49 54 56 70 76	13	10	25	247	10	6692	40	2652	1227	56
ALBION—Boone County ★ BOONE COUNTY HEALTH CENTER, 723 West Fairview Street, Zip 68620–1725, Mailing Address: P.O. Box 151, Zip 68620–0151; tel. 402/395–2191; Victor Lee, FACHE, Chief Executive Officer **A**9 10 **F**2 3 7 8 9 12 17 18 19 22 24 25 28 29 30 32 34 35 36 37 38 39 41 43 44 45 46 48 50 53 54 56 57 58 59 60 62 63 69 70 71 72 76 78 **P**6	13	10	20	764	8	49682	67	8336	4602	147
ALLIANCE—Box Butte County □ BOX BUTTE GENERAL HOSPITAL, 2101 Box Butte Avenue, Zip 69301–0810, Mailing Address: P.O. Box 810, Zip 69301–0810; tel. 308/762–6660; Terrance J. Padden, Administrator **A**1 9 10 **F**3 7 8 9 13 16 17 19 20 21 22 25 26 28 30 32 33 34 37 38 39 40 41 43 44 45 46 48 50 51 54 56 61 66 69 70 71 72 73 76 77 78 **Web address:** www.bbgh.org	13	10	44	988	11	21257	119	7621	3539	129
ALMA—Harlan County ★ HARLAN COUNTY HEALTH SYSTEM, 717 North Brown Street, Zip 68920–0836, Mailing Address: P.O. Box 836, Zip 68920–0836; tel. 308/928–2151; Allen Van Driel, Administrator **A**9 10 18 **F**7 9 17 18 22 24 25 35 36 37 38 48 49 54 76 **P**8 **S** Great Plains Health Alliance, Inc., Phillipsburg, KS **Web address:** www.gpha.com	13	10	25	262	7	6395	0	2394	1214	37
ATKINSON—Holt County WEST HOLT MEMORIAL HOSPITAL, 406 Legion Street, Zip 68713–0200, Mailing Address: Rural Route 1, Box 200, Zip 68713–0200; tel. 402/925–2811; Mel L. Snow, Administrator **A**9 10 **F**4 8 9 11 16 17 18 19 21 22 25 29 30 32 33 34 38 39 44 45 46 47 48 49 50 54 56 63 65 66 70 74 76 79 **P**6	23	10	18	419	5	9204	26	5065	1974	76
AUBURN—Nemaha County ★ NEMAHA COUNTY HOSPITAL, 2022 13th Street, Zip 68305–1799; tel. 402/274–4366; Glen E. Krueger, Administrator (Nonreporting) **A**9 10	13	10	34	—						
AURORA—Hamilton County ★ MEMORIAL HOSPITAL, 1423 Seventh Street, Zip 68818–1197; tel. 402/694–3171; Eldon A. Wall, Administrator (Total facility includes 51 beds in nursing home–type unit) **A**9 10 18 **F**7 8 9 17 22 25 27 32 34 36 37 38 40 41 43 44 45 46 48 49 54 69 70 76 **P**6 **Web address:** www.memorialfoundation.net	23	10	76	686	50	18530	95	8962	4783	150
BASSETT—Rock County ROCK COUNTY HOSPITAL, 102 East South Street, Zip 68714, Mailing Address: P.O. Box 100, Zip 68714–0100; tel. 402/684–3366; Stacey Knox, Interim Administrator (Total facility includes 30 beds in nursing home–type unit) **A**9 10 **F**1 22 25 48 69 76	13	10	47	322	37	4641	0	2561	1599	76
BEATRICE—Gage County ⊞ BEATRICE COMMUNITY HOSPITAL AND HEALTH CENTER, 1110 North Tenth Street, Zip 68310–2039, Mailing Address: P.O. Box 278, Zip 68310–0278; tel. 402/228–3344; Colleen Chapp, Interim Administrator (Total facility includes 78 beds in nursing home–type unit) **A**1 9 10 **F**7 8 9 12 17 18 19 22 24 25 26 27 28 32 34 36 37 39 40 41 44 45 48 49 54 56 67 69 70 72 76 78	23	10	126	1246	89	46507	163	18200	8913	349
BENKELMAN—Dundy County DUNDY COUNTY HOSPITAL, 1313 North Cheyenne Street, Zip 69021, Mailing Address: P.O. Box 626, Zip 69021–0626; tel. 308/423–2204; Marlo L. Miller, Administrator (Nonreporting) **A**9 10	13	10	15	—	—	—	—	—	—	—
BLAIR—Washington County ⊞ MEMORIAL COMMUNITY HOSPITAL AND HEALTH SYSTEM, 810 North 22nd Street, Zip 68008–1199, Mailing Address: P.O. Box 250, Zip 68008–0250; tel. 402/426–2182; Robert Omer, FACHE, President and Chief Executive Officer **A**1 9 10 **F**8 9 16 17 18 19 21 22 25 32 34 36 37 38 39 40 43 44 45 46 48 50 51 54 69 70 72 76 78 **P**6 **Web address:** www.mchhs.org	23	10	33	1006	10	—	117	13569	7996	262
BRIDGEPORT—Morrill County MORRILL COUNTY COMMUNITY HOSPITAL, 1313 S Street, Zip 69336–0579, Mailing Address: P.O. Box 579, Zip 69336–0579; tel. 308/262–1616; Julia Morrow, Administrator (Nonreporting) **A**9 10 18	13	10	20	—	—	—	—	—	—	—
BROKEN BOW—Custer County JENNIE M. MELHAM MEMORIAL MEDICAL CENTER, 145 Memorial Drive, Zip 68822–1378, Mailing Address: P.O. Box 250, Zip 68822–0250; tel. 308/872–6891; Michael J. Steckler, President and Chief Executive Officer (Total facility includes 77 beds in nursing home–type unit) **A**9 10 **F**6 7 8 9 19 22 24 25 28 32 34 36 37 39 48 67 69 70 76	23	10	116	1219	83	10363	107	7622	4148	177

© 2000 AHA Guide   *Many Facility Codes have changed. Please refer to the AHA Guide Code Chart.*

Hospitals, U.S. / NEBRASKA

Hospital, Address, Telephone, Administrator, Approval, Facility, and Physician Codes, Health Care System, Network

★ American Hospital Association (AHA) membership
☐ Joint Commission on Accreditation of Healthcare Organizations (JCAHO) accreditation
+ American Osteopathic Healthcare Association (AOHA) membership
○ American Osteopathic Association (AOA) accreditation
△ Commission on Accreditation of Rehabilitation Facilities (CARF) accreditation
Control codes 61, 63, 64, 71, 72 and 73 indicate hospitals listed by AOHA, but not registered by AHA. For definition of numerical codes, see page A4

Hospital	Classification Codes		Utilization Data					Expense (thousands) of dollars		Personnel
	Control	Service	Staffed Beds	Admissions	Census	Outpatient Visits	Births	Total	Payroll	
CALLAWAY—Custer County ★ CALLAWAY DISTRICT HOSPITAL, 211 Kimball, Zip 68825–0100, Mailing Address: P.O. Box 100, Zip 68825–0100; tel. 308/836–2228; Marvin Neth, Administrator **A**9 10 **F**12 17 18 22 25 37 41 44 48 76 **P**3 Web address: www.calloway–ne.com/hospital	16	10	12	288	4	—	14	1426	641	25
CAMBRIDGE—Furnas County ★ TRI–VALLEY HEALTH SYSTEM, West Highway 6 and 34, Zip 69022–0488, Mailing Address: P.O. Box 488, Zip 69022–0488; tel. 308/697–3329; Arthur H. Frable, Chief Executive Officer (Total facility includes 36 beds in nursing home–type unit) **A**9 10 **F**7 8 9 16 17 18 19 22 25 28 30 32 34 36 37 38 40 45 48 51 54 56 67 69 70 72 76 77 **P**6 **S** Brim Healthcare, Inc., Brentwood, TN	23	10	65	467	40	—	60	9956	4737	197
CENTRAL CITY—Merrick County LITZENBERG MEMORIAL COUNTY HOSPITAL, 1715 26th Street, Zip 68826–9620, Mailing Address: Route 2, Box 1, Zip 68826–0001; tel. 308/946–3015; Michael R. Bowman, Administrator (Total facility includes 46 beds in nursing home–type unit) (Nonreporting) **A**9 10	13	10	71	—	—	—	—	—	—	—
CHADRON—Dawes County ★ CHADRON COMMUNITY HOSPITAL AND HEALTH SERVICES, 821 Morehead Street, Zip 69337–2599; tel. 308/432–5586; Harold L. Krueger, Jr, Chief ExecutiveOfficer **A**9 10 **F**1 6 8 9 13 14 17 19 21 22 25 32 34 35 36 37 41 43 44 48 53 54 66 67 69 70 71 76 78 **P**5 8	23	10	32	706	8	6815	106	7043	3241	121
COLUMBUS—Platte County ✠ COLUMBUS COMMUNITY HOSPITAL, 3020 18th Street, Zip 68601–4214, Mailing Address: P.O. Box 819, Zip 68602–0819; tel. 402/564–7118; Donald H. Zornes, President and Chief Executive Officer (Total facility includes 19 beds in nursing home–type unit) **A**1 9 10 **F**8 9 11 13 17 18 19 22 23 24 25 27 32 34 35 36 37 38 39 40 43 45 48 49 50 51 54 70 72 76 78 **P**8	23	10	71	2351	39	52345	544	19845	8751	285
COZAD—Dawson County COZAD COMMUNITY HOSPITAL, 300 East 12th Street, Zip 69130–1505, Mailing Address: P.O. Box 108, Zip 69130–0108; tel. 308/784–2261; Lyle E. Davis, Administrator **A**9 10 **F**8 9 22 25 28 34 36 37 40 41 43 44 48 54 56 70 76 **P**3	16	10	21	772	3	4842	46	3947	2899	90
CREIGHTON—Knox County CREIGHTON AREA HEALTH SERVICES, 1503 Main Street, Zip 68729–0186, Mailing Address: P.O. Box 186, Zip 68729–0186; tel. 402/358–3322; Paul Hurd, Chief Executive Officer (Total facility includes 46 beds in nursing home–type unit) **A**9 10 **F**1 7 8 9 17 18 19 22 25 31 32 34 36 38 39 43 45 46 48 49 70 72 76 **P**8 Web address: www.lundsupport@cahs–ne.org	14	10	76	437	47	5702	9	3723	1934	93
CRETE—Saline County ★ CRETE MUNICIPAL HOSPITAL, 1540 Grove Street, Zip 68333–0220, Mailing Address: P.O. Box 220, Zip 68333–0220; tel. 402/826–6800; Joseph W. Lohrman, Administrator (Total facility includes 22 beds in nursing home–type unit) **A**9 10 **F**8 9 16 17 18 22 25 36 46 48 69 76 78 Web address: www.creteabc.org	14	10	57	611	42	19870	49	5682	2792	132
DAVID CITY—Butler County BUTLER COUNTY HEALTH CARE CENTER, 372 South Ninth Street, Zip 68632–2199; tel. 402/367–3115; Roger Reamer, Administrator **A**9 10 **F**1 3 8 9 15 16 17 18 19 22 23 25 28 31 32 34 36 37 38 39 40 43 44 46 48 49 50 51 54 56 63 67 69 70 71 72 76 78	13	10	29	705	9	18371	106	4264	2044	80
FAIRBURY—Jefferson County ★ JEFFERSON COMMUNITY HEALTH CENTER, 2200 H Street, Zip 68352–1119, Mailing Address: P.O. Box 277, Zip 68352–0277; tel. 402/729–3351; Bill Welch, Administrator (Total facility includes 41 beds in nursing home–type unit) **A**9 10 18 **F**1 8 9 17 18 19 22 23 25 28 31 32 33 34 38 39 43 44 45 46 48 53 54 69 70 71 72 75 76 78 **P**8	23	10	65	449	37	—	57	5886	2777	126
FALLS CITY—Richardson County ★ COMMUNITY MEDICAL CENTER, 2307 Barada Street, Zip 68355–1599; tel. 402/245–2428; Asa B. Wilson, Ph.D., Administrator **A**9 10 **F**7 8 9 17 18 19 22 24 25 30 32 34 36 37 38 39 46 48 49 54 68 69 70 71 79 **P**6 **S** Great Plains Health Alliance, Inc., Phillipsburg, KS Web address: www.gpha.com	23	10	35	989	17	22703	67	7960	2850	128
FRANKLIN—Franklin County ★ FRANKLIN COUNTY MEMORIAL HOSPITAL, 1406 Q Street, Zip 68939–0315, Mailing Address: P.O. Box 315, Zip 68939–0315; tel. 308/425–6221; Jerrell F. Gerdes, Administrator **A**9 10 18 **F**7 16 17 18 22 23 25 28 32 34 36 37 38 39 48 54 56 70 75 76 **P**6	13	10	17	272	2	4611	0	2672	1502	54
FREMONT—Dodge County ✠ FREMONT AREA MEDICAL CENTER, 450 East 23rd Street, Zip 68025–2387; tel. 402/721–1610; D. Michael Leibert, President and Chief Executive Officer (Total facility includes 162 beds in nursing home–type unit) **A**1 2 9 10 **F**1 7 8 9 12 18 19 22 24 25 30 31 32 33 34 35 36 37 38 39 41 43 44 45 46 48 50 51 54 65 68 69 70 71 72 76 77 78 **P**8 Web address: www.famc.org	13	10	259	3708	190	59518	395	40412	21175	619
FRIEND—Saline County WARREN MEMORIAL HOSPITAL, 905 Second Street, Zip 68359–1198; tel. 402/947–2541; Joseph W. Lohrman, Administrator (Total facility includes 54 beds in nursing home–type unit) **A**9 10 **F**1 16 17 18 25 32 34 36 37 38 40 43 44 48 54 62 69 76	14	10	69	68	49	4946	7	2211	1194	65

Many Facility Codes have changed. Please refer to the AHA Guide Code Chart.

© 2000 AHA Guide

Hospitals, U.S. / NEBRASKA

Hospital, Address, Telephone, Administrator, Approval, Facility, and Physician Codes, Health Care System, Network	Classification Codes		Utilization Data					Expense (thousands) of dollars		
★ American Hospital Association (AHA) membership □ Joint Commission on Accreditation of Healthcare Organizations (JCAHO) accreditation + American Osteopathic Healthcare Association (AOHA) membership ○ American Osteopathic Association (AOA) accreditation △ Commission on Accreditation of Rehabilitation Facilities (CARF) accreditation Control codes 61, 63, 64, 71, 72 and 73 indicate hospitals listed by AOHA, but not registered by AHA. For definition of numerical codes, see page A4	Control	Service	Staffed Beds	Admissions	Census	Outpatient Visits	Births	Total	Payroll	Personnel
GENEVA—Fillmore County FILLMORE COUNTY HOSPITAL, 1325 H Street, Zip 68361–1325, Mailing Address: P.O. Box 193, Zip 68361–0193; tel. 402/759–3167; Larry Eichelberger, Chief Executive Officer (Total facility includes 20 beds in nursing home–type unit) **A**9 10 18 **F**7 8 9 12 13 14 17 18 19 22 25 28 30 33 34 37 38 39 41 43 44 45 46 48 51 54 69 70 72 76 78	13	10	53	528	31	9296	43	5572	2396	88
GENOA—Nance County GENOA COMMUNITY HOSPITAL, 706 Ewing Avenue, Zip 68640, Mailing Address: P.O. Box 310, Zip 68640–0310; tel. 402/993–2283; Joyce Beck, Administrator (Total facility includes 59 beds in nursing home–type unit) (Nonreporting) **A**9 10 18	14	10	99	—	—	—	—	—	—	—
GORDON—Sheridan County ★ GORDON MEMORIAL HOSPITAL DISTRICT, 300 East Eighth Street, Zip 69343–9990; tel. 308/282–0401; Gladys Phemister, Chief Executive Officer (Total facility includes 46 beds in nursing home–type unit) **A**9 10 **F**1 6 8 9 12 17 18 19 22 25 32 34 36 41 44 48 54 66 69 76 **P**6 Web address: www.ci.gordon.ne.us/	16	10	86	849	47	17407	42	7277	3908	133
GOTHENBURG—Dawson County ★ GOTHENBURG MEMORIAL HOSPITAL, 910 20th Street, Zip 69138–1237, Mailing Address: P.O. Box 469, Zip 69138–0469; tel. 308/537–3661; John H. Johnson, Chief Executive Officer (Total facility includes 37 beds in nursing home–type unit) **A**9 10 18 **F**7 8 9 17 18 22 25 28 33 34 36 37 38 41 44 45 46 48 50 53 54 56 69 70 72 76	16	10	49	312	35	15979	53	4144	2072	88
GRAND ISLAND—Hall County ✠ ST. FRANCIS MEDICAL CENTER, (Includes Saint Francis Memorial Health Center, 2116 West Faidley Avenue, Zip 68803), 2620 West Faidley Avenue, Zip 68803–4297, Mailing Address: P.O. Box 9804, Zip 68802–9804; tel. 308/384–4600; Michael R. Gloor, FACHE, President and Chief Executive Officer (Total facility includes 36 beds in nursing home–type unit) **A**1 2 3 5 9 10 **F**2 3 4 8 9 11 12 13 17 18 19 22 23 24 25 27 31 32 34 35 36 37 38 39 41 42 43 44 45 46 48 49 54 59 63 65 67 69 70 71 72 76 78 **P**8 **S** Catholic Health Initiatives, Denver, CO Web address: www.sfmc-gi.org	23	10	198	7054	105	77905	947	71469	30169	885
GRANT—Perkins County PERKINS COUNTY HEALTH SERVICES, (Includes GOLDEN OURS CONVALESCENT HOME), 900 Lincoln Avenue, Zip 69140–9799, Mailing Address: Rural Route 1, Box 26, Zip 69140–9799; tel. 308/352–7200; Carol A. Abbuhl, Chief Executive Officer (Total facility includes 64 beds in nursing home–type unit) **A**9 10 **F**12 22 25 30 32 36 44 46 48 54 69 70 72 76	16	10	84	735	66	9786	47	5321	2783	122
HASTINGS—Adams County □ HASTINGS REGIONAL CENTER, 4200 West Second Street, Zip 68901–9700, Mailing Address: P.O. Box 579, Zip 68902–0579; tel. 402/462–1971; Michael J. Sheehan, Administrator (Nonreporting) **A**1 9 10	12	49	232	—	—	—	—	—	—	—
✠ MARY LANNING MEMORIAL HOSPITAL, 715 North St. Joseph Avenue, Zip 68901–4497; tel. 402/461–5110; W. Michael Kearney, President (Total facility includes 20 beds in nursing home–type unit) **A**1 2 9 10 **F**3 7 8 9 11 14 17 18 19 22 24 25 27 28 32 35 36 37 38 39 40 41 42 43 44 45 46 48 50 51 54 56 57 58 59 60 61 62 63 64 65 67 69 70 71 72 75 76 78 79 **P**6 Web address: www.mlmh.org	23	10	157	5057	63	43198	637	47778	22834	793
HEBRON—Thayer County ★ THAYER COUNTY HEALTH SERVICES, 120 Park Avenue, Zip 68370–2019, Mailing Address: P.O. Box 49, Zip 68370–0049; tel. 402/768–6041; Larry E. Leaming, Administrator **A**9 10 18 **F**7 8 9 14 17 19 22 28 32 34 36 37 38 39 43 44 45 46 48 50 51 54 56 70 71 72 76 78 79 **P**6	13	10	14	654	5	21149	55	6053	2639	109
HENDERSON—York County HENDERSON HEALTH CARE SERVICES, 1621 Front Street, Zip 68371–0217, Mailing Address: P.O. Box 217, Zip 68371–0217; tel. 402/723–4512; Marianna Harris, Administrator (Total facility includes 42 beds in nursing home–type unit) (Nonreporting) **A**9 10 18	23	10	51	—	—	—	—	—	—	—
HOLDREGE—Phelps County ✠ PHELPS MEMORIAL HEALTH CENTER, 1220 Miller Street, Zip 68949–0828, Mailing Address: P.O. Box 828, Zip 68949–0828; tel. 308/995–2211; Walter W. Brownlee, Interim Chief Executive Officer **A**1 9 10 **F**8 9 11 12 14 16 17 18 19 22 24 32 34 36 37 38 39 43 45 48 50 51 54 70 71 72 76 78 **S** Quorum Health Group, Brentwood, TN	23	10	31	1659	18	21471	135	10684	4645	151
IMPERIAL—Chase County CHASE COUNTY COMMUNITY HOSPITAL, 600 West 12th Street, Zip 69033–0819, Mailing Address: P.O. Box 819, Zip 69033–0819; tel. 308/882–7111; Ed Hackman, Administrator **A**9 10 **F**7 8 9 13 16 17 18 19 22 25 26 30 32 34 37 38 39 43 45 46 48 51 54 70 72 76 Web address: www.ccch.com	13	10	25	616	6	12323	61	2489	1516	54
KEARNEY—Buffalo County ✠ △ GOOD SAMARITAN HEALTH SYSTEMS, (Includes Richard H. Young Psychiatric Hospital, 4600 17th Avenue, Zip 68847; tel. 308/865–2000), 10 East 31st Street, Zip 68847–2926, Mailing Address: P.O. Box 1990, Zip 68848–1990; tel. 308/865–7100; William C. Luke, Interim President and Chief Executive Officer (Total facility includes 20 beds in nursing home–type unit) **A**1 2 3 5 7 9 10 **F**1 3 4 5 6 7 8 9 11 13 16 17 18 19 22 24 25 26 27 28 31 32 33 34 36 37 38 39 40 42 43 44 46 47 48 49 50 51 53 54 57 58 59 61 62 63 65 69 70 71 72 73 75 76 78 79 **P**6 8 **S** Catholic Health Initiatives, Denver, CO	21	10	267	8735	131	67972	836	93490	39620	1186

© 2000 AHA Guide   *Many Facility Codes have changed. Please refer to the AHA Guide Code Chart.*

Hospitals, U.S. / NEBRASKA

Hospital, Address, Telephone, Administrator, Approval, Facility, and Physician Codes, Health Care System, Network	Classification Codes		Utilization Data					Expense (thousands) of dollars		
	Control	Service	Staffed Beds	Admissions	Census	Outpatient Visits	Births	Total	Payroll	Personnel

★ American Hospital Association (AHA) membership
☐ Joint Commission on Accreditation of Healthcare Organizations (JCAHO) accreditation
+ American Osteopathic Healthcare Association (AOHA) membership
○ American Osteopathic Association (AOA) accreditation
△ Commission on Accreditation of Rehabilitation Facilities (CARF) accreditation
Control codes 61, 63, 64, 71, 72 and 73 indicate hospitals listed by AOHA, but not registered by AHA. For definition of numerical codes, see page A4

Hospital	Control	Service	Staffed Beds	Admissions	Census	Outpatient Visits	Births	Total	Payroll	Personnel
KIMBALL—Kimball County										
KIMBALL COUNTY HOSPITAL, 505 South Burg Street, Zip 69145–1398; tel. 308/235–3621; Kim Woods, Chief Executive Officer **A**9 10 18 **F**6 9 18 22 25 32 36 43 45 48 54 56 67 69 76 79 **P**5	13	10	16	196	2	4558	15	2802	1297	52
LEXINGTON—Dawson County										
☒ TRI-COUNTY AREA HOSPITAL, 13th and Erie Streets, Zip 68850–0980, Mailing Address: P.O. Box 980, Zip 68850–0980; tel. 308/324–5651; Calvin A. Hiner, Administrator **A**1 9 10 **F**7 8 9 11 12 13 16 19 22 24 25 26 28 32 34 36 37 38 39 41 43 44 45 46 48 50 54 55 67 69 70 76	16	10	25	1391	14	26198	233	9335	4164	147
LINCOLN—Lancaster County										
☒ BRYANLGH MEDICAL CENTER, (Includes Bryan Memorial–BryanLGH–East, 1600 South 48th Street; Lincoln General–BryanLGH–West, 2300 South 16th Street, Zip 68502–3781; tel. 402/475–1011), 1600 South 48th Street, Zip 68506–1299; tel. 402/489–0200; Craig M. Ames, President and Chief Operating Officer (Total facility includes 37 beds in nursing home–type unit) **A**1 2 3 5 9 10 **F**2 4 8 9 11 12 13 17 18 19 21 22 24 25 30 31 32 33 34 35 36 38 39 41 44 46 47 48 50 51 53 54 57 58 59 60 61 62 63 64 65 68 69 70 71 72 73 74 75 76 78 **P**1 6
Web address: www.bryanlgh.org
LINCOLN DIVISION See Veterans Affairs Greater Nebraska Health Care System	23	10	525	23091	297	—	1999	258822	104464	3039
☐ LINCOLN REGIONAL CENTER, West Prospector Place and Folsom, Zip 68522–2299, Mailing Address: P.O. Box 94949, Zip 68509–4949; tel. 402/471–4444; Barbara Ramsey, Ph.D., Chief Executive Officer **A**1 9 10 **F**16 17 18 23 31 45 57 58 59 60 61 62 63 70 72 78 **P**6
Web address: www.hhs.state.ne.us	12	22	194	300	184	—	—	21512	13704	469
△ MADONNA REHABILITATION HOSPITAL, 5401 South Street, Zip 68506–2134; tel. 402/489–7102; Marsha Lommel, President and Chief Executive Officer (Total facility includes 162 beds in nursing home–type unit) **A**7 9 10 **F**1 7 13 16 17 18 19 28 31 32 33 34 36 38 43 45 50 51 54 69 70 72 78 **P**6
Web address: www.madonna.org	21	46	252	1573	227	—	—	38776	23784	756
☒ SAINT ELIZABETH REGIONAL MEDICAL CENTER, 555 South 70th Street, Zip 68510–2494; tel. 402/489–7181; Robert J. Lanik, President and Chief Executive Officer **A**1 2 3 5 9 10 **F**4 7 8 9 10 11 12 13 16 17 18 19 22 25 27 31 32 34 35 36 37 39 41 42 44 45 46 47 48 49 51 54 68 70 71 72 76 77 78 **P**6 7 **S** Catholic Health Initiatives, Denver, CO
Web address: www.stez.org	23	10	197	7955	106	84354	2067	95533	34970	1264
★ VETERANS AFFAIRS GREATER NEBRASKA HEALTH CARE SYSTEM, (Includes Lincoln Division), 600 South 70th Street, Zip 68510–2493; tel. 402/489–3802; David Asper, Director (Nonreporting) **A**3 **S** Department of Veterans Affairs, Washington, DC
Web address: www.va.gov/stations97/guide/home.asp?DIVISION=ALL	45	10	191	—	—	—	—	—	—	—
LYNCH—Boyd County										
NIOBRARA VALLEY HOSPITAL, Mailing Address: P.O. Box 118, Zip 68746–0118; tel. 402/569–2451; Bruce Purviance, Administrator (Nonreporting) **A**9 10 18	23	10	29	—	—	—	—	—	—	—
MCCOOK—Red Willow County										
☒ COMMUNITY HOSPITAL, 1301 East H Street, Zip 69001–1328, Mailing Address: P.O. Box 1328, Zip 69001–1328; tel. 308/345–2650; Gary Bieganski, President **A**1 9 10 **F**7 8 9 16 17 19 22 24 25 27 32 34 36 37 38 39 45 48 50 51 54 70 76 78 79	23	10	44	1454	17	45385	130	12104	—	163
MINDEN—Kearney County										
★ KEARNEY COUNTY HEALTH SERVICES, (Formerly Kearney County Community Hospital), 727 East First Street, Zip 68959–1700; tel. 308/832–1440; David Stephenson, Administrator (Total facility includes 50 beds in nursing home–type unit) **A**9 10 18 **F**8 9 12 14 17 18 23 25 30 32 34 36 37 41 44 45 48 56 69 74 76 **P**3 6	13	10	85	242	52	6900	5	3829	2252	101
NEBRASKA CITY—Otoe County										
★ ST. MARY'S HOSPITAL, 1314 Third Avenue, Zip 68410–1999; tel. 402/873–3321; Daniel J. Kelly, President and Chief Executive Officer **A**9 10 **F**3 7 8 9 18 22 25 36 37 39 40 41 43 44 45 46 48 51 68 69 76 78 **S** Catholic Health Initiatives, Denver, CO	21	10	28	468	5	22222	124	5059	2169	92
NELIGH—Antelope County										
★ ANTELOPE MEMORIAL HOSPITAL, 102 West Ninth.Street, Zip 68756–0229, Mailing Address: P.O. Box 229, Zip 68756–0229; tel. 402/887–4151; Jack W. Green, Administrator (Nonreporting) **A**9 10	23	10	49	—	—	—	—	—	—	—
NORFOLK—Madison County										
☒ FAITH REGIONAL HEALTH SERVICES, (Includes East Campus, 1500 Koenigstein Avenue, Zip 68701, Mailing Address: East Campus, Zip 68701; tel. 402/371–3402; West Campus, 2700 Norfolk Avenue, Zip 68701; tel. 402/371–4880), 2700 Norfolk Avenue, Zip 68702–0869, Mailing Address: P.O. BOX 869, Zip 68702–0869; tel. 402/644–7201; Robert L. Driewer, Chief Executive Officer (Total facility includes 100 beds in nursing home–type unit) **A**1 9 10 **F**3 8 9 11 13 16 17 18 19 22 23 24 25 32 33 34 36 37 39 41 43 44 45 48 49 50 54 57 61 65 69 70 71 72 76 77 78 **P**8 **S** Missionary Benedictine Sisters American Province, Norfolk, NE
Web address: www.frhs.org	23	10	226	6099	150	57263	856	49207	22806	764
☐ NORFOLK REGIONAL CENTER, 1700 North Victory Road, Zip 68701–6859, Mailing Address: P.O. Box 1209, Zip 68702–1209; tel. 402/370–3400; Richard B. Gamel, Chief Executive Officer (Nonreporting) **A**1 9 10	12	22	174	—	—	—	—	—	—	—

Many Facility Codes have changed. Please refer to the AHA Guide Code Chart.

© 2000 AHA Guide

Hospitals, U.S. / NEBRASKA

Hospital, Address, Telephone, Administrator, Approval, Facility, and Physician Codes, Health Care System, Network	Classification Codes		Utilization Data					Expense (thousands) of dollars		
★ American Hospital Association (AHA) membership ☐ Joint Commission on Accreditation of Healthcare Organizations (JCAHO) accreditation + American Osteopathic Healthcare Association (AOHA) membership ○ American Osteopathic Association (AOA) accreditation △ Commission on Accreditation of Rehabilitation Facilities (CARF) accreditation Control codes 61, 63, 64, 71, 72 and 73 indicate hospitals listed by AOHA, but not registered by AHA. For definition of numerical codes, see page A4	Control	Service	Staffed Beds	Admissions	Census	Outpatient Visits	Births	Total	Payroll	Personnel

NORTH PLATTE—Lincoln County
* ✶ GREAT PLAINS REGIONAL MEDICAL CENTER, 601 West Leota Street, Zip 69101-6598, Mailing Address: P.O. Box 1167, Zip 69103-1167; tel. 308/534-9310; Lucinda A. Bradley, President **A**1 2 3 5 9 10 **F**3 7 8 9 11 13 17 18 19 22 24 25 26 27 32 34 36 37 38 39 41 43 44 45 46 48 49 51 53 54 57 61 62 63 64 65 68 70 71 72 74 76 78 **P**6 8 **S** Quorum Health Group, Brentwood, TN — 23 10 99 4897 49 154870 550 51135 20529 595

O'NEILL—Holt County
* ✶ AVERA ST. ANTHONY'S HOSPITAL, Second and Adams Streets, Zip 68763-1569; tel. 402/336-2611; Ronald J. Cork, President and Chief Executive Officer **A**1 9 10 **F**8 9 13 17 18 19 21 22 25 30 32 33 34 35 36 38 39 43 45 46 48 49 50 54 59 70 71 72 76 78 **P**1 6 **S** Avera Health, Yankton, SD
  Web address: www.avera-sta.org — 21 10 29 1028 9 17637 129 8271 3149 115

OAKLAND—Burt County
* OAKLAND MEMORIAL HOSPITAL, 601 East Second Street, Zip 68045-1499; tel. 402/685-5601; Karen Vlach, Administrator **A**9 10 18 **F**9 13 22 25 32 34 36 37 39 41 43 45 46 48 51 56 69 76 **P**5 6 — 16 10 23 210 3 6454 0 2303 1208 40

OFFUTT AFB—Sarpy County
* ✶ EHRLING BERGQUIST HOSPITAL, 2501 Capehart Road, Zip 68113-2160; tel. 402/294-7312; Colonel Thomas J. Eslick, MSC, USAF, Commander (Nonreporting) **A**1 3 5 **S** Department of the Air Force, Bowling AFB, DC — 41 10 45 — — — — — — —

OGALLALA—Keith County
* ★ OGALLALA COMMUNITY HOSPITAL, 300 East Tenth Street, Zip 69153-1509; tel. 308/284-4011; Linda Morris, Administrator **A**9 10 **F**8 9 12 13 14 17 18 19 22 25 29 32 34 36 37 41 44 46 48 49 54 56 63 69 70 72 76 77 **P**6 **S** Banner Health System, Fargo, ND — 23 10 29 662 6 29569 55 7248 3639 122

OMAHA—Douglas County
* ✶ ALEGENT HEALTH BERGAN MERCY MEDICAL CENTER, 7500 Mercy Road, Zip 68124; tel. 402/343-4410; Mike Tiesi, Administrator (Total facility includes 241 beds in nursing home-type unit) **A**1 2 3 5 9 10 **F**1 2 3 4 6 7 8 9 11 12 13 14 16 17 18 19 20 21 22 23 24 25 26 27 28 29 30 31 32 33 34 35 36 37 38 39 41 42 43 44 45 46 47 48 49 50 51 53 54 55 56 57 58 59 60 61 62 63 64 65 67 68 69 70 71 72 73 74 76 77 78 79 **P**6 8 **S** Catholic Health Initiatives, Denver, CO — 21 10 549 14358 387 125521 2220 151886 60178 2153
* ✶ △ ALEGENT HEALTH IMMANUEL MEDICAL CENTER, 6901 North 72nd Street, Zip 68122-1799; tel. 402/572-2121; Barbara K. Goodrich, R.N., Administrator (Total facility includes 197 beds in nursing home-type unit) **A**1 2 5 7 9 10 **F**2 3 4 6 7 8 9 11 12 13 16 17 18 19 21 22 23 25 26 27 28 29 30 31 32 33 34 35 36 37 38 39 41 42 43 44 45 46 47 48 49 50 51 53 54 55 56 57 58 59 60 61 62 63 64 65 67 68 69 70 71 72 73 74 76 77 78 79 **P**6 8 — 21 10 531 12284 417 159376 737 137029 53051 1727
* ☐ BOYS TOWN NATIONAL RESEARCH HOSPITAL, 555 North 30th Street, Zip 68131-2198; tel. 402/498-6511; John K. Arch, Administrator **A**1 3 9 10 **F**16 17 18 19 38 48 50 51 56 58 60 **P**6
  Web address: www.boystown.org/btnrh — 23 50 14 55 0 128450 0 — — 544
* ✶ CHILDREN'S HOSPITAL, 8301 Dodge Street, Zip 68114-4114; tel. 402/354-5400; Gary A. Perkins, President and Chief Executive Officer **A**1 3 5 9 10 **F**7 11 13 17 19 22 24 25 27 32 33 36 38 39 42 43 46 47 48 50 52 65 68 70 72 76 77 78 **P**8
  Web address: www.chsomaha.org — 23 50 100 5785 76 75772 0 70306 30326 697
* ○ DOUGLAS COUNTY HOSPITAL, 4102 Woolworth Avenue, Zip 68105-1899; tel. 402/444-7000; James C. Tourville, Administrator (Total facility includes 272 beds in nursing home-type unit) (Nonreporting) **A**9 10 11 — 13 49 329 — — — — — — —
* ☐ NEBRASKA HEALTH SYSTEM, (Includes Nebraska Health System (Formerly Bishop Clarkson Memorial Hospital), 4350 Dewey Avenue, Mailing Address: 4350 Dewey Avnue, Zip 68105-1018; Nebraska Health System (Formerly University of Nebraska Medical Center), 600 South 42nd Street, Zip 68198-4085; tel. 402/559-4000), 4350 Dewey Avenue, Zip 68105-1018; tel. 402/552-2000; Louis W. Burgher, M.D., Ph.D., President and Chief Executive Officer (Nonreporting) **A**1 2 3 5 8 9 10 — 23 10 543 — — — — — — —
* ✶ △ NEBRASKA METHODIST HOSPITAL, 8303 Dodge Street, Zip 68114-4199; tel. 402/354-4000; John Martin Fraser, President and Chief Executive Officer **A**1 2 3 7 9 10 **F**3 4 6 7 8 9 11 12 13 16 17 18 19 21 22 23 24 25 26 27 28 30 31 32 33 34 35 36 37 38 39 40 41 42 43 44 45 46 47 48 49 50 52 53 54 56 57 58 59 60 61 62 63 64 65 66 69 70 71 72 75 76 77 78 79 **P**6 7 8
  Web address: www.bestcare.org — 23 10 359 14026 173 118156 — 179205 76275 2033
* RICHARD YOUNG CENTER, (Formerly Methodist Richard Young), (Includes Richard H. Young Memorial Hospital), 515 South 26th Street, Zip 68105-4101; tel. 402/354-6600; Sandra C. Carson, FACHE, President and Chief Executive Officer **A**5 9 10 **F**3 4 8 9 11 12 17 19 21 22 24 25 26 29 30 31 32 33 34 36 37 38 39 41 42 43 44 45 46 47 48 49 50 53 54 56 57 58 60 61 62 63 64 65 67 69 70 71 72 73 75 76 77 78 **P**1
  Web address: www.bestcare.org — 21 22 97 2291 66 — 0 17369 9380 307
* ✶ ST. JOSEPH HOSPITAL, 601 North 30th Street, Zip 68131-2197; tel. 402/449-5021; J. Richard Stanko, President and Chief Executive Officer **A**1 3 5 7 9 10 **F**4 7 8 11 13 17 19 21 22 23 25 27 28 29 32 34 38 39 41 42 44 45 46 47 48 50 51 52 54 56 58 59 60 61 62 63 64 65 68 69 70 72 75 76 77 78 **P**2 7 8 **S** TENET Healthcare Corporation, Santa Barbara, CA — 33 10 278 10055 155 57666 927 101762 33852 1067

© 2000 AHA Guide *Many Facility Codes have changed. Please refer to the AHA Guide Code Chart.*

Hospitals, U.S. / NEBRASKA

Hospital, Address, Telephone, Administrator, Approval, Facility, and Physician Codes, Health Care System, Network	Classification Codes		Utilization Data					Expense (thousands) of dollars		
★ American Hospital Association (AHA) membership □ Joint Commission on Accreditation of Healthcare Organizations (JCAHO) accreditation + American Osteopathic Healthcare Association (AOHA) membership ○ American Osteopathic Association (AOA) accreditation △ Commission on Accreditation of Rehabilitation Facilities (CARF) accreditation Control codes 61, 63, 64, 71, 72 and 73 indicate hospitals listed by AOHA, but not registered by AHA. For definition of numerical codes, see page A4	Control	Service	Staffed Beds	Admissions	Census	Outpatient Visits	Births	Total	Payroll	Personnel
✠ VETERANS AFFAIRS MEDICAL CENTER, 4101 Woolworth Avenue, Zip 68105–1873; tel. 402/449–0600; John J. Phillips, Director **A**1 3 5 8 **F**2 3 4 9 11 13 19 22 23 24 25 27 30 32 34 35 38 39 41 43 45 46 47 48 50 51 54 55 56 57 59 61 62 63 64 65 68 70 72 74 76 78 79 **S** Department of Veterans Affairs, Washington, DC **Web address:** www.va.gov/stations97/guide/home.asp?DIVISION=ALL	45	10	122	4302	72	163292	—	75527	42887	804
ORD—Valley County ★ VALLEY COUNTY HOSPITAL, 217 Westridge Drive, Zip 68862–1675; tel. 308/728–3211; Colleen Chapp, Interim Chief Executive Officer and Administrator (Total facility includes 70 beds in nursing home–type unit) **A**9 10 **F**8 9 13 16 17 19 22 25 28 31 32 34 36 37 38 39 40 44 45 46 48 49 53 54 69 70 76 **P**6	13	10	96	582	69	12873	50	7237	4008	223
OSCEOLA—Polk County ANNIE JEFFREY MEMORIAL COUNTY HEALTH CENTER, 531 Beebe Street, Zip 68651, Mailing Address: P.O. Box 428, Zip 68651–0428; tel. 402/747–2031; Carol E. Jones, Administrator **A**9 10 18 **F**7 8 9 13 16 17 18 19 22 25 28 32 33 34 36 37 38 39 40 43 44 45 48 54 56 69 70 71 76	13	10	21	195	2	6528	16	2361	1151	49
OSHKOSH—Garden County GARDEN COUNTY HOSPITAL, 1100 West Second Street, Zip 69154, Mailing Address: P.O. Box 320, Zip 69154–0320; tel. 308/772–3283; Diana Stevens, Administrator (Total facility includes 36 beds in nursing home–type unit) **A**9 10 18 **F**1 7 9 12 17 19 21 22 23 25 32 36 37 38 43 48 54 69 70 76 **P**6	13	10	46	258	32	1734	0	2548	1425	69
OSMOND—Pierce County ★ OSMOND GENERAL HOSPITAL, 5th and Maple Street, Zip 68765–0429, Mailing Address: P.O. Box 429, Zip 68765–0429; tel. 402/748–3393; Celine M. Mlady, Chief Executive Officer **A**9 10 **F**1 7 9 17 18 22 25 26 32 34 37 38 39 40 48 67 69 70 72 76 **P**6	23	10	30	648	25	5666	0	3177	1814	72
PAPILLION—Sarpy County ✠ ALEGENT–HEALTH MIDLANDS COMMUNITY HOSPITAL, 11111 South 84th Street, Zip 68046–4157; tel. 402/593–3000; James P. Kelly, Administrator **A**1 2 9 10 **F**1 2 3 4 6 7 8 9 11 12 13 16 17 18 19 20 21 22 23 24 25 26 27 28 29 30 31 32 33 34 35 36 37 38 39 41 42 43 44 45 46 47 48 49 50 51 53 54 55 56 57 58 59 60 61 62 63 64 65 67 68 69 70 71 72 73 74 76 77 78 79 **P**6 8	21	10	151	2967	45	23973	381	29581	11033	498
PAWNEE CITY—Pawnee County PAWNEE COUNTY MEMORIAL HOSPITAL, 600 I Street, Zip 68420–3001, Mailing Address: P.O. Box 313, Zip 68420–0313; tel. 402/852–2231; James A. Kubik, Administrator (Nonreporting) **A**9 10 18	13	10	21	—	—	—	—	—	—	—
PENDER—Thurston County ★ PENDER COMMUNITY HOSPITAL, 603 Earl Street, Zip 68047–0100, Mailing Address: P.O. Box 100, Zip 68047–0100; tel. 402/385–3083; Roger Mazour, Administrator **A**9 10 **F**7 8 9 12 22 25 32 36 37 38 39 44 45 48 50 69 76 **P**7 **S** Trinity Health, Novi, MI	16	10	30	778	8	10146	58	4094	1675	78
PLAINVIEW—Pierce County PLAINVIEW PUBLIC HOSPITAL, 705 North Third Street, Zip 68769, Mailing Address: P.O. Box 489, Zip 68769–0489; tel. 402/582–4245; Donald T. Naiberk, Administrator and Chief Executive Officer (Nonreporting) **A**9 10	14	10	19	—	—	—	—	—	—	—
RED CLOUD—Webster County WEBSTER COUNTY COMMUNITY HOSPITAL, Sixth Avenue and Franklin Street, Zip 68970–0465; tel. 402/746–2291; Terry L. Hoffart, Administrator **A**9 10 18 **F**7 9 22 32 39 45 48 54 71 76 78 **P**3	13	10	16	249	6	575	0	1649	760	34
SAINT PAUL—Howard County ★ HOWARD COUNTY COMMUNITY HOSPITAL, 113 Sherman Street, Zip 68873–1536, Mailing Address: P.O. Box 406, Zip 68873–0406; tel. 308/754–4421; Russell W. Swigart, Administrator **A**9 10 **F**7 9 22 25 37 39 44 48 54 70 76 **P**5 6	13	10	36	540	19	26331	42	3948	2028	83
SCHUYLER—Colfax County ALEGENT HEALTH–MEMORIAL HOSPITAL, 104 West 17th Street, Zip 68661–1396; tel. 402/352–2441; Connie Peters, Operations Leader and Regional Administrator (Total facility includes 31 beds in nursing home–type unit) (Nonreporting) **A**9 10	23	10	45	—	—	—	—	—	—	—
SCOTTSBLUFF—Scotts Bluff County ✠ REGIONAL WEST MEDICAL CENTER, 4021 Avenue B, Zip 69361–4695; tel. 308/635–3711; David M. Nitschke, President and Chief Executive Officer (Total facility includes 24 beds in nursing home–type unit) **A**1 2 3 5 9 10 **F**1 7 8 9 11 13 16 17 18 19 21 22 24 25 27 28 32 34 36 37 38 39 40 41 42 43 44 45 46 48 49 50 51 53 54 57 58 59 60 61 62 63 64 65 68 69 70 71 72 75 76 78 **P**4 5 6 7	23	10	202	6659	83	38541	745	65491	28117	847
SEWARD—Seward County MEMORIAL HEALTH CARE SYSTEMS, 300 North Columbia Avenue, Zip 68434–9907; tel. 402/643–2971; Ronald D. Waltz, Chief Executive Officer (Total facility includes 120 beds in nursing home–type unit) **A**9 10 **F**1 7 8 9 13 17 18 19 22 25 28 30 31 32 36 37 38 39 40 43 48 50 51 54 56 58 60 70 71 72 76 78 **P**6 **Web address:** www.mhcs–seward.org	23	10	154	828	134	18556	117	14788	7698	279
SIDNEY—Cheyenne County ★ MEMORIAL HEALTH CENTER, 645 Osage Street, Zip 69162–1799; tel. 308/254–5825; Rex D. Walk, Chief Executive Officer (Total facility includes 70 beds in nursing home–type unit) (Nonreporting) **A**9 10	23	10	102	—	—	—	—	—	—	—

Hospitals, U.S. / NEBRASKA

Hospital, Address, Telephone, Administrator, Approval, Facility, and Physician Codes, Health Care System, Network	Classification Codes		Utilization Data					Expense (thousands) of dollars		
★ American Hospital Association (AHA) membership ☐ Joint Commission on Accreditation of Healthcare Organizations (JCAHO) accreditation + American Osteopathic Healthcare Association (AOHA) membership ○ American Osteopathic Association (AOA) accreditation △ Commission on Accreditation of Rehabilitation Facilities (CARF) accreditation Control codes 61, 63, 64, 71, 72 and 73 indicate hospitals listed by AOHA, but not registered by AHA. For definition of numerical codes, see page A4	Control	Service	Staffed Beds	Admissions	Census	Outpatient Visits	Births	Total	Payroll	Personnel
SUPERIOR—Nuckolls County MEMORIAL NUCKOLLS COUNTY HOSPITAL, (Formerly Brodstone Memorial Hospital), 520 East Tenth Street, Zip 68978–1225, Mailing Address: P.O. Box 187, Zip 68978–0187; tel. 402/879–3281; Michael J. Ellis, Administrator and Chief Executive Officer (Nonreporting) **A**9 10 18	23	10	49	—	—	—	—	—	—	—
SYRACUSE—Otoe County COMMUNITY MEMORIAL HOSPITAL, 1579 Midland Street, Zip 68446–9732, Mailing Address: P.O. Box N, Zip 68446; tel. 402/269–2011; Al Klaasmeyer, Administrator **A**9 10 18 **F**7 8 9 13 16 19 22 23 24 25 28 31 33 34 36 37 43 44 45 48 49 50 54 56 75 76 **P**6	16	10	18	187	2	17808	23	3487	1552	56
TECUMSEH—Johnson County ★ JOHNSON COUNTY HOSPITAL, 202 High Street, Zip 68450–0599, Mailing Address: P.O. Box 599, Zip 68450–0599; tel. 402/335–3361; John E. Keelan, Ph.D., Administrator **A**9 10 **F**1 8 9 16 17 18 19 22 25 32 36 38 39 41 43 44 46 48 54 56 68 76	15	10	30	419	6	9143	35	2727	1168	57
TILDEN—Antelope County TILDEN COMMUNITY HOSPITAL, Second and Pine Streets, Zip 68781, Mailing Address: P.O. Box 340, Zip 68781–0340; tel. 402/368–5343; LuAnn Barr, Administrator (Nonreporting) **A**9 10 18	23	10	20	—	—	—	—	—	—	—
VALENTINE—Cherry County ★ CHERRY COUNTY HOSPITAL, Highway 12 and Green Street, Zip 69201–0410; tel. 402/376–2525; Brent A. Peterson, Administrator **A**9 10 **F**7 9 11 16 17 18 22 25 32 33 36 38 39 41 44 46 48 51 69 75 76 78	13	10	27	716	7	8841	241	4893	2134	78
WAHOO—Saunders County SAUNDERS COUNTY HEALTH SERVICE, 805 West Tenth Street, Zip 68066–1102, Mailing Address: P.O. Box 185, Zip 68066–0185; tel. 402/443–4191; Ed Hackman, Administrator (Total facility includes 67 beds in nursing home–type unit) **A**9 10 18 **F**22 25 36 37 39 48 54 69 70 76 Web address: www.saunders–health.org	13	10	97	2731	78	11356	0	6501	3515	—
WAYNE—Wayne County ★ PROVIDENCE MEDICAL CENTER, 1200 Providence Road, Zip 68787–1299; tel. 402/375–3800; Marcile Thomas, Administrator **A**9 10 **F**8 9 16 17 18 22 25 28 36 37 39 40 46 48 54 70 71 76 **S** Missionary Benedictine Sisters American Province, Norfolk, NE	21	10	32	1026	12	11942	110	5898	2587	99
WEST POINT—Cuming County ★ ST. FRANCIS MEMORIAL HOSPITAL, 430 North Monitor Street, Zip 68788–1595; tel. 402/372–2404; Ronald O. Briggs, President (Total facility includes 70 beds in nursing home–type unit) **A**9 10 18 **F**1 6 7 8 9 17 19 22 25 28 32 34 36 37 38 39 43 44 45 46 48 49 53 54 61 63 67 69 70 71 72 76 78 **P**6 **S** Franciscan Sisters of Christian Charity HealthCare Ministry, Inc, Manitowoc, WI	21	10	102	613	76	62353	95	9735	5008	156
WINNEBAGO—Thurston County ⊞ U. S. PUBLIC HEALTH SERVICE INDIAN HOSPITAL, Highway 7577, Zip 68071; tel. 402/878–2231; Donald Lee, Service Unit Director (Nonreporting) **A**1 10 **S** U. S. Public Health Service Indian Health Service, Rockville, MD	47	10	30	—	—	—	—	—	—	—
YORK—York County ★ YORK GENERAL HOSPITAL, 2222 Lincoln Avenue, Zip 68467–1095; tel. 402/362–0445; Charles K. Schulz, Chief Executive Officer **A**9 10 **F**7 8 9 12 13 17 18 19 22 23 24 25 28 32 34 36 37 38 39 41 43 44 45 46 48 49 51 53 54 68 69 70 71 72 76 78 79 **P**5 Web address: www.yorkhospital.org	23	10	41	1127	13	31177	128	9820	4465	157

© 2000 AHA Guide   *Many Facility Codes have changed. Please refer to the AHA Guide Code Chart.*

NEVADA

Resident Population 1,747 (in thousands)
Resident population in metro areas 85.7%
Birth rate per 1,000 population 16.0
65 years and over 11.5%
Percent of persons without health insurance 17.5%

Hospital, Address, Telephone, Administrator, Approval, Facility, and Physician Codes, Health Care System, Network	Classi-fication Codes		Utilization Data					Expense (thousands) of dollars		
★ American Hospital Association (AHA) membership ☐ Joint Commission on Accreditation of Healthcare Organizations (JCAHO) accreditation + American Osteopathic Healthcare Association (AOHA) membership ○ American Osteopathic Association (AOA) accreditation △ Commission on Accreditation of Rehabilitation Facilities (CARF) accreditation Control codes 61, 63, 64, 71, 72 and 73 indicate hospitals listed by AOHA, but not registered by AHA. For definition of numerical codes, see page A4	Control	Service	Staffed Beds	Admissions	Census	Outpatient Visits	Births	Total	Payroll	Personnel
BATTLE MOUNTAIN—Lander County										
BATTLE MOUNTAIN GENERAL HOSPITAL, 535 South Humboldt Street, Zip 89820–1988; tel. 775/635–2550; Kathy Ancho, Administrator (Nonreporting) **A**10	13	10	14	—	—	—	—	—	—	—
BOULDER CITY—Clark County										
BOULDER CITY HOSPITAL, 901 Adams Boulevard, Zip 89005–2299; tel. 702/293–4111; Kim O. Crandell, Chief Executive Officer and Administrator (Total facility includes 47 beds in nursing home–type unit) **A**10 **F**6 7 9 17 22 25 32 34 36 39 48 51 54 64 69 76 77 **P**3	23	10	67	1040	54	19691	0	11719	6121	167
CARSON CITY—Carson City County										
★ CARSON TAHOE HOSPITAL, 775 Fleischmann Way, Zip 89702, Mailing Address: P.O. Box 2168, Zip 89702–2168; tel. 775/882–1361; Steve Smith, Chief Executive Officer **A**1 9 10 **F**1 2 3 7 8 11 12 13 16 17 19 21 22 24 25 26 29 30 32 33 34 35 36 38 39 41 43 44 45 46 48 50 51 54 56 57 58 59 60 61 62 63 65 68 70 72 76 77 78 79	13	10	124	7709	72	96263	851	64755	25628	684
ELKO—Elko County										
★ ELKO GENERAL HOSPITAL, 1297 College Avenue, Zip 89801–3499; tel. 775/738–5151; Fredrick W. Hodges, Chief Executive Officer (Nonreporting) **A**1 9 10 **S** Province Healthcare Corporation, Brentwood, TN Web address: www.elkogeneral.hbocvan.com	13	10	50	—	—	—	—	—	—	—
ELY—White Pine County										
☐ WILLIAM BEE RIRIE HOSPITAL, 1500 Avenue H, Zip 89301–2699; tel. 775/289–3001; Robert A. Morasko, Chief Executive Officer (Nonreporting) **A**1 9 10	13	10	40	—	—	—	—	—	—	—
FALLON—Churchill County										
★ CHURCHILL COMMUNITY HOSPITAL, 801 East Williams Avenue, Zip 89406–3052; tel. 775/423–3151; Jeffrey Feike, Administrator and Chief Executive Officer **A**1 9 10 **F**8 9 13 17 18 19 22 24 25 32 36 38 39 41 44 46 48 49 53 54 75 76 78 **P**5 6 7 **S** Banner Health System, Fargo, ND	23	10	40	2242	19	—	374	—	—	244
HAWTHORNE—Mineral County										
MOUNT GRANT GENERAL HOSPITAL, First and A Street, Zip 89415, Mailing Address: P.O. Box 1510, Zip 89415–1510; tel. 775/945–2461; Richard Munger, Administrator (Total facility includes 20 beds in nursing home–type unit) (Nonreporting) **A**9 10	46	10	35	—	—	—	—	—	—	—
HENDERSON—Clark County										
★ ST. ROSE DOMINICAN HOSPITAL, 102 Lake Mead Drive, Zip 89015–5524; tel. 702/564–2622; Rod A. Davis, President and Chief Executive Officer **A**1 9 10 **F**4 8 9 11 13 17 18 19 22 24 25 26 29 32 33 34 35 36 38 39 41 43 44 45 48 50 51 54 65 66 69 70 71 72 73 76 77 78 79 **P**7 **S** Catholic Healthcare West, San Francisco, CA Web address: www.srdh.com	23	10	143	8542	98	103474	1720	67101	29409	804
LAS VEGAS—Clark County										
☐ BHC MONTEVISTA HOSPITAL, 5900 West Rochelle Avenue, Zip 89103–3327; tel. 702/364–1111; Allan J. Kydd, Chief Executive Officer (Nonreporting) **A**1 10 **S** Behavioral Healthcare Corporation, Nashville, TN	33	22	80	—	—	—	—	—	—	—
☐ DESERT SPRINGS HOSPITAL, 2075 East Flamingo Road, Zip 89119–5121, Mailing Address: P.O. Box 19204, Zip 89132–9204; tel. 702/733–8800; John Lloyd Hummer, Chief Executive Officer (Nonreporting) **A**1 10 **S** Universal Health Services, Inc., King of Prussia, PA	33	10	225	—	—	—	—	—	—	—
★ MOUNTAINVIEW HOSPITAL, 3100 North Tenaya Way, Zip 89128; tel. 702/255–5000; Mark J. Howard, President and Chief Executive Officer **A**1 10 **F**7 8 9 11 12 13 15 17 19 20 22 23 25 30 31 32 33 34 38 39 41 43 44 45 46 48 49 50 51 54 56 65 66 70 72 76 78 79 **S** HCA – The Healthcare Company, Nashville, TN Web address: www.mountainview–hospital.com	33	10	120	10802	112	58655	1967	57843	26835	511
★ △ SUNRISE HOSPITAL AND MEDICAL CENTER, 3186 Maryland Parkway, Zip 89109–2306, Mailing Address: P.O. Box 98530, Zip 89193–8530; tel. 702/731–8000; Allan Stipe, President and Chief Executive Officer **A**1 2 3 5 7 9 10 **F**4 7 8 9 11 12 13 14 16 17 18 19 22 24 25 26 32 33 38 39 41 42 43 44 45 46 47 48 50 52 53 54 65 68 69 70 71 74 76 78 **S** HCA – The Healthcare Company, Nashville, TN Web address: www.sunrisehospital.com	33	10	675	38999	528	177023	5585	262908	110996	2682
☐ UNIVERSITY MEDICAL CENTER, 1800 West Charleston Boulevard, Zip 89102–2386; tel. 702/383–2000; William R. Hale, Chief Executive Officer **A**1 2 3 5 10 **F**4 7 8 9 10 11 12 13 17 18 19 22 24 25 27 29 30 31 32 35 36 38 41 42 43 44 45 46 47 48 51 52 53 54 56 70 72 74 75 76 77 78 79 **P**6	13	10	504	27120	431	662463	4771	294679	120288	2603
☐ VALLEY HOSPITAL MEDICAL CENTER, 620 Shadow Lane, Zip 89106–4119; tel. 702/388–4000; Roger Collins, Chief Executive Officer and Managing Director (Nonreporting) **A**1 9 10 **S** Universal Health Services, Inc., King of Prussia, PA	33	10	365	—	—	—	—	—	—	—

Hospitals, U.S. / NEVADA

Hospital, Address, Telephone, Administrator, Approval, Facility, and Physician Codes, Health Care System, Network	Classification Codes		Utilization Data					Expense (thousands) of dollars		
★ American Hospital Association (AHA) membership ☐ Joint Commission on Accreditation of Healthcare Organizations (JCAHO) accreditation + American Osteopathic Healthcare Association (AOHA) membership ○ American Osteopathic Association (AOA) accreditation △ Commission on Accreditation of Rehabilitation Facilities (CARF) accreditation Control codes 61, 63, 64, 71, 72 and 73 indicate hospitals listed by AOHA, but not registered by AHA. For definition of numerical codes, see page A4	Control	Service	Staffed Beds	Admissions	Census	Outpatient Visits	Births	Total	Payroll	Personnel
☐ VENCOR HOSPITAL–LAS VEGAS, 5100 West Sahara Avenue, Zip 89102-3436; tel. 702/871-1418; Linn P. Billingsley, Administrator (Nonreporting) **A**1 10 **S** Vencor, Incorporated, Louisville, KY	33	49	52	—	—	—	—	—	—	—
★ VETERANS AFFAIRS SOUTHERN NEVADA HEALTHCARE SYSTEM, 1700 Vegas Drive, Zip 89106; tel. 702/636-3000; Ramon J. Reevey, Director **A**5 9 **F**1 3 9 11 16 17 18 19 21 22 23 25 26 29 30 31 32 34 35 36 37 39 43 45 46 48 49 50 51 54 56 57 60 61 62 63 66 70 72 76 77 78 79 **S** Department of Veterans Affairs, Washington, DC	45	10	52	2284	39	234422	0	74275	24111	510
LOVELOCK—Pershing County										
★ PERSHING GENERAL HOSPITAL, 855 Sixth Street, Zip 89419, Mailing Address: P.O. Box 661, Zip 89419-0661; tel. 775/273-2621; Jon Smith, Interim Administrator (Total facility includes 25 beds in nursing home–type unit) (Nonreporting) **A**9 10 **S** Banner Health System, Fargo, ND	16	10	34	—	—	—	—	—	—	—
NELLIS AFB—Meade County										
☒ MIKE O'CALLAGHAN FEDERAL HOSPITAL, 4700 Las Vegas Boulevard North, Suite 2419, Zip 89191-6601; tel. 702/653-2000; Colonel John A. Butler, MSC, Administrator **A**1 **F**1 3 4 5 6 7 11 13 14 15 19 20 22 23 24 25 27 28 30 31 32 33 34 35 36 37 38 39 41 43 44 45 46 47 48 50 51 54 56 58 59 60 61 62 63 64 65 66 70 71 72 73 74 75 76 77 78 79 **P**1 **S** Department of the Air Force, Bowling AFB, DC	41	10	94	4651	61	204292	631	—	—	750
NORTH LAS VEGAS—Clark County										
☒ LAKE MEAD HOSPITAL MEDICAL CENTER, 1409 East Lake Mead Boulevard, Zip 89030-7197; tel. 702/649-7711; William P. Moore, Chief Executive Officer **A**1 10 **F**1 2 7 8 9 11 13 16 17 18 22 25 29 32 38 39 41 44 45 46 48 51 57 62 64 69 70 76 78 **S** TENET Healthcare Corporation, Santa Barbara, CA Web address: www.tenethealth.com	33	10	184	7220	110	44398	1218	45318	18803	550
OWYHEE—Elko County										
☒ U. S. PUBLIC HEALTH SERVICE OWYHEE COMMUNITY HEALTH FACILITY, Mailing Address: P.O. Box 130, Zip 89832-0130; tel. 775/757-2415; Walden Townsend, Service Unit Director (Nonreporting) **A**1 10 **S** U. S. Public Health Service Indian Health Service, Rockville, MD	46	10	15	—	—	—	—	—	—	—
RENO—Washoe County										
☐ BHC WEST HILLS HOSPITAL, 1240 East Ninth Street, Zip 89512-2997, Mailing Address: P.O. Box 30012, Zip 89520-0012; tel. 775/323-0478; Alan G. Chapman, Chief Executive Officer (Nonreporting) **A**1 3 5 10 **S** Behavioral Healthcare Corporation, Nashville, TN Web address: www.hcahealthcare.com	33	22	95	—	—	—	—	—	—	—
BHC WILLOW SPRINGS RESIDENTIAL TREATMENT CENTER, 690 Edison Way, Zip 89502-4135; tel. 775/858-3303; Nancy N. Dandliker, Executive Director (Nonreporting) **S** Behavioral Healthcare Corporation, Nashville, TN	33	52	68	—	—	—	—	—	—	—
☒ △ SAINT MARY'S REGIONAL MEDICAL CENTER, 235 West Sixth Street, Zip 89520-0108; tel. 775/323-2041; Jeff K. Bills, Chief Executive Officer (Total facility includes 16 beds in nursing home–type unit) (Nonreporting) **A**1 7 9 10 Web address: www.saintmarysreno.com	21	10	341	—	—	—	—	—	—	—
☒ VETERANS AFFAIRS SIERRA NEVADA HEALTH CARE SYSTEM, (Formerly Ioannis A. Lougaris Veterans Affairs Medical Center), 1000 Locust Street, Zip 89520-0111; tel. 775/786-7200; Gary R. Whitfield, FACHE, Director (Total facility includes 60 beds in nursing home–type unit) **A**1 3 5 **F**1 3 4 5 6 7 9 11 13 18 19 22 23 24 25 26 27 29 30 31 32 33 34 35 36 37 38 39 41 43 45 46 47 48 49 50 51 54 55 56 57 59 60 61 62 63 64 65 69 70 72 74 76 77 78 79 **P**6 **S** Department of Veterans Affairs, Washington, DC	45	10	126	3050	105	151334	0	63284	32163	689
☒ WASHOE HEALTH SYSTEM, (Formerly Washoe Medical Center), 77 Pringle Way, Zip 89502-1474; tel. 775/982-4100; James I. Miller, President and Chief Executive Officer (Total facility includes 19 beds in nursing home–type unit) (Nonreporting) **A**1 2 3 5 9 10 Web address: www.washoehealth.com	23	10	436	—	—	—	—	—	—	—
SPARKS—Washoe County										
☐ NEVADA MENTAL HEALTH INSTITUTE, 480 Galletti Way, Zip 89431-5574; tel. 775/688-2001; Harold L. Cook, Director (Nonreporting) **A**1 3 5 10	12	22	52	—	—	—	—	—	—	—
☐ NORTHERN NEVADA MEDICAL CENTER, 2375 East Prater Way, Zip 89434-9900; tel. 775/331-7000; James R. Pagels, Chief Executive Officer and Managing Director **A**1 10 **F**9 13 17 18 19 22 24 25 30 31 32 33 34 38 39 41 48 51 53 54 56 57 60 61 62 63 64 70 71 76 77 78 79 **P**5 7 **S** Universal Health Services, Inc., King of Prussia, PA Web address: www.nnmc.com	32	10	100	2663	41	48133	0	28748	11386	408
☐ TAHOE PACIFIC HOSPITAL, 2375 East Prater Way, Zip 89434; tel. 775/331-1044; Clifton Neal Orme, Administrator and Chief Executive Officer **A**1 10 **S** LifeCare Management Services, Dallas, TX	33	10	27	255	20	0	0	8479	2815	91
TONOPAH—Nye County										
NYE REGIONAL MEDICAL CENTER, 825 South Main Street, Zip 89049, Mailing Address: P.O. Box 391, Zip 89049-0391; tel. 775/482-6233; Debra Pearson, Administrator (Total facility includes 24 beds in nursing home–type unit) (Nonreporting) **A**9 10	13	10	45	—	—	—	—	—	—	—
WINNEMUCCA—Humboldt County										
★ HUMBOLDT GENERAL HOSPITAL, 118 East Haskell Street, Zip 89445-3299; tel. 775/623-5222; Byron Quinton, Administrator (Total facility includes 30 beds in nursing home–type unit) **A**9 10 **F**3 8 9 16 17 22 25 39 41 44 48 69 70 76 78 **P**5	16	10	52	763	34	25216	311	10735	4091	140

© 2000 AHA Guide   *Many Facility Codes have changed. Please refer to the AHA Guide Code Chart.*

Hospitals, U.S. / NEVADA

Hospital, Address, Telephone, Administrator, Approval, Facility, and Physician Codes, Health Care System, Network	Classi-fication Codes		Utilization Data					Expense (thousands) of dollars		
	Control	Service	Staffed Beds	Admissions	Census	Outpatient Visits	Births	Total	Payroll	Personnel

★ American Hospital Association (AHA) membership
☐ Joint Commission on Accreditation of Healthcare Organizations (JCAHO) accreditation
+ American Osteopathic Healthcare Association (AOHA) membership
○ American Osteopathic Association (AOA) accreditation
△ Commission on Accreditation of Rehabilitation Facilities (CARF) accreditation
Control codes 61, 63, 64, 71, 72 and 73 indicate hospitals listed by AOHA, but not registered by AHA. For definition of numerical codes, see page A4

YERINGTON—Lyon County

SOUTH LYON MEDICAL CENTER, Surprise at Whitacre Avenue, Zip 89447, Mailing Address: P.O. Box 940, Zip 89447–0940; tel. 775/463–2301; Joan S. Hall, R.N., Administrator (Total facility includes 29 beds in nursing home–type unit) **A**9 10 **F**7 9 12 24 25 32 36 38 39 45 48 54 56 69 77 **P**6	23	10	43	315	43	26453	—	6764	4062	138

Many Facility Codes have changed. Please refer to the AHA Guide Code Chart.   © 2000 AHA Guide

Hospitals, U.S. / NEW HAMPSHIRE

NEW HAMPSHIRE

Resident Population 1,185 (in thousands)
Resident population in metro areas 59.8%
Birth rate per 1,000 population 12.2
65 years and over 12.0%
Percent of persons without health insurance 11.8%

Hospital, Address, Telephone, Administrator, Approval, Facility, and Physician Codes, Health Care System, Network	Classification Codes		Utilization Data					Expense (thousands) of dollars		
★ American Hospital Association (AHA) membership □ Joint Commission on Accreditation of Healthcare Organizations (JCAHO) accreditation + American Osteopathic Healthcare Association (AOHA) membership ○ American Osteopathic Association (AOA) accreditation △ Commission on Accreditation of Rehabilitation Facilities (CARF) accreditation Control codes 61, 63, 64, 71, 72 and 73 indicate hospitals listed by AOHA, but not registered by AHA. For definition of numerical codes, see page A4	Control	Service	Staffed Beds	Admissions	Census	Outpatient Visits	Births	Total	Payroll	Personnel
BERLIN—Coos County ✠ ANDROSCOGGIN VALLEY HOSPITAL, 59 Page Hill Road, Zip 03570–3531; tel. 603/752–2200; Donald F. Saunders, President **A**1 9 10 **F**7 8 9 17 18 22 24 25 30 32 33 34 35 36 37 38 39 41 43 44 45 46 48 54 56 57 59 60 61 62 63 70 72 75 76 78 79 **P**3	23	10	64	2152	34	45344	127	20714	8799	269
CLAREMONT—Sullivan County ★ VALLEY REGIONAL HOSPITAL, 243 Elm Street, Zip 03743–2099; tel. 603/542–7771; Claire L. Bowen, Chief Executive Officer **A**9 10 **F**1 6 7 8 9 13 17 18 19 21 22 23 25 26 27 28 29 30 31 32 33 34 35 37 38 39 40 41 43 44 45 46 48 49 51 54 56 57 59 60 61 62 63 64 67 68 69 70 71 72 73 76 77 78 79 **P**6 Web address: www.vrh.org	23	10	59	1724	18	73266	206	23926	11513	398
COLEBROOK—Coos County ★ UPPER CONNECTICUT VALLEY HOSPITAL, Corliss Lane, Zip 03576–9533, Mailing Address: RFD 2, Box 13, Zip 03576–9533; tel. 603/237–4971; Deanna S. Howard, Chief Executive Officer (Total facility includes 16 beds in nursing home–type unit) **A**9 **F**4 8 9 10 11 12 13 14 16 17 18 19 22 24 25 26 27 30 32 33 34 35 36 37 38 39 41 42 43 44 45 46 47 48 51 52 54 55 57 58 59 61 65 66 68 69 70 72 74 75 76 Web address: www.hitchcock.org/pages/tha	23	10	46	467	5	18500	52	5780	2291	115
CONCORD—Merrimack County ✠ CONCORD HOSPITAL, 250 Pleasant Street, Zip 03301–2598; tel. 603/225–2711; Michael B. Green, President and Chief Executive Officer **A**1 2 3 5 9 10 **F**3 4 6 8 9 10 11 12 13 14 16 17 18 19 20 22 23 24 25 26 27 28 29 30 32 33 34 35 36 37 38 39 41 43 44 45 46 47 48 49 50 54 56 57 58 59 60 61 62 63 64 66 68 70 71 72 73 75 76 77 78 79 **P**6 7 Web address: www.crhc.org	23	10	179	11498	125	240457	1364	114069	52720	1436
□ △ HEALTHSOUTH REHABILITATION HOSPITAL, 254 Pleasant Street, Zip 03301–2508; tel. 603/226–9800; Lori Manor Underwood, Administrator (Nonreporting) **A**1 7 10 **S** HEALTHSOUTH Corporation, Birmingham, AL	33	46	50	—	—	—	—	—	—	—
□ NEW HAMPSHIRE HOSPITAL, 36 Clinton Street, Zip 03301–3861; tel. 603/271–5200; Chester G. Batchelder, Superintendent (Total facility includes 20 beds in nursing home–type unit) **A**1 3 5 10 **F**16 17 18 23 30 35 43 45 50 51 57 58 60 62 69 70 72 78 **P**4 6 7	12	22	232	1169	186	0	0	41038	23505	784
DERRY—Rockingham County ✠ PARKLAND MEDICAL CENTER, One Parkland Drive, Zip 03038–2750; tel. 603/432–1500; Alex M. Marceline Poirier, President and Chief Executive Officer **A**1 2 9 10 **F**7 8 9 13 18 19 22 25 27 31 32 33 34 38 39 41 43 44 46 48 49 50 51 54 56 69 70 72 75 76 78 79 **S** HCA - The Healthcare Company, Nashville, TN Web address: www.parklandmc.com	33	10	79	2892	29	59833	582	32976	14478	434
DOVER—Strafford County ✠ WENTWORTH–DOUGLASS HOSPITAL, 789 Central Avenue, Zip 03820–2589; tel. 603/740–2801; Gregory J. Walker, Chief Executive Officer **A**1 2 9 10 **F**4 7 8 9 11 13 14 16 17 18 19 20 22 24 25 28 30 32 33 34 35 36 37 38 39 41 43 44 45 46 48 49 50 51 54 56 65 66 68 70 71 72 75 76 77 78 79 **P**5 8 Web address: www.wdhospital.com	23	10	115	4259	50	80131	573	56764	23269	734
DUBLIN—Cheshire County BEECH HILL HOSPITAL, New Harrisville Road, Zip 03444, Mailing Address: P.O. Box 254, Zip 03444–0254; tel. 603/563–8511; Matt Feehery, Chief Executive Officer **A**9 **F**2 3	31	82	50	865	30	1536	0	4509	2640	74
EXETER—Rockingham County ✠ EXETER HOSPITAL, 10 Buzell Avenue, Zip 03833–2515; tel. 603/778–7311; Kevin J. Callahan, President and Chief Executive Officer **A**1 2 9 10 **F**4 7 8 9 11 13 14 17 18 19 20 22 24 25 27 28 29 30 31 32 33 34 35 37 38 39 41 43 44 45 46 48 49 50 53 54 57 66 68 69 70 72 75 76 78 79 **P**6 8 Web address: www.ehr.org	23	10	80	3991	41	61283	825	56928	22882	687
FRANKLIN—Merrimack County ✠ FRANKLIN REGIONAL HOSPITAL, 15 Aiken Avenue, Zip 03235–1299; tel. 603/934–2060; Walter A. Strauch, Executive Director **A**1 9 10 **F**8 9 16 17 18 19 22 25 26 32 33 34 36 37 38 43 44 45 48 50 51 54 56 59 61 62 69 70 72 76 78 79 **P**6 8 Web address: www.frh.org	23	10	49	1849	29	44611	95	18834	10093	290
GREENFIELD—Hillsborough County CROTCHED MOUNTAIN REHABILITATION CENTER, 1 Verney Drive, Zip 03047–5000; tel. 603/547–3311; Major W. Wheelock, President (Total facility includes 62 beds in nursing home–type unit) **F**6 13 16 17 18 19 23 28 31 32 43 53 54 58 70 72 78 Web address: www.cmf.org	23	46	146	38	102	0	0	21898	12575	452

© 2000 AHA Guide   *Many Facility Codes have changed. Please refer to the AHA Guide Code Chart.*   Hospitals **A271**

Hospitals, U.S. / NEW HAMPSHIRE

Hospital, Address, Telephone, Administrator, Approval, Facility, and Physician Codes, Health Care System, Network	Classification Codes		Utilization Data					Expense (thousands) of dollars		
★ American Hospital Association (AHA) membership. ☐ Joint Commission on Accreditation of Healthcare Organizations (JCAHO) accreditation + American Osteopathic Healthcare Association (AOHA) membership ○ American Osteopathic Association (AOA) accreditation △ Commission on Accreditation of Rehabilitation Facilities (CARF) accreditation Control codes 61, 63, 64, 71, 72 and 73 indicate hospitals listed by AOHA, but not registered by AHA. For definition of numerical codes, see page A4.	Control	Service	Staffed Beds	Admissions	Census	Outpatient Visits	Births	Total	Payroll	Personnel
HAMPSTEAD—Rockingham County ☐ HAMPSTEAD HOSPITAL, 218 East Road, Zip 03841-2228; tel. 603/329-5311; Phillip J. Kubiak, President (Nonreporting) **A**1 9 10 Web address: www.hampsteadhospital.com	33	22	99	—	—	—	—	—	—	—
KEENE—Cheshire County ★ △ CHESHIRE MEDICAL CENTER, 580 Court Street, Zip 03431-1718; tel. 603/354-5400; Robert J. Langlais, President and Chief Executive Officer (Total facility includes 8 beds in nursing home–type unit) **A**1 2 7 9 10 **F**1 8 9 12 13 16 17 18 19 20 21 22 23 24 25 26 27 28 29 31 32 33 34 35 36 37 38 39 40 41 43 44 45 46 48 49 50 51 53 54 56 57 58 59 60 61 62 63 64 65 68 69 70 71 72 75 76 77 78 79 **P**1 Web address: www.cheshire-med.com	23	10	149	4894	71	94706	467	47339	21129	686
LACONIA—Belknap County ★ LAKES REGION GENERAL HOSPITAL, 80 Highland Street, Zip 03246-3298; tel. 603/524-3211; Thomas Clairmont, President **A**2 9 10 **F**1 3 4 7 8 9 11 13 14 16 17 18 19 20 21 22 24 25 27 28 30 32 34 35 37 38 39 41 43 44 45 46 48 49 50 54 57 58 59 60 61 62 68 70 72 75 76 77 78 79 **P**6 8 Web address: www.lrgh.org	23	10	117	5008	66	42422	531	62588	29506	802
LANCASTER—Coos County ★ WEEKS MEDICAL CENTER, (Formerly Weeks Medical Hospital), 173 Middle Street, Zip 03584; tel. 603/788-4911; Scott W. Howe, Chief Executive Officer **A**1 9 10 **F**8 13 16 17 18 19 22 24 25 30 32 33 34 35 36 37 38 41 43 44 45 46 48 51 54 61 70 71 72 73 76 78 79 **P**6 Web address: www.weeks.hitchcock.org	23	10	31	1086	14	64776	88	15169	8335	264
LEBANON—Grafton County ★ ALICE PECK DAY MEMORIAL HOSPITAL, 125 Mascoma Street, Zip 03766-2650; tel. 603/448-3121; Robert A. Mesropian, President and Chief Executive Officer (Total facility includes 50 beds in nursing home–type unit) **A**9 10 **F**6 7 8 9 13 14 16 17 18 19 20 22 24 25 29 30 31 32 33 34 37 38 39 42 45 46 48 49 50 51 54 56 67 69 70 72 75 76 77 78 **P**8 Web address: www.alicepeckday.org	23	10	72	808	55	30699	233	17316	9442	265
★ MARY HITCHCOCK MEMORIAL HOSPITAL, One Medical Center Drive, Zip 03756-0001; tel. 603/650-5000; James W. Varnum, President **A**1 3 5 8 9 10 **F**3 4 7 8 9 11 12 13 17 18 19 21 22 24 25 26 27 29 30 31 32 33 34 35 36 37 38 39 40 41 42 43 44 45 46 47 48 49 50 51 52 53 54 56 57 58 59 61 62 63 64 65 66 68 70 71 72 73 74 75 76 77 78 79 **P**3 Web address: www.hitchcock.org/pages/tha/ucvh.html	23	10	315	17849	243	406455	996	258299	92784	2855
LITTLETON—Grafton County ★ LITTLETON REGIONAL HOSPITAL, 262 Cottage Street, Zip 03561-4101; tel. 603/444-7731; Robert S. Pearson, Administrator **A**1 2 9 10 **F**8 9 13 17 18 19 20 22 24 25 26 30 31 32 34 37 38 39 41 43 44 45 46 48 49 54 56 70 71 72 73 76 77 78 79 **P**6 **S** Quorum Health Group, Brentwood, TN Web address: www.littletonhospital.org	23	10	49	1318	11	36609	252	21018	9180	251
MANCHESTER—Hillsborough County ★ △ CATHOLIC MEDICAL CENTER, 100 McGregor Street, Zip 03102-3770; tel. 603/668-3545; Alyson Pitman Giles, President and Chief Executive Officer **A**1 7 9 10 **F**4 7 9 11 12 13 16 17 18 19 21 22 23 24 25 26 28 30 31 32 33 34 35 38 39 41 43 46 47 48 49 50 51 53 54 57 59 61 63 64 67 70 71 72 73 75 76 77 78 **P**4 7 8	23	10	204	7558	125	72018	0	105853	34480	1052
★ ELLIOT HOSPITAL, One Elliot Way, Zip 03103; tel. 603/669-5300; Douglas F. Dean, Jr, President and Chief Executive Officer **A**1 2 10 **F**1 5 6 7 8 9 11 13 14 15 17 18 19 20 21 22 24 25 26 27 28 29 30 31 32 33 34 35 36 37 38 39 41 42 43 44 45 46 48 49 50 51 54 56 57 59 60 61 62 63 64 65 66 67 68 70 71 72 75 76 77 78 79 **P**6 7 8	23	10	225	10620	134	93389	2650	109861	37247	1170
★ VETERANS AFFAIRS MEDICAL CENTER, 718 Smyth Road, Zip 03104-4098; tel. 603/624-4366; Marc Levenson, Administrator (Total facility includes 120 beds in nursing home–type unit) (Nonreporting) **A**1 9 **S** Department of Veterans Affairs, Washington, DC Web address: www.va.gov/stations97/guide/home.asp?DIVISION=ALL	45	10	180	—	—	—	—	—	—	—
NASHUA—Hillsborough County ★ SOUTHERN NEW HAMPSHIRE MEDICAL CENTER, 8 Prospect Street, Zip 03061, Mailing Address: P.O. Box 2014, Zip 03061-2014; tel. 603/577-2000; Thomas E. Wilhelmsen, Jr, President and Chief Executive Officer **A**1 2 9 10 **F**1 3 8 9 11 13 14 16 17 18 19 21 22 24 25 26 27 32 33 34 35 36 37 38 39 41 42 43 44 45 46 48 49 50 51 54 56 57 58 59 60 61 62 63 64 66 68 70 71 72 75 76 77 78 79 **P**6 8 Web address: www.snhmc.org	23	10	175	7203	73	155051	1472	68166	33377	963
★ △ ST. JOSEPH HOSPITAL, 172 Kinsley Street, Zip 03061; tel. 603/882-3000; Peter B. Davis, President and Chief Executive Officer **A**1 2 6 7 9 10 **F**1 3 7 8 9 11 13 14 16 17 18 19 20 21 22 23 24 25 26 27 29 30 31 32 33 34 35 36 37 38 39 40 41 43 44 45 46 48 49 50 51 53 54 56 57 62 63 65 68 70 72 75 76 77 78 79 **P**6 8 **S** Covenant Health Systems, Inc., Lexington, MA Web address: www.nh-healthcare.org	21	10	208	3405	48	97228	530	40559	18037	826
NEW LONDON—Merrimack County ★ NEW LONDON HOSPITAL, 270 County Road, Zip 03257-4570; tel. 603/526-2911; Maureen McNamara, President and Chief Executive Officer (Total facility includes 58 beds in nursing home–type unit) **A**1 9 10 **F**8 9 13 14 16 17 18 19 21 22 23 25 28 29 32 34 36 37 39 41 43 45 46 48 50 54 56 66 69 70 71 72 76 77 78 79 **P**8	23	10	93	1371	67	155150	130	19733	9862	305

Many Facility Codes have changed. Please refer to the AHA Guide Code Chart.

Hospitals, U.S. / NEW HAMPSHIRE

Hospital, Address, Telephone, Administrator, Approval, Facility, and Physician Codes, Health Care System, Network	Classification Codes		Utilization Data					Expense (thousands) of dollars		Personnel
★ American Hospital Association (AHA) membership ☐ Joint Commission on Accreditation of Healthcare Organizations (JCAHO) accreditation + American Osteopathic Healthcare Association (AOHA) membership ○ American Osteopathic Association (AOA) accreditation △ Commission on Accreditation of Rehabilitation Facilities (CARF) accreditation Control codes 61, 63, 64, 71, 72 and 73 indicate hospitals listed by AOHA, but not registered by AHA. For definition of numerical codes, see page A4	Control	Service	Staffed Beds	Admissions	Census	Outpatient Visits	Births	Total	Payroll	
NORTH CONWAY—Carroll County MEMORIAL HOSPITAL, 3073 Main Street, Zip 03860–5001, Mailing Address: P.O. Box 5001, Zip 03860–5001; tel. 603/356–5461; Gary R. Poquette, FACHE, Executive Director (Total facility includes 45 beds in nursing home–type unit) **A**9 10 **F**1 2 7 8 9 13 16 17 18 19 22 24 25 32 33 34 38 39 41 44 45 46 48 50 51 53 54 57 61 68 69 70 72 73 75 76 78 79 **P**3	23	10	80	1621	59	34419	239	20561	7846	272
PETERBOROUGH—Hillsborough County ✠ MONADNOCK COMMUNITY HOSPITAL, 452 Old Street Road, Zip 03458–1295; tel. 603/924–7191; Peter L. Gosline, Chief Executive Officer **A**1 9 10 **F**4 8 9 13 16 17 18 19 21 22 23 25 26 27 30 32 33 34 35 36 37 38 39 40 41 43 44 45 46 47 48 49 50 51 54 56 57 60 61 62 63 64 70 71 72 75 76 78 79 **P**6	23	10	62	1734	23	73863	374	18030	8592	278
PLYMOUTH—Grafton County SPEARE MEMORIAL HOSPITAL, 16 Hospital Road, Zip 03264–1199; tel. 603/536–1120; David L. Pearse, President **A**9 10 **F**8 9 12 14 16 17 19 20 22 23 25 34 37 41 43 44 45 46 48 49 54 68 70 72 76 78 **P**8 Web address: www.spearehospital.com	23	10	28	967	10	36549	113	13338	6834	183
PORTSMOUTH—Rockingham County ✠ PORTSMOUTH REGIONAL HOSPITAL AND PAVILION, 333 Borthwick Avenue, Zip 03801–7004; tel. 603/436–5110; William J. Schuler, Chief Executive Officer **A**1 9 10 **F**3 4 8 9 11 12 13 14 19 20 21 22 24 25 27 28 30 32 34 39 41 43 44 45 46 47 48 49 54 57 58 61 62 63 64 68 70 76 77 78 79 **P**8 **S** HCA - The Healthcare Company, Nashville, TN Web address: www.portsmouthhospital.com	33	10	179	7119	113	98057	911	—	—	785
ROCHESTER—Strafford County ✠ FRISBIE MEMORIAL HOSPITAL, 11 Whitehall Road, Zip 03867–3297; tel. 603/332–5211; Alvin D. Felgar, President and Chief Executive Officer **A**1 2 9 10 **F**8 9 11 12 14 17 18 19 22 23 24 25 26 30 34 35 38 39 41 43 44 45 46 48 49 51 54 55 57 59 60 62 63 64 68 70 71 72 76 78 79 **P**5 6 8 Web address: www.frisbiehospital.com	23	10	70	2933	37	58721	473	35584	15537	435
SALEM—Rockingham County ☐ △ NORTHEAST REHABILITATION HOSPITAL, 70 Butler Street, Zip 03079; tel. 603/893–2900; John F. Prochilo, Chief Executive Officer and Administrator **A**1 7 10 **F**13 16 17 18 19 32 36 38 43 45 49 50 51 53 54 70 71 72 78 79 Web address: www.rehabnet.com	33	46	80	1274	65	125651	0	27343	13253	446
WOLFEBORO—Carroll County ★ HUGGINS HOSPITAL, 240 South Main Street, Zip 03894–4411, Mailing Address: P.O. Box 912, Zip 03894–0912; tel. 603/569–7500; Leslie N. H. MacLeod, President (Total facility includes 27 beds in nursing home–type unit) **A**9 10 **F**1 6 7 8 9 18 22 25 30 32 34 38 41 43 44 45 48 49 51 54 67 69 70 72 76 79 **P**1 Web address: www.hugginshospital.org	23	10	82	1670	49	54708	121	18464	8322	273
WOODSVILLE—Grafton County ✠ COTTAGE HOSPITAL, Swiftwater Road, Zip 03785–2001, Mailing Address: P.O. Box 2001, Zip 03785–2001; tel. 603/747–2761; Reginald J. Lavoie, Administrator **A**1 2 9 10 **F**8 9 13 17 18 22 23 25 26 27 34 36 37 38 39 40 41 43 46 48 49 54 56 59 69 70 72 76 78 79 **P**8	23	10	34	944	11	37721	66	11736	6273	167

© 2000 AHA Guide   *Many Facility Codes have changed. Please refer to the AHA Guide Code Chart.*

NEW JERSEY

Resident Population 8,115 (in thousands)
Resident population in metro areas 100.0%
Birth rate per 1,000 population 14.1
65 years and over 13.6%
Percent of persons without health insurance 16.5%

★ American Hospital Association (AHA) membership
□ Joint Commission on Accreditation of Healthcare Organizations (JCAHO) accreditation
+ American Osteopathic Healthcare Association (AOHA) membership
○ American Osteopathic Association (AOA) accreditation
△ Commission on Accreditation of Rehabilitation Facilities (CARF) accreditation
Control codes 61, 63, 64, 71, 72 and 73 indicate hospitals listed by AOHA, but not registered by AHA. For definition of numerical codes, see page A4

Hospital, Address, Telephone, Administrator, Approval, Facility, and Physician Codes, Health Care System, Network	Classification Codes		Utilization Data					Expense (thousands) of dollars		
	Control	Service	Staffed Beds	Admissions	Census	Outpatient Visits	Births	Total	Payroll	Personnel
ANCORA—Atlantic County										
□ ANCORA PSYCHIATRIC HOSPITAL, 202 Spring Garden Road, Zip 08037-9699; tel. 609/561-1700; Gregory P. Roberts, Chief Executive Officer (Nonreporting) **A**1 10 **S** Division of Mental Health Services, Department of Human Services, State of New Jersey, Trenton, NJ	12	22	625	—	—	—	—	—	—	—
ATLANTIC CITY—Atlantic County										
★ ATLANTIC CITY MEDICAL CENTER, 1925 Pacific Avenue, Zip 08401-6713; tel. 609/345-4000; David P. Tilton, President and Chief Executive Officer (Total facility includes 14 beds in nursing home-type unit) **A**1 2 3 9 10 **F**3 7 9 11 12 13 14 16 17 18 19 21 22 24 25 29 30 31 32 33 34 35 36 37 38 39 41 42 44 45 46 48 49 51 52 53 54 56 57 58 59 60 61 62 63 64 65 66 68 69 70 71 72 73 75 76 77 78 79 **P**6 Web address: www.atlanticare.org	23	10	413	21027	312	248675	2112	194724	87578	2049
BAYONNE—Hudson County										
★ BAYONNE HOSPITAL, 29 East 29th Street, Zip 07002-4699; tel. 201/858-5000; Michael R. D'Agnes, President and Chief Executive Officer (Nonreporting) **A**1 2 6 9 10 Web address: www.bayonnehospital.com	23	10	261	—	—	—	—	—	—	—
BELLE MEAD—Somerset County										
★ CARRIER FOUNDATION, County Route 601, P.O. Box 147, Zip 08502-0147; tel. 908/281-1000; C. Richard Sarle, President and Chief Executive Officer (Nonreporting) **A**1 9 10 Web address: www.carrier.org	23	22	100	—	—	—	—	—	—	—
BELLEVILLE—Essex County										
★ CLARA MAASS HEALTH SYSTEM, 1 Clara Maass Drive, Zip 07109-3557; tel. 973/450-2000; Thomas A. Biga, Executive Director (Total facility includes 179 beds in nursing home-type unit) (Nonreporting) **A**1 2 9 10 **S** Saint Barnabas Health Care System, West Orange, NJ Web address: www.sbhcs.com	23	10	644	—	—	—	—	—	—	—
BERKELEY HEIGHTS—Union County										
★ RUNNELLS SPECIALIZED HOSPITAL OF UNION COUNTY, 40 Watchung Way, Zip 07922-2618; tel. 908/771-5700; Joseph W. Sharp, Administrator (Total facility includes 300 beds in nursing home-type unit) **A**9 10 **F**23 31 37 53 54 57 69 70 78 **P**6 Web address: www.unioncoutynj.org/runells	13	49	345	731	329	—	0	33508	19189	467
BERLIN—Camden County										
★ VIRTUA WEST JERSEY HOSPITAL–BERLIN, (Formerly West Jersey Hospital–Berlin), 100 Townsend Avenue, Zip 08009-9035; tel. 856/322-3100; Ellen Guarnieri, Vice President and Chief Operating Officer (Nonreporting) **A**9 **S** Virtua Health, Marlton, NJ Web address: www.virtua.org	23	10	79	—	—	—	—	—	—	—
BLACKWOOD—Camden County										
□ CAMDEN COUNTY HEALTH SERVICES CENTER, Woodbury–Turnersville Road, Zip 08012-2799, Mailing Address: P.O. Box 1639, Zip 08012-2799; tel. 856/374-6600; Stanford A. Alliker, Chief Executive Officer (Total facility includes 275 beds in nursing home-type unit) (Nonreporting) **A**1 9 10	13	49	422	—	—	—	—	—	—	—
BOONTON TOWNSHIP—Morris County										
SAINT CLARE'S HOSPITAL/BOONTON TOWNSHIP See Saint Clare's Health Services, Denville										
BRICK TOWNSHIP—Ocean County										
MEDICAL CENTER OF OCEAN COUNTY See Raritan Bay Medical Center, Perth Amboy										
BRIDGETON—Cumberland County										
★ △ SOUTH JERSEY HOSPITAL, (Includes South Jersey Hospital–Bridgeton, 333 Irving Avenue, tel. 856/451-6600; South Jersey Hospital–Elmer, West Front Street, Elmer, Zip 08318-0516, Mailing Address: P.O. Box 1090, Zip 08318-1090; tel. 856/363-1000; South Jersey Hospital–Millville, 1200 North High, Millville, Zip 08332-2586; tel. 856/825-3500), 333 Irving Avenue, Zip 08302-2100; tel. 856/451-6600; Chester B. Kaletkowski, President and Chief Executive Officer **A**1 2 7 9 10 **F**3 7 8 9 13 16 17 18 19 21 22 23 24 25 28 29 33 34 36 37 38 41 43 44 45 46 48 50 51 54 57 58 59 60 61 62 63 64 65 70 71 72 73 76 78 **S** South Jersey Health System, Bridgeton, NJ Web address: www.sjhs.com	23	10	340	12367	200	246658	817	118588	55260	1529
BROWNS MILLS—Burlington County										
★ DEBORAH HEART AND LUNG CENTER, 200 Trenton Road, Zip 08015-1799; tel. 609/893-6611; John R. Ernst, Executive Director (Nonreporting) **A**1 3 5 9 10 13 Web address: www.deborah.org	23	49	161	—	—	—	—	—	—	—

Hospitals, U.S. / NEW JERSEY

Hospital, Address, Telephone, Administrator, Approval, Facility, and Physician Codes, Health Care System, Network	Classification Codes		Utilization Data					Expense (thousands) of dollars		
★ American Hospital Association (AHA) membership □ Joint Commission on Accreditation of Healthcare Organizations (JCAHO) accreditation + American Osteopathic Healthcare Association (AOHA) membership ○ American Osteopathic Association (AOA) accreditation △ Commission on Accreditation of Rehabilitation Facilities (CARF) accreditation Control codes 61, 63, 64, 71, 72 and 73 indicate hospitals listed by AOHA, but not registered by AHA. For definition of numerical codes, see page A4	Control	Service	Staffed Beds	Admissions	Census	Outpatient Visits	Births	Total	Payroll	Personnel
CAMDEN—Camden County										
✦ △ OUR LADY OF LOURDES MEDICAL CENTER, 1600 Haddon Avenue, Zip 08103–3117; tel. 856/757–3500; Alexander J. Hatala, President and Chief Executive Officer (Nonreporting) **A**1 3 5 7 9 10 12 13 **S** Catholic Health East, Newtown Square, PA **Web address:** www.lourdesnet.org	23	10	300	—	—	—	—	—	—	—
✦ THE COOPER HEALTH SYSTEM, One Cooper Plaza, Zip 08103–1489; tel. 856/342–2000; Leslie D. Hirsch, President and Chief Executive Officer (Nonreporting) **A**1 2 3 5 8 9 10 13 **Web address:** www.cooperhealth.org	23	10	370	—	—	—	—	—	—	—
✦ VIRTUA WEST JERSEY HOSPITAL–CAMDEN, 1000 Atlantic Avenue, Zip 08104–1595; tel. 856/246–3000; Carolyn M. Ballard, Executive Director (Nonreporting) **A**1 2 3 5 9 10 **S** Virtua Health, Marlton, NJ **Web address:** www.wjhs.org	23	10	117	—	—	—	—	—	—	—
CAPE MAY COURT HOUSE—Cape May County										
✦ BURDETTE TOMLIN MEMORIAL HOSPITAL, 2 Stone Harbor Boulevard, Zip 08210–9990; tel. 609/463–2000; Thomas L. Scott, FACHE, President and Chief Executive Officer **A**1 9 10 **F**3 7 8 9 13 14 16 17 18 19 21 22 23 24 25 26 31 32 37 38 39 41 43 44 45 46 48 49 50 51 54 56 61 63 70 72 73 75 76 78 **P**7 **Web address:** www.btmh.com	23	10	206	10175	161	125520	617	70047	31988	889
CEDAR GROVE—Essex County										
□ ESSEX COUNTY HOSPITAL CENTER, 125 Fairview Avenue, Zip 07009–1399; tel. 973/228–8200; Muriel M. Shore, Ed.D., R.N., Chief Executive Officer **A**1 10 **F**10 12 22 23 24 31 32 39 41 48 51 55 57 62 68 70 72 76	13	22	400	452	335	0	0	39728	28965	496
CHERRY HILL—Camden County										
★ + ○ KENNEDY MEMORIAL HOSPITALS–UNIVERSITY MEDICAL CENTER, (Includes Kennedy Memorial Hospital, 18 East Laurel Road, Stratford, Zip 08084; tel. 609/346–6000; Kennedy Memorial Hospital, 435 Hurffville–Cross Keys Road, Turnersville, Zip 08012; tel. 609/582–2500); 2201 Chapel Avenue West, Zip 08002–2048; tel. 856/488–6500; Joseph W. Devine, Vice President, Hospital Services **A**9 10 11 12 13 **F**2 3 6 8 9 11 13 14 16 17 18 19 21 22 23 24 25 30 31 32 33 34 35 36 38 39 41 42 43 44 45 46 47 49 50 51 54 56 57 58 59 60 61 62 63 64 66 68 70 71 72 76 78 79	23	10	458	23171	277	363600	1757	194769	84152	2116
DENVILLE—Morris County										
✦ SAINT CLARE'S HEALTH SERVICES, (Includes Saint Clare's Hospital/Boonton Township, 130 Powerville Road, Boonton Township, Zip 07005; tel. 201/625–6000; Saint Clare's Hospital/Denville, 25 Pocono Road, Zip 07834; tel. 201/625–6000; Saint Clare's Hospital/Sussex, 20 Walnut Street, Sussex, Zip 07461; tel. 201/702–2200; St. Clare's Hospital/Dover, 400 West Blackwell Street, Dover, Zip 07801–3311; tel. 201/989–3000), 25 Pocono Road, Zip 07834–2995; tel. 973/625–6000; Kathryn J. McDonagh, President and Chief Executive Officer (Total facility includes 150 beds in nursing home–type unit) **A**1 2 9 10 **F**1 2 3 6 7 8 9 11 13 14 16 17 18 19 20 21 22 23 24 25 26 27 28 29 30 31 32 33 34 35 36 37 38 39 40 41 42 43 44 45 46 48 49 51 54 56 57 58 59 60 61 62 63 64 65 67 69 70 71 72 73 75 76 77 78 79 **P**1 5 7 **S** Marian Health System, Tulsa, OK **Web address:** www.saintclares.org	21	10	662	22275	330	180981	2274	226467	102413	2643
DOVER—Morris County										
ST. CLARE'S HOSPITAL/DOVER See Saint Clare's Health Services, Denville										
EAST ORANGE—Essex County										
✦ EAST ORANGE GENERAL HOSPITAL, 300 Central Avenue, Zip 07019–2819; tel. 973/672–8400; Darlene L. Cox, President and Chief Executive Officer **A**1 9 10 **F**2 3 7 9 13 14 16 17 18 19 21 22 24 25 29 30 31 34 35 36 37 38 41 45 46 48 51 54 57 58 59 60 61 62 63 64 68 70 72 76 78 79	23	10	209	7899	159	146267	0	79615	39112	842
✦ VETERANS AFFAIRS NEW JERSEY HEALTH CARE SYSTEM, (Includes East Orange Division, 385 Tremont Avenue, tel. 973/676–1000; Lyons Division, 151 Knollcroft Road, Lyons, Zip 07939–9998; tel. 908/647–0180), 385 Tremont Avenue, Zip 07018–1095; tel. 973/676–1000; Kenneth H. Mizrach, Director (Total facility includes 300 beds in nursing home–type unit) **A**1 2 3 5 8 **F**1 2 3 7 9 11 12 13 19 20 21 22 24 25 26 28 29 30 32 33 34 35 36 38 39 41 43 45 46 48 49 50 51 53 54 56 57 59 61 62 63 64 68 69 70 72 76 78 79 **P**6 **S** Department of Veterans Affairs, Washington, DC **Web address:** www.va.gov/stations97/guide/home.asp?DIVISION=ALL	45	49	934	7124	734	419571	0	236380	126051	2882
EDISON—Middlesex County										
★ △ JFK JOHNSON REHABILITATION INSTITUTE, 65 James Street, Zip 08818–3059; tel. 732/321–7050; Scott Gebhard, Senior Vice President Operations (Nonreporting) **A**7 10 **S** Solaris Health System, Edison, NJ **Web address:** www.solarishs.org	23	46	92	—	—	—	—	—	—	—
✦ JFK MEDICAL CENTER, 65 James Street, Zip 08818–3947; tel. 732/321–7000; John P. McGee, President and Chief Executive Officer (Nonreporting) **A**1 2 3 5 9 10 **S** Solaris Health System, Edison, NJ **Web address:** jfkmc.org/index.htm	23	10	380	—	—	—	—	—	—	—
ELIZABETH—Union County										
✦ ST. ELIZABETH HOSPITAL, 225 Williamson Street, Zip 07202–3600; tel. 908/527–5000; Sister Elizabeth Ann Maloney, President and Chief Executive Officer (Nonreporting) **A**1 2 3 9 10	21	10	266	—	—	—	—	—	—	—

Hospitals, U.S. / NEW JERSEY

Hospital, Address, Telephone, Administrator, Approval, Facility, and Physician Codes, Health Care System, Network	Classification Codes		Utilization Data					Expense (thousands) of dollars		
	Control	Service	Staffed Beds	Admissions	Census	Outpatient Visits	Births	Total	Payroll	Personnel

★ American Hospital Association (AHA) membership
□ Joint Commission on Accreditation of Healthcare Organizations (JCAHO) accreditation
+ American Osteopathic Healthcare Association (AOHA) membership
○ American Osteopathic Association (AOA) accreditation
△ Commission on Accreditation of Rehabilitation Facilities (CARF) accreditation
Control codes 61, 63, 64, 71, 72 and 73 indicate hospitals listed by AOHA, but not registered by AHA. For definition of numerical codes, see page A4

Hospital	Control	Service	Staffed Beds	Admissions	Census	Outpatient Visits	Births	Total	Payroll	Personnel
★ TRINITAS HOSPITAL, (Formerly Elizabeth General Medical Center), 925 East Jersey Street, Zip 07201–2728; tel. 908/289–8600; David A. Fletcher, President and Chief Executive Officer (Total facility includes 137 beds in nursing home–type unit) **A**1 2 3 5 6 9 10 **F**1 3 7 8 9 11 13 16 17 18 19 20 21 22 23 24 25 30 32 33 34 35 37 38 41 43 44 45 46 48 49 50 54 56 57 58 59 60 61 62 63 64 65 69 70 72 76 78 79 **Web address:** www.egmc.org	23	10	402	8877	298	270052	689	123878	62226	1556
ELMER—Salem County SOUTH JERSEY HOSPITAL–ELMER See South Jersey Hospital, Bridgeton										
ENGLEWOOD—Bergen County ★ ENGLEWOOD HOSPITAL AND MEDICAL CENTER, 350 Engle Street, Zip 07631–1898; tel. 201/894–3000; Daniel A. Kane, President and Chief Executive Officer (Nonreporting) **A**1 2 3 5 6 9 10	23	10	318	—	—	—	—	—	—	—
FLEMINGTON—Hunterdon County ★ HUNTERDON MEDICAL CENTER, 2100 Wescott Drive, Zip 08822–4604; tel. 908/788–6100; Robert P. Wise, President and Chief Executive Officer **A**1 2 3 5 9 10 **F**1 3 7 8 9 11 13 14 16 17 18 19 21 22 24 25 26 28 29 30 32 33 34 35 36 37 38 39 41 43 44 45 46 48 49 50 51 54 56 57 58 59 60 61 62 63 64 65 66 70 72 73 76 78 79 **P**1 5 **Web address:** www.hunterdonhealthcare.org	23	10	176	7574	104	220113	1381	94690	49376	1266
FLORHAM PARK—Morris County ★ ATLANTIC HEALTH SYSTEM, (Includes General Hospital Center at Passaic, 350 Boulevard, Passaic, Zip 07055–2800; tel. 973/365–4300; Morristown Memorial Hospital, 100 Madison Avenue, Morristown, Zip 07962–1956; tel. 973/971–5000; Mountainside Hospital, Bay and Highland Avenues, Montclair, Zip 07042–4898; tel. 973/429–6000; Overlook Hospital, 99 Beauvoir Avenue, Summit, Zip 07902–0220; tel. 908/522–2000), 325 Columbia Turnpike, Zip 07932–0959, Mailing Address: P.O. Box 959, Zip 07932–0959; tel. 973/660–3100; Richard P. Oths, President and Chief Executive Officer **A**1 2 3 5 6 8 10 **F**2 3 4 5 7 8 9 11 13 14 17 18 19 20 21 22 23 24 25 26 28 29 30 31 32 33 34 35 37 38 39 40 42 43 44 45 46 47 48 49 50 51 52 53 54 56 57 58 59 60 61 62 63 64 65 66 69 70 71 72 73 75 76 77 78 79 **P**4 5 6 7 **Web address:** www.ATLANTICHEALTH.ORG	23	10	1404	81339	1024	750161	8026	697469	332213	7999
FREEHOLD—Monmouth County ★ CENTRASTATE HEALTHCARE SYSTEM, 901 West Main Street, Zip 07728–2549; tel. 732/431–2000; Thomas H. Litz, FACHE, President and Chief Executive Officer **A**1 9 10 **F**6 7 8 9 11 12 13 14 16 17 18 19 21 22 25 27 30 32 33 34 36 37 38 39 41 43 44 45 46 48 50 51 54 55 56 57 59 60 61 66 67 69 70 71 73 74 75 76 77 78 79 **P**5 8	23	10	241	10793	147	138428	1279	88166	42848	1446
GLEN GARDNER—Hunterdon County □ SENATOR GARRETT T. W. HAGEDORN GERO PSYCHIATRIC HOSPITAL, 200 Sanitorium Road, Zip 08826–9752; tel. 908/537–2141; Donald A. Bruckman, Acting Chief Executive Officer (Nonreporting) **A**1 10 **S** Division of Mental Health Services, Department of Human Services, State of New Jersey, Trenton, NJ	12	22	181	—	—	—	—	—	—	—
GREYSTONE PARK—Morris County ★ GREYSTONE PARK PSYCHIATRIC HOSPITAL, Central Avenue, Zip 07950, Mailing Address: P.O. Box A, Zip 07950; tel. 973/538–1800; Michael Greenstein, Chief Executive Officer **A**1 10 **F**3 9 12 13 17 18 23 25 26 31 38 41 44 48 51 53 54 57 59 60 61 62 63 70 78 **P**6 **S** Division of Mental Health Services, Department of Human Services, State of New Jersey, Trenton, NJ	12	22	605	473	767	0	0	—	—	1203
HACKENSACK—Bergen County ★ HACKENSACK UNIVERSITY MEDICAL CENTER, 30 Prospect Avenue, Zip 07601–1991; tel. 201/996–2000; John P. Ferguson, FACHE, President and Chief Executive Officer **A**1 2 3 5 8 9 10 **F**3 4 5 7 8 9 11 12 13 14 16 17 18 19 20 21 22 24 25 28 29 30 31 32 33 34 35 36 37 38 39 40 41 42 43 44 45 46 47 48 49 50 51 52 54 56 57 58 59 60 61 62 63 64 65 66 70 71 72 73 74 75 76 77 78 79 **P**5 7 8 **Web address:** www.humed.com	23	10	556	60068	534	1535953	4096	490297	226082	4770
HACKETTSTOWN—Warren County ★ HACKETTSTOWN COMMUNITY HOSPITAL, 651 Willow Grove Street, Zip 07840–1798; tel. 908/852–5100; Gene C. Milton, President and Chief Executive Officer **A**1 9 10 **F**3 8 9 13 16 17 18 19 21 22 24 25 26 28 30 32 33 34 37 38 39 40 41 43 44 45 46 48 49 50 51 54 63 70 71 72 76 78 79	21	10	106	4105	53	47772	588	33995	15336	439
HAMILTON—Mercer County ★ ROBERT WOOD JOHNSON UNIVERSITY HOSPITAL AT HAMILTON, One Hamilton Health Place, Zip 08690–3599; tel. 609/586–7900; Christy Stephenson, Chief Administrative Officer **A**1 10 **F**1 7 8 9 11 12 13 14 16 17 18 19 22 23 24 25 26 30 31 32 33 34 36 37 38 39 40 41 43 44 45 46 48 49 50 51 54 56 65 66 68 69 70 72 73 76 77 78 79 **P**6 7 **Web address:** www.rwjhamilton.org	23	10	160	7370	104	77139	732	65593	26262	737
HAMMONTON—Atlantic County ★ WILLIAM B. KESSLER MEMORIAL HOSPITAL, 600 South White Horse Pike, Zip 08037–2099; tel. 609/561–6700; Warren E. Gager, President and Chief Executive Officer (Nonreporting) **A**1 9 10	23	10	96	—	—	—	—	—	—	—
HOBOKEN—Hudson County □ ST. MARY HOSPITAL, 308 Willow Avenue, Zip 07030–3889; tel. 201/418–1000; Robert S. Chaloner, President and Chief Executive Officer **A**1 3 10 **F**1 3 9 13 14 18 19 20 21 22 23 24 25 26 30 31 32 33 34 35 36 37 38 40 41 42 43 45 46 48 49 52 54 56 57 58 59 60 61 62 63 64 70 72 73 76 78 79 **P**8 **S** Franciscan Health Partnership, Inc., Latham, NY	23	10	223	9295	139	136927	—	82950	46577	878

Hospitals, U.S. / NEW JERSEY

Hospital, Address, Telephone, Administrator, Approval, Facility, and Physician Codes, Health Care System, Network	Classification Codes		Utilization Data					Expense (thousands) of dollars		
★ American Hospital Association (AHA) membership □ Joint Commission on Accreditation of Healthcare Organizations (JCAHO) accreditation + American Osteopathic Healthcare Association (AOHA) membership ○ American Osteopathic Association (AOA) accreditation △ Commission on Accreditation of Rehabilitation Facilities (CARF) accreditation Control codes 61, 63, 64, 71, 72 and 73 indicate hospitals listed by AOHA, but not registered by AHA. For definition of numerical codes, see page A4	Control	Service	Staffed Beds	Admissions	Census	Outpatient Visits	Births	Total	Payroll	Personnel
HOLMDEL—Monmouth County										
✱ BAYSHORE COMMUNITY HOSPITAL, 727 North Beers Street, Zip 07733–1598; tel. 732/739–5900; Thomas Goldman, President and Chief Executive Officer (Total facility includes 13 beds in nursing home–type unit) **A**1 9 10 **F**1 3 4 6 7 8 9 11 12 13 14 17 18 19 20 21 22 23 24 25 26 27 28 29 30 32 33 34 35 36 37 38 39 40 41 43 45 46 47 48 49 50 51 54 55 56 58 59 60 62 63 64 65 66 67 69 70 71 72 73 74 75 76 77 78 79 **P**5 7 Web address: www.bchs.com	23	10	168	8773	152	73523	0	65574	30752	1076
IRVINGTON—Essex County										
✱ IRVINGTON GENERAL HOSPITAL, 832 Chancellor Avenue, Zip 07111–0709; tel. 973/399–6000; Amit Mody, M.D., Executive Director (Nonreporting) **A**1 9 10 **S** Saint Barnabas Health Care System, West Orange, NJ Web address: www.sbhcs.com	23	10	157	—	—	—	—	—	—	—
JERSEY CITY—Hudson County										
✱ CHRIST HOSPITAL, 176 Palisade Avenue, Zip 07306–1196, Mailing Address: P.O. Box J–1, Zip 07306–1196; tel. 201/795–8200; Francis J. Cronin, President and Chief Executive Officer **A**1 2 6 9 10 13 **F**2 3 8 9 11 12 13 14 18 19 21 22 23 24 25 27 29 31 32 33 34 35 36 37 38 39 40 41 43 44 45 46 48 50 51 54 55 56 57 58 59 60 61 62 63 64 65 66 68 69 70 72 73 76 78 79 **P**3 5 8 Web address: www.christhospital.org	23	10	382	12004	204	86296	1161	103055	52584	1244
□ GREENVILLE HOSPITAL, 1825 John F. Kennedy Boulevard, Zip 07305–2198; tel. 201/547–6100; Jonathan M. Metsch, Dr.PH, President and Chief Executive Officer (Nonreporting) **A**1 9 10 **S** Liberty Healthcare System, Jersey City, NJ	23	10	86	—	—	—	—	—	—	—
✱ JERSEY CITY MEDICAL CENTER, 50 Baldwin Avenue, Zip 07304–3199; tel. 201/915–2000; Jonathan M. Metsch, Dr.PH, President and Chief Executive Officer (Nonreporting) **A**1 2 3 5 9 10 **S** Liberty Healthcare System, Jersey City, NJ	23	10	487	—	—	—	—	—	—	—
□ ST. FRANCIS HOSPITAL, 25 McWilliams Place, Zip 07302–1698; tel. 201/418–1000; Robert S. Chaloner, Chief Executive Officer **A**1 6 10 **F**1 3 9 12 13 14 18 19 21 22 23 24 25 26 30 31 32 33 34 35 36 37 38 40 41 42 43 44 45 46 48 49 52 53 54 56 58 59 60 61 62 63 64 70 72 73 76 78 79 **P**8 **S** Franciscan Health Partnership, Inc., Latham, NY	23	10	161	4688	115	52816	—	52357	28413	585
KEARNY—Hudson County										
✱ WEST HUDSON HOSPITAL, 206 Bergen Avenue, Zip 07032–3399; tel. 201/955–7051; Carmen Bruce Alecci, Executive Director (Total facility includes 46 beds in nursing home–type unit) (Nonreporting) **A**1 9 10 **S** Saint Barnabas Health Care System, West Orange, NJ	23	10	217	—	—	—	—	—	—	—
LAKEWOOD—Ocean County										
✱ KIMBALL MEDICAL CENTER, 600 River Avenue, Zip 08701–5281; tel. 732/363–1900; Joanne Carrocino, Executive Director **A**1 9 10 **F**1 2 3 4 5 6 7 8 9 10 11 12 13 14 16 17 18 19 20 21 22 23 24 25 26 27 28 29 30 31 32 33 34 35 36 37 38 39 40 41 42 43 44 45 46 47 48 49 50 51 52 54 56 57 58 59 60 61 62 63 64 65 66 69 70 71 72 73 74 75 76 77 78 79 **P**5 7 **S** Saint Barnabas Health Care System, West Orange, NJ Web address: www.sbhcs.com	23	10	300	12224	198	161369	944	108510	47357	989
LAWRENCEVILLE—Mercer County										
✱ △ ST. LAWRENCE REHABILITATION CENTER, 2381 Lawrenceville Road, Zip 08648; tel. 609/896–9500; Charles L. Brennan, Chief Executive Officer (Total facility includes 30 beds in nursing home–type unit) (Nonreporting) **A**1 7 9 10	21	46	116	—	—	—	—	—	—	—
LIVINGSTON—Essex County										
✱ ○ SAINT BARNABAS MEDICAL CENTER, 94 Old Short Hills Road, Zip 07039–5668; tel. 973/322–5000; Vincent D. Joseph, Executive Director **A**1 2 3 5 8 9 10 11 **F**3 4 5 6 7 8 9 10 11 12 13 14 15 16 17 18 19 20 21 22 23 24 25 26 27 28 29 30 32 33 34 35 36 37 38 39 40 41 42 44 45 46 47 48 49 51 52 54 56 57 58 59 60 61 62 63 64 65 66 68 69 70 71 72 74 76 78 79 **P**5 **S** Saint Barnabas Health Care System, West Orange, NJ Web address: www.sbhcs.com	23	10	581	31395	487	197715	7189	374301	166540	2786
LONG BRANCH—Monmouth County										
★ MONMOUTH MEDICAL CENTER, 300 Second Avenue, Zip 07740–6303; tel. 732/222–5200; Frank J. Vozos, M.D., FACS, Executive Director (Nonreporting) **A**2 3 5 8 9 10 **S** Saint Barnabas Health Care System, West Orange, NJ Web address: www.sbhcs.com	23	10	435	—	—	—	—	—	—	—
LYONS—Somerset County										
LYONS DIVISION See Veterans Affairs New Jersey Health Care System, East Orange										
MANAHAWKIN—Ocean County										
✱ SOUTHERN OCEAN COUNTY HOSPITAL, 1140 Route 72 West, Zip 08050–2499; tel. 609/978–8900; Joseph P. Coyle, President and Chief Executive Officer **A**1 2 9 10 **F**3 7 8 9 12 13 14 15 17 18 19 22 24 25 26 28 30 34 35 36 37 38 39 41 44 46 48 49 50 51 54 61 68 69 70 71 72 73 76 78 79 **P**1 5 7	23	10	120	6314	84	107044	193	51610	20675	515
MARLTON—Burlington County										
★ VIRRUA WEST JERSEY HOSPITAL–MARLTON, (Formerly West Jersey Hospital–Marlton), 90 Brick Road, Zip 08053–9697; tel. 856/355–6000; Leroy J. Rosenberg, Executive Director (Nonreporting) **A**9 10 **S** Virtua Health, Marlton, NJ Web address: www.wjhs.org	23	10	167	—	—	—	—	—	—	—

© 2000 AHA Guide *Many Facility Codes have changed. Please refer to the AHA Guide Code Chart.*

Hospitals, U.S. / NEW JERSEY

Hospital, Address, Telephone, Administrator, Approval, Facility, and Physician Codes, Health Care System, Network	Classification Codes		Utilization Data					Expense (thousands) of dollars		
★ American Hospital Association (AHA) membership ☐ Joint Commission on Accreditation of Healthcare Organizations (JCAHO) accreditation + American Osteopathic Healthcare Association (AOHA) membership ○ American Osteopathic Association (AOA) accreditation △ Commission on Accreditation of Rehabilitation Facilities (CARF) accreditation Control codes 61, 63, 64, 71, 72 and 73 indicate hospitals listed by AOHA, but not registered by AHA. For definition of numerical codes, see page A4	Control	Service	Staffed Beds	Admissions	Census	Outpatient Visits	Births	Total	Payroll	Personnel

MILLVILLE—Cumberland County
  SOUTH JERSEY HOSPITAL–MILLVILLE See South Jersey Hospital, Bridgeton
MONTCLAIR—Essex County
  MOUNTAINSIDE HOSPITAL See Atlantic Health System, Florham Park
MORRISTOWN—Morris County
  MORRISTOWN MEMORIAL HOSPITAL See Atlantic Health System, Florham Park
MOUNT HOLLY—Burlington County

	Control	Service	Staffed Beds	Admissions	Census	Outpatient Visits	Births	Total	Payroll	Personnel
☐ VIRTUA MEMORIAL HOSPITAL BURLINGTON COUNTY, (Formerly Memorial Hospital of Burlington County), 175 Madison Avenue, Zip 08060–2099; tel. 609/267–0700; Donald I. Brunn, Executive Vice President (Nonreporting) **A**1 2 3 5 9 10 **S** Virtua Health, Marlton, NJ **Web address:** www.virtua.org	23	10	413	—	—	—	—	—	—	—

MOUNTAINSIDE—Union County

	Control	Service	Staffed Beds	Admissions	Census	Outpatient Visits	Births	Total	Payroll	Personnel
★ △ CHILDREN'S SPECIALIZED HOSPITAL, (Includes Children's Specialized Hospital–Ocean, 94 Stevens Road, Toms River, Zip 08755–1237; tel. 732/914–1100), 150 New Providence Road, Zip 07092–2590; tel. 908/233–3720; Richard B. Ahlfeld, President (Total facility includes 41 beds in nursing home–type unit) **A**1 7 9 10 **F**13 17 19 23 29 31 33 34 38 43 50 51 53 54 56 59 69 70 72 78	23	56	117	272	85	46649	—	39543	22559	570

NEW BRUNSWICK—Middlesex County

	Control	Service	Staffed Beds	Admissions	Census	Outpatient Visits	Births	Total	Payroll	Personnel
HURTADO HEALTH CENTER, 11 Bishop Place, Zip 08901–1180; tel. 732/932–8429; Susan Skalsky, M.D., Director (Nonreporting)	12	11	27	—	—	—	—	—	—	—
★ ROBERT WOOD JOHNSON UNIVERSITY HOSPITAL, 1 Robert Wood Johnson Place, Zip 08903–2601; tel. 732/828–3000; Harvey A. Holzberg, President and Chief Executive Officer **A**1 2 3 5 8 9 10 **F**1 2 3 4 5 6 7 8 9 11 12 13 14 15 16 17 18 19 20 22 23 24 25 26 27 28 29 30 31 32 33 34 35 36 37 38 39 41 43 44 45 46 47 48 49 50 51 52 54 55 56 57 58 59 60 61 62 63 64 66 67 68 69 70 71 72 73 74 75 76 77 78 79 **Web address:** www.rwjuh.edu	23	10	445	31860	424	242229	1305	314784	126147	2908
★ ST. PETER'S UNIVERSITY HOSPITAL, (Formerly St. Peter's Medical Center), 254 Easton Avenue, Zip 08901–1780, Mailing Address: P.O. Box 591, Zip 08903–0591; tel. 732/745–8600; John E. Matuska, President and Chief Executive Officer (Total facility includes 20 beds in nursing home–type unit) **A**1 2 3 5 9 10 **F**1 7 8 9 11 12 13 14 16 17 18 19 20 22 23 24 25 26 27 29 30 31 32 33 34 36 38 39 41 42 43 44 45 46 48 49 50 51 52 54 56 59 60 61 63 65 66 67 69 70 71 72 73 76 78 79 **P**1 2 7 **Web address:** www.stpetersmc.com	21	10	416	22693	332	197707	6728	220429	107897	2069

NEWARK—Essex County

	Control	Service	Staffed Beds	Admissions	Census	Outpatient Visits	Births	Total	Payroll	Personnel
☐ COLUMBUS HOSPITAL, 495 North 13th Street, Zip 07107–1397; tel. 973/268–1400; John G. Magliaro, President and Chief Executive Officer (Nonreporting) **A**1 9 10 **S** Cathedral Healthcare System, Inc., Newark, NJ	23	10	206	—	—	—	—	—	—	—
★ ○ NEWARK BETH ISRAEL MEDICAL CENTER, 201 Lyons Avenue, Zip 07112–2027; tel. 973/926–7000; Paul A. Mertz, Executive Director **A**1 2 3 5 8 9 10 11 12 **F**1 4 6 7 9 11 12 13 14 17 18 19 20 21 22 23 25 29 30 31 32 34 35 36 37 38 39 40 41 42 43 44 45 46 47 48 49 50 51 52 54 55 56 57 58 59 60 61 63 64 65 66 68 70 72 74 75 76 78 79 **P**7 8 **S** Saint Barnabas Health Care System, West Orange, NJ **Web address:** www.saintbarnabas.com	23	10	532	22162	377	496519	2698	—	137271	3198
☐ SAINT JAMES HOSPITAL OF NEWARK, 155 Jefferson Street, Zip 07105; tel. 973/589–1300; Ceu Cirne–Neves, Administrator (Nonreporting) **A**1 3 9 10 **S** Cathedral Healthcare System, Inc., Newark, NJ	21	10	189	—	—	—	—	—	—	—
☐ SAINT MICHAEL'S MEDICAL CENTER, 268 Dr. Martin Luther King Jr. Boulevard, Zip 07102–2094; tel. 973/877–5000; Barbara Loughney, Administrator **A**1 3 5 9 10 12 13 **F**3 4 7 9 11 12 13 14 16 17 18 19 21 22 23 24 25 30 32 33 34 35 36 37 38 39 41 43 45 46 47 48 49 50 51 54 55 56 58 59 61 63 64 65 68 70 71 72 74 76 78 79 **S** Cathedral Healthcare System, Inc., Newark, NJ **Web address:** www.cathedralhealthcare.org	21	10	270	10491	189	81303	782	135597	62100	1291
★ UNIVERSITY OF MEDICINE AND DENTISTRY OF NEW JERSEY–UNIVERSITY HOSPITAL, 150 Bergen Street, Zip 07103–2406; tel. 973/972–4300; Daniel L. Marcantuono, FACHE, Acting Vice President and Chief Executive Officer (Nonreporting) **A**1 2 3 5 8 9 10	12	10	518	—	—	—	—	—	—	—

NEWTON—Sussex County

	Control	Service	Staffed Beds	Admissions	Census	Outpatient Visits	Births	Total	Payroll	Personnel
★ △ NEWTON MEMORIAL HOSPITAL, 175 High Street, Zip 07860–1004; tel. 973/383–2121; Dennis H. Collette, President and Chief Executive Officer **A**1 2 7 9 10 **F**3 8 9 13 16 17 18 19 21 22 23 24 25 31 32 33 34 35 39 40 41 43 44 45 46 48 50 51 53 54 56 57 58 59 60 61 62 63 64 66 68 70 72 76 78 **P**5 8 **Web address:** www.itsyourlife.com	23	10	162	9151	100	174706	850	63287	27306	606

NORTH BERGEN—Hudson County

	Control	Service	Staffed Beds	Admissions	Census	Outpatient Visits	Births	Total	Payroll	Personnel
★ PALISADES MEDICAL CENTER, (Formerly Palisades General Hospital), 7600 River Road, Zip 07047–6217; tel. 201/854–5000; Bruce J. Markowitz, President and Chief Executive Officer **A**1 9 10 **F**3 7 9 13 17 18 19 22 25 30 31 32 33 34 39 41 43 44 45 46 48 49 50 51 54 61 63 70 72 76 78 **P**5 **S** New York Presbyterian Healthcare System, New York, NY **Web address:** www.palisadesmedical.org	23	10	202	7804	123	43047	1394	59611	28351	671

OLD BRIDGE—Middlesex County
  OLD BRIDGE DIVISION See Raritan Bay Medical Center, Perth Amboy

Hospitals, U.S. / NEW JERSEY

Hospital, Address, Telephone, Administrator, Approval, Facility, and Physician Codes, Health Care System, Network	Classification Codes		Utilization Data					Expense (thousands) of dollars		
★ American Hospital Association (AHA) membership ☐ Joint Commission on Accreditation of Healthcare Organizations (JCAHO) accreditation + American Osteopathic Healthcare Association (AOHA) membership ○ American Osteopathic Association (AOA) accreditation △ Commission on Accreditation of Rehabilitation Facilities (CARF) accreditation Control codes 61, 63, 64, 71, 72 and 73 indicate hospitals listed by AOHA, but not registered by AHA. For definition of numerical codes, see page A4	Control	Service	Staffed Beds	Admissions	Census	Outpatient Visits	Births	Total	Payroll	Personnel
ORANGE—Essex County										
☐ HOSPITAL CENTER AT ORANGE, (Includes New Jersey Orthopedic Hospital Unit; Orange Memorial Hospital Unit), 188 South Essex Avenue, Zip 07051; tel. 973/266–2200; James E. Romer, President and Chief Executive Officer (Nonreporting) A1 2 3 5 9 10 S Cathedral Healthcare System, Inc., Newark, NJ	33	10	195	—	—	—	—	—	—	—
PARAMUS—Bergen County										
★ BERGEN REGIONAL MEDICAL CENTER, 230 East Ridgewood Avenue, Zip 07652–4131; tel. 201/967–4000; Fred S. Sganga, President and Chief Executive Officer (Total facility includes 610 beds in nursing home–type unit) A1 3 5 6 9 10 F1 3 9 10 14 15 16 17 18 19 22 23 24 25 26 30 31 32 33 34 37 38 41 46 48 49 54 56 57 58 60 61 62 63 64 69 70 72 76 78 79 Web address: www.bergenregional.com	13	22	1039	8916	840	62697	0	—	—	1486
PASSAIC—Passaic County										
★ BETH ISRAEL HOSPITAL, 70 Parker Avenue, Zip 07055–7000; tel. 973/365–5000; Jeffrey S. Moll, President and Chief Executive Officer (Total facility includes 13 beds in nursing home–type unit) A1 2 9 10 F3 9 11 12 13 14 17 18 19 22 24 25 30 31 32 33 34 35 36 37 38 39 43 45 46 48 49 50 51 54 56 65 66 68 70 73 76 77 78 79 Web address: www.pbih.org	23	10	223	6086	125	188117	0	52818	23422	858
GENERAL HOSPITAL CENTER AT PASSAIC See Atlantic Health System, Florham Park										
★ ST. MARY'S HOSPITAL, 211 Pennington Avenue, Zip 07055–4698; tel. 973/470–3000; Patricia Peterson, President and Chief Executive Officer (Nonreporting) A1 9 10	21	10	229	—	—	—	—	—	—	—
PATERSON—Passaic County										
★ BARNERT HOSPITAL, 680 Broadway Street, Zip 07514–1472; tel. 973/977–6600; Stephen M. Patz, President and Chief Executive Officer A1 9 10 F1 3 4 6 8 9 13 16 17 19 21 22 24 25 30 31 32 33 34 35 38 39 41 43 44 45 46 48 49 50 51 54 56 57 58 59 60 61 63 64 70 72 73 76 78 79 P5 Web address: www.barnerthosp.com	23	10	182	5651	94	350341	709	56014	27505	602
★ ○ ST. JOSEPH'S HOSPITAL AND MEDICAL CENTER, 703 Main Street, Zip 07503–2691; tel. 973/754–2000; Patrick R. Wardell, President and Chief Executive Officer (Total facility includes 141 beds in nursing home–type unit) (Nonreporting) A1 2 3 5 8 9 10 11 12 13 Web address: www.sjhmc.org	21	10	621	—	—	—	—	—	—	—
PEAPACK—Somerset County										
★ △ MATHENY SCHOOL AND HOSPITAL, Main Street, Zip 07977, Mailing Address: P.O. Box 339, Zip 07977–0339; tel. 908/234–0011; Steven M. Proctor, President A1 7 10 F1 6 13 17 18 19 23 31 36 38 54 56 59 69 70 78 Web address: www.matheny.org	23	49	87	58	79	500	0	18391	11680	329
PERTH AMBOY—Middlesex County										
★ RARITAN BAY MEDICAL CENTER, (Includes Old Bridge Division, One Hospital Plaza, Old Bridge, Zip 08857; tel. 732/360–1000; Perth Amboy Division, 530 New Brunswick Avenue, tel. 732/442–3700), 530 New Brunswick Avenue, Zip 08861–3685; tel. 732/442–3700; Keith H. McLaughlin, President and Chief Executive Officer A1 3 5 6 9 10 F2 3 4 6 7 8 9 11 12 13 16 17 18 19 21 22 24 25 27 29 31 32 33 34 35 36 37 38 39 41 43 44 46 48 49 51 54 56 57 59 60 61 63 66 68 70 72 73 76 77 78 79 P7 8 Web address: www.rbmc.org	23	10	365	14244	293	197060	829	138076	70819	1724
PHILLIPSBURG—Warren County										
★ WARREN HOSPITAL, 185 Roseberry Street, Zip 08865–9955; tel. 908/859–6700; Jeffrey C. Goodwin, President and Chief Executive Officer (Nonreporting) A1 2 3 5 9 10 12 13	23	10	214	—	—	—	—	—	—	—
PISCATAWAY—Middlesex County										
UNIVERSITY OF MEDICINE AND DENTISTRY OF NEW JERSEY, UNIVERSITY BEHAVIORAL HEALTHCARE, 671 Hoes Lane, Zip 08854–5633, Mailing Address: P.O. Box 1392, Zip 08855–1392; tel. 732/235–5900; Christopher O. Kosseff, Vice President and Chief Executive Officer (Nonreporting) A3 5 9 10	12	22	64	—	—	—	—	—	—	—
PLAINFIELD—Union County										
★ MUHLENBERG REGIONAL MEDICAL CENTER, 1200 Park Avenue, Zip 07061; tel. 908/668–2000; John R. Kopicki, President and Chief Executive Officer (Nonreporting) A1 3 5 6 9 10 S Solaris Health System, Edison, NJ Web address: www.solarishs.org/	23	10	261	—	—	—	—	—	—	—
POMONA—Atlantic County										
★ △ BACHARACH INSTITUTE FOR REHABILITATION, 61 West Jimmy Leeds Road, Zip 08240–0723, Mailing Address: P.O. Box 723, Zip 08240–0723; tel. 609/652–7000; Richard J. Kathrins, Administrator and Chief Executive Officer A1 7 9 10 F13 16 17 18 19 22 23 31 33 34 38 39 43 45 49 50 51 53 54 56 70 71 72 76 78 P6 Web address: www.bacharach.org	23	46	80	1497	61	56904	0	30371	17050	419
POMPTON PLAINS—Morris County										
★ CHILTON MEMORIAL HOSPITAL, 97 West Parkway, Zip 07444–1696; tel. 973/831–5000; James J. Doyle, Jr, President and Chief Executive Officer A1 2 9 10 F7 8 9 11 13 14 16 17 18 19 22 25 28 30 32 33 34 35 36 37 38 39 41 42 43 44 45 46 48 52 54 56 57 58 59 60 61 62 65 68 70 71 72 76 77 78 79 P4 5 7 8 Web address: www.chiltonmemorial.org	23	10	256	10152	63	102488	1499	85770	38346	928

Hospitals, U.S. / NEW JERSEY

Hospital, Address, Telephone, Administrator, Approval, Facility, and Physician Codes, Health Care System, Network	Classification Codes		Utilization Data					Expense (thousands) of dollars		
	Control	Service	Staffed Beds	Admissions	Census	Outpatient Visits	Births	Total	Payroll	Personnel

★ American Hospital Association (AHA) membership
□ Joint Commission on Accreditation of Healthcare Organizations (JCAHO) accreditation
+ American Osteopathic Healthcare Association (AOHA) membership
○ American Osteopathic Association (AOA) accreditation
△ Commission on Accreditation of Rehabilitation Facilities (CARF) accreditation
Control codes 61, 63, 64, 71, 72 and 73 indicate hospitals listed by AOHA, but not registered by AHA. For definition of numerical codes, see page A4

PRINCETON—Mercer County
★ MEDICAL CENTER AT PRINCETON, (Includes Acute General Hospital, Merwick Unit–Extended Care and Rehabilitation, Princeton House Unit–Community Mental Health and Substance Abuse), 253 Witherspoon Street, Zip 08540–3213; tel. 609/497–4000; Dennis W. Doody, President and Chief Executive Officer (Total facility includes 93 beds in nursing home–type unit) **A**1 2 3 5 9 10 **F**1 2 3 7 8 9 11 12 13 16 17 18 19 21 22 23 24 25 26 30 31 32 33 34 35 36 37 38 39 41 43 44 45 46 48 49 50 51 53 54 55 57 58 59 60 61 62 63 64 65 68 69 70 72 76 78 **P**7 8
Web address: www.mcp.org | 23 | 10 | 392 | 16074 | 302 | 265890 | 1610 | 135777 | 64804 | 1944 |

RAHWAY—Union County
★ RAHWAY HOSPITAL, 865 Stone Street, Zip 07065–2797; tel. 732/381–4200; Kirk C. Tice, President and Chief Executive Officer **A**1 10 **F**3 4 7 8 9 11 12 13 14 16 17 18 19 21 22 24 25 26 27 30 31 32 33 34 35 36 37 38 39 41 43 44 46 47 48 49 50 51 54 56 58 61 62 65 68 69 70 72 73 75 76 77 78 79 **P**1 5
Web address: www.rahwayhospital.com | 23 | 10 | 236 | 9328 | 174 | 65733 | 651 | 84943 | 35348 | 759 |

RED BANK—Monmouth County
RIVERVIEW MEDICAL CENTER See Raritan Bay Medical Center, Perth Amboy

RIDGEWOOD—Bergen County
★ VALLEY HOSPITAL, 223 North Van Dien Avenue, Zip 07450–9982; tel. 201/447–8000; Audrey Meyers, President and Chief Executive Officer **A**1 2 9 10 **F**4 6 7 8 9 11 12 13 14 16 17 18 19 21 22 23 24 25 26 28 29 30 31 32 33 34 35 36 37 38 39 40 41 42 43 44 45 46 47 48 49 50 51 54 56 57 58 59 60 61 62 65 66 67 69 70 71 72 73 74 75 76 77 78 79
Web address: www.valleyhealth.com | 23 | 10 | 427 | 22543 | 335 | 214597 | 3147 | 223072 | 111151 | 2473 |

SALEM—Salem County
★ MEMORIAL HOSPITAL OF SALEM COUNTY, 310 Woodstown Road, Zip 08079–2080; tel. 856/935–1000; Denise R. Williams, President and Chief Executive Officer **A**1 2 9 10 **F**7 8 9 13 16 17 18 19 22 23 24 25 26 32 34 35 36 37 38 39 40 41 43 44 45 46 48 49 51 54 59 61 69 70 72 76 78 **P**5 6
Web address: www.salemhosp.org | 23 | 10 | 122 | 4910 | 66 | 148450 | 381 | 45571 | 23259 | 581 |

SECAUCUS—Hudson County
□ MEADOWLANDS HOSPITAL MEDICAL CENTER, 55 Meadowland Parkway, Zip 07096–1580; tel. 201/392–3100; Paul V. Cavalli, M.D., President (Total facility includes 30 beds in nursing home–type unit) **A**1 9 10 **F**1 3 5 7 8 9 11 12 13 14 15 17 18 19 20 21 22 23 24 25 30 31 32 33 34 35 36 38 39 41 44 46 48 49 51 53 54 57 58 59 60 61 62 63 64 68 70 71 72 76 77 78 79
S Liberty Healthcare System, Jersey City, NJ | 23 | 10 | 173 | 6284 | 101 | 67653 | 1005 | 52688 | 21023 | 565 |

SOMERS POINT—Atlantic County
★ SHORE MEMORIAL HOSPITAL, 1 East New York Avenue, Zip 08244–2387; tel. 609/653–3500; Richard A. Pitman, President **A**1 2 9 10 **F**7 8 9 13 16 17 18 22 24 25 28 29 30 32 33 34 35 36 37 39 41 43 44 45 46 48 49 50 51 54 65 68 69 70 72 76 78 79 **P**5 7
Web address: www.shorememorial.org | 23 | 10 | 179 | 10026 | 142 | 99110 | 1181 | 104645 | 44977 | 1173 |

SOMERVILLE—Somerset County
★ SOMERSET MEDICAL CENTER, 110 Rehill Avenue, Zip 08876–2598; tel. 908/685–2200; Dennis C. Miller, President and Chief Executive Officer **A**1 2 3 5 9 10 **F**3 7 8 9 11 12 13 16 17 18 19 22 24 25 30 31 32 33 34 35 36 37 38 39 41 42 44 45 46 48 49 51 54 56 57 59 60 61 62 63 64 70 72 76 78 79 **P**5 7
Web address: www.smchealthwise.com | 23 | 10 | 261 | 12404 | 176 | 141578 | 1198 | 113346 | 54946 | 1456 |

STRATFORD—Camden County
KENNEDY MEMORIAL HOSPITAL See Kennedy Memorial Hospitals–University Medical Center, Cherry Hill

SUMMIT—Union County
□ CHARTER BEHAVIORAL HEALTH SYSTEM OF NEW JERSEY–SUMMIT, 19 Prospect Street, Zip 07902–0100; tel. 908/522–7000; Lori Ann Rizzuto, Chief Executive Officer (Nonreporting) **A**1 9 10 **S** Magellan Health Services, Atlanta, GA | 33 | 22 | 90 | — | — | — | — | — | — | — |
OVERLOOK HOSPITAL See Atlantic Health System, Florham Park

SUSSEX—Sussex County
SAINT CLARE'S HOSPITAL/SUSSEX See Saint Clare's Health Services, Denville

TEANECK—Bergen County
★ HOLY NAME HOSPITAL, 718 Teaneck Road, Zip 07666–4281; tel. 201/833–3000; Michael Maron, President and Chief Executive Officer (Nonreporting) **A**1 2 6 9 10
Web address: www.holyname.org | 23 | 10 | 323 | — | — | — | — | — | — | — |

TOMS RIVER—Ocean County
CHILDREN'S SPECIALIZED HOSPITAL–OCEAN See Children's Specialized Hospital, Mountainside
★ COMMUNITY MEDICAL CENTER, 99 Route 37 West, Zip 08755–6423; tel. 732/557–8000; Nancy L. Wollen, Executive Director **A**1 2 9 10 **F**1 3 6 7 8 9 11 12 13 14 16 17 18 19 21 22 23 24 25 26 28 29 30 31 32 33 34 35 36 37 38 39 40 41 43 44 45 46 48 49 50 51 54 56 57 59 60 61 62 63 64 65 66 68 69 70 71 72 73 76 77 78 79 **P**2 **S** Saint Barnabas Health Care System, West Orange, NJ
Web address: www.sbhcs.com | 23 | 10 | 465 | 23685 | 366 | 216819 | 1751 | 198129 | 90990 | 2158 |

Many Facility Codes have changed. Please refer to the AHA Guide Code Chart.

Hospitals, U.S. / NEW JERSEY

Hospital, Address, Telephone, Administrator, Approval, Facility, and Physician Codes, Health Care System, Network	Classification Codes		Utilization Data					Expense (thousands) of dollars		
★ American Hospital Association (AHA) membership □ Joint Commission on Accreditation of Healthcare Organizations (JCAHO) accreditation + American Osteopathic Healthcare Association (AOHA) membership ○ American Osteopathic Association (AOA) accreditation △ Commission on Accreditation of Rehabilitation Facilities (CARF) accreditation Control codes 61, 63, 64, 71, 72 and 73 indicate hospitals listed by AOHA, but not registered by AHA. For definition of numerical codes, see page A4	Control	Service	Staffed Beds	Admissions	Census	Outpatient Visits	Births	Total	Payroll	Personnel
□ △ HEALTHSOUTH REHABILITATION HOSPITAL OF NEW JERSEY, 14 Hospital Drive, Zip 08755-6470; tel. 732/244-3100; Patricia Ostaszewski, Chief Executive Officer and Administrator (Total facility includes 63 beds in nursing home–type unit) (Nonreporting) A1 7 9 10 S HEALTHSOUTH Corporation, Birmingham, AL	33	46	155	—	—	—	—	—	—	—
TRENTON—Mercer County										
★ CAPITAL HEALTH SYSTEM, (Includes Capital Health System at Fuld, 750 Brunswick Avenue, Zip 08638-4174; tel. 609/394-6000; Capital Health System at Mercer, 446 Bellevue Avenue), 446 Bellevue Avenue, Zip 08618-4597, Mailing Address: P.O. Box 1658, Zip 08607-1658; tel. 609/394-4000; Alireza Maghazehe, Chief Executive Officer A1 2 3 5 6 9 10 F1 3 5 7 8 9 11 12 13 14 15 17 18 19 21 22 23 24 25 30 31 32 33 34 35 36 37 38 39 40 41 42 43 44 45 46 48 50 51 54 56 57 59 60 61 63 64 65 66 68 70 71 72 73 76 77 78 79 Web address: www.capitalhealth.org	23	10	568	22063	348	438342	2250	239880	115423	2815
★ ST. FRANCIS MEDICAL CENTER, 601 Hamilton Avenue, Zip 08629-1986; tel. 609/599-5000; Judith M. Persichilli, President and Chief Executive Officer (Nonreporting) A1 2 3 5 6 9 10 S Catholic Health Initiatives, Denver, CO	21	10	254	—	—	—	—	—	—	—
★ TRENTON PSYCHIATRIC HOSPITAL, Sullivan Way, Zip 08625, Mailing Address: P.O. Box 7500, West Trenton, Zip 08628-7500; tel. 609/633-1500; Joseph Jupin, Jr, Chief Executive Officer A1 3 10 F3 6 7 8 9 10 11 12 13 17 18 19 21 22 24 25 26 27 28 29 30 31 32 33 34 35 36 37 38 39 40 41 43 45 46 47 48 50 51 55 57 60 61 62 63 64 65 66 68 70 71 72 74 75 76 78 79 S Division of Mental Health Services, Department of Human Services, State of New Jersey, Trenton, NJ	12	22	395	1071	390	—	—	—	—	878
TURNERSVILLE—Camden County										
KENNEDY MEMORIAL HOSPITAL See Kennedy Memorial Hospitals–University Medical Center, Cherry Hill										
UNION—Union County										
★ + ○ UNION HOSPITAL, 1000 Galloping Hill Road, Zip 07083-1652; tel. 908/687-1900; Kathryn W. Coyne, Executive Director A1 2 9 10 11 12 13 F1 2 3 4 7 8 9 10 11 12 13 16 17 19 21 22 23 24 25 29 30 31 32 33 34 35 36 37 38 39 41 42 43 44 45 46 47 48 49 50 51 52 54 57 58 59 60 61 63 65 69 70 71 74 76 77 78 P5 S Saint Barnabas Health Care System, West Orange, NJ Web address: www.sbhcs.com	23	10	148	6363	116	49659	0	63393	27801	742
VINELAND—Cumberland County										
★ SOUTH JERSEY HOSPITAL–NEWCOMB, (Formerly Newcomb Medical Center), 65 South State Street, Zip 08360-4893; tel. 856/507-8500; Chester B. Kaletkowski, President and Chief Executive Officer (Nonreporting) A1 2 9 S South Jersey Health System, Bridgeton, NJ	23	10	139	—	—	—	—	—	—	—
VINELAND DEVELOPMENTAL CENTER HOSPITAL, 1676 East Landis Avenue, Zip 08361-2992; tel. 856/696-6200; Judith L. Sisti, MS, Administrator (Nonreporting)	12	12	100	—	—	—	—	—	—	—
VOORHEES—Camden County										
★ VIRTUA WEST JERSEY HOSPITAL–VOORHEES, (Formerly West Jersey Hospital–Voorhees), 101 Carnie Boulevard, Zip 08043-1597; tel. 856/325-3000; Joan T. Meyers, R.N., Vice President and Chief Operating Officer (Nonreporting) A1 3 5 9 S Virtua Health, Marlton, NJ Web address: www.virtua.org	23	10	253	—	—	—	—	—	—	—
WAYNE—Passaic County										
★ WAYNE GENERAL HOSPITAL, 224 Hamburg Turnpike, Zip 07470-2100; tel. 973/942-6900; Geraldine Di Risic, Acting Executive Director A1 9 10 F1 7 8 9 12 13 14 17 18 19 22 24 25 27 29 30 31 32 34 35 36 37 38 39 41 43 44 45 46 48 49 50 51 54 56 65 68 70 72 76 78 P5 8 S Saint Barnabas Health Care System, West Orange, NJ Web address: www.sbhcs.com	23	10	146	7197	116	73107	792	68854	28490	769
WEST ORANGE—Essex County										
★ KESSLER INSTITUTE FOR REHABILITATION, (Includes East Orange Facility, West Orange Facility, Saddle Brook Facility and Welkind Facility), 1199 Pleasant Valley Way, Zip 07052-1419; tel. 973/731-3600; Robert Brehm, President A1 3 5 9 10 F1 13 17 18 28 36 38 45 49 53 54 70 71 72 76 78 79 P6 Web address: www.kessler-rehab.com	33	46	304	5609	289	178903	0	88077	48911	1103
WESTAMPTON TOWNSHIP—Burlington County										
□ HAMPTON HOSPITAL, Rancocas Road, Zip 08073, Mailing Address: P.O. Box 7000, Zip 08073; tel. 609/267-7000; James P. Gallagher, Chief Executive Officer (Nonreporting) A1 9 10	33	22	83	—	—	—	—	—	—	—
WESTWOOD—Bergen County										
★ PASCACK VALLEY HOSPITAL, 250 Old Hook Road, Zip 07675-3181; tel. 201/358-3000; Louis R. Ycre, Jr, FACHE, President and Chief Executive Officer (Nonreporting) A1 2 9 10 Web address: www.pvhospital.org	23	10	237	—	—	—	—	—	—	—
WILLINGBORO—Burlington County										
★ RANCOCAS HOSPITAL, 218-A Sunset Road, Zip 08046-1162; tel. 609/835-2900; Joseph Flamini, Chief Executive Officer A1 2 9 10 13 F3 4 7 8 9 11 13 17 18 19 20 22 23 24 25 26 30 32 34 37 39 41 44 45 46 47 48 49 51 54 56 57 59 61 63 64 65 66 68 70 71 72 74 76 78 79 P7 S Catholic Health East, Newtown Square, PA	23	10	237	9932	157	121191	1258	73004	36460	948

© 2000 AHA Guide   *Many Facility Codes have changed. Please refer to the AHA Guide Code Chart.*

Hospitals, U.S. / NEW JERSEY

Hospital, Address, Telephone, Administrator, Approval, Facility, and Physician Codes, Health Care System, Network	Classification Codes		Utilization Data					Expense (thousands) of dollars		
	Control	Service	Staffed Beds	Admissions	Census	Outpatient Visits	Births	Total	Payroll	Personnel

★ American Hospital Association (AHA) membership
□ Joint Commission on Accreditation of Healthcare Organizations (JCAHO) accreditation
+ American Osteopathic Healthcare Association (AOHA) membership
○ American Osteopathic Association (AOA) accreditation
△ Commission on Accreditation of Rehabilitation Facilities (CARF) accreditation
Control codes 61, 63, 64, 71, 72 and 73 indicate hospitals listed by AOHA, but not registered by AHA. For definition of numerical codes, see page A4

Hospital	Control	Service	Staffed Beds	Admissions	Census	Outpatient Visits	Births	Total	Payroll	Personnel
WOODBRIDGE—Middlesex County										
WOODBRIDGE DEVELOPMENT CENTER, Rahway Avenue, Zip 07095, Mailing Address: P.O. Box 189, Zip 07095; tel. 732/499–5951; Amy R. Bailon, M.D., Medical Director (Nonreporting)	12	12	125	—	—	—	—	—	—	—
WOODBURY—Gloucester County										
★ UNDERWOOD–MEMORIAL HOSPITAL, 509 North Broad Street, Zip 08096–1697, Mailing Address: P.O. Box 359, Zip 08096–7359; tel. 856/845–0100; Steven W. Jackmuff, President and Chief Executive Officer **A**1 3 9 10 **F**1 4 7 8 9 11 12 13 17 18 19 21 22 23 24 25 26 29 30 31 32 34 35 36 38 39 41 43 44 45 46 48 54 56 57 58 61 62 63 64 68 69 70 72 76 78 79 **P**6 Web address: www.umhospital.org	23	10	242	12178	167	114221	1323	89524	44443	1197
WYCKOFF—Bergen County										
★ CHRISTIAN HEALTH CARE CENTER, (Formerly Ramapo Ridge Psychiatric Hospital), 301 Sicomac Avenue, Zip 07481–2194; tel. 201/848–5200; Douglas A. Struyk, President and Chief Executive Officer (Nonreporting) **A**1 9 10 Web address: www.chccnj.org	23	22	80	—	—	—	—	—	—	—

NEW MEXICO

Resident Population 1,737 (in thousands)
Resident population in metro areas 56.7%
Birth rate per 1,000 population 15.5
65 years and over 11.4%
Percent of persons without health insurance 22.6%

Hospital, Address, Telephone, Administrator, Approval, Facility, and Physician Codes, Health Care System, Network

★ American Hospital Association (AHA) membership
☐ Joint Commission on Accreditation of Healthcare Organizations (JCAHO) accreditation
+ American Osteopathic Healthcare Association (AOHA) membership
○ American Osteopathic Association (AOA) accreditation
△ Commission on Accreditation of Rehabilitation Facilities (CARF) accreditation
Control codes 61, 63, 64, 71, 72 and 73 indicate hospitals listed by AOHA, but not registered by AHA. For definition of numerical codes, see page A4

Hospital	Control	Service	Staffed Beds	Admissions	Census	Outpatient Visits	Births	Total	Payroll	Personnel
ALAMOGORDO—Otero County										
★ GERALD CHAMPION REGIONAL MEDICAL CENTER, (Formerly Gerald Champion Memorial Hospital), 2669 North Scenic Drive, Zip 88310; tel. 505/439–2100; Carl W. Mantey, Administrator **A**1 9 10 **F**8 9 16 17 18 22 24 25 27 28 32 34 37 38 39 41 44 46 48 70 71 72 76 78 **P**5 **S** Quorum Health Group, Brentwood, TN	23	10	73	3666	38	46862	662	29282	9565	324
ALBUQUERQUE—Bernalillo County										
★ CARRIE TINGLEY HOSPITAL, 1127 University Boulevard N.E., Zip 87102–1715; tel. 505/272–5200; Barbara Ohm, Interim Administrator (Nonreporting) **A**3 5 9 10 **S** University of New Mexico, Albuquerque, NM	12	57	18	—	—	—	—	—	—	—
DESERT HILLS HOSPITAL, 5310 Sequoia Road N.W., Zip 87120–1249; tel. 505/836–7330; Carol Bickelman, President and Chief Executive Officer (Nonreporting) **S** Youth and Family Centered Services, Austin, TX	33	22	35	—	—	—	—	—	—	—
☐ △ HEALTHSOUTH REHABILITATION CENTER, 7000 Jefferson N.E., Zip 87109–4357; tel. 505/344–9478; Darby Brockette, Chief Executive Officer (Nonreporting) **A**1 7 9 10 **S** HEALTHSOUTH Corporation, Birmingham, AL	33	46	60	—	—	—	—	—	—	—
☐ LOVELACE HEALTH SYSTEM, 5400 Gibson Boulevard S.E., Zip 87108–4763; tel. 505/262–7000; Martin Hickey, M.D., Chief Executive Officer (Total facility includes 16 beds in nursing home–type unit) **A**1 2 3 5 9 10 **F**2 3 4 5 7 8 9 10 11 12 13 14 15 16 17 18 19 20 21 22 23 24 25 26 27 28 29 30 32 33 34 35 36 37 38 39 41 42 43 44 45 46 47 48 49 50 51 52 53 54 56 57 58 59 60 61 62 63 64 66 68 69 70 71 72 73 74 75 76 77 78 79 **P**6 Web address: www.lovelace.com	33	10	135	13444	116	992638	2163	487896	132965	2582
☐ MEMORIAL PSYCHIATRIC HOSPITAL, 806 Central Avenue S.E., Zip 87102–3671, Mailing Address: P.O. Box 26568, Zip 87125–6568; tel. 505/247–0220; Robert Lingenfelser, Administrator **A**1 10 **F**2 3 13 16 17 18 23 25 38 49 57 58 59 60 61 62 63 64 75 **P**5	32	22	58	718	35	2715	—	4886	2652	162
★ MENTAL HEALTH CENTER, (Formerly University of New Mexico Hospital), 2600 Marble N.E., Zip 87131–2600; tel. 505/272–2263; Stephen W. McKernan, Chief Executive Officer (Nonreporting) **A**5 9 10 **S** University of New Mexico, Albuquerque, NM Web address: www.mhc.unm.edu	13	22	60	—	—	—	—	—	—	—
★ PRESBYTERIAN HOSPITAL, 1100 Central Avenue S.E., Zip 87106–4934, Mailing Address: P.O. Box 26666, Zip 87125–6666; tel. 505/841–1234; Mark W. Reifsteck, Senior Vice President and Chief Operating Officer **A**1 2 3 5 9 10 **F**2 3 4 5 7 9 10 11 12 13 14 16 17 18 19 21 22 24 25 27 28 29 30 31 32 33 34 35 36 37 38 39 40 41 42 43 44 45 46 47 48 51 52 53 54 56 57 58 59 60 61 62 63 64 65 68 69 70 71 72 74 75 76 77 78 79 **P**1 4 5 6 7 **S** Presbyterian Healthcare Services, Albuquerque, NM Web address: www.phs.org	23	10	383	22360	280	43030	4503	—	—	2703
★ PRESBYTERIAN KASEMAN HOSPITAL, 8300 Constitution Avenue N.E., Zip 87110–7624, Mailing Address: P.O. Box 26666, Zip 87125–6666; tel. 505/291–2000; Robert A. Garcia, Administrative Director **A**1 9 10 **F**2 3 4 8 9 10 11 12 13 14 16 17 18 19 21 22 24 25 27 28 29 34 35 36 37 38 39 40 41 42 43 44 45 46 47 48 49 51 52 54 56 57 58 59 60 61 62 63 64 65 66 68 70 71 72 74 75 76 77 78 79 **P**1 4 5 6 7 **S** Presbyterian Healthcare Services, Albuquerque, NM	23	10	138	4638	30	32609	0	—	—	437
★ PUBLIC HEALTH SERVICE INDIAN HOSPITAL, 801 Vassar Drive N.E., Zip 87106–2799; tel. 505/248–4000; Cheri Lyon, Service Unit Director (Nonreporting) **A**1 10 **S** U. S. Public Health Service Indian Health Service, Rockville, MD	47	10	28	—	—	—	—	—	—	—
★ ST. JOSEPH MEDICAL CENTER, 601 Martin Luther King Jr. Drive N.E., Zip 87102, Mailing Address: P.O. Box 25555, Zip 87125–0555; tel. 505/727–8000; C. Vincent Townsend, Jr, Senior Vice President **A**1 2 5 9 10 **F**1 3 4 7 8 9 11 12 13 16 17 19 20 22 24 25 26 27 30 31 32 35 36 38 39 40 41 43 46 47 48 49 51 54 56 59 61 62 63 65 68 70 72 73 76 77 78 79 **P**5 **S** Catholic Health Initiatives, Denver, CO	21	10	179	10151	143	33827	—	74900	29185	865
★ ST. JOSEPH NORTHEAST HEIGHTS HOSPITAL, 4701 Montgomery Boulevard N.E., Zip 87109–1251, Mailing Address: P.O. Box 25555, Zip 87125–0555; tel. 505/727–7800; Tony Struthers, Vice President Operations and Administrator **A**1 9 10 **F**1 4 7 8 9 11 13 16 17 22 24 27 30 31 34 36 37 38 39 40 42 43 44 45 46 47 48 49 50 51 54 56 59 61 62 65 66 68 70 72 73 75 76 77 78 79 **P**5 **S** Catholic Health Initiatives, Denver, CO	21	10	78	3798	34	21285	1854	17096	7406	219
★ △ ST. JOSEPH REHABILITATION HOSPITAL AND OUTPATIENT CENTER, 505 Elm Street N.E., Zip 87102–2500, Mailing Address: P.O. Box 25555, Zip 87125–5555; tel. 505/727–4700; Mary Lou Coors, Vice President (Total facility includes 23 beds in nursing home–type unit) **A**7 9 10 **F**1 3 4 7 8 9 11 13 16 17 22 24 25 26 30 31 34 36 37 38 39 40 43 46 47 48 49 50 51 53 54 56 59 61 62 63 65 66 68 69 70 72 73 76 77 78 79 **P**5 **S** Catholic Health Initiatives, Denver, CO Web address: www.sjhs.org	21	46	62	1082	50	—	—	17351	6129	193

© 2000 AHA Guide   *Many Facility Codes have changed. Please refer to the AHA Guide Code Chart.*

Hospitals, U.S. / NEW MEXICO

	Classification Codes		Utilization Data					Expense (thousands) of dollars		
Hospital, Address, Telephone, Administrator, Approval, Facility, and Physician Codes, Health Care System, Network	Control	Service	Staffed Beds	Admissions	Census	Outpatient Visits	Births	Total	Payroll	Personnel

★ American Hospital Association (AHA) membership
☐ Joint Commission on Accreditation of Healthcare Organizations (JCAHO) accreditation
+ American Osteopathic Healthcare Association (AOHA) membership
○ American Osteopathic Association (AOA) accreditation
△ Commission on Accreditation of Rehabilitation Facilities (CARF) accreditation
Control codes 61, 63, 64, 71, 72 and 73 indicate hospitals listed by AOHA, but not registered by AHA. For definition of numerical codes, see page A4

Hospital	Control	Service	Staffed Beds	Admissions	Census	Outpatient Visits	Births	Total	Payroll	Personnel
★ ST. JOSEPH WEST MESA HOSPITAL, 10501 Golf Course Road N.W., Zip 87114–5000, Mailing Address: P.O. Box 25555, Zip 87125–0555; tel. 505/727–2000; Tony Struthers, Vice President and Administrator (Total facility includes 22 beds in nursing home–type unit) **A**1 9 10 **F**3 4 8 9 11 13 16 17 19 22 24 25 26 27 30 31 34 36 37 38 39 40 43 46 47 48 49 51 54 56 57 59 61 62 63 65 66 68 69 70 72 73 76 77 78 79 **P**5 **S** Catholic Health Initiatives, Denver, CO	21	10	74	2072	44	33826	—	13247	5740	185
★ UNIVERSITY HOSPITAL, 2211 Lomas Boulevard N.E., Zip 87106–2745; tel. 505/272–2121; Stephen W. McKernan, Chief Executive Officer **A**1 2 3 5 8 9 10 12 **F**3 4 5 7 8 9 10 11 13 16 17 18 19 22 24 25 27 28 30 32 33 34 35 36 37 38 39 41 42 44 45 46 47 48 49 50 51 52 54 59 60 63 65 66 68 70 71 72 73 74 75 76 77 78 79 **S** University of New Mexico, Albuquerque, NM Web address: www.unm.edu	12	10	261	19981	253	380867	3441	219189	82041	2480
★ UNIVERSITY OF NEW MEXICO CHILDREN'S PSYCHIATRIC HOSPITAL, 1001 Yale Boulevard N.E., Zip 87131–3830; tel. 505/272–2945; Maggie McGowan, Interim Area Director (Nonreporting) **A**5 9 **S** University of New Mexico, Albuquerque, NM Web address: www.cph.unm.edu	12	52	53	—	—	—	—	—	—	—
☐ VENCOR HOSPITAL – ALBUQUERQUE, 700 High Street N.E., Zip 87102–2565; tel. 505/242–4444; Jeanne Koester, Chief Executive Officer **A**1 5 10 **F**10 12 13 17 18 26 32 41 42 44 45 52 **P**8 **S** Vencor, Incorporated, Louisville, KY	33	10	56	422	44	0	0	12946	5248	147
★ △ VETERANS AFFAIRS MEDICAL CENTER, 1501 San Pedro S.E., Zip 87108–5138; tel. 505/265–1711; Norman E. Browne, Director (Total facility includes 47 beds in nursing home–type unit) (Nonreporting) **A**1 2 3 5 7 8 9 **S** Department of Veterans Affairs, Washington, DC Web address: www.va.gov	45	10	327	—	—	—	—	—	—	—

ARTESIA—Eddy County

Hospital	Control	Service	Staffed Beds	Admissions	Census	Outpatient Visits	Births	Total	Payroll	Personnel
★ ARTESIA GENERAL HOSPITAL, 702 North 13th Street, Zip 88210–1199; tel. 505/748–3333; Arthur R. Smith, Chief Executive Officer (Nonreporting) **A**9 10	16	10	38	—	—	—	—	—	—	—

CANNON AFB—Curry County

Hospital	Control	Service	Staffed Beds	Admissions	Census	Outpatient Visits	Births	Total	Payroll	Personnel
★ U. S. AIR FORCE HOSPITAL, 208 West Casablanca Avenue, Zip 88103–5300; tel. 505/784–6318; Major John Sell, MSC, USAF, Administrator (Nonreporting) **S** Department of the Air Force, Bowling AFB, DC	41	10	10	—	—	—	—	—	—	—

CARLSBAD—Eddy County

Hospital	Control	Service	Staffed Beds	Admissions	Census	Outpatient Visits	Births	Total	Payroll	Personnel
★ CARLSBAD MEDICAL CENTER, (Formerly Columbia Medical Center of Carlsbad), 2430 West Pierce Street, Zip 88220–3597; tel. 505/887–4100; Fred Woody, Chief Executive Officer (Nonreporting) **A**1 9 10 **S** Triad Hospitals, Inc., Dallas, TX Web address: www.hcahealthcare.com	33	10	110	—	—	—	—	—	—	—

CLAYTON—Union County

Hospital	Control	Service	Staffed Beds	Admissions	Census	Outpatient Visits	Births	Total	Payroll	Personnel
★ UNION COUNTY GENERAL HOSPITAL, 301 Harding Street, Zip 88415–3321, Mailing Address: P.O. Box 489, Zip 88415–0489; tel. 505/374–2585; W. C. McElhannon, Administrator **A**9 **F**9 22 25 32 36 38 39 44 48 54 76 **S** Brim Healthcare, Inc., Brentwood, TN	13	10	25	372	4	—	24	3572	1235	47

CLOVIS—Curry County

Hospital	Control	Service	Staffed Beds	Admissions	Census	Outpatient Visits	Births	Total	Payroll	Personnel
★ PLAINS REGIONAL MEDICAL CENTER, 2100 North Thomas Street, Zip 88101–9412, Mailing Address: P.O. Box 1688, Zip 88101–1688; tel. 505/769–2141; Richard Smith, Administrator **A**1 9 10 **F**7 8 13 22 24 25 26 27 30 32 36 37 38 39 40 41 43 44 45 46 48 54 55 61 65 66 69 70 72 76 77 78 79 **P**6 8 **S** Presbyterian Healthcare Services, Albuquerque, NM	23	10	74	6258	69	145553	1191	36826	14458	481

CROWNPOINT—McKinley County

Hospital	Control	Service	Staffed Beds	Admissions	Census	Outpatient Visits	Births	Total	Payroll	Personnel
★ U. S. PUBLIC HEALTH SERVICE INDIAN HOSPITAL, Mailing Address: P.O. Box 358, Zip 87313–0358; tel. 505/786–5291; Anita Muneta, Chief Executive Officer (Nonreporting) **A**1 10 **S** U. S. Public Health Service Indian Health Service, Rockville, MD	44	10	32	—	—	—	—	—	—	—

DEMING—Luna County

Hospital	Control	Service	Staffed Beds	Admissions	Census	Outpatient Visits	Births	Total	Payroll	Personnel
★ MIMBRES MEMORIAL HOSPITAL, 900 West Ash Street, Zip 88030–4098, Mailing Address: P.O. Box 710, Zip 88031–0710; tel. 505/546–2761; Timothy E. Schmidt, Chief Executive Officer (Total facility includes 70 beds in nursing home–type unit) (Nonreporting) **A**9 10 **S** Community Health Systems, Inc., Brentwood, TN	33	10	119	—	—	—	—	—	—	—

ESPANOLA—Rio Arriba County

Hospital	Control	Service	Staffed Beds	Admissions	Census	Outpatient Visits	Births	Total	Payroll	Personnel
★ ESPANOLA HOSPITAL, 1010 Spruce Street, Zip 87532–2746; tel. 505/753–7111; Marcella A. Romero, Administrator **A**1 9 10 **F**8 9 13 16 17 18 22 25 32 36 41 44 45 48 51 54 56 70 76 77 78 79 **P**1 3 5 **S** Presbyterian Healthcare Services, Albuquerque, NM	23	10	80	2638	20	65179	289	19317	9191	286

FARMINGTON—San Juan County

Hospital	Control	Service	Staffed Beds	Admissions	Census	Outpatient Visits	Births	Total	Payroll	Personnel
★ SAN JUAN REGIONAL MEDICAL CENTER, (Includes LifeCourse Rehabilitation Hospital, 525 South Schwartz, Zip 87401; tel. 505/327–3422), 801 West Maple Street, Zip 87401–5698; tel. 505/325–5011; Steve Altmiller, President and Chief Executive Officer (Total facility includes 15 beds in nursing home–type unit) **A**1 2 9 10 **F**3 7 8 9 11 13 14 16 17 18 19 22 24 25 26 27 29 32 33 37 38 39 41 44 45 46 48 49 50 54 58 59 61 63 64 65 68 69 70 72 75 76 77 78 79 **P**4 5 8 Web address: www.lifecoursems.com	23	10	145	8494	98	123723	1291	82958	36419	1061

FORT SUMNER—De Baca County

Hospital	Control	Service	Staffed Beds	Admissions	Census	Outpatient Visits	Births	Total	Payroll	Personnel
★ DEBACA GENERAL HOSPITAL, 500 North Tenth Street, Zip 88119, Mailing Address: P.O. Box 349, Zip 88119–0349; tel. 505/355–2414 (Nonreporting) **A**9 10	13	10	21	—	—	—	—	—	—	—

Many Facility Codes have changed. Please refer to the AHA Guide Code Chart.

© 2000 AHA Guide

Hospitals, U.S. / NEW MEXICO

Hospital, Address, Telephone, Administrator, Approval, Facility, and Physician Codes, Health Care System, Network	Classification Codes		Utilization Data					Expense (thousands) of dollars		
★ American Hospital Association (AHA) membership □ Joint Commission on Accreditation of Healthcare Organizations (JCAHO) accreditation + American Osteopathic Healthcare Association (AOHA) membership ○ American Osteopathic Association (AOA) accreditation △ Commission on Accreditation of Rehabilitation Facilities (CARF) accreditation Control codes 61, 63, 64, 71, 72 and 73 indicate hospitals listed by AOHA, but not registered by AHA. For definition of numerical codes, see page A4	Control	Service	Staffed Beds	Admissions	Census	Outpatient Visits	Births	Total	Payroll	Personnel
GALLUP—McKinley County										
✴ GALLUP INDIAN MEDICAL CENTER, 516 East Nizhoni Boulevard, Zip 87301–5748, Mailing Address: P.O. Box 1337, Zip 87305–1337; tel. 505/722–1000; Floyd Thompson, Chief Executive Officer **A**1 10 **F**8 13 18 19 22 24 25 29 39 41 44 48 51 54 56 58 61 63 **P**6 **S** U. S. Public Health Service Indian Health Service, Rockville, MD	47	10	79	4829	46	286691	924	58615	36507	852
✴ REHOBOTH MCKINLEY CHRISTIAN HOSPITAL, 1901 Red Rock Drive, Zip 87301–1901; tel. 505/863–7000; David J. Baltzer, President **A**1 9 10 **F**2 3 7 8 9 13 16 17 18 19 21 22 25 32 33 34 36 37 38 39 41 43 44 45 48 49 51 54 56 57 58 59 60 61 63 64 66 70 72 76 79 **P**5 6 Web address: www.rmch.org	23	10	118	2711	52	160618	398	45977	22024	595
GRANTS—Cibola County										
✴ CIBOLA GENERAL HOSPITAL, 1212 Bonita Avenue, Zip 87020–2104; tel. 505/287–4446; Walter Topp, II, Administrator (Nonreporting) **A**1 9 10 **S** Quorum Health Group, Brentwood, TN	23	10	22	—	—	—	—	—	—	—
HOBBS—Lea County										
✴ LEA REGIONAL MEDICAL CENTER, (Formerly Lea Regional Hospital), 5419 North Lovington Highway, Zip 88240–9125, Mailing Address: P.O. Box 3000, Zip 88240–3000; tel. 505/392–6581; William J. Gresco, Chief Executive Officer (Nonreporting) **A**1 9 10 **S** Triad Hospitals, Inc., Dallas, TX	33	10	250	—	—	—	—	—	—	—
HOLLOMAN AFB—Otero County										
✴ U. S. AIR FORCE HOSPITAL, 280 First Street, Zip 88330–8273; tel. 505/572–3777; Colonel Marilyn S. Abu-Ghusson, USAF, Commander (Nonreporting) **A**1 **S** Department of the Air Force, Bowling AFB, DC	41	10	7	—	—	—	—	—	—	—
KIRTLAND AFB—Bernalillo County										
★ U. S. AIR FORCE HOSPITAL-KIRTLAND, 1951 Second Street S.E., Zip 87117–5559; tel. 505/846–3547; Colonel Royetta Marconi-Dooley, Commander (Nonreporting) **A**3 5 **S** Department of the Air Force, Bowling AFB, DC	41	10	10	—	—	—	—	—	—	—
LAS CRUCES—Dona Ana County										
□ BHC MESILLA VALLEY HOSPITAL, 3751 Del Rey Boulevard, Zip 88012–8526, Mailing Address: P.O. Box 429, Zip 88004–0429; tel. 505/382–3500; Terry G. Johnson, Chief Executive Officer **A**1 10 **F**3 22 25 39 45 53 57 58 62 63 76 **P**8 **S** Behavioral Healthcare Corporation, Nashville, TN	32	22	115	1110	57	—	0	6475	3556	110
✴ MEMORIAL MEDICAL CENTER, 2450 South Telshor Boulevard, Zip 88011–5076; tel. 505/522–8641; Steven L. Smith, President and Chief Executive Officer **A**1 3 5 9 10 **F**4 7 8 9 11 13 17 22 24 25 29 32 36 39 41 43 44 46 47 48 49 54 55 57 61 70 75 76 77 78 79 Web address: www.mmclc.org	23	10	243	16551	189	194988	2516	120356	47033	1366
LAS VEGAS—San Miguel County										
□ LAS VEGAS MEDICAL CENTER, 3795 Hot Springs Boulevard, Zip 87701, Mailing Address: P.O. Box 1388, Zip 87701–1388; tel. 505/454–2100; Felix Alderele, Administrator (Total facility includes 176 beds in nursing home–type unit) **A**1 **F**13 16 17 18 19 21 23 30 45 50 51 54 58 59 60 61 62 63 64 70 72 **P**6	12	22	390	717	334	45609	—	36372	22595	900
✴ NORTHEASTERN REGIONAL HOSPITAL, 1235 Eighth Street, Zip 87701–4254, Mailing Address: P.O. Box 248, Zip 87701–0238; tel. 505/425–6751; Jerry B. Scott, Chief Executive Officer **A**1 9 10 **F**7 8 9 13 14 15 17 19 21 22 23 25 26 28 30 32 33 34 35 36 37 38 39 40 41 43 44 45 46 47 48 50 51 53 54 58 59 60 61 62 63 64 65 66 70 71 72 75 76 **P**7 8	23	10	54	2346	23	45938	355	15771	5694	206
LOS ALAMOS—Los Alamos County										
✴ LOS ALAMOS MEDICAL CENTER, 3917 West Road, Zip 87544–2293; tel. 505/662–4201; Paul J. Wilson, Administrator (Nonreporting) **A**1 9 10 **S** Banner Health System, Fargo, ND	23	10	47	—	—	—	—	—	—	—
LOVINGTON—Lea County										
★ NOR–LEA GENERAL HOSPITAL, 1600 North Main Avenue, Zip 88260–2871; tel. 505/396–6611; David B. Shaw, Chief Executive Officer and Administrator **A**9 10 **F**7 9 13 14 16 17 18 22 25 26 32 36 37 38 43 45 48 70 76 **P**1 4 5 8 **S** Lubbock Methodist Hospital System, Lubbock, TX Web address: www.nlgh.org	16	10	28	500	4	24920	0	7064	4093	114
MESCALERO—Otero County										
✴ U. S. PUBLIC HEALTH SERVICE INDIAN HOSPITAL, Mailing Address: Box 210, Zip 88340–0210; tel. 505/671–4441; Jo Ann Skaggs, Chief Executive Officer (Nonreporting) **A**1 10 **S** U. S. Public Health Service Indian Health Service, Rockville, MD	47	10	13	—	—	—	—	—	—	—
RATON—Colfax County										
★ MINERS' COLFAX MEDICAL CENTER, (Includes Miners' Hospital of New Mexico), 200 Hospital Drive, Zip 87740–2099; tel. 505/445–3661; David Antle, Chief Executive Officer (Total facility includes 30 beds in nursing home–type unit) (Nonreporting) **A**9 10	13	10	68	—	—	—	—	—	—	—
ROSWELL—Chaves County										
□ EASTERN NEW MEXICO MEDICAL CENTER, 405 West Country Club Road, Zip 88201–9981; tel. 505/622–8170; Ronald J. Shafer, Chief Executive Officer (Nonreporting) **A**1 9 10 **S** Community Health Systems, Inc., Brentwood, TN Web address: www.enmmc.com	13	10	168	—	—	—	—	—	—	—
□ △ SOUTHERN NEW MEXICO REHABILITATION CENTER, (Includes Pecos Valley Lodge), 31 Gail Harris Avenue, Zip 88201–8134; tel. 505/347–3400; Gary L. J. Giron, Executive Director **A**1 7 10 **F**2 3 16 17 18 53 54	12	46	35	504	24	4218	—	5156	2978	118

© 2000 AHA Guide   *Many Facility Codes have changed. Please refer to the AHA Guide Code Chart.*

Hospitals, U.S. / NEW MEXICO

Classification Codes Legend

★ American Hospital Association (AHA) membership
□ Joint Commission on Accreditation of Healthcare Organizations (JCAHO) accreditation
+ American Osteopathic Healthcare Association (AOHA) membership
○ American Osteopathic Association (AOA) accreditation
△ Commission on Accreditation of Rehabilitation Facilities (CARF) accreditation

Control codes 61, 63, 64, 71, 72 and 73 indicate hospitals listed by AOHA, but not registered by AHA. For definition of numerical codes, see page A4.

Hospital, Address, Telephone, Administrator, Approval, Facility, and Physician Codes, Health Care System, Network	Classification Codes		Utilization Data					Expense (thousands) of dollars		
	Control	Service	Staffed Beds	Admissions	Census	Outpatient Visits	Births	Total	Payroll	Personnel
RUIDOSO—Lincoln County ★ LINCOLN COUNTY MEDICAL CENTER, 211 Sudderth Drive, Zip 88345–6043, Mailing Address: P.O. Box 8000, Zip 88345–8000; tel. 505/257–7381; James P. Gibson, Administrator **A**1 9 10 **F**7 8 9 13 16 17 18 19 22 23 25 28 32 34 38 39 41 44 45 46 48 51 54 69 76 78 **P**8 **S** Presbyterian Healthcare Services, Albuquerque, NM	23	10	27	1126	6	39748	253	11945	5844	182
SAN FIDEL—Cibola County ★ ACOMA–CANONCITO–LAGUNA HOSPITAL, Mailing Address: P.O. Box 130, Zip 87049–0130; tel. 505/552–5300; R. C. Begay, Chief Executive Officer (Nonreporting) **A**1 10 **S** U. S. Public Health Service Indian Health Service, Rockville, MD	47	10	15	—	—	—	—	—	—	—
SANTA FE—Santa Fe County ★ PHS SANTA FE INDIAN HOSPITAL, 1700 Cerrillos Road, Zip 87505–3554; tel. 505/988–9821; Lawrence A. Jordan, Director (Nonreporting) **A**1 10 **S** U. S. Public Health Service Indian Health Service, Rockville, MD	47	10	39	—	—	—	—	—	—	—
★ △ ST. VINCENT HOSPITAL, 455 St. Michael's Drive, Zip 87505–7663, Mailing Address: P.O. Box 2107, Zip 87504–2107; tel. 505/983–3361; John Lucas, M.D., President and Chief Executive Officer (Nonreporting) **A**1 2 5 7 9 10 Web address: www.stvin.org	23	10	198	—	—	—	—	—	—	—
SANTA TERESA—Dona Ana County □ ALLIANCE HOSPITAL OF SANTA TERESA, 100 Laura Court, Zip 88008, Mailing Address: P.O. Box 6, Las Cruces, Zip 88008–0006; tel. 505/589–0033; Michele Irwin, Administrator (Nonreporting) **A**1 10 **S** Bowdon Corporate Offices	33	22	72	—	—	—	—	—	—	—
SHIPROCK—San Juan County ★ NORTHERN NAVAJO MEDICAL CENTER, Mailing Address: P.O. Box 160, Zip 87420–0160; tel. 505/368–6001; Dee Hutchison, Chief Executive Officer (Nonreporting) **A**1 10 **S** U. S. Public Health Service Indian Health Service, Rockville, MD	47	10	59	—	—	—	—	—	—	—
SILVER CITY—Grant County ★ GILA REGIONAL MEDICAL CENTER, 1313 East 32nd Street, Zip 88061; tel. 505/538–4000; Polly Pine, Administrator **A**1 9 10 **F**7 8 9 18 19 22 24 25 28 33 36 37 39 41 43 44 45 46 48 54 57 59 61 62 70 73 76 **P**3 5 **S** Quorum Health Group, Brentwood, TN Web address: www.grmc.org	13	10	67	2636	28	69087	548	25873	12284	389
SOCORRO—Socorro County ★ SOCORRO GENERAL HOSPITAL, 1202 Highway 60 West, Zip 87801, Mailing Address: P.O. Box 1009, Zip 87801–1009; tel. 505/835–1140; Jeff Dye, Administrator **A**1 9 10 **F**7 8 9 19 22 25 36 37 39 44 48 54 73 76 **S** Presbyterian Healthcare Services, Albuquerque, NM	23	10	24	699	6	22896	195	8483	3830	110
TAOS—Taos County ★ HOLY CROSS HOSPITAL, 1397 Weimer Road, Zip 87571, Mailing Address: P.O. Box DD, Zip 87571; tel. 505/758–8883; Warren K. Spellman, Administrator **A**1 9 10 **F**7 8 9 13 17 19 22 25 32 34 38 39 41 43 44 48 50 54 57 70 71 72 76 77 **P**3 8 **S** Quorum Health Group, Brentwood, TN Web address: www.taoshospital.org	23	10	34	1902	18	48679	252	15841	6333	251
TRUTH OR CONSEQUENCES—Sierra County ★ SIERRA VISTA HOSPITAL, 800 East Ninth Avenue, Zip 87901–1961; tel. 505/894–2111; Domenica Rush, Administrator **A**1 9 10 **F**7 13 16 17 18 19 22 25 32 34 36 38 44 48 51 54 70 76	15	10	28	443	5	18402	11	5776	3454	109
TUCUMCARI—Quay County ★ DR. DAN C. TRIGG MEMORIAL HOSPITAL, 301 East Miel De Luna Avenue, Zip 88401–3810, Mailing Address: P.O. Box 608, Zip 88401–0608; tel. 505/461–0141; Dell Willis, Administrator (Nonreporting) **A**9 10 **S** Presbyterian Healthcare Services, Albuquerque, NM	23	10	37	—	—	—	—	—	—	—
ZUNI—McKinley County ★ U. S. PUBLIC HEALTH SERVICE INDIAN HOSPITAL, Mailing Address: P.O. Box 467, Zip 87327–0467; tel. 505/782–4431; Jean Othole, Service Unit Director **A**1 10 **F**1 3 4 5 6 7 8 9 11 14 16 17 18 21 22 23 24 26 28 30 31 32 34 39 44 55 58 59 60 61 62 63 64 65 68 73 74 77 **S** U. S. Public Health Service Indian Health Service, Rockville, MD	47	10	25	819	9	70000	96	—	—	170

Hospitals, U.S. / NEW YORK

NEW YORK

Resident Population 18,175 (in thousands)
Resident population in metro areas 91.8%
Birth rate per 1,000 population 14.2
65 years and over 13.3%
Percent of persons without health insurance 17.5%

★ American Hospital Association (AHA) membership
□ Joint Commission on Accreditation of Healthcare Organizations (JCAHO) accreditation
+ American Osteopathic Healthcare Association (AOHA) membership
○ American Osteopathic Association (AOA) accreditation
△ Commission on Accreditation of Rehabilitation Facilities (CARF) accreditation
Control codes 61, 63, 64, 71, 72 and 73 indicate hospitals listed by AOHA, but not registered by AHA. For definition of numerical codes, see page A4

Hospital, Address, Telephone, Administrator, Approval, Facility, and Physician Codes, Health Care System, Network	Classification Codes		Utilization Data					Expense (thousands) of dollars		
	Control	Service	Staffed Beds	Admissions	Census	Outpatient Visits	Births	Total	Payroll	Personnel
ALBANY—Albany County										
★ ALBANY MEDICAL CENTER, (Includes Albany Medical Center South–Clinical Campus, 25 Hackett Boulevard, Zip 12208–3499; tel. 518/242–1200; Timothy W. Duffy, General Director), 43 New Scotland Avenue, Zip 12208–3478; tel. 518/262–3125; Mary A. Nolan, R.N., MS, Executive Vice President Care Delivery and General Director **A**1 2 3 5 8 9 10 **F**4 5 7 8 9 11 12 13 17 18 19 22 23 24 25 30 32 34 35 36 38 39 41 42 43 44 45 46 47 48 49 50 51 52 53 54 56 57 58 59 60 61 62 63 64 65 66 68 70 74 75 76 77 78 79 **P**6	23	10	558	23193	445	303462	2202	291697	94593	2947
★ CAPITAL DISTRICT PSYCHIATRIC CENTER, 75 New Scotland Avenue, Zip 12208–3474; tel. 518/447–9611; Jesse Nixon, Jr, Ph.D., Director (Nonreporting) **A**1 3 5 10 **S** New York State Department of Mental Health, Albany, NY	12	22	200	—	—	—	—	—	—	—
□ MEMORIAL HOSPITAL, 600 Northern Boulevard, Zip 12204–1083; tel. 518/471–3221; Norman E. Dascher, Jr, Chief Executive Officer **A**1 6 9 10 **F**1 2 3 6 7 8 9 10 12 13 14 16 17 18 19 21 22 24 25 26 27 28 29 30 31 32 33 34 35 36 37 39 41 42 43 44 45 46 48 49 50 51 52 53 54 56 57 59 60 61 62 63 65 66 67 69 70 72 73 76 78 79 **P**7 Web address: www.nehealth.com	23	10	90	5463	81	117717	0	53005	24554	647
★ ST. PETER'S HOSPITAL, 315 South Manning Boulevard, Zip 12208–1789; tel. 518/525–1550; Steven P. Boyle, President and Chief Executive Officer (Nonreporting) **A**1 2 3 5 9 10 **S** Catholic Health East, Newtown Square, PA	23	10	437	—	—	—	—	—	—	—
★ VETERANS AFFAIRS MEDICAL CENTER, 113 Holland Avenue, Zip 12208–3473; tel. 518/462–3311; Clyde L. Parkis, Director (Total facility includes 50 beds in nursing home–type unit) (Nonreporting) **A**1 2 3 5 8 9 **S** Department of Veterans Affairs, Washington, DC Web address: www.va.gov/stations97/guide/home.asp?DIVISION=ALL	45	10	298	—	—	—	—	—	—	—
ALEXANDRIA BAY—Jefferson County										
□ E. J. NOBLE HOSPITAL SAMARITAN, 19 Fuller Street, Zip 13607; tel. 315/482–2511; Donna S. MacPherson, Administrator and Chief Operating Officer (Total facility includes 27 beds in nursing home–type unit) (Nonreporting) **A**1 9 10 Web address: www.samaritanhealth.com	23	10	52	—	—	—	—	—	—	—
AMITYVILLE—Suffolk County										
□ BRUNSWICK GENERAL HOSPITAL, (Includes Brunswick Hall, 80 Louden Avenue, Zip 11701–2735; tel. 516/789–7100; Brunswick Physical Medicine and Rehabilitation Hospital, 366 Broadway), 366 Broadway, Zip 11701–9820; tel. 631/789–7000; Benjamin M. Stein, M.D., President (Total facility includes 94 beds in nursing home–type unit) **A**1 9 10 **F**7 9 12 16 17 18 19 22 24 25 30 31 32 34 36 37 39 41 43 46 48 49 51 53 57 58 59 60 61 62 63 69 70 72 76 78	33	10	474	6488	308	123920	0	70871	37857	1108
□ SOUTH OAKS HOSPITAL, 400 Sunrise Highway, Zip 11701; tel. 631/264–4000; Patrick R. Martore, Chief Executive Officer (Nonreporting) **A**1 9 10 Web address: www.southoaks.com	33	22	334	—	—	—	—	—	—	—
AMSTERDAM—Montgomery County										
★ AMSTERDAM MEMORIAL HOSPITAL, 4988 State Highway 30, Zip 12010–1699; tel. 518/842–3100; Cornelio R. Catena, President and Chief Executive Officer (Total facility includes 160 beds in nursing home–type unit) **A**1 9 10 **F**1 7 9 12 13 14 15 16 17 19 22 23 24 25 28 29 30 31 33 34 38 39 41 43 45 46 48 49 50 53 54 69 70 71 72 73 76 78 79 **S** Quorum Health Group, Brentwood, TN	23	10	242	2550	196	73522	0	31632	12526	501
★ ST. MARY'S HOSPITAL, 427 Guy Park Avenue, Zip 12010–1095; tel. 518/842–1900; Peter E. Capobianco, President and Chief Executive Officer **A**1 9 10 **F**2 3 7 8 9 12 13 14 16 17 18 19 20 21 22 25 26 29 30 31 32 33 34 35 36 37 38 39 41 43 44 45 46 48 49 50 51 54 55 57 58 59 60 61 62 63 66 70 71 72 76 78 79 **P**8 **S** Carondelet Health System, Saint Louis, MO Web address: www.smha.org	21	10	143	4723	81	186350	630	44000	23994	640
AUBURN—Cayuga County										
★ AUBURN MEMORIAL HOSPITAL, 17 Lansing Street, Zip 13021–1943; tel. 315/255–7011; Christopher J. Rogers, Administrator (Total facility includes 80 beds in nursing home–type unit) **A**1 5 9 10 **F**7 8 9 12 13 16 17 18 22 25 27 29 38 41 44 48 54 57 59 61 67 70 71 72 76 77 78 Web address: www.auburnhospital.org	23	10	244	6601	195	111005	466	54406	26863	696
BATAVIA—Genesee County										
★ UNITED MEMORIAL MEDICAL CENTER, (Includes United Memorial Medical Center–Bank Street, 127 North Street; United Memorial Medical Center–North Street, 127 North Street, Zip 14020–1697; tel. 716/343–6030), 127 North Street, Zip 14020–2260; tel. 716/343–3131; Charles S. Kinney, Chief Executive Officer **A**1 9 10 **F**2 5 8 9 12 16 17 18 19 21 25 29 31 32 33 34 37 38 39 41 43 44 45 46 48 49 50 56 66 67 70 71 72 76 78 79	23	10	119	5088	98	184549	433	43144	19554	712

© 2000 AHA Guide   *Many Facility Codes have changed. Please refer to the AHA Guide Code Chart.*   Hospitals **A287**

Hospitals, U.S. / NEW YORK

Hospital, Address, Telephone, Administrator, Approval, Facility, and Physician Codes, Health Care System, Network	Classification Codes		Utilization Data					Expense (thousands) of dollars		
★ American Hospital Association (AHA) membership □ Joint Commission on Accreditation of Healthcare Organizations (JCAHO) accreditation + American Osteopathic Healthcare Association (AOHA) membership ○ American Osteopathic Association (AOA) accreditation △ Commission on Accreditation of Rehabilitation Facilities (CARF) accreditation Control codes 61, 63, 64, 71, 72 and 73 indicate hospitals listed by AOHA, but not registered by AHA. For definition of numerical codes, see page A4	Control	Service	Staffed Beds	Admissions	Census	Outpatient Visits	Births	Total	Payroll	Personnel
★ VETERANS AFFAIRS WESTERN NEW YORK HEALTHCARE SYSTEM–BATAVIA DIVISION, 222 Richmond Avenue, Zip 14020–1288; tel. 716/343–7500; Richard S. Droske, Director (Total facility includes 70 beds in nursing home–type unit) (Nonreporting) **A**5 9 **S** Department of Veterans Affairs, Washington, DC	45	10	158	—	—	—	—	—	—	—
BATH—Steuben County										
✠ IRA DAVENPORT MEMORIAL HOSPITAL, 7571 State Route 54, Zip 14810–9533; tel. 607/776–8500; James B. Watson, Chief Executive Officer (Total facility includes 120 beds in nursing home–type unit) (Nonreporting) **A**1 9 10	23	10	186	—	—	—	—	—	—	—
✠ VETERANS AFFAIRS MEDICAL CENTER, 76 Veterans Avenue, Zip 14810–0842; tel. 607/664–4000; Joseph Striano, Acting Director (Total facility includes 125 beds in nursing home–type unit) (Nonreporting) **A**1 9 **S** Department of Veterans Affairs, Washington, DC **Web address:** www.va.gov/stations97/guide/home.asp?DIVISION=ALL	45	10	615	—	—	—	—	—	—	—
BAY SHORE—Suffolk County										
✠ SOUTHSIDE HOSPITAL, 301 East Main Street, Zip 11706–8458; tel. 631/968–3000; Theodore A. Jospe, President **A**1 3 5 9 10 **F**2 3 4 7 8 9 10 11 12 14 16 17 18 19 22 24 25 26 29 30 31 32 33 34 35 36 37 38 39 42 44 45 46 47 48 49 51 52 53 54 56 57 59 61 63 65 66 68 69 70 71 72 73 74 75 76 78 79 **P**5 7 **S** North Shore– Long Island Jewish Health System, Great Neck, NY **Web address:** www.northshorelij.com	23	10	439	15172	283	129288	2304	147829	76885	1640
BEACON—Dutchess County										
✠ CRAIG HOUSE CENTER, 7 Craig House Lane, Zip 12508; tel. 914/831–1200; Ida Tonneson, Chief Executive Officer **A**1 9 10 **F**2 16 17 18 57 58 62 **P**8	33	22	61	698	34	0	0	6218	3761	112
BELLEROSE—Queens County, See New York City										
BETHPAGE—Nassau County										
□ NEW ISLAND HOSPITAL, (Formerly Mid–Island Hospital), 4295 Hempstead Turnpike, Zip 11714–5769; tel. 516/579–6000; Paul E. Seale, Chief Executive Officer **A**1 9 10 **F**8 12 13 17 18 19 22 24 25 30 32 34 35 36 38 39 40 41 43 44 46 48 51 54 61 70 72 74 76 78	23	10	125	5317	78	28111	930	40362	17253	416
BINGHAMTON—Broome County										
BINGHAMTON GENERAL HOSPITAL See United Health Services Hospitals–Binghamton										
✠ BINGHAMTON PSYCHIATRIC CENTER, 425 Robinson Street, Zip 13901–4198; tel. 607/724–1391; Margaret R. Dugan, Executive Director **A**1 10 **F**7 17 23 29 43 51 57 58 62 63 64 70 72 78 **P**6 **S** New York State Department of Mental Health, Albany, NY	12	22	177	127	190	42204	0	23774	20308	509
✠ OUR LADY OF LOURDES MEMORIAL HOSPITAL, 169 Riverside Drive, Zip 13905–4198; tel. 607/798–5111; John D. O'Neil, President and Chief Executive Officer **A**1 2 9 10 **F**5 7 8 9 13 16 17 18 19 20 22 24 25 26 27 28 29 30 31 32 33 34 35 36 37 38 39 41 43 44 46 48 49 50 51 54 56 58 60 62 63 65 68 70 71 72 73 76 77 78 79 **P**3 5 6 7 **S** Ascension Health, Saint Louis, MO **Web address:** www.lourdes.com	21	10	184	8929	135	927493	1120	116814	51718	1099
✠ ○ UNITED HEALTH SERVICES HOSPITALS–BINGHAMTON, (Includes Binghamton General Hospital, 10–42 Mitchell Avenue; Medicenter, 600 High Avenue, Endicott, Zip 13760; tel. 607/754–7171; Wilson Memorial Regional Medical Center, 33–57 Harrison Street, Johnson City, Zip 13790; 10–42 Mitchell Avenue, Zip 13903; tel. 607/763–6000; Matthew J. Salanger, President and Chief Executive Officer **A**1 2 3 5 8 9 10 11 **F**1 2 3 4 6 7 8 9 10 11 12 13 14 16 17 18 19 21 22 23 24 25 30 32 33 34 35 36 37 38 41 42 43 44 45 46 47 48 49 50 51 53 54 55 56 57 58 59 60 61 62 63 65 66 68 69 70 71 72 75 76 77 78 79 **P**1 7 **Web address:** www.uhs.net	23	10	516	18874	344	233118	1771	201683	80925	2370
BRENTWOOD—Suffolk County										
★ PILGRIM PSYCHIATRIC CENTER, (Includes Kings Park Psychiatric Center, 998 Crooked Hill Road, tel. 516/761–3500; Alan M. Weinstock, MS, Chief Executive Officer), 998 Crooked Hill Road, Zip 11717–1087; tel. 631/761–3500; Kathleen Kelly, Chief Executive Officer (Nonreporting) **A**5 10 **S** New York State Department of Mental Health, Albany, NY	12	22	744	—	—	—	—	—	—	—
BROCKPORT—Monroe County										
✠ LAKESIDE MEMORIAL HOSPITAL, 156 West Avenue, Zip 14420–1286; tel. 716/395–6095; Robert W. Harris, President **A**1 9 10 **F**2 3 4 8 9 10 11 12 16 17 18 19 22 24 25 27 32 34 37 39 42 43 44 45 46 48 49 50 51 52 53 55 57 58 59 60 61 62 63 64 65 68 69 70 72 74 75 76 77 78 **Web address:** www.va.gov/stations97/guide/home.asp?DIVISION=ALL	23	10	72	2706	48	14540	353	—	—	324
BRONX—Bronx County, See New York City										
BRONXVILLE—Westchester County										
✠ LAWRENCE HOSPITAL, 55 Palmer Avenue, Zip 10708–3491; tel. 914/787–1000; Edward M. Dinan, President and Chief Executive Officer **A**1 2 9 10 **F**7 8 9 13 17 18 19 22 24 25 26 30 34 36 37 38 39 40 41 42 43 44 45 46 48 49 50 51 54 59 68 70 71 72 76 78 79 **P**5 **Web address:** www.lawrencehealth.org	23	10	198	8908	144	119173	1599	71112	36859	922
BROOKLYN—Kings County, See New York City										
BUFFALO—Erie County										
□ BRYLIN HOSPITALS, 1263 Delaware Avenue, Zip 14209–2497; tel. 716/886–8200; Eric D. Pleskow, President and Chief Executive Officer **A**1 9 10 **F**2 3 16 17 57 58 59 60 61 62 63 64 **Web address:** www.brylin.com	33	22	150	2856	100	—	0	13758	7246	221

Hospitals, U.S. / NEW YORK

Hospital, Address, Telephone, Administrator, Approval, Facility, and Physician Codes, Health Care System, Network	Classification Codes		Utilization Data					Expense (thousands) of dollars		
	Control	Service	Staffed Beds	Admissions	Census	Outpatient Visits	Births	Total	Payroll	Personnel

★ American Hospital Association (AHA) membership
☐ Joint Commission on Accreditation of Healthcare Organizations (JCAHO) accreditation
+ American Osteopathic Healthcare Association (AOHA) membership
○ American Osteopathic Association (AOA) accreditation
△ Commission on Accreditation of Rehabilitation Facilities (CARF) accreditation
Control codes 61, 63, 64, 71, 72 and 73 indicate hospitals listed by AOHA, but not registered by AHA. For definition of numerical codes, see page A4

Hospital	Control	Service	Staffed Beds	Admissions	Census	Outpatient Visits	Births	Total	Payroll	Personnel
★ BUFFALO GENERAL HOSPITAL, 100 High Street, Zip 14203–1154; tel. 716/845–5600; John E. Friedlander, President and Chief Executive Officer (Total facility includes 242 beds in nursing home–type unit) (Nonreporting) A1 3 5 8 9 10 S KALEIDA Health, Buffalo, NY	23	10	965	—	—	—	—	—	—	—
★ BUFFALO PSYCHIATRIC CENTER, 400 Forest Avenue, Zip 14213–1298; tel. 716/885–2261; George A. Roets, R.N., MS, Executive Director A1 10 F3 4 5 6 7 8 9 10 11 12 13 15 17 18 19 21 22 23 24 27 28 29 30 31 32 33 34 35 39 41 43 44 46 47 48 50 51 53 54 55 57 60 62 63 65 66 68 70 72 74 75 76 78 P1 S New York State Department of Mental Health, Albany, NY Web address: www.omh.state.ny.us	12	22	240	179	250	23467	0	—	—	808
☐ CHILDREN'S HOSPITAL, 219 Bryant Street, Zip 14222–2099; tel. 716/878–7000; Karen Blount, R.N., Chief Operating Officer (Nonreporting) A1 3 5 9 10 S KALEIDA Health, Buffalo, NY	23	59	313	—	—	—	—	—	—	—
☐ ERIE COUNTY MEDICAL CENTER, 462 Grider Street, Zip 14215–3098; tel. 716/898–3000; Paul J. Candino, Chief Executive Officer (Total facility includes 759 beds in nursing home–type unit) A1 3 5 9 10 F2 3 4 7 9 10 11 12 13 14 16 17 18 19 21 22 23 24 25 29 30 31 32 33 34 35 36 37 38 39 41 43 45 46 47 48 51 53 54 56 57 58 59 60 61 62 63 68 69 70 72 74 75 76 78 79 P5 Web address: www.ecmc.edu	13	10	1176	13661	1247	276756	0	226582	103392	2051
☐ MERCY HOSPITAL, 565 Abbott Road, Zip 14220–2095; tel. 716/826–7000; John P. Davanzo, President and Chief Executive Officer (Total facility includes 74 beds in nursing home–type unit) A1 3 5 9 10 F2 3 4 6 8 9 10 11 12 13 16 17 19 20 21 22 23 24 25 29 30 31 32 33 34 35 36 37 38 39 40 41 42 43 44 45 46 47 48 49 50 51 52 53 54 55 56 57 58 59 60 61 62 63 64 65 66 67 68 69 70 71 72 73 74 76 77 78 79 Web address: www.mercywny.org	21	10	350	13908	286	297481	3044	110950	48011	—
★ MILLARD FILLMORE GATES CIRCLE HOSPITAL, (Formerly Millard Fillmore Health System), (Includes Millard Fillmore Suburban Hospital, 1540 Maple Road, Williamsville, Zip 14221; tel. 716/688–3100), 3 Gates Circle, Zip 14209–9986; tel. 716/887–4600; Joyce Korzen, R.N., Chief Operating Officer (Total facility includes 75 beds in nursing home–type unit) (Nonreporting) A1 3 5 6 9 S KALEIDA Health, Buffalo, NY Web address: www.mfhs.edu	23	10	588	—	—	—	—	—	—	—
☐ ROSWELL PARK CANCER INSTITUTE, (CANCER RESEARCH & TREATMENT), Elm and Carlton Streets, Zip 14263–0001; tel. 716/845–2300; David C. Hohn, M.D., President and Chief Executive Officer A1 2 3 5 8 9 10 F9 13 16 17 18 19 22 23 24 26 32 33 34 35 37 38 39 41 43 45 46 48 49 50 51 54 59 65 68 70 72 74 76 78 79 P5 6 Web address: www.roswellpark.org	16	49	119	3901	72	100798	0	207642	81990	1300
☐ SHEEHAN MEMORIAL HOSPITAL, 425 Michigan Avenue, Zip 14203–2297; tel. 716/848–2000; Olivia Smith–Blackwell, M.D., M.P.H., President and Chief Executive Officer (Nonreporting) A1 9 10	23	10	109	—	—	—	—	—	—	—
☐ SISTERS OF CHARITY HOSPITAL OF BUFFALO, 2157 Main Street, Zip 14214–2692; tel. 716/862–1000; Patrick J. Wiles, President and Chief Executive Officer (Total facility includes 80 beds in nursing home–type unit) A1 2 3 5 6 9 10 12 13 F1 2 3 4 8 9 10 11 12 13 14 15 16 17 18 19 21 22 23 24 25 29 30 31 32 33 34 35 36 37 38 39 40 41 42 43 44 45 46 47 48 49 50 51 52 53 54 55 56 57 58 59 60 61 62 63 64 65 66 68 69 70 71 72 74 75 76 77 78 79 Web address: www.sisters–buffalo.org	21	10	295	11719	277	378979	2958	106175	49345	1520
★ VETERANS AFFAIRS WESTERN NEW YORK HEALTHCARE SYSTEM–BUFFALO DIVISION, 3495 Bailey Avenue, Zip 14215–1129; tel. 716/834–9200; William F. Feeley, Director (Total facility includes 120 beds in nursing home–type unit) A1 2 3 5 8 9 F1 2 3 4 6 9 11 12 13 19 21 22 23 24 25 26 28 29 30 31 32 33 34 35 36 37 38 39 41 43 45 46 47 48 49 50 51 54 55 56 57 59 60 61 62 63 64 65 66 68 69 70 72 74 76 77 78 79 S Department of Veterans Affairs, Washington, DC Web address: www.va.gov/stations97/guide/home.asp?DIVISION=ALL	45	10	233	4931	204	325414	0	126387	72785	1351
★ WESTERN NEW YORK CHILDREN'S PSYCHIATRIC CENTER, 1010 East and West Road, Zip 14224–3698; tel. 716/674–9730; Jed M. Cohen, Acting Executive Director (Nonreporting) A1 S New York State Department of Mental Health, Albany, NY Web address: www.omh.state.ny.us	12	52	46	—	—	—	—	—	—	—

CAMBRIDGE—Washington County

Hospital	Control	Service	Staffed Beds	Admissions	Census	Outpatient Visits	Births	Total	Payroll	Personnel
☐ MCCLELLAN HEALTH SYSTEM, (Formerly Mary McClellan Hospital), One Myrtle Avenue, Zip 12816–1098; tel. 518/677–2611; John Rugge, M.D., Chief Executive Officer A1 9 10 F7 8 9 14 17 22 24 25 29 34 37 38 41 43 44 45 48 53 54 56 69 70 71 72 76 78 79 P5 6	23	10	114	1637	55	87693	289	16434	9366	317

CANANDAIGUA—Ontario County

Hospital	Control	Service	Staffed Beds	Admissions	Census	Outpatient Visits	Births	Total	Payroll	Personnel
★ F. F. THOMPSON HEALTH SYSTEM, 350 Parrish Street, Zip 14424–1793; tel. 716/396–6000; Linda M. Janczak, President and Chief Executive Officer (Total facility includes 188 beds in nursing home–type unit) A1 3 9 10 F1 7 8 9 13 17 18 19 20 21 22 24 25 30 33 34 38 39 41 42 44 45 46 48 49 50 54 56 69 70 71 72 73 76 77 78 79 P5 6 Web address: www.ffth.com	23	10	301	4406	242	165900	644	52508	27548	889

© 2000 AHA Guide   *Many Facility Codes have changed. Please refer to the AHA Guide Code Chart.*

Hospitals, U.S. / NEW YORK

★ American Hospital Association (AHA) membership
□ Joint Commission on Accreditation of Healthcare Organizations (JCAHO) accreditation
+ American Osteopathic Healthcare Association (AOHA) membership
○ American Osteopathic Association (AOA) accreditation
△ Commission on Accreditation of Rehabilitation Facilities (CARF) accreditation

Control codes 61, 63, 64, 71, 72 and 73 indicate hospitals listed by AOHA, but not registered by AHA. For definition of numerical codes, see page A4

Hospital, Address, Telephone, Administrator, Approval, Facility, and Physician Codes, Health Care System, Network	Control	Service	Staffed Beds	Admissions	Census	Outpatient Visits	Births	Total	Payroll	Personnel
★ VETERANS AFFAIRS MEDICAL CENTER, 400 Fort Hill Avenue, Zip 14424–1197; tel. 716/394–2000; W. David Smith, Director (Total facility includes 150 beds in nursing home–type unit) (Nonreporting) **A**1 5 **S** Department of Veterans Affairs, Washington, DC Web address: www.va.gov/visns/visn02/can_nf.html	45	49	626	—	—	—	—	—	—	—
CARMEL—Putnam County										
ARMS ACRES, 75 Seminary Hill Road, Zip 10512–1921; tel. 914/225–3400; Edward Spauster, Ph.D., Executive Director (Nonreporting)	33	82	129	—	—	—	—	—	—	—
★ PUTNAM HOSPITAL CENTER, Stoneleigh Avenue, Zip 10512–9948; tel. 914/279–5711; Michael T. Weber, President and Chief Executive Officer (Nonreporting) **A**1 9 10	23	10	164	—	—	—	—	—	—	—
CARTHAGE—Jefferson County										
□ CARTHAGE AREA HOSPITAL, 1001 West Street, Zip 13619–9703; tel. 315/493–1000; Walter S. Becker, Chief Executive Officer (Total facility includes 30 beds in nursing home–type unit) **A**1 9 10 **F**7 8 9 12 13 16 17 18 19 22 25 26 30 32 33 34 43 44 48 49 50 53 54 65 69 70 72 76 78 79 **P**5	23	10	78	1869	52	52534	236	14000	7396	279
CASTLE POINT—Dutchess County										
VETERAN AFFAIRS HUDSON VALLEY HEALTH CARE SYSTEM–CASTLE POINT DIVISION See Veterans Affairs Hudson Valley Health Care System–F.D. Roosevelt Hospital, Montrose										
CHEEKTOWAGA—Erie County										
★ ST. JOSEPH HOSPITAL, 2605 Harlem Road, Zip 14225–4097; tel. 716/891–2400; Patrick J. Wiles, President and Chief Executive Officer **A**1 9 10 **F**3 4 7 8 9 11 12 13 16 17 18 19 22 23 25 32 33 34 35 36 37 39 40 41 43 45 46 47 48 49 50 51 54 55 56 58 65 68 70 74 76 78 79 **P**3 5 6 Web address: www.sjh.org	23	10	208	5738	94	170875	0	49526	22788	651
CLIFTON SPRINGS—Ontario County										
★ CLIFTON SPRINGS HOSPITAL AND CLINIC, 2 Coulter Road, Zip 14432–1189; tel. 315/462–1311; John P. Galati, President and Chief Executive Officer (Total facility includes 108 beds in nursing home–type unit) **A**1 9 10 **F**2 3 4 7 9 11 13 15 16 17 18 19 20 21 22 23 24 25 26 29 30 31 32 33 34 35 36 37 38 39 40 41 43 45 46 48 49 50 51 54 57 59 60 61 62 63 64 65 69 70 71 72 74 75 76 78 79 **P**5 7	23	10	208	2158	163	95534	0	41784	20421	655
COBLESKILL—Schoharie County										
□ BASSETT HOSPITAL OF SCHOHARIE COUNTY, 41 Grandview Drive, Zip 12043–1331; tel. 518/234–2511; Donald W. Massey, Administrator **A**1 9 10 **F**7 9 16 18 19 22 25 26 32 34 37 38 45 46 48 49 54 56 70 71 72 76 78 79 **P**6 Web address: www.bhsc.org	23	10	40	939	23	51201	0	9341	4827	181
COOPERSTOWN—Otsego County										
★ MARY IMOGENE BASSETT HOSPITAL, One Atwell Road, Zip 13326–1394; tel. 607/547–3100; William F. Streck, M.D., President and Chief Executive Officer **A**1 2 3 5 8 9 10 **F**7 8 9 11 13 14 16 17 18 19 22 23 24 25 28 29 32 33 34 35 38 39 41 43 44 45 46 48 50 51 54 56 57 58 59 60 61 62 63 64 65 66 68 70 71 72 75 76 78 79 **P**6 Web address: www.bassetthealthcare.org/	23	10	180	7947	101	452117	591	151505	81644	2047
CORNING—Steuben County										
★ CORNING HOSPITAL, 176 Denison Parkway East, Zip 14830–2899; tel. 607/937–7200; Timothy J. Dentry, President and Chief Executive Officer (Total facility includes 120 beds in nursing home–type unit) (Nonreporting) **A**1 9 10 **S** Guthrie Healthcare System, Sayre, PA Web address: www.corninghospital.com	23	10	264	—	—	—	—	—	—	—
CORNWALL—Orange County										
★ CORNWALL HOSPITAL, 19 Laurel Avenue, Zip 12518–1499; tel. 914/534–7711; Louis H. Smith, Executive Vice President and Administrator **A**1 9 10 **F**7 9 16 17 18 19 22 23 25 32 33 34 39 41 46 48 49 54 57 59 61 62 68 70 72 73 76 78 79 **S** Greater Hudson Valley Health System, Newburgh, NY	33	10	125	3521	79	58063	0	33906	18547	446
CORTLAND—Cortland County										
★ CORTLAND MEMORIAL HOSPITAL, 134 Homer Avenue, Zip 13045–0960; tel. 607/756–3500; Thomas H. Carman, President and Chief Executive Officer (Total facility includes 82 beds in nursing home–type unit) **A**1 9 10 **F**1 7 8 9 17 19 22 24 25 32 34 41 44 45 48 49 50 51 54 57 59 61 68 69 70 71 72 76 77 78 79	23	10	197	5038	155	131951	611	42441	20506	692
CORTLANDT MANOR—Westchester County										
★ HUDSON VALLEY HOSPITAL CENTER, 1980 Crompond Road, Zip 10567; tel. 914/737–9000; John C. Federspiel, President and Chief Executive Officer **A**1 9 10 **F**3 7 8 9 13 16 17 18 19 21 22 24 25 29 30 32 34 38 39 41 43 44 45 46 48 49 54 70 71 72 75 76 78 79 Web address: www.hvhc.org	23	10	92	5435	70	82884	968	52291	25732	586
CUBA—Allegany County										
□ CUBA MEMORIAL HOSPITAL, 140 West Main Street, Zip 14727–1398; tel. 716/968–2000; Darlene D. Bainbridge, Chief Executive Officer (Total facility includes 61 beds in nursing home–type unit) (Nonreporting) **A**1 9 10 18	23	10	87	—	—	—	—	—	—	—
DANSVILLE—Livingston County										
★ NICHOLAS H. NOYES MEMORIAL HOSPITAL, 111 Clara Barton Street, Zip 14437–9527; tel. 716/335–6001; James Wissler, President and Chief Executive Officer **A**1 9 10 **F**9 19 22 25 39 40 41 43 44 48 54 63 70 76 78 Web address: www.noyes-health.org/	23	10	49	2426	—	104358	250	—	9719	—

Hospitals, U.S. / NEW YORK

Hospital, Address, Telephone, Administrator, Approval, Facility, and Physician Codes, Health Care System, Network	Classification Codes		Utilization Data					Expense (thousands) of dollars		
★ American Hospital Association (AHA) membership □ Joint Commission on Accreditation of Healthcare Organizations (JCAHO) accreditation + American Osteopathic Healthcare Association (AOHA) membership ○ American Osteopathic Association (AOA) accreditation △ Commission on Accreditation of Rehabilitation Facilities (CARF) accreditation Control codes 61, 63, 64, 71, 72 and 73 indicate hospitals listed by AOHA, but not registered by AHA. For definition of numerical codes, see page A4	Control	Service	Staffed Beds	Admissions	Census	Outpatient Visits	Births	Total	Payroll	Personnel
DOBBS FERRY—Westchester County □ COMMUNITY HOSPITAL AT DOBBS FERRY, 128 Ashford Avenue, Zip 10522–1896; tel. 914/693–0700; Thomas E. Green, President and Chief Executive Officer (Nonreporting) A1 9 10	23	10	50	—	—	—	—	—	—	—
DUNKIRK—Chautauqua County ✣ BROOKS MEMORIAL HOSPITAL, 529 Central Avenue, Zip 14048–2599; tel. 716/366–1111; Richard H. Ketcham, President A1 9 10 F7 8 9 13 16 18 19 22 24 25 30 32 33 34 36 38 39 40 41 44 46 48 51 54 65 70 76 78 79 P5 Web address: www.brookshospital.org	23	10	60	3031	41	98440	489	25021	1117	346
EAST MEADOW—Nassau County □ NASSAU COUNTY MEDICAL CENTER, 2201 Hempstead Turnpike, Zip 11554–1854; tel. 516/572–6011; Jerald C. Newman, President and Chief Executive Officer (Total facility includes 809 beds in nursing home–type unit) (Nonreporting) A1 2 3 5 8 9 10 12 13	13	10	1384	—	—	—	—	—	—	—
ELIZABETHTOWN—Essex County ✣ ELIZABETHTOWN COMMUNITY HOSPITAL, Park Street, Zip 12932–0277, Mailing Address: P.O. Box 277, Zip 12932–0277; tel. 518/873–6377; Thomas A. Santoro, Administrator A1 9 18 F1 3 4 7 8 9 11 13 14 17 18 19 21 22 23 24 25 28 29 30 31 32 33 34 35 36 37 38 39 40 43 45 46 48 50 51 54 56 65 66 70 71 72 73 76 77 78 79 P3 5	23	10	25	471	14	32459	—	5134	3099	100
ELLENVILLE—Ulster County □ ELLENVILLE COMMUNITY HOSPITAL, Route 209, Zip 12428–0668, Mailing Address: P.O. Box 668, Zip 12428–0668; tel. 914/647–6400; Judith Durr, Interim Chief Executive Officer A1 9 10 F2 3 7 9 20 22 34 37 38 48 51 68 76 78	23	10	31	1037	12	—	0	—	—	—
ELMHURST—Queens County, See New York City **ELMIRA—Chemung County** ✣ ARNOT OGDEN MEDICAL CENTER, 600 Roe Avenue, Zip 14905–1629; tel. 607/737–4100; Anthony J. Cooper, President and Chief Executive Officer (Total facility includes 40 beds in nursing home–type unit) A1 2 6 9 10 F4 7 8 9 11 12 13 14 17 18 19 20 22 24 25 28 29 30 31 32 34 35 38 39 41 42 43 44 45 46 47 48 49 50 51 54 56 59 61 65 66 68 69 70 72 73 75 76 77 78 79 P6 Web address: www.aomc.org	23	10	247	7685	166	204995	1423	94552	46165	1282
✣ ELMIRA PSYCHIATRIC CENTER, 100 Washington Street, Zip 14901–2898; tel. 607/737–4739; William Benedict, Executive Director A1 10 F16 18 21 23 32 34 57 58 60 62 63 70 72 78 P1 S New York State Department of Mental Health, Albany, NY	12	22	93	226	93	46467	0	—	—	350
✣ ST. JOSEPH'S HOSPITAL, (Includes Twin Tiers Rehabilitation Center), 555 East Market Street, Zip 14902–1512; tel. 607/733–6541; Sister Marie Castagnaro, President and Chief Executive Officer (Total facility includes 71 beds in nursing home–type unit) A1 2 9 10 F2 3 7 9 10 12 13 16 17 18 19 20 21 22 24 25 26 27 30 32 33 34 35 37 38 39 41 43 45 46 48 49 50 51 53 54 56 57 59 60 61 62 63 64 67 69 70 71 72 74 75 76 78 79 P6 S Carondelet Health System, Saint Louis, MO Web address: www.stjosephs.org	21	10	240	5155	183	95490	0	—	—	771
ENDICOTT—Broome County MEDICENTER See United Health Services Hospitals–Binghamton, Binghamton **FAR ROCKAWAY—Queens County, See New York City** **FLUSHING—Queens County, See New York City** **FOREST HILLS—Queens County, See New York City** ✣ NORTH SHORE UNIVERSITY HOSPITAL–FOREST HILLS, Mailing Address: 102–01 66th Road, Zip 11375; tel. 718/830–4000; Andrew J. Mitchell, Executive Director (Nonreporting) A1 2 5 9 10 S North Shore– Long Island Jewish Health System, Great Neck, NY Web address: www.northshorelij.com	23	10	231	—	—	—	—	—	—	—
FORT DRUM—Jefferson County ★ WILCOX ARMY COMMUNITY HOSPITAL, Zip 13602–5004 (Nonreporting) S Department of the Army, Office of the Surgeon General, Falls Church, VA	42	10	30	—	—	—	—	—	—	—
FULTON—Oswego County ✣ ALBERT LINDLEY LEE MEMORIAL HOSPITAL, 510 South Fourth Street, Zip 13069–2994; tel. 315/592–2224; Dennis A. Casey, Executive Director A1 9 10 F3 4 7 9 11 18 22 24 25 29 33 34 35 36 38 39 41 45 46 48 50 56 58 59 60 61 62 63 64 68 70 71 72 74 76 78 Web address: www.leememorialhospital.com	23	10	67	2353	38	37571	—	17827	9228	286
GENEVA—Ontario County ✣ GENEVA GENERAL HOSPITAL, 196 North Street, Zip 14456–1694; tel. 315/787–4000; James J. Dooley, President and Chief Executive Officer (Total facility includes 343 beds in nursing home–type unit) A1 6 9 10 F1 2 4 7 8 9 11 13 14 16 17 18 19 22 23 24 25 29 30 31 32 33 34 35 36 37 38 39 40 41 43 44 45 46 48 49 50 51 53 54 59 61 67 68 69 70 72 74 76 77 78 79	23	10	479	4745	397	293448	654	58711	26893	690
GLEN COVE—Nassau County ✣ NORTH SHORE UNIVERSITY HOSPITAL AT GLEN COVE, 101 St. Andrews Lane, Zip 11542; tel. 516/674–7300; Mark R. Stenzler, Vice President Administration (Nonreporting) A1 2 3 5 9 10 S North Shore– Long Island Jewish Health System, Great Neck, NY Web address: www.northshorelij.com	23	10	265	—	—	—	—	—	—	—
GLEN OAKS—Queens County, See New York City										

© 2000 AHA Guide   *Many Facility Codes have changed. Please refer to the AHA Guide Code Chart.*   Hospitals **A291**

Hospitals, U.S. / NEW YORK

Hospital, Address, Telephone, Administrator, Approval, Facility, and Physician Codes, Health Care System, Network	Classification Codes		Utilization Data					Expense (thousands) of dollars		
	Control	Service	Staffed Beds	Admissions	Census	Outpatient Visits	Births	Total	Payroll	Personnel

★ American Hospital Association (AHA) membership
☐ Joint Commission on Accreditation of Healthcare Organizations (JCAHO) accreditation
+ American Osteopathic Healthcare Association (AOHA) membership
○ American Osteopathic Association (AOA) accreditation
△ Commission on Accreditation of Rehabilitation Facilities (CARF) accreditation
Control codes 61, 63, 64, 71, 72 and 73 indicate hospitals listed by AOHA, but not registered by AHA. For definition of numerical codes, see page A4

Hospital	Control	Service	Staffed Beds	Admissions	Census	Outpatient Visits	Births	Total	Payroll	Personnel
GLENS FALLS—Warren County ☐ GLENS FALLS HOSPITAL, 100 Park Street, Zip 12801-9898; tel. 518/926-1000; David G. Kruczlnicki, President and Chief Executive Officer (Nonreporting) **A**1 2 9 10 Web address: www.glensfallshosp.org	23	10	410	—	—	—	—	—	—	—
GLENVILLE—Schenectady County CONIFER PARK, 79 Glenridge Road, Zip 12302; tel. 518/399-6446; Jack Duffy, Executive Director **F**2 3 18 70 72 79 **P**6	33	82	225	2545	115	—	—	—	—	244
GLOVERSVILLE—Fulton County ☐ NATHAN LITTAUER HOSPITAL AND NURSING HOME, 99 East State Street, Zip 12078-1293; tel. 518/773-5500; Thomas J. Dowd, President (Total facility includes 84 beds in nursing home-type unit) **A**1 5 9 10 **F**3 4 7 8 9 13 16 17 18 19 22 23 24 25 30 32 33 34 35 36 37 38 39 41 43 44 45 46 48 50 51 54 56 58 59 60 61 62 63 66 69 70 72 76 78 79 Web address: www.nlh.org	23	10	208	3947	135	139235	324	39918	20771	615
GOSHEN—Orange County ★ ARDEN HILL HOSPITAL, 4 Harriman Drive, Zip 10924-2499; tel. 914/294-5441; Wayne Becker, Interim Chief Executive Officer **A**1 9 10 **F**3 7 8 9 13 19 20 22 24 25 29 30 32 33 34 39 43 44 45 46 48 49 53 54 57 58 59 60 61 62 63 64 68 70 72 76 77 78 79 Web address: www.ardenhill.org	23	10	174	6525	133	125000	739	56400	21000	655
GOUVERNEUR—St. Lawrence County ☐ EDWARD JOHN NOBLE HOSPITAL OF GOUVERNEUR, 77 West Barney Street, Zip 13642-1090; tel. 315/287-1000; Charles P. Conole, FACHE, Chief Executive Officer **A**1 9 10 **F**7 8 9 10 12 13 14 16 17 18 19 20 21 22 23 24 25 29 30 32 33 34 35 36 37 38 39 42 43 44 45 46 47 48 49 50 51 52 54 57 58 59 61 62 65 66 70 75 76 79 **P**5 Web address: www.samaritanhealth.com/EJNoble.htm	23	10	47	1371	21	30931	98	10697	5186	226
GOWANDA—Cattaraugus County ☐ TRI-COUNTY MEMORIAL HOSPITAL, 100 Memorial Drive, Zip 14070-1194; tel. 716/532-3377; Diane J. Osika, Chief Executive Officer **A**1 9 10 **F**1 2 3 4 5 6 8 9 10 11 12 13 14 16 17 18 19 21 22 23 24 25 27 28 29 30 31 32 34 35 36 37 38 39 41 42 43 44 45 46 47 48 50 51 52 53 54 55 56 57 58 59 60 61 62 63 64 65 66 69 70 72 74 75 76 77 78 79	23	10	65	1430	26	45910	0	10434	5741	201
GREENPORT—Suffolk County ☐ EASTERN LONG ISLAND HOSPITAL, 201 Manor Place, Zip 11944-1298; tel. 631/477-1000; Paul J. Connor, II, President and Chief Executive Officer **A**1 9 10 **F**2 3 7 8 9 12 13 16 17 19 22 25 27 28 30 34 35 36 39 41 44 46 48 49 50 51 54 57 59 60 61 62 63 65 66 69 70 71 72 76 78 79 Web address: www.elih.org	23	10	80	2307	56	21979	—	18298	9859	233
HAMILTON—Madison County ★ COMMUNITY MEMORIAL HOSPITAL, 150 Broad Street, Zip 13346-9518; tel. 315/824-1100; David Felton, President and Chief Executive Officer (Total facility includes 40 beds in nursing home-type unit) (Nonreporting) **A**1 9 10	23	10	84	—	—	—	—	—	—	—
HARRIS—Sullivan County ★ COMMUNITY GENERAL HOSPITAL OF SULLIVAN COUNTY, 68 Harris Bushville Road, Zip 12742, Mailing Address: P.O. Box 800, Zip 12742-0800; tel. 914/794-3300; Arthur L. Brien, Chief Executive Officer (Total facility includes 64 beds in nursing home-type unit) **A**1 2 9 10 18 **F**1 2 7 8 9 11 12 19 20 22 25 30 32 36 38 44 45 46 48 51 53 54 56 57 69 70 71 72 76 78 79	23	10	268	6699	159	277900	456	—	—	807
HARRISON—Westchester County SAINT VINCENTS HOSPITAL See Saint Vincents Hospital and Medical Center, New York City										
HEMPSTEAD—Nassau County ☐ ISLAND MEDICAL CENTER, 800 Front Street, Zip 11550-4600; tel. 516/560-1200; Leonard Polonsky, interim Chief Executive Officer (Nonreporting) **A**1 9 10	32	10	213	—	—	—	—	—	—	—
HOLLISWOOD—Queens County, See New York City										
HORNELL—Steuben County ★ ST. JAMES MERCY HOSPITAL, 411 Canisteo Street, Zip 14843-2197; tel. 607/324-8000; William G. Connors, President and Chief Executive Officer (Total facility includes 120 beds in nursing home-type unit) **A**1 6 9 10 **F**1 2 3 7 9 12 17 19 22 24 25 30 31 32 33 34 35 38 41 44 45 46 48 50 53 54 56 57 58 59 61 62 63 69 70 72 76 77 78 **P**6 7 8 **S** Catholic Health East, Newtown Square, PA Web address: www.sjmh.org	21	10	256	4186	169	246977	363	45992	22219	812
HUDSON—Columbia County ☐ COLUMBIA MEMORIAL HOSPITAL, (Includes Columbia-Greene Long Term Care, 161 Jefferson Heights, Catskill, Zip 12414; tel. 518/943-6363), 71 Prospect Avenue, Zip 12534-2900; tel. 518/828-7601; Jane Ehrlich, President and Chief Executive Officer (Total facility includes 120 beds in nursing home-type unit) **A**1 9 10 **F**7 8 9 13 17 18 22 23 25 32 34 37 38 41 44 45 48 49 50 51 54 57 65 68 69 70 76 77 **P**8 Web address: www.cmn.net.org	23	10	251	6680	214	120765	498	48924	25171	695
HUNTINGTON—Suffolk County ★ HUNTINGTON HOSPITAL, 270 Park Avenue, Zip 11743-2799; tel. 631/351-2200; J. Ronald Gaudreault, President and Chief Executive Officer **A**1 2 3 9 10 **F**4 7 8 9 12 22 24 25 29 30 32 34 38 40 41 43 44 46 48 49 51 57 59 65 66 68 70 72 75 76 78 79 **P**5 7 8 **S** North Shore- Long Island Jewish Health System, Great Neck, NY Web address: www.hunthosp.org	23	10	263	12952	217	134340	2030	111949	59846	1268

Hospitals, U.S. / NEW YORK

Hospital, Address, Telephone, Administrator, Approval, Facility, and Physician Codes, Health Care System, Network	Classification Codes		Utilization Data					Expense (thousands) of dollars		
★ American Hospital Association (AHA) membership ☐ Joint Commission on Accreditation of Healthcare Organizations (JCAHO) accreditation + American Osteopathic Healthcare Association (AOHA) membership ○ American Osteopathic Association (AOA) accreditation △ Commission on Accreditation of Rehabilitation Facilities (CARF) accreditation Control codes 61, 63, 64, 71, 72 and 73 indicate hospitals listed by AOHA, but not registered by AHA. For definition of numerical codes, see page A4	Control	Service	Staffed Beds	Admissions	Census	Outpatient Visits	Births	Total	Payroll	Personnel

HUNTINGTON STATION—Suffolk County

★ SAGAMORE CHILDREN'S PSYCHIATRIC CENTER, 197 Half Hollow Road, Zip 11746; tel. 516/673-7700; Robert Schweitzer, Ed.D., Executive Director **A**1 **F**13 16 17 18 19 22 23 24 25 36 39 43 50 51 57 58 59 60 63 64 70 76 78 **S** New York State Department of Mental Health, Albany, NY	12	52	69	296	64	17965	0	—	—	256

IRVING—Chautauqua County

○ LAKE SHORE HOSPITAL, 845 Route 5 and 20, Zip 14081-9716; tel. 716/934-2654; James B. Foster, Chief Executive Officer (Total facility includes 160 beds in nursing home–type unit) **A**9 10 11 **F**1 9 13 17 19 22 25 34 36 37 38 39 41 48 50 54 57 61 69 70 76 78 **P**8 Web address: www.lakeshorehosp.org	23	10	222	1965	297	41606	0	23827	9948	430

ITHACA—Tompkins County

★ CAYUGA MEDICAL CENTER AT ITHACA, 101 Dates Drive, Zip 14850-1383; tel. 607/274-4011; Bonnie H. Howell, FACHE, President and Chief Executive Officer **A**1 2 5 9 10 **F**8 9 13 14 16 17 18 19 21 22 24 25 27 28 29 32 35 36 37 38 39 40 41 43 44 45 46 48 49 50 51 53 54 57 59 61 62 63 65 68 70 71 72 76 77 78 79 **P**5 7 8 Web address: www.cayugamed.org	23	10	145	6469	99	131830	848	50405	22447	686

JACKSON HEIGHTS—Queens County, See New York City
JAMAICA—Queens County, See New York City
JAMESTOWN—Chautauqua County

★ WOMAN'S CHRISTIAN ASSOCIATION HOSPITAL, 207 Foote Avenue, Zip 14702-9975, Mailing Address: P.O. Box 840, Zip 14702-0840; tel. 716/487-0141; Betsy T. Wright, President and Chief Executive Officer **A**1 2 9 10 **F**2 3 7 8 9 13 14 16 17 18 19 21 22 23 24 25 26 29 31 32 33 34 35 37 38 39 41 43 44 45 46 48 49 50 51 53 54 56 57 58 59 60 61 62 63 64 65 70 71 72 73 76 78 79 **P**5 Web address: www.wcahospital.org	23	10	291	9320	160	230000	691	71587	35503	1169

JOHNSON CITY—Broome County

WILSON MEMORIAL REGIONAL MEDICAL CENTER See United Health Services Hospitals–Binghamton, Binghamton

KATONAH—Westchester County

★ FOUR WINDS HOSPITAL, 800 Cross River Road, Zip 10536-3549; tel. 914/763-8151; Samuel C. Klagsbrun, M.D., Executive Medical Director **A**1 9 10 **F**3 13 16 17 18 19 22 24 25 30 31 39 45 55 57 58 59 60 61 62 63 64 68 70 72 76 78 **P**3 4 7 Web address: www.fourwinds.com	33	22	175	2299	157	8074	0	—	—	583

KENMORE—Erie County

☐ KENMORE MERCY HOSPITAL, 2950 Elmwood Avenue, Zip 14217-1390; tel. 716/447-6100; Sister Mary Joel Schimscheiner, Chief Executive Officer (Nonreporting) **A**1 9 10	21	10	219	—	—	—	—	—	—	—

KINGSTON—Ulster County

★ BENEDICTINE HOSPITAL, 105 Marys Avenue, Zip 12401-5894; tel. 914/338-2500; Thomas A. Dee, President and Chief Executive Officer **A**1 2 3 5 9 10 **F**4 9 13 16 17 18 22 24 25 31 37 38 43 44 46 48 49 51 54 56 57 61 64 68 70 72 76 78 79 Web address: www.benedictine.org	21	10	222	6912	130	69195	779	52722	25170	719
☐ KINGSTON HOSPITAL, 396 Broadway, Zip 12401-4692; tel. 914/331-3131; Anthony P. Marmo, Chief Executive Officer (Nonreporting) **A**1 3 5 9 10	23	10	140	—	—	—	—	—	—	—

LACKAWANNA—Erie County

★ OUR LADY OF VICTORY HOSPITAL, 55 Melroy Road, Zip 14218-1687; tel. 716/825-8000; John P. Davanzo, President and Chief Executive Officer (Total facility includes 10 beds in nursing home–type unit) (Nonreporting) **A**1 9 10	21	10	232	—	—	—	—	—	—	—

LEWISTON—Niagara County

★ MOUNT ST. MARY'S HOSPITAL AND HEALTH CENTER, 5300 Military Road, Zip 14092-1997; tel. 716/297-4800; Angelo G. Calbone, President and Chief Executive Officer **A**1 9 10 **F**2 3 8 9 12 13 16 17 18 19 22 25 29 34 35 37 38 39 41 43 44 48 54 56 61 64 66 70 71 76 78 **S** Ascension Health, Saint Louis, MO	21	10	179	5421	96	226965	401	41126	19069	554

LITTLE FALLS—Herkimer County

★ LITTLE FALLS HOSPITAL, 140 Burwell Street, Zip 13365-1725; tel. 315/823-1000; David S. Armstrong, Jr, President and Chief Executive Officer (Total facility includes 34 beds in nursing home–type unit) **A**1 9 10 **F**2 4 6 7 9 11 12 13 14 16 17 18 19 20 22 24 25 26 27 28 29 30 32 33 34 36 37 38 39 40 41 43 44 45 46 47 48 49 50 51 54 56 57 58 59 60 61 62 63 65 69 70 71 72 74 75 76 77 78 79 **P**8	23	10	134	3402	86	71967	304	20344	11336	401

LITTLE NECK—Queens County, See New York City
LOCKPORT—Niagara County

LOCKPORT MEMORIAL HOSPITAL, 521 East Avenue, Zip 14094-3299; tel. 716/514-5700; Clare A. Haar, Chief Executive Officer (Nonreporting) **A**9 10	23	10	134	—	—	—	—	—	—	—

LONG BEACH—Nassau County

★ LONG BEACH MEDICAL CENTER, 455 East Bay Drive, Zip 11561-2300, Mailing Address: P.O. Box 300, Zip 11561-2300; tel. 516/897-1000; Martin F. Nester, Jr, Chief Executive Officer (Total facility includes 200 beds in nursing home–type unit) **A**1 9 10 12 13 **F**3 4 7 9 12 16 17 18 19 20 21 22 23 24 25 28 30 31 32 33 34 35 36 38 39 41 46 48 49 50 51 53 54 55 57 58 59 60 61 62 63 68 69 70 71 72 73 76 78 **P**8 Web address: www.lbmc.org	23	10	334	5845	310	258925	0	74674	38165	934

LONG ISLAND CITY—Queens County, See New York City

© 2000 AHA Guide   *Many Facility Codes have changed. Please refer to the AHA Guide Code Chart.*

Hospitals, U.S. / NEW YORK

Hospital, Address, Telephone, Administrator, Approval, Facility, and Physician Codes, Health Care System, Network	Classification Codes		Utilization Data					Expense (thousands) of dollars		
★ American Hospital Association (AHA) membership □ Joint Commission on Accreditation of Healthcare Organizations (JCAHO) accreditation + American Osteopathic Healthcare Association (AOHA) membership ○ American Osteopathic Association (AOA) accreditation △ Commission on Accreditation of Rehabilitation Facilities (CARF) accreditation Control codes 61, 63, 64, 71, 72 and 73 indicate hospitals listed by AOHA, but not registered by AHA. For definition of numerical codes, see page A4	Control	Service	Staffed Beds	Admissions	Census	Outpatient Visits	Births	Total	Payroll	Personnel
LOWVILLE—Lewis County										
★ LEWIS COUNTY GENERAL HOSPITAL, 7785 North State Street, Zip 13367–1297; tel. 315/376–5200; Mark J. Rappaport, Chief Executive Officer (Total facility includes 160 beds in nursing home–type unit) **A**1 9 10 **F**1 8 9 13 17 18 19 22 24 25 30 31 32 36 37 38 41 44 45 46 48 50 51 54 56 68 69 70 71 72 76 78 79 **P**8	13	10	214	1929	175	47559	255	21816	10131	348
MALONE—Franklin County										
★ ALICE HYDE MEDICAL CENTER, (Formerly Alice Hyde Hospital Association), 115 Park Street, Zip 12953–0729, Mailing Address: P.O. Box 729, Zip 12953–0729; tel. 518/483–3000; John W. Johnson, President (Total facility includes 75 beds in nursing home–type unit) **A**1 9 10 **F**2 4 7 8 9 10 11 12 13 14 15 16 17 18 19 21 22 23 24 25 27 30 32 34 38 39 41 42 43 44 45 46 47 48 49 50 51 52 53 54 57 59 61 62 63 65 69 70 71 72 76 78 79 **Web address:** www.alicehyde.com	23	10	155	3048	112	95625	254	28144	14799	456
MANHASSET—Nassau County										
MANHASSET AMBULATORY CARE PAVILION See Long Island Jewish Medical Center, New York										
★ NORTH SHORE UNIVERSITY HOSPITAL, 300 Community Drive, Zip 11030–3876; tel. 516/562–0100; Dennis Dowling, Executive Director (Total facility includes 256 beds in nursing home–type unit) **A**1 2 3 5 8 9 10 **F**1 3 4 5 7 8 9 10 11 12 13 14 15 16 17 18 19 20 21 22 23 24 25 26 27 29 30 31 32 33 34 35 36 37 38 39 40 41 42 43 44 45 46 47 48 49 50 51 52 54 55 56 57 58 59 60 61 62 63 65 66 68 69 70 71 72 73 74 75 76 77 78 79 **P**5 7 **S** North Shore–Long Island Jewish Health System, Great Neck, NY **Web address:** www.northshorelij.com	23	10	987	43642	932	440730	5927	673181	350632	4519
MANHATTAN—New York County, See New York City										
MARGARETVILLE—Delaware County										
□ MARGARETVILLE MEMORIAL HOSPITAL, Route 28, Zip 12455, Mailing Address: P.O. Box 200, Zip 12455–0200; tel. 914/586–2631; Roger A. Masse, Chief Executive Officer **A**1 9 10 **F**22 24 25 41 48 54 70 72 76 78 **Web address:** www.margaretville.com/hospital	23	10	22	543	8	—	0	—	—	120
MASSENA—St. Lawrence County										
□ MASSENA MEMORIAL HOSPITAL, One Hospital Drive, Zip 13662–1097; tel. 315/764–1711; Charles F. Fahd, II, Chief Executive Officer **A**1 9 10 **F**1 5 6 7 8 9 12 13 14 16 17 18 19 22 23 24 25 27 28 29 30 31 32 33 34 36 37 39 40 41 43 44 45 46 48 50 53 54 56 66 68 70 73 76 79 **P**5	14	10	50	2779	32	94912	248	22919	10929	296
MEDINA—Orleans County										
★ △ MEDINA MEMORIAL HOSPITAL, 200 Ohio Street, Zip 14103–1095; tel. 716/798–2000; James Sinner, Chief Executive Officer (Total facility includes 30 beds in nursing home–type unit) **A**1 7 9 10 **F**8 9 13 14 16 17 18 19 22 24 25 29 31 32 33 34 36 37 38 41 44 45 46 48 50 51 53 54 56 61 69 72 73 75 76 78 **P**5	23	10	101	2622	63	76458	213	22999	10194	382
MIDDLETOWN—Orange County										
★ △ HORTON MEDICAL CENTER, 60 Prospect Avenue, Zip 10940–4133; tel. 914/343–2424; Jeffrey D. Hirsch, Executive Vice President and Administrator **A**1 2 7 9 10 **F**3 7 8 9 12 13 16 17 18 19 20 22 24 25 32 34 38 39 41 43 44 46 48 51 53 54 56 61 65 66 68 70 72 76 78 79 **P**5 7 8 **S** Greater Hudson Valley Health System, Newburgh, NY	23	10	169	8400	156	134438	1392	97357	46828	804
★ MIDDLETOWN PSYCHIATRIC CENTER, 122 Dorothea Dix Drive, Zip 10940–6198; tel. 914/342–5511; James H. Bopp, Executive Director **A**1 10 **F**2 3 4 9 10 12 13 16 17 18 21 22 23 24 25 26 29 30 31 34 35 39 41 43 44 45 46 47 48 50 51 53 57 60 61 62 63 64 65 69 70 72 75 76 78 **S** New York State Department of Mental Health, Albany, NY	12	22	170	128	168	—	0	—	—	435
MINEOLA—Nassau County										
★ WINTHROP–UNIVERSITY HOSPITAL, 259 First Street, Zip 11501; tel. 516/663–2200; Daniel P. Walsh, President and Chief Executive Officer (Nonreporting) **A**1 2 3 5 8 9 10 **Web address:** www.winthrop.org	23	10	518	—						
MONTOUR FALLS—Schuyler County										
★ SCHUYLER HOSPITAL, 220 Steuben Street, Zip 14865–9709; tel. 607/535–7121; Robert Mincemoyer, President and Chief Executive Officer (Total facility includes 120 beds in nursing home–type unit) **A**1 9 10 **F**8 9 16 17 18 22 23 25 29 30 34 35 36 38 40 41 43 44 45 48 49 50 54 56 69 70 71 72 76 77 78 **P**6 **Web address:** www.schuylerhospital.org	23	10	155	1337	134	146748	207	19584	10710	467
MONTROSE—Westchester County										
★ VETERANS AFFAIRS HUDSON VALLEY HEALTH CARE SYSTEM–F.D. ROOSEVELT HOSPITAL, (COMBINED PSYCHIATRIC MED/SURG), (Includes Veteran Affairs Hudson Valley Health Care System–Castle Point Division, Castle Point, Zip 12511–9999; tel. 914/831–2000; Veterans Affairs Hudson Valley Health Care System–Montrose Division, Zip 10548), Mailing Address: P.O. Box 100, Zip 10548–0110; tel. 914/737–4400; Michael A. Sabo, Director (Total facility includes 258 beds in nursing home–type unit) **A**1 3 5 9 **F**2 13 16 17 18 19 22 23 24 25 26 28 29 30 31 33 34 35 36 38 43 45 46 48 49 50 51 54 56 57 59 60 61 62 63 64 66 68 69 70 72 76 77 78 79 **S** Department of Veterans Affairs, Washington, DC	45	49	597	3077	519	240205	0	124833	65672	1638

Hospitals, U.S. / NEW YORK

Hospital, Address, Telephone, Administrator, Approval, Facility, and Physician Codes, Health Care System, Network	Classification Codes		Utilization Data					Expense (thousands) of dollars		
★ American Hospital Association (AHA) membership ☐ Joint Commission on Accreditation of Healthcare Organizations (JCAHO) accreditation + American Osteopathic Healthcare Association (AOHA) membership ○ American Osteopathic Association (AOA) accreditation △ Commission on Accreditation of Rehabilitation Facilities (CARF) accreditation Control codes 61, 63, 64, 71, 72 and 73 indicate hospitals listed by AOHA, but not registered by AHA. For definition of numerical codes, see page A4	Control	Service	Staffed Beds	Admissions	Census	Outpatient Visits	Births	Total	Payroll	Personnel
MOUNT KISCO—Westchester County										
★ NORTHERN WESTCHESTER HOSPITAL CENTER, 400 Main Street, Zip 10549–3477; tel. 914/666–1200; Donald W. Davis, President **A**1 2 9 10 **F**4 7 8 9 12 13 17 18 19 22 24 25 29 32 33 34 38 39 41 44 45 46 48 49 51 54 56 57 61 62 63 64 65 70 72 76 78 79 **P**7 8 Web address: www.nwhc.net	23	10	239	9015	132	—	—	83123	38889	882
MOUNT VERNON—Westchester County										
☐ MOUNT VERNON HOSPITAL, 12 North Seventh Avenue, Zip 10550–2098; tel. 914/664–8000; Geroge Haskins, Senior Vice President and Chief Operating Officer (Nonreporting) **A**1 3 5 6 9 10 Web address: www.ssmc.org	23	10	182	—	—	—	—	—	—	—
NEW HAMPTON—Orange County										
☐ MID–HUDSON FORENSIC PSYCHIATRIC CENTER, (Formerly Mid–Hudson Psychiatric Center), Route 17M, Zip 10958, Mailing Address: P.O. Box 158, Zip 10958–0158; tel. 914/374–3171; Richard Bennett, Executive Director **A**1 10 **F**2 4 9 10 12 13 22 23 24 25 28 31 33 34 35 39 41 42 43 44 45 46 47 48 49 50 51 53 55 57 59 60 65 68 69 70 72 75 76 **P**6 Web address: www.omh.state.ny.us	12	22	300	317	289	0	0	27428	24428	561
NEW HYDE PARK—Queens County, See New York City										
NEW ROCHELLE—Westchester County										
★ SOUND SHORE MEDICAL CENTER OF WESTCHESTER, 16 Guion Place, Zip 10802; tel. 914/632–5000; John R. Spicer, President and Chief Executive Officer (Total facility includes 150 beds in nursing home–type unit) **A**1 2 3 5 8 9 10 **F**1 3 7 8 9 13 14 16 17 18 19 20 21 22 24 25 26 30 31 32 33 34 35 36 37 38 39 40 43 44 45 46 48 49 50 51 53 54 56 58 59 60 61 62 63 64 65 66 68 69 70 71 72 73 74 75 76 77 78 **P**4 5 6 7 8 Web address: www.ssmc.org	23	10	407	11804	310	192465	1403	111758	53478	1115
NEW YORK (Includes all hospitals located within the five boroughs) **BRONX** - Bronx County (Mailing Address - Bronx) **BROOKLYN** - Kings County (Mailing Address - Brooklyn) **MANHATTAN** - New York County (Mailing Address - New York) **QUEENS** - Queens County (Mailing Addresses - Bellerose, Elmhurst, Far Rockaway, Flushing, Forest Hills, Glen Oaks, Holliswood, Jackson Heights, Jamaica, Little Neck, Long Island City, New Hyde Park, and Queens Village) **RICHMOND VALLEY** - Richmond County (Mailing Address - Staten Island) BAYLEY SETON CAMPUS See Sisters of Charity Medical Center										
★ BELLEVUE HOSPITAL CENTER, (Includes Bellevue Comprehensive General Care, Bellevue Physical Medicine and Rehabilitation Services, Bellevue Psychiatric Services, Bellevue Tuberculosis Services, Comprehensive Ambulatory Care Services: Level I Trauma Center), 462 First Avenue, Zip 10016–9198, Mailing Address: 462 First Avenue, ME–8, Zip 10016–9198; tel. 212/562–4141; Carlos Perez, Executive Director **A**1 2 3 5 9 10 **F**1 2 3 4 7 8 9 11 12 13 14 16 17 18 19 21 22 23 24 25 26 27 29 30 31 32 33 34 35 36 38 39 41 42 43 44 45 46 47 48 49 50 51 52 53 54 56 57 58 59 60 61 62 63 64 65 66 69 70 72 73 75 76 77 78 79 **P**6 **S** New York City Health and Hospitals Corporation, New York, NY Web address: www.bellevuehospitalcenter.org/html/core.html	14	10	771	26014	683	563647	2010	325917	187881	4133
★ BETH ISRAEL MEDICAL CENTER, (Includes Beth Israel Medical Center–Herbert and Nell Singer Division, 170 East End Avenue, Zip 10128; tel. 212/870–9000; Beth Israel Medical Center–Kings Highway Division, 3201 Kings Highway, Zip 11234; tel. 718/252–3000; First Avenue and 16th Street, Zip 10003–3803; tel. 212/420–2000; Matthew E. Fink, M.D., President and Chief Executive Officer **A**1 3 5 6 8 9 10 **F**2 3 4 7 8 9 11 12 13 14 16 17 18 19 20 21 22 23 24 25 26 27 29 30 32 33 34 35 36 37 38 39 40 41 42 43 44 45 46 47 48 49 50 51 52 53 54 55 56 57 58 59 60 61 62 63 64 65 66 68 69 70 71 72 73 74 75 76 77 78 79 **P**5 6 8 **S** Continuum Health Partners, New York, NY Web address: www.bethisraelny.org	23	10	1245	53271	988	555404	4487	884914	452197	8782
★ BRONX CHILDREN'S PSYCHIATRIC CENTER, 1000 Waters Place, Bronx, Zip 10461–2799; tel. 718/239–3600; E. Richard Feinberg, M.D., Executive Director (Nonreporting) **A**1 3 **S** New York State Department of Mental Health, Albany, NY	12	52	75	—	—	—	—	—	—	—
★ BRONX PSYCHIATRIC CENTER, 1500 Waters Place, Bronx, Zip 10461–2796; tel. 718/931–0600; LeRoy Carmichael, Executive Director **A**1 3 5 10 **F**13 16 17 19 21 23 25 29 31 32 41 44 48 51 54 57 60 61 62 63 64 65 72 78 **P**6 **S** New York State Department of Mental Health, Albany, NY Web address: www.omh.state.ny.us	12	22	450	360	475	—	0	—	—	874
★ BRONX–LEBANON HOSPITAL CENTER, (Includes Concourse Division, 1650 Grand Concourse, Zip 10457; tel. 212/590–1800; Fulton Division, 1276 Fulton Avenue, Zip 10456; tel. 718/590–1800), 1276 Fulton Avenue, Bronx, Zip 10456–3499; tel. 718/590–1800; Miguel A. Fuentes, President and Chief Executive Officer **A**1 2 3 5 8 9 10 **F**1 2 3 4 8 9 11 12 13 14 17 18 19 20 22 23 24 25 29 30 31 32 33 35 38 39 41 42 43 44 46 49 50 52 54 55 57 58 59 60 61 62 63 64 65 66 70 71 72 73 74 76 77 78 79 **P**6	23	10	509	23230	426	754215	2666	350582	178711	3396
☐ BROOKDALE HOSPITAL MEDICAL CENTER, Linden Boulevard at Brookdale Plaza, Brooklyn, Zip 11212–3198; tel. 718/240–5000; Alvin I. Kahn, M.D., President and Chief Executive Officer (Total facility includes 448 beds in nursing home–type unit) **A**1 3 5 8 9 10 12 **F**1 6 8 9 11 12 13 14 19 20 21 22 23 24 25 26 29 30 32 33 34 35 36 37 38 39 41 42 43 44 45 46 47 48 49 50 51 52 54 56 57 58 59 60 61 62 63 65 66 69 70 71 72 75 76 78 79 Web address: www.brookdalehospital.com	23	10	973	24709	891	316609	2920	376432	196508	—

© 2000 AHA Guide   *Many Facility Codes have changed. Please refer to the AHA Guide Code Chart.*

Hospitals, U.S. / NEW YORK

Legend

★ American Hospital Association (AHA) membership
□ Joint Commission on Accreditation of Healthcare Organizations (JCAHO) accreditation
+ American Osteopathic Healthcare Association (AOHA) membership
○ American Osteopathic Association (AOA) accreditation
△ Commission on Accreditation of Rehabilitation Facilities (CARF) accreditation

Control codes 61, 63, 64, 71, 72 and 73 indicate hospitals listed by AOHA, but not registered by AHA. For definition of numerical codes, see page A4.

Hospital, Address, Telephone, Administrator, Approval, Facility, and Physician Codes, Health Care System, Network	Classification Codes		Utilization Data					Expense (thousands) of dollars		
	Control	Service	Staffed Beds	Admissions	Census	Outpatient Visits	Births	Total	Payroll	Personnel
★ BROOKLYN HOSPITAL CENTER, (Includes Caledonian Campus, 100 Parkside Avenue, Zip 11226; tel. 718/940–2000; Downtown Campus, 121 DeKalb Avenue, Zip 11201), 121 DeKalb Avenue, Brooklyn, Zip 11201–5493; tel. 718/250–8005; Frederick D. Alley, President and Chief Executive Officer (Nonreporting) **A**1 2 3 5 8 9 10 **S** New York Presbyterian Healthcare System, New York, NY	23	10	653	—	—	—	—	—	—	—
BROOKLYN JEWISH DIVISION See Interfaith Medical Center										
★ CABRINI MEDICAL CENTER, 227 East 19th Street, Zip 10003–2600; tel. 212/995–6000; Jeffrey Frerichs, President and Chief Executive Officer **A**1 2 3 5 8 9 10 **F**2 9 12 13 15 16 17 18 19 20 22 24 25 26 27 29 30 31 32 33 34 35 36 37 38 39 41 43 45 46 48 49 51 52 53 54 55 57 59 61 62 63 64 65 68 70 74 75 76 78 79 **P**5 8 **Web address:** www.cabrininy.org	23	10	349	11525	266	—	0	172864	91971	1725
CALEDONIAN CAMPUS See Brooklyn Hospital Center										
★ CALVARY HOSPITAL, (SPECIALTY TREATMENT ONCOLOGY), 1740 Eastchester Road, Bronx, Zip 10461–2392; tel. 718/863–6900; Frank A. Calamari, President and Chief Executive Officer **A**1 9 10 **F**9 16 18 22 23 24 25 36 37 38 43 45 46 49 50 51 59 65 70 72 78 **Web address:** www.calvaryhospital.org	21	49	200	2269	167	13806	0	53984	31348	623
★ CATHOLIC MEDICAL CENTERS, (Includes Holy Family Home, 1740 84th Street, Brooklyn, Zip 11214; tel. 718/232–3666; Mary Immaculate Hospital, 152–11 89th Avenue, Zip 11432; tel. 718/558–2000; Monsignor James H Fitzpatrick Pavilion for Skilled Nursing Care, 152–11 89th Avenue, Zip 11432; tel. 718/558–2800; St. John's Queens Hospital, 90–02 Queens Boulevard, Flushing, Zip 11373; tel. 718/558–1000; Sister ; St. Joseph's Hospital, 158–40 79th Avenue, Flushing, Zip 11366; tel. 718/558–6200; St. Mary's Hospital of Brooklyn, 170 Buffalo Avenue, Brooklyn, Zip 11213; tel. 718/221–3000), 88–25 153rd Street, Jamaica, Zip 11432–3731; tel. 718/558–6900; William D. McGuire, President and Chief Executive Officer (Total facility includes 603 beds in nursing home–type unit) **A**1 2 3 5 8 9 10 **F**2 3 5 7 9 12 13 16 17 18 19 21 22 23 24 25 27 29 30 32 34 35 36 37 38 39 41 42 43 44 45 46 48 49 50 51 52 54 56 63 64 65 69 70 71 72 73 75 76 77 78 79 **P**5 **Web address:** www.cmcny.com	21	10	1584	38159	1184	1133065	3817	564987	285295	6026
★ COLER MEMORIAL HOSPITAL, Roosevelt Island, Zip 10044; tel. 212/848–6000; Samuel Lehrfeld, Executive Director (Total facility includes 815 beds in nursing home–type unit) **A**1 10 **F**7 23 30 35 36 45 51 53 59 70 72 76 78 **S** New York City Health and Hospitals Corporation, New York, NY	14	48	1025	1183	—	0	0	—	50236	—
COLUMBIA PRESBYTERIAN MEDICAL CENTER See New York–Presbyterian Hospital										
CONCOURSE DIVISION See Bronx–Lebanon Hospital Center										
★ CONEY ISLAND HOSPITAL, 2601 Ocean Parkway, Brooklyn, Zip 11235–7795; tel. 718/616–3000; William Walsh, Executive Director **A**1 3 5 10 **F**3 5 7 9 11 12 13 16 17 18 19 21 22 23 24 25 27 29 30 31 32 34 35 36 38 39 41 42 44 45 46 48 49 51 53 54 56 57 58 59 60 61 62 63 64 65 66 70 72 73 75 76 78 79 **P**6 **S** New York City Health and Hospitals Corporation, New York, NY **Web address:** www.ci.nyc.ny.us/html/hhc/html/coneyisland.html	14	10	406	16176	333	343879	1243	204597	87130	2095
★ CORNERSTONE OF MEDICAL ARTS CENTER HOSPITAL, 57 West 57th Street, Zip 10019–2802; tel. 212/755–0200; Norman J. Sokolow, Chairman and Chief Executive Officer (Nonreporting) **A**9 **Web address:** www.nyee.edu	33	82	94	—	—	—	—	—	—	—
★ CREEDMOOR PSYCHIATRIC CENTER, Jamaica, Mailing Address: 80–45 Winchester Boulevard, Queens Village, Zip 11427–2199; tel. 718/264–3300; Charlotte Seltzer, Chief Executive Officer **A**1 3 10 **F**16 17 18 19 23 30 51 57 62 63 70 72 78 **S** New York State Department of Mental Health, Albany, NY	12	22	494	499	516	195000	—	—	—	1218
★ DOCTORS' HOSPITAL OF STATEN ISLAND, 1050 Targee Street, Staten Island, Zip 10304–4499; tel. 718/390–1400; Stephen N. F. Anderson, Director (Nonreporting) **A**1 9 10	33	10	117	—	—	—	—	—	—	—
DOWNTOWN CAMPUS See Brooklyn Hospital Center										
★ ELMHURST HOSPITAL CENTER, 79–01 Broadway, Elmhurst, Zip 11373; tel. 718/334–4000; Pete Velez, Executive Director **A**1 2 3 5 8 9 10 **F**2 3 4 5 7 8 9 10 11 12 13 14 16 17 18 19 21 22 23 24 25 27 29 30 31 32 33 34 35 36 37 38 39 41 42 43 44 45 46 47 48 49 50 51 52 53 54 55 56 57 58 59 60 61 62 63 64 65 66 68 69 70 71 72 73 74 75 76 78 79 **P**6 **S** New York City Health and Hospitals Corporation, New York, NY	14	10	506	22371	439	601699	4495	264631	127317	3115
FULTON DIVISION See Bronx–Lebanon Hospital Center										
★ △ GOLDWATER MEMORIAL HOSPITAL, Franklin D. Roosevelt Island, Zip 10044; tel. 212/318–8000; Samuel Lehrfeld, Executive Director (Total facility includes 574 beds in nursing home–type unit) **A**1 3 5 7 10 **F**7 22 23 30 45 51 53 59 70 72 78 **P**5 **S** New York City Health and Hospitals Corporation, New York, NY **Web address:** www.coler-goldwater.org	14	48	991	948	—	0	0	—	51292	—
★ GRACIE SQUARE HOSPITAL, 420 East 76th Street, Zip 10021–3104; tel. 212/988–4400; Frank Bruno, Chief Executive Officer **A**1 9 10 **F**3 16 17 18 43 51 57 62 64 70 **S** New York Presbyterian Healthcare System, New York, NY	23	22	130	2984	130	31507	0	26499	15061	318
★ △ HARLEM HOSPITAL CENTER, (Includes Harlem General Care Unit and Harlem Psychiatric Unit), 506 Lenox Avenue, Zip 10037–1894; tel. 212/939–1000; John M. Palmer, Ph.D., Executive Director **A**1 2 3 5 7 8 9 10 **F**1 2 3 4 5 6 7 8 9 10 11 12 13 14 15 16 17 18 19 20 21 22 23 24 25 27 28 29 30 31 32 34 35 36 37 38 39 40 41 42 43 44 45 46 47 48 49 50 51 52 53 54 55 56 57 58 59 60 61 62 63 64 65 66 68 69 70 72 73 74 75 76 77 78 79 **P**1 **S** New York City Health and Hospitals Corporation, New York, NY	14	10	297	12725	246	442771	1103	241769	105002	2681
HILLSIDE HOSPITAL See Long Island Jewish Medical Center										

Hospitals, U.S. / NEW YORK

Hospital, Address, Telephone, Administrator, Approval, Facility, and Physician Codes, Health Care System, Network	Classification Codes		Utilization Data					Expense (thousands) of dollars		
★ American Hospital Association (AHA) membership ☐ Joint Commission on Accreditation of Healthcare Organizations (JCAHO) accreditation + American Osteopathic Healthcare Association (AOHA) membership ○ American Osteopathic Association (AOA) accreditation △ Commission on Accreditation of Rehabilitation Facilities (CARF) accreditation Control codes 61, 63, 64, 71, 72 and 73 indicate hospitals listed by AOHA, but not registered by AHA. For definition of numerical codes, see page A4	Control	Service	Staffed Beds	Admissions	Census	Outpatient Visits	Births	Total	Payroll	Personnel
☐ HOLLISWOOD HOSPITAL, 87–37 Palermo Street, Holliswood, Zip 11423; tel. 718/776–8181; Jeffrey Borenstein, M.D., Chief Executive Officer and Medical Director (Nonreporting) **A**1 9 10 **S** Liberty Management Group, Inc., Ramsey, NJ	33	22	100	—	—	—	—	—	—	—
★ △ HOSPITAL FOR JOINT DISEASES ORTHOPAEDIC INSTITUTE, 301 East 17th Street, Zip 10003–3890; tel. 212/598–6000; John N. Kastanis, FACHE, President and Chief Executive Officer (Nonreporting) **A**1 3 5 7 9 10 **Web address:** www.hjd.edu	23	49	163	—	—	—	—	—	—	—
★ HOSPITAL FOR SPECIAL SURGERY, 535 East 70th Street, Zip 10021–4898; tel. 212/606–1000; John R. Reynolds, President and Chief Executive Officer **A**1 3 5 6 8 9 10 **F**1 2 3 4 7 8 9 10 11 12 13 14 16 17 18 19 20 21 22 23 24 25 26 27 28 29 30 31 32 33 34 35 36 38 39 40 41 42 43 44 45 46 47 48 49 50 51 52 53 54 55 56 57 58 59 60 61 62 63 64 65 66 68 69 70 71 72 73 74 75 76 77 78 79 **P**1 2 4 5 7 8 **S** New York Presbyterian Healthcare System, New York, NY **Web address:** www.hss.edu	23	47	138	7560	100	175280	0	180659	76579	1612
☐ INTERFAITH MEDICAL CENTER, (Includes Brooklyn Jewish Division, 555 Prospect Place, Zip 11238; tel. 718/935–7000; St. John's Episcopal Hospital Division, 1545 Atlantic Avenue, Zip 11213; tel. 718/604–6000), 555 Prospect Place, Brooklyn, Zip 11238–4299; tel. 718/935–7000; Corbett A. Price, Chief Executive Officer **A**1 3 5 6 9 10 **F**2 3 4 7 8 9 11 12 13 14 15 16 17 18 19 20 21 22 23 24 25 27 29 30 32 34 35 37 38 39 41 40 42 44 45 46 47 48 49 50 51 54 55 56 57 59 60 61 62 63 64 65 66 70 74 76 78 79	23	10	375	13333	332	263696	609	164923	93145	1698
★ JACOBI MEDICAL CENTER, Pelham Parkway South and Eastchester Road, Bronx, Zip 10461–1197; tel. 718/918–5000; Joseph S. Orlando, Executive Director **A**1 3 5 8 10 **F**2 3 4 7 8 9 10 11 12 13 14 16 17 18 19 20 21 22 23 24 25 26 29 30 31 32 33 34 35 36 37 38 39 40 41 42 43 44 45 46 47 48 49 50 51 52 53 54 56 57 58 59 60 61 62 63 65 66 67 69 70 72 73 75 76 77 78 79 **P**6 **S** New York City Health and Hospitals Corporation, New York, NY **Web address:** www.ci.nyc.ny.us/html/hhc/html/jacobi.html	14	10	545	19338	432	430518	2022	245983	134499	3236
★ JAMAICA HOSPITAL MEDICAL CENTER, 8900 Van Wyck Expressway, Jamaica, Zip 11418–2832; tel. 718/206–6000; David P. Rosen, President **A**1 3 5 9 10 12 13 **F**4 6 7 8 9 11 12 13 15 16 17 18 19 21 22 23 24 25 28 29 30 31 32 34 35 36 38 39 41 44 46 47 48 49 52 53 54 55 56 57 59 60 61 62 63 65 66 68 69 70 71 72 73 75 76 77 78 79 **P**5 **Web address:** www.Jamaicahospital.org	23	10	384	20869	348	352826	3525	251298	130116	2824
★ KINGS COUNTY HOSPITAL CENTER, 451 Clarkson Avenue, Brooklyn, Zip 11203–2097; tel. 718/245–3131; Jean G. Leon, R.N., Senior Vice President **A**1 2 3 5 10 **F**1 2 3 4 5 7 8 9 12 13 14 17 18 19 20 21 22 23 24 25 27 28 29 31 32 33 34 35 38 41 42 43 44 45 46 48 49 50 51 52 53 54 55 56 57 58 59 60 61 63 65 66 68 70 71 73 75 76 77 78 79 **P**6 **S** New York City Health and Hospitals Corporation, New York, NY	14	10	686	25151	589	676531	2082	238630	210557	4571
★ KINGSBORO PSYCHIATRIC CENTER, 681 Clarkson Avenue, Brooklyn, Zip 11203–2199; tel. 718/221–7395; Dean R. Weinstock, Director (Nonreporting) **A**1 3 5 10 **S** New York State Department of Mental Health, Albany, NY	12	22	400	—	—	—	—	—	—	—
★ △ KINGSBROOK JEWISH MEDICAL CENTER, 585 Schenectady Avenue, Brooklyn, Zip 11203–1891; tel. 718/604–5000; Linda Brady, M.D., President and Chief Executive Officer (Total facility includes 538 beds in nursing home–type unit) (Nonreporting) **A**1 3 5 7 9 10 **Web address:** www.kingsbrook.org	23	10	879	—	—	—	—	—	—	—
★ LENOX HILL HOSPITAL, 100 East 77th Street, Zip 10021–1883; tel. 212/434–2000; Gladys George, President and Chief Executive Officer **A**1 3 5 8 9 10 **F**3 4 5 7 8 9 11 12 13 14 15 16 17 19 21 22 23 24 25 26 28 29 30 31 32 33 34 35 36 38 39 41 42 43 44 45 46 47 48 49 50 51 52 54 56 57 58 59 60 61 62 63 65 66 70 71 72 73 76 77 78 79 **P**1 5 8 **Web address:** www.lenoxhillhospital.org	23	10	600	26923	485	288847	3480	340327	157544	2995
★ LINCOLN MEDICAL AND MENTAL HEALTH CENTER, 234 East 149th Street, Bronx, Zip 10451–9998; tel. 718/579–5700; Jose R. Sanchez, Executive Director **A**1 3 10 **F**3 7 8 9 12 13 16 17 18 19 21 24 25 29 30 31 32 33 34 35 36 38 41 42 43 44 46 48 49 50 51 52 53 54 56 57 58 59 60 61 62 65 65 70 75 76 78 79 **P**5 **S** New York City Health and Hospitals Corporation, New York, NY	14	10	438	22425	273	513832	3154	222641	117263	2867
★ LONG ISLAND COLLEGE HOSPITAL, 339 Hicks Street, Brooklyn, Zip 11201–5509; tel. 718/780–1000; Allan Gibofsky, President and Chief Executive Officer **A**1 2 3 5 8 9 10 **F**2 3 4 7 8 11 12 13 14 16 17 18 19 21 22 23 24 25 26 27 29 30 31 32 33 34 35 36 37 38 39 41 42 43 44 45 46 48 49 51 52 53 54 55 56 57 58 59 60 62 63 64 65 66 70 71 72 76 77 78 79 **P**7 8 **S** Continuum Health Partners, New York, NY **Web address:** www.lich.org	23	10	388	18551	338	263090	2527	252095	129969	2728
★ LONG ISLAND JEWISH MEDICAL CENTER, (Includes Hillside Hospital, 75–59 263rd Street, Glen Oaks, Zip 11004; tel. 718/470–8000; Manhasset Ambulatory Care Pavilion, 1554 Northern Boulevard, Manhasset, Zip 11030; tel. 516/365–2070; Schneider Children's Hospital, 270–05 76th Avenue, Zip 11040; tel. 718/470–3000), 270–05 76th Avenue, New Hyde Park, Zip 11040–1496; tel. 718/470–7000; Paul S. Hochenberg, President **A**1 2 3 5 8 9 10 13 **F**1 3 4 5 6 7 8 9 10 11 12 13 14 15 16 17 18 19 20 21 22 23 24 25 26 27 28 29 30 31 32 33 34 35 36 37 38 39 40 41 42 43 44 47 48 49 50 51 52 54 55 56 57 58 59 60 61 62 63 64 65 66 68 69 70 71 72 73 74 75 76 77 78 79 **P**5 7 **S** North Shore– Long Island Jewish Health System, Great Neck, NY **Web address:** www.lij.edu	23	10	802	36535	720	—	6044	581824	318014	5604

© 2000 AHA Guide *Many Facility Codes have changed. Please refer to the AHA Guide Code Chart.*

Hospitals, U.S. / NEW YORK

Hospital, Address, Telephone, Administrator, Approval, Facility, and Physician Codes, Health Care System, Network	Classification Codes		Utilization Data					Expense (thousands) of dollars		
★ American Hospital Association (AHA) membership ☐ Joint Commission on Accreditation of Healthcare Organizations (JCAHO) accreditation + American Osteopathic Healthcare Association (AOHA) membership ○ American Osteopathic Association (AOA) accreditation △ Commission on Accreditation of Rehabilitation Facilities (CARF) accreditation Control codes 61, 63, 64, 71, 72 and 73 indicate hospitals listed by AOHA, but not registered by AHA. For definition of numerical codes, see page A4	Control	Service	Staffed Beds	Admissions	Census	Outpatient Visits	Births	Total	Payroll	Personnel
★ LUTHERAN MEDICAL CENTER, 150 55th Street, Brooklyn, Zip 11220–2570; tel. 718/630–7000; Dominic J. Lodato, Interim President **A**1 3 5 9 10 12 13 **F**2 3 6 7 8 9 12 13 14 16 17 18 19 21 22 23 24 25 27 29 30 31 32 33 34 35 36 37 38 39 40 41 42 43 44 45 46 48 49 50 51 53 54 56 57 59 60 61 62 63 65 66 67 70 71 72 75 76 78 79 **P**8 **Web address:** www.LMCMC.COM	23	10	415	18582	344	500762	3058	223942	118583	2901
★ MAIMONIDES MEDICAL CENTER, 4802 Tenth Avenue, Brooklyn, Zip 11219–2916; tel. 718/283–6000; Stanley Brezenoff, President (Nonreporting) **A**1 3 5 8 9 10 12 13 **Web address:** www.maimonidesmed.org	23	10	626	—	—	—	—	—	—	—
★ MANHATTAN EYE, EAR AND THROAT HOSPITAL, 210 East 64th Street, Zip 10021–9885; tel. 212/838–9200; George A. Sarkar, Ph.D., JD, Executive Director (Nonreporting) **A**1 3 5 9 10 **Web address:** www.meeth.org	23	45	30	—	—	—	—	—	—	—
★ MANHATTAN PSYCHIATRIC CENTER–WARD'S ISLAND, 600 East 125th Street, Zip 10035–9998; tel. 212/369–0500; Eileen Consilvio, R.N., MS, Executive Director (Nonreporting) **A**1 3 5 10 **S** New York State Department of Mental Health, Albany, NY	12	22	745	—	—	—	—	—	—	—
MARY IMMACULATE HOSPITAL See Catholic Medical Centers										
★ MEMORIAL SLOAN–KETTERING CANCER CENTER, (Formerly Memorial Hospital for Cancer), (CANCER), 1275 York Avenue, Zip 10021–6094; tel. 212/639–2000; Harold Varmus, M.D., President and Chief Executive Officer **A**1 2 3 5 8 9 10 **F**9 13 16 17 18 19 20 22 23 24 25 29 32 33 34 35 36 37 38 39 41 43 46 48 49 50 51 54 55 59 63 65 68 70 72 74 76 77 78 79 **P**1	23	49	437	18008	359	276705	0	749650	251304	4509
★ METROPOLITAN HOSPITAL CENTER, (Includes Metropolitan General Care Unit, Metropolitan Drug Detoxification and Metropolitan Psychiatric Unit), 1901 First Avenue, Zip 10029–7496; tel. 212/423–6262; Jose R. Sanchez, Executive Director **A**1 3 5 8 9 10 **F**1 2 3 8 9 11 12 13 14 16 17 18 19 21 22 23 24 25 29 30 31 32 33 34 35 36 38 39 41 42 43 44 45 46 48 49 50 51 52 53 54 56 57 58 59 60 61 62 63 64 65 66 67 68 70 76 78 79 **S** New York City Health and Hospitals Corporation, New York, NY	14	10	325	13913	307	403844	1763	239172	10703	2457
★ MONTEFIORE MEDICAL CENTER, (Includes Jack D Weiler Hospital of Albert Einstein College of Medicine, 1825 Eastchester Road, Zip 10461–2373; tel. 718/904–2000; Loeb Center Nursing Rehabilitation, 111 East 210th Street), 111 East 210th Street, Bronx, Zip 10467–2490; tel. 718/920–4321; Spencer Foreman, M.D., President (Total facility includes 80 beds in nursing home–type unit) **A**1 2 3 5 8 9 10 **F**1 3 4 7 8 9 11 12 13 14 17 18 19 22 23 24 25 27 29 30 32 33 34 35 36 37 38 39 41 42 43 44 45 46 47 48 49 50 51 52 53 54 55 56 57 58 59 60 61 62 63 64 65 66 68 69 70 71 72 73 74 76 78 79 **P**5 7 **Web address:** www.montefiore.org	23	10	1047	48460	823	1383735	4544	1112296	580132	9880
MOUNT SINAI MEDICAL CENTER See Mount Sinai–NYU Hospitals/Health System										
★ △ MOUNT SINAI–NYU HOSPITALS/HEALTH SYSTEM, (Includes Mount Sinai Medical Center, One Gustave L. Levy Place, Zip 10029–6574; tel. 212/241–6500; Mount Sinai–NYU Medical Center, 550 First Avenue, Zip 10016–4576; tel. 212/263–7300; Rusk Institute), One Gustave Levy Place, Zip 10019–6574; tel. 212/241–6500; John W. Rowe, M.D., President (Nonreporting) **A**1 3 5 7 8 9 10	23	10	1860	—	—	—	—	—	—	—
MOUNT SINAI–NYU MEDICAL CENTER See Mount Sinai–NYU Hospitals/Health System										
★ NEW YORK COMMUNITY HOSPITAL OF BROOKLYN, 2525 Kings Highway, Brooklyn, Zip 11229–1798; tel. 718/692–5300; Lin H. Mo, President and Chief Executive Officer **A**1 9 10 **F**4 13 19 22 24 25 26 31 32 34 36 41 43 46 48 51 76 78 **S** New York Presbyterian Healthcare System, New York, NY	23	10	125	5712	112	15224	0	41834	22114	344
★ NEW YORK EYE AND EAR INFIRMARY, 310 East 14th Street, Zip 10003–4201; tel. 212/979–4000; Joseph P. Corcoran, President and Chief Executive Officer **A**1 3 5 9 10 **F**2 3 4 7 8 9 11 12 13 14 16 17 18 19 20 21 22 23 24 25 26 29 30 32 33 34 35 37 38 39 41 42 43 44 45 46 47 48 49 50 51 52 53 54 55 56 57 58 59 60 61 62 63 64 65 66 68 69 70 71 72 73 74 75 76 77 78 79 **P**5 6 8 **S** Continuum Health Partners, New York, NY **Web address:** www.nyee.edu	23	45	30	1039	8	161725	0	50583	24334	581
★ NEW YORK FLUSHING HOSPITAL MEDICAL CENTER, 45th Avenue at Parsons Boulevard, Flushing, Zip 11355–2100; tel. 718/670–5000; David P. Rosen, President and Chief Executive Officer **A**1 3 5 9 10 **F**2 3 4 7 8 9 11 12 13 14 16 17 18 19 21 22 23 24 25 29 30 32 33 34 35 36 38 39 41 42 43 44 46 47 48 50 51 54 56 58 59 60 62 63 65 66 70 72 75 76 78 **P**5	23	10	250	15364	235	151604	2500	122785	63621	1329
★ NEW YORK HOSPITAL MEDICAL CENTER OF QUEENS, 56–45 Main Street, Flushing, Zip 11355–5000; tel. 718/670–1231; Stephen S. Mills, President and Chief Executive Officer (Nonreporting) **A**1 2 3 5 9 10 **S** New York Presbyterian Healthcare System, New York, NY **Web address:** www.nyhq.org	23	10	421	—	—	—	—	—	—	—
★ NEW YORK METHODIST HOSPITAL, 506 Sixth Street, Brooklyn, Zip 11215–3645; tel. 718/780–3000; Mark J. Mundy, President and Chief Executive Officer **A**1 2 3 5 8 9 10 **F**2 3 4 5 7 8 9 10 11 12 13 18 19 22 23 25 28 29 30 32 34 35 36 38 39 41 42 43 44 46 47 48 49 51 52 53 54 55 56 57 58 59 60 61 62 63 65 66 68 69 70 71 72 73 74 75 76 78 79 **P**5 **S** New York Presbyterian Healthcare System, New York, NY **Web address:** www.nym.org	23	10	560	24226	501	329724	3192	278863	130214	2398

Many Facility Codes have changed. Please refer to the AHA Guide Code Chart.

Hospitals, U.S. / NEW YORK

Hospital, Address, Telephone, Administrator, Approval, Facility, and Physician Codes, Health Care System, Network	Classification Codes		Utilization Data					Expense (thousands) of dollars		
★ American Hospital Association (AHA) membership ☐ Joint Commission on Accreditation of Healthcare Organizations (JCAHO) accreditation + American Osteopathic Healthcare Association (AOHA) membership ○ American Osteopathic Association (AOA) accreditation △ Commission on Accreditation of Rehabilitation Facilities (CARF) accreditation Control codes 61, 63, 64, 71, 72 and 73 indicate hospitals listed by AOHA, but not registered by AHA. For definition of numerical codes, see page A4	Control	Service	Staffed Beds	Admissions	Census	Outpatient Visits	Births	Total	Payroll	Personnel
★ NEW YORK STATE PSYCHIATRIC INSTITUTE, 1051 Riverside Drive, Zip 10032-2695; tel. 212/543-5000; John M. Oldham, M.D., Director (Nonreporting) **A**1 3 5 10 **S** New York State Department of Mental Health, Albany, NY	12	22	58	—	—	—	—	—	—	—
☐ NEW YORK UNIVERSITY DOWNTOWN HOSPITAL, 170 William Street, Zip 10038-2649; tel. 212/312-5000; Leonard A. Aubrey, President and Chief Executive Officer **A**1 3 5 9 10 **F**2 3 8 9 13 15 17 18 19 22 25 26 29 30 31 32 34 35 36 38 39 41 42 43 44 45 46 47 48 49 50 51 54 56 61 70 71 74 76 78 79 **P**5 7 **Web address:** www.nyudh.med.nyu.edu NEW YORK WEILL CORNELL MEDICAL CENTER See New York–Presbyterian Hospital	23	10	149	9223	118	232124	2324	113060	59334	982
★ △ NEW YORK–PRESBYTERIAN HOSPITAL, (Includes Babies and Children's Hospital, 3959 Broadway, Zip 10032-3784; tel. 212/305-2500; Columbia Presbyterian Medical Center, Columbia–Presbyterian Medical Center, Zip 10032-3784; tel. 212/305-2500; New York Weill Cornell Medical Center, Mailing Address: 525 East 68th Street, Zip 10021-4885; New York–Presbyterian Hospital, Westchester Division, Zip 10605; Payne Whitney Psychiatric Clinic; The Allen Pavilion, 5141 Broadway, Zip 10032; tel. 212/932-5000), 525 East 68th Street, Zip 10021-4885; tel. 212/746-5454; Herbert Pardes, M.D., President and Chief Executive Officer; Michael A. Berman, M.D., Executive Vice President and Director **A**1 2 3 5 7 8 9 10 **F**1 2 3 4 5 6 7 8 9 10 11 12 13 14 16 17 18 19 20 21 22 23 24 25 26 27 28 29 30 31 32 33 34 35 36 37 38 39 40 41 42 43 44 45 46 47 48 49 50 51 52 53 54 55 56 57 58 59 60 61 62 63 64 65 66 67 68 69 70 71 72 73 74 75 76 77 78 79 **P**1 2 4 5 7 **S** New York Presbyterian Healthcare System, New York, NY **Web address:** www.nyp.org	23	10	2346	81068	1702	1018199	10284	1552324	764145	—
★ NORTH CENTRAL BRONX HOSPITAL, 3424 Kossuth Avenue, Bronx, Zip 10467-2489; tel. 718/519-3500; Arthur Wagner, Chief Operating Officer **A**1 3 5 10 **F**3 5 7 9 10 12 13 14 19 21 22 23 25 27 29 32 33 34 35 38 39 41 42 43 44 45 48 49 50 51 54 56 57 58 59 60 61 63 64 66 70 72 73 75 76 78 79 **S** New York City Health and Hospitals Corporation, New York, NY **Web address:** www.ci.nyc.ny.us/html/hhc/html/northcentralbronx.html	14	10	255	8629	181	240699	2614	122670	58678	1378
★ NORTH GENERAL HOSPITAL, 1879 Madison Avenue, Zip 10035-2745; tel. 212/423-4000; Harold Freeman, M.D., President and Chief Executive Officer **A**1 3 5 9 10 **F**2 3 9 11 12 16 17 18 19 20 22 23 25 30 34 35 36 38 41 43 44 46 48 49 50 51 54 57 58 59 61 63 70 75 76 77 78 79	23	10	160	5473	109	116002	0	101816	50592	1087
★ OUR LADY OF MERCY MEDICAL CENTER, (Includes Florence D'Urso Pavilion, 1870 Pelham Parkway South, Zip 10461; tel. 212/430-6000), 600 East 233rd Street, Bronx, Zip 10466-2697; tel. 718/920-9000; Gary S. Horan, FACHE, President and Chief Executive Officer (Nonreporting) **A**1 2 3 5 8 9 10 **S** Our Lady of Mercy Healthcare System, Inc., New York, NY **Web address:** www.ourladyofmercy.com	21	10	508	—	—	—	—	—	—	—
☐ PARKWAY HOSPITAL, 70-35 113th Street, Flushing, Zip 11375; tel. 718/990-4100; Alan P. Zeitlin, M.D., Chief Executive Officer (Nonreporting) **A**1 9 10 PAYNE WHITNEY PSYCHIATRIC CLINIC See New York–Presbyterian Hospital	33	10	251	—	—	—	—	—	—	—
☐ ○ PENINSULA HOSPITAL CENTER, 51-15 Beach Channel Drive, Far Rockaway, Zip 11691-1074; tel. 718/734-2000; Robert V. Levine, President and Chief Executive Officer **A**1 9 10 11 12 13 **F**11 12 17 18 21 22 24 25 30 31 32 34 36 37 38 39 41 43 45 46 47 48 49 50 51 52 54 56 59 61 65 68 72 74 75 76 78 **P**5 7 8	23	10	196	6297	183	83236	0	66823	37791	—
★ QUEENS CHILDREN'S PSYCHIATRIC CENTER, 74-03 Commonwealth Boulevard, Jamaica, Zip 11426-1890; tel. 718/264-4506; Robert Schweitzer, Ed.D., Executive Director **A**1 **F**13 16 17 18 19 21 23 31 32 43 45 50 51 57 58 59 60 61 63 64 70 72 73 78 **P**6 **S** New York State Department of Mental Health, Albany, NY	12	52	84	88	71	30574	0	—	—	304
★ QUEENS HOSPITAL CENTER, 82-68 164th Street, Jamaica, Zip 11432-1104; tel. 718/883-3000; Antonio D. Martin, Chief Operating Officer **A**1 2 3 5 9 10 **F**2 3 5 7 8 9 11 12 13 14 18 19 20 22 23 24 25 27 30 31 32 33 34 35 36 37 38 39 41 42 43 44 45 46 48 49 50 51 52 53 54 56 57 58 59 60 61 62 63 64 65 66 70 71 72 73 75 76 78 79 **P**6 **S** New York City Health and Hospitals Corporation, New York, NY	15	10	266	12407	235	306836	1384	147475	74236	1858
☐ ROCKEFELLER UNIVERSITY HOSPITAL, (CLINICAL RESEARCH), 1230 York Avenue, Zip 10021-6399; tel. 212/327-8000; Emil Gotschlich, M.D., Vice President Medical Sciences **A**1 3 9 10 **F**70 **Web address:** clinfo.rockefeller.edu/ RUSK INSTITUTE See Mount Sinai–NYU Hospitals/Health System	23	49	40	259	7	4704	0	—	—	60
★ SAINT VINCENTS HOSPITAL AND MEDICAL CENTER, (Includes Saint Vincents Hospital, 275 North Street, Zip 10528; tel. 914/925-5300), 170 West 12th Street, Zip 10011-8397; tel. 212/604-7000; David J. Campbell, President and Chief Executive Officer (Nonreporting) **A**1 2 3 5 6 8 9 10 **S** Sisters of Charity Center, New York, NY **Web address:** www.svh.nymc.edu/	21	10	978	—	—	—	—	—	—	—

© 2000 AHA Guide *Many Facility Codes have changed. Please refer to the AHA Guide Code Chart.*

Hospitals, U.S. / NEW YORK

Hospital, Address, Telephone, Administrator, Approval, Facility, and Physician Codes, Health Care System, Network	Classification Codes		Utilization Data					Expense (thousands) of dollars		
★ American Hospital Association (AHA) membership □ Joint Commission on Accreditation of Healthcare Organizations (JCAHO) accreditation + American Osteopathic Healthcare Association (AOHA) membership ○ American Osteopathic Association (AOA) accreditation △ Commission on Accreditation of Rehabilitation Facilities (CARF) accreditation Control codes 61, 63, 64, 71, 72 and 73 indicate hospitals listed by AOHA, but not registered by AHA. For definition of numerical codes, see page A4	Control	Service	Staffed Beds	Admissions	Census	Outpatient Visits	Births	Total	Payroll	Personnel
SCHNEIDER CHILDREN'S HOSPITAL See Long Island Jewish Medical Center										
★ SISTERS OF CHARITY MEDICAL CENTER, (Includes Bayley Seton Campus, 75 Vanderbilt Avenue, Zip 10304–3850; tel. 718/354–6000; St Vincent's Campus, 355 Bard Avenue), 355 Bard Avenue, Staten Island, Zip 10310–1699; tel. 718/876–1234; Dominick M. Stanzione, Chief Operating Officer and Executive Vice President **A**1 2 3 5 6 9 10 **F**1 2 3 4 5 6 7 8 9 11 12 13 14 16 17 18 19 20 21 22 23 24 25 26 27 29 30 31 32 33 34 35 36 37 38 39 41 42 43 44 46 47 48 49 50 51 52 53 54 56 57 58 59 60 61 62 63 64 65 66 67 69 70 71 72 73 75 76 77 78 79 **P**4 5 7 Web address: www.schsi.org	21	10	449	25397	377	479486	3797	306639	126448	2563
★ SOUTH BEACH PSYCHIATRIC CENTER, 777 Seaview Avenue, Staten Island, Zip 10305–3499; tel. 718/667–2300; Lucy Sarkis, M.D., Executive Director **A**1 10 **F**1 13 17 18 19 38 45 57 58 59 60 61 62 63 64 **S** New York State Department of Mental Health, Albany, NY	12	22	331	845	315	0	0	—	—	1038
□ ○ ST BARNABAS HOSPITAL, (Includes Union Hospital of the Bronx, 260 East 188th Street, Zip 10458; tel. 718/220–2020), 183rd Street & Third Avenue, Bronx, Zip 10457–9998; tel. 718/960–9000; Ronald Gade, M.D., President (Nonreporting) **A**1 3 5 9 10 11 12 13	23	10	655	—	—	—	—	—	—	—
ST VINCENT'S CAMPUS See Sisters of Charity Medical Center										
□ ST. CLARE'S HOSPITAL AND HEALTH CENTER, 415 West 51st Street, Zip 10019–6394; tel. 212/586–1500; James A. Rutherford, President and Chief Executive Officer (Nonreporting) **A**1 9 10 12	21	10	236	—	—	—	—	—	—	—
ST. JOHN'S EPISCOPAL HOSPITAL DIVISION See Interfaith Medical Center										
★ ○ ST. JOHN'S EPISCOPAL HOSPITAL–SOUTH SHORE, 327 Beach 19th Street, Far Rockaway, Zip 11691–4424; tel. 718/869–7000; Nancy Simmons, Administrator (Nonreporting) **A**1 3 5 9 11 12 13 **S** Episcopal Health Services Inc., Bethpage, NY	21	10	314	—	—	—	—	—	—	—
ST. JOHN'S QUEENS HOSPITAL See Catholic Medical Centers										
ST. JOSEPH'S HOSPITAL See Catholic Medical Centers										
★ ST. LUKE'S–ROOSEVELT HOSPITAL CENTER, (Includes Roosevelt Hospital, 1000 Tenth Avenue, Zip 10019; tel. 212/523–4000; St. Luke's Hospital Center, 1111 Amsterdam Avenue, tel. 212/523–4000), 1111 Amsterdam Avenue, Zip 10025; tel. 212/523–4300; Sigurd H. Ackerman, M.D., President and Chief Executive Officer (Nonreporting) **A**1 3 5 8 9 10 **S** Continuum Health Partners, New York, NY Web address: www.wehealnewyork.org	23	10	715	—	—	—	—	—	—	—
ST. MARY'S HOSPITAL OF BROOKLYN See Catholic Medical Centers										
□ △ STATEN ISLAND UNIVERSITY HOSPITAL, 475 Seaview Avenue, Staten Island, Zip 10305–9998; tel. 718/226–9000; Rick J. Varone, President (Nonreporting) **A**1 2 3 5 7 9 10 **S** North Shore– Long Island Jewish Health System, Great Neck, NY Web address: www.northshorelij.com	23	10	617	—	—	—	—	—	—	—
THE ALLEN PAVILION See New York–Presbyterian Hospital										
THE MOUNT SINAI HOSPITAL OF QUEENS, (Formerly Western Queens Community Hospital), 25–10 30th Avenue, Astoria Station, Long Island City, Zip 11102–2495; tel. 718/932–1000; Caryn A. Schwab, Executive Director (Nonreporting) **A**9 10	33	10	208	—	—	—	—	—	—	—
★ UNIVERSITY HOSPITAL OF BROOKLYN–STATE UNIVERSITY OF NEW YORK HEALTH SCIENCE CENTER AT BROOKLYN, 445 Lenox Road, Brooklyn, Zip 11203–2098; tel. 718/270–2404; John C. LaRosa, M.D., President and Chief Executive Officer **A**1 2 3 5 8 9 10 **F**4 5 8 9 11 12 13 14 16 17 18 19 21 22 23 24 25 29 31 32 33 35 36 38 39 41 42 44 45 46 47 48 49 50 51 52 53 54 55 56 57 58 59 60 61 63 64 65 66 68 70 71 72 74 76 77 78 79 Web address: www.uhb.org/	12	10	376	11861	250	188051	2238	201134	112442	1970
★ △ VETERANS ADMINISTRATION NEW YORK HARBOR HEALTHCARE SYSTEM, (Includes Veterans Affairs Medical Center, 800 Poly Place, tel. 718/630–3500; Veterans Affairs Medical Center, 423 East 23rd Street, New York, Zip 10010–5050; tel. 212/686–7500), 800 Poly Place, Brooklyn, Zip 11209–7104; tel. 718/630–3500; John J. Donnellan, Jr, Director (Total facility includes 231 beds in nursing home–type unit) **A**1 2 3 5 7 8 9 **F**1 2 3 4 11 12 13 18 19 21 22 23 24 25 26 27 28 29 30 31 32 33 34 35 37 39 41 42 43 45 46 47 48 49 50 51 53 54 56 57 59 60 61 62 63 64 65 66 68 69 70 72 76 78 79 **P**6 **S** Department of Veterans Affairs, Washington, DC	45	10	618	10960	313	731862	0	362248	185179	3667
★ VETERANS AFFAIRS MEDICAL CENTER, 130 West Kingsbridge Road, Bronx, Zip 10468–3992; tel. 718/584–9000; Maryann Musumeci, Director (Total facility includes 112 beds in nursing home–type unit) **A**1 2 3 5 8 9 **F**3 9 11 13 17 18 19 22 23 24 25 26 27 29 30 31 32 33 34 35 36 37 38 39 41 43 45 46 48 49 50 51 54 55 56 59 60 61 62 63 64 65 68 70 72 76 77 78 79 **P**6 **S** Department of Veterans Affairs, Washington, DC Web address: www.va.gov/stations97/guide/home.asp?DIVISION=ALL	45	10	328	4132	181	293676	0	132715	97976	1465
□ VICTORY MEMORIAL HOSPITAL, 9036 Seventh Avenue, Brooklyn, Zip 11228–3625; tel. 718/567–1234; Krishin L. Bhatia, Administrator (Total facility includes 150 beds in nursing home–type unit) (Nonreporting) **A**1 9 10	23	10	410	—	—	—	—	—	—	—
□ WESTCHESTER SQUARE MEDICAL CENTER, 2475 St. Raymond Avenue, Bronx, Zip 10461–3198; tel. 718/430–7300; Alan Kopman, President and Chief Executive Officer **A**1 9 10 **F**2 3 4 5 8 9 10 11 14 19 22 23 24 25 27 29 30 31 33 35 38 39 41 42 45 46 47 48 49 50 51 52 53 54 55 56 57 58 59 60 61 62 63 64 65 66 68 69 70 71 74 75 76 77 78 79 **P**1 5 **S** New York Presbyterian Healthcare System, New York, NY	33	10	205	6703	140	42523	—	53200	27100	720

Hospitals, U.S. / NEW YORK

Hospital, Address, Telephone, Administrator, Approval, Facility, and Physician Codes, Health Care System, Network	Classification Codes		Utilization Data					Expense (thousands) of dollars		
★ American Hospital Association (AHA) membership ☐ Joint Commission on Accreditation of Healthcare Organizations (JCAHO) accreditation + American Osteopathic Healthcare Association (AOHA) membership ○ American Osteopathic Association (AOA) accreditation △ Commission on Accreditation of Rehabilitation Facilities (CARF) accreditation Control codes 61, 63, 64, 71, 72 and 73 indicate hospitals listed by AOHA, but not registered by AHA. For definition of numerical codes, see page A4	Control	Service	Staffed Beds	Admissions	Census	Outpatient Visits	Births	Total	Payroll	Personnel
★ WOODHULL MEDICAL AND MENTAL HEALTH CENTER, 760 Broadway Street, Brooklyn, Zip 11206–5383; tel. 718/963–8000; Cynthia Carrington–Murray, R.N., MS, Senior Vice President **A**1 3 9 10 **F**1 2 3 7 8 9 11 13 14 16 17 18 19 20 21 22 23 24 25 28 29 30 31 32 33 34 35 38 39 41 43 44 46 48 51 53 54 56 57 58 59 60 61 62 63 64 65 66 68 70 72 73 75 76 77 78 79 **P**6 **S** New York City Health and Hospitals Corporation, New York, NY	15	10	382	16621	345	357033	1348	218596	90384	2211
★ ○ WYCKOFF HEIGHTS MEDICAL CENTER, 374 Stockholm Street, Brooklyn, Zip 11237–4099; tel. 718/963–7102; Dominick J. Gio, President and Chief Executive Officer **A**1 3 5 9 10 11 13 **F**8 9 12 17 18 19 22 23 24 25 30 31 32 34 35 36 38 41 42 43 44 46 48 51 54 56 65 70 72 74 76 77 78 **S** New York Presbyterian Healthcare System, New York, NY	23	10	324	15513	240	210746	1748	159064	74615	1600
NEWARK—Wayne County										
★ VIAHEALTH OF WAYNE, (Includes Myers Campus, 6600 Middle Road, Sodus, Zip 14551–0310; tel. 315/483–3000; Newark–Wayne Campus, Driving Park Avenue, tel. 315/332–2022), Driving Park Avenue, Zip 14513, Mailing Address: P.O. Box 111, Zip 14513–0111; tel. 315/332–2022; W. Neil Stroman, President (Total facility includes 180 beds in nursing home–type unit) **A**1 9 10 **F**1 7 8 9 13 17 18 22 24 25 39 41 43 44 45 48 49 54 57 61 69 70 71 76 78 **S** Via Health, Rochester, NY **Web address:** www.viahealth.org	23	10	255	3080	213	89374	459	44460	18532	698
NEWBURGH—Orange County										
☐ ST. LUKE'S HOSPITAL, 70 Dubois Street, Zip 12550–4898, Mailing Address: P.O. Box 631, Zip 12550–0631; tel. 914/561–4400; Laurence E. Kelly, Executive Vice President and Administrator **A**1 9 10 **F**1 3 7 8 9 13 16 17 18 19 20 22 24 25 27 29 31 33 34 38 39 41 42 43 44 45 46 48 49 50 51 53 54 56 57 59 60 61 62 63 64 65 66 68 70 71 72 76 78 79 **P**8 **S** Greater Hudson Valley Health System, Newburgh, NY **Web address:** www.stlukeshospital.org	23	10	175	9616	128	115000	1121	65616	32045	792
NEWFANE—Niagara County										
INTER-COMMUNITY MEMORIAL HOSPITAL, 2600 William Street, Zip 14108–1093; tel. 716/778–5111; Clare A. Haar, Chief Executive Officer **A**9 10 **F**7 8 9 12 16 17 18 19 22 23 24 25 29 30 32 33 34 36 38 39 41 43 44 45 46 48 49 50 51 54 56 66 69 70 76 77 78 79 **P**5 8	23	10	71	2226	31	56071	139	15002	7139	230
NIAGARA FALLS—Niagara County										
☐ NIAGARA FALLS MEMORIAL MEDICAL CENTER, 621 Tenth Street, Zip 14302–0708, Mailing Address: P.O. Box 708, Zip 14302–0708; tel. 716/278–4000; Angelo G. Calbone, President and Chief Executive Officer (Nonreporting) **A**1 3 5 9 10	23	10	288	—	—	—	—	—	—	—
NORTH TARRYTOWN—Westchester County										
PHELPS MEMORIAL HOSPITAL CENTER See Sleepy Hollow										
NORTH TONAWANDA—Niagara County										
☐ DE GRAFF MEMORIAL HOSPITAL, 445 Tremont Street, Zip 14120–0750, Mailing Address: P.O. Box 0750, Zip 14120–0750; tel. 716/694–4500; Marcia B. Gutfeld, Vice President and Chief Operating Officer (Total facility includes 80 beds in nursing home–type unit) (Nonreporting) **A**1 9 **S** KALEIDA Health, Buffalo, NY	23	10	210	—	—	—	—	—	—	—
NORTHPORT—Suffolk County										
★ VETERANS AFFAIRS MEDICAL CENTER, 79 Middleville Road, Zip 11768–2293; tel. 631/261–4400; Mary A. Dowling, Director (Total facility includes 190 beds in nursing home–type unit) (Nonreporting) **A**1 2 3 5 8 9 **S** Department of Veterans Affairs, Washington, DC **Web address:** www.va.gov/stations97/guide/home.asp?DIVISION=ALL	45	10	699	—	—	—	—	—	—	—
NORWICH—Chenango County										
☐ CHENANGO MEMORIAL HOSPITAL, 179 North Broad Street, Zip 13815–1097; tel. 607/337–4111; Frank W. Mirabito, President (Total facility includes 80 beds in nursing home–type unit) **A**1 9 10 **F**7 8 9 13 17 18 19 22 23 24 25 30 32 34 35 36 38 41 43 44 45 46 48 50 51 54 56 66 68 69 70 72 76 78 79 **P**6 7 8 **Web address:** www.uhs.net	23	10	138	1990	100	207863	276	34739	17257	491
NYACK—Rockland County										
★ NYACK HOSPITAL, 160 North Midland Avenue, Zip 10960–1998; tel. 914/348–2000; Greger C. Anderson, President and Chief Executive Officer **A**1 2 9 10 **F**2 3 7 8 9 12 13 16 17 18 19 20 21 22 24 25 32 33 34 35 36 38 39 41 43 44 45 46 48 49 50 51 54 59 65 70 72 75 76 78 79 **P**1 **Web address:** www.nyackhospital.org	23	10	317	13171	210	290949	2092	120313	51775	1065
OCEANSIDE—Nassau County										
★ SOUTH NASSAU COMMUNITIES HOSPITAL, 2445 Oceanside Road, Zip 11572–1500; tel. 516/763–2030; Joseph A. Quagliata, President and Chief Executive Officer **A**1 2 3 5 9 10 **F**4 7 8 9 10 11 12 13 16 17 18 19 21 22 24 25 30 31 32 34 35 36 37 38 39 40 41 42 43 44 45 46 47 48 49 50 51 52 54 56 57 58 59 60 61 62 63 64 65 68 70 71 72 73 74 75 76 78 79 **P**3 5 7 **Web address:** www.southnassau.org/	23	10	321	12589	262	181441	1204	117371	59963	1432
OGDENSBURG—St. Lawrence County										
☐ HEPBURN MEDICAL CENTER, 214 King Street, Zip 13669–1192; tel. 315/393–3600; Lorraine B. Kabot, FACHE, President and Chief Executive Officer (Total facility includes 29 beds in nursing home–type unit) **A**1 9 10 **F**4 7 8 9 13 16 17 18 19 21 22 24 25 26 27 28 29 30 32 33 34 35 37 38 39 43 44 46 48 49 50 51 54 56 57 59 60 61 63 65 68 69 70 72 73 74 76 78 79 **Web address:** www.hepburnmedical.com	23	10	149	4483	105	114804	316	36812	16840	476

© 2000 AHA Guide *Many Facility Codes have changed. Please refer to the AHA Guide Code Chart.*

Hospitals, U.S. / NEW YORK

Hospital, Address, Telephone, Administrator, Approval, Facility, and Physician Codes, Health Care System, Network

- ★ American Hospital Association (AHA) membership
- ☐ Joint Commission on Accreditation of Healthcare Organizations (JCAHO) accreditation
- + American Osteopathic Healthcare Association (AOHA) membership
- ○ American Osteopathic Association (AOA) accreditation
- △ Commission on Accreditation of Rehabilitation Facilities (CARF) accreditation

Control codes 61, 63, 64, 71, 72 and 73 indicate hospitals listed by AOHA, but not registered by AHA. For definition of numerical codes, see page A4.

Hospital	Control	Service	Staffed Beds	Admissions	Census	Outpatient Visits	Births	Total	Payroll	Personnel
★ ST. LAWRENCE PSYCHIATRIC CENTER, 1 Chimney Point Drive, Zip 13669–2291; tel. 315/393–3000; John R. Scott, Director **A**1 10 **F**3 4 5 6 7 8 9 11 13 14 15 21 22 23 24 25 27 28 32 35 36 37 39 40 46 47 48 50 51 54 55 58 59 61 62 63 64 65 68 74 75 76 78 **S** New York State Department of Mental Health, Albany, NY	12	22	114	210	112	26517	0	24961	18594	443
OLEAN—Cattaraugus County										
☐ OLEAN GENERAL HOSPITAL, 515 Main Street, Zip 14760–9912; tel. 716/373–2600; Robert A. Catalano, M.D., President and Chief Executive Officer **A**1 3 6 9 10 **F**7 8 9 12 13 17 18 19 21 22 24 25 27 31 32 33 34 36 37 38 39 43 44 45 46 48 49 50 51 54 56 57 59 61 62 68 70 72 76 78	23	10	209	7103	105	174931	742	48054	23767	763
ONEIDA—Madison County										
★ ONEIDA HEALTHCARE CENTER, 321 Genesee Street, Zip 13421–0321; tel. 315/363–6000; Richard G. Smith, Chief Executive Officer (Total facility includes 160 beds in nursing home–type unit) **A**1 9 10 **F**8 9 12 16 17 18 22 24 25 29 32 33 38 39 41 43 44 45 48 50 51 54 55 68 69 70 76 78 Web address: www.oneidahealthcare.org	23	10	261	3585	187	87074	477	31715	4524	619
ONEONTA—Otsego County										
★ AURELIA OSBORN FOX MEMORIAL HOSPITAL, 1 Norton Avenue, Zip 13820–2697; tel. 607/432–2000; John R. Remillard, President (Total facility includes 131 beds in nursing home–type unit) **A**1 9 10 **F**1 7 8 9 12 13 16 17 18 19 21 22 24 25 28 29 30 32 33 34 36 37 38 39 40 41 43 44 45 46 48 49 50 51 54 56 57 58 59 60 61 62 68 69 70 76 78 79 **P**5 **S** Quorum Health Group, Brentwood, TN Web address: www.foxcarenetwork.com	23	10	246	4805	205	185856	362	51907	24593	703
ORANGEBURG—Rockland County										
★ ROCKLAND CHILDREN'S PSYCHIATRIC CENTER, 599 Convent Road, Zip 10962; tel. 914/359–7400; David J. Woodlock, Executive Director (Nonreporting) **A**1 3 **S** New York State Department of Mental Health, Albany, NY	12	52	54	—	—	—	—	—	—	—
★ ROCKLAND PSYCHIATRIC CENTER, 140 Old Orangeburg Road, Zip 10962–0071; tel. 914/359–1000; James H. Bopp, Executive Director (Nonreporting) **A**1 5 10 **S** New York State Department of Mental Health, Albany, NY	12	22	525	—	—	—	—	—	—	—
OSSINING—Westchester County										
OSSINING CORRECTIONAL FACILITIES HOSPITAL, 354 Hunter Street, Zip 10562–5498; tel. 914/941–0108; Benjamin I. Dyett, M.D., Director (Nonreporting)	12	11	25	—	—	—	—	—	—	—
☐ STONY LODGE HOSPITAL, 40 Croton Dam Road, Zip 10562–2644, Mailing Address: P.O. Box 1250, Briarcliff Manor, Zip 10510–1250; tel. 914/941–7400; Kevin F. Czipo, Executive Director **A**1 10 **F**38 57 58 61 64 **P**6 Web address: www.stonylodge.com	33	22	61	1007	60	660	0	10998	6146	188
OSWEGO—Oswego County										
★ OSWEGO HOSPITAL, 110 West Sixth Street, Zip 13126–9985; tel. 315/349–5511; Corte J. Spencer, Chief Executive Officer (Total facility includes 44 beds in nursing home–type unit) **A**1 9 10 **F**1 3 7 8 9 13 16 17 18 22 24 25 29 36 37 39 41 45 46 48 49 54 55 56 57 59 61 63 64 65 67 69 70 76 78	23	10	99	4817	76	212596	748	35708	17379	522
PATCHOGUE—Suffolk County										
★ BROOKHAVEN MEMORIAL HOSPITAL MEDICAL CENTER, 101 Hospital Road, Zip 11772–9998; tel. 631/654–7100; Thomas Ockers, President and Chief Executive Officer (Nonreporting) **A**1 9 10 Web address: www.bmhmc.org	23	10	321	—	—	—	—	—	—	—
PENN YAN—Yates County										
★ SOLDIERS AND SAILORS MEMORIAL HOSPITAL OF YATES COUNTY, 418 North Main Street, Zip 14527–1085; tel. 315/531–2000; James J. Dooley, President and Chief Executive Officer (Total facility includes 152 beds in nursing home–type unit) **A**1 9 10 **F**1 7 9 13 14 16 17 18 19 22 25 29 30 32 33 34 36 37 38 41 43 45 48 54 56 57 58 59 60 61 62 63 69 70 72 76 78 79	23	10	203	1619	171	62623	0	21342	10813	400
PLAINVIEW—Nassau County										
★ NORTH SHORE UNIVERSITY HOSPITAL AT PLAINVIEW, 888 Old Country Road, Zip 11803–4978; tel. 516/719–3000; Deborah Tascone, R.N., MS, Executive Director (Nonreporting) **A**1 2 9 10 **S** North Shore–Long Island Jewish Health System, Great Neck, NY Web address: www.northshorelij.com	23	10	279	—	—	—	—	—	—	—
PLATTSBURGH—Clinton County										
★ CHAMPLAIN VALLEY PHYSICIANS HOSPITAL MEDICAL CENTER, 75 Beekman Street, Zip 12901–1493; tel. 518/561–2000; Kevin J. Carroll, President (Total facility includes 54 beds in nursing home–type unit) **A**1 2 5 9 10 **F**7 8 9 11 12 13 14 17 18 22 23 24 25 27 28 29 32 33 34 38 39 41 43 44 45 46 48 50 51 54 56 57 61 65 69 70 71 72 75 76 77 78 79 Web address: www.cvph.org	23	10	383	9607	209	228954	1010	96016	48026	1310
POMONA—Rockland County										
☐ DOCTOR ROBERT L. YEAGER HEALTH CENTER, (Includes Summit Park Hospital–Rockland County Infirmary), 50 Sanatorium Road, Zip 10970–3554; tel. 914/364–2700; Peter T. Fella, Commissioner (Total facility includes 300 beds in nursing home–type unit) (Nonreporting) **A**1 10	13	49	408	—	—	—	—	—	—	—

Hospitals, U.S. / NEW YORK

Hospital, Address, Telephone, Administrator, Approval, Facility, and Physician Codes, Health Care System, Network	Classification Codes		Utilization Data					Expense (thousands) of dollars		
★ American Hospital Association (AHA) membership □ Joint Commission on Accreditation of Healthcare Organizations (JCAHO) accreditation + American Osteopathic Healthcare Association (AOHA) membership ○ American Osteopathic Association (AOA) accreditation △ Commission on Accreditation of Rehabilitation Facilities (CARF) accreditation Control codes 61, 63, 64, 71, 72 and 73 indicate hospitals listed by AOHA, but not registered by AHA. For definition of numerical codes, see page A4	Control	Service	Staffed Beds	Admissions	Census	Outpatient Visits	Births	Total	Payroll	Personnel
PORT CHESTER—Westchester County										
★ NEW YORK UNITED HOSPITAL MEDICAL CENTER, (Formerly United Hospital Medical Center), 406 Boston Post Road, Zip 10573–7300; tel. 914/934–3000; Kevin Dahill, President and Chief Executive Officer (Total facility includes 70 beds in nursing home–type unit) **A**1 5 9 10 **F**1 2 3 7 8 9 11 12 13 16 17 18 19 20 22 24 25 26 30 31 32 34 36 37 39 40 41 42 43 44 45 46 47 48 49 50 51 52 54 57 58 59 60 61 62 63 64 69 70 76 78 79 **P**5 **S** New York Presbyterian Healthcare System, New York, NY **Web address:** www.uhmc.com	23	10	231	7203	166	44797	—	71380	34734	840
PORT JEFFERSON—Suffolk County										
★ JOHN T. MATHER MEMORIAL HOSPITAL, 75 North Country Road, Zip 11777–2190; tel. 631/473–1320; Kenneth D. Roberts, President **A**1 2 9 10 **F**2 3 7 8 9 11 12 16 18 19 22 23 24 25 30 31 34 36 37 38 39 40 41 42 43 44 45 46 48 49 50 51 53 54 57 58 61 62 63 64 65 66 68 70 71 72 76 78 79 **P**5 6 8 **Web address:** www.matherhospital.com	23	10	248	10669	219	118306	—	125125	61776	1387
★ ST. CHARLES HOSPITAL AND REHABILITATION CENTER, 200 Belle Terre Road, Zip 11777; tel. 631/474–6000; David A. Dibner, FACHE, Interim President and Chief Executive Officer (Nonreporting) **A**1 2 5 9 10 **Web address:** www.stcharles.org	21	10	235	—	—	—	—	—	—	—
PORT JERVIS—Orange County										
□ MERCY COMMUNITY HOSPITAL, 160 East Main Street, Zip 12771–2245, Mailing Address: P.O. Box 1014, Zip 12771–1014; tel. 914/856–5351; Michael Parmer, M.D., Executive Vice President and Administrator (Total facility includes 46 beds in nursing home–type unit) **A**1 2 9 10 **F**2 8 9 13 16 17 18 19 22 23 24 25 31 32 34 35 36 37 39 41 43 44 46 48 51 54 57 58 61 65 69 70 72 76 78 **P**5 **S** Franciscan Health Partnership, Inc., Latham, NY **Web address:** www.mercycommunityhospital.org	21	10	187	4124	112	67452	239	35418	16282	505
POTSDAM—St. Lawrence County										
★ CANTON–POTSDAM HOSPITAL, 50 Leroy Street, Zip 13676–1799; tel. 315/265–3300; Bruce C. Potter, President **A**1 9 10 **F**2 3 8 9 13 16 17 18 22 24 25 27 29 32 33 34 39 43 44 48 51 54 68 70 71 72 75 76 78 **Web address:** www.potsdam.ny.us/cph	23	10	94	3771	55	112425	343	29179	14394	470
POUGHKEEPSIE—Dutchess County										
★ HUDSON RIVER PSYCHIATRIC CENTER, 373 North Road, Zip 12601–1197; tel. 914/452–8000; James Regan, Ph.D., Chief Executive Officer (Nonreporting) **A**1 5 10 **S** New York State Department of Mental Health, Albany, NY	12	22	460	—	—	—	—	—	—	—
□ △ SAINT FRANCIS HOSPITAL, (Includes Saint Francis Hospital–Beacon, 60 Delavan Avenue, Beacon, Zip 12508; tel. 914/831–3500), 241 North Road, Zip 12601–1399; tel. 914/483–5000; Sister M. Ann Elizabeth, President **A**1 3 7 9 10 **F**2 3 7 8 9 11 12 13 14 19 22 23 24 25 26 27 30 31 32 33 34 35 36 37 38 39 41 43 44 45 46 48 49 50 51 53 54 55 56 57 58 59 60 61 62 63 65 66 68 70 71 72 73 75 76 77 78 79 **Web address:** www.saintfrancishospital.com	21	10	314	10838	246	286500	0	122778	61936	—
★ VASSAR BROTHERS HOSPITAL, 45 Reade Place, Zip 12601–3990; tel. 914/454–8500; Ronald T. Mullahey, President **A**1 2 3 9 10 **F**2 3 7 8 9 10 11 12 13 17 18 19 20 22 23 24 25 27 28 29 30 31 32 33 34 36 38 39 41 42 43 44 45 46 48 49 50 51 53 54 55 56 57 58 59 60 61 62 63 64 65 66 67 68 69 70 71 72 75 76 78 79 **P**7 **Web address:** www.vassarbrothers.net	23	10	249	13030	198	160927	2465	98253	48137	867
QUEENS—Queens County, See New York City										
QUEENS VILLAGE—Queens County, See New York City										
RHINEBECK—Dutchess County										
★ NORTHERN DUTCHESS HOSPITAL, 10 Springbrook Avenue, Zip 12572–5002, Mailing Address: P.O. Box 5002, Zip 12572–5002; tel. 914/876–3001; Michael C. Mazzarella, President and Chief Executive Officer **A**1 9 10 **F**2 4 7 8 9 12 13 17 18 21 22 23 24 25 28 30 34 35 36 37 38 39 41 43 44 45 46 47 48 49 51 53 54 57 67 69 70 72 74 76 78 **Web address:** www.ndhosp.com	23	10	68	2434	36	55108	466	23223	10098	353
RICHMOND VALLEY—Richmond County, See New York City										
RIVERHEAD—Suffolk County										
★ CENTRAL SUFFOLK HOSPITAL, 1300 Roanoke Avenue, Zip 11901–2028; tel. 516/548–6000; Joseph F. Turner, President (Total facility includes 60 beds in nursing home–type unit) **A**1 9 10 **F**4 7 8 9 13 16 17 18 22 24 25 32 33 34 36 38 39 41 44 45 46 48 49 50 51 54 69 70 72 76 77 78 **P**7 **Web address:** www.centralsuffolkhospital.org	23	10	196	5079	131	73965	205	55090	25568	583
ROCHESTER—Monroe County										
★ GENESEE HOSPITAL, 224 Alexander Street, Zip 14607–4055; tel. 716/922–6000; Richard S. Constantino, M.D., President (Total facility includes 40 beds in nursing home–type unit) **A**1 2 3 5 8 9 10 **F**4 6 8 9 11 12 13 16 17 18 22 23 25 26 34 35 36 37 38 39 41 42 43 44 45 46 47 48 49 52 53 54 56 57 58 59 60 61 62 63 64 65 69 70 72 74 76 78 79 **P**5 **S** Via Health, Rochester, NY	23	10	269	13144	218	142783	2337	—	—	2170
★ HIGHLAND HOSPITAL OF ROCHESTER, 1000 South Avenue, Zip 14620–2782; tel. 716/473–2200; Steven I. Goldstein, President and Chief Executive Officer **A**1 2 3 5 9 10 **F**1 4 6 8 9 10 11 12 13 14 18 19 22 24 25 26 28 30 32 33 34 35 36 37 38 39 41 42 44 45 46 47 48 49 50 51 52 53 54 55 56 57 58 59 60 61 62 63 64 65 66 68 69 70 71 72 73 74 75 76 77 78 79 **P**3 7	23	10	200	8408	111	341005	1800	104376	51174	1301

© 2000 AHA Guide   *Many Facility Codes have changed. Please refer to the AHA Guide Code Chart.*

Hospitals, U.S. / NEW YORK

Hospital, Address, Telephone, Administrator, Approval, Facility, and Physician Codes, Health Care System, Network	Classification Codes		Utilization Data					Expense (thousands) of dollars		
★ American Hospital Association (AHA) membership ☐ Joint Commission on Accreditation of Healthcare Organizations (JCAHO) accreditation + American Osteopathic Healthcare Association (AOHA) membership ○ American Osteopathic Association (AOA) accreditation △ Commission on Accreditation of Rehabilitation Facilities (CARF) accreditation Control codes 61, 63, 64, 71, 72 and 73 indicate hospitals listed by AOHA, but not registered by AHA. For definition of numerical codes, see page A4	Control	Service	Staffed Beds	Admissions	Census	Outpatient Visits	Births	Total	Payroll	Personnel
★ △ PARK RIDGE HOSPITAL, 1555 Long Pond Road, Zip 14626–4182; tel. 716/723–7000; Martin E. Carlin, President **A**1 2 3 5 7 9 10 **F**1 2 3 6 8 9 11 15 16 17 18 20 21 22 23 24 25 30 31 34 36 38 39 41 43 44 45 46 48 49 50 51 53 54 56 57 58 59 60 61 62 63 64 65 66 67 69 70 71 72 76 77 78 79 **P**5 8 **Web address:** www.parkridgehs.org	23	10	340	11876	249	783104	178	246027	87841	2334
★ ROCHESTER GENERAL HOSPITAL, 1425 Portland Avenue, Zip 14621–3099; tel. 716/338–4000; Richard S. Constantino, M.D., President (Nonreporting) **A**1 2 3 5 6 8 9 10 **S** Via Health, Rochester, NY **Web address:** www.viahealth.org/	23	10	476	—	—	—	—	—	—	—
★ ROCHESTER PSYCHIATRIC CENTER, 1111 Elmwood Avenue, Zip 14620–3005; tel. 716/473–3230; Bryan F. Rudes, Executive Director **A**1 3 5 9 10 **F**1 2 3 4 5 6 7 8 9 10 11 12 13 14 15 16 18 19 20 21 22 23 24 25 26 27 28 29 30 31 32 33 34 35 36 37 38 39 40 41 42 43 44 45 46 47 48 49 50 51 52 53 54 55 56 57 58 59 60 61 62 63 64 65 66 67 68 69 70 71 72 73 74 75 76 77 78 79 **S** New York State Department of Mental Health, Albany, NY	12	22	247	321	256	62437	0	—	—	595
★ △ STRONG MEMORIAL HOSPITAL OF THE UNIVERSITY OF ROCHESTER, 601 Elmwood Avenue, Zip 14642–0002; tel. 716/275–2100; Steven I. Goldstein, General Director and Chief Executive Officer **A**1 3 5 7 8 9 10 **F**1 2 3 4 5 6 7 8 9 10 11 12 13 14 15 16 17 18 19 20 21 22 23 24 25 26 27 28 29 30 32 33 34 35 36 37 38 39 40 41 42 43 44 45 46 47 48 49 50 51 52 53 54 55 56 57 58 59 60 61 62 63 64 65 66 67 68 69 70 71 72 73 74 75 76 77 78 79 **P**1 5 7	23	10	651	29540	547	673337	3271	426567	191169	6885
ROCKVILLE CENTRE—Nassau County										
★ MERCY MEDICAL CENTER, 1000 North Village Avenue, Zip 11570–1098; tel. 516/255–0111; Vincent DiRubbio, President and Chief Executive Officer **A**1 2 3 9 10 **F**3 4 7 8 9 11 12 13 16 17 18 19 22 24 25 27 30 32 33 34 35 36 37 38 39 41 42 44 45 46 47 48 49 51 53 54 57 59 60 61 62 63 64 65 68 70 71 72 74 75 76 78 79 **P**8	21	10	327	13825	266	192145	2081	138876	68419	1465
ROME—Oneida County										
★ ROME MEMORIAL HOSPITAL, 1500 North James Street, Zip 13440–2898; tel. 315/338–7000; Alvin C. White, President and Chief Executive Officer (Total facility includes 82 beds in nursing home–type unit) **A**1 9 10 **F**3 4 8 9 11 12 13 14 16 17 18 21 22 23 24 25 26 32 33 34 35 36 37 38 39 40 41 42 43 44 45 46 47 48 49 50 51 53 54 56 57 58 59 60 61 62 63 64 65 66 68 69 70 71 72 74 75 76 77 78 79 **P**5 **Web address:** www.romehosp.com	23	10	211	5407	157	89455	653	44323	22312	774
ROSLYN—Nassau County										
★ ST. FRANCIS HOSPITAL, (CARDIAC TERTIARY), 100 Port Washington Boulevard, Zip 11576–1348; tel. 516/562–6000; Alan D. Guerci, M.D., President and Chief Executive Officer **A**1 5 9 10 **F**2 3 4 7 8 9 11 12 13 14 16 17 18 19 21 22 23 24 25 26 27 28 30 31 32 33 34 35 36 37 39 40 41 42 43 44 45 46 47 48 49 50 51 52 55 56 57 58 59 60 61 62 63 64 65 66 67 68 70 71 72 73 76 78 79 **P**5 8 **Web address:** www.stfrancisheartcenter.com	23	49	279	15768	314	88239	0	220075	93434	1740
RYE—Westchester County										
★ RYE HOSPITAL CENTER, 754 Boston Post Road, Zip 10580–2724; tel. 914/967–4567; Jack C. Schoenholtz, M.D., Medical Director, Administrator and President **A**1 10 **F**22 23 24 25 39 55 57 58 60 62 65 68 70 76 78	33	22	34	143	26	—	0	4062	1854	48
SARANAC LAKE—Franklin County										
★ ADIRONDACK MEDICAL CENTER, Lake Colby Drive, Zip 12983, Mailing Address: P.O. Box 471, Zip 12983–0471; tel. 518/891–4141; Chandler M. Ralph, President and Chief Executive Officer **A**1 9 10 **F**8 9 16 17 18 19 22 24 32 39 41 44 45 46 48 49 54 56 57 62 64 68 70 71 75 78 **P**5 8 **S** Brim Healthcare, Inc., Brentwood, TN **Web address:** www.northnet.org/adirondackmedcenter	23	10	78	3249	49	106529	263	33396	16273	438
SARATOGA SPRINGS—Saratoga County										
★ SARATOGA HOSPITAL, 211 Church Street, Zip 12866–1003; tel. 518/587–3222; David Andersen, President and Chief Executive Officer (Total facility includes 72 beds in nursing home–type unit) **A**1 9 10 **F**8 9 12 13 16 17 18 19 21 22 24 25 30 32 34 37 38 39 41 43 44 45 46 48 51 54 56 57 58 59 60 61 62 69 70 72 76 78 79 **P**5	23	10	204	6383	166	115979	746	55169	26203	971
SCHENECTADY—Schenectady County										
☐ BELLEVUE WOMAN'S HOSPITAL, 2210 Troy Road, Zip 12309–4797; tel. 518/346–9400; Michael A. Mangini, Administrator and Chief Executive Officer (Nonreporting) **A**1 10 **Web address:** www.bellevuewoman.com	33	44	55	—	—	—	—	—	—	—
★ ELLIS HOSPITAL, 1101 Nott Street, Zip 12308–2487; tel. 518/243–4000; G. B. Serrill, President and Chief Executive Officer (Total facility includes 82 beds in nursing home–type unit) **A**1 2 3 5 6 9 10 **F**3 4 5 6 8 9 11 12 13 14 16 17 18 19 21 22 23 24 25 26 27 28 29 30 32 33 34 35 36 37 38 39 41 43 44 45 46 47 48 49 50 51 54 56 57 58 59 60 61 62 63 64 65 66 67 68 69 70 71 72 75 76 78 79 **S** Quorum Health Group, Brentwood, TN **Web address:** www.shine.org	23	10	351	12281	291	265255	433	118943	52816	1496
☐ ST. CLARE'S HOSPITAL OF SCHENECTADY, 600 McClellan Street, Zip 12304–1090; tel. 518/382–2000; Paul J. Chodkowski, President and Chief Executive Officer (Nonreporting) **A**1 3 5 9 10 12	21	10	200	—	—	—	—	—	—	—

Hospitals, U.S. / NEW YORK

Hospital, Address, Telephone, Administrator, Approval, Facility, and Physician Codes, Health Care System, Network	Classification Codes		Utilization Data					Expense (thousands) of dollars		
★ American Hospital Association (AHA) membership ☐ Joint Commission on Accreditation of Healthcare Organizations (JCAHO) accreditation + American Osteopathic Healthcare Association (AOHA) membership ○ American Osteopathic Association (AOA) accreditation △ Commission on Accreditation of Rehabilitation Facilities (CARF) accreditation Control codes 61, 63, 64, 71, 72 and 73 indicate hospitals listed by AOHA, but not registered by AHA. For definition of numerical codes, see page A4	Control	Service	Staffed Beds	Admissions	Census	Outpatient Visits	Births	Total	Payroll	Personnel
✶ △ SUNNYVIEW HOSPITAL AND REHABILITATION CENTER, 1270 Belmont Avenue, Zip 12308–2104; tel. 518/382–4500; Robert J. Bylancik, CHE, President and Chief Executive Officer **A**1 3 5 7 9 10 **F**7 13 16 17 19 22 28 29 38 39 45 50 53 54 59 70 72 78 **P**6 **Web address:** www.sunnyview.org	23	46	104	1843	79	37959	0	23450	14261	396
SEAFORD—Nassau County										
+ ○ MASSAPEQUA GENERAL HOSPITAL, 750 Hicksville Road, Zip 11783–1300, Mailing Address: P.O. Box 20, Zip 11783–0020; tel. 516/520–6000; John P. Breen, Chief Executive Officer (Nonreporting) **A**9 10 11 12 13	33	10	122	—	—	—	—	—	—	—
SIDNEY—Delaware County										
✶ THE HOSPITAL, 43 Pearl Street West, Zip 13838–1399; tel. 607/561–2153; Russell A. Test, Administrator and Chief Executive Officer (Total facility includes 40 beds in nursing home–type unit) **A**1 9 10 **F**7 8 9 16 17 18 19 22 24 25 26 29 30 32 34 35 38 41 44 45 48 51 54 56 69 70 71 72 76 77 78 79 **S** Brim Healthcare, Inc., Brentwood, TN **Web address:** www.thehospital.org	14	10	87	1699	56	41530	109	12746	6329	230
SLEEPY HOLLOW—Westchester County										
✶ PHELPS MEMORIAL HOSPITAL CENTER, 701 North Broadway, Zip 10591–1096; tel. 914/366–3000; Keith F. Safian, President and Chief Executive Officer **A**1 10 **F**3 7 8 9 12 13 14 16 17 18 19 22 23 24 25 30 31 33 34 36 37 38 39 40 41 44 45 46 48 50 51 53 54 57 59 61 62 63 65 66 68 70 72 76 77 78 79 **P**1 5 7 **Web address:** www.phelpshospital.org	23	10	235	7905	137	125500	854	74205	37472	886
SMITHTOWN—Suffolk County										
✶ ST. CATHERINE OF SIENA MEDICAL CENTER, (Formerly St. John's Episcopal Hospital–Smithtown), 50 Route 25–A, Zip 11787–1398; tel. 631/862–3000; James M. Wilson, President and Chief Executive Officer (Nonreporting) **A**1 9 **S** Episcopal Health Services Inc., Bethpage, NY	21	10	366							
SODUS—Wayne County										
MYERS CAMPUS See ViaHealth of Wayne, Newark										
SOUTHAMPTON—Suffolk County										
☐ SOUTHAMPTON HOSPITAL, 240 Meeting House Lane, Zip 11968–5090; tel. 516/726–8555; Thomas B. Doolan, Acting President and Chief Executive Officer **A**1 9 10 **F**2 3 7 8 9 10 11 12 13 16 17 18 19 21 22 23 24 25 26 27 28 29 30 31 32 33 34 35 36 37 38 39 41 42 44 45 46 47 48 49 50 51 52 53 54 56 57 59 61 63 65 68 69 70 71 72 73 74 75 76 78 79 **P**6	23	10	127	5143	74	181402	785	63238	29019	683
SPRINGVILLE—Erie County										
BERTRAND CHAFFEE HOSPITAL, 224 East Main Street, Zip 14141–1497; tel. 716/592–2871; Steve Krisiak, Chief Executive Officer (Nonreporting) **A**9 10	23	10	49	—	—	—	—	—	—	—
STAR LAKE—St. Lawrence County										
★ CLIFTON–FINE HOSPITAL, Oswegatchie Trail, Zip 13690, Mailing Address: P.O. Box 10, Zip 13690–0010; tel. 315/848–3351; Rodney C. Boula, Administrator (Nonreporting) **A**9 10 **Web address:** www.northnet.org	16	10	20							
STATEN ISLAND—Richmond County, See New York City										
STONY BROOK—Suffolk County										
✶ UNIVERSITY HOSPITAL, State University of New York, Zip 11794–8410; tel. 631/689–8333; Michael A. Maffetone, Director and Chief Executive Officer **A**1 2 3 5 8 9 10 **F**4 7 8 9 10 11 13 14 16 17 18 19 20 21 22 23 24 25 26 27 29 30 32 33 34 35 38 39 41 42 44 45 46 47 48 49 50 51 52 54 56 57 58 59 60 61 62 63 64 65 66 68 70 71 72 73 74 75 76 77 78 79 **Web address:** www.uhmc.sunysb.edu	12	10	490	24409	378	594207	3550	328903	151462	3344
SUFFERN—Rockland County										
☐ GOOD SAMARITAN HOSPITAL, 255 Lafayette Avenue, Zip 10901–4869; tel. 914/368–5000; James A. Martin, Chief Executive Officer (Nonreporting) **A**1 2 9 10 **S** Franciscan Health Partnership, Inc., Latham, NY	21	10	308	—	—	—	—	—	—	—
SYOSSET—Nassau County										
✶ NORTH SHORE UNIVERSITY HOSPITAL AT SYOSSET, 221 Jericho Turnpike, Zip 11791–4567; tel. 516/496–6400; Deborah Tascone, R.N., MS, Executive Director (Nonreporting) **A**1 3 9 **S** North Shore– Long Island Jewish Health System, Great Neck, NY **Web address:** www.northshorelij.com	23	10	186							
SYRACUSE—Onondaga County										
☐ BENJAMIN RUSH CENTER, 650 South Salina Street, Zip 13202–3524; tel. 315/476–2161; Norman J. Lesswing, Ph.D., Administrator and Chief Executive Officer (Nonreporting) **A**1 9 10	31	22	107							
✶ COMMUNITY–GENERAL HOSPITAL OF GREATER SYRACUSE, 4900 Broad Road, Zip 13215; tel. 315/492–5011; Kent A. Arnold, President (Total facility includes 40 beds in nursing home–type unit) **A**1 3 5 9 10 **F**4 7 8 9 13 16 22 24 25 29 30 32 33 34 35 37 38 41 43 44 45 46 48 54 57 58 59 60 69 70 76 78 79 **P**5 6 7 **Web address:** www.cgh.org	23	10	259	10234	156	120788	1776	81409	34872	1020
✶ CROUSE HOSPITAL, 736 Irving Avenue, Zip 13210–1690; tel. 315/470–7111; Kent A. Arnold, President and Chief Executive Officer **A**1 3 5 9 10 **F**2 3 4 7 8 9 11 13 14 16 17 19 20 21 24 25 28 29 30 31 32 33 34 35 36 37 38 39 41 42 43 44 45 46 48 49 50 51 54 55 57 59 61 65 66 68 69 70 71 72 74 75 76 77 78 79 **P**1 5 7 **Web address:** www.crouse.org	23	10	455	21965	332	235763	3611	188176	81420	2280

© 2000 AHA Guide   *Many Facility Codes have changed. Please refer to the AHA Guide Code Chart.*

Hospitals, U.S. / NEW YORK

Hospital, Address, Telephone, Administrator, Approval, Facility, and Physician Codes, Health Care System, Network	Classification Codes		Utilization Data					Expense (thousands) of dollars		
	Control	Service	Staffed Beds	Admissions	Census	Outpatient Visits	Births	Total	Payroll	Personnel

★ American Hospital Association (AHA) membership
☐ Joint Commission on Accreditation of Healthcare Organizations (JCAHO) accreditation
+ American Osteopathic Healthcare Association (AOHA) membership
○ American Osteopathic Association (AOA) accreditation
△ Commission on Accreditation of Rehabilitation Facilities (CARF) accreditation
Control codes 61, 63, 64, 71, 72 and 73 indicate hospitals listed by AOHA, but not registered by AHA. For definition of numerical codes, see page A4

Hospital	Control	Service	Staffed Beds	Admissions	Census	Outpatient Visits	Births	Total	Payroll	Personnel
★ RICHARD H. HUTCHINGS PSYCHIATRIC CENTER, 620 Madison Street, Zip 13210–2319; tel. 315/473–4980; Bryan F. Rudes, Executive Director **A**1 3 5 10 **F**13 16 17 18 21 32 57 58 59 60 61 62 63 64 70 78 **S** New York State Department of Mental Health, Albany, NY **Web address:** www.omh.state.ny.us	12	22	136	219	130	—	0	—	—	510
☐ ST. JOSEPH'S HOSPITAL HEALTH CENTER, 301 Prospect Avenue, Zip 13203–1895; tel. 315/448–5111; Theodore M. Pasinski, President (Nonreporting) **A**1 3 5 6 9 10 **S** Sisters of the 3rd Franciscan Order, Syracuse, NY **Web address:** www.SJHSYR.ORG	21	10	431	—	—	—	—	—	—	—
★ UNIVERSITY HOSPITAL–SUNY HEALTH SCIENCE CENTER AT SYRACUSE, 750 East Adams Street, Zip 13210–2399; tel. 315/464–5540; Ben Moore, II, Executive Director **A**1 3 5 8 9 10 **F**4 5 7 9 10 11 12 13 17 18 19 22 23 24 25 27 29 30 32 33 34 35 38 39 41 43 45 46 47 48 49 50 51 52 53 54 57 58 59 60 61 62 63 65 66 68 70 71 72 73 74 75 76 77 78 79 **P**7 **Web address:** www.universityhospital.org/	12	10	356	14041	295	206690	0	241021	108783	2765
★ VETERANS AFFAIRS MEDICAL CENTER, 800 Irving Avenue, Zip 13210–2796; tel. 315/476–7461; James P. Cody, Director **A**1 3 5 8 9 **F**1 3 9 11 13 19 22 25 26 27 29 30 31 32 34 35 36 38 39 41 46 48 49 50 51 53 54 56 57 60 61 62 63 64 65 68 69 70 76 77 78 79 **S** Department of Veterans Affairs, Washington, DC **Web address:** www.va.gov/stations97/guide/home.asp?DIVISION=ALL	45	10	175	3274	106	254269	0	94800	48600	987

TICONDEROGA—Essex County

Hospital	Control	Service	Staffed Beds	Admissions	Census	Outpatient Visits	Births	Total	Payroll	Personnel
☐ MOSES LUDINGTON HOSPITAL, 2 Wicker Street, Zip 12883–1097; tel. 518/585–2831; Mark R. Kubricky, Chief Executive Officer (Nonreporting) **A**1 9 10	23	10	39	—	—	—	—	—	—	—

TROY—Rensselaer County

Hospital	Control	Service	Staffed Beds	Admissions	Census	Outpatient Visits	Births	Total	Payroll	Personnel
☐ SAMARITAN HOSPITAL, 2215 Burdett Avenue, Zip 12180–2475; tel. 518/271–3300; Paul A. Milton, Chief Operating Officer **A**1 6 9 10 **F**1 2 3 6 7 8 9 12 13 14 16 17 18 19 21 22 24 25 26 28 29 30 32 34 35 36 37 39 41 42 43 44 45 46 48 49 50 51 52 53 54 56 57 59 60 61 62 63 64 65 66 67 69 70 72 73 76 78 79 **P**7 **Web address:** www.nehealth.com	23	10	135	7987	140	170367	805	61527	30934	917
★ SETON HEALTH SYSTEM, (Includes Seton Health System–St. Mary's Hospital, 1300 Massachusetts Avenue, Zip 12180), 1300 Massachusetts Avenue, Zip 12180–1695; tel. 518/268–5000; Mark A. Donovan, M.D., President and Chief Executive Officer (Nonreporting) **A**1 9 10 **S** Ascension Health, Saint Louis, MO **Web address:** www.setonhealth.org	21	10	344	—	—	—	—	—	—	—

UTICA—Oneida County

FAXTON CAMPUS See Faxton–St. Luke's Healthcare

Hospital	Control	Service	Staffed Beds	Admissions	Census	Outpatient Visits	Births	Total	Payroll	Personnel
★ △ FAXTON–ST. LUKE'S HEALTHCARE, (Includes Allen–Calder Skilled Nursing Facility; Faxton Campus, 1676 Sunset Avenue, Zip 13502–5475; tel. 315/738–6200; St. Luke's Campus, Mailing Address: P.O. Box 479, Zip 13503–0479; tel. 315/798–6000), Mailing Address: P.O. Box 479, Zip 13503–0479; tel. 315/798–6000; Andrew E. Peterson, President and Chief Executive Officer (Total facility includes 124 beds in nursing home–type unit) **A**1 2 7 9 10 **F**1 3 4 7 8 9 11 12 13 17 19 22 23 24 25 26 27 30 32 33 34 36 37 38 39 40 41 43 44 45 46 47 48 49 51 53 54 56 57 61 62 65 66 68 69 70 72 74 75 76 77 78 79	23	10	556	16879	522	269786	1940	140505	63143	1847
★ MOHAWK VALLEY PSYCHIATRIC CENTER, 1400 Noyes, Zip 13502–3803; tel. 315/797–6800; Sarah F. Rudes, Executive Director (Nonreporting) **A**1 10 **S** New York State Department of Mental Health, Albany, NY	12	22	614	—	—	—	—	—	—	—
★ ST. ELIZABETH MEDICAL CENTER, 2209 Genesee Street, Zip 13501–5999; tel. 315/798–8100; Sister Rose Vincent, President and Chief Executive Officer **A**1 3 6 9 10 12 **F**4 8 11 12 14 17 18 19 21 22 24 25 32 34 37 38 39 41 42 43 44 46 47 48 49 54 56 57 58 59 60 61 62 63 68 70 71 72 75 76 77 78 79 **P**5 6 **S** Sisters of the 3rd Franciscan Order, Syracuse, NY **Web address:** www.stemc.org	21	10	172	8517	138	298678	0	84010	41349	1274

ST. LUKE'S CAMPUS See Faxton–St. Luke's Healthcare

VALHALLA—Westchester County

Hospital	Control	Service	Staffed Beds	Admissions	Census	Outpatient Visits	Births	Total	Payroll	Personnel
★ BLYTHEDALE CHILDREN'S HOSPITAL, 95 Bradhurst Avenue, Zip 10595–1697; tel. 914/592–7555; Robert Stone, President **A**1 10 **F**16 17 18 23 28 32 33 34 36 38 45 50 51 54 58 59 60 63 70 71 72 78 **P**6 **Web address:** www.blythedale.org	23	56	92	313	77	38059	0	25270	16017	365
☐ WESTCHESTER MEDICAL CENTER, Valhalla Campus, Zip 10595; tel. 914/493–7000; Edward A. Stolzenberg, President and Chief Executive Officer (Total facility includes 355 beds in nursing home–type unit) **A**1 2 3 5 8 9 10 **F**1 3 5 7 8 9 10 11 12 13 14 15 17 18 19 21 22 23 24 25 26 27 30 31 32 33 34 35 37 38 39 41 42 43 44 45 46 47 48 49 50 51 52 53 54 55 56 57 58 59 60 61 62 63 64 65 66 68 69 70 71 72 73 74 75 76 78 79 **P**5	13	10	996	22817	919	304067	1024	—	—	3186

VALLEY STREAM—Nassau County

Hospital	Control	Service	Staffed Beds	Admissions	Census	Outpatient Visits	Births	Total	Payroll	Personnel
★ FRANKLIN HOSPITAL MEDICAL CENTER, 900 Franklin Avenue, Zip 11580–2190; tel. 516/256–6000; William Kowalewski, President and Chief Executive Officer (Total facility includes 120 beds in nursing home–type unit) **A**1 2 9 10 **F**1 2 3 4 6 7 8 9 11 12 13 14 16 17 18 19 21 22 23 24 25 26 27 29 30 31 32 33 34 35 36 37 38 39 40 41 42 43 44 45 46 47 49 50 51 52 53 54 55 57 58 59 60 61 62 63 64 65 66 67 68 69 70 71 72 73 74 75 76 77 78 79 **P**5 8 **S** North Shore– Long Island Jewish Health System, Great Neck, NY **Web address:** www.northshorelij.com	23	10	310	9968	314	37531	425	89050	40074	1041

Hospitals, U.S. / NEW YORK

Hospital, Address, Telephone, Administrator, Approval, Facility, and Physician Codes, Health Care System, Network	Classification Codes		Utilization Data					Expense (thousands) of dollars		
★ American Hospital Association (AHA) membership ☐ Joint Commission on Accreditation of Healthcare Organizations (JCAHO) accreditation + American Osteopathic Healthcare Association (AOHA) membership ○ American Osteopathic Association (AOA) accreditation △ Commission on Accreditation of Rehabilitation Facilities (CARF) accreditation Control codes 61, 63, 64, 71, 72 and 73 indicate hospitals listed by AOHA, but not registered by AHA. For definition of numerical codes, see page A4	Control	Service	Staffed Beds	Admissions	Census	Outpatient Visits	Births	Total	Payroll	Personnel
WALTON—Delaware County ☐ DELAWARE VALLEY HOSPITAL, 1 Titus Place, Zip 13856–1498; tel. 607/865–2100; David J. Polge, President and Chief Executive Officer (Nonreporting) **A**1 9 10	23	10	42	—	—	—	—	—	—	—
WARSAW—Wyoming County ☐ WYOMING COUNTY COMMUNITY HOSPITAL, 400 North Main Street, Zip 14569–1097; tel. 716/786–2233; Lucille K. Sheedy, Administrator and Chief Executive Officer (Total facility includes 160 beds in nursing home–type unit) (Nonreporting) **A**1 9 10 **Web address:** www.wycol.com/wyoming_county	13	10	262	—	—	—	—	—	—	—
WARWICK—Orange County ☐ ST. ANTHONY COMMUNITY HOSPITAL, 15 Maple Avenue, Zip 10990–5180; tel. 914/986–2276; James A. Martin, President and Chief Executive Officer **A**1 9 10 **F**1 2 6 7 8 9 12 13 16 17 18 19 22 23 24 25 32 33 34 36 37 38 39 40 41 43 44 45 46 48 49 50 51 54 57 58 59 61 62 63 64 65 68 69 70 71 72 76 78 79 **P**5 **S** Franciscan Health Partnership, Inc., Latham, NY	21	10	73	2398	37	40066	463	20639	9023	219
WATERTOWN—Jefferson County ☐ SAMARITAN MEDICAL CENTER, 830 Washington Street, Zip 13601–4066; tel. 315/785–4121; David E. Tinker, President and Chief Executive Officer **A**1 9 10 12 **F**1 7 19 25 43 50 51 54 69 70 76 **Web address:** www.samaritanhealth.com	23	10	54	397	23	16630	0	6213	3060	—
WELLSVILLE—Allegany County ✠ JONES MEMORIAL HOSPITAL, 191 North Main Street, Zip 14895–1197, Mailing Address: P.O. Box 72, Zip 14895–0072; tel. 716/593–1100; William M. DiBerardino, FACHE, President and Chief Executive Officer **A**1 9 10 **F**7 8 9 12 13 16 17 18 19 22 24 25 32 33 34 39 40 41 43 44 45 46 48 49 50 51 54 56 70 71 72 76 78 79 **P**8 **Web address:** www.jmhny.org	23	10	70	3000	32	62962	333	21674	9353	315
WEST HAVERSTRAW—Rockland County ✠ HELEN HAYES HOSPITAL, Route 9W, Zip 10993–1195; tel. 914/786–4000; Magdalena Ramirez, Chief Executive Officer **A**1 5 10 **F**13 18 23 28 34 38 45 49 50 51 53 54 70 72 78 **P**6 **Web address:** www.helenhayeshospital.org	12	46	155	2184	121	46649	0	54309	23609	787
WEST ISLIP—Suffolk County ✠ GOOD SAMARITAN HOSPITAL MEDICAL CENTER, 1000 Montauk Highway, Zip 11795–4958; tel. 631/376–3000; Richard J. Murphy, President and Chief Executive Officer (Total facility includes 100 beds in nursing home–type unit) (Nonreporting) **A**1 2 9 10 12 13	21	10	525	—	—	—	—	—	—	—
WEST POINT—Orange County ✠ KELLER ARMY COMMUNITY HOSPITAL, U.S. Military Academy, Zip 10996–1197; tel. 914/938–4837; Colonel Gordon Miller, Deputy Commander Clincial Services (Nonreporting) **A**1 3 9 **S** Department of the Army, Office of the Surgeon General, Falls Church, VA **Web address:** www.wramc.amedd.army.mil/wp	42	10	49	—	—	—	—	—	—	—
WESTFIELD—Chautauqua County ★ WESTFIELD MEMORIAL HOSPITAL, 189 East Main Street, Zip 14787–1195; tel. 716/326–4921; Mary E. LaRowe, President and Chief Executive Officer **A**9 10 **F**4 7 8 9 11 16 17 18 19 20 22 24 25 32 34 36 37 38 39 44 46 47 48 49 54 56 58 61 63 64 65 70 72 75 76 77 78 **P**1 **Web address:** www.wmhinc.org	23	10	32	902	8	36837	203	6929	3633	49
WHITE PLAINS—Westchester County ✠ △ BURKE REHABILITATION HOSPITAL, 785 Mamaroneck Avenue, Zip 10605–2593; tel. 914/597–2500; Mary Beth Walsh, M.D., Chief Executive Officer **A**1 5 7 10 **F**5 23 30 34 38 43 51 53 54 70 71 72 78 **Web address:** www.burke.org NEW YORK–PRESBYTERIAN HOSPITAL, WESTCHESTER DIVISION See New York–Presbyterian Hospital, New York	23	46	150	2339	128	—	0	40124	23010	545
☐ ST. AGNES HOSPITAL, (Includes Children's Rehabilitation Center), 305 North Street, Zip 10605–2299; tel. 914/681–4500; Gary S. Horan, FACHE, President and Chief Executive Officer (Nonreporting) **A**1 3 5 9 10 **S** Our Lady of Mercy Healthcare System, Inc., New York, NY **Web address:** www.saintagneshospital.com	21	10	184	—	—	—	—	—	—	—
✠ WHITE PLAINS HOSPITAL CENTER, Davis Avenue and Post Road, Zip 10601–4699; tel. 914/681–0600; Jon B. Schandler, President and Chief Executive Officer **A**1 2 5 9 10 **F**3 8 9 12 13 16 17 18 19 20 22 23 24 25 30 32 33 34 35 36 37 39 41 43 44 45 46 48 49 50 51 54 55 56 57 58 59 61 63 65 68 70 72 75 76 78 **P**2 5 7 8 **Web address:** www.wphospital.org	23	10	307	11931	204	119472	1798	117575	56722	1205
WILLIAMSVILLE—Erie County MILLARD FILLMORE SUBURBAN HOSPITAL See Millard Fillmore Gates Circle Hospital, Buffalo										
YONKERS—Westchester County ✠ ST. JOHN'S RIVERSIDE HOSPITAL, 967 North Broadway, Zip 10701–1399; tel. 914/964–4444; James Foy, President and Chief Executive Officer **A**1 6 9 10 **F**3 7 8 9 11 16 17 19 20 21 24 25 26 28 29 31 32 33 34 35 36 37 38 39 40 41 43 44 45 46 47 48 49 50 54 56 65 66 70 71 72 73 76 78 79 **P**5 8 **Web address:** www.riversidehealth.org	23	10	237	10002	160	86999	1842	81292	41668	999

Hospitals, U.S. / NEW YORK

Hospital, Address, Telephone, Administrator, Approval, Facility, and Physician Codes, Health Care System, Network	Classification Codes		Utilization Data					Expense (thousands) of dollars		Personnel
	Control	Service	Staffed Beds	Admissions	Census	Outpatient Visits	Births	Total	Payroll	

★ American Hospital Association (AHA) membership
□ Joint Commission on Accreditation of Healthcare Organizations (JCAHO) accreditation
+ American Osteopathic Healthcare Association (AOHA) membership
○ American Osteopathic Association (AOA) accreditation
△ Commission on Accreditation of Rehabilitation Facilities (CARF) accreditation
Control codes 61, 63, 64, 71, 72 and 73 indicate hospitals listed by AOHA, but not registered by AHA. For definition of numerical codes, see page A4

Hospital	Control	Service	Staffed Beds	Admissions	Census	Outpatient Visits	Births	Total	Payroll	Personnel
★ ST. JOSEPH'S MEDICAL CENTER, 127 South Broadway, Zip 10701–4080; tel. 914/378-7000; Michael J. Spicer, President and Chief Executive Officer **A**1 3 5 9 10 **F**1 3 4 9 10 11 12 13 14 16 17 18 19 21 22 23 24 25 27 30 31 32 34 35 36 37 38 39 41 42 43 44 45 46 47 48 49 51 52 54 55 56 57 58 59 61 62 63 64 65 69 70 72 74 75 76 77 78 **P**5 8 **S** Sisters of Charity Center, New York, NY **Web address:** www.stjosephs.org	23	10	194	6964	141	254151	0	81336	40963	873
★ YONKERS GENERAL HOSPITAL, Two Park Avenue, Zip 10703–3497; tel. 914/964-7300; Patricia Daye, Executive Vice President and Chief Operating Officer (Nonreporting) **A**1 9 10	23	10	190	—	—	—	—	—	—	—

Hospitals, U.S. / NORTH CAROLINA

NORTH CAROLINA

Resident Population 7,546 (in thousands)
Resident population in metro areas 66.8%
Birth rate per 1,000 population 14.4
65 years and over 12.5%
Percent of persons without health insurance 15.5%

★ American Hospital Association (AHA) membership
☐ Joint Commission on Accreditation of Healthcare Organizations (JCAHO) accreditation
+ American Osteopathic Healthcare Association (AOHA) membership
○ American Osteopathic Association (AOA) accreditation
△ Commission on Accreditation of Rehabilitation Facilities (CARF) accreditation
Control codes 61, 63, 64, 71, 72 and 73 indicate hospitals listed by AOHA, but not registered by AHA. For definition of numerical codes, see page A4

Hospital, Address, Telephone, Administrator, Approval, Facility, and Physician Codes, Health Care System, Network	Classification Codes		Utilization Data					Expense (thousands) of dollars		
	Control	Service	Staffed Beds	Admissions	Census	Outpatient Visits	Births	Total	Payroll	Personnel

AHOSKIE—Hertford County
★ ROANOKE–CHOWAN HOSPITAL, 500 South Academy Street, Zip 27910, Mailing Address: P.O. Box 1385, Zip 27910–1385; tel. 252/209–3000; Susan S. Lassiter, President and Chief Executive Officer **A**1 3 9 10 **F**8 9 11 13 14 17 18 22 23 24 25 28 32 34 36 37 39 41 44 45 46 48 51 54 56 57 59 61 62 63 68 70 72 76 77 78 **P**7 8 **S** University Health Systems of Eastern Carolina, Greenville, NC
Web address: www.rch.uhseast.com
| 23 | 10 | 118 | 4639 | 57 | 214233 | 473 | 29777 | 13722 | 607 |

ALBEMARLE—Stanly County
★ STANLY MEMORIAL HOSPITAL, 301 Yadkin Street, Zip 28001, Mailing Address: P.O. Box 1489, Zip 28002–1489; tel. 704/984–4000; Roy M. Hinson, CHE, President and Chief Executive Officer **A**1 9 10 **F**1 7 8 9 11 13 17 22 23 24 25 27 30 32 34 35 36 38 39 40 41 43 44 45 46 48 50 51 53 54 56 57 58 60 61 62 69 70 71 72 76 78 **P**5 6
Web address: www.stanly.org
| 23 | 10 | 119 | 4993 | 60 | 71804 | 618 | 39896 | 15700 | 517 |

ANDREWS—Cherokee County
☐ DISTRICT MEMORIAL HOSPITAL, 415 Whitaker Lane, Zip 28901–9229; tel. 828/321–1291; Allen D. Swan, Chief Executive Officer (Total facility includes 10 beds in nursing home–type unit) **A**1 10 18 **F**1 2 7 9 13 16 17 18 22 23 25 29 32 33 34 36 38 39 41 45 46 48 51 53 54 56 69 70 72 76 78 **P**5 6 8 **S** Quorum Health Group, Brentwood, TN
| 23 | 10 | 25 | 1010 | 35 | 13528 | 0 | — | — | — |

ASHEBORO—Randolph County
★ RANDOLPH HOSPITAL, 364 White Oak Street, Zip 27203, Mailing Address: P.O. Box 1048, Zip 27204–1048; tel. 336/625–5151; Robert E. Morrison, President **A**1 9 10 **F**8 9 11 13 16 17 18 19 22 23 24 25 28 31 32 34 36 39 41 43 44 45 46 48 49 50 51 54 68 70 72 76 78 **P**6
Web address: www.randolphhospital.org
| 23 | 10 | 105 | 5883 | 57 | 141061 | 834 | 46800 | 21057 | 739 |

ASHEVILLE—Buncombe County
★ MISSION ST. JOSEPH'S HEALTH, (Includes Memorial Mission Hospital, 509 Biltmore Avenue; St. Joseph's Hospital, 428 Biltmore Avenue, Zip 28801–9839; tel. 828/255–3100), 509 Biltmore Avenue, Zip 28801–4690; tel. 828/255–4000; Robert F. Burgin, President and Chief Executive Officer **A**1 2 3 5 9 10 **F**1 3 4 5 6 7 8 9 11 12 13 14 16 17 18 19 20 21 22 23 24 25 26 27 28 29 30 31 32 33 34 35 36 37 38 39 40 41 42 43 44 45 46 47 48 49 50 51 52 54 56 58 59 60 61 62 63 64 65 66 67 70 71 72 73 75 76 77 78 79 **P**5 8
Web address: www.msj.org
| 23 | 10 | 628 | 44582 | 654 | 307695 | 3402 | 339841 | 150264 | 4028 |

ST. JOSEPH'S HOSPITAL See Mission St. Joseph's Health

★ △ THOMS REHABILITATION HOSPITAL, 68 Sweeten Creek Road, Zip 28803–1599, Mailing Address: P.O. Box 15025, Zip 28813–0025; tel. 828/274–2400; Dennis A. Giles, President **A**1 7 9 10 **F**1 7 13 16 17 18 26 30 36 37 45 49 53 54 67 69 70 71 72 78 **P**1
Web address: www.carepartners.org
| 23 | 46 | 100 | 1338 | 69 | 42638 | 0 | 28368 | 13585 | 376 |

★ VETERANS AFFAIRS MEDICAL CENTER, 1100 Tunnel Road, Zip 28805–2087; tel. 828/298–7911; James A. Christian, Director (Total facility includes 120 beds in nursing home–type unit) (Nonreporting) **A**1 3 5 **S** Department of Veterans Affairs, Washington, DC
Web address: www.va.gov
| 45 | 10 | 389 | — | — | — | — | — | — | — |

BANNER ELK—Avery County
CHARLES A. CANNON JR. MEMORIAL HOSPITAL See Charles A. Cannon Jr. Memorial Hospital, Crossnore

BELHAVEN—Beaufort County
PUNGO DISTRICT HOSPITAL, 202 East Water Street, Zip 27810–9998; tel. 252/943–2111; Thomas O. Miller, Chief Executive Officer **A**9 10 **F**8 22 25 41 44 48 76 78 79
| 23 | 10 | 49 | 1700 | 31 | — | 35 | 9709 | 5081 | 189 |

BLACK MOUNTAIN—Buncombe County
JULIAN F. KEITH ALCOHOL AND DRUG ABUSE TREATMENT CENTER, 301 Tabernacle Road, Zip 28711–2599; tel. 828/669–3402; William A. Rafter, Director (Nonreporting) **A**10
Web address: www.jfkadatc.net
| 12 | 82 | 110 | | | | | | | |

BLOWING ROCK—Watauga County
★ BLOWING ROCK HOSPITAL, (Includes Dr. Charles Davant Rehabilitation and Extended Care Center), Chestnut Street, Zip 28605–0148, Mailing Address: Box 148, Zip 28605–0148; tel. 828/295–3136; Patricia Gray, Administrator and Chief Executive Officer (Total facility includes 72 beds in nursing home–type unit) **A**1 9 10 **F**1 18 23 24 25 30 31 32 36 45 48 51 54 69 70 76
| 23 | 10 | 100 | 409 | 72 | 48206 | — | 6381 | 3766 | 169 |

BOILING SPRINGS—Cleveland County
CRAWLEY MEMORIAL HOSPITAL, 315 West College Avenue, Zip 28017, Mailing Address: P.O. Box 996, Zip 28017–0996; tel. 704/434–9466; Gail McKillop, President **A**10 **F**8 9 11 12 13 14 17 19 21 22 25 29 30 31 32 33 34 35 38 41 42 43 44 45 46 48 50 51 52 53 54 56 65 69 70 72 75 76 78 **P**5 **S** Carolinas HealthCare System, Charlotte, NC
| 23 | 10 | 51 | 86 | 46 | 294 | 0 | 2214 | 965 | 41 |

© 2000 AHA Guide   *Many Facility Codes have changed. Please refer to the AHA Guide Code Chart.*

Hospitals, U.S. / NORTH CAROLINA

Hospital, Address, Telephone, Administrator, Approval, Facility, and Physician Codes, Health Care System, Network	Classification Codes		Utilization Data					Expense (thousands) of dollars		
	Control	Service	Staffed Beds	Admissions	Census	Outpatient Visits	Births	Total	Payroll	Personnel

- ★ American Hospital Association (AHA) membership
- ☐ Joint Commission on Accreditation of Healthcare Organizations (JCAHO) accreditation
- + American Osteopathic Healthcare Association (AOHA) membership
- ○ American Osteopathic Association (AOA) accreditation
- △ Commission on Accreditation of Rehabilitation Facilities (CARF) accreditation

Control codes 61, 63, 64, 71, 72 and 73 indicate hospitals listed by AOHA, but not registered by AHA. For definition of numerical codes, see page A4

BOONE—Watauga County

Hospital	Control	Service	Staffed Beds	Admissions	Census	Outpatient Visits	Births	Total	Payroll	Personnel
★ WATAUGA MEDICAL CENTER, Deerfield Road, Zip 28607–2600, Mailing Address: P.O. Box 2600, Zip 28607–2600; tel. 828/262–4100; Richard G. Sparks, President (Total facility includes 10 beds in nursing home–type unit) **A**1 2 9 10 **F**8 9 11 13 17 18 19 22 24 25 27 28 31 32 33 34 36 39 41 42 44 46 48 49 50 65 69 70 71 72 73 76 78 **P**3 8 Web address: www.wataugamc.org	23	10	105	5309	64	61443	619	43668	18845	666

BREVARD—Transylvania County

	Control	Service	Staffed Beds	Admissions	Census	Outpatient Visits	Births	Total	Payroll	Personnel
★ TRANSYLVANIA COMMUNITY HOSPITAL, Hospital Drive, Zip 28712–1116, Mailing Address: Box 1116, Zip 28712–1116; tel. 828/884–9111; Robert J. Bednarek, President and Chief Executive Officer (Total facility includes 10 beds in nursing home–type unit) **A**1 10 **F**2 3 7 8 9 12 13 16 17 18 19 22 24 25 32 33 34 36 37 38 43 44 45 46 48 51 54 68 69 70 72 76 78 79 **P**5 8	23	10	87	2477	35	42318	218	24448	12418	307

BRYSON CITY—Swain County

	Control	Service	Staffed Beds	Admissions	Census	Outpatient Visits	Births	Total	Payroll	Personnel
★ SWAIN COUNTY HOSPITAL, 45 Plateau Street, Zip 28713–6784; tel. 828/488–4013; James M. Kirby, Administrator **A**1 10 18 **F**1 7 8 9 13 16 17 18 19 22 24 25 26 27 31 33 36 37 38 39 43 45 46 48 49 50 51 54 61 65 70 76 77 78 79 **P**5 7 8 Web address: www.westcare.org	23	10	42	668	19	12094	0	6367	2726	84

BURGAW—Pender County

	Control	Service	Staffed Beds	Admissions	Census	Outpatient Visits	Births	Total	Payroll	Personnel
★ PENDER MEMORIAL HOSPITAL, 507 Freemont Street, Zip 28425; tel. 910/259–5451; Matthew Mendez, Site Administrator (Total facility includes 43 beds in nursing home–type unit) **A**9 10 **F**9 17 18 22 25 30 32 36 39 41 45 48 54 69 70 72 76 **S** New Hanover Health Network, Wilmington, NC	13	10	86	1009	93	23142	0	10835	5591	182

BURLINGTON—Alamance County

	Control	Service	Staffed Beds	Admissions	Census	Outpatient Visits	Births	Total	Payroll	Personnel
★ ALAMANCE REGIONAL MEDICAL CENTER, 1240 Huffman Mill Road, Zip 27216–0202, Mailing Address: P.O. Box 202, Zip 27216–0202; tel. 336/538–7000; Thomas E. Ryan, President (Total facility includes 81 beds in nursing home–type unit) **A**1 2 9 10 **F**2 3 4 7 8 9 11 13 16 17 18 19 22 23 24 25 26 27 30 31 32 33 34 35 36 37 38 39 41 43 44 45 46 48 49 50 51 53 54 57 58 59 60 61 62 63 64 65 66 68 69 70 71 72 73 76 78 79 **P**5 Web address: www.armc.com	23	10	319	10043	190	124315	1302	100154	40670	1109

BUTNER—Granville County

	Control	Service	Staffed Beds	Admissions	Census	Outpatient Visits	Births	Total	Payroll	Personnel
☐ JOHN UMSTEAD HOSPITAL, (Includes Alcohol and Drug Abuse Treatment Center, 205 West E Street, Zip 27509; tel. 919/575–7928; Cliff Hood, Director), 1003 12th Street, Zip 27509–1626; tel. 919/575–7211; Patricia L. Christian, R.N., Ph.D., Chief Executive Officer (Total facility includes 30 beds in nursing home–type unit) **A**1 3 5 10 **F**17 23 57 58 62 63 69 70 78 **P**1	12	22	563	4878	469	3580	0	107943	43391	1348

CAMP LEJEUNE—Onslow County

	Control	Service	Staffed Beds	Admissions	Census	Outpatient Visits	Births	Total	Payroll	Personnel
★ NAVAL HOSPITAL, Mailing Address: P.O. Box 10100, Zip 28547–0100; tel. 910/450–4300; Captain Thomas R. Collison, Commanding Officer **A**1 **F**3 9 13 14 15 17 19 21 22 23 24 25 28 29 31 32 33 34 35 38 39 41 43 44 45 48 49 50 51 54 56 57 60 61 62 66 70 71 76 78 79 **P**1 **S** Department of Navy, Washington, DC Web address: lej–www.med.navy.mil	43	10	117	3968	29	301166	1367	56285	—	363

CARY—Wake County

WESTERN WAKE MEDICAL CENTER See Wake Medical Center, Raleigh

CHAPEL HILL—Orange County

	Control	Service	Staffed Beds	Admissions	Census	Outpatient Visits	Births	Total	Payroll	Personnel
★ △ UNIVERSITY OF NORTH CAROLINA HOSPITALS, (Includes North Carolina Children's and Women's Hospital; North Carolina Neurosciences Hospital), 101 Manning Drive, Zip 27514–4220; tel. 919/966–4131; Eric B. Munson, President and Chief Executive Officer **A**1 2 3 5 7 8 9 10 **F**2 3 4 5 8 9 10 11 12 13 14 16 17 18 19 22 23 24 25 26 30 34 35 36 37 38 39 41 42 43 44 45 46 47 48 49 50 51 52 53 54 56 57 58 59 60 61 62 63 65 66 68 70 71 72 74 75 76 77 78 79 **P**5 6 7 Web address: www.med.unc.edu	12	10	677	28821	483	806174	2512	422530	169041	4234

CHARLOTTE—Mecklenburg County

	Control	Service	Staffed Beds	Admissions	Census	Outpatient Visits	Births	Total	Payroll	Personnel
AMETHYST, 1715 Sharon Road West, Zip 28210–5663, Mailing Address: P.O. Box 32861, Zip 28232–2861; tel. 704/554–8373; Steven G. Johnson, Administrator (Nonreporting) Web address: www.carolinas.org	16	82	94	—	—	—	—	—	—	—
★ CAROLINAS MEDICAL CENTER, 1000 Blythe Boulevard, Zip 28203–5871, Mailing Address: P.O. Box 32861, Zip 28232–2861; tel. 704/355–2000; Paul S. Franz, President **A**1 2 3 5 8 9 10 **F**1 2 3 4 5 6 7 8 9 10 11 12 13 14 16 17 19 20 21 22 23 24 25 26 27 28 29 30 31 32 33 34 35 36 37 38 39 40 41 42 43 44 45 46 47 48 49 50 51 52 53 54 55 56 57 58 59 60 61 62 63 64 65 66 68 69 70 71 72 73 74 75 76 77 78 79 **P**3 6 **S** Carolinas HealthCare System, Charlotte, NC Web address: www.carolinas.org	16	10	761	40043	645	416733	6347	534248	207158	7165
★ △ CHARLOTTE INSTITUTE OF REHABILITATION, 1100 Blythe Boulevard, Zip 28203–5864; tel. 704/355–4300; Cynthia King, Acting Administrator **A**1 3 7 9 10 **F**1 2 3 4 5 6 7 8 9 10 11 12 13 14 16 19 20 21 22 23 24 25 26 27 28 29 30 31 32 33 34 35 36 38 39 41 42 43 44 45 46 47 48 49 50 51 52 53 54 55 56 57 58 59 60 61 62 63 64 65 66 68 69 70 71 72 73 74 75 76 77 78 79 **P**3 6 **S** Carolinas HealthCare System, Charlotte, NC Web address: www.carolinas.org	16	46	118	1826	87	31640	0	28270	16397	392

Hospitals, U.S. / NORTH CAROLINA

Hospital, Address, Telephone, Administrator, Approval, Facility, and Physician Codes, Health Care System, Network ★ American Hospital Association (AHA) membership □ Joint Commission on Accreditation of Healthcare Organizations (JCAHO) accreditation + American Osteopathic Healthcare Association (AOHA) membership ○ American Osteopathic Association (AOA) accreditation △ Commission on Accreditation of Rehabilitation Facilities (CARF) accreditation Control codes 61, 63, 64, 71, 72 and 73 indicate hospitals listed by AOHA, but not registered by AHA. For definition of numerical codes, see page A4	Classification Codes		Utilization Data					Expense (thousands) of dollars		
	Control	Service	Staffed Beds	Admissions	Census	Outpatient Visits	Births	Total	Payroll	Personnel
✯ △ MERCY HOSPITAL, (Includes Mercy Hospital South, 10628 Park Road, Pineville, Zip 28210; tel. 704/543-2025; Bill Brown, Administrator), 2001 Vail Avenue, Zip 28207-1289; tel. 704/379-5100; C. Curtis Copenhaver, President **A**1 6 7 9 10 **F**2 4 9 11 12 13 16 17 18 22 24 25 32 34 39 41 46 47 48 49 51 53 68 70 72 76 78 **S** Carolinas HealthCare System, Charlotte, NC Web address: www.carolinas.org	16	10	224	7999	134	58376	0	74871	31110	790
✯ PRESBYTERIAN HOSPITAL, (Formerly Presbyterian Healthcare), 200 Hawthorne Lane, Zip 28204-2528, Mailing Address: P.O. Box 33549, Zip 28233-3549; tel. 704/384-4000; Thomas R. Revels, President and Chief Executive Officer (Total facility includes 289 beds in nursing home-type unit) **A**1 2 6 9 10 **F**4 5 7 8 9 11 12 13 16 18 19 20 22 24 25 26 27 29 30 32 33 34 35 36 37 38 39 41 42 43 44 45 46 47 48 49 50 51 52 54 56 57 58 59 60 61 62 63 64 65 66 68 69 70 72 73 76 78 79 **P**5 6 8 **S** Novant Health, Winston Salem, NC Web address: www.presbyterian.org	23	10	840	27883	388	140940	3961	—	—	3639
★ PRESBYTERIAN–ORTHOPAEDIC HOSPITAL, 1901 Randolph Road, Zip 28207-1195; tel. 704/375-6792; Tom McGraw, Administrator (Total facility includes 16 beds in nursing home-type unit) **A**9 10 **F**4 7 8 9 11 12 13 19 22 25 26 36 37 39 41 42 44 46 47 48 49 52 56 57 58 63 64 65 66 69 70 71 76 77 78 79 **S** Novant Health, Winston Salem, NC Web address: www.presbyterian.org	23	47	156	3192	41	—	0	—	—	—
□ UNIVERSITY HOSPITAL, 8800 North Tryon Street, Zip 28262-8415, Mailing Address: P.O. Box 560727, Zip 28256-0727; tel. 704/548-6000; W. Spencer Lilly, Administrator **A**1 9 10 **F**4 6 8 9 11 13 16 18 22 23 24 25 28 32 33 34 35 36 38 39 41 43 44 45 46 47 48 49 54 55 56 58 59 60 61 62 63 64 65 68 70 71 72 74 75 76 77 78 79 **P**6 **S** Carolinas HealthCare System, Charlotte, NC	16	10	122	6399	59	88162	1810	43752	19020	545
CHEROKEE—Swain County										
✯ U. S. PUBLIC HEALTH SERVICE INDIAN HOSPITAL, Hospital Road, Zip 28719, Mailing Address: Caller Box C-26, Zip 28719; tel. 828/497-9163; Edwin McLemore, Administrator (Nonreporting) **A**1 10 **S** U. S. Public Health Service Indian Health Service, Rockville, MD	47	10	30	—						
CHERRY POINT—Craven County										
✯ NAVAL HOSPITAL, Mailing Address: PSC Box 8023, Zip 28533-0023; tel. 252/466-0266; Captain Joan A. Bold, Commanding Officer (Nonreporting) **A**1 **S** Department of Navy, Washington, DC	43	10	23	—						
CLINTON—Sampson County										
✯ SAMPSON REGIONAL MEDICAL CENTER, (Formerly Sampson County Memorial Hospital), 607 Beaman Street, Zip 28328-2697, Mailing Address: Drawer 258, Zip 28329-0258; tel. 910/592-8511; Lee Pridgen, Jr, Administrator (Total facility includes 30 beds in nursing home-type unit) **A**1 9 10 **F**8 9 16 17 18 22 24 25 27 36 39 48 51 54 70 76 Web address: www.scmh.com	13	10	146	4405	76	197935	439	8691	16746	551
CLYDE—Haywood County										
✯ HAYWOOD REGIONAL MEDICAL CENTER, 262 Leroy George Drive, Zip 28721-9434; tel. 828/456-7311; David O. Rice, President (Total facility includes 20 beds in nursing home-type unit) **A**1 9 10 **F**7 8 9 11 13 14 16 17 18 19 22 24 25 26 27 28 32 33 34 35 36 37 38 39 41 43 44 45 46 48 49 50 51 54 55 59 61 65 70 72 76 77 78 79 **P**8 Web address: www.haymed.org	16	10	150	5451	70	46246	301	48304	21444	705
COLUMBUS—Polk County										
□ ST. LUKE'S HOSPITAL, 220 Hospital Drive, Zip 28722-9473; tel. 828/894-3311; C. Cameron Highsmith, Jr, President and Chief Executive Officer **A**1 9 10 **F**7 9 13 17 19 22 23 25 27 30 32 34 37 41 43 48 49 51 54 57 59 60 61 62 63 64 70 72 76 78 **P**6 8	23	10	73	2092	48	40606	0	13382	6129	335
CONCORD—Cabarrus County										
✯ NORTHEAST MEDICAL CENTER, 920 Church Street North, Zip 28025-2983; tel. 704/783-3000; Laurence C. Hinsdale, President and Chief Executive Officer **A**1 2 3 5 6 9 10 **F**4 8 9 11 12 13 16 17 18 19 21 22 24 25 28 32 33 34 36 37 38 39 40 41 42 44 45 46 47 48 51 54 56 57 58 59 60 61 62 63 64 65 66 70 76 77 78 79 **P**6 Web address: www.northeastmedical.org	23	10	353	18477	205	599718	2180	193224	87633	2533
CROSSNORE—Avery County										
✯ CHARLES A. CANNON JR, MEMORIAL HOSPITAL, (Includes Charles A. Cannon Jr. Memorial Hospital, 805 Shawneehaw Avenue, Banner Elk, Zip 28604-9724, Mailing Address: P.O. Box 8, Zip 28604-0008; tel. 828/898-5111), One Crossnore Drive, Zip 28616, Mailing Address: Drawer 470, Zip 28616; tel. 828/737-7000; Edward C. Greene, Jr, President (Total facility includes 10 beds in nursing home-type unit) (Nonreporting) **A**1 9	23	10	88	—	—	—	—	—	—	—
DANBURY—Stokes County										
✯ STOKES–REYNOLDS MEMORIAL HOSPITAL, Mailing Address: P.O. Box 10, Zip 27016-0010; tel. 336/593-2831; Sandra D. Priddy, President (Total facility includes 40 beds in nursing home-type unit) **A**1 9 10 **F**3 9 16 17 18 22 25 29 37 41 48 69 70 76 77 78 **P**6 Web address: www.bgsm.edu/stokes	21	10	93	784	73	20025	0	11500	5261	188
DUNN—Harnett County										
□ BETSY JOHNSON REGIONAL HOSPITAL, 800 Tilghman Drive, Zip 28334-5599, Mailing Address: Drawer 1706, Zip 28335-1706; tel. 910/892-7161; Shannon D. Brown, President **A**1 9 10 **F**7 8 9 16 22 25 32 41 43 44 45 46 48 49 54 68 70 76 78 Web address: www.bjrh.org	23	10	62	4377	45	52836	709	25449	13059	420

© 2000 AHA Guide   *Many Facility Codes have changed. Please refer to the AHA Guide Code Chart.*

Hospitals, U.S. / NORTH CAROLINA

Hospital, Address, Telephone, Administrator, Approval, Facility, and Physician Codes, Health Care System, Network

- ★ American Hospital Association (AHA) membership
- □ Joint Commission on Accreditation of Healthcare Organizations (JCAHO) accreditation
- + American Osteopathic Healthcare Association (AOHA) membership
- ○ American Osteopathic Association (AOA) accreditation
- △ Commission on Accreditation of Rehabilitation Facilities (CARF) accreditation

Control codes 61, 63, 64, 71, 72 and 73 indicate hospitals listed by AOHA, but not registered by AHA. For definition of numerical codes, see page A4

	Classification Codes		Utilization Data					Expense (thousands) of dollars		
Hospital	Control	Service	Staffed Beds	Admissions	Census	Outpatient Visits	Births	Total	Payroll	Personnel
DURHAM—Durham County										
★ DUKE UNIVERSITY MEDICAL CENTER, (Includes Duke University Hospital), Erwin Road, Zip 27710, Mailing Address: P.O. Box 3708, Zip 27710-3708; tel. 919/684-8111; Michael D. Israel, Chief Executive Officer and Vice Chancellor **A**1 2 3 5 8 9 10 **F**3 4 5 7 8 9 10 11 12 13 14 17 18 19 21 22 23 24 25 26 27 28 30 32 33 34 35 39 41 42 43 44 45 46 47 48 49 50 51 52 53 54 55 56 57 58 59 60 61 62 63 64 65 66 68 70 71 72 73 74 75 76 77 78 79 **S** Duke University Health System, Durham, NC	23	10	852	37202	664	937278	2895	682356	240436	6102
★ DURHAM REGIONAL HOSPITAL, 3643 North Roxboro Road, Zip 27704-2763; tel. 919/470-4000; Richard L. Myers, President and Chief Executive Officer **A**1 3 5 6 9 10 **F**3 4 7 8 9 11 12 13 17 18 19 22 24 25 27 28 29 30 32 33 34 35 36 38 39 41 43 44 45 46 47 48 49 50 51 54 56 57 58 59 60 61 62 63 64 65 68 70 72 76 77 78 79 **P**5 7 **S** Duke University Health System, Durham, NC Web address: www.drh.duhs.duke.edu	23	10	213	14125	176	118753	1860	165454	65750	1900
NORTH CAROLINA EYE AND EAR HOSPITAL, 1110 West Main Street, Zip 27701-2000; tel. 919/682-9341; H. Ed Jones, Chief Executive Officer (Nonreporting) **A**9 10	33	45	24	—	—	—	—	—	—	—
★ VETERANS AFFAIRS MEDICAL CENTER, 508 Fulton Street, Zip 27705-3897; tel. 919/286-0411; Michael B. Phaup, Director (Total facility includes 120 beds in nursing home-type unit) (Nonreporting) **A**1 3 5 8 9 **S** Department of Veterans Affairs, Washington, DC Web address: www.va.gov/stations97/guide/home.asp?DIVISION=ALL	45	10	382	—	—	—	—	—	—	—
EDEN—Rockingham County										
★ MOREHEAD MEMORIAL HOSPITAL, 117 East King's Highway, Zip 27288-5299; tel. 336/623-9711; Robert Enders, President (Total facility includes 128 beds in nursing home-type unit) **A**1 2 9 10 **F**6 7 8 9 17 18 19 20 22 24 25 27 30 32 33 34 36 39 43 44 45 46 48 49 50 51 54 65 68 69 70 72 73 76 78 79 **P**6 8 **S** Quorum Health Group, Brentwood, TN Web address: www.morehead.org	23	10	236	5847	187	104493	721	44661	21872	592
EDENTON—Chowan County										
★ CHOWAN HOSPITAL, 211 Virginia Road, Zip 27932-0629, Mailing Address: P.O. Box 629, Zip 27932-0629; tel. 252/482-8451; Barbara R. Cale, President (Total facility includes 40 beds in nursing home-type unit) **A**1 9 10 **F**7 8 9 13 16 17 18 19 22 24 25 32 34 35 38 39 41 43 44 45 46 49 50 51 54 69 70 72 73 76 78 79 **P**3 **S** University Health Systems of Eastern Carolina, Greenville, NC Web address: www.uhseast.com	13	10	111	3375	57	25063	383	20144	9777	375
ELIZABETH CITY—Pasquotank County										
★ ALBEMARLE HOSPITAL, 1144 North Road Street, Zip 27909, Mailing Address: P.O. Box 1587, Zip 27906-1587; tel. 252/335-0531; Philip D. Bagby, President and Chief Executive Officer **A**1 9 10 **F**7 8 9 11 13 17 18 19 22 23 24 25 27 28 32 33 34 38 39 43 45 46 48 49 50 51 54 65 70 72 76 78 Web address: www.albemarlehosp.org/	13	10	150	7642	119	90462	797	58105	24680	764
ELIZABETHTOWN—Bladen County										
★ BLADEN COUNTY HOSPITAL, 501 South Poplar Street, Zip 28337-0398, Mailing Address: P.O. Box 398, Zip 28337-0398; tel. 910/862-5100; Leo A. Petit, Jr, Chief Executive Officer (Total facility includes 10 beds in nursing home-type unit) (Nonreporting) **A**1 9 10 Web address: www.bchn.org	13	10	60	—	—	—	—	—	—	—
ELKIN—Surry County										
★ HUGH CHATHAM MEMORIAL HOSPITAL, Parkwood Drive, Zip 28621-0560, Mailing Address: P.O. Box 560, Zip 28621-0560; tel. 336/527-7000; Richard D. Osmus, Chief Executive Officer (Total facility includes 120 beds in nursing home-type unit) **A**1 9 10 **F**6 7 8 9 13 16 17 18 22 24 25 30 32 34 36 37 38 39 41 43 44 45 46 48 50 54 56 65 66 67 68 69 70 71 72 76 78 79 **P**1 **S** Quorum Health Group, Brentwood, TN Web address: www.hughchatham.org	23	10	201	3939	155	39830	471	28018	13548	601
ERWIN—Harnett County										
★ GOOD HOPE HOSPITAL, 410 Denim Drive, Zip 28339-0668, Mailing Address: P.O. Box 668, Zip 28339-0668; tel. 910/897-6151; Donald E. Annis, Chief Executive Officer **A**1 9 10 **F**7 9 13 16 19 22 24 25 39 45 48 54 59 61 62 63 64 68 70 76 77 78 **P**5 **S** Quorum Health Group, Brentwood, TN Web address: www.goodhopehospital.org	23	10	72	2716	33	36379	0	15621	8087	293
FAYETTEVILLE—Cumberland County										
BEHAVIORAL HEALTH CARE OF CAPE FEAR VALLEY HEALTH SYSTEM, (Formerly Cumberland Hospital), 3425 Melrose Road, Zip 28304-1695; tel. 910/609-3000; James P. Sprouse, Associate Administrator for Psychiatric Services (Nonreporting) **A**10 Web address: www.capefearvalley.com	23	22	110	—	—	—	—	—	—	—
★ △ CAPE FEAR VALLEY HEALTH SYSTEM, 1638 Owen Drive, Zip 28304-3431, Mailing Address: P.O. Box 2000, Zip 28302-2000; tel. 910/609-4000; John T. Carlisle, Chief Executive Officer **A**1 2 3 5 7 9 10 **F**2 3 4 7 8 9 11 12 13 16 18 19 22 24 25 26 28 29 30 32 33 35 36 37 38 39 41 42 43 44 45 46 47 48 49 50 51 54 56 57 58 59 60 61 63 64 65 68 70 71 72 76 78 79 **P**5 6 Web address: www.capefearvalley.com	23	10	619	24508	440	309311	4094	283503	115166	3743
★ HIGHSMITH–RAINEY MEMORIAL HOSPITAL, 150 Robeson Street, Zip 28301-5570; tel. 910/609-1000; Walt Rose, Associate Administrator (Nonreporting) **A**1 Web address: www.hcahealthcare.com	23	10	133	—	—	—	—	—	—	—

Hospitals, U.S. / NORTH CAROLINA

Hospital, Address, Telephone, Administrator, Approval, Facility, and Physician Codes, Health Care System, Network	Classification Codes		Utilization Data					Expense (thousands) of dollars		
★ American Hospital Association (AHA) membership □ Joint Commission on Accreditation of Healthcare Organizations (JCAHO) accreditation + American Osteopathic Healthcare Association (AOHA) membership ○ American Osteopathic Association (AOA) accreditation △ Commission on Accreditation of Rehabilitation Facilities (CARF) accreditation Control codes 61, 63, 64, 71, 72 and 73 indicate hospitals listed by AOHA, but not registered by AHA. For definition of numerical codes, see page A4	Control	Service	Staffed Beds	Admissions	Census	Outpatient Visits	Births	Total	Payroll	Personnel
★ VETERANS AFFAIRS MEDICAL CENTER, 2300 Ramsey Street, Zip 28301–3899; tel. 910/822–7059; Richard J. Baltz, Director (Total facility includes 39 beds in nursing home–type unit) (Nonreporting) **A**1 **S** Department of Veterans Affairs, Washington, DC **Web address:** www.va.gov/stations97/guide/home.asp?DIVISION=ALL	45	10	193	—	—	—	—	—	—	—
FLETCHER—Henderson County										
★ ○ PARK RIDGE HOSPITAL, Naples Road, Zip 28732, Mailing Address: P.O. Box 1569, Zip 28732–1569; tel. 828/684–8501; Michael V. Gentry, President **A**1 9 10 11 **F**8 9 11 12 13 16 17 18 22 24 25 27 36 37 39 41 43 44 45 48 51 54 57 61 62 64 70 72 76 78 **P**6 **S** Adventist Health System Sunbelt Health Care Corporation, Winter Park, FL **Web address:** www.ahss.org	23	10	96	4061	67	158045	450	40860	18505	578
FORT BRAGG—Cumberland County										
★ WOMACK ARMY MEDICAL CENTER, Normandy Drive, Zip 28307–5000; tel. 910/432–4802; Colonel Daniel F. Perugini, Commander **A**1 3 5 **F**1 2 3 4 5 6 7 8 9 10 11 12 13 14 15 17 18 19 20 21 22 23 24 25 26 27 28 29 30 31 32 33 34 35 36 37 38 39 40 41 42 43 44 45 46 47 48 49 50 51 52 53 54 55 57 58 59 60 61 62 63 64 65 66 67 70 71 72 73 74 75 76 77 78 79 **S** Department of the Army, Office of the Surgeon General, Falls Church, VA	42	10	187	8236	59	902472	2647	200590	48912	2090
FRANKLIN—Macon County										
★ ANGEL MEDICAL CENTER, Riverview and White Oak Streets, Zip 28734, Mailing Address: P.O. Box 1209, Zip 28744; tel. 828/524–8411; Michael E. Zuliani, Chief Executive Officer **A**1 9 10 **F**7 8 9 13 17 19 22 24 25 27 32 36 37 38 39 41 43 45 46 48 49 51 54 65 68 70 72 76 77 78 79 **S** Quorum Health Group, Brentwood, TN	23	10	59	2305	27	46396	178	25750	11206	362
FUQUAY–VARINA—Wake County										
SOUTHERN WAKE HOSPITAL See Wake Medical Center, Raleigh										
GASTONIA—Gaston County										
★ GASTON MEMORIAL HOSPITAL, 2525 Court Drive, Zip 28054–2142, Mailing Address: P.O. Box 1747, Zip 28053–1747; tel. 704/834–2000; Wayne F. Shovelin, President and Chief Executive Officer **A**1 2 9 10 **F**3 4 6 7 8 9 11 12 13 16 17 18 19 21 22 23 24 25 26 27 28 32 33 34 36 37 38 39 41 43 44 45 46 47 48 49 51 54 57 58 59 60 61 62 63 64 65 68 69 70 72 75 76 77 78 79 **P**6 **Web address:** www.gastonhealthcare.org	23	10	348	18809	250	—	2546	145100	61018	1779
GOLDSBORO—Wayne County										
□ CHERRY HOSPITAL, 201 Stevens Mill Road, Zip 27530–1057; tel. 919/731–3200; Liston G. Edwards, Director (Total facility includes 173 beds in nursing home–type unit) **A**1 3 5 10 **F**16 17 18 23 30 57 58 62 69 70 78 **P**6 **Web address:** www.dhhs.state.nc.us/mhddsas/cherry	12	22	662	2693	484	—	0	61050	40635	1249
★ WAYNE MEMORIAL HOSPITAL, 2700 Wayne Memorial Drive, Zip 27534–8001, Mailing Address: P.O. Box 8001, Zip 27533–8001; tel. 919/736–1110; James W. Hubbell, President and Chief Executive Officer **A**1 2 9 10 **F**8 9 11 13 16 17 19 22 24 25 27 30 33 34 35 36 37 38 39 41 42 43 44 45 46 48 50 51 54 57 58 59 60 61 62 64 65 68 70 71 72 76 78 **Web address:** www.waynehealth.org	23	10	272	11982	178	99108	2647	89508	39630	1150
GREENSBORO—Guilford County										
□ BEHAVIORAL HEALTH CENTER, 700 Walter Reed Drive, Zip 27403–1129, Mailing Address: P.O. Box 10399, Zip 27404–0399; tel. 336/852–4821; John Long, Vice President (Nonreporting) **A**1 9	33	22	68	—	—	—	—	—	—	—
★ △ MOSES CONE HEALTH SYSTEM, (Includes Moses H. Cone Memorial Hospital, 1200 North Elm Street, Zip 27401; tel. 910/574–7000; Wesley Long Community Hospital, 501 North Elam Avenue, Zip 27403–1199, Mailing Address: P.O. Box 2747, Zip 27402–2747; tel. 910/854–6100; Women's Hospital of Greensboro, 801 Green Valley Road, Zip 27408; tel. 910/574–6500), 1200 North Elm Street, Zip 27401–1020; tel. 336/832–1000; Dennis R. Barry, President (Total facility includes 290 beds in nursing home–type unit) **A**1 2 3 5 7 8 9 10 **F**4 8 9 11 12 13 14 16 17 18 19 22 23 24 25 26 27 29 30 31 32 33 34 35 36 37 38 39 41 42 43 44 45 46 47 48 49 50 51 53 54 57 59 60 62 64 65 66 68 69 70 71 72 75 76 78 79 **P**7 8 **Web address:** www.mosescone.com	23	10	1095	38647	723	362979	5486	275521	156767	5152
□ VENCOR HOSPITAL–GREENSBORO, 2401 Southside Boulevard, Zip 27406–3311; tel. 336/271–2800; Leanne Fiorentino, Chief Executive Officer (Total facility includes 65 beds in nursing home–type unit) (Nonreporting) **A**1 10 **S** Vencor, Incorporated, Louisville, KY	33	49	124	—	—	—	—	—	—	—
WESLEY LONG COMMUNITY HOSPITAL See Moses Cone Health System										
WOMEN'S HOSPITAL OF GREENSBORO See Moses Cone Health System										
GREENVILLE—Pitt County										
★ △ PITT COUNTY MEMORIAL HOSPITAL–UNIVERSITY HEALTH SYSTEMS OF EASTERN CAROLINA, 2100 Stantonsburg Road, Zip 27835–6028, Mailing Address: Box 6028, Zip 27835–6028; tel. 252/816–4451; Dave C. McRae, President and Chief Executive Officer **A**2 3 5 7 8 9 10 **F**4 8 9 11 12 13 14 16 17 18 19 22 23 24 25 27 28 29 30 31 32 33 34 35 36 37 38 39 41 42 43 44 45 46 47 48 49 50 51 52 53 54 56 57 58 59 60 61 62 63 65 66 68 70 72 74 75 76 77 78 79 **P**1 5 7 8 **S** University Health Systems of Eastern Carolina, Greenville, NC **Web address:** www.pcmh.com	23	10	695	33918	551	223150	3125	348448	155956	4227

Hospitals, U.S. / NORTH CAROLINA

Hospital, Address, Telephone, Administrator, Approval, Facility, and Physician Codes, Health Care System, Network	Classification Codes		Utilization Data					Expense (thousands) of dollars		
	Control	Service	Staffed Beds	Admissions	Census	Outpatient Visits	Births	Total	Payroll	Personnel

★ American Hospital Association (AHA) membership
☐ Joint Commission on Accreditation of Healthcare Organizations (JCAHO) accreditation
+ American Osteopathic Healthcare Association (AOHA) membership
○ American Osteopathic Association (AOA) accreditation
△ Commission on Accreditation of Rehabilitation Facilities (CARF) accreditation
Control codes 61, 63, 64, 71, 72 and 73 indicate hospitals listed by AOHA, but not registered by AHA. For definition of numerical codes, see page A4

Hospital	Control	Service	Staffed Beds	Admissions	Census	Outpatient Visits	Births	Total	Payroll	Personnel
WALTER B. JONES ALCOHOL AND DRUG ABUSE TREATMENT CENTER, 2577 West Fifth Street, Zip 27834–7813; tel. 252/830–3426; Phillip A. Mooring, Director (Nonreporting) **A**10	12	82	76	—	—	—	—	—	—	—
HAMLET—Richmond County ☐ SANDHILLS REGIONAL MEDICAL CENTER, (Formerly Hamlet Hospital), 1000 West Hamlet Avenue, Zip 28345, Mailing Address: P.O. Box 1109, Zip 28345–1109; tel. 910/205–8000; John W. McClellan, Executive Director **A**1 9 10 **F**7 13 16 17 18 22 24 25 29 30 32 34 38 39 41 43 45 48 50 51 54 57 59 62 70 71 76 78 **S** Health Management Associates, Naples, FL	33	10	64	2802	35	—	—	—	—	—
HENDERSON—Vance County ★ △ MARIA PARHAM HOSPITAL, 566 Ruin Creek Road, Zip 27536–2957; tel. 252/438–4143; Philip S. Lakernick, President and Chief Executive Officer **A**1 7 9 10 **F**7 8 9 11 13 16 17 18 19 20 22 23 24 25 27 29 32 33 34 35 36 37 38 39 41 44 45 46 48 49 50 51 53 54 58 59 61 62 63 70 71 72 75 76 77 78 79 **P**8 Web address: www.mphosp.org	23	10	102	4541	51	43137	639	36152	16339	577
HENDERSONVILLE—Henderson County ★ MARGARET R. PARDEE MEMORIAL HOSPITAL, 715 Fleming Street, Zip 28791–2563; tel. 828/696–1000; Frank J. Aaron, Jr, Chief Executive Officer (Total facility includes 20 beds in nursing home–type unit) **A**1 2 3 9 10 **F**1 8 9 12 13 16 17 18 19 22 24 25 27 30 32 33 34 36 38 39 40 41 44 45 46 48 49 50 51 54 56 57 59 62 63 65 66 68 69 70 71 72 76 77 78 79 **P**1 5 6 8 Web address: www.pardee–med.org	13	10	195	8602	135	160911	631	67720	30085	878
HICKORY—Catawba County ★ CATAWBA MEMORIAL HOSPITAL, 810 Fairgrove Church Road S.E., Zip 28602–9643; tel. 828/326–3000; J. Anthony Rose, President and Chief Executive Officer **A**1 9 10 **F**1 3 4 7 8 9 11 13 16 17 18 19 20 22 23 24 25 26 27 28 29 30 31 32 33 34 35 36 38 39 41 44 45 46 47 48 49 50 51 53 54 56 57 59 60 61 62 63 64 65 70 71 72 76 77 78 79 **P**8 Web address: www.catawbamemorial.org	13	10	187	8404	123	154889	1180	88546	40995	1074
★ △ FRYE REGIONAL MEDICAL CENTER, (Includes Frye Regional Medical Center–South Campus, tel. 704/328–2226), 420 North Center Street, Zip 28601–5049; tel. 828/322–6070; Dennis J. Phillips, Chief Executive Officer (Total facility includes 17 beds in nursing home–type unit) **A**1 7 9 10 **F**2 3 8 9 11 12 13 14 16 17 18 19 21 22 23 24 25 27 28 29 30 32 33 34 35 36 37 38 39 41 42 43 44 45 46 47 48 49 50 53 54 56 57 58 59 60 61 62 63 68 69 70 71 76 78 79 **P**1 **S** TENET Healthcare Corporation, Santa Barbara, CA	33	10	355	12095	207	—	937	—	—	—
HIGH POINT—Guilford County ★ HIGH POINT REGIONAL HEALTH SYSTEM, 601 North Elm Street, Zip 27262–4398, Mailing Address: P.O. Box HP–5, Zip 27261; tel. 336/875–6000; Jeffrey S. Miller, President (Total facility includes 30 beds in nursing home–type unit) **A**1 2 9 10 **F**2 3 4 5 7 8 9 11 12 13 14 16 17 18 19 20 21 22 23 24 25 27 28 29 30 31 32 33 34 36 37 38 39 40 41 43 44 45 46 47 48 49 50 51 54 57 59 60 61 62 63 64 65 69 70 71 72 73 76 77 78 79 **P**5 8 Web address: www.hprhs.com	23	10	341	18062	241	82490	1743	132416	54285	1586
HIGHLANDS—Macon County ★ HIGHLANDS–CASHIERS HOSPITAL, Hospital Drive, Zip 28741, Mailing Address: P.O. Drawer 190, Zip 28741–0190; tel. 828/526–1200; H. James Graham, Administrator (Total facility includes 80 beds in nursing home–type unit) **A**1 9 10 **F**7 9 13 17 22 25 32 34 37 40 45 48 49 54 69 70 76 77 78	23	10	104	654	82	91817	0	9588	5551	165
JACKSONVILLE—Onslow County ☐ BRYNN MARR BEHAVIORAL HEALTHCARE SYSTEM, 192 Village Drive, Zip 28546–7299; tel. 910/577–1400; Dale Armstrong, Chief Executive Officer (Nonreporting) **A**1 10 **S** Ramsay Youth Services, Coral Gables, FL	33	22	76	—	—	—	—	—	—	—
★ ONSLOW MEMORIAL HOSPITAL, 317 Western Boulevard, Zip 28540, Mailing Address: P.O. Box 1358, Zip 28540–1358; tel. 910/577–2281; Douglas Kramer, Chief Executive Officer (Nonreporting) **A**1 9 10	16	10	133	—	—	—	—	—	—	—
JEFFERSON—Ashe County ★ ASHE MEMORIAL HOSPITAL, 200 Hospital Avenue, Zip 28640; tel. 336/246–7101; R. D. Williams, Administrator and Chief Executive Officer (Total facility includes 60 beds in nursing home–type unit) **A**1 9 10 **F**7 8 9 10 16 17 18 19 22 24 25 28 32 33 38 39 43 44 45 48 50 54 69 70 72 76 78 **S** Quorum Health Group, Brentwood, TN Web address: www.ashememorial.org	23	10	115	1817	81	30820	123	14915	7038	271
KENANSVILLE—Duplin County ★ DUPLIN GENERAL HOSPITAL, 401 North Main Street, Zip 28349–9989, Mailing Address: P.O. Box 278, Zip 28349–0278; tel. 910/296–0941; Richard E. Harrell, President and Chief Executive Officer (Total facility includes 20 beds in nursing home–type unit) **A**1 9 10 **F**7 8 9 16 17 18 19 22 24 25 30 35 39 41 43 44 45 46 48 54 56 57 60 61 62 69 70 76 78 79 **P**6 Web address: www.dgh.org	13	10	90	3180	61	31781	552	18414	9067	354
KINGS MOUNTAIN—Cleveland County ☐ KINGS MOUNTAIN HOSPITAL, 706 West King Street, Zip 28086–2708, Mailing Address: P.O. Box 339, Zip 28086–0339; tel. 704/739–3601; Hank Neal, Administrator (Total facility includes 10 beds in nursing home–type unit) **A**1 9 10 **F**9 16 17 18 22 25 41 45 48 54 57 61 69 70 76 78 **S** Carolinas HealthCare System, Charlotte, NC	16	10	82	2466	44	28254	—	8075	5457	166

Hospitals, U.S. / NORTH CAROLINA

Hospital, Address, Telephone, Administrator, Approval, Facility, and Physician Codes, Health Care System, Network ★ American Hospital Association (AHA) membership □ Joint Commission on Accreditation of Healthcare Organizations (JCAHO) accreditation + American Osteopathic Healthcare Association (AOHA) membership ○ American Osteopathic Association (AOA) accreditation △ Commission on Accreditation of Rehabilitation Facilities (CARF) accreditation Control codes 61, 63, 64, 71, 72 and 73 indicate hospitals listed by AOHA, but not registered by AHA. For definition of numerical codes, see page A4	Classi-fication Codes		Utilization Data					Expense (thousands) of dollars		
	Control	Service	Staffed Beds	Admissions	Census	Outpatient Visits	Births	Total	Payroll	Personnel
KINSTON—Lenoir County CASWELL CENTER, 2415 West Vernon Avenue, Zip 28504–3321; tel. 252/559–5222; Michael Moseley, Director **F**1 4 6 9 12 13 16 17 18 19 22 23 24 26 30 31 32 33 34 35 39 41 43 45 48 49 50 51 53 54 55 56 59 68 69 70 76 78	12	62	785	27	612	508	0	66459	46366	1676
★ LENOIR MEMORIAL HOSPITAL, 100 Airport Road, Zip 28501, Mailing Address: P.O. Box 1678, Zip 28503–1678; tel. 252/522–7000; Gary E. Black, President and Chief Executive Officer (Total facility includes 26 beds in nursing home–type unit) **A**1 2 9 10 **F**6 7 8 11 13 16 17 18 19 22 23 24 25 27 28 30 32 33 34 35 36 38 39 41 43 44 45 46 48 49 50 51 53 54 61 65 69 70 72 75 78	13	10	196	9409	154	70936	712	67932	31742	1136
LAURINBURG—Scotland County ★ SCOTLAND MEMORIAL HOSPITAL, 500 Lauchwood Drive, Zip 28352–5599; tel. 910/291–7000; Gregory C. Wood, Chief Executive Officer (Total facility includes 50 beds in nursing home–type unit) **A**1 9 10 **F**2 3 7 8 9 11 13 14 16 17 18 19 22 25 26 27 31 32 33 34 36 37 38 39 41 42 44 45 48 49 50 51 54 56 58 59 60 61 62 63 66 69 70 71 72 73 76 77 78 79 **P**8 Web address: www.scotlandhealth.org	23	10	174	4755	100	82129	640	49366	21181	761
LENOIR—Caldwell County ★ CALDWELL MEMORIAL HOSPITAL, 321 Mulberry Street S.W., Zip 28645–5720, Mailing Address: P.O. Box 1890, Zip 28645–1890; tel. 828/757–5100; Frederick L. Soule, President and Chief Executive Officer (Total facility includes 10 beds in nursing home–type unit) **A**1 9 10 **F**4 5 7 8 9 11 13 17 18 19 22 24 25 28 29 32 33 34 36 39 41 43 44 45 46 48 51 54 64 69 70 71 72 76 77 78 79 **P**6 8	23	10	73	4134	37	189466	615	41491	21417	879
LEXINGTON—Davidson County ★ LEXINGTON MEMORIAL HOSPITAL, 250 Hospital Drive, Zip 27292, Mailing Address: P.O. Box 1817, Zip 27293–1817; tel. 336/248–5161; John A. Cashion, FACHE, President **A**1 9 10 **F**3 7 8 9 11 12 13 16 17 18 19 22 24 25 29 33 34 36 38 39 41 43 44 45 46 48 49 50 51 53 54 58 59 60 61 63 64 68 70 72 76 77 78 **P**2 3 5 7 8 Web address: www.lmh.hbocvan.com	23	10	87	3958	42	80913	737	35852	16191	486
LINCOLNTON—Lincoln County □ LINCOLN MEDICAL CENTER, 200 Gamble Drive, Zip 28092, Mailing Address: Box 677, Zip 28093–0677; tel. 704/735–3071; Peter W. Acker, President and Chief Executive Officer **A**1 9 10 **F**8 9 13 16 19 22 24 25 30 31 32 34 36 38 39 40 43 44 45 48 54 70 71 72 73 76 78 79 **P**3 5 7 Web address: www.lincolnmedical.org	23	10	75	3875	51	28258	493	36860	14984	416
LOUISBURG—Franklin County □ FRANKLIN REGIONAL MEDICAL CENTER, 100 Hospital Drive, Zip 27549–2256, Mailing Address: P.O. Box 609, Zip 27549–0609; tel. 919/497–8401; Ann Barnhart, Executive Director (Nonreporting) **A**1 9 10 **S** Health Management Associates, Naples, FL	33	10	85	—	—	—	—	—	—	—
LUMBERTON—Robeson County ★ SOUTHEASTERN REGIONAL MEDICAL CENTER, 300 West 27th Street, Zip 28358–3017, Mailing Address: P.O. Box 1408, Zip 28359–1408; tel. 910/671–5000; J. L. Welsh, Jr, President and Chief Executive Officer (Total facility includes 115 beds in nursing home–type unit) **A**1 9 10 **F**1 3 8 9 11 13 16 17 18 19 22 24 25 27 28 32 33 34 35 36 37 39 41 43 44 45 46 48 51 54 56 57 59 61 65 69 70 71 76 77 78 79 **P**8 Web address: www.srmconline.com	23	10	281	12721	309	164874	1655	97959	43599	1441
MARION—McDowell County ★ MCDOWELL HOSPITAL, 100 Rankin Drive, Zip 28752–4989, Mailing Address: P.O. Box 730, Zip 28752–0730; tel. 828/659–5000; Jeffrey M. Judd, President and Chief Executive Officer **A**1 9 10 **F**7 8 9 13 16 18 19 22 24 25 27 28 29 32 34 36 39 41 43 44 46 48 49 50 51 54 68 70 72 76 78 79 **P**6	23	10	65	2889	31	66757	361	22084	9461	379
MATTHEWS—Mecklenburg County ★ PRESBYTERIAN HOSPITAL–MATTHEWS, 1500 Matthews Township Parkway, Zip 28105, Mailing Address: P.O. Box 3310, Zip 28106–3310; tel. 704/384–6500; Mark R. Farmer, Vice President and Administrator **A**9 10 **F**4 5 7 8 9 11 12 13 19 20 22 24 25 26 27 29 30 33 34 35 36 37 38 39 41 42 43 44 45 46 47 48 49 50 51 52 54 56 57 58 59 60 61 62 63 64 65 66 68 69 70 72 73 75 76 78 79 **P**5 8 **S** Novant Health, Winston Salem, NC Web address: www.presbyterian.org	23	10	82	4507	42	51287	1063	—	—	339
MCCAIN—Hoke County MCCAIN CORRECTIONAL HOSPITAL, Mailing Address: P.O. Box 5118, Zip 28361–5118; tel. 910/944–2351; F. David Hubbard, Superintendent (Nonreporting)	12	11	81	—	—	—	—	—	—	—
MOCKSVILLE—Davie County ★ DAVIE COUNTY HOSPITAL, 223 Hospital Street, Zip 27028–2038, Mailing Address: P.O. Box 1209, Zip 27028–1209; tel. 336/751–8100; Mike Kimel, Administrator **A**1 9 10 **F**7 9 17 18 19 22 25 32 34 36 38 39 41 43 45 48 49 54 69 70 76 **P**3 5 6 8 **S** Novant Health, Winston Salem, NC Web address: www.novanthealth.org	23	10	30	274	3	14505	0	6947	4391	117
MONROE—Union County ★ UNION REGIONAL MEDICAL CENTER, 600 Hospital Drive, Zip 28112–6000, Mailing Address: P.O. Box 5003, Zip 28111–5003; tel. 704/283–3100; John W. Roberts, President and Chief Executive Officer (Total facility includes 66 beds in nursing home–type unit) **A**1 9 10 **F**2 3 4 5 6 8 9 11 12 13 14 16 17 19 21 22 23 24 25 27 28 30 31 32 33 34 35 36 38 39 40 41 43 44 45 46 47 48 49 50 51 54 55 56 58 59 60 61 62 63 64 65 66 69 70 71 72 73 74 75 76 77 78 79 **S** Carolinas HealthCare System, Charlotte, NC Web address: www.carolinas.org	16	10	223	7634	139	110526	1191	52779	24834	749

© 2000 AHA Guide *Many Facility Codes have changed. Please refer to the AHA Guide Code Chart.*

Hospitals, U.S. / NORTH CAROLINA

Hospital, Address, Telephone, Administrator, Approval, Facility, and Physician Codes, Health Care System, Network	Classification Codes		Utilization Data					Expense (thousands) of dollars		Personnel
	Control	Service	Staffed Beds	Admissions	Census	Outpatient Visits	Births	Total	Payroll	

★ American Hospital Association (AHA) membership
☐ Joint Commission on Accreditation of Healthcare Organizations (JCAHO) accreditation
+ American Osteopathic Healthcare Association (AOHA) membership
○ American Osteopathic Association (AOA) accreditation
△ Commission on Accreditation of Rehabilitation Facilities (CARF) accreditation
Control codes 61, 63, 64, 71, 72 and 73 indicate hospitals listed by AOHA, but not registered by AHA. For definition of numerical codes, see page A4.

MOORESVILLE—Iredell County
☐ LAKE NORMAN REGIONAL MEDICAL CENTER, 171 Fairview Road, Zip 28117, Mailing Address: P.O. Box 3250, Zip 28117; tel. 704/660–4000; P. Paul Smith, Jr, Executive Director **A**1 10 **F**7 8 9 11 13 16 17 18 19 22 24 25 27 29 32 34 36 38 39 40 41 43 44 45 46 48 54 70 71 72 76 78 79 **P**8 **S** Health Management Associates, Naples, FL | 33 | 10 | 105 | 4275 | 49 | 42606 | 436 | — | — | 446 |

MOREHEAD CITY—Carteret County
✠ CARTERET GENERAL HOSPITAL, 3500 Arendell Street, Zip 28557–2901, Mailing Address: P.O. Box 1619, Zip 28557–1619; tel. 252/247–1616; F. A. Odell, II, FACHE, President (Total facility includes 104 beds in nursing home–type unit) (Nonreporting) **A**1 9 10 | 13 | 10 | 225 | — | — | — | — | — | — | — |

MORGANTON—Burke County
☐ BROUGHTON HOSPITAL, 1000 South Sterling Street, Zip 28655–3999; tel. 828/433–2111; Seth P. Hunt, Jr, Director and Chief Executive Officer (Total facility includes 18 beds in nursing home–type unit) **A**1 10 **F**22 23 24 26 30 32 39 43 45 50 51 57 58 59 60 61 62 65 68 69 70 72 76 78
Web address: www.broughtonhospital.org | 12 | 22 | 538 | 4093 | 451 | 0 | 0 | 99674 | 42413 | 1354 |
✠ GRACE HOSPITAL, 2201 South Sterling Street, Zip 28655–4058; tel. 828/580–5000; V. Otis Wilson, Jr, President (Total facility includes 120 beds in nursing home–type unit) **A**1 9 10 **F**2 3 4 6 8 9 10 11 13 16 17 18 19 22 25 26 28 30 32 33 34 35 36 37 38 39 41 43 44 45 46 47 48 49 50 53 54 56 57 58 59 60 61 63 64 67 69 70 72 75 76 77 78 **P**1
Web address: www.gracehcs.org | 23 | 10 | 269 | 5625 | 180 | 102959 | 840 | 57388 | 25808 | 739 |

MOUNT AIRY—Surry County
✠ NORTHERN HOSPITAL OF SURRY COUNTY, 830 Rockford Street, Zip 27030–5365, Mailing Address: P.O. Box 1101, Zip 27030–1101; tel. 336/719–7000; William B. James, Chief Executive Officer (Total facility includes 13 beds in nursing home–type unit) **A**1 9 10 **F**7 8 9 11 13 18 19 22 23 25 30 32 33 34 36 37 38 39 41 44 45 46 48 50 51 54 61 69 70 72 76 78 79 **S** Quorum Health Group, Brentwood, TN
Web address: www.nhsc.org | 16 | 10 | 103 | 4774 | 48 | 66675 | 693 | 39359 | 16746 | 507 |

MURPHY—Cherokee County
✠ MURPHY MEDICAL CENTER, 4130 U.S. Highway 64 East, Zip 28906–7917; tel. 828/837–8161; Mike Stevenson, Administrator (Total facility includes 120 beds in nursing home–type unit) **A**1 10 **F**7 8 9 16 17 19 22 24 25 32 33 34 38 39 41 44 45 48 54 69 70 76 77 78 **P**5 8
Web address: www.grove.net/~mmc | 23 | 10 | 170 | 2881 | 140 | 33633 | 245 | 22029 | 10918 | 451 |

NEW BERN—Craven County
✠ △ CRAVEN REGIONAL MEDICAL AUTHORITY, 2000 Neuse Boulevard, Zip 28560–3499, Mailing Address: P.O. Box 12157, Zip 28561–2157; tel. 252/633–8111; Raymond Budrys, Chief Executive Officer (Total facility includes 110 beds in nursing home–type unit) **A**1 2 7 9 10 **F**4 7 8 9 11 12 13 16 17 18 22 24 25 27 29 30 31 32 33 34 35 36 38 39 41 43 44 45 46 47 48 49 53 54 57 60 61 62 64 65 68 69 70 71 76 78 79 | 16 | 10 | 365 | 13686 | 303 | 125502 | 1093 | 118920 | 49554 | 1473 |

NORTH WILKESBORO—Wilkes County
✠ WILKES REGIONAL MEDICAL CENTER, 1370 West D Street, Zip 28659–3506, Mailing Address: P.O. Box 609, Zip 28659–0609; tel. 336/651–8100; David L. Henson, Chief Executive Officer (Total facility includes 10 beds in nursing home–type unit) (Nonreporting) **A**1 9 10
Web address: www.wfubmc.edu | 14 | 10 | 130 | — | — | — | — | — | — | — |

OXFORD—Granville County
✠ GRANVILLE MEDICAL CENTER, 1010 College Street, Zip 27565–2507, Mailing Address: Box 947, Zip 27565–0947; tel. 919/690–3000; Joe W. Pollard, Jr, Chief Executive Officer (Total facility includes 80 beds in nursing home–type unit) (Nonreporting) **A**1 9 10 **S** Quorum Health Group, Brentwood, TN | 13 | 10 | 146 | — | — | — | — | — | — | — |

PINEHURST—Moore County
✠ △ FIRSTHEALTH MOORE REGIONAL HOSPITAL, (Formerly Moore Regional Hospital), 155 Memorial Drive, Zip 28374, Mailing Address: P.O. Box 3000, Zip 28374–3000; tel. 910/215–1000; Charles T. Frock, President and Chief Executive Officer **A**1 2 7 9 10 **F**2 3 4 7 8 9 11 12 13 16 17 18 19 20 22 23 24 25 27 28 29 30 31 32 33 34 35 36 37 38 39 41 42 43 44 45 46 47 48 49 50 51 53 54 57 59 60 61 62 63 64 65 68 69 70 76 77 78 79 **P**5 6 7
Web address: www.firsthealth.org | 23 | 10 | 371 | 17490 | 274 | 125206 | 1663 | 178402 | 76970 | 2367 |

PLYMOUTH—Washington County
✠ WASHINGTON COUNTY HOSPITAL, 958 U.S. Highway 64 East, Zip 27962–9591; tel. 252/793–4135; Patrick Yearty, Administrator **A**1 9 10 **F**9 13 16 17 18 22 24 25 26 39 48 76 | 13 | 10 | 33 | 986 | 12 | 17701 | — | 8188 | 3692 | 138 |

RALEIGH—Wake County
CENTRAL PRISON HOSPITAL, 1300 Western Boulevard, Zip 27606–2148; tel. 919/733–0800; Robert Reardon, Hospital Services Administrator **F**2 3 4 9 10 11 12 13 18 21 22 23 25 27 29 31 32 34 35 37 38 39 41 42 43 44 45 46 47 48 53 54 56 57 59 60 61 63 65 69 70 72 76 79 **P**6 | 12 | 11 | 229 | 3219 | 201 | 15291 | 0 | 25399 | 10515 | 193 |
☐ DOROTHEA DIX HOSPITAL, 3601 Mail Service Center, Zip 27699–3601; tel. 919/733–5324; Walter Stelle, Ph.D., Director (Nonreporting) **A**1 3 5 10 | 12 | 22 | 442 | — | — | — | — | — | — | — |
✠ HOLLY HILL/ CHARTER BEHAVIORAL HEALTH SYSTEM, 3019 Falstaff Road, Zip 27610–1812; tel. 919/250–7000; Andy Delbridge, Chief Operating Officer **A**1 9 10 **F**2 57 58 59 60 61 62 63 64 **S** Magellan Health Services, Atlanta, GA
Web address: www.hcahealthcare.com | 32 | 22 | 108 | 2514 | 58 | 9961 | 0 | — | — | 122 |

Hospitals, U.S. / NORTH CAROLINA

Hospital, Address, Telephone, Administrator, Approval, Facility, and Physician Codes, Health Care System, Network	Classification Codes		Utilization Data					Expense (thousands) of dollars		
★ American Hospital Association (AHA) membership ☐ Joint Commission on Accreditation of Healthcare Organizations (JCAHO) accreditation + American Osteopathic Healthcare Association (AOHA) membership ○ American Osteopathic Association (AOA) accreditation △ Commission on Accreditation of Rehabilitation Facilities (CARF) accreditation Control codes 61, 63, 64, 71, 72 and 73 indicate hospitals listed by AOHA, but not registered by AHA. For definition of numerical codes, see page A4	Control	Service	Staffed Beds	Admissions	Census	Outpatient Visits	Births	Total	Payroll	Personnel
☒ RALEIGH COMMUNITY HOSPITAL, 3400 Wake Forest Road, Zip 27609-7373, Mailing Address: P.O. Box 28280, Zip 27611-8280; tel. 919/954-3000; James E. Raynor, Chief Executive Officer **A**1 9 10 **F**8 13 16 17 18 22 24 25 28 34 35 38 39 41 42 43 44 45 46 48 49 54 57 62 64 69 70 71 76 78 **P**6 **S** Duke University Health System, Durham, NC	23	10	164	6595	74	74452	807	—	—	638
☒ REX HEALTHCARE, 4420 Lake Boone Trail, Zip 27607-6599; tel. 919/784-3100; James W. Albright, President and Chief Executive Officer (Total facility includes 98 beds in nursing home-type unit) **A**1 2 9 10 **F**1 4 6 9 11 12 13 16 17 18 19 22 24 25 26 28 29 30 32 33 34 36 37 38 39 41 44 46 47 48 49 54 56 65 69 71 72 76 77 78 79 **P**6 **Web address:** www.rexhealth.com	23	10	394	19399	265	101473	4996	232995	108441	3007
WAKE COUNTY ALCOHOLISM TREATMENT CENTER, 3000 Falstaff Road, Zip 27610-1897; tel. 919/250-1500; Roy Nickell, Director Substance Abuse Services **A**10 **F**2 3 13 18 31 59 61 63 70 72 **P**5 **Web address:** www.co.wake.nc.us/humnserv/alcohol/atc.htm	13	82	34	800	24	16073	0	4445	3419	124
☒ △ WAKE MEDICAL CENTER, (Includes Eastern Wake Day Hospital, 320 Hospital Road, Zebulon, Zip 27597; tel. 919/269-7406; Southern Wake Hospital, 400 West Ranson Street, Fuquay-Varina, Zip 27526; tel. 919/552-2206; Western Wake Medical Center, 1900 Kildaire Farm Road, Cary, Zip 27511; tel. 919/233-2300), 3000 New Bern Avenue, Zip 27610-1295; tel. 919/350-8000; Raymond L. Champ, President (Total facility includes 37 beds in nursing home-type unit) **A**1 3 5 7 9 10 **F**4 5 7 8 9 11 12 13 14 17 19 22 23 24 25 27 28 29 31 32 33 34 35 36 38 39 41 42 43 44 45 46 47 48 49 50 52 53 54 56 68 69 70 71 72 75 76 77 78 79 **P**3 7 **Web address:** www.wakemed.org	23	10	698	33221	520	295230	5028	320216	146768	4069
REIDSVILLE—Rockingham County										
☒ ANNIE PENN HOSPITAL, 618 South Main Street, Zip 27320-5094; tel. 336/634-1010; Susan H. Fitzgibbon, President and Chief Executive Officer (Total facility includes 42 beds in nursing home-type unit) **A**1 9 10 **F**7 8 9 13 14 16 17 18 19 22 24 25 30 33 34 35 36 38 39 41 43 44 45 46 48 50 51 54 69 70 72 73 76 78 79 **S** Carolinas HealthCare System, Charlotte, NC **Web address:** www.anniepenn.org	23	10	129	3644	78	75760	371	28600	12590	442
ROANOKE RAPIDS—Halifax County										
☒ HALIFAX REGIONAL MEDICAL CENTER, 250 Smith Church Road, Zip 27870-4914, Mailing Address: P.O. Box 1089, Zip 27870-1089; tel. 252/535-8011; M. E. Gilstrap, President and Chief Executive Officer **A**1 9 10 **F**7 8 9 13 16 17 19 20 21 22 23 24 25 27 32 33 34 35 38 39 40 41 44 46 49 50 51 54 56 57 58 60 61 62 63 65 68 70 72 76 77 78 79 **P**8 **Web address:** www.halifaxrmc.org	23	10	143	7534	111	84336	705	51521	21518	724
ROCKINGHAM—Richmond County										
☒ RICHMOND MEMORIAL HOSPITAL, 925 Long Drive, Zip 28379-4815; tel. 910/417-3000; John J. Jackson, Chief Executive Officer (Total facility includes 51 beds in nursing home-type unit) **A**1 9 10 **F**1 8 9 11 13 16 17 18 19 22 25 32 34 36 38 39 41 44 45 48 50 51 69 70 72 76 78 79 **P**7	23	10	141	5043	89	40518	513	39272	18753	615
ROCKY MOUNT—Nash County										
☒ NASH HEALTH CARE SYSTEMS, 2460 Curtis Ellis Drive, Zip 27804-2297; tel. 252/443-8000; Richard Kirk Toomey, President and Chief Executive Officer **A**1 2 9 10 **F**2 3 8 9 11 13 14 16 17 18 19 21 22 23 24 25 27 28 29 32 33 34 35 36 37 38 39 40 41 43 44 45 46 48 50 51 54 57 58 59 60 61 62 63 64 65 68 70 71 72 76 77 78 79 **P**6 7 **Web address:** www.nhcs.org	13	10	245	13274	195	183893	1602	111736	51400	1437
★ NEXTCARE SPECIALTY HOSPITAL OF NORTH CAROLINA, 1031 Noell Lane, Zip 27804; tel. 252/451-2300; Mindy S. Moore, Chief Executive Officer (Total facility includes 50 beds in nursing home-type unit) (Nonreporting) **A**10	33	49	100	—	—	—	—	—	—	—
ROXBORO—Person County										
☒ PERSON MEMORIAL HOSPITAL, (Formerly Person County Memorial Hospital), 615 Ridge Road, Zip 27573-4630; tel. 336/599-2121; Regis Cabonor, Administrator (Total facility includes 60 beds in nursing home-type unit) **A**1 9 10 **F**7 8 9 13 17 18 19 22 24 25 32 34 38 39 41 43 44 46 48 49 51 54 55 58 61 62 63 69 72 76 78	23	10	110	2156	74	36843	196	18647	7988	384
RUTHERFORDTON—Rutherford County										
☒ RUTHERFORD HOSPITAL, 288 South Ridgecrest Avenue, Zip 28139-3097; tel. 828/286-5000; Robert D. Jones, President (Total facility includes 150 beds in nursing home-type unit) **A**1 9 10 **F**7 8 9 11 16 17 18 22 24 25 27 32 34 36 38 39 41 44 45 46 48 49 50 51 54 55 57 59 60 61 63 64 69 70 72 76 78 79 **S** Quorum Health Group, Brentwood, TN **Web address:** www.rutherfordhosp.org	23	10	261	5873	201	64012	—	51881	23874	840
SALISBURY—Rowan County										
☒ ROWAN REGIONAL MEDICAL CENTER, 612 Mocksville Avenue, Zip 28144-2799; tel. 704/638-1000; James M. Freeman, Chief Executive Officer **A**1 9 10 **F**3 7 8 9 11 12 13 16 18 22 24 25 32 33 37 39 41 44 48 49 51 53 54 57 64 76 78 79 **P**1 **Web address:** www.rowan.org	23	10	222	11131	135	—	951	88877	38044	1120
☒ VETERANS AFFAIRS MEDICAL CENTER, 1601 Brenner Avenue, Zip 28144-2559; tel. 704/638-9000; Timothy May, Director (Total facility includes 300 beds in nursing home-type unit) **A**1 5 9 **F**3 4 9 11 13 16 17 18 19 22 23 24 26 28 29 30 31 32 34 35 36 38 39 45 46 49 50 51 54 56 59 61 62 63 64 68 70 72 74 75 76 77 78 79 **S** Department of Veterans Affairs, Washington, DC **Web address:** www.va.gov/stations97/guide/home.asp?DIVISION=ALL	45	22	533	3069	452	178906	0	108928	53260	1231

Hospitals, U.S. / NORTH CAROLINA

Hospital, Address, Telephone, Administrator, Approval, Facility, and Physician Codes, Health Care System, Network

- ★ American Hospital Association (AHA) membership
- ☐ Joint Commission on Accreditation of Healthcare Organizations (JCAHO) accreditation
- ＋ American Osteopathic Healthcare Association (AOHA) membership
- ○ American Osteopathic Association (AOA) accreditation
- △ Commission on Accreditation of Rehabilitation Facilities (CARF) accreditation

Control codes 61, 63, 64, 71, 72 and 73 indicate hospitals listed by AOHA, but not registered by AHA. For definition of numerical codes, see page A4.

Hospital	Classification Codes		Utilization Data					Expense (thousands) of dollars		Personnel
	Control	Service	Staffed Beds	Admissions	Census	Outpatient Visits	Births	Total	Payroll	
SANFORD—Lee County										
★ CENTRAL CAROLINA HOSPITAL, 1135 Carthage Street, Zip 27330; tel. 919/774–2100; L. Glenn Davis, Executive Director **A**1 9 10 **F**7 8 9 11 13 16 17 18 22 23 24 25 27 28 32 34 35 38 39 40 41 43 44 45 46 48 49 51 54 57 70 76 77 78 79 **P**8 **S** TENET Healthcare Corporation, Santa Barbara, CA Web address: www.centralcarolinahosp.com/	33	10	137	5886	68	58298	949	33188	15653	520
SCOTLAND NECK—Halifax County										
OUR COMMUNITY HOSPITAL, 921 Junior High Road, Zip 27874–0405, Mailing Address: Box 405, Zip 27874–0405; tel. 252/826–4144; Thomas K. Majure, Administrator (Total facility includes 60 beds in nursing home–type unit) (Nonreporting) **A**10 18	23	10	100	—	—	—	—	—	—	—
SEYMOUR JOHNSON AFB—Wayne County										
★ U. S. AIR FORCE HOSPITAL SEYMOUR JOHNSON, 1050 Curtis Avenue, Zip 27531–5300; tel. 919/722–1812; Colonel Bradford Lee, Commanding Officer (Nonreporting) **S** Department of the Air Force, Bowling AFB, DC Web address: www.med.navy.mil	41	10	41	—	—	—	—	—	—	—
SHELBY—Cleveland County										
★ CLEVELAND REGIONAL MEDICAL CENTER, 201 Grover Street, Zip 28150–3940; tel. 704/487–3000; John Young, President and Chief Executive Officer (Total facility includes 120 beds in nursing home–type unit) **A**1 2 9 10 **F**8 9 11 12 13 14 17 18 19 21 22 23 24 25 27 29 30 32 33 34 35 36 37 38 39 41 42 43 44 45 46 48 50 51 53 54 56 59 61 65 69 72 74 75 76 78 **S** Carolinas HealthCare System, Charlotte, NC Web address: www.carolinas.org	16	10	334	9234	221	74891	1023	72542	33040	1068
SILER CITY—Chatham County										
★ CHATHAM HOSPITAL, West Third Street and Ivy Avenue, Zip 27344–2343, Mailing Address: P.O. Box 649, Zip 27344; tel. 919/663–2113; Woodrow W. Hathaway, Jr, Chief Executive Officer **A**1 9 10 **F**7 13 17 19 22 25 32 39 43 48 54 64 70 75 76 78 **S** Quorum Health Group, Brentwood, TN	23	10	35	1086	13	15939	0	8751	3514	133
SMITHFIELD—Johnston County										
★ JOHNSTON MEMORIAL HOSPITAL, 509 North Bright Leaf Boulevard, Zip 27577–1376, Mailing Address: P.O. Box 1376, Zip 27577–1376; tel. 919/934–8171; Leland E. Farnell, President **A**1 9 10 **F**7 8 9 11 16 17 18 22 23 24 25 27 29 32 34 35 36 37 38 39 40 41 43 44 45 46 48 54 56 57 59 61 62 70 73 76 77 78 **P**6 **S** Quorum Health Group, Brentwood, TN Web address: www.vipmedia.com	13	10	127	5323	75	131060	758	43861	19728	647
SOUTHPORT—Brunswick County										
★ J. ARTHUR DOSHER MEMORIAL HOSPITAL, 924 Howe Street, Zip 28461–3099; tel. 910/457–3800; Edgar Haywood, II, Administrator **A**1 9 10 **F**16 17 18 22 25 30 32 36 38 39 45 48 54 70 72 76	16	10	40	1411	15	—	—	13706	5334	185
SPARTA—Alleghany County										
★ ALLEGHANY MEMORIAL HOSPITAL, 233 Doctors Street, Zip 28675–0009, Mailing Address: P.O. Box 9, Zip 28675–0009; tel. 336/372–5511; James Yarborough, Chief Executive Officer **A**1 9 10 **F**1 3 4 8 9 11 13 15 17 18 19 22 23 25 31 34 36 37 38 39 44 45 46 47 48 49 51 56 69 70 75 76 **S** Quorum Health Group, Brentwood, TN	23	10	46	1420	20	8095	53	7305	4523	177
SPRUCE PINE—Mitchell County										
☐ SPRUCE PINE COMMUNITY HOSPITAL, 125 Hospital Drive, Zip 28777–3035, Mailing Address: P.O. Drawer 9, Zip 28777–0009; tel. 828/765–4201; Keith S. Holtsclaw, Chief Executive Officer **A**1 9 10 **F**8 9 12 13 16 17 18 19 22 25 28 32 34 36 37 45 46 48 54 56 61 70 76 77 78 **P**8	23	10	42	1985	19	56668	142	—	—	247
STATESVILLE—Iredell County										
★ DAVIS MEDICAL CENTER, 218 Old Mocksville Road, Zip 28625, Mailing Address: P.O. Box 1823, Zip 28687–1823; tel. 704/873–0281; R. Alan Larson, Chief Executive Officer (Total facility includes 13 beds in nursing home–type unit) (Nonreporting) **A**1 9 10 **S** NetCare Health Systems, Inc., Nashville, TN	33	10	132	—	—	—	—	—	—	—
★ IREDELL MEMORIAL HOSPITAL, 557 Brookdale Drive, Zip 28677–1828, Mailing Address: P.O. Box 1828, Zip 28687–1828; tel. 704/873–5661; S. Arnold Nunnery, President and Chief Executive Officer (Total facility includes 48 beds in nursing home–type unit) **A**1 2 9 10 **F**7 8 9 11 12 13 14 16 17 18 19 22 24 25 28 32 33 34 35 36 37 39 41 44 45 46 48 49 50 51 54 56 58 59 60 61 62 63 64 65 68 69 70 72 76 78 79 **P**6	23	10	202	9284	141	141842	1055	77522	38369	895
SUPPLY—Brunswick County										
★ BRUNSWICK COMMUNITY HOSPITAL, (Formerly Columbia Brunswick Hospital), 1 Medical Center Drive, Zip 28462–3350, Mailing Address: P.O. Box 139, Zip 28462–0139; tel. 910/755–8121; Paul A. Schulte, Chief Executive Officer (Nonreporting) **A**1 9 10 **S** HCA – The Healthcare Company, Nashville, TN	33	10	56	—	—	—	—	—	—	—
SYLVA—Jackson County										
★ HARRIS REGIONAL HOSPITAL, 68 Hospital Road, Zip 28779–2795; tel. 828/586–7000; Mark Leonard, Chief Executive Officer (Total facility includes 100 beds in nursing home–type unit) **A**1 10 **F**1 7 8 9 13 16 17 18 19 22 24 25 26 27 31 33 36 37 38 39 41 43 44 45 46 48 49 50 51 54 61 65 68 69 70 76 77 78 79 **P**5 7 8 Web address: www.westcare.org	23	10	175	4757	138	22952	799	—	—	752
TARBORO—Edgecombe County										
★ HERITAGE HOSPITAL, 111 Hospital Drive, Zip 27886–2011; tel. 252/641–7700; Janet Mullaney, President (Total facility includes 10 beds in nursing home–type unit) **A**1 9 10 **F**7 8 9 13 17 18 22 23 25 27 32 33 34 39 41 43 44 45 46 48 51 53 54 69 70 72 76 78 **P**7 8 **S** University Health Systems of Eastern Carolina, Greenville, NC Web address: www.uhseast.com	23	10	127	5020	58	39309	641	31211	11733	397

Hospitals, U.S. / NORTH CAROLINA

Hospital, Address, Telephone, Administrator, Approval, Facility, and Physician Codes, Health Care System, Network	Classification Codes		Utilization Data					Expense (thousands) of dollars		
★ American Hospital Association (AHA) membership □ Joint Commission on Accreditation of Healthcare Organizations (JCAHO) accreditation + American Osteopathic Healthcare Association (AOHA) membership ○ American Osteopathic Association (AOA) accreditation △ Commission on Accreditation of Rehabilitation Facilities (CARF) accreditation Control codes 61, 63, 64, 71, 72 and 73 indicate hospitals listed by AOHA, but not registered by AHA. For definition of numerical codes, see page A4	Control	Service	Staffed Beds	Admissions	Census	Outpatient Visits	Births	Total	Payroll	Personnel
TAYLORSVILLE—Alexander County □ ALEXANDER COMMUNITY HOSPITAL, 326 Third Street S.W., Zip 28681–3096; tel. 828/632–4282; Bill Wilson, Chief Executive Officer **A**1 9 10 **F**9 12 17 18 19 22 24 25 32 34 39 45 48 51 54 64 70 72 76 78	23	10	39	716	8	9010	0	7404	2847	93
THOMASVILLE—Davidson County ✠ COMMUNITY GENERAL HOSPITAL OF THOMASVILLE, 207 Old Lexington Road, Zip 27360, Mailing Address: P.O. Box 789, Zip 27361–0789; tel. 336/472–2000; Lynn Ingram Boggs, President and Chief Executive Officer **A**1 9 10 **F**7 8 9 11 13 17 18 19 22 24 25 32 34 35 38 39 40 41 43 44 45 46 48 49 50 51 54 57 61 62 63 68 69 70 72 73 75 76 77 78 79 **P**5 **S** Novant Health, Winston Salem, NC **Web address:** www.cghp.org	23	10	89	4051	51	44543	627	27058	14120	407
TROY—Montgomery County □ FIRSTHEALTH MONTGOMERY MEMORIAL HOSPITAL, 520 Allen Street, Zip 27371–2802, Mailing Address: P.O. Box 486, Zip 27371–0486; tel. 910/571–5022; Kerry A. Hensley, R.N., Administrator (Total facility includes 51 beds in nursing home–type unit) **A**1 9 10 18 **F**7 9 16 17 18 19 22 23 26 28 30 31 34 36 37 45 48 54 56 58 63 69 70 76 78 79 **Web address:** www.firsthealth.org	23	10	66	799	52	19795	0	7965	3992	169
VALDESE—Burke County ✠ VALDESE GENERAL HOSPITAL, Mailing Address: P.O. Box 700, Zip 28690–0700; tel. 828/874–2251; Lloyd E. Wallace, President and Chief Executive Officer (Total facility includes 120 beds in nursing home–type unit) **A**1 2 9 10 **F**8 9 11 12 13 16 17 18 19 22 25 30 31 32 34 36 38 39 41 43 44 45 46 48 49 50 51 54 65 67 68 69 70 75 76 78 **P**8 **S** Carolinas HealthCare System, Charlotte, NC **Web address:** www.carolinas.org	16	10	199	3380	152	36409	317	30561	13679	439
WADESBORO—Anson County ✠ ANSON COMMUNITY HOSPITAL, 500 Morven Road, Zip 28170–2745; tel. 704/694–5131; Frederick G. Thompson, Ph.D., Administrator and Chief Executive Officer (Total facility includes 95 beds in nursing home–type unit) **A**1 9 10 **F**7 9 13 16 17 18 19 22 24 25 30 32 33 34 38 45 48 50 51 54 69 70 72 76 **S** Carolinas HealthCare System, Charlotte, NC **Web address:** www.carolinas.org	16	10	125	1433	106	26531	—	15461	7943	321
WASHINGTON—Beaufort County ✠ BEAUFORT COUNTY HOSPITAL, 628 East 12th Street, Zip 27889–3498; tel. 252/975–4100; Kenneth E. Ragland, Administrator **A**1 9 10 **F**3 8 9 13 16 17 18 21 22 23 24 25 28 31 32 33 34 36 37 38 39 40 43 45 46 47 48 49 50 51 54 56 59 60 61 62 67 70 71 72 73 74 75 76 77 78 79 **P**3 5	23	10	103	3495	46	—	408	29182	14163	454
WHITEVILLE—Columbus County ✠ COLUMBUS COUNTY HOSPITAL, 500 Jefferson Street, Zip 28472–9987; tel. 910/642–8011; William S. Clark, Chief Executive Officer **A**1 9 10 **F**8 11 12 13 17 18 19 22 25 27 32 38 39 40 41 43 44 48 49 50 51 54 56 70 71 76 78 **S** Quorum Health Group, Brentwood, TN **Web address:** www.cchospital.com	23	10	117	6512	80	52368	474	39993	17364	557
WILLIAMSTON—Martin County □ MARTIN GENERAL HOSPITAL, 310 South McCaskey Road, Zip 27892–2150, Mailing Address: P.O. Box 1128, Zip 27892–1128; tel. 252/809–6121; Scott M. Landrum, Chief Executive Officer (Nonreporting) **A**1 3 9 10 **S** Community Health Systems, Inc., Brentwood, TN	13	10	49	—	—	—	—	—	—	—
WILMINGTON—New Hanover County CAPE FEAR MEMORIAL HOSPITAL See New Hanover Regional Medical Center ✠ △ NEW HANOVER REGIONAL MEDICAL CENTER, (Includes Cape Fear Memorial Hospital, 5301 Wrightsville Avenue, Zip 28403–6599; tel. 910/452–8100), 2131 South 17th Street, Zip 28401–7483, Mailing Address: P.O. Box 9000, Zip 28402–9000; tel. 910/343–7000; William K. Atkinson, II, Ph.D., President and Chief Executive Officer **A**1 3 5 7 9 10 **F**4 7 8 9 11 12 13 17 18 19 20 22 23 25 26 29 30 31 32 33 34 36 37 38 39 41 42 43 44 46 47 48 49 50 51 53 54 56 57 61 62 64 65 70 72 73 75 76 78 79 **P**7 **S** New Hanover Health Network, Wilmington, NC **Web address:** www.nhrmc.org	13	10	622	27779	431	326463	3305	295266	127596	3459
WILSON—Wilson County ✠ WILSON MEMORIAL HOSPITAL, 1705 South Tarboro Street, Zip 27893–3428; tel. 252/399–8040; Christopher T. Durrer, President and Chief Executive Officer **A**1 9 10 **F**1 7 8 9 11 13 17 18 19 22 23 24 25 27 32 33 34 36 37 38 39 40 41 44 45 46 48 50 51 54 57 58 59 60 61 63 65 69 70 72 76 78 **P**6 **Web address:** www.wilsonmemorial.com	23	10	220	8131	96	102643	1309	66856	27079	950
WINDSOR—Bertie County ★ BERTIE MEMORIAL HOSPITAL, 401 Sterlingworth Street, Zip 27983–1726, Mailing Address: P.O. Box 40, Zip 27983–1726; tel. 252/794–3141; Anthony F. Mullen, Administrator **A**9 10 18 **F**9 16 17 22 25 32 38 45 48 54 76 78 79 **S** University Health Systems of Eastern Carolina, Greenville, NC **Web address:** www.bertie.uhseast.com	23	10	15	373	3	12690	0	6083	2992	117
WINSTON-SALEM—Forsyth County AMOS COTTAGE REHABILITATION HOSPITAL, 3325 Silas Creek Parkway, Zip 27103–3089; tel. 336/774–2400; Douglas M. Cody, Administrator (Nonreporting) **A**10	23	56	31	—	—	—	—	—	—	—

Hospitals, U.S. / NORTH CAROLINA

Hospital, Address, Telephone, Administrator, Approval, Facility, and Physician Codes, Health Care System, Network	Classification Codes		Utilization Data					Expense (thousands) of dollars		
★ American Hospital Association (AHA) membership ☐ Joint Commission on Accreditation of Healthcare Organizations (JCAHO) accreditation + American Osteopathic Healthcare Association (AOHA) membership ○ American Osteopathic Association (AOA) accreditation △ Commission on Accreditation of Rehabilitation Facilities (CARF) accreditation Control codes 61, 63, 64, 71, 72 and 73 indicate hospitals listed by AOHA, but not registered by AHA. For definition of numerical codes, see page A4	Control	Service	Staffed Beds	Admissions	Census	Outpatient Visits	Births	Total	Payroll	Personnel
☐ CHARTER BEHAVIORAL HEALTH SYSTEM OF WINSTON–SALEM, (Formerly Charter Hospital of Winston–Salem), 3637 Old Vineyard Road, Zip 27104–4835; tel. 336/768–7710; Marsha Olender, Chief Executive Officer (Nonreporting) **A**1 10 **S** Magellan Health Services, Atlanta, GA **Web address:** www.charterbehavioral.com	33	22	99	—	—	—	—	—	—	—
★ △ FORSYTH MEDICAL CENTER, (Formerly Forsyth Memorial Hospital), 3333 Silas Creek Parkway, Zip 27103–3090; tel. 336/718–5000; Gregory J. Beier, President (Total facility includes 22 beds in nursing home–type unit) **A**1 2 3 5 7 9 10 **F**3 4 5 7 8 9 11 12 13 14 16 17 18 19 22 23 24 25 27 28 29 30 32 33 34 36 38 39 41 42 43 44 45 46 47 48 49 50 51 53 54 56 57 59 60 61 62 63 64 65 69 70 71 72 76 77 78 79 **P**5 8 **S** Novant Health, Winston Salem, NC **Web address:** www.novanthealth.org	23	10	714	33296	539	102319	6224	265494	98580	2820
★ MEDICAL PARK HOSPITAL, 1950 South Hawthorne Road, Zip 27103–3993, Mailing Address: P.O. Box 24728, Zip 27114–4728; tel. 336/718–0600; Eduard R. Koehler, Administrator (Nonreporting) **A**1 2 9 10 **S** Novant Health, Winston Salem, NC	23	10	59	—	—	—	—	—	—	—
★ △ NORTH CAROLINA BAPTIST HOSPITAL, Medical Center Boulevard, Zip 27157; tel. 336/716–2011; Len B. Preslar, Jr, President and Chief Executive Officer (Total facility includes 49 beds in nursing home–type unit) **A**1 2 3 5 7 8 9 10 **F**1 2 3 4 5 6 7 9 10 11 12 13 14 16 17 18 19 21 22 23 24 25 26 27 28 29 30 31 32 33 34 35 36 37 38 39 40 41 42 43 44 45 46 47 48 49 50 51 52 53 54 55 56 57 58 59 60 61 62 63 64 65 66 68 69 70 71 72 73 74 75 76 77 78 79 **P**4 6 7 **Web address:** www.wfubmc.edu	23	10	814	29380	576	178433	0	435039	196330	5870
YADKINVILLE—Yadkin County										
★ HOOTS MEMORIAL HOSPITAL, 624 West Main Street, Zip 27055–7804, Mailing Address: P.O. Box 68, Zip 27055–0068; tel. 336/679–2041; Lance C. Labine, President (Nonreporting) **A**1 9 10 **Web address:** www.bgsm.edu/hoots/	13	10	30	—	—	—	—	—	—	—
ZEBULON—Wake County EASTERN WAKE DAY HOSPITAL See Wake Medical Center, Raleigh										

Hospitals, U.S. / NORTH DAKOTA

NORTH DAKOTA

Resident Population 638 (in thousands)
Resident population in metro areas 42.7%
Birth rate per 1,000 population 13.0
65 years and over 14.4%
Percent of persons without health insurance 15.2%

★ American Hospital Association (AHA) membership
☐ Joint Commission on Accreditation of Healthcare Organizations (JCAHO) accreditation
+ American Osteopathic Healthcare Association (AOHA) membership
○ American Osteopathic Association (AOA) accreditation
△ Commission on Accreditation of Rehabilitation Facilities (CARF) accreditation
Control codes 61, 63, 64, 71, 72 and 73 indicate hospitals listed by AOHA, but not registered by AHA. For definition of numerical codes, see page A4

Hospital, Address, Telephone, Administrator, Approval, Facility, and Physician Codes, Health Care System, Network	Classification Codes		Utilization Data					Expense (thousands) of dollars		
	Control	Service	Staffed Beds	Admissions	Census	Outpatient Visits	Births	Total	Payroll	Personnel
ASHLEY—McIntosh County										
★ ASHLEY MEDICAL CENTER, 612 North Center Avenue, Zip 58413-0556; tel. 701/288-3433; Lieutenant Kathleen Hoeft, Administrator and Chief Executive Officer (Total facility includes 44 beds in nursing home-type unit) **A**9 10 **F**6 7 8 9 16 17 18 19 22 23 25 28 30 31 34 36 37 38 43 44 45 48 50 51 54 56 69 70 71 75 76 78 79	23	10	70	251	45	1548	0	3954	2027	129
BELCOURT—Rolette County										
✠ U. S. PUBLIC HEALTH SERVICE INDIAN HOSPITAL, Mailing Address: P.O. Box 160, Zip 58316-0160; tel. 701/477-6111; Ray Grandbois, M.P.H., Service Unit Director (Nonreporting) **A**1 5 10 **S** U. S. Public Health Service Indian Health Service, Rockville, MD	47	10	42	—	—	—	—	—	—	—
BISMARCK—Burleigh County										
✠ △ MEDCENTER ONE, 300 North Seventh Street, Zip 58501-4439, Mailing Address: P.O. Box 5525, Zip 58506-5525; tel. 701/323-6000; Terrance G. Brosseau, President and Chief Executive Officer (Total facility includes 22 beds in nursing home-type unit) **A**1 2 3 5 7 9 10 **F**2 3 4 5 7 8 9 10 11 12 13 14 15 16 17 18 19 20 21 22 23 24 25 26 27 28 30 31 32 33 34 35 36 37 38 39 40 41 42 43 44 45 46 47 48 49 50 51 52 53 54 55 56 57 58 59 60 61 62 63 64 65 66 67 68 69 70 71 72 73 74 75 76 77 78 79 **P**6 Web address: www.medcenterone.com	23	10	208	7188	113	105089	527	131937	71387	1481
✠ △ ST. ALEXIUS MEDICAL CENTER, 900 East Broadway, Zip 58501-4586, Mailing Address: P.O. Box 5510, Zip 58506-5510; tel. 701/224-7000; Richard A. Tschider, FACHE, Administrator and Chief Executive Officer (Total facility includes 23 beds in nursing home-type unit) **A**1 2 3 5 7 9 10 **F**2 3 4 5 7 8 9 11 12 13 14 15 17 18 19 20 21 22 24 25 26 27 28 29 30 32 33 34 35 36 37 38 39 40 41 42 43 44 45 46 47 48 49 50 51 52 53 54 55 56 57 58 59 60 61 62 63 64 65 66 69 70 71 72 73 74 75 76 78 79 **P**8 **S** Benedictine Sisters of the Annunciation, Bismarck, ND Web address: www.st.alexius.org	21	10	272	10363	143	115610	1061	101512	44734	1375
BOTTINEAU—Bottineau County										
ST. ANDREW'S HEALTH CENTER, 316 Ohmer Street, Zip 58318-1018; tel. 701/228-2255; Keith Korman, President (Total facility includes 32 beds in nursing home-type unit) **A**5 9 10 **F**6 7 8 9 16 17 18 19 22 25 30 32 36 40 43 44 48 58 59 60 62 67 68 69 70 71 72 75 76 78 79 **P**5 **S** Sisters of Mary of the Presentation Health Corporation, Fargo, ND	23	10	67	439	33	7500	4	3537	1540	76
BOWMAN—Bowman County										
ST. LUKE'S TRI-STATE HOSPITAL, 202 Sixth Avenue S.W., Zip 58623-0009, Mailing Address: P.O. Drawer C, Zip 58623; tel. 701/523-5265; Darrold Bertsch, Administrator **A**9 10 **F**7 9 16 22 23 25 31 32 34 39 41 48 54 56 70 76	23	10	18	429	10	7162	0	2986	1512	47
CANDO—Towner County										
★ TOWNER COUNTY MEDICAL CENTER, Highway 281 N, Box 6888, Zip 58324-0688; tel. 701/968-4411; Timothy J. Tracy, Chief Executive Officer (Total facility includes 10 beds in nursing home-type unit) (Nonreporting) **A**9 10	23	10	32	—	—	—	—	—	—	—
CARRINGTON—Foster County										
★ CARRINGTON HEALTH CENTER, 800 North Fourth Street, Zip 58421-1217; tel. 701/652-3141; Brian J. McDermott, President and Chief Executive Officer (Total facility includes 40 beds in nursing home-type unit) (Nonreporting) **A**9 10 **S** Catholic Health Initiatives, Denver, CO	21	10	70	—	—	—	—	—	—	—
CAVALIER—Pembina County										
★ PEMBINA COUNTY MEMORIAL HOSPITAL AND WEDGEWOOD MANOR, 301 Mountain Street East, Zip 58220-4015; tel. 701/265-8461; George A. Rohrich, Administrator (Total facility includes 60 beds in nursing home-type unit) **A**9 10 **F**6 7 8 9 13 17 18 19 20 21 22 23 25 30 32 33 34 36 38 39 43 44 45 46 48 54 56 69 70 71 72 75 76 **S** Banner Health System, Fargo, ND	23	10	89	583	63	6755	25	6499	2957	104
COOPERSTOWN—Griggs County										
GRIGGS COUNTY HOSPITAL AND NURSING HOME, 1200 Roberts Avenue, Zip 58425, Mailing Address: P.O. Box 728, Zip 58425-0728; tel. 701/797-2221; Bruce D. Bowersox, Administrator and Chief Executive Officer (Total facility includes 58 beds in nursing home-type unit) **A**9 10 **F**6 9 16 17 18 19 22 23 25 30 32 33 34 36 37 38 40 43 46 51 54 62 69 70 72 76 78 **P**5	23	10	68	185	57	4732	0	4278	1951	140
CROSBY—Divide County										
ST. LUKE'S HOSPITAL, 702 First Street Southwest, Zip 58730-0010; tel. 701/965-6384; Leslie O. Urvand, Administrator **A**9 10 **F**9 12 16 22 25 32 33 34 36 38 40 48 50 51 54 76	23	10	29	301	8	3219	0	2484	994	43
DEVILS LAKE—Ramsey County										
✠ MERCY HOSPITAL, 1031 Seventh Street, Zip 58301-2798; tel. 701/662-2131; Marlene J. Krein, President and Chief Executive Officer **A**1 9 10 **F**7 8 12 16 17 18 19 20 22 24 25 32 33 35 36 37 39 41 43 44 46 48 50 51 54 70 72 73 75 76 78 **P**5 **S** Catholic Health Initiatives, Denver, CO	23	10	35	1604	18	12794	255	11027	5023	158

© 2000 AHA Guide   *Many Facility Codes have changed. Please refer to the AHA Guide Code Chart.*   Hospitals **A321**

Hospitals, U.S. / NORTH DAKOTA

Approval codes:
- ★ American Hospital Association (AHA) membership
- ☐ Joint Commission on Accreditation of Healthcare Organizations (JCAHO) accreditation
- + American Osteopathic Healthcare Association (AOHA) membership
- ○ American Osteopathic Association (AOA) accreditation
- △ Commission on Accreditation of Rehabilitation Facilities (CARF) accreditation

Control codes 61, 63, 64, 71, 72 and 73 indicate hospitals listed by AOHA, but not registered by AHA. For definition of numerical codes, see page A4

Hospital, Address, Telephone, Administrator, Approval, Facility, and Physician Codes, Health Care System, Network	Classification Codes		Utilization Data					Expense (thousands) of dollars		Personnel
	Control	Service	Staffed Beds	Admissions	Census	Outpatient Visits	Births	Total	Payroll	
DICKINSON—Stark County ★ ST. JOSEPH'S HOSPITAL AND HEALTH CENTER, 30 Seventh Street West, Zip 58601–4399; tel. 701/225–7200; Greg Hanson, President **A**1 9 10 **F**5 6 17 18 19 22 24 28 34 36 37 38 39 40 41 42 44 45 48 50 51 57 58 59 60 61 62 63 64 68 70 71 72 75 76 78 **S** Catholic Health Initiatives, Denver, CO Web address: www.stjoeshospital.org	21	10	90	2581	40	38812	317	25494	11006	366
ELGIN—Grant County JACOBSON MEMORIAL HOSPITAL CARE CENTER, 601 East Street North, Zip 58533–0376; tel. 701/584–2792; Jacqueline Seibel, Administrator (Total facility includes 25 beds in nursing home–type unit) (Nonreporting) **A**9 10	23	10	50	—	—	—	—	—	—	—
FARGO—Cass County ☐ △ DAKOTA HEARTLAND HEALTH SYSTEM, 1720 South University Drive, Zip 58103–4994; tel. 701/280–4100; Louis Kauffman, President and Chief Executive Officer (Total facility includes 16 beds in nursing home–type unit) (Nonreporting) **A**1 2 3 5 7 9 10 **S** Paracelsus Healthcare Corporation, Houston, TX Web address: www.dakotaheartland.com	32	10	203	—	—	—	—	—	—	—
★ △ MERITCARE HEALTH SYSTEM, 720 Fourth Street North, Zip 58122–0002; tel. 701/234–6000; Roger Gilbertson, M.D., President (Total facility includes 24 beds in nursing home–type unit) **A**1 2 3 5 7 8 9 10 **F**3 4 7 8 9 11 12 13 15 17 18 22 24 25 27 28 29 30 32 33 34 35 36 37 38 39 41 42 43 44 45 46 47 48 49 50 51 52 53 54 56 57 58 59 60 61 62 63 64 65 66 68 70 71 72 74 75 76 77 78 79 **P**6 Web address: www.meritcare.com	21	10	376	14755	207	252250	1625	164667	65223	2008
★ VETERANS AFFAIRS MEDICAL AND REGIONAL OFFICE CENTER, 2101 Elm Street, Zip 58102–2498; tel. 701/232–3241; Douglas M. Kenyon, Director (Total facility includes 50 beds in nursing home–type unit) **A**1 3 5 **F**2 3 7 9 13 19 21 22 23 24 25 26 30 32 33 34 35 36 37 39 41 43 45 46 48 49 50 51 53 54 56 57 59 60 61 62 63 65 66 69 70 72 76 78 79 **S** Department of Veterans Affairs, Washington, DC	45	10	109	2828	91	95473	0	48056	24980	591
FORT YATES—Sioux County ★ U. S. PUBLIC HEALTH SERVICE INDIAN HOSPITAL, N 10 North River Road, Zip 58538, Mailing Address: P.O. Box J, Zip 58538; tel. 701/854–3831; Terry Pourier, Services Unit Director (Nonreporting) **A**1 5 9 10 **S** U. S. Public Health Service Indian Health Service, Rockville, MD	47	10	14	—	—	—	—	—	—	—
GARRISON—McLean County ★ GARRISON MEMORIAL HOSPITAL, 407 Third Avenue S.E., Zip 58540–0039; tel. 701/463–2275; Dennis Goebel, Administrator (Total facility includes 24 beds in nursing home–type unit) (Nonreporting) **A**5 9 10 18 **S** Benedictine Sisters of the Annunciation, Bismarck, ND	21	10	54	—	—	—	—	—	—	—
GRAFTON—Walsh County ★ UNITY MEDICAL CENTER, 164 West 13th Street, Zip 58237–1896; tel. 701/352–1620; Everett A. Butler, Chief Executive Officer **A**1 5 9 10 **F**7 8 9 12 18 19 22 25 29 32 34 36 37 38 39 43 44 48 54 56 70 72 76 **P**6	23	10	17	381	5	29347	37	4821	2338	77
GRAND FORKS—Grand Forks County ★ △ ALTRU HEALTH SYSTEM, (Includes Altru Hospital, 1200 South Columbia Road, tel. 701/780–5000; Altrua Health Institute, 1300 South Columbia Road, tel. 701/780–2311), 1000 South Columbia Road, Zip 58201; tel. 701/780–5000 (Nonreporting) **A**1 2 3 5 7 9 10 Web address: www.altru.org	23	10	291	—	—	—	—	—	—	—
GRAND FORKS AFB—Grand Forks County ★ U. S. AIR FORCE HOSPITAL, 220 G Street, Zip 58205–6332; tel. 701/747–5391; Lieutenant Colonel Robert J. Rennie, Administrator (Nonreporting) **A**1 5 **S** Department of the Air Force, Bowling AFB, DC	41	10	15	—	—	—	—	—	—	—
HARVEY—Wells County ★ ST. ALOISIUS MEDICAL CENTER, 325 East Brewster Street, Zip 58341–1605; tel. 701/324–4651; Ronald J. Volk, President (Total facility includes 116 beds in nursing home–type unit) **A**5 9 10 **F**3 8 9 19 22 23 25 32 34 36 37 39 41 44 45 46 48 54 58 59 62 63 67 69 70 71 72 76 78 79 **S** Sisters of Mary of the Presentation Health Corporation, Fargo, ND	21	10	141	849	128	7808	18	7889	4381	131
HAZEN—Mercer County ★ SAKAKAWEA MEDICAL CENTER, 510 Eighth Avenue N.E., Zip 58545–4637; tel. 701/748–2225; Edwin E. Hurysz, Chief Executive Officer **A**5 9 10 **F**3 7 8 9 12 15 17 18 22 25 30 32 34 36 37 39 41 43 44 48 50 53 67 70 71 72 76 78 **P**6	23	10	29	492	7	11992	41	4133	2012	105
HETTINGER—Adams County ☐ WEST RIVER REGIONAL MEDICAL CENTER, 1000 Highway 12, Zip 58639–7530; tel. 701/567–4561; James K. Long, CPA, Administrator and Chief Executive Officer **A**1 5 9 10 **F**6 8 9 12 13 14 15 17 18 19 21 22 23 24 25 26 30 31 32 33 34 36 38 39 41 43 44 45 46 48 49 50 51 54 56 63 67 68 70 71 72 75 76 78 79 **P**3 Web address: www.wrhs.com	23	10	43	1652	18	9035	125	15291	5212	201
HILLSBORO—Traill County HILLSBORO MEDICAL CENTER, 12 Third Street S.E., Zip 58045–4821, Mailing Address: P.O. Box 609, Zip 58045–0609; tel. 701/436–4501; Bruce D. Bowersox, Administrator (Total facility includes 50 beds in nursing home–type unit) (Nonreporting) **A**5 9 10	23	10	74	—	—	—	—	—	—	—

Hospitals, U.S. / NORTH DAKOTA

Hospital, Address, Telephone, Administrator, Approval, Facility, and Physician Codes, Health Care System, Network

- ★ American Hospital Association (AHA) membership
- ☐ Joint Commission on Accreditation of Healthcare Organizations (JCAHO) accreditation
- + American Osteopathic Healthcare Association (AOHA) membership
- ○ American Osteopathic Association (AOA) accreditation
- △ Commission on Accreditation of Rehabilitation Facilities (CARF) accreditation

Control codes 61, 63, 64, 71, 72 and 73 indicate hospitals listed by AOHA, but not registered by AHA. For definition of numerical codes, see page A4.

Hospital	Control	Service	Staffed Beds	Admissions	Census	Outpatient Visits	Births	Total	Payroll	Personnel
JAMESTOWN—Stutsman County										
✠ JAMESTOWN HOSPITAL, 419 Fifth Street N.E., Zip 58401-3360; tel. 701/252-1050; Richard W. Hall, President **A**1 5 9 10 **F**8 9 17 18 22 24 25 34 35 36 37 38 39 41 43 44 45 48 49 50 51 54 61 66 68 69 70 72 75 76 78 Web address: www.jamestownhospital.com	23	10	56	1975	25	22701	230	14274	7393	242
☐ NORTH DAKOTA STATE HOSPITAL, 2605 Circle Drive, Zip 58401-6905; tel. 701/253-3964; Alex Schweitzer, Superintendent and Chief Executive Officer **A**1 5 9 10 **F**2 3 17 23 43 45 57 58 62 70 78 **P**6	12	22	200	1069	179	—	0	22483	15596	505
KENMARE—Ward County										
★ KENMARE COMMUNITY HOSPITAL, 317 First Avenue N.W., Zip 58746-7104, Mailing Address: P.O. Box 697, Zip 58746-0697; tel. 701/385-4296; Jared Ferguson, Administrator and Chief Executive Officer (Total facility includes 12 beds in nursing home–type unit) (Nonreporting) **A**9 10 **S** Quorum Health Group, Brentwood, TN	33	48	42	—	—	—	—	—	—	—
LANGDON—Cavalier County										
★ CAVALIER COUNTY MEMORIAL HOSPITAL, 909 Second Street, Zip 58249-2499; tel. 701/256-6100; Robert N. Jenkins, Interim Administrator **A**5 9 10 **F**7 8 9 12 16 17 22 25 32 33 34 36 37 38 41 43 44 46 48 54 56 70 76 77 **P**6	23	10	28	578	6	10954	25	3274	1779	69
LINTON—Emmons County										
LINTON HOSPITAL, 518 North Broadway, Zip 58552-7308, Mailing Address: P.O. Box 850, Zip 58552-0850; tel. 701/254-4511; Dale Aman, Administrator **A**5 9 10 **F**6 7 9 18 22 24 25 34 36 37 39 40 41 44 48 54 67 70 75 76 78	23	10	25	337	4	—	1	—	—	49
LISBON—Ransom County										
★ LISBON MEDICAL CENTER, 905 Main Street, Zip 58054-0353, Mailing Address: P.O. Box 353, Zip 58054-0353; tel. 701/683-5241; Michael Matthews, Administrator (Total facility includes 45 beds in nursing home–type unit) (Nonreporting) **A**5 9 10 **S** Banner Health System, Fargo, ND Web address: www.lhsnet.com	23	10	70	—	—	—	—	—	—	—
MAYVILLE—Traill County										
★ UNION HOSPITAL, 42 Sixth Avenue S.E., Zip 58257-1598; tel. 701/786-3800; Roger Baier, Chief Executive Officer **A**5 9 10 **F**3 8 9 16 17 18 22 24 25 28 30 35 36 38 43 44 45 53 63 66 69 70 75 76 Web address: www.unionhospital.com	23	10	28	427	7	10643	20	2819	1327	55
MCVILLE—Nelson County										
COMMUNITY HOSPITAL IN NELSON COUNTY, 200 Main Street, Zip 58254, Mailing Address: P.O. Box 367, Zip 58254-0367; tel. 701/322-4328; Jim Obdahl, Administrator (Nonreporting) **A**9 10	23	10	19	—	—	—	—	—	—	—
MINOT—Ward County										
✠ △ TRINITY HEALTH, (Formerly Trinity Medical Center), Burdick Expressway at Main Street, Zip 58701-5020, Mailing Address: P.O. Box 5020, Zip 58702-5020; tel. 701/857-5000; Terry G. Hoff, President (Total facility includes 294 beds in nursing home–type unit) **A**1 2 3 5 7 9 10 **F**1 3 4 7 8 9 11 13 14 16 17 18 19 20 21 22 24 25 26 27 28 29 30 32 34 35 36 37 38 39 41 42 43 44 45 46 47 48 49 50 51 53 54 56 58 59 60 61 62 63 64 65 66 67 68 69 70 71 72 73 75 76 77 78 79 **P**1 4 5 6 7	23	10	472	5953	362	46440	662	103081	53366	1072
★ U. S. AIR FORCE REGIONAL HOSPITAL, 10 Missile Avenue, Zip 58705-5024; tel. 701/723-5103; Colonel David L. Clark, Commander (Nonreporting) **A**5 **S** Department of the Air Force, Bowling AFB, DC	41	10	39	—	—	—	—	—	—	—
✠ UNIMED MEDICAL CENTER, 407 3rd Street S.E., Zip 58702-5001; tel. 701/857-2000; Michael L. Mullins, Chief Executive Officer **A**1 2 3 5 9 10 **F**2 4 8 9 11 13 16 19 21 22 23 24 25 32 33 34 36 37 39 45 46 47 48 49 50 51 54 58 59 60 61 62 63 64 65 70 72 76 78 79 **P**6 **S** Quorum Health Group, Brentwood, TN Web address: www.unimedmedical.com	33	10	160	4760	62	46263	447	49168	20609	589
NORTHWOOD—Grand Forks County										
★ NORTHWOOD DEACONESS HEALTH CENTER, 4 North Park Street, Zip 58267-0190; tel. 701/587-6060; Pete Antonson, Chief Executive Officer (Total facility includes 112 beds in nursing home–type unit) (Nonreporting) **A**9 10	21	10	124	—	—	—	—	—	—	—
OAKES—Dickey County										
✠ OAKES COMMUNITY HOSPITAL, 314 South Eighth Street, Zip 58474-2099; tel. 701/742-3291; Bradley D. Burris, President and Chief Executive Officer **A**1 9 10 **F**7 8 9 12 14 17 19 22 24 25 28 32 36 37 39 44 45 46 48 50 54 59 68 70 71 76 **P**5 **S** Catholic Health Initiatives, Denver, CO	21	10	25	818	9	17371	47	8973	2839	75
PARK RIVER—Walsh County										
★ ST. ANSGAR'S HEALTH CENTER, 115 Vivian Street, Zip 58270-0708; tel. 701/284-7500; Michael D. Mahrer, President **A**9 10 **F**7 8 9 17 22 25 31 34 36 37 38 43 44 48 59 70 73 76 **P**5 **S** Catholic Health Initiatives, Denver, CO	21	10	20	509	9	10258	27	3862	1619	60
RICHARDTON—Stark County										
RICHARDTON HEALTH CENTER, 212 Third Avenue West, Zip 58652-7103, Mailing Address: P.O. Box H, Zip 58652; tel. 701/974-3304; Kurt Waldbillig, Chief Executive Officer (Nonreporting) **A**9 10	23	10	26	—	—	—	—	—	—	—
ROLLA—Rolette County										
PRESENTATION MEDICAL CENTER, 213 Second Avenue N.E., Zip 58367-7153, Mailing Address: P.O. Box 759, Zip 58367-0759; tel. 701/477-3161; Kimber Wraalstad, President and Chief Executive Officer (Total facility includes 48 beds in nursing home–type unit) **A**9 10 **F**7 8 9 14 17 19 22 25 28 32 34 36 38 40 43 44 45 46 48 50 51 54 58 59 62 63 69 70 71 75 76 78 79 **S** Sisters of Mary of the Presentation Health Corporation, Fargo, ND	21	10	102	900	56	6977	69	6724	3556	146

© 2000 AHA Guide   *Many Facility Codes have changed. Please refer to the AHA Guide Code Chart.*

Hospitals, U.S. / NORTH DAKOTA

Hospital, Address, Telephone, Administrator, Approval, Facility, and Physician Codes, Health Care System, Network	Classification Codes		Utilization Data					Expense (thousands) of dollars		Personnel
★ American Hospital Association (AHA) membership ☐ Joint Commission on Accreditation of Healthcare Organizations (JCAHO) accreditation + American Osteopathic Healthcare Association (AOHA) membership ○ American Osteopathic Association (AOA) accreditation △ Commission on Accreditation of Rehabilitation Facilities (CARF) accreditation Control codes 61, 63, 64, 71, 72 and 73 indicate hospitals listed by AOHA, but not registered by AHA. For definition of numerical codes, see page A4	Control	Service	Staffed Beds	Admissions	Census	Outpatient Visits	Births	Total	Payroll	
RUGBY—Pierce County ★ HEART OF AMERICA MEDICAL CENTER, 800 Main Avenue South, Zip 58368–2198; tel. 701/776–5261; Jerry E. Jurena, Executive Director (Total facility includes 198 beds in nursing home–type unit) **A**9 10 **F**3 7 8 9 22 24 25 28 30 32 35 36 37 38 40 41 43 44 45 48 49 54 67 69 70 71 72 76 78 **Web address:** www.hamc.com	23	10	218	1152	192	22145	71	12205	6160	246
STANLEY—Mountrail County MOUNTRAIL COUNTY MEDICAL CENTER, 502 Third Street S.E., Zip 58784–4323, Mailing Address: P.O. Box 399, Zip 58784–0399; tel. 701/628–2424; Mitch Leupp, Administrator (Nonreporting) **A**9 10 18	23	10	25	—	—	—	—	—	—	—
TIOGA—Williams County ★ TIOGA MEDICAL CENTER, 810 North Welo Street, Zip 58852–0159, Mailing Address: P.O. Box 159, Zip 58852–0159; tel. 701/664–3305; Lowell D. Herfindahl, President and Chief Executive Officer (Total facility includes 30 beds in nursing home–type unit) **A**9 10 18 **F**7 9 17 22 24 25 30 32 36 44 46 48 49 50 54 62 69 70 75 76 78 **P**6	23	10	55	434	37	21139	9	3287	1739	48
TURTLE LAKE—McLean County COMMUNITY MEMORIAL HOSPITAL, 220 Fifth Avenue, Zip 58575, Mailing Address: P.O. Box 280, Zip 58575–0280; tel. 701/448–2331; Dennis Goebel, Administrator (Nonreporting) **A**9 10 18	21	10	29	—	—	—	—	—	—	—
VALLEY CITY—Barnes County ✠ MERCY HOSPITAL, 570 Chautauqua Boulevard, Zip 58072–3199; tel. 701/845–6400; Jane Bissel, President and Chief Executive Officer **A**1 9 10 **F**1 7 8 9 12 13 17 22 25 30 33 34 36 37 38 39 41 43 44 48 54 70 71 72 75 76 78 **S** Catholic Health Initiatives, Denver, CO	21	10	50	972	28	15648	91	7003	3729	137
WATFORD CITY—McKenzie County ★ MCKENZIE COUNTY MEMORIAL HOSPITAL, 516 North Main Street, Zip 58854–0548, Mailing Address: P.O. Box 548, Zip 58854–0548; tel. 701/842–3000; Colette Anderson, Administrator **A**9 10 18 **F**7 9 17 18 22 25 28 36 43 45 48 54 69 70 71 76 **P**5	23	10	24	139	4	—	0	1747	865	34
WILLISTON—Williams County ✠ MERCY MEDICAL CENTER, 1301 15th Avenue West, Zip 58801–3896; tel. 701/774–7400; M. Thomas Mitchell, President and Chief Executive Officer **A**1 9 10 **F**2 3 7 8 9 13 17 19 22 24 25 27 28 32 34 36 37 38 39 41 43 44 45 46 48 51 54 56 57 58 59 60 61 62 63 64 65 68 69 70 71 72 76 78 **P**6 **S** Catholic Health Initiatives, Denver, CO **Web address:** www.dia.net/mercy	21	10	93	2614	37	31195	321	26282	12798	374
WISHEK—McIntosh County ★ WISHEK COMMUNITY HOSPITAL AND CLINICS, 1007 Fourth Avenue South, Zip 58495, Mailing Address: P.O. Box 647, Zip 58495–0647; tel. 701/452–2326; C. Gary Kopp, Administrator **A**9 10 **F**7 12 16 17 18 19 22 24 25 29 32 34 36 38 41 48 50 53 54 68 69 75 79 **P**6 8 **Web address:** www.wchc.com	23	10	22	497	4	13219	0	4014	2088	81

Hospitals, U.S. / OHIO

OHIO

Resident Population 11,209 (in thousands)
Resident population in metro areas 81.1%
Birth rate per 1,000 population 13.6
65 years and over 13.4%
Percent of persons without health insurance 11.5%

Hospital, Address, Telephone, Administrator, Approval, Facility, and Physician Codes, Health Care System, Network	Classification Codes		Utilization Data					Expense (thousands) of dollars		
	Control	Service	Staffed Beds	Admissions	Census	Outpatient Visits	Births	Total	Payroll	Personnel

★ American Hospital Association (AHA) membership
☐ Joint Commission on Accreditation of Healthcare Organizations (JCAHO) accreditation
+ American Osteopathic Healthcare Association (AOHA) membership
○ American Osteopathic Association (AOA) accreditation
△ Commission on Accreditation of Rehabilitation Facilities (CARF) accreditation
Control codes 61, 63, 64, 71, 72 and 73 indicate hospitals listed by AOHA, but not registered by AHA. For definition of numerical codes, see page A4

AKRON—Summit County

AKRON CITY HOSPITAL See Summa Health System

★ AKRON GENERAL MEDICAL CENTER, 400 Wabash Avenue, Zip 44307–2433; tel. 330/384–6000; Alan J. Bleyer, President **A**1 2 3 5 9 10 **F**1 2 3 4 5 7 8 9 10 11 12 13 14 16 17 18 19 20 21 22 23 24 25 26 27 28 29 30 31 32 33 34 35 36 37 38 39 40 41 42 43 44 45 46 47 48 49 50 51 52 53 54 55 56 57 58 59 60 61 62 63 64 65 66 68 69 70 71 72 73 74 75 76 77 78 79 **P**1 2 7
Web address: www.agmc.org ... 23 10 473 24118 315 393486 3031 262781 118134 2641

★ CHILDREN'S HOSPITAL MEDICAL CENTER OF AKRON, One Perkins Square, Zip 44308–1062; tel. 330/543–1000; William H. Considine, President **A**1 3 5 8 9 10 **F**1 2 3 4 8 9 10 11 12 13 14 16 17 18 19 21 22 23 24 25 26 27 28 29 30 31 32 33 34 35 36 37 38 39 40 41 42 43 44 45 46 47 48 49 50 51 52 53 54 55 56 57 58 59 60 61 62 63 64 65 66 68 69 70 71 72 73 74 75 76 77 78 79 **P**6 8
Web address: www.akronchildrens.org ... 23 50 200 7170 101 233481 0 126968 59596 1480

★ △ EDWIN SHAW HOSPITAL FOR REHABILITATION, 1621 Flickinger Road, Zip 44312–4495; tel. 330/784–1271; Daniel K. Church, Ph.D., President and Chief Executive Officer (Total facility includes 49 beds in nursing home–type unit) **A**1 7 9 10 **F**2 3 16 17 19 23 28 38 40 51 53 54 69 70 72 78 ... 13 46 112 2167 88 — 0 27117 13826 421

SAINT THOMAS HOSPITAL See Summa Health System

★ SUMMA HEALTH SYSTEM, (Includes Akron City Hospital, 525 East Market Street, Zip 44309–2090, Mailing Address: P.O. Box 2090, Zip 44309–2090; tel. 330/375–3000; Saint Thomas Hospital, 444 North Main Street, Zip 44310; tel. 330/375–3000), Thomas J. Strauss, President and Chief Executive Officer (Total facility includes 12 beds in nursing home–type unit) **A**1 2 3 5 8 9 10 **F**2 3 4 5 8 9 10 11 12 13 14 15 16 17 18 19 20 21 22 23 24 25 26 27 28 29 30 31 32 33 34 35 36 37 38 39 40 41 42 43 44 45 46 47 48 50 51 52 53 54 55 56 57 58 59 61 62 63 64 65 66 68 69 70 71 72 73 74 75 76 77 78 79 **P**6 8
Web address: www.summahealth.org ... 23 10 548 32458 422 391160 3564 — — 3517

ALLIANCE—Stark County

☐ △ ALLIANCE COMMUNITY HOSPITAL, 264 East Rice Street, Zip 44601–4399; tel. 330/829–4000; Stanley W. Jonas, Chief Executive Officer (Total facility includes 78 beds in nursing home–type unit) **A**1 2 7 9 10 **F**7 8 9 13 17 18 19 22 24 25 26 29 30 31 32 33 34 36 37 38 39 40 41 43 44 45 46 48 49 50 51 53 54 68 69 70 72 75 76 77 78 79 **P**1 6
Web address: www.achosp.org ... 23 10 206 5256 117 121194 546 46872 22611 615

AMHERST—Lorain County

☐ EMH AMHERST HOSPITAL, 254 Cleveland Avenue, Zip 44001–1699; tel. 440/988–6000; Kevin C. Martin, President and Chief Executive Officer **A**1 10 **F**4 7 8 9 11 12 13 16 17 18 22 24 25 28 30 31 32 34 36 37 38 39 40 41 42 43 44 45 46 47 48 49 50 54 56 57 59 60 61 68 70 71 72 74 76 77 78 79 **P**7 8 ... 23 10 29 889 11 22479 16 9330 4217 125

ASHLAND—Ashland County

★ △ SAMARITAN REGIONAL HEALTH SYSTEM, 1025 Center Street, Zip 44805–4098; tel. 419/289–0491; William C. Kelley, Jr, FACHE, President and Chief Executive Officer **A**1 7 9 10 **F**7 8 9 13 14 17 18 19 22 24 25 26 29 32 34 36 38 39 41 44 45 46 48 49 50 51 54 57 62 64 68 70 71 72 76 78
Web address: www.samho.org ... 23 10 70 2880 32 114840 559 38193 14494 464

ASHTABULA—Ashtabula County

★ ASHTABULA COUNTY MEDICAL CENTER, 2420 Lake Avenue, Zip 44004–4993; tel. 440/997–2262; R. D. Richardson, President and Chief Executive Officer (Total facility includes 15 beds in nursing home–type unit) **A**1 9 10 **F**3 4 7 8 9 13 16 17 18 19 22 25 26 27 30 32 34 36 37 39 41 44 45 46 48 49 51 54 56 57 58 59 62 63 64 68 69 70 71 76 78 **P**6
Web address: www.acmchealth.org ... 23 10 152 5690 74 103625 656 47341 21088 1069

ATHENS—Athens County

★ + O'BLENESS MEMORIAL HOSPITAL, 55 Hospital Drive, Zip 45701–2302; tel. 740/593–5551; Richard F. Castrop, President **A**1 9 10 12 13 **F**8 9 16 19 22 23 24 25 26 27 30 32 34 35 36 37 38 39 41 43 44 46 48 50 51 53 54 56 61 68 70 72 76 77 78
Web address: www.obleness.org ... 23 10 75 2494 23 63632 458 26134 11009 321

SOUTHEAST PSYCHIATRIC HOSPITAL See Appalachian Psychiatric Healthcare System, Cambridge

BARBERTON—Summit County

★ △ BARBERTON CITIZENS HOSPITAL, 155 Fifth Street N.E., Zip 44203–3398; tel. 330/745–1611; Ronald J. Elder, Chief Executive Officer (Total facility includes 50 beds in nursing home–type unit) **A**1 2 3 5 7 9 10 **F**8 9 11 12 13 17 18 19 22 25 27 30 32 33 36 38 39 41 43 44 46 48 49 51 53 54 57 61 62 70 72 76 78 79 **P**8 **S** Quorum Health Group, Brentwood, TN
Web address: www.barbhosp.com ... 33 10 255 8762 165 342214 834 69526 35547 904

Hospitals, U.S. / OHIO

Legend

★ American Hospital Association (AHA) membership
☐ Joint Commission on Accreditation of Healthcare Organizations (JCAHO) accreditation
+ American Osteopathic Healthcare Association (AOHA) membership
○ American Osteopathic Association (AOA) accreditation
△ Commission on Accreditation of Rehabilitation Facilities (CARF) accreditation

Control codes 61, 63, 64, 71, 72 and 73 indicate hospitals listed by AOHA, but not registered by AHA. For definition of numerical codes, see page A4.

Hospital, Address, Telephone, Administrator, Approval, Facility, and Physician Codes, Health Care System, Network	Classification Codes		Utilization Data					Expense (thousands) of dollars		
	Control	Service	Staffed Beds	Admissions	Census	Outpatient Visits	Births	Total	Payroll	Personnel
BARNESVILLE—Belmont County										
★ BARNESVILLE HOSPITAL ASSOCIATION, 639 West Main Street, Zip 43713–0309; Mailing Address: P.O. Box 309, Zip 43713–0309; tel. 740/425–3941; Richard L. Doan, Chief Executive Officer **A**1 9 10 **F**7 12 17 18 19 22 24 25 32 34 36 37 38 40 41 43 46 48 50 51 54 69 70 76 78 **P**6	23	10	56	2189	27	27576	0	11680	5965	243
BATAVIA—Clermont County										
☐ MERCY HOSPITAL CLERMONT, (Formerly Clermont Mercy Hospital), 3000 Hospital Drive, Zip 45103–1998; tel. 513/732–8200; John M. Dawes, Vice President Operations **A**1 9 10 **F**6 8 9 11 13 15 16 17 18 19 20 22 24 25 28 30 32 33 34 36 38 39 41 45 46 48 49 50 51 54 57 58 62 63 64 65 67 68 70 71 72 76 77 78 79 **P**6 8 **S** Catholic Healthcare Partners, Cincinnati, OH Web address: www.mercy.health-partners.org	21	10	85	4862	58	122384	0	47844	20311	422
BEDFORD—Cuyahoga County										
★ UHHS BEDFORD MEDICAL CENTER, 44 Blaine Avenue, Zip 44146–2799; tel. 440/439–2000; Arlene A. Rak, President **A**1 9 10 **F**2 3 4 5 7 8 9 11 12 13 14 16 17 18 19 20 21 22 23 24 25 26 27 28 29 30 31 32 33 34 35 36 37 38 39 40 41 42 43 44 45 46 47 48 49 50 51 52 53 54 55 56 57 58 59 60 61 62 63 64 65 66 68 69 70 71 72 73 74 75 76 77 78 79 **P**1 5 7 **S** University Hospitals Health System, Cleveland, OH	23	10	99	3720	48	173052	456	29459	12958	344
BELLAIRE—Belmont County										
★ BELMONT COMMUNITY HOSPITAL, 4697 Harrison Street, Zip 43906, Mailing Address: P.O. Box 653, Zip 43906–0653; tel. 740/671–1200; Gary R. Gould, FACHE, Chief Executive Officer **A**1 9 10 **F**4 7 8 9 11 13 14 17 18 19 20 22 23 25 27 28 29 30 31 32 33 34 36 38 39 41 43 44 45 46 47 48 49 50 53 54 56 57 61 64 65 66 70 71 72 75 76 78 79 **P**6	23	10	81	2206	33	37158	70	15148	7835	267
BELLEFONTAINE—Logan County										
★ MARY RUTAN HOSPITAL, 205 Palmer Avenue, Zip 43311–2298; tel. 937/592–4015; Ewing H. Crawfis, President (Nonreporting) **A**1 3 9 10	23	10	72	—	—	—	—	—	—	—
BELLEVUE—Sandusky County										
★ BELLEVUE HOSPITAL, 811 Northwest Street, Zip 44811, Mailing Address: P.O. Box 8004, Zip 44811–8004; tel. 419/483–4040; Michael K. Winthrop, President **A**1 2 9 10 **F**7 8 9 17 18 22 24 25 26 30 31 34 35 36 37 39 41 44 45 46 48 54 62 68 70 71 72 76 78 **P**7 8 Web address: www.bellevuehospital.com	23	10	48	2185	22	41672	349	20721	8629	261
BLUFFTON—Allen County										
BLANCHARD VALLEY REGIONAL HEALTH CENTER–BLUFFTON CAMPUS See Blanchard Valley Health Association System, Findlay										
BOWLING GREEN—Wood County										
★ WOOD COUNTY HOSPITAL, 950 West Wooster Street, Zip 43402–2699; tel. 419/354–8900; Michael A. Miesle, Administrator **A**1 9 10 **F**7 8 9 19 22 24 25 27 32 34 35 37 38 39 40 41 43 44 45 48 54 55 65 68 70 71 72 76 78 79 **P**8 Web address: www.wch.net	23	10	80	3270	37	92899	427	30058	14335	432
BRYAN—Williams County										
☐ COMMUNITY HOSPITALS OF WILLIAMS COUNTY, (Includes Bryan Hospital, 433 West High Street, Zip 43506; tel. 419/636–1131; Montpelier Hospital, Snyder and Lincoln Avenue, Montpelier, Zip 43543; tel. 419/485–3154), 433 West High Street, Zip 43506–1680; tel. 419/636–1131; Rusty O. Brunicardi, President (Nonreporting) **A**1 2 9 10	23	10	121	—	—	—	—	—	—	—
BUCYRUS—Crawford County										
★ BUCYRUS COMMUNITY HOSPITAL, 629 North Sandusky Avenue, Zip 44820–0627, Mailing Address: Box 627, Zip 44820–0627; tel. 419/562–4677; Nellie Clady, R.N., Interim Administrator **A**1 9 10 **F**9 17 19 22 24 25 32 34 39 40 41 45 46 48 54 70 71 76 78 **P**6	23	10	25	901	10	23534	0	10732	4270	168
CADIZ—Harrison County										
★ HARRISON COMMUNITY HOSPITAL, 951 East Market Street, Zip 43907–9749; tel. 740/942–4631; Terry Carson, Chief Executive Officer **A**1 9 10 **F**7 9 12 19 22 23 24 25 28 32 34 36 38 39 41 43 48 50 53 54 70 72 75 76 78 79 Web address: www.harrisoncommunity.com	23	10	48	835	25	11146	—	7481	3413	155
CAMBRIDGE—Guernsey County										
☐ APPALACHIAN PSYCHIATRIC HEALTHCARE SYSTEM, (Includes Southeast Psychiatric Hospital, 100 Hospital Drive, Athens, Zip 45701–2301; tel. 614/594–5000; Mark F. McGee, M.D., Chief Clinical Officer), 66737 Old 21 Road North, Zip 43725–9298; tel. 740/439–1371; Don W. Mobley, Chief Executive Officer (Nonreporting) **A**1 10	12	22	224	—	—	—	—	—	—	—
★ SOUTHEASTERN OHIO REGIONAL MEDICAL CENTER, 1341 North Clark Street, Zip 43725–0610, Mailing Address: P.O. Box 610, Zip 43725–0610; tel. 740/439–3561; Philip E. Hearing, President and Chief Executive Officer (Total facility includes 20 beds in nursing home–type unit) **A**1 2 9 10 **F**7 8 9 13 16 17 18 19 22 25 32 33 34 36 38 39 40 41 43 44 45 48 49 51 54 68 69 70 71 72 76 78 79 **P**6 8	23	10	113	4719	53	80876	425	37158	15111	550
CANTON—Stark County										
★ AULTMAN HOSPITAL, 2600 Sixth Street S.W., Zip 44710–1799; tel. 330/452–9911; Richard J. Pryce, President (Nonreporting) **A**1 2 3 5 6 9 10	23	10	736	—	—	—	—	—	—	—
★ △ MERCY MEDICAL CENTER, 1320 Mercy Drive N.W., Zip 44708–2641; tel. 330/489–1000; Christopher M. Dadlez, President and Chief Executive Officer **A**1 2 3 5 7 9 10 **F**3 4 8 9 11 12 13 17 18 19 22 26 28 30 31 32 33 34 36 37 38 39 41 43 46 47 48 49 50 51 53 54 55 57 58 59 60 61 62 63 64 65 68 70 71 72 74 75 76 77 78 79 **S** University Hospitals Health System, Cleveland, OH	23	10	374	16485	246	479682	1877	158254	66449	2167

Hospitals, U.S. / OHIO

Hospital, Address, Telephone, Administrator, Approval, Facility, and Physician Codes, Health Care System, Network	Classification Codes		Utilization Data					Expense (thousands) of dollars		
	Control	Service	Staffed Beds	Admissions	Census	Outpatient Visits	Births	Total	Payroll	Personnel

★ American Hospital Association (AHA) membership
□ Joint Commission on Accreditation of Healthcare Organizations (JCAHO) accreditation
+ American Osteopathic Healthcare Association (AOHA) membership
○ American Osteopathic Association (AOA) accreditation
△ Commission on Accreditation of Rehabilitation Facilities (CARF) accreditation
Control codes 61, 63, 64, 71, 72 and 73 indicate hospitals listed by AOHA, but not registered by AHA. For definition of numerical codes, see page A4

CHAGRIN FALLS—Cuyahoga County

□ BHC WINDSOR HOSPITAL, 115 East Summit Street, Zip 44022–2750; tel. 440/247-5300; Donald K. Sykes, Jr, Chief Executive Officer (Nonreporting) **A**1 10 **S** Behavioral Healthcare Corporation, Nashville, TN | 33 | 22 | 50 | — | — | — | — | — | — | — |

CHARDON—Geauga County

□ HEATHER HILL HOSPITAL, HEALTH AND CARE CENTER, (LONG TERM ACUTE), 12340 Bass Lake Road, Zip 44024–8327; tel. 440/285–4040; Robert Glenn Harr, President (Total facility includes 194 beds in nursing home–type unit) **A**1 7 10 **F**6 13 16 17 19 20 22 23 24 30 31 32 34 36 38 39 53 54 55 62 68 69 70 72 76 78
Web address: www.heatherhill.org | 23 | 49 | 250 | 1176 | 206 | 1392 | — | 25070 | 13328 | 436 |

★ UHHS GEAUGA REGIONAL HOSPITAL, 13207 Ravenna Road, Zip 44024–9012; tel. 440/269–6000; Richard J. Frenchie, President and Chief Executive Officer (Total facility includes 21 beds in nursing home–type unit) **A**1 2 9 10 **F**7 8 9 12 13 16 17 18 19 22 23 24 25 26 30 32 34 36 37 38 39 40 41 43 44 45 46 48 49 50 51 54 57 59 61 62 68 69 70 71 72 76 78 79 **P**4 5 7 8 **S** University Hospitals Health System, Cleveland, OH
Web address: www.uhhs.com/uhhs/geauga/index.html | 23 | 10 | 142 | 5333 | 72 | 64511 | 685 | 41899 | 17499 | 380 |

CHILLICOTHE—Ross County

★ ADENA HEALTH SYSTEM, 272 Hospital Road, Zip 45601–0708; tel. 740/779–7500; Allen V. Rupiper, President **A**1 2 9 10 **F**3 8 9 11 13 16 17 18 19 22 24 25 29 30 34 35 36 37 38 39 41 43 44 45 46 48 49 50 51 53 54 56 57 58 59 60 61 62 63 64 65 68 70 71 72 73 76 77 78 79 **P**6 8
Web address: www.adena.org | 23 | 10 | 187 | 9803 | 91 | 264976 | 1136 | 94238 | 42993 | 1181 |

★ VETERANS AFFAIRS MEDICAL CENTER, 17273 State Route 104, Zip 45601–0999; tel. 740/773–1141; Michael W. Walton, Director (Total facility includes 162 beds in nursing home–type unit) **A**1 5 9 **F**1 3 9 12 13 17 19 22 23 24 30 31 32 33 34 35 36 37 39 41 45 48 50 51 54 56 57 59 60 61 62 63 64 69 70 72 76 78 79 **P**6 **S** Department of Veterans Affairs, Washington, DC
Web address: www.bright.net/~vachilli | 45 | 22 | 304 | 3997 | 262 | 141277 | 0 | 75154 | 45398 | 1112 |

CINCINNATI—Hamilton County

□ BETHESDA NORTH HOSPITAL, 10500 Montgomery Road, Zip 45242–4415; tel. 513/745–1111; John S. Prout, President and Chief Executive Officer **A**1 9 10 **F**1 3 4 6 7 8 9 11 12 13 14 15 17 19 21 22 24 25 26 27 28 29 30 31 32 33 34 35 36 37 38 39 40 41 42 43 44 45 46 48 50 54 55 56 57 58 59 60 61 62 63 65 66 67 68 69 70 71 72 73 74 75 76 77 78 **P**3 7
Web address: www.trihealth.com | 23 | 10 | 261 | 15414 | 155 | 191799 | 2761 | — | — | — |

★ △ CHILDREN'S HOSPITAL MEDICAL CENTER, (Includes Division of Adolescent Medicine, Cincinnati Center for Developmental Disorders, and Convalescent Hospital for Children; Children's Hospital), 3333 Burnet Avenue, Zip 45229–3039; tel. 513/636–4200; James M. Anderson, President and Chief Executive Officer **A**1 2 3 5 7 8 9 10 **F**3 5 7 11 12 13 14 17 18 19 20 21 22 23 24 25 29 32 33 34 35 36 37 38 39 42 43 46 47 48 49 50 51 52 53 54 56 57 58 59 60 61 63 65 68 70 71 72 73 74 75 76 77 78 **P**1
Web address: www.chmcc.org | 23 | 50 | 307 | 13902 | 203 | 442198 | 0 | 253914 | 94834 | 3639 |

★ △ CHRIST HOSPITAL, 2139 Auburn Avenue, Zip 45219–2989; tel. 513/585–2000; Richard L. Seim, Senior Vice President (Total facility includes 20 beds in nursing home–type unit) **A**1 2 3 5 6 7 9 10 **F**2 3 4 5 7 8 9 10 11 12 13 14 15 16 17 18 19 20 21 22 23 24 25 26 27 28 29 30 31 32 33 34 35 36 37 38 39 40 41 42 43 44 45 46 47 48 49 50 51 53 54 55 56 57 58 59 60 61 62 63 64 65 66 68 69 70 71 72 73 74 75 76 77 78 79 **P**6 8 **S** Health Alliance of Greater Cincinnati, Cincinnati, OH
Web address: www.health–alliance.com | 23 | 10 | 431 | 24429 | 307 | 150444 | 3484 | 268862 | 103848 | 2586 |

□ △ DEACONESS HOSPITAL, 311 Straight Street, Zip 45219–1099; tel. 513/559–2100; E. Anthony Woods, President (Total facility includes 20 beds in nursing home–type unit) (Nonreporting) **A**1 7 9 10
Web address: www.Deaconess–healthcare.com | 23 | 10 | 219 | — | — | — | — | — | — | — |

★ DRAKE CENTER, 151 West Galbraith Road, Zip 45216–1096; tel. 513/948–2500; Roberta J. Bradford, President and Chief Executive Officer (Total facility includes 204 beds in nursing home–type unit) **A**1 3 5 7 9 10 **F**7 13 15 16 17 18 19 22 23 28 29 30 31 32 33 34 35 39 43 45 50 51 53 54 55 59 60 62 63 69 70 71 72 76 78 **P**5 6
Web address: www.drakecenter.com | 23 | 46 | 288 | 1318 | 231 | 27183 | 0 | 44925 | 22071 | 680 |

□ FRANCISCAN HOSPITAL—WESTERN HILLS, 3131 Queen City Avenue, Zip 45238–2396; tel. 513/389–5000; Charles C. Lobeck, President (Total facility includes 34 beds in nursing home–type unit) **A**1 2 7 9 10 **F**2 3 6 7 8 9 11 12 13 17 20 22 23 24 25 26 28 29 30 32 34 36 37 38 39 40 41 43 44 45 46 48 51 53 54 56 57 58 61 62 63 64 67 69 70 71 72 76 77 78 **P**1 5 7 **S** Catholic Healthcare Partners, Cincinnati, OH
Web address: www.mercy.health–partners.org | 21 | 10 | 223 | 6371 | 124 | 40477 | 0 | 51182 | 21424 | 686 |

★ △ GOOD SAMARITAN HOSPITAL, 375 Dixmyth Avenue, Zip 45220–2489; tel. 513/872–1400; John S. Prout, President and Chief Executive Officer (Total facility includes 15 beds in nursing home–type unit) **A**1 2 3 5 6 7 8 9 10 **F**1 3 4 6 7 8 9 11 12 13 14 17 18 19 20 21 22 23 25 26 27 28 29 30 31 32 33 34 35 36 37 38 39 41 42 43 44 45 46 47 48 49 50 51 53 54 55 56 57 58 59 61 62 63 64 65 66 67 68 69 70 71 72 73 74 75 76 77 78 **P**3 7 **S** Catholic Health Initiatives, Denver, CO
Web address: www.trihealth.com | 21 | 10 | 419 | 20577 | 260 | 136947 | 4730 | 192506 | 86475 | 1960 |

© 2000 AHA Guide   *Many Facility Codes have changed. Please refer to the AHA Guide Code Chart.*

Hospitals, U.S. / OHIO

Hospital, Address, Telephone, Administrator, Approval, Facility, and Physician Codes, Health Care System, Network	Classification Codes		Utilization Data					Expense (thousands) of dollars		Personnel
	Control	Service	Staffed Beds	Admissions	Census	Outpatient Visits	Births	Total	Payroll	

★ American Hospital Association (AHA) membership
□ Joint Commission on Accreditation of Healthcare Organizations (JCAHO) accreditation
+ American Osteopathic Healthcare Association (AOHA) membership
○ American Osteopathic Association (AOA) accreditation
△ Commission on Accreditation of Rehabilitation Facilities (CARF) accreditation
Control codes 61, 63, 64, 71, 72 and 73 indicate hospitals listed by AOHA, but not registered by AHA. For definition of numerical codes, see page A4

Hospital	Control	Service	Staffed Beds	Admissions	Census	Outpatient Visits	Births	Total	Payroll	Personnel
★ JEWISH HOSPITAL KENWOOD, 4777 East Galbraith Road, Zip 45236; tel. 513/686–3000; M. Aurora Lambert, Senior Vice President **A**1 2 3 5 9 10 **F**2 3 4 5 7 8 9 10 11 12 13 14 15 16 17 18 19 20 21 22 23 24 25 26 27 28 29 30 31 32 33 34 35 36 37 38 39 40 41 42 43 44 45 46 47 48 49 50 51 53 54 55 56 57 58 59 60 61 62 63 64 65 66 68 69 70 71 72 73 74 75 76 77 78 79 **P**6 8 **S** Health Alliance of Greater Cincinnati, Cincinnati, OH Web address: www.health-alliance.com	23	10	169	10509	133	126813	966	131392	46683	950
□ △ MERCY FRANCISCAN HOSPITAL–MOUNT AIRY, (Formerly Franciscan Hospital–Mount Airy), 2446 Kipling Avenue, Zip 45239–6650; tel. 513/853–5000; Steven Grinnell, President (Total facility includes 20 beds in nursing home–type unit) **A**1 2 3 5 7 9 10 **F**2 3 6 7 8 9 11 12 13 17 20 22 23 24 25 26 28 29 32 34 36 37 38 39 40 41 43 44 45 46 48 51 53 54 56 57 58 61 62 63 64 67 69 70 71 72 76 77 78 **P**1 5 7 **S** Catholic Healthcare Partners, Cincinnati, OH Web address: www.mercy.health-partners.org	21	10	246	7734	122	60513	709	63273	28406	1023
□ MERCY HOSPITAL ANDERSON, 7500 State Road, Zip 45255–2492; tel. 513/624–4500; Fred L. Kolb, President **A**1 2 9 10 **F**6 7 8 9 11 14 15 16 17 18 19 22 24 25 28 30 32 33 34 36 37 39 41 43 44 45 46 48 49 50 51 54 65 67 68 70 71 72 76 77 78 79 **P**6 8 **S** Catholic Healthcare Partners, Cincinnati, OH Web address: www.mercy.health-partners.org	21	10	151	9628	95	96693	2136	75775	28215	679
□ PAULINE WARFIELD LEWIS CENTER, 1101 Summit Road, Zip 45237–2652; tel. 513/948–3600; Elizabeth Banks, Chief Executive Officer (Nonreporting) **A**1 10 Web address: www.prime/prime.htm	12	22	357	—	—	—	—	—	—	—
□ SHRINERS HOSPITALS FOR CHILDREN, SHRINERS BURNS HOSPITAL, CINCINNATI, (PEDIATRIC BURN INJURIES), 3229 Burnet Avenue, Zip 45229–3095; tel. 513/872–6000; Ronald R. Hitzler, Administrator **A**1 **F**10 13 22 24 31 39 45 48 49 50 51 55 59 61 68 70 72 76 78 **S** Shriners Hospitals for Children, Tampa, FL Web address: www.shrinershq.org	23	59	30	804	19	4988	0	—	—	304
★ UNIVERSITY HOSPITAL, 234 Goodman Street, Zip 45219–2316; tel. 513/584–1000; Elliot G. Cohen, Senior Vice President **A**1 2 3 5 8 9 10 **F**2 3 4 5 7 8 9 10 11 12 13 14 15 16 17 18 19 20 21 22 23 24 25 26 27 28 29 30 31 32 33 34 35 36 37 38 39 40 41 42 43 44 45 46 47 48 49 51 52 53 54 55 56 57 58 59 60 61 62 63 64 65 66 68 69 70 71 72 73 74 75 76 77 78 79 **P**6 8 **S** Health Alliance of Greater Cincinnati, Cincinnati, OH Web address: www.health-alliance.com	23	10	429	21349	317	232679	2362	309584	114854	3931
★ VETERANS AFFAIRS MEDICAL CENTER, 3200 Vine Street, Zip 45220–2288; tel. 513/861–3100; Gary N. Nugent, Medical Director (Total facility includes 64 beds in nursing home–type unit) (Nonreporting) **A**1 3 5 8 9 **S** Department of Veterans Affairs, Washington, DC Web address: www.va.gov/stations97/guide/home.asp?DIVISION=ALL	45	10	240	—	—	—	—	—	—	—

CIRCLEVILLE—Pickaway County

Hospital	Control	Service	Staffed Beds	Admissions	Census	Outpatient Visits	Births	Total	Payroll	Personnel
★ △ BERGER HEALTH SYSTEM, 600 North Pickaway Street, Zip 43113–1499; tel. 740/420–8231; Brian R. Colfack, CHE, President and Chief Executive Officer **A**1 7 9 10 **F**8 9 13 16 17 18 19 22 24 25 26 29 30 31 32 33 34 36 37 38 39 41 43 44 45 46 48 49 50 51 53 54 56 70 71 72 75 76 77 78 79 **P**3 Web address: www.bergerhealth.com	15	10	75	2453	26	70442	209	27181	8554	234

CLEVELAND—Cuyahoga County

CLEVELAND CAMPUS See Northcoast Behavioral Healthcare System, Northfield

Hospital	Control	Service	Staffed Beds	Admissions	Census	Outpatient Visits	Births	Total	Payroll	Personnel
★ △ CLEVELAND CLINIC CHILDREN'S HOSPITAL FOR REHABILITATION, (Formerly Health Hill Hospital for Children), Mailing Address: 2801 Martin Luther King Jr. Drive, Zip 44104–3865; tel. 216/721–5400; Thomas A. Rathbone, President (Nonreporting) **A**1 7 10 **S** Cleveland Clinic Health System, Cleveland, OH Web address: www.clevelandclinic.org/childrensrehab	23	56	46	—	—	—	—	—	—	—
★ △ CLEVELAND CLINIC FOUNDATION, 9500 Euclid Avenue, Zip 44195–5108; tel. 216/444–2200; Frank L. Lordeman, Chief Operating Officer (Total facility includes 59 beds in nursing home–type unit) **A**1 2 3 5 7 8 9 10 **F**2 3 4 5 8 9 11 12 13 14 16 17 18 19 20 22 23 24 25 26 27 28 29 30 31 32 33 34 35 36 37 38 39 41 43 44 45 46 47 48 49 50 51 52 53 54 55 56 57 58 59 60 61 62 63 64 65 66 68 69 70 71 72 74 75 76 77 78 79 **P**1 3 5 6 **S** Cleveland Clinic Health System, Cleveland, OH Web address: www.ccf.org	23	10	1001	49779	792	1664063	2347	736076	260494	12794
□ DEACONESS HOSPITAL OF CLEVELAND, 4229 Pearl Road, Zip 44109–4218; tel. 216/459–6300; Geoffrey D. Moebius, Chief Executive Officer (Total facility includes 15 beds in nursing home–type unit) (Nonreporting) **A**1 2 9 10	32	10	212	—	—	—	—	—	—	—
★ FAIRVIEW HOSPITAL, 18101 Lorain Avenue, Zip 44111–5656; tel. 216/476–7000; Louis P. Caravella, M.D., Chief Executive Officer (Total facility includes 20 beds in nursing home–type unit) (Nonreporting) **A**1 2 3 5 6 9 10 **S** Cleveland Clinic Health System, Cleveland, OH	23	10	428	—	—	—	—	—	—	—
★ GRACE HOSPITAL, 2307 West 14th Street, Zip 44113–3698; tel. 216/687–1500; Robert P. Range, President and Chief Executive Officer **A**1 9 10 **F**16 17 18 30 31 32 33 34 36 38 41 43 45 48 49 50 51 54 56 70 76 77 Web address: www.transcare.org	23	10	57	404	34	12013	0	14401	6716	232

HEALTH HILL HOSPITAL FOR CHILDREN See Cleveland Clinic Children's Hospital for Rehabilitation

Hospitals, U.S. / OHIO

Hospital, Address, Telephone, Administrator, Approval, Facility, and Physician Codes, Health Care System, Network	Classification Codes		Utilization Data					Expense (thousands) of dollars		
★ American Hospital Association (AHA) membership □ Joint Commission on Accreditation of Healthcare Organizations (JCAHO) accreditation + American Osteopathic Healthcare Association (AOHA) membership ○ American Osteopathic Association (AOA) accreditation △ Commission on Accreditation of Rehabilitation Facilities (CARF) accreditation Control codes 61, 63, 64, 71, 72 and 73 indicate hospitals listed by AOHA, but not registered by AHA. For definition of numerical codes, see page A4	Control	Service	Staffed Beds	Admissions	Census	Outpatient Visits	Births	Total	Payroll	Personnel
□ △ LUTHERAN HOSPITAL, 1730 West 25th Street, Zip 44113; tel. 216/696-4300; John Brocketi, Associate Vice President (Total facility includes 35 beds in nursing home-type unit) (Nonreporting) **A**1 7 9 10 **S** Cleveland Clinic Health System, Cleveland, OH	23	10	219	—	—	—	—	—	—	—
□ MERIDIA HILLCREST HOSPITAL, 6780 Mayfield Road, Zip 44124-2202; tel. 440/449-4500; Catherine B. Leary, R.N., Chief Operating Officer **A**1 2 3 9 10 **F**2 3 4 7 8 9 11 12 13 14 16 17 18 19 22 24 25 27 28 29 30 31 32 33 34 35 37 38 39 40 41 42 43 44 45 46 47 48 49 50 51 52 53 54 56 57 59 60 61 62 63 64 65 66 68 69 70 71 72 73 75 76 77 78 79 **P**1 3 4 7 8 **S** Cleveland Clinic Health System, Cleveland, OH Web address: www.meridia.org	23	10	305	15915	201	249552	2814	143909	53905	1400
□ MERIDIA HURON HOSPITAL, 13951 Terrace Road, Zip 44112-4399; tel. 216/761-3300; Beverly Lozar, Chief Operating Officer (Total facility includes 20 beds in nursing home-type unit) **A**1 2 3 5 6 9 10 **F**2 3 4 7 8 9 11 12 13 14 16 17 18 19 22 24 25 27 28 29 30 31 32 33 34 35 37 38 39 40 41 42 44 45 47 48 49 50 51 52 53 54 56 57 59 60 61 62 63 64 65 66 68 69 70 71 72 73 75 76 77 78 79 **P**1 3 4 7 8 **S** Cleveland Clinic Health System, Cleveland, OH Web address: www.meridia.org	23	10	163	5595	92	47065	0	58618	26265	646
★ △ METROHEALTH MEDICAL CENTER, 2500 MetroHealth Drive, Zip 44109-1998; tel. 216/778-7800; Terry R. White, President and Chief Executive Officer (Total facility includes 497 beds in nursing home-type unit) **A**1 2 3 5 7 8 9 10 **F**1 2 3 4 5 8 9 10 11 12 13 15 17 18 19 22 23 24 25 29 30 31 32 33 34 35 37 38 39 41 42 43 44 45 46 47 48 49 50 51 52 53 54 56 57 58 59 60 61 62 63 64 65 66 68 69 70 71 72 74 75 76 77 78 79 **P**6 Web address: www.metrohealth.org RAINBOW BABIES AND CHILDREN'S HOSPITAL See University Hospitals of Cleveland SAINT LUKE'S MEDICAL CENTER See St. Vincent Charity Hospital	13	10	980	22318	743	585978	3250	432879	237014	5314
□ SAINT MICHAEL HOSPITAL, 5163 Broadway Avenue, Zip 44127-1532; tel. 216/429-8000; Richard J. Frenchie, Chief Executive Officer (Total facility includes 55 beds in nursing home-type unit) (Nonreporting) **A**1 2 9 10 **S** University Hospitals Health System, Cleveland, OH	33	10	199	—	—	—	—	—	—	—
★ ○ ST. JOHN WEST SHORE HOSPITAL, 29000 Center Ridge Road, Zip 44145-5219; tel. 440/835-8000; Fred M. DeGrandis, President (Nonreporting) **A**1 9 10 11 12 **S** University Hospitals Health System, Cleveland, OH	23	10	183	—	—	—	—	—	—	—
★ ST. VINCENT CHARITY HOSPITAL, (Includes Saint Luke's Medical Center, 11311 Shaker Boulevard, Zip 44104-3805; tel. 216/368-7000), 2351 East 22nd Street, Zip 44115-3111; tel. 216/861-6200; Alan H. Channing, Chief Executive Officer (Nonreporting) **A**1 2 3 5 9 10 **S** University Hospitals Health System, Cleveland, OH	23	10	471	—	—	—	—	—	—	—
★ △ UNIVERSITY HOSPITALS OF CLEVELAND, (Includes Alfred and Norma Lerner Tower, Bolwell Health Center, Hanna Pavilion, Lakeside Hospital, Samuel Mather Pavilion; Rainbow Babies and Children's Hospital; University MacDonald Women's Hospital), 11100 Euclid Avenue, Zip 44106-2602; tel. 216/844-1000; Farah M. Walters, President and Chief Executive Officer (Total facility includes 50 beds in nursing home-type unit) **A**1 2 3 5 7 8 9 10 **F**3 4 5 8 9 11 12 14 16 18 19 21 22 23 24 25 26 27 28 29 30 31 32 33 34 35 36 37 38 39 41 42 43 45 46 47 48 49 50 51 52 53 54 55 56 57 58 59 60 61 62 63 64 65 66 68 69 70 71 72 73 74 75 76 77 78 79 **P**3 5 6 7 **S** University Hospitals Health System, Cleveland, OH Web address: www.uhhs.com/uhhs/ UNIVERSITY MACDONALD WOMEN'S HOSPITAL See University Hospitals of Cleveland	23	10	752	39520	615	666668	4818	509889	210940	5539
★ VETERANS AFFAIRS MEDICAL CENTER, 10701 East Boulevard, Zip 44106-1702; tel. 216/791-3800; William D. Montague, Director (Total facility includes 195 beds in nursing home-type unit) (Nonreporting) **A**1 3 5 8 9 **S** Department of Veterans Affairs, Washington, DC Web address: www.va.gov/stations97/guide/home.asp?DIVISION=ALL	45	10	817	—	—	—	—	—	—	—
COLDWATER—Mercer County										
★ MERCER COUNTY JOINT TOWNSHIP COMMUNITY HOSPITAL, 800 West Main Street, Zip 45828-1698; tel. 419/678-2341; James W. Isaacs, Chief Executive Officer **A**1 9 10 **F**7 8 9 17 18 19 22 24 25 29 32 34 36 37 39 41 44 45 48 51 68 70 71 72 76 77 78	16	10	59	2365	23	69103	379	21019	9382	290
COLUMBUS—Franklin County										
★ ARTHUR G. JAMES CANCER HOSPITAL AND RICHARD J. SOLOVE RESEARCH INSTITUTE, (Formerly Arthur G. James Cancer Hospital and Research Institute), (ACUTE CARE CANCER HOSP & RSRCH), 300 West Tenth Avenue, Zip 43210-1240; tel. 614/293-5485; David E. Schuller, M.D., Chief Executive Officer **A**1 2 3 5 8 9 10 **F**1 2 3 4 5 6 7 8 10 11 12 13 14 15 16 17 18 19 20 21 22 23 24 25 26 28 29 30 31 32 33 34 35 36 37 38 39 41 42 43 44 45 46 47 48 49 50 51 52 53 54 56 57 58 59 60 62 63 64 65 66 67 68 69 70 71 72 73 74 75 76 77 78 79 **P**5 Web address: www.jamesline.com	12	49	120	6661	108	110654	0	114120	26475	1506
★ △ CHILDREN'S HOSPITAL, 700 Children's Drive, Zip 43205-2696; tel. 614/722-2000; Thomas N. Hansen, M.D., Chief Executive Officer **A**1 2 3 5 7 9 10 **F**4 11 13 14 16 17 18 19 20 22 23 28 29 31 32 33 34 35 37 38 39 42 43 45 46 47 48 50 51 52 53 54 56 58 59 60 61 63 68 70 72 73 74 75 76 77 78 **P**8 Web address: www.childrenscolumbus.org COLUMBUS CAMPUS See Twin Valley Psychiatric System, Dayton	23	50	281	11100	159	364931	0	—	—	2280

© 2000 AHA Guide   *Many Facility Codes have changed. Please refer to the AHA Guide Code Chart.*

Hospitals, U.S. / OHIO

	Key
★	American Hospital Association (AHA) membership
☐	Joint Commission on Accreditation of Healthcare Organizations (JCAHO) accreditation
+	American Osteopathic Healthcare Association (AOHA) membership
○	American Osteopathic Association (AOA) accreditation
△	Commission on Accreditation of Rehabilitation Facilities (CARF) accreditation

Control codes 61, 63, 64, 71, 72 and 73 indicate hospitals listed by AOHA, but not registered by AHA. For definition of numerical codes, see page A4

Hospital, Address, Telephone, Administrator, Approval, Facility, and Physician Codes, Health Care System, Network	Classification Codes		Utilization Data					Expense (thousands) of dollars		
	Control	Service	Staffed Beds	Admissions	Census	Outpatient Visits	Births	Total	Payroll	Personnel
☐ △ **COLUMBUS COMMUNITY HOSPITAL**, 1430 South High Street, Zip 43207–1093; tel. 614/437–5000; Michael L. Brown, Interim Chief Executive Officer (Total facility includes 10 beds in nursing home–type unit) **A**1 7 9 10 **F**7 11 13 15 22 24 25 31 34 36 39 41 45 48 49 50 53 54 57 62 68 69 70 76 78 **Web address:** www.columbuscommunity.com	32	10	140	4366	66	—	0	—	—	522
✠ + ○ △ **DOCTORS HOSPITAL**, (Includes Doctors Hospital West, 5100 West Broad Street, Zip 43228; tel. 614/297–4000), 1087 Dennison Avenue, Zip 43201–3496; tel. 614/297–4000; Dennis J. Freudeman, President (Nonreporting) **A**1 7 9 10 11 12 13 **S** OhioHealth, Columbus, OH **Web address:** www.doctorshospital.org	23	10	380	—	—	—	—	—	—	—
✠ △ **GRANT/RIVERSIDE METHODIST HOSPITALS–GRANT CAMPUS**, 111 South Grant Avenue, Zip 43215–1898; tel. 614/566–9000; Mark H. Shuter, President (Nonreporting) **A**1 3 5 7 8 9 10 **S** OhioHealth, Columbus, OH **Web address:** www.ohiohealth.com	21	10	460	—	—	—	—	—	—	—
✠ △ **GRANT/RIVERSIDE METHODIST HOSPITALS–RIVERSIDE CAMPUS**, 3535 Olentangy River Road, Zip 43214–3998; tel. 614/566–5000; Mark H. Shuter, President (Nonreporting) **A**1 2 3 5 7 8 9 10 **S** OhioHealth, Columbus, OH **Web address:** www.ohiohealth.com	21	10	778	—	—	—	—	—	—	—
✠ △ **MOUNT CARMEL HEALTH SYSTEM**, (Includes Mount Carmel East Hospital, 6001 East Broad Street, Zip 43213; tel. 614/234–6000; Mount Carmel Medical Center, 793 West State Street, Zip 43222; tel. 614/234–5000; St. Ann's Hospital, 500 South Cleveland Avenue, Westerville, Zip 43081–8998; tel. 614/898–4000), Mailing Address: 793 West State Street, Zip 43222–1551; tel. 614/234–5423; Joseph T. Calvaruso, President and Chief Executive Officer (Total facility includes 14 beds in nursing home–type unit) (Nonreporting) **A**1 2 3 5 7 9 10 **S** Trinity Health, Novi, MI **Web address:** www.mchs.org	21	10	929	—	—	—	—	—	—	—
✠ **OHIO STATE UNIVERSITY HOSPITAL EAST**, (Formerly Park Medical Center), 1492 East Broad Street, Zip 43205–1546; tel. 614/251–3000; Larry Anstine, Chief Operating Officer (Total facility includes 20 beds in nursing home–type unit) **A**1 2 3 9 10 **F**1 2 3 4 5 8 9 10 11 12 13 15 16 17 18 19 21 22 23 24 25 28 29 30 31 32 33 34 35 36 37 38 39 41 42 43 44 45 46 47 48 49 50 51 53 54 56 57 58 59 60 61 62 63 64 65 66 68 69 70 71 72 74 75 76 77 78 79	12	10	150	5172	75	42216	0	—	—	542
✠ △ **OHIO STATE UNIVERSITY MEDICAL CENTER**, 410 West 10th Avenue, Zip 43210–1240; tel. 614/293–8000; R. Reed Fraley, Vice President for Health Services **A**1 3 5 7 8 9 10 **F**1 3 4 5 8 9 10 11 12 13 16 17 18 19 20 21 22 24 25 27 28 29 30 32 33 34 35 36 37 38 39 41 42 43 44 45 46 47 48 49 50 51 53 54 56 57 58 59 60 61 62 63 64 65 66 68 70 71 72 74 75 76 77 78 79	12	10	550	25327	389	298291	3253	351217	125122	3514
CONNEAUT—Ashtabula County										
✠ **UHHS BROWN MEMORIAL HOSPITAL**, 158 West Main Road, Zip 44030–2039, Mailing Address: P.O. Box 648, Zip 44030–0648; tel. 440/593–1131; William P. Lawrence, Chief Executive Officer **A**1 9 10 **F**7 8 9 13 16 17 19 22 25 30 32 34 36 38 39 41 44 46 48 49 50 54 57 59 62 63 64 68 70 72 75 76 78 79 **P**6 7 **S** University Hospitals Health System, Cleveland, OH	23	10	51	1794	22	141227	259	15247	6506	175
COSHOCTON—Coshocton County										
☐ **COSHOCTON COUNTY MEMORIAL HOSPITAL**, 1460 Orange Street, Zip 43812–6330, Mailing Address: P.O. Box 1330, Zip 43812–6330; tel. 740/622–6411; Gregory M. Nowak, Administrator and Chief Executive Officer (Total facility includes 61 beds in nursing home–type unit) (Nonreporting) **A**1 9 10 **Web address:** www.ccmh.com	23	10	151	—	—	—	—	—	—	—
CRESTLINE—Crawford County CRESTLINE HOSPITAL See MedCentral Health System, Mansfield										
CUYAHOGA FALLS—Summit County										
+ ○ △ **CUYAHOGA FALLS GENERAL HOSPITAL**, 1900 23rd Street, Zip 44223–1499; tel. 330/971–7000; Fred Anthony, President and Chief Executive Officer **A**7 9 10 11 12 13 **F**7 8 9 13 16 17 18 19 20 22 24 25 31 32 34 36 38 39 41 43 44 45 46 48 49 54 56 57 61 62 63 64 70 72 73 76 77 78 79 **P**6 8 **Web address:** www.cfgh.org	23	10	135	3975	54	84711	549	50861	23052	634
DAYTON—Montgomery County										
✠ **CHILDREN'S MEDICAL CENTER**, One Children's Plaza, Zip 45404–1815; tel. 937/226–8300; Laurence P. Harkness, President and Chief Executive Officer **A**1 3 5 8 9 10 **F**7 11 13 14 16 17 18 19 22 23 25 26 29 31 32 33 34 35 36 37 38 39 42 43 45 46 48 49 50 51 52 56 58 59 60 63 70 72 73 76 77 78 **Web address:** www.cmc-dayton.org/ DAYTON CAMPUS See Twin Valley Psychiatric System	23	50	123	6148	77	226693	0	83835	37556	1093
☐ △ **FRANCISCAN MEDICAL CENTER–DAYTON CAMPUS**, One Franciscan Way, Zip 45408–1498; tel. 937/229–6000; James E. Grobmyer, Interim Chief Executive Officer (Total facility includes 30 beds in nursing home–type unit) **A**1 2 3 5 7 9 10 **F**1 6 8 9 11 13 16 17 18 19 20 21 22 23 24 25 26 28 29 30 31 32 33 34 35 36 37 38 39 41 42 43 44 45 46 48 49 50 51 53 54 56 57 58 59 60 61 63 64 65 67 69 70 71 72 73 75 76 77 78 79 **P**1 4 7 **S** Franciscan Health Partnership, Inc., Latham, NY	21	10	317	12276	193	267591	890	130800	61400	1672

Many Facility Codes have changed. Please refer to the AHA Guide Code Chart.

© 2000 AHA Guide

Hospitals, U.S. / OHIO

Hospital, Address, Telephone, Administrator, Approval, Facility, and Physician Codes, Health Care System, Network	Classification Codes		Utilization Data					Expense (thousands) of dollars		
★ American Hospital Association (AHA) membership ☐ Joint Commission on Accreditation of Healthcare Organizations (JCAHO) accreditation + American Osteopathic Healthcare Association (AOHA) membership ○ American Osteopathic Association (AOA) accreditation △ Commission on Accreditation of Rehabilitation Facilities (CARF) accreditation Control codes 61, 63, 64, 71, 72 and 73 indicate hospitals listed by AOHA, but not registered by AHA. For definition of numerical codes, see page A4	Control	Service	Staffed Beds	Admissions	Census	Outpatient Visits	Births	Total	Payroll	Personnel
★ GOOD SAMARITAN HOSPITAL AND HEALTH CENTER, 2222 Philadelphia Drive, Zip 45406-1813; tel. 937/278-2612; K. Douglas Deck, President and Chief Executive Officer **A**1 2 3 5 9 10 **F**2 3 4 6 7 8 9 10 11 12 13 16 17 18 19 20 21 22 23 24 25 27 29 30 31 32 33 34 35 36 38 39 41 42 43 44 45 46 47 48 49 50 51 53 54 56 57 58 59 60 61 62 63 64 65 67 69 70 71 72 74 75 76 77 78 79 **P**6 8 **S** Catholic Health Initiatives, Denver, CO GRANDVIEW HOSPITAL AND MEDICAL CENTER See Kettering Medical Center-Network, Kettering KETTERING YOUTH SERVICES See Kettering Medical Center-Network, Kettering	21	10	496	16785	210	208303	1428	174577	76832	2310
★ △ MIAMI VALLEY HOSPITAL, One Wyoming Street, Zip 45409-2793; tel. 937/208-8000; William M. Thornton, Presdent and Chief Executive Officer **A**1 2 3 5 7 8 9 10 **F**1 3 4 8 9 10 11 12 13 16 17 18 19 21 22 23 24 25 26 27 28 29 30 31 32 33 34 35 36 38 39 40 41 42 43 44 45 46 47 48 49 50 51 53 54 56 57 58 59 60 61 62 63 64 65 66 68 70 71 72 73 74 75 76 77 78 **P**5 8 SOUTHVIEW HOSPITAL AND FAMILY HEALTH CENTER See Kettering Medical Center-Network, Kettering	23	10	603	28382	385	568302	5309	319510	139129	4102
☐ TWIN VALLEY PSYCHIATRIC SYSTEM, (Includes Columbus Campus, 2200 West Broad Street, Columbus, Zip 43223-1295; tel. 614/752-0333; Dayton Campus, 2611 Wayne Avenue, tel. 937/258-0440), 2611 Wayne Avenue, Zip 45420-1800; tel. 937/258-0440; James Ignelzi, Chief Executive Officer **A**1 10 **F**13 16 17 18 23 57 63 70 72 78 **P**6	12	22	438	938	344	—	—	51979	35269	810
★ VETERANS AFFAIRS MEDICAL CENTER, 4100 West Third Street, Zip 45428-1002; tel. 937/268-6511; Steven M. Cohen, M.D., Director (Total facility includes 282 beds in nursing home-type unit) (Nonreporting) **A**1 3 5 8 9 **S** Department of Veterans Affairs, Washington, DC **Web address:** www.va.gov/stations97/guide/home.asp?DIVISION=ALL	45	10	835	—	—	—	—	—	—	—
DEFIANCE—Defiance County										
★ DEFIANCE HOSPITAL, 1206 East Second Street, Zip 43512-2495; tel. 419/783-6955; Robert J. Coholich, President **A**1 9 10 **F**7 8 9 12 17 18 22 24 25 31 32 33 34 36 39 40 41 43 44 45 46 48 50 51 54 57 60 61 62 63 64 68 70 72 76 78 **P**6 7 8 **S** ProMedica Health System, Toledo, OH **Web address:** www.promedica.org	23	10	80	2888	30	32370	535	25027	9637	287
DELAWARE—Delaware County										
☐ △ GRADY MEMORIAL HOSPITAL, 561 West Central Avenue, Zip 43015-1485; tel. 740/369-8711; Everett P. Weber, Jr, President and Chief Executive Officer (Nonreporting) **A**1 2 7 9 10	23	10	84	—	—	—	—	—	—	—
DENNISON—Tuscarawas County										
★ TWIN CITY HOSPITAL, 819 North First Street, Zip 44621-1098; tel. 740/922-2800; Cheryl Hicks, Chief Executive Officer **A**1 9 10 **F**7 9 12 13 16 18 19 22 23 24 25 32 33 34 36 37 38 41 43 45 48 50 51 53 54 55 56 69 70 71 76 78 79 **P**7 **Web address:** www.twincityhospital.org	23	10	30	678	9	73355	0	6709	3149	123
DOVER—Tuscarawas County										
★ UNION HOSPITAL, 659 Boulevard, Zip 44622-2077; tel. 330/343-3311; William W. Harding, President and Chief Executive Officer **A**1 9 10 **F**7 8 9 16 17 18 19 22 24 25 32 34 36 38 39 41 43 44 46 48 49 54 59 61 68 70 71 72 76 78	23	10	104	4980	52	190464	834	37897	17372	532
EAST LIVERPOOL—Columbiana County										
★ EAST LIVERPOOL CITY HOSPITAL, 425 West Fifth Street, Zip 43920-2498; tel. 330/385-7200; Melvin R. Creeley, President (Total facility includes 20 beds in nursing home-type unit) **A**1 9 10 **F**1 7 8 9 12 14 17 18 22 23 24 25 26 30 31 32 33 36 38 39 41 43 44 45 46 48 50 51 54 57 59 61 62 63 68 69 70 72 76 77 **P**8 **Web address:** www.eastliverpoolhospital.baweb.com/	23	10	160	6627	92	68282	400	40583	18443	574
ELYRIA—Lorain County										
★ EMH REGIONAL MEDICAL CENTER, 630 East River Street, Zip 44035-5902; tel. 440/329-7500; Kevin C. Martin, President and Chief Executive Officer **A**1 2 9 10 **F**4 7 8 9 11 12 13 16 17 18 22 24 25 27 28 30 31 32 34 36 37 38 39 41 42 43 44 45 46 47 48 54 56 57 59 60 61 68 70 71 72 74 76 77 78 79 **P**7 8 **Web address:** www.emh-healthcare.org	23	10	266	12329	138	213402	1057	107594	37715	1068
EUCLID—Cuyahoga County										
☐ △ EUCLID HOSPITAL, (Formerly Meridia Euclid Hospital), 18901 Lake Shore Boulevard, Zip 44119-1090; tel. 216/531-9000; Lauren Rock, Chief Operating Officer (Total facility includes 40 beds in nursing home-type unit) **A**1 2 7 9 10 **F**2 3 4 7 8 9 11 12 13 14 16 17 18 19 22 24 25 28 29 30 31 32 33 34 35 37 38 39 40 41 42 44 45 46 47 48 49 50 51 52 53 54 55 57 59 60 61 62 63 64 65 66 68 69 70 71 72 73 75 76 77 78 79 **P**1 3 4 7 8 **S** Cleveland Clinic Health System, Cleveland, OH **Web address:** www.meridia.org	23	10	187	6867	141	59705	416	50745	24337	645
FAIRFIELD—Butler County										
MERCY HOSPITAL OF FAIRFIELD See Mercy Hospital, Hamilton										

© 2000 AHA Guide   *Many Facility Codes have changed. Please refer to the AHA Guide Code Chart.*

Hospitals, U.S. / OHIO

Hospital, Address, Telephone, Administrator, Approval, Facility, and Physician Codes, Health Care System, Network

- ★ American Hospital Association (AHA) membership
- ☐ Joint Commission on Accreditation of Healthcare Organizations (JCAHO) accreditation
- + American Osteopathic Healthcare Association (AOHA) membership
- ○ American Osteopathic Association (AOA) accreditation
- △ Commission on Accreditation of Rehabilitation Facilities (CARF) accreditation

Control codes 61, 63, 64, 71, 72 and 73 indicate hospitals listed by AOHA, but not registered by AHA. For definition of numerical codes, see page A4.

Hospital	Control	Service	Staffed Beds	Admissions	Census	Outpatient Visits	Births	Total	Payroll	Personnel
FINDLAY—Hancock County ★ BLANCHARD VALLEY HEALTH ASSOCIATION SYSTEM, (Includes Blanchard Valley Regional Health Center–Bluffton Campus, 139 Garau Street, Bluffton, Zip 45817-0048; tel. 419/358-9010; Blanchard Valley Regional Health Center–Findlay Campus, 145 West Wallace Street, tel. 419/423-4500; Clifford R. Lehman, President), 145 West Wallace Street, Zip 45840-1299; tel. 419/423-4500; William E. Ruse, FACHE, President and Chief Executive Officer **A**1 9 10 **F**1 6 7 8 9 11 13 14 16 17 18 19 22 24 25 26 29 30 31 32 33 34 35 36 37 38 39 40 41 43 44 45 46 48 49 50 51 54 56 57 61 62 64 65 67 69 70 71 72 76 77 78 79 **P**5 Web address: www.bvha.org	23	10	133	7753	83	184732	1273	62700	29216	986
FOSTORIA—Hancock County ★ FOSTORIA COMMUNITY HOSPITAL, 501 Van Buren Street, Zip 44830-0907, Mailing Address: P.O. Box 907, Zip 44830-0907; tel. 419/435-7734; Brad A. Higgins, President **A**1 9 10 **F**7 8 9 12 16 17 18 19 22 24 25 31 32 33 34 35 36 38 39 40 41 43 44 45 46 48 49 50 51 54 68 70 71 72 75 76 78 **S** ProMedica Health System, Toledo, OH Web address: www.fchosp.org	23	10	39	1348	12	44223	180	16976	6636	204
FREMONT—Sandusky County ★ MEMORIAL HOSPITAL, 715 South Taft Avenue, Zip 43420-3200; tel. 419/332-7321; John A. Gorman, Chief Executive Officer **A**1 9 10 **F**1 8 9 16 17 18 19 22 24 31 33 34 36 37 38 39 40 41 43 44 45 46 48 50 54 57 59 60 62 63 64 70 76 78 79 **P**6 8 **S** Quorum Health Group, Brentwood, TN Web address: www.fremontmemorial.org	23	10	121	3036	29	37650	503	32178	13014	377
GALION—Crawford County ★ GALION COMMUNITY HOSPITAL, 269 Portland Way South, Zip 44833-2399; tel. 419/468-4841; Lyndon J. Christman, President and Chief Executive Officer (Total facility includes 33 beds in nursing home–type unit) **A**1 9 10 **F**7 8 9 16 17 18 19 22 24 25 32 34 36 37 39 40 41 43 44 45 46 48 54 68 69 70 72 76 78 79 **P**3 **S** OhioHealth, Columbus, OH Web address: www.galionhospital.org	23	10	108	2150	36	38146	483	19203	7349	262
GALLIPOLIS—Gallia County ★ △ HOLZER MEDICAL CENTER, 100 Jackson Pike, Zip 45631-1563; tel. 740/446-5000; LaMar L. Wyse, President and Chief Executive Officer **A**1 2 7 9 10 **F**8 9 12 13 18 19 22 24 25 27 28 29 30 33 34 36 37 39 41 43 44 45 46 48 51 53 54 63 65 68 69 70 72 76 78 79 **P**5 6 Web address: www.holzer.org	23	10	149	6233	59	84103	812	52555	20997	799
GARFIELD HEIGHTS—Cuyahoga County ★ △ MARYMOUNT HOSPITAL, 12300 McCracken Road, Zip 44125-2975; tel. 216/581-0500; Thomas J. Trudell, President and Chief Executive Officer (Nonreporting) **A**1 2 6 7 10 **S** Cleveland Clinic Health System, Cleveland, OH	21	10	213	—	—	—	—	—	—	—
GENEVA—Ashtabula County ★ UHHS–MEMORIAL HOSPITAL OF GENEVA, 870 West Main Street, Zip 44041-1295; tel. 440/466-1141; William P. Lawrence, President and Chief Executive Officer **A**1 9 10 **F**7 9 12 13 16 17 18 19 22 25 32 34 38 39 43 45 46 48 49 50 51 54 68 70 72 75 76 78 79 **P**7 **S** University Hospitals Health System, Cleveland, OH Web address: www.uhhs.com	23	10	40	1237	12	—	0	14583	5195	152
GEORGETOWN—Brown County ★ BROWN COUNTY GENERAL HOSPITAL, 425 Home Street, Zip 45121-1407; tel. 937/378-6121; David T. Wallace, President and Chief Executive Officer **A**1 9 10 **F**3 7 8 9 16 17 22 24 25 32 34 36 37 39 41 44 45 46 48 50 51 58 59 60 61 62 63 64 68 70 74 76 78 **P**6 **S** Quorum Health Group, Brentwood, TN Web address: www.bcgh.org	13	10	53	1654	14	52180	435	15579	6610	269
GREEN SPRINGS—Sandusky County ★ △ ST. FRANCIS HEALTH CARE CENTRE, 401 North Broadway, Zip 44836-9653; tel. 419/639-2626; Dan Schwanke, Executive Director (Total facility includes 150 beds in nursing home–type unit) **A**1 7 9 10 **F**13 16 17 18 26 30 31 35 38 43 45 51 54 69 70 72 78	21	49	186	546	102	6781	—	12600	4675	160
GREENFIELD—Highland County ★ △ GREENFIELD AREA MEDICAL CENTER, 550 Mirabeau Street, Zip 45123; tel. 937/981-2116; Mark E. Marchetti, Chief Executive Officer (Nonreporting) **A**1 7 9 10	23	10	36	—	—	—	—	—	—	—
GREENVILLE—Darke County ☐ WAYNE HOSPITAL, 835 Sweitzer Street, Zip 45331-1077; tel. 937/548-1141; Raymond E. Laughlin, Jr, President and Chief Executive Officer **A**1 9 10 **F**7 8 9 17 18 19 22 24 25 32 38 39 41 43 44 48 49 50 54 68 70 76 78 **P**5 6	23	10	92	2820	32	79482	464	27432	12055	415
HAMILTON—Butler County ★ FORT HAMILTON HOSPITAL, 630 Eaton Avenue, Zip 45013-2770; tel. 513/867-2000; James A. Kingsbury, President and Chief Executive Officer **A**1 2 9 10 **F**2 3 4 5 7 8 9 10 11 12 13 14 15 16 17 18 19 20 21 22 23 24 25 26 27 28 29 30 31 32 33 34 35 36 37 38 39 40 41 42 43 44 45 46 47 48 49 50 51 53 54 55 56 57 58 59 60 61 62 63 64 65 66 67 68 69 70 71 72 73 74 75 76 77 78 79 **P**7 8 **S** Health Alliance of Greater Cincinnati, Cincinnati, OH Web address: www.health–alliance.com	23	10	181	8349	100	98074	1229	74915	35480	844

Hospitals, U.S. / OHIO

Hospital, Address, Telephone, Administrator, Approval, Facility, and Physician Codes, Health Care System, Network	Classification Codes		Utilization Data					Expense (thousands) of dollars		
★ American Hospital Association (AHA) membership ☐ Joint Commission on Accreditation of Healthcare Organizations (JCAHO) accreditation + American Osteopathic Healthcare Association (AOHA) membership ○ American Osteopathic Association (AOA) accreditation △ Commission on Accreditation of Rehabilitation Facilities (CARF) accreditation Control codes 61, 63, 64, 71, 72 and 73 indicate hospitals listed by AOHA, but not registered by AHA. For definition of numerical codes, see page A4	Control	Service	Staffed Beds	Admissions	Census	Outpatient Visits	Births	Total	Payroll	Personnel
☐ △ MERCY HOSPITAL, (Includes Mercy Hospital of Fairfield, 3000 Mack Road, Fairfield; Mercy Hospital of Hamilton, 100 Riverfront Plaza), Mailing Address: P.O. Box 418, Zip 45012-0418; tel. 513/867-6400; David A. Ferrell, President (Total facility includes 32 beds in nursing home–type unit) **A**1 2 7 9 10 **F**1 4 6 8 9 11 13 15 16 17 18 19 20 22 24 25 28 29 30 31 32 33 34 36 38 39 40 41 43 44 45 46 48 49 50 51 53 54 67 68 69 70 71 72 76 77 78 79 **P**6 8 **S** Catholic Healthcare Partners, Cincinnati, OH Web address: www.mercy.health-partners.org	21	10	205	10712	143	181942	1436	96419	39215	1080
HICKSVILLE—Defiance County										
☐ COMMUNITY MEMORIAL HOSPITAL, 208 North Columbus Street, Zip 43526-1299; tel. 419/542-6692; Olas A. Hubbs, Chief Executive Officer **A**1 9 10 **F**7 9 13 16 17 19 21 22 25 28 29 32 34 37 38 39 40 43 44 48 54 56 70 71 72 76 77 78 Web address: www.cmhosp.com	16	10	22	485	5	16183	108	6704	2426	108
HILLSBORO—Highland County										
★ HIGHLAND DISTRICT HOSPITAL, 1275 North High Street, Zip 45133-8571; tel. 937/393-6100; Charles H. Bair, Chief Executive Officer **A**1 9 10 **F**7 8 9 13 16 17 18 19 22 39 44 45 46 48 51 54 70 71 73 76 78	16	10	51	2243	23	55129	365	22705	9109	304
IRONTON—Lawrence County										
☐ RIVER VALLEY HEALTH SYSTEM, (Includes Behavioral Health–Portsmouth Campus, 2201 25th Street, Portsmouth, Zip 45662-3252; tel. 614/354-2804; Rick E. Harlow, Vice President Behavioral Health), 2228 South Ninth Street, Zip 45638-2526; tel. 740/532-3231; Terry L. Vanderhoof, President and Chief Executive Officer (Total facility includes 11 beds in nursing home–type unit) (Nonreporting) **A**1 9 10	13	10	219	—	—	—	—	—	—	—
KENTON—Hardin County										
★ HARDIN MEMORIAL HOSPITAL, 921 East Franklin Street, Zip 43326-2099, Mailing Address: P.O. Box 710, Zip 43326-0710; tel. 419/673-0761; Don J. Sabol, Chief Executive Officer **A**1 9 10 **F**1 3 4 5 7 8 9 11 13 14 15 16 17 18 19 20 21 22 23 24 25 26 27 28 29 30 31 32 33 34 35 36 37 38 39 40 41 43 44 45 46 47 48 49 50 51 54 55 56 58 59 60 61 62 63 64 65 66 67 68 70 71 72 73 74 76 77 78 79 **P**3 5 **S** OhioHealth, Columbus, OH	23	10	51	1837	24	53372	158	14753	6082	243
KETTERING—Montgomery County										
CHARLES F. KETTERING MEMORIAL CENTER See Kettering Medical Center–Network										
★ ○ △ KETTERING MEDICAL CENTER–NETWORK, (Formerly Kettering Adventist Health), (Includes Charles F. Kettering Memorial Center, 3535 Southern Boulevard, Zip 45429; tel. 513/298-4331; Grandview Hospital and Medical Center, 405 Grand Avenue, Dayton, Zip 45405-4796; tel. 937/226-3200; Roy G. Chew, Ph.D., President; Kettering Youth Services, 5350 Lamme Road, Dayton, Zip 45439; tel. 513/299-9511; Southview Hospital and Family Health Center, 1997 Miamisburg–Centerville Road, Dayton, Zip 45459-3800; tel. 937/439-6000; Sycamore Hospital, 2150 Leiter Road, Miamisburg, Zip 45342; tel. 513/866-0551), 3535 Southern Boulevard, Zip 45429-1221; tel. 937/298-4331; Francisco J. Perez, FACHE, President **A**1 2 3 5 7 8 9 10 11 12 13 **F**3 4 5 6 8 9 11 13 14 16 17 18 19 21 22 24 25 27 29 30 31 32 33 34 35 36 37 38 39 40 41 42 43 44 45 46 47 48 49 50 51 53 54 55 56 57 58 59 60 61 62 63 64 65 66 67 68 70 71 72 76 78 79 **P**6 8 Web address: www.ketthealth.com	21	10	626	28157	347	284984	2959	386924	173030	4227
LAKEWOOD—Cuyahoga County										
★ △ LAKEWOOD HOSPITAL, 14519 Detroit Avenue, Zip 44107-4383; tel. 216/521-4200; V. Richard Stelzer, Jr, Chief Administrative Officer (Total facility includes 45 beds in nursing home–type unit) **A**1 2 7 9 10 **F**1 2 3 4 5 8 9 10 11 12 13 14 16 17 18 19 22 24 25 27 28 29 30 31 32 33 34 35 36 37 38 39 40 41 42 43 44 45 46 47 48 49 50 51 52 53 54 55 56 57 58 59 60 61 62 63 64 65 66 68 69 70 71 72 73 74 75 76 77 78 79 **P**2 6 7 8 **S** Cleveland Clinic Health System, Cleveland, OH	23	10	328	11099	182	133373	498	96845	46836	1080
LANCASTER—Fairfield County										
★ △ FAIRFIELD MEDICAL CENTER, 401 North Ewing Street, Zip 43130-3371; tel. 740/687-8000; Creighton E. Likes, Jr, President and Chief Executive Officer (Total facility includes 24 beds in nursing home–type unit) **A**1 7 9 10 **F**3 7 8 9 11 13 16 17 18 19 20 21 22 24 25 28 29 30 32 33 34 36 38 39 41 43 44 45 46 48 49 51 53 54 56 57 59 60 61 63 64 65 68 69 70 71 72 75 76 78 **P**4 7 Web address: www.fmchealth.org	23	10	196	11558	135	255181	1403	96592	41235	1158
LIMA—Allen County										
★ △ LIMA MEMORIAL HOSPITAL, 1001 Bellefontaine Avenue, Zip 45804-2899; tel. 419/228-3335; John B. White, President and Chief Executive Officer **A**1 2 7 9 10 **F**4 7 8 9 11 12 13 16 17 19 22 24 25 27 28 30 32 33 34 35 36 38 39 40 41 43 44 45 46 47 48 49 50 51 54 62 65 68 70 71 72 76 78 79 **P**3 7 8	23	10	162	8379	122	158817	547	90310	36073	1016
☐ OAKWOOD CORRECTIONAL FACILITY, 3200 North West Street, Zip 45801-2000; tel. 419/225-8052; Christopher Yanai, M.D., Warden and Chief Executive Officer **A**1 **F**13 16 17 18 19 21 31 34 35 43 49 50 51 56 57 59 60 61 62 63 70 72 78 79 Web address: www.drc.ohio.gov/web/ocf.htm	12	22	131	312	98	—	0	20843	13979	313
☐ △ ST. RITA'S MEDICAL CENTER, 730 West Market Street, Zip 45801-4670; tel. 419/227-3361; James P. Reber, President **A**1 2 7 9 10 **F**2 3 4 8 9 11 12 13 16 17 19 21 22 23 24 25 26 27 28 29 30 31 34 35 36 37 38 39 41 43 44 45 46 47 48 49 50 51 54 55 56 57 58 59 60 61 62 63 65 68 69 70 71 76 77 78 79 **P**8 **S** Catholic Healthcare Partners, Cincinnati, OH Web address: www.mercy.com\srmc	21	10	351	14215	171	279456	2025	155865	65676	1837

Hospitals, U.S. / OHIO

Hospital, Address, Telephone, Administrator, Approval, Facility, and Physician Codes, Health Care System, Network	Classification Codes		Utilization Data					Expense (thousands) of dollars		
★ American Hospital Association (AHA) membership ☐ Joint Commission on Accreditation of Healthcare Organizations (JCAHO) accreditation + American Osteopathic Healthcare Association (AOHA) membership ○ American Osteopathic Association (AOA) accreditation △ Commission on Accreditation of Rehabilitation Facilities (CARF) accreditation Control codes 61, 63, 64, 71, 72 and 73 indicate hospitals listed by AOHA, but not registered by AHA. For definition of numerical codes, see page A4	Control	Service	Staffed Beds	Admissions	Census	Outpatient Visits	Births	Total	Payroll	Personnel
LODI—Medina County ✣ LODI COMMUNITY HOSPITAL, 225 Elyria Street, Zip 44254–1096; tel. 330/948-1222; Thomas L. Lockard, President and Chief Executive Officer (Total facility includes 7 beds in nursing home–type unit) (Nonreporting) **A**1 5 9 10	23	10	21	—	—	—	—	—	—	—
LOGAN—Hocking County ✣ HOCKING VALLEY COMMUNITY HOSPITAL, Route 2, State Route 664, Zip 43138–0966, Mailing Address: Box 966, Zip 43138–0966; tel. 740/385-5631; Larry Willard, Administrator (Total facility includes 30 beds in nursing home–type unit) **A**1 9 10 **F**7 8 9 13 16 17 18 22 25 30 32 34 38 39 44 45 46 48 50 54 55 57 62 68 69 70 71 72 76 78 79 **P**1 3	13	10	92	1725	42	48336	126	18911	6491	238
LONDON—Madison County ✣ MADISON COUNTY HOSPITAL, 210 North Main Street, Zip 43140–1115; tel. 740/852-1372; Stuart W. Williams, Interim Chief Executive Officer (Total facility includes 11 beds in nursing home–type unit) **A**1 9 10 **F**3 8 9 12 16 17 18 19 22 25 28 29 30 32 33 34 35 36 37 38 39 40 41 43 44 45 46 48 49 53 54 57 58 59 63 64 69 70 71 72 73 76 78 79 **P**6	23	10	46	1736	30	13832	176	22736	9928	384
LORAIN—Lorain County ☐ △ LORAIN COMMUNITY/ST. JOSEPH REGIONAL HEALTH CENTER, (Includes Lorain Community/St. Joseph Health Center—East Campus, 205 West 20th Street, Zip 44052–3794; tel. 216/233-1000; Lorain Community/St. Joseph Regional Health Center–West Campus, tel. 216/960-3000), 3700 Kolbe Road, Zip 44053–1697; tel. 440/960-3000; Brian C. Lockwood, President and Chief Executive Officer **A**1 2 7 9 10 **F**4 7 8 9 10 11 12 13 14 16 17 18 19 20 22 24 25 26 27 28 29 30 31 32 33 34 35 36 37 38 39 41 42 43 44 45 46 48 49 50 51 53 54 55 56 57 58 59 60 61 62 63 64 65 69 70 71 72 73 75 76 78 79 **P**5 6 7 **S** Catholic Healthcare Partners, Cincinnati, OH	21	10	282	13217	192	195613	1321	133819	60746	832
MANSFIELD—Richland County ✣ MEDCENTRAL HEALTH SYSTEM, (Includes Crestline Hospital, 291 Heiser Court, Crestline, Zip 44827–1453; tel. 419/683-1212; Susan Brown, Site Administrator and Nursing Director; Mansfield Hospital, 335 Glessner Avenue, tel. 419/526-8000; Shelby Hospital, 20 Morris Road, Shelby, Zip 44875–0608; tel. 419/342-5015; Ron Distl, Vice President and Chief Operating Officer), 335 Glessner Avenue, Zip 44903–2265; tel. 419/526-8000; James E. Meyer, President and Chief Executive Officer **A**1 2 6 9 10 **F**2 3 4 7 8 9 11 12 13 17 18 19 22 23 24 25 26 27 28 29 32 33 34 35 36 37 38 39 41 43 44 45 46 47 48 49 50 51 53 54 57 58 59 60 61 62 63 65 68 70 71 72 75 76 77 78 79 **P**5 7 8 Web address: www.medcentral.org	23	10	350	13304	213	164532	1175	132767	61735	1730
✣ RICHLAND HOSPITAL, 1451 Lucas Road, Zip 44901–0637, Mailing Address: P.O. Box 637, Zip 44901–0637; tel. 419/589-5511; Bruce Waldo, Chief Executive Officer **A**1 9 10 **F**57	23	22	44	397	10	0	0	3844	212	89
MARIETTA—Washington County ✣ △ MARIETTA MEMORIAL HOSPITAL, 401 Matthew Street, Zip 45750–1699; tel. 740/374-1400; Larry J. Unroe, President **A**1 7 9 10 **F**2 3 4 8 9 13 16 17 18 19 22 24 25 27 28 30 31 32 33 34 35 36 37 38 39 41 43 44 45 46 48 50 51 53 54 57 59 60 61 63 64 65 68 69 70 71 72 76 77 78 79 **P**8 Web address: www.mmhospital.org	23	10	135	5903	77	101743	668	53752	23700	785
★ + ○ SELBY GENERAL HOSPITAL, 1106 Colegate Drive, Zip 45750–1323; tel. 740/373-0582; Maryann J. Greenwell, Chief Executive Officer **A**9 10 11 12 13 **F**8 9 13 17 18 19 22 25 30 34 38 39 40 41 43 44 45 46 48 51 54 57 59 62 63 64 66 70 75 76 78 79 **P**6 8 **S** Quorum Health Group, Brentwood, TN Web address: www.selby.wscc.edu	23	10	54	1752	22	27002	110	15725	6547	166
MARION—Marion County ✣ △ MARION GENERAL HOSPITAL, 1000 McKinley Park Drive, Zip 43302–6397; tel. 740/383-8400; Ronald J. Bachman, Interim President and Chief Executive Officer **A**1 2 7 9 10 **F**1 8 9 11 17 18 19 22 24 25 32 34 35 36 37 38 39 41 43 44 45 46 48 49 50 51 53 54 57 58 59 60 61 62 63 64 65 70 71 72 78 79 **P**7 8 **S** OhioHealth, Columbus, OH Web address: www.mariongeneral.com	23	10	188	8772	99	146112	1000	79778	33594	997
MEDCENTER HOSPITAL, 1050 Delaware Avenue, Zip 43302–6459; tel. 740/383-8000; Cheryl Herbert, President (Nonreporting) **A**9	23	10	86	—	—	—	—	—	—	—
MARTINS FERRY—Belmont County ✣ EAST OHIO REGIONAL HOSPITAL, 90 North Fourth Street, Zip 43935–1648; tel. 740/633-1100; Brian K. Felici, Vice President and Administrator (Total facility includes 94 beds in nursing home–type unit) **A**1 9 10 **F**2 3 5 7 8 9 11 12 13 16 17 18 19 20 21 22 23 24 25 27 28 29 30 31 32 33 34 35 36 38 39 41 43 44 45 46 48 49 50 51 52 53 54 56 57 58 59 60 61 62 63 64 65 66 68 69 70 71 72 76 77 78 79 **P**6 8 **S** Ohio Valley Health Services, Wheeling, WV Web address: www.evha.com/web/ovmc/	23	10	165	4180	131	141641	274	41422	17347	509
MARYSVILLE—Union County ✣ MEMORIAL HOSPITAL, 500 London Avenue, Zip 43040–1594; tel. 937/644-6115; Danny L. Boggs, President and Chief Executive Officer (Total facility includes 112 beds in nursing home–type unit) **A**1 9 10 **F**7 8 9 12 13 15 16 17 18 19 22 31 32 34 35 36 38 39 40 43 44 45 46 48 51 54 68 69 70 71 72 76 77 78 **P**2 7	13	10	162	2534	97	109035	655	38378	17663	527
MASSILLON—Stark County ★ + ○ △ DOCTORS HOSPITAL OF STARK COUNTY, 400 Austin Avenue N.W., Zip 44646–3554; tel. 330/837-7200; Thomas E. Cecconi, Chief Executive Officer **A**2 7 9 10 11 12 13 **F**8 9 11 13 16 17 18 22 25 27 30 31 34 36 38 39 41 43 44 45 46 48 51 53 54 56 57 59 62 64 70 72 76 78 79 **P**7 8 **S** Quorum Health Group, Brentwood, TN Web address: www.drshospital.com	33	10	110	3983	59	62460	346	42482	18297	508

Hospitals, U.S. / OHIO

Hospital, Address, Telephone, Administrator, Approval, Facility, and Physician Codes, Health Care System, Network	Classification Codes		Utilization Data					Expense (thousands) of dollars		
★ American Hospital Association (AHA) membership □ Joint Commission on Accreditation of Healthcare Organizations (JCAHO) accreditation + American Osteopathic Healthcare Association (AOHA) membership ○ American Osteopathic Association (AOA) accreditation △ Commission on Accreditation of Rehabilitation Facilities (CARF) accreditation Control codes 61, 63, 64, 71, 72 and 73 indicate hospitals listed by AOHA, but not registered by AHA. For definition of numerical codes, see page A4	Control	Service	Staffed Beds	Admissions	Census	Outpatient Visits	Births	Total	Payroll	Personnel
★ △ MASSILLON COMMUNITY HOSPITAL, 875 Eighth Street N.E., Zip 44646-8503, Mailing Address: P.O. Box 805, Zip 44648-8503; tel. 330/832-8761; Mervin F. Strine, President and Chief Executive Officer (Total facility includes 20 beds in nursing home–type unit) **A**1 7 9 10 **F**2 3 4 8 9 13 17 18 19 20 22 23 24 25 28 30 32 33 34 35 36 38 39 41 43 44 45 48 49 50 51 53 54 57 62 64 68 69 70 72 76 78 **P**4 6 7 8 **Web address:** www.mchosp.org	23	10	159	4719	70	102622	190	41332	19358	644
□ MASSILLON PSYCHIATRIC CENTER, 3000 Erie Street, Zip 44646-7993, Mailing Address: Box 540, Zip 44648-0540; tel. 330/833-3135; Cathy L. Cincinat, Chief Executive Officer (Nonreporting) **A**1 10	12	22	184	—	—	—	—	—	—	—
MAUMEE—Lucas County										
□ FOCUS HEALTHCARE OF OHIO, (Formerly Charter Hospital of Toledo), 1725 Timber Line Road, Zip 43537-4015; tel. 419/891-9333; Joseph R. Hartel, Chief Executive Officer **A**1 10 **F**2 17 18 57 58 61 64	33	52	42	891	22	166	0	—	—	58
★ ST. LUKE'S HOSPITAL, 5901 Monclova Road, Zip 43537-1899; tel. 419/893-5911; Frank J. Bartell, II, President and Chief Executive Officer (Total facility includes 26 beds in nursing home–type unit) **A**1 2 9 10 **F**8 9 11 13 16 17 18 19 22 24 25 31 32 34 38 39 40 45 46 48 50 51 54 59 68 69 70 71 72 73 76 78 **P**8 **Web address:** www.stlukeshospital.com	23	10	170	10288	127	146212	763	89493	40564	998
MEDINA—Medina County										
□ △ MEDINA GENERAL HOSPITAL, 1000 East Washington Street, Zip 44256-2170; tel. 330/725-1000; Gary D. Hallman, President and Chief Executive Officer **A**1 2 7 9 10 **F**8 9 13 14 16 17 19 22 23 24 25 29 32 34 38 39 41 43 44 46 48 54 56 66 70 71 72 76 78 79 **P**8 **Web address:** www.medinahospital.org	23	10	118	4951	56	174593	908	58514	25988	866
MIAMISBURG—Montgomery County SYCAMORE HOSPITAL See Kettering Medical Center–Network, Kettering										
MIDDLEBURG HEIGHTS—Cuyahoga County										
□ SOUTHWEST GENERAL HEALTH CENTER, 18697 Bagley Road, Zip 44130-3497; tel. 440/816-8000; L. Jon Schurmeier, President and Chief Executive Officer **A**1 2 9 10 **F**2 3 4 7 8 9 11 12 13 14 16 17 18 19 20 21 22 23 24 25 28 29 30 31 32 33 34 35 37 38 39 41 43 44 45 46 47 48 49 50 51 53 54 57 58 59 60 61 62 63 64 65 69 70 71 72 73 75 76 77 78 79 **P**6 8 **Web address:** www.swgeneral.com	23	10	293	13172	192	279037	1477	142061	63336	1776
MIDDLETOWN—Butler County										
★ △ MIDDLETOWN REGIONAL HOSPITAL, 105 McKnight Drive, Zip 45044-4838; tel. 513/424-2111; Douglas W. McNeill, FACHE, President and Chief Executive Officer **A**1 2 7 9 10 **F**4 6 8 9 11 13 14 16 17 18 19 21 22 24 25 27 28 30 32 33 34 36 37 39 40 43 45 46 48 49 51 54 58 59 60 61 62 63 64 65 68 70 71 72 76 77 78 79 **P**6 8 **Web address:** www.middletownhospital.org	23	10	183	9065	101	—	1129	83439	35993	1311
MILLERSBURG—Holmes County										
□ JOEL POMERENE MEMORIAL HOSPITAL, 981 Wooster Road, Zip 44654-1094; tel. 330/674-1015; P. W. Smith, Jr, Administrator and Chief Executive Officer **A**1 9 10 **F**8 9 16 17 22 25 29 32 39 41 44 45 48 54 70 71 76 78 **P**5	13	10	38	2030	15	27086	589	15543	5936	179
MONTPELIER—Williams County MONTPELIER HOSPITAL See Community Hospitals of Williams County, Bryan										
MOUNT GILEAD—Morrow County										
★ MORROW COUNTY HOSPITAL, 651 West Marion Road, Zip 43338-1096; tel. 419/946-5015; Alan C. Pauley, Administrator (Total facility includes 38 beds in nursing home–type unit) **A**1 9 10 **F**1 7 8 9 16 17 19 22 24 25 32 34 36 38 39 40 41 43 44 46 48 54 56 69 70 71 76 78 **P**7 8 **S** OhioHealth, Columbus, OH **Web address:** www.mtgilead.com	13	10	75	1067	41	31652	96	12269	4564	172
MOUNT VERNON—Knox County										
★ KNOX COMMUNITY HOSPITAL, 1330 Coshocton Road, Zip 43050-1495; tel. 740/393-9000; Robert G. Polahar, Chief Executive Officer **A**1 9 10 **F**7 8 16 17 18 22 25 36 39 40 41 44 46 48 51 57 64 70 76 78 **S** Quorum Health Group, Brentwood, TN	23	10	75	4352	46	75927	414	22034	14789	503
NAPOLEON—Henry County										
★ HENRY COUNTY HOSPITAL, 11600 State Route 424, Zip 43545-9399; tel. 419/592-4015; Kimberly Bordenkircher, Chief Executive Officer **A**1 9 10 **F**3 7 8 9 17 18 22 24 25 34 38 39 43 44 46 48 50 51 54 58 59 60 62 63 70 71 72 76 78 **P**3	23	10	39	868	7	28986	136	10712	4309	107
NELSONVILLE—Athens County										
★ + ○ DOCTORS HOSPITAL OF NELSONVILLE, 1950 Mount Saint Mary Drive, Zip 45764-1193; tel. 740/753-1931; Joel Kaiser, Chief Executive Officer (Total facility includes 45 beds in nursing home–type unit) (Nonreporting) **A**9 10 11 **S** OhioHealth, Columbus, OH	23	10	70	—	—	—	—	—	—	—
NEWARK—Licking County										
★ LICKING MEMORIAL HOSPITAL, 1320 West Main Street, Zip 43055-3699; tel. 740/348-4000; William J. Andrews, President **A**1 9 10 **F**1 2 3 7 8 9 11 13 14 16 17 18 19 20 21 22 24 25 32 33 34 36 38 39 41 43 44 45 46 48 49 50 51 54 56 57 59 60 61 62 63 64 65 66 68 70 72 76 77 78 79 **P**6	23	10	165	7057	69	—	1059	62370	30035	914

Hospitals, U.S. / OHIO

Hospital, Address, Telephone, Administrator, Approval, Facility, and Physician Codes, Health Care System, Network	Classification Codes		Utilization Data					Expense (thousands) of dollars		
	Control	Service	Staffed Beds	Admissions	Census	Outpatient Visits	Births	Total	Payroll	Personnel

★ American Hospital Association (AHA) membership
□ Joint Commission on Accreditation of Healthcare Organizations (JCAHO) accreditation
+ American Osteopathic Healthcare Association (AOHA) membership
○ American Osteopathic Association (AOA) accreditation
△ Commission on Accreditation of Rehabilitation Facilities (CARF) accreditation
Control codes 61, 63, 64, 71, 72 and 73 indicate hospitals listed by AOHA, but not registered by AHA. For definition of numerical codes, see page A4

NORTHFIELD—Summit County
□ NORTHCOAST BEHAVIORAL HEALTHCARE SYSTEM, (Includes Cleveland Campus, 1708 Southpoint Drive, Cleveland, Zip 44109-1999; tel. 216/787-0500; Northfield Campus, 1756 Sagamore Road, tel. 330/467-7131; Toledo Campus, 930 South Detroit Avenue, Toledo, Zip 43614-2701; tel. 419/381-1881), 1756 Sagamore Road, Zip 44067; tel. 330/467-7131; George P. Gintoli, Chief Executive Officer **A**1 5 10 **F**16 17 23 31 51 57 59 60 62 70 72 78 **P**6 — 12 22 333 2559 380 0 0 — — 923

NORWALK—Huron County
★ + ○ FISHER–TITUS MEDICAL CENTER, 272 Benedict Avenue, Zip 44857-2374; tel. 419/668-8101; Patrick J. Martin, President and Chief Executive Officer (Total facility includes 69 beds in nursing home–type unit) **A**1 2 9 10 11 **F**4 6 7 8 9 13 17 18 19 22 23 24 25 27 30 31 32 33 34 36 39 40 41 43 44 45 46 48 50 54 59 61 67 68 69 70 71 72 76 78 79 **P**2 7
Web address: www.fisher-titus.com — 23 10 134 3882 99 103478 682 42631 18583 548

OAK HILL—Jackson County
★ OAK HILL COMMUNITY MEDICAL CENTER, 350 Charlotte Avenue, Zip 45656-1326; tel. 740/682-7717; Robert A. Bowers, Chief Executive Officer (Total facility includes 24 beds in nursing home–type unit) (Nonreporting) **A**9 10 12 — 23 10 68 — — — — — — —

OBERLIN—Lorain County
★ ALLEN MEMORIAL HOSPITAL, 200 West Lorain Street, Zip 44074-1077; tel. 440/775-1211; James H. Schaum, President and Chief Executive Officer (Total facility includes 16 beds in nursing home–type unit) **A**1 9 10 **F**7 8 9 13 14 16 17 18 19 20 22 23 24 25 30 32 33 34 35 36 38 39 40 41 43 44 45 46 48 49 50 54 66 69 70 71 76 77 78 — 23 10 91 1839 24 21609 271 16409 7278 201

OREGON—Lucas County
□ △ ST. CHARLES MERCY HOSPITAL, 2600 Navarre Avenue, Zip 43616-3297; tel. 419/696-7200; Cathleen K. Nelson, President and Chief Executive Officer (Total facility includes 20 beds in nursing home–type unit) **A**1 2 7 9 10 **F**2 3 4 7 8 9 10 11 12 13 14 16 17 18 19 20 22 24 25 26 27 28 29 30 31 32 34 35 36 37 38 39 40 41 42 43 44 45 46 47 48 49 50 51 52 53 54 56 57 58 59 61 62 63 64 65 67 68 69 70 71 72 73 74 75 76 77 78 **P**1 3 6 **S** Catholic Healthcare Partners, Cincinnati, OH
Web address: www.mercyweb.org — 21 10 309 11280 160 134594 865 107464 53454 1473

ORRVILLE—Wayne County
★ DUNLAP MEMORIAL HOSPITAL, 832 South Main Street, Zip 44667-2208; tel. 330/682-3010; Lynn V. Horner, President and Chief Executive Officer (Nonreporting) **A**1 9 10 — 23 10 38 — — — — — — —

OXFORD—Butler County
★ MCCULLOUGH–HYDE MEMORIAL HOSPITAL, 110 North Poplar Street, Zip 45056-1292; tel. 513/523-2111; Richard A. Daniels, President and Chief Executive Officer **A**1 9 10 **F**7 8 9 13 16 17 18 19 22 24 25 31 32 34 36 37 38 39 40 41 43 44 45 46 48 54 68 70 71 72 76 77 78
Web address: www.mhmh.org/ — 23 10 44 2723 21 59210 489 26675 11736 294

PAINESVILLE—Lake County
★ △ LAKE HOSPITAL SYSTEM, 10 East Washington, Zip 44077-3472; tel. 440/354-2400; Cynthia Ann Moore–Hardy, President and Chief Executive Officer **A**1 2 7 9 10 **F**4 7 8 9 11 13 14 16 17 18 19 21 22 23 24 25 29 30 31 32 33 34 35 36 37 38 39 41 42 43 44 45 46 47 48 49 50 51 54 57 62 65 68 69 70 71 72 76 77 78 79 **P**1 3
Web address: www.lhs.net — 23 10 374 13538 170 429153 1497 139828 55613 1478

PARMA—Cuyahoga County
★ △ PARMA COMMUNITY GENERAL HOSPITAL, 7007 Powers Boulevard, Zip 44129-5495; tel. 440/743-3000; Thomas A. Selden, President and Chief Executive Officer (Total facility includes 27 beds in nursing home–type unit) **A**1 2 7 9 10 **F**1 4 7 8 9 11 12 13 14 16 17 18 19 22 24 25 26 28 30 31 32 33 34 36 37 38 39 40 41 43 44 45 46 47 48 49 50 51 53 54 57 60 62 63 64 69 70 71 72 76 78 **P**1 6
Web address: www.parmahospital.org — 23 10 283 13213 215 184717 774 111925 49754 1394

PAULDING—Paulding County
□ PAULDING COUNTY HOSPITAL, 1035 West Wayne Street, Zip 45879-9220; tel. 419/399-4080; Larry Thornhill, Chief Executive Officer (Nonreporting) **A**1 9 10
Web address: www.bright.net/~pch/ — 13 10 51 — — — — — — —

POMEROY—Meigs County
VETERANS MEMORIAL HOSPITAL OF MEIGS COUNTY, 115 East Memorial Drive, Zip 45769-9572; tel. 740/992-2104; Robert Bowers, Chief Executive Officer (Total facility includes 40 beds in nursing home–type unit) **A**9 10 12 **F**16 17 18 22 25 32 36 37 38 43 45 46 48 50 57 62 69 70 76 78 — 23 10 69 178 40 16331 0 — — —

PORT CLINTON—Ottawa County
□ H. B. MAGRUDER MEMORIAL HOSPITAL, 615 Fulton Street, Zip 43452-2034; tel. 419/734-3131; David R. Norwine, President and Chief Executive Officer **A**1 9 10 **F**7 9 13 16 17 18 19 22 24 25 32 34 38 40 43 46 50 51 54 56 68 70 71 72 76 78 **P**6 7 8 — 23 10 33 1655 16 66399 0 17009 7332 225

PORTSMOUTH—Scioto County
BEHAVIORAL HEALTH–PORTSMOUTH CAMPUS See River Valley Health System, Ironton

Hospitals, U.S. / OHIO

Hospital, Address, Telephone, Administrator, Approval, Facility, and Physician Codes, Health Care System, Network	Classification Codes		Utilization Data					Expense (thousands) of dollars		
★ American Hospital Association (AHA) membership □ Joint Commission on Accreditation of Healthcare Organizations (JCAHO) accreditation + American Osteopathic Healthcare Association (AOHA) membership ○ American Osteopathic Association (AOA) accreditation △ Commission on Accreditation of Rehabilitation Facilities (CARF) accreditation Control codes 61, 63, 64, 71, 72 and 73 indicate hospitals listed by AOHA, but not registered by AHA. For definition of numerical codes, see page A4	Control	Service	Staffed Beds	Admissions	Census	Outpatient Visits	Births	Total	Payroll	Personnel
★ △ SOUTHERN OHIO MEDICAL CENTER, (Includes Mercy Hospital, 1248 Kinneys Lane, Zip 45662; Scioto Memorial Hospital, 1805 27th Street, Zip 45662), 1805 27th Street, Zip 45662-2400; tel. 740/354-5000; Randal M. Arnett, President and Chief Executive Officer **A**1 7 9 10 12 13 **F**1 7 8 9 16 17 19 20 21 22 23 24 25 26 27 28 29 30 32 33 34 35 36 37 38 39 40 41 43 44 45 46 48 49 50 51 53 54 56 59 60 61 63 65 66 67 68 70 71 72 73 76 77 78 79 **P**3 **S** OhioHealth, Columbus, OH **Web address:** www.somc.org	23	10	205	10858	148	214823	1481	103991	45806	1630
RAVENNA—Portage County										
★ ROBINSON MEMORIAL HOSPITAL, 6847 North Chestnut Street, Zip 44266-1204, Mailing Address: P.O. Box 1204, Zip 44266-1204; tel. 330/297-0811; Stephen Colecchi, President and Chief Executive Officer **A**1 2 5 9 10 **F**7 8 9 11 12 13 14 17 18 19 22 24 25 26 27 28 29 30 32 33 34 35 36 37 38 39 41 43 44 45 46 48 49 50 51 54 56 57 59 60 61 64 65 66 68 70 71 72 76 77 78 79 **P**6 8 **Web address:** www.robinsonmemorial.org	13	10	131	8545	100	117018	805	92035	39979	1005
RICHMOND HEIGHTS—Cuyahoga County										
+ ○ UHHS RICHMOND HEIGHTS HOSPITAL, (Formerly PHS Mt. Sinai Medical Center), 27100 Chardon Road, Zip 44143-1198; tel. 440/585-6500; William P. Lawrence, President and Chief Executive Officer (Nonreporting) **A**9 11 13 **S** University Hospitals Health System, Cleveland, OH	23	10	98	—	—	—	—	—	—	—
ROCK CREEK—Ashtabula County										
GLENBEIGH HEALTH SOURCES, Route 45, Zip 44084, Mailing Address: P.O. Box 298, Zip 44084-0298; tel. 440/563-3400; Patricia Weston-Hall, Executive Director **A**9 10 **F**2 3 17 18 **P**5 **Web address:** www.glenbeigh.com	23	82	80	948	23	18333	0	—	—	63
SAINT CLAIRSVILLE—Belmont County										
□ BHC FOX RUN HOSPITAL, 67670 Traco Drive, Zip 43950-9375; tel. 740/695-2131; R. Dale Reynolds, Chief Executive Officer (Nonreporting) **A**1 9 10 **S** Behavioral Healthcare Corporation, Nashville, TN	33	22	65	—	—	—	—	—	—	—
SAINT MARYS—Auglaize County										
★ JOINT TOWNSHIP DISTRICT MEMORIAL HOSPITAL, 200 St. Clair Street, Zip 45885-2400; tel. 419/394-3387; James R. Chick, President (Total facility includes 23 beds in nursing home-type unit) **A**1 9 10 **F**7 8 9 13 16 17 18 19 22 24 25 29 31 32 33 36 37 38 39 40 41 43 44 45 46 48 49 50 51 54 56 69 70 71 72 76 78 **Web address:** www.jtdmh.com	23	10	106	4014	53	71500	350	31330	12893	454
SALEM—Columbiana County										
★ SALEM COMMUNITY HOSPITAL, 1995 East State Street, Zip 44460-0121; tel. 330/332-1551; Howard E. Rohleder, Administrator and Chief Executive Officer (Total facility includes 15 beds in nursing home-type unit) **A**1 5 9 10 **F**8 9 11 13 16 17 18 22 24 25 32 34 38 41 43 44 45 46 48 49 54 56 68 69 70 72 76 78	23	10	123	5574	72	106284	511	50005	24361	687
SANDUSKY—Erie County										
□ + ○ △ FIRELANDS COMMUNITY HOSPITAL, 1101 Decatur Street, Zip 44870-3335; tel. 419/626-7795; Dennis A. Sokol, President and Chief Executive Officer **A**1 2 7 9 10 11 12 13 **F**2 3 22 24 25 27 39 41 44 45 46 48 53 54 57 58 59 61 63 64 65 69 70 76 78	23	10	200	6048	91	283264	750	71073	29625	785
★ PROVIDENCE HOSPITAL, 1912 Hayes Avenue, Zip 44870-4736; tel. 419/621-7000; Sister Nancy Linenkugel, FACHE, President and Chief Executive Officer (Total facility includes 46 beds in nursing home-type unit) **A**1 2 6 9 10 **F**2 3 6 7 8 9 11 12 13 16 17 18 19 20 21 22 24 25 26 27 29 30 31 32 33 34 35 36 37 38 39 41 43 44 45 46 48 49 50 51 53 54 57 58 59 60 61 62 63 64 65 67 68 69 70 71 72 75 76 78 79 **P**3 8 **S** Franciscan Services Corporation, Sylvania, OH **Web address:** www.providencehealth.org	21	10	170	4052	83	62145	252	43668	19392	609
SHELBY—Richland County										
SHELBY HOSPITAL See MedCentral Health System, Mansfield										
SIDNEY—Shelby County										
★ WILSON MEMORIAL HOSPITAL, 915 West Michigan Street, Zip 45365-2491; tel. 937/498-2311; Thomas J. Boecker, President and Chief Executive Officer (Total facility includes 62 beds in nursing home-type unit) **A**1 9 10 **F**7 8 9 13 16 17 18 22 24 25 30 32 34 36 37 39 41 44 45 48 51 54 57 62 69 70 72 76 **P**6 **Web address:** www.wilsonhospital.com	23	10	143	3691	97	130836	576	39098	14810	510
SPRINGFIELD—Clark County										
★ COMMUNITY HOSPITAL, 2615 East High Street, Zip 45505-1422, Mailing Address: Box 1228, Zip 45501-1228; tel. 937/325-0531; Neal E. Kresheck, President (Total facility includes 41 beds in nursing home-type unit) **A**1 6 9 10 **F**4 6 7 8 9 11 12 13 14 16 17 18 19 20 22 24 25 26 28 30 32 33 34 35 36 37 38 39 40 41 43 44 45 46 47 48 49 50 51 54 56 65 68 69 70 71 72 73 76 77 78 79 **Web address:** www.communityhospital.com	23	10	201	9074	133	126128	1586	84845	36747	1171
□ △ MERCY MEDICAL CENTER, 1343 North Fountain Boulevard, Zip 45501-1380; tel. 937/390-5000; Marian R. Purdue, Senior Vice President and Chief Operating Officer (Total facility includes 20 beds in nursing home-type unit) (Nonreporting) **A**1 2 5 7 9 10 **S** Catholic Healthcare Partners, Cincinnati, OH	21	10	218	—	—	—	—	—	—	—

Hospitals, U.S. / OHIO

Hospital, Address, Telephone, Administrator, Approval, Facility, and Physician Codes, Health Care System, Network

★ American Hospital Association (AHA) membership
☐ Joint Commission on Accreditation of Healthcare Organizations (JCAHO) accreditation
+ American Osteopathic Healthcare Association (AOHA) membership
○ American Osteopathic Association (AOA) accreditation
△ Commission on Accreditation of Rehabilitation Facilities (CARF) accreditation
Control codes 61, 63, 64, 71, 72 and 73 indicate hospitals listed by AOHA, but not registered by AHA. For definition of numerical codes, see page A4

Hospital	Control	Service	Staffed Beds	Admissions	Census	Outpatient Visits	Births	Total	Payroll	Personnel
STEUBENVILLE—Jefferson County										
★ TRINITY HEALTH SYSTEM, (Includes Trinity Medical Center East, 380 Summit Avenue, tel. 740/283-7000; Trinity Medical Center West, 4000 Johnson Road, Zip 43952-2393; tel. 740/264-8000), 380 Summit Avenue, Zip 43952-2699; tel. 740/283-7000; Fred B. Brower, President and Chief Executive Officer **A**1 2 6 9 10 **F**2 3 7 8 9 11 12 13 14 16 17 18 19 21 22 23 25 27 28 30 31 32 33 34 36 37 38 39 40 41 43 44 45 46 48 49 50 51 52 53 54 56 57 58 59 60 61 62 63 64 65 69 70 71 72 75 76 77 78 79 **P**3 7 **S** Franciscan Services Corporation, Sylvania, OH Web address: www.trinityhealth.com	21	10	355	11052	194	190415	584	107772	49429	1563
SYLVANIA—Lucas County										
★ △ FLOWER HOSPITAL, 5200 Harroun Road, Zip 43560-2196; tel. 419/824-1444; Randall Kelley, President (Total facility includes 244 beds in nursing home-type unit) **A**1 3 5 7 9 10 **F**2 3 4 5 6 7 8 9 11 12 13 14 16 17 18 19 20 21 22 23 24 25 27 28 29 30 31 32 33 34 35 36 38 39 41 42 43 44 45 46 47 48 49 50 51 52 53 54 56 57 58 59 60 61 62 63 64 65 66 67 68 69 70 71 72 73 75 76 77 78 79 **P**6 7 8 **S** ProMedica Health System, Toledo, OH Web address: www.promedica.org	23	10	468	11238	374	87176	1204	96108	46566	1112
TIFFIN—Seneca County										
☐ MERCY HOSPITAL, 485 West Market Street, Zip 44883-0727; tel. 419/448-3133; Mark Shugarman, President **A**1 9 10 **F**4 7 8 9 12 13 16 17 18 19 20 22 24 25 26 30 31 32 33 34 35 36 38 40 43 44 45 46 48 50 51 56 68 70 72 73 75 76 78 **P**8 **S** Catholic Healthcare Partners, Cincinnati, OH Web address: www.mhsnr.org	21	10	66	2379	23	88698	402	27335	11703	342
TOLEDO—Lucas County										
☐ △ MEDICAL COLLEGE OF OHIO HOSPITALS, 3000 Arlington Avenue, Zip 43614-5805; tel. 419/383-4000; Frank S. McCullough, M.D., President (Nonreporting) **A**1 2 3 5 7 8 9 10 Web address: www.mco.edu	12	10	240	—	—	—	—	—	—	—
☐ ○ RIVERSIDE MERCY HOSPITAL, (Formerly Riverside Hospital), 1600 North Superior Street, Zip 43604-2199; tel. 419/729-6000; Scott E. Shook, President (Total facility includes 12 beds in nursing home-type unit) (Nonreporting) **A**1 2 9 10 11 **S** Catholic Healthcare Partners, Cincinnati, OH Web address: www.mhsnr.org	23	10	162	—	—	—	—	—	—	—
☐ ○ ST. VINCENT MERCY MEDICAL CENTER, 2213 Cherry Street, Zip 43608-2691; tel. 419/251-3232; Steven L. Mickus, President and Chief Executive Officer (Nonreporting) **A**1 2 3 5 6 9 10 11 12 13 **S** Catholic Healthcare Partners, Cincinnati, OH Web address: www.mercyweb.org	21	10	459	—	—	—	—	—	—	—
★ THE TOLEDO HOSPITAL, (Includes Toledo Children's Hospital, 2142 North Cove Boulevard, Zip 43606; Janice E. McBride, President), 2142 North Cove Boulevard, Zip 43606-3896; tel. 419/471-4000; Barbara Steele, President (Total facility includes 25 beds in nursing home-type unit) **A**1 2 3 5 8 9 10 **F**2 3 4 5 6 7 8 9 11 12 13 14 16 17 18 19 20 21 22 23 24 25 27 28 29 30 31 32 33 34 35 36 38 39 41 42 43 44 45 46 47 48 49 50 51 52 53 54 56 57 58 59 60 61 62 64 65 66 67 68 69 70 71 72 73 75 76 77 78 79 **P**6 7 8 **S** ProMedica Health System, Toledo, OH Web address: www.promedica.org	23	10	673	25786	351	270181	3846	300225	126165	3641
TOLEDO CAMPUS See Northcoast Behavioral Healthcare System, Northfield										
TOLEDO CHILDREN'S HOSPITAL See The Toledo Hospital										
TROY—Miami County										
☐ △ UPPER VALLEY MEDICAL CENTER, (Includes Dettmer Hospital, 3130 North Dixie Highway, Zip 45373-1039; tel. 937/440-7500), 3130 North Dixie Highway, Zip 45373; tel. 937/440-7500; David J. Meckstroth, President and Chief Executive Officer (Total facility includes 16 beds in nursing home-type unit) (Nonreporting) **A**1 2 7 9 10 Web address: www.uvmc.com	23	10	392	—	—	—	—	—	—	—
UPPER SANDUSKY—Wyandot County										
★ WYANDOT MEMORIAL HOSPITAL, 885 North Sandusky Avenue, Zip 43351-1098; tel. 419/294-4991; Joseph A. D'Ettorre, Chief Executive Officer **A**9 10 **F**7 8 9 12 13 17 18 22 24 25 32 34 37 38 39 40 44 45 46 48 49 50 51 61 68 76 78 **P**6	16	10	31	861	9	41532	96	11859	4512	144
URBANA—Champaign County										
MERCY MEMORIAL HOSPITAL, 904 Scioto Street, Zip 43078-2200; tel. 937/653-5231; Karl Zalar, Administrator (Nonreporting) **A**9 10 **S** Catholic Healthcare Partners, Cincinnati, OH	21	10	20	—	—	—	—	—	—	—
VAN WERT—Van Wert County										
★ VAN WERT COUNTY HOSPITAL, 1250 South Washington Street, Zip 45891-2599; tel. 419/238-2390; Mark J. Minick, President and Chief Executive Officer **A**1 9 10 **F**8 9 12 13 14 16 17 18 19 22 25 30 32 33 34 39 41 43 44 45 46 48 51 68 70 71 76 78 **P**8 Web address: www.vanwerthospital.org	23	10	99	2240	19	153569	363	22950	9157	272
WADSWORTH—Medina County										
☐ WADSWORTH-RITTMAN HOSPITAL, 195 Wadsworth Road, Zip 44281-9505; tel. 330/334-1504; James W. Brumlow, Jr, President and Chief Executive Officer **A**1 9 10 **F**7 9 22 24 25 30 32 34 36 38 39 41 44 45 46 48 49 50 51 53 54 61 68 70 72 76 79 **P**1 2 5 7 8	23	10	67	2350	31	65971	130	21781	10007	309

Hospitals, U.S. / OHIO

	Symbol Key
★	American Hospital Association (AHA) membership
□	Joint Commission on Accreditation of Healthcare Organizations (JCAHO) accreditation
+	American Osteopathic Healthcare Association (AOHA) membership
○	American Osteopathic Association (AOA) accreditation
△	Commission on Accreditation of Rehabilitation Facilities (CARF) accreditation

Control codes 61, 63, 64, 71, 72 and 73 indicate hospitals listed by AOHA, but not registered by AHA. For definition of numerical codes, see page A4

Hospital, Address, Telephone, Administrator, Approval, Facility, and Physician Codes, Health Care System, Network	Classification Codes		Utilization Data					Expense (thousands) of dollars		Personnel
	Control	Service	Staffed Beds	Admissions	Census	Outpatient Visits	Births	Total	Payroll	
WARREN—Trumbull County										
★ HILLSIDE REHABILITATION HOSPITAL, 8747 Squires Lane N.E., Zip 44484-1649; tel. 330/841-3700; Rodney Jones, Chief Operating Officer **A**1 5 9 10 **F**4 6 7 8 9 11 12 13 14 16 17 18 19 22 24 25 26 29 30 31 32 33 34 35 36 37 38 39 40 41 42 43 44 45 46 47 48 49 50 51 52 53 54 56 57 58 59 60 61 62 63 65 66 69 70 71 72 73 76 77 78 79 **P**7 8 **S** Forum Health, Youngstown, OH Web address: www.forumhealth.org	23	46	47	1007	45	0	0	13720	6757	221
□ ○ ST. JOSEPH HEALTH CENTER, 667 Eastland Avenue S.E., Zip 44484-4531; tel. 330/841-4000; Michael Terrance Rowan, President and Chief Executive Officer (Total facility includes 11 beds in nursing home–type unit) **A**1 2 9 10 11 12 13 **F**2 3 6 7 8 9 11 13 16 17 18 19 20 22 23 24 25 26 27 28 29 30 31 32 33 34 35 36 37 38 39 41 43 44 45 46 47 48 49 50 51 54 56 57 59 60 61 63 64 65 66 68 69 70 71 72 74 75 76 77 78 79 **P**8 **S** Catholic Healthcare Partners, Cincinnati, OH Web address: www.hmhs.org	21	10	136	6938	97	131555	799	61621	26041	748
★ TRUMBULL MEMORIAL HOSPITAL, (Formerly Forum Health–Trumbull Memorial Hospital), 1350 East Market Street, Zip 44482-6628; tel. 330/841-9011; N. Kristopher Hoce, Interim President and Chief Executive Officer **A**1 2 5 9 10 **F**2 3 4 6 7 8 9 11 12 13 14 16 17 18 19 21 22 24 25 26 27 28 29 30 32 33 34 35 36 37 38 39 41 42 43 44 45 46 47 48 49 52 53 54 56 57 58 61 62 63 64 65 68 69 70 71 72 76 78 79 **P**7 8 **S** Forum Health, Youngstown, OH Web address: www.forumhealth.org	23	10	284	13448	140	214524	987	116799	55256	1520
WARRENSVILLE HEIGHTS—Morgan County										
□ + ○ △ MERIDIA SOUTH POINTE HOSPITAL, 4110 Warrensville Center Road, Zip 44122-7099; tel. 216/491-6000; Kathleen A. Rice, Chief Operating Officer **A**1 2 7 10 11 12 13 **F**2 3 4 7 8 9 11 12 13 14 15 16 17 18 19 20 21 22 24 25 27 28 29 30 31 32 33 34 35 36 37 38 39 40 41 42 43 44 45 46 47 48 49 50 51 52 53 54 55 56 57 59 60 61 62 63 64 65 66 68 69 70 73 74 75 76 77 78 79 **P**1 3 4 7 8 **S** Cleveland Clinic Health System, Cleveland, OH Web address: www.meridia.com	23	10	198	6823	105	123364	0	73734	32108	833
WASHINGTON COURT HOUSE—Fayette County										
★ FAYETTE COUNTY MEMORIAL HOSPITAL, 1430 Columbus Avenue, Zip 43160-1791; tel. 740/335-1210; Francis G. Albarano, Administrator **A**1 9 10 **F**7 8 9 13 16 17 19 22 23 24 25 27 32 33 34 35 37 38 39 40 41 43 44 45 46 48 49 50 51 54 61 70 71 72 75 76 78 **S** Quorum Health Group, Brentwood, TN Web address: www.fcmh.org	13	10	35	1321	12	66099	338	17033	6884	254
WAUSEON—Fulton County										
★ FULTON COUNTY HEALTH CENTER, 725 South Shoop Avenue, Zip 43567-1701; tel. 419/335-2015; E. Dean Beck, Administrator (Total facility includes 86 beds in nursing home–type unit) **A**1 2 9 10 **F**3 6 7 8 9 16 17 22 24 25 28 32 34 39 40 41 43 44 45 46 48 54 57 60 61 63 64 68 69 70 71 72 76 78	23	10	172	2520	103	115537	298	23246	11406	452
WAVERLY—Pike County										
□ PIKE COMMUNITY HOSPITAL, 100 Dawn Lane, Zip 45690-9664; tel. 740/947-2186; Richard E. Sobota, President and Chief Executive Officer **A**1 9 10 **F**7 9 17 18 19 22 24 25 26 30 31 32 33 34 36 37 38 43 45 48 50 51 54 68 70 76 77 78 **P**6	23	10	35	878	7	25279	0	7790	4334	193
WEST UNION—Adams County										
□ ADAMS COUNTY HOSPITAL, 210 North Wilson Drive, Zip 45693-1574; tel. 937/544-5571; Linda Niles, Interim Chief Executive Officer (Total facility includes 18 beds in nursing home–type unit) (Nonreporting) **A**1 9 10 **S** Brim Healthcare, Inc., Brentwood, TN	13	10	49	—	—	—	—	—	—	—
WESTERVILLE—Franklin County										
ST. ANN'S HOSPITAL See Mount Carmel Health System, Columbus										
WILLARD—Huron County										
□ MERCY HOSPITAL OF WILLARD, 110 East Howard Street, Zip 44890-1611; tel. 419/964-5000; Dale E. Thornton, M.P.H., CHE, President and Chief Executive Officer **A**1 9 10 **F**8 9 17 18 19 22 25 27 33 34 36 37 38 39 40 41 44 45 46 48 51 54 63 70 72 76 78 **P**8 **S** Catholic Healthcare Partners, Cincinnati, OH Web address: www.mhsnr.org	21	10	30	826	7	47140	148	13364	6017	192
WILLOUGHBY—Lake County										
□ UHHS LAURELWOOD HOSPITAL, 35900 Euclid Avenue, Zip 44094-4648; tel. 440/953-3000; Farshid Afsarifar, Ph.D., President **A**1 9 10 **F**2 3 4 9 11 13 17 18 19 20 21 22 24 25 26 34 38 39 46 47 48 49 50 51 54 55 56 57 58 59 60 61 62 63 64 65 68 70 71 72 74 76 78 **P**5 6 **S** University Hospitals Health System, Cleveland, OH Web address: www.laurelwoodhospital.com	23	22	120	3636	85	17831	0	13609	8213	359
WILMINGTON—Clinton County										
□ CLINTON MEMORIAL HOSPITAL, 610 West Main Street, Zip 45177-2194; tel. 937/382-6611; Thomas F. Kurtz, Jr, President and Chief Executive Officer (Total facility includes 12 beds in nursing home–type unit) **A**1 2 3 9 10 **F**7 8 9 13 17 19 21 22 23 24 25 27 28 29 30 32 33 34 36 38 39 40 41 43 44 45 46 48 50 51 54 56 59 63 65 69 70 71 72 76 77 78 79 **P**1	13	10	93	4411	50	161544	654	51129	22418	557
WOOSTER—Wayne County										
□ WOOSTER COMMUNITY HOSPITAL, 1761 Beall Avenue, Zip 44691-2342; tel. 330/263-8100; William E. Sheron, Chief Executive Officer (Nonreporting) **A**1 2 9 10 **S** Quorum Health Group, Brentwood, TN	14	10	90	—	—	—	—	—	—	—

Hospitals, U.S. / OHIO

Hospital, Address, Telephone, Administrator, Approval, Facility, and Physician Codes, Health Care System, Network	Classification Codes		Utilization Data					Expense (thousands) of dollars		
	Control	Service	Staffed Beds	Admissions	Census	Outpatient Visits	Births	Total	Payroll	Personnel

★ American Hospital Association (AHA) membership
☐ Joint Commission on Accreditation of Healthcare Organizations (JCAHO) accreditation
+ American Osteopathic Healthcare Association (AOHA) membership
○ American Osteopathic Association (AOA) accreditation
△ Commission on Accreditation of Rehabilitation Facilities (CARF) accreditation
Control codes 61, 63, 64, 71, 72 and 73 indicate hospitals listed by AOHA, but not registered by AHA. For definition of numerical codes, see page A4

WORTHINGTON—Franklin County
☐ OSU&HARDING BEHAVIORAL HEALTHCARE AND MEDICINE, (Formerly Harding Hospital), 445 East Granville Road, Zip 43085–3195; tel. 614/293–9450; S. R. Thorward, M.D., Chief Operating Officer (Nonreporting) **A**1 3 5 9 10
— Control 23, Service 22, Staffed Beds 56

WRIGHT-PATTERSON AFB—Greene County
★ U. S. AIR FORCE MEDICAL CENTER WRIGHT-PATTERSON, 4881 Sugar Maple Drive, Zip 45433–5529; tel. 937/257–8762; Brigadier General Joseph Kelley, Commander **A**1 2 3 5 9 **F**2 3 4 8 9 10 11 12 13 14 16 18 21 22 23 24 25 27 28 32 33 34 38 39 41 42 43 44 45 46 47 48 49 50 51 52 53 54 55 56 57 58 59 61 62 63 64 65 66 68 70 71 72 74 75 76 78 79 **P**1 5 **S** Department of the Air Force, Bowling AFB, DC
Web address: www.wpmc1.wpafb.af.mil
— Control 41, Service 10, Staffed Beds 65, Admissions 3047, Census 34, Outpatient Visits 402793, Births 550, Total 162416, Payroll 94263, Personnel 1772

XENIA—Greene County
★ △ GREENE MEMORIAL HOSPITAL, 1141 North Monroe Drive, Zip 45385–1600; tel. 937/372–8011; Michael R. Stephens, President (Total facility includes 12 beds in nursing home–type unit) **A**1 2 5 7 9 10 **F**2 3 6 7 8 9 11 13 17 18 19 22 24 25 29 30 31 32 34 36 37 38 39 40 41 43 44 45 46 48 50 51 53 54 56 57 58 59 60 61 62 63 64 65 67 68 69 70 71 72 75 76 77 78 79 **P**6 7 8
Web address: www.greene-memorial.org
— Control 23, Service 10, Staffed Beds 150, Admissions 4363, Census 64, Outpatient Visits 119617, Births 196, Total 46557, Payroll 18690, Personnel 643

YOUNGSTOWN—Mahoning County
☐ BHC BELMONT PINES HOSPITAL, 615 Churchill–Hubbard Road, Zip 44505–1379; tel. 330/759–2700; Richard I. Feldman, Chief Executive Officer **A**1 10 **F**16 17 18 21 25 57 58 60 61 62 64 70 75 **S** Behavioral Healthcare Corporation, Nashville, TN
Web address: www.belmontpines.com
— Control 33, Service 22, Staffed Beds 77, Admissions 691, Census 15, Outpatient Visits 0, Births 0, Total 5906, Payroll 3002, Personnel 74

NORTHSIDE MEDICAL CENTER See Western Reserve Care System

☐ △ ST. ELIZABETH HEALTH CENTER, 1044 Belmont Avenue, Zip 44501, Mailing Address: P.O. Box 1790, Zip 44501–1790; tel. 330/746–7211; Michael Terrance Rowan, President and Chief Executive Officer (Total facility includes 30 beds in nursing home–type unit) **A**1 2 3 5 6 7 8 9 10 **F**3 4 6 7 8 9 11 12 13 16 17 18 19 21 22 23 24 25 26 27 28 29 30 31 32 33 34 35 36 37 38 39 41 42 43 44 45 46 47 48 49 51 54 56 57 59 60 61 62 63 64 65 66 68 69 70 71 72 74 75 76 78 79 **P**8 **S** Catholic Healthcare Partners, Cincinnati, OH
Web address: www.hmhs.org
— Control 21, Service 10, Staffed Beds 339, Admissions 17823, Census 309, Outpatient Visits 254234, Births 1972, Total 192984, Payroll 87335, Personnel 2205

TOD CHILDREN'S HOSPITAL See Western Reserve Care System

★ WESTERN RESERVE CARE SYSTEM, (Includes Northside Medical Center, tel. 330/747–1444; Tod Children's Hospital, tel. 330/747–6700), 500 Gypsy Lane, Zip 44501–0240, Mailing Address: P.O. Box 990, Zip 44501–0990; tel. 330/747–0777; N. Kristopher Hoce, Interim President and Chief Executive Officer (Total facility includes 26 beds in nursing home–type unit) **A**1 2 3 8 9 10 **F**2 3 4 6 7 8 9 11 12 13 14 16 17 18 19 20 21 22 23 24 25 26 27 28 29 30 31 32 33 34 35 36 37 38 39 40 41 42 43 44 45 46 47 48 49 50 51 52 53 54 56 57 58 59 60 61 62 63 64 65 68 69 70 71 72 73 76 77 78 79 **P**7 8 **S** Forum Health, Youngstown, OH
Web address: www.forumhealth.org
— Control 23, Service 10, Staffed Beds 361, Admissions 17518, Census 247, Outpatient Visits 275438, Births 1834, Total 207852, Payroll 85539, Personnel 2377

+ ○ YOUNGSTOWN OSTEOPATHIC HOSPITAL, 1319 Florencedale Avenue, Zip 44505–2795, Mailing Address: P.O. Box 1258, Zip 44501–1258; tel. 330/744–9200; Sean McKibben, President and Chief Executive Officer (Nonreporting) **A**9 10 11 13
— Control 23, Service 10, Staffed Beds 88

ZANESVILLE—Muskingum County
★ △ GENESIS HEALTHCARE SYSTEM, (Includes Bethesda Hospital, 2951 Maple Avenue, Zip 43701–1465; tel. 614/454–4000); Good Samaritan Medical and Rehabilitation Center, 800 Forest Avenue), 2951 Maple Avenue, Zip 43701–2881; tel. 740/454–5000); Thomas L. Sieber, President and Chief Executive Officer (Total facility includes 44 beds in nursing home–type unit) **A**1 2 7 9 10 **F**1 3 7 8 9 11 12 13 14 16 17 18 19 22 24 25 26 28 29 30 31 32 33 34 35 36 37 38 39 40 41 43 44 45 46 48 49 50 51 52 53 54 56 57 58 59 60 61 62 63 64 65 66 69 70 71 72 76 77 78 79 **P**8 **S** Franciscan Sisters of Christian Charity HealthCare Ministry, Inc, Manitowoc, WI
— Control 21, Service 10, Staffed Beds 433, Admissions 17417, Census 225, Outpatient Visits 288678, Births 1830, Total 138330, Payroll 61210, Personnel 1984

Hospitals, U.S. / OKLAHOMA

OKLAHOMA

Resident Population 3,347 (in thousands)
Resident population in metro areas 60.2%
Birth rate per 1,000 population 14.6
65 years and over 13.4%
Percent of persons without health insurance 17.8%

Hospital, Address, Telephone, Administrator, Approval, Facility, and Physician Codes, Health Care System, Network	Classi-fication Codes		Utilization Data					Expense (thousands) of dollars		
★ American Hospital Association (AHA) membership ☐ Joint Commission on Accreditation of Healthcare Organizations (JCAHO) accreditation + American Osteopathic Healthcare Association (AOHA) membership ○ American Osteopathic Association (AOA) accreditation △ Commission on Accreditation of Rehabilitation Facilities (CARF) accreditation Control codes 61, 63, 64, 71, 72 and 73 indicate hospitals listed by AOHA, but not registered by AHA. For definition of numerical codes, see page A4	Control	Service	Staffed Beds	Admissions	Census	Outpatient Visits	Births	Total	Payroll	Personnel
ADA—Pontotoc County										
✠ CARL ALBERT INDIAN HEALTH FACILITY, 1001 North Country Club Road, Zip 74820-2847; tel. 580/436-3980; Bruce A. Bennett, Administrator **A**1 10 **F**1 3 13 16 17 18 19 25 51 57 58 59 60 61 62 63 64 70 72 78 **P**1 **S** U. S. Public Health Service Indian Health Service, Rockville, MD	12	22	28	860	21	0	0	6295	3957	126
☐ ROLLING HILLS HOSPITAL, 1000 Rolling Hills Lane, Zip 74820-9415; tel. 580/436-3600; Darnell Powell, Executive Director (Nonreporting) **A**1 9 10 **S** Liberty Management Group, Inc., Ramsey, NJ	33	22	40	—	—	—	—	—	—	—
✠ △ VALLEY VIEW REGIONAL HOSPITAL, 430 North Monta Vista, Zip 74820-4610; tel. 580/332-2323; Philip Fisher, President and Chief Executive Officer **A**1 2 7 9 10 **F**8 9 16 17 19 22 24 25 27 31 32 34 36 38 39 40 41 42 43 44 46 48 50 51 53 54 65 68 70 72 75 76 77 78	14	10	153	6230	83	49799	607	45462	16726	651
ALTUS—Jackson County										
✠ JACKSON COUNTY MEMORIAL HOSPITAL, 1200 East Pecan Street, Zip 73521-6192, Mailing Address: Box 8190, Zip 73522-8190; tel. 580/482-4781; William G. Wilson, President and Chief Executive Officer (Total facility includes 25 beds in nursing home-type unit) **A**1 9 10 **F**6 7 8 9 16 17 18 19 22 24 25 33 34 36 37 38 39 40 41 43 44 45 46 48 49 50 51 53 54 61 63 64 67 69 70 71 72 75 76 78 **Web address:** www.jcmh.com	16	10	101	4475	67	49826	322	36084	15863	692
★ U. S. AIR FORCE HOSPITAL ALTUS, 301 North First Street, Zip 73523-5005; tel. 580/481-7347; Colonel David L. Clark, USAF, Commander (Nonreporting) **S** Department of the Air Force, Bowling AFB, DC	41	10	14	—	—	—	—	—	—	—
ALVA—Woods County										
★ SHARE MEDICAL CENTER, 800 Share Drive, Zip 73717-3699, Mailing Address: P.O. Box 727, Zip 73717-0727; tel. 580/327-2800; Barbara Oestmann, Chief Executive Officer (Total facility includes 80 beds in nursing home-type unit) **A**9 10 **F**1 8 13 16 17 18 22 23 24 25 30 32 36 37 38 40 44 46 48 51 56 58 60 61 62 69 72 78 **S** Quorum Health Group, Brentwood, TN	16	10	117	968	79	13092	57	7363	3590	136
ANADARKO—Caddo County										
ANADARKO MUNICIPAL HOSPITAL, 1002 Central Boulevard East, Zip 73005-4496; tel. 405/247-2551; Alan Riffel, Acting Administrator **A**9 10 **F**7 17 22 24 25 31 39 44 48 56 67 6 78 **P**5	14	49	45	383	4	3499	4	2814	1206	49
ANTLERS—Pushmataha County										
PUSHMATAHA COUNTY–TOWN OF ANTLERS HOSPITAL AUTHORITY, 510 East Main Street, Zip 74523-3262, Mailing Address: P.O. Box 518, Zip 74523-3262; tel. 580/298-3342; Chris Mattingly, Chief Executive Officer **A**9 10 **F**2 3 4 5 7 8 9 10 11 12 13 22 24 25 27 32 33 35 36 38 39 40 41 42 44 46 47 48 49 51 53 54 55 57 58 59 60 61 62 63 64 65 68 69 70 71 74 75 76 79 **P**5	16	10	46	1583	20	7311	0	7278	3508	154
ARDMORE—Carter County										
✠ MERCY MEMORIAL HEALTH CENTER, 1011 14th Street N.W., Zip 73401-1889; tel. 580/223-5400; Bobby G. Thompson, President and Chief Executive Officer **A**1 9 10 **F**3 8 9 11 13 16 17 18 19 22 23 24 25 27 30 32 33 34 35 36 38 39 41 44 45 46 48 49 50 51 53 54 57 59 60 61 62 64 65 69 70 72 76 77 78 **P**8 **S** Sisters of Mercy Health System–St. Louis, Saint Louis, MO **Web address:** www.mercyok.com	21	10	199	6631	107	122695	880	52842	19171	843
ATOKA—Atoka County										
★ ATOKA MEMORIAL HOSPITAL, 1501 South Virginia Avenue, Zip 74525-3298; tel. 580/889-3333; Paul David Moore, Administrator **A**9 10 18 **F**7 13 16 17 22 23 25 31 36 54 76 **Web address:** www.atoka-hosp.otnnet.net	13	10	25	764	9	7118	1	4255	2502	99
BARTLESVILLE—Washington County										
✠ JANE PHILLIPS MEDICAL CENTER, 3500 East Frank Phillips Boulevard, Zip 74006-2409; tel. 918/333-7200; Larry Minden, Chief Executive Officer (Total facility includes 69 beds in nursing home-type unit) **A**1 2 5 9 10 **F**4 8 9 11 12 13 17 18 22 24 25 26 27 28 30 32 33 34 36 37 38 39 41 44 45 46 48 49 50 51 53 54 55 57 61 62 65 68 69 70 71 75 76 77 78 79 **P**6	23	10	227	6675	154	59637	794	55505	22775	1000
BEAVER—Beaver County										
BEAVER COUNTY MEMORIAL HOSPITAL, 212 East Eighth Street, Zip 73932, Mailing Address: P.O. Box 640, Zip 73932-0640; tel. 580/625-4551; Brent Meyers, Administrator **A**9 10 **F**8 9 25 31 37 48 70 76 **P**6	16	10	24	168	1	9924	34	1978	987	50
BLACKWELL—Kay County										
★ BLACKWELL REGIONAL HOSPITAL, 710 South 13th Street, Zip 74631-3700; tel. 580/363-2311; Cindy White, Chief Financial Officer **A**9 10 **F**7 8 9 17 18 22 36 38 39 44 48 54 70 76 78 **P**7 **S** INTEGRIS Health, Oklahoma City, OK	23	10	34	1380	16	13410	103	7753	3316	113
BOISE CITY—Cimarron County										
CIMARRON MEMORIAL HOSPITAL, 100 South Ellis Street, Zip 73933; tel. 580/544-2501; Ronny Lathrop, Chief Executive Officer and Administrator (Total facility includes 44 beds in nursing home-type unit) (Nonreporting) **A**9 10	13	10	64	—	—	—	—	—	—	—

© 2000 AHA Guide *Many Facility Codes have changed. Please refer to the AHA Guide Code Chart.*

Hospitals, U.S. / OKLAHOMA

Hospital, Address, Telephone, Administrator, Approval, Facility, and Physician Codes, Health Care System, Network	Classification Codes		Utilization Data					Expense (thousands) of dollars		
	Control	Service	Staffed Beds	Admissions	Census	Outpatient Visits	Births	Total	Payroll	Personnel

★ American Hospital Association (AHA) membership
☐ Joint Commission on Accreditation of Healthcare Organizations (JCAHO) accreditation
+ American Osteopathic Healthcare Association (AOHA) membership
○ American Osteopathic Association (AOA) accreditation
△ Commission on Accreditation of Rehabilitation Facilities (CARF) accreditation
Control codes 61, 63, 64, 71, 72 and 73 indicate hospitals listed by AOHA, but not registered by AHA. For definition of numerical codes, see page A4

Hospital	Control	Service	Beds	Adm	Census	OPV	Births	Total	Payroll	Personnel
BRISTOW—Creek County ★ BRISTOW MEMORIAL HOSPITAL, Seventh and Spruce Streets, Zip 74010, Mailing Address: P.O. Box 780, Zip 74010–0780; tel. 918/367–2215; Ron Cackler, President and Chief Executive Officer (Nonreporting) A9 10 S Hillcrest HealthCare System, Tulsa, OK	23	10	22	—	—	—	—	—	—	—
BROKEN ARROW—Tulsa County ☐ BROKEN ARROW MEDICAL CENTER, 3000 South Elm Place, Zip 74012–7952; tel. 918/455–3535; Bruce Switzer, Administrator A1 10 F7 9 13 22 23 24 25 36 37 39 41 43 45 46 48 49 50 53 54 65 70 72 76 78 Web address: www.stfrancis.com	23	10	62	2027	38	35075	3	20562	9472	349
BUFFALO—Harper County ★ HARPER COUNTY COMMUNITY HOSPITAL, Highway 64 North, Zip 73834, Mailing Address: P.O. Box 60, Zip 73834–0060; tel. 580/735–2555; Karen Ives, Interim Administrator A9 10 F9 17 19 25 32 33 34 37 40 43 48 51 54 76	13	10	25	298	5	1151	6	1646	851	49
CARNEGIE—Caddo County ★ CARNEGIE TRI–COUNTY MUNICIPAL HOSPITAL, 102 North Broadway, Zip 73015, Mailing Address: P.O. Box 97, Zip 73015–0097; tel. 580/654–1050; Phil Hawkins, Administrator A9 10 F17 18 25 31 36 44 76 P6	14	10	28	694	7	1715	14	2267	1239	61
CHEYENNE—Roger Mills County ★ ROGER MILLS MEMORIAL HOSPITAL, Fifth and L. L Males Avenue, Zip 73628, Mailing Address: P.O. Box 219, Zip 73628–0219; tel. 580/497–3336; Marilyn Bryan, Administrator A9 10 18 F25 26 32 34 36 37 70	13	10	15	155	2	14846	0	2107	1236	37
CHICKASHA—Grady County ⊞ GRADY MEMORIAL HOSPITAL, 2220 North Iowa Avenue, Zip 73018–2738; tel. 405/224–2300; E. Michael Nunamaker, Chief Executive Officer A1 9 10 F7 8 13 22 24 25 27 34 36 38 40 41 43 44 45 48 54 61 68 70 72 76 78 Web address: www.gradymemhosp.org	16	10	123	3267	38	24039	369	25190	11990	347
CLAREMORE—Rogers County ⊞ CLAREMORE REGIONAL HOSPITAL, 1202 North Muskogee Place, Zip 74017–3036; tel. 918/341–2556; Ken Seidel, Chief Executive Officer A1 9 10 F2 4 8 9 11 12 13 14 16 17 18 19 20 21 22 23 25 26 27 29 30 31 32 33 34 37 38 39 41 42 44 45 46 47 48 50 52 53 54 55 56 57 59 60 61 62 63 64 68 70 71 72 74 76 77 78 79 P6 S Triad Hospitals, Inc., Dallas, TX	33	10	68	3733	47	37598	593	22930	9936	379
⊞ U. S. PUBLIC HEALTH SERVICE COMPREHENSIVE INDIAN HEALTH FACILITY, 101 South Moore Avenue, Zip 74017–5091; tel. 918/342–6434; John Daugherty, Jr, Service Unit Director A1 5 10 F9 17 18 23 25 38 41 44 48 54 56 66 70 76 P6 S U. S. Public Health Service Indian Health Service, Rockville, MD	47	10	46	1993	22	151191	511	4367	2869	326
CLEVELAND—Pawnee County ★ CLEVELAND AREA HOSPITAL, 1401 West Pawnee Street, Zip 74020–3019; tel. 918/358–2501; Thomas Henton, Chief Executive Officer A9 10 F7 17 18 22 25 28 32 34 36 38 45 48 54 70 71 76 S Hillcrest HealthCare System, Tulsa, OK	23	10	19	328	4	6519	0	3886	2071	80
CLINTON—Custer County ⊞ INTEGRIS CLINTON REGIONAL HOSPITAL, 100 North 30th Street, Zip 73601–3117, Mailing Address: P.O. Box 1569, Zip 73601–1569; tel. 580/323–2363; Jerry Jones, Administrator (Nonreporting) A1 9 10 S INTEGRIS Health, Oklahoma City, OK Web address: www.integris–health.com	14	10	49	—	—	—	—	—	—	—
⊞ U. S. PUBLIC HEALTH SERVICE INDIAN HOSPITAL, Mailing Address: Route 1, Box 3060, Zip 73601–9303; tel. 580/323–2884; Thedis V. Mitchell, Director A1 10 F1 2 3 4 5 6 8 9 10 11 12 13 14 15 16 17 18 19 22 23 24 25 31 32 34 35 38 39 40 41 42 43 44 46 47 48 49 51 52 53 54 55 56 57 58 59 60 61 62 63 64 65 68 69 70 74 75 76 79 P6 S U. S. Public Health Service Indian Health Service, Rockville, MD	47	10	11	265	3	29737	0	4351	3083	103
COALGATE—Coal County ★ HURLEY HEALTH CENTER, 6 North Covington Street, Zip 74538–2002, Mailing Address: P.O. Box 326, Zip 74538; tel. 580/927–2327; Dan A. Clements, Chief Executive Officer (Total facility includes 75 beds in nursing home–type unit) A9 10 F13 18 19 22 32 34 36 38 48 54 69 70 71 75 76 S Hillcrest HealthCare System, Tulsa, OK	23	10	95	598	76	4518	0	2807	1743	151
CORDELL—Washita County ★ CORDELL MEMORIAL HOSPITAL, 1220 North Glenn English Street, Zip 73632–2099; tel. 580/832–3339; Charles H. Greene, Jr, Administrator A9 10 F12 17 25 32 34 48 76	14	10	28	533	5	4194	0	2228	967	46
CUSHING—Payne County ⊞ CUSHING REGIONAL HOSPITAL, 1027 East Cherry Street, Zip 74023–4101, Mailing Address: P.O. Box 1409, Zip 74023–1409; tel. 918/225–2915; Ron Cackler, President and Chief Executive Officer A1 9 10 F7 8 9 13 17 18 19 22 24 25 27 30 32 33 34 36 38 39 40 41 43 44 45 46 48 50 51 54 57 59 60 61 62 63 64 67 69 70 71 72 76 78 S Quorum Health Group, Brentwood, TN	14	10	75	2794	36	18510	388	13222	6332	218
DRUMRIGHT—Creek County ★ DRUMRIGHT MEMORIAL HOSPITAL, 501 South Lou Allard Drive, Zip 74030–4899; tel. 918/352–2525; James L. Clough, Administrator (Nonreporting) A9 10 S INTEGRIS Health, Oklahoma City, OK	23	10	15	—	—	—	—	—	—	—
DUNCAN—Stephens County ⊞ DUNCAN REGIONAL HOSPITAL, 1407 North Whisenant Drive, Zip 73533–1650, Mailing Address: P.O. Box 2000, Zip 73534–2000; tel. 580/252–5300; David Robertson, Chief Executive Officer (Total facility includes 16 beds in nursing home–type unit) A1 9 10 F7 8 9 12 16 17 18 19 22 24 25 27 31 32 33 34 36 37 39 41 43 44 45 48 49 50 53 54 64 69 70 71 72 76 78 P8	23	10	98	4305	51	53886	462	30660	13925	504

Hospitals, U.S. / OKLAHOMA

Hospital, Address, Telephone, Administrator, Approval, Facility, and Physician Codes, Health Care System, Network	Classification Codes		Utilization Data					Expense (thousands) of dollars		
★ American Hospital Association (AHA) membership ☐ Joint Commission on Accreditation of Healthcare Organizations (JCAHO) accreditation + American Osteopathic Healthcare Association (AOHA) membership ○ American Osteopathic Association (AOA) accreditation △ Commission on Accreditation of Rehabilitation Facilities (CARF) accreditation Control codes 61, 63, 64, 71, 72 and 73 indicate hospitals listed by AOHA, but not registered by AHA. For definition of numerical codes, see page A4	Control	Service	Staffed Beds	Admissions	Census	Outpatient Visits	Births	Total	Payroll	Personnel

DURANT—Bryan County
★ MEDICAL CENTER OF SOUTHEASTERN OKLAHOMA, 1800 University Boulevard, Zip 74701-3006, Mailing Address: P.O. Box 1207, Zip 74702-1207; tel. 580/924-3080; Jacquelyn Harms, R.N., Executive Director **A**1 9 10 **F**7 8 9 11 13 14 15 16 19 22 23 24 25 27 28 32 33 34 35 36 37 38 39 40 41 43 44 45 46 48 49 50 51 54 68 70 71 72 75 76 78 79 **P**8 **S** Health Management Associates, Naples, FL

| 33 | 10 | 103 | 6125 | 60 | 31665 | 731 | — | — | 336 |

EDMOND—Oklahoma County
★ EDMOND MEDICAL CENTER, 1 South Bryant Street, Zip 73034-4798; tel. 405/341-6100; Stanley D. Tatum, Chief Executive Officer **A**1 9 10 **F**4 5 7 8 9 10 11 12 13 16 17 18 19 21 22 23 24 25 28 29 30 32 33 34 35 37 38 39 41 42 45 46 47 48 49 50 51 53 54 56 58 59 60 61 62 63 64 65 66 69 70 71 72 73 74 76 77 78 79 **P**1 5 7 8 **S** HCA – The Healthcare Company, Nashville, TN
Web address: www.edmondmedctr.com

| 33 | 10 | 84 | 2609 | 42 | 32845 | 0 | 29147 | 10278 | 259 |

INTEGRATED SPECIALTY HOSPITAL, (Formerly Horizon Specialty Hospital), 1100 East Ninth Street, Zip 73034-5755; tel. 405/341-8150; Joe Smithers, Administrator (Nonreporting) **A**10 **S** Integrated Health Services, Sparks Glencoe, MD

| 33 | 49 | 43 | — | — | — | — | — | — | — |

EL RENO—Canadian County
★ PARK VIEW HOSPITAL, 2115 Parkview Drive, Zip 73036-2199, Mailing Address: P.O. Box 129, Zip 73036-0129; tel. 405/262-2640; Lex Smith, Administrator **A**9 10 **F**7 8 13 16 17 18 19 22 23 25 32 33 34 36 37 38 39 40 41 43 44 48 49 50 53 54 61 69 70 72 76 78

| 16 | 10 | 54 | 1717 | 20 | 25606 | 165 | 12751 | 6678 | 257 |

ELK CITY—Beckham County
★ GREAT PLAINS REGIONAL MEDICAL CENTER, 1705 West Second Street, Zip 73644-4496, Mailing Address: P.O. Box 2339, Zip 73648-2339; tel. 580/225-2511; Robin E. Lake, Chief Executive Officer **A**1 9 10 **F**7 9 12 13 16 17 18 19 20 22 23 24 25 30 31 32 34 36 38 39 41 43 44 45 46 48 50 51 54 56 57 59 60 61 62 65 68 69 70 71 72 75 76 78 79 **P**8
Web address: www.gprmc-ok.com

| 23 | 10 | 76 | 3829 | 43 | 55095 | 413 | 23606 | 10689 | 356 |

ENID—Garfield County
INTEGRIS BASS BEHAVIORAL HEALTH SYSTEM, 2216 South Van Buren Street, Zip 73703-8299; tel. 580/234-2220; James Hutchison, Director (Nonreporting) **S** INTEGRIS Health, Oklahoma City, OK

| 33 | 22 | 50 | — | — | — | — | — | — | — |

★ △ INTEGRIS BASS BAPTIST HEALTH CENTER, 600 South Monroe Street, Zip 73701, Mailing Address: P.O. Box 3168, Zip 73702-3168; tel. 580/233-2300; Thomas Schmitt, Administrator (Nonreporting) **A**1 3 5 7 9 10 **S** INTEGRIS Health, Oklahoma City, OK
Web address: www.integris-health.com

| 23 | 10 | 119 | — | — | — | — | — | — | — |

★ △ ST. MARY'S MERCY HOSPITAL, 305 South Fifth Street, Zip 73701-5899, Mailing Address: Box 232, Zip 73702-0232; tel. 580/233-6100; Frank Lopez, FACHE, President and Chief Executive Officer **A**1 2 3 5 7 9 10 **F**7 8 9 11 13 16 17 18 19 22 24 25 27 28 29 32 33 34 35 36 38 39 40 43 45 46 48 49 50 54 70 72 76 78 79 **P**4 5
Web address: www.mercyok.com

| 21 | 10 | 137 | 5314 | 96 | 69713 | 239 | 47529 | 17517 | 584 |

EUFAULA—Mcintosh County
COMMUNITY HOSPITAL–LAKEVIEW, 1 Hospital Drive, Zip 74432, Mailing Address: P.O. Box 629, Zip 74432-0629; tel. 918/689-2535; Daniel J. Schaetzle, Administrator **A**9 10 **F**7 9 16 17 18 22 24 25 32 36 38 48 51 72 76 78

| 33 | 10 | 33 | 428 | 4 | 11225 | 0 | 3286 | 1163 | 59 |

FAIRFAX—Osage County
★ FAIRFAX MEMORIAL HOSPITAL, Taft Avenue and Highway 18, Zip 74637, Mailing Address: P.O. Box 219, Zip 74637-0219; tel. 918/642-3291; Xavier Villarreal, Chief Executive Officer **A**9 10 **F**9 22 25 36 37 38 48 54 76 **P**6 **S** Hillcrest HealthCare System, Tulsa, OK

| 23 | 10 | 15 | 301 | 3 | 3942 | 0 | 2298 | 1100 | 48 |

FAIRVIEW—Major County
FAIRVIEW HOSPITAL, 523 East State Road, Zip 73737-1498; tel. 580/227-3721; Mark Harrel, Administrator **A**9 10 **F**8 9 12 13 17 22 25 32 36 40 41 44 48 54 70 76 **P**6

| 14 | 10 | 31 | 486 | 4 | 3499 | 4 | 3756 | 2121 | 69 |

FORT SILL—Comanche County
★ REYNOLDS ARMY COMMUNITY HOSPITAL, 4301 Mow-way Street, Zip 73503-6300; tel. 580/458-3000; Colonel Alice Demarais, Commander **A**1 **F**2 3 8 9 13 14 15 16 17 18 19 21 22 23 24 25 28 29 32 33 34 38 41 43 44 45 46 48 49 50 51 54 54 59 61 63 65 68 70 72 76 77 78 **S** Department of the Army, Office of the Surgeon General, Falls Church, VA

| 42 | 10 | 73 | 2077 | 16 | 389816 | 856 | 61741 | 16999 | — |

FREDERICK—Tillman County
★ MEMORIAL HOSPITAL, 319 East Josephine, Zip 73542-2299; tel. 580/335-7565; Al Allee, Chief Executive Officer (Total facility includes 30 beds in nursing home–type unit) **A**9 10 **F**7 13 17 19 22 25 30 31 34 36 37 38 48 51 56 67 69 70 76

| 16 | 10 | 60 | 850 | 38 | 12156 | 2 | 4568 | 1895 | 86 |

GROVE—Delaware County
★ INTEGRIS GROVE GENERAL HOSPITAL, 1310 South Main Street, Zip 74344-1310; tel. 918/786-2243; Greg Martin, Administrator and Chief Executive Officer **A**1 9 10 **F**7 8 9 11 12 15 17 18 19 22 25 32 34 36 39 46 48 49 50 54 67 69 70 72 76 78 **P**5 8 **S** INTEGRIS Health, Oklahoma City, OK
Web address: www.integris-health.com

| 23 | 10 | 72 | 3303 | 36 | 58321 | 192 | 22620 | 10325 | 331 |

© 2000 AHA Guide   *Many Facility Codes have changed. Please refer to the AHA Guide Code Chart.*   Hospitals **A343**

Hospitals, U.S. / OKLAHOMA

Hospital, Address, Telephone, Administrator, Approval, Facility, and Physician Codes, Health Care System, Network

- ★ American Hospital Association (AHA) membership
- ☐ Joint Commission on Accreditation of Healthcare Organizations (JCAHO) accreditation
- + American Osteopathic Healthcare Association (AOHA) membership
- ○ American Osteopathic Association (AOA) accreditation
- △ Commission on Accreditation of Rehabilitation Facilities (CARF) accreditation
  Control codes 61, 63, 64, 71, 72 and 73 indicate hospitals listed by AOHA, but not registered by AHA. For definition of numerical codes, see page A4

Hospital	Control	Service	Staffed Beds	Admissions	Census	Outpatient Visits	Births	Total	Payroll	Personnel
GUTHRIE—Logan County ✠ LOGAN HOSPITAL AND MEDICAL CENTER, Highway 33 West at Academy Road, Zip 73044, Mailing Address: P.O. Box 1017, Zip 73044-1017; tel. 405/282-6700; Judith K. Feuquay, Chief Executive Officer **A**1 9 10 **F**7 9 16 17 18 22 23 24 25 32 34 36 45 48 54 56 69 70 72 76 78 **S** Quorum Health Group, Brentwood, TN	13	10	32	1207	17	11736	0	9194	4259	124
GUYMON—Texas County ★ MEMORIAL HOSPITAL OF TEXAS COUNTY, 520 Medical Drive, Zip 73942-4438; tel. 580/338-6515; Kevin Cox, Administrator **A**9 10 **F**7 8 9 13 14 16 17 19 21 22 24 25 32 33 34 35 36 37 39 40 41 43 44 48 51 54 68 70 71 76 79	13	10	40	2247	19	16389	327	12222	4695	164
HENRYETTA—Okmulgee County ✠ HENRYETTA MEDICAL CENTER, Dewey Bartlett and Main Streets, Zip 74437, Mailing Address: P.O. Box 1269, Zip 74437-1269; tel. 918/652-4463; James P. Bailey, President and Chief Executive Officer (Nonreporting) **A**1 9 10 **S** Quorum Health Group, Brentwood, TN	16	10	28	—	—	—	—	—	—	—
HOBART—Kiowa County ✠ ELKVIEW GENERAL HOSPITAL, 429 West Elm Street, Zip 73651-1699; tel. 580/726-3324; J. W. Finch, Jr, Administrator **A**9 10 **F**8 9 13 17 22 23 24 25 30 34 36 46 48 54 61 68 70 76 78	16	10	30	1380	19	8008	88	6623	3513	165
HOLDENVILLE—Hughes County ★ HOLDENVILLE GENERAL HOSPITAL, 100 McDougal Drive, Zip 74848-9700; tel. 405/379-6631; Shawn Morrow, Chief Executive Officer and Administrator **A**9 10 **F**22 25 36 38 46 48 76 78 **P**1 **S** Quorum Health Group, Brentwood, TN	16	10	22	624	7	—	0	4921	1816	84
HOLLIS—Harmon County ★ HARMON MEMORIAL HOSPITAL, 400 East Chestnut Street, Zip 73550-2030, Mailing Address: P.O. Box 791, Zip 73550-0791; tel. 580/688-3363; James Koulovatos, Chief Executive Officer **A**9 10 **F**7 25 36 54 76	16	10	16	394	4	2974	0	1525	930	38
HUGO—Choctaw County ★ CHOCTAW MEMORIAL HOSPITAL, 1405 East Kirk Road, Zip 74743-3603; tel. 580/326-6414; Emmett C. Schuster, Chief Executive Officer and Administrator **A**9 10 **F**7 17 22 25 32 34 36 48 70 76 **S** Quorum Health Group, Brentwood, TN	16	10	34	1485	17	9546	71	5738	2425	108
IDABEL—Mccurtain County ★ MCCURTAIN MEMORIAL HOSPITAL, 1301 Lincoln Road, Zip 74745-7341; tel. 580/286-7623; Claude E. Camp, II, Chief Executive Officer **A**9 10 **F**7 8 22 24 25 32 34 36 39 41 44 48 54 57 62 72 76 78 **P**8 **S** Quorum Health Group, Brentwood, TN	23	10	81	2473	28	18301	363	16675	8174	240
KINGFISHER—Kingfisher County ★ KINGFISHER REGIONAL HOSPITAL, 500 South Ninth Street, Zip 73750-3528, Mailing Address: P.O. Box 59, Zip 73750-0059; tel. 405/375-3141; Daryle Voss, Chief Executive Officer **A**9 10 **F**7 8 9 22 25 32 34 36 38 44 48 51 54 56 58 70 76 78 79 **S** Quorum Health Group, Brentwood, TN Web address: www.kingfisherhospital.com	23	10	27	1048	9	7802	138	6331	2870	94
LAWTON—Comanche County ✠ △ COMANCHE COUNTY MEMORIAL HOSPITAL, 3401 Gore Boulevard, Zip 73505-0129, Mailing Address: Box 129, Zip 73502-0129; tel. 580/355-8620; Randall K. Segler, Chief Executive Officer **A**1 2 7 9 10 **F**4 7 8 9 11 12 13 16 17 18 21 22 23 24 25 29 30 31 32 33 34 35 36 37 38 39 41 43 44 45 46 47 48 49 50 51 53 54 55 57 59 61 62 63 65 68 69 70 71 72 73 75 76 78 79	16	10	283	7999	97	64590	2469	122768	49030	1506
MEMORIAL PAVILION, 1602 S.W. 82nd Street, Zip 73505-9099; tel. 580/357-7827; Kim Holland, Interim Administrator (Nonreporting) **A**10	33	22	99	—	—	—	—	—	—	—
✠ △ SOUTHWESTERN MEDICAL CENTER, 5602 S.W. Lee Boulevard, Zip 73505-9635, Mailing Address: P.O. Box 7290, Zip 73506-7290; tel. 580/531-4700; Thomas L. Rine, President and Chief Executive Officer **A**1 2 7 9 10 **F**7 8 9 11 13 16 17 18 19 22 24 25 27 30 32 34 38 39 41 43 44 45 46 48 53 54 56 57 58 59 61 62 64 65 68 70 72 75 76 77 78 79 **P**1 7 **S** HCA – The Healthcare Company, Nashville, TN Web address: www.hcahealthcare.com	33	10	158	3880	50	64736	345	39485	11845	428
✠ U. S. PUBLIC HEALTH SERVICE INDIAN HOSPITAL, 1515 Lawrie Tatum Road, Zip 73507-3099; tel. 580/353-0350 (Nonreporting) **A**1 10 **S** U. S. Public Health Service Indian Health Service, Rockville, MD	47	10	44	—	—	—	—	—	—	—
MADILL—Marshall County ★ MARSHALL MEMORIAL HOSPITAL, 1 Hospital Drive, Zip 73446, Mailing Address: P.O. Box 827, Zip 73446-0827; tel. 580/795-3384; Norma Howard, Administrator **A**9 10 **F**7 9 17 18 25 26 32 34 36 37 44 48 51 54 67 70 72 76 **S** INTEGRIS Health, Oklahoma City, OK	13	10	25	749	9	11426	22	4203	2145	—
MANGUM—Greer County MANGUM CITY HOSPITAL, One Wickersham Drive, Zip 73554, Mailing Address: P.O. Box 280, Zip 73554-0280; tel. 580/782-3353; Ben White, Administrator (Nonreporting) **A**9 10	14	10	40	—	—	—	—	—	—	—
MARIETTA—Love County ★ MERCY HEALTH LOVE COUNTY, 300 Wanda Street, Zip 73448-1200; tel. 580/276-3347; Richard Barker, Administrator **A**9 10 18 **F**7 16 17 18 32 76	13	10	25	438	5	—	0	3264	2161	51
MCALESTER—Pittsburg County ✠ △ MCALESTER REGIONAL HEALTH CENTER, One Clark Bass Boulevard, Zip 74501-4267, Mailing Address: P.O. Box 1228, Zip 74502-1228; tel. 918/426-1800; Joel W. Tate, FACHE, Chief Executive Officer **A**1 7 9 10 **F**2 3 4 6 7 8 9 11 13 17 18 19 21 22 24 25 26 27 30 31 32 33 35 36 37 38 39 40 41 43 44 45 46 48 49 50 51 53 54 57 68 69 70 71 72 76 78	16	10	197	5477	88	44569	637	40878	16826	629

Hospitals, U.S. / OKLAHOMA

Hospital, Address, Telephone, Administrator, Approval, Facility, and Physician Codes, Health Care System, Network	Classification Codes		Utilization Data					Expense (thousands) of dollars		
★ American Hospital Association (AHA) membership ☐ Joint Commission on Accreditation of Healthcare Organizations (JCAHO) accreditation + American Osteopathic Healthcare Association (AOHA) membership ○ American Osteopathic Association (AOA) accreditation △ Commission on Accreditation of Rehabilitation Facilities (CARF) accreditation Control codes 61, 63, 64, 71, 72 and 73 indicate hospitals listed by AOHA, but not registered by AHA. For definition of numerical codes, see page A4	Control	Service	Staffed Beds	Admissions	Census	Outpatient Visits	Births	Total	Payroll	Personnel
MIAMI—Ottawa County										
★ INTEGRIS BAPTIST REGIONAL HEALTH CENTER, 200 Second Street S.W., Zip 74354–6830, Mailing Address: P.O. Box 1207, Zip 74355–1207; tel. 918/542–6611; W. Eugene Baxter, Dr.PH, FACHE, Interim Administrator **A**1 9 10 **F**7 8 9 13 14 16 17 18 19 22 24 25 30 31 32 33 34 35 36 39 40 41 43 44 45 46 48 49 50 51 54 56 57 61 62 64 67 68 69 70 71 72 76 77 78 79 **P**4 5 8 **S** INTEGRIS Health, Oklahoma City, OK Web address: www.integris–health.com	23	10	113	4702	70	56865	310	33685	15638	497
WILLOW CREST HOSPITAL, 130 A Street S.W., Zip 74354–6800; tel. 918/542–1836; Anne G. Anthony, Administrator and Chief Executive Officer **A**9 10 **F**18 29 31 57 58 61 Web address: www.willowcresthospital.com	33	22	50	299	48	0	0	6408	4060	133
MIDWEST CITY—Oklahoma County										
★ INTEGRATED SPECIALTY HOSPITAL, 8210 National Avenue, Zip 73110; tel. 405/739–0800; Gayla Campbell, Administrator (Nonreporting) **A**10 **S** Integrated Health Services, Sparks Glencoe, MD	33	46	31	—	—	—	—	—	—	—
★ MIDWEST REGIONAL MEDICAL CENTER, 2825 Parklawn Drive, Zip 73110–4258; tel. 405/610–4411; Tim Parker, Chief Executive Officer (Total facility includes 20 beds in nursing home–type unit) **A**1 2 9 10 **F**4 8 9 11 12 13 16 17 18 22 24 25 30 31 32 33 34 36 39 41 44 45 46 47 48 51 54 55 56 57 59 60 61 62 69 70 71 72 75 76 78 79 **S** Health Management Associates, Naples, FL	33	10	247	11916	161	103907	1015	72639	28867	1011
MUSKOGEE—Muskogee County										
★ △ MUSKOGEE REGIONAL MEDICAL CENTER, 300 Rockefeller Drive, Zip 74401–5081; tel. 918/682–5501; Bill R. Kennedy, President and Chief Executive Officer **A**1 2 7 9 10 **F**7 16 17 18 22 24 25 32 33 34 36 38 39 41 43 44 45 46 48 49 51 53 54 57 62 63 64 65 70 73 77 78	16	10	225	11419	170	81392	1063	68152	29210	968
★ VETERANS AFFAIRS MEDICAL CENTER, 1011 Honor Heights Drive, Zip 74401–1399; tel. 918/683–3261 **A**1 3 5 **F**9 13 18 22 23 24 25 26 31 34 35 37 39 46 48 51 54 56 70 76 77 78 79 **S** Department of Veterans Affairs, Washington, DC Web address: www.visn16.med.va.gov	45	10	50	2231	43	157452	0	58833	33711	573
NORMAN—Cleveland County										
☐ GRIFFIN MEMORIAL HOSPITAL, 900 East Main Street, Zip 73071–5305, Mailing Address: P.O. Box 151, Zip 73070–0151; tel. 405/321–4880; Don Bowen, Superintendent (Nonreporting) **A**1 3 5 10 **S** Oklahoma State Department of Mental Health and Substance Abuse Services, Oklahoma City, OK	12	22	182	—	—	—	—	—	—	—
J. D. MCCARTY CENTER FOR CHILDREN WITH DEVELOPMENTAL DISABILITIES, 1125 East Alameda, Zip 73071–5264; tel. 405/321–4830; Curtis A. Peters, Chief Executive Officer **A**10 **F**13 23 45 53 54 63 70 72 78 Web address: www.jdmc.org	12	56	32	260	31	4548	0	5958	3677	128
★ NORMAN REGIONAL HOSPITAL, 901 North Porter Street, Zip 73071–6482, Mailing Address: P.O. Box 1308, Zip 73070–1308; tel. 405/307–1000; David D. Whitaker, FACHE, President and Chief Executive Officer **A**1 2 9 10 **F**3 4 7 8 9 11 13 16 17 18 19 21 22 23 25 28 29 31 32 33 34 35 36 38 39 40 43 44 45 46 47 48 50 51 53 54 56 57 58 59 60 62 63 64 65 68 69 70 71 72 75 76 77 78 79 **P**1 7 Web address: www.normanregional.com	16	10	271	12926	182	256983	1685	107233	44717	611
NOWATA—Nowata County										
JANE PHILLIPS NOWATA HEALTH CENTER, 237 South Locust Street, Zip 74048–0426, Mailing Address: P.O. Box 426, Zip 74048–0426; tel. 918/273–3102; Maggie Blevins, Administrator **A**9 10 18 **F**25 48 76 78	33	10	34	403	4	2529	0	1591	641	30
OKEENE—Blaine County										
OKEENE MUNICIPAL HOSPITAL, 207 East F Street, Zip 73763, Mailing Address: P.O. Box 489, Zip 73763–0489; tel. 580/822–4417; Debbie Howe, Administrator (Total facility includes 20 beds in nursing home–type unit) **A**9 10 **F**6 8 9 13 17 22 25 32 34 36 40 44 48 54 69 75 76 Web address: www.okeenehospital.com	16	10	70	476	19	—	84	2615	1337	55
OKEMAH—Okfuskee County										
★ CREEK NATION COMMUNITY HOSPITAL, 309 North 14th Street, Zip 74859–2099; tel. 918/623–1424; Frank H. Wahpepah, M.P.H., Administrator (Nonreporting) **A**9 10 **S** U. S. Public Health Service Indian Health Service, Rockville, MD	47	10	34	—	—	—	—	—	—	—
OKLAHOMA CITY—Oklahoma County										
★ △ BONE AND JOINT HOSPITAL, 1111 North Dewey Avenue, Zip 73103–2615; tel. 405/552–9100; James A. Hyde, Administrator (Nonreporting) **A**1 3 5 7 9 10 **S** SSM Health Care, Saint Louis, MO	23	47	89	—	—	—	—	—	—	—
CHILDREN'S HOSPITAL OF OKLAHOMA See University Health Partners										
★ DEACONESS HOSPITAL, 5501 North Portland Avenue, Zip 73112–2099; tel. 405/604–6000; Paul Dougherty, President and Chief Executive Officer (Total facility includes 22 beds in nursing home–type unit) (Nonreporting) **A**1 2 9 10 Web address: www.deaconessokc.com	23	10	226	—	—	—	—	—	—	—
☐ △ HEALTHSOUTH REHABILITATION HOSPITAL, 700 N.W. Seventh Street, Zip 73102–1295; tel. 405/553–1192; Hank Ross, Chief Executive Officer (Nonreporting) **A**1 7 10 **S** HEALTHSOUTH Corporation, Birmingham, AL	33	46	46	—	—	—	—	—	—	—
★ + ○ HILLCREST HEALTH CENTER, 2129 S.W. 59th Street, Zip 73119–7001; tel. 405/685–6671; Ray Brazier, President (Nonreporting) **A**1 9 10 11 12 13 **S** SSM Health Care, Saint Louis, MO	23	10	181	—	—	—	—	—	—	—

Hospitals, U.S. / OKLAHOMA

Hospital, Address, Telephone, Administrator, Approval, Facility, and Physician Codes, Health Care System, Network	Classification Codes		Utilization Data					Expense (thousands) of dollars		
★ American Hospital Association (AHA) membership ☐ Joint Commission on Accreditation of Healthcare Organizations (JCAHO) accreditation + American Osteopathic Healthcare Association (AOHA) membership ○ American Osteopathic Association (AOA) accreditation △ Commission on Accreditation of Rehabilitation Facilities (CARF) accreditation Control codes 61, 63, 64, 71, 72 and 73 indicate hospitals listed by AOHA, but not registered by AHA. For definition of numerical codes, see page A4	Control	Service	Staffed Beds	Admissions	Census	Outpatient Visits	Births	Total	Payroll	Personnel
✣ INTEGRIS BAPTIST MEDICAL CENTER, 3300 N.W. Expressway, Zip 73112–4481; tel. 405/949–3011; Thomas R. Rice, FACHE, President and Chief Operating Officer **A**1 2 3 5 9 10 **F**1 2 3 4 7 8 9 10 11 12 13 14 16 17 18 19 20 21 22 23 24 25 26 27 28 29 30 31 32 33 34 35 36 37 38 39 41 42 43 44 45 46 47 48 50 51 52 54 56 57 58 59 60 61 62 63 64 65 66 68 69 70 71 72 73 74 75 76 77 78 79 **P**8 **S** INTEGRIS Health, Oklahoma City, OK Web address: www.integris–health.com	23	10	503	22419	325	—	2212	251258	92731	2282
✣ △ INTEGRIS SOUTHWEST MEDICAL CENTER, 4401 South Western, Zip 73109–3441; tel. 405/636–7000; Thomas R. Rice, FACHE, President and Chief Operating Officer **A**1 2 7 9 10 **F**2 3 4 7 8 9 10 11 12 13 14 16 17 18 19 20 22 24 25 27 28 30 31 32 33 34 36 37 38 39 40 41 42 43 44 45 46 47 48 49 50 51 52 53 54 55 56 57 58 59 60 61 62 63 64 65 66 68 69 70 71 72 74 76 78 79 **P**6 7 8 **S** INTEGRIS Health, Oklahoma City, OK Web address: www.integris–health.com	23	10	325	11932	244	137514	999	115341	48229	1307
✣ △ MERCY HEALTH CENTER, 4300 West Memorial Road, Zip 73120–8362; tel. 405/755–1515; Michael J. Packnett, President and Chief Executive Officer (Nonreporting) **A**1 2 7 9 10 **S** Sisters of Mercy Health System–St. Louis, Saint Louis, MO Web address: www.mercyok.com	21	10	363	—	—	—	—	—	—	—
☐ NORTHWEST SURGICAL HOSPITAL, 9204 North May Avenue, Zip 73120–4419; tel. 405/848–1918; William Federman, Chief Executive Officer **A**1 10 **F**25 48 49	33	49	9	352	2	1830	0	5385	2259	36
PRESBYTERIAN HOSPITAL See University Health Partners										
✣ △ ST. ANTHONY HOSPITAL, 1000 North Lee Street, Zip 73102–1080, Mailing Address: P.O. Box 205, Zip 73101–0205; tel. 405/272–7000; Valinda Rutledge, President (Total facility includes 20 beds in nursing home–type unit) **A**1 2 3 5 7 9 10 **F**2 3 4 7 8 9 11 12 13 16 17 18 19 22 23 24 25 28 29 31 33 34 35 38 39 41 43 44 45 46 47 48 50 51 53 54 55 56 57 58 59 60 61 62 63 64 65 68 69 70 71 72 74 76 78 79 **P**8 **S** SSM Health Care, Saint Louis, MO	21	10	362	15266	244	173392	1174	137491	49745	1706
✣ UNIVERSITY HEALTH PARTNERS, (Includes Children's Hospital of Oklahoma, 940 N.E. 13th Street, Zip 73104; tel. 405/271–6165; Presbyterian Hospital, 700 N.E. 13th Street, Zip 73104–5070; tel. 405/271–5100; University Hospital, 920 N.E. 13th Street, Zip 73104; tel. 405/271–4700), 6501 North Broadway, Suite 200, Zip 73116; tel. 405/879–0900; Jeffrey A. Dorsey, Chief Executive Officer **A**1 2 3 5 8 9 10 **F**4 7 8 9 11 12 13 14 17 18 19 22 23 24 25 27 28 29 30 31 32 33 34 35 38 39 41 42 43 44 45 46 47 48 49 50 51 52 53 54 56 57 58 59 60 62 63 66 69 70 71 72 74 76 78 79 **P**1 5 7 8 **S** HCA – The Healthcare Company, Nashville, TN	33	10	621	28521	426	291421	3603	326545	105185	2661
UNIVERSITY HOSPITAL See University Health Partners										
✣ VETERANS AFFAIRS MEDICAL CENTER, 921 N.E. 13th Street, Zip 73104–5028; tel. 405/270–0501; Steven J. Gentling, Director (Total facility includes 40 beds in nursing home–type unit) (Nonreporting) **A**1 3 5 8 **S** Department of Veterans Affairs, Washington, DC Web address: www.va.gov/stations97/guide/home.asp?DIVISION=ALL	45	10	277	—	—	—	—	—	—	—
OKMULGEE—Okmulgee County										
GEORGE NIGH REHABILITATION CENTER, (Formerly George Nigh Rehabilitation Institute), 900 East Airport Road, Zip 74447–9762, Mailing Address: P.O. Box 1118, Zip 74447–1118; tel. 918/756–9211; Michael J. Duncan, Chief Executive Officer (Nonreporting) **A**10	12	46	26	—	—	—	—	—	—	—
☐ OKMULGEE MEMORIAL HOSPITAL, 1401 Morris Drive, Zip 74447–6419, Mailing Address: P.O. Box 1038, Zip 74447–1038; tel. 918/756–4233; David D. Rasmussen, Administrator **A**1 9 10 **F**7 8 9 13 17 18 22 24 25 30 32 34 36 37 44 48 57 62 68 70 76 78	23	10	66	2488	33	25292	380	14262	6324	196
PAULS VALLEY—Garvin County										
★ PAULS VALLEY GENERAL HOSPITAL, 100 Valley Drive, Zip 73075–0368, Mailing Address: Box 368, Zip 73075–0368; tel. 405/238–5501; Charles Johnston, Administrator (Total facility includes 8 beds in nursing home–type unit) **A**9 10 **F**7 9 22 25 26 31 32 36 37 41 44 45 48 54 69 70 76 Web address: www.telepath.com/pvgh/	14	10	50	1425	20	11978	67	7802	3971	162
PAWHUSKA—Osage County										
PAWHUSKA HOSPITAL, 1101 East 15th Street, Zip 74056–1920; tel. 918/287–3232; Samuel T. Guild, Administrator (Nonreporting) **A**9 10	14	10	19	—	—	—	—	—	—	—
PAWNEE—Pawnee County										
★ PAWNEE MUNICIPAL HOSPITAL, 1212 Fourth Street, Zip 74058–4046, Mailing Address: P.O. Box 467, Zip 74058–0467; tel. 918/762–2577; John H. Ketring, Administrator (Nonreporting) **A**9 10 **S** INTEGRIS Health, Oklahoma City, OK	23	10	40	—	—	—	—	—	—	—
PERRY—Noble County										
✣ PERRY MEMORIAL HOSPITAL, 501 14th Street, Zip 73077–5099; tel. 580/336–3541; Joe Duerr, Chief Executive Officer **A**1 9 10 **F**7 9 13 17 22 25 32 34 36 37 45 46 48 54 70 76 78 **P**8 **S** Quorum Health Group, Brentwood, TN	16	10	28	724	12	20985	0	5242	2390	78
PONCA CITY—Kay County										
✣ ST. JOSEPH REGIONAL MEDICAL CENTER OF NORTHERN OKLAHOMA, 14th Street and Hartford Avenue, Zip 74601–2035, Mailing Address: Box 1270, Zip 74602–1270; tel. 580/765–3321; Garry L. England, President and Chief Executive Officer (Total facility includes 10 beds in nursing home–type unit) **A**1 9 10 **F**6 8 9 16 17 18 19 21 22 25 27 28 31 32 33 34 35 36 37 38 39 40 41 44 45 46 48 49 54 57 65 67 68 69 70 71 72 76 78 **P**5 6 **S** Via Christi Health System, Wichita, KS Web address: www.sjrmcpc.com	21	10	100	4151	56	58108	620	27342	10959	379

Hospitals, U.S. / OKLAHOMA

Hospital, Address, Telephone, Administrator, Approval, Facility, and Physician Codes, Health Care System, Network	Classification Codes		Utilization Data					Expense (thousands) of dollars		
★ American Hospital Association (AHA) membership □ Joint Commission on Accreditation of Healthcare Organizations (JCAHO) accreditation + American Osteopathic Healthcare Association (AOHA) membership ○ American Osteopathic Association (AOA) accreditation △ Commission on Accreditation of Rehabilitation Facilities (CARF) accreditation Control codes 61, 63, 64, 71, 72 and 73 indicate hospitals listed by AOHA, but not registered by AHA. For definition of numerical codes, see page A4	Control	Service	Staffed Beds	Admissions	Census	Outpatient Visits	Births	Total	Payroll	Personnel
POTEAU—Le Flore County										
☒ EASTERN OKLAHOMA MEDICAL CENTER, 105 Wall Street, Zip 74953, Mailing Address: P.O. Box 1148, Zip 74953–1148; tel. 918/647–8161; L. Gene Matthews, Chief Executive Officer **A**1 9 10 **F**7 8 9 16 19 22 24 25 27 30 32 34 36 38 41 43 44 46 48 54 58 60 68 76 78 **P**6 **S** Hillcrest HealthCare System, Tulsa, OK	23	10	72	3326	28	16424	395	13026	6402	223
PRAGUE—Lincoln County										
★ PRAGUE MUNICIPAL HOSPITAL, 1322 Klabzuba Avenue, Zip 74864, Mailing Address: P.O. Drawer S, Zip 74864; tel. 405/567–4922; Chris Mattingly, Chief Executive Officer (Nonreporting) **A**9 10 18 **S** Hillcrest HealthCare System, Tulsa, OK	14	10	19	—	—	—	—	—	—	—
PRYOR—Mayes County										
☒ MAYES COUNTY MEDICAL CENTER, 129 North Kentucky Street, Zip 74361–4211, Mailing Address: P.O. Box 278, Zip 74362–0278; tel. 918/825–1600; W. Charles Jordan, Administrator **A**1 9 10 **F**8 9 13 18 19 22 25 32 34 36 37 38 39 45 46 48 51 70 71 72 76 78 **P**5 **S** INTEGRIS Health, Oklahoma City, OK	23	10	38	1545	16	21967	163	11526	5782	177
PURCELL—McClain County										
★ PURCELL MUNICIPAL HOSPITAL, 1500 North Green Avenue, Zip 73080–1699, Mailing Address: P.O. Box 511, Zip 73080–0511; tel. 405/527–6524; Curtis R. Pryor, Administrator **A**9 10 **F**7 8 9 13 16 18 19 22 25 29 32 34 36 44 48 50 51 54 70 72 76 **P**8 **S** Quorum Health Group, Brentwood, TN	14	10	22	1576	16	30128	95	8077	3527	140
SALLISAW—Sequoyah County										
SEQUOYAH MEMORIAL HOSPITAL, 213 East Redwood Street, Zip 74955–2811, Mailing Address: P.O. Box 505, Zip 74955–0505; tel. 918/774–1100; Ruth Ann Roark, Administrator (Nonreporting) **A**9 10	15	10	41	—	—	—	—	—	—	—
SAPULPA—Creek County										
★ ST. JOHN SAPULPA, (Formerly Bartlett Memorial Medical Center), 519 South Division Street, Zip 74066–4501, Mailing Address: P.O. Box 1368, Zip 74067–1368; tel. 918/224–4280; Raymond L. Replogle, President and Chief Executive Officer **A**9 10 **F**7 9 17 18 19 22 23 24 25 32 34 38 41 48 50 51 53 54 69 70 73 76 78 **P**5 **S** Marian Health System, Tulsa, OK	21	10	113	1741	23	13379	0	13878	6777	160
SAYRE—Beckham County										
★ SAYRE MEMORIAL HOSPITAL, 501 East Washington Street, Zip 73662, Mailing Address: P.O. Box 680, Zip 73662; tel. 580/928–5541; Larry Anderson, Administrator **A**9 10 **F**8 9 11 18 22 25 34 36 38 45 48 54 58 70 76 78 **P**6 **S** Quorum Health Group, Brentwood, TN	23	10	46	1158	12	14847	111	6471	3452	112
SEILING—Dewey County										
SEILING HOSPITAL, Highway 60 N.E., Zip 73663, Mailing Address: P.O. Box 720, Zip 73663–0720; tel. 580/922–7361; Jane McDowell, Administrator **A**9 10 **F**9 17 22 25 32 36 76 **P**5 6	14	10	18	490	6	6510	0	2041	1140	63
SEMINOLE—Seminole County										
★ SEMINOLE MEDICAL CENTER, (Formerly Seminole Municipal Hospital), 2401 Wrangler Boulevard, Zip 74868; tel. 405/303–4000; Janet Jackman, Chief Executive Officer (Nonreporting) **A**9 10 **S** HCA – The Healthcare Company, Nashville, TN	14	10	39	—	—	—	—	—	—	—
SHATTUCK—Ellis County										
★ NEWMAN MEMORIAL HOSPITAL, 905 South Main Street, Zip 73858–9802; tel. 580/938–2551; Gary W. Mitchell, Chief Executive Officer **A**9 10 **F**7 8 9 14 17 19 22 25 28 36 38 39 40 41 44 46 48 54 70 75 76	23	10	27	1007	10	24300	90	6297	2714	103
SHAWNEE—Pottawatomie County										
☒ MISSION HILL MEMORIAL HOSPITAL, 1900 Gordon Cooper Drive, Zip 74801–8600; tel. 405/273–2240; Gray Cox, President **A**1 9 10 **F**8 9 11 13 15 17 19 22 23 24 25 26 34 36 37 38 39 41 43 44 45 48 54 66 70 76 78 79 **P**1 8 **S** SSM Health Care, Saint Louis, MO	21	10	49	1731	18	17941	189	10561	4608	159
☒ SHAWNEE REGIONAL HOSPITAL, 1102 West MacArthur Street, Zip 74804–1744; tel. 405/273–2270; Charles E. Skillings, President and Chief Executive Officer (Nonreporting) **A**1 2 9 10	23	10	116	—	—	—	—	—	—	—
SPENCER—Oklahoma County										
☒ INTEGRIS MENTAL HEALTH SYSTEM–SPENCER, 2601 North Spencer Road, Zip 73084–3699, Mailing Address: P.O. Box 11137, Oklahoma City, Zip 73136–0137; tel. 405/427–2441; Murali Krishna, M.D., President and Chief Operating Officer (Nonreporting) **A**1 **S** INTEGRIS Health, Oklahoma City, OK Web address: www.integris–health.com	23	22	44	—	—	—	—	—	—	—
STIGLER—Haskell County										
★ HASKELL COUNTY HEALTHCARE SYSTEM, 401 N.W. H Street, Zip 74462–1625; tel. 918/967–4682; Stacy D. Holland, Administrator and Chief Executive Officer **A**9 10 **F**7 9 19 22 29 31 32 34 36 37 38 43 45 46 48 54 70 75 76 77 78 **P**5	13	10	31	942	13	13250	0	6477	3647	176
STILLWATER—Payne County										
☒ STILLWATER MEDICAL CENTER, 1323 West Sixth Avenue, Zip 74074–4399, Mailing Address: P.O. Box 2408, Zip 74076–2408; tel. 405/372–1480; Jerry G. Moeller, President and Chief Executive Officer (Total facility includes 30 beds in nursing home–type unit) **A**1 9 10 **F**4 7 8 9 11 16 17 18 22 23 24 25 27 35 36 37 38 39 40 41 44 46 48 49 51 54 61 64 65 68 69 70 74 76 78 79 **P**8 Web address: www.stillwater–medical.org	16	10	119	4771	68	67591	766	42939	17309	582
SULPHUR—Murray County										
ARBUCKLE MEMORIAL HOSPITAL, 2011 West Broadway Street, Zip 73086–4221; tel. 580/622–2161; Kenneth A. Ross, Chief Executive Officer **A**9 10 **F**7 9 16 17 18 25 38 57 61 70 76	13	10	35	1422	16	5138	1	3376	1827	72

© 2000 AHA Guide   *Many Facility Codes have changed. Please refer to the AHA Guide Code Chart.*

Hospitals, U.S. / OKLAHOMA

	Classification Codes		Utilization Data					Expense (thousands) of dollars		
Hospital, Address, Telephone, Administrator, Approval, Facility, and Physician Codes, Health Care System, Network	Control	Service	Staffed Beds	Admissions	Census	Outpatient Visits	Births	Total	Payroll	Personnel

Approval codes:
- ★ American Hospital Association (AHA) membership
- □ Joint Commission on Accreditation of Healthcare Organizations (JCAHO) accreditation
- + American Osteopathic Healthcare Association (AOHA) membership
- ○ American Osteopathic Association (AOA) accreditation
- △ Commission on Accreditation of Rehabilitation Facilities (CARF) accreditation

Control codes 61, 63, 64, 71, 72 and 73 indicate hospitals listed by AOHA, but not registered by AHA. For definition of numerical codes, see page A4.

TAHLEQUAH—Cherokee County

Hospital	Control	Service	Staffed Beds	Admissions	Census	Outpatient Visits	Births	Total	Payroll	Personnel
✠ TAHLEQUAH CITY HOSPITAL, 1400 East Downing Street, Zip 74464-3324, Mailing Address: P.O. Box 1008, Zip 74465-1008; tel. 918/456-0641; Gary L. Jepson, Chief Executive Officer **A**1 9 10 **F**7 8 9 11 16 17 18 22 24 25 30 32 34 36 38 39 41 44 48 50 54 57 62 68 70 76 78 Web address: www.tahlequahcityhospital.com	16	10	75	2614	29	40309	284	17574	8413	313
✠ WILLIAM W. HASTINGS INDIAN HOSPITAL, 100 South Bliss Avenue, Zip 74464-3399; tel. 918/458-3100; Hickory Starr, Jr, Administrator **A**1 10 **F**8 11 13 14 17 22 23 25 32 35 38 41 43 44 48 57 58 59 60 61 62 63 64 76 78 **P**6 **S** U. S. Public Health Service Indian Health Service, Rockville, MD	47	10	60	3341	28	210546	1027	27032	16229	438

TALIHINA—La Flore County

Hospital	Control	Service	Staffed Beds	Admissions	Census	Outpatient Visits	Births	Total	Payroll	Personnel
✠ CHOCTAW NATION HEALTH CARE CENTER, (Formerly Choctaw Nation Indian Hospital), One Choctaw Way, Zip 74571-9517; tel. 918/567-7000; Robert W. Blum, FACHE, Administrator **A**1 10 **F**8 9 11 13 15 17 22 23 24 25 27 29 30 31 32 33 34 35 36 37 38 39 40 43 45 46 47 48 49 50 51 54 55 56 58 59 60 61 62 63 64 65 66 67 68 70 71 72 73 74 76 77 79 **S** U. S. Public Health Service Indian Health Service, Rockville, MD Web address: www.choctawnation.com	47	10	37	1476	15	69303	278	—	—	310

TISHOMINGO—Johnston County

Hospital	Control	Service	Staffed Beds	Admissions	Census	Outpatient Visits	Births	Total	Payroll	Personnel
JOHNSTON MEMORIAL HOSPITAL, 1000 South Byrd Street, Zip 73460-3299; tel. 580/371-2327; Jack D. Martin, Interim Administrator (Nonreporting) **A**9 10 18	13	10	30	—	—	—	—	—	—	—

TULSA—Tulsa County

Hospital	Control	Service	Staffed Beds	Admissions	Census	Outpatient Visits	Births	Total	Payroll	Personnel
BROOKHAVEN HOSPITAL, 201 South Garnett Road, Zip 74128-1800; tel. 918/438-4257; Rolf B. Gainer, Chief Executive Officer and Administrator (Nonreporting) **A**10 Web address: www.brookhavenhospital.com	31	22	40	—	—	—	—	—	—	—
□ CANCER TREATMENT CENTERS OF AMERICA–TULSA, 2408 East 81st Street, Zip 74137-4210; tel. 918/496-5000; Joseph A. Gagliardi, President and Chief Executive Officer **A**1 2 10 **F**9 12 13 15 16 17 18 19 20 21 22 23 24 32 33 34 38 39 41 43 45 46 48 49 50 51 54 55 60 63 65 68 70 72 76 78 79 **P**6 **S** Cancer Treatment Centers of America, Arlington Heights, IL Web address: www.cancercenter.com	33	10	40	702	13	—	0	42268	9419	333
✠ CHILDREN'S MEDICAL CENTER, 5300 East Skelly Drive, Zip 74135-6599, Mailing Address: P.O. Box 35648, Zip 74153-0648; tel. 918/664-6600; Gerald Rothlein, Chief Executive Officer (Nonreporting) **A**1 3 5 10 **S** Hillcrest HealthCare System, Tulsa, OK	23	59	108	—	—	—	—	—	—	—
★ CONTINUOUS CARE CENTER OF TULSA, 1923 South Utica Avenue, Zip 74105, Mailing Address: 1755 South Utica Avenue, Zip 74105; tel. 918/749-8930; Raymond L. Replogle, President and Chief Executive Officer **A**10 **F**12 13 16 17 18 22 24 25 39 41 45 70 76	23	49	28	368	26	0	0	8512	3193	70
✠ DOCTORS HOSPITAL, 2323 South Harvard Avenue, Zip 74114-3370; tel. 918/744-4000; Kenneth Noteboom, Chief Executive Officer **A**1 9 10 **F**8 9 11 13 16 19 22 24 25 27 28 30 31 34 36 38 39 41 44 45 46 47 48 49 51 53 54 57 58 62 64 65 68 69 70 72 76 78 **P**6 8 **S** Hillcrest HealthCare System, Tulsa, OK Web address: www.hillcrest.com	23	10	121	2922	52	19074	721	22378	10450	373
✠ HILLCREST MEDICAL CENTER, 1120 South Utica, Zip 74104-4090; tel. 918/579-1000; Donald A. Lorack, Jr, President and Chief Executive Officer **A**1 2 3 5 9 10 **F**2 3 4 6 7 8 9 10 11 12 13 14 16 17 18 19 21 22 24 25 28 29 30 31 32 33 34 35 36 37 38 39 41 42 43 44 45 46 47 48 49 50 52 53 54 55 56 57 58 59 60 61 62 63 64 65 66 67 68 69 70 71 72 73 74 76 77 78 79 **P**5 6 8 **S** Hillcrest HealthCare System, Tulsa, OK Web address: www.hillcrest.com	23	10	421	21539	296	103780	3866	177036	69861	1942
✠ HILLCREST SPECIALTY HOSPITAL, (Formerly Specialty Hospital of Tulsa), 2408 East 81st Street, 2500, Zip 74137-4210; tel. 918/491-2400; Kenneth Noteboom, Chief Executive Officer (Nonreporting) **A**1 10 **S** Hillcrest HealthCare System, Tulsa, OK Web address: www.hcahealthcare.com	33	49	22	—	—	—	—	—	—	—
□ LAUREATE PSYCHIATRIC CLINIC AND HOSPITAL, 6655 South Yale Avenue, Zip 74136-3329; tel. 918/481-4000; John L. Fleming, M.D., Interim Chief Executive Officer (Nonreporting) **A**1 3 5 9 10	23	22	75	—	—	—	—	—	—	—
PARKSIDE HOSPITAL, 1620 East 12th Street, Zip 74120-5499; tel. 918/582-2131; Paul Greever, Chief Executive Officer **A**3 5 10 **F**1 2 3 13 16 19 21 34 57 58 59 60 61 63 64 70 72 78 **P**6	23	22	40	1602	23	109180	0	12900	7468	216
□ SAINT FRANCIS HOSPITAL, 6161 South Yale Avenue, Zip 74136-1992; tel. 918/494-2200; Donna Rheault, Chief Operating Officer (Total facility includes 40 beds in nursing home–type unit) **A**1 2 3 5 8 10 **F**2 3 4 8 9 11 12 13 14 17 18 19 21 22 23 24 25 26 27 28 32 33 34 35 36 37 38 39 40 41 42 43 44 45 46 47 48 49 50 51 52 53 54 57 58 59 60 61 62 63 64 65 68 69 70 71 72 73 74 75 76 78 79 **P**6 8 Web address: www.saintfrancis.com	23	10	624	36334	457	507585	3750	254133	107677	4213
✠ SOUTHCREST HOSPITAL, 8801 South 101st East Avenue, Zip 74133; tel. 918/294-4000; Anthony R. Young, Chief Executive Officer (Nonreporting) **A**1 9 **S** Triad Hospitals, Inc., Dallas, TX Web address: www.southcresthospital.com	33	10	119	—	—	—	—	—	—	—

Hospitals, U.S. / OKLAHOMA

Hospital, Address, Telephone, Administrator, Approval, Facility, and Physician Codes, Health Care System, Network	Classification Codes		Utilization Data					Expense (thousands) of dollars		
★ American Hospital Association (AHA) membership □ Joint Commission on Accreditation of Healthcare Organizations (JCAHO) accreditation + American Osteopathic Healthcare Association (AOHA) membership ○ American Osteopathic Association (AOA) accreditation △ Commission on Accreditation of Rehabilitation Facilities (CARF) accreditation Control codes 61, 63, 64, 71, 72 and 73 indicate hospitals listed by AOHA, but not registered by AHA. For definition of numerical codes, see page A4.	Control	Service	Staffed Beds	Admissions	Census	Outpatient Visits	Births	Total	Payroll	Personnel
★ △ ST. JOHN MEDICAL CENTER, 1923 South Utica Avenue, Zip 74104–5445; tel. 918/744–2345; David Pynn, President and Chief Executive Officer **A**1 2 3 5 7 9 10 **F**2 3 4 7 8 9 11 12 13 16 17 18 19 21 22 23 24 25 26 27 28 29 30 31 32 33 34 35 37 38 39 41 42 43 44 45 46 47 48 49 50 52 53 54 56 57 59 60 61 62 63 64 65 67 69 70 71 72 73 74 75 76 77 78 79 **S** Marian Health System, Tulsa, OK **Web address:** www.sjmc.org	21	10	556	24106	382	—	2466	213025	78653	3675
□ THE BROWN SCHOOLS AT SHADOW MOUNTAIN, 6262 South Sheridan Road, Zip 74133–4099; tel. 918/492–8200; Sharon Worsham, Chief Executive Officer (Nonreporting) **A**1 **S** Brown Schools, Inc., Austin, TX	33	52	100	—	—	—	—	—	—	—
★ + ○ △ TULSA REGIONAL MEDICAL CENTER, 744 West Ninth Street, Zip 74127–9990; tel. 918/599–5900; Steve Dobbs, Chief Executive Officer **A**1 7 9 10 11 12 13 **F**3 4 7 8 9 10 11 12 13 17 18 22 25 27 30 31 34 36 37 39 41 42 43 44 46 47 48 52 53 54 56 57 58 59 60 61 62 63 64 65 69 70 71 72 74 75 76 77 78 **P**5 7 8 **S** Hillcrest HealthCare System, Tulsa, OK	23	10	255	10029	166	27857	680	83184	36706	916
VINITA—Craig County										
★ CRAIG GENERAL HOSPITAL, 735 North Foreman Street, Zip 74301–1418, Mailing Address: Box 326, Zip 74301–0326; tel. 918/256–7551; B. Joe Gunn, FACHE, Administrator and Chief Executive Officer (Nonreporting) **A**1 9 10	16	10	28	—	—	—	—	—	—	—
□ EASTERN STATE HOSPITAL, Mailing Address: P.O. Box 69, Zip 74301–0069; tel. 918/256–7841; William T. Burkett, Chief Executive Officer **A**1 10 **F**16 17 18 23 25 28 31 32 33 34 35 43 45 50 51 60 61 70 78 **P**1 **S** Oklahoma State Department of Mental Health and Substance Abuse Services, Oklahoma City, OK	12	22	314	1733	280	0	0	29848	19180	567
WAGONER—Wagoner County										
★ WAGONER COMMUNITY HOSPITAL, 1200 West Cherokee, Zip 74467–4681, Mailing Address: Box 407, Zip 74477–0407; tel. 918/485–5514; John W. Crawford, Chief Executive Officer **A**1 9 10 **F**9 13 16 17 18 22 23 24 25 28 32 33 34 35 38 41 44 46 48 50 54 56 57 59 60 61 70 76 78 79 **P**3 8 **S** Hillcrest HealthCare System, Tulsa, OK	23	10	100	1552	25	7543	0	6834	3349	135
WATONGA—Blaine County										
★ WATONGA MUNICIPAL HOSPITAL, 500 North Nash Boulevard, Zip 73772–0370, Mailing Address: Box 370, Zip 73772–0370; tel. 580/623–7211; David R. Jordan, Ph.D., Chief Executive Officer (Nonreporting) **A**9 10 18 **S** Quorum Health Group, Brentwood, TN **Web address:** www.watongahospital.com	16	10	24	—	—	—	—	—	—	—
WAURIKA—Jefferson County										
★ JEFFERSON COUNTY HOSPITAL, Highway 70 and 81, Zip 73573, Mailing Address: P.O. Box 90, Zip 73573–0090; tel. 580/228–2344; Buck McKinney, Jr, Chief Executive Officer (Nonreporting) **A**9 10	13	10	29	—	—	—	—	—	—	—
WEATHERFORD—Custer County										
★ SOUTHWESTERN MEMORIAL HOSPITAL, 215 North Kansas Street, Zip 73096–5499; tel. 580/772–5551; Ronnie D. Walker, President **A**9 10 **F**7 8 9 22 25 32 38 39 48 76 78	16	10	46	789	6	11207	190	5549	2488	86
WILBURTON—Latimer County										
LATIMER COUNTY GENERAL HOSPITAL, 806 Highway 2 North, Zip 74578–3698; tel. 918/465–2391; M. Sue Turner, Administrator **A**9 10 **F**7 22 25 32 36 76 78 **P**5	13	10	33	479	5	—	0	2459	1183	61
WOODWARD—Woodward County										
WESTERN STATE PSYCHIATRIC CENTER, 1222 10th Street, Suite 211, Zip 73801; tel. 580/571–3233; Steve Norwood, Executive Director **A**10 **F**7 13 16 17 21 23 29 30 32 34 35 43 51 58 59 60 61 62 63 64 70 72 **S** Oklahoma State Department of Mental Health and Substance Abuse Services, Oklahoma City, OK	12	22	102	745	70	52270	0	12809	7024	209
★ WOODWARD HOSPITAL AND HEALTH CENTER, 900 17th Street, Zip 73801–2423; tel. 580/256–5511; Joel A. Hart, Chief Executive Officer **A**1 9 10 **F**7 8 9 12 13 16 17 18 22 24 25 27 32 34 36 37 39 41 43 44 45 46 48 49 54 62 65 69 70 72 76 77 **S** Quorum Health Group, Brentwood, TN	23	10	68	1850	27	13045	264	20167	6997	268

© 2000 AHA Guide   *Many Facility Codes have changed. Please refer to the AHA Guide Code Chart.*

Hospitals, U.S. / OREGON

OREGON

Resident Population 3,282 (in thousands)
Resident population in metro areas 70.2%
Birth rate per 1,000 population 13.5
65 years and over 13.2%
Percent of persons without health insurance 13.3%

★ American Hospital Association (AHA) membership
☐ Joint Commission on Accreditation of Healthcare Organizations (JCAHO) accreditation
+ American Osteopathic Healthcare Association (AOHA) membership
○ American Osteopathic Association (AOA) accreditation
△ Commission on Accreditation of Rehabilitation Facilities (CARF) accreditation
Control codes 61, 63, 64, 71, 72 and 73 indicate hospitals listed by AOHA, but not registered by AHA. For definition of numerical codes, see page A4

Hospital, Address, Telephone, Administrator, Approval, Facility, and Physician Codes, Health Care System, Network	Classification Codes		Utilization Data					Expense (thousands) of dollars		
	Control	Service	Staffed Beds	Admissions	Census	Outpatient Visits	Births	Total	Payroll	Personnel
ALBANY—Linn County ★ ALBANY GENERAL HOSPITAL, 1046 West Sixth Avenue, Zip 97321–1999; tel. 541/812–4000; Richard J. Delano, President **A**1 2 9 10 **F**8 9 11 13 17 19 22 24 25 32 33 34 36 37 38 39 41 43 44 45 46 48 51 54 56 59 64 65 70 71 72 73 75 76 77 78 79 **P**6 **S** Samaritan Health Services, Corvallis, OR	23	10	71	3636	29	40376	697	30917	13644	397
ASHLAND—Jackson County ★ ASHLAND COMMUNITY HOSPITAL, 280 Maple Street, Zip 97520, Mailing Address: P.O. Box 98, Zip 97520; tel. 541/482–2441; James R. Watson, Administrator **A**1 9 10 **F**1 6 7 8 9 13 16 18 19 22 25 27 32 34 36 37 38 39 40 41 43 44 45 48 49 50 51 69 70 71 72 75 76 **P**5 Web address: www.ashlandhospital.org	23	10	49	1557	15	28725	277	17368	8243	187
ASTORIA—Clatsop County ★ COLUMBIA MEMORIAL HOSPITAL, 2111 Exchange Street, Zip 97103; tel. 503/325–4321; Terry O. Finklein, Chief Executive Officer **A**1 9 10 **F**7 8 9 18 19 22 24 25 32 34 36 37 38 41 43 44 45 46 48 49 54 70 72 73 75 76 78 79 **P**8 Web address: www.columbiamemorial.org	23	10	37	2396	20	41799	334	19379	8977	251
BAKER CITY—Baker County ★ ST. ELIZABETH HEALTH SERVICES, 3325 Pocahontas Road, Zip 97814; tel. 541/523–6461; John R. Perushek, President and Chief Executive Officer (Total facility includes 98 beds in nursing home–type unit) (Nonreporting) **A**1 9 10 **S** Catholic Health Initiatives, Denver, CO	21	10	134	—	—	—	—	—	—	—
BANDON—Coos County ★ SOUTHERN COOS HOSPITAL AND HEALTH CENTER, (Formerly Southern Coos General Hospital), 900 11th Street S.E., Zip 97411; tel. 541/347–2426; James A. Wathen, Chief Executive Officer **A**9 10 **F**7 9 22 25 32 33 34 36 48 70 76	16	10	18	274	4	13133	0	3083	1558	54
BEND—Deschutes County ★ ST. CHARLES MEDICAL CENTER, 2500 N.E. Neff Road, Zip 97701–6015; tel. 541/382–4321; James T. Lussier, President and Chief Executive Officer (Nonreporting) **A**1 2 3 9 10 Web address: www.scmc.org	23	10	181	—	—	—	—	—	—	—
BURNS—Harney County HARNEY DISTRICT HOSPITAL, 557 West Washington Street, Zip 97720–1497; tel. 541/573–7281; David L. Harman, Administrator **A**9 10 **F**8 18 19 22 25 34 44 48 54 57 61 69 75 76 **P**5	16	10	44	660	5	20678	53	5056	2192	61
CLACKAMAS—Clackamas County ★ KAISER SUNNYSIDE MEDICAL CENTER, 10180 S.E. Sunnyside Road, Zip 97015–9303; tel. 503/652–2880; Kathleen S. Wegener, Administrator **A**1 2 10 **F**2 3 4 7 8 9 10 11 12 13 14 15 16 17 18 19 20 21 22 23 24 25 26 27 28 30 31 32 33 34 35 36 37 38 39 41 42 43 44 45 46 47 48 49 50 51 52 53 54 55 57 58 59 60 61 62 63 64 65 66 68 69 70 71 72 74 75 76 77 78 79 **P**6 **S** Kaiser Foundation Hospitals, Oakland, CA	23	10	178	12230	132	271673	1588	—	—	1202
COOS BAY—Coos County ★ BAY AREA HOSPITAL, 1775 Thompson Road, Zip 97420–2198; tel. 541/269–8111; Dale Jessup, President and Chief Executive Officer (Nonreporting) **A**1 2 9 10	16	10	114	—	—	—	—	—	—	—
COQUILLE—Coos County COQUILLE VALLEY HOSPITAL, 940 East Fifth Street, Zip 97423; tel. 541/396–3101; Edna J. Cotner, Administrator **A**9 10 **F**7 8 9 17 18 22 25 36 44 48 72 76	16	10	20	511	5	13891	70	5001	1997	83
CORVALLIS—Benton County ★ GOOD SAMARITAN HOSPITAL CORVALLIS, 3600 N.W. Samaritan Drive, Zip 97330, Mailing Address: P.O. Box 1068, Zip 97339; tel. 541/757–5111; Steven W. Jasperson, Executive Vice President Operations (Nonreporting) **A**1 2 9 10 **S** Samaritan Health Services, Corvallis, OR Web address: www.goodsam.com	23	10	124	—	—	—	—	—	—	—
DALLAS—Polk County ☐ VALLEY COMMUNITY HOSPITAL, 550 S.E. Clay Street, Zip 97338, Mailing Address: P.O. Box 378, Zip 97338; tel. 503/623–8301; Kim Flitcroft, President **A**1 9 10 **F**7 8 13 16 17 19 22 44 48 54 69 71 75 76 78	23	10	36	1184	11	29364	186	13887	7868	174
ENTERPRISE—Wallowa County ★ WALLOWA MEMORIAL HOSPITAL, 401 East First Street, Zip 97828, Mailing Address: P.O. Box 460, Zip 97828; tel. 541/426–3111; Kim Dahlman, Chief Executive Officer (Total facility includes 32 beds in nursing home–type unit) (Nonreporting) **A**9 10	16	10	55	—	—	—	—	—	—	—
EUGENE—Lane County ★ △ SACRED HEART MEDICAL CENTER, 1255 Hilyard Street, Zip 97401, Mailing Address: P.O. Box 10905, Zip 97440; tel. 541/686–7300; Judy Hodgson, Administrator **A**1 2 7 9 10 **F**4 8 9 11 12 13 16 17 18 19 22 24 25 26 28 29 30 32 33 34 35 38 39 41 42 44 45 46 47 48 49 50 53 54 56 57 61 65 66 70 72 75 76 77 78 79 **P**6 **S** PeaceHealth, Bellevue, WA Web address: www.peacehealth.com	21	10	404	20420	248	105098	2480	227774	86057	2087

Hospitals, U.S. / OREGON

Hospital, Address, Telephone, Administrator, Approval, Facility, and Physician Codes, Health Care System, Network	Classification Codes		Utilization Data					Expense (thousands) of dollars		
★ American Hospital Association (AHA) membership □ Joint Commission on Accreditation of Healthcare Organizations (JCAHO) accreditation + American Osteopathic Healthcare Association (AOHA) membership ○ American Osteopathic Association (AOA) accreditation △ Commission on Accreditation of Rehabilitation Facilities (CARF) accreditation Control codes 61, 63, 64, 71, 72 and 73 indicate hospitals listed by AOHA, but not registered by AHA. For definition of numerical codes, see page A4	Control	Service	Staffed Beds	Admissions	Census	Outpatient Visits	Births	Total	Payroll	Personnel
SERENITY LANE, 616 East 16th, Zip 97401; tel. 541/687-1110; Neil H. McNaughton, Executive Director and Administrator (Nonreporting) **Web address:** www.serenitylane.org	23	82	55	—	—	—	—	—	—	—
FLORENCE—Lane County										
✯ PEACE HARBOR HOSPITAL, 400 Ninth Street, Zip 97439, Mailing Address: P.O. Box 580, Zip 97439; tel. 541/997-8412; James Barnhart, Chief Executive Officer **A**1 9 10 **F**3 7 8 9 16 17 18 19 22 24 25 32 34 36 37 39 41 44 48 54 68 70 72 75 76 **P**6 **S** PeaceHealth, Bellevue, WA **Web address:** www.peacehealth.org	21	10	21	1363	13	34172	67	15574	6826	156
FOREST GROVE—Washington County										
TUALITY FOREST GROVE HOSPITAL See Tuality Healthcare, Hillsboro										
GOLD BEACH—Curry County										
CURRY GENERAL HOSPITAL, 94220 Fourth Street, Zip 97444-9990; tel. 541/247-6621; Ginny Hochberg, Clinical Administrator **A**9 10 **F**7 8 9 14 16 17 18 19 22 25 29 31 32 34 38 44 48 51 56 61 72 75 76 77 78 79 **P**1	16	10	24	544	4	18671	95	5006	2323	85
GRANTS PASS—Josephine County										
✯ THREE RIVERS COMMUNITY HOSPITAL AND HEALTH CENTER, (Includes Dimmick Campus, 715 N.W. Dimmick Street, tel. 541/476-6831; Washington Campus, 1505 N.W. Washington Boulevard, Zip 97526; tel. 541/479-7531), 715 N.W. Dimmick Street, Zip 97526-1596; tel. 541/476-6831; Paul Janke, Senior Vice President **A**1 9 10 **F**7 8 9 13 16 17 18 19 21 22 24 25 27 28 32 34 36 39 41 44 45 46 48 51 54 57 61 68 70 72 76 77 78 **P**6 **S** Asante Health System, Medford, OR	23	10	71	6632	60	262890	642	53207	24066	598
GRESHAM—Multnomah County										
✯ LEGACY MOUNT HOOD MEDICAL CENTER, 24800 S.E. Stark, Zip 97030-0154; tel. 503/667-1122; Thomas S. Parker, Site Administrator **A**1 2 9 10 **F**1 2 3 4 7 8 9 10 11 13 14 16 17 18 19 20 21 22 23 24 25 26 27 28 29 30 32 33 34 35 36 37 38 39 41 42 43 44 45 46 47 48 49 50 51 52 53 54 56 57 58 59 60 61 62 64 65 68 69 70 72 74 75 76 77 78 79 **S** Legacy Health System, Portland, OR **Web address:** www.legacyhealth.org	23	10	58	3576	32	50749	753	30910	13998	357
HEPPNER—Morrow County										
PIONEER MEMORIAL HOSPITAL, 564 East Pioneer Drive, Zip 97836, Mailing Address: P.O. Box 9, Zip 97836; tel. 541/676-9133; Victor Vander Does, Administrator (Total facility includes 32 beds in nursing home-type unit) **A**9 10 **F**12 25 29 36 40 43 54 58 59 60 61 62 63 69 70 76 **Web address:** www.ucinet.com/~mchd	16	10	44	125	20	15158	0	4543	2111	66
HERMISTON—Umatilla County										
✯ GOOD SHEPHERD MEDICAL CENTER, (Formerly Good Shepherd Community Hospital), 610 N.W. 11th Street, Zip 97838-9696; tel. 541/667-3400; Dennis E. Burke, President **A**1 9 10 **F**7 8 9 16 17 18 22 24 25 27 32 33 34 36 37 38 39 41 43 44 45 48 50 51 56 70 72 75 76 78 **P**5 6 **Web address:** www.gshealth.org	23	10	45	2617	22	43382	498	22254	10123	287
HILLSBORO—Washington County										
✯ TUALITY HEALTHCARE, (Includes Tuality Community Hospital, 335 S.E. Eighth Avenue, Mailing Address: P.O. Box 309, Zip 97123; tel. 503/681-1111; Tuality Forest Grove Hospital, 1809 Maple Street, Forest Grove, Zip 97116-1995; tel. 503/357-2173), 335 S.E. Eighth Avenue, Zip 97123; tel. 503/681-1111; Richard Stenson, President and Chief Executive Officer (Total facility includes 18 beds in nursing home-type unit) **A**1 9 10 **F**3 4 7 8 9 11 13 14 16 18 19 22 24 25 26 27 28 29 30 31 32 33 34 36 37 38 39 41 43 44 46 48 50 54 57 62 69 70 71 72 76 77 78 79 **P**1 6 7 **Web address:** www.tuality.com	23	10	147	6846	73	134847	1496	72295	31945	821
HOOD RIVER—Hood River County										
✯ PROVIDENCE HOOD RIVER MEMORIAL HOSPITAL, (Formerly Hood River Memorial Hospital), 13th and May Streets, Zip 97031, Mailing Address: P.O. Box 149, Zip 97031; tel. 541/386-3911; Larry Bowe, JD, Chief Executive Officer **A**1 9 10 **F**1 2 3 8 9 12 17 18 22 23 24 25 28 33 35 36 38 41 44 45 46 48 49 72 75 76 77 78 **P**8 **S** Providence Health System, Seattle, WA **Web address:** www.hrmh.org	23	10	31	1500	12	41580	408	16613	7241	215
JOHN DAY—Grant County										
★ BLUE MOUNTAIN HOSPITAL, 170 Ford Road, Zip 97845; tel. 541/575-1311; Robert Houser, Chief Executive Officer (Total facility includes 52 beds in nursing home-type unit) **A**9 10 **F**1 3 6 7 8 10 12 16 17 18 19 21 22 23 25 32 33 36 37 38 41 42 44 48 49 50 51 52 53 54 58 59 60 61 62 63 69 70 71 72 75 76 **P**5 **S** Brim Healthcare, Inc., Brentwood, TN	16	10	73	515	43	15406	62	6232	3249	117
KLAMATH FALLS—Klamath County										
✯ MERLE WEST MEDICAL CENTER, 2865 Daggett Street, Zip 97601-1180; tel. 541/882-6311; Paul R. Stewart, President and Chief Executive Officer (Total facility includes 107 beds in nursing home-type unit) **A**1 2 3 9 10 **F**4 6 7 8 9 11 13 17 18 19 22 23 25 27 28 31 32 34 35 36 39 41 44 45 46 48 54 56 57 61 63 65 67 69 70 71 72 75 76 77 78 **P**6 8 **Web address:** www.mwmc.org	23	10	243	7235	139	143698	871	65174	30055	802
LA GRANDE—Union County										
✯ GRANDE RONDE HOSPITAL, 900 Sunset Drive, Zip 97850, Mailing Address: P.O. Box 3290, Zip 97850; tel. 541/963-8421; James A. Mattes, President (Total facility includes 13 beds in nursing home-type unit) **A**1 9 10 **F**7 8 9 13 14 16 17 18 22 24 25 26 27 28 36 37 39 40 41 43 44 45 46 48 49 54 58 59 61 62 63 68 69 70 71 72 75 76 78 **P**1	23	10	62	2060	23	39187	310	20784	10133	296

Hospitals, U.S. / OREGON

Hospital, Address, Telephone, Administrator, Approval, Facility, and Physician Codes, Health Care System, Network	Classification Codes		Utilization Data					Expense (thousands) of dollars		Personnel
	Control	Service	Staffed Beds	Admissions	Census	Outpatient Visits	Births	Total	Payroll	

★ American Hospital Association (AHA) membership
☐ Joint Commission on Accreditation of Healthcare Organizations (JCAHO) accreditation
+ American Osteopathic Healthcare Association (AOHA) membership
○ American Osteopathic Association (AOA) accreditation
△ Commission on Accreditation of Rehabilitation Facilities (CARF) accreditation
Control codes 61, 63, 64, 71, 72 and 73 indicate hospitals listed by AOHA, but not registered by AHA. For definition of numerical codes, see page A4

Hospital	Control	Service	Staffed Beds	Admissions	Census	Outpatient Visits	Births	Total	Payroll	Personnel
LAKEVIEW—Lake County LAKE DISTRICT HOSPITAL, 700 South J Street, Zip 97630–1679; tel. 541/947-2114; Gordon Ensley, Acting Administrator (Total facility includes 47 beds in nursing home–type unit) **A**9 10 **F**2 7 8 9 12 22 25 32 36 41 44 45 48 54 61 69 70 72 75 76 **P**5	16	10	68	461	40	15403	55	—	—	—
LEBANON—Linn County ★ LEBANON COMMUNITY HOSPITAL, 525 North Santiam Highway, Zip 97355, Mailing Address: P.O. Box 739, Zip 97355–0739; tel. 541/258-2101; Steven W. Jasperson, Executive Vice President Operations **A**1 9 10 **F**6 8 9 13 16 17 22 25 28 32 33 34 36 37 38 39 41 43 44 45 46 48 50 51 54 67 70 72 75 76 78 **P**6 **S** Samaritan Health Services, Corvallis, OR	23	10	49	2876	29	64725	386	24292	13054	359
LINCOLN CITY—Lincoln County ★ NORTH LINCOLN HOSPITAL, 3043 N.E. 28th Street, Zip 97367–4523, Mailing Address: P.O. Box 767, Zip 97367–0767; tel. 541/994-3661; David C. Bigelow, Chief Executive Officer **A**1 9 10 **F**7 8 9 22 24 25 27 36 37 39 41 44 48 54 69 70 72 75 76 **P**5 **S** Samaritan Health Services, Corvallis, OR	16	10	30	1410	12	35791	198	18128	9408	229
MADRAS—Jefferson County ★ MOUNTAIN VIEW HOSPITAL DISTRICT, 470 N.E. A Street, Zip 97741; tel. 541/475-3882; Susan McGough, Administrator (Total facility includes 68 beds in nursing home–type unit) **A**9 10 **F**7 8 9 12 17 18 19 22 25 34 36 37 41 44 45 48 56 69 76 **P**6	16	10	102	874	51	28660	179	10315	5361	167
MCMINNVILLE—Yamhill County ★ WILLAMETTE VALLEY MEDICAL CENTER, 2700 Three Mile Lane, Zip 97128–6498; tel. 503/472-6131; Rosemari Davis, Chief Executive Officer **A**1 9 10 **F**8 9 11 13 19 22 24 25 27 30 32 34 38 39 41 44 45 48 53 54 70 72 75 76 78 79 **P**5 6 **S** Triad Hospitals, Inc., Dallas, TX Web address: www.hcahealthcare.com	33	10	67	3856	36	56112	722	31123	13114	307
MEDFORD—Jackson County ★ △ PROVIDENCE MEDFORD MEDICAL CENTER, 1111 Crater Lake Avenue, Zip 97504–6241; tel. 541/732-5000; Charles T. Wright, Chief Executive, Southern Oregon Service Area **A**1 2 7 9 10 **F**1 4 8 9 11 13 14 16 17 18 19 22 24 25 27 30 31 32 33 34 35 36 37 38 39 41 43 44 45 46 48 49 50 51 53 54 56 61 65 68 70 72 75 76 78 79 **P**4 5 6 7 **S** Providence Health System, Seattle, WA Web address: www.providence.org	21	10	121	5506	64	310054	504	57787	26518	741
★ ROGUE VALLEY MEDICAL CENTER, 2825 East Barnett Road, Zip 97504–8332; tel. 541/608-4900; Roseanne McLaren, Senior Vice President **A**1 2 9 10 **F**2 3 4 7 8 9 11 12 13 14 16 17 18 19 22 23 24 25 26 27 31 32 33 34 36 37 38 39 41 42 43 44 45 46 47 48 49 50 51 54 57 59 61 65 68 69 70 72 75 76 78 79 **P**6 8 **S** Asante Health System, Medford, OR	23	10	264	12478	151	499497	1421	137564	51987	1399
MILWAUKIE—Clackamas County ★ PROVIDENCE MILWAUKIE HOSPITAL, 10150 S.E. 32nd Avenue, Zip 97222–6593; tel. 503/513-8300; Janice Burger, Operations Administrator (Total facility includes 29 beds in nursing home–type unit) **A**1 2 9 10 **F**1 2 3 4 5 7 8 9 10 11 12 13 16 17 18 19 21 22 23 25 26 27 28 30 33 35 36 37 38 39 41 42 43 44 45 46 47 48 49 53 54 55 56 57 58 59 60 61 62 63 64 65 67 69 70 71 72 73 75 76 77 78 79 **P**5 6 **S** Providence Health System, Seattle, WA Web address: www.providence.org	21	10	56	3494	49	127784	407	31623	13224	276
NEWBERG—Yamhill County ★ PROVIDENCE NEWBERG HOSPITAL, 501 Villa Road, Zip 97132; tel. 503/537-1555; Mark W. Meinert, CHE, Chief Executive, Yamhill Service Area **A**1 9 10 **F**1 7 8 9 16 17 18 19 22 24 25 32 33 34 36 37 38 39 41 43 44 45 46 48 50 51 54 59 61 70 72 75 76 78 **P**5 **S** Providence Health System, Seattle, WA Web address: www.phsor.org	21	10	35	1318	11	77647	292	18395	8676	221
NEWPORT—Lincoln County ★ PACIFIC COMMUNITIES HEALTH DISTRICT, 930 S.W. Abbey Street, Zip 97365–4820, Mailing Address: P.O. Box 945, Zip 97365–4820; tel. 541/265-2244; Michael R. Fraser, Administrator (Nonreporting) **A**1 9 10 Web address: www.pchd.net	16	10	41	—	—	—	—	—	—	—
ONTARIO—Malheur County ★ HOLY ROSARY MEDICAL CENTER, 351 S.W. Ninth Street, Zip 97914–2693; tel. 541/881-7000; Bruce C. Jensen, President and Chief Executive Officer **A**1 9 10 **F**7 8 9 12 16 18 22 24 25 29 32 34 35 36 37 39 43 44 45 46 48 49 50 51 54 68 70 71 75 76 77 78 **P**5 **S** Catholic Health Initiatives, Denver, CO	21	10	74	3753	33	57787	737	30945	11852	327
OREGON CITY—Clackamas County ★ WILLAMETTE FALLS HOSPITAL, 1500 Division Street, Zip 97045–1597; tel. 503/656-1631; Robert A. Steed, President **A**1 2 9 10 **F**7 8 9 17 18 22 23 24 25 29 33 34 36 37 38 39 41 43 44 45 46 48 49 50 54 56 68 70 72 76 77 78 **P**5 8	23	10	91	5835	44	87447	1101	47524	22937	446
PENDLETON—Umatilla County EASTERN OREGON PSYCHIATRIC CENTER, 2575 Westgate, Zip 97801; tel. 541/276-4511; Maxine Stone, Superintendent (Nonreporting) **A**10	12	22	60	—	—	—	—	—	—	—
★ ST. ANTHONY HOSPITAL, 1601 S.E. Court Avenue, Zip 97801–3297; tel. 541/276-5121; Jeffrey S. Drop, President and Chief Executive Officer **A**1 2 9 10 **F**8 9 13 16 17 18 19 22 23 24 25 27 28 30 32 33 34 36 37 38 39 43 44 45 46 48 51 54 56 68 70 72 75 76 78 **P**5 **S** Catholic Health Initiatives, Denver, CO	21	10	49	2044	19	22069	455	24527	9236	277

Many Facility Codes have changed. Please refer to the AHA Guide Code Chart.

Hospitals, U.S. / OREGON

Hospital, Address, Telephone, Administrator, Approval, Facility, and Physician Codes, Health Care System, Network	Classification Codes		Utilization Data					Expense (thousands) of dollars		
★ American Hospital Association (AHA) membership □ Joint Commission on Accreditation of Healthcare Organizations (JCAHO) accreditation + American Osteopathic Healthcare Association (AOHA) membership ○ American Osteopathic Association (AOA) accreditation △ Commission on Accreditation of Rehabilitation Facilities (CARF) accreditation Control codes 61, 63, 64, 71, 72 and 73 indicate hospitals listed by AOHA, but not registered by AHA. For definition of numerical codes, see page A4	Control	Service	Staffed Beds	Admissions	Census	Outpatient Visits	Births	Total	Payroll	Personnel
PORTLAND—Multnomah County										
★ ADVENTIST MEDICAL CENTER, 10123 S.E. Market, Zip 97216–2599; tel. 503/257–2500; Deryl L. Jones, President **A**1 2 3 9 10 **F**2 3 4 7 8 9 11 13 16 17 18 19 22 24 25 26 27 28 32 33 34 36 37 38 39 41 43 44 45 46 48 49 50 51 54 57 58 59 60 61 62 63 64 65 66 70 71 72 76 77 78 79 **P**5 6 7 **S** Adventist Health, Roseville, CA **Web address:** www.adventisthealthnw.com	21	10	214	9767	120	299669	1439	114179	59155	1602
DOERNBECHER CHILDREN'S HOSPITAL See OHSU Hospital										
○ EASTMORELAND HOSPITAL, (Osteopathic), 2900 S.E. Steele Street, Zip 97202; tel. 503/234–0411; J. Phillip Young, Chief Executive Officer **A**9 10 11 12 13 **F**15 25 48 **S** New American Healthcare Corporation, Brentwood, TN **Web address:** www.eastmorelandhospital.net	33	49	77	1331	21	0	0	15170	7440	188
GOOD SAMARITAN HOSPITAL AND MEDICAL CENTER See Legacy Good Samaritan Hospital and Medical Center										
★ △ LEGACY EMANUEL HOSPITAL AND HEALTH CENTER, 2801 North Gantenbein Avenue, Zip 97227–1674; tel. 503/413–2200; Stephani White, Vice President and Site Administrator (Total facility includes 27 beds in nursing home–type unit) **A**1 3 5 7 9 10 **F**1 2 3 4 7 8 9 10 11 13 14 16 17 18 19 21 22 24 25 26 27 28 29 30 32 33 34 35 36 37 38 39 41 42 43 44 45 46 47 48 49 50 51 52 53 54 56 57 58 59 60 61 62 65 68 69 70 72 74 75 76 77 78 79 **S** Legacy Health System, Portland, OR **Web address:** www.legacyhealth.org	23	10	356	18501	255	173381	2310	211998	98844	2460
★ LEGACY GOOD SAMARITAN HOSPITAL AND MEDICAL CENTER, (Includes Good Samaritan Hospital and Medical Center; Rehabilitation Institute of Oregon), 1015 N.W. 22nd Avenue, Zip 97210; tel. 503/413–7711; Martha C. Wangenstein, Vice President and Site Administrator (Total facility includes 40 beds in nursing home–type unit) **A**1 2 3 5 9 10 **F**1 2 3 4 7 8 9 10 11 13 14 16 17 18 19 21 22 24 25 26 27 28 29 30 32 33 34 35 36 37 38 39 41 42 43 44 45 46 47 48 49 50 51 52 53 54 55 56 57 58 59 60 62 64 65 66 67 69 70 72 74 75 76 77 78 79 **S** Legacy Health System, Portland, OR **Web address:** www.legacyhealth.org	23	10	279	12119	185	119918	1546	144139	60130	1454
★ OHSU HOSPITAL, (Includes Doernbecher Children's Hospital), 3181 S.W. Sam Jackson Park Road, Zip 97201–3098; tel. 503/494–8311; Timothy M. Goldfarb, Director Health Systems **A**1 2 3 5 8 9 10 **F**1 3 4 5 7 8 9 11 12 13 14 15 16 17 18 19 20 21 22 23 24 25 26 27 28 29 30 31 32 33 34 35 36 37 38 39 41 42 43 44 46 47 48 49 50 51 52 54 55 56 57 58 59 60 61 62 63 65 66 68 70 71 72 73 74 75 76 77 78 79 **P**3 6 7 8 **Web address:** www.ohsu.edu	16	10	373	21292	301	470956	2536	377268	132671	3417
□ PACIFIC GATEWAY HOSPITAL AND COUNSELING CENTER, 1345 S.E. Harney, Zip 97202; tel. 503/234–5353; Karl R. Brady, Chief Executive Officer (Nonreporting) **A**1 10 **S** Behavioral Healthcare Corporation, Nashville, TN **Web address:** www.pacificgate.com	33	22	66	—	—	—	—	—	—	—
★ PROVIDENCE PORTLAND MEDICAL CENTER, 4805 N.E. Glisan Street, Zip 97213–2967; tel. 503/215–1111; David T. Underriner, Operations Administrator **A**1 2 3 5 9 10 **F**1 3 4 5 6 7 8 9 11 12 13 16 17 18 19 21 22 24 25 26 27 28 29 30 32 33 34 35 36 37 38 39 41 42 43 44 45 46 47 48 49 50 53 54 55 56 57 58 59 60 61 62 63 64 65 67 69 70 71 72 73 74 76 77 78 79 **P**5 6 **S** Providence Health System, Seattle, WA **Web address:** www.providence.org	21	10	380	22025	243	647744	2340	245245	97007	2024
★ PROVIDENCE ST. VINCENT MEDICAL CENTER, 9205 S.W. Barnes Road, Zip 97225–6661; tel. 503/216–1234; Donald Elsom, Operations Administrator **A**1 2 3 5 9 10 **F**1 2 3 4 5 6 7 8 9 11 12 13 16 17 18 19 21 22 24 25 26 27 28 29 30 32 33 34 35 36 37 38 39 41 42 43 44 45 46 47 48 49 50 51 53 54 55 56 57 58 59 61 62 63 65 67 68 69 70 71 72 73 76 77 78 79 **P**5 6 **S** Providence Health System, Seattle, WA **Web address:** www.providence.org/portland/hospitals	21	10	389	28139	295	768303	5262	282363	109382	2197
REHABILITATION INSTITUTE OF OREGON See Legacy Good Samaritan Hospital and Medical Center										
□ SHRINERS HOSPITALS FOR CHILDREN, PORTLAND, 3101 S.W. Sam Jackson Park Road, Zip 97201; tel. 503/241–5090; C. Thomas D'Esmond, Administrator **A**1 3 5 **F**13 19 28 43 45 49 54 70 71 78 **S** Shriners Hospitals for Children, Tampa, FL **Web address:** www.shcc.org	23	57	40	1391	13	11482	0	—	—	301
★ △ VETERANS AFFAIRS MEDICAL CENTER, 3710 S.W. U.S. Veterans Hospital Road, Zip 97201; tel. 503/220–8262; James Tuchschmidt, M.D., Chief Executive Officer (Total facility includes 120 beds in nursing home–type unit) (Nonreporting) **A**1 2 3 5 7 8 **S** Department of Veterans Affairs, Washington, DC **Web address:** www.va.gov/stations97/guide/home.asp?DIVISION=ALL	45	10	591	—	—	—	—	—	—	—
□ WOODLAND PARK HOSPITAL, 10300 N.E. Hancock, Zip 97220; tel. 503/257–5500; J. Phillip Young, Chief Executive Officer **A**1 9 10 **F**41 44 48 **S** New American Healthcare Corporation, Brentwood, TN **Web address:** www.woodlandparkhospital.net	33	10	121	2108	29	27033	206	19057	10836	280
PRINEVILLE—Crook County										
★ PIONEER MEMORIAL HOSPITAL, 1201 N.E. Elm Street, Zip 97754; tel. 541/447–6254; Donald J. Wee, Executive Director **A**9 10 **F**8 9 17 18 19 22 25 26 36 37 41 43 44 45 48 51 54 66 70 75 76 78 **P**5 **S** Banner Health System, Fargo, ND **Web address:** www.pmhprineville.org	23	10	30	977	9	26252	121	10028	4563	124

© 2000 AHA Guide *Many Facility Codes have changed. Please refer to the AHA Guide Code Chart.*

Hospitals, U.S. / OREGON

Legend (Classification Codes):
- ★ American Hospital Association (AHA) membership
- ☐ Joint Commission on Accreditation of Healthcare Organizations (JCAHO) accreditation
- + American Osteopathic Healthcare Association (AOHA) membership
- ○ American Osteopathic Association (AOA) accreditation
- △ Commission on Accreditation of Rehabilitation Facilities (CARF) accreditation

Control codes 61, 63, 64, 71, 72 and 73 indicate hospitals listed by AOHA, but not registered by AHA. For definition of numerical codes, see page A4

Hospital, Address, Telephone, Administrator, Approval, Facility, and Physician Codes, Health Care System, Network	Classification Codes		Utilization Data					Expense (thousands) of dollars		Personnel
	Control	Service	Staffed Beds	Admissions	Census	Outpatient Visits	Births	Total	Payroll	
REDMOND—Deschutes County ★ CENTRAL OREGON DISTRICT HOSPITAL, 1253 North Canal Boulevard, Zip 97756–1395; tel. 541/548–8131; James A. Diegel, CHE, Executive Director **A**1 9 10 **F**7 8 9 13 16 17 18 19 22 24 25 29 32 33 34 35 36 38 41 43 44 48 49 50 54 61 70 71 75 76 78 79 **P**5 7 **S** Banner Health System, Fargo, ND Web address: www.codh.org	16	10	48	2047	15	26684	289	18369	8743	248
REEDSPORT—Douglas County LOWER UMPQUA HOSPITAL DISTRICT, 600 Ranch Road, Zip 97467–1795; tel. 541/271–2171; Sandra Reese, Administrator (Total facility includes 28 beds in nursing home–type unit) **A**9 10 **F**7 8 9 12 17 22 25 30 32 36 37 38 39 41 44 48 54 69 70 75 76 78	16	10	49	948	35	14970	42	9154	4139	119
ROSEBURG—Douglas County ★ MERCY MEDICAL CENTER, 2700 Stewart Parkway, Zip 97470–1297; tel. 541/673–0611; Victor J. Fresolone, FACHE, President and Chief Executive Officer **A**1 2 9 10 **F**6 7 8 9 11 12 13 17 18 19 22 24 25 27 31 32 34 35 36 37 39 41 44 45 46 48 49 51 54 57 58 59 60 61 62 63 64 65 67 69 70 71 72 73 75 76 78 79 **S** Catholic Health Initiatives, Denver, CO Web address: www.mercyrose.org	21	10	114	7914	81	164102	866	56920	22744	695
★ VETERANS AFFAIRS ROSEBURG HEALTHCARE SYSTEM, 913 N.W. Garden Valley Boulevard, Zip 97470–6513; tel. 541/440–1000; George Marnell, Director **A**1 9 **F**2 3 13 16 18 19 20 21 22 23 24 25 26 29 30 31 32 33 34 35 36 38 41 43 45 48 49 50 51 54 56 57 59 60 61 62 63 64 68 69 70 72 76 77 78 79 **P**1 **S** Department of Veterans Affairs, Washington, DC	45	10	132	615	22	48111	0	57815	30149	592
SALEM—Marion County ☐ OREGON STATE HOSPITAL, 2600 Center Street N.E., Zip 97310–0530; tel. 503/945–2870; Stanley F. Mazur-Hart, Ph.D., Superintendent (Nonreporting) **A**1 3 5 10 PSYCHIATRIC MEDICINE CENTER See Salem Hospital REGIONAL REHABILITATION CENTER See Salem Hospital	12	22	546	—	—	—	—	—	—	—
★ SALEM HOSPITAL, (Includes Psychiatric Medicine Center, 1127 Oak Street S.E., Zip 97301; Regional Rehabilitation Center, 2561 Center Street N.E., Zip 97301; 665 Winter Street S.E., Zip 97301–3959, Mailing Address: Box 14001, Zip 97309–5014; tel. 503/370–5200; Dennis Noonan, President and Chief Executive Officer (Total facility includes 35 beds in nursing home–type unit) **A**1 2 9 10 **F**4 7 8 9 11 12 13 14 16 17 19 22 24 25 30 31 32 33 34 35 36 38 39 41 43 44 46 47 48 50 51 53 54 57 58 59 60 61 62 63 65 66 68 69 70 71 72 74 75 76 77 78 Web address: www.salemhospital.org	23	10	437	18092	246	285990	3505	179732	91749	2176
SEASIDE—Clatsop County ★ PROVIDENCE SEASIDE HOSPITAL, 725 South Wahanna Road, Zip 97138–7735; tel. 503/717–7000; Gail Harper, R.N., Chief Executive (Total facility includes 22 beds in nursing home–type unit) **A**1 10 **F**7 8 9 12 13 14 15 16 17 18 19 20 21 22 23 24 25 26 29 31 32 33 34 36 37 41 43 44 45 46 48 50 54 56 69 70 72 76 78 79 **P**6 7 **S** Providence Health System, Seattle, WA Web address: www.providence.org	21	10	45	1115	25	71905	99	13493	7795	187
SILVERTON—Marion County ★ SILVERTON HOSPITAL, 342 Fairview Street, Zip 97381; tel. 503/873–1500; William E. Winter, Administrative Director **A**9 10 **F**5 7 8 9 12 13 16 18 19 22 24 25 29 31 32 33 34 38 41 43 44 45 48 50 51 72 75 76 78 **P**6 Web address: www.silvertonhospital.org	23	10	38	2512	22	42288	877	17748	7440	221
SPRINGFIELD—Lane County ★ MCKENZIE-WILLAMETTE HOSPITAL, 1460 G Street, Zip 97477–4197; tel. 541/726–4400; Roy J. Orr, President and Chief Executive Officer **A**1 9 10 **F**1 8 13 16 17 18 19 20 22 24 25 30 32 33 34 36 37 41 43 44 45 48 50 54 68 70 72 75 76 77 78 79 **P**1 Web address: www.mckweb.com	23	10	106	6036	62	128628	1256	59226	28293	828
STAYTON—Marion County ★ SANTIAM MEMORIAL HOSPITAL, 1401 North 10th Avenue, Zip 97383; tel. 503/769–2175; Terry L. Fletchall, Administrator **A**1 9 10 **F**7 8 9 16 17 18 19 22 25 38 39 44 45 48 49 54 70 75 76 Web address: www.santiamhospital.com	23	10	40	912	8	23806	151	8119	3386	118
THE DALLES—Wasco County ★ MID-COLUMBIA MEDICAL CENTER, 1700 East 19th Street, Zip 97058–3316; tel. 541/296–1111; Mark D. Scott, President (Nonreporting) **A**1 9 10 Web address: www.mcmc.net	23	10	49	—	—	—	—	—	—	—
TILLAMOOK—Tillamook County ★ TILLAMOOK COUNTY GENERAL HOSPITAL, 1000 Third Street, Zip 97141–3430; tel. 503/842–4444; Wendell Hesseltine, President (Nonreporting) **A**1 9 10 **S** Adventist Health, Roseville, CA	21	10	33	—	—	—	—	—	—	—
TUALATIN—Clackamas County ★ LEGACY MERIDIAN PARK HOSPITAL, 19300 S.W. 65th Avenue, Zip 97062–9741; tel. 503/692–1212; Jeff Cushing, Vice President and Site Administrator **A**1 2 9 10 **F**1 2 3 4 7 8 9 10 11 13 14 16 17 18 19 21 22 24 25 26 27 28 29 30 32 33 34 35 36 37 38 39 41 42 43 44 45 46 47 48 49 50 51 52 53 54 56 57 58 59 60 61 62 64 65 68 69 70 72 74 75 76 77 78 79 **S** Legacy Health System, Portland, OR Web address: www.legacyhealth.org	23	10	117	7614	68	78650	1400	53646	22322	561

Hospitals, U.S. / PENNSYLVANIA

PENNSYLVANIA

Resident Population 12,001 (in thousands)
Resident population in metro areas 84.6%
Birth rate per 1,000 population 12.0
65 years and over 15.9%
Percent of persons without health insurance 10.1%

Hospital, Address, Telephone, Administrator, Approval, Facility, and Physician Codes, Health Care System, Network	Classification Codes		Utilization Data					Expense (thousands) of dollars		
★ American Hospital Association (AHA) membership ☐ Joint Commission on Accreditation of Healthcare Organizations (JCAHO) accreditation + American Osteopathic Healthcare Association (AOHA) membership ○ American Osteopathic Association (AOA) accreditation △ Commission on Accreditation of Rehabilitation Facilities (CARF) accreditation Control codes 61, 63, 64, 71, 72 and 73 indicate hospitals listed by AOHA, but not registered by AHA. For definition of numerical codes, see page A4	Control	Service	Staffed Beds	Admissions	Census	Outpatient Visits	Births	Total	Payroll	Personnel

ABINGTON—Montgomery County
★ ABINGTON MEMORIAL HOSPITAL, 1200 Old York Road, Zip 19001–3720; tel. 215/481–2000; Richard L. Jones, Jr, President and Chief Executive Officer **A**1 2 3 5 10 **F**1 4 8 9 11 12 13 16 17 18 19 22 23 24 25 27 28 29 30 31 32 33 34 35 36 37 38 39 40 41 42 43 44 45 46 47 48 49 51 52 53 54 56 57 58 61 62 63 64 65 66 68 69 70 71 72 74 75 76 78 79 **P**6
Web address: www.amh.org | 23 | 10 | 424 | 25100 | 329 | 457402 | 4392 | 291054 | 145536 | 3357

ALIQUIPPA—Beaver County
★ UPMC BEAVER VALLEY, 2500 Hospital Drive, Zip 15001–2123; tel. 724/857–1212; Susan Dachille, Interim President (Total facility includes 16 beds in nursing home–type unit) **A**1 9 10 **F**1 3 4 5 6 7 9 11 13 14 16 17 18 19 20 21 22 23 24 25 26 27 29 30 31 32 33 34 35 36 37 38 39 40 41 43 45 46 47 48 49 50 51 53 54 55 56 57 58 59 60 61 62 63 64 65 66 67 68 69 70 71 72 73 74 75 76 77 78 79 **P**1 6 7 **S** UPMC Health System, Pittsburgh, PA
Web address: www.upmc.edu | 23 | 10 | 112 | 5012 | 88 | — | 0 | 40806 | 18156 | 439

ALLENTOWN—Lehigh County
☐ ALLENTOWN STATE HOSPITAL, 1600 Hanover Avenue, Zip 18103–2408; tel. 610/740–3200; Gregory M. Smith, Chief Executive Officer (Nonreporting) **A**1 10 | 12 | 22 | 415 | — | — | — | — | — | — | —

☐ △ GOOD SHEPHERD REHABILITATION HOSPITAL, 543 St. John Street, Zip 18103–3295; tel. 610/776–3120; Sara Gammon, President and Chief Executive Officer (Nonreporting) **A**1 7 10
Web address: www.goodshepherdrehab.org | 23 | 46 | 75 | — | — | — | — | — | — | —

★ LEHIGH VALLEY HOSPITAL, Cedar Crest Boulevard and 1–78, Zip 18103, Mailing Address: P.O. Box 689, Zip 18105–1556; tel. 610/402–8000; Elliot J. Sussman, M.D., President and Chief Executive Officer (Total facility includes 42 beds in nursing home–type unit) **A**1 2 3 5 8 9 10 **F**4 5 6 7 8 9 10 11 12 13 14 16 17 18 19 21 22 23 24 25 27 28 30 32 33 34 35 36 37 38 39 40 41 42 43 44 45 46 47 48 49 50 51 54 56 57 58 59 60 61 62 63 64 65 66 69 70 71 72 73 74 75 76 78 79 **P**3 5 7 8
Web address: www.lvhhn.org | 23 | 10 | 540 | 31865 | 452 | 172662 | 3436 | 331343 | 131529 | 3368

★ SACRED HEART HOSPITAL, 421 Chew Street, Zip 18102–3490; tel. 610/776–4500; Joseph M. Cimerola, FACHE, President and Chief Executive Officer (Total facility includes 22 beds in nursing home–type unit) (Nonreporting) **A**1 2 3 5 9 10
Web address: www.shh.org
ST LUKE'S HOSPITAL-ALLENTOWN CAMPUS See St. Luke's Hospital and Health Network, Bethlehem | 23 | 10 | 245 | — | — | — | — | — | — | —

ALTOONA—Blair County
ALTOONA CENTER, 1515 Fourth Street, Zip 16601–4595; tel. 814/946–6900; Barry C. Benford, Director (Nonreporting) | 12 | 62 | 138 | — | — | — | — | — | — | —

★ ○ ALTOONA HOSPITAL, 620 Howard Avenue, Zip 16601–4899; tel. 814/946–2011; James W. Barner, President and Chief Executive Officer **A**1 2 3 5 9 10 11 12 **F**2 3 4 6 7 8 9 11 12 13 16 17 18 21 22 24 25 27 29 30 32 34 36 37 38 39 40 41 42 43 44 45 46 47 48 49 50 51 54 57 58 59 60 61 62 63 64 65 66 69 70 72 76 78 79 **P**1
Web address: www.altoonahosp.com | 23 | 10 | 189 | 13333 | 183 | 336787 | 1269 | 131918 | 58141 | 1476

★ BON SECOURS–HOLY FAMILY REGIONAL HEALTH SYSTEM, 2500 Seventh Avenue, Zip 16602–2099; tel. 814/944–1681; Barbara H. Biehner, Chief Executive Officer (Total facility includes 17 beds in nursing home–type unit) **A**1 2 9 10 **F**7 8 9 11 13 16 17 18 19 20 22 24 25 26 30 31 32 34 35 37 39 41 44 45 46 48 50 51 53 54 57 59 62 64 65 69 70 71 72 76 78 **P**8 **S** Bon Secours Health System, Inc., Marriottsville, MD
Web address: www.mercynet.org | 23 | 10 | 153 | 4976 | 88 | 116710 | 416 | 48385 | 22014 | 584

☐ HEALTHSOUTH REHABILITATION HOSPITAL OF ALTOONA, 2005 Valley View Boulevard, Zip 16602–4598; tel. 814/944–3535; Scott Filler, Chief Executive Officer **A**1 9 10 **F**13 16 17 30 49 53 54 71 **S** HEALTHSOUTH Corporation, Birmingham, AL | 33 | 46 | 70 | 1260 | 63 | 40796 | — | 14066 | 7946 | 256

★ JAMES E. VAN ZANDT VETERANS AFFAIRS MEDICAL CENTER, 2907 Pleasant Valley Boulevard, Zip 16602–4377; tel. 814/943–8164; Gerald L. Williams, Director and Chief Executive Officer (Total facility includes 40 beds in nursing home–type unit) **A**1 9 **F**3 9 13 16 17 18 19 22 23 25 26 29 30 31 32 33 34 35 36 37 38 41 43 48 50 51 54 56 59 63 69 70 72 76 78 79 **P**6
S Department of Veterans Affairs, Washington, DC
Web address: www.va.gov/stations97/guide/home.asp?DIVISION=ALL | 45 | 10 | 68 | 1533 | 63 | 103216 | 0 | 33683 | 14436 | 362

AMBLER—Montgomery County
☐ HORSHAM CLINIC, 722 East Butler Pike, Zip 19002–2398; tel. 215/643–7800; David A. Baron, D.O., Medical Director (Nonreporting) **A**1 5 9 10 **S** Universal Health Services, Inc., King of Prussia, PA | 33 | 22 | 138 | — | — | — | — | — | — | —

© 2000 AHA Guide *Many Facility Codes have changed. Please refer to the AHA Guide Code Chart.*

Hospitals, U.S. / PENNSYLVANIA

Hospital, Address, Telephone, Administrator, Approval, Facility, and Physician Codes, Health Care System, Network	Classification Codes		Utilization Data					Expense (thousands) of dollars		
	Control	Service	Staffed Beds	Admissions	Census	Outpatient Visits	Births	Total	Payroll	Personnel

★ American Hospital Association (AHA) membership
☐ Joint Commission on Accreditation of Healthcare Organizations (JCAHO) accreditation
+ American Osteopathic Healthcare Association (AOHA) membership
○ American Osteopathic Association (AOA) accreditation
△ Commission on Accreditation of Rehabilitation Facilities (CARF) accreditation
Control codes 61, 63, 64, 71, 72 and 73 indicate hospitals listed by AOHA, but not registered by AHA. For definition of numerical codes, see page A4

Hospital	Control	Service	Staffed Beds	Admissions	Census	Outpatient Visits	Births	Total	Payroll	Personnel
ASHLAND—Schuylkill County ☐ ASHLAND REGIONAL MEDICAL CENTER, 101 Broad Street, Zip 17921–2198; tel. 717/875–2000; Michael J. Callan, Sr, Chief Executive Officer (Total facility includes 20 beds in nursing home–type unit) (Nonreporting) **A**1 9 10	23	10	97	—	—	—	—	—	—	—
BENSALEM—Bucks County LIVENGRIN FOUNDATION, 4833 Hulmeville Road, Zip 19020–3099; tel. 215/638–5200; Richard M. Pine, President and Chief Executive Officer (Nonreporting)	23	82	76	—	—	—	—	—	—	—
BERWICK—Columbia County ☐ BERWICK HOSPITAL CENTER, 701 East 16th Street, Zip 18603–2397; tel. 570/759–5000; Donald Henderson, President and Chief Executive Officer (Total facility includes 240 beds in nursing home–type unit) **A**1 9 10 **F**8 22 25 31 36 37 39 41 44 45 48 49 54 62 69 70 76 78 **S** Community Health Systems, Inc., Brentwood, TN	33	10	340	2680	252	86975	140	—	—	592
BETHLEHEM—Northampton County ★ △ MUHLENBERG HOSPITAL CENTER, 2545 Schoenersville Road, Zip 18017–7384; tel. 610/861–2200; Elliot J. Sussman, M.D., President and Chief Executive Officer **A**1 7 9 10 **F**6 8 9 10 11 12 13 14 16 17 18 19 22 23 24 25 26 27 29 30 31 32 33 34 35 36 37 38 39 41 42 43 44 45 46 47 48 49 50 51 52 53 54 57 58 61 62 63 64 65 66 69 70 71 72 74 75 76 78 79 **P**8	23	10	148	6861	101	116702	0	52715	22071	587
☐ + ○ ST. LUKE'S HOSPITAL AND HEALTH NETWORK, (Includes St Luke's Hospital–Allentown Campus, 1736 Hamilton Street, Allentown, Zip 18104–5656; tel. 610/770–8300; Elaine Thompson, President; St. Luke's Quakertown Hospital, 1021 Park Avenue, Quakertown, Zip 18951–9003; tel. 215/538–4510; Frederick P. Sprissler, President), 801 Ostrum Street, Zip 18015–1014; tel. 610/954–4000; Richard A. Anderson, President and Chief Executive Officer (Total facility includes 18 beds in nursing home–type unit) **A**1 2 3 5 6 8 9 10 11 12 13 **F**3 4 7 8 9 11 12 13 14 16 17 18 19 22 24 25 27 28 29 30 32 33 34 35 36 37 38 39 41 42 43 45 46 47 48 49 50 54 56 57 59 63 64 65 66 68 69 70 72 75 76 77 78 79 **P**8 Web address: www.slhn–lehighvalley.org	23	10	549	24902	356	421799	2907	217344	102449	2769
BLOOMSBURG—Columbia County ★ BLOOMSBURG HOSPITAL, 549 East Fair Street, Zip 17815–0340; tel. 570/387–2100; Robert J. Spinelli, Administrator and Chief Executive Officer **A**1 9 10 **F**2 3 7 8 9 16 17 19 22 24 25 26 31 32 33 34 36 37 38 39 41 44 45 46 48 49 51 57 59 60 61 63 68 69 70 71 72 76 78	23	10	266	3313	38	87627	532	26137	10492	502
BRADDOCK—Allegheny County ★ UPMC BRADDOCK, 400 Holland Avenue, Zip 15104–1599; tel. 412/636–5000; Margaret Priselac, R.N., Chief Executive Officer (Total facility includes 20 beds in nursing home–type unit) **A**1 9 10 **F**3 9 13 14 16 17 18 19 21 22 24 25 27 31 32 33 34 35 36 37 39 40 41 46 48 57 59 60 61 62 68 69 70 72 73 76 78 **P**8 **S** UPMC Health System, Pittsburgh, PA Web address: www.upmc.edu	23	10	148	6897	110	86129	0	38851	17784	532
BRADFORD—McKean County ★ BRADFORD REGIONAL MEDICAL CENTER, 116 Interstate Parkway, Zip 16701–0218; tel. 814/368–4143; George E. Leonhardt, President and Chief Executive Officer (Total facility includes 95 beds in nursing home–type unit) **A**1 9 10 **F**7 8 9 13 16 17 18 19 22 23 24 25 27 28 30 32 34 36 37 38 39 41 43 44 45 46 48 49 50 51 54 56 57 59 60 61 62 64 68 69 70 71 72 76 78 79 **P**8	23	10	200	4765	157	123326	338	43985	19845	650
BRIDGEVILLE—Allegheny County ☐ MAYVIEW STATE HOSPITAL, 1601 Mayview Road, Zip 15017–1547; tel. 412/257–6500; David W. P. Jones, Chief Executive Officer **A**1 5 9 10 **F**23 57 62 70 78 **P**6	12	22	509	601	471	0	0	62719	35975	894
BRISTOL—Bucks County ☐ LOWER BUCKS HOSPITAL, 501 Bath Road, Zip 19007–3190; tel. 215/785–9200; Nathan Bosk, FACHE, Chief Executive Officer (Nonreporting) **A**1 9 10 **S** Temple University Health System, Philadelphia, PA	23	10	166	—	—	—	—	—	—	—
BROOKVILLE—Jefferson County ★ BROOKVILLE HOSPITAL, 100 Hospital Road, Zip 15825–1367; tel. 814/849–2312; William J. Polito, President and Chief Executive Officer **A**1 9 10 **F**8 9 12 16 17 18 19 22 23 24 25 32 34 36 43 44 45 48 50 54 68 70 71 74 76 78 **P**5 Web address: www.brookvillehospital.org	23	10	63	2178	22	103573	120	20961	8643	329
BROWNSVILLE—Fayette County ★ BROWNSVILLE GENERAL HOSPITAL, 125 Simpson Road, Zip 15417–9699; tel. 724/785–7200; Richard D. Constantine, Chief Executive Officer (Total facility includes 21 beds in nursing home–type unit) **A**1 9 10 **F**9 17 18 19 22 24 25 27 30 32 33 34 35 38 39 41 43 45 48 50 51 54 57 60 61 62 64 69 70 72 76 **P**8 **S** Quorum Health Group, Brentwood, TN Web address: www.bghlink.com	23	10	115	3016	72	42465	—	20435	9197	266

Hospitals, U.S. / PENNSYLVANIA

Hospital, Address, Telephone, Administrator, Approval, Facility, and Physician Codes, Health Care System, Network	Control	Service	Staffed Beds	Admissions	Census	Outpatient Visits	Births	Total	Payroll	Personnel
★ American Hospital Association (AHA) membership □ Joint Commission on Accreditation of Healthcare Organizations (JCAHO) accreditation + American Osteopathic Healthcare Association (AOHA) membership ○ American Osteopathic Association (AOA) accreditation △ Commission on Accreditation of Rehabilitation Facilities (CARF) accreditation Control codes 61, 63, 64, 71, 72 and 73 indicate hospitals listed by AOHA, but not registered by AHA. For definition of numerical codes, see page A4										
BRYN MAWR—Montgomery County										
BRYN MAWR COLLEGE INFIRMARY, Bryn Mawr College Campus, Zip 19010; tel. 610/526–7360; Kay Kerr, M.D., Medical Director (Nonreporting)	23	11	7	—	—	—	—	—	—	—
★ BRYN MAWR HOSPITAL, 130 South Bryn Mawr Avenue, Zip 19010–3160; tel. 610/526–3000; Andrea F. Gilbert, Senior Vice President (Total facility includes 17 beds in nursing home–type unit) A1 2 3 5 9 10 F1 3 4 5 6 7 8 9 11 12 13 16 17 18 19 20 21 22 23 24 25 27 28 29 30 31 32 33 34 35 36 37 38 39 40 41 42 43 44 45 46 47 48 49 50 51 53 54 55 56 57 58 59 60 61 62 63 64 65 66 67 68 69 70 71 72 74 76 78 79 P2 5 6 7 S Jefferson Health System, Wayne, PA **Web address:** www.jeffersonhealth.org	23	10	277	14777	196	141720	2009	147327	62738	1597
BUTLER—Butler County										
★ BUTLER HEALTH SYSTEM, 911 East Brady Street, Zip 16001–4646; tel. 724/283–6666; Joseph A. Stewart, Chief Executive Officer (Total facility includes 23 beds in nursing home–type unit) A1 9 10 F2 3 4 8 9 11 12 13 14 16 17 18 19 22 24 25 27 28 31 32 35 36 37 39 41 44 47 48 51 54 57 59 61 62 68 69 70 72 76 79 P4 5 7	23	10	240	10026	151	242667	871	73218	33451	1021
★ VETERANS AFFAIRS MEDICAL CENTER, (EXTENDED CARE & PRIMARY MED), 325 New Castle Road, Zip 16001–2480; tel. 724/287–4781; Michael E. Moreland, Director (Total facility includes 106 beds in nursing home–type unit) A1 9 F1 3 4 9 11 12 16 17 18 19 22 23 24 25 26 27 28 30 31 32 34 35 36 37 38 39 41 43 45 46 47 48 49 50 51 54 56 57 59 61 62 63 65 69 70 72 74 76 78 79 P6 S Department of Veterans Affairs, Washington, DC **Web address:** www.va.gov/station/529–butler	45	49	170	834	93	93541	0	42756	21546	515
CAMP HILL—Cumberland County										
★ HOLY SPIRIT HEALTH SYSTEM, (Formerly Holy Spirit Hospital), 503 North 21st Street, Zip 17011–2288; tel. 717/763–2100; Sister Romaine Niemeyer, President A1 5 9 10 F2 3 4 7 8 9 11 13 17 18 19 21 22 24 25 31 32 33 34 35 36 37 38 39 41 42 43 44 46 48 51 54 56 57 58 59 60 61 62 63 64 65 68 70 72 73 74 76 78 79 P1 **Web address:** www.hsh.org	21	10	263	12745	188	160551	930	93870	47647	1483
STATE CORRECTIONAL INSTITUTION AT CAMP HILL, 2500 Lisbon Road, Zip 17011, Mailing Address: P.O. Box 200, Zip 17011–0200; tel. 717/737–4531; Kathy Montag, Administrator Health Care (Nonreporting)	12	49	34	—	—	—	—	—	—	—
CANONSBURG—Washington County										
★ CANONSBURG GENERAL HOSPITAL, (Formerly Allegheny University Hospitals, Canonsburg), 100 Medical Boulevard, Zip 15317–9762; tel. 724/745–6100; Barbara A. Bensaia, Chief Executive Officer (Total facility includes 28 beds in nursing home–type unit) (Nonreporting) A1 9 10 S West Penn Allegheny Health System, Pittsburgh, PA	23	10	120	—	—	—	—	—	—	—
CARBONDALE—Lackawanna County										
★ MARIAN COMMUNITY HOSPITAL, 100 Lincoln Avenue, Zip 18407–2170; tel. 570/281–1000; Sister Jean Coughlin, President and Chief Executive Officer A1 9 10 F1 9 13 16 17 18 19 22 24 25 30 32 33 34 35 39 41 45 46 48 49 50 54 57 61 62 70 72 74 76 78 79 P1	21	10	104	3581	54	56562	0	27176	11134	418
CARLISLE—Cumberland County										
★ CARLISLE HOSPITAL AND HEALTH SERVICES, 246 Parker Street, Zip 17013–3618; tel. 717/249–1212; Michael J. Halstead, President and Chief Executive Officer A1 9 10 F6 7 8 9 10 12 13 14 16 17 18 19 22 23 24 25 26 35 36 37 38 39 41 42 43 44 46 48 49 50 51 52 53 54 56 65 66 67 69 70 72 75 76 77 78 79 P8 S Quorum Health Group, Brentwood, TN **Web address:** www.chhs.org	23	10	110	6556	75	154245	618	56881	25218	721
CENTRE HALL—Centre County										
□ MEADOWS PSYCHIATRIC CENTER, 132 The Meadows Drive, Zip 16828–9798; tel. 814/364–2161; Joseph Barszczewski, Chief Executive Officer and Managing Director A1 9 10 F17 18 57 58 59 60 61 62 63 64 P7 S Universal Health Services, Inc., King of Prussia, PA	33	22	101	1789	82	—	—	14279	7238	315
CHAMBERSBURG—Franklin County										
★ △ CHAMBERSBURG HOSPITAL, 112 North Seventh Street, Zip 17201–6005, Mailing Address: P.O. Box 6005, Zip 17201–6005; tel. 717/267–3000; Norman B. Epstein, President (Total facility includes 18 beds in nursing home–type unit) A1 2 7 9 10 F1 2 3 7 8 9 11 12 13 16 17 18 19 20 21 22 23 24 25 26 27 28 29 30 31 32 33 34 35 36 37 38 39 41 42 43 44 45 46 48 49 50 51 52 53 54 56 57 58 59 60 61 62 63 65 68 69 70 71 72 73 74 75 76 78 79 P6 8 S Summit Health, Chambersburg, PA **Web address:** www.summithealth.org	23	10	223	11207	149	200519	1133	90028	41050	996
CHESTER—Delaware County										
KEYSTONE CENTER, 2001 Providence Avenue, Zip 19013–5504; tel. 610/876–9000; Jimmy Patton, Chief Executive Officer and Managing Director A9 F2 3 29 70 S Universal Health Services, Inc., King of Prussia, PA	33	82	84	1941	74	4340	0	4165	2507	78
CLARION—Clarion County										
★ + ○ CLARION HOSPITAL, One Hospital Drive, Zip 16214–8599; tel. 814/226–9500; Donald D. Evans, President and Chief Executive Officer A9 10 11 12 13 F8 9 19 22 24 25 28 32 34 37 38 39 41 44 45 46 48 54 70 76 78 P7 S Quorum Health Group, Brentwood, TN **Web address:** www.clarionhospital.org	23	10	77	3480	32	84021	362	25721	10742	368

© 2000 AHA Guide *Many Facility Codes have changed. Please refer to the AHA Guide Code Chart.*

Hospitals, U.S. / PENNSYLVANIA

	★	American Hospital Association (AHA) membership
	☐	Joint Commission on Accreditation of Healthcare Organizations (JCAHO) accreditation
	+	American Osteopathic Healthcare Association (AOHA) membership
	○	American Osteopathic Association (AOA) accreditation
	△	Commission on Accreditation of Rehabilitation Facilities (CARF) accreditation

Control codes 61, 63, 64, 71, 72 and 73 indicate hospitals listed by AOHA, but not registered by AHA. For definition of numerical codes, see page A4.

Hospital, Address, Telephone, Administrator, Approval, Facility, and Physician Codes, Health Care System, Network	Classification Codes		Utilization Data					Expense (thousands) of dollars		Personnel
	Control	Service	Staffed Beds	Admissions	Census	Outpatient Visits	Births	Total	Payroll	
☐ CLARION PSYCHIATRIC CENTER, 2 Hospital Drive, Zip 16214–9424; tel. 814/226–9545; Michael R. Keefer, CHE, Chief Executive Officer and Managing Director (Nonreporting) **A**1 10 **S** Universal Health Services, Inc., King of Prussia, PA	33	22	52	—	—	—	—	—	—	—
CLARKS SUMMIT—Lackawanna County										
☐ CLARKS SUMMIT STATE HOSPITAL, 1451 Hillside Drive, Zip 18411–9505; tel. 570/586–2011; Thomas P. Comerford, Jr, Superintendent **A**1 10 **F**1 2 9 10 11 12 13 16 18 19 20 21 22 23 24 30 31 32 34 39 41 43 44 46 48 50 51 53 55 57 59 60 61 62 65 66 68 70 72 76 78 **P**6	12	22	300	80	241	0	0	32867	19605	480
CLEARFIELD—Clearfield County										
☐ CLEARFIELD HOSPITAL, 809 Turnpike Avenue, Zip 16830–1232, Mailing Address: P.O. Box 992, Zip 16830–0992; tel. 814/765–5341; Kent C. Hess, Chief Executive Officer (Nonreporting) **A**1 9 10 Web address: www.clearfieldhospital.org	23	10	92	—	—	—	—	—	—	—
COAL TOWNSHIP—Northumberland County										
★ SHAMOKIN AREA COMMUNITY HOSPITAL, 4200 Hospital Road, Zip 17866–9697; tel. 570/644–4200; John P. Wiercinski, President and Chief Executive Officer (Total facility includes 15 beds in nursing home–type unit) **A**1 9 10 **F**6 7 9 13 16 17 18 19 20 21 22 24 25 30 32 34 35 39 41 43 45 48 49 51 54 57 59 62 64 69 70 71 72 76 78 **P**1 Web address: www.shamokinhospital.org	23	10	61	1953	31	44633	0	14625	5515	217
COALDALE—Schuylkill County										
★ MINER'S MEMORIAL MEDICAL CENTER, 360 West Ruddle Street, Zip 18218–0067, Mailing Address: P.O. Box 67, Zip 18218–0067; tel. 570/645–2131; William J. Crossin, President and Chief Executive Officer (Total facility includes 48 beds in nursing home–type unit) **A**1 9 10 **F**9 16 17 18 22 24 25 30 34 36 38 39 46 48 51 54 61 64 70 71 76 78	23	10	114	2253	76	39786	0	23595	11528	328
COATESVILLE—Chester County										
★ BRANDYWINE HOSPITAL, 201 Reeceville Road, Zip 19320–1536; tel. 610/383–8000; Marion A. McGowan, President and Chief Executive Officer (Total facility includes 12 beds in nursing home–type unit) **A**1 2 9 10 **F**8 9 11 13 14 16 17 18 19 21 22 23 24 25 26 28 29 30 31 32 33 34 35 36 37 38 39 40 41 43 44 45 46 48 49 50 51 53 54 55 56 57 61 62 64 65 66 68 69 70 71 72 73 75 76 77 78 79 **P**8 Web address: www.brandywinehospital.org	23	10	176	7827	102	120132	696	67893	30284	945
★ VETERANS AFFAIRS MEDICAL CENTER, 1400 Black Horse Hill Road, Zip 19320–2097; tel. 610/384–7711; Gary W. Devansky, Chief Executive Officer (Total facility includes 299 beds in nursing home–type unit) **A**1 9 **F**1 2 3 4 5 6 7 8 9 10 11 12 13 16 17 18 19 22 23 24 25 26 28 30 31 32 33 34 35 36 39 41 43 44 45 46 47 48 50 51 53 54 55 56 57 59 60 61 62 63 64 65 66 68 69 70 72 74 75 76 77 78 79 **P**6 **S** Department of Veterans Affairs, Washington, DC Web address: www.coatesville.med.va.gov	45	22	607	3620	542	94391	0	—	—	1093
COLUMBIA—Lancaster County										
★ LANCASTER GENERAL HOSPITAL–SUSQUEHANNA DIVISION, 306 North Seventh Street, Zip 17512–2132, Mailing Address: P.O. Box 926, Zip 17512–0926; tel. 717/684–2841; Scott A. Berlucchi, President and Chief Executive Officer **A**1 9 10 **F**2 3 9 16 17 18 19 22 25 32 34 38 43 45 48 50 51 54 63 70 71 72 76 78 79 **P**5 Web address: www.lha.org	23	10	62	1582	32	—	0	9285	3941	167
CONNELLSVILLE—Fayette County										
★ HIGHLANDS HOSPITAL, 401 East Murphy Avenue, Zip 15425–2700; tel. 724/628–1500; Michelle Cunningham, Chief Executive Officer **A**1 9 10 **F**7 8 9 13 18 19 22 24 25 30 32 33 34 35 36 37 39 41 43 44 45 46 48 51 54 55 57 58 59 60 61 62 64 65 68 69 70 72 76 78 79 **P**8 **S** Fay–West Health System, Mount Pleasant, PA	23	10	87	3024	52	48869	0	18695	7684	233
CONSHOHOCKEN—Montgomery County										
★ MERCY HEALTH SYSTEM OF SOUTHEASTERN PENNSYLVANIA, (Includes Mercy Fitzgerald Hospital, 1500 South Lansdowne Avenue, Darby, Zip 19023; tel. 610/237–4000; Mercy Hospital of Philadelphia, 501 South 54th Street, Philadelphia, Zip 19143; tel. 215/748–9000), 1 West Elm Street, Zip 19428–2007; tel. 610/567–6000; Mark T. O'Neil, Jr, President and Chief Executive Officer (Total facility includes 38 beds in nursing home–type unit) (Nonreporting) **A**1 2 3 5 9 10 **S** Catholic Health East, Newtown Square, PA Web address: www.mercyhealth.org	21	10	536	—	—	—	—	—	—	—
CORRY—Erie County										
★ CORRY MEMORIAL HOSPITAL, 612 West Smith Street, Zip 16407–1152; tel. 814/664–4641; Barbara Nichols, Acting President (Nonreporting) **A**1 9 10	23	10	55	—	—	—	—	—	—	—
COUDERSPORT—Potter County										
★ CHARLES COLE MEMORIAL HOSPITAL, 1001 East Second Street, Zip 16915–9762; tel. 814/274–9300; David B. Acker, Chief Executive Officer (Total facility includes 55 beds in nursing home–type unit) **A**1 9 10 **F**3 6 7 8 9 12 13 16 17 18 19 21 22 24 25 28 29 30 32 34 36 37 38 39 43 44 45 46 48 54 55 56 58 59 60 61 62 63 64 68 69 70 71 72 76 78 79	23	10	125	2522	80	102100	321	35864	15134	475
CRANBERRY—Butler County										
★ ST. FRANCIS HOSPITAL CRANBERRY, (Formerly St. Francis Medical Center North), One St. Francis Way, Zip 16066; tel. 724/772–5300; John L. Spieler, Dr.PH, FACHE, Executive Director (Total facility includes 150 beds in nursing home–type unit) (Nonreporting) **A**9 **S** St. Francis Health System, Pittsburgh, PA	23	10	185	—	—	—	—	—	—	—

Hospitals, U.S. / PENNSYLVANIA

Hospital, Address, Telephone, Administrator, Approval, Facility, and Physician Codes, Health Care System, Network	Classification Codes		Utilization Data					Expense (thousands) of dollars		
★ American Hospital Association (AHA) membership □ Joint Commission on Accreditation of Healthcare Organizations (JCAHO) accreditation + American Osteopathic Healthcare Association (AOHA) membership ○ American Osteopathic Association (AOA) accreditation △ Commission on Accreditation of Rehabilitation Facilities (CARF) accreditation Control codes 61, 63, 64, 71, 72 and 73 indicate hospitals listed by AOHA, but not registered by AHA. For definition of numerical codes, see page A4	Control	Service	Staffed Beds	Admissions	Census	Outpatient Visits	Births	Total	Payroll	Personnel

DANVILLE—Montour County
- □ DANVILLE STATE HOSPITAL, 200 State Hospital Drive, Zip 17821-9198; tel. 570/271-4500; Paul J. Gritman, Superintendent **A**1 10 **F**1 2 3 4 5 6 7 8 9 10 11 12 13 14 15 19 20 21 22 23 24 25 26 27 28 29 30 31 32 33 34 35 36 37 38 39 40 41 42 43 44 45 46 47 48 49 50 51 52 53 54 55 56 58 59 60 61 62 63 64 65 66 67 68 69 70 71 72 73 74 75 76 77 78 79 **P**6 | 12 22 | 242 | 105 | 223 | 0 | 0 | 29392 | 18536 | 428
- ★ GEISINGER MEDICAL CENTER, 100 North Academy Avenue, Zip 17822-0150; tel. 570/271-6211; Nancy L. Rizzo, Senior Vice President, Operations **A**1 2 3 5 6 8 9 10 12 13 **F**3 4 5 7 8 9 11 12 13 14 16 17 18 19 21 22 23 24 25 26 27 29 30 33 34 35 38 39 41 42 43 44 45 46 47 48 49 50 51 52 53 54 56 57 58 59 60 61 62 63 64 65 66 70 71 72 74 75 76 77 78 79 **P**4 **S** Geisinger Health System, Danville, PA
Web address: www.ghs.edu | 23 10 | 333 | 16539 | 238 | 466109 | 1028 | 241968 | 71846 | 2208

DARBY—Delaware County
- MERCY FITZGERALD HOSPITAL See Mercy Health System of Southeastern Pennsylvania, Conshohocken

DOWNINGTOWN—Chester County
- ★ ST. JOHN VIANNEY HOSPITAL, 151 Woodbine Road, Zip 19335-3057; tel. 610/269-2600; Thomas F. Dugan, Administrator (Nonreporting) **A**9
Web address: www.sjvcenter.org | 21 22 | 54 | — | — | — | — | — | — | —

DOYLESTOWN—Bucks County
- ★ △ DOYLESTOWN HOSPITAL, 595 West State Street, Zip 18901-2597; tel. 215/345-2200; Richard A. Reif, President and Chief Executive Officer (Total facility includes 297 beds in nursing home-type unit) **A**1 7 9 10 **F**1 4 6 8 9 11 13 14 16 17 18 19 20 21 22 23 24 25 26 27 29 30 31 32 33 34 35 36 37 38 39 40 41 42 43 44 45 46 47 48 49 50 51 53 54 56 57 59 60 61 62 64 66 67 69 70 72 73 76 78 79 **P**5 7 8
Web address: www.dh.org | 23 10 | 475 | 10054 | 398 | 236944 | 1182 | 106898 | 49953 | 1606
- □ FOUNDATIONS BEHAVIORAL HEALTH, 833 East Butler Avenue, Zip 18901-2280; tel. 215/345-0444; Ronald T. Bernstein, Chief Executive Officer (Nonreporting) **A**1 10 | 23 22 | 45 | — | — | — | — | — | — | —

DREXEL HILL—Delaware County
- ★ ○ △ DELAWARE COUNTY MEMORIAL HOSPITAL, 501 North Lansdowne Avenue, Zip 19026-1114; tel. 610/284-8100; Joan K. Richards, President **A**1 2 5 7 9 10 11 12 **F**1 2 3 4 5 7 8 9 11 12 13 14 15 16 17 18 19 20 21 22 24 25 26 27 28 29 30 31 32 33 34 35 37 38 39 40 41 42 43 44 45 46 47 48 49 50 51 53 54 56 58 59 60 61 62 64 65 66 69 70 71 72 73 75 76 77 78 79 **P**5 6 **S** Crozer-Keystone Health System, Springfield, PA | 23 10 | 231 | 10850 | 163 | 83902 | 1113 | 93656 | 37595 | 1007

DU BOIS—Clearfield County
- □ DUBOIS REGIONAL MEDICAL CENTER, 100 Hospital Avenue, Zip 15801-1440, Mailing Address: P.O. Box 447, Zip 15801-0447; tel. 814/371-2200; Raymond A. Graeca, President and Chief Executive Officer **A**1 2 9 10 **F**7 8 9 11 14 15 16 17 18 19 20 22 24 25 27 29 30 31 32 33 34 36 37 38 39 41 42 43 44 45 46 48 49 51 53 54 56 57 58 59 60 61 62 63 65 70 71 72 76 78 79 **P**6 8
Web address: www.drmc.org | 23 10 | 189 | 7715 | 109 | 149647 | 605 | 74113 | 37071 | 1050

EAGLEVILLE—Montgomery County
- ★ EAGLEVILLE HOSPITAL, 100 Eagleville Road, Zip 19408-0045, Mailing Address: P.O. Box 45, Zip 19408-0045; tel. 610/539-6000; Kendria Kurtz, Chief Executive Officer **A**10 **F**2 13 16 17 19 25 33 35 43 45 50 59 60 61 70 72 78 79 **P**6
Web address: www.eaglevillehospital.org/ | 23 82 | 100 | 1662 | 53 | 0 | 0 | 13606 | 7459 | 249

EAST STROUDSBURG—Monroe County
- ★ POCONO MEDICAL CENTER, 206 East Brown Street, Zip 18301-3006; tel. 570/421-4000; Jane Stuckey, Interim Chief Executive Officer (Nonreporting) **A**1 2 9 10
Web address: www.pmchealthsystem.org | 23 10 | 226 | — | — | — | — | — | — | —

EASTON—Northampton County
- ★ EASTON HOSPITAL, 250 South 21st Street, Zip 18042-3892; tel. 610/250-4000; Donna Mulholland, President and Chief Executive Officer **A**1 2 3 5 9 10 12 13 **F**4 8 9 11 13 16 17 18 19 22 23 24 25 32 33 34 35 38 39 40 41 42 43 44 45 46 47 48 49 50 51 53 54 59 60 61 63 64 65 68 70 72 76 78 79 **P**6 8
Web address: www.eastonhospital.org | 23 10 | 233 | 12484 | 184 | 226442 | 657 | 119114 | 53612 | 1381

ELKINS PARK—Montgomery County
- ★ ELKINS PARK HOSPITAL, 60 East Township Line Road, Zip 19027-2220; tel. 215/663-6000; Richard Centafont, Chief Executive Officer (Nonreporting) **A**1 3 5 9 10 **S** TENET Healthcare Corporation, Santa Barbara, CA
Web address: www.auhs.edu | 23 10 | 158 | — | — | — | — | — | — | —

ELLWOOD CITY—Lawrence County
- ELLWOOD CITY HOSPITAL, 724 Pershing Street, Zip 16117-1474; tel. 724/752-0081; Herbert S. Skuba, President and Chief Executive Officer (Total facility includes 23 beds in nursing home-type unit) (Nonreporting) **A**9 10 | 23 10 | 118 | — | — | — | — | — | — | —

EPHRATA—Lancaster County
- □ EPHRATA COMMUNITY HOSPITAL, 169 Martin Avenue, Zip 17522-1724, Mailing Address: P.O. Box 1002, Zip 17522-1002; tel. 717/733-0311; John M. Porter, Jr., President and Chief Executive Officer (Total facility includes 15 beds in nursing home-type unit) **A**1 9 10 **F**7 8 9 12 16 17 18 19 22 24 25 26 27 30 34 35 36 37 38 39 40 41 43 44 45 46 48 50 51 54 55 56 57 58 59 60 61 62 63 68 69 70 72 76 78 79 **P**6 8 | 23 10 | 129 | 6624 | 80 | 202884 | 656 | 53679 | 26366 | 838

Hospitals, U.S. / PENNSYLVANIA

Hospital, Address, Telephone, Administrator, Approval, Facility, and Physician Codes, Health Care System, Network	Classification Codes		Utilization Data					Expense (thousands) of dollars		
	Control	Service	Staffed Beds	Admissions	Census	Outpatient Visits	Births	Total	Payroll	Personnel

★ American Hospital Association (AHA) membership
□ Joint Commission on Accreditation of Healthcare Organizations (JCAHO) accreditation
+ American Osteopathic Healthcare Association (AOHA) membership
○ American Osteopathic Association (AOA) accreditation
△ Commission on Accreditation of Rehabilitation Facilities (CARF) accreditation
Control codes 61, 63, 64, 71, 72 and 73 indicate hospitals listed by AOHA, but not registered by AHA. For definition of numerical codes, see page A4

ERIE—Erie County

☆ HAMOT MEDICAL CENTER, 201 State Street, Zip 16550-0002; tel. 814/877-6000; John T. Malone, President and Chief Executive Officer (Total facility includes 35 beds in nursing home–type unit) **A**1 2 3 5 9 10 **F**3 4 6 7 8 9 11 12 13 14 16 17 18 19 20 21 22 24 25 26 27 28 29 30 31 32 33 34 36 37 38 39 40 41 42 43 44 45 46 47 48 49 50 51 54 56 57 58 59 60 61 63 64 65 67 68 69 70 71 72 75 76 77 79 **P**6 8
Web address: www.hamot.org — 23 10 344 14104 190 99284 1357 140560 54612 2243

□ HEALTHSOUTH LAKE ERIE INSTITUTE OF REHABILITATION, 143 East Second Street, Zip 16507-1403; tel. 814/453-5602; Louis M. Condrasky, Chief Executive Officer (Total facility includes 27 beds in nursing home–type unit) (Nonreporting) **A**1 10 **S** HEALTHSOUTH Corporation, Birmingham, AL — 33 46 99 — — — — — — —

□ HEALTHSOUTH REHABILITATION HOSPITAL OF ERIE, (Formerly HEALTHSOUTH Great Lakes Hospital), 143 East Second Street, Zip 16507-1595; tel. 814/878-1200; Louis M. Condrasky, Chief Executive Officer (Nonreporting) **A**1 10 **S** HEALTHSOUTH Corporation, Birmingham, AL — 33 46 108 — — — — — — —

★ ○ METRO HEALTH CENTER, 252 West 11th Street, Zip 16501-9964; tel. 814/870-3400; Debra M. Dragovan, Chief Executive Officer **A**10 11 12 13 **F**8 9 16 17 18 22 24 25 34 38 39 41 44 48 54 56 57 62 64 68 70 76 78 **P**8
Web address: www.metrohealth.org — 23 10 111 2154 28 39390 160 18764 6001 198

+ ○ MILLCREEK COMMUNITY HOSPITAL, 5515 Peach Street, Zip 16509-2695; tel. 814/864-4031; Mary L. Eckert, President and Chief Executive Officer **A**9 10 11 12 13 **F**2 8 9 11 15 16 17 18 22 25 39 41 44 48 56 70 76 77 78
Web address: www.lecom.edu/millcreek-community-hospital/index.html — 23 10 101 2984 35 43766 192 19768 7820 266

□ SAINT VINCENT HEALTH CENTER, 232 West 25th Street, Zip 16544-0001; tel. 814/452-5000; Sister Catherine Manning, President and Chief Executive Officer (Total facility includes 14 beds in nursing home–type unit) **A**1 3 5 9 10 **F**3 4 7 8 9 11 12 13 14 16 17 18 19 20 21 22 23 24 25 26 27 29 30 32 33 34 35 36 37 38 39 41 42 44 45 46 47 48 49 50 51 53 54 56 57 59 60 61 62 63 65 69 70 71 72 75 76 77 78 79 **P**5 6
Web address: www.svhs.org — 23 10 436 14577 230 197024 1811 144238 61750 1868

□ SHRINERS HOSPITALS FOR CHILDREN, ERIE, 1645 West 8th Street, Zip 16505-5007; tel. 814/875-8700; Richard W. Brzuz, Administrator (Nonreporting) **A**1 3 9 **S** Shriners Hospitals for Children, Tampa, FL — 23 57 30 — — — — — — —

☆ VETERANS AFFAIRS MEDICAL CENTER, 135 East 38th Street, Zip 16504-1559; tel. 814/860-2576; Stephen M. Lucas, Chief Executive Officer (Total facility includes 9 beds in nursing home–type unit) **A**1 **F**2 3 4 9 11 12 13 16 17 18 19 21 22 23 24 25 26 30 31 32 33 34 35 36 37 38 39 41 43 45 46 47 48 49 50 51 53 54 56 57 59 60 61 62 63 64 65 66 69 70 72 74 76 78 79 **P**6
S Department of Veterans Affairs, Washington, DC
Web address: www.erie.net/~vamcerie — 45 10 61 1366 34 108241 0 41583 17352 419

EVERETT—Bedford County

☆ UPMC BEDFORD MEMORIAL, 10455 Lincoln Highway, Zip 15537-7046; tel. 814/623-6161; James C. Vreeland, FACHE, President and Chief Executive Officer **A**1 9 10 **F**3 4 6 7 8 9 11 13 14 15 16 17 18 19 20 21 22 23 24 25 26 27 30 31 32 33 34 35 36 37 38 39 40 41 43 44 45 46 47 48 49 50 51 55 56 58 59 60 61 62 63 64 65 67 68 70 71 72 75 76 78 **P**3 7 8 **S** UPMC Health System, Pittsburgh, PA
Web address: www.bedford.org — 23 10 27 2266 21 77803 294 19650 8537 277

FARRELL—Mercer County
SHENANGO VALLEY CAMPUS See UPMC Horizon, Greenville

FORT WASHINGTON—Montgomery County

□ NORTHWESTERN INSTITUTE, 450 Bethlehem Pike, Zip 19034-0209; tel. 215/641-5300; Joseph Roynan, Administrator (Nonreporting) **A**1 9 10 **S** Progressions Group, Inc., Fort Washington, PA — 33 22 146 — — — — — — —

GETTYSBURG—Adams County

☆ GETTYSBURG HOSPITAL, 147 Gettys Street, Zip 17325-0786; tel. 717/334-2121; Steven W. Renner, CPA, President and Chief Executive Officer (Total facility includes 23 beds in nursing home–type unit) **A**1 9 10 **F**3 4 8 9 16 17 18 19 22 24 25 27 32 34 36 37 38 39 41 43 44 45 46 48 49 51 54 59 61 69 70 71 72 76 78 79 **P**6 7 8 **S** South Central Community Health, York, PA
Web address: www.gettysburghosp.org — 23 10 99 4684 58 115555 512 41273 19294 575

GLENSIDE—Montgomery County

☆ CHESTNUT HILL REHABILITATION HOSPITAL, 8601 Stenton Avenue, Zip 19038-8312; tel. 215/233-6200; James B. McCaslin, Director (Total facility includes 34 beds in nursing home–type unit) **A**1 10 **F**1 5 6 7 8 9 11 13 14 16 17 18 19 22 23 24 25 26 30 31 32 35 36 37 38 39 40 43 45 46 48 49 50 51 53 54 55 56 59 61 62 65 66 67 68 69 70 71 72 73 74 76 78 79 **P**4 5 7
Web address: www.chh.org/rehab_hospital.html — 23 46 82 1552 63 14016 0 14359 6255 238

GREENSBURG—Westmoreland County

☆ WESTMORELAND REGIONAL HOSPITAL, 532 West Pittsburgh Street, Zip 15601-2239; tel. 724/832-4000; Joseph J. Peluso, President and Chief Executive Officer (Total facility includes 46 beds in nursing home–type unit) **A**1 2 10 **F**1 2 3 4 5 7 8 9 11 12 13 14 16 18 19 20 22 23 24 25 26 27 29 30 31 32 33 34 35 36 37 38 39 41 42 43 44 45 46 47 48 49 50 51 53 54 57 58 59 60 61 62 63 64 65 66 68 69 70 72 73 75 76 78 79 **P**1
Web address: www.westmoreland.org — 23 10 309 13457 200 361200 792 99092 47120 1434

Hospitals, U.S. / PENNSYLVANIA

Hospital, Address, Telephone, Administrator, Approval, Facility, and Physician Codes, Health Care System, Network ★ American Hospital Association (AHA) membership ☐ Joint Commission on Accreditation of Healthcare Organizations (JCAHO) accreditation + American Osteopathic Healthcare Association (AOHA) membership ○ American Osteopathic Association (AOA) accreditation △ Commission on Accreditation of Rehabilitation Facilities (CARF) accreditation Control codes 61, 63, 64, 71, 72 and 73 indicate hospitals listed by AOHA, but not registered by AHA. For definition of numerical codes, see page A4	Classification Codes		Utilization Data					Expense (thousands) of dollars		
	Control	Service	Staffed Beds	Admissions	Census	Outpatient Visits	Births	Total	Payroll	Personnel
GREENVILLE—Mercer County										
★ UPMC HORIZON, (Includes Greenville Campus, 110 North Main Street, Zip 16125–1795; tel. 724/588-2100; Shenango Valley Campus, 2200 Memorial Drive, Farrell, Zip 16121–1398; tel. 724/981-3500), J. Larry Heinike, President and Chief Executive Officer (Total facility includes 38 beds in nursing home–type unit) **A**1 2 9 10 12 **F**2 3 5 7 8 9 11 13 14 16 17 18 19 22 23 24 25 26 27 28 29 30 31 32 33 34 36 37 38 39 41 43 44 45 46 48 49 50 51 53 54 59 60 61 62 63 65 68 69 70 71 72 73 76 77 78 79 **P**4 7 8 **S** UPMC Health System, Pittsburgh, PA **Web address:** www.hhs.org	23	10	243	9624	135	199727	611	68028	31827	995
GROVE CITY—Mercer County										
+ ○ UNITED COMMUNITY HOSPITAL, 631 North Broad Street Extension, Zip 16127–9703; tel. 724/458-5442; Edward J. Reiss, Interim Administrator (Total facility includes 20 beds in nursing home–type unit) **A**10 11 **F**3 7 8 9 16 17 18 19 22 23 24 25 32 34 36 37 38 39 41 43 44 45 46 48 49 50 54 61 65 68 69 70 72 75 76 78 **Web address:** www.uchpa.org	23	10	104	3603	51	65349	333	24183	10492	326
HANOVER—York County										
☐ HANOVER HOSPITAL, 300 Highland Avenue, Zip 17331–2297; tel. 717/637-3711; William R. Walb, President and Chief Executive Officer **A**1 9 10 **F**4 7 8 9 11 12 13 14 17 18 19 21 22 23 24 25 29 31 32 34 35 36 37 38 39 41 43 44 45 46 48 49 50 51 54 68 70 71 72 76 78 **P**8 **Web address:** www.hanoverhospital.org	23	10	101	5370	64	144011	646	51443	23574	716
HARRISBURG—Dauphin County										
☐ EDGEWATER PSYCHIATRIC CENTER, 1829 North Front Street, Zip 17102–2213; tel. 717/238-8666; Stephen C. Blanchard, Director (Nonreporting) **A**1 9 10	23	22	26	—	—	—	—	—	—	—
☐ HARRISBURG STATE HOSPITAL, Mailing Address: P.O. Box 61260, Zip 17106–1260; tel. 717/772-7455; Bruce Darney, Superintendent (Nonreporting) **A**1 9 10	12	22	392	—	—	—	—	—	—	—
★ + ○ PINNACLEHEALTH SYSTEM, (Includes PinnacleHealth at Community General Osteopathic Hospital, 4300 Londonderry Road, Zip 17109–5397; tel. 717/652-3000; PinnacleHealth at Harrisburg Hospital, 111 South Front Street, Zip 17101–2099; tel. 717/782-3131; PinnacleHealth at Polyclinic Hospital, 2601 North Third Street, Zip 17110–2098; tel. 717/782-4141; PinnacleHealth at Seidle Memorial Hospital, 120 South Filbert Street, Mechanicsburg, Zip 17055–6591; tel. 717/795-6760; Susan A. Edwards, Senior Vice President for Operations), 17 South Market Square, Zip 17101–2003, Mailing Address: P.O. Box 8700, Zip 17105–8700; tel. 717/782-5678; John S. Cramer, FACHE, President and Chief Executive Officer (Total facility includes 123 beds in nursing home–type unit) **A**1 2 3 5 9 10 11 12 13 **F**1 3 4 6 7 8 9 11 13 17 18 19 20 22 23 24 25 27 30 31 32 33 34 35 36 37 38 39 41 42 43 44 45 46 47 48 49 50 51 53 54 55 56 57 58 59 60 62 63 64 65 66 68 69 70 72 73 76 77 78 79 **P**8 **Web address:** www.pinnaclehealth.org	23	10	782	34201	614	358640	4211	325543	149163	4732
HASTINGS—Cambria County										
★ MINERS HOSPITAL NORTHERN CAMBRIA, 290 Haida Avenue, Zip 16646, Mailing Address: P.O. Box 689, Zip 16646; tel. 814/247-3100; Roger P. Winn, Administrator **A**1 9 10 **F**9 16 17 22 24 25 30 32 34 37 38 39 41 43 45 46 48 54 61 70 76 **P**1	23	10	40	1478	18	30324	0	11503	4767	173
HAVERTOWN—Delaware County										
★ MERCY COMMUNITY HOSPITAL, 2000 Old West Chester Pike, Zip 19083–2712; tel. 610/853-7000; Mary C. Morrison, R.N., Chief Executive Officer (Nonreporting) **A**1 9 10 **S** Catholic Health East, Newtown Square, PA	23	10	107	—	—	—	—	—	—	—
HAZLETON—Luzerne County										
★ HAZLETON GENERAL HOSPITAL, 700 East Broad Street, Zip 18201–6897; tel. 570/501-4357; E. Richard Moore, President **A**1 9 10 **F**7 8 9 13 16 17 18 19 22 24 25 28 31 32 33 34 35 36 38 39 40 41 43 44 45 46 48 49 50 51 53 54 56 57 59 60 61 62 66 68 69 70 71 72 76 78 79 **Web address:** www.ghha.org	23	10	152	5812	108	117605	0	37977	15244	550
★ HAZLETON–ST. JOSEPH MEDICAL CENTER, 687 North Church Street, Zip 18201–3198; tel. 570/501-6000; Bernard C. Rudegeair, President and Chief Executive Officer (Total facility includes 11 beds in nursing home–type unit) **A**1 9 10 **F**3 8 9 13 14 16 17 18 19 22 24 25 27 28 29 31 32 33 34 36 37 38 39 40 41 43 44 45 46 48 49 50 51 54 56 59 60 61 62 63 64 68 69 70 72 76 78 79 **Web address:** www.ghha.org	23	10	120	4210	70	152765	459	36282	16683	559
HERSHEY—Dauphin County										
★ △ PENN STATE GEISINGER HEALTH SYSTEM–MILTON S. HERSHEY MEDICAL CENTER, 500 University Drive, Zip 17033–0850, Mailing Address: P.O. Box 850, Zip 17033–0850; tel. 717/531-8521; John E. May, II, Senior Vice President Operations **A**1 2 3 5 7 8 9 10 **F**4 5 8 9 11 13 14 16 17 19 20 22 24 25 26 27 28 29 30 31 32 33 34 35 36 38 39 41 42 43 44 45 46 47 48 49 50 51 52 53 54 56 57 58 59 60 61 62 63 64 65 66 68 69 70 71 72 73 74 75 76 77 78 79 **P**1 6 **Web address:** www.collmed.psu.edu/	23	10	415	19998	360	345487	1238	327884	129614	4733
HONESDALE—Wayne County										
★ WAYNE MEMORIAL HOSPITAL, 601 Park Street, Zip 18431–1445; tel. 570/253-8100; G. Richard Garman, Executive Director **A**1 9 10 **F**1 7 8 9 17 18 19 20 22 23 24 25 31 32 34 35 36 37 39 43 44 45 46 48 49 50 54 58 60 61 62 65 69 70 71 72 73 76 78 **P**5 **Web address:** www.wmh.org	23	10	78	4173	57	82199	486	35952	14716	477

© 2000 AHA Guide *Many Facility Codes have changed. Please refer to the AHA Guide Code Chart.*

Hospitals, U.S. / PENNSYLVANIA

Hospital, Address, Telephone, Administrator, Approval, Facility, and Physician Codes, Health Care System, Network	Classification Codes		Utilization Data					Expense (thousands) of dollars		
	Control	Service	Staffed Beds	Admissions	Census	Outpatient Visits	Births	Total	Payroll	Personnel

★ American Hospital Association (AHA) membership
☐ Joint Commission on Accreditation of Healthcare Organizations (JCAHO) accreditation
+ American Osteopathic Healthcare Association (AOHA) membership
○ American Osteopathic Association (AOA) accreditation
△ Commission on Accreditation of Rehabilitation Facilities (CARF) accreditation
Control codes 61, 63, 64, 71, 72 and 73 indicate hospitals listed by AOHA, but not registered by AHA. For definition of numerical codes, see page A4

HUNTINGDON—Huntingdon County

★ J. C. BLAIR MEMORIAL HOSPITAL, 1225 Warm Springs Avenue, Zip 16652-2398; tel. 814/643-2290; Richard E. D'Alberto, Chief Executive Officer **A**1 9 10 **F**7 8 9 13 16 17 18 22 24 25 32 39 41 44 48 51 54 57 62 63 64 70 71 76 78 **S** Quorum Health Group, Brentwood, TN Web address: www.JCBlair.Org	23	10	104	4063	50	91632	337	28371	12292	347

INDIANA—Indiana County

★ INDIANA HOSPITAL, 835 Hospital Road, Zip 15701-3650, Mailing Address: P.O. Box 788, Zip 15701-0788; tel. 724/357-7000; Stephen A. Wolfe, President and Chief Executive Officer (Total facility includes 18 beds in nursing home-type unit) **A**1 9 10 **F**7 8 9 13 14 16 17 18 19 22 23 24 25 28 29 30 32 34 38 41 44 45 46 48 50 51 54 57 59 61 62 63 65 68 69 70 72 76 78 **P**6	23	10	148	6871	93	193986	701	54350	28836	801

JEANNETTE—Westmoreland County

☐ JEANNETTE DISTRICT MEMORIAL HOSPITAL, 600 Jefferson Avenue, Zip 15644-2504; tel. 724/527-3551; Robert J. Bulger, President and Chief Executive Officer (Total facility includes 11 beds in nursing home-type unit) **A**1 9 10 **F**7 8 9 13 17 18 22 24 25 29 31 32 33 39 41 44 48 50 53 54 69 70 72 76 78 **P**8 Web address: www.jdmh.org/	23	10	137	5578	76	89659	490	35945	16829	554
☐ MONSOUR MEDICAL CENTER, 70 Lincoln Way East, Zip 15644-3167; tel. 724/527-1511; Geraldine Pozzuto, Acting Chief Executive Officer (Nonreporting) **A**1 9 10	23	10	146	—	—	—	—	—	—	—

JERSEY SHORE—Lycoming County

★ JERSEY SHORE HOSPITAL, 1020 Thompson Street, Zip 17740-1794; tel. 570/398-0100; Louis A. Ditzel, Jr, President and Chief Executive Officer **A**1 9 10 **F**9 12 13 14 16 17 18 19 22 24 25 27 32 33 34 37 38 39 40 41 43 45 48 49 50 54 56 68 69 70 71 72 74 76 78 **P**6 **S** Quorum Health Group, Brentwood, TN	23	10	49	1146	11	74657	0	12732	5429	198

JOHNSTOWN—Cambria County

★ CONEMAUGH MEMORIAL MEDICAL CENTER, (Includes Good Samaritan Medical Center, 1020 Franklin Street, Zip 15905-4186; tel. 814/533-1000), 1086 Franklin Street, Zip 15905-4305; tel. 814/534-9000; Richard Salluzzo, Chief Executive Officer **A**1 2 3 5 6 9 10 12 **F**2 3 4 6 7 8 9 11 12 13 14 16 17 18 19 21 22 23 24 25 27 28 29 30 31 32 33 34 35 36 37 39 41 42 43 44 45 46 47 48 49 50 51 53 54 56 57 58 59 60 62 63 64 65 67 68 70 72 75 76 77 78 79 **P**4 6 8 Web address: www.conemaugh.org	23	10	400	16646	277	432472	626	184240	69547	2157
GOOD SAMARITAN MEDICAL CENTER See Conemaugh Memorial Medical Center										
★ UPMC LEE REGIONAL, 320 Main Street, Zip 15901-1694; tel. 814/533-0123; David R. Davis, President and Chief Executive Officer (Total facility includes 15 beds in nursing home-type unit) **A**1 2 9 10 **F**4 7 8 9 11 12 13 16 17 18 19 22 23 24 25 29 30 31 32 33 34 36 37 38 39 41 42 43 44 45 46 47 48 50 53 54 56 61 65 69 70 72 76 77 78 79 **P**8 **S** UPMC Health System, Pittsburgh, PA Web address: www.upmc.edu/lee/	23	10	217	8745	142	133692	758	77267	31919	1065

KANE—McKean County

KANE COMMUNITY HOSPITAL, North Fraley Street, Zip 16735, Mailing Address: Rural Route 2, Box 230, Zip 16733-9654; tel. 814/837-8585; J. Gary Rhodes, Chief Executive Officer **A**9 10 **F**9 13 16 19 22 25 31 32 34 36 38 41 45 46 48 49 54 56 61 66 70 71 72 76 78 **P**6 Web address: www.kanehosp.com	23	10	39	1329	16	23586	0	9273	4336	148

KINGSTON—Luzerne County

NESBITT MEMORIAL HOSPITAL See Wyoming Valley Health Care System, Wilkes-Barre

KITTANNING—Armstrong County

☐ ARMSTRONG COUNTY MEMORIAL HOSPITAL, One Nolte Drive, Zip 16201-8808; tel. 724/543-8500; Jack D. Hoard, President and Chief Executive Officer (Total facility includes 25 beds in nursing home-type unit) **A**1 2 9 10 **F**7 8 9 11 12 13 16 17 19 22 24 25 27 32 33 34 36 38 39 41 43 44 45 46 48 49 51 54 55 56 57 58 59 60 61 62 65 68 69 70 71 72 76 78 **P**5	23	10	210	6700	103	162230	583	47013	22609	737

LAFAYETTE HILL—Montgomery County

☐ EUGENIA HOSPITAL, 660 Thomas Road, Zip 19444-1199; tel. 215/836-7700; John P. Ash, FACHE, President and Chief Executive Officer (Nonreporting) **A**1 9 10 **S** Progressions Group, Inc., Fort Washington, PA	33	22	126	—	—	—	—	—	—	—

LANCASTER—Lancaster County

+ ○ COMMUNITY HOSPITAL OF LANCASTER, 1100 East Orange Street, Zip 17602-3218, Mailing Address: P.O. Box 3002, Zip 17604-3002; tel. 717/397-3711; Maureen Gallo, Administrator (Nonreporting) **A**9 10 11 12 13 **S** Health Management Associates, Naples, FL Web address: www.chol.org	23	10	142	—	—	—	—	—	—	—
☐ △ LANCASTER GENERAL HOSPITAL, 555 North Duke Street, Zip 17604-3555, Mailing Address: P.O. Box 3555, Zip 17604-3555; tel. 717/290-5511; Mark A. Brazitis, President (Total facility includes 30 beds in nursing home-type unit) (Nonreporting) **A**1 2 3 5 6 7 9 10 Web address: www.lha.org	23	10	493	—	—	—	—	—	—	—
★ △ ST. JOSEPH HOSPITAL, 250 College Avenue, Zip 17604, Mailing Address: P.O. Box 3509, Zip 17604-3509; tel. 717/291-8211; John Kerr Tolmie, President and Chief Executive Officer (Total facility includes 21 beds in nursing home-type unit) **A**1 2 7 9 10 **F**1 4 7 8 9 11 12 13 16 17 18 19 20 22 24 25 26 28 30 31 32 33 34 35 36 37 38 39 41 42 43 44 45 46 47 48 49 51 53 54 56 57 58 59 63 65 66 68 69 70 72 76 78 **P**2 6 7 **S** Catholic Health Initiatives, Denver, CO Web address: www.chieast.org	23	10	208	10005	122	252877	1280	77805	30516	746

Hospitals, U.S. / PENNSYLVANIA

Hospital, Address, Telephone, Administrator, Approval, Facility, and Physician Codes, Health Care System, Network	Classification Codes		Utilization Data					Expense (thousands) of dollars		
★ American Hospital Association (AHA) membership □ Joint Commission on Accreditation of Healthcare Organizations (JCAHO) accreditation + American Osteopathic Healthcare Association (AOHA) membership ○ American Osteopathic Association (AOA) accreditation △ Commission on Accreditation of Rehabilitation Facilities (CARF) accreditation Control codes 61, 63, 64, 71, 72 and 73 indicate hospitals listed by AOHA, but not registered by AHA. For definition of numerical codes, see page A4	Control	Service	Staffed Beds	Admissions	Census	Outpatient Visits	Births	Total	Payroll	Personnel

LANGHORNE—Bucks County

BUCKS COUNTY CAMPUS See Frankford Hospital of the City of Philadelphia, Philadelphia

☆ ST. MARY MEDICAL CENTER, Langhorne–Newtown Road, Zip 19047–1295; tel. 215/750–2000; Gregory T. Wozniak, President and Chief Executive Officer **A**1 2 9 10 **F**8 9 11 12 13 14 16 17 18 19 22 24 25 28 33 34 36 38 39 41 42 44 45 46 47 48 49 51 53 54 65 68 70 71 75 76 78 79 **P**8 **S** Catholic Health Initiatives, Denver, CO   23 10 257 13864 176 102839 1389 104644 43244 1216

LANSDALE—Montgomery County

☆ NORTH PENN HOSPITAL, 100 Medical Campus Drive, Zip 19446–1200; tel. 215/368–2100; Robert H. McKay, President (Nonreporting) **A**1 2 9 10
Web address: www.nph.org   23 10 150 — — — — — — —

LATROBE—Westmoreland County

☆ LATROBE AREA HOSPITAL, 121 West Second Avenue, Zip 15650–1096; tel. 724/537–1000; Douglas A. Clark, Executive Director (Total facility includes 20 beds in nursing home–type unit) **A**1 2 3 5 9 10 **F**5 7 8 9 11 12 13 14 16 17 18 19 21 22 24 25 26 27 28 29 31 32 33 34 35 36 37 38 39 41 43 44 45 46 49 50 54 56 57 58 59 60 61 63 64 65 68 69 70 72 73 76 78 79 **P**6
Web address: www.lah.com   23 10 215 12102 155 318641 839 101266 47146 1255

LEBANON—Lebanon County

☆ GOOD SAMARITAN HOSPITAL, Fourth and Walnut Streets, Zip 17042, Mailing Address: P.O. Box 1281, Zip 17042–1281; tel. 717/270–7500; Robert J. Longo, President and Chief Executive Officer (Total facility includes 19 beds in nursing home–type unit) **A**1 3 5 9 10 **F**3 4 8 9 11 13 16 17 19 21 22 23 24 25 28 31 34 35 36 37 39 41 43 44 45 46 48 53 54 56 58 59 60 61 62 63 64 65 68 70 71 72 76 77 78 79 **P**8
Web address: www.gshleb.com   23 10 178 9469 134 199125 1016 76786 34849 952

☆ VETERANS AFFAIRS MEDICAL CENTER, 1700 South Lincoln Avenue, Zip 17042–7529; tel. 717/272–6621; Charleen R. Szabo, FACHE, Chief Executive Officer (Total facility includes 114 beds in nursing home–type unit) **A**1 3 5 9 **F**2 3 4 13 17 18 19 22 25 26 29 30 31 34 35 37 38 41 43 45 46 48 50 51 54 56 57 59 61 62 63 64 69 70 72 73 76 77 78 79 **S** Department of Veterans Affairs, Washington, DC
Web address: www.va.gov   45 10 285 2461 221 168783 0 77561 40131 967

LEHIGHTON—Carbon County

☆ GNADEN HUETTEN MEMORIAL HOSPITAL, 211 North 12th Street, Zip 18235–1138; tel. 610/377–1300; Robert J. Clark, FACHE, President and Chief Executive Officer (Total facility includes 91 beds in nursing home–type unit) **A**1 9 10 **F**7 8 9 13 16 17 18 19 22 23 24 25 29 30 31 32 33 34 36 37 39 40 41 43 44 45 46 48 49 50 51 53 54 57 58 59 60 61 62 63 64 66 69 70 72 76 78 79 **P**8   23 10 202 3810 138 121157 275 31497 14139 470

LEWISBURG—Union County

EVANGELICAL COMMUNITY HOSPITAL, One Hospital Drive, Zip 17837–9314; tel. 570/522–2000; Michael Daniloff, President (Nonreporting) **A**9 10   23 10 115 — — — — — — —

U. S. PENITENTIARY INFIRMARY, Route 7, Zip 17837–9303; tel. 570/523–1251; Arnold Reyes, Administrator (Nonreporting)   48 11 17 — — — — — — —

LEWISTOWN—Mifflin County

☆ LEWISTOWN HOSPITAL, 400 Highland Avenue, Zip 17044–1198; tel. 717/248–5411; A. Gordon McAleer, FACHE, President and Chief Executive Officer **A**1 2 9 10 **F**1 3 7 8 9 12 13 16 17 18 19 20 21 22 23 24 25 26 29 30 32 34 35 36 37 38 39 41 43 44 45 46 48 49 54 56 57 58 59 60 61 62 63 64 65 68 70 72 76 78 **P**3 6
Web address: www.lewistownhospital.org   23 10 158 7184 80 151682 619 44449 21891 795

LOCK HAVEN—Clinton County

☆ LOCK HAVEN HOSPITAL, 24 Cree Drive, Zip 17745–2699; tel. 570/893–5000; Gary R. Rhoads, President and Chief Executive Officer (Total facility includes 120 beds in nursing home–type unit) **A**1 9 10 **F**8 9 17 18 19 22 24 29 30 32 33 34 38 39 43 46 48 50 51 54 56 59 63 66 67 68 69 70 76 78 **P**5 **S** Quorum Health Group, Brentwood, TN   23 10 195 2634 138 49042 348 23166 10296 380

MALVERN—Chester County

☆ △ BRYN MAWR REHABILITATION HOSPITAL, 414 Paoli Pike, Zip 19355–3300, Mailing Address: P.O. Box 3007, Zip 19355–3300; tel. 610/251–5400; Patricia Ryan, Senior Vice President (Total facility includes 23 beds in nursing home–type unit) **A**1 7 9 10 **F**2 3 4 5 8 9 10 11 12 13 14 16 17 18 19 22 24 25 26 29 30 32 33 34 35 36 37 38 39 41 42 43 44 45 46 47 48 49 50 52 53 54 55 56 57 58 59 60 61 62 63 64 65 66 68 69 70 71 72 74 76 78 79 **P**5 **S** Jefferson Health System, Wayne, PA
Web address: www.jeffersonhealth.org   23 46 141 3417 136 27553 0 32402 16754 430

□ DEVEREUX MAPLETON PSYCHIATRIC INSTITUTE–MAPLETON CENTER, 655 Sugartown Road, Zip 19355–0297, Mailing Address: Box 297, Zip 19355–0297; tel. 610/296–6974; James M. Cole, Executive Director (Nonreporting) **A**1 **S** Devereux Foundation, Villanova, PA   23 22 13 — — — — — — —

MALVERN INSTITUTE, 940 King Road, Zip 19355–3167; tel. 610/647–0330; Thomas Cain, Administrator and Chief Executive Officer (Nonreporting) **A**9 **S** Progressions Group, Inc., Fort Washington, PA   33 82 40 — — — — — — —

MCCONNELLSBURG—Fulton County

★ FULTON COUNTY MEDICAL CENTER, 216 South First Street, Zip 17233–1399; tel. 717/485–3155; Robert B. Murray, II, President and Chief Executive Officer (Total facility includes 57 beds in nursing home–type unit) **A**9 10 **F**7 8 9 17 22 25 32 34 36 38 39 41 44 48 51 68 69 70 76   23 10 96 1529 75 38803 127 14625 7566 274

© 2000 AHA Guide   *Many Facility Codes have changed. Please refer to the AHA Guide Code Chart.*

Hospitals, U.S. / PENNSYLVANIA

Hospital, Address, Telephone, Administrator, Approval, Facility, and Physician Codes, Health Care System, Network	Classification Codes		Utilization Data					Expense (thousands) of dollars		
	Control	Service	Staffed Beds	Admissions	Census	Outpatient Visits	Births	Total	Payroll	Personnel

★ American Hospital Association (AHA) membership
□ Joint Commission on Accreditation of Healthcare Organizations (JCAHO) accreditation
+ American Osteopathic Healthcare Association (AOHA) membership
○ American Osteopathic Association (AOA) accreditation
△ Commission on Accreditation of Rehabilitation Facilities (CARF) accreditation
Control codes 61, 63, 64, 71, 72 and 73 indicate hospitals listed by AOHA, but not registered by AHA. For definition of numerical codes, see page A4

Hospital	Control	Service	Staffed Beds	Admissions	Census	Outpatient Visits	Births	Total	Payroll	Personnel
MCKEES ROCKS—Allegheny County ★ OHIO VALLEY GENERAL HOSPITAL, 25 Heckel Road, Zip 15136–1694; tel. 412/777–6161; William F. Provenzano, President **A**1 6 9 10 **F**6 7 8 9 12 13 18 22 24 25 27 32 34 39 43 44 45 46 48 53 54 70 76 **S** Quorum Health Group, Brentwood, TN	23	10	118	4551	66	94569	361	40839	15135	449
MCKEESPORT—Allegheny County ★ UPMC MCKEESPORT, 1500 Fifth Avenue, Zip 15132–2482; tel. 412/664–2000; Ronald H. Ott, President and Chief Executive Officer (Total facility includes 28 beds in nursing home–type unit) (Nonreporting) **A**1 3 5 9 10 **S** UPMC Health System, Pittsburgh, PA Web address: www.upmc.edu/mckeesport	23	10	320	—	—	—	—	—	—	—
MEADOWBROOK—Montgomery County ★ HOLY REDEEMER HOSPITAL AND MEDICAL CENTER, 1648 Huntingdon Pike, Zip 19046–8099; tel. 215/947–3000; Mark T. Jones, President (Total facility includes 15 beds in nursing home–type unit) (Nonreporting) **A**1 5 9 10 Web address: www.holyredeemer.com	23	10	217	—	—	—	—	—	—	—
MEADVILLE—Crawford County ★ MEADVILLE MEDICAL CENTER, 751 Liberty Street, Zip 16335–2555; tel. 814/333–5000; Anthony J. DeFail, President and Chief Executive Officer (Total facility includes 32 beds in nursing home–type unit) **A**1 2 9 10 **F**2 3 8 9 13 17 18 19 20 22 24 25 28 30 36 37 39 41 44 45 46 48 49 50 51 53 54 56 57 58 62 68 69 70 71 72 76 78 79 **P**6 7 8 Web address: www.mmchs.org	23	10	240	8457	129	150707	605	64257	28178	802
MECHANICSBURG—Cumberland County □ △ HEALTHSOUTH REHABILITATION OF MECHANICSBURG, 175 Lancaster Boulevard, Zip 17055–0736, Mailing Address: P.O. Box 2016, Zip 17055–2016; tel. 717/691–3700; Melissa Kutz, Administrator and Chief Executive Officer (Nonreporting) **A**1 7 10 **S** HEALTHSOUTH Corporation, Birmingham, AL PINNACLEHEALTH AT SEIDLE MEMORIAL HOSPITAL See PinnacleHealth System, Harrisburg	33	46	103	—	—	—	—	—	—	—
MEDIA—Delaware County ★ RIDDLE MEMORIAL HOSPITAL, 1068 West Baltimore Pike, Zip 19063–5177; tel. 610/566–9400; Donald L. Laughlin, President (Total facility includes 23 beds in nursing home–type unit) **A**1 2 9 10 **F**3 5 6 7 8 9 11 13 14 16 17 18 19 20 22 23 24 25 28 30 32 34 35 36 37 38 39 41 42 43 44 45 46 48 49 50 51 54 55 65 66 67 69 70 71 72 76 78 79 **P**5 6 7 Web address: www.riddlehospital.org	23	10	198	10461	147	105369	1053	69062	32924	880
MEYERSDALE—Somerset County □ MEYERSDALE MEDICAL CENTER, 200 Hospital Drive, Zip 15552–1247; tel. 814/634–5911; Mary L. Libengood, President **A**1 9 10 **F**7 16 17 18 19 22 25 32 34 36 41 48 54 68 70 72 76 78	23	10	20	622	8	22690	0	5422	2370	91
MONONGAHELA—Washington County ★ MONONGAHELA VALLEY HOSPITAL, 1163 Country Club Road, Rt 88, Zip 15063–1095; tel. 724/258–1000; Anthony M. Lombardi, President and Chief Executive Officer (Total facility includes 15 beds in nursing home–type unit) **A**1 2 9 10 **F**2 5 6 7 8 9 11 12 16 17 18 19 22 23 24 25 26 27 30 31 32 33 34 35 36 37 38 39 41 43 44 45 46 48 49 50 51 53 54 57 58 59 60 61 62 65 66 68 69 70 71 72 73 76 78 79 **P**8 Web address: www.monvalleyhospital.com	23	10	255	11591	194	185030	483	74941	36165	994
MONROEVILLE—Allegheny County ★ FORBES REGIONAL HOSPITAL (Formerly Allegheny University Hospitals, Forbes Regional), 2570 Haymaker Road, Zip 15146–3592; tel. 412/858–2000; Barry H. Roth, President and Chief Executive Officer (Total facility includes 25 beds in nursing home–type unit) **A**1 2 3 5 9 10 **F**7 8 9 11 13 16 17 18 19 22 24 25 27 28 30 31 32 34 36 37 38 39 40 41 43 44 45 46 48 49 50 51 54 57 61 62 64 65 66 68 69 70 71 72 75 76 78 **S** West Penn Allegheny Health System, Pittsburgh, PA	23	10	335	14091	195	84955	1400	104335	39987	1136
□ HEALTHSOUTH GREATER PITTSBURGH REHABILITATION HOSPITAL, 2380 McGinley Road, Zip 15146–4400; tel. 412/856–2400; Faith A. Deigan, Administrator and Chief Executive Officer (Nonreporting) **A**1 9 10 **S** HEALTHSOUTH Corporation, Birmingham, AL Web address: www.healthsouth.com	33	46	89	—	—	—	—	—	—	—
MONTROSE—Susquehanna County ENDLESS MOUNTAIN HEALTH SYSTEMS, 1 Grow Avenue, Zip 18801–1199; tel. 570/278–3801; Rex Catlin, Chief Executive Officer **A**9 10 **F**9 16 18 19 22 25 30 37 41 48 54 70 72 76 **P**4 7 Web address: www.emhs.org	23	10	32	896	9	54181	0	7480	2883	133
MOUNT GRETNA—Lebanon County □ PHILHAVEN, BAHAVIORAL HEALTHCARE SERVICES, 283 South Butler Road, Zip 17064, Mailing Address: P.O. Box 550, Zip 17064–0550; tel. 717/273–8871; LaVern J. Yutzy, Chief Executive Officer **A**1 9 10 **F**16 17 36 57 58 59 60 61 62 63 64 78 79 **P**6 Web address: www.philhaven.com	21	22	83	1716	53	45812	0	23866	15428	604
MOUNT PLEASANT—Westmoreland County ★ FRICK HOSPITAL, 508 South Church Street, Zip 15666–1790; tel. 724/547–1500; Rodney L. Gunderson, Chief Executive Officer (Total facility includes 18 beds in nursing home–type unit) **A**1 2 9 10 **F**7 8 9 11 12 13 16 17 18 19 21 22 23 24 25 30 32 34 35 36 37 38 39 41 43 44 45 46 48 49 50 51 54 58 59 60 61 62 63 64 65 69 70 71 72 74 76 78 79 **P**8 **S** Fay-West Health System, Mount Pleasant, PA	23	10	171	5842	92	125960	350	40997	19141	523

Hospitals, U.S. / PENNSYLVANIA

Hospital, Address, Telephone, Administrator, Approval, Facility, and Physician Codes, Health Care System, Network	Classification Codes		Utilization Data					Expense (thousands) of dollars		
★ American Hospital Association (AHA) membership □ Joint Commission on Accreditation of Healthcare Organizations (JCAHO) accreditation + American Osteopathic Healthcare Association (AOHA) membership ○ American Osteopathic Association (AOA) accreditation △ Commission on Accreditation of Rehabilitation Facilities (CARF) accreditation Control codes 61, 63, 64, 71, 72 and 73 indicate hospitals listed by AOHA, but not registered by AHA. For definition of numerical codes, see page A4	Control	Service	Staffed Beds	Admissions	Census	Outpatient Visits	Births	Total	Payroll	Personnel

MUNCY—Lycoming County
MUNCY VALLEY HOSPITAL See Susquehanna Health System, Williamsport

NANTICOKE—Luzerne County

	Control	Service	Staffed Beds	Admissions	Census	Outpatient Visits	Births	Total	Payroll	Personnel
MERCY SPECIAL CARE HOSPITAL, 128 West Washington Street, Zip 18634–3113; tel. 570/735-5000; Robert D. Williams, Administrator (Nonreporting) **A**10 **S** Catholic Healthcare Partners, Cincinnati, OH	23	49	38	—	—	—	—	—	—	—

NATRONA HEIGHTS—Allegheny County

	Control	Service	Staffed Beds	Admissions	Census	Outpatient Visits	Births	Total	Payroll	Personnel
✠ ALLEGHENY UNIVERSITY HOSPITALS, ALLEGHENY VALLEY, 1301 Carlisle Street, Zip 15065–1192; tel. 724/224-5100; Joseph Calig, President and Chief Executive Officer (Total facility includes 21 beds in nursing home–type unit) **A**1 2 9 10 **F**3 7 8 9 11 12 13 17 18 19 22 24 25 32 33 34 36 37 38 39 40 41 43 44 45 46 48 49 50 54 56 57 59 61 62 63 65 66 68 69 70 71 72 76 77 78 79 **S** West Penn Allegheny Health System, Pittsburgh, PA	23	10	258	9426	148	—	538	73838	30750	785

NEW CASTLE—Lawrence County

	Control	Service	Staffed Beds	Admissions	Census	Outpatient Visits	Births	Total	Payroll	Personnel
✠ △ JAMESON HOSPITAL, 1211 Wilmington Avenue, Zip 16105–2595; tel. 724/658-9001; Thomas White, President and Chief Executive Officer (Total facility includes 20 beds in nursing home–type unit) **A**1 2 6 7 9 10 **F**6 7 8 9 11 12 13 14 16 17 18 19 22 23 24 25 26 27 30 32 33 34 36 38 39 41 43 44 45 46 48 49 50 53 54 57 62 64 65 66 68 69 70 71 72 76 77 78 79 **P**7 8 Web address: www.jamesonhealthsystem.com	23	10	195	7119	113	195488	456	61154	27027	1007
✠ ST. FRANCIS HOSPITAL OF NEW CASTLE, 1000 South Mercer Street, Zip 16101–4673; tel. 724/658-3511; Sister Patricia Fogle, Chief Executive Officer (Total facility includes 45 beds in nursing home–type unit) (Nonreporting) **A**1 6 9 10 **S** St. Francis Health System, Pittsburgh, PA Web address: www.sfhs.edu	23	10	193	—	—	—	—	—	—	—

NEW KENSINGTON—Westmoreland County

	Control	Service	Staffed Beds	Admissions	Census	Outpatient Visits	Births	Total	Payroll	Personnel
□ CITIZENS GENERAL HOSPITAL, 651 Fourth Avenue, Zip 15068–6591; tel. 724/337-3541; Edward M. Klaman, Acting Chief Executive Officer (Total facility includes 20 beds in nursing home–type unit) **A**1 2 6 9 10 **F**6 7 8 9 13 16 18 22 23 24 25 26 27 31 32 33 34 36 37 39 40 43 44 45 46 48 49 54 57 62 64 65 69 70 72 75 76 78 **P**5 Web address: www.citizensgeneralhospital.baweb.com	23	10	200	5304	79	81687	278	42829	17050	474

NORRISTOWN—Montgomery County

	Control	Service	Staffed Beds	Admissions	Census	Outpatient Visits	Births	Total	Payroll	Personnel
★ + ○ MERCY SUBURBAN HOSPITAL, (Formerly Mercy Suburban General Hospital), 2701 DeKalb Pike, Zip 19401–1820; tel. 610/278-2000; Edward R. Solvibile, Chief Executive Officer **A**2 9 10 11 12 13 **F**7 8 9 13 16 17 18 22 23 24 25 30 33 34 35 36 38 39 41 43 44 45 46 48 49 50 51 54 56 57 62 65 68 70 71 72 76 78 79 **P**6 **S** Catholic Health East, Newtown Square, PA Web address: www.mercyhealth.org	21	10	115	5821	71	84759	458	51533	21921	—
□ MONTGOMERY COUNTY EMERGENCY SERVICE, 50 Beech Drive, Zip 19403–5421; tel. 610/279-6100; Rocio Nell, M.D., Chief Executive Officer and Medical Director (Nonreporting) **A**1 9 10	23	22	53	—	—	—	—	—	—	—
✠ MONTGOMERY HOSPITAL, 1301 Powell Street, Zip 19401, Mailing Address: P.O. Box 992, Zip 19404–0992; tel. 610/270-2000; Timothy M. Casey, President and Chief Executive Officer (Total facility includes 19 beds in nursing home–type unit) **A**1 2 3 5 9 10 **F**4 7 8 9 11 12 13 16 17 18 19 20 22 24 25 27 31 32 34 36 37 38 39 41 43 44 45 46 48 49 51 54 56 57 64 65 68 69 70 72 76 78 79 **P**6 Web address: www.mont-hosp.com	23	10	201	9115	133	—	673	73361	35140	964
□ NORRISTOWN STATE HOSPITAL, 1001 Sterigere Street, Zip 19401–5399; tel. 610/270-1000; Albert R. Di Dario, Superintendent (Nonreporting) **A**1 5 9 10	12	22	664	—	—	—	—	—	—	—
✠ VALLEY FORGE MEDICAL CENTER AND HOSPITAL, 1033 West Germantown Pike, Zip 19403–3998; tel. 610/539-8500; Marian W. Colcher, President (Nonreporting) **A**1 9 10	33	10	70	—	—	—	—	—	—	—

NORTH WARREN—Warren County

	Control	Service	Staffed Beds	Admissions	Census	Outpatient Visits	Births	Total	Payroll	Personnel
□ WARREN STATE HOSPITAL, 33 Main Drive, Zip 16365–5099; tel. 814/723-5500; Carmen N. Ferranto, Chief Executive Officer **A**1 9 10 **F**9 12 18 22 23 25 30 34 35 37 39 41 43 44 46 48 49 53 54 57 60 65 70 72 76 78 79 Web address: www.hslc.org/~warmedlib/	12	22	333	284	252	0	0	32610	19977	536

OAKDALE—Allegheny County

	Control	Service	Staffed Beds	Admissions	Census	Outpatient Visits	Births	Total	Payroll	Personnel
✠ VENCOR HOSPITAL–PITTSBURGH, 7777 Steubenville Pike, Zip 15071–3409; tel. 412/494-5500; Judy Weaver, Administrator (Nonreporting) **A**1 10 **S** Vencor, Incorporated, Louisville, KY Web address: www.vencor.com	33	49	63	—	—	—	—	—	—	—

OIL CITY—Venango County
NORTHWEST MEDICAL CENTER–OIL CITY CAMPUS See Northwest Medical Centers

	Control	Service	Staffed Beds	Admissions	Census	Outpatient Visits	Births	Total	Payroll	Personnel
□ NORTHWEST MEDICAL CENTERS, (Includes Northwest Medical Center–Franklin Campus, Franklin; Northwest Medical Center–Oil City Campus, 174 East Bissell Avenue, Mailing Address: P.O. Box 1068, Zip 16301–0568; tel. 814/677-1711), 174 Bissell Avenue, Zip 16301–0568; tel. 814/437-7000; Neil E. Todhunter, Chief Executive Officer (Total facility includes 16 beds in nursing home–type unit) **A**1 2 10 **F**6 8 9 16 17 19 22 24 25 32 34 36 37 38 39 40 41 43 44 45 46 48 49 53 54 56 57 61 63 64 65 68 69 70 71 75 76 77 78 **P**8 Web address: www.northwesthealthsystem.org	23	10	214	8156	104	—	426	60324	27035	816

© 2000 AHA Guide *Many Facility Codes have changed. Please refer to the AHA Guide Code Chart.*

Hospitals, U.S. / PENNSYLVANIA

Hospital, Address, Telephone, Administrator, Approval, Facility, and Physician Codes, Health Care System, Network	Classification Codes		Utilization Data					Expense (thousands) of dollars		
★ American Hospital Association (AHA) membership □ Joint Commission on Accreditation of Healthcare Organizations (JCAHO) accreditation + American Osteopathic Healthcare Association (AOHA) membership ○ American Osteopathic Association (AOA) accreditation △ Commission on Accreditation of Rehabilitation Facilities (CARF) accreditation Control codes 61, 63, 64, 71, 72 and 73 indicate hospitals listed by AOHA, but not registered by AHA. For definition of numerical codes, see page A4	Control	Service	Staffed Beds	Admissions	Census	Outpatient Visits	Births	Total	Payroll	Personnel
OREFIELD—Lehigh County ★ NATIONAL HOSPITAL FOR KIDS IN CRISIS, 5300 Kids Peace Drive, Zip 18069–9101; tel. 610/799–8800; John P. Peter, President and Chief Executive Officer **A**9 10 **F**17 18 57 58 64 **P**6 Web address: www.kidspeace.org	23	52	72	1133	52	2560	0	14236	5899	162
PALMERTON—Carbon County □ PALMERTON HOSPITAL, 135 Lafayette Avenue, Zip 18071–9990; tel. 610/826–3141; Peter L. Kern, President and Chief Executive Officer (Nonreporting) **A**1 9 10 Web address: www.palmertonhospital.com	23	10	70	—	—	—	—	—	—	—
PAOLI—Chester County ★ PAOLI MEMORIAL HOSPITAL, 255 West Lancaster Avenue, Zip 19301–1792; tel. 610/648–1000; Barbara Tachovsky, Senior Vice President **A**2 9 10 **F**1 3 4 5 6 7 8 9 11 12 13 16 17 18 19 20 21 22 23 24 25 27 28 29 30 31 32 33 34 35 36 37 38 39 40 41 42 43 44 45 46 47 48 49 50 51 52 53 54 55 56 57 58 59 60 61 62 63 64 65 66 67 68 69 70 71 72 73 74 76 78 79 **P**2 5 6 7 **S** Jefferson Health System, Wayne, PA Web address: www.jeffersonhealth.org/paoli/index.html	23	10	138	7716	81	110683	903	57276	22492	596
PECKVILLE—Lackawanna County MID-VALLEY HOSPITAL, 1400 Main Street, Zip 18452–2009; tel. 570/383–5500; Gerard H. Warner, Jr, Chief Executive Officer **A**9 10 **F**9 16 17 18 19 22 24 25 30 32 34 36 37 38 41 43 46 48 51 54 70 76 78 **P**8 Web address: www.mid-valleyhospital.baweb.com/	23	10	40	1211	18	29829	0	10561	4381	163
PHILADELPHIA—Philadelphia County □ △ ALBERT EINSTEIN MEDICAL CENTER, (Includes Moss Rehabilitation Hospital, 1200 West Tabor Road, Zip 19141–3099; tel. 215/456–9070), 5501 Old York Road, Zip 19141–3098; tel. 215/456–7890; Martin Goldsmith, President (Total facility includes 102 beds in nursing home–type unit) (Nonreporting) **A**1 2 3 5 7 8 9 10 13 **S** Albert Einstein Healthcare Network, Philadelphia, PA	23	10	701	—	—	—	—	—	—	—
□ BELMONT CENTER FOR COMPREHENSIVE TREATMENT, 4200 Monument Road, Zip 19131–1625; tel. 215/877–2000; Jack H. Dembow, General Director and Vice President (Nonreporting) **A**1 3 5 9 10 **S** Albert Einstein Healthcare Network, Philadelphia, PA	23	22	146	—	—	—	—	—	—	—
□ CHARTER FAIRMOUNT BEHAVIORAL HEALTH SYSTEM, 561 Fairthorne Avenue, Zip 19128–2499; tel. 215/487–4000; Diane Kiddy, Chief Executive Officer (Nonreporting) **A**1 9 10 **S** Magellan Health Services, Atlanta, GA Web address: www.charterbehavioral.com	33	22	146	—	—	—	—	—	—	—
⊠ CHESTNUT HILL HEALTHCARE, 8835 Germantown Avenue, Zip 19118–2765; tel. 215/248–8200; Cary F. Leptuck, President and Chief Executive Officer (Nonreporting) **A**1 3 5 9 10 Web address: www.chh.org	23	10	165	—	—	—	—	—	—	—
□ CHILDREN'S HOSPITAL OF PHILADELPHIA, (GEN MED/SURG REHAB PSYCH), (Includes Children's Seashore House, 3405 Civic Center Boulevard, Zip 19104–4302), 34th Street and Civic Center Boulevard, Zip 19104–4399; tel. 215/590–1000; Steven M. Altschuler, President and Chief Executive Officer **A**1 2 3 5 8 9 10 **F**4 11 12 13 14 16 17 18 19 22 23 24 25 27 29 31 32 33 34 35 36 38 39 42 43 46 47 48 49 50 51 52 53 54 56 57 58 59 68 70 71 72 73 74 75 76 78 **P**1 Web address: www.chop.edu EASTERN PENNSYLVANIA PSYCHIATRIC INSTITUTE See Medical College of Pennsylvania Hospital	23	59	387	17765	227	623439	0	321494	155216	4692
□ EPISCOPAL HOSPITAL, (Includes George L. Harrison Memorial House), 100 East Lehigh Avenue, Zip 19125–1098; tel. 215/427–7000; Kathleen Barron, Executive Director (Total facility includes 35 beds in nursing home–type unit) (Nonreporting) **A**1 2 3 5 6 9 10 **S** Temple University Health System, Philadelphia, PA	23	10	218	—	—	—	—	—	—	—
⊠ FOX CHASE CANCER CENTER–AMERICAN ONCOLOGIC HOSPITAL, (ONCOLOGY), 7701 Burholme Avenue, Zip 19111–2412; tel. 215/728–6900; Robert C. Young, M.D., President **A**1 2 3 5 8 9 10 **F**9 13 16 17 18 19 20 21 22 23 24 26 32 33 34 35 36 37 38 39 41 43 45 46 48 49 50 51 54 59 65 68 70 72 74 76 78 79 **P**6 Web address: www.fccc.edu	23	49	76	3660	52	44146	0	64746	20396	534
⊠ + ○ FRANKFORD HOSPITAL OF THE CITY OF PHILADELPHIA, (Includes Bucks County Campus, 380 North Oxford Valley Road, Langhorne, Zip 19047–8399; tel. 215/949–5000; Frankford Campus, Frankford Avenue and Wakeling Street, Zip 19124; tel. 215/831–2000), Knights and Red Lion Roads, Zip 19114–1486; tel. 215/612–4000; Roy A. Powell, President (Total facility includes 30 beds in nursing home–type unit) **A**1 3 5 8 9 10 11 13 **F**1 2 3 4 7 8 9 10 11 13 14 16 17 18 19 20 22 23 24 25 26 27 28 29 30 31 32 33 34 35 36 37 38 39 40 41 42 43 44 45 46 47 48 49 50 51 53 54 55 56 57 58 59 60 61 62 63 64 65 68 69 70 71 72 74 75 76 77 78 79 **P**3 **S** Jefferson Health System, Wayne, PA Web address: www.jeffersonhealth.org/frankford/index.html	23	10	567	22172	305	241403	2207	176539	82776	2897
FRIEDMAN HOSPITAL OF THE HOME FOR THE JEWISH AGED, 5301 Old York Road, Zip 19141–2996; tel. 215/456–2900; Frank Podietz, President (Total facility includes 538 beds in nursing home–type unit) (Nonreporting) Web address: www.pgc.org	23	10	566	—	—	—	—	—	—	—

Hospitals, U.S. / PENNSYLVANIA

Hospital, Address, Telephone, Administrator, Approval, Facility, and Physician Codes, Health Care System, Network	Control	Service	Staffed Beds	Admissions	Census	Outpatient Visits	Births	Total	Payroll	Personnel
★ American Hospital Association (AHA) membership □ Joint Commission on Accreditation of Healthcare Organizations (JCAHO) accreditation + American Osteopathic Healthcare Association (AOHA) membership ○ American Osteopathic Association (AOA) accreditation △ Commission on Accreditation of Rehabilitation Facilities (CARF) accreditation Control codes 61, 63, 64, 71, 72 and 73 indicate hospitals listed by AOHA, but not registered by AHA. For definition of numerical codes, see page A4										
⊠ FRIENDS HOSPITAL, 4641 Roosevelt Boulevard, Zip 19124–2399; tel. 215/831–4600; Wayne A. Mugrauer, Chief Executive Officer (Nonreporting) **A**1 3 9 10 **Web address:** www.med.upenn.edu/health/ms.html	23	22	192	—	—	—	—	—	—	—
□ GERMANTOWN HOSPITAL AND COMMUNITY HEALTH SERVICES, One Penn Boulevard, Zip 19144–1498; tel. 215/951–8000; Cynthia McGlone, Chief Operating Officer (Total facility includes 22 beds in nursing home–type unit) (Nonreporting) **A**1 5 9 10 **S** Jefferson Health System, Wayne, PA GIRARD MEDICAL CENTER See North Philadelphia Health System	23	10	158	—	—	—	—	—	—	—
⊠ GRADUATE HOSPITAL, One Graduate Plaza, Zip 19146–1407; tel. 215/893–2000; Christopher DiCicco, Chief Executive Officer (Nonreporting) **A**1 2 3 5 8 9 10 **S** TENET Healthcare Corporation, Santa Barbara, CA	23	10	198	—	—	—	—	—	—	—
⊠ HAHNEMANN UNIVERSITY HOSPITAL, Broad and Vine Streets, Zip 19102–1192; tel. 215/762–7000; Michael P. Halter, Chief Executive Officer (Nonreporting) **A**1 2 3 5 8 9 10 **S** TENET Healthcare Corporation, Santa Barbara, CA **Web address:** www.auhs.edu	23	10	540	—	—	—	—	—	—	—
⊠ △ HOSPITAL OF THE UNIVERSITY OF PENNSYLVANIA, 3400 Spruce Street, Zip 19104–4385; tel. 215/662–4000; Peter G. Traber, M.D., Chief Executive Officer and Dean **A**1 3 5 7 8 9 10 **F**1 3 4 5 7 8 9 11 12 13 14 15 16 17 18 19 20 21 22 23 24 25 26 27 29 30 31 32 33 34 35 36 37 38 39 41 42 43 44 45 46 47 48 49 50 51 53 54 55 56 57 58 59 60 61 62 63 64 65 66 68 70 71 72 73 74 75 76 78 79 **P**1 4 5 6 7 **S** University of Pennsylvania Health System, Philadelphia, PA **Web address:** www.med.upenn.edu	23	10	659	33473	557	583036	3092	717973	240337	6315
□ JEANES HOSPITAL, 7600 Central Avenue, Zip 19111–2499; tel. 215/728–2000; G. Roger Martin, President and Chief Executive Officer (Nonreporting) **A**1 9 10 **S** Temple University Health System, Philadelphia, PA **Web address:** www.jeanes.com	23	10	188	—	—	—	—	—	—	—
□ JOHN F. KENNEDY MEMORIAL HOSPITAL, Langdon Street and Cheltenham Avenue, Zip 19124–1098; tel. 215/831–7000; Stephen H. Saks, Chief Executive Officer (Nonreporting) **A**1 9 10	23	10	141	—	—	—	—	—	—	—
□ KENSINGTON HOSPITAL, 136 West Diamond Street, Zip 19122–1721; tel. 215/426–8100; Eileen Hause, Chief Executive Officer **A**1 9 10 **F**2 3 9 16 17 18 23 35 38 48 70 76	23	10	45	3897	30	6503	0	4650	2876	120
⊠ △ MAGEE REHABILITATION HOSPITAL, Six Franklin Plaza, Zip 19102–1177; tel. 215/587–3099; William E. Staas, Jr, President and Medical Director **A**1 3 7 10 **F**13 16 17 18 29 32 43 45 49 50 53 54 70 72 **P**4 7 **S** Jefferson Health System, Wayne, PA **Web address:** www.mageerehab.org	23	46	96	1366	73	32573	0	27781	15726	409
⊠ MEDICAL COLLEGE OF PENNSYLVANIA HOSPITAL, (Includes Eastern Pennsylvania Psychiatric Institute, 3200 Henry Avenue, Zip 19129; tel. 215/842–4000), 3300 Henry Avenue, Zip 19129–1121; tel. 215/842–6000; Richard S. Freeman, Chief Executive Officer (Nonreporting) **A**1 2 3 5 8 9 10 **S** TENET Healthcare Corporation, Santa Barbara, CA MERCY HOSPITAL OF PHILADELPHIA See Mercy Health System of Southeastern Pennsylvania, Conshohocken METHODIST HOSPITAL See Thomas Jefferson University Hospital	23	10	369	—	—	—	—	—	—	—
⊠ △ NAZARETH HOSPITAL, 2601 Holme Avenue, Zip 19152–2007; tel. 215/335–6000; Patricia B. DeAngelis, President and Chief Operating Officer (Nonreporting) **A**1 7 9 10 **S** Catholic Health Initiatives, Denver, CO MOSS REHABILITATION HOSPITAL See Albert Einstein Medical Center	21	10	236	—	—	—	—	—	—	—
⊠ NORTH PHILADELPHIA HEALTH SYSTEM, (Includes Girard Medical Center, Girard Avenue at Eighth Street, Zip 19122; tel. 215/787–2000; St. Joseph's Hospital, 16th Street and Girard Avenue, Zip 19130; tel. 215/787–9000; Catherine Kutzler, R.N., Senior Vice President and Chief Executive Officer), 16th Street and Girard Avenue, Zip 19130–1615; tel. 215/787–9000; George J. Walmsley, II, President and Chief Executive Officer (Nonreporting) **A**1 5 9 10 12 13 **S** Catholic Health East, Newtown Square, PA	23	10	315	—	—	—	—	—	—	—
NORTHEASTERN HOSPITAL OF PHILADELPHIA, 2301 East Allegheny Avenue, Zip 19134–4497; tel. 215/291–3000; Lynn Holder, Executive Director (Nonreporting) **A**5 6 9 **S** Temple University Health System, Philadelphia, PA	23	10	166	—	—	—	—	—	—	—
★ ○ PARKVIEW HOSPITAL, 1331 East Wyoming Avenue, Zip 19124–3808; tel. 215/537–7400; David J. Fikse, Chief Executive Officer (Total facility includes 19 beds in nursing home–type unit) (Nonreporting) **A**9 11 13 **S** TENET Healthcare Corporation, Santa Barbara, CA	23	10	165	—	—	—	—	—	—	—
⊠ PENNSYLVANIA HOSPITAL, 800 Spruce Street, Zip 19107–6192; tel. 215/829–3000; Timothy O. Morgan, Executive Director (Total facility includes 29 beds in nursing home–type unit) (Nonreporting) **A**1 2 3 5 8 9 10 **S** University of Pennsylvania Health System, Philadelphia, PA **Web address:** www.pahosp.com	23	10	414	—	—	—	—	—	—	—
□ PRESBYTERIAN MEDICAL CENTER OF THE UNIVERSITY OF PENNSYLVANIA HEALTH SYSTEM, 51 North 39th Street, Zip 19104–2640; tel. 215/662–8000; Michele M. Volpe, Executive Director (Total facility includes 20 beds in nursing home–type unit) (Nonreporting) **A**1 3 5 6 9 10 **S** University of Pennsylvania Health System, Philadelphia, PA **Web address:** www.health.upenn.edu/pmc	23	10	325	—	—	—	—	—	—	—

Hospitals, U.S. / PENNSYLVANIA

Legend for Classification Codes:
- ★ American Hospital Association (AHA) membership
- ☐ Joint Commission on Accreditation of Healthcare Organizations (JCAHO) accreditation
- + American Osteopathic Healthcare Association (AOHA) membership
- ○ American Osteopathic Association (AOA) accreditation
- △ Commission on Accreditation of Rehabilitation Facilities (CARF) accreditation

Control codes 61, 63, 64, 71, 72 and 73 indicate hospitals listed by AOHA, but not registered by AHA. For definition of numerical codes, see page A4.

Hospital, Address, Telephone, Administrator, Approval, Facility, and Physician Codes, Health Care System, Network	Control	Service	Staffed Beds	Admissions	Census	Outpatient Visits	Births	Total	Payroll	Personnel
☐ ROXBOROUGH MEMORIAL HOSPITAL, 5800 Ridge Avenue, Zip 19128–1737; tel. 215/483–9900; John J. Donnelly, Jr, President and Chief Executive Officer (Total facility includes 24 beds in nursing home–type unit) (Nonreporting) **A**1 6 9 10	23	10	129	—	—	—	—	—	—	—
☐ SHRINERS HOSPITALS FOR CHILDREN, PHILADELPHIA, 3551 North Broad Street, Zip 19140–4105; tel. 215/430–4000; Sharon J. Rajnic, Administrator (Nonreporting) **A**1 3 5 **S** Shriners Hospitals for Children, Tampa, FL	23	57	80	—	—	—	—	—	—	—
★ ○ ST. AGNES MEDICAL CENTER, 1900 South Broad Street, Zip 19145–2304; tel. 215/339–4100; Sister Margaret T. Sullivan, President and Chief Executive Officer (Total facility includes 19 beds in nursing home–type unit) **A**1 3 5 9 10 11 **F**10 13 17 18 19 20 22 25 28 31 32 34 36 37 38 41 45 46 48 53 54 69 70 76 78 79 **S** Catholic Health Initiatives, Denver, CO Web address: www.chi–east.org	21	10	172	5434	102	76422	0	53157	24890	513
★ ST. CHRISTOPHER'S HOSPITAL FOR CHILDREN, Erie Avenue at Front Street, Zip 19134–1095; tel. 215/427–5000; Jeffrey Green, Chief Executive Officer (Nonreporting) **A**1 3 5 8 9 10 **S** TENET Healthcare Corporation, Santa Barbara, CA	23	50	178	—	—	—	—	—	—	—
ST. JOSEPH'S HOSPITAL See North Philadelphia Health System										
☐ TEMPLE EAST, NEUMANN MEDICAL CENTER, 1741 Frankford Avenue, Zip 19125–2495; tel. 215/291–2000; Robert P. Perry, Executive Director and Chief Executive Officer (Nonreporting) **A**1 9 10 **S** Temple University Health System, Philadelphia, PA Web address: www.neumann.org	23	10	166	—	—	—	—	—	—	—
☐ TEMPLE UNIVERSITY HOSPITAL, Broad and Ontario Streets, Zip 19140–5192; tel. 215/707–2000; Paul Boehringer, Executive Director (Total facility includes 16 beds in nursing home–type unit) **A**1 2 3 5 8 9 10 **F**1 4 5 6 7 8 9 11 12 13 14 16 17 18 19 20 21 22 23 24 25 27 28 29 30 31 32 33 34 35 36 37 38 39 41 42 43 44 45 46 47 48 49 50 51 52 53 54 55 56 57 59 60 61 62 63 64 65 66 67 68 69 70 71 72 74 75 76 77 78 79 **P**3 4 5 6 7 **S** Temple University Health System, Philadelphia, PA Web address: www.allcet.com/tuhs/index.htm	23	10	439	20579	347	153400	2130	292777	102286	2685
★ △ THOMAS JEFFERSON UNIVERSITY HOSPITAL, (Includes Methodist Hospital, 2301 South Broad Street, Zip 19148; tel. 215/952–9000; Thomas Jefferson University Hospital–Ford Road Campus, 3905 Ford Road, Zip 19131; tel. 215/578–3630), 111 South 11th Street, Zip 19107–5096; tel. 215/955–7022; Thomas J. Lewis, President and Chief Executive Officer (Total facility includes 210 beds in nursing home–type unit) **A**1 2 3 5 6 7 8 9 10 **F**1 2 3 4 5 6 7 8 9 11 12 13 14 15 17 18 19 20 21 22 23 24 25 26 27 28 29 30 31 32 33 34 35 36 37 38 39 40 41 42 43 44 45 46 47 48 49 50 51 52 53 54 56 57 58 59 60 61 62 63 64 65 66 68 69 70 71 72 73 74 75 76 78 79 **P**2 8 **S** Jefferson Health System, Wayne, PA Web address: www.jeffersonhealth.org	23	10	981	38002	790	823810	3222	619158	249493	5671
☐ VENCOR HOSPITAL–PHILADELPHIA, 6129 Palmetto Street, Zip 19111–5729; tel. 215/722–8555; Garrett Arneson, Administrator (Nonreporting) **A**1 9 10 **S** Vencor, Incorporated, Louisville, KY Web address: www.vencor.com	33	49	52	—	—	—	—	—	—	—
★ VETERANS AFFAIRS MEDICAL CENTER, University and Woodland Avenues, Zip 19104–4594; tel. 215/823–5800; Michael J. Sullivan, Director (Total facility includes 240 beds in nursing home–type unit) **A**1 3 5 9 **F**3 9 10 11 12 19 21 22 23 24 25 26 29 30 31 32 33 34 35 36 37 38 39 41 43 44 45 46 47 48 49 50 51 53 54 56 57 62 63 64 65 68 69 70 72 74 76 78 79 **S** Department of Veterans Affairs, Washington, DC Web address: www.va.gov/stations97/guide/home.asp?DIVISION=ALL	45	10	389	5707	343	403647	0	146199	79365	1860
★ WILLS EYE HOSPITAL, (EYE HOSPITAL), 900 Walnut Street, Zip 19107–5598; tel. 215/928–3000; D. McWilliams Kessler, Executive Director and Chief Executive Officer **A**1 3 5 9 10 **F**3 4 5 7 8 9 11 13 14 15 16 17 18 19 20 21 22 23 24 25 26 27 28 29 30 31 32 33 34 35 36 37 38 39 41 43 45 46 47 48 49 50 51 54 55 56 57 58 59 60 61 62 63 64 65 66 68 70 71 72 73 74 75 76 77 78 79 Web address: www.wills.com	23	49	115	4946	47	57939	0	66156	25687	601

PHOENIXVILLE—Chester County

Hospital	Control	Service	Staffed Beds	Admissions	Census	Outpatient Visits	Births	Total	Payroll	Personnel
★ PHOENIXVILLE HOSPITAL OF THE UNIVERSITY OF PENNSYLVANIA HEALTH SYSTEM, 140 Nutt Road, Zip 19460–0809, Mailing Address: P.O. Box 809, Zip 19460–0809; tel. 610/983–1000; Richard E. Seagrave, Executive Director and Chief Operating Officer (Total facility includes 20 beds in nursing home–type unit) **A**1 9 10 **F**3 4 7 8 9 11 12 14 16 17 18 19 20 22 23 24 25 27 30 33 34 35 36 37 38 39 41 42 44 45 46 47 48 49 51 54 59 60 61 65 66 68 69 70 71 72 74 75 76 78 79 **P**4 6 **S** University of Pennsylvania Health System, Philadelphia, PA Web address: www.med.upenn.edu/health/ms.html	23	10	126	6928	79	102863	1203	48485	21343	607

PITTSBURGH—Allegheny County

Hospital	Control	Service	Staffed Beds	Admissions	Census	Outpatient Visits	Births	Total	Payroll	Personnel
ALLEGHENY UNIVERSITY HOSPITAL–FORBES See LifeCare Hospital of Pittsburgh										
★ ALLEGHENY GENERAL HOSPITAL, (Formerly Allegheny University Hospitals, Allegheny General), 320 East North Avenue, Zip 15212–4756; tel. 412/359–3131; Connie M. Cibrone, President and Chief Executive Officer (Total facility includes 49 beds in nursing home–type unit) **A**1 2 3 5 8 9 10 **F**3 4 7 8 9 11 12 13 14 16 17 18 19 20 21 22 23 24 25 26 27 28 29 30 31 32 34 35 36 37 38 39 41 42 43 44 45 46 47 48 49 51 54 55 56 57 58 59 60 61 63 64 65 66 69 70 71 72 73 74 75 76 77 78 79 **S** West Penn Allegheny Health System, Pittsburgh, PA Web address: www.allhealth.edu	23	10	492	32519	505	431985	2081	442677	160087	5184

Hospitals, U.S. / PENNSYLVANIA

Hospital, Address, Telephone, Administrator, Approval, Facility, and Physician Codes, Health Care System, Network	Classification Codes		Utilization Data					Expense (thousands) of dollars		
★ American Hospital Association (AHA) membership □ Joint Commission on Accreditation of Healthcare Organizations (JCAHO) accreditation + American Osteopathic Healthcare Association (AOHA) membership ○ American Osteopathic Association (AOA) accreditation △ Commission on Accreditation of Rehabilitation Facilities (CARF) accreditation Control codes 61, 63, 64, 71, 72 and 73 indicate hospitals listed by AOHA, but not registered by AHA. For definition of numerical codes, see page A4	Control	Service	Staffed Beds	Admissions	Census	Outpatient Visits	Births	Total	Payroll	Personnel
★ CHILDREN'S HOME OF PITTSBURGH, (NEONATAL PEDIATRIC SPECIALTY), 5618 Kentucky Avenue, Zip 15232-2606; tel. 412/441-4884; Pamela R. Schanwald, Chief Executive Officer **A**9 10 **F**22 24 35 36 37 39 45 50 51 55 68 70 76 78 **Web address:** www.almost-home.org	23	59	9	136	7	0	—	2039	1166	38
□ CHILDREN'S HOSPITAL OF PITTSBURGH, 3705 Fifth Avenue at De Soto Street, Zip 15213-2583; tel. 412/692-5325; Ronald L. Violi, President and Chief Executive Officer (Nonreporting) **A**1 2 3 5 8 9 10	23	50	235	—	—	—	—	—	—	—
EYE AND EAR HOSPITAL OF PITTSBURGH See UPMC Presbyterian										
□ △ HEALTHSOUTH HARMARVILLE REHABILITATION HOSPITAL, Guys Run Road, Zip 15238-0460, Mailing Address: Box 11460, Guys Run Road, Zip 15238-0460; tel. 412/781-5700; Faith A. Deigan, Interim Administrator (Total facility includes 40 beds in nursing home-type unit) **A**1 3 7 10 **F**9 13 16 17 18 22 30 32 34 38 43 45 46 49 50 51 54 70 71 72 76 78 **S** HEALTHSOUTH Corporation, Birmingham, AL	33	46	202	2081	133	39705	0	24020	15349	493
⊞ LIFECARE HOSPITAL OF PITTSBURGH, (Formerly Allegheny University Hospital-Forbes), 225 Penn Avenue, Zip 15221-2173; tel. 412/247-2424; April A. Stevens, R.N., Chief Executive Officer (Nonreporting) **A**1 9 10 **S** LifeCare Management Services, Dallas, TX	33	49	152	—	—	—	—	—	—	—
⊞ MAGEE-WOMENS HOSPITAL, 300 Halket Street, Zip 15213-3180; tel. 412/641-1000; Irma E. Goertzen, President and Chief Executive Officer (Nonreporting) **A**1 2 3 5 8 9 10 **S** UPMC Health System, Pittsburgh, PA **Web address:** www.magee.edu	23	44	263	—	—	—	—	—	—	—
⊞ △ MERCY HOSPITAL OF PITTSBURGH, 1400 Locust Street, Zip 15219-5166; tel. 412/232-8111; Gregg G. Zoller, FACHE, President and Chief Executive Officer (Total facility includes 30 beds in nursing home-type unit) **A**1 2 3 5 6 7 8 9 10 12 **F**1 3 4 6 8 9 10 11 12 13 14 16 17 18 19 21 22 23 24 25 26 27 29 30 32 33 34 35 36 37 38 39 41 42 43 44 45 46 47 48 49 50 51 52 53 54 56 57 58 59 60 61 62 63 64 65 66 69 70 72 73 75 76 77 78 79 **P**7 8 **S** Catholic Health East, Newtown Square, PA **Web address:** www.mercylink.org	23	10	399	17641	293	—	1023	205735	66045	2085
⊞ MERCY PROVIDENCE HOSPITAL, 1004 Arch Street, Zip 15212-5235; tel. 412/323-5600; Gregg G. Zoller, FACHE, President and Chief Executive Officer **A**1 9 10 **F**1 3 4 9 13 16 17 18 19 21 22 23 24 25 26 31 32 33 34 35 36 37 38 41 43 46 48 49 50 51 53 54 55 56 57 58 59 60 61 62 63 64 70 72 73 76 78 **P**7 8 **S** Catholic Health East, Newtown Square, PA **Web address:** www.mercylink.org	23	10	146	4016	65	12381	0	23944	8488	249
MONTEFIORE HOSPITAL See UPMC Presbyterian										
PITTSBURGH SPECIALTY HOSPITAL, (Formerly Podiatry Hospital of Pittsburgh), 215 South Negley Avenue, Zip 15206-3594; tel. 412/661-0814; Chelle Verk, Executive Administrator (Nonreporting) **A**9 10	23	49	13	—	—	—	—	—	—	—
SOUTH HILLS HEALTH SYSTEM, 565 Coal Valley Road, Zip 15236-0119, Mailing Address: Box 18119, Zip 15236-0119; tel. 412/469-5000; William R. Jennings, President and Chief Executive Officer (Total facility includes 74 beds in nursing home-type unit) (Nonreporting) **A**9 10 **Web address:** www.shhspgh.org	23	10	466	—	—	—	—	—	—	—
□ SOUTHWOOD PSYCHIATRIC HOSPITAL, 2575 Boyce Plaza Road, Zip 15241-3925; tel. 412/257-2290; Lynne M. Struble, MSN, Chief Executive Officer (Nonreporting) **A**1 **S** Youth and Family Centered Services, Austin, TX	33	52	50	—	—	—	—	—	—	—
⊞ ST. CLAIR MEMORIAL HOSPITAL, 1000 Bower Hill Road, Zip 15243-1873; tel. 412/561-4900; Benjamin E. Snead, President and Chief Executive Officer (Total facility includes 26 beds in nursing home-type unit) **A**1 2 9 10 **F**1 2 4 5 6 7 8 9 11 12 13 14 16 17 18 19 21 22 24 25 27 28 29 30 31 32 33 34 35 36 37 38 39 41 43 44 45 46 47 48 49 50 51 54 57 59 60 61 62 63 64 65 66 69 69 70 72 73 76 78 79 **P**8 **Web address:** www.stclair.org	23	10	292	13073	186	142741	1498	97384	43869	1299
⊞ ○ ST. FRANCIS CENTRAL HOSPITAL, 1200 Centre Avenue, Zip 15219-3507; tel. 412/562-3000; Robin Z. Mohr, Chief Executive Officer (Total facility includes 19 beds in nursing home-type unit) **A**1 9 10 11 12 **F**2 3 4 5 8 9 11 12 13 14 16 19 21 22 23 24 25 27 29 30 31 32 33 34 35 36 38 39 41 43 44 45 46 47 48 50 51 53 54 55 56 57 58 59 60 61 62 63 64 65 66 67 68 69 70 71 72 73 76 77 78 79 **P**5 6 **S** St. Francis Health System, Pittsburgh, PA **Web address:** www.sfhs.edu	23	10	136	4196	72	69939	0	41260	16087	433
⊞ △ ST. FRANCIS MEDICAL CENTER, 400 45th Street, Zip 15201-1198; tel. 412/622-4343; Sister Donna Zwigart, FACHE, Chief Executive Officer (Total facility includes 220 beds in nursing home-type unit) **A**1 2 3 5 6 7 8 9 10 **F**2 3 4 5 7 8 9 11 12 13 16 19 21 22 24 25 26 27 28 29 30 31 32 34 36 38 39 41 43 44 45 46 47 48 49 50 51 53 54 55 56 57 58 59 60 61 62 63 64 65 68 69 70 72 73 76 78 **P**6 7 **S** St. Francis Health System, Pittsburgh, PA **Web address:** www.sfhs.edu	23	10	715	17298	482	—	549	184145	76750	2014
STATE CORRECTIONAL INSTITUTION HOSPITAL, Doerr Street, Zip 15233, Mailing Address: Box 99901, Zip 15233; tel. 412/761-1955; Joseph Morrash, Administrator (Nonreporting)	12	11	27	—	—	—	—	—	—	—
□ SUBURBAN GENERAL HOSPITAL, 100 South Jackson Avenue, Zip 15202-3428; tel. 412/734-6000; Frank G. DeLisi, II, CHE, President and Chief Executive Officer (Total facility includes 26 beds in nursing home-type unit) (Nonreporting) **A**1 9 10 **S** West Penn Allegheny Health System, Pittsburgh, PA **Web address:** www.wphs.org/westpennhospital.htm	23	10	144	—	—	—	—	—	—	—

Hospitals, U.S. / PENNSYLVANIA

Hospital, Address, Telephone, Administrator, Approval, Facility, and Physician Codes, Health Care System, Network

★ American Hospital Association (AHA) membership
□ Joint Commission on Accreditation of Healthcare Organizations (JCAHO) accreditation
+ American Osteopathic Healthcare Association (AOHA) membership
○ American Osteopathic Association (AOA) accreditation
△ Commission on Accreditation of Rehabilitation Facilities (CARF) accreditation
Control codes 61, 63, 64, 71, 72 and 73 indicate hospitals listed by AOHA, but not registered by AHA. For definition of numerical codes, see page A4

Hospital	Control	Service	Staffed Beds	Admissions	Census	Outpatient Visits	Births	Total	Payroll	Personnel
★ △ THE CHILDREN'S INSTITUTE OF PITTSBURGH, 6301 Northumberland Street, Zip 15217–1396; tel. 412/420–2400; John A. Wilson, President and Chief Executive Officer **A**7 9 10 **F**13 16 17 18 19 38 45 51 53 54 58 78 **Web address:** www.amazingkids.org	23	56	38	180	22	16694	—	12408	6678	168
✶ UPMC PASSAVANT, 9100 Babcock Boulevard, Zip 15237–5815; tel. 412/367–6700; Raymond J. Beck, President and Chief Executive Officer (Total facility includes 24 beds in nursing home–type unit) **A**1 9 10 **F**1 2 3 4 5 6 7 8 9 11 12 13 14 15 16 17 18 19 20 21 22 23 24 25 26 27 28 29 30 31 32 33 34 35 36 37 38 39 40 41 42 43 44 45 46 47 48 49 50 51 52 53 54 55 56 57 58 59 60 61 62 63 64 65 66 67 68 69 70 71 72 73 74 75 76 77 78 79 **P**1 5 6 7 **S** UPMC Health System, Pittsburgh, PA **Web address:** www.upmc.edu/passavant	23	10	199	9953	155	172422	0	84949	40284	1195
✶ UPMC PRESBYTERIAN, (Includes Eye and Ear Hospital of Pittsburgh, 200 Lothrop Street, Zip 15213–2592; tel. 412/647–2345; Montefiore Hospital, 200 Lothrop Street, Zip 15213; tel. 412/647–2345; UPMC Presbyterian Hospital, 200 Lothrop Street, Zip 15213; tel. 412/647–2345; Western Psychiatric Institute and Clinic, 3811 O'Hara Street, Zip 15213–2593; tel. 412/624–2100), Henry A. Mordoh, President (Total facility includes 30 beds in nursing home–type unit) **A**1 2 3 5 8 9 **F**1 2 3 4 5 6 7 8 9 11 12 13 14 16 17 18 19 20 21 22 23 24 25 27 28 29 30 31 32 33 34 35 36 37 38 39 40 41 42 43 44 45 46 47 48 49 50 51 52 53 54 55 56 57 58 59 60 61 62 63 64 65 66 67 68 69 70 71 72 73 74 75 76 77 78 79 **P**1 6 7 **S** UPMC Health System, Pittsburgh, PA **Web address:** www.upmc.edu	23	10	752	34097	651	335045	0	678488	200743	7065
✶ UPMC SHADYSIDE, 5230 Centre Avenue, Zip 15232–1304; tel. 412/623–2121; Henry A. Mordoh, President (Total facility includes 145 beds in nursing home–type unit) **A**1 2 3 5 9 10 **F**1 2 3 4 5 6 7 8 9 11 12 13 14 15 17 18 19 20 21 22 23 24 25 26 27 28 29 30 31 32 33 34 35 36 37 38 39 40 41 42 43 44 45 46 47 48 49 50 51 52 53 54 55 56 57 58 59 60 61 62 63 64 65 66 67 68 69 70 71 72 73 74 75 76 77 78 79 **P**1 2 5 6 7 **S** UPMC Health System, Pittsburgh, PA **Web address:** www.upmc.edu	23	10	502	20084	410	79873	794	234472	86271	2059
✶ UPMC SOUTH SIDE, 2000 Mary Street, Zip 15203–2095; tel. 412/488–5550; Marcie S. Caplan, Chief Executive Officer (Total facility includes 23 beds in nursing home–type unit) **A**1 9 10 **F**1 2 3 4 5 6 7 8 9 11 12 13 14 15 16 17 18 19 20 21 22 23 24 25 30 31 32 34 38 39 41 42 43 44 45 46 48 49 50 51 52 53 54 55 56 57 58 59 60 61 62 63 64 65 66 67 68 69 70 71 72 73 74 76 77 78 79 **P**1 6 7 **S** UPMC Health System, Pittsburgh, PA **Web address:** www.upmc.edu/southside/	21	10	136	5740	106	20637	0	36202	15077	447
✶ UPMC ST. MARGARET, 815 Freeport Road, Zip 15215–3301; tel. 412/784–4000; Richard E. Sobehart, President (Total facility includes 22 beds in nursing home–type unit) **A**1 2 3 5 6 8 9 10 **F**5 6 7 9 11 13 17 18 19 22 23 24 25 26 28 29 30 32 33 34 35 36 37 38 39 41 43 45 46 48 49 50 51 53 54 56 61 62 63 65 69 70 71 72 73 76 78 **P**8 **S** UPMC Health System, Pittsburgh, PA **Web address:** www.upmc.edu	23	10	223	9297	142	142738	0	85161	30379	946
✶ VETERANS AFFAIRS PITTSBURGH HEALTHCARE SYSTEM, Includes Veterans Affairs Medical Center, 7180 Highland Drive, Zip 15206–1297; tel. 412/365–4900; Veterans Affairs Medical Center, University Drive C, tel. 412/688–6000), Delafield Road, Zip 15240–1001; tel. 412/784–3900; John C. Lowe, Acting Director (Total facility includes 316 beds in nursing home–type unit) **A**1 2 3 5 8 9 **F**1 3 4 5 9 10 11 12 13 16 18 19 21 22 23 24 25 26 27 28 30 31 32 33 34 35 36 37 38 39 41 43 44 45 46 47 48 49 50 51 54 55 56 57 59 60 61 62 63 64 65 68 69 70 72 74 76 77 78 79 **P**6 **S** Department of Veterans Affairs, Washington, DC **Web address:** www.pitt.edu	45	49	809	8038	636	356249	0	218285	113180	2328
✶ WESTERN PENNSYLVANIA HOSPITAL, 4800 Friendship Avenue, Zip 15224–1722; tel. 412/578–5000; James M. Collins, President and Chief Executive Officer (Nonreporting) **A**1 2 3 5 6 8 9 10 12 **S** West Penn Allegheny Health System, Pittsburgh, PA **Web address:** www.westpennhospital.org	23	10	462	—	—	—	—	—	—	—
WESTERN PSYCHIATRIC INSTITUTE AND CLINIC See UPMC Presbyterian										
PLEASANT GAP—Centre County										
□ HEALTHSOUTH NITTANY VALLEY REHABILITATION HOSPITAL, 550 West College Avenue, Zip 16823–8808; tel. 814/359–3421; Tom Swavely, Administrator and Chief Executive Officer **A**1 10 **F**13 22 24 39 45 49 53 54 70 71 72 76 **S** HEALTHSOUTH Corporation, Birmingham, AL	33	46	87	1167	53	34150	—	12428	6679	213
POTTSTOWN—Montgomery County										
✶ POTTSTOWN MEMORIAL MEDICAL CENTER, 1600 East High Street, Zip 19464–5008; tel. 610/327–7000; John J. Buckley, President and Chief Executive Officer (Total facility includes 21 beds in nursing home–type unit) **A**1 2 9 10 **F**7 8 9 11 13 17 18 19 22 23 24 25 27 28 29 30 31 32 33 34 36 38 39 40 41 43 44 45 46 48 49 51 54 57 59 61 62 65 68 69 70 71 72 73 76 78 79 **P**6 **Web address:** www.pmmctr.org	23	10	222	9334	118	142691	863	74215	33547	901
POTTSVILLE—Schuylkill County										
✶ GOOD SAMARITAN REGIONAL MEDICAL CENTER, 700 East Norwegian Street, Zip 17901–2798; tel. 570/621–4000; Gino J. Pazzaglini, President and Chief Executive Officer **A**1 2 5 9 10 **F**3 4 7 8 9 12 13 16 17 18 22 25 30 32 34 35 36 37 38 39 40 41 43 44 45 46 48 49 50 51 65 70 72 76 78 79 **P**6 **S** Ascension Health, Saint Louis, MO **Web address:** www.goodsamrmc.com	21	10	153	7389	112	61874	283	50204	24818	690

Many Facility Codes have changed. Please refer to the AHA Guide Code Chart.

© 2000 AHA Guide

Hospitals, U.S. / PENNSYLVANIA

Hospital, Address, Telephone, Administrator, Approval, Facility, and Physician Codes, Health Care System, Network	Classification Codes		Utilization Data					Expense (thousands) of dollars		
★ American Hospital Association (AHA) membership □ Joint Commission on Accreditation of Healthcare Organizations (JCAHO) accreditation + American Osteopathic Healthcare Association (AOHA) membership ○ American Osteopathic Association (AOA) accreditation △ Commission on Accreditation of Rehabilitation Facilities (CARF) accreditation Control codes 61, 63, 64, 71, 72 and 73 indicate hospitals listed by AOHA, but not registered by AHA. For definition of numerical codes, see page A4	Control	Service	Staffed Beds	Admissions	Census	Outpatient Visits	Births	Total	Payroll	Personnel
★ △ POTTSVILLE HOSPITAL AND WARNE CLINIC, 420 South Jackson Street, Zip 17901–3692; tel. 570/621–5000; Donald R. Gintzig, President and Chief Executive Officer **A**1 2 6 7 9 10 **F**7 8 9 13 14 16 17 18 19 22 23 24 25 27 30 31 32 34 35 36 37 38 39 41 43 44 45 46 48 49 50 53 54 57 58 60 61 62 63 64 65 70 71 74 76 78 79 **P**8 **S** Quorum Health Group, Brentwood, TN Web address: www.pottsville.com/hospital	23	10	197	6431	118	84051	694	48221	21909	651
PUNXSUTAWNEY—Jefferson County										
□ PUNXSUTAWNEY AREA HOSPITAL, 81 Hillcrest Drive, Zip 15767–2616; tel. 814/938–1881; Daniel D. Blough, Jr, Chief Executive Officer **A**1 9 10 **F**8 9 16 17 18 22 23 24 25 34 35 36 38 41 43 44 45 46 48 49 54 64 70 76 **P**6 Web address: www.pah.org	23	10	51	2286	25	94644	211	19102	7501	277
QUAKERTOWN—Bucks County ST. LUKE'S QUAKERTOWN HOSPITAL See St. Luke's Hospital and Health Network, Bethlehem										
READING—Berks County										
□ HEALTHSOUTH READING REHABILITATION HOSPITAL, 1623 Morgantown Road, Zip 19607–9455; tel. 610/796–6000; Tammy L. Ober, Administrator and Chief Executive Officer **A**1 9 10 **F**13 28 29 30 31 32 34 38 43 49 50 53 54 62 63 78 **S** HEALTHSOUTH Corporation, Birmingham, AL Web address: www.healthsouth.com	12	46	76	1359	56	18096	—	10783	8839	254
★ READING HOSPITAL AND MEDICAL CENTER, Sixth Avenue and Spruce Street, Zip 19611–1428, Mailing Address: P.O. Box 16052, Zip 19612–6052; tel. 610/988–8000; Charles Sullivan, President and Chief Executive Officer **A**1 2 3 5 9 10 **F**3 4 7 8 9 11 13 14 16 17 18 19 21 22 23 24 25 27 29 30 32 33 34 35 38 39 41 42 43 44 45 46 47 48 49 50 51 53 54 56 57 58 59 60 61 62 63 64 65 66 67 70 71 72 73 76 77 78 79 **P**8 Web address: www.readinghospital.org	23	10	594	29844	415	636387	2948	238325	107651	2954
★ ST. JOSEPH MEDICAL CENTER, 215 North 12th Street, Zip 19603–0316, Mailing Address: P.O. Box 316, Zip 19603–0316; tel. 610/378–2000; John R. Morahan, President (Total facility includes 24 beds in nursing home–type unit) **A**3 5 9 10 12 **F**1 3 4 7 8 9 11 13 14 16 17 18 19 22 23 24 25 29 34 35 36 38 39 41 42 43 44 45 46 47 48 51 54 56 57 58 59 60 61 62 64 65 67 69 70 71 76 78 79 **P**8 **S** Catholic Health Initiatives, Denver, CO Web address: www.chi–east.org/	21	10	269	11840	164	246601	849	95319	38053	1083
RENOVO—Clinton County										
BUCKTAIL MEDICAL CENTER, 1001 Pine Street, Zip 17764–1618; tel. 570/923–1000; Lennea F. Brown, Administrator (Total facility includes 41 beds in nursing home–type unit) (Nonreporting) **A**9 10	23	10	50	—	—	—	—	—	—	—
RIDGWAY—Elk County										
RIDGWAY HEALTH CENTER, (Formerly Elk County Regional Medical Center), 94 Hospital Street, Zip 15853–0190, Mailing Address: P.O. Box M., Zip 15853–0190; tel. 814/776–6111; Paul A. DeSantis, President and Chief Executive Officer **A**9 **F**7 9 16 17 18 22 25 45 48 56 57 62 70 76 77 78	23	10	18	668	11	—	0	7489	3127	87
RIDLEY PARK—Delaware County TAYLOR HOSPITAL See Crozer–Chester Medical Center, Upland										
ROARING SPRING—Blair County										
★ NASON HOSPITAL, 105 Nason Drive, Zip 16673–1202; tel. 814/224–2141; Garrett W. Hoover, President and Chief Executive Officer (Nonreporting) **A**1 5 9 10	23	10	50	—	—	—	—	—	—	—
SAINT MARYS—Elk County										
★ ELK REGIONAL HEALTH CENTER, (Formerly St. Marys Health Center), 763 Johnsonburg Road, Zip 15857–3417; tel. 814/781–7500; Paul A. DeSantis, President (Total facility includes 138 beds in nursing home–type unit) **A**1 9 10 **F**7 8 9 13 16 17 18 19 22 24 25 27 32 33 34 36 37 39 41 43 44 45 46 48 49 50 51 54 67 69 70 71 76 78 79	23	10	204	3413	162	73945	356	30872	15449	637
SAYRE—Bradford County										
★ ROBERT PACKER HOSPITAL, 1 Guthrie Square, Zip 18840–1698; tel. 570/888–6666; William F. Vanaskie, President and Chief Executive Officer (Total facility includes 14 beds in nursing home–type unit) **A**1 2 3 5 9 10 **F**1 4 6 7 8 9 11 13 14 16 17 18 19 21 22 24 25 26 27 31 32 33 34 35 36 37 39 40 41 44 45 46 47 48 51 53 57 61 64 65 68 69 70 71 72 75 76 77 78 79 **S** Guthrie Healthcare System, Sayre, PA Web address: www.guthrie.org	23	10	252	10900	149	122012	735	112494	37472	1353
SCRANTON—Lackawanna County										
★ △ ALLIED SERVICES REHABILITATION HOSPITAL, 475 Morgan Highway, Zip 18501–1130; tel. 570/348–1300; William J. Schoen, Vice President (Nonreporting) **A**1 7 9 10 Web address: www.allied–services.org	23	46	98	—	—	—	—	—	—	—
★ COMMUNITY MEDICAL CENTER, 1800 Mulberry Street, Zip 18510; tel. 570/969–8000; C. Richard Hartman, M.D., President and Chief Executive Officer (Total facility includes 20 beds in nursing home–type unit) **A**1 3 9 10 **F**1 4 7 8 9 11 12 13 14 16 17 18 19 21 22 24 25 26 27 29 30 31 32 33 34 35 37 38 39 41 42 44 45 46 47 48 50 51 54 55 57 58 59 60 61 62 63 64 65 66 69 70 72 73 75 76 77 78 79 **P**5 8 Web address: www.cmchealthsys.com	23	10	278	13486	210	110125	1530	107211	44115	1525
□ MERCY HOSPITAL OF SCRANTON, 746 Jefferson Avenue, Zip 18501–1624; tel. 570/348–7100; Susan Petula, President (Total facility includes 22 beds in nursing home–type unit) **A**1 2 3 5 9 10 **F**4 7 8 9 11 12 13 14 16 17 18 19 22 24 25 29 30 34 37 38 41 43 44 45 46 47 48 49 50 51 54 56 65 69 70 76 77 78 79 **P**8 **S** Catholic Healthcare Partners, Cincinnati, OH Web address: www.mhs–nepa.com	21	10	265	11741	190	227430	981	100550	40893	1311

© 2000 AHA Guide *Many Facility Codes have changed. Please refer to the AHA Guide Code Chart.*

Hospitals, U.S. / PENNSYLVANIA

Hospital, Address, Telephone, Administrator, Approval, Facility, and Physician Codes, Health Care System, Network	Classification Codes		Utilization Data					Expense (thousands) of dollars		
★ American Hospital Association (AHA) membership □ Joint Commission on Accreditation of Healthcare Organizations (JCAHO) accreditation + American Osteopathic Healthcare Association (AOHA) membership ○ American Osteopathic Association (AOA) accreditation △ Commission on Accreditation of Rehabilitation Facilities (CARF) accreditation Control codes 61, 63, 64, 71, 72 and 73 indicate hospitals listed by AOHA, but not registered by AHA. For definition of numerical codes, see page A4	Control	Service	Staffed Beds	Admissions	Census	Outpatient Visits	Births	Total	Payroll	Personnel
★ MOSES TAYLOR HOSPITAL, 700 Quincy Avenue, Zip 18510–1724; tel. 570/340–2100; Harold E. Anderson, Chief Executive Officer (Total facility includes 32 beds in nursing home–type unit) **A**1 3 5 9 10 **F**7 9 13 16 17 18 22 24 25 27 30 33 36 38 39 41 45 46 48 49 50 51 54 57 62 64 69 70 76 78 79 **P**1 6 7 Web address: www.mth.org	23	10	176	6995	131	103424	0	67873	25230	792
SELLERSVILLE—Bucks County										
★ △ GRAND VIEW HOSPITAL, 700 Lawn Avenue, Zip 18960–1576; tel. 215/453–4000; Stuart H. Fine, Chief Executive Officer (Total facility includes 20 beds in nursing home–type unit) **A**1 2 7 9 10 **F**2 3 7 8 9 12 13 14 17 18 19 20 22 24 25 26 27 28 30 32 33 34 35 36 37 38 40 41 44 45 46 48 49 50 51 54 57 58 59 61 62 63 64 65 68 69 70 71 72 76 78 79 **P**1 Web address: www.gvh.org	23	10	194	9123	113	199434	1176	71913	32807	1141
SEWICKLEY—Allegheny County										
□ △ HEALTHSOUTH REHABILITATION HOSPITAL, (Formerly D. T. Watson Rehabilitation Hospital), 303 Camp Meeting Road, Zip 15143–8348; tel. 412/741–9500; Kenneth J. Anthony, President and Chief Executive Officer **A**1 7 9 10 **F**13 18 22 45 53 54 71 72 78 **S** HEALTHSOUTH Corporation, Birmingham, AL Web address: www.healthsouth.com	33	46	25	50	16	1141	—	1108	576	105
★ VALLEY MEDICAL FACILITIES, (Includes Sewickley Valley Hospital, 720 Blackburn Road, Zip 15143–1459; tel. 412/741–6600; The Medical Center, Beaver, 1000 Dutch Ridge Road, Beaver, Zip 15009–9727; tel. 724/728–7000), 720 Blackburn Road, Zip 15143–1498; tel. 412/741–6600; James C. Cooper, Chief Operating Officer (Total facility includes 18 beds in nursing home–type unit) **A**1 2 5 6 9 10 **F**4 7 8 9 11 13 17 18 22 23 24 25 30 32 33 34 35 36 38 41 44 45 46 47 48 51 53 54 57 58 59 60 61 62 63 64 65 70 72 76 78 79 **P**1 6	23	10	186	9830	114	209833	748	86261	39552	1052
SHARON—Mercer County										
★ △ SHARON REGIONAL HEALTH SYSTEM, 740 East State Street, Zip 16146–3395; tel. 724/983–3911; Wayne W. Johnston, President and Chief Executive Officer (Total facility includes 38 beds in nursing home–type unit) **A**1 2 6 7 9 10 **F**3 7 8 9 11 12 13 14 17 18 19 22 24 25 27 28 29 30 32 33 34 36 37 38 39 41 43 44 45 46 48 49 50 53 54 56 57 58 59 60 61 62 63 64 65 68 69 70 71 72 75 76 77 78 79 **P**6 7 8 Web address: www.sharonregional.com	23	10	232	9763	162	—	630	83870	40005	1381
SHICKSHINNY—Luzerne County										
CLEAR BROOK LODGE, Bethel Road, Zip 18655, Mailing Address: Rural Delivery 2, Box 2166, Zip 18655; tel. 570/864–3116; Dave Lombard, President and Chief Executive Officer (Nonreporting)	23	82	65	—	—	—	—	—	—	—
SOMERSET—Somerset County										
★ SOMERSET HOSPITAL CENTER FOR HEALTH, 225 South Center Avenue, Zip 15501–2088; tel. 814/443–5000; Michael J. Farrell, Chief Executive Officer (Total facility includes 15 beds in nursing home–type unit) **A**1 2 9 10 **F**1 3 7 8 9 11 13 14 16 17 18 19 21 22 24 25 27 30 32 33 34 35 36 37 38 39 41 43 44 45 46 48 49 51 54 57 58 59 60 61 62 63 64 69 70 71 72 76 77 78 79 **P**6 Web address: www.somersethospital.com	23	10	130	4913	76	123539	537	36344	14923	526
SPRINGFIELD—Delaware County										
SPRINGFIELD HOSPITAL See Crozer–Chester Medical Center, Upland										
STATE COLLEGE—Centre County										
★ CENTRE COMMUNITY HOSPITAL, 1800 East Park Avenue, Zip 16803–6797; tel. 814/231–7000; Lance H. Rose, FACHE, President and Chief Executive Officer (Total facility includes 16 beds in nursing home–type unit) **A**1 2 9 10 **F**7 8 9 12 16 17 18 19 22 24 25 32 34 35 36 37 38 39 41 43 44 45 46 48 51 54 57 59 61 62 65 66 68 69 70 75 76 78 Web address: www.cch1.org	23	10	186	8259	105	132960	1146	57802	26603	692
SUNBURY—Northumberland County										
★ SUNBURY COMMUNITY HOSPITAL, 350 North Eleventh Street, Zip 17801–0737; tel. 570/286–3333; Nicholas A. Prisco, Chief Executive Officer (Total facility includes 29 beds in nursing home–type unit) (Nonreporting) **A**1 9 10 Web address: www.sunburyhospital.com	23	10	101	—	—	—	—	—	—	—
SUSQUEHANNA—Susquehanna County										
BARNES–KASSON COUNTY HOSPITAL, 400 Turnpike Street, Zip 18847–1638; tel. 570/853–3135; Sara C. Iveson, Executive Director (Total facility includes 58 beds in nursing home–type unit) **A**9 10 **F**7 8 9 13 14 18 19 22 23 25 31 34 36 38 39 40 41 44 45 46 48 49 54 56 68 69 70 73 76 78 Web address: www.barnes–kasson.org	23	10	107	1724	78	24110	113	12956	6053	247
TITUSVILLE—Crawford County										
★ TITUSVILLE AREA HOSPITAL, 406 West Oak Street, Zip 16354–1404; tel. 814/827–1851; Anthony J. Nasralla, FACHE, President and Chief Executive Officer **A**9 10 **F**7 9 16 22 25 27 32 34 36 39 40 41 44 45 46 48 49 50 53 54 76 Web address: www.titusvillehospital.org	23	10	60	2988	32	70315	330	21015	8475	259
TORRANCE—Westmoreland County										
□ TORRANCE STATE HOSPITAL, Torrance Road, Zip 15779–0111, Mailing Address: P.O. Box 111, Zip 15779–0111; tel. 724/459–8000; Richard A. Stillwagon, Superintendent **A**1 10 **F**9 12 16 17 18 23 25 31 41 57 62 70 78	12	22	335	159	321	—	—	35192	21056	551

Hospitals, U.S. / PENNSYLVANIA

Hospital, Address, Telephone, Administrator, Approval, Facility, and Physician Codes, Health Care System, Network ★ American Hospital Association (AHA) membership □ Joint Commission on Accreditation of Healthcare Organizations (JCAHO) accreditation + American Osteopathic Healthcare Association (AOHA) membership ○ American Osteopathic Association (AOA) accreditation △ Commission on Accreditation of Rehabilitation Facilities (CARF) accreditation Control codes 61, 63, 64, 71, 72 and 73 indicate hospitals listed by AOHA, but not registered by AHA. For definition of numerical codes, see page A4	Classification Codes		Utilization Data					Expense (thousands) of dollars		
	Control	Service	Staffed Beds	Admissions	Census	Outpatient Visits	Births	Total	Payroll	Personnel
TOWANDA—Bradford County ✠ MEMORIAL HOSPITAL, One Hospital Drive, Zip 18848–9702; tel. 570/265–2191; Gary A. Baker, President (Total facility includes 44 beds in nursing home–type unit) **A**1 9 10 **F**7 8 9 12 13 17 19 22 24 25 32 34 36 37 39 41 43 44 45 48 51 54 69 70 75 76 78 **S** Quorum Health Group, Brentwood, TN Web address: www.memorialhospital.org	23	10	93	2443	68	31759	287	19288	8802	283
TROY—Bradford County ★ ○ TROY COMMUNITY HOSPITAL, 100 John Street, Zip 16947–0036; tel. 570/297–2121; Mark Webster, President **A**9 10 11 **F**1 4 6 7 8 9 11 12 13 16 17 19 20 22 23 24 25 26 27 28 30 31 32 33 34 35 36 37 39 41 44 45 46 47 48 49 50 51 52 54 55 57 59 60 63 65 66 68 69 70 71 72 75 76 78 79 **S** Guthrie Healthcare System, Sayre, PA Web address: www.guthrie.org	23	10	32	520	22	16093	1	9356	4243	92
TUNKHANNOCK—Wyoming County ✠ TYLER MEMORIAL HOSPITAL, 880 State Road 6 West, Zip 18657–6149; tel. 570/836–2161; William M. Milligan, Jr, President and Chief Executive Officer **A**1 2 9 10 **F**7 8 9 13 16 17 18 19 22 24 25 28 34 36 37 39 41 43 44 45 46 48 50 51 54 69 70 76 78 79	23	10	60	2333	23	43946	272	16003	6768	248
TYRONE—Blair County ✠ TYRONE HOSPITAL, One Hospital Drive, Zip 16686–1810; tel. 814/684–1255; Thomas G. Bartlett, II, Chief Executive Officer (Nonreporting) **A**1 9 10 **S** Quorum Health Group, Brentwood, TN	23	10	59	—	—	—	—	—	—	—
UNION CITY—Erie County ✠ UNION CITY MEMORIAL HOSPITAL, 130 North Main Street, Zip 16438–1094, Mailing Address: P.O. Box 111, Zip 16438–0111; tel. 814/438–1000; Thomas McLoughlin, President and Chief Executive Officer **A**1 9 10 **F**9 13 14 16 17 18 20 21 22 23 25 29 32 33 34 36 37 38 41 43 45 48 50 51 54 70 72 76 78 **P**3 7 Web address: www.svhs.org	23	10	23	680	11	19266	0	5128	2462	83
UNIONTOWN—Fayette County ✠ UNIONTOWN HOSPITAL, 500 West Berkeley Street, Zip 15401–5596; tel. 724/430–5000; Paul Bacharach, President and Chief Executive Officer (Total facility includes 19 beds in nursing home–type unit) **A**1 2 9 10 **F**7 8 9 11 16 17 18 22 24 25 27 34 36 37 38 39 41 43 44 46 48 53 54 68 69 70 76 77 78	23	10	206	9745	139	161742	924	64006	26949	876
UPLAND—Delaware County ✠ ○ △ CROZER–CHESTER MEDICAL CENTER, (Includes Springfield Hospital, 190 West Sproul Road, Springfield, Zip 19064–2097; tel. 610/328–8700; Gwendolyn A. Smith, R.N., Vice President; Taylor Hospital, 175 East Chester Pike, Ridley Park, Zip 19078–2212; tel. 610/595–6000; Diane C. Miller, President and Chief Operating Officer), One Medical Center Boulevard, Zip 19013–3995; tel. 610/447–2000; Joan K. Richards, President **A**1 2 3 5 7 8 9 10 11 12 13 **F**1 3 4 5 7 8 9 10 11 12 13 14 16 17 18 19 20 21 22 24 25 26 27 28 29 30 32 33 34 35 36 37 38 39 40 41 42 43 44 45 46 47 48 49 50 51 53 54 56 57 58 59 60 61 62 63 64 65 66 69 70 71 72 73 75 76 78 79 **P**5 6 **S** Crozer–Keystone Health System, Springfield, PA	23	10	574	26767	419	329205	2139	306024	124832	3510
WARMINSTER—Bucks County ✠ WARMINSTER HOSPITAL, 225 Newtown Road, Zip 18974–5221; tel. 215/441–6600; Jeffrey Yarmel, Chief Executive Officer (Nonreporting) **A**1 3 5 9 10 **S** TENET Healthcare Corporation, Santa Barbara, CA Web address: www.warminsterhospital.com	23	10	132	—	—	—	—	—	—	—
WARREN—Warren County WARREN GENERAL HOSPITAL, 2 Crescent Park West, Zip 16365–2111, Mailing Address: P.O. Box 68, Zip 16365–2111; tel. 814/723–4973; Alton M. Schadt, Executive Director (Total facility includes 16 beds in nursing home–type unit) **A**9 10 **F**3 7 8 9 16 22 23 24 25 26 27 31 34 36 37 38 39 41 44 45 46 48 51 54 56 57 58 59 60 61 62 63 64 65 68 69 70 71 76 78 Web address: www.wgh.org WARREN STATE HOSPITAL See North Warren	23	10	105	3777	57	80287	351	33866	15428	467
WASHINGTON—Washington County ✠ WASHINGTON HOSPITAL, 155 Wilson Avenue, Zip 15301–3398; tel. 724/225–7000; Telford W. Thomas, President and Chief Executive Officer (Total facility includes 17 beds in nursing home–type unit) **A**1 2 3 5 6 9 10 **F**4 7 8 9 11 12 13 14 16 17 18 19 22 23 24 25 26 29 30 32 34 36 37 38 39 41 43 44 45 46 47 48 49 50 54 56 57 59 60 61 62 64 65 66 68 69 70 71 72 73 76 78 79 **P**1 7 Web address: www.washingtonhospital.org	23	10	237	13428	180	—	1104	131239	62061	1596
WAYNESBORO—Franklin County ✠ WAYNESBORO HOSPITAL, 501 East Main Street, Zip 17268–2394; tel. 717/765–4000; Rita C. Brizzee, Chief Operating Officer **A**1 5 9 10 **F**7 8 9 13 17 18 19 22 24 25 32 33 34 38 43 45 46 48 49 50 51 61 70 72 76 78 79 **P**8 **S** Summit Health, Chambersburg, PA Web address: www.summithealth.org	23	10	62	3029	34	60021	477	27662	14217	339
WAYNESBURG—Greene County ✠ GREENE COUNTY MEMORIAL HOSPITAL, Seventh Street and Bonar Avenue, Zip 15370–1697; tel. 724/627–3101; Raoul Walsh, Chief Executive Officer (Total facility includes 20 beds in nursing home–type unit) **A**1 9 10 **F**7 14 16 17 18 22 24 25 26 27 30 32 34 35 36 38 39 41 45 46 48 50 51 54 57 60 62 69 70 72 76 78 79 **P**1 **S** Quorum Health Group, Brentwood, TN	23	10	65	2883	46	41115	0	24754	9181	295

Hospitals, U.S. / PENNSYLVANIA

Hospital, Address, Telephone, Administrator, Approval, Facility, and Physician Codes, Health Care System, Network	Classification Codes		Utilization Data					Expense (thousands) of dollars		Personnel
★ American Hospital Association (AHA) membership □ Joint Commission on Accreditation of Healthcare Organizations (JCAHO) accreditation + American Osteopathic Healthcare Association (AOHA) membership ○ American Osteopathic Association (AOA) accreditation △ Commission on Accreditation of Rehabilitation Facilities (CARF) accreditation Control codes 61, 63, 64, 71, 72 and 73 indicate hospitals listed by AOHA, but not registered by AHA. For definition of numerical codes, see page A4	Control	Service	Staffed Beds	Admissions	Census	Outpatient Visits	Births	Total	Payroll	
WELLSBORO—Tioga County ★ SOLDIERS AND SAILORS MEMORIAL HOSPITAL, 32–36 Central Avenue, Zip 16901–1899; tel. 570/724–1631; Jan E. Fisher, R.N., Executive Director **A**1 9 10 **F**1 2 3 5 6 7 8 9 12 13 14 15 16 17 18 19 22 24 25 28 29 30 32 33 34 35 36 37 38 39 40 41 43 44 45 48 50 51 54 56 57 58 59 60 61 62 63 64 66 68 70 71 72 76 78 **P**4 5 7 **Web address:** www.laurelhs.org/Service%20Sites/Service%20Sites.htm	23	10	83	3479	40	74150	253	23200	10294	394
WERNERSVILLE—Berks County □ WERNERSVILLE STATE HOSPITAL, Route 422, Zip 19565–0300, Mailing Address: P.O. Box 300, Zip 19565–0300; tel. 610/670–4111; Kenneth W. Ehrhart, Superintendent **A**1 10 **F**4 9 11 22 23 24 28 35 39 43 46 47 48 50 51 54 57 59 65 70 76 78 **Web address:** www.geocities.com/Heartland/Valley/8638/	12	22	320	151	249	0	0	—	—	513
WEST CHESTER—Chester County ★ CHESTER COUNTY HOSPITAL, 701 East Marshall Street, Zip 19380–4412; tel. 610/431–5000; H. L. Perry Pepper, President (Total facility includes 20 beds in nursing home–type unit) **A**1 2 6 9 10 **F**8 9 11 12 13 16 17 18 19 22 24 25 28 30 32 33 34 36 37 38 39 40 41 42 43 44 45 46 48 49 50 51 52 54 65 68 69 70 71 72 76 78 79 **P**4 6 7 8 **Web address:** www.med.upenn.edu/health/ms.html	23	10	215	11294	135	335874	2083	86777	40566	1183
WEST GROVE—Chester County □ SOUTHERN CHESTER COUNTY MEDICAL CENTER, 1015 West Baltimore Pike, Zip 19390–9499; tel. 610/869–1000; Scott K. Phillips, President and Chief Executive Officer (Total facility includes 25 beds in nursing home–type unit) **A**1 9 10 **F**3 8 9 13 16 17 19 22 24 25 34 35 36 37 38 39 41 43 44 45 46 48 54 56 58 59 60 61 62 63 70 72 76 78 79 **Web address:** www.sccmc.com	23	10	56	2685	37	76127	0	29355	11910	474
WILKES–BARRE—Luzerne County CLEAR BROOK MANOR, Road 10 East Northampton Street, Zip 18702; tel. 570/823–1171; Donald Noll, Director (Nonreporting)	23	82	50	—	—	—	—	—	—	—
□ FIRST HOSPITAL WYOMING VALLEY, 149 Dana Street, Zip 18702–4825; tel. 570/829–7900; John Malia, Director (Nonreporting) **A**1 10	33	22	96	—	—	—	—	—	—	—
★ △ JOHN HEINZ INSTITUTE OF REHABILITATION MEDICINE, 150 Mundy Street, Zip 18702–6830; tel. 570/826–3800; Thomas E. Pugh, Vice President Rehabilitation Services **A**1 7 9 10 **F**7 13 16 17 18 19 22 24 31 32 38 39 43 45 50 51 53 54 70 72 76 78 **Web address:** www.alliedservices.org	23	46	112	2096	96	98832	—	31590	14861	445
□ MERCY HOSPITAL OF WILKES–BARRE, 25 Church Street, Zip 18765–0999, Mailing Address: P.O. Box 658, Zip 18765–0658; tel. 570/826–3100; V. Gail Blaum, President (Total facility includes 20 beds in nursing home–type unit) **A**1 9 10 **F**4 7 8 9 11 12 13 16 17 18 19 21 22 24 25 26 27 33 34 36 37 38 39 41 43 44 45 46 47 48 49 50 51 54 57 58 61 65 69 70 71 72 73 76 78 **P**1 2 3 4 5 6 7 8 **S** Catholic Healthcare Partners, Cincinnati, OH **Web address:** www.mhs-nepa.com	21	10	215	9091	142	103239	427	68923	27765	731
★ PENN STATE GEISINGER WYOMING VALLEY MEDICAL CENTER, 1000 East Mountain Drive, Zip 18711–0027; tel. 570/826–7300; Conrad W. Schintz, Senior Vice–President Operations **A**1 2 9 10 **F**3 7 8 9 13 16 17 18 22 24 25 30 32 33 38 39 43 45 46 48 50 51 54 56 59 61 65 68 70 72 75 78 **P**3 6 8 **S** Geisinger Health System, Danville, PA **Web address:** www.psghs.edu	23	10	132	5369	73	192453	516	34314	16351	672
★ VETERANS AFFAIRS MEDICAL CENTER, 1111 East End Boulevard, Zip 18711–0026; tel. 570/824–3521; Reedes Hurt, Chief Executive Officer (Total facility includes 180 beds in nursing home–type unit) (Nonreporting) **A**1 2 3 5 9 **S** Department of Veterans Affairs, Washington, DC **Web address:** www.va.gov/stations97/guide/home.asp?DIVISION=ALL WILKES–BARRE GENERAL HOSPITAL See Wyoming Valley Health Care System	45	10	339	—	—	—	—	—	—	—
★ WYOMING VALLEY HEALTH CARE SYSTEM, (Includes Nesbitt Memorial Hospital, 562 Wyoming Avenue, Kingston, Zip 18704–3784; tel. 717/283–7000; Wilkes–Barre General Hospital, 575 North River Street, Zip 18764), 575 North River Street, Zip 18764–0001; tel. 570/829–8111; Patricia Finan, President and Chief Executive Officer (Total facility includes 26 beds in nursing home–type unit) **A**1 5 9 10 **F**3 4 6 7 8 9 11 12 13 16 17 18 19 21 22 23 24 25 27 28 29 31 32 33 34 36 37 38 39 41 43 44 45 46 47 48 50 51 54 57 58 59 60 61 62 63 64 65 68 69 70 71 72 73 76 77 78 79 **P**1 **Web address:** www.wvhc.org	23	10	435	19797	293	434465	1803	217812	81390	2384
WILLIAMSBURG—Blair County ★ COVE FORGE BEHAVIORAL HEALTH SYSTEM, (Formerly Charter Behavioral Health System), New Beginnings Road, P.O. Box B, Zip 16693; tel. 814/832–2121; Mark Sarneso, Chief Executive Officer (Nonreporting) **Web address:** www.charterbehavioral.com	33	82	100	—	—	—	—	—	—	—

Hospitals, U.S. / PENNSYLVANIA

Hospital, Address, Telephone, Administrator, Approval, Facility, and Physician Codes, Health Care System, Network	Classi-fication Codes		Utilization Data					Expense (thousands) of dollars		
★ American Hospital Association (AHA) membership ☐ Joint Commission on Accreditation of Healthcare Organizations (JCAHO) accreditation + American Osteopathic Healthcare Association (AOHA) membership ○ American Osteopathic Association (AOA) accreditation △ Commission on Accreditation of Rehabilitation Facilities (CARF) accreditation Control codes 61, 63, 64, 71, 72 and 73 indicate hospitals listed by AOHA, but not registered by AHA. For definition of numerical codes, see page A4	Control	Service	Staffed Beds	Admissions	Census	Outpatient Visits	Births	Total	Payroll	Personnel

WILLIAMSPORT—Lycoming County

✦ △ SUSQUEHANNA HEALTH SYSTEM, (Includes Divine Providence Hospital, 1100 Grampian Boulevard, Zip 17701–1995; tel. 570/320–7000; Muncy Valley Hospital, 215 East Water Street, Muncy, Zip 17756–8700; tel. 570/546–8282; Williamsport Hospital and Medical Center, 777 Rural Avenue, Zip 17701–3198; tel. 570/321–1000; Steven P. Johnson, Senior Vice President and Chief Operating Officer), 1001 Grampian Boulevard, Zip 17701–1946; tel. 570/320–7000; Donald R. Creamer, President and Chief Executive Officer (Total facility includes 139 beds in nursing home–type unit) **A**1 2 3 5 6 7 9 10 **F**1 4 5 6 7 8 9 11 12 13 14 16 17 18 19 22 23 24 25 27 28 29 30 31 32 33 34 35 36 37 38 39 41 43 44 45 46 47 48 49 50 51 53 54 56 57 58 59 60 61 62 63 64 65 66 68 69 70 71 72 73 76 77 78 79 **P**3 7 8
Web address: www.shscares.org | 23 | 10 | 424 | 13754 | 294 | 488197 | 1377 | 145532 | 59555 | 2060 |

WINDBER—Somerset County

✦ WINDBER MEDICAL CENTER, (Formerly Windber Hospital), 600 Somerset Avenue, Zip 15963–1331; tel. 814/467–6611; Nicholas Jacobs, Executive Director **A**1 9 10 **F**2 3 4 6 7 8 9 10 11 12 13 14 16 17 18 19 20 21 22 23 24 25 26 27 28 29 30 31 32 33 34 36 37 38 39 40 41 42 43 44 45 46 47 48 49 50 51 52 53 54 57 58 59 60 61 62 63 64 65 66 67 68 69 70 72 73 75 76 77 78 79 **P**7 8
Web address: www.conemaugh.org | 23 | 10 | 67 | 2345 | 25 | 49088 | 146 | 19706 | 7583 | 315 |

WYNNEWOOD—Montgomery County

★ LANKENAU HOSPITAL, 100 Lancaster Avenue West, Zip 19096–3411; tel. 610/645–2000; C. Barry Dykes, Senior Vice President (Total facility includes 22 beds in nursing home–type unit) **A**2 3 5 9 10 **F**1 3 4 5 6 7 8 9 11 12 13 16 17 18 19 20 21 22 23 24 25 27 28 29 30 31 32 33 34 35 36 37 38 39 40 41 42 43 44 45 46 47 48 49 50 51 53 54 56 57 58 59 60 61 62 63 64 65 66 68 69 70 71 72 73 74 76 78 79 **P**1 2 5 6 7 **S** Jefferson Health System, Wayne, PA
Web address: www.jeffersonhealth.org | 23 | 10 | 309 | 15394 | 246 | 133283 | 1525 | 157004 | 63288 | 1699 |

YORK—York County

☐ △ HEALTHSOUTH REHABILITATION HOSPITAL OF YORK, 1850 Normandie Drive, Zip 17404–1534; tel. 717/767–6941; Cheryl Fleming, Chief Executive Officer (Nonreporting) **A**1 7 10 **S** HEALTHSOUTH Corporation, Birmingham, AL | 33 | 48 | 88 | — | — | — | — | — | — | — |

★ + ○ MEMORIAL HOSPITAL, 325 South Belmont Street, Zip 17403–2609, Mailing Address: P.O. Box 15118, Zip 17405–5118; tel. 717/843–8623; Sally J. Dixon, President and Chief Executive Officer **A**9 10 11 12 13 **F**7 8 9 11 13 16 17 18 19 22 24 25 26 27 29 30 32 33 34 35 36 37 38 39 40 41 43 44 45 46 48 49 50 51 54 56 57 58 61 62 63 65 68 70 71 72 76 78 79 **P**6
Web address: www.mhyork.org | 23 | 10 | 119 | 5760 | 67 | 85785 | 501 | 44471 | 21220 | 824 |

✦ YORK HOSPITAL, 1001 South George Street, Zip 17405–3645; tel. 717/851–2345; Brian A. Gragnolati, President **A**1 2 3 5 8 9 10 **F**3 4 7 8 9 11 12 13 14 16 17 18 19 20 22 23 24 25 26 27 29 30 32 33 34 35 36 37 38 39 41 42 43 44 45 46 47 48 49 50 51 54 55 56 57 58 59 60 61 62 63 64 65 66 68 70 71 72 73 75 76 78 79 **P**6 8 **S** South Central Community Health, York, PA
Web address: www.yorkhealth.org | 23 | 10 | 437 | 23835 | 329 | — | 2724 | 248413 | 114721 | 3529 |

RHODE ISLAND

Resident Population 988 (in thousands)
Resident population in metro areas 93.8%
Birth rate per 1,000 population 12.6
65 years and over 15.6%
Percent of persons without health insurance 10.2%

Hospital, Address, Telephone, Administrator, Approval, Facility, and Physician Codes, Health Care System, Network	Classification Codes		Utilization Data					Expense (thousands) of dollars		
	Control	Service	Staffed Beds	Admissions	Census	Outpatient Visits	Births	Total	Payroll	Personnel

★ American Hospital Association (AHA) membership
☐ Joint Commission on Accreditation of Healthcare Organizations (JCAHO) accreditation
+ American Osteopathic Healthcare Association (AOHA) membership
○ American Osteopathic Association (AOA) accreditation
△ Commission on Accreditation of Rehabilitation Facilities (CARF) accreditation
Control codes 61, 63, 64, 71, 72 and 73 indicate hospitals listed by AOHA, but not registered by AHA. For definition of numerical codes, see page A4

CRANSTON—Providence County

☐ ELEANOR SLATER HOSPITAL, (Includes Institute of Mental Health–Rhode Island Medical Center, Howard Avenue, Howard, Zip 02920, Mailing Address: Box 8281, Cranston, Zip 02920–0281; tel. 401/464–2495; Betty A. Fielder, Clinical Administrative Officer; Rhode Island Medical Center, Mailing Address: Box 8269, Zip 02920; tel. 401/464–3085), 111 Howard Avenue, Zip 02920–3001, Mailing Address: P.O. Box 8269, Zip 02920–8269; tel. 401/462–3085; Richard H. Freeman, Chief Executive Officer (Nonreporting) **A**1 9 10 — 12 48 507 — — — — — — — —

EAST PROVIDENCE—Providence County

★ EMMA PENDLETON BRADLEY HOSPITAL, 1011 Veterans Memorial Parkway, Zip 02915–5099; tel. 401/432–1000; Daniel J. Wall, President and Chief Executive Officer **A**1 3 5 9 10 **F**2 4 5 9 10 11 12 13 14 16 17 18 19 21 22 23 24 25 27 28 30 32 33 34 35 36 37 38 39 41 43 45 46 47 48 49 50 52 54 56 57 58 59 60 61 62 63 64 65 68 69 70 71 72 74 75 76 78 79 **P**3 6 8 **S** Lifespan Corporation, Providence, RI
Web address: www.lifespan.org — 23 52 60 858 53 48357 0 27991 16672 484

HOWARD—Providence County

INSTITUTE OF MENTAL HEALTH–RHODE ISLAND MEDICAL CENTER See Eleanor Slater Hospital, Cranston

NEWPORT—Newport County

★ △ NEWPORT HOSPITAL, 11 Friendship Street, Zip 02840–2299; tel. 401/846–6400; Arthur J. Sampson, President and Chief Executive Officer **A**1 2 7 9 10 **F**7 8 9 12 13 14 18 19 22 25 29 30 32 33 34 38 39 40 41 43 44 45 46 48 49 50 51 53 54 56 57 61 62 69 70 72 76 78 **P**3 6 7 **S** Lifespan Corporation, Providence, RI
Web address: www.lifespan.org — 23 10 116 5877 81 108666 708 58064 25711 580

NORTH PROVIDENCE—Providence County

OUR LADY OF FATIMA HOSPITAL See St. Joseph Health Services of Rhode Island
☐ ST. JOSEPH HEALTH SERVICES OF RHODE ISLAND, (Includes Our Lady of Fatima Hospital, 200 High Service Avenue, Zip 02904; St. Joseph Hospital for Specialty Care, 21 Peace Street, Providence, Zip 02907; tel. 401/456–3000), 200 High Service Avenue, Zip 02904–5199; tel. 401/456–3000; H. John Keimig, President and Chief Executive Officer (Total facility includes 20 beds in nursing home–type unit) **A**1 6 9 10 **F**6 7 9 13 18 19 21 22 23 24 25 27 30 31 32 34 38 39 43 45 46 48 51 53 54 56 57 59 61 62 63 64 65 69 70 72 74 76 77 78 79 **P**5
Web address: www.saintjosephri.com — 21 10 281 10747 213 243020 0 111816 59608 1398

PAWTUCKET—Providence County

★ △ MEMORIAL HOSPITAL OF RHODE ISLAND, 111 Brewster Street, Zip 02860–4499; tel. 401/729–2000; Francis R. Dietz, President **A**1 2 3 5 7 8 9 10 **F**1 2 3 4 7 8 9 10 11 12 13 14 16 17 19 22 24 25 26 27 29 30 31 32 34 35 36 37 38 39 40 41 42 43 44 45 46 47 48 49 50 52 53 54 56 57 58 59 61 62 63 64 65 69 70 71 72 74 75 76 77 78 79 **P**1 — 23 10 199 7617 111 140177 738 112336 62445 1194

PROVIDENCE—Providence County

★ BUTLER HOSPITAL, 345 Blackstone Boulevard, Zip 02906–4829; tel. 401/455–6200; Patricia R. Recupero, JD, M.D., President and Chief Executive Officer **A**1 3 5 9 10 **F**2 3 4 7 8 9 11 13 17 19 20 21 22 23 24 25 26 29 30 31 32 33 34 35 36 37 38 39 41 42 43 44 45 46 48 49 50 51 53 54 56 57 58 59 60 61 62 63 64 66 68 70 71 72 73 76 78 79 **P**6 8 **S** Care New England Health System, Providence, RI
Web address: www.butler.org — 23 22 105 4899 97 52580 0 41855 27418 571

★ MIRIAM HOSPITAL, 164 Summit Avenue, Zip 02906–2895; tel. 401/793–2500; Kathleen C. Hittner, M.D., President and Chief Executive Officer **A**1 2 3 5 8 9 10 **F**2 4 5 9 10 11 12 13 14 16 17 18 19 21 22 23 24 25 27 28 29 30 32 33 34 35 36 37 38 39 41 43 45 46 47 48 49 50 52 54 56 57 58 59 60 61 62 63 64 65 68 69 70 71 72 74 75 76 78 79 **P**3 8 **S** Lifespan Corporation, Providence, RI
Web address: www.lifespan.org — 23 10 227 11981 162 54508 0 132059 55215 1231

★ RHODE ISLAND HOSPITAL, 593 Eddy Street, Zip 02903–4900; tel. 401/444–4000; Joseph E. Amaral, M.D., President and Chief Executive Officer **A**1 2 3 5 8 9 10 **F**2 4 5 9 11 12 13 14 16 17 18 19 21 22 23 24 25 27 28 30 32 33 34 35 36 37 38 39 41 43 45 46 47 48 49 50 51 52 53 54 56 57 58 59 60 61 62 63 64 65 68 69 70 71 72 74 75 76 78 79 **P**3 6 8 **S** Lifespan Corporation, Providence, RI
Web address: www.lifespan.org — 23 10 529 29660 451 247618 — 397870 176233 4279

★ ROGER WILLIAMS MEDICAL CENTER, 825 Chalkstone Avenue, Zip 02908–4735; tel. 401/456–2000; Robert A. Urciuoli, President and Chief Executive Officer **A**1 2 3 5 8 9 10 **F**3 6 7 9 11 13 16 17 18 19 22 24 25 27 30 32 33 34 35 36 38 39 41 45 46 48 49 51 54 56 59 63 65 68 69 70 72 74 76 78 **P**3 5 8
Web address: www.rwmc.com — 23 10 146 7954 119 224522 0 90915 42787 1253

ST. JOSEPH HOSPITAL FOR SPECIALTY CARE See St. Joseph Health Services of Rhode Island, North Providence

Hospitals, U.S. / RHODE ISLAND

Hospital, Address, Telephone, Administrator, Approval, Facility, and Physician Codes, Health Care System, Network	Classification Codes		Utilization Data					Expense (thousands) of dollars		
★ American Hospital Association (AHA) membership ☐ Joint Commission on Accreditation of Healthcare Organizations (JCAHO) accreditation + American Osteopathic Healthcare Association (AOHA) membership ○ American Osteopathic Association (AOA) accreditation △ Commission on Accreditation of Rehabilitation Facilities (CARF) accreditation Control codes 61, 63, 64, 71, 72 and 73 indicate hospitals listed by AOHA, but not registered by AHA. For definition of numerical codes, see page A4	Control	Service	Staffed Beds	Admissions	Census	Outpatient Visits	Births	Total	Payroll	Personnel
★ VETERANS AFFAIRS MEDICAL CENTER, 830 Chalkstone Avenue, Zip 02908-4799; tel. 401/457-3042; Louise McMahon, Acting Director **A**1 3 5 9 **F**3 4 9 11 13 16 17 18 19 21 22 23 24 25 27 29 30 31 32 33 34 35 36 37 38 39 41 43 45 46 47 48 49 51 54 55 56 57 59 60 61 63 65 66 68 69 70 72 74 76 77 78 79 **S** Department of Veterans Affairs, Washington, DC **Web address:** www.va.gov/stations97/guide/home.asp?DIVISION=ALL	45	10	66	3003	61	225605	0	73014	34417	768
★ WOMEN AND INFANTS HOSPITAL OF RHODE ISLAND, 101 Dudley Street, Zip 02905-2499; tel. 401/274-1100; Thomas G. Parris, Jr, President **A**1 3 5 8 9 10 **F**2 3 4 5 7 8 9 11 12 13 14 17 18 19 20 21 22 23 24 25 26 27 28 29 30 31 32 33 34 35 36 37 38 39 41 42 43 44 47 48 49 50 51 52 53 54 56 57 58 59 60 61 62 63 64 65 66 68 70 71 72 73 75 76 78 79 **P**6 8 **S** Care New England Health System, Providence, RI **Web address:** www.womenandinfants.com	23	44	197	13591	163	60266	9245	154882	80290	1734
WAKEFIELD—Washington County										
★ SOUTH COUNTY HOSPITAL, 100 Kenyon Avenue, Zip 02879-4299; tel. 401/782-8000; Patrick L. Muldoon, President and Chief Executive Officer **A**1 9 10 **F**1 3 7 8 9 12 13 14 16 17 18 19 21 22 23 24 25 28 29 30 31 32 33 34 35 36 37 38 39 40 41 43 44 45 46 48 49 50 51 54 56 58 59 60 61 62 63 64 68 70 71 72 76 77 78 79 **P**5 7 8 **Web address:** www.schospital.com	23	10	83	5014	59	95556	565	50159	24053	613
WARWICK—Kent County										
★ △ KENT COUNTY MEMORIAL HOSPITAL, 455 Tollgate Road, Zip 02886-2770; tel. 401/737-7000; Robert E. Baute, M.D., President and Chief Executive Officer **A**1 2 7 9 10 **F**2 3 4 7 8 9 11 13 17 18 19 20 21 22 23 24 25 26 29 30 31 32 33 34 35 36 37 38 39 41 42 43 44 45 46 48 49 50 51 53 54 56 57 58 59 60 61 62 63 64 66 68 70 71 72 73 76 78 79 **P**6 8 **S** Care New England Health System, Providence, RI **Web address:** www.kentri.org	23	10	339	13445	199	172814	1152	131911	68436	1395
WESTERLY—Washington County										
★ WESTERLY HOSPITAL, 25 Wells Street, Zip 02891-2934; tel. 401/596-6000; Michael K. Lally, President and Chief Executive Officer **A**1 9 10 **F**1 7 8 9 13 19 22 24 25 30 32 34 35 38 39 40 41 43 44 45 46 48 49 50 51 54 56 59 61 62 68 70 71 72 73 76 77 78 79 **P**8 **Web address:** www.westerlyhospital.com	23	10	125	4354	52	355161	481	47676	21901	413
WOONSOCKET—Providence County										
★ LANDMARK MEDICAL CENTER, (Includes Landmark Medical Center–Fogarty Unit, Eddie Dowling Highway, North Smithfield, Zip 02896; tel. 401/766-0800; Landmark Medical Center–Woonsocket Unit, 115 Cass Avenue, Zip 02895; tel. 401/769-4100), 115 Cass Avenue, Zip 02895-4731; tel. 401/769-4100; Gary J. Gaube, President (Total facility includes 19 beds in nursing home–type unit) **A**1 9 10 **F**7 8 9 12 13 17 18 19 22 24 25 26 27 28 30 32 33 34 39 41 43 44 45 46 48 49 50 53 54 57 58 59 60 61 62 63 68 69 70 72 76 77 78 **P**6 7 8	23	10	158	6923	98	209249	431	74451	33640	683

Hospitals, U.S. / SOUTH CAROLINA

SOUTH CAROLINA

Resident Population 3,836 (in thousands)
Resident population in metro areas 69.6%
Birth rate per 1,000 population 13.9
65 years and over 12.2%
Percent of persons without health insurance 16.8%

Hospital, Address, Telephone, Administrator, Approval, Facility, and Physician Codes, Health Care System, Network	Classification Codes		Utilization Data					Expense (thousands) of dollars		
	Control	Service	Staffed Beds	Admissions	Census	Outpatient Visits	Births	Total	Payroll	Personnel

★ American Hospital Association (AHA) membership
☐ Joint Commission on Accreditation of Healthcare Organizations (JCAHO) accreditation
+ American Osteopathic Healthcare Association (AOHA) membership
○ American Osteopathic Association (AOA) accreditation
△ Commission on Accreditation of Rehabilitation Facilities (CARF) accreditation
Control codes 61, 63, 64, 71, 72 and 73 indicate hospitals listed by AOHA, but not registered by AHA. For definition of numerical codes, see page A4

ABBEVILLE—Abbeville County
★ ABBEVILLE COUNTY MEMORIAL HOSPITAL, 901 West Greenwood Street, Zip 29620-0887, Mailing Address: P.O. Box 887, Zip 29620-0887; tel. 864/459-5011; Alvin Hoover, CHE, Administrator (Total facility includes 18 beds in nursing home–type unit) **A**9 10 **F**8 9 12 13 17 19 22 25 30 31 32 34 36 38 39 41 44 45 48 49 50 51 53 54 61 68 70 74 76 78 79 **P**8 **S** Quorum Health Group, Brentwood, TN | 13 | 10 | 60 | 1386 | 14 | 25019 | 202 | 11203 | 5735 | 180 |

AIKEN—Aiken County
AIKEN REGIONAL MEDICAL CENTERS, (Includes Aurora Pavilion, 655 Medical Park Drive, Zip 29801, Mailing Address: P.O. Box 1073, Zip 29802; tel. 803/641-5900), 302 University Parkway, Zip 29801-2757, Mailing Address: P.O. Box 1117, Zip 29802-1117; tel. 803/641-5000; Richard H. Satcher, Chief Executive Officer **A**1 2 9 10 **F**2 3 4 7 8 9 11 12 13 16 17 18 19 22 24 25 27 29 30 31 32 35 36 38 39 40 41 43 44 45 46 47 48 49 50 51 53 54 57 58 59 60 61 62 63 64 65 68 70 72 73 74 75 76 78 79 **P**8 **S** Universal Health Services, Inc., King of Prussia, PA | 33 | 10 | 269 | 12098 | 150 | 60655 | 1052 | 98885 | 31275 | 770 |

ANDERSON—Anderson County
ANDERSON AREA MEDICAL CENTER, 800 North Fant Street, Zip 29621-5793; tel. 864/261-1000; John A. Miller, Jr, President **A**1 2 3 5 9 10 **F**2 3 7 8 9 11 12 13 14 16 17 18 19 22 24 25 27 28 29 30 31 32 33 34 35 36 38 39 41 42 44 45 46 48 49 50 51 52 53 54 58 59 60 61 62 63 65 66 67 68 70 71 72 74 75 76 78 79 **P**1 | 23 | 10 | 369 | 19216 | 274 | 456473 | 1911 | 183470 | 79422 | 2799 |

BAMBERG—Bamberg County
BAMBERG COUNTY MEMORIAL HOSPITAL AND NURSING CENTER, North and McGee Streets, Zip 29003-0507, Mailing Address: P.O. Box 507, Zip 29003-0507; tel. 803/245-4321; Warren E. Hammett, Administrator (Total facility includes 44 beds in nursing home–type unit) (Nonreporting) **A**1 9 10 | 13 | 10 | 84 | — | | | | | | |

BARNWELL—Barnwell County
BARNWELL COUNTY HOSPITAL, 811 Reynolds Road, Zip 29812; tel. 803/259-1000; J. Larry Dozier, Jr, FACHE, Chief Executive Officer (Total facility includes 12 beds in nursing home–type unit) **A**1 9 10 **F**9 13 17 18 19 22 24 25 30 32 34 35 37 38 41 45 48 50 53 54 70 74 76 78 | 13 | 10 | 45 | 868 | 12 | 24172 | 0 | — | 2658 | 143 |

BEAUFORT—Beaufort County
BEAUFORT MEMORIAL HOSPITAL, 955 Ribaut Road, Zip 29902-5441, Mailing Address: P.O. Box 1068, Zip 29901-1068; tel. 843/522-5200; David E. Brown, President and Chief Executive Officer (Total facility includes 44 beds in nursing home–type unit) **A**1 9 10 **F**7 8 9 16 17 18 19 22 24 25 27 28 32 34 35 36 37 38 39 40 41 44 45 48 50 51 54 59 60 61 62 64 68 70 71 74 76 78 79 | 13 | 10 | 179 | 8828 | 109 | 29258 | 1620 | 59496 | 23133 | 750 |

NAVAL HOSPITAL, 1 Pinckney Boulevard, Zip 29902-6148; tel. 843/525-5301; Captain Gary W. Zuckerman, MSC, USN, Commanding Officer (Nonreporting) **A**1 5 **S** Department of Navy, Washington, DC | 43 | 10 | 20 | — | | | | | | |

BENNETTSVILLE—Marlboro County
☐ MARLBORO PARK HOSPITAL, 1138 Cheraw Highway, Zip 29512-0738, Mailing Address: P.O. Box 738, Zip 29512-0738; tel. 843/479-2881; William M. Donohoo, FACHE, Chief Executive Officer (Total facility includes 7 beds in nursing home–type unit) **A**1 9 10 **F**8 9 12 17 19 22 24 25 27 32 34 35 37 39 41 44 48 50 54 55 60 62 64 68 70 74 76 78 79 **P**2 8 **S** Community Health Systems, Inc., Brentwood, TN | 32 | 10 | 111 | 2361 | 35 | 15575 | 204 | 19770 | 7739 | 201 |

CAMDEN—Kershaw County
KERSHAW COUNTY MEDICAL CENTER, Haile and Roberts Streets, Zip 29020-7003, Mailing Address: P.O. Box 7003, Zip 29020-7003; tel. 803/432-4311; Donnie J. Weeks, President and Chief Executive Officer (Total facility includes 88 beds in nursing home–type unit) **A**1 9 10 **F**1 2 3 4 6 7 8 9 10 11 12 15 16 17 18 19 22 23 24 25 29 30 31 32 33 34 35 36 37 38 39 41 42 43 44 45 46 47 48 49 50 52 53 54 56 58 59 60 61 62 63 64 65 67 68 70 72 73 74 76 78 79 | 13 | 10 | 188 | 4554 | 146 | 81531 | 336 | 41467 | 18115 | 569 |

CHARLESTON—Charleston County
BON SECOURS–ST. FRANCIS XAVIER HOSPITAL, 2095 Henry Tecklenburg Drive, Zip 29414-0001, Mailing Address: P.O. Box 160001, Zip 29414-0001; tel. 843/402-1000; Allen P. Carroll, Chief Executive Officer **A**1 9 10 **F**2 4 8 9 11 12 16 17 18 19 22 24 25 27 28 29 30 31 32 34 35 36 37 38 39 41 42 44 45 47 48 50 51 54 59 60 61 62 63 64 65 66 70 71 74 76 78 79 **S** Carolinas HealthCare System, Charlotte, NC
Web address: www.sfxhospital.com | 23 | 10 | 145 | 7716 | 98 | 74609 | 1241 | 56965 | 23344 | 743 |

△ CHARLESTON MEMORIAL HOSPITAL, 326 Calhoun Street, Zip 29401-1189; tel. 843/953-8300; Thomas F. Moore, Administrator **A**1 3 5 7 9 10 **F**4 9 11 12 17 18 19 22 25 27 35 36 39 41 50 54 59 61 65 70 74 76 78 79 **P**6
Web address: www.musc.edu | 13 | 10 | 113 | 1185 | 46 | 37710 | 0 | 39153 | 11834 | 352 |

A378 Hospitals   *Many Facility Codes have changed. Please refer to the AHA Guide Code Chart.*   © 2000 AHA Guide

Hospitals, U.S. / SOUTH CAROLINA

Hospital, Address, Telephone, Administrator, Approval, Facility, and Physician Codes, Health Care System, Network	Classification Codes		Utilization Data					Expense (thousands) of dollars		
	Control	Service	Staffed Beds	Admissions	Census	Outpatient Visits	Births	Total	Payroll	Personnel

★ American Hospital Association (AHA) membership
☐ Joint Commission on Accreditation of Healthcare Organizations (JCAHO) accreditation
+ American Osteopathic Healthcare Association (AOHA) membership
○ American Osteopathic Association (AOA) accreditation
△ Commission on Accreditation of Rehabilitation Facilities (CARF) accreditation
Control codes 61, 63, 64, 71, 72 and 73 indicate hospitals listed by AOHA, but not registered by AHA. For definition of numerical codes, see page A4

Hospital	Control	Service	Staffed Beds	Admissions	Census	Outpatient Visits	Births	Total	Payroll	Personnel
☐ CHARTER CHARLESTON BEHAVIORAL HEALTH SYSTEM, (Formerly Charter Hospital of Charleston), 2777 Speissegger Drive, Zip 29405–8299; tel. 843/747–5830; Anne Battin, Administrator (Nonreporting) A1 10 S Magellan Health Services, Atlanta, GA	33	22	70	—	—	—	—	—	—	—
★ △ MUSC MEDICAL CENTER OF MEDICAL UNIVERSITY OF SOUTH CAROLINA, 171 Ashley Avenue, Zip 29425; tel. 843/792–2300; Stuart Smith, Vice President Clinical Operations and Executive Director A1 2 3 5 7 8 9 10 F2 3 4 5 6 7 8 9 10 11 12 13 14 16 17 18 19 21 22 23 24 25 27 28 29 30 31 32 33 34 35 36 37 38 39 40 41 42 43 44 45 46 47 48 49 50 51 52 53 54 55 56 57 58 59 60 61 62 63 64 65 66 67 68 70 71 72 73 74 75 76 78 79 Web address: www.musc.edu	12	10	572	26371	449	585435	1912	411825	154038	3672
NAVAL HOSPITAL See North Charleston										
★ RALPH H. JOHNSON VETERANS AFFAIRS MEDICAL CENTER, 109 Bee Street, Zip 29401–5703; tel. 843/577–5011 (Nonreporting) A1 2 3 5 8 S Department of Veterans Affairs, Washington, DC	45	10	161	—	—	—	—	—	—	—
★ ROPER HOSPITAL, 316 Calhoun Street, Zip 29401–1125; tel. 843/724–2000; Matt Severance, Administrator A1 2 6 9 10 F2 3 4 7 8 9 11 12 13 14 16 17 18 19 21 22 24 25 27 28 29 31 32 33 34 35 36 37 38 39 40 41 42 44 45 46 47 48 49 50 51 53 54 55 56 57 58 59 60 61 62 63 64 65 68 70 71 72 74 75 76 78 79 S Carolinas HealthCare System, Charlotte, NC Web address: www.carealliance.com	23	10	375	16896	300	256950	1228	203688	77861	2013
★ ROPER HOSPITAL NORTH, 2750 Speissegger Drive, Zip 29405–8294; tel. 843/745–2800; John C. Hales, Jr FACHE, President and Chief Executive Officer A1 9 10 F2 3 7 9 11 13 14 16 17 18 19 21 22 24 25 27 28 29 31 32 33 34 35 37 38 39 41 42 43 44 45 46 47 48 49 50 51 53 54 56 58 59 60 61 62 63 64 65 68 70 71 72 74 76 78 79 S Carolinas HealthCare System, Charlotte, NC Web address: www.carealliance.com	23	10	104	1482	20	55742	—	22049	8828	226
★ TRIDENT MEDICAL CENTER, 9330 Medical Plaza Drive, Zip 29406–9195; tel. 843/797–7000; Michael P. Joyce, President and Chief Executive Officer (Total facility includes 25 beds in nursing home–type unit) A1 2 9 10 F2 4 5 8 9 10 11 12 13 18 19 22 23 24 25 26 27 28 29 30 31 32 33 34 35 36 37 38 39 41 42 43 44 45 46 47 48 49 50 51 52 53 54 58 59 60 61 62 63 64 65 68 69 70 71 72 74 75 76 78 79 P7 S HCA – The Healthcare Company, Nashville, TN Web address: www.tridenthealthsystem.com	33	10	305	14695	196	162559	2089	—	—	951

CHERAW—Chesterfield County

Hospital	Control	Service	Staffed Beds	Admissions	Census	Outpatient Visits	Births	Total	Payroll	Personnel
☐ CHESTERFIELD GENERAL HOSPITAL, Highway 9 West, Zip 29520, Mailing Address: P.O. Box 151, Zip 29520-0151; tel. 843/537–7881; Chris Wolf, Chief Executive Officer A1 9 10 F6 7 8 9 12 14 17 18 19 22 24 25 27 30 31 32 34 35 36 37 38 39 41 42 43 44 45 48 50 51 52 53 54 56 68 70 74 76 78 S Community Health Systems, Inc., Brentwood, TN Web address: www.chs.net/chesterfield.html	33	10	58	2195	20	65495	262	20059	7902	256

CHESTER—Chester County

Hospital	Control	Service	Staffed Beds	Admissions	Census	Outpatient Visits	Births	Total	Payroll	Personnel
★ CHESTER COUNTY HOSPITAL AND NURSING CENTER, 1 Medical Park Drive, Zip 29706–9799; tel. 803/581–9400; William H. Bundy, Chief Executive Officer (Total facility includes 100 beds in nursing home–type unit) A1 9 10 F4 8 9 11 12 17 18 19 21 22 24 25 30 31 32 34 35 36 37 38 39 40 41 42 43 44 45 46 47 48 50 51 54 55 58 65 67 68 70 72 73 74 76 78 79	13	10	154	3340	134	17559	226	24212	10473	356

CLINTON—Laurens County

Hospital	Control	Service	Staffed Beds	Admissions	Census	Outpatient Visits	Births	Total	Payroll	Personnel
★ LAURENS COUNTY HEALTHCARE SYSTEM, (Includes Laurens County Hospital, Mailing Address: P.O. Box 976, Zip 29325; tel. 803/833–9100), Highway 76 West, Zip 29325, Mailing Address: P.O. Box 976, Zip 29325–0976; tel. 864/833–9100; Michael A. Kozar, Chief Executive Officer A1 9 10 F7 8 9 12 13 14 16 17 18 19 22 24 25 27 32 34 35 36 37 38 39 41 43 44 45 48 49 50 51 54 60 61 62 64 70 72 74 76 79 P8 S Quorum Health Group, Brentwood, TN Web address: www.lchcs.org	16	10	85	3724	52	69802	419	28706	11796	398
WHITTEN CENTER INFIRMARY, Whitten Center, Zip 29325, Mailing Address: Drawer 239, Zip 29325; tel. 864/833–2733; George Dellaportas, M.D., Director Professional Services F24 45 54 58 59 69	12	62	22	209	12	0	0	—	—	37

COLUMBIA—Richland County

Hospital	Control	Service	Staffed Beds	Admissions	Census	Outpatient Visits	Births	Total	Payroll	Personnel
★ △ HEALTHSOUTH REHABILITATION HOSPITAL, 2935 Colonial Drive, Zip 29203–6811; tel. 803/254–7777; Debbie W. Johnston, Director Operations A1 7 10 F13 19 28 30 31 38 43 45 49 50 51 53 54 70 71 72 74 76 S HEALTHSOUTH Corporation, Birmingham, AL Web address: www.healthsouth.com	33	46	87	1391	73	12894	0	14806	7156	227
MIDLANDS CENTER, 8301 Farrow Road, Zip 29203–3294; tel. 803/935–7508; Ronald P. Childs, FACHE, Health Services Administrator (Nonreporting)	12	12	24	—	—	—	—	—	—	—
★ PALMETTO BAPTIST MEDICAL CENTER/COLUMBIA, Taylor at Marion Street, Zip 29220; tel. 803/296–5010; James M. Bridges, Executive Vice President and Chief Operating Officer (Total facility includes 22 beds in nursing home–type unit) A1 2 9 10 F2 7 8 9 11 12 13 16 17 18 19 22 24 25 27 29 30 32 35 36 37 38 39 41 42 43 44 45 46 48 49 50 51 52 53 54 58 59 60 61 62 63 64 65 68 70 72 74 76 78 79 P7 S Palmetto Health Alliance, Columbia, SC Web address: www.palmettohealth.org/	23	10	383	18534	273	202438	3114	190351	80290	2042

© 2000 AHA Guide *Many Facility Codes have changed. Please refer to the AHA Guide Code Chart.*

Hospitals, U.S. / SOUTH CAROLINA

Hospital, Address, Telephone, Administrator, Approval, Facility, and Physician Codes, Health Care System, Network	Classification Codes		Utilization Data					Expense (thousands) of dollars		
★ American Hospital Association (AHA) membership □ Joint Commission on Accreditation of Healthcare Organizations (JCAHO) accreditation + American Osteopathic Healthcare Association (AOHA) membership ○ American Osteopathic Association (AOA) accreditation △ Commission on Accreditation of Rehabilitation Facilities (CARF) accreditation Control codes 61, 63, 64, 71, 72 and 73 indicate hospitals listed by AOHA, but not registered by AHA. For definition of numerical codes, see page A4	Control	Service	Staffed Beds	Admissions	Census	Outpatient Visits	Births	Total	Payroll	Personnel
★ PALMETTO RICHLAND MEMORIAL HOSPITAL, Five Richland Medical Park Drive, Zip 29203, Mailing Address: P.O. Box 2266, Zip 29203–2266; tel. 803/434–7000; B. Daniel Paysinger, M.D., Chief Operating Officer **A**1 2 3 5 8 9 10 **F**1 2 3 4 7 8 9 10 11 12 13 17 18 19 22 23 24 25 27 28 29 30 31 32 33 34 35 38 39 41 42 43 44 45 46 47 48 50 51 52 53 54 56 58 59 60 61 62 63 64 65 66 68 70 71 72 73 74 75 76 77 78 79 **S** Palmetto Health Alliance, Columbia, SC **Web address:** www.rmh.edu	13	10	612	30418	521	88045	—	380890	157915	4224
★ PROVIDENCE HOSPITAL, (Includes Providence Hospital Northeast, 120 Gateway Corporate Boulevard, Zip 29203–9611; tel. 803/865–4500; Anne Marie Moncure, Executive Director), 2435 Forest Drive, Zip 29204–2098; tel. 803/256–5300; Stephen A. Purves, CHE, President and Chief Executive Officer **A**1 9 10 **F**4 7 9 11 12 16 17 18 19 22 23 24 25 29 32 33 34 35 38 39 41 44 45 47 48 50 51 54 59 68 70 72 74 76 78 79 **S** Sisters of Charity of St. Augustine Health System, Cleveland, OH **Web address:** www.provhosp.com	32	10	228	11395	176	71717	—	—	—	1066
PROVIDENCE HOSPITAL NORTHEAST See Providence Hospital										
□ SOUTH CAROLINA STATE HOSPITAL, 2100 Bull Street, Zip 29202, Mailing Address: P.O. Box 119, Zip 29202–0119; tel. 803/898–2261; Jaime E. Condom, M.D., Director (Nonreporting) **A**1 **F**2 3 9 10 21 22 23 24 30 35 39 41 44 53 56 57 58 59 60 61 62 76	12	22	350	—	—	—	—	—	—	—
□ WILLIAM S. HALL PSYCHIATRIC INSTITUTE, 1800 Colonial Drive, Zip 29203–6827, Mailing Address: P.O. Box 202, Zip 29202–0202; tel. 803/898–1725; Dalmer P. Sercy, Director **A**1 3 5 10 **F**1 3 4 5 6 9 10 11 12 13 14 19 20 21 22 24 25 26 27 28 29 30 31 32 33 34 35 36 37 38 39 40 41 43 44 45 46 47 48 49 50 51 52 54 55 56 57 58 59 60 61 62 63 64 65 68 70 71 72 73 74 76 78 79	12	22	232	1083	189	0	0	28890	23111	546
★ WM. JENNINGS BRYAN DORN VETERANS AFFAIRS MEDICAL CENTER, 6439 Garners Ferry Road, Zip 29209–1639; tel. 803/776–4000; Brian Heckert, Medical Center Director (Total facility includes 121 beds in nursing home–type unit) **A**1 2 3 5 **F**1 2 3 4 6 9 11 12 13 18 19 22 23 24 25 26 29 30 31 32 34 35 36 37 38 39 41 43 45 46 47 48 49 50 51 53 54 56 57 59 60 61 62 63 64 65 68 69 70 72 74 76 78 79 **S** Department of Veterans Affairs, Washington, DC	45	10	280	4357	217	247508	0	115951	66992	1089
CONWAY—Horry County										
★ CONWAY HOSPITAL, 300 Singleton Ridge Road, Zip 29526, Mailing Address: P.O. Box 829, Zip 29528–0829; tel. 843/347–7111; Philip A. Clayton, President and Chief Executive Officer (Total facility includes 88 beds in nursing home–type unit) **A**1 9 10 **F**8 9 11 16 17 18 19 22 24 25 27 32 34 35 36 37 39 41 43 44 48 50 53 54 68 69 70 72 74 75 76 78 79	23	10	225	9727	183	82074	1073	—	—	773
DARLINGTON—Darlington County										
WILSON MEDICAL CENTER See McLeod Regional Medical Center, Florence										
DILLON—Dillon County										
★ SAINT EUGENE MEDICAL CENTER, 301 East Jackson Street, Zip 29536–2509, Mailing Address: P.O. Box 1327, Zip 29536–1327; tel. 843/774–4111 (Total facility includes 13 beds in nursing home–type unit) **A**1 9 10 **F**7 8 9 14 17 18 19 22 24 25 27 28 32 33 34 35 37 38 39 44 45 48 50 51 52 53 54 56 68 70 71 72 73 74 76 78 79 **P**8	23	10	109	4115	43	30681	315	21900	9454	306
EASLEY—Pickens County										
★ PALMETTO BAPTIST MEDICAL CENTER EASLEY, 200 Fleetwood Drive, Zip 29640–2076, Mailing Address: P.O. Box 2129, Zip 29641–2129; tel. 864/855–7200; Roddey E. Gettys, II, Executive Vice President (Total facility includes 13 beds in nursing home–type unit) **A**1 9 10 **F**7 8 9 12 14 16 17 18 19 22 23 24 25 27 30 32 33 34 35 38 39 40 41 43 44 45 48 50 51 53 54 67 70 72 74 76 78 79 **S** Palmetto Health Alliance, Columbia, SC **Web address:** www.palmettohealth.org/	23	10	106	4452	53	31191	651	35898	14330	481
EDGEFIELD—Edgefield County										
★ EDGEFIELD COUNTY HOSPITAL, 300 Ridge Medical Plaza, Zip 29824; tel. 803/637–3174; W. Joseph Seel, Administrator (Total facility includes 19 beds in nursing home–type unit) **A**1 9 10 **F**7 9 14 16 18 19 22 25 30 31 32 34 36 37 43 45 48 50 53 54 56 72 73 74 76 **P**1 5	13	10	59	880	8	10276	0	6292	2887	145
FAIRFAX—Allendale County										
★ ALLENDALE COUNTY HOSPITAL, Highway 278 West, Zip 29827–0278, Mailing Address: Box 218, Zip 29827–0218; tel. 803/632–3311; M. K. Hiatt, Administrator (Total facility includes 44 beds in nursing home–type unit) **A**9 10 **F**8 9 17 18 22 23 25 32 34 35 37 44 45 48 54 70 72 74 76 79	13	10	80	562	48	21373	139	5972	2499	111
FLORENCE—Florence County										
★ △ CAROLINAS HOSPITAL SYSTEM, (Includes Bruce Hospital System, 121 East Cedar Street, Zip 29501; Florence General Hospital, 512 South Irby Street, Zip 29501–5210; tel. 803/661–3000), 805 Pamplico Highway, Zip 29505, Mailing Address: P.O. Box 100550, Zip 29501–0550; tel. 843/674–5000; David A. McClellan, Chief Executive Officer (Total facility includes 24 beds in nursing home–type unit) **A**1 7 9 10 **F**2 3 4 9 11 12 13 14 16 17 18 19 22 23 24 25 27 28 29 30 32 33 34 35 36 37 38 39 41 42 43 44 45 47 48 49 50 52 53 54 56 65 67 68 69 70 71 72 74 75 76 78 79 **S** Quorum Health Group, Brentwood, TN **Web address:** www.carolinashospital.com	33	10	320	12800	209	109617	—	121949	43284	1196

Hospitals, U.S. / SOUTH CAROLINA

Hospital, Address, Telephone, Administrator, Approval, Facility, and Physician Codes, Health Care System, Network	Classification Codes		Utilization Data					Expense (thousands) of dollars		
★ American Hospital Association (AHA) membership ☐ Joint Commission on Accreditation of Healthcare Organizations (JCAHO) accreditation + American Osteopathic Healthcare Association (AOHA) membership ○ American Osteopathic Association (AOA) accreditation △ Commission on Accreditation of Rehabilitation Facilities (CARF) accreditation Control codes 61, 63, 64, 71, 72 and 73 indicate hospitals listed by AOHA, but not registered by AHA. For definition of numerical codes, see page A4	Control	Service	Staffed Beds	Admissions	Census	Outpatient Visits	Births	Total	Payroll	Personnel
☐ HEALTHSOUTH REHABILITATION HOSPITAL, 900 East Cheves Street, Zip 29506-2704; tel. 843/679-9000; Dennis A. Lofe, FACHE, Chief Executive Officer **A**1 10 **F**4 5 7 9 11 12 13 14 17 18 19 22 25 27 28 29 30 31 32 33 34 35 37 38 39 41 42 43 44 45 47 48 49 50 51 52 53 54 58 60 61 62 63 65 70 71 72 74 76 78 **S** HEALTHSOUTH Corporation, Birmingham, AL Web address: www.healthsouth.com	33	46	88	1282	72	9073	0	13027	6264	214
✣ MCLEOD REGIONAL MEDICAL CENTER, (Includes Wilson Medical Center, 701 Cashua Ferry Road, Darlington, Zip 29532, Mailing Address: Box 1859, Zip 29540; tel. 803/395-1100; Tom Hartley, Administrator), 555 East Cheves Street, Zip 29506-2617, Mailing Address: P.O. Box 100551, Zip 29501-0551; tel. 843/667-2000; J. Bruce Barragan, President and Chief Executive Officer **A**1 2 3 5 9 10 **F**2 3 4 7 8 9 10 11 12 13 14 16 17 18 19 22 23 24 25 26 27 28 29 31 32 33 34 35 36 37 38 39 40 41 42 43 44 45 46 47 48 49 50 51 52 53 54 56 57 58 59 60 61 62 63 64 65 68 70 71 72 73 74 75 76 78 79 **P**7 Web address: www.mcleodregional.org	23	10	411	23001	324	188528	2000	249288	90829	2544

FORT JACKSON—Richland County

✣ MONCRIEF ARMY COMMUNITY HOSPITAL, 4500 Stuart Street, Zip 29207-5720; tel. 803/751-2284; Colonel Stephen G. Oswald, Commander (Nonreporting) **A**1 2 **S** Department of the Army, Office of the Surgeon General, Falls Church, VA	42	10	91	—	—	—	—	—	—	—

GAFFNEY—Cherokee County

☐ UPSTATE CAROLINA MEDICAL CENTER, 1530 North Limestone Street, Zip 29340-4738; tel. 864/487-4271; Joe D. Howell, Executive Director **A**1 9 10 **F**7 8 9 13 16 17 19 22 24 25 28 32 34 37 39 43 44 45 48 49 50 51 53 54 70 71 76 78 79 **P**8 **S** Health Management Associates, Naples, FL	33	10	125	3761	42	43542	352	23328	9299	292

GEORGETOWN—Georgetown County

✣ GEORGETOWN MEMORIAL HOSPITAL, 606 Black River Road, Zip 29440-3368, Mailing Address: Drawer 1718, Zip 29442-1718; tel. 843/527-7000; Paul D. Gatens, Sr, Administrator **A**1 9 10 **F**2 5 7 8 9 10 11 12 13 16 17 18 19 22 24 25 27 28 29 30 32 33 34 35 38 39 41 44 45 46 48 49 50 51 52 53 54 59 61 64 65 66 68 70 71 72 73 74 75 76 78 79 **P**1 **S** Quorum Health Group, Brentwood, TN Web address: www.gmhsc.com	23	10	141	7951	98	98373	787	56352	19988	585

GREENVILLE—Greenville County

✣ △ GREENVILLE MEMORIAL HOSPITAL, (Includes Marshall I. Pickens Hospital; Roger C. Peace Rehabilitation Hospital), 701 Grove Road, Zip 29605-4295; tel. 864/455-7000; J. Bland Burkhardt, Jr, Senior Vice President and Administrator (Total facility includes 32 beds in nursing home–type unit) **A**1 2 5 7 8 9 10 **F**2 3 4 7 8 9 11 12 13 14 16 17 18 19 22 24 25 28 29 30 31 32 33 34 35 36 37 38 39 41 42 43 44 45 46 47 48 50 51 52 53 54 56 57 58 59 60 61 62 63 65 66 68 69 70 71 72 73 74 75 76 78 79 **P**1 2 6 **S** Greenville Hospital System, Greenville, SC Web address: www.ghs.org	23	10	809	35560	637	415318	5136	—	—	3969
☐ SHRINERS HOSPITALS FOR CHILDREN, GREENVILLE, 950 West Faris Road, Zip 29605-4277; tel. 864/271-3444; Gary F. Fraley, Administrator **A**1 3 5 **F**7 17 22 24 25 31 32 34 38 41 42 45 50 52 53 54 55 58 68 70 74 75 76 78 **S** Shriners Hospitals for Children, Tampa, FL Web address: www.shrinershq.org	23	57	50	305	4	13378	0	—	—	211
✣ △ ST. FRANCIS HEALTH SYSTEM, One St. Francis Drive, Zip 29601-3207; tel. 864/255-1000; Richard C. Neugent, Chief Executive Officer **A**1 2 7 10 **F**2 3 4 9 11 12 13 14 17 18 19 22 24 25 27 29 32 33 34 35 36 37 38 39 41 42 43 44 45 47 48 49 50 51 53 54 57 59 60 62 63 64 65 69 70 71 72 74 76 78 79 **P**1 2 6 Web address: www.stfrancishealth.com	23	10	225	9554	162	188231	0	—	—	1392
W. J. BARGE MEMORIAL HOSPITAL, Wade Hampton Boulevard, Zip 29614; tel. 864/242-5100; Aras Pundys, Administrator **F**8 25 31 34 38 44 48 50 54 79	23	11	79	1450	8	7189	0	3437	752	45

GREENWOOD—Greenwood County

✣ SELF MEMORIAL HOSPITAL, 1325 Spring Street, Zip 29646-3860; tel. 864/227-4111; M. John Heydel, President and Chief Executive Officer **A**1 2 3 5 9 10 **F**2 8 9 11 12 14 15 16 17 18 19 21 22 23 24 25 26 27 28 29 30 32 33 34 35 36 37 38 39 41 42 43 44 45 46 48 49 50 51 52 54 56 58 59 60 61 62 64 65 68 70 71 72 73 74 75 76 78 79 **P**5 8	23	10	339	10922	158	154167	1505	106041	50157	1512

GREER—Greenville County

★ ALLEN BENNETT HOSPITAL, (Includes Roger Huntington Nursing Center), 313 Memorial Drive, Zip 29650-1521; tel. 864/848-8200; Michael W. Massey, Administrator (Total facility includes 88 beds in nursing home–type unit) **A**9 10 **F**2 3 4 7 8 9 11 12 13 14 16 17 18 19 20 21 22 24 25 26 28 29 30 31 32 33 34 35 36 37 38 39 41 42 43 44 45 46 47 48 49 50 51 53 54 56 57 59 60 61 62 63 64 65 66 68 69 70 71 72 73 74 75 76 78 79 **P**1 2 6 **S** Greenville Hospital System, Greenville, SC Web address: www.ghs.org	16	10	146	2983	126	87332	382	26886	11167	302
☐ CHARTER GREENVILLE BEHAVIORAL HEALTH SYSTEM, 2700 East Phillips Road, Zip 29650-4816; tel. 864/968-6300; William L. Callison, Chief Executive Officer **A**1 10 **F**2 3 17 18 19 31 32 34 38 50 58 59 60 61 62 63 64 70 72 **S** Magellan Health Services, Atlanta, GA Web address: www.charterbehavioral.com/locations/sc_gville.html	33	22	66	1837	40	0	0	8654	3893	69

© 2000 AHA Guide   *Many Facility Codes have changed. Please refer to the AHA Guide Code Chart.*   Hospitals **A381**

Hospitals, U.S. / SOUTH CAROLINA

Hospital, Address, Telephone, Administrator, Approval, Facility, and Physician Codes, Health Care System, Network	Classification Codes		Utilization Data					Expense (thousands) of dollars		
★ American Hospital Association (AHA) membership ☐ Joint Commission on Accreditation of Healthcare Organizations (JCAHO) accreditation + American Osteopathic Healthcare Association (AOHA) membership ○ American Osteopathic Association (AOA) accreditation △ Commission on Accreditation of Rehabilitation Facilities (CARF) accreditation Control codes 61, 63, 64, 71, 72 and 73 indicate hospitals listed by AOHA, but not registered by AHA. For definition of numerical codes, see page A4	Control	Service	Staffed Beds	Admissions	Census	Outpatient Visits	Births	Total	Payroll	Personnel
HARTSVILLE—Darlington County										
☐ CAROLINA PINES REGIONAL MEDICAL CENTER, (Formerly Byerly Hospital), 1304 West BoBo Newsom Highway, Zip 29550; tel. 843/339-2100; Page Vaughan, Executive Director **A**1 9 10 **F**7 8 9 12 14 17 19 22 24 25 28 32 34 35 39 40 41 44 48 50 51 54 68 70 71 72 73 74 75 76 78 **S** Health Management Associates, Naples, FL **Web address:** www.hartsvillesc.com/byerly.html	33	10	116	5773	66	50917	582	28545	10815	459
HILTON HEAD ISLAND—Beaufort County										
✠ HILTON HEAD MEDICAL CENTER AND CLINICS, 25 Hospital Center Boulevard, Zip 29926, Mailing Address: P.O. Box 21117, Zip 29925-1117; tel. 843/681-6122; Dennis Ray Bruns, President and Chief Executive Officer **A**1 9 10 **F**1 4 6 7 8 9 10 11 12 13 17 19 22 23 24 25 27 28 29 30 31 32 33 34 35 36 37 38 39 40 41 42 43 44 45 46 48 49 50 51 52 53 54 57 58 59 60 61 62 63 64 70 71 72 74 75 76 78 79 **S** TENET Healthcare Corporation, Santa Barbara, CA **Web address:** www.tenethealth.com	32	10	79	4556	51	88329	380	42155	13694	433
KINGSTREE—Williamsburg County										
✠ CAROLINAS HOSPITAL SYSTEM–KINGSTREE, 500 Nelson Boulevard, Zip 29556-4027, Mailing Address: P.O. Drawer 568, Zip 29556-0568; tel. 843/354-9661; Clarence W. Bowman, Chief Executive Officer (Nonreporting) **A**1 9 10 **S** Quorum Health Group, Brentwood, TN **Web address:** www.carolinashospital.com	33	10	47	—	—	—	—	—	—	—
LAKE CITY—Florence County										
✠ CAROLINAS HOSPITAL SYSTEM–LAKE CITY, 258 North Ron McNair Boulevard, Zip 29560-1029, Mailing Address: P.O. Box 1029, Zip 29560-1029; tel. 843/394-2036; Clarence W. Bowman, Chief Executive Officer (Nonreporting) **A**1 9 10 **S** Quorum Health Group, Brentwood, TN	33	10	40	—	—	—	—	—	—	—
LANCASTER—Lancaster County										
☐ SPRINGS MEMORIAL HOSPITAL, 800 West Meeting Street, Zip 29720-2298; tel. 803/286-1214; Daniel E. McKay, Chief Executive Officer (Total facility includes 14 beds in nursing home–type unit) **A**1 9 10 **F**2 3 7 8 9 11 17 18 19 22 24 25 27 32 34 35 36 37 38 39 41 44 45 48 52 54 65 69 70 74 76 78 79 **P**8 **S** Community Health Systems, Inc., Brentwood, TN	33	10	208	8159	113	54030	672	—	—	512
LOCKHART—Union County										
★ HOPE HOSPITAL, 102 Hope Drive, Zip 29364, Mailing Address: P.O. Box 280, Zip 29364-0280; tel. 864/545-6500; Jimmie Ruth Gibson, Administrator **F**32 50	13	10	10	116	2	0	0	613	335	11
LORIS—Horry County										
✠ LORIS COMMUNITY HOSPITAL, 3655 Mitchell Street, Zip 29569-2827; tel. 843/716-7000; J. Timothy Browne, Chief Executive Officer (Total facility includes 88 beds in nursing home–type unit) **A**1 9 10 **F**7 8 9 12 14 16 17 18 19 22 24 25 27 28 32 33 34 36 37 38 39 41 43 44 45 48 49 50 51 54 68 70 71 73 74 75 76 79 **Web address:** www.lorishealthcaresystem.com	16	10	193	4489	136	71859	397	38635	15821	589
MANNING—Clarendon County										
✠ CLARENDON MEMORIAL HOSPITAL, 10 Hospital Street, Zip 29102, Mailing Address: P.O. Box 550, Zip 29102-0550; tel. 803/435-8463; Edward R. Frye, Jr, Administrator **A**1 9 10 **F**3 7 8 9 12 15 16 17 18 19 21 22 23 24 25 29 30 31 32 34 35 36 37 38 39 40 41 43 44 45 48 49 50 54 59 70 73 74 76 78 79	16	10	56	2213	33	88836	412	18619	8782	318
MOUNT PLEASANT—Charleston County										
✠ EAST COOPER REGIONAL MEDICAL CENTER, 1200 Johnnie Dodds Boulevard, Zip 29464-3294; tel. 843/881-0100; Jack Dusenbery, President **A**1 9 10 **F**8 9 11 12 16 17 18 19 22 25 27 28 29 32 34 35 36 38 39 41 43 44 45 48 50 53 54 61 66 70 71 74 75 76 78 79 **P**6 **S** TENET Healthcare Corporation, Santa Barbara, CA **Web address:** www.tenethealth.com	33	10	112	4440	44	76837	1378	—	—	422
MULLINS—Marion County										
✠ MARION COUNTY MEDICAL CENTER, 2829 East Highway 76, Zip 29574, Mailing Address: P.O. Drawer 1150, Marion, Zip 29571-1150; tel. 843/431-2000; Thomas E. Fuller, Executive Director (Total facility includes 92 beds in nursing home–type unit) **A**1 9 10 **F**2 3 4 6 8 9 11 12 14 17 18 19 21 22 23 24 25 27 28 29 30 31 32 34 35 36 37 38 39 40 41 42 43 44 45 46 47 48 50 52 53 54 56 57 58 59 60 61 62 63 64 65 70 71 72 73 74 76 78 79 **P**5 **Web address:** www.mcmed.org	16	10	216	7597	89	25109	504	36643	13920	526
MYRTLE BEACH—Horry County										
✠ GRAND STRAND REGIONAL MEDICAL CENTER, 809 82nd Parkway, Zip 29572-1413; tel. 803/692-1100; Doug White, Chief Executive Officer (Total facility includes 18 beds in nursing home–type unit) **A**1 2 9 10 **F**4 7 8 9 11 12 13 14 18 19 22 24 25 27 28 29 30 32 34 35 36 37 38 39 41 43 44 45 46 47 48 49 50 51 53 54 65 68 69 70 71 72 74 75 76 78 79 **P**6 **S** HCA – The Healthcare Company, Nashville, TN **Web address:** www.medtropolis.com/medtropolis/fac_right.asp?facility_id=3	33	10	186	11542	129	132118	834	—	—	897
NEWBERRY—Newberry County										
✠ NEWBERRY COUNTY MEMORIAL HOSPITAL, 2669 Kinard Street, Zip 29108-0497, Mailing Address: P.O. Box 497, Zip 29108-0497; tel. 803/276-7570; Lynn W. Beasley, President and Chief Executive Officer **A**1 9 10 **F**8 9 12 13 14 16 17 18 19 22 24 25 29 30 31 32 33 34 35 41 43 44 45 48 49 50 52 53 54 64 70 74 76 78 79 **P**6 **S** Quorum Health Group, Brentwood, TN	13	10	77	2350	28	29355	262	—	—	295

Many Facility Codes have changed. Please refer to the AHA Guide Code Chart.   © 2000 AHA Guide

Hospitals, U.S. / SOUTH CAROLINA

Hospital, Address, Telephone, Administrator, Approval, Facility, and Physician Codes, Health Care System, Network ★ American Hospital Association (AHA) membership □ Joint Commission on Accreditation of Healthcare Organizations (JCAHO) accreditation + American Osteopathic Healthcare Association (AOHA) membership ○ American Osteopathic Association (AOA) accreditation △ Commission on Accreditation of Rehabilitation Facilities (CARF) accreditation Control codes 61, 63, 64, 71, 72 and 73 indicate hospitals listed by AOHA, but not registered by AHA. For definition of numerical codes, see page A4	Classification Codes		Utilization Data					Expense (thousands) of dollars		
	Control	Service	Staffed Beds	Admissions	Census	Outpatient Visits	Births	Total	Payroll	Personnel
NORTH CHARLESTON—Charleston County ★ NAVAL HOSPITAL, 3600 Rivers Avenue, Zip 29405; tel. 843/743–7000; Captain John M. Mateczun, Commanding Officer **A**3 5 **F**2 3 4 9 10 11 12 13 14 16 17 18 19 22 23 24 25 27 28 29 31 32 33 34 36 37 38 39 41 42 43 44 45 46 47 48 49 50 51 52 53 54 55 56 57 58 59 60 61 62 63 64 65 68 70 71 72 73 74 76 78 79 **S** Department of Navy, Washington, DC Web address: www.nhchasn.med.navy.mil	43	10	15	945	9	164744	—	28294	10379	679
ORANGEBURG—Orangeburg County ☒ REGIONAL MEDICAL CENTER OF ORANGEBURG AND CALHOUN COUNTIES, 3000 St. Matthews Road, Zip 29118–1470; tel. 803/533–2200; Thomas C. Dandridge, President **A**1 2 9 10 **F**2 3 4 5 6 7 8 9 11 12 14 17 18 19 21 22 23 24 25 27 28 30 31 32 34 35 36 37 38 39 40 41 42 43 44 45 46 47 48 49 50 51 52 53 54 55 58 59 60 61 62 63 65 66 67 68 70 71 72 73 74 75 76 78 79 **S** Quorum Health Group, Brentwood, TN Web address: www.regmed.com	13	10	295	10736	184	56453	1505	86729	37319	1025
PICKENS—Pickens County ☒ CANNON MEMORIAL HOSPITAL, 123 West G. Acker Drive, Zip 29671, Mailing Address: P.O. Box 188, Zip 29671–0188; tel. 864/878–4791; Norman G. Rentz, President and Chief Executive Officer **A**1 9 10 **F**7 9 12 16 17 19 22 25 27 30 32 34 35 38 41 48 50 54 69 70 74 76 **P**8 Web address: www.cannonhospital.org	23	10	42	1229	17	28583	0	10398	4538	157
RIDGELAND—Jasper County LOW COUNTRY GENERAL HOSPITAL, Highway 278, Zip 29936, Mailing Address: Drawer 400, Zip 29936–0400; tel. 843/717–3300; Jeffrey L. White, Chief Executive Officer **A**9 10 **F**2 3 4 5 6 7 9 10 11 12 14 18 19 21 22 23 24 25 27 28 29 30 31 32 34 35 36 37 38 39 40 41 42 43 44 45 46 47 48 50 51 52 53 54 55 56 57 58 59 60 61 62 63 64 65 66 68 70 71 72 73 74 75 76 78 79	23	10	31	536	7	7966	—	3805	1801	48
ROCK HILL—York County ☒ PIEDMONT HEALTHCARE SYSTEM, 222 Herlong Avenue, Zip 29732–1952; tel. 803/329–1234; Charles F. Miller, President and Chief Executive Officer **A**1 9 10 **F**3 4 7 8 9 11 12 13 17 18 19 22 24 25 27 29 30 31 32 34 35 38 39 41 42 43 44 45 47 48 49 50 51 54 56 58 59 60 61 62 63 64 65 70 72 74 75 76 78 79 **S** TENET Healthcare Corporation, Santa Barbara, CA Web address: www.tenethealth.com	33	10	276	13786	181	131314	1521	122274	42271	1231
SENECA—Oconee County ☒ OCONEE MEMORIAL HOSPITAL, (Includes Lila Doyle Nursing Care Facility), 298 Memorial Drive, Zip 29672; tel. 864/882–3351; W. H. Hudson, President (Total facility includes 79 beds in nursing home–type unit) **A**1 9 10 **F**3 7 8 9 11 12 13 14 16 17 18 19 22 23 24 25 26 27 28 30 31 32 33 34 35 36 37 38 39 40 41 43 44 45 48 49 50 51 54 56 59 61 64 68 69 70 71 72 74 76 78 Web address: www.oconeememorial.org	23	10	190	7781	165	97526	625	62480	25427	932
SHAW A F B—Greenville County ☒ U. S. AIR FORCE HOSPITAL SHAW, 431 Meadowlark Street, Zip 29152–5019; tel. 803/895–6324; Lieutenant Colonel Daniel P. Dickinson, Administrator **A**1 **F**1 2 3 4 5 6 7 8 9 10 11 12 13 14 15 16 17 18 19 20 21 22 23 24 25 26 27 28 29 30 31 32 33 34 35 36 37 38 39 40 41 42 43 44 45 46 47 48 49 50 51 52 53 54 55 56 57 60 62 63 64 65 66 67 68 69 70 71 72 73 74 75 76 77 78 79 **P**6 **S** Department of the Air Force, Bowling AFB, DC Web address: www.shaw.af.mil	41	10	35	824	4	113482	295	10049	1700	44
SIMPSONVILLE—Greenville County ★ HILLCREST HOSPITAL, 729 S.E. Main Street, Zip 29681–3280; tel. 864/967–6100; Mark Slyter, Administrator **A**9 10 **F**2 3 4 7 9 11 12 13 14 16 17 18 19 22 24 25 26 28 29 31 32 33 34 35 36 37 38 39 41 42 43 44 45 46 47 48 50 51 52 53 54 57 58 59 60 61 62 63 64 65 66 68 70 71 72 73 74 76 78 79 **P**1 2 6 **S** Greenville Hospital System, Greenville, SC Web address: www.ghs.org	23	10	46	1732	22	71229	0	18403	6934	156
SPARTANBURG—Spartanburg County ☒ △ MARY BLACK HEALTH SYSTEM, 1700 Skylyn Drive, Zip 29307–1061, Mailing Address: P.O. Box 3217, Zip 29304–3217; tel. 864/573–3000; William W. Fox, Chief Executive Officer **A**1 7 9 10 **F**7 8 9 11 12 13 14 16 17 18 19 22 24 25 27 29 32 34 35 38 39 41 43 44 45 46 48 50 51 53 54 62 68 70 72 74 76 78 79 **P**2 **S** Quorum Health Group, Brentwood, TN	33	10	212	7068	94	125798	987	—		674
★ SPARTANBURG HOSPITAL FOR RESTORATIVE CARE, 389 Serpentine Drive, Zip 29303; tel. 864/560–3280; Anita M. Butler, Chief Executive Officer **F**3 4 5 6 7 9 10 11 12 13 19 21 28 29 30 31 32 33 35 36 37 38 39 40 41 42 43 44 45 46 47 48 49 50 51 52 53 54 55 56 57 58 59 60 61 62 63 64 65 66 67 70 71 72 73 74 75 76 78 79 **P**1 **S** Spartanburg Regional Healthcare System, Spartanburg, SC Web address: www.srhs.com	16	10	63	365	32	11898	—	14910	5363	143
☒ SPARTANBURG REGIONAL MEDICAL CENTER, 101 East Wood Street, Zip 29303–3016; tel. 864/560–6000; Joseph Michael Oddis, President **A**1 2 3 5 9 10 **F**4 8 9 11 12 16 17 18 19 22 24 25 27 28 29 30 31 32 34 35 36 37 38 39 41 42 43 44 45 47 48 49 50 51 52 53 54 55 56 57 58 59 60 61 62 63 64 65 66 67 68 70 71 72 74 75 76 78 79 **P**5 **S** Spartanburg Regional Healthcare System, Spartanburg, SC Web address: www.srhs.com	16	10	408	22457	316	390121	2541	284960	120485	3206

© 2000 AHA Guide — *Many Facility Codes have changed. Please refer to the AHA Guide Code Chart.*

Hospitals, U.S. / SOUTH CAROLINA

Hospital, Address, Telephone, Administrator, Approval, Facility, and Physician Codes, Health Care System, Network	Classification Codes		Utilization Data					Expense (thousands) of dollars		
	Control	Service	Staffed Beds	Admissions	Census	Outpatient Visits	Births	Total	Payroll	Personnel

★ American Hospital Association (AHA) membership
☐ Joint Commission on Accreditation of Healthcare Organizations (JCAHO) accreditation
+ American Osteopathic Healthcare Association (AOHA) membership
○ American Osteopathic Association (AOA) accreditation
△ Commission on Accreditation of Rehabilitation Facilities (CARF) accreditation
Control codes 61, 63, 64, 71, 72 and 73 indicate hospitals listed by AOHA, but not registered by AHA. For definition of numerical codes, see page A4

SUMMERVILLE—Dorchester County

★ SUMMERVILLE MEDICAL CENTER, 295 Midland Parkway, Zip 29485–8104; tel. 843/832–5100; Steven M. Anderson, Chief Executive Officer (Total facility includes 20 beds in nursing home–type unit) **A**9 **F**4 8 9 10 11 12 14 18 19 21 22 24 25 26 27 28 29 30 31 32 33 34 35 38 39 41 42 43 44 45 46 47 48 49 50 51 52 54 55 58 60 61 62 63 64 65 68 69 70 71 72 74 76 78 79 **P**7 **S** HCA – The Healthcare Company, Nashville, TN

| 33 | 10 | 85 | 3687 | 44 | 76390 | 564 | — | — | 227 |

SUMTER—Sumter County

☒ TUOMEY HEALTHCARE SYSTEM, 129 North Washington Street, Zip 29150–4983; tel. 803/778–9000; Jay Cox, President and Chief Executive Officer (Total facility includes 18 beds in nursing home–type unit) **A**1 9 10 **F**2 4 8 9 11 12 13 16 17 18 19 22 24 25 26 27 28 29 30 32 33 34 36 37 38 39 41 42 43 44 45 46 47 48 50 51 52 53 54 56 57 58 61 62 65 68 69 70 71 72 74 76 78 79 **P**8 **S** Quorum Health Group, Brentwood, TN
Web address: www.tuomey.com

| 23 | 10 | 251 | 10910 | 179 | 108874 | 1227 | — | — | 1125 |

TRAVELERS REST—Greenville County

☐ SPRING BROOK BEHAVIORAL HEALTHCARE SYSTEM, One Chestnut Way, Zip 29690–1005, Mailing Address: P.O. Box 1005, Zip 29690–1005; tel. 864/834–8013; Thomas Barnard, Chief Executive Officer **A**1 10 **F**19 22 24 25 31 38 39 50 51 53 54 57 58 59 60 61 62 63 64 70 75 76

| 33 | 22 | 44 | 180 | 9 | 0 | 0 | 3491 | 2015 | 77 |

UNION—Union County

☒ WALLACE THOMSON HOSPITAL, 322 West South Street, Zip 29379–2857, Mailing Address: P.O. Box 789, Zip 29379–0789; tel. 864/429–2600; Harrell L. Connelly, Chief Executive Officer (Total facility includes 113 beds in nursing home–type unit) **A**1 9 10 **F**9 16 17 18 19 22 25 31 32 34 36 38 39 40 41 43 44 45 48 50 51 54 65 68 69 70 74 76 78 79 **P**3 8 **S** Quorum Health Group, Brentwood, TN
Web address: www.wallacethomson.com/index.htm/default.htm

| 16 | 10 | 220 | 4239 | 159 | 45216 | 182 | — | — | 435 |

VARNVILLE—Hampton County

★ HAMPTON REGIONAL MEDICAL CENTER, 503 Carolina Avenue West, Zip 29944, Mailing Address: P.O. Box 338, Zip 29944–0338; tel. 803/943–2771; Dave H. Hamill, President and Chief Executive Officer **A**9 10 **F**9 18 19 22 25 32 34 38 45 48 50 54 70 74 76 78 79

| 23 | 10 | 36 | 738 | 9 | 8231 | — | 7188 | 3166 | 119 |

WALTERBORO—Colleton County

☒ COLLETON MEDICAL CENTER, 501 Robertson Boulevard, Zip 29488–5714; tel. 843/549–2000; Rebecca T. Brewer, CHE, Chief Executive Officer (Total facility includes 15 beds in nursing home–type unit) **A**1 9 10 **F**7 8 9 11 13 14 16 17 18 19 20 22 24 25 27 28 29 30 32 34 38 39 43 44 45 48 49 50 51 53 54 56 68 70 71 72 73 74 76 78 79 **S** HCA – The Healthcare Company, Nashville, TN

| 33 | 10 | 131 | 4964 | 78 | 25545 | 398 | — | — | 401 |

WEST COLUMBIA—Lexington County

☐ CHARTER RIVERS BEHAVIORAL HEALTH SYSTEM, 2900 Sunset Boulevard, Zip 29169–3422; tel. 803/796–9911; R. Andy Hanner, Chief Executive Officer **A**1 10 **F**2 3 6 19 22 29 31 32 38 39 50 54 57 58 59 60 61 62 63 64 70 **S** Magellan Health Services, Atlanta, GA
Web address: www.charterbehavioral.com

| 33 | 22 | 66 | 1583 | 32 | 3633 | 0 | — | — | 113 |

☒ LEXINGTON MEDICAL CENTER, 2720 Sunset Boulevard, Zip 29169–4816; tel. 803/791–2000; Michael J. Biediger, President **A**1 9 10 **F**7 8 9 11 12 13 14 17 18 19 21 22 23 24 25 26 28 29 30 31 32 34 35 38 39 41 42 43 44 45 48 49 50 51 53 54 56 65 68 70 71 72 74 75 76 78 79
Web address: www.lexmed.com

| 16 | 10 | 275 | 14902 | 193 | 573153 | 2341 | 168363 | 77200 | 1971 |

WINNSBORO—Fairfield County

☒ FAIRFIELD MEMORIAL HOSPITAL, 102 U.S. Highway 321 By-Pass North, Zip 29180, Mailing Address: P.O. Box 620, Zip 29180–0620; tel. 803/635–5548; J. Larry Dozier, Jr, FACHE, Chief Executive Officer **A**1 9 10 **F**7 9 17 18 19 22 25 32 34 36 37 38 43 45 46 48 50 51 54 72 74 76

| 13 | 10 | 33 | 973 | 12 | 22889 | 0 | 10137 | 4853 | 197 |

WOODRUFF—Spartanburg County

★ B.J. WORKMAN MEMORIAL HOSPITAL, 751 East Georgia Street, Zip 29388, Mailing Address: P.O. Box 699, Zip 29388–0699; tel. 864/476–8122; Alan Caldwell, Administrator **A**9 10 **F**2 7 9 16 17 18 22 25 38 48 54 76 79 **S** Spartanburg Regional Healthcare System, Spartanburg, SC
Web address: www.srhs.com

| 13 | 10 | 43 | 1210 | 8 | 15518 | 0 | 6698 | 2918 | 87 |

Hospitals, U.S. / SOUTH DAKOTA

SOUTH DAKOTA

Resident Population 738 (in thousands)
Resident population in metro areas 33.3%
Birth rate per 1,000 population 13.8
65 years and over 14.3%
Percent of persons without health insurance 11.8%

Hospital, Address, Telephone, Administrator, Approval, Facility, and Physician Codes, Health Care System, Network	Classification Codes		Utilization Data					Expense (thousands) of dollars		
★ American Hospital Association (AHA) membership □ Joint Commission on Accreditation of Healthcare Organizations (JCAHO) accreditation + American Osteopathic Healthcare Association (AOHA) membership ○ American Osteopathic Association (AOA) accreditation △ Commission on Accreditation of Rehabilitation Facilities (CARF) accreditation Control codes 61, 63, 64, 71, 72 and 73 indicate hospitals listed by AOHA, but not registered by AHA. For definition of numerical codes, see page A4	Control	Service	Staffed Beds	Admissions	Census	Outpatient Visits	Births	Total	Payroll	Personnel
ABERDEEN—Brown County										
★ △ AVERA ST. LUKE'S, 305 South State Street, Zip 57402–4450; tel. 605/622–5000; Dale J. Stein, President and Chief Executive Officer (Total facility includes 81 beds in nursing home–type unit) **A**1 2 7 9 10 **F**1 2 3 6 7 8 9 11 12 13 16 17 18 19 20 22 23 24 25 26 27 30 32 34 35 36 37 38 39 40 41 43 44 45 46 48 49 50 51 53 54 56 57 58 59 60 61 62 63 64 65 66 67 69 70 71 72 76 78 **P**6 8 **S** Avera Health, Yankton, SD Web address: www.averastlukes.org	21	10	224	6063	159	174973	712	71346	30482	852
ARMOUR—Douglas County										
DOUGLAS COUNTY MEMORIAL HOSPITAL, 708 Eighth Street, Zip 57313–2102; tel. 605/724–2159; Heath Brouwer, Administrator (Nonreporting) **A**10 18	23	10	9	—	—	—	—	—	—	—
BOWDLE—Edmunds County										
★ BOWDLE HOSPITAL, 8001 West Fifth Street, Zip 57428–0566; tel. 605/285–6146; Bryan Breitling, Administrator and Chief Executive Officer (Total facility includes 41 beds in nursing home–type unit) **A**9 10 **F**7 9 17 22 25 28 31 34 36 37 38 48 69 70 76	14	10	61	343	45	5643	9	2963	1604	83
BRITTON—Marshall County										
MARSHALL COUNTY HEALTHCARE CENTER/AVERA HEALTH, 413 Ninth Street, Zip 57430–0230, Mailing Address: Box 230, Zip 57430–0230; tel. 605/448–2253; Stephanie Lulewicz, Administrator **A**9 10 18 **F**6 9 17 18 22 25 32 34 36 49 54 76 **P**5 **S** Avera Health, Yankton, SD	23	10	20	429	6	8920	0	3591	1061	74
BROOKINGS—Brookings County										
★ BROOKINGS HOSPITAL, 300 22nd Avenue, Zip 57006–2496; tel. 605/696–9000; David B. Johnson, Administrator (Total facility includes 79 beds in nursing home–type unit) **A**9 10 **F**7 8 13 16 18 19 22 25 30 31 32 34 36 37 39 40 41 43 44 48 50 51 69 72 76 78	14	10	140	2018	97	52759	315	15081	7952	257
BURKE—Gregory County										
COMMUNITY MEMORIAL HOSPITAL/AVERA HEALTH, Eighth and Jackson, Zip 57523, Mailing Address: P.O. Box 319, Zip 57523–0319; tel. 605/775–2621; Carol A. Varland, Administrator **A**9 10 18 **F**18 22 25 37 39 76 **S** Avera Health, Yankton, SD	23	10	16	334	9	2212	0	2085	910	50
CANTON—Lincoln County										
★ CANTON–INWOOD MEMORIAL HOSPITAL, 440 North Hiawatha Drive, Zip 57013–9404; tel. 605/987–2621; Larry W. Veitz, Chief Executive Officer **A**9 10 **F**6 8 9 17 18 22 24 25 27 32 35 37 39 41 44 48 54 55 65 68 76 **S** Sioux Valley Hospitals and Health System, Sioux Falls, SD	23	10	25	510	5	38237	0	3206	1448	65
CHAMBERLAIN—Brule County										
★ MID DAKOTA HOSPITAL, 300 South Byron Boulevard, Zip 57325–9741; tel. 605/734–5511; Earl N. Sheehy, Administrator **A**9 10 **F**7 8 9 17 18 19 22 25 32 34 36 37 39 41 45 46 48 54 70 76 **P**6 **S** Sioux Valley Hospitals and Health System, Sioux Falls, SD	23	10	36	1352	11	8898	72	6572	3094	104
CLEAR LAKE—Deuel County										
★ DEUEL COUNTY MEMORIAL HOSPITAL, 701 Third Avenue South, Zip 57226–1037, Mailing Address: P.O. Box 1037, Zip 57226–1037; tel. 605/874–2141; Robert J. Salmon, Administrator (Nonreporting) **A**9 10 18 **S** Sioux Valley Hospitals and Health System, Sioux Falls, SD	23	10	20	—	—	—	—	—	—	—
CUSTER—Custer County										
CUSTER COMMUNITY HOSPITAL, 1039 Montgomery Street, Zip 57730–1397; tel. 605/673–2229; Jason Petik, Administrator **A**9 10 **F**6 7 8 9 16 17 22 25 29 32 36 37 43 44 45 54 56 63 70 76 77 **P**7 8 Web address: www.rcrh.org	23	10	11	240	4	7836	9	2981	1864	62
DE SMET—Kingsbury County										
DE SMET MEMORIAL HOSPITAL, 306 Prairie Avenue S.W., Zip 57231–9499; tel. 605/854–3329; John L. Single, Chief Executive Officer and Administrator **A**9 10 **F**9 16 17 18 22 25 34 36 37 48 54 70 76	14	10	13	283	4	8491	0	1478	719	19
DEADWOOD—Lawrence County										
★ NORTHERN HILLS GENERAL HOSPITAL, 61 Charles Street, Zip 57732–1303; tel. 605/578–2313; Jack Brinkers, CHE, Interim Chief Executive Officer **A**9 10 **F**1 3 7 8 9 17 18 22 25 28 32 33 34 36 37 39 40 41 43 44 45 48 54 58 59 60 62 63 70 71 73 76 Web address: www.rcrh.org	23	10	18	483	7	15232	25	4855	2245	77
DELL RAPIDS—Minnehaha County										
DELLS AREA HEALTH CENTER, (Formerly Dell Rapids Community Hospital), 909 North Iowa Avenue, Zip 57022–1231; tel. 605/428–5431; James A. Faulwell, Chief Executive Officer and Administrator (Total facility includes 50 beds in nursing home–type unit) **A**9 10 **F**8 9 12 19 22 23 24 25 28 34 37 38 39 43 44 48 54 69 76 78	23	10	68	688	54	6913	36	5012	2520	62
EAGLE BUTTE—Dewey County										
U. S. PUBLIC HEALTH SERVICE INDIAN HOSPITAL, Mailing Address: P.O. Box 1012, Zip 57625–1012; tel. 605/964–3001; Donald D. Annis, Service Unit Director (Nonreporting) **A**1 10 **S** U. S. Public Health Service Indian Health Service, Rockville, MD	44	10	27	—	—	—	—	—	—	—

© 2000 AHA Guide   *Many Facility Codes have changed. Please refer to the AHA Guide Code Chart.*   Hospitals **A385**

Hospitals, U.S. / SOUTH DAKOTA

- ★ American Hospital Association (AHA) membership
- ☐ Joint Commission on Accreditation of Healthcare Organizations (JCAHO) accreditation
- + American Osteopathic Healthcare Association (AOHA) membership
- ○ American Osteopathic Association (AOA) accreditation
- △ Commission on Accreditation of Rehabilitation Facilities (CARF) accreditation

Control codes 61, 63, 64, 71, 72 and 73 indicate hospitals listed by AOHA, but not registered by AHA. For definition of numerical codes, see page A4

Hospital, Address, Telephone, Administrator, Approval, Facility, and Physician Codes, Health Care System, Network	Classification Codes		Utilization Data					Expense (thousands) of dollars		
	Control	Service	Staffed Beds	Admissions	Census	Outpatient Visits	Births	Total	Payroll	Personnel
ELLSWORTH AFB—Meade County										
★ U. S. AIR FORCE HOSPITAL, 2900 Doolittle Drive, Zip 57706–4821; tel. 605/385–3201; Colonel Farley Howell, Commanding Officer (Nonreporting) **A**1 **S** Department of the Air Force, Bowling AFB, DC Web address: www.elsworth.af.mil/~medge/index.htm	41	10	31	—	—	—	—	—	—	—
EUREKA—McPherson County										
EUREKA COMMUNITY HEALTH SERVICES/AVERA HEALTH, 410 Ninth Street, Zip 57437–0517, Mailing Address: P.O. Box 517, Zip 57437–0517; tel. 605/284–2661; Robert A. Dockter, Administrator **A**9 10 18 **F**6 9 17 18 19 22 25 36 39 48 54 70 71 76 **S** Avera Health, Yankton, SD	23	10	6	184	1	6533	0	1213	568	30
FAULKTON—Faulk County										
FAULK COUNTY MEMORIAL HOSPITAL, 911 St. John Street, Zip 57438, Mailing Address: P.O. Box 100, Zip 57438–0100; tel. 605/598–6263; Patricia Kadlec, Administrator **A**9 10 18 **F**6 12 13 15 16 17 18 22 25 31 34 36 38 45 54 56 67 69 70 76	13	10	13	217	6	6764	0	1489	700	30
FLANDREAU—Moody County										
★ FLANDREAU MUNICIPAL HOSPITAL/AVERA HEALTH, 214 North Prairie Avenue, Zip 57028–1243; tel. 605/997–2433; John E. Barrett, Administrator (Nonreporting) **A**9 10 18 **S** Avera Health, Yankton, SD	14	10	18	—	—	—	—	—	—	—
FORT MEADE—Meade County										
★ VETERANS AFFAIRS BLACK HILLS HEALTH CARE SYSTEM, (Includes Veterans Affairs Medical Center, 500 North Fifth Street, Hot Springs, Zip 57747; tel. 605/745–2052), 113 Comanche Road, Zip 57741–1099; tel. 605/347–2511; Peter P. Henry, Director (Total facility includes 104 beds in nursing home–type unit) **A**1 5 **F**3 9 11 13 18 19 22 23 24 26 29 30 31 32 33 34 36 37 38 39 43 45 46 48 49 50 51 54 56 57 61 62 63 64 69 70 72 74 76 77 78 79 **S** Department of Veterans Affairs, Washington, DC Web address: www.va.gov/stations97/guide/home.asp?DIVISION=ALL	45	10	163	2915	147	177746	0	84458	41170	935
FREEMAN—Hutchinson County										
★ FREEMAN COMMUNITY HOSPITAL, 510 East Eighth Street, Zip 57029–0370, Mailing Address: P.O. Box 370, Zip 57029–0370; tel. 605/925–4000; Daniel Gran, Chief Executive Officer (Total facility includes 59 beds in nursing home–type unit) **A**9 10 **F**1 8 16 17 18 19 25 30 31 32 33 34 38 40 41 43 44 45 46 48 50 53 54 67 69 70 72 76 78 **P**4 7 Web address: www.fchnh.com	23	10	85	401	62	9839	30	5012	2642	105
GETTYSBURG—Potter County										
★ GETTYSBURG MEDICAL CENTER, 606 East Garfield, Zip 57442–1398; tel. 605/765–2480; Mark Schmidt, President and Chief Executive Officer (Total facility includes 54 beds in nursing home–type unit) **A**9 10 18 **F**1 6 7 9 13 17 18 22 23 25 26 28 32 33 34 36 37 38 39 43 48 50 54 67 69 70 72 75 76 78 **P**5 **S** Catholic Health Initiatives, Denver, CO	21	10	61	145	40	8503	0	2154	1159	—
GREGORY—Gregory County										
★ GREGORY COMMUNITY HOSPITAL, 400 Park Avenue, Zip 57533–0400, Mailing Address: P.O. Box 408, Zip 57533–0408; tel. 605/835–8394; Carol A. Varland, Chief Executive Officer (Total facility includes 58 beds in nursing home–type unit) **A**9 10 **F**1 8 9 12 13 16 17 18 22 23 24 25 30 31 32 33 34 36 39 44 45 46 48 49 50 51 62 69 70 71 72 76 **S** Banner Health System, Fargo, ND	23	10	84	866	65	20662	44	6166	2948	121
HOT SPRINGS—Fall River County										
VETERANS AFFAIRS MEDICAL CENTER See Veterans Affairs Black Hills Health Care System, Fort Meade										
HOVEN—Potter County										
★ HOLY INFANT HOSPITAL, Main Street, Zip 57450–0158, Mailing Address: P.O. Box 158, Zip 57450–0158; tel. 605/948–2262; Jeff Marlette, Administrator **A**9 10 **F**12 17 18 22 34 36 37 41 48 70 75 76	23	10	22	148	13	2857	0	1115	498	36
HURON—Beadle County										
★ HURON REGIONAL MEDICAL CENTER, 172 Fourth Street S.E., Zip 57350–2590; tel. 605/353–6200; John L. Single, Chief Executive Officer **A**1 9 10 **F**8 9 16 17 18 22 24 25 28 34 36 37 38 39 41 43 44 45 48 50 54 61 70 71 76 78 **S** Quorum Health Group, Brentwood, TN	23	10	61	2494	29	45557	270	19437	7960	240
LEMMON—Perkins County										
FIVE COUNTIES HOSPITAL, 405 Sixth Avenue West, Zip 57638–1318, Mailing Address: P.O. Box 479, Zip 57638–0479; tel. 605/374–3871; James Haeder, Interim Administrator (Total facility includes 52 beds in nursing home–type unit) **A**9 10 18 **F**25 69	23	10	56	57	41	3499	0	1732	868	44
MADISON—Lake County										
★ MADISON COMMUNITY HOSPITAL, 917 North Washington Avenue, Zip 57042–1696; tel. 605/256–6551; Tamara Miller, Administrator **A**1 9 10 **F**7 8 9 16 17 19 22 25 32 34 36 37 39 40 41 43 44 45 48 54 69 70 72 76	23	10	49	839	15	16213	72	5665	2999	115
MARTIN—Bennett County										
BENNETT COUNTY HEALTHCARE CENTER, 102 Major Allen Street, Zip 57551, Mailing Address: P.O. Box 70–D, Zip 57551; tel. 605/685–6622; John L. Jacobs, Administrator (Total facility includes 48 beds in nursing home–type unit) **A**9 10 **F**6 8 12 25 36 44 69 **P**8	13	10	64	425	46	2034	6	2903	1662	73
MILBANK—Grant County										
☐ ST. BERNARD'S PROVIDENCE HOSPITAL, (Includes St. William Home for the Aged), 901 East Virgil Avenue, Zip 57252–2124, Mailing Address: P.O. Box 432, Zip 57252–0432; tel. 605/432–4538; Sister Genevieve Karels, Administrator (Total facility includes 82 beds in nursing home–type unit) **A**1 9 10 **F**6 8 9 16 17 18 22 25 34 36 37 38 39 41 44 54 69 76	21	10	117	654	85	—	52	6072	2375	151

Hospitals, U.S. / SOUTH DAKOTA

Hospital, Address, Telephone, Administrator, Approval, Facility, and Physician Codes, Health Care System, Network	Classification Codes		Utilization Data					Expense (thousands) of dollars		
★ American Hospital Association (AHA) membership ☐ Joint Commission on Accreditation of Healthcare Organizations (JCAHO) accreditation + American Osteopathic Healthcare Association (AOHA) membership ○ American Osteopathic Association (AOA) accreditation △ Commission on Accreditation of Rehabilitation Facilities (CARF) accreditation Control codes 61, 63, 64, 71, 72 and 73 indicate hospitals listed by AOHA, but not registered by AHA. For definition of numerical codes, see page A4	Control	Service	Staffed Beds	Admissions	Census	Outpatient Visits	Births	Total	Payroll	Personnel
MILLER—Hand County ★ HAND COUNTY MEMORIAL HOSPITAL/AVERA HEALTH, 300 West Fifth Street, Zip 57362-1238; tel. 605/853-2421; Clarence A. Lee, Administrator (Total facility includes 22 beds in nursing home-type unit) **A**9 10 **F**3 6 7 9 12 13 14 16 17 18 19 22 23 24 25 30 31 32 33 34 36 38 40 43 45 46 48 50 51 54 58 59 63 68 69 70 71 72 73 75 76 78 79 **P**1 3 4 5 6 8 **S** Avera Health, Yankton, SD	23	10	43	552	29	3318	0	2766	1208	60
MITCHELL—Davison County ✣ AVERA QUEEN OF PEACE, 525 North Foster, Zip 57301-2999; tel. 605/995-2000; Ronald L. Jacobson, President and Chief Executive Officer (Total facility includes 84 beds in nursing home-type unit) **A**1 9 10 **F**1 3 7 8 9 13 16 17 18 19 22 23 25 26 27 28 30 31 32 34 36 37 38 39 40 41 43 44 45 46 48 49 50 54 61 67 69 70 71 72 76 78 79 **P**6 **S** Avera Health, Yankton, SD **Web address:** www.averaqueenofpeace.org	21	10	183	4115	128	76911	496	36124	16688	469
MOBRIDGE—Walworth County ★ MOBRIDGE REGIONAL HOSPITAL, 1401 Tenth Avenue West, Zip 57601-1199, Mailing Address: P.O. Box 580, Zip 57601-0580; tel. 605/845-3693; Marlene Odde, Chief Executive Officer (Total facility includes 16 beds in nursing home-type unit) **A**9 10 **F**6 7 8 9 16 17 18 22 25 28 30 32 33 34 35 36 37 38 39 41 43 44 48 50 54 61 62 67 69 70 71 72 75 76 **P**6 **Web address:** www.cam-walnet.com/~mrh/index.htm	23	10	47	826	22	14707	64	7322	3883	126
PARKSTON—Hutchinson County ★ AVERA ST. BENEDICT HEALTH CENTER, (Formerly St. Benedict Health Center), Glynn Drive, Zip 57366, Mailing Address: P.O. Box B, Zip 57366; tel. 605/928-3311; Gale Walker, Administrator (Total facility includes 75 beds in nursing home-type unit) **A**9 10 **F**1 6 8 9 13 17 18 19 22 25 28 30 32 33 34 36 37 38 39 40 41 44 46 48 54 56 69 70 71 72 76 78 **S** Avera Health, Yankton, SD **Web address:** www.parkston.com	21	10	105	740	75	23511	57	6292	2829	124
PHILIP—Haakon County HANS P. PETERSON MEMORIAL HOSPITAL, 503 West Pine Street, Zip 57567, Mailing Address: P.O. Box 790, Zip 57567-0790; tel. 605/859-2511; David Dick, Administrator (Total facility includes 46 beds in nursing home-type unit) **A**9 10 **F**6 22 23 24 25 36 43 69 70 71 **P**6	23	10	66	340	53	1530	4	2430	1222	104
PIERRE—Hughes County ✣ ST. MARY'S HEALTHCARE CENTER, 800 East Dakota Avenue, Zip 57501-3313; tel. 605/224-3100; James D. M. Russell, Chief Executive Officer (Total facility includes 105 beds in nursing home-type unit) **A**1 9 10 **F**7 8 9 16 17 18 22 25 34 36 37 38 39 40 41 44 45 46 48 54 67 69 70 71 76 78 **P**5 **S** Catholic Health Initiatives, Denver, CO **Web address:** www.st-marys.com	23	10	191	2904	132	15122	293	22823	11071	312
PINE RIDGE—Shannon County ✣ U. S. PUBLIC HEALTH SERVICE INDIAN HOSPITAL, Mailing Address: P.O. Box 1201, Zip 57770-1201; tel. 605/867-5131; Vern F. Donnell, Service Unit Director (Nonreporting) **A**1 10 **S** U. S. Public Health Service Indian Health Service, Rockville, MD	47	10	46	—	—	—	—	—	—	—
PLATTE—Charles Mix County ★ PLATTE HEALTH CENTER/AVERA HEALTH, (Formerly Platte Community Memorial Hospital), 601 East Seventh, Zip 57369-2123, Mailing Address: P.O. Box 200, Zip 57369-0200; tel. 605/337-3364; Mark Burket, Chief Executive Officer (Total facility includes 48 beds in nursing home-type unit) (Nonreporting) **A**9 10 18 **S** Avera Health, Yankton, SD	23	10	63	—	—	—	—	—	—	—
RAPID CITY—Pennington County ✣ INDIAN HEALTH SERVICE HOSPITAL, 3200 Canyon Lake Drive, Zip 57702-8197; tel. 605/355-2280; Michelle Leach, Director **A**1 10 **F**1 2 9 10 12 14 17 18 22 23 24 25 26 27 31 32 33 34 35 36 38 39 40 41 42 44 45 46 47 48 49 50 51 52 53 54 55 56 57 58 59 60 61 62 63 64 65 66 67 68 69 70 71 72 73 74 75 76 77 78 79 **S** U. S. Public Health Service Indian Health Service, Rockville, MD	47	10	32	523	10	60148	0	10809	6418	—
✣ RAPID CITY REGIONAL HOSPITAL SYSTEM OF CARE, 353 Fairmont Boulevard, Zip 57701-7393, Mailing Address: P.O. Box 6000, Zip 57709-6000; tel. 605/341-1000; Adil M. Ameer, President and Chief Executive Officer **A**1 2 3 5 9 10 **F**1 4 6 7 8 9 11 13 16 17 18 22 24 25 27 32 34 36 37 38 39 41 42 44 45 46 47 48 52 53 54 57 58 60 62 63 64 65 70 71 72 76 78 **P**1 6 7 **Web address:** www.rcrh.org	23	10	360	16207	238	115324	1688	153904	70919	1773
REDFIELD—Spink County COMMUNITY MEMORIAL HOSPITAL, 110 West Tenth Avenue, Zip 57469-0420, Mailing Address: P.O. Box 420, Zip 57469-0420; tel. 605/472-1111; Dan Odegaard, Administrator (Nonreporting) **A**9 10	14	10	25	—	—	—	—	—	—	—
ROSEBUD—Todd County ✣ U. S. PUBLIC HEALTH SERVICE INDIAN HOSPITAL, Highway 18, Soldier Creek Road, Zip 57570; tel. 605/747-2231; Gayla J. Twiss, Service Unit Director (Nonreporting) **A**1 10 **S** U. S. Public Health Service Indian Health Service, Rockville, MD	47	10	35	—	—	—	—	—	—	—
SCOTLAND—Bon Homme County ★ LANDMANN-JUNGMAN MEMORIAL HOSPITAL, 600 Billars Street, Zip 57059-2026; tel. 605/583-2226; Philip Hibnick, Administrator **A**9 10 **F**7 9 16 17 18 22 25 32 36 37 39 40 45 48 51 54 56 67 70 76 78 **S** Avera Health, Yankton, SD	23	10	19	317	4	4390	7	2341	1096	48

Hospitals, U.S. / SOUTH DAKOTA

Hospital, Address, Telephone, Administrator, Approval, Facility, and Physician Codes, Health Care System, Network	Classification Codes		Utilization Data					Expense (thousands) of dollars		
★ American Hospital Association (AHA) membership ☐ Joint Commission on Accreditation of Healthcare Organizations (JCAHO) accreditation + American Osteopathic Healthcare Association (AOHA) membership ○ American Osteopathic Association (AOA) accreditation △ Commission on Accreditation of Rehabilitation Facilities (CARF) accreditation Control codes 61, 63, 64, 71, 72 and 73 indicate hospitals listed by AOHA, but not registered by AHA. For definition of numerical codes, see page A4	Control	Service	Staffed Beds	Admissions	Census	Outpatient Visits	Births	Total	Payroll	Personnel
SIOUX FALLS—Minnehaha County ※ △ AVERA MCKENNAN HOSPITAL, 800 East 21st Street, Zip 57105–1096, Mailing Address: P.O. Box 5045, Zip 57117–5045; tel. 605/322–8000; Fredrick Slunecka, President and Chief Executive Officer (Total facility includes 196 beds in nursing home–type unit) **A**1 2 3 5 7 9 10 **F**3 4 6 7 8 9 10 11 12 13 14 17 18 19 20 21 22 24 25 26 28 29 30 31 32 33 34 35 36 37 38 39 41 43 44 45 46 47 48 49 50 51 52 53 54 56 57 58 59 60 61 62 63 64 65 66 67 68 69 70 71 72 73 74 75 76 78 79 **P**1 6 **S** Avera Health, Yankton, SD Web address: www.mckennan.org	21	10	521	15362	418	433539	1205	199577	87445	2447
△ CHILDRENS CARE HOSPITAL AND SCHOOL, (CHILDREN'S SPECIALTY HOSPITAL), 2501 West 26th Street, Zip 57105–2498; tel. 605/782–2300; Charisse S. Oland, President and Chief Executive Officer **A**7 9 **F**7 13 16 17 18 19 26 29 31 38 53 54 69 70 78 Web address: www.cchs.org	23	59	96	53	77	0	0	11271	7109	298
※ ROYAL C. JOHNSON VETERANS MEMORIAL HOSPITAL, 2501 West 22nd Street, Zip 57105–9920, Mailing Address: P.O. Box 5046, Zip 57117–9920; tel. 605/336–3230; Ronald T. Porzio, Chief Operating Officer (Total facility includes 65 beds in nursing home–type unit) **A**1 3 5 **F**1 2 3 6 9 11 13 16 17 18 19 22 23 24 25 26 30 31 32 33 34 35 36 37 38 39 41 43 45 46 48 49 50 51 53 54 56 57 59 61 62 63 65 68 69 70 72 76 77 78 79 **P**6 **S** Department of Veterans Affairs, Washington, DC Web address: www.va.gov/stations97/guide/home.asp?DIVISION=ALL	45	10	84	2497	75	106926	0	50840	24382	654
※ △ SIOUX VALLEY HOSPITAL AND UNIVERSITY MEDICAL CENTER, (Includes Sioux Valley Behavioral Health, 2812 South Louise Avenue, Zip 57106–4309; tel. 605/361–8111), 1100 South Euclid Avenue, Zip 57105–0496, Mailing Address: P.O. Box 5039, Zip 57117–5039; tel. 605/333–1000; Becky Nelson, President **A**1 2 3 5 7 9 10 **F**3 4 7 8 9 11 12 13 16 17 18 19 21 22 23 24 25 26 28 29 30 31 32 33 34 35 36 37 38 39 41 42 43 44 45 46 47 48 49 50 51 52 53 54 55 56 57 58 59 60 61 62 63 66 68 70 71 72 75 76 77 78 79 **P**6 **S** Sioux Valley Hospitals and Health System, Sioux Falls, SD Web address: www.siouxvalley.org	23	10	496	19400	304	161003	1825	195861	88234	3103
SISSETON—Roberts County ★ COTEAU DES PRAIRIES HOSPITAL, 205 Orchard Drive, Zip 57262–2398; tel. 605/698–7647; Bill Nelson, Administrator and Chief Executive Officer **A**9 10 **F**8 9 12 18 19 22 23 25 28 31 34 36 37 41 44 48 54 76	23	10	27	379	4	8305	74	2832	1273	50
※ U. S. PUBLIC HEALTH SERVICE INDIAN HOSPITAL, Chestnut Street, Zip 57262, Mailing Address: P.O. Box 189, Zip 57262–0189; tel. 605/698–7606; Richard Huff, Administrator (Nonreporting) **A**1 10 **S** U. S. Public Health Service Indian Health Service, Rockville, MD Web address: www.home.aberdeen.his.gov	47	10	18	—	—	—	—	—	—	—
SPEARFISH—Lawrence County ★ LOOKOUT MEMORIAL HOSPITAL, 1440 North Main Street, Zip 57783–1504; tel. 605/642–2617; Deb J. Krmpotic, R.N., Administrator **A**9 10 **F**1 6 7 8 9 12 13 16 17 18 22 25 26 31 32 34 36 37 38 39 40 41 43 44 45 46 48 49 50 51 54 66 67 69 70 71 72 76 78 **S** Banner Health System, Fargo, ND	23	10	32	1691	15	38495	308	10802	4657	224
STURGIS—Meade County ★ STURGIS COMMUNITY HEALTH CARE CENTER, 949 Harmon Street, Zip 57785–2452; tel. 605/347–2536; Roger R. Heidt, Administrator (Total facility includes 84 beds in nursing home–type unit) **A**9 10 **F**7 8 9 13 16 17 18 22 36 37 39 44 45 48 69 70 72 76 **S** Banner Health System, Fargo, ND	23	10	114	1094	96	7696	90	9052	4357	114
TYNDALL—Bon Homme County ★ ST. MICHAEL'S HOSPITAL, Douglas Street and Broadway, Zip 57066, Mailing Address: P.O. Box 27, Zip 57066–0027; tel. 605/589–3341; Carol Deurmier, Chief Executive Officer (Total facility includes 9 beds in nursing home–type unit) **A**10 **F**8 9 16 17 18 22 25 34 36 39 41 44 48 50 69 70 71 76	21	10	34	452	14	15798	22	2906	1602	59
VERMILLION—Clay County ★ SIOUX VALLEY VERMILLION CAMPUS, 20 South Plum Street, Zip 57069–3346; tel. 605/624–2611; John E. Paulson, Chief Executive Officer (Total facility includes 89 beds in nursing home–type unit) **A**9 10 **F**9 22 25 36 37 39 41 44 48 56 69 70 71 72 76 **P**6 8 **S** Sioux Valley Hospitals and Health System, Sioux Falls, SD Web address: www.siouxvalley.org	23	10	118	964	71	16248	81	8706	4423	118
VIBORG—Turner County ★ PIONEER MEMORIAL HOSPITAL AND HEALTH SERVICES, 315 North Washington Street, Zip 57070, Mailing Address: P.O. Box 368, Zip 57070–0368; tel. 605/326–5161; Georgia Pokorney, Chief Executive Officer (Total facility includes 52 beds in nursing home–type unit) **A**9 10 **F**1 2 3 4 6 8 9 10 11 12 14 17 18 22 23 24 25 28 32 34 36 37 38 39 40 41 42 43 44 45 46 47 48 49 50 52 53 54 56 57 65 67 69 70 71 72 75 76 79 **P**5 **S** Sioux Valley Hospitals and Health System, Sioux Falls, SD	23	10	64	401	54	11759	3	5148	2637	106
WAGNER—Charles Mix County ★ WAGNER COMMUNITY MEMORIAL HOSPITAL, Third and Walnut, Zip 57380, Mailing Address: P.O. Box 280, Zip 57380–0280; tel. 605/384–3611; Arlene C. Bich, Administrator **A**9 10 **F**8 9 12 17 18 22 25 30 32 33 34 36 37 38 39 41 44 48 50 51 54 56 67 69 70 75 76	23	10	20	678	6	7330	0	3091	1428	48

Hospitals, U.S. / SOUTH DAKOTA

Hospital, Address, Telephone, Administrator, Approval, Facility, and Physician Codes, Health Care System, Network	Classification Codes		Utilization Data					Expense (thousands) of dollars		
★ American Hospital Association (AHA) membership □ Joint Commission on Accreditation of Healthcare Organizations (JCAHO) accreditation + American Osteopathic Healthcare Association (AOHA) membership ○ American Osteopathic Association (AOA) accreditation △ Commission on Accreditation of Rehabilitation Facilities (CARF) accreditation Control codes 61, 63, 64, 71, 72 and 73 indicate hospitals listed by AOHA, but not registered by AHA. For definition of numerical codes, see page A4	Control	Service	Staffed Beds	Admissions	Census	Outpatient Visits	Births	Total	Payroll	Personnel

WATERTOWN—Codington County

★ PRAIRIE LAKES HOSPITAL AND CARE CENTER, 400 Tenth Avenue N.W., Zip 57201–6210, Mailing Address: P.O. Box 1210, Zip 57201–1210; tel. 605/882–7000; Paul A. Hanson, Chief Executive Officer (Total facility includes 51 beds in nursing home–type unit) **A**1 2 9 10 **F**7 8 9 16 17 18 19 22 25 33 36 37 38 39 41 43 44 45 46 48 49 50 51 54 61 63 69 70 71 72 76 78 79 **S** Sioux Valley Hospitals and Health System, Sioux Falls, SD
Web address: www.prairielakes.com

| 23 | 10 | 119 | 3152 | 82 | 55097 | 603 | 28530 | 11604 | 388 |

WEBSTER—Day County

★ LAKE AREA HOSPITAL, North First Street, Zip 57274, Mailing Address: P.O. Box 489, Zip 57274–0489; tel. 605/345–3336; Donald J. Finn, Administrator (Nonreporting) **A**9 10 18 **S** Sioux Valley Hospitals and Health System, Sioux Falls, SD

| 23 | 10 | 26 | — | — | — | — | — | — | — |

WESSINGTON SPRINGS—Jerauld County

WESKOTA MEMORIAL MEDICAL CENTER, 604 First Street N.E., Zip 57382, Mailing Address: P.O. Box 429, Zip 57382; tel. 605/539–1201; Kayleen R. Lee, Chief Executive Officer **A**9 10 **F**7 8 9 16 17 18 22 23 24 25 30 32 34 36 37 38 40 43 45 48 50 54 70 71 72 76 **P**5

| 23 | 10 | 28 | 385 | 7 | 3606 | 14 | 1524 | 807 | 32 |

WINNER—Tripp County

★ WINNER REGIONAL HEALTHCARE CENTER, 745 East Eighth Street, Zip 57580–2677, Mailing Address: P.O. Box 745, Zip 57580–0745; tel. 605/842–7100; Michael M. Penticoff, Administrator (Total facility includes 81 beds in nursing home–type unit) **A**9 10 **F**8 9 12 16 17 18 19 22 24 25 28 30 32 33 34 36 37 38 39 40 43 44 46 48 49 54 55 66 69 71 74 76 **S** Sioux Valley Hospitals and Health System, Sioux Falls, SD

| 23 | 10 | 116 | 818 | 88 | 9199 | 135 | 9522 | 4833 | 189 |

YANKTON—Yankton County

★ △ AVERA SACRED HEART, (Formerly Sacred Heart Health Services), 501 Summit Avenue, Zip 57078–3899; tel. 605/668–8000; Pamela J. Rezac, President and Chief Executive Officer (Total facility includes 113 beds in nursing home–type unit) **A**1 2 7 9 10 **F**1 7 8 9 11 12 13 16 17 18 19 22 24 25 27 28 30 32 33 34 36 37 38 39 40 41 43 44 45 46 48 49 50 51 53 65 68 69 70 71 72 76 78 **P**3 7 **S** Avera Health, Yankton, SD
Web address: www.shhservices.com

| 21 | 10 | 257 | 5341 | 175 | 23342 | 691 | 42232 | 18065 | 582 |

© 2000 AHA Guide *Many Facility Codes have changed. Please refer to the AHA Guide Code Chart.*

Hospitals, U.S. / TENNESSEE

TENNESSEE

Resident Population 5,431 (in thousands)
Resident population in metro areas 68.0%
Birth rate per 1,000 population 13.9
65 years and over 12.5%
Percent of persons without health insurance 13.6%

★ American Hospital Association (AHA) membership
□ Joint Commission on Accreditation of Healthcare Organizations (JCAHO) accreditation
+ American Osteopathic Healthcare Association (AOHA) membership
○ American Osteopathic Association (AOA) accreditation
△ Commission on Accreditation of Rehabilitation Facilities (CARF) accreditation
Control codes 61, 63, 64, 71, 72 and 73 indicate hospitals listed by AOHA, but not registered by AHA. For definition of numerical codes, see page A4

Hospital, Address, Telephone, Administrator, Approval, Facility, and Physician Codes, Health Care System, Network	Classification Codes		Utilization Data					Expense (thousands) of dollars		
	Control	Service	Staffed Beds	Admissions	Census	Outpatient Visits	Births	Total	Payroll	Personnel
ASHLAND CITY—Cheatham County										
★ CHEATHAM MEDICAL CENTER, 313 North Main Street, Zip 37015-1358; tel. 615/792-3030; Michael W. Garfield, Administrator (Nonreporting) **A**9 **S** HCA – The Healthcare Company, Nashville, TN Web address: www.hcahealthcare.com	33	10	29	—	—	—	—	—	—	—
ATHENS—McMinn County										
★ ATHENS REGIONAL MEDICAL CENTER, 1114 West Madison Avenue, Zip 37303-4150, Mailing Address: P.O. Box 250, Zip 37371-0250; tel. 423/745-1411; John R. Workman, Chief Executive Officer **A**1 9 10 **F**8 9 12 13 16 17 18 19 22 24 25 26 27 28 30 32 34 38 39 41 42 43 44 45 46 48 50 54 63 64 68 70 72 75 76 78 **P**7 **S** HCA – The Healthcare Company, Nashville, TN Web address: www.columbiachat.com/athens	33	10	91	2202	21	44773	357	16662	7824	260
BOLIVAR—Hardeman County										
★ BOLIVAR GENERAL HOSPITAL, 650 Nuckolls Road, Zip 38008-1500; tel. 901/658-3100; Rosamond Tyler, Administrator (Nonreporting) **A**1 9 10 **S** West Tennessee Healthcare, Jackson, TN Web address: www.wth.net	23	10	47	—	—	—	—	—	—	—
□ WESTERN MENTAL HEALTH INSTITUTE, 11100 Old Highway 64, Zip 38008; tel. 901/658-5141; Elizabeth Littlefield, Ed.D., Superintendent **A**1 10 **F**16 17 18 57	12	22	247	1638	228	0	0	26392	17413	601
BRISTOL—Sullivan County										
★ WELLMONT BRISTOL REGIONAL MEDICAL CENTER, 1 Medical Park Boulevard, Zip 37620-7434; tel. 423/844-4200; Randall M. Olson, President (Total facility includes 30 beds in nursing home–type unit) **A**1 2 3 5 9 10 **F**1 4 6 7 8 9 11 12 13 16 17 18 19 22 23 24 25 27 28 29 30 32 33 34 35 36 37 38 39 41 43 44 45 46 47 48 49 50 51 54 55 56 57 58 60 61 62 63 64 65 68 69 70 71 72 75 76 77 78 79 **P**5 **S** Wellmont Health System, Kingsport, TN Web address: www.wellmont.org	23	10	348	12124	174	177113	814	117453	45320	—
BROWNSVILLE—Haywood County										
★ METHODIST HEALTHCARE–BROWNSVILLE, 2545 North Washington Avenue, Zip 38012-1697; tel. 901/772-4110; Sandra Bailey, Administrator **A**1 9 10 **F**3 4 7 8 9 11 13 14 17 18 22 25 26 27 30 32 34 38 44 45 46 47 48 51 54 58 59 60 61 62 63 64 65 69 76 78 79 **P**3 8 **S** Methodist Healthcare, Memphis, TN Web address: www.methodisthealth.org	23	10	44	1169	14	12664	212	9028	2255	88
CAMDEN—Benton County										
★ CAMDEN GENERAL HOSPITAL, 175 Hospital Drive, Zip 38320-1617; tel. 901/584-6135; John M. Carruth, Administrator (Nonreporting) **A**1 9 10 **S** West Tennessee Healthcare, Jackson, TN Web address: www.wth.net	16	10	40	—	—	—	—	—	—	—
CARTHAGE—Smith County										
★ CARTHAGE GENERAL HOSPITAL, 130 Lebanon Highway, Zip 37030-2955, Mailing Address: P.O. Box 319, Zip 37030-0319; tel. 615/735-9815; Scott Tongate, Chief Administrative Officer **A**1 9 10 **F**2 8 9 13 17 18 19 22 25 32 34 36 39 43 44 48 50 54 68 70 72 73 76 78 Web address: www.ftrmh.com	23	10	50	2163	23	27648	101	13709	6612	297
★ SMITH COUNTY MEMORIAL HOSPITAL, 158 Hospital Drive, Zip 37030-1096; tel. 615/735-1560; Jerry H. Futrell, Chief Executive Officer **A**1 9 10 **F**8 9 13 16 17 18 22 25 30 32 39 44 48 54 57 62 69 70 76 78 **P**8 **S** LifePoint Hospitals, Inc., Brentwood, TN	33	10	40	1506	20	15448	49	9424	3584	121
CELINA—Clay County										
□ CUMBERLAND RIVER HOSPITAL, (Formerly Cumberland River Hospital North), 100 Old Jefferson Street, Zip 38551, Mailing Address: P. O. Box 427, Zip 38551-0427; tel. 931/243-3581; Patrick J. Gray, President and Chief Executive Officer (Total facility includes 8 beds in nursing home–type unit) (Nonreporting) **A**1 9 10 **S** Paracelsus Healthcare Corporation, Houston, TX	33	10	66	—	—	—	—	—	—	—
CENTERVILLE—Hickman County										
□ BAPTIST HICKMAN COMMUNITY HOSPITAL, 135 East Swan Street, Zip 37033-1446; tel. 931/729-4271; Jack M. Keller, Administrator (Total facility includes 40 beds in nursing home–type unit) **A**1 9 18 **F**9 16 17 18 22 25 32 34 36 37 38 45 48 54 64 69 70 76	23	10	55	369	42	8254	0	6592	2590	80
CHATTANOOGA—Hamilton County										
★ ERLANGER HEALTH SYSTEM, (Includes Erlanger North Hospital, 632 Morrison Springs Road, Zip 37415; tel. 615/778-3300; T. C. Thompson Children's Hospital, 910 Blackford Street, Zip 37403; tel. 615/778-6011; Willie D. Miller Eye Center), 975 East Third Street, Zip 37403-2112; tel. 423/778-7000; Dennis Pettigrew, President and Chief Executive Officer (Nonreporting) **A**1 2 3 5 9 10 Web address: www.erlanger.org	16	10	536	—	—	—	—	—	—	—

Many Facility Codes have changed. Please refer to the AHA Guide Code Chart.

© 2000 AHA Guide

Hospitals, U.S. / TENNESSEE

Hospital, Address, Telephone, Administrator, Approval, Facility, and Physician Codes, Health Care System, Network	Classification Codes		Utilization Data					Expense (thousands) of dollars		
★ American Hospital Association (AHA) membership □ Joint Commission on Accreditation of Healthcare Organizations (JCAHO) accreditation + American Osteopathic Healthcare Association (AOHA) membership ○ American Osteopathic Association (AOA) accreditation △ Commission on Accreditation of Rehabilitation Facilities (CARF) accreditation Control codes 61, 63, 64, 71, 72 and 73 indicate hospitals listed by AOHA, but not registered by AHA. For definition of numerical codes, see page A4	Control	Service	Staffed Beds	Admissions	Census	Outpatient Visits	Births	Total	Payroll	Personnel
□ HEALTHSOUTH CHATTANOOGA REHABILITATION HOSPITAL, 2412 McCallie Avenue, Zip 37404–3398; tel. 423/698–0221; Donna Bourdon, Chief Operating Officer (Nonreporting) **A**1 10 **S** HEALTHSOUTH Corporation, Birmingham, AL Web address: www.healthsouth.com	33	46	69	—	—	—	—	—	—	—
★ MEMORIAL HOSPITAL, (Includes Memorial North Park Hospital, 2051 Hamill Road, Zip 37343–4096; tel. 423/870–6100), 2525 De Sales Avenue, Zip 37404–3322; tel. 423/495–2525; L. Clark Taylor, Jr, Ph.D., President and Chief Executive Officer (Total facility includes 15 beds in nursing home–type unit) **A**1 2 3 5 9 10 **F**1 4 9 11 13 16 17 18 19 22 24 25 29 30 32 33 34 35 36 38 39 41 43 44 45 46 47 48 51 54 55 56 65 69 70 71 72 73 76 78 79 **P**1 7 **S** Catholic Health Initiatives, Denver, CO	23	10	370	19172	257	185526	0	212350	80255	2272
MEMORIAL NOTH PARK HOSPITAL See Memorial Hospital										
□ MOCCASIN BEND MENTAL HEALTH INSTITUTE, 100 Moccasin Bend Road, Zip 37405–4496; tel. 423/785–3400; Russell K. Vatter, Superintendent **A**1 10 **F**16 17 18 35 57 59 60 61 62	12	22	172	1769	147	0	0	17810	11267	414
★ PARKRIDGE MEDICAL CENTER, (Includes East Ridge Hospital, 941 Spring Creek Road, East Ridge, Zip 37412; tel. 423/855–3500; Brenda M. Waltz, CHE, Chief Executive Officer; Valley Behavioral Health System, 2200 Morris Hill Road, Zip 37421; tel. 423/499–1204; Philip R. Cook, Chief Executive Officer), 2333 McCallie Avenue, Zip 37404–3285; tel. 423/698–6061; Niels P. Vernegaard, Chief Executive Officer (Total facility includes 28 beds in nursing home–type unit) (Nonreporting) **A**1 9 10 **S** HCA – The Healthcare Company, Nashville, TN Web address: www.hcahealthcare.com	33	10	517	—	—	—	—	—	—	—
★ △ SISKIN HOSPITAL FOR PHYSICAL REHABILITATION, One Siskin Plaza, Zip 37403–1306; tel. 423/634–1200; Robert P. Main, President and Chief Executive Officer **A**1 7 10 **F**13 16 18 20 23 29 30 38 43 45 49 50 53 54 70 71 72 78 **P**5 Web address: www.siskinrehab.org	23	46	80	1399	69	16830	0	24018	12912	302
T. C. THOMPSON CHILDREN'S HOSPITAL See Erlanger Health System										
VALLEY BEHAVIORAL HEALTH SYSTEM See Parkridge Medical Center										
□ VENCOR HOSPITAL–CHATTANOOGA, (LONG TERM ACUTE CARE), 709 Walnut Street, Zip 37402–1961; tel. 423/266–7721; Steven E. McGraw, Administrator **A**1 10 **F**13 18 22 24 25 31 39 41 49 70 76 **S** Vencor, Incorporated, Louisville, KY Web address: www.vencor.com	33	49	44	287	34	0	0	—	—	121
WILLIE D. MILLER EYE CENTER See Erlanger Health System										
CLARKSVILLE—Montgomery County										
★ GATEWAY HEALTH SYSTEM, (Formerly Clarksville Memorial Hospital), 1771 Madison Street, Zip 37043–4900, Mailing Address: P.O. Box 3160, Zip 37043–3160; tel. 931/552–6622; James Lee Decker, President and Chief Executive Officer (Total facility includes 29 beds in nursing home–type unit) **A**1 9 10 **F**7 8 9 11 22 24 25 27 32 34 35 36 37 38 39 41 43 44 45 46 48 50 51 54 57 59 60 61 62 63 65 66 68 69 70 72 76 78 **P**2 Web address: www.crhs.com	23	10	165	9607	116	108129	1336	73962	30365	931
CLEVELAND—Bradley County										
★ BRADLEY MEMORIAL HOSPITAL, 2305 Chambliss Avenue N.W., Zip 37311, Mailing Address: P.O. Box 3060, Zip 37320–3060; tel. 423/559–6000; John Barnes, Administrator **A**1 9 10 **F**7 8 9 11 13 16 17 18 22 24 25 32 34 36 37 38 39 41 43 44 45 46 48 50 54 65 70 72 76 78 79 Web address: www.bmhosp.org	13	10	174	7110	73	108467	1239	64808	27216	815
□ CLEVELAND COMMUNITY HOSPITAL, 2800 Westside Drive N.W., Zip 37312–3599; tel. 423/339–4100; Martin D. Smith, Chief Executive Officer (Nonreporting) **A**1 9 10 **S** Community Health Systems, Inc., Brentwood, TN	33	10	70	—	—	—	—	—	—	—
COLLIERVILLE—Shelby County										
BAPTIST MEMORIAL HOSPITAL–COLLIERVILLE See Baptist Memorial Hospital, Memphis										
COLUMBIA—Maury County										
★ MAURY REGIONAL HOSPITAL, 1224 Trotwood Avenue, Zip 38401–4823; tel. 931/381–1111; William R. Walter, Chief Executive Officer (Nonreporting) **A**1 9 10 Web address: www.mauryregional.com	13	10	275	—	—	—	—	—	—	—
COOKEVILLE—Putnam County										
★ COOKEVILLE REGIONAL MEDICAL CENTER, 142 West Fifth Street, Zip 38501–1760, Mailing Address: P.O. Box 340, Zip 38503–0340; tel. 931/528–2541; Tod N. Lambert, Administrator and Chief Executive Officer **A**1 9 10 **F**4 7 8 9 11 12 13 16 17 19 22 25 27 29 32 33 34 36 39 41 44 45 46 47 48 50 51 54 55 65 70 71 72 76 78 79	14	10	168	7816	97	103064	1240	71375	30192	977
COPPERHILL—Polk County										
□ COPPER BASIN MEDICAL CENTER, State Highway 68, Zip 37317, Mailing Address: P.O. Box 990, Zip 37317–0990; tel. 423/496–5511; Grady Scott, President and Chief Executive Officer (Nonreporting) **A**1 9 10	23	10	44	—	—	—	—	—	—	—
COVINGTON—Tipton County										
★ BAPTIST MEMORIAL HOSPITAL–TIPTON, 1995 Highway 51 South, Zip 38019–3635; tel. 901/476–2621; Glenn Baker, Administrator **A**1 9 10 **F**7 8 9 13 16 17 18 19 20 22 25 29 33 34 35 36 37 39 41 43 44 45 48 49 50 51 54 70 72 76 78 **S** Baptist Memorial Health Care Corporation, Memphis, TN Web address: www.bmhcc.org	23	10	70	2635	28	36875	427	18246	6319	241

© 2000 AHA Guide   *Many Facility Codes have changed. Please refer to the AHA Guide Code Chart.*

Hospitals, U.S. / TENNESSEE

Hospital, Address, Telephone, Administrator, Approval, Facility, and Physician Codes, Health Care System, Network	Classification Codes		Utilization Data					Expense (thousands) of dollars		
★ American Hospital Association (AHA) membership □ Joint Commission on Accreditation of Healthcare Organizations (JCAHO) accreditation + American Osteopathic Healthcare Association (AOHA) membership ○ American Osteopathic Association (AOA) accreditation △ Commission on Accreditation of Rehabilitation Facilities (CARF) accreditation Control codes 61, 63, 64, 71, 72 and 73 indicate hospitals listed by AOHA, but not registered by AHA. For definition of numerical codes, see page A4	Control	Service	Staffed Beds	Admissions	Census	* Outpatient Visits	Births	Total	Payroll	Personnel

CROSSVILLE—Cumberland County
★ CUMBERLAND MEDICAL CENTER, 421 South Main Street, Zip 38555–5031; tel. 931/484–9511; Edwin S. Anderson, President (Total facility includes 20 beds in nursing home–type unit) **A**1 9 10 **F**7 8 9 11 12 13 17 18 22 24 25 27 28 32 33 34 36 39 41 43 44 45 46 48 53 54 56 65 69 70 72 76 78
Web address: www.cmchealthcare.org
23 10 166 6641 73 63012 628 41186 21091 755

DAYTON—Rhea County
★ RHEA MEDICAL CENTER, 7900 Rhea County Highway, Zip 37321–5912; tel. 423/775–1121; Kennedy L. Croom, Jr, Administrator and Chief Executive Officer (Total facility includes 89 beds in nursing home–type unit) **A**1 9 10 **F**17 22 25 39 41 48 54 69 76 **S** Quorum Health Group, Brentwood, TN
13 10 131 1117 96 30933 0 12143 4514 162

DICKSON—Dickson County
★ HORIZON MEDICAL CENTER, 111 Highway 70 East, Zip 37055–2033; tel. 615/441–2357; Benjamin J. Everett, Chief Executive Officer (Total facility includes 26 beds in nursing home–type unit) **A**1 9 10 **F**8 9 11 13 16 17 18 22 24 25 30 32 34 38 39 41 43 44 46 48 49 50 51 54 56 57 61 62 69 70 71 76 77 78 79 **P**7 **S** HCA – The Healthcare Company, Nashville, TN
Web address: www.hcahealthcare.com
33 10 168 3986 50 54879 500 28715 12351 368

DYERSBURG—Dyer County
★ METHODIST HEALTHCARE– DYERSBURG HOSPITAL, (Formerly Methodist Hospital of Dyersburg), 400 Tickle Street, Zip 38024–3182; tel. 901/285–2410; R. Coleman Foss, Chief Executive Officer **A**1 9 10 **F**5 7 8 9 13 16 17 22 24 25 27 32 34 36 37 39 41 43 48 50 51 54 65 70 76 78 **P**5 7 8 **S** Methodist Healthcare, Memphis, TN
Web address: www.methodisthealth.org
23 10 105 3577 39 44665 640 27668 10828 389

EAST RIDGE—Hamilton County
EAST RIDGE HOSPITAL See Parkridge Medical Center, Chattanooga

ELIZABETHTON—Carter County
□ SYCAMORE SHOALS HOSPITAL, 1501 West Elk Avenue, Zip 37643–1368; tel. 423/542–1300; Scott Williams, Chief Executive Officer (Total facility includes 12 beds in nursing home–type unit) **A**1 9 10 **F**1 2 3 4 6 7 8 9 11 13 14 16 17 18 19 21 22 23 24 25 26 27 28 29 30 31 32 33 34 35 36 37 38 39 41 42 43 44 45 46 47 48 49 50 51 52 53 54 56 57 58 59 60 61 62 63 64 65 66 68 69 70 71 72 73 74 75 76 77 78 79 **P**5 7 8 **S** Mountain States Health Alliance, Johnson City, TN
23 10 105 2372 26 52033 445 20296 6829 247

ERIN—Houston County
★ TRINITY HOSPITAL, 353 Main Street, Zip 37061–0489, Mailing Address: P.O. Box 489, Zip 37061–0489; tel. 931/289–4211; Jay Woodall, Chief Executive Officer **A**1 9 10 **F**16 17 18 19 22 23 25 29 32 34 48 49 54 70 71 76
33 10 31 1309 12 17332 42 5993 2586 93

ERWIN—Unicoi County
★ UNICOI COUNTY MEMORIAL HOSPITAL, 100 Greenway Circle, Zip 37650–2196, Mailing Address: P.O. Box 802, Zip 37650–0802; tel. 423/743–3141; Jim S. Pate, Acting Chief Executive Officer (Total facility includes 46 beds in nursing home–type unit) **A**1 9 10 **F**7 9 16 17 18 22 24 25 32 34 36 39 41 43 45 48 54 69 70 71 76 **P**5
15 10 74 1117 58 23294 0 10330 4603 188

ETOWAH—McMinn County
★ WOODS MEMORIAL HOSPITAL DISTRICT, Highway 411 North, Zip 37331, Mailing Address: P.O. Box 410, Zip 37331–0410; tel. 423/263–3600; Guy Hazlett, FACHE, Chief Executive Officer (Total facility includes 88 beds in nursing home–type unit) (Nonreporting) **A**1 9 10
13 10 160 — — — — — — —

FAYETTEVILLE—Lincoln County
★ LINCOLN COUNTY HEALTH FACILITIES, 700 West Maple Street, Zip 37334–3202; tel. 931/438–1111; Gary G. Kendrick, Chief Executive Officer **A**1 9 10 **F**7 8 9 17 19 22 24 25 28 30 31 32 36 37 38 39 41 44 45 46 48 54 62 72 76 78 **S** Quorum Health Group, Brentwood, TN
13 10 51 2015 21 34991 234 12638 6370 270

FRANKLIN—Williamson County
★ WILLIAMSON MEDICAL CENTER, 2021 Carothers Road, Zip 37067–5822, Mailing Address: P.O. Box 681600, Zip 37068–1600; tel. 615/791–0500; Ronald G. Joyner, Chief Executive Officer **A**1 9 10 **F**4 7 8 9 11 22 24 25 27 32 34 37 38 39 41 44 46 48 50 51 54 59 61 68 70 71 72 76 78 **P**6
Web address: www.williamsonmedicalcntr.org
13 10 126 5635 61 119400 670 59472 25076 750

GALLATIN—Sumner County
★ △ SUMNER REGIONAL MEDICAL CENTER, 555 Hartsville Pike, Zip 37066–2449, Mailing Address: P.O. Box 1558, Zip 37066–1558; tel. 615/452–4210; William T. Sugg, President and Chief Executive Officer (Total facility includes 10 beds in nursing home–type unit) **A**1 7 9 10 **F**7 8 9 11 13 14 16 17 18 19 22 24 25 26 27 28 31 32 36 37 38 39 41 42 43 44 45 46 48 49 50 51 53 54 61 65 69 70 71 72 74 76 78 79 **P**5
23 10 150 4258 60 95472 766 47199 19549 539

GERMANTOWN—Shelby County
□ BAPTIST REHABILITATION–GERMANTOWN, 2100 Exeter Road, Zip 38138; tel. 901/757–1350; Paula Gisler, Administrator **A**1 9 10 **F**2 3 4 5 8 9 10 11 12 13 14 16 17 18 19 21 22 23 24 25 26 27 28 29 30 31 32 33 34 36 37 38 39 41 42 43 44 45 46 47 48 49 50 51 52 53 54 56 57 58 59 60 61 62 63 64 65 66 68 69 70 71 72 74 75 76 77 78 79 **S** Baptist Memorial Health Care Corporation, Memphis, TN
Web address: www.bmhcc.org
METHODIST HOSPITAL GERMANTOWN See Methodist Healthcare–Memphis Hospital, Memphis
21 46 63 1396 42 — 0 20465 8020 180

Hospitals, U.S. / TENNESSEE

Hospital, Address, Telephone, Administrator, Approval, Facility, and Physician Codes, Health Care System, Network	Classification Codes		Utilization Data					Expense (thousands) of dollars		
★ American Hospital Association (AHA) membership □ Joint Commission on Accreditation of Healthcare Organizations (JCAHO) accreditation + American Osteopathic Healthcare Association (AOHA) membership ○ American Osteopathic Association (AOA) accreditation △ Commission on Accreditation of Rehabilitation Facilities (CARF) accreditation Control codes 61, 63, 64, 71, 72 and 73 indicate hospitals listed by AOHA, but not registered by AHA. For definition of numerical codes, see page A4	Control	Service	Staffed Beds	Admissions	Census	Outpatient Visits	Births	Total	Payroll	Personnel

GREENEVILLE—Greene County

☒ LAUGHLIN MEMORIAL HOSPITAL, 1420 Tusculum Boulevard, Zip 37745; tel. 423/787-5000; Charles H. Whitfield, Jr, President and Chief Executive Officer (Total facility includes 90 beds in nursing home-type unit) **A**1 9 10 **F**8 9 15 17 18 19 22 24 25 30 32 36 38 39 41 44 45 46 48 50 51 54 65 68 69 70 71 72 76 78 79 | 23 | 10 | 230 | 5122 | 142 | 57575 | 524 | 34392 | 13288 | 446

☒ TAKOMA ADVENTIST HOSPITAL, 401 Takoma Avenue, Zip 37743-4647; tel. 423/639-3151; Carlyle L. E. Walton, President (Nonreporting) **A**1 9 10 **S** Adventist Health System Sunbelt Health Care Corporation, Winter Park, FL | 21 | 10 | 80 | — | — | — | — | — | — | —

HARRIMAN—Roane County

□ ROANE MEDICAL CENTER, 412 Devonia Street, Zip 37748, Mailing Address: P.O. Box 489, Zip 37748-0489; tel. 423/882-1323; Jim Gann, Administrator **A**1 9 10 **F**7 9 11 17 18 19 22 25 28 31 32 33 34 39 41 48 70 72 76 78 79 **P**8
Web address: www.kornet.org/r_health | 14 | 10 | 85 | 3583 | 35 | 50324 | 3 | 22997 | 10011 | 380

HENDERSONVILLE—Sumner County

☒ HENDERSONVILLE HOSPITAL, 355 New Shackle Island Road, Zip 37075-2393; tel. 615/264-4000; Robert Klein, Chief Executive Officer (Total facility includes 10 beds in nursing home-type unit) **A**1 9 10 **F**8 9 11 13 16 18 19 22 24 25 30 32 33 34 38 39 41 44 48 49 50 51 54 58 59 60 61 62 63 65 68 69 70 71 72 76 78 79 **P**7 **S** HCA – The Healthcare Company, Nashville, TN
Web address: www.hvillehospital.com | 33 | 10 | 66 | 3234 | 35 | 68368 | 617 | 23763 | 10834 | 231

HERMITAGE—Davidson County

☒ SUMMIT MEDICAL CENTER, 5655 Frist Boulevard, Zip 37076-2053; tel. 615/316-3000; Bryan K. Dearing, Chief Executive Officer (Total facility includes 16 beds in nursing home-type unit) **A**1 9 10 **F**3 4 6 8 9 10 11 12 13 16 17 18 19 21 22 23 25 27 30 31 32 33 34 35 37 38 39 41 42 44 45 46 47 48 49 50 51 52 53 54 55 56 57 58 59 60 61 62 63 64 65 66 67 69 70 71 72 73 74 76 77 78 79 **P**5 7 **S** HCA – The Healthcare Company, Nashville, TN
Web address: www.summitmedctr.com | 33 | 10 | 204 | 9660 | 123 | 100328 | 1396 | 60599 | 27517 | 790

HUMBOLDT—Gibson County

☒ HUMBOLDT GENERAL HOSPITAL, 3525 Chere Carol Road, Zip 38343-3699; tel. 901/784-0301; Bill Kail, Administrator **A**1 9 10 **F**8 9 13 16 17 18 19 22 25 32 34 36 37 44 48 49 54 70 71 76 78 **S** West Tennessee Healthcare, Jackson, TN
Web address: www.wth.net | 15 | 10 | 42 | 1332 | 16 | 21043 | 130 | 5229 | 2573 | 83

HUNTINGDON—Carroll County

☒ BAPTIST MEMORIAL HOSPITAL–HUNTINGDON, 631 R. B. Wilson Drive, Zip 38344-1675; tel. 901/986-4461; Susan M. Breeden, Administrator (Nonreporting) **A**1 9 10 **S** Baptist Memorial Health Care Corporation, Memphis, TN
Web address: www.bmhcc.org | 21 | 10 | 70 | — | — | — | — | — | — | —

JACKSON—Madison County

☒ △ JACKSON–MADISON COUNTY GENERAL HOSPITAL, 708 West Forest Avenue, Zip 38301-3855; tel. 901/425-5000; James T. Moss, President and Chief Executive Officer (Total facility includes 85 beds in nursing home-type unit) (Nonreporting) **A**1 2 3 5 7 9 10 **S** West Tennessee Healthcare, Jackson, TN
Web address: www.wth.net | 16 | 10 | 567 | — | — | — | — | — | — | —

☒ METHODIST LEBONHEUR HEALTHCARE–JACKSON, 367 Hospital Boulevard, Zip 38305-4518, Mailing Address: P.O. Box 3310, Zip 38303-0310; tel. 901/661-2000; Richard M. McCormick, Administrator **A**1 9 10 **F**3 4 8 9 11 12 13 14 16 17 18 19 22 24 25 26 27 32 34 36 37 39 41 43 44 45 46 47 48 50 51 54 58 59 60 61 62 63 64 65 70 71 76 78 79 **P**6 **S** Methodist Healthcare, Memphis, TN
Web address: www.regionalhospital.com | 21 | 10 | 120 | 4107 | 59 | 29849 | 257 | 41856 | 14217 | 386

★ PATHWAYS, (Formerly Pathways of Tennessee), 238 Summar Drive, Zip 38301-3982; tel. 901/935-8200; Karen Utley, Executive Director **A**10 **F**2 3 6 13 16 17 18 21 57 58 59 60 61 62 63 64 70 72 **S** West Tennessee Healthcare, Jackson, TN | 23 | 22 | 25 | 1220 | 19 | 74291 | 0 | 9415 | 8343 | 243

JAMESTOWN—Fentress County

□ FENTRESS COUNTY GENERAL HOSPITAL, Highway 52 West, Zip 38556, Mailing Address: P.O. Box 1500, Zip 38556; tel. 931/879-8171; Patrick J. Gray, Chief Executive Officer (Total facility includes 13 beds in nursing home-type unit) (Nonreporting) **A**1 9 10 **S** Paracelsus Healthcare Corporation, Houston, TX | 33 | 10 | 73 | — | — | — | — | — | — | —

JASPER—Marion County

☒ GRANDVIEW MEDICAL CENTER, 1000 Highway 28, Zip 37347; tel. 423/837-9500; Phil Rowland, Chief Executive Officer **A**1 9 10 **F**2 3 4 7 8 9 11 12 13 17 18 22 24 25 28 29 30 32 34 38 39 41 42 44 46 47 48 50 51 54 55 57 58 59 60 61 62 63 64 65 66 67 70 71 76 78 79 **S** HCA – The Healthcare Company, Nashville, TN
Web address: www.hcahealthcare.com | 33 | 10 | 50 | 2022 | 18 | 38984 | 204 | 18988 | 5822 | 204

JEFFERSON CITY—Jefferson County

□ JEFFERSON MEMORIAL HOSPITAL, 1800 Bishop Avenue, Zip 37760-1992, Mailing Address: P.O. Box 560, Zip 37760-0560; tel. 865/475-2091; Michael C. Hicks, President and Chief Executive Officer **A**1 9 10 **F**7 9 13 17 18 22 24 25 29 36 38 41 43 44 45 48 51 54 56 70 72 76 **S** Catholic Healthcare Partners, Cincinnati, OH
Web address: www.jeffersonhealthinc.com | 23 | 10 | 29 | 1792 | 19 | 42579 | 0 | 11819 | 5080 | 195

© 2000 AHA Guide *Many Facility Codes have changed. Please refer to the AHA Guide Code Chart.*

Hospitals, U.S. / TENNESSEE

Hospital, Address, Telephone, Administrator, Approval, Facility, and Physician Codes, Health Care System, Network

- ★ American Hospital Association (AHA) membership
- □ Joint Commission on Accreditation of Healthcare Organizations (JCAHO) accreditation
- + American Osteopathic Healthcare Association (AOHA) membership
- ○ American Osteopathic Association (AOA) accreditation
- △ Commission on Accreditation of Rehabilitation Facilities (CARF) accreditation

Control codes 61, 63, 64, 71, 72 and 73 indicate hospitals listed by AOHA, but not registered by AHA. For definition of numerical codes, see page A4

Hospital	Control	Service	Staffed Beds	Admissions	Census	Outpatient Visits	Births	Total	Payroll	Personnel
JELLICO—Campbell County										
★ JELLICO COMMUNITY HOSPITAL, 188 Hospital Lane, Zip 37762–4400; tel. 423/784–7252; Jimm Bunch, President and Chief Executive Officer **A**1 9 10 **F**7 8 11 13 16 17 18 19 21 22 23 24 25 32 36 37 39 41 44 45 48 51 54 70 73 76 78 **P**8 **S** Adventist Health System Sunbelt Health Care Corporation, Winter Park, FL Web address: www.ahss.org	23	10	54	2146	20	43716	249	16858	5774	241
JOHNSON CITY—Washington County										
★ JOHNSON CITY MEDICAL CENTER, 400 North State of Franklin Road, Zip 37604–6094; tel. 423/431–6111; Dennis Vonderfecht, President and Chief Executive Officer (Total facility includes 34 beds in nursing home–type unit) **A**1 2 3 5 8 9 10 **F**1 2 3 4 6 7 8 9 11 13 14 16 17 18 19 21 22 23 24 25 27 28 29 30 31 32 33 34 35 36 37 38 39 41 42 43 44 45 46 47 48 49 50 51 52 53 54 55 56 57 58 59 60 61 62 63 64 65 66 68 69 70 71 72 73 74 75 76 77 78 79 **P**5 7 8 **S** Mountain States Health Alliance, Johnson City, TN Web address: www.jcmc.com	23	10	410	19018	281	172154	1484	179357	68330	2697
□ JOHNSON CITY SPECIALTY HOSPITAL, 203 East Watauga Avenue, Zip 37601–4651; tel. 423/926–1111; Carolyn Gemmell, Director Operations and Chief Nursing Officer **A**1 9 10 **F**1 2 3 4 6 7 8 9 11 12 13 14 16 17 18 19 21 22 23 24 25 27 28 29 30 31 32 33 34 35 36 37 38 39 41 42 43 44 45 46 47 48 49 50 51 52 53 54 55 56 57 58 59 60 61 62 63 64 65 66 68 69 70 71 72 73 74 75 76 77 78 79 **P**5 7 8 **S** Mountain States Health Alliance, Johnson City, TN Web address: www.MSHA.com	23	45	49	1121	8	12396	675	6861	3189	107
□ △ QUILLEN REHABILITATION HOSPITAL, (Formerly James H. and Cecile C Quillen Rehabilitation Hospital), 2511 Wesley Street, Zip 37601–1723; tel. 423/283–0700; John Turner, Chief Executive Officer **A**1 7 9 **F**8 9 10 11 12 13 14 16 17 19 22 24 25 26 28 29 30 32 35 36 37 38 39 41 42 43 44 45 46 47 48 49 50 51 52 53 54 55 56 65 68 69 70 71 72 73 74 75 76 77 78 79 **P**3 5 7 8 **S** Mountain States Health Alliance, Johnson City, TN	23	46	60	817	31	52000	0	—	—	—
WOODRIDGE HOSPITAL, 403 State of Franklin Road, Zip 37604–6009, Mailing Address: P.O. Box 2226, Zip 37604–2226; tel. 423/928–7111; Donald Larkin, Ph.D., Administrator **A**3 5 9 10 **F**1 2 3 13 16 17 18 21 50 57 58 59 60 61 62 63 64 70 72 **P**6 Web address: www.frontierhealth.org	23	22	75	3704	55	0	0	6689	3561	134
KINGSPORT—Sullivan County										
□ HEALTHSOUTH REHABILITATION HOSPITAL, 113 Cassel Drive, Zip 37660–3775; tel. 423/246–7240; Terry R. Maxhimer, Administrator and Chief Executive Officer (Nonreporting) **A**1 9 10 **S** HEALTHSOUTH Corporation, Birmingham, AL Web address: www.healthsouth.com	33	46	50	—	—	—	—	—	—	—
□ INDIAN PATH MEDICAL CENTER, (Includes Indian Path Pavilion, 2300 Pavilion Drive, Zip 37660–4672; tel. 423/378–7500), 2000 Brookside Drive, Zip 37660–4604; tel. 423/392–7000; Randy Cook, Administrator and Chief Executive Officer (Total facility includes 30 beds in nursing home–type unit) **A**1 9 10 **F**1 2 3 4 6 7 8 9 11 13 14 16 17 18 19 21 22 23 24 25 26 27 28 29 30 31 32 33 34 35 36 37 38 39 41 42 43 44 45 46 47 48 49 50 51 52 53 54 56 57 58 59 60 61 62 63 64 65 66 68 69 70 71 72 73 74 75 76 77 78 79 **P**5 7 8 **S** Mountain States Health Alliance, Johnson City, TN	23	10	196	5229	85	89547	320	47922	17155	525
★ WELLMONT HOLSTON VALLEY MEDICAL CENTER, West Ravine Street, Zip 37662–0224, Mailing Address: Box 238, Zip 37662–0224; tel. 423/224–4000; Louis H. Bremer, President and Chief Executive Officer (Total facility includes 39 beds in nursing home–type unit) **A**1 2 3 5 9 10 **F**1 4 6 8 9 11 12 13 16 17 18 19 22 24 25 27 30 32 34 35 36 37 38 39 41 42 43 44 45 46 47 48 49 51 52 54 68 69 70 71 74 75 76 78 79 **P**5 **S** Wellmont Health System, Kingsport, TN Web address: www.wellmont.org	23	10	375	15621	216	200783	1726	168382	63933	1655
KNOXVILLE—Knox County										
★ △ BAPTIST HOSPITAL OF EAST TENNESSEE, 137 Blount Avenue S.E., Zip 37920–1643, Mailing Address: P.O. Box 1788, Zip 37901–1788; tel. 865/632–5011; Jon Foster, Executive Vice President and Administrator (Nonreporting) **A**1 2 7 9 10 **S** Baptist Health System of Tennessee, Knoxville, TN Web address: www.bhset.org	21	10	316	—	—	—	—	—	—	—
□ EAST TENNESSEE CHILDREN'S HOSPITAL, 2018 Clinch Avenue, Zip 37916–2393, Mailing Address: P.O. Box 15010, Zip 37901–5010; tel. 865/541–8000; Robert F. Koppel, President and Chief Executive Officer **A**1 9 10 **F**11 17 18 22 25 36 38 39 42 43 45 46 48 50 51 52 54 56 65 70 75 76 78 **P**8 Web address: www.etch.com	23	50	103	5111	71	90307	0	53178	25290	737
★ △ FORT SANDERS REGIONAL MEDICAL CENTER, 1901 Clinch Avenue S.W., Zip 37916–2394; tel. 865/541–1111; Richard Rose, M.D., President and Chief Administrative Officer (Total facility includes 24 beds in nursing home–type unit) **A**1 2 6 7 9 10 **F**2 3 4 7 8 9 11 12 13 16 17 18 19 20 21 22 24 25 27 28 29 30 31 32 33 34 35 36 37 38 39 41 43 44 45 46 47 48 49 50 51 53 54 57 58 59 60 61 62 63 64 65 66 68 69 70 71 72 73 76 77 78 79 **P**6 7 **S** Covenant Health, Knoxville, TN Web address: www.covenanthealth.com	23	10	422	13495	248	286883	2605	134834	54576	1764

Hospitals, U.S. / TENNESSEE

Hospital, Address, Telephone, Administrator, Approval, Facility, and Physician Codes, Health Care System, Network	Classification Codes		Utilization Data					Expense (thousands) of dollars		
★ American Hospital Association (AHA) membership ☐ Joint Commission on Accreditation of Healthcare Organizations (JCAHO) accreditation + American Osteopathic Healthcare Association (AOHA) membership ○ American Osteopathic Association (AOA) accreditation △ Commission on Accreditation of Rehabilitation Facilities (CARF) accreditation Control codes 61, 63, 64, 71, 72 and 73 indicate hospitals listed by AOHA, but not registered by AHA. For definition of numerical codes, see page A4	Control	Service	Staffed Beds	Admissions	Census	Outpatient Visits	Births	Total	Payroll	Personnel
★ FORT SANDERS–PARKWEST MEDICAL CENTER, 9352 Park West Boulevard, Zip 37923-4387, Mailing Address: P.O. Box 22993, Zip 37933-0993; tel. 865/693-5151; Wayne S. Heatherly, President and Chief Administrative Officer (Nonreporting) **A**1 2 9 10 **S** Covenant Health, Knoxville, TN **Web address:** www.covenanthealth.com	23	10	262	—	—	—	—	—	—	—
☐ LAKESHORE MENTAL HEALTH INSTITUTE, 5908 Lyons View Drive, Zip 37919-7598; tel. 865/450-5200; Richard Lee Thomas, Superintendent (Nonreporting) **A**1 10	12	22	277	—	—	—	—	—	—	—
☐ △ ST. MARY'S HEALTH SYSTEM, 900 East Oak Hill Avenue, Zip 37917-4556; tel. 865/545-8000; Richard C. Williams, President and Chief Executive Officer (Total facility includes 25 beds in nursing home–type unit) (Nonreporting) **A**1 2 3 7 9 10 **S** Catholic Healthcare Partners, Cincinnati, OH **Web address:** www.mercy.com/stmarys	21	10	300	—	—	—	—	—	—	—
★ UNIVERSITY OF TENNESSEE MEMORIAL HOSPITAL, 1924 Alcoa Highway, Zip 37920-6900; tel. 865/544-9000; Thomas M. Kish, Senior Vice President (Total facility includes 21 beds in nursing home–type unit) **A**1 2 3 9 10 **F**4 7 8 9 10 11 12 13 16 18 19 22 23 24 25 26 27 28 33 36 37 38 39 41 42 44 45 46 47 48 49 51 52 54 55 56 65 66 69 70 74 75 76 77 78 79 **P**5 6 7	12	10	443	19487	304	430340	3041	265456	113093	3292
LA FOLLETTE—Campbell County										
★ LA FOLLETTE MEDICAL CENTER, East Avenue, Zip 37766, Mailing Address: P.O. Box 1301, Zip 37766-1301; tel. 423/562-2211; Nicholas P. Lewis, Administrator (Total facility includes 98 beds in nursing home–type unit) **A**1 9 10 **F**12 17 18 22 24 25 29 31 32 36 43 45 48 69 70 72 76 78	14	10	165	2532	125	46256	0	13066	6685	481
LAFAYETTE—Macon County										
★ MACON COUNTY GENERAL HOSPITAL, 204 Medical Drive, Zip 37083-1799, Mailing Address: P.O. Box 378, Zip 37083-0378; tel. 615/666-2147; Dennis A. Wolford, FACHE, Administrator (Nonreporting) **A**1 9 10 **S** Quorum Health Group, Brentwood, TN	23	10	43	—	—	—	—	—	—	—
LAWRENCEBURG—Lawrence County										
★ CROCKETT HOSPITAL, U.S. Highway 43 South, Zip 38464-0847, Mailing Address: P.O. Box 847, Zip 38464-0847; tel. 931/762-6571; Jack S. Buck, Chief Executive Officer **A**1 9 10 **F**8 9 13 14 16 17 18 19 21 22 23 24 25 32 33 34 38 39 41 43 44 45 48 49 50 51 53 54 56 70 71 72 73 76 79 **P**7 **S** LifePoint Hospitals, Inc., Brentwood, TN **Web address:** www.crocketthospital.com	33	10	98	2970	34	41030	205	16262	6972	250
LEBANON—Wilson County										
★ UNIVERSITY MEDICAL CENTER/MCFARLAND HOSPITAL, (Includes McFarland Specialty Hospital, 500 Park Avenue, Zip 37087-3720; tel. 615/449-0500), 1411 Baddour Parkway, Zip 37087-2573; tel. 615/444-8262; Larry W. Keller, Chief Executive Officer (Total facility includes 12 beds in nursing home–type unit) **A**1 9 10 **F**7 8 9 11 13 17 22 23 24 25 34 36 39 41 44 45 46 48 49 51 53 54 57 59 60 61 62 64 65 68 69 70 71 72 76 78 79 **P**5 6 7 **S** TENET Healthcare Corporation, Santa Barbara, CA	33	10	225	7585	113	96792	815	65638	20488	672
LEWISBURG—Marshall County										
☐ MARSHALL MEDICAL CENTER, 1080 North Ellington Parkway, Zip 37091-2227, Mailing Address: P.O. Box 1609, Zip 37091-1609; tel. 931/359-6241; Steve C. Hoelscher, Administrator **A**1 9 10 **F**9 13 16 17 18 22 24 25 32 34 37 38 39 41 48 70 71 74 76 78	33	10	77	1160	12	29793	2	10216	4314	147
LEXINGTON—Henderson County										
★ METHODIST HEALTHCARE–LEXINGTON HOSPITAL, 200 West Church Street, Zip 38351-2014; tel. 901/968-3646; Eugene Ragghianti, Administrator (Nonreporting) **A**1 9 10 **S** Methodist Healthcare, Memphis, TN **Web address:** www.methodisthealth.org	21	10	32	—	—	—	—	—	—	—
LINDEN—Perry County										
PERRY COMMUNITY HOSPITAL, (Formerly Baptist Perry Community Hospital), 805 Squirrel Hollow Road, Zip 37096; tel. 931/589-2121; Gary C. Morse, Chief Executive Officer and Administrator (Nonreporting) **A**9 10	23	10	53	—	—	—	—	—	—	—
LIVINGSTON—Overton County										
★ LIVINGSTON REGIONAL HOSPITAL, 315 Oak Street, Zip 38570, Mailing Address: P.O. Box 550, Zip 38570-0550; tel. 931/823-5611; Timothy W. McGill, Chief Executive Officer (Total facility includes 15 beds in nursing home–type unit) (Nonreporting) **A**1 9 10 **S** LifePoint Hospitals, Inc., Brentwood, TN	33	10	85	—	—	—	—	—	—	—
LOUDON—Loudon County										
★ FORT SANDERS LOUDON MEDICAL CENTER, 1125 Grove Street, Zip 37774-1512, Mailing Address: P.O. Box 217, Zip 37774-0217; tel. 865/458-8222; Martha O'Regan Chill, Administrator **A**1 9 10 **F**8 9 17 18 22 25 32 34 36 37 39 41 43 44 45 48 51 54 61 63 68 70 76 78 **S** Covenant Health, Knoxville, TN **Web address:** www.covenanthealth.com	23	10	50	1253	10	36144	1	—	—	165
LOUISVILLE—Blount County										
PENINSULA HOSPITAL, 2347 Jones Bend Road, Zip 37777-5213, Mailing Address: P.O. Box 2000, Zip 37777-2000; tel. 865/970-9800; Barbara S. Blevins, President (Nonreporting) **A**9 10	33	22	159	—	—	—	—	—	—	—
MADISON—Davidson County										
★ NASHVILLE MEMORIAL HOSPITAL, 612 West Due West Avenue, Zip 37115-4474; tel. 615/865-3511; Allyn R. Harris, Chief Executive Officer (Nonreporting) **A**1 2 5 9 10 **S** HCA – The Healthcare Company, Nashville, TN **Web address:** www.hcahealthcare.com	33	10	250	—	—	—	—	—	—	—

Hospitals, U.S. / TENNESSEE

Hospital, Address, Telephone, Administrator, Approval, Facility, and Physician Codes, Health Care System, Network

- ★ American Hospital Association (AHA) membership
- □ Joint Commission on Accreditation of Healthcare Organizations (JCAHO) accreditation
- + American Osteopathic Healthcare Association (AOHA) membership
- ○ American Osteopathic Association (AOA) accreditation
- △ Commission on Accreditation of Rehabilitation Facilities (CARF) accreditation

Control codes 61, 63, 64, 71, 72 and 73 indicate hospitals listed by AOHA, but not registered by AHA. For definition of numerical codes, see page A4

Hospital	Classification Codes		Utilization Data					Expense (thousands) of dollars		
	Control	Service	Staffed Beds	Admissions	Census	Outpatient Visits	Births	Total	Payroll	Personnel
★ △ TENNESSEE CHRISTIAN MEDICAL CENTER, (Includes Tennessee Christian Medical Center – Portland, 105 Redbud Drive, Portland, Zip 37148), 500 Hospital Drive, Zip 37115–5032; tel. 615/865–2373; Clint Kreitner, President and Chief Executive Officer (Total facility includes 50 beds in nursing home–type unit) (Nonreporting) **A**1 7 9 10 **S** Adventist Health System Sunbelt Health Care Corporation, Winter Park, FL	21	10	288	—	—	—	—	—	—	—
MANCHESTER—Coffee County										
COFFEE MEDICAL CENTER, 1001 McArthur Drive, Zip 37355–2455, Mailing Address: P.O. Box 1079, Zip 37349–1079; tel. 931/728–3586; James L. Muse, Administrator (Total facility includes 72 beds in nursing home–type unit) **A**9 10 **F**9 19 22 25 30 37 38 45 48 54 69 70 72 76	16	10	108	816	76	12478	0	4105	1782	90
★ ○ MEDICAL CENTER OF MANCHESTER, 481 Interstate Drive, Zip 37355–3108, Mailing Address: P.O. Box 1409, Zip 37349–1409; tel. 931/728–6354; Robert C. Couch, Chief Executive Officer (Nonreporting) **A**9 10 11 **S** TENET Healthcare Corporation, Santa Barbara, CA	33	10	49	—	—	—	—	—	—	—
MARTIN—Weakley County										
★ METHODIST HEALTHCARE–VOLUNTEER HOSPITAL, 161 Mount Pelia Road, Zip 38237–0967, Mailing Address: P.O. Box 967, Zip 38237–0967; tel. 901/587–4261; Eugene Ragghianti, Administrator (Nonreporting) **A**1 9 10 **S** Methodist Healthcare, Memphis, TN Web address: www.methodisthealth.org	33	10	65	—	—	—	—	—	—	—
MARYVILLE—Blount County										
★ BLOUNT MEMORIAL HOSPITAL, 907 East Lamar Alexander Parkway, Zip 37804–5016; tel. 423/983–7211; Joseph M. Dawson, Administrator (Total facility includes 50 beds in nursing home–type unit) **A**1 2 6 9 10 **F**2 3 4 8 9 11 12 13 14 16 17 18 19 21 22 24 25 27 28 29 32 33 34 35 36 37 38 39 41 43 44 45 46 48 51 54 57 59 60 61 63 64 65 68 69 70 71 72 75 76 78 **P**8	13	10	173	7576	87	151608	610	78477	34034	1180
MCKENZIE—Carroll County										
★ METHODIST HEALTHCARE – MCKENZIE, 161 Hospital Drive, Zip 38201–1636; tel. 901/352–5344; Richard M. McCormick, Administrator **A**1 9 10 **F**8 9 17 18 22 25 28 31 32 34 36 43 44 45 46 48 51 54 70 71 76 78 **S** Methodist Healthcare, Memphis, TN Web address: www.methodisthealth.org	21	10	29	938	8	16472	301	6383	2829	98
MCMINNVILLE—Warren County										
★ RIVER PARK HOSPITAL, 1559 Sparta Road, Zip 37110–1316; tel. 931/815–4000; Terry J. Gunn, Chief Executive Officer (Nonreporting) **A**1 9 10 **S** HCA – The Healthcare Company, Nashville, TN Web address: www.hcahealthcare.com	33	10	90	—	—	—	—	—	—	—
MEMPHIS—Shelby County										
★ BAPTIST MEMORIAL HOSPITAL, (Includes Baptist Memorial Hospital East, 6019 Walnut Grove Road, Zip 38119; tel. 901/226–5000; Baptist Memorial Hospital Rehabilitation Center; Baptist Memorial Hospital–Collierville, 1500 West Poplar Avenue, Collierville, Zip 38017; tel. 901/227–8140; James Vandersteeg, Vice President and Administrator), 899 Madison Avenue, Zip 38146–0002; tel. 901/227–2727; Stephen Curtis Reynolds, President and Chief Executive Officer (Total facility includes 28 beds in nursing home–type unit) **A**1 2 3 5 6 9 10 **F**4 7 8 9 11 12 13 14 16 17 18 19 21 22 24 25 27 28 29 30 32 34 36 37 38 39 41 42 43 44 45 46 47 48 49 53 54 55 56 57 58 62 63 65 68 69 70 71 72 74 75 76 77 78 79 **P**1 2 3 4 5 6 7 8 **S** Baptist Memorial Health Care Corporation, Memphis, TN Web address: www.baptistonline.org	21	10	1054	47823	841	247478	5948	445915	151594	4476
□ CHARTER LAKESIDE BEHAVIORAL HEALTH SYSTEM, 2911 Brunswick Road, Zip 38133–4199, Mailing Address: P.O. Box 341308, Zip 38134–1308; tel. 901/377–4700; Rob S. Waggener, Chief Executive Officer (Nonreporting) **A**1 9 10 **S** Magellan Health Services, Atlanta, GA	33	22	174	—	—	—	—	—	—	—
□ DELTA MEDICAL CENTER, 3000 Getwell Road, Zip 38118–2299; tel. 901/369–8500; Craig B. Watson, Chief Executive Officer (Nonreporting) **A**1 9 10	33	10	209	—	—	—	—	—	—	—
□ HEALTHSOUTH REHABILITATION HOSPITAL, 1282 Union Avenue, Zip 38104–3414; tel. 901/722–2000; Jerry Gray, Administrator **A**1 9 10 **F**5 13 18 22 24 25 36 38 39 50 53 54 55 63 68 70 76 **S** HEALTHSOUTH Corporation, Birmingham, AL Web address: www.healthsouth.com	32	46	80	1614	79	16760	0	14288	6696	237
LE BONHEUR CHILDREN'S MEDICAL CENTER See Methodist Healthcare–Memphis Hospital										
□ MEMPHIS MENTAL HEALTH INSTITUTE, 865 Poplar Avenue, Zip 38105–4626, Mailing Address: P.O. Box 40966, Zip 38174–0966; tel. 901/524–1201; Thomas V. Sellars, Superintendent **A**1 5 10 **F**16 17 18 57	12	22	98	2010	102	0	0	15340	8722	296

Hospitals, U.S. / TENNESSEE

Hospital, Address, Telephone, Administrator, Approval, Facility, and Physician Codes, Health Care System, Network	Classification Codes		Utilization Data					Expense (thousands) of dollars		
★ American Hospital Association (AHA) membership □ Joint Commission on Accreditation of Healthcare Organizations (JCAHO) accreditation + American Osteopathic Healthcare Association (AOHA) membership ○ American Osteopathic Association (AOA) accreditation △ Commission on Accreditation of Rehabilitation Facilities (CARF) accreditation Control codes 61, 63, 64, 71, 72 and 73 indicate hospitals listed by AOHA, but not registered by AHA. For definition of numerical codes, see page A4	Control	Service	Staffed Beds	Admissions	Census	Outpatient Visits	Births	Total	Payroll	Personnel
★ METHODIST HEALTHCARE–MEMPHIS HOSPITAL, (Includes Le Bonheur Children's Medical Center, One Children's Plaza, Zip 38103–2893; tel. 901/572–3000; James E. Shmerling, President; Methodist Hospital Germantown, 7691 Poplar, Germantown, Zip 38138, Mailing Address: P.O. Box 381588, Zip 38138; tel. 901/754–6418; David G. Baytos, Administrator; Methodist Hospitals of Memphis–Central, 1265 Union Avenue, Zip 38104; Methodist Hospitals of Memphis–South Unit, 1300 Wesley Drive, Zip 38116; tel. 901/346–3700; Cecelia Sawyer, Administrator; Methodist North–J. Harris Hospital, 3960 New Covington Pike, Zip 38128; tel. 901/372–5200), 1265 Union Avenue, Zip 38104–3499; tel. 901/726–7000; David L. Ramsey, President (Total facility includes 24 beds in nursing home–type unit) **A**1 2 3 5 6 9 10 **F**2 3 4 5 7 8 9 11 12 13 14 17 18 19 21 22 23 24 25 27 28 29 30 31 32 34 35 36 37 38 39 41 42 43 44 45 46 47 48 49 50 51 52 54 56 57 58 59 60 62 63 64 65 66 68 69 70 71 72 74 75 76 77 78 79 **P**6 7 8 **S** Methodist Healthcare, Memphis, TN **Web address:** www.methodisthealth.org	23	10	1272	56855	892	411513	7267	525816	222553	6881
□ REGIONAL MEDICAL CENTER AT MEMPHIS, 877 Jefferson Avenue, Zip 38103–2897; tel. 901/545–7100; Bruce W. Steinhauer, M.D., President and Chief Executive Officer (Nonreporting) **A**1 2 3 5 6 8 9 10 **Web address:** www.the-med.org	23	10	361	—	—	—	—	—	—	—
★ SAINT FRANCIS HOSPITAL, 5959 Park Avenue, Zip 38119–5198, Mailing Address: P.O. Box 171808, Zip 38187–1808; tel. 901/765–1000; David L. Archer, Chief Executive Officer (Total facility includes 42 beds in nursing home–type unit) **A**1 2 3 5 9 10 **F**2 3 4 7 8 9 11 12 13 16 18 22 24 25 28 30 31 32 34 35 36 37 38 39 41 44 46 47 48 50 51 53 54 57 58 62 64 65 68 69 70 71 72 75 76 78 79 **P**5 7 8 **S** TENET Healthcare Corporation, Santa Barbara, CA **Web address:** www.tenethealth.com/saintfrancis	33	10	503	18681	341	173544	1246	155808	57467	1539
★ ST. JUDE CHILDREN'S RESEARCH HOSPITAL, (PEDIATRIC HEMATOLOGY–ONCOLOGY), 332 North Lauderdale Street, Zip 38105–2794; tel. 901/495–3300; Arthur W. Nienhuis, M.D., Director **A**1 2 3 5 9 10 **F**7 18 21 22 23 24 35 38 39 43 46 48 49 50 51 52 54 59 61 65 68 70 72 74 76 78 **P**6 **Web address:** www.stjude.org	23	59	54	2207	42	41517	—	188005	80740	2023
□ UNIVERSITY OF TENNESSEE BOWLD HOSPITAL, 951 Court Avenue, Zip 38103–2898; tel. 901/448–4000; Jeffrey R. Woodside, M.D., Executive Director **A**1 2 3 5 9 10 **F**4 11 12 22 23 24 25 27 30 35 38 39 41 43 46 47 48 51 55 59 65 66 68 70 74 76 78	12	10	101	3394	65	21036	0	50545	17232	530
★ VETERANS AFFAIRS MEDICAL CENTER, 1030 Jefferson Avenue, Zip 38104–2193; tel. 901/523–8990; K. L. Mulholland, Jr, Director **A**1 2 3 5 8 **F**1 3 4 5 6 7 8 9 11 12 13 15 16 17 18 19 21 22 23 24 25 26 27 30 31 32 33 34 35 36 37 38 39 41 43 46 47 48 49 50 51 54 56 57 59 60 61 62 63 64 65 69 70 72 74 75 76 78 79 **P**6 **S** Department of Veterans Affairs, Washington, DC **Web address:** www.va.gov/stations97/guide/home.asp?DIVISION=ALL	45	10	293	7150	211	—	0	154371	77625	1772
MILAN—Gibson County										
★ MILAN GENERAL HOSPITAL, 4039 South Highland, Zip 38358; tel. 901/686–1591; Alfred P. Taylor, Administrator and Chief Executive Officer (Total facility includes 13 beds in nursing home–type unit) **A**1 9 10 **F**9 16 17 18 22 38 45 48 54 57 62 69 70 71 76 78 **S** West Tennessee Healthcare, Jackson, TN **Web address:** www.wth.net	16	10	62	986	25	12602	0	6058	1090	85
MORRISTOWN—Hamblen County										
□ △ LAKEWAY REGIONAL HOSPITAL, 726 McFarland Street, Zip 37814–3990; tel. 423/586–2302; Michael I. Terry, Chief Executive Officer (Nonreporting) **A**1 7 9 10 **S** Community Health Systems, Inc., Brentwood, TN	33	10	135	—	—	—	—	—	—	—
□ MORRISTOWN–HAMBLEN HOSPITAL, 908 West Fourth North Street, Zip 37816–1178, Mailing Address: P.O. Box 1178, Zip 37816–1178; tel. 423/586–4231; Richard L. Clark, Administrator and Chief Executive Officer (Nonreporting) **A**1 9 10 **Web address:** www.mhhs1.org	23	10	143	—	—	—	—	—	—	—
MOUNTAIN HOME—Washington County										
★ JAMES H. QUILLEN VETERANS AFFAIRS MEDICAL CENTER, Zip 37684–4000; tel. 423/926–1171; Carl J. Gerber, M.D., Ph.D., Director (Total facility includes 120 beds in nursing home–type unit) (Nonreporting) **A**1 2 3 5 8 9 **S** Department of Veterans Affairs, Washington, DC	45	10	390	—	—	—	—	—	—	—
MURFREESBORO—Rutherford County										
★ ALVIN C. YORK VETERANS AFFAIRS MEDICAL CENTER, 3400 Lebanon Pike, Zip 37129–1236; tel. 615/867–6100; Lea Swafford, Acting Director (Total facility includes 135 beds in nursing home–type unit) **A**1 3 5 9 **F**1 3 4 7 9 11 12 13 18 22 23 24 25 27 28 29 30 31 32 33 34 35 36 37 38 39 41 43 45 46 47 48 49 50 51 53 54 55 56 57 59 61 62 63 64 65 68 69 70 72 75 76 78 79 **P**6 **S** Department of Veterans Affairs, Washington, DC **Web address:** www.va.gov/murfreesboro	45	10	372	3794	338	188184	0	84443	48244	1301
★ MIDDLE TENNESSEE MEDICAL CENTER, 400 North Highland Avenue, Zip 37130–3854, Mailing Address: P.O. Box 1178, Zip 37133–1178; tel. 615/849–4100; Arthur W. Hastings, President and Chief Executive Officer **A**1 9 10 **F**1 4 7 8 9 10 11 12 13 17 18 19 22 23 24 27 28 30 31 32 33 34 35 36 37 38 39 41 43 44 45 46 48 49 50 51 54 64 65 70 71 72 74 75 76 78 79 **Web address:** www.mtmc.org	21	10	184	10941	117	138614	1944	77497	31287	813

Hospitals, U.S. / TENNESSEE

Hospital, Address, Telephone, Administrator, Approval, Facility, and Physician Codes, Health Care System, Network	Classification Codes		Utilization Data					Expense (thousands) of dollars		
	Control	Service	Staffed Beds	Admissions	Census	Outpatient Visits	Births	Total	Payroll	Personnel

★ American Hospital Association (AHA) membership
☐ Joint Commission on Accreditation of Healthcare Organizations (JCAHO) accreditation
+ American Osteopathic Healthcare Association (AOHA) membership
○ American Osteopathic Association (AOA) accreditation
△ Commission on Accreditation of Rehabilitation Facilities (CARF) accreditation
Control codes 61, 63, 64, 71, 72 and 73 indicate hospitals listed by AOHA, but not registered by AHA. For definition of numerical codes, see page A4

Hospital	Control	Service	Staffed Beds	Admissions	Census	Outpatient Visits	Births	Total	Payroll	Personnel
NASHVILLE—Davidson County										
★ BAPTIST HOSPITAL, 2000 Church Street, Zip 37236-0002; tel. 615/329-5555; Erie Chapman, II, President and Chief Executive Officer (Nonreporting) **A**1 2 3 5 9 10 Web address: www.baptist-hosp.org/	23	10	545	—	—	—	—	—	—	—
★ △ CENTENNIAL MEDICAL CENTER AND PARTHENON PAVILION, 2300 Patterson Street, Zip 37203-1528; tel. 615/342-1000; Lawrence Kloess, President (Total facility includes 24 beds in nursing home-type unit) (Nonreporting) **A**1 2 3 5 7 9 10 **S** HCA - The Healthcare Company, Nashville, TN Web address: www.hcahealthcare.com	33	10	680	—	—	—	—	—	—	—
★ METROPOLITAN NASHVILLE GENERAL HOSPITAL, 1818 Albion Street, Zip 37208; tel. 615/341-4000; Roxane Stitzer, Ph.D., Chief Executive Officer (Nonreporting) **A**1 2 3 5 6 9 10	15	10	105	—	—	—	—	—	—	—
☐ MIDDLE TENNESSEE MENTAL HEALTH INSTITUTE, 221 Stewarts Ferry Pike, Zip 37214-3325; tel. 615/902-7535; Joseph W. Carobene, Superintendent **A**1 3 10 **F**16 17 18 24 43 45 49 50 57 58 59 60 61 62 70 78	12	22	283	2430	208	0	0	30179	18473	670
★ NASHVILLE METROPOLITAN BORDEAUX HOSPITAL, 1414 County Hospital Road, Zip 37218-3001; tel. 615/862-7000; Richard D. Alston, Administrator (Total facility includes 525 beds in nursing home-type unit) **A**10 **F**17 23 30 31 32 45 51 69 70 72 78	23	48	565	661	484	0	0	32065	19726	563
☐ △ NASHVILLE REHABILITATION HOSPITAL, 610 Gallatin Avenue, Zip 37206-3225; tel. 615/226-4330; Jane Andrews, Chief Executive Officer **A**1 7 10 **F**13 16 22 25 31 39 45 53 54 57 62 70 72 76 78	33	46	46	697	32	4472	0	9246	4668	128
☐ PSYCHIATRIC HOSPITAL AT VANDERBILT, 1601 23rd Avenue South, Zip 37212-3198; tel. 615/320-7770; Lynn E. Webb, Chief Executive Officer and Administrator **A**1 3 10 **F**2 3 17 18 19 22 24 25 39 55 57 58 59 60 61 63 64 68 70 75 76	23	22	88	2765	54	6192	0	10825	5696	148
★ SOUTHERN HILLS MEDICAL CENTER, 391 Wallace Road, Zip 37211-4859; tel. 615/781-4000; Jeffrey Whitehorn, Chief Executive Officer (Total facility includes 20 beds in nursing home-type unit) **A**1 9 10 **F**1 2 3 4 5 8 9 11 12 13 14 16 17 18 19 20 21 22 23 24 25 26 27 28 29 30 32 33 34 35 37 39 41 42 43 44 45 46 47 48 50 51 53 54 56 57 58 59 60 61 63 64 68 69 70 71 72 74 75 76 77 78 79 **P**7 **S** HCA - The Healthcare Company, Nashville, TN Web address: www.hcahealthcare.com	33	10	140	6485	83	72161	1096	48277	22897	597
★ ST. THOMAS HEALTH SERVICES, 4220 Harding Road, Zip 37205-2095, Mailing Address: P.O. Box 380, Zip 37202-0380; tel. 615/222-2111; Thomas E. Beeman, President and Chief Executive Officer **A**1 2 3 5 9 10 **F**4 7 8 9 11 12 13 16 17 19 22 24 25 28 29 31 32 33 34 35 36 38 39 43 45 46 47 48 50 51 54 57 59 62 63 64 65 67 **P**3 5 6 7 **S** Ascension Health, Saint Louis, MO	21	10	523	27807	399	150407	884	289736	118512	3475
★ VANDERBILT UNIVERSITY HOSPITAL, 1161 21st Avenue South, Zip 37232; tel. 615/322-5000; Mark L. Penkhus, Chief Executive Officer (Total facility includes 23 beds in nursing home-type unit) (Nonreporting) **A**1 2 3 5 8 9 10 Web address: www.mc.vanderbilt.edu	23	10	576	—	—	—	—	—	—	—
★ VETERANS AFFAIRS MEDICAL CENTER, 1310 24th Avenue South, Zip 37212-2637; tel. 615/327-4751; William A. Mountcastle, Director **A**1 2 3 5 8 9 **F**1 2 3 4 9 11 13 18 19 21 22 23 24 25 26 29 30 31 32 33 34 35 36 37 38 39 41 43 44 45 46 47 48 49 50 51 53 54 55 56 57 61 62 63 64 65 68 69 70 72 74 76 78 79 **P**6 **S** Department of Veterans Affairs, Washington, DC Web address: www.nashville.med.va.gov	45	10	137	6046	123	232659	0	135838	51364	1497
NEWPORT—Cocke County										
☐ BAPTIST HOSPITAL OF COCKE COUNTY, 435 Second Street, Zip 37821-3799; tel. 423/625-2200; Wayne Buckner, Administrator (Total facility includes 56 beds in nursing home-type unit) (Nonreporting) **A**1 9 10 **S** Baptist Health System of Tennessee, Knoxville, TN Web address: www.baptistoneword.org/	21	10	109	—	—	—	—	—	—	—
OAK RIDGE—Anderson County										
☐ METHODIST MEDICAL CENTER OF OAK RIDGE, 990 Oak Ridge Turnpike, Zip 37830-6976, Mailing Address: P.O. Box 2529, Zip 37831-2529; tel. 865/481-1000; George A. Mathews, President and Chief Administrative Officer **A**1 2 9 10 **F**2 3 4 7 8 9 11 12 13 16 17 18 19 20 21 22 25 26 29 32 33 34 36 37 38 39 41 43 44 45 46 47 48 49 50 51 53 54 57 61 63 65 66 71 72 76 77 78 79 **S** Covenant Health, Knoxville, TN Web address: www.mmcoakridge.com	23	10	290	12723	169	156358	1177	103826	41217	—
RIDGEVIEW PSYCHIATRIC HOSPITAL AND CENTER, 240 West Tyrone Road, Zip 37830-6571; tel. 423/482-1076; Robert J. Benning, Chief Executive Officer (Nonreporting) **A**10	23	22	20	—	—	—	—	—	—	—
ONEIDA—Scott County										
☐ SCOTT COUNTY HOSPITAL, 18797 Alberta Avenue, Zip 37841-4939, Mailing Address: P.O. Box 4939, Zip 37841-4939; tel. 423/569-8521; Peter T. Petruzzi, Chief Executive Officer **A**1 9 10 **F**2 3 7 8 9 12 13 17 18 21 22 25 32 41 44 45 48 51 53 54 57 58 60 63 64 69 70 71 76 78 **S** Community Health Systems, Inc., Brentwood, TN Web address: www.scottcountyhospital.com	33	10	77	2790	28	19863	20	9809	4790	176
PARIS—Henry County										
★ HENRY COUNTY MEDICAL CENTER, 301 Tyson Avenue, Zip 38242-4544, Mailing Address: Box 1030, Zip 38242-1030; tel. 901/642-1220; Thomas H. Gee, Administrator (Total facility includes 174 beds in nursing home-type unit) **A**1 9 10 **F**7 8 9 12 11 18 22 23 24 25 27 28 30 31 32 34 36 37 38 39 41 43 44 45 46 48 51 54 57 58 59 60 61 62 64 65 68 69 70 71 72 74 76 78 **P**5 Web address: www.hcmc-tn.org	16	10	269	4493	220	62801	378	31656	15042	582

Hospitals, U.S. / TENNESSEE

Hospital, Address, Telephone, Administrator, Approval, Facility, and Physician Codes, Health Care System, Network	Classification Codes		Utilization Data					Expense (thousands) of dollars		
★ American Hospital Association (AHA) membership □ Joint Commission on Accreditation of Healthcare Organizations (JCAHO) accreditation + American Osteopathic Healthcare Association (AOHA) membership ○ American Osteopathic Association (AOA) accreditation △ Commission on Accreditation of Rehabilitation Facilities (CARF) accreditation Control codes 61, 63, 64, 71, 72 and 73 indicate hospitals listed by AOHA, but not registered by AHA. For definition of numerical codes, see page A4	Control	Service	Staffed Beds	Admissions	Census	Outpatient Visits	Births	Total	Payroll	Personnel
PARSONS—Decatur County										
□ DECATUR COUNTY GENERAL HOSPITAL, 969 Tennessee Avenue South, Zip 38363–0250, Mailing Address: Box 250, Zip 38363–0250; tel. 901/847–3031; Larry N. Lindsey, Administrator and Chief Executive Officer (Nonreporting) A1 9 10	13	10	40	—	—	—	—	—	—	—
PIKEVILLE—Bledsoe County										
□ BLEDSOE COMMUNITY MEDICAL CENTER, (Formerly Bledsoe County General Hospital), 128 Wheelertown Road, Zip 37367, Mailing Address: P.O. Box 699, Zip 37367–0699; tel. 423/447–2112; Keith Smith, Chief Executive Officer (Nonreporting) A1 9 10 S Associates Capital Group, LLC, Birmingham, AL	33	10	26	—	—	—	—	—	—	—
PORTLAND—Sumner County										
TENNESSEE CHRISTIAN MEDICAL CENTER – PORTLAND See Tennessee Christian Medical Center, Madison										
PULASKI—Giles County										
★ HILLSIDE HOSPITAL, 1265 East College Street, Zip 38478–4541; tel. 931/363–7531; James H. Edmondson, Chief Executive Officer and Administrator A1 9 10 F8 9 11 14 17 18 19 20 22 24 25 30 31 32 34 38 39 41 43 44 45 46 48 50 54 62 70 71 72 76 78 P7 S LifePoint Hospitals, Inc., Brentwood, TN	33	10	86	2408	26	27683	156	12601	5818	89
RIPLEY—Lauderdale County										
★ BAPTIST MEMORIAL HOSPITAL–LAUDERDALE, 326 Asbury Road, Zip 38063–9701; tel. 901/221–2200; Zach Chandler, Administrator A1 9 10 F2 3 7 9 17 18 22 25 30 32 34 36 37 38 41 43 48 50 51 54 57 58 59 60 61 62 63 64 70 76 78 S Baptist Memorial Health Care Corporation, Memphis, TN Web address: www.baptistonline.org	21	10	60	943	13	18985	0	8874	3419	133
ROGERSVILLE—Hawkins County										
★ HAWKINS COUNTY MEMORIAL HOSPITAL, 851 Locust Street, Zip 37857; tel. 423/272–2671; R. Frank Testerman, Administrator A1 9 10 F9 17 19 22 25 32 34 36 39 48 50 54 69 70 74 76 78	13	10	50	977	11	34456	0	6747	3133	146
SAVANNAH—Hardin County										
□ HARDIN COUNTY GENERAL HOSPITAL, 2006 Wayne Road, Zip 38372–2294; tel. 901/925–4954; Charlotte Burns, Administrator and Chief Executive Officer (Total facility includes 73 beds in nursing home–type unit) A1 9 10 F8 9 16 17 22 24 25 32 34 36 43 44 46 48 51 54 56 68 69 70 76 78	13	10	123	1591	86	58466	117	8802	5298	260
SELMER—McNairy County										
★ METHODIST HEALTHCARE–MCNAIRY HOSPITAL, 705 East Poplar Avenue, Zip 38375–1748; tel. 901/645–3221; John R. Borden, Administrator A1 9 10 F7 8 9 19 22 24 25 31 32 36 37 38 43 44 46 48 50 51 54 58 59 70 76 78 S Methodist Healthcare, Memphis, TN Web address: www.methodisthealth.org	21	10	48	1526	16	23640	243	8286	3827	162
SEVIERVILLE—Sevier County										
★ FORT SANDERS–SEVIER MEDICAL CENTER, 709 Middle Creek Road, Zip 37862–5016, Mailing Address: P.O. Box 8005, Zip 37864–8005; tel. 865/429–6100; Ellen Wilhoit, President and Chief Administrative Officer (Total facility includes 54 beds in nursing home–type unit) A1 9 10 F3 4 7 8 9 11 13 17 18 19 21 22 24 25 26 27 28 30 32 34 35 36 37 38 39 41 43 44 45 46 47 48 50 54 58 62 63 66 68 69 70 71 72 73 76 78 79 P7 S Covenant Health, Knoxville, TN Web address: www.covenanthealth.com	23	10	104	2742	80	72933	582	22120	8940	344
SEWANEE—Franklin County										
EMERALD–HODGSON HOSPITAL See Southern Tennessee Medical Center, Winchester										
SHELBYVILLE—Bedford County										
★ BEDFORD COUNTY MEDICAL CENTER, 845 Union Street, Zip 37160–9971; tel. 931/685–5433; David M. Snyder, Chief Executive Officer (Total facility includes 107 beds in nursing home–type unit) (Nonreporting) A1 9 10 S Quorum Health Group, Brentwood, TN	13	10	180	—	—	—	—	—	—	—
SMITHVILLE—DeKalb County										
★ BAPTIST DEKALB HOSPITAL, 520 West Main Street, Zip 37166–0840, Mailing Address: P.O. Box 640, Zip 37166–0640; tel. 615/597–7171; Dennis Smock, Chief Executive Officer A1 9 10 F8 9 13 17 18 19 21 22 25 30 32 33 34 39 41 43 44 46 48 51 54 62 69 70 76 78	32	10	52	1713	16	15250	43	10226	4129	146
SOMERVILLE—Fayette County										
★ METHODIST HEALTHCARE–SOMERVILLE, (Formerly Methodist Healthcare–Fayette Hospital), 214 Lakeview Drive, Zip 38068; tel. 901/465–0532; Michael Blome', Administrator A1 9 10 F1 2 3 4 5 6 7 8 9 10 11 12 13 14 15 16 17 18 19 20 21 22 24 25 26 27 28 29 30 31 32 33 34 35 36 37 38 39 40 41 42 43 44 45 46 47 48 49 50 51 52 53 54 55 56 57 58 59 60 61 62 63 64 65 66 67 68 69 70 71 72 73 74 75 76 77 78 79 P1 2 4 5 6 7 8 S Methodist Healthcare, Memphis, TN Web address: www.methodisthealth.org	21	10	38	799	85	7422	80	3815	3110	96
SPARTA—White County										
□ WHITE COUNTY COMMUNITY HOSPITAL, 401 Sewell Road, Zip 38583–1299; tel. 931/738–9211; Mark Cain, Chief Executive Officer (Nonreporting) A1 9 10 S Community Health Systems, Inc., Brentwood, TN	33	10	60	—	—	—	—	—	—	—
SPRINGFIELD—Robertson County										
□ NORTH CREST MEDICAL CENTER, 100 North Crest Drive, Zip 37172–2984; tel. 615/384–2411; William A. Kenley, President A1 9 10 F4 7 8 9 11 13 16 17 18 22 25 32 34 36 37 39 44 45 48 50 51 54 59 63 70 72 76 77 78 79 P6 Web address: www.hcahealthcare.com	23	10	100	3884	47	56509	516	32583	12088	373

© 2000 AHA Guide   *Many Facility Codes have changed. Please refer to the AHA Guide Code Chart.*

Hospitals, U.S. / TENNESSEE

Hospital, Address, Telephone, Administrator, Approval, Facility, and Physician Codes, Health Care System, Network	Classification Codes		Utilization Data					Expense (thousands) of dollars		Personnel
	Control	Service	Staffed Beds	Admissions	Census	Outpatient Visits	Births	Total	Payroll	

- ★ American Hospital Association (AHA) membership
- ☐ Joint Commission on Accreditation of Healthcare Organizations (JCAHO) accreditation
- + American Osteopathic Healthcare Association (AOHA) membership
- ○ American Osteopathic Association (AOA) accreditation
- △ Commission on Accreditation of Rehabilitation Facilities (CARF) accreditation

Control codes 61, 63, 64, 71, 72 and 73 indicate hospitals listed by AOHA, but not registered by AHA. For definition of numerical codes, see page A4

Hospital	Control	Service	Staffed Beds	Admissions	Census	Outpatient Visits	Births	Total	Payroll	Personnel
SWEETWATER—Monroe County ★ SWEETWATER HOSPITAL, 304 Wright Street, Zip 37874–2897; tel. 423/337–6171; Scott Bowman, Administrator (Nonreporting) A1 9 10	23	10	59	—	—	—	—	—	—	—
TAZEWELL—Claiborne County ★ CLAIBORNE COUNTY HOSPITAL, 1850 Old Knoxville Road, Zip 37879–3625, Mailing Address: P.O. Box 219, Zip 37879–0219; tel. 423/626–4211; Michael T. Hutchins, Administrator (Total facility includes 100 beds in nursing home–type unit) A1 9 10 F9 13 17 18 19 22 25 31 34 36 37 38 39 41 43 45 46 48 49 50 51 54 65 69 70 76 78 Web address: www.clairbornehospital.org	13	10	165	2637	95	23831	0	13168	7013	357
TRENTON—Gibson County ★ GIBSON GENERAL HOSPITAL, 200 Hospital Drive, Zip 38382–3313; tel. 901/855–7900; Kelly R. Yenawine, Administrator A1 9 10 F9 13 16 17 18 22 24 25 32 34 36 37 38 48 54 70 76 78 P1 S West Tennessee Healthcare, Jackson, TN Web address: www.wth.net	15	10	42	804	9	—	0	4140	1947	64
TULLAHOMA—Coffee County ★ HARTON REGIONAL MEDICAL CENTER, 1801 North Jackson Street, Zip 37388–2201, Mailing Address: P.O. Box 460, Zip 37388–0460; tel. 931/393–3000; David C. Wilson, Chief Executive Officer (Nonreporting) A1 9 10 S TENET Healthcare Corporation, Santa Barbara, CA Web address: www.tenethealth.com\harton\	33	10	137	—	—	—	—	—	—	—
UNION CITY—Obion County ★ BAPTIST MEMORIAL HOSPITAL–UNION CITY, 1201 Bishop Street, Zip 38261–5403, Mailing Address: P.O. Box 310, Zip 38281–0310; tel. 901/884–8601; Mike Perryman, Administrator A1 9 10 F2 3 8 9 11 13 16 17 18 19 22 24 25 28 32 36 37 39 41 43 44 46 48 51 54 57 58 61 63 65 68 70 72 76 78 S Baptist Memorial Health Care Corporation, Memphis, TN Web address: www.bmhcc.org	23	10	133	4591	53	37551	340	26866	10027	385
WAVERLY—Humphreys County ☐ THREE RIVERS HOSPITAL, (Formerly Baptist Three Rivers Hospital), 451 Highway 13 South, Zip 37185–2149, Mailing Address: P.O. Box 437, Zip 37185–2149; tel. 931/296–4203; Donald W. James, Ph.D., Administrator and Chief Executive Officer (Total facility includes 2 beds in nursing home–type unit) A1 9 10 F9 13 16 17 18 22 25 32 34 48 51 56 62 69 76 78	32	10	52	518	8	28784	0	5876	2925	90
WAYNESBORO—Wayne County ☐ WAYNE MEDICAL CENTER, 103 J. V. Mangubat Drive, Zip 38485, Mailing Address: P.O. Box 580, Zip 38485–0580; tel. 931/722–5411; Shirley Harder, Chief Executive Officer (Total facility includes 61 beds in nursing home–type unit) (Nonreporting) A1 9 10	23	10	110	—	—	—	—	—	—	—
WINCHESTER—Franklin County ★ SOUTHERN TENNESSEE MEDICAL CENTER, (Includes Emerald–Hodgson Hospital, University Avenue, Sewanee, Zip 37375; tel. 615/598–5691), 185 Hospital Road, Zip 37398–2468; tel. 931/967–8200; William Russell Spray, Chief Executive Officer (Total facility includes 71 beds in nursing home–type unit) A1 9 10 F8 9 13 17 22 24 25 30 33 34 38 39 43 44 45 46 48 50 54 57 62 69 70 71 72 76 78 P6 7 8 S LifePoint Hospitals, Inc., Brentwood, TN	33	10	211	4582	95	52240	503	21590	9894	386
WOODBURY—Cannon County ★ STONES RIVER HOSPITAL, 324 Doolittle Road, Zip 37190; tel. 615/563–4001; Bill Patterson, Administrator (Nonreporting) A1 9 10 Web address: www.wth.net	33	10	55	—	—	—	—	—	—	—

Hospitals, U.S. / TEXAS

TEXAS

Resident Population 19,760 (in thousands)
Resident population in metro areas 84.2%
Birth rate per 1,000 population 17.2
65 years and over 10.1%
Percent of persons without health insurance 24.5%

Hospital, Address, Telephone, Administrator, Approval, Facility, and Physician Codes, Health Care System, Network	Classification Codes		Utilization Data					Expense (thousands) of dollars		
★ American Hospital Association (AHA) membership ☐ Joint Commission on Accreditation of Healthcare Organizations (JCAHO) accreditation + American Osteopathic Healthcare Association (AOHA) membership ○ American Osteopathic Association (AOA) accreditation △ Commission on Accreditation of Rehabilitation Facilities (CARF) accreditation Control codes 61, 63, 64, 71, 72 and 73 indicate hospitals listed by AOHA, but not registered by AHA. For definition of numerical codes, see page A4	Control	Service	Staffed Beds	Admissions	Census	Outpatient Visits	Births	Total	Payroll	Personnel

ABILENE—Taylor County

✠ ABILENE REGIONAL MEDICAL CENTER, 6250 Highway 83–84 at Antilley Road, Zip 79606–5299; tel. 915/695–9900; Mary T. Brasseaux, Chief Executive Officer (Total facility includes 25 beds in nursing home–type unit) **A**1 9 10 **F**4 7 8 9 11 12 13 16 17 18 19 22 24 27 28 29 30 31 32 33 34 36 37 38 39 41 42 43 44 46 47 48 49 50 51 54 56 66 68 69 70 72 75 76 77 78 79 **P**3 **S** Quorum Health Group, Brentwood, TN
Web address: www.abilene.com/armc | 33 | 10 | 187 | 7486 | 105 | 65294 | 1293 | 56806 | 22108 | 620 |

✠ △ HENDRICK HEALTH SYSTEM, 1242 North 19th Street, Zip 79601–2316; tel. 915/670–2000; Michael C. Waters, FACHE, President (Total facility includes 41 beds in nursing home–type unit) **A**1 7 9 10 **F**4 6 7 8 9 11 12 13 17 18 19 22 23 24 25 26 27 28 29 30 31 32 33 34 35 36 37 38 39 41 43 44 45 46 47 48 49 50 51 52 53 54 56 61 65 67 68 69 70 71 72 75 76 78 79 **P**6 7 8
Web address: www.abilene.com/hmc/ | 21 | 10 | 410 | 14505 | 250 | 122288 | 1309 | 149447 | 62367 | 2132 |

✠ U. S. AIR FORCE HOSPITAL, 7th Medical Group, Dyess AFB, Zip 79607–1367; tel. 915/696–5429; Major John G. Wiseman, Administrator (Nonreporting) **A**1 **S** Department of the Air Force, Bowling AFB, DC | 41 | 10 | 20 | — | — | — | — | — | — | — |

ALICE—Jim Wells County

✠ ALICE REGIONAL HOSPITAL, 2500 East Main Street, Zip 78332–4794; tel. 361/664–4376; Bradley E. Jones, Chief Executive Officer (Total facility includes 22 beds in nursing home–type unit) **A**1 9 10 **F**4 7 8 9 11 13 16 17 18 19 21 22 24 25 27 29 30 32 33 34 38 39 41 43 44 45 46 48 49 51 54 56 57 59 60 62 63 66 69 70 71 75 76 78 79 **P**8 **S** Triad Hospitals, Inc., Dallas, TX | 32 | 10 | 112 | 4581 | 65 | 72687 | 241 | 30862 | 10891 | 365 |

+ CHRISTUS SPOHN HOSPITAL ALICE, 700 North Flournoy Road, Zip 78332; tel. 361/661–8000 (Nonreporting) **A**10 | 21 | 10 | 49 | — | — | — | — | — | — | — |

ALPINE—Brewster County

★ BIG BEND REGIONAL MEDICAL CENTER, 2600 Highway 118 North, Zip 79830; tel. 915/837–3447; David Conejo, Chief Executive Officer **A**9 **F**7 8 13 16 17 18 19 22 25 31 32 36 38 44 48 54 76 **S** Community Health Systems, Inc., Brentwood, TN
Web address: www.overland.net/bbrmc | 33 | 10 | 36 | 305 | 9 | 11481 | 42 | 1546 | 1216 | 135 |

AMARILLO—Potter County

✠ BAPTIST ST. ANTHONY HEALTH SYSTEM, 1600 Wallace Boulevard, Zip 79106–1799; tel. 806/212–2000; John D. Hicks, President and Chief Executive Officer (Total facility includes 99 beds in nursing home–type unit) **A**1 2 3 5 9 10 **F**4 7 8 9 11 12 13 16 17 18 19 22 23 24 25 26 27 29 30 31 32 34 36 37 38 39 40 41 42 43 44 45 46 47 48 49 50 51 52 53 54 56 68 69 70 71 72 74 75 76 77 78 79 **P**3 7
Web address: www.bsahs.org | 21 | 10 | 526 | 24081 | 359 | 154379 | 2079 | 198552 | 82405 | 2654 |

☐ IHS OF AMARILLO, 5601 Plum Creek Drive, Zip 79124; tel. 806/351–1000; Neal Duncan, Executive Director **A**1 10 **F**7 13 16 17 18 31 32 38 45 54 70 72 78 **S** Integrated Health Services, Sparks Glencoe, MD
Web address: www.ihs–inc.com | 33 | 10 | 20 | 271 | 17 | 2030 | 0 | 5694 | 2188 | 184 |

✠ NORTHWEST TEXAS HEALTHCARE SYSTEM, (Includes Psychiatric Pavilion, 7201 Evans, Zip 79106), 1501 South Coulter Avenue, Zip 79106–1790, Mailing Address: P.O. Box 1110, Zip 79175–1110; tel. 806/354–1000; Moody L. Chisholm, Chief Executive Officer and Managing Director **A**1 3 5 9 10 **F**2 3 4 7 8 9 11 12 13 14 16 17 18 19 21 22 24 25 29 30 33 34 35 38 39 41 42 43 44 45 46 47 48 49 50 51 52 54 56 57 58 59 60 61 62 63 64 68 70 71 72 75 76 78 79 **P**6 **S** Universal Health Services, Inc., King of Prussia, PA
Web address: www.nwths.com | 33 | 10 | 353 | 13978 | 191 | 244028 | 2195 | 150741 | 47743 | 1488 |

✠ VETERANS AFFAIRS MEDICAL CENTER, 6010 Amarillo Boulevard West, Zip 79106–1992; tel. 806/354–7801; Wallace M. Hopkins, FACHE, Chief Executive Officer (Total facility includes 120 beds in nursing home–type unit) (Nonreporting) **A**1 2 3 5 **S** Department of Veterans Affairs, Washington, DC | 45 | 10 | 218 | — | — | — | — | — | — | — |

ANAHUAC—Chambers County

BAYSIDE COMMUNITY HOSPITAL, 200 Hospital Drive, Zip 77514, Mailing Address: P.O. Box 398, Zip 77514–0398; tel. 409/267–3143; Stephen M. Goode, Executive Director **A**9 10 **F**25 32 38 48 **P**6 | 16 | 10 | 12 | 240 | 2 | 13602 | 0 | 3254 | 1599 | 54 |

ANDREWS—Andrews County

✠ PERMIAN GENERAL HOSPITAL, Northeast By–Pass, Zip 79714, Mailing Address: P.O. Box 2108, Zip 79714–2108; tel. 915/523–2200; Randy R. Richards, Chief Executive Officer **A**1 9 10 **F**7 8 9 13 16 17 18 19 21 22 23 24 25 28 32 34 36 38 39 41 43 44 45 48 50 51 54 56 70 72 75 76 78 | 13 | 10 | 74 | 1313 | 12 | 54918 | 231 | 12908 | 5911 | 233 |

ANGLETON—Brazoria County

✠ ANGLETON–DANBURY GENERAL HOSPITAL, 132 East Hospital Drive, Zip 77515–4197; tel. 409/849–7721; David A. Bleakney, Administrator **A**1 9 10 **F**7 8 9 11 13 17 18 22 24 25 28 32 33 34 35 38 39 41 44 48 50 51 54 70 71 72 76 78 **P**8
Web address: www.adgh.org | 16 | 10 | 49 | 3161 | 24 | 33524 | 511 | 21179 | 6700 | 256 |

© 2000 AHA Guide *Many Facility Codes have changed. Please refer to the AHA Guide Code Chart.* Hospitals **A401**

Hospitals, U.S. / TEXAS

Hospital, Address, Telephone, Administrator, Approval, Facility, and Physician Codes, Health Care System, Network

- ★ American Hospital Association (AHA) membership
- ☐ Joint Commission on Accreditation of Healthcare Organizations (JCAHO) accreditation
- \+ American Osteopathic Healthcare Association (AOHA) membership
- ○ American Osteopathic Association (AOA) accreditation
- △ Commission on Accreditation of Rehabilitation Facilities (CARF) accreditation

Control codes 61, 63, 64, 71, 72 and 73 indicate hospitals listed by AOHA, but not registered by AHA. For definition of numerical codes, see page A4

Hospital	Classification Codes		Utilization Data					Expense (thousands) of dollars		Personnel
	Control	Service	Staffed Beds	Admissions	Census	Outpatient Visits	Births	Total	Payroll	
ANSON—Jones County										
★ ANSON GENERAL HOSPITAL, 101 Avenue J, Zip 79501–2198; tel. 915/823–3231; Dudley R. White, Administrator (Total facility includes 8 beds in nursing home–type unit) **A**9 10 **F**7 22 23 25 28 36 39 45 48 49 54 69 70 76 78 **P**3 8	14	10	30	728	12	25922	0	5358	2733	—
ARANSAS PASS—San Patricio County										
✠ NORTH BAY HOSPITAL, 1711 West Wheeler Avenue, Zip 78336–4536; tel. 361/758–8585; John Krogness, Chief Executive Officer **A**1 9 10 **F**7 13 17 18 22 25 32 34 38 39 41 43 48 56 57 59 62 63 70 76 78 79 **P**7 8 **S** HCA – The Healthcare Company, Nashville, TN Web address: www.hcahealthcare.com	33	10	69	2554	32	42186	76	16544	7440	177
ARLINGTON—Tarrant County										
✠ ARLINGTON MEMORIAL HOSPITAL, 800 West Randol Mill Road, Zip 76012–2503; tel. 817/548–6100; Wayne N. Clark, President and Chief Executive Officer **A**1 9 10 **F**4 7 8 9 11 12 13 16 17 18 22 24 25 28 29 39 41 42 44 46 47 48 54 70 72 76 77 78 79 **P**1 **S** Texas Health Resources, Irving, TX	23	10	339	17806	210	119377	3253	127418	49085	1553
☐ BHC MILLWOOD HOSPITAL, 1011 North Cooper Street, Zip 76011–5517; tel. 817/261–3121; Wayne Hallford, Chief Executive Officer **A**1 9 10 **F**2 3 13 16 25 29 38 51 57 58 59 61 63 64 70 72 **P**8 **S** Behavioral Healthcare Corporation, Nashville, TN	33	22	82	1614	29	9179	0	5867	3035	106
☐ △ HEALTHSOUTH REHABILITATION HOSPITAL OF ARLINGTON, 3200 Matlock Road, Zip 76015–2911; tel. 817/468–4000; Philip Patterson, Administrator and Chief Operating Officer **A**1 7 10 **F**9 11 13 22 28 29 30 38 39 45 48 49 50 53 54 70 71 72 75 78 **S** HEALTHSOUTH Corporation, Birmingham, AL Web address: www.healthsouth.com	33	46	65	983	53	15456	0	9790	5157	204
✠ △ MEDICAL CENTER OF ARLINGTON, 3301 Matlock Road, Zip 76015–2998; tel. 817/465–3241; Michael R. Burroughs, FACHE, President and Chief Executive Officer **A**1 7 9 10 **F**1 2 3 4 7 8 9 11 13 16 17 19 22 23 24 25 30 31 32 33 34 38 39 41 42 43 44 45 46 47 48 50 51 53 54 57 58 59 60 61 62 63 64 70 76 78 79 **P**6 **S** HCA – The Healthcare Company, Nashville, TN Web address: www.medicalcenterarlington.com	33	10	188	8506	114	73141	2188	75483	24898	540
☐ VENCOR ARLINGTON, TEXAS, (LONG–TERM ACUTE CARE FACILITY), 1000 North Cooper Street, Zip 76011–5540; tel. 817/543–0200; Joy Dier, Administrator **A**1 9 10 **F**13 16 18 19 30 32 43 54 70 75 76 **S** Vencor, Incorporated, Louisville, KY	33	49	63	390	32	—	0	9479	4081	148
ASPERMONT—Stonewall County										
★ STONEWALL MEMORIAL HOSPITAL, U.S. Highway 380 & 83 North, Zip 79502, Mailing Address: P.O. Box C, Zip 79502; tel. 940/989–3551; Walt Haislip, Administrator **A**9 10 **F**25 56 69	16	10	18	206	2	4428	0	1735	557	40
ATHENS—Henderson County										
✠ EAST TEXAS MEDICAL CENTER ATHENS, 2000 South Palestine Street, Zip 75751–5610; tel. 903/676–1000; Patrick L. Wallace, Administrator **A**1 9 10 **F**7 9 13 22 25 27 32 34 36 38 41 44 48 54 64 75 76 **P**7 **S** East Texas Medical Center Regional Healthcare System, Tyler, TX	23	10	108	6402	76	67938	873	36029	11990	380
ATLANTA—Cass County										
★ ATLANTA MEMORIAL HOSPITAL, Highway 77 at South William, Zip 75551, Mailing Address: P.O. Box 1049, Zip 75551–1049; tel. 903/799–3000; Tom Crow, Administrator **A**9 10 **F**7 8 9 17 18 22 25 28 30 31 32 34 36 37 41 43 44 45 46 47 48 49 51 54 57 59 62 64 66 70 74 75 76 **P**8 Web address: www.atlantamemorial.com	16	10	44	1952	26	12069	163	10525	4697	173
BROOKS HOSPITAL, 230 North Louise Street, Zip 75551–2589, Mailing Address: P.O. Box 1069, Zip 75551–1069; tel. 903/796–2873; Jesse Brooks, M.D., Administrator **F**1 3 4 5 6 7 8 9 11 13 14 15 19 20 21 22 23 24 25 26 27 28 29 30 31 32 33 34 35 36 37 38 39 40 43 45 46 47 48 49 50 51 54 55 56 58 59 60 61 62 63 64 65 66 67 68 70 71 72 73 74 75 76 77 78 79 **P**1 2 3 4 5 6 8	33	10	22	36	0	0	0	1161	658	30
AUSTIN—Travis County										
☐ AUSTIN STATE HOSPITAL, 4110 Guadalupe Street, Zip 78751–4296; tel. 512/452–0381; Carl Schock, Superintendent **A**1 3 10 **F**12 23 41 44 45 57 58 60 61 62 70 78 Web address: www.mhmr.state.tx.us	12	22	308	2578	241	0	0	42549	22013	779
✠ BRACKENRIDGE HOSPITAL, (Includes Children's Hospital of Austin, tel. 512/324–8000; Patrick Shumaker, Administrator), 601 East 15th Street, Zip 78701–1996; tel. 512/324–7000; Susan McClernon, Administrator **A**1 2 3 9 10 **F**2 3 4 7 8 9 11 12 13 14 17 18 19 20 22 24 25 26 27 29 30 32 33 34 35 36 38 39 41 42 43 44 45 46 47 48 49 51 52 54 56 57 58 59 61 62 63 64 65 66 68 69 70 71 72 74 75 76 77 78 79 **P**5 6 8 **S** Ascension Health, Saint Louis, MO Web address: www.goodhealth.com	21	10	312	14871	191	158027	2926	136960	52808	1516
☐ △ BROWN SCHOOLS REHABILITATION CENTER, 1106 West Dittmar, Zip 78745–9990, Mailing Address: P.O. Box 150459, Zip 78715–0459; tel. 512/444–4835; Kay Peck, Chief Executive Officer **A**1 7 9 10 **F**13 17 18 38 43 45 50 51 54 70 **S** Brown Schools, Inc., Austin, TX Web address: www.brownschools.com	33	46	30	267	28	0	0	5451	1218	52
CHRISTOPHER HOUSE, 2820 East Martin Luther King, Zip 78702; tel. 512/322–0747; Marjorie Mulanax, Executive Director (Nonreporting)	23	49	15	—	—	—	—	—	—	—

Hospitals, U.S. / TEXAS

Hospital, Address, Telephone, Administrator, Approval, Facility, and Physician Codes, Health Care System, Network	Classification Codes		Utilization Data					Expense (thousands) of dollars		
★ American Hospital Association (AHA) membership □ Joint Commission on Accreditation of Healthcare Organizations (JCAHO) accreditation + American Osteopathic Healthcare Association (AOHA) membership ○ American Osteopathic Association (AOA) accreditation △ Commission on Accreditation of Rehabilitation Facilities (CARF) accreditation Control codes 61, 63, 64, 71, 72 and 73 indicate hospitals listed by AOHA, but not registered by AHA. For definition of numerical codes, see page A4	Control	Service	Staffed Beds	Admissions	Census	Outpatient Visits	Births	Total	Payroll	Personnel
□ HEALTHSOUTH REHABILITATION HOSPITAL OF AUSTIN, 1215 Red River Street, Zip 78701; tel. 512/474-5700; Laurie Bajich, Chief Executive Officer **A**1 9 10 **F**13 17 18 25 38 43 51 53 54 72 75 78 **S** HEALTHSOUTH Corporation, Birmingham, AL Web address: www.healthsouth.com	33	46	79	1598	67	34325	0	14872	7573	264
★ NORTH AUSTIN MEDICAL CENTER, 12221 MoPac Expressway North, Zip 78758-2483; tel. 512/901-1000; Donald H. Wilkerson, Chief Executive Officer **A**1 9 10 **F**2 4 7 8 9 11 12 13 16 17 18 19 21 22 23 24 25 26 27 28 29 30 32 33 34 35 36 38 39 41 42 43 44 45 46 47 48 49 50 51 53 54 57 59 60 62 63 64 65 66 68 69 70 71 72 73 74 76 77 78 79 **P**1 3 7 8 **S** HCA - The Healthcare Company, Nashville, TN Web address: www.hcahealthcare.com	32	10	128	7132	84	105599	654	67749	26854	697
□ RENAISSANCE WOMEN'S CENTER OF AUSTIN, 3003 Bee Cave Road, Zip 78746-5561; tel. 512/858-7155; Edward Gray, Chief Executive Officer **A**1 9 **F**8 9 16 18 25 43 48 50 51 76 79 **P**1 2 3 4 5 6 7 8	33	10	24	4376	19	1529	1807	9880	4474	96
★ SETON MEDICAL CENTER, (Includes Seton Northwest Hospital, 11113 Research Boulevard, Zip 78759-7513; tel. 512/324-6000; Charles E. Durant, Jr, FACHE, Administrator), 1201 West 38th Street, Zip 78705-1056; tel. 512/324-1000; Gregory R. Angle, Administrator **A**1 2 9 10 **F**2 3 4 7 8 9 11 12 13 14 17 18 19 20 22 24 25 26 27 29 30 32 33 34 35 36 38 39 41 42 43 44 45 46 47 48 49 51 52 54 56 57 58 59 61 62 63 64 65 66 68 69 70 71 72 74 75 76 77 78 79 **P**5 6 8 **S** Ascension Health, Saint Louis, MO Web address: www.goodhealth.com	21	10	527	26039	355	469953	5680	278305	130657	2946
★ SETON SHOAL CREEK HOSPITAL, 3501 Mills Avenue, Zip 78731-6391; tel. 512/452-0361; Armin L. Steege, Interim Administrator **A**1 9 10 **F**2 3 4 7 8 9 11 12 13 14 17 18 19 20 22 24 25 26 27 29 30 32 33 34 35 36 38 39 41 42 43 44 45 46 47 48 49 51 52 54 56 57 58 59 61 62 63 64 65 66 68 69 70 71 72 74 75 76 77 78 79 **P**1 5 6 8 **S** Ascension Health, Saint Louis, MO Web address: www.goodhealth.com	21	22	118	1841	29	11603	0	5766	3257	99
★ SOUTH AUSTIN HOSPITAL, (Formerly St. David's South Hospital), 901 West Ben White Boulevard, Zip 78704-6903; tel. 512/447-2211; Richard W. Klusmann, Chief Executive Officer **A**1 9 10 **F**4 5 8 9 11 12 13 17 22 24 25 27 32 34 36 39 41 44 45 46 47 48 49 54 69 70 76 78 79 **P**1 **S** HCA - The Healthcare Company, Nashville, TN	32	10	200	9951	122	124915	1246	74131	29474	719
□ SPECIALTY HOSPITAL OF AUSTIN, (LONG TERM ACUTE CARE HOSPITAL), 4207 Burnet Road, Zip 78756-3396; tel. 512/706-1900; Robert F. Berry, Chief Executive Officer **A**1 9 10 **F**22 25 31 39 65 70 76 **S** Mariner Post-Acute Network, Inc., Atlanta, GA	33	49	133	1060	76	0	0	18793	7136	262
★ ST. DAVID'S MEDICAL CENTER, 919 East 32nd Street, Zip 78705-2709, Mailing Address: P.O. Box 4039, Zip 78765-4039; tel. 512/476-7111; Cole C. Eslyn, Chief Executive Officer **A**1 2 9 10 **F**2 3 4 7 8 9 11 13 16 17 18 19 20 22 24 25 27 28 29 30 31 32 33 34 35 36 38 39 41 42 43 44 45 46 47 48 49 50 51 53 54 57 58 59 60 62 63 64 65 66 68 69 70 71 72 74 75 76 77 78 79 **P**8 **S** HCA - The Healthcare Company, Nashville, TN Web address: www.hcahealthcare.com	32	10	298	16561	229	75142	4200	129074	52888	1777
★ ST. DAVID'S PAVILION, 1025 East 32nd Street, Zip 78765; tel. 512/867-5800; Cole C. Eslyn, Chief Executive Officer **A**1 9 10 **F**3 4 8 9 11 13 16 17 18 19 20 22 24 25 27 28 29 30 31 32 33 34 35 36 38 39 41 42 43 44 45 46 47 48 49 50 51 53 54 57 58 59 60 62 63 64 66 68 69 70 71 72 74 75 76 77 78 79 **P**8 **S** HCA - The Healthcare Company, Nashville, TN Web address: www.hcahealthcare.com	32	22	38	1607	26	14138	0	9289	3107	112
★ △ ST. DAVID'S REHABILITATION CENTER, 1005 East 32nd Street, Zip 78705-2705, Mailing Address: P.O. Box 4270, Zip 78765-4270; tel. 512/867-5100; Cole C. Eslyn, Chief Executive Officer **A**1 7 9 10 **F**2 3 4 7 8 9 11 13 16 17 18 19 20 21 22 24 25 27 28 29 30 32 33 34 35 36 38 39 41 42 43 44 45 46 47 48 49 50 51 53 54 57 58 59 60 62 63 64 65 66 68 69 70 71 72 74 75 76 77 78 79 **P**8 **S** HCA - The Healthcare Company, Nashville, TN Web address: www.hcahealthcare.com	32	46	67	1497	58	30344	0	19412	9215	317
AZLE—Tarrant County										
★ HARRIS METHODIST NORTHWEST, 108 Denver Trail, Zip 76020-3697; tel. 817/444-8600; Larry Thompson, Vice President and Administrator **A**1 9 10 **F**1 2 3 4 7 8 9 10 11 12 13 14 16 17 18 19 20 21 22 23 24 25 26 27 28 29 30 32 33 34 35 36 37 39 41 42 43 44 45 46 47 48 49 50 51 52 53 54 55 57 58 59 60 61 62 63 64 65 66 68 69 70 71 72 74 75 76 77 78 79 **S** Texas Health Resources, Irving, TX Web address: www.hmhs.com	23	10	36	1215	12	23885	0	11992	5239	167
BALLINGER—Runnels County										
BALLINGER MEMORIAL HOSPITAL, 608 Avenue B, Zip 76821-2499; tel. 915/365-2531; Lance W. Keilers, Administrator **A**9 10 **F**7 16 17 18 25 28 30 32 35 70 75 78 79	16	10	16	316	4	5740	2	2493	1228	57
BAY CITY—Matagorda County										
★ MATAGORDA GENERAL HOSPITAL, 1115 Avenue G, Zip 77414-3544; tel. 979/245-6383; Wendell H. Baker, Jr, Chief Executive Officer **A**1 9 10 **F**4 7 8 9 11 17 18 21 22 24 25 28 30 31 32 34 35 36 37 39 41 43 44 45 48 53 54 57 59 62 63 70 72 75 76 78 79 **P**5 **S** Matagorda County Hospital District, Bay City, TX	16	10	67	2065	18	28553	371	25538	9293	460

Hospitals, U.S. / TEXAS

Hospital, Address, Telephone, Administrator, Approval, Facility, and Physician Codes, Health Care System, Network	Classification Codes		Utilization Data					Expense (thousands) of dollars		
★ American Hospital Association (AHA) membership ☐ Joint Commission on Accreditation of Healthcare Organizations (JCAHO) accreditation + American Osteopathic Healthcare Association (AOHA) membership ○ American Osteopathic Association (AOA) accreditation △ Commission on Accreditation of Rehabilitation Facilities (CARF) accreditation Control codes 61, 63, 64, 71, 72 and 73 indicate hospitals listed by AOHA, but not registered by AHA. For definition of numerical codes, see page A4	Control	Service	Staffed Beds	Admissions	Census	Outpatient Visits	Births	Total	Payroll	Personnel
BAYTOWN—Harris County										
☐ BAYCOAST MEDICAL CENTER, 1700 James Bowie Drive, Zip 77520–3386; tel. 281/420–6100; Walter J. Ornsteen, President and Chief Executive Officer (Total facility includes 20 beds in nursing home–type unit) **A**1 9 10 **F**7 8 9 12 13 17 18 22 24 25 27 31 32 37 38 41 43 45 46 48 51 54 61 69 70 76 78 **P**3 **S** Paracelsus Healthcare Corporation, Houston, TX	33	10	191	2516	30	23642	438	20492	7550	218
★ △ SAN JACINTO METHODIST HOSPITAL, 4401 Garth Road, Zip 77521–3160; tel. 281/420–8600; William Simmons, President and Chief Executive Officer (Total facility includes 45 beds in nursing home–type unit) **A**1 3 5 7 9 10 **F**4 8 9 11 13 17 19 21 22 23 24 25 27 30 31 32 34 36 37 38 39 41 43 44 45 46 48 50 51 53 54 56 57 59 60 61 62 64 65 68 69 70 72 74 76 78 **P**3 7 8 **S** Methodist Health Care System, Houston, TX **Web address:** www.sanjacintomethodisthospital.com	21	10	231	11491	153	147901	1327	86000	37309	1065
BEAUMONT—Jefferson County										
★ CHRISTUS ST. ELIZABETH HOSPITAL, 2830 Calder Avenue, Zip 77702, Mailing Address: P.O. Box 5405, Zip 77726–5405; tel. 409/892–7171; Edward W. Myers, Chief Executive Officer (Total facility includes 27 beds in nursing home–type unit) **A**1 2 5 9 10 **F**4 8 9 11 12 13 14 16 17 18 19 20 22 23 24 25 28 30 31 32 33 34 35 36 38 39 41 42 43 44 45 46 47 48 50 51 52 53 54 56 65 68 69 70 75 76 77 78 79 **P**3 5 6 7 8 **S** Christus Health, Irving, TX **Web address:** www.sch.org FANNIN PAVILION OF BEAUMONT REGIONAL MEDICAL CENTER See Memorial Hermann Baptist Hospital–East Campus	21	10	447	21932	324	173154	2468	182855	72399	2332
☐ △ HEALTHSOUTH REHABILITATION HOSPITAL OF BEAUMONT, 3340 Plaza 10 Boulevard, Zip 77707; tel. 409/835–0835; Michael Hagen, Administrator **A**1 7 10 **F**13 19 28 29 31 32 38 49 53 54 70 72 78 **P**5 **S** HEALTHSOUTH Corporation, Birmingham, AL **Web address:** www.healthsouth.com	32	46	61	885	39	18589	0	9892	4582	122
★ MEMORIAL HERMANN BAPTIST HOSPITAL–EAST CAMPUS, (Formerly Beaumont Medical and Surgical Hospital), (Includes Fannin Pavilion of Beaumont Regional Medical Center, 3250 Fannin Street, Zip 77701; tel. 409/833–1411), 3080 College Street, Zip 77701–4689, Mailing Address: P.O. Box 5817, Zip 77726–5817; tel. 409/833–1411; David N. Parmer, President and Chief Executive Officer **A**1 9 10 **F**2 3 4 6 8 9 11 13 16 17 18 19 20 22 23 24 25 26 27 28 29 30 31 32 33 34 35 36 37 38 39 40 41 43 44 45 46 47 48 49 50 51 54 55 56 57 58 59 60 61 62 63 64 65 66 67 68 69 70 71 72 73 74 75 76 77 78 79 **P**5 7 **S** Memorial Hermann Healthcare System, Houston, TX	23	10	372	5382	84	53124	1057	38745	15331	—
★ MEMORIAL HERMANN BAPTIST HOSPITAL–WEST CAMPUS, (Formerly Baptist Hospital of Southeast Texas), College and 11th Streets, Zip 77701, Mailing Address: Drawer 1591, Zip 77704–1591; tel. 409/835–3781; David N. Parmer, President and Chief Executive Officer (Total facility includes 31 beds in nursing home–type unit) **A**1 5 9 10 **F**2 3 4 6 7 8 9 10 11 12 13 19 20 22 23 24 25 26 27 28 29 30 31 32 33 34 35 36 37 38 39 40 41 42 43 44 45 46 47 48 49 50 51 52 53 54 55 56 57 58 59 60 61 62 63 64 65 66 67 68 69 70 71 72 73 74 75 76 77 78 79 **P**3 5 **S** Memorial Hermann Healthcare System, Houston, TX	23	10	184	6367	96	46240	0	54507	18168	642
BEDFORD—Tarrant County										
★ HARRIS METHODIST–HEB, (Includes Harris Methodist–Springwood, 1608 Hospital Parkway, Zip 76022; tel. 817/355–7700), 1600 Hospital Parkway, Zip 76022–6913, Mailing Address: P.O. Box 669, Zip 76095–0669; tel. 817/685–4000; Jack McCabe, President and Chief Executive Officer (Total facility includes 15 beds in nursing home–type unit) **A**1 2 9 10 **F**2 3 4 7 8 9 11 13 16 17 18 19 21 22 24 25 27 28 30 31 32 34 35 36 37 38 41 42 43 44 45 46 47 48 49 50 51 53 54 57 58 59 60 61 62 63 64 65 69 70 72 76 78 79 **P**2 5 7 **S** Texas Health Resources, Irving, TX **Web address:** www.hmhs.com	21	10	180	11442	127	88095	1437	94896	40789	1177
BEEVILLE—Bee County										
★ CHRISTUS SPOHN HOSPITAL BEEVILLE, (Formerly Spohn Bee County Hospital), 1500 East Houston Street, Zip 78102; tel. 361/354–2000; David S. Wagner, Vice President and Administrator **A**1 9 10 **F**8 9 16 17 18 19 22 24 25 27 32 36 37 38 39 41 44 48 50 51 54 62 70 71 72 75 76 78 **P**3 5 8 **S** Christus Health, Irving, TX **Web address:** www.sch.org	21	10	67	4152	41	92323	452	22990	9972	275
BELLVILLE—Austin County										
☐ BELLVILLE GENERAL HOSPITAL, 44 North Cummings Street, Zip 77418–1347; tel. 409/865–3141; Bob Ellzey, Administrator **A**1 9 10 **F**7 8 9 13 16 17 18 22 25 28 32 34 36 38 39 45 48 54 70 76 78 **P**3	16	10	26	851	9	18749	46	6165	2265	77
BIG LAKE—Reagan County										
REAGAN MEMORIAL HOSPITAL, 805 North Main Street, Zip 76932–3999; tel. 915/884–2561; Ron Galloway, Administrator (Total facility includes 48 beds in nursing home–type unit) (Nonreporting) **A**9 10 18	16	10	62	—	—	—	—	—	—	—
BIG SPRING—Howard County										
☐ BIG SPRING STATE HOSPITAL, Lamesa Highway, Zip 79720, Mailing Address: P.O. Box 231, Zip 79721–0231; tel. 915/267–8216; Edward Moughon, Superintendent **A**1 10 **F**16 17 18 19 21 22 23 25 30 39 48 50 54 57 58 60 61 62 70 76 78 **Web address:** www.mhmr.state.tx.us/hospitals/bigspringSH/bigspringsh.html	12	22	234	919	186	0	0	48112	16441	638

Many Facility Codes have changed. Please refer to the AHA Guide Code Chart.

Hospitals, U.S. / TEXAS

Hospital, Address, Telephone, Administrator, Approval, Facility, and Physician Codes, Health Care System, Network	Classification Codes		Utilization Data					Expense (thousands) of dollars		
★ American Hospital Association (AHA) membership □ Joint Commission on Accreditation of Healthcare Organizations (JCAHO) accreditation + American Osteopathic Healthcare Association (AOHA) membership ○ American Osteopathic Association (AOA) accreditation △ Commission on Accreditation of Rehabilitation Facilities (CARF) accreditation Control codes 61, 63, 64, 71, 72 and 73 indicate hospitals listed by AOHA, but not registered by AHA. For definition of numerical codes, see page A4	Control	Service	Staffed Beds	Admissions	Census	Outpatient Visits	Births	Total	Payroll	Personnel
☒ SCENIC MOUNTAIN MEDICAL CENTER, 1601 West 11th Place, Zip 79720–4198; tel. 915/263–1211; Loren F. Chandler, Chief Executive Officer (Total facility includes 18 beds in nursing home–type unit) **A**1 9 10 **F**8 9 11 12 13 18 19 22 24 25 30 32 34 36 38 39 41 44 45 48 50 51 54 57 62 68 69 70 75 76 78 **S** Community Health Systems, Inc., Brentwood, TN **Web address:** www.smmccares.com	33	10	128	3967	46	20649	259	19385	8767	425
☒ VETERANS AFFAIRS MEDICAL CENTER, 300 Veterans Boulevard, Zip 79720–5500; tel. 915/263–7361; Cary D. Brown, Director (Total facility includes 40 beds in nursing home–type unit) (Nonreporting) **A**1 2 3 5 **S** Department of Veterans Affairs, Washington, DC	45	10	189	—	—	—	—	—	—	—
BONHAM—Fannin County □ NORTHEAST MEDICAL CENTER, 504 Lipscomb Boulevard, Zip 75418–4096; Mailing Address: P.O. Drawer C, Zip 75418–4096; tel. 903/583–8585; Kenneth May, Chief Executive Officer **A**1 9 10 **F**7 9 13 17 22 24 25 32 34 36 38 39 41 45 48 49 54 68 70 72 74 76 **S** Community Health Systems, Inc., Brentwood, TN SAM RAYBURN MEMORIAL VETERANS CENTER See Veterans Affairs North Texas Health Care System, Dallas	32	10	39	1320	15	12200	0	11108	4233	102
BORGER—Hutchinson County ☒ GOLDEN PLAINS COMMUNITY HOSPITAL, 200 South McGee Street, Zip 79007–0495; tel. 806/273–1100; Norman Lambert, Chief Executive Officer **A**1 9 10 **F**7 8 9 13 17 18 22 25 27 32 36 39 41 43 44 48 51 54 70 71 75 76 78 **Web address:** www.borger.com	16	10	48	1220	11	25260	110	12515	5366	186
BOWIE—Montague County ★ BOWIE MEMORIAL HOSPITAL, 705 East Greenwood Avenue, Zip 76230–3199; tel. 940/872–1126; Joyce Crumpler, R.N., Administrator **A**9 10 **F**16 17 18 22 25 32 36 37 39 41 48 54 67 70 75 76	16	10	44	1544	20	27996	0	9977	4789	183
BRADY—McCulloch County HEART OF TEXAS MEMORIAL HOSPITAL, Nine Road, Zip 76825–1150, Mailing Address: P.O. Box 1150, Zip 76825–1150; tel. 915/597–2901; Windell M. McCord, Administrator **A**9 10 **F**7 9 22 24 25 28 32 36 48 54 62 75 76	16	10	27	874	9	17653	0	5185	2345	88
BRECKENRIDGE—Stephens County STEPHENS MEMORIAL HOSPITAL, 200 South Geneva Street, Zip 76424–4799; tel. 254/559–2241; James Reese, CHE, Administrator **A**9 10 **F**8 9 17 18 22 25 30 32 34 36 38 39 40 44 45 46 48 49 54 56 70 75 76	13	10	33	750	9	16938	30	5906	2779	119
BRENHAM—Washington County ☒ TRINITY COMMUNITY MEDICAL CENTER OF BRENHAM, 700 Medical Parkway, Zip 77833–5498; tel. 979/836–6173; John L. Simms, President and Chief Executive Officer **A**1 9 10 **F**7 8 16 17 18 19 22 24 27 30 32 34 36 41 44 48 54 69 70 75 76 **S** Franciscan Services Corporation, Sylvania, OH **Web address:** www.trinitymed.com	21	10	60	2009	22	38695	363	16308	6680	224
BROWNFIELD—Terry County ☒ BROWNFIELD REGIONAL MEDICAL CENTER, 705 East Felt, Zip 79316–3439; tel. 806/637–3551; Mike Click, Administrator **A**1 9 10 **F**8 9 16 17 18 19 22 25 28 32 33 34 35 36 38 44 48 51 54 70 75 76 78	16	10	42	708	8	40826	104	8255	4001	168
BROWNSVILLE—Cameron County ☒ BROWNSVILLE MEDICAL CENTER, 1040 West Jefferson Street, Zip 78520–5829, Mailing Address: P.O. Box 3590, Zip 78523–3590; tel. 956/544–1400; John M. Chubb, Chief Executive Officer **A**1 9 10 **F**4 7 8 9 11 13 17 18 19 22 25 27 28 32 34 39 41 42 44 45 47 48 49 50 51 54 56 58 59 60 61 63 64 70 75 76 78 79 **P**4 7 **S** TENET Healthcare Corporation, Santa Barbara, CA **Web address:** www.tenethealth.com	32	10	219	11241	153	59084	2652	57788	24883	791
☒ VALLEY REGIONAL MEDICAL CENTER, 100A Alton Gloor Boulevard, Zip 78526, Mailing Address: P.O. Box 3710, Zip 78521–3710; tel. 956/350–7101; Charles F. Sexton, Chief Executive Officer **A**1 9 10 **F**4 8 9 11 13 16 17 18 19 22 24 25 31 32 34 38 39 41 42 43 46 47 48 51 54 70 72 75 76 78 79 **P**7 **S** HCA – The Healthcare Company, Nashville, TN **Web address:** www.valleyregionalmedicalcenter.com	32	10	177	8827	120	70706	2521	58585	23731	691
BROWNWOOD—Brown County ☒ BROWNWOOD REGIONAL MEDICAL CENTER, 1501 Burnet Drive, Zip 76801–5933, Mailing Address: P.O. Box 760, Zip 76804–0760; tel. 915/646–8541; Tim Lancaster, Chief Executive Officer (Total facility includes 20 beds in nursing home–type unit) **A**1 9 10 **F**7 8 9 11 13 16 17 18 19 22 24 25 27 28 29 30 32 34 38 39 40 41 43 44 45 46 48 49 50 51 53 54 56 57 59 62 65 68 69 70 72 76 78 79 **P**3 8 **S** Triad Hospitals, Inc., Dallas, TX **Web address:** www.brmc–cares.com	32	10	163	7250	100	125352	703	43007	17821	626
BRYAN—Brazos County ☒ ST. JOSEPH REGIONAL HEALTH CENTER, 2801 Franciscan Drive, Zip 77802–2599; tel. 979/776–3777; Daniel L. Buche, Chief Executive Officer (Total facility includes 30 beds in nursing home–type unit) **A**1 3 5 9 10 **F**4 6 7 8 9 11 12 13 14 16 17 18 19 22 24 25 27 28 29 30 31 32 33 34 35 36 37 39 41 43 44 45 46 47 48 49 50 51 53 54 55 57 59 60 62 63 64 65 68 69 70 71 72 76 77 78 **P**8 **S** Franciscan Services Corporation, Sylvania, OH **Web address:** www.st–joseph.org	21	10	289	15176	205	183721	2430	121845	48285	1854
BURNET—Burnet County ☒ SETON HIGHLAND LAKES, Highway 281 South, Zip 78611, Mailing Address: P.O. Box 1219, Zip 78611–0840; tel. 512/756–6000; Janna Maturo, R.N., Administrator and Vice President Operations **A**1 9 10 **F**7 9 13 17 18 22 24 25 26 32 34 36 37 38 43 46 48 49 54 68 70 72 76 **P**5 6 8 **S** Ascension Health, Saint Louis, MO **Web address:** www.goodhealth.com/fac/highlandlakes.html	21	10	26	900	9	57400	0	9662	4623	157

© 2000 AHA Guide   *Many Facility Codes have changed. Please refer to the AHA Guide Code Chart.*

Hospitals, U.S. / TEXAS

Hospital, Address, Telephone, Administrator, Approval, Facility, and Physician Codes, Health Care System, Network	Classification Codes		Utilization Data					Expense (thousands) of dollars		Personnel
★ American Hospital Association (AHA) membership ☐ Joint Commission on Accreditation of Healthcare Organizations (JCAHO) accreditation + American Osteopathic Healthcare Association (AOHA) membership ○ American Osteopathic Association (AOA) accreditation △ Commission on Accreditation of Rehabilitation Facilities (CARF) accreditation Control codes 61, 63, 64, 71, 72 and 73 indicate hospitals listed by AOHA, but not registered by AHA. For definition of numerical codes, see page A4	Control	Service	Staffed Beds	Admissions	Census	Outpatient Visits	Births	Total	Payroll	
CALDWELL—Burleson County										
★ BURLESON ST. JOSEPH HEALTH CENTER, 1101 Woodson Drive, Zip 77836–1052, Mailing Address: P.O. Drawer 360, Zip 77836–0360; tel. 409/567–3245; Reed Edmundson, Administrator **A**9 10 **F**9 14 16 17 18 19 22 24 25 29 30 32 33 34 36 38 51 54 70 76 78 **P**5 7 8 **S** Franciscan Services Corporation, Sylvania, OH **Web address:** www.st–joseph.org/	21	10	30	345	7	13681	0	5071	2042	68
CAMERON—Milam County										
CENTRAL TEXAS HOSPITAL, 806 North Crockett Avenue, Zip 76520–2599; tel. 254/697–6591; Tariq Mahmood, Chief Executive Officer **A**9 10 **F**7 13 19 22 24 25 29 31 32 34 37 41 48 54 76 77 78	33	10	34	693	9	14429	0	—	—	55
CANADIAN—Hemphill County										
HEMPHILL COUNTY HOSPITAL, 1020 South Fourth Street, Zip 79014–3315; tel. 806/323–6422; Robert Ezzell, Administrator **A**9 **F**1 9 13 14 19 21 23 24 25 26 30 31 32 33 34 36 37 38 40 50 51 54 56 61 70 72 75 76 78	16	10	19	246	3	10544	0	3464	1509	64
CARRIZO SPRINGS—Dimmit County										
DIMMIT COUNTY MEMORIAL HOSPITAL, 704 Hospital Drive, Zip 78834–3836; tel. 830/876–2424; Ernesto G. Flores, Jr, Administrator **A**9 10 **F**8 9 12 16 17 18 22 25 32 36 38 44 48 51 54 66 75 76	13	10	35	977	9	26459	83	7304	3222	131
CARROLLTON—Denton County										
✠ TRINITY MEDICAL CENTER, 4343 North Josey Lane, Zip 75010–4691; tel. 972/492–1010; Craig E. Sims, President (Total facility includes 12 beds in nursing home–type unit) **A**1 9 10 **F**4 7 8 9 11 13 16 17 18 19 22 23 24 25 27 29 30 32 33 34 36 37 38 39 41 42 43 44 45 46 47 48 49 51 54 59 66 68 69 70 71 72 74 75 76 77 78 79 **P**5 **S** TENET Healthcare Corporation, Santa Barbara, CA **Web address:** www.tenethealth.com	33	10	137	6137	60	94095	1922	54409	18721	429
CARTHAGE—Panola County										
☐ EAST TEXAS MEDICAL CENTER CARTHAGE, 409 Cottage Road, Zip 75633–1466, Mailing Address: P.O. Box 549, Zip 75633–0549; tel. 903/693–3841; Gary Mikeal Hudson, Administrator **A**1 9 10 **F**7 9 18 22 25 32 39 41 48 54 70 75 76 **S** East Texas Medical Center Regional Healthcare System, Tyler, TX **Web address:** www.etmc.org	23	10	30	1032	10	27425	0	10529	3958	117
CENTER—Shelby County										
☐ MEMORIAL HOSPITAL OF CENTER, 602 Hurst Street, Zip 75935–3414, Mailing Address: P.O. Box 1749, Zip 75935–1749; tel. 409/598–2781; John A. Tucker, Chief Executive Officer **A**1 9 10 **F**8 9 16 17 18 22 24 25 36 40 44 45 46 48 54 70 75 76 78 **P**8 **S** New American Healthcare Corporation, Brentwood, TN **Web address:** www.memorial.nahc.net	33	10	46	1729	17	28556	111	11198	4400	145
CHILDRESS—Childress County										
☐ CHILDRESS REGIONAL MEDICAL CENTER, Highway 83 North, Zip 79201, Mailing Address: P.O. Box 1030, Zip 79201–1030; tel. 940/937–6371; Frances T. Smith, Administrator **A**1 9 10 **F**9 13 14 15 16 17 18 19 22 24 25 30 31 32 33 34 35 36 37 38 43 44 48 50 51 54 56 70 71 72 75 76 78 79	16	10	35	1018	9	29247	210	8367	4130	164
CHILLICOTHE—Hardeman County										
☐ CHILLICOTHE HOSPITAL DISTRICT, 303 Avenue I, Zip 79225, Mailing Address: P.O. Box 370, Zip 79225–0370; tel. 940/852–5131; Linda Hall, Administrator **A**9 10 **F**13 16 17 18 22 24 25 32 34 39 48 74 75 76 **Web address:** www.chillicothehospital.com	16	10	12	96	1	449	0	1161	573	25
CLARKSVILLE—Red River County										
✠ EAST TEXAS MEDICAL CENTER–CLARKSVILLE, 3000 Highway 82 West, Zip 75426, Mailing Address: P.O. Box 1270, Zip 75426–1270; tel. 903/427–3851; Terry Cutler, Administrator and Chief Operating Officer **A**1 9 10 **F**7 9 16 17 22 24 25 32 34 38 41 43 48 50 51 54 70 72 75 76 78 **P**8 **S** East Texas Medical Center Regional Healthcare System, Tyler, TX	23	10	36	1708	17	12472	0	7292	2748	108
CLEBURNE—Johnson County										
✠ WALLS REGIONAL HOSPITAL, 201 Walls Drive, Zip 76031–1008; tel. 817/641–2551; Brent D. Magers, FACHE, President (Total facility includes 11 beds in nursing home–type unit) **A**1 9 10 **F**3 4 7 8 9 11 13 14 17 18 19 20 22 23 24 25 26 28 30 31 32 33 34 35 36 37 38 39 41 43 44 45 46 47 48 49 50 51 54 56 58 59 60 61 63 64 65 66 68 69 70 71 72 74 75 76 78 79 **P**5 **S** Texas Health Resources, Irving, TX **Web address:** www.hmhs.com	21	10	137	4622	52	73533	620	32345	13073	361
CLEVELAND—Liberty County										
☐ CLEVELAND REGIONAL MEDICAL CENTER, 300 East Crockett Street, Zip 77327–4062, Mailing Address: P.O. Box 1688, Zip 77328–1688; tel. 281/593–1811; Ron J. MacLaren, Chief Executive Officer (Total facility includes 11 beds in nursing home–type unit) **A**1 9 10 **F**4 7 8 9 11 13 17 18 19 21 22 24 25 29 32 34 37 38 39 41 44 46 48 49 50 51 54 61 68 69 70 71 72 76 78 79 **P**7 **S** Community Health Systems, Inc., Brentwood, TN **Web address:** www.crmcr.com	32	10	115	3339	39	48070	404	26922	9833	258
CLIFTON—Bosque County										
★ GOODALL–WITCHER HEALTHCARE, 101 South Avenue T, Zip 76634–1897, Mailing Address: P.O. Box 549, Zip 76634–0549; tel. 254/675–8322; Jim B. Smith, President and Chief Executive Officer (Total facility includes 30 beds in nursing home–type unit) **A**9 10 **F**8 9 17 22 24 25 34 36 38 41 44 48 54 69 70 75 76 78 **P**3 **Web address:** www.gwhf.org	23	10	70	1292	43	67329	215	12730	5366	185

Hospitals, U.S. / TEXAS

Hospital, Address, Telephone, Administrator, Approval, Facility, and Physician Codes, Health Care System, Network ★ American Hospital Association (AHA) membership □ Joint Commission on Accreditation of Healthcare Organizations (JCAHO) accreditation + American Osteopathic Healthcare Association (AOHA) membership ○ American Osteopathic Association (AOA) accreditation △ Commission on Accreditation of Rehabilitation Facilities (CARF) accreditation Control codes 61, 63, 64, 71, 72 and 73 indicate hospitals listed by AOHA, but not registered by AHA. For definition of numerical codes, see page A4	Classification Codes		Utilization Data					Expense (thousands) of dollars		
	Control	Service	Staffed Beds	Admissions	Census	Outpatient Visits	Births	Total	Payroll	Personnel
COLEMAN—Coleman County COLEMAN COUNTY MEDICAL CENTER, 310 South Pecos Street, Zip 76834–4159; tel. 915/625-2135; Michael Morris, Administrator **A**9 10 **F**7 16 17 18 22 25 28 34 39 40 43 46 48 54 76 78	16	10	27	1566	15	21341	44	6890	3102	178
COLLEGE STATION—Brazos County ✠ COLLEGE STATION MEDICAL CENTER, 1604 Rock Prairie Road, Zip 77845–8345, Mailing Address: P.O. Box 10000, Zip 77842–3500; tel. 979/764–5100; Thomas W. Jackson, Chief Executive Officer **A**1 5 9 10 **F**4 7 8 9 11 13 17 18 22 24 25 27 28 32 34 35 39 41 44 45 47 48 53 54 69 70 76 78 **P**7 8 **S** Triad Hospitals, Inc., Dallas, TX **Web address:** www.csmedcenter.com	32	10	119	3624	43	34582	650	27846	12632	369
COLORADO CITY—Mitchell County ★ MITCHELL COUNTY HOSPITAL, 1543 Chestnut Street, Zip 79512–3998; tel. 915/728–3431; Roland K. Rickard, Administrator **A**9 10 **F**7 8 9 13 16 17 18 19 22 25 28 33 34 36 48 51 54 70 72 75 76 78 **P**5 **S** Lubbock Methodist Hospital System, Lubbock, TX	16	10	25	772	10	42438	54	11128	5572	199
COLUMBUS—Colorado County □ COLUMBUS COMMUNITY HOSPITAL, 110 Shult Drive, Zip 78934–3010, Mailing Address: P.O. Box 865, Zip 78934–0865; tel. 409/732–2371; Robert Thomas, Administrator (Nonreporting) **A**1 9 10	23	10	36	—	—	—	—	—	—	—
COMANCHE—Comanche County COMANCHE COMMUNITY HOSPITAL, 211 South Austin Street, Zip 76442–3224; tel. 915/356–5241; W. Evan Moore, Administrator **A**9 10 **F**17 18 22 25 28 34 36 38 44 48 54 56 61 63 69 70 75 76 **P**4 7	16	10	19	631	8	40169	7	5522	2639	107
COMMERCE—Hunt County PRESBYTERIAN HOSPITAL OF COMMERCE See Hunt Memorial Hospital District, Greenville										
CONROE—Montgomery County ✠ CONROE REGIONAL MEDICAL CENTER, 504 Medical Boulevard, Zip 77304, Mailing Address: P.O. Box 1538, Zip 77305–1538; tel. 936/539–1111; Russell Meyers, Chief Executive Officer (Total facility includes 12 beds in nursing home–type unit) **A**1 3 9 10 **F**4 8 9 11 12 13 16 17 18 22 24 25 30 32 33 34 38 39 41 42 43 44 45 46 47 48 49 50 53 54 56 65 68 69 70 72 75 76 78 79 **P**7 8 **S** HCA – The Healthcare Company, Nashville, TN **Web address:** www.conroeregional.com	33	10	244	13114	159	98449	1795	82053	33997	902
CORPUS CHRISTI—Nueces County ✠ CHRISTUS SPOHN HOSPITAL MEMORIAL, 2606 Hospital Boulevard, Zip 78405–1818, Mailing Address: Box 5280, Zip 78465–5280; tel. 361/902–4000; Thomas G. Neff, Vice President and Administrator **A**1 3 9 10 **F**3 4 7 8 9 10 11 12 13 16 17 18 19 21 22 23 24 25 27 28 30 31 32 33 34 35 36 37 38 39 41 43 44 46 47 48 49 51 54 56 57 58 59 60 61 62 63 64 65 69 70 71 72 73 74 75 76 77 78 79 **P**3 5 8 **S** Christus Health, Irving, TX **Web address:** www.sch.org	21	10	270	9842	158	166976	948	99311	39871	1245
✠ △ CHRISTUS SPOHN HOSPITAL SHORELINE, (Formerly Christus Spohn Health System), 600 Elizabeth Street, Zip 78404; tel. 361/881–3000; Andrew M. Harris, Vice President and Administrator (Total facility includes 36 beds in nursing home–type unit) **A**1 2 7 9 10 **F**4 7 8 9 11 12 13 16 17 18 19 22 24 25 27 28 30 32 33 34 36 37 38 39 41 42 43 44 45 46 47 48 50 51 53 54 56 57 62 65 68 69 70 71 72 75 76 78 79 **P**3 5 8 **S** Christus Health, Irving, TX **Web address:** www.sch.org	21	10	377	14730	251	137377	0	131032	48155	1113
CHRISTUS SPOHN HOSPITAL SOUTH, 5950 Saratoga, Zip 78414; tel. 361/985–5000 (Nonreporting)	21	10	95	—	—	—	—	—	—	—
✠ CORPUS CHRISTI MEDICAL CENTER, 3315 South Alameda Street, Zip 78411–1883, Mailing Address: P.O. Box 8991, Zip 78468–8991; tel. 361/857–1400; Steven Woerner, Chief Executive Officer (Total facility includes 26 beds in nursing home–type unit) (Nonreporting) **A**1 9 **S** HCA – The Healthcare Company, Nashville, TN **Web address:** www.hcahealthcare.com	32	10	237	—	—	—	—	—	—	—
✠ CORPUS CHRISTI MEDICAL CENTER BAY AREA, 7101 South Padre Island Drive, Zip 78412–4999; tel. 361/985–1200; Steven Woerner, Chief Executive Officer (Total facility includes 26 beds in nursing home–type unit) **A**1 9 10 12 13 **F**4 8 9 11 12 13 16 17 18 19 22 23 24 25 27 29 30 31 32 33 34 35 38 39 41 42 43 44 45 46 47 48 50 51 54 65 66 69 70 71 73 74 76 78 79 **P**3 5 7 8 **S** HCA – The Healthcare Company, Nashville, TN	32	10	398	18945	252	67813	3533	115483	46264	1890
✠ DRISCOLL CHILDREN'S HOSPITAL, 3533 South Alameda Street, Zip 78411–1785, Mailing Address: P.O. Box 6530, Zip 78466–6530; tel. 361/694–5000; Rick W. Merrill, President and Chief Executive Officer **A**1 3 5 9 10 **F**4 5 7 11 13 16 17 18 19 22 24 25 29 31 32 33 34 35 36 37 38 39 42 43 45 46 47 48 50 51 52 54 56 58 59 60 61 62 63 64 65 66 68 70 71 72 73 74 76 77 78 79 **Web address:** www.driscollchildrens.org	23	50	200	6824	120	82265	0	77327	37293	1243
★ NAVAL HOSPITAL, 10651 E Street, Zip 78419–5131; tel. 361/961–2688; Captain Elizabeth R. Barker, Commanding Officer (Nonreporting) **S** Department of Navy, Washington, DC **Web address:** www.nhcc.med.navy.mil	43	10	25	—	—	—	—	—	—	—
✠ NORTHWEST REGIONAL HOSPITAL, 13725 Northwest Boulevard, Zip 78410–5199; tel. 361/241–4243; Winston Borland, Chief Executive Officer **A**1 9 10 **F**7 9 17 22 23 24 25 28 30 32 35 39 45 48 49 50 53 54 69 70 71 72 76 78 **S** HCA – The Healthcare Company, Nashville, TN **Web address:** www.hcahealthcare.com	33	10	73	2930	43	76014	0	24553	10732	335

© 2000 AHA Guide *Many Facility Codes have changed. Please refer to the AHA Guide Code Chart.*

Hospitals, U.S. / TEXAS

Hospital, Address, Telephone, Administrator, Approval, Facility, and Physician Codes, Health Care System, Network	Classification Codes		Utilization Data					Expense (thousands) of dollars		Personnel
	Control	Service	Staffed Beds	Admissions	Census	Outpatient Visits	Births	Total	Payroll	

★ American Hospital Association (AHA) membership
☐ Joint Commission on Accreditation of Healthcare Organizations (JCAHO) accreditation
+ American Osteopathic Healthcare Association (AOHA) membership
○ American Osteopathic Association (AOA) accreditation
△ Commission on Accreditation of Rehabilitation Facilities (CARF) accreditation
Control codes 61, 63, 64, 71, 72 and 73 indicate hospitals listed by AOHA, but not registered by AHA. For definition of numerical codes, see page A4

Hospital	Control	Service	Staffed Beds	Admissions	Census	Outpatient Visits	Births	Total	Payroll	Personnel
CORSICANA—Navarro County ★ NAVARRO REGIONAL HOSPITAL, 3201 West State Highway 22, Zip 75110; tel. 903/654–6800; Nancy A. Byrnes, Chief Executive Officer **A**1 9 10 **F**4 7 8 9 11 13 16 17 18 22 23 25 27 32 34 35 37 39 41 43 44 45 46 48 53 54 69 70 76 78 **P**7 8 **S** Triad Hospitals, Inc., Dallas, TX Web address: www.hcahealthcare.com	32	10	144	4250	60	35193	522	28010	9929	332
CRANE—Crane County ★ CRANE MEMORIAL HOSPITAL, 1310 South Alford Street, Zip 79731–3899; tel. 915/558–3555; Stan Wiley, Administrator **A**9 10 **F**14 16 17 18 19 25 30 32 33 34 35 38 43 48 50 56 76 77 79	13	10	28	218	2	8677	0	2910	1298	37
CROCKETT—Houston County ★ EAST TEXAS MEDICAL CENTER CROCKETT, 1100 Loop 304 East, Zip 75835–1810; tel. 936/546–3862; Nelda K. Welch, Administrator **A**1 9 10 **F**7 8 9 14 16 17 18 19 22 24 25 26 29 31 32 34 35 36 38 39 41 43 44 45 46 48 51 54 56 68 70 71 72 75 76 78 **P**3 7 **S** East Texas Medical Center Regional Healthcare System, Tyler, TX	23	10	68	2127	26	44060	97	15190	6031	196
CROSBYTON—Crosby County ★ CROSBYTON CLINIC HOSPITAL, (SPECIALTY MEDICAL ONLY), 710 West Main Street, Zip 79322–2143; tel. 806/675–2382; Jeffrey Madison, Administrator and Chief Executive Officer **A**9 10 **F**3 4 6 7 8 9 11 13 17 18 19 21 22 23 24 25 28 30 32 33 34 36 38 39 43 45 46 47 48 49 50 51 54 56 58 59 60 62 63 64 65 70 76 78 79 **P**6 **S** St. Joseph Health System, Orange, CA	23	49	30	758	11	23323	0	4216	1904	88
CUERO—De Witt County ★ CUERO COMMUNITY HOSPITAL, 2550 North Esplanade Street, Zip 77954–4716; tel. 361/275–6191; James E. Buckner, Jr, Administrator **A**1 9 10 **F**7 8 9 16 17 18 22 24 25 29 32 34 35 36 39 43 44 45 48 49 50 54 56 64 70 71 75 76 78 Web address: www.cuerohosp.org	16	10	60	3255	39	165171	181	21358	9152	358
DALHART—Dallam County COON MEMORIAL HOSPITAL AND HOME, 1411 Denver Avenue, Zip 79022–4809; tel. 806/244–4571; Leroy Schaffner, Chief Executive Officer **A**9 10 **F**7 8 9 22 30 32 36 37 38 40 44 45 48 50 54 75 76 78	16	10	23	575	7	14611	67	7275	3330	103
DALLAS—Dallas County A. WEBB ROBERTS HOSPITAL See Baylor University Medical Center										
★ BAYLOR CENTER FOR RESTORATIVE CARE, (LONG TERM ACUTE CARE HOSPITAL), 3504 Swiss Avenue, Zip 75204–6224; tel. 214/820–9700; Geraldine Brueckner, R.N., Executive Director **A**9 10 **F**4 7 8 9 10 11 12 13 16 17 18 19 22 24 25 28 29 30 32 34 36 39 41 42 44 47 48 49 50 52 53 54 55 56 65 66 68 69 70 71 72 74 75 76 77 78 **P**1 3 5 7 **S** Baylor Health Care System, Dallas, TX Web address: www.baylordallas.edu/	23	49	72	766	58	0	0	10826	4873	168
★ △ BAYLOR INSTITUTE FOR REHABILITATION, 3505 Gaston Avenue, Zip 75246–2018; tel. 214/826–7030; Laura J. Lycan, Executive Director **A**3 7 10 **F**2 3 4 5 8 9 10 11 12 13 16 17 18 19 21 24 25 27 28 29 30 31 32 33 34 35 36 37 38 39 41 42 43 44 45 46 47 48 49 50 51 52 53 54 56 57 58 61 62 63 65 66 69 70 71 72 74 75 76 78 79 **P**5 7 **S** Baylor Health Care System, Dallas, TX Web address: www.bhcs.com	21	46	92	1424	77	28252	0	21232	10684	355
★ BAYLOR UNIVERSITY MEDICAL CENTER, (Includes A. Webb Roberts Hospital; Erik and Margaret Jonsson Hospital; George W. Truett Memorial Hospital; Karl and Esther Hoblitzelle Memorial Hospital), 3500 Gaston Avenue, Zip 75246–2088; tel. 214/820–0111; Boone Powell, Jr, President and Chief Executive Officer (Total facility includes 29 beds in nursing home–type unit) **A**1 2 3 5 8 9 10 **F**3 4 5 7 8 9 11 12 13 14 16 17 18 19 20 21 22 23 24 25 27 28 29 30 32 33 34 35 36 37 38 39 40 41 42 43 44 45 46 47 48 49 50 51 54 55 56 57 59 60 61 62 64 65 66 69 70 71 72 74 75 76 77 78 79 **P**5 6 7 **S** Baylor Health Care System, Dallas, TX Web address: www.bhcs.com	23	10	876	36789	598	277267	4388	442059	177224	4709
★ CHARLTON METHODIST HOSPITAL, 3500 West Wheatland Road, Zip 75237, Mailing Address: Box 225357, Zip 75222–5357; tel. 214/947–7500; David L. Knocke, CHE, Executive Director **A**1 3 9 10 **F**3 4 5 6 8 9 11 12 13 16 17 18 19 21 22 24 25 27 28 30 31 32 33 34 35 38 39 41 42 43 44 45 46 47 48 49 50 53 54 56 59 60 61 65 66 68 69 70 71 72 74 75 76 78 79 **P**1 7 **S** Methodist Hospitals of Dallas, Dallas, TX Web address: www.mhd.com	23	10	130	8828	96	121057	1678	58480	26605	747
★ CHILDREN'S MEDICAL CENTER OF DALLAS, 1935 Motor Street, Zip 75235–7794; tel. 214/456–7000; George D. Farr, President and Chief Executive Officer **A**1 2 3 5 8 9 10 **F**4 11 13 14 15 16 17 18 19 21 22 23 24 25 26 29 31 32 33 35 36 38 39 43 45 46 47 48 49 50 51 52 54 55 56 57 58 59 60 61 62 63 64 68 70 71 72 74 75 76 77 78 Web address: www.childrens.com	23	50	224	13315	166	276164	0	201438	97721	1963
★ ○ DALLAS SOUTHWEST MEDICAL CENTER, 2929 South Hampton Road, Zip 75224–3026; tel. 214/330–4611; Carolyn Caldwell, Chief Executive Officer **A**1 9 10 11 12 13 **F**1 2 3 4 5 6 7 8 9 10 11 12 13 14 15 17 18 19 20 21 22 23 24 25 26 27 28 29 30 32 33 34 35 36 37 38 39 40 41 42 43 44 45 46 47 48 49 50 51 52 53 54 55 56 57 58 59 60 62 63 64 65 66 67 68 69 70 72 73 74 75 76 77 78 79 **P**5 **S** HCA – The Healthcare Company, Nashville, TN Web address: www.hcahealthcare.com	32	10	107	3149	32	21698	496	31039	9243	249

Hospitals, U.S. / TEXAS

Hospital, Address, Telephone, Administrator, Approval, Facility, and Physician Codes, Health Care System, Network	Classification Codes		Utilization Data					Expense (thousands) of dollars		
★ American Hospital Association (AHA) membership □ Joint Commission on Accreditation of Healthcare Organizations (JCAHO) accreditation + American Osteopathic Healthcare Association (AOHA) membership ○ American Osteopathic Association (AOA) accreditation △ Commission on Accreditation of Rehabilitation Facilities (CARF) accreditation Control codes 61, 63, 64, 71, 72 and 73 indicate hospitals listed by AOHA, but not registered by AHA. For definition of numerical codes, see page A4	Control	Service	Staffed Beds	Admissions	Census	Outpatient Visits	Births	Total	Payroll	Personnel
★ DOCTORS HOSPITAL OF DALLAS, 9440 Poppy Drive, Zip 75218-3694; tel. 214/324-6100; Robert S. Freymuller, Chief Executive Officer (Total facility includes 19 beds in nursing home-type unit) **A**1 9 10 **F**4 8 9 11 13 16 17 18 19 22 23 24 25 27 30 31 32 33 34 35 36 37 38 39 41 44 45 46 47 48 49 50 51 54 57 60 61 62 63 64 65 68 69 70 71 72 75 76 77 78 79 **P**5 7 **S** TENET Healthcare Corporation, Santa Barbara, CA Web address: www.tenethealth.com/ ERIK AND MARGARET JONSSON HOSPITAL See Baylor University Medical Center GEORGE W. TRUETT MEMORIAL HOSPITAL See Baylor University Medical Center	32	10	198	8093	116	92617	535	59533	23885	669
★ GREEN OAKS HOSPITAL, 7808 Clodus Fields Drive, Zip 75251-2206; tel. 972/991-9504; Thomas M. Collins, Chief Executive Officer (Nonreporting) **A**1 9 **S** HCA – The Healthcare Company, Nashville, TN Web address: www.greenoakspsych.com	33	22	106	—	—	—	—	—	—	—
□ HEALTHSOUTH MEDICAL CENTER, 2124 Research Row, Zip 75235-2504; tel. 214/904-6100; Robert M. Smart, Area Manager and Chief Executive Officer **A**1 9 10 **F**5 13 17 18 22 30 31 32 34 35 36 37 38 39 43 45 48 49 50 53 54 70 71 72 76 **S** HEALTHSOUTH Corporation, Birmingham, AL Web address: www.healthsouth.com KARL AND ESTHER HOBLITZELLE MEMORIAL HOSPITAL See Baylor University Medical Center	33	46	86	1124	52	11201	0	15181	7943	235
★ MARY SHIELS HOSPITAL, 3515 Howell Street, Zip 75204-2895; tel. 214/443-3000; Rob Shiels, Administrator **A**1 9 10 **F**38 48 49 51 54	32	10	15	280	1	2655	0	6622	2851	67
★ △ MEDICAL CITY DALLAS HOSPITAL, 7777 Forest Lane, Zip 75230-2598; tel. 972/566-7000; Britt Berrett, President and Chief Executive Officer (Total facility includes 34 beds in nursing home-type unit) **A**1 2 7 9 10 **F**2 3 4 7 8 9 11 12 13 16 18 19 21 22 23 25 26 27 28 30 32 33 34 35 37 38 39 41 42 43 44 45 46 47 48 49 50 51 52 53 54 55 57 58 59 60 61 62 63 64 65 66 68 69 70 71 72 74 76 78 79 **S** HCA – The Healthcare Company, Nashville, TN Web address: www.medicalcityhospital.com	33	10	530	21822	324	122696	3703	239387	83953	1816
★ △ METHODIST MEDICAL CENTER, 1441 North Beckley Avenue, Zip 75203-1201, Mailing Address: Box 655999, Zip 75265-5999; tel. 214/947-8181; Kim N. Hollon, FACHE, Executive Director **A**1 2 3 5 7 8 9 10 **F**4 7 8 9 11 12 13 16 17 18 19 22 24 25 26 27 28 29 30 31 32 33 34 35 38 39 41 42 43 44 45 46 47 48 49 50 51 53 54 56 65 66 68 69 70 71 72 74 75 76 78 79 **P**1 7 **S** Methodist Hospitals of Dallas, Dallas, TX Web address: www.mhd.com	23	10	362	15584	273	129023	2168	153339	63427	2015
□ △ NORTH DALLAS REHABILITATION HOSPITAL, 8383 Meadow Road, Zip 75231-3798; tel. 214/891-0880; Pam Duhon, Administrator and Chief Executive Officer **A**1 7 10 **F**13 16 17 18 31 43 45 53 54 70 **P**6	33	46	36	320	15	0	0	3421	1647	86
OUR CHILDREN'S HOUSE AT BAYLOR, (Formerly Pediatric Center Care), (CHILDREN'S HOSP FOR CHRONI), 3301 Swiss Avenue, Zip 75204-6219; tel. 214/820-9838; Geraldine Brueckner, R.N., Executive Director **A**9 10 **F**4 7 8 9 10 11 12 13 14 16 17 18 19 22 24 25 28 29 30 32 34 36 39 41 42 44 46 47 48 49 50 51 52 53 54 55 56 65 66 68 69 70 71 72 74 75 76 77 78 **P**1 3 5 7 Web address: www.baylordallas.edu/	23	59	21	170	14	13232	0	5479	3115	112
★ PARKLAND HEALTH AND HOSPITAL SYSTEM, 5201 Harry Hines Boulevard, Zip 75235-7731; tel. 214/590-8000; Ron J. Anderson, M.D., President and Chief Executive Officer (Nonreporting) **A**1 2 3 5 8 9 10 Web address: www.swmed.edv/home_pages/parkland/	16	10	702	—	—	—	—	—	—	—
★ △ PRESBYTERIAN HOSPITAL OF DALLAS, 8200 Walnut Hill Lane, Zip 75231-4402; tel. 214/345-6789; Mark H. Merrill, President (Total facility includes 52 beds in nursing home-type unit) **A**1 2 3 5 7 9 10 **F**1 3 4 5 6 7 8 9 11 12 13 14 16 17 18 19 21 22 23 24 25 26 27 28 29 30 31 32 33 34 35 36 38 39 40 41 42 43 44 45 46 47 48 49 50 51 53 54 56 57 58 59 60 61 62 63 64 65 66 67 68 69 70 72 73 74 76 77 78 79 **P**2 5 6 **S** Texas Health Resources, Irving, TX Web address: www.texashealth.org	23	10	656	26551	405	301597	5172	287129	111890	3386
★ RHD MEMORIAL MEDICAL CENTER, Seven Medical Parkway, Zip 75381, Mailing Address: P.O. Box 819094, Zip 75381-9094; tel. 972/247-1000; Craig E. Sims, President and Chief Executive Officer **A**1 9 10 **F**4 7 8 9 11 13 16 17 18 19 22 23 24 25 27 29 30 32 33 34 36 37 38 39 41 43 44 45 46 47 48 49 50 51 53 54 59 66 68 70 71 72 74 75 76 78 79 **P**5 **S** TENET Healthcare Corporation, Santa Barbara, CA Web address: www.tenethealth.com	33	10	141	4336	57	58002	523	58122	18267	427
□ SELECT SPECIALTY HOSPITAL–DALLAS/FORTH WORTH, 10 Medical Parkway, Suite 205, Zip 75234; tel. 972/488-9167; LouAnn O. Mathews, Administrator **A**1 9 10 **F**13 22 25 35 39 70 76 **S** Select Medical Corporation, Mechanicsburg, PA	33	49	36	298	21	0	0	5914	2175	38
★ ST. PAUL MEDICAL CENTER, 5909 Harry Hines Boulevard, Zip 75235-6285; tel. 214/879-1000; Frank Tiedemann, President **A**1 2 3 5 8 9 10 **F**1 3 4 5 7 8 9 11 12 13 14 17 18 19 21 22 23 24 25 26 27 28 29 30 31 32 33 34 35 36 37 38 39 41 42 43 44 45 46 47 48 49 50 51 53 54 55 56 57 58 59 60 61 62 63 64 65 66 67 68 69 70 72 73 74 76 78 79 **P**2 5 7 **S** Texas Health Resources, Irving, TX Web address: www.texashealth.com	21	10	339	13937	224	141279	2553	151463	59019	1561

© 2000 AHA Guide *Many Facility Codes have changed. Please refer to the AHA Guide Code Chart.*

Hospitals, U.S. / TEXAS

Hospital, Address, Telephone, Administrator, Approval, Facility, and Physician Codes, Health Care System, Network	Classification Codes		Utilization Data					Expense (thousands) of dollars		
★ American Hospital Association (AHA) membership □ Joint Commission on Accreditation of Healthcare Organizations (JCAHO) accreditation + American Osteopathic Healthcare Association (AOHA) membership ○ American Osteopathic Association (AOA) accreditation △ Commission on Accreditation of Rehabilitation Facilities (CARF) accreditation Control codes 61, 63, 64, 71, 72 and 73 indicate hospitals listed by AOHA, but not registered by AHA. For definition of numerical codes, see page A4	Control	Service	Staffed Beds	Admissions	Census	Outpatient Visits	Births	Total	Payroll	Personnel
★ TEXAS SCOTTISH RITE HOSPITAL FOR CHILDREN, (PED ORTHO & LEARNING DIS), 2222 Welborn Street, Zip 75219–9982, Mailing Address: P.O. Box 190567, Zip 75219–0567; tel. 214/559–5000; J. C. Montgomery, Jr, President **A**1 3 5 **F**5 13 22 23 31 33 49 50 51 70 72 76 78 **P**6	23	59	52	2540	26	41068	0	—	—	584
□ TIMBERLAWN MENTAL HEALTH SYSTEM, 4600 Samuell Boulevard, Zip 75228–6800; tel. 214/381–7181; Craig Nuckles, Group Director **A**1 9 10 **F**3 17 18 19 29 33 34 51 57 58 59 60 61 62 63 64 70 72 **S** Universal Health Services, Inc., King of Prussia, PA **Web address:** www.timberlawn.com	33	22	92	3216	65	24014	0	11865	5865	151
□ VENCOR HOSPITAL – DALLAS, (LONG TERM ACUTE CARE), 9525 Greenville Avenue, Zip 75243–4116; tel. 214/355–2600; Dorothy J. Elford, Executive Director and Administrator **A**1 9 10 **F**22 39 41 70 75 76 **S** Vencor, Incorporated, Louisville, KY	32	49	125	598	60	0	0	20220	8758	171
★ VETERANS AFFAIRS NORTH TEXAS HEALTH CARE SYSTEM, (Includes Sam Rayburn Memorial Veterans Center, 1201 East Ninth Street, Bonham, Zip 75418–4091; tel. 903/583–2111), 4500 South Lancaster Road, Zip 75216–7167; tel. 214/742–8387; Alan G. Harper, Director (Total facility includes 240 beds in nursing home–type unit) (Nonreporting) **A**1 2 3 5 8 **S** Department of Veterans Affairs, Washington, DC	45	10	1031	—	—	—	—	—	—	—
□ △ ZALE LIPSHY UNIVERSITY HOSPITAL, 5151 Harry Hines Boulevard, Zip 75235–7786; tel. 214/590–3000; Robert B. Smith, President and Chief Executive Officer **A**1 3 5 7 8 9 10 **F**4 9 11 13 16 22 25 32 34 36 38 39 45 46 47 48 50 59 61 62 64 65 70 72 76 78 **Web address:** www.zluh.org	23	10	145	5954	106	11757	0	92425	35349	820
DE LEON—Comanche County										
★ DE LEON HOSPITAL, 407 South Texas Street, Zip 76444–1947; tel. 254/893–2011; Michael K. Hare, Administrator **A**9 10 **F**7 9 16 17 18 22 25 32 36 38 41 48 54 70 76 **S** Brim Healthcare, Inc., Brentwood, TN	16	10	14	839	11	22043	1	5168	2047	77
DE SOTO—Dallas County										
□ CEDARS HOSPITAL, 2000 North Old Hickory Trail, Zip 75115–2242; tel. 972/298–7323; Don P. Johnson, Administrator **A**1 9 10 **F**2 3 30 35 38 50 57 58 59 60 61 62 63 64 70	33	22	76	905	24	2730	0	4958	2683	89
DECATUR—Wise County										
★ DECATUR COMMUNITY HOSPITAL, 2000 South FM 51, Zip 76234–9295; tel. 940/627–5921; Stephen M. Summers, CPA, CHE, Chief Executive Officer (Total facility includes 10 beds in nursing home–type unit) **A**1 9 10 **F**7 8 9 13 16 17 18 22 25 28 29 32 36 41 44 45 48 49 54 68 69 70 71 72 75 76 **P**5 7 **Web address:** www.decaturcommunity.com	16	10	69	3207	34	68964	449	19930	9904	356
DEL RIO—Val Verde County										
★ VAL VERDE REGIONAL MEDICAL CENTER, 801 Bedell Avenue, Zip 78840–4185, Mailing Address: P.O. Box 1527, Zip 78840–1527; tel. 830/775–8566; Patrick J. Jacobus, Chief Executive Officer **A**1 9 10 **F**7 8 9 11 13 17 18 22 24 25 32 34 36 37 38 39 40 41 43 44 45 48 50 51 54 56 70 75 76 77 78 79 **P**5	16	10	81	3849	38	27662	954	24516	10927	416
DENISON—Grayson County										
★ TEXOMA HEALTHCARE SYSTEM, 1000 Memorial Drive, Zip 75020–2035, Mailing Address: P.O. Box 890, Zip 75021–9988; tel. 903/416–4000; Arthur L. Hohenberger, FACHE, President and Chief Executive Officer **A**1 2 9 10 **F**3 4 7 8 9 11 13 16 17 18 19 22 24 25 26 27 29 30 31 32 33 34 36 37 38 39 41 43 44 45 46 47 48 50 51 53 54 56 57 58 59 61 62 63 64 65 70 71 72 75 76 78 79 **P**3 5 **Web address:** www.thcs.org	23	10	206	8617	122	228032	456	77081	32566	1178
DENTON—Denton County										
★ DENTON COMMUNITY HOSPITAL, 207 North Bonnie Brae Street, Zip 76201–3798; tel. 940/898–7000; Timothy Charles, Chief Executive Officer **A**1 9 10 **F**4 7 8 9 11 13 16 18 22 24 25 32 34 35 37 39 41 43 44 45 46 47 48 49 54 61 68 70 71 72 76 78 79 **S** NetCare Health Systems, Inc., Nashville, TN **Web address:** www.dentonhospital.com	16	10	122	5729	63	44550	942	34765	13985	428
★ DENTON REGIONAL MEDICAL CENTER, 3535 South I–35 East, Zip 76205; tel. 940/384–3535; Bob Haley, Chief Executive Officer (Total facility includes 25 beds in nursing home–type unit) **A**1 9 10 **F**4 8 9 11 13 18 22 23 24 25 27 37 39 41 44 46 47 48 53 54 57 62 64 65 69 70 76 78 79 **P**5 **S** HCA – The Healthcare Company, Nashville, TN **Web address:** www.dentonregional.com	32	10	222	6994	112	84875	925	54819	24194	738
DENVER CITY—Yoakum County										
★ YOAKUM COUNTY HOSPITAL, 412 Mustang Avenue, Zip 79323–2750, Mailing Address: P.O. Drawer 1130, Zip 79323–1130; tel. 806/592–5484; Edward Rodgers, Chief Executive Officer **A**9 10 **F**6 8 13 17 19 25 32 33 34 38 41 43 44 48 54 69 70 75 76 78 **P**5 **S** St. Joseph Health System, Orange, CA	13	10	21	374	3	20164	73	4467	1561	60
DIMMITT—Castro County										
PLAINS MEMORIAL HOSPITAL, 310 West Halsell Street, Zip 79027–1846, Mailing Address: P.O. Box 278, Zip 79027–0278; tel. 806/647–2191; Joseph F. Sloan, CHE, Chief Executive Officer **A**9 10 **F**7 9 13 16 17 19 20 22 25 26 30 32 34 36 37 38 40 43 44 45 48 54 57 62 63 64 69 70 75 76 78	16	10	36	522	8	38548	52	7885	3581	173
DUMAS—Moore County										
★ MOORE COUNTY HOSPITAL DISTRICT, 224 East Second Street, Zip 79029–3808; tel. 806/935–7171; Scott R. Brown, Administrator and Chief Executive Officer **A**1 9 10 **F**7 8 9 16 17 18 19 22 23 25 30 31 32 34 36 37 39 41 43 44 45 48 50 51 54 56 70 75 76 77 78 79 **P**8	16	10	58	2032	25	19392	385	14347	5887	286

Many Facility Codes have changed. Please refer to the AHA Guide Code Chart.

Hospitals, U.S. / TEXAS

Hospital, Address, Telephone, Administrator, Approval, Facility, and Physician Codes, Health Care System, Network	Classification Codes		Utilization Data					Expense (thousands) of dollars		
★ American Hospital Association (AHA) membership □ Joint Commission on Accreditation of Healthcare Organizations (JCAHO) accreditation + American Osteopathic Healthcare Association (AOHA) membership ○ American Osteopathic Association (AOA) accreditation △ Commission on Accreditation of Rehabilitation Facilities (CARF) accreditation Control codes 61, 63, 64, 71, 72 and 73 indicate hospitals listed by AOHA, but not registered by AHA. For definition of numerical codes, see page A4	Control	Service	Staffed Beds	Admissions	Census	Outpatient Visits	Births	Total	Payroll	Personnel
EAGLE LAKE—Colorado County										
□ RICE MEDICAL CENTER, 600 South Austin Road, Zip 77434–3298, Mailing Address: P.O. Box 277, Zip 77434–0277; tel. 409/234–5571; David N. Keith, Chief Executive Officer **A**1 9 10 **F**2 7 8 9 16 17 18 22 25 30 32 34 36 39 48 63 70 75 76 78 **P**6	16	10	30	764	8	6205	73	5746	2476	93
EAGLE PASS—Maverick County										
⊞ FORT DUNCAN MEDICAL CENTER, 350 South Adams Street, Zip 78852; tel. 830/773–5321; Don Spaulding, Administrator and Chief Executive Officer **A**1 6 9 10 **F**7 9 17 18 19 22 25 29 32 34 36 38 39 41 44 48 50 51 54 70 75 76 78	16	10	69	4373	46	25402	1024	24360	9096	346
EASTLAND—Eastland County										
EASTLAND MEMORIAL HOSPITAL, 304 South Daugherty Street, Zip 76448–2609, Mailing Address: P.O. Box 897, Zip 76448–0897; tel. 254/629–2601; John M. Yeary, FACHE, Administrator **A**9 10 **F**7 8 9 16 17 18 22 24 25 28 30 32 33 34 36 38 39 44 45 48 51 54 75 76 Web address: www.eastland.net	16	10	40	1424	12	18329	128	6994	3496	148
EDEN—Concho County										
CONCHO COUNTY HOSPITAL, 614 Eaker Street, Zip 76837–0359, Mailing Address: P.O. Box 987, Zip 76837–0359; tel. 915/869–5911; Joe Brosig, Administrator **A**9 10 **F**16 17 18 25 32 33 34 36 75 76 **P**5	16	10	20	216	2	6010	0	1654	889	35
EDINBURG—Hidalgo County										
⊞ CORNERSTONE REGIONAL HOSPITAL, 2302 Cornerstone Boulevard, Zip 78539; tel. 956/618–4444; Linda Resendez, R.N., Administrator **A**1 **F**38 48 50	32	10	6	286	2	3007	0	6790	1541	67
⊞ EDINBURG REGIONAL MEDICAL CENTER, 1102 West Trenton Road, Zip 78539–6199; tel. 956/388–6000; Chris Smolik, Chief Executive Officer **A**1 9 10 **F**1 2 4 6 7 8 9 11 13 16 17 18 19 22 24 25 28 32 33 34 38 39 41 43 44 45 46 47 48 50 51 53 54 56 57 58 59 60 61 62 63 64 65 68 70 71 72 75 76 78 79 **P**3 7 8 **S** Universal Health Services, Inc., King of Prussia, PA Web address: www.uhsermc.com	32	10	163	8240	114	33437	2302	50036	18165	451
EDNA—Jackson County										
JACKSON COUNTY HOSPITAL, 1013 South Wells Street, Zip 77957–4098; tel. 361/782–5241; Marcella V. Henke, Administrator and Chief Executive Officer **A**9 10 **F**9 16 17 18 22 25 30 36 38 39 43 48 62 75 76 78	16	10	19	546	5	19354	0	3767	1506	86
EL CAMPO—Wharton County										
□ EL CAMPO MEMORIAL HOSPITAL, 303 Sandy Corner Road, Zip 77437–9535; tel. 409/543–6251; Steve Gularte, Administrator **A**1 9 10 **F**9 13 17 18 19 20 22 24 25 28 30 31 32 33 34 36 38 39 41 43 45 48 49 50 51 54 56 64 70 71 72 76 78 **P**1	16	10	42	831	1	45093	0	9960	3891	132
EL PASO—El Paso County										
★ COLUMBIA BEHAVIORAL CENTER, 1155 Idaho Street, Zip 79902–1699; tel. 915/544–4000; Serena Pickman, Director **A**9 **F**2 3 4 7 8 9 11 12 13 16 17 18 20 21 22 23 24 25 27 29 30 32 34 35 37 38 39 41 42 43 44 45 46 47 48 49 50 51 52 53 54 57 58 59 60 61 62 63 64 65 68 69 70 71 72 75 78 79 **S** HCA – The Healthcare Company, Nashville, TN Web address: www.hcahealthcare.com	32	22	49	902	10	3016	0	3891	2213	53
⊞ COLUMBIA MEDICAL CENTER WEST, 1801 North Oregon Street, Zip 79902–3591; tel. 915/521–1200; Hank Hernandez, Chief Executive Officer **A**1 2 9 10 **F**3 4 7 8 9 11 12 13 16 17 18 19 20 21 22 23 24 25 27 28 29 30 32 34 37 38 39 41 42 44 45 46 47 48 49 51 52 54 58 59 60 61 62 63 64 65 68 69 70 71 72 74 76 78 79 **S** HCA – The Healthcare Company, Nashville, TN Web address: www.hcahealthcare.com	32	10	228	9005	117	87011	1361	80899	29069	820
★ △ COLUMBIA REHABILITATION HOSPITAL, 300 Waymore Drive, Zip 77902–1628; tel. 915/577–2600; Cristina Huerta, Administrative Director (Nonreporting) **A**7	33	46	40	—	—	—	—	—	—	—
⊞ DEL SOL MEDICAL CENTER, (Formerly Columbia Medical Center–East), 10301 Gateway West, Zip 79925–7798; tel. 915/595–9000; Douglas A. Matney, Chief Executive Officer (Total facility includes 29 beds in nursing home–type unit) **A**1 9 10 **F**2 3 4 7 8 9 10 11 12 13 15 17 18 19 20 21 22 23 24 25 27 28 29 30 31 32 33 34 35 36 37 38 39 41 42 43 44 45 46 47 48 49 50 51 52 53 54 57 58 59 60 61 62 63 64 65 68 69 70 71 72 73 74 76 78 79 **P**5 7 **S** HCA – The Healthcare Company, Nashville, TN Web address: www.hcahealthcare.com	32	10	299	14421	207	121942	2297	105947	40764	947
⊞ PROVIDENCE MEMORIAL HOSPITAL, 2001 North Oregon Street, Zip 79902–3368; tel. 915/577–6011; Thomas E. Casaday, President and Chief Executive Officer (Total facility includes 64 beds in nursing home–type unit) **A**1 2 5 9 10 **F**4 7 8 9 11 12 13 17 18 19 22 23 29 32 33 34 37 38 39 40 41 42 43 44 45 46 47 48 49 50 51 52 55 66 65 69 70 72 74 75 76 78 79 **P**7 **S** TENET Healthcare Corporation, Santa Barbara, CA Web address: www.tenethealh.com	32	10	392	16285	243	169976	3145	143376	58786	1611
□ R. E. THOMASON GENERAL HOSPITAL, 4815 Alameda Avenue, Zip 79905–2794, Mailing Address: P.O. Box 20009, Zip 79998–0009; tel. 915/544–1200; Pete T. Duarte, Chief Executive Officer **A**1 2 3 5 9 10 **F**4 9 11 16 17 18 19 22 23 24 25 27 29 31 32 34 35 37 39 41 42 43 44 45 46 47 48 49 50 51 54 56 59 65 66 68 70 71 73 75 76 77 78	16	10	267	12542	178	488371	4956	137976	49392	1548
⊞ △ RIO VISTA PHYSICAL REHABILITATION HOSPITAL, 1740 Curie Drive, Zip 79902–2900; tel. 915/544–3399; Teresa C. Urquhart, Administrator and Chief Operating Officer (Total facility includes 24 beds in nursing home–type unit) **A**1 7 10 **F**4 5 8 9 10 11 12 13 16 17 18 19 22 24 25 29 31 32 34 37 38 39 41 42 44 45 46 47 48 49 51 52 53 54 65 68 69 70 72 74 76 78 79 **P**7 8 **S** TENET Healthcare Corporation, Santa Barbara, CA Web address: www.tenethealh.com	33	46	100	1505	55	36889	0	19263	11532	202

Hospitals, U.S. / TEXAS

Hospital, Address, Telephone, Administrator, Approval, Facility, and Physician Codes, Health Care System, Network

- ★ American Hospital Association (AHA) membership
- ☐ Joint Commission on Accreditation of Healthcare Organizations (JCAHO) accreditation
- + American Osteopathic Healthcare Association (AOHA) membership
- ○ American Osteopathic Association (AOA) accreditation
- △ Commission on Accreditation of Rehabilitation Facilities (CARF) accreditation

Control codes 61, 63, 64, 71, 72 and 73 indicate hospitals listed by AOHA, but not registered by AHA. For definition of numerical codes, see page A4

Hospital	Control	Service	Staffed Beds	Admissions	Census	Outpatient Visits	Births	Total	Payroll	Personnel
★ SIERRA MEDICAL CENTER, 1625 Medical Center Drive, Zip 79902–5044; tel. 915/747–4000; Thomas E. Casaday, President and Chief Executive Officer A1 2 9 10 F4 7 8 9 11 12 13 17 18 19 22 23 24 25 32 33 34 35 37 38 39 40 41 42 43 44 45 46 47 48 49 50 51 52 53 54 65 66 68 69 70 71 72 74 76 78 79 P7 8 S TENET Healthcare Corporation, Santa Barbara, CA Web address: www.tenethealh.com	32	10	328	12250	167	97793	2226	111175	40657	1178
☐ SOUTHWESTERN GENERAL HOSPITAL, 1221 North Cotton, Zip 79902–3096; tel. 915/496–9600; Sharon Peterson, Administrator A1 9 10 F3 7 8 9 13 17 18 19 22 24 25 32 34 37 38 39 41 43 44 45 46 48 54 68 70 75 76 79	32	10	102	2395	25	21785	242	15467	6793	202
★ WILLIAM BEAUMONT ARMY MEDICAL CENTER, 5005 North Piedras Street, Zip 79920–5001; tel. 915/569–2121; Lieutenant Colonel William Barrett, Jr, Chief of Staff (Nonreporting) A1 2 3 5 S Department of the Army, Office of the Surgeon General, Falls Church, VA	42	10	209	—	—	—	—	—	—	—
ELDORADO—Schleicher County										
★ SCHLEICHER COUNTY MEDICAL CENTER, 400 West Murchison, Zip 76936, Mailing Address: Box V, Zip 76936; tel. 915/853–2507; Ann Fagan–Cook, Administrator and Chief Executive Officer A9 10 F7 22 23 25 30 32 37 43 45 54 70 75 P6	16	10	16	82	1	3070	0	1506	667	30
ELECTRA—Wichita County										
ELECTRA MEMORIAL HOSPITAL, 1207 South Bailey Street, Zip 76360–3221, Mailing Address: P.O. Box 1112, Zip 76360–1112; tel. 940/495–3981; Jan A. Reed, CPA, Administrator and Chief Executive Officer A9 10 F7 9 14 17 22 24 25 30 32 34 36 38 45 48 54 56 70 71 73 74 75 76 78 79	16	10	23	620	7	7646	0	3679	1793	87
FAIRFIELD—Freestone County										
★ EAST TEXAS MEDICAL CENTER FAIRFIELD, 125 Newman Street, Zip 75840–1499; tel. 903/389–2121; Ruth Cook, Administrator A9 10 F8 17 18 22 24 25 32 34 37 41 44 48 54 70 75 76 P7 S East Texas Medical Center Regional Healthcare System, Tyler, TX	23	10	19	387	5	18308	48	5089	1820	73
FLORESVILLE—Wilson County										
WILSON MEMORIAL HOSPITAL, 1301 Hospital Boulevard, Zip 78114–2798; tel. 830/393–3122; Robert Duffield, Administrator A9 10 F7 9 13 16 18 19 22 24 25 32 33 34 36 37 38 39 43 48 50 51 54 70 71 72 76 78	16	10	30	809	11	40424	0	7542	3354	114
FORT HOOD—Bell County										
★ DARNALL ARMY COMMUNITY HOSPITAL, 36000 Darnall Loop, Zip 76544–4752; tel. 254/288–8000; Colonel Gerald M. Cross, USA, Commander A1 2 3 5 F2 3 8 9 12 13 14 17 18 22 23 24 25 29 30 33 34 35 38 39 41 42 43 44 45 46 48 49 50 51 53 54 56 57 58 59 60 61 63 64 65 66 70 71 72 75 76 77 78 79 P5 S Department of the Army, Office of the Surgeon General, Falls Church, VA Web address: www.hood–meddac.army.mil	42	10	109	8524	68	818379	2617	126916	56595	1823
FORT STOCKTON—Pecos County										
★ PECOS COUNTY MEMORIAL HOSPITAL, Sanderson Highway, Zip 79735, Mailing Address: P.O. Box 1648, Zip 79735–1648; tel. 915/336–2241; Nicholas R. Blythe, Interim Administrator and Chief Executive Officer A1 9 10 F7 8 9 13 16 17 18 19 22 25 28 32 34 43 44 48 54 56 62 75 76	13	10	31	910	11	33427	187	9437	4528	163
FORT WORTH—Tarrant County										
☐ ALL SAINTS EPISCOPAL HOSPITAL OF FORT WORTH, 1400 Eighth Avenue, Zip 76104–4192, Mailing Address: P.O. Box 31, Zip 76101–0031; tel. 817/926–2544; Patrick D. Flynn, President and Chief Executive Officer (Total facility includes 32 beds in nursing home–type unit) A1 2 9 10 F3 4 7 8 9 11 12 13 16 17 18 19 20 22 25 27 28 29 30 32 33 34 36 37 38 39 41 42 43 44 45 46 47 48 50 51 53 54 57 59 60 61 62 63 64 65 66 67 68 69 70 71 72 74 76 78 79 P6 7 8 Web address: www.allsaints.com	23	10	281	12883	180	72220	1267	116372	46701	1089
ALL SAINTS HOSPITAL–CITYVIEW, 7100 Oakmont Boulevard, Zip 76132–3999; tel. 817/346–5870; Patrick D. Flynn, President and Chief Executive Officer F2 3 4 7 8 9 11 12 13 14 16 17 18 19 22 23 24 25 26 28 29 30 32 33 34 36 37 38 39 41 42 44 45 46 47 48 49 50 51 53 54 56 57 58 59 60 61 62 63 64 65 69 70 71 72 76 78 79 P5 6 7 Web address: www.allsaints.com	23	10	42	2055	18	17137	1780	11883	5366	147
☐ COOK CHILDREN'S MEDICAL CENTER, (PEDIATRIC HOSPITAL), 801 Seventh Avenue, Zip 76104–2796; tel. 817/885–4000; Russell K. Tolman, President and Chief Executive Officer A1 2 3 9 10 F11 13 14 16 17 18 19 21 22 23 24 25 29 31 32 33 34 35 36 38 39 42 43 46 47 48 49 50 51 52 53 54 56 57 58 60 61 63 64 65 68 70 71 72 73 74 75 76 77 78 P3 4 6 Web address: www.cookchildrens.org	23	59	181	7127	124	192224	0	146379	59966	1846
★ △ HARRIS CONTINUED CARE HOSPITAL, (LONG TERM ADULT CARE), 1301 Pennsylvania Avenue, 4th Floor, Zip 76104–2190, Mailing Address: P.O. Box 3471, Zip 76113–3471; tel. 817/878–5500; Larry Thompson, Senior Vice President and Executive Director A7 10 F2 3 4 8 9 11 12 13 18 19 21 22 24 25 26 27 28 30 31 32 33 34 35 36 37 38 39 41 42 43 44 45 46 47 48 49 50 51 53 54 55 57 58 59 60 61 63 64 65 68 69 70 71 72 74 75 76 77 78 79 P2 5 7 S Texas Health Resources, Irving, TX Web address: www.hmhs.com	21	49	10	78	7	0	0	5089	1196	29
★ HARRIS METHODIST FORT WORTH, 1301 Pennsylvania Avenue, Zip 76104–2895; tel. 817/882–2000; Barclay E. Berdan, President (Total facility includes 11 beds in nursing home–type unit) A1 2 3 9 10 F2 3 4 7 8 9 11 12 13 16 17 18 19 21 22 23 24 25 26 27 28 29 30 32 33 34 35 36 37 38 39 41 42 43 44 45 46 47 48 49 50 51 53 54 55 58 59 60 61 62 63 64 65 69 70 72 74 75 76 78 79 P3 5 S Texas Health Resources, Irving, TX Web address: www.texashealth.org	21	10	518	27163	392	228142	5684	267055	114335	3219

Hospitals, U.S. / TEXAS

Hospital, Address, Telephone, Administrator, Approval, Facility, and Physician Codes, Health Care System, Network	Classification Codes		Utilization Data					Expense (thousands) of dollars		
★ American Hospital Association (AHA) membership □ Joint Commission on Accreditation of Healthcare Organizations (JCAHO) accreditation + American Osteopathic Healthcare Association (AOHA) membership ○ American Osteopathic Association (AOA) accreditation △ Commission on Accreditation of Rehabilitation Facilities (CARF) accreditation Control codes 61, 63, 64, 71, 72 and 73 indicate hospitals listed by AOHA, but not registered by AHA. For definition of numerical codes, see page A4	Control	Service	Staffed Beds	Admissions	Census	Outpatient Visits	Births	Total	Payroll	Personnel
★ HARRIS METHODIST SOUTHWEST, 6100 Harris Parkway, Zip 76132–4199; tel. 817/346–5050; Stansel Harvey, Senior Executive Vice President, Executive Director/Administrator **A**1 9 10 **F**2 3 4 8 9 11 13 14 16 17 18 19 21 22 23 24 25 26 27 28 30 31 32 33 34 35 36 37 38 39 41 42 43 44 45 46 47 48 49 50 51 53 54 55 56 57 58 59 60 61 62 63 64 65 66 67 68 69 70 71 72 73 74 76 77 78 79 **P**2 3 5 7 8 **S** Texas Health Resources, Irving, TX **Web address:** www.hmhs.com	21	10	83	5072	45	101136	1816	45841	15823	467
□ HEALTHSOUTH REHABILITATION HOSPITAL OF FORT WORTH, 1212 West Lancaster Avenue, Zip 76102–4510; tel. 817/870–2336; S. Denise Borroni, Administrator and Chief Executive Officer **A**1 10 **F**13 18 31 38 45 46 49 53 54 59 70 71 72 **S** HEALTHSOUTH Corporation, Birmingham, AL **Web address:** www.healthsouth.com	33	46	60	801	38	9395	0	4485	4088	173
□ HEALTHSOUTH REHABILITATION HOSPITAL–CITYVIEW, 6701 Oakmont Boulevard, Zip 76132–2957; tel. 817/370–4700; Mark Bennett, Administrator and Chief Executive Officer **A**1 10 **F**5 13 16 17 18 29 30 31 38 43 45 46 49 51 53 54 70 71 72 78 **S** HEALTHSOUTH Corporation, Birmingham, AL **Web address:** www.healthsouth.com	33	46	62	735	42	12124	0	9562	4983	173
★ HUGULEY MEMORIAL MEDICAL CENTER, 11801 South Freeway, Zip 76115, Mailing Address: P.O. Box 6337, Zip 76115–6337; tel. 817/293–9110; Peter M. Weber, President and Chief Executive Officer (Total facility includes 33 beds in nursing home–type unit) **A**1 9 10 **F**3 8 9 11 13 14 16 17 18 19 22 24 25 27 28 30 32 33 34 36 37 38 39 41 43 44 45 46 48 49 50 51 54 56 57 59 60 61 62 64 65 67 68 69 70 72 76 78 79 **P**7 8 **S** Adventist Health System Sunbelt Health Care Corporation, Winter Park, FL	21	10	189	8345	111	72812	1060	64543	25849	943
□ JPS HEALTH NETWORK, (Includes John Peter Smith Hospital), 1500 South Main Street, Zip 76104–4941; tel. 817/921–3431; Anthony J. Alcini, President and Chief Executive Officer (Total facility includes 15 beds in nursing home–type unit) **A**1 3 5 6 9 10 **F**4 8 9 11 13 16 17 18 19 22 23 24 25 29 31 32 33 34 35 36 38 39 41 42 44 45 46 47 48 49 50 51 54 55 56 57 59 60 61 63 64 68 69 70 72 73 75 76 77 78 79 **P**3 **S** Tarrant County Hospital District, Fort Worth, TX **Web address:** www.jpshealthnet.org	16	10	293	15216	206	439367	4877	248447	115230	3845
□ + ○ △ OSTEOPATHIC MEDICAL CENTER OF TEXAS, 1000 Montgomery Street, Zip 76107–2691; tel. 817/731–4311; Ron Stephen, Executive Vice President and Administrator (Total facility includes 12 beds in nursing home–type unit) **A**1 7 9 10 11 12 13 **F**4 7 8 9 11 12 13 14 16 17 18 19 20 22 24 25 27 28 29 30 31 32 33 34 35 36 38 39 41 43 44 45 46 47 48 51 53 54 57 58 59 60 61 62 64 66 69 70 71 72 75 76 77 78 **P**5 7 **Web address:** www.ohst.com	23	10	209	8148	146	87072	662	89126	33250	905
★ △ PLAZA MEDICAL CENTER OF FORT WORTH, 900 Eighth Avenue, Zip 76104–3986; tel. 817/347–5857; Stephen Bernstein, FACHE, Chief Executive Officer (Total facility includes 26 beds in nursing home–type unit) **A**1 7 9 10 13 **F**2 4 7 8 9 10 11 12 13 22 23 24 25 27 30 32 33 34 35 36 39 40 41 42 43 44 45 46 47 48 50 52 53 54 57 58 59 60 61 62 63 64 66 68 69 70 71 76 78 79 **S** HCA – The Healthcare Company, Nashville, TN **Web address:** www.hcahealthcare.com	33	10	261	9489	146	45405	639	68021	28747	789
TARRANT COUNTY PSYCHIATRIC CENTER, 1527 Hemphill Street, Zip 76104–4789; tel. 817/927–3437; Connie Oliverson Perra, Director (Nonreporting)	16	22	39	—	—	—	—	—	—	—
TRINITY SPRINGS PAVILION, 1500 South Main Street, Zip 76104–4917; tel. 817/927–3636; Robert N. Bourassa, Executive Director (Nonreporting) **A**9 **S** Tarrant County Hospital District, Fort Worth, TX	16	52	34	—	—	—	—	—	—	—
VENCOR HOSPITAL–FORT WORTH SOUTHWEST, (LTAC), 7800 Oakmont Boulevard, Zip 76132–4299; tel. 817/346–0094; Robert L. McNew, Administrator **A**9 **F**18 31 54 69 70 75 **S** Vencor, Incorporated, Louisville, KY	33	49	41	383	34	0	0	7674	4110	161
FREDERICKSBURG—Gillespie County										
★ HILL COUNTRY MEMORIAL HOSPITAL, 1020 Kerrville Road, Zip 78624, Mailing Address: P.O. Box 835, Zip 78624–0835; tel. 830/997–4353; Jeff A. Bourgeois, Chief Executive Officer **A**1 9 10 **F**7 8 9 11 17 18 19 22 24 25 27 28 32 34 36 37 38 39 41 43 44 45 46 48 51 54 55 68 70 71 72 75 76 78 **P**8 **Web address:** www.hillcountrymemorial.com	23	10	59	3587	38	60930	452	24106	10114	395
FRIONA—Parmer County										
PARMER COUNTY COMMUNITY HOSPITAL, 1307 Cleveland Street, Zip 79035–1121; tel. 806/250–2754; Bill J. Neely, Administrator **A**9 10 18 **F**9 17 22 25 34 36 37 38 40 43 76	23	10	25	399	2	8246	0	2920	1209	53
GAINESVILLE—Cooke County										
GAINESVILLE MEMORIAL HOSPITAL, 1016 Ritchey Street, Zip 76240–3539; tel. 940/665–1751; Andrew E. Anderson, Jr, Administrator (Total facility includes 10 beds in nursing home–type unit) **A**9 10 **F**7 8 9 16 17 18 22 24 25 34 36 38 39 41 43 44 45 46 48 49 54 68 69 70 75 76 78 **P**1	16	10	54	2152	24	—	276	14417	7445	273
GALVESTON—Galveston County										
□ SHRINERS HOSPITALS FOR CHILDREN, GALVESTON BURNS HOSPITAL, (PEDIATRIC BURN CARE), 815 Market Street, Zip 77550–2725; tel. 409/770–6600; John A. Swartwout, Administrator **A**1 3 5 **F**7 10 13 22 38 39 48 49 59 70 76 78 **S** Shriners Hospitals for Children, Tampa, FL **Web address:** www.shrinershq.org	23	59	30	1378	21	3709	0	23812	10285	283
★ △ UNIVERSITY OF TEXAS MEDICAL BRANCH HOSPITALS, 301 University Boulevard, Zip 77555–0138; tel. 409/772–1011; David S. Lopez, FACHE, Senior Executive Director **A**1 2 3 5 7 8 9 10 **F**4 7 8 10 11 12 13 14 17 18 19 22 24 25 26 27 28 29 30 31 33 34 35 38 39 40 41 42 43 44 45 46 47 48 49 50 51 52 53 54 54 55 56 57 58 59 60 61 62 63 64 65 66 69 70 71 72 73 74 75 76 77 78 79 **P**6 **S** University of Texas System, Austin, TX **Web address:** www.utmb.edu	12	10	776	29194	452	848696	4346	472095	181459	5042

© 2000 AHA Guide *Many Facility Codes have changed. Please refer to the AHA Guide Code Chart.*

Hospitals, U.S. / TEXAS

Hospital, Address, Telephone, Administrator, Approval, Facility, and Physician Codes, Health Care System, Network	Classification Codes		Utilization Data					Expense (thousands) of dollars		Personnel
★ American Hospital Association (AHA) membership □ Joint Commission on Accreditation of Healthcare Organizations (JCAHO) accreditation + American Osteopathic Healthcare Association (AOHA) membership ○ American Osteopathic Association (AOA) accreditation △ Commission on Accreditation of Rehabilitation Facilities (CARF) accreditation Control codes 61, 63, 64, 71, 72 and 73 indicate hospitals listed by AOHA, but not registered by AHA. For definition of numerical codes, see page A4	Control	Service	Staffed Beds	Admissions	Census	Outpatient Visits	Births	Total	Payroll	Personnel
GARLAND—Dallas County										
★ BAYLOR MEDICAL CENTER AT GARLAND, 2300 Marie Curie Boulevard, Zip 75042–5706; tel. 972/487–5000; John B. McWhorter, II, Executive Director (Total facility includes 20 beds in nursing home–type unit) **A**1 3 9 10 **F**4 5 7 8 9 11 12 13 17 18 19 22 23 24 25 26 27 28 30 31 32 33 34 35 36 37 38 39 41 42 43 44 45 46 47 48 49 50 51 52 53 54 55 56 58 59 60 61 65 66 68 69 70 71 72 73 74 75 76 77 79 **P**6 7 8 **S** Baylor Health Care System, Dallas, TX **Web address:** www.baylordallas.edu	23	10	195	10257	132	100187	1725	82058	37016	955
★ GARLAND COMMUNITY HOSPITAL, 2696 West Walnut Street, Zip 75042–6499; tel. 972/276–7116; Gene Miller, Chief Executive Officer **A**1 9 10 **F**1 2 3 9 13 15 18 19 22 24 25 30 31 32 33 34 36 37 39 41 43 45 46 48 49 51 57 59 60 61 62 63 64 68 70 72 75 76 78 **P**4 7 **S** TENET Healthcare Corporation, Santa Barbara, CA **Web address:** www.tenethealh.com	32	10	113	2722	40	40866	0	27128	12308	326
GATESVILLE—Coryell County										
□ CORYELL MEMORIAL HOSPITAL, 1507 West Main Street, Zip 76528–1098, Mailing Address: P.O. Box 659, Zip 76528–0659; tel. 254/248–6300; David Byrom, Administrator **A**1 9 10 **F**6 7 16 17 18 22 32 36 41 48 54 56 67 70 72 75 76 78 **P**4 **Web address:** www.cmhos.org	16	10	48	1079	12	39778	0	10565	5206	244
GEORGETOWN—Williamson County										
★ GEORGETOWN HEALTHCARE SYSTEM, 2000 Scenic Drive, Zip 78626–7793; tel. 512/943–3000; Kenneth W. Poteete, President and Chief Executive Officer (Total facility includes 9 beds in nursing home–type unit) **A**1 9 10 **F**8 9 16 17 18 22 24 25 32 34 36 38 39 41 43 44 45 46 48 54 65 69 70 71 72 75 76 78 **Web address:** www.georgetownhealthcare.org	23	10	65	3399	31	54303	813	26451	11839	354
GLEN ROSE—Somervell County										
★ GLEN ROSE MEDICAL CENTER, 1021 Holden Street, Zip 76043–4937, Mailing Address: P.O. Box 2099, Zip 76043–2099; tel. 254/897–2215; Gary A. Marks, Administrator **A**1 9 10 **F**9 16 17 22 24 25 26 27 30 31 32 34 37 38 39 45 48 54 55 56 61 69 70 72 75 76	16	10	16	778	7	20262	1	7926	3150	128
GONZALES—Gonzales County										
★ MEMORIAL HOSPITAL, Highway 90A By–Pass, Zip 78629, Mailing Address: P.O. Box 587, Zip 78629–0587; tel. 830/672–7581; Douglas Langley, Administrator **A**9 10 **F**7 9 16 17 18 19 21 22 25 32 33 34 36 37 38 39 41 43 44 45 46 48 51 54 56 64 70 71 72 75 76	16	10	34	1223	13	30808	149	11090	4867	186
□ WARM SPRINGS REHABILITATION HOSPITAL, Mailing Address: P.O. Box 58, Zip 78629–0058; tel. 830/672–6592; John W. Davis, Administrator **A**1 10 **F**17 18 45 53 54 70 **Web address:** www.warmsprings.org	23	46	68	626	47	11296	0	10801	4618	197
GRAHAM—Young County										
★ GRAHAM REGIONAL MEDICAL CENTER, (Formerly Graham General Hospital), 1301 Montgomery Road, Zip 76450–4224, Mailing Address: P.O. Box 1390, Zip 76450–1390; tel. 940/549–3400; Blake Kretz, Administrator **A**9 10 **F**7 8 9 13 17 18 22 25 32 34 36 37 39 40 44 45 46 48 54 62 70 71 73 75 76 **P**5 **Web address:** www.grahamrmc.com	14	10	38	1422	14	80056	225	12366	5320	179
GRANBURY—Hood County										
□ LAKE GRANBURY MEDICAL CENTER, 1310 Paluxy Road, Zip 76048–5699; tel. 817/573–2683; Mike Pruitt, Chief Executive Officer **A**1 9 10 **F**7 8 13 16 17 18 22 24 25 28 32 34 39 41 43 44 48 54 68 70 76 78 **S** Community Health Systems, Inc., Brentwood, TN	33	10	34	1894	22	25077	145	18739	7247	209
GRAND PRAIRIE—Dallas County										
★ + ○ DALLAS–FORT WORTH MEDICAL CENTER, 2709 Hospital Boulevard, Zip 75051–1083; tel. 972/641–5000; Robert A. Ficken, Chief Executive Officer (Total facility includes 11 beds in nursing home–type unit) **A**1 9 10 11 13 **F**4 7 8 9 11 13 17 18 19 22 24 25 27 28 30 31 32 34 36 38 41 42 43 44 45 48 51 53 54 56 62 66 69 70 76 78 79 **P**5 **S** Quorum Health Group, Brentwood, TN **Web address:** www.dfwmedicalcenter.com	23	10	147	3849	58	33501	797	45367	16274	408
GRAND SALINE—Van Zandt County										
★ COZBY–GERMANY HOSPITAL, 707 North Waldrip Street, Zip 75140–1555; tel. 903/962–4242; William Rowton, Chief Executive Officer **A**9 10 **F**9 22 23 25 32 36 37 38 48 64 70 75 76	23	10	20	517	5	6966	0	3370	1696	87
GRAPEVINE—Tarrant County										
★ BAYLOR MEDICAL CENTER AT GRAPEVINE, 1650 West College Street, Zip 76051–1650; tel. 817/481–1588; Mark C. Hood, Executive Director (Total facility includes 9 beds in nursing home–type unit) **A**1 9 10 **F**8 9 13 16 17 18 19 22 24 25 30 31 32 33 34 36 37 38 39 41 43 44 45 46 48 49 50 51 54 68 69 70 71 72 74 76 77 78 79 **P**7 **S** Baylor Health Care System, Dallas, TX **Web address:** www.bhcs.com	21	10	97	7301	69	81812	2114	24826	21631	701
GREENVILLE—Hunt County										
□ GLEN OAKS HOSPITAL, 301 East Division, Zip 75402; tel. 903/454–6000; Thomas E. Rourke, Administrator **A**1 9 10 **F**2 18 25 57 58 59 60 61 62 63 64 70 72 **S** Universal Health Services, Inc., King of Prussia, PA	33	22	54	1333	29	4986	0	4898	2641	86
★ HUNT MEMORIAL HOSPITAL DISTRICT, (Includes Presbyterian Hospital of Commerce, 2900 Sterling Hart Drive, Commerce, Zip 75428; tel. 903/886–3161; Presbyterian Hospital of Greenville), 4215 Joe Ramsey Boulevard, Zip 75401–7899, Mailing Address: P.O. Drawer 1059, Zip 75403–1059; tel. 903/408–5000; Richard Carter, Chief Executive Officer (Total facility includes 15 beds in nursing home–type unit) **A**1 9 10 **F**7 8 9 13 16 17 18 19 22 24 25 27 32 33 34 36 39 41 43 44 45 48 49 50 51 54 69 70 72 75 76 78 **P**8 **Web address:** www.hmhd.org	16	10	139	7206	85	107582	941	53096	23208	672

Hospitals, U.S. / TEXAS

Hospital, Address, Telephone, Administrator, Approval, Facility, and Physician Codes, Health Care System, Network	Classification Codes		Utilization Data					Expense (thousands) of dollars		
★ American Hospital Association (AHA) membership □ Joint Commission on Accreditation of Healthcare Organizations (JCAHO) accreditation + American Osteopathic Healthcare Association (AOHA) membership ○ American Osteopathic Association (AOA) accreditation △ Commission on Accreditation of Rehabilitation Facilities (CARF) accreditation Control codes 61, 63, 64, 71, 72 and 73 indicate hospitals listed by AOHA, but not registered by AHA. For definition of numerical codes, see page A4	Control	Service	Staffed Beds	Admissions	Census	Outpatient Visits	Births	Total	Payroll	Personnel
GROESBECK—Limestone County LIMESTONE MEDICAL CENTER, 701 McClintic Street, Zip 76642–2105; tel. 254/729–3281; Penny Gray, Administrator and Chief Executive Officer **A**9 10 **F**7 14 17 18 19 22 24 25 32 33 34 36 38 43 54 56 64 66 70 75 76 78	16	10	15	271	2	13066	0	4273	1853	70
GROVES—Jefferson County ★ + ○ DOCTORS HOSPITAL, 5500 39th Street, Zip 77619–9805; tel. 409/962–5733; David Cottey, Chief Executive Officer (Total facility includes 6 beds in nursing home–type unit) **A**9 10 11 12 13 **F**9 11 13 16 17 22 24 25 32 34 38 39 41 45 48 51 54 56 65 68 69 70 76 78 **P**8	23	10	78	2155	26	33372	0	20595	7362	247
HALE CENTER—Hale County ⊞ HI–PLAINS HOSPITAL, 203 West Fourth Street, Zip 79041, Mailing Address: P.O. Box 1260, Zip 79041–1260; tel. 806/839–2471; Gordon H. Russell, Administrator (Total facility includes 44 beds in nursing home–type unit) **A**1 9 10 **F**7 8 18 22 24 36 44 48 69 70 75 76 **P**8	23	10	84	456	46	—	73	6762	2753	143
HALLETTSVILLE—Lavaca County LAVACA MEDICAL CENTER, 1400 North Texana Street, Zip 77964–2099; tel. 361/798–3671; James Vanek, Administrator (Nonreporting) **A**9 10	16	10	36	—	—	—	—	—	—	—
HAMILTON—Hamilton County HAMILTON GENERAL HOSPITAL, 400 North Brown Street, Zip 76531–1598; tel. 254/386–3151; Michael R. Graham, Administrator **A**9 10 **F**7 8 13 16 17 18 22 24 25 30 44 48 54 62 64 65 70 76	16	10	22	1019	10	33344	57	5958	2222	92
HAMLIN—Jones County HAMLIN MEMORIAL HOSPITAL, 632 Northwest Second Street, Zip 79520–3831, Mailing Address: P.O. Box 400, Zip 79520–0400; tel. 915/576–3646; James L. Barnett, Administrator **A**9 10 **F**7 17 18 22 25 28 30 32 36 37 38 39 40 45 48 54 56 70 76 **P**6	16	10	23	347	8	7147	1	7435	1469	89
HARLINGEN—Cameron County □ RIO GRANDE STATE CENTER, 1401 South Rangerville Road, Zip 78552–7638; tel. 956/425–8900; Sonia Hernandez–Keeble, Director **A**1 **F**28 32 43 50 51 57 60 61 62 70 72 78 **Web address:** www.mhmr.state.tx.us	12	22	55	1255	42	0	0	15003	8404	305
□ SOUTH TEXAS HOSPITAL, 1301 Rangerville Road, Zip 78552–7609, Mailing Address: P.O. Box 592, Zip 78551–0592; tel. 956/423–3420; Mary Diaz, R.N., Ed.D., Director **A**1 10 **F**9 13 16 17 18 19 22 23 24 31 32 33 34 35 38 39 43 45 48 50 51 54 56 70 76 78 79 **P**6 **S** Texas Department of Health, Austin, TX **Web address:** www.tdh.texas.gov	12	10	60	455	21	36777	0	13306	6519	239
⊞ VALLEY BAPTIST MEDICAL CENTER, 2101 Pease Street, Zip 78550–8307, Mailing Address: P.O. Drawer 2588, Zip 78551–2588; tel. 956/389–1100; Ben M. McKibbens, President **A**1 2 3 5 9 10 **F**4 6 7 8 9 11 12 13 14 15 17 18 19 21 22 24 25 27 30 32 33 34 36 37 39 41 42 43 44 45 46 47 48 49 50 51 52 53 54 56 58 59 60 62 63 64 65 67 68 70 72 75 76 78 79 **P**8 **Web address:** www.vbmc.org	21	10	343	22111	252	173957	3864	190341	76594	2281
HASKELL—Haskell County HASKELL MEMORIAL HOSPITAL, 1 North Avenue N, Zip 79521–5499, Mailing Address: P.O. Box 1117, Zip 79521–1117; tel. 940/864–2621; Bill Nemir, Administrator **A**9 10 **F**16 17 18 19 22 25 28 29 31 32 33 34 36 39 40 48 49 51 54 71 76 78 **P**1	16	10	30	399	4	2057	0	2732	1279	57
HEMPHILL—Sabine County ★ SABINE COUNTY HOSPITAL, Highway 83 West, Zip 75948, Mailing Address: P.O. Box 750, Zip 75948–0750; tel. 409/787–3300; Edith McCauley, Administrator **A**9 10 **F**17 22 23 25 32 36 38 44 45 48 54 60 61 62 63 70 75 76	16	10	36	511	5	4106	36	3595	1299	52
HENDERSON—Rusk County ⊞ HENDERSON MEMORIAL HOSPITAL, 300 Wilson Street, Zip 75652–5956; tel. 903/657–7541; George T. Roberts, Jr, FACHE, Chief Executive Officer (Total facility includes 16 beds in nursing home–type unit) **A**1 9 10 **F**7 8 9 13 17 18 19 22 23 25 32 33 34 35 36 38 39 41 43 44 48 49 50 51 54 68 69 70 75 76 79 **P**8 **S** Quorum Health Group, Brentwood, TN	23	10	96	3541	39	48708	458	21713	10412	323
HENRIETTA—Clay County CLAY COUNTY MEMORIAL HOSPITAL, 310 West South Street, Zip 76365–3399; tel. 940/538–5621; Jimmy Ben Gill, Chief Executive Officer and Administrator **A**9 10 **F**8 22 25 30 34 36 37 44 48 54 62 75 76 **P**1	16	10	25	424	5	41380	18	3331	1386	57
HEREFORD—Deaf Smith County ⊞ HEREFORD REGIONAL MEDICAL CENTER, 801 East Third Street, Zip 79045–5727, Mailing Address: P.O. Box 1858, Zip 79045–1858; tel. 806/364–2141; J. O. Lewis, Acting Administrator **A**1 9 10 **F**7 9 13 14 17 18 19 21 22 24 25 32 34 36 37 38 39 41 43 44 45 48 50 54 66 68 70 71 75 76 78 79 **P**5	16	10	40	1049	9	47460	268	10808	4739	202
HILLSBORO—Hill County □ HILL REGIONAL HOSPITAL, 101 Circle Drive, Zip 76645–2670; tel. 254/582–8425; Jan McClure, Chief Executive Officer (Total facility includes 17 beds in nursing home–type unit) **A**1 9 10 **F**8 9 13 17 18 22 25 30 34 38 39 41 44 45 48 50 51 54 57 62 68 69 75 76 78 **S** Community Health Systems, Inc., Brentwood, TN	33	10	80	2192	26	21639	240	12266	4710	157
HONDO—Medina County ★ MEDINA COMMUNITY HOSPITAL, 3100 Avenue East, Zip 78861–3599; tel. 830/741–4677; Elwood E. Currier, Jr, CHE, Administrator **A**9 10 **F**8 9 13 16 17 22 24 28 32 33 36 38 44 45 46 48 49 54 70 75 76 **P**4 7	15	10	32	916	8	83433	148	14868	7181	271

© 2000 AHA Guide *Many Facility Codes have changed. Please refer to the AHA Guide Code Chart.*

Hospitals, U.S. / TEXAS

Hospital, Address, Telephone, Administrator, Approval, Facility, and Physician Codes, Health Care System, Network	Classification Codes		Utilization Data					Expense (thousands) of dollars		
	Control	Service	Staffed Beds	Admissions	Census	Outpatient Visits	Births	Total	Payroll	Personnel

★ American Hospital Association (AHA) membership
☐ Joint Commission on Accreditation of Healthcare Organizations (JCAHO) accreditation
+ American Osteopathic Healthcare Association (AOHA) membership
○ American Osteopathic Association (AOA) accreditation
△ Commission on Accreditation of Rehabilitation Facilities (CARF) accreditation
Control codes 61, 63, 64, 71, 72 and 73 indicate hospitals listed by AOHA, but not registered by AHA. For definition of numerical codes, see page A4.

HOUSTON—Harris County

Hospital	Control	Service	Staffed Beds	Admissions	Census	Outpatient Visits	Births	Total	Payroll	Personnel
★ BAYOU CITY MEDICAL CENTER, (Includes North Campus, 4200 Portsmouth Street, tel. 713/623–2500; South Campus, 6700 Bellaire at Tarnef, Zip 77074–4999, Mailing Address: P.O. Box 740389, Zip 77274–0389; tel. 713/774–7611), 4200 Portsmouth Street, Zip 77027–6899; tel. 713/623–2500; Iris Simonis, Chief Executive Officer (Total facility includes 15 beds in nursing home–type unit) **A**1 9 10 **F**4 7 8 9 11 13 16 17 18 19 22 23 24 25 28 30 31 32 33 34 35 37 38 39 41 42 44 45 46 47 48 49 50 53 54 56 57 58 59 60 61 62 65 69 70 72 75 76 78 79 **P**5 7 **S** TENET Healthcare Corporation, Santa Barbara, CA	32	10	356	7800	122	38102	1630	69223	26289	707
★ BELLAIRE MEDICAL CENTER, 5314 Dashwood Street, Zip 77081–4689; tel. 713/512–1200; Walter Leleux, Chief Executive Officer (Total facility includes 15 beds in nursing home–type unit) **A**1 9 10 **F**1 2 3 4 5 8 9 11 12 13 16 17 18 19 20 22 24 25 26 27 28 29 30 32 33 34 36 37 38 39 41 42 43 44 45 46 47 48 49 50 51 52 53 54 56 57 58 59 60 61 62 63 64 65 66 69 70 71 72 73 76 77 78 79 **P**1 2 4 5 6 7 8 **S** HCA – The Healthcare Company, Nashville, TN Web address: www.hcahealthcare.com	33	10	209	4960	82	33966	1327	38602	16836	431
BEN TAUB GENERAL HOSPITAL See Harris County Hospital District										
CASA, A SPECIAL HOSPITAL, (SPECIAL HOSPITAL SUBACUTE CARE), 1803 Old Spanish Trail, Zip 77054–2001; tel. 713/796–2272; Gretchen Thorp, R.N., Administrator **A**9 10 **F**13 17 26 35 46 70 78	32	49	40	772	22	0	0	3153	1539	70
★ △ CHRISTUS ST. JOSEPH HOSPITAL, (Formerly St. Joseph Hospital), 1919 LaBranch Street, Zip 77002; tel. 713/757–1000; Sally E. Jeffcoat, Chief Executive Officer (Total facility includes 29 beds in nursing home–type unit) **A**1 2 3 5 7 9 10 **F**3 4 7 8 9 11 13 14 16 17 18 19 21 22 24 25 26 27 30 32 33 34 35 36 37 38 39 41 42 43 44 45 46 47 48 50 51 53 54 56 57 59 60 61 62 64 65 66 68 69 70 71 72 73 75 76 77 78 79 **P**1 5 **S** Christus Health, Irving, TX Web address: www.sch.org	21	10	424	18333	261	125213	—	160920	73584	1738
☐ CYPRESS CREEK HOSPITAL, 17750 Cali Drive, Zip 77090–2700; tel. 281/586–7600; Lawrence Story, Administrator **A**1 9 10 **F**2 3 16 17 18 57 58 61 62 63 64 **S** Brown Schools, Inc., Austin, TX Web address: www.brownschools.com	33	22	94	2828	57	9262	0	11601	5571	173
★ △ CYPRESS FAIRBANKS MEDICAL CENTER, 10655 Steepletop Drive, Zip 77065–4297; tel. 281/890–4285; Elizabeth A. Primeaux, Chief Executive Officer **A**1 7 9 10 **F**2 8 9 11 13 16 18 22 24 25 32 33 34 35 36 38 39 41 45 48 49 51 53 54 55 57 68 69 70 71 72 76 78 79 **P**5 7 8 **S** TENET Healthcare Corporation, Santa Barbara, CA Web address: www.tenethealth.com/cypressfairbanks	33	10	140	8044	82	86544	1300	51851	22570	753
★ DIAGNOSTIC CENTER HOSPITAL, 6447 Main Street, Zip 77030–1595; tel. 713/790–0790; Marc Boom, M.D., Chief Executive Officer (Total facility includes 25 beds in nursing home–type unit) **A**1 9 10 **F**2 4 8 9 10 11 12 13 15 17 18 19 21 22 23 24 25 27 28 30 31 32 34 35 36 37 38 39 41 42 43 44 45 46 47 48 49 50 51 52 53 54 55 57 59 60 62 63 65 66 69 70 71 72 74 76 78 **P**1 3 **S** Methodist Health Care System, Houston, TX Web address: www.tmh.tmc.edi/	23	10	109	3499	60	15711	0	33426	16026	354
★ DOCTORS HOSPITAL PARKWAY, (Formerly North Houston Medical Center), 233 West Parker Road, Zip 77076–2999; tel. 281/765–2600; John H. Styles, Jr, Administrator **A**1 9 10 **F**4 7 8 9 11 13 16 17 18 22 24 25 31 32 34 37 39 41 44 45 46 48 49 51 54 70 75 76 78 79	32	10	134	2224	50	15956	563	12376	5465	399
★ DOCTORS HOSPITAL–TIDWELL, 510 West Tidwell Road, Zip 77091–4399; tel. 713/691–1111; John H. Styles, Jr, Administrator **A**1 9 10 **F**4 7 8 9 11 13 16 17 18 22 24 25 31 32 34 37 39 41 44 45 46 48 49 51 52 54 70 74 76 78 79 Web address: www.health–plus.net	32	10	101	4681	61	23959	348	37049	13465	444
★ EAST HOUSTON REGIONAL MEDICAL CENTER, 13111 East Freeway, Zip 77015; tel. 713/393–2000; Terry Hutton, Chief Executive Officer **A**1 9 10 **F**7 8 9 11 13 17 18 19 22 24 25 26 27 30 32 34 37 38 39 41 44 45 48 51 54 55 68 70 71 72 75 76 78 79 **P**5 **S** HCA – The Healthcare Company, Nashville, TN Web address: www.hcahealthcare.com	33	10	121	6347	65	56109	1463	39320	16809	—
☐ HARRIS COUNTY HOSPITAL DISTRICT, (Includes Ben Taub General Hospital, 1504 Taub Loop, Zip 77030; tel. 713/793–2300; Lyndon B Johnson General Hospital, 5656 Kelley, Zip 77026; tel. 713/636–5000; Margo Hilliard, M.D., Senior Vice President; Quentin Mease Hospital, 3601 North MacGregor, Zip 77004; tel. 713/528–1499), 2525 Holly Hall Street, Zip 77054–4108, Mailing Address: P.O. Box 66769, Zip 77266–6769; tel. 713/746–6400; John A. Guest, President and Chief Executive Officer (Total facility includes 24 beds in nursing home–type unit) **A**1 2 3 5 8 9 10 **F**4 8 9 11 12 13 16 17 19 21 22 24 25 29 30 31 34 35 36 38 39 41 42 44 46 47 48 52 53 54 57 61 63 64 65 66 68 69 70 72 73 75 76 78 **P**6 Web address: www.tmc.edu/hchd	16	10	825	39820	645	868662	10717	462605	—	5424
★ HARRIS COUNTY PSYCHIATRIC CENTER, 2800 South MacGregor Way, Zip 77021–1000, Mailing Address: P.O. Box 20249, Zip 77225–0249; tel. 713/741–5000; Robert W. Guynn, M.D., Executive Director **A**1 3 5 9 10 **F**3 13 16 17 18 22 24 31 39 45 51 55 57 58 59 60 61 62 63 64 68 70 72 76 78 **S** University of Texas System, Austin, TX Web address: www.uth.tmc.edu	12	22	193	5263	146	0	0	32595	16285	411

Hospitals, U.S. / TEXAS

Hospital, Address, Telephone, Administrator, Approval, Facility, and Physician Codes, Health Care System, Network	Classification Codes		Utilization Data					Expense (thousands) of dollars		
★ American Hospital Association (AHA) membership □ Joint Commission on Accreditation of Healthcare Organizations (JCAHO) accreditation + American Osteopathic Healthcare Association (AOHA) membership ○ American Osteopathic Association (AOA) accreditation △ Commission on Accreditation of Rehabilitation Facilities (CARF) accreditation Control codes 61, 63, 64, 71, 72 and 73 indicate hospitals listed by AOHA, but not registered by AHA. For definition of numerical codes, see page A4	Control	Service	Staffed Beds	Admissions	Census	Outpatient Visits	Births	Total	Payroll	Personnel
□ △ HEALTHSOUTH HOUSTON REHABILITATION INSTITUTE, 17506 Red Oak Drive, Zip 77090–7721, Mailing Address: P.O. Box 73684, Zip 77273–3684; tel. 281/580–1212; Anne R. Leon, Chief Executive Officer (Total facility includes 14 beds in nursing home–type unit) **A**1 7 10 **F**5 13 16 17 18 22 24 30 31 37 38 39 45 48 49 51 53 54 69 70 71 72 76 78 **S** HEALTHSOUTH Corporation, Birmingham, AL Web address: www.healthsouth.com	32	46	79	868	59	16100	0	12220	5895	153
✻ △ HERMANN HOSPITAL, 6411 Fannin, Zip 77030–1501; tel. 713/704–4000; James E. Eastham, Senior Vice President and Chief Executive Officer (Total facility includes 15 beds in nursing home–type unit) **A**1 3 5 7 8 9 10 **F**2 3 4 6 8 9 10 11 12 13 16 17 18 19 20 22 23 24 25 26 27 28 29 30 31 32 33 34 35 36 37 38 39 40 41 42 43 44 45 46 47 48 49 50 51 52 53 54 55 56 57 58 59 60 61 62 63 64 65 66 67 68 69 70 71 72 73 74 75 76 77 78 79 **P**5 **S** Memorial Hermann Healthcare System, Houston, TX Web address: www.mhhs.org	23	10	625	25654	455	327322	3042	366449	127048	3162
✻ HOUSTON NORTHWEST MEDICAL CENTER, 710 FM 1960 West, Zip 77090–3496; tel. 281/440–1000; James Kelly, Chief Executive Officer (Total facility includes 20 beds in nursing home–type unit) **A**1 2 9 10 **F**3 4 7 8 9 11 13 17 18 19 22 23 24 25 27 28 31 32 33 34 35 36 38 39 41 42 44 45 46 47 48 49 50 51 54 57 59 61 62 63 64 65 68 69 70 72 76 77 78 79 **P**1 **S** TENET Healthcare Corporation, Santa Barbara, CA Web address: www.hnmc.com/home/home.cfm	32	10	386	19465	236	272305	3654	144965	58303	1558
□ INTRACARE MEDICAL CENTER HOSPITAL, 7601 Fannin Street, Zip 77054–1905; tel. 713/790–0949; Alice Hiniker, Ph.D., Administrator **A**1 9 10 **F**2 3 17 18 22 24 31 39 57 58 59 60 61 63 64 70 **S** Cambridge International, Inc, Houston, TX	33	22	100	1086	34	6308	0	8352	3912	119
INTRACARE NORTH HOSPITAL, (Formerly Forest Springs Hospital), 1120 Cypress Station, Zip 77090–3031; tel. 281/893–7200; Deo Shanker, CPA, Chief Executive Officer **A**9 **F**2 3 22 24 31 39 57 58 59 60 61 62 63 64 70 **S** Cambridge International, Inc, Houston, TX	33	22	48	443	11	1581	0	3212	1658	60
LYNDON B JOHNSON GENERAL HOSPITAL See Harris County Hospital District										
□ MEMORIAL HERMANN BEHAVIORAL HEALTH CENTER, (Formerly Memorial Spring Shadows Glen), 2801 Gessner, Zip 77080–2599; tel. 713/462–4000; Sue E. Green, Vice President and Chief Executive Officer **A**1 9 **F**2 3 4 6 8 9 10 11 12 13 16 17 18 19 20 22 23 24 25 26 27 28 29 30 31 32 33 34 35 36 37 38 39 40 41 42 43 44 45 46 47 48 49 50 51 52 53 54 55 56 57 58 59 60 61 62 63 64 65 66 67 68 69 70 71 72 73 74 75 76 77 78 79 **P**5 Web address: www.mhhs.org	23	22	106	2774	49	538	0	14934	6363	189
✻ MEMORIAL HERMANN MEMORIAL CITY HOSPITAL, 920 Frostwood Drive, Zip 77024–9173; tel. 713/932–3000; Wayne M. Voss, Chief Executive Officer (Total facility includes 24 beds in nursing home–type unit) **A**1 2 6 9 10 **F**2 3 4 6 8 9 10 11 12 13 16 17 18 19 20 22 23 24 25 26 27 28 29 30 31 32 33 34 35 36 37 38 39 40 41 42 43 44 45 46 47 48 49 50 51 52 53 54 55 56 57 58 59 60 61 62 63 64 65 66 67 68 69 70 71 72 73 74 75 76 77 78 79 **P**5 **S** Memorial Hermann Healthcare System, Houston, TX Web address: www.mhhs.org	23	10	324	18103	205	106271	3694	130183	35750	1088
★ MEMORIAL HERMANN REHABILITATION HOSPITAL, (Formerly Memorial Rehabilitation Hospital), 3043 Gessner Drive, Zip 77080–2597; tel. 713/462–2515; Roger Truskoloski, Vice President and Chief Executive Officer (Total facility includes 24 beds in nursing home–type unit) **F**2 3 4 6 8 9 10 11 12 13 16 17 18 19 20 22 23 24 25 26 27 28 29 30 31 32 33 34 35 36 37 38 39 40 41 42 43 44 45 46 47 48 49 50 51 52 53 54 55 56 57 58 59 60 61 62 63 64 65 66 67 68 69 70 71 72 73 74 75 76 77 78 79 **P**5 **S** Memorial Hermann Healthcare System, Houston, TX Web address: www.mhhs.org	23	46	106	787	42	3244	0	14563	4876	152
✻ MEMORIAL HERMANN SOUTHWEST HOSPITAL, (Formerly Memorial Hospital Southwest), 7600 Beechnut, Zip 77074–1850; tel. 713/776–5000; Jerel T. Humphrey, Chief Executive Officer (Total facility includes 89 beds in nursing home–type unit) **A**1 2 3 5 9 10 **F**2 3 4 6 8 9 10 11 12 13 16 17 18 19 20 22 23 24 25 26 27 28 29 30 31 32 33 34 35 36 37 38 39 40 41 42 43 44 45 46 47 48 49 50 51 52 53 54 55 56 57 58 59 60 61 62 63 64 65 66 67 68 69 70 71 72 73 74 75 76 77 78 79 **P**5 **S** Memorial Hermann Healthcare System, Houston, TX Web address: www.mhhs.org	23	10	877	45512	610	300111	6913	273415	114880	3499
NORTHSIDE GENERAL HOSPITAL, 2807 Little York Road, Zip 77093–3495; tel. 713/697–7777; Dac Vu, M.D., Chief Executive Officer **A**9 10 **F**13 16 17 18 19 22 24 32 34 38 41 48 49 51 54 70 75 76	33	10	39	1516	14	13862	0	4908	3610	107
✻ △ PARK PLAZA HOSPITAL, 1313 Hermann Drive, Zip 77004–7092; tel. 713/527–5000; Robert L. Quist, Chief Executive Officer (Total facility includes 40 beds in nursing home–type unit) **A**1 2 3 5 7 9 10 **F**2 4 8 9 11 13 16 17 18 19 20 21 22 24 26 30 32 34 35 39 41 44 45 46 47 48 50 51 52 53 54 57 62 65 68 70 72 76 78 79 **P**5 7 **S** TENET Healthcare Corporation, Santa Barbara, CA Web address: www.parkplazahospital.com	32	10	299	9653	173	66986	1306	91256	34868	1044
QUENTIN MEASE HOSPITAL See Harris County Hospital District										
□ RIVERSIDE GENERAL HOSPITAL, 3204 Ennis Street, Zip 77004–3299; tel. 713/526–2441; Earnest Gibson, II, Administrator **A**1 9 10 **F**1 2 3 14 17 18 19 25 29 30 31 34 38 41 44 48 55 58 59 60 61 62 63 64 70 72 75 78 **P**5	23	22	69	785	16	512	0	10079	4517	142

© 2000 AHA Guide *Many Facility Codes have changed. Please refer to the AHA Guide Code Chart.*

Hospitals, U.S. / TEXAS

Hospital, Address, Telephone, Administrator, Approval, Facility, and Physician Codes, Health Care System, Network	Classification Codes		Utilization Data					Expense (thousands) of dollars		
★ American Hospital Association (AHA) membership □ Joint Commission on Accreditation of Healthcare Organizations (JCAHO) accreditation + American Osteopathic Healthcare Association (AOHA) membership ○ American Osteopathic Association (AOA) accreditation △ Commission on Accreditation of Rehabilitation Facilities (CARF) accreditation Control codes 61, 63, 64, 71, 72 and 73 indicate hospitals listed by AOHA, but not registered by AHA. For definition of numerical codes, see page A4	Control	Service	Staffed Beds	Admissions	Census	Outpatient Visits	Births	Total	Payroll	Personnel
□ SELECT SPECIALTY HOSPITAL–HOUSTON HEIGHTS, (Formerly SSH Heights Hospital), (LONG TERM ACUTE CARE), 1917 Ashland Street, Zip 77008–3994; tel. 713/861–6161 **A**1 9 10 **F**13 18 22 24 30 31 39 41 45 46 48 49 53 55 70 72 76 **S** Select Medical Corporation, Mechanicsburg, PA	33	49	170	1131	100	329	0	25525	12351	393
□ SELECT SPECIALTY HOSPITAL–HOUSTON MEDICAL CENTER, 6447 Main Street, Zip 77030, Mailing Address: 6500 Fannin Street, Suite 907, Zip 77030; tel. 713/791–9393; Guido J. Cubellis, Chief Executive Officer (Nonreporting) **A**1 9 10 **S** Select Medical Corporation, Mechanicsburg, PA	33	49	34	—	—	—	—	—	—	—
□ SHRINERS HOSPITALS FOR CHILDREN, HOUSTON, (PEDIATRIC ORTHOPAEDIC HOSP), 6977 Main Street, Zip 77030–3701; tel. 713/797–1616; Steven B. Reiter, Administrator **A**1 3 5 **F**5 10 13 19 22 23 32 33 38 39 43 48 50 51 52 54 56 59 70 72 76 78 **P**6 **S** Shriners Hospitals for Children, Tampa, FL Web address: www.shc–houston.org	23	59	40	747	18	10182	0	—	—	211
★ SPECIALTY HOSPITAL OF HOUSTON, 5556 Gasmer Drive, Zip 77035–4598; tel. 713/551–5300; Ronald J. Castagno, FACHE, Chief Executive Officer **A**1 9 10 **F**4 11 13 16 17 18 22 24 26 29 30 31 37 39 41 46 47 48 49 50 51 54 55 56 65 68 70 76 **S** Mariner Post–Acute Network, Inc., Atlanta, GA	33	10	106	705	72	0	0	29300	8779	296
★ △ SPRING BRANCH MEDICAL CENTER, 8850 Long Point Road, Zip 77055–3082; tel. 713/467–6555; Patricia Currie, Chief Executive Officer (Total facility includes 25 beds in nursing home–type unit) (Nonreporting) **A**1 2 7 9 10 **S** HCA – The Healthcare Company, Nashville, TN Web address: www.hcahealthcare.com	33	10	345	—	—	—	—	—	—	—
★ △ ST. LUKE'S EPISCOPAL HEALTH SYSTEM, 6720 Bertner Avenue, Zip 77030–2697, Mailing Address: Box 20269, Zip 77225–0269; tel. 713/791–1000; Michael K. Jhin, President and Chief Executive Officer **A**1 2 3 5 7 8 9 10 **F**4 7 8 9 11 12 13 16 17 18 19 20 22 24 25 26 29 30 32 33 34 36 38 39 41 43 44 45 46 47 48 50 51 53 54 56 59 61 66 68 70 72 73 74 76 78 79 **P**5 7 8 Web address: www.sleh.com	21	10	648	32518	473	188771	2582	391586	154250	3704
★ TEXAS CHILDREN'S HOSPITAL, 6621 Fannin Street, Zip 77030–2399, Mailing Address: Box 300630, Zip 77230–0630; tel. 713/770–1000; Mark A. Wallace, Executive Director and Chief Executive Officer **A**1 3 5 8 9 10 **F**4 5 7 11 13 14 17 18 19 22 23 24 25 28 29 31 33 34 35 36 38 39 42 43 45 46 47 48 49 50 51 52 54 56 59 60 63 65 68 70 71 72 73 74 76 77 78 **P**7 Web address: www.txchildrens.org	23	50	378	18572	333	394852	0	314427	139476	3130
★ TEXAS ORTHOPEDIC HOSPITAL, 7401 South Main Street, Zip 77030–4509; tel. 713/799–8600; Beryl Ramsey, Chief Executive Officer (Total facility includes 9 beds in nursing home–type unit) **A**1 9 10 **F**2 3 4 5 8 9 11 12 13 16 18 19 20 22 24 25 26 27 28 29 30 32 33 34 36 37 38 39 41 42 43 44 45 46 47 48 49 50 51 52 53 54 56 57 58 60 61 62 63 64 65 66 69 70 71 72 73 76 77 78 79 **P**2 4 5 6 7 8 **S** HCA – The Healthcare Company, Nashville, TN Web address: www.hcahealthcare.com	32	47	49	1787	17	32671	0	24588	9884	301
★ △ THE INSTITUTE FOR REHABILITATION AND RESEARCH, 1333 Moursund, Zip 77030–3405; tel. 713/799–5000; Louisa F. Adelung, President and Chief Executive Officer **A**1 3 5 7 9 10 **F**13 18 22 24 25 33 38 39 45 48 50 51 53 54 70 71 72 76 78 **P**5 Web address: www.tirr.org	23	46	70	759	57	25304	0	34471	13252	317
★ △ THE METHODIST HOSPITAL, 6565 Fannin Street, Zip 77030–2707; tel. 713/790–3311; Lynn Schroth, Dr.PH, Executive Vice President (Total facility includes 25 beds in nursing home–type unit) **A**1 2 3 5 7 8 9 10 **F**2 3 4 5 8 9 10 11 12 13 16 17 18 19 21 22 23 24 25 26 27 30 31 32 33 34 35 36 37 38 39 41 42 43 44 45 46 47 48 49 50 51 52 53 54 56 57 59 60 61 62 63 64 65 66 68 69 70 71 72 74 76 78 79 **P**2 3 5 **S** Methodist Health Care System, Houston, TX Web address: www.methodisthealth.com	23	10	879	35205	616	313493	2501	533022	184801	4253
★ THE WOMAN'S HOSPITAL OF TEXAS, 7600 Fannin Street, Zip 77054–1900; tel. 713/790–1234; Linda B. Russell, President **A**1 5 9 10 **F**2 3 4 5 8 9 11 13 19 20 22 24 25 26 27 28 29 30 32 33 34 36 37 38 39 41 42 43 44 45 46 47 48 49 50 51 53 54 56 57 58 60 61 62 63 64 65 66 69 70 71 72 73 76 77 78 79 **S** HCA – The Healthcare Company, Nashville, TN Web address: www.hcahealthcare.com	33	44	199	11589	139	32289	7239	70940	33118	813
★ UNIVERSITY OF TEXAS M. D. ANDERSON CANCER CENTER, (COMPREHENSIVE CANCER CENTER), 1515 Holcombe Boulevard, Box 91, Zip 77030–4095; tel. 713/792–6000; John Mendelsohn, M.D., President and Chief Executive Officer **A**1 2 3 5 8 9 10 **F**9 13 16 18 19 20 22 23 24 25 26 29 32 33 34 38 39 41 43 45 46 48 49 50 51 53 54 58 59 60 61 63 65 69 70 72 74 76 78 **P**5 6 **S** University of Texas System, Austin, TX Web address: www.mdanderson.org	12	49	437	16499	347	609862	0	880662	410359	8927
★ VENCOR HOSPITAL–HOUSTON, 6441 Main Street, Zip 77030–1596; tel. 713/790–0500; Bob Stein, Executive Director **A**1 9 10 **F**13 22 24 25 32 36 37 39 41 46 48 51 54 65 69 75 76 77 **S** Vencor, Incorporated, Louisville, KY Web address: www.vencor.com	32	10	110	536	59	—	0	17804	7429	209
★ VETERANS AFFAIRS MEDICAL CENTER, 2002 Holcombe Boulevard, Zip 77030–4298; tel. 713/791–1414; David Whatley, Director (Total facility includes 120 beds in nursing home–type unit) (Nonreporting) **A**1 3 5 8 **S** Department of Veterans Affairs, Washington, DC Web address: www.va.gov/stations97/guide/home.asp?DIVISION=ALL	45	10	859	—	—	—	—	—	—	—

Hospitals, U.S. / TEXAS

Hospital, Address, Telephone, Administrator, Approval, Facility, and Physician Codes, Health Care System, Network	Classification Codes		Utilization Data					Expense (thousands) of dollars		
★ American Hospital Association (AHA) membership □ Joint Commission on Accreditation of Healthcare Organizations (JCAHO) accreditation + American Osteopathic Healthcare Association (AOHA) membership ○ American Osteopathic Association (AOA) accreditation △ Commission on Accreditation of Rehabilitation Facilities (CARF) accreditation Control codes 61, 63, 64, 71, 72 and 73 indicate hospitals listed by AOHA, but not registered by AHA. For definition of numerical codes, see page A4	Control	Service	Staffed Beds	Admissions	Census	Outpatient Visits	Births	Total	Payroll	Personnel
★ △ WEST HOUSTON MEDICAL CENTER, 12141 Richmond Avenue, Zip 77082–2499; tel. 281/558–3444; Jeffrey S. Holland, Chief Executive Officer (Total facility includes 18 beds in nursing home–type unit) **A**1 7 9 10 **F**2 3 4 5 7 8 9 11 12 13 16 19 20 22 23 24 25 26 27 28 29 30 32 33 34 36 37 38 39 41 42 43 44 45 46 47 48 49 50 51 52 53 54 56 57 58 60 61 62 63 64 65 66 69 70 71 72 73 76 77 78 79 **P**2 4 5 6 7 8 **S** HCA – The Healthcare Company, Nashville, TN **Web address:** www.hcahealthcare.com	33	10	169	7136	96	56697	1328	55084	21595	449
□ WEST OAKS HOSPITAL, 6500 Hornwood Drive, Zip 77074–5095; tel. 713/995–0909; Charlene Arnett, Chief Executive Officer **A**1 10 **F**2 17 18 22 24 25 39 55 57 58 59 60 65 68 72 75 **S** Brown Schools, Inc., Austin, TX **Web address:** www.brownschools.com/services/westoaks.html	33	22	40	2177	52	11929	0	11693	5478	214
HUMBLE—Harris County										
□ HEALTHSOUTH REHABILITATION HOSPITAL, 19002 McKay Drive, Zip 77338–5701; tel. 281/446–6148; Darrell L. Pile, Regional Vice President **A**1 10 **F**13 16 17 18 22 24 25 30 31 36 38 39 43 48 49 50 51 53 54 70 71 72 76 **S** HEALTHSOUTH Corporation, Birmingham, AL **Web address:** www.healthsouth.com	33	46	60	661	34	11250	0	6036	3662	114
★ NORTHEAST MEDICAL CENTER HOSPITAL, 18951 Memorial North, Zip 77338–4297; tel. 281/540–7700; Syble F. Missildine, Administrator (Total facility includes 16 beds in nursing home–type unit) **A**1 2 9 10 **F**1 3 4 5 7 8 9 11 13 14 15 17 18 19 20 22 23 24 25 27 28 29 30 31 32 33 34 35 36 37 38 39 40 41 43 44 45 46 47 48 49 50 51 54 56 58 59 60 62 63 64 65 66 67 68 69 70 72 73 74 75 76 77 78 79 **P**1 8 **Web address:** www.nemch.org	16	10	204	10399	132	138589	1448	80975	32028	860
HUNT—Kerr County										
LA HACIENDA TREATMENT CENTER, FM 1340, Zip 78024, Mailing Address: P.O. Box 1, Zip 78024–0001; tel. 830/238–4222; Frank J. Sadlack, Ph.D., Executive Director **F**2 3 13 51 72 **Web address:** www.lahacienda.com	32	82	97	1046	73	—	0	9057	4228	145
HUNTSVILLE—Walker County										
★ HUNTSVILLE MEMORIAL HOSPITAL, 485 I–45 South, Zip 77340–4362, Mailing Address: P.O. Box 4001, Zip 77342–4001; tel. 409/291–3411; Ralph E. Beaty, Administrator **A**1 6 9 10 **F**8 9 16 18 22 24 25 26 32 34 36 38 39 41 44 48 49 54 63 69 70 71 72 76 78 79 **S** Quorum Health Group, Brentwood, TN **Web address:** www.huntsvillememorial.com	23	10	104	3149	37	77983	491	30883	13443	422
IRAAN—Pecos County										
□ PECOS COUNTY GENERAL HOSPITAL, 305 West Fifth Street, Zip 79744, Mailing Address: P.O. Box 665, Zip 79744–2057; tel. 915/639–2871; Nicholas R. Blythe, Interim Administrator and Chief Executive Officer **A**1 9 10 **F**9 16 17 18 25 32 34 38 43 48 50 56 70 75	13	10	14	254	3	5273	0	2324	1281	24
IRVING—Dallas County										
★ BAYLOR MEDICAL CENTER AT IRVING, 1901 North MacArthur Boulevard, Zip 75061–2291; tel. 972/579–8100; Michael F. O'Keefe, FACHE, Executive Director (Total facility includes 18 beds in nursing home–type unit) **A**1 2 9 10 **F**4 7 8 9 11 12 13 15 17 18 19 22 23 24 25 27 29 30 31 32 33 34 35 36 37 38 39 41 43 44 45 46 47 48 50 51 53 54 56 59 61 65 68 70 71 72 76 77 78 79 **P**6 **S** Baylor Health Care System, Dallas, TX **Web address:** www.bhcs.com/irving	21	10	235	13358	168	104832	2108	117431	50927	1362
★ LAS COLINAS MEDICAL CENTER, 6800 North MacArthur Boulevard, Zip 75039–2422; tel. 972/969–2000; Stan Morton, Chief Executive Officer **A**1 9 **F**2 3 4 8 9 11 12 13 16 17 18 22 24 25 27 32 34 39 41 42 43 44 45 46 47 48 49 51 52 53 54 55 57 61 62 63 64 65 69 70 71 74 76 78 79 **P**5 **S** HCA – The Healthcare Company, Nashville, TN **Web address:** www.lascolinasmedical.com	33	10	77	2394	18	22991	943	19852	7435	198
JACKSBORO—Jack County										
FAITH COMMUNITY HOSPITAL, 717 Magnolia Street, Zip 76458–1111; tel. 940/567–6633; Don Hopkins, Administrator **A**9 10 **F**7 17 22 25 36 37 45 48 54 69 70 75 76 **P**6	16	10	17	570	6	15908	0	4007	1776	92
JACKSONVILLE—Cherokee County										
★ EAST TEXAS MEDICAL CENTER JACKSONVILLE, 501 South Ragsdale Street, Zip 75766–2413; tel. 903/541–5000; Steve Bowen, President (Total facility includes 18 beds in nursing home–type unit) **A**9 10 **F**7 8 9 17 19 22 23 24 25 27 28 32 38 39 41 44 45 48 51 54 56 57 62 69 70 71 72 76 78 79 **P**8 **S** East Texas Medical Center Regional Healthcare System, Tyler, TX	23	10	83	2716	42	52007	424	25004	9689	299
JASPER—Jasper County										
★ CHRISTUS JASPER MEMORIAL HOSPITAL, (Formerly Jasper Memorial Hospital), 1275 Marvin Hancock Drive, Zip 75951–4995; tel. 409/384–5461; George N. Miller, Jr, Chief Executive Officer **A**1 6 9 10 **F**7 8 9 13 17 18 19 22 25 29 30 32 33 34 36 38 39 41 44 45 48 50 51 53 54 70 75 76 78 **P**7 8 **S** Christus Health, Irving, TX	21	10	57	2638	27	52501	410	16232	7092	227
JOURDANTON—Atascosa County										
□ SOUTH TEXAS REGIONAL MEDICAL CENTER, (Formerly Tri-City Community Hospital), 1905 Highway 97 East, Zip 78026, Mailing Address: P.O. Box 189, Zip 78026–0189; tel. 830/769–3515; Stephen B. Hill, Chief Executive Officer **A**1 10 **F**9 18 21 22 23 24 25 30 32 34 36 37 38 39 43 45 46 48 51 54 62 63 70 71 72 76 77 79 **P**5	32	10	30	1640	15	48119	12	14094	6418	248

© 2000 AHA Guide   *Many Facility Codes have changed. Please refer to the AHA Guide Code Chart.*

Hospitals, U.S. / TEXAS

Hospital, Address, Telephone, Administrator, Approval, Facility, and Physician Codes, Health Care System, Network	Classification Codes		Utilization Data					Expense (thousands) of dollars		
★ American Hospital Association (AHA) membership ☐ Joint Commission on Accreditation of Healthcare Organizations (JCAHO) accreditation + American Osteopathic Healthcare Association (AOHA) membership ○ American Osteopathic Association (AOA) accreditation △ Commission on Accreditation of Rehabilitation Facilities (CARF) accreditation Control codes 61, 63, 64, 71, 72 and 73 indicate hospitals listed by AOHA, but not registered by AHA. For definition of numerical codes, see page A4	Control	Service	Staffed Beds	Admissions	Census	Outpatient Visits	Births	Total	Payroll	Personnel
JUNCTION—Kimble County										
KIMBLE HOSPITAL, 2101 Main Street, Zip 76849–2101; tel. 915/446–3321; Jamie R. Jacoby, Administrator **A**9 10 **F**25 28 30 32 36 38 43 54 75 76	16	10	15	308	3	19105	0	2974	1421	52
KATY—Fort Bend County										
★ KATY MEDICAL CENTER, 5602 Medical Center Drive, Zip 77494–6399; tel. 281/392–1111; Brian S. Barbe, Chief Executive Officer **A**1 9 10 **F**2 3 4 6 7 8 9 10 11 12 13 16 17 18 19 20 22 23 24 25 26 28 29 30 31 32 33 34 35 36 37 38 39 40 41 42 43 44 45 46 47 48 49 50 51 52 53 54 55 56 57 58 59 60 61 62 63 64 65 66 67 68 69 70 71 72 73 74 75 76 77 78 79 **P**5 **S** Memorial Hermann Healthcare System, Houston, TX	23	10	80	4620	43	48154	776	22102	11239	305
KAUFMAN—Kaufman County										
★ PRESBYTERIAN HOSPITAL OF KAUFMAN, 850 Highway 243 West, Zip 75142–9998, Mailing Address: P.O. Box 310, Zip 75142–0310; tel. 972/932–7200; Kirk King, Senior Vice President and Executive Director (Total facility includes 6 beds in nursing home–type unit) **A**1 9 10 **F**7 8 9 13 17 18 19 22 25 32 34 39 41 43 44 48 51 54 69 70 76 78 **S** Texas Health Resources, Irving, TX Web address: www.phscare.org	23	10	62	2459	29	37853	311	19390	7696	225
KENEDY—Karnes County										
OTTO KAISER MEMORIAL HOSPITAL, 3349 South Highway 181, Zip 78119–5240; tel. 830/583–3401; Nancy Kinkler, Administrator **A**9 10 **F**22 25 36 39 41 48 54 76 **P**8	16	10	30	438	5	26409	0	4568	1932	82
KERMIT—Winkler County										
MEMORIAL HOSPITAL, 821 Jeffee Drive, Zip 79745–4696, Mailing Address: Drawer H, Zip 79745–6008; tel. 915/586–5864; Judene Willhelm, Administrator **A**9 10 **F**7 14 22 25 54 75 76	13	10	16	523	7	12536	0	3762	1643	69
KERRVILLE—Kerr County										
☐ KERRVILLE STATE HOSPITAL, 721 Thompson Drive, Zip 78028–5154; tel. 830/896–2211; Gloria P. Olsen, Ph.D., Chief Executive Officer **A**1 10 **F**16 17 18 23 25 30 34 43 50 57 61 62 70 72 78 Web address: www.mhmr.state.tx.us	12	22	224	489	139	0	0	27244	14799	567
KERVILLE DIVISION See South Texas Veterans Health Care System, San Antonio										
★ SID PETERSON MEMORIAL HOSPITAL, 710 Water Street, Zip 78028–5398; tel. 830/896–4200; James Patrick Murray, Chief Executive Officer (Total facility includes 28 beds in nursing home–type unit) **A**1 9 10 **F**7 8 9 12 13 16 17 18 22 24 25 26 27 32 34 36 37 38 39 44 45 46 48 49 50 51 54 67 69 70 76 78 79 **P**8 Web address: www.spmh.com	23	10	132	6227	85	94637	454	41564	17383	513
KILGORE—Gregg County										
★ ROY H. LAIRD MEMORIAL HOSPITAL, 1612 South Henderson Boulevard, Zip 75662–3594; tel. 903/984–3505; Roderick G. La Grone, President and Chief Executive Officer **A**9 10 **F**7 8 9 22 24 25 30 34 36 39 43 44 45 48 50 54 75 76 78 79	14	10	50	1574	13	26090	316	13275	6059	193
KILLEEN—Bell County										
★ METROPLEX ADVENTIST HOSPITAL, 2201 South Clear Creek Road, Zip 76542–9305; tel. 254/526–7523; Kenneth A. Finch, Chief Executive Officer (Total facility includes 13 beds in nursing home–type unit) **A**1 9 10 **F**8 9 11 13 16 17 18 19 22 24 25 27 29 32 33 34 35 36 37 38 39 41 43 44 45 46 48 49 50 51 54 57 58 59 60 61 62 64 65 68 69 70 72 76 77 78 **P**8 **S** Adventist Health System Sunbelt Health Care Corporation, Winter Park, FL	21	10	213	7316	86	96547	955	52413	18803	668
KINGSVILLE—Kleberg County										
★ CHRISTUS SPOHN HOSPITAL KLEBERG, (Formerly Spohn Kleberg Memorial Hospital), 1311 General Cavazos Boulevard, Zip 78363–1197, Mailing Address: P.O. Box 1197, Zip 78363–1197; tel. 361/595–1661; Ernesto G. Flores, Jr, Administrator (Total facility includes 15 beds in nursing home–type unit) **A**1 9 10 **F**7 8 9 13 16 17 18 22 24 25 26 32 34 37 41 44 45 46 51 54 58 59 61 62 63 64 69 72 75 76 78 79 **P**3 5 8 **S** Christus Health, Irving, TX Web address: www.sch.org	21	10	100	5813	75	79348	434	29749	13950	397
KINGWOOD—Harris County										
★ KINGWOOD MEDICAL CENTER, 22999 U.S. Highway 59, Zip 77339; tel. 281/359–7500; Charles D. Schuetz, Chief Executive Officer **A**1 9 10 **F**1 2 3 4 6 7 8 9 10 11 12 13 14 15 16 17 18 19 20 21 22 23 24 25 26 27 28 29 30 31 32 33 34 35 36 37 38 39 40 41 42 43 44 45 46 47 48 49 50 51 52 53 54 55 56 57 58 59 60 61 62 63 64 65 66 67 68 69 70 71 72 73 74 75 76 77 78 79 **P**1 5 7 **S** HCA – The Healthcare Company, Nashville, TN Web address: www.hcahealthcare.com	33	10	153	7149	88	52157	954	45128	20549	426
LA GRANGE—Fayette County										
★ FAYETTE MEMORIAL HOSPITAL, 543 North Jackson Street, Zip 78945–2040; tel. 409/968–3166; Kelley Oliphint, Chief Executive Officer and Administrator **A**1 9 10 **F**7 8 9 13 16 17 18 19 22 24 25 30 32 33 34 36 38 39 43 44 45 46 48 49 51 54 56 70 76 78 79 Web address: www.fmh-lagrange.org	23	10	45	1885	25	46588	66	13516	5248	178
LACKLAND AFB—Bexar County										
★ WILFORD HALL MEDICAL CENTER, 2200 Bergquist Drive, Suite 1, Zip 78236–5300; tel. 210/292–7353; Colonel Arthur E. Aenchbacher, Jr, Administrator **A**1 2 3 5 **F**1 3 4 5 6 9 11 12 13 14 15 18 20 21 22 23 24 25 26 27 28 29 30 31 32 34 35 36 37 38 39 41 42 43 44 45 46 47 48 49 50 51 52 54 55 56 57 58 59 60 61 62 63 64 65 69 70 71 72 74 75 76 77 78 79 **P**6 **S** Department of the Air Force, Bowling AFB, DC	41	10	284	14904	179	908111	1902	149823	28047	803

Many Facility Codes have changed. Please refer to the AHA Guide Code Chart.

© 2000 AHA Guide

Hospitals, U.S. / TEXAS

Hospital, Address, Telephone, Administrator, Approval, Facility, and Physician Codes, Health Care System, Network	Classification Codes		Utilization Data					Expense (thousands) of dollars		
★ American Hospital Association (AHA) membership ☐ Joint Commission on Accreditation of Healthcare Organizations (JCAHO) accreditation + American Osteopathic Healthcare Association (AOHA) membership ○ American Osteopathic Association (AOA) accreditation △ Commission on Accreditation of Rehabilitation Facilities (CARF) accreditation Control codes 61, 63, 64, 71, 72 and 73 indicate hospitals listed by AOHA, but not registered by AHA. For definition of numerical codes, see page A4	Control	Service	Staffed Beds	Admissions	Census	Outpatient Visits	Births	Total	Payroll	Personnel
LAKE JACKSON—Brazoria County ✦ △ BRAZOSPORT MEMORIAL HOSPITAL, 100 Medical Drive, Zip 77566–9983; tel. 979/297–4411; Wesley W. Oswald, Chief Executive Officer **A**1 2 7 9 10 **F**2 3 8 9 11 13 17 18 22 24 25 27 34 36 39 40 41 44 45 46 48 53 54 57 58 61 62 63 64 65 69 70 72 76 78 79 **P**8 **S** Quorum Health Group, Brentwood, TN **Web address:** www.brazosportmemorial.com	23	10	156	5561	67	65741	755	41943	17419	516
LAMESA—Dawson County ★ MEDICAL ARTS HOSPITAL, 1600 North Bryan Avenue, Zip 79331; tel. 806/872–2183; Karl R. Stinson, CHE, Chief Executive Officer **A**9 10 **F**7 8 9 13 16 17 18 19 22 25 32 34 36 38 39 44 48 51 54 70 75 76 77	13	10	38	905	11	18585	102	8446	4054	148
LANCASTER—Dallas County ✦ MEDICAL CENTER AT LANCASTER, 2600 West Pleasant Run Road, Zip 75146–1199; tel. 972/223–9600; Ernest C. Lynch, II, Chief Executive Officer **A**1 9 10 **F**3 4 8 9 11 12 13 16 17 18 19 22 23 24 25 27 29 30 31 32 34 37 38 39 43 45 46 47 48 49 51 54 57 58 59 60 61 62 63 64 65 66 68 70 71 72 74 76 77 78 79 **P**1 **S** HCA – The Healthcare Company, Nashville, TN **Web address:** www.hcahealthcare.com	33	10	79	2591	35	32493	135	22009	10763	199
LAREDO—Webb County ✦ DOCTORS HOSPITAL OF LAREDO, 500 East Mann Road, Zip 78041–2699; tel. 956/723–1131; Abraham Martinez, Chief Executive Officer (Total facility includes 6 beds in nursing home–type unit) **A**1 9 10 **F**9 13 17 18 21 22 24 25 29 32 33 34 38 39 41 42 43 44 45 46 48 50 51 54 56 65 68 69 70 75 76 78 **P**5 8 **S** Universal Health Services, Inc., King of Prussia, PA **Web address:** www.hcahealthcare.com	32	10	114	6171	66	38287	1879	37539	14772	467
✦ △ MERCY HEALTH CENTER, (Formerly Mercy Regional Medical Center), 1700 East Saunders Avenue, Zip 78041, Mailing Address: Drawer 2068, Zip 78044–2068; tel. 956/718–6222; Mark S. Stauder, President and Chief Executive Officer (Total facility includes 30 beds in nursing home–type unit) (Nonreporting) **A**1 7 9 10 **S** Sisters of Mercy Health System–St. Louis, Saint Louis, MO **Web address:** www.mhst.smhs.com	21	10	320	—	—	—	—	—	—	—
LEAGUE CITY—Galveston County ☐ DEVEREUX TEXAS TREATMENT NETWORK, 1150 Devereux Drive, Zip 77573–2043; tel. 281/335–1000; L. Gail Atkinson, Executive Director **A**1 9 10 **F**2 13 14 17 18 19 21 23 25 28 29 30 34 36 38 43 45 48 50 51 57 58 59 60 61 62 63 64 70 72 73 75 **S** Devereux Foundation, Villanova, PA **Web address:** www.devereux.org	23	22	88	1336	57	10089	0	10230	2476	77
LEVELLAND—Hockley County ✦ COVENANT HOSPITAL–LEVELLAND, (Formerly Methodist Hospital–Levelland), 1900 South College Avenue, Zip 79336–6508; tel. 806/894–4963; Jerry Osburn, Administrator **A**1 9 10 **F**1 3 6 8 9 14 15 16 17 18 19 20 22 23 24 25 28 31 32 33 34 35 36 38 40 43 44 48 49 50 51 53 54 56 58 59 60 61 62 63 69 70 75 76 78 **P**7 **S** St. Joseph Health System, Orange, CA	21	10	49	1323	12	38470	322	10894	3948	147
LEWISVILLE—Denton County ✦ MEDICAL CENTER OF LEWISVILLE, 500 West Main, Zip 75057–3699; tel. 972/420–1000; Raymond M. Dunning, Jr, Chief Executive Officer (Total facility includes 16 beds in nursing home–type unit) **A**1 9 10 **F**4 8 9 13 22 24 25 27 34 37 39 41 44 45 46 48 50 54 68 69 70 71 72 75 76 78 79 **S** HCA – The Healthcare Company, Nashville, TN **Web address:** www.lewisvillemedical.com	33	10	116	7551	87	58251	1287	48178	21991	650
LIBERTY—Liberty County ☐ LIBERTY–DAYTON HOSPITAL, 1353 North Travis Street, Zip 77575–1353; tel. 409/336–7316; Sean Stricker, Administrator **A**1 9 10 **F**7 17 18 22 24 25 29 33 34 36 37 48 49 54 76 78 **S** Northeast Health Management, Inc., Stevensville, MD	33	10	29	957	8	14964	0	6529	2554	101
LIBERTY HILL—Williamson County MERIDELL ACHIEVEMENT CENTER, 12550 West Highway 29, Zip 78642, Mailing Address: P.O. Box 87, Zip 78642–0087; tel. 800/366–8656; Trish Mitchell, Chief Executive Officer (Nonreporting) **A**9 **S** Universal Health Services, Inc., King of Prussia, PA	33	52	78	—	—	—	—	—	—	—
LINDEN—Cass County LINDEN MUNICIPAL HOSPITAL, 404 North Kaufman Street, Zip 75563–5235; tel. 903/756–5561; Richard D. Arnold, CHE, Administrator and Chief Executive Officer **A**9 10 18 **F**9 18 22 23 25 36 41 48 51 53 54 69 70 75 76 78	16	10	39	630	9	10008	0	5015	2414	78
LITTLEFIELD—Lamb County ✦ LAMB HEALTHCARE CENTER, 1500 South Sunset, Zip 79339–4899; tel. 806/385–6411; Randall A. Young, Administrator **A**1 9 10 **F**8 17 18 19 22 25 32 34 36 37 38 40 43 44 48 50 51 69 70 72 73 75 76 79 **S** Lubbock Methodist Hospital System, Lubbock, TX	13	10	41	1048	12	13744	108	5862	2923	117
LIVINGSTON—Polk County ☐ MEMORIAL MEDICAL CENTER, 602 East Church Street, Zip 77351–1257, Mailing Address: P.O. Box 1257, Zip 77351–1257; tel. 936/327–4381; James C. Dickson, Administrator **A**1 9 10 **F**7 8 9 17 19 22 25 32 34 39 41 48 70 76 78 **S** Memorial Health System of East Texas, Lufkin, TX	23	10	31	1753	13	48662	155	10017	4306	111
LLANO—Llano County ✦ LLANO MEMORIAL HEALTHCARE SYSTEM, 200 West Ollie Street, Zip 78643–2628; tel. 915/247–5040; Ernest Parisi, Administrator and Chief Executive Officer **A**1 9 10 **F**7 8 9 17 18 19 22 24 25 34 36 37 45 46 48 54 56 70 76 **Web address:** www.llanomemorial.org	16	10	30	1914	16	99183	329	16388	6397	237

© 2000 AHA Guide *Many Facility Codes have changed. Please refer to the AHA Guide Code Chart.* Hospitals **A421**

Hospitals, U.S. / TEXAS

- ★ American Hospital Association (AHA) membership
- ☐ Joint Commission on Accreditation of Healthcare Organizations (JCAHO) accreditation
- + American Osteopathic Healthcare Association (AOHA) membership
- ○ American Osteopathic Association (AOA) accreditation
- △ Commission on Accreditation of Rehabilitation Facilities (CARF) accreditation

Control codes 61, 63, 64, 71, 72 and 73 indicate hospitals listed by AOHA, but not registered by AHA. For definition of numerical codes, see page A4

Hospital, Address, Telephone, Administrator, Approval, Facility, and Physician Codes, Health Care System, Network	Classification Codes		Utilization Data					Expense (thousands) of dollars		Personnel
	Control	Service	Staffed Beds	Admissions	Census	Outpatient Visits	Births	Total	Payroll	
LOCKNEY—Floyd County										
W. J. MANGOLD MEMORIAL HOSPITAL, 320 North Main Street, Zip 79241–0037; Mailing Address: Box 37, Zip 79241–0037; tel. 806/652-3373; Sharon Hunt, Administrator **A**9 10 **F**8 17 18 19 22 25 28 32 34 36 37 38 44 48 54 56 66 75 76	16	10	27	592	6	23239	106	3677	1808	84
LONGVIEW—Gregg County										
★ △ GOOD SHEPHERD MEDICAL CENTER, 700 East Marshall Avenue, Zip 75601–5571; tel. 903/236-2000; Jerry D. Adair, President and Chief Executive Officer (Total facility includes 25 beds in nursing home–type unit) **A**1 7 9 10 **F**4 7 8 9 11 13 16 17 18 19 22 23 24 25 27 29 30 31 32 33 34 35 36 38 39 41 43 44 45 46 47 48 49 50 51 52 53 54 56 61 65 68 70 71 72 74 76 77 78 79 **P**1 Web address: www.gsmc.org	23	10	320	17241	241	153618	1648	132296	54549	1699
★ LONGVIEW REGIONAL MEDICAL CENTER, 2901 North Fourth Street, Zip 75605–5191, Mailing Address: P.O. Box 14000, Zip 75607–4000; tel. 903/758-1818; Vicki L. Romero, Chief Executive Officer (Total facility includes 15 beds in nursing home–type unit) **A**1 9 10 **F**4 7 8 9 11 13 16 17 18 19 22 24 25 27 32 34 35 38 39 41 43 44 45 46 47 48 49 50 51 53 54 65 68 69 70 71 72 76 78 79 **P**1 **S** Triad Hospitals, Inc., Dallas, TX Web address: www.longviewregional.com	33	10	164	5746	74	44144	742	42361	18340	636
LUBBOCK—Lubbock County										
★ COVENANT CHILDREN'S HOSPITAL, 3610 21st Street, Zip 79410–1218; tel. 806/725-1011; Charley O. Trimble, President and Chief Executive Officer (Nonreporting) **A**9 10 **S** St. Joseph Health System, Orange, CA Web address: www.covenanthealth.org	23	50	65	—	—	—	—	—	—	—
★ △ COVENANT MEDICAL CENTER, (Formerly Methodist Hospital), 3615 19th Street, Zip 79410–1201, Mailing Address: P.O. Box 1201, Zip 79408–1201; tel. 806/725-1011; Charley O. Trimble, President and Chief Executive Officer (Nonreporting) **A**1 2 6 7 9 10 **S** St. Joseph Health System, Orange, CA Web address: www.covenanthealth.org	23	10	520	—	—	—	—	—	—	—
★ △ COVENANT MEDICAL CENTER–LAKESIDE, (Formerly St. Mary of the Plains Hospital), 4000 24th Street, Zip 79410–1894; tel. 806/725-6000; Charley O. Trimble, President and Chief Executive Officer (Nonreporting) **A**1 3 5 7 9 10 **S** St. Joseph Health System, Orange, CA	21	10	410	—	—	—	—	—	—	—
☐ HIGHLAND MEDICAL CENTER, 2412 50th Street, Zip 79412–2494; tel. 806/788-4060; John D. Brock, Chief Executive Officer (Total facility includes 8 beds in nursing home–type unit) **A**1 2 9 10 **F**7 8 9 13 17 18 19 22 23 24 25 32 34 38 39 43 44 45 46 48 51 53 54 69 70 72 76 77 78 79 **S** Community Health Systems, Inc., Brentwood, TN	33	10	123	1778	21	16131	525	17596	6151	174
IHS HOSPITAL OF LUBBOCK, (Formerly Horizon Specialty Hospital), (LONG TERM ACUTE CARE), 1409 9th Street, Zip 79401–2601; tel. 806/767-9133; Steve Grappe, Administrator (Total facility includes 58 beds in nursing home–type unit) **A**9 10 **F**13 31 38 43 45 69 70 **S** Integrated Health Services, Sparks Glencoe, MD Web address: www.ihs-inc.com	33	49	88	496	45	100	0	6715	2944	122
★ UNIVERSITY MEDICAL CENTER, 602 Indiana Avenue, Zip 79415–3364, Mailing Address: P.O. Box 5980, Zip 79408–5980; tel. 806/743-3111; James P. Courtney, President and Chief Executive Officer (Total facility includes 17 beds in nursing home–type unit) **A**1 2 3 5 9 10 **F**4 7 8 9 10 11 12 13 17 19 22 23 24 25 27 32 33 34 35 36 37 39 41 42 43 44 45 46 47 48 49 51 52 53 54 61 65 68 69 70 71 72 74 75 76 78 79 Web address: www.teamumc.org	16	10	318	15346	192	169211	2008	111815	49755	1653
LUFKIN—Angelina County										
★ MEMORIAL HEALTH SYSTEM OF EAST TEXAS, (Formerly Memorial Medical Center of East Texas), 1201 West Frank Avenue, Zip 75904–3357, Mailing Address: P.O. Box 1447, Zip 75902–1447; tel. 936/634-8111; Gary Lex Whatley, President and Chief Executive Officer (Total facility includes 31 beds in nursing home–type unit) **A**1 2 9 10 **F**7 8 9 11 13 16 17 18 19 21 22 24 25 27 28 30 31 32 33 34 35 36 37 38 39 41 43 44 45 46 48 49 50 51 53 54 56 57 59 60 61 63 69 70 72 75 76 77 78 79 **P**5 6 7 8 **S** Memorial Health System of East Texas, Lufkin, TX Web address: www.memorialhealth.org	23	10	234	10842	172	100560	568	72597	29990	975
★ WOODLAND HEIGHTS MEDICAL CENTER, 505 South John Redditt Drive, Zip 75904, Mailing Address: P.O. Box 150610, Zip 75915–0610; tel. 936/634-8311; Don H. McBride, Chief Executive Officer (Total facility includes 16 beds in nursing home–type unit) **A**1 9 10 **F**4 8 9 11 12 13 16 17 18 22 24 25 27 29 32 34 38 39 43 44 45 47 48 50 51 54 69 70 71 76 78 79 **P**5 8 **S** Triad Hospitals, Inc., Dallas, TX	32	10	138	6442	89	41564	657	36099	14740	484
LULING—Caldwell County										
★ SETON EDGAR B. DAVIS HOSPITAL, (Formerly Edgar B. Davis Memorial Hospital), 130 Hays Street, Zip 78648–3207; tel. 830/875-5643; Neal Kelley, Administrator (Total facility includes 6 beds in nursing home–type unit) **A**9 10 **F**17 18 22 24 25 36 38 39 48 54 62 69 70 75 76 78 **P**5 6 8 **S** Ascension Health, Saint Louis, MO Web address: www.goodhealth.com	21	10	21	1039	11	—	54	7116	3128	117
MADISONVILLE—Madison County										
★ MADISON ST. JOSEPH HEALTH CENTER, 100 West Cross Street, Zip 77864–0698, Mailing Address: Box 698, Zip 77864–0698; tel. 409/348-2631; Reed Edmundson, Administrator **A**1 9 10 **F**7 8 9 16 17 18 22 23 25 29 32 38 44 48 54 56 63 70 76 78 **P**6 **S** Franciscan Services Corporation, Sylvania, OH	21	10	35	988	12	36423	74	8653	4557	178

Many Facility Codes have changed. Please refer to the AHA Guide Code Chart.

© 2000 AHA Guide

Hospitals, U.S. / TEXAS

Hospital, Address, Telephone, Administrator, Approval, Facility, and Physician Codes, Health Care System, Network ★ American Hospital Association (AHA) membership ☐ Joint Commission on Accreditation of Healthcare Organizations (JCAHO) accreditation + American Osteopathic Healthcare Association (AOHA) membership ○ American Osteopathic Association (AOA) accreditation △ Commission on Accreditation of Rehabilitation Facilities (CARF) accreditation Control codes 61, 63, 64, 71, 72 and 73 indicate hospitals listed by AOHA, but not registered by AHA. For definition of numerical codes, see page A4	Classification Codes		Utilization Data					Expense (thousands) of dollars		
	Control	Service	Staffed Beds	Admissions	Census	Outpatient Visits	Births	Total	Payroll	Personnel
MANSFIELD—Tarrant County										
☐ VENCOR HOSPITAL–MANSFIELD, (Formerly Mansfield General Hospital), (LONG TERM ACUTE CARE), (Includes Vencor Hospital – Fort Worth West, 815 Eighth Avenue, Fort Worth, Zip 76104; tel. 817/332–4812), 1802 Highway 157 North, Zip 76063–9555; tel. 817/473–6101; M. Joanne Saltzman, Interim Administrator **A**1 9 10 **F**13 18 22 30 41 43 45 48 54 70 78 **S** Vencor, Incorporated, Louisville, KY	33	49	122	637	56	2074	0	22220	8295	253
MARLIN—Falls County										
CENTRAL TEXAS VETERANS AFFAIRS HEALTH CARE SYSTEM, MARLIN INTEGRATED CLINICAL FACILITY See Central Texas Veterans Affairs Healthcare System, Temple										
FALLS COMMUNITY HOSPITAL AND CLINIC, (GENERAL MEDICAL), 322 Coleman Street, Zip 76661–2358, Mailing Address: Box 60, Zip 76661–0060; tel. 254/803–3561; Willis L. Reese, Administrator **A**9 10 **F**9 15 17 18 22 24 25 29 30 32 34 37 38 39 43 45 64 75 76 **P**5	23	49	36	1157	12	42612	4	7639	2278	130
MARSHALL—Harrison County										
✠ MARSHALL REGIONAL MEDICAL CENTER, 811 South Washington Avenue, Zip 75670–5336, Mailing Address: P.O. Box 1599, Zip 75671–1599; tel. 903/927–6000; James E. Hodges, Chief Operating Officer (Total facility includes 10 beds in nursing home–type unit) **A**1 9 10 **F**7 8 9 13 17 18 19 22 24 25 27 28 32 34 36 38 39 41 43 44 45 46 48 51 54 68 69 70 76 79 **P**3 7 8	23	10	101	3148	39	82331	579	28619	13415	398
MCALLEN—Hidalgo County										
☐ MCALLEN HEART HOSPITAL, (SPECIALIZED CARDIOVASCULAR), 1900 South D. Street, Zip 78503; tel. 956/994–2000; Roy C. Vinson, President **A**1 10 **F**4 11 12 13 17 18 19 22 25 32 34 47 48 50 72 76 78 **S** MedCath, Inc., Charlotte, NC	32	49	60	3017	46	15490	0	37019	11050	234
☐ MCALLEN MEDICAL CENTER, 301 West Expressway 83, Zip 78503; tel. 956/632–4000; Daniel P. McLean, Executive Director (Total facility includes 32 beds in nursing home–type unit) **A**1 3 9 10 **F**2 4 6 7 8 9 11 13 16 17 18 22 24 25 32 33 34 38 39 41 42 43 44 45 46 47 48 50 51 52 54 56 57 58 59 60 61 62 63 64 65 66 69 70 71 75 76 78 **P**3 7 8 **S** Universal Health Services, Inc., King of Prussia, PA **Web address:** www.uhsmmc.com	32	10	467	26308	338	83059	4940	146546	51704	1472
✠ RIO GRANDE REGIONAL HOSPITAL, 101 East Ridge Road, Zip 78503–1299; tel. 956/632–6000; William A. Burns, Chief Executive Officer **A**1 9 10 **F**4 7 8 9 11 12 13 18 19 22 23 24 25 27 29 30 32 33 34 38 39 41 42 43 44 45 46 47 48 51 54 65 70 72 76 78 79 **S** HCA – The Healthcare Company, Nashville, TN **Web address:** www.riohealth.com	33	10	230	11662	141	93618	2716	67506	27212	753
MCCAMEY—Upton County										
MCCAMEY HOSPITAL, Highway 305 South, Zip 79752, Mailing Address: P.O. Box 1200, Zip 79752–1200; tel. 915/652–8626; Bill Boswell, Chief Executive Officer (Total facility includes 30 beds in nursing home–type unit) **A**9 10 **F**7 25 32 36 38 48 54 69	16	10	46	95	25	14225	0	4101	1808	78
MCKINNEY—Collin County										
✠ △ NORTH CENTRAL MEDICAL CENTER, (Formerly Medical Center of McKinney), (Includes Westpark Surgery Center, 130 South Central Expressway, Zip 75070; tel. 972/548–5300), 4500 Medical Center Drive, Zip 75069–3499; tel. 972/547–8000; John F. Adams, Chief Executive Officer **A**1 7 9 10 **F**7 8 9 11 13 17 18 19 22 24 25 27 29 30 31 37 38 39 41 44 45 46 48 53 54 57 62 63 64 69 70 76 78 79 **P**7 **S** HCA – The Healthcare Company, Nashville, TN **Web address:** www.hcahealthcare.com	32	10	159	6909	88	77835	1070	47126	20556	499
MEMPHIS—Hall County										
HALL COUNTY HOSPITAL, 1800 North Boykin Drive, Zip 79245–2039; tel. 806/259–3504; Ted Kubicki, Administrator **A**9 10 **F**7 9 17 18 22 25 36 37 43 54 56 76 **P**6	16	10	20	366	5	12608	0	2308	1099	44
MESQUITE—Dallas County										
☐ MEDICAL CENTER OF MESQUITE, 1011 North Galloway Avenue, Zip 75149–2433; tel. 972/320–7000; Terry J. Fontenot, President and Chief Executive Officer (Total facility includes 10 beds in nursing home–type unit) **A**1 9 10 **F**4 7 8 9 11 12 13 17 19 22 23 24 25 26 27 28 30 31 32 33 34 37 38 39 41 43 44 45 46 47 48 49 50 51 54 55 57 61 62 64 65 66 68 69 70 74 76 78 79 **P**5 **S** Paracelsus Healthcare Corporation, Houston, TX	33	10	176	6409	83	53940	400	43802	17888	544
☐ MESQUITE COMMUNITY HOSPITAL, 3500 Interstate 30, Zip 75150–2696; tel. 972/698–3300; Raymond P. De Blasi, Chief Executive Officer (Total facility includes 13 beds in nursing home–type unit) **A**1 9 10 **F**8 9 11 16 17 18 22 23 24 25 27 31 37 39 41 43 44 48 54 56 57 62 64 69 70 75 76 78	32	10	128	6161	66	55025	1357	34594	15339	517
MEXIA—Limestone County										
☐ PARKVIEW REGIONAL HOSPITAL, 312 East Glendale Street, Zip 76667–3608; tel. 254/562–5332; Tim Adams, CHE, Administrator and Chief Executive Officer **A**1 9 10 **F**8 9 13 16 17 18 22 24 25 28 30 32 33 34 38 39 41 44 45 48 51 53 54 70 71 75 76 **P**4 7 **S** Province Healthcare Corporation, Brentwood, TN **Web address:** www.parkviewregional.com	32	10	44	2217	30	29698	180	16840	6290	218
MIDLAND—Midland County										
☐ DESERT SPRINGS MEDICAL CENTER, 3300 South FM 1788, Zip 79711–2699, Mailing Address: P.O. Box 60608, Zip 79711–0608; tel. 915/563–1200; Marjorie McLoughlin, Chief Executive Officer **A**1 9 10 **F**2 3 13 17 18 19 29 30 57 58 59 60 61 62 63 64 70 72 **S** Health Systems America, Sunrise, FL	33	22	48	1059	16	1587	0	3184	1635	65

© 2000 AHA Guide   *Many Facility Codes have changed. Please refer to the AHA Guide Code Chart.*   Hospitals **A423**

Hospitals, U.S. / TEXAS

Hospital, Address, Telephone, Administrator, Approval, Facility, and Physician Codes, Health Care System, Network	Classification Codes		Utilization Data					Expense (thousands) of dollars		
	Control	Service	Staffed Beds	Admissions	Census	Outpatient Visits	Births	Total	Payroll	Personnel

- ★ American Hospital Association (AHA) membership
- ☐ Joint Commission on Accreditation of Healthcare Organizations (JCAHO) accreditation
- + American Osteopathic Healthcare Association (AOHA) membership
- ○ American Osteopathic Association (AOA) accreditation
- △ Commission on Accreditation of Rehabilitation Facilities (CARF) accreditation

Control codes 61, 63, 64, 71, 72 and 73 indicate hospitals listed by AOHA, but not registered by AHA. For definition of numerical codes, see page A4

Hospital	Control	Service	Staffed Beds	Admissions	Census	Outpatient Visits	Births	Total	Payroll	Personnel
★ △ MIDLAND MEMORIAL HOSPITAL, (Formerly Memorial Hospital and Medical Center), (Includes Memorial Rehabilitation Hospital, Zip 79704; tel. 915/520-2333), 2200 West Illinois Avenue, Zip 79701-6499; tel. 915/685-1111; Harold Rubin, FACHE, President and Chief Executive Officer (Total facility includes 13 beds in nursing home-type unit) **A**1 2 3 5 7 9 10 **F**3 4 7 8 9 11 13 14 16 17 18 19 22 24 25 27 29 31 32 33 34 37 38 39 42 45 46 47 48 49 53 54 56 58 59 61 62 65 68 69 70 71 72 73 76 77 78 79 **P**3 8 **Web address:** www.midland-memorial.com	16	10	268	10782	176	139131	1409	120999	41423	1281
☐ WESTWOOD MEDICAL CENTER, 4214 Andrews Highway, Zip 79703-4861; tel. 915/522-2273; Dan Gideon, President and Chief Executive Officer **A**1 9 10 **F**7 8 9 11 13 16 18 22 24 25 27 32 35 38 39 41 43 44 48 49 51 54 68 70 72 76 **P**1 2 3 4 5 6 7 8 **S** Paracelsus Healthcare Corporation, Houston, TX **Web address:** www.westwoodmed.com	33	10	86	2433	25	17724	405	18399	7291	216
MINERAL WELLS—Palo Pinto County										
★ PALO PINTO GENERAL HOSPITAL, 400 S.W. 25th Avenue, Zip 76067-9685; tel. 940/325-7891; Patricia Dorris, Chief Executive Officer **A**1 9 10 **F**4 7 8 9 13 14 16 17 18 22 24 25 28 33 34 36 41 43 44 45 48 49 50 51 54 56 70 71 72 75 76 78 79	16	10	44	2867	30	94312	403	23617	10735	328
MISSION—Hidalgo County										
★ MISSION HOSPITAL, 900 South Bryan Road, Zip 78572-6613; tel. 956/580-9000; Paul H. Ballard, Chief Executive Officer **A**1 9 10 **F**4 8 9 11 12 13 17 18 19 22 24 25 30 32 33 34 39 41 42 43 44 45 46 48 50 51 52 53 54 56 57 70 75 76 78 **P**3 8 **S** Quorum Health Group, Brentwood, TN **Web address:** www.missionhosp.com	23	10	138	6750	81	48634	1481	48132	17453	559
MISSOURI CITY—Fort Bend County										
★ MEMORIAL HERMANN FORT BEND HOSPITAL, (Formerly Fort Bend Medical Center), 3803 FM 1092 at Highway 6, Zip 77459; tel. 281/499-4800; Rod Brace, Chief Executive Officer **A**1 9 10 **F**2 3 4 6 7 8 9 10 11 12 13 16 17 18 19 20 22 23 24 25 26 28 29 30 31 32 33 34 35 36 37 38 39 40 41 42 43 44 45 46 47 48 49 50 51 52 53 54 55 56 57 58 59 60 61 62 63 64 65 66 67 68 69 70 71 72 73 74 75 76 77 78 79 **P**5 7 **S** Memorial Hermann Healthcare System, Houston, TX **Web address:** www.mhhs.org	23	10	65	2691	31	46937	414	21481	9048	262
MONAHANS—Ward County										
★ WARD MEMORIAL HOSPITAL, 406 South Gary Street, Zip 79756-4798, Mailing Address: P.O. Box 40, Zip 79756-0040; tel. 915/943-2511; Joseph Wright, Administrator **A**9 10 **F**1 3 4 5 6 7 8 9 11 13 14 15 16 17 18 19 20 21 22 23 24 25 26 27 28 29 30 31 32 33 34 35 36 37 38 39 40 43 44 45 46 47 48 49 50 51 54 55 56 58 59 60 61 62 63 64 65 66 67 68 70 71 72 73 74 75 76 77 78 79	13	10	36	917	7	15079	50	6682	2815	118
MORTON—Cochran County										
★ COCHRAN MEMORIAL HOSPITAL, 201 East Grant Street, Zip 79346-3444; tel. 806/266-5565; Paul McKinney, Administrator **A**9 10 **F**25 32 36 75 **P**5	16	10	15	144	1	—	0	2433	1214	40
MOUNT PLEASANT—Titus County										
★ TITUS REGIONAL MEDICAL CENTER, 2001 North Jefferson Avenue, Zip 75455-2398; tel. 903/577-6000; Steven K. Jacobson, Chief Executive Officer (Total facility includes 14 beds in nursing home-type unit) **A**1 9 10 **F**7 8 9 11 17 18 19 22 24 25 27 32 34 36 38 39 41 43 48 53 54 69 70 75 76 78 79 **P**8 **S** Quorum Health Group, Brentwood, TN	16	10	165	6684	88	76191	908	44044	18982	564
MOUNT VERNON—Franklin County										
★ EAST TEXAS MEDICAL CENTER—MOUNT VERNON, 500 Highway 37 South, Zip 75457, Mailing Address: P.O. Box 477, Zip 75457-0477; tel. 903/537-4552; Perry Henderson, Administrator **A**1 9 10 **F**9 13 14 17 18 19 22 23 25 32 33 34 36 38 43 48 75 76 **P**7 8 **S** East Texas Medical Center Regional Healthcare System, Tyler, TX **Web address:** www.etmc.org	23	10	30	810	8	11177	0	4179	1992	47
MUENSTER—Cooke County										
MUENSTER MEMORIAL HOSPITAL, 605 North Maple Street, Zip 76252-2424, Mailing Address: P.O. Box 370, Zip 76252-0370; tel. 940/759-2271; Jack R. Endres, Administrator **A**9 10 **F**7 8 9 17 22 24 25 32 34 36 37 38 44 48 54 70 72 75 76 **P**8	16	10	18	473	4	20177	84	3949	1968	73
MULESHOE—Bailey County										
★ MULESHOE AREA MEDICAL CENTER, 708 South First Street, Zip 79347-3627; tel. 806/272-4524; Jim G. Bone, Interim Administrator (Total facility includes 54 beds in nursing home-type unit) **A**9 10 **F**8 18 22 25 29 32 33 34 36 39 44 48 69 75 76 78 **S** Lubbock Methodist Hospital System, Lubbock, TX	16	10	79	642	57	42089	62	4863	2314	119
NACOGDOCHES—Nacogdoches County										
★ NACOGDOCHES MEDICAL CENTER, 4920 N.E. Stallings, Zip 75961-1200, Mailing Address: P.O. Box 631604, Zip 75963-1604; tel. 409/568-3380; Glenn A. Robinson, Chief Executive Officer **A**1 9 10 **F**4 7 8 9 11 13 18 19 22 23 24 25 27 30 32 33 34 36 38 39 41 43 44 45 46 47 48 49 51 53 54 65 70 72 76 77 78 79 **P**5 **S** TENET Healthcare Corporation, Santa Barbara, CA **Web address:** www.tenethealth.com/nacogdoches	32	10	124	6753	75	68227	755	38452	16466	515
☐ △ NACOGDOCHES MEMORIAL HOSPITAL, 1204 North Mound Street, Zip 75961-4061; tel. 409/568-8520; G. W. Jones, Administrator (Total facility includes 11 beds in nursing home-type unit) **A**1 7 9 10 **F**4 8 9 11 16 17 18 22 24 25 32 34 35 36 37 38 39 41 44 45 46 47 48 50 53 54 68 69 70 72 76 78 **P**8	16	10	151	5760	89	51190	709	47900	19622	645

Hospitals, U.S. / TEXAS

Hospital, Address, Telephone, Administrator, Approval, Facility, and Physician Codes, Health Care System, Network	Classification Codes		Utilization Data					Expense (thousands) of dollars		
★ American Hospital Association (AHA) membership ☐ Joint Commission on Accreditation of Healthcare Organizations (JCAHO) accreditation + American Osteopathic Healthcare Association (AOHA) membership ○ American Osteopathic Association (AOA) accreditation △ Commission on Accreditation of Rehabilitation Facilities (CARF) accreditation Control codes 61, 63, 64, 71, 72 and 73 indicate hospitals listed by AOHA, but not registered by AHA. For definition of numerical codes, see page A4	Control	Service	Staffed Beds	Admissions	Census	Outpatient Visits	Births	Total	Payroll	Personnel
PINELANDS HOSPITAL, 4632 Northeast Stallings Drive, Zip 75961–1617, Mailing Address: P.O. Box 1004, Zip 79563–1004; tel. 409/560–5900; Steve Scott, Chief Executive Officer (Nonreporting) **A**10 **S** Progressions Group, Inc., Fort Washington, PA	33	22	38	—	—	—	—	—	—	—
NASSAU BAY—Harris County										
✠ CHRISTUS ST. JOHN HOSPITAL, (Formerly St. John Hospital), 18300 St. John Drive, Zip 77058; tel. 281/333–5503; Thomas Permetti, Chief Executive Officer **A**1 9 10 **F**2 3 5 7 8 9 10 11 12 13 16 17 18 19 21 22 24 25 28 32 34 35 36 37 38 39 40 41 42 43 44 45 46 48 49 50 51 52 53 54 55 56 57 58 59 60 61 62 63 64 65 66 68 69 70 71 72 74 76 77 78 79 **P**5 6 7 8 **S** Christus Health, Irving, TX	23	10	135	5167	51	108880	827	44978	22384	555
NAVASOTA—Grimes County										
GRIMES ST. JOSEPH HEALTH CENTER, 210 South Judson Street, Zip 77868–3704, Mailing Address: P.O. Box 1390, Zip 77868–1390; tel. 409/825–6585; Molly Hurst, Administrative Director (Total facility includes 12 beds in nursing home–type unit) (Nonreporting) **A**9 Web address: www.st–joseph.org	33	10	47	—	—	—	—	—	—	—
NEDERLAND—Jefferson County										
✠ MID–JEFFERSON HOSPITAL, Highway 365 and 27th Street, Zip 77627–6288, Mailing Address: P.O. Box 1917, Zip 77627–1917; tel. 409/727–2321; Michael Miller, Chief Executive Officer (Total facility includes 18 beds in nursing home–type unit) **A**1 5 9 10 **F**8 9 13 14 17 18 19 22 24 25 32 33 34 35 36 39 41 44 48 50 51 56 69 76 78 79 **P**3 7 **S** IASIS Healthcare, Nashville, TN Web address: www.tenethealth.com	32	10	138	2925	31	36554	443	15354	6637	207
NEW BRAUNFELS—Comal County										
✠ MCKENNA MEMORIAL HOSPITAL, 600 North Union Avenue, Zip 78130; tel. 830/606–9111; Tim Brierty, Chief Executive Officer **A**1 9 10 **F**8 9 11 12 13 17 18 19 22 23 24 25 27 28 32 34 36 37 38 39 41 43 44 45 46 48 49 50 51 53 54 56 59 61 68 70 76 77 78 79 **P**1	23	10	114	5071	58	88253	754	43413	19380	571
NOCONA—Montague County										
★ NOCONA GENERAL HOSPITAL, 100 Park Street, Zip 76255–3616; tel. 940/825–3235; Charles Norris, Administrator **A**9 10 **F**8 9 13 16 17 18 22 25 32 36 38 39 43 46 48 54 56 70 75 76 78 **P**5	16	10	33	997	11	10878	72	6014	3035	121
NORTH RICHLAND HILLS—Tarrant County										
✠ NORTH HILLS HOSPITAL, 4401 Booth Calloway Road, Zip 76180–7399; tel. 817/255–1000; Randolph Moresi, Chief Executive Officer (Total facility includes 14 beds in nursing home–type unit) **A**1 9 10 **F**4 7 8 9 10 11 12 13 17 18 22 24 25 26 28 30 32 33 34 38 39 41 43 44 45 46 47 48 49 50 51 52 53 54 69 76 78 79 **P**3 5 **S** HCA – The Healthcare Company, Nashville, TN Web address: www.northhillshospital.com	32	10	129	5823	76	66650	824	48259	19366	561
ODESSA—Ector County										
✠ MEDICAL CENTER HOSPITAL, 500 West Fourth Street, Zip 79761–5059, Mailing Address: P.O. Drawer 7239, Zip 79760–7239; tel. 915/640–4000; J. Michael Stephans, Administrator (Total facility includes 25 beds in nursing home–type unit) **A**1 2 3 5 9 10 **F**4 7 8 9 11 12 13 18 19 22 24 25 27 29 32 34 37 38 39 41 42 43 44 46 47 48 51 52 54 55 56 58 61 63 64 65 68 69 70 75 76 78 **P**8	16	10	334	14318	234	149324	1620	151538	50389	1620
✠ ODESSA REGIONAL HOSPITAL, 520 East Sixth Street, Zip 79761–4565, Mailing Address: P.O. Box 4859, Zip 79760–4859; tel. 915/334–8200; Michael S. Potter, FACHE, President and Chief Executive Officer **A**1 9 10 **F**7 8 9 11 13 17 18 19 22 24 25 31 32 33 34 38 40 41 42 43 44 48 50 51 70 75 76 78 79 **P**8 **S** IASIS Healthcare, Nashville, TN Web address: www.orh.net	32	10	100	3835	42	39995	1459	25627	9679	339
OLNEY—Young County										
★ HAMILTON HOSPITAL, 903 West Hamilton Street, Zip 76374–1725, Mailing Address: P.O. Box 158, Zip 76374–0158; tel. 940/564–5521; William R. Smith, Administrator (Nonreporting) **A**9 10	16	10	46	—	—	—	—	—	—	—
ORANGE—Orange County										
☐ BAPTIST HOSPITAL–ORANGE, 608 Strickland Drive, Zip 77630–4717; tel. 409/883–9361; Kevin T. Coleman, Administrator (Total facility includes 16 beds in nursing home–type unit) **A**1 9 10 **F**2 3 4 6 7 8 9 10 11 12 13 19 20 22 23 24 25 26 27 28 29 30 31 32 33 34 35 36 37 38 39 40 41 42 43 44 45 46 47 48 49 50 51 52 53 54 55 56 57 58 59 60 61 62 63 64 65 66 67 68 69 70 71 72 73 74 75 76 77 78 79 **P**5 Web address: www.mhhs.org	23	10	120	3420	32	53143	169	27821	9060	372
PALACIOS—Matagorda County										
WAGNER GENERAL HOSPITAL, 310 Green Street, Zip 77465–3214, Mailing Address: P.O. Box 859, Zip 77465–0859; tel. 361/972–2511; Kevin Hecht, Director **A**9 10 **F**17 18 25 32 34 36 38 54 **P**6 **S** Matagorda County Hospital District, Bay City, TX	16	10	6	28	0	3444	0	1267	778	16
PALESTINE—Anderson County										
☐ PALESTINE REGIONAL MEDICAL CENTER, (Formerly Memorial Mother Frances Hospital), 4000 South Loop 256, Zip 75801–8467, Mailing Address: P.O. Box 4070, Zip 75802–4070; tel. 903/731–1000; Randell G. Stokes, Chief Executive Officer (Nonreporting) **A**1 9 10 **S** Province Healthcare Corporation, Brentwood, TN Web address: www.palestineregional.com	33	10	97	—	—	—	—	—	—	—
✠ △ TRINITY VALLEY MEDICAL CENTER, 2900 South Loop 256, Zip 75801–6958; tel. 903/731–1000; Larry C. Bozeman, Chief Executive Officer (Total facility includes 12 beds in nursing home–type unit) (Nonreporting) **A**1 7 9 10	33	10	150	—	—	—	—	—	—	—

© 2000 AHA Guide *Many Facility Codes have changed. Please refer to the AHA Guide Code Chart.*

Hospitals, U.S. / TEXAS

Hospital, Address, Telephone, Administrator, Approval, Facility, and Physician Codes, Health Care System, Network	Classification Codes		Utilization Data					Expense (thousands) of dollars		
★ American Hospital Association (AHA) membership ☐ Joint Commission on Accreditation of Healthcare Organizations (JCAHO) accreditation + American Osteopathic Healthcare Association (AOHA) membership ○ American Osteopathic Association (AOA) accreditation △ Commission on Accreditation of Rehabilitation Facilities (CARF) accreditation Control codes 61, 63, 64, 71, 72 and 73 indicate hospitals listed by AOHA, but not registered by AHA. For definition of numerical codes, see page A4	Control	Service	Staffed Beds	Admissions	Census	Outpatient Visits	Births	Total	Payroll	Personnel
PAMPA—Gray County ✠ PAMPA REGIONAL MEDICAL CENTER, (Formerly Columbia Medical Center), One Medical Plaza, Zip 79065; tel. 806/665–3721; Mike Munnerlyn, Chief Executive Officer (Total facility includes 16 beds in nursing home–type unit) **A**1 9 10 **F**7 8 9 11 13 17 18 22 24 25 27 30 32 34 38 39 41 43 44 45 48 51 54 57 62 66 69 70 76 78 **P**8 **S** Triad Hospitals, Inc., Dallas, TX **Web address:** www.cmcp.com	32	10	107	3021	39	18333	286	17863	7463	268
PARIS—Lamar County ✠ CHRISTUS ST. JOSEPH'S HEALTH SYSTEM, (Formerly Christus St. Joseph's Hospital and Health Center), 820 Clarksville Street, Zip 75460–9070, Mailing Address: P.O. Box 9070, Zip 75461–9070; tel. 903/785–4521; Monty E. McLaurin, President **A**1 9 10 **F**4 7 9 11 13 16 17 18 19 20 22 24 25 27 28 30 32 33 34 35 36 37 38 39 41 43 45 46 47 48 51 53 54 56 57 59 60 61 62 63 64 65 70 71 72 76 78 **P**3 7 8 **S** Christus Health, Irving, TX **Web address:** www.stjosephhc.com	21	10	175	7160	111	44390	0	50639	19792	760
✠ MCCUISTION REGIONAL MEDICAL CENTER, 865 Deshong Drive, Zip 75462–2097; tel. 903/737–1111; Michael J. McBride, FACHE, President **A**1 9 10 **F**8 9 11 13 16 17 18 19 22 24 25 26 27 28 31 32 33 34 35 36 37 38 39 41 44 45 46 48 50 51 54 65 70 71 72 76 78 79 **P**1 2 6 7 8 **S** Texas Health Resources, Irving, TX **Web address:** www.texashealth.com	23	10	152	6423	63	64279	635	35337	15388	469
PASADENA—Harris County ✠ △ BAYSHORE MEDICAL CENTER, 4000 Spencer Highway, Zip 77504–1294; tel. 713/359–2000; Donald L. Stewart, Chief Executive Officer (Total facility includes 36 beds in nursing home–type unit) **A**1 2 7 9 10 **F**4 8 9 11 13 16 17 18 19 22 23 24 25 27 28 30 31 32 33 34 36 37 38 39 41 44 45 46 47 48 49 50 51 53 54 56 58 60 61 62 63 64 65 66 69 70 71 72 73 76 77 78 79 **P**1 2 4 5 6 7 8 **S** HCA – The Healthcare Company, Nashville, TN **Web address:** www.bayshoremedical.com	33	10	307	15173	176	137775	2234	98444	35851	1042
PEARSALL—Frio County FRIO HOSPITAL, 320 Berry Ranch Road, Zip 78061–3998; tel. 830/334–3617; Alan D. Holmes, Chief Executive Officer **A**9 10 **F**8 9 17 18 22 25 32 36 38 48 54 68 75	23	10	22	882	9	26250	227	5505	2407	88
PECOS—Reeves County ★ REEVES COUNTY HOSPITAL, 2323 Texas Street, Zip 79772–7338; tel. 915/447–3551; Charles N. Butts, Chief Executive Officer **A**9 10 **F**8 9 16 17 22 25 32 36 38 41 44 48 51 54 70 71 75 76 79 **S** Lubbock Methodist Hospital System, Lubbock, TX **Web address:** www.rchd.org	16	10	44	767	10	20486	101	6925	2764	109
PERRYTON—Ochiltree County OCHILTREE GENERAL HOSPITAL, 3101 Garrett Drive, Zip 79070–5393; tel. 806/435–3606; Wallace N. Boyd, Administrator **A**9 10 **F**7 8 9 13 17 18 19 22 24 25 32 33 34 36 37 38 40 41 44 48 54 70 72 75 76 78 79 **P**1	16	10	45	965	11	22521	206	6576	3419	105
PITTSBURG—Camp County ✠ EAST TEXAS MEDICAL CENTER PITTSBURG, 414 Quitman Street, Zip 75686–1032; tel. 903/856–6663; W. Perry Henderson, Administrator **A**1 9 10 **F**7 9 22 25 29 36 48 75 76 **P**5 7 **S** East Texas Medical Center Regional Healthcare System, Tyler, TX **Web address:** www.etmc.org	23	10	42	1407	20	69519	0	11888	5535	210
PLAINVIEW—Hale County ✠ COVENANT HOSPITAL PLAINVIEW, 2601 Dimmitt Road, Zip 79072–1833; tel. 806/296–5531; Joe S. Langford, Chief Executive Officer **A**1 9 10 **F**2 3 7 8 9 11 13 16 17 18 19 21 22 23 24 25 27 29 32 34 35 38 39 40 41 43 44 45 46 48 49 50 51 54 56 57 59 60 61 62 63 64 70 71 72 75 76 77 78 **P**3 7 **S** St. Joseph Health System, Orange, CA	21	10	36	2555	27	52415	556	21228	7268	291
PLANO—Collin County ☐ HEALTHSOUTH PLANO REHABILITATION HOSPITAL, 2800 West 15th Street, Zip 75075–7526; tel. 972/612–9000; Tracey Nixon, Chief Executive Officer **A**1 10 **F**1 13 17 18 28 30 31 40 43 45 49 53 54 59 63 70 72 78 **P**5 **S** HEALTHSOUTH Corporation, Birmingham, AL **Web address:** www.healthsouth.com	32	46	62	1474	53	26781	0	10816	5782	195
✠ MEDICAL CENTER OF PLANO, 3901 West 15th Street, Zip 75075–7799; tel. 972/596–6800; Harvey L. Fishero, President and Chief Executive Officer (Total facility includes 20 beds in nursing home–type unit) **A**1 2 9 10 **F**4 8 9 11 12 13 16 17 19 21 22 23 24 25 26 27 29 30 32 34 35 37 38 39 41 42 44 45 46 47 48 49 50 51 54 65 68 69 70 71 72 76 78 79 **P**3 **S** HCA – The Healthcare Company, Nashville, TN **Web address:** www.hcahealthcare.com	32	10	265	14743	181	67532	3976	107245	41486	1087
✠ PRESBYTERIAN HOSPITAL OF PLANO, 6200 West Parker Road, Zip 75093–7914; tel. 972/981–8000; Philip M. Wentworth, FACHE, President **A**1 9 10 **F**8 9 11 13 16 17 18 19 22 24 25 32 33 34 38 39 41 43 44 45 47 48 49 54 66 68 70 71 72 76 78 79 **P**8 **S** Texas Health Resources, Irving, TX **Web address:** www.texashealth.org	23	10	155	8205	73	68597	2313	81137	28842	763
PORT ARTHUR—Jefferson County ✠ CHRISTUS ST. MARY HOSPITAL, (Formerly St. Mary Hospital), 3600 Gates Boulevard, Zip 77642–3601, Mailing Address: P.O. Box 3696, Zip 77643–3696; tel. 409/985–7431; Alice Baker, Chief Executive Officer (Total facility includes 19 beds in nursing home–type unit) **A**1 3 5 9 10 **F**3 4 7 8 9 11 13 16 17 18 19 22 24 25 28 29 31 34 36 37 38 39 41 43 44 45 46 47 48 50 51 54 57 59 60 61 62 63 64 65 69 70 76 78 79 **P**6 7 8 **S** Christus Health, Irving, TX **Web address:** www.sch.org	21	10	242	9243	116	109233	850	65383	25051	789

Hospitals, U.S. / TEXAS

Hospital, Address, Telephone, Administrator, Approval, Facility, and Physician Codes, Health Care System, Network	Classification Codes		Utilization Data					Expense (thousands) of dollars		
★ American Hospital Association (AHA) membership ☐ Joint Commission on Accreditation of Healthcare Organizations (JCAHO) accreditation + American Osteopathic Healthcare Association (AOHA) membership ○ American Osteopathic Association (AOA) accreditation △ Commission on Accreditation of Rehabilitation Facilities (CARF) accreditation Control codes 61, 63, 64, 71, 72 and 73 indicate hospitals listed by AOHA, but not registered by AHA. For definition of numerical codes, see page A4	Control	Service	Staffed Beds	Admissions	Census	Outpatient Visits	Births	Total	Payroll	Personnel
★ PARK PLACE MEDICAL CENTER, 3050 39th Street, Zip 77642-5535, Mailing Address: P.O. Box 1648, Zip 77641-1648; tel. 409/983-4951; Michael S. Miller, Chief Executive Officer (Total facility includes 21 beds in nursing home-type unit) **A**1 9 10 **F**4 8 9 11 13 17 18 19 22 24 25 27 31 32 33 34 38 39 41 42 44 45 46 47 48 49 50 51 53 54 56 65 69 70 72 76 77 78 79 **P**3 7 **S** IASIS Healthcare, Nashville, TN Web address: www.tenethealth.com	32	10	219	4111	56	24648	627	29384	13195	399
PORT LAVACA—Calhoun County										
★ MEMORIAL MEDICAL CENTER, 815 North Virginia Street, Zip 77979-3025, Mailing Address: P.O. Box 25, Zip 77979-0025; tel. 361/552-6713; Bob L. Bybee, President and Chief Executive Officer **A**1 9 10 **F**7 8 9 16 17 18 22 24 25 30 32 34 36 37 38 39 41 42 43 44 45 48 49 54 62 63 70 72 73 75 76 Web address: www.mmcportlavaca.com	13	10	56	1506	17	37098	237	7559	7220	265
QUANAH—Hardeman County										
HARDEMAN COUNTY MEMORIAL HOSPITAL, 402 Mercer Street, Zip 79252-4026, Mailing Address: P.O. Box 90, Zip 79252-0090; tel. 940/663-2795; Jerry C. Varnado, Administrator **A**9 10 **F**17 22 24 25 31 34 36 38 45 48 54 70 75 76 78 **P**5 6	16	10	23	175	6	16001	0	2367	1064	52
QUITMAN—Wood County										
☐ EAST TEXAS MEDICAL CENTER–QUITMAN, (Formerly ETMC – Wood County at Quitman), 117 Winnsboro Street, Zip 75783-2144, Mailing Address: P.O. Box 1000, Zip 75783-1000; tel. 903/763-4505; Michael J. McCoy, Administrator **A**1 9 10 **F**8 9 13 16 17 18 22 25 32 34 39 46 48 51 72 75 76 78 **P**2 3 7 8 **S** East Texas Medical Center Regional Healthcare System, Tyler, TX Web address: www.etmc.org	23	10	15	1303	15	32780	95	8541	3572	107
RANKIN—Upton County										
RANKIN HOSPITAL DISTRICT, 1105 Elizabeth Street, Zip 79778, Mailing Address: P.O. Box 327, Zip 79778-0327; tel. 915/693-2443; John Paul Loyless, Administrator **A**9 10 **F**16 17 18 19 25 38 43 51 56	16	10	20	60	0	1410	0	1413	670	24
REFUGIO—Refugio County										
★ REFUGIO COUNTY MEMORIAL HOSPITAL, 107 Swift Street, Zip 78377-2425; tel. 361/526-2321; Louis R. Willeke, Administrator **A**1 9 10 **F**1 16 17 18 19 22 25 32 35 37 38 40 43 48 50 51 54 56 62 70 75 76 78 **P**6	16	10	20	253	3	15856	0	6538	2111	87
RICHARDSON—Dallas County										
☐ BAYLOR/ RICHARDSON MEDICAL CENTER, 401 West Campbell Road, Zip 75080-3499; tel. 972/498-4000; Ronald L. Boring, President and Chief Executive Officer (Total facility includes 16 beds in nursing home-type unit) **A**1 9 10 **F**2 3 4 7 8 9 10 11 12 13 14 18 19 21 22 23 25 26 27 29 32 34 35 36 37 38 39 41 42 43 44 45 46 47 48 50 51 52 53 54 57 58 59 60 61 63 64 66 68 69 70 71 72 74 75 76 77 78 79 **P**6 8 Web address: www.baylordallas.edu	16	10	113	6393	67	65650	847	53992	21005	521
RICHMOND—Fort Bend County										
☐ POLLY RYON MEMORIAL HOSPITAL, 1705 Jackson Street, Zip 77469-3289; tel. 281/341-3000; Sam L. Steffee, Executive Director and Chief Executive Officer (Total facility includes 34 beds in nursing home-type unit) **A**1 9 10 **F**7 8 9 16 17 18 22 24 25 27 35 36 37 38 39 41 44 45 46 48 51 54 69 70 71 72 75 76 78 **P**5 8 Web address: www.pollyryon.org	16	10	178	4783	69	49644	781	33017	14865	600
RIO GRANDE CITY—Starr County										
★ STARR COUNTY MEMORIAL HOSPITAL, Rural Route 1, Zip 78582-9801, Mailing Address: P.O. Box 78, Zip 78582-0078; tel. 956/487-5561; Thalia H. Munoz, Administrator **A**9 10 **F**8 16 17 18 22 23 25 32 34 48 70 75 76	16	10	44	1950	18	27219	877	10573	5009	214
ROCKDALE—Milam County										
RICHARDS MEMORIAL HOSPITAL, 1700 Brazos Street, Zip 76567-2517, Mailing Address: Drawer 1010, Zip 76567-1010; tel. 512/446-2513; Edward F. Lynch, Administrator **A**9 10 **F**7 13 17 18 22 24 25 26 29 30 31 35 36 37 38 48 54 56 75 76	16	10	47	421	5	16203	0	5673	1916	100
ROTAN—Fisher County										
FISHER COUNTY HOSPITAL DISTRICT, Roby Highway, Zip 79546, Mailing Address: Drawer F, Zip 79546; tel. 915/735-2256; Ella Raye Helms, Administrator (Total facility includes 10 beds in nursing home-type unit) **A**9 10 **F**6 14 17 18 19 22 28 32 34 36 38 39 43 54 56 69 70 75 76 78 **P**6 **S** Lubbock Methodist Hospital System, Lubbock, TX	16	10	23	367	10	19557	1	4218	1775	73
ROUND ROCK—Williamson County										
★ ROUND ROCK HOSPITAL, 2400 Round Rock Avenue, Zip 78681-4097; tel. 512/341-1000; Deborah L. Ryle, Chief Executive Officer (Total facility includes 7 beds in nursing home-type unit) **A**1 9 10 **F**8 9 13 16 17 18 22 24 25 27 32 33 34 38 39 40 41 43 44 46 48 51 54 69 70 76 78 79 **P**1 5 7 **S** HCA – The Healthcare Company, Nashville, TN Web address: www.hcahealthcare.com	32	10	103	4164	39	48700	1173	29040	12411	337
ROWLETT—Rockwall County										
★ LAKE POINTE MEDICAL CENTER, 6800 Scenic Drive, Zip 75088, Mailing Address: P.O. Box 1550, Zip 75030-1550; tel. 972/412-2273; Kenneth R. Teel, Administrator (Total facility includes 10 beds in nursing home-type unit) **A**1 9 10 **F**4 8 9 12 13 18 19 22 23 25 28 32 37 38 39 43 44 45 46 48 49 50 51 69 70 71 72 74 76 77 78 79 **P**8 **S** TENET Healthcare Corporation, Santa Barbara, CA Web address: www.lakepointemedical.com	33	10	97	4633	44	43335	685	23255	11772	358

© 2000 AHA Guide   *Many Facility Codes have changed. Please refer to the AHA Guide Code Chart.*

Hospitals, U.S. / TEXAS

Hospital, Address, Telephone, Administrator, Approval, Facility, and Physician Codes, Health Care System, Network	Classification Codes		Utilization Data					Expense (thousands) of dollars		
★ American Hospital Association (AHA) membership □ Joint Commission on Accreditation of Healthcare Organizations (JCAHO) accreditation + American Osteopathic Healthcare Association (AOHA) membership ○ American Osteopathic Association (AOA) accreditation △ Commission on Accreditation of Rehabilitation Facilities (CARF) accreditation Control codes 61, 63, 64, 71, 72 and 73 indicate hospitals listed by AOHA, but not registered by AHA. For definition of numerical codes, see page A4	Control	Service	Staffed Beds	Admissions	Census	Outpatient Visits	Births	Total	Payroll	Personnel

RUSK—Cherokee County

□ RUSK STATE HOSPITAL, Jacksonville Highway North, Zip 75785, Mailing Address: P.O. Box 318, Zip 75785–0318; tel. 903/683–3421; Harold R. Parrish, Superintendent **A**1 9 10 **F**16 17 18 22 23 24 30 31 32 34 35 39 48 50 51 57 59 60 61 62 70 72 76 78
Web address: www.mhmr.state.tx.us | 12 | 22 | 375 | 1531 | 301 | 0 | 0 | 38457 | 22679 | 925 |

SAN ANGELO—Tom Green County

□ RIVER CREST HOSPITAL, 1636 Hunters Glen Road, Zip 76901–5016; tel. 915/949–5722; Larry Grimes, Managing Director **A**1 9 10 **F**2 3 13 14 17 18 19 22 24 25 30 31 32 34 39 45 51 54 55 57 58 59 60 61 62 63 64 68 70 72 73 76 **P**5 **S** Universal Health Services, Inc., King of Prussia, PA | 33 | 22 | 80 | 1517 | 27 | 1163 | 0 | 4596 | 2304 | 75 |

★ △ SAN ANGELO COMMUNITY MEDICAL CENTER, 3501 Knickerbocker Road, Zip 76904–7698; tel. 915/949–9511; Samuel G. Feazell, Chief Executive Officer **A**1 2 7 9 10 **F**2 3 5 7 8 9 11 13 14 15 16 17 18 19 22 23 24 25 26 27 30 31 32 33 34 35 36 37 38 39 41 42 43 44 45 46 47 48 49 50 51 52 53 54 56 57 58 59 60 61 62 63 64 65 66 68 69 70 71 72 76 77 78 79 **P**8 **S** Triad Hospitals, Inc., Dallas, TX | 32 | 10 | 136 | 6857 | 70 | 76496 | 896 | 43803 | 15657 | 526 |

★ △ SHANNON MEDICAL CENTER, (Includes Shannon Medical Center– St. John's Campus, 2018 Pulliam Street, Zip 76905–5197; tel. 915/659–7100), 120 East Harris Street, Zip 76903–5976; tel. 915/653–6741; Lawrence Leonard, President and Chief Executive Officer (Total facility includes 22 beds in nursing home–type unit) **A**1 2 7 9 10 **F**2 3 4 7 8 9 11 13 16 17 18 19 21 22 24 25 27 28 29 30 32 33 34 36 38 39 41 42 43 44 45 46 47 48 49 50 51 53 54 57 59 60 61 62 63 65 68 69 70 71 72 76 77 78 79 **P**3
Web address: www.shannonhealth.com | 23 | 10 | 246 | 12227 | 171 | 115392 | 1211 | 109892 | 41546 | 1383 |

SAN ANTONIO—Bexar County

★ BAPTIST MEDICAL CENTER, 111 Dallas Street, Zip 78205–1230; tel. 210/297–7000; Perry Willmore, Vice President Operations (Total facility includes 31 beds in nursing home–type unit) **A**1 2 3 5 6 9 10 **F**2 3 4 8 9 11 12 13 16 17 18 19 22 24 25 26 27 28 30 32 33 34 35 36 37 38 39 41 42 43 44 45 46 47 48 49 50 51 52 53 54 57 59 60 61 62 64 65 68 69 70 72 75 76 78 79 **P**7 8 **S** Baptist Health System, San Antonio, TX
Web address: www.baptisthealthsystem.org | 21 | 10 | 445 | 16881 | 296 | 97458 | 1923 | 155699 | 84224 | 1616 |

★ BROOKE ARMY MEDICAL CENTER, Fort Sam Houston, Zip 78234–6200; tel. 210/916–2225; Colonel Martin J. Fisher, MSC, USA, Deputy Commander for Administration **A**1 2 3 5 9 **F**3 4 5 7 8 9 10 11 12 13 14 15 16 17 18 19 20 21 22 23 24 25 26 27 28 29 31 32 33 34 35 36 37 38 39 41 42 43 44 45 46 47 48 49 50 51 52 53 54 55 56 57 58 59 60 61 62 63 64 65 66 68 70 71 72 73 74 75 76 77 78 79 **P**6 **S** Department of the Army, Office of the Surgeon General, Falls Church, VA | 42 | 10 | 226 | 9267 | 132 | 713538 | 0 | — | — | 3082 |

CHARTER REAL BEHAVIORAL HEALTH SYSTEM See Covenant Behavioral Health System

★ △ CHRISTUS SANTA ROSA HEALTH CARE, (Formerly Santa Rosa Health Care Corporation), 519 West Houston Street, Zip 78207–3108; tel. 210/704–2011; James P. Houser, President and Chief Executive Officer (Nonreporting) **A**1 2 3 5 7 9 10 **S** Christus Health, Irving, TX
Web address: www.sch.org | 21 | 10 | 636 | — | — | — | — | — | — | — |

□ COVENANT BEHAVIORAL HEALTH SYSTEM, (Formerly Charter Real Behavioral Health System), 8550 Huebner Road, Zip 78240–1897, Mailing Address: P.O. Box 380157, Zip 78280–0157; tel. 210/699–8585; James M. Hunt, Chief Executive Officer **A**1 9 10 **F**1 2 3 4 5 6 7 8 9 10 11 12 13 14 15 17 19 20 21 22 23 24 25 26 27 28 29 30 31 32 33 34 35 36 37 38 39 40 41 42 43 44 45 46 47 48 49 50 51 52 53 54 55 56 57 58 59 60 61 62 63 64 65 66 67 68 69 70 71 72 73 74 75 76 77 78 79
Web address: www.charterbehavioral.com | 32 | 22 | 84 | 1258 | 47 | 4048 | 0 | 4193 | 2185 | 125 |

□ △ HEALTHSOUTH REHABILITATION INSTITUTE OF SAN ANTONIO, 9119 Cinnamon Hill, Zip 78240–5401; tel. 210/691–0737; Diane B. Lampe, Administrator and Chief Executive Officer **A**1 7 10 **F**5 13 16 17 18 22 24 29 30 31 39 45 46 48 49 51 53 54 55 68 70 71 72 76 78 **S** HEALTHSOUTH Corporation, Birmingham, AL
Web address: www.healthsouth.com | 33 | 46 | 108 | 1397 | 69 | 22024 | 0 | 14501 | 7003 | 241 |

□ IHS HOSPITAL AT SAN ANTONIO, (Formerly Horizon Specialty Hospital), (LONG–TERM ACUTE CARE LTAC), 7310 Oak Manor Drive, Zip 78229–4509; tel. 210/308–0261; Peggy Cliff, Administrator **A**1 10 **F**13 16 18 22 24 26 30 31 32 37 39 43 49 50 51 54 55 68 69 70 76 **S** Integrated Health Services, Sparks Glencoe, MD
Web address: www.ihs–inc.com | 33 | 49 | 27 | 336 | 27 | 0 | 0 | 6133 | 2842 | 71 |

★ METHODIST AMBULATORY SURGERY HOSPITAL, (SURGICAL SPECIALTY HOSPITAL), 9150 Huebner Road, Suite 100, Zip 78240–1545; tel. 210/691–8000; Elaine F. Morris, Administrator **A**1 10 **F**1 2 3 4 8 9 11 12 13 14 16 17 18 19 21 22 23 24 25 27 28 29 30 31 32 33 34 35 37 41 42 43 44 45 46 47 48 50 51 52 53 54 57 59 60 61 62 63 64 65 66 68 69 70 71 72 74 75 76 77 78 79 **P**2 5 7 8 **S** HCA – The Healthcare Company, Nashville, TN
Web address: www.hcahealthcare.com | 32 | 49 | 37 | 525 | 5 | 11250 | 0 | 16413 | 4889 | 135 |

★ METHODIST CHILDREN'S HOSPITAL OF SOUTH TEXAS, (Formerly Methodist Women's and Children's Hospital), 7700 Floyd Curl Drive, Zip 78229–3383; tel. 210/575–7138; Arthur E. Marlin, M.D., Chief Executive Officer (Nonreporting) **A**9 10 **S** HCA – The Healthcare Company, Nashville, TN
Web address: www.mhshealthcare.com | 32 | 10 | 150 | — | — | — | — | — | — | — |

Many Facility Codes have changed. Please refer to the AHA Guide Code Chart.

Hospitals, U.S. / TEXAS

Hospital, Address, Telephone, Administrator, Approval, Facility, and Physician Codes, Health Care System, Network	Classification Codes		Utilization Data					Expense (thousands) of dollars		
★ American Hospital Association (AHA) membership □ Joint Commission on Accreditation of Healthcare Organizations (JCAHO) accreditation + American Osteopathic Healthcare Association (AOHA) membership ○ American Osteopathic Association (AOA) accreditation △ Commission on Accreditation of Rehabilitation Facilities (CARF) accreditation Control codes 61, 63, 64, 71, 72 and 73 indicate hospitals listed by AOHA, but not registered by AHA. For definition of numerical codes, see page A4	Control	Service	Staffed Beds	Admissions	Census	Outpatient Visits	Births	Total	Payroll	Personnel
★ METHODIST SPECIALTY AND TRANSPLANT HOSPITAL, (Formerly San Antonio Community Hospital), 8026 Floyd Curl Drive, Zip 78229–3915; tel. 210/575–8110; John E. Hornbeak, Chief Executive Officer (Total facility includes 20 beds in nursing home–type unit) **A**1 3 5 9 10 **F**1 2 3 4 8 9 11 12 13 14 16 17 18 19 21 22 23 24 25 27 28 29 30 31 32 33 34 35 37 38 39 41 42 43 44 45 46 47 48 50 51 52 53 54 57 59 60 61 62 63 64 65 66 68 69 70 71 72 74 75 76 77 78 79 **P**2 5 7 8 **S** HCA – The Healthcare Company, Nashville, TN **Web address:** www.mhshealthcare.com	32	10	218	6232	101	45198	0	63386	24838	555
★ METROPOLITAN METHODIST HOSPITAL, 1310 McCullough Avenue, Zip 78212–2617; tel. 210/208–2200; Mark L. Bernard, Chief Executive Officer (Total facility includes 16 beds in nursing home–type unit) **A**9 **F**1 2 3 4 8 9 11 12 13 14 16 17 18 19 21 22 23 24 25 27 28 29 30 31 32 33 34 35 37 38 39 41 42 43 44 45 46 47 48 50 51 52 53 54 57 59 60 61 62 63 64 65 66 68 69 70 71 72 74 75 76 77 78 79 **P**2 5 7 8 **S** HCA – The Healthcare Company, Nashville, TN **Web address:** www.mhshealthcare.com	32	10	228	11335	139	38450	2481	70787	28202	691
□ MISSION VISTA BEHAVIORAL HEALTH SYSTEM, 14747 Jones Maltsberger, Zip 78247–3713; tel. 210/490–0000; Holly Minnis, Chief Executive Officer **A**1 9 10 **F**2 3 13 16 17 18 25 30 38 50 51 57 59 61 62 63 64 70 72 **P**6 **S** Ramsay Youth Services, Coral Gables, FL	33	22	16	560	12	4480	0	2800	1369	43
□ NIX HEALTH CARE SYSTEM, 414 Navarro Street, Zip 78205–2522; tel. 210/271–1800; John F. Strieby, Chief Executive Officer (Total facility includes 17 beds in nursing home–type unit) **A**1 3 9 10 **F**4 8 9 11 13 22 24 30 31 32 34 36 37 38 39 41 43 44 46 47 48 49 50 51 54 55 56 57 60 62 63 64 65 68 69 70 71 72 74 76 78 79 **P**1	33	10	169	4170	74	62071	654	43570	18148	469
NORTH CENTRAL BAPTIST HOSPITAL, 520 Madison Oak Drive, Zip 78258–3912; tel. 210/297–4000; Kim Murphy–Abdouch, Vice President Operations **A**9 **F**2 3 4 8 9 11 12 13 16 17 18 19 22 23 24 25 27 28 29 30 31 32 33 34 35 36 37 38 39 41 42 43 44 45 46 47 48 49 50 51 52 53 54 57 59 60 61 62 64 65 66 70 72 75 76 78 79 **P**7 8 **S** Baptist Health System, San Antonio, TX	21	10	126	6145	66	44735	983	41826	17098	402
NORTHEAST BAPTIST HOSPITAL, 8811 Village Drive, Zip 78217–5440; tel. 210/297–2000; Dan Brown, Vice President Operations **A**3 9 **F**2 3 4 8 9 11 12 13 16 17 18 19 22 23 24 25 27 28 29 30 31 32 33 34 35 36 37 39 41 42 43 44 45 46 47 48 49 50 51 52 53 54 57 58 59 60 61 62 63 64 65 66 68 70 72 74 75 76 78 79 **P**7 8 **S** Baptist Health System, San Antonio, TX **Web address:** www.baptisthealthsystem.org	21	10	234	11343	142	54845	1894	76212	28220	824
★ NORTHEAST METHODIST HOSPITAL, 12412 Judson Road, Zip 78233–3272, Mailing Address: P.O. Box 659510, Zip 78265–9510; tel. 210/650–4949; Mark L. Bernard, Chief Executive Officer (Total facility includes 10 beds in nursing home–type unit) **A**1 9 10 **F**1 2 3 4 8 9 11 12 13 14 16 17 18 19 21 22 23 24 25 27 28 29 30 31 32 33 34 35 37 38 39 41 42 43 44 45 46 47 48 50 51 52 53 54 57 59 60 61 62 63 64 65 66 68 69 70 71 72 74 75 76 77 78 79 **P**2 5 7 8 **S** HCA – The Healthcare Company, Nashville, TN **Web address:** www.mhshealthcare.com	32	10	99	3692	53	40400	0	30963	12334	285
□ SAN ANTONIO STATE HOSPITAL, 6711 South New Braunfels, Zip 78223–3009, Mailing Address: Box 23991, Highland Hills Station, Zip 78223–0991; tel. 210/531–7711; Robert C. Arizpe, Superintendent **A**1 10 **F**6 9 13 19 21 23 25 31 32 33 34 50 51 57 58 59 60 61 70 72 78 **Web address:** www.mhmr.state.tx.us	12	22	401	1940	339	0	0	48351	27978	1057
★ SOUTH TEXAS VETERANS HEALTH CARE SYSTEM, (Includes Kerville Division, 3600 Memorial Boulevard, Kerrville, Zip 78028; tel. 210/896–2020; San Antonio Division, 7400 Merton Minter Boulevard, tel. 210/617–5300), 7400 Merton Minter Boulevard, Zip 78284–5799; tel. 210/617–5140; Jose R. Coronado, FACHE, Director (Total facility includes 274 beds in nursing home–type unit) (Nonreporting) **A**1 2 5 8 **S** Department of Veterans Affairs, Washington, DC **Web address:** www.vasthcs.med.va.gov	45	10	1112	—	—	—	—	—	—	—
SOUTHEAST BAPTIST HOSPITAL, 4214 East Southcross Boulevard, Zip 78222–3740; tel. 210/297–3000; Kevin Walters, Administrator (Total facility includes 14 beds in nursing home–type unit) **A**9 **F**2 3 4 8 9 11 12 13 16 17 18 19 22 24 25 26 27 28 30 32 33 34 35 36 37 38 39 41 42 43 44 45 46 47 48 49 50 51 52 53 54 57 59 60 61 62 63 64 65 66 68 69 70 72 75 76 78 79 **P**7 8 **S** Baptist Health System, San Antonio, TX **Web address:** www.baptisthealthsystem.org	21	10	167	6467	99	39588	410	42033	17293	463
★ △ SOUTHWEST GENERAL HOSPITAL, 7400 Barlite Boulevard, Zip 78224–1399; tel. 210/921–2000; Keith Swinney, Chief Executive Officer (Total facility includes 25 beds in nursing home–type unit) **A**1 7 10 **F**4 8 9 11 13 16 17 18 19 22 24 25 31 32 33 34 37 39 41 43 44 45 46 48 50 51 53 54 57 60 61 62 63 65 69 70 72 75 76 77 78 79 **S** IASIS Healthcare, Nashville, TN **Web address:** www.tenethealth.comswgh	32	10	200	6083	110	61033	1235	40007	19158	609
SOUTHWEST MENTAL HEALTH CENTER, 8535 Tom Slick, Zip 78229–3363; tel. 210/616–0300; Frederick W. Hines, President **A**5 9 **F**17 18 23 25 31 34 57 58 59 60 61 63 64 70 **P**8 **Web address:** www.smhc.org	23	52	40	1360	25	639	0	4520	2528	260
★ SOUTHWEST TEXAS METHODIST HOSPITAL, 7700 Floyd Curl Drive, Zip 78229–3993; tel. 210/575–4000; John E. Hornbeak, Chief Executive Officer (Total facility includes 38 beds in nursing home–type unit) **A**1 2 3 5 9 10 **F**1 2 3 4 8 9 11 12 13 14 16 17 18 19 21 22 23 24 25 27 28 29 30 31 32 33 34 35 37 38 39 41 42 43 44 45 46 47 48 50 51 52 53 54 57 59 60 61 62 63 64 65 66 68 69 70 71 72 74 75 76 77 78 79 **P**2 5 7 8 **S** HCA – The Healthcare Company, Nashville, TN **Web address:** www.mhshealthcare.com	32	10	774	34201	460	169305	7610	273596	110014	2816

© 2000 AHA Guide   *Many Facility Codes have changed. Please refer to the AHA Guide Code Chart.*

Hospitals, U.S. / TEXAS

Hospital, Address, Telephone, Administrator, Approval, Facility, and Physician Codes, Health Care System, Network

- ★ American Hospital Association (AHA) membership
- ☐ Joint Commission on Accreditation of Healthcare Organizations (JCAHO) accreditation
- + American Osteopathic Healthcare Association (AOHA) membership
- ○ American Osteopathic Association (AOA) accreditation
- △ Commission on Accreditation of Rehabilitation Facilities (CARF) accreditation

Control codes 61, 63, 64, 71, 72 and 73 indicate hospitals listed by AOHA, but not registered by AHA. For definition of numerical codes, see page A4.

Hospital	Classification Codes		Utilization Data					Expense (thousands) of dollars		Personnel
	Control	Service	Staffed Beds	Admissions	Census	Outpatient Visits	Births	Total	Payroll	
ST. LUKE'S BAPTIST HOSPITAL, 7930 Floyd Curl Drive, Zip 78229–0100; tel. 210/297–5000; Virginia Dempsey, Vice President Operations (Total facility includes 29 beds in nursing home–type unit) **A**3 5 9 **F**1 2 4 8 9 11 12 13 16 17 18 19 22 23 24 25 26 27 28 30 32 33 34 35 36 37 38 39 41 42 43 44 45 46 47 48 49 50 51 52 53 54 57 58 59 60 61 62 64 65 68 69 70 72 75 76 78 79 **P**7 8 **S** Baptist Health System, San Antonio, TX Web address: www.baptisthealthsystem.org	21	10	195	7567	101	25789	0	65301	20629	550
☐ TEXAS CENTER FOR INFECTIOUS DISEASE, 2303 S.E. Military Drive, Zip 78223–3597; tel. 210/534–8857; James N. Elkins, FACHE, Director **A**1 9 10 **F**7 16 17 18 22 23 24 31 35 38 51 70 72 76 78 **P**4 7 **S** Texas Department of Health, Austin, TX Web address: www.tdh.state.tx.us	12	33	109	168	59	6119	0	14038	7169	250
⊠ UNIVERSITY HEALTH SYSTEM, (Includes University Health Center – Downtown, tel. 210/358–3400; University Hospital, tel. 210/358–4000), 4502 Medical Drive, Zip 78229–4493; tel. 210/358–4000; Jeff Turner, President and Chief Executive Officer **A**1 2 3 5 8 9 10 **F**1 3 4 7 8 9 11 12 13 14 16 17 18 19 21 22 23 24 27 28 29 30 31 32 33 34 35 36 38 39 41 42 43 44 45 46 47 48 49 50 51 52 53 54 56 57 58 59 60 61 62 63 65 66 68 70 71 72 73 74 75 76 77 78 79 **P**4 7 Web address: www.universityhealthsystem.com	16	10	547	19930	325	512725	2869	367313	117147	4301
☐ △ WARM SPRINGS REHABILITATION HOSPITAL, (Formerly Warm Springs and Baptist Rehabilitation Hospital), 5101 Medical Drive, Zip 78229–6098; tel. 210/616–0100; Girard Seitter, IV, CHE, Administrator **A**1 3 7 10 **F**7 13 17 18 19 22 31 39 45 49 50 53 54 70 72 76 78 Web address: www.warmsprings.org	23	46	64	1112	55	36296	0	17089	6513	193
SAN AUGUSTINE—San Augustine County										
MEMORIAL MEDICAL CENTER OF SAN AUGUSTINE, 511 East Hospital Street, Zip 75972–2121, Mailing Address: P.O. Box 658, Zip 75972–0658; tel. 409/275–3446; Terry Napper, Administrator (Nonreporting) **A**9 10 **S** Memorial Health System of East Texas, Lufkin, TX Web address: www.memorialhealth.org	16	10	16	—	—	—	—	—	—	—
SAN BENITO—Cameron County										
☐ DOLLY VINSANT MEMORIAL HOSPITAL, 400 East U.S. Highway 77, Zip 78586–5310, Mailing Address: P.O. Box 42, Zip 78586–0042; tel. 956/399–1313; Mark Dooley, Chief Executive Officer **A**1 9 10 **F**7 13 16 17 18 22 23 24 25 32 34 38 39 43 48 50 54 71 76 77 78 **S** New American Healthcare Corporation, Brentwood, TN Web address: www.dollyvinsant.nahc.net	33	10	33	1269	11	9918	0	7241	3117	103
SAN MARCOS—Hays County										
⊠ CENTRAL TEXAS MEDICAL CENTER, 1301 Wonder World Drive, Zip 78666–7544; tel. 512/353–8979; Ken Bacon, President and Chief Executive Officer (Total facility includes 5 beds in nursing home–type unit) **A**1 9 10 **F**8 9 11 13 16 17 18 19 22 23 24 25 28 32 33 34 36 37 39 41 43 44 45 48 49 50 51 54 69 70 71 72 76 78 **P**6 8 **S** Adventist Health System Sunbelt Health Care Corporation, Winter Park, FL	21	10	113	4688	47	—	1001	17330	13603	493
SEGUIN—Guadalupe County										
⊠ GUADALUPE VALLEY HOSPITAL, 1215 East Court Street, Zip 78155–5189; tel. 830/379–2411; Don L. Richey, Administrator **A**1 9 10 **F**3 7 8 9 13 16 17 21 22 24 25 26 30 32 35 36 37 38 39 41 44 45 46 48 50 51 54 58 60 62 63 64 68 70 71 72 75 76 78 **P**1 Web address: www.gvh.com	15	10	105	4647	51	52824	693	32026	14690	615
SEMINOLE—Gaines County										
★ MEMORIAL HOSPITAL, 209 N.W. Eighth Street, Zip 79360–3447; tel. 915/758–5811; Steve Beck, Chief Executive Officer and Administrator **A**9 10 **F**3 7 8 9 13 14 16 17 18 19 21 22 23 24 25 26 28 30 32 33 34 36 37 38 39 43 44 45 48 50 51 54 56 58 59 60 61 64 66 70 71 72 75 76 78 79	16	10	33	873	9	30089	177	10163	3355	143
SEYMOUR—Baylor County										
★ SEYMOUR HOSPITAL, 200 Stadium Drive, Zip 76380–2344; tel. 940/888–5572; Robert E. Vernor, Administrator **A**9 10 **F**22 25 30 32 34 36 38 41 44 45 48 54 69 70 72 75 **P**6	16	10	34	655	11	20340	37	5521	2223	93
SHAMROCK—Wheeler County										
SHAMROCK GENERAL HOSPITAL, 1000 South Main Street, Zip 79079–2896; tel. 806/256–2114; Wiley M. Fires, Administrator (Total facility includes 11 beds in nursing home–type unit) **A**9 10 **F**13 25 37 48 69 75 76 78	13	10	27	504	13	20929	1	2558	102	61
SHEPPARD AFB—Wichita County										
⊠ U. S. AIR FORCE REGIONAL HOSPITAL–SHEPPARD, 149 Hart Street, Suite 1, Zip 76311–3478; tel. 940/676–2010; Lieutenant Colonel Karen A. Bradway, MSC, USAF, Administrator (Nonreporting) **A**1 **S** Department of the Air Force, Bowling AFB, DC	41	10	65	—	—	—	—	—	—	—
SHERMAN—Grayson County										
⊠ COMMUNITY MEDICAL CENTER SHERMAN, (Formerly Medical Center of Sherman), 1111 Gallagher Road, Zip 75090–1798; tel. 903/870–7000; William A. Keaton, Chief Executive Officer (Total facility includes 23 beds in nursing home–type unit) **A**1 9 10 **F**8 9 13 17 22 24 25 27 30 32 33 34 35 37 38 39 41 44 45 46 48 49 50 51 53 54 55 68 69 70 72 76 78 79 **P**5 **S** Triad Hospitals, Inc., Dallas, TX Web address: www.hcahealthcare.com	33	10	128	3434	49	45695	306	26860	10314	360

Hospitals, U.S. / TEXAS

Hospital, Address, Telephone, Administrator, Approval, Facility, and Physician Codes, Health Care System, Network	Classification Codes		Utilization Data					Expense (thousands) of dollars		
★ American Hospital Association (AHA) membership □ Joint Commission on Accreditation of Healthcare Organizations (JCAHO) accreditation + American Osteopathic Healthcare Association (AOHA) membership ○ American Osteopathic Association (AOA) accreditation △ Commission on Accreditation of Rehabilitation Facilities (CARF) accreditation Control codes 61, 63, 64, 71, 72 and 73 indicate hospitals listed by AOHA, but not registered by AHA. For definition of numerical codes, see page A4	Control	Service	Staffed Beds	Admissions	Census	Outpatient Visits	Births	Total	Payroll	Personnel
★ △ WILSON N. JONES MEDICAL CENTER, (Formerly Wilson N. Jones Regional Health System), 500 North Highland Avenue, Zip 75092-7354; tel. 903/870-4611; K. Steven Rowley, CHE, President and Chief Executive Officer (Total facility includes 29 beds in nursing home-type unit) (Nonreporting) **A**1 7 9 10 Web address: www.wnj.org	23	10	190	—	—	—	—	—	—	—
SMITHVILLE—Bastrop County SMITHVILLE REGIONAL HOSPITAL, (Formerly Smithville Hospital), Ninth and Mills Streets, Zip 78957, Mailing Address: P.O. Box 359, Zip 78957-0359; tel. 512/237-3214; James W. Langford, Administrator **A**9 10 **F**9 22 25 38 39 48 76 78	16	10	24	1518	12	9989	159	12561	5467	207
SNYDER—Scurry County ★ D. M. COGDELL MEMORIAL HOSPITAL, 1700 Cogdell Boulevard, Zip 79549-6198; tel. 915/573-6374; Jeff Reecer, Chief Executive Officer (Total facility includes 25 beds in nursing home-type unit) **A**1 9 10 **F**7 8 9 13 16 17 18 19 22 23 24 25 28 29 30 32 34 36 37 38 41 43 44 45 48 50 51 54 69 70 71 72 75 76 78 **P**6 **S** St. Joseph Health System, Orange, CA	13	10	64	1191	37	51829	127	12900	5630	239
SONORA—Sutton County LILLIAN M. HUDSPETH MEMORIAL HOSPITAL, 308 Hudspeth Avenue, Zip 76950-3399, Mailing Address: P.O. Box 455, Zip 76950-0455; tel. 915/387-2521; Dianne Dower, Administrator **A**9 10 **F**16 17 25 32 54 75	16	10	13	227	4	3814	0	1810	748	37
SPEARMAN—Hansford County ★ HANSFORD HOSPITAL, 707 South Roland Street, Zip 79081-3441; tel. 806/659-2535; Allen R. Alberty, Chief Executive Officer (Total facility includes 84 beds in nursing home-type unit) **A**9 10 **F**7 9 14 16 17 18 25 26 32 34 36 37 38 40 46 54 69 76 78 **P**6	16	10	112	357	69	18103	0	6693	3206	153
STAMFORD—Jones County STAMFORD MEMORIAL HOSPITAL, Highway 6 East, Zip 79553, Mailing Address: P.O. Box 911, Zip 79553-0911; tel. 915/773-2725; Sam H. Raney, Interim Administrator **A**9 10 **F**7 9 17 22 23 25 28 36 37 39 48 49 54 75 76 **P**5	16	10	26	424	4	3835	0	4014	1862	74
STANTON—Martin County MARTIN COUNTY HOSPITAL DISTRICT, 610 North St. Peter Street, Zip 79782, Mailing Address: P.O. Box 640, Zip 79782-0640; tel. 915/756-3345; Doris Bergerson, Interim Administrator **A**9 10 **F**17 18 25 48 75 76 **P**5	16	10	21	418	6	4228	17	4342	1765	60
STEPHENVILLE—Erath County ★ HARRIS METHODIST-ERATH COUNTY, 411 North Belknap Street, Zip 76401-3415, Mailing Address: P.O. Box 1399, Zip 76401-1399; tel. 254/965-1500; Ronald E. Dorris, Senior Vice President and Executive Director **A**1 9 10 **F**7 8 13 17 18 22 25 32 34 36 37 38 39 41 43 44 48 49 50 51 54 70 75 76 78 79 **P**5 **S** Texas Health Resources, Irving, TX Web address: www.hmhs.com	21	10	75	3207	34	16381	484	18434	7368	227
SUGAR LAND—Fort Bend County ★ METHODIST HEALTH CENTER-SUGAR LAND, 16655 S.W. Freeway, Zip 77479; tel. 281/274-8000; Joan Damon, Administrator **A**1 9 **F**8 9 13 17 18 22 25 27 34 36 38 39 44 48 51 76 78 79 **S** Methodist Health Care System, Houston, TX Web address: www.methodisthealth.com	21	10	22	1068	7	23501	423	18497	6210	136
SULPHUR SPRINGS—Hopkins County ★ HOPKINS COUNTY MEMORIAL HOSPITAL, 115 Airport Road, Zip 75482-0115; tel. 903/885-7671; Richard L. Goddard, Chief Executive Officer **A**1 9 10 **F**8 9 16 17 18 19 22 25 30 32 34 35 36 37 39 41 44 48 51 54 62 64 70 75 76 78 Web address: www.hcmhospital.org	16	10	94	3945	38	39620	967	21325	10159	326
SWEENY—Brazoria County □ SWEENY COMMUNITY HOSPITAL, 305 North McKinney Street, Zip 77480-2895; tel. 409/548-3311; Herbert A. Turk, FACHE, Administrator **A**9 10 **F**7 16 17 19 22 25 26 28 36 40 41 48 51 54 64 70 72 76	16	10	18	212	2	5249	2	6445	3184	105
SWEETWATER—Nolan County ★ ROLLING PLAINS MEMORIAL HOSPITAL, 200 East Arizona Street, Zip 79556-7199, Mailing Address: P.O. Box 690, Zip 79556-0690; tel. 915/235-1701; Thomas F. Kennedy, Administrator **A**1 9 10 **F**7 8 9 16 17 18 22 23 25 28 36 37 39 41 44 48 54 56 70 72 75 76	16	10	54	1943	27	28630	228	12702	5768	213
TAHOKA—Lynn County LYNN COUNTY HOSPITAL DISTRICT, Brownfield Highway, Zip 79373-1310, Mailing Address: Box 1310, Zip 79373-1310; tel. 806/998-4533; Louise Landers, Administrator (Nonreporting) **A**9 10	16	10	24	—	—	—	—	—	—	—
TAYLOR—Williamson County □ JOHNS COMMUNITY HOSPITAL, 305 Mallard Lane, Zip 76574-1208; tel. 512/352-7611; Ernest Balla, R.N., Administrator **A**1 9 10 **F**7 9 16 17 18 22 24 25 31 34 36 38 41 48 50 54 70 76 **P**6 Web address: www.spinoza.pub-lib.ci.taylor.tx.us	23	10	50	1294	29	41674	0	8745	4780	162
TEMPLE—Bell County ★ CENTRAL TEXAS VETERANS AFFAIRS HEALTHCARE SYSTEM, (Includes Central Texas Veterans Affairs Health Care System, 4800 Memorial Drive, Waco, Zip 76711-1397; tel. 817/752-6581; Central Texas Veterans Affairs Health Care System, Marlin Integrated Clinical Facility, 1016 Ward Street, Marlin, Zip 76661-2162; tel. 817/778-4811; Olin E. Teague Veterans' Center), 1901 South First Street, Zip 76504-7493; tel. 254/778-4811; Dean S. Billik, Director (Total facility includes 320 beds in nursing home-type unit) (Nonreporting) **A**1 2 3 5 **S** Department of Veterans Affairs, Washington, DC	45	10	1852	—	—	—	—	—	—	—

© 2000 AHA Guide   *Many Facility Codes have changed. Please refer to the AHA Guide Code Chart.*

Hospitals, U.S. / TEXAS

Hospital, Address, Telephone, Administrator, Approval, Facility, and Physician Codes, Health Care System, Network	Classification Codes		Utilization Data					Expense (thousands) of dollars		
★ American Hospital Association (AHA) membership ☐ Joint Commission on Accreditation of Healthcare Organizations (JCAHO) accreditation + American Osteopathic Healthcare Association (AOHA) membership ○ American Osteopathic Association (AOA) accreditation △ Commission on Accreditation of Rehabilitation Facilities (CARF) accreditation Control codes 61, 63, 64, 71, 72 and 73 indicate hospitals listed by AOHA, but not registered by AHA. For definition of numerical codes, see page A4	Control	Service	Staffed Beds	Admissions	Census	Outpatient Visits	Births	Total	Payroll	Personnel
★ KING'S DAUGHTERS HOSPITAL, 1901 S.W. H. K. Dodgen Loop, Zip 76502–1896; tel. 254/771–8600; Tucker Bonner, President (Total facility includes 8 beds in nursing home–type unit) **A**1 9 10 **F**7 8 16 17 18 22 23 24 25 31 32 34 35 36 37 38 39 41 43 44 45 46 48 49 50 54 61 68 69 70 72 76 78 Web address: www.kdhosp.org	23	10	116	2595	27	30192	479	24212	10615	349
OLIN E. TEAGUE VETERANS' CENTER See Central Texas Veterans Affairs Healthcare System										
★ △ SCOTT AND WHITE MEMORIAL HOSPITAL, 2401 South 31st Street, Zip 76508–0002; tel. 254/724–2111; Dick Sweeden, Administrator (Total facility includes 49 beds in nursing home–type unit) **A**1 2 3 5 7 8 9 10 **F**2 7 8 9 11 12 13 16 17 18 19 22 23 24 25 27 29 30 31 32 33 34 35 36 37 39 41 42 44 45 46 47 48 49 50 51 52 53 54 57 58 59 61 62 63 64 65 66 69 70 71 72 74 75 76 77 78 79 Web address: www.sw.org	23	10	460	21153	318	105356	2376	265858	169269	3237
TERRELL—Kaufman County										
★ MEDICAL CENTER AT TERRELL, 1551 Highway 34 South, Zip 75160–4833; tel. 972/563–7611; Ronald J. Ensor, Chief Executive Officer (Total facility includes 18 beds in nursing home–type unit) **A**1 9 10 **F**8 9 13 17 18 22 24 25 38 39 41 43 44 45 48 49 50 51 53 54 69 70 76 78 **S** Triad Hospitals, Inc., Dallas, TX	32	10	130	3011	35	34817	274	18146	8752	254
☐ TERRELL STATE HOSPITAL, 1200 East Brin Street, Zip 75160–2938, Mailing Address: P.O. Box 70, Zip 75160–0070; tel. 972/563–6452; Beatrice Butler, Chief Executive Officer **A**1 3 5 9 10 **F**1 3 4 5 6 8 9 10 11 12 13 16 17 18 19 21 22 23 24 25 27 30 31 32 33 34 35 39 40 41 42 43 44 45 46 47 48 49 50 52 53 54 55 57 58 59 60 61 62 64 65 68 70 72 73 78 Web address: www.mhmr.state.tx.us	12	22	364	1993	328	0	0	41289	22927	886
TEXARKANA—Bowie County										
★ △ CHRISTUS ST. MICHAEL HEALTH SYSTEM, (Includes Christus St. Michael Rehabilitation Hospital, 2400 St. Michael Drive, Zip 75503; tel. 903/614–4000; Claudia Ann Eisenmann, Administrator), 2600 St. Michael Drive, Zip 75503–2372; tel. 903/614–1000; Don A. Beeler, President and Chief Executive Officer **A**1 2 7 9 10 **F**4 7 8 9 11 12 13 14 16 17 18 19 22 24 25 26 27 28 29 30 31 32 33 34 36 37 38 39 41 43 44 45 46 47 48 49 51 53 54 56 62 65 66 69 70 71 72 74 76 77 78 79 **P**8 **S** Christus Health, Irving, TX Web address: www.smhcc.org	21	10	239	14147	183	157229	1004	109974	46379	1334
☐ △ HEALTHSOUTH REHABILITATION HOSPITAL OF TEXARKANA, 515 West 12th Street, Zip 75501–4416; tel. 903/793–0088; Nate Miller, Chief Executive Officer **A**1 7 9 10 **F**16 17 18 25 49 51 53 54 71 **S** HEALTHSOUTH Corporation, Birmingham, AL Web address: www.healthsouth.com	33	46	60	922	53	13058	0	9830	5746	237
★ WADLEY REGIONAL MEDICAL CENTER, 1000 Pine Street, Zip 75501–5170, Mailing Address: Box 1878, Zip 75504–1878; tel. 903/798–8000; James A. Summersett, II, FACHE, President and Chief Executive Officer (Total facility includes 26 beds in nursing home–type unit) **A**1 2 3 5 9 10 **F**4 7 8 9 11 13 14 17 18 19 22 23 24 25 27 28 32 33 34 35 37 38 39 41 43 44 45 46 47 48 50 51 54 55 56 65 68 69 70 71 72 76 78 79 **P**8 Web address: www.wadleyrmc.com	23	10	361	10874	151	105822	1376	98678	38340	1112
TEXAS CITY—Galveston County										
★ △ MAINLAND MEDICAL CENTER, 6801 E F Lowry Expressway, Zip 77591; tel. 409/938–5000; Maura Walsh, Chief Executive Officer (Total facility includes 28 beds in nursing home–type unit) **A**1 5 7 9 10 **F**3 4 7 8 9 11 12 13 16 17 18 21 22 23 24 25 30 32 33 34 35 37 38 39 41 43 44 45 46 47 48 49 50 51 53 54 55 57 59 60 61 62 63 64 65 66 69 70 71 72 76 77 78 79 **P**5 7 **S** HCA – The Healthcare Company, Nashville, TN Web address: www.mainlandmedical.com	32	10	180	8254	99	92040	490	42050	21720	592
THE WOODLANDS—Montgomery County										
★ MEMORIAL HERMANN THE WOODLANDS HOSPITAL, (Formerly Memorial Hospital–The Woodlands), 9250 Pinecroft Drive, Zip 77380–3225; tel. 281/364–2300; Steve Sanders, Vice President and Chief Executive Officer **A**1 9 10 **F**2 3 4 6 8 9 10 11 12 13 16 17 18 19 20 22 23 24 25 26 27 28 29 30 31 32 33 34 35 36 37 38 39 40 41 42 43 44 45 46 47 48 49 50 51 52 53 54 55 56 57 58 59 60 61 62 63 64 65 66 67 68 69 70 71 72 73 74 75 76 77 78 79 **P**5 **S** Memorial Hermann Healthcare System, Houston, TX Web address: www.mhhs.org	23	10	90	6457	44	46129	2193	29524	12870	453
THROCKMORTON—Throckmorton County										
THROCKMORTON COUNTY MEMORIAL HOSPITAL, 802 North Minter Street, Zip 76483, Mailing Address: P.O. Box 729, Zip 76483–0729; tel. 940/849–2151; Stasha Siegert, Administrator **A**9 10 **F**17 24 25 31 36 38 64 72	13	10	25	234	2	5739	0	1611	534	32
TOMBALL—Harris County										
★ △ TOMBALL REGIONAL HOSPITAL, 605 Holderrieth Street, Zip 77375–0889, Mailing Address: Box 889, Zip 77377–0889; tel. 281/351–1623; Robert F. Schaper, President and Chief Executive Officer (Total facility includes 17 beds in nursing home–type unit) (Nonreporting) **A**1 7 9 10 Web address: www.tomballhospital.org	16	10	92	—	—	—	—	—	—	—
TRINITY—Trinity County										
EAST TEXAS MEDICAL CENTER TRINITY, 900 Prospect Drive, Zip 75862–0471, Mailing Address: P.O. Box 471, Zip 75862–0471; tel. 409/594–3541; Grady Hooper, Chief Executive Officer **A**9 10 **F**17 18 22 25 32 36 37 38 70 75 78 **P**3 7 **S** East Texas Medical Center Regional Healthcare System, Tyler, TX	23	10	22	564	7	28853	0	4744	1867	66

Hospitals, U.S. / TEXAS

Hospital, Address, Telephone, Administrator, Approval, Facility, and Physician Codes, Health Care System, Network	Classification Codes		Utilization Data					Expense (thousands) of dollars		Personnel
★ American Hospital Association (AHA) membership □ Joint Commission on Accreditation of Healthcare Organizations (JCAHO) accreditation + American Osteopathic Healthcare Association (AOHA) membership ○ American Osteopathic Association (AOA) accreditation △ Commission on Accreditation of Rehabilitation Facilities (CARF) accreditation Control codes 61, 63, 64, 71, 72 and 73 indicate hospitals listed by AOHA, but not registered by AHA. For definition of numerical codes, see page A4	Control	Service	Staffed Beds	Admissions	Census	Outpatient Visits	Births	Total	Payroll	
TULIA—Swisher County										
★ SWISHER MEMORIAL HOSPITAL DISTRICT, 539 Southeast Second, Zip 79088–2403, Mailing Address: P.O. Box 808, Zip 79088–0808; tel. 806/995–8200; Steve S. Holmes, Chief Executive Officer **A**9 10 **F**6 7 9 13 14 15 17 19 21 22 25 26 29 30 32 33 34 35 36 37 38 49 50 51 54 70 76 78 **P**6 **S** St. Joseph Health System, Orange, CA	16	10	26	224	11	13096	0	3260	1494	59
TYLER—Smith County										
DOCTORS MEMORIAL HOSPITAL, 1400 West Southwest Loop 323, Zip 75701; tel. 903/561–3771; Olie E. Clem, Chief Executive Officer (Nonreporting) **A**9 10	23	10	46	—	—	—	—	—	—	—
□ EAST TEXAS MEDICAL CENTER REHABILITATION CENTER, 701 Olympic Plaza Circle, Zip 75701–1996; tel. 903/596–3000; Eddie L. Howard, Vice President and Chief Operating Officer **A**1 10 **F**2 3 4 5 7 8 9 10 11 12 13 17 20 21 22 24 25 26 27 29 30 32 33 34 35 36 37 38 39 41 43 44 45 46 47 48 49 50 51 53 54 57 58 59 60 61 62 63 64 65 69 70 71 72 74 75 76 78 79 **P**7 **S** East Texas Medical Center Regional Healthcare System, Tyler, TX **Web address:** www.etmc.org	23	46	49	1009	44	56433	0	15281	7257	199
⊠ △ EAST TEXAS MEDICAL CENTER TYLER, (Includes East Texas Medical Center Behavioral Health Center, 4101 University Boulevard, Zip 75701–6600; tel. 903/566–8668), 1000 South Beckham Street, Zip 75701–1996, Mailing Address: Box 6400, Zip 75711–6400; tel. 903/597–0351; Robert B. Evans, Administrator and Chief Executive Officer (Total facility includes 22 beds in nursing home–type unit) **A**1 2 7 9 10 **F**2 3 4 7 8 9 11 12 13 16 18 22 24 25 27 28 30 31 32 34 36 38 39 41 43 44 45 46 47 48 49 54 57 58 59 60 61 62 63 64 65 68 69 70 71 74 75 76 77 78 **P**6 7 8 **S** East Texas Medical Center Regional Healthcare System, Tyler, TX **Web address:** www.etmc.org	23	10	362	17280	242	179114	556	187137	67128	2818
□ △ HEALTHSOUTH REHABILITATION HOSPITAL–TYLER, 3131 Troup Highway, Zip 75701–8352; tel. 903/510–7000; Sharla Anderson, Interim Chief Executive Officer **A**1 7 10 **F**13 16 17 18 22 24 25 32 34 38 39 43 45 51 53 54 70 71 72 76 78 **S** HEALTHSOUTH Corporation, Birmingham, AL **Web address:** www.healthsouth.com	32	46	63	1065	54	10438	0	10800	5415	179
⊠ TRINITY MOTHER FRANCES HEALTH SYSTEM, 910 East Houston, Zip 75702; tel. 903/531–4445; J. Lindsey Bradley, Jr, FACHE, President and Chief Administrative Officer (Total facility includes 17 beds in nursing home–type unit) **A**1 2 3 9 10 **F**4 8 9 11 12 13 14 16 17 19 21 22 23 24 25 26 27 28 29 32 33 34 35 36 38 39 41 44 45 46 47 48 49 50 51 53 54 56 57 61 63 65 66 69 70 71 72 73 75 76 77 78 79 **P**2 5 6 7 8 **Web address:** www.trimofran.org	23	10	312	17361	219	256822	2431	205523	75689	1944
⊠ UNIVERSITY OF TEXAS HEALTH CENTER AT TYLER, 11937 Highway 271, Zip 75708–3154; tel. 903/877–3451; Ronald F. Garvey, M.D., President (Nonreporting) **A**1 3 9 10 **S** University of Texas System, Austin, TX **Web address:** www.uthct.edu	12	10	117	—	—	—	—	—	—	—
UVALDE—Uvalde County										
⊠ UVALDE COUNTY HOSPITAL AUTHORITY, 1025 Garner Field Road, Zip 78801–1025; tel. 830/278–6251; Ben M. Durr, Administrator **A**1 9 10 **F**7 8 9 11 13 17 18 22 24 25 29 32 36 37 38 39 41 44 45 48 50 54 62 68 70 75 76 77 78 **P**5	16	10	54	2850	30	58170	650	19783	9057	366
VAN HORN—Culberson County										
CULBERSON HOSPITAL DISTRICT, Eisenhower–Farm Market Road 2185, Zip 79855, Mailing Address: P.O. Box 609, Zip 79855–0609; tel. 915/283–2760; Margie Hinojos, Administrator **A**9 10 **F**7 16 17 18 25 35 44 48 54 75 76	16	10	25	66	1	—	12	3194	1015	42
VERNON—Wilbarger County										
□ WILBARGER GENERAL HOSPITAL, 920 Hillcrest Drive, Zip 76384–3196; tel. 940/552–9351; Larry Parsons, Administrator **A**1 9 10 **F**7 8 9 13 16 17 18 22 25 30 32 33 34 36 38 43 44 48 50 51 54 56 62 70 72 76 **P**5	16	10	49	2186	28	119700	123	11277	4645	205
VICTORIA—Victoria County										
⊠ CITIZENS MEDICAL CENTER, 2701 Hospital Drive, Zip 77901–5749; tel. 361/573–9181; David P. Brown, Administrator (Total facility includes 20 beds in nursing home–type unit) **A**1 2 9 10 **F**4 7 8 9 11 12 13 16 17 18 19 21 22 24 25 27 29 30 32 33 34 35 36 37 38 39 41 43 44 45 46 47 48 49 50 51 52 54 55 57 59 60 61 62 64 65 68 69 70 72 76 78 **P**8 **Web address:** www.citizensmedicalcenter.org	13	10	251	9697	131	75063	721	73449	29455	2092
⊠ DETAR HOSPITAL, 506 East San Antonio Street, Zip 77901–6060, Mailing Address: Box 2089, Zip 77902–2089; tel. 361/575–7441; William R. Blanchard, Chief Executive Officer (Total facility includes 20 beds in nursing home–type unit) **A**1 9 10 **F**4 7 8 9 11 12 13 16 18 22 25 26 28 30 31 32 34 37 39 43 44 45 46 48 51 53 54 57 69 70 76 77 78 79 **P**3 8 **S** Triad Hospitals, Inc., Dallas, TX **Web address:** www.detar.com	32	10	211	7298	89	129776	0	53894	19345	588
⊠ REGIONAL MEDICAL CENTER, (Formerly Victoria Regional Medical Center), 101 Medical Drive, Zip 77904–3198; tel. 361/573–6100; William R. Blancher, Chief Executive Officer (Nonreporting) **A**1 9 10 **S** Triad Hospitals, Inc., Dallas, TX **Web address:** www.detar.com	33	10	108	—	—	—	—	—	—	—
WACO—McLennan County										
CENTRAL TEXAS VETERANS AFFAIRS HEALTH CARE SYSTEM See Central Texas Veterans Affairs Healthcare System, Temple										

© 2000 AHA Guide   *Many Facility Codes have changed. Please refer to the AHA Guide Code Chart.*

Hospitals, U.S. / TEXAS

Hospital, Address, Telephone, Administrator, Approval, Facility, and Physician Codes, Health Care System, Network	Classification Codes		Utilization Data					Expense (thousands) of dollars		
★ American Hospital Association (AHA) membership □ Joint Commission on Accreditation of Healthcare Organizations (JCAHO) accreditation + American Osteopathic Healthcare Association (AOHA) membership ○ American Osteopathic Association (AOA) accreditation △ Commission on Accreditation of Rehabilitation Facilities (CARF) accreditation Control codes 61, 63, 64, 71, 72 and 73 indicate hospitals listed by AOHA, but not registered by AHA. For definition of numerical codes, see page A4	Control	Service	Staffed Beds	Admissions	Census	Outpatient Visits	Births	Total	Payroll	Personnel
★ △ HILLCREST BAPTIST MEDICAL CENTER, 3000 Herring Avenue, Zip 76708-3299, Mailing Address: Box 5100, Zip 76708-0100; tel. 254/202-2000; Richard E. Scott, President **A**1 2 3 5 7 9 10 **F**1 4 5 7 8 9 11 12 13 14 17 18 19 20 22 24 25 26 27 28 29 30 31 32 33 34 35 36 37 38 39 41 42 43 44 45 46 47 48 50 51 53 54 56 61 65 68 70 71 72 73 75 76 77 78 79 **P**6 7 8 Web address: www.hillcrest.net	21	10	272	13886	176	204605	2998	120441	44610	1496
★ PROVIDENCE HEALTH CENTER, 6901 Medical Parkway, Zip 76712-7998, Mailing Address: P.O. Box 2589, Zip 76702-2589; tel. 254/751-4000; Kent A. Keahey, President and Chief Executive Officer (Total facility includes 209 beds in nursing home-type unit) **A**1 2 3 5 9 10 **F**2 3 4 6 7 8 9 11 13 16 17 18 19 21 22 24 25 27 30 31 32 34 35 36 37 38 39 41 43 44 45 46 47 48 51 54 56 57 58 59 60 61 62 63 64 65 68 69 70 72 76 77 78 79 **P**6 8 **S** Ascension Health, Saint Louis, MO Web address: www.providence-waco.org	21	10	427	10334	321	170845	491	93577	37326	1296
WAXAHACHIE—Ellis County ★ BAYLOR MEDICAL CENTER–ELLIS COUNTY, 1405 West Jefferson Street, Zip 75165-2275; tel. 972/923-7000; Ronald Hudspeth, Executive Director (Total facility includes 15 beds in nursing home-type unit) **A**1 9 10 **F**7 8 9 11 13 22 25 28 31 32 36 37 39 40 41 43 44 45 46 48 54 69 70 76 79 **P**3 5 6 **S** Baylor Health Care System, Dallas, TX Web address: www.baylordallas.edu	23	10	81	4950	48	80670	1033	39949	16871	500
WEATHERFORD—Parker County ★ CAMPBELL HEALTH SYSTEM, 713 East Anderson Street, Zip 76086-9971; tel. 817/596-8751; John B. Millstead, Chief Executive Officer **A**1 9 10 **F**7 8 9 13 16 17 18 19 22 24 25 27 28 34 36 37 39 40 41 43 44 45 46 48 54 70 72 75 76 78 **P**8 **S** Quorum Health Group, Brentwood, TN	16	10	67	3797	35	55462	579	28060	10825	399
WEBSTER—Harris County ★ CLEAR LAKE REGIONAL MEDICAL CENTER, (Includes Alvin Diagnostic and Urgent Care Center, 301 Medic Lane, Alvin, Zip 77511-5597; tel. 281/331-6141), 500 Medical Center Boulevard, Zip 77598-4286; tel. 281/338-3110; Donald A. Shaffett, Chief Executive Officer (Total facility includes 39 beds in nursing home-type unit) **A**1 2 9 10 **F**2 3 4 5 7 8 9 10 11 12 13 16 17 18 19 20 22 24 25 26 27 28 29 30 32 33 34 36 37 38 39 41 42 43 44 45 46 47 48 49 50 51 52 53 54 55 56 57 58 60 61 62 63 64 65 66 69 70 71 72 73 76 77 78 79 **P**5 7 **S** HCA – The Healthcare Company, Nashville, TN Web address: www.hcahealthcare.com	33	10	377	17415	204	90228	2769	88679	39868	1171
WEIMAR—Colorado County □ COLORADO-FAYETTE MEDICAL CENTER, 400 Youens Drive, Zip 78962-9561; tel. 409/725-9531; Randy Bacus, Chief Executive Officer (Total facility includes 14 beds in nursing home-type unit) **A**1 9 10 **F**7 9 13 22 25 32 36 39 45 48 54 63 69 70 76	23	10	38	1398	21	28208	0	9816	3579	143
WELLINGTON—Collingsworth County COLLINGSWORTH GENERAL HOSPITAL, 1014 15th Street, Zip 79095-3704; tel. 806/447-2521; S. Beth Caison, Administrator **A**9 10 **F**7 14 17 22 25 30 32 34 36 43 48 51 54 76 79 **P**6	16	10	20	362	5	17434	0	2713	1353	63
WESLACO—Hidalgo County ★ KNAPP MEDICAL CENTER, 1401 East Eighth Street, Zip 78596-6640, Mailing Address: P.O. Box 1110, Zip 78599-1110; tel. 956/968-8567; Robert W. Vanderveer, President and Chief Executive Officer **A**1 9 10 **F**7 8 9 16 17 18 19 22 23 24 25 30 31 32 34 36 37 38 39 41 43 44 46 48 49 50 51 54 68 70 72 75 76 78 79 **P**3	23	10	233	13131	132	86805	1861	70785	28935	969
WEST—McLennan County □ HILLCREST MEDICAL CENTER AT WEST, (Formerly West Community Hospital), 501 Meadow Drive, Zip 76691-1018, Mailing Address: P.O. Box 478, Zip 76691-0478; tel. 254/202-7000; Marilyn K. Lord, Administrator **A**1 9 10 **F**7 17 18 22 25 32 34 36 38 51 56 70 76 78 **P**6 7 8	21	10	19	247	4	15211	0	3389	1637	56
WHARTON—Wharton County ★ GULF COAST MEDICAL CENTER, 1400 Highway 59, Zip 77488-3004, Mailing Address: P.O. Box 3004, Zip 77488-3004; tel. 409/532-2500; Michael D. Murphy, Chief Executive Officer (Total facility includes 20 beds in nursing home-type unit) **A**1 2 9 10 **F**7 8 11 13 16 17 18 22 24 25 34 41 44 45 46 48 50 51 53 55 65 68 69 70 74 75 76 78 79 **S** Triad Hospitals, Inc., Dallas, TX Web address: www.gulfcoastmedical.com	32	10	161	3546	53	28932	634	23686	11376	338
WHEELER—Wheeler County PARKVIEW HOSPITAL, 1000 Sweetwater Street, Zip 79096, Mailing Address: P.O. Box 1030, Zip 79096-1030; tel. 806/826-5581; B. W. Robertson, Administrator and Chief Executive Officer **A**9 10 **F**9 16 17 18 19 22 25 36 44 51 69 70 76	16	10	25	454	11	5920	0	3145	1497	62
WHITNEY—Hill County LAKE WHITNEY MEDICAL CENTER, 200 North San Jacinto Street, Zip 76692-2388, Mailing Address: P.O. Box 458, Zip 76692-0458; tel. 254/694-3165; Ruth Ann Crow, Administrator (Nonreporting) **A**9 10	16	10	48	—	—	—	—	—	—	—
WICHITA FALLS—Wichita County □ △ HEALTHSOUTH REHABILITATION HOSPITAL–WICHITA FALLS, 3901 Armory Road, Zip 76302-2204; tel. 940/720-5700; Martin A. Lautner, Chief Executive Officer **A**1 7 10 **F**13 17 18 22 25 31 38 39 45 48 49 50 51 53 54 70 71 72 76 **S** HEALTHSOUTH Corporation, Birmingham, AL Web address: www.healthsouth.com	32	46	63	825	43	8086	0	8754	4045	138

Hospitals, U.S. / TEXAS

Hospital, Address, Telephone, Administrator, Approval, Facility, and Physician Codes, Health Care System, Network	Control	Service	Staffed Beds	Admissions	Census	Outpatient Visits	Births	Total	Payroll	Personnel
★ American Hospital Association (AHA) membership □ Joint Commission on Accreditation of Healthcare Organizations (JCAHO) accreditation + American Osteopathic Healthcare Association (AOHA) membership ○ American Osteopathic Association (AOA) accreditation △ Commission on Accreditation of Rehabilitation Facilities (CARF) accreditation Control codes 61, 63, 64, 71, 72 and 73 indicate hospitals listed by AOHA, but not registered by AHA. For definition of numerical codes, see page A4										
✦ KELL WEST REGIONAL HOSPITAL, 5420 Kell West Boulevard, Zip 76310; tel. 940/692-5888; Anthony German, Administrator and Chief Executive Officer **A**1 9 10 **F**9 22 25 27 36 37 39 43 45 46 48 49 54 76 **P**5	32	10	27	829	8	10610	0	11560	2708	121
□ NORTH TEXAS STATE HOSPITAL, WICHITA FALLS CAMPUS, (Formerly Wichita Falls State Hospital), 6515 Lake Road, Zip 76308-5419, Mailing Address: Box 300, Zip 76307-0300; tel. 940/692-1220; James E. Smith, Superintendent (Nonreporting) **A**1 10 Web address: www.mhmr.state.tx.us	12	22	381	—	—	—	—	—	—	—
□ RED RIVER HOSPITAL, 1505 Eighth Street, Zip 76301-3106; tel. 940/322-3171; Ricky Powell, Chief Executive Officer **A**1 9 10 **F**1 2 3 17 57 58 62 63 64	31	22	62	959	26	—	0	5136	2616	95
✦ UNITED REGIONAL HEALTH CARE SYSTEM, (Includes United Regional Health Care System–Eighth Street Campus, 1600 Eighth Street, Zip 76301-3164; United Regional Health Care System–Eleventh Street Campus, 1600 11th Street, Zip 76301-9988; tel. 940/764-0055), 1600 Tenth Street, Zip 76301; tel. 940/764-3055; Mindy Burdick, Executive Vice President and Chief Operating Officer **A**1 2 3 5 9 10 **F**4 7 8 9 11 12 13 14 16 17 18 19 22 23 24 25 26 27 31 32 33 34 35 36 37 38 39 41 43 44 45 46 47 48 49 50 51 54 61 65 66 68 69 70 71 72 73 76 77 78 79 Web address: www.urhcs.org	23	10	385	16622	237	125104	1856	133586	54479	1610
WINNIE—Chambers County										
□ MEDICAL CENTER OF WINNIE, Broadway at Campbell Road, Zip 77665, Mailing Address: P.O. Box 208, Zip 77665-0208; tel. 409/296-2131; John W. Beauchamp, Chief Executive Officer (Nonreporting) **A**1	23	10	49	—	—	—	—	—	—	—
WINNSBORO—Wood County										
✦ PRESBYTERIAN HOSPITAL OF WINNSBORO, 719 West Coke Road, Zip 75494-3098, Mailing Address: P.O. Box 628, Zip 75494-0628; tel. 903/342-5227; Dan Noteware, Senior Vice President and Executive Director (Total facility includes 8 beds in nursing home–type unit) **A**1 9 10 **F**9 13 17 18 19 22 24 25 31 32 33 34 39 41 43 48 51 54 69 70 72 75 76 78 **P**1 2 3 **S** Texas Health Resources, Irving, TX Web address: www.phscare.org	23	10	46	1356	20	33413	0	12362	5222	140
WINTERS—Runnels County										
NORTH RUNNELS HOSPITAL, East Highway 53, Zip 79567, Mailing Address: P.O. Box 185, Zip 79567-0185; tel. 915/754-4553; Dick L. Stout, Administrator (Nonreporting) **A**9 10	16	10	21	—	—	—	—	—	—	—
WOODVILLE—Tyler County										
TYLER COUNTY HOSPITAL, 1100 West Bluff Street, Zip 75979-4799, Mailing Address: P.O. Box 549, Zip 75979-0549; tel. 409/283-8141; James W. Gainey, R.N., Administrator **A**6 9 10 **F**6 7 8 9 16 22 25 32 34 36 38 48 54 76 78	16	10	26	1047	12	15240	0	5040	2212	95
YOAKUM—Lavaca County										
✦ YOAKUM COMMUNITY HOSPITAL, 1200 Carl Ramert Drive, Zip 77995-4198, Mailing Address: P.O. Box 753, Zip 77995-0753; tel. 361/293-2321; Jeff R. Egbert, Chief Executive Officer **A**1 9 10 **F**7 8 9 13 16 17 18 19 22 23 25 30 32 34 36 38 39 41 43 44 48 49 50 54 56 70 72 73 75 76 78 Web address: www.yoakumhospital.com	23	10	28	1241	13	12381	141	9080	3269	107

Hospitals, U.S. / UTAH

UTAH

Resident Population 2,100 (in thousands)
Resident population in metro areas 77.1%
Birth rate per 1,000 population 20.9
65 years and over 8.8%
Percent of persons without health insurance 13.4%

- ★ American Hospital Association (AHA) membership
- ☐ Joint Commission on Accreditation of Healthcare Organizations (JCAHO) accreditation
- + American Osteopathic Healthcare Association (AOHA) membership
- ○ American Osteopathic Association (AOA) accreditation
- △ Commission on Accreditation of Rehabilitation Facilities (CARF) accreditation

Control codes 61, 63, 64, 71, 72 and 73 indicate hospitals listed by AOHA, but not registered by AHA. For definition of numerical codes, see page A4

Hospital, Address, Telephone, Administrator, Approval, Facility, and Physician Codes, Health Care System, Network	Classification Codes		Utilization Data					Expense (thousands) of dollars		
	Control	Service	Staffed Beds	Admissions	Census	Outpatient Visits	Births	Total	Payroll	Personnel
AMERICAN FORK—Utah County ★ AMERICAN FORK HOSPITAL, 170 North 1100 East, Zip 84003–2096; tel. 801/763–3300; Keith N. Alexander, Administrator and Chief Operating Officer (Nonreporting) **A**1 9 10 **S** Intermountain Health Care, Inc., Salt Lake City, UT **Web address:** www.ihc.com	23	10	66	—	—	—	—	—	—	—
BEAVER—Beaver County BEAVER VALLEY HOSPITAL, 85 North 400 East, Zip 84713, Mailing Address: P.O. Box 1670, Zip 84713–1670; tel. 435/438–2531; Craig Val Davidson, CHE, Administrator (Total facility includes 24 beds in nursing home–type unit) **A**9 10 **F**8 16 22 25 36 48 51 54 70 76 78	14	10	36	852	30	8234	97	4732	2027	88
BOUNTIFUL—Davis County ★ LAKEVIEW HOSPITAL, 630 East Medical Drive, Zip 84010–4996; tel. 801/292–6231; Craig Preston, Chief Executive Officer (Total facility includes 10 beds in nursing home–type unit) **A**1 9 10 **F**2 8 9 11 12 13 16 17 18 21 22 24 25 28 30 32 34 37 39 41 43 44 45 46 48 49 50 51 54 57 58 61 62 69 70 72 76 78 79 **P**5 **S** HCA – The Healthcare Company, Nashville, TN **Web address:** www.hcahealthcare.com	33	10	128	3640	46	50264	688	26422	12145	426
BRIGHAM CITY—Box Elder County ★ BRIGHAM CITY COMMUNITY HOSPITAL, 950 South Medical Drive, Zip 84302; tel. 435/734–9471; Tad A. Morley, Chief Executive Officer **A**1 9 10 **F**8 9 12 13 16 17 22 24 25 32 34 38 39 41 43 44 45 48 70 78 **S** HCA – The Healthcare Company, Nashville, TN **Web address:** www.brighamcityhospital.com	33	10	49	1296	8	16496	490	10252	4357	162
CEDAR CITY—Iron County ★ VALLEY VIEW MEDICAL CENTER, 595 South 75 East, Zip 84720–3462; tel. 435/586–6587; Craig M. Smedley, Administrator **A**1 9 10 **F**8 9 13 17 22 24 25 32 33 36 41 44 45 48 51 54 69 70 72 76 78 79 **P**6 **S** Intermountain Health Care, Inc., Salt Lake City, UT **Web address:** www.ihc.com	23	10	36	2096	15	66424	640	17492	6647	—
DELTA—Millard County ★ DELTA COMMUNITY MEDICAL CENTER, 126 South White Sage Avenue, Zip 84624–8928; tel. 435/864–5591; James E. Beckstrand, Administrator **A**9 10 **F**1 3 6 8 9 16 19 20 25 30 32 33 36 37 38 43 44 48 50 51 53 54 58 59 60 61 62 63 69 71 76 78 79 **P**5 **S** Intermountain Health Care, Inc., Salt Lake City, UT **Web address:** www.ihc.com	23	10	20	398	4	14505	105	3055	1249	35
FILLMORE—Millard County ★ FILLMORE COMMUNITY MEDICAL CENTER, 674 South Highway 99, Zip 84631–9701; tel. 435/743–5591; James E. Beckstrand, Administrator **A**9 10 **F**8 9 12 16 17 21 25 30 32 33 36 37 38 41 43 44 48 49 52 53 54 56 69 70 76 78 **P**6 **S** Intermountain Health Care, Inc., Salt Lake City, UT **Web address:** www.ihc.com	23	10	20	269	14	21824	51	2662	1006	47
GUNNISON—Sanpete County ★ GUNNISON VALLEY HOSPITAL, 64 East 100 North, Zip 84634, Mailing Address: P.O. Box 759, Zip 84634–0759; tel. 435/528–7246; Greg Rosenvall, Administrator **A**9 10 **F**8 22 25 36 37 38 48 76 **P**5 **S** Rural Health Management Corporation, Nephi, UT	16	10	20	881	11	31417	224	6485	2684	113
HEBER CITY—Wasatch County ★ HEBER VALLEY MEDICAL CENTER, (Formerly Wasatch County Hospital), 1485 South Highway 40, Zip 84032–3522; tel. 435/654–2500; Randall K. Probst, Administrator (Nonreporting) **A**9 10 **S** Intermountain Health Care, Inc., Salt Lake City, UT **Web address:** www.ihc.com	23	10	25	—	—	—	—	—	—	—
KANAB—Kane County KANE COUNTY HOSPITAL, 355 North Main Street, Zip 84741–3238; tel. 435/644–5811; Mike Sinclair, Administrator (Nonreporting) **A**9 10	16	10	33	—	—	—	—	—	—	—
LAYTON—Davis County ★ DAVIS HOSPITAL AND MEDICAL CENTER, 1600 West Antelope Drive, Zip 84041–1142; tel. 801/825–9561; Bruce A. Baldwin, Chief Executive Officer **A**1 9 10 **F**4 7 8 9 11 13 16 17 18 19 22 24 25 30 32 33 34 37 38 39 41 42 43 44 46 48 49 50 51 54 57 62 69 70 71 76 77 78 79 **P**6 **S** IASIS Healthcare, Nashville, TN	33	10	126	6182	62	77446	2036	33410	14714	—
LOGAN—Cache County ★ LOGAN REGIONAL HOSPITAL, 1400 North 500 East, Zip 84341–2499; tel. 435/716–1000; Richard Smith, Administrator (Total facility includes 15 beds in nursing home–type unit) **A**1 9 10 **F**3 8 9 11 12 13 17 18 22 24 25 28 30 32 33 34 36 37 38 39 41 43 44 45 46 48 49 50 54 56 57 58 59 61 62 64 69 70 71 72 75 76 77 78 79 **P**6 **S** Intermountain Health Care, Inc., Salt Lake City, UT **Web address:** www.ihc.com	23	10	112	8072	66	176532	2276	49273	24035	680

Many Facility Codes have changed. Please refer to the AHA Guide Code Chart.

© 2000 AHA Guide

Hospitals, U.S. / UTAH

Hospital, Address, Telephone, Administrator, Approval, Facility, and Physician Codes, Health Care System, Network	Classification Codes		Utilization Data					Expense (thousands) of dollars		
★ American Hospital Association (AHA) membership □ Joint Commission on Accreditation of Healthcare Organizations (JCAHO) accreditation + American Osteopathic Healthcare Association (AOHA) membership ○ American Osteopathic Association (AOA) accreditation △ Commission on Accreditation of Rehabilitation Facilities (CARF) accreditation Control codes 61, 63, 64, 71, 72 and 73 indicate hospitals listed by AOHA, but not registered by AHA. For definition of numerical codes, see page A4	Control	Service	Staffed Beds	Admissions	Census	Outpatient Visits	Births	Total	Payroll	Personnel
MIDVALE—Salt Lake County										
HIGHLAND RIDGE HOSPITAL, 175 West 7200 South, Zip 84047; tel. 801/569–2153; Michael S. Talmo, Chief Executive Officer **F**2 3 17 **P**6 **S** Pioneer Behavioral Health, Peabody, MA	33	82	32	464	19	3867	0	2722	1022	40
MILFORD—Beaver County										
★ MILFORD VALLEY MEMORIAL HOSPITAL, 451 North Main Street, Zip 84751–0640, Mailing Address: P.O. Box 640, Zip 84751–0640; tel. 435/387–2411; John E. Gledhill, Administrator **A**9 10 **F**1 2 3 4 5 6 7 8 9 10 11 12 13 14 15 16 17 18 19 20 21 22 23 24 25 26 27 28 29 30 31 32 33 34 35 36 37 38 39 40 41 42 43 44 45 46 47 48 49 50 51 52 53 54 55 56 57 58 59 60 61 62 63 64 65 66 67 68 69 70 71 72 73 74 75 76 77 78 79 **P**5 6 **S** Rural Health Management Corporation, Nephi, UT	16	10	34	628	24	—	18	3710	1974	86
MOAB—Grand County										
★ ALLEN MEMORIAL HOSPITAL. 719 West 400 North Street, Zip 84532–2297, Mailing Address: P.O. Box 998, Zip 84532–0998; tel. 435/259–7191; Charles A. Davis, Administrator and Chief Executive Officer **A**9 10 **F**1 7 8 9 15 16 22 23 25 29 30 32 34 36 37 38 43 44 48 49 54 70 75 76 78 **S** Rural Health Management Corporation, Nephi, UT	16	10	38	574	13	13570	101	7036	3287	92
MONTICELLO—San Juan County										
★ SAN JUAN HOSPITAL, 364 West First North, Zip 84535, Mailing Address: P.O. Box 308, Zip 84535–0308; tel. 435/587–2116; Cleal Bradford, Executive Director (Nonreporting) **A**9 10	16	10	26	—	—	—	—	—	—	—
MOUNT PLEASANT—Sanpete County										
★ SANPETE VALLEY HOSPITAL, 1100 South Medical Drive, Zip 84647–2222; tel. 435/462–2441; George Winn, Administrator **A**9 10 **F**8 9 13 16 17 18 19 22 25 30 32 34 36 37 43 48 49 51 54 61 69 70 72 76 **P**6 **S** Intermountain Health Care, Inc., Salt Lake City, UT **Web address:** www.ihc.com	23	10	20	591	10	89000	159	6858	2701	114
MURRAY—Salt Lake County										
✠ COTTONWOOD HOSPITAL MEDICAL CENTER, 5770 South 300 East, Zip 84107–6186, Mailing Address: P.O. Box 57800, Salt Lake City, Zip 84107–0800; tel. 801/262–3461; Douglas R. Fonnesbeck, Administrator and Chief Executive Officer **A**1 2 9 10 **F**2 3 4 5 8 9 10 11 12 13 14 16 17 18 19 21 22 24 25 26 28 29 30 32 33 34 35 36 37 38 39 40 41 42 43 44 45 46 47 48 49 50 51 52 53 54 56 57 58 59 60 61 62 63 64 65 66 68 69 70 71 72 73 74 75 76 77 78 79 **P**5 6 **S** Intermountain Health Care, Inc., Salt Lake City, UT **Web address:** www.ihc.com	23	10	182	11391	96	391347	3492	102933	43194	1436
NEPHI—Juab County										
★ CENTRAL VALLEY MEDICAL CENTER, 549 North 400 East, Zip 84648–1226; tel. 435/623–1242; Mark R. Stoddard, President **A**9 10 **F**8 9 22 25 34 36 38 43 44 48 54 56 75 76 **P**6 **S** Rural Health Management Corporation, Nephi, UT	23	10	20	575	5	58506	95	7063	2620	105
OGDEN—Weber County										
✠ MCKAY–DEE HOSPITAL CENTER, 3939 Harrison Boulevard, Zip 84409–0370, Mailing Address: Box 9370, Zip 84409–0370; tel. 801/398–2800; Thomas F. Hanrahan, FACHE, Chief Executive Officer and Regional Vice President **A**1 2 3 5 9 10 **F**2 3 4 8 9 11 12 13 16 17 19 22 24 25 28 29 30 32 33 34 35 36 37 38 39 41 42 43 44 45 46 47 48 49 50 53 54 56 57 58 59 60 61 62 63 64 66 70 71 72 75 76 77 78 79 **S** Intermountain Health Care, Inc., Salt Lake City, UT **Web address:** www.ihc.com	23	10	293	13895	184	450622	3042	149266	67353	1881
✠ OGDEN REGIONAL MEDICAL CENTER, 5475 South 500 East, Zip 84405–6978; tel. 801/479–2111; Steven B. Bateman, Chief Executive Officer **A**1 2 9 10 **F**2 3 4 7 8 9 11 12 13 14 15 16 17 18 19 20 21 22 23 24 25 26 28 30 32 33 34 35 38 39 41 42 43 44 45 46 47 48 49 50 51 53 56 57 58 59 60 61 62 63 64 65 68 69 70 72 73 75 76 77 78 79 **P**5 6 7 8 **S** HCA – The Healthcare Company, Nashville, TN **Web address:** www.hcahealthcare.com	33	10	179	6821	81	73836	1871	60687	22641	760
OREM—Utah County										
★ OREM COMMUNITY HOSPITAL, 331 North 400 West, Zip 84057–1999; tel. 801/224–4080; Kim Nielsen, Administrator and Chief Operating Officer (Nonreporting) **A**9 10 **S** Intermountain Health Care, Inc., Salt Lake City, UT **Web address:** www.ihc.com	23	10	20	—	—	—	—	—	—	—
★ TIMPANOGOS REGIONAL HOSPITAL, 750 West 800 North, Zip 84059; tel. 801/714–6000; Kenneth Armstrong, Chief Executive Officer **A**9 10 **F**8 9 12 16 17 18 22 24 25 32 34 39 41 44 48 51 59 61 70 75 78 **S** HCA – The Healthcare Company, Nashville, TN **Web address:** www.hcahealthcare.com	33	10	51	2344	18	30735	2031	16601	7555	235
PANGUITCH—Garfield County										
★ GARFIELD MEMORIAL HOSPITAL AND CLINICS, 200 North 400 East, Zip 84759; Mailing Address: P.O. Box 389, Zip 84759–0389; tel. 435/676–8811; Eric Packer, Administrator **A**9 10 **F**8 13 16 17 19 25 32 36 38 43 44 48 51 53 54 69 76 78 **P**6 **S** Intermountain Health Care, Inc., Salt Lake City, UT **Web address:** www.ihc.com	23	10	44	370	2	26083	31	4433	2247	75
PAYSON—Utah County										
✠ MOUNTAIN VIEW HOSPITAL, 1000 East 100 North, Zip 84651–1690; tel. 801/465–9201; Kevin Johnson, Chief Executive Officer **A**1 9 10 **F**3 4 6 7 8 9 11 13 16 17 18 19 22 26 27 30 32 34 35 37 38 39 40 43 45 48 50 51 54 58 59 60 61 62 63 65 67 70 75 76 78 79 **P**5 **S** HCA – The Healthcare Company, Nashville, TN **Web address:** www.hcahealthcare.com	33	10	126	3742	39	47307	959	27999	10477	289

Hospitals, U.S. / UTAH

Hospital, Address, Telephone, Administrator, Approval, Facility, and Physician Codes, Health Care System, Network	Classification Codes		Utilization Data					Expense (thousands) of dollars		
	Control	Service	Staffed Beds	Admissions	Census	Outpatient Visits	Births	Total	Payroll	Personnel

★ American Hospital Association (AHA) membership
□ Joint Commission on Accreditation of Healthcare Organizations (JCAHO) accreditation
+ American Osteopathic Healthcare Association (AOHA) membership
○ American Osteopathic Association (AOA) accreditation
△ Commission on Accreditation of Rehabilitation Facilities (CARF) accreditation
Control codes 61, 63, 64, 71, 72 and 73 indicate hospitals listed by AOHA, but not registered by AHA. For definition of numerical codes, see page A4

Hospital	Control	Service	Staffed Beds	Admissions	Census	Outpatient Visits	Births	Total	Payroll	Personnel
PRICE—Carbon County										
★ CASTLEVIEW HOSPITAL, 300 North Hospital Drive, Zip 84501–4200; tel. 435/637–4800; Jeff Frandsen, Chief Executive Officer (Total facility includes 10 beds in nursing home–type unit) (Nonreporting) A1 9 10 S LifePoint Hospitals, Inc., Brentwood, TN	33	10	84	—	—	—	—	—	—	—
PROVO—Utah County										
□ UTAH STATE HOSPITAL, 1300 East Center Street, Zip 84606–3554, Mailing Address: P.O. Box 270, Zip 84603–0270; tel. 801/344–4400; Mark I. Payne, Superintendent (Nonreporting) A1 10	12	22	343	—	—	—	—	—	—	—
★ △ UTAH VALLEY REGIONAL MEDICAL CENTER, 1034 North 500 West, Zip 84604–3337; tel. 801/373–7850; Mary Ann Young, R.N., Administrator (Total facility includes 14 beds in nursing home–type unit) (Nonreporting) A1 2 3 7 9 10 S Intermountain Health Care, Inc., Salt Lake City, UT Web address: www.ihc.com	23	10	343	—	—	—	—	—	—	—
RICHFIELD—Sevier County										
★ SEVIER VALLEY HOSPITAL, 1100 North Main Street, Zip 84701–1843; tel. 435/896–8271; Gary E. Beck, Administrator A1 9 10 F8 9 13 16 17 18 19 22 24 25 32 33 34 36 37 38 39 43 44 45 48 53 54 56 68 69 70 76 78 P3 5 6 S Intermountain Health Care, Inc., Salt Lake City, UT Web address: www.ihc.com	23	10	26	1236	8	29809	256	9612	3194	—
ROOSEVELT—Duchesne County										
★ UINTAH BASIN MEDICAL CENTER, 250 West 300 North, 75–2, Zip 84066; tel. 435/722–6163; Bradley D. LeBaron, Administrator and Chief Executive Officer A9 10 F7 8 9 16 17 18 22 24 25 26 32 34 35 36 37 39 41 43 44 48 51 54 56 61 69 71 72 76 78 79 P5 7 8	13	10	42	2077	17	32677	392	18779	6524	266
SAINT GEORGE—Washington County										
★ DIXIE REGIONAL MEDICAL CENTER, 544 South 400 East, Zip 84770–3799; tel. 435/634–4000; L. Steven Wilson, Administrator (Nonreporting) A1 2 9 10 S Intermountain Health Care, Inc., Salt Lake City, UT Web address: www.ihc.com	23	10	137	—	—	—	—	—	—	—
SALT LAKE CITY—Salt Lake County										
★ △ LDS HOSPITAL, Eighth Avenue and C Street, Zip 84143–0001; tel. 801/408–1100; Richard M. Cagen, Chief Executive Officer and Administrator (Total facility includes 32 beds in nursing home–type unit) A1 2 3 5 7 9 10 F2 3 4 7 8 9 11 12 13 14 15 16 17 18 19 21 22 24 25 26 28 29 30 32 33 34 35 37 38 39 41 42 43 44 45 46 47 48 49 50 51 52 53 54 56 57 58 59 60 61 62 63 64 65 66 69 70 71 72 74 75 76 77 78 79 P5 6 S Intermountain Health Care, Inc., Salt Lake City, UT Web address: www.ihcweb.co.ihc.com	23	10	433	21964	319	589534	4556	290838	127705	3277
PIONEER VALLEY HOSPITAL See West Valley City										
★ PRIMARY CHILDREN'S MEDICAL CENTER, 100 North Medical Drive, Zip 84113–1100; tel. 801/588–2000; Joseph R. Horton, Chief Executive Officer and Administrator A1 3 5 9 10 F2 3 4 5 8 9 11 12 13 16 17 18 19 22 23 24 25 26 28 29 30 34 35 36 38 39 41 42 43 44 45 46 47 48 49 50 51 52 53 54 56 57 58 59 60 61 62 63 64 65 66 68 69 70 71 72 74 75 76 77 78 79 P6 S Intermountain Health Care, Inc., Salt Lake City, UT Web address: www.ihc.com	23	50	191	10054	154	112498	0	148762	72509	2106
□ SALT LAKE REGIONAL MEDICAL CENTER, 1050 East South Temple, Zip 84102–1599; tel. 801/350–4111; Kay Matsumura, Chief Executive Officer A1 2 3 5 9 10 F4 8 9 11 12 13 16 17 20 30 35 38 39 41 42 43 44 45 46 47 48 49 50 51 53 54 55 56 65 68 70 72 76 78 79 P7 S IASIS Healthcare, Nashville, TN	33	10	138	5438	57	99734	1652	54183	17049	486
□ SHRINERS HOSPITALS FOR CHILDREN–INTERMOUNTAIN, Fairfax Road and Virginia Street, Zip 84103–4399; tel. 801/536–3500; J. Craig Patchin, Administrator A1 3 5 F13 22 38 39 43 45 52 54 59 70 72 76 78 P5 6 S Shriners Hospitals for Children, Tampa, FL Web address: www.shriners.com	23	57	40	1223	23	6012	0	—	—	188
★ ST. MARK'S HOSPITAL, 1200 East 3900 South, Zip 84124–1390; tel. 801/268–7111; John Hanshaw, Chief Executive Officer A1 2 3 9 10 F4 7 8 9 11 12 13 14 15 16 17 18 19 22 24 25 27 29 30 31 32 33 34 36 38 39 41 42 43 44 45 46 47 48 49 50 51 58 60 63 64 65 68 69 70 76 77 78 79 P4 5 7 S HCA – The Healthcare Company, Nashville, TN Web address: www.stmarkshospital.com	33	10	229	15082	176	161396	3089	94118	42243	1118
★ △ UNIVERSITY OF UTAH HOSPITALS AND CLINICS, 50 North Medical Drive, Zip 84132–0002; tel. 801/581–2380; Richard A. Fullmer, Interim Administrator A1 2 3 5 7 8 9 10 F4 7 8 9 10 11 12 13 16 17 18 19 21 22 23 24 25 26 27 29 30 32 34 35 36 38 39 41 42 43 44 45 46 47 48 49 50 51 53 54 56 57 59 61 62 65 66 68 69 70 71 72 73 74 75 76 77 78 79 P5 Web address: www.med.utah.edu/	12	10	346	16157	277	493673	2998	289346	104473	3177
□ UNIVERSITY OF UTAH NEUROPSYCHIATRIC INSTITUTE, 501 Chipeta Way, Zip 84108–1225; tel. 801/583–2500; Ross Van Vranken, Chief Executive Officer A1 3 5 10 F1 2 3 24 42 30 39 50 57 58 59 60 61 62 63 64 70 72 73 P1 5 6 Web address: www.med.utah.edu/uni	23	22	90	2139	53	7633	0	13645	6829	220
★ VETERANS AFFAIRS MEDICAL CENTER, 500 Foothill Drive, Zip 84148–0002; tel. 801/582–1565; James R. Floyd, Director A1 2 3 5 8 9 F3 4 9 11 13 16 17 18 19 21 22 23 24 25 26 27 28 29 30 31 32 33 34 35 36 37 38 39 41 43 45 46 47 48 49 50 51 53 54 55 56 57 59 60 61 62 63 65 66 68 69 70 73 74 76 77 78 79 P6 S Department of Veterans Affairs, Washington, DC Web address: www.va.gov/stations97/guide/home.asp?DIVISION=ALL	45	10	121	4890	98	255311	0	122432	58179	1267

Hospitals, U.S. / UTAH

Hospital, Address, Telephone, Administrator, Approval, Facility, and Physician Codes, Health Care System, Network	Classification Codes		Utilization Data					Expense (thousands) of dollars		
★ American Hospital Association (AHA) membership □ Joint Commission on Accreditation of Healthcare Organizations (JCAHO) accreditation + American Osteopathic Healthcare Association (AOHA) membership ○ American Osteopathic Association (AOA) accreditation △ Commission on Accreditation of Rehabilitation Facilities (CARF) accreditation Control codes 61, 63, 64, 71, 72 and 73 indicate hospitals listed by AOHA, but not registered by AHA. For definition of numerical codes, see page A4	Control	Service	Staffed Beds	Admissions	Census	Outpatient Visits	Births	Total	Payroll	Personnel
SANDY—Salt Lake County										
✣ ALTA VIEW HOSPITAL, 9660 South 1300 East, Zip 84094-3793; tel. 801/501-2600; Wes Thompson, Administrator and Chief Executive Officer **A**1 9 10 **F**2 3 4 5 7 8 9 11 12 13 14 16 17 18 19 21 22 24 25 26 28 29 30 32 33 34 35 36 37 38 39 41 42 43 44 45 46 47 48 49 50 51 52 53 54 56 57 58 59 60 61 62 63 64 65 66 68 69 70 71 72 74 75 76 77 78 79 **P**5 6 **S** Intermountain Health Care, Inc., Salt Lake City, UT **Web address:** www.ihc.com	23	10	72	5416	39	194221	1994	43399	19707	472
□ △ HEALTHSOUTH REHABILITATION HOSPITAL OF UTAH, 8074 South 1300 East, Zip 84094-0743; tel. 801/561-3400; Richard M. Richards, Administrator **A**1 7 10 **F**1 13 17 18 30 31 34 36 45 46 49 50 51 53 54 71 78 **P**5 **S** HEALTHSOUTH Corporation, Birmingham, AL	33	46	86	1046	49	—	0	6657	5861	175
TOOELE—Tooele County										
TOOELE VALLEY REGIONAL MEDICAL CENTER, 211 South 100 East, Zip 84074-2794; tel. 435/843-3611; Brent Cope, Chief Executive Officer (Total facility includes 84 beds in nursing home-type unit) **A**9 10 **F**8 9 13 16 17 21 22 23 25 26 32 34 36 37 38 41 43 44 45 48 49 54 56 58 59 61 69 70 72 75 76 79 **S** Community Health Systems, Inc., Brentwood, TN	16	10	108	1318	76	—	190	16864	6486	281
TREMONTON—Box Elder County										
★ BEAR RIVER VALLEY HOSPITAL, 440 West 600 North, Zip 84337-2497; tel. 435/257-7441; Robert F. Jex, Administrator (Total facility includes 38 beds in nursing home-type unit) **A**9 10 **F**7 8 13 16 17 19 23 25 32 34 36 37 44 48 51 54 69 76 78 **S** Intermountain Health Care, Inc., Salt Lake City, UT **Web address:** www.ihc.com	23	10	58	514	4	13822	83	3518	1566	33
VERNAL—Uintah County										
✣ ASHLEY VALLEY MEDICAL CENTER, (Formerly Columbia Ashley Valley Medical Center), 151 West 200 North, Zip 84078-1907; tel. 435/789-3342; Ronald J. Perry, Chief Executive Officer (Nonreporting) **A**1 9 10 **S** LifePoint Hospitals, Inc., Brentwood, TN **Web address:** www.avmc-hospital.com	33	10	29	—	—	—	—	—	—	—
WEST JORDAN—Salt Lake County										
COPPER HILLS YOUTH CENTER, 5899 West Rivendell Drive, Zip 84088-5700; tel. 801/561-3377; David Damshen, Chief Executive Officer **A**9 10 **F**16 17 18 57 58 64 **S** Children's Comprehensive Services, Inc., Nashville, TN	33	52	98	262	73	0	0	4855	2928	130
□ JORDAN VALLEY HOSPITAL, 3580 West 9000 South, Zip 84088-8811; tel. 801/561-8888; Jeffrey J. Manley, Chief Executive Officer **A**1 9 10 **F**8 9 16 17 18 22 24 25 27 32 34 39 41 44 48 51 68 70 76 78 79 **P**1 6 7 8 **S** IASIS Healthcare, Nashville, TN	33	10	50	3400	25	51276	1643	24993	9284	280
WEST VALLEY CITY—Salt Lake County										
PIONEER VALLEY HOSPITAL, 3460 South Pioneer Parkway, Zip 84120-2648; tel. 801/964-3100; Keith Tintle, Chief Executive Officer (Nonreporting) **A**1 2 9 10 **S** IASIS Healthcare, Nashville, TN	33	10	127	—	—	—	—	—	—	—
WOODS CROSS—Davis County										
□ BENCHMARK BEHAVIORAL HEALTH SYSTEMS, 592 West 1350 South, Zip 84087-1665; tel. 801/299-5300; Richard O. Hurt, Ph.D., Chief Executive Officer (Nonreporting) **A**1 10 **S** Ramsay Youth Services, Coral Gables, FL	33	22	68	—	—	—	—	—	—	—

© 2000 AHA Guide   *Many Facility Codes have changed. Please refer to the AHA Guide Code Chart.*

Hospitals, U.S. / VERMONT

VERMONT

Resident Population 591 (in thousands)
Resident population in metro areas 27.7%
Birth rate per 1,000 population 11.2
65 years and over 12.3%
Percent of persons without health insurance 9.5%

★ American Hospital Association (AHA) membership
☐ Joint Commission on Accreditation of Healthcare Organizations (JCAHO) accreditation
+ American Osteopathic Healthcare Association (AOHA) membership
○ American Osteopathic Association (AOA) accreditation
△ Commission on Accreditation of Rehabilitation Facilities (CARF) accreditation
Control codes 61, 63, 64, 71, 72 and 73 indicate hospitals listed by AOHA, but not registered by AHA. For definition of numerical codes, see page A4

Hospital, Address, Telephone, Administrator, Approval, Facility, and Physician Codes, Health Care System, Network	Classification Codes		Utilization Data					Expense (thousands) of dollars		
	Control	Service	Staffed Beds	Admissions	Census	Outpatient Visits	Births	Total	Payroll	Personnel
BARRE—Washington County ★ CENTRAL VERMONT MEDICAL CENTER, Fisher Road, Zip 05641–9060, Mailing Address: P.O. Box 547, Zip 05641–0547; tel. 802/371–4100; Daria V. Mason, Chief Executive Officer (Total facility includes 153 beds in nursing home–type unit) **A**1 9 10 **F**16 17 18 22 24 31 39 41 44 46 48 50 51 53 54 56 57 59 61 62 66 68 69 70 71 72 76 77 78 79 **P**1 6 Web address: www.cvmc.hitchcock.org/	23	10	294	3878	197	87850	505	50943	22549	563
BENNINGTON—Bennington County ★ SOUTHWESTERN VERMONT MEDICAL CENTER, 100 Hospital Drive East, Zip 05201–5013; tel. 802/442–6361; Harvey M. Yorke, President and Chief Executive Officer **A**1 2 9 10 **F**1 2 3 4 7 8 9 11 12 13 14 15 16 17 18 19 20 22 24 25 29 30 31 32 33 34 36 37 38 39 40 41 43 44 45 46 48 49 50 51 53 54 56 57 58 59 60 61 62 63 64 65 68 69 70 71 72 73 74 75 76 77 78 79 **P**6 8	23	10	76	4382	48	120531	407	43018	20192	608
BRATTLEBORO—Windham County ★ BRATTLEBORO MEMORIAL HOSPITAL, 17 Belmont Avenue, Zip 05301–3498; tel. 802/257–0341; Brian R. Mitteer, President **A**1 9 10 **F**7 8 9 12 16 17 18 19 22 24 25 27 28 32 34 35 39 41 43 44 45 46 48 51 54 68 70 72 76 78 **P**7 Web address: www.bmhvt.org	23	10	61	2398	28	66068	310	24432	9964	271
★ BRATTLEBORO RETREAT, Anna Marsh Lane, Zip 05301, Mailing Address: P.O. Box 803, Zip 05302–0803; tel. 802/257–7785; Richard T. Palmisano, II, R.N., MS, Chief Executive Officer (Total facility includes 92 beds in nursing home–type unit) **A**1 5 9 10 **F**3 30 49 57 58 59 60 61 62 63 64 69 72 **P**6 7 Web address: www.bratretreat.org	23	22	163	1865	140	14036	0	31782	13861	419
BURLINGTON—Chittenden County ★ FLETCHER ALLEN HEALTH CARE, (Includes Fanny Allen Campus, 101 College Parkway, Colchester, Zip 05446–3035; tel. 802/655–1234; Medical Center Hospital Campus, Colchester Avenue, Zip 05401; tel. 802/847–2345), 111 Colchester Avenue, Zip 05401–1429; tel. 802/847–2345; William V. Boettcher, Chief Executive Officer **A**1 2 3 5 8 9 10 **F**2 3 4 7 8 9 10 11 12 13 14 15 16 17 18 19 21 22 23 24 25 26 27 28 29 30 32 33 34 35 36 37 38 39 41 42 43 44 45 46 47 48 49 50 51 52 53 54 56 57 58 59 60 61 62 63 64 65 68 69 70 71 72 74 75 76 77 78 **P**1 8 Web address: www.fahc.org	23	10	508	19268	337	384727	2270	282756	116820	3639
COLCHESTER—Chittenden County FANNY ALLEN CAMPUS See Fletcher Allen Health Care, Burlington										
MIDDLEBURY—Addison County ★ PORTER HOSPITAL, 115 Porter Drive, Zip 05753–8606; tel. 802/388–4701; James L. Daily, President (Total facility includes 118 beds in nursing home–type unit) **A**1 9 10 **F**9 17 19 22 24 25 30 32 33 34 37 39 41 43 44 46 48 51 54 56 68 69 70 72 76 78 79 Web address: www.addisonindependent.com/porter	23	10	163	1607	127	68119	359	24849	11516	440
MORRISVILLE—Lamoille County ★ COPLEY HOSPITAL, 528 Washington Highway, Zip 05661–9209; tel. 802/888–4231; Warren K. West, President **A**1 9 10 **F**8 9 12 16 17 18 19 22 24 25 32 33 34 37 38 40 41 42 43 44 46 48 51 53 54 58 63 69 70 71 72 76 78 **P**8 Web address: www.copleyhealthsystems.org	23	10	41	1684	22	50979	239	20978	8177	256
NEWPORT—Orleans County ★ NORTH COUNTRY HOSPITAL AND HEALTH CENTER, 189 Prouty Drive, Zip 05855–9329; tel. 802/334–7331; Sidney A. Toll, President **A**1 9 10 **F**7 8 11 18 19 22 24 25 32 33 34 39 41 43 44 45 46 48 49 50 51 54 56 63 70 72 76 78 79 **P**6 Web address: www.nchsi.org	23	10	27	2182	20	303080	198	23748	12439	325
RANDOLPH—Orange County ★ GIFFORD MEDICAL CENTER, 44 South Main Street, Zip 05060, Mailing Address: P.O. Box 2000, Zip 05060–2000; tel. 802/728–4441; Joseph L. Woodin, President and Chief Executive Officer **A**1 2 9 10 **F**1 7 8 9 12 13 14 16 17 18 19 20 22 24 25 26 29 30 31 32 33 34 36 37 38 43 44 45 46 48 49 50 51 54 56 58 59 60 61 62 63 64 70 71 72 73 76 77 78 79 **P**6 Web address: www.giffordmed.org	23	10	49	1242	36	25560	251	18132	9366	259
RUTLAND—Rutland County ★ RUTLAND REGIONAL MEDICAL CENTER, 160 Allen Street, Zip 05701–4595; tel. 802/775–7111; Thomas W. Huebner, President and Chief Executive Officer **A**1 2 9 10 **F**4 6 7 8 9 13 14 15 16 17 18 22 24 25 27 32 34 35 38 39 41 43 44 45 46 48 50 51 53 54 57 59 60 61 63 64 65 68 70 71 72 75 76 77 78 **P**5 8 Web address: www.rrmc.org	23	10	132	6469	85	118089	613	67789	30253	828

Many Facility Codes have changed. Please refer to the AHA Guide Code Chart.

Hospitals, U.S. / VERMONT

Hospital, Address, Telephone, Administrator, Approval, Facility, and Physician Codes, Health Care System, Network	Classification Codes		Utilization Data					Expense (thousands) of dollars		
★ American Hospital Association (AHA) membership □ Joint Commission on Accreditation of Healthcare Organizations (JCAHO) accreditation + American Osteopathic Healthcare Association (AOHA) membership ○ American Osteopathic Association (AOA) accreditation △ Commission on Accreditation of Rehabilitation Facilities (CARF) accreditation Control codes 61, 63, 64, 71, 72 and 73 indicate hospitals listed by AOHA, but not registered by AHA. For definition of numerical codes, see page A4	Control	Service	Staffed Beds	Admissions	Census	Outpatient Visits	Births	Total	Payroll	Personnel
SAINT ALBANS—Franklin County ✠ NORTHWESTERN MEDICAL CENTER, 131 Fairfield Street, Zip 05478–1734, Mailing Address: P.O. Box 1370, Zip 05478–1370; tel. 802/524–5911; Peter A. Hofstetter, Chief Executive Officer **A**1 2 9 10 **F**8 9 13 16 17 18 19 22 25 26 32 33 34 38 39 40 41 43 44 45 48 50 51 54 70 72 76 77 78 **P**8 **S** Quorum Health Group, Brentwood, TN **Web address:** www.nmcinc.org	23	10	53	2217	22	26198	885	25613	11985	320
SAINT JOHNSBURY—Caledonia County ✠ NORTHEASTERN VERMONT REGIONAL HOSPITAL, Hospital Drive, Zip 05819–9962, Mailing Address: P.O. Box 905, Zip 05819–9962; tel. 802/748–8141; Paul R. Bengtson, Chief Executive Officer **A**1 9 10 **F**7 8 9 12 13 16 17 18 19 22 24 25 26 33 34 35 38 39 43 44 45 48 50 51 54 58 59 61 63 68 70 71 76 77 78 79 **P**7 **S** Quorum Health Group, Brentwood, TN	23	10	49	1508	16	83752	223	22329	9037	259
SPRINGFIELD—Windsor County ✠ SPRINGFIELD HOSPITAL, 25 Ridgewood Road, Zip 05156–2003, Mailing Address: P.O. Box 2003, Zip 05156–2003; tel. 802/885–2151; Glenn D. Cordner, Chief Executive Officer **A**1 9 10 **F**1 8 9 13 16 17 18 19 20 22 24 25 26 28 29 30 32 33 35 37 38 39 41 43 44 46 48 49 50 51 54 56 57 59 61 62 64 70 72 76 77 78 **P**4 7 **Web address:** www.springfieldhospital.org	23	10	69	2575	31	45115	240	23543	8890	293
TOWNSHEND—Windham County ★ GRACE COTTAGE HOSPITAL, (Includes Stratton House Nursing Home), Route 35, Zip 05353–0216, Mailing Address: P.O. Box 216, Zip 05353–0216; tel. 802/365–7357; Albert LaRochelle, Administrator (Total facility includes 30 beds in nursing home–type unit) (Nonreporting) **A**9 10 **Web address:** www.gracecottage.org	23	10	45	—	—	—	—	—	—	—
WATERBURY—Washington County VERMONT STATE HOSPITAL, 103 South Main Street, Zip 05671–2501; tel. 802/241–1000; Bertold Francke, M.D., Interim Executive Director **A**9 10 **F**23 57 70 78 **P**6	12	22	54	224	45	0	—	9087	5261	162
WHITE RIVER JUNCTION—Windsor County ✠ VETERANS AFFAIRS MEDICAL CENTER, North Hartland Road, Zip 05009–0001; tel. 802/295–9363; Gary M. De Gasta, Center Director **A**1 3 5 8 **F**1 3 4 5 6 9 11 13 16 17 18 19 20 21 22 23 24 25 26 29 30 31 32 33 34 35 36 37 38 39 41 43 45 46 48 49 50 51 54 56 57 59 60 62 63 65 70 72 76 78 79 **P**6 **S** Department of Veterans Affairs, Washington, DC **Web address:** www.va.gov	45	10	60	2306	43	130443	0	59986	26300	587
WINDSOR—Windsor County ★ MT. ASCUTNEY HOSPITAL AND HEALTH CENTER, 289 County Road, Zip 05089–9702; tel. 802/674–6711; Richard Slusky, Administrator (Total facility includes 66 beds in nursing home–type unit) **A**9 10 **F**7 9 13 16 17 18 19 20 23 25 26 30 31 33 34 35 36 37 38 40 41 43 45 48 50 51 53 54 56 59 61 63 67 69 70 72 76 78 **P**6 **Web address:** www.mtascutneyhosp.hitchcock.org	23	10	99	1040	73	22189	0	14073	6484	253

© 2000 AHA Guide   *Many Facility Codes have changed. Please refer to the AHA Guide Code Chart.*

Hospitals, U.S. / VIRGINIA

VIRGINIA

Resident Population 6,791 (in thousands)
Resident population in metro areas 77.9%
Birth rate per 1,000 population 13.6
65 years and over 11.3%
Percent of persons without health insurance 12.6%

★ American Hospital Association (AHA) membership
☐ Joint Commission on Accreditation of Healthcare Organizations (JCAHO) accreditation
+ American Osteopathic Healthcare Association (AOHA) membership
○ American Osteopathic Association (AOA) accreditation
△ Commission on Accreditation of Rehabilitation Facilities (CARF) accreditation
Control codes 61, 63, 64, 71, 72 and 73 indicate hospitals listed by AOHA, but not registered by AHA. For definition of numerical codes, see page A4

Hospital, Address, Telephone, Administrator, Approval, Facility, and Physician Codes, Health Care System, Network	Classification Codes		Utilization Data					Expense (thousands) of dollars		Personnel
	Control	Service	Staffed Beds	Admissions	Census	Outpatient Visits	Births	Total	Payroll	
ABINGDON—Washington County										
★ JOHNSTON MEMORIAL HOSPITAL, 351 Court Street N.E., Zip 24210–2921; tel. 540/676–7000; Clark R. Beil, Chief Executive Officer **A**1 2 9 10 **F**3 4 8 9 11 12 13 16 17 18 19 22 23 24 25 26 30 32 34 35 36 37 38 39 41 42 43 44 45 46 48 49 50 51 53 54 56 57 61 62 64 68 70 71 72 76 77 78 79 **P**8 Web address: www.jmh.org	23	10	135	5539	71	83618	725	41627	17427	603
ALEXANDRIA—Independent City County										
★ INOVA ALEXANDRIA HOSPITAL, 4320 Seminary Road, Zip 22304–1594; tel. 703/504–3000; Kenneth H. Kozloff, FACHE, Administrator **A**1 2 3 5 9 10 **F**3 4 6 7 8 9 11 12 13 14 17 18 19 20 22 24 25 28 29 30 31 32 34 35 36 38 39 41 42 43 44 45 46 47 48 49 51 52 53 54 56 57 58 59 60 61 62 63 64 65 66 68 69 70 71 72 73 74 75 76 77 78 79 **P**4 5 6 **S** Inova Health System, Falls Church, VA Web address: www.inova.com	23	10	311	15300	225	97417	3344	124371	59035	1299
★ △ INOVA MOUNT VERNON HOSPITAL, 2501 Parker's Lane, Zip 22306–3209; tel. 703/664–7000; Susan Herbert, Administrator **A**1 2 3 7 9 10 **F**1 2 3 4 6 7 8 9 11 12 13 14 16 17 18 19 20 22 24 25 26 27 29 30 31 32 34 35 36 37 38 39 40 41 42 43 44 45 46 47 48 49 50 51 52 53 54 56 57 58 59 60 61 62 63 64 65 66 67 68 69 70 71 72 73 74 75 76 77 78 79 **P**4 5 6 **S** Inova Health System, Falls Church, VA Web address: www.inova.org	23	10	229	8408	157	66897	0	83427	35273	900
ARLINGTON—Arlington County										
★ ARLINGTON HOSPITAL, 1701 North George Mason Drive, Zip 22205–3698; tel. 703/558–5000; James B. Cole, Chief Executive Officer (Nonreporting) **A**1 9	32	10	256	—	—	—	—	—	—	—
☐ NORTHERN VIRGINIA COMMUNITY HOSPITAL, (Formerly Vencor Hospital-Arlington), 601 South Carlin Springs Road, Zip 22204–1096; tel. 703/671–1200; Mark Aanonson, Administrator **A**1 5 9 10 **F**4 9 11 13 19 22 25 27 34 38 39 41 43 45 48 51 54 57 60 61 63 64 70 72 76 78 **S** Vencor, Incorporated, Louisville, KY Web address: www.nvchospital.com	33	10	96	3320	69	18018	0	38319	16685	319
BEDFORD—Independent City County										
★ CARILION BEDFORD MEMORIAL HOSPITAL, 1613 Oakwood Street, Zip 24523–0688, Mailing Address: P.O. Box 688, Zip 24523–0688; tel. 540/586–2441; Howard Ainsley, Vice President and Hospital Director (Total facility includes 111 beds in nursing home–type unit) **A**1 9 10 **F**1 7 8 9 13 16 17 18 19 21 22 23 25 26 30 31 32 33 34 36 37 41 43 44 46 48 49 54 56 57 58 59 60 61 62 63 65 68 69 70 72 76 78 79 **P**6 **S** Carilion Health System, Roanoke, VA Web address: www.carilion.com	23	10	160	1928	121	25493	203	18739	8458	259
BIG STONE GAP—Wise County										
★ WELLMONT LONESOME PINE HOSPITAL, 1990 Holton Avenue East, Zip 24219–0230; tel. 540/523–3111; Paul A. Bishop, Administrator **A**1 9 10 **F**7 8 9 13 16 17 18 19 20 21 22 25 26 27 28 30 31 32 34 35 36 37 38 39 40 41 43 44 45 46 48 49 50 51 54 65 68 70 71 72 73 74 76 78 79 **P**1 5 6 7 **S** Wellmont Health System, Kingsport, TN	23	10	49	2026	21	20554	212	14858	6697	198
BLACKSBURG—Montgomery County										
★ MONTGOMERY REGIONAL HOSPITAL, 3700 South Main Street, Zip 24060–7081, Mailing Address: P.O. Box 90004, Zip 24062–9004; tel. 540/951–1111; David R. Williams, Chief Executive Officer (Total facility includes 11 beds in nursing home–type unit) **A**1 9 10 **F**2 3 4 8 9 11 13 16 17 18 19 21 22 24 25 26 27 28 30 32 33 34 35 38 39 41 43 44 45 46 47 48 49 50 51 52 53 54 56 57 58 59 60 61 62 63 64 65 66 68 69 70 71 72 75 76 77 78 79 **P**8 **S** HCA – The Healthcare Company, Nashville, TN Web address: www.montreghosp.com	33	10	115	4582	58	36506	597	37147	13438	444
BURKEVILLE—Nottoway County										
☐ PIEDMONT GERIATRIC HOSPITAL, 900 East Patrick Henry, Zip 23922–0427, Mailing Address: P.O. Box 427, Zip 23922–0427; tel. 804/767–4401; Willard R. Pierce, Jr, Director (Nonreporting) **A**1 9 10 **S** Virginia Department of Mental Health, Richmond, VA	12	49	210	—	—	—	—	—	—	—
CATAWBA—Roanoke County										
☐ CATAWBA HOSPITAL, 5525 Catawba Hospital Drive, Zip 24070, Mailing Address: P.O. Box 200, Zip 24070–0200; tel. 540/375–4200; James S. Reinhard, M.D., Director **A**1 9 10 **F**16 17 18 22 23 30 39 50 51 57 62 70 78 **P**6 **S** Virginia Department of Mental Health, Richmond, VA	12	22	171	380	104	0	0	10160	9624	320
CHARLOTTESVILLE—Independent City County										
☐ CHARTER BEHAVIORAL HEALTH SYSTEM OF CHARLOTTESVILLE, 2101 Arlington Boulevard, Zip 22903–1593; tel. 804/977–1120; David Carlini, Chief Executive Officer (Nonreporting) **A**1 10 **S** Magellan Health Services, Atlanta, GA	33	22	62	—	—	—	—	—	—	—

Hospitals, U.S. / VIRGINIA

Hospital, Address, Telephone, Administrator, Approval, Facility, and Physician Codes, Health Care System, Network	Classification Codes		Utilization Data					Expense (thousands) of dollars		
★ American Hospital Association (AHA) membership □ Joint Commission on Accreditation of Healthcare Organizations (JCAHO) accreditation + American Osteopathic Healthcare Association (AOHA) membership ○ American Osteopathic Association (AOA) accreditation △ Commission on Accreditation of Rehabilitation Facilities (CARF) accreditation Control codes 61, 63, 64, 71, 72 and 73 indicate hospitals listed by AOHA, but not registered by AHA. For definition of numerical codes, see page A4	Control	Service	Staffed Beds	Admissions	Census	Outpatient Visits	Births	Total	Payroll	Personnel
★ MARTHA JEFFERSON HOSPITAL, 459 Locust Avenue, Zip 22902–9940; tel. 804/982–7000; James E. Haden, President and Chief Executive Officer **A**1 2 9 10 **F**6 7 8 9 11 13 16 17 18 19 22 24 25 26 27 30 32 33 34 35 36 37 39 41 43 44 45 46 48 49 50 51 54 65 70 72 76 78 79 **P**1 4 6 7 Web address: www.marthajefferson.org	23	10	156	9005	91	246472	1585	83104	38920	1024
★ UNIVERSITY OF VIRGINIA MEDICAL CENTER, Jefferson Park Avenue, Zip 22908, Mailing Address: P.O. Box 800788, Zip 22908–0788; tel. 804/924–0211; William E. Carter, Jr, Senior Associate Vice President for Operations **A**1 2 3 5 8 9 10 **F**3 4 5 6 7 8 9 10 11 12 13 14 17 18 19 20 21 22 23 24 25 26 27 29 31 32 33 34 35 36 37 38 39 41 42 43 44 45 46 47 48 49 50 51 52 53 54 56 57 58 59 60 61 62 63 64 65 66 68 70 71 72 73 74 75 76 77 78 79 **P**3 Web address: www.med.virginia.edu	12	10	555	28984	423	532597	1412	454032	164945	4534
CHESAPEAKE—Independent City County										
★ CHESAPEAKE GENERAL HOSPITAL, 736 Battlefield Boulevard North, Zip 23320–4941, Mailing Address: P.O. Box 2028, Zip 23327–2028; tel. 757/312–8121; Donald S. Buckley, FACHE, President **A**1 2 5 9 10 **F**1 6 7 8 9 11 13 18 19 20 22 23 24 25 26 27 28 30 32 33 34 36 37 38 39 40 41 43 44 45 46 48 49 51 54 57 62 64 65 66 68 70 72 76 78 79 Web address: www.chealth.org	16	10	260	15033	221	149642	3170	118634	50893	1640
CLINTWOOD—Dickenson County										
□ DICKENSON COUNTY MEDICAL CENTER, Hospital Drive, Zip 24228, Mailing Address: P.O. Box 1390, Zip 24228–1390; tel. 540/926–0300; Benjamin A. Peak, Chief Executive Officer **A**1 9 10 **F**9 16 22 25 30 32 34 36 41 48 56 70 72 76 78 79 **P**6	33	10	41	1226	16	40146	0	7710	3910	169
CULPEPER—Culpeper County										
★ CULPEPER REGIONAL HOSPITAL, (Formerly Culpeper Memorial Hospital), 501 Sunset Lane, Zip 22701–3917, Mailing Address: Box 592, Zip 22701–0592; tel. 540/829–4100; H. Lee Kirk, Jr, President and Chief Executive Officer (Nonreporting) **A**1 9 10 Web address: www.culmem.com	23	10	70	—	—	—	—	—	—	—
DANVILLE—Independent City County										
★ DANVILLE REGIONAL MEDICAL CENTER, 142 South Main Street, Zip 24541–2922; tel. 804/799–2100; William R. Isemann, Interim President (Total facility includes 60 beds in nursing home–type unit) **A**1 2 3 5 6 9 10 **F**2 3 6 7 8 9 11 12 13 16 17 18 19 22 24 25 26 28 29 31 32 33 34 35 36 37 38 39 41 43 44 45 46 48 49 50 51 53 54 56 57 59 60 61 63 65 66 67 68 69 70 72 76 77 78 79 **P**6 8 Web address: www.danvilleregional.org	23	10	203	11352	199	123311	1205	97184	42402	1178
□ SOUTHERN VIRGINIA MENTAL HEALTH INSTITUTE, 382 Taylor Drive, Zip 24541–4023; tel. 804/799–6220; Constance N. Fletcher, Ph.D., Director **A**1 9 10 **F**2 10 12 13 16 17 18 28 41 44 50 51 52 53 57 59 60 61 69 70 72 78 **S** Virginia Department of Mental Health, Richmond, VA	12	22	96	655	87	0	0	8995	5631	165
EMPORIA—Independent City County										
□ GREENSVILLE MEMORIAL HOSPITAL, 214 Weaver Avenue, Zip 23847–1482; tel. 804/348–2000; Gene Faile, Chief Executive Officer (Total facility includes 65 beds in nursing home–type unit) **A**1 9 10 **F**7 8 13 17 18 22 24 25 28 32 34 36 38 39 41 43 44 45 46 48 54 69 70 75 76 **S** Community Health Systems, Inc., Brentwood, TN	33	10	154	3253	102	36274	159	21986	9534	301
FAIRFAX—Independent City County										
★ INOVA FAIR OAKS HOSPITAL, 3600 Joseph Siewick Drive, Zip 22033–1709; tel. 703/391–3600; William A. Brown, CHE, Vice President and Administrator **A**1 2 5 9 10 **F**3 4 6 7 8 9 11 13 14 16 18 19 22 23 24 25 26 32 33 34 35 36 37 38 39 40 41 43 44 45 46 47 48 51 54 58 63 65 66 67 68 70 72 74 75 76 77 78 79 **P**4 5 6 **S** Inova Health System, Falls Church, VA Web address: www.inova.com	23	10	151	11182	102	72605	3183	80918	31675	802
FALLS CHURCH—Independent City County										
★ DOMINION HOSPITAL, 2960 Sleepy Hollow Road, Zip 22044–2001; tel. 703/536–2000; Barbara D. S. Hekimian, Chief Executive Officer **A**1 9 10 **F**17 19 21 57 58 59 60 61 62 63 64 70 72 **P**2 4 7 **S** HCA – The Healthcare Company, Nashville, TN Web address: www.dominionhospital.com	33	22	100	2182	59	—	0	11842	6111	167
□ HOSPICE OF NORTHERN VIRGINIA, 6565 Arlington Boulevard, Suite 500, Zip 22042; tel. 703/534–7070; David J. English, President and Chief Executive Officer (Nonreporting) **A**1 10 Web address: www.hospiceonline.org	23	49	15	—	—	—	—	—	—	—
★ INOVA FAIRFAX HOSPITAL, 3300 Gallows Road, Zip 22042–3300; tel. 703/698–1110; Steven E. Brown, Administrator **A**1 2 3 5 8 9 10 **F**1 3 4 6 7 8 9 11 12 13 14 16 18 19 22 24 25 29 32 33 34 35 36 38 39 40 41 42 43 44 45 46 47 48 49 50 51 52 54 56 57 58 59 60 61 62 63 64 65 66 68 70 71 72 73 74 75 76 77 78 79 **P**4 5 6 **S** Inova Health System, Falls Church, VA Web address: www.inova.com	23	10	656	46973	617	121479	9814	428016	176682	4069
□ NORTHERN VIRGINIA MENTAL HEALTH INSTITUTE, 3302 Gallows Road, Zip 22042–3398; tel. 703/207–7110; Mohamed El-Sabaawi, M.D., Acting Facility Director **A**1 9 10 **F**17 22 23 24 25 39 57 59 61 62 63 65 70 76 78 **S** Virginia Department of Mental Health, Richmond, VA	12	22	137	449	125	0	0	20863	12664	330
FARMVILLE—Prince Edward County										
★ SOUTHSIDE COMMUNITY HOSPITAL, 800 Oak Street, Zip 23901–1199; tel. 804/392–8811; John H. Greer, President **A**1 9 10 **F**8 9 16 17 18 22 23 25 36 39 41 44 45 46 48 49 50 54 70 71 75 76 78 **S** Carilion Health System, Roanoke, VA	23	10	88	4982	46	46659	370	28959	13012	432

© 2000 AHA Guide   *Many Facility Codes have changed. Please refer to the AHA Guide Code Chart.*

Hospitals, U.S. / VIRGINIA

Hospital, Address, Telephone, Administrator, Approval, Facility, and Physician Codes, Health Care System, Network	Classification Codes		Utilization Data					Expense (thousands) of dollars		Personnel
★ American Hospital Association (AHA) membership ☐ Joint Commission on Accreditation of Healthcare Organizations (JCAHO) accreditation + American Osteopathic Healthcare Association (AOHA) membership ○ American Osteopathic Association (AOA) accreditation △ Commission on Accreditation of Rehabilitation Facilities (CARF) accreditation Control codes 61, 63, 64, 71, 72 and 73 indicate hospitals listed by AOHA, but not registered by AHA. For definition of numerical codes, see page A4	Control	Service	Staffed Beds	Admissions	Census	Outpatient Visits	Births	Total	Payroll	
FISHERSVILLE—Augusta County ☐ AUGUSTA HEALTH CARE, 96 Medical Center Drive, Zip 22939, Mailing Address: P.O. Box 1000, Zip 22939–1000; tel. 540/932–4000; Richard H. Graham, President and Chief Executive Officer **A**1 2 9 10 **F**1 2 3 7 8 9 11 13 16 17 18 19 22 23 24 25 27 28 30 31 32 33 34 35 36 37 38 39 40 41 43 44 45 46 48 49 50 51 53 54 56 57 58 59 60 61 62 63 64 68 69 70 71 72 75 76 77 78 **Web address:** www.augustamed.com	23	10	205	11776	136	269904	1000	96923	43167	1376
△ WOODROW WILSON REHABILITATION CENTER, Mailing Address: P.O. Box 1500, Zip 22939–1500; tel. 540/332–7000; David J. Schwemer, Administrator (Nonreporting) **A**7 10	12	46	30	—	—	—	—	—	—	—
FORT BELVOIR—Fairfax County ★ DEWITT ARMY COMMUNITY HOSPITAL, 9501 Farrell Road, Zip 22060–5901; tel. 703/805–0510; Colonel James W. Martin, Commander (Nonreporting) **A**1 3 5 9 **S** Department of the Army, Office of the Surgeon General, Falls Church, VA **Web address:** www.dewitt.wramc.amedd.army.mil	42	10	62	—	—	—	—	—	—	—
FORT EUSTIS—Independent City County ★ MCDONALD ARMY COMMUNITY HOSPITAL, Jefferson Avenue, Zip 23604–5548; tel. 757/314–7501; Colonel George Weightman, Commander (Nonreporting) **A**1 **S** Department of the Army, Office of the Surgeon General, Falls Church, VA	42	10	30	—	—	—	—	—	—	—
FRANKLIN—Independent City County ☐ SOUTHAMPTON MEMORIAL HOSPITAL, 100 Fairview Drive, Zip 23851–1206, Mailing Address: P.O. Box 817, Zip 23851–0817; tel. 757/569–6100; Gwen S. Eddleman, R.N., Interim Chief Executive Officer (Total facility includes 131 beds in nursing home–type unit) **A**1 9 10 **F**3 6 7 8 9 13 16 17 18 19 22 24 25 27 32 34 36 37 38 39 41 43 44 45 46 48 51 54 58 59 60 61 62 63 67 64 69 70 71 72 76 78 79 **P**8	23	10	203	2824	155	54001	280	27306	11691	476
FREDERICKSBURG—Independent City County ★ MARY WASHINGTON HOSPITAL, 1001 Sam Perry Boulevard, Zip 22401–3354; tel. 540/899–1100; Fred M. Rankin, II, President and Chief Executive Officer **A**1 2 9 10 **F**3 4 6 7 8 9 11 12 13 14 17 19 21 22 23 25 26 27 30 31 32 33 34 35 36 37 38 39 40 41 42 43 44 45 46 47 48 49 50 51 53 54 57 58 59 60 61 62 63 64 65 67 68 69 70 71 72 73 76 77 78 79 **P**7 8	23	10	318	16771	211	177356	2473	146605	55848	1569
FRONT ROYAL—Warren County ★ △ WARREN MEMORIAL HOSPITAL, 1000 Shenandoah Avenue, Zip 22630–3598; tel. 540/636–0300; Charlie M. Horton, President (Total facility includes 40 beds in nursing home–type unit) **A**1 7 9 10 **F**7 8 9 13 17 19 22 24 25 31 32 34 36 37 38 41 43 44 45 48 49 50 51 54 68 69 70 72 76 77 78 79 **P**8 **S** Valley Health System, Winchester, VA **Web address:** www.valleyhealthlink.com	23	10	91	1889	65	39794	120	19399	10406	289
GALAX—Independent City County ★ TWIN COUNTY REGIONAL HOSPITAL, 200 Hospital Drive, Zip 24333–2283; tel. 540/236–8181; Marcus G. Kuhn, President and Chief Executive Officer **A**1 9 10 **F**8 9 12 13 16 17 18 22 25 28 32 34 36 37 38 39 43 44 45 48 50 51 54 56 57 59 61 62 63 64 70 71 72 76 78 79 **P**5 8 **Web address:** www.tcrh.org	23	10	76	4690	55	18519	421	35513	14675	545
GLOUCESTER—Gloucester County ☐ RIVERSIDE WALTER REED HOSPITAL, 7519 Hospital Drive, Zip 23061–4178, Mailing Address: P.O. Box 1130, Zip 23061–1130; tel. 804/693–8800; Grady W. Philips, II, Vice President and Administrator **A**1 9 10 **F**1 2 3 4 6 7 8 9 11 12 13 14 16 17 18 19 21 22 24 25 26 27 28 29 30 31 32 33 34 35 36 37 38 39 41 43 44 45 46 47 48 49 50 51 53 54 56 57 58 59 60 61 62 63 64 65 66 67 68 69 70 71 72 75 76 77 78 79 **P**6 **S** Riverside Health System, Newport News, VA **Web address:** www.riverside-online.com	23	10	71	1875	28	—	—	13257	6592	249
GRUNDY—Buchanan County ★ BUCHANAN GENERAL HOSPITAL, Mailing Address: Route 5, Box 20, Zip 24614–9611; tel. 540/935–1000; Randy Brown, Interim Administrator **A**1 9 10 **F**7 9 17 18 22 24 25 27 32 34 36 39 41 45 46 48 54 68 70 76 78 79 **P**8 **S** Quorum Health Group, Brentwood, TN	23	10	144	4554	51	56325	0	24067	11516	323
HAMPTON—Independent City County ★ PENINSULA BEHAVIORAL CENTER, 2244 Executive Drive, Zip 23666–2430; tel. 757/827–1001; Steuart A. Kimmeth, Vice President and Administrator **A**1 9 10 **F**2 13 17 18 22 39 57 58 59 60 61 62 64 70 **P**6 **S** HCA - The Healthcare Company, Nashville, TN **Web address:** www.hcahealthcare.com	33	22	115	2762	65	5587	—	10263	6143	262
★ SENTARA HAMPTON GENERAL HOSPITAL, 3120 Victoria Boulevard, Zip 23661–1585, Mailing Address: Drawer 640, Zip 23669–0640; tel. 757/727–7000; Megan Perry, Administrator (Total facility includes 26 beds in nursing home–type unit) **A**1 2 9 10 **F**1 4 6 7 8 9 10 11 12 13 14 15 16 17 18 19 20 21 22 23 24 25 26 27 28 29 30 31 32 33 34 35 36 37 38 39 40 41 42 43 44 45 46 47 48 49 50 51 53 54 56 57 58 59 60 61 62 63 64 65 66 67 68 69 70 71 72 73 74 75 76 77 78 79 **P**6 7 8 **S** Sentara Healthcare, Norfolk, VA **Web address:** www.sentara.com	23	10	193	8319	136	142428	990	77397	29686	987
★ U. S. AIR FORCE HOSPITAL, 45 Pine Street, Zip 23665–2080; tel. 757/764–6969; Colonel Glenn R. Willauer, Administrator (Nonreporting) **A**1 **S** Department of the Air Force, Bowling AFB, DC	41	10	59	—	—	—	—	—	—	—

Hospitals, U.S. / VIRGINIA

Hospital, Address, Telephone, Administrator, Approval, Facility, and Physician Codes, Health Care System, Network	Classification Codes		Utilization Data					Expense (thousands) of dollars		
	Control	Service	Staffed Beds	Admissions	Census	Outpatient Visits	Births	Total	Payroll	Personnel

★ American Hospital Association (AHA) membership
☐ Joint Commission on Accreditation of Healthcare Organizations (JCAHO) accreditation
+ American Osteopathic Healthcare Association (AOHA) membership
○ American Osteopathic Association (AOA) accreditation
△ Commission on Accreditation of Rehabilitation Facilities (CARF) accreditation
Control codes 61, 63, 64, 71, 72 and 73 indicate hospitals listed by AOHA, but not registered by AHA. For definition of numerical codes, see page A4

✠ VETERANS AFFAIRS MEDICAL CENTER, 100 Emancipation Drive, Zip 23667-0001; tel. 757/722-9961; Bettye W. Story, Ph.D., Director (Total facility includes 104 beds in nursing home-type unit) **A**1 2 3 5 8 **F**3 9 11 13 17 18 19 20 22 23 24 25 26 27 30 31 32 33 34 35 36 37 38 39 41 43 45 46 47 48 49 50 51 54 56 57 59 60 61 62 63 64 65 66 68 69 70 72 74 75 76 77 78 79 **P**6 **S** Department of Veterans Affairs, Washington, DC Web address: www.va.gov	45	10	470	3927	244	205259	0	85005	59715	818

HARRISONBURG—Independent City County

✠ ROCKINGHAM MEMORIAL HOSPITAL, 235 Cantrell Avenue, Zip 22801-3293; tel. 540/433-4100; T. Carter Melton, Jr, President **A**1 2 9 10 **F**3 7 8 9 11 12 13 14 16 17 18 19 20 21 22 23 24 25 27 28 29 32 33 34 35 36 37 38 39 43 44 45 46 48 49 50 51 54 57 59 60 61 62 63 64 65 68 70 71 72 73 76 78 79 **P**8	23	10	251	12011	141	134249	1743	106387	48512	1301

HOPEWELL—Independent City County

✠ JOHN RANDOLPH MEDICAL CENTER, 411 West Randolph Road, Zip 23860, Mailing Address: P.O. Box 971, Zip 23860; tel. 804/541-1600; Daniel J. Wetta, Jr, Chief Executive Officer (Total facility includes 124 beds in nursing home-type unit) **A**1 9 10 **F**2 3 4 7 8 9 11 12 13 14 16 17 18 19 21 22 23 24 25 26 27 28 30 32 33 34 35 37 38 39 40 41 42 43 44 45 46 47 48 49 50 51 52 53 54 56 57 58 59 60 61 62 63 64 65 68 69 70 71 72 73 74 75 76 78 79 **P**1 2 4 5 6 7 8 **S** HCA – The Healthcare Company, Nashville, TN Web address: www.hcahealthcare.com	33	10	222	6981	210	88643	458	47663	25318	726

HOT SPRINGS—Bath County

★ BATH COUNTY COMMUNITY HOSPITAL, Route 220, Zip 24445, Mailing Address: Drawer Z, Zip 24445; tel. 540/839-7000; Harry M. Lowd, II, President **A**9 10 **F**9 17 19 25 34 36 37 38 40 41 43 48 50 54 61 70 72 76	23	10	25	457	6	14102	0	5832	2570	85

KILMARNOCK—Lancaster County

✠ RAPPAHANNOCK GENERAL HOSPITAL, 101 Harris Drive, Zip 22482, Mailing Address: P.O. Box 1449, Zip 22482-1449; tel. 804/435-8000; James M. Holmes, President and Chief Executive Officer **A**1 9 10 **F**7 8 9 13 16 17 18 19 22 23 24 25 27 28 30 32 34 35 36 38 39 41 43 44 45 46 48 49 50 51 54 59 61 64 70 71 72 76 78 **P**3 4 7	23	10	76	2825	33	26811	297	22136	10672	347

LEBANON—Russell County

☐ RUSSELL COUNTY MEDICAL CENTER, Carroll and Tate Streets, Zip 24266-4510; tel. 540/889-1224; David L. Brash, Chief Executive Officer **A**1 9 10 **F**7 8 9 13 16 17 18 21 22 25 29 30 32 36 38 39 41 43 44 45 48 54 56 57 59 61 62 70 75 76 78 **S** Community Health Systems, Inc., Brentwood, TN Web address: www.rcmc.net	33	10	78	3284	39	66327	0	22844	6671	275

LEESBURG—Loudoun County

★ GRAYDON MANOR, 801 Children's Center Road S.W., Zip 20175-2598; tel. 703/777-3485; Bernard J. Haberlein, Executive Director **F**57 58 60 63 Web address: www.graydonmanor.org	23	52	43	48	39	1336	0	5364	3542	121
✠ LOUDOUN HOSPITAL CENTER, 44045 Riverside Parkway, Zip 20176-2799; tel. 703/858-6000; Rodney N. Huebbers, President and Chief Executive Officer **A**1 2 9 10 **F**8 9 13 16 17 18 19 22 24 25 30 34 35 38 41 43 44 45 48 49 54 57 59 60 61 62 63 64 65 68 70 72 76 77 78 **P**1 Web address: www.loudounhospital.org	23	10	92	6243	84	58276	1141	74299	28448	643
☐ PIEDMONT BEHAVIORAL HEALTH CENTER, 42009 Victory Lane, Zip 20176-6269; tel. 703/777-0800; Michael Beavers, Chief Executive Officer (Nonreporting) **A**1 10	33	22	77	—	—	—	—	—	—	—

LEXINGTON—Independent City County

✠ STONEWALL JACKSON HOSPITAL, 1 Health Circle, Zip 24450-2492; tel. 540/462-1200; Robert E. Huch, President (Total facility includes 50 beds in nursing home-type unit) **A**1 9 10 **F**7 8 9 16 17 18 22 24 25 31 32 34 36 37 38 39 40 41 43 44 45 48 51 54 68 69 70 71 76 78 Web address: www.sjhospital.com	23	10	130	2124	70	56158	253	17449	8364	326

LOW MOOR—Alleghany County

✠ ALLEGHANY REGIONAL HOSPITAL, One ARH Lane, Zip 24457, Mailing Address: P.O. Box 7, Zip 24457-0007; tel. 540/862-6011; Ward W. Stevens, CHE, Chief Executive Officer **A**1 9 10 12 13 **F**7 8 9 13 16 17 18 19 22 23 24 25 27 32 34 38 39 40 41 44 46 48 51 61 68 70 76 78 **S** HCA – The Healthcare Company, Nashville, TN Web address: www.hcahealthcare.com	33	10	156	4025	50	57792	278	26405	11036	311

LURAY—Page County

✠ PAGE MEMORIAL HOSPITAL, 200 Memorial Drive, Zip 22835-1005; tel. 540/743-4561; Donald J. Morgan, President and Chief Executive Officer **A**1 9 10 **F**9 16 17 19 22 25 32 34 36 37 39 43 48 50 51 54 68 70 72 76 78 79 **P**6	23	10	54	1466	13	29082	0	12219	7217	198

LYNCHBURG—Independent City County

✠ LYNCHBURG GENERAL HOSPITAL, 1901 Tate Springs Road, Zip 24501-1167; tel. 804/947-3000; L. Darrell Powers, Senior Vice President (Total facility includes 130 beds in nursing home-type unit) **A**1 2 5 6 9 10 **F**1 3 4 8 9 11 16 17 18 19 21 22 23 24 25 26 27 28 29 30 32 33 34 36 37 38 39 45 46 47 48 49 54 58 59 60 61 62 63 64 65 68 70 72 76 77 78 79 **P**6 7 8 **S** Centra Health, Inc., Lynchburg, VA Web address: www.centrahealth.com	23	10	350	12520	305	133230	0	—	—	1314

Hospitals, U.S. / VIRGINIA

Hospital, Address, Telephone, Administrator, Approval, Facility, and Physician Codes, Health Care System, Network	Classification Codes		Utilization Data					Expense (thousands) of dollars		
	Control	Service	Staffed Beds	Admissions	Census	Outpatient Visits	Births	Total	Payroll	Personnel

- ★ American Hospital Association (AHA) membership
- ☐ Joint Commission on Accreditation of Healthcare Organizations (JCAHO) accreditation
- + American Osteopathic Healthcare Association (AOHA) membership
- ○ American Osteopathic Association (AOA) accreditation
- △ Commission on Accreditation of Rehabilitation Facilities (CARF) accreditation

Control codes 61, 63, 64, 71, 72 and 73 indicate hospitals listed by AOHA, but not registered by AHA. For definition of numerical codes, see page A4

Hospital	Control	Service	Staffed Beds	Admissions	Census	Outpatient Visits	Births	Total	Payroll	Personnel
★ △ VIRGINIA BAPTIST HOSPITAL, 3300 Rivermont Avenue, Zip 24503–9989; tel. 804/947–4000; Thomas C. Jividen, Senior Vice President **A**1 5 7 9 10 **F**1 2 3 4 9 11 12 16 17 18 19 21 22 23 24 25 28 29 30 31 32 33 34 36 37 38 39 41 42 44 45 46 47 50 53 54 57 58 59 60 61 62 63 64 65 68 69 70 72 76 77 78 79 **P**6 7 8 **S** Centra Health, Inc., Lynchburg, VA Web address: www.centrahealth.com	23	10	323	9999	229	—	2381	—	—	1667
MADISON HEIGHTS—Amherst County										
CENTRAL VIRGINIA TRAINING CENTER, 210 East Colony Road, Zip 24572–2005, Mailing Address: P.O. Box 1098, Lynchburg, Zip 24505–1098; tel. 804/947–6326; Judy Dudley, Director (Total facility includes 104 beds in nursing home–type unit) (Nonreporting) **A**10 **S** Virginia Department of Mental Health, Richmond, VA	12	62	1112	—	—	—	—	—	—	—
MANASSAS—Independent City County										
★ PRINCE WILLIAM HOSPITAL, 8700 Sudley Road, Zip 20110–4418, Mailing Address: Box 2610, Zip 20108–0867; tel. 703/369–8000; Michael J. Schwartz, President and Chief Executive Officer **A**1 2 9 10 **F**3 6 7 8 9 12 13 16 17 18 19 21 22 24 25 27 28 30 32 33 34 36 37 39 44 45 46 48 49 50 51 54 57 58 59 60 61 62 63 64 67 68 70 72 76 79 **P**8 Web address: www.pwhs.org	23	10	135	8378	80	103809	1582	66893	28304	789
MARION—Smyth County										
★ SMYTH COUNTY COMMUNITY HOSPITAL, 565 Radio Hill Road, Zip 24354–3526, Mailing Address: P.O. Box 880, Zip 24354–0880; tel. 540/782–1234; William Mahone, V, Interim President and Chief Executive Officer (Total facility includes 125 beds in nursing home–type unit) (Nonreporting) **A**1 9 10 **S** Carilion Health System, Roanoke, VA	23	10	285	—	—	—	—	—	—	—
☐ SOUTHWESTERN VIRGINIA MENTAL HEALTH INSTITUTE, 340 Bagley Circle, Zip 24354–3390; tel. 540/783–1200; Gerald E. Deans, Director (Nonreporting) **A**1 9 10 **S** Virginia Department of Mental Health, Richmond, VA	12	22	266	—	—	—	—	—	—	—
MARTINSVILLE—Independent City County										
★ MEMORIAL HOSPITAL OF MARTINSVILLE AND HENRY COUNTY, 320 Hospital Drive, Zip 24112–1981, Mailing Address: Box 4788, Zip 24115–4788; tel. 540/666–7200; Joseph Roach, Chief Executive Officer **A**1 2 9 10 **F**7 8 9 11 16 17 18 22 24 25 27 32 33 34 35 36 37 39 43 44 45 46 48 49 50 51 54 57 59 60 61 63 64 65 68 70 72 76 78 79 **S** Quorum Health Group, Brentwood, TN Web address: www.martinsvillehospital.org	23	10	152	7162	90	200754	558	60337	26355	835
MECHANICSVILLE—Hanover County										
★ MEMORIAL REGIONAL MEDICAL CENTER, 8260 Atlee Road, Zip 23116, Mailing Address: P.O. Box 26783, Richmond, Zip 23261–6783; tel. 804/764–6102; Michael Robinson, Executive Vice President and Administrator (Total facility includes 20 beds in nursing home–type unit) **A**1 2 5 6 9 10 **F**1 2 3 4 5 6 7 8 9 10 11 12 13 14 16 17 18 19 20 21 22 23 24 25 26 27 28 29 30 32 33 34 35 36 37 38 39 40 41 42 43 44 45 46 47 48 49 50 51 52 53 54 55 56 57 58 59 60 61 62 63 64 65 66 68 69 70 71 72 73 75 76 78 79 **S** Bon Secours Health System, Inc., Marriottsville, MD	21	10	200	8205	115	80349	503	76739	22842	1102
NASSAWADOX—Northampton County										
★ SHORE MEMORIAL HOSPITAL, 9507 Hospital Avenue, Zip 23413–1821, Mailing Address: P.O. Box 17, Zip 23413–0017; tel. 757/414–8000; Alan Markowitz, Ph.D., FACHE, President and Chief Executive Officer (Total facility includes 13 beds in nursing home–type unit) **A**1 5 9 10 **F**7 8 9 13 14 16 17 18 19 21 22 24 25 29 30 31 32 33 34 35 36 37 38 39 40 41 43 44 45 46 48 49 50 51 53 54 56 57 59 60 61 62 63 66 68 69 70 71 72 74 76 77 78 79 **P**6 Web address: www.shorehealthservices.org	23	10	143	5181	198	57513	512	37665	16873	657
NEW KENT—New Kent County										
☐ △ CUMBERLAND, A BROWN SCHOOLS HOSPITAL FOR CHILDREN AND ADOLESCENTS, 9407 Cumberland Road, Zip 23124–2029; tel. 804/966–2242; Ernest C. Priddy, II, Chief Executive Officer **A**1 7 10 **F**13 18 53 54 **S** Brown Schools, Inc., Austin, TX	33	56	84	187	88	382	0	13748	7064	220
NEWPORT NEWS—Independent City County										
★ MARY IMMACULATE HOSPITAL, (Includes St. Francis Nursing Center), 2 Bernardine Drive, Zip 23602–4499; tel. 757/886–6000; Cynthia B. Farrand, Executive Vice President and Administrator (Total facility includes 115 beds in nursing home–type unit) (Nonreporting) **A**1 5 9 10 **S** Bon Secours Health System, Inc., Marriottsville, MD Web address: www.mihospital.com	21	10	225	—	—	—	—	—	—	—
★ RIVERSIDE REGIONAL MEDICAL CENTER, (Includes Riverside Psychiatric Institute), 500 J. Clyde Morris Boulevard, Zip 23601–1976; tel. 757/594–2000; M. Caroline Martin, President **A**1 2 3 5 6 9 10 **F**1 2 3 4 6 7 8 9 11 12 13 14 16 17 18 19 20 21 22 23 24 25 26 27 28 29 30 31 32 33 34 35 36 37 38 39 41 43 44 45 46 47 48 49 50 51 53 54 56 57 58 59 60 61 62 63 64 65 66 67 68 69 70 71 72 75 76 77 78 79 **P**6 **S** Riverside Health System, Newport News, VA Web address: www.riverside–online.com	23	10	360	17465	246	268085	2215	141316	57554	2023
☐ WOODSIDE HOSPITAL, 17579 Warwick Boulevard, Zip 23603–1343; tel. 757/888–0400; Mark S. Roth, Chief Executive Officer (Nonreporting) **A**1 9 10	33	22	68	—	—	—	—	—	—	—
NORFOLK—Independent City County										
★ △ BON SECOURS–DEPAUL MEDICAL CENTER, 150 Kingsley Lane, Zip 23505–4650; tel. 757/889–5000; David J. McCombs, Executive Vice President and Administrator **A**1 2 3 5 7 9 10 **F**2 6 7 8 9 11 13 14 16 17 18 19 20 21 22 24 26 29 30 34 35 36 37 38 39 40 41 43 44 45 46 48 50 51 53 54 58 59 60 61 62 63 64 65 66 68 70 72 76 77 78 79 **P**6 **S** Bon Secours Health System, Inc., Marriottsville, MD	23	10	293	7102	102	112125	801	75344	31719	1157

Many Facility Codes have changed. Please refer to the AHA Guide Code Chart.

Hospitals, U.S. / VIRGINIA

Hospital, Address, Telephone, Administrator, Approval, Facility, and Physician Codes, Health Care System, Network	Classification Codes		Utilization Data					Expense (thousands) of dollars		
★ American Hospital Association (AHA) membership ☐ Joint Commission on Accreditation of Healthcare Organizations (JCAHO) accreditation + American Osteopathic Healthcare Association (AOHA) membership ○ American Osteopathic Association (AOA) accreditation △ Commission on Accreditation of Rehabilitation Facilities (CARF) accreditation Control codes 61, 63, 64, 71, 72 and 73 indicate hospitals listed by AOHA, but not registered by AHA. For definition of numerical codes, see page A4	Control	Service	Staffed Beds	Admissions	Census	Outpatient Visits	Births	Total	Payroll	Personnel
☒ CHILDREN'S HOSPITAL OF THE KING'S DAUGHTERS, 601 Children's Lane, Zip 23507–1971; tel. 757/668–7700; Robert I. Bonar, Jr, President and Chief Executive Officer **A**1 2 3 5 9 10 **F**7 10 11 13 14 18 19 22 23 24 25 26 29 31 34 35 36 37 38 39 42 43 45 46 47 48 49 51 52 53 54 56 58 59 60 61 63 65 70 71 72 74 76 78 **Web address:** www.chkd.org	23	50	151	5519	117	126025	—	104311	46505	1270
★ LAKE TAYLOR HOSPITAL, 1309 Kempsville Road, Zip 23502–2286; tel. 757/461–5001; Thomas J. Orsini, Chief Executive Officer (Total facility includes 226 beds in nursing home–type unit) **A**9 10 **F**7 16 23 35 59 62 69 70 78 **Web address:** www.laketaylor.org	16	48	330	386	227	0	0	15781	7971	352
☐ NORFOLK PSYCHIATRIC CENTER, 860 Kempsville Road, Zip 23502–3980; tel. 757/461–4565; Arlene Manzella, Administrator (Nonreporting) **A**1 9 10 **S** Magellan Health Services, Atlanta, GA	33	22	77	—	—	—	—	—	—	—
☒ SENTARA LEIGH HOSPITAL, 830 Kempsville Road, Zip 23502–3981; tel. 757/466–6000; Darleen S. Anderson, R.N., MSN, Site Administrator **A**1 3 5 9 10 **F**1 4 6 7 8 9 10 11 12 13 14 15 16 17 18 19 20 21 22 23 24 25 26 27 28 29 30 31 32 33 34 35 36 37 38 39 40 41 42 43 44 45 46 47 48 49 50 51 52 53 54 56 57 58 59 60 61 62 63 64 65 66 67 68 69 70 71 72 73 74 75 76 77 78 79 **P**6 7 8 **S** Sentara Healthcare, Norfolk, VA **Web address:** www.sentara.com	23	10	212	12271	147	106678	2073	82929	29187	876
☒ SENTARA NORFOLK GENERAL HOSPITAL, 600 Gresham Drive, Zip 23507–1999; tel. 757/668–3000; Mark R. Gavens, President **A**1 2 3 5 6 8 9 10 **F**1 4 6 7 8 9 10 11 12 13 14 15 16 17 18 19 20 21 22 23 24 25 26 27 28 29 30 31 32 33 34 35 36 37 38 39 40 41 42 43 44 45 46 47 48 49 50 51 52 53 54 56 57 58 59 60 61 62 63 64 65 66 67 68 69 70 71 72 73 74 75 76 77 78 79 **P**6 7 8 **S** Sentara Healthcare, Norfolk, VA **Web address:** www.sentara.com	23	10	478	22697	346	204669	2514	246996	91424	2878

NORTON—Independent City County

☐ NORTON COMMUNITY HOSPITAL, 100 15th Street N.W., Zip 24273–1699; tel. 540/679–9600; Ricky D. Napper, Chief Executive Officer **A**1 9 10 **F**7 8 9 13 16 17 18 19 22 24 25 27 28 29 30 32 34 35 36 37 38 39 41 43 44 45 48 49 50 51 53 54 65 68 70 71 72 73 76 78 79 **P**6 8 **Web address:** www.nchosp.org	23	10	55	4467	53	83673	452	27358	10444	337
☒ ST. MARY'S HOSPITAL, Third Street N.E., Zip 24273–1131, Mailing Address: P.O. Box 620, Zip 24273–0620; tel. 540/679–9100; Gary L. DelForge, Administrator (Total facility includes 44 beds in nursing home–type unit) **A**1 9 10 **F**7 8 9 13 17 18 22 25 29 32 34 36 38 39 41 44 45 48 49 51 57 61 63 68 69 70 72 76 78 **P**6 **Web address:** www.st–maryshospital.com	23	10	133	3438	76	67452	77	26089	10926	412

PEARISBURG—Giles County

☒ CARILION GILES MEMORIAL HOSPITAL, 1 Taylor Avenue, Zip 24134–1932; tel. 540/921–6000; Morris D. Reece, Administrator and Chief Executive Officer (Total facility includes 21 beds in nursing home–type unit) **A**1 9 10 **F**9 13 16 17 18 19 22 24 31 32 33 34 36 37 38 39 41 43 45 46 48 50 51 54 55 56 61 62 63 64 65 66 67 68 70 71 72 73 74 75 76 78 79 **P**1 2 3 4 5 6 7 8 **S** Carilion Health System, Roanoke, VA **Web address:** www.carilion.com	23	10	52	1312	35	30811	—	14568	7468	229

PENNINGTON GAP—Lee County

☒ LEE COUNTY COMMUNITY HOSPITAL, West Morgan Avenue, Zip 24277–0070, Mailing Address: P.O. Box 70, Zip 24277–0070; tel. 540/546–1440; Gowdagere Udayakumar, Chief Executive Officer (Nonreporting) **A**1 9 10	23	10	80	—	—	—	—	—	—	—

PETERSBURG—Independent City County

☐ CENTRAL STATE HOSPITAL, 26317 West Washington Street, Zip 23803, Mailing Address: P.O. Box 4030, Zip 23803–4030; tel. 804/524–7000; Larry L. Latham, Director **A**1 5 9 10 **F**16 17 18 57 61 **P**6 **S** Virginia Department of Mental Health, Richmond, VA **Web address:** www.csh.state.va.us	12	22	366	901	382	0	0	43494	—	827
☒ POPLAR SPRINGS HOSPITAL, 350 Poplar Drive, Zip 23805–4657; tel. 804/733–6874; Anthony J. Vadella, Chief Executive Officer **A**1 9 10 **F**3 13 17 18 21 57 58 59 60 61 62 63 64 69 **Web address:** www.poplarsprings.com	33	22	111	1648	86	3001	0	10817	5763	191
☒ SOUTHSIDE REGIONAL MEDICAL CENTER, 801 South Adams Street, Zip 23803–5133; tel. 804/862–5000; David S. Dunham, President (Total facility includes 20 beds in nursing home–type unit) **A**1 6 9 10 **F**7 8 9 11 13 16 17 18 22 23 24 25 27 29 32 33 34 36 38 39 41 43 44 45 46 48 49 50 51 54 57 59 60 61 62 64 65 68 69 70 72 75 76 77 78 **P**8 **S** Quorum Health Group, Brentwood, TN **Web address:** www.srmconline.com	16	10	292	13490	191	159907	1415	91615	42860	1333

PORTSMOUTH—Independent City County

☒ △ MARYVIEW MEDICAL CENTER, (Formerly Maryview Hospital), 3636 High Street, Zip 23707–3236; tel. 757/398–2200; Wayne Jones, Executive Vice President and Administrator (Total facility includes 120 beds in nursing home–type unit) **A**1 2 3 5 7 9 10 **F**3 4 6 7 8 9 11 12 13 16 17 18 19 20 21 22 24 26 29 30 32 33 34 35 36 37 38 39 40 41 43 44 45 46 47 48 49 50 51 54 57 58 59 60 61 62 63 64 65 66 68 69 70 71 72 73 76 77 78 79 **P**6 8 **S** Bon Secours Health System, Inc., Marriottsville, MD **Web address:** www.bonsecours.com	23	10	466	15436	340	—	1317	130420	53706	1906

© 2000 AHA Guide   *Many Facility Codes have changed. Please refer to the AHA Guide Code Chart.*

Hospitals, U.S. / VIRGINIA

Hospital, Address, Telephone, Administrator, Approval, Facility, and Physician Codes, Health Care System, Network	Classification Codes		Utilization Data					Expense (thousands) of dollars		
	Control	Service	Staffed Beds	Admissions	Census	Outpatient Visits	Births	Total	Payroll	Personnel

★ American Hospital Association (AHA) membership
☐ Joint Commission on Accreditation of Healthcare Organizations (JCAHO) accreditation
+ American Osteopathic Healthcare Association (AOHA) membership
○ American Osteopathic Association (AOA) accreditation
△ Commission on Accreditation of Rehabilitation Facilities (CARF) accreditation
Control codes 61, 63, 64, 71, 72 and 73 indicate hospitals listed by AOHA, but not registered by AHA. For definition of numerical codes, see page A4

Hospital	Control	Service	Staffed Beds	Admissions	Census	Outpatient Visits	Births	Total	Payroll	Personnel
★ NAVAL MEDICAL CENTER, 620 John Paul Jones Circle, Zip 23708–2197; tel. 757/953–7424; Rear Admiral Marion Balsam, MC, USN, Commander (Nonreporting) A1 2 3 5 S Department of Navy, Washington, DC Web address: www.164.167.49.190/	43	10	330	—	—	—	—	—	—	—
PULASKI—Independent City County										
★ PULASKI COMMUNITY HOSPITAL, 2400 Lee Highway, Zip 24301–0759, Mailing Address: P.O. Box 759, Zip 24301–0759; tel. 540/994–8100; Jack Nunley, Chief Executive Officer (Total facility includes 12 beds in nursing home–type unit) A1 9 10 F8 9 13 16 17 18 22 24 25 32 34 39 41 44 45 46 48 50 61 65 68 69 70 76 78 P8 S HCA – The Healthcare Company, Nashville, TN Web address: www.pch–va.com	33	10	99	3474	49	53421	190	19660	9636	332
RADFORD—Independent City County										
★ △ CARILION NEW RIVER VALLEY MEDICAL CENTER, 2900 Tyler Road, Zip 24073, Mailing Address: P.O. Box 5, Zip 24141–0005; tel. 540/731–2000; Virginia Ousley, Vice President and Hospital Director (Total facility includes 27 beds in nursing home–type unit) A1 7 9 10 F2 3 4 7 8 9 11 12 13 14 16 17 18 19 20 21 22 23 24 25 26 27 28 31 32 34 35 36 37 38 39 40 41 43 44 45 46 48 49 50 53 54 56 57 58 59 60 61 62 63 64 69 70 72 75 76 77 78 79 P8 S Carilion Health System, Roanoke, VA Web address: www.carilion.com	23	10	97	5441	76	132545	867	53624	19712	650
★ △ CARILION SAINT ALBANS HOSPITAL, Route 11, Lee Highway, Zip 24143, Mailing Address: P.O. Box 3608, Zip 24143–3608; tel. 540/639–2481; Janet McKinney Crawford, Vice President and Administrator A1 7 9 10 F3 13 16 17 18 57 58 59 61 62 63 70 78 P8 S Carilion Health System, Roanoke, VA Web address: www.carilion.com	23	22	60	1799	30	—	0	9107	4655	142
RESTON—Fairfax County										
★ RESTON HOSPITAL CENTER, (Formerly Columbia Reston Hospital Center), 1850 Town Center Parkway, Zip 20190–3298; tel. 703/689–9000; William A. Adams, President and Chief Executive Officer A1 2 5 9 10 F8 9 11 13 16 17 18 22 24 25 27 28 34 36 37 39 43 44 45 46 48 50 54 65 68 70 71 72 76 78 S HCA – The Healthcare Company, Nashville, TN Web address: www.restonhospital.net	33	10	121	8777	95	138340	2124	76553	27242	600
RICHLANDS—Tazewell County										
★ CLINCH VALLEY MEDICAL CENTER, 2949 West Front Street, Zip 24641–2099; tel. 540/596–6000; James W. Thweatt, Chief Executive Officer (Total facility includes 22 beds in nursing home–type unit) A1 9 10 F3 7 8 9 11 12 13 16 17 19 22 23 24 25 27 32 33 34 35 38 39 41 43 44 45 46 48 50 51 53 54 63 65 66 69 70 72 76 78 S HCA – The Healthcare Company, Nashville, TN Web address: www.ccvmc.com	33	10	200	6296	71	48726	546	36090	13230	489
RICHMOND—Independent City County										
★ BON SECOURS ST. MARY'S HOSPITAL, 5801 Bremo Road, Zip 23226–1900; tel. 804/285–2011; Ann E. Honeycutt, Executive Vice President and Administrator A1 2 3 5 9 10 F3 4 6 7 8 9 11 13 16 17 18 19 20 21 22 24 25 26 27 29 30 32 33 34 35 36 37 38 39 41 42 43 44 45 46 47 48 49 54 56 57 58 59 60 61 62 63 64 67 68 70 71 72 76 78 79 P1 6 8 S Bon Secours Health System, Inc., Marriottsville, MD	21	10	348	21164	269	204629	3020	152335	49623	1496
★ BON SECOURS–RICHMOND COMMUNITY HOSPITAL, 1500 North 28th Street, Zip 23223–5396, Mailing Address: Box 27184, Zip 23261–7184; tel. 804/225–1700; Eugene Toomer, Chief Operating Officer (Nonreporting) A1 9 10 S Bon Secours Health System, Inc., Marriottsville, MD	23	10	88	—	—	—	—	—	—	—
★ BON SECOURS–STUART CIRCLE, 413 Stuart Circle, Zip 23220–3799; tel. 804/358–7051; Ann E. Honeycutt, Executive Vice President and Administrator (Nonreporting) A1 9 10 S Bon Secours Health System, Inc., Marriottsville, MD	21	10	158	—	—	—	—	—	—	—
☐ CAPITOL MEDICAL CENTER, 701 West Grace Street, Zip 23220–4191; tel. 804/775–4100; Priscilla J. Shuler, Chief Executive Officer A1 9 10 F7 16 17 18 25 36 39 41 45 48 57 64 70 P7 S Paracelsus Healthcare Corporation, Houston, TX	33	10	135	3416	70	41022	0	25732	14040	437
★ △ CHILDREN'S HOSPITAL, 2924 Brook Road, Zip 23220–1298; tel. 804/321–7474; Leslie G. Wyatt, Administrator (Nonreporting) A1 3 5 7 9 Web address: www.childrenshosp–richmond.org	23	57	18	—	—	—	—	—	—	—
★ △ CHIPPENHAM MEDICAL CENTER/JOHNSTON–WILLIS HOSPITAL, (Formerly Chippenham and Johnston–Willis Hospital), (Includes Chippenham Medical Center, 7101 Jahnke Road, Zip 23225; tel. 804/320–3911; Johnston–Willis Hospital, 1401 Johnston–Willis Drive, Zip 23235; tel. 804/330–2000), 7101 Jahnke Road, Zip 23225–4044; tel. 804/320–3911; Marilyn B. Tavenner, Chief Executive Officer A1 2 3 5 7 9 10 F1 3 4 7 8 9 11 12 13 16 17 18 19 21 22 23 24 25 26 27 28 29 30 31 32 33 34 37 38 39 41 42 43 44 45 46 47 48 50 51 52 53 54 55 56 57 58 59 60 61 62 63 64 65 66 68 70 71 72 73 74 75 76 78 79 P6 7 S HCA – The Healthcare Company, Nashville, TN	33	10	748	30078	466	211778	3704	199168	87059	2379
☐ △ HEALTHSOUTH MEDICAL CENTER, 7700 East Parham Road, Zip 23294–4301; tel. 804/747–5600; Charles A. Stark, CHE, Administrator, Chief Executive Officer and Regional Vice President A1 2 5 7 10 F5 9 11 12 13 16 17 18 19 22 23 24 25 26 27 29 30 31 32 33 34 35 37 38 39 41 43 45 46 48 49 50 51 53 54 56 59 60 61 62 63 68 70 71 72 76 77 78 79 S HEALTHSOUTH Corporation, Birmingham, AL Web address: www.healthsouth–richmond.com	33	10	147	4552	78	37625	—	37335	15205	395

Hospitals, U.S. / VIRGINIA

Hospital, Address, Telephone, Administrator, Approval, Facility, and Physician Codes, Health Care System, Network	Classification Codes		Utilization Data					Expense (thousands) of dollars		
★ American Hospital Association (AHA) membership ☐ Joint Commission on Accreditation of Healthcare Organizations (JCAHO) accreditation + American Osteopathic Healthcare Association (AOHA) membership ○ American Osteopathic Association (AOA) accreditation △ Commission on Accreditation of Rehabilitation Facilities (CARF) accreditation Control codes 61, 63, 64, 71, 72 and 73 indicate hospitals listed by AOHA, but not registered by AHA. For definition of numerical codes, see page A4	Control	Service	Staffed Beds	Admissions	Census	Outpatient Visits	Births	Total	Payroll	Personnel
☐ HEALTHSOUTH REHABILITATION HOSPITAL OF VIRGINIA, 5700 Fitzhugh Avenue, Zip 23226–1800; tel. 804/288–5700; Jeff Ruskan, Administrator (Nonreporting) **A**1 9 10 **S** HEALTHSOUTH Corporation, Birmingham, AL Web address: www.healthsouth.com	33	46	40	—	—	—	—	—	—	—
★ HENRICO DOCTORS' HOSPITAL, 1602 Skipwith Road, Zip 23229–5298; tel. 804/289–4500; Patrick W. Farrell, Chief Executive Officer **A**1 2 9 10 **F**2 3 4 5 7 8 9 11 12 13 16 17 18 19 21 22 24 25 27 28 31 32 33 34 37 38 39 40 41 42 43 44 45 46 47 48 49 51 52 53 54 57 58 59 60 61 62 63 64 65 66 68 69 70 71 72 74 75 76 78 79 **P**5 **S** HCA – The Healthcare Company, Nashville, TN Web address: www.hcahealthcare.com	33	10	340	14674	206	107179	3404	—	—	976
★ HUNTER HOLMES MCGUIRE VETERANS AFFAIRS MEDICAL CENTER, 1201 Broad Rock Boulevard, Zip 23249–0002; tel. 804/675–5000; James W. Dudley, Director (Total facility includes 80 beds in nursing home–type unit) (Nonreporting) **A**1 2 3 5 8 9 **S** Department of Veterans Affairs, Washington, DC JOHNSTON–WILLIS HOSPITAL See Chippenham Medical Center/Johnston–Willis Hospital	45	10	616	—	—	—	—	—	—	—
★ △ MEDICAL COLLEGE OF VIRGINIA HOSPITALS, VIRGINIA COMMONWEALTH UNIVERSITY, 401 North 12th Street, Zip 23219, Mailing Address: P.O. Box 980510, Zip 23298–0510; tel. 804/828–9000; Carl R. Fischer, Associate Vice President and Chief Executive Officer **A**1 2 3 5 7 8 9 10 **F**3 4 7 8 9 10 11 12 13 16 17 18 19 20 21 22 23 24 25 28 29 30 31 32 33 34 35 36 38 39 41 42 43 44 45 46 47 48 49 50 51 52 54 56 57 58 59 61 62 63 64 65 66 68 70 71 72 73 74 75 76 77 78 79 **P**4 7 Web address: www.mcvh.org	16	10	714	28718	493	432350	2345	420932	174214	5043
★ RETREAT HOSPITAL, 2621 Grove Avenue, Zip 23220–4308; tel. 804/254–5100; Paul L. Baldwin, Chief Executive Officer **A**1 2 9 10 **F**2 3 8 9 10 11 12 13 16 17 18 19 20 22 25 26 28 29 30 32 34 37 38 39 41 42 43 44 45 46 47 48 49 51 52 54 57 66 69 70 71 74 75 76 78 79 **P**1 2 4 5 6 7 **S** HCA – The Healthcare Company, Nashville, TN	33	10	100	2472	43	36707	0	27496	13000	354
★ RICHMOND EYE AND EAR HOSPITAL, 1001 East Marshall Street, Zip 23219–1993; tel. 804/775–4500; James W. Worrell, Chief Executive Officer (Nonreporting) **A**1 9 10 **S** Quorum Health Group, Brentwood, TN	23	45	32	—	—	—	—	—	—	—
☐ △ SHELTERING ARMS REHABILITATION HOSPITAL, 1311 Palmyra Avenue, Zip 23227–4418; tel. 804/342–4100; Jack A. Carroll, Ph.D., President and Chief Executive Officer **A**1 7 9 10 **F**16 17 20 22 28 29 31 32 33 34 39 45 49 51 53 54 70 71 76 **P**6 Web address: www.shelteringarms.com	23	46	40	1097	33	64026	0	23449	13053	274
☐ VALUEMARK WEST END BEHAVIORAL HEALTHCARE SYSTEM, 12800 West Creek Parkway, Zip 23238–1116; tel. 804/784–2200; Wanda H. Sadler, Chief Executive Officer (Nonreporting) **A**1 9 10 **S** ValueMark Healthcare Systems, Inc., Atlanta, GA	33	22	84	—	—	—	—	—	—	—

ROANOKE—Independent City County

★ △ CARILION MEDICAL CENTER, (Formerly Carilion Roanoke Memorial Hospital), (Includes Carilion Roanoke Community Hospital, 101 Elm Avenue S.E., Zip 24013–2230, Mailing Address: P.O. Box 12946, Zip 24029–2946; tel. 540/985–8000; Roanoke Memorial Rehabilitation Center, South Jefferson and McClanahan Streets, Mailing Address: P.O. Box 13367, Zip 24033), Belleview at Jefferson Street, Zip 24014, Mailing Address: P.O. Box 13367, Zip 24033–3367; tel. 540/981–7000; Lucas A. Snipes, FACHE, Director **A**1 2 3 5 6 7 9 10 **F**2 3 4 7 8 9 11 12 13 14 17 18 19 21 22 23 24 25 26 27 28 29 30 31 32 33 34 35 36 37 38 39 41 42 43 44 45 46 47 48 49 50 51 52 53 54 56 57 58 59 60 61 62 63 64 65 66 68 69 70 71 72 73 75 76 77 78 79 **P**2 7 8 **S** Carilion Health System, Roanoke, VA Web address: www.carilion.com	23	10	740	30757	458	246762	2681	349575	126175	3837

ROCKY MOUNT—Franklin County

★ CARILION FRANKLIN MEMORIAL HOSPITAL, 180 Floyd Avenue, Zip 24151–1389; tel. 540/483–5277; Matthew J. Perry, Director (Nonreporting) **A**1 9 10 **S** Carilion Health System, Roanoke, VA Web address: www.carilion.com	23	10	37	—	—	—	—	—	—	—

SALEM—Independent City County

★ △ LEWIS–GALE MEDICAL CENTER, (Includes Lewis–Gale Pavilion, 1902 Braeburn Drive, Zip 24153–7391; tel. 703/772–2800), 1900 Electric Road, Zip 24153–7494; tel. 540/776–4000; William B. Downey, President and Chief Executive Officer (Nonreporting) **A**1 2 7 9 10 **S** HCA – The Healthcare Company, Nashville, TN Web address: www.lewis–gale.com	33	10	521	—	—	—	—	—	—	—
MOUNT REGIS CENTER, 405 Kimball Avenue, Zip 24153–6299; tel. 540/389–4761; Gail S. Basham, Chief Executive Officer **F**2 3 **S** Pioneer Behavioral Health, Peabody, MA	33	82	25	378	13	—	0	2111	772	29
★ VETERANS AFFAIRS MEDICAL CENTER, 1970 Roanoke Boulevard, Zip 24153; tel. 540/982–2463; Stephen L. Lemons, Ed.D., Director (Total facility includes 90 beds in nursing home–type unit) **A**1 2 3 5 8 9 **F**1 2 3 4 9 11 12 13 16 17 18 19 22 23 25 27 28 29 30 31 34 35 38 39 41 43 45 46 47 48 49 50 51 54 56 57 59 60 61 62 63 64 65 69 70 72 73 75 76 79 **S** Department of Veterans Affairs, Washington, DC Web address: www.va.gov	45	10	268	4653	247	219870	0	66005	—	1270

© 2000 AHA Guide   *Many Facility Codes have changed. Please refer to the AHA Guide Code Chart.*

Hospitals, U.S. / VIRGINIA

Hospital, Address, Telephone, Administrator, Approval, Facility, and Physician Codes, Health Care System, Network	Classification Codes		Utilization Data					Expense (thousands) of dollars		Personnel
	Control	Service	Staffed Beds	Admissions	Census	Outpatient Visits	Births	Total	Payroll	

★ American Hospital Association (AHA) membership
☐ Joint Commission on Accreditation of Healthcare Organizations (JCAHO) accreditation
+ American Osteopathic Healthcare Association (AOHA) membership
○ American Osteopathic Association (AOA) accreditation
△ Commission on Accreditation of Rehabilitation Facilities (CARF) accreditation
Control codes 61, 63, 64, 71, 72 and 73 indicate hospitals listed by AOHA, but not registered by AHA. For definition of numerical codes, see page A4

SOUTH BOSTON—Independent City County

★ HALIFAX REGIONAL HEALTH SYSTEM, (Formerly Halifax Regional Hospital), 2204 Wilborn Avenue, Zip 24592-1638; tel. 804/517-3100; Chris A. Lumsden, Chief Executive Officer **A**1 9 10 **F**3 7 8 9 11 13 16 17 18 19 22 23 24 25 32 33 34 35 36 37 38 39 43 45 46 48 50 51 54 62 64 70 71 72 76 78 79 **P**2 7 8 **S** Quorum Health Group, Brentwood, TN
Web address: www.hrhs.org
— 23 10 138 5515 76 66485 560 41597 16825 547

SOUTH HILL—Mecklenburg County

★ COMMUNITY MEMORIAL HEALTHCENTER, 125 Buena Vista Circle, Zip 23970-0090, Mailing Address: P.O. Box 90, Zip 23970-0090; tel. 804/447-3151; W. Scott Burnette, President (Total facility includes 161 beds in nursing home-type unit) **A**1 9 10 **F**2 3 7 8 9 13 14 16 17 18 19 22 24 25 26 27 30 32 34 35 36 37 38 39 40 41 43 44 45 46 48 49 50 51 54 56 57 61 62 63 64 68 69 70 71 72 76 77 78 79 **P**3 8
Web address: www.cmh-sh.org
— 23 10 284 5067 214 87517 258 37662 22031 622

STAUNTON—Independent City County

DE JARNETTE CENTER, 1355 Richmond Road, Zip 24401-1091, Mailing Address: Box 2309, Zip 24402-2309; tel. 540/332-2100; William J. Tuell, Director (Nonreporting) **A**3 9 **S** Virginia Department of Mental Health, Richmond, VA
— 12 59 60 — — — — — — —

☐ WESTERN STATE HOSPITAL, 1301 Richmond Avenue, Zip 24401-9146, Mailing Address: P.O. Box 2500, Zip 24402-2500; tel. 540/332-8000; Jack W. Barber, M.D., Director (Nonreporting) **A**1 9 10 **S** Virginia Department of Mental Health, Richmond, VA
Web address: www.wsh.state.va.us
— 12 22 488 — — — — — — —

STUART—Patrick County

★ R. J. REYNOLDS-PATRICK COUNTY MEMORIAL HOSPITAL, (Formerly Patrick Community Hospital), 18688 Jeb Stuart Highway, Zip 24171-9512; tel. 540/694-3151; Norman E. Walters, Administrator (Total facility includes 25 beds in nursing home-type unit) **A**1 9 10 **F**7 8 9 13 18 19 22 25 32 34 36 37 40 41 43 44 45 48 51 54 69 70 76 78
— 23 10 58 1287 34 32390 139 — 7285 168

SUFFOLK—Independent City County

★ LOUISE OBICI MEMORIAL HOSPITAL, 1900 North Main Street, Zip 23434-4323, Mailing Address: P.O. Box 1100, Zip 23439-1100; tel. 757/934-4000; William C. Giermak, President and Chief Executive Officer **A**1 2 5 6 9 10 **F**7 8 9 11 13 15 17 19 22 25 28 31 32 34 35 38 39 40 41 43 44 45 46 48 49 50 54 57 59 60 65 70 72 76 78 79
Web address: www.obici.com
— 23 10 160 7442 108 100101 867 59152 26517 840

TAPPAHANNOCK—Essex County

☐ RIVERSIDE TAPPAHANNOCK HOSPITAL, 618 Hospital Road, Zip 22560; tel. 804/443-3311; Elizabeth J. Martin, Vice President and Administrator (Total facility includes 25 beds in nursing home-type unit) **A**1 9 10 **F**7 9 11 13 16 17 18 19 22 24 25 27 28 30 31 32 33 34 36 37 38 39 41 43 45 46 48 50 51 53 54 56 66 69 70 71 72 76 77 78 **P**6 **S** Riverside Health System, Newport News, VA
Web address: www.riverside-online.com
— 23 10 44 2101 44 — — 13724 6748 242

TAZEWELL—Tazewell County

★ TAZEWELL COMMUNITY HOSPITAL, 141 Ben Bolt Avenue, Zip 24651-9700; tel. 540/988-2506; Craig B. James, President and Chief Executive Officer **A**1 9 10 **F**7 9 17 22 25 34 36 38 39 48 51 76 78 **P**1 **S** Carilion Health System, Roanoke, VA
Web address: www.tazecommhospital.org
— 23 10 38 1257 14 27161 0 8393 3474 141

VIRGINIA BEACH—Independent City County

★ SENTARA BAYSIDE HOSPITAL, 800 Independence Boulevard, Zip 23455-6076; tel. 757/363-6100; Rosemary C. Check, Administrator **A**1 5 9 10 **F**1 4 6 7 8 9 10 11 12 13 14 15 16 17 18 19 20 21 22 23 24 25 26 27 28 29 30 31 32 33 34 35 36 37 38 39 40 41 42 43 44 45 46 47 48 49 50 51 52 53 54 56 57 58 59 60 61 62 63 64 65 66 67 68 69 70 71 72 73 74 75 76 77 78 79 **P**6 7 8 **S** Sentara Healthcare, Norfolk, VA
Web address: www.sentara.com
— 23 10 100 4439 56 60668 38 41039 12801 439

★ SENTARA VIRGINIA BEACH GENERAL HOSPITAL, (Formerly Virginia Beach General Hospital), 1060 First Colonial Road, Zip 23454-9000; tel. 757/395-8000; Robert L. Graves, Administrator **A**1 2 3 5 9 10 **F**1 4 6 7 8 9 10 11 12 13 14 15 16 17 18 19 20 21 22 23 24 25 26 27 28 29 30 31 32 33 34 35 36 37 38 39 40 41 42 43 44 45 46 47 48 49 50 51 52 53 54 56 57 58 59 60 61 62 63 64 65 66 67 68 69 70 71 72 73 74 75 76 77 78 79 **P**6 7 8 **S** Sentara Healthcare, Norfolk, VA
Web address: www.sentara.com
— 23 10 193 12700 166 176369 2637 103136 40031 1097

WARRENTON—Fauquier County

★ FAUQUIER HOSPITAL, 500 Hospital Drive, Zip 20186-3099; tel. 540/349-0531; Rodger H. Baker, President and Chief Executive Officer **A**1 9 10 **F**6 7 8 9 13 16 17 18 19 22 24 25 26 30 32 33 34 36 37 38 39 41 43 44 45 46 48 50 51 54 57 68 69 70 71 72 76 78
Web address: www.fauquierhospital.org
— 23 10 83 4765 49 58395 511 42482 20469 594

WILLIAMSBURG—Independent City County

☐ EASTERN STATE HOSPITAL, (PSYCHIATRIC), 4601 Ironbound Road, Zip 23187-8791, Mailing Address: P.O. Box 8791, Zip 23187-8791; tel. 757/253-5161; John M. Favret, Director (Total facility includes 285 beds in nursing home-type unit) **A**1 5 9 10 **F**13 16 17 18 22 23 24 28 30 31 32 33 34 39 43 45 49 50 51 57 59 60 61 62 64 69 70 78 **P**6 **S** Virginia Department of Mental Health, Richmond, VA
Web address: www.easternstatehospital.org
— 12 22 581 1157 496 0 0 62789 38420 1228

Hospitals, U.S. / VIRGINIA

Hospital, Address, Telephone, Administrator, Approval, Facility, and Physician Codes, Health Care System, Network	Classification Codes		Utilization Data					Expense (thousands) of dollars		
★ American Hospital Association (AHA) membership □ Joint Commission on Accreditation of Healthcare Organizations (JCAHO) accreditation + American Osteopathic Healthcare Association (AOHA) membership ○ American Osteopathic Association (AOA) accreditation △ Commission on Accreditation of Rehabilitation Facilities (CARF) accreditation Control codes 61, 63, 64, 71, 72 and 73 indicate hospitals listed by AOHA, but not registered by AHA. For definition of numerical codes, see page A4	Control	Service	Staffed Beds	Admissions	Census	Outpatient Visits	Births	Total	Payroll	Personnel
☒ WILLIAMSBURG COMMUNITY HOSPITAL, 301 Monticello Avenue, Zip 23187–8700, Mailing Address: Box 8700, Zip 23187–8700; tel. 757/259–6000; Les A. Donahue, President and Chief Executive Officer (Nonreporting) **A**1 2 5 9 10 **S** Sentara Healthcare, Norfolk, VA **Web address:** www.sentara.com	23	10	100	—	—	—	—	—	—	—
WINCHESTER—Independent City County ☒ WINCHESTER MEDICAL CENTER, 1840 Amherst Street, Zip 22601–2540, Mailing Address: P.O. Box 3340, Zip 22604–3340; tel. 540/722–8000; George B. Caley, President **A**1 2 9 10 **F**4 7 8 9 11 12 13 16 17 18 19 22 24 25 27 32 33 34 35 36 37 38 39 40 41 42 43 44 45 46 47 48 49 51 53 54 57 58 59 60 61 63 64 65 68 70 72 76 77 78 **P**5 7 8 **S** Valley Health System, Winchester, VA **Web address:** www.valleyhealthlink.com	23	10	387	22100	284	132006	1966	176423	79512	1852
WOODBRIDGE—Prince William County ☒ POTOMAC HOSPITAL, 2300 Opitz Boulevard, Zip 22191–3399; tel. 703/670–1313; William Mason Moss, President **A**1 2 9 10 **F**6 7 8 9 11 13 14 16 17 18 19 22 24 25 26 30 31 32 33 34 35 36 37 38 39 41 42 43 44 45 46 48 51 54 56 57 58 59 61 62 64 65 68 70 72 76 78 79 **P**6 **Web address:** www.potomachospital.com	23	10	137	8564	93	146546	1874	71259	31228	681
WOODSTOCK—Shenandoah County ☒ SHENANDOAH MEMORIAL HOSPITAL, 759 South Main Street, Zip 22664–1127, Mailing Address: P.O. Box 508, Zip 22664–0508; tel. 540/459–4021; Floyd Heater, Chief Executive Officer (Total facility includes 34 beds in nursing home–type unit) **A**1 9 10 **F**3 4 7 8 9 11 13 16 17 18 19 22 24 25 26 27 28 30 31 32 34 36 37 38 39 41 43 44 45 46 48 49 50 51 54 55 56 57 58 59 60 61 62 63 68 69 70 71 72 74 75 76 78 79 **Web address:** www.shenmemhosp.com	23	10	129	2446	57	66316	234	22555	9538	302
WYTHEVILLE—Wythe County ☒ WYTHE COUNTY COMMUNITY HOSPITAL, 600 West Ridge Road, Zip 24382–1099; tel. 540/228–0200; Larry H. Chewning, II, Chief Executive Officer (Total facility includes 8 beds in nursing home–type unit) **A**1 2 9 10 **F**7 8 9 12 13 14 16 17 18 19 20 22 24 25 29 30 31 32 33 34 36 37 38 39 41 43 44 45 46 48 49 50 53 54 56 66 69 70 71 72 76 78 79 **S** Carilion Health System, Roanoke, VA **Web address:** www.wcch.org	23	10	90	2709	37	33887	245	24528	10871	—

© 2000 AHA Guide   *Many Facility Codes have changed. Please refer to the AHA Guide Code Chart.*

WASHINGTON

Resident Population 5,689 (in thousands)
Resident population in metro areas 82.8%
Birth rate per 1,000 population 13.9
65 years and over 11.5%
Percent of persons without health insurance 11.4%

Hospital, Address, Telephone, Administrator, Approval, Facility, and Physician Codes, Health Care System, Network	Classification Codes		Utilization Data					Expense (thousands) of dollars		
	Control	Service	Staffed Beds	Admissions	Census	Outpatient Visits	Births	Total	Payroll	Personnel

★ American Hospital Association (AHA) membership
□ Joint Commission on Accreditation of Healthcare Organizations (JCAHO) accreditation
+ American Osteopathic Healthcare Association (AOHA) membership
○ American Osteopathic Association (AOA) accreditation
△ Commission on Accreditation of Rehabilitation Facilities (CARF) accreditation
Control codes 61, 63, 64, 71, 72 and 73 indicate hospitals listed by AOHA, but not registered by AHA. For definition of numerical codes, see page A4

Hospital	Control	Service	Staffed Beds	Admissions	Census	Outpatient Visits	Births	Total	Payroll	Personnel
ABERDEEN—Grays Harbor County										
★ GRAYS HARBOR COMMUNITY HOSPITAL, 915 Anderson Drive, Zip 98520; tel. 360/532-8330; Thomas J. Troy, President and Chief Executive Officer (Total facility includes 60 beds in nursing home–type unit) **A**1 9 10 **F**2 3 7 8 13 18 19 22 25 27 30 36 39 41 44 46 48 49 54 59 61 69 70 75 76 77 78 **P**8	23	10	172	4513	107	72536	504	44019	20156	483
ANACORTES—Skagit County										
★ ISLAND HEALTH NORTHWEST, 1211 24th Street, Zip 98221-2590; tel. 360/299-1300; Vince Oliver, Chief Executive Officer (Nonreporting) **A**1 2 9 10 Web address: www.island-health.org	16	10	43	—	—	—	—	—	—	—
ARLINGTON—Snohomish County										
★ CASCADE VALLEY HOSPITAL, NORTH SNOHOMISH COUNTY HEALTH SYSTEM, (Formerly North Snohomish County Health System), 330 South Stillaguamish Avenue, Zip 98223-1642; tel. 360/435-2133; Robert D. Campbell, Jr, Administrator (Nonreporting) **A**1 9 10	16	10	48	—	—	—	—	—	—	—
AUBURN—King County										
□ AUBURN REGIONAL MEDICAL CENTER, 202 North Division, Plaza One, Zip 98001-4908; tel. 253/833-7711; Michael M. Gherardini, Chief Executive Officer and Managing Director (Nonreporting) **A**1 2 9 10 **S** Universal Health Services, Inc., King of Prussia, PA	33	10	100	—	—	—	—	—	—	—
BELLEVUE—King County										
★ OVERLAKE HOSPITAL MEDICAL CENTER, 1035 116th Avenue N.E., Zip 98004; tel. 425/688-5000; Kenneth D. Graham, President and Chief Executive Officer **A**1 2 9 10 **F**4 7 8 9 11 12 13 16 17 18 19 22 24 25 27 30 38 41 43 44 45 46 47 48 49 50 51 53 54 57 58 59 62 63 64 65 70 71 72 75 76 77 78 79 Web address: www.overlakehospital.org	23	10	218	14577	151	160997	3270	133211	60535	—
BELLINGHAM—Whatcom County										
★ △ ST. JOSEPH HOSPITAL, 2901 Squalicum Parkway, Zip 98225-1898; tel. 360/734-5400; Nancy J. Bitting, Regional Chief Executive Officer **A**1 2 7 9 10 **F**1 2 3 4 5 7 8 9 11 12 13 14 16 17 19 22 24 25 26 27 30 31 32 33 34 38 39 41 42 43 44 45 46 47 48 49 50 51 52 53 54 55 56 57 60 61 63 65 66 68 70 71 72 73 75 76 77 78 **P**7 **S** PeaceHealth, Bellevue, WA Web address: www.peacehealth.org	23	10	189	12234	132	91571	1955	111394	49298	1081
BREMERTON—Kitsap County										
★ HARRISON MEMORIAL HOSPITAL, 2520 Cherry Street, Zip 98310-4270; tel. 360/377-3911; David W. Gitch, President and Chief Executive Officer **A**1 2 9 10 **F**4 7 8 9 11 13 16 17 18 19 22 24 25 26 27 29 30 31 32 33 34 35 36 37 38 39 41 43 44 45 46 48 49 50 51 54 57 58 59 60 61 62 63 65 66 70 72 75 76 77 78 79 **P**1 Web address: www.harrisonhospital.org	23	10	219	11274	111	111706	1617	91747	46155	941
★ NAVAL HOSPITAL, Boone Road, Zip 98312-1898; tel. 360/475-4000; Captain Gregg S. Parker, Commanding Officer **A**1 5 **F**3 8 9 12 13 14 22 23 24 25 28 31 32 34 38 39 41 43 44 45 46 48 49 50 51 53 54 56 59 60 61 63 64 68 70 72 76 78 79 **S** Department of Navy, Washington, DC Web address: www.nh_bremerton.med.navy.mil	43	10	91	2647	21	349095	729	44346	—	—
BREWSTER—Okanogan County										
★ OKANOGAN–DOUGLAS COUNTY HOSPITAL, 507 Hospital Way, Zip 98812-0577; Mailing Address: P.O. Box 577, Zip 98812-0577; tel. 509/689-2517; Martin Nolan, Administrator (Nonreporting) **A**9 10	16	10	43	—	—	—	—	—	—	—
CENTRALIA—Lewis County										
★ PROVIDENCE CENTRALIA HOSPITAL, 914 South Scheuber Road, Zip 98531; tel. 360/736-2803; Steve Burdick, Administrator (Total facility includes 63 beds in nursing home–type unit) **A**1 2 9 10 **F**3 7 8 9 12 13 16 17 18 22 23 24 25 30 32 33 34 36 37 38 39 44 45 48 50 51 53 54 56 61 67 69 70 71 72 75 76 77 78 79 **P**8 **S** Providence Health System, Seattle, WA Web address: www.providence.org	21	10	142	4965	94	163494	636	44626	22591	552
CHELAN—Chelan County										
★ LAKE CHELAN COMMUNITY HOSPITAL, 503 East Highland Avenue, Zip 98816-0908, Mailing Address: P.O. Box 908, Zip 98816-0908; tel. 509/682-2531; Larry Peterson, Chief Executive Officer (Nonreporting) **A**9 10	16	10	30	—	—	—	—	—	—	—
CHEWELAH—Stevens County										
★ ST. JOSEPH'S HOSPITAL, 500 East Webster Street, Zip 99109-0197, Mailing Address: P.O. Box 197, Zip 99109-0197; tel. 509/935-8211; Gary V. Peck, Chief Executive Officer (Total facility includes 40 beds in nursing home–type unit) (Nonreporting) **A**9 10 **S** Providence Services, Spokane, WA	21	10	65	—	—	—	—	—	—	—
CLARKSTON—Asotin County										
★ TRI-STATE MEMORIAL HOSPITAL, 1221 Highland Avenue, Zip 99403-0189, Mailing Address: P.O. Box 189, Zip 99403-0189; tel. 509/758-5511; Joseph K. Lillard, Administrator **A**1 9 10 **F**6 7 9 12 16 17 18 19 22 24 25 27 32 34 36 37 38 39 41 48 49 51 54 67 70 72 74 75 76 77 78 **P**8 Web address: www.tri-statehospital.com	23	10	41	1467	16	39546	0	16962	6421	214

Hospitals, U.S. / WASHINGTON

Hospital, Address, Telephone, Administrator, Approval, Facility, and Physician Codes, Health Care System, Network	Classification Codes		Utilization Data					Expense (thousands) of dollars		
★ American Hospital Association (AHA) membership ☐ Joint Commission on Accreditation of Healthcare Organizations (JCAHO) accreditation + American Osteopathic Healthcare Association (AOHA) membership ○ American Osteopathic Association (AOA) accreditation △ Commission on Accreditation of Rehabilitation Facilities (CARF) accreditation Control codes 61, 63, 64, 71, 72 and 73 indicate hospitals listed by AOHA, but not registered by AHA. For definition of numerical codes, see page A4	Control	Service	Staffed Beds	Admissions	Census	Outpatient Visits	Births	Total	Payroll	Personnel
COLFAX—Whitman County ★ WHITMAN HOSPITAL AND MEDICAL CENTER, 1200 West Fairview, Zip 99111–9579; tel. 509/397–3435; Gordon C. McLean, Administrator **A**9 10 **F**6 7 8 9 13 16 17 22 25 26 36 37 40 43 44 45 46 48 54 69 70 71 76 **Web address:** www.whitmanhospital.com	16	10	31	931	8	10572	64	7422	3685	120
COLVILLE—Stevens County ✠ MOUNT CARMEL HOSPITAL, 982 East Columbia Street, Zip 99114–0351, Mailing Address: Box 351, Zip 99114–0351; tel. 509/684–2561; Gloria Cooper, Chief Executive Officer **A**1 3 9 10 **F**8 9 13 16 17 18 22 25 38 39 41 44 45 48 50 51 54 61 72 75 76 **P**8 **S** Providence Services, Spokane, WA	21	10	33	1584	14	21988	234	14015	6161	140
COUPEVILLE—Island County ✠ WHIDBEY GENERAL HOSPITAL, 101 North Main Street, Zip 98239–0400, Mailing Address: P.O. Box 400, Zip 98239–0400; tel. 360/678–7656; Scott Rhine, Administrator and Chief Executive Officer (Nonreporting) **A**1 2 9 10 **Web address:** www.whidbeygen.comwghosp	16	10	51	—	—	—	—	—	—	—
DAVENPORT—Lincoln County ★ LINCOLN HOSPITAL, 10 Nichols Street, Zip 99122; tel. 509/725–7101; Thomas J. Martin, Administrator (Total facility includes 71 beds in nursing home–type unit) **A**9 10 **F**6 7 8 9 13 17 18 19 22 25 30 32 34 37 43 48 51 54 69 70 75 76 77 78 **P**7	16	10	95	480	62	9973	19	7944	4204	155
DAYTON—Columbia County DAYTON GENERAL HOSPITAL, 1012 South Third Street, Zip 99328; tel. 509/382–2531; Oral R. Compson, Administrator (Nonreporting) **A**9 10 18	16	10	18	—	—	—	—	—	—	—
DEER PARK—Spokane County ★ DEER PARK HOSPITAL, (Formerly Deer Park Health Center and Hospital), East 1015 D Street, Zip 99006–0742, Mailing Address: P.O. Box 742, Zip 99006–0742; tel. 509/276–5061; Garvin Olson, Chief Operating Officer (Nonreporting) **A**9 10 **S** Providence Services, Spokane, WA	33	10	26	—	—	—	—	—	—	—
EDMONDS—Snohomish County ✠ STEVENS HEALTHCARE, 21601 76th Avenue West, Zip 98026–7506; tel. 425/640–4000; Steve C. McCary, President and Chief Executive Officer **A**1 2 9 10 **F**1 4 7 8 9 11 18 19 20 21 22 23 24 25 26 27 30 31 32 33 34 35 38 39 41 43 44 45 46 48 49 50 51 54 56 57 58 59 60 61 62 63 64 65 70 71 72 76 78 79 **P**1 6 7 **Web address:** www.stevenshealthcare.org	16	10	124	8154	91	366527	1643	97787	45258	1067
ELLENSBURG—Kittitas County KITTITAS VALLEY COMMUNITY HOSPITAL, 603 South Chestnut Street, Zip 98926; tel. 509/962–7302; Eric Jensen, Administrator **A**3 9 10 **F**7 8 9 12 17 18 19 22 25 28 30 33 36 37 39 40 41 43 44 45 48 54 70 72 75 76 78	16	10	32	1677	14	49636	315	16535	7608	194
ENUMCLAW—King County ENUMCLAW COMMUNITY HOSPITAL, (Formerly Community Memorial Hospital), 1450 Battersby Avenue, Zip 98022, Mailing Address: P.O. Box 218, Zip 98022–0218; tel. 360/825–2505; Dennis A. Popp, Administrator and Chief Executive Officer **A**9 10 **F**8 9 13 14 16 17 19 22 24 25 31 32 33 34 35 37 39 41 43 44 46 48 68 72 73 76 78	23	10	27	1060	8	23127	245	12676	5366	138
EPHRATA—Grant County ★ COLUMBIA BASIN HOSPITAL, 200 Southeast Boulevard, Zip 98823–1997; tel. 509/754–4631; Allen L. Beach, Administrator (Total facility includes 29 beds in nursing home–type unit) **A**9 10 **F**6 9 17 18 22 23 24 25 29 32 34 54 69 70 76 **P**6	16	10	59	312	70	19435	0	6172	3057	128
EVERETT—Snohomish County ✠ △ PROVIDENCE EVERETT MEDICAL CENTER, (Formerly Providence General Medical Center), (Includes Providence Everett Medical Center – Colby Campus, 14th and Colby Avenue, Mailing Address: P.O. Box 1147, Zip 98206; tel. 206/261–2000; Providence Everett Medical Center – Pacific Campus, Pacific and Nassau Streets, Zip 98201; tel. 206/258–7123), 1321 Colby Street, Zip 98206, Mailing Address: P.O. Box 1147, Zip 98206–1147; tel. 425/261–2000; Mel Pyne, Administrator **A**1 2 7 9 10 **F**2 3 4 8 9 11 13 16 17 18 19 21 22 25 28 29 30 32 33 34 35 36 37 38 39 41 43 44 45 46 47 48 49 50 51 53 54 55 56 58 61 65 66 68 70 71 72 73 75 76 78 79 **P**6 **S** Providence Health System, Seattle, WA **Web address:** www.providence.org	21	10	283	17626	167	489751	3120	170430	72963	1789
FAIRCHILD AFB—Spokane County ★ U. S. AIR FORCE HOSPITAL, 701 Hospital Loop, Suite 102, Zip 99011–8701; tel. 509/247–5217; Major Scott F. Wardell, Administrator (Nonreporting) **S** Department of the Air Force, Bowling AFB, DC	41	10	35	—	—	—	—	—	—	—
FEDERAL WAY—King County ★ ST. FRANCIS HOSPITAL, 34515 Ninth Avenue South, Zip 98003–9710; tel. 253/927–9700; Joseph W. Wilczek, President and Chief Executive Officer **A**2 9 10 **F**4 8 9 10 11 13 14 17 18 19 21 22 23 24 25 26 27 28 30 32 33 34 36 37 38 39 41 42 43 44 45 46 47 48 53 54 57 58 60 61 62 69 70 72 73 74 75 76 77 78 79 **P**2 5 8 **S** Catholic Health Initiatives, Denver, CO	21	10	99	5473	46	60956	1601	47571	21116	417
FORKS—Clallam County FORKS COMMUNITY HOSPITAL, 530 Bogachiel Way, Zip 98331–9699; tel. 360/374–6271; Janet A. Hays, Administrator (Total facility includes 36 beds in nursing home–type unit) **A**9 10 **F**3 8 9 14 16 17 18 19 23 24 25 30 32 33 34 35 43 44 45 48 49 50 54 56 63 69 70 72 75 76 78 79 **P**6 **Web address:** www.forkshospital.org	16	10	53	390	32	40875	58	10359	5429	166

© 2000 AHA Guide *Many Facility Codes have changed. Please refer to the AHA Guide Code Chart.*

Hospitals, U.S. / WASHINGTON

Hospital, Address, Telephone, Administrator, Approval, Facility, and Physician Codes, Health Care System, Network	Classification Codes		Utilization Data					Expense (thousands) of dollars		
★ American Hospital Association (AHA) membership ☐ Joint Commission on Accreditation of Healthcare Organizations (JCAHO) accreditation + American Osteopathic Healthcare Association (AOHA) membership ○ American Osteopathic Association (AOA) accreditation △ Commission on Accreditation of Rehabilitation Facilities (CARF) accreditation Control codes 61, 63, 64, 71, 72 and 73 indicate hospitals listed by AOHA, but not registered by AHA. For definition of numerical codes, see page A4	Control	Service	Staffed Beds	Admissions	Census	Outpatient Visits	Births	Total	Payroll	Personnel
GOLDENDALE—Klickitat County										
KLICKITAT VALLEY HOSPITAL, 310 South Roosevelt, Zip 98620, Mailing Address: P.O. Box 5, Zip 98620; tel. 509/773–4022; Ron Ingraham, Administrator **A**3 9 10 **F**6 8 9 17 22 25 31 32 34 35 36 37 39 44 45 48 54 61 63 70 73 76 77 79 **P**8	16	10	15	474	3	17693	50	4702	2703	68
GRAND COULEE—Grant County										
★ COULEE COMMUNITY HOSPITAL, 411 Fortuyn Road, Zip 99133–8718; tel. 509/633–1753; Michael C. Wiltermood, Chief Executive Officer (Total facility includes 29 beds in nursing home–type unit) (Nonreporting) **A**9 10	16	10	48	—	—	—	—	—	—	—
ILWACO—Pacific County										
★ OCEAN BEACH HOSPITAL, First and Fir, Zip 98624, Mailing Address: P.O. Drawer H, Zip 98624; tel. 360/642–3181; Pamela Ott, R.N., Chief Executive Officer (Nonreporting) **A**9 10	16	10	14	—	—	—	—	—	—	—
KENNEWICK—Benton County										
✥ KENNEWICK GENERAL HOSPITAL, 900 South Auburn Street, Zip 99336–0128, Mailing Address: Box 6128, Zip 99336; tel. 509/586–6111; Tom Nielsen, Administrator **A**1 2 9 10 **F**1 7 8 9 11 13 17 18 22 24 25 27 34 35 36 38 39 41 43 44 45 46 48 50 51 64 65 70 75 76 77 78 79 **P**7 Web address: www.kennewickgeneral.com	16	10	71	4674	41	86924	1106	43227	16985	424
KIRKLAND—King County										
☐ BHC FAIRFAX HOSPITAL, 10200 N.E. 132nd Street, Zip 98034; tel. 425/821–2000; Ron Escarda, Chief Executive Officer (Nonreporting) **A**1 9 10 **S** Behavioral Healthcare Corporation, Nashville, TN	33	22	133	—	—	—	—	—	—	—
✥ EVERGREEN COMMUNITY HEALTH CENTER, 12040 N.E. 128th Street, Zip 98034; tel. 425/899–1000; Andrew Fallat, FACHE, Chief Executive Officer (Total facility includes 17 beds in nursing home–type unit) **A**1 2 9 10 **F**1 4 8 9 11 12 13 16 17 18 22 24 25 26 27 28 30 31 33 34 36 37 38 39 41 43 44 45 46 48 49 50 54 55 59 61 62 63 65 69 70 72 73 75 76 77 78 **P**6 Web address: www.evergreenghealthnet.org	16	10	166	11329	109	212919	3582	128821	58520	1574
LAKEWOOD—Pierce County										
★ ST. CLARE HOSPITAL, 11315 Bridgeport Way S.W., Zip 98499–0998, Mailing Address: P.O. Box 99998, Zip 98499–0998; tel. 253/588–1711; Syd Bersante, Chief of Operations **A**9 10 **F**2 3 4 6 8 9 10 11 12 13 16 17 18 19 21 22 23 24 25 26 27 29 30 31 32 33 34 35 36 37 38 39 41 42 43 44 45 46 47 48 49 50 51 52 53 54 57 58 59 60 61 62 63 64 65 66 69 70 71 72 73 74 75 76 77 78 79 **P**5 6 7 8 **S** Catholic Health Initiatives, Denver, CO	21	10	60	3821	36	53969	558	34753	15515	369
LONGVIEW—Cowlitz County										
✥ ST. JOHN MEDICAL CENTER, 1615 Delaware Street, Zip 98632, Mailing Address: P.O. Box 3002, Zip 98632–0302; tel. 360/414–2000; Mark E. McGourty, Regional Chief Executive Officer (Nonreporting) **A**1 2 9 10 **S** PeaceHealth, Bellevue, WA Web address: www.peacehealth.org	23	10	178	—	—	—	—	—	—	—
MCCLEARY—Grays Harbor County										
★ MARK REED HOSPITAL, 322 South Birch Street, Zip 98557; tel. 360/495–3244; Jean E. Roberts, Administrator (Nonreporting) **A**9 10 **S** Providence Health System, Seattle, WA	16	10	7	—	—	—	—	—	—	—
MEDICAL LAKE—Spokane County										
☐ EASTERN STATE HOSPITAL, Maple Street, Zip 99022–0045, Mailing Address: P.O. Box A, Zip 99022–0045; tel. 509/299–3121; C. Jan Gregg, Chief Executive Officer **A**1 10 **F**16 17 18 23 31 57 59 60 61 62 70 **P**6	12	22	302	1001	299	—	—	43530	25283	579
MONROE—Snohomish County										
✥ VALLEY GENERAL HOSPITAL, 14701 179th S.E., Zip 98272, Mailing Address: P.O. Box 646, Zip 98272–0646; tel. 360/794–7497; Mark D. Judy, Chief Executive Officer **A**1 9 10 **F**2 3 7 8 9 12 17 18 22 24 25 27 28 30 32 34 35 38 41 44 48 51 54 57 61 62 63 70 71 72 73 75 76 78	16	10	69	2489	37	32894	460	21022	9596	264
MORTON—Lewis County										
★ MORTON GENERAL HOSPITAL, 521 Adams Street, Zip 98356, Mailing Address: Drawer C, Zip 98356–0019; tel. 360/496–5112; Mike Lee, Superintendent (Total facility includes 30 beds in nursing home–type unit) (Nonreporting) **A**9 10 **S** Providence Health System, Seattle, WA	16	10	50	—	—	—	—	—	—	—
MOSES LAKE—Grant County										
✥ SAMARITAN HEALTHCARE, 801 East Wheeler Road, Zip 98837–1899; tel. 509/765–5606; Keith J. Baldwin, Chief Executive Officer and Administrator **A**1 9 10 **F**8 9 12 17 18 19 22 24 25 29 32 33 34 38 39 41 43 44 45 46 48 50 51 54 56 70 71 72 75 77 78 **P**6 Web address: www.samaritanhealthcare.com	16	10	50	2881	25	61115	961	32469	15112	396
MOUNT VERNON—Skagit County										
✥ AFFILIATED HEALTH SERVICES, (Includes Skagit Valley Hospital, Gregg A. Davidson, Associate Administrator and Chief Operating Officer; United General Hospital, 1971 Highway 20, Sedro Woolley, Zip 98284, Mailing Address: P.O. Box 1376, Zip 98273–1376; tel. 360/856–6021), 1415 Kincaid Street, Zip 98274, Mailing Address: P.O. Box 1376, Zip 98273–1376; tel. 360/424–4111; Patrick R. Mahoney, Administrator and Chief Executive Officer **A**1 9 10 **F**4 5 8 9 11 12 13 16 17 18 19 22 24 25 26 27 30 32 33 34 36 37 38 39 41 43 44 45 46 48 51 54 57 59 61 62 63 64 65 68 70 72 75 76 78 79 Web address: www.affiliatedhealth.org	16	10	166	6939	73	91533	1290	82599	36142	841

Hospitals, U.S. / WASHINGTON

Hospital, Address, Telephone, Administrator, Approval, Facility, and Physician Codes, Health Care System, Network	Classification Codes		Utilization Data					Expense (thousands) of dollars		
★ American Hospital Association (AHA) membership ☐ Joint Commission on Accreditation of Healthcare Organizations (JCAHO) accreditation + American Osteopathic Healthcare Association (AOHA) membership ○ American Osteopathic Association (AOA) accreditation △ Commission on Accreditation of Rehabilitation Facilities (CARF) accreditation Control codes 61, 63, 64, 71, 72 and 73 indicate hospitals listed by AOHA, but not registered by AHA. For definition of numerical codes, see page A4	Control	Service	Staffed Beds	Admissions	Census	Outpatient Visits	Births	Total	Payroll	Personnel
NEWPORT—Pend Oreille County NEWPORT COMMUNITY HOSPITAL, 714 West Pine, Zip 99156; tel. 509/447–2441; John R. White, Chief Executive Officer and Superintendent (Total facility includes 50 beds in nursing home–type unit) **A**9 10 **F**8 9 16 17 25 32 34 38 43 44 48 54 56 69 70 75 76 78 **P**6 Web address: www.phd1.org	16	10	74	555	50	22984	95	9093	4975	148
OAK HARBOR—Island County ✠ NAVAL HOSPITAL, 3475 North Saratoga Street, Zip 98278–8800; tel. 360/257–9500; Captain John Tracy, Commander (Nonreporting) **A**1 **S** Department of Navy, Washington, DC	43	10	25	—	—	—	—	—	—	—
ODESSA—Lincoln County ★ ODESSA MEMORIAL HOSPITAL, 502 East Amende, Zip 99159–0368, Mailing Address: P.O. Box 368, Zip 99159–0368; tel. 509/982–2611; Jon R. Davis, Administrator (Total facility includes 23 beds in nursing home–type unit) **A**10 **F**6 7 9 17 18 23 25 30 31 32 34 38 45 48 54 56 69 70 71 72 76 **P**6	16	10	38	136	24	3007	0	2878	1296	68
OLYMPIA—Thurston County ✠ CAPITAL MEDICAL CENTER, 3900 Capital Mall Drive S.W., Zip 98502–5026, Mailing Address: P.O. Box 19002, Zip 98507–9002; tel. 360/754–5858; Joseph Sharp, Chief Executive Officer (Total facility includes 9 beds in nursing home–type unit) **A**1 2 9 10 **F**4 7 8 9 11 12 13 16 17 18 19 22 24 25 27 29 32 34 35 38 39 41 44 45 46 48 49 54 65 69 71 72 75 76 78 79 **P**5 8 **S** HCA – The Healthcare Company, Nashville, TN Web address: www.capitalmedical.com	32	10	110	4028	34	81884	623	—	—	410
✠ △ PROVIDENCE ST. PETER HOSPITAL, 413 Lilly Road N.E., Zip 98506–5116; tel. 360/491–9480; C. Scott Bond, Administrator and Chief Executive Officer **A**1 2 3 5 7 9 10 **F**2 3 8 9 11 12 13 14 15 16 17 19 21 22 23 24 25 26 27 28 29 31 32 33 34 35 36 37 38 39 41 43 44 45 46 47 48 50 51 53 54 56 57 58 59 60 61 62 63 64 65 67 68 69 70 72 75 76 78 **P**7 8 **S** Providence Health System, Seattle, WA Web address: www.providence.org	21	10	314	16026	173	285498	2030	165177	77630	1755
OMAK—Okanogan County MID–VALLEY HOSPITAL, 810 Jasmine, Zip 98841–0793, Mailing Address: P.O. Box 793, Zip 98841–0793; tel. 509/826–1760; Michael D. Billing, Administrator **A**3 9 10 **F**7 8 9 13 22 24 25 38 39 48 49 51 54 75 76	16	10	30	1426	11	14399	289	10407	4507	131
OTHELLO—Adams County ★ OTHELLO COMMUNITY HOSPITAL, 315 North 14th Street, Zip 99344; tel. 509/488–2636; Jerry Lane, Administrator **A**9 10 **F**8 9 22 25 32 38 40 41 44 45 48 75 76	16	10	32	936	6	27503	414	6706	3262	89
PASCO—Franklin County ✠ △ LOURDES MEDICAL CENTER, 520 North Fourth Avenue, Zip 99301–2568, Mailing Address: P.O. Box 2568, Zip 99302–2568; tel. 509/547–7704; James F. Dover, FACHE, Chief Executive Officer (Total facility includes 21 beds in nursing home–type unit) (Nonreporting) **A**1 2 7 9 10 **S** Carondelet Health System, Saint Louis, MO Web address: www.cbvcp.com\healthcenter	21	10	132	—	—	—	—	—	—	—
POMEROY—Garfield County GARFIELD COUNTY MEMORIAL HOSPITAL, 66th North Sixth Street, Zip 99347–0880, Mailing Address: P.O. Box 880, Zip 99347; tel. 509/843–1591; Gail McDowell, Administrator (Total facility includes 40 beds in nursing home–type unit) (Nonreporting) **A**10 18	16	10	54	—	—	—	—	—	—	—
PORT ANGELES—Clallam County ☐ OLYMPIC MEMORIAL HOSPITAL, 939 Caroline Street, Zip 98362–3997; tel. 360/417–7000; Michael Glenn, Administrator and Chief Executive Officer (Total facility includes 125 beds in nursing home–type unit) **A**1 2 9 10 **F**7 8 9 12 14 16 17 18 19 22 24 25 28 32 33 34 36 38 41 43 44 45 46 48 50 51 54 65 69 70 75 76 78 79 **P**3 Web address: www.OMHNET.COM	16	10	203	5052	146	96249	522	51374	24189	652
PORT TOWNSEND—Jefferson County ★ JEFFERSON GENERAL HOSPITAL, 834 Sheridan Road, Zip 98368–2443; tel. 360/385–2200; Victor J. Dirksen, Administrator (Nonreporting) **A**9 10 Web address: www.jgh.org	16	10	31	—	—	—	—	—	—	—
PROSSER—Benton County ★ PROSSER MEMORIAL HOSPITAL, 723 Memorial Street, Zip 99350–1593; tel. 509/786–2222; James Tavary, Administrator (Total facility includes 36 beds in nursing home–type unit) **A**9 10 **F**8 9 22 25 30 35 36 44 45 46 48 54 69 70 76 78 79	16	10	60	710	36	10958	379	7666	3481	132
PULLMAN—Whitman County ☐ PULLMAN MEMORIAL HOSPITAL, N.E. 1125 Washington Avenue, Zip 99163–4742; tel. 509/332–2541; Scott K. Adams, Chief Executive Officer **A**1 9 10 **F**1 2 3 4 5 6 8 9 10 11 12 13 15 19 21 22 23 24 25 27 28 30 32 33 34 35 37 38 39 40 41 42 43 44 45 46 47 48 49 50 51 52 53 54 56 58 59 60 61 62 63 64 65 66 67 68 69 70 71 72 74 75 76 77 78 Web address: www.pullmanhospital.org	16	10	24	1010	8	178204	271	14687	6364	152
PUYALLUP—Pierce County ✠ △ GOOD SAMARITAN COMMUNITY HEALTHCARE, 407 14th Avenue S.E., Zip 98372–0118, Mailing Address: P.O. Box 1247, Zip 98371–1247; tel. 253/848–6661; Edwin L. Miller, FACHE, President **A**1 2 7 9 10 **F**1 6 7 8 12 13 16 17 18 19 21 24 25 26 28 29 30 32 33 34 35 36 37 38 41 42 43 44 45 46 48 49 50 51 54 56 58 59 60 61 62 63 64 65 68 70 71 72 73 75 76 77 78 **P**1 6 7	21	10	211	10029	126	426519	1434	124052	73455	1848

© 2000 AHA Guide *Many Facility Codes have changed. Please refer to the AHA Guide Code Chart.*

Hospitals, U.S. / WASHINGTON

Hospital, Address, Telephone, Administrator, Approval, Facility, and Physician Codes, Health Care System, Network

- ★ American Hospital Association (AHA) membership
- ☐ Joint Commission on Accreditation of Healthcare Organizations (JCAHO) accreditation
- + American Osteopathic Healthcare Association (AOHA) membership
- ○ American Osteopathic Association (AOA) accreditation
- △ Commission on Accreditation of Rehabilitation Facilities (CARF) accreditation

Control codes 61, 63, 64, 71, 72 and 73 indicate hospitals listed by AOHA, but not registered by AHA. For definition of numerical codes, see page A4.

Hospital	Classification Codes		Utilization Data					Expense (thousands of dollars)		Personnel
	Control	Service	Staffed Beds	Admissions	Census	Outpatient Visits	Births	Total	Payroll	
QUINCY—Grant County QUINCY VALLEY MEDICAL CENTER, 908 Tenth Avenue S.W., Zip 98848–1376; tel. 509/787–3531; Alan MacPhee, Administrator (Total facility includes 22 beds in nursing home–type unit) (Nonreporting) **A**9 10	13	10	38	—	—	—	—	—	—	—
REDMOND—King County THE EASTSIDE HOSPITAL, 2700 152nd Avenue N.E., Zip 98052–5560; tel. 425/883–5151; Patricia Kennedy-Scott, Northern Region Vice President (Nonreporting)	23	10	125	—	—	—	—	—	—	—
RENTON—King County ★ VALLEY MEDICAL CENTER, 400 South 43rd Street, Zip 98055–5784; tel. 425/228–3450; Richard D. Roodman, Chief Executive Officer (Total facility includes 39 beds in nursing home–type unit) (Nonreporting) **A**1 2 3 5 9 10 Web address: www.valleymed.org	16	10	196	—	—	—	—	—	—	—
REPUBLIC—Ferry County FERRY COUNTY MEMORIAL HOSPITAL, 36 Klondike Road, Zip 99166–9701; tel. 509/775–3333; Nancy McIntyre, Administrator (Total facility includes 14 beds in nursing home–type unit) **A**9 10 **F**8 9 10 11 12 13 15 17 18 19 20 21 22 23 25 30 31 32 33 34 35 36 37 39 40 41 42 43 44 45 48 49 50 52 54 56 57 58 59 60 61 62 63 64 65 66 67 69 70 71 72 73 76 78 79 Web address: www.ferryco.com/hospital	16	10	25	345	14	7927	11	3229	1469	55
RICHLAND—Benton County ★ △ KADLEC MEDICAL CENTER, 888 Swift Boulevard, Zip 99352–3542; tel. 509/946–4611; Marcel Loh, President and Chief Executive Officer **A**1 2 7 9 10 **F**1 7 8 9 11 13 16 17 18 22 24 25 26 27 36 39 41 42 43 44 45 46 48 50 51 53 54 56 65 70 75 76 77 78 **S** Quorum Health Group, Brentwood, TN Web address: www.kadlecmed.com	23	10	124	6424	73	61731	1262	69250	28292	573
★ LOURDES COUNSELING CENTER, 1175 Carondelet Drive, Zip 99352–1175; tel. 509/943–9104; James F. Dover, FACHE, Chief Executive Officer (Nonreporting) **A**1 9 10 **S** Carondelet Health System, Saint Louis, MO Web address: www.lourdesonline.com	21	22	32	—	—	—	—	—	—	—
RITZVILLE—Adams County EAST ADAMS RURAL HOSPITAL, 903 South Adams Street, Zip 99169–2298; tel. 509/659–1200; James G. Parrish, Administrator (Nonreporting) **A**9 10	16	10	17	—	—	—	—	—	—	—
SEATTLE—King County ★ △ CHILDREN'S HOSPITAL AND REGIONAL MEDICAL CENTER, 4800 Sand Point Way N.E., Zip 98105–0371, Mailing Address: Box 5371, Zip 98105–0371; tel. 206/526–2000; Treuman Katz, President and Chief Executive Officer **A**1 2 3 5 7 8 9 10 **F**5 11 13 14 16 17 18 19 22 23 24 25 26 29 32 33 38 39 42 43 45 46 47 48 49 50 51 52 53 54 56 57 58 59 60 61 63 64 65 66 70 71 72 73 74 75 76 77 78 **P**4	23	50	208	11253	150	168534	—	173091	70702	1595
★ △ HARBORVIEW MEDICAL CENTER, 325 Ninth Avenue, Box 359717, Zip 98104–2499; tel. 206/731–3000; David E. Jaffe, Executive Director **A**1 3 5 7 8 9 10 **F**3 4 5 8 9 10 11 12 13 14 16 17 18 19 20 21 22 23 24 25 27 29 30 31 32 33 34 35 37 38 39 41 43 44 45 46 47 48 49 50 51 53 54 55 56 57 58 59 60 61 62 63 64 65 70 71 72 73 74 75 76 77 78 79 **P**3 Web address: www.washington.edu/medical/hmc/index.html	13	10	348	15096	295	357002	0	312519	132855	3091
★ △ HIGHLINE COMMUNITY HOSPITAL, (Includes Highline Specialty Center, 12844 Military Road Fork, Tukwila, Zip 98168; Mark Benedum, Administrator), 16251 Sylvester Road S.W., Zip 98166–0657; tel. 206/244–9970; Paul Tucker, Administrator (Total facility includes 30 beds in nursing home–type unit) (Nonreporting) **A**1 2 7 9 10	23	10	203	—	—	—	—	—	—	—
★ △ NORTHWEST HOSPITAL, 1550 North 115th Street, Zip 98133–0806; tel. 206/364–0500; C. W. Schneider, President and Chief Executive Officer (Total facility includes 42 beds in nursing home–type unit) (Nonreporting) **A**1 2 3 7 9 10 Web address: www.nwhospital.org	23	10	238	—	—	—	—	—	—	—
★ △ PROVIDENCE SEATTLE MEDICAL CENTER, 500 17th Avenue, Zip 98122–1008, Mailing Address: P.O. Box 34008, Zip 98124–1008; tel. 206/320–2000; Craig L. Hendrickson, Chief Operating Officer (Total facility includes 51 beds in nursing home–type unit) **A**1 2 3 5 7 9 10 **F**1 2 4 6 7 8 9 10 11 12 13 16 17 18 19 22 24 25 26 30 31 32 33 34 35 36 37 38 39 41 42 43 44 45 46 47 48 49 50 51 52 53 54 56 57 59 60 61 62 63 64 65 66 67 69 70 71 72 73 76 78 79 **P**5 6 7 **S** Providence Health System, Seattle, WA Web address: www.providence.org	21	10	296	12841	165	130655	1560	174574	77114	1624
☐ REGIONAL HOSPITAL FOR RESPIRATORY AND COMPLEX CARE, 12844 Military Road South, Zip 98168–9981; tel. 206/248–4548; James C. Cannon, Administrator and Chief Executive Officer (Nonreporting) **A**1 10 Web address: www.regionalhospital.org	23	49	27	—	—	—	—	—	—	—
☐ SCHICK SHADEL HOSPITAL, 12101 Ambaum Boulevard S.W., Zip 98146–2699, Mailing Address: Box 48149, Zip 98148–0149; tel. 206/244–8100; Marvy Schmidt, Administrator **A**1 9 10 **F**2	33	82	63	446	12	0	0	—	—	—
★ SWEDISH HEALTH SERVICES, (Includes Swedish Medical Center–Ballard, Northwest Market and Barnes, Zip 98107–1507, Mailing Address: Box 70707, Zip 98107; tel. 206/782–2700), 747 Broadway Avenue, Zip 98122–4307; tel. 206/386–6000; Richard H. Peterson, President and Chief Executive Officer **A**1 2 3 5 9 10 **F**2 3 4 7 8 10 11 12 13 14 16 17 18 19 20 22 24 25 27 28 31 32 33 34 35 36 37 38 39 41 42 43 44 45 46 47 48 49 50 51 52 53 54 56 57 58 59 60 61 63 65 66 68 69 70 71 72 73 74 75 76 78 79 **P**6 Web address: www.swedish.org	23	10	601	30606	425	462319	4846	446688	186346	3865

Many Facility Codes have changed. Please refer to the AHA Guide Code Chart.

Hospitals, U.S. / WASHINGTON

Hospital, Address, Telephone, Administrator, Approval, Facility, and Physician Codes, Health Care System, Network	Classification Codes		Utilization Data					Expense (thousands) of dollars		
★ American Hospital Association (AHA) membership □ Joint Commission on Accreditation of Healthcare Organizations (JCAHO) accreditation + American Osteopathic Healthcare Association (AOHA) membership ○ American Osteopathic Association (AOA) accreditation △ Commission on Accreditation of Rehabilitation Facilities (CARF) accreditation Control codes 61, 63, 64, 71, 72 and 73 indicate hospitals listed by AOHA, but not registered by AHA. For definition of numerical codes, see page A4	Control	Service	Staffed Beds	Admissions	Census	Outpatient Visits	Births	Total	Payroll	Personnel
✠ △ UNIVERSITY OF WASHINGTON MEDICAL CENTER, 1959 Northeast Pacific Street, Box 356151, Zip 98195–6151; tel. 206/598–3300; Robert H. Muilenburg, Executive Director **A**1 2 3 5 7 8 9 10 **F**4 5 7 8 9 11 16 17 18 22 23 24 25 27 29 32 33 34 35 38 39 41 42 43 44 45 46 47 48 49 50 51 53 54 55 56 57 59 60 61 62 63 64 65 66 68 70 71 72 74 76 77 78 79 **P**6 **Web address:** www.washington.edu/medical	12	10	376	15548	273	353782	1339	320749	126846	2859
□ VENCOR HOSPITAL SEATTLE, (LONG TERM ACUTE CARE), 10560 Fifth Avenue N.E., Zip 98125–0977; tel. 206/364–2050; Jim Steinruck, CHE, Administrator and Chief Executive Officer **A**1 9 10 **F**13 18 70 76 **S** Vencor, Incorporated, Louisville, KY **Web address:** www.vencor.com	33	49	42	248	26	32	0	10373	3939	104
✠ △ VETERANS AFFAIRS PUGET SOUND HEALTH CARE SYSTEM, (Includes Veterans Affairs Puget Sound Health Care System–American Lake Division, Tacoma, Zip 98493; tel. 253/582–8440), 1660 South Columbian Way, Zip 98108–1597; tel. 206/762–1010; Timothy B. Williams, Director (Total facility includes 132 beds in nursing home–type unit) (Nonreporting) **A**1 3 5 7 8 9 **S** Department of Veterans Affairs, Washington, DC	45	10	557	—	—	—	—	—	—	—
✠ △ VIRGINIA MASON MEDICAL CENTER, 1100 Ninth Avenue, Zip 98101, Mailing Address: P.O. Box 900, Zip 98111–0900; tel. 206/223–6600; J. Michael Rona, President (Total facility includes 23 beds in nursing home–type unit) **A**1 2 3 5 7 9 10 **F**1 3 4 5 7 8 9 11 12 13 16 18 20 21 22 24 25 27 30 33 34 35 38 39 41 43 45 46 47 48 49 50 51 53 54 56 58 59 61 63 65 66 69 70 71 72 74 76 77 78 79 **P**6 **Web address:** www.vmmc.org	23	10	305	16271	241	—	0	442845	226363	4737
SEDRO WOOLLEY—Skagit County UNITED GENERAL HOSPITAL See Affiliated Health Services, Mount Vernon										
SHELTON—Mason County □ MASON GENERAL HOSPITAL, 901 Mountainview Drive, Zip 98584–1668, Mailing Address: P.O. Box 1668, Zip 98584–1668; tel. 360/426–1611; G. Robert Appel, Administrator **A**1 9 10 **F**8 12 13 17 18 22 24 25 32 41 44 45 46 48 54 69 70 76 78 **P**3	16	10	51	2430	20	48011	293	20423	9836	222
SOUTH BEND—Pacific County WILLAPA HARBOR HOSPITAL, 800 Alder Street, Zip 98586–0438, Mailing Address: P.O. Box 438, Zip 98586–0438; tel. 360/875–4502; Moe Chaudry, Chief Executive Officer **A**9 10 **F**6 7 8 9 11 13 14 16 17 18 19 22 25 31 32 34 46 48 50 51 56 70 75 76 77	16	10	18	589	5	8833	55	6744	3458	94
SPOKANE—Spokane County ✠ DEACONESS MEDICAL CENTER–SPOKANE, 800 West Fifth Avenue, Zip 99204, Mailing Address: P.O. Box 248, Zip 99210–0248; tel. 509/458–5800; Thomas J. Zellers, Chief Operating Officer **A**1 2 3 5 10 **F**1 2 3 4 5 6 7 8 9 10 11 12 13 15 16 17 18 19 20 21 22 23 24 25 26 27 28 29 30 31 32 33 34 35 36 37 38 39 40 41 42 43 44 45 46 47 48 49 50 52 53 54 55 58 59 60 61 62 63 64 65 66 67 68 69 70 71 72 73 74 75 76 77 78 79 **P**8 **S** Empire Health Services, Spokane, WA **Web address:** www.deaconess–spokane.org	23	10	326	13609	174	150395	2650	143085	55048	1410
✠ HOLY FAMILY HOSPITAL, North 5633 Lidgerwood Avenue, Zip 99207–2533; tel. 509/482–0111; Thomas Corley, President and Chief Executive Officer **A**1 2 9 10 **F**1 2 3 4 6 7 8 9 10 11 12 13 17 18 19 22 24 25 26 27 30 31 32 33 34 36 37 39 41 42 43 44 45 46 47 48 49 50 51 52 53 54 56 57 58 59 60 61 62 63 64 65 68 69 70 71 72 73 74 75 76 77 78 79 **P**5 **S** Providence Services, Spokane, WA **Web address:** www.holy–family.org	21	10	190	8089	85	75469	1024	68497	29270	707
✠ SACRED HEART MEDICAL CENTER, West 101 Eighth Avenue, Zip 99220–2555, Mailing Address: P.O. Box 2555, Zip 99220–2555; tel. 509/474–3040; Ryland P. Davis, President and Chief Executive Officer **A**1 2 3 5 9 10 **F**1 2 4 6 7 8 9 10 11 13 17 18 22 24 25 26 28 29 31 32 36 38 39 41 42 44 46 47 48 49 50 51 52 53 54 55 57 58 61 62 63 64 65 68 69 70 74 75 76 78 79 **P**6 **S** Providence Services, Spokane, WA **Web address:** www.shmc.org	21	10	607	23255	341	—	2016	289632	127974	2690
□ SHRINERS HOSPITALS FOR CHILDREN–SPOKANE, 911 West Fifth Avenue, Zip 99204–2901, Mailing Address: P.O. Box 2472, Zip 99210–2472; tel. 509/455–7844; Charles R. Young, Administrator **A**1 3 **F**13 16 17 18 19 38 43 49 50 51 53 54 70 71 78 **S** Shriners Hospitals for Children, Tampa, FL **Web address:** www.shrinershq.org	23	50	30	680	10	8087	0	—	—	—
□ △ ST. LUKES REHABILITATION INSTITUTE, 711 South Cowley Street, Zip 99202; tel. 509/838–4771; Thomas M. Fritz, Administrator (Nonreporting) **A**1 7 10 **Web address:** www.stlukesrehab.org	23	46	72	—	—	—	—	—	—	—
✠ VALLEY HOSPITAL AND MEDICAL CENTER, 12606 East Mission Avenue, Zip 99216–1090; tel. 509/924–6650; Michael T. Liepman, Chief Operating Officer (Nonreporting) **A**1 2 10 **S** Empire Health Services, Spokane, WA	23	10	117	—	—	—	—	—	—	—
✠ VETERANS AFFAIRS MEDICAL CENTER, North 4815 Assembly Street, Zip 99205–6197; tel. 509/434–7200; Joseph M. Manley, Director (Total facility includes 44 beds in nursing home–type unit) **A**1 **F**1 3 4 9 11 13 16 22 23 24 25 26 27 30 31 35 36 37 38 39 41 46 47 48 49 50 51 54 55 56 58 59 60 61 62 63 64 65 66 69 70 72 74 76 77 78 79 **P**6 **S** Department of Veterans Affairs, Washington, DC **Web address:** www.va.gov/stations97/guide/home.asp?DIVISION=ALL	45	10	86	2033	62	132806	0	—	—	519

© 2000 AHA Guide *Many Facility Codes have changed. Please refer to the AHA Guide Code Chart.*

Hospitals, U.S. / WASHINGTON

★ American Hospital Association (AHA) membership
☐ Joint Commission on Accreditation of Healthcare Organizations (JCAHO) accreditation
+ American Osteopathic Healthcare Association (AOHA) membership
○ American Osteopathic Association (AOA) accreditation
△ Commission on Accreditation of Rehabilitation Facilities (CARF) accreditation
Control codes 61, 63, 64, 71, 72 and 73 indicate hospitals listed by AOHA, but not registered by AHA. For definition of numerical codes, see page A4

Hospital, Address, Telephone, Administrator, Approval, Facility, and Physician Codes, Health Care System, Network	Classification Codes		Utilization Data					Expense (thousands) of dollars		
	Control	Service	Staffed Beds	Admissions	Census	Outpatient Visits	Births	Total	Payroll	Personnel

SUNNYSIDE—Yakima County

★ + ○ SUNNYSIDE COMMUNITY HOSPITAL, 10th and Tacoma Avenue, Zip 98944–0719, Mailing Address: P.O. Box 719, Zip 98944–0719; tel. 509/837–1650; Jon D. Smiley, Chief Executive Officer **A**2 9 10 11 **F**7 8 9 13 19 22 24 25 27 32 33 34 36 37 38 39 41 43 44 46 48 50 51 56 70 72 73 75 76 78 **S** Brim Healthcare, Inc., Brentwood, TN
Web address: www.televar.com/sch — 23 10 38 1890 17 51589 540 — 7490 175

TACOMA—Pierce County

ALLENMORE HOSPITAL See Tacoma General Hospital

★ MADIGAN ARMY MEDICAL CENTER, Zip 98431–5000; tel. 253/968–1110; Brigadier General Mack C. Hill, Commanding General (Nonreporting) **A**1 2 3 5 **S** Department of the Army, Office of the Surgeon General, Falls Church, VA
Web address: www.mamc.amedd.army.mil — 42 10 216 — — — — — — —

☐ MARY BRIDGE CHILDREN'S HOSPITAL AND HEALTH CENTER, 317 Martin Luther King Jr. Way, Zip 98405–0299, Mailing Address: Box 5299, Zip 98405–0299; tel. 253/403–1400; Diane Cecchettini, President and Chief Executive Officer **A**1 3 5 9 10 **F**1 4 8 9 11 12 13 14 19 20 21 22 24 25 29 30 32 33 34 35 36 37 38 39 41 42 43 44 45 46 47 48 49 52 54 55 56 59 65 66 68 70 72 73 75 76 77 78 79 **P**1 5 6 **S** MultiCare Health System, Tacoma, WA
Web address: www.multicare.com — 23 50 72 3194 34 177944 0 39661 18656 403

★ PUGET SOUND HOSPITAL, 215 South 36th Street, Zip 98408–6853, Mailing Address: P.O. Box 11412, Zip 98411–0412; tel. 253/474–0561; C. Mark Gregson, Chief Executive Officer (Nonreporting) **A**1 9 10 **S** New American Healthcare Corporation, Brentwood, TN
Web address: www.puretsound.nahc.net — 33 10 146 — — — — — — —

ST. CLARE HOSPITAL See Lakewood

★ △ ST. JOSEPH MEDICAL CENTER, 1717 South J Street, Zip 98405–3004, Mailing Address: P.O. Box 2197, Zip 98401–2197; tel. 253/627–4101; June C. Bowman, R.N., Chief Operating Officer and Nurse Executive **A**1 2 7 9 10 **F**2 4 6 7 8 9 10 11 12 13 16 17 18 19 20 21 22 23 24 25 26 27 28 29 30 31 32 33 34 35 36 37 38 39 41 43 44 45 46 47 48 49 50 51 53 54 56 57 59 61 62 63 64 65 66 68 69 70 72 74 75 76 77 78 79 **P**2 5 8 **S** Catholic Health Initiatives, Denver, CO — 21 10 283 15349 182 196987 2707 181466 73126 1868

★ TACOMA GENERAL HOSPITAL, (Includes Allenmore Hospital, South 19th and Union Avenue, Zip 98405, Mailing Address: P.O. Box 11414, Zip 98411–0414; tel. 253/403–2323), 315 Martin Luther King Jr. Way, Zip 98405–0299, Mailing Address: P.O. Box 5299, Zip 98405–0299; tel. 253/403–1000; Diane Cecchettini, President and Chief Executive Officer **A**1 2 3 5 9 10 **F**1 4 8 9 11 12 13 14 19 21 22 24 25 29 30 32 33 34 35 36 37 38 39 41 42 43 44 45 46 47 48 49 50 51 52 54 55 56 59 65 66 68 70 72 73 75 76 77 78 79 **P**1 5 6 **S** MultiCare Health System, Tacoma, WA
Web address: www.multicare.org — 23 10 377 17015 226 366641 3439 216379 83073 1862

VETERANS AFFAIRS PUGET SOUND HEALTH CARE SYSTEM–AMERICAN LAKE DIVISION See Veterans Affairs Puget Sound Health Care System, Seattle

☐ WESTERN STATE HOSPITAL, 9601 Steilacoom Boulevard S.W., Zip 98498; tel. 253/582–8900; Jerry Lovrien, Chief Executive Officer (Nonreporting) **A**1 10 — 12 22 835 — — — — — — —

TONASKET—Okanogan County

NORTH VALLEY HOSPITAL, 203 South Western Avenue, Zip 98855; tel. 509/486–2151; Warner H. Bartleson, Administrator (Total facility includes 70 beds in nursing home–type unit) (Nonreporting) **A**9 10 — 16 10 92 — — — — — — —

TOPPENISH—Yakima County

★ PROVIDENCE TOPPENISH HOSPITAL, 502 West Fourth Avenue, Zip 98948–0672, Mailing Address: P.O. Box 672, Zip 98948–0672; tel. 509/865–3105; Larry Anthony, Administrator **A**1 9 10 **F**7 8 9 16 17 18 19 22 24 25 36 37 38 41 44 45 48 51 56 70 72 75 76 78 79 **S** Providence Health System, Seattle, WA
Web address: www.providence.org — 21 10 48 2079 17 54634 565 14533 5967 160

VANCOUVER—Clark County

★ △ SOUTHWEST WASHINGTON MEDICAL CENTER, (Includes Vancouver Memorial Campus, 3400 Main Street, Zip 98663; tel. 206/696–5000), 400 N.E. Mother Joseph Place, Zip 98664, Mailing Address: P.O. Box 1600, Zip 98668; tel. 360/256–2000; Geoffrey N. Lang, President and Chief Executive Officer **A**1 2 3 7 9 10 **F**4 7 8 9 11 13 16 17 18 19 22 24 25 26 27 32 33 34 35 36 37 38 39 41 43 44 45 46 47 48 49 50 51 53 54 55 56 57 60 61 62 63 64 65 70 71 72 75 76 77 78 **P**1 5 7
Web address: www.swmedctr.com — 23 10 279 18355 177 199416 4397 181638 86362 1944

WALLA WALLA—Walla Walla County

★ JONATHAN M. WAINWRIGHT MEMORIAL VA MEDICAL CENTER, 77 Wainwright Drive, Zip 99362–3994; tel. 509/525–5200; Roxanne Sisemore, Acting Director (Total facility includes 30 beds in nursing home–type unit) **A**1 **F**2 3 9 12 13 16 18 19 22 23 25 26 29 31 34 35 39 41 43 46 48 50 51 54 57 59 61 63 64 65 66 69 70 72 76 78 79 **P**6 **S** Department of Veterans Affairs, Washington, DC
Web address: www.va.gov/stations97/guide/home.asp?DIVISION=ALL — 45 10 76 1054 39 56671 — — — 307

★ △ ST. MARY MEDICAL CENTER, 401 West Poplar Street, Zip 99362–1477, Mailing Address: Box 1477, Zip 99362–1477; tel. 509/525–3320; John A. Isely, President **A**1 2 7 9 10 **F**8 9 16 22 25 32 34 35 36 39 41 42 43 44 45 46 48 53 54 57 61 62 63 65 70 75 76 77 78 79 **P**6 **S** Providence Services, Spokane, WA — 21 10 107 4036 55 79718 515 57421 28691 750

Hospitals, U.S. / WASHINGTON

Hospital, Address, Telephone, Administrator, Approval, Facility, and Physician Codes, Health Care System, Network	Classification Codes		Utilization Data					Expense (thousands) of dollars		
★ American Hospital Association (AHA) membership ☐ Joint Commission on Accreditation of Healthcare Organizations (JCAHO) accreditation + American Osteopathic Healthcare Association (AOHA) membership ○ American Osteopathic Association (AOA) accreditation △ Commission on Accreditation of Rehabilitation Facilities (CARF) accreditation Control codes 61, 63, 64, 71, 72 and 73 indicate hospitals listed by AOHA, but not registered by AHA. For definition of numerical codes, see page A4	Control	Service	Staffed Beds	Admissions	Census	Outpatient Visits	Births	Total	Payroll	Personnel
STATE PENITENTIARY HOSPITAL, Mailing Address: Box 520, Zip 99362; tel. 509/525-3610; Pat Rima, Health Care Manager (Nonreporting)	12	11	36	—	—	—	—	—	—	—
★ WALLA WALLA GENERAL HOSPITAL, 1025 South Second Avenue, Zip 99362-1398, Mailing Address: Box 1398, Zip 99362-1398; tel. 509/525-0480; Morre Dean, President (Nonreporting) **A**1 2 9 10 **S** Adventist Health, Roseville, CA **Web address:** www.wwgh.com	21	10	72	—	—	—	—	—	—	—
WENATCHEE—Chelan County										
★ CENTRAL WASHINGTON HOSPITAL, 1201 South Miller Street, Zip 98801-1948, Mailing Address: P.O. Box 1887, Zip 98807-1887; tel. 509/662-1511; John T. Evans, Jr, President and Chief Executive Officer (Total facility includes 22 beds in nursing home-type unit) **A**1 9 10 **F**4 7 8 9 11 12 13 16 17 18 19 22 25 26 27 32 33 36 37 38 39 40 41 42 43 44 45 46 48 49 50 51 56 69 70 72 75 76 78 79 **P**8 **Web address:** www.cwhs.com	23	10	133	7724	87	119114	1336	71060	34111	753
WHITE SALMON—Klickitat County										
SKYLINE HOSPITAL, 211 Skyline Drive, Zip 98672-0099, Mailing Address: Box 99, Zip 98672-0099; tel. 509/493-1101; Michael J. Madden, Superintendent and Chief Executive Officer **A**9 10 **F**8 9 10 11 12 17 18 25 37 38 41 42 44 48 52 56 69 75 **P**5 **Web address:** www.skylinehospital.com	16	10	24	731	6	13520	114	6385	3523	113
YAKIMA—Yakima County										
★ △ PROVIDENCE YAKIMA MEDICAL CENTER, 110 South Ninth Avenue, Zip 98902-3397; tel. 509/575-5000; Andrew S. Robertson, M.D., Chief Executive Officer **A**1 2 3 7 9 10 **F**4 8 9 11 12 16 17 18 19 22 24 25 27 32 33 34 36 37 38 39 41 44 45 46 47 48 49 50 51 53 54 56 67 64 68 69 70 72 75 76 78 79 **P**6 **S** Providence Health System, Seattle, WA **Web address:** www.providence.org	21	10	197	6530	78	213750	630	91008	38298	896
★ YAKIMA VALLEY MEMORIAL HOSPITAL, 2811 Tieton Drive, Zip 98902-3761; tel. 509/575-8000; Richard W. Linneweh, Jr, President and Chief Executive Officer (Total facility includes 86 beds in nursing home-type unit) **A**1 2 3 9 10 **F**7 8 9 11 13 14 16 17 18 19 22 26 32 33 34 36 37 38 39 41 42 43 44 45 46 48 50 51 54 57 59 61 63 65 68 69 70 71 72 75 76 78 79 **P**4 **Web address:** www.yvmh.org	23	10	296	11095	187	163366	2408	96210	20514	1055

Hospitals, U.S. / WEST VIRGINIA

WEST VIRGINIA

Resident Population 1,811 (in thousands)
Resident population in metro areas 41.8%
Birth rate per 1,000 population 11.4
65 years and over 15.2%
Percent of persons without health insurance 17.2%

Hospital, Address, Telephone, Administrator, Approval, Facility, and Physician Codes, Health Care System, Network	Classification Codes		Utilization Data					Expense (thousands) of dollars		
	Control	Service	Staffed Beds	Admissions	Census	Outpatient Visits	Births	Total	Payroll	Personnel

★ American Hospital Association (AHA) membership
☐ Joint Commission on Accreditation of Healthcare Organizations (JCAHO) accreditation
+ American Osteopathic Healthcare Association (AOHA) membership
○ American Osteopathic Association (AOA) accreditation
△ Commission on Accreditation of Rehabilitation Facilities (CARF) accreditation
Control codes 61, 63, 64, 71, 72 and 73 indicate hospitals listed by AOHA, but not registered by AHA. For definition of numerical codes, see page A4

BECKLEY—Raleigh County

☐ BECKLEY APPALACHIAN REGIONAL HOSPITAL, 306 Stanaford Road, Zip 25801-3142; tel. 304/255-3000; David R. Lyon, Administrator **A**1 9 10 **F**1 3 4 9 12 13 17 18 19 21 22 24 25 30 32 33 34 35 36 39 41 43 46 48 49 54 57 58 59 60 61 62 63 64 68 70 76 78 **P**6 **S** Appalachian Regional Healthcare, Lexington, KY	23	10	173	8400	136	26400	0	50899	20884	654
✠ RALEIGH GENERAL HOSPITAL, (Formerly Columbia Raleigh General Hospital), 1710 Harper Road, Zip 25801-3397; tel. 304/256-4100; David B. Darden, Chief Executive Officer **A**1 9 10 13 **F**8 9 11 13 17 18 19 22 24 25 27 29 32 34 37 38 39 41 43 44 45 46 48 51 54 68 70 71 72 75 76 77 78 79 **S** HCA - The Healthcare Company, Nashville, TN Web address: www.raleighgeneral.com	33	10	325	12224	164	98414	1658	68147	27906	959
✠ VETERANS AFFAIRS MEDICAL CENTER, 200 Veterans Avenue, Zip 25801-6499; tel. 304/255-2121; Gerard P. Husson, Director (Total facility includes 50 beds in nursing home-type unit) **A**1 **F**3 22 23 25 31 32 33 34 35 41 45 46 48 51 54 56 63 65 70 76 78 79 **S** Department of Veterans Affairs, Washington, DC Web address: www.va.gov/stations97/guide/home.asp?DIVISION=ALL	45	10	90	2059	78	85345	0	37825	17293	413

BERKELEY SPRINGS—Morgan County

★ MORGAN COUNTY WAR MEMORIAL HOSPITAL, 1124 Fairfax Street, Zip 25411-1718; tel. 304/258-1234; Patrick Nolan, Administrator (Total facility includes 16 beds in nursing home-type unit) **A**9 10 **F**9 17 18 22 23 25 31 32 34 36 37 38 48 50 51 54 69 70 72 76 78 **S** Valley Health System, Winchester, VA Web address: www.valleyhealthlink.com	13	10	44	949	29	19250	0	8010	3104	105

BLUEFIELD—Mercer County

✠ BLUEFIELD REGIONAL MEDICAL CENTER, 500 Cherry Street, Zip 24701-3390; tel. 304/327-1100; Eugene P. Pawlowski, President **A**1 9 10 **F**8 9 11 12 13 14 16 17 18 22 24 25 28 34 36 38 39 41 43 44 45 46 48 49 54 55 65 68 69 70 76 77 78 **P**8 Web address: www.bluefield.org	23	10	265	8394	137	125451	812	71769	30815	948
✠ ST. LUKE'S HOSPITAL, 1333 Southview Drive, Zip 24701-4399, Mailing Address: P.O. Box 1190, Zip 24701-1190; tel. 304/327-2900; Deane E. Beamer, President and Chief Executive Officer **A**1 9 10 **F**9 13 16 17 18 22 24 25 27 34 39 41 43 45 48 54 59 61 68 70 72 76 78 Web address: www.columbiastlukes.com	33	10	52	857	28	8983	—	5901	2295	217

BUCKEYE—Pocahontas County

★ POCAHONTAS MEMORIAL HOSPITAL, Mailing Address: Rural Route 2, Box 52 W, Zip 24924; tel. 304/799-7400; Ivan Withers, Chief Executive Officer **A**9 10 **F**7 9 16 17 18 22 24 25 30 32 33 34 36 38 45 48 50 51 54 56 70 76 77 78	13	10	27	761	15	21364	0	4398	1788	85

BUCKHANNON—Upshur County

✠ ST. JOSEPH'S HOSPITAL OF BUCKHANNON, Amalia Drive, Zip 26201-2222; tel. 304/473-2000; Wayne B. Griffith, FACHE, Chief Executive Officer (Total facility includes 16 beds in nursing home-type unit) **A**1 9 10 **F**2 7 8 9 13 16 17 18 19 22 25 26 31 32 33 34 36 37 38 39 43 48 50 51 54 57 60 61 62 63 69 70 72 75 76 77 78 **P**7 8 Web address: www.stj.net	23	10	95	2499	38	38666	251	18238	7411	287

CHARLESTON—Kanawha County

✠ △ CHARLESTON AREA MEDICAL CENTER, (Includes General Division, 501 Morris Street, Zip 25301, Mailing Address: Box 1393, Zip 25325; tel. 304/348-5432; Memorial Division, 3200 MacCorkle Avenue S.E., Zip 25304; tel. 304/348-5432; Women and Children's Hospital, 800 Pennsylvania Avenue, Zip 25302; tel. 304/348-5432), 501 Morris Street, Zip 25301-1300, Mailing Address: P.O. Box 1547, Zip 25326-1547; tel. 304/348-5432; Phillip H. Goodwin, FACHE, President and Chief Executive Officer **A**1 2 3 5 7 8 9 10 **F**3 4 5 6 7 8 9 11 12 13 14 16 17 18 19 20 21 22 23 24 25 26 27 28 29 30 31 32 33 34 35 37 38 39 40 41 42 43 44 45 46 47 48 49 50 51 52 53 54 56 57 58 59 60 61 62 63 64 65 66 68 69 70 71 72 73 74 75 76 77 78 79 **P**3 6 7 **S** Camcare, Inc., Charleston, WV Web address: www.camcare.com	23	10	765	34838	547	416603	3159	400172	135462	4429
✠ EYE AND EAR CLINIC OF CHARLESTON, 1306 Kanawha Boulevard East, Zip 25301, Mailing Address: P.O. Box 2271, Zip 25328-2271; tel. 304/343-4371; W. Allen Shelton, II, Administrator and Chief Executive Officer **A**1 9 10 **F**48 74 **P**6 Web address: www.eyeandearclinicwv.com	33	45	26	35	0	5062	0	4400	1729	60
GENERAL DIVISION See Charleston Area Medical Center										
✠ HIGHLAND HOSPITAL, 300 56th Street S.E., Zip 25304-2361, Mailing Address: P.O. Box 4107, Zip 25364-4107; tel. 304/926-1600; David M. McWatters, Administrator **A**1 5 9 10 **F**18 29 30 32 33 36 43 57 58 59 60 61 62 63 64 70 **P**6 Web address: www.highlandhosp.com	23	22	58	967	24	1587	—	8686	4348	171
MEMORIAL DIVISION See Charleston Area Medical Center										

Hospitals, U.S. / WEST VIRGINIA

Hospital, Address, Telephone, Administrator, Approval, Facility, and Physician Codes, Health Care System, Network	Classification Codes		Utilization Data					Expense (thousands) of dollars		
★ American Hospital Association (AHA) membership □ Joint Commission on Accreditation of Healthcare Organizations (JCAHO) accreditation + American Osteopathic Healthcare Association (AOHA) membership ○ American Osteopathic Association (AOA) accreditation △ Commission on Accreditation of Rehabilitation Facilities (CARF) accreditation Control codes 61, 63, 64, 71, 72 and 73 indicate hospitals listed by AOHA, but not registered by AHA. For definition of numerical codes, see page A4	Control	Service	Staffed Beds	Admissions	Census	Outpatient Visits	Births	Total	Payroll	Personnel
✦ SAINT FRANCIS HOSPITAL, 333 Laidley Street, Zip 25301-1628, Mailing Address: P.O. Box 471, Zip 25322-0471; tel. 304/347-6500; Dan Lauffer, Chief Executive Officer (Total facility includes 30 beds in nursing home–type unit) **A**1 9 10 **F**9 11 13 16 17 18 22 24 25 29 32 33 34 37 38 39 40 41 43 45 48 49 50 51 54 56 65 69 70 71 76 78 **S** HCA – The Healthcare Company, Nashville, TN WOMEN AND CHILDREN'S HOSPITAL See Charleston Area Medical Center	33	10	151	5055	86	61917	0	43335	17263	561
CLARKSBURG—Harrison County										
✦ LOUIS A. JOHNSON VETERANS AFFAIRS MEDICAL CENTER, 1 Medical Center Drive, Zip 26301-4199; tel. 304/623-3461; Michael W. Neusch, FACHE, Director (Nonreporting) **A**1 2 3 5 9 **S** Department of Veterans Affairs, Washington, DC	45	10	160	—	—	—	—	—	—	—
✦ UNITED HOSPITAL CENTER, Route 19 South, Zip 26301, Mailing Address: P.O. Box 1680, Zip 26302-1680; tel. 304/624-2121; Bruce C. Carter, President (Total facility includes 51 beds in nursing home–type unit) **A**1 2 3 5 9 10 12 13 **F**3 6 7 8 9 11 12 13 17 18 20 21 22 23 24 25 26 27 29 32 34 36 37 38 39 41 44 45 46 48 49 50 51 54 56 57 58 59 60 61 62 63 65 67 68 69 70 72 76 78 **P**6 8 **S** West Virginia United Health System, Fairmont, WV Web address: www.uhcwv.org	23	10	367	13569	256	336311	897	99528	43696	1340
ELKINS—Randolph County										
✦ DAVIS MEMORIAL HOSPITAL, Gorman Avenue and Reed Street, Zip 26241, Mailing Address: P.O. Box 1484, Zip 26241-1484; tel. 304/636-3300; Robert L. Hammer, II, Chief Executive Officer **A**1 9 10 **F**2 3 4 6 7 8 9 10 11 12 13 16 18 22 24 25 27 28 29 30 31 32 33 34 35 36 37 38 39 40 41 42 43 44 45 46 47 48 51 52 53 54 55 57 58 59 60 61 62 63 64 65 68 69 70 74 75 76 78 **P**7 8 **S** West Virginia United Health System, Fairmont, WV Web address: www.davishealthcare.com	23	10	115	6141	64	120221	540	45358	19241	580
FAIRMONT—Marion County										
✦ FAIRMONT GENERAL HOSPITAL, 1325 Locust Avenue, Zip 26554-1435; tel. 304/367-7100; Richard W. Graham, FACHE, President and Chief Executive Officer (Total facility includes 25 beds in nursing home–type unit) **A**1 9 10 **F**2 3 8 9 11 12 13 18 19 22 24 25 27 31 32 33 34 35 37 39 40 43 44 45 46 48 51 54 57 59 60 61 62 63 64 68 69 70 71 72 76 78 79 **P**4 7 **S** Quorum Health Group, Brentwood, TN Web address: www.fghi.com	23	10	181	6723	101	142092	507	46255	19134	576
GASSAWAY—Braxton County										
★ BRAXTON COUNTY MEMORIAL HOSPITAL, 100 Hoylman Drive, Zip 26624-9320; tel. 304/364-5156; Tony E. Atkins, Administrator **A**9 10 **F**7 9 14 17 18 19 22 24 25 28 32 33 35 36 38 39 48 54 56 66 70 71 76 79 **S** Camcare, Inc., Charleston, WV Web address: www.pihn.org	23	10	25	746	7	19091	—	6861	2933	124
GLEN DALE—Marshall County										
✦ REYNOLDS MEMORIAL HOSPITAL, 800 Wheeling Avenue, Zip 26038-1697; tel. 304/845-3211; John Sicurella, Chief Executive Officer (Total facility includes 20 beds in nursing home–type unit) **A**1 6 9 10 **F**1 3 7 8 9 16 17 18 22 24 25 26 28 30 32 33 34 36 37 38 39 41 43 44 45 46 48 49 50 51 54 58 59 60 61 62 63 64 65 68 69 70 75 76 78 **P**8 Web address: www.reymem.com	23	10	140	3185	56	74412	83	27850	12373	416
GRAFTON—Taylor County										
□ GRAFTON CITY HOSPITAL, 500 Market Street, Zip 26354-1187; tel. 304/265-0400; Gary R. Willmon, Administrator (Total facility includes 76 beds in nursing home–type unit) **A**1 9 18 **F**7 9 12 13 16 17 18 22 24 25 28 29 30 31 32 33 34 36 37 38 41 43 45 46 48 50 51 54 56 69 70 71 73 75 76 77 78 79 **P**6 Web address: www.gchospital@aol.com	14	10	110	1366	85	16160	0	11245	5099	256
GRANTSVILLE—Calhoun County										
MINNIE HAMILTON HEALTHCARE CENTER, High Street, Zip 26147, Mailing Address: Route 1, Box 1A, Zip 26147; tel. 304/354-9244; Barbara Lay, Administrator (Total facility includes 24 beds in nursing home–type unit) **A**9 10 18 **F**7 9 14 17 18 19 21 22 23 24 25 28 29 32 33 34 35 38 43 50 54 56 58 59 60 61 62 63 69 70 72 73 75 76 78 79 **P**6	23	10	42	335	26	35279	0	7471	3994	133
HINTON—Summers County										
SUMMERS COUNTY APPALACHIAN REGIONAL HOSPITAL, Terrace Street, Zip 25951, Mailing Address: Drawer 940, Zip 25951-0940; tel. 304/466-1000; Rocco K. Massey, Administrator (Total facility includes 24 beds in nursing home–type unit) **A**9 10 **F**7 9 13 16 17 18 19 22 25 32 34 38 41 48 51 54 56 69 70 76 78 79 **S** Appalachian Regional Healthcare, Lexington, KY Web address: www.arh.org	23	10	50	853	34	50773	0	8992	4669	138
HUNTINGTON—Cabell County										
✦ CABELL HUNTINGTON HOSPITAL, 1340 Hal Greer Boulevard, Zip 25701-0195; tel. 304/526-2000; W. Don Smith, II, President and Chief Executive Officer (Total facility includes 15 beds in nursing home–type unit) **A**1 3 5 9 10 **F**2 3 4 7 8 9 10 11 12 13 17 18 19 22 23 24 25 26 27 30 32 33 34 35 36 37 38 39 41 42 43 44 45 46 47 48 49 50 51 52 54 56 57 58 59 60 61 62 64 65 66 68 69 70 71 72 75 76 78 79 **P**8 Web address: www.chhi.org	23	10	293	15404	185	235672	2275	118734	51519	1384

Hospitals, U.S. / WEST VIRGINIA

Hospital, Address, Telephone, Administrator, Approval, Facility, and Physician Codes, Health Care System, Network	Classification Codes		Utilization Data					Expense (thousands) of dollars		
★ American Hospital Association (AHA) membership ☐ Joint Commission on Accreditation of Healthcare Organizations (JCAHO) accreditation + American Osteopathic Healthcare Association (AOHA) membership ○ American Osteopathic Association (AOA) accreditation △ Commission on Accreditation of Rehabilitation Facilities (CARF) accreditation Control codes 61, 63, 64, 71, 72 and 73 indicate hospitals listed by AOHA, but not registered by AHA. For definition of numerical codes, see page A4	Control	Service	Staffed Beds	Admissions	Census	Outpatient Visits	Births	Total	Payroll	Personnel
★ COLUMBIA RIVER PARK HOSPITAL, 1230 Sixth Avenue, Zip 25701–2312, Mailing Address: P.O. Box 1875, Zip 25719–1875; tel. 304/526–9111; Scott C. Stamm, Chief Executive Officer **A**1 9 10 **F**18 19 21 25 32 34 57 58 59 60 61 62 63 **S** HCA – The Healthcare Company, Nashville, TN Web address: www.hcahealthcare.com	33	22	125	1747	65	—	—	11184	5022	196
☐ △ HEALTHSOUTH HUNTINGTON REHABILITATION HOSPITAL, 6900 West Country Club Drive, Zip 25705–2000; tel. 304/733–1060; John Forester, Chief Operating Officer **A**1 7 10 **F**13 16 17 18 30 32 45 49 53 54 70 71 **S** HEALTHSOUTH Corporation, Birmingham, AL	33	46	40	737	37	8637	0	10530	3835	120
☐ MILDRED MITCHELL–BATEMAN HOSPITAL, (Formerly Huntington State Hospital), 1530 Norway Avenue, Zip 25705–1358, Mailing Address: P.O. Box 448, Zip 25709–0448; tel. 304/525–7801; Jack C. Clohan, Jr, Interim Administrator **A**1 9 10 **F**3 13 16 17 18 29 50 57 58 60 61 62 70 72 78 Web address: www.state.wv.us/newhh/	12	22	90	626	78	0	0	12781	6713	303
★ ST. MARY'S HOSPITAL, 2900 First Avenue, Zip 25702–1272; tel. 304/526–1234; J. Thomas Jones, Executive Director (Total facility includes 38 beds in nursing home–type unit) **A**1 2 3 5 6 9 10 **F**3 4 7 8 9 11 12 13 17 18 19 22 24 25 27 30 32 33 34 36 38 39 41 43 44 45 46 47 48 49 50 51 54 56 57 58 59 60 61 62 64 65 68 69 70 72 75 76 78 79 **P**2 8 Web address: www.st-marys.org	21	10	403	17824	280	147424	693	158926	64600	1810
★ VETERANS AFFAIRS MEDICAL CENTER, 1540 Spring Valley Drive, Zip 25704–9300; tel. 304/429–6741; David N. Pennington, FACHE, Chief Executive Officer **A**1 3 5 9 **F**3 4 9 11 13 16 17 18 19 22 23 24 25 26 27 29 30 31 32 33 34 35 36 37 38 39 41 43 44 46 47 48 49 50 51 54 56 59 61 62 63 65 70 72 74 76 77 78 79 **P**6 **S** Department of Veterans Affairs, Washington, DC Web address: www.va.gov	45	10	80	3297	61	170649	—	—	—	705
HURRICANE—Putnam County										
★ PUTNAM GENERAL HOSPITAL, 1400 Hospital Drive, Zip 25526–9210, Mailing Address: P.O. Box 900, Zip 25526–0900; tel. 304/757–1700; Patsy Hardy, Administrator **A**1 9 10 **F**8 9 11 13 16 17 18 22 24 25 27 32 34 38 39 41 43 44 45 48 49 51 54 70 71 76 78 **S** HCA – The Healthcare Company, Nashville, TN Web address: www.hcahealthcare.com	33	10	64	3023	43	51033	92	23293	9805	—
KEYSER—Mineral County										
☐ POTOMAC VALLEY HOSPITAL, 167 South Mineral Street, Zip 26726–2699; tel. 304/788–3141; Larry Abrams, Administrator **A**1 9 10 **F**9 12 16 22 24 25 33 34 35 36 37 41 48 49 54 68 70 72 76 78 **S** Northeast Health Management, Inc., Stevensville, MD	33	10	42	1728	16	45715	—	13248	4691	186
KINGWOOD—Preston County										
★ PRESTON MEMORIAL HOSPITAL, 300 South Price Street, Zip 26537–1495; tel. 304/329–1400; Charles Lonchar, President and Chief Executive Officer **A**1 9 10 **F**2 3 7 8 9 13 19 22 24 25 32 34 36 38 39 43 44 45 48 54 56 68 70 72 76 78 79 **S** Quorum Health Group, Brentwood, TN	23	10	56	1116	14	47570	137	10889	5061	239
LOGAN—Logan County										
GUYAN VALLEY HOSPITAL, 396 Dingess Street, Zip 25601–3695; tel. 304/792–1700; Linda Saunders, Administrator **A**10 18 **F**7 8 9 12 13 14 16 17 18 19 22 23 25 30 32 34 35 36 38 39 41 44 45 48 51 53 54 70 75 76 78 79	23	49	15	315	9	29467	0	4448	2325	84
☐ LOGAN GENERAL HOSPITAL, 20 Hospital Drive, Zip 25601–3473; tel. 304/792–1101; Thomas J. Senker, Interim Chief Executive Officer **A**1 10 13 **F**7 17 22 24 25 26 28 34 36 37 38 39 41 44 45 46 48 49 54 56 63 70 75 76 **P**6	23	10	132	6596	81	178814	411	72533	34663	833
MADISON—Boone County										
★ BOONE MEMORIAL HOSPITAL, 701 Madison Avenue, Zip 25130–1699; tel. 304/369–1230; Tommy H. Mullins, Administrator **A**1 9 10 **F**7 16 17 18 22 24 25 36 37 39 48 54 70 76 Web address: www.wvbmh.com	13	10	38	712	13	28552	0	7388	2922	114
MAN—Logan County										
☐ MAN ARH HOSPITAL, 700 East McDonald Avenue, Zip 25635–1011; tel. 304/583–8421; Erica McDonald, Administrator **A**1 9 10 **F**9 13 16 17 18 22 24 25 29 32 33 34 35 37 38 39 41 48 54 56 60 63 68 70 76 78 **P**6 **S** Appalachian Regional Healthcare, Lexington, KY Web address: www.arh.org	23	10	46	829	8	62648	0	—	—	195
MARTINSBURG—Berkeley County										
★ CITY HOSPITAL, Dry Run Road, Zip 25401, Mailing Address: P.O. Box 1418, Zip 25402–1418; tel. 304/264–1000; Jon D. Applebaum, Chief Executive Officer (Total facility includes 19 beds in nursing home–type unit) **A**1 2 3 9 10 **F**1 2 3 7 8 9 13 18 19 21 22 24 25 27 28 30 32 33 34 35 36 37 38 39 41 43 44 45 46 48 49 50 51 54 55 57 58 59 62 63 64 65 69 70 71 72 76 78 79 **P**8	23	10	164	6873	101	86045	842	51714	21339	674
★ VETERANS AFFAIRS MEDICAL CENTER, Charles Town Road, Zip 25401–0205; tel. 304/263–0811; George Moore, Director (Total facility includes 150 beds in nursing home–type unit) (Nonreporting) **A**1 3 5 9 **S** Department of Veterans Affairs, Washington, DC Web address: www.va.gov/visn5	45	10	370	—	—	—	—	—	—	—

Hospitals, U.S. / WEST VIRGINIA

Hospital, Address, Telephone, Administrator, Approval, Facility, and Physician Codes, Health Care System, Network	Classification Codes		Utilization Data					Expense (thousands) of dollars		
★ American Hospital Association (AHA) membership □ Joint Commission on Accreditation of Healthcare Organizations (JCAHO) accreditation + American Osteopathic Healthcare Association (AOHA) membership ○ American Osteopathic Association (AOA) accreditation △ Commission on Accreditation of Rehabilitation Facilities (CARF) accreditation Control codes 61, 63, 64, 71, 72 and 73 indicate hospitals listed by AOHA, but not registered by AHA. For definition of numerical codes, see page A4	Control	Service	Staffed Beds	Admissions	Census	Outpatient Visits	Births	Total	Payroll	Personnel
MONTGOMERY—Fayette County										
✠ MONTGOMERY GENERAL HOSPITAL, 401 Sixth Avenue, Zip 25136–0270, Mailing Address: P.O. Box 270, Zip 25136–0270; tel. 304/442–5151; William R. Laird, IV, President and Chief Executive Officer (Total facility includes 44 beds in nursing home–type unit) **A**1 9 10 **F**7 9 17 18 19 22 25 26 33 36 38 39 41 48 49 51 54 56 62 69 70 71 72 78 **P**6 8 Web address: www.mghwv.org	23	10	99	1736	57	58521	0	20668	8385	255
MORGANTOWN—Monongalia County										
CHESTNUT RIDGE HOSPITAL See West Virginia University Hospitals										
□ △ HEALTHSOUTH MOUNTAINVIEW REGIONAL REHABILITATION HOSPITAL, 1160 Van Voorhis Road, Zip 26505–3435; tel. 304/598–1100; Teresa K. Stranko, Chief Executive Officer **A**1 7 10 **F**5 13 14 16 18 19 34 38 43 45 46 49 53 54 70 71 79 **S** HEALTHSOUTH Corporation, Birmingham, AL Web address: www.healthsouth.com	33	46	80	1196	76	11375	0	15173	7509	233
✠ MONONGALIA GENERAL HOSPITAL, 1200 J. D. Anderson Drive, Zip 26505–3486; tel. 304/598–1200; Robert P. Ritz, Chief Executive Officer **A**1 3 5 9 10 **F**4 6 7 8 9 11 12 13 14 15 16 17 18 19 22 24 25 26 27 28 29 32 33 34 35 36 37 38 39 41 43 46 47 48 51 54 56 59 65 66 68 70 71 72 76 77 78 79 Web address: www.monhealthsys.org	23	10	207	7742	103	95140	564	74561	31219	910
✠ WEST VIRGINIA UNIVERSITY HOSPITALS, (Includes Chestnut Ridge Hospital, 930 Chestnut Ridge Road, Zip 26505–2854; tel. 304/293–4000), Medical Center Drive, Zip 26506–4749; tel. 304/598–4000; Bruce McClymonds, President (Total facility includes 20 beds in nursing home–type unit) **A**1 2 3 5 8 9 10 **F**2 3 4 7 8 9 11 12 13 19 21 22 23 24 25 26 27 29 30 32 33 34 35 36 37 38 39 41 42 44 45 46 47 48 49 50 51 52 54 55 56 57 58 59 60 61 62 63 64 65 66 68 69 70 71 72 74 75 76 78 79 **P**6 8 **S** West Virginia United Health System, Fairmont, WV Web address: www.wvhealth.wvu.edu	23	10	401	14500	273	395200	1346	208681	77755	2426
NEW MARTINSVILLE—Wetzel County										
✠ WETZEL COUNTY HOSPITAL, 3 East Benjamin Drive, Zip 26155–2758; tel. 304/455–8000; Alvin R. Lawson, JD, CHE, Chief Executive Officer (Total facility includes 10 beds in nursing home–type unit) **A**1 9 10 **F**7 8 9 13 16 17 18 19 22 24 25 30 32 33 34 36 38 39 41 43 44 45 48 49 50 51 54 56 69 70 75 76 78 79 **P**6	13	10	49	1667	23	68948	113	14327	5716	175
OAK HILL—Fayette County										
✠ PLATEAU MEDICAL CENTER, 430 Main Street, Zip 25901–3455; tel. 304/469–8600; Hank Woodson, Administrator **A**1 9 10 **F**7 16 17 18 19 22 24 25 28 30 32 39 41 45 48 50 53 54 55 64 68 69 70 76 **P**8 **S** Camcare, Inc., Charleston, WV	23	10	74	2663	43	24953	0	16638	6926	283
PARKERSBURG—Wood County										
✠ CAMDEN–CLARK MEMORIAL HOSPITAL, 800 Garfield Avenue, Zip 26101, Mailing Address: P.O. Box 718, Zip 26102–0718; tel. 304/424–2111; Thomas J. Corder, President and Chief Executive Officer (Total facility includes 25 beds in nursing home–type unit) **A**1 2 9 10 **F**7 8 9 13 16 17 18 19 22 24 25 27 28 32 33 34 36 37 38 39 43 44 46 48 49 50 51 54 65 68 69 70 72 76 78 79 **P**7 Web address: www.ccmh.org	23	10	239	12760	160	249801	1018	89096	35110	1188
□ HEALTHSOUTH WESTERN HILLS REGIONAL REHABILITATION HOSPITAL, 3 Western Hills Drive, Zip 26101–8122; tel. 304/420–1300; Thomas Heller, Administrator **A**1 10 **F**13 16 18 19 30 31 32 34 38 43 45 49 53 54 71 72 78 **S** HEALTHSOUTH Corporation, Birmingham, AL	33	46	40	730	36	10016	0	5856	3796	125
✠ ST. JOSEPH'S HOSPITAL, 1824 Murdoch Avenue, Zip 26101–3246, Mailing Address: P.O. Box 327, Zip 26102–0327; tel. 304/424–4111; Stephens M. Mundy, Chief Executive Officer (Total facility includes 35 beds in nursing home–type unit) **A**1 9 10 **F**2 3 8 9 11 12 13 16 17 18 19 22 25 27 29 30 31 32 33 34 35 36 38 39 41 43 44 45 46 48 49 50 51 53 54 57 58 60 61 62 64 68 69 70 71 72 76 77 78 79 **P**7 Web address: www.wvha.com/web/sjh	32	10	294	8454	120	146004	498	62324	24399	911
PETERSBURG—Grant County										
★ GRANT MEMORIAL HOSPITAL, Route 55 West, Zip 26847, Mailing Address: P.O. Box 1019, Zip 26847–1019; tel. 304/257–1026; Robert L. Harman, Administrator (Total facility includes 10 beds in nursing home–type unit) **A**9 10 **F**8 9 13 14 17 19 22 23 24 25 28 30 32 34 36 37 39 41 44 46 48 49 54 69 70 72 75 76 79	13	10	61	2368	36	82140	296	20129	8423	323
PHILIPPI—Barbour County										
★ BROADDUS HOSPITAL, College Hill, Zip 26416–1051; tel. 304/457–1760; Susannah Higgins, Chief Executive Officer (Total facility includes 60 beds in nursing home–type unit) **A**10 18 **F**9 13 14 16 17 18 19 22 25 30 31 32 36 37 38 46 48 54 56 59 62 63 69 70 78 79 **P**7 8 **S** West Virginia United Health System, Fairmont, WV	23	10	72	378	58	20524	0	5955	3011	140
POINT PLEASANT—Mason County										
✠ PLEASANT VALLEY HOSPITAL, 2520 Valley Drive, Zip 25550–2083; tel. 304/675–4340; Michael G. Sellards, Executive Director (Total facility includes 100 beds in nursing home–type unit) **A**1 9 10 **F**7 8 9 13 16 17 18 19 22 25 27 28 32 33 36 37 38 39 41 43 44 45 46 47 48 49 50 51 54 56 59 63 68 69 70 72 76 77 78 **P**8 Web address: www.pvalley.org	23	10	202	4990	139	80658	171	43103	20666	746

© 2000 AHA Guide   *Many Facility Codes have changed. Please refer to the AHA Guide Code Chart.*

Hospitals, U.S. / WEST VIRGINIA

Hospital, Address, Telephone, Administrator, Approval, Facility, and Physician Codes, Health Care System, Network	Classification Codes		Utilization Data					Expense (thousands) of dollars		Personnel
★ American Hospital Association (AHA) membership □ Joint Commission on Accreditation of Healthcare Organizations (JCAHO) accreditation + American Osteopathic Healthcare Association (AOHA) membership ○ American Osteopathic Association (AOA) accreditation △ Commission on Accreditation of Rehabilitation Facilities (CARF) accreditation Control codes 61, 63, 64, 71, 72 and 73 indicate hospitals listed by AOHA, but not registered by AHA. For definition of numerical codes, see page A4	Control	Service	Staffed Beds	Admissions	Census	Outpatient Visits	Births	Total	Payroll	
PRINCETON—Mercer County										
□ △ HEALTHSOUTH SOUTHERN HILLS REHABILITATION HOSPITAL, 120 Twelfth Street, Zip 24740–2312; tel. 304/487–8000; Ken Howell, Administrator **A**1 7 10 **F**5 13 16 17 18 19 22 23 25 28 29 30 31 32 33 34 38 39 45 48 49 50 51 53 54 59 60 62 63 70 71 72 76 78 79 **S** HEALTHSOUTH Corporation, Birmingham, AL Web address: www.healthsouth.com	33	46	54	895	48	17379	0	8192	4093	131
★ PRINCETON COMMUNITY HOSPITAL, 12th Street, Zip 24740–1369, Mailing Address: P.O. Box 1369, Zip 24740–1369; tel. 304/487–7000; Daniel C. Dunmyer, Chief Executive Officer (Total facility includes 23 beds in nursing home–type unit) **A**1 2 9 10 **F**3 4 8 9 12 13 16 17 18 19 22 23 24 25 27 28 30 32 34 35 36 37 38 39 41 43 44 45 46 48 50 51 54 56 57 59 60 61 62 63 65 67 68 69 70 71 72 73 74 76 78 **P**1 4 7	14	10	211	9103	137	134857	427	67712	30440	976
RANSON—Jefferson County										
★ JEFFERSON MEMORIAL HOSPITAL, 300 South Preston Street, Zip 25438–1699; tel. 304/728–1600; John M. Sherwood, FACHE, Chief Executive Officer **A**1 5 9 10 **F**8 9 13 16 17 18 19 22 25 32 36 38 41 43 44 45 46 48 50 51 54 69 70 71 72 75 76 77 78 **P**8	23	10	62	2316	29	49269	226	20653	10187	298
RICHWOOD—Nicholas County										
RICHWOOD AREA COMMUNITY HOSPITAL, Riverside Addition, Zip 26261; tel. 304/846–2573; Eugene Underwood, Chief Executive Officer **A**9 10 18 **F**7 9 14 25 32 34 37 38 48 56 74 76 79 Web address: www.pihn.org	23	10	25	223	5	8816	0	—	—	67
RIPLEY—Jackson County										
★ JACKSON GENERAL HOSPITAL, Pinnell Street, Zip 25271, Mailing Address: P.O. Box 720, Zip 25271–0720; tel. 304/372–2731; Richard L. Rohaley, President and Chief Executive Officer **A**1 9 10 **F**7 8 9 13 16 17 18 22 24 25 32 38 39 45 48 54 70 71 76 77	23	10	74	2775	33	51500	116	20628	9601	314
ROMNEY—Hampshire County										
□ HAMPSHIRE MEMORIAL HOSPITAL, 549 Center Avenue, Zip 26757–1199; tel. 304/822–4561; Roberta D. McCauley, Chief Executive Officer (Total facility includes 30 beds in nursing home–type unit) **A**1 9 10 **F**9 16 17 18 22 25 35 36 48 54 69 70 76 **P**4 7 **S** Northeast Health Management, Inc., Stevensville, MD	33	10	47	809	35	27161	0	4826	2180	109
RONCEVERTE—Greenbrier County										
★ ○ GREENBRIER VALLEY MEDICAL CENTER, 202 Maplewood Avenue, Zip 24970–0497, Mailing Address: P.O. Box 497, Zip 24970–0497; tel. 304/647–4411; Stephen Brandt, Interim Chief Executive Officer **A**1 9 10 11 13 **F**1 8 9 13 15 16 17 18 22 23 24 25 27 30 32 33 34 35 36 37 39 40 41 43 44 46 48 50 51 54 58 59 60 61 62 63 65 67 68 70 71 72 76 78 **S** NetCare Health Systems, Inc., Nashville, TN Web address: www.gvmc.com	33	10	122	4175	52	38221	393	26183	10538	368
SISTERSVILLE—Tyler County										
SISTERSVILLE GENERAL HOSPITAL, 314 South Wells Street, Zip 26175–1098; tel. 304/652–2611; F. David Richardson, Ph.D., Chief Executive Officer **A**9 10 18 **F**9 17 18 25 28 32 34 36 37 45 48 54 69 70 76 78 Web address: www.wvha.com/web/sjh	14	10	12	175	2	22776	0	3686	1994	76
SOUTH CHARLESTON—Kanawha County										
★ THOMAS MEMORIAL HOSPITAL, 4605 MacCorkle Avenue S.W., Zip 25309–1398; tel. 304/766–3600; Stephen P. Dexter, Chief Executive Officer (Total facility includes 19 beds in nursing home–type unit) **A**1 3 5 9 10 **F**2 3 7 8 9 12 16 17 18 19 22 24 25 28 29 30 32 33 34 36 37 38 39 40 41 42 43 44 45 46 48 49 50 54 57 58 59 60 61 62 63 64 65 69 70 71 72 76 77 78 79 **P**7 Web address: www.thomaswv.org	23	10	231	9639	147	186823	669	82231	31914	1018
SPENCER—Roane County										
★ ROANE GENERAL HOSPITAL, 200 Hospital Drive, Zip 25276–1060; tel. 304/927–4444; Lewis Newberry, Chief Executive Officer (Total facility includes 35 beds in nursing home–type unit) **A**10 18 **F**8 9 19 22 24 28 32 34 36 38 44 48 50 69 70 75 76 78 Web address: www.roanegeneralhospital.com	23	10	60	1043	24	26108	124	11058	6000	183
SUMMERSVILLE—Nicholas County										
★ SUMMERSVILLE MEMORIAL HOSPITAL, 400 Fairview Heights Road, Zip 26651–0400; tel. 304/872–2891; Dennis R. Burns, FACHE, Chief Executive Officer (Total facility includes 52 beds in nursing home–type unit) **A**9 10 **F**4 8 9 19 22 24 25 29 30 38 39 41 44 48 54 69 70 72 75 76 77 78	14	10	109	2309	76	62211	225	20723	9312	328
WEBSTER SPRINGS—Webster County										
★ WEBSTER COUNTY MEMORIAL HOSPITAL, 324 Miller Mountain Drive, Zip 26288–1087; tel. 304/847–5682; Stephen M. Gavalchik, Administrator **A**9 18 **F**16 17 18 19 25 28 32 33 34 36 38 45 48 56 70 76 **P**6	13	10	15	222	1	32283	0	5146	2958	91
WEIRTON—Brooke County										
★ WEIRTON MEDICAL CENTER, 601 Colliers Way, Zip 26062–5091; tel. 304/797–6000; Donald Muhlenthaler, FACHE, President and Chief Executive Officer (Total facility includes 33 beds in nursing home–type unit) **A**1 9 10 **F**3 5 7 8 9 11 12 13 14 16 17 18 19 22 23 24 25 28 29 30 31 32 33 34 35 36 37 38 39 43 44 45 46 48 49 50 54 56 57 58 59 60 61 62 63 64 68 69 70 71 72 75 76 78 79 **P**8 Web address: www.weirtonmedical.com	23	10	238	7249	104	128449	244	54579	24777	829

Hospitals, U.S. / WEST VIRGINIA

Hospital, Address, Telephone, Administrator, Approval, Facility, and Physician Codes, Health Care System, Network	Classification Codes		Utilization Data					Expense (thousands) of dollars		
★ American Hospital Association (AHA) membership ☐ Joint Commission on Accreditation of Healthcare Organizations (JCAHO) accreditation + American Osteopathic Healthcare Association (AOHA) membership ○ American Osteopathic Association (AOA) accreditation △ Commission on Accreditation of Rehabilitation Facilities (CARF) accreditation Control codes 61, 63, 64, 71, 72 and 73 indicate hospitals listed by AOHA, but not registered by AHA. For definition of numerical codes, see page A4	Control	Service	Staffed Beds	Admissions	Census	Outpatient Visits	Births	Total	Payroll	Personnel

WESTON—Lewis County

✣ STONEWALL JACKSON MEMORIAL HOSPITAL, Mailing Address: Route 4, Box 10, Zip 26452; tel. 304/269–8000; David D. Shaffer, Chief Executive Officer **A**1 9 10 **F**7 8 9 16 17 18 22 23 25 30 32 34 36 38 39 41 44 45 46 48 50 54 69 70 71 72 75 76 78 **P**8	23	10	70	3453	50	71375	279	18769	9084	283
☐ WILLIAM R. SHARPE JR. HOSPITAL, Route 33 West, Zip 26452, Mailing Address: P.O. Box 1127, Zip 26452–1127; tel. 304/269–1210; Jack C. Clohan, Jr, Administrator **A**1 5 10 **F**16 17 18 31 50 51 57 59 60 61 62 70 72 78 **P**6	12	22	150	1100	130	0	0	19823	7932	377

WHEELING—Ohio County

✣ OHIO VALLEY MEDICAL CENTER, 2000 Eoff Street, Zip 26003–3870; tel. 304/234–0123; Thomas P. Galinski, President and Chief Executive Officer (Total facility includes 172 beds in nursing home–type unit) **A**1 2 3 5 9 10 13 **F**3 5 7 8 9 11 12 13 16 17 18 19 20 21 22 24 25 27 28 29 30 31 32 33 34 35 36 37 38 39 41 43 44 45 46 48 49 50 51 52 53 54 56 57 58 59 60 61 62 63 64 65 66 68 69 70 71 72 76 77 78 79 **P**6 8 **S** Ohio Valley Health Services, Wheeling, WV	23	10	363	7256	235	127195	586	69709	29965	959
✣ WHEELING HOSPITAL, 1 Medical Park, Zip 26003–0708; tel. 304/243–3000; Donald H. Hofreuter, M.D., Administrator and Chief Executive Officer (Total facility includes 24 beds in nursing home–type unit) **A**) 1 2 3 5 9 10 **F**3 4 7 8 9 10 11 12 13 14 17 18 19 22 24 25 27 28 29 30 31 32 33 34 35 36 38 39 41 43 44 45 46 47 48 50 51 54 56 58 59 60 61 62 63 64 65 68 69 70 71 72 75 76 77 78 79 **P**8 Web address: www.wheelinghosp.com	23	10	276	11699	165	281524	1039	135669	58055	1713

WILLIAMSON—Mingo County

☐ WILLIAMSON MEMORIAL HOSPITAL, 859 Alderson Street, Zip 25661–3215, Mailing Address: P.O. Box 1980, Zip 25661–1980; tel. 304/235–2500; Andrew Knizley, Chief Executive Officer **A**1 9 10 **F**8 9 13 17 18 22 24 25 27 32 34 35 36 39 41 43 45 46 48 51 54 70 71 76 78 **P**6 8 **S** Health Management Associates, Naples, FL	33	10	76	3587	44	35317	94	21700	7734	263

© 2000 AHA Guide *Many Facility Codes have changed. Please refer to the AHA Guide Code Chart.*

Hospitals, U.S. / WISCONSIN

WISCONSIN

Resident Population 5,224 (in thousands)
Resident population in metro areas 67.7%
Birth rate per 1,000 population 12.9
65 years and over 13.2%
Percent of persons without health insurance 8.0%

Hospital, Address, Telephone, Administrator, Approval, Facility, and Physician Codes, Health Care System, Network	Classification Codes		Utilization Data					Expense (thousands) of dollars		
★ American Hospital Association (AHA) membership ☐ Joint Commission on Accreditation of Healthcare Organizations (JCAHO) accreditation + American Osteopathic Healthcare Association (AOHA) membership ○ American Osteopathic Association (AOA) accreditation △ Commission on Accreditation of Rehabilitation Facilities (CARF) accreditation Control codes 61, 63, 64, 71, 72 and 73 indicate hospitals listed by AOHA, but not registered by AHA. For definition of numerical codes, see page A4	Control	Service	Staffed Beds	Admissions	Census	Outpatient Visits	Births	Total	Payroll	Personnel
AMERY—Polk County ★ AMERY REGIONAL MEDICAL CENTER, 225 Scholl Court, Zip 54001–1292; tel. 715/268–8000; Michael Karuschak, Jr, Chief Executive Officer **A**1 9 10 **F**7 8 9 12 18 19 22 24 25 31 34 36 37 38 39 41 43 44 45 46 48 50 53 54 56 70 71 72 76 78 **S** Quorum Health Group, Brentwood, TN	23	10	15	1167	11	54859	130	14139	4832	148
ANTIGO—Langlade County ☐ LANGLADE MEMORIAL HOSPITAL, 112 East Fifth Avenue, Zip 54409–2796; tel. 715/623–2331; David R. Schneider, Executive Director **A**1 9 10 **F**1 2 3 4 5 6 8 9 10 11 12 13 14 15 18 19 21 22 23 24 25 26 27 28 31 32 34 35 36 37 38 39 40 41 42 43 44 45 46 47 48 50 51 52 53 54 55 56 57 58 59 60 61 62 63 64 65 67 68 70 71 72 73 74 75 76 77 78 79	21	10	43	1788	19	36056	185	21914	9329	294
APPLETON—Outagamie County ★ APPLETON MEDICAL CENTER, 1818 North Meade Street, Zip 54911–3496; tel. 920/731–4101; Robert H. Malte, Senior Vice President **A**2 3 5 9 10 **F**1 4 5 8 9 10 11 12 13 14 15 16 18 19 22 23 24 25 26 27 28 31 32 34 35 36 37 38 39 40 41 43 44 45 46 47 48 50 51 52 54 55 56 65 67 68 70 71 72 73 74 75 76 77 78 79 **P**6 8 **S** ThedaCare, Inc., Appleton, WI Web address: www.thedacare.com	23	10	146	7127	79	91822	1203	75012	32789	725
★ △ ST. ELIZABETH HOSPITAL, 1506 South Oneida Street, Zip 54915–1397; tel. 920/738–2000; Robert J. Turner, Chief Operating Officer **A**1 2 3 5 7 9 10 **F**1 2 3 4 5 6 7 8 9 10 11 12 13 18 20 21 22 24 25 27 36 37 38 39 40 41 42 43 44 45 46 47 48 49 50 51 52 53 54 57 58 59 60 61 62 63 64 65 67 68 69 70 71 75 76 77 79 **P**6 **S** Wheaton Franciscan Services, Inc., Wheaton, IL	21	10	166	8247	96	202531	1429	79057	34464	861
ARCADIA—Trempealeau County ★ FRANCISCAN SKEMP HEALTHCARE–ARCADIA CAMPUS, 464 South St. Joseph Avenue, Zip 54612–1401; tel. 608/323–3341; Robert M. Tracey, Administrator (Total facility includes 75 beds in nursing home–type unit) **A**1 9 10 **F**1 2 3 4 5 6 8 9 10 11 12 13 14 16 18 22 23 24 25 27 28 32 34 35 36 37 38 39 40 41 42 43 44 45 46 47 48 50 51 52 53 54 55 56 57 58 59 60 61 62 63 64 65 67 68 69 70 71 72 74 75 76 77 78 79 **P**6 **S** Franciscan Skemp Healthcare, La Crosse, WI Web address: www.mayo.edu/fsh	21	10	101	348	75	15940	41	3739	2215	119
ASHLAND—Ashland County ★ MEMORIAL MEDICAL CENTER, 1615 Maple Lane, Zip 54806–3689; tel. 715/682–4563; Daniel J. Hymans, President **A**1 9 10 **F**2 3 7 8 9 12 16 22 24 25 26 32 34 37 38 39 41 43 44 45 46 48 50 53 54 57 58 59 60 61 62 63 64 68 70 71 72 76 77 78 Web address: www.ashlandmmc.com	23	10	101	3066	35	29551	315	26493	13521	365
BALDWIN—St. Croix County ★ BALDWIN AREA MEDICAL CENTER, (Formerly Baldwin Hospital), 730 10th Avenue, Zip 54002–0300, Mailing Address: P.O. Box 300, Zip 54002–0300; tel. 715/684–3311; Richard L. Range, Chief Executive Officer **A**9 10 **F**7 8 9 12 13 20 22 25 32 34 38 39 41 43 44 45 46 48 50 51 53 54 56 60 63 70 76 78 Web address: www.baldwin-hospital.com	23	10	27	1124	9	27477	98	12165	4942	128
BARABOO—Sauk County ★ ST. CLARE HOSPITAL AND HEALTH SERVICES, 707 14th Street, Zip 53913–1597; tel. 608/356–1400; David B. Jordahl, FACHE, President **A**1 3 9 10 **F**1 2 3 4 5 6 8 9 10 11 12 13 16 18 21 22 24 25 27 28 35 36 37 38 39 40 41 42 43 44 45 46 47 48 50 51 52 53 54 55 57 58 59 60 61 62 63 64 65 67 68 70 71 74 75 76 77 79 **S** SSM Health Care, Saint Louis, MO Web address: www.stclare.com	21	10	82	2505	23	49298	300	21509	10114	268
BARRON—Barron County ☐ BARRON MEDICAL CENTER–MAYO HEALTH SYSTEM, (Formerly Barron Memorial Medical Center), 1222 Woodland Avenue, Zip 54812–1798; tel. 715/537–3186; Mark D. Wilson, Administrator (Total facility includes 50 beds in nursing home–type unit) (Nonreporting) **A**1 9 10 **S** Mayo Foundation, Rochester, MN	23	10	92	—	—	—	—	—	—	—
BEAVER DAM—Dodge County ★ BEAVER DAM COMMUNITY HOSPITALS, 707 South University Avenue, Zip 53916–3089; tel. 920/887–7181; John R. Landdeck, President (Total facility includes 123 beds in nursing home–type unit) **A**1 9 10 **F**2 6 7 9 12 13 16 18 22 25 26 32 34 38 39 40 41 42 43 44 45 46 48 50 51 53 54 56 57 67 69 70 71 72 76 77 78 79	23	10	216	3009	145	69033	384	35796	16896	905
BELOIT—Rock County ☐ △ BELOIT MEMORIAL HOSPITAL, 1969 West Hart Road, Zip 53511–2299; tel. 608/364–5011; Gregory K. Britton, President and Chief Executive Officer **A**1 7 9 10 **F**1 2 3 4 5 6 8 9 10 11 12 13 18 19 21 22 24 25 27 28 31 32 34 35 36 37 38 39 40 41 42 43 44 45 46 47 48 50 51 52 53 54 55 57 58 59 60 61 62 63 64 65 67 68 70 71 72 74 75 76 77 78 79 **P**1 7 Web address: www.beloitmemorialhospital.org	23	10	124	4820	64	158761	666	49826	23434	717

Hospitals, U.S. / WISCONSIN

Hospital, Address, Telephone, Administrator, Approval, Facility, and Physician Codes, Health Care System, Network	Classification Codes		Utilization Data					Expense (thousands) of dollars		
★ American Hospital Association (AHA) membership ☐ Joint Commission on Accreditation of Healthcare Organizations (JCAHO) accreditation + American Osteopathic Healthcare Association (AOHA) membership ○ American Osteopathic Association (AOA) accreditation △ Commission on Accreditation of Rehabilitation Facilities (CARF) accreditation Control codes 61, 63, 64, 71, 72 and 73 indicate hospitals listed by AOHA, but not registered by AHA. For definition of numerical codes, see page A4	Control	Service	Staffed Beds	Admissions	Census	Outpatient Visits	Births	Total	Payroll	Personnel
BERLIN—Green Lake County ☐ BERLIN MEMORIAL HOSPITAL, (Includes Juliette Manor Nursing Home, Community Clinics), 225 Memorial Drive, Zip 54923–1295; tel. 920/361–1313; Craig W. C. Schmidt, President and Chief Executive Officer (Total facility includes 104 beds in nursing home–type unit) **A**1 9 10 **F**2 3 4 6 7 8 9 10 11 12 13 16 18 20 22 24 25 28 36 37 38 39 40 41 43 44 45 46 48 49 50 52 53 54 57 58 59 60 61 62 63 64 67 68 69 70 71 75 76 77 79 **P**1 6 8 **Web address:** www.partnershealthsystem.org	23	10	165	1918	122	72265	208	21432	9641	247
BLACK RIVER FALLS—Jackson County ☐ BLACK RIVER MEMORIAL HOSPITAL, 711 West Adams Street, Zip 54615–9113; tel. 715/284–5361; Stanley J. Gaynor, Chief Executive Officer and Administrator **A**1 9 10 **F**2 3 7 8 13 19 22 25 26 32 34 38 39 40 44 45 48 50 54 57 59 70 71 75 76 77 78 **Web address:** discover–net.net/~brmh/	23	10	38	1201	11	9874	161	9108	4141	126
BLOOMER—Chippewa County ☐ BLOOMER MEMORIAL MEDICAL CENTER, (Formerly Bloomer Community Memorial Hospital and MapleWood), 1501 Thompson Street, Zip 54724–1299; tel. 715/568–2000; Mary Kerg, Administrator (Total facility includes 75 beds in nursing home–type unit) **A**1 9 10 **F**1 2 3 4 5 6 8 9 10 11 12 13 16 18 19 21 22 24 25 27 28 31 32 34 35 36 37 38 39 40 41 42 43 44 45 46 47 48 50 51 52 53 54 55 57 58 59 60 61 62 63 64 65 67 68 69 70 71 72 74 75 76 77 78 79 **S** Mayo Foundation, Rochester, MN	23	10	107	586	80	7960	43	3897	1744	134
BOSCOBEL—Grant County BOSCOBEL AREA HEALTH CARE, 205 Parker Street, Zip 53805–1698; tel. 608/375–4112; Steven T. Moburg, Administrator (Total facility includes 79 beds in nursing home–type unit) **A**9 10 **F**1 3 7 8 9 12 18 19 21 22 23 25 26 28 32 34 36 38 39 41 44 45 48 50 53 54 57 58 59 60 61 62 63 69 70 72 75 76 77 78 **P**6	23	10	123	1273	70	10401	80	8863	4768	176
BROOKFIELD—Waukesha County ★ △ ELMBROOK MEMORIAL HOSPITAL, 19333 West North Avenue, Zip 53045–4198; tel. 262/785–2000; Kimry A. Johnsrud, President **A**1 7 9 10 **F**2 3 4 5 6 7 8 9 11 12 13 14 19 20 21 22 23 24 25 26 27 31 32 34 35 36 37 38 39 40 41 42 43 44 45 46 47 48 49 50 51 53 54 55 56 58 59 60 61 62 63 64 65 67 68 70 71 72 74 75 76 77 78 79 **P**2 5 8 **S** Wheaton Franciscan Services, Inc., Wheaton, IL **Web address:** www.covhealth.org	21	10	136	6231	73	80447	984	58667	24875	439
BURLINGTON—Racine County ★ MEMORIAL HOSPITAL CORPORATION OF BURLINGTON, (Includes Aurora Medical Center, 10400 75th Street, Kenosha, Zip 53142; tel. 414/697–7000; Seonaid A. Ritz, R.N., Site Administrator), 252 McHenry Street, Zip 53105–1828; tel. 262/767–6000; Lief Erickson, M.D., President **A**1 9 10 **F**1 2 5 6 8 9 10 11 12 13 18 21 22 24 25 27 28 35 38 39 40 41 42 43 44 48 50 51 52 53 54 60 61 62 65 68 70 71 76 79 **P**4 6 **S** Aurora Health Care, Milwaukee, WI **Web address:** www.aurorahealthcare.org	23	10	87	2801	32	74102	569	36742	13733	381
CHILTON—Calumet County ★ CALUMET MEDICAL CENTER, 614 Memorial Drive, Zip 53014–1597; tel. 920/849–2386; Lea Whitby, Administrator **A**1 9 10 **F**3 7 9 11 12 13 18 19 21 22 24 25 26 32 33 34 36 37 38 39 40 41 43 45 46 48 50 51 54 56 58 59 60 61 62 63 64 70 72 75 76 78	23	10	26	641	8	31897	0	9371	4244	138
CHIPPEWA FALLS—Chippewa County ★ ST. JOSEPH'S HOSPITAL, 2661 County Highway I, Zip 54729–1498; tel. 715/723–1811; David B. Fish, Executive Vice President **A**1 9 10 **F**2 3 7 8 9 12 13 14 15 16 18 20 22 24 26 32 34 36 37 38 40 41 43 44 45 46 48 50 51 52 56 61 70 72 73 76 78 **S** Hospital Sisters Health System, Springfield, IL **Web address:** www.stjoeschipfalls.com	21	10	127	3303	51	58062	437	28901	14174	410
COLUMBUS—Columbia County ★ COLUMBUS COMMUNITY HOSPITAL, 1515 Park Avenue, Zip 53925; tel. 920/623–2200; Edward A. Harding, President and Chief Executive Officer **A**1 9 10 **F**8 9 10 12 13 16 18 22 24 25 38 39 41 43 44 45 46 48 50 52 54 68 70 76 77 79	23	10	34	1685	21	29376	135	12685	5696	164
CUBA CITY—Grant County SOUTHWEST HEALTH CENTER NURSING HOME See Southwest Health Center, Platteville										
CUMBERLAND—Barron County ☐ CUMBERLAND MEMORIAL HOSPITAL, 1110 Seventh Avenue, Zip 54829; tel. 715/822–2741; Robert Hansen, Chief Executive Officer (Total facility includes 71 beds in nursing home–type unit) **A**1 9 10 **F**2 7 8 9 13 14 15 18 19 22 23 24 25 26 31 32 34 36 38 39 43 44 46 48 50 51 54 56 57 59 61 62 63 67 68 69 70 71 72 73 75 76 78 **P**5 6	23	10	111	1542	86	8001	70	9203	5271	188
DARLINGTON—Lafayette County MEMORIAL HOSPITAL OF LAFAYETTE COUNTY, 800 Clay Street, Zip 53530–1228, Mailing Address: P.O. Box 70, Zip 53530–0070; tel. 608/776–4466; Sherry Kudronowicz, Administrator **A**9 10 **F**1 2 3 4 5 6 8 9 10 11 12 13 16 19 21 22 24 25 27 28 35 36 37 38 39 40 41 43 44 45 46 47 48 50 51 52 53 54 55 57 58 59 60 61 62 63 64 65 67 68 70 71 74 75 76 77 78 79	13	10	28	441	4	18508	40	4533	1595	61

Hospitals, U.S. / WISCONSIN

Hospital, Address, Telephone, Administrator, Approval, Facility, and Physician Codes, Health Care System, Network	Control	Service	Staffed Beds	Admissions	Census	Outpatient Visits	Births	Total	Payroll	Personnel
★ American Hospital Association (AHA) membership ☐ Joint Commission on Accreditation of Healthcare Organizations (JCAHO) accreditation + American Osteopathic Healthcare Association (AOHA) membership ○ American Osteopathic Association (AOA) accreditation △ Commission on Accreditation of Rehabilitation Facilities (CARF) accreditation Control codes 61, 63, 64, 71, 72 and 73 indicate hospitals listed by AOHA, but not registered by AHA. For definition of numerical codes, see page A4										
DODGEVILLE—Iowa County ★ MEMORIAL HOSPITAL OF IOWA COUNTY, 825 South Iowa Street, Zip 53533–1999; tel. 608/935–2711; Ray Marmorstone, Administrator and Chief Executive Officer (Total facility includes 44 beds in nursing home–type unit) **A**1 9 10 **F**1 6 7 8 9 12 13 18 22 25 36 37 38 39 41 43 44 45 46 48 49 50 51 52 53 54 61 69 70 71 76 77 79 Web address: www.mhihealth.org	23	10	84	1405	46	36524	237	13364	5517	171
DURAND—Pepin County CHIPPEWA VALLEY HOSPITAL AND OAKVIEW CARE CENTER, 1220 Third Avenue West, Zip 54736–1600, Mailing Address: P.O. Box 224, Zip 54736–0224; tel. 715/672–4211; Douglas R. Peterson, President and Chief Executive Officer (Total facility includes 58 beds in nursing home–type unit) **A**9 10 **F**1 2 3 4 5 6 8 9 10 11 12 13 19 21 22 24 25 27 28 35 36 37 38 39 40 41 42 43 44 45 46 47 48 50 51 52 53 54 55 57 58 59 60 61 62 63 64 65 67 68 69 70 71 74 75 76 77 79 **S** Adventist Health System Sunbelt Health Care Corporation, Winter Park, FL	21	10	83	742	62	9161	29	6410	3089	162
EAGLE RIVER—Vilas County ★ EAGLE RIVER MEMORIAL HOSPITAL, 201 Hospital Road, Zip 54521–8835; tel. 715/479–7411; Tim Gengler, Administrator **A**9 10 18 **F**2 3 6 7 8 9 12 13 16 18 20 22 24 25 28 36 37 38 39 40 41 43 44 45 46 48 49 50 51 53 54 57 67 70 71 76 77 79	23	10	8	427	5	42681	0	9455	4773	116
EAU CLAIRE—Eau Claire County ☐ LUTHER HOSPITAL, 1221 Whipple Street, Zip 54702–4105, Mailing Address: P.O. Box 5, Zip 54702–0005; tel. 715/838–3311; William Rupp, M.D., President and Chief Executive Officer **A**1 2 3 5 9 10 **F**1 2 3 4 5 6 8 9 10 11 12 13 21 22 24 25 27 28 35 36 37 38 39 40 41 42 43 44 45 46 47 48 50 51 52 53 54 55 57 58 59 60 61 62 63 64 65 67 68 70 71 74 75 76 77 79 **S** Mayo Foundation, Rochester, MN	23	10	179	8070	92	137978	889	74589	31576	1060
★ △ SACRED HEART HOSPITAL, 900 West Clairemont Avenue, Zip 54701–6122; tel. 715/839–4121; Stephen F. Ronstrom, Executive Vice President and Administrator **A**1 2 3 5 7 9 10 **F**7 8 9 11 12 13 16 18 21 22 24 25 27 28 33 34 36 37 38 39 40 41 42 43 44 45 46 48 49 50 52 53 54 56 57 58 59 60 61 62 63 64 65 67 68 70 72 75 76 78 **S** Hospital Sisters Health System, Springfield, IL Web address: www.sacredhearthospital–ec.org	21	10	179	7530	97	101225	787	63609	28207	812
EDGERTON—Rock County MEMORIAL COMMUNITY HOSPITAL, 313 Stoughton Road, Zip 53534–1198; tel. 608/884–3441; Steven H. Spencer, Chief Executive Officer (Total facility includes 61 beds in nursing home–type unit) **A**9 10 **F**1 2 3 4 5 6 8 9 10 11 12 13 14 15 21 22 23 24 25 26 27 28 31 32 34 35 36 37 38 39 40 41 43 44 45 46 47 48 50 51 52 53 54 55 56 57 58 59 60 61 62 63 64 65 67 68 69 70 71 72 73 74 75 76 77 78 79 **P**5 7 **S** Brim Healthcare, Inc., Brentwood, TN	23	10	125	894	79	14467	0	14722	6884	187
ELKHORN—Walworth County ★ △ LAKELAND MEDICAL CENTER, West 3985 County Road NN, Zip 53121, Mailing Address: P.O. Box 1002, Zip 53121–1002; tel. 262/741–2000; Kathleen Skowlund, Site Administrator and Chief Nurse Executive **A**1 7 9 10 **F**1 2 5 6 8 9 12 13 18 21 22 24 25 27 28 35 38 39 40 41 42 43 44 48 50 51 52 53 54 57 60 61 62 65 68 70 71 76 77 79 **P**4 6 **S** Aurora Health Care, Milwaukee, WI Web address: www.aurorahealthcare.org	23	10	78	3655	38	58502	524	33163	13144	414
FOND DU LAC—Fond Du Lac County ☐ △ AGNESIAN HEALTHCARE, 430 East Division Street, Zip 54935–0385, Mailing Address: P.O. Box 385, Zip 54936–0385; tel. 920/929–2300; Robert A. Fale, President and Chief Executive Officer **A**1 2 7 9 10 **F**1 2 3 4 6 7 8 9 11 12 13 18 20 21 22 24 25 27 36 37 38 39 40 41 43 44 45 46 47 48 49 50 51 52 53 54 57 58 59 60 61 62 63 64 65 67 68 70 71 75 76 77 79 **P**3 Web address: www.agnesian.com	21	10	90	6788	87	192446	973	103212	36972	849
FORT ATKINSON—Jefferson County ★ FORT ATKINSON MEMORIAL HEALTH SERVICES, 611 East Sherman Avenue, Zip 53538–1998; tel. 920/568–5000; John C. Albaugh, President and Chief Executive Officer (Total facility includes 28 beds in nursing home–type unit) **A**1 9 10 **F**3 7 8 9 10 12 13 18 22 23 24 25 26 27 28 31 32 34 36 37 38 39 41 43 44 45 46 48 49 50 51 52 53 54 59 63 68 69 70 71 72 76 77 78 79 **P**6 7 Web address: www.famhs.org	23	10	102	4204	52	87656	452	41822	20122	540
FRIENDSHIP—Adams County ☐ ADAMS COUNTY MEMORIAL HOSPITAL AND NURSING CARE UNIT, 402 West Lake Street, Zip 53934–9699, Mailing Address: P.O. Box 40, Zip 53934–0040; tel. 608/339–3331; Steven R. Nockerts, Administrator and Chief Executive Officer (Total facility includes 18 beds in nursing home–type unit) **A**1 9 10 **F**1 3 9 13 18 21 22 25 36 38 39 43 45 48 50 53 54 68 69 70 71 76 **P**5	23	10	58	820	29	35111	0	8576	4385	135
GRANTSBURG—Burnett County ★ BURNETT MEDICAL CENTER, 257 West St. George Avenue, Zip 54840–7827; tel. 715/463–5353; Timothy J. Wick, Chief Executive Officer (Total facility includes 53 beds in nursing home–type unit) **A**9 10 **F**1 8 9 16 18 22 23 24 25 26 34 38 39 43 44 46 48 50 51 53 54 69 70 71 76 77 **S** Brim Healthcare, Inc., Brentwood, TN	23	10	70	675	58	11002	45	6791	2769	109

Hospitals, U.S. / WISCONSIN

Hospital, Address, Telephone, Administrator, Approval, Facility, and Physician Codes, Health Care System, Network	Classification Codes		Utilization Data					Expense (thousands) of dollars		
	Control	Service	Staffed Beds	Admissions	Census	Outpatient Visits	Births	Total	Payroll	Personnel

★ American Hospital Association (AHA) membership
□ Joint Commission on Accreditation of Healthcare Organizations (JCAHO) accreditation
+ American Osteopathic Healthcare Association (AOHA) membership
○ American Osteopathic Association (AOA) accreditation
△ Commission on Accreditation of Rehabilitation Facilities (CARF) accreditation
Control codes 61, 63, 64, 71, 72 and 73 indicate hospitals listed by AOHA, but not registered by AHA. For definition of numerical codes, see page A4

GREEN BAY—Brown County

Hospital	Control	Service	Staffed Beds	Admissions	Census	Outpatient Visits	Births	Total	Payroll	Personnel
★ BELLIN HOSPITAL, 744 South Webster Avenue, Zip 54301–3581, Mailing Address: P.O. Box 23400, Zip 54305–3400; tel. 920/433–3500; George Kerwin, President **A**1 9 10 **F**4 7 8 9 11 12 13 16 18 19 22 24 26 27 28 31 32 36 37 38 39 41 43 44 45 46 47 48 49 50 51 52 56 68 70 71 72 76 77 78 **P**5 6 8 Web address: www.bellin.org	21	10	179	9613	93	420682	1909	139603	67808	1662
□ BELLIN PSYCHIATRIC CENTER, 301 East St. Joseph Street, Zip 54301–2241, Mailing Address: P.O. Box 23725, Zip 54305–3725; tel. 920/433–3630; Robert W. Fry, President **A**1 10 **F**2 3 12 16 22 24 38 39 41 50 53 55 57 58 59 60 61 62 63 64 68 70 76 Web address: www.bellin.org	21	22	60	1485	26	25885	0	7929	4634	101
BROWN COUNTY HUMAN SERVICES MENTAL HEALTH CENTER, (Formerly Brown County Mental Health Center), 2900 St. Anthony Drive, Zip 54311–5899; tel. 920/468–1136; Mark Quam, Director **A**10 **F**1 2 3 4 5 6 8 9 10 12 13 21 22 24 25 26 27 28 35 36 37 38 39 40 41 42 43 44 45 46 47 48 50 51 52 53 54 55 57 58 59 60 61 62 63 64 65 67 68 70 71 74 75 76 77 78 79	13	22	74	1582	30	15461	0	7133	4344	240
★ ST. MARY'S HOSPITAL MEDICAL CENTER, 1726 Shawano Avenue, Zip 54303–3282; tel. 920/498–4200; James G. Coller, Executive Vice President and Administrator **A**1 9 10 **F**7 8 9 12 13 18 22 24 25 26 34 37 38 39 40 41 43 44 45 49 50 51 52 61 68 70 72 73 75 76 77 78 79 **S** Hospital Sisters Health System, Springfield, IL Web address: www.stmgb.org	21	10	119	4666	47	80239	562	43464	18973	491
★ △ ST. VINCENT HOSPITAL, 835 South Van Buren Street, Zip 54307–3508, Mailing Address: P.O. Box 13508, Zip 54307–3508; tel. 920/433–0111; Joseph J. Neidenbach, Administrator and Chief Executive Officer **A**1 2 7 9 10 **F**4 7 8 9 11 12 13 14 18 19 22 23 24 25 27 31 32 33 34 36 37 38 39 40 41 42 43 44 45 46 48 49 50 51 53 54 65 68 70 71 72 73 75 76 78 **P**2 **S** Hospital Sisters Health System, Springfield, IL Web address: www.stvgb.org	21	10	285	11881	167	107204	1614	125373	59531	1602

GREENFIELD—Milwaukee County

Hospital	Control	Service	Staffed Beds	Admissions	Census	Outpatient Visits	Births	Total	Payroll	Personnel
□ VENCOR HOSPITAL–MILWAUKEE, 5017 South 110th Street, Zip 53228; tel. 414/427–8282; Daniel R. West, Administrator **A**1 9 10 **F**1 2 3 4 5 6 8 9 10 11 12 13 14 18 19 21 22 23 24 25 27 28 31 32 35 36 37 38 39 40 42 43 44 45 46 47 48 50 51 52 54 55 57 58 59 60 61 62 63 64 65 67 68 70 71 74 75 76 77 79 **S** Vencor, Incorporated, Louisville, KY Web address: www.vencor.com	33	10	34	191	22	0	0	9562	3567	94

HARTFORD—Washington County

Hospital	Control	Service	Staffed Beds	Admissions	Census	Outpatient Visits	Births	Total	Payroll	Personnel
★ HARTFORD MEMORIAL HOSPITAL, 1032 East Sumner Street, Zip 53027–1698; tel. 262/673–2300; Mark Schwartz, Administrator **A**1 9 10 **F**1 2 3 4 5 6 8 9 10 11 12 13 16 18 22 24 25 27 28 35 38 39 40 41 42 43 44 45 47 48 50 51 52 53 55 57 58 59 60 61 62 63 64 65 67 68 70 71 74 75 76 77 **P**4 6 **S** Aurora Health Care, Milwaukee, WI Web address: www.aurorahealthcare.org	23	10	71	1732	31	53682	209	23932	9438	285

HAYWARD—Sawyer County

Hospital	Control	Service	Staffed Beds	Admissions	Census	Outpatient Visits	Births	Total	Payroll	Personnel
★ HAYWARD AREA MEMORIAL HOSPITAL AND NURSING HOME, 11040 North State Road 77, Zip 54843; tel. 715/634–8911; Barbara A. Peickert, R.N., Chief Executive Officer (Total facility includes 76 beds in nursing home–type unit) **A**1 9 10 **F**7 8 9 16 18 19 22 23 24 25 26 32 34 37 38 44 48 50 56 61 68 69 70 72 76 78	23	10	117	1374	86	20845	117	9518	4882	220

HAZEL GREEN—Grant County
EVERGREEN ADULT CENTER See Southwest Health Center, Platteville

HILLSBORO—Vernon County

Hospital	Control	Service	Staffed Beds	Admissions	Census	Outpatient Visits	Births	Total	Payroll	Personnel
★ ST. JOSEPH'S COMMUNITY HEALTH SERVICES, (Formerly St. Joseph's Memorial Hospital and Nursing Home), 400 Water Avenue, Zip 54634–0527, Mailing Address: P.O. Box 527, Zip 54634–0527; tel. 608/489–2211; Billy F. Bruce, Jr, Chief Executive Officer (Total facility includes 65 beds in nursing home–type unit) **A**9 10 **F**7 8 9 13 22 24 25 28 36 37 38 39 40 43 44 45 48 50 53 54 59 61 62 69 70 71 75 76 77 **S** Brim Healthcare, Inc., Brentwood, TN	21	10	80	461	66	25862	30	5081	1945	61

HUDSON—St. Croix County

Hospital	Control	Service	Staffed Beds	Admissions	Census	Outpatient Visits	Births	Total	Payroll	Personnel
□ HUDSON MEDICAL CENTER, 400 Wisconsin Street, Zip 54016–1600; tel. 715/386–9321; Marian M. Furlong, R.N., Chief Executive Officer **A**1 9 10 **F**1 2 3 4 5 6 8 9 10 11 12 13 15 16 18 19 21 22 23 24 25 26 27 28 31 32 34 35 36 37 38 39 40 41 42 43 44 45 46 47 48 50 51 52 53 54 55 57 58 59 60 61 62 63 64 65 67 68 70 71 72 73 74 75 76 77 78 79 **P**4	23	10	39	867	14	18107	170	10197	4719	141

JANESVILLE—Rock County

Hospital	Control	Service	Staffed Beds	Admissions	Census	Outpatient Visits	Births	Total	Payroll	Personnel
★ MERCY HEALTH SYSTEM, 1000 Mineral Point Avenue, Zip 53547–5003, Mailing Address: P.O. Box 5003, Zip 53547–5003; tel. 608/756–6000; Javon R. Bea, President and Chief Executive Officer (Total facility includes 81 beds in nursing home–type unit) **A**1 2 3 9 10 **F**1 2 3 4 5 6 7 8 9 10 11 12 13 14 15 16 18 19 20 21 22 24 25 26 27 28 31 32 34 35 36 37 38 39 40 41 42 43 44 45 46 47 48 49 50 51 52 53 54 57 58 59 60 61 62 63 64 65 67 68 69 70 71 72 73 75 76 77 78 79 **P**2 Web address: www.mercyhealthsystem.org	23	10	273	9152	172	585602	1352	166189	89834	1834

KENOSHA—Kenosha County

Hospital	Control	Service	Staffed Beds	Admissions	Census	Outpatient Visits	Births	Total	Payroll	Personnel
★ KENOSHA HOSPITAL AND MEDICAL CENTER, 6308 Eighth Avenue, Zip 53143–5082; tel. 262/656–2011; Richard O. Schmidt, Jr, President and Chief Executive Officer **A**1 9 10 **F**2 3 4 7 8 9 10 11 12 13 16 18 21 22 24 25 27 28 35 36 38 39 40 41 42 43 44 45 46 47 48 49 50 51 52 53 54 57 58 59 60 61 62 63 64 65 68 70 71 75 76 77 79 **P**6 8 **S** Horizon Healthcare, Inc., Milwaukee, WI	23	10	143	6826	72	150906	636	86720	42375	959

© 2000 AHA Guide   *Many Facility Codes have changed. Please refer to the AHA Guide Code Chart.*

Hospitals, U.S. / WISCONSIN

	Classification Codes		Utilization Data					Expense (thousands) of dollars		
Hospital, Address, Telephone, Administrator, Approval, Facility, and Physician Codes, Health Care System, Network	Control	Service	Staffed Beds	Admissions	Census	Outpatient Visits	Births	Total	Payroll	Personnel

★ American Hospital Association (AHA) membership
☐ Joint Commission on Accreditation of Healthcare Organizations (JCAHO) accreditation
+ American Osteopathic Healthcare Association (AOHA) membership
○ American Osteopathic Association (AOA) accreditation
△ Commission on Accreditation of Rehabilitation Facilities (CARF) accreditation
Control codes 61, 63, 64, 71, 72 and 73 indicate hospitals listed by AOHA, but not registered by AHA. For definition of numerical codes, see page A4

Hospital	Control	Service	Staffed Beds	Admissions	Census	Outpatient Visits	Births	Total	Payroll	Personnel
★ ST. CATHERINE'S HOSPITAL, 3556 Seventh Avenue, Zip 53140–2595; tel. 262/656–2011; Richard O. Schmidt, Jr, President and Chief Executive Officer **A**1 2 3 9 10 **F**2 3 7 8 9 10 11 12 13 16 18 21 22 24 25 36 37 38 39 40 41 43 44 45 46 48 50 51 53 54 57 59 60 61 62 63 64 65 68 70 71 74 75 76 79 **P**6 **S** Wheaton Franciscan Services, Inc., Wheaton, IL Web address: www.acronet.net/~stcath	21	10	114	4333	58	51036	763	40635	17372	432
KEWAUNEE—Kewaunee County										
★ ST. MARY'S KEWAUNEE AREA MEMORIAL HOSPITAL, 810 Lincoln Street, Zip 54216; tel. 920/388–2210; Cathie A. Kocourek, Acting Administrator **A**1 9 10 **F**1 2 3 4 5 8 9 10 11 12 13 19 21 22 24 25 27 28 32 34 35 36 37 38 39 40 41 42 43 44 45 46 47 48 50 51 52 53 54 55 56 57 58 59 60 61 62 63 64 65 67 68 70 71 72 74 75 76 77 79 **S** Aurora Health Care, Milwaukee, WI	23	10	18	267	3	18489	14	3643	2115	62
LA CROSSE—La Crosse County										
★ FRANCISCAN SKEMP HEALTHCARE–LA CROSSE CAMPUS, 700 West Avenue South, Zip 54601–4783; tel. 608/785–0940; Glenn Forbes, M.D., President and Chief Executive Officer **A**1 2 3 9 10 **F**1 2 4 5 8 9 10 11 12 18 22 24 25 27 28 35 38 39 40 41 42 43 44 46 47 48 51 52 53 54 55 57 58 59 60 61 62 63 64 65 66 68 70 74 75 76 **P**8 **S** Franciscan Skemp Healthcare, La Crosse, WI Web address: www.mayo.edu/fsh/	21	10	213	8558	98	81003	736	71856	32469	1038
★ △ GUNDERSEN LUTHERAN, (Formerly Lutheran Hospital–La Crosse), 1910 South Avenue, Zip 54601–9980; tel. 608/785–0530; Philip J. Dahlberg, M.D., Chief Executive Officer **A**1 2 5 7 8 9 10 **F**1 2 3 4 5 8 9 10 11 12 13 14 16 18 19 21 22 23 24 25 26 27 28 31 32 34 35 38 39 40 41 43 44 45 46 47 48 50 51 52 53 54 55 56 57 58 59 60 61 62 63 64 65 67 68 70 71 72 73 74 75 76 77 78 79 Web address: www.gundluth.org	23	10	277	13465	154	110663	1508	148345	60204	1786
LADYSMITH—Rusk County										
RUSK COUNTY MEMORIAL HOSPITAL AND NURSING HOME, 900 College Avenue West, Zip 54848–2116; tel. 715/532–5561; J. Michael Shaw, Administrator (Total facility includes 99 beds in nursing home–type unit) **A**9 10 **F**1 2 3 4 5 6 8 9 10 11 12 13 14 15 19 21 22 24 25 26 27 28 31 32 34 35 36 37 38 39 40 41 42 43 44 45 46 47 48 49 50 51 52 53 54 55 56 57 58 59 60 61 62 63 64 65 67 68 69 70 71 72 74 75 76 77 78 79	13	10	134	1005	98	29213	119	11238	4779	241
LANCASTER—Grant County										
★ GRANT REGIONAL HEALTH CENTER, 507 South Monroe Street, Zip 53813–2099; tel. 608/723–2143; Larry D. Rentfro, FACHE, President and Chief Executive Officer **A**1 9 10 **F**1 2 3 4 5 8 9 10 11 12 13 16 18 21 22 23 24 25 26 27 28 32 34 35 36 37 38 39 40 41 42 43 44 45 46 47 48 50 51 52 53 54 55 56 57 58 59 60 61 62 63 64 65 67 68 70 71 72 74 75 76 77 78 79 **P**5 **S** Brim Healthcare, Inc., Brentwood, TN Web address: www.grantregionalhealthctr.com	23	10	28	916	6	20623	106	7872	3031	96
MADISON—Dane County										
☐ MENDOTA MENTAL HEALTH INSTITUTE, 301 Troy Drive, Zip 53704–1599; tel. 608/243–2500; Steve Watters, Chief Executive Officer **A**1 3 5 10 **F**2 13 21 25 38 43 50 51 57 58 59 60 61 63 64 70 **P**6	12	22	257	831	220	13330	0	41964	24801	682
★ △ MERITER HOSPITAL, (Includes Meriter–Capitol), 202 South Park Street, Zip 53715–1599; tel. 608/267–6000; Terri L. Potter, President and Chief Executive Officer **A**1 3 5 7 9 10 **F**2 3 4 5 8 9 11 12 14 15 18 19 21 22 23 24 25 26 27 28 31 32 35 37 38 39 41 42 43 44 45 46 47 48 50 51 52 53 54 55 56 57 58 59 60 61 62 63 64 65 67 68 70 71 72 73 74 75 76 77 78 79 Web address: www.meriter.com	23	10	369	14532	193	136308	3338	160927	65625	1574
★ ST. MARYS HOSPITAL MEDICAL CENTER, 707 South Mills Street, Zip 53715–0450; tel. 608/251–6100; Gerald W. Lefert, President **A**1 3 5 9 10 **F**1 2 3 4 5 8 9 10 11 12 13 14 15 16 18 19 21 22 23 24 25 26 27 28 32 34 35 36 37 38 39 40 41 42 43 44 46 47 48 50 51 52 53 54 55 56 57 58 59 60 61 62 63 64 65 67 68 70 71 72 73 74 75 76 77 78 79 **S** SSM Health Care, Saint Louis, MO Web address: www.stmarysmadison.com	23	10	287	16866	203	55846	2939	140109	55095	1167
★ △ UNIVERSITY OF WISCONSIN HOSPITAL AND CLINICS, (Includes University of Wisconsin Children's Hospital), 600 Highland Avenue, Zip 53792–0002; tel. 608/263–6400; Gordon M. Derzon, Chief Executive Officer **A**1 3 5 7 8 9 10 **F**3 4 5 7 9 10 11 12 13 16 18 22 24 25 27 28 35 36 38 39 41 43 44 45 46 47 48 49 50 51 52 53 54 55 57 58 59 60 61 62 63 65 67 68 70 71 74 75 76 77 79 **P**3 Web address: www.biostat.wisc.edu/	23	10	467	21039	352	482546	0	346672	140101	4148
★ WILLIAM S. MIDDLETON MEMORIAL VETERANS HOSPITAL, 2500 Overlook Terrace, Zip 53705–2286; tel. 608/256–1901; Nathan L. Geraths, Director (Nonreporting) **A**1 3 5 9 **S** Department of Veterans Affairs, Washington, DC	45	10	200	—	—	—	—	—	—	—
MANITOWOC—Manitowoc County										
★ △ HOLY FAMILY MEMORIAL MEDICAL CENTER, 2300 Western Avenue, Zip 54220, Mailing Address: P.O. Box 1450, Zip 54221–1450; tel. 920/684–2011; Daniel B. McGinty, President and Chief Executive Officer **A**1 7 10 **F**2 3 4 5 8 9 10 11 12 13 16 18 19 21 22 24 25 26 27 28 31 32 34 35 37 38 39 40 41 42 43 44 45 46 47 48 50 51 52 53 54 55 56 57 58 59 60 61 62 64 65 66 68 70 71 72 74 75 76 77 78 79 **P**6 7 **S** Franciscan Sisters of Christian Charity HealthCare Ministry, Inc, Manitowoc, WI Web address: www.hfmhealth.org	21	10	176	5645	70	177945	453	67815	33640	857

Hospitals, U.S. / WISCONSIN

Hospital, Address, Telephone, Administrator, Approval, Facility, and Physician Codes, Health Care System, Network	Classification Codes		Utilization Data					Expense (thousands) of dollars		
★ American Hospital Association (AHA) membership ☐ Joint Commission on Accreditation of Healthcare Organizations (JCAHO) accreditation + American Osteopathic Healthcare Association (AOHA) membership ○ American Osteopathic Association (AOA) accreditation △ Commission on Accreditation of Rehabilitation Facilities (CARF) accreditation Control codes 61, 63, 64, 71, 72 and 73 indicate hospitals listed by AOHA, but not registered by AHA. For definition of numerical codes, see page A4	Control	Service	Staffed Beds	Admissions	Census	Outpatient Visits	Births	Total	Payroll	Personnel
MARINETTE—Marinette County ★ BAY AREA MEDICAL CENTER, 3100 Shore Drive, Zip 54143–4297; tel. 715/735–6621; David Olson, Chief Executive Officer **A**1 9 10 **F**3 7 8 9 12 13 21 22 24 25 27 38 39 41 43 44 45 46 48 49 50 51 54 57 59 60 62 63 65 68 70 71 76 77 79 Web address: www.bayareamedical.com	23	10	115	4663	53	60374	376	43243	20662	499
MARSHFIELD—Wood County NORWOOD HEALTH CENTER, 1600 North Chestnut Avenue, Zip 54449–1499; tel. 715/384–2188; Randy Bestul, Administrator **A**10 **F**1 2 3 4 5 6 8 9 10 11 12 13 21 22 24 25 27 28 35 36 37 38 39 40 41 42 43 44 45 46 47 48 50 51 52 53 54 55 57 58 59 60 61 62 63 64 65 67 68 70 71 74 75 76 77 79	13	22	19	516	8	0	0	1556	966	43
★ △ SAINT JOSEPH'S HOSPITAL, 611 St. Joseph Avenue, Zip 54449–1898; tel. 715/387–1713; Michael A. Schmidt, President and Chief Executive Officer **A**1 2 3 5 7 9 10 **F**2 3 4 5 6 7 8 10 11 12 14 15 16 17 19 22 23 24 25 26 27 32 34 35 36 37 38 39 41 42 43 44 45 46 47 48 49 50 51 52 53 54 56 57 58 61 62 63 64 65 68 70 71 72 73 75 76 78 79 **P**1 8 **S** Marian Health System, Tulsa, OK Web address: www.stjosephs-marshfield.org	21	10	524	17190	259	84195	1166	168474	65062	1936
MAUSTON—Juneau County ☐ MILE BLUFF MEDICAL CENTER, 1050 Division Street, Zip 53948–1997; tel. 608/847–6161; Daniel N. Manders, President and Chief Executive Officer (Total facility includes 60 beds in nursing home–type unit) **A**1 9 10 **F**7 8 9 18 22 24 25 32 34 36 37 38 39 43 44 45 46 48 49 50 51 54 56 67 68 69 70 71 76 77 78 **P**5	23	10	97	2147	77	75637	231	22102	11953	330
MEDFORD—Taylor County ★ MEMORIAL HOSPITAL OF TAYLOR COUNTY, (Includes Memorial Nursing Home), 135 South Gibson Street, Zip 54451–1696; tel. 715/748–8100; Greg Roraff, President and Chief Executive Officer (Total facility includes 104 beds in nursing home–type unit) **A**1 9 10 **F**1 6 7 8 9 12 18 19 22 24 25 26 32 34 36 38 39 41 43 44 45 48 50 51 54 56 59 61 67 68 69 70 71 72 76 78 **P**4	23	10	153	1069	100	28034	172	23784	11759	690
MENOMONEE FALLS—Waukesha County ★ △ COMMUNITY MEMORIAL HOSPITAL, W180 N8085 Town Hall Road, Zip 53051, Mailing Address: P.O. Box 408, Zip 53052–0408; tel. 262/251–1000; Robert E. Drisner, President and Chief Executive Officer **A**1 2 7 9 10 **F**2 3 4 5 6 7 8 9 10 11 12 16 18 19 20 21 22 23 24 25 27 28 31 34 36 37 38 39 40 41 42 43 44 45 46 47 48 49 50 52 53 54 57 59 60 61 62 63 64 65 70 71 72 74 75 76 78 79 **S** Horizon Healthcare, Inc., Milwaukee, WI Web address: www.communitymemorial.com	23	10	142	6789	79	58144	887	60520	26763	778
MENOMONIE—Dunn County ☐ MYRTLE WERTH HOSPITAL–MAYO HEALTH SYSTEM, 2321 Stout Road, Zip 54751–2397; tel. 715/235–5531; Thomas Miller, II, Chief Executive Officer **A**1 3 9 10 **F**1 2 3 4 5 6 7 8 9 10 11 12 13 18 21 22 24 25 27 28 35 36 37 38 39 40 41 42 43 44 45 46 47 48 49 50 51 52 53 54 55 57 58 59 60 61 62 63 64 65 67 68 70 71 72 75 76 77 79	23	10	55	1611	13	46131	268	12236	5225	187
MEQUON—Ozaukee County ★ ST. MARY'S HOSPITAL OZAUKEE, 13111 North Port Washington Road, Zip 53097–2416; tel. 262/243–7300; Therese B. Pandl, Executive Vice President and Chief Operating Officer **A**1 9 10 **F**2 3 4 5 7 8 9 10 11 12 13 14 15 16 18 19 20 21 22 23 25 26 31 32 34 35 36 37 38 39 41 44 45 46 47 48 49 50 51 52 53 54 56 57 58 59 60 61 62 63 64 67 70 71 72 73 75 76 77 78 79 **P**8 **S** Ascension Health, Saint Louis, MO Web address: www.columbia-stmarys.com	21	10	82	4751	52	171536	729	52444	26467	605
MERRILL—Lincoln County ★ GOOD SAMARITAN HEALTH CENTER OF MERRILL, 601 Center Avenue South, Zip 54452–3404; tel. 715/536–5511; Michael Hammer, President and Chief Executive Officer **A**1 10 **F**1 2 3 4 5 6 7 8 9 10 11 12 13 14 15 16 19 20 21 22 23 24 25 26 27 28 31 32 34 35 36 37 38 39 40 41 42 43 44 45 46 47 48 49 50 51 52 53 54 55 56 57 58 59 60 61 62 63 64 65 67 68 70 71 72 73 74 75 76 77 78 79 **S** Catholic Health Initiatives, Denver, CO	21	10	63	1463	22	44291	144	12662	5564	170
MILWAUKEE—Milwaukee County CHARTER HOSPITAL OF MILWAUKEE, 11101 West Lincoln Avenue, Zip 53227–1166; tel. 414/327–3000; William E. Henricks, Ph.D., Chief Operating Officer (Nonreporting) **A**10	33	22	80	—	—	—	—	—	—	—
★ CHILDREN'S HOSPITAL OF WISCONSIN, 9000 West Wisconsin Avenue, Zip 53226–4810, Mailing Address: P.O. Box 1997, Zip 53201–1997; tel. 414/266–2000; Jon E. Vice, President and Chief Executive Officer **A**1 3 5 8 9 10 **F**1 2 3 4 5 6 8 9 10 11 12 13 14 16 18 19 21 22 23 25 27 28 32 34 35 36 37 38 39 40 41 42 43 44 45 46 47 48 50 51 52 53 54 55 56 57 58 59 60 61 62 63 64 65 68 70 71 72 73 74 75 76 77 78 79 **P**4 Web address: www.chw.org	23	50	222	18397	163	190199	0	174088	56633	1476
★ △ CLEMENT J. ZABLOCKI VETERANS AFFAIRS MEDICAL CENTER, 5000 West National Avenue, Zip 53295; tel. 414/384–2000; Glen W. Grippen, Director (Total facility includes 196 beds in nursing home–type unit) (Nonreporting) **A**1 2 3 5 7 8 9 **S** Department of Veterans Affairs, Washington, DC	45	10	566	—	—	—	—	—	—	—
★ COLUMBIA HOSPITAL, 2025 East Newport Avenue, Zip 53211–2990; tel. 414/961–3300; Susan Henckel, Executive Vice President and Chief Operating Officer **A**1 2 3 5 7 9 10 **F**2 3 4 5 8 9 10 11 12 13 15 16 19 21 22 23 24 25 27 28 31 32 34 35 36 37 38 39 41 42 43 44 45 46 47 48 49 50 51 52 53 54 56 57 58 59 60 61 62 63 64 65 70 71 72 74 75 76 77 78 79 **P**6 **S** Horizon Healthcare, Inc., Milwaukee, WI Web address: www.columbia-stmarys.com	23	10	328	10401	141	298335	1117	139978	56247	1452

© 2000 AHA Guide   *Many Facility Codes have changed. Please refer to the AHA Guide Code Chart.*

Hospitals, U.S. / WISCONSIN

Hospital, Address, Telephone, Administrator, Approval, Facility, and Physician Codes, Health Care System, Network	Classification Codes		Utilization Data					Expense (thousands) of dollars		
★ American Hospital Association (AHA) membership ☐ Joint Commission on Accreditation of Healthcare Organizations (JCAHO) accreditation + American Osteopathic Healthcare Association (AOHA) membership ○ American Osteopathic Association (AOA) accreditation △ Commission on Accreditation of Rehabilitation Facilities (CARF) accreditation Control codes 61, 63, 64, 71, 72 and 73 indicate hospitals listed by AOHA, but not registered by AHA. For definition of numerical codes, see page A4	Control	Service	Staffed Beds	Admissions	Census	Outpatient Visits	Births	Total	Payroll	Personnel
★ △ FROEDTERT MEMORIAL LUTHERAN HOSPITAL, 9200 West Wisconsin Avenue, Zip 53226–3596, Mailing Address: P.O. Box 26099, Zip 53226–3596; tel. 414/259–3000; William D. Petasnick, President **A**1 2 3 5 7 8 9 10 **F**1 2 3 4 5 6 8 9 10 11 12 13 14 16 18 21 22 24 25 27 28 35 36 37 38 39 40 41 42 43 44 45 46 47 48 50 51 52 53 54 55 57 58 59 60 61 62 63 64 65 67 68 70 71 74 75 76 77 79 **S** Horizon Healthcare, Inc., Milwaukee, WI **Web address:** www.froedtert.com	23	10	472	17842	316	375683	967	288163	81931	2221
★ MILWAUKEE COUNTY MENTAL HEALTH DIVISION, 9455 Watertown Plank Road, Zip 53226–3559; tel. 414/257–6995; M. Kathleen Eilers, Administrator (Total facility includes 216 beds in nursing home–type unit) **A**1 3 5 10 **F**1 2 3 4 5 6 8 9 10 11 12 13 15 16 21 22 23 24 25 27 28 31 35 36 37 38 39 40 41 42 43 44 45 46 47 48 50 51 52 53 54 55 57 58 59 60 61 62 63 64 65 67 68 69 70 71 72 74 75 76 77 78 79	13	22	372	3014	319	—	0	120280	42463	1210
MILWAUKEE PSYCHIATRIC HOSPITAL See Wauwatosa										
○ NORTHWEST GENERAL HOSPITAL, 5310 West Capitol Drive, Zip 53216–2299; tel. 414/447–8543; Ed Reger, President and Chief Executive Officer **A**10 11 **F**1 2 3 4 5 6 8 9 10 11 12 13 21 22 24 25 27 28 35 36 37 38 39 40 43 44 45 46 47 48 50 51 52 53 54 55 57 58 59 60 61 62 63 64 65 67 68 70 71 76 77 79	23	10	98	2246	30	25014	0	12704	6444	212
★ △ SACRED HEART REHABILITATION INSTITUTE, 2350 North Lake Drive, Zip 53211–4507, Mailing Address: P.O. Box 392, Zip 53201–0392; tel. 414/298–6700; Nancy D. Kuelz, Administrator **A**1 7 10 **F**13 14 16 18 19 22 24 26 31 32 34 38 39 45 50 51 53 54 59 62 70 71 72 76 78 **P**6 **S** Ascension Health, Saint Louis, MO **Web address:** www.columbia-stmarys.com	21	46	45	673	24	20158	0	15888	8585	156
★ △ SINAI SAMARITAN MEDICAL CENTER, 945 North 12th Street, Zip 53233–1337, Mailing Address: P.O. Box 342, Zip 53201–0342; tel. 414/219–2000; Leonard E. Wilk, Administrator **A**1 2 3 5 7 8 9 **F**1 2 3 4 5 6 8 9 10 11 12 13 14 16 18 19 21 22 24 25 26 28 31 32 34 35 37 38 39 41 42 43 44 45 46 47 48 51 52 53 54 55 56 57 58 59 60 61 62 63 64 65 67 68 70 71 72 73 74 75 76 77 78 79 **P**4 6 **S** Aurora Health Care, Milwaukee, WI **Web address:** www.aurorahealthcare.org	23	10	255	12764	156	259117	3062	169890	62932	1623
★ △ ST. FRANCIS HOSPITAL, 3237 South 16th Street, Zip 53215–4592; tel. 414/647–5000; Jerrold A. Maki, President **A**1 2 5 7 9 10 **F**1 4 5 8 9 10 11 12 13 14 16 18 19 21 22 24 25 26 28 31 32 34 35 37 38 39 41 42 43 44 45 46 47 48 50 51 52 53 54 55 56 59 60 68 70 71 72 73 74 76 78 79 **P**1 4 5 6 7 **S** Wheaton Franciscan Services, Inc., Wheaton, IL **Web address:** www.covhealth.org	23	10	212	12955	157	112529	1639	110721	41091	1097
★ △ ST. JOSEPH'S HOSPITAL, 5000 West Chambers Street, Zip 53210–9988; tel. 414/447–2000; Patricia A. Kaldor, R.N., President (Total facility includes 28 beds in nursing home–type unit) **A**1 2 3 5 7 9 10 **F**2 3 4 5 6 7 8 9 10 11 12 13 14 19 20 21 22 24 25 26 27 31 32 34 35 37 38 39 40 41 42 44 45 46 47 48 49 50 51 52 53 54 55 56 57 58 59 60 62 63 64 65 67 68 69 70 71 72 73 74 75 76 77 78 79 **P**5 **S** Wheaton Franciscan Services, Inc., Wheaton, IL **Web address:** www.covhealth.org	21	10	473	17392	313	162794	3740	185667	77319	2155
★ ST. LUKE'S MEDICAL CENTER, (Includes St. Luke's South Shore, 5900 South Lake Drive, Cudahy, Zip 53110–8903; tel. 414/769–9000), 2900 West Oklahoma Avenue, Zip 53215–4330, Mailing Address: P.O. Box 2901, Zip 53201–2901; tel. 414/649–6000; Mark S. Wiener, Administrator **A**1 2 3 5 7 8 9 10 **F**2 3 4 5 8 9 10 11 12 13 14 16 18 19 21 22 24 25 26 27 28 31 32 34 35 36 37 38 39 41 43 44 45 46 47 48 50 51 53 54 55 56 57 58 59 60 61 62 63 64 65 67 68 70 71 72 73 74 75 76 77 78 79 **P**4 6 **S** Aurora Health Care, Milwaukee, WI **Web address:** www.aurorahealthcare.org	23	10	747	32119	494	401813	1385	458696	141298	3788
★ ST. MARY'S HOSPITAL, 2323 North Lake Drive, Zip 53211–9682, Mailing Address: P.O. Box 503, Zip 53201–0503; tel. 414/291–1000; Susan Henckel, Chief Operating Officer **A**1 2 3 5 9 10 **F**3 4 8 9 10 11 12 13 15 16 18 19 20 21 22 23 24 25 26 31 32 34 36 38 39 41 42 43 44 45 46 47 48 49 50 56 58 59 62 63 64 68 70 71 72 76 77 78 79 **P**8 **S** Ascension Health, Saint Louis, MO **Web address:** www.columbia-stmarys.com	21	10	241	9440	129	394543	2605	138990	71129	1618
★ △ ST. MICHAEL HOSPITAL, 2400 West Villard Avenue, Zip 53209–4999; tel. 414/527–8000; Jeffrey K. Jenkins, President **A**1 2 3 5 7 9 10 **F**1 2 3 4 7 8 9 11 12 13 14 16 18 19 20 21 22 24 25 26 27 28 31 32 34 36 37 38 39 41 42 43 44 45 46 47 48 50 51 53 54 57 58 59 60 61 62 63 64 65 68 70 71 72 75 76 77 78 79 **P**4 6 7 **S** Wheaton Franciscan Services, Inc., Wheaton, IL **Web address:** www.covhealth.org	21	10	179	7884	119	166783	1014	82524	32071	895
VENCOR HOSPITAL–MILWAUKEE, 5700 West Layton Avenue, Zip 53202; tel. 414/427–8282; E. Kay Gray, Interim Administrator (Nonreporting) **S** Vencor, Incorporated, Louisville, KY	33	49	60	—	—	—	—	—	—	—
MONROE—Green County										
☐ THE MONROE CLINIC, 515 22nd Avenue, Zip 53566–1598; tel. 608/324–1000; Kenneth Blount, President and Chief Executive Officer **A**1 10 **F**1 2 3 4 5 6 8 9 10 11 12 13 14 16 18 19 21 22 24 25 26 27 28 32 34 35 36 37 38 39 40 41 42 43 44 45 46 47 48 50 51 52 53 54 55 56 57 58 59 60 61 62 63 64 65 67 68 70 71 72 74 75 76 77 78 79 **P**6 8 **Web address:** www.themonroeclinic.org	21	10	117	3587	36	234048	446	61568	33112	754

Hospitals, U.S. / WISCONSIN

Hospital, Address, Telephone, Administrator, Approval, Facility, and Physician Codes, Health Care System, Network	Classification Codes		Utilization Data					Expense (thousands) of dollars		
★ American Hospital Association (AHA) membership □ Joint Commission on Accreditation of Healthcare Organizations (JCAHO) accreditation + American Osteopathic Healthcare Association (AOHA) membership ○ American Osteopathic Association (AOA) accreditation △ Commission on Accreditation of Rehabilitation Facilities (CARF) accreditation Control codes 61, 63, 64, 71, 72 and 73 indicate hospitals listed by AOHA, but not registered by AHA. For definition of numerical codes, see page A4	Control	Service	Staffed Beds	Admissions	Census	Outpatient Visits	Births	Total	Payroll	Personnel
NEENAH—Winnebago County ★ △ THEDA CLARK MEDICAL CENTER, 130 Second Street, Zip 54956-2883, Mailing Address: P.O. Box 2021, Zip 54957-2021; tel. 920/729-3100; Robert H. Malte, Senior Vice President **A**1 7 9 10 **F**1 2 3 4 5 8 9 10 11 12 13 14 15 16 18 19 22 23 24 25 26 27 28 31 32 34 35 36 37 38 39 40 41 42 43 44 45 46 47 48 50 51 52 53 54 55 56 57 58 60 61 62 63 64 67 68 70 71 72 73 74 75 76 77 78 79 **P**6 8 **S** ThedaCare, Inc., Appleton, WI **Web address:** www.thedacare.org	23	10	216	8937	118	77537	1019	76764	35504	785
NEILLSVILLE—Clark County MEMORIAL MEDICAL CENTER, (Includes Neillsville Memorial Home), 216 Sunset Place, Zip 54456-1799; tel. 715/743-3101; Glen E. Grady, Administrator (Total facility includes 137 beds in nursing home-type unit) **A**10 **F**1 2 3 4 5 6 8 9 10 11 12 13 14 18 19 21 22 23 24 25 26 27 28 32 33 34 35 36 37 38 39 40 41 42 43 44 45 46 47 48 50 51 52 53 54 55 56 57 58 59 60 61 62 63 64 65 67 68 69 70 71 72 74 75 76 77 78 79 **P**6	23	10	166	1092	116	44623	38	10233	5541	358
NEW LONDON—Outagamie County ★ NEW LONDON FAMILY MEDICAL CENTER, 1405 Mill Street, Zip 54961-2155, Mailing Address: P.O. Box 307, Zip 54961-0307; tel. 920/982-5330; Paul E. Gurgel, President and Chief Executive Officer **A**1 9 10 **F**7 8 9 12 19 22 24 25 26 32 38 39 41 43 44 45 48 49 50 53 54 71 72 76 77 78	23	10	39	1329	12	56695	198	11388	5158	132
NEW RICHMOND—St. Croix County ★ HOLY FAMILY HOSPITAL, 535 Hospital Road, Zip 54017-1495; tel. 715/246-2101; Jean M. Needham, President **A**9 10 **F**1 2 3 4 5 6 8 9 10 11 12 13 14 16 18 21 22 23 24 25 27 28 32 34 35 36 37 38 39 40 41 42 43 44 45 46 47 48 50 51 52 53 54 55 57 58 59 60 61 62 63 64 65 67 68 70 71 72 74 75 76 77 78 79	21	10	20	962	11	12573	124	7420	4094	100
OCONOMOWOC—Waukesha County ★ △ OCONOMOWOC MEMORIAL HOSPITAL, 791 Summit Avenue, Zip 53066-3896; tel. 262/569-9400; Douglas Guy, President and Chief Executive Officer **A**1 7 9 10 **F**1 2 3 6 7 8 9 12 16 18 22 24 25 27 28 35 36 37 38 39 41 43 44 45 46 48 49 50 51 53 54 61 68 70 75 76 79 **S** ProHealth Care, Waukesha, WI	23	10	72	3533	34	91418	649	41716	17634	452
□ ROGERS MEMORIAL HOSPITAL, 34700 Valley Road, Zip 53066-4599; tel. 262/646-4411; David L. Moulthrop, Ph.D., President and Chief Executive Officer **A**1 10 **F**3 13 18 21 22 31 38 39 43 50 51 57 58 59 60 61 62 63 64 70 73 **Web address:** www.rogershospital.org	23	22	90	1131	61	21180	0	15124	8798	265
OCONTO—Oconto County OCONTO MEMORIAL HOSPITAL, 405 First Street, Zip 54153-1299; tel. 920/834-8806; David McMahon, Chief Executive Officer **A**9 10 **F**1 2 3 4 5 6 8 9 10 11 12 13 21 22 24 25 27 28 35 36 37 38 39 40 41 42 43 44 45 46 47 48 50 51 52 53 54 55 57 58 59 60 61 62 63 64 65 67 68 70 71 74 75 76 77 79 **P**6	23	10	17	348	5	13002	0	3114	1572	50
OCONTO FALLS—Oconto County ★ COMMUNITY MEMORIAL HOSPITAL, 855 South Main Street, Zip 54154-1296; tel. 920/846-3444; Jim Van Dornick, Administrator **A**10 **F**3 7 8 9 13 18 22 25 38 39 43 44 45 48 49 50 51 52 53 54 59 60 63 70 71 75 76 79 **P**6 **S** Brim Healthcare, Inc., Brentwood, TN **Web address:** www.cmhospital.org	23	10	27	792	10	26931	54	9007	4384	114
OSCEOLA—Polk County OSCEOLA MEDICAL CENTER, 301 River Street, Zip 54020, Mailing Address: P.O. Box 218, Zip 54020-0218; tel. 715/294-2111; Jeffrey K. Meyer, Chief Executive Officer (Total facility includes 40 beds in nursing home-type unit) **A**9 10 **F**1 2 3 4 5 6 8 9 10 11 12 13 21 22 24 25 27 28 35 36 37 38 39 40 41 42 43 44 45 46 47 48 50 51 52 53 54 55 57 58 59 60 61 62 63 64 65 67 68 69 70 71 74 75 76 77 79 **P**5 **Web address:** www.centurytel.net/omc	23	10	59	694	45	22481	86	4582	2510	89
OSHKOSH—Winnebago County ★ △ MERCY MEDICAL CENTER, 631 Hazel Street, Zip 54901-4680, Mailing Address: P.O. Box 1100, Zip 54902-1100; tel. 920/236-2000; Otto L. Cox, President **A**1 2 7 9 10 **F**2 3 4 5 7 8 9 10 11 12 13 18 19 20 21 22 24 25 26 27 32 34 36 37 38 39 40 41 42 44 45 48 49 50 51 52 53 54 56 57 58 59 60 61 62 63 65 67 68 70 71 72 73 75 76 77 78 79 **P**6	21	10	175	7367	95	335924	961	91876	42516	914
OSSEO—Trempealeau County OSSEO AREA HOSPITAL AND NURSING HOME, 13025 Eighth Street, Zip 54758, Mailing Address: P.O. Box 70, Zip 54758-0070; tel. 715/597-3121; Bradley D. Groseth, Administrator (Total facility includes 61 beds in nursing home-type unit) **A**9 10 18 **F**1 2 3 4 5 6 8 9 10 11 12 13 14 19 21 22 23 24 25 27 28 31 32 34 35 36 37 38 39 40 41 42 43 44 45 46 47 48 50 51 52 53 54 55 56 57 58 59 60 61 62 63 64 65 67 68 69 70 71 72 73 74 75 76 77 78 79 **S** Mayo Foundation, Rochester, MN	23	10	77	169	39	9243	0	4055	2126	139
PARK FALLS—Price County ★ FLAMBEAU HOSPITAL, 98 Sherry Avenue, Zip 54552-1467, Mailing Address: P.O. Box 310, Zip 54552-0310; tel. 715/762-2484; Curtis A. Johnson, Administrator **A**1 9 10 **F**7 8 9 12 13 14 18 19 22 24 25 26 28 32 34 36 37 38 40 41 43 44 45 48 49 50 51 53 54 56 70 71 72 76 77 78 **S** Marian Health System, Tulsa, OK **Web address:** www.ministryhealth.org/facility/fh.html	23	10	42	1394	13	24921	82	11252	4940	170

Hospitals, U.S. / WISCONSIN

Hospital, Address, Telephone, Administrator, Approval, Facility, and Physician Codes, Health Care System, Network	Classification Codes		Utilization Data					Expense (thousands) of dollars		
	Control	Service	Staffed Beds	Admissions	Census	Outpatient Visits	Births	Total	Payroll	Personnel

★ American Hospital Association (AHA) membership
☐ Joint Commission on Accreditation of Healthcare Organizations (JCAHO) accreditation
✛ American Osteopathic Healthcare Association (AOHA) membership
○ American Osteopathic Association (AOA) accreditation
△ Commission on Accreditation of Rehabilitation Facilities (CARF) accreditation
Control codes 61, 63, 64, 71, 72 and 73 indicate hospitals listed by AOHA, but not registered by AHA. For definition of numerical codes, see page A4

PLATTEVILLE—Grant County

★ SOUTHWEST HEALTH CENTER, (Includes Evergreen Adult Center, 2110 Church Street, Hazel Green, Zip 53811; tel. 608/854-2231; Southwest Health Center Nursing Home, 808 South Washington Street, Cuba City, Zip 53807; tel. 608/744-2161), 250 Camp Street, Zip 53818-1703; tel. 608/348-2331; Anne K. Klawiter, President and Chief Executive Officer (Total facility includes 110 beds in nursing home–type unit) **A**1 9 10 **F**6 7 8 9 16 18 19 22 25 26 31 32 34 36 37 38 39 40 43 44 48 50 53 54 57 59 60 62 63 64 69 70 72 76 79 **S** Brim Healthcare, Inc., Brentwood, TN
Web address: www.southwesthealth.org | 23 | 10 | 143 | 1414 | 114 | 20576 | 139 | 12986 | 4985 | 183 |

PLYMOUTH—Sheboygan County

★ VALLEY VIEW MEDICAL CENTER, 901 Reed Street, Zip 53073-2409; tel. 920/893-1771; T. Gregg Watson, Administrator (Total facility includes 60 beds in nursing home–type unit) (Nonreporting) **A**1 9 10 **S** Aurora Health Care, Milwaukee, WI
Web address: www.aurorahealthcare.org | 23 | 10 | 92 | — | — | — | — | — | — | — |

PORT WASHINGTON—Ozaukee County

ST. MARY'S HOSPITAL OZAUKEE See Mequon

PORTAGE—Columbia County

☐ DIVINE SAVIOR HEALTHCARE, (Formerly Divine Savior Hospital Healthcare), 1015 West Pleasant Street, Zip 53901-9987, Mailing Address: P.O. Box 387, Zip 53901-0387; tel. 608/742-4131; Michael Decker, President and Chief Executive Officer (Total facility includes 114 beds in nursing home–type unit) **A**1 9 10 **F**2 3 7 8 9 15 16 18 19 20 22 23 24 25 26 31 32 34 36 38 39 40 41 43 44 45 46 48 50 51 53 54 56 61 68 69 70 71 72 75 76 78 **P**6 8 | 21 | 10 | 156 | 1786 | 133 | 45319 | 204 | 25480 | 11850 | 409 |

PRAIRIE DU CHIEN—Crawford County

★ PRAIRIE DU CHIEN MEMORIAL HOSPITAL, 705 East Taylor Street, Zip 53821-2196; tel. 608/326-2431; Harold W. Brown, Chief Executive Officer **A**1 9 10 **F**1 2 3 6 7 8 9 12 13 16 18 22 25 36 37 38 39 40 41 43 44 45 46 48 50 51 54 58 59 61 63 64 67 70 71 76 77
Web address: www.pdcmem@pdhhospital.org | 23 | 10 | 43 | 1563 | 33 | 20605 | 143 | 12530 | 6559 | 203 |

PRAIRIE DU SAC—Sauk County

☐ SAUK PRAIRIE MEMORIAL HOSPITAL, 80 First Street, Zip 53578-1550; tel. 608/643-7166; Bobbe Teigen, Administrator **A**1 9 10 **F**1 2 3 4 5 6 8 9 10 11 12 13 16 18 21 22 24 25 27 28 35 36 37 38 39 40 41 42 43 44 45 46 47 48 50 51 52 53 54 55 57 58 59 60 61 62 63 64 65 67 68 70 71 74 75 76 77 79 **P**6
Web address: www.spmh.org | 23 | 10 | 36 | 2196 | 19 | 42639 | 230 | 24051 | 12043 | 323 |

RACINE—Racine County

★ △ ALL SAINT'S HEALTHCARE SYSTEM, (Formerly Saint Mary's Medical Center), 3801 Spring Street, Zip 53405-1690; tel. 262/636-4011; Kenneth R. Buser, President and Chief Executive Officer **A**1 2 3 7 9 10 **F**2 3 4 7 8 9 11 12 13 14 16 18 19 22 24 25 26 27 28 32 34 36 37 38 39 41 42 43 44 45 46 47 48 49 50 51 52 53 54 56 57 58 59 60 61 62 63 64 65 70 71 72 73 76 77 78 79 **P**6 **S** Wheaton Franciscan Services, Inc., Wheaton, IL | 21 | 10 | 215 | 9784 | 145 | 229556 | 0 | 99392 | 43899 | 1360 |

★ ST. LUKE'S MEMORIAL HOSPITAL, 1320 Wisconsin Avenue, Zip 53403-1987; tel. 262/636-2011; Kenneth R. Buser, President and Chief Executive Officer (Total facility includes 50 beds in nursing home–type unit) **A**5 9 10 **F**2 3 4 7 8 9 11 12 13 16 18 21 22 24 25 27 28 36 37 38 39 41 42 43 44 45 46 47 48 49 50 51 52 53 54 57 58 59 60 61 62 63 64 65 69 70 71 76 77 79 **P**6 **S** Wheaton Franciscan Services, Inc., Wheaton, IL | 23 | 10 | 151 | 4276 | 100 | 97455 | 1945 | 42392 | 18484 | 418 |

REEDSBURG—Sauk County

★ REEDSBURG AREA MEDICAL CENTER, 2000 North Dewey Street, Zip 53959-1097; tel. 608/524-6487; George L. Johnson, President (Total facility includes 50 beds in nursing home–type unit) **A**1 9 10 **F**4 7 8 9 11 12 13 18 20 21 22 24 25 28 32 36 37 38 39 40 41 43 44 45 46 48 49 50 52 54 69 70 71 75 76 77 78 **P**6 | 23 | 10 | 88 | 1905 | 69 | 36507 | 170 | 20153 | 9145 | 338 |

RHINELANDER—Oneida County

★ SACRED HEART–ST. MARY'S HOSPITALS, (Includes Sacred Heart Hospital, 216 North Seventh Street, Tomahawk, Zip 54487; tel. 715/453-7700; St. Mary's Hospital, 1044 Kabel Avenue, Zip 54501-3998; tel. 715/369-6600; Kevin J. O'Donnell, President and Chief Executive Officer **A**1 10 **F**2 3 8 9 12 13 18 22 25 27 28 31 32 34 36 37 38 39 40 41 43 44 45 46 48 49 50 51 54 57 58 59 60 61 62 63 64 65 68 70 71 76 78 79 **S** Marian Health System, Tulsa, OK
Web address: www.ministryhealth.org | 21 | 10 | 53 | 4950 | 52 | 56642 | 401 | 41895 | 20150 | 601 |

RICE LAKE—Barron County

★ LAKEVIEW MEDICAL CENTER, 1100 North Main Street, Zip 54868-1238; tel. 715/234-1515; Edward H. Wolf, President and Chief Executive Officer **A**1 9 10 **F**7 8 12 14 18 19 22 25 26 27 28 32 36 37 38 39 40 41 43 44 45 46 48 49 50 54 68 70 71 72 76 78 | 23 | 10 | 69 | 2759 | 26 | 26909 | 409 | 21315 | 10428 | 272 |

RICHLAND CENTER—Richland County

☐ RICHLAND HOSPITAL, 431 North Park Street, Zip 53581-1899; tel. 608/647-6321; Thomas J. Werner, Chief Executive Officer **A**1 9 10 **F**1 2 3 4 5 6 8 9 10 11 12 13 19 21 22 24 25 26 27 28 32 34 35 36 37 38 39 40 41 42 43 44 45 46 47 48 50 51 52 53 54 55 57 58 59 60 61 62 63 64 65 67 68 70 71 72 74 75 76 77 79
Web address: www.richlandhospital.com | 23 | 10 | 38 | 1604 | 18 | 18100 | 175 | 14432 | 6899 | 229 |

Hospitals, U.S. / WISCONSIN

Hospital, Address, Telephone, Administrator, Approval, Facility, and Physician Codes, Health Care System, Network	Classification Codes		Utilization Data					Expense (thousands) of dollars		Personnel
★ American Hospital Association (AHA) membership □ Joint Commission on Accreditation of Healthcare Organizations (JCAHO) accreditation + American Osteopathic Healthcare Association (AOHA) membership ○ American Osteopathic Association (AOA) accreditation △ Commission on Accreditation of Rehabilitation Facilities (CARF) accreditation Control codes 61, 63, 64, 71, 72 and 73 indicate hospitals listed by AOHA, but not registered by AHA. For definition of numerical codes, see page A4	Control	Service	Staffed Beds	Admissions	Census	Outpatient Visits	Births	Total	Payroll	Personnel
RIPON—Fond Du Lac County ★ RIPON MEDICAL CENTER, 933 Newbury Street, Zip 54971-1798, Mailing Address: P.O. Box 390, Zip 54971-0390; tel. 920/748-3101; Jon W. Baker, Chief Executive Officer **A**1 9 10 **F**7 8 9 12 13 18 22 24 25 28 31 32 34 38 39 40 41 43 44 45 46 48 50 51 52 54 56 59 63 68 70 71 72 75 76 77 78 79 **S** Brim Healthcare, Inc., Brentwood, TN Web address: www.riponmedicalcenter.com	23	10	29	993	11	30034	103	11346	4696	138
RIVER FALLS—St. Croix County ★ RIVER FALLS AREA HOSPITAL, 1629 East Division Street, Zip 54022-1571; tel. 715/425-6155; Sharon Whelan, Administrator **A**1 9 10 **F**1 2 3 4 5 6 8 9 10 11 12 13 14 15 16 18 19 21 22 23 24 25 26 27 28 31 32 34 35 36 37 38 39 40 41 43 44 45 46 47 48 50 51 52 53 54 55 56 57 58 59 60 61 62 63 64 65 67 68 70 71 72 73 74 75 76 77 78 79 **S** Allina Health System, Minneapolis, MN Web address: www.allina.com	23	10	31	1224	11	11437	268	11220	4444	101
SAINT CROIX FALLS—Polk County □ ST. CROIX REGIONAL MEDICAL CENTER, (Formerly St. Croix Valley Memorial Hospital), 204 South Adams Street, Zip 54024-9400; tel. 715/483-3261; Steve L. Urosevich, Chief Executive Officer **A**1 9 10 **F**2 3 6 7 8 9 12 13 19 21 22 24 25 26 28 31 32 34 36 37 38 39 41 44 45 46 48 50 51 52 54 55 56 57 58 59 61 62 63 67 68 70 71 72 73 75 76 77 78 79 Web address: www.scrmc.org	23	10	69	2322	18	16516	273	16246	6675	373
SHAWANO—Shawano County ★ SHAWANO MEDICAL CENTER, 309 North Bartlette Street, Zip 54166-0477; tel. 715/526-2111; John J. Kestly, Administrator **A**1 9 10 **F**8 9 11 12 14 16 18 19 22 24 25 26 31 32 34 36 37 38 39 41 43 44 48 50 51 53 54 56 61 68 70 71 72 76 78 **P**5 **S** Brim Healthcare, Inc., Brentwood, TN Web address: www.shawanomed.com	23	10	46	2147	20	41999	364	16253	7263	227
SHEBOYGAN—Sheboygan County ★ △ SHEBOYGAN MEMORIAL MEDICAL CENTER, 2629 North Seventh Street, Zip 53083-4998; tel. 920/451-5000; T. Gregg Watson, Administrator (Total facility includes 60 beds in nursing home-type unit) **A**1 2 7 9 10 **F**1 2 3 4 5 6 8 9 10 11 12 13 18 21 22 24 25 27 28 35 38 39 41 42 43 44 45 46 47 48 50 51 52 53 54 55 57 58 59 60 61 62 63 64 65 67 68 69 70 71 74 75 76 77 79 **S** Aurora Health Care, Milwaukee, WI Web address: www.aurorahealthcare.org	23	10	217	6081	122	60068	1056	51624	20546	691
★ △ ST. NICHOLAS HOSPITAL, 1601 North Taylor Drive, Zip 53081-2496; tel. 920/459-8300; Michael J. Stenger, Executive Vice President and Administrator **A**1 2 7 9 10 **F**7 8 9 11 12 13 14 16 18 19 20 21 22 23 24 25 26 27 28 31 32 34 36 37 38 39 40 41 43 44 45 46 48 49 50 51 53 54 56 58 59 60 61 65 68 70 71 72 73 74 75 76 77 78 79 **P**5 **S** Hospital Sisters Health System, Springfield, IL Web address: www.stnicholashospital.org	21	10	185	3232	42	54016	315	33132	13455	361
SHELL LAKE—Washburn County □ INDIANHEAD MEDICAL CENTER, 113 Fourth Avenue West, Zip 54871; tel. 715/468-7833; Paul Naglosky, Administrator **A**1 9 10 **F**1 2 3 4 5 6 8 9 10 11 12 13 19 21 22 23 24 25 28 31 34 35 36 37 38 39 40 41 42 43 44 45 46 47 48 50 51 52 53 54 55 56 57 58 59 60 61 62 63 64 65 67 68 70 71 72 74 75 76 77 78 79 **P**5 **S** Northeast Health Management, Inc., Stevensville, MD	33	10	49	618	6	8962	22	3997	1884	70
SPARTA—Monroe County ★ FRANCISCAN SKEMP HEALTHCARE–SPARTA CAMPUS, 310 West Main Street, Zip 54656-2171; tel. 608/269-2132; William P. Sexton, Administrator (Total facility includes 30 beds in nursing home-type unit) **A**1 10 **F**1 2 3 4 5 6 8 9 10 11 12 13 16 18 21 22 24 25 27 28 35 36 37 38 39 40 41 42 43 44 45 46 47 48 50 51 52 53 54 55 57 58 59 60 61 62 63 65 67 68 69 70 71 74 75 76 77 79 **P**8 **S** Franciscan Skemp Healthcare, La Crosse, WI Web address: www.mayo.edu/fsh	21	10	59	708	37	41743	124	5604	2899	92
SPOONER—Washburn County ★ SPOONER HEALTH SYSTEM, 819 Ash Street, Zip 54801-1299; tel. 715/635-2111; Michael Schafer, Chief Executive Officer (Total facility includes 90 beds in nursing home-type unit) **A**1 9 10 **F**2 7 8 9 12 13 18 19 22 24 25 26 31 32 34 36 37 38 40 41 44 45 48 49 50 51 53 54 55 56 68 69 70 71 72 76 78 **S** Brim Healthcare, Inc., Brentwood, TN	23	10	136	1208	99	24844	81	9543	4347	192
STANLEY—Chippewa County ★ VICTORY MEDICAL CENTER, 230 East Fourth Avenue, Zip 54768-1298; tel. 715/644-5571; Cynthia Eichman, Chief Executive Officer and Administrator (Total facility includes 70 beds in nursing home-type unit) **A**1 9 10 **F**1 7 9 12 18 19 22 23 24 25 26 32 34 38 41 43 45 48 50 51 54 56 63 69 70 71 72 74 75 76 77 78 **P**6 **S** Marian Health System, Tulsa, OK Web address: www.victorymedicalcenter.org	23	10	111	731	75	21250	0	9396	4746	171
STEVENS POINT—Portage County ★ SAINT MICHAEL'S HOSPITAL, 900 Illinois Avenue, Zip 54481-3196; tel. 715/346-5000; Jeffrey L. Martin, President and Chief Executive Officer **A**1 9 10 **F**2 3 7 8 12 13 15 16 19 22 24 25 26 27 32 34 36 37 38 39 40 41 42 43 44 45 46 48 50 51 52 54 55 57 58 59 60 61 62 64 65 68 70 71 72 76 77 78 **S** Marian Health System, Tulsa, OK Web address: www.smhosp.org	21	10	114	4408	46	122216	738	55921	28663	671

Hospitals, U.S. / WISCONSIN

Hospital, Address, Telephone, Administrator, Approval, Facility, and Physician Codes, Health Care System, Network	Classification Codes		Utilization Data					Expense (thousands) of dollars		
★ American Hospital Association (AHA) membership ☐ Joint Commission on Accreditation of Healthcare Organizations (JCAHO) accreditation + American Osteopathic Healthcare Association (AOHA) membership ○ American Osteopathic Association (AOA) accreditation △ Commission on Accreditation of Rehabilitation Facilities (CARF) accreditation Control codes 61, 63, 64, 71, 72 and 73 indicate hospitals listed by AOHA, but not registered by AHA. For definition of numerical codes, see page A4	Control	Service	Staffed Beds	Admissions	Census	Outpatient Visits	Births	Total	Payroll	Personnel
STOUGHTON—Dane County ☐ STOUGHTON HOSPITAL ASSOCIATION, 900 Ridge Street, Zip 53589–1896; tel. 608/873–6611; Terrence Brenny, President and Chief Executive Officer **A**1 9 10 **F**1 3 6 7 9 12 13 16 19 22 25 28 32 34 36 37 38 39 40 41 43 45 48 50 53 54 57 59 60 62 63 64 67 70 71 72 76 77 78 79	23	10	38	1286	19	32425	0	15221	5927	200
STURGEON BAY—Door County ★ DOOR COUNTY MEMORIAL HOSPITAL, 323 South 18th Avenue, Zip 54235–1495; tel. 920/743–5566; Gerald M. Worrick, President and Chief Executive Officer (Total facility includes 30 beds in nursing home–type unit) **A**1 9 10 **F**1 4 7 8 9 11 12 16 18 19 22 23 24 25 26 32 34 35 36 37 38 39 41 43 44 45 46 47 48 49 50 51 53 54 56 58 59 60 63 69 70 72 74 75 76 77 78 **P**6 **S** Marian Health System, Tulsa, OK Web address: www.doorcounty–wi.com	23	10	75	2099	50	36832	179	26034	13299	376
SUPERIOR—Douglas County ☐ ST. MARY'S HOSPITAL OF SUPERIOR, 3500 Tower Avenue, Zip 54880–5395; tel. 715/392–8281; Terry Jacobson, Administrator **A**1 9 10 **F**7 9 12 13 14 16 18 19 22 25 26 31 32 34 36 37 38 39 41 43 45 46 48 50 51 53 54 56 70 72 76 77 78 **S** Benedictine Health System, Duluth, MN Web address: www.smdc.org	23	10	42	1002	10	60844	0	12188	5865	145
TOMAH—Monroe County ★ TOMAH MEMORIAL HOSPITAL, 321 Butts Avenue, Zip 54660–1412; tel. 608/372–2181; Philip Stuart, Administrator **A**1 9 10 **F**2 3 7 8 9 13 18 19 22 25 26 28 37 38 39 40 44 45 46 48 51 57 63 70 71 76 77 **S** Brim Healthcare, Inc., Brentwood, TN	23	10	45	912	10	27539	182	10182	4518	147
★ VETERANS AFFAIRS MEDICAL CENTER, 500 East Veterans Street, Zip 54660; tel. 608/372–3971; Stan Johnson, Medical Center Director (Total facility includes 100 beds in nursing home–type unit) (Nonreporting) **A**1 **S** Department of Veterans Affairs, Washington, DC	45	22	569	—	—	—	—	—	—	—
TOMAHAWK—Lincoln County SACRED HEART HOSPITAL See Sacred Heart–St. Mary's Hospitals, Rhinelander										
TWO RIVERS—Manitowoc County ★ TWO RIVERS COMMUNITY HOSPITAL AND HAMILTON MEMORIAL HOME, 2500 Garfield Street, Zip 54241–2399; tel. 920/793–1178; Patrick J. Trotter, Chief Executive Officer (Total facility includes 85 beds in nursing home–type unit) **A**1 9 10 **F**1 2 3 4 5 6 8 9 10 11 12 13 16 18 19 21 22 24 25 27 28 35 38 39 40 41 42 43 44 46 47 48 50 51 52 53 54 55 57 58 59 60 61 62 63 64 65 67 68 69 70 71 74 75 76 77 79 **S** Aurora Health Care, Milwaukee, WI Web address: www.aurorahealthcare.org	23	10	138	1516	98	26817	301	13698	6144	201
VIROQUA—Vernon County VERNON MEMORIAL HOSPITAL, 507 South Main Street, Zip 54665–2096; tel. 608/637–2101; Garith W. Steiner, Chief Executive Officer and Administrator **A**10 **F**2 3 7 8 9 13 16 18 19 20 22 25 28 36 37 38 43 44 45 46 48 50 51 54 59 60 61 62 63 70 71 74 75 76 77	23	10	17	1869	16	58817	191	15214	7501	167
WATERTOWN—Dodge County ★ WATERTOWN MEMORIAL HOSPITAL, 125 Hospital Drive, Zip 53098–3384; tel. 920/261–4210; John P. Kosanovich, President **A**1 10 **F**1 2 3 4 5 6 7 8 9 11 12 13 18 19 20 21 22 24 25 26 27 28 31 32 34 35 36 37 38 39 40 41 42 43 44 45 46 47 48 49 50 51 52 53 54 55 57 58 59 60 61 62 63 64 65 67 68 70 71 72 74 75 76 77 78 79 **P**6 8 Web address: www.wahs.com	23	10	45	2404	32	88708	214	27891	12899	353
WAUKESHA—Waukesha County ★ △ WAUKESHA MEMORIAL HOSPITAL, 725 American Avenue, Zip 53188–5099; tel. 262/928–1000; Rexford W. Titus, II, President and Chief Executive Officer **A**1 2 3 5 7 9 10 **F**2 3 4 6 7 8 9 11 12 13 14 15 16 18 19 20 22 24 25 27 28 31 32 34 36 37 38 39 40 41 42 43 44 45 46 47 48 49 50 53 54 56 57 58 59 60 61 62 63 64 65 67 68 70 71 72 75 76 77 78 79 **P**5 6 7 **S** ProHealth Care, Waukesha, WI Web address: www.phci.org	23	10	288	12912	177	252200	2295	161572	58352	1556
WAUPACA—Waupaca County ★ RIVERSIDE MEDICAL CENTER, 800 Riverside Drive, Zip 54981–1999; tel. 715/258–1000; Craig A. Kantos, Chief Executive Officer **A**1 9 10 **F**7 8 9 10 11 12 22 24 25 27 38 39 41 44 45 46 48 50 51 52 53 68 70 76 77 79 **S** Quorum Health Group, Brentwood, TN Web address: www.riversidemedical.org	23	10	32	1644	16	47956	259	17447	7604	205
WAUPUN—Fond Du Lac County ★ WAUPUN MEMORIAL HOSPITAL, 620 West Brown Street, Zip 53963–1799; tel. 920/324–5581; James E. Baer, FACHE, President **A**1 10 **F**1 2 3 4 5 6 7 8 9 10 11 12 13 16 18 20 21 22 24 25 27 36 37 38 39 40 41 42 43 44 45 46 47 48 49 50 51 52 53 54 57 58 59 60 61 62 63 64 65 70 71 74 75 76 77 79	21	10	30	1007	10	39389	125	12092	4633	131
WAUSAU—Marathon County NORTH CENTRAL HEALTH CARE FACILITIES, 1100 Lakeview Drive, Zip 54403–6799; tel. 715/848–4600; Tim Steller, Chief Executive Officer (Total facility includes 338 beds in nursing home–type unit) **A**10 **F**1 2 3 4 5 6 8 9 10 11 12 13 19 21 22 24 25 27 28 31 35 36 37 38 39 40 41 42 43 44 45 46 47 48 50 51 52 53 54 55 57 58 59 60 61 62 63 64 65 66 67 68 69 70 71 72 74 75 76 77 78 79	13	22	388	1179	343	124593	0	43804	22587	774

Hospitals, U.S. / WISCONSIN

Hospital, Address, Telephone, Administrator, Approval, Facility, and Physician Codes, Health Care System, Network	Classification Codes		Utilization Data					Expense (thousands) of dollars		
★ American Hospital Association (AHA) membership ☐ Joint Commission on Accreditation of Healthcare Organizations (JCAHO) accreditation + American Osteopathic Healthcare Association (AOHA) membership ○ American Osteopathic Association (AOA) accreditation △ Commission on Accreditation of Rehabilitation Facilities (CARF) accreditation Control codes 61, 63, 64, 71, 72 and 73 indicate hospitals listed by AOHA, but not registered by AHA. For definition of numerical codes, see page A4	Control	Service	Staffed Beds	Admissions	Census	Outpatient Visits	Births	Total	Payroll	Personnel
★ △ WAUSAU HOSPITAL, 333 Pine Ridge Boulevard, Zip 54401-4187, Mailing Address: P.O. Box 1847, Zip 54402-1847; tel. 715/847-2121; Paul A. Spaude, President and Chief Executive Officer **A**1 2 3 5 7 9 10 **F**2 3 4 7 8 9 10 11 12 16 18 22 24 25 26 27 32 33 34 35 36 37 38 39 40 41 43 44 45 46 47 48 49 50 51 52 53 54 57 58 59 61 62 63 64 65 68 70 72 75 76 77 78 **P**1 6 **Web address:** www.wausauhospital.org	23	10	218	11454	132	77695	1384	120749	47145	1372
WAUWATOSA—Milwaukee County										
★ MILWAUKEE PSYCHIATRIC HOSPITAL, 1220 Dewey Avenue, Zip 53213-2598; tel. 414/454-6600; James A. Moore, Chief Operating Officer and Chief Financial Officer **A**1 3 5 10 **F**2 3 13 16 18 38 43 50 51 57 58 59 60 63 64 70 **P**4 6 **S** Aurora Health Care, Milwaukee, WI **Web address:** www.aurorahealthcare.org	23	22	75	1592	50	27146	0	13278	6094	202
+ ○ ST. JOSEPH'S HOSPITAL BLUEMOUND, (Formerly Lakeview Hospital), 10010 West Bluemound Road, Zip 53226; tel. 414/259-7200; J. E. Race, Administrator and Chief Executive Officer (Nonreporting) **A**11	23	10	72	—	—	—	—	—	—	—
WEST ALLIS—Milwaukee County										
☐ CHARTER BEHAVIORAL HEALTH SYSTEM OF MILWAUKEE/WEST ALLIS, 11101 West Lincoln Avenue, Zip 53227; tel. 414/327-3000; Ron Escarda, Chief Executive Officer **A**1 10 **F**1 2 3 13 16 18 21 38 43 50 51 57 58 59 60 61 62 63 64 70 74	33	22	80	1730	37	61677	0	—	—	157
★ WEST ALLIS MEMORIAL HOSPITAL, 8901 West Lincoln Avenue, Zip 53227-0901, Mailing Address: P.O. Box 27901, Zip 53227-0901; tel. 414/328-6000; Richard A. Kellar, Administrator **A**1 2 9 10 **F**5 8 9 10 11 12 13 18 19 22 24 25 27 28 31 34 35 38 39 41 43 44 46 48 50 51 52 54 55 65 68 70 71 72 75 76 78 79 **P**4 6 **S** Aurora Health Care, Milwaukee, WI **Web address:** www.aurorahealthcare.org	23	10	147	7159	104	67826	679	77749	28120	754
WEST BEND—Washington County										
★ ST. JOSEPH'S COMMUNITY HOSPITAL OF WEST BEND, 551 South Silverbrook Drive, Zip 53095-3898; tel. 414/334-5533; Gregory T. Burns, Executive Director **A**1 9 10 **F**2 7 8 9 12 13 16 18 20 21 22 24 25 27 38 39 40 41 43 44 45 46 48 50 52 54 57 59 62 68 70 75 76	23	10	103	5086	56	49088	781	32906	15748	443
WHITEHALL—Trempealeau County										
TRI-COUNTY MEMORIAL HOSPITAL, 18601 Lincoln Street, Zip 54773-0065; tel. 715/538-4361; Ronald B. Fields, President (Total facility includes 68 beds in nursing home-type unit) **A**9 10 **F**2 3 4 5 6 7 8 9 10 11 12 14 15 16 18 19 22 23 24 25 26 31 32 34 35 36 37 38 39 40 41 44 45 46 47 48 49 50 51 52 53 54 55 56 57 58 59 60 61 62 63 64 65 66 68 69 70 71 72 73 74 75 76 77 78 79	23	10	92	633	76	11715	0	7960	3726	208
WILD ROSE—Waushara County										
WILD ROSE COMMUNITY MEMORIAL HOSPITAL, 601 Grove Avenue, Zip 54984, Mailing Address: P.O. Box 243, Zip 54984-0243; tel. 920/622-3257; Craig W. C. Schmidt, President and Chief Executive Officer **A**9 10 **F**1 2 3 4 5 6 8 9 10 11 12 13 15 18 19 21 22 23 24 25 27 31 32 34 35 37 38 39 40 41 42 43 44 45 46 47 48 50 51 52 53 54 55 56 57 58 59 60 61 62 63 64 65 67 68 70 72 74 75 76 77 78 **P**6	23	10	26	350	4	9158	9	4532	1837	77
WINNEBAGO—Winnebago County										
☐ WINNEBAGO MENTAL HEALTH INSTITUTE, Mailing Address: P.O. Box 9, Zip 54985-0009; tel. 920/235-4910; Joann O'Connor, Director **A**1 10 **F**2 4 8 11 12 22 25 28 39 41 44 45 48 50 51 52 53 55 57 58 60 61 68 70 75 76 77 **P**6	12	22	330	936	270	273	0	37272	21730	701
WISCONSIN RAPIDS—Wood County										
★ RIVERVIEW HOSPITAL ASSOCIATION, (Includes Riverview Manor), 410 Dewey Street, Zip 54494-4724, Mailing Address: P.O. Box 8080, Zip 54495-8080; tel. 715/423-6060; Celse A. Berard, President (Total facility includes 118 beds in nursing home-type unit) **A**1 9 10 **F**2 7 8 9 11 12 22 24 25 38 39 40 41 43 44 46 48 50 52 53 54 57 59 68 69 70 71 75 76 **Web address:** www.rhahealthcare.org	23	10	197	3515	137	37027	533	28203	12372	386
WOODRUFF—Oneida County										
★ HOWARD YOUNG MEDICAL CENTER, 240 Maple Street, Zip 54568, Mailing Address: P.O. Box 470, Zip 54568-0470; tel. 715/356-8000; Patricia L. Richardson, President and Chief Executive Officer **A**1 9 10 **F**3 6 7 8 9 10 12 13 16 18 20 21 22 24 25 27 28 36 37 38 39 41 43 44 45 46 48 49 50 51 52 53 54 61 63 68 70 71 76	23	10	65	4093	42	74626	239	39602	17547	540

Hospitals, U.S. / WYOMING

WYOMING

Resident Population 481 (in thousands)
Resident population in metro areas 29.7%
Birth rate per 1,000 population 13.3
65 years and over 11.5%
Percent of persons without health insurance 15.5%

Hospital, Address, Telephone, Administrator, Approval, Facility, and Physician Codes, Health Care System, Network	Classification Codes		Utilization Data					Expense (thousands) of dollars		
	Control	Service	Staffed Beds	Admissions	Census	Outpatient Visits	Births	Total	Payroll	Personnel

★ American Hospital Association (AHA) membership
□ Joint Commission on Accreditation of Healthcare Organizations (JCAHO) accreditation
+ American Osteopathic Healthcare Association (AOHA) membership
○ American Osteopathic Association (AOA) accreditation
△ Commission on Accreditation of Rehabilitation Facilities (CARF) accreditation
Control codes 61, 63, 64, 71, 72 and 73 indicate hospitals listed by AOHA, but not registered by AHA. For definition of numerical codes, see page A4

AFTON—Lincoln County
★ STAR VALLEY MEDICAL CENTER, (Formerly Star Valley Hospital), 110 Hospital Lane, Zip 83110–0579, Mailing Address: P.O. Box 579, Zip 83110–0579; tel. 307/885–5800; J. Steve Perry, Chief Executive Officer (Total facility includes 24 beds in nursing home–type unit) **A**9 10 **F**8 9 13 16 17 18 22 25 32 45 48 69 70 76 78 **P**5
Web address: www.ihc.com
16 10 36 616 28 9833 91 4899 2593 98

BUFFALO—Johnson County
□ JOHNSON COUNTY HEALTHCARE CENTER, 497 West Lott Street, Zip 82834–1691; tel. 307/684–5521; Sandy Ward, Administrator (Total facility includes 50 beds in nursing home–type unit) **A**1 9 10 **F**1 7 8 9 22 25 30 32 36 37 39 41 44 46 48 50 54 69 70 76
16 10 65 640 53 11202 57 7349 3960 158

CASPER—Natrona County
✻ △ WYOMING MEDICAL CENTER, 1233 East Second Street, Zip 82601–2988; tel. 307/577–7201; Michael E. Schrader, President and Chief Executive Officer (Total facility includes 15 beds in nursing home–type unit) **A**1 3 7 9 10 **F**3 4 8 9 11 13 16 17 18 19 22 24 25 27 29 31 32 34 35 38 39 43 44 45 46 47 48 50 51 53 54 56 65 66 68 69 70 72 76 78 79 **P**6
Web address: www.wmcnet.org
23 10 216 7778 92 66691 857 86400 33067 934

CHEYENNE—Laramie County
✻ △ UNITED MEDICAL CENTER, (Includes De Paul Hospital, 2600 East 18th Street, Zip 82001–5511; tel. 307/634–2273), 214 East 23rd Street, Zip 82001–3790; tel. 307/634–2273; Jon M. Gates, Chief Executive Officer (Total facility includes 10 beds in nursing home–type unit) **A**1 3 7 9 10 **F**2 3 4 7 8 9 11 12 13 16 17 18 19 22 23 24 25 26 27 28 32 34 36 37 39 41 43 44 45 46 47 48 49 51 54 57 58 59 60 61 62 63 65 68 69 70 71 72 76 78 79
Web address: www.umcwy.org
13 10 188 7690 95 103410 826 67091 28873 1059

✻ VETERANS AFFAIRS MEDICAL CENTER, 2360 East Pershing Boulevard, Zip 82001–5392; tel. 307/778–7550; Richard Fry, Director (Total facility includes 50 beds in nursing home–type unit) **A**1 9 **F**2 3 4 9 11 12 13 18 19 21 22 23 24 25 26 27 30 31 32 34 35 36 37 38 39 41 43 45 46 47 48 49 51 53 54 56 57 59 60 61 63 65 66 69 70 72 74 76 78 79 **P**6 **S** Department of Veterans Affairs, Washington, DC
Web address: www.va.gov/stations97/guide/home.asp?DIVISION=ALL
45 10 71 1004 60 81262 0 28945 — 329

CODY—Park County
✻ WEST PARK HOSPITAL, 707 Sheridan Avenue, Zip 82414; tel. 307/527–7501; Douglas A. McMillan, Administrator and Chief Executive Officer (Total facility includes 90 beds in nursing home–type unit) **A**1 9 10 **F**2 3 7 8 9 13 17 18 19 21 22 23 24 25 26 30 31 32 34 36 37 38 39 41 43 44 45 46 48 49 50 51 53 54 56 58 59 61 63 65 69 70 71 72 75 76 77 78 **P**8 **S** Quorum Health Group, Brentwood, TN
Web address: www.westparkhospital.org
16 10 122 1691 111 100338 193 27438 12082 411

DOUGLAS—Converse County
★ MEMORIAL HOSPITAL OF CONVERSE COUNTY, 111 South Fifth Street, Zip 82633–1450, Mailing Address: P.O. Box 1450, Zip 82633–1450; tel. 307/358–2122; Sam D. Radke, Interim Chief Executive Officer **A**9 10 **F**1 2 3 4 5 6 8 9 10 11 13 14 15 17 18 19 20 21 22 23 24 25 26 27 28 29 30 32 33 34 35 36 37 38 39 40 43 44 45 46 47 48 49 50 51 52 53 54 55 56 57 58 59 60 61 62 63 64 65 66 67 69 70 71 72 73 74 75 76 78 79 **P**5
Web address: www.mhccdouglaswy.com
13 10 34 641 5 19654 89 7701 3492 144

EVANSTON—Uinta County
✻ EVANSTON REGIONAL HOSPITAL, 190 Arrowhead Drive, Zip 82930–9266; tel. 307/789–3636; Robert W. Allen, Chief Executive Officer **A**1 9 10 **F**8 9 12 13 17 18 19 22 25 26 32 33 34 36 37 38 45 48 50 51 54 56 69 70 72 75 76 77 78 79 **S** Community Health Systems, Inc., Brentwood, TN
Web address: www.ihc.com
33 10 38 999 8 44460 239 8923 4016 143

WYOMING STATE HOSPITAL, 830 Highway 150 South, Zip 82931–5341, Mailing Address: P.O. Box 177, Zip 82931–0177; tel. 307/789–3464; Pablo Hernandez, M.D., Administrator **A**9 10 **F**3 13 16 17 18 19 23 31 33 38 45 50 51 57 58 59 60 61 62 63 64 70 72 78 **P**6
12 22 122 404 36 0 0 16305 10282 452

GILLETTE—Campbell County
✻ CAMPBELL COUNTY MEMORIAL HOSPITAL, 501 South Burma Avenue, Zip 82716–3426, Mailing Address: P.O. Box 3011, Zip 82717–3011; tel. 307/682–8811; David Crow, Chief Executive Officer **A**1 9 10 **F**3 8 9 13 16 17 18 19 22 25 28 32 34 36 39 41 43 44 45 46 48 49 50 51 52 54 57 58 60 61 62 63 64 70 71 72 75 76 78
Web address: www.ccmh.net
16 10 76 2664 31 87725 490 32488 15383 456

Hospitals, U.S. / WYOMING

Hospital, Address, Telephone, Administrator, Approval, Facility, and Physician Codes, Health Care System, Network	Classification Codes		Utilization Data					Expense (thousands) of dollars		
★ American Hospital Association (AHA) membership ☐ Joint Commission on Accreditation of Healthcare Organizations (JCAHO) accreditation + American Osteopathic Healthcare Association (AOHA) membership ○ American Osteopathic Association (AOA) accreditation △ Commission on Accreditation of Rehabilitation Facilities (CARF) accreditation Control codes 61, 63, 64, 71, 72 and 73 indicate hospitals listed by AOHA, but not registered by AHA. For definition of numerical codes, see page A4	Control	Service	Staffed Beds	Admissions	Census	Outpatient Visits	Births	Total	Payroll	Personnel
JACKSON—Teton County ☐ ST. JOHN'S HOSPITAL AND LIVING CENTER, 625 East Broadway Street, Zip 83001, Mailing Address: P.O. Box 428, Zip 83001-0428; tel. 307/733-3636; John Valiante, Chief Executive Officer (Total facility includes 60 beds in nursing home–type unit) **A**1 9 10 **F**7 8 9 13 16 17 18 19 20 22 25 26 27 28 31 32 34 36 37 38 39 41 43 44 45 46 48 49 51 53 54 56 57 61 68 69 70 72 76 78 79 **Web address:** www.tetonhospital.org	16	10	102	2294	72	10184	271	31835	14047	392
KEMMERER—Lincoln County ★ SOUTH LINCOLN MEDICAL CENTER, 711 Onyx Street, Zip 83101-3214, Mailing Address: P.O. Box 390, Zip 83101-0390; tel. 307/877-4401; Marla Shelby, Administrator and Chief Executive Officer (Total facility includes 24 beds in nursing home–type unit) **A**9 10 **F**25 32 36 44 48 54 69 76	16	10	40	254	7	24080	27	5479	2896	92
LANDER—Fremont County ☐ LANDER VALLEY MEDICAL CENTER, 1320 Bishop Randall Drive, Zip 82520-3996; tel. 307/335-6330; Andrew Gramlich, Chief Executive Officer (Total facility includes 21 beds in nursing home–type unit) **A**1 9 10 **F**2 3 7 8 9 11 12 13 17 18 19 22 23 24 25 30 36 38 39 41 43 44 45 48 51 54 58 59 60 61 62 63 68 69 70 72 76 78 79 **P**5 **S** New American Healthcare Corporation, Brentwood, TN **Web address:** www.landerhospital.com	33	10	102	2358	28	8614	187	14271	7750	245
LARAMIE—Albany County ✯ IVINSON MEMORIAL HOSPITAL, 255 North 30th Street, Zip 82070-5195; tel. 307/742-2141; Thomas A. Nord, FACHE, Chief Executive Officer **A**1 9 10 **F**7 8 9 13 16 17 18 19 21 24 22 25 27 30 32 33 34 37 38 39 41 43 44 45 46 48 49 50 54 55 57 58 59 60 62 63 69 70 72 73 75 76 78 79 **P**6 8 **Web address:** www.ivinsonhospital.org	16	10	72	2793	28	58482	350	27712	12489	341
LOVELL—Big Horn County ★ NORTH BIG HORN HOSPITAL, 1115 Lane 12, Zip 82431-9580, Mailing Address: P.O. Box 518, Zip 82431-0518; tel. 307/548-2771; Walter S. Busch, Administrator (Total facility includes 85 beds in nursing home–type unit) **A**9 10 **F**6 9 13 16 17 18 19 22 25 28 30 32 34 35 36 37 38 41 43 48 49 50 51 54 56 69 70 71 72 76 78 **Web address:** www.nbhh.com	16	10	98	389	83	8973	0	6898	3887	155
NEWCASTLE—Weston County WESTON COUNTY HEALTH SERVICES, 1124 Washington Street, Zip 82701-2996; tel. 307/746-4491; Greg Nielsen, Administrator (Total facility includes 51 beds in nursing home–type unit) **A**9 10 **F**8 12 17 18 25 30 32 34 36 41 43 44 48 54 69 70 72 76	16	10	74	419	48	10478	40	4806	2361	98
POWELL—Park County ✯ POWELL HOSPITAL, 777 Avenue H, Zip 82435-2296; tel. 307/754-2267; Rod Barton, Chief Executive Officer (Total facility includes 100 beds in nursing home–type unit) **A**1 9 10 **F**7 8 9 16 18 19 22 24 25 26 30 32 33 34 36 37 38 39 41 43 44 45 48 54 55 56 69 70 71 72 76 78 **P**1 **S** Brim Healthcare, Inc., Brentwood, TN **Web address:** www.wir.net/powell–hospital	23	10	130	928	104	15643	193	12334	6672	237
RAWLINS—Carbon County MEMORIAL HOSPITAL OF CARBON COUNTY, 2221 West Elm Street, Zip 82301-0460, Mailing Address: P.O. Box 460, Zip 82301-0460; tel. 307/324-8213; Patricia L. Carter, Chief Executive Officer **A**9 10 **F**7 8 9 13 16 17 18 22 25 30 32 34 36 38 39 40 41 43 44 45 48 51 54 61 69 70 75 76	13	10	35	1481	14	36477	116	13318	6000	192
RIVERTON—Fremont County ✯ RIVERTON MEMORIAL HOSPITAL, 2100 West Sunset Drive, Zip 82501-2274; tel. 307/856-4161; William Russell, Chief Executive Officer **A**1 9 10 **F**8 9 12 16 17 18 22 24 25 32 34 35 41 43 44 45 48 50 51 54 70 75 76 78 **P**7 **S** LifePoint Hospitals, Inc., Brentwood, TN **Web address:** www.riverton–hospital.com	33	10	59	1878	17	30607	259	12695	5090	188
ROCK SPRINGS—Sweetwater County ✯ MEMORIAL HOSPITAL OF SWEETWATER COUNTY, 1200 College Drive, Zip 82901-5868, Mailing Address: Box 1359, Zip 82902-1359; tel. 307/362-3711; John M. Ferry, Executive Director **A**1 9 10 **F**22 39 48 54 70 76 78	13	10	99	2731	20	71719	536	24334	9946	324
SHERIDAN—Sheridan County ☐ MEMORIAL HOSPITAL OF SHERIDAN COUNTY, 1401 West Fifth Street, Zip 82801-2799; tel. 307/672-1000; T. Marvin Goldman, Administrator **A**1 9 10 **F**7 8 9 12 16 17 22 25 27 32 34 37 39 41 44 46 48 51 54 61 65 70 72 76 78 **Web address:** www.sheridanhospital.org	13	10	60	2764	31	—	294	22763	10909	350
✯ VETERANS AFFAIRS MEDICAL CENTER, 1898 Fort Road, Zip 82801-8320; tel. 307/672-3473; Maureen Humphrys, Director (Total facility includes 50 beds in nursing home–type unit) **A**1 9 **F**3 9 12 16 17 18 22 23 24 30 31 32 34 36 38 39 43 45 48 50 51 54 56 57 59 61 62 63 64 65 69 70 76 78 79 **P**6 **S** Department of Veterans Affairs, Washington, DC **Web address:** www.va.gov/stations97/guide/home.asp?DIVISION=ALL	45	22	114	1104	103	60441	0	31979	17946	389
SUNDANCE—Crook County CROOK COUNTY MEDICAL SERVICES DISTRICT, 713 Oak Street, Zip 82729, Mailing Address: P.O. Box 517, Zip 82729-0517; tel. 307/283-3501; Don A. Nelson, Administrator (Total facility includes 32 beds in nursing home–type unit) **A**9 10 **F**1 16 17 18 23 25 32 36 37 50 51 54 69 70 76 **P**6	16	10	48	248	31	4949	0	3943	1672	90

© 2000 AHA Guide   *Many Facility Codes have changed. Please refer to the AHA Guide Code Chart.*

Hospitals, U.S. / WYOMING

Hospital, Address, Telephone, Administrator, Approval, Facility, and Physician Codes, Health Care System, Network	Classification Codes		Utilization Data					Expense (thousands) of dollars		
★ American Hospital Association (AHA) membership ☐ Joint Commission on Accreditation of Healthcare Organizations (JCAHO) accreditation + American Osteopathic Healthcare Association (AOHA) membership ○ American Osteopathic Association (AOA) accreditation △ Commission on Accreditation of Rehabilitation Facilities (CARF) accreditation Control codes 61, 63, 64, 71, 72 and 73 indicate hospitals listed by AOHA, but not registered by AHA. For definition of numerical codes, see page A4	Control	Service	Staffed Beds	Admissions	Census	Outpatient Visits	Births	Total	Payroll	Personnel
THERMOPOLIS—Hot Springs County ★ HOT SPRINGS COUNTY MEMORIAL HOSPITAL, 150 East Arapahoe Street, Zip 82443–2498; tel. 307/864–3121; Edward G. Leake, Chief Executive Officer **A**1 9 10 **F**7 8 9 17 22 25 32 38 41 44 48 49 50 53 68 70 76	13	10	49	921	9	7759	52	7003	2864	95
TORRINGTON—Goshen County ★ COMMUNITY HOSPITAL, 2000 Campbell Drive, Zip 82240–1597; tel. 307/532–4181; Charles Myers, Administrator **A**1 9 10 **F**8 9 12 13 19 22 25 26 30 32 33 34 36 38 39 40 41 43 46 48 54 69 70 71 72 76 **S** Banner Health System, Fargo, ND	23	10	36	1359	19	36361	96	7639	3489	168
WHEATLAND—Platte County ★ PLATTE COUNTY MEMORIAL HOSPITAL, 201 14th Street, Zip 82201–3201, Mailing Address: P.O. Box 848, Zip 82201–0848; tel. 307/322–3636; Steve Hannah, Administrator (Total facility includes 43 beds in nursing home–type unit) **A**1 9 10 **F**8 9 13 16 17 18 22 25 32 33 38 39 41 48 69 70 76 78 **S** Banner Health System, Fargo, ND	23	10	86	1170	66	29329	64	6441	2860	159
WORLAND—Washakie County ★ WASHAKIE MEDICAL CENTER, (Formerly Washakie Memorial Hospital), 400 South 15th Street, Zip 82401–3531, Mailing Address: P.O. Box 700, Zip 82401–0700; tel. 307/347–3221; Kent Aland, Interim Administrator **A**1 9 10 **F**8 9 13 16 17 18 19 22 25 32 34 36 38 39 40 41 43 44 45 46 48 49 50 51 53 54 70 72 76 78 **S** Banner Health System, Fargo, ND	23	10	30	1146	12	39801	106	9349	4060	122

Hospitals in Areas Associated with the United States, by Area

	Classification Codes		Utilization Data					Expense (thousands) of dollars		
Hospital, Address, Telephone, Administrator, Approval, Facility, and Physician Codes, Health Care System, Network	Control	Service	Staffed Beds	Admissions	Census	Outpatient Visits	Births	Total	Payroll	Personnel

★ American Hospital Association (AHA) membership
☐ Joint Commission on Accreditation of Healthcare Organizations (JCAHO) accreditation
+ American Osteopathic Healthcare Association (AOHA) membership
○ American Osteopathic Association (AOA) accreditation
△ Commission on Accreditation of Rehabilitation Facilities (CARF) accreditation
Control codes 61, 63, 64, 71, 72 and 73 indicate hospitals listed by AOHA, but not registered by AHA. For definition of numerical codes, see page A4

AMERICAN SAMOA

PAGO PAGO—American Samoa County
LYNDON B. JOHNSON TROPICAL MEDICAL CENTER, Zip 96799; tel. 684/633–1222; Iotamo T. Saleapaga, M.D., Director Health (Nonreporting) **A**10

12	10	125	—	—	—	—	—	—	—

GUAM

AGANA—Guam County
★ U. S. NAVAL HOSPITAL, Mailing Address: PSC 490, Box 7607, FPO, AP, Zip 96538–1600; tel. 671/344–9340; Captain J. L. Ulmer, Sr, Commanding Officer (Nonreporting) **S** Department of Navy, Washington, DC

| 43 | 10 | 55 | — | — | — | — | — | — | — |

TAMUNING—Guam County
GUAM MEMORIAL HOSPITAL AUTHORITY, 850 Governor Carlos G. Camacho Road, Zip 96911; tel. 671/647–2108; Tyrone J. Taitano, Administrator (Total facility includes 29 beds in nursing home–type unit) **F**8 9 18 22 24 25 35 38 39 41 42 43 44 48 50 51 52 53 54 69 70 76 78
Web address: www.gmha.org

| 12 | 10 | 187 | 11369 | 149 | 106911 | 3673 | 63159 | 34106 | 932 |

MARSHALL ISLANDS

KWAJALEIN ISLAND—Marshall Islands County
KWAJALEIN HOSPITAL, U.S. Army Kwajalein Atoll, Zip 96960, Mailing Address: Box 1702, APO, AP, Zip 96555–5000; tel. 805/355–2225; Elaine McMahon, Administrator (Nonreporting) **S** Department of the Army, Office of the Surgeon General, Falls Church, VA

| 42 | 10 | 14 | — | — | — | — | — | — | — |

PUERTO RICO

AGUADILLA—Aguadilla County
✠ AGUADILLA GENERAL HOSPITAL, Carr Aguadilla San Juan, Zip 00605, Mailing Address: P.O. Box 4036, Zip 00605; tel. 787/891–3534; Marco Reyes, Executive Director (Nonreporting) **A**1 9 10 **S** Puerto Rico Department of Health, San Juan, PR

| 12 | 10 | 110 | — | — | — | — | — | — | — |

AIBONITO—Aibonito County
★ MENNONITE GENERAL HOSPITAL, Jose Vasquez, Zip 00705, Mailing Address: P.O. Box 1379, Zip 00705; tel. 787/735–8001; Domingo Torres Zayas, CHE, Executive Director (Nonreporting) **A**9 10

| 23 | 10 | 131 | — | — | — | — | — | — | — |

ARECIBO—Arecibo County
★ ARECIBO REGIONAL HOSPITAL, 129 San Luis Avenue, Zip 00612, Mailing Address: P.O. Box 659, Zip 00613; tel. 787/878–7272; Samuel Monroig, Vice President for Administration **A**9 10 **F**12 16 22 25 41 42 44 48 70 76 77 78 **S** Puerto Rico Department of Health, San Juan, PR

| 33 | 10 | 188 | 9847 | 161 | — | 1467 | 19030 | 8905 | 729 |

HOSPITAL DR. SUSONI, 55 Nicomedes Rivera Street, Zip 00612, Mailing Address: P.O. Box 145200, Zip 00614; tel. 787/878–1010; Hector Barreto, M.D., Director (Nonreporting) **A**9 10

| 33 | 10 | 138 | — | — | — | — | — | — | — |

★ HOSPITAL EL BUEN PASTOR, 52 De Diego, Zip 00612, Mailing Address: P.O. Box 413, Zip 00612; tel. 787/878–2730; Julio Galarce, Administrator (Nonreporting)

| 33 | 10 | 72 | — | — | — | — | — | — | — |

ARROYO—Arroyo County
★ LAFAYETTE HOSPITAL, Central Lafayette, Zip 00714, Mailing Address: P.O. Box 207, Zip 00714; tel. 787/839–3232; Francisco Santiago–Vega, Consultor **A**9 10 **F**16 17 18 22 25 38 48 69 70 76 **P**8

| 33 | 10 | 41 | 2710 | 27 | 21041 | 150 | 5184 | 1958 | 126 |

BAYAMON—Bayamon County
✠ HOSPITAL HERMANOS MELENDEZ, Route 2, KM 11–7, Zip 00960, Mailing Address: P.O. Box 306, Zip 00960; tel. 787/620–8181; Tomas Martinez, Administrator **A**1 9 10 **F**11 12 17 18 22 25 41 44 48 54 70 76 78 **P**8

| 33 | 10 | 211 | 14997 | 186 | 57951 | 3804 | 41012 | 12620 | 656 |

★ HOSPITAL MATILDE BRENES, Extension Hermanas Davila, Zip 00960, Mailing Address: P.O. Box 2957, Zip 00960; tel. 787/786–0050; Manuel J. Vazquez, Administrator (Nonreporting) **A**9 10

| 33 | 10 | 95 | — | — | — | — | — | — | — |

© 2000 AHA Guide   *Many Facility Codes have changed. Please refer to the AHA Guide Code Chart.*   Hospitals **A481**

Hospitals, U.S. / PUERTO RICO

Hospital, Address, Telephone, Administrator, Approval, Facility, and Physician Codes, Health Care System, Network	Classification Codes		Utilization Data					Expense (thousands) of dollars		
	Control	Service	Staffed Beds	Admissions	Census	Outpatient Visits	Births	Total	Payroll	Personnel

★ American Hospital Association (AHA) membership
☐ Joint Commission on Accreditation of Healthcare Organizations (JCAHO) accreditation
+ American Osteopathic Healthcare Association (AOHA) membership
○ American Osteopathic Association (AOA) accreditation
△ Commission on Accreditation of Rehabilitation Facilities (CARF) accreditation
Control codes 61, 63, 64, 71, 72 and 73 indicate hospitals listed by AOHA, but not registered by AHA. For definition of numerical codes, see page A4.

Hospital	Control	Service	Staffed Beds	Admissions	Census	Outpatient Visits	Births	Total	Payroll	Personnel
★ HOSPITAL SAN PABLO, Calle Santa Cruz 70, Zip 00961, Mailing Address: P.O. Box 236, Zip 00960; tel. 787/740–4747; Jorge Matta, Associate Administrator (Nonreporting) **A**1 3 5 9 10 **S** Universal Health Services, Inc., King of Prussia, PA **Web address:** www.sanpablo.com	33	10	364	—	—	—	—	—	—	—
★ HOSPITAL UNIVERSITARIO DR. RAMON RUIZ ARNAU, Avenue Laurel, Santa Juanita, Zip 00956; tel. 787/787–5151; Nilda E. Diaz, Executive Director **A**1 3 5 9 10 **F**2 3 4 5 6 7 8 9 10 11 13 14 15 17 18 19 20 21 22 23 24 25 26 27 28 29 30 31 32 33 34 35 36 37 38 39 40 41 42 43 44 45 46 47 48 49 50 51 52 53 54 55 56 57 58 59 60 61 62 63 64 65 66 67 68 69 70 71 72 73 74 75 76 77 78 79 **P**6 8 **S** Puerto Rico Department of Health, San Juan, PR	12	10	341	8930	158	84688	1915	—	—	1046
★ MEPSI CENTER, Carretera Numero 2 K 8–2, Zip 00959–6089, Mailing Address: Carretera Numero 2 K. 8–2, Zip 00960–6089; tel. 787/793–3030; Manuel Diaz Ruiz, President **A**1 9 10 **F**2 17 18 22 39 51 54 55 57 58 59 60 62 64 68 70 76	33	22	450	4875	140	0	0	17608	7405	386
CAGUAS—Caguas County										
★ CAGUAS REGIONAL HOSPITAL, Carretera Caguas A Cidra, Zip 00725, Mailing Address: Call Box 4964, Zip 00726–4964; tel. 787/744–2500; Pedro Juan Santiago, Executive Director (Nonreporting) **A**1 3 5 9 10 **S** Puerto Rico Department of Health, San Juan, PR	12	10	256	—	—	—	—	—	—	—
☐ HOSPITAL INTERAMERICANO DE MEDICINA AVANZADA, Avenida Luis Munoz Marin, Zip 00726, Mailing Address: Apartado 4980, Zip 00726; tel. 787/743–3434; Carlos M. Pineiro, President (Nonreporting) **A**1 10	32	10	300	—	—	—	—	—	—	—
CAROLINA—Carolina County										
★ HOSPITAL DR. FEDERICO TRILLA, 65th Infanteria, KM 8 3, Zip 00984, Mailing Address: P.O. Box 3869, Zip 00984; tel. 787/757–1800; Domingo Nevarez, Administrator (Nonreporting) **A**1 3 5 9 10	33	10	220	—	—	—	—	—	—	—
CASTANER—Lares County										
★ CASTANER GENERAL HOSPITAL, KM 64–2, Route 135, Zip 00631, Mailing Address: P.O. Box 1003, Zip 00631; tel. 787/829–5010; Domingo Monroig, Administrator (Nonreporting) **A**9 10	23	10	24	—	—	—	—	—	—	—
CAYEY—Cayey County										
★ HOSPITAL MENONITA DE CAYEY, 4 H. Mendoza Street, Zip 00737, Mailing Address: P.O. Box 373130, Zip 00737; tel. 787/263–1001; Domingo Torres–Zayas, Executive Director (Nonreporting) **A**9 10	23	10	50	—	—	—	—	—	—	—
CIDRA—Cidra County										
★ FIRST HOSPITAL PANAMERICANO, State Road 787 KM 1 5, Zip 00739, Mailing Address: P.O. Box 1398, Zip 00739; tel. 787/739–5555; Jorge Torres, Vice President and Chief Executive Officer (Nonreporting) **A**1 5 9 10 **S** FHC Health Systems, Norfolk, VA	33	22	165	—	—	—	—	—	—	—
FAJARDO—Fajardo County										
★ HOSPITAL DOCTOR GUBERN, (Formerly Doctors Gubern's Hospital), (Includes Dr. Gubern's Hospital, General Valero Avenue 267 & 261, Mailing Address: Box 846, Zip 00738; tel. 809/792–3495; Antonio R. Barcelo, Director), 110 Antonio R. Barcelo, Zip 00738, Mailing Address: P.O. Box 846, Zip 00738–0846; tel. 787/863–0669; Edwin Sueiro, Executive Director (Nonreporting) **A**9 10 **S** United Medical Corporation, Windermere, FL	33	10	51	—	—	—	—	—	—	—
HOSPITAL SAN PABLO DEL ESTE, (Formerly Dr. Jose Ramos Lebron Hospital), Avenida General Valero, 404, Zip 00738, Mailing Address: P.O. Box 1028, Zip 00738–1028; tel. 787/863–0505; Maria Elena Rodriguez, Executive Administrator (Nonreporting) **A**9 10 **F**2 9 18 22 25 41 43 44 48 70 76 **S** Universal Health Services, Inc., King of Prussia, PA **Web address:** www.sanpablo.com	33	10	107	4436	73	30285	131	16347	4819	293
GUAYAMA—Guayama County										
★ HOSPITAL EPISCOPAL CRISTO REDENTOR, (Formerly Dr. Alejandro Buitrago–Guayama Hospital), Avenue Pedro Albesus, Zip 00784, Mailing Address: Call Box 1006, Zip 00785–1006; tel. 787/864–4300; Jose Joaquin Cora, Executive Director (Nonreporting) **A**1 9 10	12	10	155	—	—	—	—	—	—	—
★ HOSPITAL SANTA ROSA, Veterans Avenue, Zip 00784, Mailing Address: P.O. Box 10008, Zip 00785; tel. 787/864–0101; Herson E. Morales, Executive Director (Nonreporting) **A**9 10	23	10	89	—	—	—	—	—	—	—
HUMACAO—Humacao County										
☐ FONT MARTELO HOSPITAL, 3 Font Martelo Street, Zip 00792, Mailing Address: P.O. Box 639, Zip 00792–0639; tel. 787/852–2424; Julio A. Ortiz, M.D., Chairman (Nonreporting) **A**1 9 10	33	10	64	—	—	—	—	—	—	—
HOSPITAL DR. DOMINGUEZ, 300 Font Martelo Street, Zip 00791, Mailing Address: P.O. Box 699, Zip 00792; tel. 787/852–0505; Rogelio Diaz–Reyes, Administrator (Nonreporting) **A**9 10	33	10	54	—	—	—	—	—	—	—
★ HOSPITAL SUB-REGIONAL DR. VICTOR R. NUNEZ, Avenida Tejas, Expreso Cruz Ortiz Stella, Zip 00791; tel. 787/852–2727; Ahmed Alvarez Pabon, Executive Director (Nonreporting) **A**10 **S** Puerto Rico Department of Health, San Juan, PR	12	10	83	—	—	—	—	—	—	—
★ RYDER MEMORIAL HOSPITAL, 355 Font Martelo Street, Zip 00792, Mailing Address: P.O. Box 859, Zip 00792–0859; tel. 787/852–0768; Jose R. Feliciano, Executive Director (Total facility includes 62 beds in nursing home–type unit) **A**9 10 **F**1 9 12 16 18 19 22 23 25 29 32 34 35 37 38 39 41 43 44 45 46 48 50 51 54 56 63 67 68 69 70 74 76 78 **P**8	23	10	206	9535	120	162158	—	44946	20487	1178
MANATI—Manati County										
★ CLINICA SAN AGUSTIN, Route 2, KM 49–5, Zip 00674, Mailing Address: P.O. Box 991, Zip 00674; tel. 787/854–2091; Astrid Abreu, Administrator **A**9 10 **F**17 18 25 43 48 50 56 63 70 76 **P**5 8	33	10	12	1144	19	—	66	3005	958	55

Hospitals, U.S. / PUERTO RICO

Hospital, Address, Telephone, Administrator, Approval, Facility, and Physician Codes, Health Care System, Network	Classification Codes		Utilization Data					Expense (thousands) of dollars		
★ American Hospital Association (AHA) membership □ Joint Commission on Accreditation of Healthcare Organizations (JCAHO) accreditation + American Osteopathic Healthcare Association (AOHA) membership ○ American Osteopathic Association (AOA) accreditation △ Commission on Accreditation of Rehabilitation Facilities (CARF) accreditation Control codes 61, 63, 64, 71, 72 and 73 indicate hospitals listed by AOHA, but not registered by AHA. For definition of numerical codes, see page A4	Control	Service	Staffed Beds	Admissions	Census	Outpatient Visits	Births	Total	Payroll	Personnel
✴ DOCTORS CENTER, KM 47–7, Zip 00674, Mailing Address: P.O. Box 30532, Zip 00674; tel. 787/854–3322; Pedro Rivera, Administrator (Nonreporting) **A**1 3 9 10	33	10	150	—	—	—	—	—	—	—
MAYAGUEZ—Mayaguez County										
✴ BELLA VISTA HOSPITAL, State Road 349, Zip 00680, Mailing Address: P.O. Box 1750, Zip 00681; tel. 787/834–6000; Ruth M. Ortiz, Chief Operating Officer (Nonreporting) **A**1 3 9 10 **S** Adventist Health System Sunbelt Health Care Corporation, Winter Park, FL	21	10	157	—	—	—	—	—	—	—
CLINICA ESPANOLA, Barrio La Quinta, Zip 00680, Mailing Address: P.O. Box 490, Zip 00681–0490; tel. 787/832–0442; Emigdio Inigo–Agostini, M.D., Board President (Nonreporting) **A**9 10	33	10	69	—	—	—	—	—	—	—
✴ DR. RAMON E. BETANCES HOSPITAL–MAYAGUEZ MEDICAL CENTER BRANCH, 410 Hostos Avenue, Zip 00680; tel. 787/834–8686; Maria Del Pilar Rodriguez, Chief Executive Officer (Nonreporting) **A**1 3 5 10 **S** Puerto Rico Department of Health, San Juan, PR	12	10	253	—	—	—	—	—	—	—
★ HOSPITAL PEREA, 15 Basora Street, Zip 00681, Mailing Address: P.O. Box 170, Zip 00681; tel. 787/834–0101; Ramon Lopez, Administrator (Nonreporting) **A**10 **S** United Medical Corporation, Windermere, FL	33	10	82	—	—	—	—	—	—	—
PONCE—Ponce County										
✴ DR. PILA'S HOSPITAL, Avenida Las Americas, Zip 00731, Mailing Address: P.O. Box 1910, Zip 00733–1910; tel. 787/848–5600; Miguel J. Bustelo, Executive Director **A**1 3 5 9 10 **F**4 7 8 13 16 17 18 21 22 23 25 27 29 32 33 34 36 38 41 44 45 48 50 51 54 56 59 68 70 76 77 78	23	10	177	9252	128	115768	981	33954	11202	587
✴ HOSPITAL DE DAMAS, Ponce by Pass, Zip 00731; tel. 787/840–8686; Roberto A. Rentas, Administrator **A**1 3 5 9 10 **F**2 3 4 9 11 12 16 17 18 22 24 25 32 34 36 37 39 41 42 44 46 48 49 51 52 58 59 60 61 62 63 64 65 69 70 74 76 78	23	10	267	15039	198	464515	1672	43759	20040	—
✴ HOSPITAL EPISCOPAL SAN LUCAS, Guadalupe Street, Zip 00731, Mailing Address: P.O. Box 2027, Zip 00733; tel. 787/840–4545; Guillermo J. Martin, Executive Director **A**1 3 5 10 **F**4 8 11 12 17 18 22 24 25 31 36 37 38 41 42 44 48 51 54 68 69 70 76 **P**8	21	10	168	8969	141	30758	677	40441	13265	697
✴ HOSPITAL ONCOLOGICO ANDRES GRILLASCA, (ONCOLOGIC), Centro Medico De Ponce, Zip 00733, Mailing Address: P.O. Box 1324, Zip 00733; tel. 787/848–0800; Santiago Rivera, Executive Administrator **A**1 2 5 9 10 **F**9 17 18 22 24 35 37 38 39 46 48 49 51 55 59 65 68 70 75 76 78 **P**5 6	23	49	50	1446	18	16632	0	5663	1936	129
✴ PONCE REGIONAL HOSPITAL, 917 Tito Castro Avenue, Zip 00731; tel. 787/844–2080; Julio Andino Rodriguez, Executive Director **A**1 3 5 9 10 **F**12 17 18 25 38 41 42 43 44 52 53 54 70 **S** Puerto Rico Department of Health, San Juan, PR	12	10	324	15144	220	359846	2423	—	—	—
SAN GERMAN—San German County										
✴ HOSPITAL DE LA CONCEPCION, 41 Luna Street, Zip 00683, Mailing Address: P.O. Box 285, Zip 00683–0285; tel. 787/892–1860; Jaime F. Maestre Grau, Executive Director (Nonreporting) **A**1 2 3 5 9 10	21	10	167	—	—	—	—	—	—	—
SAN JUAN—San Juan County										
✴ ASHFORD PRESBYTERIAN COMMUNITY HOSPITAL, 1451 Ashford Avenue Condado, Zip 00907, Mailing Address: P.O. Box 9020032, Zip 00902–0032; tel. 787/721–2160; Pedro J. Gonzalez, Executive Director **A**1 9 10 **F**8 16 17 18 22 25 39 41 42 43 44 48 51 56 68 76 78	23	10	187	11578	145	30145	3400	30845	10339	694
✴ AUXILIO MUTUO HOSPITAL, Ponce De Leon Avenue, Zip 00919, Mailing Address: P.O. Box 191227, Zip 00919–1227; tel. 787/758–2000; Ivan E. Colon, Administrator (Nonreporting) **A**1 9 10	23	10	402	—	—	—	—	—	—	—
✴ BHC HOSPITAL SAN JUAN CAPESTRANO, Mailing Address: Rural Route 2, Box 11, Zip 00926; tel. 787/760–0222; Laura Vargas, Administrator and Chief Executive Officer (Nonreporting) **A**1 10 **S** Behavioral Healthcare Corporation, Nashville, TN	33	22	88	—	—	—	—	—	—	—
✴ CARDIOVASCULAR CENTER OF PUERTO RICO AND THE CARIBBEAN, Americo Miranda Centro Medico, Zip 00936, Mailing Address: P.O. Box 366528, Zip 00936–6528; tel. 787/754–8500; Marilyn Perez de Vazquez, Executive Director (Nonreporting) **A**1	12	49	192	—	—	—	—	—	—	—
DOCTORS HOSPITAL, 1395 San Rafael Street, Zip 00910, Mailing Address: Box 11338, Santurce Station, Zip 00910; tel. 787/723–2950; Teodoro Muniz, Administrator **A**9 10 **F**22 25 32 36 37 39 44 70 76 **P**5	33	10	89	4007	48	7292	322	8885	2430	119
✴ HOSPITAL DEL MAESTRO, 550 Sergio Cuevas, Zip 00918, Mailing Address: P.O. Box 364708, Zip 00936–4708; tel. 787/758–8383; William Rodriguez Castro, Administrator **A**1 10 **F**8 9 22 25 41 43 44 48 53 54 70 76 78 **P**8	23	10	247	9861	10	33647	928	27190	9658	604
✴ HOSPITAL METROPOLITAN, (Formerly Fundacion Hospital Metropolitan), 1785 Route 21, Zip 00922, Mailing Address: P.O. Box 11981, Zip 00922; tel. 787/782–9999; Henry Ruberte, Executive Director (Nonreporting) **A**1 9	23	10	119	—	—	—	—	—	—	—
★ HOSPITAL PAVIA–HATO REY, (Formerly Hato Rey Community Hospital), Mailing Address: 435 Ponce De Leon, Hato Rey, Zip 00917; tel. 787/754–0909; Alfredo Bolchers, Executive Vice President (Nonreporting) **A**9 **S** United Medical Corporation, Windermere, FL	33	10	105	—	—	—	—	—	—	—
✴ HOSPITAL PAVIA–SANTURCE, 1462 Asia Street, Zip 00909, Mailing Address: Box 11137, Santurce Station, Zip 00910; tel. 787/727–6060; Alfredo Volckers, Executive Director (Nonreporting) **A**1 9 10 **S** United Medical Corporation, Windermere, FL	33	10	183	—	—	—	—	—	—	—

© 2000 AHA Guide *Many Facility Codes have changed. Please refer to the AHA Guide Code Chart.*

Hospitals, U.S. / PUERTO RICO—VIRGIN ISLANDS

Approval, Facility, and Physician Code Key:
- ★ American Hospital Association (AHA) membership
- ☐ Joint Commission on Accreditation of Healthcare Organizations (JCAHO) accreditation
- + American Osteopathic Healthcare Association (AOHA) membership
- ○ American Osteopathic Association (AOA) accreditation
- △ Commission on Accreditation of Rehabilitation Facilities (CARF) accreditation

Control codes 61, 63, 64, 71, 72 and 73 indicate hospitals listed by AOHA, but not registered by AHA. For definition of numerical codes, see page A4.

Hospital, Address, Telephone, Administrator, Approval, Facility, and Physician Codes, Health Care System, Network	Classification Codes		Utilization Data					Expense (thousands) of dollars		Personnel
	Control	Service	Staffed Beds	Admissions	Census	Outpatient Visits	Births	Total	Payroll	
★ HOSPITAL SAN FRANCISCO, 371 Avenida De Diego, Rio Piedras, Zip 00923, Mailing Address: P.O. Box 29025, San Juan, Zip 00929–0025; tel. 787/767–2528; Eric Grafals, Executive Director **A**1 10 **F**4 9 11 12 13 16 17 18 22 25 32 39 41 42 44 46 47 48 50 51 52 70 76 78 **S** Universal Health Services, Inc., King of Prussia, PA **Web address:** www.sanpablo.com	33	10	160	7870	127	74020	0	27518	11288	569
★ I. GONZALEZ MARTINEZ ONCOLOGIC HOSPITAL, (ONCOLOGY), Puerto Rico Medical Center, Hato Rey, Zip 00935, Mailing Address: P.O. Box 191811, Zip 00919–1811; tel. 787/765–2382; Celia Molano, Executive Director **A**1 2 3 5 9 10 **F**22 23 24 25 39 41 46 48 53 54 64 70 76	23	49	85	1834	33	27854	—	11405	5030	276
★ INDUSTRIAL HOSPITAL, Puerto Rico Medical Center, Zip 00936, Mailing Address: P.O. Box 365028, Zip 00936; tel. 787/764–3660; Domingo Velez, Administrator (Nonreporting) **A**5	12	10	125	—	—	—	—	—	—	—
★ SAN CARLOS GENERAL HOSPITAL, 1822 Ponce De Leon Avenue, Zip 00919, Mailing Address: Call Box 8410, Zip 00910–8410; tel. 787/727–5858; Pedro J. Gonzalez, Executive Director (Total facility includes 8 beds in nursing home–type unit) (Nonreporting) **A**9 10	33	10	66	—	—	—	—	—	—	—
★ SAN JORGE CHILDREN'S HOSPITAL, 258 San Jorge Avenue, Zip 00912; tel. 787/727–1000; Domingo Cruz Vivaldi, Administrator (Nonreporting) **A**9 **S** United Medical Corporation, Windermere, FL	33	50	85	—	—	—	—	—	—	—
★ SAN JUAN CITY HOSPITAL, Puerto Rico Medical Center, Zip 00928, Mailing Address: PMB 79, P.O. Box 70344, Zip 00936–8344; tel. 787/766–1298; Sylvette Clovet, Chief Executive Officer (Nonreporting) **A**1 3 5 10	14	10	267	—	—	—	—	—	—	—
★ STATE PSYCHIATRIC HOSPITAL, Monacillos Avenue, Zip 00936, Mailing Address: Call Box 2100, Caparra Heights Station, Zip 00922–2100; tel. 787/766–4646; Ivette Molena, Administrator (Nonreporting) **A**3 **S** Puerto Rico Department of Health, San Juan, PR	12	22	425	—	—	—	—	—	—	—
★ U. S. NAVAL HOSPITAL, Roosevelt Roads, Mailing Address: P.O. Box 3007, FPO, AA, Zip 34051–8100; tel. 787/865–5762; Captain G. R. Brown, Commanding Officer (Nonreporting) **S** Department of Navy, Washington, DC	43	10	35	—	—	—	—	—	—	—
★ UNIVERSITY HOSPITAL, Puerto Rico Medical Center, Rio Piedras Station, Zip 00920–2116; tel. 787/777–3535; Betty Ocasio, Executive Director (Nonreporting) **A**1 2 3 5 9 10 **S** Puerto Rico Department of Health, San Juan, PR	12	10	297	—	—	—	—	—	—	—
★ UNIVERSITY PEDIATRIC HOSPITAL, Mailing Address: Call Box 191079, Zip 00910–1079; tel. 787/756–3198; Sylvia Mercado, Chief Executive Officer (Nonreporting) **A**1 3 5 9 10	12	50	135	—	—	—	—	—	—	—
★ VETERANS AFFAIRS MEDICAL CENTER, One Veterans Plaza, Zip 00936–5800; tel. 787/641–7582; James A. Palmer, Director (Total facility includes 120 beds in nursing home–type unit) (Nonreporting) **A**1 2 3 5 8 9 **S** Department of Veterans Affairs, Washington, DC **Web address:** www.va.gov/stations97/guide/home.asp?DIVISION=ALL	45	10	693	—	—	—	—	—	—	—
VEGA BAJA—Vega Baja County										
★ WILMA N. VAZQUEZ MEDICAL CENTER, KM 39.5 Road 2, Call Box 7001, Zip 00694; tel. 787/858–1580; Ramon J. Vilar, Administrator (Total facility includes 20 beds in nursing home–type unit) **A**9 10 **F**22 25 31 39 41 48 54 69 70 76 **P**8	33	10	130	4478	55	27731	22	11110	4120	255
YAUCO—Yauco County										
★ BELLA VISTA SOUTHWEST HOSPITAL, Carretera 128 KM 1.0, Zip 00698, Mailing Address: P.O. Box 68, Zip 00698; tel. 787/856–1000; Nemuel O. Artiles, Chief Executive Officer **A**1 5 10 **F**16 17 18 22 25 41 44 48 70 76	21	10	111	4279	53	36143	1004	—	—	334

VIRGIN ISLANDS

CHRISTIANSTED—St. Croix County

★ GOVERNOR JUAN F. LOUIS HOSPITAL, 4007 Estate Diamond Ruby, Zip 00820–4421; tel. 340/778–6311; Thomas D. Robinson, FACHE, Chief Executive Officer (Nonreporting) **A**1 10	12	10	87	—	—	—	—	—	—	—

SAINT THOMAS—St. Thomas County

★ ROY LESTER SCHNEIDER HOSPITAL, 9048 Sugar Estate, Charlotte Amalie, Zip 00802; tel. 340/776–8311; Eugene A. Woods, Chief Executive Officer (Nonreporting) **A**10 **Web address:** www.rlshospital.org	12	10	133	—	—	—	—	—	—	—

U.S. Government Hospitals Outside the United States, by Area

GERMANY
Heidelberg: ★ U. S. Army Hospital, APO, USAMEDDAC HEIDELBERG, AE 09042
Landstuhl: ★ Landstuhl Army Regional Medical Center, APO, AE 09180
Wurzburg: ★ U. S. Army Hospital, APO, USAMEDDAC Wurzburg, AE 09244

ICELAND
Keflavilk: ★ U. S. Naval Hospital–Keflavilk, FPO, PSC 1003, Box 8, AE 09728–0308

ITALY
Naples: ★ U. S. Naval Hospital, FPO, AE 09619

JAPAN
Yokosuka: ★ U. S. Naval Hospital, FPO, Box 1487, AP 96350

KOREA
Seoul: ★ U. S. Army Community Hospital Seoul, APO, AP 96205
Yongsan: Medcom 18th Commander, Facilities Division Eamc L EM, APO, AP 96205

PANAMA
Ancon: ★ Gorgas Army Hospital, APO, AA 34004

SPAIN
Rota: ★ U. S. Naval Hospital, Rota, FPO, PSC 819, Box 18, AE 09645–2500

TAIWAN
Taipei: U. S. Naval Hospital Taipei, Taipei, No 300 Shin–Pai Road, Sec 2

★Indicates membership in the American Hospital Association

Index of Hospitals

This section is an index of all hospitals in alphabetical order by hospital name, followed by the city, state and page reference to the hospital's listing in Section A.

A

A. G. HOLLEY STATE HOSPITAL, LANTANA, FL, p. A88
A. WEBB ROBERTS HOSPITAL, DALLAS, TEXAS, p. A408
ABBEVILLE COUNTY MEMORIAL HOSPITAL, ABBEVILLE, SC, p. A378
ABBEVILLE GENERAL HOSPITAL, ABBEVILLE, LA, p. A180
ABBOTT NORTHWESTERN HOSPITAL, MINNEAPOLIS, MN, p. A230
ABERDEEN-MONROE COUNTY HOSPITAL, ABERDEEN, MS, p. A236
ABILENE REGIONAL MEDICAL CENTER, ABILENE, TX, p. A401
ABINGTON MEMORIAL HOSPITAL, ABINGTON, PA, p. A355
ABRAHAM LINCOLN MEMORIAL HOSPITAL, LINCOLN, IL, p. A129
ABROM KAPLAN MEMORIAL HOSPITAL, KAPLAN, LA, p. A183
ACADIA HOSPITAL, BANGOR, ME, p. A191
ACADIA-ST. LANDRY HOSPITAL, CHURCH POINT, LA, p. A181
ACOMA-CANONCITO-LAGUNA HOSPITAL, SAN FIDEL, NM, p. A286
ACUTE GENERAL HOSPITAL, MERWICK UNIT-EXTENDED CARE AND REHABILITATION, PRINCETON HOUSE UNIT-COMMUNITY MENTAL HEALTH AND SUBSTANCE ABUSE, p. A280
ADAIR COUNTY MEMORIAL HOSPITAL, GREENFIELD, IA, p. A152
ADAMS COUNTY HOSPITAL, WEST UNION, OH, p. A339
ADAMS COUNTY MEMORIAL HOSPITAL, DECATUR, IN, p. A139
ADAMS COUNTY MEMORIAL HOSPITAL AND NURSING CARE UNIT, FRIENDSHIP, WI, p. A468
ADCARE HOSPITAL OF WORCESTER, WORCESTER, MA, p. A210
ADDISON COMMUNITY HOSPITAL, ADDISON, MI, p. A211
ADDISON GILBERT HOSPITAL, GLOUCESTER, MASSACHUSETTS, p. A201
ADENA HEALTH SYSTEM, CHILLICOTHE, OH, p. A327
ADIRONDACK MEDICAL CENTER, SARANAC LAKE, NY, p. A304
ADVENTIST MEDICAL CENTER, PORTLAND, OR, p. A353
AFFILIATED HEALTH SERVICES, MOUNT VERNON, WA, p. A454
AGNESIAN HEALTHCARE, FOND DU LAC, WI, p. A468
AGUADILLA GENERAL HOSPITAL, AGUADILLA, PR, p. A481
AIKEN REGIONAL MEDICAL CENTERS, AIKEN, SC, p. A378
AKRON CITY HOSPITAL, AKRON, OHIO, p. A325
AKRON GENERAL MEDICAL CENTER, AKRON, OH, p. A325
ALAMANCE REGIONAL MEDICAL CENTER, BURLINGTON, NC, p. A310
ALAMEDA COUNTY MEDICAL CENTER, SAN LEANDRO, CA, p. A61
ALAMEDA COUNTY MEDICAL CENTER-HIGHLAND CAMPUS, OAKLAND, CA, p. A53
ALAMEDA HOSPITAL, ALAMEDA, CA, p. A35
ALASKA NATIVE MEDICAL CENTER, ANCHORAGE, AK, p. A20
ALASKA PSYCHIATRIC INSTITUTE, ANCHORAGE, AK, p. A20
ALASKA REGIONAL HOSPITAL, ANCHORAGE, AK, p. A20
ALBANY AREA HOSPITAL AND MEDICAL CENTER, ALBANY, MN, p. A225
ALBANY GENERAL HOSPITAL, ALBANY, OR, p. A350
ALBANY MEDICAL CENTER, ALBANY, NY, p. A287
ALBANY MEDICAL CENTER SOUTH-CLINICAL CAMPUS, ALBANY, NEW YORK, p. A287
ALBEMARLE HOSPITAL, ELIZABETH CITY, NC, p. A312
ALBERT EINSTEIN MEDICAL CENTER, PHILADELPHIA, PA, p. A366
ALBERT LEA MEDICAL CENTER, ALBERT LEA, MN, p. A225
ALBERT LINDLEY LEE MEMORIAL HOSPITAL, FULTON, NY, p. A291
ALCOHOL AND DRUG ABUSE TREATMENT CENTER, BUTNER, NORTH CAROLINA, p. A310
ALEDA E. LUTZ VETERANS AFFAIRS MEDICAL CENTER, SAGINAW, MI, p. A221
ALEGENT HEALTH BERGAN MERCY MEDICAL CENTER, OMAHA, NE, p. A265
ALEGENT HEALTH COMMUNITY MEMORIAL HOSPITAL, MISSOURI VALLEY, IA, p. A154
ALEGENT HEALTH IMMANUEL MEDICAL CENTER, OMAHA, NE, p. A265
ALEGENT HEALTH MERCY HOSPITAL, CORNING, IA, p. A149
ALEGENT HEALTH MERCY HOSPITAL, COUNCIL BLUFFS, IA, p. A150
ALEGENT HEALTH-MEMORIAL HOSPITAL, SCHUYLER, NE, p. A266

ALEGENT-HEALTH MIDLANDS COMMUNITY HOSPITAL, PAPILLION, NE, p. A266
ALEXANDER COMMUNITY HOSPITAL, TAYLORSVILLE, NC, p. A319
ALEXIAN BROTHERS BEHAVIORAL HEALTH HOSPITAL, HOFFMAN ESTATES, IL, p. A128
ALEXIAN BROTHERS HOSPITAL, SAINT LOUIS, MO, p. A252
ALEXIAN BROTHERS MEDICAL CENTER, ELK GROVE VILLAGE, IL, p. A125
ALFRED AND NORMA LERNER TOWER, BOLWELL HEALTH CENTER, HANNA PAVILION, LAKESIDE HOSPITAL, SAMUEL MATHER PAVILION, RAINBOW BABIES AND CHILDREN'S HOSPITAL, CLEVELAND, OHIO, p. A329
UNIVERSITY MACDONALD WOMEN'S HOSPITAL, CLEVELAND, OHIO, p. A329
ALFRED I. DUPONT HOSPITAL FOR CHILDREN, WILMINGTON, DE, p. A78
ALHAMBRA HOSPITAL MEDICAL CENTER, ALHAMBRA, CA, p. A35
ALICE HYDE MEDICAL CENTER, MALONE, NY, p. A294
ALICE PECK DAY MEMORIAL HOSPITAL, LEBANON, NH, p. A272
ALICE REGIONAL HOSPITAL, ALICE, TX, p. A401
ALL CHILDREN'S HOSPITAL, SAINT PETERSBURG, FL, p. A94
ALL SAINT'S HEALTHCARE SYSTEM, RACINE, WI, p. A474
ALL SAINTS EPISCOPAL HOSPITAL OF FORT WORTH, FORT WORTH, TX, p. A412
ALL SAINTS HOSPITAL-CITYVIEW, FORT WORTH, TX, p. A412
ALL SAINTS SPECIAL CARE HOSPITAL, BRIDGETON, MO, p. A244
ALLEGAN GENERAL HOSPITAL, ALLEGAN, MI, p. A211
ALLEGHANY MEMORIAL HOSPITAL, SPARTA, NC, p. A318
ALLEGHANY REGIONAL HOSPITAL, LOW MOOR, VA, p. A445
ALLEGHENY UNIVERSITY HOSPITALS, ALLEGHENY GENERAL, PITTSBURGH, PA, p. A368
ALLEGHENY UNIVERSITY HOSPITALS, ALLEGHENY VALLEY, NATRONA HEIGHTS, PA, p. A365
ALLEGHENY UNIVERSITY HOSPITALS, FORBES REGIONAL, MONROEVILLE, PA, p. A364
ALLEN BENNETT HOSPITAL, GREER, SC, p. A381
ALLEN COUNTY HOSPITAL, IOLA, KS, p. A163
ALLEN MEMORIAL HOSPITAL, OBERLIN, OH, p. A336
ALLEN MEMORIAL HOSPITAL, WATERLOO, IA, p. A157
ALLEN MEMORIAL HOSPITAL, MOAB, UT, p. A437
ALLEN PARISH HOSPITAL, KINDER, LA, p. A184
ALLEN-CALDER SKILLED NURSING FACILITY, FAXTON CAMPUS, UTICA, NEW YORK, p. A306
ST. LUKE'S CAMPUS, UTICA, NEW YORK, p. A306
ALLENDALE COUNTY HOSPITAL, FAIRFAX, SC, p. A380
ALLENMORE HOSPITAL, TACOMA, WASHINGTON, p. A458
ALLENTOWN STATE HOSPITAL, ALLENTOWN, PA, p. A355
ALLIANCE COMMUNITY HOSPITAL, ALLIANCE, OH, p. A325
ALLIANCE HEALTHCARE SYSTEM, HOLLY SPRINGS, MS, p. A238
ALLIANCE HOSPITAL OF SANTA TERESA, SANTA TERESA, NM, p. A286
ALLIED SERVICES REHABILITATION HOSPITAL, SCRANTON, PA, p. A371
ALPENA GENERAL HOSPITAL, ALPENA, MI, p. A211
ALTA BATES MEDICAL CENTER-ASHBY CAMPUS, BERKELEY, CA, p. A37
ALTA BATES MEDICAL CENTER-HERRICK CAMPUS, BERKELEY, CALIFORNIA, p. A37
ALTA DISTRICT HOSPITAL, DINUBA, CA, p. A40
ALTA VIEW HOSPITAL, SANDY, UT, p. A439
ALTON MEMORIAL HOSPITAL, ALTON, IL, p. A119
ALTON MENTAL HEALTH CENTER, ALTON, IL, p. A119
ALTOONA CENTER, ALTOONA, PA, p. A355
ALTOONA HOSPITAL, ALTOONA, PA, p. A355
ALTRU HEALTH SYSTEM, GRAND FORKS, ND, p. A322
ALTRU HOSPITAL, GRAND FORKS, NORTH DAKOTA, p. A322
ALTRUA HEALTH INSTITUTE, GRAND FORKS, NORTH DAKOTA, p. A322
ALVARADO HOSPITAL MEDICAL CENTER, SAN DIEGO, CA, p. A58
ALVIN C. YORK VETERANS AFFAIRS MEDICAL CENTER, MURFREESBORO, TN, p. A397
ALVIN DIAGNOSTIC AND URGENT CARE CENTER, ALVIN, TEXAS, p. A434
AMERICAN FORK HOSPITAL, AMERICAN FORK, UT, p. A436
AMERICAN LEGION HOSPITAL, CROWLEY, LA, p. A182
AMERY REGIONAL MEDICAL CENTER, AMERY, WI, p. A466
AMETHYST, CHARLOTTE, NC, p. A310

AMOS COTTAGE REHABILITATION HOSPITAL, WINSTON-SALEM, NC, p. A319
AMSTERDAM MEMORIAL HOSPITAL, AMSTERDAM, NY, p. A287
ANACAPA HOSPITAL, PORT HUENEME, CA, p. A56
ANADARKO MUNICIPAL HOSPITAL, ANADARKO, OK, p. A341
ANAHEIM GENERAL HOSPITAL, ANAHEIM, CA, p. A35
ANAHEIM MEMORIAL MEDICAL CENTER, ANAHEIM, CA, p. A35
ANAHEIM MEMORIAL OUTPATIENT TOWER, ANAHEIM, CALIFORNIA, p. A35
ANCORA PSYCHIATRIC HOSPITAL, ANCORA, NJ, p. A274
ANDALUSIA REGIONAL HOSPITAL, ANDALUSIA, AL, p. A11
ANDERSON AREA MEDICAL CENTER, ANDERSON, SC, p. A378
ANDERSON COUNTY HOSPITAL, GARNETT, KS, p. A161
ANDERSON HOSPITAL, MARYVILLE, IL, p. A130
ANDREW MCFARLAND MENTAL HEALTH CENTER, SPRINGFIELD, IL, p. A135
ANDROSCOGGIN VALLEY HOSPITAL, BERLIN, NH, p. A271
ANGEL MEDICAL CENTER, FRANKLIN, NC, p. A313
ANGLETON-DANBURY GENERAL HOSPITAL, ANGLETON, TX, p. A401
ANNA JAQUES HOSPITAL, NEWBURYPORT, MA, p. A207
ANNE ARUNDEL MEDICAL CENTER, ANNAPOLIS, MD, p. A195
ANNIE JEFFREY MEMORIAL COUNTY HEALTH CENTER, OSCEOLA, NE, p. A266
ANNIE PENN HOSPITAL, REIDSVILLE, NC, p. A317
ANOKA-METROPOLITAN REGIONAL TREATMENT CENTER, ANOKA, MN, p. A225
ANSON COMMUNITY HOSPITAL, WADESBORO, NC, p. A319
ANSON GENERAL HOSPITAL, ANSON, TX, p. A402
ANTELOPE MEMORIAL HOSPITAL, NELIGH, NE, p. A264
ANTELOPE VALLEY HOSPITAL, LANCASTER, CA, p. A45
APPALACHIAN PSYCHIATRIC HEALTHCARE SYSTEM, CAMBRIDGE, OH, p. A326
APPLETON MEDICAL CENTER, APPLETON, WI, p. A466
APPLETON MUNICIPAL HOSPITAL AND NURSING HOME, APPLETON, MN, p. A225
APPLING HEALTHCARE SYSTEM, BAXLEY, GA, p. A101
ARBORVIEW HOSPITAL, WARREN, MI, p. A223
ARBOUR H. R. I. HOSPITAL, BROOKLINE, MA, p. A203
ARBOUR HOSPITAL, BOSTON, MA, p. A201
ARBOUR-FULLER HOSPITAL, ATTLEBORO, MA, p. A201
ARBUCKLE MEMORIAL HOSPITAL, SULPHUR, OK, p. A347
ARDEN HILL HOSPITAL, GOSHEN, NY, p. A292
ARECIBO REGIONAL HOSPITAL, ARECIBO, PR, p. A481
ARH REGIONAL MEDICAL CENTER, HAZARD, KY, p. A173
ARIZONA HEART HOSPITAL, PHOENIX, AZ, p. A24
ARIZONA STATE HOSPITAL, PHOENIX, AZ, p. A24
ARKANSAS CHILDREN'S HOSPITAL, LITTLE ROCK, AR, p. A31
ARKANSAS HEART HOSPITAL, LITTLE ROCK, AR, p. A31
ARKANSAS METHODIST HOSPITAL, PARAGOULD, AR, p. A33
ARKANSAS STATE HOSPITAL, LITTLE ROCK, AR, p. A31
ARKANSAS VALLEY REGIONAL MEDICAL CENTER, LA JUNTA, CO, p. A71
ARLINGTON HOSPITAL, ARLINGTON, VA, p. A442
ARLINGTON MEMORIAL HOSPITAL, ARLINGTON, TX, p. A402
ARLINGTON MUNICIPAL HOSPITAL, ARLINGTON, MN, p. A225
ARMS ACRES, CARMEL, NY, p. A290
ARMSTRONG COUNTY MEMORIAL HOSPITAL, KITTANNING, PA, p. A362
ARNOLD MEMORIAL HEALTH CARE CENTER, ADRIAN, MN, p. A225
ARNOLD PALMER HOSPITAL FOR CHILDREN AND WOMEN; M. D. ANDERSON CANCER CENTER AND SAND LAKE HOSPITAL, p. A92
ARNOT OGDEN MEDICAL CENTER, ELMIRA, NY, p. A291
AROOSTOOK HEALTH CENTER, MARS HILL, MAINE, p. A193
AROOSTOOK MEDICAL CENTER, PRESQUE ISLE, ME, p. A193
ARROWHEAD COMMUNITY HOSPITAL AND MEDICAL CENTER, GLENDALE, AZ, p. A22
ARROWHEAD REGIONAL MEDICAL CENTER, COLTON, CA, p. A39
ARROYO GRANDE COMMUNITY HOSPITAL, ARROYO GRANDE, CA, p. A35
ARTESIA GENERAL HOSPITAL, ARTESIA, NM, p. A284
ARTHUR G. JAMES CANCER HOSPITAL AND RICHARD J. SOLOVE RESEARCH INSTITUTE, COLUMBUS, OH, p. A329
ARTHUR R. GOULD MEMORIAL HOSPITAL, PRESQUE ISLE, MAINE, p. A193
ASCENSION HOSPITAL AND BEHAVIORAL HEALTH SERVICES, GONZALES, LA, p. A182
ASHE MEMORIAL HOSPITAL, JEFFERSON, NC, p. A314
ASHFORD PRESBYTERIAN COMMUNITY HOSPITAL, SAN JUAN, PR, p. A483

Index of Hospitals / Behavioral Health–Portsmouth Campus

ASHLAND COMMUNITY HOSPITAL, ASHLAND, OR, p. A350
ASHLAND HEALTH CENTER, ASHLAND, KS, p. A159
ASHLAND REGIONAL MEDICAL CENTER, ASHLAND, PA, p. A356
ASHLEY COUNTY MEDICAL CENTER, CROSSETT, AR, p. A29
ASHLEY MEDICAL CENTER, ASHLEY, ND, p. A321
ASHLEY VALLEY MEDICAL CENTER, VERNAL, UT, p. A439
ASHTABULA COUNTY MEDICAL CENTER, ASHTABULA, OH, p. A325
ASPEN HILL BEHAVIORAL HEALTH SYSTEM, FLAGSTAFF, ARIZONA, p. A22
ASPEN VALLEY HOSPITAL DISTRICT, ASPEN, CO, p. A68
ATASCADERO STATE HOSPITAL, ATASCADERO, CA, p. A36
ATCHISON HOSPITAL, ATCHISON, KS, p. A159
ATHENS REGIONAL MEDICAL CENTER, ATHENS, GA, p. A99
ATHENS REGIONAL MEDICAL CENTER, ATHENS, TN, p. A390
ATHENS–LIMESTONE HOSPITAL, ATHENS, AL, p. A11
ATHOL MEMORIAL HOSPITAL, ATHOL, MA, p. A201
ATLANTA MEDICAL CENTER, ATLANTA, GA, p. A99
ATLANTA MEMORIAL HOSPITAL, ATLANTA, TX, p. A402
ATLANTIC CITY MEDICAL CENTER, ATLANTIC CITY, NJ, p. A274
ATLANTIC GENERAL HOSPITAL, BERLIN, MD, p. A196
ATLANTIC HEALTH SYSTEM, FLORHAM PARK, NJ, p. A276
ATLANTIC MEDICAL CENTER, DAYTONA BEACH, FL, p. A83
ATLANTIC SHORES HOSPITAL, FORT LAUDERDALE, FL, p. A84
ATMORE COMMUNITY HOSPITAL, ATMORE, AL, p. A11
ATOKA MEMORIAL HOSPITAL, ATOKA, OK, p. A341
AUBURN MEMORIAL HOSPITAL, AUBURN, NY, p. A287
AUBURN REGIONAL MEDICAL CENTER, AUBURN, WA, p. A452
AUDRAIN MEDICAL CENTER, MEXICO, MO, p. A250
AUDUBON COUNTY MEMORIAL HOSPITAL, AUDUBON, IA, p. A148
AUGUSTA HEALTH CARE, FISHERSVILLE, VA, p. A444
AUGUSTA MEDICAL COMPLEX, AUGUSTA, KS, p. A159
AUGUSTA MENTAL HEALTH INSTITUTE, AUGUSTA, ME, p. A191
AULTMAN HOSPITAL, CANTON, OH, p. A326
AURELIA OSBORN FOX MEMORIAL HOSPITAL, ONEONTA, NY, p. A302
AURORA COMMUNITY HOSPITAL, AURORA, MO, p. A244
AURORA MEDICAL CENTER, KENOSHA, WISCONSIN, p. A467
AURORA PAVILION, AIKEN, SOUTH CAROLINA, p. A378
AUSTEN RIGGS CENTER, STOCKBRIDGE, MA, p. A208
AUSTIN MEDICAL CENTER, AUSTIN, MN, p. A225
AUSTIN STATE HOSPITAL, AUSTIN, TX, p. A402
AUXILIO MUTUO HOSPITAL, SAN JUAN, PR, p. A483
AVALON MUNICIPAL HOSPITAL AND CLINIC, AVALON, CA, p. A36
AVENTURA HOSPITAL AND MEDICAL CENTER, MIAMI, FL, p. A89
AVERA HOLY FAMILY HOSPITAL, ESTHERVILLE, IA, p. A151
AVERA MCKENNAN HOSPITAL, SIOUX FALLS, SD, p. A388
AVERA QUEEN OF PEACE, MITCHELL, SD, p. A387
AVERA SACRED HEART, YANKTON, SD, p. A389
AVERA ST. ANTHONY'S HOSPITAL, O'NEILL, NE, p. A265
AVERA ST. BENEDICT HEALTH CENTER, PARKSTON, SD, p. A387
AVERA ST. LUKE'S, ABERDEEN, SD, p. A385
AVISTA ADVENTIST HOSPITAL, LOUISVILLE, CO, p. A72
AVOYELLES HOSPITAL, MARKSVILLE, LA, p. A185

B

B.J. WORKMAN MEMORIAL HOSPITAL, WOODRUFF, SC, p. A384
BABIES AND CHILDREN'S HOSPITAL, NEW YORK, NEW YORK, p. A299
BACHARACH INSTITUTE FOR REHABILITATION, POMONA, NJ, p. A279
BACON COUNTY HOSPITAL, ALMA, GA, p. A99
BAKER COMMUNITY HOSPITAL AND HEALTH CENTER, MACCLENNY, FL, p. A89
BAKERSFIELD MEMORIAL HOSPITAL, BAKERSFIELD, CA, p. A36
BALDPATE HOSPITAL, HAVERHILL, MA, p. A205
BALDWIN AREA MEDICAL CENTER, BALDWIN, WI, p. A466
BALL MEMORIAL HOSPITAL, MUNCIE, IN, p. A144
BALLINGER MEMORIAL HOSPITAL, BALLINGER, TX, p. A403
BAMBERG COUNTY MEMORIAL HOSPITAL AND NURSING CENTER, BAMBERG, SC, p. A378
BANGOR MENTAL HEALTH INSTITUTE, BANGOR, ME, p. A191
BANNOCK REGIONAL MEDICAL CENTER, POCATELLO, ID, p. A117
BAPTIST BEHAVIORAL HEALTH, JACKSON, MISSISSIPPI, p. A239
BAPTIST DEKALB HOSPITAL, SMITHVILLE, TN, p. A399
BAPTIST HEALTH BAPTIST MEMORIAL MEDICAL CENTER, NORTH LITTLE ROCK, AR, p. A32
BAPTIST HEALTH MEDICAL CENTER–ARKADELPHIA, ARKADELPHIA, AR, p. A28
BAPTIST HEALTH MEDICAL CENTER–HEBER SPRINGS, HEBER SPRINGS, AR, p. A30

BAPTIST HEALTH MEDICAL CENTER–LITTLE ROCK, LITTLE ROCK, AR, p. A31
BAPTIST HEALTH REHABILITATION INSTITUTE, LITTLE ROCK, AR, p. A31
BAPTIST HICKMAN COMMUNITY HOSPITAL, CENTERVILLE, TN, p. A390
BAPTIST HOSPITAL, PENSACOLA, FL, p. A92
BAPTIST HOSPITAL, NASHVILLE, TN, p. A398
BAPTIST HOSPITAL EAST, LOUISVILLE, KY, p. A175
BAPTIST HOSPITAL OF COCKE COUNTY, NEWPORT, TN, p. A398
BAPTIST HOSPITAL OF EAST TENNESSEE, KNOXVILLE, TN, p. A394
BAPTIST HOSPITAL OF MIAMI, MIAMI, FL, p. A89
BAPTIST HOSPITAL, WORTH COUNTY, SYLVESTER, GA, p. A110
BAPTIST HOSPITAL–ORANGE, ORANGE, TX, p. A425
BAPTIST MEDICAL CENTER, CUMMING, GA, p. A103
BAPTIST MEDICAL CENTER, JACKSONVILLE, FL, p. A86
BAPTIST MEDICAL CENTER, MONTGOMERY, AL, p. A16
BAPTIST MEDICAL CENTER, KANSAS CITY, MO, p. A248
BAPTIST MEDICAL CENTER, SAN ANTONIO, TX, p. A428
BAPTIST MEDICAL CENTER EAST, MONTGOMERY, AL, p. A16
BAPTIST MEDICAL CENTER–BEACHES, JACKSONVILLE BEACH, FL, p. A87
BAPTIST MEDICAL CENTER–NASSAU, FERNANDINA BEACH, FL, p. A84
BAPTIST MEMORIAL HOSPITAL, MEMPHIS, TN, p. A396
BAPTIST MEMORIAL HOSPITAL EAST, MEMPHIS, TENNESSEE, p. A396
BAPTIST MEMORIAL HOSPITAL REHABILITATION CENTER, MEMPHIS, TENNESSEE, p. A396
BAPTIST MEMORIAL HOSPITAL–BLYTHEVILLE, BLYTHEVILLE, AR, p. A28
BAPTIST MEMORIAL HOSPITAL–BOONEVILLE, BOONEVILLE, MS, p. A236
BAPTIST MEMORIAL HOSPITAL–COLLIERVILLE, COLLIERVILLE, TENNESSEE, p. A396
BAPTIST MEMORIAL HOSPITAL–DESOTO, SOUTHAVEN, MS, p. A242
BAPTIST MEMORIAL HOSPITAL–FORREST CITY, FORREST CITY, AR, p. A29
BAPTIST MEMORIAL HOSPITAL–GOLDEN TRIANGLE, COLUMBUS, MS, p. A237
BAPTIST MEMORIAL HOSPITAL–HUNTINGDON, HUNTINGDON, TN, p. A393
BAPTIST MEMORIAL HOSPITAL–LAUDERDALE, RIPLEY, TN, p. A399
BAPTIST MEMORIAL HOSPITAL–NORTH MISSISSIPPI, OXFORD, MS, p. A241
BAPTIST MEMORIAL HOSPITAL–OSCEOLA, OSCEOLA, AR, p. A33
BAPTIST MEMORIAL HOSPITAL–TIPTON, COVINGTON, TN, p. A391
BAPTIST MEMORIAL HOSPITAL–UNION CITY, UNION CITY, TN, p. A400
BAPTIST MEMORIAL HOSPITAL–UNION COUNTY, NEW ALBANY, MS, p. A241
BAPTIST MERIWETHER HOSPITAL, WARM SPRINGS, GA, p. A111
BAPTIST REGIONAL MEDICAL CENTER, CORBIN, KY, p. A171
BAPTIST REHABILITATION–GERMANTOWN, GERMANTOWN, TN, p. A392
BAPTIST ST. ANTHONY HEALTH SYSTEM, AMARILLO, TX, p. A401
BARAGA COUNTY MEMORIAL HOSPITAL, L'ANSE, MI, p. A218
BARBERTON CITIZENS HOSPITAL, BARBERTON, OH, p. A325
BARLOW RESPIRATORY HOSPITAL, LOS ANGELES, CA, p. A47
BARNERT HOSPITAL, PATERSON, NJ, p. A279
BARNES–JEWISH HOSPITAL, SAINT LOUIS, MO, p. A252
BARNES–JEWISH ST. PETERS HOSPITAL, SAINT PETERS, MO, p. A254
BARNES–JEWISH WEST COUNTY HOSPITAL, SAINT LOUIS, MO, p. A252
BARNES–KASSON COUNTY HOSPITAL, SUSQUEHANNA, PA, p. A372
BARNESVILLE HOSPITAL ASSOCIATION, BARNESVILLE, OH, p. A326
BARNSTABLE COUNTY HOSPITAL, POCASSET, MA, p. A208
BARNWELL COUNTY HOSPITAL, BARNWELL, SC, p. A378
BARRETT MEMORIAL HOSPITAL, DILLON, MT, p. A257
BARRON MEDICAL CENTER–MAYO HEALTH SYSTEM, BARRON, WI, p. A466
BARROW MEDICAL CENTER, WINDER, GA, p. A111
BARSTOW COMMUNITY HOSPITAL, BARSTOW, CA, p. A36
BARTLETT REGIONAL HOSPITAL, JUNEAU, AK, p. A21
BARTON COUNTY MEMORIAL HOSPITAL, LAMAR, MO, p. A249
BARTON MEMORIAL HOSPITAL, SOUTH LAKE TAHOE, CA, p. A64
BARTOW MEMORIAL HOSPITAL, BARTOW, FL, p. A81

BASCOM PALMER EYE INSTITUTE–ANNE BATES LEACH EYE HOSPITAL, MIAMI, FL, p. A89
BASSETT ARMY COMMUNITY HOSPITAL, FORT WAINWRIGHT, AK, p. A20
BASSETT HOSPITAL OF SCHOHARIE COUNTY, COBLESKILL, NY, p. A290
BATES COUNTY MEMORIAL HOSPITAL, BUTLER, MO, p. A245
BATH COUNTY COMMUNITY HOSPITAL, HOT SPRINGS, VA, p. A445
BATH HEALTH CARE CENTER, BATH, MAINE, p. A191
BATON ROUGE GENERAL HEALTH CENTER, BATON ROUGE, LOUISIANA, p. A180
BATON ROUGE GENERAL MEDICAL CENTER, BATON ROUGE, LA, p. A180
BATTLE CREEK HEALTH SYSTEM, BATTLE CREEK, MI, p. A212
BATTLE MOUNTAIN GENERAL HOSPITAL, BATTLE MOUNTAIN, NV, p. A268
BAUM HARMON MERCY HOSPITAL, PRIMGHAR, IA, p. A156
BAXTER REGIONAL MEDICAL CENTER, MOUNTAIN HOME, AR, p. A32
BAY AREA HOSPITAL, COOS BAY, OR, p. A350
BAY AREA MEDICAL CENTER, MARINETTE, WI, p. A471
BAY MEDICAL CENTER, PANAMA CITY, FL, p. A92
BAY MEDICAL CENTER, BAY CITY, MI, p. A212
BAY MEDICAL CENTER–WEST CAMPUS, BAY CITY, MICHIGAN, p. A212
BAY SPECIAL CARE, BAY CITY, MI, p. A212
BAYCOAST MEDICAL CENTER, BAYTOWN, TX, p. A404
BAYFRONT MEDICAL CENTER, SAINT PETERSBURG, FL, p. A94
BAYHEALTH MEDICAL CENTER, DOVER, DE, p. A78
BAYHEALTH MEDICAL CENTER AT KENT GENERAL, DOVER, DELAWARE, p. A78
BAYHEALTH MEDICAL CENTER, MILFORD MEMORIAL HOSPITAL, MILFORD, DELAWARE, p. A78
BAYLEY SETON CAMPUS, NEW YORK, NEW YORK, p. A300
BAYLOR CENTER FOR RESTORATIVE CARE, DALLAS, TX, p. A408
BAYLOR INSTITUTE FOR REHABILITATION, DALLAS, TX, p. A408
BAYLOR MEDICAL CENTER AT GARLAND, GARLAND, TX, p. A414
BAYLOR MEDICAL CENTER AT GRAPEVINE, GRAPEVINE, TX, p. A414
BAYLOR MEDICAL CENTER AT IRVING, IRVING, TX, p. A419
BAYLOR MEDICAL CENTER–ELLIS COUNTY, WAXAHACHIE, TX, p. A434
BAYLOR UNIVERSITY MEDICAL CENTER, DALLAS, TX, p. A408
BAYLOR/ RICHARDSON MEDICAL CENTER, RICHARDSON, TX, p. A427
BAYNE–JONES ARMY COMMUNITY HOSPITAL, FORT POLK, LA, p. A182
BAYONNE HOSPITAL, BAYONNE, NJ, p. A274
BAYOU CITY MEDICAL CENTER, HOUSTON, TX, p. A416
BAYOU OAKS BEHAVIORAL HEALTH SYSTEM, HOUMA, LA, p. A183
BAYSHORE COMMUNITY HOSPITAL, HOLMDEL, NJ, p. A277
BAYSHORE MEDICAL CENTER, PASADENA, TX, p. A426
BAYSIDE COMMUNITY HOSPITAL, ANAHUAC, TX, p. A401
BAYSTATE MEDICAL CENTER, SPRINGFIELD, MA, p. A208
BAYVIEW HOSPITAL AND MENTAL HEALTH SYSTEM, CHULA VISTA, CA, p. A38
BEACHAM MEMORIAL HOSPITAL, MAGNOLIA, MS, p. A240
BEAR LAKE MEMORIAL HOSPITAL, MONTPELIER, ID, p. A117
BEAR RIVER VALLEY HOSPITAL, TREMONTON, UT, p. A439
BEAR VALLEY COMMUNITY HOSPITAL, BIG BEAR LAKE, CA, p. A37
BEARTOOTH HOSPITAL AND HEALTH CENTER, RED LODGE, MT, p. A259
BEATRICE COMMUNITY HOSPITAL AND HEALTH CENTER, BEATRICE, NE, p. A261
BEAUFORT COUNTY HOSPITAL, WASHINGTON, NC, p. A319
BEAUFORT MEMORIAL HOSPITAL, BEAUFORT, SC, p. A378
BEAUREGARD MEMORIAL HOSPITAL, DE RIDDER, LA, p. A182
BEAVER COUNTY MEMORIAL HOSPITAL, BEAVER, OK, p. A341
BEAVER DAM COMMUNITY HOSPITALS, BEAVER DAM, WI, p. A466
BEAVER VALLEY HOSPITAL, BEAVER, UT, p. A436
BECKLEY APPALACHIAN REGIONAL HOSPITAL, BECKLEY, WV, p. A460
BEDFORD COUNTY MEDICAL CENTER, SHELBYVILLE, TN, p. A399
BEDFORD REGIONAL MEDICAL CENTER, BEDFORD, IN, p. A137
BEEBE MEDICAL CENTER, LEWES, DE, p. A78
BEECH HILL HOSPITAL, DUBLIN, NH, p. A271
BEHAVIORAL HEALTH CARE OF CAPE FEAR VALLEY HEALTH SYSTEM, FAYETTEVILLE, NC, p. A312
BEHAVIORAL HEALTH CENTER, GREENSBORO, NC, p. A313
BEHAVIORAL HEALTH CENTER, WINFIELD, ILLINOIS, p. A136
BEHAVIORAL HEALTH–PORTSMOUTH CAMPUS, PORTSMOUTH, OHIO, p. A333

© 2000 AHA Guide   Index of Hospitals **A487**

Index of Hospitals / Behavioral Healthcare of Northern Indiana

BEHAVIORAL HEALTHCARE OF NORTHERN INDIANA, PLYMOUTH, IN, p. A145
BEHAVIORAL HEALTHCARE–COLUMBUS, COLUMBUS, IN, p. A138
BELL MEMORIAL HOSPITAL, ISHPEMING, MI, p. A217
BELLA VISTA HOSPITAL, MAYAGUEZ, PR, p. A483
BELLA VISTA SOUTHWEST HOSPITAL, YAUCO, PR, p. A484
BELLAIRE MEDICAL CENTER, HOUSTON, TX, p. A416
BELLEVUE COMPREHENSIVE GENERAL CARE, BELLEVUE PHYSICAL MEDICINE AND REHABILITATION SERVICES, BELLEVUE PSYCHIATRIC SERVICES, BELLEVUE TUBERCULOSIS SERVICES, COMPREHENSIVE AMBULATORY CARE SERVICES: LEVEL I TRAUMA CENTER, p. A295
BELLEVUE HOSPITAL, BELLEVUE, OH, p. A326
BELLEVUE HOSPITAL CENTER, NEW YORK, NY, p. A295
BELLEVUE WOMAN'S HOSPITAL, SCHENECTADY, NY, p. A304
BELLFLOWER MEDICAL CENTER, BELLFLOWER, CA, p. A36
BELLIN HOSPITAL, GREEN BAY, WI, p. A469
BELLIN PSYCHIATRIC CENTER, GREEN BAY, WI, p. A469
BELLVILLE GENERAL HOSPITAL, BELLVILLE, TX, p. A404
BELLWOOD GENERAL HOSPITAL, BELLFLOWER, CA, p. A36
BELMOND MEDICAL CENTER, BELMOND, IA, p. A148
BELMONT CENTER FOR COMPREHENSIVE TREATMENT, PHILADELPHIA, PA, p. A366
BELMONT COMMUNITY HOSPITAL, BELLAIRE, OH, p. A326
BELOIT MEMORIAL HOSPITAL, BELOIT, WI, p. A466
BEN TAUB GENERAL HOSPITAL, HOUSTON, TEXAS, p. A416
BENCHMARK BEHAVIORAL HEALTH SYSTEMS, WOODS CROSS, UT, p. A439
BENEDICTINE HOSPITAL, KINGSTON, NY, p. A293
BENEFIS HEALTH CARE–EAST CAMPUS, GREAT FALLS, MONTANA, p. A257
BENEFIS HEALTH CARE–WEST CAMPUS, GREAT FALLS, MONTANA, p. A257
BENEFIS HEALTHCARE, GREAT FALLS, MT, p. A257
BENEWAH COMMUNITY HOSPITAL, SAINT MARIES, ID, p. A117
BENJAMIN RUSH CENTER, SYRACUSE, NY, p. A305
BENNETT COUNTY HEALTHCARE CENTER, MARTIN, SD, p. A386
BENSON HOSPITAL, BENSON, AZ, p. A22
BEREA HOSPITAL, BEREA, KY, p. A170
BERGEN REGIONAL MEDICAL CENTER, PARAMUS, NJ, p. A279
BERGER HEALTH SYSTEM, CIRCLEVILLE, OH, p. A328
BERKSHIRE MEDICAL CENTER, PITTSFIELD, MA, p. A207
BERLIN MEMORIAL HOSPITAL, BERLIN, WI, p. A467
BERNARD MITCHELL HOSPITAL, CHICAGO, ILLINOIS, p. A124
BERRIEN COUNTY HOSPITAL, NASHVILLE, GA, p. A108
BERT FISH MEDICAL CENTER, NEW SMYRNA BEACH, FL, p. A91
BERTIE MEMORIAL HOSPITAL, WINDSOR, NC, p. A319
BERTRAND CHAFFEE HOSPITAL, SPRINGVILLE, NY, p. A305
BERWICK HOSPITAL CENTER, BERWICK, PA, p. A356
BESSEMER CARRAWAY MEDICAL CENTER, BESSEMER, AL, p. A11
BETH ISRAEL DEACONESS MEDICAL CENTER, BOSTON, MA, p. A201
BETH ISRAEL HOSPITAL, PASSAIC, NJ, p. A279
BETH ISRAEL MEDICAL CENTER, NEW YORK, NY, p. A295
BETH ISRAEL MEDICAL CENTER–HERBERT AND NELL SINGER DIVISION, NEW YORK, NEW YORK, p. A295
BETH ISRAEL MEDICAL CENTER–KINGS HIGHWAY DIVISION, NEW YORK, NEW YORK, p. A295
BETHANY HOSPITAL, CHICAGO, IL, p. A121
BETHANY MEDICAL CENTER, KANSAS CITY, KS, p. A163
BETHESDA HOSPITAL, ZANESVILLE, OHIO, p. A340
BETHESDA MEMORIAL HOSPITAL, BOYNTON BEACH, FL, p. A81
BETHESDA NORTH HOSPITAL, CINCINNATI, OH, p. A327
BETHESDA REHABILITATION HOSPITAL, SAINT PAUL, MN, p. A233
BETSY JOHNSON REGIONAL HOSPITAL, DUNN, NC, p. A311
BEVERLY HOSPITAL, BEVERLY, MA, p. A201
BEVERLY HOSPITAL, MONTEBELLO, CA, p. A52
BHC ALHAMBRA HOSPITAL, ROSEMEAD, CA, p. A57
BHC BELMONT PINES HOSPITAL, YOUNGSTOWN, OH, p. A340
BHC CEDAR VISTA HOSPITAL, FRESNO, CA, p. A41
BHC EAST LAKE HOSPITAL, NEW ORLEANS, LA, p. A186
BHC FAIRFAX HOSPITAL, KIRKLAND, WA, p. A454
BHC FORT LAUDERDALE HOSPITAL, FORT LAUDERDALE, FL, p. A84
BHC FOX RUN HOSPITAL, SAINT CLAIRSVILLE, OH, p. A337
BHC FREMONT HOSPITAL, FREMONT, CA, p. A41
BHC HERITAGE OAKS HOSPITAL, SACRAMENTO, CA, p. A57
BHC HOSPITAL SAN JUAN CAPESTRANO, SAN JUAN, PR, p. A483
BHC INTERMOUNTAIN HOSPITAL, BOISE, ID, p. A115
BHC MEADOW WOOD HOSPITAL, BATON ROUGE, LA, p. A180
BHC MESILLA VALLEY HOSPITAL, LAS CRUCES, NM, p. A285
BHC MILLWOOD HOSPITAL, ARLINGTON, TX, p. A402
BHC MONTEVISTA HOSPITAL, LAS VEGAS, NV, p. A268
BHC PINNACLE POINTE HOSPITAL, LITTLE ROCK, AR, p. A31
BHC ROSS HOSPITAL, KENTFIELD, CA, p. A44

BHC SAN LUIS REY HOSPITAL, ENCINITAS, CA, p. A40
BHC SIERRA VISTA HOSPITAL, SACRAMENTO, CA, p. A57
BHC SPIRIT OF ST. LOUIS HOSPITAL, SAINT CHARLES, MO, p. A252
BHC STREAMWOOD HOSPITAL, STREAMWOOD, IL, p. A135
BHC VALLE VISTA HOSPITAL, GREENWOOD, IN, p. A140
BHC VISTA DEL MAR HOSPITAL, VENTURA, CA, p. A66
BHC WALNUT CREEK HOSPITAL, WALNUT CREEK, CA, p. A66
BHC WEST HILLS HOSPITAL, RENO, NV, p. A269
BHC WILLOW SPRINGS RESIDENTIAL TREATMENT CENTER, RENO, NV, p. A269
BHC WINDSOR HOSPITAL, CHAGRIN FALLS, OH, p. A327
BI-COUNTY COMMUNITY HOSPITAL, WARREN, MI, p. A223
BIBB MEDICAL CENTER, CENTREVILLE, AL, p. A13
BIG BEND REGIONAL MEDICAL CENTER, ALPINE, TX, p. A401
BIG HORN COUNTY MEMORIAL HOSPITAL, HARDIN, MT, p. A258
BIG SANDY MEDICAL CENTER, BIG SANDY, MT, p. A256
BIG SPRING STATE HOSPITAL, BIG SPRING, TX, p. A404
BIGGS–GRIDLEY MEMORIAL HOSPITAL, GRIDLEY, CA, p. A43
BILOXI REGIONAL MEDICAL CENTER, BILOXI, MS, p. A236
BINGHAM MEMORIAL HOSPITAL, BLACKFOOT, ID, p. A115
BINGHAMTON GENERAL HOSPITAL, BINGHAMTON, NEW YORK, p. A288
BINGHAMTON PSYCHIATRIC CENTER, BINGHAMTON, NY, p. A288
BIXBY MEDICAL CENTER, LENAWEE HEALTH ALLIANCE, ADRIAN, MI, p. A211
BJC MEDICAL CENTER, COMMERCE, GA, p. A103
BLACK RIVER MEMORIAL HOSPITAL, BLACK RIVER FALLS, WI, p. A467
BLACKFORD COUNTY HOSPITAL, HARTFORD CITY, IN, p. A141
BLACKWELL REGIONAL HOSPITAL, BLACKWELL, OK, p. A341
BLADEN COUNTY HOSPITAL, ELIZABETHTOWN, NC, p. A312
BLAINE COUNTY MEDICAL CENTER, HAILEY, IDAHO, p. A118
BLAKE MEDICAL CENTER, BRADENTON, FL, p. A82
BLANCHARD VALLEY HEALTH ASSOCIATION SYSTEM, FINDLAY, OH, p. A332
BLANCHARD VALLEY REGIONAL HEALTH CENTER–BLUFFTON CAMPUS, BLUFFTON, OHIO, p. A332
BLANCHARD VALLEY REGIONAL HEALTH CENTER–FINDLAY CAMPUS, FINDLAY, OHIO, p. A332
BLECKLEY MEMORIAL HOSPITAL, COCHRAN, GA, p. A102
BLEDSOE COMMUNITY MEDICAL CENTER, PIKEVILLE, TN, p. A399
BLESSING HOSPITAL, QUINCY, IL, p. A133
BLESSING HOSPITAL, QUINCY, ILLINOIS, p. A133
BLOOMER MEMORIAL MEDICAL CENTER, BLOOMER, WI, p. A467
BLOOMINGTON HOSPITAL, BLOOMINGTON, IN, p. A137
BLOOMINGTON HOSPITAL OF ORANGE COUNTY, PAOLI, IN, p. A144
BLOOMSBURG HOSPITAL, BLOOMSBURG, PA, p. A356
BLOUNT MEMORIAL HOSPITAL, MARYVILLE, TN, p. A396
BLOWING ROCK HOSPITAL, BLOWING ROCK, NC, p. A309
BLUE HILL MEMORIAL HOSPITAL, BLUE HILL, ME, p. A191
BLUE MOUNTAIN HOSPITAL, JOHN DAY, OR, p. A351
BLUEFIELD REGIONAL MEDICAL CENTER, BLUEFIELD, WV, p. A460
BLYTHEDALE CHILDREN'S HOSPITAL, VALHALLA, NY, p. A306
BOB WILSON MEMORIAL GRANT COUNTY HOSPITAL, ULYSSES, KS, p. A168
BOCA RATON COMMUNITY HOSPITAL, BOCA RATON, FL, p. A81
BOGALUSA COMMUNITY MEDICAL CENTER, BOGALUSA, LA, p. A181
BOLIVAR GENERAL HOSPITAL, BOLIVAR, TN, p. A390
BOLIVAR MEDICAL CENTER, CLEVELAND, MS, p. A237
BON SECOURS BALTIMORE HEALTH SYSTEM, BALTIMORE, MD, p. A195
BON SECOURS COTTAGE HEALTH SERVICES–BON SECOURS HOSPITAL, GROSSE POINTE, MI, p. A216
BON SECOURS COTTAGE HEALTH SERVICES–COTTAGE HOSPITAL, GROSSE POINTE FARMS, MI, p. A216
BON SECOURS ST. MARY'S HOSPITAL, RICHMOND, VA, p. A448
BON SECOURS–DEPAUL MEDICAL CENTER, NORFOLK, VA, p. A446
BON SECOURS–HOLY FAMILY REGIONAL HEALTH SYSTEM, ALTOONA, PA, p. A355
BON SECOURS–RICHMOND COMMUNITY HOSPITAL, RICHMOND, VA, p. A448
BON SECOURS–ST. FRANCIS XAVIER HOSPITAL, CHARLESTON, SC, p. A378
BON SECOURS–ST. JOSEPH HEALTHCARE GROUP, PORT CHARLOTTE, FL, p. A93
BON SECOURS–STUART CIRCLE, RICHMOND, VA, p. A448
BON SECOURS–VENICE HOSPITAL, VENICE, FL, p. A97
BONE AND JOINT HOSPITAL, OKLAHOMA CITY, OK, p. A345
BONNER GENERAL HOSPITAL, SANDPOINT, ID, p. A117
BOONE COUNTY HEALTH CENTER, ALBION, NE, p. A261
BOONE COUNTY HOSPITAL, BOONE, IA, p. A148

BOONE HOSPITAL CENTER, COLUMBIA, MO, p. A245
BOONE MEMORIAL HOSPITAL, MADISON, WV, p. A462
BOONEVILLE COMMUNITY HOSPITAL, BOONEVILLE, AR, p. A28
BORGESS MEDICAL CENTER, KALAMAZOO, MI, p. A217
BORGESS–PIPP HEALTH CENTER, PLAINWELL, MICHIGAN, p. A217
BOSCOBEL AREA HEALTH CARE, BOSCOBEL, WI, p. A467
BOSTON MEDICAL CENTER, BOSTON, MA, p. A202
BOTHWELL REGIONAL HEALTH CENTER, SEDALIA, MO, p. A254
BOTSFORD GENERAL HOSPITAL, FARMINGTON HILLS, MI, p. A214
BOULDER CITY HOSPITAL, BOULDER CITY, NV, p. A268
BOULDER COMMUNITY HOSPITAL, BOULDER, CO, p. A68
BOUNDARY COMMUNITY HOSPITAL, BONNERS FERRY, ID, p. A115
BOUNDARY COUNTY NURSING HOME, p. A115
BOURBON COMMUNITY HOSPITAL, PARIS, KY, p. A177
BOURNEWOOD HOSPITAL, BROOKLINE, MA, p. A203
BOWDLE HOSPITAL, BOWDLE, SD, p. A385
BOWIE MEMORIAL HOSPITAL, BOWIE, TX, p. A405
BOX BUTTE GENERAL HOSPITAL, ALLIANCE, NE, p. A261
BOYS TOWN NATIONAL RESEARCH HOSPITAL, OMAHA, NE, p. A265
BOZEMAN DEACONESS HOSPITAL, BOZEMAN, MT, p. A256
BRACKENRIDGE HOSPITAL, AUSTIN, TX, p. A402
BRADFORD HEALTH SERVICES AT HUNTSVILLE, MADISON, AL, p. A16
BRADFORD HEALTH SERVICES AT OAK MOUNTAIN, PELHAM, AL, p. A17
BRADFORD REGIONAL MEDICAL CENTER, BRADFORD, PA, p. A356
BRADLEY CENTER OF ST. FRANCIS, COLUMBUS, GEORGIA, p. A103
BRADLEY COUNTY MEDICAL CENTER, WARREN, AR, p. A34
BRADLEY MEMORIAL HOSPITAL, CLEVELAND, TN, p. A391
BRADLEY MEMORIAL HOSPITAL AND HEALTH CENTER, SOUTHINGTON, CT, p. A77
BRAINERD REGIONAL HUMAN SERVICES CENTER, BRAINERD, MN, p. A226
BRANDON REGIONAL HOSPITAL, BRANDON, FL, p. A82
BRANDYWINE HOSPITAL, COATESVILLE, PA, p. A358
BRATTLEBORO MEMORIAL HOSPITAL, BRATTLEBORO, VT, p. A440
BRATTLEBORO RETREAT, BRATTLEBORO, VT, p. A440
BRAXTON COUNTY MEMORIAL HOSPITAL, GASSAWAY, WV, p. A461
BRAZOSPORT MEMORIAL HOSPITAL, LAKE JACKSON, TX, p. A421
BREA COMMUNITY HOSPITAL, BREA, CA, p. A37
BRECKINRIDGE MEMORIAL HOSPITAL, HARDINSBURG, KY, p. A172
BREECH REGIONAL MEDICAL CENTER, LEBANON, MO, p. A249
BRENTWOOD, A BEHAVIORAL HEALTH COMPANY, SHREVEPORT, LA, p. A188
BRIDGEPORT HOSPITAL, BRIDGEPORT, CT, p. A74
BRIDGES MEDICAL SERVICES, ADA, MN, p. A225
BRIDGEWATER STATE HOSPITAL, BRIDGEWATER, MA, p. A203
BRIDGEWAY, NORTH LITTLE ROCK, AR, p. A33
BRIDGTON HOSPITAL, BRIDGTON, ME, p. A192
BRIGHAM AND WOMEN'S HOSPITAL, BOSTON, MA, p. A202
BRIGHAM CITY COMMUNITY HOSPITAL, BRIGHAM CITY, UT, p. A436
BRIGHTON HOSPITAL, BRIGHTON, MI, p. A212
BRISTOL HOSPITAL, BRISTOL, CT, p. A74
BRISTOW MEMORIAL HOSPITAL, BRISTOW, OK, p. A342
BROADDUS HOSPITAL, PHILIPPI, WV, p. A463
BROADLAWNS MEDICAL CENTER, DES MOINES, IA, p. A150
BROADWATER HEALTH CENTER, TOWNSEND, MT, p. A260
BROCKTON HOSPITAL, BROCKTON, MA, p. A203
BROCKTON VETERANS AFFAIRS MEDICAL CENTER, BROCKTON, MA, p. A203
BROKEN ARROW MEDICAL CENTER, BROKEN ARROW, OK, p. A342
BROMENN HEALTHCARE, NORMAL, IL, p. A131
BROMENN REGIONAL MEDICAL CENTER, NORMAL, ILLINOIS, p. A131
BRONSON METHODIST HOSPITAL, KALAMAZOO, MI, p. A218
BRONSON VICKSBURG HOSPITAL, VICKSBURG, MI, p. A223
BRONX CHILDREN'S PSYCHIATRIC CENTER, NEW YORK, NY, p. A295
BRONX PSYCHIATRIC CENTER, NEW YORK, NY, p. A295
BRONX–LEBANON HOSPITAL CENTER, NEW YORK, NY, p. A295
BROOK LANE HEALTH SERVICES, HAGERSTOWN, MD, p. A198
BROOKDALE HOSPITAL MEDICAL CENTER, NEW YORK, NY, p. A295
BROOKE ARMY MEDICAL CENTER, SAN ANTONIO, TX, p. A428
BROOKHAVEN HOSPITAL, TULSA, OK, p. A348
BROOKHAVEN MEMORIAL HOSPITAL MEDICAL CENTER, PATCHOGUE, NY, p. A302
BROOKINGS HOSPITAL, BROOKINGS, SD, p. A385

Index of Hospitals / Central Arkansas Hospital

BROOKLYN HOSPITAL CENTER, NEW YORK, NY, p. A296
BROOKLYN JEWISH DIVISION, NEW YORK, NEW YORK, p. A297
BROOKS COUNTY HOSPITAL, QUITMAN, GA, p. A108
BROOKS HOSPITAL, ATLANTA, TX, p. A402
BROOKS MEMORIAL HOSPITAL, DUNKIRK, NY, p. A291
BROOKS REHABILITATION HOSPITAL, JACKSONVILLE, FL, p. A86
BROOKSVILLE REGIONAL HOSPITAL, BROOKSVILLE, FL, p. A82
BROOKVILLE HOSPITAL, BROOKVILLE, PA, p. A356
BROOKWOOD MEDICAL CENTER, BIRMINGHAM, AL, p. A11
BROTMAN MEDICAL CENTER, CULVER CITY, CA, p. A39
BROUGHTON HOSPITAL, MORGANTON, NC, p. A316
BROWARD GENERAL MEDICAL CENTER, FORT LAUDERDALE, FL, p. A84
BROWN COUNTY GENERAL HOSPITAL, GEORGETOWN, OH, p. A332
BROWN COUNTY HOSPITAL, AINSWORTH, NE, p. A261
BROWN COUNTY HUMAN SERVICES MENTAL HEALTH CENTER, GREEN BAY, WI, p. A469
BROWN MEMORIAL CONVALESCENT CENTER, COBB HEALTH CARE CENTER AND COBB TERRACE PERSONAL CARE CENTER, p. A109
BROWN SCHOOLS REHABILITATION CENTER, AUSTIN, TX, p. A402
BROWNFIELD REGIONAL MEDICAL CENTER, BROWNFIELD, TX, p. A405
BROWNSVILLE GENERAL HOSPITAL, BROWNSVILLE, PA, p. A356
BROWNSVILLE MEDICAL CENTER, BROWNSVILLE, TX, p. A405
BROWNWOOD REGIONAL MEDICAL CENTER, BROWNWOOD, TX, p. A405
BRUCE HOSPITAL SYSTEM, FLORENCE, SOUTH CAROLINA, p. A380
BRUNSWICK COMMUNITY HOSPITAL, SUPPLY, NC, p. A318
BRUNSWICK GENERAL HOSPITAL, AMITYVILLE, NY, p. A287
BRUNSWICK HALL, AMITYVILLE, NEW YORK, p. A287
BRUNSWICK PHYSICAL MEDICINE AND REHABILITATION HOSPITAL, AMITYVILLE, NEW YORK, p. A287
BRYAN HOSPITAL, BRYAN, OHIO, p. A326
BRYAN MEMORIAL–BRYANLGH–EAST, LINCOLN, NEBRASKA, p. A264
BRYAN W. WHITFIELD MEMORIAL HOSPITAL, DEMOPOLIS, AL, p. A14
BRYANLGH MEDICAL CENTER, LINCOLN, NE, p. A264
BRYCE HOSPITAL, TUSCALOOSA, AL, p. A18
BRYLIN HOSPITALS, BUFFALO, NY, p. A288
BRYN MAWR COLLEGE INFIRMARY, BRYN MAWR, PA, p. A357
BRYN MAWR HOSPITAL, BRYN MAWR, PA, p. A357
BRYN MAWR REHABILITATION HOSPITAL, MALVERN, PA, p. A363
BRYNN MARR BEHAVIORAL HEALTHCARE SYSTEM, JACKSONVILLE, NC, p. A314
BUCHANAN GENERAL HOSPITAL, GRUNDY, VA, p. A444
BUCKS COUNTY CAMPUS, LANGHORNE, PENNSYLVANIA, p. A366
BUCKTAIL MEDICAL CENTER, RENOVO, PA, p. A371
BUCYRUS COMMUNITY HOSPITAL, BUCYRUS, OH, p. A326
BUENA VISTA COUNTY HOSPITAL, STORM LAKE, IA, p. A157
BUFFALO GENERAL HOSPITAL, BUFFALO, NY, p. A289
BUFFALO HOSPITAL, BUFFALO, MN, p. A226
BUFFALO PSYCHIATRIC CENTER, BUFFALO, NY, p. A289
BULLOCH MEMORIAL HOSPITAL, STATESBORO, GA, p. A110
BULLOCK COUNTY HOSPITAL, UNION SPRINGS, AL, p. A19
BUNKIE GENERAL HOSPITAL, BUNKIE, LA, p. A181
BURDETTE TOMLIN MEMORIAL HOSPITAL, CAPE MAY COURT HOUSE, NJ, p. A275
BURGESS HEALTH CENTER, ONAWA, IA, p. A155
BURKE COUNTY HOSPITAL, WAYNESBORO, GA, p. A111
BURKE REHABILITATION HOSPITAL, WHITE PLAINS, NY, p. A307
BURLESON ST. JOSEPH HEALTH CENTER, CALDWELL, TX, p. A406
BURNETT MEDICAL CENTER, GRANTSBURG, WI, p. A468
BUTLER COUNTY HEALTH CARE CENTER, DAVID CITY, NE, p. A262
BUTLER HEALTH SYSTEM, BUTLER, PA, p. A357
BUTLER HOSPITAL, PROVIDENCE, RI, p. A376
BYRD REGIONAL HOSPITAL, LEESVILLE, LA, p. A185

C

C. F. MENNINGER MEMORIAL HOSPITAL, TOPEKA, KS, p. A168
CABELL HUNTINGTON HOSPITAL, HUNTINGTON, WV, p. A461
CABRINI MEDICAL CENTER, NEW YORK, NY, p. A296
CAGUAS REGIONAL HOSPITAL, CAGUAS, PR, p. A482
CALAIS REGIONAL HOSPITAL, CALAIS, ME, p. A192
CALDWELL COUNTY HOSPITAL, PRINCETON, KY, p. A178
CALDWELL MEMORIAL HOSPITAL, LENOIR, NC, p. A315
CALDWELL MEMORIAL HOSPITAL, COLUMBIA, LA, p. A181
CALEDONIAN CAMPUS, NEW YORK, NEW YORK, p. A296
CALHOUN MEMORIAL HOSPITAL, ARLINGTON, GA, p. A99
CALHOUN–LIBERTY HOSPITAL, BLOUNTSTOWN, FL, p. A81
CALIFORNIA HOSPITAL MEDICAL CENTER, LOS ANGELES, CA, p. A47
CALIFORNIA MEDICAL FACILITY, VACAVILLE, CA, p. A65
CALIFORNIA MENS COLONY HOSPITAL, SAN LUIS OBISPO, CA, p. A61
CALIFORNIA PACIFIC MEDICAL CENTER, SAN FRANCISCO, CA, p. A59
CALIFORNIA PACIFIC MEDICAL CENTER–DAVIES CAMPUS, SAN FRANCISCO, CALIFORNIA, p. A59
CALIFORNIA SPECIALTY HOSPITAL, VALLEJO, CA, p. A66
CALLAHAN EYE FOUNDATION HOSPITAL, BIRMINGHAM, AL, p. A12
CALLAWAY COMMUNITY HOSPITAL, FULTON, MO, p. A247
CALLAWAY DISTRICT HOSPITAL, CALLAWAY, NE, p. A262
CALUMET MEDICAL CENTER, CHILTON, WI, p. A467
CALVARY HOSPITAL, NEW YORK, NY, p. A296
CALVERT MEMORIAL HOSPITAL, PRINCE FREDERICK, MD, p. A199
CAMBRIDGE HEALTH ALLIANCE, CAMBRIDGE, MA, p. A204
CAMBRIDGE HOSPITAL, CAMBRIDGE, MASSACHUSETTS, p. A204
CAMBRIDGE MEDICAL CENTER, CAMBRIDGE, MN, p. A226
CAMDEN COUNTY HEALTH SERVICES CENTER, BLACKWOOD, NJ, p. A274
CAMDEN GENERAL HOSPITAL, CAMDEN, TN, p. A390
CAMDEN MEDICAL CENTER, SAINT MARYS, GA, p. A109
CAMDEN–CLARK MEMORIAL HOSPITAL, PARKERSBURG, WV, p. A463
CAMERON COMMUNITY HOSPITAL, CAMERON, MO, p. A245
CAMERON MEMORIAL COMMUNITY HOSPITAL, ANGOLA, IN, p. A137
CAMPBELL COUNTY MEMORIAL HOSPITAL, GILLETTE, WY, p. A478
CAMPBELL HEALTH SYSTEM, WEATHERFORD, TX, p. A434
CAMPBELLTON GRACEVILLE HOSPITAL, GRACEVILLE, FL, p. A85
CANCER TREATMENT CENTERS OF AMERICA–TULSA, TULSA, OK, p. A348
CANDLER COUNTY HOSPITAL, METTER, GA, p. A107
CANDLER HOSPITAL, SAVANNAH, GA, p. A109
CANNON MEMORIAL HOSPITAL, PICKENS, SC, p. A383
CANONSBURG GENERAL HOSPITAL, CANONSBURG, PA, p. A357
CANTON–INWOOD MEMORIAL HOSPITAL, CANTON, SD, p. A385
CANTON–POTSDAM HOSPITAL, POTSDAM, NY, p. A303
CANYON RIDGE HOSPITAL, CHINO, CA, p. A38
CAPE COD HOSPITAL, HYANNIS, MA, p. A205
CAPE CORAL HOSPITAL, CAPE CORAL, FL, p. A82
CAPE FEAR MEMORIAL HOSPITAL, WILMINGTON, NORTH CAROLINA, p. A319
CAPE FEAR VALLEY HEALTH SYSTEM, FAYETTEVILLE, NC, p. A312
CAPITAL DISTRICT PSYCHIATRIC CENTER, ALBANY, NY, p. A287
CAPITAL HEALTH SYSTEM, TRENTON, NJ, p. A281
CAPITAL HEALTH SYSTEM AT FULD, TRENTON, NEW JERSEY, p. A281
CAPITAL HEALTH SYSTEM AT MERCER, TRENTON, NEW JERSEY, p. A281
CAPITAL MEDICAL CENTER, OLYMPIA, WA, p. A455
CAPITAL REGION MEDICAL CENTER, JEFFERSON CITY, MO, p. A247
CAPITOL MEDICAL CENTER, RICHMOND, VA, p. A448
CARDINAL GLENNON CHILDREN'S HOSPITAL, SAINT LOUIS, MO, p. A252
CARDINAL HILL REHABILITATION HOSPITAL, LEXINGTON, KY, p. A174
CARDIOVASCULAR CENTER OF PUERTO RICO AND THE CARIBBEAN, SAN JUAN, PR, p. A483
CARIBOU MEMORIAL HOSPITAL AND LIVING CENTER, SODA SPRINGS, ID, p. A118
CARILION BEDFORD MEMORIAL HOSPITAL, BEDFORD, VA, p. A442
CARILION FRANKLIN MEMORIAL HOSPITAL, ROCKY MOUNT, VA, p. A449
CARILION GILES MEMORIAL HOSPITAL, PEARISBURG, VA, p. A447
CARILION MEDICAL CENTER, ROANOKE, VA, p. A449
CARILION NEW RIVER VALLEY MEDICAL CENTER, RADFORD, VA, p. A448
CARILION ROANOKE COMMUNITY HOSPITAL, ROANOKE, VIRGINIA, p. A449
CARILION SAINT ALBANS HOSPITAL, RADFORD, VA, p. A448
CARITAS GOOD SAMARITAN MEDICAL CENTER, BROCKTON, MA, p. A203
CARITAS MEDICAL CENTER, LOUISVILLE, KY, p. A175
CARITAS NORWOOD HOSPITAL, NORWOOD, MA, p. A207
CARITAS PEACE CENTER, LOUISVILLE, KY, p. A175
CARL ALBERT INDIAN HEALTH FACILITY, ADA, OK, p. A341
CARL T. HAYDEN VETERANS AFFAIRS MEDICAL CENTER, PHOENIX, AZ, p. A24
CARLE FOUNDATION HOSPITAL, URBANA, IL, p. A135
CARLINVILLE AREA HOSPITAL, CARLINVILLE, IL, p. A120
CARLISLE HOSPITAL AND HEALTH SERVICES, CARLISLE, PA, p. A357
CARLSBAD MEDICAL CENTER, CARLSBAD, NM, p. A284
CARNEGIE TRI–COUNTY MUNICIPAL HOSPITAL, CARNEGIE, OK, p. A342
CARNEY HOSPITAL, DORCHESTER, MA, p. A204
CARO CENTER, CARO, MI, p. A212
CARO COMMUNITY HOSPITAL, CARO, MI, p. A212
CAROLINA PINES REGIONAL MEDICAL CENTER, HARTSVILLE, SC, p. A382
CAROLINAS HOSPITAL SYSTEM, FLORENCE, SC, p. A380
CAROLINAS HOSPITAL SYSTEM–KINGSTREE, KINGSTREE, SC, p. A382
CAROLINAS HOSPITAL SYSTEM–LAKE CITY, LAKE CITY, SC, p. A382
CAROLINAS MEDICAL CENTER, CHARLOTTE, NC, p. A310
CARONDELET HOLY CROSS HOSPITAL, NOGALES, AZ, p. A23
CARONDELET ST. JOSEPH'S HOSPITAL, TUCSON, AZ, p. A26
CARONDELET ST. MARY'S HOSPITAL, TUCSON, AZ, p. A26
CARRAWAY BURDICK WEST MEDICAL CENTER, HALEYVILLE, AL, p. A15
CARRAWAY METHODIST MEDICAL CENTER, BIRMINGHAM, AL, p. A12
CARRAWAY NORTHWEST MEDICAL CENTER, WINFIELD, AL, p. A19
CARRIE TINGLEY HOSPITAL, ALBUQUERQUE, NM, p. A283
CARRIER FOUNDATION, BELLE MEAD, NJ, p. A274
CARRINGTON HEALTH CENTER, CARRINGTON, ND, p. A321
CARROLL COUNTY GENERAL HOSPITAL, WESTMINSTER, MD, p. A200
CARROLL COUNTY HOSPITAL, CARROLLTON, KY, p. A171
CARROLL COUNTY MEMORIAL HOSPITAL, CARROLLTON, MO, p. A245
CARROLL REGIONAL MEDICAL CENTER, BERRYVILLE, AR, p. A28
CARSON CITY HOSPITAL, CARSON CITY, MI, p. A212
CARSON TAHOE HOSPITAL, CARSON CITY, NV, p. A268
CARTERET GENERAL HOSPITAL, MOREHEAD CITY, NC, p. A316
CARTHAGE AREA HOSPITAL, CARTHAGE, NY, p. A290
CARTHAGE GENERAL HOSPITAL, CARTHAGE, TN, p. A390
CARY MEDICAL CENTER, CARIBOU, ME, p. A192
CASA COLINA HOSPITAL FOR REHABILITATIVE MEDICINE, POMONA, CA, p. A55
CASA GRANDE REGIONAL MEDICAL CENTER, CASA GRANDE, AZ, p. A22
CASA, A SPECIAL HOSPITAL, HOUSTON, TX, p. A416
CASCADE MEDICAL CENTER, CASCADE, ID, p. A116
CASCADE VALLEY HOSPITAL, NORTH SNOHOMISH COUNTY HEALTH SYSTEM, ARLINGTON, WA, p. A452
CASS COUNTY MEMORIAL HOSPITAL, ATLANTIC, IA, p. A148
CASS MEDICAL CENTER, HARRISONVILLE, MO, p. A247
CASSIA REGIONAL MEDICAL CENTER, BURLEY, ID, p. A115
CASTANER GENERAL HOSPITAL, CASTANER, PR, p. A482
CASTLE MEDICAL CENTER, KAILUA, HI, p. A113
CASTLEVIEW HOSPITAL, PRICE, UT, p. A438
CASWELL CENTER, KINSTON, NC, p. A315
CATAWBA HOSPITAL, CATAWBA, VA, p. A442
CATAWBA MEMORIAL HOSPITAL, HICKORY, NC, p. A314
CATHOLIC MEDICAL CENTER, MANCHESTER, NH, p. A272
CATHOLIC MEDICAL CENTERS, NEW YORK, NY, p. A296
CAVALIER COUNTY MEMORIAL HOSPITAL, LANGDON, ND, p. A323
CAVERNA MEMORIAL HOSPITAL, HORSE CAVE, KY, p. A173
CAYLOR–NICKEL MEDICAL CENTER, BLUFFTON, IN, p. A137
CAYUGA MEDICAL CENTER AT ITHACA, ITHACA, NY, p. A293
CEDAR COUNTY MEMORIAL HOSPITAL, EL DORADO SPRINGS, MO, p. A246
CEDAR SPRINGS BEHAVIORAL HEALTH SYSTEM, COLORADO SPRINGS, CO, p. A68
CEDAR VALE COMMUNITY HOSPITAL, CEDAR VALE, KS, p. A159
CEDARCREST HOSPITAL, NEWINGTON, CT, p. A76
CEDARS HOSPITAL, DE SOTO, TX, p. A410
CEDARS MEDICAL CENTER, MIAMI, FL, p. A89
CEDARS–SINAI MEDICAL CENTER, LOS ANGELES, CA, p. A47
CENTENNIAL MEDICAL CENTER AND PARTHENON PAVILION, NASHVILLE, TN, p. A398
CENTENNIAL PEAKS HEALTH, LOUISVILLE, CO, p. A72
CENTINELA HOSPITAL MEDICAL CENTER, INGLEWOOD, CA, p. A44
CENTRAL ALABAMA VETERAN AFFAIRS HEALTH CARE SYSTEM, MONTGOMERY, AL, p. A17
CENTRAL ARKANSAS HOSPITAL, SEARCY, AR, p. A33

© 2000 AHA Guide

Index of Hospitals / Central Arkansas Veterans Affairs Healthcare System

CENTRAL ARKANSAS VETERANS AFFAIRS HEALTHCARE SYSTEM, LITTLE ROCK, AR, p. A31
CENTRAL BAPTIST HOSPITAL, LEXINGTON, KY, p. A174
CENTRAL CAROLINA HOSPITAL, SANFORD, NC, p. A318
CENTRAL COMMUNITY HOSPITAL, ELKADER, IA, p. A151
CENTRAL DUPAGE HOSPITAL, WINFIELD, IL, p. A136
CENTRAL FLORIDA REGIONAL HOSPITAL, SANFORD, FL, p. A95
CENTRAL KANSAS MEDICAL CENTER, GREAT BEND, KS, p. A161
CENTRAL KANSAS MEDICAL CENTER-ST. JOSEPH CAMPUS, LARNED, KANSAS, p. A161
CENTRAL LOUISIANA STATE HOSPITAL, PINEVILLE, LA, p. A188
CENTRAL MAINE MEDICAL CENTER, LEWISTON, ME, p. A193
CENTRAL MICHIGAN COMMUNITY HOSPITAL, MOUNT PLEASANT, MI, p. A219
CENTRAL MISSISSIPPI MEDICAL CENTER, JACKSON, MS, p. A239
CENTRAL MONTANA MEDICAL CENTER, LEWISTOWN, MT, p. A258
CENTRAL OREGON DISTRICT HOSPITAL, REDMOND, OR, p. A354
CENTRAL PENINSULA GENERAL HOSPITAL, SOLDOTNA, AK, p. A21
CENTRAL PRISON HOSPITAL, RALEIGH, NC, p. A316
CENTRAL STATE HOSPITAL, PETERSBURG, VA, p. A447
CENTRAL STATE HOSPITAL, MILLEDGEVILLE, GA, p. A107
CENTRAL STATE HOSPITAL, LOUISVILLE, KY, p. A175
CENTRAL SUFFOLK HOSPITAL, RIVERHEAD, NY, p. A303
CENTRAL TEXAS HOSPITAL, CAMERON, TX, p. A406
CENTRAL TEXAS MEDICAL CENTER, SAN MARCOS, TX, p. A430
CENTRAL TEXAS VETERANS AFFAIRS HEALTH CARE SYSTEM, WACO, TEXAS, p. A431
CENTRAL TEXAS VETERANS AFFAIRS HEALTH CARE SYSTEM, MARLIN INTEGRATED CLINICAL FACILITY, MARLIN, TEXAS, p. A431
CENTRAL TEXAS VETERANS AFFAIRS HEALTHCARE SYSTEM, TEMPLE, TX, p. A431
CENTRAL VALLEY GENERAL HOSPITAL, HANFORD, CA, p. A43
CENTRAL VALLEY MEDICAL CENTER, NEPHI, UT, p. A437
CENTRAL VERMONT MEDICAL CENTER, BARRE, VT, p. A440
CENTRAL VIRGINIA TRAINING CENTER, MADISON HEIGHTS, VA, p. A446
CENTRAL WASHINGTON HOSPITAL, WENATCHEE, WA, p. A459
CENTRASTATE HEALTHCARE SYSTEM, FREEHOLD, NJ, p. A276
CENTRE COMMUNITY HOSPITAL, STATE COLLEGE, PA, p. A372
CENTURA SPECIAL CARE HOSPITAL, DENVER, CO, p. A69
CENTURY CITY HOSPITAL, LOS ANGELES, CA, p. A47
CGH MEDICAL CENTER, STERLING, IL, p. A135
CHADRON COMMUNITY HOSPITAL AND HEALTH SERVICES, CHADRON, NE, p. A262
CHALMETTE MEDICAL CENTER, CHALMETTE, LA, p. A181
CHAMBERS MEMORIAL HOSPITAL, DANVILLE, AR, p. A29
CHAMBERSBURG HOSPITAL, CHAMBERSBURG, PA, p. A357
CHAMPLAIN VALLEY PHYSICIANS HOSPITAL MEDICAL CENTER, PLATTSBURGH, NY, p. A302
CHANDLER REGIONAL HOSPITAL, CHANDLER, AZ, p. A22
CHAPMAN MEDICAL CENTER, ORANGE, CA, p. A54
CHARITY CAMPUS, NEW ORLEANS, LOUISIANA, p. A186
CHARLES A. CANNON JR, MEMORIAL HOSPITAL, CROSSNORE, NC, p. A311
CHARLES A. CANNON JR. MEMORIAL HOSPITAL, BANNER ELK, NORTH CAROLINA, p. A311
CHARLES A. DEAN MEMORIAL HOSPITAL, GREENVILLE, ME, p. A192
CHARLES COLE MEMORIAL HOSPITAL, COUDERSPORT, PA, p. A358
CHARLES F. KETTERING MEMORIAL CENTER, KETTERING, OHIO, p. A333
CHARLES RIVER HOSPITAL, WELLESLEY, MA, p. A209
CHARLESTON AREA MEDICAL CENTER, CHARLESTON, WV, p. A460
CHARLESTON MEMORIAL HOSPITAL, CHARLESTON, SC, p. A378
CHARLEVOIX AREA HOSPITAL, CHARLEVOIX, MI, p. A212
CHARLOTTE HUNGERFORD HOSPITAL, TORRINGTON, CT, p. A77
CHARLOTTE INSTITUTE OF REHABILITATION, CHARLOTTE, NC, p. A310
CHARLOTTE REGIONAL MEDICAL CENTER, PUNTA GORDA, FL, p. A94
CHARLTON MEMORIAL HOSPITAL, FALL RIVER, MASSACHUSETTS, p. A204
CHARLTON MEMORIAL HOSPITAL, FOLKSTON, GA, p. A105
CHARLTON METHODIST HOSPITAL, DALLAS, TX, p. A408
CHARTER ANCHOR HOSPITAL, ATLANTA, GA, p. A99
CHARTER BEACON, FORT WAYNE, IN, p. A139
CHARTER BEHAVIORAL HEALTH SYSTEM OF ATLANTA, ATLANTA, GA, p. A99
CHARTER BEHAVIORAL HEALTH SYSTEM OF ATLANTA AT PEACHFORD, ATLANTA, GA, p. A99

CHARTER BEHAVIORAL HEALTH SYSTEM OF CHARLOTTESVILLE, CHARLOTTESVILLE, VA, p. A442
CHARTER BEHAVIORAL HEALTH SYSTEM OF MILWAUKEE/WEST ALLIS, WEST ALLIS, WI, p. A477
CHARTER BEHAVIORAL HEALTH SYSTEM OF NEW JERSEY-SUMMIT, SUMMIT, NJ, p. A280
CHARTER BEHAVIORAL HEALTH SYSTEM OF NORTHWEST ARKANSAS, FAYETTEVILLE, AR, p. A29
CHARTER BEHAVIORAL HEALTH SYSTEM OF SAN DIEGO, SAN DIEGO, CA, p. A58
CHARTER BEHAVIORAL HEALTH SYSTEM OF SOUTHERN CALIFORNIA-CHARTER OAK, COVINA, CA, p. A39
CHARTER BEHAVIORAL HEALTH SYSTEM OF WINSTON-SALEM, WINSTON-SALEM, NC, p. A320
CHARTER BY-THE-SEA BEHAVIORAL HEALTH SYSTEM, SAINT SIMONS ISLAND, GA, p. A109
CHARTER CHARLESTON BEHAVIORAL HEALTH SYSTEM, CHARLESTON, SC, p. A379
CHARTER FAIRMOUNT BEHAVIORAL HEALTH SYSTEM, PHILADELPHIA, PA, p. A366
CHARTER GREENVILLE BEHAVIORAL HEALTH SYSTEM, GREER, SC, p. A381
CHARTER HOSPITAL OF MILWAUKEE, MILWAUKEE, WI, p. A471
CHARTER LAKESIDE BEHAVIORAL HEALTH SYSTEM, MEMPHIS, TN, p. A396
CHARTER NORTH STAR BEHAVIORAL HEALTH SYSTEM, ANCHORAGE, AK, p. A20
CHARTER NORTH STAR BEHAVIORAL HEALTH SYSTEM, ANCHORAGE, AK, p. A20
CHARTER RIDGE BEHAVIORAL HEALTH SYSTEM, LEXINGTON, KY, p. A174
CHARTER RIVERS BEHAVIORAL HEALTH SYSTEM, WEST COLUMBIA, SC, p. A384
CHARTER SAVANNAH BEHAVIORAL HEALTH SYSTEM, SAVANNAH, GA, p. A109
CHARTER SPRINGS HOSPITAL, OCALA, FL, p. A91
CHASE COUNTY COMMUNITY HOSPITAL, IMPERIAL, NE, p. A263
CHATHAM HOSPITAL, SILER CITY, NC, p. A318
CHATUGE REGIONAL HOSPITAL AND NURSING HOME, HIAWASSEE, GA, p. A106
CHEATHAM MEDICAL CENTER, ASHLAND CITY, TN, p. A390
CHELSEA COMMUNITY HOSPITAL, CHELSEA, MI, p. A213
CHEMICAL DEPENDENCY CENTER, IOWA CITY, IOWA, p. A153
CHENANGO MEMORIAL HOSPITAL, NORWICH, NY, p. A301
CHEROKEE BAPTIST MEDICAL CENTER, CENTRE, AL, p. A13
CHERRY COUNTY HOSPITAL, VALENTINE, NE, p. A267
CHERRY HOSPITAL, GOLDSBORO, NC, p. A313
CHESAPEAKE GENERAL HOSPITAL, CHESAPEAKE, VA, p. A443
CHESHIRE MEDICAL CENTER, KEENE, NH, p. A272
CHESTATEE REGIONAL HOSPITAL, DAHLONEGA, GA, p. A103
CHESTER COUNTY HOSPITAL, WEST CHESTER, PA, p. A374
CHESTER COUNTY HOSPITAL AND NURSING CENTER, CHESTER, SC, p. A379
CHESTER MENTAL HEALTH CENTER, CHESTER, IL, p. A121
CHESTERFIELD GENERAL HOSPITAL, CHERAW, SC, p. A379
CHESTNUT HILL HEALTHCARE, PHILADELPHIA, PA, p. A366
CHESTNUT HILL REHABILITATION HOSPITAL, GLENSIDE, PA, p. A360
CHESTNUT LODGE HOSPITAL, ROCKVILLE, MD, p. A199
CHESTNUT RIDGE HOSPITAL, MORGANTOWN, WEST VIRGINIA, p. A463
CHEYENNE COUNTY HOSPITAL, SAINT FRANCIS, KS, p. A167
CHICAGO LAKESHORE HOSPITAL, CHICAGO, IL, p. A121
CHICAGO LYING-IN HOSPITAL, CHICAGO, ILLINOIS, p. A124
CHICAGO-READ MENTAL HEALTH CENTER, CHICAGO, IL, p. A121
CHICOT MEMORIAL HOSPITAL, LAKE VILLAGE, AR, p. A31
CHILD AND ADOLESCENT SERVICES OF THE MENNINGER CLINIC, TOPEKA, KANSAS, p. A168
CHILDREN'S HEALTHCARE OF ATLANTA AT EGLESTON, ATLANTA, GA, p. A99
CHILDREN'S HEALTHCARE OF ATLANTA AT SCOTTISH RITE, ATLANTA, GA, p. A100
CHILDREN'S HOME OF PITTSBURGH, PITTSBURGH, PA, p. A369
CHILDREN'S HOSPITAL, BOSTON, MA, p. A202
CHILDREN'S HOSPITAL, BUFFALO, NY, p. A289
CHILDREN'S HOSPITAL, RICHMOND, VA, p. A448
CHILDREN'S HOSPITAL, COLUMBUS, OH, p. A329
CHILDREN'S HOSPITAL, CHICAGO, ILLINOIS, p. A124
CHILDREN'S HOSPITAL, OMAHA, NE, p. A265
CHILDREN'S HOSPITAL, NEW ORLEANS, LA, p. A186
CHILDREN'S HOSPITAL, DENVER, CO, p. A69
CHILDREN'S HOSPITAL AND CLINICS, SAINT PAUL, MN, p. A233
CHILDREN'S HOSPITAL AND HEALTH CENTER, SAN DIEGO, CA, p. A58
CHILDREN'S HOSPITAL AND REGIONAL MEDICAL CENTER, SEATTLE, WA, p. A456
CHILDREN'S HOSPITAL AT SINAI, p. A196

CHILDREN'S HOSPITAL MEDICAL CENTER, CINCINNATI, OH, p. A327
CHILDREN'S HOSPITAL MEDICAL CENTER OF AKRON, AKRON, OH, p. A325
CHILDREN'S HOSPITAL OAKLAND, OAKLAND, CA, p. A53
CHILDREN'S HOSPITAL OF ALABAMA, BIRMINGHAM, AL, p. A12
CHILDREN'S HOSPITAL OF AUSTIN, AUSTIN, TEXAS, p. A402
CHILDREN'S HOSPITAL OF MICHIGAN, DETROIT, MI, p. A213
CHILDREN'S HOSPITAL OF OKLAHOMA, OKLAHOMA CITY, OKLAHOMA, p. A346
CHILDREN'S HOSPITAL OF ORANGE COUNTY, ORANGE, CA, p. A54
CHILDREN'S HOSPITAL OF PHILADELPHIA, PHILADELPHIA, PA, p. A366
CHILDREN'S HOSPITAL OF PITTSBURGH, PITTSBURGH, PA, p. A369
CHILDREN'S HOSPITAL OF THE KING'S DAUGHTERS, NORFOLK, VA, p. A447
CHILDREN'S HOSPITAL OF WISCONSIN, MILWAUKEE, WI, p. A471
CHILDREN'S HOSPITALS AND CLINICS, MINNEAPOLIS, MINNEAPOLIS, MN, p. A230
CHILDREN'S MEDICAL CENTER, DAYTON, OH, p. A330
CHILDREN'S MEDICAL CENTER, TULSA, OK, p. A348
CHILDREN'S MEDICAL CENTER OF DALLAS, DALLAS, TX, p. A408
CHILDREN'S MEMORIAL HOSPITAL, CHICAGO, IL, p. A121
CHILDREN'S MERCY HOSPITAL, KANSAS CITY, MO, p. A248
CHILDREN'S MERCY SOUTH, KANSAS CITY, KANSAS, p. A248
CHILDREN'S NATIONAL MEDICAL CENTER, WASHINGTON, DC, p. A79
CHILDREN'S REHABILITATION CENTER, p. A307
CHILDREN'S SEASHORE HOUSE, 3405 CIVIC CENTER BOULEVARD, ZIP 19104-4302, p. A366
CHILDREN'S SPECIALIZED HOSPITAL, MOUNTAINSIDE, NJ, p. A278
CHILDREN'S SPECIALIZED HOSPITAL-OCEAN, TOMS RIVER, NEW JERSEY, p. A278
CHILDRENS CARE HOSPITAL AND SCHOOL, SIOUX FALLS, SD, p. A388
CHILDRENS HOSPITAL OF LOS ANGELES, LOS ANGELES, CA, p. A47
CHILDRESS REGIONAL MEDICAL CENTER, CHILDRESS, TX, p. A406
CHILLICOTHE HOSPITAL DISTRICT, CHILLICOTHE, TX, p. A406
CHILTON MEDICAL CENTER, CLANTON, AL, p. A13
CHILTON MEMORIAL HOSPITAL, POMPTON PLAINS, NJ, p. A279
CHINESE HOSPITAL, SAN FRANCISCO, CA, p. A59
CHINLE COMPREHENSIVE HEALTH CARE FACILITY, CHINLE, AZ, p. A22
CHINO VALLEY MEDICAL CENTER, CHINO, CA, p. A38
CHIPPENHAM MEDICAL CENTER, RICHMOND, VIRGINIA, p. A448
CHIPPENHAM MEDICAL CENTER/JOHNSTON-WILLIS HOSPITAL, RICHMOND, VA, p. A448
CHIPPEWA COUNTY MONTEVIDEO HOSPITAL, MONTEVIDEO, MN, p. A231
CHIPPEWA COUNTY WAR MEMORIAL HOSPITAL, SAULT STE. MARIE, MI, p. A222
CHIPPEWA VALLEY HOSPITAL AND OAKVIEW CARE CENTER, DURAND, WI, p. A468
CHOATE MENTAL HEALTH CENTER, ANNA, IL, p. A119
CHOCTAW COUNTY MEDICAL CENTER, ACKERMAN, MS, p. A236
CHOCTAW HEALTH CENTER, PHILADELPHIA, MS, p. A241
CHOCTAW MEMORIAL HOSPITAL, HUGO, OK, p. A344
CHOCTAW NATION HEALTH CARE CENTER, TALIHINA, OK, p. A348
CHOWAN HOSPITAL, EDENTON, NC, p. A312
CHOWCHILLA DISTRICT MEMORIAL HOSPITAL, CHOWCHILLA, CA, p. A38
CHRIST HOSPITAL, JERSEY CITY, NJ, p. A277
CHRIST HOSPITAL, CINCINNATI, OH, p. A327
CHRIST HOSPITAL AND MEDICAL CENTER, OAK LAWN, IL, p. A131
CHRISTIAN HEALTH CARE CENTER, WYCKOFF, NJ, p. A282
CHRISTIAN HOSPITAL NORTHEAST-NORTHWEST, SAINT LOUIS, MO, p. A252
CHRISTIAN HOSPITAL NORTHWEST, FLORISSANT, MISSOURI, p. A252
CHRISTIANA HOSPITAL, NEWARK, DE, p. A78
CHRISTOPHER HOUSE, AUSTIN, TX, p. A402
CHRISTUS COUSHATTA HEALTH CARE CENTER, COUSHATTA, LA, p. A181
CHRISTUS JASPER MEMORIAL HOSPITAL, JASPER, TX, p. A419
CHRISTUS SANTA ROSA HEALTH CARE, SAN ANTONIO, TX, p. A428
CHRISTUS SCHUMPERT BOSSIER, BOSSIER CITY, LA, p. A181
CHRISTUS SCHUMPERT MEDICAL CENTER, SHREVEPORT, LA, p. A188
CHRISTUS SPOHN HOSPITAL ALICE, ALICE, TX, p. A401

Index of Hospitals / Conejos County Hospital

CHRISTUS SPOHN HOSPITAL BEEVILLE, BEEVILLE, TX, p. A404
CHRISTUS SPOHN HOSPITAL KLEBERG, KINGSVILLE, TX, p. A420
CHRISTUS SPOHN HOSPITAL MEMORIAL, CORPUS CHRISTI, TX, p. A407
CHRISTUS SPOHN HOSPITAL SHORELINE, CORPUS CHRISTI, TX, p. A407
CHRISTUS SPOHN HOSPITAL SOUTH, CORPUS CHRISTI, TX, p. A407
CHRISTUS ST. ELIZABETH HOSPITAL, BEAUMONT, TX, p. A404
CHRISTUS ST. FRANCES CABRINI HOSPITAL, ALEXANDRIA, LA, p. A180
CHRISTUS ST. JOHN HOSPITAL, NASSAU BAY, TX, p. A425
CHRISTUS ST. JOSEPH HOSPITAL, HOUSTON, TX, p. A416
CHRISTUS ST. JOSEPH'S HEALTH SYSTEM, PARIS, TX, p. A426
CHRISTUS ST. MARY HOSPITAL, PORT ARTHUR, TX, p. A426
CHRISTUS ST. MICHAEL HEALTH SYSTEM, TEXARKANA, TX, p. A432
CHRISTUS ST. MICHAEL REHABILITATION HOSPITAL, TEXARKANA, TEXAS, p. A432
CHRISTUS ST. PATRICK HOSPITAL, LAKE CHARLES, LA, p. A184
CHURCHILL COMMUNITY HOSPITAL, FALLON, NV, p. A268
CIBOLA GENERAL HOSPITAL, GRANTS, NM, p. A285
CIMARRON MEMORIAL HOSPITAL, BOISE CITY, OK, p. A341
CIRCLES OF CARE, MELBOURNE, FL, p. A89
CITIZENS BAPTIST MEDICAL CENTER, TALLADEGA, AL, p. A18
CITIZENS GENERAL HOSPITAL, NEW KENSINGTON, PA, p. A365
CITIZENS MEDICAL CENTER, COLBY, KS, p. A160
CITIZENS MEDICAL CENTER, VICTORIA, TX, p. A433
CITIZENS MEMORIAL HOSPITAL, BOLIVAR, MO, p. A244
CITRUS MEMORIAL HOSPITAL, INVERNESS, FL, p. A86
CITRUS VALLEY MEDICAL CENTER INTER-COMMUNITY CAMPUS, COVINA, CA, p. A39
CITRUS VALLEY MEDICAL CENTER-QUEEN OF THE VALLEY CAMPUS, WEST COVINA, CA, p. A67
CITY HOSPITAL, MARTINSBURG, WV, p. A462
CITY OF HOPE NATIONAL MEDICAL CENTER, DUARTE, CA, p. A40
CIVISTA HEALTH, LA PLATA, MD, p. A199
CLAIBORNE COUNTY HOSPITAL, TAZEWELL, TN, p. A400
CLAIBORNE COUNTY HOSPITAL, PORT GIBSON, MS, p. A242
CLARA BARTON HOSPITAL, HOISINGTON, KS, p. A162
CLARA MAASS HEALTH SYSTEM, BELLEVILLE, NJ, p. A274
CLAREMORE REGIONAL HOSPITAL, CLAREMORE, OK, p. A342
CLARENDON MEMORIAL HOSPITAL, MANNING, SC, p. A382
CLARIAN HEALTH PARTNERS, INDIANAPOLIS, IN, p. A141
CLARINDA REGIONAL HEALTH CENTER, CLARINDA, IA, p. A149
CLARION HOSPITAL, CLARION, PA, p. A357
CLARION PSYCHIATRIC CENTER, CLARION, PA, p. A358
CLARK FORK VALLEY HOSPITAL, PLAINS, MT, p. A259
CLARK MEMORIAL HOSPITAL, JEFFERSONVILLE, IN, p. A142
CLARK REGIONAL MEDICAL CENTER, WINCHESTER, KY, p. A179
CLARKE COUNTY HOSPITAL, OSCEOLA, IA, p. A155
CLARKS SUMMIT STATE HOSPITAL, CLARKS SUMMIT, PA, p. A358
CLAY COUNTY HOSPITAL, BRAZIL, IN, p. A138
CLAY COUNTY HOSPITAL, FLORA, IL, p. A126
CLAY COUNTY HOSPITAL, ASHLAND, AL, p. A11
CLAY COUNTY MEDICAL CENTER, WEST POINT, MS, p. A243
CLAY COUNTY MEDICAL CENTER, CLAY CENTER, KS, p. A160
CLAY COUNTY MEMORIAL HOSPITAL, HENRIETTA, TX, p. A415
CLEAR BROOK LODGE, SHICKSHINNY, PA, p. A372
CLEAR BROOK MANOR, WILKES-BARRE, PA, p. A374
CLEAR LAKE REGIONAL MEDICAL CENTER, WEBSTER, TX, p. A434
CLEARFIELD HOSPITAL, CLEARFIELD, PA, p. A358
CLEARWATER HEALTH SERVICES, BAGLEY, MN, p. A225
CLEARWATER VALLEY HOSPITAL AND CLINICS, OROFINO, ID, p. A117
CLEMENT J. ZABLOCKI VETERANS AFFAIRS MEDICAL CENTER, MILWAUKEE, WI, p. A471
CLEO WALLACE CENTERS HOSPITAL, WESTMINSTER, CO, p. A73
CLEVELAND AREA HOSPITAL, CLEVELAND, OK, p. A342
CLEVELAND CAMPUS, CLEVELAND, OHIO, p. A336
CLEVELAND CLINIC CHILDREN'S HOSPITAL FOR REHABILITATION, CLEVELAND, OH, p. A328
CLEVELAND CLINIC FOUNDATION, CLEVELAND, OH, p. A328
CLEVELAND CLINIC HOSPITAL, FORT LAUDERDALE, FL, p. A84
CLEVELAND COMMUNITY HOSPITAL, CLEVELAND, TN, p. A391
CLEVELAND REGIONAL MEDICAL CENTER, SHELBY, NC, p. A318
CLEVELAND REGIONAL MEDICAL CENTER, CLEVELAND, TX, p. A406
CLIFTON SPRINGS HOSPITAL AND CLINIC, CLIFTON SPRINGS, NY, p. A290
CLIFTON T. PERKINS HOSPITAL CENTER, JESSUP, MD, p. A199
CLIFTON-FINE HOSPITAL, STAR LAKE, NY, p. A305

CLINCH MEMORIAL HOSPITAL, HOMERVILLE, GA, p. A106
CLINCH VALLEY MEDICAL CENTER, RICHLANDS, VA, p. A448
CLINICA ESPANOLA, MAYAGUEZ, PR, p. A483
CLINICA SAN AGUSTIN, MANATI, PR, p. A482
CLINTON COUNTY HOSPITAL, ALBANY, KY, p. A170
CLINTON HOSPITAL, CLINTON, MA, p. A204
CLINTON MEMORIAL HOSPITAL, WILMINGTON, OH, p. A339
CLINTON MEMORIAL HOSPITAL, SAINT JOHNS, MI, p. A222
CLOQUET COMMUNITY MEMORIAL HOSPITAL, CLOQUET, MN, p. A226
CLOUD COUNTY HEALTH CENTER, CONCORDIA, KS, p. A160
COALINGA REGIONAL MEDICAL CENTER, COALINGA, CA, p. A39
COAST PLAZA DOCTORS HOSPITAL, NORWALK, CA, p. A53
COASTAL COMMUNITIES HOSPITAL, SANTA ANA, CA, p. A61
COBB MEMORIAL HOSPITAL, ROYSTON, GA, p. A109
COBRE VALLEY COMMUNITY HOSPITAL, GLOBE, AZ, p. A23
COCHRAN MEMORIAL HOSPITAL, MORTON, TX, p. A424
COFFEE MEDICAL CENTER, MANCHESTER, TN, p. A396
COFFEE REGIONAL MEDICAL CENTER, DOUGLAS, GA, p. A104
COFFEY COUNTY HOSPITAL, BURLINGTON, KS, p. A159
COFFEYVILLE REGIONAL MEDICAL CENTER, COFFEYVILLE, KS, p. A160
COLEMAN COUNTY MEDICAL CENTER, COLEMAN, TX, p. A407
COLER MEMORIAL HOSPITAL, NEW YORK, NY, p. A296
COLISEUM MEDICAL CENTERS, MACON, GA, p. A107
COLISEUM PSYCHIATRIC CENTER, MACON, GA, p. A107
COLLEGE HOSPITAL, CERRITOS, CA, p. A38
COLLEGE HOSPITAL COSTA MESA, COSTA MESA, CA, p. A39
COLLEGE STATION MEDICAL CENTER, COLLEGE STATION, TX, p. A407
COLLETON MEDICAL CENTER, WALTERBORO, SC, p. A384
COLLINGSWORTH GENERAL HOSPITAL, WELLINGTON, TX, p. A434
COLMERY-O'NEIL VETERANS AFFAIRS MEDICAL CENTER, TOPEKA, KANSAS, p. A168
COLONEL FLORENCE A. BLANCHFIELD ARMY COMMUNITY HOSPITAL, FORT CAMPBELL, KY, p. A172
COLORADO MENTAL HEALTH INSTITUTE AT FORT LOGAN, DENVER, CO, p. A69
COLORADO MENTAL HEALTH INSTITUTE AT PUEBLO, PUEBLO, CO, p. A72
COLORADO PLAINS MEDICAL CENTER, FORT MORGAN, CO, p. A70
COLORADO RIVER MEDICAL CENTER, NEEDLES, CA, p. A53
COLORADO-FAYETTE MEDICAL CENTER, WEIMAR, TX, p. A434
COLQUITT REGIONAL MEDICAL CENTER, MOULTRIE, GA, p. A108
COLUMBIA BASIN HOSPITAL, EPHRATA, WA, p. A453
COLUMBIA BEHAVIORAL CENTER, EL PASO, TX, p. A411
COLUMBIA GARDEN PARK HOSPITAL, GULFPORT, MS, p. A238
COLUMBIA HOSPITAL, WEST PALM BEACH, FL, p. A97
COLUMBIA HOSPITAL, MILWAUKEE, WI, p. A471
COLUMBIA HOSPITAL FOR WOMEN MEDICAL CENTER, WASHINGTON, DC, p. A79
COLUMBIA MEDICAL CENTER WEST, EL PASO, TX, p. A411
COLUMBIA MEMORIAL HOSPITAL, HUDSON, NY, p. A292
COLUMBIA MEMORIAL HOSPITAL, ASTORIA, OR, p. A350
COLUMBIA PRESBYTERIAN MEDICAL CENTER, NEW YORK, NEW YORK, p. A299
COLUMBIA REGIONAL HOSPITAL, COLUMBIA, MO, p. A245
COLUMBIA REGIONAL MEDICAL CENTER-SOUTH CAMPUS, AURORA, COLORADO, p. A68
COLUMBIA REHABILITATION HOSPITAL, EL PASO, TX, p. A411
COLUMBIA RIVER PARK HOSPITAL, HUNTINGTON, WV, p. A462
COLUMBIA-GREENE LONG TERM CARE, CATSKILL, NEW YORK, p. A292
COLUMBUS CAMPUS, COLUMBUS, OHIO, p. A331
COLUMBUS COMMUNITY HOSPITAL, COLUMBUS, OH, p. A330
COLUMBUS COMMUNITY HOSPITAL, COLUMBUS, WI, p. A467
COLUMBUS COMMUNITY HOSPITAL, COLUMBUS, NE, p. A262
COLUMBUS COMMUNITY HOSPITAL, COLUMBUS, TX, p. A407
COLUMBUS COUNTY HOSPITAL, WHITEVILLE, NC, p. A319
COLUMBUS HOSPITAL, NEWARK, NJ, p. A278
COLUMBUS HOSPITAL, CHICAGO, IL, p. A121
COLUMBUS REGIONAL HOSPITAL, COLUMBUS, IN, p. A138
COLUSA COMMUNITY HOSPITAL, COLUSA, CA, p. A39
COMANCHE COMMUNITY HOSPITAL, COMANCHE, TX, p. A407
COMANCHE COUNTY HOSPITAL, COLDWATER, KS, p. A160
COMANCHE COUNTY MEMORIAL HOSPITAL, LAWTON, OK, p. A344
COMMMUNITY HOSPITAL OF SAN BERNARDINO, SAN BERNARDINO, CA, p. A58
COMMUNITY GENERAL HEALTH CENTER, FORT FAIRFIELD, MAINE, p. A193
COMMUNITY GENERAL HOSPITAL OF SULLIVAN COUNTY, HARRIS, NY, p. A292
COMMUNITY GENERAL HOSPITAL OF THOMASVILLE, THOMASVILLE, NC, p. A319
COMMUNITY HEALTH CENTER, VISALIA, CALIFORNIA, p. A66

COMMUNITY HEALTH CENTER OF BRANCH COUNTY, COLDWATER, MI, p. A213
COMMUNITY HOSPITAL, SPRINGFIELD, OH, p. A337
COMMUNITY HOSPITAL, MUNSTER, IN, p. A144
COMMUNITY HOSPITAL, BATTLE CREEK, MICHIGAN, p. A212
COMMUNITY HOSPITAL, WATERVLIET, MI, p. A224
COMMUNITY HOSPITAL, TALLASSEE, AL, p. A18
COMMUNITY HOSPITAL, CANNON FALLS, MN, p. A226
COMMUNITY HOSPITAL, MCCOOK, NE, p. A264
COMMUNITY HOSPITAL, TORRINGTON, WY, p. A480
COMMUNITY HOSPITAL, GRAND JUNCTION, CO, p. A70
COMMUNITY HOSPITAL AND HEALTH CARE CENTER, SAINT PETER, MN, p. A233
COMMUNITY HOSPITAL ASSOCIATION, FAIRFAX, MO, p. A246
COMMUNITY HOSPITAL AT DOBBS FERRY, DOBBS FERRY, NY, p. A291
COMMUNITY HOSPITAL EAST, INDIANAPOLIS, INDIANA, p. A141
COMMUNITY HOSPITAL IN NELSON COUNTY, MCVILLE, ND, p. A323
COMMUNITY HOSPITAL MEDICAL CENTER, PHOENIX, AZ, p. A24
COMMUNITY HOSPITAL NORTH, INDIANAPOLIS, INDIANA, p. A141
COMMUNITY HOSPITAL OF ANACONDA, ANACONDA, MT, p. A256
COMMUNITY HOSPITAL OF ANDERSON AND MADISON COUNTY, ANDERSON, INDIANA, p. A141
COMMUNITY HOSPITAL OF BREMEN, BREMEN, IN, p. A138
COMMUNITY HOSPITAL OF GARDENA, GARDENA, CA, p. A42
COMMUNITY HOSPITAL OF HUNTINGTON PARK, HUNTINGTON PARK, CA, p. A44
COMMUNITY HOSPITAL OF LANCASTER, LANCASTER, PA, p. A362
COMMUNITY HOSPITAL OF LOS GATOS, LOS GATOS, CA, p. A50
COMMUNITY HOSPITAL OF NEW PORT RICHEY, NEW PORT RICHEY, FL, p. A91
COMMUNITY HOSPITAL OF NOBLE COUNTY, KENDALLVILLE, IN, p. A142
COMMUNITY HOSPITAL OF OTTAWA, OTTAWA, IL, p. A132
COMMUNITY HOSPITAL OF THE MONTEREY PENINSULA, MONTEREY, CA, p. A52
COMMUNITY HOSPITAL ONAGA, ONAGA, KS, p. A166
COMMUNITY HOSPITAL SOUTH, INDIANAPOLIS, INDIANA, p. A141
COMMUNITY HOSPITAL-LAKEVIEW, EUFAULA, OK, p. A343
COMMUNITY HOSPITALS INDIANAPOLIS, INDIANAPOLIS, IN, p. A141
COMMUNITY HOSPITALS OF WILLIAMS COUNTY, BRYAN, OH, p. A326
COMMUNITY MEDICAL CENTER, TOMS RIVER, NJ, p. A280
COMMUNITY MEDICAL CENTER, SCRANTON, PA, p. A371
COMMUNITY MEDICAL CENTER, FALLS CITY, NE, p. A262
COMMUNITY MEDICAL CENTER, MISSOULA, MT, p. A259
COMMUNITY MEDICAL CENTER AT WESTERN ILLINOIS, MONMOUTH, IL, p. A130
COMMUNITY MEDICAL CENTER SHERMAN, SHERMAN, TX, p. A430
COMMUNITY MEDICAL CENTER-CLOVIS, CLOVIS, CA, p. A38
COMMUNITY MEDICAL CENTER-FRESNO, FRESNO, CA, p. A42
COMMUNITY MEMORIAL HEALTHCARE, MARYSVILLE, KS, p. A165
COMMUNITY MEMORIAL HEALTHCENTER, SOUTH HILL, VA, p. A450
COMMUNITY MEMORIAL HOSPITAL, HAMILTON, NY, p. A292
COMMUNITY MEMORIAL HOSPITAL, HICKSVILLE, OH, p. A333
COMMUNITY MEMORIAL HOSPITAL, STAUNTON, IL, p. A135
COMMUNITY MEMORIAL HOSPITAL, CHEBOYGAN, MI, p. A213
COMMUNITY MEMORIAL HOSPITAL, MENOMONEE FALLS, WI, p. A471
COMMUNITY MEMORIAL HOSPITAL, OCONTO FALLS, WI, p. A473
COMMUNITY MEMORIAL HOSPITAL, CLARION, IA, p. A149
COMMUNITY MEMORIAL HOSPITAL, SUMNER, IA, p. A157
COMMUNITY MEMORIAL HOSPITAL, TURTLE LAKE, ND, p. A324
COMMUNITY MEMORIAL HOSPITAL, REDFIELD, SD, p. A387
COMMUNITY MEMORIAL HOSPITAL, SYRACUSE, NE, p. A267
COMMUNITY MEMORIAL HOSPITAL OF SAN BUENAVENTURA, VENTURA, CA, p. A66
COMMUNITY MEMORIAL HOSPITAL/AVERA HEALTH, BURKE, SD, p. A385
COMMUNITY-GENERAL HOSPITAL OF GREATER SYRACUSE, SYRACUSE, NY, p. A305
COMPTON HEIGHTS HOSPITAL, SAINT LOUIS, MO, p. A252
CONCHO COUNTY HOSPITAL, EDEN, TX, p. A411
CONCORD HOSPITAL, CONCORD, NH, p. A271
CONCOURSE DIVISION, NEW YORK, NEW YORK, p. A295
CONDELL MEDICAL CENTER, LIBERTYVILLE, IL, p. A129
CONEJOS COUNTY HOSPITAL, LA JARA, CO, p. A71

Index of Hospitals / Conemaugh Memorial Medical Center

CONEMAUGH MEMORIAL MEDICAL CENTER, JOHNSTOWN, PA, p. A362
CONEY ISLAND HOSPITAL, NEW YORK, NY, p. A296
CONIFER PARK, GLENVILLE, NY, p. A292
CONNECTICUT CHILDREN'S MEDICAL CENTER, HARTFORD, CT, p. A74
CONNECTICUT DEPARTMENT OF CORRECTION'S HOSPITAL, SOMERS, CT, p. A77
CONNECTICUT MENTAL HEALTH CENTER, NEW HAVEN, CT, p. A75
CONNECTICUT VALLEY HOSPITAL, MIDDLETOWN, CT, p. A75
CONROE REGIONAL MEDICAL CENTER, CONROE, TX, p. A407
CONTINUOUS CARE CENTER OF TULSA, TULSA, OK, p. A348
CONTRA COSTA REGIONAL MEDICAL CENTER, MARTINEZ, CA, p. A51
CONWAY HOSPITAL, CONWAY, SC, p. A380
CONWAY REGIONAL MEDICAL CENTER, CONWAY, AR, p. A29
COOK CHILDREN'S MEDICAL CENTER, FORT WORTH, TX, p. A412
COOK COUNTY HOSPITAL, CHICAGO, IL, p. A121
COOK COUNTY NORTH SHORE HOSPITAL, GRAND MARAIS, MN, p. A228
COOK HOSPITAL AND CONVALESCENT NURSING CARE UNIT, COOK, MN, p. A227
COOKEVILLE REGIONAL MEDICAL CENTER, COOKEVILLE, TN, p. A391
COOLEY DICKINSON HOSPITAL, NORTHAMPTON, MA, p. A207
COON MEMORIAL HOSPITAL AND HOME, DALHART, TX, p. A408
COOPER COUNTY MEMORIAL HOSPITAL, BOONVILLE, MO, p. A244
COOPER GREEN HOSPITAL, BIRMINGHAM, AL, p. A12
COOSA VALLEY BAPTIST MEDICAL CENTER, SYLACAUGA, AL, p. A18
COPLEY HOSPITAL, MORRISVILLE, VT, p. A440
COPPER BASIN MEDICAL CENTER, COPPERHILL, TN, p. A391
COPPER HILLS YOUTH CENTER, WEST JORDAN, UT, p. A439
COPPER QUEEN COMMUNITY HOSPITAL, BISBEE, AZ, p. A22
COQUILLE VALLEY HOSPITAL, COQUILLE, OR, p. A350
CORAL GABLES HOSPITAL, CORAL GABLES, FL, p. A83
CORAL SPRINGS MEDICAL CENTER, CORAL SPRINGS, FL, p. A83
CORCORAN DISTRICT HOSPITAL, CORCORAN, CA, p. A39
CORDELL MEMORIAL HOSPITAL, CORDELL, OK, p. A342
CORDOVA COMMUNITY MEDICAL CENTER, CORDOVA, AK, p. A20
CORNERSTONE OF MEDICAL ARTS CENTER HOSPITAL, NEW YORK, NY, p. A296
CORNERSTONE REGIONAL HOSPITAL, EDINBURG, TX, p. A411
CORNING HOSPITAL, CORNING, NY, p. A290
CORNWALL HOSPITAL, CORNWALL, NY, p. A290
CORONA REGIONAL MEDICAL CENTER, CORONA, CA, p. A39
CORONA REGIONAL MEDICAL CENTER–REHABILITATION, CORONA, CALIFORNIA, p. A39
CORPUS CHRISTI MEDICAL CENTER, CORPUS CHRISTI, TX, p. A407
CORPUS CHRISTI MEDICAL CENTER BAY AREA, CORPUS CHRISTI, TX, p. A407
CORRY MEMORIAL HOSPITAL, CORRY, PA, p. A358
CORTLAND MEMORIAL HOSPITAL, CORTLAND, NY, p. A290
CORYELL MEMORIAL HOSPITAL, GATESVILLE, TX, p. A414
COSHOCTON COUNTY MEMORIAL HOSPITAL, COSHOCTON, OH, p. A330
COTEAU DES PRAIRIES HOSPITAL, SISSETON, SD, p. A388
COTTAGE HOSPITAL, WOODSVILLE, NH, p. A273
COTTONWOOD HOSPITAL MEDICAL CENTER, MURRAY, UT, p. A437
COULEE COMMUNITY HOSPITAL, GRAND COULEE, WA, p. A454
COUNCIL COMMUNITY HOSPITAL AND NURSING HOME, COUNCIL, ID, p. A116
COVE FORGE BEHAVIORAL HEALTH SYSTEM, WILLIAMSBURG, PA, p. A374
COVENANT BEHAVIORAL HEALTH SYSTEM, SAN ANTONIO, TX, p. A428
COVENANT CHILDREN'S HOSPITAL, LUBBOCK, TX, p. A422
COVENANT HEALTHCARE, SAGINAW, MI, p. A221
COVENANT HOSPITAL PLAINVIEW, PLAINVIEW, TX, p. A426
COVENANT HOSPITAL–LEVELLAND, LEVELLAND, TX, p. A421
COVENANT MEDICAL CENTER, WATERLOO, IA, p. A157
COVENANT MEDICAL CENTER, LUBBOCK, TX, p. A422
COVENANT MEDICAL CENTER–COOPER, SAGINAW, MICHIGAN, p. A221
COVENANT MEDICAL CENTER–HARRISON, SAGINAW, MICHIGAN, p. A221
COVENANT MEDICAL CENTER–LAKESIDE, LUBBOCK, TX, p. A422
COVINGTON COUNTY HOSPITAL, COLLINS, MS, p. A237
COX MONETT HOSPITAL, MONETT, MO, p. A250
COZAD COMMUNITY HOSPITAL, COZAD, NE, p. A262
COZBY–GERMANY HOSPITAL, GRAND SALINE, TX, p. A414

CRAIG GENERAL HOSPITAL, VINITA, OK, p. A349
CRAIG HOSPITAL, ENGLEWOOD, CO, p. A70
CRAIG HOUSE CENTER, BEACON, NY, p. A288
CRANE MEMORIAL HOSPITAL, CRANE, TX, p. A408
CRAVEN REGIONAL MEDICAL AUTHORITY, NEW BERN, NC, p. A316
CRAWFORD COUNTY HOSPITAL DISTRICT ONE, GIRARD, KS, p. A161
CRAWFORD COUNTY MEMORIAL HOSPITAL, DENISON, IA, p. A150
CRAWFORD LONG HOSPITAL OF EMORY UNIVERSITY, ATLANTA, GA, p. A100
CRAWFORD MEMORIAL HOSPITAL, ROBINSON, IL, p. A133
CRAWFORD MEMORIAL HOSPITAL, VAN BUREN, AR, p. A34
CRAWLEY MEMORIAL HOSPITAL, BOILING SPRINGS, NC, p. A309
CREEDMOOR PSYCHIATRIC CENTER, NEW YORK, NY, p. A296
CREEK NATION COMMUNITY HOSPITAL, OKEMAH, OK, p. A345
CREIGHTON AREA HEALTH SERVICES, CREIGHTON, NE, p. A262
CRENSHAW BAPTIST HOSPITAL, LUVERNE, AL, p. A16
CRESTLINE HOSPITAL, CRESTLINE, OHIO, p. A334
CRESTWOOD MEDICAL CENTER, HUNTSVILLE, AL, p. A15
CRETE MUNICIPAL HOSPITAL, CRETE, NE, p. A262
CRISP REGIONAL HOSPITAL, CORDELE, GA, p. A103
CRITTENDEN COUNTY HOSPITAL, MARION, KY, p. A176
CRITTENDEN MEMORIAL HOSPITAL, WEST MEMPHIS, AR, p. A34
CRITTENTON, KANSAS CITY, MO, p. A248
CRITTENTON HOSPITAL, ROCHESTER, MI, p. A221
CROCKETT HOSPITAL, LAWRENCEBURG, TN, p. A395
CROOK COUNTY MEDICAL SERVICES DISTRICT, SUNDANCE, WY, p. A479
CROSBY MEMORIAL HOSPITAL, PICAYUNE, MS, p. A241
CROSBYTON CLINIC HOSPITAL, CROSBYTON, TX, p. A408
CROSSBRIDGE COMMUNITY HOSPITAL, WYNNE, AR, p. A34
CROSSROADS COMMUNITY HOSPITAL, MOUNT VERNON, IL, p. A131
CROTCHED MOUNTAIN REHABILITATION CENTER, GREENFIELD, NH, p. A271
CROUSE HOSPITAL, SYRACUSE, NY, p. A305
CROWNSVILLE HOSPITAL CENTER, CROWNSVILLE, MD, p. A197
CROZER–CHESTER MEDICAL CENTER, UPLAND, PA, p. A373
CUBA MEMORIAL HOSPITAL, CUBA, NY, p. A290
CUERO COMMUNITY HOSPITAL, CUERO, TX, p. A408
CULBERSON HOSPITAL DISTRICT, VAN HORN, TX, p. A433
CULLMAN REGIONAL MEDICAL CENTER, CULLMAN, AL, p. A13
CULPEPER REGIONAL HOSPITAL, CULPEPER, VA, p. A443
CUMBERLAND COUNTY HOSPITAL, BURKESVILLE, KY, p. A170
CUMBERLAND HALL HOSPITAL, HOPKINSVILLE, KY, p. A173
CUMBERLAND MEDICAL CENTER, CROSSVILLE, TN, p. A392
CUMBERLAND MEMORIAL HOSPITAL, CUMBERLAND, WI, p. A467
CUMBERLAND RIVER HOSPITAL, CELINA, TN, p. A390
CUMBERLAND, A BROWN SCHOOLS HOSPITAL FOR CHILDREN AND ADOLESCENTS, NEW KENT, VA, p. A446
CURRY GENERAL HOSPITAL, GOLD BEACH, OR, p. A351
CUSHING MEMORIAL HOSPITAL, LEAVENWORTH, KS, p. A164
CUSHING REGIONAL HOSPITAL, CUSHING, OK, p. A342
CUSTER COMMUNITY HOSPITAL, CUSTER, SD, p. A385
CUYAHOGA FALLS GENERAL HOSPITAL, CUYAHOGA FALLS, OH, p. A330
CUYUNA REGIONAL MEDICAL CENTER, CROSBY, MN, p. A227
CYPRESS CREEK HOSPITAL, HOUSTON, TX, p. A416
CYPRESS FAIRBANKS MEDICAL CENTER, HOUSTON, TX, p. A416

D

D. M. COGDELL MEMORIAL HOSPITAL, SNYDER, TX, p. A431
D. W. MCMILLAN MEMORIAL HOSPITAL, BREWTON, AL, p. A13
DAKOTA HEARTLAND HEALTH SYSTEM, FARGO, ND, p. A322
DALE MEDICAL CENTER, OZARK, AL, p. A17
DALLAS COUNTY HOSPITAL, PERRY, IA, p. A155
DALLAS COUNTY HOSPITAL, FORDYCE, AR, p. A29
DALLAS SOUTHWEST MEDICAL CENTER, DALLAS, TX, p. A408
DALLAS–FORT WORTH MEDICAL CENTER, GRAND PRAIRIE, TX, p. A414
DAMERON HOSPITAL, STOCKTON, CA, p. A64
DANA–FARBER CANCER INSTITUTE, BOSTON, MA, p. A202
DANBURY HOSPITAL, DANBURY, CT, p. A74
DANIEL FREEMAN MARINA HOSPITAL, VENICE, CA, p. A66
DANIEL FREEMAN MEMORIAL HOSPITAL, INGLEWOOD, CA, p. A44
DANIELS MEMORIAL HOSPITAL, SCOBEY, MT, p. A259
DANVILLE REGIONAL MEDICAL CENTER, DANVILLE, VA, p. A443
DANVILLE STATE HOSPITAL, DANVILLE, PA, p. A359

DARDANELLE HOSPITAL, DARDANELLE, AR, p. A29
DARNALL ARMY COMMUNITY HOSPITAL, FORT HOOD, TX, p. A412
DAUTERIVE HOSPITAL, NEW IBERIA, LA, p. A186
DAVID GRANT MEDICAL CENTER, TRAVIS AFB, CA, p. A65
DAVIE COUNTY HOSPITAL, MOCKSVILLE, NC, p. A315
DAVIESS COUNTY HOSPITAL, WASHINGTON, IN, p. A147
DAVIS COUNTY HOSPITAL, BLOOMFIELD, IA, p. A148
DAVIS HOSPITAL AND MEDICAL CENTER, LAYTON, UT, p. A436
DAVIS MEDICAL CENTER, STATESVILLE, NC, p. A318
DAVIS MEMORIAL HOSPITAL, ELKINS, WV, p. A461
DAY KIMBALL HOSPITAL, PUTNAM, CT, p. A76
DAYTON CAMPUS, DAYTON, OHIO, p. A331
DAYTON GENERAL HOSPITAL, DAYTON, WA, p. A453
DCH REGIONAL MEDICAL CENTER, TUSCALOOSA, AL, p. A19
DE GRAFF MEMORIAL HOSPITAL, NORTH TONAWANDA, NY, p. A301
DE JARNETTE CENTER, STAUNTON, VA, p. A450
DE LEON HOSPITAL, DE LEON, TX, p. A410
DE PAUL HOSPITAL, CHEYENNE, WYOMING, p. A478
DE POO HOSPITAL, KEY WEST, FLORIDA, p. A87
DE QUEEN REGIONAL MEDICAL CENTER, DE QUEEN, AR, p. A29
DE SMET MEMORIAL HOSPITAL, DE SMET, SD, p. A385
DE SOTO REGIONAL HEALTH SYSTEM, MANSFIELD, LA, p. A185
DEACONESS BILLINGS CLINIC, BILLINGS, MT, p. A256
DEACONESS HOSPITAL, CINCINNATI, OH, p. A327
DEACONESS HOSPITAL, EVANSVILLE, IN, p. A139
DEACONESS HOSPITAL, OKLAHOMA CITY, OK, p. A345
DEACONESS HOSPITAL OF CLEVELAND, CLEVELAND, OH, p. A328
DEACONESS MEDICAL CENTER–SPOKANE, SPOKANE, WA, p. A457
DEACONESS ST. JOSEPH'S HOSPITAL, HUNTINGBURG, IN, p. A141
DEACONESS WALTHAM HOSPITAL, WALTHAM, MA, p. A209
DEACONESS–GLOVER HOSPITAL CORPORATION, NEEDHAM, MA, p. A207
DEACONESS–NASHOBA HOSPITAL, AYER, MA, p. A201
DEARBORN COUNTY HOSPITAL, LAWRENCEBURG, IN, p. A143
DEATON SPECIALTY HOSPITAL AND HOME, BALTIMORE, MD, p. A195
DEBACA GENERAL HOSPITAL, FORT SUMNER, NM, p. A284
DEBORAH HEART AND LUNG CENTER, BROWNS MILLS, NJ, p. A274
DECATUR COMMUNITY HOSPITAL, DECATUR, TX, p. A410
DECATUR COUNTY GENERAL HOSPITAL, PARSONS, TN, p. A399
DECATUR COUNTY HOSPITAL, LEON, IA, p. A154
DECATUR COUNTY HOSPITAL AND CEDAR LIVING CENTER, OBERLIN, KS, p. A165
DECATUR COUNTY MEMORIAL HOSPITAL, GREENSBURG, IN, p. A140
DECATUR GENERAL HOSPITAL, DECATUR, AL, p. A13
DECATUR GENERAL HOSPITAL, DECATUR, ALABAMA, p. A13
DECATUR GENERAL HOSPITAL–WEST, DECATUR, ALABAMA, p. A13
DECATUR HOSPITAL, DECATUR, GA, p. A103
DECATUR MEMORIAL HOSPITAL, DECATUR, IL, p. A124
DECKERVILLE COMMUNITY HOSPITAL, DECKERVILLE, MI, p. A213
DEER PARK HOSPITAL, DEER PARK, WA, p. A453
DEER RIVER HEALTHCARE CENTER, DEER RIVER, MN, p. A227
DEER'S HEAD CENTER, SALISBURY, MD, p. A200
DEERING HOSPITAL, MIAMI, FL, p. A89
DEFIANCE HOSPITAL, DEFIANCE, OH, p. A331
DEKALB BAPTIST MEDICAL CENTER, FORT PAYNE, AL, p. A14
DEKALB MEDICAL CENTER, DECATUR, GA, p. A103
DEKALB MEMORIAL HOSPITAL, AUBURN, IN, p. A137
DEL AMO HOSPITAL, TORRANCE, CA, p. A64
DEL E. WEBB MEMORIAL HOSPITAL, SUN CITY WEST, AZ, p. A26
DEL SOL MEDICAL CENTER, EL PASO, TX, p. A411
DELANO REGIONAL MEDICAL CENTER, DELANO, CA, p. A40
DELAWARE COUNTY MEMORIAL HOSPITAL, DREXEL HILL, PA, p. A359
DELAWARE PSYCHIATRIC CENTER, NEW CASTLE, DE, p. A78
DELAWARE VALLEY HOSPITAL, WALTON, NY, p. A307
DELLS AREA HEALTH CENTER, DELL RAPIDS, SD, p. A385
DELNOR–COMMUNITY HOSPITAL, GENEVA, IL, p. A126
DELRAY MEDICAL CENTER, DELRAY BEACH, FL, p. A83
DELTA COMMUNITY MEDICAL CENTER, DELTA, UT, p. A436
DELTA COUNTY MEMORIAL HOSPITAL, DELTA, CO, p. A69
DELTA MEDICAL CENTER, MEMPHIS, TN, p. A396
DELTA MEMORIAL HOSPITAL, DUMAS, AR, p. A29
DELTA REGIONAL MEDICAL CENTER, GREENVILLE, MS, p. A238
DENTON COMMUNITY HOSPITAL, DENTON, TX, p. A410
DENTON REGIONAL MEDICAL CENTER, DENTON, TX, p. A410
DENVER HEALTH MEDICAL CENTER, DENVER, CO, p. A69

DEPAUL HEALTH CENTER, SAINT LOUIS, MO, p. A253
DEPAUL/TULANE BEHAVIORAL HEALTH CENTER, NEW ORLEANS, LOUISIANA, p. A187
DEQUINCY MEMORIAL HOSPITAL, DEQUINCY, LA, p. A182
DES MOINES DIVISION, DES MOINES, IOWA, p. A151
DES MOINES GENERAL HOSPITAL, DES MOINES, IA, p. A150
DES PERES HOSPITAL, SAINT LOUIS, MO, p. A253
DESERT HILLS HOSPITAL, ALBUQUERQUE, NM, p. A283
DESERT REGIONAL MEDICAL CENTER, PALM SPRINGS, CA, p. A54
DESERT SAMARITAN MEDICAL CENTER, MESA, AZ, p. A23
DESERT SPRINGS HOSPITAL, LAS VEGAS, NV, p. A268
DESERT SPRINGS MEDICAL CENTER, MIDLAND, TX, p. A423
DESERT VALLEY HOSPITAL, VICTORVILLE, CA, p. A66
DESOTO MEMORIAL HOSPITAL, ARCADIA, FL, p. A81
DETAR HOSPITAL, VICTORIA, TX, p. A433
DETROIT RECEIVING HOSPITAL AND UNIVERSITY HEALTH CENTER, DETROIT, MI, p. A213
DETTMER HOSPITAL, TROY, OHIO, p. A338
DEUEL COUNTY MEMORIAL HOSPITAL, CLEAR LAKE, SD, p. A385
DEVEREUX GEORGIA TREATMENT NETWORK, KENNESAW, GA, p. A106
DEVEREUX HOSPITAL AND CHILDREN'S CENTER OF FLORIDA, MELBOURNE, FL, p. A89
DEVEREUX MAPLETON PSYCHIATRIC INSTITUTE-MAPLETON CENTER, MALVERN, PA, p. A363
DEVEREUX TEXAS TREATMENT NETWORK, LEAGUE CITY, TX, p. A421
DEWITT ARMY COMMUNITY HOSPITAL, FORT BELVOIR, VA, p. A444
DEWITT CITY HOSPITAL, DE WITT, AR, p. A29
DEWITT COMMUNITY HOSPITAL, DE WITT, IA, p. A150
DEXTER MEMORIAL HOSPITAL, DEXTER, MO, p. A246
DIAGNOSTIC CENTER HOSPITAL, HOUSTON, TX, p. A416
DICKENSON COUNTY MEDICAL CENTER, CLINTWOOD, VA, p. A443
DICKINSON COUNTY HEALTHCARE SYSTEM, IRON MOUNTAIN, MI, p. A217
DICKINSON COUNTY MEMORIAL HOSPITAL, SPIRIT LAKE, IA, p. A157
DIMMICK CAMPUS, GRANTS PASS, OREGON, p. A351
DIMMIT COUNTY MEMORIAL HOSPITAL, CARRIZO SPRINGS, TX, p. A406
DISTRICT MEMORIAL HOSPITAL, ANDREWS, NC, p. A309
DISTRICT OF COLUMBIA GENERAL HOSPITAL, WASHINGTON, DC, p. A79
DISTRICT ONE HOSPITAL, FARIBAULT, MN, p. A227
DIVINE PROVIDENCE HEALTH CENTER/AVERA HEALTH, IVANHOE, MN, p. A229
DIVINE PROVIDENCE HOSPITAL, WILLIAMSPORT, PENNSYLVANIA, p. A375
DIVINE SAVIOR HEALTHCARE, PORTAGE, WI, p. A474
DIVISION OF ADOLESCENT MEDICINE, CINCINNATI CENTER FOR DEVELOPMENTAL DISORDERS, AND CONVALESCENT HOSPITAL FOR CHILDREN, CHILDREN'S HOSPITAL, CINCINNATI, OHIO, p. A327
DIXIE REGIONAL MEDICAL CENTER, SAINT GEORGE, UT, p. A438
DOCTOR ROBERT L. YEAGER HEALTH CENTER, POMONA, NY, p. A302
DOCTOR'S MEMORIAL HOSPITAL, PERRY, FL, p. A93
DOCTORS CENTER, MANATI, PR, p. A483
DOCTORS COMMUNITY HOSPITAL, LANHAM, MD, p. A199
DOCTORS HOSPITAL, SAN JUAN, PR, p. A483
DOCTORS HOSPITAL, AUGUSTA, GA, p. A100
DOCTORS HOSPITAL, COLUMBUS, GA, p. A102
DOCTORS HOSPITAL, COLUMBUS, OH, p. A330
DOCTORS HOSPITAL, SPRINGFIELD, IL, p. A135
DOCTORS HOSPITAL, WENTZVILLE, MO, p. A255
DOCTORS HOSPITAL, TULSA, OK, p. A348
DOCTORS HOSPITAL, GROVES, TX, p. A415
DOCTORS HOSPITAL OF DALLAS, DALLAS, TX, p. A409
DOCTORS HOSPITAL OF JACKSON, JACKSON, MI, p. A217
DOCTORS HOSPITAL OF JEFFERSON, METAIRIE, LA, p. A185
DOCTORS HOSPITAL OF LAREDO, LAREDO, TX, p. A421
DOCTORS HOSPITAL OF MANTECA, MANTECA, CA, p. A51
DOCTORS HOSPITAL OF NELSONVILLE, NELSONVILLE, OH, p. A335
DOCTORS HOSPITAL OF SARASOTA, SARASOTA, FL, p. A95
DOCTORS HOSPITAL OF SPRINGFIELD, SPRINGFIELD, MO, p. A254
DOCTORS HOSPITAL OF STARK COUNTY, MASSILLON, OH, p. A334
DOCTORS HOSPITAL OF WEST COVINA, WEST COVINA, CA, p. A67
DOCTORS HOSPITAL PARKWAY, HOUSTON, TX, p. A416
DOCTORS HOSPITAL WEST, COLUMBUS, OHIO, p. A330
DOCTORS HOSPITAL-TIDWELL, HOUSTON, TX, p. A416
DOCTORS MEDICAL CENTER, MODESTO, CA, p. A51

DOCTORS MEDICAL CENTER-PINOLE CAMPUS, PINOLE, CA, p. A55
DOCTORS MEDICAL CENTER-SAN PABLO CAMPUS, SAN PABLO, CA, p. A61
DOCTORS MEMORIAL HOSPITAL, BONIFAY, FL, p. A81
DOCTORS MEMORIAL HOSPITAL, TYLER, TX, p. A433
DOCTORS REGIONAL MEDICAL CENTER, POPLAR BLUFF, MO, p. A251
DOCTORS' HOSPITAL OF OPELOUSAS, OPELOUSAS, LA, p. A187
DOCTORS' HOSPITAL OF SHREVEPORT, SHREVEPORT, LA, p. A188
DOCTORS' HOSPITAL OF STATEN ISLAND, NEW YORK, NY, p. A296
DODGE COUNTY HOSPITAL, EASTMAN, GA, p. A104
DOERNBECHER CHILDREN'S HOSPITAL, PORTLAND, OREGON, p. A353
DOLLY VINSANT MEMORIAL HOSPITAL, SAN BENITO, TX, p. A430
DOMINICAN HOSPITAL, SANTA CRUZ, CA, p. A62
DOMINION HOSPITAL, FALLS CHURCH, VA, p. A443
DONALSONVILLE HOSPITAL, DONALSONVILLE, GA, p. A104
DOOLY MEDICAL CENTER, VIENNA, GA, p. A111
DOOR COUNTY MEMORIAL HOSPITAL, STURGEON BAY, WI, p. A476
DORCHESTER GENERAL HOSPITAL, CAMBRIDGE, MD, p. A197
DORMINY MEDICAL CENTER, FITZGERALD, GA, p. A105
DOROTHEA DIX HOSPITAL, RALEIGH, NC, p. A316
DOS PALOS MEMORIAL HOSPITAL, DOS PALOS, CA, p. A40
DOUGLAS COUNTY HOSPITAL, ALEXANDRIA, MN, p. A225
DOUGLAS COUNTY HOSPITAL, OMAHA, NE, p. A265
DOUGLAS COUNTY MEMORIAL HOSPITAL, ARMOUR, SD, p. A385
DOWN EAST COMMUNITY HOSPITAL, MACHIAS, ME, p. A193
DOWNEY COMMUNITY HOSPITAL, DOWNEY, CALIFORNIA, p. A40
DOWNEY REGIONAL MEDICAL CENTER, DOWNEY, CA, p. A40
DOWNTOWN CAMPUS, NEW YORK, NEW YORK, p. A296
DOYLESTOWN HOSPITAL, DOYLESTOWN, PA, p. A359
DR. CHARLES DAVANT REHABILITATION AND EXTENDED CARE CENTER, p. A309
DR. DAN C. TRIGG MEMORIAL HOSPITAL, TUCUMCARI, NM, p. A286
DR. GUBERN'S HOSPITAL, FAJARDO, PUERTO RICO, p. A482
DR. JOHN WARNER HOSPITAL, CLINTON, IL, p. A124
DR. PILA'S HOSPITAL, PONCE, PR, p. A483
DR. RAMON E. BETANCES HOSPITAL-MAYAGUEZ MEDICAL CENTER BRANCH, MAYAGUEZ, PR, p. A483
DRAKE CENTER, CINCINNATI, OH, p. A327
DREW MEMORIAL HOSPITAL, MONTICELLO, AR, p. A32
DRISCOLL CHILDREN'S HOSPITAL, CORPUS CHRISTI, TX, p. A407
DRUMRIGHT MEMORIAL HOSPITAL, DRUMRIGHT, OK, p. A342
DUANE L. WATERS HOSPITAL, JACKSON, MI, p. A217
DUBOIS REGIONAL MEDICAL CENTER, DU BOIS, PA, p. A359
DUBUIS HOSPITAL FOR CONTINUING CARE, LAKE CHARLES, LA, p. A184
DUKE UNIVERSITY HOSPITAL, DURHAM, NORTH CAROLINA, p. A312
DUKE UNIVERSITY MEDICAL CENTER, DURHAM, NC, p. A312
DUKES MEMORIAL HOSPITAL, PERU, IN, p. A145
DUNCAN REGIONAL HOSPITAL, DUNCAN, OK, p. A342
DUNDY COUNTY HOSPITAL, BENKELMAN, NE, p. A261
DUNLAP MEMORIAL HOSPITAL, ORRVILLE, OH, p. A336
DUNN MEMORIAL HOSPITAL, BEDFORD, IN, p. A137
DUPLIN GENERAL HOSPITAL, KENANSVILLE, NC, p. A314
DURHAM REGIONAL HOSPITAL, DURHAM, NC, p. A312
DWIGHT D. EISENHOWER VETERANS AFFAIRS MEDICAL CENTER, LEAVENWORTH, KANSAS, p. A168
DWIGHT DAVID EISENHOWER ARMY MEDICAL CENTER, FORT GORDON, GA, p. A105

E

E. A. CONWAY MEDICAL CENTER, MONROE, LA, p. A185
E. J. NOBLE HOSPITAL SAMARITAN, ALEXANDRIA BAY, NY, p. A287
EAGLE RIVER MEMORIAL HOSPITAL, EAGLE RIVER, WI, p. A468
EAGLEVILLE HOSPITAL, EAGLEVILLE, PA, p. A359
EARL K. LONG MEDICAL CENTER, BATON ROUGE, LA, p. A180
EARLY MEMORIAL HOSPITAL, BLAKELY, GA, p. A101
EAST ADAMS RURAL HOSPITAL, RITZVILLE, WA, p. A456
EAST ALABAMA MEDICAL CENTER, OPELIKA, AL, p. A17
EAST CAMPUS, MERIDEN, CONNECTICUT, p. A75
EAST CAMPUS, NORFOLK, NEBRASKA, p. A264
EAST CARROLL PARISH HOSPITAL, LAKE PROVIDENCE, LA, p. A184

EAST COOPER REGIONAL MEDICAL CENTER, MOUNT PLEASANT, SC, p. A382
EAST HOUSTON REGIONAL MEDICAL CENTER, HOUSTON, TX, p. A416
EAST JEFFERSON GENERAL HOSPITAL, METAIRIE, LA, p. A185
EAST LIVERPOOL CITY HOSPITAL, EAST LIVERPOOL, OH, p. A331
EAST LOS ANGELES DOCTORS HOSPITAL, LOS ANGELES, CA, p. A47
EAST LOUISIANA STATE HOSPITAL, JACKSON, LA, p. A183
EAST MISSISSIPPI STATE HOSPITAL, MERIDIAN, MS, p. A240
EAST MORGAN COUNTY HOSPITAL, BRUSH, CO, p. A68
EAST OHIO REGIONAL HOSPITAL, MARTINS FERRY, OH, p. A334
EAST ORANGE DIVISION, EAST ORANGE, NEW JERSEY, p. A275
EAST ORANGE FACILITY, WEST ORANGE FACILITY, SADDLE BROOK FACILITY AND WELKIND FACILITY, p. A281
EAST ORANGE GENERAL HOSPITAL, EAST ORANGE, NJ, p. A275
EAST PASCO MEDICAL CENTER, ZEPHYRHILLS, FL, p. A98
EAST POINTE HOSPITAL, LEHIGH ACRES, FL, p. A88
EAST RIDGE HOSPITAL, EAST RIDGE, TENNESSEE, p. A391
EAST TENNESSEE CHILDREN'S HOSPITAL, KNOXVILLE, TN, p. A394
EAST TEXAS MEDICAL CENTER ATHENS, ATHENS, TX, p. A402
EAST TEXAS MEDICAL CENTER BEHAVIORAL HEALTH CENTER, TYLER, TEXAS, p. A433
EAST TEXAS MEDICAL CENTER CARTHAGE, CARTHAGE, TX, p. A406
EAST TEXAS MEDICAL CENTER CROCKETT, CROCKETT, TX, p. A408
EAST TEXAS MEDICAL CENTER FAIRFIELD, FAIRFIELD, TX, p. A412
EAST TEXAS MEDICAL CENTER JACKSONVILLE, JACKSONVILLE, TX, p. A419
EAST TEXAS MEDICAL CENTER PITTSBURG, PITTSBURG, TX, p. A426
EAST TEXAS MEDICAL CENTER REHABILITATION CENTER, TYLER, TX, p. A433
EAST TEXAS MEDICAL CENTER TRINITY, TRINITY, TX, p. A432
EAST TEXAS MEDICAL CENTER TYLER, TYLER, TX, p. A433
EAST TEXAS MEDICAL CENTER-CLARKSVILLE, CLARKSVILLE, TX, p. A406
EAST TEXAS MEDICAL CENTER-MOUNT VERNON, MOUNT VERNON, TX, p. A424
EAST TEXAS MEDICAL CENTER-QUITMAN, QUITMAN, TX, p. A427
EASTERN IDAHO REGIONAL MEDICAL CENTER, IDAHO FALLS, ID, p. A116
EASTERN LONG ISLAND HOSPITAL, GREENPORT, NY, p. A292
EASTERN LOUISIANA MENTAL HEALTH SYSTEM/GREENWELL SPRING CAMPUS, GREENWELL SPRINGS, LA, p. A183
EASTERN MAINE MEDICAL CENTER, BANGOR, ME, p. A191
EASTERN NEW MEXICO MEDICAL CENTER, ROSWELL, NM, p. A285
EASTERN OKLAHOMA MEDICAL CENTER, POTEAU, OK, p. A347
EASTERN OREGON PSYCHIATRIC CENTER, PENDLETON, OR, p. A352
EASTERN OZARKS REGIONAL HEALTH SYSTEM, CHEROKEE VILLAGE, AR, p. A28
EASTERN PENNSYLVANIA PSYCHIATRIC INSTITUTE, PHILADELPHIA, PENNSYLVANIA, p. A367
EASTERN PLUMAS DISTRICT HOSPITAL, PORTOLA, CA, p. A56
EASTERN SHORE HOSPITAL CENTER, CAMBRIDGE, MD, p. A197
EASTERN STATE HOSPITAL, WILLIAMSBURG, VA, p. A450
EASTERN STATE HOSPITAL, LEXINGTON, KY, p. A174
EASTERN STATE HOSPITAL, VINITA, OK, p. A349
EASTERN STATE HOSPITAL, MEDICAL LAKE, WA, p. A454
EASTERN WAKE DAY HOSPITAL, ZEBULON, NORTH CAROLINA, p. A317
EASTLAND MEMORIAL HOSPITAL, EASTLAND, TX, p. A411
EASTMORELAND HOSPITAL, PORTLAND, OR, p. A353
EASTON HOSPITAL, EASTON, PA, p. A359
EATON RAPIDS MEDICAL CENTER, EATON RAPIDS, MI, p. A214
EDEN MEDICAL CENTER, CASTRO VALLEY, CA, p. A38
EDGE REGIONAL MEDICAL CENTER, TROY, AL, p. A18
EDGEFIELD COUNTY HOSPITAL, EDGEFIELD, SC, p. A380
EDGEMONT HOSPITAL, LOS ANGELES, CA, p. A47
EDGEWATER MEDICAL CENTER, CHICAGO, IL, p. A121
EDGEWATER PSYCHIATRIC CENTER, HARRISBURG, PA, p. A361
EDINBURG REGIONAL MEDICAL CENTER, EDINBURG, TX, p. A411
EDITH NOURSE ROGERS MEMORIAL VETERANS HOSPITAL, BEDFORD, MA, p. A201
EDMOND MEDICAL CENTER, EDMOND, OK, p. A343
EDWARD A. UTLAUT MEMORIAL HOSPITAL, GREENVILLE, IL, p. A127
EDWARD HOSPITAL, NAPERVILLE, IL, p. A131
EDWARD JOHN NOBLE HOSPITAL OF GOUVERNEUR, GOUVERNEUR, NY, p. A292

EDWARD W. MCCREADY MEMORIAL HOSPITAL, CRISFIELD, MD, p. A197
EDWARD WHITE HOSPITAL, SAINT PETERSBURG, FL, p. A94
EDWIN SHAW HOSPITAL FOR REHABILITATION, AKRON, OH, p. A325
EFFINGHAM HOSPITAL, SPRINGFIELD, GA, p. A110
EHRLING BERGQUIST HOSPITAL, OFFUTT AFB, NE, p. A265
EISENHOWER MEMORIAL HOSPITAL AND BETTY FORD CENTER AT EISENHOWER, RANCHO MIRAGE, CA, p. A56
EL CAMINO HOSPITAL, MOUNTAIN VIEW, CA, p. A52
EL CAMPO MEMORIAL HOSPITAL, EL CAMPO, TX, p. A411
EL CENTRO REGIONAL MEDICAL CENTER, EL CENTRO, CA, p. A40
EL DORADO HOSPITAL, TUCSON, AZ, p. A26
ELBA GENERAL HOSPITAL, ELBA, AL, p. A14
ELBERT MEMORIAL HOSPITAL, ELBERTON, GA, p. A104
ELEANOR SLATER HOSPITAL, CRANSTON, RI, p. A376
ELECTRA MEMORIAL HOSPITAL, ELECTRA, TX, p. A412
ELGIN MENTAL HEALTH CENTER, ELGIN, IL, p. A125
ELIZA COFFEE MEMORIAL HOSPITAL, FLORENCE, AL, p. A14
ELIZABETHTOWN COMMUNITY HOSPITAL, ELIZABETHTOWN, NY, p. A291
ELK REGIONAL HEALTH CENTER, SAINT MARYS, PA, p. A371
ELKHART GENERAL HOSPITAL, ELKHART, IN, p. A139
ELKINS PARK HOSPITAL, ELKINS PARK, PA, p. A359
ELKO GENERAL HOSPITAL, ELKO, NV, p. A268
ELKVIEW GENERAL HOSPITAL, HOBART, OK, p. A344
ELLENVILLE COMMUNITY HOSPITAL, ELLENVILLE, NY, p. A291
ELLETT MEMORIAL HOSPITAL, APPLETON CITY, MO, p. A244
ELLINWOOD DISTRICT HOSPITAL, ELLINWOOD, KS, p. A160
ELLIOT HOSPITAL, MANCHESTER, NH, p. A272
ELLIS FISCHEL CANCER CENTER, COLUMBIA, MISSOURI, p. A246
ELLIS HOSPITAL, SCHENECTADY, NY, p. A304
ELLSWORTH COUNTY MEDICAL CENTER, ELLSWORTH, KS, p. A161
ELLSWORTH MUNICIPAL HOSPITAL, IOWA FALLS, IA, p. A153
ELLWOOD CITY HOSPITAL, ELLWOOD CITY, PA, p. A359
ELMBROOK MEMORIAL HOSPITAL, BROOKFIELD, WI, p. A467
ELMHURST HOSPITAL CENTER, NEW YORK, NY, p. A296
ELMHURST MEMORIAL HOSPITAL, NEW YORK, IL, p. A125
ELMIRA PSYCHIATRIC CENTER, ELMIRA, NY, p. A291
ELMORE COMMUNITY HOSPITAL, WETUMPKA, AL, p. A19
ELMORE MEDICAL CENTER, MOUNTAIN HOME, ID, p. A117
ELY-BLOOMENSON COMMUNITY HOSPITAL, ELY, MN, p. A227
EMANUEL COUNTY HOSPITAL, SWAINSBORO, GA, p. A110
EMANUEL MEDICAL CENTER, TURLOCK, CA, p. A65
EMERALD-HODGSON HOSPITAL, SEWANEE, TENNESSEE, p. A400
EMERSON HOSPITAL, CONCORD, MA, p. A204
EMH AMHERST HOSPITAL, AMHERST, OH, p. A325
EMH REGIONAL MEDICAL CENTER, ELYRIA, OH, p. A331
EMMA PENDLETON BRADLEY HOSPITAL, EAST PROVIDENCE, RI, p. A376
EMORY CARTERSVILLE MEDICAL CENTER, CARTERSVILLE, GA, p. A102
EMORY DUNWOODY MEDICAL CENTER, ATLANTA, GA, p. A100
EMORY EASTSIDE MEDICAL CENTER, SNELLVILLE, GA, p. A109
EMORY NORTHLAKE REGIONAL MEDICAL CENTER, TUCKER, GA, p. A110
EMORY PARKWAY MEDICAL CENTER, LITHIA SPRINGS, GA, p. A106
EMORY PEACHTREE REGIONAL HOSPITAL, NEWNAN, GA, p. A108
EMORY UNIVERSITY HOSPITAL, ATLANTA, GA, p. A100
EMORY-ADVENTIST HOSPITAL, SMYRNA, GA, p. A109
ENCINO-TARZANA REGIONAL MEDICAL CENTER ENCINO CAMPUS, LOS ANGELES, CA, p. A47
ENCINO-TARZANA REGIONAL MEDICAL CENTER TARZANA CAMPUS, LOS ANGELES, CA, p. A47
ENDLESS MOUNTAIN HEALTH SYSTEMS, MONTROSE, PA, p. A364
ENGLEWOOD COMMUNITY HOSPITAL, ENGLEWOOD, FL, p. A84
ENGLEWOOD HOSPITAL AND MEDICAL CENTER, ENGLEWOOD, NJ, p. A276
ENLOE MEDICAL CENTER, CHICO, CA, p. A38
ENLOE MEDICAL CENTER-COHASSET, CHICO, CALIFORNIA, p. A38
ENUMCLAW COMMUNITY HOSPITAL, ENUMCLAW, WA, p. A453
EPHRAIM MCDOWELL REGIONAL MEDICAL CENTER, DANVILLE, KY, p. A171
EPHRATA COMMUNITY HOSPITAL, EPHRATA, PA, p. A359
EPISCOPAL HOSPITAL, PHILADELPHIA, PA, p. A366
ERIE COUNTY MEDICAL CENTER, BUFFALO, NY, p. A289
ERIK AND MARGARET JONSSON HOSPITAL, DALLAS, TEXAS, p. A408
ERLANGER HEALTH SYSTEM, CHATTANOOGA, TN, p. A390
ERLANGER NORTH HOSPITAL, CHATTANOOGA, TENNESSEE, p. A390
ESPANOLA HOSPITAL, ESPANOLA, NM, p. A284

ESSEX COUNTY HOSPITAL CENTER, CEDAR GROVE, NJ, p. A275
ESTES PARK MEDICAL CENTER, ESTES PARK, CO, p. A70
EUCLID HOSPITAL, EUCLID, OH, p. A331
EUGENIA HOSPITAL, LAFAYETTE HILL, PA, p. A362
EUNICE COMMUNITY MEDICAL CENTER, EUNICE, LA, p. A182
EUREKA COMMUNITY HEALTH SERVICES/AVERA HEALTH, EUREKA, SD, p. A386
EUREKA COMMUNITY HOSPITAL, EUREKA, ILLINOIS, p. A131
EUREKA SPRINGS HOSPITAL, EUREKA SPRINGS, AR, p. A29
EVANGELICAL COMMUNITY HOSPITAL, LEWISBURG, PA, p. A363
EVANS MEMORIAL HOSPITAL, CLAXTON, GA, p. A102
EVANS U. S. ARMY COMMUNITY HOSPITAL, FORT CARSON, CO, p. A70
EVANSTON NORTHWESTERN HEALTHCARE CORPORATION, EVANSTON, IL, p. A126
EVANSTON NORTHWESTERN HEALTHCARE CORPORATION, EVANSTON, ILLINOIS, p. A126
EVANSTON REGIONAL HOSPITAL, EVANSTON, WY, p. A478
EVANSVILLE STATE HOSPITAL, EVANSVILLE, IN, p. A139
EVERGREEN ADULT CENTER, HAZEL GREEN, WISCONSIN, p. A474
EVERGREEN COMMUNITY HEALTH CENTER, KIRKLAND, WA, p. A454
EXCELSIOR SPRINGS MEDICAL CENTER, EXCELSIOR SPRINGS, MO, p. A246
EXEMPLA LUTHERAN MEDICAL CENTER, WHEAT RIDGE, CO, p. A73
EXEMPLA SAINT JOSEPH HOSPITAL, DENVER, CO, p. A69
EXEMPLA WEST PINES, WHEAT RIDGE, COLORADO, p. A73
EXETER HOSPITAL, EXETER, NH, p. A271
EYE AND EAR CLINIC OF CHARLESTON, CHARLESTON, WV, p. A460
EYE AND EAR HOSPITAL OF PITTSBURGH, PITTSBURGH, PENNSYLVANIA, p. A370

F

F. F. THOMPSON HEALTH SYSTEM, CANANDAIGUA, NY, p. A289
FAIR OAKS, p. A127
FAIR OAKS HOSPITAL, DELRAY BEACH, FLORIDA, p. A83
FAIRBANKS HOSPITAL, INDIANAPOLIS, IN, p. A141
FAIRBANKS MEMORIAL HOSPITAL, FAIRBANKS, AK, p. A20
FAIRCHILD MEDICAL CENTER, YREKA, CA, p. A67
FAIRFAX MEMORIAL HOSPITAL, FAIRFAX, OK, p. A343
FAIRFIELD MEDICAL CENTER, LANCASTER, OH, p. A333
FAIRFIELD MEMORIAL HOSPITAL, WINNSBORO, SC, p. A384
FAIRFIELD MEMORIAL HOSPITAL, FAIRFIELD, IL, p. A126
FAIRLAWN REHABILITATION HOSPITAL, WORCESTER, MA, p. A210
FAIRMONT COMMUNITY HOSPITAL, FAIRMONT, MN, p. A227
FAIRMONT GENERAL HOSPITAL, FAIRMONT, WV, p. A461
FAIRVIEW HOSPITAL, GREAT BARRINGTON, MA, p. A205
FAIRVIEW HOSPITAL, CLEVELAND, OH, p. A328
FAIRVIEW HOSPITAL, FAIRVIEW, OK, p. A343
FAIRVIEW LAKES REGIONAL MEDICAL CENTER, WYOMING, MN, p. A235
FAIRVIEW NORTHLAND REGIONAL HEALTH CARE, PRINCETON, MN, p. A232
FAIRVIEW PARK HOSPITAL, DUBLIN, GA, p. A104
FAIRVIEW RED WING HOSPITAL, RED WING, MN, p. A232
FAIRVIEW RIDGES HOSPITAL, BURNSVILLE, MN, p. A226
FAIRVIEW RIVERSIDE HOSPITAL, MINNEAPOLIS, MINNESOTA, p. A230
FAIRVIEW SOUTHDALE HOSPITAL, MINNEAPOLIS, MN, p. A230
FAIRVIEW-UNIVERSITY MEDICAL CENTER, MINNEAPOLIS, MN, p. A230
FAITH COMMUNITY HOSPITAL, JACKSBORO, TX, p. A419
FAITH REGIONAL HEALTH SERVICES, NORFOLK, NE, p. A264
FALLBROOK HOSPITAL DISTRICT, FALLBROOK, CA, p. A41
FALLON MEDICAL COMPLEX, BAKER, MT, p. A256
FALLS COMMUNITY HOSPITAL AND CLINIC, MARLIN, TX, p. A423
FALLS MEMORIAL HOSPITAL, INTERNATIONAL FALLS, MN, p. A229
FALLSTON GENERAL HOSPITAL, FALLSTON, MD, p. A198
FALMOUTH HOSPITAL, FALMOUTH, MA, p. A204
FAMILY HEALTH WEST, FRUITA, CO, p. A70
FANNIN PAVILION OF BEAUMONT REGIONAL MEDICAL CENTER, BEAUMONT, TEXAS, p. A404
FANNIN REGIONAL HOSPITAL, BLUE RIDGE, GA, p. A101
FANNY ALLEN CAMPUS, COLCHESTER, VERMONT, p. A440
FAULK COUNTY MEMORIAL HOSPITAL, FAULKTON, SD, p. A386
FAULKNER HOSPITAL, BOSTON, MA, p. A202
FAUQUIER HOSPITAL, WARRENTON, VA, p. A450

FAWCETT MEMORIAL HOSPITAL, PORT CHARLOTTE, FL, p. A93
FAXTON-ST. LUKE'S HEALTHCARE, UTICA, NY, p. A306
FAYETTE COUNTY HOSPITAL, VANDALIA, IL, p. A135
FAYETTE COUNTY MEMORIAL HOSPITAL, WASHINGTON COURT HOUSE, OH, p. A339
FAYETTE MEDICAL CENTER, FAYETTE, AL, p. A14
FAYETTE MEMORIAL HOSPITAL, CONNERSVILLE, IN, p. A138
FAYETTE MEMORIAL HOSPITAL, LA GRANGE, TX, p. A420
FEATHER RIVER HOSPITAL, PARADISE, CA, p. A54
FEDERAL MEDICAL CENTER, LEXINGTON, KY, p. A174
FENTRESS COUNTY GENERAL HOSPITAL, JAMESTOWN, TN, p. A393
FERGUS FALLS REGIONAL TREATMENT CENTER, FERGUS FALLS, MN, p. A228
FERGUSON CAMPUS, GRAND RAPIDS, MICHIGAN, p. A216
FERRELL HOSPITAL, ELDORADO, IL, p. A125
FERRY COUNTY MEMORIAL HOSPITAL, REPUBLIC, WA, p. A456
FIELD MEMORIAL COMMUNITY HOSPITAL, CENTREVILLE, MS, p. A237
FIELDSTONE CENTER, BATTLE CREEK, MICHIGAN, p. A212
FILLMORE COMMUNITY MEDICAL CENTER, FILLMORE, UT, p. A436
FILLMORE COUNTY HOSPITAL, GENEVA, NE, p. A263
FINLEY HOSPITAL, DUBUQUE, IA, p. A151
FIRELANDS COMMUNITY HOSPITAL, SANDUSKY, OH, p. A337
FIRST CARE MEDICAL SERVICES, FOSSTON, MN, p. A228
FIRST HOSPITAL PANAMERICANO, CIDRA, PR, p. A482
FIRST HOSPITAL WYOMING VALLEY, WILKES-BARRE, PA, p. A374
FIRSTHEALTH MONTGOMERY MEMORIAL HOSPITAL, TROY, NC, p. A319
FIRSTHEALTH MOORE REGIONAL HOSPITAL, PINEHURST, NC, p. A316
FISHER COUNTY HOSPITAL DISTRICT, ROTAN, TX, p. A427
FISHER-TITUS MEDICAL CENTER, NORWALK, OH, p. A336
FISHERMEN'S HOSPITAL, MARATHON, FL, p. A89
FITZGIBBON HOSPITAL, MARSHALL, MO, p. A250
FIVE COUNTIES HOSPITAL, LEMMON, SD, p. A386
FLAGET MEMORIAL HOSPITAL, BARDSTOWN, KY, p. A170
FLAGLER HOSPITAL, SAINT AUGUSTINE, FL, p. A94
FLAGSTAFF MEDICAL CENTER, FLAGSTAFF, AZ, p. A22
FLAMBEAU HOSPITAL, PARK FALLS, WI, p. A473
FLANDREAU MUNICIPAL HOSPITAL/AVERA HEALTH, FLANDREAU, SD, p. A386
FLEMING COUNTY HOSPITAL, FLEMINGSBURG, KY, p. A171
FLETCHER ALLEN HEALTH CARE, BURLINGTON, VT, p. A440
FLINT RIVER COMMUNITY HOSPITAL, MONTEZUMA, GA, p. A108
FLORALA MEMORIAL HOSPITAL, FLORALA, AL, p. A14
FLORENCE D'URSO PAVILION, NEW YORK, NEW YORK, p. A299
FLORENCE GENERAL HOSPITAL, FLORENCE, SOUTH CAROLINA, p. A380
FLORIDA CENTER FOR ADDICTIONS AND DUAL DISORDERS, AVON PARK, FL, p. A81
FLORIDA HOSPITAL, ORLANDO, FL, p. A91
FLORIDA HOSPITAL CELEBRATION, CELEBRATION, FLORIDA, p. A91
FLORIDA HOSPITAL EAST ORLANDO, ORLANDO, FLORIDA, p. A91
FLORIDA HOSPITAL HEARTLAND DIVISION, SEBRING, FL, p. A95
FLORIDA HOSPITAL KISSIMMEE, KISSIMMEE, FLORIDA, p. A91
FLORIDA HOSPITAL WATERMAN, EUSTIS, FL, p. A84
FLORIDA HOSPITAL-ALTAMONTE, ALTAMONTE SPRINGS, FLORIDA, p. A91
FLORIDA HOSPITAL-APOPKA, APOPKA, FLORIDA, p. A91
FLORIDA KEYS MEMORIAL HOSPITAL, KEY WEST, FLORIDA, p. A87
FLORIDA MEDICAL CENTER, FORT LAUDERDALE, FL, p. A84
FLORIDA STATE HOSPITAL, CHATTAHOOCHEE, FL, p. A82
FLOWER HOSPITAL, SYLVANIA, OH, p. A338
FLOWERS HOSPITAL, DOTHAN, AL, p. A14
FLOYD COUNTY MEMORIAL HOSPITAL, CHARLES CITY, IA, p. A149
FLOYD MEDICAL CENTER, ROME, GA, p. A108
FLOYD MEMORIAL HOSPITAL AND HEALTH SERVICES, NEW ALBANY, IN, p. A144
FLOYD VALLEY HOSPITAL/AVERA HEALTH, LE MARS, IA, p. A154
FOCUS HEALTHCARE OF OHIO, MAUMEE, OH, p. A335
FONT MARTELO HOSPITAL, HUMACAO, PR, p. A482
FOOTHILL PRESBYTERIAN HOSPITAL-MORRIS L. JOHNSTON MEMORIAL, GLENDORA, CA, p. A43
FOREST PARK HOSPITAL, SAINT LOUIS, MO, p. A253
FOREST VIEW HOSPITAL, GRAND RAPIDS, MI, p. A215
FORKS COMMUNITY HOSPITAL, FORKS, WA, p. A453
FORREST GENERAL HOSPITAL, HATTIESBURG, MS, p. A238
FORSYTH MEDICAL CENTER, WINSTON-SALEM, NC, p. A320
FORT ATKINSON MEMORIAL HEALTH SERVICES, FORT ATKINSON, WI, p. A468
FORT DEFIANCE INDIAN HEALTH SERVICE HOSPITAL, FORT DEFIANCE, AZ, p. A22

Index of Hospitals / Good Samaritan Hospital of Maryland

FORT DUNCAN MEDICAL CENTER, EAGLE PASS, TX, p. A411
FORT HAMILTON HOSPITAL, HAMILTON, OH, p. A332
FORT LOGAN HOSPITAL, STANFORD, KY, p. A178
FORT MADISON COMMUNITY HOSPITAL, FORT MADISON, IA, p. A152
FORT SANDERS LOUDON MEDICAL CENTER, LOUDON, TN, p. A395
FORT SANDERS REGIONAL MEDICAL CENTER, KNOXVILLE, TN, p. A394
FORT SANDERS–PARKWEST MEDICAL CENTER, KNOXVILLE, TN, p. A395
FORT SANDERS–SEVIER MEDICAL CENTER, SEVIERVILLE, TN, p. A399
FORT WALTON BEACH MEDICAL CENTER, FORT WALTON BEACH, FL, p. A85
FORT WASHINGTON HOSPITAL, FORT WASHINGTON, MD, p. A198
FOSTORIA COMMUNITY HOSPITAL, FOSTORIA, OH, p. A332
FOUNDATIONS BEHAVIORAL HEALTH, DOYLESTOWN, PA, p. A359
FOUNTAIN VALLEY REGIONAL HOSPITAL AND MEDICAL CENTER, FOUNTAIN VALLEY, CA, p. A41
FOUR WINDS HOSPITAL, KATONAH, NY, p. A293
45TH STREET MENTAL HEALTH CENTER, WEST PALM BEACH, FL, p. A97
FOX CHASE CANCER CENTER–AMERICAN ONCOLOGIC HOSPITAL, PHILADELPHIA, PA, p. A366
FRAMINGHAM UNION HOSPITAL, FRAMINGHAM, MASSACHUSETTS, p. A205
FRANCES MAHON DEACONESS HOSPITAL, GLASGOW, MT, p. A257
FRANCISCAN CHILDREN'S HOSPITAL AND REHABILITATION CENTER, BOSTON, MA, p. A202
FRANCISCAN HOSPITAL–WESTERN HILLS, CINCINNATI, OH, p. A327
FRANCISCAN MEDICAL CENTER–DAYTON CAMPUS, DAYTON, OH, p. A330
FRANCISCAN SKEMP HEALTHCARE–ARCADIA CAMPUS, ARCADIA, WI, p. A466
FRANCISCAN SKEMP HEALTHCARE–LA CROSSE CAMPUS, LA CROSSE, WI, p. A470
FRANCISCAN SKEMP HEALTHCARE–SPARTA CAMPUS, SPARTA, WI, p. A475
FRANK R. HOWARD MEMORIAL HOSPITAL, WILLITS, CA, p. A67
FRANKFORD CAMPUS, PHILADELPHIA, PENNSYLVANIA, p. A366
FRANKFORD HOSPITAL OF THE CITY OF PHILADELPHIA, PHILADELPHIA, PA, p. A366
FRANKFORT REGIONAL MEDICAL CENTER, FRANKFORT, KY, p. A172
FRANKLIN COUNTY MEDICAL CENTER, PRESTON, ID, p. A117
FRANKLIN COUNTY MEMORIAL HOSPITAL, MEADVILLE, MS, p. A240
FRANKLIN COUNTY MEMORIAL HOSPITAL, FRANKLIN, NE, p. A262
FRANKLIN FOUNDATION HOSPITAL, FRANKLIN, LA, p. A182
FRANKLIN GENERAL HOSPITAL, HAMPTON, IA, p. A152
FRANKLIN HOSPITAL AND SKILLED NURSING CARE UNIT, BENTON, IL, p. A120
FRANKLIN HOSPITAL MEDICAL CENTER, VALLEY STREAM, NY, p. A306
FRANKLIN MEDICAL CENTER, GREENFIELD, MA, p. A205
FRANKLIN MEDICAL CENTER, WINNSBORO, LA, p. A189
FRANKLIN MEMORIAL HOSPITAL, FARMINGTON, ME, p. A192
FRANKLIN REGIONAL HOSPITAL, FRANKLIN, NH, p. A271
FRANKLIN REGIONAL HOSPITAL, LOUISBURG, NC, p. A315
FRANKLIN SQUARE HOSPITAL CENTER, BALTIMORE, MD, p. A195
FRAZIER REHABILITATION CENTER, LOUISVILLE, KY, p. A175
FREDERICK MEMORIAL HOSPITAL, FREDERICK, MD, p. A198
FREDONIA REGIONAL HOSPITAL, FREDONIA, KS, p. A161
FREEMAN COMMUNITY HOSPITAL, FREEMAN, SD, p. A386
FREEMAN HEALTH SYSTEM, JOPLIN, MO, p. A247
FREEMAN HOSPITAL EAST, JOPLIN, MISSOURI, p. A247
FREEMAN HOSPITAL WEST, JOPLIN, MISSOURI, p. A247
FREEMAN NEOSHO HOSPITAL, NEOSHO, MO, p. A251
FREEPORT MEMORIAL HOSPITAL, FREEPORT, IL, p. A126
FREMONT AREA MEDICAL CENTER, FREMONT, NE, p. A262
FREMONT MEDICAL CENTER, YUBA CITY, CA, p. A67
FRENCH HOSPITAL MEDICAL CENTER, SAN LUIS OBISPO, CA, p. A61
FRESNO SURGERY CENTER–THE HOSPITAL FOR SURGERY, FRESNO, CA, p. A42
FRICK HOSPITAL, MOUNT PLEASANT, PA, p. A364
FRIEDMAN HOSPITAL OF THE HOME FOR THE JEWISH AGED, PHILADELPHIA, PA, p. A366
FRIENDS HOSPITAL, PHILADELPHIA, PA, p. A367
FRIO HOSPITAL, PEARSALL, TX, p. A426
FRISBIE MEMORIAL HOSPITAL, ROCHESTER, NH, p. A273

FROEDTERT MEMORIAL LUTHERAN HOSPITAL, MILWAUKEE, WI, p. A472
FRYE REGIONAL MEDICAL CENTER, HICKORY, NC, p. A314
FRYE REGIONAL MEDICAL CENTER–SOUTH CAMPUS, HICKORY, NORTH CAROLINA, p. A314
FULTON COUNTY HEALTH CENTER, WAUSEON, OH, p. A339
FULTON COUNTY HOSPITAL, SALEM, AR, p. A33
FULTON COUNTY MEDICAL CENTER, MCCONNELLSBURG, PA, p. A363
FULTON DIVISION, NEW YORK, NEW YORK, p. A295
FULTON STATE HOSPITAL, FULTON, MO, p. A247

G

G. PIERCE WOOD MEMORIAL HOSPITAL, ARCADIA, FL, p. A81
G.V. MONTGOMERY VETERANS AFFAIRS MEDICAL CENTER, JACKSON, MS, p. A239
GADSDEN COMMUNITY HOSPITAL, QUINCY, FL, p. A94
GADSDEN REGIONAL MEDICAL CENTER, GADSDEN, AL, p. A15
GAINESVILLE MEMORIAL HOSPITAL, GAINESVILLE, TX, p. A413
GALENA-STAUSS HOSPITAL, GALENA, IL, p. A126
GALESBURG COTTAGE HOSPITAL, GALESBURG, IL, p. A126
GALION COMMUNITY HOSPITAL, GALION, OH, p. A332
GALLUP INDIAN MEDICAL CENTER, GALLUP, NM, p. A285
GARDEN CITY HOSPITAL, GARDEN CITY, MI, p. A215
GARDEN COUNTY HOSPITAL, OSHKOSH, NE, p. A266
GARDEN GROVE HOSPITAL AND MEDICAL CENTER, GARDEN GROVE, CA, p. A42
GARDENVIEW NURSING HOME, p. A229
GARFIELD COUNTY MEMORIAL HOSPITAL, POMEROY, WA, p. A455
GARFIELD MEDICAL CENTER, MONTEREY PARK, CA, p. A52
GARFIELD MEMORIAL HOSPITAL AND CLINICS, PANGUITCH, UT, p. A437
GARLAND COMMUNITY HOSPITAL, GARLAND, TX, p. A414
GARRARD COUNTY MEMORIAL HOSPITAL, LANCASTER, KY, p. A173
GARRETT COUNTY MEMORIAL HOSPITAL, OAKLAND, MD, p. A199
GARRISON MEMORIAL HOSPITAL, GARRISON, ND, p. A322
GARY MEMORIAL HOSPITAL, BREAUX BRIDGE, LA, p. A181
GASTON MEMORIAL HOSPITAL, GASTONIA, NC, p. A313
GATEWAY HEALTH SYSTEM, CLARKSVILLE, TN, p. A391
GATEWAY REGIONAL HEALTH SYSTEM, MOUNT STERLING, KY, p. A177
GATEWAYS HOSPITAL AND MENTAL HEALTH CENTER, LOS ANGELES, CA, p. A47
GAYLORD HOSPITAL, WALLINGFORD, CT, p. A77
GEARY COMMUNITY HOSPITAL, JUNCTION CITY, KS, p. A163
GEISINGER MEDICAL CENTER, DANVILLE, PA, p. A359
GENERAL DIVISION, CHARLESTON, WEST VIRGINIA, p. A460
GENERAL HOSPITAL, EUREKA, CA, p. A40
GENERAL HOSPITAL, LOS ANGELES, CALIFORNIA, p. A48
GENERAL HOSPITAL CENTER AT PASSAIC, PASSAIC, NEW JERSEY, p. A276
GENERAL JOHN J. PERSHING MEMORIAL HOSPITAL, BROOKFIELD, MO, p. A244
GENERAL LEONARD WOOD ARMY COMMUNITY HOSPITAL, FORT LEONARD WOOD, MO, p. A246
GENESEE HOSPITAL, ROCHESTER, NY, p. A303
GENESIS HEALTHCARE SYSTEM, ZANESVILLE, OH, p. A340
GENESIS MEDICAL CENTER, DAVENPORT, IA, p. A150
GENESIS MEDICAL CENTER–EAST CAMPUS, DAVENPORT, IOWA, p. A150
GENESIS MEDICAL CENTER–WEST CAMPUS, DAVENPORT, IOWA, p. A150
GENESYS REGIONAL MEDICAL CENTER, GRAND BLANC, MI, p. A215
GENEVA GENERAL HOSPITAL, GENEVA, NY, p. A291
GENOA COMMUNITY HOSPITAL, GENOA, NE, p. A263
GENTRY COUNTY MEMORIAL HOSPITAL, ALBANY, MO, p. A244
GEORGE A. ZELLER MENTAL HEALTH CENTER, PEORIA, IL, p. A132
GEORGE COUNTY HOSPITAL, LUCEDALE, MS, p. A240
GEORGE E. WEEMS MEMORIAL HOSPITAL, APALACHICOLA, FL, p. A81
GEORGE L. HARRISON MEMORIAL HOUSE, p. A366
GEORGE L. MEE MEMORIAL HOSPITAL, KING CITY, CA, p. A45
GEORGE NIGH REHABILITATION CENTER, OKMULGEE, OK, p. A346
GEORGE W. TRUETT MEMORIAL HOSPITAL, DALLAS, TEXAS, p. A408
GEORGE WASHINGTON UNIVERSITY HOSPITAL, WASHINGTON, DC, p. A79
GEORGETOWN COMMUNITY HOSPITAL, GEORGETOWN, KY, p. A172

GEORGETOWN HEALTHCARE SYSTEM, GEORGETOWN, TX, p. A414
GEORGETOWN MEMORIAL HOSPITAL, GEORGETOWN, SC, p. A381
GEORGETOWN UNIVERSITY HOSPITAL, WASHINGTON, DC, p. A79
GEORGIA REGIONAL HOSPITAL AT ATLANTA, DECATUR, GA, p. A104
GEORGIA REGIONAL HOSPITAL AT AUGUSTA, AUGUSTA, GA, p. A101
GEORGIA REGIONAL HOSPITAL AT SAVANNAH, SAVANNAH, GA, p. A109
GEORGIANA HOSPITAL, GEORGIANA, AL, p. A15
GERALD CHAMPION REGIONAL MEDICAL CENTER, ALAMOGORDO, NM, p. A283
GERBER MEMORIAL HEALTH SERVICES, FREMONT, MI, p. A215
GERMANTOWN HOSPITAL AND COMMUNITY HEALTH SERVICES, PHILADELPHIA, PA, p. A367
GETTYSBURG HOSPITAL, GETTYSBURG, PA, p. A360
GETTYSBURG MEDICAL CENTER, GETTYSBURG, SD, p. A386
GIBSON AREA HOSPITAL AND HEALTH SERVICES, GIBSON CITY, IL, p. A127
GIBSON COMMUNITY HOSPITAL NURSING HOME, p. A127
GIBSON GENERAL HOSPITAL, PRINCETON, IN, p. A145
GIBSON GENERAL HOSPITAL, TRENTON, TN, p. A400
GIFFORD MEDICAL CENTER, RANDOLPH, VT, p. A440
GILA REGIONAL MEDICAL CENTER, SILVER CITY, NM, p. A286
GILLETTE CHILDREN'S SPECIALTY HEALTHCARE, SAINT PAUL, MN, p. A233
GILMORE MEMORIAL HOSPITAL, AMORY, MS, p. A236
GIRARD MEDICAL CENTER, PHILADELPHIA, PENNSYLVANIA, p. A367
GLACIAL RIDGE HOSPITAL AND HEALTHCARE SERVICES, GLENWOOD, MN, p. A228
GLACIER COUNTY MEDICAL CENTER, CUT BANK, MT, p. A257
GLADES GENERAL HOSPITAL, BELLE GLADE, FL, p. A81
GLADYS SPELLMAN SPECIALTY HOSPITAL AND NURSING CENTER, CHEVERLY, MD, p. A197
GLEN OAKS HOSPITAL, GREENVILLE, TX, p. A414
GLEN ROSE MEDICAL CENTER, GLEN ROSE, TX, p. A414
GLENBEIGH HEALTH SOURCES, ROCK CREEK, OH, p. A337
GLENBROOK HOSPITAL, GLENVIEW, ILLINOIS, p. A126
GLENCOE REGIONAL HEALTH SERVICES, GLENCOE, MN, p. A228
GLENDALE ADVENTIST MEDICAL CENTER, GLENDALE, CA, p. A42
GLENDALE MEMORIAL HOSPITAL AND HEALTH CENTER, GLENDALE, CA, p. A42
GLENDIVE MEDICAL CENTER, GLENDIVE, MT, p. A257
GLENN MEDICAL CENTER, WILLOWS, CA, p. A67
GLENOAKS HOSPITAL, GLENDALE HEIGHTS, IL, p. A127
GLENS FALLS HOSPITAL, GLENS FALLS, NY, p. A292
GLENWOOD REGIONAL MEDICAL CENTER, WEST MONROE, LA, p. A189
GLENWOOD STATE HOSPITAL SCHOOL, GLENWOOD, IA, p. A152
GNADEN HUETTEN MEMORIAL HOSPITAL, LEHIGHTON, PA, p. A363
GOLDEN OURS CONVALESCENT HOME, p. A263
GOLDEN PLAINS COMMUNITY HOSPITAL, BORGER, TX, p. A405
GOLDEN VALLEY MEMORIAL HOSPITAL, CLINTON, MO, p. A245
GOLDWATER MEMORIAL HOSPITAL, NEW YORK, NY, p. A296
GOLETA VALLEY COTTAGE HOSPITAL, SANTA BARBARA, CA, p. A62
GOLI MEDICAL CENTER, SARGENT, NE, p. A
GOOD HOPE HOSPITAL, ERWIN, NC, p. A312
GOOD SAMARITAN COMMUNITY HEALTHCARE, PUYALLUP, WA, p. A455
GOOD SAMARITAN HEALTH CENTER OF MERRILL, MERRILL, WI, p. A471
GOOD SAMARITAN HEALTH SYSTEMS, KEARNEY, NE, p. A263
GOOD SAMARITAN HOSPITAL, SUFFERN, NY, p. A305
GOOD SAMARITAN HOSPITAL, LEBANON, PA, p. A363
GOOD SAMARITAN HOSPITAL, CINCINNATI, OH, p. A327
GOOD SAMARITAN HOSPITAL, VINCENNES, IN, p. A146
GOOD SAMARITAN HOSPITAL, DOWNERS GROVE, IL, p. A125
GOOD SAMARITAN HOSPITAL, SAN JOSE, CA, p. A60
GOOD SAMARITAN HOSPITAL, BAKERSFIELD, CA, p. A36
GOOD SAMARITAN HOSPITAL, LOS ANGELES, CA, p. A47
GOOD SAMARITAN HOSPITAL AND HEALTH CENTER, DAYTON, OH, p. A331
GOOD SAMARITAN HOSPITAL AND MEDICAL CENTER, PORTLAND, OREGON, p. A353
GOOD SAMARITAN HOSPITAL CORVALLIS, CORVALLIS, OR, p. A350
GOOD SAMARITAN HOSPITAL MEDICAL CENTER, WEST ISLIP, NY, p. A307
GOOD SAMARITAN HOSPITAL OF MARYLAND, BALTIMORE, MD, p. A195

© 2000 AHA Guide

Index of Hospitals / Good Samaritan Medical and Rehabilitation Center

GOOD SAMARITAN MEDICAL AND REHABILITATION CENTER, ZANESVILLE, OHIO, p. A340
GOOD SAMARITAN MEDICAL CENTER, JOHNSTOWN, PENNSYLVANIA, p. A362
GOOD SAMARITAN MEDICAL CENTER, WEST PALM BEACH, FL, p. A97
GOOD SAMARITAN MEDICAL CENTER – CUSHING CAMPUS, BROCKTON, MASSACHUSETTS, p. A203
GOOD SAMARITAN REGIONAL HEALTH CENTER, MOUNT VERNON, IL, p. A131
GOOD SAMARITAN REGIONAL MEDICAL CENTER, POTTSVILLE, PA, p. A370
GOOD SAMARITAN REGIONAL MEDICAL CENTER, PHOENIX, AZ, p. A24
GOOD SHEPHERD HOSPITAL, BARRINGTON, IL, p. A119
GOOD SHEPHERD MEDICAL CENTER, LONGVIEW, TX, p. A422
GOOD SHEPHERD MEDICAL CENTER, HERMISTON, OR, p. A351
GOOD SHEPHERD REHABILITATION HOSPITAL, ALLENTOWN, PA, p. A355
GOODALL-WITCHER HEALTHCARE, CLIFTON, TX, p. A406
GOODING COUNTY MEMORIAL HOSPITAL, GOODING, ID, p. A116
GOODLAND REGIONAL MEDICAL CENTER, GOODLAND, KS, p. A161
GORDON HOSPITAL, CALHOUN, GA, p. A102
GORDON MEMORIAL HOSPITAL DISTRICT, GORDON, NE, p. A263
GOSHEN GENERAL HOSPITAL, GOSHEN, IN, p. A140
GOTHENBURG MEMORIAL HOSPITAL, GOTHENBURG, NE, p. A263
GOTTLIEB MEMORIAL HOSPITAL, MELROSE PARK, IL, p. A130
GOVE COUNTY MEDICAL CENTER, QUINTER, KS, p. A167
GOVERNOR JUAN F. LOUIS HOSPITAL, CHRISTIANSTED, VI, p. A484
GRACE COTTAGE HOSPITAL, TOWNSHEND, VT, p. A441
GRACE HOSPITAL, MORGANTON, NC, p. A316
GRACE HOSPITAL, CLEVELAND, OH, p. A328
GRACEVILLE HEALTH CENTER, GRACEVILLE, MN, p. A228
GRACEWOOD STATE SCHOOL AND HOSPITAL, GRACEWOOD, GA, p. A105
GRACIE SQUARE HOSPITAL, NEW YORK, NY, p. A296
GRADUATE HOSPITAL, PHILADELPHIA, PA, p. A367
GRADY GENERAL HOSPITAL, CAIRO, GA, p. A102
GRADY MEMORIAL HOSPITAL, ATLANTA, GA, p. A100
GRADY MEMORIAL HOSPITAL, DELAWARE, OH, p. A331
GRADY MEMORIAL HOSPITAL, CHICKASHA, OK, p. A342
GRAFTON CITY HOSPITAL, GRAFTON, WV, p. A461
GRAHAM COUNTY HOSPITAL, HILL CITY, KS, p. A162
GRAHAM HOSPITAL, CANTON, IL, p. A120
GRAHAM REGIONAL MEDICAL CENTER, GRAHAM, TX, p. A414
GRANADA HILLS COMMUNITY HOSPITAL, LOS ANGELES, CA, p. A47
GRAND RIVER HOSPITAL DISTRICT, RIFLE, CO, p. A72
GRAND STRAND REGIONAL MEDICAL CENTER, MYRTLE BEACH, SC, p. A382
GRAND VIEW HOSPITAL, SELLERSVILLE, PA, p. A372
GRAND VIEW HOSPITAL, IRONWOOD, MI, p. A217
GRANDE RONDE HOSPITAL, LA GRANDE, OR, p. A351
GRANDVIEW HOSPITAL AND MEDICAL CENTER, DAYTON, OHIO, p. A333
GRANDVIEW MEDICAL CENTER, JASPER, TN, p. A393
GRANITE COUNTY MEMORIAL HOSPITAL AND NURSING HOME, PHILIPSBURG, MT, p. A259
GRANITE FALLS MUNICIPAL HOSPITAL AND MANOR, GRANITE FALLS, MN, p. A228
GRANT COUNTY HEALTH CENTER, ELBOW LAKE, MN, p. A227
GRANT HOSPITAL, CHICAGO, IL, p. A121
GRANT MEMORIAL HOSPITAL, PETERSBURG, WV, p. A463
GRANT REGIONAL HEALTH CENTER, LANCASTER, WI, p. A470
GRANT/RIVERSIDE METHODIST HOSPITALS-GRANT CAMPUS, COLUMBUS, OH, p. A330
GRANT/RIVERSIDE METHODIST HOSPITALS-RIVERSIDE CAMPUS, COLUMBUS, OH, p. A330
GRANVILLE MEDICAL CENTER, OXFORD, NC, p. A316
GRAPE COMMUNITY HOSPITAL, HAMBURG, IA, p. A152
GRATIOT COMMUNITY HOSPITAL, ALMA, MI, p. A211
GRAVETTE MEDICAL CENTER HOSPITAL, GRAVETTE, AR, p. A30
GRAYDON MANOR, LEESBURG, VA, p. A445
GRAYS HARBOR COMMUNITY HOSPITAL, ABERDEEN, WA, p. A452
GREAT LAKES REHABILITATION HOSPITAL, SOUTHFIELD, MI, p. A222
GREAT PLAINS REGIONAL MEDICAL CENTER, NORTH PLATTE, NE, p. A265
GREAT PLAINS REGIONAL MEDICAL CENTER, ELK CITY, OK, p. A343
GREAT RIVER MEDICAL CENTER, WEST BURLINGTON, IA, p. A157
GREATER BALTIMORE MEDICAL CENTER, BALTIMORE, MD, p. A195

GREATER COMMUNITY HOSPITAL, CRESTON, IA, p. A150
GREATER EL MONTE COMMUNITY HOSPITAL, SOUTH EL MONTE, CA, p. A63
GREATER LAFAYETTE HEALTH SERVICE, LAFAYETTE, IN, p. A143
GREATER SOUTHEAST COMMUNITY HOSPITAL, WASHINGTON, DC, p. A79
GREELEY COUNTY HOSPITAL, TRIBUNE, KS, p. A168
GREEN OAKS HOSPITAL, DALLAS, TX, p. A409
GREENBRIER VALLEY MEDICAL CENTER, RONCEVERTE, WV, p. A464
GREENE COUNTY GENERAL HOSPITAL, LINTON, IN, p. A143
GREENE COUNTY HOSPITAL, EUTAW, AL, p. A14
GREENE COUNTY MEDICAL CENTER, JEFFERSON, IA, p. A153
GREENE COUNTY MEMORIAL HOSPITAL, WAYNESBURG, PA, p. A373
GREENE MEMORIAL HOSPITAL, XENIA, OH, p. A340
GREENFIELD AREA MEDICAL CENTER, GREENFIELD, OH, p. A332
GREENLEAF CENTER, VALDOSTA, GA, p. A111
GREENSVILLE MEMORIAL HOSPITAL, EMPORIA, VA, p. A443
GREENVIEW REGIONAL HOSPITAL, BOWLING GREEN, KY, p. A170
GREENVILLE CAMPUS, GREENVILLE, PENNSYLVANIA, p. A361
GREENVILLE HOSPITAL, JERSEY CITY, NJ, p. A277
GREENVILLE MEMORIAL HOSPITAL, GREENVILLE, SC, p. A381
GREENWICH HOSPITAL, GREENWICH, CT, p. A74
GREENWOOD COUNTY HOSPITAL, EUREKA, KS, p. A161
GREENWOOD LEFLORE HOSPITAL, GREENWOOD, MS, p. A238
GREGORY COMMUNITY HOSPITAL, GREGORY, SD, p. A386
GRENADA LAKE MEDICAL CENTER, GRENADA, MS, p. A238
GREYSTONE PARK PSYCHIATRIC HOSPITAL, GREYSTONE PARK, NJ, p. A276
GRIFFIN HOSPITAL, DERBY, CT, p. A74
GRIFFIN MEMORIAL HOSPITAL, NORMAN, OK, p. A345
GRIGGS COUNTY HOSPITAL AND NURSING HOME, COOPERSTOWN, ND, p. A321
GRIMES ST. JOSEPH HEALTH CENTER, NAVASOTA, TX, p. A425
GRINNELL REGIONAL MEDICAL CENTER, GRINNELL, IA, p. A152
GRISELL MEMORIAL HOSPITAL DISTRICT ONE, RANSOM, KS, p. A167
GRITMAN MEDICAL CENTER, MOSCOW, ID, p. A117
GROSSMONT HOSPITAL, LA MESA, CA, p. A45
GROVE HILL MEMORIAL HOSPITAL, GROVE HILL, AL, p. A15
GRUNDY COUNTY MEMORIAL HOSPITAL, GRUNDY CENTER, IA, p. A152
GUADALUPE VALLEY HOSPITAL, SEGUIN, TX, p. A430
GUAM MEMORIAL HOSPITAL AUTHORITY, TAMUNING, GU, p. A481
GULF BREEZE HOSPITAL, GULF BREEZE, FL, p. A86
GULF COAST HOSPITAL, FORT MYERS, FL, p. A85
GULF COAST MEDICAL CENTER, PANAMA CITY, FL, p. A92
GULF COAST MEDICAL CENTER, BILOXI, MS, p. A236
GULF COAST MEDICAL CENTER, WHARTON, TX, p. A434
GULF COAST TREATMENT CENTER, FORT WALTON BEACH, FL, p. A85
GULF OAKS HOSPITAL, BILOXI, MISSISSIPPI, p. A236
GULF PINES HOSPITAL, PORT SAINT JOE, FL, p. A93
GUNDERSEN LUTHERAN, LA CROSSE, WI, p. A470
GUNNISON VALLEY HOSPITAL, GUNNISON, CO, p. A71
GUNNISON VALLEY HOSPITAL, GUNNISON, UT, p. A436
GUTHRIE COUNTY HOSPITAL, GUTHRIE CENTER, IA, p. A152
GUTTENBERG MUNICIPAL HOSPITAL, GUTTENBERG, IA, p. A152
GUYAN VALLEY HOSPITAL, LOGAN, WV, p. A462
GWINNETT MEDICAL CENTER, LAWRENCEVILLE, GEORGIA, p. A106

H

H. B. MAGRUDER MEMORIAL HOSPITAL, PORT CLINTON, OH, p. A336
H. C. WATKINS MEMORIAL HOSPITAL, QUITMAN, MS, p. A242
H. DOUGLAS SINGER MENTAL HEALTH AND DEVELOPMENTAL CENTER, ROCKFORD, IL, p. A134
H. LEE MOFFITT CANCER CENTER AND RESEARCH INSTITUTE, TAMPA, FL, p. A96
H. O. DILLEY SKILLED NURSING FACILITY, p. A231
H.S.C. MEDICAL CENTER, MALVERN, AR, p. A32
HABERSHAM COUNTY MEDICAL CENTER, DEMOREST, GA, p. A104
HACKENSACK UNIVERSITY MEDICAL CENTER, HACKENSACK, NJ, p. A276
HACKETTSTOWN COMMUNITY HOSPITAL, HACKETTSTOWN, NJ, p. A276
HACKLEY HEALTH, MUSKEGON, MI, p. A219
HADLEY CAMPUS, HAYS, KANSAS, p. A162
HADLEY MEMORIAL HOSPITAL, WASHINGTON, DC, p. A79

HAHNEMANN CAMPUS, WORCESTER, MASSACHUSETTS, p. A210
HAHNEMANN UNIVERSITY HOSPITAL, PHILADELPHIA, PA, p. A367
HALE COUNTY HOSPITAL, GREENSBORO, AL, p. A15
HALE HO'OLA HAMAKUA, HONOKAA, HI, p. A112
HALE HOSPITAL, HAVERHILL, MA, p. A205
HALIFAX BEHAVIORAL SERVICES, DAYTONA BEACH, FLORIDA, p. A83
HALIFAX MEDICAL CENTER, DAYTONA BEACH, FL, p. A83
HALIFAX REGIONAL HEALTH SYSTEM, SOUTH BOSTON, VA, p. A450
HALIFAX REGIONAL MEDICAL CENTER, ROANOKE RAPIDS, NC, p. A317
HALL COUNTY HOSPITAL, MEMPHIS, TX, p. A423
HALL-BROOKE HOSPITAL, A DIVISION OF HALL-BROOKE FOUNDATION, WESTPORT, CONNECTICUT, p. A74
HALLMARK HEALTH SYSTEM, MALDEN, MA, p. A206
HALLMARK YOUTHCARE OF KANSAS CITY, KANSAS CITY, MO, p. A248
HALSTEAD HOSPITAL, HALSTEAD, KS, p. A162
HAMILTON CENTER, TERRE HAUTE, IN, p. A146
HAMILTON COUNTY HOSPITAL, SYRACUSE, KS, p. A168
HAMILTON COUNTY PUBLIC HOSPITAL, WEBSTER CITY, IA, p. A157
HAMILTON GENERAL HOSPITAL, HAMILTON, TX, p. A415
HAMILTON HOSPITAL, OLNEY, TX, p. A425
HAMILTON MEDICAL CENTER, DALTON, GA, p. A103
HAMILTON MEMORIAL HOSPITAL DISTRICT, MCLEANSBORO, IL, p. A130
HAMLIN MEMORIAL HOSPITAL, HAMLIN, TX, p. A415
HAMMOND-HENRY HOSPITAL, GENESEO, IL, p. A126
HAMOT MEDICAL CENTER, ERIE, PA, p. A360
HAMPSHIRE MEMORIAL HOSPITAL, ROMNEY, WV, p. A464
HAMPSTEAD HOSPITAL, HAMPSTEAD, NH, p. A272
HAMPTON HOSPITAL, WESTAMPTON TOWNSHIP, NJ, p. A281
HAMPTON REGIONAL MEDICAL CENTER, VARNVILLE, SC, p. A384
HANCOCK COUNTY MEMORIAL HOSPITAL, BRITT, IA, p. A148
HANCOCK MEDICAL CENTER, BAY SAINT LOUIS, MS, p. A236
HANCOCK MEMORIAL HOSPITAL, SPARTA, GA, p. A110
HANCOCK MEMORIAL HOSPITAL AND HEALTH SERVICES, GREENFIELD, IN, p. A140
HAND COUNTY MEMORIAL HOSPITAL/AVERA HEALTH, MILLER, SD, p. A387
HANFORD COMMUNITY MEDICAL CENTER, HANFORD, CA, p. A43
HANNIBAL REGIONAL HOSPITAL, HANNIBAL, MO, p. A247
HANOVER HOSPITAL, HANOVER, PA, p. A361
HANOVER HOSPITAL, HANOVER, KS, p. A162
HANS P. PETERSON MEMORIAL HOSPITAL, PHILIP, SD, p. A387
HANSFORD HOSPITAL, SPEARMAN, TX, p. A431
HARBOR BEACH COMMUNITY HOSPITAL, HARBOR BEACH, MI, p. A216
HARBOR HOSPITAL CENTER, BALTIMORE, MD, p. A195
HARBOR OAKS HOSPITAL, NEW BALTIMORE, MI, p. A220
HARBOR VIEW MERCY HOSPITAL, FORT SMITH, AR, p. A30
HARBORVIEW MEDICAL CENTER, SEATTLE, WA, p. A456
HARDEMAN COUNTY MEMORIAL HOSPITAL, QUANAH, TX, p. A427
HARDIN COUNTY GENERAL HOSPITAL, ROSICLARE, IL, p. A134
HARDIN COUNTY GENERAL HOSPITAL, SAVANNAH, TN, p. A399
HARDIN MEMORIAL HOSPITAL, KENTON, OH, p. A333
HARDIN MEMORIAL HOSPITAL, ELIZABETHTOWN, KY, p. A171
HARDTNER MEDICAL CENTER, OLLA, LA, p. A187
HARDY WILSON MEMORIAL HOSPITAL, HAZLEHURST, MS, p. A238
HARFORD MEMORIAL HOSPITAL, HAVRE DE GRACE, MD, p. A199
HARLAN ARH HOSPITAL, HARLAN, KY, p. A172
HARLAN COUNTY HEALTH SYSTEM, ALMA, NE, p. A261
HARLEM GENERAL CARE UNIT AND HARLEM PSYCHIATRIC UNIT, p. A296
HARLEM HOSPITAL CENTER, NEW YORK, NY, p. A296
HARMON MEMORIAL HOSPITAL, HOLLIS, OK, p. A344
HARMS MEMORIAL HOSPITAL DISTRICT, AMERICAN FALLS, ID, p. A115
HARNEY DISTRICT HOSPITAL, BURNS, OR, p. A350
HARPER COUNTY COMMUNITY HOSPITAL, BUFFALO, OK, p. A342
HARPER HOSPITAL, DETROIT, MI, p. A
HARPER HOSPITAL, DETROIT, MI, p. A213
HARRINGTON MEMORIAL HOSPITAL, SOUTHBRIDGE, MA, p. A208
HARRIS CONTINUED CARE HOSPITAL, FORT WORTH, TX, p. A412
HARRIS COUNTY HOSPITAL DISTRICT, HOUSTON, TX, p. A416
HARRIS COUNTY PSYCHIATRIC CENTER, HOUSTON, TX, p. A416
HARRIS HOSPITAL, NEWPORT, AR, p. A32

Index of Hospitals / HI–Desert Medical Center

HARRIS METHODIST FORT WORTH, FORT WORTH, TX, p. A412
HARRIS METHODIST NORTHWEST, AZLE, TX, p. A403
HARRIS METHODIST SOUTHWEST, FORT WORTH, TX, p. A413
HARRIS METHODIST-ERATH COUNTY, STEPHENVILLE, TX, p. A431
HARRIS METHODIST-HEB, BEDFORD, TX, p. A404
HARRIS METHODIST-SPRINGWOOD, BEDFORD, TEXAS, p. A404
HARRIS REGIONAL HOSPITAL, SYLVA, NC, p. A318
HARRISBURG MEDICAL CENTER, HARRISBURG, IL, p. A127
HARRISBURG STATE HOSPITAL, HARRISBURG, PA, p. A361
HARRISON COMMUNITY HOSPITAL, CADIZ, OH, p. A326
HARRISON COUNTY COMMUNITY HOSPITAL, BETHANY, MO, p. A244
HARRISON COUNTY HOSPITAL, CORYDON, IN, p. A138
HARRISON MEMORIAL HOSPITAL, CYNTHIANA, KY, p. A171
HARRISON MEMORIAL HOSPITAL, BREMERTON, WA, p. A452
HARRY S. TRUMAN MEMORIAL VETERANS HOSPITAL, COLUMBIA, MO, p. A245
HART COUNTY HOSPITAL, HARTWELL, GA, p. A105
HARTFORD HOSPITAL, HARTFORD, CT, p. A75
HARTFORD MEMORIAL HOSPITAL, HARTFORD, WI, p. A469
HARTGROVE HOSPITAL, CHICAGO, IL, p. A121
HARTON REGIONAL MEDICAL CENTER, TULLAHOMA, TN, p. A400
HARTSELLE MEDICAL CENTER, HARTSELLE, AL, p. A15
HARVARD MEMORIAL HOSPITAL, HARVARD, IL, p. A127
HASKELL COUNTY HEALTHCARE SYSTEM, STIGLER, OK, p. A347
HASKELL MEMORIAL HOSPITAL, HASKELL, TX, p. A415
HASTINGS REGIONAL CENTER, HASTINGS, NE, p. A263
HAVASU REGIONAL MEDICAL CENTER, LAKE HAVASU CITY, AZ, p. A23
HAVENWYCK HOSPITAL, AUBURN HILLS, MI, p. A211
HAWAII STATE HOSPITAL, KANEOHE, HI, p. A113
HAWARDEN COMMUNITY HOSPITAL, HAWARDEN, IA, p. A152
HAWKINS COUNTY MEMORIAL HOSPITAL, ROGERSVILLE, TN, p. A399
HAWTHORN CENTER, NORTHVILLE, MI, p. A220
HAWTHORNE HOSPITAL, LOS ANGELES, CALIFORNIA, p. A48
HAXTUN HOSPITAL DISTRICT, HAXTUN, CO, p. A71
HAYES-GREEN-BEACH MEMORIAL HOSPITAL, CHARLOTTE, MI, p. A212
HAYS MEDICAL CENTER, HAYS, KS, p. A162
HAYWARD AREA MEMORIAL HOSPITAL AND NURSING HOME, HAYWARD, WI, p. A469
HAYWOOD REGIONAL MEDICAL CENTER, CLYDE, NC, p. A311
HAZEL HAWKINS CONVALESCENT HOSPITAL-SOUTHSIDE, HOLLISTER, CALIFORNIA, p. A44
HAZEL HAWKINS MEMORIAL HOSPITAL, HOLLISTER, CA, p. A44
HAZLETON GENERAL HOSPITAL, HAZLETON, PA, p. A361
HAZLETON-ST. JOSEPH MEDICAL CENTER, HAZLETON, PA, p. A361
HEALDSBURG GENERAL HOSPITAL, HEALDSBURG, CA, p. A43
HEALTH ALLIANCE HOSPITALS, LEOMINSTER, MA, p. A205
HEALTH ALLIANCE-BURBANK HOSPITAL, FITCHBURG, MASSACHUSETTS, p. A205
HEALTH CENTRAL, OCOEE, FL, p. A91
HEALTH FIRST/CAPE CANAVERAL HOSPITAL, COCOA BEACH, FL, p. A82
HEALTHMARK REGIONAL MEDICAL CENTER, DE FUNIAK SPRINGS, FL, p. A83
HEALTHPARK, OWENSBORO, KENTUCKY, p. A177
HEALTHSOURCE SAGINAW, SAGINAW, MI, p. A221
HEALTHSOUTH BAKERSFIELD REHABILITATION HOSPITAL, BAKERSFIELD, CA, p. A36
HEALTHSOUTH BRAINTREE REHABILITATION HOSPITAL, BRAINTREE, MA, p. A203
HEALTHSOUTH CENTRAL GEORGIA REHABILITATION HOSPITAL, MACON, GA, p. A107
HEALTHSOUTH CHATTANOOGA REHABILITATION HOSPITAL, CHATTANOOGA, TN, p. A391
HEALTHSOUTH CHESAPEAKE REHABILITATION HOSPITAL, SALISBURY, MD, p. A200
HEALTHSOUTH DOCTORS' HOSPITAL, CORAL GABLES, FL, p. A83
HEALTHSOUTH GREATER PITTSBURGH REHABILITATION HOSPITAL, MONROEVILLE, PA, p. A364
HEALTHSOUTH HARMARVILLE REHABILITATION HOSPITAL, PITTSBURGH, PA, p. A369
HEALTHSOUTH HOUSTON REHABILITATION INSTITUTE, HOUSTON, TX, p. A417
HEALTHSOUTH HUNTINGTON REHABILITATION HOSPITAL, HUNTINGTON, WV, p. A462
HEALTHSOUTH LAKE ERIE INSTITUTE OF REHABILITATION, ERIE, PA, p. A360
HEALTHSOUTH LAKESHORE REHABILITATION HOSPITAL, BIRMINGHAM, AL, p. A12
HEALTHSOUTH MEDICAL CENTER, RICHMOND, VA, p. A448
HEALTHSOUTH MEDICAL CENTER, BIRMINGHAM, AL, p. A12
HEALTHSOUTH MEDICAL CENTER, DALLAS, TX, p. A409
HEALTHSOUTH MERIDIAN POINT REHABILITATION HOSPITAL, SCOTTSDALE, AZ, p. A25
HEALTHSOUTH METRO WEST HOSPITAL, FAIRFIELD, AL, p. A14
HEALTHSOUTH MOUNTAINVIEW REGIONAL REHABILITATION HOSPITAL, MORGANTOWN, WV, p. A463
HEALTHSOUTH NEW ENGLAND REHABILITATION HOSPITAL, WOBURN, MA, p. A210
HEALTHSOUTH NITTANY VALLEY REHABILITATION HOSPITAL, PLEASANT GAP, PA, p. A370
HEALTHSOUTH NORTH LOUISIANA REHABILITATION HOSPITAL, RUSTON, LA, p. A188
HEALTHSOUTH NORTHERN KENTUCKY REHABILITATION HOSPITAL, COVINGTON, KY, p. A171
HEALTHSOUTH PLANO REHABILITATION HOSPITAL, PLANO, TX, p. A426
HEALTHSOUTH READING REHABILITATION HOSPITAL, READING, PA, p. A371
HEALTHSOUTH REHABILITATION CENTER, ALBUQUERQUE, NM, p. A283
HEALTHSOUTH REHABILITATION HOSPITAL, CONCORD, NH, p. A271
HEALTHSOUTH REHABILITATION HOSPITAL, SEWICKLEY, PA, p. A372
HEALTHSOUTH REHABILITATION HOSPITAL, COLUMBIA, SC, p. A379
HEALTHSOUTH REHABILITATION HOSPITAL, FLORENCE, SC, p. A381
HEALTHSOUTH REHABILITATION HOSPITAL, LARGO, FL, p. A88
HEALTHSOUTH REHABILITATION HOSPITAL, MIAMI, FL, p. A89
HEALTHSOUTH REHABILITATION HOSPITAL, KINGSPORT, TN, p. A394
HEALTHSOUTH REHABILITATION HOSPITAL, MEMPHIS, TN, p. A396
HEALTHSOUTH REHABILITATION HOSPITAL, FAYETTEVILLE, AR, p. A29
HEALTHSOUTH REHABILITATION HOSPITAL, OKLAHOMA CITY, OK, p. A345
HEALTHSOUTH REHABILITATION HOSPITAL, HUMBLE, TX, p. A419
HEALTHSOUTH REHABILITATION HOSPITAL OF ALTOONA, ALTOONA, PA, p. A355
HEALTHSOUTH REHABILITATION HOSPITAL OF ARLINGTON, ARLINGTON, TX, p. A402
HEALTHSOUTH REHABILITATION HOSPITAL OF AUSTIN, AUSTIN, TX, p. A403
HEALTHSOUTH REHABILITATION HOSPITAL OF BATON ROUGE, BATON ROUGE, LA, p. A180
HEALTHSOUTH REHABILITATION HOSPITAL OF BEAUMONT, BEAUMONT, TX, p. A404
HEALTHSOUTH REHABILITATION HOSPITAL OF CENTRAL KENTUCKY, ELIZABETHTOWN, KY, p. A171
HEALTHSOUTH REHABILITATION HOSPITAL OF ERIE, ERIE, PA, p. A360
HEALTHSOUTH REHABILITATION HOSPITAL OF FORT SMITH, FORT SMITH, AR, p. A30
HEALTHSOUTH REHABILITATION HOSPITAL OF FORT WORTH, FORT WORTH, TX, p. A413
HEALTHSOUTH REHABILITATION HOSPITAL OF JONESBORO, JONESBORO, AR, p. A30
HEALTHSOUTH REHABILITATION HOSPITAL OF KOKOMO, KOKOMO, IN, p. A142
HEALTHSOUTH REHABILITATION HOSPITAL OF MONTGOMERY, MONTGOMERY, AL, p. A17
HEALTHSOUTH REHABILITATION HOSPITAL OF NEW JERSEY, TOMS RIVER, NJ, p. A281
HEALTHSOUTH REHABILITATION HOSPITAL OF NORTH ALABAMA, HUNTSVILLE, AL, p. A15
HEALTHSOUTH REHABILITATION HOSPITAL OF SARASOTA, SARASOTA, FL, p. A95
HEALTHSOUTH REHABILITATION HOSPITAL OF TALLAHASSEE, TALLAHASSEE, FL, p. A96
HEALTHSOUTH REHABILITATION HOSPITAL OF TEXARKANA, TEXARKANA, TX, p. A432
HEALTHSOUTH REHABILITATION HOSPITAL OF UTAH, SANDY, UT, p. A439
HEALTHSOUTH REHABILITATION HOSPITAL OF VIRGINIA, RICHMOND, VA, p. A449
HEALTHSOUTH REHABILITATION HOSPITAL OF WESTERN MASSACHUSETTS, LUDLOW, MA, p. A206
HEALTHSOUTH REHABILITATION HOSPITAL OF YORK, YORK, PA, p. A375
HEALTHSOUTH REHABILITATION HOSPITAL-CITYVIEW, FORT WORTH, TX, p. A413
HEALTHSOUTH REHABILITATION HOSPITAL-TYLER, TYLER, TX, p. A433
HEALTHSOUTH REHABILITATION HOSPITAL-WICHITA FALLS, WICHITA FALLS, TX, p. A434
HEALTHSOUTH REHABILITATION INSTITUTE OF SAN ANTONIO, SAN ANTONIO, TX, p. A428
HEALTHSOUTH REHABILITATION INSTITUTE OF TUCSON, TUCSON, AZ, p. A26
HEALTHSOUTH REHABILITATION OF MECHANICSBURG, MECHANICSBURG, PA, p. A364
HEALTHSOUTH SEA PINES REHABILITATION HOSPITAL, MELBOURNE, FL, p. A89
HEALTHSOUTH SOUTHERN HILLS REHABILITATION HOSPITAL, PRINCETON, WV, p. A464
HEALTHSOUTH SUNRISE REHABILITATION HOSPITAL, FORT LAUDERDALE, FL, p. A84
HEALTHSOUTH TREASURE COAST REHABILITATION HOSPITAL, VERO BEACH, FL, p. A97
HEALTHSOUTH TRI-STATE REHABILITATION HOSPITAL, EVANSVILLE, IN, p. A139
HEALTHSOUTH VALLEY OF THE SUN REHABILITATION HOSPITAL, GLENDALE, AZ, p. A23
HEALTHSOUTH WESTERN HILLS REGIONAL REHABILITATION HOSPITAL, PARKERSBURG, WV, p. A463
HEART OF AMERICA MEDICAL CENTER, RUGBY, ND, p. A324
HEART OF FLORIDA BEHAVIORAL CENTER, LAKELAND, FL, p. A88
HEART OF FLORIDA REGIONAL MEDICAL CENTER, DAVENPORT, FL, p. A83
HEART OF TEXAS MEMORIAL HOSPITAL, BRADY, TX, p. A405
HEART OF THE ROCKIES REGIONAL MEDICAL CENTER, SALIDA, CO, p. A72
HEARTLAND BEHAVIORAL HEALTH SERVICES, NEVADA, MO, p. A251
HEARTLAND HOSPITAL EAST, SAINT JOSEPH, MISSOURI, p. A252
HEARTLAND HOSPITAL WEST, SAINT JOSEPH, MISSOURI, p. A252
HEARTLAND REGIONAL MEDICAL CENTER, SAINT JOSEPH, MO, p. A252
HEATHER HILL HOSPITAL, HEALTH AND CARE CENTER, CHARDON, OH, p. A327
HEBER VALLEY MEDICAL CENTER, HEBER CITY, UT, p. A436
HEBREW HOME AND HOSPITAL, WEST HARTFORD, CT, p. A77
HEBREW REHABILITATION CENTER FOR AGED, BOSTON, MA, p. A202
HEDRICK MEDICAL CENTER, CHILLICOTHE, MO, p. A245
HEGG MEMORIAL HEALTH CENTER/AVERA HEALTH, ROCK VALLEY, IA, p. A156
HELEN ELLIS MEMORIAL HOSPITAL, TARPON SPRINGS, FL, p. A97
HELEN HAYES HOSPITAL, WEST HAVERSTRAW, NY, p. A307
HELEN KELLER HOSPITAL, SHEFFIELD, AL, p. A18
HELEN NEWBERRY JOY HOSPITAL, NEWBERRY, MI, p. A220
HELEN NEWBERRY JOY HOSPITAL ANNEX, p. A220
HELENA REGIONAL MEDICAL CENTER, HELENA, AR, p. A30
HEMET VALLEY MEDICAL CENTER, HEMET, CA, p. A44
HEMPHILL COUNTY HOSPITAL, CANADIAN, TX, p. A406
HENDERSON HEALTH CARE SERVICES, HENDERSON, NE, p. A263
HENDERSON MEMORIAL HOSPITAL, HENDERSON, TX, p. A415
HENDERSONVILLE HOSPITAL, HENDERSONVILLE, TN, p. A393
HENDRICK HEALTH SYSTEM, ABILENE, TX, p. A401
HENDRICKS COMMUNITY HOSPITAL, DANVILLE, IN, p. A139
HENDRICKS COMMUNITY HOSPITAL, HENDRICKS, MN, p. A229
HENDRY REGIONAL MEDICAL CENTER, CLEWISTON, FL, p. A82
HENNEPIN COUNTY MEDICAL CENTER, MINNEAPOLIS, MN, p. A230
HENRICO DOCTORS' HOSPITAL, RICHMOND, VA, p. A449
HENRIETTA D. GOODALL HOSPITAL, SANFORD, ME, p. A194
HENRY COUNTY HEALTH CENTER, MOUNT PLEASANT, IA, p. A154
HENRY COUNTY HOSPITAL, NAPOLEON, OH, p. A335
HENRY COUNTY MEDICAL CENTER, PARIS, TN, p. A398
HENRY COUNTY MEMORIAL HOSPITAL, NEW CASTLE, IN, p. A144
HENRY FORD HOSPITAL, DETROIT, MI, p. A213
HENRY FORD KINGSWOOD HOSPITAL, FERNDALE, MI, p. A214
HENRY FORD WYANDOTTE HOSPITAL, WYANDOTTE, MI, p. A224
HENRY MAYO NEWHALL MEMORIAL HOSPITAL, VALENCIA, CA, p. A66
HENRY MEDICAL CENTER, STOCKBRIDGE, GA, p. A110
HENRYETTA MEDICAL CENTER, HENRYETTA, OK, p. A344
HEPBURN MEDICAL CENTER, OGDENSBURG, NY, p. A301
HEREFORD REGIONAL MEDICAL CENTER, HEREFORD, TX, p. A415
HERINGTON MUNICIPAL HOSPITAL, HERINGTON, KS, p. A162
HERITAGE HOSPITAL, TARBORO, NC, p. A318
HERMANN AREA DISTRICT HOSPITAL, HERMANN, MO, p. A247
HERMANN HOSPITAL, HOUSTON, TX, p. A417
HERRICK MEMORIAL HOSPITAL, LENAWEE HEALTH ALLIANCE, TECUMSEH, MI, p. A223
HERRIN HOSPITAL, HERRIN, IL, p. A127
HEYWOOD HOSPITAL, GARDNER, MA, p. A205
HI-DESERT MEDICAL CENTER, JOSHUA TREE, CA, p. A44

© 2000 AHA Guide   Index of Hospitals   **A497**

Index of Hospitals / HI–Plains Hospital

HI-PLAINS HOSPITAL, HALE CENTER, TX, p. A415
HIALEAH HOSPITAL, HIALEAH, FL, p. A86
HIAWATHA COMMUNITY HOSPITAL, HIAWATHA, KS, p. A162
HIGGINS GENERAL HOSPITAL, BREMEN, GA, p. A101
HIGH POINT REGIONAL HEALTH SYSTEM, HIGH POINT, NC, p. A314
HIGH POINTE, OKLAHOMA CITY, OK, p. A
HIGHLAND DISTRICT HOSPITAL, HILLSBORO, OH, p. A333
HIGHLAND HOSPITAL, CHARLESTON, WV, p. A460
HIGHLAND HOSPITAL, SHREVEPORT, LA, p. A188
HIGHLAND HOSPITAL OF ROCHESTER, ROCHESTER, NY, p. A303
HIGHLAND MEDICAL CENTER, LUBBOCK, TX, p. A422
HIGHLAND PARK HOSPITAL, MIAMI, FLORIDA, p. A89
HIGHLAND PARK HOSPITAL, HIGHLAND PARK, ILLINOIS, p. A126
HIGHLAND RIDGE HOSPITAL, MIDVALE, UT, p. A437
HIGHLANDS HOSPITAL, CONNELLSVILLE, PA, p. A358
HIGHLANDS REGIONAL MEDICAL CENTER, SEBRING, FL, p. A95
HIGHLANDS REGIONAL MEDICAL CENTER, PRESTONSBURG, KY, p. A178
HIGHLANDS–CASHIERS HOSPITAL, HIGHLANDS, NC, p. A314
HIGHLINE COMMUNITY HOSPITAL, SEATTLE, WA, p. A456
HIGHLINE SPECIALTY CENTER, 12844 MILITARY ROAD FORK, TUKWILA, ZIP 98168; MARK BENEDUM, ADMINISTRATOR, p. A456
HIGHSMITH–RAINEY MEMORIAL HOSPITAL, FAYETTEVILLE, NC, p. A312
HILL COUNTRY MEMORIAL HOSPITAL, FREDERICKSBURG, TX, p. A413
HILL CREST BEHAVIORAL HEALTH SERVICES, BIRMINGHAM, AL, p. A12
HILL REGIONAL HOSPITAL, HILLSBORO, TX, p. A415
HILLCREST BAPTIST MEDICAL CENTER, WACO, TX, p. A434
HILLCREST HEALTH CENTER, OKLAHOMA CITY, OK, p. A345
HILLCREST HOSPITAL, PITTSFIELD, MASSACHUSETTS, p. A207
HILLCREST HOSPITAL, SIMPSONVILLE, SC, p. A383
HILLCREST HOSPITAL, CALHOUN CITY, MS, p. A237
HILLCREST MEDICAL CENTER, TULSA, OK, p. A348
HILLCREST MEDICAL CENTER AT WEST, WEST, TX, p. A434
HILLCREST SPECIALTY HOSPITAL, TULSA, OK, p. A348
HILLS AND DALES GENERAL HOSPITAL, CASS CITY, MI, p. A212
HILLSBORO AREA HOSPITAL, HILLSBORO, IL, p. A128
HILLSBORO COMMUNITY MEDICAL CENTER, HILLSBORO, KS, p. A162
HILLSBORO MEDICAL CENTER, HILLSBORO, ND, p. A322
HILLSDALE COMMUNITY HEALTH CENTER, HILLSDALE, MI, p. A217
HILLSIDE HOSPITAL, NEW YORK, NEW YORK, p. A297
HILLSIDE HOSPITAL, ATLANTA, GA, p. A100
HILLSIDE HOSPITAL, PULASKI, TN, p. A399
HILLSIDE REHABILITATION HOSPITAL, WARREN, OH, p. A339
HILO MEDICAL CENTER, HILO, HI, p. A112
HILTON HEAD MEDICAL CENTER AND CLINICS, HILTON HEAD ISLAND, SC, p. A382
HINSDALE HOSPITAL, HINSDALE, IL, p. A128
HOAG MEMORIAL HOSPITAL PRESBYTERIAN, NEWPORT BEACH, CA, p. A53
HOCKING VALLEY COMMUNITY HOSPITAL, LOGAN, OH, p. A334
HODGEMAN COUNTY HEALTH CENTER, JETMORE, KS, p. A163
HOLDENVILLE GENERAL HOSPITAL, HOLDENVILLE, OK, p. A344
HOLLAND COMMUNITY HOSPITAL, HOLLAND, MI, p. A217
HOLLISWOOD HOSPITAL, NEW YORK, NY, p. A297
HOLLY HILL/ CHARTER BEHAVIORAL HEALTH SYSTEM, RALEIGH, NC, p. A316
HOLLYWOOD COMMUNITY HOSPITAL OF HOLLYWOOD, LOS ANGELES, CA, p. A47
HOLLYWOOD COMMUNITY HOSPITAL OF VAN NUYS, LOS ANGELES, CALIFORNIA, p. A47
HOLLYWOOD MEDICAL CENTER, LOS ANGELES, FL, p. A86
HOLLYWOOD PAVILION, LOS ANGELES, FL, p. A86
HOLMES REGIONAL MEDICAL CENTER, MELBOURNE, FL, p. A89
HOLTON COMMUNITY HOSPITAL, HOLTON, KS, p. A162
HOLY CROSS HOSPITAL, FORT LAUDERDALE, FL, p. A84
HOLY CROSS HOSPITAL, CHICAGO, IL, p. A121
HOLY CROSS HOSPITAL, TAOS, NM, p. A286
HOLY CROSS HOSPITAL OF SILVER SPRING, SILVER SPRING, MD, p. A200
HOLY FAMILY HOME, NEW YORK, NEW YORK, p. A296
HOLY FAMILY HOSPITAL, NEW RICHMOND, WI, p. A473
HOLY FAMILY HOSPITAL, SPOKANE, WA, p. A457
HOLY FAMILY HOSPITAL AND MEDICAL CENTER, METHUEN, MA, p. A206
HOLY FAMILY MEDICAL CENTER, DES PLAINES, IL, p. A125
HOLY FAMILY MEMORIAL MEDICAL CENTER, MANITOWOC, WI, p. A470
HOLY INFANT HOSPITAL, HOVEN, SD, p. A386
HOLY NAME HOSPITAL, TEANECK, NJ, p. A280

HOLY REDEEMER HOSPITAL AND MEDICAL CENTER, MEADOWBROOK, PA, p. A364
HOLY ROSARY HEALTH CENTER, MILES CITY, MT, p. A258
HOLY ROSARY MEDICAL CENTER, ONTARIO, OR, p. A352
HOLY SPIRIT HEALTH SYSTEM, CAMP HILL, PA, p. A357
HOLYOKE HOSPITAL, HOLYOKE, MA, p. A205
HOLZER MEDICAL CENTER, GALLIPOLIS, OH, p. A332
HOMER MEMORIAL HOSPITAL, HOMER, LA, p. A183
HOMESTEAD HOSPITAL, HOMESTEAD, FL, p. A86
HOOD MEMORIAL HOSPITAL, AMITE, LA, p. A180
HOOPESTON COMMUNITY MEMORIAL HOSPITAL, HOOPESTON, IL, p. A128
HOOTS MEMORIAL HOSPITAL, YADKINVILLE, NC, p. A320
HOPE CHILDREN'S HOSPITAL, p. A131
HOPE HOSPITAL, LOCKHART, SC, p. A382
HOPEDALE MEDICAL COMPLEX, HOPEDALE, IL, p. A128
HOPKINS COUNTY MEMORIAL HOSPITAL, SULPHUR SPRINGS, TX, p. A431
HORIZON MEDICAL CENTER, DICKSON, TN, p. A392
HORN MEMORIAL HOSPITAL, IDA GROVE, IA, p. A153
HORSHAM CLINIC, AMBLER, PA, p. A355
HORTON MEDICAL CENTER, MIDDLETOWN, NY, p. A294
HOSPICE OF NORTHERN VIRGINIA, FALLS CHURCH, VA, p. A443
HOSPICE OF PALM BEACH COUNTY, WEST PALM BEACH, FL, p. A97
HOSPITAL CENTER AT ORANGE, ORANGE, NJ, p. A279
HOSPITAL DE DAMAS, PONCE, PR, p. A483
HOSPITAL DE LA CONCEPCION, SAN GERMAN, PR, p. A483
HOSPITAL DEL MAESTRO, SAN JUAN, PR, p. A483
HOSPITAL DISTRICT NUMBER FIVE OF HARPER COUNTY, HARPER, KS, p. A162
HOSPITAL DISTRICT NUMBER SIX OF HARPER COUNTY, ANTHONY, KS, p. A159
HOSPITAL DOCTOR GUBERN, FAJARDO, PR, p. A482
HOSPITAL DR. DOMINGUEZ, HUMACAO, PR, p. A482
HOSPITAL DR. FEDERICO TRILLA, CAROLINA, PR, p. A482
HOSPITAL DR. SUSONI, ARECIBO, PR, p. A481
HOSPITAL EL BUEN PASTOR, ARECIBO, PR, p. A481
HOSPITAL EPISCOPAL CRISTO REDENTOR, GUAYAMA, PR, p. A482
HOSPITAL EPISCOPAL SAN LUCAS, PONCE, PR, p. A483
HOSPITAL FOR JOINT DISEASES ORTHOPAEDIC INSTITUTE, NEW YORK, NY, p. A297
HOSPITAL FOR SICK CHILDREN, WASHINGTON, DC, p. A79
HOSPITAL FOR SPECIAL CARE, NEW BRITAIN, CT, p. A75
HOSPITAL FOR SPECIAL SURGERY, NEW YORK, NY, p. A297
HOSPITAL HERMANOS MELENDEZ, BAYAMON, PR, p. A481
HOSPITAL INTERAMERICANO DE MEDICINA AVANZADA, CAGUAS, PR, p. A482
HOSPITAL MATILDE BRENES, BAYAMON, PR, p. A481
HOSPITAL MENONITA DE CAYEY, CAYEY, PR, p. A482
HOSPITAL METROPOLITAN, SAN JUAN, PR, p. A483
HOSPITAL OF SAINT RAPHAEL, NEW HAVEN, CT, p. A76
HOSPITAL OF THE UNIVERSITY OF PENNSYLVANIA, PHILADELPHIA, PA, p. A367
HOSPITAL ONCOLOGICO ANDRES GRILLASCA, PONCE, PR, p. A483
HOSPITAL PAVIA–HATO REY, SAN JUAN, PR, p. A483
HOSPITAL PAVIA–SANTURCE, SAN JUAN, PR, p. A483
HOSPITAL PEREA, MAYAGUEZ, PR, p. A483
HOSPITAL SAN FRANCISCO, RIO PIEDRAS, PR, p. A484
HOSPITAL SAN PABLO, BAYAMON, PR, p. A482
HOSPITAL SAN PABLO DEL ESTE, FAJARDO, PR, p. A482
HOSPITAL SANTA ROSA, GUAYAMA, PR, p. A482
HOSPITAL SUB–REGIONAL DR. VICTOR R. NUNEZ, HUMACAO, PR, p. A482
HOSPITAL UNIVERSITARIO DR. RAMON RUIZ ARNAU, BAYAMON, PR, p. A482
HOT SPRINGS COUNTY MEMORIAL HOSPITAL, THERMOPOLIS, WY, p. A480
HOULTON REGIONAL HOSPITAL, HOULTON, ME, p. A192
HOUSTON MEDICAL CENTER, WARNER ROBINS, GA, p. A111
HOUSTON NORTHWEST MEDICAL CENTER, HOUSTON, TX, p. A417
HOWARD COMMUNITY HOSPITAL, KOKOMO, IN, p. A142
HOWARD COUNTY COMMUNITY HOSPITAL, SAINT PAUL, NE, p. A266
HOWARD COUNTY GENERAL HOSPITAL, COLUMBIA, MD, p. A197
HOWARD MEMORIAL HOSPITAL, NASHVILLE, AR, p. A32
HOWARD UNIVERSITY HOSPITAL, WASHINGTON, DC, p. A79
HOWARD YOUNG MEDICAL CENTER, WOODRUFF, WI, p. A477
HUBBARD REGIONAL HOSPITAL, WEBSTER, MA, p. A209
HUDSON MEDICAL CENTER, HUDSON, WI, p. A469
HUDSON RIVER PSYCHIATRIC CENTER, POUGHKEEPSIE, NY, p. A303
HUDSON VALLEY HOSPITAL CENTER, CORTLANDT MANOR, NY, p. A290
HUERFANO MEDICAL CENTER, WALSENBURG, CO, p. A73
HUEY P. LONG MEDICAL CENTER, PINEVILLE, LA, p. A188

HUGGINS HOSPITAL, WOLFEBORO, NH, p. A273
HUGH CHATHAM MEMORIAL HOSPITAL, ELKIN, NC, p. A312
HUGHSTON SPORTS MEDICINE HOSPITAL, COLUMBUS, GA, p. A102
HUGULEY MEMORIAL MEDICAL CENTER, FORT WORTH, TX, p. A413
HUHUKAM MEMORIAL HOSPITAL, SACATON, AZ, p. A25
HUMBOLDT COUNTY MEMORIAL HOSPITAL, HUMBOLDT, IA, p. A153
HUMBOLDT GENERAL HOSPITAL, HUMBOLDT, TN, p. A393
HUMBOLDT GENERAL HOSPITAL, WINNEMUCCA, NV, p. A269
HUMPHREYS COUNTY MEMORIAL HOSPITAL, BELZONI, MS, p. A236
HUNT MEMORIAL HOSPITAL DISTRICT, GREENVILLE, TX, p. A414
HUNTER HOLMES MCGUIRE VETERANS AFFAIRS MEDICAL CENTER, RICHMOND, VA, p. A449
HUNTERDON MEDICAL CENTER, FLEMINGTON, NJ, p. A276
HUNTINGTON BEACH HOSPITAL, HUNTINGTON BEACH, CA, p. A44
HUNTINGTON EAST VALLEY HOSPITAL, GLENDORA, CA, p. A43
HUNTINGTON HOSPITAL, HUNTINGTON, NY, p. A292
HUNTINGTON MEMORIAL HOSPITAL, HUNTINGTON, IN, p. A141
HUNTINGTON MEMORIAL HOSPITAL, PASADENA, CA, p. A55
HUNTSVILLE HOSPITAL, HUNTSVILLE, AL, p. A15
HUNTSVILLE HOSPITAL EAST, HUNTSVILLE, ALABAMA, p. A15
HUNTSVILLE MEMORIAL HOSPITAL, HUNTSVILLE, TX, p. A419
HURLEY HEALTH CENTER, COALGATE, OK, p. A342
HURLEY MEDICAL CENTER, FLINT, MI, p. A215
HURON MEMORIAL HOSPITAL, BAD AXE, MI, p. A211
HURON REGIONAL MEDICAL CENTER, HURON, SD, p. A386
HURON VALLEY–SINAI HOSPITAL, COMMERCE TOWNSHIP, MI, p. A213
HURTADO HEALTH CENTER, NEW BRUNSWICK, NJ, p. A278
HUTCHESON MEDICAL CENTER, FORT OGLETHORPE, GA, p. A105
HUTCHINSON AREA HEALTH CARE, HUTCHINSON, MN, p. A229
HUTCHINSON HOSPITAL CORPORATION, HUTCHINSON, KS, p. A163
HUTZEL HOSPITAL, DETROIT, MI, p. A214

I

I. GONZALEZ MARTINEZ ONCOLOGIC HOSPITAL, HATO REY, PR, p. A484
IBERIA MEDICAL CENTER, NEW IBERIA, LA, p. A186
IDAHO ELKS REHABILITATION HOSPITAL, BOISE, ID, p. A115
IDAHO FALLS RECOVERY CENTER, IDAHO FALLS, ID, p. A116
IHS HOSPITAL AT SAN ANTONIO, SAN ANTONIO, TX, p. A428
IHS HOSPITAL OF LUBBOCK, LUBBOCK, TX, p. A422
IHS OF AMARILLO, AMARILLO, TX, p. A401
ILLINI COMMUNITY HOSPITAL, PITTSFIELD, IL, p. A133
ILLINI HOSPITAL, SILVIS, IL, p. A134
ILLINOIS MASONIC MEDICAL CENTER, CHICAGO, IL, p. A121
ILLINOIS VALLEY COMMUNITY HOSPITAL, PERU, IL, p. A133
IMMANUEL ST. JOSEPH'S–MAYO HEALTH SYSTEM, MANKATO, MN, p. A230
IMPACT DRUG AND ALCOHOL TREATMENT CENTER, PASADENA, CA, p. A55
IMPERIAL POINT MEDICAL CENTER, FORT LAUDERDALE, FL, p. A84
INDEPENDENCE REGIONAL HEALTH CENTER, INDEPENDENCE, MO, p. A247
INDIAN HEALTH SERVICE HOSPITAL, RAPID CITY, SD, p. A387
INDIAN PATH MEDICAL CENTER, KINGSPORT, TN, p. A394
INDIAN PATH PAVILION, KINGSPORT, TENNESSEE, p. A394
INDIAN RIVER MEMORIAL HOSPITAL, VERO BEACH, FL, p. A97
INDIAN VALLEY HOSPITAL DISTRICT, GREENVILLE, CA, p. A43
INDIANA HOSPITAL, INDIANA, PA, p. A362
INDIANA UNIVERSITY MEDICAL CENTER, INDIANAPOLIS, INDIANA, p. A141
INDIANHEAD MEDICAL CENTER, SHELL LAKE, WI, p. A475
INDUSTRIAL HOSPITAL, SAN JUAN, PR, p. A484
INGALLS HOSPITAL, HARVEY, IL, p. A127
INGHAM REGIONAL MEDICAL CENTER, LANSING, MI, p. A218
INGHAM REGIONAL MEDICAL CENTER, GREENLAWN CAMPUS, LANSING, MICHIGAN, p. A218
INGHAM REGIONAL MEDICAL CENTER, PENNSYLVANIA CAMPUS, LANSING, MICHIGAN, p. A218
INLAND HOSPITAL, WATERVILLE, ME, p. A194
INLAND VALLEY REGIONAL MEDICAL CENTER, WILDOMAR, CA, p. A67
INNER HARBOUR HOSPITALS, DOUGLASVILLE, GA, p. A104
INOVA ALEXANDRIA HOSPITAL, ALEXANDRIA, VA, p. A442
INOVA FAIR OAKS HOSPITAL, FAIRFAX, VA, p. A443
INOVA FAIRFAX HOSPITAL, FALLS CHURCH, VA, p. A443
INOVA MOUNT VERNON HOSPITAL, ALEXANDRIA, VA, p. A442

INSTITUTE OF LIVING, HARTFORD, CONNECTICUT, p. A75
INSTITUTE OF MENTAL HEALTH–RHODE ISLAND MEDICAL CENTER, HOWARD, RHODE ISLAND, p. A376
INTEGRATED SPECIALTY HOSPITAL, EDMOND, OK, p. A343
INTEGRATED SPECIALTY HOSPITAL, MIDWEST CITY, OK, p. A345
INTEGRIS BAPTIST MEDICAL CENTER, OKLAHOMA CITY, OK, p. A346
INTEGRIS BAPTIST REGIONAL HEALTH CENTER, MIAMI, OK, p. A345
INTEGRIS BASS BEHAVIORAL HEALTH SYSTEM, ENID, OK, p. A343
INTEGRIS BASS BAPTIST HEALTH CENTER, ENID, OK, p. A343
INTEGRIS GROVE GENERAL HOSPITAL, GROVE, OK, p. A343
INTEGRIS MENTAL HEALTH SYSTEM–SPENCER, SPENCER, OK, p. A347
INTEGRIS SOUTHWEST MEDICAL CENTER, OKLAHOMA CITY, OK, p. A346
INTER–COMMUNITY MEMORIAL HOSPITAL, NEWFANE, NY, p. A301
INTERFAITH MEDICAL CENTER, NEW YORK, NY, p. A297
INTERGRIS CLINTON REGIONAL HOSPITAL, CLINTON, OK, p. A342
INTRACARE MEDICAL CENTER HOSPITAL, HOUSTON, TX, p. A417
INTRACARE NORTH HOSPITAL, HOUSTON, TX, p. A417
IONIA COUNTY MEMORIAL HOSPITAL, IONIA, MI, p. A217
IOWA LUTHERAN HOSPITAL, DES MOINES, IA, p. A151
IOWA MEDICAL AND CLASSIFICATION CENTER, OAKDALE, IA, p. A155
IOWA METHODIST MEDICAL CENTER, DES MOINES, IA, p. A151
IRA DAVENPORT MEMORIAL HOSPITAL, BATH, NY, p. A288
IREDELL MEMORIAL HOSPITAL, STATESVILLE, NC, p. A318
IRELAND ARMY COMMUNITY HOSPITAL, FORT KNOX, KY, p. A172
IRON COUNTY COMMUNITY HOSPITAL, IRON RIVER, MI, p. A217
IROQUOIS MEMORIAL HOSPITAL AND RESIDENT HOME, WATSEKA, IL, p. A136
IRVINE REGIONAL HOSPITAL AND MEDICAL CENTER, IRVINE, CA, p. A44
IRVINGTON GENERAL HOSPITAL, IRVINGTON, NJ, p. A277
IRWIN ARMY COMMUNITY HOSPITAL, FORT RILEY, KS, p. A161
IRWIN COUNTY HOSPITAL, OCILLA, GA, p. A108
ISHAM HEALTH CENTER, ANDOVER, MA, p. A201
ISLAND HEALTH NORTHWEST, ANACORTES, WA, p. A452
ISLAND MEDICAL CENTER, HEMPSTEAD, NY, p. A292
ITASCA MEDICAL CENTER, GRAND RAPIDS, MN, p. A228
IUKA HOSPITAL, IUKA, MS, p. A239
IVINSON MEMORIAL HOSPITAL, LARAMIE, WY, p. A479

J

J. ARTHUR DOSHER MEMORIAL HOSPITAL, SOUTHPORT, NC, p. A318
J. C. BLAIR MEMORIAL HOSPITAL, HUNTINGDON, PA, p. A362
J. D. MCCARTY CENTER FOR CHILDREN WITH DEVELOPMENTAL DISABILITIES, NORMAN, OK, p. A345
J. F. K. MEDICAL CENTER, ATLANTIS, FL, p. A81
J. PAUL JONES HOSPITAL, CAMDEN, AL, p. A13
JACK D WEILER HOSPITAL OF ALBERT EINSTEIN COLLEGE OF MEDICINE, NEW YORK, NEW YORK, p. A298
JACKSON COUNTY HOSPITAL, SCOTTSBORO, AL, p. A18
JACKSON COUNTY HOSPITAL, EDNA, TX, p. A411
JACKSON COUNTY MEMORIAL HOSPITAL, ALTUS, OK, p. A341
JACKSON COUNTY PUBLIC HOSPITAL, MAQUOKETA, IA, p. A154
JACKSON GENERAL HOSPITAL, RIPLEY, WV, p. A464
JACKSON HOSPITAL, MARIANNA, FL, p. A89
JACKSON HOSPITAL AND CLINIC, MONTGOMERY, AL, p. A17
JACKSON MEDICAL CENTER, JACKSON, AL, p. A16
JACKSON MEDICAL CENTER, JACKSON, MN, p. A229
JACKSON MEMORIAL HOSPITAL, MIAMI, FL, p. A89
JACKSON PARISH HOSPITAL, JONESBORO, LA, p. A183
JACKSON PARK HOSPITAL AND MEDICAL CENTER, CHICAGO, IL, p. A122
JACKSON PURCHASE MEDICAL CENTER, MAYFIELD, KY, p. A176
JACKSON–MADISON COUNTY GENERAL HOSPITAL, JACKSON, TN, p. A393
JACKSONVILLE HOSPITAL, JACKSONVILLE, AL, p. A16
JACOBI MEDICAL CENTER, NEW YORK, NY, p. A297
JACOBSON MEMORIAL HOSPITAL CARE CENTER, ELGIN, ND, p. A322
JAMAICA HOSPITAL MEDICAL CENTER, NEW YORK, NY, p. A297
JAMES A. HALEY VETERANS HOSPITAL, TAMPA, FL, p. A96
JAMES E. VAN ZANDT VETERANS AFFAIRS MEDICAL CENTER, ALTOONA, PA, p. A355
JAMES H. QUILLEN VETERANS AFFAIRS MEDICAL CENTER, MOUNTAIN HOME, TN, p. A397
JAMES LAWRENCE KERNAN HOSPITAL, BALTIMORE, MD, p. A195
JAMESON HOSPITAL, NEW CASTLE, PA, p. A365
JAMESTOWN HOSPITAL, JAMESTOWN, ND, p. A323
JANE PHILLIPS MEDICAL CENTER, BARTLESVILLE, OK, p. A341
JANE PHILLIPS NOWATA HEALTH CENTER, NOWATA, OK, p. A345
JANE TODD CRAWFORD HOSPITAL, GREENSBURG, KY, p. A172
JASPER COUNTY HOSPITAL, RENSSELAER, IN, p. A145
JASPER COUNTY NURSING HOME, p. A236
JASPER GENERAL HOSPITAL, BAY SPRINGS, MS, p. A236
JASPER MEMORIAL HOSPITAL, MONTICELLO, GA, p. A108
JAY COUNTY HOSPITAL, PORTLAND, IN, p. A145
JAY HOSPITAL, JAY, FL, p. A87
JEANES HOSPITAL, PHILADELPHIA, PA, p. A367
JEANNETTE DISTRICT MEMORIAL HOSPITAL, JEANNETTE, PA, p. A362
JEFF ANDERSON REGIONAL MEDICAL CENTER, MERIDIAN, MS, p. A240
JEFF DAVIS HOSPITAL, HAZLEHURST, GA, p. A106
JEFFERSON COMMUNITY HEALTH CENTER, FAIRBURY, NE, p. A262
JEFFERSON COUNTY HOSPITAL, FAYETTE, MS, p. A238
JEFFERSON COUNTY HOSPITAL, FAIRFIELD, IA, p. A152
JEFFERSON COUNTY HOSPITAL, WAURIKA, OK, p. A349
JEFFERSON COUNTY MEMORIAL HOSPITAL, WINCHESTER, KS, p. A169
JEFFERSON GENERAL HOSPITAL, PORT TOWNSEND, WA, p. A455
JEFFERSON HOSPITAL, LOUISVILLE, GA, p. A106
JEFFERSON MEMORIAL HOSPITAL, RANSON, WV, p. A464
JEFFERSON MEMORIAL HOSPITAL, JEFFERSON CITY, TN, p. A393
JEFFERSON MEMORIAL HOSPITAL, CRYSTAL CITY, MO, p. A246
JEFFERSON REGIONAL MEDICAL CENTER, PINE BLUFF, AR, p. A33
JELLICO COMMUNITY HOSPITAL, JELLICO, TN, p. A394
JENKINS COMMUNITY HOSPITAL, JENKINS, KY, p. A173
JENKINS COUNTY HOSPITAL, MILLEN, GA, p. A107
JENNIE EDMUNDSON MEMORIAL HOSPITAL, COUNCIL BLUFFS, IA, p. A150
JENNIE M. MELHAM MEMORIAL MEDICAL CENTER, BROKEN BOW, NE, p. A261
JENNIE STUART MEDICAL CENTER, HOPKINSVILLE, KY, p. A173
JENNINGS AMERICAN LEGION HOSPITAL, JENNINGS, LA, p. A183
JERRY L. PETTIS MEMORIAL VETERANS MEDICAL CENTER, LOMA LINDA, CA, p. A46
JERSEY CITY MEDICAL CENTER, JERSEY CITY, NJ, p. A277
JERSEY COMMUNITY HOSPITAL, JERSEYVILLE, IL, p. A128
JERSEY SHORE HOSPITAL, JERSEY SHORE, PA, p. A362
JEWELL COUNTY HOSPITAL, MANKATO, KS, p. A164
JEWISH HOSPITAL, LOUISVILLE, KY, p. A175
JEWISH HOSPITAL KENWOOD, CINCINNATI, OH, p. A328
JEWISH HOSPITAL–SHELBYVILLE, SHELBYVILLE, KY, p. A178
JEWISH MEMORIAL HOSPITAL AND REHABILITATION CENTER, BOSTON, MA, p. A202
JFK JOHNSON REHABILITATION INSTITUTE, EDISON, NJ, p. A275
JFK MEDICAL CENTER, EDISON, NJ, p. A275
JM/MD HEALTH SYSTEM, WALNUT CREEK, CA, p. A66
JOAN GLANCY MEMORIAL HOSPITAL, DULUTH, GEORGIA, p. A106
JOE DIMAGGIO CHILDREN'S HOSPITAL, p. A86
JOEL POMERENE MEMORIAL HOSPITAL, MILLERSBURG, OH, p. A335
JOHN AND MARY KIRBY HOSPITAL, MONTICELLO, IL, p. A131
JOHN C LINCOLN HOSPITAL–DEER VALLEY, PHOENIX, AZ, p. A24
JOHN C. FREMONT HEALTHCARE DISTRICT, MARIPOSA, CA, p. A51
JOHN C. LINCOLN HOSPITAL – NORTH MOUNTAIN, PHOENIX, AZ, p. A24
JOHN D. ARCHBOLD MEMORIAL HOSPITAL, THOMASVILLE, GA, p. A110
JOHN D. DINGELL VETERANS AFFAIRS MEDICAL CENTER, DETROIT, MI, p. A214
JOHN F. KENNEDY MEMORIAL HOSPITAL, PHILADELPHIA, PA, p. A367
JOHN F. KENNEDY MEMORIAL HOSPITAL, INDIO, CA, p. A44
JOHN HEINZ INSTITUTE OF REHABILITATION MEDICINE, WILKES-BARRE, PA, p. A374
JOHN J. MADDEN MENTAL HEALTH CENTER, HINES, IL, p. A128
JOHN J. PERSHING VETERANS AFFAIRS MEDICAL CENTER, POPLAR BLUFF, MO, p. A251
JOHN MUIR MEDICAL CENTER, WALNUT CREEK, CALIFORNIA, p. A66
JOHN PETER SMITH HOSPITAL, FORT WORTH, TEXAS, p. A413
JOHN RANDOLPH MEDICAL CENTER, HOPEWELL, VA, p. A445
JOHN T. MATHER MEMORIAL HOSPITAL, PORT JEFFERSON, NY, p. A303
JOHN UMSTEAD HOSPITAL, BUTNER, NC, p. A310
JOHNS COMMUNITY HOSPITAL, TAYLOR, TX, p. A431
JOHNS HOPKINS BAYVIEW MEDICAL CENTER, BALTIMORE, MD, p. A195
JOHNS HOPKINS HOSPITAL, BALTIMORE, MD, p. A195
JOHNSON CITY MEDICAL CENTER, JOHNSON CITY, TN, p. A394
JOHNSON CITY SPECIALTY HOSPITAL, JOHNSON CITY, TN, p. A394
JOHNSON COUNTY HEALTHCARE CENTER, BUFFALO, WY, p. A478
JOHNSON COUNTY HOSPITAL, TECUMSEH, NE, p. A267
JOHNSON MEMORIAL HEALTH SERVICES, DAWSON, MN, p. A227
JOHNSON MEMORIAL HOSPITAL, STAFFORD SPRINGS, CT, p. A77
JOHNSON MEMORIAL HOSPITAL, FRANKLIN, IN, p. A140
JOHNSON REGIONAL MEDICAL CENTER, CLARKSVILLE, AR, p. A28
JOHNSON–MATHERS NURSING HOME, p. A171
JOHNSTON MEMORIAL HOSPITAL, ABINGDON, VA, p. A442
JOHNSTON MEMORIAL HOSPITAL, SMITHFIELD, NC, p. A318
JOHNSTON MEMORIAL HOSPITAL, TISHOMINGO, OK, p. A348
JOHNSTON R. BOWMAN HEALTH CENTER, CHICAGO, ILLINOIS, p. A123
JOHNSTON–WILLIS HOSPITAL, RICHMOND, VIRGINIA, p. A448
JOINT TOWNSHIP DISTRICT MEMORIAL HOSPITAL, SAINT MARYS, OH, p. A337
JONATHAN M. WAINWRIGHT MEMORIAL VA MEDICAL CENTER, WALLA WALLA, WA, p. A458
JONES MEMORIAL HOSPITAL, WELLSVILLE, NY, p. A307
JONES REGIONAL MEDICAL CENTER, ANAMOSA, IA, p. A148
JORDAN HOSPITAL, PLYMOUTH, MA, p. A208
JORDAN VALLEY HOSPITAL, WEST JORDAN, UT, p. A439
JPS HEALTH NETWORK, FORT WORTH, TX, p. A413
JULIAN F. KEITH ALCOHOL AND DRUG ABUSE TREATMENT CENTER, BLACK MOUNTAIN, NC, p. A309
JULIETTE MANOR NURSING HOME, COMMUNITY CLINICS, p. A467
JUPITER MEDICAL CENTER, JUPITER, FL, p. A87

K

KADLEC MEDICAL CENTER, RICHLAND, WA, p. A456
KAHI MOHALA, EWA BEACH, HI, p. A112
KAHUKU HOSPITAL, KAHUKU, HI, p. A113
KAISER FOUNDATION HOSPITAL, SAN FRANCISCO, CA, p. A59
KAISER FOUNDATION HOSPITAL, SANTA ROSA, CA, p. A62
KAISER FOUNDATION HOSPITAL, LOS ANGELES, CA, p. A48
KAISER FOUNDATION HOSPITAL, FRESNO, CA, p. A42
KAISER FOUNDATION HOSPITAL, OAKLAND, CA, p. A53
KAISER FOUNDATION HOSPITAL, WALNUT CREEK, CA, p. A67
KAISER FOUNDATION HOSPITAL, MARTINEZ, CALIFORNIA, p. A67
KAISER FOUNDATION HOSPITAL, ANAHEIM, CA, p. A35
KAISER FOUNDATION HOSPITAL, BALDWIN PARK, CA, p. A36
KAISER FOUNDATION HOSPITAL, FONTANA, CA, p. A41
KAISER FOUNDATION HOSPITAL, LOS ANGELES, CA, p. A48
KAISER FOUNDATION HOSPITAL, HAYWARD, CA, p. A43
KAISER FOUNDATION HOSPITAL, SAN DIEGO, CA, p. A58
KAISER FOUNDATION HOSPITAL, EL CAJON, CALIFORNIA, p. A58
KAISER FOUNDATION HOSPITAL, REDWOOD CITY, CA, p. A56
KAISER FOUNDATION HOSPITAL, SACRAMENTO, CA, p. A57
KAISER FOUNDATION HOSPITAL, SACRAMENTO, CA, p. A57
KAISER FOUNDATION HOSPITAL, SAN RAFAEL, CA, p. A61
KAISER FOUNDATION HOSPITAL, SANTA CLARA, CA, p. A62
KAISER FOUNDATION HOSPITAL, SOUTH SAN FRANCISCO, CA, p. A64
KAISER FOUNDATION HOSPITAL, LOS ANGELES, CA, p. A48
KAISER FOUNDATION HOSPITAL, LOS ANGELES, CA, p. A48
KAISER FOUNDATION HOSPITAL, HONOLULU, HI, p. A112
KAISER FOUNDATION HOSPITAL AND REHABILITATION CENTER, VALLEJO, CA, p. A66
KAISER FOUNDATION HOSPITAL–BELLFLOWER, BELLFLOWER, CA, p. A36
KAISER FOUNDATION HOSPITAL–RIVERSIDE, RIVERSIDE, CA, p. A57
KAISER FOUNDATION HOSPITAL–WEST LOS ANGELES, LOS ANGELES, CA, p. A48
KAISER FOUNDATION MENTAL HEALTH CENTER, LOS ANGELES, CALIFORNIA, p. A48
KAISER SUNNYSIDE MEDICAL CENTER, CLACKAMAS, OR, p. A350

Index of Hospitals / Kalamazoo Regional Psychiatric Hospital

KALAMAZOO REGIONAL PSYCHIATRIC HOSPITAL, KALAMAZOO, MI, p. A218
KALISPELL REGIONAL MEDICAL CENTER, KALISPELL, MT, p. A258
KALKASKA MEMORIAL HEALTH CENTER, KALKASKA, MI, p. A218
KANABEC HOSPITAL, MORA, MN, p. A231
KANAKANAK HOSPITAL, DILLINGHAM, AK, p. A20
KANE COMMUNITY HOSPITAL, KANE, PA, p. A362
KANE COUNTY HOSPITAL, KANAB, UT, p. A436
KANSAS NEUROLOGICAL INSTITUTE, TOPEKA, KS, p. A168
KANSAS REHABILITATION HOSPITAL, TOPEKA, KS, p. A168
KAPIOLANI MEDICAL CENTER FOR WOMEN AND CHILDREN, HONOLULU, HI, p. A112
KARL AND ESTHER HOBLITZELLE MEMORIAL HOSPITAL, DALLAS, TEXAS, p. A408
KATHERINE SHAW BETHEA HOSPITAL, DIXON, IL, p. A125
KATY MEDICAL CENTER, KATY, TX, p. A420
KAU HOSPITAL, PAHALA, HI, p. A113
KAUAI VETERANS MEMORIAL HOSPITAL, WAIMEA, HI, p. A114
KAWEAH DELTA HEALTH CARE DISTRICT, VISALIA, CA, p. A66
KEARNEY COUNTY HEALTH SERVICES, MINDEN, NE, p. A264
KEARNY COUNTY HOSPITAL, LAKIN, KS, p. A163
KEEFE MEMORIAL HOSPITAL, CHEYENNE WELLS, CO, p. A68
KELL WEST REGIONAL HOSPITAL, WICHITA FALLS, TX, p. A435
KELLER ARMY COMMUNITY HOSPITAL, WEST POINT, NY, p. A307
KELSEY MEMORIAL HOSPITAL, LAKEVIEW, MICHIGAN, p. A216
KENDALL MEDICAL CENTER, MIAMI, FL, p. A89
KENMARE COMMUNITY HOSPITAL, KENMARE, ND, p. A323
KENMORE MERCY HOSPITAL, KENMORE, NY, p. A293
KENNEDY KRIEGER CHILDREN'S HOSPITAL, BALTIMORE, MD, p. A196
KENNEDY MEMORIAL HOSPITAL, STRATFORD, NEW JERSEY, p. A275
KENNEDY MEMORIAL HOSPITAL, TURNERSVILLE, NEW JERSEY, p. A275
KENNEDY MEMORIAL HOSPITALS–UNIVERSITY MEDICAL CENTER, CHERRY HILL, NJ, p. A275
KENNER REGIONAL MEDICAL CENTER, KENNER, LA, p. A183
KENNEWICK GENERAL HOSPITAL, KENNEWICK, WA, p. A454
KENOSHA HOSPITAL AND MEDICAL CENTER, KENOSHA, WI, p. A469
KENSINGTON HOSPITAL, PHILADELPHIA, PA, p. A367
KENT & QUEEN ANNE'S HOSPITAL, CHESTERTOWN, MD, p. A197
KENT COUNTY MEMORIAL HOSPITAL, WARWICK, RI, p. A377
KENTFIELD REHABILITATION HOSPITAL, KENTFIELD, CA, p. A44
KENTUCKY RIVER MEDICAL CENTER, JACKSON, KY, p. A173
KEOKUK AREA HOSPITAL, KEOKUK, IA, p. A153
KEOKUK COUNTY HEALTH CENTER, SIGOURNEY, IA, p. A156
KERN HOSPITAL AND MEDICAL CENTER, WARREN, MI, p. A224
KERN MEDICAL CENTER, BAKERSFIELD, CA, p. A36
KERN VALLEY HEALTHCARE DISTRICT, LAKE ISABELLA, CA, p. A45
KERRVILLE STATE HOSPITAL, KERRVILLE, TX, p. A420
KERSHAW COUNTY MEDICAL CENTER, CAMDEN, SC, p. A378
KERVILLE DIVISION, KERRVILLE, TEXAS, p. A429
KESSLER INSTITUTE FOR REHABILITATION, WEST ORANGE, NJ, p. A281
KETCHIKAN GENERAL HOSPITAL, KETCHIKAN, AK, p. A21
KETTERING MEDICAL CENTER–NETWORK, KETTERING, OH, p. A333
KETTERING YOUTH SERVICES, DAYTON, OHIO, p. A333
KEWANEE HOSPITAL, KEWANEE, IL, p. A129
KEWEENAW MEMORIAL MEDICAL CENTER, LAURIUM, MI, p. A218
KEYSTONE CENTER, CHESTER, PA, p. A357
KILMICHAEL HOSPITAL, KILMICHAEL, MS, p. A239
KIMBALL COUNTY HOSPITAL, KIMBALL, NE, p. A264
KIMBALL MEDICAL CENTER, LAKEWOOD, NJ, p. A277
KIMBALL–RIDGE CENTER, WATERLOO, IOWA, p. A157
KIMBLE HOSPITAL, JUNCTION, TX, p. A420
KING'S DAUGHTERS HOSPITAL, GREENVILLE, MS, p. A238
KING'S DAUGHTERS HOSPITAL, YAZOO CITY, MS, p. A243
KING'S DAUGHTERS HOSPITAL, TEMPLE, TX, p. A432
KING'S DAUGHTERS MEDICAL CENTER, ASHLAND, KY, p. A170
KING'S DAUGHTERS MEDICAL CENTER, BROOKHAVEN, MS, p. A236
KING'S DAUGHTERS' HOSPITAL AND HEALTH SERVICES, MADISON, IN, p. A143
KINGFISHER REGIONAL HOSPITAL, KINGFISHER, OK, p. A344
KINGMAN REGIONAL MEDICAL CENTER, KINGMAN, AZ, p. A23
KINGS COUNTY HOSPITAL CENTER, NEW YORK, NY, p. A297
KINGS MOUNTAIN HOSPITAL, KINGS MOUNTAIN, NC, p. A314
KINGS PARK PSYCHIATRIC CENTER, BRENTWOOD, NEW YORK, p. A288
KINGSBORO PSYCHIATRIC CENTER, NEW YORK, NY, p. A297
KINGSBROOK JEWISH MEDICAL CENTER, NEW YORK, NY, p. A297

KINGSBURG MEDICAL CENTER, KINGSBURG, CA, p. A45
KINGSTON HOSPITAL, KINGSTON, NY, p. A293
KINGWOOD MEDICAL CENTER, KINGWOOD, TX, p. A420
KINO COMMUNITY HOSPITAL, TUCSON, AZ, p. A26
KIOWA COUNTY MEMORIAL HOSPITAL, GREENSBURG, KS, p. A161
KIOWA DISTRICT HOSPITAL, KIOWA, KS, p. A163
KISHWAUKEE COMMUNITY HOSPITAL, DE KALB, IL, p. A124
KIT CARSON COUNTY MEMORIAL HOSPITAL, BURLINGTON, CO, p. A68
KITTITAS VALLEY COMMUNITY HOSPITAL, ELLENSBURG, WA, p. A453
KITTSON MEMORIAL HEALTHCARE CENTER, HALLOCK, MN, p. A228
KLICKITAT VALLEY HOSPITAL, GOLDENDALE, WA, p. A454
KNAPP MEDICAL CENTER, WESLACO, TX, p. A434
KNOX COMMUNITY HOSPITAL, MOUNT VERNON, OH, p. A335
KNOX COUNTY HOSPITAL, BARBOURVILLE, KY, p. A170
KNOXVILLE AREA COMMUNITY HOSPITAL, KNOXVILLE, IA, p. A153
KNOXVILLE DIVISION, KNOXVILLE, IOWA, p. A151
KOHALA HOSPITAL, KOHALA, HI, p. A113
KONA COMMUNITY HOSPITAL, KEALAKEKUA, HI, p. A113
KOOTENAI MEDICAL CENTER, COEUR D'ALENE, ID, p. A116
KOSAIR CHILDREN'S HOSPITAL, LOUISVILLE, KENTUCKY, p. A175
KOSCIUSKO COMMUNITY HOSPITAL, WARSAW, IN, p. A146
KOSSUTH REGIONAL HEALTH CENTER, ALGONA, IA, p. A148
KPC GLOBAL MEDICAL CENTER, MONTCLAIR, CA, p. A52
KREMMLING MEMORIAL HOSPITAL, KREMMLING, CO, p. A71
KUAKINI MEDICAL CENTER, HONOLULU, HI, p. A112
KULA HOSPITAL, KULA, HI, p. A113
KWAJALEIN HOSPITAL, KWAJALEIN ISLAND, MH, p. A481

L

L. V. STABLER MEMORIAL HOSPITAL, GREENVILLE, AL, p. A15
LA FOLLETTE MEDICAL CENTER, LA FOLLETTE, TN, p. A395
LA GRANGE MEMORIAL HOSPITAL, LA GRANGE, IL, p. A129
LA HACIENDA TREATMENT CENTER, HUNT, TX, p. A419
LA PALMA INTERCOMMUNITY HOSPITAL, LA PALMA, CA, p. A45
LA PAZ REGIONAL HOSPITAL, PARKER, AZ, p. A23
LA PORTE REGIONAL HEALTH SYSTEM, LA PORTE, IN, p. A143
LABETTE COUNTY MEDICAL CENTER, PARSONS, KS, p. A166
LAC–HARBOR-UNIVERSITY OF CALIFORNIA AT LOS ANGELES MEDICAL CENTER, TORRANCE, CA, p. A65
LAC–HIGH DESERT HOSPITAL, LANCASTER, CA, p. A45
LAC–KING-DREW MEDICAL CENTER, LOS ANGELES, CA, p. A48
LAC–OLIVE VIEW-UCLA MEDICAL CENTER, LOS ANGELES, CA, p. A48
LAC-RANCHO LOS AMIGOS NATIONAL REHABILITATION CENTER, DOWNEY, CA, p. A40
LAC/UNIVERSITY OF SOUTHERN CALIFORNIA MEDICAL CENTER, LOS ANGELES, CA, p. A48
LACKEY MEMORIAL HOSPITAL, FOREST, MS, p. A238
LADY OF THE SEA GENERAL HOSPITAL, CUT OFF, LA, p. A182
LAFAYETTE GENERAL MEDICAL CENTER, LAFAYETTE, LA, p. A184
LAFAYETTE HOME HOSPITAL, LAFAYETTE, INDIANA, p. A143
LAFAYETTE HOSPITAL, ARROYO, PR, p. A481
LAFAYETTE REGIONAL HEALTH CENTER, LEXINGTON, MO, p. A250
LAGUNA HONDA HOSPITAL AND REHABILITATION CENTER, SAN FRANCISCO, CA, p. A60
LAHEY CLINIC HOSPITAL, BURLINGTON, MA, p. A203
LAIRD HOSPITAL, UNION, MS, p. A242
LAKE AREA HOSPITAL, WEBSTER, SD, p. A389
LAKE CHARLES MEMORIAL HOSPITAL, LAKE CHARLES, LA, p. A184
LAKE CHELAN COMMUNITY HOSPITAL, CHELAN, WA, p. A452
LAKE CITY MEDICAL CENTER, LAKE CITY, FL, p. A87
LAKE CITY MEDICAL CENTER, LAKE CITY, MN, p. A229
LAKE CUMBERLAND REGIONAL HOSPITAL, SOMERSET, KY, p. A178
LAKE DISTRICT HOSPITAL, LAKEVIEW, OR, p. A352
LAKE FOREST HOSPITAL, LAKE FOREST, IL, p. A129
LAKE GRANBURY MEDICAL CENTER, GRANBURY, TX, p. A414
LAKE HOSPITAL SYSTEM, PAINESVILLE, OH, p. A336
LAKE MEAD HOSPITAL MEDICAL CENTER, NORTH LAS VEGAS, NV, p. A269
LAKE NORMAN REGIONAL MEDICAL CENTER, MOORESVILLE, NC, p. A316
LAKE POINTE MEDICAL CENTER, ROWLETT, TX, p. A427
LAKE REGION HEALTHCARE CORPORATION, FERGUS FALLS, MN, p. A228
LAKE REGIONAL HEALTH SYSTEM, OSAGE BEACH, MO, p. A251

LAKE SHORE HOSPITAL, IRVING, NY, p. A293
LAKE TAYLOR HOSPITAL, NORFOLK, VA, p. A447
LAKE VIEW MEMORIAL HOSPITAL, TWO HARBORS, MN, p. A234
LAKE WALES MEDICAL CENTERS, LAKE WALES, FLORIDA, p. A98
LAKE WHITNEY MEDICAL CENTER, WHITNEY, TX, p. A434
LAKELAND MEDICAL CENTER, ELKHORN, WI, p. A468
LAKELAND MEDICAL CENTER, NEW ORLEANS, LA, p. A186
LAKELAND MEDICAL CENTER, BERRIEN CENTER, BERRIEN CENTER, MICHIGAN, p. A222
LAKELAND MEDICAL CENTER–NILES, NILES, MICHIGAN, p. A222
LAKELAND MEDICAL CENTER–ST. JOSEPH, SAINT JOSEPH, MI, p. A222
LAKELAND REGIONAL HOSPITAL, SPRINGFIELD, MO, p. A254
LAKELAND REGIONAL MEDICAL CENTER, LAKELAND, FL, p. A88
LAKES REGION GENERAL HOSPITAL, LACONIA, NH, p. A272
LAKESHORE COMMUNITY HOSPITAL, SHELBY, MI, p. A222
LAKESHORE COMMUNITY HOSPITAL, DADEVILLE, AL, p. A13
LAKESHORE MENTAL HEALTH INSTITUTE, KNOXVILLE, TN, p. A395
LAKESIDE HOSPITAL, METAIRIE, LA, p. A185
LAKESIDE MEMORIAL HOSPITAL, BROCKPORT, NY, p. A288
LAKEVIEW COMMUNITY HOSPITAL, PAW PAW, MI, p. A220
LAKEVIEW COMMUNITY HOSPITAL, EUFAULA, AL, p. A14
LAKEVIEW HOSPITAL, STILLWATER, MN, p. A234
LAKEVIEW HOSPITAL, BOUNTIFUL, UT, p. A436
LAKEVIEW MEDICAL CENTER, RICE LAKE, WI, p. A474
LAKEVIEW REGIONAL MEDICAL CENTER, COVINGTON, LA, p. A181
LAKEWAY REGIONAL HOSPITAL, MORRISTOWN, TN, p. A397
LAKEWOOD HEALTH CENTER, BAUDETTE, MN, p. A225
LAKEWOOD HEALTH SYSTEM, STAPLES, MN, p. A234
LAKEWOOD HOSPITAL, LAKEWOOD, OH, p. A333
LAKEWOOD MEDICAL CENTER, MORGAN CITY, LA, p. A186
LAKEWOOD REGIONAL MEDICAL CENTER, LAKEWOOD, CA, p. A45
LALLIE KEMP MEDICAL CENTER, INDEPENDENCE, LA, p. A183
LAMB HEALTHCARE CENTER, LITTLEFIELD, TX, p. A421
LANAI COMMUNITY HOSPITAL, LANAI CITY, HI, p. A113
LANCASTER COMMUNITY HOSPITAL, LANCASTER, CA, p. A45
LANCASTER GENERAL HOSPITAL, LANCASTER, PA, p. A362
LANCASTER GENERAL HOSPITAL–SUSQUEHANNA DIVISION, COLUMBIA, PA, p. A358
LANDER VALLEY MEDICAL CENTER, LANDER, WY, p. A479
LANDMANN–JUNGMAN MEMORIAL HOSPITAL, SCOTLAND, SD, p. A387
LANDMARK MEDICAL CENTER, WOONSOCKET, RI, p. A377
LANDMARK MEDICAL CENTER–FOGARTY UNIT, NORTH SMITHFIELD, RHODE ISLAND, p. A377
LANDMARK MEDICAL CENTER–WOONSOCKET UNIT, WOONSOCKET, RHODE ISLAND, p. A377
LANE COUNTY HOSPITAL, DIGHTON, KS, p. A160
LANE MEMORIAL HOSPITAL, ZACHARY, LA, p. A190
LANGLADE MEMORIAL HOSPITAL, ANTIGO, WI, p. A466
LANIER HEALTH SERVICES, VALLEY, AL, p. A19
LANIER PARK HOSPITAL, GAINESVILLE, GA, p. A105
LANKENAU HOSPITAL, WYNNEWOOD, PA, p. A375
LANTERMAN DEVELOPMENTAL CENTER, POMONA, CA, p. A55
LAPEER REGIONAL HOSPITAL, LAPEER, MI, p. A218
LARABIDA CHILDREN'S HOSPITAL AND RESEARCH CENTER, CHICAGO, IL, p. A122
LARGO MEDICAL CENTER, LARGO, FL, p. A88
LARKIN COMMUNITY HOSPITAL, SOUTH MIAMI, FL, p. A95
LARNED STATE HOSPITAL, LARNED, KS, p. A164
LARUE D. CARTER MEMORIAL HOSPITAL, INDIANAPOLIS, IN, p. A141
LAS COLINAS MEDICAL CENTER, IRVING, TX, p. A419
LAS ENCINAS HOSPITAL, PASADENA, CA, p. A55
LAS VEGAS MEDICAL CENTER, LAS VEGAS, NM, p. A285
LASALLE GENERAL HOSPITAL, JENA, LA, p. A183
LASSEN COMMUNITY HOSPITAL, SUSANVILLE, CA, p. A64
LATIMER COUNTY GENERAL HOSPITAL, WILBURTON, OK, p. A349
LATROBE AREA HOSPITAL, LATROBE, PA, p. A363
LAUGHLIN MEMORIAL HOSPITAL, GREENEVILLE, TN, p. A393
LAUREATE PSYCHIATRIC CLINIC AND HOSPITAL, TULSA, OK, p. A348
LAUREL REGIONAL HOSPITAL, LAUREL, MD, p. A199
LAUREL WOOD CENTER, MERIDIAN, MS, p. A240
LAURENS COUNTY HEALTHCARE SYSTEM, CLINTON, SC, p. A379
LAURENS COUNTY HOSPITAL, CLINTON, SOUTH CAROLINA, p. A379
LAVACA MEDICAL CENTER, HALLETTSVILLE, TX, p. A415
LAWNWOOD PAVILION, FORT PIERCE, FLORIDA, p. A85
LAWNWOOD REGIONAL MEDICAL CENTER, FORT PIERCE, FL, p. A85
LAWRENCE & MEMORIAL HOSPITAL, NEW LONDON, CT, p. A76

LAWRENCE BAPTIST MEDICAL CENTER, MOULTON, AL, p. A17
LAWRENCE COUNTY HOSPITAL, MONTICELLO, MS, p. A241
LAWRENCE COUNTY MEMORIAL HOSPITAL, LAWRENCEVILLE, IL, p. A129
LAWRENCE F. QUIGLEY MEMORIAL HOSPITAL, CHELSEA, MA, p. A204
LAWRENCE GENERAL HOSPITAL, LAWRENCE, MA, p. A205
LAWRENCE HALL NURSING HOME, p. A34
LAWRENCE HOSPITAL, BRONXVILLE, NY, p. A288
LAWRENCE MEMORIAL HOSPITAL, LAWRENCE, KS, p. A164
LAWRENCE MEMORIAL HOSPITAL, WALNUT RIDGE, AR, p. A34
LAWRENCE MEMORIAL HOSPITAL OF MEDFORD, MEDFORD, MASSACHUSETTS, p. A206
LDS HOSPITAL, SALT LAKE CITY, UT, p. A438
LE BONHEUR CHILDREN'S MEDICAL CENTER, MEMPHIS, TENNESSEE, p. A397
LEA REGIONAL MEDICAL CENTER, HOBBS, NM, p. A285
LEAHI HOSPITAL, HONOLULU, HI, p. A112
LEAKE MEMORIAL HOSPITAL, CARTHAGE, MS, p. A237
LEBANON COMMUNITY HOSPITAL, LEBANON, OR, p. A352
LEE COUNTY COMMUNITY HOSPITAL, PENNINGTON GAP, VA, p. A447
LEE MEMORIAL HEALTH SYSTEM, FORT MYERS, FL, p. A85
LEE MEMORIAL HOSPITAL, DOWAGIAC, MI, p. A214
LEE'S SUMMIT HOSPITAL, LEES SUMMIT, MO, p. A249
LEELANAU MEMORIAL HEALTH CENTER, NORTHPORT, MI, p. A220
LEESBURG REGIONAL MEDICAL CENTER, LEESBURG, FL, p. A88
LEGACY EMANUEL HOSPITAL AND HEALTH CENTER, PORTLAND, OR, p. A353
LEGACY GOOD SAMARITAN HOSPITAL AND MEDICAL CENTER, PORTLAND, OR, p. A353
LEGACY MERIDIAN PARK HOSPITAL, TUALATIN, OR, p. A354
LEGACY MOUNT HOOD MEDICAL CENTER, GRESHAM, OR, p. A351
LEHIGH VALLEY HOSPITAL, ALLENTOWN, PA, p. A355
LEILA HOSPITAL, BATTLE CREEK, MICHIGAN, p. A212
LEMUEL SHATTUCK HOSPITAL, BOSTON, MA, p. A202
LENOIR MEMORIAL HOSPITAL, KINSTON, NC, p. A315
LENOX HILL HOSPITAL, NEW YORK, NY, p. A297
LEONARD J. CHABERT MEDICAL CENTER, HOUMA, LA, p. A183
LEONARD MORSE HOSPITAL, NATICK, MASSACHUSETTS, p. A205
LESTER E. COX MEDICAL CENTER NORTH, SPRINGFIELD, MISSOURI, p. A254
LESTER E. COX MEDICAL CENTER SOUTH, SPRINGFIELD, MISSOURI, p. A254
LESTER E. COX MEDICAL CENTERS, SPRINGFIELD, MO, p. A254
LEVI HOSPITAL, HOT SPRINGS NATIONAL PARK, AR, p. A30
LEVINDALE HEBREW GERIATRIC CENTER AND HOSPITAL, BALTIMORE, MD, p. A196
LEWIS COUNTY GENERAL HOSPITAL, LOWVILLE, NY, p. A294
LEWIS-GALE MEDICAL CENTER, SALEM, VA, p. A449
LEWIS-GALE PAVILION, SALEM, VIRGINIA, p. A449
LEWISTOWN HOSPITAL, LEWISTOWN, PA, p. A363
LEXINGTON MEDICAL CENTER, WEST COLUMBIA, SC, p. A384
LEXINGTON MEMORIAL HOSPITAL, LEXINGTON, NC, p. A315
LIBERTY COUNTY HOSPITAL AND NURSING HOME, CHESTER, MT, p. A256
LIBERTY HOSPITAL, LIBERTY, MO, p. A250
LIBERTY REGIONAL MEDICAL CENTER, HINESVILLE, GA, p. A106
LIBERTY-DAYTON HOSPITAL, LIBERTY, TX, p. A421
LICKING MEMORIAL HOSPITAL, NEWARK, OH, p. A335
LIFECARE HOSPITAL OF PITTSBURGH, PITTSBURGH, PA, p. A369
LIFECARE HOSPITALS, SHREVEPORT, LA, p. A188
LIFECOURSE REHABILITATION HOSPITAL, FARMINGTON, NEW MEXICO, p. A284
LILA DOYLE NURSING CARE FACILITY, p. A383
LILLIAN M. HUDSPETH MEMORIAL HOSPITAL, SONORA, TX, p. A431
LIMA MEMORIAL HOSPITAL, LIMA, OH, p. A333
LIMESTONE MEDICAL CENTER, GROESBECK, TX, p. A415
LINCOLN COMMUNITY HOSPITAL AND NURSING HOME, HUGO, CO, p. A71
LINCOLN COUNTY HEALTH FACILITIES, FAYETTEVILLE, TN, p. A392
LINCOLN COUNTY HOSPITAL, LINCOLN, KS, p. A164
LINCOLN COUNTY MEDICAL CENTER, RUIDOSO, NM, p. A286
LINCOLN COUNTY MEMORIAL HOSPITAL, TROY, MO, p. A255
LINCOLN DEVELOPMENTAL CENTER, LINCOLN, IL, p. A129
LINCOLN DIVISION, LINCOLN, NEBRASKA, p. A264
LINCOLN GENERAL HOSPITAL, RUSTON, LA, p. A188
LINCOLN GENERAL-BRYANLGH-WEST, LINCOLN, NEBRASKA, p. A264
LINCOLN HOSPITAL, DAVENPORT, WA, p. A453

LINCOLN HOSPITAL MEDICAL CENTER, LOS ANGELES, CA, p. A48
LINCOLN MEDICAL AND MENTAL HEALTH CENTER, NEW YORK, NY, p. A297
LINCOLN MEDICAL CENTER, LINCOLNTON, NC, p. A315
LINCOLN REGIONAL CENTER, LINCOLN, NE, p. A264
LINCOLN TRAIL BEHAVIORAL HEALTH SYSTEM, RADCLIFF, KY, p. A178
LINDEN MUNICIPAL HOSPITAL, LINDEN, TX, p. A421
LINDSAY DISTRICT HOSPITAL, LINDSAY, CA, p. A46
LINDSBORG COMMUNITY HOSPITAL, LINDSBORG, KS, p. A164
LINTON HOSPITAL, LINTON, ND, p. A323
LISBON MEDICAL CENTER, LISBON, ND, p. A323
LITTLE COMPANY OF MARY HEALTH SERVICES, TORRANCE, CA, p. A65
LITTLE COMPANY OF MARY HOSPITAL AND HEALTH CARE CENTERS, EVERGREEN PARK, IL, p. A126
LITTLE FALLS HOSPITAL, LITTLE FALLS, NY, p. A293
LITTLE RIVER MEMORIAL HOSPITAL, ASHDOWN, AR, p. A28
LITTLETON ADVENTIST HOSPITAL, LITTLETON, CO, p. A72
LITTLETON REGIONAL HOSPITAL, LITTLETON, NH, p. A272
LITZENBERG MEMORIAL COUNTY HOSPITAL, CENTRAL CITY, NE, p. A262
LIVENGRIN FOUNDATION, BENSALEM, PA, p. A356
LIVINGSTON HOSPITAL AND HEALTHCARE SERVICES, SALEM, KY, p. A178
LIVINGSTON MEMORIAL HOSPITAL, LIVINGSTON, MT, p. A258
LIVINGSTON REGIONAL HOSPITAL, LIVINGSTON, TN, p. A395
LLANO MEMORIAL HEALTHCARE SYSTEM, LLANO, TX, p. A421
LOCK HAVEN HOSPITAL, LOCK HAVEN, PA, p. A363
LOCKPORT MEMORIAL HOSPITAL, LOCKPORT, NY, p. A293
LODI COMMUNITY HOSPITAL, LODI, OH, p. A334
LODI MEMORIAL HOSPITAL, LODI, CA, p. A46
LODI MEMORIAL HOSPITAL WEST, LODI, CALIFORNIA, p. A46
LOEB CENTER NURSING REHABILITATION, NEW YORK, NEW YORK, p. A298
LOGAN COUNTY HOSPITAL, OAKLEY, KS, p. A165
LOGAN GENERAL HOSPITAL, LOGAN, WV, p. A462
LOGAN HOSPITAL AND MEDICAL CENTER, GUTHRIE, OK, p. A344
LOGAN MEMORIAL HOSPITAL, RUSSELLVILLE, KY, p. A178
LOGAN REGIONAL HOSPITAL, LOGAN, UT, p. A436
LOGANSPORT STATE HOSPITAL, LOGANSPORT, IN, p. A143
LOMA LINDA UNIVERSITY BEHAVIORAL MEDICINE CENTER, REDLANDS, CA, p. A56
LOMA LINDA UNIVERSITY COMMUNITY MEDICAL CENTER, LOMA LINDA, CALIFORNIA, p. A46
LOMA LINDA UNIVERSITY MEDICAL CENTER, LOMA LINDA, CA, p. A46
LOMPOC HEALTHCARE DISTRICT, LOMPOC, CA, p. A46
LONG BEACH COMMUNITY MEDICAL CENTER, LONG BEACH, CA, p. A46
LONG BEACH MEDICAL CENTER, LONG BEACH, NY, p. A293
LONG BEACH MEMORIAL MEDICAL CENTER, LONG BEACH, CA, p. A46
LONG ISLAND COLLEGE HOSPITAL, NEW YORK, NY, p. A297
LONG ISLAND JEWISH MEDICAL CENTER, NEW YORK, NY, p. A297
LONG PRAIRIE MEMORIAL HOSPITAL AND HOME, LONG PRAIRIE, MN, p. A229
LONG TERM CARE HOSPITAL AT JACKSON, MONTGOMERY, AL, p. A17
LONGMONT UNITED HOSPITAL, LONGMONT, CO, p. A72
LONGVIEW REGIONAL MEDICAL CENTER, LONGVIEW, TX, p. A422
LOOKOUT MEMORIAL HOSPITAL, SPEARFISH, SD, p. A388
LORAIN COMMUNITY/ST. JOSEPH HEALTH CENTER—EAST CAMPUS, LORAIN, OHIO, p. A334
LORAIN COMMUNITY/ST. JOSEPH REGIONAL HEALTH CENTER, LORAIN, OH, p. A334
LORAIN COMMUNITY/ST. JOSEPH REGIONAL HEALTH CENTER-WEST CAMPUS, LORAIN, OHIO, p. A334
LORETTO HOSPITAL, CHICAGO, IL, p. A122
LORING HOSPITAL, SAC CITY, IA, p. A156
LORIS COMMUNITY HOSPITAL, LORIS, SC, p. A382
LOS ALAMITOS MEDICAL CENTER, LOS ALAMITOS, CA, p. A47
LOS ALAMOS MEDICAL CENTER, LOS ALAMOS, NM, p. A285
LOS ANGELES COMMUNITY HOSPITAL, LOS ANGELES, CA, p. A48
LOS ANGELES COMMUNITY HOSPITAL OF NORWALK, LOS ANGELES, CALIFORNIA, p. A48
LOS ANGELES COUNTY CENTRAL JAIL HOSPITAL, LOS ANGELES, CA, p. A48
LOS ANGELES METROPOLITAN MEDICAL CENTER, LOS ANGELES, CA, p. A48
LOS ROBLES REGIONAL MEDICAL CENTER, THOUSAND OAKS, CA, p. A64
LOST RIVERS DISTRICT HOSPITAL, ARCO, ID, p. A115
LOUDOUN HOSPITAL CENTER, LEESBURG, VA, p. A445

LOUIS A. JOHNSON VETERANS AFFAIRS MEDICAL CENTER, CLARKSBURG, WV, p. A461
LOUIS A. WEISS MEMORIAL HOSPITAL, CHICAGO, IL, p. A122
LOUIS SMITH MEMORIAL HOSPITAL, LAKELAND, GA, p. A106
LOUISE OBICI MEMORIAL HOSPITAL, SUFFOLK, VA, p. A450
LOURDES COUNSELING CENTER, RICHLAND, WA, p. A456
LOURDES HOSPITAL, PADUCAH, KY, p. A177
LOURDES MEDICAL CENTER, PASCO, WA, p. A455
LOVELACE HEALTH SYSTEM, ALBUQUERQUE, NM, p. A283
LOW COUNTRY GENERAL HOSPITAL, RIDGELAND, SC, p. A383
LOWELL GENERAL HOSPITAL, LOWELL, MA, p. A206
LOWER BUCKS HOSPITAL, BRISTOL, PA, p. A356
LOWER KEYS MEDICAL CENTER, KEY WEST, FL, p. A87
LOWER UMPQUA HOSPITAL DISTRICT, REEDSPORT, OR, p. A354
LOYOLA UNIVERSITY MEDICAL CENTER, MAYWOOD, IL, p. A130
LSU MEDICAL CENTER-UNIVERSITY HOSPITAL, SHREVEPORT, LA, p. A188
LUCAS COUNTY HEALTH CENTER, CHARITON, IA, p. A149
LUCILE SALTER PACKARD CHILDREN'S HOSPITAL AT STANFORD, PALO ALTO, CA, p. A54
LUCY LEE HOSPITAL, POPLAR BLUFF, MO, p. A251
LUTHER HOSPITAL, EAU CLAIRE, WI, p. A468
LUTHERAN GENERAL HOSPITAL, PARK RIDGE, IL, p. A132
LUTHERAN HOSPITAL, CLEVELAND, OH, p. A329
LUTHERAN HOSPITAL OF INDIANA, FORT WAYNE, IN, p. A139
LUTHERAN MEDICAL CENTER, NEW YORK, NY, p. A298
LUTZ WING CONVALESCENT AND NURSING CARE UNIT, p. A227
LUVERNE COMMUNITY HOSPITAL, LUVERNE, MN, p. A229
LYNCHBURG GENERAL HOSPITAL, LYNCHBURG, VA, p. A445
LYNDON B JOHNSON GENERAL HOSPITAL, HOUSTON, TEXAS, p. A416
LYNDON B. JOHNSON TROPICAL MEDICAL CENTER, PAGO PAGO, AS, p. A481
LYNN COUNTY HOSPITAL DISTRICT, TAHOKA, TX, p. A431
LYONS DIVISION, LYONS, NEW JERSEY, p. A275
LYSTER U. S. ARMY COMMUNITY HOSPITAL, FORT RUCKER, AL, p. A15

M

M. I. T. MEDICAL DEPARTMENT, CAMBRIDGE, MA, p. A204
MACKINAC STRAITS HOSPITAL AND HEALTH CENTER, SAINT IGNACE, MI, p. A221
MACNEAL HOSPITAL, BERWYN, IL, p. A120
MACON COUNTY GENERAL HOSPITAL, LAFAYETTE, TN, p. A395
MACON NORTHSIDE HOSPITAL, MACON, GA, p. A107
MAD RIVER COMMUNITY HOSPITAL, ARCATA, CA, p. A35
MADELIA COMMUNITY HOSPITAL, MADELIA, MN, p. A229
MADERA COMMUNITY HOSPITAL, MADERA, CA, p. A50
MADIGAN ARMY MEDICAL CENTER, TACOMA, WA, p. A458
MADISON COMMUNITY HOSPITAL, MADISON HEIGHTS, MI, p. A218
MADISON COMMUNITY HOSPITAL, MADISON, SD, p. A386
MADISON COUNTY HOSPITAL, LONDON, OH, p. A334
MADISON COUNTY MEDICAL CENTER, CANTON, MS, p. A237
MADISON COUNTY MEMORIAL HOSPITAL, MADISON, FL, p. A89
MADISON COUNTY MEMORIAL HOSPITAL, WINTERSET, IA, p. A158
MADISON HOSPITAL, MADISON, MN, p. A229
MADISON MEDICAL CENTER, FREDERICKTOWN, MO, p. A246
MADISON MEMORIAL HOSPITAL, REXBURG, ID, p. A117
MADISON PARISH HOSPITAL, TALLULAH, LA, p. A189
MADISON ST. JOSEPH HEALTH CENTER, MADISONVILLE, TX, p. A422
MADISON STATE HOSPITAL, MADISON, IN, p. A143
MADISON VALLEY HOSPITAL, ENNIS, MT, p. A257
MADONNA REHABILITATION HOSPITAL, LINCOLN, NE, p. A264
MAGEE GENERAL HOSPITAL, MAGEE, MS, p. A240
MAGEE REHABILITATION HOSPITAL, PHILADELPHIA, PA, p. A367
MAGEE-WOMENS HOSPITAL, PITTSBURGH, PA, p. A369
MAGIC VALLEY REGIONAL MEDICAL CENTER, TWIN FALLS, ID, p. A118
MAGNOLIA HOSPITAL, MAGNOLIA, AR, p. A32
MAGNOLIA REGIONAL HEALTH CENTER, CORINTH, MS, p. A237
MAHASKA COUNTY HOSPITAL, OSKALOOSA, IA, p. A155
MAHNOMEN HEALTH CENTER, MAHNOMEN, MN, p. A230
MAIMONIDES MEDICAL CENTER, NEW YORK, NY, p. A298
MAINE COAST MEMORIAL HOSPITAL, ELLSWORTH, ME, p. A192
MAINE MEDICAL CENTER, PORTLAND, ME, p. A193
MAINE MEDICAL CENTER, BRIGHTON CAMPUS, PORTLAND, MAINE, p. A193
MAINEGENERAL MEDICAL CENTER–AUGUSTA CAMPUS, AUGUSTA, MAINE, p. A194
MAINEGENERAL MEDICAL CENTER–WATERVILLE CAMPUS, WATERVILLE, ME, p. A194

Index of Hospitals / Mainland Medical Center

MAINLAND MEDICAL CENTER, TEXAS CITY, TX, p. A432
MAJOR HOSPITAL, SHELBYVILLE, IN, p. A145
MALCOLM GROW MEDICAL CENTER, ANDREWS AFB, MD, p. A195
MALCOM RANDALL VETERANS AFFAIRS MEDICAL CENTER, GAINESVILLE, FL, p. A85
MALDEN MEDICAL CENTER, MALDEN, MASSACHUSETTS, p. A206
MALVERN INSTITUTE, MALVERN, PA, p. A363
MAMMOTH HOSPITAL, MAMMOTH LAKES, CA, p. A51
MAN ARH HOSPITAL, MAN, WV, p. A462
MANATEE MEMORIAL HOSPITAL, BRADENTON, FL, p. A82
MANCHESTER MEMORIAL HOSPITAL, MANCHESTER, CT, p. A75
MANGUM CITY HOSPITAL, MANGUM, OK, p. A344
MANHASSET AMBULATORY CARE PAVILION, MANHASSET, NEW YORK, p. A297
MANHATTAN EYE, EAR AND THROAT HOSPITAL, NEW YORK, NY, p. A298
MANHATTAN PSYCHIATRIC CENTER-WARD'S ISLAND, NEW YORK, NY, p. A298
MANIILAQ HEALTH CENTER, KOTZEBUE, AK, p. A21
MANNING REGIONAL HEALTHCARE CENTER, MANNING, IA, p. A154
MANSFIELD HOSPITAL, MANSFIELD, OHIO, p. A334
MARCUM AND WALLACE MEMORIAL HOSPITAL, IRVINE, KY, p. A173
MARCUS DALY MEMORIAL HOSPITAL, HAMILTON, MT, p. A258
MARENGO MEMORIAL HOSPITAL, MARENGO, IA, p. A154
MARGARET MARY COMMUNITY HOSPITAL, BATESVILLE, IN, p. A137
MARGARET R. PARDEE MEMORIAL HOSPITAL, HENDERSONVILLE, NC, p. A314
MARGARETVILLE MEMORIAL HOSPITAL, MARGARETVILLE, NY, p. A294
MARIA PARHAM HOSPITAL, HENDERSON, NC, p. A314
MARIAN COMMUNITY HOSPITAL, CARBONDALE, PA, p. A357
MARIAN MEDICAL CENTER, SANTA MARIA, CA, p. A62
MARIANJOY REHABILITATION HOSPITAL, WHEATON, IL, p. A136
MARIAS MEDICAL CENTER, SHELBY, MT, p. A259
MARICOPA MEDICAL CENTER, PHOENIX, AZ, p. A24
MARIETTA MEMORIAL HOSPITAL, MARIETTA, OH, p. A334
MARIN GENERAL HOSPITAL, GREENBRAE, CA, p. A43
MARINERS HOSPITAL, TAVERNIER, FL, p. A97
MARION BAPTIST MEDICAL CENTER, HAMILTON, AL, p. A15
MARION COUNTY MEDICAL CENTER, MULLINS, SC, p. A382
MARION GENERAL HOSPITAL, MARION, OH, p. A334
MARION GENERAL HOSPITAL, MARION, IN, p. A143
MARION GENERAL HOSPITAL, COLUMBIA, MS, p. A237
MARION MEMORIAL HOSPITAL, MARION, IL, p. A130
MARK REED HOSPITAL, MCCLEARY, WA, p. A454
MARK TWAIN ST. JOSEPH'S HOSPITAL, SAN ANDREAS, CA, p. A58
MARLBORO PARK HOSPITAL, BENNETTSVILLE, SC, p. A378
MARLETTE COMMUNITY HOSPITAL, MARLETTE, MI, p. A219
MARQUETTE GENERAL HEALTH SYSTEM, MARQUETTE, MI, p. A219
MARSHALL BROWNING HOSPITAL, DU QUOIN, IL, p. A125
MARSHALL COUNTY HEALTHCARE CENTER/AVERA HEALTH, BRITTON, SD, p. A385
MARSHALL COUNTY HOSPITAL, BENTON, KY, p. A170
MARSHALL HOSPITAL, PLACERVILLE, CA, p. A55
MARSHALL I. PICKENS HOSPITAL, GREENVILLE, SOUTH CAROLINA, p. A381
MARSHALL MEDICAL CENTER, LEWISBURG, TN, p. A395
MARSHALL MEDICAL CENTER NORTH, GUNTERSVILLE, AL, p. A15
MARSHALL MEDICAL CENTER SOUTH, BOAZ, AL, p. A12
MARSHALL MEMORIAL HOSPITAL, MADILL, OK, p. A344
MARSHALL REGIONAL MEDICAL CENTER, MARSHALL, TX, p. A423
MARSHALLTOWN MEDICAL AND SURGICAL CENTER, MARSHALLTOWN, IA, p. A154
MARTHA JEFFERSON HOSPITAL, CHARLOTTESVILLE, VA, p. A443
MARTHA'S VINEYARD HOSPITAL, OAK BLUFFS, MA, p. A207
MARTIN ARMY COMMUNITY HOSPITAL, FORT BENNING, GA, p. A105
MARTIN COUNTY HOSPITAL DISTRICT, STANTON, TX, p. A431
MARTIN GENERAL HOSPITAL, WILLIAMSTON, NC, p. A319
MARTIN MEMORIAL HEALTH SYSTEMS, STUART, FL, p. A95
MARTIN MEMORIAL HOSPITAL SOUTH, STUART, FLORIDA, p. A95
MARY BLACK HEALTH SYSTEM, SPARTANBURG, SC, p. A383
MARY BRECKINRIDGE HOSPITAL, HYDEN, KY, p. A173
MARY BRIDGE CHILDREN'S HOSPITAL AND HEALTH CENTER, TACOMA, WA, p. A458
MARY FREE BED HOSPITAL AND REHABILITATION CENTER, GRAND RAPIDS, MI, p. A215
MARY GREELEY MEDICAL CENTER, AMES, IA, p. A148

MARY HITCHCOCK MEMORIAL HOSPITAL, LEBANON, NH, p. A272
MARY IMMACULATE HOSPITAL, NEW YORK, NEW YORK, p. A296
MARY IMMACULATE HOSPITAL, NEWPORT NEWS, VA, p. A446
MARY IMOGENE BASSETT HOSPITAL, COOPERSTOWN, NY, p. A290
MARY LANE HOSPITAL, WARE, MA, p. A209
MARY LANNING MEMORIAL HOSPITAL, HASTINGS, NE, p. A263
MARY RUTAN HOSPITAL, BELLEFONTAINE, OH, p. A326
MARY SHIELS HOSPITAL, DALLAS, TX, p. A409
MARY WASHINGTON HOSPITAL, FREDERICKSBURG, VA, p. A444
MARYLAND GENERAL HOSPITAL, BALTIMORE, MD, p. A196
MARYMOUNT HOSPITAL, GARFIELD HEIGHTS, OH, p. A332
MARYMOUNT MEDICAL CENTER, LONDON, KY, p. A174
MARYVALE HOSPITAL MEDICAL CENTER, PHOENIX, AZ, p. A24
MARYVIEW MEDICAL CENTER, PORTSMOUTH, VA, p. A447
MASON DISTRICT HOSPITAL, HAVANA, IL, p. A127
MASON GENERAL HOSPITAL, SHELTON, WA, p. A457
MASONIC GERIATRIC HEALTHCARE CENTER, WALLINGFORD, CT, p. A77
MASSAC MEMORIAL HOSPITAL, METROPOLIS, IL, p. A130
MASSACHUSETTS EYE AND EAR INFIRMARY, BOSTON, MA, p. A202
MASSACHUSETTS GENERAL HOSPITAL, BOSTON, MA, p. A202
MASSACHUSETTS HOSPITAL SCHOOL, CANTON, MA, p. A204
MASSACHUSETTS RESPIRATORY HOSPITAL, BRAINTREE, MA, p. A203
MASSAPEQUA GENERAL HOSPITAL, SEAFORD, NY, p. A305
MASSENA MEMORIAL HOSPITAL, MASSENA, NY, p. A294
MASSILLON COMMUNITY HOSPITAL, MASSILLON, OH, p. A335
MASSILLON PSYCHIATRIC CENTER, MASSILLON, OH, p. A335
MATAGORDA GENERAL HOSPITAL, BAY CITY, TX, p. A403
MATHENY SCHOOL AND HOSPITAL, PEAPACK, NJ, p. A279
MAUI MEMORIAL MEDICAL CENTER, WAILUKU, HI, p. A114
MAURY REGIONAL HOSPITAL, COLUMBIA, TN, p. A391
MAYERS MEMORIAL HOSPITAL DISTRICT, FALL RIVER MILLS, CA, p. A41
MAYES COUNTY MEDICAL CENTER, PRYOR, OK, p. A347
MAYO CLINIC HOSPITAL, PHOENIX, AZ, p. A24
MAYO REGIONAL HOSPITAL, DOVER-FOXCROFT, ME, p. A192
MAYVIEW STATE HOSPITAL, BRIDGEVILLE, PA, p. A356
MCALESTER REGIONAL HEALTH CENTER, MCALESTER, OK, p. A344
MCALLEN HEART HOSPITAL, MCALLEN, TX, p. A423
MCALLEN MEDICAL CENTER, MCALLEN, TX, p. A423
MCCAIN CORRECTIONAL HOSPITAL, MCCAIN, NC, p. A315
MCCALL MEMORIAL HOSPITAL, MCCALL, ID, p. A117
MCCAMEY HOSPITAL, MCCAMEY, TX, p. A423
MCCLELLAN HEALTH SYSTEM, CAMBRIDGE, NY, p. A289
MCCONE COUNTY MEDICAL ASSISTANCE FACILITY, CIRCLE, MT, p. A256
MCCUISTION REGIONAL MEDICAL CENTER, PARIS, TX, p. A426
MCCULLOUGH-HYDE MEMORIAL HOSPITAL, OXFORD, OH, p. A336
MCCUNE-BROOKS HOSPITAL, CARTHAGE, MO, p. A245
MCCURTAIN MEMORIAL HOSPITAL, IDABEL, OK, p. A344
MCDONALD ARMY COMMUNITY HOSPITAL, FORT EUSTIS, VA, p. A444
MCDONOUGH DISTRICT HOSPITAL, MACOMB, IL, p. A129
MCDOWELL ARH HOSPITAL, MCDOWELL, KY, p. A176
MCDOWELL HOSPITAL, MARION, NC, p. A315
MCDUFFIE REGIONAL MEDICAL CENTER, THOMSON, GA, p. A110
MCFARLAND SPECIALTY HOSPITAL, LEBANON, TENNESSEE, p. A395
MCGEHEE-DESHA COUNTY HOSPITAL, MCGEHEE, AR, p. A32
MCKAY-DEE HOSPITAL CENTER, OGDEN, UT, p. A437
MCKEE MEDICAL CENTER, LOVELAND, CO, p. A72
MCKENNA MEMORIAL HOSPITAL, NEW BRAUNFELS, TX, p. A425
MCKENZIE COUNTY MEMORIAL HOSPITAL, WATFORD CITY, ND, p. A324
MCKENZIE MEMORIAL HOSPITAL, SANDUSKY, MI, p. A222
MCKENZIE-WILLAMETTE HOSPITAL, SPRINGFIELD, OR, p. A354
MCLAREN REGIONAL MEDICAL CENTER, FLINT, MI, p. A215
MCLEAN HOSPITAL, BELMONT, MA, p. A201
MCLEOD REGIONAL MEDICAL CENTER, FLORENCE, SC, p. A381
MCPHERSON HOSPITAL, HOWELL, MI, p. A217
MCREYNOLDS HALL, p. A215
MEADE DISTRICT HOSPITAL, MEADE, KS, p. A165
MEADOW WOOD BEHAVIORAL HEALTH SYSTEM, NEW CASTLE, DE, p. A78
MEADOWBROOK REHABILITATION HOSPITAL, GARDNER, KS, p. A161
MEADOWCREST HOSPITAL, GRETNA, LA, p. A183
MEADOWLANDS HOSPITAL MEDICAL CENTER, SECAUCUS, NJ, p. A280
MEADOWS PSYCHIATRIC CENTER, CENTRE HALL, PA, p. A357

MEADOWS REGIONAL MEDICAL CENTER, VIDALIA, GA, p. A111
MEADOWVIEW REGIONAL MEDICAL CENTER, MAYSVILLE, KY, p. A176
MEADVILLE MEDICAL CENTER, MEADVILLE, PA, p. A364
MEASE COUNTRYSIDE HOSPITAL, SAFETY HARBOR, FL, p. A94
MEASE HOSPITAL DUNEDIN, DUNEDIN, FL, p. A84
MECOSTA COUNTY GENERAL HOSPITAL, BIG RAPIDS, MI, p. A212
MEDCENTER HOSPITAL, MARION, OH, p. A334
MEDCENTER ONE, BISMARCK, ND, p. A321
MEDCENTRAL HEALTH SYSTEM, MANSFIELD, OH, p. A334
MEDFIELD STATE HOSPITAL, MEDFIELD, MA, p. A206
MEDICAL ARTS HOSPITAL, LAMESA, TX, p. A421
MEDICAL CENTER AT LANCASTER, LANCASTER, TX, p. A421
MEDICAL CENTER AT PRINCETON, PRINCETON, NJ, p. A280
MEDICAL CENTER AT SCOTTSVILLE, SCOTTSVILLE, KENTUCKY, p. A170
MEDICAL CENTER AT TERRELL, TERRELL, TX, p. A432
MEDICAL CENTER BLOUNT, ONEONTA, AL, p. A17
MEDICAL CENTER EAST, BIRMINGHAM, AL, p. A12
MEDICAL CENTER ENTERPRISE, ENTERPRISE, AL, p. A14
MEDICAL CENTER HOSPITAL, ODESSA, TX, p. A425
MEDICAL CENTER HOSPITAL CAMPUS, BURLINGTON, VERMONT, p. A440
MEDICAL CENTER OF ARLINGTON, ARLINGTON, TX, p. A402
MEDICAL CENTER OF AURORA-SOUTH, AURORA, CO, p. A68
MEDICAL CENTER OF CALICO ROCK, CALICO ROCK, AR, p. A28
MEDICAL CENTER OF CENTRAL GEORGIA, MACON, GA, p. A107
MEDICAL CENTER OF INDEPENDENCE, INDEPENDENCE, MO, p. A247
MEDICAL CENTER OF LEWISVILLE, LEWISVILLE, TX, p. A421
MEDICAL CENTER OF LOUISIANA AT NEW ORLEANS, NEW ORLEANS, LA, p. A186
MEDICAL CENTER OF MANCHESTER, MANCHESTER, TN, p. A396
MEDICAL CENTER OF MESQUITE, MESQUITE, TX, p. A423
MEDICAL CENTER OF PLANO, PLANO, TX, p. A426
MEDICAL CENTER OF SOUTH ARKANSAS, EL DORADO, AR, p. A29
MEDICAL CENTER OF SOUTHEASTERN OKLAHOMA, DURANT, OK, p. A343
MEDICAL CENTER OF SOUTHERN INDIANA, CHARLESTOWN, IN, p. A138
MEDICAL CENTER OF SOUTHWEST LOUISIANA, LAFAYETTE, LA, p. A184
MEDICAL CENTER OF WINNIE, WINNIE, TX, p. A435
MEDICAL CITY DALLAS HOSPITAL, DALLAS, TX, p. A409
MEDICAL COLLEGE OF GEORGIA HOSPITAL AND CLINICS, AUGUSTA, GA, p. A101
MEDICAL COLLEGE OF OHIO HOSPITALS, TOLEDO, OH, p. A338
MEDICAL COLLEGE OF PENNSYLVANIA HOSPITAL, PHILADELPHIA, PA, p. A367
MEDICAL COLLEGE OF VIRGINIA HOSPITALS, VIRGINIA COMMONWEALTH UNIVERSITY, RICHMOND, VA, p. A449
MEDICAL PARK HOSPITAL, WINSTON-SALEM, NC, p. A320
MEDICAL PARK HOSPITAL, HOPE, AR, p. A30
MEDICENTER, ENDICOTT, NEW YORK, p. A288
MEDICINE LODGE MEMORIAL HOSPITAL, MEDICINE LODGE, KS, p. A165
MEDINA COMMUNITY HOSPITAL, HONDO, TX, p. A415
MEDINA GENERAL HOSPITAL, MEDINA, OH, p. A335
MEDINA MEMORIAL HOSPITAL, MEDINA, NY, p. A294
MEDIPLEX REHABILITATION HOSPITAL, BOWLING GREEN, KY, p. A170
MEDLINK HOSPITAL AND NURSING CENTER AT CAPITOL HILL, WASHINGTON, DC, p. A79
MEEKER COUNTY MEMORIAL HOSPITAL, LITCHFIELD, MN, p. A229
MELISSA MEMORIAL HOSPITAL, HOLYOKE, CO, p. A71
MELROSE AREA HOSPITAL, MELROSE, MN, p. A230
MELROSE-WAKEFIELD HOSPITAL, MELROSE, MASSACHUSETTS, p. A206
MEMORIAL BEHAVIORAL HEALTH, GULFPORT, MS, p. A238
MEMORIAL CAMPUS, WORCESTER, MASSACHUSETTS, p. A210
MEMORIAL CENTER, BAKERSFIELD, CALIFORNIA, p. A36
MEMORIAL COMMUNITY HOSPITAL, EDGERTON, WI, p. A468
MEMORIAL COMMUNITY HOSPITAL AND HEALTH SYSTEM, BLAIR, NE, p. A261
MEMORIAL DIVISION, CHARLESTON, WEST VIRGINIA, p. A460
MEMORIAL HEALTH, SAVANNAH, GA, p. A109
MEMORIAL HEALTH CARE SYSTEMS, SEWARD, NE, p. A266
MEMORIAL HEALTH CENTER, SIDNEY, NE, p. A266
MEMORIAL HEALTH SYSTEM OF EAST TEXAS, LUFKIN, TX, p. A422
MEMORIAL HEALTHCARE CENTER, OWOSSO, MI, p. A220
MEMORIAL HERMANN BAPTIST HOSPITAL-EAST CAMPUS, BEAUMONT, TX, p. A404
MEMORIAL HERMANN BAPTIST HOSPITAL-WEST CAMPUS, BEAUMONT, TX, p. A404

Index of Hospitals / Mesa Lutheran Hospital

MEMORIAL HERMANN BEHAVIORAL HEALTH CENTER, HOUSTON, TX, p. A417
MEMORIAL HERMANN FORT BEND HOSPITAL, MISSOURI CITY, TX, p. A424
MEMORIAL HERMANN MEMORIAL CITY HOSPITAL, HOUSTON, TX, p. A417
MEMORIAL HERMANN REHABILITATION HOSPITAL, HOUSTON, TX, p. A417
MEMORIAL HERMANN SOUTHWEST HOSPITAL, HOUSTON, TX, p. A417
MEMORIAL HERMANN THE WOODLANDS HOSPITAL, THE WOODLANDS, TX, p. A432
MEMORIAL HOSPITAL, NORTH CONWAY, NH, p. A273
MEMORIAL HOSPITAL, ALBANY, NY, p. A287
MEMORIAL HOSPITAL, TOWANDA, PA, p. A373
MEMORIAL HOSPITAL, YORK, PA, p. A375
MEMORIAL HOSPITAL, FREMONT, OH, p. A332
MEMORIAL HOSPITAL, MARYSVILLE, OH, p. A334
MEMORIAL HOSPITAL, LOGANSPORT, IN, p. A143
MEMORIAL HOSPITAL, SEYMOUR, IN, p. A145
MEMORIAL HOSPITAL, BELLEVILLE, IL, p. A119
MEMORIAL HOSPITAL, CARTHAGE, IL, p. A120
MEMORIAL HOSPITAL, CHESTER, IL, p. A121
MEMORIAL HOSPITAL, MANCHESTER, KY, p. A176
MEMORIAL HOSPITAL, CHATTANOOGA, TN, p. A391
MEMORIAL HOSPITAL, AURORA, NE, p. A261
MEMORIAL HOSPITAL, ABILENE, KS, p. A159
MEMORIAL HOSPITAL, NEW YORK, KANSAS, p. A164
MEMORIAL HOSPITAL, MCPHERSON, KS, p. A165
MEMORIAL HOSPITAL, FREDERICK, OK, p. A343
MEMORIAL HOSPITAL, GONZALES, TX, p. A414
MEMORIAL HOSPITAL, KERMIT, TX, p. A420
MEMORIAL HOSPITAL, SEMINOLE, TX, p. A430
MEMORIAL HOSPITAL, WEISER, ID, p. A118
MEMORIAL HOSPITAL, COLORADO SPRINGS, CO, p. A68
MEMORIAL HOSPITAL, CRAIG, CO, p. A69
MEMORIAL HOSPITAL AND HEALTH CARE CENTER, JASPER, IN, p. A142
MEMORIAL HOSPITAL AND MANOR, BAINBRIDGE, GA, p. A101
MEMORIAL HOSPITAL AND MEDICAL CENTER OF CUMBERLAND, CUMBERLAND, MD, p. A197
MEMORIAL HOSPITAL AT EASTON MARYLAND, EASTON, MD, p. A198
MEMORIAL HOSPITAL AT EXETER, EXETER, CA, p. A40
MEMORIAL HOSPITAL AT GULFPORT, GULFPORT, MS, p. A238
MEMORIAL HOSPITAL CORPORATION OF BURLINGTON, BURLINGTON, WI, p. A467
MEMORIAL HOSPITAL LOS BANOS, LOS BANOS, CALIFORNIA, p. A51
MEMORIAL HOSPITAL OF ADEL, ADEL, GA, p. A99
MEMORIAL HOSPITAL OF CARBON COUNTY, RAWLINS, WY, p. A479
MEMORIAL HOSPITAL OF CARBONDALE, CARBONDALE, IL, p. A120
MEMORIAL HOSPITAL OF CENTER, CENTER, TX, p. A406
MEMORIAL HOSPITAL OF CONVERSE COUNTY, DOUGLAS, WY, p. A478
MEMORIAL HOSPITAL OF GARDENA, GARDENA, CA, p. A42
MEMORIAL HOSPITAL OF IOWA COUNTY, DODGEVILLE, WI, p. A468
MEMORIAL HOSPITAL OF JACKSONVILLE, JACKSONVILLE, FL, p. A86
MEMORIAL HOSPITAL OF LAFAYETTE COUNTY, DARLINGTON, WI, p. A467
MEMORIAL HOSPITAL OF MARTINSVILLE AND HENRY COUNTY, MARTINSVILLE, VA, p. A446
MEMORIAL HOSPITAL OF MICHIGAN CITY, MICHIGAN CITY, INDIANA, p. A144
MEMORIAL HOSPITAL OF RHODE ISLAND, PAWTUCKET, RI, p. A376
MEMORIAL HOSPITAL OF SALEM COUNTY, SALEM, NJ, p. A280
MEMORIAL HOSPITAL OF SHERIDAN COUNTY, SHERIDAN, WY, p. A479
MEMORIAL HOSPITAL OF SOUTH BEND, SOUTH BEND, IN, p. A146
MEMORIAL HOSPITAL OF SWEETWATER COUNTY, ROCK SPRINGS, WY, p. A479
MEMORIAL HOSPITAL OF TAMPA, TAMPA, FL, p. A96
MEMORIAL HOSPITAL OF TAYLOR COUNTY, MEDFORD, WI, p. A471
MEMORIAL HOSPITAL OF TEXAS COUNTY, GUYMON, OK, p. A344
MEMORIAL HOSPITAL PEMBROKE, PEMBROKE PINES, FL, p. A92
MEMORIAL HOSPITAL WEST, PEMBROKE PINES, FL, p. A92
MEMORIAL HOSPITAL-FLAGLER, BUNNELL, FL, p. A82
MEMORIAL HOSPITAL-ORMOND BEACH, ORMOND BEACH, FL, p. A92
MEMORIAL HOSPITAL-PENINSULA, ORMOND BEACH, FL, p. A92
MEMORIAL HOSPITAL-WEST VOLUSIA, DE LAND, FL, p. A83

MEMORIAL HOSPITALS ASSOCIATION, MODESTO, CA, p. A51
MEMORIAL MEDICAL CENTER, SPRINGFIELD, IL, p. A135
MEMORIAL MEDICAL CENTER, WOODSTOCK, IL, p. A136
MEMORIAL MEDICAL CENTER, ASHLAND, WI, p. A466
MEMORIAL MEDICAL CENTER, NEILLSVILLE, WI, p. A473
MEMORIAL MEDICAL CENTER, NEW ORLEANS, LA, p. A186
MEMORIAL MEDICAL CENTER, LIVINGSTON, TX, p. A421
MEMORIAL MEDICAL CENTER, PORT LAVACA, TX, p. A427
MEMORIAL MEDICAL CENTER, LAS CRUCES, NM, p. A285
MEMORIAL MEDICAL CENTER, MODESTO, CALIFORNIA, p. A51
MEMORIAL MEDICAL CENTER OF SAN AUGUSTINE, SAN AUGUSTINE, TX, p. A430
MEMORIAL MEDICAL CENTER OF WEST MICHIGAN, LUDINGTON, MI, p. A218
MEMORIAL MEDICAL CENTER–BAPTIST CAMPUS, NEW ORLEANS, LOUISIANA, p. A186
MEMORIAL MEDICAL CENTER–MERCY CAMPUS, NEW ORLEANS, LOUISIANA, p. A186
MEMORIAL MISSION HOSPITAL, ASHEVILLE, NORTH CAROLINA, p. A309
MEMORIAL NORTH PARK HOSPITAL, CHATTANOOGA, TENNESSEE, p. A391
MEMORIAL NUCKOLLS COUNTY HOSPITAL, SUPERIOR, NE, p. A267
MEMORIAL NURSING HOME, p. A471
MEMORIAL PAVILION, LAWTON, OK, p. A344
MEMORIAL PSYCHIATRIC HOSPITAL, ALBUQUERQUE, NM, p. A283
MEMORIAL REGIONAL HOSPITAL, LOS ANGELES, FL, p. A86
MEMORIAL REGIONAL MEDICAL CENTER, MECHANICSVILLE, VA, p. A446
MEMORIAL REHABILITATION HOSPITAL, MIDLAND, TEXAS, p. A424
MEMORIAL SLOAN-KETTERING CANCER CENTER, NEW YORK, NY, p. A298
MEMPHIS MENTAL HEALTH INSTITUTE, MEMPHIS, TN, p. A396
MENA MEDICAL CENTER, MENA, AR, p. A32
MENDOCINO COAST DISTRICT HOSPITAL, FORT BRAGG, CA, p. A41
MENDOTA COMMUNITY HOSPITAL, MENDOTA, IL, p. A130
MENDOTA MENTAL HEALTH INSTITUTE, MADISON, WI, p. A470
MENIFEE VALLEY MEDICAL CENTER, SUN CITY, CA, p. A64
MENNONITE GENERAL HOSPITAL, AIBONITO, PR, p. A481
MENORAH MEDICAL CENTER, SHAWNEE MISSION, KS, p. A167
MENTAL HEALTH CENTER, ALBUQUERQUE, NM, p. A283
MENTAL HEALTH INSTITUTE, CHEROKEE, IA, p. A149
MENTAL HEALTH INSTITUTE, CLARINDA, IA, p. A149
MENTAL HEALTH INSTITUTE, INDEPENDENCE, IA, p. A153
MENTAL HEALTH INSTITUTE, MOUNT PLEASANT, IA, p. A154
MEPSI CENTER, BAYAMON, PR, p. A482
MERCER COUNTY HOSPITAL, ALEDO, IL, p. A119
MERCER COUNTY JOINT TOWNSHIP COMMUNITY HOSPITAL, COLDWATER, OH, p. A329
MERCY AMERICAN RIVER HOSPITAL, CARMICHAEL, CALIFORNIA, p. A37
MERCY AMERICAN RIVER/MERCY SAN JUAN HOSPITAL, CARMICHAEL, CA, p. A37
MERCY BEHAVIORAL HEALTH CENTER, SIOUX CITY, IOWA, p. A156
MERCY COMMUNITY HOSPITAL, PORT JERVIS, NY, p. A303
MERCY COMMUNITY HOSPITAL, HAVERTOWN, PA, p. A361
MERCY FITZGERALD HOSPITAL, DARBY, PENNSYLVANIA, p. A358
MERCY FRANCISCAN HOSPITAL-MOUNT AIRY, CINCINNATI, OH, p. A328
MERCY FRANKLIN CENTER, DES MOINES, IOWA, p. A151
MERCY GENERAL HEALTH PARTNERS, MUSKEGON, MI, p. A220
MERCY GENERAL HEALTH PARTNERS-OAK AVENUE CAMPUS, MUSKEGON, MICHIGAN, p. A220
MERCY GENERAL HEALTH PARTNERS-SHERMAN BOULEVARD CAMPUS, MUSKEGON, MICHIGAN, p. A220
MERCY GENERAL HOSPITAL, SACRAMENTO, CA, p. A57
MERCY HEALTH CENTER, OKLAHOMA CITY, OK, p. A346
MERCY HEALTH CENTER, LAREDO, TX, p. A421
MERCY HEALTH CENTER OF MANHATTAN, NEW YORK, KS, p. A164
MERCY HEALTH LOVE COUNTY, MARIETTA, OK, p. A344
MERCY HEALTH SERVICES NORTH-GRAYLING, GRAYLING, MI, p. A216
MERCY HEALTH SYSTEM, JANESVILLE, WI, p. A469
MERCY HEALTH SYSTEM OF KANSAS, FORT SCOTT, KS, p. A161
MERCY HEALTH SYSTEM OF KANSAS, INDEPENDENCE, KS, p. A163
MERCY HEALTH SYSTEM OF SOUTHEASTERN PENNSYLVANIA, CONSHOHOCKEN, PA, p. A358
MERCY HOSPITAL, SPRINGFIELD, MA, p. A208
MERCY HOSPITAL, BUFFALO, NY, p. A289
MERCY HOSPITAL, CHARLOTTE, NC, p. A311
MERCY HOSPITAL, MIAMI, FL, p. A90

MERCY HOSPITAL, HAMILTON, OH, p. A333
MERCY HOSPITAL, PORTSMOUTH, OHIO, p. A337
MERCY HOSPITAL, TIFFIN, OH, p. A338
MERCY HOSPITAL, CADILLAC, MI, p. A212
MERCY HOSPITAL, PORT HURON, MI, p. A221
MERCY HOSPITAL, COON RAPIDS, MN, p. A227
MERCY HOSPITAL, IOWA CITY, IA, p. A153
MERCY HOSPITAL, DEVILS LAKE, ND, p. A321
MERCY HOSPITAL, VALLEY CITY, ND, p. A324
MERCY HOSPITAL, MOUNDRIDGE, KS, p. A165
MERCY HOSPITAL, BAKERSFIELD, CA, p. A36
MERCY HOSPITAL AND HEALTH CARE CENTER, MOOSE LAKE, MN, p. A231
MERCY HOSPITAL AND HEALTH SERVICES, MERCED, CA, p. A51
MERCY HOSPITAL AND MEDICAL CENTER, CHICAGO, IL, p. A122
MERCY HOSPITAL ANDERSON, CINCINNATI, OH, p. A328
MERCY HOSPITAL CLERMONT, BATAVIA, OH, p. A326
MERCY HOSPITAL OF FAIRFIELD, FAIRFIELD, OHIO, p. A333
MERCY HOSPITAL OF FOLSOM, FOLSOM, CA, p. A41
MERCY HOSPITAL OF FRANCISCAN SISTERS, OELWEIN, IA, p. A155
MERCY HOSPITAL OF HAMILTON, HAMILTON, OHIO, p. A333
MERCY HOSPITAL OF PHILADELPHIA, PHILADELPHIA, PENNSYLVANIA, p. A358
MERCY HOSPITAL OF PITTSBURGH, PITTSBURGH, PA, p. A369
MERCY HOSPITAL OF PORTLAND, PORTLAND, ME, p. A193
MERCY HOSPITAL OF SCOTT COUNTY, WALDRON, AR, p. A34
MERCY HOSPITAL OF SCRANTON, SCRANTON, PA, p. A371
MERCY HOSPITAL OF WILKES-BARRE, WILKES-BARRE, PA, p. A374
MERCY HOSPITAL OF WILLARD, WILLARD, OH, p. A339
MERCY HOSPITAL SOUTH, PINEVILLE, NORTH CAROLINA, p. A311
MERCY HOSPITAL-TURNER MEMORIAL, OZARK, AR, p. A33
MERCY MEDICAL, DAPHNE, AL, p. A13
MERCY MEDICAL CENTER, ROCKVILLE CENTRE, NY, p. A304
MERCY MEDICAL CENTER, BALTIMORE, MD, p. A196
MERCY MEDICAL CENTER, CANTON, OH, p. A326
MERCY MEDICAL CENTER, SPRINGFIELD, OH, p. A337
MERCY MEDICAL CENTER, OSHKOSH, WI, p. A473
MERCY MEDICAL CENTER, CEDAR RAPIDS, IA, p. A149
MERCY MEDICAL CENTER, WILLISTON, ND, p. A324
MERCY MEDICAL CENTER, NAMPA, ID, p. A117
MERCY MEDICAL CENTER, DURANGO, CO, p. A70
MERCY MEDICAL CENTER, ROSEBURG, OR, p. A354
MERCY MEDICAL CENTER – NORTH IOWA, MASON CITY, IA, p. A154
MERCY MEDICAL CENTER MOUNT SHASTA, MOUNT SHASTA, CA, p. A52
MERCY MEDICAL CENTER REDDING, REDDING, CA, p. A56
MERCY MEDICAL CENTER-CENTERVILLE, CENTERVILLE, IA, p. A149
MERCY MEDICAL CENTER-CLINTON, CLINTON, IA, p. A149
MERCY MEDICAL CENTER-DES MOINES, DES MOINES, IA, p. A151
MERCY MEDICAL CENTER-DUBUQUE, DUBUQUE, IA, p. A151
MERCY MEDICAL CENTER-DYERSVILLE, DYERSVILLE, IOWA, p. A151
MERCY MEDICAL CENTER-NEW HAMPTON, NEW HAMPTON, IA, p. A155
MERCY MEDICAL CENTER-SIOUX CITY, SIOUX CITY, IA, p. A156
MERCY MEMORIAL HEALTH CENTER, ARDMORE, OK, p. A341
MERCY MEMORIAL HOSPITAL, URBANA, OH, p. A338
MERCY MEMORIAL HOSPITAL, MONROE, MI, p. A219
MERCY PROVIDENCE HOSPITAL, PITTSBURGH, PA, p. A369
MERCY SAN JUAN HOSPITAL, CARMICHAEL, CALIFORNIA, p. A37
MERCY SERVICES FOR AGING, CLINTON, IOWA, p. A149
MERCY SOUTHWEST HOSPITAL, BAKERSFIELD, CALIFORNIA, p. A36
MERCY SPECIAL CARE HOSPITAL, NANTICOKE, PA, p. A365
MERCY SUBURBAN HOSPITAL, NORRISTOWN, PA, p. A365
MERCY WESTBROOK, WESTBROOK, MAINE, p. A193
MERCY WESTSIDE HOSPITAL, TAFT, CA, p. A64
MERIDELL ACHIEVEMENT CENTER, LIBERTY HILL, TX, p. A421
MERIDIA HILLCREST HOSPITAL, CLEVELAND, OH, p. A329
MERIDIA HURON HOSPITAL, CLEVELAND, OH, p. A329
MERIDIA SOUTH POINTE HOSPITAL, WARRENSVILLE HEIGHTS, OH, p. A339
MERITCARE HEALTH SYSTEM, FARGO, ND, p. A322
MERITER HOSPITAL, MADISON, WI, p. A470
MERITER-CAPITOL, MADISON, WISCONSIN, p. A470
MERLE WEST MEDICAL CENTER, KLAMATH FALLS, OR, p. A351
MERRILL PIONEER COMMUNITY HOSPITAL, ROCK RAPIDS, IA, p. A156
MESA GENERAL HOSPITAL MEDICAL CENTER, MESA, AZ, p. A23
MESA LUTHERAN HOSPITAL, MESA, AZ, p. A23

© 2000 AHA Guide

Index of Hospitals / Mesquite Community Hospital

MESQUITE COMMUNITY HOSPITAL, MESQUITE, TX, p. A423
METHODIST AMBULATORY SURGERY HOSPITAL, SAN ANTONIO, TX, p. A428
METHODIST BEHAVIORAL RESOURCES, NEW ORLEANS, LA, p. A187
METHODIST CHILDREN'S HOSPITAL OF SOUTH TEXAS, SAN ANTONIO, TX, p. A428
METHODIST HEALTH CENTER–SUGAR LAND, SUGAR LAND, TX, p. A431
METHODIST HEALTHCARE – MCKENZIE, MCKENZIE, TN, p. A396
METHODIST HEALTHCARE– DYERSBURG HOSPITAL, DYERSBURG, TN, p. A392
METHODIST HEALTHCARE–BROWNSVILLE, BROWNSVILLE, TN, p. A390
METHODIST HEALTHCARE–LEXINGTON HOSPITAL, LEXINGTON, TN, p. A395
METHODIST HEALTHCARE–MCNAIRY HOSPITAL, SELMER, TN, p. A399
METHODIST HEALTHCARE–MEMPHIS HOSPITAL, MEMPHIS, TN, p. A397
METHODIST HEALTHCARE–SOMERVILLE, SOMERVILLE, TN, p. A399
METHODIST HEALTHCARE–VOLUNTEER HOSPITAL, MARTIN, TN, p. A396
METHODIST HOSPITAL, PHILADELPHIA, PENNSYLVANIA, p. A368
METHODIST HOSPITAL, HENDERSON, KY, p. A173
METHODIST HOSPITAL GERMANTOWN, GERMANTOWN, TENNESSEE, p. A397
METHODIST HOSPITAL HEALTHSYSTEM MINNESOTA, SAINT LOUIS PARK, MN, p. A233
METHODIST HOSPITAL OF CHICAGO, CHICAGO, IL, p. A122
METHODIST HOSPITAL OF INDIANA, INDIANAPOLIS, INDIANA, p. A141
METHODIST HOSPITAL OF SACRAMENTO, SACRAMENTO, CA, p. A57
METHODIST HOSPITAL OF SOUTHERN CALIFORNIA, ARCADIA, CA, p. A35
METHODIST HOSPITAL UNION COUNTY, MORGANFIELD, KY, p. A177
METHODIST HOSPITALS, GARY, IN, p. A140
METHODIST HOSPITALS OF MEMPHIS–CENTRAL, MEMPHIS, TENNESSEE, p. A397
METHODIST HOSPITALS OF MEMPHIS–SOUTH UNIT, MEMPHIS, TENNESSEE, p. A397
METHODIST LEBONHEUR HEALTHCARE–JACKSON, JACKSON, TN, p. A393
METHODIST MEDICAL CENTER, JACKSONVILLE, FLORIDA, p. A87
METHODIST MEDICAL CENTER, DALLAS, TX, p. A409
METHODIST MEDICAL CENTER OF ILLINOIS, PEORIA, IL, p. A132
METHODIST MEDICAL CENTER OF OAK RIDGE, OAK RIDGE, TN, p. A398
METHODIST NORTH–J. HARRIS HOSPITAL, MEMPHIS, TENNESSEE, p. A397
METHODIST SPECIALTY AND TRANSPLANT HOSPITAL, SAN ANTONIO, TX, p. A429
METRO HEALTH CENTER, ERIE, PA, p. A360
METROHEALTH MEDICAL CENTER, CLEVELAND, OH, p. A329
METROPLEX ADVENTIST HOSPITAL, KILLEEN, TX, p. A420
METROPOLITAN GENERAL CARE UNIT, METROPOLITAN DRUG DETOXIFICATION AND METROPOLITAN PSYCHIATRIC UNIT, p. A298
METROPOLITAN HOSPITAL, ATLANTA, GA, p. A100
METROPOLITAN HOSPITAL, GRAND RAPIDS, MI, p. A215
METROPOLITAN HOSPITAL CENTER, NEW YORK, NY, p. A298
METROPOLITAN MEDICAL CENTER–WEST, SAINT LOUIS, MISSOURI, p. A253
METROPOLITAN METHODIST HOSPITAL, SAN ANTONIO, TX, p. A429
METROPOLITAN NASHVILLE GENERAL HOSPITAL, NASHVILLE, TN, p. A398
METROPOLITAN ST. LOUIS PSYCHIATRIC CENTER, SAINT LOUIS, MO, p. A253
METROPOLITAN STATE HOSPITAL, NORWALK, CA, p. A53
METROWEST MEDICAL CENTER, FRAMINGHAM, MA, p. A205
MEYERSDALE MEDICAL CENTER, MEYERSDALE, PA, p. A364
MIAMI CHILDREN'S HOSPITAL, MIAMI, FL, p. A90
MIAMI COUNTY MEDICAL CENTER, PAOLA, KS, p. A166
MIAMI HEART INSTITUTE AND MEDICAL CENTER, MIAMI, FL, p. A90
MIAMI JEWISH HOME AND HOSPITAL FOR AGED, MIAMI, FL, p. A90
MIAMI VALLEY HOSPITAL, DAYTON, OH, p. A331
MICHAEL REESE HOSPITAL AND MEDICAL CENTER, CHICAGO, IL, p. A122
MID COAST HOSPITAL, BATH, ME, p. A191
MID COAST HOSPITAL, BRUNSWICK, MAINE, p. A191

MID DAKOTA HOSPITAL, CHAMBERLAIN, SD, p. A385
MID MISSOURI MENTAL HEALTH CENTER, COLUMBIA, MO, p. A246
MID-AMERICA REHABILITATION HOSPITAL, OVERLAND PARK, KS, p. A166
MID-COLUMBIA MEDICAL CENTER, THE DALLES, OR, p. A354
MID-HUDSON FORENSIC PSYCHIATRIC CENTER, NEW HAMPTON, NY, p. A295
MID-JEFFERSON HOSPITAL, NEDERLAND, TX, p. A425
MID-VALLEY HOSPITAL, PECKVILLE, PA, p. A366
MID-VALLEY HOSPITAL, OMAK, WA, p. A455
MIDDLE GEORGIA HOSPITAL, MACON, GA, p. A107
MIDDLE TENNESSEE MEDICAL CENTER, MURFREESBORO, TN, p. A397
MIDDLE TENNESSEE MENTAL HEALTH INSTITUTE, NASHVILLE, TN, p. A398
MIDDLESBORO APPALACHIAN REGIONAL HOSPITAL, MIDDLESBORO, KY, p. A176
MIDDLESEX HOSPITAL, MIDDLETOWN, CT, p. A75
MIDDLETOWN PSYCHIATRIC CENTER, MIDDLETOWN, NY, p. A294
MIDDLETOWN REGIONAL HOSPITAL, MIDDLETOWN, OH, p. A335
MIDLAND MEMORIAL HOSPITAL, MIDLAND, TX, p. A424
MIDLANDS CENTER, COLUMBIA, SC, p. A379
MIDMICHIGAN MEDICAL CENTER–CLARE, CLARE, MI, p. A213
MIDMICHIGAN MEDICAL CENTER–GLADWIN, GLADWIN, MI, p. A215
MIDMICHIGAN MEDICAL CENTER–MIDLAND, MIDLAND, MI, p. A219
MIDSTATE MEDICAL CENTER, MERIDEN, CT, p. A75
MIDWAY HOSPITAL MEDICAL CENTER, LOS ANGELES, CA, p. A48
MIDWEST REGIONAL MEDICAL CENTER, MIDWEST CITY, OK, p. A345
MIDWESTERN REGIONAL MEDICAL CENTER, ZION, IL, p. A136
MIKE O'CALLAGHAN FEDERAL HOSPITAL, NELLIS AFB, NV, p. A269
MILAN GENERAL HOSPITAL, MILAN, TN, p. A397
MILDRED MITCHELL–BATEMAN HOSPITAL, HUNTINGTON, WV, p. A462
MILE BLUFF MEDICAL CENTER, MAUSTON, WI, p. A471
MILES MEMORIAL HOSPITAL, DAMARISCOTTA, ME, p. A192
MILFORD HOSPITAL, MILFORD, CT, p. A75
MILFORD VALLEY MEMORIAL HOSPITAL, MILFORD, UT, p. A437
MILFORD–WHITINSVILLE REGIONAL HOSPITAL, MILFORD, MA, p. A206
MILLARD FILLMORE GATES CIRCLE HOSPITAL, BUFFALO, NY, p. A289
MILLARD FILLMORE SUBURBAN HOSPITAL, WILLIAMSVILLE, NEW YORK, p. A289
MILLCREEK COMMUNITY HOSPITAL, ERIE, PA, p. A360
MILLE LACS HEALTH SYSTEM, ONAMIA, MN, p. A231
MILLER COUNTY HOSPITAL, COLQUITT, GA, p. A102
MILLER DWAN MEDICAL CENTER, DULUTH, MN, p. A227
MILLINOCKET REGIONAL HOSPITAL, MILLINOCKET, ME, p. A193
MILLS HOSPITAL, SAN MATEO, CALIFORNIA, p. A37
MILLS–PENINSULA HEALTH SERVICES, BURLINGAME, CA, p. A37
MILTON HOSPITAL, MILTON, MA, p. A206
MILWAUKEE COUNTY MENTAL HEALTH DIVISION, MILWAUKEE, WI, p. A472
MILWAUKEE PSYCHIATRIC HOSPITAL, WAUWATOSA, WI, p. A477
MIMBRES MEMORIAL HOSPITAL, DEMING, NM, p. A284
MINDEN MEDICAL CENTER, MINDEN, LA, p. A185
MINER'S MEMORIAL MEDICAL CENTER, COALDALE, PA, p. A358
MINERAL AREA REGIONAL MEDICAL CENTER, FARMINGTON, MO, p. A246
MINERAL COMMUNITY HOSPITAL, SUPERIOR, MT, p. A259
MINERS HOSPITAL NORTHERN CAMBRIA, HASTINGS, PA, p. A361
MINERS' COLFAX MEDICAL CENTER, RATON, NM, p. A285
MINERS' HOSPITAL OF NEW MEXICO, RATON, NEW MEXICO, p. A285
MINIDOKA MEMORIAL HOSPITAL AND EXTENDED CARE FACILITY, RUPERT, ID, p. A117
MINNEOLA DISTRICT HOSPITAL, MINNEOLA, KS, p. A165
MINNESOTA SECURITY HOSPITAL, SAINT PETER, MINNESOTA, p. A233
MINNESOTA VALLEY HEALTH CENTER, LE SUEUR, MN, p. A229
MINNEWASKA DISTRICT HOSPITAL, STARBUCK, MN, p. A234
MINNIE G. BOSWELL MEMORIAL HOSPITAL, GREENSBORO, GA, p. A105
MINNIE HAMILTON HEALTHCARE CENTER, GRANTSVILLE, WV, p. A461
MIRIAM HOSPITAL, PROVIDENCE, RI, p. A376
MISSION BAY HOSPITAL, SAN DIEGO, CA, p. A58
MISSION COMMUNITY HOSPITAL–PANORAMA CITY CAMPUS, LOS ANGELES, CALIFORNIA, p. A59

MISSION COMMUNITY HOSPITAL–SAN FERNANDO CAMPUS, SAN FERNANDO, CA, p. A59
MISSION HILL MEMORIAL HOSPITAL, SHAWNEE, OK, p. A347
MISSION HOSPITAL, MISSION, TX, p. A424
MISSION HOSPITAL OF HUNTINGTON PARK, HUNTINGTON PARK, CALIFORNIA, p. A44
MISSION HOSPITAL REGIONAL MEDICAL CENTER, MISSION VIEJO, CA, p. A51
MISSION ST. JOSEPH'S HEALTH, ASHEVILLE, NC, p. A309
MISSION VISTA BEHAVIORAL HEALTH SYSTEM, SAN ANTONIO, TX, p. A429
MISSISSIPPI BAPTIST HEALTH SYSTEMS, JACKSON, MS, p. A239
MISSISSIPPI HOSPITAL RESTORATIVE CARE, JACKSON, MS, p. A239
MISSISSIPPI METHODIST HOSPITAL AND REHABILITATION CENTER, JACKSON, MS, p. A239
MISSISSIPPI STATE HOSPITAL, WHITFIELD, MS, p. A243
MISSOURI BAPTIST HOSPITAL OF SULLIVAN, SULLIVAN, MO, p. A255
MISSOURI BAPTIST MEDICAL CENTER, TOWN AND COUNTRY, MO, p. A255
MISSOURI DELTA MEDICAL CENTER, SIKESTON, MO, p. A254
MISSOURI REHABILITATION CENTER, MOUNT VERNON, MO, p. A250
MISSOURI RIVER MEDICAL CENTER, FORT BENTON, MT, p. A257
MITCHELL COUNTY HOSPITAL, CAMILLA, GA, p. A102
MITCHELL COUNTY HOSPITAL, BELOIT, KS, p. A159
MITCHELL COUNTY HOSPITAL, COLORADO CITY, TX, p. A407
MITCHELL COUNTY REGIONAL HEALTH CENTER, OSAGE, IA, p. A155
MITCHELL–HOLLINGSWORTH ANNEX, p. A14
MIZELL MEMORIAL HOSPITAL, OPP, AL, p. A17
MOBERLY REGIONAL MEDICAL CENTER, MOBERLY, MO, p. A250
MOBILE INFIRMARY MEDICAL CENTER, MOBILE, AL, p. A16
MOBRIDGE REGIONAL HOSPITAL, MOBRIDGE, SD, p. A387
MOCCASIN BEND MENTAL HEALTH INSTITUTE, CHATTANOOGA, TN, p. A391
MODOC MEDICAL CENTER, ALTURAS, CA, p. A35
MOHAVE VALLEY HOSPITAL AND MEDICAL CENTER, BULLHEAD CITY, AZ, p. A22
MOHAWK VALLEY PSYCHIATRIC CENTER, UTICA, NY, p. A306
MOLOKAI GENERAL HOSPITAL, KAUNAKAKAI, HI, p. A113
MONADNOCK COMMUNITY HOSPITAL, PETERBOROUGH, NH, p. A273
MONCRIEF ARMY COMMUNITY HOSPITAL, FORT JACKSON, SC, p. A381
MONMOUTH MEDICAL CENTER, LONG BRANCH, NJ, p. A277
MONONGAHELA VALLEY HOSPITAL, MONONGAHELA, PA, p. A364
MONONGALIA GENERAL HOSPITAL, MORGANTOWN, WV, p. A463
MONROE COUNTY HOSPITAL, FORSYTH, GA, p. A105
MONROE COUNTY HOSPITAL, MONROEVILLE, AL, p. A16
MONROE COUNTY HOSPITAL, ALBIA, IA, p. A148
MONROE COUNTY MEDICAL CENTER, TOMPKINSVILLE, KY, p. A178
MONROVIA COMMUNITY HOSPITAL, MONROVIA, CA, p. A51
MONSIGNOR JAMES H FITZPATRICK PAVILION FOR SKILLED NURSING CARE, NEW YORK, NEW YORK, p. A296
MONSOUR MEDICAL CENTER, JEANNETTE, PA, p. A362
MONTANA STATE HOSPITAL, WARM SPRINGS, MT, p. A260
MONTCLAIR BAPTIST MEDICAL CENTER, BIRMINGHAM, AL, p. A12
MONTEFIORE HOSPITAL, PITTSBURGH, PENNSYLVANIA, p. A370
MONTEFIORE MEDICAL CENTER, NEW YORK, NY, p. A298
MONTEREY PARK HOSPITAL, MONTEREY PARK, CA, p. A52
MONTFORT JONES MEMORIAL HOSPITAL, KOSCIUSKO, MS, p. A240
MONTGOMERY COUNTY EMERGENCY SERVICE, NORRISTOWN, PA, p. A365
MONTGOMERY COUNTY MEMORIAL HOSPITAL, RED OAK, IA, p. A156
MONTGOMERY DIVISION, MONTGOMERY, ALABAMA, p. A17
MONTGOMERY GENERAL HOSPITAL, OLNEY, MD, p. A199
MONTGOMERY GENERAL HOSPITAL, MONTGOMERY, WV, p. A463
MONTGOMERY HOSPITAL, NORRISTOWN, PA, p. A365
MONTGOMERY REGIONAL HOSPITAL, BLACKSBURG, VA, p. A442
MONTICELLO BIG LAKE HOSPITAL, MONTICELLO, MN, p. A231
MONTPELIER HOSPITAL, MONTPELIER, OHIO, p. A326
MONTROSE MEMORIAL HOSPITAL, MONTROSE, CO, p. A72
MOORE COUNTY HOSPITAL DISTRICT, DUMAS, TX, p. A410
MOREHEAD MEMORIAL HOSPITAL, EDEN, NC, p. A312
MOREHOUSE GENERAL HOSPITAL, BASTROP, LA, p. A180

MORENO VALLEY COMMUNITY HOSPITAL, MORENO VALLEY, CA, p. A52
MORGAN COUNTY APPALACHIAN REGIONAL HOSPITAL, WEST LIBERTY, KY, p. A179
MORGAN COUNTY MEMORIAL HOSPITAL, MARTINSVILLE, IN, p. A143
MORGAN COUNTY WAR MEMORIAL HOSPITAL, BERKELEY SPRINGS, WV, p. A460
MORGAN MEMORIAL HOSPITAL, MADISON, GA, p. A107
MORITZ COMMUNITY HOSPITAL, LOS ANGELES, IDAHO, p. A118
MORRILL COUNTY COMMUNITY HOSPITAL, BRIDGEPORT, NE, p. A261
MORRIS COUNTY HOSPITAL, COUNCIL GROVE, KS, p. A160
MORRIS HOSPITAL, MORRIS, IL, p. A131
MORRISON COMMUNITY HOSPITAL, MORRISON, IL, p. A131
MORRISTOWN MEMORIAL HOSPITAL, MORRISTOWN, NEW JERSEY, p. A276
MORRISTOWN–HAMBLEN HOSPITAL, MORRISTOWN, TN, p. A397
MORROW COUNTY HOSPITAL, MOUNT GILEAD, OH, p. A335
MORTON COUNTY HEALTH SYSTEM, ELKHART, KS, p. A160
MORTON GENERAL HOSPITAL, MORTON, WA, p. A454
MORTON HOSPITAL AND MEDICAL CENTER, TAUNTON, MA, p. A209
MORTON PLANT HOSPITAL, CLEARWATER, FL, p. A82
MORTON PLANT MEASE–NORTH BAY HOSPITAL, NEW PORT RICHEY, FL, p. A91
MOSES CONE HEALTH SYSTEM, GREENSBORO, NC, p. A313
MOSES H. CONE MEMORIAL HOSPITAL, GREENSBORO, NORTH CAROLINA, p. A313
MOSES LUDINGTON HOSPITAL, TICONDEROGA, NY, p. A306
MOSES TAYLOR HOSPITAL, SCRANTON, PA, p. A372
MOSS REHABILITATION HOSPITAL, PHILADELPHIA, PENNSYLVANIA, p. A366
MOTION PICTURE AND TELEVISION FUND HOSPITAL AND RESIDENTIAL SERVICES, LOS ANGELES, CA, p. A49
MOUNT AUBURN HOSPITAL, CAMBRIDGE, MA, p. A204
MOUNT CARMEL EAST HOSPITAL, COLUMBUS, OHIO, p. A330
MOUNT CARMEL HEALTH SYSTEM, COLUMBUS, OH, p. A330
MOUNT CARMEL HOSPITAL, COLVILLE, WA, p. A453
MOUNT CARMEL MEDICAL CENTER, COLUMBUS, OHIO, p. A330
MOUNT CARMEL MEDICAL CENTER, PITTSBURG, KS, p. A166
MOUNT CLEMENS GENERAL HOSPITAL, MOUNT CLEMENS, MI, p. A219
MOUNT DESERT ISLAND HOSPITAL, BAR HARBOR, ME, p. A191
MOUNT DIABLO MEDICAL CENTER, CONCORD, CALIFORNIA, p. A66
MOUNT GRAHAM COMMUNITY HOSPITAL, SAFFORD, AZ, p. A25
MOUNT GRANT GENERAL HOSPITAL, HAWTHORNE, NV, p. A268
MOUNT REGIS CENTER, SALEM, VA, p. A449
MOUNT SINAI HOSPITAL MEDICAL CENTER OF CHICAGO, CHICAGO, IL, p. A122
MOUNT SINAI MEDICAL CENTER, NEW YORK, NEW YORK, p. A298
MOUNT SINAI MEDICAL CENTER, MIAMI BEACH, FL, p. A90
MOUNT SINAI–NYU HOSPITALS/HEALTH SYSTEM, NEW YORK, NY, p. A298
MOUNT SINAI–NYU MEDICAL CENTER, NEW YORK, NEW YORK, p. A298
MOUNT ST. MARY'S HOSPITAL AND HEALTH CENTER, LEWISTON, NY, p. A293
MOUNT VERNON HOSPITAL, MOUNT VERNON, NY, p. A295
MOUNTAIN CREST HOSPITAL, FORT COLLINS, COLORADO, p. A70
MOUNTAIN MANOR TREATMENT CENTER, EMMITSBURG, MD, p. A198
MOUNTAIN VIEW HOSPITAL, GADSDEN, AL, p. A15
MOUNTAIN VIEW HOSPITAL, PAYSON, UT, p. A437
MOUNTAIN VIEW HOSPITAL DISTRICT, MADRAS, OR, p. A352
MOUNTAINSIDE HOSPITAL, MONTCLAIR, NEW JERSEY, p. A276
MOUNTAINVIEW HOSPITAL, LAS VEGAS, NV, p. A268
MOUNTAINVIEW MEDICAL CENTER, WHITE SULPHUR SPRINGS, MT, p. A260
MOUNTRAIL COUNTY MEDICAL CENTER, STANLEY, ND, p. A324
MT. ASCUTNEY HOSPITAL AND HEALTH CENTER, WINDSOR, VT, p. A441
MT. SAN RAFAEL HOSPITAL, TRINIDAD, CO, p. A73
MT. WASHINGTON PEDIATRIC HOSPITAL, BALTIMORE, MD, p. A196
MUENSTER MEMORIAL HOSPITAL, MUENSTER, TX, p. A424
MUHLENBERG COMMUNITY HOSPITAL, GREENVILLE, KY, p. A172
MUHLENBERG HOSPITAL CENTER, BETHLEHEM, PA, p. A356
MUHLENBERG REGIONAL MEDICAL CENTER, PLAINFIELD, NJ, p. A279
MULESHOE AREA MEDICAL CENTER, MULESHOE, TX, p. A424
MUNCY VALLEY HOSPITAL, MUNCY, PENNSYLVANIA, p. A375
MUNISING MEMORIAL HOSPITAL, MUNISING, MI, p. A219
MUNROE REGIONAL MEDICAL CENTER, OCALA, FL, p. A91
MUNSON MEDICAL CENTER, TRAVERSE CITY, MI, p. A223
MURPHY MEDICAL CENTER, MURPHY, NC, p. A316
MURRAY COUNTY MEMORIAL HOSPITAL, SLAYTON, MN, p. A233
MURRAY MEDICAL CENTER, CHATSWORTH, GA, p. A102
MURRAY–CALLOWAY COUNTY HOSPITAL, MURRAY, KY, p. A177
MUSC MEDICAL CENTER OF MEDICAL UNIVERSITY OF SOUTH CAROLINA, CHARLESTON, SC, p. A379
MUSKOGEE REGIONAL MEDICAL CENTER, MUSKOGEE, OK, p. A345
MYERS CAMPUS, SODUS, NEW YORK, p. A301
MYRTLE WERTH HOSPITAL–MAYO HEALTH SYSTEM, MENOMONIE, WI, p. A471

N

NACOGDOCHES MEDICAL CENTER, NACOGDOCHES, TX, p. A424
NACOGDOCHES MEMORIAL HOSPITAL, NACOGDOCHES, TX, p. A424
NANTICOKE MEMORIAL HOSPITAL, SEAFORD, DE, p. A78
NANTUCKET COTTAGE HOSPITAL, NANTUCKET, MA, p. A206
NAPA STATE HOSPITAL, NAPA, CA, p. A52
NAPLES COMMUNITY HOSPITAL, NAPLES, FL, p. A90
NASH HEALTH CARE SYSTEMS, ROCKY MOUNT, NC, p. A317
NASHVILLE MEMORIAL HOSPITAL, MADISON, TN, p. A395
NASHVILLE METROPOLITAN BORDEAUX HOSPITAL, NASHVILLE, TN, p. A398
NASHVILLE REHABILITATION HOSPITAL, NASHVILLE, TN, p. A398
NASON HOSPITAL, ROARING SPRING, PA, p. A371
NASSAU COUNTY MEDICAL CENTER, EAST MEADOW, NY, p. A291
NATCHAUG HOSPITAL, MANSFIELD CENTER, CT, p. A75
NATCHEZ COMMUNITY HOSPITAL, NATCHEZ, MS, p. A241
NATCHEZ REGIONAL MEDICAL CENTER, NATCHEZ, MS, p. A241
NATCHITOCHES PARISH HOSPITAL, NATCHITOCHES, LA, p. A186
NATHAN LITTAUER HOSPITAL AND NURSING HOME, GLOVERSVILLE, NY, p. A292
NATIONAL HOSPITAL FOR KIDS IN CRISIS, OREFIELD, PA, p. A366
NATIONAL JEWISH MEDICAL AND RESEARCH CENTER, DENVER, CO, p. A69
NATIONAL NAVAL MEDICAL CENTER, BETHESDA, MD, p. A197
NATIONAL PARK MEDICAL CENTER, HOT SPRINGS, AR, p. A30
NATIONAL REHABILITATION HOSPITAL, WASHINGTON, DC, p. A79
NATIVIDAD MEDICAL CENTER, SALINAS, CA, p. A58
NATURE COAST REGIONAL HOSPITAL, WILLISTON, FL, p. A98
NAVAL HOSPITAL, CAMP LEJEUNE, NC, p. A310
NAVAL HOSPITAL, CHERRY POINT, NC, p. A311
NAVAL HOSPITAL, BEAUFORT, SC, p. A378
NAVAL HOSPITAL, NORTH CHARLESTON, SC, p. A383
NAVAL HOSPITAL, JACKSONVILLE, FL, p. A86
NAVAL HOSPITAL, PENSACOLA, FL, p. A93
NAVAL HOSPITAL, GREAT LAKES, IL, p. A127
NAVAL HOSPITAL, CORPUS CHRISTI, TX, p. A407
NAVAL HOSPITAL, BREMERTON, WA, p. A452
NAVAL HOSPITAL, OAK HARBOR, WA, p. A455
NAVAL HOSPITAL, LEMOORE, CA, p. A46
NAVAL HOSPITAL, CAMP PENDLETON, CA, p. A37
NAVAL HOSPITAL, TWENTYNINE PALMS, CA, p. A65
NAVAL MEDICAL CENTER, PORTSMOUTH, VA, p. A448
NAVAL MEDICAL CENTER, SAN DIEGO, CA, p. A59
NAVAPACHE REGIONAL MEDICAL CENTER, SHOW LOW, AZ, p. A26
NAVARRO REGIONAL HOSPITAL, CORSICANA, TX, p. A408
NAZARETH HOSPITAL, PHILADELPHIA, PA, p. A367
NEBRASKA HEALTH SYSTEM, OMAHA, NE, p. A265
NEBRASKA HEALTH SYSTEM, OMAHA, NEBRASKA, p. A265
NEBRASKA HEALTH SYSTEM, OMAHA, NEBRASKA, p. A265
NEBRASKA METHODIST HOSPITAL, OMAHA, NE, p. A265
NEILLSVILLE MEMORIAL HOME, p. A473
NEMAHA COUNTY HOSPITAL, AUBURN, NE, p. A261
NEMAHA VALLEY COMMUNITY HOSPITAL, SENECA, KS, p. A167
NEOSHO MEMORIAL REGIONAL MEDICAL CENTER, CHANUTE, KS, p. A160
NESBITT MEMORIAL HOSPITAL, KINGSTON, PENNSYLVANIA, p. A374
NESHOBA COUNTY GENERAL HOSPITAL, PHILADELPHIA, MS, p. A241
NESS COUNTY HOSPITAL, NESS CITY, KS, p. A165
NEVADA MENTAL HEALTH INSTITUTE, SPARKS, NV, p. A269
NEVADA REGIONAL MEDICAL CENTER, NEVADA, MO, p. A251
NEW BRITAIN GENERAL HOSPITAL, NEW BRITAIN, CT, p. A75

NEW ENGLAND BAPTIST HOSPITAL, BOSTON, MA, p. A202
NEW ENGLAND MEDICAL CENTER, BOSTON, MA, p. A202
NEW ENGLAND REHABILITATION HOSPITAL OF PORTLAND, PORTLAND, ME, p. A193
NEW ENGLAND SINAI HOSPITAL AND REHABILITATION CENTER, STOUGHTON, MA, p. A209
NEW HAMPSHIRE HOSPITAL, CONCORD, NH, p. A271
NEW HANOVER REGIONAL MEDICAL CENTER, WILMINGTON, NC, p. A319
NEW ISLAND HOSPITAL, BETHPAGE, NY, p. A288
NEW JERSEY ORTHOPEDIC HOSPITAL UNIT, ORANGE, NEW JERSEY, p. A279
NEW LONDON FAMILY MEDICAL CENTER, NEW LONDON, WI, p. A473
NEW LONDON HOSPITAL, NEW LONDON, NH, p. A272
NEW MILFORD HOSPITAL, NEW MILFORD, CT, p. A76
NEW ORLEANS ADOLESCENT HOSPITAL, NEW ORLEANS, LA, p. A187
NEW ULM MEDICAL CENTER, NEW ULM, MN, p. A231
NEW YORK COMMUNITY HOSPITAL OF BROOKLYN, NEW YORK, NY, p. A298
NEW YORK EYE AND EAR INFIRMARY, NEW YORK, NY, p. A298
NEW YORK FLUSHING HOSPITAL MEDICAL CENTER, NEW YORK, NY, p. A298
NEW YORK HOSPITAL MEDICAL CENTER OF QUEENS, NEW YORK, NY, p. A298
NEW YORK METHODIST HOSPITAL, NEW YORK, NY, p. A298
NEW YORK STATE PSYCHIATRIC INSTITUTE, NEW YORK, NY, p. A299
NEW YORK UNITED HOSPITAL MEDICAL CENTER, PORT CHESTER, NY, p. A303
NEW YORK UNIVERSITY DOWNTOWN HOSPITAL, NEW YORK, NY, p. A299
NEW YORK WEILL CORNELL MEDICAL CENTER, NEW YORK, NEW YORK, p. A299
NEW YORK–PRESBYTERIAN HOSPITAL, NEW YORK, NY, p. A299
NEW YORK–PRESBYTERIAN HOSPITAL, WESTCHESTER DIVISION, NEW YORK, NEW YORK, p. A299
NEWARK BETH ISRAEL MEDICAL CENTER, NEWARK, NJ, p. A278
NEWARK–WAYNE CAMPUS, NEWARK, NEW YORK, p. A301
NEWBERRY COUNTY MEMORIAL HOSPITAL, NEWBERRY, SC, p. A382
NEWMAN MEMORIAL COUNTY HOSPITAL, EMPORIA, KS, p. A161
NEWMAN MEMORIAL HOSPITAL, SHATTUCK, OK, p. A347
NEWNAN HOSPITAL, NEWNAN, GA, p. A108
NEWPORT COMMUNITY HOSPITAL, NEWPORT, WA, p. A455
NEWPORT HOSPITAL, NEWPORT, RI, p. A376
NEWPORT HOSPITAL AND CLINIC, NEWPORT, AR, p. A32
NEWTON GENERAL HOSPITAL, COVINGTON, GA, p. A103
NEWTON MEDICAL CENTER, NEWTON, KS, p. A165
NEWTON MEMORIAL HOSPITAL, NEWTON, NJ, p. A278
NEWTON–WELLESLEY HOSPITAL, NEWTON LOWER FALLS, MA, p. A207
NEXTCARE SPECIALTY HOSPITAL OF NORTH CAROLINA, ROCKY MOUNT, NC, p. A317
NIAGARA FALLS MEMORIAL MEDICAL CENTER, NIAGARA FALLS, NY, p. A301
NICHOLAS COUNTY HOSPITAL, CARLISLE, KY, p. A171
NICHOLAS H. NOYES MEMORIAL HOSPITAL, DANSVILLE, NY, p. A290
NINNESCAH VALLEY HEALTH SYSTEM, KINGMAN, KS, p. A163
NIOBRARA VALLEY HOSPITAL, LYNCH, NE, p. A264
NIX HEALTH CARE SYSTEM, SAN ANTONIO, TX, p. A429
NOBLE HOSPITAL, WESTFIELD, MA, p. A209
NOCONA GENERAL HOSPITAL, NOCONA, TX, p. A425
NOR–LEA GENERAL HOSPITAL, LOVINGTON, NM, p. A285
NORFOLK PSYCHIATRIC CENTER, NORFOLK, VA, p. A447
NORFOLK REGIONAL CENTER, NORFOLK, NE, p. A264
NORMAN AND IDA STONE INSTITUTE OF PSYCHIATRY, CHICAGO, ILLINOIS, p. A122
NORMAN REGIONAL HOSPITAL, NORMAN, OK, p. A345
NORRISTOWN STATE HOSPITAL, NORRISTOWN, PA, p. A365
NORTH ADAMS REGIONAL HOSPITAL, NORTH ADAMS, MA, p. A207
NORTH ALABAMA REGIONAL HOSPITAL, DECATUR, AL, p. A13
NORTH ARKANSAS REGIONAL MEDICAL CENTER, HARRISON, AR, p. A30
NORTH ARUNDEL HOSPITAL, GLEN BURNIE, MD, p. A198
NORTH AUSTIN MEDICAL CENTER, AUSTIN, TX, p. A403
NORTH BALDWIN HOSPITAL, BAY MINETTE, AL, p. A11
NORTH BAY HOSPITAL, ARANSAS PASS, TX, p. A402
NORTH BIG HORN HOSPITAL, LOVELL, WY, p. A479
NORTH BROWARD MEDICAL CENTER, POMPANO BEACH, FL, p. A93
NORTH CADDO MEDICAL CENTER, VIVIAN, LA, p. A189
NORTH CAMPUS, HOUSTON, TEXAS, p. A416
NORTH CAMPUS AND COLUMBIA AURORA PRESBYTERIAN TRANSITIONAL CARE CENTER, AURORA, COLORADO, p. A68

Index of Hospitals / North Carolina Baptist Hospital

NORTH CAROLINA BAPTIST HOSPITAL, WINSTON-SALEM, NC, p. A320
NORTH CAROLINA CHILDREN'S AND WOMEN'S HOSPITAL, NORTH CAROLINA NEUROSCIENCES HOSPITAL, CHAPEL HILL, NORTH CAROLINA, p. A310
NORTH CAROLINA EYE AND EAR HOSPITAL, DURHAM, NC, p. A312
NORTH CENTRAL BAPTIST HOSPITAL, SAN ANTONIO, TX, p. A429
NORTH CENTRAL BRONX HOSPITAL, NEW YORK, NY, p. A299
NORTH CENTRAL HEALTH CARE FACILITIES, WAUSAU, WI, p. A476
NORTH CENTRAL MEDICAL CENTER, MCKINNEY, TX, p. A423
NORTH COAST HEALTH CARE CENTERS, SANTA ROSA, CA, p. A63
NORTH COLORADO MEDICAL CENTER, GREELEY, CO, p. A71
NORTH COUNTRY HOSPITAL AND HEALTH CENTER, NEWPORT, VT, p. A440
NORTH COUNTRY REGIONAL HOSPITAL, BEMIDJI, MN, p. A226
NORTH CREST MEDICAL CENTER, SPRINGFIELD, TN, p. A399
NORTH DAKOTA STATE HOSPITAL, JAMESTOWN, ND, p. A323
NORTH DALLAS REHABILITATION HOSPITAL, DALLAS, TX, p. A409
NORTH FLORIDA RECEPTION CENTER HOSPITAL, LAKE BUTLER, FL, p. A87
NORTH FLORIDA REGIONAL MEDICAL CENTER, GAINESVILLE, FL, p. A85
NORTH FULTON REGIONAL HOSPITAL, ROSWELL, GA, p. A109
NORTH GENERAL HOSPITAL, NEW YORK, NY, p. A299
NORTH GEORGIA MEDICAL CENTER, ELLIJAY, GA, p. A104
NORTH HILLS HOSPITAL, NORTH RICHLAND HILLS, TX, p. A425
NORTH IDAHO BEHAVIORAL HEALTH, DIVISION OF KOOTENAI MEDICAL CENTER, COEUR D'ALENE, IDAHO, p. A116
NORTH JACKSON HOSPITAL, BRIDGEPORT, AL, p. A13
NORTH KANSAS CITY HOSPITAL, NORTH KANSAS CITY, MO, p. A251
NORTH LINCOLN HOSPITAL, LINCOLN CITY, OR, p. A352
NORTH LITTLE ROCK DIVISION, NORTH LITTLE ROCK, ARKANSAS, p. A31
NORTH LOGAN MERCY HOSPITAL, PARIS, AR, p. A33
NORTH MEMORIAL HEALTH CARE, ROBBINSDALE, MN, p. A232
NORTH MISSISSIPPI MEDICAL CENTER, TUPELO, MS, p. A242
NORTH MONROE HOSPITAL, MONROE, LA, p. A186
NORTH OAK REGIONAL MEDICAL CENTER, SENATOBIA, MS, p. A242
NORTH OAKLAND MEDICAL CENTERS, PONTIAC, MI, p. A220
NORTH OAKS MEDICAL CENTER, HAMMOND, LA, p. A183
NORTH OKALOOSA MEDICAL CENTER, CRESTVIEW, FL, p. A83
NORTH OTTAWA COMMUNITY HOSPITAL, GRAND HAVEN, MI, p. A215
NORTH PENN HOSPITAL, LANSDALE, PA, p. A363
NORTH PHILADELPHIA HEALTH SYSTEM, PHILADELPHIA, PA, p. A367
NORTH RIDGE MEDICAL CENTER, FORT LAUDERDALE, FL, p. A84
NORTH RUNNELS HOSPITAL, WINTERS, TX, p. A435
NORTH SHORE CHILDREN'S HOSPITAL, SALEM, MASSACHUSETTS, p. A208
NORTH SHORE MEDICAL CENTER, MIAMI, FL, p. A90
NORTH SHORE UNIVERSITY HOSPITAL, MANHASSET, NY, p. A294
NORTH SHORE UNIVERSITY HOSPITAL AT GLEN COVE, GLEN COVE, NY, p. A291
NORTH SHORE UNIVERSITY HOSPITAL AT PLAINVIEW, PLAINVIEW, NY, p. A302
NORTH SHORE UNIVERSITY HOSPITAL AT SYOSSET, SYOSSET, NY, p. A305
NORTH SHORE UNIVERSITY HOSPITAL-FOREST HILLS, NEW YORK, NY, p. A291
NORTH SUBURBAN MEDICAL CENTER, THORNTON, CO, p. A73
NORTH SUNFLOWER COUNTY HOSPITAL, RULEVILLE, MS, p. A242
NORTH TEXAS STATE HOSPITAL, WICHITA FALLS CAMPUS, WICHITA FALLS, TX, p. A435
NORTH VALLEY HEALTH CENTER, WARREN, MN, p. A234
NORTH VALLEY HOSPITAL, WHITEFISH, MT, p. A260
NORTH VALLEY HOSPITAL, TONASKET, WA, p. A458
NORTHBAY MEDICAL CENTER, FAIRFIELD, CA, p. A41
NORTHCOAST BEHAVIORAL HEALTHCARE SYSTEM, NORTHFIELD, OH, p. A336
NORTHEAST ALABAMA REGIONAL MEDICAL CENTER, ANNISTON, AL, p. A11
NORTHEAST BAPTIST HOSPITAL, SAN ANTONIO, TX, p. A429
NORTHEAST GEORGIA MEDICAL CENTER, GAINESVILLE, GA, p. A105
NORTHEAST KANSAS CENTER FOR HEALTH AND WELLNESS, HORTON, KS, p. A162
NORTHEAST MEDICAL CENTER, CONCORD, NC, p. A311
NORTHEAST MEDICAL CENTER, BONHAM, TX, p. A405

NORTHEAST MEDICAL CENTER HOSPITAL, HUMBLE, TX, p. A419
NORTHEAST METHODIST HOSPITAL, SAN ANTONIO, TX, p. A429
NORTHEAST MONTANA HEALTH SERVICES, WOLF POINT, MT, p. A260
NORTHEAST REGIONAL MEDICAL CENTER-JEFFERSON CAMPUS, KIRKSVILLE, MO, p. A249
NORTHEAST REGIONAL MEDICAL CENTER-PATTERSON CAMPUS, KIRKSVILLE, MISSOURI, p. A249
NORTHEAST REHABILITATION HOSPITAL, SALEM, NH, p. A273
NORTHEASTERN HOSPITAL OF PHILADELPHIA, PHILADELPHIA, PA, p. A367
NORTHEASTERN REGIONAL HOSPITAL, LAS VEGAS, NM, p. A285
NORTHEASTERN VERMONT REGIONAL HOSPITAL, SAINT JOHNSBURY, VT, p. A441
NORTHERN ARIZONA VA HEALTH CARE SYSTEM, PRESCOTT, AZ, p. A25
NORTHERN COCHISE COMMUNITY HOSPITAL, WILLCOX, AZ, p. A27
NORTHERN DUTCHESS HOSPITAL, RHINEBECK, NY, p. A303
NORTHERN HILLS GENERAL HOSPITAL, DEADWOOD, SD, p. A385
NORTHERN HOSPITAL OF SURRY COUNTY, MOUNT AIRY, NC, p. A316
NORTHERN ILLINOIS MEDICAL CENTER, MCHENRY, IL, p. A130
NORTHERN INYO HOSPITAL, BISHOP, CA, p. A37
NORTHERN ITASCA HEALTH CARE CENTER, BIGFORK, MN, p. A226
NORTHERN MAINE MEDICAL CENTER, FORT KENT, ME, p. A192
NORTHERN MICHIGAN REGIONAL HEALTH SYSTEM, PETOSKEY, MI, p. A220
NORTHERN MONTANA HOSPITAL, HAVRE, MT, p. A258
NORTHERN NAVAJO MEDICAL CENTER, SHIPROCK, NM, p. A286
NORTHERN NEVADA MEDICAL CENTER, SPARKS, NV, p. A269
NORTHERN VIRGINIA COMMUNITY HOSPITAL, ARLINGTON, VA, p. A442
NORTHERN VIRGINIA MENTAL HEALTH INSTITUTE, FALLS CHURCH, VA, p. A443
NORTHERN WESTCHESTER HOSPITAL CENTER, MOUNT KISCO, NY, p. A295
NORTHFIELD CAMPUS, NORTHFIELD, OHIO, p. A336
NORTHFIELD HOSPITAL, NORTHFIELD, MN, p. A231
NORTHKEY COMMUNITY CARE, COVINGTON, KY, p. A171
NORTHLAKE CAMPUS, GARY, INDIANA, p. A140
NORTHPORT MEDICAL CENTER, NORTHPORT, AL, p. A17
NORTHRIDGE HOSPITAL AND MEDICAL CENTER, SHERMAN WAY CAMPUS, LOS ANGELES, CA, p. A49
NORTHRIDGE HOSPITAL MEDICAL CENTER-ROSCOE BOULEVARD CAMPUS, LOS ANGELES, CA, p. A49
NORTHSHORE PSYCHIATRIC HOSPITAL, SLIDELL, LA, p. A189
NORTHSHORE REGIONAL MEDICAL CENTER, SLIDELL, LA, p. A189
NORTHSIDE GENERAL HOSPITAL, HOUSTON, TX, p. A417
NORTHSIDE HOSPITAL, ATLANTA, GA, p. A100
NORTHSIDE HOSPITAL – CHEROKEE, CANTON, GA, p. A102
NORTHSIDE HOSPITAL AND HEART INSTITUTE, SAINT PETERSBURG, FL, p. A94
NORTHSIDE MEDICAL CENTER, YOUNGSTOWN, OHIO, p. A340
NORTHVILLE PSYCHIATRIC HOSPITAL, NORTHVILLE, MI, p. A220
NORTHWEST COMMUNITY HEALTHCARE, ARLINGTON HEIGHTS, IL, p. A119
NORTHWEST FLORIDA COMMUNITY HOSPITAL, CHIPLEY, FL, p. A82
NORTHWEST GENERAL HOSPITAL, MILWAUKEE, WI, p. A472
NORTHWEST GEORGIA REGIONAL HOSPITAL, ROME, GA, p. A109
NORTHWEST HOSPITAL, SEATTLE, WA, p. A456
NORTHWEST HOSPITAL CENTER, RANDALLSTOWN, MD, p. A199
NORTHWEST IOWA HEALTH CENTER, SHELDON, IA, p. A156
NORTHWEST MEDICAL CENTER, POMPANO BEACH, FL, p. A93
NORTHWEST MEDICAL CENTER, THIEF RIVER FALLS, MN, p. A234
NORTHWEST MEDICAL CENTER, SPRINGDALE, AR, p. A34
NORTHWEST MEDICAL CENTER, TUCSON, AZ, p. A26
NORTHWEST MEDICAL CENTER-FRANKLIN CAMPUS, FRANKLIN, PENNSYLVANIA, p. A365
NORTHWEST MEDICAL CENTER-OIL CITY CAMPUS, OIL CITY, PENNSYLVANIA, p. A365
NORTHWEST MEDICAL CENTERS, OIL CITY, PA, p. A365
NORTHWEST MISSISSIPPI REGIONAL MEDICAL CENTER, CLARKSDALE, MS, p. A237
NORTHWEST MISSOURI PSYCHIATRIC REHABILITATION CENTER, SAINT JOSEPH, MO, p. A252
NORTHWEST REGIONAL HOSPITAL, CORPUS CHRISTI, TX, p. A407

NORTHWEST SUBURBAN COMMUNITY HOSPITAL, BELVIDERE, IL, p. A120
NORTHWEST SURGICAL HOSPITAL, OKLAHOMA CITY, OK, p. A346
NORTHWEST TEXAS HEALTHCARE SYSTEM, AMARILLO, TX, p. A401
NORTHWESTERN INSTITUTE, FORT WASHINGTON, PA, p. A360
NORTHWESTERN MEDICAL CENTER, SAINT ALBANS, VT, p. A441
NORTHWESTERN MEMORIAL HOSPITAL, CHICAGO, IL, p. A122
NORTHWOOD DEACONESS HEALTH CENTER, NORTHWOOD, ND, p. A323
NORTON AUDUBON HOSPITAL, LOUISVILLE, KY, p. A175
NORTON COMMUNITY HOSPITAL, NORTON, VA, p. A447
NORTON COUNTY HOSPITAL, NORTON, KS, p. A165
NORTON HEALTHCARE PAVILION, LOUISVILLE, KY, p. A175
NORTON HOSPITAL, LOUISVILLE, KY, p. A175
NORTON SOUND REGIONAL HOSPITAL, NOME, AK, p. A21
NORTON SOUTHWEST HOSPITAL, LOUISVILLE, KY, p. A175
NORTON SPRING VIEW HOSPITAL, LEBANON, KY, p. A174
NORTON SUBURBAN HOSPITAL, LOUISVILLE, KY, p. A175
NORWALK HOSPITAL, NORWALK, CT, p. A76
NORWEGIAN-AMERICAN HOSPITAL, CHICAGO, IL, p. A122
NORWOOD HEALTH CENTER, MARSHFIELD, WI, p. A471
NOVATO COMMUNITY HOSPITAL, NOVATO, CA, p. A53
NOXUBEE GENERAL HOSPITAL, MACON, MS, p. A240
NYACK HOSPITAL, NYACK, NY, p. A301
NYE REGIONAL MEDICAL CENTER, TONOPAH, NV, p. A269

O

O'BLENESS MEMORIAL HOSPITAL, ATHENS, OH, p. A325
O'CONNOR HOSPITAL, SAN JOSE, CA, p. A60
OAK FOREST HOSPITAL OF COOK COUNTY, OAK FOREST, IL, p. A131
OAK HILL COMMUNITY MEDICAL CENTER, OAK HILL, OH, p. A336
OAK HILL HOSPITAL, SPRING HILL, FL, p. A95
OAK PARK HOSPITAL, OAK PARK, IL, p. A132
OAK VALLEY DISTRICT HOSPITAL, OAKDALE, CA, p. A53
OAKDALE COMMUNITY HOSPITAL, OAKDALE, LA, p. A187
OAKES COMMUNITY HOSPITAL, OAKES, ND, p. A323
OAKLAND MEMORIAL HOSPITAL, OAKLAND, NE, p. A265
OAKLAWN HOSPITAL, MARSHALL, MI, p. A219
OAKLAWN PSYCHIATRIC CENTER, INC., GOSHEN, IN, p. A140
OAKWOOD ANNAPOLIS HOSPITAL, WAYNE, MI, p. A224
OAKWOOD CORRECTIONAL FACILITY, LIMA, OH, p. A333
OAKWOOD HERITAGE HOSPITAL, TAYLOR, MI, p. A223
OAKWOOD HOSPITAL AND MEDICAL CENTER-DEARBORN, DEARBORN, MI, p. A213
OAKWOOD HOSPITAL MERRIMAN CENTER-WESTLAND, WESTLAND, MICHIGAN, p. A224
OAKWOOD SEAWAY HOSPITAL, TRENTON, MI, p. A223
OCALA REGIONAL MEDICAL CENTER, OCALA, FL, p. A91
OCEAN BEACH HOSPITAL, ILWACO, WA, p. A454
OCEAN SPRINGS HOSPITAL, OCEAN SPRINGS, MS, p. A241
OCHILTREE GENERAL HOSPITAL, PERRYTON, TX, p. A426
OCHSNER FOUNDATION HOSPITAL, NEW ORLEANS, LA, p. A187
OCONEE MEMORIAL HOSPITAL, SENECA, SC, p. A383
OCONEE REGIONAL MEDICAL CENTER, MILLEDGEVILLE, GA, p. A107
OCONOMOWOC MEMORIAL HOSPITAL, OCONOMOWOC, WI, p. A473
OCONTO MEMORIAL HOSPITAL, OCONTO, WI, p. A473
ODESSA MEMORIAL HOSPITAL, ODESSA, WA, p. A455
ODESSA REGIONAL HOSPITAL, ODESSA, TX, p. A425
OGALLALA COMMUNITY HOSPITAL, OGALLALA, NE, p. A265
OGDEN REGIONAL MEDICAL CENTER, OGDEN, UT, p. A437
OHIO COUNTY HOSPITAL, HARTFORD, KY, p. A173
OHIO STATE UNIVERSITY HOSPITAL EAST, COLUMBUS, OH, p. A330
OHIO STATE UNIVERSITY MEDICAL CENTER, COLUMBUS, OH, p. A330
OHIO VALLEY GENERAL HOSPITAL, MCKEES ROCKS, PA, p. A364
OHIO VALLEY MEDICAL CENTER, WHEELING, WV, p. A465
OHSU HOSPITAL, PORTLAND, OR, p. A353
OJAI VALLEY COMMUNITY HOSPITAL, OJAI, CA, p. A53
OKANOGAN-DOUGLAS COUNTY HOSPITAL, BREWSTER, WA, p. A452
OKEENE MUNICIPAL HOSPITAL, OKEENE, OK, p. A345
OKMULGEE MEMORIAL HOSPITAL, OKMULGEE, OK, p. A346
OKOLONA COMMUNITY HOSPITAL, OKOLONA, MS, p. A241
OKTIBBEHA COUNTY HOSPITAL, STARKVILLE, MS, p. A242
OLATHE MEDICAL CENTER, OLATHE, KS, p. A166
OLD BRIDGE DIVISION, OLD BRIDGE, NEW JERSEY, p. A279

Index of Hospitals / Philhaven, Bahavioral Healthcare Services

OLEAN GENERAL HOSPITAL, OLEAN, NY, p. A302
OLIN E. TEAGUE VETERANS' CENTER, TEMPLE, TEXAS, p. A431
OLMSTED MEDICAL CENTER, ROCHESTER, MN, p. A232
OLYMPIC MEMORIAL HOSPITAL, PORT ANGELES, WA, p. A455
OLYMPUS SPECIALTY HOSPITAL, WALTHAM, MA, p. A209
OLYMPUS SPECIALTY HOSPITAL-SPRINGFIELD, SPRINGFIELD, MA, p. A208
ONEIDA COUNTY HOSPITAL, MALAD CITY, ID, p. A116
ONEIDA HEALTHCARE CENTER, ONEIDA, NY, p. A302
ONSLOW MEMORIAL HOSPITAL, JACKSONVILLE, NC, p. A314
ONTONAGON MEMORIAL HOSPITAL, ONTONAGON, MI, p. A220
OPELOUSAS GENERAL HOSPITAL, OPELOUSAS, LA, p. A188
ORANGE CITY HEALTH SYSTEM, ORANGE CITY, IA, p. A155
ORANGE COAST MEMORIAL MEDICAL CENTER, FOUNTAIN VALLEY, CA, p. A41
ORANGE COUNTY COMMUNITY HOSPITAL OF BUENA PARK, BUENA PARK, CA, p. A37
ORANGE MEMORIAL HOSPITAL UNIT, ORANGE, NEW JERSEY, p. A279
ORANGE PARK MEDICAL CENTER, ORANGE PARK, FL, p. A91
OREGON STATE HOSPITAL, SALEM, OR, p. A354
OREM COMMUNITY HOSPITAL, OREM, UT, p. A437
ORLANDO REGIONAL MEDICAL CENTER, ORLANDO, FL, p. A92
ORLANDO REGIONAL SOUTH SEMINOLE HOSPITAL, LONGWOOD, FL, p. A88
ORLANDO REGIONAL-LUCERNE, ORLANDO, FL, p. A92
OROVILLE HOSPITAL, OROVILLE, CA, p. A54
ORTHOPAEDIC HOSPITAL, LOS ANGELES, CA, p. A49
ORTONVILLE AREA HEALTH SERVICES, ORTONVILLE, MN, p. A231
OSAWATOMIE STATE HOSPITAL, OSAWATOMIE, KS, p. A166
OSBORNE COUNTY MEMORIAL HOSPITAL, OSBORNE, KS, p. A166
OSCEOLA COMMUNITY HOSPITAL, SIBLEY, IA, p. A156
OSCEOLA MEDICAL CENTER, OSCEOLA, WI, p. A473
OSCEOLA REGIONAL MEDICAL CENTER, KISSIMMEE, FL, p. A87
OSF SAINT FRANCIS MEDICAL CENTER, PEORIA, IL, p. A132
OSF SAINT JAMES HOSPITAL, PONTIAC, IL, p. A133
OSF ST. JOSEPH MEDICAL CENTER, BLOOMINGTON, IL, p. A120
OSF ST. MARY MEDICAL CENTER, GALESBURG, IL, p. A126
OSMOND GENERAL HOSPITAL, OSMOND, NE, p. A266
OSSEO AREA HOSPITAL AND NURSING HOME, OSSEO, WI, p. A473
OSSINING CORRECTIONAL FACILITIES HOSPITAL, OSSINING, NY, p. A302
OSTEOPATHIC MEDICAL CENTER OF TEXAS, FORT WORTH, TX, p. A413
OSU&HARDING BEHAVIORAL HEALTHCARE AND MEDICINE, WORTHINGTON, OH, p. A340
OSWEGO HOSPITAL, OSWEGO, NY, p. A302
OTHELLO COMMUNITY HOSPITAL, OTHELLO, WA, p. A455
OTSEGO MEMORIAL HOSPITAL, GAYLORD, MI, p. A215
OTTAWA COUNTY HEALTH CENTER, MINNEAPOLIS, KS, p. A165
OTTO KAISER MEMORIAL HOSPITAL, KENEDY, TX, p. A420
OTTUMWA REGIONAL HEALTH CENTER, OTTUMWA, IA, p. A155
OUACHITA MEDICAL CENTER, CAMDEN, AR, p. A28
OUR CHILDREN'S HOUSE AT BAYLOR, DALLAS, TX, p. A409
OUR COMMUNITY HOSPITAL, SCOTLAND NECK, NC, p. A318
OUR LADY OF BELLEFONTE HOSPITAL, ASHLAND, KY, p. A170
OUR LADY OF FATIMA HOSPITAL, NORTH PROVIDENCE, RHODE ISLAND, p. A376
OUR LADY OF LOURDES MEDICAL CENTER, CAMDEN, NJ, p. A275
OUR LADY OF LOURDES MEMORIAL HOSPITAL, BINGHAMTON, NY, p. A288
OUR LADY OF LOURDES REGIONAL MEDICAL CENTER, LAFAYETTE, LA, p. A184
OUR LADY OF MERCY MEDICAL CENTER, NEW YORK, NY, p. A299
OUR LADY OF THE LAKE REGIONAL MEDICAL CENTER, BATON ROUGE, LA, p. A180
OUR LADY OF THE LAKE-ASSUMPTION, NAPOLEONVILLE, LOUISIANA, p. A180
OUR LADY OF THE RESURRECTION MEDICAL CENTER, CHICAGO, IL, p. A122
OUR LADY OF THE WAY HOSPITAL, MARTIN, KY, p. A176
OUR LADY OF VICTORY HOSPITAL, LACKAWANNA, NY, p. A293
OVERLAKE HOSPITAL MEDICAL CENTER, BELLEVUE, WA, p. A452
OVERLAND PARK REGIONAL MEDICAL CENTER, SHAWNEE MISSION, KS, p. A168
OVERLOOK HOSPITAL, SUMMIT, NEW JERSEY, p. A276
OVERTON BROOKS VETERANS AFFAIRS MEDICAL CENTER, SHREVEPORT, LA, p. A188
OWATONNA HOSPITAL, OWATONNA, MN, p. A231
OWEN COUNTY MEMORIAL HOSPITAL, OWENTON, KY, p. A177
OWENSBORO MERCY HEALTH SYSTEM, OWENSBORO, KY, p. A177

OZARK HEALTH MEDICAL CENTER, CLINTON, AR, p. A29
OZARKS MEDICAL CENTER, WEST PLAINS, MO, p. A255

P

PACIFIC ALLIANCE MEDICAL CENTER, LOS ANGELES, CA, p. A49
PACIFIC COAST HOSPITAL, SAN FRANCISCO, CA, p. A60
PACIFIC COMMUNITIES HEALTH DISTRICT, NEWPORT, OR, p. A352
PACIFIC GATEWAY HOSPITAL AND COUNSELING CENTER, PORTLAND, OR, p. A353
PACIFIC HOSPITAL OF LONG BEACH, LONG BEACH, CA, p. A46
PACIFICA HOSPITAL OF THE VALLEY, LOS ANGELES, CA, p. A49
PAGE HOSPITAL, PAGE, AZ, p. A23
PAGE MEMORIAL HOSPITAL, LURAY, VA, p. A445
PALESTINE REGIONAL MEDICAL CENTER, PALESTINE, TX, p. A425
PALISADES MEDICAL CENTER, NORTH BERGEN, NJ, p. A278
PALM BEACH GARDENS MEDICAL CENTER, PALM BEACH GARDENS, FL, p. A92
PALM DRIVE HOSPITAL, SEBASTOPOL, CA, p. A63
PALM SPRINGS GENERAL HOSPITAL, HIALEAH, FL, p. A86
PALMER LUTHERAN HEALTH CENTER, WEST UNION, IA, p. A158
PALMERTON HOSPITAL, PALMERTON, PA, p. A366
PALMETTO BAPTIST MEDICAL CENTER EASLEY, EASLEY, SC, p. A380
PALMETTO BAPTIST MEDICAL CENTER/COLUMBIA, COLUMBIA, SC, p. A379
PALMETTO GENERAL HOSPITAL, HIALEAH, FL, p. A86
PALMETTO RICHLAND MEMORIAL HOSPITAL, COLUMBIA, SC, p. A380
PALMS OF PASADENA HOSPITAL, SAINT PETERSBURG, FL, p. A94
PALMS WEST HOSPITAL, LOXAHATCHEE, FL, p. A88
PALMYRA MEDICAL CENTERS, ALBANY, GA, p. A99
PALO ALTO DIVISION, PALO ALTO, CALIFORNIA, p. A54
PALO ALTO HEALTH SYSTEM, EMMETSBURG, IA, p. A151
PALO PINTO GENERAL HOSPITAL, MINERAL WELLS, TX, p. A424
PALO VERDE HOSPITAL, BLYTHE, CA, p. A37
PALO VERDE MENTAL HEALTH SERVICES, TUCSON, ARIZONA, p. A27
PALOMAR MEDICAL CENTER, ESCONDIDO, CA, p. A40
PALOS COMMUNITY HOSPITAL, PALOS HEIGHTS, IL, p. A132
PAMPA REGIONAL MEDICAL CENTER, PAMPA, TX, p. A426
PAN AMERICAN HOSPITAL, MIAMI, FL, p. A90
PANA COMMUNITY HOSPITAL, PANA, IL, p. A132
PAOLI MEMORIAL HOSPITAL, PAOLI, PA, p. A366
PARADISE VALLEY HOSPITAL, PHOENIX, AZ, p. A24
PARADISE VALLEY HOSPITAL, NATIONAL CITY, CA, p. A53
PARIS COMMUNITY HOSPITAL, PARIS, IL, p. A132
PARK PLACE MEDICAL CENTER, PORT ARTHUR, TX, p. A427
PARK PLAZA HOSPITAL, HOUSTON, TX, p. A417
PARK RIDGE HOSPITAL, ROCHESTER, NY, p. A304
PARK RIDGE HOSPITAL, FLETCHER, NC, p. A313
PARK VIEW HOSPITAL, EL RENO, OK, p. A343
PARKLAND HEALTH AND HOSPITAL SYSTEM, DALLAS, TX, p. A409
PARKLAND HEALTH CENTER, FARMINGTON, MO, p. A246
PARKLAND HEALTH CENTER-BONNE TERRE, BONNE TERRE, MISSOURI, p. A246
PARKLAND MEDICAL CENTER, DERRY, NH, p. A271
PARKRIDGE MEDICAL CENTER, CHATTANOOGA, TN, p. A391
PARKSIDE HOSPITAL, TULSA, OK, p. A348
PARKVIEW COMMUNITY HOSPITAL MEDICAL CENTER, RIVERSIDE, CA, p. A57
PARKVIEW HOSPITAL, BRUNSWICK, ME, p. A192
PARKVIEW HOSPITAL, PHILADELPHIA, PA, p. A367
PARKVIEW HOSPITAL, FORT WAYNE, IN, p. A139
PARKVIEW HOSPITAL, WHEELER, TX, p. A434
PARKVIEW MEDICAL CENTER, PUEBLO, CO, p. A72
PARKVIEW REGIONAL HOSPITAL, MEXIA, TX, p. A423
PARKVIEW REGIONAL MEDICAL CENTER, VICKSBURG, MS, p. A242
PARKWAY HOSPITAL, NEW YORK, NY, p. A299
PARKWAY MEDICAL CENTER HOSPITAL, DECATUR, AL, p. A14
PARKWAY REGIONAL HOSPITAL, FULTON, KY, p. A172
PARKWAY REGIONAL MEDICAL CENTER, NORTH MIAMI BEACH, FL, p. A91
PARKWOOD BEHAVIORAL HEALTH SYSTEM, OLIVE BRANCH, MS, p. A241
PARMA COMMUNITY GENERAL HOSPITAL, PARMA, OH, p. A336
PARMER COUNTY COMMUNITY HOSPITAL, FRIONA, TX, p. A413
PARRISH MEDICAL CENTER, TITUSVILLE, FL, p. A97

PARSONS STATE HOSPITAL AND TRAINING CENTER, PARSONS, KS, p. A166
PASCACK VALLEY HOSPITAL, WESTWOOD, NJ, p. A281
PASCO COMMUNITY HOSPITAL, DADE CITY, FL, p. A83
PASSAVANT AREA HOSPITAL, JACKSONVILLE, IL, p. A128
PATHWAYS, JACKSON, TN, p. A393
PATHWAYS TREATMENT CENTER, KALISPELL, MONTANA, p. A258
PATTIE A. CLAY HOSPITAL, RICHMOND, KY, p. A178
PATTON STATE HOSPITAL, PATTON, CA, p. A55
PAUL B. HALL REGIONAL MEDICAL CENTER, PAINTSVILLE, KY, p. A177
PAUL OLIVER MEMORIAL HOSPITAL, FRANKFORT, MI, p. A215
PAULDING COUNTY HOSPITAL, PAULDING, OH, p. A336
PAULINE WARFIELD LEWIS CENTER, CINCINNATI, OH, p. A328
PAULS VALLEY GENERAL HOSPITAL, PAULS VALLEY, OK, p. A346
PAWHUSKA HOSPITAL, PAWHUSKA, OK, p. A346
PAWNEE COUNTY MEMORIAL HOSPITAL, PAWNEE CITY, NE, p. A266
PAWNEE MUNICIPAL HOSPITAL, PAWNEE, OK, p. A346
PAYNE WHITNEY PSYCHIATRIC CLINIC, NEW YORK, NEW YORK, p. A299
PAYNESVILLE AREA HEALTH CARE SYSTEM, PAYNESVILLE, MN, p. A232
PAYSON REGIONAL MEDICAL CENTER, PAYSON, AZ, p. A24
PEACE HARBOR HOSPITAL, FLORENCE, OR, p. A351
PEACH REGIONAL MEDICAL CENTER, FORT VALLEY, GA, p. A105
PEARL RIVER COUNTY HOSPITAL, POPLARVILLE, MS, p. A241
PECOS COUNTY GENERAL HOSPITAL, IRAAN, TX, p. A419
PECOS COUNTY MEMORIAL HOSPITAL, FORT STOCKTON, TX, p. A412
PECOS VALLEY LODGE, ROSWELL, NEW MEXICO, p. A285
PEKIN HOSPITAL, PEKIN, IL, p. A132
PELLA REGIONAL HEALTH CENTER, PELLA, IA, p. A155
PEMBINA COUNTY MEMORIAL HOSPITAL AND WEDGEWOOD MANOR, CAVALIER, ND, p. A321
PEMBROKE HOSPITAL, PEMBROKE, MA, p. A207
PEMISCOT MEMORIAL HEALTH SYSTEM, HAYTI, MO, p. A247
PENDER COMMUNITY HOSPITAL, PENDER, NE, p. A266
PENDER MEMORIAL HOSPITAL, BURGAW, NC, p. A310
PENDLETON MEMORIAL METHODIST HOSPITAL, NEW ORLEANS, LA, p. A187
PENINSULA BEHAVIORAL CENTER, HAMPTON, VA, p. A444
PENINSULA HOSPITAL, LOUISVILLE, TN, p. A395
PENINSULA HOSPITAL, BURLINGAME, CALIFORNIA, p. A37
PENINSULA HOSPITAL CENTER, NEW YORK, NY, p. A299
PENINSULA REGIONAL HEALTH SYSTEM, SALISBURY, MD, p. A200
PENN STATE GEISINGER HEALTH SYSTEM-MILTON S. HERSHEY MEDICAL CENTER, HERSHEY, PA, p. A361
PENN STATE GEISINGER WYOMING VALLEY MEDICAL CENTER, WILKES-BARRE, PA, p. A374
PENNOCK HOSPITAL, HASTINGS, MI, p. A216
PENNSYLVANIA HOSPITAL, PHILADELPHIA, PA, p. A367
PENOBSCOT BAY MEDICAL CENTER, ROCKPORT, ME, p. A193
PENOBSCOT VALLEY HOSPITAL, LINCOLN, ME, p. A193
PENROSE COMMUNITY HOSPITAL, COLORADO SPRINGS, COLORADO, p. A69
PENROSE HOSPITAL, COLORADO SPRINGS, COLORADO, p. A69
PENROSE-ST. FRANCIS HEALTH SERVICES, COLORADO SPRINGS, CO, p. A69
PEOPLE'S MEMORIAL HOSPITAL OF BUCHANAN COUNTY, INDEPENDENCE, IA, p. A153
PERHAM MEMORIAL HOSPITAL AND HOME, PERHAM, MN, p. A232
PERKINS COUNTY HEALTH SERVICES, GRANT, NE, p. A263
PERMIAN GENERAL HOSPITAL, ANDREWS, TX, p. A401
PERRY COMMUNITY HOSPITAL, LINDEN, TN, p. A395
PERRY COUNTY GENERAL HOSPITAL, RICHTON, MS, p. A242
PERRY COUNTY MEMORIAL HOSPITAL, TELL CITY, IN, p. A146
PERRY COUNTY MEMORIAL HOSPITAL, PERRYVILLE, MO, p. A251
PERRY HOSPITAL, PERRY, GA, p. A108
PERRY MEMORIAL HOSPITAL, PRINCETON, IL, p. A133
PERRY MEMORIAL HOSPITAL, PERRY, OK, p. A346
PERSHING GENERAL HOSPITAL, LOVELOCK, NV, p. A269
PERSON MEMORIAL HOSPITAL, ROXBORO, NC, p. A317
PERTH AMBOY DIVISION, PERTH AMBOY, NEW JERSEY, p. A279
PETALUMA VALLEY HOSPITAL, PETALUMA, CA, p. A55
PETERSBURG MEDICAL CENTER, PETERSBURG, AK, p. A21
PHELPS COUNTY REGIONAL MEDICAL CENTER, ROLLA, MO, p. A252
PHELPS MEMORIAL HEALTH CENTER, HOLDREGE, NE, p. A263
PHELPS MEMORIAL HOSPITAL CENTER, SLEEPY HOLLOW, NY, p. A305
PHENIX REGIONAL HOSPITAL, PHENIX CITY, AL, p. A18
PHILHAVEN, BAHAVIORAL HEALTHCARE SERVICES, MOUNT GRETNA, PA, p. A364

© 2000 AHA Guide Index of Hospitals **A507**

Index of Hospitals / Phillips County Hospital

PHILLIPS COUNTY HOSPITAL, PHILLIPSBURG, KS, p. A166
PHILLIPS COUNTY MEDICAL CENTER, MALTA, MT, p. A258
PHILLIPS EYE INSTITUTE, MINNEAPOLIS, MN, p. A230
PHOEBE PUTNEY MEMORIAL HOSPITAL, ALBANY, GA, p. A99
PHOENIX BAPTIST HOSPITAL AND MEDICAL CENTER, PHOENIX, AZ, p. A24
PHOENIX CHILDREN'S HOSPITAL, PHOENIX, AZ, p. A24
PHOENIX MEMORIAL HEALTH SYSTEM, PHOENIX, AZ, p. A25
PHOENIXVILLE HOSPITAL OF THE UNIVERSITY OF PENNSYLVANIA HEALTH SYSTEM, PHOENIXVILLE, PA, p. A368
PHS SANTA FE INDIAN HOSPITAL, SANTA FE, NM, p. A286
PHYSICIANS HOSPITAL, NEW ORLEANS, LA, p. A187
PICKENS COUNTY MEDICAL CENTER, CARROLLTON, AL, p. A13
PIEDMONT BEHAVIORAL HEALTH CENTER, LEESBURG, VA, p. A445
PIEDMONT GERIATRIC HOSPITAL, BURKEVILLE, VA, p. A442
PIEDMONT HEALTHCARE SYSTEM, ROCK HILL, SC, p. A383
PIEDMONT HOSPITAL, ATLANTA, GA, p. A100
PIGGOTT COMMUNITY HOSPITAL, PIGGOTT, AR, p. A33
PIKE COMMUNITY HOSPITAL, WAVERLY, OH, p. A339
PIKE COUNTY MEMORIAL HOSPITAL, LOUISIANA, MO, p. A250
PIKE COUNTY MEMORIAL HOSPITAL, MURFREESBORO, AR, p. A32
PIKEVILLE UNITED METHODIST HOSPITAL OF KENTUCKY, PIKEVILLE, KY, p. A177
PILGRIM PSYCHIATRIC CENTER, BRENTWOOD, NY, p. A288
PINCKNEYVILLE COMMUNITY HOSPITAL, PINCKNEYVILLE, IL, p. A133
PINE GROVE HOSPITAL, LOS ANGELES, CA, p. A49
PINE MEDICAL CENTER, SANDSTONE, MN, p. A233
PINE REST CHRISTIAN MENTAL HEALTH SERVICES, GRAND RAPIDS, MI, p. A216
PINECREST REHABILITATION HOSPITAL, DELRAY BEACH, FL, p. A84
PINELANDS HOSPITAL, NACOGDOCHES, TX, p. A425
PINEVILLE COMMUNITY HOSPITAL ASSOCIATION, PINEVILLE, KY, p. A178
PINNACLEHEALTH AT COMMUNITY GENERAL OSTEOPATHIC HOSPITAL, HARRISBURG, PENNSYLVANIA, p. A361
PINNACLEHEALTH AT HARRISBURG HOSPITAL, HARRISBURG, PENNSYLVANIA, p. A361
PINNACLEHEALTH AT POLYCLINIC HOSPITAL, HARRISBURG, PENNSYLVANIA, p. A361
PINNACLEHEALTH AT SEIDLE MEMORIAL HOSPITAL, MECHANICSBURG, PENNSYLVANIA, p. A361
PINNACLEHEALTH SYSTEM, HARRISBURG, PA, p. A361
PIONEER MEDICAL CENTER, BIG TIMBER, MT, p. A256
PIONEER MEMORIAL HOSPITAL, HEPPNER, OR, p. A351
PIONEER MEMORIAL HOSPITAL, PRINEVILLE, OR, p. A353
PIONEER MEMORIAL HOSPITAL AND HEALTH SERVICES, VIBORG, SD, p. A388
PIONEER VALLEY HOSPITAL, SALT LAKE CITY, UT, p. A439
PIONEERS HOSPITAL OF RIO BLANCO COUNTY, MEEKER, CO, p. A72
PIONEERS MEMORIAL HEALTHCARE DISTRICT, BRAWLEY, CA, p. A37
PIPESTONE COUNTY MEDICAL CENTER/AVERA HEALTH, PIPESTONE, MN, p. A232
PITT COUNTY MEMORIAL HOSPITAL–UNIVERSITY HEALTH SYSTEMS OF EASTERN CAROLINA, GREENVILLE, NC, p. A313
PITTSBURGH SPECIALTY HOSPITAL, PITTSBURGH, PA, p. A369
PLACENTIA LINDA HOSPITAL, PLACENTIA, CA, p. A55
PLAINS MEMORIAL HOSPITAL, DIMMITT, TX, p. A410
PLAINS REGIONAL MEDICAL CENTER, CLOVIS, NM, p. A284
PLAINVIEW PUBLIC HOSPITAL, PLAINVIEW, NE, p. A266
PLAINVILLE RURAL HOSPITAL DISTRICT NUMBER ONE, PLAINVILLE, KS, p. A166
PLANTATION GENERAL HOSPITAL, PLANTATION, FL, p. A93
PLATEAU MEDICAL CENTER, OAK HILL, WV, p. A463
PLATTE COUNTY MEMORIAL HOSPITAL, WHEATLAND, WY, p. A480
PLATTE HEALTH CENTER/AVERA HEALTH, PLATTE, SD, p. A387
PLATTE VALLEY MEDICAL CENTER, BRIGHTON, CO, p. A68
PLAZA MEDICAL CENTER OF FORT WORTH, FORT WORTH, TX, p. A413
PLEASANT VALLEY HOSPITAL, POINT PLEASANT, WV, p. A463
PLUMAS DISTRICT HOSPITAL, QUINCY, CA, p. A56
POCAHONTAS COMMUNITY HOSPITAL, POCAHONTAS, IA, p. A156
POCAHONTAS MEMORIAL HOSPITAL, BUCKEYE, WV, p. A460
POCATELLO REGIONAL MEDICAL CENTER, POCATELLO, ID, p. A117
POCONO MEDICAL CENTER, EAST STROUDSBURG, PA, p. A359
POH MEDICAL CENTER, PONTIAC, MI, p. A220
POINTE COUPEE GENERAL HOSPITAL, NEW ROADS, LA, p. A187
POLK MEDICAL CENTER, CEDARTOWN, GA, p. A102

POLLY RYON MEMORIAL HOSPITAL, RICHMOND, TX, p. A427
POMERADO HOSPITAL, POWAY, CA, p. A56
POMONA VALLEY HOSPITAL MEDICAL CENTER, POMONA, CA, p. A55
PONCE REGIONAL HOSPITAL, PONCE, PR, p. A483
PONDERA MEDICAL CENTER, CONRAD, MT, p. A257
PONTOTOC HOSPITAL AND EXTENDED CARE FACILITY, PONTOTOC, MS, p. A241
POPLAR COMMUNITY HOSPITAL, POPLAR, MONTANA, p. A260
POPLAR SPRINGS HOSPITAL, PETERSBURG, VA, p. A447
PORT HURON HOSPITAL, PORT HURON, MI, p. A221
PORTAGE HEALTH SYSTEM, HANCOCK, MI, p. A216
PORTER ADVENTIST HOSPITAL, DENVER, CO, p. A69
PORTER HOSPITAL, MIDDLEBURY, VT, p. A440
PORTER MEMORIAL HOSPITAL, VALPARAISO, IN, p. A146
PORTERVILLE DEVELOPMENTAL CENTER, PORTERVILLE, CA, p. A56
PORTSMOUTH REGIONAL HOSPITAL AND PAVILION, PORTSMOUTH, NH, p. A273
POTOMAC HOSPITAL, WOODBRIDGE, VA, p. A451
POTOMAC RIDGE, ROCKVILLE, MD, p. A200
POTOMAC VALLEY HOSPITAL, KEYSER, WV, p. A462
POTTSTOWN MEMORIAL MEDICAL CENTER, POTTSTOWN, PA, p. A370
POTTSVILLE HOSPITAL AND WARNE CLINIC, POTTSVILLE, PA, p. A371
POUDRE VALLEY HOSPITAL, FORT COLLINS, CO, p. A70
POWELL CONVALESCENT CENTER, DES MOINES, IOWA, p. A151
POWELL COUNTY MEMORIAL HOSPITAL, DEER LODGE, MT, p. A257
POWELL HOSPITAL, POWELL, WY, p. A479
PRAGUE MUNICIPAL HOSPITAL, PRAGUE, OK, p. A347
PRAIRIE COMMUNITY MEDICAL ASSISTANCE FACILITY, TERRY, MT, p. A260
PRAIRIE DU CHIEN MEMORIAL HOSPITAL, PRAIRIE DU CHIEN, WI, p. A474
PRAIRIE LAKES HOSPITAL AND CARE CENTER, WATERTOWN, SD, p. A389
PRAIRIE VIEW, NEWTON, KS, p. A165
PRATT REGIONAL MEDICAL CENTER, PRATT, KS, p. A166
PRATTVILLE BAPTIST HOSPITAL, PRATTVILLE, AL, p. A18
PRENTICE WOMEN'S HOSPITAL, CHICAGO, ILLINOIS, p. A122
PRENTISS REGIONAL HOSPITAL AND EXTENDED CARE FACILITIES, PRENTISS, MS, p. A242
PRESBYTERIAN HOSPITAL, CHARLOTTE, NC, p. A311
PRESBYTERIAN HOSPITAL, OKLAHOMA CITY, OKLAHOMA, p. A346
PRESBYTERIAN HOSPITAL, ALBUQUERQUE, NM, p. A283
PRESBYTERIAN HOSPITAL OF COMMERCE, COMMERCE, TEXAS, p. A414
PRESBYTERIAN HOSPITAL OF DALLAS, DALLAS, TX, p. A409
PRESBYTERIAN HOSPITAL OF GREENVILLE, GREENVILLE, TEXAS, p. A414
PRESBYTERIAN HOSPITAL OF KAUFMAN, KAUFMAN, TX, p. A420
PRESBYTERIAN HOSPITAL OF PLANO, PLANO, TX, p. A426
PRESBYTERIAN HOSPITAL OF WINNSBORO, WINNSBORO, TX, p. A435
PRESBYTERIAN HOSPITAL–MATTHEWS, MATTHEWS, NC, p. A315
PRESBYTERIAN INTERCOMMUNITY HOSPITAL, WHITTIER, CA, p. A67
PRESBYTERIAN KASEMAN HOSPITAL, ALBUQUERQUE, NM, p. A283
PRESBYTERIAN MEDICAL CENTER OF THE UNIVERSITY OF PENNSYLVANIA HEALTH SYSTEM, PHILADELPHIA, PA, p. A367
PRESBYTERIAN–DENVER HOSPITAL, DENVER, COLORADO, p. A69
PRESBYTERIAN–ORTHOPAEDIC HOSPITAL, CHARLOTTE, NC, p. A311
PRESBYTERIAN–ST. LUKE'S MEDICAL CENTER, DENVER, CO, p. A69
PRESENTATION MEDICAL CENTER, ROLLA, ND, p. A323
PRESTON MEMORIAL HOSPITAL, KINGWOOD, WV, p. A462
PREVOST MEMORIAL HOSPITAL, DONALDSONVILLE, LA, p. A182
PRIMARY CHILDREN'S MEDICAL CENTER, SALT LAKE CITY, UT, p. A438
PRINCE GEORGE'S HOSPITAL CENTER, CHEVERLY, MD, p. A197
PRINCE WILLIAM HOSPITAL, MANASSAS, VA, p. A446
PRINCETON BAPTIST MEDICAL CENTER, BIRMINGHAM, AL, p. A12
PRINCETON COMMUNITY HOSPITAL, PRINCETON, WV, p. A464
PROCTOR HOSPITAL, PEORIA, IL, p. A133
PROFESSIONAL REHABILITATION HOSPITAL, FERRIDAY, LA, p. A182

PROMINA GWINNETT HOSPITAL SYSTEM, LAWRENCEVILLE, GA, p. A106
PROSSER MEMORIAL HOSPITAL, PROSSER, WA, p. A455
PROVENA COVENANT MEDICAL CENTER, URBANA, IL, p. A135
PROVENA MERCY CENTER, AURORA, IL, p. A119
PROVENA SAINT JOSEPH HOSPITAL, ELGIN, IL, p. A125
PROVENA SAINT JOSEPH MEDICAL CENTER, JOLIET, IL, p. A128
PROVENA SAINT THERESE MEDICAL CENTER, WAUKEGAN, IL, p. A136
PROVENA ST. MARY'S HOSPITAL, KANKAKEE, IL, p. A129
PROVENA UNITED SAMARITANS MEDICAL CENTER, DANVILLE, IL, p. A124
PROVIDENCE ALASKA MEDICAL CENTER, ANCHORAGE, AK, p. A20
PROVIDENCE CENTRALIA HOSPITAL, CENTRALIA, WA, p. A452
PROVIDENCE EVERETT MEDICAL CENTER, EVERETT, WA, p. A453
PROVIDENCE EVERETT MEDICAL CENTER – COLBY CAMPUS, EVERETT, WASHINGTON, p. A453
PROVIDENCE EVERETT MEDICAL CENTER – PACIFIC CAMPUS, EVERETT, WASHINGTON, p. A453
PROVIDENCE HEALTH CENTER, WACO, TX, p. A434
PROVIDENCE HOLY CROSS MEDICAL CENTER, LOS ANGELES, CA, p. A49
PROVIDENCE HOOD RIVER MEMORIAL HOSPITAL, HOOD RIVER, OR, p. A351
PROVIDENCE HOSPITAL, WASHINGTON, DC, p. A79
PROVIDENCE HOSPITAL, COLUMBIA, SC, p. A380
PROVIDENCE HOSPITAL, SANDUSKY, OH, p. A337
PROVIDENCE HOSPITAL, MOBILE, AL, p. A16
PROVIDENCE HOSPITAL AND MEDICAL CENTERS, SOUTHFIELD, MI, p. A222
PROVIDENCE HOSPITAL NORTHEAST, COLUMBIA, SOUTH CAROLINA, p. A380
PROVIDENCE KODIAK ISLAND MEDICAL CENTER, KODIAK, AK, p. A21
PROVIDENCE MEDFORD MEDICAL CENTER, MEDFORD, OR, p. A352
PROVIDENCE MEDICAL CENTER, WAYNE, NE, p. A267
PROVIDENCE MEDICAL CENTER, KANSAS CITY, KS, p. A163
PROVIDENCE MEMORIAL HOSPITAL, EL PASO, TX, p. A411
PROVIDENCE MILWAUKIE HOSPITAL, MILWAUKIE, OR, p. A352
PROVIDENCE NEWBERG HOSPITAL, NEWBERG, OR, p. A352
PROVIDENCE PORTLAND MEDICAL CENTER, PORTLAND, OR, p. A353
PROVIDENCE SAINT JOSEPH MEDICAL CENTER, BURBANK, CA, p. A37
PROVIDENCE SEASIDE HOSPITAL, SEASIDE, OR, p. A354
PROVIDENCE SEATTLE MEDICAL CENTER, SEATTLE, WA, p. A456
PROVIDENCE SEWARD MEDICAL CENTER, SEWARD, AK, p. A21
PROVIDENCE ST. PETER HOSPITAL, OLYMPIA, WA, p. A455
PROVIDENCE ST. VINCENT MEDICAL CENTER, PORTLAND, OR, p. A353
PROVIDENCE TOPPENISH HOSPITAL, TOPPENISH, WA, p. A458
PROVIDENCE YAKIMA MEDICAL CENTER, YAKIMA, WA, p. A459
PROVIDENT HOSPITAL OF COOK COUNTY, CHICAGO, IL, p. A122
PROWERS MEDICAL CENTER, LAMAR, CO, p. A71
PSYCHIATRIC HOSPITAL AT VANDERBILT, NASHVILLE, TN, p. A398
PSYCHIATRIC INSTITUTE OF WASHINGTON, WASHINGTON, DC, p. A79
PSYCHIATRIC MEDICINE CENTER, SALEM, OREGON, p. A354
PSYCHIATRIC PAVILION, AMARILLO, TEXAS, p. A401
PUBLIC HEALTH SERVICE INDIAN HOSPITAL, ALBUQUERQUE, NM, p. A283
PUGET SOUND HOSPITAL, TACOMA, WA, p. A458
PULASKI COMMUNITY HOSPITAL, PULASKI, VA, p. A448
PULASKI MEMORIAL HOSPITAL, WINAMAC, IN, p. A147
PULLMAN MEMORIAL HOSPITAL, PULLMAN, WA, p. A455
PUNGO DISTRICT HOSPITAL, BELHAVEN, NC, p. A309
PUNXSUTAWNEY AREA HOSPITAL, PUNXSUTAWNEY, PA, p. A371
PURCELL MUNICIPAL HOSPITAL, PURCELL, OK, p. A347
PUSHMATAHA COUNTY–TOWN OF ANTLERS HOSPITAL AUTHORITY, ANTLERS, OK, p. A341
PUTNAM COMMUNITY MEDICAL CENTER, PALATKA, FL, p. A92
PUTNAM COUNTY HOSPITAL, GREENCASTLE, IN, p. A140
PUTNAM COUNTY MEMORIAL HOSPITAL, UNIONVILLE, MO, p. A255
PUTNAM GENERAL HOSPITAL, HURRICANE, WV, p. A462
PUTNAM GENERAL HOSPITAL, EATONTON, GA, p. A104
PUTNAM HOSPITAL CENTER, CARMEL, NY, p. A290

Q

QUEEN OF ANGELS–HOLLYWOOD PRESBYTERIAN MEDICAL CENTER, LOS ANGELES, CA, p. A49
QUEEN OF PEACE HOSPITAL, NEW PRAGUE, MN, p. A231
QUEEN OF THE VALLEY HOSPITAL, NAPA, CA, p. A52
QUEEN'S MEDICAL CENTER, HONOLULU, HI, p. A112
QUEENS CHILDREN'S PSYCHIATRIC CENTER, NEW YORK, NY, p. A299
QUEENS HOSPITAL CENTER, NEW YORK, NY, p. A299
QUENTIN MEASE HOSPITAL, HOUSTON, TEXAS, p. A416
QUILLEN REHABILITATION HOSPITAL, JOHNSON CITY, TN, p. A394
QUINCY MEDICAL CENTER, QUINCY, MA, p. A208
QUINCY VALLEY MEDICAL CENTER, QUINCY, WA, p. A456
QUITMAN COUNTY HOSPITAL AND NURSING HOME, MARKS, MS, p. A240

R

R. E. THOMASON GENERAL HOSPITAL, EL PASO, TX, p. A411
R. J. REYNOLDS–PATRICK COUNTY MEMORIAL HOSPITAL, STUART, VA, p. A450
R. M. L. SPECIALTY HOSPITAL, HINSDALE, IL, p. A128
RABUN COUNTY MEMORIAL HOSPITAL, CLAYTON, GA, p. A102
RAHWAY HOSPITAL, RAHWAY, NJ, p. A280
RALEIGH COMMUNITY HOSPITAL, RALEIGH, NC, p. A317
RALEIGH GENERAL HOSPITAL, BECKLEY, WV, p. A460
RALPH H. JOHNSON VETERANS AFFAIRS MEDICAL CENTER, CHARLESTON, SC, p. A379
RANCHO SPRINGS MEDICAL CENTER, MURRIETA, CA, p. A52
RANCOCAS HOSPITAL, WILLINGBORO, NJ, p. A281
RANDOLPH COUNTY HOSPITAL, ROANOKE, AL, p. A18
RANDOLPH COUNTY MEDICAL CENTER, POCAHONTAS, AR, p. A33
RANDOLPH HOSPITAL, ASHEBORO, NC, p. A309
RANGELY DISTRICT HOSPITAL, RANGELY, CO, p. A72
RANKIN HOSPITAL DISTRICT, RANKIN, TX, p. A427
RANKIN MEDICAL CENTER, BRANDON, MS, p. A236
RANSOM MEMORIAL HOSPITAL, OTTAWA, KS, p. A166
RAPID CITY REGIONAL HOSPITAL SYSTEM OF CARE, RAPID CITY, SD, p. A387
RAPIDES REGIONAL MEDICAL CENTER, ALEXANDRIA, LA, p. A180
RAPPAHANNOCK GENERAL HOSPITAL, KILMARNOCK, VA, p. A445
RARITAN BAY MEDICAL CENTER, PERTH AMBOY, NJ, p. A279
RAULERSON HOSPITAL, OKEECHOBEE, FL, p. A91
RAVENSWOOD HOSPITAL MEDICAL CENTER, CHICAGO, IL, p. A122
RAWLINS COUNTY HEALTH CENTER, ATWOOD, KS, p. A159
RAY COUNTY MEMORIAL HOSPITAL, RICHMOND, MO, p. A251
RAYMOND BLANK MEMORIAL HOSPITAL FOR CHILDREN, DES MOINES, IOWA, p. A151
READING HOSPITAL AND MEDICAL CENTER, READING, PA, p. A371
REAGAN MEMORIAL HOSPITAL, BIG LAKE, TX, p. A404
REBSAMEN MEDICAL CENTER, JACKSONVILLE, AR, p. A30
RECOVERY INN OF MENLO PARK, MENLO PARK, CA, p. A51
RED BAY HOSPITAL, RED BAY, AL, p. A18
RED RIVER HOSPITAL, WICHITA FALLS, TX, p. A435
REDBUD COMMUNITY HOSPITAL, CLEARLAKE, CA, p. A38
REDDING MEDICAL CENTER, REDDING, CA, p. A56
REDGATE MEMORIAL HOSPITAL, LONG BEACH, CA, p. A46
REDINGTON–FAIRVIEW GENERAL HOSPITAL, SKOWHEGAN, ME, p. A194
REDLANDS COMMUNITY HOSPITAL, REDLANDS, CA, p. A56
REDMOND REGIONAL MEDICAL CENTER, ROME, GA, p. A109
REDWOOD FALLS MUNICIPAL HOSPITAL, REDWOOD FALLS, MN, p. A232
REDWOOD MEMORIAL HOSPITAL, FORTUNA, CA, p. A41
REEDSBURG AREA MEDICAL CENTER, REEDSBURG, WI, p. A474
REEVES COUNTY HOSPITAL, PECOS, TX, p. A426
REFUGIO COUNTY MEMORIAL HOSPITAL, REFUGIO, TX, p. A427
REGINA MEDICAL CENTER, HASTINGS, MN, p. A229
REGIONAL HEALTH SERVICES OF HOWARD COUNTY, CRESCO, IA, p. A150
REGIONAL HOSPITAL FOR RESPIRATORY AND COMPLEX CARE, SEATTLE, WA, p. A456
REGIONAL MEDICAL CENTER, VICTORIA, TX, p. A433
REGIONAL MEDICAL CENTER AT MEMPHIS, MEMPHIS, TN, p. A397
REGIONAL MEDICAL CENTER OF HOPKINS COUNTY, MADISONVILLE, KY, p. A176
REGIONAL MEDICAL CENTER OF NORTHEAST ARKANSAS, JONESBORO, AR, p. A31
REGIONAL MEDICAL CENTER OF NORTHEAST IOWA AND DELAWARE COUNTY, MANCHESTER, IA, p. A154
REGIONAL MEDICAL CENTER OF ORANGEBURG AND CALHOUN COUNTIES, ORANGEBURG, SC, p. A383
REGIONAL MEDICAL CENTER OF SAN JOSE, SAN JOSE, CA, p. A60
REGIONAL MEDICAL CENTER–BAYONET POINT, HUDSON, FL, p. A86
REGIONAL REHABILITATION CENTER, SALEM, OREGON, p. A354
REGIONAL WEST MEDICAL CENTER, SCOTTSBLUFF, NE, p. A266
REGIONS HOSPITAL, SAINT PAUL, MN, p. A233
REHABILITATION HOSPITAL OF FORT WAYNE, FORT WAYNE, IN, p. A140
REHABILITATION HOSPITAL OF INDIANA, INDIANAPOLIS, IN, p. A141
REHABILITATION HOSPITAL OF THE PACIFIC, HONOLULU, HI, p. A112
REHABILITATION INSTITUTE, KANSAS CITY, MO, p. A248
REHABILITATION INSTITUTE AT SANTA BARBARA, SANTA BARBARA, CA, p. A62
REHABILITATION INSTITUTE OF CHICAGO, CHICAGO, IL, p. A122
REHABILITATION INSTITUTE OF MICHIGAN, DETROIT, MI, p. A214
REHABILITATION INSTITUTE OF OREGON, PORTLAND, OREGON, p. A353
REHABILITATION INSTITUTE OF WEST FLORIDA, PENSACOLA, FLORIDA, p. A93
REHOBOTH MCKINLEY CHRISTIAN HOSPITAL, GALLUP, NM, p. A285
REID HOSPITAL AND HEALTH CARE SERVICES, RICHMOND, IN, p. A145
REISCH MEMORIAL NURSING HOME, p. A120
RENAISSANCE WOMEN'S CENTER OF AUSTIN, AUSTIN, TX, p. A403
RENVILLE COUNTY HOSPITAL, OLIVIA, MN, p. A231
REPUBLIC COUNTY HOSPITAL, BELLEVILLE, KS, p. A159
RESEARCH BELTON HOSPITAL, BELTON, MO, p. A244
RESEARCH MEDICAL CENTER, KANSAS CITY, MO, p. A248
RESEARCH PSYCHIATRIC CENTER, KANSAS CITY, MO, p. A248
RESTON HOSPITAL CENTER, RESTON, VA, p. A448
RESURRECTION MEDICAL CENTER, CHICAGO, IL, p. A123
RETREAT HOSPITAL, RICHMOND, VA, p. A449
REX HEALTHCARE, RALEIGH, NC, p. A317
REYNOLDS ARMY COMMUNITY HOSPITAL, FORT SILL, OK, p. A343
REYNOLDS MEMORIAL HOSPITAL, GLEN DALE, WV, p. A461
RHD MEMORIAL MEDICAL CENTER, DALLAS, TX, p. A409
RHEA MEDICAL CENTER, DAYTON, TN, p. A392
RHODE ISLAND HOSPITAL, PROVIDENCE, RI, p. A376
RHODE ISLAND MEDICAL CENTER, CRANSTON, RHODE ISLAND, p. A376
RICE COUNTY HOSPITAL DISTRICT NUMBER ONE, LYONS, KS, p. A164
RICE MEDICAL CENTER, EAGLE LAKE, TX, p. A411
RICE MEMORIAL HOSPITAL, WILLMAR, MN, p. A235
RICHARD H. HUTCHINGS PSYCHIATRIC CENTER, SYRACUSE, NY, p. A306
RICHARD H. YOUNG MEMORIAL HOSPITAL, OMAHA, NEBRASKA, p. A265
RICHARD H. YOUNG PSYCHIATRIC HOSPITAL, KEARNEY, NEBRASKA, p. A263
RICHARD L. ROUDEBUSH VETERANS AFFAIRS MEDICAL CENTER, INDIANAPOLIS, IN, p. A141
RICHARD YOUNG CENTER, OMAHA, NE, p. A265
RICHARDS MEMORIAL HOSPITAL, ROCKDALE, TX, p. A427
RICHARDSON MEDICAL CENTER, RAYVILLE, LA, p. A188
RICHARDTON HEALTH CENTER, RICHARDTON, ND, p. A323
RICHLAND HOSPITAL, MANSFIELD, OH, p. A334
RICHLAND HOSPITAL, RICHLAND CENTER, WI, p. A474
RICHLAND MEMORIAL HOSPITAL, OLNEY, IL, p. A132
RICHLAND PARISH HOSPITAL–DELHI, DELHI, LA, p. A182
RICHMOND EYE AND EAR HOSPITAL, RICHMOND, VA, p. A449
RICHMOND MEMORIAL HOSPITAL, ROCKINGHAM, NC, p. A317
RICHMOND STATE HOSPITAL, RICHMOND, IN, p. A145
RICHWOOD AREA COMMUNITY HOSPITAL, RICHWOOD, WV, p. A464
RIDDLE MEMORIAL HOSPITAL, MEDIA, PA, p. A364
RIDEOUT MEMORIAL HOSPITAL, MARYSVILLE, CA, p. A51
RIDGECREST REGIONAL HOSPITAL, RIDGECREST, CA, p. A57
RIDGEVIEW INSTITUTE, SMYRNA, GA, p. A109
RIDGEVIEW MEDICAL CENTER, WACONIA, MN, p. A234
RIDGEVIEW PSYCHIATRIC HOSPITAL AND CENTER, OAK RIDGE, TN, p. A398
RIDGWAY HEALTH CENTER, RIDGWAY, PA, p. A371
RILEY HOSPITAL FOR CHILDREN, INDIANAPOLIS, INDIANA, p. A141
RILEY MEMORIAL HOSPITAL, MERIDIAN, MS, p. A240
RINGGOLD COUNTY HOSPITAL, MOUNT AYR, IA, p. A154
RIO GRANDE HOSPITAL, DEL NORTE, CO, p. A69
RIO GRANDE REGIONAL HOSPITAL, MCALLEN, TX, p. A423
RIO GRANDE STATE CENTER, HARLINGEN, TX, p. A415
RIO VISTA PHYSICAL REHABILITATION HOSPITAL, EL PASO, TX, p. A411
RIPLEY COUNTY MEMORIAL HOSPITAL, DONIPHAN, MO, p. A246
RIPON MEDICAL CENTER, RIPON, WI, p. A475
RIVENDELL BEHAVIORAL HEALTH SERVICES, BENTON, AR, p. A28
RIVENDELL OF MICHIGAN, SAINT JOHNS, MI, p. A222
RIVER CREST HOSPITAL, SAN ANGELO, TX, p. A428
RIVER FALLS AREA HOSPITAL, RIVER FALLS, WI, p. A475
RIVER OAKS HOSPITAL, JACKSON, MS, p. A239
RIVER OAKS HOSPITAL, NEW ORLEANS, LA, p. A187
RIVER PARISHES HOSPITAL, LA PLACE, LA, p. A184
RIVER PARK HOSPITAL, MCMINNVILLE, TN, p. A396
RIVER VALLEY HEALTH SYSTEM, IRONTON, OH, p. A333
RIVER WEST MEDICAL CENTER, PLAQUEMINE, LA, p. A188
RIVEREDGE HOSPITAL, FOREST PARK, IL, p. A126
RIVERLAND MEDICAL CENTER, FERRIDAY, LA, p. A182
RIVERSIDE COMMUNITY HOSPITAL, RIVERSIDE, CA, p. A57
RIVERSIDE COUNTY REGIONAL MEDICAL CENTER, MORENO VALLEY, CA, p. A52
RIVERSIDE GENERAL HOSPITAL, HOUSTON, TX, p. A417
RIVERSIDE HEALTH SYSTEM, WICHITA, KS, p. A169
RIVERSIDE MEDICAL CENTER, KANKAKEE, IL, p. A129
RIVERSIDE MEDICAL CENTER, WAUPACA, WI, p. A476
RIVERSIDE MEDICAL CENTER, FRANKLINTON, LA, p. A182
RIVERSIDE MERCY HOSPITAL, TOLEDO, OH, p. A338
RIVERSIDE OSTEOPATHIC HOSPITAL, TRENTON, MI, p. A223
RIVERSIDE PSYCHIATRIC INSTITUTE, p. A446
RIVERSIDE REGIONAL MEDICAL CENTER, NEWPORT NEWS, VA, p. A446
RIVERSIDE TAPPAHANNOCK HOSPITAL, TAPPAHANNOCK, VA, p. A450
RIVERSIDE WALTER REED HOSPITAL, GLOUCESTER, VA, p. A444
RIVERTON MEMORIAL HOSPITAL, RIVERTON, WY, p. A479
RIVERVALLEY BEHAVIORAL HEALTH HOSPITAL, OWENSBORO, KY, p. A177
RIVERVIEW HEALTHCARE ASSOCIATION, CROOKSTON, MN, p. A227
RIVERVIEW HOSPITAL, NOBLESVILLE, IN, p. A144
RIVERVIEW HOSPITAL ASSOCIATION, WISCONSIN RAPIDS, WI, p. A477
RIVERVIEW HOSPITAL FOR CHILDREN, MIDDLETOWN, CT, p. A75
RIVERVIEW MANOR, p. A477
RIVERVIEW MEDICAL CENTER, GONZALES, LA, p. A182
RIVERVIEW REGIONAL MEDICAL CENTER, GADSDEN, AL, p. A15
RIVERWOOD HEALTHCARE CENTER, AITKIN, MN, p. A225
ROANE GENERAL HOSPITAL, SPENCER, WV, p. A464
ROANE MEDICAL CENTER, HARRIMAN, TN, p. A393
ROANOKE MEMORIAL REHABILITATION CENTER, ROANOKE, VIRGINIA, p. A449
ROANOKE–CHOWAN HOSPITAL, AHOSKIE, NC, p. A309
ROBERT F. KENNEDY MEDICAL CENTER, HAWTHORNE, CA, p. A43
ROBERT PACKER HOSPITAL, SAYRE, PA, p. A371
ROBERT WOOD JOHNSON UNIVERSITY HOSPITAL, NEW BRUNSWICK, NJ, p. A278
ROBERT WOOD JOHNSON UNIVERSITY HOSPITAL AT HAMILTON, HAMILTON, NJ, p. A276
ROBINSON MEMORIAL HOSPITAL, RAVENNA, OH, p. A337
ROCHELLE COMMUNITY HOSPITAL, ROCHELLE, IL, p. A133
ROCHESTER GENERAL HOSPITAL, ROCHESTER, NY, p. A304
ROCHESTER METHODIST HOSPITAL, ROCHESTER, MN, p. A232
ROCHESTER PSYCHIATRIC CENTER, ROCHESTER, NY, p. A304
ROCK COUNTY HOSPITAL, BASSETT, NE, p. A261
ROCK CREEK CENTER, LEMONT, IL, p. A129
ROCKCASTLE HOSPITAL AND RESPIRATORY CARE CENTER, MOUNT VERNON, KY, p. A177
ROCKDALE HOSPITAL AND HEALTH SYSTEM, CONYERS, GA, p. A103
ROCKEFELLER UNIVERSITY HOSPITAL, NEW YORK, NY, p. A299
ROCKFORD CENTER, NEWARK, DE, p. A78
ROCKFORD MEMORIAL HOSPITAL, ROCKFORD, IL, p. A134
ROCKINGHAM MEMORIAL HOSPITAL, HARRISONBURG, VA, p. A445
ROCKLAND CHILDREN'S PSYCHIATRIC CENTER, ORANGEBURG, NY, p. A302
ROCKLAND PSYCHIATRIC CENTER, ORANGEBURG, NY, p. A302
ROCKVILLE GENERAL HOSPITAL, VERNON ROCKVILLE, CT, p. A77

Index of Hospitals / Roger C. Peace Rehabilitation Hospital

ROGER C. PEACE REHABILITATION HOSPITAL, GREENVILLE, SOUTH CAROLINA, p. A381
ROGER HUNTINGTON NURSING CENTER, p. A381
ROGER MILLS MEMORIAL HOSPITAL, CHEYENNE, OK, p. A342
ROGER WILLIAMS MEDICAL CENTER, PROVIDENCE, RI, p. A376
ROGERS CITY REHABILITATION HOSPITAL, ROGERS CITY, MI, p. A221
ROGERS MEMORIAL HOSPITAL, OCONOMOWOC, WI, p. A473
ROGUE VALLEY MEDICAL CENTER, MEDFORD, OR, p. A352
ROLLING HILLS HOSPITAL, ADA, OK, p. A341
ROLLING PLAINS MEMORIAL HOSPITAL, SWEETWATER, TX, p. A431
ROME MEMORIAL HOSPITAL, ROME, NY, p. A304
ROOSEVELT HOSPITAL, NEW YORK, NEW YORK, p. A300
ROOSEVELT MEMORIAL MEDICAL CENTER, CULBERTSON, MT, p. A257
ROOSEVELT WARM SPRINGS INSTITUTE FOR REHABILITATION, WARM SPRINGS, GA, p. A111
ROPER HOSPITAL, CHARLESTON, SC, p. A379
ROPER HOSPITAL NORTH, CHARLESTON, SC, p. A379
ROSE MEDICAL CENTER, DENVER, CO, p. A69
ROSEAU AREA HOSPITAL AND HOMES, ROSEAU, MN, p. A232
ROSEBUD HEALTH CARE CENTER, FORSYTH, MT, p. A257
ROSELAND COMMUNITY HOSPITAL, CHICAGO, IL, p. A123
ROSS SKILLED NURSING FACILITY, p. A191
ROSWELL PARK CANCER INSTITUTE, BUFFALO, NY, p. A289
ROTARY REHABILITATION HOSPITAL, MOBILE, ALABAMA, p. A16
ROUND ROCK HOSPITAL, ROUND ROCK, TX, p. A427
ROUNDUP MEMORIAL HOSPITAL, ROUNDUP, MT, p. A259
ROWAN REGIONAL MEDICAL CENTER, SALISBURY, NC, p. A317
ROXBOROUGH MEMORIAL HOSPITAL, PHILADELPHIA, PA, p. A368
ROY H. LAIRD MEMORIAL HOSPITAL, KILGORE, TX, p. A420
ROY LESTER SCHNEIDER HOSPITAL, SAINT THOMAS, VI, p. A484
ROYAL C. JOHNSON VETERANS MEMORIAL HOSPITAL, SIOUX FALLS, SD, p. A388
RUBY VALLEY HOSPITAL, SHERIDAN, MT, p. A259
RUMFORD HOSPITAL, RUMFORD, ME, p. A194
RUNNELLS SPECIALIZED HOSPITAL OF UNION COUNTY, BERKELEY HEIGHTS, NJ, p. A274
RUSH COUNTY MEMORIAL HOSPITAL, LA CROSSE, KS, p. A163
RUSH FOUNDATION HOSPITAL, MERIDIAN, MS, p. A240
RUSH MEMORIAL HOSPITAL, RUSHVILLE, IN, p. A145
RUSH NORTH SHORE MEDICAL CENTER, SKOKIE, IL, p. A134
RUSH–COPLEY MEDICAL CENTER, AURORA, IL, p. A119
RUSH–PRESBYTERIAN–ST. LUKE'S MEDICAL CENTER, CHICAGO, IL, p. A123
RUSK COUNTY MEMORIAL HOSPITAL AND NURSING HOME, LADYSMITH, WI, p. A470
RUSK INSTITUTE, NEW YORK, NEW YORK, p. A298
RUSK STATE HOSPITAL, RUSK, TX, p. A428
RUSSELL COUNTY HOSPITAL, RUSSELL SPRINGS, KY, p. A178
RUSSELL COUNTY MEDICAL CENTER, LEBANON, VA, p. A445
RUSSELL MEDICAL CENTER, ALEXANDER CITY, AL, p. A11
RUSSELL REGIONAL HOSPITAL, RUSSELL, KS, p. A167
RUSSELLVILLE HOSPITAL, RUSSELLVILLE, AL, p. A18
RUTHERFORD HOSPITAL, RUTHERFORDTON, NC, p. A317
RUTLAND REGIONAL MEDICAL CENTER, RUTLAND, VT, p. A440
RYDER MEMORIAL HOSPITAL, HUMACAO, PR, p. A482
RYE HOSPITAL CENTER, RYE, NY, p. A304

S

SABETHA COMMUNITY HOSPITAL, SABETHA, KS, p. A167
SABINE COUNTY HOSPITAL, HEMPHILL, TX, p. A415
SABINE MEDICAL CENTER, MANY, LA, p. A185
SAC-OSAGE HOSPITAL, OSCEOLA, MO, p. A251
SACRED HEART HEALTH SYSTEM, PENSACOLA, FL, p. A93
SACRED HEART HOSPITAL, ALLENTOWN, PA, p. A355
SACRED HEART HOSPITAL, CUMBERLAND, MD, p. A198
SACRED HEART HOSPITAL, CHICAGO, IL, p. A123
SACRED HEART HOSPITAL, EAU CLAIRE, WI, p. A468
SACRED HEART HOSPITAL, TOMAHAWK, WISCONSIN, p. A474
SACRED HEART MEDICAL CENTER, SPOKANE, WA, p. A457
SACRED HEART MEDICAL CENTER, EUGENE, OR, p. A350
SACRED HEART REHABILITATION INSTITUTE, MILWAUKEE, WI, p. A472
SACRED HEART–ST. MARY'S HOSPITALS, RHINELANDER, WI, p. A474
SADDLEBACK MEMORIAL MEDICAL CENTER, LAGUNA HILLS, CA, p. A45
SAGAMORE CHILDREN'S PSYCHIATRIC CENTER, HUNTINGTON STATION, NY, p. A293
SAGE MEMORIAL HOSPITAL, GANADO, AZ, p. A22
SAINT AGNES MEDICAL CENTER, FRESNO, CA, p. A42

SAINT ALPHONSUS REGIONAL MEDICAL CENTER, BOISE, ID, p. A115
SAINT ANNE'S HOSPITAL, FALL RIVER, MA, p. A204
SAINT ANTHONY HOSPITAL, CHICAGO, IL, p. A123
SAINT ANTHONY MEDICAL CENTER, ROCKFORD, IL, p. A134
SAINT ANTHONY MEMORIAL HEALTH CENTERS, MICHIGAN CITY, IN, p. A144
SAINT ANTHONY'S HEALTH CENTER, ALTON, IL, p. A119
SAINT BARNABAS MEDICAL CENTER, LIVINGSTON, NJ, p. A277
SAINT CLARE'S HEALTH SERVICES, DENVILLE, NJ, p. A275
SAINT CLARE'S HOSPITAL, ALTON, ILLINOIS, p. A119
SAINT CLARE'S HOSPITAL/BOONTON TOWNSHIP, BOONTON TOWNSHIP, NEW JERSEY, p. A275
SAINT CLARE'S HOSPITAL/DENVILLE, DENVILLE, NEW JERSEY, p. A275
SAINT CLARE'S HOSPITAL/SUSSEX, SUSSEX, NEW JERSEY, p. A275
SAINT ELIZABETH REGIONAL MEDICAL CENTER, LINCOLN, NE, p. A264
SAINT EUGENE MEDICAL CENTER, DILLON, SC, p. A380
SAINT FRANCIS CARE BEHAVIORAL HEALTH, PORTLAND, CT, p. A76
SAINT FRANCIS HOSPITAL, POUGHKEEPSIE, NY, p. A303
SAINT FRANCIS HOSPITAL, CHARLESTON, WV, p. A461
SAINT FRANCIS HOSPITAL, MEMPHIS, TN, p. A397
SAINT FRANCIS HOSPITAL, TULSA, OK, p. A348
SAINT FRANCIS HOSPITAL AND HEALTH CENTER, BLUE ISLAND, IL, p. A120
SAINT FRANCIS HOSPITAL AND MEDICAL CENTER, HARTFORD, CT, p. A75
SAINT FRANCIS HOSPITAL–BEACON, BEACON, NEW YORK, p. A303
SAINT FRANCIS MEDICAL CENTER, CAPE GIRARDEAU, MO, p. A245
SAINT FRANCIS MEMORIAL HEALTH CENTER, GRAND ISLAND, NEBRASKA, p. A263
SAINT FRANCIS MEMORIAL HOSPITAL, SAN FRANCISCO, CA, p. A60
SAINT JAMES HOSPITAL OF NEWARK, NEWARK, NJ, p. A278
SAINT JOHN HOSPITAL, LEAVENWORTH, KS, p. A164
SAINT JOHN'S HEALTH SYSTEM, ANDERSON, IN, p. A137
SAINT JOHN'S HOSPITAL AND HEALTH CENTER, SANTA MONICA, CA, p. A62
SAINT JOSEPH HEALTH CENTER, KANSAS CITY, MO, p. A248
SAINT JOSEPH HOSPITAL, LEXINGTON, KY, p. A174
SAINT JOSEPH HOSPITAL, EUREKA, CA, p. A40
SAINT JOSEPH HOSPITAL EAST, LEXINGTON, KY, p. A174
SAINT JOSEPH MERCY HEALTH SYSTEM, ANN ARBOR, MI, p. A211
SAINT JOSEPH'S HOSPITAL, MARSHFIELD, WI, p. A471
SAINT JOSEPH'S HOSPITAL OF ATLANTA, ATLANTA, GA, p. A100
SAINT JOSEPH'S REGIONAL MEDICAL CENTER–PLYMOUTH CAMPUS, PLYMOUTH, IN, p. A145
SAINT JOSEPH'S REGIONAL MEDICAL CENTER–SOUTH BEND CAMPUS, SOUTH BEND, IN, p. A146
SAINT LOUIS UNIVERSITY HOSPITAL, SAINT LOUIS, MO, p. A253
SAINT LUKE INSTITUTE, SILVER SPRING, MD, p. A200
SAINT LUKE'S HOSPITAL, KANSAS CITY, MO, p. A248
SAINT LUKE'S MEDICAL CENTER, CLEVELAND, OHIO, p. A329
SAINT LUKE'S NORTHLAND HOSPITAL, KANSAS CITY, MO, p. A248
SAINT LUKE'S NORTHLAND HOSPITAL–SMITHVILLE CAMPUS, SMITHVILLE, MO, p. A254
SAINT LUKE'S SOUTH HOSPITAL, OVERLAND PARK, KS, p. A166
SAINT MARGARET MERCY HEALTHCARE CENTERS, HAMMOND, IN, p. A141
SAINT MARGARET MERCY HEALTHCARE CENTERS–NORTH CAMPUS, HAMMOND, INDIANA, p. A141
SAINT MARGARET MERCY HEALTHCARE CENTERS–SOUTH CAMPUS, DYER, INDIANA, p. A141
SAINT MARY HOSPITAL, NEW YORK, KANSAS, p. A164
SAINT MARY OF NAZARETH HOSPITAL CENTER, CHICAGO, IL, p. A123
SAINT MARY REGIONAL MEDICAL CENTER, APPLE VALLEY, CA, p. A35
SAINT MARY'S MERCY MEDICAL CENTER, GRAND RAPIDS, MI, p. A216
SAINT MARY'S REGIONAL MEDICAL CENTER, RUSSELLVILLE, AR, p. A33
SAINT MARY'S REGIONAL MEDICAL CENTER, RENO, NV, p. A269
SAINT MARYS HOSPITAL, ROCHESTER, MN, p. A232
SAINT MICHAEL HOSPITAL, CLEVELAND, OH, p. A329
SAINT MICHAEL'S HOSPITAL, STEVENS POINT, WI, p. A475
SAINT MICHAEL'S MEDICAL CENTER, NEWARK, NJ, p. A278
SAINT THOMAS HOSPITAL, AKRON, OHIO, p. A325
SAINT VINCENT HEALTH CENTER, ERIE, PA, p. A360

SAINT VINCENT HOSPITAL, WORCESTER, MA, p. A210
SAINT VINCENT HOSPITAL AND HEALTH CENTER, BILLINGS, MT, p. A256
SAINT VINCENTS HOSPITAL, NEW YORK, NEW YORK, p. A299
SAINT VINCENTS HOSPITAL AND MEDICAL CENTER, NEW YORK, NY, p. A299
SAINTS MEMORIAL MEDICAL CENTER, LOWELL, MA, p. A206
SAKAKAWEA MEDICAL CENTER, HAZEN, ND, p. A322
SALEM COMMUNITY HOSPITAL, SALEM, OH, p. A337
SALEM HOSPITAL, SALEM, MA, p. A208
SALEM HOSPITAL, SALEM, OR, p. A354
SALEM MEMORIAL DISTRICT HOSPITAL, SALEM, MO, p. A254
SALEM TOWNSHIP HOSPITAL, SALEM, IL, p. A134
SALINA REGIONAL HEALTH CENTER, SALINA, KS, p. A167
SALINA REGIONAL HEALTH CENTER– PENN CAMPUS, SALINA, KANSAS, p. A167
SALINA REGIONAL HEALTH CENTER–SANTA FE CAMPUS, SALINA, KANSAS, p. A167
SALINAS VALLEY MEMORIAL HEALTHCARE SYSTEM, SALINAS, CA, p. A58
SALINE COMMUNITY HOSPITAL, SALINE, MI, p. A222
SALINE MEMORIAL HOSPITAL, BENTON, AR, p. A28
SALT LAKE REGIONAL MEDICAL CENTER, SALT LAKE CITY, UT, p. A438
SAM RAYBURN MEMORIAL VETERANS CENTER, BONHAM, TEXAS, p. A410
SAMARITAN BEHAVIORAL HEALTH CENTER–DESERT SAMARITAN MEDICAL CENTER, MESA, ARIZONA, p. A23
SAMARITAN BEHAVIORAL HEALTH CENTER–SCOTTSDALE, SCOTTSDALE, AZ, p. A25
SAMARITAN BEHAVIORAL HEALTH CENTER–THUNDERBIRD SAMARITAN CAMPUS, GLENDALE, ARIZONA, p. A23
SAMARITAN HEALTH CENTER, BAY CITY, MICHIGAN, p. A212
SAMARITAN HEALTHCARE, MOSES LAKE, WA, p. A454
SAMARITAN HOSPITAL, TROY, NY, p. A306
SAMARITAN HOSPITAL, LEXINGTON, KY, p. A174
SAMARITAN MEDICAL CENTER, WATERTOWN, NY, p. A307
SAMARITAN MEMORIAL HOSPITAL, MACON, MO, p. A250
SAMARITAN REGIONAL HEALTH SYSTEM, ASHLAND, OH, p. A325
SAMPSON REGIONAL MEDICAL CENTER, CLINTON, NC, p. A311
SAMUEL MAHELONA MEMORIAL HOSPITAL, KAPAA, HI, p. A113
SAMUEL SIMMONDS MEMORIAL HOSPITAL, BARROW, AK, p. A20
SAN ANGELO COMMUNITY MEDICAL CENTER, SAN ANGELO, TX, p. A428
SAN ANTONIO COMMUNITY HOSPITAL, UPLAND, CA, p. A65
SAN ANTONIO DIVISION, SAN ANTONIO, TEXAS, p. A429
SAN ANTONIO STATE HOSPITAL, SAN ANTONIO, TX, p. A429
SAN BERNARDINO MOUNTAINS COMMUNITY HOSPITAL DISTRICT, LAKE ARROWHEAD, CA, p. A45
SAN CARLOS GENERAL HOSPITAL, SAN JUAN, PR, p. A484
SAN CLEMENTE HOSPITAL AND MEDICAL CENTER, SAN CLEMENTE, CA, p. A58
SAN DIEGO COUNTY PSYCHIATRIC HOSPITAL, SAN DIEGO, CA, p. A59
SAN DIEGO HOSPICE, SAN DIEGO, CA, p. A59
SAN DIMAS COMMUNITY HOSPITAL, SAN DIMAS, CA, p. A59
SAN FRANCISCO GENERAL HOSPITAL MEDICAL CENTER, SAN FRANCISCO, CA, p. A60
SAN GABRIEL VALLEY MEDICAL CENTER, SAN GABRIEL, CA, p. A60
SAN GORGONIO MEMORIAL HOSPITAL, BANNING, CA, p. A36
SAN JACINTO METHODIST HOSPITAL, BAYTOWN, TX, p. A404
SAN JOAQUIN COMMUNITY HOSPITAL, BAKERSFIELD, CA, p. A36
SAN JOAQUIN GENERAL HOSPITAL, FRENCH CAMP, CA, p. A41
SAN JOAQUIN VALLEY REHABILITATION HOSPITAL, FRESNO, CA, p. A42
SAN JORGE CHILDREN'S HOSPITAL, SAN JUAN, PR, p. A484
SAN JOSE MEDICAL CENTER, SAN JOSE, CA, p. A60
SAN JUAN CITY HOSPITAL, SAN JUAN, PR, p. A484
SAN JUAN HOSPITAL, MONTICELLO, UT, p. A437
SAN JUAN REGIONAL MEDICAL CENTER, FARMINGTON, NM, p. A284
SAN LEANDRO HOSPITAL, SAN LEANDRO, CA, p. A61
SAN LUIS OBISPO GENERAL HOSPITAL, SAN LUIS OBISPO, CA, p. A61
SAN LUIS VALLEY REGIONAL MEDICAL CENTER, ALAMOSA, CO, p. A68
SAN MATEO COUNTY GENERAL HOSPITAL AND CLINICS, SAN MATEO, CA, p. A61
SAN PEDRO PENINSULA HOSPITAL, LOS ANGELES, CA, p. A49
SAN RAMON REGIONAL MEDICAL CENTER, SAN RAMON, CA, p. A61
SAN VICENTE HOSPITAL, LOS ANGELES, CA, p. A49
SANDHILLS REGIONAL MEDICAL CENTER, HAMLET, NC, p. A314
SANDYPINES, TEQUESTA, FL, p. A97
SANGER GENERAL HOSPITAL, SANGER, CA, p. A61

A510 Index of Hospitals © 2000 AHA Guide

Index of Hospitals / Sisters of Charity Hospital of Buffalo

SANPETE VALLEY HOSPITAL, MOUNT PLEASANT, UT, p. A437
SANTA ANA HOSPITAL MEDICAL CENTER, SANTA ANA, CA, p. A61
SANTA BARBARA COTTAGE CARE CENTER, SANTA BARBARA, CALIFORNIA, p. A62
SANTA BARBARA COTTAGE HOSPITAL, SANTA BARBARA, CA, p. A62
SANTA CLARA VALLEY MEDICAL CENTER, SAN JOSE, CA, p. A61
SANTA MARTA HOSPITAL, LOS ANGELES, CA, p. A49
SANTA MONICA-UCLA MEDICAL CENTER, SANTA MONICA, CA, p. A62
SANTA PAULA MEMORIAL HOSPITAL, SANTA PAULA, CA, p. A62
SANTA ROSA MEDICAL CENTER, MILTON, FL, p. A90
SANTA ROSA MEMORIAL HOSPITAL, SANTA ROSA, CA, p. A63
SANTA TERESA COMMUNITY MEDICAL CENTER, SAN JOSE, CA, p. A61
SANTA TERESITA HOSPITAL, DUARTE, CA, p. A40
SANTA YNEZ VALLEY COTTAGE HOSPITAL, SOLVANG, CA, p. A63
SANTIAM MEMORIAL HOSPITAL, STAYTON, OR, p. A354
SARAH BUSH LINCOLN HEALTH CENTER, MATTOON, IL, p. A130
SARAH D. CULBERTSON MEMORIAL HOSPITAL, RUSHVILLE, IL, p. A134
SARASOTA MEMORIAL HOSPITAL, SARASOTA, FL, p. A95
SARATOGA HOSPITAL, SARATOGA SPRINGS, NY, p. A304
SARTORI MEMORIAL HOSPITAL, CEDAR FALLS, IA, p. A148
SATANTA DISTRICT HOSPITAL, SATANTA, KS, p. A167
SATILLA REGIONAL MEDICAL CENTER, WAYCROSS, GA, p. A111
SAUK PRAIRIE MEMORIAL HOSPITAL, PRAIRIE DU SAC, WI, p. A474
SAUNDERS COUNTY HEALTH SERVICE, WAHOO, NE, p. A267
SAVANNAS HOSPITAL, PORT ST. LUCIE, FL, p. A93
SAVOY MEDICAL CENTER, MAMOU, LA, p. A185
SAYRE MEMORIAL HOSPITAL, SAYRE, OK, p. A347
SCCI HOSPITAL OF KOKOMO, KOKOMO, IN, p. A142
SCENIC MOUNTAIN MEDICAL CENTER, BIG SPRING, TX, p. A405
SCHEURER HOSPITAL, PIGEON, MI, p. A220
SCHICK SHADEL HOSPITAL, SEATTLE, WA, p. A456
SCHLEICHER COUNTY MEDICAL CENTER, ELDORADO, TX, p. A412
SCHNEIDER CHILDREN'S HOSPITAL, NEW YORK, NEW YORK, p. A297
SCHOOLCRAFT MEMORIAL HOSPITAL, MANISTIQUE, MI, p. A219
SCHUYLER HOSPITAL, MONTOUR FALLS, NY, p. A294
SCHWAB REHABILITATION HOSPITAL AND CARE NETWORK, CHICAGO, IL, p. A123
SCIOTO MEMORIAL HOSPITAL, PORTSMOUTH, OHIO, p. A337
SCOTLAND COUNTY MEMORIAL HOSPITAL, MEMPHIS, MO, p. A250
SCOTLAND MEMORIAL HOSPITAL, LAURINBURG, NC, p. A315
SCOTT AND WHITE MEMORIAL HOSPITAL, TEMPLE, TX, p. A432
SCOTT COUNTY HOSPITAL, ONEIDA, TN, p. A398
SCOTT COUNTY HOSPITAL, SCOTT CITY, KS, p. A167
SCOTT MEDICAL CENTER, SCOTT AFB, IL, p. A134
SCOTT MEMORIAL HOSPITAL, SCOTTSBURG, IN, p. A145
SCOTTSDALE HEALTHCARE-OSBORN, SCOTTSDALE, AZ, p. A25
SCOTTSDALE HEALTHCARE-SHEA, SCOTTSDALE, AZ, p. A25
SCREVEN COUNTY HOSPITAL, SYLVANIA, GA, p. A110
SCRIPPS GREEN HOSPITAL, LA JOLLA, CA, p. A45
SCRIPPS MEMORIAL HOSPITAL CHULA VISTA, CHULA VISTA, CA, p. A38
SCRIPPS MEMORIAL HOSPITAL-ENCINITAS, ENCINITAS, CA, p. A40
SCRIPPS MEMORIAL HOSPITAL-LA JOLLA, LA JOLLA, CA, p. A45
SCRIPPS MERCY HOSPITAL, SAN DIEGO, CA, p. A59
SEARCY HOSPITAL, MOUNT VERNON, AL, p. A17
SEARHC MT. EDGECUMBE HOSPITAL, SITKA, AK, p. A21
SEBASTIAN RIVER MEDICAL CENTER, SEBASTIAN, FL, p. A95
SEBASTICOOK VALLEY HOSPITAL, PITTSFIELD, ME, p. A193
SEDAN CITY HOSPITAL, SEDAN, KS, p. A167
SEDGWICK COUNTY HEALTH CENTER, JULESBURG, CO, p. A71
SEILING HOSPITAL, SEILING, OK, p. A347
SELBY GENERAL HOSPITAL, MARIETTA, OH, p. A334
SELECT SPECIALTY HOSPITAL-DALLAS/FORTH WORTH, DALLAS, TX, p. A409
SELECT SPECIALTY HOSPITAL-HOUSTON HEIGHTS, HOUSTON, TX, p. A418
SELECT SPECIALTY HOSPITAL-HOUSTON MEDICAL CENTER, HOUSTON, TX, p. A418
SELF MEMORIAL HOSPITAL, GREENWOOD, SC, p. A381
SELMA BAPTIST HOSPITAL, SELMA, AL, p. A18
SELMA COMMUNITY HOSPITAL, SELMA, CA, p. A63
SEMINOLE MEDICAL CENTER, SEMINOLE, OK, p. A347

SENATOR GARRETT T. W. HAGEDORN GERO PSYCHIATRIC HOSPITAL, GLEN GARDNER, NJ, p. A276
SENECA DISTRICT HOSPITAL, CHESTER, CA, p. A38
SENIOR HAVEN CONVALESCENT NURSING CENTER, p. A226
SENTARA BAYSIDE HOSPITAL, VIRGINIA BEACH, VA, p. A450
SENTARA HAMPTON GENERAL HOSPITAL, HAMPTON, VA, p. A444
SENTARA LEIGH HOSPITAL, NORFOLK, VA, p. A447
SENTARA NORFOLK GENERAL HOSPITAL, NORFOLK, VA, p. A447
SENTARA VIRGINIA BEACH GENERAL HOSPITAL, VIRGINIA BEACH, VA, p. A450
SEQUOIA HOSPITAL, REDWOOD CITY, CA, p. A56
SEQUOYAH MEMORIAL HOSPITAL, SALLISAW, OK, p. A347
SERENITY LANE, EUGENE, OR, p. A351
SETON EDGAR B. DAVIS HOSPITAL, LULING, TX, p. A422
SETON HEALTH SYSTEM, TROY, NY, p. A306
SETON HEALTH SYSTEM-ST. MARY'S HOSPITAL, TROY, NEW YORK, p. A306
SETON HIGHLAND LAKES, BURNET, TX, p. A405
SETON MEDICAL CENTER, AUSTIN, TX, p. A403
SETON MEDICAL CENTER, DALY CITY, CA, p. A39
SETON MEDICAL CENTER COASTSIDE, MOSS BEACH, CA, p. A52
SETON NORTHWEST HOSPITAL, AUSTIN, TEXAS, p. A403
SETON SHOAL CREEK HOSPITAL, AUSTIN, TX, p. A403
SEVEN RIVERS COMMUNITY HOSPITAL, CRYSTAL RIVER, FL, p. A83
SEVIER VALLEY HOSPITAL, RICHFIELD, UT, p. A438
SEWICKLEY VALLEY HOSPITAL, (A DIVISION OF VALLEY MEDICAL FACILITIES), SEWICKLEY, PENNSYLVANIA, p. A372
SEYMOUR HOSPITAL, SEYMOUR, TX, p. A430
SHADY GROVE ADVENTIST HOSPITAL, ROCKVILLE, MD, p. A200
SHAMOKIN AREA COMMUNITY HOSPITAL, COAL TOWNSHIP, PA, p. A358
SHAMROCK GENERAL HOSPITAL, SHAMROCK, TX, p. A430
SHANDS AT AGH, GAINESVILLE, FL, p. A85
SHANDS AT LAKE SHORE, LAKE CITY, FL, p. A88
SHANDS AT LIVE OAK, LIVE OAK, FL, p. A88
SHANDS AT STARKE, STARKE, FL, p. A95
SHANDS AT THE UNIVERSITY OF FLORIDA, GAINESVILLE, FL, p. A85
SHANDS AT VISTA, GAINESVILLE, FLORIDA, p. A85
SHANDS JACKSONVILLE MEDICAL CENTER, JACKSONVILLE, FL, p. A87
SHANDS REHAB HOSPITAL, GAINESVILLE, FL, p. A85
SHANNON MEDICAL CENTER, SAN ANGELO, TX, p. A428
SHANNON MEDICAL CENTER- ST. JOHN'S CAMPUS, SAN ANGELO, TEXAS, p. A428
SHARE MEDICAL CENTER, ALVA, OK, p. A341
SHARON HOSPITAL, SHARON, CT, p. A76
SHARON REGIONAL HEALTH SYSTEM, SHARON, PA, p. A372
SHARP CABRILLO HOSPITAL, SAN DIEGO, CA, p. A59
SHARP CHULA VISTA MEDICAL CENTER, CHULA VISTA, CA, p. A38
SHARP CORONADO HOSPITAL, CORONADO, CA, p. A39
SHARP MEMORIAL HOSPITAL, SAN DIEGO, CA, p. A59
SHARP MESA VISTA HOSPITAL, SAN DIEGO, CA, p. A59
SHAUGHNESSY-KAPLAN REHABILITATION HOSPITAL, SALEM, MA, p. A208
SHAWANO MEDICAL CENTER, SHAWANO, WI, p. A475
SHAWNEE MISSION MEDICAL CENTER, SHAWNEE MISSION, KS, p. A168
SHAWNEE REGIONAL HOSPITAL, SHAWNEE, OK, p. A347
SHEARER-RICHARDSON MEMORIAL NURSING HOME, p. A241
SHEBOYGAN MEMORIAL MEDICAL CENTER, SHEBOYGAN, WI, p. A475
SHEEHAN MEMORIAL HOSPITAL, BUFFALO, NY, p. A289
SHELBY BAPTIST MEDICAL CENTER, ALABASTER, AL, p. A11
SHELBY COUNTY MYRTUE MEMORIAL HOSPITAL, HARLAN, IA, p. A152
SHELBY HOSPITAL, SHELBY, OHIO, p. A334
SHELBY MEMORIAL HOSPITAL, SHELBYVILLE, IL, p. A134
SHELTERING ARMS REHABILITATION HOSPITAL, RICHMOND, VA, p. A449
SHENANDOAH MEDICAL CENTER, SHENANDOAH, IA, p. A156
SHENANDOAH MEMORIAL HOSPITAL, WOODSTOCK, VA, p. A451
SHENANGO VALLEY CAMPUS, FARRELL, PENNSYLVANIA, p. A361
SHEPHERD CENTER, ATLANTA, GA, p. A100
SHEPPARD AND ENOCH PRATT HOSPITAL, BALTIMORE, MD, p. A196
SHERIDAN COMMUNITY HOSPITAL, SHERIDAN, MI, p. A222
SHERIDAN COUNTY HEALTH COMPLEX, HOXIE, KS, p. A162
SHERIDAN MEMORIAL HOSPITAL, PLENTYWOOD, MT, p. A259
SHERMAN HOSPITAL, ELGIN, IL, p. A125
SHERMAN OAKS HOSPITAL AND HEALTH CENTER, LOS ANGELES, CA, p. A49
SHOALS HOSPITAL, MUSCLE SHOALS, AL, p. A17

SHODAIR CHILDREN'S HOSPITAL, HELENA, MT, p. A258
SHORE MEMORIAL HOSPITAL, SOMERS POINT, NJ, p. A280
SHORE MEMORIAL HOSPITAL, NASSAWADOX, VA, p. A446
SHOSHONE MEDICAL CENTER, KELLOGG, ID, p. A116
SHRINERS HOSPITALS FOR CHILDREN, ERIE, ERIE, PA, p. A360
SHRINERS HOSPITALS FOR CHILDREN, GALVESTON BURNS HOSPITAL, GALVESTON, TX, p. A413
SHRINERS HOSPITALS FOR CHILDREN, GREENVILLE, GREENVILLE, SC, p. A381
SHRINERS HOSPITALS FOR CHILDREN, HONOLULU, HONOLULU, HI, p. A112
SHRINERS HOSPITALS FOR CHILDREN, HOUSTON, HOUSTON, TX, p. A418
SHRINERS HOSPITALS FOR CHILDREN, LOS ANGELES, LOS ANGELES, CA, p. A49
SHRINERS HOSPITALS FOR CHILDREN, NORTHERN CALIFORNIA, SACRAMENTO, CA, p. A57
SHRINERS HOSPITALS FOR CHILDREN, PHILADELPHIA, PHILADELPHIA, PA, p. A368
SHRINERS HOSPITALS FOR CHILDREN, PORTLAND, PORTLAND, OR, p. A353
SHRINERS HOSPITALS FOR CHILDREN, SHREVEPORT, SHREVEPORT, LA, p. A189
SHRINERS HOSPITALS FOR CHILDREN, SHRINERS BURNS HOSPITAL, CINCINNATI, CINCINNATI, OH, p. A328
SHRINERS HOSPITALS FOR CHILDREN, SHRINERS BURNS HOSPITAL-BOSTON, BOSTON, MA, p. A202
SHRINERS HOSPITALS FOR CHILDREN, SPRINGFIELD, SPRINGFIELD, MA, p. A208
SHRINERS HOSPITALS FOR CHILDREN, ST. LOUIS, SAINT LOUIS, MO, p. A253
SHRINERS HOSPITALS FOR CHILDREN, TAMPA, TAMPA, FL, p. A96
SHRINERS HOSPITALS FOR CHILDREN, TWIN CITIES, MINNEAPOLIS, MN, p. A231
SHRINERS HOSPITALS FOR CHILDREN-CHICAGO, CHICAGO, IL, p. A123
SHRINERS HOSPITALS FOR CHILDREN-INTERMOUNTAIN, SALT LAKE CITY, UT, p. A438
SHRINERS HOSPITALS FOR CHILDREN-LEXINGTON, LEXINGTON, KY, p. A174
SHRINERS HOSPITALS FOR CHILDREN-SPOKANE, SPOKANE, WA, p. A457
SIBLEY MEMORIAL HOSPITAL, WASHINGTON, DC, p. A80
SID PETERSON MEMORIAL HOSPITAL, KERRVILLE, TX, p. A420
SIDNEY HEALTH CENTER, SIDNEY, MT, p. A259
SIERRA MEDICAL CENTER, EL PASO, TX, p. A412
SIERRA NEVADA MEMORIAL HOSPITAL, GRASS VALLEY, CA, p. A43
SIERRA TUCSON, TUCSON, AZ, p. A27
SIERRA VALLEY DISTRICT HOSPITAL, LOYALTON, CA, p. A50
SIERRA VIEW DISTRICT HOSPITAL, PORTERVILLE, CA, p. A56
SIERRA VISTA HOSPITAL, TRUTH OR CONSEQUENCES, NM, p. A286
SIERRA VISTA REGIONAL HEALTH CENTER, SIERRA VISTA, AZ, p. A26
SIERRA VISTA REGIONAL MEDICAL CENTER, SAN LUIS OBISPO, CA, p. A61
SIERRA-KINGS DISTRICT HOSPITAL, REEDLEY, CA, p. A57
SILOAM SPRINGS MEMORIAL HOSPITAL, SILOAM SPRINGS, AR, p. A34
SILVER CROSS HOSPITAL, JOLIET, IL, p. A129
SILVER HILL HOSPITAL, NEW CANAAN, CT, p. A75
SILVERTON HOSPITAL, SILVERTON, OR, p. A354
SIMI VALLEY HOSPITAL AND HEALTH CARE SERVICES, SIMI VALLEY, CA, p. A63
SIMI VALLEY HOSPITAL AND HEALTH CARE SERVICES-SOUTH CAMPUS, SIMI VALLEY, CALIFORNIA, p. A63
SIMPSON GENERAL HOSPITAL, MENDENHALL, MS, p. A240
SIMPSON INFIRMARY, WELLESLEY COLLEGE, WELLESLEY, MA, p. A209
SINAI HOSPITAL OF BALTIMORE, BALTIMORE, MD, p. A196
SINAI SAMARITAN MEDICAL CENTER, MILWAUKEE, WI, p. A472
SINAI/GRACE HOSPITAL, DETROIT, MI, p. A214
SINGING RIVER HOSPITAL, PASCAGOULA, MS, p. A241
SIOUX CENTER COMMUNITY HOSPITAL AND HEALTH CENTER/AVERA HEALTH, SIOUX CENTER, IA, p. A156
SIOUX VALLEY BEHAVIORAL HEALTH, SIOUX FALLS, SOUTH DAKOTA, p. A388
SIOUX VALLEY CANBY CAMPUS, CANBY, MN, p. A226
SIOUX VALLEY HOSPITAL AND UNIVERSITY MEDICAL CENTER, SIOUX FALLS, SD, p. A388
SIOUX VALLEY MEMORIAL HOSPITAL, CHEROKEE, IA, p. A149
SIOUX VALLEY VERMILLION CAMPUS, VERMILLION, SD, p. A388
SISKIN HOSPITAL FOR PHYSICAL REHABILITATION, CHATTANOOGA, TN, p. A391
SISTER KENNY INSTITUTE, MINNEAPOLIS, MINNESOTA, p. A230
SISTERS OF CHARITY HOSPITAL OF BUFFALO, BUFFALO, NY, p. A289

© 2000 AHA Guide

Index of Hospitals / Sisters of Charity Medical Center

SISTERS OF CHARITY MEDICAL CENTER, NEW YORK, NY, p. A300
SISTERSVILLE GENERAL HOSPITAL, SISTERSVILLE, WV, p. A464
SITKA COMMUNITY HOSPITAL, SITKA, AK, p. A21
SKAGGS COMMUNITY HEALTH CENTER, BRANSON, MO, p. A244
SKAGIT VALLEY HOSPITAL, MOUNT VERNON, WASHINGTON, p. A454
SKIFF MEDICAL CENTER, NEWTON, IA, p. A155
SKYLINE HOSPITAL, WHITE SALMON, WA, p. A459
SLEEPY EYE MUNICIPAL HOSPITAL, SLEEPY EYE, MN, p. A233
SLIDELL MEMORIAL HOSPITAL AND MEDICAL CENTER, SLIDELL, LA, p. A189
SMITH COUNTY MEMORIAL HOSPITAL, CARTHAGE, TN, p. A390
SMITH COUNTY MEMORIAL HOSPITAL, SMITH CENTER, KS, p. A168
SMITH HOSPITAL, HAHIRA, GA, p. A105
SMITHVILLE REGIONAL HOSPITAL, SMITHVILLE, TX, p. A431
SMYTH COUNTY COMMUNITY HOSPITAL, MARION, VA, p. A446
SOCORRO GENERAL HOSPITAL, SOCORRO, NM, p. A286
SOLDIERS AND SAILORS MEMORIAL HOSPITAL, WELLSBORO, PA, p. A374
SOLDIERS AND SAILORS MEMORIAL HOSPITAL OF YATES COUNTY, PENN YAN, NY, p. A302
SOLDIERS' HOME IN HOLYOKE, HOLYOKE, MA, p. A205
SOMERSET HOSPITAL CENTER FOR HEALTH, SOMERSET, PA, p. A372
SOMERSET MEDICAL CENTER, SOMERVILLE, NJ, p. A280
SOMERVILLE HOSPITAL, SOMERVILLE, MASSACHUSETTS, p. A204
SONOMA DEVELOPMENTAL CENTER, ELDRIDGE, CA, p. A40
SONOMA VALLEY HOSPITAL, SONOMA, CA, p. A63
SONORA COMMUNITY HOSPITAL, SONORA, CA, p. A63
SOUND SHORE MEDICAL CENTER OF WESTCHESTER, NEW ROCHELLE, NY, p. A295
SOUTH AUSTIN HOSPITAL, AUSTIN, TX, p. A403
SOUTH BALDWIN REGIONAL MEDICAL CENTER, FOLEY, AL, p. A14
SOUTH BARRY COUNTY MEMORIAL HOSPITAL, CASSVILLE, MO, p. A245
SOUTH BAY HOSPITAL, SUN CITY CENTER, FL, p. A95
SOUTH BEACH PSYCHIATRIC CENTER, NEW YORK, NY, p. A300
SOUTH CAMERON MEMORIAL HOSPITAL, CAMERON, LA, p. A181
SOUTH CAMPUS, HOUSTON, TEXAS, p. A416
SOUTH CAROLINA STATE HOSPITAL, COLUMBIA, SC, p. A380
SOUTH CENTRAL EXTENDED CARE, ELLISVILLE, MISSISSIPPI, p. A239
SOUTH CENTRAL KANSAS REGIONAL MEDICAL CENTER, ARKANSAS CITY, KS, p. A159
SOUTH CENTRAL REGIONAL MEDICAL CENTER, LAUREL, MS, p. A239
SOUTH COAST MEDICAL CENTER, SOUTH LAGUNA, CA, p. A63
SOUTH COUNTY HOSPITAL, WAKEFIELD, RI, p. A377
SOUTH FLORIDA BAPTIST HOSPITAL, PLANT CITY, FL, p. A93
SOUTH FLORIDA EVALUATION AND TREATMENT CENTER, MIAMI, FL, p. A90
SOUTH FLORIDA STATE HOSPITAL, PEMBROKE PINES, FL, p. A92
SOUTH FULTON MEDICAL CENTER, EAST POINT, GA, p. A104
SOUTH GEORGIA MEDICAL CENTER, VALDOSTA, GA, p. A111
SOUTH HAVEN COMMUNITY HOSPITAL, SOUTH HAVEN, MI, p. A222
SOUTH HILLS HEALTH SYSTEM, PITTSBURGH, PA, p. A369
SOUTH JERSEY HOSPITAL, BRIDGETON, NJ, p. A274
SOUTH JERSEY HOSPITAL–BRIDGETON, BRIDGETON, NEW JERSEY, p. A274
SOUTH JERSEY HOSPITAL–ELMER, ELMER, NEW JERSEY, p. A274
SOUTH JERSEY HOSPITAL–MILLVILLE, MILLVILLE, NEW JERSEY, p. A274
SOUTH JERSEY HOSPITAL–NEWCOMB, VINELAND, NJ, p. A281
SOUTH LAKE HOSPITAL, CLERMONT, FL, p. A82
SOUTH LINCOLN MEDICAL CENTER, KEMMERER, WY, p. A479
SOUTH LYON MEDICAL CENTER, YERINGTON, NV, p. A270
SOUTH MIAMI HOSPITAL, MIAMI, FL, p. A90
SOUTH NASSAU COMMUNITIES HOSPITAL, OCEANSIDE, NY, p. A301
SOUTH OAKS HOSPITAL, AMITYVILLE, NY, p. A287
SOUTH PANOLA COMMUNITY HOSPITAL, BATESVILLE, MS, p. A236
SOUTH PENINSULA HOSPITAL, HOMER, AK, p. A20
SOUTH SEMINOLE COMMUNITY HOSPITAL, LONGWOOD, FLORIDA, p. A88
SOUTH SHORE HOSPITAL, SOUTH WEYMOUTH, MA, p. A208
SOUTH SHORE HOSPITAL, CHICAGO, IL, p. A123
SOUTH SHORE HOSPITAL AND MEDICAL CENTER, MIAMI BEACH, FL, p. A90
SOUTH SUBURBAN HOSPITAL, HAZEL CREST, IL, p. A127

SOUTH SUNFLOWER COUNTY HOSPITAL, INDIANOLA, MS, p. A238
SOUTH TEXAS HOSPITAL, HARLINGEN, TX, p. A415
SOUTH TEXAS REGIONAL MEDICAL CENTER, JOURDANTON, TX, p. A419
SOUTH TEXAS VETERANS HEALTH CARE SYSTEM, SAN ANTONIO, TX, p. A429
SOUTHAMPTON HOSPITAL, SOUTHAMPTON, NY, p. A305
SOUTHAMPTON MEMORIAL HOSPITAL, FRANKLIN, VA, p. A444
SOUTHCOAST HOSPITALS GROUP, FALL RIVER, MA, p. A204
SOUTHCREST HOSPITAL, TULSA, OK, p. A348
SOUTHEAST ALABAMA MEDICAL CENTER, DOTHAN, AL, p. A14
SOUTHEAST ARIZONA MEDICAL CENTER, DOUGLAS, AZ, p. A22
SOUTHEAST BAPTIST HOSPITAL, SAN ANTONIO, TX, p. A429
SOUTHEAST COLORADO HOSPITAL AND LONG TERM CARE, SPRINGFIELD, CO, p. A73
SOUTHEAST GEORGIA REGIONAL MEDICAL CENTER, BRUNSWICK, GA, p. A101
SOUTHEAST LOUISIANA HOSPITAL, MANDEVILLE, LA, p. A185
SOUTHEAST MISSOURI HOSPITAL, CAPE GIRARDEAU, MO, p. A245
SOUTHEAST MISSOURI MENTAL HEALTH CENTER, FARMINGTON, MO, p. A246
SOUTHEAST PSYCHIATRIC HOSPITAL, ATHENS, OHIO, p. A326
SOUTHEASTERN OHIO REGIONAL MEDICAL CENTER, CAMBRIDGE, OH, p. A326
SOUTHEASTERN REGIONAL MEDICAL CENTER, LUMBERTON, NC, p. A315
SOUTHERN ARIZONA VETERANS AFFAIRS HEALTHCARE SYSTEM, TUCSON, AZ, p. A27
SOUTHERN CHESTER COUNTY MEDICAL CENTER, WEST GROVE, PA, p. A374
SOUTHERN COOS HOSPITAL AND HEALTH CENTER, BANDON, OR, p. A350
SOUTHERN HILLS MEDICAL CENTER, NASHVILLE, TN, p. A398
SOUTHERN HUMBOLDT COMMUNITY HEALTHCARE DISTRICT, GARBERVILLE, CA, p. A42
SOUTHERN INDIANA REHABILITATION HOSPITAL, NEW ALBANY, IN, p. A144
SOUTHERN INYO COUNTY LOCAL HEALTH CARE DISTRICT, LONE PINE, CA, p. A46
SOUTHERN MAINE MEDICAL CENTER, BIDDEFORD, ME, p. A191
SOUTHERN MARYLAND HOSPITAL, CLINTON, MD, p. A197
SOUTHERN NEW HAMPSHIRE MEDICAL CENTER, NASHUA, NH, p. A272
SOUTHERN NEW MEXICO REHABILITATION CENTER, ROSWELL, NM, p. A285
SOUTHERN OCEAN COUNTY HOSPITAL, MANAHAWKIN, NJ, p. A277
SOUTHERN OHIO MEDICAL CENTER, PORTSMOUTH, OH, p. A337
SOUTHERN REGIONAL MEDICAL CENTER, RIVERDALE, GA, p. A108
SOUTHERN TENNESSEE MEDICAL CENTER, WINCHESTER, TN, p. A400
SOUTHERN VIRGINIA MENTAL HEALTH INSTITUTE, DANVILLE, VA, p. A443
SOUTHERN WAKE HOSPITAL, FUQUAY-VARINA, NORTH CAROLINA, p. A317
SOUTHERN WINDS HOSPITAL, HIALEAH, FL, p. A86
SOUTHLAKE CAMPUS, MERRILLVILLE, INDIANA, p. A140
SOUTHPOINTE HOSPITAL, SAINT LOUIS, MO, p. A253
SOUTHSIDE COMMUNITY HOSPITAL, FARMVILLE, VA, p. A443
SOUTHSIDE HOSPITAL, BAY SHORE, NY, p. A288
SOUTHSIDE REGIONAL MEDICAL CENTER, PETERSBURG, VA, p. A447
SOUTHVIEW HOSPITAL AND FAMILY HEALTH CENTER, DAYTON, OHIO, p. A333
SOUTHWEST CONNECTICUT MENTAL HEALTH SYSTEM, BRIDGEPORT, CT, p. A74
SOUTHWEST FLORIDA REGIONAL MEDICAL CENTER, FORT MYERS, FL, p. A85
SOUTHWEST GENERAL HEALTH CENTER, MIDDLEBURG HEIGHTS, OH, p. A335
SOUTHWEST GENERAL HOSPITAL, SAN ANTONIO, TX, p. A429
SOUTHWEST GEORGIA REGIONAL MEDICAL CENTER, CUTHBERT, GA, p. A103
SOUTHWEST HEALTH CENTER, PLATTEVILLE, WI, p. A474
SOUTHWEST HEALTH CENTER NURSING HOME, CUBA CITY, WISCONSIN, p. A474
SOUTHWEST HOSPITAL AND MEDICAL CENTER, ATLANTA, GA, p. A100
SOUTHWEST MEDICAL CENTER, LIBERAL, KS, p. A164
SOUTHWEST MEMORIAL HOSPITAL, CORTEZ, CO, p. A69
SOUTHWEST MENTAL HEALTH CENTER, SAN ANTONIO, TX, p. A429
SOUTHWEST MISSISSIPPI REGIONAL MEDICAL CENTER, MCCOMB, MS, p. A240
SOUTHWEST REGIONAL MEDICAL CENTER, LITTLE ROCK, AR, p. A31

SOUTHWEST REHABILITATION HOSPITAL, BATTLE CREEK, MI, p. A212
SOUTHWEST TEXAS METHODIST HOSPITAL, SAN ANTONIO, TX, p. A429
SOUTHWEST WASHINGTON MEDICAL CENTER, VANCOUVER, WA, p. A458
SOUTHWESTERN GENERAL HOSPITAL, EL PASO, TX, p. A412
SOUTHWESTERN MEDICAL CENTER, LAWTON, OK, p. A344
SOUTHWESTERN MEMORIAL HOSPITAL, WEATHERFORD, OK, p. A349
SOUTHWESTERN VERMONT MEDICAL CENTER, BENNINGTON, VT, p. A440
SOUTHWESTERN VIRGINIA MENTAL HEALTH INSTITUTE, MARION, VA, p. A446
SOUTHWOOD PSYCHIATRIC HOSPITAL, PITTSBURGH, PA, p. A369
SPALDING REGIONAL HOSPITAL, GRIFFIN, GA, p. A105
SPALDING REHABILITATION HOSPITAL, AURORA, CO, p. A68
SPARKS REGIONAL MEDICAL CENTER, FORT SMITH, AR, p. A30
SPARROW HEALTH SYSTEM, LANSING, MI, p. A218
SPARTA COMMUNITY HOSPITAL, SPARTA, IL, p. A134
SPARTANBURG HOSPITAL FOR RESTORATIVE CARE, SPARTANBURG, SC, p. A383
SPARTANBURG REGIONAL MEDICAL CENTER, SPARTANBURG, SC, p. A383
SPAULDING REHABILITATION HOSPITAL, BOSTON, MA, p. A203
SPEARE MEMORIAL HOSPITAL, PLYMOUTH, NH, p. A273
SPECIALTY HOSPITAL, WEST COVINA, CA, p. A67
SPECIALTY HOSPITAL JACKSONVILLE, JACKSONVILLE, FL, p. A87
SPECIALTY HOSPITAL OF AUSTIN, AUSTIN, TX, p. A403
SPECIALTY HOSPITAL OF HOUSTON, HOUSTON, TX, p. A418
SPECIALTY HOSPITAL OF MERIDIAN, MERIDIAN, MS, p. A240
SPECIALTY HOSPITAL OF SANTA ANA, SANTA ANA, CA, p. A62
SPECTRUM HEALTH, GRAND RAPIDS, MI, p. A216
SPECTRUM HEALTH–DOWNTOWN CAMPUS, GRAND RAPIDS, MICHIGAN, p. A216
SPECTRUM HEALTH–KENT COMMUNITY CAMPUS, GRAND RAPIDS, MI, p. A216
SPECTRUM HEALTH–REED CITY CAMPUS, REED CITY, MI, p. A221
SPENCER MUNICIPAL HOSPITAL, SPENCER, IA, p. A157
SPOONER HEALTH SYSTEM, SPOONER, WI, p. A475
SPRING BRANCH MEDICAL CENTER, HOUSTON, TX, p. A418
SPRING BROOK BEHAVIORAL HEALTHCARE SYSTEM, TRAVELERS REST, SC, p. A384
SPRING GROVE HOSPITAL CENTER, BALTIMORE, MD, p. A196
SPRING HARBOR HOSPITAL, SOUTH PORTLAND, ME, p. A194
SPRING HILL REGIONAL HOSPITAL, SPRING HILL, FL, p. A95
SPRINGBROOK HOSPITAL, BROOKSVILLE, FL, p. A82
SPRINGFIELD HOSPITAL, SPRINGFIELD, VT, p. A441
SPRINGFIELD HOSPITAL, SPRINGFIELD, PENNSYLVANIA, p. A373
SPRINGFIELD HOSPITAL CENTER, SYKESVILLE, MD, p. A200
SPRINGFIELD MEDICAL CENTER–MAYO HEALTH SYSTEM, SPRINGFIELD, MN, p. A233
SPRINGHILL MEDICAL CENTER, SPRINGHILL, LA, p. A189
SPRINGHILL MEMORIAL HOSPITAL, MOBILE, AL, p. A16
SPRINGS MEMORIAL HOSPITAL, LANCASTER, SC, p. A382
SPRUCE PINE COMMUNITY HOSPITAL, SPRUCE PINE, NC, p. A318
SSM REHAB, SAINT LOUIS, MO, p. A253
ST BARNABAS HOSPITAL, NEW YORK, NY, p. A300
ST FRANCIS HEALTH CENTER, COLORADO SPRINGS, COLORADO, p. A69
ST LUKE'S HOSPITAL–ALLENTOWN CAMPUS, ALLENTOWN, PENNSYLVANIA, p. A356
ST MARY'S HEALTH SERVICES–WELBORN CAMPUS, EVANSVILLE, INDIANA, p. A139
ST VINCENT'S CAMPUS, NEW YORK, NEW YORK, p. A300
ST, ANNE'S SKILLED NURSING DIVISION, DEPAUL HOSPITAL, BRIDGETON, MISSOURI, p. A253
ST. VINCENT'S PSYCHIATRIC DIVISION, BRIDGETON, MISSOURI, p. A253
ST. AGNES HEALTHCARE, BALTIMORE, MD, p. A196
ST. AGNES HOSPITAL, WHITE PLAINS, NY, p. A307
ST. AGNES MEDICAL CENTER, PHILADELPHIA, PA, p. A368
ST. ALEXIUS MEDICAL CENTER, HOFFMAN ESTATES, IL, p. A128
ST. ALEXIUS MEDICAL CENTER, BISMARCK, ND, p. A321
ST. ALOISIUS MEDICAL CENTER, HARVEY, ND, p. A322
ST. ANDREW'S HEALTH CENTER, BOTTINEAU, ND, p. A321
ST. ANDREWS HOSPITAL AND HEALTHCARE CENTER, BOOTHBAY HARBOR, ME, p. A191
ST. ANN'S HOSPITAL, WESTERVILLE, OHIO, p. A330
ST. ANNE GENERAL HOSPITAL, RACELAND, LA, p. A188
ST. ANSGAR'S HEALTH CENTER, PARK RIVER, ND, p. A323
ST. ANTHONY CAMPUS, HAYS, KANSAS, p. A162
ST. ANTHONY CENTRAL HOSPITAL, DENVER, CO, p. A69
ST. ANTHONY COMMUNITY HOSPITAL, WARWICK, NY, p. A307

Index of Hospitals / St. Joseph's Mercy Hospitals and Health Services

ST. ANTHONY HOSPITAL, OKLAHOMA CITY, OK, p. A346
ST. ANTHONY HOSPITAL, PENDLETON, OR, p. A352
ST. ANTHONY MEDICAL CENTER, CROWN POINT, IN, p. A138
ST. ANTHONY NORTH HOSPITAL, WESTMINSTER, CO, p. A73
ST. ANTHONY REGIONAL HOSPITAL, CARROLL, IA, p. A148
ST. ANTHONY'S HEALTHCARE CENTER, MORRILTON, AR, p. A32
ST. ANTHONY'S HOSPITAL, SAINT PETERSBURG, FL, p. A94
ST. ANTHONY'S MEDICAL CENTER, SAINT LOUIS, MO, p. A253
ST. ANTHONY'S MEMORIAL HOSPITAL, EFFINGHAM, IL, p. A125
ST. BENEDICTS FAMILY MEDICAL CENTER, JEROME, ID, p. A116
ST. BERNARD HOSPITAL AND HEALTH CARE CENTER, CHICAGO, IL, p. A123
ST. BERNARD'S BEHAVIORAL HEALTH, JONESBORO, AR, p. A31
ST. BERNARD'S PROVIDENCE HOSPITAL, MILBANK, SD, p. A386
ST. BERNARDINE MEDICAL CENTER, SAN BERNARDINO, CA, p. A58
ST. BERNARDS REGIONAL MEDICAL CENTER, JONESBORO, AR, p. A31
ST. CATHERINE HOSPITAL, EAST CHICAGO, IN, p. A139
ST. CATHERINE HOSPITAL, GARDEN CITY, KS, p. A161
ST. CATHERINE OF SIENA MEDICAL CENTER, SMITHTOWN, NY, p. A305
ST. CATHERINE'S HOSPITAL, KENOSHA, WI, p. A470
ST. CHARLES GENERAL HOSPITAL, NEW ORLEANS, LA, p. A187
ST. CHARLES HOSPITAL AND REHABILITATION CENTER, PORT JEFFERSON, NY, p. A303
ST. CHARLES MEDICAL CENTER, BEND, OR, p. A350
ST. CHARLES MERCY HOSPITAL, OREGON, OH, p. A336
ST. CHARLES PARISH HOSPITAL, LULING, LA, p. A185
ST. CHRISTOPHER'S HOSPITAL FOR CHILDREN, PHILADELPHIA, PA, p. A368
ST. CLAIR MEMORIAL HOSPITAL, PITTSBURGH, PA, p. A369
ST. CLAIR REGIONAL HOSPITAL, PELL CITY, AL, p. A17
ST. CLAIRE MEDICAL CENTER, MOREHEAD, KY, p. A177
ST. CLARE HOSPITAL, LAKEWOOD, WA, p. A454
ST. CLARE HOSPITAL AND HEALTH SERVICES, BARABOO, WI, p. A466
ST. CLARE MEDICAL CENTER, CRAWFORDSVILLE, IN, p. A138
ST. CLARE'S HOSPITAL AND HEALTH CENTER, NEW YORK, NY, p. A300
ST. CLARE'S HOSPITAL OF SCHENECTADY, SCHENECTADY, NY, p. A304
ST. CLARE'S HOSPITAL/DOVER, DOVER, NEW JERSEY, p. A275
ST. CLAUDE MEDICAL CENTER, NEW ORLEANS, LA, p. A187
ST. CLEMENT HEALTH SERVICES, RED BUD, IL, p. A133
ST. CLOUD HOSPITAL, SAINT CLOUD, MN, p. A232
ST. CLOUD HOSPITAL, A DIVISION OF ORLANDO REGIONAL HEALTHCARE SYSTEM, SAINT CLOUD, FL, p. A94
ST. CROIX REGIONAL MEDICAL CENTER, SAINT CROIX FALLS, WI, p. A475
ST. DAVID'S MEDICAL CENTER, AUSTIN, TX, p. A403
ST. DAVID'S PAVILION, AUSTIN, TX, p. A403
ST. DAVID'S REHABILITATION CENTER, AUSTIN, TX, p. A403
ST. DOMINIC'S HOSPITAL, MANTECA, CA, p. A51
ST. DOMINIC-JACKSON MEMORIAL HOSPITAL, JACKSON, MS, p. A239
ST. EDWARD MERCY MEDICAL CENTER, FORT SMITH, AR, p. A30
ST. ELIZABETH ANN SETON HOSPITAL, BOONVILLE, IN, p. A138
ST. ELIZABETH COMMUNITY HOSPITAL, RED BLUFF, CA, p. A56
ST. ELIZABETH HEALTH CENTER, YOUNGSTOWN, OH, p. A340
ST. ELIZABETH HEALTH SERVICES, BAKER CITY, OR, p. A350
ST. ELIZABETH HOSPITAL, ELIZABETH, NJ, p. A275
ST. ELIZABETH HOSPITAL, APPLETON, WI, p. A466
ST. ELIZABETH HOSPITAL, WABASHA, MN, p. A234
ST. ELIZABETH MEDICAL CENTER, UTICA, NY, p. A306
ST. ELIZABETH MEDICAL CENTER, LAFAYETTE, INDIANA, p. A143
ST. ELIZABETH MEDICAL CENTER, GRANITE CITY, IL, p. A127
ST. ELIZABETH MEDICAL CENTER-GRANT COUNTY, WILLIAMSTOWN, KY, p. A179
ST. ELIZABETH MEDICAL CENTER-NORTH, COVINGTON, KENTUCKY, p. A171
ST. ELIZABETH MEDICAL CENTER-SOUTH, EDGEWOOD, KY, p. A171
ST. ELIZABETH'S HOSPITAL, BELLEVILLE, IL, p. A120
ST. ELIZABETH'S HOSPITAL, CHICAGO, IL, p. A123
ST. ELIZABETH'S MEDICAL CENTER OF BOSTON, BRIGHTON, MA, p. A203
ST. ELIZABETHS HOSPITAL, WASHINGTON, DC, p. A80
ST. FRANCIS AT SALINA, SALINA, KS, p. A167
ST. FRANCIS CAMPUS, WICHITA, KANSAS, p. A169
ST. FRANCIS CENTRAL HOSPITAL, PITTSBURGH, PA, p. A369
ST. FRANCIS HEALTH CARE CENTRE, GREEN SPRINGS, OH, p. A332
ST. FRANCIS HEALTH SYSTEM, GREENVILLE, SC, p. A381
ST. FRANCIS HOSPITAL, ROSLYN, NY, p. A304
ST. FRANCIS HOSPITAL, JERSEY CITY, NJ, p. A277
ST. FRANCIS HOSPITAL, WILMINGTON, DE, p. A78
ST. FRANCIS HOSPITAL, COLUMBUS, GA, p. A103
ST. FRANCIS HOSPITAL, EVANSTON, IL, p. A126
ST. FRANCIS HOSPITAL, LITCHFIELD, IL, p. A129
ST. FRANCIS HOSPITAL, ESCANABA, MI, p. A214
ST. FRANCIS HOSPITAL, MILWAUKEE, WI, p. A472
ST. FRANCIS HOSPITAL, MOUNTAIN VIEW, MO, p. A250
ST. FRANCIS HOSPITAL, FEDERAL WAY, WA, p. A453
ST. FRANCIS HOSPITAL AND HEALTH CENTERS – NORTH CAMPUS, BEECH GROVE, IN, p. A137
ST. FRANCIS HOSPITAL AND HEALTH CENTERS – SOUTH CAMPUS, INDIANAPOLIS, INDIANA, p. A137
ST. FRANCIS HOSPITAL AND HEALTH SERVICES, MARYVILLE, MO, p. A250
ST. FRANCIS HOSPITAL AND MEDICAL CENTER, TOPEKA, KS, p. A168
ST. FRANCIS HOSPITAL CRANBERRY, CRANBERRY, PA, p. A358
ST. FRANCIS HOSPITAL OF NEW CASTLE, NEW CASTLE, PA, p. A365
ST. FRANCIS HOSPITAL–MOORESVILLE, MOORESVILLE, IN, p. A144
ST. FRANCIS MEDICAL CENTER, TRENTON, NJ, p. A281
ST. FRANCIS MEDICAL CENTER, PITTSBURGH, PA, p. A369
ST. FRANCIS MEDICAL CENTER, BRECKENRIDGE, MN, p. A226
ST. FRANCIS MEDICAL CENTER, GRAND ISLAND, NE, p. A263
ST. FRANCIS MEDICAL CENTER, MONROE, LA, p. A186
ST. FRANCIS MEDICAL CENTER, LYNWOOD, CA, p. A50
ST. FRANCIS MEDICAL CENTER, HONOLULU, HI, p. A112
ST. FRANCIS MEDICAL CENTER OF SANTA BARBARA, SANTA BARBARA, CA, p. A62
ST. FRANCIS MEDICAL CENTER–WEST, EWA BEACH, HI, p. A112
ST. FRANCIS MEMORIAL HOSPITAL, WEST POINT, NE, p. A267
ST. FRANCIS NURSING CENTER, p. A446
ST. FRANCIS REGIONAL MEDICAL CENTER, SHAKOPEE, MN, p. A233
ST. FRANCIS SPECIALTY HOSPITAL, MONROE, LA, p. A186
ST. GABRIEL'S HOSPITAL, LITTLE FALLS, MN, p. A229
ST. HELENA HOSPITAL, DEER PARK, CA, p. A39
ST. HELENA PARISH HOSPITAL, GREENSBURG, LA, p. A182
ST. JAMES COMMUNITY HOSPITAL, BUTTE, MT, p. A256
ST. JAMES HEALTH SERVICES, SAINT JAMES, MN, p. A233
ST. JAMES HOSPITAL AND HEALTH CENTERS – CHICAGO HEIGHTS CAMPUS, CHICAGO HEIGHTS, IL, p. A124
ST. JAMES HOSPITALS AND HEALTH CENTERS – OLYMPIA FIELDS CAMPUS, OLYMPIA FIELDS, IL, p. A132
ST. JAMES MERCY HOSPITAL, HORNELL, NY, p. A292
ST. JAMES PARISH HOSPITAL, LUTCHER, LA, p. A185
ST. JOHN DETROIT RIVERVIEW HOSPITAL, DETROIT, MI, p. A214
ST. JOHN HOSPITAL AND MEDICAL CENTER, DETROIT, MI, p. A214
ST. JOHN HOSPITAL–MACOMB CENTER, HARRISON TOWNSHIP, MICHIGAN, p. A214
ST. JOHN MACOMB HOSPITAL, WARREN, MI, p. A224
ST. JOHN MEDICAL CENTER, TULSA, OK, p. A349
ST. JOHN MEDICAL CENTER, LONGVIEW, WA, p. A454
ST. JOHN NORTHEAST COMMUNITY HOSPITAL, DETROIT, MI, p. A214
ST. JOHN OAKLAND HOSPITAL, MADISON HEIGHTS, MI, p. A219
ST. JOHN RIVER DISTRICT HOSPITAL, EAST CHINA, MI, p. A214
ST. JOHN SAPULPA, SAPULPA, OK, p. A347
ST. JOHN VIANNEY HOSPITAL, DOWNINGTOWN, PA, p. A359
ST. JOHN WEST SHORE HOSPITAL, CLEVELAND, OH, p. A329
ST. JOHN'S EPISCOPAL HOSPITAL DIVISION, NEW YORK, NEW YORK, p. A297
ST. JOHN'S EPISCOPAL HOSPITAL–SOUTH SHORE, NEW YORK, NY, p. A300
ST. JOHN'S HOSPITAL, SPRINGFIELD, IL, p. A135
ST. JOHN'S HOSPITAL, MAPLEWOOD, MN, p. A230
ST. JOHN'S HOSPITAL AND LIVING CENTER, JACKSON, WY, p. A479
ST. JOHN'S LUTHERAN HOSPITAL, LIBBY, MT, p. A258
ST. JOHN'S MAUDE NORTON MEMORIAL HOSPITAL, COLUMBUS, KS, p. A160
ST. JOHN'S MERCY HOSPITAL, WASHINGTON, MISSOURI, p. A253
ST. JOHN'S MERCY MEDICAL CENTER, SAINT LOUIS, MO, p. A253
ST. JOHN'S PLEASANT VALLEY HOSPITAL, CAMARILLO, CA, p. A37
ST. JOHN'S QUEENS HOSPITAL, NEW YORK, NEW YORK, p. A296
ST. JOHN'S REGIONAL HEALTH CENTER, SPRINGFIELD, MO, p. A254
ST. JOHN'S REGIONAL MEDICAL CENTER, JOPLIN, MO, p. A248
ST. JOHN'S REGIONAL MEDICAL CENTER, OXNARD, CA, p. A54
ST. JOHN'S RIVERSIDE HOSPITAL, YONKERS, NY, p. A307
ST. JOSEPH CAMPUS, WICHITA, KANSAS, p. A169
ST. JOSEPH COMMUNITY HOSPITAL, MISHAWAKA, IN, p. A144
ST. JOSEPH HEALTH CENTER, WARREN, OH, p. A339
ST. JOSEPH HEALTH CENTER, SAINT CHARLES, MO, p. A252
ST. JOSEPH HEALTH SERVICES OF RHODE ISLAND, NORTH PROVIDENCE, RI, p. A376
ST. JOSEPH HEALTH SYSTEM, TAWAS CITY, MI, p. A223
ST. JOSEPH HOSPITAL, BANGOR, ME, p. A191
ST. JOSEPH HOSPITAL, NASHUA, NH, p. A272
ST. JOSEPH HOSPITAL, CHEEKTOWAGA, NY, p. A290
ST. JOSEPH HOSPITAL, LANCASTER, PA, p. A362
ST. JOSEPH HOSPITAL, AUGUSTA, GA, p. A101
ST. JOSEPH HOSPITAL, FORT WAYNE, IN, p. A140
ST. JOSEPH HOSPITAL, CHICAGO, IL, p. A123
ST. JOSEPH HOSPITAL, OMAHA, NE, p. A265
ST. JOSEPH HOSPITAL, POLSON, MT, p. A259
ST. JOSEPH HOSPITAL, BELLINGHAM, WA, p. A452
ST. JOSEPH HOSPITAL, ORANGE, CA, p. A54
ST. JOSEPH HOSPITAL & HEALTH CENTER, KOKOMO, IN, p. A142
ST. JOSEPH HOSPITAL FOR SPECIALTY CARE, PROVIDENCE, RHODE ISLAND, p. A376
ST. JOSEPH HOSPITAL OF KIRKWOOD, SAINT LOUIS, MO, p. A253
ST. JOSEPH HOSPITAL WEST, LAKE SAINT LOUIS, MO, p. A249
ST. JOSEPH MEDICAL CENTER, READING, PA, p. A371
ST. JOSEPH MEDICAL CENTER, TOWSON, MD, p. A200
ST. JOSEPH MEDICAL CENTER, ALBUQUERQUE, NM, p. A283
ST. JOSEPH MEDICAL CENTER, TACOMA, WA, p. A458
ST. JOSEPH MEMORIAL HOSPITAL, MURPHYSBORO, IL, p. A131
ST. JOSEPH MERCY HOSPITAL, ANN ARBOR, MICHIGAN, p. A211
ST. JOSEPH MERCY OAKLAND, PONTIAC, MI, p. A221
ST. JOSEPH NORTHEAST HEIGHTS HOSPITAL, ALBUQUERQUE, NM, p. A283
ST. JOSEPH REGIONAL HEALTH CENTER, BRYAN, TX, p. A405
ST. JOSEPH REGIONAL MEDICAL CENTER, LEWISTON, ID, p. A116
ST. JOSEPH REGIONAL MEDICAL CENTER OF NORTHERN OKLAHOMA, PONCA CITY, OK, p. A346
ST. JOSEPH REHABILITATION HOSPITAL AND OUTPATIENT CENTER, ALBUQUERQUE, NM, p. A283
ST. JOSEPH WEST MESA HOSPITAL, ALBUQUERQUE, NM, p. A284
ST. JOSEPH'S AREA HEALTH SERVICES, PARK RAPIDS, MN, p. A232
ST. JOSEPH'S BEHAVIORAL HEALTH CENTER, STOCKTON, CA, p. A64
ST. JOSEPH'S CANDLER HEALTH SYSTEM, SAVANNAH, GA, p. A109
ST. JOSEPH'S COMMUNITY HEALTH SERVICES, HILLSBORO, WI, p. A469
ST. JOSEPH'S COMMUNITY HOSPITAL OF WEST BEND, WEST BEND, WI, p. A477
ST. JOSEPH'S HOSPITAL, NEW YORK, NEW YORK, p. A296
ST. JOSEPH'S HOSPITAL, ELMIRA, NY, p. A291
ST. JOSEPH'S HOSPITAL, PHILADELPHIA, PENNSYLVANIA, p. A367
ST. JOSEPH'S HOSPITAL, PARKERSBURG, WV, p. A463
ST. JOSEPH'S HOSPITAL, ASHEVILLE, NORTH CAROLINA, p. A309
ST. JOSEPH'S HOSPITAL, TAMPA, FL, p. A96
ST. JOSEPH'S HOSPITAL, BREESE, IL, p. A120
ST. JOSEPH'S HOSPITAL, HIGHLAND, IL, p. A128
ST. JOSEPH'S HOSPITAL, CHIPPEWA FALLS, WI, p. A467
ST. JOSEPH'S HOSPITAL, MILWAUKEE, WI, p. A472
ST. JOSEPH'S HOSPITAL, SAINT PAUL, MN, p. A233
ST. JOSEPH'S HOSPITAL, CHEWELAH, WA, p. A452
ST. JOSEPH'S HOSPITAL AND HEALTH CENTER, DICKINSON, ND, p. A322
ST. JOSEPH'S HOSPITAL AND MEDICAL CENTER, PATERSON, NJ, p. A279
ST. JOSEPH'S HOSPITAL AND MEDICAL CENTER, PHOENIX, AZ, p. A25
ST. JOSEPH'S HOSPITAL BLUEMOUND, WAUWATOSA, WI, p. A477
ST. JOSEPH'S HOSPITAL HEALTH CENTER, SYRACUSE, NY, p. A306
ST. JOSEPH'S HOSPITAL OF BUCKHANNON, BUCKHANNON, WV, p. A460
ST. JOSEPH'S MEDICAL CENTER, YONKERS, NY, p. A308
ST. JOSEPH'S MEDICAL CENTER, BRAINERD, MN, p. A226
ST. JOSEPH'S MEDICAL CENTER, STOCKTON, CA, p. A64
ST. JOSEPH'S MERCY HOSPITAL–EAST, MOUNT CLEMENS, MICHIGAN, p. A213
ST. JOSEPH'S MERCY HOSPITAL–WEST, CLINTON TOWNSHIP, MICHIGAN, p. A213
ST. JOSEPH'S MERCY HOSPITALS AND HEALTH SERVICES, CLINTON TOWNSHIP, MI, p. A213

© 2000 AHA Guide

Index of Hospitals / St. Joseph's Mercy–North

ST. JOSEPH'S MERCY–NORTH, ROMEO, MICHIGAN, p. A213
ST. JOSEPH'S REGIONAL HEALTH CENTER, HOT SPRINGS NATIONAL PARK, AR, p. A30
ST. JUDE CHILDREN'S RESEARCH HOSPITAL, MEMPHIS, TN, p. A397
ST. JUDE MEDICAL CENTER, FULLERTON, CA, p. A42
ST. LAWRENCE HOSPITAL AND HEALTHCARE SERVICES, LANSING, MICHIGAN, p. A218
ST. LAWRENCE PSYCHIATRIC CENTER, OGDENSBURG, NY, p. A302
ST. LAWRENCE REHABILITATION CENTER, LAWRENCEVILLE, NJ, p. A277
ST. LOUIS CHILDREN'S HOSPITAL, SAINT LOUIS, MO, p. A253
ST. LOUIS PSYCHIATRIC REHABILITATION CENTER, SAINT LOUIS, MO, p. A254
ST. LOUISE REGIONAL HOSPITAL, GILROY, CA, p. A42
ST. LUCIE MEDICAL CENTER, PORT ST. LUCIE, FL, p. A94
ST. LUKE COMMUNITY HOSPITAL, RONAN, MT, p. A259
ST. LUKE HOSPITAL AND LIVING CENTER, MARION, KS, p. A164
ST. LUKE HOSPITAL EAST, FORT THOMAS, KY, p. A172
ST. LUKE HOSPITAL WEST, FLORENCE, KY, p. A172
ST. LUKE MEDICAL CENTER, PASADENA, CA, p. A55
ST. LUKE'S BAPTIST HOSPITAL, SAN ANTONIO, TX, p. A430
ST. LUKE'S BEHAVIORAL HEALTH CENTER, PHOENIX, AZ, p. A25
ST. LUKE'S EPISCOPAL HEALTH SYSTEM, HOUSTON, TX, p. A418
ST. LUKE'S HOSPITAL, NEWBURGH, NY, p. A301
ST. LUKE'S HOSPITAL, BLUEFIELD, WV, p. A460
ST. LUKE'S HOSPITAL, COLUMBUS, NC, p. A311
ST. LUKE'S HOSPITAL, JACKSONVILLE, FL, p. A87
ST. LUKE'S HOSPITAL, MAUMEE, OH, p. A335
ST. LUKE'S HOSPITAL, DULUTH, MN, p. A227
ST. LUKE'S HOSPITAL, CEDAR RAPIDS, IA, p. A149
ST. LUKE'S HOSPITAL, CHESTERFIELD MO, p. A245
ST. LUKE'S HOSPITAL, CROSBY, ND, p. A321
ST. LUKE'S HOSPITAL, SAN FRANCISCO, CA, p. A60
ST. LUKE'S HOSPITAL AND HEALTH NETWORK, BETHLEHEM, PA, p. A356
ST. LUKE'S HOSPITAL CENTER, NEW YORK, NEW YORK, p. A300
ST. LUKE'S HOSPITAL OF NEW BEDFORD, NEW BEDFORD, MASSACHUSETTS, p. A204
ST. LUKE'S MEDICAL CENTER, MILWAUKEE, WI, p. A472
ST. LUKE'S MEDICAL CENTER, PHOENIX, AZ, p. A25
ST. LUKE'S MEMORIAL HOSPITAL, RACINE, WI, p. A474
ST. LUKE'S QUAKERTOWN HOSPITAL, QUAKERTOWN, PENNSYLVANIA, p. A356
ST. LUKE'S REGIONAL MEDICAL CENTER, SIOUX CITY, IA, p. A157
ST. LUKE'S REGIONAL MEDICAL CENTER, BOISE, ID, p. A115
ST. LUKE'S SOUTH SHORE, CUDAHY, WISCONSIN, p. A472
ST. LUKE'S TRI-STATE HOSPITAL, BOWMAN, ND, p. A321
ST. LUKE'S–ROOSEVELT HOSPITAL CENTER, NEW YORK, NY, p. A300
ST. LUKES REHABILITATION INSTITUTE, SPOKANE, WA, p. A457
ST. MARGARET'S HOSPITAL, SPRING VALLEY, IL, p. A134
ST. MARK'S HOSPITAL, SALT LAKE CITY, UT, p. A438
ST. MARY HOSPITAL, HOBOKEN, NJ, p. A276
ST. MARY HOSPITAL, LIVONIA, MI, p. A218
ST. MARY MEDICAL CENTER, LANGHORNE, PA, p. A363
ST. MARY MEDICAL CENTER, HOBART, IN, p. A141
ST. MARY MEDICAL CENTER, WALLA WALLA, WA, p. A458
ST. MARY MEDICAL CENTER, LONG BEACH, CA, p. A46
ST. MARY'S WARRICK, BOONVILLE, IN, p. A138
ST. MARY'S HEALTH CARE SYSTEM, ATHENS, GA, p. A99
ST. MARY'S HEALTH CENTER, SAINT LOUIS, MO, p. A254
ST. MARY'S HEALTH SYSTEM, KNOXVILLE, TN, p. A395
ST. MARY'S HEALTHCARE CENTER, PIERRE, SD, p. A387
ST. MARY'S HOSPITAL, WATERBURY, CT, p. A77
ST. MARY'S HOSPITAL, AMSTERDAM, NY, p. A287
ST. MARY'S HOSPITAL, PASSAIC, NJ, p. A279
ST. MARY'S HOSPITAL, LEONARDTOWN, MD, p. A199
ST. MARY'S HOSPITAL, NORTON, VA, p. A447
ST. MARY'S HOSPITAL, HUNTINGTON, WV, p. A462
ST. MARY'S HOSPITAL, WEST PALM BEACH, FL, p. A97
ST. MARY'S HOSPITAL, CENTRALIA, IL, p. A121
ST. MARY'S HOSPITAL, DECATUR, IL, p. A125
ST. MARY'S HOSPITAL, STREATOR, IL, p. A135
ST. MARY'S HOSPITAL, MILWAUKEE, WI, p. A472
ST. MARY'S HOSPITAL, RHINELANDER, WISCONSIN, p. A474
ST. MARY'S HOSPITAL, KANSAS CITY, MISSOURI, p. A249
ST. MARY'S HOSPITAL, NEBRASKA CITY, NE, p. A264
ST. MARY'S HOSPITAL, COTTONWOOD, ID, p. A116
ST. MARY'S HOSPITAL AND MEDICAL CENTER, GRAND JUNCTION, CO, p. A71
ST. MARY'S HOSPITAL AND REHABILITATION CENTER, MINNEAPOLIS, MINNESOTA, p. A230
ST. MARY'S HOSPITAL MEDICAL CENTER, GREEN BAY, WI, p. A469
ST. MARY'S HOSPITAL OF BLUE SPRINGS, BLUE SPRINGS, MO, p. A244
ST. MARY'S HOSPITAL OF BROOKLYN, NEW YORK, NEW YORK, p. A296
ST. MARY'S HOSPITAL OF EAST ST. LOUIS, EAST ST. LOUIS, IL, p. A125
ST. MARY'S HOSPITAL OF SUPERIOR, SUPERIOR, WI, p. A476
ST. MARY'S HOSPITAL OZAUKEE, MEQUON, WI, p. A471
ST. MARY'S KEWAUNEE AREA MEMORIAL HOSPITAL, KEWAUNEE, WI, p. A470
ST. MARY'S MEDICAL CENTER, EVANSVILLE, IN, p. A139
ST. MARY'S MEDICAL CENTER, SAGINAW, MI, p. A221
ST. MARY'S MEDICAL CENTER, DULUTH, MN, p. A227
ST. MARY'S MEDICAL CENTER, SAN FRANCISCO, CA, p. A60
ST. MARY'S MERCY HOSPITAL, ENID, OK, p. A343
ST. MARY'S REGIONAL HEALTH CENTER, DETROIT LAKES, MN, p. A227
ST. MARY'S REGIONAL MEDICAL CENTER, LEWISTON, ME, p. A193
ST. MARY-CORWIN MEDICAL CENTER, PUEBLO, CO, p. A72
ST. MARY-ROGERS MEMORIAL HOSPITAL, ROGERS, AR, p. A33
ST. MARYS HEALTH CENTER, JEFFERSON CITY, MO, p. A247
ST. MARYS HOSPITAL MEDICAL CENTER, MADISON, WI, p. A470
ST. MICHAEL HOSPITAL, MILWAUKEE, WI, p. A472
ST. MICHAEL'S HOSPITAL, SAUK CENTRE, MN, p. A233
ST. MICHAEL'S HOSPITAL, TYNDALL, SD, p. A388
ST. NICHOLAS HOSPITAL, SHEBOYGAN, WI, p. A475
ST. PATRICK HOSPITAL, MISSOULA, MT, p. A259
ST. PAUL MEDICAL CENTER, DALLAS, TX, p. A409
ST. PETER REGIONAL TREATMENT CENTER, SAINT PETER, MN, p. A233
ST. PETER'S HOSPITAL, ALBANY, NY, p. A287
ST. PETER'S HOSPITAL, HELENA, MT, p. A258
ST. PETER'S UNIVERSITY HOSPITAL, NEW BRUNSWICK, NJ, p. A278
ST. PETERSBURG GENERAL HOSPITAL, SAINT PETERSBURG, FL, p. A94
ST. RITA'S MEDICAL CENTER, LIMA, OH, p. A333
ST. ROSE DOMINICAN HOSPITAL, HENDERSON, NV, p. A268
ST. ROSE HOSPITAL, HAYWARD, CA, p. A43
ST. TAMMANY PARISH HOSPITAL, COVINGTON, LA, p. A181
ST. THOMAS HEALTH SERVICES, NASHVILLE, TN, p. A398
ST. THOMAS MORE HOSPITAL AND PROGRESSIVE CARE CENTER, CANON CITY, CO, p. A68
ST. VINCENT CARMEL HOSPITAL, CARMEL, INDIANA, p. A142
ST. VINCENT CHARITY HOSPITAL, CLEVELAND, OH, p. A329
ST. VINCENT DOCTORS HOSPITAL, LITTLE ROCK, AR, p. A31
ST. VINCENT FRANKFORT HOSPITAL, FRANKFORT, IN, p. A140
ST. VINCENT GENERAL HOSPITAL, LEADVILLE, CO, p. A71
ST. VINCENT HOSPITAL, GREEN BAY, WI, p. A469
ST. VINCENT HOSPITAL, SANTA FE, NM, p. A286
ST. VINCENT HOSPITALS AND HEALTH SERVICES, INDIANAPOLIS, IN, p. A142
ST. VINCENT INFIRMARY MEDICAL CENTER, LITTLE ROCK, AR, p. A32
ST. VINCENT JENNINGS HOSPITAL, NORTH VERNON, IN, p. A144
ST. VINCENT MEDICAL CENTER, LOS ANGELES, CA, p. A49
ST. VINCENT MEMORIAL HOSPITAL, TAYLORVILLE, IL, p. A135
ST. VINCENT MERCY HOSPITAL, ELWOOD, IN, p. A139
ST. VINCENT MERCY MEDICAL CENTER, TOLEDO, OH, p. A338
ST. VINCENT RANDOLPH HOSPITAL, WINCHESTER, IN, p. A147
ST. VINCENT REHABILITATION HOSPITAL, SHERWOOD, AR, p. A33
ST. VINCENT STRESS CENTER, INDIANAPOLIS, INDIANA, p. A142
ST. VINCENT WILLIAMSPORT HOSPITAL, WILLIAMSPORT, IN, p. A147
ST. VINCENT'S HOSPITAL, BIRMINGHAM, AL, p. A12
ST. VINCENT'S MEDICAL CENTER, BRIDGEPORT, CT, p. A74
ST. VINCENT'S MEDICAL CENTER, JACKSONVILLE, FL, p. A87
ST. WILLIAM HOME FOR THE AGED, p. A386
STAFFORD DISTRICT HOSPITAL, STAFFORD, KS, p. A168
STAMFORD HEALTH SYSTEM, STAMFORD, CT, p. A77
STAMFORD MEMORIAL HOSPITAL, STAMFORD, TX, p. A431
STANDISH COMMUNITY HOSPITAL, STANDISH, MI, p. A222
STANFORD HOSPITAL AND CLINICS, STANFORD, CA, p. A64
STANLY MEMORIAL HOSPITAL, ALBEMARLE, NC, p. A309
STANTON COUNTY HEALTH CARE FACILITY, JOHNSON, KS, p. A163
STAR VALLEY MEDICAL CENTER, AFTON, WY, p. A478
STARKE MEMORIAL HOSPITAL, KNOX, IN, p. A142
STARR COUNTY MEMORIAL HOSPITAL, RIO GRANDE CITY, TX, p. A427
STATE CORRECTIONAL INSTITUTION AT CAMP HILL, CAMP HILL, PA, p. A357
STATE CORRECTIONAL INSTITUTION HOSPITAL, PITTSBURGH, PA, p. A369
STATE HOSPITAL NORTH, OROFINO, ID, p. A117
STATE HOSPITAL SOUTH, BLACKFOOT, ID, p. A115
STATE PENITENTIARY HOSPITAL, WALLA WALLA, WA, p. A459
STATE PSYCHIATRIC HOSPITAL, SAN JUAN, PR, p. A484
STATE PSYCHIATRIC HOSPITAL, IOWA CITY, IOWA, p. A153
STATEN ISLAND UNIVERSITY HOSPITAL, NEW YORK, NY, p. A300
STE. GENEVIEVE COUNTY MEMORIAL HOSPITAL, STE. GENEVIEVE, MO, p. A255
STEELE MEMORIAL HOSPITAL, SALMON, ID, p. A117
STEPHENS COUNTY HOSPITAL, TOCCOA, GA, p. A110
STEPHENS MEMORIAL HOSPITAL, NORWAY, ME, p. A193
STEPHENS MEMORIAL HOSPITAL, BRECKENRIDGE, TX, p. A405
STERLING REGIONAL MEDCENTER, STERLING, CO, p. A73
STEVENS COMMUNITY MEDICAL CENTER, MORRIS, MN, p. A231
STEVENS COUNTY HOSPITAL, HUGOTON, KS, p. A162
STEVENS HEALTHCARE, EDMONDS, WA, p. A453
STEWART MEMORIAL COMMUNITY HOSPITAL, LAKE CITY, IA, p. A154
STEWART–WEBSTER HOSPITAL, RICHLAND, GA, p. A108
STILLMAN INFIRMARY, HARVARD UNIVERSITY HEALTH SERVICES, CAMBRIDGE, MA, p. A204
STILLWATER COMMUNITY HOSPITAL, COLUMBUS, MT, p. A257
STILLWATER MEDICAL CENTER, STILLWATER, OK, p. A347
STOKES–REYNOLDS MEMORIAL HOSPITAL, DANBURY, NC, p. A311
STONE COUNTY MEDICAL CENTER, MOUNTAIN VIEW, AR, p. A32
STONES RIVER HOSPITAL, WOODBURY, TN, p. A400
STONEWALL JACKSON HOSPITAL, LEXINGTON, VA, p. A445
STONEWALL JACKSON MEMORIAL HOSPITAL, WESTON, WV, p. A465
STONEWALL MEDICAL CENTER, STONEWALL, LA, p. A189
STONEWALL MEMORIAL HOSPITAL, ASPERMONT, TX, p. A402
STONY LODGE HOSPITAL, OSSINING, NY, p. A302
STORMONT–VAIL HEALTHCARE, TOPEKA, KS, p. A168
STORY COUNTY HOSPITAL AND LONG TERM CARE FACILITY, NEVADA, IA, p. A155
STOUGHTON HOSPITAL ASSOCIATION, STOUGHTON, WI, p. A476
STRAITH HOSPITAL FOR SPECIAL SURGERY, SOUTHFIELD, MI, p. A222
STRATTON HOUSE NURSING HOME, p. A441
STRAUB CLINIC AND HOSPITAL, HONOLULU, HI, p. A112
STRINGFELLOW MEMORIAL HOSPITAL, ANNISTON, AL, p. A11
STRONG MEMORIAL HOSPITAL OF THE UNIVERSITY OF ROCHESTER, ROCHESTER, NY, p. A304
STURDY MEMORIAL HOSPITAL, ATTLEBORO, MA, p. A201
STURGIS COMMUNITY HEALTH CARE CENTER, STURGIS, SD, p. A388
STURGIS HOSPITAL, STURGIS, MI, p. A222
STUTTGART REGIONAL MEDICAL CENTER, STUTTGART, AR, p. A34
SUBURBAN GENERAL HOSPITAL, PITTSBURGH, PA, p. A369
SUBURBAN HOSPITAL, BETHESDA, MD, p. A197
SUBURBAN MEDICAL CENTER, PARAMOUNT, CA, p. A55
SULLIVAN COUNTY COMMUNITY HOSPITAL, SULLIVAN, IN, p. A146
SULLIVAN COUNTY MEMORIAL HOSPITAL, MILAN, MO, p. A250
SUMMA HEALTH SYSTEM, AKRON, OH, p. A325
SUMMERS COUNTY APPALACHIAN REGIONAL HOSPITAL, HINTON, WV, p. A461
SUMMERSVILLE MEMORIAL HOSPITAL, SUMMERSVILLE, WV, p. A464
SUMMERVILLE MEDICAL CENTER, SUMMERVILLE, SC, p. A384
SUMMIT HOSPITAL, BATON ROUGE, LA, p. A181
SUMMIT HOSPITAL OF NORTHWEST LOUISIANA, BOSSIER CITY, LA, p. A181
SUMMIT MEDICAL CENTER, HERMITAGE, TN, p. A393
SUMMIT MEDICAL CENTER, OAKLAND, CA, p. A53
SUMMIT PARK HOSPITAL–ROCKLAND COUNTY INFIRMARY, p. A302
SUMNER COUNTY HOSPITAL DISTRICT ONE, CALDWELL, KS, p. A159
SUMNER REGIONAL MEDICAL CENTER, GALLATIN, TN, p. A392
SUMNER REGIONAL MEDICAL CENTER, WELLINGTON, KS, p. A169
SUMTER REGIONAL HOSPITAL, AMERICUS, GA, p. A99
SUN COAST HOSPITAL, LARGO, FL, p. A88
SUNBURY COMMUNITY HOSPITAL, SUNBURY, PA, p. A372
SUNHEALTH SPECIALTY HOSPITAL FOR DENVER, THORNTON, CO, p. A73
SUNNYSIDE COMMUNITY HOSPITAL, SUNNYSIDE, WA, p. A458
SUNNYVIEW HOSPITAL AND REHABILITATION CENTER, SCHENECTADY, NY, p. A305
SUNRISE HOSPITAL AND MEDICAL CENTER, LAS VEGAS, NV, p. A268

SUNRISE REGIONAL MEDICAL CENTER, SUNRISE, FL, p. A96
SURPRISE VALLEY COMMUNITY HOSPITAL, CEDARVILLE, CA, p. A38
SUSAN B. ALLEN MEMORIAL HOSPITAL, EL DORADO, KS, p. A160
SUSQUEHANNA HEALTH SYSTEM, WILLIAMSPORT, PA, p. A375
SUTTER AMADOR HOSPITAL, JACKSON, CA, p. A44
SUTTER AUBURN FAITH COMMUNITY HOSPITAL, AUBURN, CA, p. A36
SUTTER CENTER FOR PSYCHIATRY, SACRAMENTO, CA, p. A57
SUTTER COAST HOSPITAL, CRESCENT CITY, CA, p. A39
SUTTER DAVIS HOSPITAL, DAVIS, CA, p. A39
SUTTER DELTA MEDICAL CENTER, ANTIOCH, CA, p. A35
SUTTER GENERAL HOSPITAL, SACRAMENTO, CALIFORNIA, p. A58
SUTTER LAKESIDE HOSPITAL, LAKEPORT, CA, p. A45
SUTTER MATERNITY AND SURGERY CENTER OF SANTA CRUZ, SANTA CRUZ, CA, p. A62
SUTTER MEDICAL CENTER, SACRAMENTO, CA, p. A58
SUTTER MEDICAL CENTER, SANTA ROSA, SANTA ROSA, CA, p. A63
SUTTER MEMORIAL HOSPITAL, SACRAMENTO, CALIFORNIA, p. A58
SUTTER MERCED MEDICAL CENTER, MERCED, CA, p. A51
SUTTER ROSEVILLE MEDICAL CENTER, ROSEVILLE, CA, p. A57
SUTTER SOLANO MEDICAL CENTER, VALLEJO, CA, p. A66
SUTTER TRACY COMMUNITY HOSPITAL, TRACY, CA, p. A65
SWAIN COUNTY HOSPITAL, BRYSON CITY, NC, p. A310
SWEDISH COVENANT HOSPITAL, CHICAGO, IL, p. A123
SWEDISH HEALTH SERVICES, SEATTLE, WA, p. A456
SWEDISH MEDICAL CENTER, ENGLEWOOD, CO, p. A70
SWEDISH MEDICAL CENTER–BALLARD, SEATTLE, WASHINGTON, p. A456
SWEDISHAMERICAN HEALTH SYSTEM, ROCKFORD, IL, p. A134
SWEENY COMMUNITY HOSPITAL, SWEENY, TX, p. A431
SWEETWATER HOSPITAL, SWEETWATER, TN, p. A400
SWIFT COUNTY–BENSON HOSPITAL, BENSON, MN, p. A226
SWISHER MEMORIAL HOSPITAL DISTRICT, TULIA, TX, p. A433
SYCAMORE HOSPITAL, MIAMISBURG, OHIO, p. A333
SYCAMORE SHOALS HOSPITAL, ELIZABETHTON, TN, p. A392
SYLVAN GROVE HOSPITAL, JACKSON, GA, p. A106
SYRINGA GENERAL HOSPITAL, GRANGEVILLE, ID, p. A116

T

T. C. THOMPSON CHILDREN'S HOSPITAL, CHATTANOOGA, TENNESSEE, p. A390
T. J. SAMSON COMMUNITY HOSPITAL, GLASGOW, KY, p. A172
TACOMA GENERAL HOSPITAL, TACOMA, WA, p. A458
TAHLEQUAH CITY HOSPITAL, TAHLEQUAH, OK, p. A348
TAHOE FOREST HOSPITAL DISTRICT, TRUCKEE, CA, p. A65
TAHOE PACIFIC HOSPITAL, SPARKS, NV, p. A269
TAKOMA ADVENTIST HOSPITAL, GREENEVILLE, TN, p. A393
TALLAHASSEE COMMUNITY HOSPITAL, TALLAHASSEE, FL, p. A96
TALLAHASSEE MEMORIAL HEALTHCARE, TALLAHASSEE, FL, p. A96
TALLAHATCHIE GENERAL HOSPITAL, CHARLESTON, MS, p. A237
TAMPA CHILDREN'S HOSPITAL AT ST. JOSEPH'S, ST. JOSEPH'S WOMEN'S HOSPITAL – TAMPA, TAMPA, FLORIDA, p. A96
TAMPA GENERAL HEALTHCARE, TAMPA, FL, p. A96
TANNER MEDICAL CENTER, CARROLLTON, GA, p. A102
TANNER MEDICAL CENTER–VILLA RICA, VILLA RICA, GA, p. A111
TARRANT COUNTY PSYCHIATRIC CENTER, FORT WORTH, TX, p. A413
TATTNALL MEMORIAL HOSPITAL, REIDSVILLE, GA, p. A108
TAUNTON STATE HOSPITAL, TAUNTON, MA, p. A209
TAYLOR COUNTY HOSPITAL, CAMPBELLSVILLE, KY, p. A171
TAYLOR HOSPITAL, RIDLEY PARK, PENNSYLVANIA, p. A373
TAYLOR MANOR HOSPITAL, ELLICOTT CITY, MD, p. A198
TAYLOR REGIONAL HOSPITAL, HAWKINSVILLE, GA, p. A106
TAZEWELL COMMUNITY HOSPITAL, TAZEWELL, VA, p. A450
TEHACHAPI VALLEY HEALTHCARE DISTRICT, TEHACHAPI, CA, p. A64
TELFAIR COUNTY HOSPITAL, MCRAE, GA, p. A107
TEMPE ST. LUKE'S HOSPITAL, TEMPE, AZ, p. A26
TEMPLE COMMUNITY HOSPITAL, LOS ANGELES, CA, p. A49
TEMPLE EAST, NEUMANN MEDICAL CENTER, PHILADELPHIA, PA, p. A368
TEMPLE UNIVERSITY HOSPITAL, PHILADELPHIA, PA, p. A368
TEN BROECK HOSPITAL, LOUISVILLE, KY, p. A176
TEN BROECK HOSPITAL JACKSONVILLE, JACKSONVILLE, FL, p. A87
TENNESSEE CHRISTIAN MEDICAL CENTER, MADISON, TN, p. A396
TENNESSEE CHRISTIAN MEDICAL CENTER – PORTLAND, PORTLAND, TENNESSEE, p. A396
TERRE HAUTE REGIONAL HOSPITAL, TERRE HAUTE, IN, p. A146
TERREBONNE GENERAL MEDICAL CENTER, HOUMA, LA, p. A183
TERRELL STATE HOSPITAL, TERRELL, TX, p. A432
TETON MEDICAL CENTER, CHOTEAU, MT, p. A256
TETON VALLEY HOSPITAL, DRIGGS, ID, p. A116
TEWKSBURY HOSPITAL, TEWKSBURY, MA, p. A209
TEXAS CENTER FOR INFECTIOUS DISEASE, SAN ANTONIO, TX, p. A430
TEXAS CHILDREN'S HOSPITAL, HOUSTON, TX, p. A418
TEXAS COUNTY MEMORIAL HOSPITAL, HOUSTON, MO, p. A247
TEXAS ORTHOPEDIC HOSPITAL, HOUSTON, TX, p. A418
TEXAS SCOTTISH RITE HOSPITAL FOR CHILDREN, DALLAS, TX, p. A410
TEXOMA HEALTHCARE SYSTEM, DENISON, TX, p. A410
THAYER COUNTY HEALTH SERVICES, HEBRON, NE, p. A263
THE ALLEN PAVILION, NEW YORK, NEW YORK, p. A299
THE BROWN SCHOOLS AT SHADOW MOUNTAIN, TULSA, OK, p. A349
THE CHILDREN'S INSTITUTE OF PITTSBURGH, PITTSBURGH, PA, p. A370
THE CONNECTICUT HOSPICE, BRANFORD, CT, p. A74
THE COOPER HEALTH SYSTEM, CAMDEN, NJ, p. A275
THE EASTSIDE HOSPITAL, REDMOND, WA, p. A456
THE FRIARY OF BAPTIST HEALTH CENTER, GULF BREEZE, FL, p. A86
THE HOSPITAL, SIDNEY, NY, p. A305
THE INSTITUTE FOR REHABILITATION AND RESEARCH, HOUSTON, TX, p. A418
THE JAMES B. HAGGIN MEMORIAL HOSPITAL, HARRODSBURG, KY, p. A173
THE MEDICAL CENTER, COLUMBUS, GA, p. A103
THE MEDICAL CENTER AT BOWLING GREEN, BOWLING GREEN, KY, p. A170
THE MEDICAL CENTER AT FRANKLIN, FRANKLIN, KY, p. A172
THE MEDICAL CENTER, BEAVER, BEAVER, PENNSYLVANIA, p. A372
THE METHODIST HOSPITAL, HOUSTON, TX, p. A418
THE MONROE CLINIC, MONROE, WI, p. A472
THE MOUNT SINAI HOSPITAL OF QUEENS, NEW YORK, NY, p. A300
THE PAVILION, PENSACOLA, FLORIDA, p. A93
THE PAVILION, CHAMPAIGN, IL, p. A121
THE TOLEDO HOSPITAL, TOLEDO, OH, p. A338
THE UNION HOSPITAL, LYNN, MA, p. A206
THE WILLIAM W. BACKUS HOSPITAL, NORWICH, CT, p. A76
THE WOMAN'S HOSPITAL OF TEXAS, HOUSTON, TX, p. A418
THEDA CLARK MEDICAL CENTER, NEENAH, WI, p. A473
THIBODAUX REGIONAL MEDICAL CENTER, THIBODAUX, LA, p. A189
THOMAS B. FINAN CENTER, CUMBERLAND, MD, p. A198
THOMAS H. BOYD MEMORIAL HOSPITAL, CARROLLTON, IL, p. A120
THOMAS HOSPITAL, FAIRHOPE, AL, p. A14
THOMAS JEFFERSON UNIVERSITY HOSPITAL, PHILADELPHIA, PA, p. A368
THOMAS JEFFERSON UNIVERSITY HOSPITAL–FORD ROAD CAMPUS, PHILADELPHIA, PENNSYLVANIA, p. A368
THOMAS MEMORIAL HOSPITAL, SOUTH CHARLESTON, WV, p. A464
THOMASVILLE INFIRMARY, THOMASVILLE, AL, p. A18
THOMS REHABILITATION HOSPITAL, ASHEVILLE, NC, p. A309
THOREK HOSPITAL AND MEDICAL CENTER, CHICAGO, IL, p. A124
THREE RIVERS AREA HOSPITAL, THREE RIVERS, MI, p. A223
THREE RIVERS COMMUNITY HOSPITAL AND HEALTH CENTER, GRANTS PASS, OR, p. A351
THREE RIVERS HOSPITAL, WAVERLY, TN, p. A400
THREE RIVERS MEDICAL CENTER, LOUISA, KY, p. A175
THROCKMORTON COUNTY MEMORIAL HOSPITAL, THROCKMORTON, TX, p. A432
THUNDERBIRD SAMARITAN MEDICAL CENTER, GLENDALE, AZ, p. A23
TIFT GENERAL HOSPITAL, TIFTON, GA, p. A110
TILDEN COMMUNITY HOSPITAL, TILDEN, NE, p. A267
TILLAMOOK COUNTY GENERAL HOSPITAL, TILLAMOOK, OR, p. A354
TIMBERLAWN MENTAL HEALTH SYSTEM, DALLAS, TX, p. A410
TIMPANOGOS REGIONAL HOSPITAL, OREM, UT, p. A437
TINLEY PARK MENTAL HEALTH CENTER, TINLEY PARK, IL, p. A135
TIOGA MEDICAL CENTER, TIOGA, ND, p. A324
TIPPAH COUNTY HOSPITAL, RIPLEY, MS, p. A242
TIPTON COUNTY MEMORIAL HOSPITAL, TIPTON, IN, p. A146
TITUS REGIONAL MEDICAL CENTER, MOUNT PLEASANT, TX, p. A424
TITUSVILLE AREA HOSPITAL, TITUSVILLE, PA, p. A372
TOBEY HOSPITAL, WAREHAM, MASSACHUSETTS, p. A204
TOD CHILDREN'S HOSPITAL, YOUNGSTOWN, OHIO, p. A340
TOLEDO CAMPUS, TOLEDO, OHIO, p. A336
TOLEDO CHILDREN'S HOSPITAL, TOLEDO, OHIO, p. A338
TOMAH MEMORIAL HOSPITAL, TOMAH, WI, p. A476
TOMBALL REGIONAL HOSPITAL, TOMBALL, TX, p. A432
TOOELE VALLEY REGIONAL MEDICAL CENTER, TOOELE, UT, p. A439
TORRANCE MEMORIAL MEDICAL CENTER, TORRANCE, CA, p. A65
TORRANCE STATE HOSPITAL, TORRANCE, PA, p. A372
TOUCHETTE REGIONAL HOSPITAL, CENTREVILLE, IL, p. A121
TOURO INFIRMARY, NEW ORLEANS, LA, p. A187
TOWN AND COUNTRY HOSPITAL, TAMPA, FL, p. A96
TOWNER COUNTY MEDICAL CENTER, CANDO, ND, p. A321
TRACE REGIONAL HOSPITAL, HOUSTON, MS, p. A238
TRACY AREA MEDICAL SERVICES, TRACY, MN, p. A234
TRANSYLVANIA COMMUNITY HOSPITAL, BREVARD, NC, p. A310
TREGO COUNTY–LEMKE MEMORIAL HOSPITAL, WAKEENEY, KS, p. A169
TRENTON PSYCHIATRIC HOSPITAL, TRENTON, NJ, p. A281
TRI COUNTY BAPTIST HOSPITAL, LA GRANGE, KY, p. A173
TRI–CITY MEDICAL CENTER, OCEANSIDE, CA, p. A53
TRI–COUNTY AREA HOSPITAL, LEXINGTON, NE, p. A264
TRI–COUNTY HOSPITAL, WADENA, MN, p. A234
TRI–COUNTY MEMORIAL HOSPITAL, GOWANDA, NY, p. A292
TRI–COUNTY MEMORIAL HOSPITAL, WHITEHALL, WI, p. A477
TRI–STATE MEMORIAL HOSPITAL, CLARKSTON, WA, p. A452
TRI–VALLEY HEALTH SYSTEM, CAMBRIDGE, NE, p. A262
TRI–WARD GENERAL HOSPITAL, BERNICE, LA, p. A181
TRIDENT MEDICAL CENTER, CHARLESTON, SC, p. A379
TRIGG COUNTY HOSPITAL, CADIZ, KY, p. A170
TRILLIUM HOSPITAL, ALBION, MI, p. A211
TRINITAS HOSPITAL, ELIZABETH, NJ, p. A276
TRINITY COMMUNITY HOSPITAL, JASPER, FL, p. A87
TRINITY COMMUNITY MEDICAL CENTER OF BRENHAM, BRENHAM, TX, p. A405
TRINITY HEALTH, MINOT, ND, p. A323
TRINITY HEALTH SYSTEM, STEUBENVILLE, OH, p. A338
TRINITY HOSPITAL, CHICAGO, IL, p. A124
TRINITY HOSPITAL, ERIN, TN, p. A392
TRINITY HOSPITAL, FARMINGTON, MN, p. A228
TRINITY HOSPITAL, WOLF POINT, MONTANA, p. A260
TRINITY HOSPITAL, WEAVERVILLE, CA, p. A67
TRINITY LUTHERAN HOSPITAL, KANSAS CITY, MO, p. A249
TRINITY MEDICAL CENTER, CARROLLTON, TX, p. A406
TRINITY MEDICAL CENTER EAST, STEUBENVILLE, OHIO, p. A338
TRINITY MEDICAL CENTER WEST, STEUBENVILLE, OHIO, p. A338
TRINITY MEDICAL CENTER–NORTH CAMPUS, DAVENPORT, IA, p. A150
TRINITY MEDICAL CENTER–SEVENTH STREET CAMPUS, MOLINE, ILLINOIS, p. A133
TRINITY MEDICAL CENTER–WEST CAMPUS, ROCK ISLAND, IL, p. A133
TRINITY MOTHER FRANCES HEALTH SYSTEM, TYLER, TX, p. A433
TRINITY REGIONAL HOSPITAL, FORT DODGE, IA, p. A152
TRINITY SPRINGS PAVILION, FORT WORTH, TX, p. A413
TRINITY VALLEY MEDICAL CENTER, PALESTINE, TX, p. A425
TRIPLER ARMY MEDICAL CENTER, HONOLULU, HI, p. A113
TROY COMMUNITY HOSPITAL, TROY, PA, p. A373
TRUMAN MEDICAL CENTER–EAST, KANSAS CITY, MO, p. A249
TRUMAN MEDICAL CENTER–HOSPITAL HILL, KANSAS CITY, MO, p. A249
TRUMBULL MEMORIAL HOSPITAL, WARREN, OH, p. A339
TUALITY COMMUNITY HOSPITAL, HILLSBORO, OREGON, p. A351
TUALITY FOREST GROVE HOSPITAL, FOREST GROVE, OREGON, p. A351
TUALITY HEALTHCARE, HILLSBORO, OR, p. A351
TUBA CITY INDIAN MEDICAL CENTER, TUBA CITY, AZ, p. A26
TUCSON GENERAL HOSPITAL, TUCSON, AZ, p. A27
TUCSON MEDICAL CENTER, TUCSON, AZ, p. A27
TULANE UNIVERSITY HOSPITAL AND CLINIC, NEW ORLEANS, LA, p. A187
TULARE LOCAL HEALTH CARE DISTRICT, TULARE, CA, p. A65
TULSA REGIONAL MEDICAL CENTER, TULSA, OK, p. A349
TUOLUMNE GENERAL HOSPITAL, SONORA, CA, p. A63
TUOMEY HEALTHCARE SYSTEM, SUMTER, SC, p. A384
TURNING POINT HOSPITAL, MOULTRIE, GA, p. A108
TUSTIN HOSPITAL AND MEDICAL CENTER, TUSTIN, CA, p. A65
TUSTIN REHABILITATION HOSPITAL, TUSTIN, CA, p. A65
TWEETEN HEALTH SERVICES, SPRING GROVE, MN, p. A233
TWIN CITIES COMMUNITY HOSPITAL, TEMPLETON, CA, p. A64
TWIN CITIES HOSPITAL, NICEVILLE, FL, p. A91
TWIN CITY HOSPITAL, DENNISON, OH, p. A331
TWIN COUNTY REGIONAL HOSPITAL, GALAX, VA, p. A444
TWIN FALLS CLINIC AND HOSPITAL, TWIN FALLS, ID, p. A118

Index of Hospitals / Twin Lakes Regional Medical Center

TWIN LAKES REGIONAL MEDICAL CENTER, LEITCHFIELD, KY, p. A174
TWIN RIVERS REGIONAL MEDICAL CENTER, KENNETT, MO, p. A249
TWIN TIERS REHABILITATION CENTER, p. A291
TWIN VALLEY PSYCHIATRIC SYSTEM, DAYTON, OH, p. A331
TWO RIVERS COMMUNITY HOSPITAL AND HAMILTON MEMORIAL HOME, TWO RIVERS, WI, p. A476
TWO RIVERS PSYCHIATRIC HOSPITAL, KANSAS CITY, MO, p. A249
TYLER COUNTY HOSPITAL, WOODVILLE, TX, p. A435
TYLER HEALTHCARE CENTER/AVERA HEALTH, TYLER, MN, p. A234
TYLER HOLMES MEMORIAL HOSPITAL, WINONA, MS, p. A243
TYLER MEMORIAL HOSPITAL, TUNKHANNOCK, PA, p. A373
TYRONE HOSPITAL, TYRONE, PA, p. A373

U

U. S. AIR FORCE ACADEMY HOSPITAL, USAF ACADEMY, CO, p. A73
U. S. AIR FORCE HOSPITAL, HAMPTON, VA, p. A444
U. S. AIR FORCE HOSPITAL, TYNDALL AFB, FL, p. A97
U. S. AIR FORCE HOSPITAL, MACDILL AFB, FL, p. A89
U. S. AIR FORCE HOSPITAL, COLUMBUS, MS, p. A237
U. S. AIR FORCE HOSPITAL, GRAND FORKS AFB, ND, p. A322
U. S. AIR FORCE HOSPITAL, ELLSWORTH AFB, SD, p. A386
U. S. AIR FORCE HOSPITAL, BARKSDALE AFB, LA, p. A180
U. S. AIR FORCE HOSPITAL, ABILENE, TX, p. A401
U. S. AIR FORCE HOSPITAL, HOLLOMAN AFB, NM, p. A285
U. S. AIR FORCE HOSPITAL, CANNON AFB, NM, p. A284
U. S. AIR FORCE HOSPITAL, DAVIS–MONTHAN AFB, AZ, p. A22
U. S. AIR FORCE HOSPITAL, FAIRCHILD AFB, WA, p. A453
U. S. AIR FORCE HOSPITAL, VANDENBERG AFB, CA, p. A66
U. S. AIR FORCE HOSPITAL, EDWARDS AFB, CA, p. A40
U. S. AIR FORCE HOSPITAL ALTUS, ALTUS, OK, p. A341
U. S. AIR FORCE HOSPITAL LUKE, GLENDALE, AZ, p. A23
U. S. AIR FORCE HOSPITAL MOUNTAIN HOME, MOUNTAIN HOME AFB, ID, p. A117
U. S. AIR FORCE HOSPITAL ROBINS, ROBINS AFB, GA, p. A108
U. S. AIR FORCE HOSPITAL SEYMOUR JOHNSON, SEYMOUR JOHNSON AFB, NC, p. A318
U. S. AIR FORCE HOSPITAL SHAW, SHAW A F B, SC, p. A383
U. S. AIR FORCE HOSPITAL–KIRTLAND, KIRTLAND AFB, NM, p. A285
U. S. AIR FORCE MEDICAL CENTER KEESLER, KEESLER AFB, MS, p. A239
U. S. AIR FORCE MEDICAL CENTER WRIGHT–PATTERSON, WRIGHT–PATTERSON AFB, OH, p. A340
U. S. AIR FORCE REGIONAL HOSPITAL, EGLIN AFB, FL, p. A84
U. S. AIR FORCE REGIONAL HOSPITAL, MINOT, ND, p. A323
U. S. AIR FORCE REGIONAL HOSPITAL, ELMENDORF AFB, AK, p. A20
U. S. AIR FORCE REGIONAL HOSPITAL–SHEPPARD, SHEPPARD AFB, TX, p. A430
U. S. MEDICAL CENTER FOR FEDERAL PRISONERS, SPRINGFIELD, MO, p. A254
U. S. NAVAL HOSPITAL, ROOSEVELT ROADS, PR, p. A484
U. S. NAVAL HOSPITAL, AGANA, GU, p. A481
U. S. PENITENTIARY INFIRMARY, LEWISBURG, PA, p. A363
U. S. PUBLIC HEALTH SERVICE BLACKFEET COMMUNITY HOSPITAL, BROWNING, MT, p. A256
U. S. PUBLIC HEALTH SERVICE COMPREHENSIVE INDIAN HEALTH FACILITY, CLAREMORE, OK, p. A342
U. S. PUBLIC HEALTH SERVICE INDIAN HOSPITAL, CHEROKEE, NC, p. A311
U. S. PUBLIC HEALTH SERVICE INDIAN HOSPITAL, CASS LAKE, MN, p. A226
U. S. PUBLIC HEALTH SERVICE INDIAN HOSPITAL, BELCOURT, ND, p. A321
U. S. PUBLIC HEALTH SERVICE INDIAN HOSPITAL, FORT YATES, ND, p. A322
U. S. PUBLIC HEALTH SERVICE INDIAN HOSPITAL, EAGLE BUTTE, SD, p. A385
U. S. PUBLIC HEALTH SERVICE INDIAN HOSPITAL, PINE RIDGE, SD, p. A387
U. S. PUBLIC HEALTH SERVICE INDIAN HOSPITAL, ROSEBUD, SD, p. A387
U. S. PUBLIC HEALTH SERVICE INDIAN HOSPITAL, SISSETON, SD, p. A388
U. S. PUBLIC HEALTH SERVICE INDIAN HOSPITAL, WINNEBAGO, NE, p. A267
U. S. PUBLIC HEALTH SERVICE INDIAN HOSPITAL, CLINTON, OK, p. A342
U. S. PUBLIC HEALTH SERVICE INDIAN HOSPITAL, LAWTON, OK, p. A344
U. S. PUBLIC HEALTH SERVICE INDIAN HOSPITAL, CROW AGENCY, MT, p. A257
U. S. PUBLIC HEALTH SERVICE INDIAN HOSPITAL, HARLEM, MT, p. A258
U. S. PUBLIC HEALTH SERVICE INDIAN HOSPITAL, CROWNPOINT, NM, p. A284
U. S. PUBLIC HEALTH SERVICE INDIAN HOSPITAL, MESCALERO, NM, p. A285
U. S. PUBLIC HEALTH SERVICE INDIAN HOSPITAL, ZUNI, NM, p. A286
U. S. PUBLIC HEALTH SERVICE INDIAN HOSPITAL, PARKER, AZ, p. A23
U. S. PUBLIC HEALTH SERVICE INDIAN HOSPITAL, SELLS, AZ, p. A26
U. S. PUBLIC HEALTH SERVICE INDIAN HOSPITAL, SAN CARLOS, AZ, p. A25
U. S. PUBLIC HEALTH SERVICE INDIAN HOSPITAL, WHITERIVER, AZ, p. A27
U. S. PUBLIC HEALTH SERVICE INDIAN HOSPITAL, WINTERHAVEN, CA, p. A67
U. S. PUBLIC HEALTH SERVICE OWYHEE COMMUNITY HEALTH FACILITY, OWYHEE, NV, p. A269
U. S. PUBLIC HEALTH SERVICE PHOENIX INDIAN MEDICAL CENTER, PHOENIX, AZ, p. A25
U. S. PUBLIC HEALTH SERVICES INDIAN HOSPITAL, KEAMS CANYON, AZ, p. A23
U.S. PUBLIC HEALTH SERVICE INDIAN HOSPITAL, REDLAKE, MN, p. A232
UHHS BEDFORD MEDICAL CENTER, BEDFORD, OH, p. A326
UHHS BROWN MEMORIAL HOSPITAL, CONNEAUT, OH, p. A330
UHHS GEAUGA REGIONAL HOSPITAL, CHARDON, OH, p. A327
UHHS LAURELWOOD HOSPITAL, WILLOUGHBY, OH, p. A339
UHHS RICHMOND HEIGHTS HOSPITAL, RICHMOND HEIGHTS, OH, p. A337
UHHS–MEMORIAL HOSPITAL OF GENEVA, GENEVA, OH, p. A332
UINTAH BASIN MEDICAL CENTER, ROOSEVELT, UT, p. A438
UKIAH VALLEY MEDICAL CENTER, UKIAH, CA, p. A65
UKIAH VALLEY MEDICAL CENTER–DORA STREET, UKIAH, CALIFORNIA, p. A65
UKIAH VALLEY MEDICAL CENTER–HOSPITAL DRIVE, UKIAH, CALIFORNIA, p. A65
UMASS MARLBOROUGH HOSPITAL, MARLBOROUGH, MA, p. A206
UMASS MEMORIAL HEALTH CARE, WORCESTER, MA, p. A210
UNDERWOOD–MEMORIAL HOSPITAL, WOODBURY, NJ, p. A282
UNICOI COUNTY MEMORIAL HOSPITAL, ERWIN, TN, p. A392
UNIMED MEDICAL CENTER, MINOT, ND, p. A323
UNION CITY MEMORIAL HOSPITAL, UNION CITY, PA, p. A373
UNION COUNTY GENERAL HOSPITAL, CLAYTON, NM, p. A284
UNION COUNTY HOSPITAL DISTRICT, ANNA, IL, p. A119
UNION GENERAL HOSPITAL, BLAIRSVILLE, GA, p. A101
UNION GENERAL HOSPITAL, FARMERVILLE, LA, p. A182
UNION HOSPITAL, UNION, NJ, p. A281
UNION HOSPITAL, ELKTON, MD, p. A198
UNION HOSPITAL, DOVER, OH, p. A331
UNION HOSPITAL, TERRE HAUTE, IN, p. A146
UNION HOSPITAL, MAYVILLE, ND, p. A323
UNION HOSPITAL OF THE BRONX, NEW YORK, NEW YORK, p. A300
UNION MEDICAL CENTER, EL DORADO, ARKANSAS, p. A29
UNION MEMORIAL HOSPITAL, BALTIMORE, MD, p. A196
UNION REGIONAL MEDICAL CENTER, MONROE, NC, p. A315
UNIONTOWN HOSPITAL, UNIONTOWN, PA, p. A373
UNITED COMMUNITY HOSPITAL, GROVE CITY, PA, p. A361
UNITED GENERAL HOSPITAL, SEDRO WOOLLEY, WASHINGTON, p. A454
UNITED HEALTH SERVICES HOSPITALS–BINGHAMTON, BINGHAMTON, NY, p. A288
UNITED HOSPITAL, SAINT PAUL, MN, p. A233
UNITED HOSPITAL CENTER, CLARKSBURG, WV, p. A461
UNITED HOSPITAL DISTRICT, BLUE EARTH, MN, p. A226
UNITED MEDICAL CENTER, CHEYENNE, WY, p. A478
UNITED MEMORIAL HEALTH CENTER, GREENVILLE, MI, p. A216
UNITED MEMORIAL MEDICAL CENTER, BATAVIA, NY, p. A287
UNITED MEMORIAL MEDICAL CENTER–BANK STREET, BATAVIA, NEW YORK, p. A287
UNITED MEMORIAL MEDICAL CENTER–NORTH STREET, BATAVIA, NEW YORK, p. A287
UNITED MINE WORKERS OF AMERICA UNION HOSPITAL, WEST FRANKFORT, IL, p. A136
UNITED REGIONAL HEALTH CARE SYSTEM, WICHITA FALLS, TX, p. A435
UNITED REGIONAL HEALTH CARE SYSTEM–EIGHTH STREET CAMPUS, WICHITA FALLS, TEXAS, p. A435
UNITED REGIONAL HEALTH CARE SYSTEM–ELEVENTH STREET CAMPUS, WICHITA FALLS, TEXAS, p. A435
UNITED SAMARITANS MEDICAL CENTER, DANVILLE, ILLINOIS, p. A124
UNITY HOSPITAL, FRIDLEY, MN, p. A228
UNITY HOSPITAL, MUSCATINE, IA, p. A154
UNITY MEDICAL CENTER, GRAFTON, ND, p. A322
UNIVERSITY OF COLORADO HOSPITAL, DENVER, CO, p. A70
UNIVERSITY BEHAVIORAL CENTER, ORLANDO, FL, p. A92
UNIVERSITY CAMPUS, WORCESTER, MASSACHUSETTS, p. A210
UNIVERSITY CAMPUS, NEW ORLEANS, LOUISIANA, p. A186
UNIVERSITY COMMUNITY HOSPITAL, TAMPA, FL, p. A96
UNIVERSITY COMMUNITY HOSPITAL–CARROLLWOOD, TAMPA, FL, p. A96
UNIVERSITY HEALTH CARE SYSTEM, AUGUSTA, GA, p. A101
UNIVERSITY HEALTH CENTER – DOWNTOWN, SAN ANTONIO, TEXAS, p. A430
UNIVERSITY HEALTH PARTNERS, OKLAHOMA CITY, OK, p. A346
UNIVERSITY HEALTH SERVICES, AMHERST, MA, p. A201
UNIVERSITY HEALTH SYSTEM, SAN ANTONIO, TX, p. A430
UNIVERSITY HOSPITAL, SAN JUAN, PR, p. A484
UNIVERSITY HOSPITAL, STONY BROOK, NY, p. A305
UNIVERSITY HOSPITAL, CHARLOTTE, NC, p. A311
UNIVERSITY HOSPITAL, CINCINNATI, OH, p. A328
UNIVERSITY HOSPITAL, OKLAHOMA CITY, OKLAHOMA, p. A346
UNIVERSITY HOSPITAL, SAN ANTONIO, TEXAS, p. A430
UNIVERSITY HOSPITAL, ALBUQUERQUE, NM, p. A284
UNIVERSITY HOSPITAL AND MEDICAL CENTER, TAMARAC, FL, p. A96
UNIVERSITY HOSPITAL OF ARKANSAS, LITTLE ROCK, AR, p. A32
UNIVERSITY HOSPITAL OF BROOKLYN–STATE UNIVERSITY OF NEW YORK HEALTH SCIENCE CENTER AT BROOKLYN, NEW YORK, NY, p. A300
UNIVERSITY HOSPITAL SCHOOL, IOWA CITY, IOWA, p. A153
UNIVERSITY HOSPITAL–SUNY HEALTH SCIENCE CENTER AT SYRACUSE, SYRACUSE, NY, p. A306
UNIVERSITY HOSPITALS AND CLINICS, COLUMBIA, MO, p. A246
UNIVERSITY HOSPITALS AND CLINICS – HOLMES COUNTY, LEXINGTON, MS, p. A240
UNIVERSITY HOSPITALS AND CLINICS OF HOLMES COUNTY–DURANT, DURANT, MS, p. A237
UNIVERSITY HOSPITALS AND CLINICS, UNIVERSITY OF MISSISSIPPI MEDICAL CENTER, JACKSON, MS, p. A239
UNIVERSITY HOSPITALS OF CLEVELAND, CLEVELAND, OH, p. A329
UNIVERSITY MEDICAL CENTER, LAFAYETTE, LA, p. A184
UNIVERSITY MEDICAL CENTER, LUBBOCK, TX, p. A422
UNIVERSITY MEDICAL CENTER, TUCSON, AZ, p. A27
UNIVERSITY MEDICAL CENTER, LAS VEGAS, NV, p. A268
UNIVERSITY MEDICAL CENTER, FRESNO, CA, p. A42
UNIVERSITY MEDICAL CENTER–MESABI, HIBBING, MN, p. A229
UNIVERSITY MEDICAL CENTER/MCFARLAND HOSPITAL, LEBANON, TN, p. A395
UNIVERSITY OF ALABAMA HOSPITAL, BIRMINGHAM, AL, p. A12
UNIVERSITY OF CALIFORNIA LOS ANGELES MEDICAL CENTER, LOS ANGELES, CA, p. A50
UNIVERSITY OF CALIFORNIA LOS ANGELES NEUROPSYCHIATRIC HOSPITAL, LOS ANGELES, CA, p. A50
UNIVERSITY OF CALIFORNIA SAN DIEGO MEDICAL CENTER, SAN DIEGO, CA, p. A59
UNIVERSITY OF CALIFORNIA SAN FRANCISCO MEDICAL CENTER, SAN FRANCISCO, CA, p. A60
UNIVERSITY OF CALIFORNIA, DAVIS MEDICAL CENTER, SACRAMENTO, CA, p. A58
UNIVERSITY OF CALIFORNIA, IRVINE MEDICAL CENTER, ORANGE, CA, p. A54
UNIVERSITY OF CALIFORNIA–SAN FRANCISCO MOUNT ZION MEDICAL CENTER, SAN FRANCISCO, CALIFORNIA, p. A60
UNIVERSITY OF CHICAGO HOSPITALS, CHICAGO, IL, p. A124
UNIVERSITY OF CONNECTICUT HEALTH CENTER, JOHN DEMPSEY HOSPITAL, FARMINGTON, CT, p. A74
UNIVERSITY OF ILLINOIS AT CHICAGO MEDICAL CENTER, CHICAGO, IL, p. A124
UNIVERSITY OF IOWA HOSPITALS AND CLINICS, IOWA CITY, IA, p. A153
UNIVERSITY OF KANSAS MEDICAL CENTER, KANSAS CITY, KS, p. A163
UNIVERSITY OF KENTUCKY HOSPITAL, LEXINGTON, KY, p. A174
UNIVERSITY OF LOUISVILLE HOSPITAL, LOUISVILLE, KY, p. A176
UNIVERSITY OF MARYLAND MEDICAL CENTER, BALTIMORE, MD, p. A196
UNIVERSITY OF MEDICINE AND DENTISTRY OF NEW JERSEY, UNIVERSITY BEHAVIORAL HEALTHCARE, PISCATAWAY, NJ, p. A279
UNIVERSITY OF MEDICINE AND DENTISTRY OF NEW JERSEY–UNIVERSITY HOSPITAL, NEWARK, NJ, p. A278
UNIVERSITY OF MIAMI HOSPITAL AND CLINICS, MIAMI, FL, p. A90
UNIVERSITY OF MICHIGAN HOSPITALS AND HEALTH CENTERS, ANN ARBOR, MI, p. A211
UNIVERSITY OF MINNESOTA HOSPITAL AND CLINIC, MINNEAPOLIS, MINNESOTA, p. A230

Index of Hospitals / Veterans Affairs Medical Center

UNIVERSITY OF NEW MEXICO CHILDREN'S PSYCHIATRIC HOSPITAL, ALBUQUERQUE, NM, p. A284
UNIVERSITY OF NORTH CAROLINA HOSPITALS, CHAPEL HILL, NC, p. A310
UNIVERSITY OF SOUTH ALABAMA KNOLLWOOD PARK HOSPITAL, MOBILE, AL, p. A16
UNIVERSITY OF SOUTH ALABAMA MEDICAL CENTER, MOBILE, AL, p. A16
UNIVERSITY OF SOUTHERN CALIFORNIA–KENNETH NORRIS JR. CANCER HOSPITAL, LOS ANGELES, CA, p. A50
UNIVERSITY OF TENNESSEE BOWLD HOSPITAL, MEMPHIS, TN, p. A397
UNIVERSITY OF TENNESSEE MEMORIAL HOSPITAL, KNOXVILLE, TN, p. A395
UNIVERSITY OF TEXAS HEALTH CENTER AT TYLER, TYLER, TX, p. A433
UNIVERSITY OF TEXAS M. D. ANDERSON CANCER CENTER, HOUSTON, TX, p. A418
UNIVERSITY OF TEXAS MEDICAL BRANCH HOSPITALS, GALVESTON, TX, p. A413
UNIVERSITY OF UTAH HOSPITALS AND CLINICS, SALT LAKE CITY, UT, p. A438
UNIVERSITY OF UTAH NEUROPSYCHIATRIC INSTITUTE, SALT LAKE CITY, UT, p. A438
UNIVERSITY OF VIRGINIA MEDICAL CENTER, CHARLOTTESVILLE, VA, p. A443
UNIVERSITY OF WASHINGTON MEDICAL CENTER, SEATTLE, WA, p. A457
UNIVERSITY OF WISCONSIN CHILDREN'S HOSPITAL, p. A470
UNIVERSITY OF WISCONSIN HOSPITAL AND CLINICS, MADISON, WI, p. A470
UNIVERSITY PAVILION, TAMARAC, FLORIDA, p. A96
UNIVERSITY PEDIATRIC HOSPITAL, SAN JUAN, PR, p. A484
UPMC BEAVER VALLEY, ALIQUIPPA, PA, p. A355
UPMC BEDFORD MEMORIAL, EVERETT, PA, p. A360
UPMC BRADDOCK, BRADDOCK, PA, p. A356
UPMC HORIZON, GREENVILLE, PA, p. A361
UPMC LEE REGIONAL, JOHNSTOWN, PA, p. A362
UPMC MCKEESPORT, MCKEESPORT, PA, p. A364
UPMC PASSAVANT, PITTSBURGH, PA, p. A370
UPMC PRESBYTERIAN, PITTSBURGH, PA, p. A370
UPMC PRESBYTERIAN HOSPITAL, PITTSBURGH, PENNSYLVANIA, p. A370
UPMC SHADYSIDE, PITTSBURGH, PA, p. A370
UPMC SOUTH SIDE, PITTSBURGH, PA, p. A370
UPMC ST. MARGARET, PITTSBURGH, PA, p. A370
UPPER CONNECTICUT VALLEY HOSPITAL, COLEBROOK, NH, p. A271
UPPER SHORE COMMUNITY MENTAL HEALTH CENTER, CHESTERTOWN, MD, p. A197
UPPER VALLEY MEDICAL CENTER, TROY, OH, p. A338
UPSON REGIONAL MEDICAL CENTER, THOMASTON, GA, p. A110
UPSTATE CAROLINA MEDICAL CENTER, GAFFNEY, SC, p. A381
USA CHILDREN'S AND WOMEN'S HOSPITAL, MOBILE, AL, p. A16
USC UNIVERSITY HOSPITAL, LOS ANGELES, CA, p. A50
UTAH STATE HOSPITAL, PROVO, UT, p. A438
UTAH VALLEY REGIONAL MEDICAL CENTER, PROVO, UT, p. A438
UVALDE COUNTY HOSPITAL AUTHORITY, UVALDE, TX, p. A433

V

VA GULF COAST VETERANS HEALTH CARE SYSTEM, BILOXI, MS, p. A236
VACAVALLEY HOSPITAL, VACAVILLE, CA, p. A66
VAIL VALLEY MEDICAL CENTER, VAIL, CO, p. A73
VAL VERDE REGIONAL MEDICAL CENTER, DEL RIO, TX, p. A410
VALDESE GENERAL HOSPITAL, VALDESE, NC, p. A319
VALDEZ COMMUNITY HOSPITAL, VALDEZ, AK, p. A21
VALLEY BAPTIST MEDICAL CENTER, HARLINGEN, TX, p. A415
VALLEY BEHAVIORAL HEALTH SYSTEM, CHATTANOOGA, TENNESSEE, p. A391
VALLEY CHILDREN'S HOSPITAL, MADERA, CA, p. A50
VALLEY COMMUNITY HOSPITAL, DALLAS, OR, p. A350
VALLEY COUNTY HOSPITAL, ORD, NE, p. A266
VALLEY FORGE MEDICAL CENTER AND HOSPITAL, NORRISTOWN, PA, p. A365
VALLEY GENERAL HOSPITAL, MONROE, WA, p. A454
VALLEY HOSPITAL, RIDGEWOOD, NJ, p. A280
VALLEY HOSPITAL, PALMER, AK, p. A21
VALLEY HOSPITAL AND MEDICAL CENTER, SPOKANE, WA, p. A457
VALLEY HOSPITAL MEDICAL CENTER, LAS VEGAS, NV, p. A268
VALLEY LUTHERAN HOSPITAL, MESA, AZ, p. A23
VALLEY MEDICAL CENTER, RENTON, WA, p. A456
VALLEY MEDICAL FACILITIES, SEWICKLEY, PA, p. A372
VALLEY PRESBYTERIAN HOSPITAL, LOS ANGELES, CA, p. A50
VALLEY REGIONAL HOSPITAL, CLAREMONT, NH, p. A271
VALLEY REGIONAL MEDICAL CENTER, BROWNSVILLE, TX, p. A405
VALLEY VIEW HOSPITAL, GLENWOOD SPRINGS, CO, p. A70
VALLEY VIEW MEDICAL CENTER, PLYMOUTH, WI, p. A474
VALLEY VIEW MEDICAL CENTER, CEDAR CITY, UT, p. A436
VALLEY VIEW REGIONAL HOSPITAL, ADA, OK, p. A341
VALLEY WEST COMMUNITY HOSPITAL, SANDWICH, IL, p. A134
VALLEYCARE MEDICAL CENTER, PLEASANTON, CA, p. A55
VALLEYCARE MEMORIAL HOSPITAL, LIVERMORE, CA, p. A46
VALUEMARK WEST END BEHAVIORAL HEALTHCARE SYSTEM, RICHMOND, VA, p. A449
VAN BUREN COUNTY HOSPITAL, KEOSAUQUA, IA, p. A153
VAN NUYS HOSPITAL, LOS ANGELES, CA, p. A50
VAN WERT COUNTY HOSPITAL, VAN WERT, OH, p. A338
VANCOUVER MEMORIAL CAMPUS, VANCOUVER, WASHINGTON, p. A458
VANDERBILT UNIVERSITY HOSPITAL, NASHVILLE, TN, p. A398
VASSAR BROTHERS HOSPITAL, POUGHKEEPSIE, NY, p. A303
VAUGHAN REGIONAL MEDICAL CENTER, SELMA, AL, p. A18
VENCOR ARLINGTON, TEXAS, ARLINGTON, TX, p. A402
VENCOR HOSPITAL – ALBUQUERQUE, ALBUQUERQUE, NM, p. A284
VENCOR HOSPITAL – CENTRAL TAMPA, TAMPA, FL, p. A97
VENCOR HOSPITAL – DALLAS, DALLAS, TX, p. A410
VENCOR HOSPITAL – FORT WORTH WEST, FORT WORTH, TEXAS, p. A423
VENCOR HOSPITAL – NEW ORLEANS, NEW ORLEANS, LA, p. A187
VENCOR HOSPITAL – TUCSON, TUCSON, AZ, p. A27
VENCOR HOSPITAL NORTH SHORE, PEABODY, MA, p. A207
VENCOR HOSPITAL SEATTLE, SEATTLE, WA, p. A457
VENCOR HOSPITAL–ATLANTA, ATLANTA, GA, p. A100
VENCOR HOSPITAL–BOSTON, BOSTON, MA, p. A203
VENCOR HOSPITAL–BREA, BREA, CA, p. A37
VENCOR HOSPITAL–CHATTANOOGA, CHATTANOOGA, TN, p. A391
VENCOR HOSPITAL–CHICAGO CENTRAL, CHICAGO, IL, p. A124
VENCOR HOSPITAL–CHICAGO NORTH, CHICAGO, IL, p. A124
VENCOR HOSPITAL–CORAL GABLES, CORAL GABLES, FL, p. A83
VENCOR HOSPITAL–FORT LAUDERDALE, FORT LAUDERDALE, FL, p. A84
VENCOR HOSPITAL–FORT WORTH SOUTHWEST, FORT WORTH, TX, p. A413
VENCOR HOSPITAL–GREENSBORO, GREENSBORO, NC, p. A313
VENCOR HOSPITAL–HOUSTON, HOUSTON, TX, p. A418
VENCOR HOSPITAL–KANSAS CITY, KANSAS CITY, MO, p. A249
VENCOR HOSPITAL–LAGRANGE, LAGRANGE, IN, p. A143
VENCOR HOSPITAL–LAS VEGAS, LAS VEGAS, NV, p. A269
VENCOR HOSPITAL–LOS ANGELES, LOS ANGELES, CA, p. A50
VENCOR HOSPITAL–LOUISVILLE, LOUISVILLE, KY, p. A176
VENCOR HOSPITAL–MANSFIELD, MANSFIELD, TX, p. A423
VENCOR HOSPITAL–METRO DETROIT, DETROIT, MI, p. A214
VENCOR HOSPITAL–MILWAUKEE, GREENFIELD, WI, p. A469
VENCOR HOSPITAL–MILWAUKEE, MILWAUKEE, WI, p. A472
VENCOR HOSPITAL–MINNEAPOLIS, GOLDEN VALLEY, MN, p. A228
VENCOR HOSPITAL–ONTARIO, ONTARIO, CA, p. A54
VENCOR HOSPITAL–PHILADELPHIA, PHILADELPHIA, PA, p. A368
VENCOR HOSPITAL–PHOENIX, PHOENIX, AZ, p. A25
VENCOR HOSPITAL–PITTSBURGH, OAKDALE, PA, p. A365
VENCOR HOSPITAL–SACRAMENTO, FOLSOM, CA, p. A41
VENCOR HOSPITAL–SAN DIEGO, SAN DIEGO, CA, p. A59
VENCOR HOSPITAL–SAN LEANDRO, SAN LEANDRO, CA, p. A61
VENCOR HOSPITAL–ST PETERSBURG, SAINT PETERSBURG, FL, p. A94
VENCOR HOSPITAL–SYCAMORE, SYCAMORE, IL, p. A135
VENCOR HOSPITAL–TAMPA, TAMPA, FL, p. A97
VENCOR–NORTH FLORIDA, GREEN COVE SPRINGS, FL, p. A85
VENTURA COUNTY MEDICAL CENTER, VENTURA, CA, p. A66
VERDE VALLEY MEDICAL CENTER, COTTONWOOD, AZ, p. A22
VERDUGO HILLS HOSPITAL, GLENDALE, CA, p. A43
VERMILION HOSPITAL FOR PSYCHIATRIC AND ADDICTIVE MEDICINE, LAFAYETTE, LA, p. A184
VERMONT STATE HOSPITAL, WATERBURY, VT, p. A441
VERNON MEMORIAL HOSPITAL, VIROQUA, WI, p. A476
VETERAN AFFAIRS HUDSON VALLEY HEALTH CARE SYSTEM–CASTLE POINT DIVISION, CASTLE POINT, NEW YORK, p. A294
VETERANS ADMINISTRATION NEW YORK HARBOR HEALTHCARE SYSTEM, NEW YORK, NY, p. A300
VETERANS AFFAIRS BLACK HILLS HEALTH CARE SYSTEM, FORT MEADE, SD, p. A386
VETERANS AFFAIRS BOSTON HEALTHCARE SYSTEM, BOSTON, MA, p. A203
VETERANS AFFAIRS CENTRAL IOWA HEALTH CARE SYSTEM, DES MOINES, IA, p. A151
VETERANS AFFAIRS CHICAGO HEALTH CARE SYSTEM, CHICAGO, IL, p. A124
VETERANS AFFAIRS CHICAGO HEALTH CARE SYSTEM, CHICAGO, ILLINOIS, p. A124
VETERANS AFFAIRS CHICAGO HEALTH CARE SYSTEM, CHICAGO, ILLINOIS, p. A124
VETERANS AFFAIRS CONNECTICUT HEALTHCARE SYSTEM–WEST HAVEN DIVISION, NEW HAVEN, CT, p. A76
VETERANS AFFAIRS EASTERN KANSAS HEALTH CARE SYSTEM, TOPEKA, KS, p. A168
VETERANS AFFAIRS EDWARD HINES, JR. HOSPITAL, HINES, IL, p. A128
VETERANS AFFAIRS GREATER NEBRASKA HEALTH CARE SYSTEM, LINCOLN, NE, p. A264
VETERANS AFFAIRS HEALTH CARE SYSTEM–TUSKEGEE DIVISION, TUSKEGEE, ALABAMA, p. A17
VETERANS AFFAIRS HUDSON VALLEY HEALTH CARE SYSTEM–F.D. ROOSEVELT HOSPITAL, MONTROSE, NY, p. A294
VETERANS AFFAIRS HUDSON VALLEY HEALTH CARE SYSTEM–MONTROSE DIVISION, MONTROSE, NEW YORK, p. A294
VETERANS AFFAIRS MARYLAND HEALTH CARE SYSTEM–BALTIMORE DIVISION, BALTIMORE, MD, p. A196
VETERANS AFFAIRS MARYLAND HEALTH CARE SYSTEM–FORT HOWARD DIVISION, FORT HOWARD, MD, p. A198
VETERANS AFFAIRS MARYLAND HEALTH CARE SYSTEM–PERRY POINT DIVISION, PERRY POINT, MD, p. A199
VETERANS AFFAIRS MEDICAL AND REGIONAL OFFICE CENTER, FARGO, ND, p. A322
VETERANS AFFAIRS MEDICAL AND REGIONAL OFFICE CENTER, WICHITA, KS, p. A169
VETERANS AFFAIRS MEDICAL CENTER, SAN JUAN, PR, p. A484
VETERANS AFFAIRS MEDICAL CENTER, TOGUS, ME, p. A194
VETERANS AFFAIRS MEDICAL CENTER, MANCHESTER, NH, p. A272
VETERANS AFFAIRS MEDICAL CENTER, WHITE RIVER JUNCTION, VT, p. A441
VETERANS AFFAIRS MEDICAL CENTER, LEEDS, MA, p. A205
VETERANS AFFAIRS MEDICAL CENTER, PROVIDENCE, RI, p. A377
VETERANS AFFAIRS MEDICAL CENTER, NEW YORK, NEW YORK, p. A300
VETERANS AFFAIRS MEDICAL CENTER, NEW YORK, NEW YORK, p. A300
VETERANS AFFAIRS MEDICAL CENTER, ALBANY, NY, p. A287
VETERANS AFFAIRS MEDICAL CENTER, BATH, NY, p. A288
VETERANS AFFAIRS MEDICAL CENTER, CANANDAIGUA, NY, p. A290
VETERANS AFFAIRS MEDICAL CENTER, NEW YORK, NY, p. A300
VETERANS AFFAIRS MEDICAL CENTER, NORTHPORT, NY, p. A301
VETERANS AFFAIRS MEDICAL CENTER, SYRACUSE, NY, p. A306
VETERANS AFFAIRS MEDICAL CENTER, PITTSBURGH, PENNSYLVANIA, p. A370
VETERANS AFFAIRS MEDICAL CENTER, PITTSBURGH, PENNSYLVANIA, p. A370
VETERANS AFFAIRS MEDICAL CENTER, BUTLER, PA, p. A357
VETERANS AFFAIRS MEDICAL CENTER, COATESVILLE, PA, p. A358
VETERANS AFFAIRS MEDICAL CENTER, ERIE, PA, p. A360
VETERANS AFFAIRS MEDICAL CENTER, LEBANON, PA, p. A363
VETERANS AFFAIRS MEDICAL CENTER, PHILADELPHIA, PA, p. A368
VETERANS AFFAIRS MEDICAL CENTER, WILKES–BARRE, PA, p. A374
VETERANS AFFAIRS MEDICAL CENTER, WILMINGTON, DE, p. A78
VETERANS AFFAIRS MEDICAL CENTER, WASHINGTON, DC, p. A80
VETERANS AFFAIRS MEDICAL CENTER, HAMPTON, VA, p. A445
VETERANS AFFAIRS MEDICAL CENTER, SALEM, VA, p. A449
VETERANS AFFAIRS MEDICAL CENTER, BECKLEY, WV, p. A460
VETERANS AFFAIRS MEDICAL CENTER, HUNTINGTON, WV, p. A462
VETERANS AFFAIRS MEDICAL CENTER, MARTINSBURG, WV, p. A462
VETERANS AFFAIRS MEDICAL CENTER, DURHAM, NC, p. A312
VETERANS AFFAIRS MEDICAL CENTER, FAYETTEVILLE, NC, p. A313
VETERANS AFFAIRS MEDICAL CENTER, ASHEVILLE, NC, p. A309
VETERANS AFFAIRS MEDICAL CENTER, SALISBURY, NC, p. A317
VETERANS AFFAIRS MEDICAL CENTER, DECATUR, GA, p. A104
VETERANS AFFAIRS MEDICAL CENTER, AUGUSTA, GA, p. A101
VETERANS AFFAIRS MEDICAL CENTER, DUBLIN, GA, p. A104
VETERANS AFFAIRS MEDICAL CENTER, BAY PINES, FL, p. A81

© 2000 AHA Guide

Index of Hospitals / Veterans Affairs Medical Center

VETERANS AFFAIRS MEDICAL CENTER, WEST PALM BEACH, FL, p. A98
VETERANS AFFAIRS MEDICAL CENTER, MIAMI, FL, p. A90
VETERANS AFFAIRS MEDICAL CENTER, LAKE CITY, FL, p. A88
VETERANS AFFAIRS MEDICAL CENTER, CLEVELAND, OH, p. A329
VETERANS AFFAIRS MEDICAL CENTER, CHILLICOTHE, OH, p. A327
VETERANS AFFAIRS MEDICAL CENTER, CINCINNATI, OH, p. A328
VETERANS AFFAIRS MEDICAL CENTER, DAYTON, OH, p. A331
VETERANS AFFAIRS MEDICAL CENTER, DANVILLE, IL, p. A124
VETERANS AFFAIRS MEDICAL CENTER, NORTH CHICAGO, IL, p. A131
VETERANS AFFAIRS MEDICAL CENTER, MARION, IL, p. A130
VETERANS AFFAIRS MEDICAL CENTER, ANN ARBOR, MI, p. A211
VETERANS AFFAIRS MEDICAL CENTER, BATTLE CREEK, MI, p. A212
VETERANS AFFAIRS MEDICAL CENTER, IRON MOUNTAIN, MI, p. A217
VETERANS AFFAIRS MEDICAL CENTER, TOMAH, WI, p. A476
VETERANS AFFAIRS MEDICAL CENTER, MEMPHIS, TN, p. A397
VETERANS AFFAIRS MEDICAL CENTER, NASHVILLE, TN, p. A398
VETERANS AFFAIRS MEDICAL CENTER, BIRMINGHAM, AL, p. A12
VETERANS AFFAIRS MEDICAL CENTER, TUSCALOOSA, AL, p. A19
VETERANS AFFAIRS MEDICAL CENTER, MINNEAPOLIS, MN, p. A231
VETERANS AFFAIRS MEDICAL CENTER, SAINT CLOUD, MN, p. A232
VETERANS AFFAIRS MEDICAL CENTER, IOWA CITY, IA, p. A153
VETERANS AFFAIRS MEDICAL CENTER, SAINT LOUIS, MO, p. A254
VETERANS AFFAIRS MEDICAL CENTER, KANSAS CITY, MO, p. A249
VETERANS AFFAIRS MEDICAL CENTER, HOT SPRINGS, SOUTH DAKOTA, p. A386
VETERANS AFFAIRS MEDICAL CENTER, OMAHA, NE, p. A266
VETERANS AFFAIRS MEDICAL CENTER, FAYETTEVILLE, AR, p. A29
VETERANS AFFAIRS MEDICAL CENTER, ALEXANDRIA, LA, p. A180
VETERANS AFFAIRS MEDICAL CENTER, NEW ORLEANS, LA, p. A187
VETERANS AFFAIRS MEDICAL CENTER, MUSKOGEE, OK, p. A345
VETERANS AFFAIRS MEDICAL CENTER, OKLAHOMA CITY, OK, p. A346
VETERANS AFFAIRS MEDICAL CENTER, AMARILLO, TX, p. A401
VETERANS AFFAIRS MEDICAL CENTER, BIG SPRING, TX, p. A405
VETERANS AFFAIRS MEDICAL CENTER, HOUSTON, TX, p. A418
VETERANS AFFAIRS MEDICAL CENTER, BOISE, ID, p. A115
VETERANS AFFAIRS MEDICAL CENTER, CHEYENNE, WY, p. A478
VETERANS AFFAIRS MEDICAL CENTER, SHERIDAN, WY, p. A479
VETERANS AFFAIRS MEDICAL CENTER, DENVER, CO, p. A70
VETERANS AFFAIRS MEDICAL CENTER, GRAND JUNCTION, CO, p. A71
VETERANS AFFAIRS MEDICAL CENTER, ALBUQUERQUE, NM, p. A284
VETERANS AFFAIRS MEDICAL CENTER, SALT LAKE CITY, UT, p. A438
VETERANS AFFAIRS MEDICAL CENTER, SPOKANE, WA, p. A457
VETERANS AFFAIRS MEDICAL CENTER, PORTLAND, OR, p. A353
VETERANS AFFAIRS MEDICAL CENTER, FRESNO, CA, p. A42
VETERANS AFFAIRS MEDICAL CENTER, LONG BEACH, CA, p. A47
VETERANS AFFAIRS MEDICAL CENTER, SAN DIEGO, CA, p. A59
VETERANS AFFAIRS MEDICAL CENTER, SAN FRANCISCO, CA, p. A60
VETERANS AFFAIRS MEDICAL CENTER, GULFPORT DIVISION, GULFPORT, MISSISSIPPI, p. A236
VETERANS AFFAIRS MEDICAL CENTER–LEXINGTON, LEXINGTON, KY, p. A174
VETERANS AFFAIRS MEDICAL CENTER–LOUISVILLE, LOUISVILLE, KY, p. A176
VETERANS AFFAIRS MEDICAL CENTER–WEST LOS ANGELES, LOS ANGELES, CA, p. A50
VETERANS AFFAIRS MONTANA HEALTHCARE SYSTEM, FORT HARRISON, MT, p. A257
VETERANS AFFAIRS NEW JERSEY HEALTH CARE SYSTEM, EAST ORANGE, NJ, p. A275
VETERANS AFFAIRS NORTH TEXAS HEALTH CARE SYSTEM, DALLAS, TX, p. A410
VETERANS AFFAIRS NORTHERN INDIANA HEALTH CARE SYSTEM, FORT WAYNE, IN, p. A140
VETERANS AFFAIRS NORTHERN INDIANA HEALTH CARE SYSTEM–MARION CAMPUS, MARION, INDIANA, p. A140
VETERANS AFFAIRS PALO ALTO HEALTH CARE SYSTEM, PALO ALTO, CA, p. A54
VETERANS AFFAIRS PALO ALTO HEALTH CARE SYSTEM, LIVERMORE DIVISION, LIVERMORE, CALIFORNIA, p. A54
VETERANS AFFAIRS PITTSBURGH HEALTHCARE SYSTEM, PITTSBURGH, PA, p. A370
VETERANS AFFAIRS PUGET SOUND HEALTH CARE SYSTEM, SEATTLE, WA, p. A457
VETERANS AFFAIRS PUGET SOUND HEALTH CARE SYSTEM–AMERICAN LAKE DIVISION, TACOMA, WASHINGTON, p. A457
VETERANS AFFAIRS ROSEBURG HEALTHCARE SYSTEM, ROSEBURG, OR, p. A354
VETERANS AFFAIRS SIERRA NEVADA HEALTH CARE SYSTEM, RENO, NV, p. A269
VETERANS AFFAIRS SOUTHERN NEVADA HEALTHCARE SYSTEM, LAS VEGAS, NV, p. A269
VETERANS AFFAIRS WESTERN NEW YORK HEALTHCARE SYSTEM–BATAVIA DIVISION, BATAVIA, NY, p. A288
VETERANS AFFAIRS WESTERN NEW YORK HEALTHCARE SYSTEM–BUFFALO DIVISION, BUFFALO, NY, p. A289
VETERANS HOME AND HOSPITAL, ROCKY HILL, CT, p. A76
VETERANS HOME OF CALIFORNIA, YOUNTVILLE, CA, p. A67
VETERANS MEMORIAL HOSPITAL, WAUKON, IA, p. A157
VETERANS MEMORIAL HOSPITAL OF MEIGS COUNTY, POMEROY, OH, p. A336
VIA CHRISTI REGIONAL MEDICAL CENTER, WICHITA, KS, p. A169
VIA CHRISTI REHABILITATION CENTER, WICHITA, KS, p. A169
VIAHEALTH OF WAYNE, NEWARK, NY, p. A301
VICKSBURG MEDICAL CENTER, VICKSBURG, MS, p. A242
VICTOR VALLEY COMMUNITY HOSPITAL, VICTORVILLE, CA, p. A66
VICTORY MEDICAL CENTER, STANLEY, WI, p. A475
VICTORY MEMORIAL HOSPITAL, NEW YORK, NY, p. A300
VICTORY MEMORIAL HOSPITAL, WAUKEGAN, IL, p. A136
VILLA FELICIANA MEDICAL COMPLEX, JACKSON, LA, p. A183
VILLA MARIA HOSPITAL, NORTH MIAMI, FL, p. A91
VILLAVIEW COMMUNITY HOSPITAL, SAN DIEGO, CA, p. A59
VILLE PLATTE MEDICAL CENTER, VILLE PLATTE, LA, p. A189
VINELAND DEVELOPMENTAL CENTER HOSPITAL, VINELAND, NJ, p. A281
VIRGINIA BAPTIST HOSPITAL, LYNCHBURG, VA, p. A446
VIRGINIA GAY HOSPITAL, VINTON, IA, p. A157
VIRGINIA MASON MEDICAL CENTER, SEATTLE, WA, p. A457
VIRGINIA REGIONAL MEDICAL CENTER, VIRGINIA, MN, p. A234
VIRRUA WEST JERSEY HOSPITAL–MARLTON, MARLTON, NJ, p. A277
VIRTUA MEMORIAL HOSPITAL BURLINGTON COUNTY, MOUNT HOLLY, NJ, p. A278
VIRTUA WEST JERSEY HOSPITAL–BERLIN, BERLIN, NJ, p. A274
VIRTUA WEST JERSEY HOSPITAL–CAMDEN, CAMDEN, NJ, p. A275
VIRTUA WEST JERSEY HOSPITAL–VOORHEES, VOORHEES, NJ, p. A281
VIRTUE STREET MEDICAL PAVILION, CHALMETTE, LOUISIANA, p. A181

W

W. A. FOOTE MEMORIAL HOSPITAL, JACKSON, MI, p. A217
W. J. BARGE MEMORIAL HOSPITAL, GREENVILLE, SC, p. A381
W. J. MANGOLD MEMORIAL HOSPITAL, LOCKNEY, TX, p. A422
WABASH COUNTY HOSPITAL, WABASH, IN, p. A146
WABASH GENERAL HOSPITAL DISTRICT, MOUNT CARMEL, IL, p. A131
WABASH VALLEY HOSPITAL, WEST LAFAYETTE, IN, p. A147
WADLEY REGIONAL MEDICAL CENTER, TEXARKANA, TX, p. A432
WADSWORTH–RITTMAN HOSPITAL, WADSWORTH, OH, p. A338
WAGNER COMMUNITY MEMORIAL HOSPITAL, WAGNER, SD, p. A388
WAGNER GENERAL HOSPITAL, PALACIOS, TX, p. A425
WAGONER COMMUNITY HOSPITAL, WAGONER, OK, p. A349
WAHIAWA GENERAL HOSPITAL, WAHIAWA, HI, p. A113
WAKE COUNTY ALCOHOLISM TREATMENT CENTER, RALEIGH, NC, p. A317
WAKE MEDICAL CENTER, RALEIGH, NC, p. A317
WALBRIDGE MEMORIAL CONVALESCENT WING, p. A72
WALDO COUNTY GENERAL HOSPITAL, BELFAST, ME, p. A191
WALKER BAPTIST MEDICAL CENTER, JASPER, AL, p. A16
WALLA WALLA GENERAL HOSPITAL, WALLA WALLA, WA, p. A459
WALLACE THOMSON HOSPITAL, UNION, SC, p. A384
WALLOWA MEMORIAL HOSPITAL, ENTERPRISE, OR, p. A350
WALLS REGIONAL HOSPITAL, CLEBURNE, TX, p. A406
WALTER B. JONES ALCOHOL AND DRUG ABUSE TREATMENT CENTER, GREENVILLE, NC, p. A314
WALTER KNOX MEMORIAL HOSPITAL, EMMETT, ID, p. A116
WALTER O. BOSWELL MEMORIAL HOSPITAL, SUN CITY, AZ, p. A26
WALTER OLIN MOSS REGIONAL MEDICAL CENTER, LAKE CHARLES, LA, p. A184
WALTER P. REUTHER PSYCHIATRIC HOSPITAL, WESTLAND, MI, p. A224
WALTER REED ARMY MEDICAL CENTER, WASHINGTON, DC, p. A80
WALTHALL COUNTY GENERAL HOSPITAL, TYLERTOWN, MS, p. A242
WALTON MEDICAL CENTER, MONROE, GA, p. A107
WALTON REHABILITATION HOSPITAL, AUGUSTA, GA, p. A101
WAMEGO CITY HOSPITAL, WAMEGO, KS, p. A169
WARD MEMORIAL HOSPITAL, MONAHANS, TX, p. A424
WARM SPRINGS REHABILITATION HOSPITAL, GONZALES, TX, p. A414
WARM SPRINGS REHABILITATION HOSPITAL, SAN ANTONIO, TX, p. A430
WARMINSTER HOSPITAL, WARMINSTER, PA, p. A373
WARNER BROWN HOSPITAL, EL DORADO, ARKANSAS, p. A29
WARRACK MEDICAL CENTER HOSPITAL, SANTA ROSA, CA, p. A63
WARREN G. MAGNUSON CLINICAL CENTER, NATIONAL INSTITUTES OF HEALTH, BETHESDA, MD, p. A197
WARREN GENERAL HOSPITAL, WARREN, PA, p. A373
WARREN HOSPITAL, PHILLIPSBURG, NJ, p. A279
WARREN MEMORIAL HOSPITAL, FRONT ROYAL, VA, p. A444
WARREN MEMORIAL HOSPITAL, FRIEND, NE, p. A262
WARREN STATE HOSPITAL, NORTH WARREN, PA, p. A365
WARWICK MANOR BEHAVIORAL HEALTH, EAST NEW MARKET, MD, p. A198
WASECA MEDICAL CENTER, WASECA, MN, p. A234
WASHAKIE MEDICAL CENTER, WORLAND, WY, p. A480
WASHINGTON ADVENTIST HOSPITAL, TAKOMA PARK, MD, p. A200
WASHINGTON CAMPUS, GRANTS PASS, OREGON, p. A351
WASHINGTON COUNTY HEALTH SYSTEM, HAGERSTOWN, MD, p. A198
WASHINGTON COUNTY HOSPITAL, PLYMOUTH, NC, p. A316
WASHINGTON COUNTY HOSPITAL, NASHVILLE, IL, p. A131
WASHINGTON COUNTY HOSPITAL, WASHINGTON, IA, p. A157
WASHINGTON COUNTY HOSPITAL, WASHINGTON, KS, p. A169
WASHINGTON COUNTY INFIRMARY AND NURSING HOME, CHATOM, AL, p. A13
WASHINGTON COUNTY MEMORIAL HOSPITAL, SALEM, IN, p. A145
WASHINGTON COUNTY MEMORIAL HOSPITAL, POTOSI, MO, p. A251
WASHINGTON COUNTY REGIONAL MEDICAL CENTER, SANDERSVILLE, GA, p. A109
WASHINGTON HOSPITAL, WASHINGTON, PA, p. A373
WASHINGTON HOSPITAL CENTER, WASHINGTON, DC, p. A80
WASHINGTON REGIONAL MEDICAL CENTER, FAYETTEVILLE, AR, p. A29
WASHINGTON TOWNSHIP HEALTH CARE DISTRICT, FREMONT, CA, p. A41
WASHINGTON–ST. TAMMANY REGIONAL MEDICAL CENTER, BOGALUSA, LA, p. A181
WASHOE HEALTH SYSTEM, RENO, NV, p. A269
WATAUGA MEDICAL CENTER, BOONE, NC, p. A310
WATERBURY HOSPITAL, WATERBURY, CT, p. A77
WATERTOWN MEMORIAL HOSPITAL, WATERTOWN, WI, p. A476
WATONGA MUNICIPAL HOSPITAL, WATONGA, OK, p. A349
WATSONVILLE COMMUNITY HOSPITAL, WATSONVILLE, CA, p. A67
WAUKESHA MEMORIAL HOSPITAL, WAUKESHA, WI, p. A476
WAUPUN MEMORIAL HOSPITAL, WAUPUN, WI, p. A476
WAUSAU HOSPITAL, WAUSAU, WI, p. A477
WAVERLY MUNICIPAL HOSPITAL, WAVERLY, IA, p. A157
WAYNE COUNTY HOSPITAL, MONTICELLO, KY, p. A176
WAYNE COUNTY HOSPITAL, CORYDON, IA, p. A149
WAYNE GENERAL HOSPITAL, WAYNE, NJ, p. A281
WAYNE GENERAL HOSPITAL, WAYNESBORO, MS, p. A243
WAYNE HOSPITAL, GREENVILLE, OH, p. A332
WAYNE MEDICAL CENTER, WAYNESBORO, TN, p. A400
WAYNE MEMORIAL HOSPITAL, HONESDALE, PA, p. A361
WAYNE MEMORIAL HOSPITAL, GOLDSBORO, NC, p. A313
WAYNE MEMORIAL HOSPITAL, JESUP, GA, p. A106
WAYNESBORO HOSPITAL, WAYNESBORO, PA, p. A373
WEBSTER COUNTY COMMUNITY HOSPITAL, RED CLOUD, NE, p. A266
WEBSTER COUNTY MEMORIAL HOSPITAL, WEBSTER SPRINGS, WV, p. A464
WEBSTER HEALTH SERVICES, EUPORA, MS, p. A237

WEDOWEE HOSPITAL, WEDOWEE, AL, p. A19
WEED ARMY COMMUNITY HOSPITAL, FORT IRWIN, CA, p. A41
WEEKS MEDICAL CENTER, LANCASTER, NH, p. A272
WEINER MEMORIAL MEDICAL CENTER, MARSHALL, MN, p. A230
WEIRTON MEDICAL CENTER, WEIRTON, WV, p. A464
WEISBROD MEMORIAL COUNTY HOSPITAL, EADS, CO, p. A70
WELLINGTON REGIONAL MEDICAL CENTER, WEST PALM BEACH, FL, p. A98
WELLMONT BRISTOL REGIONAL MEDICAL CENTER, BRISTOL, TN, p. A390
WELLMONT HOLSTON VALLEY MEDICAL CENTER, KINGSPORT, TN, p. A394
WELLMONT LONESOME PINE HOSPITAL, BIG STONE GAP, VA, p. A442
WELLS COMMUNITY HOSPITAL, BLUFFTON, IN, p. A137
WELLSPRING FOUNDATION, BETHLEHEM, CT, p. A74
WELLSTAR COBB HOSPITAL, AUSTELL, GA, p. A101
WELLSTAR DOUGLAS HOSPITAL, DOUGLASVILLE, GA, p. A104
WELLSTAR KENNESTONE HOSPITAL, MARIETTA, GA, p. A107
WELLSTAR PAULDING HOSPITAL, DALLAS, GA, p. A103
WELLSTAR WINDY HILL HOSPITAL, MARIETTA, GA, p. A107
WENTWORTH-DOUGLASS HOSPITAL, DOVER, NH, p. A271
WERNERSVILLE STATE HOSPITAL, WERNERSVILLE, PA, p. A374
WESKOTA MEMORIAL MEDICAL CENTER, WESSINGTON SPRINGS, SD, p. A389
WESLEY LONG COMMUNITY HOSPITAL, GREENSBORO, NORTH CAROLINA, p. A313
WESLEY MEDICAL CENTER, HATTIESBURG, MS, p. A238
WESLEY MEDICAL CENTER, WICHITA, KS, p. A169
WESLEY REHABILITATION HOSPITAL, WICHITA, KS, p. A169
WESLEY WOODS CENTER OF EMORY UNIVERSITY, ATLANTA, GA, p. A100
WEST ALLIS MEMORIAL HOSPITAL, WEST ALLIS, WI, p. A477
WEST ANAHEIM MEDICAL CENTER, ANAHEIM, CA, p. A35
WEST BOCA MEDICAL CENTER, BOCA RATON, FL, p. A81
WEST BRANCH REGIONAL MEDICAL CENTER, WEST BRANCH, MI, p. A224
WEST CALCASIEU CAMERON HOSPITAL, SULPHUR, LA, p. A189
WEST CAMPUS, NORFOLK, NEBRASKA, p. A264
WEST CARROLL MEMORIAL HOSPITAL, OAK GROVE, LA, p. A187
WEST CENTRAL COMMUNITY HOSPITAL, CLINTON, IN, p. A138
WEST FELICIANA PARISH HOSPITAL, SAINT FRANCISVILLE, LA, p. A188
WEST FLORIDA REGIONAL MEDICAL CENTER, PENSACOLA, FL, p. A93
WEST GEORGIA HEALTH SYSTEM, LA GRANGE, GA, p. A106
WEST HAVEN DIVISION, WEST HAVEN, CONNECTICUT, p. A76
WEST HILLS HOSPITAL AND MEDICAL CENTER, LOS ANGELES, CA, p. A50
WEST HOLT MEMORIAL HOSPITAL, ATKINSON, NE, p. A261
WEST HOUSTON MEDICAL CENTER, HOUSTON, TX, p. A419
WEST HUDSON HOSPITAL, KEARNY, NJ, p. A277
WEST JEFFERSON MEDICAL CENTER, MARRERO, LA, p. A185
WEST OAKS HOSPITAL, HOUSTON, TX, p. A419
WEST PARK HOSPITAL, CODY, WY, p. A478
WEST RIVER REGIONAL MEDICAL CENTER, HETTINGER, ND, p. A322
WEST SHORE MEDICAL CENTER, MANISTEE, MI, p. A219
WEST SUBURBAN HOSPITAL MEDICAL CENTER, OAK PARK, IL, p. A132
WEST VALLEY MEDICAL CENTER, CALDWELL, ID, p. A115
WEST VIRGINIA UNIVERSITY HOSPITALS, MORGANTOWN, WV, p. A463
WESTBOROUGH STATE HOSPITAL, WESTBOROUGH, MA, p. A209
WESTBRIDGE TREATMENT CENTER, PHOENIX, AZ, p. A25
WESTBROOK HEALTH CENTER, WESTBROOK, MN, p. A234
WESTCHESTER GENERAL HOSPITAL, MIAMI, FL, p. A90
WESTCHESTER MEDICAL CENTER, VALHALLA, NY, p. A306
WESTCHESTER SQUARE MEDICAL CENTER, NEW YORK, NY, p. A300
WESTERLY HOSPITAL, WESTERLY, RI, p. A377
WESTERN ARIZONA REGIONAL MEDICAL CENTER, BULLHEAD CITY, AZ, p. A22
WESTERN BAPTIST HOSPITAL, PADUCAH, KY, p. A177
WESTERN MARYLAND CENTER, HAGERSTOWN, MD, p. A199
WESTERN MEDICAL CENTER HOSPITAL ANAHEIM, ANAHEIM, CA, p. A35
WESTERN MEDICAL CENTER-SANTA ANA, SANTA ANA, CA, p. A62
WESTERN MENTAL HEALTH INSTITUTE, BOLIVAR, TN, p. A390
WESTERN MISSOURI MEDICAL CENTER, WARRENSBURG, MO, p. A255
WESTERN MISSOURI MENTAL HEALTH CENTER, KANSAS CITY, MO, p. A249
WESTERN NEW YORK CHILDREN'S PSYCHIATRIC CENTER, BUFFALO, NY, p. A289
WESTERN PENNSYLVANIA HOSPITAL, PITTSBURGH, PA, p. A370
WESTERN PLAINS MEDICAL COMPLEX, DODGE CITY, KS, p. A160
WESTERN PSYCHIATRIC INSTITUTE AND CLINIC, PITTSBURGH, PENNSYLVANIA, p. A370
WESTERN RESERVE CARE SYSTEM, YOUNGSTOWN, OH, p. A340
WESTERN STATE HOSPITAL, STAUNTON, VA, p. A450
WESTERN STATE HOSPITAL, HOPKINSVILLE, KY, p. A173
WESTERN STATE HOSPITAL, TACOMA, WA, p. A458
WESTERN STATE PSYCHIATRIC CENTER, WOODWARD, OK, p. A349
WESTERN WAKE MEDICAL CENTER, CARY, NORTH CAROLINA, p. A317
WESTFIELD MEMORIAL HOSPITAL, WESTFIELD, NY, p. A307
WESTLAKE HOSPITAL, MELROSE PARK, IL, p. A130
WESTLAKE REGIONAL HOSPITAL, COLUMBIA, KY, p. A171
WESTMORELAND REGIONAL HOSPITAL, GREENSBURG, PA, p. A360
WESTON COUNTY HEALTH SERVICES, NEWCASTLE, WY, p. A479
WESTPARK SURGERY CENTER, MCKINNEY, TEXAS, p. A423
WESTSIDE REGIONAL MEDICAL CENTER, PLANTATION, FL, p. A93
WESTVIEW HOSPITAL, INDIANAPOLIS, IN, p. A142
WESTWOOD LODGE HOSPITAL, WESTWOOD, MA, p. A209
WESTWOOD MEDICAL CENTER, MIDLAND, TX, p. A424
WETZEL COUNTY HOSPITAL, NEW MARTINSVILLE, WV, p. A463
WHEATLAND MEMORIAL HOSPITAL, HARLOWTON, MT, p. A258
WHEATON COMMUNITY HOSPITAL, WHEATON, MN, p. A235
WHEELER COUNTY HOSPITAL, GLENWOOD, GA, p. A105
WHEELING HOSPITAL, WHEELING, WV, p. A465
WHIDBEY GENERAL HOSPITAL, COUPEVILLE, WA, p. A453
WHIDDEN MEMORIAL HOSPITAL, EVERETT, MASSACHUSETTS, p. A206
WHITE COMMUNITY HOSPITAL, AURORA, MN, p. A225
WHITE COUNTY COMMUNITY HOSPITAL, SPARTA, TN, p. A399
WHITE COUNTY MEDICAL CENTER, CARMI, IL, p. A120
WHITE COUNTY MEDICAL CENTER, SEARCY, AR, p. A33
WHITE COUNTY MEMORIAL HOSPITAL, MONTICELLO, IN, p. A144
WHITE MEMORIAL MEDICAL CENTER, LOS ANGELES, CA, p. A50
WHITE MOUNTAIN REGIONAL MEDICAL CENTER, SPRINGERVILLE, AZ, p. A26
WHITE PLAINS HOSPITAL CENTER, WHITE PLAINS, NY, p. A307
WHITE RIVER MEDICAL CENTER, BATESVILLE, AR, p. A28
WHITESBURG APPALACHIAN REGIONAL HOSPITAL, WHITESBURG, KY, p. A179
WHITFIELD MEDICAL SURGICAL HOSPITAL, WHITFIELD, MISSISSIPPI, p. A243
WHITING FORENSIC DIVISION OF CONNECTICUT VALLEY HOSPITAL, MIDDLETOWN, CONNECTICUT, p. A75
WHITINSVILLE MEDICAL CENTER, WHITINSVILLE, MASSACHUSETTS, p. A206
WHITLEY MEMORIAL HOSPITAL, COLUMBIA CITY, IN, p. A138
WHITMAN HOSPITAL AND MEDICAL CENTER, COLFAX, WA, p. A453
WHITTEN CENTER INFIRMARY, CLINTON, SC, p. A379
WHITTIER HOSPITAL MEDICAL CENTER, WHITTIER, CA, p. A67
WHITTIER REHABILITATION HOSPITAL, HAVERHILL, MA, p. A205
WICHITA COUNTY HEALTH CENTER, LEOTI, KS, p. A164
WICHITA COUNTY HOSPITAL LONG TERM CARE, LEOTI, KANSAS, p. A164
WICKENBURG REGIONAL HOSPITAL, WICKENBURG, AZ, p. A27
WILBARGER GENERAL HOSPITAL, VERNON, TX, p. A433
WILCOX ARMY COMMUNITY HOSPITAL, FORT DRUM, NY, p. A291
WILCOX MEMORIAL HOSPITAL, LIHUE, HI, p. A113
WILD ROSE COMMUNITY MEMORIAL HOSPITAL, WILD ROSE, WI, p. A477
WILDWOOD LIFESTYLE CENTER AND HOSPITAL, WILDWOOD, GA, p. A111
WILFORD HALL MEDICAL CENTER, LACKLAND AFB, TX, p. A420
WILKES REGIONAL MEDICAL CENTER, NORTH WILKESBORO, NC, p. A316
WILKES-BARRE GENERAL HOSPITAL, WILKES-BARRE, PENNSYLVANIA, p. A374
WILLAMETTE FALLS HOSPITAL, OREGON CITY, OR, p. A352
WILLAMETTE VALLEY MEDICAL CENTER, MCMINNVILLE, OR, p. A352
WILLAPA HARBOR HOSPITAL, SOUTH BEND, WA, p. A457
WILLIAM B. KESSLER MEMORIAL HOSPITAL, HAMMONTON, NJ, p. A276
WILLIAM BEAUMONT ARMY MEDICAL CENTER, EL PASO, TX, p. A412
WILLIAM BEAUMONT HOSPITAL-ROYAL OAK, ROYAL OAK, MI, p. A221
WILLIAM BEAUMONT HOSPITAL-TROY, TROY, MI, p. A223
WILLIAM BEE RIRIE HOSPITAL, ELY, NV, p. A268
WILLIAM NEWTON MEMORIAL HOSPITAL, WINFIELD, KS, p. A169
WILLIAM R. SHARPE JR. HOSPITAL, WESTON, WV, p. A465
WILLIAM S. HALL PSYCHIATRIC INSTITUTE, COLUMBIA, SC, p. A380
WILLIAM S. MIDDLETON MEMORIAL VETERANS HOSPITAL, MADISON, WI, p. A470
WILLIAM W. HASTINGS INDIAN HOSPITAL, TAHLEQUAH, OK, p. A348
WILLIAMSBURG COMMUNITY HOSPITAL, WILLIAMSBURG, VA, p. A451
WILLIAMSON ARH HOSPITAL, SOUTH WILLIAMSON, KY, p. A178
WILLIAMSON MEDICAL CENTER, FRANKLIN, TN, p. A392
WILLIAMSON MEMORIAL HOSPITAL, WILLIAMSON, WV, p. A465
WILLIAMSPORT HOSPITAL AND MEDICAL CENTER, WILLIAMSPORT, PENNSYLVANIA, p. A375
WILLIE D. MILLER EYE CENTER, CHATTANOOGA, TENNESSEE, p. A390
WILLINGWAY HOSPITAL, STATESBORO, GA, p. A110
WILLIS-KNIGHTON MEDICAL CENTER, SHREVEPORT, LA, p. A189
WILLMAR REGIONAL TREATMENT CENTER, WILLMAR, MN, p. A235
WILLOUGH HEALTHCARE SYSTEM, NAPLES, FL, p. A91
WILLOW CREST HOSPITAL, MIAMI, OK, p. A345
WILLS EYE HOSPITAL, PHILADELPHIA, PA, p. A368
WILLS MEMORIAL HOSPITAL, WASHINGTON, GA, p. A111
WILMA N. VAZQUEZ MEDICAL CENTER, VEGA BAJA, PR, p. A484
WILMINGTON HOSPITAL, WILMINGTON, DELAWARE, p. A78
WILSON CENTER PSYCHIATRIC FACILITY FOR CHILDREN AND ADOLESCENTS, FARIBAULT, MN, p. A228
WILSON COUNTY HOSPITAL, NEODESHA, KS, p. A165
WILSON MEDICAL CENTER, DARLINGTON, SOUTH CAROLINA, p. A381
WILSON MEMORIAL HOSPITAL, WILSON, NC, p. A319
WILSON MEMORIAL HOSPITAL, SIDNEY, OH, p. A337
WILSON MEMORIAL HOSPITAL, FLORESVILLE, TX, p. A412
WILSON MEMORIAL REGIONAL MEDICAL CENTER, JOHNSON CITY, NEW YORK, p. A288
WILSON N. JONES MEDICAL CENTER, SHERMAN, TX, p. A431
WINCHESTER HOSPITAL, WINCHESTER, MA, p. A209
WINCHESTER MEDICAL CENTER, WINCHESTER, VA, p. A451
WINDBER MEDICAL CENTER, WINDBER, PA, p. A375
WINDHAM COMMUNITY MEMORIAL HOSPITAL, WILLIMANTIC, CT, p. A77
WINDMOOR HEALTHCARE OF CLEARWATER, CLEARWATER, FL, p. A82
WINDMOOR HEALTHCARE OF MIAMI, MIAMI, FL, p. A90
WINDOM AREA HOSPITAL, WINDOM, MN, p. A235
WING MEMORIAL HOSPITAL AND MEDICAL CENTERS, PALMER, MA, p. A207
WINN ARMY COMMUNITY HOSPITAL, HINESVILLE, GA, p. A106
WINN PARISH MEDICAL CENTER, WINNFIELD, LA, p. A189
WINNEBAGO MENTAL HEALTH INSTITUTE, WINNEBAGO, WI, p. A477
WINNER REGIONAL HEALTHCARE CENTER, WINNER, SD, p. A389
WINNESHIEK COUNTY MEMORIAL HOSPITAL, DECORAH, IA, p. A150
WINONA COMMUNITY MEMORIAL HOSPITAL, WINONA, MN, p. A235
WINONA MEMORIAL HOSPITAL, INDIANAPOLIS, IN, p. A142
WINSLOW MEMORIAL HOSPITAL, WINSLOW, AZ, p. A27
WINSTON MEDICAL CENTER, LOUISVILLE, MS, p. A240
WINTER HAVEN HOSPITAL, WINTER HAVEN, FL, p. A98
WINTER PARK MEMORIAL HOSPITAL, WINTER PARK, FL, p. A98
WINTER PARK PSYCHIATRIC CARE CENTER, WINTER PARK, FLORIDA, p. A98
WINTHROP-UNIVERSITY HOSPITAL, MINEOLA, NY, p. A294
WIREGRASS MEDICAL CENTER, GENEVA, AL, p. A15
WIRTH REGIONAL HOSPITAL, OAKLAND CITY, IN, p. A144
WISHARD HEALTH SERVICES, INDIANAPOLIS, IN, p. A142
WISHEK COMMUNITY HOSPITAL AND CLINICS, WISHEK, ND, p. A324
WITHAM MEMORIAL HOSPITAL, LEBANON, IN, p. A143
WM. JENNINGS BRYAN DORN VETERANS AFFAIRS MEDICAL CENTER, COLUMBIA, SC, p. A380
WOMACK ARMY MEDICAL CENTER, FORT BRAGG, NC, p. A313
WOMAN'S CHRISTIAN ASSOCIATION HOSPITAL, JAMESTOWN, NY, p. A293
WOMAN'S HOSPITAL, BATON ROUGE, LA, p. A181
WOMAN'S HOSPITAL AT RIVER OAKS, JACKSON, MS, p. A239
WOMEN AND CHILDREN'S HOSPITAL, CHARLESTON, WEST VIRGINIA, p. A460
WOMEN AND CHILDREN'S HOSPITAL-LAKE CHARLES, LAKE CHARLES, LA, p. A184
WOMEN AND INFANTS HOSPITAL OF RHODE ISLAND, PROVIDENCE, RI, p. A377

Index of Hospitals / Women's and Children's Hospital

WOMEN'S AND CHILDREN'S HOSPITAL, LAFAYETTE, LA, p. A184
WOMEN'S AND CHILDREN'S HOSPITAL, LOS ANGELES, CALIFORNIA, p. A48
WOMEN'S HOSPITAL OF GREENSBORO, GREENSBORO, NORTH CAROLINA, p. A313
WOMEN'S HOSPITAL–INDIANAPOLIS, INDIANAPOLIS, IN, p. A142
WOOD COUNTY HOSPITAL, BOWLING GREEN, OH, p. A326
WOOD RIVER MEDICAL CENTER, LOS ANGELES, ID, p. A118
WOOD RIVER TOWNSHIP HOSPITAL, WOOD RIVER, IL, p. A136
WOODBRIDGE DEVELOPMENT CENTER, WOODBRIDGE, NJ, p. A282
WOODHULL MEDICAL AND MENTAL HEALTH CENTER, NEW YORK, NY, p. A301
WOODLAND HEALTHCARE, WOODLAND, CA, p. A67
WOODLAND HEIGHTS MEDICAL CENTER, LUFKIN, TX, p. A422
WOODLAND MEDICAL CENTER, CULLMAN, AL, p. A13
WOODLAND PARK HOSPITAL, PORTLAND, OR, p. A353
WOODLAWN HOSPITAL, ROCHESTER, IN, p. A145
WOODRIDGE HOSPITAL, JOHNSON CITY, TN, p. A394
WOODROW WILSON REHABILITATION CENTER, FISHERSVILLE, VA, p. A444
WOODS MEMORIAL HOSPITAL DISTRICT, ETOWAH, TN, p. A392
WOODSIDE HOSPITAL, NEWPORT NEWS, VA, p. A446
WOODSON CHILDRENS PSYCHIATRIC HOSPITAL, SAINT JOSEPH, MISSOURI, p. A252
WOODWARD HOSPITAL AND HEALTH CENTER, WOODWARD, OK, p. A349
WOODWARD STATE HOSPITAL–SCHOOL, WOODWARD, IA, p. A158
WOOSTER COMMUNITY HOSPITAL, WOOSTER, OH, p. A339
WORCESTER STATE HOSPITAL, WORCESTER, MA, p. A210
WORTHINGTON REGIONAL HOSPITAL, WORTHINGTON, MN, p. A235
WRANGELL MEDICAL CENTER, WRANGELL, AK, p. A21
WRAY COMMUNITY DISTRICT HOSPITAL, WRAY, CO, p. A73
WRIGHT MEMORIAL HOSPITAL, TRENTON, MO, p. A255
WUESTHOFF HEALTH SYSTEM, ROCKLEDGE, FL, p. A94
WYANDOT MEMORIAL HOSPITAL, UPPER SANDUSKY, OH, p. A338
WYCKOFF HEIGHTS MEDICAL CENTER, NEW YORK, NY, p. A301
WYOMING COUNTY COMMUNITY HOSPITAL, WARSAW, NY, p. A307
WYOMING MEDICAL CENTER, CASPER, WY, p. A478
WYOMING STATE HOSPITAL, EVANSTON, WY, p. A478
WYOMING VALLEY HEALTH CARE SYSTEM, WILKES-BARRE, PA, p. A374
WYTHE COUNTY COMMUNITY HOSPITAL, WYTHEVILLE, VA, p. A451

Y

YAKIMA VALLEY MEMORIAL HOSPITAL, YAKIMA, WA, p. A459
YALE PSYCHIATRIC INSTITUTE, NEW HAVEN, CT, p. A76
YALE–NEW HAVEN HOSPITAL, NEW HAVEN, CT, p. A76
YALOBUSHA GENERAL HOSPITAL, WATER VALLEY, MS, p. A243
YAMPA VALLEY MEDICAL CENTER, STEAMBOAT SPRINGS, CO, p. A73
YAVAPAI REGIONAL MEDICAL CENTER, PRESCOTT, AZ, p. A25
YOAKUM COMMUNITY HOSPITAL, YOAKUM, TX, p. A435
YOAKUM COUNTY HOSPITAL, DENVER CITY, TX, p. A410
YONKERS GENERAL HOSPITAL, YONKERS, NY, p. A308
YORK GENERAL HOSPITAL, YORK, NE, p. A267
YORK HOSPITAL, YORK, ME, p. A194
YORK HOSPITAL, YORK, PA, p. A375
YOUNGSTOWN OSTEOPATHIC HOSPITAL, YOUNGSTOWN, OH, p. A340
YOUNKER MEMORIAL REHABILITATION CENTER, DES MOINES, IOWA, p. A151
YOUVILLE LIFECARE, CAMBRIDGE, MA, p. A204
YUKON–KUSKOKWIM DELTA REGIONAL HOSPITAL, BETHEL, AK, p. A20
YUMA DISTRICT HOSPITAL, YUMA, CO, p. A73
YUMA REGIONAL MEDICAL CENTER, YUMA, AZ, p. A27

Z

ZALE LIPSHY UNIVERSITY HOSPITAL, DALLAS, TX, p. A410
ZEELAND COMMUNITY HOSPITAL, ZEELAND, MI, p. A224
ZUMBROTA HEALTH CARE, ZUMBROTA, MN, p. A235

Index of Health Care Professionals

This section is an index of the key health care professionals for the hospitals and/or health care systems listed in this publication. The index is in alphabetical order, by individual, followed by the title, institutional affiliation, city, state and page reference to the hospital and/or health care system listing in section A and/or B.

A

AANONSON, Mark, Administrator, Northern Virginia Community Hospital, Arlington, VA, p. A442
AARON, Jr, Frank J., Chief Executive Officer, Margaret R. Pardee Memorial Hospital, Hendersonville, NC, p. A314
AASVED, Craig E.
  Chief Executive Officer, North Valley Hospital, Whitefish, MT, p. A260
  Administrator, Wheatland Memorial Hospital, Harlowton, MT, p. A258
ABBOTT, Stephen L., President and Chief Executive Officer, Cape Cod Healthcare, Inc., Hyannis, MA, p. B64
ABBUHL, Carol A., Chief Executive Officer, Perkins County Health Services, Grant, NE, p. A263
ABOUD, Alberto J., Administrator, Fishermen's Hospital, Marathon, FL, p. A89
ABRAHAM, Mathew, Chief Executive Officer, Antelope Valley Hospital, Lancaster, CA, p. A45
ABRAMS, Larry, Administrator, Potomac Valley Hospital, Keyser, WV, p. A462
ABREU, Astrid, Administrator, Clinica San Agustin, Manati, PR, p. A482
ABRUTZ, Jr, Joseph F., Administrator, Cameron Community Hospital, Cameron, MO, p. A245
ABU–GHUSSON, Marilyn S., USAF, Commander, U. S. Air Force Hospital, Holloman AFB, NM, p. A285
ACKER, David B., Chief Executive Officer, Charles Cole Memorial Hospital, Coudersport, PA, p. A358
ACKER, Peter W., President and Chief Executive Officer, Lincoln Medical Center, Lincolnton, NC, p. A315
ACKERMAN, Sigurd H., M.D., President and Chief Executive Officer, St. Luke's–Roosevelt Hospital Center, New York, NY, p. A300
ADAIR, Jerry D., President and Chief Executive Officer, Good Shepherd Medical Center, Longview, TX, p. A422
ADAMS, Charles T., Chief Executive Officer, Chestatee Regional Hospital, Dahlonega, GA, p. A103
ADAMS, Daniel F., President and Chief Executive Officer, Presbyterian Intercommunity Hospital, Whittier, CA, p. A67
ADAMS, Gregory A., Senior Vice President and Service Area Manager, Kaiser Foundation Hospital, Baldwin Park, CA, p. A36
ADAMS, Jerry W., President, Sumter Regional Hospital, Americus, GA, p. A99
ADAMS, John F., Chief Executive Officer, North Central Medical Center, McKinney, TX, p. A423
ADAMS, Judy, Administrator and Chief Executive Officer, Little River Memorial Hospital, Ashdown, AR, p. A28
ADAMS, Mark, Chief Executive Officer, West Valley Medical Center, Caldwell, ID, p. A115
ADAMS, Mark A., President and Chief Executive Officer, Mississippi Methodist Hospital and Rehabilitation Center, Jackson, MS, p. A239
ADAMS, Robert W., President and Chief Executive Officer, St. Agnes Healthcare, Baltimore, MD, p. A196
ADAMS, Scott K., Chief Executive Officer, Pullman Memorial Hospital, Pullman, WA, p. A455
ADAMS, Tim, CHE, Administrator and Chief Executive Officer, Parkview Regional Hospital, Mexia, TX, p. A423
ADAMS, William A., President and Chief Executive Officer, Reston Hospital Center, Reston, VA, p. A448
ADAMS, Nancy R., Commander, Tripler Army Medical Center, Honolulu, HI, p. A113
ADDISON, Wilfred J., President and Chief Executive Officer, Inland Hospital, Waterville, ME, p. A194
ADELUNG, Louisa F., President and Chief Executive Officer, The Institute for Rehabilitation and Research, Houston, TX, p. A418
AENCHBACHER, Jr, Arthur E., Administrator, Wilford Hall Medical Center, Lackland AFB, TX, p. A420
AFSARIFARD, Farshid, Ph.D., President, UHHS Laurelwood Hospital, Willoughby, OH, p. A339
AHLFELD, Richard B., President, Children's Specialized Hospital, Mountainside, NJ, p. A278
AINSLEY, Howard, Vice President and Hospital Director, Carilion Bedford Memorial Hospital, Bedford, VA, p. A442
AINSWORTH, Larry K., President and Chief Executive Officer, St. Joseph Hospital, Orange, CA, p. A54
AKERS, Cynthia D., R.N., Administrator, Hamilton County Hospital, Syracuse, KS, p. A168
AKIN, Dan H., Interim Chief Executive Officer, Wesley Medical Center, Hattiesburg, MS, p. A238
ALAND, Kent, Interim Administrator, Washakie Medical Center, Worland, WY, p. A480
ALBARANO, Francis G., Administrator, Fayette County Memorial Hospital, Washington Court House, OH, p. A339
ALBAUGH, John C., President and Chief Executive Officer, Fort Atkinson Memorial Health Services, Fort Atkinson, WI, p. A468
ALBERT, Anna, Chief Executive Officer, U. S. Public Health Service Phoenix Indian Medical Center, Phoenix, AZ, p. A25
ALBERTY, Allen R., Chief Executive Officer, Hansford Hospital, Spearman, TX, p. A431
ALBIS, Harry, Interim Chief Executive Officer, Crosby Memorial Hospital, Picayune, MS, p. A241
ALBRIGHT, James W., President and Chief Executive Officer, Rex Healthcare, Raleigh, NC, p. A317
ALCHESAY–NACHU, Carla, Service Unit Director, U. S. Public Health Service Indian Hospital, Whiteriver, AZ, p. A27
ALCINI, Anthony J.
  President and Chief Executive Officer, JPS Health Network, Fort Worth, TX, p. A413
  President and Chief Executive Officer, Tarrant County Hospital District, Fort Worth, TX, p. B139
ALDERELE, Felix, Administrator, Las Vegas Medical Center, Las Vegas, NM, p. A285
ALECCI, Carmen Bruce, Executive Director, West Hudson Hospital, Kearny, NJ, p. A277
ALEMAN, Ralph A., Chief Executive Officer, Miami Heart Institute and Medical Center, Miami, FL, p. A90
ALENDER, James, President and Chief Executive Officer, Howard Community Hospital, Kokomo, IN, p. A142
ALEXANDER, Alan B., Administrator, Caverna Memorial Hospital, Horse Cave, KY, p. A173
ALEXANDER, Gordon L., M.D., Senior Vice President and Chief Executive Officer, Fairview–University Medical Center, Minneapolis, MN, p. A230
ALEXANDER, Keith N., Administrator and Chief Operating Officer, American Fork Hospital, American Fork, UT, p. A436
ALEXANDER, Michael, President and Chief Executive Officer, Candler County Hospital, Metter, GA, p. A107
ALFORD, Wendell, Administrator, Madison Parish Hospital, Tallulah, LA, p. A189
ALLEE, Al, Chief Executive Officer, Memorial Hospital, Frederick, OK, p. A343
ALLEN, John, President and Chief Executive Officer, Spencer Municipal Hospital, Spencer, IA, p. A157
ALLEN, John E., Chief Executive Officer, Northwest Florida Community Hospital, Chipley, FL, p. A82
ALLEN, Richard L., President and Chief Executive Officer, Mercy Health Center of Manhattan, New York, KS, p. A164
ALLEN, Robert W., Chief Executive Officer, Evanston Regional Hospital, Evanston, WY, p. A478
ALLEN, Sam J., Chief Executive Officer, Community Hospital of Anaconda, Anaconda, MT, p. A256
ALLEN, Terry H., Executive Director, 45th Street Mental Health Center, West Palm Beach, FL, p. A97
ALLEN, Mark L., USAF, Administrator, U. S. Air Force Hospital, Columbus, MS, p. A237
ALLEN, II, Percy, FACHE, Chief Executive Officer, Bon Secours Baltimore Health System, Baltimore, MD, p. A195
ALLEY, Frederick D., President and Chief Executive Officer, Brooklyn Hospital Center, New York, NY, p. A296
ALLEY, Richard S., Executive Vice President and Chief Executive Officer, Arrowhead Community Hospital and Medical Center, Glendale, AZ, p. A22
ALLIKER, Stanford A., Chief Executive Officer, Camden County Health Services Center, Blackwood, NJ, p. A274
ALLISON, Joel T., President and Chief Executive Officer, Baylor Health Care System, Dallas, TX, p. B59
ALLMAN, Roger J., Chief Executive Officer, King's Daughters' Hospital and Health Services, Madison, IN, p. A143
ALSTON, Richard D., Administrator, Nashville Metropolitan Bordeaux Hospital, Nashville, TN, p. A398
ALTMILLER, Steve, President and Chief Executive Officer, San Juan Regional Medical Center, Farmington, NM, p. A284
ALTON, Aaron, President, Sisters of Mary of the Presentation Health Corporation, Fargo, ND, p. B133
ALTSCHULER, Steven M., President and Chief Executive Officer, Children's Hospital of Philadelphia, Philadelphia, PA, p. A366
ALVAREZ, Frank D., President and Chief Executive Officer, Tucson Medical Center, Tucson, AZ, p. A27
ALVIN, William R., President, Henry Ford Wyandotte Hospital, Wyandotte, MI, p. A224
AMAN, Dale, Administrator, Linton Hospital, Linton, ND, p. A323
AMARAL, Joseph E., M.D., President and Chief Executive Officer, Rhode Island Hospital, Providence, RI, p. A376
AMEEN, David J., President and Chief Executive Officer, Santa Rosa Memorial Hospital, Santa Rosa, CA, p. A63
AMEER, Adil M., President and Chief Executive Officer, Rapid City Regional Hospital System of Care, Rapid City, SD, p. A387
AMES, Craig M., President and Chief Operating Officer, BryanLGH Medical Center, Lincoln, NE, p. A264
AMMON, Donald R., President, Adventist Health, Roseville, CA, p. B50
AMOS, James L., President, Margaret Mary Community Hospital, Batesville, IN, p. A137
AMSTUTZ, Terry L., CHE, Chief Executive Officer and Administrator, Medical Center of Calico Rock, Calico Rock, AR, p. A28
ANAEBONAM, Nneka, Administrator, Isham Health Center, Andover, MA, p. A201
ANASTASIO, Lance W., President, Winter Haven Hospital, Winter Haven, FL, p. A97
ANCELL, Charles D., President, Missouri Delta Medical Center, Sikeston, MO, p. A254
ANCHO, Kathy, Administrator, Battle Mountain General Hospital, Battle Mountain, NV, p. A268

ANDERSEN, David, President and Chief Executive Officer, Saratoga Hospital, Saratoga Springs, NY, p. A304
ANDERSEN, Edward, President and Chief Executive Officer, CGH Medical Center, Sterling, IL, p. A135
ANDERSON, Chris, Chief Executive Officer, Singing River Hospital System, Gautier, MS, p. B132
ANDERSON, Colette, Administrator, McKenzie County Memorial Hospital, Watford City, ND, p. A324
ANDERSON, Daniel K., Senior Vice President and Administrator, Fairview Lakes Regional Medical Center, Wyoming, MN, p. A235
ANDERSON, Darleen S., MSN, Site Administrator, Sentara Leigh Hospital, Norfolk, VA, p. A447
ANDERSON, David S., FACHE, Administrator, Lassen Community Hospital, Susanville, CA, p. A64
ANDERSON, Edwin S., President, Cumberland Medical Center, Crossville, TN, p. A392
ANDERSON, Greger C., President and Chief Executive Officer, Nyack Hospital, Nyack, NY, p. A301
ANDERSON, Harold E., Chief Executive Officer, Moses Taylor Hospital, Scranton, PA, p. A372
ANDERSON, J. Kendall, President and Chief Executive Officer, JM/MD Health System, Walnut Creek, CA, p. A66
ANDERSON, James M., President and Chief Executive Officer, Children's Hospital Medical Center, Cincinnati, OH, p. A327
ANDERSON, John D., Chief Executive Officer, Emory Parkway Medical Center, Lithia Springs, GA, p. A106
ANDERSON, Larry, Administrator, Sayre Memorial Hospital, Sayre, OK, p. A347
ANDERSON, Melinda, Administrator, LAC–Olive View–UCLA Medical Center, Los Angeles, CA, p. A48
ANDERSON, Richard A., President and Chief Executive Officer, St. Luke's Hospital and Health Network, Bethlehem, PA, p. A356
ANDERSON, Ron J., M.D., President and Chief Executive Officer, Parkland Health and Hospital System, Dallas, TX, p. A409
ANDERSON, Scott R., President and Chief Executive Officer, North Memorial Health Care, Robbinsdale, MN, p. A232
ANDERSON, Sharla, Interim Chief Executive Officer, HEALTHSOUTH Rehabilitation Hospital–Tyler, Tyler, TX, p. A433
ANDERSON, Stephen N. F., Director, Doctors' Hospital of Staten Island, New York, NY, p. A296
ANDERSON, Steven M., Chief Executive Officer, Summerville Medical Center, Summerville, SC, p. A384
ANDERSON, Thomas E., Chief Executive Officer, St. Mary–Corwin Medical Center, Pueblo, CO, p. A72
ANDERSON, William H., President, Helen Keller Hospital, Sheffield, AL, p. A18
ANDERSON , Jr, Andrew E., Administrator, Gainesville Memorial Hospital, Gainesville, TX, p. A413
ANDREWS, Jane, Chief Executive Officer, Nashville Rehabilitation Hospital, Nashville, TN, p. A398
ANDREWS, William J., President, Licking Memorial Hospital, Newark, OH, p. A335
ANDRON, Thomas, Administrator and Chief Executive Officer, Kremmling Memorial Hospital, Kremmling, CO, p. A71
ANDRUS, Michael G., Administrator and Chief Executive Officer, Franklin County Medical Center, Preston, ID, p. A117
ANDRUS, Terry W., President, East Alabama Medical Center, Opelika, AL, p. A17
ANGERMEIER, Ingo, FACHE, Administrator and Chief Executive Officer, LSU Medical Center–University Hospital, Shreveport, LA, p. A188
ANGLE, Gregory R., Administrator, Seton Medical Center, Austin, TX, p. A403
ANGLE, Toni, Administrator, Fresno Surgery Center–The Hospital for Surgery, Fresno, CA, p. A42
ANNIS, Donald D., Service Unit Director, U. S. Public Health Service Indian Hospital, Eagle Butte, SD, p. A385
ANNIS, Donald E., Chief Executive Officer, Good Hope Hospital, Erwin, NC, p. A312
ANSTINE, Larry, Chief Operating Officer, Ohio State University Hospital East, Columbus, OH, p. A330

ANTHONY, Anne G., Administrator and Chief Executive Officer, Willow Crest Hospital, Miami, OK, p. A345
ANTHONY, Fred, President and Chief Executive Officer, Cuyahoga Falls General Hospital, Cuyahoga Falls, OH, p. A330
ANTHONY, Kenneth J., President and Chief Executive Officer, HEALTHSOUTH Rehabilitation Hospital, Sewickley, PA, p. A372
ANTHONY, Larry, Administrator, Providence Toppenish Hospital, Toppenish, WA, p. A458
ANTLE, David, Chief Executive Officer, Miners' Colfax Medical Center, Raton, NM, p. A285
ANTONSON, Pete, Chief Executive Officer, Northwood Deaconess Health Center, Northwood, ND, p. A323
ANTWINE, Brenda, Administrator, HEALTHSOUTH Rehabilitation Hospital of Jonesboro, Jonesboro, AR, p. A30
APPEL, G. Robert, Administrator, Mason General Hospital, Shelton, WA, p. A457
APPLEBAUM, Jon D., Chief Executive Officer, City Hospital, Martinsburg, WV, p. A462
APRATO, Peter P., President, Robert F. Kennedy Medical Center, Hawthorne, CA, p. A43
ARBUCKLE, Barry S., Ph.D.
  Chief Executive Officer, Orange Coast Memorial Medical Center, Fountain Valley, CA, p. A41
  Chief Executive Officer, Saddleback Memorial Medical Center, Laguna Hills, CA, p. A45
ARCH, John K., Administrator, Boys Town National Research Hospital, Omaha, NE, p. A265
ARCHBELL, Larry J., Vice President Operations, University Community Hospital–Carrollwood, Tampa, FL, p. A96
ARCHER, David L., Chief Executive Officer, Saint Francis Hospital, Memphis, TN, p. A397
ARCHER, Kenneth W., Administrator, Ortonville Area Health Services, Ortonville, MN, p. A231
ARCHER, Lorne J., Chief Executive Officer, United Memorial Health Center, Greenville, MI, p. A216
ARCHER , II, William R., M.D., Commissioner, Texas Department of Health, Austin, TX, p. B142
ARCIDI, Alfred J., M.D., Senior Vice President, Whittier Rehabilitation Hospital, Haverhill, MA, p. A205
AREHART, Michael, Chief Executive Officer, Twin Falls Clinic and Hospital, Twin Falls, ID, p. A118
ARISMENDI, Christopher, M.D., Administrator, Dameron Hospital, Stockton, CA, p. A64
ARIZPE, Robert C., Superintendent, San Antonio State Hospital, San Antonio, TX, p. A429
ARMADA, Anthony A., Senior Vice President and Service Area Manager, Kaiser Foundation Hospital, Los Angeles, CA, p. A48
ARMINGTON, Denny, Chief Executive Officer, Rehabilitation Hospital of Indiana, Indianapolis, IN, p. A141
ARMSTRONG, Dale, Chief Executive Officer, Brynn Marr Behavioral Healthcare System, Jacksonville, NC, p. A314
ARMSTRONG, Kenneth, Chief Executive Officer, Timpanogos Regional Hospital, Orem, UT, p. A437
ARMSTRONG , Jr, David S., President and Chief Executive Officer, Little Falls Hospital, Little Falls, NY, p. A293
ARNESON, Garrett, Administrator, Vencor Hospital–Philadelphia, Philadelphia, PA, p. A368
ARNETT, Charlene, Chief Executive Officer, West Oaks Hospital, Houston, TX, p. A419
ARNETT, Randal M., President and Chief Executive Officer, Southern Ohio Medical Center, Portsmouth, OH, p. A337
ARNOLD, Kent A.
  President, Community–General Hospital of Greater Syracuse, Syracuse, NY, p. A305
  President and Chief Executive Officer, Crouse Hospital, Syracuse, NY, p. A305
ARNOLD, Margo, Administrator, Mercy Westside Hospital, Taft, CA, p. A64
ARNOLD, Nancy, Director, John J. Pershing Veterans Affairs Medical Center, Poplar Bluff, MO, p. A251
ARNOLD, Richard D., CHE, Administrator and Chief Executive Officer, Linden Municipal Hospital, Linden, TX, p. A421
ARP, James, Chief Executive Officer, Colorado River Medical Center, Needles, CA, p. A53

ARTILES, Nemuel O., Chief Executive Officer, Bella Vista Southwest Hospital, Yauco, PR, p. A484
ASBE, Vickie, Administrator, Jones Regional Medical Center, Anamosa, IA, p. A148
ASH, James L., President and Chief Executive Officer, Goleta Valley Cottage Hospital, Santa Barbara, CA, p. A62
ASH, John P., FACHE, President and Chief Executive Officer, Eugenia Hospital, Lafayette Hill, PA, p. A362
ASH, Richard M., Chief Executive Officer, Northern Itasca Health Care Center, Bigfork, MN, p. A226
ASHBURY, Lee, Chief Executive Officer, Selma Baptist Hospital, Selma, AL, p. A18
ASHKIN, David, M.D., Medical Executive Director, A. G. Holley State Hospital, Lantana, FL, p. A88
ASHTON, Becky
  Administrator, Franklin Hospital and Skilled Nursing Care Unit, Benton, IL, p. A120
  Senior Vice President and Administrator, United Mine Workers of America Union Hospital, West Frankfort, IL, p. A136
ASHWORTH, Ronald B., Chief Executive Officer, Sisters of Mercy Health System–St. Louis, Saint Louis, MO, p. B134
ASPER, David, Director, Veterans Affairs Greater Nebraska Health Care System, Lincoln, NE, p. A264
ASSELL, William C., President and Chief Executive Officer, Mercy Medical Center–Centerville, Centerville, IA, p. A149
ATKINS, Tony E., Administrator, Braxton County Memorial Hospital, Gassaway, WV, p. A461
ATKINSON, Allan, Chief Executive Officer, Winneshiek County Memorial Hospital, Decorah, IA, p. A150
ATKINSON, L. Gail, Executive Director, Devereux Texas Treatment Network, League City, TX, p. A421
ATKINSON, Robert P., President and Chief Executive Officer, Jefferson Regional Medical Center, Pine Bluff, AR, p. A33
ATKINSON , II, William K., Ph.D.
  President and Chief Executive Officer, New Hanover Health Network, Wilmington, NC, p. B113
  President and Chief Executive Officer, New Hanover Regional Medical Center, Wilmington, NC, p. A319
ATZROTT, Allan E., President and Chief Executive Officer, North Shore Medical Center, Miami, FL, p. A90
AUBERT, Harry, Chief Executive Officer, Lost Rivers District Hospital, Arco, ID, p. A115
AUBREY, Leonard A., President and Chief Executive Officer, New York University Downtown Hospital, New York, NY, p. A299
AUSMAN, Dan F., Chief Executive Officer, Irvine Regional Hospital and Medical Center, Irvine, CA, p. A44
AUSTIN, James D., CHE
  Administrator, Kalkaska Memorial Health Center, Kalkaska, MI, p. A218
  Administrator, Paul Oliver Memorial Hospital, Frankfort, MI, p. A215
AUSTIN, L. Joe, Chief Executive Officer, Huntsville Hospital, Huntsville, AL, p. A15
AUSTIN, Robert S., President, Gunnison Valley Hospital, Gunnison, CO, p. A71
AVERS, John M., Chief Executive Officer, White County Memorial Hospital, Monticello, IN, p. A144
AYRES, Larry J., Administrator and Chief Executive Officer, Pointe Coupee General Hospital, New Roads, LA, p. A187

B

BABB, Donald J., Chief Executive Officer, Citizens Memorial Hospital, Bolivar, MO, p. A244
BACHARACH, Paul, President and Chief Executive Officer, Uniontown Hospital, Uniontown, PA, p. A373
BACHMAN, Ronald J., Interim President and Chief Executive Officer, Marion General Hospital, Marion, OH, p. A334
BACON, Ken, President and Chief Executive Officer, Central Texas Medical Center, San Marcos, TX, p. A430

BACUS, Randy, Chief Executive Officer, Colorado–Fayette Medical Center, Weimar, TX, p. A434
BADGER, Jr, Theodore J., Chief Executive Officer, Beauregard Memorial Hospital, De Ridder, LA, p. A182
BAER, James E., FACHE, President, Waupun Memorial Hospital, Waupun, WI, p. A476
BAGBY, Philip D., President and Chief Executive Officer, Albemarle Health Group, Elizabeth City, NC, p. A312
BAGGERLY, Gregory C., USAF, Commander, U. S. Air Force Hospital, MacDill AFB, FL, p. A89
BAHL, Barry I., Director, Veterans Affairs Medical Center, Saint Cloud, MN, p. A232
BAIER, Roger, Chief Executive Officer, Union Hospital, Mayville, ND, p. A323
BAILEY, Carl W., President and Chief Executive Officer, Coffee Health Group, Florence, AL, p. B73
BAILEY, G. Owen, Administrator, Thomas Hospital, Fairhope, AL, p. A14
BAILEY, James P., President and Chief Executive Officer, Henryetta Medical Center, Henryetta, OK, p. A344
BAILEY, Sandra, Administrator, Methodist Healthcare–Brownsville, Brownsville, TN, p. A390
BAILON, Amy R., M.D., Medical Director, Woodbridge Development Center, Woodbridge, NJ, p. A282
BAINBRIDGE, Darlene D., Chief Executive Officer, Cuba Memorial Hospital, Cuba, NY, p. A290
BAIR, Charles H., Chief Executive Officer, Highland District Hospital, Hillsboro, OH, p. A333
BAIRD, Marvin L., Executive Director, Adams County Memorial Hospital, Decatur, IN, p. A139
BAJICH, Laurie, Chief Executive Officer, HEALTHSOUTH Rehabilitation Hospital of Austin, Austin, TX, p. A403
BAKER, Alice, Chief Executive Officer, Christus St. Mary Hospital, Port Arthur, TX, p. A426
BAKER, Bob M., President and Chief Executive Officer, Gratiot Community Hospital, Alma, MI, p. A211
BAKER, Gary A., President, Memorial Hospital, Towanda, PA, p. A373
BAKER, Glenn, Administrator, Baptist Memorial Hospital–Tipton, Covington, TN, p. A391
BAKER, Jeannie, Administrator, Shands at Starke, Starke, FL, p. A95
BAKER, Jon W., Chief Executive Officer, Ripon Medical Center, Ripon, WI, p. A475
BAKER, Rod L., President and Chief Executive Officer, Parrish Medical Center, Titusville, FL, p. A97
BAKER, Rodger H., President and Chief Executive Officer, Fauquier Hospital, Warrenton, VA, p. A450
BAKER, Ronald D., Administrator, Minneola District Hospital, Minneola, KS, p. A165
BAKER, Jr, Wendell H.
  District Administrator, Matagorda County Hospital District, Bay City, TX, p. B108
  Chief Executive Officer, Matagorda General Hospital, Bay City, TX, p. A403
BAKST, Michael D., Ph.D., Executive Director, Community Memorial Hospital of San Buenaventura, Ventura, CA, p. A66
BALDWIN, Bruce A., Chief Executive Officer, Davis Hospital and Medical Center, Layton, UT, p. A436
BALDWIN, Gilda
  Chief Executive Officer, Southern Winds Hospital, Hialeah, FL, p. A86
  Chief Executive Officer, Westchester General Hospital, Miami, FL, p. A90
BALDWIN, Keith J., Chief Executive Officer and Administrator, Samaritan Healthcare, Moses Lake, WA, p. A454
BALDWIN, Paul L., Chief Executive Officer, Retreat Hospital, Richmond, VA, p. A449
BALIK, M. Barbara, Ed.D., Administrator, United Hospital, Saint Paul, MN, p. A233
BALL, Donald M., President and Chief Executive Officer, Jackson Hospital and Clinic, Montgomery, AL, p. A17
BALLA, Ernest, R.N., Administrator, Johns Community Hospital, Taylor, TX, p. A431
BALLANTYNE, II, Reginald M., President, PMH Health Resources, Inc., Phoenix, AZ, p. B119
BALLARD, Bryan M., Chief Executive Officer, Mendocino Coast District Hospital, Fort Bragg, CA, p. A41
BALLARD, Carolyn M., Executive Director, Virtua West Jersey Hospital–Camden, Camden, NJ, p. A275
BALLARD, Paul H., Chief Executive Officer, Mission Hospital, Mission, TX, p. A424
BALLARD, Susan, Administrator, Menifee Valley Medical Center, Sun City, CA, p. A64
BALLARD, William J., Chief Executive Officer, Children's Comprehensive Services, Inc., Nashville, TN, p. B71
BALSAM, Marion, USN, Commander, Naval Medical Center, Portsmouth, VA, p. A448
BALTZ, Richard J., Director, Veterans Affairs Medical Center, Fayetteville, NC, p. A313
BALTZER, David J., President, Rehoboth McKinley Christian Hospital, Gallup, NM, p. A285
BAMBERG, Barbara, Chief Administrative Officer, Sonoma Valley Hospital, Sonoma, CA, p. A63
BAN, Jr, Albert, Administrator, Thomasville Infirmary, Thomasville, AL, p. A18
BANE, Raymond, Executive Director, Natchez Community Hospital, Natchez, MS, p. A241
BANGS, Kathryn A., President and Chief Executive Officer, Clinton Memorial Hospital, Saint Johns, MI, p. A222
BANK, Kendall C., Administrator, Northfield Hospital, Northfield, MN, p. A231
BANKS, Elizabeth, Chief Executive Officer, Pauline Warfield Lewis Center, Cincinnati, OH, p. A328
BARB, Thomas D., Executive Director, Brooksville Regional Hospital, Brooksville, FL, p. A82
BARBAKOW, Jeffrey, Chairman and Chief Executive Officer, TENET Healthcare Corporation, Santa Barbara, CA, p. B139
BARBATO, Anthony L., M.D., President and Chief Executive Officer, Loyola University Medical Center, Maywood, IL, p. A130
BARBE, Brian S., Chief Executive Officer, Katy Medical Center, Katy, TX, p. A420
BARBER, Jack W., M.D., Director, Western State Hospital, Staunton, VA, p. A450
BARBER, Jeffrey B., Dr.PH
  President and Chief Executive Officer, North Mississippi Health Services, Inc., Tupelo, MS, p. B115
  President and Chief Executive Officer, North Mississippi Medical Center, Tupelo, MS, p. A242
BARBER, Steve, Administrator, Dorminy Medical Center, Fitzgerald, GA, p. A105
BARBERA, Sal A., FACHE, Administrator, South Florida State Hospital, Pembroke Pines, FL, p. A92
BARBINI, Gerald J., Administrator and Chief Executive Officer, Hubbard Regional Hospital, Webster, MA, p. A209
BARCO, Lawrence F., President, MidMichigan Medical Center–Clare, Clare, MI, p. A213
BARD, Thomas, Chief Executive Officer, Spring Hill Regional Hospital, Spring Hill, FL, p. A95
BARKER, Richard, Administrator, Mercy Health Love County, Marietta, OK, p. A344
BARKER, Elizabeth R., Commanding Officer, Naval Hospital, Corpus Christi, TX, p. A407
BARNARD, Thomas, Chief Executive Officer, Spring Brook Behavioral Healthcare System, Travelers Rest, SC, p. A384
BARNER, James W., President and Chief Executive Officer, Altoona Hospital, Altoona, PA, p. A355
BARNES, John, Administrator, Bradley Memorial Hospital, Cleveland, TN, p. A391
BARNETT, Gary L., President and Chief Executive Officer, Sarah Bush Lincoln Health Center, Mattoon, IL, p. A130
BARNETT, James L., Administrator, Hamlin Memorial Hospital, Hamlin, TX, p. A415
BARNETT, Richard J., Executive Vice President and Chief Operating Officer, Mercy Medical Center Mount Shasta, Mount Shasta, CA, p. A52
BARNETT, Timothy, Chief Executive Officer, Yavapai Regional Medical Center, Prescott, AZ, p. A25
BARNHART, Ann, Executive Director, Franklin Regional Medical Center, Louisburg, NC, p. A315
BARNHART, James, Chief Executive Officer, Peace Harbor Hospital, Florence, OR, p. A351
BARON, David A., D.O., Medical Director, Horsham Clinic, Ambler, PA, p. A355
BARR, LuAnn, Administrator, Tilden Community Hospital, Tilden, NE, p. A267
BARRAGAN, J. Bruce, President and Chief Executive Officer, McLeod Regional Medical Center, Florence, SC, p. A381
BARRETO, Hector, M.D., Director, Hospital Dr. Susoni, Arecibo, PR, p. A481
BARRETT, David M., M.D., Chief Executive Officer, Lahey Clinic Hospital, Burlington, MA, p. A203
BARRETT, John E., Administrator, Flandreau Municipal Hospital/Avera Health, Flandreau, SD, p. A386
BARRETT, Susan, President and Chief Executive Officer, St. Mary–Rogers Memorial Hospital, Rogers, AR, p. A33
BARRETT, Jr, William, Chief of Staff, William Beaumont Army Medical Center, El Paso, TX, p. A412
BARRON, Kathleen, Executive Director, Episcopal Hospital, Philadelphia, PA, p. A366
BARRON, Steven R.
  President and Chief Executive Officer, Regional Medical Center of San Jose, San Jose, CA, p. A60
  President, St. Bernardine Medical Center, San Bernardino, CA, p. A58
BARROW, William F., President and Chief Executive Officer, De Soto Regional Health System, Mansfield, LA, p. A185
BARRY, Dennis R., President, Moses Cone Health System, Greensboro, NC, p. A313
BARRY, R. Michael
  Chief Executive Officer, Jupiter Medical Center, Jupiter, FL, p. A87
  Administrator, Plumas District Hospital, Quincy, CA, p. A56
BARRY, Suzanne, Administrator and Chief Operating Officer, Hartgrove Hospital, Chicago, IL, p. A121
BARSZCZEWSKI, Joseph, Chief Executive Officer and Managing Director, Meadows Psychiatric Center, Centre Hall, PA, p. A357
BARTELL, II, Frank J., President and Chief Executive Officer, St. Luke's Hospital, Maumee, OH, p. A335
BARTELS, Bruce M., President, South Central Community Health, York, PA, p. B135
BARTLESON, Warner H., Administrator, North Valley Hospital, Tonasket, WA, p. A458
BARTLETT, John D., Chief Executive Officer, Palms of Pasadena Hospital, Saint Petersburg, FL, p. A94
BARTLETT, John T., Director, Searcy Hospital, Mount Vernon, AL, p. A17
BARTLETT, II, Thomas G., Chief Executive Officer, Tyrone Hospital, Tyrone, PA, p. A373
BARTO, Jr, John K., Interim President and Chief Executive Officer, Provena Mercy Center, Aurora, IL, p. A119
BARTON, Donald L., Superintendent, Southeast Missouri Mental Health Center, Farmington, MO, p. A246
BARTON, Larry O., President, Western Baptist Hospital, Paducah, KY, p. A177
BARTON, Rod, Chief Executive Officer, Powell Hospital, Powell, WY, p. A479
BARTOS, John M., Administrator, Marcus Daly Memorial Hospital, Hamilton, MT, p. A258
BARTZ, Daniel R., Chief Executive Officer, Cloud County Health Center, Concordia, KS, p. A160
BASH, Robert R., Administrator, Booneville Community Hospital, Booneville, AR, p. A28
BASHAM, Gail S., Chief Executive Officer, Mount Regis Center, Salem, VA, p. A449
BASLER, Jack, President, Henry County Memorial Hospital, New Castle, IN, p. A144
BASTONE, Peter F., President and Chief Executive Officer, Mission Hospital Regional Medical Center, Mission Viejo, CA, p. A51
BATAL, Lucille M., Administrator, Baldpate Hospital, Haverhill, MA, p. A205
BATCHELDER, Chester G., Superintendent, New Hampshire Hospital, Concord, NH, p. A271
BATEMAN, Steven B., Chief Executive Officer, Ogden Regional Medical Center, Ogden, UT, p. A437
BATES, Jonathan R., M.D., President and Chief Executive Officer, Arkansas Children's Hospital, Little Rock, AR, p. A31
BATES, Rodney, Administrator, Logan County Hospital, Oakley, KS, p. A165

Index of Health Care Professionals / Batt

BATT, Richard A., President and Chief Executive Officer, Franklin Memorial Hospital, Farmington, ME, p. A192
BATTIN, Anne, Administrator, Charter Charleston Behavioral Health System, Charleston, SC, p. A379
BATTISTA, Donald P., President and Chief Executive Officer, Garrett County Memorial Hospital, Oakland, MD, p. A199
BATULIS, Scott, Vice President and Administrator, Bethesda Rehabilitation Hospital, Saint Paul, MN, p. A233
BAUER, Clifford J., Chief Executive Officer, North Ridge Medical Center, Fort Lauderdale, FL, p. A84
BAUER, Robert, Administrator, Smith Hospital, Hahira, GA, p. A105
BAUM, Carla S., President, St. Joseph Hospital of Kirkwood, Saint Louis, MO, p. A253
BAUMGARDNER, Brian P., Administrator, Bartow Memorial Hospital, Bartow, FL, p. A81
BAUMGART, Kris, Chief Executive Officer, Stewart Memorial Community Hospital, Lake City, IA, p. A154
BAUMGARTNER, Michael, President, St. Francis Hospital and Health Services, Maryville, MO, p. A250
BAUTE, Robert E., M.D., President and Chief Executive Officer, Kent County Memorial Hospital, Warwick, RI, p. A377
BAXTER, W. Eugene, FACHE, Interim Administrator, Integris Baptist Regional Health Center, Miami, OK, p. A345
BEA, Javon R., President and Chief Executive Officer, Mercy Health System, Janesville, WI, p. A469
BEACH, Allen L., Administrator, Columbia Basin Hospital, Ephrata, WA, p. A453
BEAMAN, Jr, Charles D., President, Palmetto Health Alliance, Columbia, SC, p. B118
BEAMER, Deane E., President and Chief Executive Officer, St. Luke's Hospital, Bluefield, WV, p. A460
BEAR, Lawrence P., Administrator, Jersey Community Hospital, Jerseyville, IL, p. A128
BEARD, Les, Chief Executive Officer, Emory Eastside Medical Center, Snellville, GA, p. A109
BEARDSLEY, David L., Administrator, University Behavioral Center, Orlando, FL, p. A92
BEASLEY, Lynn W., President and Chief Executive Officer, Newberry County Memorial Hospital, Newberry, SC, p. A382
BEATY, Ralph E., Administrator, Huntsville Memorial Hospital, Huntsville, TX, p. A419
BEAUCHAMP, John W., Chief Executive Officer, Medical Center of Winnie, Winnie, TX, p. A435
BEAUCHAMP, Philip K., FACHE
President and Chief Executive Officer, Morton Plant Hospital, Clearwater, FL, p. A82
President and Chief Executive Officer, Morton Plant Mease Health Care, Dunedin, FL, p. B112
BEAUREGARD, Jodi, Chief Executive Officer, North Georgia Medical Center, Ellijay, GA, p. A104
BEAUVAIS, Richard E., Ph.D., Chief Executive Officer, Wellspring Foundation, Bethlehem, CT, p. A74
BEAVERS, Michael, Chief Executive Officer, Piedmont Behavioral Health Center, Leesburg, VA, p. A445
BEBOW, Gary, Administrator and Chief Executive Officer, White River Medical Center, Batesville, AR, p. A28
BECHTOLD, Gregg A., President and Chief Executive Officer, Johnson Memorial Hospital, Franklin, IN, p. A140
BECK, E. Dean, Administrator, Fulton County Health Center, Wauseon, OH, p. A339
BECK, Gary E., Administrator, Sevier Valley Hospital, Richfield, UT, p. A438
BECK, Joyce, Administrator, Genoa Community Hospital, Genoa, NE, p. A263
BECK, Judi, Administrator and Chief Executive Officer, Mayers Memorial Hospital District, Fall River Mills, CA, p. A41
BECK, Lawrence M., President and Chief Executive Officer, Good Samaritan Hospital of Maryland, Baltimore, MD, p. A195
BECK, Raymond J., President and Chief Executive Officer, UPMC Passavant, Pittsburgh, PA, p. A370
BECK, Steve, Chief Executive Officer and Administrator, Memorial Hospital, Seminole, TX, p. A430
BECK, Walter G., Chief Executive Officer, George L. Mee Memorial Hospital, King City, CA, p. A45

BECKER, Michael, Executive Director, Devereux Hospital and Children's Center of Florida, Melbourne, FL, p. A89
BECKER, Walter S., Chief Executive Officer, Carthage Area Hospital, Carthage, NY, p. A290
BECKER, Wayne, Interim Chief Executive Officer, Arden Hill Hospital, Goshen, NY, p. A292
BECKMAN, Gregory L., President and Chief Executive Officer, McLaren Regional Medical Center, Flint, MI, p. A215
BECKSTRAND, James E.
Administrator, Delta Community Medical Center, Delta, UT, p. A436
Administrator, Fillmore Community Medical Center, Fillmore, UT, p. A436
BEDNAREK, Robert J., President and Chief Executive Officer, Transylvania Community Hospital, Brevard, NC, p. A310
BEEKMAN, Marge, Facility Director, Community Medical Center–Fresno, Fresno, CA, p. A42
BEELER, Don A., President and Chief Executive Officer, Christus St. Michael Health System, Texarkana, TX, p. A432
BEEMAN, Barry G., President and Chief Executive Officer, Atlantic General Hospital, Berlin, MD, p. A196
BEEMAN, Thomas E., President and Chief Executive Officer, St. Thomas Health Services, Nashville, TN, p. A398
BEGAY, R. C., Chief Executive Officer, Acoma–Canoncito–Laguna Hospital, San Fidel, NM, p. A286
BEGLEY, Bruce D., Executive Director, Methodist Hospital, Henderson, KY, p. A173
BEHRENS, B. Lyn
President, Loma Linda University Health Sciences Center, Loma Linda, CA, p. B106
President and Chief Executive Officer, Loma Linda University Medical Center, Loma Linda, CA, p. A46
BEIER, Gregory J., President, Forsyth Medical Center, Winston–Salem, NC, p. A320
BEIL, Clark R., Chief Executive Officer, Johnston Memorial Hospital, Abingdon, VA, p. A442
BEIRNE, Frank, Chief Executive Officer, Samaritan Hospital, Lexington, KY, p. A174
BELMONT, Terry A., Administrator, Kaiser Foundation Hospital, San Diego, CA, p. A58
BEN, Nella, Chief Executive Officer, U. S. Public Health Service Indian Hospital, San Carlos, AZ, p. A25
BENDER, Ronald, Chief Executive Officer, Clay County Medical Center, Clay Center, KS, p. A160
BENEDICT, William, Executive Director, Elmira Psychiatric Center, Elmira, NY, p. A291
BENFER, David W., FACHE, President and Chief Executive Officer, Hospital of Saint Raphael, New Haven, CT, p. A76
BENFORD, Barry C., Director, Altoona Center, Altoona, PA, p. A355
BENGTSON, Paul R., Chief Executive Officer, Northeastern Vermont Regional Hospital, Saint Johnsbury, VT, p. A441
BENN, David P., President and Chief Executive Officer, Memorial Hospitals Association, Modesto, CA, p. A51
BENNETT, Bruce A., Administrator, Carl Albert Indian Health Facility, Ada, OK, p. A341
BENNETT, John, President and Chief Executive Officer, Shelby Memorial Hospital, Shelbyville, IL, p. A134
BENNETT, Mark, Administrator and Chief Executive Officer, HEALTHSOUTH Rehabilitation Hospital–Cityview, Fort Worth, TX, p. A413
BENNETT, Richard, Executive Director, Mid–Hudson Forensic Psychiatric Center, New Hampton, NY, p. A295
BENNING, Robert J., Chief Executive Officer, Ridgeview Psychiatric Hospital and Center, Oak Ridge, TN, p. A398
BENSAIA, Barbara A., Chief Executive Officer, Canonsburg General Hospital, Canonsburg, PA, p. A357
BENTON, Lowell S., Executive Director, Woodland Medical Center, Cullman, AL, p. A13
BERARD, Celse A., President, Riverview Hospital Association, Wisconsin Rapids, WI, p. A477

BERAULT, John S., Chief Executive Officer, Medical Center of Louisiana at New Orleans, New Orleans, LA, p. A186
BERDAN, Barclay E., President, Harris Methodist Fort Worth, Fort Worth, TX, p. A412
BERGENFELD, Joel, Chief Executive Officer, Florida Medical Center, Fort Lauderdale, FL, p. A84
BERGER, Susan, Prioress, Benedictine Sisters of the Annunciation, Bismarck, ND, p. B60
BERGERSON, Doris, Interim Administrator, Martin County Hospital District, Stanton, TX, p. A431
BERGLING, Richard Q., Administrator and Chief Executive Officer, Plainville Rural Hospital District Number One, Plainville, KS, p. A166
BERGREN, Jeff, Chief Executive Officer and Administrator, BHC Streamwood Hospital, Streamwood, IL, p. A135
BERLUCCHI, Scott A., President and Chief Executive Officer, Lancaster General Hospital–Susquehanna Division, Columbia, PA, p. A358
BERMAN, Michael A., M.D., Executive Vice President and Director, New York–Presbyterian Hospital, New York, NY, p. A299
BERNARD, Mark L.
Chief Executive Officer, Metropolitan Methodist Hospital, San Antonio, TX, p. A429
Chief Executive Officer, Northeast Methodist Hospital, San Antonio, TX, p. A429
BERNARD, Patricia, R.N., Administrator, Osborne County Memorial Hospital, Osborne, KS, p. A166
BERNARD, Peter J.
President and Chief Executive Officer, CARITAS Medical Center, Louisville, KY, p. A175
President and Chief Executive Officer, CARITAS Peace Center, Louisville, KY, p. A175
BERND, David L., Chief Executive Officer, Sentara Healthcare, Norfolk, VA, p. B131
BERNIER, Mark F., Director, Naval Hospital, Pensacola, FL, p. A93
BERNSTEIN, Martin B., Chief Executive Officer, Northern Maine Medical Center, Fort Kent, ME, p. A192
BERNSTEIN, Ronald T., Chief Executive Officer, Foundations Behavioral Health, Doylestown, PA, p. A359
BERNSTEIN, Stephen, FACHE, Chief Executive Officer, Plaza Medical Center of Fort Worth, Fort Worth, TX, p. A413
BERO, Joan A., Regional Vice President and Chief Operating Officer, O'Connor Hospital, San Jose, CA, p. A60
BERRETT, Britt, President and Chief Executive Officer, Medical City Dallas Hospital, Dallas, TX, p. A409
BERRIDGE, Linda, Chief Executive Officer, Two Rivers Psychiatric Hospital, Kansas City, MO, p. A249
BERRY, Robert F., Chief Executive Officer, Specialty Hospital of Austin, Austin, TX, p. A403
BERRY, Stan B., FACHE, Administrator, Sierra–Kings District Hospital, Reedley, CA, p. A57
BERSANTE, Syd, Chief of Operations, St. Clare Hospital, Lakewood, WA, p. A454
BERTSCH, Darrold, Administrator, St. Luke's Tri–State Hospital, Bowman, ND, p. A321
BESTUL, Randy, Administrator, Norwood Health Center, Marshfield, WI, p. A471
BESWICK, Melinda D., President, California Hospital Medical Center, Los Angeles, CA, p. A47
BETJEMANN, John H., President, Methodist Hospitals, Gary, IN, p. A140
BETTS, Peter J., President and Chief Executive Officer, East Jefferson General Hospital, Metairie, LA, p. A185
BEUTLER, Geri, Chief Executive Officer, Edgemont Hospital, Los Angeles, CA, p. A47
BEVERLY, Ken B., President and Chief Executive Officer, Archbold Medical Center, Thomasville, GA, p. B53
BEVINS, O. David, Chief Executive Officer, Kentucky River Medical Center, Jackson, KY, p. A173
BEYER, Robert L., President and Chief Executive Officer, Saint Joseph's Regional Medical Center–South Bend Campus, South Bend, IN, p. A146
BHATIA, Krishin L., Administrator, Victory Memorial Hospital, New York, NY, p. A300
BIANCHI, Charles A., President, Hillsdale Community Health Center, Hillsdale, MI, p. A217

BICH, Arlene C., Administrator, Wagner Community Memorial Hospital, Wagner, SD, p. A388
BICKELMAN, Carol, President and Chief Executive Officer, Desert Hills Hospital, Albuquerque, NM, p. A283
BICKLING, J. Allan, Chief Executive Officer, Edward W. McCready Memorial Hospital, Crisfield, MD, p. A197
BIEDIGER, Michael J., President, Lexington Medical Center, West Columbia, SC, p. A384
BIEGANSKI, Gary, President, Community Hospital, McCook, NE, p. A264
BIEHNER, Barbara H., Chief Executive Officer, Bon Secours–Holy Family Regional Health System, Altoona, PA, p. A355
BIERMAN, Ronald L., Chief Executive Officer, Lower Keys Medical Center, Key West, FL, p. A87
BIESTER, Doris J., R.N., President and Chief Executive Officer, Children's Hospital, Denver, CO, p. A69
BIGA, Thomas A., Executive Director, Clara Maass Health System, Belleville, NJ, p. A274
BIGELOW, David C., Chief Executive Officer, North Lincoln Hospital, Lincoln City, OR, p. A352
BIGLEY, Robert F., Administrator, Dale Medical Center, Ozark, AL, p. A17
BIHLDORFF, John P., President and Chief Executive Officer, Newton–Wellesley Hospital, Newton Lower Falls, MA, p. A207
BILBO, Dorothy C., Administrator, Pearl River County Hospital, Poplarville, MS, p. A241
BILL, Charles E., CHE, Chief Executive Officer, Cobre Valley Community Hospital, Globe, AZ, p. A23
BILLIK, Dean S., Director, Central Texas Veterans Affairs Healthcare System, Temple, TX, p. A431
BILLING, Michael D., Administrator, Mid–Valley Hospital, Omak, WA, p. A455
BILLINGSLEY, Linn P., Administrator, Vencor Hospital–Las Vegas, Las Vegas, NV, p. A269
BILLS, Jeff K., Chief Executive Officer, Saint Mary's Regional Medical Center, Reno, NV, p. A269
BILLS, Robert C., President and Vice Chairman, Valley Presbyterian Hospital, Los Angeles, CA, p. A50
BING, William W., Administrator, Morehouse General Hospital, Bastrop, LA, p. A180
BIRCHELL, Bruce K.
  Administrator and Chief Executive Officer, Greenwood County Hospital, Eureka, KS, p. A161
  Chief Executive Officer, Morton County Health System, Elkhart, KS, p. A160
BIRDZELL, JoAnn
  President and Chief Executive Officer, St. Catherine Hospital, East Chicago, IN, p. A139
  President and Chief Executive Officer, St. Elizabeth's Hospital, Chicago, IL, p. A123
BISCARO, Ron, Administrator and Chief Operating Officer, St. Francis Medical Center of Santa Barbara, Santa Barbara, CA, p. A62
BISCHALANEY, George, President and Chief Executive Officer, Eden Medical Center, Castro Valley, CA, p. A38
BISCONE, Mark A., Executive Director, Waldo County General Hospital, Belfast, ME, p. A191
BISHOP, Marvin O., Chief Executive Officer and Administrator, Weisbrod Memorial County Hospital, Eads, CO, p. A70
BISHOP, Paul A., Administrator, Wellmont Lonesome Pine Hospital, Big Stone Gap, VA, p. A442
BISSEL, Jane, President and Chief Executive Officer, Mercy Hospital, Valley City, ND, p. A324
BITTING, Nancy J., Regional Chief Executive Officer, St. Joseph Hospital, Bellingham, WA, p. A452
BJELICH, Steven E., President and Chief Executive Officer, Saint Francis Medical Center, Cape Girardeau, MO, p. A245
BJELLA, Karmon T., Chief Executive Officer, Unity Hospital, Muscatine, IA, p. A154
BLACK, Gary E., President and Chief Executive Officer, Lenoir Memorial Hospital, Kinston, NC, p. A315
BLACK, Glenn, Associate Vice President and Chief Operating Officer, Henry Ford Kingswood Hospital, Ferndale, MI, p. A214
BLACKBURN, David, President, Arkansas Heart Hospital, Little Rock, AR, p. A31
BLAIR, John E., Chief Executive, Ravenswood Hospital Medical Center, Chicago, IL, p. A122

BLAKLEY, Scott F., Chief Executive Officer, Brentwood, a Behavioral Health Company, Shreveport, LA, p. A188
BLANCHARD, Stephen C., Director, Edgewater Psychiatric Center, Harrisburg, PA, p. A361
BLANCHARD, William R., Chief Executive Officer, DeTar Hospital, Victoria, TX, p. A433
BLANCHER, William R., Chief Executive Officer, Regional Medical Center, Victoria, TX, p. A433
BLANCHETTE, Edward A., M.D., Director, Connecticut Department of Correction's Hospital, Somers, CT, p. A77
BLAND, Edward C., President and Chief Executive Officer, Healdsburg General Hospital, Healdsburg, CA, p. A43
BLAND, Thomas, Administrator, Montfort Jones Memorial Hospital, Kosciusko, MS, p. A239
BLANK, Arthur, Chief Executive Officer, Mount Desert Island Hospital, Bar Harbor, ME, p. A191
BLASBAND, Charles A., Chief Executive Officer, Citrus Memorial Hospital, Inverness, FL, p. A86
BLAUM, V. Gail, President, Mercy Hospital of Wilkes–Barre, Wilkes–Barre, PA, p. A374
BLEAKNEY, David A., Administrator, Angleton–Danbury General Hospital, Angleton, TX, p. A401
BLEIBERG, Efrain, M.D., President and Chief of Staff, C. F. Menninger Memorial Hospital, Topeka, KS, p. A168
BLESSING, William H., President, Mary Free Bed Hospital and Rehabilitation Center, Grand Rapids, MI, p. A215
BLESSITT, H. J., Administrator, South Sunflower County Hospital, Indianola, MS, p. A238
BLEVINS, Barbara S., President, Peninsula Hospital, Louisville, TN, p. A395
BLEVINS, Maggie, Administrator, Jane Phillips Nowata Health Center, Nowata, OK, p. A345
BLEYER, Alan J., President, Akron General Medical Center, Akron, OH, p. A325
BLODGETT, Ruth P., Chief Operating Officer, Berkshire Medical Center, Pittsfield, MA, p. A207
BLOME', Michael, Administrator, Methodist Healthcare–Somerville, Somerville, TN, p. A399
BLOOM, Russell, Chief Executive Officer, Alta District Hospital, Dinuba, CA, p. A40
BLOUGH, Jr, Daniel D., Chief Executive Officer, Punxsutawney Area Hospital, Punxsutawney, PA, p. A371
BLOUNT, Karen, R.N., Chief Operating Officer, Children's Hospital, Buffalo, NY, p. A289
BLOUNT, Kenneth, President and Chief Executive Officer, The Monroe Clinic, Monroe, WI, p. A472
BLUFORD, John W., Executive Director and Chief Executive Officer, Truman Health System, Kansas City, MO, p. B145
BLUM, Joanne M., Administrator, Veterans Home and Hospital, Rocky Hill, CT, p. A76
BLUM, Robert W., FACHE, Administrator, Choctaw Nation Health Care Center, Talihina, OK, p. A348
BLYTHE, Nicholas R.
  Interim Administrator and Chief Executive Officer, Pecos County General Hospital, Iraan, TX, p. A419
  Interim Administrator and Chief Executive Officer, Pecos County Memorial Hospital, Fort Stockton, TX, p. A412
BOARDMAN, Debra, Chief Executive Officer, Riverwood HealthCare Center, Aitkin, MN, p. A225
BOBBS, Kathy J., Chief Executive Officer, Riverview Medical Center, Gonzales, LA, p. A182
BOBELDYK, Jerry, Administrator, Murray County Memorial Hospital, Slayton, MN, p. A233
BOECKER, Thomas J., President and Chief Executive Officer, Wilson Memorial Hospital, Sidney, OH, p. A337
BOEHLER, Sharron D., Commissioner, Oklahoma State Department of Mental Health and Substance Abuse Services, Oklahoma City, OK, p. B117
BOEHRINGER, Paul, Executive Director, Temple University Hospital, Philadelphia, PA, p. A368
BOERBOOM, Jerry, Chief Executive Officer, Minnesota Valley Health Center, Le Sueur, MN, p. A229
BOETTCHER, William V., Chief Executive Officer, Fletcher Allen Health Care, Burlington, VT, p. A440
BOFF, Michael G., President, Trillium Hospital, Albion, MI, p. A211

BOGAN, James, Chief Executive Officer, Portage Health System, Hancock, MI, p. A216
BOGGS, Danny L., President and Chief Executive Officer, Memorial Hospital, Marysville, OH, p. A334
BOGGS, Lynn Ingram, President and Chief Executive Officer, Community General Hospital of Thomasville, Thomasville, NC, p. A319
BOGGUS, Jr, Solon H., Interim Chief Executive Officer, Colorado Plains Medical Center, Fort Morgan, CO, p. A70
BOHL, Jim, President and Chief Executive Officer, Doctors Hospital, Springfield, IL, p. A135
BOHNE', Mary S., Administrator, Sandypines, Tequesta, FL, p. A97
BOLANDIS, Jerry L., CPA, Administrator and Chief Executive Officer, Pinckneyville Community Hospital, Pinckneyville, IL, p. A133
BOLCHERS, Alfredo, Executive Vice President, Hospital Pavia–Hato Rey, San Juan, PR, p. A483
BOLD, Harry, Administrator, Big Sandy Medical Center, Big Sandy, MT, p. A256
BOLD, Joan A., Commanding Officer, Naval Hospital, Cherry Point, NC, p. A311
BOLEWARE, Mike, Administrator, Prentiss Regional Hospital and Extended Care Facilities, Prentiss, MS, p. A242
BONAR, Jr, Robert I., President and Chief Executive Officer, Children's Hospital of The King's Daughters, Norfolk, VA, p. A447
BOND, C. Scott, Administrator and Chief Executive Officer, Providence St. Peter Hospital, Olympia, WA, p. A455
BONE, Jim G., Interim Administrator, Muleshoe Area Medical Center, Muleshoe, TX, p. A424
BONNER, Tucker, President, King's Daughters Hospital, Temple, TX, p. A432
BOOKER, Oliver J., Chief Executive Officer, Bacon County Hospital, Alma, GA, p. A99
BOOM, Marc, M.D., Chief Executive Officer, Diagnostic Center Hospital, Houston, TX, p. A416
BOONE, Richard, Executive Director, Crawford Memorial Hospital, Van Buren, AR, p. A34
BOOR, Leon J., Chief Executive Officer and Administrator, Memorial Hospital, Abilene, KS, p. A159
BOOTH, Patrick M., President, Winona Community Memorial Hospital, Winona, MN, p. A235
BOOTH, Peter G., President, Henrietta D. Goodall Hospital, Sanford, ME, p. A194
BOPP, James H.
  Executive Director, Middletown Psychiatric Center, Middletown, NY, p. A294
  Executive Director, Rockland Psychiatric Center, Orangeburg, NY, p. A302
BORDEN, John R., Administrator, Methodist Healthcare–McNairy Hospital, Selmer, TN, p. A399
BORDENKIRCHER, Kimberly, Chief Executive Officer, Henry County Hospital, Napoleon, OH, p. A335
BORENSTEIN, Jeffrey, M.D., Chief Executive Officer and Medical Director, Holliswood Hospital, New York, NY, p. A297
BORIES, Jr, Robert F., FACHE, Administrator, Shriners Hospitals for Children, Shriners Burns Hospital–Boston, Boston, MA, p. A202
BORING, Ronald L., President and Chief Executive Officer, Baylor/ Richardson Medical Center, Richardson, TX, p. A427
BORLAND, Winston, Chief Executive Officer, Northwest Regional Hospital, Corpus Christi, TX, p. A407
BORRONI, S. Denise, Administrator and Chief Executive Officer, HEALTHSOUTH Rehabilitation Hospital of Fort Worth, Fort Worth, TX, p. A413
BOSK, Nathan, FACHE, Chief Executive Officer, Lower Bucks Hospital, Bristol, PA, p. A356
BOSSARD, Karen L., Administrator and Chief Executive Officer, Greene County Medical Center, Jefferson, IA, p. A153
BOSWELL, Bill, Chief Executive Officer, McCamey Hospital, McCamey, TX, p. A423
BOUFFARD, Rodney, Superintendent, Augusta Mental Health Institute, Augusta, ME, p. A191
BOUGHTON, Charles M., Chief Executive Officer, Northeast Regional Medical Center–Jefferson Campus, Kirksville, MO, p. A249

BOUIS, Charles, President and Chief Executive Officer, Edward A. Utlaut Memorial Hospital, Greenville, IL, p. A127

BOULA, Rodney C., Administrator, Clifton-Fine Hospital, Star Lake, NY, p. A305

BOULENGER, Bo, Chief Executive Officer, Homestead Hospital, Homestead, FL, p. A86

BOUNDS, Floyd D., Administrator, Madison Medical Center, Fredericktown, MO, p. A246

BOUR, Thomas C., Administrator, Mayo Clinic Hospital, Phoenix, AZ, p. A24

BOURASSA, Robert N., Executive Director, Trinity Springs Pavilion, Fort Worth, TX, p. A413

BOURDON, Donna, Chief Operating Officer, HEALTHSOUTH Chattanooga Rehabilitation Hospital, Chattanooga, TN, p. A391

BOURGEOIS, Jeff A., Chief Executive Officer, Hill Country Memorial Hospital, Fredericksburg, TX, p. A413

BOURGEOIS, Jr, Milton D., Administrator, St. Anne General Hospital, Raceland, LA, p. A188

BOVENDER, Jr, Jack O., President and Chief Operating Officer, HCA – The Healthcare Company, Nashville, TN, p. B88

BOWE, Larry, JD, Chief Executive Officer, Providence Hood River Memorial Hospital, Hood River, OR, p. A351

BOWEN, Claire L., Chief Executive Officer, Valley Regional Hospital, Claremont, NH, p. A271

BOWEN, Don, Superintendent, Griffin Memorial Hospital, Norman, OK, p. A345

BOWEN, Steve, President, East Texas Medical Center Jacksonville, Jacksonville, TX, p. A419

BOWERS, Robert, Chief Executive Officer, Veterans Memorial Hospital of Meigs County, Pomeroy, OH, p. A336

BOWERS, Robert A., Chief Executive Officer, Oak Hill Community Medical Center, Oak Hill, OH, p. A336

BOWERS, Susan P., Acting Director, Richard L. Roudebush Veterans Affairs Medical Center, Indianapolis, IN, p. A141

BOWERSOX, Bruce D.
Administrator and Chief Executive Officer, Griggs County Hospital and Nursing Home, Cooperstown, ND, p. A321
Administrator, Hillsboro Medical Center, Hillsboro, ND, p. A322

BOWMAN, Clarence W.
Chief Executive Officer, Carolinas Hospital System–Kingstree, Kingstree, SC, p. A382
Chief Executive Officer, Carolinas Hospital System–Lake City, Lake City, SC, p. A382

BOWMAN, June C., R.N., Chief Operating Officer and Nurse Executive, St. Joseph Medical Center, Tacoma, WA, p. A458

BOWMAN, Leslie C., Senior Vice President Operations, Detroit Receiving Hospital and University Health Center, Detroit, MI, p. A213

BOWMAN, Michael R., Administrator, Litzenberg Memorial County Hospital, Central City, NE, p. A262

BOWMAN, Scott, Administrator, Sweetwater Hospital, Sweetwater, TN, p. A400

BOXX, Sue, Administrator, Lakeshore Community Hospital, Dadeville, AL, p. A13

BOYD, Charles E., Chief Executive Officer and Managing Director, Doctors' Hospital of Shreveport, Shreveport, LA, p. A188

BOYD, Christopher L., Chief Executive Officer and Managing Director, Inland Valley Regional Medical Center, Wildomar, CA, p. A67

BOYD, Wallace N., Administrator, Ochiltree General Hospital, Perryton, TX, p. A426

BOYER, Gregory E., Chief Executive Officer, Wellington Regional Medical Center, West Palm Beach, FL, p. A98

BOYLE, Steven P., President and Chief Executive Officer, St. Peter's Hospital, Albany, NY, p. A287

BOYLES, Jackie, Administrator, Cedar County Memorial Hospital, El Dorado Springs, MO, p. A246

BOYLES, Michael E., Chief Executive Officer, Citizens Medical Center, Colby, KS, p. A160

BOZEMAN, Larry C., Chief Executive Officer, Trinity Valley Medical Center, Palestine, TX, p. A425

BRABAND, Jon D., President and Chief Executive Officer, Glencoe Regional health Services, Glencoe, MN, p. A228

BRACE, Rod, Chief Executive Officer, Memorial Hermann Fort Bend Hospital, Missouri City, TX, p. A424

BRACHT, Gerald E., Vice President and Administrator, Palomar Medical Center, Escondido, CA, p. A40

BRACKIN, D. Wayne, Chief Executive Officer, South Miami Hospital, Miami, FL, p. A90

BRADDOM, Randall L., M.D., Chief Executive Officer and Medical Director, Wishard Health Services, Indianapolis, IN, p. A142

BRADFORD, Cleal, Executive Director, San Juan Hospital, Monticello, UT, p. A437

BRADFORD, Donald L., Chief Executive Officer, Gadsden Community Hospital, Quincy, FL, p. A94

BRADFORD, Roberta J., President and Chief Executive Officer, Drake Center, Cincinnati, OH, p. A327

BRADLEY, David K., CHE, Chief Executive Officer, Geary Community Hospital, Junction City, KS, p. A163

BRADLEY, Lucinda A., President, Great Plains Regional Medical Center, North Platte, NE, p. A265

BRADLEY, Jr, J. Lindsey, FACHE, President and Chief Administrative Officer, Trinity Mother Frances Health System, Tyler, TX, p. A433

BRADSHAW, Dorothy A., Director, Deer's Head Center, Salisbury, MD, p. A200

BRADWAY, Karen A., USAF, Administrator, U. S. Air Force Regional Hospital-Sheppard, Sheppard AFB, TX, p. A430

BRADY, Karl R., Chief Executive Officer, Pacific Gateway Hospital and Counseling Center, Portland, OR, p. A353

BRADY, Linda, M.D., President and Chief Executive Officer, Kingsbrook Jewish Medical Center, New York, NY, p. A297

BRADY, Patrick R., Chief Executive Officer, Sutter Roseville Medical Center, Roseville, CA, p. A57

BRADY, Timothy F., FACHE
Chief Executive Officer, Doctors Regional Medical Center, Poplar Bluff, MO, p. A251
Chief Executive Officer, Lucy Lee Hospital, Poplar Bluff, MO, p. A251

BRAMLETT, Jr, E. Chandler
President and Chief Executive Officer, Infirmary Health System, Inc., Mobile, AL, p. B100
President and Chief Executive Officer, Mobile Infirmary Medical Center, Mobile, AL, p. A16

BRANCO, Patrick, Administrator, Divine Providence Health Center/Avera Health, Ivanhoe, MN, p. A229

BRANDON, David R., Chief Executive Officer, Fayette Memorial Hospital, Connersville, IN, p. A138

BRANDT, Stephen, Interim Chief Executive Officer, Greenbrier Valley Medical Center, Ronceverte, WV, p. A464

BRANTLEY, Cheryl Y., Administrator, South Florida Evaluation and Treatment Center, Miami, FL, p. A90

BRASH, David L., Chief Executive Officer, Russell County Medical Center, Lebanon, VA, p. A445

BRASS, Alan W., FACHE, President and Chief Executive Officer, ProMedica Health System, Toledo, OH, p. B120

BRASSEAUX, Mary T., Chief Executive Officer, Abilene Regional Medical Center, Abilene, TX, p. A401

BRAZIER, Ray, President, Hillcrest Health Center, Oklahoma City, OK, p. A345

BRAZITIS, Mark A., President, Lancaster General Hospital, Lancaster, PA, p. A362

BREEDEN, Susan M., Administrator, Baptist Memorial Hospital–Huntingdon, Huntingdon, TN, p. A393

BREEN, John P., Chief Executive Officer, Massapequa General Hospital, Seaford, NY, p. A305

BREEN, Michael F., President, St. John NorthEast Community Hospital, Detroit, MI, p. A214

BREHE, Deborah, Chief Executive Officer, Mission Bay Hospital, San Diego, CA, p. A58

BREHM, Robert, President, Kessler Institute for Rehabilitation, West Orange, NJ, p. A281

BREITLING, Bryan, Administrator and Chief Executive Officer, Bowdle Hospital, Bowdle, SD, p. A385

BREKHUS, Pete, Chief Executive Officer, Madison Valley Hospital, Ennis, MT, p. A257

BREMER, Louis H., President and Chief Executive Officer, Wellmont Holston Valley Medical Center, Kingsport, TN, p. A394

BRENNAN, Charles L., Chief Executive Officer, St. Lawrence Rehabilitation Center, Lawrenceville, NJ, p. A277

BRENNAN, Darlene, Chief Executive Officer, BHC East Lake Hospital, New Orleans, LA, p. A186

BRENNAN, Donald A., President and Chief Executive Officer, Ascension Health, Saint Louis, MO, p. B53

BRENNY, Terrence, President and Chief Executive Officer, Stoughton Hospital Association, Stoughton, WI, p. A476

BRESSANELLI, Leo A., President and Chief Executive Officer, Genesis Medical Center, Davenport, IA, p. A150

BRETT, C. William, Ph.D., President and Chief Executive Officer, Windmoor Healthcare of Clearwater, Clearwater, FL, p. A82

BREWER, Gary L., Chief Executive Officer, Valley View Hospital, Glenwood Springs, CO, p. A70

BREWER, Rebecca T., CHE, Chief Executive Officer, Colleton Medical Center, Walterboro, SC, p. A384

BREXLER, James L., President and Chief Executive Officer, LSU Medical Center Health Care Services Division, Baton Rouge, LA, p. B106

BREZENOFF, Stanley, President, Maimonides Medical Center, New York, NY, p. A298

BRIDGES, James M., Executive Vice President and Chief Operating Officer, Palmetto Baptist Medical Center/Columbia, Columbia, SC, p. A379

BRIEN, Arthur L., Chief Executive Officer, Community General Hospital of Sullivan County, Harris, NY, p. A292

BRIERTY, Tim, Chief Executive Officer, McKenna Memorial Hospital, New Braunfels, TX, p. A425

BRIGGS, Ronald O., President, St. Francis Memorial Hospital, West Point, NE, p. A267

BRILEY, Ellen C., Administrator and Chief Executive Officer, Elba General Hospital, Elba, AL, p. A14

BRIMHALL, Dennis C., President, University of Colorado Hospital, Denver, CO, p. A70

BRINGHURST, John F., Administrator, Petersburg Medical Center, Petersburg, AK, p. A21

BRINKERS, Jack, CHE, Interim Chief Executive Officer, Northern Hills General Hospital, Deadwood, SD, p. A385

BRINSON, Patricia, Administrator, Wayne County Hospital, Monticello, KY, p. A176

BRITT, John H., Executive Director, Massachusetts Hospital School, Canton, MA, p. A204

BRITTON, Gregory K., President and Chief Executive Officer, Beloit Memorial Hospital, Beloit, WI, p. A466

BRIZZEE, Rita C., Chief Operating Officer, Waynesboro Hospital, Waynesboro, PA, p. A373

BROCCOLINO, Victor A., President and Chief Executive Officer, Howard County General Hospital, Columbia, MD, p. A197

BROCK, John D., Chief Executive Officer, Highland Medical Center, Lubbock, TX, p. A422

BROCKETI, John, Associate Vice President, Lutheran Hospital, Cleveland, OH, p. A329

BROCKETTE, Darby, Chief Executive Officer, HEALTHSOUTH Rehabilitation Center, Albuquerque, NM, p. A283

BROCKMANN, William F., President and Chief Executive Officer, Caylor-Nickel Medical Center, Bluffton, IN, p. A137

BRODEUR, Mark S., Chief Executive Officer, Jefferson Memorial Hospital, Crystal City, MO, p. A246

BRODHEAD, Robert T., President, St. John's Regional Health Center, Springfield, MO, p. A254

BRODY, Robert J., President and Chief Executive Officer, St. Francis Hospital and Health Centers – North Campus, Beech Grove, IN, p. A137

BRODY, Sue G.
President and Chief Executive Officer, Bayfront Medical Center, Saint Petersburg, FL, p. A94
President and Chief Executive Officer, St. Anthony's Hospital, Saint Petersburg, FL, p. A94

BROOKS, Jesse, M.D., Administrator, Brooks Hospital, Atlanta, TX, p. A402

BROOKS , II, J. Milton, Administrator, Pineville Community Hospital Association, Pineville, KY, p. A178
BROSIG, Joe, Administrator, Concho County Hospital, Eden, TX, p. A411
BROSSEAU, Terrance G., President and Chief Executive Officer, MedCenter One, Bismarck, ND, p. A321
BROTHERTON, Thomas J., Administrator, Shriners Hospitals for Children, Honolulu, Honolulu, HI, p. A112
BROTHMAN, Daniel, Chief Executive Officer, Western Medical Center–Santa Ana, Santa Ana, CA, p. A62
BROTMAN, Martin, M.D., President and Chief Executive Officer, California Pacific Medical Center, San Francisco, CA, p. A59
BROUSSARD, Clifford M., Chief Executive Officer, Lakewood Medical Center, Morgan City, LA, p. A186
BROUWER, Heath, Administrator, Douglas County Memorial Hospital, Armour, SD, p. A385
BROWER, Fred B., President and Chief Executive Officer, Trinity Health System, Steubenville, OH, p. A338
BROWN, Carl A., Administrator, Lakeview Community Hospital, Eufaula, AL, p. A14
BROWN, Cary D., Director, Veterans Affairs Medical Center, Big Spring, TX, p. A405
BROWN, Dan, Vice President Operations, Northeast Baptist Hospital, San Antonio, TX, p. A429
BROWN, David E., President and Chief Executive Officer, Beaufort Memorial Hospital, Beaufort, SC, p. A378
BROWN, David P., Administrator, Citizens Medical Center, Victoria, TX, p. A433
BROWN, Donald G., Chief Executive Officer, Community Medical Center at Western Illinois, Monmouth, IL, p. A130
BROWN, Harold W., Chief Executive Officer, Prairie du Chien Memorial Hospital, Prairie Du Chien, WI, p. A474
BROWN, Lennea F., Administrator, Bucktail Medical Center, Renovo, PA, p. A371
BROWN, Luella, Service Unit Director, U. S. Public Health Service Indian Hospital, Cass Lake, MN, p. A226
BROWN, Michael L., Interim Chief Executive Officer, Columbus Community Hospital, Columbus, OH, p. A330
BROWN, Murray L., Administrator, Neosho Memorial Regional Medical Center, Chanute, KS, p. A160
BROWN, Patricia W., Ph.D., Executive Director, Savannas Hospital, Port St. Lucie, FL, p. A93
BROWN, Randy, Interim Administrator, Buchanan General Hospital, Grundy, VA, p. A444
BROWN, Rex H., President, Hillsboro Area Hospital, Hillsboro, IL, p. A128
BROWN, Richard V., Chief Executive Officer, Livingston Memorial Hospital, Livingston, MT, p. A258
BROWN, Richard W., President and Chief Executive Officer, Health Midwest, Kansas City, MO, p. B95
BROWN, Robert A., Senior Vice President and Chief Operating Officer, Addison Community Hospital, Addison, MI, p. A211
BROWN, Scott R., Administrator and Chief Executive Officer, Moore County Hospital District, Dumas, TX, p. A410
BROWN, Shannon D., President, Betsy Johnson Regional Hospital, Dunn, NC, p. A311
BROWN, Steven E., Administrator, Inova Fairfax Hospital, Falls Church, VA, p. A443
BROWN, Terry, Administrator and Chief Executive Officer, HEALTHSOUTH Lakeshore Rehabilitation Hospital, Birmingham, AL, p. A12
BROWN, William A., CHE, Vice President and Administrator, Inova Fair Oaks Hospital, Fairfax, VA, p. A443
BROWN, G. R., Commanding Officer, U. S. Naval Hospital, Roosevelt Roads, PR, p. A484
BROWNE, J. Timothy, Chief Executive Officer, Loris Community Hospital, Loris, SC, p. A382
BROWNE, James N., Interim Chief Executive Officer, Sturgis Hospital, Sturgis, MI, p. A222
BROWNE, Norman E., Director, Veterans Affairs Medical Center, Albuquerque, NM, p. A284
BROWNLEE, Walter W., Interim Chief Executive Officer, Phelps Memorial Health Center, Holdrege, NE, p. A263
BROYLES, Dan P., CHE, Administrator, Harrison County Community Hospital, Bethany, MO, p. A244
BRUCE, Sandra B., President and Chief Executive Officer, Saint Alphonsus Regional Medical Center, Boise, ID, p. A115
BRUCE , Jr, Billy J., Chief Executive Officer, St. Joseph's Community Health Services, Hillsboro, WI, p. A469
BRUCKMAN, Donald A., Acting Chief Executive Officer, Senator Garrett T. W. Hagedorn Gero Psychiatric Hospital, Glen Gardner, NJ, p. A276
BRUECKNER, Geraldine, R.N.
Executive Director, Baylor Center for Restorative Care, Dallas, TX, p. A408
Executive Director, Our Children's House at Baylor, Dallas, TX, p. A409
BRUM, Joseph G., President and Chief Executive Officer, Henry Medical Center, Stockbridge, GA, p. A110
BRUMITT, Jerry D., President and Chief Executive Officer, Saint John's Health System, Anderson, IN, p. A137
BRUMLOW , Jr, James W., President and Chief Executive Officer, Wadsworth–Rittman Hospital, Wadsworth, OH, p. A338
BRUNDIGE, James E., Administrator, Haxtun Hospital District, Haxtun, CO, p. A71
BRUNICARDI, Rusty O., President, Community Hospitals of Williams County, Bryan, OH, p. A326
BRUNN, Donald I., Executive Vice President, Virtua Memorial Hospital Burlington County, Mount Holly, NJ, p. A278
BRUNO, Frank, Chief Executive Officer, Gracie Square Hospital, New York, NY, p. A296
BRUNS, Dennis Ray, President and Chief Executive Officer, Hilton Head Medical Center and Clinics, Hilton Head Island, SC, p. A382
BRUSS, Jonathan R., Chief Executive, Good Samaritan Hospital, Downers Grove, IL, p. A125
BRUZEK–KOHLER, Christine M., Commanding Officer, Naval Hospital, Lemoore, CA, p. A46
BRVENIK, Richard A., President and Chief Executive Officer, Windham Community Memorial Hospital, Willimantic, CT, p. A77
BRYAN, Jay, Chief Executive Officer, Lakeshore Community Hospital, Shelby, MI, p. A222
BRYAN, Margaret, Administrator, Shriners Hospitals for Children, Northern California, Sacramento, CA, p. A57
BRYAN, Marilyn, Administrator, Roger Mills Memorial Hospital, Cheyenne, OK, p. A342
BRYAN, Peter K., Chief Executive Officer, Kern Medical Center, Bakersfield, CA, p. A36
BRYANT, Len, Chief Executive Officer, Associates Capital Group, LLC, Birmingham, AL, p. B55
BRYANT, W. Michael, President and Chief Executive Officer, Methodist Medical Center of Illinois, Peoria, IL, p. A132
BRZUZ, Richard W., Administrator, Shriners Hospitals for Children, Erie, Erie, PA, p. A360
BUCHANAN, A. C., President and Chief Executive Officer, Rapides Regional Medical Center, Alexandria, LA, p. A180
BUCHANAN, Bruce F., FACHE, President and Chief Executive Officer, Atlanta Medical Center, Atlanta, GA, p. A99
BUCHANAN, Don, Chief Operating Officer, Aurora Community Hospital, Aurora, MO, p. A244
BUCHANAN, Georgia, President, Laird Hospital, Union, MS, p. A242
BUCHE, Daniel L., Chief Executive Officer, St. Joseph Regional Health Center, Bryan, TX, p. A405
BUCK, Jack S., Chief Executive Officer, Crockett Hospital, Lawrenceburg, TN, p. A395
BUCK, William G., Chief Executive Officer, Pasco Community Hospital, Dade City, FL, p. A83
BUCKLEY, Donald S., FACHE, President, Chesapeake General Hospital, Chesapeake, VA, p. A443
BUCKLEY, Howard R., President, Mercy Hospital of Portland, Portland, ME, p. A193
BUCKLEY, John J., President and Chief Executive Officer, Pottstown Memorial Medical Center, Pottstown, PA, p. A370
BUCKLEY , Jr, John J., President, Southern Illinois Hospital Services, Carbondale, IL, p. B135
BUCKNER, Wayne, Administrator, Baptist Hospital of Cocke County, Newport, TN, p. A398
BUCKNER , Jr, James E., Administrator, Cuero Community Hospital, Cuero, TX, p. A408
BUDNICK, Michael J., FACHE, Administrator and Chief Executive Officer, Gibson General Hospital, Princeton, IN, p. A145
BUDRYS, Raymond, Chief Executive Officer, Craven Regional Medical Authority, New Bern, NC, p. A316
BUHRMANN, Henry J., President and Chief Executive Officer, Marin General Hospital, Greenbrae, CA, p. A43
BULGER, Robert J., President and Chief Executive Officer, Jeannette District Memorial Hospital, Jeannette, PA, p. A362
BULL, Jayne R., Administrator, Leelanau Memorial Health Center, Northport, MI, p. A220
BULLOCK, Scott B., President, MaineGeneral Medical Center–Waterville Campus, Waterville, ME, p. A194
BUMGARNER, William, Chief Executive Officer, Avera Holy Family Hospital, Estherville, IA, p. A151
BUNCH, Jimm
President and Chief Executive Officer, Jellico Community Hospital, Jellico, TN, p. A394
President and Chief Executive Officer, Memorial Hospital, Manchester, KY, p. A176
BUNDY, William H., Chief Executive Officer, Chester County Hospital and Nursing Center, Chester, SC, p. A379
BUNKER, Stephen P., President, Holmes Regional Medical Center, Melbourne, FL, p. A89
BURCHILL, Kevin R., Chief Executive Officer, Martha's Vineyard Hospital, Oak Bluffs, MA, p. A207
BURD, Ronald P., President and Chief Executive Officer, Devereux Foundation, Villanova, PA, p. B82
BURDICK, Mindy, Executive Vice President and Chief Operating Officer, United Regional Health Care System, Wichita Falls, TX, p. A435
BURDICK, Steve, Administrator, Providence Centralia Hospital, Centralia, WA, p. A452
BURFEIND, Raymond F., President, Covenant Medical Center, Waterloo, IA, p. A157
BURGER, Janice, Operations Administrator, Providence Milwaukie Hospital, Milwaukie, OR, p. A352
BURGER, Ken, Superintendent, Mental Health Institute, Mount Pleasant, IA, p. A154
BURGESS, Roger M., Administrator, St. Francis Hospital, Escanaba, MI, p. A214
BURGHER, Louis W., Ph.D., President and Chief Executive Officer, Nebraska Health System, Omaha, NE, p. A265
BURGIN, Robert F., President and Chief Executive Officer, Mission St. Joseph's Health, Asheville, NC, p. A309
BURGIO, David E., FACHE, President and Chief Executive Officer, Berea Hospital, Berea, KY, p. A170
BURK, Judith, Administrator, Fort Washington Hospital, Fort Washington, MD, p. A198
BURKE, Dennis E., President, Good Shepherd Medical Center, Hermiston, OR, p. A351
BURKET, Mark, Chief Executive Officer, Platte Health Center/Avera Health, Platte, SD, p. A387
BURKETT, William T., Chief Executive Officer, Eastern State Hospital, Vinita, OK, p. A349
BURKHARD, Thomas, Commanding Officer, Naval Hospital, Camp Pendleton, CA, p. A37
BURKHARDT , Jr, J. Bland, Senior Vice President and Administrator, Greenville Memorial Hospital, Greenville, SC, p. A381
BURKLOW, Bryan D., Chief Executive Officer, Community Hospital Medical Center, Phoenix, AZ, p. A24
BURNETTE, W. Scott, President, Community Memorial Healthcenter, South Hill, VA, p. A450
BURNHAM, Ben, Administrator, Calhoun–Liberty Hospital, Blountstown, FL, p. A81
BURNS, Charlotte, Administrator and Chief Executive Officer, Hardin County General Hospital, Savannah, TN, p. A399
BURNS, Dennis R., FACHE, Chief Executive Officer, Summersville Memorial Hospital, Summersville, WV, p. A464

Index of Health Care Professionals / Burns

BURNS, Gregory T., Executive Director, St. Joseph's Community Hospital of West Bend, West Bend, WI, p. A477
BURNS, Randall P., Chief Executive Officer, Alaska Psychiatric Institute, Anchorage, AK, p. A20
BURNS, William A., Chief Executive Officer, Rio Grande Regional Hospital, McAllen, TX, p. A423
BURRIS, Bradley D., President and Chief Executive Officer, Oakes Community Hospital, Oakes, ND, p. A323
BURROUGHS, Michael R., FACHE, President and Chief Executive Officer, Medical Center of Arlington, Arlington, TX, p. A402
BURROWS, Jack A., Administrator, Hemet Valley Medical Center, Hemet, CA, p. A44
BURTON, W. R., Administrator, Memorial Hospital at Gulfport, Gulfport, MS, p. A238
BURZYNSKI, Cheryl A., President, Bay Special Care, Bay City, MI, p. A212
BUSCH, Walter S., Administrator, North Big Horn Hospital, Lovell, WY, p. A479
BUSER, Kenneth R.
  President and Chief Executive Officer, All Saint's Healthcare System, Racine, WI, p. A474
  President and Chief Executive Officer, St. Luke's Memorial Hospital, Racine, WI, p. A474
BUSH, Mark E., Executive Vice President, MidMichigan Medical Center–Gladwin, Gladwin, MI, p. A215
BUSHART, Phyllis, R.N., Chief Executive Officer, St. Luke Medical Center, Pasadena, CA, p. A55
BUSTELO, Miguel J., Executive Director, Dr. Pila's Hospital, Ponce, PR, p. A483
BUTIKOFER, Lon D., Ph.D., Chief Executive Officer, Regional Medical Center of Northeast Iowa and Delaware County, Manchester, IA, p. A154
BUTLER, Anita M., Chief Executive Officer, Spartanburg Hospital for Restorative Care, Spartanburg, SC, p. A383
BUTLER, Barbara, Administrator and Chief Operating Officer, HEALTHSOUTH Tri–State Rehabilitation Hospital, Evansville, IN, p. A139
BUTLER, Beatrice, Chief Executive Officer, Terrell State Hospital, Terrell, TX, p. A432
BUTLER, David, Chief Executive Officer, Paradise Valley Hospital, National City, CA, p. A53
BUTLER, Everett A., Chief Executive Officer, Unity Medical Center, Grafton, ND, p. A322
BUTLER, Frank, Director, University of Kentucky Hospital, Lexington, KY, p. A174
BUTLER, Jeffrey, Acting Superintendent, Richmond State Hospital, Richmond, IN, p. A145
BUTLER, Peter W., President and Chief Executive Officer, Methodist Health Care System, Houston, TX, p. B110
BUTLER, Victor D.
  Acting President and Chief Executive Officer, Baptist Health, Montgomery, AL, p. B57
  President and Chief Executive Officer, Baptist Medical Center, Montgomery, AL, p. A16
BUTLER, Jeffrey L., Administrator, Malcolm Grow Medical Center, Andrews AFB, MD, p. A195
BUTLER, John A., MSC, Administrator, Mike O'Callaghan Federal Hospital, Nellis AFB, NV, p. A269
BUTLER, Joe W., Deputy Commander for Administration, Martin Army Community Hospital, Fort Benning, GA, p. A105
BUTTS, Charles N., Chief Executive Officer, Reeves County Hospital, Pecos, TX, p. A426
BUURMAN, Rita K., Chief Executive Officer, Sabetha Community Hospital, Sabetha, KS, p. A167
BYBEE, Bob L., President and Chief Executive Officer, Memorial Medical Center, Port Lavaca, TX, p. A427
BYLANCIK, Robert J., CHE, President and Chief Executive Officer, Sunnyview Hospital and Rehabilitation Center, Schenectady, NY, p. A305
BYRNE, Frank D., M.D., President, Parkview Hospital, Fort Wayne, IN, p. A139
BYRNES, Nancy A., Chief Executive Officer, Navarro Regional Hospital, Corsicana, TX, p. A408
BYROM, David, Administrator, Coryell Memorial Hospital, Gatesville, TX, p. A414

C

CABONOR, Regis, Administrator, Person Memorial Hospital, Roxboro, NC, p. A317
CACKLER, Ron
  President and Chief Executive Officer, Bristow Memorial Hospital, Bristow, OK, p. A342
  President and Chief Executive Officer, Cushing Regional Hospital, Cushing, OK, p. A342
CAGEN, Richard M., Chief Executive Officer and Administrator, LDS Hospital, Salt Lake City, UT, p. A438
CAHILL, Patricia A., President and Chief Executive Officer, Catholic Health Initiatives, Denver, CO, p. B67
CAIN, Margaret C., President and Chief Executive Officer, North Suburban Medical Center, Thornton, CO, p. A73
CAIN, Mark, Chief Executive Officer, White County Community Hospital, Sparta, TN, p. A399
CAIN, Thomas, Administrator and Chief Executive Officer, Malvern Institute, Malvern, PA, p. A363
CAISON, S. Beth, Administrator, Collingsworth General Hospital, Wellington, TX, p. A434
CALAMARI, Frank A., President and Chief Executive Officer, Calvary Hospital, New York, NY, p. A296
CALBONE, Angelo G.
  President and Chief Executive Officer, Mount St. Mary's Hospital and Health Center, Lewiston, NY, p. A293
  President and Chief Executive Officer, Niagara Falls Memorial Medical Center, Niagara Falls, NY, p. A301
CALDERONE, John A., Ph.D., Chief Executive Officer, Corona Regional Medical Center, Corona, CA, p. A39
CALDWELL, Alan, Administrator, B.J. Workman Memorial Hospital, Woodruff, SC, p. A384
CALDWELL, Carolyn, Chief Executive Officer, Dallas Southwest Medical Center, Dallas, TX, p. A408
CALDWELL, Darren, Chief Executive Officer, Drew Memorial Hospital, Monticello, AR, p. A32
CALDWELL, Harvey G., Administrator and Chief Executive Officer, Brainerd Regional Human Services Center, Brainerd, MN, p. A226
CALDWELL, Robert C.
  Chief Executive Officer, Coastal Communities Hospital, Santa Ana, CA, p. A61
  Chief Executive Officer, Santa Ana Hospital Medical Center, Santa Ana, CA, p. A61
CALE, Barbara R., President, Chowan Hospital, Edenton, NC, p. A312
CALEY, George B., President, Winchester Medical Center, Winchester, VA, p. A451
CALHOUN, Jean, Administrator, Metropolitan Hospital, Atlanta, GA, p. A100
CALHOUN, Kevin P., President and Chief Executive Officer, Bell Memorial Hospital, Ishpeming, MI, p. A217
CALIG, Joseph, President and Chief Executive Officer, Allegheny University Hospitals, Allegheny Valley, Natrona Heights, PA, p. A365
CALLAHAN, Kevin J., President and Chief Executive Officer, Exeter Hospital, Exeter, NH, p. A271
CALLAHAN, Michael A., Chief Executive Officer, Highlands Regional Medical Center, Sebring, FL, p. A95
CALLAN, Sr, Michael J., Chief Executive Officer, Ashland Regional Medical Center, Ashland, PA, p. A356
CALLANDER, Bruce D., Ed.D., Superintendent, Gracewood State School and Hospital, Gracewood, GA, p. A105
CALLECOD, David L., CHE, Chief Executive Officer, Winona Memorial Hospital, Indianapolis, IN, p. A142
CALLISON, William L., Chief Executive Officer, Charter Greenville Behavioral Health System, Greer, SC, p. A381
CALVARUSO, Joseph T., President and Chief Executive Officer, Mount Carmel Health System, Columbus, OH, p. A330
CAMERON, Marie, FACHE, President and Chief Executive Officer, Southwest Hospital and Medical Center, Atlanta, GA, p. A100

CAMERON, Richard, M.D., Administrator, Harbor View Mercy Hospital, Fort Smith, AR, p. A30
CAMP, II, Claude E., Chief Executive Officer, McCurtain Memorial Hospital, Idabel, OK, p. A344
CAMPBELL, Al, Chief Executive Officer, Southeast Colorado Hospital and Long Term Care, Springfield, CO, p. A73
CAMPBELL, Bruce C., President and Chief Executive Officer, Illinois Masonic Medical Center, Chicago, IL, p. A121
CAMPBELL, C. Scott, Executive Director, Bulloch Memorial Hospital, Statesboro, GA, p. A110
CAMPBELL, David J., President and Chief Executive Officer, Saint Vincents Hospital and Medical Center, New York, NY, p. A299
CAMPBELL, Deborah, Administrator, Thomas H. Boyd Memorial Hospital, Carrollton, IL, p. A120
CAMPBELL, Gary L., Director, Harry S. Truman Memorial Veterans Hospital, Columbia, MO, p. A245
CAMPBELL, Gayla, Administrator, Integrated Specialty Hospital, Midwest City, OK, p. A345
CAMPBELL, Katharine Ann, Administrator, Mountainview Medical Center, White Sulphur Springs, MT, p. A260
CAMPBELL, Ronald L., Chief Executive Officer, Walton Medical Center, Monroe, GA, p. A107
CAMPBELL, Wayne, Chief Executive Officer, Fort Walton Beach Medical Center, Fort Walton Beach, FL, p. A85
CAMPBELL, William E., Ph.D., Superintendent, Glenwood State Hospital School, Glenwood, IA, p. A152
CAMPBELL, Jr, Robert D., Administrator, Cascade Valley Hospital, North Snohomish County Health System, Arlington, WA, p. A452
CANDINO, Paul J., Chief Executive Officer, Erie County Medical Center, Buffalo, NY, p. A289
CANNON, James C., Administrator and Chief Executive Officer, Regional Hospital for Respiratory and Complex Care, Seattle, WA, p. A456
CANOTE, Dennis R., Chief Executive Officer, Mid Missouri Mental Health Center, Columbia, MO, p. A246
CANTER, Jay M., Chief Executive Officer, Community Memorial Healthcare, Marysville, KS, p. A165
CANTRELL, Gary, President and Chief Executive Officer, St. Lucie Medical Center, Port St. Lucie, FL, p. A94
CANTRELL, Gregory Z., Chief Executive Officer, Laurel Wood Center, Meridian, MS, p. A240
CAPLAN, Marcie S., Chief Executive Officer, UPMC South Side, Pittsburgh, PA, p. A370
CAPOBIANCO, Peter E., President and Chief Executive Officer, St. Mary's Hospital, Amsterdam, NY, p. A287
CARAVELLA, Louis P., M.D., Chief Executive Officer, Fairview Hospital, Cleveland, OH, p. A328
CARBONE, Davide M., Chief Executive Officer, Aventura Hospital and Medical Center, Miami, FL, p. A89
CARDA, Vern, Administrator, Hegg Memorial Health Center/Avera Health, Rock Valley, IA, p. A156
CARL, Gerald E.
  Administrator, Arnold Memorial Health Care Center, Adrian, MN, p. A225
  Administrator, Luverne Community Hospital, Luverne, MN, p. A229
CARLE, Chris, Administrator, St. Elizabeth Medical Center–Grant County, Williamstown, KY, p. A179
CARLIN, Martin E., President, Park Ridge Hospital, Rochester, NY, p. A304
CARLINI, David, Chief Executive Officer, Charter Behavioral Health System of Charlottesville, Charlottesville, VA, p. A442
CARLISLE, John T., Chief Executive Officer, Cape Fear Valley Health System, Fayetteville, NC, p. A312
CARLSON, Brian J., FACHE, President and Chief Executive Officer, Lake View Memorial Hospital, Two Harbors, MN, p. A234
CARLSON, Greg L., President and Chief Executive Officer, Owensboro Mercy Health System, Owensboro, KY, p. A177
CARLSON, Stephen G., President and Chief Operating Officer, Flagstaff Medical Center, Flagstaff, AZ, p. A22
CARLSTEDT, Nancy S., President and Chief Executive Officer, Bloomington Hospital, Bloomington, IN, p. A137
CARLTON, Paul, M.D., Surgeon General, Department of the Air Force, Bowling AFB, DC, p. B77

CARMAN, Thomas H., President and Chief Executive Officer, Cortland Memorial Hospital, Cortland, NY, p. A290
CARMICHAEL, LeRoy, Executive Director, Bronx Psychiatric Center, New York, NY, p. A295
CARNEY, Christopher M., President and Chief Executive Officer, Bon Secours Health System, Inc., Marriottsville, MD, p. B61
CAROBENE, Joseph W., Superintendent, Middle Tennessee Mental Health Institute, Nashville, TN, p. A398
CAROSELLI, Joseph P., Administrator, Idaho Elks Rehabilitation Hospital, Boise, ID, p. A115
CARPENTER, David R., FACHE, President and Chief Executive Officer, North Kansas City Hospital, North Kansas City, MO, p. A251
CARR, C. Larry, Regional Executive Vice President and President, Bakersfield Memorial Hospital, Bakersfield, CA, p. A36
CARR, Wiley N., President and Chief Executive Officer, Porter Memorial Hospital, Valparaiso, IN, p. A146
CARRAWAY, Robert M., M.D., Chairman and Chief Executive Officer, Carraway Methodist Health System, Birmingham, AL, p. B66
CARRINGTON–MURRAY, Cynthia, MS, Senior Vice President, Woodhull Medical and Mental Health Center, New York, NY, p. A301
CARROCINO, Joanne, Executive Director, Kimball Medical Center, Lakewood, NJ, p. A277
CARROLL, Allen P., Chief Executive Officer, Bon Secours–St. Francis Xavier Hospital, Charleston, SC, p. A378
CARROLL, Jack A., Ph.D., President and Chief Executive Officer, Sheltering Arms Rehabilitation Hospital, Richmond, VA, p. A449
CARROLL, James J., Administrator, Cloquet Community Memorial Hospital, Cloquet, MN, p. A226
CARROLL, Kevin J., President, Champlain Valley Physicians Hospital Medical Center, Plattsburgh, NY, p. A302
CARROLL, Michael W., Administrator, Richland Parish Hospital–Delhi, Delhi, LA, p. A182
CARRUTH, John M., Administrator, Camden General Hospital, Camden, TN, p. A390
CARSON, Mitchell C., President, Ball Memorial Hospital, Muncie, IN, p. A144
CARSON, Sandra C., FACHE, President and Chief Executive Officer, Richard Young Center, Omaha, NE, p. A265
CARSON, Terry, Chief Executive Officer, Harrison Community Hospital, Cadiz, OH, p. A326
CARTER, Bruce C., President, United Hospital Center, Clarksburg, WV, p. A461
CARTER, Michael C., Chief Executive Officer, Anaheim Memorial Medical Center, Anaheim, CA, p. A35
CARTER, Patricia L., Chief Executive Officer, Memorial Hospital of Carbon County, Rawlins, WY, p. A479
CARTER, Richard, Chief Executive Officer, Hunt Memorial Hospital District, Greenville, TX, p. A414
CARTER , Jr, William E., Senior Associate Vice President for Operations, University of Virginia Medical Center, Charlottesville, VA, p. A443
CARUSO, Frank T., Chief Executive Officer, Hoopeston Community Memorial Hospital, Hoopeston, IL, p. A128
CARY, Roger C., President and Chief Executive Officer, Midwestern Regional Medical Center, Zion, IL, p. A136
CASADAY, Thomas E.
  President and Chief Executive Officer, Providence Memorial Hospital, El Paso, TX, p. A411
  President and Chief Executive Officer, Sierra Medical Center, El Paso, TX, p. A412
CASALOU, Robert F., President, Providence Hospital and Medical Centers, Southfield, MI, p. A222
CASELDINE, Robbee, Administrator, HEALTHSOUTH Rehabilitation Institute of Tucson, Tucson, AZ, p. A26
CASEY, Dennis A., Executive Director, Albert Lindley Lee Memorial Hospital, Fulton, NY, p. A291
CASEY, Jack, Administrator, Shodair Children's Hospital, Helena, MT, p. A258
CASEY, Marsha N., President, St. Vincent Hospitals and Health Services, Indianapolis, IN, p. A142

CASEY, Timothy M., President and Chief Executive Officer, Montgomery Hospital, Norristown, PA, p. A365
CASEY, William J., Administrator, Kingsburg Medical Center, Kingsburg, CA, p. A45
CASHION, John A., FACHE, President, Lexington Memorial Hospital, Lexington, NC, p. A315
CASON, Randall R., Chief Executive Officer, Southwest Regional Medical Center, Little Rock, AR, p. A31
CASSELS, William H., Administrator, DCH Regional Medical Center, Tuscaloosa, AL, p. A19
CASSIDY, James E., President and Chief Executive Officer, St. Mary's Regional Medical Center, Lewiston, ME, p. A193
CASTAGNARO, Marie, President and Chief Executive Officer, St. Joseph's Hospital, Elmira, NY, p. A291
CASTAGNO, Ronald J., FACHE, Chief Executive Officer, Specialty Hospital of Houston, Houston, TX, p. A418
CASTRO, William Rodriguez, Administrator, Hospital Del Maestro, San Juan, PR, p. A483
CASTROP, Richard F., President, O'Bleness Memorial Hospital, Athens, OH, p. A325
CATALANO, Robert A., M.D., President and Chief Executive Officer, Olean General Hospital, Olean, NY, p. A302
CATALDO, Vince A., Administrator, Prevost Memorial Hospital, Donaldsonville, LA, p. A182
CATELLIER, Julie A., Director, VA Gulf Coast Veterans Health Care System, Biloxi, MS, p. A236
CATENA, Cornelio R., President and Chief Executive Officer, Amsterdam Memorial Hospital, Amsterdam, NY, p. A287
CATHEY, Shawn, Administrator, Dardanelle Hospital, Dardanelle, AR, p. A29
CATHEY , Jr, James E., Chief Executive Officer, North Oaks Medical Center, Hammond, LA, p. A183
CATLIN, Rex, Chief Executive Officer, Endless Mountain Health Systems, Montrose, PA, p. A364
CAULK, Susan, Director Operations, Kaiser Foundation Hospital, Fontana, CA, p. A41
CAVAGNARO, Charles E., M.D., President and Chief Executive Officer, Wing Memorial Hospital and Medical Centers, Palmer, MA, p. A207
CAVALLI, Paul V., M.D., President, Meadowlands Hospital Medical Center, Secaucus, NJ, p. A280
CECCHETTINI, Diane
  President and Chief Executive Officer, Mary Bridge Children's Hospital and Health Center, Tacoma, WA, p. A458
  President and Chief Executive Officer, MultiCare Health System, Tacoma, WA, p. B112
  President and Chief Executive Officer, Tacoma General Hospital, Tacoma, WA, p. A458
CECCHINI, Marina, Chief Executive Officer, Charter Springs Hospital, Ocala, FL, p. A91
CECCONI, Thomas E., Chief Executive Officer, Doctors Hospital of Stark County, Massillon, OH, p. A334
CENTAFONT, Richard, Chief Executive Officer, Elkins Park Hospital, Elkins Park, PA, p. A359
CERCEO, Richard, Administrator, Vencor Hospital–Chicago Central, Chicago, IL, p. A124
CERNY, Ralph J., President and Chief Executive Officer, Munson Medical Center, Traverse City, MI, p. A223
CETTI, Janet E., President and Chief Executive Officer, San Diego Hospice, San Diego, CA, p. A59
CHADDIC, Jim, Chief Executive Officer, Goodland Regional Medical Center, Goodland, KS, p. A161
CHADWICK, Elizabeth M., JD, Executive Director, Devereux Georgia Treatment Network, Kennesaw, GA, p. A106
CHADWICK, Robyn, Administrator, Wesley Rehabilitation Hospital, Wichita, KS, p. A169
CHALKE, Peter E., President and Chief Executive Officer, Central Maine Medical Center, Lewiston, ME, p. A193
CHALONER, Robert S.
  Chief Executive Officer, St. Francis Hospital, Jersey City, NJ, p. A277
  President and Chief Executive Officer, St. Mary Hospital, Hoboken, NJ, p. A276
CHAMBERS, Cory, President and Chief Executive Officer, Shady Grove Adventist Hospital, Rockville, MD, p. A200

CHAMBERS, Matthew, Chief Executive Officer, Three Rivers Area Hospital, Three Rivers, MI, p. A223
CHAMP, Raymond L., President, Wake Medical Center, Raleigh, NC, p. A317
CHANDLER, Brue, President and Chief Executive Officer, Saint Joseph's Hospital of Atlanta, Atlanta, GA, p. A100
CHANDLER, Loren F., Chief Executive Officer, Scenic Mountain Medical Center, Big Spring, TX, p. A405
CHANDLER, Zach, Administrator, Baptist Memorial Hospital–Lauderdale, Ripley, TN, p. A399
CHANEY, Dennis R., Administrator, Morgan County Appalachian Regional Hospital, West Liberty, KY, p. A179
CHANNING, Alan H., Chief Executive Officer, St. Vincent Charity Hospital, Cleveland, OH, p. A329
CHAPMAN, Alan G., Chief Executive Officer, BHC West Hills Hospital, Reno, NV, p. A269
CHAPMAN, Richard, Administrator, Trigg County Hospital, Cadiz, KY, p. A170
CHAPMAN, Robert C., FACHE, President and Chief Executive Officer, Eastern Health System, Inc., Birmingham, AL, p. B84
CHAPMAN, Thomas W., President and Chief Executive Officer, Hospital for Sick Children, Washington, DC, p. A79
CHAPMAN , II, Erie, President and Chief Executive Officer, Baptist Hospital, Nashville, TN, p. A398
CHAPP, Colleen
  Interim Administrator, Beatrice Community Hospital and Health Center, Beatrice, NE, p. A261
  Interim Chief Executive Officer and Administrator, Valley County Hospital, Ord, NE, p. A266
CHAPPELOW, Michael W., President and Chief Executive Officer, Independence Regional Health Center, Independence, MO, p. A247
CHARLES, Timothy, Chief Executive Officer, Denton Community Hospital, Denton, TX, p. A410
CHARMEL, Patrick, President and Chief Executive Officer, Griffin Hospital, Derby, CT, p. A74
CHASE, Howard M., FACHE, President and Chief Executive Officer, Methodist Hospitals of Dallas, Dallas, TX, p. B111
CHASTAIN, James G., Director, Mississippi State Hospital, Whitfield, MS, p. A243
CHATTERTON, Claude, Administrator, Harrisburg Medical Center, Harrisburg, IL, p. A127
CHAUDRY, Moe, Chief Executive Officer, Willapa Harbor Hospital, South Bend, WA, p. A457
CHECK, Rosemary C., Administrator, Sentara Bayside Hospital, Virginia Beach, VA, p. A450
CHENSVOLD, Debrah, President, Palmer Lutheran Health Center, West Union, IA, p. A158
CHERAMIE, Lane M., Chief Executive Officer, Lady of the Sea General Hospital, Cut Off, LA, p. A182
CHERRY , Jr, Vincent T., Administrator, Stringfellow Memorial Hospital, Anniston, AL, p. A11
CHESNUT, Arden, Administrator, J. Paul Jones Hospital, Camden, AL, p. A13
CHESTER, Sandra M., Chief Executive Officer, Whittier Hospital Medical Center, Whittier, CA, p. A67
CHEWNING , II, Larry H., Chief Executive Officer, Wythe County Community Hospital, Wytheville, VA, p. A451
CHIARAMONTE, Francis P., M.D., Chief Executive Officer, Southern Maryland Hospital, Clinton, MD, p. A197
CHICK, James R., President, Joint Township District Memorial Hospital, Saint Marys, OH, p. A337
CHILDERS , Jr, Leo F., FACHE, President, Good Samaritan Regional Health Center, Mount Vernon, IL, p. A131
CHILDS, Ronald P., FACHE, Health Services Administrator, Midlands Center, Columbia, SC, p. A379
CHILL, Martha O'Regan, Administrator, Fort Sanders Loudon Medical Center, Loudon, TN, p. A395
CHILTON, Harold E., Chief Executive Officer, Twin Cities Community Hospital, Templeton, CA, p. A64
CHIOUTSIS, John M., Chief Executive Officer, Rosebud Health Care Center, Forsyth, MT, p. A257
CHISHOLM, Moody L., Chief Executive Officer and Managing Director, Northwest Texas Healthcare System, Amarillo, TX, p. A401

Index of Health Care Professionals / Chmiel

CHMIEL, Katherine, MS, Administrator and Chief Operating Officer, Taunton State Hospital, Taunton, MA, p. A209

CHODKOWSKI, Paul J., President and Chief Executive Officer, St. Clare's Hospital of Schenectady, Schenectady, NY, p. A304

CHRISTENSEN, Jay, Administrator, Mahaska County Hospital, Oskaloosa, IA, p. A155

CHRISTIAN, James A., Director, Veterans Affairs Medical Center, Asheville, NC, p. A309

CHRISTIAN, Patricia L., Ph.D., Chief Executive Officer, John Umstead Hospital, Butner, NC, p. A310

CHRISTIANSEN, Gary, President and Chief Executive Officer, Carondelet Health System, Saint Louis, MO, p. B65

CHRISTIANSEN, Kevin, Administrator, Vencor Hospital – Tucson, Tucson, AZ, p. A27

CHRISTIANSON, Clark P.
  Senior Vice President and Administrator, Memorial Hospital–Flagler, Bunnell, FL, p. A82
  Senior Vice President and Administrator, Memorial Hospital–Ormond Beach, Ormond Beach, FL, p. A92
  Senior Vice President and Administrator, Memorial Hospital–Peninsula, Ormond Beach, FL, p. A92

CHRISTIANSON, Delano, Administrator, St. Michael's Hospital, Sauk Centre, MN, p. A233

CHRISTIE, Arthur P., Administrator, Houston Medical Center, Warner Robins, GA, p. A111

CHRISTMAN, Lyndon J., President and Chief Executive Officer, Galion Community Hospital, Galion, OH, p. A332

CHRISTOPHER, William T., President and Chief Executive Officer, Lawrence & Memorial Hospital, New London, CT, p. A76

CHROMIK, James R., Regional Vice President, Administration, North Broward Medical Center, Pompano Beach, FL, p. A93

CHUBB, John M., Chief Executive Officer, Brownsville Medical Center, Brownsville, TX, p. A405

CHURCH, Daniel K., Ph.D., President and Chief Executive Officer, Edwin Shaw Hospital for Rehabilitation, Akron, OH, p. A325

CHURCH , Jr, John D., Director, Veterans Affairs Medical Center, New Orleans, LA, p. A187

CHURCHILL, Timothy A., President, Stephens Memorial Hospital, Norway, ME, p. A193

CIBRAN, Bert, President and Chief Operating Officer, Ramsay Youth Services, Coral Gables, FL, p. B128

CIBRONE, Connie M., President and Chief Executive Officer, Allegheny University Hospitals, Allegheny General, Pittsburgh, PA, p. A368

CIMEROLA, Joseph M., FACHE, President and Chief Executive Officer, Sacred Heart Hospital, Allentown, PA, p. A355

CINCINAT, Cathy L., Chief Executive Officer, Massillon Psychiatric Center, Massillon, OH, p. A335

CIRNE–NEVES, Ceu, Administrator, Saint James Hospital of Newark, Newark, NJ, p. A278

CITRON, Richard S., Director, Veterans Affairs Chicago Health Care System, Chicago, IL, p. A124

CLADY, Nellie, R.N., Interim Administrator, Bucyrus Community Hospital, Bucyrus, OH, p. A326

CLAFFEY, Patricia, Executive Director, McPherson Hospital, Howell, MI, p. A217

CLAIRMONT, Thomas, President, Lakes Region General Hospital, Laconia, NH, p. A272

CLARK, Douglas A., Executive Director, Latrobe Area Hospital, Latrobe, PA, p. A363

CLARK, Frank, Chief Executive Officer, Cascade Medical Center, Cascade, ID, p. A116

CLARK, Ira C., President, Jackson Memorial Hospital, Miami, FL, p. A89

CLARK, M. Victoria, Chief Executive Officer, Palo Verde Hospital, Blythe, CA, p. A37

CLARK, Melinda, President, SSM Rehab, Saint Louis, MO, p. A253

CLARK, Michael, Chief Executive Officer, Logan Memorial Hospital, Russellville, KY, p. A178

CLARK, Richard L., Administrator and Chief Executive Officer, Morristown–Hamblen Hospital, Morristown, TN, p. A397

CLARK, Robert J., FACHE, President and Chief Executive Officer, Gnaden Huetten Memorial Hospital, Lehighton, PA, p. A363

CLARK, Thomas, President and Chief Executive Officer, Saints Memorial Medical Center, Lowell, MA, p. A206

CLARK, Thomas A., Chief Executive Officer, Wells Community Hospital, Bluffton, IN, p. A137

CLARK, Wayne N., President and Chief Executive Officer, Arlington Memorial Hospital, Arlington, TX, p. A402

CLARK, William S., Chief Executive Officer, Columbus County Hospital, Whiteville, NC, p. A319

CLARK, David L., USAF, Commander, U. S. Air Force Hospital Altus, Altus, OK, p. A341

CLARK, David L., Commander, U. S. Air Force Regional Hospital, Minot, ND, p. A323

CLARKE, Robert T.
  President and Chief Executive Officer, Memorial Health System, Springfield, IL, p. B109
  President and Chief Executive Officer, Memorial Medical Center, Springfield, IL, p. A135

CLASSEN, Howard H., Chief Executive Officer, Natividad Medical Center, Salinas, CA, p. A58

CLAYTON, Philip A., President and Chief Executive Officer, Conway Hospital, Conway, SC, p. A380

CLEARWATER, William J., Vice President and Site Administrator, St. John's Pleasant Valley Hospital, Camarillo, CA, p. A37

CLEARY, John J., President and Chief Executive Officer, River Oaks Hospital, Jackson, MS, p. A239

CLEARY, Margaret, Chief Executive Officer, Woodland Healthcare, Woodland, CA, p. A67

CLEM, Olie E., Chief Executive Officer, Doctors Memorial Hospital, Tyler, TX, p. A433

CLEMENTS, Dan A., Chief Executive Officer, Hurley Health Center, Coalgate, OK, p. A342

CLEMENTS, Larry E., Administrator, Wildwood Lifestyle Center and Hospital, Wildwood, GA, p. A111

CLENDENIN, Phillip A., Chief Executive Officer, Greenview Regional Hospital, Bowling Green, KY, p. A170

CLICK, Mike, Administrator, Brownfield Regional Medical Center, Brownfield, TX, p. A405

CLIFF, Peggy, Administrator, IHS Hospital at San Antonio, San Antonio, TX, p. A428

CLINE, Phillip E., Administrator, Providence Kodiak Island Medical Center, Kodiak, AK, p. A21

CLOHAN , Jr, Jack C.
  Interim Administrator, Mildred Mitchell–Bateman Hospital, Huntington, WV, p. A462
  Administrator, William R. Sharpe Jr. Hospital, Weston, WV, p. A465

CLOUGH, James L., Administrator, Drumright Memorial Hospital, Drumright, OK, p. A342

CLOUGH, Jeanette G., President and Chief Executive Officer, Mount Auburn Hospital, Cambridge, MA, p. A204

CLOVET, Sylvette, Chief Executive Officer, San Juan City Hospital, San Juan, PR, p. A484

COATES, Cliff, Chief Executive Officer, Sutter Medical Center, Santa Rosa, Santa Rosa, CA, p. A63

COATES, David M., Ph.D., Chief Executive Officer, Clarke County Hospital, Osceola, IA, p. A155

COATS, Rodney M., President and Chief Executive Officer, Washington County Memorial Hospital, Salem, IN, p. A145

COBB, Terrell M., Executive Director, Greenwood Leflore Hospital, Greenwood, MS, p. A238

COCHRAN, Barry S.
  President, Cherokee Baptist Medical Center, Centre, AL, p. A13
  President, DeKalb Baptist Medical Center, Fort Payne, AL, p. A14

CODY, Douglas M., Administrator, Amos Cottage Rehabilitation Hospital, Winston–Salem, NC, p. A319

CODY, James P., Director, Veterans Affairs Medical Center, Syracuse, NY, p. A306

COE, Isaac S., President, Murray–Calloway County Hospital, Murray, KY, p. A177

COE, William G., Executive Vice President and Chief Executive Officer, La Paz Regional Hospital, Parker, AZ, p. A23

COHEN, Bruce M., Ph.D., President and Psychiatrist–in–Chief, McLean Hospital, Belmont, MA, p. A201

COHEN, Elliot G., Senior Vice President, University Hospital, Cincinnati, OH, p. A328

COHEN, Jed M., Acting Executive Director, Western New York Children's Psychiatric Center, Buffalo, NY, p. A289

COHEN, Kenneth B., Director, Riverside County Regional Medical Center, Moreno Valley, CA, p. A52

COHEN, Philip A.
  Chief Executive Officer, Garfield Medical Center, Monterey Park, CA, p. A52
  Chief Executive Officer, Monterey Park Hospital, Monterey Park, CA, p. A52

COHEN, Steven M., M.D., Director, Veterans Affairs Medical Center, Dayton, OH, p. A331

COHOLICH, Robert J., President, Defiance Hospital, Defiance, OH, p. A331

COKER , Jr, Robert J., Administrator, Greene County Hospital, Eutaw, AL, p. A14

COLBERG, Gary R., CHE, Chief Executive Officer, Medical Center East, Birmingham, AL, p. A12

COLBY, Dan, President and Chief Executive Officer, Harvard Memorial Hospital, Harvard, IL, p. A127

COLCHER, Marian W., President, Valley Forge Medical Center and Hospital, Norristown, PA, p. A365

COLE, Geoffrey F., President and Chief Executive Officer, Emerson Hospital, Concord, MA, p. A204

COLE, Harry, Interim Administrator, Georgiana Hospital, Georgiana, AL, p. A15

COLE, James B., Chief Executive Officer, Arlington Hospital, Arlington, VA, p. A442

COLE, James M., Executive Director, Devereux Mapleton Psychiatric Institute–Mapleton Center, Malvern, PA, p. A363

COLECCHI, Stephen, President and Chief Executive Officer, Robinson Memorial Hospital, Ravenna, OH, p. A337

COLEMAN, Curt, Chief Executive Officer, Jackson County Public Hospital, Maquoketa, IA, p. A154

COLEMAN, Dan C.
  President and Chief Executive Officer, John C Lincoln Health Network, Phoenix, AZ, p. B103
  President and Chief Executive Officer, John C. Lincoln Hospital – North Mountain, Phoenix, AZ, p. A24

COLEMAN, James, Director, Kalamazoo Regional Psychiatric Hospital, Kalamazoo, MI, p. A218

COLEMAN, Kevin T., Administrator, Baptist Hospital–Orange, Orange, TX, p. A425

COLES, Bettie L., R.N., Administrator, Kaiser Foundation Hospital, Oakland, CA, p. A53

COLFACK, Brian R., CHE, President and Chief Executive Officer, Berger Health System, Circleville, OH, p. A328

COLLER, James G., Executive Vice President and Administrator, St. Mary's Hospital Medical Center, Green Bay, WI, p. A469

COLLETTE, Dennis H., President and Chief Executive Officer, Newton Memorial Hospital, Newton, NJ, p. A278

COLLIER, C. Thomas, President and Chief Executive Officer, Sierra Nevada Memorial Hospital, Grass Valley, CA, p. A43

COLLINS, Dale, President and Chief Executive Officer, Baptist Health System of Tennessee, Knoxville, TN, p. B58

COLLINS, James M., President and Chief Executive Officer, Western Pennsylvania Hospital, Pittsburgh, PA, p. A370

COLLINS, Jeffrey A., Chief Executive Officer, Sun Coast Hospital, Largo, FL, p. A88

COLLINS, Michael F., M.D.
  President, Caritas Christi Health Care, Boston, MA, p. B64
  President, St. Elizabeth's Medical Center of Boston, Brighton, MA, p. A203

COLLINS, Roger, Chief Executive Officer and Managing Director, Valley Hospital Medical Center, Las Vegas, NV, p. A268

COLLINS, Thomas J., President and Chief Executive Officer, Memorial Health Services, Long Beach, CA, p. B109

COLLINS, Thomas M., Chief Executive Officer, Green Oaks Hospital, Dallas, TX, p. A409
COLLISON, Thomas R., Commanding Officer, Naval Hospital, Camp Lejeune, NC, p. A310
COLOMBO, Armando, Chief Executive Officer, HEALTHSOUTH Rehabilitation Hospital of Tallahassee, Tallahassee, FL, p. A96
COLON, Ivan E., Administrator, Auxilio Mutuo Hospital, San Juan, PR, p. A483
COLSTON, Allen J., Director, Veterans Affairs Medical Center, Alexandria, LA, p. A180
COLVERT, Charles C., President, Shelby Baptist Medical Center, Alabaster, AL, p. A11
COLVIN, Robert A., President and Chief Executive Officer, Memorial Health, Savannah, GA, p. A109
COLVIN, Wesley E., Senior Vice President and Chief Executive Officer, Carondelet St. Joseph's Hospital, Tucson, AZ, p. A26
COLWELL, Loretto Marie, President and Chief Executive Officer, St. Francis Hospital and Medical Center, Topeka, KS, p. A168
COMER, W. Jefferson, FACHE, Chief Executive Officer, Northwest Medical Center, Tucson, AZ, p. A26
COMERFORD, Jr, Thomas P., Superintendent, Clarks Summit State Hospital, Clarks Summit, PA, p. A358
COMPSON, Oral R., Administrator, Dayton General Hospital, Dayton, WA, p. A453
COMSTOCK, John M., Chief Executive Officer, Sioux Valley Memorial Hospital, Cherokee, IA, p. A149
CONAWAY, Jr, Robert J., Chief Executive Officer, Phoenix Memorial Health System, Phoenix, AZ, p. A25
CONDOM, Jaime E., M.D., Director, South Carolina State Hospital, Columbia, SC, p. A380
CONDRASKY, Louis M.
Chief Executive Officer, HEALTHSOUTH Lake Erie Institute of Rehabilitation, Erie, PA, p. A360
Chief Executive Officer, HEALTHSOUTH Rehabilitation Hospital of Erie, Erie, PA, p. A360
CONEJO, David, Chief Executive Officer, Big Bend Regional Medical Center, Alpine, TX, p. A401
CONELL, Marge, Administrator, Ellinwood District Hospital, Ellinwood, KS, p. A160
CONGER, Rex D., President and Chief Executive Officer, Iroquois Memorial Hospital and Resident Home, Watseka, IL, p. A136
CONKLIN, Richard L., President, Parkland Health Center, Farmington, MO, p. A246
CONN, Kevin R., Administrator, HEALTHSOUTH Sunrise Rehabilitation Hospital, Fort Lauderdale, FL, p. A84
CONNELLY, Harrell L., Chief Executive Officer, Wallace Thomson Hospital, Union, SC, p. A384
CONNELLY, Michael D., President and Chief Executive Officer, Catholic Healthcare Partners, Cincinnati, OH, p. B69
CONNOR, II, Paul J., President and Chief Executive Officer, Eastern Long Island Hospital, Greenport, NY, p. A292
CONNORS, William G., President and Chief Executive Officer, St. James Mercy Hospital, Hornell, NY, p. A292
CONOLE, Charles P., FACHE, Chief Executive Officer, Edward John Noble Hospital of Gouverneur, Gouverneur, NY, p. A292
CONSIDINE, William H., President, Children's Hospital Medical Center of Akron, Akron, OH, p. A325
CONSILVIO, Eileen, MS, Executive Director, Manhattan Psychiatric Center-Ward's Island, New York, NY, p. A298
CONSTANTINE, Richard D., Chief Executive Officer, Brownsville General Hospital, Brownsville, PA, p. A356
CONSTANTINO, Richard S., M.D.
President, Genesee Hospital, Rochester, NY, p. A303
President, Rochester General Hospital, Rochester, NY, p. A304
CONTE, William A., Director, Edith Nourse Rogers Memorial Veterans Hospital, Bedford, MA, p. A201
CONTI, Vincent S., President and Chief Executive Officer, Maine Medical Center, Portland, ME, p. A193
CONTRATTO, Blair, President and Chief Executive Officer, Little Company of Mary Health Services, Torrance, CA, p. A65
CONZEMIUS, James D., President, Flagler Hospital, Saint Augustine, FL, p. A94
COOK, Bill, President and Chief Executive Officer, Specialty Hospital Group, Atlanta, GA, p. B136
COOK, E. Tim, Chief Executive Officer, Osceola Regional Medical Center, Kissimmee, FL, p. A87
COOK, Harold L., Director, Nevada Mental Health Institute, Sparks, NV, p. A269
COOK, Jack M., President and Chief Executive Officer, Health Alliance of Greater Cincinnati, Cincinnati, OH, p. B94
COOK, Patricia F., R.N., Vice President Operations, Alexian Brothers Hospital, Saint Louis, MO, p. A252
COOK, Randy, Administrator and Chief Executive Officer, Indian Path Medical Center, Kingsport, TN, p. A394
COOK, Ruth, Administrator, East Texas Medical Center Fairfield, Fairfield, TX, p. A412
COOKE, Paula Tamme, Chief Executive Officer, Central State Hospital, Louisville, KY, p. A175
COOPER, Anthony J., President and Chief Executive Officer, Arnot Ogden Medical Center, Elmira, NY, p. A291
COOPER, Chad, Administrator, United Hospital District, Blue Earth, MN, p. A226
COOPER, Donald C., Director, Veterans Affairs Central Iowa Health Care System, Des Moines, IA, p. A151
COOPER, Gerson I., President, Botsford General Hospital, Farmington Hills, MI, p. A214
COOPER, Gloria, Chief Executive Officer, Mount Carmel Hospital, Colville, WA, p. A453
COOPER, James C., Chief Operating Officer, Valley Medical Facilities, Sewickley, PA, p. A372
COOPER, Maxine T.
Chief Executive Officer, Chapman Medical Center, Orange, CA, p. A54
Chief Executive Officer, Placentia Linda Hospital, Placentia, CA, p. A55
COOPER, Paul S., Chief Executive Officer, South Jersey Health System, Bridgeton, NJ, p. B135
COOPER, Robert, Chief Executive Officer, Marshalltown Medical and Surgical Center, Marshalltown, IA, p. A154
COOPER, Roger W., Chief Executive Officer, Biggs-Gridley Memorial Hospital, Gridley, CA, p. A43
COORS, Mary Lou, Vice President, St. Joseph Rehabilitation Hospital and Outpatient Center, Albuquerque, NM, p. A283
COPE, Brent, Chief Executive Officer, Tooele Valley Regional Medical Center, Tooele, UT, p. A439
COPELAN, H. Neil, President and Chief Executive Officer, South Fulton Medical Center, East Point, GA, p. A104
COPELAND, Jr, Robert Y., Chief Executive Officer, McCune-Brooks Hospital, Carthage, MO, p. A245
COPENHAVER, C. Curtis, President, Mercy Hospital, Charlotte, NC, p. A311
COPPLE, Brad, Administrator, Kishwaukee Community Hospital, De Kalb, IL, p. A124
CORA, Jose Joaquin, Executive Director, Hospital Episcopal Cristo Redentor, Guayama, PR, p. A482
CORBETT, Clifford L., President and Chief Executive Officer, Morris Hospital, Morris, IL, p. A131
CORCORAN, Joseph P., President and Chief Executive Officer, New York Eye and Ear Infirmary, New York, NY, p. A298
CORDER, Thomas J., President and Chief Executive Officer, Camden-Clark Memorial Hospital, Parkersburg, WV, p. A463
CORDNER, Glenn D., Chief Executive Officer, Springfield Hospital, Springfield, VT, p. A441
COREY, Jack M., President, DeKalb Memorial Hospital, Auburn, IN, p. A137
CORK, Ronald J., President and Chief Executive Officer, Avera St. Anthony's Hospital, O'Neill, NE, p. A265
CORLEY, Thomas, President and Chief Executive Officer, Holy Family Hospital, Spokane, WA, p. A457
CORLEY, William E., President, Community Hospitals Indianapolis, Indianapolis, IN, p. A141
CORLISS, Pam, Chief Executive Officer, Atlantic Medical Center, Daytona Beach, FL, p. A83
CORMIER, Richard, Ph.D., Chief Executive Officer, Conejos County Hospital, La Jara, CO, p. A71
CORNISH, Helen K., Director, Veterans Affairs Medical Center-Lexington, Lexington, KY, p. A174
CORONADO, Jose R., FACHE, Director, South Texas Veterans Health Care System, San Antonio, TX, p. A429
CORVINO, Frank A., President and Chief Executive Officer, Greenwich Hospital, Greenwich, CT, p. A74
COSTA, David, Administrator, David Grant Medical Center, Travis AFB, CA, p. A65
COSTELLO, Bud, Administrator and Chief Executive Officer, Macon Northside Hospital, Macon, GA, p. A107
COTNER, Edna J., Administrator, Coquille Valley Hospital, Coquille, OR, p. A350
COTTEY, David, Chief Executive Officer, Doctors Hospital, Groves, TX, p. A415
COUCH, Robert C., Chief Executive Officer, Medical Center of Manchester, Manchester, TN, p. A396
COUGHLIN, Jean, President and Chief Executive Officer, Marian Community Hospital, Carbondale, PA, p. A357
COURAGE, Kenneth F., Chief Executive Officer and Chairman of the Board, Psychiatric Institute of Washington, Washington, DC, p. A79
COURTNEY, Curtis B., Chief Executive Officer, Meadowview Regional Medical Center, Maysville, KY, p. A176
COURTNEY, James P., President and Chief Executive Officer, University Medical Center, Lubbock, TX, p. A422
COVA, Charles J., Executive Vice President and Chief Operating Officer, Marian Medical Center, Santa Maria, CA, p. A62
COVERT, David G., President and Chief Administrative Officer, Chandler Regional Hospital, Chandler, AZ, p. A22
COVERT, Michael H., FACHE, President, Washington Hospital Center, Washington, DC, p. A80
COVERT, Rob, President and Chief Executive Officer, Oaklawn Hospital, Marshall, MI, p. A219
COVEY, Laird P., President and Chief Executive Officer, Bridgton Hospital, Bridgton, ME, p. A192
COX, Darlene L., President and Chief Executive Officer, East Orange General Hospital, East Orange, NJ, p. A275
COX, Gray, President, Mission Hill Memorial Hospital, Shawnee, OK, p. A347
COX, Jay, President and Chief Executive Officer, Tuomey Healthcare System, Sumter, SC, p. A384
COX, Kevin, Administrator, Memorial Hospital of Texas County, Guymon, OK, p. A344
COX, Leigh, Chief Executive Officer, Navapache Regional Medical Center, Show Low, AZ, p. A26
COX, Otto L., President, Mercy Medical Center, Oshkosh, WI, p. A473
COX, Sr, Arthur J., Director, Florida Center for Addictions and Dual Disorders, Avon Park, FL, p. A81
COYLE, Joseph P., President and Chief Executive Officer, Southern Ocean County Hospital, Manahawkin, NJ, p. A277
COYNE, Kathryn W., Executive Director, Union Hospital, Union, NJ, p. A281
CRABTREE, Douglas, Chief Executive Officer, Eastern Idaho Regional Medical Center, Idaho Falls, ID, p. A116
CRAIGIN, Jane, Chief Executive Officer, St. Vincent Williamsport Hospital, Williamsport, IN, p. A147
CRAIN, Stephen L., Chief Executive Officer, Mineral Area Regional Medical Center, Farmington, MO, p. A246
CRAMER, John S., FACHE, President and Chief Executive Officer, PinnacleHealth System, Harrisburg, PA, p. A361
CRANDALL, David, President and Chief Executive Officer, Hospital for Special Care, New Britain, CT, p. A75
CRANDELL, Kim O., Chief Executive Officer and Administrator, Boulder City Hospital, Boulder City, NV, p. A268
CRANE, Margaret W., Chief Executive Officer, Barlow Respiratory Hospital, Los Angeles, CA, p. A47
CRAWFIS, Ewing H., President, Mary Rutan Hospital, Bellefontaine, OH, p. A326
CRAWFORD, Janet McKinney, Vice President and Administrator, Carilion Saint Albans Hospital, Radford, VA, p. A448
CRAWFORD, John W., Chief Executive Officer, Wagoner Community Hospital, Wagoner, OK, p. A349

CREAMER, Donald R., President and Chief Executive Officer, Susquehanna Health System, Williamsport, PA, p. A375
CREEDEN, Jr., Francis V., Senior Executive Officer, Providence Medical Center, Kansas City, KS, p. A163
CREELEY, Melvin R., President, East Liverpool City Hospital, East Liverpool, OH, p. A331
CRIPE, Kimberly C., Chief Executive Officer, Children's Hospital of Orange County, Orange, CA, p. A54
CRONBERG, Chris, Chief Executive Officer, Northern Cochise Community Hospital, Willcox, AZ, p. A27
CRONE, William G., President and Chief Executive Officer, Naples Community Hospital, Naples, FL, p. A90
CRONEN, Kathleen
 Chief Executive Officer, Charter North Star Behavioral Health System, Anchorage, AK, p. A20
 Chief Executive Officer, Charter North Star Behavioral Health System, Anchorage, AK, p. A20
CRONIN, Francis J., President and Chief Executive Officer, Christ Hospital, Jersey City, NJ, p. A277
CRONIN, John C. J., President and Chief Executive Officer, North Adams Regional Hospital, North Adams, MA, p. A207
CROOM, Jr., Kennedy L., Administrator and Chief Executive Officer, Rhea Medical Center, Dayton, TN, p. A392
CROPPER, Douglas P.
 Vice President and Administrator, St. John's Hospital, Maplewood, MN, p. A230
 Vice President and Administrator, St. Joseph's Hospital, Saint Paul, MN, p. A233
CROSS, Gerald M., USA, Commander, Darnall Army Community Hospital, Fort Hood, TX, p. A412
CROSSETT, Joseph W., Administrator, Liberty Hospital, Liberty, MO, p. A250
CROSSIN, William J., President and Chief Executive Officer, Miner's Memorial Medical Center, Coaldale, PA, p. A358
CROUCH, Matthew, Chief Executive Officer, Charter Anchor Hospital, Atlanta, GA, p. A99
CROW, David, Chief Executive Officer, Campbell County Memorial Hospital, Gillette, WY, p. A478
CROW, Ruth Ann, Administrator, Lake Whitney Medical Center, Whitney, TX, p. A434
CROW, Tom, Administrator, Atlanta Memorial Hospital, Atlanta, TX, p. A402
CROWDER, Jerry W., President and Chief Executive Officer, Bradford Health Services, Birmingham, AL, p. B62
CROWE, Danny, Interim Chief Executive Officer, Parkway Medical Center Hospital, Decatur, AL, p. A14
CROWELL, Eric, President and Chief Executive Officer, Trinity Medical Center–West Campus, Rock Island, IL, p. A133
CROWELL, Lynn, Chief Executive Officer, Arkansas Valley Regional Medical Center, La Junta, CO, p. A71
CROWLEY, Thomas, President, St. Elizabeth Hospital, Wabasha, MN, p. A234
CROWTHER, Bruce K., President and Chief Executive Officer, Northwest Community Healthcare, Arlington Heights, IL, p. A119
CRUICKSHANK, James A., Chief Executive Officer, University Hospital and Medical Center, Tamarac, FL, p. A96
CRUMPLER, Joyce, R.N., Administrator, Bowie Memorial Hospital, Bowie, TX, p. A405
CRUMPTON, Althea H., Administrator, Magee General Hospital, Magee, MS, p. A240
CUBELLIS, Guido J., Chief Executive Officer, Select Specialty Hospital–Houston Medical Center, Houston, TX, p. A418
CUCCI, Edward A., President, Louis A. Weiss Memorial Hospital, Chicago, IL, p. A122
CUDWORTH, Craig R., Chief Executive Officer, De Queen Regional Medical Center, De Queen, AR, p. A29
CULBERSON, David K.
 Chief Executive Officer, Huntington Beach Hospital, Huntington Beach, CA, p. A44
 Chief Executive Officer, La Palma Intercommunity Hospital, La Palma, CA, p. A45
 Chief Executive Officer, West Anaheim Medical Center, Anaheim, CA, p. A35

CULLEN, James J., President and Chief Executive Officer, St. Joseph Medical Center, Towson, MD, p. A200
CULLEN, Sheila M., Director, Veterans Affairs Medical Center, San Francisco, CA, p. A60
CULLEY, James R., Administrator, Valdez Community Hospital, Valdez, AK, p. A21
CULVERN, Rita, Administrator, Jefferson Hospital, Louisville, GA, p. A106
CUMMING, Irene M., Chief Executive Officer, University of Kansas Medical Center, Kansas City, KS, p. A163
CUMMINGS, Bruce D., Chief Executive Officer, Blue Hill Memorial Hospital, Blue Hill, ME, p. A191
CUNNINGHAM, Michelle, Chief Executive Officer, Highlands Hospital, Connellsville, PA, p. A358
CUPPLES, John E., President, Spaulding Rehabilitation Hospital, Boston, MA, p. A203
CURE, DeAnn K., Chief Executive Officer, Rangely District Hospital, Rangely, CO, p. A72
CURRIE, Patricia, Chief Executive Officer, Spring Branch Medical Center, Houston, TX, p. A418
CURRIER, Jr., Elwood E., CHE, Administrator, Medina Community Hospital, Hondo, TX, p. A415
CURRY, Robert H., Senior Vice President and Chief Executive Officer, Thunderbird Samaritan Medical Center, Glendale, AZ, p. A23
CURTIS, Jeff, President and Chief Executive Officer, H.S.C. Medical Center, Malvern, AR, p. A32
CURTIS, Scott, Administrator and Chief Executive Officer, Kossuth Regional Health Center, Algona, IA, p. A148
CUSANO, Philip D., President and Chief Executive Officer, Stamford Health System, Stamford, CT, p. A77
CUSHING, Jeff, Vice President and Site Administrator, Legacy Meridian Park Hospital, Tualatin, OR, p. A354
CUSTER-MITCHELL, Marilyn J., Administrator, West Central Community Hospital, Clinton, IN, p. A138
CUTLER, Terry, Administrator and Chief Operating Officer, East Texas Medical Center–Clarksville, Clarksville, TX, p. A406
CYGAN, Ralph, M.D., Interim Director, University of California, Irvine Medical Center, Orange, CA, p. A54
CZIPO, Kevin F., Executive Director, Stony Lodge Hospital, Ossining, NY, p. A302

D

D'AGNES, Michael R., President and Chief Executive Officer, Bayonne Hospital, Bayonne, NJ, p. A274
D'ALBERTO, Richard E., Chief Executive Officer, J. C. Blair Memorial Hospital, Huntingdon, PA, p. A362
D'ERAMO, David, President and Chief Executive Officer, Saint Francis Hospital and Medical Center, Hartford, CT, p. A75
D'ESMOND, C. Thomas, Administrator, Shriners Hospitals for Children, Portland, Portland, OR, p. A353
D'ETTORRE, Joseph A., Chief Executive Officer, Wyandot Memorial Hospital, Upper Sandusky, OH, p. A338
DACHILLE, Susan, Interim President, UPMC Beaver Valley, Aliquippa, PA, p. A355
DADLEZ, Christopher M., President and Chief Executive Officer, Mercy Medical Center, Canton, OH, p. A326
DAGUE, James O., President and Chief Executive Officer, Goshen General Hospital, Goshen, IN, p. A140
DAHILL, Kevin, President and Chief Executive Officer, New York United Hospital Medical Center, Port Chester, NY, p. A303
DAHLBERG, Edwin E., President, St. Luke's Regional Medical Center, Boise, ID, p. A115
DAHLBERG, Philip J., M.D., Chief Executive Officer, Gundersen Lutheran, La Crosse, WI, p. A470
DAHLMAN, Kim, Chief Executive Officer, Wallowa Memorial Hospital, Enterprise, OR, p. A350
DAIGLE, Anthony A., Administrator, Southwest Medical Center, Liberal, KS, p. A164
DAILY, James L., President, Porter Hospital, Middlebury, VT, p. A440
DAL CIELO, William J., Chief Executive Officer, Alameda Hospital, Alameda, CA, p. A35

DALTON, John, President and Chief Executive Officer, Deaconess–Glover Hospital Corporation, Needham, MA, p. A207
DALTON, Jr., James E., President and Chief Executive Officer, Quorum Health Group, Brentwood, TN, p. B122
DALY, Michael J., President, Baystate Health System, Inc., Springfield, MA, p. B59
DAMON, Joan, Administrator, Methodist Health Center–Sugar Land, Sugar Land, TX, p. A431
DAMORE, Joseph F., President and Chief Executive Officer, Sparrow Health System, Lansing, MI, p. A218
DAMPIER, Bobby H., Chief Executive Officer, Regional Medical Center of Hopkins County, Madisonville, KY, p. A176
DAMSHEN, David, Chief Executive Officer, Copper Hills Youth Center, West Jordan, UT, p. A439
DANDLIKER, Nancy N., Executive Director, BHC Willow Springs Residential Treatment Center, Reno, NV, p. A269
DANDRIDGE, Thomas C., President, Regional Medical Center of Orangeburg and Calhoun Counties, Orangeburg, SC, p. A383
DANIEL, Steven G., Administrator, Bob Wilson Memorial Grant County Hospital, Ulysses, KS, p. A168
DANIEL, William W., Chief Executive Officer, Mission Community Hospital–San Fernando Campus, San Fernando, CA, p. A59
DANIELS, Gary J., Ph.D., Superintendent, Parsons State Hospital and Training Center, Parsons, KS, p. A166
DANIELS, John D., President and Chief Executive Officer, St. Luke's Regional Medical Center, Sioux City, IA, p. A157
DANIELS, Richard A., President and Chief Executive Officer, McCullough–Hyde Memorial Hospital, Oxford, OH, p. A336
DANILOFF, Michael, President, Evangelical Community Hospital, Lewisburg, PA, p. A363
DANKINS, Jeff, Vice President Operations, Harper Hospital, Detroit, MI, p. A213
DARDEN, David B., Chief Executive Officer, Raleigh General Hospital, Beckley, WV, p. A460
DARLING, Rudy, President and Chief Executive Officer, Carroll Regional Medical Center, Berryville, AR, p. A28
DARNEY, Bruce, Superintendent, Harrisburg State Hospital, Harrisburg, PA, p. A361
DASCHER, Jr., Norman E., Chief Executive Officer, Memorial Hospital, Albany, NY, p. A287
DAUBY, Randall W., Chief Executive Officer, Hamilton Memorial Hospital District, McLeansboro, IL, p. A130
DAUGHERTY, Charles R., Administrator, Baptist Memorial Hospital–Forrest City, Forrest City, AR, p. A29
DAUGHERTY, R. Allan, Chief Executive Officer, Parkview Regional Medical Center, Vicksburg, MS, p. A242
DAUGHERTY, Thomas E., Administrator, Mecosta County General Hospital, Big Rapids, MI, p. A212
DAUGHERTY, Jr., John, Service Unit Director, U. S. Public Health Service Comprehensive Indian Health Facility, Claremore, OK, p. A342
DAVANZO, John P.
 President and Chief Executive Officer, Mercy Hospital, Buffalo, NY, p. A289
 President and Chief Executive Officer, Our Lady of Victory Hospital, Lackawanna, NY, p. A293
DAVE, Bhasker J., M.D., Superintendent, Mental Health Institute, Independence, IA, p. A153
DAVIDGE, Robert C., Chief Executive Officer, Our Lady of the Lake Regional Medical Center, Baton Rouge, LA, p. A180
DAVIDSON, Craig Val, CHE, Administrator, Beaver Valley Hospital, Beaver, UT, p. A436
DAVIS, Charles A., Administrator and Chief Executive Officer, Allen Memorial Hospital, Moab, UT, p. A437
DAVIS, David R., President and Chief Executive Officer, UPMC Lee Regional, Johnstown, PA, p. A362
DAVIS, Donald W., President, Northern Westchester Hospital Center, Mount Kisco, NY, p. A295
DAVIS, Gary, Service Unit Director, U. S. Public Health Service Indian Hospital, Parker, AZ, p. A23
DAVIS, Glen C., Administrator, Grady General Hospital, Cairo, GA, p. A102

DAVIS, Gregg, Interim Chief Executive Officer, Perry Memorial Hospital, Princeton, IL, p. A133
DAVIS, Hervey, Administrator, Dr. John Warner Hospital, Clinton, IL, p. A124
DAVIS, John W., Administrator, Warm Springs Rehabilitation Hospital, Gonzales, TX, p. A414
DAVIS, Jon R., Administrator, Odessa Memorial Hospital, Odessa, WA, p. A455
DAVIS, Karen, Chief Executive Officer, HealthSouth Metro West Hospital, Fairfield, AL, p. A14
DAVIS, Kenneth A.
  Chief Executive Officer, Pembroke Hospital, Pembroke, MA, p. A207
  Chief Executive Officer, Westwood Lodge Hospital, Westwood, MA, p. A209
DAVIS, L. Glenn, Executive Director, Central Carolina Hospital, Sanford, NC, p. A318
DAVIS, Larry R., President and Chief Executive Officer, Huron Memorial Hospital, Bad Axe, MI, p. A211
DAVIS, Lary, President, Sonora Community Hospital, Sonora, CA, p. A63
DAVIS, Lora, Administrator, Perry Hospital, Perry, GA, p. A108
DAVIS, Lyle E., Administrator, Cozad Community Hospital, Cozad, NE, p. A262
DAVIS, Michael J., Ph.D., Superintendent, Woodward State Hospital–School, Woodward, IA, p. A158
DAVIS, Pamela Meyer, President and Chief Executive Officer, Edward Hospital, Naperville, IL, p. A131
DAVIS, Paul, Administrator, Gove County Medical Center, Quinter, KS, p. A167
DAVIS, Peter B., President and Chief Executive Officer, St. Joseph Hospital, Nashua, NH, p. A272
DAVIS, Robert L., President and Chief Executive Officer, North Oakland Medical Centers, Pontiac, MI, p. A220
DAVIS, Rod A., President and Chief Executive Officer, St. Rose Dominican Hospital, Henderson, NV, p. A268
DAVIS, Ronald D., Chief Executive Officer, Greater Community Hospital, Creston, IA, p. A150
DAVIS, Rosemari, Chief Executive Officer, Willamette Valley Medical Center, McMinnville, OR, p. A352
DAVIS, Ryland P., President and Chief Executive Officer, Sacred Heart Medical Center, Spokane, WA, p. A457
DAVIS , Jr, Ray H., Chief Executive Officer, Calais Regional Hospital, Calais, ME, p. A192
DAWES, Christopher G., President, Lucile Salter Packard Children's Hospital at Stanford, Palo Alto, CA, p. A54
DAWES, Dennis W., President, Hendricks Community Hospital, Danville, IN, p. A139
DAWES, John M., Vice President Operations, Mercy Hospital Clermont, Batavia, OH, p. A326
DAWSON, George W., President, Centra Health, Inc., Lynchburg, VA, p. B71
DAWSON, Joseph M., Administrator, Blount Memorial Hospital, Maryville, TN, p. A396
DAYE, Patricia, Executive Vice President and Chief Operating Officer, Yonkers General Hospital, Yonkers, NY, p. A308
DE BLASI, Raymond P., Chief Executive Officer, Mesquite Community Hospital, Mesquite, TX, p. A423
DE GASTA, Gary M., Center Director, Veterans Affairs Medical Center, White River Junction, VT, p. A441
DE JEAN, Julie, Administrator and Chief Executive Officer, Kansas Rehabilitation Hospital, Topeka, KS, p. A168
DE MELECIO, Carmen Feliciano, M.D., Secretary of Health, Puerto Rico Department of Health, San Juan, PR, p. B122
DE VOSS, Gerald, Acting Administrator, Duane L. Waters Hospital, Jackson, MI, p. A217
DEAL, Virgil T., Commander, Colonel Florence A. Blanchfield Army Community Hospital, Fort Campbell, KY, p. A172
DEAN, Harrison M., Senior Vice President and Administrator, Baptist Health Baptist Memorial Medical Center, North Little Rock, AR, p. A32
DEAN, Lloyd H., President and Chief Executive Officer, Catholic Healthcare West, San Francisco, CA, p. B69
DEAN, Morre, President, Walla Walla General Hospital, Walla Walla, WA, p. A459
DEAN, Rhonda, Chief Executive Officer, El Dorado Hospital, Tucson, AZ, p. A26

DEAN , Jr, Douglas F., President and Chief Executive Officer, Elliot Hospital, Manchester, NH, p. A272
DEANGELIS, Patricia B., President and Chief Operating Officer, Nazareth Hospital, Philadelphia, PA, p. A367
DEANS, Gerald E., Director, Southwestern Virginia Mental Health Institute, Marion, VA, p. A446
DEARING, Bryan R., Chief Executive Officer, Summit Medical Center, Hermitage, TN, p. A393
DEARTH, Jim, M.D., Chief Executive Officer, Children's Hospital of Alabama, Birmingham, AL, p. A12
DEBRUCE, Lucinda, Chief Executive Officer, BHC Pinnacle Pointe Hospital, Little Rock, AR, p. A31
DECK, K. Douglas, President and Chief Executive Officer, Good Samaritan Hospital and Health Center, Dayton, OH, p. A331
DECKER, James Lee, President and Chief Executive Officer, Gateway Health System, Clarksville, TN, p. A391
DECKER, Michael, President and Chief Executive Officer, Divine Savior Healthcare, Portage, WI, p. A474
DEE, Thomas A., President and Chief Executive Officer, Benedictine Hospital, Kingston, NY, p. A293
DEEMS, Andrew W., President and Chief Executive Officer, Eisenhower Memorial Hospital and Betty Ford Center at Eisenhower, Rancho Mirage, CA, p. A56
DEEN, Robert V., Interim Chief Executive Officer, Flint River Community Hospital, Montezuma, GA, p. A108
DEFAIL, Anthony J., President and Chief Executive Officer, Meadville Medical Center, Meadville, PA, p. A364
DEGEORGE–SMITH, Ellen, FACHE, Director, Veterans Affairs Medical Center, Augusta, GA, p. A101
DEGINA , Jr, Anthony M., Chief Executive Officer, Plantation General Hospital, Plantation, FL, p. A93
DEGRAAF, Douglas P., Chief Executive Officer, Winter Park Memorial Hospital, Winter Park, FL, p. A98
DEGRANDIS, Fred M., President, St. John West Shore Hospital, Cleveland, OH, p. A329
DEGROOT, Randy, Chief Executive Officer, Community Health Center of Branch County, Coldwater, MI, p. A213
DEHNE, Marvin L., Executive Officer, Mercy Hospital, Coon Rapids, MN, p. A227
DEIGAN, Faith A.
  Administrator and Chief Executive Officer, HEALTHSOUTH Greater Pittsburgh Rehabilitation Hospital, Monroeville, PA, p. A364
  Interim Administrator, HEALTHSOUTH Harmarville Rehabilitation Hospital, Pittsburgh, PA, p. A369
DEIKER, Tom, Ph.D., Superintendent, Mental Health Institute, Cherokee, IA, p. A149
DEL MAURO, Ronald J., President and Chief Executive Officer, Saint Barnabas Health Care System, West Orange, NJ, p. B129
DELA CRUZ, Romel, Administrator, Hale Ho'ola Hamakua, Honokaa, HI, p. A112
DELANO, Richard J., President, Albany General Hospital, Albany, OR, p. A350
DELBRIDGE, Andy, Chief Operating Officer, Holly Hill/ Charter Behavioral Health System, Raleigh, NC, p. A316
DELFORGE, Gary L., Administrator, St. Mary's Hospital, Norton, VA, p. A447
DELGADO, Audrey, Administrator, Windmoor Healthcare of Miami, Miami, FL, p. A90
DELISI , II, Frank G., CHE, President and Chief Executive Officer, Suburban General Hospital, Pittsburgh, PA, p. A369
DELLAPORTAS, George, M.D., Director Professional Services, Whitten Center Infirmary, Clinton, SC, p. A379
DELLAROCCO, Paul J.
  President and Chief Executive Officer, Franciscan Children's Hospital and Rehabilitation Center, Boston, MA, p. A202
  President and Chief Executive Officer, Jewish Memorial Hospital and Rehabilitation Center, Boston, MA, p. A202
DELLEA, Eugene A., Interim President, Fairview Hospital, Great Barrington, MA, p. A205
DEMARAIS, Alice, Commander, Reynolds Army Community Hospital, Fort Sill, OK, p. A343

DEMBOW, Jack H., General Director and Vice President, Belmont Center for Comprehensive Treatment, Philadelphia, PA, p. A366
DEMORALES, Jon, Executive Director, Atascadero State Hospital, Atascadero, CA, p. A36
DEMPSEY, Virginia, Vice President Operations, St. Luke's Baptist Hospital, San Antonio, TX, p. A430
DENARDO, John J., Executive Director, University of Illinois at Chicago Medical Center, Chicago, IL, p. A124
DENEY, Robert A., Chief Executive Officer, Charter Behavioral Health System of San Diego, San Diego, CA, p. A58
DENNIS, Daniel, Administrator, Wray Community District Hospital, Wray, CO, p. A73
DENTON, Jack L., President, Eaton Rapids Medical Center, Eaton Rapids, MI, p. A214
DENTRY, Timothy J., President and Chief Executive Officer, Corning Hospital, Corning, NY, p. A290
DEPUTAT, Robert, President, St. John Oakland Hospital, Madison Heights, MI, p. A219
DERNIER, J. Marty, President and Chief Executive Officer, Casa Grande Regional Medical Center, Casa Grande, AZ, p. A22
DERZON, Gordon M., Chief Executive Officer, University of Wisconsin Hospital and Clinics, Madison, WI, p. A470
DESANTIS, Paul A.
  President, Elk Regional Health Center, Saint Marys, PA, p. A371
  President and Chief Executive Officer, Ridgway Health Center, Ridgway, PA, p. A371
DESCHAINE, Terry, Chief Executive Officer, Fredonia Regional Hospital, Fredonia, KS, p. A161
DEUEL, Teresa L., Administrator and Chief Executive Officer, Rush County Memorial Hospital, La Crosse, KS, p. A163
DEURMIER, Carol, Chief Executive Officer, St. Michael's Hospital, Tyndall, SD, p. A388
DEVANSKY, Gary W., Chief Executive Officer, Veterans Affairs Medical Center, Coatesville, PA, p. A358
DEVILLE, Linda F., Chief Executive Officer, Ville Platte Medical Center, Ville Platte, LA, p. A189
DEVINE, Joseph W., Vice President, Hospital Services, Kennedy Memorial Hospitals–University Medical Center, Cherry Hill, NJ, p. A275
DEVINS, Thomas, President, Clinton Hospital, Clinton, MA, p. A204
DEVOCELLE, Frank H., President and Chief Executive Officer, Olathe Medical Center, Olathe, KS, p. A166
DEXTER, Stephen P., Chief Executive Officer, Thomas Memorial Hospital, South Charleston, WV, p. A464
DEXTROM, Nancy, Executive Director, Rogers City Rehabilitation Hospital, Rogers City, MI, p. A221
DEYOUNG, Andrew, Administrator, St. Bernard's Behavioral Health, Jonesboro, AR, p. A31
DI DARIO, Albert R., Superintendent, Norristown State Hospital, Norristown, PA, p. A365
DI PERRY , Jr, John, Executive Vice President and Chief Operating Officer, Mercy Medical Center Redding, Redding, CA, p. A56
DI RISIC, Geraldine, Acting Executive Director, Wayne General Hospital, Wayne, NJ, p. A281
DIAL, Marcia R., Administrator, Scotland County Memorial Hospital, Memphis, MO, p. A250
DIAMOND, Eugene C., President and Chief Executive Officer, Saint Margaret Mercy Healthcare Centers, Hammond, IN, p. A141
DIAZ, Consuelo C., Chief Executive Officer, LAC–Rancho Los Amigos National Rehabilitation Center, Downey, CA, p. A40
DIAZ, Mary, Ed.D., Director, South Texas Hospital, Harlingen, TX, p. A415
DIAZ, Nilda E., Executive Director, Hospital Universitario Dr. Ramon Ruiz Arnau, Bayamon, PR, p. A482
DIAZ , Jr, Alberto, USN, Commander, Naval Medical Center, San Diego, CA, p. A59
DIAZ–REYES, Rogelio, Administrator, Hospital Dr. Dominguez, Humacao, PR, p. A482
DIBERARDINO, William M., FACHE, President and Chief Executive Officer, Jones Memorial Hospital, Wellsville, NY, p. A307

Index of Health Care Professionals / Dibner

DIBNER, David A., FACHE, Interim President and Chief Executive Officer, St. Charles Hospital and Rehabilitation Center, Port Jefferson, NY, p. A303

DICESARE, Gayle, President and Chief Officer, RiverValley Behavioral Health Hospital, Owensboro, KY, p. A177

DICICCO, Christopher, Chief Executive Officer, Graduate Hospital, Philadelphia, PA, p. A367

DICK, David, Administrator, Hans P. Peterson Memorial Hospital, Philip, SD, p. A387

DICKINSON, Daniel P., Administrator, U. S. Air Force Hospital Shaw, Shaw A F B, SC, p. A383

DICKSON, James C., Administrator, Memorial Medical Center, Livingston, TX, p. A421

DICKSON, James J., Administrator and Chief Executive Officer, Copper Queen Community Hospital, Bisbee, AZ, p. A22

DICKSON, Thomas C., Executive Vice President and Chief Operating Officer, Del E. Webb Memorial Hospital, Sun City West, AZ, p. A26

DIEGEL, James A., CHE, Executive Director, Central Oregon District Hospital, Redmond, OR, p. A354

DIER, Joy, Administrator, Vencor Arlington, Texas, Arlington, TX, p. A402

DIETZ, Brian E., FACHE, Executive Vice President, Saint Joseph's Regional Medical Center–Plymouth Campus, Plymouth, IN, p. A145

DIETZ, Francis R., President, Memorial Hospital of Rhode Island, Pawtucket, RI, p. A376

DIFEDERICO, William J., Chief Executive Officer, Olympus Specialty Hospital, Waltham, MA, p. A209

DIFRANCO, Bonnie, Chief Executive Officer, Metropolitan St. Louis Psychiatric Center, Saint Louis, MO, p. A253

DIGNUM, Kirk, Ph.D., President and Chief Executive Officer, Mercy Medical Center, Durango, CO, p. A70

DILLARD, Evan S., President, Walker Baptist Medical Center, Jasper, AL, p. A16

DINAN, Edward M., President and Chief Executive Officer, Lawrence Hospital, Bronxville, NY, p. A288

DINTER, Richard W., M.D., Chief Operating Officer, University Medical Center–Mesabi, Hibbing, MN, p. A229

DIRKSEN, Victor J., Administrator, Jefferson General Hospital, Port Townsend, WA, p. A455

DIRUBBIO, Vincent, President and Chief Executive Officer, Mercy Medical Center, Rockville Centre, NY, p. A304

DISCH, Catherine D., Chief Operating Officer, Truman Medical Center–Hospital Hill, Kansas City, MO, p. A249

DITCH, Donna, Interim President and Chief Executive Officer, Athol Memorial Hospital, Athol, MA, p. A201

DITZEL, Jr, Louis A., President and Chief Executive Officer, Jersey Shore Hospital, Jersey Shore, PA, p. A362

DIX, Dexter D., Director, Veterans Affairs Medical Center, Wilmington, DE, p. A78

DIXON, Mark, Administrator, Abbott Northwestern Hospital, Minneapolis, MN, p. A230

DIXON, Robert, President and Chief Executive Officer, Riverside Health System, Wichita, KS, p. A169

DIXON, Sally J., President and Chief Executive Officer, Memorial Hospital, York, PA, p. A375

DIXON, Stephen E., Chief Executive Officer, Chino Valley Medical Center, Chino, CA, p. A38

DIXON, Thomas D., Administrator, John and Mary Kirby Hospital, Monticello, IL, p. A131

DIZNEY, Donald R., Chairman, United Medical Corporation, Windermere, FL, p. B147

DOAN, Richard L., Chief Executive Officer, Barnesville Hospital Association, Barnesville, OH, p. A326

DOBBS, Steve, Chief Executive Officer, Tulsa Regional Medical Center, Tulsa, OK, p. A349

DOBBS–JOHNSON, Lena, Chief Executive, Bethany Hospital, Chicago, IL, p. A121

DOCKING, Gordon, Chief Executive Officer, St. Mary's Hospital of Blue Springs, Blue Springs, MO, p. A244

DOCKTER, Robert A., Administrator, Eureka Community Health Services/Avera Health, Eureka, SD, p. A386

DODSON, Jean, Administrator, Sylvan Grove Hospital, Jackson, GA, p. A106

DOEDEN, Lynn, Administrator, Decatur County Hospital and Cedar Living Center, Oberlin, KS, p. A165

DOERR, David R., Chief Executive Officer, Union Hospital, Terre Haute, IN, p. A146

DOHERTY, Thomas C., Medical Director, Veterans Affairs Medical Center, Miami, FL, p. A90

DOISE, Daryl J., Administrator, Opelousas General Hospital, Opelousas, LA, p. A188

DONAHUE, Les A., President and Chief Executive Officer, Williamsburg Community Hospital, Williamsburg, VA, p. A451

DONAHUE, Patrick, Administrator, Methodist Hospital Union County, Morganfield, KY, p. A177

DONALD, Donna M., Administrator, Southern Inyo County Local Health Care District, Lone Pine, CA, p. A46

DONEPUDI, Suresh, M.D., Chief Executive Officer, Stonewall Medical Center, Stonewall, LA, p. A189

DONEY, Tennyson, Service Unit Director, U. S. Public Health Service Indian Hospital, Crow Agency, MT, p. A257

DONLIN, Michael, Administrator, Floyd Valley Hospital/Avera Health, Le Mars, IA, p. A154

DONNELL, Vern F., Service Unit Director, U. S. Public Health Service Indian Hospital, Pine Ridge, SD, p. A387

DONNELLAN, Jr, John J., Director, Veterans Administration New York Harbor Healthcare System, New York, NY, p. A300

DONNELLY, Leo J., Executive Director, The Friary of Baptist Health Center, Gulf Breeze, FL, p. A86

DONNELLY, Jr, John J., President and Chief Executive Officer, Roxborough Memorial Hospital, Philadelphia, PA, p. A368

DONOHOO, William M., FACHE, Chief Executive Officer, Marlboro Park Hospital, Bennettsville, SC, p. A378

DONOVAN, Mark A., M.D., President and Chief Executive Officer, Seton Health System, Troy, NY, p. A306

DONOVAN, Robert A., President and Chief Executive Officer, Lowell General Hospital, Lowell, MA, p. A206

DOODY, Dennis W., President and Chief Executive Officer, Medical Center at Princeton, Princeton, NJ, p. A280

DOODY–CHABRE, Kris, Chief Executive Officer, Cary Medical Center, Caribou, ME, p. A192

DOOLAN, Thomas B., Acting President and Chief Executive Officer, Southampton Hospital, Southampton, NY, p. A305

DOOLEY, James J.
President and Chief Executive Officer, Geneva General Hospital, Geneva, NY, p. A291
President and Chief Executive Officer, Soldiers and Sailors Memorial Hospital of Yates County, Penn Yan, NY, p. A302

DOOLEY, Jerry, Chief Executive Officer, Terre Haute Regional Hospital, Terre Haute, IN, p. A146

DOOLEY, Mark, Chief Executive Officer, Dolly Vinsant Memorial Hospital, San Benito, TX, p. A430

DOORDAN, Martin L., President, Anne Arundel Medical Center, Annapolis, MD, p. A195

DOORE, Daniel P., Chief Executive Officer, Community Hospital of Los Gatos, Los Gatos, CA, p. A50

DORAN, Dennis J., Administrator, Cambridge Medical Center, Cambridge, MN, p. A226

DORAN, Hugh F., Director, Veterans Affairs Medical Center, Kansas City, MO, p. A249

DORIS, Doug, Chief Executive Officer, SouthPointe Hospital, Saint Louis, MO, p. A253

DORRIS, Patricia, Chief Executive Officer, Palo Pinto General Hospital, Mineral Wells, TX, p. A424

DORRIS, Ronald E., Senior Vice President and Executive Director, Harris Methodist–Erath County, Stephenville, TX, p. A431

DORSEY, Jeffrey A., Chief Executive Officer, University Health Partners, Oklahoma City, OK, p. A346

DORSEY, Lawrence T., Administrator, University Medical Center, Lafayette, LA, p. A184

DOTSON, Philip E., Chief Executive Officer, Athens–Limestone Hospital, Athens, AL, p. A11

DOTY, Elizabeth A., President and Chief Executive Officer, Regional Health Services of Howard County, Cresco, IA, p. A150

DOUCET, Leonard W.
Interim Chief Executive Officer, Bayou Oaks Behavioral Health System, Houma, LA, p. A183
Interim Chief Executive Officer, Terrebonne General Medical Center, Houma, LA, p. A183

DOUGHERTY, Paul, President and Chief Executive Officer, Deaconess Hospital, Oklahoma City, OK, p. A345

DOVER, James F., FACHE
Chief Executive Officer, Lourdes Counseling Center, Richland, WA, p. A456
Chief Executive Officer, Lourdes Medical Center, Pasco, WA, p. A455

DOVER, Jerry, Chief Executive Officer, Carroll County Memorial Hospital, Carrollton, MO, p. A245

DOWD, Thomas J., President, Nathan Littauer Hospital and Nursing Home, Gloversville, NY, p. A292

DOWDELL, Thomas C., Executive Director and Senior Vice President, Memorial Hospital and Medical Center of Cumberland, Cumberland, MD, p. A197

DOWELL, Jr, Floyd B., Administrator, Lincoln County Memorial Hospital, Troy, MO, p. A255

DOWER, Dianne, Administrator, Lillian M. Hudspeth Memorial Hospital, Sonora, TX, p. A431

DOWLING, Dennis, Executive Director, North Shore University Hospital, Manhasset, NY, p. A294

DOWLING, Mary A., Director, Veterans Affairs Medical Center, Northport, NY, p. A301

DOWN, Philip B., President, Doctors Community Hospital, Lanham, MD, p. A199

DOWNEY, William B., President and Chief Executive Officer, Lewis–Gale Medical Center, Salem, VA, p. A449

DOWNING, Samuel W., Chief Executive Officer, Salinas Valley Memorial Healthcare System, Salinas, CA, p. A58

DOWNS, Martin, Facility Director, Lincoln Developmental Center, Lincoln, IL, p. A129

DOYLE, Jr, James J., President and Chief Executive Officer, Chilton Memorial Hospital, Pompton Plains, NJ, p. A279

DOZIER, Jr, J. Larry, FACHE
Chief Executive Officer, Barnwell County Hospital, Barnwell, SC, p. A378
Chief Executive Officer, Fairfield Memorial Hospital, Winnsboro, SC, p. A384

DOZORETZ, Ronald I., M.D., Chairman, FHC Health Systems, Norfolk, VA, p. B85

DRAGOVAN, Debra M., Chief Executive Officer, Metro Health Center, Erie, PA, p. A360

DRENNAN, Annette V., R.N., President, Specialty Hospital of Meridian, Meridian, MS, p. A240

DREW, John A., President and Chief Executive Officer, Athens Regional Medical Center, Athens, GA, p. A99

DREW, W. David, President and Chief Executive Officer, Atchison Hospital, Atchison, KS, p. A159

DRIEWER, Robert L., Chief Executive Officer, Faith Regional Health Services, Norfolk, NE, p. A264

DRISKILL, Jr, Thomas M., President and Chief Executive Officer, Hawaii Health Systems Corporation, Honolulu, HI, p. B88

DRISNER, Robert E., President and Chief Executive Officer, Community Memorial Hospital, Menomonee Falls, WI, p. A471

DROBOT, Michael D., President and Chief Executive Officer, Pacific Hospital of Long Beach, Long Beach, CA, p. A46

DROP, Jeffrey S., President and Chief Executive Officer, St. Anthony Hospital, Pendleton, OR, p. A352

DROSKE, Richard S., Director, Veterans Affairs Western New York Healthcare System–Batavia Division, Batavia, NY, p. A288

DRUCKER, Steve C., President and Chief Executive Officer, Loretto Hospital, Chicago, IL, p. A122

DRUE, Margi, Administrator, Kahi Mohala, Ewa Beach, HI, p. A112

DUARTE, Pete T., Chief Executive Officer, R. E. Thomason General Hospital, El Paso, TX, p. A411

DUDLEY, James W., Director, Hunter Holmes McGuire Veterans Affairs Medical Center, Richmond, VA, p. A449

DUDLEY, Judy, Director, Central Virginia Training Center, Madison Heights, VA, p. A446

DUERR, Joe, Chief Executive Officer, Perry Memorial Hospital, Perry, OK, p. A346
DUFFIELD, Robert, Administrator, Wilson Memorial Hospital, Floresville, TX, p. A412
DUFFY, Jack, Executive Director, Conifer Park, Glenville, NY, p. A292
DUGAN, Margaret R., Executive Director, Binghamton Psychiatric Center, Binghamton, NY, p. A288
DUGAN, Thomas F., Administrator, St. John Vianney Hospital, Downingtown, PA, p. A359
DUHON, Pam, Administrator and Chief Executive Officer, North Dallas Rehabilitation Hospital, Dallas, TX, p. A409
DUKE, Lance B., FACHE
President and Chief Executive Officer, Phenix Regional Hospital, Phenix City, AL, p. A18
President and Chief Executive Officer, The Medical Center, Columbus, GA, p. A103
DUNAWAY, Clay, Administrator, Walter Olin Moss Regional Medical Center, Lake Charles, LA, p. A184
DUNCAN, Gary D., President and Chief Executive Officer, Freeman Health System, Joplin, MO, p. A247
DUNCAN, Michael J., Chief Executive Officer, George Nigh Rehabilitation Center, Okmulgee, OK, p. A346
DUNCAN, Neal, Executive Director, IHS of Amarillo, Amarillo, TX, p. A401
DUNHAM, David S., President, Southside Regional Medical Center, Petersburg, VA, p. A447
DUNMYER, Daniel C., Chief Executive Officer, Princeton Community Hospital, Princeton, WV, p. A464
DUNN, Joseph W., Ph.D.
Chief Executive Officer, Daniel Freeman Marina Hospital, Venice, CA, p. A66
President and Chief Executive Officer, Daniel Freeman Memorial Hospital, Inglewood, CA, p. A44
DUNN, Michael A., Commander, Walter Reed Army Medical Center, Washington, DC, p. A80
DUNNING, Jr, Raymond M., Chief Executive Officer, Medical Center of Lewisville, Lewisville, TX, p. A421
DUPUIS, Burton, Chief Executive Officer, Gary Memorial Hospital, Breaux Bridge, LA, p. A181
DURHAM, Jeffrey L., Chief Executive Officer, The Medical Center at Franklin, Franklin, KY, p. A172
DURR, Ben M., Administrator, Uvalde County Hospital Authority, Uvalde, TX, p. A433
DURR, Judith, Interim Chief Executive Officer, Ellenville Community Hospital, Ellenville, NY, p. A291
DURRER, Christopher T., President and Chief Executive Officer, Wilson Memorial Hospital, Wilson, NC, p. A319
DUSENBERY, Jack, President, East Cooper Regional Medical Center, Mount Pleasant, SC, p. A382
DWOZAN, C. Richard, President, Habersham County Medical Center, Demorest, GA, p. A104
DYAR, David C., Chief Executive Officer, Westview Hospital, Indianapolis, IN, p. A142
DYE, Jeff, Administrator, Socorro General Hospital, Socorro, NM, p. A286
DYER, Paul F., Administrator, Sutter Merced Medical Center, Merced, CA, p. A51
DYER, Rebecca T., Administrator, Union General Hospital, Blairsville, GA, p. A101
DYETT, Benjamin I., M.D., Director, Ossining Correctional Facilities Hospital, Ossining, NY, p. A302
DYKES, Bradford W., President and Chief Executive Officer, Bedford Regional Medical Center, Bedford, IN, p. A137
DYKES, C. Barry, Senior Vice President, Lankenau Hospital, Wynnewood, PA, p. A375
DYKES , Sr, Kenneth E., Administrator, Trinity Community Hospital, Jasper, FL, p. A87
DYKSTERHOUSE, Trevor J., President and Chief Executive Officer, Northwest Suburban Community Hospital, Belvidere, IL, p. A120
DYKSTRA, Janet, Administrator, Osceola Community Hospital, Sibley, IA, p. A156

E

EADS, John S., Administrator, Washington County Infirmary and Nursing Home, Chatom, AL, p. A13
EAGAR , Jr, Dan M., Administrator, Bessemer Carraway Medical Center, Bessemer, AL, p. A11
EASTHAM, James E., Senior Vice President and Chief Executive Officer, Hermann Hospital, Houston, TX, p. A417
EATON, Fred R., Administrator, Bannock Regional Medical Center, Pocatello, ID, p. A117
EATON, R. Philip, M.D., Vice President Health Scences, University of New Mexico, Albuquerque, NM, p. B149
EBAUGH, Elaine D., Chief Executive Officer, HEALTHSOUTH Rehabilitation Hospital, Largo, FL, p. A88
ECHELARD, Paul D., Administrator, Pinecrest Rehabilitation Hospital, Delray Beach, FL, p. A84
ECKENHOFF, Edward A., President and Chief Executive Officer, National Rehabilitation Hospital, Washington, DC, p. A79
ECKERT, Mary L., President and Chief Executive Officer, Millcreek Community Hospital, Erie, PA, p. A360
ECTON, Doris, Administrator and Chief Executive Officer, Nicholas County Hospital, Carlisle, KY, p. A171
EDDLEMAN, Gwen S., R.N., Interim Chief Executive Officer, Southampton Memorial Hospital, Franklin, VA, p. A444
EDMONDSON, James H., Chief Executive Officer and Administrator, Hillside Hospital, Pulaski, TN, p. A399
EDMUNDSON, Reed
Administrator, Burleson St. Joseph Health Center, Caldwell, TX, p. A406
Administrator, Madison St. Joseph Health Center, Madisonville, TX, p. A422
EDWARDS, John R., Administrator and Chief Executive Officer, Pacific Alliance Medical Center, Los Angeles, CA, p. A49
EDWARDS, Liston G., Director, Cherry Hospital, Goldsboro, NC, p. A313
EDWARDS, Mark, Chief Executive Officer, Massac Memorial Hospital, Metropolis, IL, p. A130
EDWARDS, Samuel, Associate Administrator Hospital Services, Ventura County Medical Center, Ventura, CA, p. A66
EDWARDS , Jr, Bob S., Chief Executive Officer, Bates County Memorial Hospital, Butler, MO, p. A245
EGBERT, Jeff R., Chief Executive Officer, Yoakum Community Hospital, Yoakum, TX, p. A435
EHRHART, Kenneth W., Superintendent, Wernersville State Hospital, Wernersville, PA, p. A374
EHRLICH, Jane, President and Chief Executive Officer, Columbia Memorial Hospital, Hudson, NY, p. A292
EICHELBERGER, Larry, Chief Executive Officer, Fillmore County Hospital, Geneva, NE, p. A263
EICHMAN, Cynthia, Chief Executive Officer and Administrator, Victory Medical Center, Stanley, WI, p. A475
EILERMAN, Ted, President, St. Elizabeth Medical Center, Granite City, IL, p. A127
EILERS, M. Kathleen, Administrator, Milwaukee County Mental Health Division, Milwaukee, WI, p. A472
EISNER, Nina W., Chief Executive Officer, The Pavilion, Champaign, IL, p. A121
EKDAHL, Patricia, President and Chief Executive Officer, Russell County Hospital, Russell Springs, KY, p. A178
EL–SABAAWI, Mohamed, M.D., Acting Facility Director, Northern Virginia Mental Health Institute, Falls Church, VA, p. A443
ELDER, Ronald J., Chief Executive Officer, Barberton Citizens Hospital, Barberton, OH, p. A325
ELDREDGE, Clifford M., President and Chief Executive Officer, Vail Valley Medical Center, Vail, CO, p. A73
ELEGANT, Bruce M., President and Chief Executive Officer, Oak Park Hospital, Oak Park, IL, p. A132
ELFORD, Dorothy J., Executive Director and Administrator, Vencor Hospital – Dallas, Dallas, TX, p. A410
ELHAJ, Ali A., President and Chief Exective Officer, Acadia Hospital, Bangor, ME, p. A191
ELIZABETH, M. Ann, President, Saint Francis Hospital, Poughkeepsie, NY, p. A303
ELKINS, James N., FACHE, Director, Texas Center for Infectious Disease, San Antonio, TX, p. A430
ELKINS, Robert, M.D., Chairman and Chief Exective Officer, Integrated Health Services, Sparks Glencoe, MD, p. B100
ELLERMANN, Michael P., President and Chief Executive Officer, Washington County Hospital, Nashville, IL, p. A131
ELLIOTT, Maurice W., Chief Executive Officer, Methodist Healthcare, Memphis, TN, p. B111
ELLIS, Dan, Administrator, Horn Memorial Hospital, Ida Grove, IA, p. A153
ELLIS, Elmer G., President and Chief Executive Officer, East Texas Medical Center Regional Healthcare System, Tyler, TX, p. B83
ELLIS, Hayden, Administrator, Villa Feliciana Medical Complex, Jackson, LA, p. A183
ELLIS, Michael J., Administrator and Chief Executive Officer, Memorial Nuckolls County Hospital, Superior, NE, p. A267
ELLZEY, Bob, Administrator, Bellville General Hospital, Bellville, TX, p. A404
ELROD, James K., President and Chief Executive Officer, Willis–Knighton Medical Center, Shreveport, LA, p. A189
ELSOM, Donald, Operations Administrator, Providence St. Vincent Medical Center, Portland, OR, p. A353
EMGE, Joann, Chief Executive Officer, Sparta Community Hospital, Sparta, IL, p. A134
ENDERS, Robert, President, Morehead Memorial Hospital, Eden, NC, p. A312
ENDRES, Jack R., Administrator, Muenster Memorial Hospital, Muenster, TX, p. A424
ENG, Bland, Interim Chief Executive Officer, Putnam Community Medical Center, Palatka, FL, p. A92
ENGELKEN, Joseph T., Chief Executive Officer, Community Hospital Onaga, Onaga, KS, p. A166
ENGER, Mark M.
Senior Vice President and Administrator, Fairview Ridges Hospital, Burnsville, MN, p. A226
Senior Vice President and Administrator, Fairview Southdale Hospital, Minneapolis, MN, p. A230
ENGHOLM, Kari L., Administrator and Chief Executive Officer, Dallas County Hospital, Perry, IA, p. A155
ENGLAND, Garry L., President and Chief Executive Officer, St. Joseph Regional Medical Center of Northern Oklahoma, Ponca City, OK, p. A346
ENGLERTH, Ladonna, Administrator, East Carroll Parish Hospital, Lake Providence, LA, p. A184
ENGLES, Joel F., Administrator, Tempe St. Luke's Hospital, Tempe, AZ, p. A26
ENGLISH, David J., President and Chief Executive Officer, Hospice of Northern Virginia, Falls Church, VA, p. A443
ENSLEY, Gordon, Acting Administrator, Lake District Hospital, Lakeview, OR, p. A352
ENSOR, Ronald J., Chief Executive Officer, Medical Center at Terrell, Terrell, TX, p. A432
EPPLEY, Daniel A., FACHE, Executive Director, Vencor Hospital–Metro Detroit, Detroit, MI, p. A214
EPSTEIN, Norman B.
President, Chambersburg Hospital, Chambersburg, PA, p. A357
President, Summit Health, Chambersburg, PA, p. B138
ERB–GUNDEL, Myrna, Administrator, Adair County Memorial Hospital, Greenfield, IA, p. A152
ERGLE , Jr, F. W., Administrator, Tallahatchie General Hospital, Charleston, MS, p. A237
ERICH, Kevin R., President, Frank R. Howard Memorial Hospital, Willits, CA, p. A67
ERICKSON, Lief, M.D., President, Memorial Hospital Corporation of Burlington, Burlington, WI, p. A467
ERICKSON, Tyler A., Chief Executive Officer, Wahiawa General Hospital, Wahiawa, HI, p. A113
ERIXON, Stephen M., Chief Executive Officer, Baxter Regional Medical Center, Mountain Home, AR, p. A32
ERNE, Michael H., President and Chief Executive Officer, Mercy American River/Mercy San Juan Hospital, Carmichael, CA, p. A37
ERNST, John R., Executive Director, Deborah Heart and Lung Center, Browns Mills, NJ, p. A274
ERWINE, Terry E., Administrator, Sac–Osage Hospital, Osceola, MO, p. A251

Index of Health Care Professionals / Escarda

ESCARDA, Ron
　Chief Executive Officer, BHC Fairfax Hospital, Kirkland, WA, p. A454
　Chief Executive Officer, Charter Behavioral Health System of Milwaukee/West Allis, West Allis, WI, p. A477
ESLICK, Thomas J., USAF, Commander, Ehrling Bergquist Hospital, Offutt AFB, NE, p. A265
ESLYN, Cole C.
　Chief Executive Officer, St. David's Medical Center, Austin, TX, p. A403
　Chief Executive Officer, St. David's Pavilion, Austin, TX, p. A403
　Chief Executive Officer, St. David's Rehabilitation Center, Austin, TX, p. A403
ESPELAND, David, Chief Executive Officer, Fallon Medical Complex, Baker, MT, p. A256
ESTUDILLO, Nenda, Administrator, Specialty Hospital, West Covina, CA, p. A67
ETHEREDGE, H. Rex, President and Chief Executive Officer, Memorial Hospital of Jacksonville, Jacksonville, FL, p. A86
ETTER, Carl J., Chief Executive Officer, Riley Memorial Hospital, Meridian, MS, p. A240
ETTLINGER, Roy A.
　Chief Executive Officer, Arbour H. R. I. Hospital, Brookline, MA, p. A203
　Chief Executive Officer, Arbour Hospital, Boston, MA, p. A201
EUSTIS, Mark A.
　President, Christian Hospital Northeast–Northwest, Saint Louis, MO, p. A252
　President and Senior Executive Officer, Missouri Baptist Medical Center, Town and Country, MO, p. A255
EVANS, Donald D., President and Chief Executive Officer, Clarion Hospital, Clarion, PA, p. A357
EVANS, Kelley, Administrator, Beartooth Hospital and Health Center, Red Lodge, MT, p. A259
EVANS, Robert B., Administrator and Chief Executive Officer, East Texas Medical Center Tyler, Tyler, TX, p. A433
EVANS , Jr, John T., President and Chief Executive Officer, Central Washington Hospital, Wenatchee, WA, p. A459
EVENS, Ronald G., M.D.
　President, Barnes–Jewish Hospital, Saint Louis, MO, p. A252
　Interim President and Senior Executive Officer, Barnes–Jewish West County Hospital, Saint Louis, MO, p. A252
EVERETT, Benjamin J., Chief Executive Officer, Horizon Medical Center, Dickson, TN, p. A392
EZZELL, Robert, Administrator, Hemphill County Hospital, Canadian, TX, p. A406

F

FAAS, Michael D., President and Chief Executive Officer, Metropolitan Hospital, Grand Rapids, MI, p. A215
FAGAN–COOK, Ann, Administrator and Chief Executive Officer, Schleicher County Medical Center, Eldorado, TX, p. A412
FAGERSTROM, Charles, Vice President, Norton Sound Regional Hospital, Nome, AK, p. A21
FAHD , II, Charles F., Chief Executive Officer, Massena Memorial Hospital, Massena, NY, p. A294
FAHRENBACHER, Fritz, President and Chief Executive Officer, Lee Memorial Hospital, Dowagiac, MI, p. A214
FAILE, Gene, Chief Executive Officer, Greensville Memorial Hospital, Emporia, VA, p. A443
FAILING, Richard J., Chief Executive Officer, Kittson Memorial Healthcare Center, Hallock, MN, p. A228
FAILLA, Richard, Chief Executive Officer, Centennial Peaks Health, Louisville, CO, p. A72
FAIRCHILD, Wayne, Chief Executive Officer, Kahuku Hospital, Kahuku, HI, p. A113
FAIRMAN, John A., Chief Executive Officer, District of Columbia General Hospital, Washington, DC, p. A79

FAITH, Ramona, MS, Site Administrator and Chief Nurse Executive, Petaluma Valley Hospital, Petaluma, CA, p. A55
FAJA, Garry C.
　President and Chief Executive Officer, Saint Joseph Mercy Health System, Ann Arbor, MI, p. A211
　President and Chief Executive Officer, Saline Community Hospital, Saline, MI, p. A222
FAJT, John D., FACHE, President and Chief Operating Officer, Paris Community Hospital, Paris, IL, p. A132
FAKINOS, Maureen, Administrator, Tustin Rehabilitation Hospital, Tustin, CA, p. A65
FALAST, Earl F., Director, Veterans Affairs Medical Center, Marion, IL, p. A130
FALATKO, Michael J., President and Chief Executive Officer, Doctors Hospital of Jackson, Jackson, MI, p. A217
FALE, Randall J., FACHE, President and Chief Executive Officer, St. Joseph's Regional Health Center, Hot Springs National Park, AR, p. A30
FALE, Robert A., President and Chief Executive Officer, Agnesian HealthCare, Fond Du Lac, WI, p. A468
FALLAT, Andrew, FACHE, Chief Executive Officer, Evergreen Community Health Center, Kirkland, WA, p. A454
FALLER, Barbara, Administrator, Chowchilla District Memorial Hospital, Chowchilla, CA, p. A38
FAMA, Cheryl A., Administrator, Vice President and Chief Operating Officer, Saint Francis Memorial Hospital, San Francisco, CA, p. A60
FANNING , Jr, Robert R., President and Chief Executive Officer, Beverly Hospital, Beverly, MA, p. A201
FANTASIA, Saverio C., Chief Financial Officer, St. Elizabeths Hospital, Washington, DC, p. A80
FARBER, Nancy D., Chief Executive Officer, Washington Township Health Care District, Fremont, CA, p. A41
FARMER, Mark R., Vice President and Administrator, Presbyterian Hospital–Matthews, Matthews, NC, p. A315
FARNELL, Leland E., President, Johnston Memorial Hospital, Smithfield, NC, p. A318
FARNSWORTH, Edward F., President, Capital Region Medical Center, Jefferson City, MO, p. A247
FARNSWORTH, Tracy J., Administrator, Pocatello Regional Medical Center, Pocatello, ID, p. A117
FARR, George D., President and Chief Executive Officer, Children's Medical Center of Dallas, Dallas, TX, p. A408
FARRAND, Cynthia B., Executive Vice President and Administrator, Mary Immaculate Hospital, Newport News, VA, p. A446
FARRELL, Michael J., Chief Executive Officer, Somerset Hospital Center for Health, Somerset, PA, p. A372
FARRELL, Patrick W., Chief Executive Officer, Henrico Doctors' Hospital, Richmond, VA, p. A449
FARRIS, James R., CHE, Chief Executive Officer, Wabash General Hospital District, Mount Carmel, IL, p. A131
FARROW, Randall A., Administrator, Mille Lacs Health System, Onamia, MN, p. A231
FARROW, Shelby, Administrator, California Medical Facility, Vacaville, CA, p. A65
FATCH, Casey, Administrator and Chief Operating Officer, Pacifica Hospital of the Valley, Los Angeles, CA, p. A49
FAULK, A. Donald, FACHE, President, Medical Center of Central Georgia, Macon, GA, p. A107
FAULKNER, Charlie, President, Princeton Baptist Medical Center, Birmingham, AL, p. A12
FAULKNER, David M., Chief Executive Officer, Central Montana Medical Center, Lewistown, MT, p. A258
FAULKNER, John M., Executive Director, Northwest Mississippi Regional Medical Center, Clarksdale, MS, p. A237
FAULKNER, Mark, Administrator, Jay Hospital, Jay, FL, p. A87
FAULKNER, Tom, Chief Executive Officer, Hillsboro Community Medical Center, Hillsboro, KS, p. A162
FAULWELL, James A., Chief Executive Officer and Administrator, Dells Area Health Center, Dell Rapids, SD, p. A385

FAUS, Douglas
　Chief Executive Officer, Jefferson County Hospital, Fairfield, IA, p. A152
　Chief Executive Officer, Liberty County Hospital and Nursing Home, Chester, MT, p. A256
FAUST, Bill D., Administrator, Floyd County Memorial Hospital, Charles City, IA, p. A149
FAVRET, John M., Director, Eastern State Hospital, Williamsburg, VA, p. A450
FAWZY, Fawzy I., M.D., Medical Director, University of California Los Angeles Neuropsychiatric Hospital, Los Angeles, CA, p. A50
FEARS, John R.
　Director, Carl T. Hayden Veterans Affairs Medical Center, Phoenix, AZ, p. A24
　Acting Director, Veterans Affairs Edward Hines, Jr. Hospital, Hines, IL, p. A128
FEAZELL, Samuel G., Chief Executive Officer, San Angelo Community Medical Center, San Angelo, TX, p. A428
FEDERMAN, William, Chief Executive Officer, Northwest Surgical Hospital, Oklahoma City, OK, p. A346
FEDERSPIEL, John C., President and Chief Executive Officer, Hudson Valley Hospital Center, Cortlandt Manor, NY, p. A290
FEDYK, Mark F., Administrator, Morrison Community Hospital, Morrison, IL, p. A131
FEEHERY, Matt, Chief Executive Officer, Beech Hill Hospital, Dublin, NH, p. A271
FEELEY, William F., Director, Veterans Affairs Western New York Healthcare System–Buffalo Division, Buffalo, NY, p. A289
FEIKE, Jeffrey, Administrator and Chief Executive Officer, Churchill Community Hospital, Fallon, NV, p. A268
FEILER, Kenneth H., President and Chief Executive Officer, Rose Medical Center, Denver, CO, p. A69
FEINBERG, E. Richard, M.D., Executive Director, Bronx Children's Psychiatric Center, New York, NY, p. A295
FEIT, Marcy L.
　Chief Executive Officer, ValleyCare Health System, Pleasanton, CA, p. B151
　Chief Executive Officer, ValleyCare Medical Center, Pleasanton, CA, p. A55
　Chief Executive Officer, ValleyCare Memorial Hospital, Livermore, CA, p. A46
FELDMAN, Mitchell S., Chief Executive Officer, Delray Medical Center, Delray Beach, FL, p. A83
FELDMAN, Richard I., Chief Executive Officer, BHC Belmont Pines Hospital, Youngstown, OH, p. A340
FELDT, Roger D., FACHE, President and Chief Executive Officer, Saline Memorial Hospital, Benton, AR, p. A28
FELGAR, Alvin D., President and Chief Executive Officer, Frisbie Memorial Hospital, Rochester, NH, p. A273
FELICI, Brian K., Vice President and Administrator, East Ohio Regional Hospital, Martins Ferry, OH, p. A334
FELICIANO, Jose R., Executive Director, Ryder Memorial Hospital, Humacao, PR, p. A482
FELIX, Larry A., CHE, Administrator, Ransom Memorial Hospital, Ottawa, KS, p. A166
FELLA, Peter T., Commissioner, Doctor Robert L. Yeager Health Center, Pomona, NY, p. A302
FELLOWS, Steven A., President, San Gabriel Valley Medical Center, San Gabriel, CA, p. A60
FELTON, David, President and Chief Executive Officer, Community Memorial Hospital, Hamilton, NY, p. A292
FENCEL, Michael M., Chief Executive Officer, Brandon Regional Hospital, Brandon, FL, p. A82
FENSKE, Candace, Administrator, Madelia Community Hospital, Madelia, MN, p. A229
FERGUSON, James E., Interim Administrator, Stanton County Health Care Facility, Johnson, KS, p. A163
FERGUSON, Jared, Administrator and Chief Executive Officer, Kenmare Community Hospital, Kenmare, ND, p. A323
FERGUSON, John P., FACHE, President and Chief Executive Officer, Hackensack University Medical Center, Hackensack, NJ, p. A276
FERGUSON, Joseph W., Vice President of Administration, Crittenton Hospital, Rochester, MI, p. A221
FERNANDEZ, Andres, Director, University Medical Center, Fresno, CA, p. A42

FERNENDEZ, Aurelio, Chief Executive Officer, Hialeah Hospital, Hialeah, FL, p. A86
FERRANTO, Carmen N., Chief Executive Officer, Warren State Hospital, North Warren, PA, p. A365
FERRELL, David A., President, Mercy Hospital, Hamilton, OH, p. A333
FERRY, John M., Executive Director, Memorial Hospital of Sweetwater County, Rock Springs, WY, p. A479
FERRY, Thomas P., Administrator and Chief Executive, Alfred I. duPont Hospital for Children, Wilmington, DE, p. A78
FERRY, William A., Administrator, Vermilion Hospital for Psychiatric and Addictive Medicine, Lafayette, LA, p. A184
FETH, Joseph S., Chief Executive Officer, Provena Health, Frankfort, IL, p. B120
FETTERS, Larry S., Administrator and Chief Operating Officer, Foothill Presbyterian Hospital–Morris L. Johnston Memorial, Glendora, CA, p. A43
FEUQUAY, Judith K., Chief Executive Officer, Logan Hospital and Medical Center, Guthrie, OK, p. A344
FEURIG, Thomas L., President and Chief Executive Officer, St. Joseph Mercy Oakland, Pontiac, MI, p. A221
FICKEN, Robert A., Chief Executive Officer, Dallas–Fort Worth Medical Center, Grand Prairie, TX, p. A414
FICKLEN, Susan, Administrator and Chief Operating Officer, George E. Weems Memorial Hospital, Apalachicola, FL, p. A81
FICKLIN, Dennis E., Chief Executive Officer, Family Health West, Fruita, CO, p. A70
FIDUCIA, Karen A., Interim Chief Executive Officer, Natchez Regional Medical Center, Natchez, MS, p. A241
FIELD, Robyn, Ph.D., Chief Operating Officer, HEALTHSOUTH Bakersfield Rehabilitation Hospital, Bakersfield, CA, p. A36
FIELDS, Donald, Administrator, Whitesburg Appalachian Regional Hospital, Whitesburg, KY, p. A179
FIELDS, Ronald B., President, Tri–County Memorial Hospital, Whitehall, WI, p. A477
FIGUN, Monica A., USAF, Administrator, U. S. Air Force Regional Hospital, Eglin AFB, FL, p. A84
FIKE, Ruthita J.
  Administrator, Littleton Adventist Hospital, Littleton, CO, p. A72
  Administrator, Porter Adventist Hospital, Denver, CO, p. A69
FIKSE, David J., Chief Executive Officer, Parkview Hospital, Philadelphia, PA, p. A367
FILLER, Scott, Chief Executive Officer, HEALTHSOUTH Rehabilitation Hospital of Altoona, Altoona, PA, p. A355
FINAN, Patricia, President and Chief Executive Officer, Wyoming Valley Health Care System, Wilkes–Barre, PA, p. A374
FINAN , Jr, John J., President and Chief Executive Officer, Franciscan Missionaries of Our Lady Health System, Inc., Baton Rouge, LA, p. B85
FINCH, Kenneth A., Chief Executive Officer, Metroplex Adventist Hospital, Killeen, TX, p. A420
FINCH , Jr, J. W., Administrator, Elkview General Hospital, Hobart, OK, p. A344
FINCHER, Ron, Chief Executive Officer, Charter Behavioral Health System of Atlanta at Peachford, Atlanta, GA, p. A99
FINE, David J., Chief Executive Officer, University of Alabama System, Birmingham, AL, p. B149
FINE, Stuart H., Chief Executive Officer, Grand View Hospital, Sellersville, PA, p. A372
FINK, Matthew E., M.D., President and Chief Executive Officer, Beth Israel Medical Center, New York, NY, p. A295
FINKLEIN, Terry O., Chief Executive Officer, Columbia Memorial Hospital, Astoria, OR, p. A350
FINLEY, Edward, Administrator, Wichita County Health Center, Leoti, KS, p. A164
FINN, Donald J., Administrator, Lake Area Hospital, Webster, SD, p. A389
FINN, Michael J., Acting Vice President and Chief Operating Officer, Methodist Hospital of Sacramento, Sacramento, CA, p. A57
FINNEGAN, John R., Chief Executive Officer, Central Mississippi Medical Center, Jackson, MS, p. A239

FINNEY, Michele, Chief Executive Officer, Los Alamitos Medical Center, Los Alamitos, CA, p. A47
FINUCANE, Mark, Director Health Services, Los Angeles County–Department of Health Services, Los Angeles, CA, p. B106
FINZEN, Terry S., President, Regions Hospital, Saint Paul, MN, p. A233
FIORENTINO, Leanne, Chief Executive Officer, Vencor Hospital–Greensboro, Greensboro, NC, p. A313
FIRES, Wiley M., Administrator, Shamrock General Hospital, Shamrock, TX, p. A430
FISCHER, Carl R., Associate Vice President and Chief Executive Officer, Medical College of Virginia Hospitals, Virginia Commonwealth University, Richmond, VA, p. A449
FISCHER, Robert W., President, Northwest Hospital Center, Randallstown, MD, p. A199
FISH, David R., Executive Vice President, St. Joseph's Hospital, Chippewa Falls, WI, p. A467
FISHER, Donald Joe, Administrator, King's Daughters Hospital, Greenville, MS, p. A238
FISHER, Jan E., R.N., Executive Director, Soldiers and Sailors Memorial Hospital, Wellsboro, PA, p. A374
FISHER, Philip, President and Chief Executive Officer, Valley View Regional Hospital, Ada, OK, p. A341
FISHER, Reis, Service Unit Director, U. S. Public Health Service Blackfeet Community Hospital, Browning, MT, p. A256
FISHER, Martin J., USA, Deputy Commander for Administration, Brooke Army Medical Center, San Antonio, TX, p. A428
FISHERO, Harvey L., President and Chief Executive Officer, Medical Center of Plano, Plano, TX, p. A426
FITCH , Sr, Carl W., President and Chief Executive Officer, Wesley Medical Center, Wichita, KS, p. A169
FITZ , Jr, Thomas E., FACHE, President and Chief Executive Officer, St. Mary's Health Care System, Athens, GA, p. A99
FITZGERALD, Gerald D., President and Chief Executive Officer, Oakwood Healthcare, Inc., Dearborn, MI, p. B116
FITZGIBBON, Susan H., President and Chief Executive Officer, Annie Penn Hospital, Reidsville, NC, p. A317
FITZPATRICK, Daniel, Chief Executive Officer, Harlan ARH Hospital, Harlan, KY, p. A172
FITZPATRICK, Susan, Administrator, Meadowbrook Rehabilitation Hospital, Gardner, KS, p. A161
FLAHERTY, Tom, Assistant Administrator, Los Angeles County Central Jail Hospital, Los Angeles, CA, p. A48
FLAIG, William G., Administrator, Douglas County Hospital, Alexandria, MN, p. A225
FLAKE, Glenn M., Executive Director, Newnan Hospital, Newnan, GA, p. A108
FLAMINI, Joseph, Chief Executive Officer, Rancocas Hospital, Willingboro, NJ, p. A281
FLEETWOOD , Jr, James M., Chairman, President, Chief Executive Officer and Chief Operating Officer, LifePoint Hospitals, Inc., Brentwood, TN, p. B105
FLEISCHMANN, Larry, M.D., President, Children's Hospital of Michigan, Detroit, MI, p. A213
FLEMING, Cheryl, Chief Executive Officer, HEALTHSOUTH Rehabilitation Hospital of York, York, PA, p. A375
FLEMING, John L., M.D., Interim Chief Executive Officer, Laureate Psychiatric Clinic and Hospital, Tulsa, OK, p. A348
FLEMING, Leslie K., CPA, Co–Chief Executive Officer, San Luis Valley Regional Medical Center, Alamosa, CO, p. A68
FLEMING, Wanda C., Administrator and Chief Executive Officer, Claiborne County Hospital, Port Gibson, MS, p. A242
FLESSNER, Arnold, Administrator, Waverly Municipal Hospital, Waverly, IA, p. A157
FLETCHALL, Terry L., Administrator, Santiam Memorial Hospital, Stayton, OR, p. A354
FLETCHER, Allen P., President and Chief Executive Officer, Northeast Alabama Regional Medical Center, Anniston, AL, p. A11
FLETCHER, Constance N., Ph.D., Director, Southern Virginia Mental Health Institute, Danville, VA, p. A443
FLETCHER, David A., President and Chief Executive Officer, Trinitas Hospital, Elizabeth, NJ, p. A276

FLETCHER, Donald C.
  President and Chief Executive Officer, Blue Water Health Services Corporation, Port Huron, MI, p. B61
  President and Chief Executive Officer, Port Huron Hospital, Port Huron, MI, p. A221
FLITCROFT, Kim, President, Valley Community Hospital, Dallas, OR, p. A350
FLOCKEN, Jeffrey, Interim President and Chief Executive Officer, North Coast Health Care Centers, Santa Rosa, CA, p. A63
FLODEN, Scott, Administrator, Kino Community Hospital, Tucson, AZ, p. A26
FLORES, Toni, Director Operations, Kaiser Foundation Hospital, Fresno, CA, p. A42
FLORES , Jr, Ernesto G.
  Administrator, Christus Spohn Hospital Kleberg, Kingsville, TX, p. A420
  Administrator, Dimmit County Memorial Hospital, Carrizo Springs, TX, p. A406
FLORO, Mark K., Chief Operating Officer, HEALTHSOUTH Rehabilitation Hospital of Central Kentucky, Elizabethtown, KY, p. A171
FLOWERS, Randel, Ph.D., Administrator, Clinton County Hospital, Albany, KY, p. A170
FLOYD, James R., Director, Veterans Affairs Medical Center, Salt Lake City, UT, p. A438
FLYNN, Patrick D.
  President and Chief Executive Officer, All Saints Episcopal Hospital of Fort Worth, Fort Worth, TX, p. A412
  President and Chief Executive Officer, All Saints Hospital–Cityview, Fort Worth, TX, p. A412
FLYNN , Jr, James H., President and Chief Executive Officer, Franciscan Health Partnership, Inc., Latham, NY, p. B85
FOGLE, Patricia, Chief Executive Officer, St. Francis Hospital of New Castle, New Castle, PA, p. A365
FOJTASEK, Georgia R., President and Chief Executive Officer, W. A. Foote Memorial Hospital, Jackson, MI, p. A217
FOLGER, W. Neath, M.D., President and Chief Executive Officer, Immanuel St. Joseph's–Mayo Health System, Mankato, MN, p. A230
FOLLOWELL, Rob, Chief Operating Officer and Administrator, Vicksburg Medical Center, Vicksburg, MS, p. A242
FONNESBECK, Douglas R., Administrator and Chief Executive Officer, Cottonwood Hospital Medical Center, Murray, UT, p. A437
FONTENOT, Teri G., President and Chief Executive Officer, Woman's Hospital, Baton Rouge, LA, p. A181
FONTENOT, Terry J., President and Chief Executive Officer, Medical Center of Mesquite, Mesquite, TX, p. A423
FORBES, Glenn, M.D.
  President and Chief Executive Officer, Franciscan Skemp Healthcare, La Crosse, WI, p. B86
  President and Chief Executive Officer, Franciscan Skemp Healthcare–La Crosse Campus, La Crosse, WI, p. A470
FORD, Raymond L., President and Chief Executive Officer, Glenwood Regional Medical Center, West Monroe, LA, p. A189
FORD, W. Raymond C., Chief Executive Officer, Specialty Hospital Jacksonville, Jacksonville, FL, p. A87
FOREMAN, Spencer, M.D., President, Montefiore Medical Center, New York, NY, p. A298
FORESTER, John, Chief Operating Officer, HEALTHSOUTH Huntington Rehabilitation Hospital, Huntington, WV, p. A462
FORMIGONI, Ugo, Metro–West Network Manager, John J. Madden Mental Health Center, Hines, IL, p. A128
FORNOFF, Gerald A., Chief Executive Officer, Lakeside Hospital, Metairie, LA, p. A185
FOSDICK, Glenn A., President and Chief Executive Officer, Hurley Medical Center, Flint, MI, p. A215
FOSS, R. Coleman, Chief Executive Officer, Methodist Healthcare– Dyersburg Hospital, Dyersburg, TN, p. A392
FOSSUM, John, Administrator, Ely–Bloomenson Community Hospital, Ely, MN, p. A227

Index of Health Care Professionals / Foster

FOSTER, Allen, Administrator, Mizell Memorial Hospital, Opp, AL, p. A17
FOSTER, James B., Chief Executive Officer, Lake Shore Hospital, Irving, NY, p. A293
FOSTER, James R., President, Bert Fish Medical Center, New Smyrna Beach, FL, p. A91
FOSTER, Jon, Executive Vice President and Administrator, Baptist Hospital of East Tennessee, Knoxville, TN, p. A394
FOSTER, Randall S., Administrator and Chief Executive Officer, LAC–King–Drew Medical Center, Los Angeles, CA, p. A48
FOSTER, Jr, Charles L., FACHE, President and Chief Executive Officer, West Georgia Health System, La Grange, GA, p. A106
FOWLER, Kevin N., Chief Executive Officer, Oakdale Community Hospital, Oakdale, LA, p. A187
FOX, Chris, Executive Director, Professional Rehabilitation Hospital, Ferriday, LA, p. A182
FOX, David S., President, Central DuPage Hospital, Winfield, IL, p. A136
FOX, Rosemary, Vice President and Chief Operating Officer, St. Mary's Medical Center, San Francisco, CA, p. A60
FOX, Ted, Administrator and Chief Executive Officer, El Centro Regional Medical Center, El Centro, CA, p. A40
FOX, William W., Chief Executive Officer, Mary Black Health System, Spartanburg, SC, p. A383
FOY, James, President and Chief Executive Officer, St. John's Riverside Hospital, Yonkers, NY, p. A307
FRABLE, Arthur H., Chief Executive Officer, Tri–Valley Health System, Cambridge, NE, p. A262
FRAGALA, M. Richard, M.D., Superintendent, Clifton T. Perkins Hospital Center, Jessup, MD, p. A199
FRAIZER, Frederic L., President and Chief Executive Officer, St. Mary's Medical Center, Saginaw, MI, p. A221
FRALEY, Gary F., Administrator, Shriners Hospitals for Children, Greenville, Greenville, SC, p. A381
FRALEY, R. Reed, Vice President for Health Services, Ohio State University Medical Center, Columbus, OH, p. A330
FRANCES, Richard J., M.D., President and Medical Director, Silver Hill Hospital, New Canaan, CT, p. A75
FRANCIS, M. Lynne, Chief Executive Officer, Massachusetts Respiratory Hospital, Braintree, MA, p. A203
FRANCKE, Bertold, M.D., Interim Executive Director, Vermont State Hospital, Waterbury, VT, p. A441
FRANDSEN, Jeff, Chief Executive Officer, Castleview Hospital, Price, UT, p. A438
FRANKLIN, James P., Administrator, Hillcrest Hospital, Calhoun City, MS, p. A237
FRANZ, Charles C., Chief Executive Officer, South Peninsula Hospital, Homer, AK, p. A20
FRANZ, Paul S., President, Carolinas Medical Center, Charlotte, NC, p. A310
FRARACCIO, Robert D., Chief Executive Officer, Clark Regional Medical Center, Winchester, KY, p. A179
FRASCHETTI, Robert J., President and Chief Executive Officer, St. Jude Medical Center, Fullerton, CA, p. A42
FRASER, John Martin, President and Chief Executive Officer, Nebraska Methodist Hospital, Omaha, NE, p. A265
FRASER, Michael R., Administrator, Pacific Communities Health District, Newport, OR, p. A352
FRAY, George S., Administrator, Ozark Health Medical Center, Clinton, AR, p. A29
FRECH, Terrance R., Chief Executive Officer, Effingham Hospital, Springfield, GA, p. A110
FREEBORN, Lisa J., R.N., Administrator, Trego County–Lemke Memorial Hospital, Wakeeney, KS, p. A169
FREEBURG, Eric, Administrator, Memorial Hospital, Chester, IL, p. A121
FREELAND, Franklin, Ed.D., Chief Executive Officer, Fort Defiance Indian Health Service Hospital, Fort Defiance, AZ, p. A22
FREEMAN, Alan O., Chief Executive Officer, Cass Medical Center, Harrisonville, MO, p. A247
FREEMAN, Carol B., Interim Chief Executive Officer, San Leandro Hospital, San Leandro, CA, p. A61
FREEMAN, Charles Ray, Administrator, Ripley County Memorial Hospital, Doniphan, MO, p. A246
FREEMAN, Harold, M.D., President and Chief Executive Officer, North General Hospital, New York, NY, p. A299
FREEMAN, James M., Chief Executive Officer, Rowan Regional Medical Center, Salisbury, NC, p. A317
FREEMAN, Richard H., Chief Executive Officer, Eleanor Slater Hospital, Cranston, RI, p. A376
FREEMAN, Richard S., Chief Executive Officer, Medical College of Pennsylvania Hospital, Philadelphia, PA, p. A367
FRENCH, II, George E., Chief Executive Officer, Minden Medical Center, Minden, LA, p. A185
FRENCHIE, Richard J.
 Chief Executive Officer, Saint Michael Hospital, Cleveland, OH, p. A329
 President and Chief Executive Officer, UHHS Geauga Regional Hospital, Chardon, OH, p. A327
FRERICHS, Jeffrey, President and Chief Executive Officer, Cabrini Medical Center, New York, NY, p. A296
FRESOLONE, Victor J., FACHE, President and Chief Executive Officer, Mercy Medical Center, Roseburg, OR, p. A354
FREUDEMAN, Dennis J., President, Doctors Hospital, Columbus, OH, p. A330
FREY, Mark A., President and Chief Executive Officer, Alexian Brothers Behavioral Health Hospital, Hoffman Estates, IL, p. A128
FREY, Ted W., President and Senior Executive Officer, St. Louis Children's Hospital, Saint Louis, MO, p. A253
FREYMULLER, Robert S., Chief Executive Officer, Doctors Hospital of Dallas, Dallas, TX, p. A409
FREYSINGER, Edward E., Administrator, Oakwood Heritage Hospital, Taylor, MI, p. A223
FRIED, Jeffrey M., FACHE, President and Chief Executive Officer, Beebe Medical Center, Lewes, DE, p. A78
FRIEDELL, Peter E., M.D., President, Jackson Park Hospital and Medical Center, Chicago, IL, p. A122
FRIEDLANDER, John E.
 President and Chief Executive Officer, Buffalo General Hospital, Buffalo, NY, p. A289
 President and Chief Executive Officer, KALEIDA Health, Buffalo, NY, p. B104
FRIEDMAN, Diane, R.N., President and Chief Executive Officer, Provena Covenant Medical Center, Urbana, IL, p. A135
FRIEDMAN, Steven H., Ph.D., Executive Vice President, Methodist Hospital of Chicago, Chicago, IL, p. A122
FRIEDRICH, II, Daniel J., President and Chief Executive Officer, St. Petersburg General Hospital, Saint Petersburg, FL, p. A94
FRIES, Jack E., President, St. Luke's Hospital, San Francisco, CA, p. A60
FRIESWICK, Gail M., Ed.D., Executive Vice President, Cape Cod Hospital, Hyannis, MA, p. A205
FRIGO, John S., President, Rush North Shore Medical Center, Skokie, IL, p. A134
FRITTS, Rosemary, Administrator, Pike County Memorial Hospital, Murfreesboro, AR, p. A32
FRITZ, Thomas M., Administrator, St. Lukes Rehabilitation Institute, Spokane, WA, p. A457
FROBENIUS, John, President and Chief Executive Officer, St. Cloud Hospital, Saint Cloud, MN, p. A232
FROCK, Charles T., President and Chief Executive Officer, FirstHealth Moore Regional Hospital, Pinehurst, NC, p. A316
FRONZA, Jr, Leo F., President and Chief Executive Officer, Elmhurst Memorial Hospital, New York, IL, p. A125
FRY, Richard, Director, Veterans Affairs Medical Center, Cheyenne, WY, p. A478
FRY, Robert W., President, Bellin Psychiatric Center, Green Bay, WI, p. A469
FRY, Willis F., Administrator, Illinois Valley Community Hospital, Peru, IL, p. A133
FRYE, R. Mark, Chief Executive Officer, Barton County Memorial Hospital, Lamar, MO, p. A249
FRYE, Jr, Edward R., Administrator, Clarendon Memorial Hospital, Manning, SC, p. A382
FUENTES, Miguel A., President and Chief Executive Officer, Bronx–Lebanon Hospital Center, New York, NY, p. A295
FUHRMAN, Andrew, Chief Executive Officer, BHC Fort Lauderdale Hospital, Fort Lauderdale, FL, p. A84
FULFORD, Richard C., Administrator, Gulf Breeze Hospital, Gulf Breeze, FL, p. A86
FULKS, Gerald N., Chief Executive Officer, Lanier Park Hospital, Gainesville, GA, p. A105
FULL, James M., FACHE, Chief Executive Officer, St. Vincent Randolph Hospital, Winchester, IN, p. A147
FULLER, David W., Chief Executive Officer, Harris Hospital, Newport, AR, p. A32
FULLER, Thomas E., Executive Director, Marion County Medical Center, Mullins, SC, p. A382
FULLMER, Richard A., Interim Administrator, University of Utah Hospitals and Clinics, Salt Lake City, UT, p. A438
FULTON, Matthew S., Senior Vice President and Administrator, St. Anthony Central Hospital, Denver, CO, p. A69
FULTS, Kendall R., Chief Operating Officer, Central Valley General Hospital, Hanford, CA, p. A43
FUMAI, Frank L., President and Chief Executive Officer, Cathedral Healthcare System, Inc., Newark, NJ, p. B66
FUNDINGSLAND, Donald W., Chief Executive Officer, ProHealth Care, Waukesha, WI, p. B120
FUNK, Lawrence J., Executive Administrator, Laguna Honda Hospital and Rehabilitation Center, San Francisco, CA, p. A60
FUNK, Michael J., Chief Executive Officer, North Ottawa Community Hospital, Grand Haven, MI, p. A215
FUQUA, David G., R.N., Chief Executive Officer, Daviess County Hospital, Washington, IN, p. A147
FURLONG, Marian M., R.N., Chief Executive Officer, Hudson Medical Center, Hudson, WI, p. A469
FURSTMAN, Marc A., Chief Executive Officer, Los Angeles Metropolitan Medical Center, Los Angeles, CA, p. A48
FUTRELL, Jerry H., Chief Executive Officer, Smith County Memorial Hospital, Carthage, TN, p. A390

G

GABARRO, Ralph, Chief Executive Officer, Mayo Regional Hospital, Dover–Foxcroft, ME, p. A192
GABOW, Patricia A., M.D., Chief Executive Officer and Medical Director, Denver Health Medical Center, Denver, CO, p. A69
GADE, Ronald, M.D., President, St Barnabas Hospital, New York, NY, p. A300
GAFFNEY, Betty, Senior Vice President and Administrator, St. Joseph Memorial Hospital, Murphysboro, IL, p. A131
GAGEN, Thomas C.
 Senior Vice President and Regional Administrator, Scripps Green Hospital, La Jolla, CA, p. A45
 Senior Vice President and Regional Administrator, Scripps Memorial Hospital–La Jolla, La Jolla, CA, p. A45
GAGER, Warren E., President and Chief Executive Officer, William B. Kessler Memorial Hospital, Hammonton, NJ, p. A276
GAGLIARDI, Joseph A., President and Chief Executive Officer, Cancer Treatment Centers of America–Tulsa, Tulsa, OK, p. A348
GAINER, Rolf B., Chief Executive Officer and Administrator, Brookhaven Hospital, Tulsa, OK, p. A348
GAINEY, James W., R.N., Administrator, Tyler County Hospital, Woodville, TX, p. A435
GAINTNER, J. Richard, M.D., Chief Executive Officer, Shands HealthCare, Gainesville, FL, p. B131
GALARCE, Julio, Administrator, Hospital El Buen Pastor, Arecibo, PR, p. A481
GALATI, John P., President and Chief Executive Officer, Clifton Springs Hospital and Clinic, Clifton Springs, NY, p. A290

GALINSKI, Thomas P.
  President and Chief Executive Officer, Ohio Valley Health Services, Wheeling, WV, p. B116
  President and Chief Executive Officer, Ohio Valley Medical Center, Wheeling, WV, p. A465
GALLACHER, Michael R., President and Chief Executive Officer, Sharon Hospital, Sharon, CT, p. A76
GALLAGHER, James P., Chief Executive Officer, Hampton Hospital, Westampton Township, NJ, p. A281
GALLAGHER, John S. T., Chief Executive Officer, North Shore– Long Island Jewish Health System, Great Neck, NY, p. B115
GALLATI, Todd, Chief Executive Officer, Lake City Medical Center, Lake City, FL, p. A87
GALLIN, John I., M.D., Director, Warren G. Magnuson Clinical Center, National Institutes of Health, Bethesda, MD, p. A197
GALLO, Maureen, Administrator, Community Hospital of Lancaster, Lancaster, PA, p. A362
GALLOWAY, Ron, Administrator, Reagan Memorial Hospital, Big Lake, TX, p. A404
GAMACHE, Edward L., Administrator, Deckerville Community Hospital, Deckerville, MI, p. A213
GAMBRELL , Jr, Edward C., Administrator, Stephens County Hospital, Toccoa, GA, p. A110
GAMEL, Richard B., Chief Executive Officer, Norfolk Regional Center, Norfolk, NE, p. A264
GAMMIERE, Thomas A., Senior Vice President and Regional Administrator, Scripps Mercy Hospital, San Diego, CA, p. A59
GAMMON, Sara, President and Chief Executive Officer, Good Shepherd Rehabilitation Hospital, Allentown, PA, p. A355
GANDY, Patrick W., Chief Executive Officer, Sabine Medical Center, Many, LA, p. A185
GANDY , Jr, M. P., Chief Executive Officer, Santa Rosa Medical Center, Milton, FL, p. A90
GANN, Jim, Administrator, Roane Medical Center, Harriman, TN, p. A393
GANTZ, Daniel L., President, Fayette County Hospital, Vandalia, IL, p. A135
GARBER, Jeff, Administrator and Chief Executive Officer, HEALTHSOUTH Rehabilitation Hospital of Sarasota, Sarasota, FL, p. A95
GARCIA, Kay, Interim Administrator, Council Community Hospital and Nursing Home, Council, ID, p. A116
GARCIA, Martha, Chief Executive Officer, Coral Gables Hospital, Coral Gables, FL, p. A83
GARCIA, Robert A., Administrative Director, Presbyterian Kaseman Hospital, Albuquerque, NM, p. A283
GARDINE, Roberta, Chief Executive Officer, St. Louis Psychiatric Rehabilitation Center, Saint Louis, MO, p. A254
GARDNER, Jonathan H., Chief Executive Officer, Southern Arizona Veterans Affairs Healthcare System, Tucson, AZ, p. A27
GARDNER, Paul A., CPA, Administrator, George County Hospital, Lucedale, MS, p. A240
GARDNER , Jr, James E., Chief Executive Officer, Christus St. Patrick Hospital, Lake Charles, LA, p. A184
GARFIELD, Michael W., Administrator, Cheatham Medical Center, Ashland City, TN, p. A390
GARFUNKEL, Sanford M., Director, Veterans Affairs Medical Center, Washington, DC, p. A80
GARMAN, G. Richard, Executive Director, Wayne Memorial Hospital, Honesdale, PA, p. A361
GARNAS, David, Administrator, Wickenburg Regional Hospital, Wickenburg, AZ, p. A27
GARNER, Douglas, Chief Executive Officer, Magnolia Regional Health Center, Corinth, MS, p. A237
GARNER, Gerald J., Chief Executive Officer, Coast Plaza Doctors Hospital, Norwalk, CA, p. A53
GARRETT, Bruce, R.N., Administrator and Chief Executive Officer, Russell Regional Hospital, Russell, KS, p. A167
GARRETT, Patrick R., Chief Executive Officer, Battle Creek Health System, Battle Creek, MI, p. A212
GARRETT, Vernon G., Chief Executive Officer, BHC Intermountain Hospital, Boise, ID, p. A115
GARRIGAN, Michael E., FACHE, President and Chief Executive Officer, St. Francis Hospital, Columbus, GA, p. A103

GARTHWAITE, Thomas L., M.D., Acting Undersecretary for Health, Department of Veterans Affairs, Washington, DC, p. B78
GARVEY, Ronald F., M.D., President, University of Texas Health Center at Tyler, Tyler, TX, p. A433
GASCHO, Dwight, President and Chief Executive Officer, Scheurer Hospital, Pigeon, MI, p. A220
GASCHO, Gale E.
  Chief Executive Officer, Arroyo Grande Community Hospital, Arroyo Grande, CA, p. A35
  Chief Executive Officer, French Hospital Medical Center, San Luis Obispo, CA, p. A61
GASSAWAY, Ross, Executive Director and Chief Executive Officer, Desert Valley Hospital, Victorville, CA, p. A66
GAST, Edwin A., Chief Executive Officer and Administrator, Crawford County Memorial Hospital, Denison, IA, p. A150
GATENS , Sr, Paul D., Administrator, Georgetown Memorial Hospital, Georgetown, SC, p. A381
GATES, Jon M., Chief Executive Officer, United Medical Center, Cheyenne, WY, p. A478
GATES, Monica P., FACHE, Chief Executive Officer, Slidell Memorial Hospital and Medical Center, Slidell, LA, p. A189
GATES, Truman L.
  President and Chief Executive Officer, Desert Regional Medical Center, Palm Springs, CA, p. A54
  President and Chief Executive Officer, John F. Kennedy Memorial Hospital, Indio, CA, p. A44
GATHRIGHT, Dan, Senior Vice President and Administrator, Baptist Health Medical Center–Arkadelphia, Arkadelphia, AR, p. A28
GATMAITAN, Alfonso W., Chief Executive Officer, Tipton County Memorial Hospital, Tipton, IN, p. A146
GAU, Kim, Interim Chief Executive Officer, Guttenberg Municipal Hospital, Guttenberg, IA, p. A152
GAUBE, Gary J., President, Landmark Medical Center, Woonsocket, RI, p. A377
GAUDREAULT, J. Ronald, President and Chief Executive Officer, Huntington Hospital, Huntington, NY, p. A292
GAUTHIER, Bonnie B., President and Chief Executive Officer, Hebrew Home and Hospital, West Hartford, CT, p. A77
GAVALCHIK, Stephen M., Administrator, Webster County Memorial Hospital, Webster Springs, WV, p. A464
GAVENS, Mark R., President, Sentara Norfolk General Hospital, Norfolk, VA, p. A447
GAY , Jr, David E., Director, Bryce Hospital, Tuscaloosa, AL, p. A18
GAYNOR, Stanley J., Chief Executive Officer and Administrator, Black River Memorial Hospital, Black River Falls, WI, p. A467
GEARY, George A., President, Milton Hospital, Milton, MA, p. A206
GEBHARD, Scott, Senior Vice President Operations, JFK Johnson Rehabilitation Institute, Edison, NJ, p. A275
GEE, Thomas H., Administrator, Henry County Medical Center, Paris, TN, p. A398
GEHANT, David P., President and Chief Executive Officer, Boulder Community Hospital, Boulder, CO, p. A68
GEISSLER, Frederick, Chief Executive Officer, Grand View Hospital, Ironwood, MI, p. A217
GEMMELL, Carolyn, Director Operations and Chief Nursing Officer, Johnson City Specialty Hospital, Johnson City, TN, p. A394
GENGLER, Tim, Administrator, Eagle River Memorial Hospital, Eagle River, WI, p. A468
GENTILE, Lawrence, Chief Executive Officer, Redgate Memorial Hospital, Long Beach, CA, p. A46
GENTLING, Steven J., Director, Veterans Affairs Medical Center, Oklahoma City, OK, p. A346
GENTRY, Lee, President, Lawrence Memorial Hospital, Walnut Ridge, AR, p. A34
GENTRY, Michael V., President, Park Ridge Hospital, Fletcher, NC, p. A313
GEORGE, Alan E., Administrator, Camden Medical Center, Saint Marys, GA, p. A109
GEORGE, Dennis L., Chief Executive Officer, Coffey County Hospital, Burlington, KS, p. A159
GEORGE, Eddie A., President and Chief Executive Officer, Wellmont Health System, Kingsport, TN, p. B153

GEORGE, Elnora, Administrator, Chief Executive Officer and Chief Financial Officer, John C. Fremont Healthcare District, Mariposa, CA, p. A51
GEORGE, Gladys, President and Chief Executive Officer, Lenox Hill Hospital, New York, NY, p. A297
GEPFORD, Jon W., President and Chief Executive Officer, Parkview Hospital, Brunswick, ME, p. A192
GERATHS, Nathan L., Director, William S. Middleton Memorial Veterans Hospital, Madison, WI, p. A470
GERBER, Carl J., Ph.D., Director, James H. Quillen Veterans Affairs Medical Center, Mountain Home, TN, p. A397
GERDES, Jerrell F., Administrator, Franklin County Memorial Hospital, Franklin, NE, p. A262
GERLACH, George, Administrator, Granite Falls Municipal Hospital and Manor, Granite Falls, MN, p. A228
GERLACH, John R., Chief Executive Officer and Administrator, DeKalb Medical Center, Decatur, GA, p. A103
GERLACH, Matthew S., Chief Executive Officer and President, Beverly Hospital, Montebello, CA, p. A52
GERMAN, Anthony, Administrator and Chief Executive Officer, Kell West Regional Hospital, Wichita Falls, TX, p. A435
GETTYS , II, Roddey E., Executive Vice President, Palmetto Baptist Medical Center Easley, Easley, SC, p. A380
GHERARDINI, Michael M., Chief Executive Officer and Managing Director, Auburn Regional Medical Center, Auburn, WA, p. A452
GHOLSTON, Linda J., Chief Executive Officer, Grenada Lake Medical Center, Grenada, MS, p. A238
GIANNUNZIO, Diane D., President, Southwest Rehabilitation Hospital, Battle Creek, MI, p. A212
GIBBS, Henry T., Administrator and Chief Executive Officer, Hancock Memorial Hospital, Sparta, GA, p. A110
GIBOFSKY, Allan, President and Chief Executive Officer, Long Island College Hospital, New York, NY, p. A297
GIBSON, James P., Administrator, Lincoln County Medical Center, Ruidoso, NM, p. A286
GIBSON, Jimmie Ruth, Administrator, Hope Hospital, Lockhart, SC, p. A382
GIBSON, Reginald P., FACHE, Executive Director, St. Elizabeth Ann Seton Hospital, Boonville, IN, p. A138
GIBSON, Thomas J., Administrator, University of South Alabama Knollwood Park Hospital, Mobile, AL, p. A16
GIBSON , II, Earnest, Administrator, Riverside General Hospital, Houston, TX, p. A417
GIDDINGS, Lucille C., CHE, President and Chief Executive Officer, Nantucket Cottage Hospital, Nantucket, MA, p. A206
GIDEON, Dan, President and Chief Executive Officer, Westwood Medical Center, Midland, TX, p. A424
GIERMAK, William C., President and Chief Executive Officer, Louise Obici Memorial Hospital, Suffolk, VA, p. A450
GILBERT, Andrea F., Senior Vice President, Bryn Mawr Hospital, Bryn Mawr, PA, p. A357
GILBERT, Berry, Administrator, Choctaw County Medical Center, Ackerman, MS, p. A236
GILBERT, Brian D., Chief Executive Officer, Wrangell Medical Center, Wrangell, AK, p. A21
GILBERT, Thomas D.
  President and Chief Executive Officer, Emory Dunwoody Medical Center, Atlanta, GA, p. A100
  Chief Executive Officer, Emory Northlake Regional Medical Center, Tucker, GA, p. A110
GILBERT, Tim J., Administrator, Maniilaq Health Center, Kotzebue, AK, p. A21
GILBERT, William L., Chief Executive Officer, San Jose Medical Center, San Jose, CA, p. A60
GILBERTI, Gary M., Chief Executive Officer, Arbour–Fuller Hospital, Attleboro, MA, p. A201
GILBERTSON, Gerry, Administrator, Fairmont Community Hospital, Fairmont, MN, p. A227
GILBERTSON, Roger, M.D., President, MeritCare Health System, Fargo, ND, p. A322
GILES, Alyson Pitman, President and Chief Executive Officer, Catholic Medical Center, Manchester, NH, p. A272
GILES, Dennis A., President, Thoms Rehabilitation Hospital, Asheville, NC, p. A309

Index of Health Care Professionals / Gill

GILL, Jimmy Ben, Chief Executive Officer and Administrator, Clay County Memorial Hospital, Henrietta, TX, p. A415

GILLEN, Michael J., Administrator, Sterling Regional MedCenter, Sterling, CO, p. A73

GILLIARD, Ronald M., FACHE, Administrator, Mitchell County Hospital, Camilla, GA, p. A102

GILLIHAN, Kerry G., FACHE, President and Chief Executive Officer, Cardinal Hill Rehabilitation Hospital, Lexington, KY, p. A174

GILLMAN, Jerry E., Chief Executive Officer, Sanger General Hospital, Sanger, CA, p. A61

GILMORE, Beverly, Chief Executive Officer, Sutter Solano Medical Center, Vallejo, CA, p. A66

GILSTRAP, M. E., President and Chief Executive Officer, Halifax Regional Medical Center, Roanoke Rapids, NC, p. A317

GINGERICH, James, Senior Vice President and Chief Executive Officer, Mesa Lutheran Hospital, Mesa, AZ, p. A23

GINTOLI, George P., Chief Executive Officer, Northcoast Behavioral Healthcare System, Northfield, OH, p. A336

GINTZIG, Donald R., President and Chief Executive Officer, Pottsville Hospital and Warne Clinic, Pottsville, PA, p. A371

GIO, Dominick J., President and Chief Executive Officer, Wyckoff Heights Medical Center, New York, NY, p. A301

GIRON, Gary L. J., Executive Director, Southern New Mexico Rehabilitation Center, Roswell, NM, p. A285

GISLER, Paula, Administrator, Baptist Rehabilitation–Germantown, Germantown, TN, p. A392

GITCH, David W., President and Chief Executive Officer, Harrison Memorial Hospital, Bremerton, WA, p. A452

GIULITTO, Dean R., Commander, Irwin Army Community Hospital, Fort Riley, KS, p. A161

GLAVIS, Edward S.
 Administrator, Kaiser Foundation Hospital, Sacramento, CA, p. A57
 Administrator, Kaiser Foundation Hospital, Sacramento, CA, p. A57

GLAZIER, Stephen M., Executive Director, Orlando Regional South Seminole Hospital, Longwood, FL, p. A88

GLEDHILL, John E., Administrator, Milford Valley Memorial Hospital, Milford, UT, p. A437

GLENN, Michael, Administrator and Chief Executive Officer, Olympic Memorial Hospital, Port Angeles, WA, p. A455

GLOOR, Michael R., FACHE, President and Chief Executive Officer, St. Francis Medical Center, Grand Island, NE, p. A263

GLOSSY, Bernard, President and Chief Executive Officer, Verdugo Hills Hospital, Glendale, CA, p. A43

GLUECKERT, John W., President, St. Joseph Hospital, Polson, MT, p. A259

GOBLE, Jonathan R., President and Chief Executive Officer, La Porte Regional Health System, La Porte, IN, p. A143

GODDARD, Richard L., Chief Executive Officer, Hopkins County Memorial Hospital, Sulphur Springs, TX, p. A431

GOEBEL, Dennis
 Administrator, Community Memorial Hospital, Turtle Lake, ND, p. A324
 Administrator, Garrison Memorial Hospital, Garrison, ND, p. A322

GOERING, Melvin, Chief Executive Officer, Prairie View, Newton, KS, p. A165

GOERTZEN, Irma E., President and Chief Executive Officer, Magee–Womens Hospital, Pittsburgh, PA, p. A369

GOESER, Stephen L., Administrator, Shelby County Myrtue Memorial Hospital, Harlan, IA, p. A152

GOFF, James A., FACHE, Director, Veterans Affairs Palo Alto Health Care System, Palo Alto, CA, p. A54

GOFORTH, Sheri, Chief Executive Officer, Jay County Hospital, Portland, IN, p. A145

GOLD, Larry M., President and Chief Executive Officer, Connecticut Children's Medical Center, Hartford, CT, p. A74

GOLD, Richard, Chief Executive Officer, West Boca Medical Center, Boca Raton, FL, p. A81

GOLDBERG, Donald H., President, New England Sinai Hospital and Rehabilitation Center, Stoughton, MA, p. A209

GOLDBERG, Edward M., President and Chief Executive Officer, St. Alexius Medical Center, Hoffman Estates, IL, p. A128

GOLDEN, Carolyn P., Administrator, Shriners Hospitals for Children, St. Louis, Saint Louis, MO, p. A253

GOLDFARB, Saul, President and Chief Executive Officer, Gateways Hospital and Mental Health Center, Los Angeles, CA, p. A47

GOLDFARB, Timothy M., Director Health Systems, OHSU Hospital, Portland, OR, p. A353

GOLDMAN, Eric, Chief Operating Officer, Columbia Hospital, West Palm Beach, FL, p. A97

GOLDMAN, T. Marvin, Administrator, Memorial Hospital of Sheridan County, Sheridan, WY, p. A479

GOLDMAN, Thomas, President and Chief Executive Officer, Bayshore Community Hospital, Holmdel, NJ, p. A277

GOLDSMITH, Martin
 President, Albert Einstein Healthcare Network, Philadelphia, PA, p. B51
 President, Albert Einstein Medical Center, Philadelphia, PA, p. A366

GOLDSTEIN, Gary W., M.D., President, Kennedy Krieger Children's Hospital, Baltimore, MD, p. A196

GOLDSTEIN, Steven, Ph.D., President and Chief Executive Officer, Chestnut Lodge Hospital, Rockville, MD, p. A199

GOLDSTEIN, Steven I.
 President and Chief Executive Officer, Highland Hospital of Rochester, Rochester, NY, p. A303
 General Director and Chief Executive Officer, Strong Memorial Hospital of the University of Rochester, Rochester, NY, p. A304

GOLI, Rajitha, M.D., Administrator and Chief Executive Officer, Goli Medical Center, Sargent, NE, p. A

GOLSON, Allen, Chief Executive Officer, Palmyra Medical Centers, Albany, GA, p. A99

GONZALES, Joseph, Chief Executive Officer, Hendry Regional Medical Center, Clewiston, FL, p. A82

GONZALEZ, Arthur A., Dr.PH, President and Chief Executive Officer, Tri–City Medical Center, Oceanside, CA, p. A53

GONZALEZ, Pedro J.
 Executive Director, Ashford Presbyterian Community Hospital, San Juan, PR, p. A483
 Executive Director, San Carlos General Hospital, San Juan, PR, p. A484

GOODE, Galen, Chief Executive Officer, Hamilton Center, Terre Haute, IN, p. A146

GOODE, Stephen M., Executive Director, Bayside Community Hospital, Anahuac, TX, p. A401

GOODLOE, Larry S., Administrator, Community Hospital Association, Fairfax, MO, p. A246

GOODMAN, Carol L., Administrator and Chief Executive Officer, Union County Hospital District, Anna, IL, p. A119

GOODMAN, Norman B., President and Chief Executive Officer, Brockton Hospital, Brockton, MA, p. A203

GOODMAN, Terry, Chief Operating Officer, Miami Jewish Home and Hospital for Aged, Miami, FL, p. A90

GOODRICH, Barbara K., R.N., Administrator, Alegent Health Immanuel Medical Center, Omaha, NE, p. A265

GOODRICH, Ralph G., Chief Executive Officer, Wright Memorial Hospital, Trenton, MO, p. A255

GOODSPEED, Ronald B., M.P.H., President, Southcoast Hospitals Group, Fall River, MA, p. A204

GOODSPEED, Scott W., FACHE, President and Chief Executive Officer, Anna Jaques Hospital, Newburyport, MA, p. A207

GOODWIN, Jeffrey C., President and Chief Executive Officer, Warren Hospital, Phillipsburg, NJ, p. A279

GOODWIN, Phillip H., FACHE
 President and Chief Executive Officer, Camcare, Inc., Charleston, WV, p. B63
 President and Chief Executive Officer, Charleston Area Medical Center, Charleston, WV, p. A460

GOODWIN, Robert P., President and Chief Executive Officer, Lourdes Hospital, Paducah, KY, p. A177

GORDON, Bruce A., Director, Veterans Affairs Medical Center, Leeds, MA, p. A205

GORDON, William G., Chief Executive Officer, Barton Memorial Hospital, South Lake Tahoe, CA, p. A64

GORE, Gary R., Chief Executive Officer, Marshall Medical Center North, Guntersville, AL, p. A15

GORMAN, John A., Chief Executive Officer, Memorial Hospital, Fremont, OH, p. A332

GOSLINE, Peter L., Chief Executive Officer, Monadnock Community Hospital, Peterborough, NH, p. A273

GOTSCHLICH, Emil, M.D., Vice President Medical Sciences, Rockefeller University Hospital, New York, NY, p. A299

GOTTSCHALK, M. Therese, President, Marian Health System, Tulsa, OK, p. B107

GOULD, Gary R., FACHE, Chief Executive Officer, Belmont Community Hospital, Bellaire, OH, p. A326

GOULET, Diana L., Administrator and Chief Executive Officer, BHC Vista Del Mar Hospital, Ventura, CA, p. A66

GOUX, L. Rene'
 Chief Executive Officer, NorthShore Regional Medical Center, Slidell, LA, p. A189
 Chief Executive Officer, St. Charles General Hospital, New Orleans, LA, p. A187

GOWER, Wayne, President and Chief Executive Officer, IASIS Healthcare, Nashville, TN, p. B99

GOWING, Robert E., Administrator, Atmore Community Hospital, Atmore, AL, p. A11

GRADY, Glen E., Administrator, Memorial Medical Center, Neillsville, WI, p. A473

GRADY, Phillip L., Chief Executive Officer, King's Daughters Medical Center, Brookhaven, MS, p. A236

GRAEBER, Lawrence, Administrator, Neshoba County General Hospital, Philadelphia, MS, p. A241

GRAECA, Raymond A., President and Chief Executive Officer, DuBois Regional Medical Center, Du Bois, PA, p. A359

GRAFALS, Eric, Executive Director, Hospital San Francisco, Rio Piedras, PR, p. A484

GRAGG, Martha, Chief Executive Officer, Sullivan County Memorial Hospital, Milan, MO, p. A250

GRAGNOLATI, Brian A., President, York Hospital, York, PA, p. A375

GRAH, John, Administrator, Scripps Memorial Hospital Chula Vista, Chula Vista, CA, p. A38

GRAHAM, George W., President and Chief Executive Officer, Torrance Memorial Medical Center, Torrance, CA, p. A65

GRAHAM, H. James, Administrator, Highlands–Cashiers Hospital, Highlands, NC, p. A314

GRAHAM, John A., President and Chief Executive Officer, Sherman Hospital, Elgin, IL, p. A125

GRAHAM, Kenneth D., President and Chief Executive Officer, Overlake Hospital Medical Center, Bellevue, WA, p. A452

GRAHAM, Larry M., Chief Executive Officer, Chalmette Medical Center, Chalmette, LA, p. A181

GRAHAM, Michael R., Administrator, Hamilton General Hospital, Hamilton, TX, p. A415

GRAHAM, Richard H., President and Chief Executive Officer, Augusta Health Care, Fishersville, VA, p. A444

GRAHAM, Richard W., FACHE, President and Chief Executive Officer, Fairmont General Hospital, Fairmont, WV, p. A461

GRAJEWSKI, Timothy J., President and Chief Executive Officer, St. John Hospital and Medical Center, Detroit, MI, p. A214

GRAMLICH, Andrew, Chief Executive Officer, Lander Valley Medical Center, Lander, WY, p. A479

GRAN, Daniel, Chief Executive Officer, Freeman Community Hospital, Freeman, SD, p. A386

GRAND, Gary S., Chief Executive Officer, Central Louisiana State Hospital, Pineville, LA, p. A188

GRANDBOIS, Ray, M.P.H., Service Unit Director, U. S. Public Health Service Indian Hospital, Belcourt, ND, p. A321

GRANGER, Keith
 President and Chief Executive Officer, Flowers Hospital, Dothan, AL, p. A14
 President and Chief Executive Officer, Medical Center Enterprise, Enterprise, AL, p. A14

GRAPPE, Steve, Administrator, IHS Hospital of Lubbock, Lubbock, TX, p. A422
GRAVES, Jimmy, Administrator, Walthall County General Hospital, Tylertown, MS, p. A242
GRAVES, John T., President and Chief Executive Officer, Deaconess St. Joseph's Hospital, Huntingburg, IN, p. A141
GRAVES, Philip G., Administrator, Hutchinson Area Health Care, Hutchinson, MN, p. A229
GRAVES, Robert L., Administrator, Sentara Virginia Beach General Hospital, Virginia Beach, VA, p. A450
GRAY, David L., President, Hardin Memorial Hospital, Elizabethtown, KY, p. A171
GRAY, E. Kay, Interim Administrator, Vencor Hospital–Milwaukee, Milwaukee, WI, p. A472
GRAY, Edward, Chief Executive Officer, Renaissance Women's Center of Austin, Austin, TX, p. A403
GRAY, Jerry, Administrator, HEALTHSOUTH Rehabilitation Hospital, Memphis, TN, p. A396
GRAY, Patricia, Administrator and Chief Executive Officer, Blowing Rock Hospital, Blowing Rock, NC, p. A309
GRAY, Patrick J.
  President and Chief Executive Officer, Cumberland River Hospital, Celina, TN, p. A390
  Chief Executive Officer, Fentress County General Hospital, Jamestown, TN, p. A393
GRAY, Penny, Administrator and Chief Executive Officer, Limestone Medical Center, Groesbeck, TX, p. A415
GRAY, Val S., Interim President and Chief Executive Officer, Greater Hudson Valley Health System, Newburgh, NY, p. B87
GRAY , Jr, George H., Director, Central Arkansas Veterans Affairs Healthcare System, Little Rock, AR, p. A31
GRAYBILL, Scott R., Chief Executive Officer and Administrator, Community Hospital of Bremen, Bremen, IN, p. A138
GRAZIANI, Dave, Acting Executive Director, Napa State Hospital, Napa, CA, p. A52
GREEN, David R., Chief Executive Officer, Corcoran District Hospital, Corcoran, CA, p. A39
GREEN, Jack W., Administrator, Antelope Memorial Hospital, Neligh, NE, p. A264
GREEN, Jeffrey, Chief Executive Officer, St. Christopher's Hospital for Children, Philadelphia, PA, p. A368
GREEN, Jerry, Administrator, Tippah County Hospital, Ripley, MS, p. A242
GREEN, John H., Administrator, West Feliciana Parish Hospital, Saint Francisville, LA, p. A188
GREEN, Michael B., President and Chief Executive Officer, Concord Hospital, Concord, NH, p. A271
GREEN, Patrick, Administrator, Morgan Memorial Hospital, Madison, GA, p. A107
GREEN, Sue E., Vice President and Chief Executive Officer, Memorial Hermann Behavioral Health Center, Houston, TX, p. A417
GREEN, Thomas E., President and Chief Executive Officer, Community Hospital at Dobbs Ferry, Dobbs Ferry, NY, p. A291
GREEN, Warren A., President and Chief Executive Officer, LifeBridge Health, Baltimore, MD, p. B104
GREENE, William M., FACHE, President and Chief Executive Officer, Santa Paula Memorial Hospital, Santa Paula, CA, p. A62
GREENE , Jr, Charles H., Administrator, Cordell Memorial Hospital, Cordell, OK, p. A342
GREENE , Jr, Edward C., President, Charles A. Cannon Jr, Memorial Hospital, Crossnore, NC, p. A311
GREENSTEIN, Michael, Chief Executive Officer, Greystone Park Psychiatric Hospital, Greystone Park, NJ, p. A276
GREENWELL, Maryann J., Chief Executive Officer, Selby General Hospital, Marietta, OH, p. A334
GREENWOOD, Kay, MS, Facility Director, North Alabama Regional Hospital, Decatur, AL, p. A13
GREER, John H., President, Southside Community Hospital, Farmville, VA, p. A443
GREEVER, Paul, Chief Executive Officer, Parkside Hospital, Tulsa, OK, p. A348
GREGG, C. Jan, Chief Executive Officer, Eastern State Hospital, Medical Lake, WA, p. A454

GREGORY, Mary Jo, Chief Executive Officer, MetroWest Medical Center, Framingham, MA, p. A205
GREGORY, Samuel S., Administrator, Upson Regional Medical Center, Thomaston, GA, p. A110
GREGSON, C. Mark, Chief Executive Officer, Puget Sound Hospital, Tacoma, WA, p. A458
GRESCO, William J., Chief Executive Officer, Lea Regional Medical Center, Hobbs, NM, p. A285
GREY, William, President and Chief Executive Officer, Century Healthcare Development Corporation, Tulsa, OK, p. B71
GRIFFIN, Dean A., Chief Executive Officer, Baptist Memorial Hospital–Golden Triangle, Columbus, MS, p. A237
GRIFFIN, Debra L., Administrator, Humphreys County Memorial Hospital, Belzoni, MS, p. A236
GRIFFIN, Don, Ph.D., President and Chief Executive Officer, Regional Medical Center–Bayonet Point, Hudson, FL, p. A86
GRIFFITH, Greg, Chief Executive Officer, Memorial Hospital of Adel, Adel, GA, p. A99
GRIFFITH, Richard L., President and Chief Executive Officer, Queen's Health Systems, Honolulu, HI, p. B122
GRIFFITH, Wayne B., FACHE, Chief Executive Officer, St. Joseph's Hospital of Buckhannon, Buckhannon, WV, p. A460
GRIFFITHS, Kathleen S., President and Chief Executive Officer, Chelsea Community Hospital, Chelsea, MI, p. A213
GRIMES, Jonathan D., Chief Executive Officer, Straub Clinic and Hospital, Honolulu, HI, p. A112
GRIMES, Larry, Managing Director, River Crest Hospital, San Angelo, TX, p. A428
GRIMES, Teresa F., Administrator, Jackson Medical Center, Jackson, AL, p. A16
GRIMES , II, Thomas F., Executive Vice President and Chief Operating Officer, St. Elizabeth Community Hospital, Red Bluff, CA, p. A56
GRIMM, Steve, CHE, Chief Executive Officer, Summit Hospital, Baton Rouge, LA, p. A181
GRINNELL, Steven, President, Mercy Franciscan Hospital–Mount Airy, Cincinnati, OH, p. A328
GRIPPEN, Glen W., Director, Clement J. Zablocki Veterans Affairs Medical Center, Milwaukee, WI, p. A471
GRISSLER, Brian G., President and Chief Executive Officer, Suburban Hospital, Bethesda, MD, p. A197
GRISWOLD, Rosanne U., President and Chief Executive Officer, Charlotte Hungerford Hospital, Torrington, CT, p. A77
GRITMAN, Paul J., Superintendent, Danville State Hospital, Danville, PA, p. A359
GROBMYER, James E., Interim Chief Executive Officer, Franciscan Medical Center–Dayton Campus, Dayton, OH, p. A330
GRONEWALD, John E., Chief Operating Officer, Ridgeview Institute, Smyrna, GA, p. A109
GROSETH, Bradley D., Administrator, Osseo Area Hospital and Nursing Home, Osseo, WI, p. A473
GROSS, Dan, Chief Executive Officer, Sharp Memorial Hospital, San Diego, CA, p. A59
GROSS, Joseph W., President and Chief Executive Officer, St. Elizabeth Medical Center–South, Edgewood, KY, p. A171
GROSSMEIER, John C., President and Chief Executive Officer, Hannibal Regional Hospital, Hannibal, MO, p. A247
GROVER , Sr, Bradley K., FACHE, President and Chief Executive Officer, Northside Hospital and Heart Institute, Saint Petersburg, FL, p. A94
GRUBER, Norman F., President and Chief Executive Officer, Palomar Pomerado Health System, San Diego, CA, p. B118
GRUNDSTROM, David A., Chief Executive Officer, Trinity Hospital, Farmington, MN, p. A228
GRUSSING, Mel, Administrator, LAC–High Desert Hospital, Lancaster, CA, p. A45
GUARNIERI, Ellen, Vice President and Chief Operating Officer, Virtua West Jersey Hospital–Berlin, Berlin, NJ, p. A274
GUENTHER, Charles R., Administrator, Eastern Plumas District Hospital, Portola, CA, p. A56

GUERCI, Alan D., M.D., President and Chief Executive Officer, St. Francis Hospital, Roslyn, NY, p. A304
GUEST, John A., President and Chief Executive Officer, Harris County Hospital District, Houston, TX, p. A416
GUILD, Samuel T., Administrator, Pawhuska Hospital, Pawhuska, OK, p. A346
GUINN, Lex A., Chief Executive Officer, Spalding Regional Hospital, Griffin, GA, p. A105
GULARTE, Steve, Administrator, El Campo Memorial Hospital, El Campo, TX, p. A411
GULEY, Michael G., Chief Executive Officer, Bon Secours–Venice Hospital, Venice, FL, p. A97
GULICK, Margaret S., President and Chief Executive Officer, Memorial Healthcare Center, Owosso, MI, p. A220
GULLIFORD, Deryl E., Ph.D., Chief Executive Officer, Stevens County Hospital, Hugoton, KS, p. A162
GUNABALAN, Ram, M.D., Chief Executive Officer, Madison Community Hospital, Madison Heights, MI, p. A218
GUNDERSON, Robert A., Executive Vice President, Falmouth Hospital, Falmouth, MA, p. A204
GUNDERSON, Rodney L.
  Chief Executive Officer, Fay–West Health System, Mount Pleasant, PA, p. B85
  Chief Executive Officer, Frick Hospital, Mount Pleasant, PA, p. A364
GUNN, B. Joe, FACHE, Administrator and Chief Executive Officer, Craig General Hospital, Vinita, OK, p. A349
GUNN, Terry J., Chief Executive Officer, River Park Hospital, McMinnville, TN, p. A396
GURGEL, Paul E., President and Chief Executive Officer, New London Family Medical Center, New London, WI, p. A473
GUSTAFSON, Peggy, Administrator, St. Anthony North Hospital, Westminster, CO, p. A73
GUSTAFSON, Philip P., Administrator, San Ramon Regional Medical Center, San Ramon, CA, p. A61
GUTFELD, Marcia B., Vice President and Chief Operating Officer, De Graff Memorial Hospital, North Tonawanda, NY, p. A301
GUTHMILLER, Martin W., Administrator and Chief Executive Officer, Orange City Health System, Orange City, IA, p. A155
GUTTZEIT, Lauren, Acting Chief Executive Officer, Eastern Louisiana Mental Health System/Greenwell Spring Campus, Greenwell Springs, LA, p. A183
GUTZKE, Ella, Administrator, Sheridan Memorial Hospital, Plentywood, MT, p. A259
GUY, Alan C., President and Chief Executive Officer, Covenant Health, Knoxville, TN, p. B75
GUY, Douglas, President and Chief Executive Officer, Oconomowoc Memorial Hospital, Oconomowoc, WI, p. A473
GUYNN, Robert W., M.D., Executive Director, Harris County Psychiatric Center, Houston, TX, p. A416
GYSIN, Joyce I., Administrator, Surprise Valley Community Hospital, Cedarville, CA, p. A38

H

HAAR, Clare A.
  Chief Executive Officer, Inter–Community Memorial Hospital, Newfane, NY, p. A301
  Chief Executive Officer, Lockport Memorial Hospital, Lockport, NY, p. A293
HABERLEIN, Bernard J., Executive Director, Graydon Manor, Leesburg, VA, p. A445
HACHENBERG, Dennis A., CHE, Chief Executive Officer, Anderson County Hospital, Garnett, KS, p. A161
HACKMAN, Ed
  Administrator, Chase County Community Hospital, Imperial, NE, p. A263
  Administrator, Saunders County Health Service, Wahoo, NE, p. A267
HADDLE, Michael A., CPA, Chief Executive Officer and Chief Financial Officer, Burke County Hospital, Waynesboro, GA, p. A111
HADEN, James E., President and Chief Executive Officer, Martha Jefferson Hospital, Charlottesville, VA, p. A443

HAEDER, James, Interim Administrator, Five Counties Hospital, Lemmon, SD, p. A386
HAGEL, Sonja, Chief Executive Officer, Brotman Medical Center, Culver City, CA, p. A39
HAGEN, David F., President and Chief Executive Officer, Roseau Area Hospital and Homes, Roseau, MN, p. A232
HAGEN, Michael, Administrator, HEALTHSOUTH Rehabilitation Hospital of Beaumont, Beaumont, TX, p. A404
HAHN, James, Administrator, Baptist Memorial Hospital–North Mississippi, Oxford, MS, p. A241
HAILS, Robert, Chief Executive Officer, Charter Beacon, Fort Wayne, IN, p. A139
HAISLIP, Walt, Administrator, Stonewall Memorial Hospital, Aspermont, TX, p. A402
HALE, William R., Chief Executive Officer, University Medical Center, Las Vegas, NV, p. A268
HALES , Jr, John C., FACHE, President and Chief Executive Officer, Roper Hospital North, Charleston, SC, p. A379
HALEY, Bob, Chief Executive Officer, Denton Regional Medical Center, Denton, TX, p. A410
HALL, Cindy, Administrator, Eastern Ozarks Regional Health System, Cherokee Village, AR, p. A28
HALL, Dennis A., President, Baptist Health System, Birmingham, AL, p. B57
HALL, Joan S., R.N., Administrator, South Lyon Medical Center, Yerington, NV, p. A270
HALL, Linda, Administrator, Chillicothe Hospital District, Chillicothe, TX, p. A406
HALL, Marcia K., Chief Executive Officer, Sharp Coronado Hospital, Coronado, CA, p. A39
HALL, Philo D., Chief Executive Officer, Down East Community Hospital, Machias, ME, p. A193
HALL, Richard W., President, Jamestown Hospital, Jamestown, ND, p. A323
HALL, Roger L., Chief Executive Officer, North Okaloosa Medical Center, Crestview, FL, p. A83
HALLFORD, Wayne, Chief Executive Officer, BHC Millwood Hospital, Arlington, TX, p. A402
HALLMAN, Gary D., President and Chief Executive Officer, Medina General Hospital, Medina, OH, p. A335
HALLONQUIST, Frances A., Chief Executive Officer, Kapiolani Medical Center for Women and Children, Honolulu, HI, p. A112
HALM, Barry J., President and Chief Executive Officer, Benedictine Health System, Duluth, MN, p. B60
HALSETH, Michael J., President and Chief Executive Officer, Valley Health System, Winchester, VA, p. B150
HALSTEAD, Michael J., President and Chief Executive Officer, Carlisle Hospital and Health Services, Carlisle, PA, p. A357
HALTER, Michael P., Chief Executive Officer, Hahnemann University Hospital, Philadelphia, PA, p. A367
HAMES, Deena, Administrator, Madison County Memorial Hospital, Madison, FL, p. A89
HAMILL, Dave H., President and Chief Executive Officer, Hampton Regional Medical Center, Varnville, SC, p. A384
HAMILTON, Daniel, Chief Executive Officer, Pennock Hospital, Hastings, MI, p. A216
HAMILTON, Dennis L., Chief Executive Officer, Freeport Memorial Hospital, Freeport, IL, p. A126
HAMILTON, Phil, R.N., Chief Executive Officer, General John J. Pershing Memorial Hospital, Brookfield, MO, p. A244
HAMMACK, Stanley K., Administrator, USA Children's and Women's Hospital, Mobile, AL, p. A16
HAMMER, Michael, President, Good Samaritan Health Center of Merrill, Merrill, WI, p. A471
HAMMER, Pat, Chief Executive Officer, Ten Broeck Hospital, Louisville, KY, p. A176
HAMMER, Patrick, Chief Executive Officer, Ten Broeck Hospital Jacksonville, Jacksonville, FL, p. A87
HAMMER , II, Robert L., Chief Executive Officer, Davis Memorial Hospital, Elkins, WV, p. A461
HAMMETT, Warren E., Administrator, Bamberg County Memorial Hospital and Nursing Center, Bamberg, SC, p. A378
HAMMOND, Joseph, CHE, Administrator, North Sunflower County Hospital, Ruleville, MS, p. A242
HAMMOND , Jr, Robert L., Executive Director, Rankin Medical Center, Brandon, MS, p. A236
HAMNER, David, Administrator, Hardtner Medical Center, Olla, LA, p. A187
HANCOCK, Edward H., President, Nanticoke Memorial Hospital, Seaford, DE, p. A78
HANKO, James F., President and Chief Executive Officer, North Country Regional Hospital, Bemidji, MN, p. A226
HANNA, Mitch, Chief Administrative Officer, Sutter Auburn Faith Community Hospital, Auburn, CA, p. A36
HANNAH, Steve, Administrator, Platte County Memorial Hospital, Wheatland, WY, p. A480
HANNAN, David T., President and Chief Executive Officer, South Shore Hospital, South Weymouth, MA, p. A208
HANNEKEN, Maureen E., Chief Executive Officer, All Saints Special Care Hospital, Bridgeton, MO, p. A244
HANNER, R. Andy, Chief Executive Officer, Charter Rivers Behavioral Health System, West Columbia, SC, p. A384
HANNIG, Virgil, Senior Vice President and Administrator, Herrin Hospital, Herrin, IL, p. A127
HANNON, Edward J., President and Chief Executive Officer, DeSoto Memorial Hospital, Arcadia, FL, p. A81
HANRAHAN, Thomas F., FACHE, Chief Executive Officer and Regional Vice President, McKay–Dee Hospital Center, Ogden, UT, p. A437
HANSEN, Edwin L., Vice President, Yukon–Kuskokwim Delta Regional Hospital, Bethel, AK, p. A20
HANSEN, Irwin C., President and Chief Executive Officer, Summit Medical Center, Oakland, CA, p. A53
HANSEN, Robert, Chief Executive Officer, Cumberland Memorial Hospital, Cumberland, WI, p. A467
HANSEN, Thomas N., M.D., Chief Executive Officer, Children's Hospital, Columbus, OH, p. A329
HANSHAW, John, Chief Executive Officer, St. Mark's Hospital, Salt Lake City, UT, p. A438
HANSON, Bryant R., President and Chief Executive Officer, Floyd Memorial Hospital and Health Services, New Albany, IN, p. A144
HANSON, Carl, Administrator, Minidoka Memorial Hospital and Extended Care Facility, Rupert, ID, p. A117
HANSON, Craig, Administrator, St. Luke Hospital and Living Center, Marion, KS, p. A164
HANSON, Greg, President, St. Joseph's Hospital and Health Center, Dickinson, ND, p. A322
HANSON, J. Marlin, Administrator, Marshall Medical Center South, Boaz, AL, p. A12
HANSON, Paul A., Chief Executive Officer, Prairie Lakes Hospital and Care Center, Watertown, SD, p. A389
HANSON, Stephen C., President, Appalachian Regional Healthcare, Lexington, KY, p. B53
HANSON, Timothy H., President and Chief Executive Officer, HealthEast, Saint Paul, MN, p. B96
HANYAK, Diana C., Chief Executive Officer, Canyon Ridge Hospital, Chino, CA, p. A38
HARBARGER, Claude W., President, St. Dominic–Jackson Memorial Hospital, Jackson, MS, p. A239
HARBIN, Henry, M.D., President and Chief Executive Officer, Magellan Health Services, Atlanta, GA, p. B107
HARDER, Shirley, Chief Executive Officer, Wayne Medical Center, Waynesboro, TN, p. A400
HARDING, Edward A., President and Chief Executive Officer, Columbus Community Hospital, Columbus, WI, p. A467
HARDING, John R., President and Chief Executive Officer, Florida Hospital Heartland Division, Sebring, FL, p. A95
HARDING, William W., President and Chief Executive Officer, Union Hospital, Dover, OH, p. A331
HARDY, Patsy, Administrator, Putnam General Hospital, Hurricane, WV, p. A462
HARDY, Stephen L., Ph.D., Facility Director, Chester Mental Health Center, Chester, IL, p. A121
HARE, Michael K., Administrator, De Leon Hospital, De Leon, TX, p. A410
HARKNESS, Laurence P., President and Chief Executive Officer, Children's Medical Center, Dayton, OH, p. A330
HARMAN, David L., Administrator, Harney District Hospital, Burns, OR, p. A350
HARMAN, Gerald M., Executive Vice President and Administrator, St. Elizabeth's Hospital, Belleville, IL, p. A120
HARMAN, Richmond M., President and Chief Executive Officer, Martin Memorial Health Systems, Stuart, FL, p. A95
HARMAN, Robert L., Administrator, Grant Memorial Hospital, Petersburg, WV, p. A463
HARMON, Ronald A., M.D., Chief Executive Officer, Albert Lea Medical Center, Albert Lea, MN, p. A225
HARMS, Charles F., Administrator, McKee Medical Center, Loveland, CO, p. A72
HARMS, Jacquelyn, R.N., Executive Director, Medical Center of Southeastern Oklahoma, Durant, OK, p. A343
HARPER, Alan G., Director, Veterans Affairs North Texas Health Care System, Dallas, TX, p. A410
HARPER, Gail, R.N., Chief Executive, Providence Seaside Hospital, Seaside, OR, p. A354
HARR, Robert Glenn, President, Heather Hill Hospital, Health and Care Center, Chardon, OH, p. A327
HARREL, Mark, Administrator, Fairview Hospital, Fairview, OK, p. A343
HARRELL, David E., Chief Executive Officer, Georgia Baptist Health Care System, Atlanta, GA, p. B86
HARRELL, Richard E., President and Chief Executive Officer, Duplin General Hospital, Kenansville, NC, p. A314
HARRINGTON, Frank, Administrator, Aberdeen–Monroe County Hospital, Aberdeen, MS, p. A236
HARRINGTON, Joseph P., Chief Executive Officer, Lodi Memorial Hospital, Lodi, CA, p. A46
HARRINGTON, Michael L., Chief Executive Officer, Bon Secours–St. Joseph Healthcare Group, Port Charlotte, FL, p. A93
HARRINGTON, Timothy, President, Victory Memorial Hospital, Waukegan, IL, p. A136
HARRINGTON , Jr, Allan, Chief Executive Officer, Tucson General Hospital, Tucson, AZ, p. A27
HARRINGTON , Jr, John L., FACHE, President, Arizona Heart Hospital, Phoenix, AZ, p. A24
HARRINGTON , Jr, Russell D., President, Baptist Health, Little Rock, AR, p. B57
HARRIS, Allyn R., Chief Executive Officer, Nashville Memorial Hospital, Madison, TN, p. A395
HARRIS, Andrew M., Vice President and Administrator, Christus Spohn Hospital Shoreline, Corpus Christi, TX, p. A407
HARRIS, Frank W., President and Chief Executive Officer, Russell Medical Center, Alexander City, AL, p. A11
HARRIS, Marianna, Administrator, Henderson Health Care Services, Henderson, NE, p. A263
HARRIS, Robert L., President and Chief Executive Officer, Ingalls Hospital, Harvey, IL, p. A127
HARRIS, Robert W., President, Lakeside Memorial Hospital, Brockport, NY, p. A288
HARRIS, Stephen J., President and Chief Executive Officer, Des Moines General Hospital, Des Moines, IA, p. A150
HARRIS, Wayne, Administrator, Simpson General Hospital, Mendenhall, MS, p. A240
HARRISON, Dan M., Executive Vice President and Administrator, Rush Foundation Hospital, Meridian, MS, p. A240
HARRYMAN, John D., President and Chief Executive Officer, Norton Suburban Hospital, Louisville, KY, p. A175
HART, Gerald L., Chief Executive Officer, Magic Valley Regional Medical Center, Twin Falls, ID, p. A118
HART, Joel A., Chief Executive Officer, Woodward Hospital and Health Center, Woodward, OK, p. A349
HART, Noel W., Administrator, King's Daughters Hospital, Yazoo City, MS, p. A243
HART, Remy, Chief Executive Officer, Los Angeles Community Hospital, Los Angeles, CA, p. A48
HARTBERG, David, Administrator, Sleepy Eye Municipal Hospital, Sleepy Eye, MN, p. A233

HARTEL, Joseph R., Chief Executive Officer, Focus Healthcare of Ohio, Maumee, OH, p. A335
HARTIGAN, William J., President and Chief Executive Officer, Liberty Management Group, Inc., Ramsey, NJ, p. B104
HARTLEY, William, Administrator, Ferrell Hospital, Eldorado, IL, p. A125
HARTLEY, Randall W., Administrator, U. S. Air Force Medical Center Keesler, Keesler AFB, MS, p. A239
HARTMAN, C. Richard, M.D., President and Chief Executive Officer, Community Medical Center, Scranton, PA, p. A371
HARVEY, Stansel, Senior Executive Vice President, Executive Director/Administrator, Harris Methodist Southwest, Fort Worth, TX, p. A413
HASKINS, Geroge, Senior Vice President and Chief Operating Officer, Mount Vernon Hospital, Mount Vernon, NY, p. A295
HASTINGS, Arthur W., President and Chief Executive Officer, Middle Tennessee Medical Center, Murfreesboro, TN, p. A397
HASTINGS, G. Richard
  President and Chief Executive Officer, Saint Luke's Hospital, Kansas City, MO, p. A248
  President and Chief Executive Officer, Saint Luke's Shawnee Mission Health System, Kansas City, MO, p. B130
HATALA, Alexander J., President and Chief Executive Officer, Our Lady of Lourdes Medical Center, Camden, NJ, p. A275
HATCHER, John M.
  President, Community Hospital of Noble County, Kendallville, IN, p. A142
  President, Whitley Memorial Hospital, Columbia City, IN, p. A138
HATHAWAY, Richard D., Chief Operating Officer, Redbud Community Hospital, Clearlake, CA, p. A38
HATHAWAY , Jr, Woodrow W., Chief Executive Officer, Chatham Hospital, Siler City, NC, p. A318
HATTON, William R., Chief Executive Officer and Administrator, Bogalusa Community Medical Center, Bogalusa, LA, p. A181
HAUG, William F., FACHE
  President and Chief Executive Officer, Motion Picture and Television Fund Hospital and Residential Services, Los Angeles, CA, p. A49
  President and Chief Executive Officer, Valley Children's Hospital, Madera, CA, p. A50
HAUGH, Diana, MS, Superintendent, Larue D. Carter Memorial Hospital, Indianapolis, IN, p. A141
HAUGO, Glenn, Administrator, Daniels Memorial Hospital, Scobey, MT, p. A259
HAUSE, Eileen, Chief Executive Officer, Kensington Hospital, Philadelphia, PA, p. A367
HAWKINS, Phil, Administrator, Carnegie Tri–County Municipal Hospital, Carnegie, OK, p. A342
HAWKINS, Robert L., Superintendent, Colorado Mental Health Institute at Pueblo, Pueblo, CO, p. A72
HAWKINSON, Curtis, Chief Executive Officer, Keefe Memorial Hospital, Cheyenne Wells, CO, p. A68
HAWLEY, Jess, Administrator, Syringa General Hospital, Grangeville, ID, p. A116
HAWLEY , Jr, Robert L., Chief Executive Officer, Bolivar Medical Center, Cleveland, MS, p. A237
HAWTHORNE, Connie, Chief Executive Officer, Shoals Hospital, Muscle Shoals, AL, p. A17
HAWTHORNE, Douglas D., President and Chief Executive Officer, Texas Health Resources, Irving, TX, p. B142
HAYES, Billy, Administrator, Baptist Hospital, Worth County, Sylvester, GA, p. A110
HAYES, David R., President, Taylor County Hospital, Campbellsville, KY, p. A171
HAYES, Howard A., President and Chief Executive Officer, St. Joseph Regional Medical Center, Lewiston, ID, p. A116
HAYES, James M., Executive Vice President and Administrator, St. Mary's Warrick, Boonville, IN, p. A138
HAYES, T. Farrell, President, Healthcorp of Tennessee, Inc., Chattanooga, TN, p. B96

HAYES, Thomas P.
  Chief Executive Officer, Fremont Medical Center, Yuba City, CA, p. A67
  Chief Executive Officer, Fremont–Rideout Health Group, Yuba City, CA, p. B86
  Chief Executive Officer, Rideout Memorial Hospital, Marysville, CA, p. A51
HAYS, Janet A., Administrator, Forks Community Hospital, Forks, WA, p. A453
HAYWARD, John, President and Chief Executive Officer, PeaceHealth, Bellevue, WA, p. B119
HAYWOOD, Thomas L., Chief Executive Officer, Southeast Arizona Medical Center, Douglas, AZ, p. A22
HAYWOOD , II, Edgar, Administrator, J. Arthur Dosher Memorial Hospital, Southport, NC, p. A318
HAZLETT, Guy, FACHE, Chief Executive Officer, Woods Memorial Hospital District, Etowah, TN, p. A392
HEAD, Janice, Administrator, Kaiser Foundation Hospital, Anaheim, CA, p. A35
HEADDING, John, Chief Administrative Officer, Mercy Hospital and Health Services, Merced, CA, p. A51
HEADLEY, Elwood J., M.D., System Director, Malcom Randall Veterans Affairs Medical Center, Gainesville, FL, p. A85
HEARD, William C., Administrator and Chief Executive Officer, Cumberland Hall Hospital, Hopkinsville, KY, p. A173
HEARING, Philip E., President and Chief Executive Officer, Southeastern Ohio Regional Medical Center, Cambridge, OH, p. A326
HEATER, Floyd, Chief Executive Officer, Shenandoah Memorial Hospital, Woodstock, VA, p. A451
HEATHERLY, Wayne S., President and Chief Administrative Officer, Fort Sanders–Parkwest Medical Center, Knoxville, TN, p. A395
HECHT, Kevin, Director, Wagner General Hospital, Palacios, TX, p. A425
HECK , II, George L., President and Chief Executive Officer, Coffee Regional Medical Center, Douglas, GA, p. A104
HECKERT, Brian, Medical Center Director, Wm. Jennings Bryan Dorn Veterans Affairs Medical Center, Columbia, SC, p. A380
HEDRIX, Michael D., Administrator, Pine Medical Center, Sandstone, MN, p. A233
HEER, John R., Administrator, Baptist Hospital, Pensacola, FL, p. A92
HEIDT, Roger R., Administrator, Sturgis Community Health Care Center, Sturgis, SD, p. A388
HEINIKE, J. Larry, President and Chief Executive Officer, UPMC Horizon, Greenville, PA, p. A361
HEISE, Patrick B., Chief Executive Officer, Community Memorial Hospital, Staunton, IL, p. A135
HEITKAMP, Charlotte, Chief Executive Officer, Jackson Medical Center, Jackson, MN, p. A229
HEITZENRATER, James F., President and Chief Executive Officer, Marcum and Wallace Memorial Hospital, Irvine, KY, p. A173
HEKIMIAN, Barbara D. S., Chief Executive Officer, Dominion Hospital, Falls Church, VA, p. A443
HELLER, Thomas, Administrator, HEALTHSOUTH Western Hills Regional Rehabilitation Hospital, Parkersburg, WV, p. A463
HELLERSTEDT, Wayne P., Chief Executive Officer, Helen Newberry Joy Hospital, Newberry, MI, p. A220
HELLYER, Nancy R., President and Chief Executive Officer, Alexian Brothers Medical Center, Elk Grove Village, IL, p. A125
HELM, Michael D., President, Sparks Regional Medical Center, Fort Smith, AR, p. A30
HELMS, Ella Raye, Administrator, Fisher County Hospital District, Rotan, TX, p. A427
HELMS, Joyce A., Interim President and Chief Executive Officer, Saint Mary's Mercy Medical Center, Grand Rapids, MI, p. A216
HEMETER, Donald, Administrator, Wayne General Hospital, Waynesboro, MS, p. A243
HENCKEL, Susan
  Executive Vice President and Chief Operating Officer, Columbia Hospital, Milwaukee, WI, p. A471
  Chief Operating Officer, St. Mary's Hospital, Milwaukee, WI, p. A472

HENDERSCHEDT, Robert, Chief Executive Officer, Adventist Healthcare, Rockville, MD, p. B51
HENDERSON, Cynthia T., M.P.H., Director and Chief Operating Officer, Oak Forest Hospital of Cook County, Oak Forest, IL, p. A131
HENDERSON, Donald, President and Chief Executive Officer, Berwick Hospital Center, Berwick, PA, p. A356
HENDERSON, Perry, Administrator, East Texas Medical Center–Mount Vernon, Mount Vernon, TX, p. A424
HENDERSON, W. Perry, Administrator, East Texas Medical Center Pittsburg, Pittsburg, TX, p. A426
HENDERSON , Jr, Donald, Deputy Commander for Administration, Lyster U. S. Army Community Hospital, Fort Rucker, AL, p. A15
HENDLER, Ronald, Chief Executive Officer, Crownsville Hospital Center, Crownsville, MD, p. A197
HENDRICKSON, Craig L., Chief Operating Officer, Providence Seattle Medical Center, Seattle, WA, p. A456
HENDRIX, Wayne, Chief Executive Officer, Kosciusko Community Hospital, Warsaw, IN, p. A146
HENGER, Robert E., Administrator, Carraway Northwest Medical Center, Winfield, AL, p. A19
HENIKOFF, Leo M., M.D.
  President and Chief Executive Officer, Rush–Presbyterian–St. Luke's Medical Center, Chicago, IL, p. A123
  President, Rush–Presbyterian–St. Luke's Medical Center, Chicago, IL, p. B129
HENKE, Marcella V., Administrator and Chief Executive Officer, Jackson County Hospital, Edna, TX, p. A411
HENLEY, Darryl E., Administrator, Dos Palos Memorial Hospital, Dos Palos, CA, p. A40
HENNESSY, Thomas G.
  President and Chief Executive Officer, Long Beach Community Medical Center, Long Beach, CA, p. A46
  President and Chief Executive Officer, St. Mary Medical Center, Long Beach, CA, p. A46
HENRICKS, William E., Ph.D., Chief Operating Officer, Charter Hospital of Milwaukee, Milwaukee, WI, p. A471
HENRY, David, Chief Executive Officer, Northern Montana Hospital, Havre, MT, p. A258
HENRY, Peter P., Director, Veterans Affairs Black Hills Health Care System, Fort Meade, SD, p. A386
HENRY , Sr, John Dunklin, FACHE
  Chief Executive Officer, Crawford Long Hospital of Emory University, Atlanta, GA, p. A100
  Chief Executive Officer, Emory University Hospital, Atlanta, GA, p. A100
HENSHAW, Jim, President and Chief Executive Officer, Gooding County Memorial Hospital, Gooding, ID, p. A116
HENSLEY, Kerry A., R.N., Administrator, FirstHealth Montgomery Memorial Hospital, Troy, NC, p. A319
HENSON, Blair W., Administrator, Florala Memorial Hospital, Florala, AL, p. A14
HENSON, David L., Chief Executive Officer, Wilkes Regional Medical Center, North Wilkesboro, NC, p. A316
HENSON, James C., President, United Hospital Corporation, Memphis, TN, p. B147
HENSON, John S., President, Baptist Regional Medical Center, Corbin, KY, p. A171
HENTON, Thomas, Chief Executive Officer, Cleveland Area Hospital, Cleveland, OK, p. A342
HENZE, Michael E., Chief Executive Officer, Lake Regional Health System, Osage Beach, MO, p. A251
HEPBURN, Margaret, Chief Administrative Officer and Chief Nurse Executive, St. Dominic's Hospital, Manteca, CA, p. A51
HERBERT, Cheryl, President, MedCenter Hospital, Marion, OH, p. A334
HERBERT, Susan, Administrator, Inova Mount Vernon Hospital, Alexandria, VA, p. A442
HERFINDAHL, Lowell D., President and Chief Executive Officer, Tioga Medical Center, Tioga, ND, p. A324
HERMAN, Bernard J., President and Chief Executive Officer, Mercy Hospital, Bakersfield, CA, p. A36
HERMAN, Paul L., Chief Executive Officer, Mt. San Rafael Hospital, Trinidad, CO, p. A73

HERMANSON, Patrick M., Senior Executive Officer, Saint Vincent Hospital and Health Center, Billings, MT, p. A256
HERNANDEZ, Hank, Chief Executive Officer, Columbia Medical Center West, El Paso, TX, p. A411
HERNANDEZ, Leonard, Chief Executive Officer, Holton Community Hospital, Holton, KS, p. A162
HERNANDEZ, Pablo, M.D., Administrator, Wyoming State Hospital, Evanston, WY, p. A478
HERNANDEZ-KEEBLE, Sonia, Director, Rio Grande State Center, Harlingen, TX, p. A415
HERRICK, Ronald L., President, Rehabilitation Institute, Kansas City, MO, p. A248
HERRING, Michael S., Administrator, Samuel Simmonds Memorial Hospital, Barrow, AK, p. A20
HERRON, John M., Chief Executive Officer, Minnie G. Boswell Memorial Hospital, Greensboro, GA, p. A105
HERRON, Thomas L., FACHE, President and Chief Executive Officer, Largo Medical Center, Largo, FL, p. A88
HERVEY, Roger D., Administrator, Galena-Stauss Hospital, Galena, IL, p. A126
HESS, Carolyn K., Administrator and Chief Executive Officer, Grape Community Hospital, Hamburg, IA, p. A152
HESS, Kent C., Chief Executive Officer, Clearfield Hospital, Clearfield, PA, p. A358
HESSELMANN, Thomas J., President and Chief Executive Officer, Mercy Medical Center-Clinton, Clinton, IA, p. A149
HESSELTINE, Wendell, President, Tillamook County General Hospital, Tillamook, OR, p. A354
HESTER, Forrest G., President and Chief Executive Officer, Abraham Lincoln Memorial Hospital, Lincoln, IL, p. A129
HETLAGE, C. Kennon, Administrator, Memorial Regional Hospital, Los Angeles, FL, p. A86
HEUSER, Keith E., Chief Executive Officer, Memorial Hospital, Carthage, IL, p. A120
HEYBOER , Jr, Lester, President and Chief Executive Officer, HealthSource Saginaw, Saginaw, MI, p. A221
HEYDEL, M. John, President and Chief Executive Officer, Self Memorial Hospital, Greenwood, SC, p. A381
HIATT, M. K., Administrator, Allendale County Hospital, Fairfax, SC, p. A380
HIBBS, Cathryn A., Chief Executive Officer, Moberly Regional Medical Center, Moberly, MO, p. A250
HIBNICK, Philip, Administrator, Landmann-Jungman Memorial Hospital, Scotland, SD, p. A387
HICKEY, Martin, M.D., Chief Executive Officer, Lovelace Health System, Albuquerque, NM, p. A283
HICKS, Cheryl, Chief Executive Officer, Twin City Hospital, Dennison, OH, p. A331
HICKS, John D., President and Chief Executive Officer, Baptist St. Anthony Health System, Amarillo, TX, p. A401
HICKS, John R., President and Chief Executive Officer, Platte Valley Medical Center, Brighton, CO, p. A68
HICKS, Kevin J., President and Chief Executive Officer, Overland Park Regional Medical Center, Shawnee Mission, KS, p. A168
HICKS, Michael C., President and Chief Executive Officer, Jefferson Memorial Hospital, Jefferson City, TN, p. A393
HICKS, Shelleye, Administrator, Vencor Hospital-LaGrange, LaGrange, IN, p. A143
HICKS, Tommy L., Administrator, Ray County Memorial Hospital, Richmond, MO, p. A251
HIDDE, A. John, President and Chief Executive Officer, Good Samaritan Hospital, Vincennes, IN, p. A146
HIETPAS, Bernard G.
  Chief Executive Officer, Glenn Medical Center, Willows, CA, p. A67
  Chief Executive Officer, Seneca District Hospital, Chester, CA, p. A38
HIGGINBOTHAM, G. Douglas, Executive Director, South Central Regional Medical Center, Laurel, MS, p. A239
HIGGINS, Brad A., President, Fostoria Community Hospital, Fostoria, OH, p. A332
HIGGINS, Susannah, Chief Executive Officer, Broaddus Hospital, Philippi, WV, p. A463
HIGHSMITH, Jr, C. Cameron, President and Chief Executive Officer, St. Luke's Hospital, Columbus, NC, p. A311

HIGHTOWER, George W., CHE, President and Chief Executive Officer, St. Francis Specialty Hospital, Monroe, LA, p. A186
HILL, Kent D., Director, Veterans Affairs Medical and Regional Office Center, Wichita, KS, p. A169
HILL, Robert B., President and Chief Executive Officer, Bethesda Memorial Hospital, Boynton Beach, FL, p. A81
HILL, Stephen B., Chief Executive Officer, South Texas Regional Medical Center, Jourdanton, TX, p. A419
HILL, Thomas E.
  Chief Executive Officer, WellStar Cobb Hospital, Austell, GA, p. A101
  Chief Executive Officer, WellStar Douglas Hospital, Douglasville, GA, p. A104
  Chief Executive Officer, WellStar Health System, Marietta, GA, p. B153
  Chief Executive Officer, WellStar Kennestone Hospital, Marietta, GA, p. A107
  Chief Executive Officer, WellStar Paulding Hospital, Dallas, GA, p. A103
  Chief Executive Officer, WellStar Windy Hill Hospital, Marietta, GA, p. A107
HILL, Timothy E., Chief Executive Officer, North Arkansas Regional Medical Center, Harrison, AR, p. A30
HILL, Mack C., Commanding General, Madigan Army Medical Center, Tacoma, WA, p. A458
HILLARD, Mark, Chief Executive Officer, Maricopa Medical Center, Phoenix, AZ, p. A24
HILLENMEYER, John, President and Chief Executive Officer, Orlando Regional Healthcare, Orlando, FL, p. B117
HILLIS, David W., President and Chief Executive Officer, Adcare Hospital of Worcester, Worcester, MA, p. A210
HILTZ, Richard S., President and Chief Executive Officer, Mercy Memorial Hospital, Monroe, MI, p. A219
HINCHEY, Paul P.
  President and Chief Executive Officer, Candler Hospital, Savannah, GA, p. A109
  President and Chief Executive Officer, St. Joseph's Candler Health System, Savannah, GA, p. A109
HINDS, Bob, Executive Director, Bradford Health Services at Huntsville, Madison, AL, p. A16
HINER, Calvin A., Administrator, Tri-County Area Hospital, Lexington, NE, p. A264
HINES, Frederick W., President, Southwest Mental Health Center, San Antonio, TX, p. A429
HINES, William E., Administrator, Prattville Baptist Hospital, Prattville, AL, p. A18
HINIKER, Alice, Ph.D., Administrator, Intracare Medical Center Hospital, Houston, TX, p. A417
HINO, Raymond T., Chief Executive Officer, Tehachapi Valley Healthcare District, Tehachapi, CA, p. A64
HINOJOS, Margie, Administrator, Culberson Hospital District, Van Horn, TX, p. A433
HINSDALE, Laurence C., President and Chief Executive Officer, NorthEast Medical Center, Concord, NC, p. A311
HINSON, Roy M., CHE, President and Chief Executive Officer, Stanly Memorial Hospital, Albemarle, NC, p. A309
HINTON, Brad, Administrator, North Jackson Hospital, Bridgeport, AL, p. A13
HINTON, J. Philip, M.D.
  President and Chief Executive Officer, Community Medical Center-Clovis, Clovis, CA, p. A38
  President and Chief Executive Officer, Community Medical Centers, Fresno, CA, p. B74
HINTON, James H., President and Chief Executive Officer, Presbyterian Healthcare Services, Albuquerque, NM, p. B119
HIRSCH, Jeffrey D., Executive Vice President and Administrator, Horton Medical Center, Middletown, NY, p. A294
HIRSCH, Leslie D., President and Chief Executive Officer, The Cooper Health System, Camden, NJ, p. A275
HITCHINGS , Jr, Roy A., FACHE, President and Chief Executive Officer, Penobscot Bay Medical Center, Rockport, ME, p. A193
HITT, Irving, Administrator, Covington County Hospital, Collins, MS, p. A237

HITTNER, Kathleen C., M.D., President and Chief Executive Officer, Miriam Hospital, Providence, RI, p. A376
HITZLER, Ronald R., Administrator, Shriners Hospitals for Children, Shriners Burns Hospital, Cincinnati, Cincinnati, OH, p. A328
HOARD, Jack D., President and Chief Executive Officer, Armstrong County Memorial Hospital, Kittanning, PA, p. A362
HOCE, N. Kristopher
  Interim President and Chief Executive Officer, Trumbull Memorial Hospital, Warren, OH, p. A339
  Interim President and Chief Executive Officer, Western Reserve Care System, Youngstown, OH, p. A340
HOCHBERG, Ginny, Clinical Administrator, Curry General Hospital, Gold Beach, OR, p. A351
HOCHENBERG, Paul S., President, Long Island Jewish Medical Center, New York, NY, p. A297
HODGE , Jr, Joseph T., Facility Administrator, Central State Hospital, Milledgeville, GA, p. A107
HODGES, Fredrick W., Chief Executive Officer, Elko General Hospital, Elko, NV, p. A268
HODGES, James E., Chief Operating Officer, Marshall Regional Medical Center, Marshall, TX, p. A423
HODGSON, Judy, Administrator, Sacred Heart Medical Center, Eugene, OR, p. A350
HOEFT, Kathleen, Administrator and Chief Executive Officer, Ashley Medical Center, Ashley, ND, p. A321
HOELSCHER, Steve C., Administrator, Marshall Medical Center, Lewisburg, TN, p. A395
HOFER, Kathleen, President, St. Mary's Medical Center, Duluth, MN, p. A227
HOFF, David L., Chief Executive Officer, Iron County Community Hospital, Iron River, MI, p. A217
HOFF, Terry G., President, Trinity Health, Minot, ND, p. A323
HOFFART, Terry L., Administrator, Webster County Community Hospital, Red Cloud, NE, p. A266
HOFIUS, Chuck, Administrator, Perham Memorial Hospital and Home, Perham, MN, p. A232
HOFREUTER, Donald H., M.D., Administrator and Chief Executive Officer, Wheeling Hospital, Wheeling, WV, p. A465
HOFSTETTER, Peter A., Chief Executive Officer, Northwestern Medical Center, Saint Albans, VT, p. A441
HOGAN, Karen C., Administrator and Chief Executive Officer, San Diego County Psychiatric Hospital, San Diego, CA, p. A59
HOGAN, Ronald C., Superintendent, Georgia Regional Hospital at Atlanta, Decatur, GA, p. A104
HOH, Bonnie, MSN, Administrator, Avalon Municipal Hospital and Clinic, Avalon, CA, p. A36
HOHENBERGER, Arthur L., FACHE, President and Chief Executive Officer, Texoma Healthcare System, Denison, TX, p. A410
HOHN, David C., M.D., President and Chief Executive Officer, Roswell Park Cancer Institute, Buffalo, NY, p. A289
HOLCOMB, David M., President and Chief Executive Officer, Jennie Edmundson Memorial Hospital, Council Bluffs, IA, p. A150
HOLDEN, Peter J., President, Caritas Good Samaritan Medical Center, Brockton, MA, p. A203
HOLDER, Lynn, Executive Director, Northeastern Hospital of Philadelphia, Philadelphia, PA, p. A367
HOLLAND, Jeffrey S., Chief Executive Officer, West Houston Medical Center, Houston, TX, p. A419
HOLLAND, John F., President, North Fulton Regional Hospital, Roswell, GA, p. A109
HOLLAND, Kim, Interim Administrator, Memorial Pavilion, Lawton, OK, p. A344
HOLLAND, Stacy D., Administrator and Chief Executive Officer, Haskell County Healthcare System, Stigler, OK, p. A347
HOLLANDER, Sharon Flynn, Chief Executive Officer, Georgetown University Hospital, Washington, DC, p. A79
HOLLON, Kim N., FACHE, Executive Director, Methodist Medical Center, Dallas, TX, p. A409
HOLLOWAY, Roger L., Administrator, Valley West Community Hospital, Sandwich, IL, p. A134

Index of Health Care Professionals / Hupfeld

HOLMAN, Donna, Administrator, Jasper Memorial Hospital, Monticello, GA, p. A108
HOLMES, Alan D., Chief Executive Officer, Frio Hospital, Pearsall, TX, p. A426
HOLMES, James M., President and Chief Executive Officer, Rappahannock General Hospital, Kilmarnock, VA, p. A445
HOLMES, James R., President and Chief Executive Officer, Redlands Community Hospital, Redlands, CA, p. A56
HOLMES, Steve S., Chief Executive Officer, Swisher Memorial Hospital District, Tulia, TX, p. A433
HOLMES, Elaine C., USN, Commanding Officer, Naval Hospital, Great Lakes, IL, p. A127
HOLOM, Randall G., Chief Executive Officer, Frances Mahon Deaconess Hospital, Glasgow, MT, p. A257
HOLTER, Lee, Chief Executive Officer, St. James Health Services, Saint James, MN, p. A233
HOLTHAUS, Vickie, Interim Chief Executive Officer, Pana Community Hospital, Pana, IL, p. A132
HOLTSCLAW, Keith S., Chief Executive Officer, Spruce Pine Community Hospital, Spruce Pine, NC, p. A318
HOLTZ, John, Administrator, Shriners Hospitals for Children, Tampa, Tampa, FL, p. A96
HOLWERDA, Daniel L., President and Chief Executive Officer, Pine Rest Christian Mental Health Services, Grand Rapids, MI, p. A216
HOLZBERG, Harvey A., President and Chief Executive Officer, Robert Wood Johnson University Hospital, New Brunswick, NJ, p. A278
HONACKER, Thomas, Interim Chief Executive Officer, University Hospitals and Clinics – Holmes County, Lexington, MS, p. A240
HONAKER, C. Ray, Chief Executive Officer, St. Thomas More Hospital and Progressive Care Center, Canon City, CO, p. A68
HONAKER , II, Thomas G., FACHE, Administrator, University Hospitals and Clinics of Holmes County–Durant, Durant, MS, p. A237
HONEYCUTT, Ann E.
 Executive Vice President and Administrator, Bon Secours St. Mary's Hospital, Richmond, VA, p. A448
 Executive Vice President and Administrator, Bon Secours–Stuart Circle, Richmond, VA, p. A448
HONEYCUTT, Steven, Administrator, Lawrence Baptist Medical Center, Moulton, AL, p. A17
HOOD, Fred B., Administrator, Pontotoc Hospital and Extended Care Facility, Pontotoc, MS, p. A241
HOOD, M. Michelle
 Chief Administrative Officer, Norton Healthcare Pavilion, Louisville, KY, p. A175
 Chief Administrative Officer, Norton Hospital, Louisville, KY, p. A175
HOOD, Mark C., Executive Director, Baylor Medical Center at Grapevine, Grapevine, TX, p. A414
HOOPER, Grady, Chief Executive Officer, East Texas Medical Center Trinity, Trinity, TX, p. A432
HOOPER, Ross, Chief Executive Officer, Crittenden Memorial Hospital, West Memphis, AR, p. A34
HOOPES, John L., Chief Executive Officer, Caribou Memorial Hospital and Living Center, Soda Springs, ID, p. A118
HOOSE, Gregory R., Chief Executive Officer, Straith Hospital for Special Surgery, Southfield, MI, p. A222
HOOVER, Alvin, CHE, Administrator, Abbeville County Memorial Hospital, Abbeville, SC, p. A378
HOOVER, Garrett W., President and Chief Executive Officer, Nason Hospital, Roaring Spring, PA, p. A371
HOOVER, Randall L., Chief Executive Officer, Memorial Medical Center, New Orleans, LA, p. A186
HOPKINS, Don, Administrator, Faith Community Hospital, Jacksboro, TX, p. A419
HOPKINS, Wallace M., FACHE, Chief Executive Officer, Veterans Affairs Medical Center, Amarillo, TX, p. A401
HOPPER, Cornelius L., M.D., Vice President Health Affairs, University of California–Systemwide Administration, Oakland, CA, p. B149
HOPPER, Stephen R., President and Chief Executive Officer, McDonough District Hospital, Macomb, IL, p. A129
HOPSTAD, Kyle, Administrator, Virginia Regional Medical Center, Virginia, MN, p. A234

HORAN, Gary S., FACHE
 President and Chief Executive Officer, Our Lady of Mercy Healthcare System, Inc., New York, NY, p. B118
 President and Chief Executive Officer, Our Lady of Mercy Medical Center, New York, NY, p. A299
 President and Chief Executive Officer, St. Agnes Hospital, White Plains, NY, p. A307
HORN, Jerome H., President and Chief Executive Officer, Vaughan Regional Medical Center, Selma, AL, p. A18
HORN, Linda, Chief Executive Officer, Sutter Delta Medical Center, Antioch, CA, p. A35
HORNBEAK, John E.
 Chief Executive Officer, Methodist Specialty and Transplant Hospital, San Antonio, TX, p. A429
 Chief Executive Officer, Southwest Texas Methodist Hospital, San Antonio, TX, p. A429
HORNER, Lynn V., President and Chief Executive Officer, Dunlap Memorial Hospital, Orrville, OH, p. A336
HORNER, Seward, President, Riverview Hospital, Noblesville, IN, p. A144
HORTON, Charlie M., President, Warren Memorial Hospital, Front Royal, VA, p. A444
HORTON, Jerrell J., Chief Executive Officer, Greeley County Hospital, Tribune, KS, p. A168
HORTON, Joseph R., Chief Executive Officer and Administrator, Primary Children's Medical Center, Salt Lake City, UT, p. A438
HOSFELD, Anne L., Chief Administrative Officer, Novato Community Hospital, Novato, CA, p. A53
HOSS, James R., Chief Executive Officer, San Bernardino Mountains Community Hospital District, Lake Arrowhead, CA, p. A45
HOUSE, Judy G., Chief Executive Officer, BHC Ross Hospital, Kentfield, CA, p. A44
HOUSER, James P., President and Chief Executive Officer, Christus Santa Rosa Health Care, San Antonio, TX, p. A428
HOUSER, Robert, Chief Executive Officer, Blue Mountain Hospital, John Day, OR, p. A351
HOUSLEY, Charles E., FACHE, Administrator, ARH Regional Medical Center, Hazard, KY, p. A173
HOVE, Barton A., Chief Executive Officer, Delta Regional Medical Center, Greenville, MS, p. A238
HOWARD, Deanna S., Chief Executive Officer, Upper Connecticut Valley Hospital, Colebrook, NH, p. A271
HOWARD, Eddie L., Vice President and Chief Operating Officer, East Texas Medical Center Rehabilitation Center, Tyler, TX, p. A433
HOWARD, J. Kent, President and Chief Executive Officer, Medical Center of Independence, Independence, MO, p. A247
HOWARD, Loy M., Chief Executive Officer, Tanner Medical Center, Carrollton, GA, p. A102
HOWARD, Mark J., President and Chief Executive Officer, Mountainview Hospital, Las Vegas, NV, p. A268
HOWARD, Norma, Administrator, Marshall Memorial Hospital, Madill, OK, p. A344
HOWE, Debbie, Administrator, Okeene Municipal Hospital, Okeene, OK, p. A345
HOWE, G. Edwin, President, Aurora Health Care, Milwaukee, WI, p. B55
HOWE, Scott W., Chief Executive Officer, Weeks Medical Center, Lancaster, NH, p. A272
HOWELL, Bonnie H., FACHE, President and Chief Executive Officer, Cayuga Medical Center at Ithaca, Ithaca, NY, p. A293
HOWELL, Jerry M., Chief Operating Officer, Marion General Hospital, Columbia, MS, p. A237
HOWELL, Joe D., Executive Director, Upstate Carolina Medical Center, Gaffney, SC, p. A381
HOWELL, Ken, Administrator, HEALTHSOUTH Southern Hills Rehabilitation Hospital, Princeton, WV, p. A464
HOWELL, R. Edward, Director and Chief Executive Officer, University of Iowa Hospitals and Clinics, Iowa City, IA, p. A153
HOWELL, Farley, Commanding Officer, U. S. Air Force Hospital, Ellsworth AFB, SD, p. A386
HOWERY, Patrick, Chief Executive Officer, Grand River Hospital District, Rifle, CO, p. A72
HUBBARD, F. David, Superintendent, McCain Correctional Hospital, McCain, NC, p. A315

HUBBARD , II, Richard B., President and Chief Executive Officer, Piedmont Hospital, Atlanta, GA, p. A100
HUBBELL, James W., President and Chief Executive Officer, Wayne Memorial Hospital, Goldsboro, NC, p. A313
HUBBS, Olas A., Chief Executive Officer, Community Memorial Hospital, Hicksville, OH, p. A333
HUBER, Joan M., Commanding Officer, Naval Hospital, Twentynine Palms, CA, p. A65
HUCH, Robert E., President, Stonewall Jackson Hospital, Lexington, VA, p. A445
HUDDLESTON, David, Deputy Commander for Administration, Ireland Army Community Hospital, Fort Knox, KY, p. A172
HUDGINS, Thomas J., Administrator, Sullivan County Community Hospital, Sullivan, IN, p. A146
HUDSON, Donald C., Vice President and Chief Operating Officer, Mercy Hospital of Folsom, Folsom, CA, p. A41
HUDSON, Gary Mikeal, Administrator, East Texas Medical Center Carthage, Carthage, TX, p. A406
HUDSON, W. H., President, Oconee Memorial Hospital, Seneca, SC, p. A383
HUDSPETH, Ronald, Executive Director, Baylor Medical Center–Ellis County, Waxahachie, TX, p. A434
HUDSPETH, Todd, Administrator and Chief Executive Officer, Guthrie County Hospital, Guthrie Center, IA, p. A152
HUEBBERS, Rodney N., President and Chief Executive Officer, Loudoun Hospital Center, Leesburg, VA, p. A445
HUEBNER, Thomas W., President and Chief Executive Officer, Rutland Regional Medical Center, Rutland, VT, p. A440
HUERTA, Cristina, Administrative Director, Columbia Rehabilitation Hospital, El Paso, TX, p. A411
HUEY, Kenneth R., President and Chief Executive Officer, Longmont United Hospital, Longmont, CO, p. A72
HUFF, David A., Administrator, Good Samaritan Hospital, Bakersfield, CA, p. A36
HUFF, Richard, Administrator, U. S. Public Health Service Indian Hospital, Sisseton, SD, p. A388
HUFF, William J., Chief Executive Officer, Marshall Browning Hospital, Du Quoin, IL, p. A125
HUGHES, David T., FACHE, Chief Executive Officer, Sutter Maternity and Surgery Center of Santa Cruz, Santa Cruz, CA, p. A62
HUGHES , Jr, Ned B., President, Gerber Memorial Health Services, Fremont, MI, p. A215
HUMMER, John Lloyd, Chief Executive Officer, Desert Springs Hospital, Las Vegas, NV, p. A268
HUMPHREY, Jerel T., Chief Executive Officer, Memorial Hermann Southwest Hospital, Houston, TX, p. A417
HUMPHREY, Robert J., Administrator, Lanier Health Services, Valley, AL, p. A19
HUMPHRYS, Maureen, Director, Veterans Affairs Medical Center, Sheridan, WY, p. A479
HUNKINS, Theresa, Administrator, Vencor Hospital–Tampa, Tampa, FL, p. A97
HUNN, Michael F., Chief Executive Officer, Anaheim General Hospital, Anaheim, CA, p. A35
HUNSAKER, Susan L., CHE, Director and Chief Executive Officer, Broadlawns Medical Center, Des Moines, IA, p. A150
HUNT, James M., Chief Executive Officer, Covenant Behavioral Health System, San Antonio, TX, p. A428
HUNT, Linda A., President and Chief Administrative Officer, St. Joseph's Hospital and Medical Center, Phoenix, AZ, p. A25
HUNT, Sharon, Administrator, W. J. Mangold Memorial Hospital, Lockney, TX, p. A422
HUNT , Jr, Seth P., Director and Chief Executive Officer, Broughton Hospital, Morganton, NC, p. A316
HUNTER, David, Interim President and Chief Executive Officer, UCSF Stanford Health Care, San Francisco, CA, p. B137
HUNTER, David C., Chief Executive Officer, Wabash County Hospital, Wabash, IN, p. A146
HUNTLEY, Lee S., Chief Executive Officer, Baptist Hospital of Miami, Miami, FL, p. A89
HUPFELD, Stanley F., President and Chief Executive Officer, INTEGRIS Health, Oklahoma City, OK, p. B100

© 2000 AHA Guide

HURD, Paul, Chief Executive Officer, Creighton Area Health Services, Creighton, NE, p. A262
HURST, Molly, Administrative Director, Grimes St. Joseph Health Center, Navasota, TX, p. A425
HURT, Reedes, Chief Executive Officer, Veterans Affairs Medical Center, Wilkes-Barre, PA, p. A374
HURT, Richard O., Ph.D., Chief Executive Officer, Benchmark Behavioral Health Systems, Woods Cross, UT, p. A439
HURYSZ, Edwin E., Chief Executive Officer, Sakakawea Medical Center, Hazen, ND, p. A322
HURZELER, Rosemary Johnson, President and Chief Executive Officer, The Connecticut Hospice, Branford, CT, p. A74
HUSSON, Gerard P., Director, Veterans Affairs Medical Center, Beckley, WV, p. A460
HUSTON, Joye H., Acting Chief Executive Officer, Jefferson County Memorial Hospital, Winchester, KS, p. A169
HUTCHENRIDER, Ken, President and Chief Executive Officer, Western Plains Medical Complex, Dodge City, KS, p. A160
HUTCHINS, Michael T., Administrator, Claiborne County Hospital, Tazewell, TN, p. A400
HUTCHISON, Dee, Chief Executive Officer, Northern Navajo Medical Center, Shiprock, NM, p. A286
HUTCHISON, James, Director, Integris Bass Behavioral Health System, Enid, OK, p. A343
HUTTON, Terry, Chief Executive Officer, East Houston Regional Medical Center, Houston, TX, p. A416
HYDE, James A., Administrator, Bone and Joint Hospital, Oklahoma City, OK, p. A345
HYER, Julie, President and Chief Executive Officer, Dominican Hospital, Santa Cruz, CA, p. A62
HYMANS, Daniel J., President, Memorial Medical Center, Ashland, WI, p. A466
HYNES, John J., President and Chief Executive Officer, Care New England Health System, Providence, RI, p. B64
HYTOFF, Ronald A., President and Chief Executive Officer, Tampa General Healthcare, Tampa, FL, p. A96

I

IACOBELL, Frank P., Interim President, Brighton Hospital, Brighton, MI, p. A212
ICHINOSE, Calvin M., Administrator, Molokai General Hospital, Kaunakakai, HI, p. A113
IFILL, Gordon L., M.D., Acting Facility Administrator, Georgia Regional Hospital at Savannah, Savannah, GA, p. A109
IFTINIUK, Alan, Chief Executive, Good Shepherd Hospital, Barrington, IL, p. A119
IGNELZI, James, Chief Executive Officer, Twin Valley Psychiatric System, Dayton, OH, p. A331
INGALA, Robert J., Chief Executive Officer, Hale Hospital, Haverhill, MA, p. A205
INGHAM, Raymond V., President and Chief Executive Officer, Witham Memorial Hospital, Lebanon, IN, p. A143
INGRAHAM, Ron, Administrator, Klickitat Valley Hospital, Goldendale, WA, p. A454
INIGO-AGOSTINI, Emigdio, M.D., Board President, Clinica Espanola, Mayaguez, PR, p. A483
IRBY, Frank, Chief Executive Officer, Raulerson Hospital, Okeechobee, FL, p. A91
IRWIN, Michele, Administrator, Alliance Hospital of Santa Teresa, Santa Teresa, NM, p. A286
IRWIN , Jr, Richard M., President and Chief Executive Officer, Health Central, Ocoee, FL, p. A91
ISAACS, James W., Chief Executive Officer, Mercer County Joint Township Community Hospital, Coldwater, OH, p. A329
ISANI, Alice, Acting Administrator, Kaiser Foundation Hospital–West Los Angeles, Los Angeles, CA, p. A48
ISELY, John A., President, St. Mary Medical Center, Walla Walla, WA, p. A458
ISEMANN, William R., Interim President, Danville Regional Medical Center, Danville, VA, p. A443
ISRAEL, Michael D., Chief Executive Officer and Vice Chancellor, Duke University Medical Center, Durham, NC, p. A312
IVERSEN, Dale E., President and Chief Executive Officer, Warrack Medical Center Hospital, Santa Rosa, CA, p. A63
IVES, Karen, Interim Administrator, Harper County Community Hospital, Buffalo, OK, p. A342
IVES, R. Wayne, Administrator, San Vicente Hospital, Los Angeles, CA, p. A49
IVESON, Sara C., Executive Director, Barnes-Kasson County Hospital, Susquehanna, PA, p. A372

J

JACKMAN, Janet, Chief Executive Officer, Seminole Medical Center, Seminole, OK, p. A347
JACKMUFF, Steven W., President and Chief Executive Officer, Underwood-Memorial Hospital, Woodbury, NJ, p. A282
JACKSON, Cecil, Co-Administrator, Steele Memorial Hospital, Salmon, ID, p. A117
JACKSON, Fred L., Chief Executive Officer, King's Daughters Medical Center, Ashland, KY, p. A170
JACKSON, Jane, Chief Executive Officer, Vencor Hospital–Coral Gables, Coral Gables, FL, p. A83
JACKSON, Joan, Administrator, Melrose Area Hospital, Melrose, MN, p. A230
JACKSON, John J., Chief Executive Officer, Richmond Memorial Hospital, Rockingham, NC, p. A317
JACKSON, Thomas W., Chief Executive Officer, College Station Medical Center, College Station, TX, p. A407
JACKSON, Valerie A.
  Chief Executive Officer, East Pointe Hospital, Lehigh Acres, FL, p. A88
  Chief Executive Officer, Gulf Coast Hospital, Fort Myers, FL, p. A85
JACKSON, William, President, Charlevoix Area Hospital, Charlevoix, MI, p. A212
JACOBI, Paula, President and Chief Executive Officer, Provena St. Mary's Hospital, Kankakee, IL, p. A129
JACOBS, John L., Administrator, Bennett County Healthcare Center, Martin, SD, p. A386
JACOBS, Nicholas, Executive Director, Windber Medical Center, Windber, PA, p. A375
JACOBS, Selby, M.D., Director, Connecticut Mental Health Center, New Haven, CT, p. A75
JACOBSEN, David P., Administrator/Chief Executive Officer, Coalinga Regional Medical Center, Coalinga, CA, p. A39
JACOBSON, John L., President and Chief Executive Officer, Lee's Summit Hospital, Lees Summit, MO, p. A249
JACOBSON, Peter, President and Chief Executive Officer, St. Joseph's Area Health Services, Park Rapids, MN, p. A232
JACOBSON, Rod, Administrator, Bear Lake Memorial Hospital, Montpelier, ID, p. A117
JACOBSON, Ronald L., President and Chief Executive Officer, Avera Queen of Peace, Mitchell, SD, p. A387
JACOBSON, Steven K., Chief Executive Officer, Titus Regional Medical Center, Mount Pleasant, TX, p. A424
JACOBSON, Terry, Administrator, St. Mary's Hospital of Superior, Superior, WI, p. A476
JACOBUS, Patrick J., Chief Executive Officer, Val Verde Regional Medical Center, Del Rio, TX, p. A410
JACOBY, Jamie R., Administrator, Kimble Hospital, Junction, TX, p. A420
JACQUES, Teresa, Chief Executive Officer, Modoc Medical Center, Alturas, CA, p. A35
JAEGER, Mark J., CHE, President and Chief Executive Officer, Saint John Hospital, Leavenworth, KS, p. A164
JAFFE, David E., Executive Director, Harborview Medical Center, Seattle, WA, p. A456
JAHN, David B., Administrator and Chief Financial Officer, Schoolcraft Memorial Hospital, Manistique, MI, p. A219
JAMERSON, Carlene, President and Chief Executive Officer, Gordon Hospital, Calhoun, GA, p. A102
JAMES, Craig B., President and Chief Executive Officer, Tazewell Community Hospital, Tazewell, VA, p. A450
JAMES, Curtis, President and Chief Executive Officer, St. Vincent's Hospital, Birmingham, AL, p. A12
JAMES, Diane R., Administrator, Florida State Hospital, Chattahoochee, FL, p. A82
JAMES, Donald W., Ph.D., Administrator and Chief Executive Officer, Three Rivers Hospital, Waverly, TN, p. A400
JAMES, William B., Chief Executive Officer, Northern Hospital of Surry County, Mount Airy, NC, p. A316
JAMES , Jr, George H., President and Chief Executive Officer, Memorial Hospital, Seymour, IN, p. A145
JANATKA, Lucille A., President and Chief Executive Officer, MidState Medical Center, Meriden, CT, p. A75
JANCZAK, Linda M., President and Chief Executive Officer, F. F. Thompson Health System, Canandaigua, NY, p. A289
JANKE, Paul, Senior Vice President, Three Rivers Community Hospital and Health Center, Grants Pass, OR, p. A351
JARM, Timothy L., President, Jewish Hospital–Shelbyville, Shelbyville, KY, p. A178
JARRETT, James L., Chief Executive Officer, Berrien County Hospital, Nashville, GA, p. A108
JARRY, Jacques, Administrator, Bullock County Hospital, Union Springs, AL, p. A19
JASPERSON, Steven W.
  Executive Vice President Operations, Good Samaritan Hospital Corvallis, Corvallis, OR, p. A350
  Executive Vice President Operations, Lebanon Community Hospital, Lebanon, OR, p. A352
JAUDES, Paula Kienberger, M.D., President and Chief Executive Officer, LaRabida Children's Hospital and Research Center, Chicago, IL, p. A122
JAVOIS, Laurent D., Superintendent, Northwest Missouri Psychiatric Rehabilitation Center, Saint Joseph, MO, p. A252
JEAN, Darrell, Administrator and Chief Executive Officer, Pemiscot Memorial Health System, Hayti, MO, p. A247
JEANMARD, William C., Chief Executive Officer, Allen Parish Hospital, Kinder, LA, p. A184
JEFFCOAT, Sally E., Chief Executive Officer, Christus St. Joseph Hospital, Houston, TX, p. A416
JENKINS, Jeffrey K., President, St. Michael Hospital, Milwaukee, WI, p. A472
JENKINS, Robert N., Interim Administrator, Cavalier County Memorial Hospital, Langdon, ND, p. A323
JENNINGS, Jacki, Chief Executive Officer, Medical Center Blount, Oneonta, AL, p. A17
JENNINGS, William M., Administrator and Chief Operating Officer, Morton Plant Mease–North Bay Hospital, New Port Richey, FL, p. A91
JENNINGS, William R., President and Chief Executive Officer, South Hills Health System, Pittsburgh, PA, p. A369
JENSEN, Bruce C., President and Chief Executive Officer, Holy Rosary Medical Center, Ontario, OR, p. A352
JENSEN, Eric, Administrator, Kittitas Valley Community Hospital, Ellensburg, WA, p. A453
JEPSON, Gary L., Chief Executive Officer, Tahlequah City Hospital, Tahlequah, OK, p. A348
JERNIGAN, Donald L., President, Florida Hospital, Orlando, FL, p. A91
JESIOLOWSKI, Craig A., Chief Executive Officer, Gibson Area Hospital and Health Services, Gibson City, IL, p. A127
JESSEN, Georgianne
  Chief Executive Officer, Providence Holy Cross Medical Center, Los Angeles, CA, p. A49
  Chief Executive Officer, Providence Saint Joseph Medical Center, Burbank, CA, p. A37
JESSUP, Dale, President and Chief Executive Officer, Bay Area Hospital, Coos Bay, OR, p. A350
JETER, John H., M.D., President and Chief Executive Officer, Hays Medical Center, Hays, KS, p. A162
JEX, Robert F., Administrator, Bear River Valley Hospital, Tremonton, UT, p. A439
JHIN, Michael K., President and Chief Executive Officer, St. Luke's Episcopal Health System, Houston, TX, p. A418

JIVIDEN, Thomas C., Senior Vice President, Virginia Baptist Hospital, Lynchburg, VA, p. A446
JOHN, Roger S., President and Chief Executive Officer, Great Plains Health Alliance, Inc., Phillipsburg, KS, p. B87
JOHN, Susie, M.D., Chief Executive Officer, Tuba City Indian Medical Center, Tuba City, AZ, p. A26
JOHNSON, Calvin D., Chief Executive Officer, Kilmichael Hospital, Kilmichael, MS, p. A239
JOHNSON, Curtis A., Administrator, Flambeau Hospital, Park Falls, WI, p. A473
JOHNSON, David B., Administrator, Brookings Hospital, Brookings, SD, p. A385
JOHNSON, Dennis B., Administrator, Tri County Baptist Hospital, La Grange, KY, p. A173
JOHNSON, Don P., Administrator, Cedars Hospital, De Soto, TX, p. A410
JOHNSON, Doyle K., Administrator, Mercy Hospital, Moundridge, KS, p. A165
JOHNSON, Elizabeth B., Chief Executive Officer, Sage Memorial Hospital, Ganado, AZ, p. A22
JOHNSON, George L., President, Reedsburg Area Medical Center, Reedsburg, WI, p. A474
JOHNSON, Gregory D., Administrator, Cox Monett Hospital, Monett, MO, p. A250
JOHNSON, James K., Chief Executive Officer, Hedrick Medical Center, Chillicothe, MO, p. A245
JOHNSON, John C., Chief Executive Officer, Holy Cross Hospital, Fort Lauderdale, FL, p. A84
JOHNSON, John H., Chief Executive Officer, Gothenburg Memorial Hospital, Gothenburg, NE, p. A263
JOHNSON, John W., President, Alice Hyde Medical Center, Malone, NY, p. A294
JOHNSON, Karl E., Chief Executive Officer, Mount Graham Community Hospital, Safford, AZ, p. A25
JOHNSON, Kevin, Chief Executive Officer, Mountain View Hospital, Payson, UT, p. A437
JOHNSON, L. Barney, President and Chief Executive Officer, Harbor Hospital Center, Baltimore, MD, p. A195
JOHNSON, Laurence E., Administrator, Shriners Hospitals for Children, Twin Cities, Minneapolis, MN, p. A231
JOHNSON, Paul H., President and Chief Executive Officer, Gaylord Hospital, Wallingford, CT, p. A77
JOHNSON, Ronald E., Administrator, Meeker County Memorial Hospital, Litchfield, MN, p. A229
JOHNSON, Stan, Medical Center Director, Veterans Affairs Medical Center, Tomah, WI, p. A476
JOHNSON, Steven G., Administrator, Amethyst, Charlotte, NC, p. A310
JOHNSON, Steven M.
President, Citizens Baptist Medical Center, Talladega, AL, p. A18
President, Coosa Valley Baptist Medical Center, Sylacauga, AL, p. A18
JOHNSON, Terry G., Chief Executive Officer, BHC Mesilla Valley Hospital, Las Cruces, NM, p. A285
JOHNSON, Thomas M.
Chief Executive Officer, Kaweah Delta Health Care District, Visalia, CA, p. A66
Chief Executive Officer, Memorial Hospital at Exeter, Exeter, CA, p. A40
JOHNSON, Timothy, M.D., President, Austin Medical Center, Austin, MN, p. A225
JOHNSON, Van R., President and Chief Executive Officer, Sutter Health, Sacramento, CA, p. B138
JOHNSON, Viola L., M.P.H., Chief Executive Officer, Huhukam Memorial Hospital, Sacaton, AZ, p. A25
JOHNSON–PHILLIPPE, Sue E., Chief Executive Officer, LakeView Community Hospital, Paw Paw, MI, p. A220
JOHNSRUD, Kimry A., President, Elmbrook Memorial Hospital, Brookfield, WI, p. A467
JOHNSTON, Charles, Administrator, Pauls Valley General Hospital, Pauls Valley, OK, p. A346
JOHNSTON, Debbie W., Director Operations, HEALTHSOUTH Rehabilitation Hospital, Columbia, SC, p. A379
JOHNSTON, R. Joe, President and Chief Executive Officer, Dukes Memorial Hospital, Peru, IN, p. A145
JOHNSTON, Wayne W., President and Chief Executive Officer, Sharon Regional Health System, Sharon, PA, p. A372
JOLLY, Jay P., Administrator and Chief Executive Officer, Clay County Hospital, Brazil, IN, p. A138
JONAS, Stanley W., Chief Executive Officer, Alliance Community Hospital, Alliance, OH, p. A325
JONES, Bradley E., Chief Executive Officer, Alice Regional Hospital, Alice, TX, p. A401
JONES, Carol E., Administrator, Annie Jeffrey Memorial County Health Center, Osceola, NE, p. A266
JONES, David W. P., Chief Executive Officer, Mayview State Hospital, Bridgeville, PA, p. A356
JONES, Deryl L., President, Adventist Medical Center, Portland, OR, p. A353
JONES, Donald J., Administrator, Carraway Burdick West Medical Center, Haleyville, AL, p. A15
JONES, Douglas T., Chief Executive Officer, Maine Coast Memorial Hospital, Ellsworth, ME, p. A192
JONES, Dwayne, Chief Executive Officer, Fairchild Medical Center, Yreka, CA, p. A67
JONES, G. W., Administrator, Nacogdoches Memorial Hospital, Nacogdoches, TX, p. A424
JONES, H. Ed, Chief Executive Officer, North Carolina Eye and Ear Hospital, Durham, NC, p. A312
JONES, J. Thomas, Executive Director, St. Mary's Hospital, Huntington, WV, p. A462
JONES, Jerry, Administrator, Intergris Clinton Regional Hospital, Clinton, OK, p. A342
JONES, John R., Administrator, Yalobusha General Hospital, Water Valley, MS, p. A243
JONES, Lowell
President and Chief Executive Officer, Marymount Medical Center, London, KY, p. A174
Chief Executive Officer, Our Lady of the Way Hospital, Martin, KY, p. A176
JONES, Mark T., President, Holy Redeemer Hospital and Medical Center, Meadowbrook, PA, p. A364
JONES, Maurice, Administrator, Inner Harbour Hospitals, Douglasville, GA, p. A104
JONES, Rex, Chief Executive Officer, Howard Memorial Hospital, Nashville, AR, p. A32
JONES, Robert D., President, Rutherford Hospital, Rutherfordton, NC, p. A317
JONES, Robert T., M.D., President and Chief Executive Officer, Hutcheson Medical Center, Fort Oglethorpe, GA, p. A105
JONES, Rodney, Chief Operating Officer, Hillside Rehabilitation Hospital, Warren, OH, p. A339
JONES, Wayne, Executive Vice President and Administrator, Maryview Medical Center, Portsmouth, VA, p. A447
JONES , Jr., Richard L., President and Chief Executive Officer, Abington Memorial Hospital, Abington, PA, p. A355
JONES , Jr., Stephen K., Chief Executive Officer, Medical Center of Southwest Louisiana, Lafayette, LA, p. A184
JORDAHL, David B., FACHE, President, St. Clare Hospital and Health Services, Baraboo, WI, p. A466
JORDAN, Bobby, Chief Executive Officer, Winn Parish Medical Center, Winnfield, LA, p. A189
JORDAN, David R., Ph.D., Chief Executive Officer, Watonga Municipal Hospital, Watonga, OK, p. A349
JORDAN, Gary W., President and Chief Executive Officer, St. Francis Hospital, Mountain View, MO, p. A250
JORDAN, Lawrence A., Director, PHS Santa Fe Indian Hospital, Santa Fe, NM, p. A286
JORDAN, Linda U., Administrator, Clay County Hospital, Ashland, AL, p. A11
JORDAN, W. Charles, Administrator, Mayes County Medical Center, Pryor, OK, p. A347
JORDEN, James, Chief Executive Officer, Kit Carson County Memorial Hospital, Burlington, CO, p. A68
JORVE, Helen, Chief Executive Officer, Graceville Health Center, Graceville, MN, p. A228
JOSEF, Norma C., M.D., Director, Walter P. Reuther Psychiatric Hospital, Westland, MI, p. A224
JOSEPH, Elliot T., President and Chief Executive Officer, Genesys Regional Medical Center, Grand Blanc, MI, p. A215
JOSEPH, Gloria, Superintendent, Western Missouri Mental Health Center, Kansas City, MO, p. A249
JOSEPH, Michael G., Chief Executive Officer, Westside Regional Medical Center, Plantation, FL, p. A93
JOSEPH, Vincent D., Executive Director, Saint Barnabas Medical Center, Livingston, NJ, p. A277
JOSEY, Brenda, Administrator, Wheeler County Hospital, Glenwood, GA, p. A105
JOSHI, Shobhana, M.D., Director, Northville Psychiatric Hospital, Northville, MI, p. A220
JOSLIN, Tim A.
Chief Executive Officer, Doctors Hospital of Manteca, Manteca, CA, p. A51
Chief Executive Officer, Doctors Medical Center, Modesto, CA, p. A51
JOSPE, Theodore A., President, Southside Hospital, Bay Shore, NY, p. A288
JOYCE, Michael P., President and Chief Executive Officer, Trident Medical Center, Charleston, SC, p. A379
JOYNER, Ronald G., Chief Executive Officer, Williamson Medical Center, Franklin, TN, p. A392
JUBINSKY, Linda, Chief Executive Officer, Emory Peachtree Regional Hospital, Newnan, GA, p. A108
JUDD, Jeffrey M., President and Chief Executive Officer, McDowell Hospital, Marion, NC, p. A315
JUDD, Russell V., Chief Executive Officer, Payson Regional Medical Center, Payson, AZ, p. A24
JUDY, Mark D., Chief Executive Officer, Valley General Hospital, Monroe, WA, p. A454
JUENEMANN, Jean, Chief Executive Officer, Queen of Peace Hospital, New Prague, MN, p. A231
JUENGLING, Craig S., Chief Executive Officer, Potomac Ridge, Rockville, MD, p. A200
JUPIN , Jr, Joseph, Chief Executive Officer, Trenton Psychiatric Hospital, Trenton, NJ, p. A281
JURENA, Jerry E., Executive Director, Heart of America Medical Center, Rugby, ND, p. A324

K

KAATZ, Gary E., Chief Executive Officer, Forum Health, Youngstown, OH, p. B85
KABOT, Lorraine B., FACHE, President and Chief Executive Officer, Hepburn Medical Center, Ogdensburg, NY, p. A301
KADLEC, Patricia, Administrator, Faulk County Memorial Hospital, Faulkton, SD, p. A386
KAHN, Alvin I., M.D., President and Chief Executive Officer, Brookdale Hospital Medical Center, New York, NY, p. A295
KAIL, Bill, Administrator, Humboldt General Hospital, Humboldt, TN, p. A393
KAISER, Joel, Chief Executive Officer, Doctors Hospital of Nelsonville, Nelsonville, OH, p. A335
KAJIWARA, Gary K., President and Chief Executive Officer, Kuakini Medical Center, Honolulu, HI, p. A112
KALDOR, Patricia A., R.N., President, St. Joseph's Hospital, Milwaukee, WI, p. A472
KALETKOWSKI, Chester B.
President and Chief Executive Officer, South Jersey Hospital, Bridgeton, NJ, p. A274
President and Chief Executive Officer, South Jersey Hospital–Newcomb, Vineland, NJ, p. A281
KALLEN–ZURY, Karen, Chief Executive Officer, Hollywood Pavilion, Los Angeles, FL, p. A86
KAMINSKI, Elizabeth K., President and Chief Executive Officer, Ancilla Systems Inc., Hobart, IN, p. B52
KANE, Daniel A., President and Chief Executive Officer, Englewood Hospital and Medical Center, Englewood, NJ, p. A276
KANNADY, Donald L., Chief Executive Officer, Bunkie General Hospital, Bunkie, LA, p. A181
KANTOS, Craig A., Chief Executive Officer, Riverside Medical Center, Waupaca, WI, p. A476
KARAM, Judith Ann, President and Chief Executive Officer, Sisters of Charity of St. Augustine Health System, Cleveland, OH, p. B133
KARELS, Genevieve, Administrator, St. Bernard's Providence Hospital, Milbank, SD, p. A386
KARPF, Michael, M.D., Vice Provost Hospital System and Director Medical Center, University of California Los Angeles Medical Center, Los Angeles, CA, p. A50
KARUSCHAK , Jr, Michael, Chief Executive Officer, Amery Regional Medical Center, Amery, WI, p. A466

KASEY, Jay D., President, St. Mary's Medical Center, Evansville, IN, p. A139

KAST, Kevin F.
  President, Chief Executive Officer and Market Executive, St. Joseph Health Center, Saint Charles, MO, p. A252
  President, Chief Executive Officer and Market Executive, St. Joseph Hospital West, Lake Saint Louis, MO, p. A249

KASTANIS, John N., FACHE, President and Chief Executive Officer, Hospital for Joint Diseases Orthopaedic Institute, New York, NY, p. A297

KASTELIC, Sumiyo E., Director, University of California San Diego Medical Center, San Diego, CA, p. A59

KATHRINS, Richard J., Administrator and Chief Executive Officer, Bacharach Institute for Rehabilitation, Pomona, NJ, p. A279

KATSUDA, Frank
  Administrator and Chief Executive Officer, East Los Angeles Doctors Hospital, Los Angeles, CA, p. A47
  Administrator and Chief Executive Officer, Memorial Hospital of Gardena, Gardena, CA, p. A42

KATZ, Stuart A., FACHE, Chief Executive Officer, Hawarden Community Hospital, Hawarden, IA, p. A152

KATZ, Treuman, President and Chief Executive Officer, Children's Hospital and Regional Medical Center, Seattle, WA, p. A456

KAUFFMAN, Louis, President and Chief Executive Officer, Dakota Heartland Health System, Fargo, ND, p. A322

KAUFMAN, Alan G., Director, Division of Mental Health Services, Department of Human Services, State of New Jersey, Trenton, NJ, p. B83

KAUFMAN, Thomas D., Administrator, Kanabec Hospital, Mora, MN, p. A231

KAUFMANN, Paul M., Ph.D., Chief Operating Officer, Choate Mental Health Center, Anna, IL, p. A119

KEAHEY, Kent A., President and Chief Executive Officer, Providence Health Center, Waco, TX, p. A434

KEARNEY, W. Michael, President, Mary Lanning Memorial Hospital, Hastings, NE, p. A263

KEARS, David J., Director, Alameda County Health Care Services Agency, San Leandro, CA, p. B51

KEATON, William A., Chief Executive Officer, Community Medical Center Sherman, Sherman, TX, p. A430

KECK, Wade E., Chief Executive Officer, Memorial Health Services, Adel, GA, p. B109

KEEFER, Michael R., CHE, Chief Executive Officer and Managing Director, Clarion Psychiatric Center, Clarion, PA, p. A358

KEEHAN, Carol, President and Chief Executive Officer, Providence Hospital, Washington, DC, p. A79

KEEL, Barry L., Chief Executive Officer, Andalusia Regional Hospital, Andalusia, AL, p. A11

KEEL, Deborah C., Chief Executive Officer, Kenner Regional Medical Center, Kenner, LA, p. A183

KEELAN, John E., Ph.D., Administrator, Johnson County Hospital, Tecumseh, NE, p. A267

KEELEY, Brian E., President and Chief Executive Officer, Baptist Health System of South Florida, Coral Gables, FL, p. B58

KEEN, Robert C., CHE, President and Chief Executive Officer, Hancock Memorial Hospital and Health Services, Greenfield, IN, p. A140

KEENE, Lee D., President and Chief Executive Officer, Rockcastle Hospital and Respiratory Care Center, Mount Vernon, KY, p. A177

KEENER, Carl, M.D., Medical Director, Montana State Hospital, Warm Springs, MT, p. A260

KEILERS, Lance W., Administrator, Ballinger Memorial Hospital, Ballinger, TX, p. A403

KEIMIG, H. John, President and Chief Executive Officer, St. Joseph Health Services of Rhode Island, North Providence, RI, p. A376

KEIR, Douglas C., Chief Executive Officer, McDuffie Regional Medical Center, Thomson, GA, p. A110

KEITH, David N., Chief Executive Officer, Rice Medical Center, Eagle Lake, TX, p. A411

KELLAR, Richard A., Administrator, West Allis Memorial Hospital, West Allis, WI, p. A477

KELLER, Jack M., Administrator, Baptist Hickman Community Hospital, Centerville, TN, p. A390

KELLER, Larry W., Chief Executive Officer, University Medical Center/McFarland Hospital, Lebanon, TN, p. A395

KELLEY, Lewis, Administrator, Chatuge Regional Hospital and Nursing Home, Hiawassee, GA, p. A106

KELLEY, Neal, Administrator, Seton Edgar B. Davis Hospital, Luling, TX, p. A422

KELLEY, Randall, President, Flower Hospital, Sylvania, OH, p. A338

KELLEY, Robert C., President and Chief Executive Officer, Madera Community Hospital, Madera, CA, p. A50

KELLEY, Joseph, Commander, U. S. Air Force Medical Center Wright–Patterson, Wright–Patterson AFB, OH, p. A340

KELLEY, Jr, William C., FACHE, President and Chief Executive Officer, Samaritan Regional Health System, Ashland, OH, p. A325

KELLIE, Karen J., President, McCall Memorial Hospital, McCall, ID, p. A117

KELLISON, Jay R., Chief Executive Officer, BHC Walnut Creek Hospital, Walnut Creek, CA, p. A66

KELLOGG, Richard E., Commissioner, Virginia Department of Mental Health, Richmond, VA, p. B153

KELLY, Arthur C., Administrator and Chief Executive Officer, Oktibbeha County Hospital, Starkville, MS, p. A242

KELLY, Daniel J., President and Chief Executive Officer, St. Mary's Hospital, Nebraska City, NE, p. A264

KELLY, Daniel R., President and Chief Executive Officer, Halstead Hospital, Halstead, KS, p. A162

KELLY, Frank J., President and Chief Executive Officer, Danbury Hospital, Danbury, CT, p. A74

KELLY, James, Chief Executive Officer, Houston Northwest Medical Center, Houston, TX, p. A417

KELLY, James P., Administrator, Alegent–Health Midlands Community Hospital, Papillion, NE, p. A266

KELLY, James R., Chief Operating Officer, Truman Medical Center–East, Kansas City, MO, p. A249

KELLY, Jeffrey R., President and Chief Executive Officer, Deaconess–Nashoba Hospital, Ayer, MA, p. A201

KELLY, Kathleen, Chief Executive Officer, Pilgrim Psychiatric Center, Brentwood, NY, p. A288

KELLY, Laurence E., Executive Vice President and Administrator, St. Luke's Hospital, Newburgh, NY, p. A301

KELLY, Patrick, Chief Executive Officer, Charter Behavioral Health System of Northwest Arkansas, Fayetteville, AR, p. A29

KELLY, Steven G., President and Chief Executive Officer, Newton Medical Center, Newton, KS, p. A165

KELLY, Timothy J., M.D., President, Fairbanks Hospital, Indianapolis, IN, p. A141

KELLY, Jr, Winfield M., President and Chief Executive Officer, Dimensions Health Corporation, Largo, MD, p. B83

KENDRICK, Gary G., Chief Executive Officer, Lincoln County Health Facilities, Fayetteville, TN, p. A392

KENLEY, William A., President, North Crest Medical Center, Springfield, TN, p. A399

KENNEDY, Bill R., President and Chief Executive Officer, Muskogee Regional Medical Center, Muskogee, OK, p. A345

KENNEDY, Christopher S., President and Chief Operating Officer, Health First/Cape Canaveral Hospital, Cocoa Beach, FL, p. A82

KENNEDY, Jerry, Administrator, Jefferson County Hospital, Fayette, MS, p. A238

KENNEDY, Thomas F., Administrator, Rolling Plains Memorial Hospital, Sweetwater, TX, p. A431

KENNEDY , II, Thomas D., President and Chief Executive Officer, Bristol Hospital, Bristol, CT, p. A74

KENNEDY–SCOTT, Patricia, Northern Region Vice President, The Eastside Hospital, Redmond, WA, p. A456

KENNER, Gary, President and Chief Executive Officer, Itasca Medical Center, Grand Rapids, MN, p. A228

KENT, Alan, Interim Chief Executive Officer, Meadows Regional Medical Center, Vidalia, GA, p. A111

KENYON, Douglas M., Director, Veterans Affairs Medical and Regional Office Center, Fargo, ND, p. A322

KERCORIAN, Robert A., Chief Executive Officer, Havenwyck Hospital, Auburn Hills, MI, p. A211

KERG, Mary, Administrator, Bloomer Memorial Medical Center, Bloomer, WI, p. A467

KERN, Peter L., President and Chief Executive Officer, Palmerton Hospital, Palmerton, PA, p. A366

KERNER, Michael K., President and Chief Executive Officer, Doctors Hospital, Augusta, GA, p. A100

KERR, Gary, Administrator, Christus Schumpert Bossier, Bossier City, LA, p. A181

KERR, Kay, M.D., Medical Director, Bryn Mawr College Infirmary, Bryn Mawr, PA, p. A357

KERR, Michael
  Chief Executive Officer, Bellwood General Hospital, Bellflower, CA, p. A36
  Chief Executive Officer, Orange County Community Hospital of Buena Park, Buena Park, CA, p. A37

KERVIN, David D., Administrator, Richardson Medical Center, Rayville, LA, p. A188

KERWIN, George, President, Bellin Hospital, Green Bay, WI, p. A469

KESSEN, Donald J., Administrator and Chief Executive Officer, Rawlins County Health Center, Atwood, KS, p. A159

KESSINGER, A. Jay, Administrative Director, State Hospital North, Orofino, ID, p. A117

KESSLER, D. McWilliams, Executive Director and Chief Executive Officer, Wills Eye Hospital, Philadelphia, PA, p. A368

KESSLER, William E., President, Saint Anthony's Health Center, Alton, IL, p. A119

KESTLY, John J., Administrator, Shawano Medical Center, Shawano, WI, p. A475

KETCHAM, Michael S., Chief Executive Officer, Manning Regional Healthcare Center, Manning, IA, p. A154

KETCHAM, Richard H., President, Brooks Memorial Hospital, Dunkirk, NY, p. A291

KETRING, John H., Administrator, Pawnee Municipal Hospital, Pawnee, OK, p. A346

KEUSENKOTHEN, Thomas, President and Chief Executive Officer, Alexian Brothers Health System, Inc., Elk Grove Village, IL, p. B52

KHAN, Nasir A., M.D., Director, Bournewood Hospital, Brookline, MA, p. A203

KIDDY, Diane, Chief Executive Officer, Charter Fairmount Behavioral Health System, Philadelphia, PA, p. A366

KIEF, Brian, Administrator, New Ulm Medical Center, New Ulm, MN, p. A231

KIEFER, Joseph N., Administrator, Helen Ellis Memorial Hospital, Tarpon Springs, FL, p. A97

KIELANOWICZ, Marie, Provincial Superior, Sisters of the Holy Family of Nazareth–Sacred Heart Province, Des Plaines, IL, p. B135

KIELMAN, Richard C., President and Chief Executive Officer, Dickinson County Memorial Hospital, Spirit Lake, IA, p. A157

KIELY, Robert Gerard, President and Chief Executive Officer, Middlesex Hospital, Middletown, CT, p. A75

KIEPURA, Sally Marie, President and Chief Executive Officer, Saint Mary of Nazareth Hospital Center, Chicago, IL, p. A123

KIER, Aloha, Administrator, Jewell County Hospital, Mankato, KS, p. A164

KIKUKAWA, Marion, General Minister, Sisters of the 3rd Franciscan Order, Syracuse, NY, p. B135

KILEY, Dennis, President, Emory–Adventist Hospital, Smyrna, GA, p. A109

KIMEL, Mike, Administrator, Davie County Hospital, Mocksville, NC, p. A315

KIMMEL, Arnie, President and Chief Executive Officer, Catholic Health Partners, Chicago, IL, p. B69

KIMMEL, Arnold
  Interim President and Chief Executive Officer, Columbus Hospital, Chicago, IL, p. A121
  Interim President and Chief Executive Officer, Saint Anthony Hospital, Chicago, IL, p. A123
  Interim President and Chief Executive Officer, St. Joseph Hospital, Chicago, IL, p. A123

KIMMETH, Steuart A., Vice President and Administrator, Peninsula Behavioral Center, Hampton, VA, p. A444

KINDRED, Bryan N., President and Chief Executive Officer, DCH Health System, Tuscaloosa, AL, p. B76

KING, Cynthia, Acting Administrator, Charlotte Institute of Rehabilitation, Charlotte, NC, p. A310

KING, Dennis, President and Chief Executive Officer, Spring Harbor Hospital, South Portland, ME, p. A194

KING, Kirk, Senior Vice President and Executive Director, Presbyterian Hospital of Kaufman, Kaufman, TX, p. A420

KING, Larry R., Administrator, Washington-St. Tammany Regional Medical Center, Bogalusa, LA, p. A181

KINGSBURY, James A., President and Chief Executive Officer, Fort Hamilton Hospital, Hamilton, OH, p. A332

KINKLER, Nancy, Administrator, Otto Kaiser Memorial Hospital, Kenedy, TX, p. A420

KINNEY, Charles S., Chief Executive Officer, United Memorial Medical Center, Batavia, NY, p. A287

KIRBY, Dale A.
President, College Health Enterprises, Downey, CA, p. B73
Chief Executive Officer, College Hospital Costa Mesa, Costa Mesa, CA, p. A39

KIRBY, James M., Administrator, Swain County Hospital, Bryson City, NC, p. A310

KIRK, Brian, Chief Executive Officer, Sheridan County Health Complex, Hoxie, KS, p. A162

KIRK, Warren J., President and Chief Administrative Officer, Alta Bates Medical Center-Ashby Campus, Berkeley, CA, p. A37

KIRK, Jr, H. Lee, President and Chief Executive Officer, Culpeper Regional Hospital, Culpeper, VA, p. A443

KIRK, Jr, Thomas A., Ph.D., Commissioner, Connecticut Department of Mental Health and Addiction Services, Hartford, CT, p. B75

KIRK, Jr, William R., President and Chief Executive Officer, Kent & Queen Anne's Hospital, Chestertown, MD, p. A197

KIRN, Galen, Administrator, California Mens Colony Hospital, San Luis Obispo, CA, p. A61

KIROUSIS, Theodore E., Area Director, Westborough State Hospital, Westborough, MA, p. A209

KIRSCHNER, Sidney, President and Chief Executive Officer, Northside Hospital, Atlanta, GA, p. A100

KISER, Greg, Chief Executive Officer, Three Rivers Medical Center, Louisa, KY, p. A175

KISH, Thomas M., Senior Vice President, University of Tennessee Memorial Hospital, Knoxville, TN, p. A395

KITCHEN, Barbara, Chief Executive Officer, Charter Ridge Behavioral Health System, Lexington, KY, p. A174

KLAASMEYER, Al, Administrator, Community Memorial Hospital, Syracuse, NE, p. A267

KLAGSBRUN, Samuel C., M.D., Executive Medical Director, Four Winds Hospital, Katonah, NY, p. A293

KLAMAN, Edward M., Acting Chief Executive Officer, Citizens General Hospital, New Kensington, PA, p. A365

KLAWITER, Anne K., President and Chief Executive Officer, Southwest Health Center, Platteville, WI, p. A474

KLEEFISCH, William B., Chief Executive Officer, Maui Memorial Medical Center, Wailuku, HI, p. A114

KLEIN, Robert, Chief Executive Officer, Hendersonville Hospital, Hendersonville, TN, p. A393

KLEINGLASS, Steven, Acting Director, Veterans Affairs Medical Center, Minneapolis, MN, p. A231

KLIMA, Dennis E., President and Chief Executive Officer, Bayhealth Medical Center, Dover, DE, p. A78

KLIMP, Mary, Administrator and Chief Executive Officer, Falls Memorial Hospital, International Falls, MN, p. A229

KLINT, Robert B., M.D., President and Chief Executive Officer, SwedishAmerican Health System, Rockford, IL, p. A134

KLOESS, Lawrence, President, Centennial Medical Center and Parthenon Pavilion, Nashville, TN, p. A398

KLUN, James A., President, Allegan General Hospital, Allegan, MI, p. A211

KLUSMANN, Richard W., Chief Executive Officer, South Austin Hospital, Austin, TX, p. A403

KLUTTS, Robert, Chief Executive Officer, Touchette Regional Hospital, Centreville, IL, p. A121

KLUTTZ, James K., President and Chief Executive Officer, Frederick Memorial Hospital, Frederick, MD, p. A198

KMETZ, Thomas D., Chief Administrative Officer, Norton Audubon Hospital, Louisville, KY, p. A175

KNAPP, Dennis L., President, Cameron Memorial Community Hospital, Angola, IN, p. A137

KNAUSS, Albert C., President and Chief Executive Officer, Marion General Hospital, Marion, IN, p. A143

KNEPP, Gerald E., Chief Executive Officer, Rabun County Memorial Hospital, Clayton, GA, p. A102

KNIGHT, Alan D., President and Chief Executive Officer, Jordan Hospital, Plymouth, MA, p. A208

KNIGHT, Russell M., President and Chief Executive Officer, Mercy Medical Center-Dubuque, Dubuque, IA, p. A151

KNIZLEY, Andrew, Chief Executive Officer, Williamson Memorial Hospital, Williamson, WV, p. A465

KNOCKE, David L., CHE, Executive Director, Charlton Methodist Hospital, Dallas, TX, p. A408

KNOX, John E., President, St. John Macomb Hospital, Warren, MI, p. A224

KNOX, Jud, President, York Hospital, York, ME, p. A194

KNOX, Stacey, Interim Administrator, Rock County Hospital, Bassett, NE, p. A261

KNUTSON, Fred, Administrator, Chippewa County Montevideo Hospital, Montevideo, MN, p. A231

KOBAN, Jr, Michael A., Chief Executive Officer, NetCare Health Systems, Inc., Nashville, TN, p. B112

KOCHIS, Thomas, Chief Administrative Officer, Oakwood Annapolis Hospital, Wayne, MI, p. A224

KOCOUREK, Cathie A., Acting Administrator, St. Mary's Kewaunee Area Memorial Hospital, Kewaunee, WI, p. A470

KOEHLER, Eduard R., Administrator, Medical Park Hospital, Winston-Salem, NC, p. A320

KOENIG, David Scott, Chief Executive Officer, St. James Hospitals and Health Centers – Olympia Fields Campus, Olympia Fields, IL, p. A132

KOENIG, Harris, Chief Executive Officer, Rancho Springs Medical Center, Murrieta, CA, p. A52

KOESTER, Jeanne, Chief Executive Officer, Vencor Hospital - Albuquerque, Albuquerque, NM, p. A284

KOLB, Fred L., President, Mercy Hospital Anderson, Cincinnati, OH, p. A328

KOLLARS, Tim, Administrator and Chief Executive Officer, Lincoln Hospital Medical Center, Los Angeles, CA, p. A48

KOLLER, George J., President and Chief Executive Officer, Noble Hospital, Westfield, MA, p. A209

KOORTBOJIAN, George, Interim Administrator, Southern Humboldt Community Healthcare District, Garberville, CA, p. A42

KOOY, Donald C., President and Chief Executive Officer, Lapeer Regional Hospital, Lapeer, MI, p. A218

KOPICKI, John R., President and Chief Executive Officer, Muhlenberg Regional Medical Center, Plainfield, NJ, p. A279

KOPMAN, Alan, President and Chief Executive Officer, Westchester Square Medical Center, New York, NY, p. A300

KOPP, C. Gary, Administrator, Wishek Community Hospital and Clinics, Wishek, ND, p. A324

KOPPEL, Robert F., President and Chief Executive Officer, East Tennessee Children's Hospital, Knoxville, TN, p. A394

KOPPELMAN, Ben, Administrator, Albany Area Hospital and Medical Center, Albany, MN, p. A225

KORBELAK, Kathleen M., President, St. Joseph Hospital & Health Center, Kokomo, IN, p. A142

KORDICK, Jill, Administrator, Madison County Memorial Hospital, Winterset, IA, p. A158

KORMAN, Keith, President, St. Andrew's Health Center, Bottineau, ND, p. A321

KORNBLATT, Michael J., Chief Executive Officer, South Cameron Memorial Hospital, Cameron, LA, p. A181

KORZEN, Joyce, R.N., Chief Operating Officer, Millard Fillmore Gates Circle Hospital, Buffalo, NY, p. A289

KOSANOVICH, John P., President, Watertown Memorial Hospital, Watertown, WI, p. A476

KOSCHALKE, Patricia Ann, President and Chief Executive Officer, Holy Family Medical Center, Des Plaines, IL, p. A125

KOSSEFF, Christopher O., Vice President and Chief Executive Officer, University of Medicine and Dentistry of New Jersey, University Behavioral Healthcare, Piscataway, NJ, p. A279

KOULOVATOS, James, Chief Executive Officer, Harmon Memorial Hospital, Hollis, OK, p. A344

KOWALEWSKI, William, President and Chief Executive Officer, Franklin Hospital Medical Center, Valley Stream, NY, p. A306

KOWALSKI, Richard S., Administrator and Chief Executive Officer, OSF St. Mary Medical Center, Galesburg, IL, p. A126

KOZAI, Gerald T., President, St. Francis Medical Center, Lynwood, CA, p. A50

KOZAR, Michael A., Chief Executive Officer, Laurens County Healthcare System, Clinton, SC, p. A379

KOZLOFF, Kenneth H., FACHE, Administrator, Inova Alexandria Hospital, Alexandria, VA, p. A442

KRABBENHOFT, Kelby K., President, Sioux Valley Hospitals and Health System, Sioux Falls, SD, p. B132

KRAGE, Oliver D., President and Chief Executive Officer, Roseland Community Hospital, Chicago, IL, p. A123

KRAMER, Douglas, Chief Executive Officer, Onslow Memorial Hospital, Jacksonville, NC, p. A314

KRAMER, Norm, Executive Director, Porterville Developmental Center, Porterville, CA, p. A56

KRAMER, Thomas H., President and Chief Executive Officer, Deaconess Hospital, Evansville, IN, p. A139

KRAML, Louis, Chief Executive Officer, Bingham Memorial Hospital, Blackfoot, ID, p. A115

KRASS, Todd, Administrator and Chief Executive Officer, Research Psychiatric Center, Kansas City, MO, p. A248

KREIN, Marlene J., President and Chief Executive Officer, Mercy Hospital, Devils Lake, ND, p. A321

KREITNER, Clint, President and Chief Executive Officer, Tennessee Christian Medical Center, Madison, TN, p. A396

KRESHECK, Neal E., President, Community Hospital, Springfield, OH, p. A337

KRETZ, Blake, Administrator, Graham Regional Medical Center, Graham, TX, p. A414

KREUZER, Jay E., FACHE, President, Saint Francis Hospital and Health Center, Blue Island, IL, p. A120

KRIEGER, Robert M., Chief Executive Officer, Orange Park Medical Center, Orange Park, FL, p. A91

KRISHNA, Murali, M.D., President and Chief Operating Officer, Integris Mental Health System-Spencer, Spencer, OK, p. A347

KRISIAK, Steve, Chief Executive Officer, Bertrand Chaffee Hospital, Springville, NY, p. A305

KRMPOTIC, Deb J., R.N., Administrator, Lookout Memorial Hospital, Spearfish, SD, p. A388

KROELL, Jr, H. Scott, Chief Executive Officer, Liberty Regional Medical Center, Hinesville, GA, p. A106

KROESE, Robert D., Chief Executive Officer, Pella Regional Health Center, Pella, IA, p. A155

KROGNESS, John, Chief Executive Officer, North Bay Hospital, Aransas Pass, TX, p. A402

KROHN, Judith, Ph.D., Chief Executive Officer, Anoka-Metropolitan Regional Treatment Center, Anoka, MN, p. A225

KRUCKEBERG, Karl, Director and Network Manager, Alton Mental Health Center, Alton, IL, p. A119

KRUCZLNICKI, David G., President and Chief Executive Officer, Glens Falls Hospital, Glens Falls, NY, p. A292

KRUEGER, Glen E., Administrator, Nemaha County Hospital, Auburn, NE, p. A261

KRUEGER, Jr, Harold L., Chief ExecutiveOfficer, Chadron Community Hospital and Health Services, Chadron, NE, p. A262

KRUSE, Lowell C., Chief Executive Officer, Heartland Regional Medical Center, Saint Joseph, MO, p. A252

KUBIAK, Phillip J., President, Hampstead Hospital, Hampstead, NH, p. A272

KUBICKI, Ted, Administrator, Hall County Hospital, Memphis, TX, p. A423

KUBIK, James A., Administrator, Pawnee County Memorial Hospital, Pawnee City, NE, p. A266

KUBRICKY, Mark R., Chief Executive Officer, Moses Ludington Hospital, Ticonderoga, NY, p. A306

KUCZKOWSKI, Claire, Chief Executive Officer, Pioneers Memorial Healthcare District, Brawley, CA, p. A37

KUDRLE, Venetia, Administrator, St. Francis Regional Medical Center, Shakopee, MN, p. A233

KUDRONOWICZ, Sherry, Administrator, Memorial Hospital of Lafayette County, Darlington, WI, p. A467

KUELZ, Nancy D., Administrator, Sacred Heart Rehabilitation Institute, Milwaukee, WI, p. A472

KUHN, John F., Chief Executive Officer, Forest View Hospital, Grand Rapids, MI, p. A215
KUHN, Marcus G., President and Chief Executive Officer, Twin County Regional Hospital, Galax, VA, p. A444
KUHN, Rebecca C., Chief Executive Officer, Paradise Valley Hospital, Phoenix, AZ, p. A24
KUNTZ, Edward L., Board Chairman, President and Chief Executive Officer, Vencor, Incorporated, Louisville, KY, p. B151
KUNZ, Susan, Administrator, Teton Valley Hospital, Driggs, ID, p. A116
KURTZ, Kendria, Chief Executive Officer, Eagleville Hospital, Eagleville, PA, p. A359
KURTZ, Jr, Thomas F., President and Chief Executive Officer, Clinton Memorial Hospital, Wilmington, OH, p. A339
KURZ, Linda, CHE, Director, Veterans Affairs Medical Center, Saint Louis, MO, p. A254
KUSS, B. Ann, Chief Executive Officer and Managing Director, River Parishes Hospital, La Place, LA, p. A184
KUTZ, Melissa, Administrator and Chief Executive Officer, HEALTHSOUTH Rehabilitation of Mechanicsburg, Mechanicsburg, PA, p. A364
KUYKENDALL, George A., President and Chief Executive Officer, San Antonio Community Hospital, Upland, CA, p. A65
KYDD, Allan J., Chief Executive Officer, BHC Montevista Hospital, Las Vegas, NV, p. A268

L

LA GRONE, Roderick G., President and Chief Executive Officer, Roy H. Laird Memorial Hospital, Kilgore, TX, p. A420
LAABS, Allison C., Executive Vice President and Administrator, St. John's Hospital, Springfield, IL, p. A135
LABARCA, Laurie, Chief Operating Officer, Via Christi Rehabilitation Center, Wichita, KS, p. A169
LABINE, Lance C., President, Hoots Memorial Hospital, Yadkinville, NC, p. A320
LABONTE, Frank, FACHE, Administrator, Shriners Hospitals for Children, Los Angeles, Los Angeles, CA, p. A49
LABRIOLA, John D., Senior Vice President and Hospital Director, William Beaumont Hospital–Royal Oak, Royal Oak, MI, p. A221
LACKEY, Thomas O., Chief Executive Officer, Jackson County Hospital, Scottsboro, AL, p. A18
LACONTE, Norman H., President and Chief Executive Officer, Proctor Hospital, Peoria, IL, p. A133
LACROIX, William M., Administrator, Paynesville Area Health Care System, Paynesville, MN, p. A232
LACY, Edward L., Administrator, Baptist Health Medical Center–Heber Springs, Heber Springs, AR, p. A30
LACY, Leslie, Administrator, Cheyenne County Hospital, Saint Francis, KS, p. A167
LADA, Stephen C., President, Central Michigan Community Hospital, Mount Pleasant, MI, p. A219
LADENBURGER, Robert W., President and Chief Executive Officer, St. Mary's Hospital and Medical Center, Grand Junction, CO, p. A71
LAFFERTY, Douglas L., President and Chief Executive Officer, San Joaquin Community Hospital, Bakersfield, CA, p. A36
LAFFOON, David C., CHE, Chief Executive Officer, Central Arkansas Hospital, Searcy, AR, p. A33
LAIBLE, Ray, Administrative Director, State Hospital South, Blackfoot, ID, p. A115
LAIRD, Michael J., FACHE, Chief Executive Officer, Ste. Genevieve County Memorial Hospital, Ste. Genevieve, MO, p. A255
LAIRD, Stewart, Interim Chief Executive Officer, Regina Medical Center, Hastings, MN, p. A229
LAIRD, IV, William R., President and Chief Executive Officer, Montgomery General Hospital, Montgomery, WV, p. A463
LAKE, Robin E., Chief Executive Officer, Great Plains Regional Medical Center, Elk City, OK, p. A343

LAKE, Thomas E., Administrator and Chief Executive Officer, Pioneers Hospital of Rio Blanco County, Meeker, CO, p. A72
LAKERNICK, Philip S., President and Chief Executive Officer, Maria Parham Hospital, Henderson, NC, p. A314
LALLY, Jeanne, Senior Vice President and Administrator, Fairview Northland Regional Health Care, Princeton, MN, p. A232
LALLY, Michael K., President and Chief Executive Officer, Westerly Hospital, Westerly, RI, p. A377
LAMB, Brent, Administrator, Van Nuys Hospital, Los Angeles, CA, p. A50
LAMB, Edward H., President and Chief Executive Officer, Alaska Regional Hospital, Anchorage, AK, p. A20
LAMBERT, M. Aurora, Senior Vice President, Jewish Hospital Kenwood, Cincinnati, OH, p. A328
LAMBERT, Norman, Chief Executive Officer, Golden Plains Community Hospital, Borger, TX, p. A405
LAMBERT, Terry R., CHE, Chief Executive Officer, Newman Memorial County Hospital, Emporia, KS, p. A161
LAMBERT, Tod N., Administrator and Chief Executive Officer, Cookeville Regional Medical Center, Cookeville, TN, p. A391
LAMBERTI, Patrick, Chief Executive Officer, POH Medical Center, Pontiac, MI, p. A220
LAMKIN, Elizabeth, Administrator, HEALTHSOUTH Meridian Point Rehabilitation Hospital, Scottsdale, AZ, p. A25
LAMONTAGNE, Margaret E., R.N., Chief Operating Officer, Medfield State Hospital, Medfield, MA, p. A206
LAMOUREUX, Bruce, Chief Executive Officer, Saint John's Hospital and Health Center, Santa Monica, CA, p. A62
LAMPE, Diane B., Administrator and Chief Executive Officer, HEALTHSOUTH Rehabilitation Institute of San Antonio, San Antonio, TX, p. A428
LANCASTER, Tim, Chief Executive Officer, Brownwood Regional Medical Center, Brownwood, TX, p. A405
LANDDECK, John R., President, Beaver Dam Community Hospitals, Beaver Dam, WI, p. A466
LANDERS, Louise, Administrator, Lynn County Hospital District, Tahoka, TX, p. A431
LANDRUM, Scott M., Chief Executive Officer, Martin General Hospital, Williamston, NC, p. A319
LANDRY, Ray A., Chief Executive Officer, Abbeville General Hospital, Abbeville, LA, p. A180
LANDSMAN, Robert E., Interim President and Chief Executive Officer, West Suburban Hospital Medical Center, Oak Park, IL, p. A132
LANE, Jerry, Administrator, Othello Community Hospital, Othello, WA, p. A455
LANE, Michael, Administrator and Chief Executive Officer, Greenleaf Center, Valdosta, GA, p. A111
LANE, William L., President, Holy Family Hospital and Medical Center, Methuen, MA, p. A206
LANG, Geoffrey N., President and Chief Executive Officer, Southwest Washington Medical Center, Vancouver, WA, p. A458
LANG, Steve, Administrator, Ruby Valley Hospital, Sheridan, MT, p. A259
LANGBEHN, Cody, Administrator, Pioneer Medical Center, Big Timber, MT, p. A256
LANGFORD, James W., Administrator, Smithville Regional Hospital, Smithville, TX, p. A431
LANGFORD, Joe S., Chief Executive Officer, Covenant Hospital Plainview, Plainview, TX, p. A426
LANGLAIS, Robert J., President and Chief Executive Officer, Cheshire Medical Center, Keene, NH, p. A272
LANGLEY, Douglas, Administrator, Memorial Hospital, Gonzales, TX, p. A414
LANGMEAD, Paula A., Chief Executive Officer, Springfield Hospital Center, Sykesville, MD, p. A200
LANIK, Robert J., President and Chief Executive Officer, Saint Elizabeth Regional Medical Center, Lincoln, NE, p. A264
LARCEN, Stephen W., Ph.D., Chief Executive Officer, Natchaug Hospital, Mansfield Center, CT, p. A75
LARET, Mark R., Chief Executive Officer, University of California San Francisco Medical Center, San Francisco, CA, p. A60

LARKIN, Donald, Ph.D., Administrator, Woodridge Hospital, Johnson City, TN, p. A394
LARKIN, Donald N., Chief Executive Officer, San Gorgonio Memorial Hospital, Banning, CA, p. A36
LAROCHELLE, Albert, Administrator, Grace Cottage Hospital, Townshend, VT, p. A441
LAROSA, John C., M.D., President and Chief Executive Officer, University Hospital of Brooklyn–State University of New York Health Science Center at Brooklyn, New York, NY, p. A300
LAROWE, Mary E., President and Chief Executive Officer, Westfield Memorial Hospital, Westfield, NY, p. A307
LARSON, Dale, Chief Executive Officer, Doctors Memorial Hospital, Bonifay, FL, p. A81
LARSON, Gary E., Chief Executive Officer, Illini Hospital, Silvis, IL, p. A134
LARSON, R. Alan, Chief Executive Officer, Davis Medical Center, Statesville, NC, p. A318
LARSON, II, George V., Administrator, Melissa Memorial Hospital, Holyoke, CO, p. A71
LARSSON, Randi, Vice President, Sharp Cabrillo Hospital, San Diego, CA, p. A59
LASKOWSKI, Rose, R.N., Hospital Director, Caro Center, Caro, MI, p. A212
LASSITER, Susan S., President and Chief Executive Officer, Roanoke–Chowan Hospital, Ahoskie, NC, p. A309
LATHAM, Larry L., Director, Central State Hospital, Petersburg, VA, p. A447
LATHROP, Ronny, Chief Executive Officer and Administrator, Cimarron Memorial Hospital, Boise City, OK, p. A341
LAUDERDALE, Max, Chief Executive Officer, Lakeview Regional Medical Center, Covington, LA, p. A181
LAUDICK, Paul E.
President and Chief Executive Officer, Memorial Medical Center, Woodstock, IL, p. A136
President and Chief Executive Officer, Northern Illinois Medical Center, McHenry, IL, p. A130
LAUDON, Larry, Administrator, Clearwater Health Services, Bagley, MN, p. A225
LAUFFER, Dan, Chief Executive Officer, Saint Francis Hospital, Charleston, WV, p. A461
LAUGHLIN, Donald L., President, Riddle Memorial Hospital, Media, PA, p. A364
LAUGHLIN, Jr, Raymond E., President and Chief Executive Officer, Wayne Hospital, Greenville, OH, p. A332
LAUGHNAN, Woody J., Interim Chief Executive Officer, Colusa Community Hospital, Colusa, CA, p. A39
LAURI, John P., Chief Executive Officer, Valley Health System, Hemet, CA, p. B150
LAUTNER, Martin A., Chief Executive Officer, HEALTHSOUTH Rehabilitation Hospital–Wichita Falls, Wichita Falls, TX, p. A434
LAVENDER, Tunisia, R.N., Chief Operating Officer, Pickens County Medical Center, Carrollton, AL, p. A13
LAVOIE, Reginald J., Administrator, Cottage Hospital, Woodsville, NH, p. A273
LAW, Wayne P., Acting Administrator, Hawaii State Hospital, Kaneohe, HI, p. A113
LAWATSCH, Frank, Chief Executive Officer, Swift County–Benson Hospital, Benson, MN, p. A226
LAWRENCE, David M., M.D., Chairman and Chief Executive Officer, Kaiser Foundation Hospitals, Oakland, CA, p. B103
LAWRENCE, William P.
Chief Executive Officer, UHHS Brown Memorial Hospital, Conneaut, OH, p. A330
President and Chief Executive Officer, UHHS Richmond Heights Hospital, Richmond Heights, OH, p. A337
President and Chief Executive Officer, UHHS–Memorial Hospital of Geneva, Geneva, OH, p. A332
LAWRENCE, Jr, J. David, Chief Executive Officer, BJC Medical Center, Commerce, GA, p. A103
LAWS, James R., Chief Executive Officer, Hallmark Youthcare of Kansas City, Kansas City, MO, p. A248
LAWSON, Alvin R., CHE, Chief Executive Officer, Wetzel County Hospital, New Martinsville, WV, p. A463

LAWSON, Michael E., Director, Veterans Affairs Boston Healthcare System, Boston, MA, p. A203
LAWSON, Michael P., Administrator, Mark Twain St. Joseph's Hospital, San Andreas, CA, p. A58
LAY, Barbara, Administrator, Minnie Hamilton HealthCare Center, Grantsville, WV, p. A461
LAY, Clarence E., Administrator, Washington County Memorial Hospital, Potosi, MO, p. A251
LAYFIELD, Michael G., Chief Executive Officer, Randolph County Medical Center, Pocahontas, AR, p. A33
LAYNE, Art, Chief Executive Officer, Maryvale Hospital Medical Center, Phoenix, AZ, p. A24
LAZATIN, Lou, Chief Executive Officer, Queen of Angels–Hollywood Presbyterian Medical Center, Los Angeles, CA, p. A49
LAZO, Nelson, Chief Executive Officer, HEALTHSOUTH Rehabilitation Hospital, Miami, FL, p. A89
LEACH, Kiltie, Chief Operating Officer, Washington Adventist Hospital, Takoma Park, MD, p. A200
LEACH, Michelle, Director, Indian Health Service Hospital, Rapid City, SD, p. A387
LEAHEY, Daniel P., President and Chief Executive Officer, Youville Lifecare, Cambridge, MA, p. A204
LEAHY, Annette B., President and Chief Executive Officer, UMass Marlborough Hospital, Marlborough, MA, p. A206
LEAHY, Kevin D., President and Chief Executive Officer, Sisters of St. Francis Health Services, Inc., Mishawaka, IN, p. B134
LEAKE, Edward G., Chief Executive Officer, Hot Springs County Memorial Hospital, Thermopolis, WY, p. A480
LEAMING, Larry E., Administrator, Thayer County Health Services, Hebron, NE, p. A263
LEARY, Catherine B., R.N., Chief Operating Officer, Meridia Hillcrest Hospital, Cleveland, OH, p. A329
LEARY, Edward B., President, Barnstable County Hospital, Pocasset, MA, p. A208
LEBARON, Bradley D., Administrator and Chief Executive Officer, Uintah Basin Medical Center, Roosevelt, UT, p. A438
LEBLANC, David B., President, LifeCare Management Services, Dallas, TX, p. B105
LEBLANC, Keith G., Chief Executive Officer, Biloxi Regional Medical Center, Biloxi, MS, p. A236
LEBLOND, Eugene A., FACHE, President and Chief Executive Officer, Southern Regional Medical Center, Riverdale, GA, p. A108
LECONTE, Chantal, Administrator, Cleveland Clinic Hospital, Fort Lauderdale, FL, p. A84
LEDOUX, Roger C., Chief Executive Officer, Byrd Regional Hospital, Leesville, LA, p. A185
LEDWIN, Norman A.
  President and Chief Executive Officer, Eastern Maine Healthcare, Bangor, ME, p. B84
  President and Chief Executive Officer, Eastern Maine Medical Center, Bangor, ME, p. A191
LEE, Alan G., Administrator, Kula Hospital, Kula, HI, p. A113
LEE, Clarence A., Administrator, Hand County Memorial Hospital/Avera Health, Miller, SD, p. A387
LEE, Dennis M., President, Methodist Hospital of Southern California, Arcadia, CA, p. A35
LEE, Donald, Service Unit Director, U. S. Public Health Service Indian Hospital, Winnebago, NE, p. A267
LEE, Kayleen R., Chief Executive Officer, Weskota Memorial Medical Center, Wessington Springs, SD, p. A389
LEE, Mani, Ph.D., Superintendent, Larned State Hospital, Larned, KS, p. A164
LEE, Mike, Superintendent, Morton General Hospital, Morton, WA, p. A454
LEE, T. G., Administrator, Satanta District Hospital, Satanta, KS, p. A167
LEE, Victor, FACHE
  Chief Executive Officer, Boone County Health Center, Albion, NE, p. A261
  Interim Administrator, Brown County Hospital, Ainsworth, NE, p. A261
LEE, Bradford, Commanding Officer, U. S. Air Force Hospital Seymour Johnson, Seymour Johnson AFB, NC, p. A318
LEE, John A., MSC, Commander, U. S. Air Force Hospital Robins, Robins AFB, GA, p. A108

LEE–EDDIE, Deborah M.
  Administrator, Kaiser Foundation Hospital, Los Angeles, CA, p. A48
  Administrator, Kaiser Foundation Hospital, Los Angeles, CA, p. A48
LEEKA, Andrew B., President and Chief Executive Officer, Good Samaritan Hospital, Los Angeles, CA, p. A47
LEFERT, Gerald W., President, St. Marys Hospital Medical Center, Madison, WI, p. A470
LEFTWICH, Hal W., FACHE, Administrator, Hancock Medical Center, Bay Saint Louis, MS, p. A236
LEGG, Susan, Administrator, Vencor Hospital–Chicago North, Chicago, IL, p. A124
LEGGETT, Gail, Administrator, Telfair County Hospital, McRae, GA, p. A107
LEHRFELD, Samuel
  Executive Director, Coler Memorial Hospital, New York, NY, p. A296
  Executive Director, Goldwater Memorial Hospital, New York, NY, p. A296
LEIBERT, D. Michael, President and Chief Executive Officer, Fremont Area Medical Center, Fremont, NE, p. A262
LEIBERT, Fritz, Interim Chief Executive Officer, Via Health, Rochester, NY, p. B152
LELEUX, Walter, Chief Executive Officer, Bellaire Medical Center, Houston, TX, p. A416
LEMANSKI, Dennis A., D.O., Vice President and Chief Executive Officer, Riverside Osteopathic Hospital, Trenton, MI, p. A223
LEMON, Brian J., President, MacNeal Hospital, Berwyn, IL, p. A120
LEMON, Thomas R., Chief Executive Officer, Otsego Memorial Hospital, Gaylord, MI, p. A215
LEMONS, Stephen L., Ed.D., Director, Veterans Affairs Medical Center, Salem, VA, p. A449
LENEAVE, Mark, Chief Executive Officer, Elbert Memorial Hospital, Elberton, GA, p. A104
LENERTZ, Thomas C., President and Chief Executive Officer, Riverview Healthcare Association, Crookston, MN, p. A227
LENNEN, Anthony B., President and Chief Executive Officer, Major Hospital, Shelbyville, IN, p. A145
LENZ, Raymond, Director Operations, HEALTHSOUTH Rehabilitation Hospital of Fort Smith, Fort Smith, AR, p. A30
LENZ, Roger W., Administrator, Hamilton County Public Hospital, Webster City, IA, p. A157
LEON, Anne R., Chief Executive Officer, HEALTHSOUTH Houston Rehabilitation Institute, Houston, TX, p. A417
LEON, Jean G., R.N., Senior Vice President, Kings County Hospital Center, New York, NY, p. A297
LEONARD, Douglas J., Chief Executive Officer, Columbus Regional Hospital, Columbus, IN, p. A138
LEONARD, James, M.D., Interim Administrator, Carle Foundation Hospital, Urbana, IL, p. A135
LEONARD, Lawrence, President and Chief Executive Officer, Shannon Medical Center, San Angelo, TX, p. A428
LEONARD, Mark, Chief Executive Officer, Harris Regional Hospital, Sylva, NC, p. A318
LEONHARDT, George E., President and Chief Executive Officer, Bradford Regional Medical Center, Bradford, PA, p. A356
LEOPARD, Jimmy, Chief Executive Officer, Medical Park Hospital, Hope, AR, p. A30
LEPE, Patty, Administrator, Pine Grove Hospital, Los Angeles, CA, p. A49
LEPTUCK, Cary F., President and Chief Executive Officer, Chestnut Hill HealthCare, Philadelphia, PA, p. A366
LERNER, Wayne M., DPH, President and Chief Executive Officer, Rehabilitation Institute of Chicago, Chicago, IL, p. A122
LERZ, Alfred A., President and Chief Executive Officer, Johnson Memorial Hospital, Stafford Springs, CT, p. A77
LESSWING, Norman J., Ph.D., Administrator and Chief Executive Officer, Benjamin Rush Center, Syracuse, NY, p. A305
LETSON, Robert F., President and Chief Executive Officer, Gilmore Memorial Hospital, Amory, MS, p. A236

LETT, Bryan W., Chief Executive Officer, Behavioral Healthcare–Columbus, Columbus, IN, p. A138
LEUPP, Mitch, Administrator, Mountrail County Medical Center, Stanley, ND, p. A324
LEURCK, Stephen O., President and Chief Executive Officer, St. Anthony Medical Center, Crown Point, IN, p. A138
LEVENSON, Marc, Administrator, Veterans Affairs Medical Center, Manchester, NH, p. A272
LEVENSON, Marvin W., M.D., Administrator and Chief Operating Officer, Pomerado Hospital, Poway, CA, p. A56
LEVINE, Alan M., Chief Executive Officer, South Bay Hospital, Sun City Center, FL, p. A95
LEVINE, Peter H., M.D., President and Chief Executive Officer, UMass Memorial Health Care, Worcester, MA, p. A210
LEVINE, Robert V., President and Chief Executive Officer, Peninsula Hospital Center, New York, NY, p. A299
LEVINSONN, David, Chief Executive Officer, Sherman Oaks Hospital and Health Center, Los Angeles, CA, p. A49
LEVITSKY, Steven E., Administrator, Vencor Hospital North Shore, Peabody, MA, p. A207
LEVY, Shari E., Administrator, Phillips Eye Institute, Minneapolis, MN, p. A230
LEWGOOD, Tony, Administrator, Shriners Hospitals for Children–Lexington, Lexington, KY, p. A174
LEWIS, Brinsley, Senior Executive Officer, GlenOaks Hospital, Glendale Heights, IL, p. A127
LEWIS, J. O., Acting Administrator, Hereford Regional Medical Center, Hereford, TX, p. A415
LEWIS, Luther J., Chief Executive Officer, Medical Center of South Arkansas, El Dorado, AR, p. A29
LEWIS, Mary Jo, Chief Executive Officer, Jackson Purchase Medical Center, Mayfield, KY, p. A176
LEWIS, Nicholas P., Administrator, La Follette Medical Center, La Follette, TN, p. A395
LEWIS, Theodore M., Chief Executive Officer, Riverside Medical Center, Franklinton, LA, p. A182
LEWIS, Thomas J., President and Chief Executive Officer, Thomas Jefferson University Hospital, Philadelphia, PA, p. A368
LEY, Gary R., President and Chief Executive Officer, Garden City Hospital, Garden City, MI, p. A215
LIBENGOOD, Mary L., President, Meyersdale Medical Center, Meyersdale, PA, p. A364
LIEPMAN, Michael T., Chief Operating Officer, Valley Hospital and Medical Center, Spokane, WA, p. A457
LIKES, Jr., Creighton E., President and Chief Executive Officer, Fairfield Medical Center, Lancaster, OH, p. A333
LILLARD, Joseph K., Administrator, Tri–State Memorial Hospital, Clarkston, WA, p. A452
LILLY, W. Spencer, Administrator, University Hospital, Charlotte, NC, p. A311
LINCOLN, David R., President and Chief Executive Officer, Covenant Health Systems, Inc., Lexington, MA, p. B75
LIND, Richard A., President and Chief Executive Officer, Memorial Health Systems, Ormond Beach, FL, p. B110
LINDEN, Todd C., President and Chief Executive Officer, Grinnell Regional Medical Center, Grinnell, IA, p. A152
LINDSEY, John, Administrator and Chief Executive Officer, Charlton Memorial Hospital, Folkston, GA, p. A105
LINDSEY, Larry N., Administrator and Chief Executive Officer, Decatur County General Hospital, Parsons, TN, p. A399
LINENKUGEL, Nancy, FACHE, President and Chief Executive Officer, Providence Hospital, Sandusky, OH, p. A337
LINGENFELSER, Robert, Administrator, Memorial Psychiatric Hospital, Albuquerque, NM, p. A283
LINGOR, John Daniel, President and Chief Executive Officer, Mount Carmel Medical Center, Pittsburg, KS, p. A166
LINNELL, Jon, Administrator, North Valley Health Center, Warren, MN, p. A234
LINNEWEH, Jr., Richard W., President and Chief Executive Officer, Yakima Valley Memorial Hospital, Yakima, WA, p. A459

LINTJER, Gregory W., President, Elkhart General Hospital, Elkhart, IN, p. A139
LIPSTEIN, Steven H., President and Chief Operating Officer, BJC Health System, Saint Louis, MO, p. B61
LISCHAK, Michael, USAF, Commander, U. S. Air Force Hospital Luke, Glendale, AZ, p. A23
LITCHFORD, Jim, Administrator, Baptist Medical Center, Cumming, GA, p. A103
LITOS, Dennis M., President and Chief Executive Officer, Ingham Regional Medical Center, Lansing, MI, p. A218
LITTLEFIELD, Elizabeth, Ed.D., Superintendent, Western Mental Health Institute, Bolivar, TN, p. A390
LITZ, Thomas H., FACHE, President and Chief Executive Officer, CentraState Healthcare System, Freehold, NJ, p. A276
LIVERMORE, Craig A., President and Chief Executive Officer, Delnor–Community Hospital, Geneva, IL, p. A126
LOBECK, Charles C., President, Franciscan Hospital–Western Hills, Cincinnati, OH, p. A327
LOCKARD, Thomas L., President and Chief Executive Officer, Lodi Community Hospital, Lodi, OH, p. A334
LOCKWOOD, Brian C., President and Chief Executive Officer, Lorain Community/St. Joseph Regional Health Center, Lorain, OH, p. A334
LODATO, Dominic J., Interim President, Lutheran Medical Center, New York, NY, p. A298
LODGE, Dale A., President and Chief Executive Officer, Winchester Hospital, Winchester, MA, p. A209
LOEBIG , Jr, Wilfred F., President and Chief Executive Officer, Wheaton Franciscan Services, Inc., Wheaton, IL, p. B154
LOEPP , Jr, Robert A., CHE, Administrator, Lifecare Hospitals, Shreveport, LA, p. A188
LOEWEN, Harold C., President, Oaklawn Psychiatric Center, Inc., Goshen, IN, p. A140
LOFE, Dennis A., FACHE, Chief Executive Officer, HEALTHSOUTH Rehabilitation Hospital, Florence, SC, p. A381
LOGUE, John W., Executive Vice President and Chief Operating Officer, St. Vincent's Medical Center, Jacksonville, FL, p. A87
LOH, Marcel, President and Chief Executive Officer, Kadlec Medical Center, Richland, WA, p. A456
LOHRMAN, Joseph W.
  Administrator, Crete Municipal Hospital, Crete, NE, p. A262
  Administrator, Warren Memorial Hospital, Friend, NE, p. A262
LOMBARD, Dave, President and Chief Executive Officer, Clear Brook Lodge, Shickshinny, PA, p. A372
LOMBARDI, Anthony M., President and Chief Executive Officer, Monongahela Valley Hospital, Monongahela, PA, p. A364
LOMMEL, Marsha, President and Chief Executive Officer, Madonna Rehabilitation Hospital, Lincoln, NE, p. A264
LONCHAR, Charles, President and Chief Executive Officer, Preston Memorial Hospital, Kingwood, WV, p. A462
LONG, Faye, Administrator, Caldwell Memorial Hospital, Columbia, LA, p. A181
LONG, James K., CPA, Administrator and Chief Executive Officer, West River Regional Medical Center, Hettinger, ND, p. A322
LONG, Jan Robert, Chief Executive Officer, Chinese Hospital, San Francisco, CA, p. A59
LONG, John, Vice President, Behavioral Health Center, Greensboro, NC, p. A313
LONG, Kathy, Chief Executive Officer, Marshall County Hospital, Benton, KY, p. A170
LONG, Lawrence C., Chief Executive Officer, Tahoe Forest Hospital District, Truckee, CA, p. A65
LONG, Max, Chief Executive Officer, Walter Knox Memorial Hospital, Emmett, ID, p. A116
LONGACRE, Leslie, Executive Director and Chief Executive Officer, South Lake Hospital, Clermont, FL, p. A82
LONGO, Robert J., President and Chief Executive Officer, Good Samaritan Hospital, Lebanon, PA, p. A363
LOOP, Fred, M.D., President, Cleveland Clinic Health System, Cleveland, OH, p. B72

LOPEZ, David S., FACHE, Senior Executive Director, University of Texas Medical Branch Hospitals, Galveston, TX, p. A413
LOPEZ, Frank, FACHE, President and Chief Executive Officer, St. Mary's Mercy Hospital, Enid, OK, p. A343
LOPEZ, Ramon, Administrator, Hospital Perea, Mayaguez, PR, p. A483
LOPMAN, Abe, Executive Director, Orlando Regional Medical Center, Orlando, FL, p. A92
LORACK , Jr, Donald A.
  President and Chief Executive Officer, Hillcrest HealthCare System, Tulsa, OK, p. B98
  President and Chief Executive Officer, Hillcrest Medical Center, Tulsa, OK, p. A348
LORD, Marilyn K., Administrator, Hillcrest Medical Center at West, West, TX, p. A434
LORDEMAN, Frank L., Chief Operating Officer, Cleveland Clinic Foundation, Cleveland, OH, p. A328
LORY, Marc H.
  President and Chief Executive Officer, Manchester Memorial Hospital, Manchester, CT, p. A75
  President and Chief Executive Officer, Rockville General Hospital, Vernon Rockville, CT, p. A77
LOSOFF, Martin, President and Chief Executive Officer, Rush–Copley Medical Center, Aurora, IL, p. A119
LOTHE, Eric L., President and Chief Executive Officer, Skiff Medical Center, Newton, IA, p. A155
LOTT , Jr, Carlos B., Director, John D. Dingell Veterans Affairs Medical Center, Detroit, MI, p. A214
LOUGHNEY, Barbara, Administrator, Saint Michael's Medical Center, Newark, NJ, p. A278
LOVE, Martin, Chief Executive Officer, General Hospital, Eureka, CA, p. A40
LOVEDAY, William J., President and Chief Executive Officer, Clarian Health Partners, Indianapolis, IN, p. A141
LOVERSO, Felice, Ph.D., President and Chief Executive Officer, Casa Colina Hospital for Rehabilitative Medicine, Pomona, CA, p. A55
LOVING, David E., Chief Executive Officer, Edge Regional Medical Center, Troy, AL, p. A18
LOVRIEN, Jerry, Chief Executive Officer, Western State Hospital, Tacoma, WA, p. A458
LOWD , II, Harry M., President, Bath County Community Hospital, Hot Springs, VA, p. A445
LOWE, John C., Acting Director, Veterans Affairs Pittsburgh Healthcare System, Pittsburgh, PA, p. A370
LOWE, Phillip, Chief Executive Officer, St. Vincent General Hospital, Leadville, CO, p. A71
LOWRANCE, Bill, Administrator, Hodgeman County Health Center, Jetmore, KS, p. A163
LOWRY, James R., FACHE, Chief Executive Officer, Colquitt Regional Medical Center, Moultrie, GA, p. A108
LOYLESS, John Paul, Administrator, Rankin Hospital District, Rankin, TX, p. A427
LOZAR, Beverly, Chief Operating Officer, Meridia Huron Hospital, Cleveland, OH, p. A329
LUCAS, John, M.D., President and Chief Executive Officer, St. Vincent Hospital, Santa Fe, NM, p. A286
LUCAS, Stephen M., Chief Executive Officer, Veterans Affairs Medical Center, Erie, PA, p. A360
LUCK , Jr, James V., M.D., Chief Executive Officer and Medical Director, Orthopaedic Hospital, Los Angeles, CA, p. A49
LUKE, William C., Interim President and Chief Executive Officer, Good Samaritan Health Systems, Kearney, NE, p. A263
LUKER, Patricia, Chief Executive Officer, Franklin Foundation Hospital, Franklin, LA, p. A182
LULEWICZ, Stephanie, Administrator, Marshall County Healthcare Center/Avera Health, Britton, SD, p. A385
LUMSDEN, Chris A., Chief Executive Officer, Halifax Regional Health System, South Boston, VA, p. A450
LUNA, Richard, Chief Executive Officer, Specialty Hospital of Santa Ana, Santa Ana, CA, p. A62
LUND, Mark, Superintendent, Mental Health Institute, Clarinda, IA, p. A149
LUNDIN , II, Robert J., Chief Executive Officer, Trinity Medical Center–North Campus, Davenport, IA, p. A150

LUNDSTROM, Greg, Administrator and Chief Executive Officer, Lindsborg Community Hospital, Lindsborg, KS, p. A164
LUSE, Robert H., Chief Executive Officer, Mariners Hospital, Tavernier, FL, p. A97
LUSSIER, James T., President and Chief Executive Officer, St. Charles Medical Center, Bend, OR, p. A350
LUTHER, Robert M., Chief Executive Officer, St. Luke's Medical Center, Phoenix, AZ, p. A25
LUTJEMEIER, Everett, Administrator, Washington County Hospital, Washington, KS, p. A169
LYBARGER, William A., Ph.D., Administrator, Cedar Vale Community Hospital, Cedar Vale, KS, p. A159
LYCAN, Laura J., Executive Director, Baylor Institute for Rehabilitation, Dallas, TX, p. A408
LYNCH, Edward F., Administrator, Richards Memorial Hospital, Rockdale, TX, p. A427
LYNCH , II, Ernest C., Chief Executive Officer, Medical Center at Lancaster, Lancaster, TX, p. A421
LYON, Cheri, Service Unit Director, Public Health Service Indian Hospital, Albuquerque, NM, p. A283
LYON, David R., Administrator, Beckley Appalachian Regional Hospital, Beckley, WV, p. A460
LYONS, Richard D.
  Senior Vice President and Chief Operating Officer, Northridge Hospital and Medical Center, Sherman Way Campus, Los Angeles, CA, p. A49
  Interim President and Chief Executive Officer, Northridge Hospital Medical Center–Roscoe Boulevard Campus, Los Angeles, CA, p. A49
LYSINGER, R. Craig, Administrator, Wabash Valley Hospital, West Lafayette, IN, p. A147

M

MAAS, Lawrence A., Chief Executive Officer, Sutter Medical Center, Sacramento, CA, p. A58
MABRY, Jerry D., Executive Director, National Park Medical Center, Hot Springs, AR, p. A30
MAC DEVITT, Robert E., Chief Executive Officer, Labette County Medical Center, Parsons, KS, p. A166
MACDOWELL, Barry S., President, Reid Hospital and Health Care Services, Richmond, IN, p. A145
MACKAY, Lorin C., Administrator, Teton Medical Center, Choteau, MT, p. A256
MACLAREN, Ron J., Chief Executive Officer, Cleveland Regional Medical Center, Cleveland, TX, p. A406
MACLAUCHLAN, Steven, Chief Executive Officer, Hollywood Medical Center, Los Angeles, FL, p. A86
MACLEOD, John L., Chief Executive Officer, Mercy Hospital, Cadillac, MI, p. A212
MACLEOD, Leslie N. H., President, Huggins Hospital, Wolfeboro, NH, p. A273
MACPHEE, Alan, Administrator, Quincy Valley Medical Center, Quincy, WA, p. A456
MACPHERSON, Donna S., Administrator and Chief Operating Officer, E. J. Noble Hospital Samaritan, Alexandria Bay, NY, p. A287
MACRI, William P., Chief Executive Officer, Caldwell County Hospital, Princeton, KY, p. A178
MACRITCHIE, Anne M., Chief Executive Officer, HEALTHSOUTH Braintree Rehabilitation Hospital, Braintree, MA, p. A203
MADALAO, Michael, Interim Administrator, Veterans Home of California, Yountville, CA, p. A67
MADDEN, Michael J., Superintendent and Chief Executive Officer, Skyline Hospital, White Salmon, WA, p. A459
MADDEN, Patrick J., President and Chief Executive Officer, Sacred Heart Health System, Pensacola, FL, p. A93
MADDOCK, Dan S., President, Taylor Regional Hospital, Hawkinsville, GA, p. A106
MADDOX, Jim L.
  Administrator, Mercy Hospital of Scott County, Waldron, AR, p. A34
  Regional Administrator, Mercy Hospital–Turner Memorial, Ozark, AR, p. A33
MADDUX, Yvonne, Interim Chief Executive Officer, Livingston Hospital and Healthcare Services, Salem, KY, p. A178

MADISON, Jeffrey, Administrator and Chief Executive Officer, Crosbyton Clinic Hospital, Crosbyton, TX, p. A408
MAESTRE GRAU, Jaime F., Executive Director, Hospital De La Concepcion, San German, PR, p. A483
MAFFETONE, Michael A., Director and Chief Executive Officer, University Hospital, Stony Brook, NY, p. A305
MAGEE, James L., Executive Director, Piggott Community Hospital, Piggott, AR, p. A33
MAGERS, Brent D., FACHE, President, Walls Regional Hospital, Cleburne, TX, p. A406
MAGERS, Ray, Administrator, Putnam County Memorial Hospital, Unionville, MO, p. A255
MAGHAZEHE, Alireza, Chief Executive Officer, Capital Health System, Trenton, NJ, p. A281
MAGLIARO, John G., President and Chief Executive Officer, Columbus Hospital, Newark, NJ, p. A278
MAGOON, Patrick M., President and Chief Executive Officer, Children's Memorial Hospital, Chicago, IL, p. A121
MAHADEVAN, Dev, Chief Executive Officer, Oak Valley District Hospital, Oakdale, CA, p. A53
MAHAFFEY, Robert, Administrator, Heart of Florida Regional Medical Center, Davenport, FL, p. A83
MAHAN, Stephen, Chief Executive Officer, Ocala Regional Medical Center, Ocala, FL, p. A91
MAHER, Robert J., President, Our Lady of Bellefonte Hospital, Ashland, KY, p. A170
MAHER , Jr, Robert E., President and Chief Executive Officer, Saint Vincent Hospital, Worcester, MA, p. A210
MAHMOOD, Tariq, Chief Executive Officer, Central Texas Hospital, Cameron, TX, p. A406
MAHN, Edward F., Chief Executive Officer, Ketchikan General Hospital, Ketchikan, AK, p. A21
MAHONE , V, William, Interim President and Chief Executive Officer, Smyth County Community Hospital, Marion, VA, p. A446
MAHONEY, Michael P., President and Chief Executive Officer, St. Rose Hospital, Hayward, CA, p. A43
MAHONEY, Patrick R., Administrator and Chief Executive Officer, Affiliated Health Services, Mount Vernon, WA, p. A454
MAHONEY, William K., Chief Executive Officer, Wamego City Hospital, Wamego, KS, p. A169
MAHRER, Michael D., President, St. Ansgar's Health Center, Park River, ND, p. A323
MAIDLOW, Spencer, President, Covenant HealthCare, Saginaw, MI, p. A221
MAIER, Harry R., President, Memorial Hospital, Belleville, IL, p. A119
MAIER, Vonnie, President and Chief Executive Officer, Huerfano Medical Center, Walsenburg, CO, p. A73
MAIN, Robert P., President and Chief Executive Officer, Siskin Hospital for Physical Rehabilitation, Chattanooga, TN, p. A391
MAINIERI, John, Interim Chief Executive Officer, Memorial Hospital of Tampa, Tampa, FL, p. A96
MAJURE, Thomas K., Administrator, Our Community Hospital, Scotland Neck, NC, p. A318
MAKI, James W., Chief Executive Officer, Huntington East Valley Hospital, Glendora, CA, p. A43
MAKI, Jerrold A., President, St. Francis Hospital, Milwaukee, WI, p. A472
MAKOWSKI, Peter E.
President and Chief Executive Officer, Citrus Valley Health Partners, Covina, CA, p. B72
President and Chief Executive Officer, Citrus Valley Medical Center Inter–Community Campus, Covina, CA, p. A39
MALIA, John, Director, First Hospital Wyoming Valley, Wilkes-Barre, PA, p. A374
MALINOWSKI, Mary Norberta, President, St. Joseph Hospital, Bangor, ME, p. A191
MALLAH, Isaac, President and Chief Executive Officer, St. Joseph's Hospital, Tampa, FL, p. A96
MALLORY, Kaye, Administrator, Stone County Medical Center, Mountain View, AR, p. A32
MALMUD, Leon S., M.D., President, Temple University Health System, Philadelphia, PA, p. B139
MALONE, John T., President and Chief Executive Officer, Hamot Medical Center, Erie, PA, p. A360

MALONE, William J., M.P.H., Acting Chief Executive Officer, New Orleans Adolescent Hospital, New Orleans, LA, p. A187
MALONEY, Elizabeth Ann, President and Chief Executive Officer, St. Elizabeth Hospital, Elizabeth, NJ, p. A275
MALTE, Robert H.
Senior Vice President, Appleton Medical Center, Appleton, WI, p. A466
Senior Vice President, Theda Clark Medical Center, Neenah, WI, p. A473
MAMOON, Wendy, Chief Executive Officer, Rock Creek Center, Lemont, IL, p. A129
MANCHUR, Fred M.
President and Chief Executive Officer, Glendale Adventist Medical Center, Glendale, CA, p. A42
President and Chief Executive Officer, White Memorial Medical Center, Los Angeles, CA, p. A50
MANCINI, Dorothy J., R.N., Regional Vice President Administration, Imperial Point Medical Center, Fort Lauderdale, FL, p. A84
MANDERNACH, Dianne, Chief Executive Officer, Mercy Hospital and Health Care Center, Moose Lake, MN, p. A231
MANDERS, Daniel N., President and Chief Executive Officer, Mile Bluff Medical Center, Mauston, WI, p. A471
MANDSAGER, Richard, M.D., Administrator, Alaska Native Medical Center, Anchorage, AK, p. A20
MANGINI, Michael A., Administrator and Chief Executive Officer, Bellevue Woman's Hospital, Schenectady, NY, p. A304
MANGION, Richard M., President and Chief Executive Officer, Harrington Memorial Hospital, Southbridge, MA, p. A208
MANLEY, Jeffrey J., Chief Executive Officer, Jordan Valley Hospital, West Jordan, UT, p. A439
MANLEY, Joseph M., Director, Veterans Affairs Medical Center, Spokane, WA, p. A457
MANN, Emily S., MSN, Acting Administrator, Elmore Community Hospital, Wetumpka, AL, p. A19
MANNING, Richard W., Administrator, South Panola Community Hospital, Batesville, MS, p. A236
MANNING, Catherine, President and Chief Executive Officer, Saint Vincent Health Center, Erie, PA, p. A360
MANOR UNDERWOOD, Lori, Administrator, Healthsouth Rehabilitation Hospital, Concord, NH, p. A271
MANSFIELD, Jodi J., Executive Vice President and Chief Operating Officer, Shands at the University of Florida, Gainesville, FL, p. A85
MANTEGAZZA, Peter M., President and Chief Executive Officer, Fairlawn Rehabilitation Hospital, Worcester, MA, p. A210
MANTEY, Carl W., Administrator, Gerald Champion Regional Medical Center, Alamogordo, NM, p. A283
MANTZ, James R., Administrator, Prairie Community Medical Assistance Facility, Terry, MT, p. A260
MANZELLA, Arlene, Administrator, Norfolk Psychiatric Center, Norfolk, VA, p. A447
MAPLES, Ruth, Executive Director, Lanterman Developmental Center, Pomona, CA, p. A55
MARCANTUONO, Daniel L., FACHE, Acting Vice President and Chief Executive Officer, University of Medicine and Dentistry of New Jersey–University Hospital, Newark, NJ, p. A278
MARCHETTI, Mark E., Chief Executive Officer, Greenfield Area Medical Center, Greenfield, OH, p. A332
MARCONI–DOOLEY, Royetta, Commander, U. S. Air Force Hospital–Kirtland, Kirtland AFB, NM, p. A285
MARCOS, Luis R., M.D., President, New York City Health and Hospitals Corporation, New York, NY, p. B113
MARIE, Donna, Executive Vice President and Chief Executive Officer, Resurrection Medical Center, Chicago, IL, p. A123
MARION, Ben, Chief Executive Officer, Turning Point Hospital, Moultrie, GA, p. A108
MARK, Richard J., President and Chief Executive Officer, St. Mary's Hospital of East St. Louis, East St. Louis, IL, p. A125
MARKHAM, Patricia, Administrator, Cass County Memorial Hospital, Atlantic, IA, p. A148
MARKOS, Dennis R., Chief Executive Officer, Baker Community Hospital and Health Center, MacClenny, FL, p. A89

MARKOWITZ, Alan, FACHE, President and Chief Executive Officer, Shore Memorial Hospital, Nassawadox, VA, p. A446
MARKOWITZ, Bruce J., President and Chief Executive Officer, Palisades Medical Center, North Bergen, NJ, p. A278
MARKS, Craig J., President and Chief Executive Officer, South Haven Community Hospital, South Haven, MI, p. A222
MARKS, Gary A., Administrator, Glen Rose Medical Center, Glen Rose, TX, p. A414
MARKS, Victor, M.D., Interim President and Chief Executive Officer, Geisinger Health System, Danville, PA, p. B86
MARLETTE, Jeff, Administrator, Holy Infant Hospital, Hoven, SD, p. A386
MARLEY, Mark E., Chief Executive Officer, Natchitoches Parish Hospital, Natchitoches, LA, p. A186
MARLIN, Arthur E., M.D., Chief Executive Officer, Methodist Children's Hospital of South Texas, San Antonio, TX, p. A428
MARMERSTEIN, Peter A., Chief Executive Officer, Parkway Regional Medical Center, North Miami Beach, FL, p. A91
MARMO, Anthony P., Chief Executive Officer, Kingston Hospital, Kingston, NY, p. A293
MARMORSTONE, Ray, Administrator and Chief Executive Officer, Memorial Hospital of Iowa County, Dodgeville, WI, p. A468
MARNELL, George, Director, Veterans Affairs Roseburg Healthcare System, Roseburg, OR, p. A354
MARON, Michael, President and Chief Executive Officer, Holy Name Hospital, Teaneck, NJ, p. A280
MARONEY, George, Senior Vice President and Administrator, Memorial Hospital of Carbondale, Carbondale, IL, p. A120
MARQUARDT, Robert C., FACHE, President and Chief Executive Officer, Memorial Medical Center of West Michigan, Ludington, MI, p. A218
MARQUARDT, Dennis, USAF, Commander, U. S. Air Force Hospital, Barksdale AFB, LA, p. A180
MARQUETTE , Jr, Gerald J., Chief Executive Officer, Coffeyville Regional Medical Center, Coffeyville, KS, p. A160
MARQUEZ, Michael, Chief Executive Officer, Manatee Memorial Hospital, Bradenton, FL, p. A82
MARR, Charles J., Chief Executive Officer, Alegent Health Mercy Hospital, Council Bluffs, IA, p. A150
MARR, Larry, Senior Vice President and Administrator, St. Vincent Doctors Hospital, Little Rock, AR, p. A31
MARSH, Martha H., Director, University of California, Davis Medical Center, Sacramento, CA, p. A58
MARSHALL, Anthony, Service Unit Director, U. S. Public Health Services Indian Hospital, Keams Canyon, AZ, p. A23
MARSHALL, Michael D., Chief Executive Officer, HEALTHSOUTH Rehabilitation Hospital of Baton Rouge, Baton Rouge, LA, p. A180
MARSHALL, Philomena A., R.N., President and Chief Executive Officer, Charles A. Dean Memorial Hospital, Greenville, ME, p. A192
MARSTELLER, Brent A., Chief Executive Officer, Gulf Coast Medical Center, Panama City, FL, p. A92
MARTIN, Antonio D., Chief Operating Officer, Queens Hospital Center, New York, NY, p. A299
MARTIN, Cary, Administrator, Bleckley Memorial Hospital, Cochran, GA, p. A102
MARTIN, D. Wayne, President and Chief Executive Officer, Crisp Regional Hospital, Cordele, GA, p. A103
MARTIN, Elizabeth J., Vice President and Administrator, Riverside Tappahannock Hospital, Tappahannock, VA, p. A450
MARTIN, G. Roger, President and Chief Executive Officer, Jeanes Hospital, Philadelphia, PA, p. A367
MARTIN, Greg, Administrator and Chief Executive Officer, Integris Grove General Hospital, Grove, OK, p. A343
MARTIN, Guillermo J., Executive Director, Hospital Episcopal San Lucas, Ponce, PR, p. A483
MARTIN, Jack D., Interim Administrator, Johnston Memorial Hospital, Tishomingo, OK, p. A348

MARTIN, James A.
　Chief Executive Officer, Good Samaritan Hospital, Suffern, NY, p. A305
　President and Chief Executive Officer, St. Anthony Community Hospital, Warwick, NY, p. A307
MARTIN, Jeffrey L., President and Chief Executive Officer, Saint Michael's Hospital, Stevens Point, WI, p. A475
MARTIN, Kevin C.
　President and Chief Executive Officer, EMH Amherst Hospital, Amherst, OH, p. A325
　President and Chief Executive Officer, EMH Regional Medical Center, Elyria, OH, p. A331
MARTIN, M. Caroline, President, Riverside Regional Medical Center, Newport News, VA, p. A446
MARTIN, Norman, President and Chief Executive Officer, Parkview Community Hospital Medical Center, Riverside, CA, p. A57
MARTIN, Patricia A., Chief Executive, South Suburban Hospital, Hazel Crest, IL, p. A127
MARTIN, Patrick J., President and Chief Executive Officer, Fisher–Titus Medical Center, Norwalk, OH, p. A336
MARTIN, Thomas J., Administrator, Lincoln Hospital, Davenport, WA, p. A453
MARTIN, James W., Commander, DeWitt Army Community Hospital, Fort Belvoir, VA, p. A444
MARTIN, Julie, Chief Operating Officer, Dwight David Eisenhower Army Medical Center, Fort Gordon, GA, p. A105
MARTIN , Jr, Charles N., President and Chief Executive Officer, Vanguard Health System, Nashville, TN, p. B151
MARTIN–SHAW, Carolyn, President, Mercy Medical Center–New Hampton, New Hampton, IA, p. A155
MARTINEZ, Abraham, Chief Executive Officer, Doctors Hospital of Laredo, Laredo, TX, p. A421
MARTINEZ, Charles, Ph.D., Chief Executive Officer, Community Hospital of Huntington Park, Huntington Park, CA, p. A44
MARTINEZ, Ramiro J., M.D., Director, East Mississippi State Hospital, Meridian, MS, p. A240
MARTINEZ, Tomas, Administrator, Hospital Hermanos Melendez, Bayamon, PR, p. A481
MARTINEZ , Jr, Fred, Chief Executive Officer, St. Charles Parish Hospital, Luling, LA, p. A185
MARTORE, Patrick R., Chief Executive Officer, South Oaks Hospital, Amityville, NY, p. A287
MARTZ, Jodi M., Administrator, Granite County Memorial Hospital and Nursing Home, Philipsburg, MT, p. A259
MASCHING, Frances Marie, President, OSF Healthcare System, Peoria, IL, p. B117
MASI, George V., Commander, Winn Army Community Hospital, Hinesville, GA, p. A106
MASON, Bill A., President, Springhill Memorial Hospital, Mobile, AL, p. A16
MASON, Daria V., Chief Executive Officer, Central Vermont Medical Center, Barre, VT, p. A440
MASON , Jr, Charles H., President and Chief Executive Officer, Parkview Health System, Fort Wayne, IN, p. B118
MASSA, Lawrence J., Chief Executive Officer, Rice Memorial Hospital, Willmar, MN, p. A235
MASSE, Roger A., Chief Executive Officer, Margaretville Memorial Hospital, Margaretville, NY, p. A294
MASSEY, Donald W., Administrator, Bassett Hospital of Schoharie County, Cobleskill, NY, p. A290
MASSEY, Michael W., Administrator, Allen Bennett Hospital, Greer, SC, p. A381
MASSEY, Rocco K., Administrator, Summers County Appalachian Regional Hospital, Hinton, WV, p. A461
MASTERSON, David, Administrator, St. Vincent Mercy Hospital, Elwood, IN, p. A139
MASTRANGELO, Anthony G., Executive Vice President and Administrator, St. Joseph's Hospital, Highland, IL, p. A128
MATECZUN, John M., Commanding Officer, Naval Hospital, North Charleston, SC, p. A383
MATHERLEE, Tom, Interim Chief Executive Officer, Saint Joseph Hospital, Lexington, KY, p. A174
MATHESON, John A., Administrator, DeQuincy Memorial Hospital, DeQuincy, LA, p. A182

MATHEWS, George A., President and Chief Administrative Officer, Methodist Medical Center of Oak Ridge, Oak Ridge, TN, p. A398
MATHEWS, LouAnn O., Administrator, Select Specialty Hospital–Dallas/Forth Worth, Dallas, TX, p. A409
MATNEY, Douglas A., Chief Executive Officer, Del Sol Medical Center, El Paso, TX, p. A411
MATSUMURA, Kay, Chief Executive Officer, Salt Lake Regional Medical Center, Salt Lake City, UT, p. A438
MATSUWAKA, Robert, Regional Administrator, Kaiser Foundation Hospital, Honolulu, HI, p. A112
MATTA, Jorge, Associate Administrator, Hospital San Pablo, Bayamon, PR, p. A482
MATTES, James A., President, Grande Ronde Hospital, La Grande, OR, p. A351
MATTHEWS, Clint, Chief Executive Officer, Palm Beach Gardens Medical Center, Palm Beach Gardens, FL, p. A92
MATTHEWS, L. Gene, Chief Executive Officer, Eastern Oklahoma Medical Center, Poteau, OK, p. A347
MATTHEWS, Michael, Administrator, Lisbon Medical Center, Lisbon, ND, p. A323
MATTINGLY, Chris
　Chief Executive Officer, Prague Municipal Hospital, Prague, OK, p. A347
　Chief Executive Officer, Pushmataha County–Town of Antlers Hospital Authority, Antlers, OK, p. A341
MATTISON, Kenneth R., President and Chief Executive Officer, Florida Hospital Waterman, Eustis, FL, p. A84
MATTISON, Lynne M., FACHE, Interim Administrator, St. Benedicts Family Medical Center, Jerome, ID, p. A116
MATURO, Janna, R.N., Administrator and Vice President Operations, Seton Highland Lakes, Burnet, TX, p. A405
MATUSKA, John E., President and Chief Executive Officer, St. Peter's University Hospital, New Brunswick, NJ, p. A278
MAURER, Gregory L., Administrator, Elmore Medical Center, Mountain Home, ID, p. A117
MAXHIMER, Terry R., Administrator and Chief Executive Officer, HEALTHSOUTH Rehabilitation Hospital, Kingsport, TN, p. A394
MAY, Bill, Chief Executive Officer, Allen County Hospital, Iola, KS, p. A163
MAY, John C., Chief Executive Officer, Sebasticook Valley Hospital, Pittsfield, ME, p. A193
MAY, Kenneth, Chief Executive Officer, Northeast Medical Center, Bonham, TX, p. A405
MAY, Maurice I., President and Chief Executive Officer, Hebrew Rehabilitation Center for Aged, Boston, MA, p. A202
MAY, Timothy, Director, Veterans Affairs Medical Center, Salisbury, NC, p. A317
MAY, Walter E., Interim Administrator, Pikeville United Methodist Hospital of Kentucky, Pikeville, KY, p. A177
MAY , II, John E., Senior Vice President Operations, Penn State Geisinger Health System–Milton S. Hershey Medical Center, Hershey, PA, p. A361
MAYA, Victor, Chief Executive Officer, Kendall Medical Center, Miami, FL, p. A89
MAYO, Jim L., Administrator, Baptist Medical Center–Nassau, Fernandina Beach, FL, p. A84
MAYO, M. Andrew, Chief Executive Officer, Parkwood Behavioral Health System, Olive Branch, MS, p. A241
MAZOUR, Roger, Administrator, Pender Community Hospital, Pender, NE, p. A266
MAZUR–HART, Stanley F., Ph.D., Superintendent, Oregon State Hospital, Salem, OR, p. A354
MAZZARELLA, Michael C., President and Chief Executive Officer, Northern Dutchess Hospital, Rhinebeck, NY, p. A303
MAZZUCA, Phillip J., Chief Executive Officer, Town and Country Hospital, Tampa, FL, p. A96
MCAFEE , Jr, James T., Chairman, President and Chief Executive Officer, ValueMark Healthcare Systems, Inc., Atlanta, GA, p. B151
MCALEER, A. Gordon, FACHE, President and Chief Executive Officer, Lewistown Hospital, Lewistown, PA, p. A363
MCALLISTER, C. C., President and Chief Executive Officer, Ouachita Medical Center, Camden, AR, p. A28

MCANDREW, Michael, Chief Executive Officer, Lancaster Community Hospital, Lancaster, CA, p. A45
MCAVOY, Lawrence H., Interim President and Chief Executive Officer, H. C. Watkins Memorial Hospital, Quitman, MS, p. A242
MCBEE, Harold A., President, Northeast Health Management, Inc., Stevensville, MD, p. B115
MCBEE, Marie, Chief Executive Officer, Warwick Manor Behavioral Health, East New Market, MD, p. A198
MCBRIDE, Don H., Chief Executive Officer, Woodland Heights Medical Center, Lufkin, TX, p. A422
MCBRIDE, Michael J., FACHE, President, McCuistion Regional Medical Center, Paris, TX, p. A426
MCCABE, Jack, President and Chief Executive Officer, Harris Methodist–HEB, Bedford, TX, p. A404
MCCABE, Steve, Chief Executive Officer, Hill Crest Behavioral Health Services, Birmingham, AL, p. A12
MCCABE , Jr, Patrick, Executive Director, Levi Hospital, Hot Springs National Park, AR, p. A30
MCCAFFREY, Michael, Commander, Weed Army Community Hospital, Fort Irwin, CA, p. A41
MCCALL, Gerald A., Chief Executive Officer, Kaiser Foundation Hospital–Riverside, Riverside, CA, p. A57
MCCART, Janice, Chief Executive Officer, Grundy County Memorial Hospital, Grundy Center, IA, p. A152
MCCARY, Steve C., President and Chief Executive Officer, Stevens Healthcare, Edmonds, WA, p. A453
MCCASLIN, James B., Director, Chestnut Hill Rehabilitation Hospital, Glenside, PA, p. A360
MCCAULEY, Edith, Administrator, Sabine County Hospital, Hemphill, TX, p. A415
MCCAULEY, Roberta D., Chief Executive Officer, Hampshire Memorial Hospital, Romney, WV, p. A464
MCCLELLAN, David A., Chief Executive Officer, Carolinas Hospital System, Florence, SC, p. A380
MCCLELLAN, John W., Executive Director, Sandhills Regional Medical Center, Hamlet, NC, p. A314
MCCLERNON, Susan, Administrator, Brackenridge Hospital, Austin, TX, p. A402
MCCLESKEY, George H., President and Chief Executive Officer, Lubbock Methodist Hospital System, Lubbock, TX, p. B107
MCCLINTOCK, William T., FACHE, Chief Executive Officer, Boundary Community Hospital, Bonners Ferry, ID, p. A115
MCCLUNG, James W., Acting Administrator, Homer Memorial Hospital, Homer, LA, p. A183
MCCLURE, Jan, Chief Executive Officer, Hill Regional Hospital, Hillsboro, TX, p. A415
MCCLURE, Gwenda, USAF, Commanding Officer, U. S. Air Force Hospital Mountain Home, Mountain Home AFB, ID, p. A117
MCCLYMONDS, Bruce, President, West Virginia University Hospitals, Morgantown, WV, p. A463
MCCOMBS, David J., Executive Vice President and Administrator, Bon Secours–DePaul Medical Center, Norfolk, VA, p. A446
MCCONAHY, Richard L., Chief Executive Officer, Middle Georgia Hospital, Macon, GA, p. A107
MCCOOL, Paul J., Director, Veterans Affairs Connecticut Healthcare System–West Haven Division, New Haven, CT, p. A76
MCCORD, Windell M., Administrator, Heart of Texas Memorial Hospital, Brady, TX, p. A405
MCCORKLE, Vincent J., President, Mercy Hospital, Springfield, MA, p. A208
MCCORMACK, J. David, Executive Director, Riverview Regional Medical Center, Gadsden, AL, p. A15
MCCORMICK, John J., Interim Chief Executive Officer, Hi-Desert Medical Center, Joshua Tree, CA, p. A44
MCCORMICK, Richard M.
　Administrator, Methodist Healthcare – McKenzie, McKenzie, TN, p. A396
　Administrator, Methodist LeBonheur Healthcare–Jackson, Jackson, TN, p. A393
MCCOY, L. Kent, President, Huntington Memorial Hospital, Huntington, IN, p. A141
MCCOY, Michael J., Administrator, East Texas Medical Center–Quitman, Quitman, TX, p. A427
MCCOY, Mike, Chief Executive Officer, Saint Mary's Regional Medical Center, Russellville, AR, p. A33
MCCOY, Sherman P., Executive Director and Chief Executive Officer, Howard University Hospital, Washington, DC, p. A79

MCCRACKEN, Clyde T., Administrator, Ness County Hospital, Ness City, KS, p. A165
MCCRAY, Cindy M., Administrator and Chief Executive Officer, Hospital District Number Six of Harper County, Anthony, KS, p. A159
MCCULLOUGH, Frank S., M.D., President, Medical College of Ohio Hospitals, Toledo, OH, p. A338
MCCURDY, Judith, Administrator and Chief Executive Officer, Vencor Hospital–Los Angeles, Los Angeles, CA, p. A50
MCDANIEL, John P., Chief Executive Officer, MedStar Health, Columbia, MD, p. B109
MCDANIEL, Ruth, Chief Executive Officer, Crossroads Community Hospital, Mount Vernon, IL, p. A131
MCDERMOTT, Brian J., President and Chief Executive Officer, Carrington Health Center, Carrington, ND, p. A321
MCDONAGH, Kathryn J., President and Chief Executive Officer, Saint Clare's Health Services, Denville, NJ, p. A275
MCDONALD, Erica, Administrator, Man ARH Hospital, Man, WV, p. A462
MCDONALD, William A., President and Chief Executive Officer, St. Vincent Infirmary Medical Center, Little Rock, AR, p. A32
MCDOUGAL, Jr, Tom R., Chief Executive Officer, L. V. Stabler Memorial Hospital, Greenville, AL, p. A15
MCDOWELL, Gail, Administrator, Garfield County Memorial Hospital, Pomeroy, WA, p. A455
MCDOWELL, James W., President, St. Mary's Hospital, Centralia, IL, p. A121
MCDOWELL, Jane, Administrator, Seiling Hospital, Seiling, OK, p. A347
MCELHANNON, W. C., Administrator, Union County General Hospital, Clayton, NM, p. A284
MCEWEN, David S., Chief Executive Officer, Marlette Community Hospital, Marlette, MI, p. A219
MCGAHEE, James, Administrator and Chief Executive Officer, South Georgia Medical Center, Valdosta, GA, p. A111
MCGEACHEY, Edward J., President and Chief Executive Officer, Southern Maine Medical Center, Biddeford, ME, p. A191
MCGEE, John P.
President and Chief Executive Officer, JFK Medical Center, Edison, NJ, p. A275
President and Chief Executive Officer, Solaris Health System, Edison, NJ, p. B135
MCGILL, Richard M., Administrator, Hale County Hospital, Greensboro, AL, p. A15
MCGILL, Sandy D., Administrator, South Baldwin Regional Medical Center, Foley, AL, p. A14
MCGILL, Timothy W., Chief Executive Officer, Livingston Regional Hospital, Livingston, TN, p. A395
MCGINTY, Daniel B., President and Chief Executive Officer, Holy Family Memorial Medical Center, Manitowoc, WI, p. A470
MCGLASHAN, Thomas H., M.D., Director and Psychiatrist–in–Chief, Yale Psychiatric Institute, New Haven, CT, p. A76
MCGLONE, Cynthia, Chief Operating Officer, Germantown Hospital and Community Health Services, Philadelphia, PA, p. A367
MCGOUGH, Susan, Administrator, Mountain View Hospital District, Madras, OR, p. A352
MCGOURTY, Mark E., Regional Chief Executive Officer, St. John Medical Center, Longview, WA, p. A454
MCGOWAN, Donna, Administrator, Lane County Hospital, Dighton, KS, p. A160
MCGOWAN, Maggie, Interim Area Director, University of New Mexico Children's Psychiatric Hospital, Albuquerque, NM, p. A284
MCGOWAN, Marion A., President and Chief Executive Officer, Brandywine Hospital, Coatesville, PA, p. A358
MCGRATH, Denise B., Chief Executive Officer, HEALTHSOUTH Sea Pines Rehabilitation Hospital, Melbourne, FL, p. A89
MCGRAW, Steven E., Administrator, Vencor Hospital–Chattanooga, Chattanooga, TN, p. A391
MCGRAW, Tom, Administrator, Presbyterian–Orthopaedic Hospital, Charlotte, NC, p. A311
MCGUIRE, Aryon, Acting Administrator, E. A. Conway Medical Center, Monroe, LA, p. A185

MCGUIRE, William D., President and Chief Executive Officer, Catholic Medical Centers, New York, NY, p. A296
MCINNIS, Gwendolyn M., R.N., Chief Executive Officer, St. Claude Medical Center, New Orleans, LA, p. A187
MCINTYRE, Nancy, Administrator, Ferry County Memorial Hospital, Republic, WA, p. A456
MCINTYRE, Kathleen, President, Little Company of Mary Hospital and Health Care Centers, Evergreen Park, IL, p. A126
MCIVOR, Dave, Administrator, Roundup Memorial Hospital, Roundup, MT, p. A259
MCKAY, Daniel E., Chief Executive Officer, Springs Memorial Hospital, Lancaster, SC, p. A382
MCKAY, Robert H., President, North Penn Hospital, Lansdale, PA, p. A363
MCKENNA, Donald, Chief Executive Officer, Seven Rivers Community Hospital, Crystal River, FL, p. A83
MCKENNA, John, Administrator, Charter Behavioral Health System of Atlanta, Atlanta, GA, p. A99
MCKERNAN, Stephen W.
Chief Executive Officer, Mental health Center, Albuquerque, NM, p. A283
Chief Executive Officer, University Hospital, Albuquerque, NM, p. A284
MCKIBBEN, Sean, President and Chief Executive Officer, Youngstown Osteopathic Hospital, Youngstown, OH, p. A340
MCKIBBENS, Ben M., President, Valley Baptist Medical Center, Harlingen, TX, p. A415
MCKILLOP, Gail, President, Crawley Memorial Hospital, Boiling Springs, NC, p. A309
MCKINNEY, Dan, Administrator, Hermann Area District Hospital, Hermann, MO, p. A247
MCKINNEY, Paul, Administrator, Cochran Memorial Hospital, Morton, TX, p. A424
MCKINNEY, Jr, Buck, Chief Executive Officer, Jefferson County Hospital, Waurika, OK, p. A349
MCKINNON, Ronald A., Chief Executive Officer, Benson Hospital, Benson, AZ, p. A22
MCKLEM, Patricia A., Chief Executive Officer, Northern Arizona VA Health Care System, Prescott, AZ, p. A25
MCKNIGHT, James, Interim Chief Executive Officer, Doctor's Memorial Hospital, Perry, FL, p. A93
MCKROW, Dee, Chief Executive Officer, Hills and Dales General Hospital, Cass City, MI, p. A212
MCLAREN, Roseanne, Senior Vice President, Rogue Valley Medical Center, Medford, OR, p. A352
MCLAUGHLIN, Keith H., President and Chief Executive Officer, Raritan Bay Medical Center, Perth Amboy, NJ, p. A279
MCLAURIN, Monty E., President, Christus St. Joseph's Health System, Paris, TX, p. A426
MCLEAN, Daniel P., Executive Director, McAllen Medical Center, McAllen, TX, p. A423
MCLEAN, Gordon C., Administrator, Whitman Hospital and Medical Center, Colfax, WA, p. A453
MCLEMORE, Edwin, Administrator, U. S. Public Health Service Indian Hospital, Cherokee, NC, p. A311
MCLEOD, Richard D., Administrator, Owen County Memorial Hospital, Owenton, KY, p. A177
MCLOUGHLIN, Marjorie, Chief Executive Officer, Desert Springs Medical Center, Midland, TX, p. A423
MCLOUGHLIN, Thomas, President and Chief Executive Officer, Union City Memorial Hospital, Union City, PA, p. A373
MCMAHON, David, Chief Executive Officer, Oconto Memorial Hospital, Oconto, WI, p. A473
MCMAHON, Elaine, Administrator, Kwajalein Hospital, Kwajalein Island, MH, p. A481
MCMAHON, Louise, Acting Director, Veterans Affairs Medical Center, Providence, RI, p. A377
MCMANN, David L., Chief Executive Officer, Community Hospital, Watervliet, MI, p. A224
MCMANUS, Joseph S., President and Chief Executive Officer, Lawrence General Hospital, Lawrence, MA, p. A205
MCMANUS, Michael T., Administrator, St. Clement Health Services, Red Bud, IL, p. A133
MCMEEKIN, John C., President and Chief Executive Officer, Crozer–Keystone Health System, Springfield, PA, p. B76

MCMILLAN, Douglas A., Administrator and Chief Executive Officer, West Park Hospital, Cody, WY, p. A478
MCMULLEN, Ronald B., President, Alton Memorial Hospital, Alton, IL, p. A119
MCMURDO, Timothy B., Chief Executive Officer, San Mateo County General Hospital and Clinics, San Mateo, CA, p. A61
MCMURTRY, Roger, Chief Mental Health Bureau, Mississippi State Department of Mental Health, Jackson, MS, p. B111
MCNAIR, Mike H., Chief Executive Officer, Hartselle Medical Center, Hartselle, AL, p. A15
MCNAMARA, Maureen, President and Chief Executive Officer, New London Hospital, New London, NH, p. A272
MCNASH, Mark, Vice President Operations, Hutzel Hospital, Detroit, MI, p. A214
MCNAUGHTON, Neil H., Executive Director and Administrator, Serenity Lane, Eugene, OR, p. A351
MCNEIL, Greg R., Administrator, Dallas County Hospital, Fordyce, AR, p. A29
MCNEILL, Douglas W., FACHE, President and Chief Executive Officer, Middletown Regional Hospital, Middletown, OH, p. A335
MCNEW, Robert L., Administrator, Vencor Hospital–Fort Worth Southwest, Fort Worth, TX, p. A413
MCPHAIL, Mark D., Chief Executive Officer, Jeff Anderson Regional Medical Center, Meridian, MS, p. A240
MCQUEEN, Elbert T., Chief Executive Officer, HEALTHSOUTH Central Georgia Rehabilitation Hospital, Macon, GA, p. A107
MCRAE, Dave C.
President and Chief Executive Officer, Pitt County Memorial Hospital–University Health Systems of Eastern Carolina, Greenville, NC, p. A313
President and Chief Executive Officer, University Health Systems of Eastern Carolina, Greenville, NC, p. B148
MCVEETY, John A., Chief Executive Officer, Alpena General Hospital, Alpena, MI, p. A211
MCWATTERS, David M., Administrator, Highland Hospital, Charleston, WV, p. A460
MCWHORTER, II, John B., Executive Director, Baylor Medical Center at Garland, Garland, TX, p. A414
MEADE, Robert C., Chief Executive Officer, Englewood Community Hospital, Englewood, FL, p. A84
MEADES, LeVern S., Administrator, Lallie Kemp Medical Center, Independence, LA, p. A183
MEARIAN, Chase, Administrator, Sierra Valley District Hospital, Loyalton, CA, p. A50
MECHTENBERG, David A., Chief Executive Officer, Ridgecrest Regional Hospital, Ridgecrest, CA, p. A57
MECKLENBURG, Gary A., President and Chief Executive Officer, Northwestern Memorial Hospital, Chicago, IL, p. A122
MECKSTROTH, David J., President and Chief Executive Officer, Upper Valley Medical Center, Troy, OH, p. A338
MEEHAN, John J., President and Chief Executive Officer, Hartford Hospital, Hartford, CT, p. A75
MEEKER, Timothy L., Executive Director, Sonoma Developmental Center, Eldridge, CA, p. A40
MEHL, Edward J., Chief Executive Officer, Lake Region Healthcare Corporation, Fergus Falls, MN, p. A228
MEIER, Ernie, Administrator, Community Hospital of New Port Richey, New Port Richey, FL, p. A91
MEINERT, Mark W., CHE, Chief Executive, Yamhill Service Area, Providence Newberg Hospital, Newberg, OR, p. A352
MEIS, Fred J., Administrator and Chief Executive Officer, Graham County Hospital, Hill City, KS, p. A162
MELBY, Bernette A., Executive Director, University Health Services, Amherst, MA, p. A201
MELBY, Gina, Chief Executive Officer, Northwest Medical Center, Pompano Beach, FL, p. A93
MELCHIORRE, Jr, Joseph E., CHE, Executive Administrator, Shriners Hospitals for Children, Tampa, FL, p. B131
MELIN, Craig N., President and Chief Executive Officer, Cooley Dickinson Hospital, Northampton, MA, p. A207

Index of Health Care Professionals / Melton

MELTON, John W., Administrator, Baptist Medical Center East, Montgomery, AL, p. A16
MELTON, Jr, T. Carter, President, Rockingham Memorial Hospital, Harrisonburg, VA, p. A445
MELTZER, Neil M., President and Chief Operating Officer, Sinai Hospital of Baltimore, Baltimore, MD, p. A196
MENAUGH, John E., Chief Executive Officer, Sutter Coast Hospital, Crescent City, CA, p. A39
MENDELSOHN, John, M.D., President and Chief Executive Officer, University of Texas M. D. Anderson Cancer Center, Houston, TX, p. A418
MENDELSON, Peter, Superintendent, Cedarcrest Hospital, Newington, CT, p. A76
MENDEZ, Lincoln S., Chief Executive Officer, HEALTHSOUTH Doctors' Hospital, Coral Gables, FL, p. A83
MENDEZ, Matthew, Site Administrator, Pender Memorial Hospital, Burgaw, NC, p. A310
MENTON, Timothy P., Administrator, Broward General Medical Center, Fort Lauderdale, FL, p. A84
MERCADO, Sylvia, Chief Executive Officer, University Pediatric Hospital, San Juan, PR, p. A484
MEREDITH, Stephen L., Chief Executive Officer, Twin Lakes Regional Medical Center, Leitchfield, KY, p. A174
MERLIS, Laurence M., President and Chief Executive Officer, Greater Baltimore Medical Center, Baltimore, MD, p. A195
MERRILL, Mark H., President, Presbyterian Hospital of Dallas, Dallas, TX, p. A409
MERRILL, Rick W., President and Chief Executive Officer, Driscoll Children's Hospital, Corpus Christi, TX, p. A407
MERRITT, Tim E., Chief Executive Officer, Wills Memorial Hospital, Washington, GA, p. A111
MERTZ, Paul A., Executive Director, Newark Beth Israel Medical Center, Newark, NJ, p. A278
MERWIN, Robert W., Chief Executive Officer, Mills-Peninsula Health Services, Burlingame, CA, p. A37
MESMER, Keith, Chief Executive Officer, Hazel Hawkins Memorial Hospital, Hollister, CA, p. A44
MESROPIAN, Robert A., President and Chief Executive Officer, Alice Peck Day Memorial Hospital, Lebanon, NH, p. A272
MESSMER, Joseph, President and Chief Executive Officer, Mercy Medical Center, Nampa, ID, p. A117
METIVIER, Roland, Chief Executive Officer, Las Encinas Hospital, Pasadena, CA, p. A55
METSCH, Jonathan M., Dr.PH
   President and Chief Executive Officer, Greenville Hospital, Jersey City, NJ, p. A277
   President and Chief Executive Officer, Jersey City Medical Center, Jersey City, NJ, p. A277
   President and Chief Executive Officer, Liberty Healthcare System, Jersey City, NJ, p. B104
METZLER, Michael W., President, Saint Anne's Hospital, Fall River, MA, p. A204
METZNER, Kurt W., President and Chief Executive Officer, Mississippi Baptist Health Systems, Jackson, MS, p. A239
MEYER, Eugene W., President and Chief Executive Officer, Lawrence Memorial Hospital, Lawrence, KS, p. A164
MEYER, James E., President and Chief Executive Officer, MedCentral Health System, Mansfield, OH, p. A334
MEYER, Jeffrey K., Chief Executive Officer, Osceola Medical Center, Osceola, WI, p. A473
MEYER, Kurt, Administrator, Delta Memorial Hospital, Dumas, AR, p. A29
MEYER, Marlis, Division Director, Veterans Affairs Medical Center, Lake City, FL, p. A88
MEYER, Michele C., Chief Executive Officer, Des Peres Hospital, Saint Louis, MO, p. A253
MEYER, Robert F., M.D., Chief Executive Officer, Samaritan Behavioral Health Center-Scottsdale, Scottsdale, AZ, p. A25
MEYER, Wilbert E., Administrator and Chief Executive Officer, Cooper County Memorial Hospital, Boonville, MO, p. A244
MEYERS, Audrey, President and Chief Executive Officer, Valley Hospital, Ridgewood, NJ, p. A280

MEYERS, Brent, Administrator, Beaver County Memorial Hospital, Beaver, OK, p. A341
MEYERS, Joan T., R.N., Vice President and Chief Operating Officer, Virtua West Jersey Hospital-Voorhees, Voorhees, NJ, p. A281
MEYERS, Mark A.
   President and Chief Executive Officer, Garden Grove Hospital and Medical Center, Garden Grove, CA, p. A42
   President and Chief Executive Officer, Western Medical Center Hospital Anaheim, Anaheim, CA, p. A35
MEYERS, Russell, Chief Executive Officer, Conroe Regional Medical Center, Conroe, TX, p. A407
MICHAEL, Max, M.D., Chief Executive Officer and Medical Director, Cooper Green Hospital, Birmingham, AL, p. A12
MICHALSKI, Eugene F., Senior Vice President and Director, William Beaumont Hospital-Troy, Troy, MI, p. A223
MICHEL, Jack, M.D., Chief Executive Officer, Larkin Community Hospital, South Miami, FL, p. A95
MICHELL, Dyer T., President, Munroe Regional Medical Center, Ocala, FL, p. A91
MICKOSEFF, Tecla A., Administrator, LAC-Harbor-University of California at Los Angeles Medical Center, Torrance, CA, p. A65
MICKUS, Steven L., President and Chief Executive Officer, St. Vincent Mercy Medical Center, Toledo, OH, p. A338
MIDDLEBROOK, Randy, Chief Executive Officer and Administrator, Aspen Valley Hospital District, Aspen, CO, p. A68
MIESLE, Michael A., Administrator, Wood County Hospital, Bowling Green, OH, p. A326
MIGUEL, Hortense, R.N., Service Unit Director, U. S. Public Health Service Indian Hospital, Winterhaven, CA, p. A67
MILANES, Carlos, Executive Vice President and Administrator, Palm Springs General Hospital, Hialeah, FL, p. A86
MILBRATH, Michael, Administrator, Waseca Medical Center, Waseca, MN, p. A234
MILES, Paul V., Administrator, Middlesboro Appalachian Regional Hospital, Middlesboro, KY, p. A176
MILEWSKI, Robert, President and Chief Executive Officer, Mount Clemens General Hospital, Mount Clemens, MI, p. A219
MILEY, Dennis C., Administrator, Tri-County Hospital, Wadena, MN, p. A234
MILLBURG, Charles L., CHE, Chief Executive Officer, Shenandoah Medical Center, Shenandoah, IA, p. A156
MILLER, Alan B., President and Chief Executive Officer, Universal Health Services, Inc., King of Prussia, PA, p. B147
MILLER, Blaine K., Administrator, Republic County Hospital, Belleville, KS, p. A159
MILLER, Charles F., President and Chief Executive Officer, Piedmont Healthcare System, Rock Hill, SC, p. A383
MILLER, Charles R., Chief Executive Officer, Northwest Iowa Health Center, Sheldon, IA, p. A156
MILLER, Dennis C., President and Chief Executive Officer, Somerset Medical Center, Somerville, NJ, p. A280
MILLER, Donald H., Chief Operation Officer, Downey Regional Medical Center, Downey, CA, p. A40
MILLER, Edwin L., FACHE, President, Good Samaritan Community Healthcare, Puyallup, WA, p. A455
MILLER, Emil P., President and Chief Executive Officer, Wuesthoff Health System, Rockledge, FL, p. A94
MILLER, Gene, Chief Executive Officer, Garland Community Hospital, Garland, TX, p. A414
MILLER, George E., Chief Executive Officer, North Monroe Hospital, Monroe, LA, p. A186
MILLER, James I., President and Chief Executive Officer, Washoe Health System, Reno, NV, p. A269
MILLER, Jeffrey S., President, High Point Regional Health System, High Point, NC, p. A314
MILLER, Kevin J., FACHE, President and Chief Executive Officer, Medical Center of Southern Indiana, Charlestown, IN, p. A138

MILLER, Kimberly J., CHE, Administrator and Chief Executive Officer, Mitchell County Regional Health Center, Osage, IA, p. A155
MILLER, Marlo L., Administrator, Dundy County Hospital, Benkelman, NE, p. A261
MILLER, Michael, Chief Executive Officer, Mid-Jefferson Hospital, Nederland, TX, p. A425
MILLER, Michael S., Chief Executive Officer, Park Place Medical Center, Port Arthur, TX, p. A427
MILLER, Nate, Chief Executive Officer, HEALTHSOUTH Rehabilitation Hospital of Texarkana, Texarkana, TX, p. A432
MILLER, Peter J., Administrator, Long Term Care Hospital at Jackson, Montgomery, AL, p. A17
MILLER, Richard, Administrator and Chief Executive Officer, Norton County Hospital, Norton, KS, p. A165
MILLER, Richard F., Director, G.V. Montgomery Veterans Affairs Medical Center, Jackson, MS, p. A239
MILLER, Richard P., President and Chief Executive Officer, Virtua Health, Marlton, NJ, p. B153
MILLER, Robert, Chief Executive Officer, Henry County Health Center, Mount Pleasant, IA, p. A154
MILLER, Tamara, Administrator, Madison Community Hospital, Madison, SD, p. A386
MILLER, Thomas D., President and Chief Executive Officer, Lutheran Hospital of Indiana, Fort Wayne, IN, p. A139
MILLER, Thomas O., Chief Executive Officer, Pungo District Hospital, Belhaven, NC, p. A309
MILLER, Wayne T., Administrator, Behavioral Healthcare of Northern Indiana, Plymouth, IN, p. A145
MILLER, William P., President and Chief Executive Officer, Caro Community Hospital, Caro, MI, p. A212
MILLER, Gordon, Deputy Commander Clincial Services, Keller Army Community Hospital, West Point, NY, p. A307
MILLER, Mark A., Deputy Commander for Administration, General Leonard Wood Army Community Hospital, Fort Leonard Wood, MO, p. A246
MILLER, II, Thomas, Chief Executive Officer, Myrtle Werth Hospital-Mayo Health System, Menomonie, WI, p. A471
MILLER, Jr, George N., Chief Executive Officer, Christus Jasper Memorial Hospital, Jasper, TX, p. A419
MILLER, Jr, John A., President, Anderson Area Medical Center, Anderson, SC, p. A378
MILLIGAN, Jr, William M., President and Chief Executive Officer, Tyler Memorial Hospital, Tunkhannock, PA, p. A373
MILLIRONS, Dennis C., President and Chief Executive Officer, Riverside Medical Center, Kankakee, IL, p. A129
MILLS, Fred R., President and Chief Executive Officer, Baptist Health System, San Antonio, TX, p. B57
MILLS, Pete, Chief Executive Officer, Jenkins County Hospital, Millen, GA, p. A107
MILLS, Randy, Chief Executive Officer, Barrow Medical Center, Winder, GA, p. A111
MILLS, Stephen S., President and Chief Executive Officer, New York Hospital Medical Center of Queens, New York, NY, p. A298
MILLSTEAD, John B., Chief Executive Officer, Campbell Health System, Weatherford, TX, p. A434
MILNER, Susan, Administrator, Baptist Meriwether Hospital, Warm Springs, GA, p. A111
MILTON, Gene C., President and Chief Executive Officer, Hackettstown Community Hospital, Hackettstown, NJ, p. A276
MILTON, Paul A., Chief Operating Officer, Samaritan Hospital, Troy, NY, p. A306
MINCEMOYER, Robert, President and Chief Executive Officer, Schuyler Hospital, Montour Falls, NY, p. A294
MINDEN, Larry, Chief Executive Officer, Jane Phillips Medical Center, Bartlesville, OK, p. A341
MINER, Greg, Administrator, Loring Hospital, Sac City, IA, p. A156
MINICK, Mark J., President and Chief Executive Officer, Van Wert County Hospital, Van Wert, OH, p. A338
MINNICK, Peggy, R.N., Chief Executive Officer, BHC Alhambra Hospital, Rosemead, CA, p. A57
MINNIS, Holly, Chief Executive Officer, Mission Vista Behavioral Health System, San Antonio, TX, p. A429

MINNIS, Vernon, Administrator and Chief Executive Officer, Stafford District Hospital, Stafford, KS, p. A168
MINNIX, Jr, William L., President and Chief Executive Officer, Wesley Woods Center of Emory University, Atlanta, GA, p. A100
MIRABITO, Frank W., President, Chenango Memorial Hospital, Norwich, NY, p. A301
MISSILDINE, Syble F., Administrator, Northeast Medical Center Hospital, Humble, TX, p. A419
MITCHEL, David M., Chief Executive Officer, Avoyelles Hospital, Marksville, LA, p. A185
MITCHELL, Andrew J., Executive Director, North Shore University Hospital–Forest Hills, New York, NY, p. A291
MITCHELL, Gary W., Chief Executive Officer, Newman Memorial Hospital, Shattuck, OK, p. A347
MITCHELL, Jack C., Interim President and Chief Executive Officer, Washington Regional Medical Center, Fayetteville, AR, p. A29
MITCHELL, Jerald F., President and Chief Executive Officer, West Florida Regional Medical Center, Pensacola, FL, p. A93
MITCHELL, Joseph K., Administrator, Tuolumne General Hospital, Sonora, CA, p. A63
MITCHELL, Kerlene, Administrator, Wedowee Hospital, Wedowee, AL, p. A19
MITCHELL, M. Thomas, President and Chief Executive Officer, Mercy Medical Center, Williston, ND, p. A324
MITCHELL, Malinda S., President and Chief Executive Officer, Stanford Hospital and Clinics, Stanford, CA, p. A64
MITCHELL, Thedis V., Director, U. S. Public Health Service Indian Hospital, Clinton, OK, p. A342
MITCHELL, Timothy W., Chief Executive Officer, HEALTHSOUTH Northern Kentucky Rehabilitation Hospital, Covington, KY, p. A171
MITCHELL, Trish, Chief Executive Officer, Meridell Achievement Center, Liberty Hill, TX, p. A421
MITCHELL, William, Administrator, Vencor Hospital–San Diego, San Diego, CA, p. A59
MITCHENER, Jr, Charles, Chief Executive Officer, Jacksonville Hospital, Jacksonville, AL, p. A16
MITRICK, Joseph, Administrator, Baptist Medical Center–Beaches, Jacksonville Beach, FL, p. A87
MITTEER, Brian R., President, Brattleboro Memorial Hospital, Brattleboro, VT, p. A440
MIZRACH, Kenneth H., Director, Veterans Affairs New Jersey Health Care System, East Orange, NJ, p. A275
MLADY, Celine M., Chief Executive Officer, Osmond General Hospital, Osmond, NE, p. A266
MO, Lin H., President and Chief Executive Officer, New York Community Hospital of Brooklyn, New York, NY, p. A298
MOAKLER, Thomas J., Chief Executive Officer, Houlton Regional Hospital, Houlton, ME, p. A192
MOBLEY, Don W., Chief Executive Officer, Appalachian Psychiatric Healthcare System, Cambridge, OH, p. A326
MOBURG, Steven T., Administrator, Boscobel Area Health Care, Boscobel, WI, p. A467
MOCERI, Carmelo J., President, Barnes–Jewish St. Peters Hospital, Saint Peters, MO, p. A254
MODDERMAN, Melvin E., Administrator, Lincoln Trail Behavioral Health System, Radcliff, KY, p. A178
MODY, Amit, M.D., Executive Director, Irvington General Hospital, Irvington, NJ, p. A277
MOEBIUS, Geoffrey D., Chief Executive Officer, Deaconess Hospital of Cleveland, Cleveland, OH, p. A328
MOED, Richard, President and Chief Executive Officer, Saint Francis Care Behavioral Health, Portland, CT, p. A76
MOELLER, Jerry G., President and Chief Executive Officer, Stillwater Medical Center, Stillwater, OK, p. A347
MOEN, Daniel P., President and Chief Executive Officer, Heywood Hospital, Gardner, MA, p. A205
MOEN, Robert A., President and Chief Executive Officer, Emanuel Medical Center, Turlock, CA, p. A65
MOFFETT, Mary B., Administrator, LaSalle General Hospital, Jena, LA, p. A183

MOHR, Robin Z., Chief Executive Officer, St. Francis Central Hospital, Pittsburgh, PA, p. A369
MOLANO, Celia, Executive Director, I. Gonzalez Martinez Oncologic Hospital, Hato Rey, PR, p. A484
MOLENA, Ivette, Administrator, State Psychiatric Hospital, San Juan, PR, p. A484
MOLL, Jeffrey S., President and Chief Executive Officer, Beth Israel Hospital, Passaic, NJ, p. A279
MONGAN, James J., M.D., President, Massachusetts General Hospital, Boston, MA, p. A202
MONGE, Peter W., President and Chief Executive Officer, Montgomery General Hospital, Olney, MD, p. A199
MONNAHAN, John E., Administrator, Davis County Hospital, Bloomfield, IA, p. A148
MONROIG, Domingo, Administrator, Castaner General Hospital, Castaner, PR, p. A482
MONROIG, Samuel, Vice President for Administration, Arecibo Regional Hospital, Arecibo, PR, p. A481
MONTAG, Kathy, Administrator Health Care, State Correctional Institution at Camp Hill, Camp Hill, PA, p. A357
MONTAGUE, William D., Director, Veterans Affairs Medical Center, Cleveland, OH, p. A329
MONTES, Lisa K., Administrator and Chief Executive Officer, Del Amo Hospital, Torrance, CA, p. A64
MONTGOMERY, Michael J., President and Chief Executive Officer, Cleo Wallace Centers Hospital, Westminster, CO, p. A73
MONTGOMERY, II, Raymond W., President and Chief Executive Officer, White County Medical Center, Searcy, AR, p. A33
MONTGOMERY, Jr, J. C., President, Texas Scottish Rite Hospital for Children, Dallas, TX, p. A410
MONTION, Robert M., Chief Executive Officer, Tulare Local Health Care District, Tulare, CA, p. A65
MOONEY, Jimmy, Chief Executive Officer, Willingway Hospital, Statesboro, GA, p. A110
MOORE, Darrell W., President and Chief Executive Officer, Baptist Medical Center, Kansas City, MO, p. A248
MOORE, Duncan, President and Chief Executive Officer, Tallahassee Memorial HealthCare, Tallahassee, FL, p. A96
MOORE, E. Richard, President, Hazleton General Hospital, Hazleton, PA, p. A361
MOORE, Gary, Chief Executive Officer, Shoshone Medical Center, Kellogg, ID, p. A116
MOORE, George, Director, Veterans Affairs Medical Center, Martinsburg, WV, p. A462
MOORE, Greg, Chief Executive Officer, Crittenden County Hospital, Marion, KY, p. A176
MOORE, James A., Chief Operating Officer and Chief Financial Officer, Milwaukee Psychiatric Hospital, Wauwatosa, WI, p. A477
MOORE, John, Administrator, Hiawatha Community Hospital, Hiawatha, KS, p. A162
MOORE, Mindy S., Chief Executive Officer, NextCARE Specialty Hospital of North Carolina, Rocky Mount, NC, p. A317
MOORE, Paul David, Administrator, Atoka Memorial Hospital, Atoka, OK, p. A341
MOORE, Robert J., CHE, Chief Executive Officer, Pekin Hospital, Pekin, IL, p. A132
MOORE, Roland E., Director, Brockton Veterans Affairs Medical Center, Brockton, MA, p. A203
MOORE, Terence F., President, MidMichigan Health, Midland, MI, p. B111
MOORE, Thomas F., Administrator, Charleston Memorial Hospital, Charleston, SC, p. A378
MOORE, W. Evan, Administrator, Comanche Community Hospital, Comanche, TX, p. A407
MOORE, William P., Chief Executive Officer, Lake Mead Hospital Medical Center, North Las Vegas, NV, p. A269
MOORE, Mark D., Deputy Commander and Administrator, Bayne–Jones Army Community Hospital, Fort Polk, LA, p. A182
MOORE, II, Ben, Executive Director, University Hospital–SUNY Health Science Center at Syracuse, Syracuse, NY, p. A306
MOORE–HARDY, Cynthia Ann, President and Chief Executive Officer, Lake Hospital System, Painesville, OH, p. A336

MOORING, Phillip A., Director, Walter B. Jones Alcohol and Drug Abuse Treatment Center, Greenville, NC, p. A314
MOOTRY, John M., Chief Executive Officer, Barrett Memorial Hospital, Dillon, MT, p. A257
MORAHAN, John R., President, St. Joseph Medical Center, Reading, PA, p. A371
MORALES, Herson E., Executive Director, Hospital Santa Rosa, Guayama, PR, p. A482
MORAN, John, Chief Executive Officer, Doctors Hospital of Springfield, Springfield, MO, p. A254
MORAN, Michael D., FACHE, Administrator, Methodist Behavioral Resources, New Orleans, LA, p. A187
MORASKO, Jerry, Administrator, Marias Medical Center, Shelby, MT, p. A259
MORASKO, Robert A., Chief Executive Officer, William Bee Ririe Hospital, Ely, NV, p. A268
MORDOH, Henry A.
President, UPMC Presbyterian, Pittsburgh, PA, p. A370
President, UPMC Shadyside, Pittsburgh, PA, p. A370
MORELAND, L. Pat, Administrator, Hardy Wilson Memorial Hospital, Hazlehurst, MS, p. A238
MORELAND, Michael E., Director, Veterans Affairs Medical Center, Butler, PA, p. A357
MORESI, Randolph, Chief Executive Officer, North Hills Hospital, North Richland Hills, TX, p. A425
MORGAN, Charles R., Administrator, Wayne Memorial Hospital, Jesup, GA, p. A106
MORGAN, Craig, Administrator, Knox County Hospital, Barbourville, KY, p. A170
MORGAN, Donald J., President and Chief Executive Officer, Page Memorial Hospital, Luray, VA, p. A445
MORGAN, James E., Administrator, Huey P. Long Medical Center, Pineville, LA, p. A188
MORGAN, John, President, Gottlieb Memorial Hospital, Melrose Park, IL, p. A130
MORGAN, Kelly C.
President and Chief Executive Officer, Lindsay District Hospital, Lindsay, CA, p. A46
President and Chief Executive Officer, Sierra View District Hospital, Porterville, CA, p. A56
MORGAN, Michael L., President and Chief Executive Officer, St. Edward Mercy Medical Center, Fort Smith, AR, p. A30
MORGAN, Timothy O., Executive Director, Pennsylvania Hospital, Philadelphia, PA, p. A367
MORIN, Paul A., Superintendent, Soldiers' Home in Holyoke, Holyoke, MA, p. A205
MORLEY, Tad A., Chief Executive Officer, Brigham City Community Hospital, Brigham City, UT, p. A436
MORRASH, Joseph, Administrator, State Correctional Institution Hospital, Pittsburgh, PA, p. A369
MORRELL, Nikki, Acting Superintendent, Madison State Hospital, Madison, IN, p. A143
MORRIS, Elaine F., Administrator, Methodist Ambulatory Surgery Hospital, San Antonio, TX, p. A428
MORRIS, Jack, Administrator, Eureka Springs Hospital, Eureka Springs, AR, p. A29
MORRIS, Joe, Chief Executive Officer, Kootenai Medical Center, Coeur D'Alene, ID, p. A116
MORRIS, Linda, Administrator, Ogallala Community Hospital, Ogallala, NE, p. A265
MORRIS, Michael, Administrator, Coleman County Medical Center, Coleman, TX, p. A407
MORRIS, R. Randall, Administrator, West Carroll Memorial Hospital, Oak Grove, LA, p. A187
MORRISON, David, Chief Executive Officer, Heartland Behavioral Health Services, Nevada, MO, p. A251
MORRISON, Mary C., R.N., Chief Executive Officer, Mercy Community Hospital, Havertown, PA, p. A361
MORRISON, Robert E., President, Randolph Hospital, Asheboro, NC, p. A309
MORROW, Julia, Administrator, Morrill County Community Hospital, Bridgeport, NE, p. A261
MORROW, Shawn, Chief Executive Officer and Administrator, Holdenville General Hospital, Holdenville, OK, p. A344
MORSE, Amy, Chief Executive Officer, New England Rehabilitation Hospital of Portland, Portland, ME, p. A193
MORSE, Gary C., Chief Executive Officer and Administrator, Perry Community Hospital, Linden, TN, p. A395

MORTON, Stan, Chief Executive Officer, Las Colinas Medical Center, Irving, TX, p. A419
MOSCATO, Mary, Chief Executive Officer, HEALTHSOUTH New England Rehabilitation Hospital, Woburn, MA, p. A210
MOSELEY, Michael, Director, Caswell Center, Kinston, NC, p. A315
MOSES, Jon, Administrator, Wood River Medical Center, Los Angeles, ID, p. A118
MOSS, Dwayne, Chief Executive Officer, T. J. Samson Community Hospital, Glasgow, KY, p. A172
MOSS, James T.
  President and Chief Executive Officer, Jackson–Madison County General Hospital, Jackson, TN, p. A393
  President, West Tennessee Healthcare, Jackson, TN, p. B154
MOSS, Joseph, Administrator, Ellett Memorial Hospital, Appleton City, MO, p. A244
MOSS, Paul E., President, Milford Hospital, Milford, CT, p. A75
MOSS, Rod, Chief Executive Officer, HEALTHSOUTH Rehabilitation Hospital of North Alabama, Huntsville, AL, p. A15
MOSS, William Mason, President, Potomac Hospital, Woodbridge, VA, p. A451
MOTZER, Earl James, FACHE, Chief Executive Officer, The James B. Haggin Memorial Hospital, Harrodsburg, KY, p. A173
MOUGHON, Edward, Superintendent, Big Spring State Hospital, Big Spring, TX, p. A404
MOULTHROP, David L., Ph.D., President and Chief Executive Officer, Rogers Memorial Hospital, Oconomowoc, WI, p. A473
MOUNTCASTLE, William A., Director, Veterans Affairs Medical Center, Nashville, TN, p. A398
MOUSA, Barry L., Chief Executive Officer, Fannin Regional Hospital, Blue Ridge, GA, p. A101
MUDLER, Gordon A., President and Chief Executive Officer, Hackley Health, Muskegon, MI, p. A219
MUELLER, Jens, Chairman, Pacific Health Corporation, Tustin, CA, p. B118
MUGRAUER, Wayne A., Chief Executive Officer, Friends Hospital, Philadelphia, PA, p. A367
MUHLENTHALER, Donald, FACHE, President and Chief Executive Officer, Weirton Medical Center, Weirton, WV, p. A464
MUILENBURG, Robert H., Executive Director, University of Washington Medical Center, Seattle, WA, p. A457
MULANAX, Marjorie, Executive Director, Christopher House, Austin, TX, p. A402
MULDER, Dale R., Chief Executive Officer, Twin Rivers Regional Medical Center, Kennett, MO, p. A249
MULDOON, Patrick L., President and Chief Executive Officer, South County Hospital, Wakefield, RI, p. A377
MULHOLLAND, Donna, President and Chief Executive Officer, Easton Hospital, Easton, PA, p. A359
MULHOLLAND , Jr, K. L., Director, Veterans Affairs Medical Center, Memphis, TN, p. A397
MULL, Connie, Chief Executive Officer, Cedar Springs Behavioral Health System, Colorado Springs, CO, p. A68
MULLAHEY, Ronald T., President, Vassar Brothers Hospital, Poughkeepsie, NY, p. A303
MULLANEY, Garrell S., Chief Executive Officer, Connecticut Valley Hospital, Middletown, CT, p. A75
MULLANEY, Janet, President, Heritage Hospital, Tarboro, NC, p. A318
MULLEN, Anthony F., Administrator, Bertie Memorial Hospital, Windsor, NC, p. A319
MULLEN, Gregory S., Administrator, Tyler Holmes Memorial Hospital, Winona, MS, p. A243
MULLEN, Robert L., Chief Executive Officer, Rice County Hospital District Number One, Lyons, KS, p. A164
MULLEN, Thomas R., President and Chief Executive Officer, Mercy Medical Center, Baltimore, MD, p. A196
MULLER, A. Gary, FACHE, President and Chief Executive Officer, West Jefferson Medical Center, Marrero, LA, p. A185

MULLER, Ralph W.
  President and Chief Executive Officer, The University of Chicago Hospitals and Health System, Chicago, IL, p. B143
  President and Chief Executive Officer, University of Chicago Hospitals, Chicago, IL, p. A124
MULLER, Thomas W., M.D., Superintendent, Northwest Georgia Regional Hospital, Rome, GA, p. A109
MULLINS, Charles B., M.D., Executive Vice Chancellor, University of Texas System, Austin, TX, p. B150
MULLINS, Larry A., President and Chief Executive Officer, Samaritan Health Services, Corvallis, OR, p. B130
MULLINS, Michael L., Chief Executive Officer, UniMed Medical Center, Minot, ND, p. A323
MULLINS, Tommy H., Administrator, Boone Memorial Hospital, Madison, WV, p. A462
MULVIHILL, Deborah, Regional Vice President and Administrator, Coral Springs Medical Center, Coral Springs, FL, p. A83
MUNDY, Mark J., President and Chief Executive Officer, New York Methodist Hospital, New York, NY, p. A298
MUNDY, Stephens M., Chief Executive Officer, St. Joseph's Hospital, Parkersburg, WV, p. A463
MUNETA, Anita, Chief Executive Officer, U. S. Public Health Service Indian Hospital, Crownpoint, NM, p. A284
MUNGER, Richard, Administrator, Mount Grant General Hospital, Hawthorne, NV, p. A268
MUNIZ, Teodoro, Administrator, Doctors Hospital, San Juan, PR, p. A483
MUNNERLYN, Mike, Chief Executive Officer, Pampa Regional Medical Center, Pampa, TX, p. A426
MUNOZ, Humberto J., Chief Executive Officer, Sunrise Regional Medical Center, Sunrise, FL, p. A96
MUNOZ, Thalia H., Administrator, Starr County Memorial Hospital, Rio Grande City, TX, p. A427
MUNSON, Eric B., President and Chief Executive Officer, University of North Carolina Hospitals, Chapel Hill, NC, p. A310
MUNTEL, Edward G., Ph.D., President and Chief Executive Officer, NorthKey Community Care, Covington, KY, p. A171
MUNTZ, Tim, President, St. Margaret's Hospital, Spring Valley, IL, p. A134
MURPHY, Horace W., President, Washington County Health System, Hagerstown, MD, p. A198
MURPHY, Jim, Chief Executive Officer, Knoxville Area Community Hospital, Knoxville, IA, p. A153
MURPHY, Joyce A., President, Carney Hospital, Dorchester, MA, p. A204
MURPHY, Michael, President and Chief Executive Officer, Sharp Healthcare, San Diego, CA, p. B131
MURPHY, Michael D., Chief Executive Officer, Gulf Coast Medical Center, Wharton, TX, p. A434
MURPHY, Michael W., Ph.D., Director and Chief Executive Officer, Veterans Affairs Northern Indiana Health Care System, Fort Wayne, IN, p. A140
MURPHY, Mike, Acting Administrator, G. Pierce Wood Memorial Hospital, Arcadia, FL, p. A81
MURPHY, Peter J., President and Chief Executive Officer, St. James Hospital and Health Centers – Chicago Heights Campus, Chicago Heights, IL, p. A124
MURPHY, Richard J., President and Chief Executive Officer, Good Samaritan Hospital Medical Center, West Islip, NY, p. A307
MURPHY, Susan, Director, Santa Clara Valley Medical Center, San Jose, CA, p. A61
MURPHY, Michael J., Commander, U. S. Air Force Hospital, Tyndall AFB, FL, p. A97
MURPHY–ABDOUCH, Kim, Vice President Operations, North Central Baptist Hospital, San Antonio, TX, p. A429
MURRAY, James Patrick, Chief Executive Officer, Sid Peterson Memorial Hospital, Kerrville, TX, p. A420
MURRAY, Joan Z., R.N., Administrator and Chief Executive Officer, St. James Parish Hospital, Lutcher, LA, p. A185
MURRAY, T. Michael, President, South Coast Medical Center, South Laguna, CA, p. A63
MURRAY, William M., President, Sisters of Charity of Leavenworth Health Services Corporation, Leavenworth, KS, p. B133

MURRAY , II, Robert B., President and Chief Executive Officer, Fulton County Medical Center, McConnellsburg, PA, p. A363
MURTHA, Patrick, President and Chief Executive Officer, St. Joseph Health System, Tawas City, MI, p. A223
MUSE, James L., Administrator, Coffee Medical Center, Manchester, TN, p. A396
MUSUMECI, Maryann, Director, Veterans Affairs Medical Center, New York, NY, p. A300
MUTCH, Patrick F., President, Laurel Regional Hospital, Laurel, MD, p. A199
MYERS, Charles, Administrator, Community Hospital, Torrington, WY, p. A480
MYERS, Edward W., Chief Executive Officer, Christus St. Elizabeth Hospital, Beaumont, TX, p. A404
MYERS, Gary, Administrator, Mammoth Hospital, Mammoth Lakes, CA, p. A51
MYERS, Michael D., Administrator, Veterans Memorial Hospital, Waukon, IA, p. A157
MYERS, Richard L., President and Chief Executive Officer, Durham Regional Hospital, Durham, NC, p. A312
MYNARK, Richard H., Chief Executive Officer, Pulaski Memorial Hospital, Winamac, IN, p. A147

N

NABORS, Charles E., FACHE, Administrator and Chief Executive Officer, Bryan W. Whitfield Memorial Hospital, Demopolis, AL, p. A14
NACHTMAN, Frank, Administrator, Marshall Hospital, Placerville, CA, p. A55
NAGLOSKY, Paul, Administrator, Indianhead Medical Center, Shell Lake, WI, p. A475
NAIBERK, Donald T., Administrator and Chief Executive Officer, Plainview Public Hospital, Plainview, NE, p. A266
NANCE, Sally S., Chief Executive Officer, Excelsior Springs Medical Center, Excelsior Springs, MO, p. A246
NAPIER, Randy L., President and Chief Executive Officer, Southern Indiana Rehabilitation Hospital, New Albany, IN, p. A144
NAPPER, Ricky D., Chief Executive Officer, Norton Community Hospital, Norton, VA, p. A447
NAPPER, Terry, Administrator, Memorial Medical Center of San Augustine, San Augustine, TX, p. A430
NARBUTAS, Virgis, Executive Director, Vencor Hospital–Brea, Brea, CA, p. A37
NARUM, Larry, President, Provena Saint Joseph Hospital, Elgin, IL, p. A125
NASEM, Charles, Chief Executive Officer, Trace Regional Hospital, Houston, MS, p. A238
NASRALLA, Anthony J., FACHE, President and Chief Executive Officer, Titusville Area Hospital, Titusville, PA, p. A372
NATHAN, David G., M.D., President and Chief Executive Officer, Dana–Farber Cancer Institute, Boston, MA, p. A202
NATHAN, James R., Chief Executive Officer, Lee Memorial Health System, Fort Myers, FL, p. A85
NATHAN, Steven R.
  President and Chief Executive Officer, Good Samaritan Medical Center, West Palm Beach, FL, p. A97
  President and Chief Executive Officer, St. Mary's Hospital, West Palm Beach, FL, p. A97
NATZKE, Kenneth J., Administrator, OSF St. Joseph Medical Center, Bloomington, IL, p. A120
NAY, Clifford D., Executive Director, Scott Memorial Hospital, Scottsburg, IN, p. A145
NAYLOR , II, George F., CHE, Chief Executive Officer, Barstow Community Hospital, Barstow, CA, p. A36
NEAL, Hank, Administrator, Kings Mountain Hospital, Kings Mountain, NC, p. A314
NEAL, John C., Chief Executive Officer, Stuttgart Regional Medical Center, Stuttgart, AR, p. A34
NEAMAN, Mark R., President and Chief Executive Officer, Evanston Northwestern Healthcare Corporation, Evanston, IL, p. A126
NEEDHAM, Jean M., President, Holy Family Hospital, New Richmond, WI, p. A473

NEEDMAN, Herbert G., Administrator and Chief Executive Officer, Temple Community Hospital, Los Angeles, CA, p. A49
NEELY, Bill J., Administrator, Parmer County Community Hospital, Friona, TX, p. A413
NEELY, Cindy, Administrator, St. John's Maude Norton Memorial Hospital, Columbus, KS, p. A160
NEFF, Mark J., President and Chief Executive Officer, St. Claire Medical Center, Morehead, KY, p. A177
NEFF, Thomas G., Vice President and Administrator, Christus Spohn Hospital Memorial, Corpus Christi, TX, p. A407
NEHLS, Dennis E., Administrator and Chief Executive Officer, Crawford County Hospital District One, Girard, KS, p. A161
NEIDENBACH, Joseph J., Administrator and Chief Executive Officer, St. Vincent Hospital, Green Bay, WI, p. A469
NEITZEL, Monte, Administrator and Chief Executive Officer, Humboldt County Memorial Hospital, Humboldt, IA, p. A153
NELL, Rocio, M.D., Chief Executive Officer and Medical Director, Montgomery County Emergency Service, Norristown, PA, p. A365
NELSON, Becky, President, Sioux Valley Hospital and University Medical Center, Sioux Falls, SD, p. A388
NELSON, Bill, Administrator and Chief Executive Officer, Coteau Des Prairies Hospital, Sisseton, SD, p. A388
NELSON, Brock D.
  Chief Executive Officer, Children's Hospital and Clinics, Saint Paul, MN, p. A233
  Chief Executive Officer, Children's Hospitals and Clinics, Minneapolis, Minneapolis, MN, p. A230
NELSON, Cathleen K., President and Chief Executive Officer, St. Charles Mercy Hospital, Oregon, OH, p. A336
NELSON, David A., President and Chief Executive Officer, St. Francis Medical Center, Breckenridge, MN, p. A226
NELSON, Don A., Administrator, Crook County Medical Services District, Sundance, WY, p. A479
NELSON, Fred, Administrator, Ontonagon Memorial Hospital, Ontonagon, MI, p. A220
NELSON, Kenneth W., Superintendent, Bridgewater State Hospital, Bridgewater, MA, p. A203
NELSON, Rodney M., President and Chief Executive Officer, Mackinac Straits Hospital and Health Center, Saint Ignace, MI, p. A221
NELSON, William H., President and Chief Executive Officer, Intermountain Health Care, Inc., Salt Lake City, UT, p. B101
NELSON, Richard A., Surgeon General, Department of Navy, Washington, DC, p. B76
NEMACHECK, William, Chief Executive Officer, Marquette General Health System, Marquette, MI, p. A219
NEMIR, Bill, Administrator, Haskell Memorial Hospital, Haskell, TX, p. A415
NESTER , Jr, Arthur, Administrator, Noxubee General Hospital, Macon, MS, p. A240
NESTER , Jr, Martin F., Chief Executive Officer, Long Beach Medical Center, Long Beach, NY, p. A293
NETH, Marvin, Administrator, Callaway District Hospital, Callaway, NE, p. A262
NETHERLAND, Ann, Administrator, Franklin Medical Center, Winnsboro, LA, p. A189
NETTLES, Sheila, Administrator, Sedan City Hospital, Sedan, KS, p. A167
NEUGENT, Richard C., Chief Executive Officer, St. Francis Health System, Greenville, SC, p. A381
NEUSCH, Michael W., FACHE, Director, Louis A. Johnson Veterans Affairs Medical Center, Clarksburg, WV, p. A461
NEUSE, Barbara, Chief Executive Officer, Rockford Center, Newark, DE, p. A78
NEVAREZ, Domingo, Administrator, Hospital Dr. Federico Trilla, Carolina, PR, p. A482
NEWBERRY, Lewis, Chief Executive Officer, Roane General Hospital, Spencer, WV, p. A464
NEWBERRY, R. Alan, President and Chief Executive Officer, Peninsula Regional Health System, Salisbury, MD, p. A200

NEWBOLD, Philip A., President and Chief Executive Officer, Memorial Hospital of South Bend, South Bend, IN, p. A146
NEWCOMB, Sherrie, Administrator, Jenkins Community Hospital, Jenkins, KY, p. A173
NEWHAM, Judeth, R.N., President and Chief Executive Officer, Holland Community Hospital, Holland, MI, p. A217
NEWMAN, Delores, MS, Network Manager, Metro South Network, Tinley Park Mental Health Center, Tinley Park, IL, p. A135
NEWMAN, Jerald C., President and Chief Executive Officer, Nassau County Medical Center, East Meadow, NY, p. A291
NEWMAN, Robert G., M.D., President, Continuum Health Partners, New York, NY, p. B75
NEWMILLER, Vicky, Interim Chief Executive Officer, Pondera Medical Center, Conrad, MT, p. A257
NEWTON, Mark, President and Chief Executive Officer, Swedish Covenant Hospital, Chicago, IL, p. A123
NEWTON, Steven R., President and Chief Executive Officer, Research Medical Center, Kansas City, MO, p. A248
NEWTON, Alan D., Commander, U. S. Air Force Hospital, Vandenberg AFB, CA, p. A66
NICHOLS, Barbara, Acting President, Corry Memorial Hospital, Corry, PA, p. A358
NICHOLS, Mark, Chief Executive Officer, Polk Medical Center, Cedartown, GA, p. A102
NICHOLS, Ralph, Superintendent, Evansville State Hospital, Evansville, IN, p. A139
NICKELL, Roy, Director Substance Abuse Services, Wake County Alcoholism Treatment Center, Raleigh, NC, p. A317
NICKENS , II, John R., Chief Executive Officer, Brookwood Medical Center, Birmingham, AL, p. A11
NICKERSON, Ruth Marie, President and Chief Executive Officer, Saint Agnes Medical Center, Fresno, CA, p. A42
NIEDERPRUEM, Mark L., Administrator, Shriners Hospitals for Children, Springfield, Springfield, MA, p. A208
NIELSEN, Greg, Administrator, Weston County Health Services, Newcastle, WY, p. A479
NIELSEN, Kim, Administrator and Chief Operating Officer, Orem Community Hospital, Orem, UT, p. A437
NIELSEN, Tom, Administrator, Kennewick General Hospital, Kennewick, WA, p. A454
NIEMEYER, Romaine, President, Holy Spirit Health System, Camp Hill, PA, p. A357
NIENHUIS, Arthur W., M.D., Director, St. Jude Children's Research Hospital, Memphis, TN, p. A397
NILES, Linda, Interim Chief Executive Officer, Adams County Hospital, West Union, OH, p. A339
NILLES, Edward L., President and Chief Executive Officer, Bradley County Medical Center, Warren, AR, p. A34
NITSCHKE, David M., President and Chief Executive Officer, Regional West Medical Center, Scottsbluff, NE, p. A266
NIXON, Tracey, Chief Executive Officer, HEALTHSOUTH Plano Rehabilitation Hospital, Plano, TX, p. A426
NIXON , Jr, Jesse, Ph.D., Director, Capital District Psychiatric Center, Albany, NY, p. A287
NOBLE, Mallie S., Administrator, Mary Breckinridge Hospital, Hyden, KY, p. A173
NOBLE, Stephen H.
  President, Accord Health Care Corporation, Clearwater, FL, p. B50
  President, Stewart–Webster Hospital, Richland, GA, p. A108
NOCE , Jr, Walter W., President and Chief Executive Officer, Childrens Hospital of Los Angeles, Los Angeles, CA, p. A47
NOCKERTS, Steven R., Administrator and Chief Executive Officer, Adams County Memorial Hospital and Nursing Care Unit, Friendship, WI, p. A468
NOLAN, Martin, Administrator, Okanogan–Douglas County Hospital, Brewster, WA, p. A452
NOLAN, Mary A., MS, Executive Vice President Care Delivery and General Director, Albany Medical Center, Albany, NY, p. A287

NOLAN, Michael J., Chief Executive Officer, Ascension Hospital and Behavioral Health Services, Gonzales, LA, p. A182
NOLAN, Patrick, Administrator, Morgan County War Memorial Hospital, Berkeley Springs, WV, p. A460
NOLAND, Christopher, Chief Executive Officer, Sheridan Community Hospital, Sheridan, MI, p. A222
NOLL, Cecilia, Administrator, Kiowa County Memorial Hospital, Greensburg, KS, p. A161
NOLL, Donald, Director, Clear Brook Manor, Wilkes–Barre, PA, p. A374
NOONAN, Dennis, President and Chief Executive Officer, Salem Hospital, Salem, OR, p. A354
NORD, Thomas A., FACHE, Chief Executive Officer, Ivinson Memorial Hospital, Laramie, WY, p. A479
NORDWICK, John A., President and Chief Executive Officer, Bozeman Deaconess Hospital, Bozeman, MT, p. A256
NOREM, Kathryn J., Chief Executive Officer, Starke Memorial Hospital, Knox, IN, p. A142
NOREN, Mary Kay
  Superintendent, Eastern Shore Hospital Center, Cambridge, MD, p. A197
  Chief Executive Officer, Upper Shore Community Mental Health Center, Chestertown, MD, p. A197
NORGAARD, Margaret, Administrator, Northeast Montana Health Services, Wolf Point, MT, p. A260
NORMAN, Jeffrey K., Executive Vice President and Chief Executive Officer, Phoenix Baptist Hospital and Medical Center, Phoenix, AZ, p. A24
NORMAN, Mary, Administrator and Chief Executive Officer, Bear Valley Community Hospital, Big Bear Lake, CA, p. A37
NORMAN, Paul Michael, President, East Pasco Medical Center, Zephyrhills, FL, p. A98
NORRIS, Charles, Administrator, Nocona General Hospital, Nocona, TX, p. A425
NORRIS, Jim A., Executive Director, St. Cloud Hospital, A Division of Orlando Regional Healthcare System, Saint Cloud, FL, p. A94
NORTH, Joel E., Administrator, Baptist Memorial Hospital–Osceola, Osceola, AR, p. A33
NORTON, Robert G., President and Chief Executive Officer, Shands Jacksonville Medical Center, Jacksonville, FL, p. A87
NORWINE, David R., President and Chief Executive Officer, H. B. Magruder Memorial Hospital, Port Clinton, OH, p. A336
NORWOOD, Steve, Executive Director, Western State Psychiatric Center, Woodward, OK, p. A349
NOSACKA, Mark, Chief Executive Officer, River West Medical Center, Plaquemine, LA, p. A188
NOTARIANNI, Robert G., Chief Executive Officer, Big Horn County Memorial Hospital, Hardin, MT, p. A258
NOTEBOOM, Kenneth
  Chief Executive Officer, Doctors Hospital, Tulsa, OK, p. A348
  Chief Executive Officer, Hillcrest Specialty Hospital, Tulsa, OK, p. A348
NOTEWARE, Dan, Senior Vice President and Executive Director, Presbyterian Hospital of Winnsboro, Winnsboro, TX, p. A435
NOVAK, Edward, President and Chief Executive Officer, Sacred Heart Hospital, Chicago, IL, p. A123
NOWAK, Gregory M., Administrator and Chief Executive Officer, Coshocton County Memorial Hospital, Coshocton, OH, p. A330
NOWAK, Martin, Interim Executive Director, University of Alabama Hospital, Birmingham, AL, p. A12
NUCKLES, Craig, Group Director, Timberlawn Mental Health System, Dallas, TX, p. A410
NUGENT, Gary N., Medical Director, Veterans Affairs Medical Center, Cincinnati, OH, p. A328
NUNAMAKER, E. Michael, Chief Executive Officer, Grady Memorial Hospital, Chickasha, OK, p. A342
NUNLEY, Jack, Chief Executive Officer, Pulaski Community Hospital, Pulaski, VA, p. A448
NUNNERY, S. Arnold, President and Chief Executive Officer, Iredell Memorial Hospital, Statesville, NC, p. A318
NURKIN, Harry A., Ph.D., President, Carolinas HealthCare System, Charlotte, NC, p. B65

Index of Health Care Professionals / Nyp

NYP, Randall G., President and Chief Executive Officer, Via Christi Regional Medical Center, Wichita, KS, p. A169

O

O'BRIEN, John, Administrator, Ellsworth Municipal Hospital, Iowa Falls, IA, p. A153
O'BRIEN, John G., Chief Executive Officer, Cambridge Health Alliance, Cambridge, MA, p. A204
O'BRIEN, Michael C., Administrator, Sarah D. Culbertson Memorial Hospital, Rushville, IL, p. A134
O'BRIEN, Jr, Charles M., President and Chief Executive Officer, West Penn Allegheny Health System, Pittsburgh, PA, p. B154
O'CONNELL, Gene, Executive Administrator and Director Patient Care Services Community Health Network, San Francisco General Hospital Medical Center, San Francisco, CA, p. A60
O'CONNELL, John W., President, Franciscan Services Corporation, Sylvania, OH, p. B85
O'CONNELL, Rick, President and Chief Executive Officer, Penrose–St. Francis Health Services, Colorado Springs, CO, p. A69
O'CONNOR, Delia, President, Caritas Norwood Hospital, Norwood, MA, p. A207
O'CONNOR, Joann, Director, Winnebago Mental Health Institute, Winnebago, WI, p. A477
O'CONNOR, Shawn J., Chief Executive Officer, Anacapa Hospital, Port Hueneme, CA, p. A56
O'CONNOR, William D., President and Chief Executive Officer, Rehabilitation Hospital of the Pacific, Honolulu, HI, p. A112
O'DONNELL, Kevin J., President and Chief Executive Officer, Sacred Heart–St. Mary's Hospitals, Rhinelander, WI, p. A474
O'DONNELL, Randall L., Ph.D., President and Chief Executive Officer, Children's Mercy Hospital, Kansas City, MO, p. A248
O'DONNELL, Jr, Thomas F., FACS, President and Chief Executive Officer, New England Medical Center, Boston, MA, p. A202
O'GRADY, Jr, Michael J., Interim President and Chief Executive Officer, Norwegian–American Hospital, Chicago, IL, p. A122
O'HALLARON, Ronald, Administrator, Harms Memorial Hospital District, American Falls, ID, p. A115
O'HARA, Gene L., Administrator, Providence Alaska Medical Center, Anchorage, AK, p. A20
O'KEEFE, James M., President and Chief Executive Officer, Woodlawn Hospital, Rochester, IN, p. A145
O'KEEFE, Michael F., FACHE, Executive Director, Baylor Medical Center at Irving, Irving, TX, p. A419
O'LOUGHLIN, James F., Chief Executive Officer, Gadsden Regional Medical Center, Gadsden, AL, p. A15
O'MALLEY, Dennis, President, Craig Hospital, Englewood, CO, p. A70
O'MARA, Richard P., Chief Executive Officer, Hospital District Number Five of Harper County, Harper, KS, p. A162
O'NEAL, Graham J., Interim Chief Executive Officer, Ozarks Medical Center, West Plains, MO, p. A255
O'NEAL, Sean, Administrator, Sierra Vista Regional Medical Center, San Luis Obispo, CA, p. A61
O'NEIL, John D., President and Chief Executive Officer, Our Lady of Lourdes Memorial Hospital, Binghamton, NY, p. A288
O'NEIL, Jr, Mark T., President and Chief Executive Officer, Mercy Health System of Southeastern Pennsylvania, Conshohocken, PA, p. A358
O'ROURKE, Terrence M.
 President, Spectrum Health, Grand Rapids, MI, p. A216
 Interim Chief Executive Officer, Spectrum Health, Grand Rapids, MI, p. B136
O'SHAUGHNESSY, Jon C., President and Chief Executive Officer, Lake Cumberland Regional Hospital, Somerset, KY, p. A178
OBDAHL, Jim, Administrator, Community Hospital in Nelson County, McVille, ND, p. A323

OBER, Tammy L., Administrator and Chief Executive Officer, HEALTHSOUTH Reading Rehabilitation Hospital, Reading, PA, p. A371
OCASIO, Betty, Executive Director, University Hospital, San Juan, PR, p. A484
OCHS, David T., Administrator, OSF Saint James Hospital, Pontiac, IL, p. A133
OCHS, Kristine, R.N., Administrator, Grisell Memorial Hospital District One, Ransom, KS, p. A167
OCKERS, Thomas, President and Chief Executive Officer, Brookhaven Memorial Hospital Medical Center, Patchogue, NY, p. A302
ODDE, Marlene, Chief Executive Officer, Mobridge Regional Hospital, Mobridge, SD, p. A387
ODDIS, Joseph Michael
 President, Spartanburg Regional Healthcare System, Spartanburg, SC, p. B136
 President, Spartanburg Regional Medical Center, Spartanburg, SC, p. A383
ODEGAARD, Dan, Administrator, Community Memorial Hospital, Redfield, SD, p. A387
ODELL, II, F. A., FACHE, President, Carteret General Hospital, Morehead City, NC, p. A316
OESTMANN, Barbara, Chief Executive Officer, Share Medical Center, Alva, OK, p. A341
OGLESBY, Darrell M., Administrator, Putnam General Hospital, Eatonton, GA, p. A104
OGLEVIE, Anne, Administrator, Memorial Hospital, Weiser, ID, p. A118
OHLEN, Robert B., President and Chief Executive Officer, Nevada Regional Medical Center, Nevada, MO, p. A251
OHM, Barbara, Interim Administrator, Carrie Tingley Hospital, Albuquerque, NM, p. A283
OKINAKA, Cynthia, Administrator, St. Francis Medical Center, Honolulu, HI, p. A112
OLAND, Charisse S., President and Chief Executive Officer, Childrens Care Hospital and School, Sioux Falls, SD, p. A388
OLDHAM, John M., M.D., Director, New York State Psychiatric Institute, New York, NY, p. A299
OLENDER, Marsha, Chief Executive Officer, Charter Behavioral Health System of Winston–Salem, Winston–Salem, NC, p. A320
OLIPHINT, Kelley, Chief Executive Officer and Administrator, Fayette Memorial Hospital, La Grange, TX, p. A420
OLIVER, Michael J., Administrator, HEALTHSOUTH Valley of the Sun Rehabilitation Hospital, Glendale, AZ, p. A23
OLIVER, Vince, Chief Executive Officer, Island Health Northwest, Anacortes, WA, p. A452
OLIVER, William C., President, Forrest General Hospital, Hattiesburg, MS, p. A238
OLIVERIUS, Maynard F., President and Chief Executive Officer, Stormont–Vail HealthCare, Topeka, KS, p. A168
OLNEY, Garry M., R.N., Chief Executive Officer, San Dimas Community Hospital, San Dimas, CA, p. A59
OLSEN, Gloria P., Ph.D., Chief Executive Officer, Kerrville State Hospital, Kerrville, TX, p. A420
OLSEN, Robert T., CHE, President and Chief Executive Officer, Yuma Regional Medical Center, Yuma, AZ, p. A27
OLSON, David, Chief Executive Officer, Bay Area Medical Center, Marinette, WI, p. A471
OLSON, Garvin, Chief Operating Officer, Deer Park Hospital, Deer Park, WA, p. A453
OLSON, Gary R., President, St. Luke's Hospital, Chesterfield, MO, p. A245
OLSON, Gregg, Interim Chief Executive Officer, Rochelle Community Hospital, Rochelle, IL, p. A133
OLSON, JoAline, R.N.
 President and Chief Executive Officer, California Specialty Hospital, Vallejo, CA, p. A66
 President and Chief Executive Officer, St. Helena Hospital, Deer Park, CA, p. A39
OLSON, Lynn W., President, Ottumwa Regional Health Center, Ottumwa, IA, p. A155
OLSON, Michael R., Administrator, Cassia Regional Medical Center, Burley, ID, p. A115
OLSON, Nathan C., President and Chief Executive Officer, Hammond–Henry Hospital, Geneseo, IL, p. A126

OLSON, Randall M., President, Wellmont Bristol Regional Medical Center, Bristol, TN, p. A390
OMER, Robert, FACHE, President and Chief Executive Officer, Memorial Community Hospital and Health System, Blair, NE, p. A261
OMMEN, Ronald A., President and Chief Executive Officer, Trinity Lutheran Hospital, Kansas City, MO, p. A249
ONG, Jesus M., President, South Shore Hospital, Chicago, IL, p. A123
OPIRHORY, Gloria J., Ph.D., Director, University of Connecticut Health Center, John Dempsey Hospital, Farmington, CT, p. A74
ORLANDO, Joseph S., Executive Director, Jacobi Medical Center, New York, NY, p. A297
ORLOWSKI, Carolyn, Director Operations, Kaiser Foundation Hospital, Los Angeles, CA, p. A48
ORMAN, Jr, Bernard A., Administrator, Samaritan Memorial Hospital, Macon, MO, p. A250
ORME, Clifton Neal, Administrator and Chief Executive Officer, Tahoe Pacific Hospital, Sparks, NV, p. A269
ORMOND, Evalyn, Administrator, Union General Hospital, Farmerville, LA, p. A182
ORNSTEEN, Walter J., President and Chief Executive Officer, Baycoast Medical Center, Baytown, TX, p. A404
ORR, Lindell W., Chief Executive Officer, Blake Medical Center, Bradenton, FL, p. A82
ORR, Roy J., President and Chief Executive Officer, McKenzie–Willamette Hospital, Springfield, OR, p. A354
ORR, Steven R., Chairman and Chief Executive Officer, Banner Health System, Fargo, ND, p. B56
ORRICK, Charles H., Administrator, Donalsonville Hospital, Donalsonville, GA, p. A104
ORSINI, Thomas J., Chief Executive Officer, Lake Taylor Hospital, Norfolk, VA, p. A447
ORTENZIO, Rocco A., Chief Executive Officer, Select Medical Corporation, Mechanicsburg, PA, p. B130
ORTIZ, Julio A., M.D., Chairman, Font Martelo Hospital, Humacao, PR, p. A482
ORTIZ, Ruth M., Chief Operating Officer, Bella Vista Hospital, Mayaguez, PR, p. A483
OSBORNE, David W., President and Chief Executive Officer, Norwalk Hospital, Norwalk, CT, p. A76
OSBORNE, Terry W., Chief Executive Officer, American Legion Hospital, Crowley, LA, p. A182
OSBURN, Jerry, Administrator, Covenant Hospital-Levelland, Levelland, TX, p. A421
OSIKA, Diane J., Chief Executive Officer, Tri–County Memorial Hospital, Gowanda, NY, p. A292
OSMUS, Richard D., Chief Executive Officer, Hugh Chatham Memorial Hospital, Elkin, NC, p. A312
OSSE, John M., Administrator, Mitchell County Hospital, Beloit, KS, p. A159
OSTASZEWSKI, Patricia, Chief Executive Officer and Administrator, HEALTHSOUTH Rehabilitation Hospital of New Jersey, Toms River, NJ, p. A281
OSWALD, Wesley W., Chief Executive Officer, Brazosport Memorial Hospital, Lake Jackson, TX, p. A421
OSWALD, Stephen G., Commander, Moncrief Army Community Hospital, Fort Jackson, SC, p. A381
OTAKE, Stanley, Administrator and Chief Executive Officer, Bellflower Medical Center, Bellflower, CA, p. A36
OTHOLE, Jean, Service Unit Director, U. S. Public Health Service Indian Hospital, Zuni, NM, p. A286
OTHS, Richard P., President and Chief Executive Officer, Atlantic Health System, Florham Park, NJ, p. A276
OTT, Pamela, R.N., Chief Executive Officer, Ocean Beach Hospital, Ilwaco, WA, p. A454
OTT, Ronald A., Chief Executive Officer, Fitzgibbon Hospital, Marshall, MO, p. A250
OTT, Ronald H., President and Chief Executive Officer, UPMC McKeesport, McKeesport, PA, p. A364
OTTEN, Jeffrey, President, Brigham and Women's Hospital, Boston, MA, p. A202
OUSLEY, Virginia, Vice President and Hospital Director, Carilion New River Valley Medical Center, Radford, VA, p. A448
OWEN, Edward, Chief Executive Officer, BHC Fremont Hospital, Fremont, CA, p. A41

OWEN, Ronald S., Chief Executive Officer, Southeast Alabama Medical Center, Dothan, AL, p. A14
OWENS, Ben E., President, St. Bernards Regional Medical Center, Jonesboro, AR, p. A31
OWENS, Craig A., President and Chief Operating Officer, Verde Valley Medical Center, Cottonwood, AZ, p. A22
OWENS, Leon, Superintendent, Kansas Neurological Institute, Topeka, KS, p. A168

P

PAAP, Antonie H., President and Chief Executive Officer, Children's Hospital Oakland, Oakland, CA, p. A53
PABON, Ahmed Alvarez, Executive Director, Hospital Sub-Regional Dr. Victor R. Nunez, Humacao, PR, p. A482
PACINI, Carol, Provincialate Superior, Little Company of Mary Sisters Healthcare System, Evergreen Park, IL, p. B106
PACKER, Eric, Administrator, Garfield Memorial Hospital and Clinics, Panguitch, UT, p. A437
PACKER, Steven J., M.D., Chief Executive Officer, Community Hospital of the Monterey Peninsula, Monterey, CA, p. A52
PACKNETT, Michael J., President and Chief Executive Officer, Mercy Health Center, Oklahoma City, OK, p. A346
PADDEN, Terrance J., Administrator, Box Butte General Hospital, Alliance, NE, p. A261
PADILLA, Charles E., Administrator and Chief Operating Officer, St. John's Regional Medical Center, Oxnard, CA, p. A54
PAGE, David R., President and Chief Executive Officer, Fairview Health Services, Minneapolis, MN, p. B84
PAGE, Susan M., President and Chief Executive Officer, Pratt Regional Medical Center, Pratt, KS, p. A166
PAGELS, James R., Chief Executive Officer and Managing Director, Northern Nevada Medical Center, Sparks, NV, p. A269
PAINTER, Laureen, Chief Executive Officer, Christus Coushatta Health Care Center, Coushatta, LA, p. A181
PALAGI, Richard L., Chief Executive Officer, St. John's Lutheran Hospital, Libby, MT, p. A258
PALLARI, Robert, President and Chief Executive Officer, Legacy Health System, Portland, OR, p. B104
PALLOS, Steve E., Administrator, Physicians Hospital, New Orleans, LA, p. A187
PALM, SharRay, President and Chief Executive Officer, Lakewood Health Center, Baudette, MN, p. A225
PALMER, James A., Director, Veterans Affairs Medical Center, San Juan, PR, p. A484
PALMER, John M., Ph.D., Executive Director, Harlem Hospital Center, New York, NY, p. A296
PALMER, William H., President, Miller Dwan Medical Center, Duluth, MN, p. A227
PALMISANO , II, Richard T., MS, Chief Executive Officer, Brattleboro Retreat, Brattleboro, VT, p. A440
PANDL, Therese B., Executive Vice President and Chief Operating Officer, St. Mary's Hospital Ozaukee, Mequon, WI, p. A471
PANICEK, John M.
  Administrator, Rochester Methodist Hospital, Rochester, MN, p. A232
  Administrator, Saint Marys Hospital, Rochester, MN, p. A232
PANIS, Reggie, Chief Executive Officer, Victor Valley Community Hospital, Victorville, CA, p. A66
PAPANIA, Barry A., Chief Executive Officer, Norton Spring View Hospital, Lebanon, KY, p. A174
PAPPELBAUM, Stan, M.D., President and Chief Executive Officer, Scripps Health, San Diego, CA, p. B130
PARDES, Herbert, M.D.
  Chief Executive Officer, New York Presbyterian Healthcare System, New York, NY, p. B113
  President and Chief Executive Officer, New York-Presbyterian Hospital, New York, NY, p. A299
PARENTE, William D., President, St. Vincent Medical Center, Los Angeles, CA, p. A49

PARIS, Gregory A., Administrator, Monroe County Hospital, Albia, IA, p. A148
PARIS, Herbert, President, Mid Coast Hospital, Bath, ME, p. A191
PARISI, Ernest, Administrator and Chief Executive Officer, Llano Memorial Healthcare System, Llano, TX, p. A421
PARKER, Douglas M., Chief Executive Officer, Northside Hospital – Cherokee, Canton, GA, p. A102
PARKER, Phillip L., Administrator, D. W. McMillan Memorial Hospital, Brewton, AL, p. A13
PARKER, Thomas S., Site Administrator, Legacy Mount Hood Medical Center, Gresham, OR, p. A351
PARKER, Tim, Chief Executive Officer, Midwest Regional Medical Center, Midwest City, OK, p. A345
PARKER, Gregg S., Commanding Officer, Naval Hospital, Bremerton, WA, p. A452
PARKIS, Clyde L., Director, Veterans Affairs Medical Center, Albany, NY, p. A287
PARKS , II, Burton O., President, West Shore Medical Center, Manistee, MI, p. A219
PARMER, David N.
  President and Chief Executive Officer, Memorial Hermann Baptist Hospital-East Campus, Beaumont, TX, p. A404
  President and Chief Executive Officer, Memorial Hermann Baptist Hospital-West Campus, Beaumont, TX, p. A404
PARMER, Michael, M.D., Executive Vice President and Administrator, Mercy Community Hospital, Port Jervis, NY, p. A303
PARRIS, Y. C., Director, Veterans Affairs Medical Center, Birmingham, AL, p. A12
PARRIS , Jr, Thomas G., President, Women and Infants Hospital of Rhode Island, Providence, RI, p. A377
PARRISH, Harold R., Superintendent, Rusk State Hospital, Rusk, TX, p. A428
PARRISH, James G., Administrator, East Adams Rural Hospital, Ritzville, WA, p. A456
PARSONS, Larry, Administrator, Wilbarger General Hospital, Vernon, TX, p. A433
PARTON, Gerald L., Chief Executive Officer, Meadowcrest Hospital, Gretna, LA, p. A183
PASINSKI, Theodore M., President, St. Joseph's Hospital Health Center, Syracuse, NY, p. A306
PASSAMA, Gary J., President and Chief Executive Officer, NorthBay Healthcare System, Fairfield, CA, p. B115
PATCHIN, J. Craig, Administrator, Shriners Hospitals for Children-Intermountain, Salt Lake City, UT, p. A438
PATE, Alfred S., Director, Veterans Affairs Medical Center, North Chicago, IL, p. A131
PATE, Jim S., Acting Chief Executive Officer, Unicoi County Memorial Hospital, Erwin, TN, p. A392
PATTEN, Bill, Administrator, Sedgwick County Health Center, Julesburg, CO, p. A71
PATTERSON, Bill, Administrator, Stones River Hospital, Woodbury, TN, p. A400
PATTERSON, Dennis, Interim President and Chief Executive Officer, Mercy Hospital and Medical Center, Chicago, IL, p. A122
PATTERSON, Donald E., Chief Executive Officer, Washington County Hospital, Washington, IA, p. A157
PATTERSON, Michael, Chief Executive Officer, Parkway Regional Hospital, Fulton, KY, p. A172
PATTERSON, Philip, Administrator and Chief Operating Officer, HEALTHSOUTH Rehabilitation Hospital of Arlington, Arlington, TX, p. A402
PATTERSON, Rebecca, Administrator, Rio Grande Hospital, Del Norte, CO, p. A69
PATTON, David W., Ph.D., President and Chief Executive Officer, Wilcox Memorial Hospital, Lihue, HI, p. A113
PATTON, Jimmy, Chief Executive Officer and Managing Director, KeyStone Center, Chester, PA, p. A357
PATTULLO, Douglas E., Chief Executive Officer, West Branch Regional Medical Center, West Branch, MI, p. A224
PATZ, Stephen M., President and Chief Executive Officer, Barnert Hospital, Paterson, NJ, p. A279
PAUGH, J. William, President and Chief Executive Officer, St. Joseph Hospital, Augusta, GA, p. A101
PAULDING, Ralph, President and Chief Executive Officer, Perry County Memorial Hospital, Perryville, MO, p. A251

PAULEY, Alan C., Administrator, Morrow County Hospital, Mount Gilead, OH, p. A335
PAULSON, John E., Chief Executive Officer, Sioux Valley Vermillion Campus, Vermillion, SD, p. A388
PAULSON, Mark E., Administrator, Appleton Municipal Hospital and Nursing Home, Appleton, MN, p. A225
PAWLAK, Paul, President and Chief Executive Officer, Silver Cross Hospital, Joliet, IL, p. A129
PAWLOWSKI, Eugene P., President, Bluefield Regional Medical Center, Bluefield, WV, p. A460
PAYNE, Mark I., Superintendent, Utah State Hospital, Provo, UT, p. A438
PAYSINGER, B. Daniel, M.D., Chief Operating Officer, Palmetto Richland Memorial Hospital, Columbia, SC, p. A380
PAZZAGLINI, Gino J., President and Chief Executive Officer, Good Samaritan Regional Medical Center, Pottsville, PA, p. A370
PEAK, Benjamin A., Chief Executive Officer, Dickenson County Medical Center, Clintwood, VA, p. A443
PEAK, James G., Chief Executive Officer, Memorial Hospital and Manor, Bainbridge, GA, p. A101
PEAKS, William E., Chief Executive Officer, Columbia Garden Park Hospital, Gulfport, MS, p. A238
PEARCE, Richard J., President and Chief Operating Officer, Riverside Health System, Newport News, VA, p. B129
PEARSE, David L., President, Speare Memorial Hospital, Plymouth, NH, p. A273
PEARSON, Bruce E., Senior Vice President and Chief Executive Officer, Desert Samaritan Medical Center, Mesa, AZ, p. A23
PEARSON, Debra, Administrator, Nye Regional Medical Center, Tonopah, NV, p. A269
PEARSON, Diane, Administrator, Cook County North Shore Hospital, Grand Marais, MN, p. A228
PEARSON, Robert S., Administrator, Littleton Regional Hospital, Littleton, NH, p. A272
PEARSON, Roger W., Administrator, Ellsworth County Medical Center, Ellsworth, KS, p. A161
PECEVICH, Mark, M.D., Superintendent, Spring Grove Hospital Center, Baltimore, MD, p. A196
PECK, Gary V., Chief Executive Officer, St. Joseph's Hospital, Chewelah, WA, p. A452
PECK, Kay, Chief Executive Officer, Brown Schools Rehabilitation Center, Austin, TX, p. A402
PECK, Richard H., President and Chief Executive Officer, Eliza Coffee Memorial Hospital, Florence, AL, p. A14
PECOT, L. J., Administrator, Jackson Parish Hospital, Jonesboro, LA, p. A183
PEDERSEN, William L., Chief Executive Officer, St. Peter Regional Treatment Center, Saint Peter, MN, p. A233
PEED, Nancy, Administrator, Peach Regional Medical Center, Fort Valley, GA, p. A105
PEEK, Scott, Administrator, Chambers Memorial Hospital, Danville, AR, p. A29
PEEPLES, Lewis T., Chief Executive Officer, Jennie Stuart Medical Center, Hopkinsville, KY, p. A173
PEICKERT, Barbara A., R.N., Chief Executive Officer, Hayward Area Memorial Hospital and Nursing Home, Hayward, WI, p. A469
PELHAM, Judith, President and Chief Executive Officer, Trinity Health, Novi, MI, p. B144
PELLEGRINO, Cynthia Miller, Director and Chief Executive Officer, Western Maryland Center, Hagerstown, MD, p. A199
PELLEY, Catherine M., President and Chief Executive Officer, Saint Mary Regional Medical Center, Apple Valley, CA, p. A35
PELTZ, Brian, Administrator, Oakwood Seaway Hospital, Trenton, MI, p. A223
PELUSO, Joseph J., President and Chief Executive Officer, Westmoreland Regional Hospital, Greensburg, PA, p. A360
PENKHUS, Mark L., Chief Executive Officer, Vanderbilt University Hospital, Nashville, TN, p. A398
PENNINGTON, David N., FACHE, Chief Executive Officer, Veterans Affairs Medical Center, Huntington, WV, p. A462
PENTICOFF, Michael M., Administrator, Winner Regional Healthcare Center, Winner, SD, p. A389
PENTZ, Thomas R., President and Executive Officer, Lawnwood Regional Medical Center, Fort Pierce, FL, p. A85

Index of Health Care Professionals / Pepper

PEPPER, H. L. Perry, President, Chester County Hospital, West Chester, PA, p. A374
PEREZ, Carlos, Executive Director, Bellevue Hospital Center, New York, NY, p. A295
PEREZ, Francisco J., FACHE, President, Kettering Medical Center–Network, Kettering, OH, p. A333
PEREZ, George, Executive Vice President and Chief Operating Officer, Walter O. Boswell Memorial Hospital, Sun City, AZ, p. A26
PEREZ DE VAZQUEZ, Marilyn, Executive Director, Cardiovascular Center of Puerto Rico and the Caribbean, San Juan, PR, p. A483
PERFETTO, Patricia, MSN, Executive Director, Willough Healthcare System, Naples, FL, p. A91
PERKINS, Gary A., President and Chief Executive Officer, Children's Hospital, Omaha, NE, p. A265
PERMETTI, Thomas, Chief Executive Officer, Christus St. John Hospital, Nassau Bay, TX, p. A425
PERRA, Connie Oliverson, Director, Tarrant County Psychiatric Center, Fort Worth, TX, p. A413
PERREAULT, Robert A., Director, Veterans Affairs Medical Center, Decatur, GA, p. A104
PERRY, Alan S., Director, Veterans Affairs Medical Center, Fresno, CA, p. A42
PERRY, Bruce M., Chief Executive Officer, Mount Sinai Medical Center, Miami Beach, FL, p. A90
PERRY, George H., Ph.D., Chief Executive Officer, NorthShore Psychiatric Hospital, Slidell, LA, p. A189
PERRY, J. Steve, Chief Executive Officer, Star Valley Medical Center, Afton, WY, p. A478
PERRY, L. Gene, Chief Executive Officer, Bloomington Hospital of Orange County, Paoli, IN, p. A144
PERRY, Matthew J., Director, Carilion Franklin Memorial Hospital, Rocky Mount, VA, p. A449
PERRY, Megan, Administrator, Sentara Hampton General Hospital, Hampton, VA, p. A444
PERRY, Mike, Chief Executive Officer, Westbridge Treatment Center, Phoenix, AZ, p. A25
PERRY, Robert P., Executive Director and Chief Executive Officer, Temple East, Neumann Medical Center, Philadelphia, PA, p. A368
PERRY, Ronald J., Chief Executive Officer, Ashley Valley Medical Center, Vernal, UT, p. A439
PERRYMAN, Daniel, Administrator, Iuka Hospital, Iuka, MS, p. A239
PERRYMAN, Margaret, Chief Executive Officer, Gillette Children's Specialty Healthcare, Saint Paul, MN, p. A233
PERRYMAN, Mike, Administrator, Baptist Memorial Hospital–Union City, Union City, TN, p. A400
PERSICHILLI, Judith M., President and Chief Executive Officer, St. Francis Medical Center, Trenton, NJ, p. A281
PERUGINI, Daniel F., Commander, Womack Army Medical Center, Fort Bragg, NC, p. A313
PERUSHEK, John R., President and Chief Executive Officer, St. Elizabeth Health Services, Baker City, OR, p. A350
PETASNICK, William D., President, Froedtert Memorial Lutheran Hospital, Milwaukee, WI, p. A472
PETER, John P., President and Chief Executive Officer, National Hospital for Kids in Crisis, Orefield, PA, p. A366
PETERS, Connie, Operations Leader and Regional Administrator, Alegent Health–Memorial Hospital, Schuyler, NE, p. A266
PETERS, Curtis A., Chief Executive Officer, J. D. McCarty Center for Children With Developmental Disabilities, Norman, OK, p. A345
PETERS, Douglas S., President and Chief Executive Officer, Jefferson Health System, Wayne, PA, p. B102
PETERS, J. Robert, Executive Director, Memorial Hospital, Colorado Springs, CO, p. A68
PETERSEN, Gary L., President and Chief Executive Officer, Spectrum Health–Reed City Campus, Reed City, MI, p. A221
PETERSEN, Keith J., Chief Executive Officer, Southwest Georgia Regional Medical Center, Cuthbert, GA, p. A103
PETERSEN, Thomas A., Vice President and Chief Operating Officer, Mercy General Hospital, Sacramento, CA, p. A57

PETERSON, Andrew E., President and Chief Executive Officer, Faxton–St. Luke's Healthcare, Utica, NY, p. A306
PETERSON, Brent A., Administrator, Cherry County Hospital, Valentine, NE, p. A267
PETERSON, Bruce D., Administrator, Mercer County Hospital, Aledo, IL, p. A119
PETERSON, Clayton R.
 President, CentraCare, Long Prairie, MN, p. B71
 President, Long Prairie Memorial Hospital and Home, Long Prairie, MN, p. A229
PETERSON, David A., President and Chief Executive Officer, Aroostook Medical Center, Presque Isle, ME, p. A193
PETERSON, Douglas R., President and Chief Executive Officer, Chippewa Valley Hospital and Oakview Care Center, Durand, WI, p. A468
PETERSON, Larry, Chief Executive Officer, Lake Chelan Community Hospital, Chelan, WA, p. A452
PETERSON, Leland W., President and Chief Executive Officer, Sun Health Corporation, Sun City, AZ, p. B138
PETERSON, Michael J., Interim Chief Executive Officer, Holy Cross Hospital, Chicago, IL, p. A121
PETERSON, Noel, M.D., President and Chief Executive Officer, Olmsted Medical Center, Rochester, MN, p. A232
PETERSON, Patricia, President and Chief Executive Officer, St. Mary's Hospital, Passaic, NJ, p. A279
PETERSON, Randy, President and Chief Executive Officer, Salina Regional Health Center, Salina, KS, p. A167
PETERSON, Richard H., President and Chief Executive Officer, Swedish Health Services, Seattle, WA, p. A456
PETERSON, Robert M., President and Chief Executive Officer, Southwest Memorial Hospital, Cortez, CO, p. A69
PETERSON, Ronald R.
 President, Johns Hopkins Health System, Baltimore, MD, p. B103
 President, Johns Hopkins Hospital, Baltimore, MD, p. A195
PETERSON, Sharon, Administrator, Southwestern General Hospital, El Paso, TX, p. A412
PETERSON, William D., Administrator, Herington Municipal Hospital, Herington, KS, p. A162
PETIK, Jason, Administrator, Custer Community Hospital, Custer, SD, p. A385
PETIT, Jr, Leo A., Chief Executive Officer, Bladen County Hospital, Elizabethtown, NC, p. A312
PETRINI, Julie A.
 Administrator, Kaiser Foundation Hospital, San Francisco, CA, p. A59
 Administrator, Kaiser Foundation Hospital, San Rafael, CA, p. A61
 Administrator, Kaiser Foundation Hospital, Santa Rosa, CA, p. A62
 Administrator, Kaiser Foundation Hospital, South San Francisco, CA, p. A64
PETRUZZI, Peter T., Chief Executive Officer, Scott County Hospital, Oneida, TN, p. A398
PETTIGREW, Dennis, President and Chief Executive Officer, Erlanger Health System, Chattanooga, TN, p. A390
PETTRY, Harvey H., President and Chief Executive Officer, Richland Memorial Hospital, Olney, IL, p. A132
PETULA, Susan, President, Mercy Hospital of Scranton, Scranton, PA, p. A371
PFAFF, Tony, Chief Executive Officer, Powell County Memorial Hospital, Deer Lodge, MT, p. A257
PFEIFER, Dave, Chief Executive Officer, Valley Hospital, Palmer, AK, p. A21
PFEIFFER, James A.
 Chief Operating Officer, Mease Countryside Hospital, Safety Harbor, FL, p. A94
 Chief Operating Officer, Mease Hospital Dunedin, Dunedin, FL, p. A84
PFEIFFER, Trudy, Administrator, Baum Harmon Mercy Hospital, Primghar, IA, p. A156
PFITZER, Anthony D., Executive Vice President and Administrator, St. Mary's Hospital, Decatur, IL, p. A125

PHAUP, Michael B., Director, Veterans Affairs Medical Center, Durham, NC, p. A312
PHELPS, David E., President and Chief Executive Officer, Berkshire Health Systems, Inc., Pittsfield, MA, p. B60
PHELPS, M. Randell, Administrator, Memorial Hospital, Craig, CO, p. A69
PHEMISTER, Gladys, Chief Executive Officer, Gordon Memorial Hospital District, Gordon, NE, p. A263
PHILIPS, II, Grady W., Vice President and Administrator, Riverside Walter Reed Hospital, Gloucester, VA, p. A444
PHILLIPS, Bob D., Administrator, Skaggs Community Health Center, Branson, MO, p. A244
PHILLIPS, Dennis J., Chief Executive Officer, Frye Regional Medical Center, Hickory, NC, p. A314
PHILLIPS, Joan, R.N., Interim Chief Executive Officer, Doctors Hospital, Wentzville, MO, p. A255
PHILLIPS, John F., Administrator, Gravette Medical Center Hospital, Gravette, AR, p. A30
PHILLIPS, John J., Director, Veterans Affairs Medical Center, Omaha, NE, p. A266
PHILLIPS, Randall M., President and Chief Executive Officer, Community Hospital, Grand Junction, CO, p. A70
PHILLIPS, Scott K., President and Chief Executive Officer, Southern Chester County Medical Center, West Grove, PA, p. A374
PICHE, William K., Chief Executive Officer, Good Samaritan Hospital, San Jose, CA, p. A60
PICKENS, Paula, Interim Chief Executive Officer, Kiowa District Hospital, Kiowa, KS, p. A163
PICKMAN, Serena, Director, Columbia Behavioral Center, El Paso, TX, p. A411
PIEPER, Blaine, Administrator, Ohio County Hospital, Hartford, KY, p. A173
PIERCE, Peggy, Administrator, Calhoun Memorial Hospital, Arlington, GA, p. A99
PIERCE, Randolph J., President and Chief Executive Officer, Boca Raton Community Hospital, Boca Raton, FL, p. A81
PIERCE, Jr, Willard R., Director, Piedmont Geriatric Hospital, Burkeville, VA, p. A442
PIERCEY, Michael, M.D., President and Chief Executive Officer, Health Systems America, Sunrise, FL, p. B95
PIERSON, Richard, Executive Director, Clinical Programs, University Hospital of Arkansas, Little Rock, AR, p. A32
PILE, Darrell L., Regional Vice President, HEALTHSOUTH Rehabilitation Hospital, Humble, TX, p. A419
PILKINGTON, II, Albert, Chief Executive Officer, Muhlenberg Community Hospital, Greenville, KY, p. A172
PINCKNEY, Frank D., President, Greenville Hospital System, Greenville, SC, p. B88
PINE, Polly, Administrator, Gila Regional Medical Center, Silver City, NM, p. A286
PINE, Richard M., President and Chief Executive Officer, Livengrin Foundation, Bensalem, PA, p. A356
PINEIRO, Carlos M., President, Hospital Interamericano De Medicina Avanzada, Caguas, PR, p. A482
PINIZZOTTO, Tom, Administrator and Chief Executive Officer, BHC Sierra Vista Hospital, Sacramento, CA, p. A57
PINKHAM, Margaret G., President and Chief Executive Officer, St. Andrews Hospital and Healthcare Center, Boothbay Harbor, ME, p. A191
PIPICELLI, Thomas P., President and Chief Executive Officer, The William W. Backus Hospital, Norwich, CT, p. A76
PIPKIN, Barry, Chief Executive Officer and Managing Director, BridgeWay, North Little Rock, AR, p. A33
PIRIZ, J. E., Administrator, Memorial Hospital Pembroke, Pembroke Pines, FL, p. A92
PISCIOTTA, James M., Chief Executive Officer, Southwest Connecticut Mental Health System, Bridgeport, CT, p. A74
PITMAN, Richard A., President, Shore Memorial Hospital, Somers Point, NJ, p. A280
PITTMAN, Deanna, Administrator, Wilson County Hospital, Neodesha, KS, p. A165
PIVIROTTO, Gregory A., President and Chief Executive Officer, University Medical Center, Tucson, AZ, p. A27

PLANT, Robert, Ph.D., Superintendent, Riverview Hospital for Children, Middletown, CT, p. A75
PLANTZ, Thomas D., Interim Chief Executive Officer, Kern Valley Healthcare District, Lake Isabella, CA, p. A45
PLATOU, Kenneth E. S., Chief Executive Officer, Montrose Memorial Hospital, Montrose, CO, p. A72
PLATT, Anne, Administrator, East Morgan County Hospital, Brush, CO, p. A68
PLATT, C. James, Chief Executive Officer, Fort Madison Community Hospital, Fort Madison, IA, p. A152
PLATT, Melvin J., Administrator, Worthington Regional Hospital, Worthington, MN, p. A235
PLESKOW, Eric D., President and Chief Executive Officer, Brylin Hospitals, Buffalo, NY, p. A288
PLOWDEN, Moultrie D., CHE, Administrator, Crenshaw Baptist Hospital, Luverne, AL, p. A16
PLUMAGE, Charles D., Director, U. S. Public Health Service Indian Hospital, Harlem, MT, p. A258
PLUMMER, James S., Chief Executive Officer, BHC San Luis Rey Hospital, Encinitas, CA, p. A40
PODIETZ, Frank, President, Friedman Hospital of the Home for the Jewish Aged, Philadelphia, PA, p. A366
POEHLING, James C., Director, Columbia Regional Hospital, Columbia, MO, p. A245
POHREN, Allen E., Administrator, Montgomery County Memorial Hospital, Red Oak, IA, p. A156
POIRIER, Alex M. Marceline, President and Chief Executive Officer, Parkland Medical Center, Derry, NH, p. A271
POISSON, Keith R., President and Chief Executive Officer, Bethany Medical Center, Kansas City, KS, p. A163
POKORNEY, Georgia, Chief Executive Officer, Pioneer Memorial Hospital and Health Services, Viborg, SD, p. A388
POLAHAR, Robert G., Chief Executive Officer, Knox Community Hospital, Mount Vernon, OH, p. A335
POLGE, David J., President and Chief Executive Officer, Delaware Valley Hospital, Walton, NY, p. A307
POLHEBER, Richard
  Interim Vice President and Chief Executive Officer, Carondelet Holy Cross Hospital, Nogales, AZ, p. A23
  Chief Executive Officer, Page Hospital, Page, AZ, p. A23
POLITO, William J., President and Chief Executive Officer, Brookville Hospital, Brookville, PA, p. A356
POLL, Max, President and Chief Executive Officer, Scottsdale Healthcare, Scottsdale, AZ, p. B130
POLLA, Dale E., Chief Executive Officer, Glacier County Medical Center, Cut Bank, MT, p. A257
POLLACK, Ellen, R.N., Interim Chief Operating Officer and Director Nursing, Santa Monica–UCLA Medical Center, Santa Monica, CA, p. A62
POLLARD, Jr, Joe W., Chief Executive Officer, Granville Medical Center, Oxford, NC, p. A316
POLLOCK, Rusty, President and Chief Executive Officer, Rehabilitation Institute at Santa Barbara, Santa Barbara, CA, p. A62
POLONSKY, Leonard, interim Chief Executive Officer, Island Medical Center, Hempstead, NY, p. A292
POLUNAS, David M., Administrator and Chief Executive Officer, Heart of Florida Behavioral Center, Lakeland, FL, p. A88
POMA, Frank W., President, St. John River District Hospital, East China, MI, p. A214
POMMETT, Jr, Francis A., Executive Director and Senior Vice President, Sacred Heart Hospital, Cumberland, MD, p. A198
POORTEN, Kevin P., Chief Executive Officer, Havasu Regional Medical Center, Lake Havasu City, AZ, p. A23
POPE, James W.
  Chief Executive Officer, Norton Southwest Hospital, Louisville, KY, p. A175
  President and Chief Executive Officer, Provena United Samaritans Medical Center, Danville, IL, p. A124
POPIEL, Gary W., Executive Vice President and Chief Executive Officer, Bi–County Community Hospital, Warren, MI, p. B23
POPP, Dennis A., Administrator and Chief Executive Officer, Enumclaw Community Hospital, Enumclaw, WA, p. A453

POQUETTE, Gary R., FACHE, Executive Director, Memorial Hospital, North Conway, NH, p. A273
PORTEN, Hank J., President and Chief Executive Officer, Holyoke Hospital, Holyoke, MA, p. A205
PORTER, Arthur, M.D., President and Chief Executive Officer, Detroit Medical Center, Detroit, MI, p. B82
PORTER, John T., President and Chief Executive Officer, Avera Health, Yankton, SD, p. B55
PORTER, Robert G., President, DePaul Health Center, Saint Louis, MO, p. A253
PORTER, Ronald W., Chief Executive Officer, KPC Global Medical Center, Montclair, CA, p. A52
PORTER, Thomas C., President, Morton Hospital and Medical Center, Taunton, MA, p. A209
PORTER, Jr, John M., President and Chief Executive Officer, Ephrata Community Hospital, Ephrata, PA, p. A359
PORTEUS, Robert W., President and Chief Executive Officer, Carlinville Area Hospital, Carlinville, IL, p. A120
PORTFLEET, Lori, Chief Executive Officer, Spectrum Health–Kent Community Campus, Grand Rapids, MI, p. A216
PORZIO, Ronald T., Chief Operating Officer, Royal C. Johnson Veterans Memorial Hospital, Sioux Falls, SD, p. A388
POSEY, M. Kenneth, FACHE, Administrator, Jasper General Hospital, Bay Springs, MS, p. A236
POTEETE, Kenneth W., President and Chief Executive Officer, Georgetown Healthcare System, Georgetown, TX, p. A414
POTTENGER, Jay, Administrator, Missouri River Medical Center, Fort Benton, MT, p. A257
POTTER, Bruce C., President, Canton–Potsdam Hospital, Potsdam, NY, p. A303
POTTER, Michael S., FACHE, President and Chief Execfutive Officer, Odessa Regional Hospital, Odessa, TX, p. A425
POTTER, Terri L., President and Chief Executive Officer, Meriter Hospital, Madison, WI, p. A470
POTTER, Bonnie B., Commander, National Naval Medical Center, Bethesda, MD, p. A197
POURIER, Terry, Services Unit Director, U. S. Public Health Service Indian Hospital, Fort Yates, ND, p. A322
POWELL, Darnell, Executive Director, Rolling Hills Hospital, Ada, OK, p. A341
POWELL, Ricky, Chief Executive Officer, Red River Hospital, Wichita Falls, TX, p. A435
POWELL, Roy A., President, Frankford Hospital of the City of Philadelphia, Philadelphia, PA, p. A366
POWELL, Jr, Boone, President and Chief Executive Officer, Baylor University Medical Center, Dallas, TX, p. A408
POWERS, L. Darrell, Senior Vice President, Lynchburg General Hospital, Lynchburg, VA, p. A445
POWERS, Michael K., Administrator, Fairbanks Memorial Hospital, Fairbanks, AK, p. A20
POWERS, Terry C., Administrator, Fort Logan Hospital, Stanford, KY, p. A178
POZZUTO, Geraldine, Acting Chief Executive Officer, Monsour Medical Center, Jeannette, PA, p. A362
PRASAD, Manoj K., M.D., President and Chief Executive Officer, Kern Hospital and Medical Center, Warren, MI, p. A224
PRESLAR, Jr, Len B., President and Chief Executive Officer, North Carolina Baptist Hospital, Winston–Salem, NC, p. A320
PRESTON, Craig, Chief Executive Officer, Lakeview Hospital, Bountiful, UT, p. A436
PRICE, Corbett A.
  Chief Executive Officer, Episcopal Health Services Inc., Bethpage, NY, p. B84
  Chief Executive Officer, Interfaith Medical Center, New York, NY, p. A297
PRICE, Kim, Administrator, Belmond Medical Center, Belmond, IA, p. A148
PRICE, Norman M., FACHE, Administrator, Southwest Mississippi Regional Medical Center, McComb, MS, p. A240
PRICE, Jr, Eston, Administrator, Evans Memorial Hospital, Claxton, GA, p. A102
PRICE, Jr, Warren T., Chief Executive Officer, East Louisiana State Hospital, Jackson, LA, p. A183

PRIDDY, Sandra D., President, Stokes–Reynolds Memorial Hospital, Danbury, NC, p. A311
PRIDDY, II, Ernest C., Chief Executive Officer, Cumberland, A Brown Schools Hospital for Children and Adolescents, New Kent, VA, p. A446
PRIDGEN, Jr, Lee, Administrator, Sampson Regional Medical Center, Clinton, NC, p. A311
PRIMEAUX, Elizabeth A., Chief Executive Officer, Cypress Fairbanks Medical Center, Houston, TX, p. A416
PRISCO, Nicholas A., Chief Executive Officer, Sunbury Community Hospital, Sunbury, PA, p. A372
PRISELAC, Margaret, R.N., Chief Executive Officer, UPMC Braddock, Braddock, PA, p. A356
PRISELAC, Thomas M., President and Chief Executive Officer, Cedars–Sinai Medical Center, Los Angeles, CA, p. A47
PRISTER, James Richard, President, R. M. L. Specialty Hospital, Hinsdale, IL, p. A128
PRITCHARD, Eugene, President, Condell Medical Center, Libertyville, IL, p. A129
PROBST, Randall K., Administrator, Heber Valley Medical Center, Heber City, UT, p. A436
PROBUS, Jeff, Interim Chief Exective Officer, Wirth Regional Hospital, Oakland City, IN, p. A144
PROCHILO, John F., Chief Executive Officer and Administrator, Northeast Rehabilitation Hospital, Salem, NH, p. A273
PROCTOR, Randy, Superintendent, Osawatomie State Hospital, Osawatomie, KS, p. A166
PROCTOR, Steven M., President, Matheny School and Hospital, Peapack, NJ, p. A279
PROUT, John S.
  President and Chief Executive Officer, Bethesda North Hospital, Cincinnati, OH, p. A327
  President and Chief Executive Officer, Good Samaritan Hospital, Cincinnati, OH, p. A327
PROVENZANO, William F., President, Ohio Valley General Hospital, McKees Rocks, PA, p. A364
PRUITT, Mike, Chief Executive Officer, Lake Granbury Medical Center, Granbury, TX, p. A414
PRUSAK, Thomas K., President, St. Joseph's Medical Center, Brainerd, MN, p. A226
PRYCE, Richard J., President, Aultman Hospital, Canton, OH, p. A326
PRYOR, Curtis R., Administrator, Purcell Municipal Hospital, Purcell, OK, p. A347
PRYOR, Dennis P., Administrator, Salem Memorial District Hospital, Salem, MO, p. A254
PUCCI, Duayna, Director Operations, Kaiser Foundation Hospital, Hayward, CA, p. A43
PUCKETT, Stephen R., Chairman, President and Chief Executive Officer, MedCath, Inc., Charlotte, NC, p. B109
PUGH, Richard E., President and Chief Executive Officer, New Milford Hospital, New Milford, CT, p. A76
PUGH, Thomas E., Vice President Rehabilitation Services, John Heinz Institute of Rehabilitation Medicine, Wilkes–Barre, PA, p. A374
PUGLISI, Jr, Frank J., Executive Director, Contra Costa Regional Medical Center, Martinez, CA, p. A51
PULSIPHER, Gary W., President, Breech Regional Medical Center, Lebanon, MO, p. A249
PUNDYS, Aras, Administrator, W. J. Barge Memorial Hospital, Greenville, SC, p. A381
PUNG, Dawn S., Administrator, Kau Hospital, Pahala, HI, p. A113
PURCELL, II, James E., Chief Executive Officer, Glades General Hospital, Belle Glade, FL, p. A81
PURCELL, Jr, Howard J., President, Community Memorial Hospital, Cheboygan, MI, p. A213
PURDUE, Marian R., Senior Vice President and Chief Operating Officer, Mercy Medical Center, Springfield, OH, p. A337
PURVES, Stephen A., CHE, President and Chief Executive Officer, Providence Hospital, Columbia, SC, p. A380
PURVIANCE, Bruce, Administrator, Niobrara Valley Hospital, Lynch, NE, p. A264
PURVIS, J. Jay, Interim Chief Executive Officer, Rush Memorial Hospital, Rushville, IN, p. A145

PURVIS, Michael L.
  President and Chief Executive Officer, Redwood Memorial Hospital, Fortuna, CA, p. A41
  President and Chief Executive Officer, Saint Joseph Hospital, Eureka, CA, p. A40
PUTNAM, Larry E., Administrator, Phillips County Medical Center, Malta, MT, p. A258
PUTTER, Joshua S., Executive Director, Charlotte Regional Medical Center, Punta Gorda, FL, p. A94
PYLE, Joseph, Administrator, Meadow Wood Behavioral Health System, New Castle, DE, p. A78
PYNE, Mel, Administrator, Providence Everett Medical Center, Everett, WA, p. A453
PYNN, David, President and Chief Executive Officer, St. John Medical Center, Tulsa, OK, p. A349

Q

QUAGLIATA, Joseph A., President and Chief Executive Officer, South Nassau Communities Hospital, Oceanside, NY, p. A301
QUAM, Mark, Director, Brown County Human Services Mental Health Center, Green Bay, WI, p. A469
QUINLAN, Richard S., President and Chief Executive Officer, Hallmark Health System, Malden, MA, p. A206
QUINN, Deborah, Administrator, BHC Cedar Vista Hospital, Fresno, CA, p. A41
QUINTON, Byron, Administrator, Humboldt General Hospital, Winnemucca, NV, p. A269
QUIST, Robert L., Chief Executive Officer, Park Plaza Hospital, Houston, TX, p. A417

R

RAAB, Daniel J., President and Chief Executive Officer, St. Vincent Memorial Hospital, Taylorville, IL, p. A135
RABUKA, Mickey, Administrator, Murray Medical Center, Chatsworth, GA, p. A102
RACE, J. E., Administrator and Chief Executive Officer, St. Joseph's Hospital Bluemound, Wauwatosa, WI, p. A477
RADKE, Sam D., Interim Chief Executive Officer, Memorial Hospital of Converse County, Douglas, WY, p. A478
RAFTER, William A., Director, Julian F. Keith Alcohol and Drug Abuse Treatment Center, Black Mountain, NC, p. A309
RAGGHIANTI, Eugene
  Administrator, Methodist Healthcare–Lexington Hospital, Lexington, TN, p. A395
  Administrator, Methodist Healthcare–Volunteer Hospital, Martin, TN, p. A396
RAGGIO, James J., Administrator, Lompoc Healthcare District, Lompoc, CA, p. A46
RAGLAND, Kenneth E., Administrator, Beaufort County Hospital, Washington, NC, p. A319
RAHM, Linda K., Chief Executive Officer, Olympus Specialty Hospital–Springfield, Springfield, MA, p. A208
RAJNIC, Sharon J., Administrator, Shriners Hospitals for Children, Philadelphia, Philadelphia, PA, p. A368
RAK, Arlene A., President, UHHS Bedford Medical Center, Bedford, OH, p. A326
RALEY, Ana, Chief Executive Officer, Greater Southeast Community Hospital, Washington, DC, p. A79
RALPH, Chandler M., President and Chief Executive Officer, Adirondack Medical Center, Saranac Lake, NY, p. A304
RALPH, Stephen A.
  President and Chief Executive Officer, Huntington Memorial Hospital, Pasadena, CA, p. A55
  President and Chief Executive Officer, Southern California Healthcare Systems, Pasadena, CA, p. B135
RAMIREZ, Magdalena, Chief Executive Officer, Helen Hayes Hospital, West Haverstraw, NY, p. A307
RAMISH, Dana W., FACHE, President and Chief Executive Officer, Deaconess Waltham Hospital, Waltham, MA, p. A209
RAMPAGE, Bruce E., President and Chief Executive Officer, Saint Anthony Memorial Health Centers, Michigan City, IN, p. A144
RAMSEY, Barbara, Ph.D., Chief Executive Officer, Lincoln Regional Center, Lincoln, NE, p. A264
RAMSEY, Beryl, Chief Executive Officer, Texas Orthopedic Hospital, Houston, TX, p. A418
RAMSEY, David L., President, Methodist Healthcare–Memphis Hospital, Memphis, TN, p. A397
RANEY, Sam H., Interim Administrator, Stamford Memorial Hospital, Stamford, TX, p. A431
RANGE, Richard L., Chief Executive Officer, Baldwin Area Medical Center, Baldwin, WI, p. A466
RANGE, Robert P., President and Chief Executive Officer, Grace Hospital, Cleveland, OH, p. A328
RANK, James T., Administrator, Bothwell Regional Health Center, Sedalia, MO, p. A254
RANKIN , II, Fred M., President and Chief Executive Officer, Mary Washington Hospital, Fredericksburg, VA, p. A444
RANSDELL, Lewis A., Administrator, Vencor Hospital–Fort Lauderdale, Fort Lauderdale, FL, p. A84
RAPAPORT, Gary D., Chief Executive Officer, Sutter Tracy Community Hospital, Tracy, CA, p. A65
RAPOPORT, Morton I., M.D., President and Chief Executive Officer, University of Maryland Medical System, Baltimore, MD, p. B149
RAPP, Larry, M.D., Chief Medical and Executive Officer, Grant County Health Center, Elbow Lake, MN, p. A227
RAPP, Phillip J., President and Chief Executive Officer, St. Francis at Salina, Salina, KS, p. A167
RAPPAPORT, Mark J., Chief Executive Officer, Lewis County General Hospital, Lowville, NY, p. A294
RASH, Marty, President and Chief Executive Officer, Province Healthcare Corporation, Brentwood, TN, p. B121
RASMUSSEN, David D., Administrator, Okmulgee Memorial Hospital, Okmulgee, OK, p. A346
RASMUSSEN, Kyle, Administrator, Bridges Medical Services, Ada, MN, p. A225
RATHBONE, Thomas A., President, Cleveland Clinic Children's Hospital for Rehabilitation, Cleveland, OH, p. A328
RATHJE, Judy Christine, Administrator, Providence Seward Medical Center, Seward, AK, p. A21
RAU, John, Administrator, Stevens Community Medical Center, Morris, MN, p. A231
RAVENBERG, Larry, Administrator, White Community Hospital, Aurora, MN, p. A225
RAWSON, Richard L., President, Selma Community Hospital, Selma, CA, p. A63
RAYNER, Evan, Administrator, Hollywood Community Hospital of Hollywood, Los Angeles, CA, p. A47
RAYNOR, James E., Chief Executive Officer, Raleigh Community Hospital, Raleigh, NC, p. A317
READ, J. Larry, President and Chief Executive Officer, University Health Care System, Augusta, GA, p. A101
REAGAN , Jr, James H., Ph.D., Chief Executive Officer, Morris County Hospital, Council Grove, KS, p. A160
REAMER, Roger, Administrator, Butler County Health Care Center, David City, NE, p. A262
REAMEY, Kirk, Chief Executive Officer, Magnolia Hospital, Magnolia, AR, p. A32
REARDON, Robert, Hospital Services Administrator, Central Prison Hospital, Raleigh, NC, p. A316
REARDON, Timothy F., FACHE, Chief Executive Officer, Yuma District Hospital, Yuma, CO, p. A73
REASBECK, Suzanne, President and Chief Executive Officer, Flaget Memorial Hospital, Bardstown, KY, p. A170
REBER, James P., President, St. Rita's Medical Center, Lima, OH, p. A333
RECUPERO, Patricia R., M.D., President and Chief Executive Officer, Butler Hospital, Providence, RI, p. A376
REDDISH, Robert R., Administrator and Chief Executive Officer, Chicot Memorial Hospital, Lake Village, AR, p. A31
REDMAN, Melvin, President and Chief Operating Officer, Doctors Community Healthcare Corporation, Scottsdale, AZ, p. B83
REECE, David A., President, MidMichigan Medical Center–Midland, Midland, MI, p. A219
REECE, Morris D., Administrator and Chief Executive Officer, Carilion Giles Memorial Hospital, Pearisburg, VA, p. A447
REECER, Jeff, Chief Executive Officer, D. M. Cogdell Memorial Hospital, Snyder, TX, p. A431
REED, Gregory C., Administrator, Pike County Memorial Hospital, Louisiana, MO, p. A250
REED, Harold, Administrator, Fayette Medical Center, Fayette, AL, p. A14
REED, Jan A., CPA, Administrator and Chief Executive Officer, Electra Memorial Hospital, Electra, TX, p. A412
REED, Joy, R.N., Administrator, Ottawa County Health Center, Minneapolis, KS, p. A165
REED, Ronald R., President and Chief Executive Officer, Mercy Hospital, Iowa City, IA, p. A153
REED, Steven B., President and Chief Executive Officer, Women's Hospital–Indianapolis, Indianapolis, IN, p. A142
REEDER, Steve, Chief Executive Officer, Helena Regional Medical Center, Helena, AR, p. A30
REEK, Thomas F., Chief Executive Officer, Cuyuna Regional Medical Center, Crosby, MN, p. A227
REES, Ron R., President and Chief Executive Officer, Halifax Medical Center, Daytona Beach, FL, p. A83
REESE, James, CHE, Administrator, Stephens Memorial Hospital, Breckenridge, TX, p. A405
REESE, Sandra, Administrator, Lower Umpqua Hospital District, Reedsport, OR, p. A354
REESE, Willis L., Administrator, Falls Community Hospital and Clinic, Marlin, TX, p. A423
REEVES, Luther E., Chief Executive Officer, Fleming County Hospital, Flemingsburg, KY, p. A171
REEVEY, Ramon J., Director, Veterans Affairs Southern Nevada Healthcare System, Las Vegas, NV, p. A269
REGAN, James, Ph.D., Chief Executive Officer, Hudson River Psychiatric Center, Poughkeepsie, NY, p. A303
REGEHR, Stan, President and Chief Executive Officer, Memorial Hospital, McPherson, KS, p. A165
REGER, Ed, President and Chief Executive Officer, Northwest General Hospital, Milwaukee, WI, p. A472
REGLING, Anne M., Senior Vice President, Sinai/Grace Hospital, Detroit, MI, p. A214
REID, David M., Administrator, Clay County Medical Center, West Point, MS, p. A243
REIF, Richard A., President and Chief Executive Officer, Doylestown Hospital, Doylestown, PA, p. A359
REIFSTECK, Mark W., Senior Vice President and Chief Operating Officer, Presbyterian Hospital, Albuquerque, NM, p. A283
REILEY, Peggy, Senior Vice President and Chief Clinical Officer, Scottsdale Healthcare–Osborn, Scottsdale, AZ, p. A25
REINER, Dan
  Administrator and Chief Executive Officer, Tracy Area Medical Services, Tracy, MN, p. A234
  Administrator and Chief Executive Officer, Westbrook Health Center, Westbrook, MN, p. A234
REINER, Steven S., Administrator, Kearny County Hospital, Lakin, KS, p. A163
REINERTSEN, James, M.D.
  Chief Executive Officer, Beth Israel Deaconess Medical Center, Boston, MA, p. A201
  Chief Executive Officer, CareGroup, Boston, MA, p. B64
REINHARD, James S., M.D., Director, Catawba Hospital, Catawba, VA, p. A442
REISS, Edward J., Interim Administrator, United Community Hospital, Grove City, PA, p. A361
REITER, Steven B., Administrator, Shriners Hospitals for Children, Houston, Houston, TX, p. A418
REITINGER, Thomas A., Chief Executive Officer, Provena Saint Joseph Medical Center, Joliet, IL, p. A128
REKER, Douglas J., Administrator and Chief Executive Officer, Glacial Ridge Hospital and Healthcare Services, Glenwood, MN, p. A228
REMBIS, Michael A., FACHE, Chief Executive Officer, Centinela Hospital Medical Center, Inglewood, CA, p. A44

Index of Health Care Professionals / Roberts

REMBOLDT, Darwin R., President and Chief Executive Officer, Hanford Community Medical Center, Hanford, CA, p. A43

REMILLARD, John R., President, Aurelia Osborn Fox Memorial Hospital, Oneonta, NY, p. A302

RENANDER, Dennis J., President and Chief Executive Officer, Galesburg Cottage Hospital, Galesburg, IL, p. A126

RENFORD, Edward J., President and Chief Executive Officer, Grady Memorial Hospital, Atlanta, GA, p. A100

RENNER, Steven W., CPA, President and Chief Executive Officer, Gettysburg Hospital, Gettysburg, PA, p. A360

RENNIE, Robert J., Administrator, U. S. Air Force Hospital, Grand Forks AFB, ND, p. A322

RENTAS, Roberto A., Administrator, Hospital De Damas, Ponce, PR, p. A483

RENTFRO, Larry D., FACHE, President and Chief Executive Officer, Grant Regional Health Center, Lancaster, WI, p. A470

RENTZ, Norman G., President and Chief Executive Officer, Cannon Memorial Hospital, Pickens, SC, p. A383

REPLOGLE, Raymond L.
President and Chief Executive Officer, Continuous Care Center of Tulsa, Tulsa, OK, p. A348
President and Chief Executive Officer, St. John Sapulpa, Sapulpa, OK, p. A347

RESCA, Michael, Chief Executive Officer, Lawrence F. Quigley Memorial Hospital, Chelsea, MA, p. A204

RESENDEZ, Linda, R.N., Administrator, Cornerstone Regional Hospital, Edinburg, TX, p. A411

RESNICK, Peter V., Executive Director, Dearborn County Hospital, Lawrenceburg, IN, p. A143

RESSLER, David R., President and Chief Executive Officer, Sierra Vista Regional Health Center, Sierra Vista, AZ, p. A26

RESTUM, William H., Ph.D., President and Chief Executive Officer, Great Lakes Rehabilitation Hospital, Southfield, MI, p. A222

REVELS, Thomas R., President and Chief Executive Officer, Presbyterian Hospital, Charlotte, NC, p. A311

REYES, Arnold, Administrator, U. S. Penitentiary Infirmary, Lewisburg, PA, p. A363

REYES, Marco, Executive Director, Aguadilla General Hospital, Aguadilla, PR, p. A481

REYNOLDS, John R., President and Chief Executive Officer, Hospital for Special Surgery, New York, NY, p. A297

REYNOLDS, R. Dale, Chief Executive Officer, BHC Fox Run Hospital, Saint Clairsville, OH, p. A337

REYNOLDS, Stephen Curtis
President and Chief Executive Officer, Baptist Memorial Health Care Corporation, Memphis, TN, p. B58
President and Chief Executive Officer, Baptist Memorial Hospital, Memphis, TN, p. A396

REZAC, Pamela J., President and Chief Executive Officer, Avera Sacred Heart, Yankton, SD, p. A389

RHEAULT, Donna, Chief Operating Officer, Saint Francis Hospital, Tulsa, OK, p. A348

RHEAULT, LeRoy E., President and Chief Executive Officer, Via Christi Health System, Wichita, KS, p. B152

RHINE, Scott, Administrator and Chief Executive Officer, Whidbey General Hospital, Coupeville, WA, p. A453

RHINEHART, Jennie R., Administrator and Chief Executive Officer, Community Hospital, Tallassee, AL, p. A18

RHOADS, Gary R., President and Chief Executive Officer, Lock Haven Hospital, Lock Haven, PA, p. A363

RHODES, J. Gary, Chief Executive Officer, Kane Community Hospital, Kane, PA, p. A362

RHUDY, Kenneth D., Chief Executive Officer, Dooly Medical Center, Vienna, GA, p. A111

RICE, Alan J., President, Simi Valley Hospital and Health Care Services, Simi Valley, CA, p. A63

RICE, David O., President, Haywood Regional Medical Center, Clyde, NC, p. A311

RICE, Kathleen A., Chief Operating Officer, Meridia South Pointe Hospital, Warrensville Heights, OH, p. A339

RICE, Mark, Chief Executive Officer, HEALTHSOUTH North Louisiana Rehabilitation Hospital, Ruston, LA, p. A188

RICE, Thomas J., President and Chief Executive Officer, Fawcett Memorial Hospital, Port Charlotte, FL, p. A93

RICE, Thomas R., FACHE
President and Chief Operating Officer, Integris Baptist Medical Center, Oklahoma City, OK, p. A346
President and Chief Operating Officer, Integris Southwest Medical Center, Oklahoma City, OK, p. A346

RICE, Tim, President, Lakewood Health System, Staples, MN, p. A234

RICHARD, Robert J., Administrator, People's Memorial Hospital of Buchanan County, Independence, IA, p. A153

RICHARD, Tracey S., Administrator, Dubuis Hospital for Continuing Care, Lake Charles, LA, p. A184

RICHARDS, Joan K.
President, Crozer-Chester Medical Center, Upland, PA, p. A373
President, Delaware County Memorial Hospital, Drexel Hill, PA, p. A359

RICHARDS, Randy R., Chief Executive Officer, Permian General Hospital, Andrews, TX, p. A401

RICHARDS, Richard M., Administrator, HEALTHSOUTH Rehabilitation Hospital of Utah, Sandy, UT, p. A439

RICHARDSON, A. D., Administrator, Hood Memorial Hospital, Amite, LA, p. A180

RICHARDSON, Darrel C., Chief Operating Officer, Kanakanak Hospital, Dillingham, AK, p. A20

RICHARDSON, F. David, Ph.D., Chief Executive Officer, Sistersville General Hospital, Sistersville, WV, p. A464

RICHARDSON, J. E., Chief Executive Officer, Savoy Medical Center, Mamou, LA, p. A185

RICHARDSON, Mark D., President and Chief Executive Officer, Great River Medical Center, West Burlington, IA, p. A157

RICHARDSON, Patricia L., President and Chief Executive Officer, Howard Young Medical Center, Woodruff, WI, p. A477

RICHARDSON, R. D., President and Chief Executive Officer, Ashtabula County Medical Center, Ashtabula, OH, p. A325

RICHARDSON, William T., President and Chief Executive Officer, Tift General Hospital, Tifton, GA, p. A110

RICHER, R. David, Administrator, Healthsouth Rehabilitation Hospital of Western Massachusetts, Ludlow, MA, p. A206

RICHEY, Don L., Administrator, Guadalupe Valley Hospital, Seguin, TX, p. A430

RICHMAN, Martin I., Chief Executive Officer, Central Peninsula General Hospital, Soldotna, AK, p. A21

RICHMOND, John W., President and Chief Executive Officer, Gentry County Memorial Hospital, Albany, MO, p. A244

RICHMOND, Kenneth A., President and Chief Executive Officer, Mount Sinai Hospital Medical Center of Chicago, Chicago, IL, p. A122

RICHTER, Thomas, Chief Executive Officer, Madison Hospital, Madison, MN, p. A229

RICKARD, Roland K., Administrator, Mitchell County Hospital, Colorado City, TX, p. A407

RIDDLE, Brian L., President and Chief Executive Officer, Oconee Regional Medical Center, Milledgeville, GA, p. A107

RIDER , II, Harrison J., President, Union Memorial Hospital, Baltimore, MD, p. A196

RIEDMANN, Gary P., President and Chief Executive Officer, St. Anthony Regional Hospital, Carroll, IA, p. A148

RIEGE, Michael J., Chief Executive Officer, Virginia Gay Hospital, Vinton, IA, p. A157

RIEMER-MATUZAK, Stephanie J., Chief Executive Officer, Mercy Health Services North-Grayling, Grayling, MI, p. A216

RIES, Douglas A., President, Cardinal Glennon Children's Hospital, Saint Louis, MO, p. A252

RIES, William G., President, Lake Forest Hospital, Lake Forest, IL, p. A129

RIFE, Roger, Co-Administrator, Steele Memorial Hospital, Salmon, ID, p. A117

RIFFEL, Alan, Acting Administrator, Anadarko Municipal Hospital, Anadarko, OK, p. A341

RIGBY, James B., Interim President, St. Mary's Health Center, Saint Louis, MO, p. A254

RIGDON, Henry, Executive Vice President, Northeast Georgia Medical Center, Gainesville, GA, p. A105

RIGSBY, John P., Administrator, Garrard County Memorial Hospital, Lancaster, KY, p. A173

RILEY, Jim, Administrator, Tattnall Memorial Hospital, Reidsville, GA, p. A108

RILEY, Thomas, Chief Executive Officer, Brown Schools, Inc., Austin, TX, p. B63

RIMA, Pat, Health Care Manager, State Penitentiary Hospital, Walla Walla, WA, p. A459

RIMES, Dwight, Administrator, Ocean Springs Hospital, Ocean Springs, MS, p. A241

RINE, Thomas L., President and Chief Executive Officer, Southwestern Medical Center, Lawton, OK, p. A344

RINEHARDT, Mark, Administrator, Lake City Medical Center, Lake City, MN, p. A229

RINGL, Karen K., Director Hospital Operations, Kaiser Foundation Hospital-Bellflower, Bellflower, CA, p. A36

RINKER, Franklin M., President and Chief Executive Officer, Promina Gwinnett Hospital System, Lawrenceville, GA, p. A106

RIORDAN, William J., President and Chief Executive Officer, St. Vincent's Medical Center, Bridgeport, CT, p. A74

RISER, Donna, Administrator, Lackey Memorial Hospital, Forest, MS, p. A238

RISK, Richard R., President and Chief Executive Officer, Advocate Health Care, Oak Brook, IL, p. B51

RISON, R. H., Warden, U. S. Medical Center for Federal Prisoners, Springfield, MO, p. A254

RITCHIE, Judith
President and Chief Executive Officer, Salem Hospital, Salem, MA, p. A208
President and Chief Executive Officer, The Union Hospital, Lynn, MA, p. A206

RITER, Pamela M., R.N., Administrator, Vencor Hospital-St Petersburg, Saint Petersburg, FL, p. A94

RITZ, Robert P., Chief Executive Officer, Monongalia General Hospital, Morgantown, WV, p. A463

RIVERA, Pedro, Administrator, Doctors Center, Manati, PR, p. A483

RIVERA, Santiago, Executive Administrator, Hospital Oncologico Andres Grillasca, Ponce, PR, p. A483

RIVERS, Kenneth I.
Chief Executive Officer, Lakewood Regional Medical Center, Lakewood, CA, p. A45
Chief Executive Officer, Suburban Medical Center, Paramount, CA, p. A55

RIZZO, Nancy L., Senior Vice President, Operations, Geisinger Medical Center, Danville, PA, p. A359

RIZZUTO, Lori Ann, Chief Executive Officer, Charter Behavioral Health System of New Jersey-Summit, Summit, NJ, p. A280

ROACH, Joseph, Chief Executive Officer, Memorial Hospital of Martinsville and Henry County, Martinsville, VA, p. A446

ROARK, Ruth Ann, Administrator, Sequoyah Memorial Hospital, Sallisaw, OK, p. A347

ROBBINS, Alan H., M.D., President, New England Baptist Hospital, Boston, MA, p. A202

ROBBINS, John N., President and Chief Executive Officer, Conway Regional Medical Center, Conway, AR, p. A29

ROBBINS, Jonathan H., M.D., President and Chief Executive Officer, Health Alliance Hospitals, Leominster, MA, p. A205

ROBBINS, Wes, Chief Executive Officer, Charter by-the-Sea Behavioral Health System, Saint Simons Island, GA, p. A109

ROBERSON, Madeleine, President and Chief Executive Officer, Presbyterian-St. Luke's Medical Center, Denver, CO, p. A69

ROBERTS, Deborah, Administrator, Lawrence County Hospital, Monticello, MS, p. A241

ROBERTS, Gregory P., Chief Executive Officer, Ancora Psychiatric Hospital, Ancora, NJ, p. A274

ROBERTS, Jean E., Administrator, Mark Reed Hospital, McCleary, WA, p. A454

ROBERTS, John W., President and Chief Executive Officer, Union Regional Medical Center, Monroe, NC, p. A315

© 2000 AHA Guide

ROBERTS, Jonathan, Dr.PH, Administrator, Earl K. Long Medical Center, Baton Rouge, LA, p. A180
ROBERTS, Kenneth D., President, John T. Mather Memorial Hospital, Port Jefferson, NY, p. A303
ROBERTS, Robert D., President, Pacific Coast Hospital, San Francisco, CA, p. A60
ROBERTS, Shane, Administrator, St. Luke Community Hospital, Ronan, MT, p. A259
ROBERTS, Jr, George T., FACHE, Chief Executive Officer, Henderson Memorial Hospital, Henderson, TX, p. A415
ROBERTSON, Andrew S., M.D., Chief Executive Officer, Providence Yakima Medical Center, Yakima, WA, p. A459
ROBERTSON, B. W., Administrator and Chief Executive Officer, Parkview Hospital, Wheeler, TX, p. A434
ROBERTSON, David, Chief Executive Officer, Duncan Regional Hospital, Duncan, OK, p. A342
ROBERTSON, Jeffrey J., Chief Executive Officer, Lakeview Hospital, Stillwater, MN, p. A234
ROBERTSON, John L., Chief Executive Officer, Wiregrass Medical Center, Geneva, AL, p. A15
ROBERTSON, Thomas L., President and Chief Executive Officer, Carilion Health System, Roanoke, VA, p. B64
ROBERTSON, William G.
  Chief Executive Officer, Saint Luke's South Hospital, Overland Park, KS, p. A166
  Chief Executive Officer, Shawnee Mission Medical Center, Shawnee Mission, KS, p. A168
ROBERTSON , Jr, James E., President, Salem Township Hospital, Salem, IL, p. A134
ROBERTSTAD, John R.
  President and Chief Executive Officer, Bixby Medical Center, Lenawee Health Alliance, Adrian, MI, p. A211
  President and Chief Executive Officer, Herrick Memorial Hospital, Lenawee Health Alliance, Tecumseh, MI, p. A223
ROBINSON, Brian C., Chief Executive Officer, North Florida Regional Medical Center, Gainesville, FL, p. A85
ROBINSON, Edward P., Administrator, Community Hospital, Munster, IN, p. A144
ROBINSON, Glenn A., Chief Executive Officer, Nacogdoches Medical Center, Nacogdoches, TX, p. A424
ROBINSON, Karenlee, Chief Operating Officer, Sharp Mesa Vista Hospital, San Diego, CA, p. A59
ROBINSON, Michael, Executive Vice President and Administrator, Memorial Regional Medical Center, Mechanicsville, VA, p. A446
ROBINSON, Phillip D., Chief Executive Officer, J. F. K. Medical Center, Atlantis, FL, p. A81
ROBINSON, Raymond, Chief Executive Officer, Worcester State Hospital, Worcester, MA, p. A210
ROBINSON, Richard F., Director, Veterans Affairs Medical Center, Fayetteville, AR, p. A29
ROBINSON, Thomas D., FACHE, Chief Executive Officer, Governor Juan F. Louis Hospital, Christiansted, VI, p. A484
ROBY, William J., Executive Vice President, Mountain Manor Treatment Center, Emmitsburg, MD, p. A198
ROCHE, Joseph, Administrator, St. Vincent Jennings Hospital, North Vernon, IN, p. A144
ROCK, Lauren, Chief Operating Officer, Euclid Hospital, Euclid, OH, p. A331
ROCKWOOD , Jr, John M., President and Chief Executive Officer, Munson Healthcare, Traverse City, MI, p. B112
RODERICK, Travis W., Administrator and Chief Executive Officer, Mena Medical Center, Mena, AR, p. A32
RODGERS, Edward, Chief Executive Officer, Yoakum County Hospital, Denver City, TX, p. A410
RODGERS, Robert, Administrator and Senior Executive Officer, St. James Community Hospital, Butte, MT, p. A256
RODRIGUEZ, Julio Andino, Executive Director, Ponce Regional Hospital, Ponce, PR, p. A483
RODRIGUEZ, Maria Del Pilar, Chief Executive Officer, Dr. Ramon E. Betances Hospital–Mayaguez Medical Center Branch, Mayaguez, PR, p. A483
RODRIGUEZ, Maria Elena, Executive Administrator, Hospital San Pablo Del Este, Fajardo, PR, p. A482
RODRIGUEZ, Roberto, Executive Director and Chief Executive Officer, LAC/University of Southern California Medical Center, Los Angeles, CA, p. A48
RODRIGUEZ, Roy, Ph.D.
  Chief Executive Officer, Bayview Hospital and Mental Health System, Chula Vista, CA, p. A38
  Chief Executive Officer, Villaview Community Hospital, San Diego, CA, p. A59
ROE , Jr, Louis G., Administrator, Williamson ARH Hospital, South Williamson, KY, p. A178
ROEBUCK, Jason N., Chief Executive Officer, HEALTHSOUTH Treasure Coast Rehabilitation Hospital, Vero Beach, FL, p. A97
ROEDER, John R., President and Chief Executive Officer, Providence Hospital, Mobile, AL, p. A16
ROETS, George A., MS, Executive Director, Buffalo Psychiatric Center, Buffalo, NY, p. A289
ROGERS, Bryan R., President and Chief Executive Officer, Riverside Community Hospital, Riverside, CA, p. A57
ROGERS, Charles L., President, Cushing Memorial Hospital, Leavenworth, KS, p. A164
ROGERS, Christopher J., Administrator, Auburn Memorial Hospital, Auburn, NY, p. A287
ROGERS, Tracy A., Chief Executive Officer, Lakeland Medical Center, New Orleans, LA, p. A186
ROGERSON, Russell E., Warden, Iowa Medical and Classification Center, Oakdale, IA, p. A155
ROGOLS, Kevin L., President and Chief Executive Officer, Finley Hospital, Dubuque, IA, p. A151
ROHALEY, Richard L., President and Chief Executive Officer, Jackson General Hospital, Ripley, WV, p. A464
ROHALL, Roger, Chief Executive Officer, Rivendell of Michigan, Saint Johns, MI, p. A222
ROHAN, Heather J., Chief Executive Officer, Palms West Hospital, Loxahatchee, FL, p. A88
ROHLEDER, Howard E., Administrator and Chief Executive Officer, Salem Community Hospital, Salem, OH, p. A337
ROHRICH, George A., Administrator, Pembina County Memorial Hospital and Wedgewood Manor, Cavalier, ND, p. A321
ROJEK, Kenneth J., Chief Executive, Lutheran General Hospital, Park Ridge, IL, p. A132
ROMANO, John A., Chief Executive Officer, Mountain View Hospital, Gadsden, AL, p. A15
ROMANO, Patrick A., Interim Chief Executive Officer, Gateway Regional Health System, Mount Sterling, KY, p. A177
ROMER, James E., President and Chief Executive Officer, Hospital Center at Orange, Orange, NJ, p. A279
ROMERO, Marcella A., Administrator, Espanola Hospital, Espanola, NM, p. A284
ROMERO, Vicki L., Chief Executive Officer, Longview Regional Medical Center, Longview, TX, p. A422
ROMOFF, Jeffrey A., President, UPMC Health System, Pittsburgh, PA, p. B150
RONA, J. Michael, President, Virginia Mason Medical Center, Seattle, WA, p. A457
RONSTROM, Stephen F., Executive Vice President and Administrator, Sacred Heart Hospital, Eau Claire, WI, p. A468
ROODMAN, Richard D., Chief Executive Officer, Valley Medical Center, Renton, WA, p. A456
ROONEY, Ronald K., President, Arkansas Methodist Hospital, Paragould, AR, p. A33
ROOS, Mary, President and Chief Executive Officer, St. Joseph Community Hospital, Mishawaka, IN, p. A144
ROOT, Darwin E., Administrator, Harrison Memorial Hospital, Cynthiana, KY, p. A171
ROPCHAN, Rebecca, Administrator, Scripps Memorial Hospital–Encinitas, Encinitas, CA, p. A40
RORAFF, Greg, President and Chief Executive Officer, Memorial Hospital of Taylor County, Medford, WI, p. A471
ROSASCO , Jr, Edward J., President and Chief Executive Officer, Mercy Hospital, Miami, FL, p. A90
ROSE, J. Anthony, President and Chief Executive Officer, Catawba Memorial Hospital, Hickory, NC, p. A314
ROSE, Lance H., FACHE, President and Chief Executive Officer, Centre Community Hospital, State College, PA, p. A372
ROSE, Richard, M.D., President and Chief Administrative Officer, Fort Sanders Regional Medical Center, Knoxville, TN, p. A394
ROSE, Walt, Associate Administrator, Highsmith–Rainey Memorial Hospital, Fayetteville, NC, p. A312
ROSE, Renee, President and Chief Executive Officer, Horizon Healthcare, Inc., Milwaukee, WI, p. B99
ROSEBOROUGH, James W., CHE, Director, Veterans Affairs Medical Center, Ann Arbor, MI, p. A211
ROSEN, David P.
  President, Jamaica Hospital Medical Center, New York, NY, p. A297
  President and Chief Executive Officer, New York Flushing Hospital Medical Center, New York, NY, p. A298
ROSENBERG, Leroy J., Executive Director, Virrua West Jersey Hospital–Marlton, Marlton, NJ, p. A277
ROSENTHAL, David S., M.D., Director, Stillman Infirmary, Harvard University Health Services, Cambridge, MA, p. A204
ROSENVALL, Greg, Administrator, Gunnison Valley Hospital, Gunnison, UT, p. A436
ROSS, David, Chief Executive Officer, Phelps County Regional Medical Center, Rolla, MO, p. A252
ROSS, Hank, Chief Executive Officer, HEALTHSOUTH Rehabilitation Hospital, Oklahoma City, OK, p. A345
ROSS, James E., FACHE
  Chief Executive Officer, Deaton Specialty Hospital and Home, Baltimore, MD, p. A195
  Chief Executive Officer, James Lawrence Kernan Hospital, Baltimore, MD, p. A195
ROSS, Joseph P.
  President and Chief Executive Officer, Dorchester General Hospital, Cambridge, MD, p. A197
  President and Chief Executive Officer, Memorial Hospital at Easton Maryland, Easton, MD, p. A198
ROSS, Kenneth R., Chief Executive Officer, Arbuckle Memorial Hospital, Sulphur, OK, p. A347
ROSS, Zeff, Administrator, Memorial Hospital West, Pembroke Pines, FL, p. A92
ROSS , Jr, Semmes, Administrator, Franklin County Memorial Hospital, Meadville, MS, p. A240
ROSSETTI, Stephen J., Ph.D., President and Chief Executive Officer, Saint Luke Institute, Silver Spring, MD, p. A200
ROSSFELD, John, Administrator, University of Miami Hospital and Clinics, Miami, FL, p. A90
ROSSI, L. J., M.D., Chief Executive Officer, Hopedale Medical Complex, Hopedale, IL, p. A128
ROSSIO, Gary J., Director and Chief Executive Officer, Veterans Affairs Medical Center, San Diego, CA, p. A59
ROTH, Barry H., President and Chief Executive Officer, Allegheny University Hospitals, Forbes Regional, Monroeville, PA, p. A364
ROTH, Mark S., Chief Executive Officer, Woodside Hospital, Newport News, VA, p. A446
ROTH, William, Chief Executive Officer, HEALTHSOUTH Chesapeake Rehabilitation Hospital, Salisbury, MD, p. A200
ROTHLEIN, Gerald, Chief Executive Officer, Children's Medical Center, Tulsa, OK, p. A348
ROTHSTEIN, Ronald, President and Chief Executive Officer, Levindale Hebrew Geriatric Center and Hospital, Baltimore, MD, p. A196
ROTHSTEIN, Ruth M., Chief, Cook County Bureau of Health Services, Chicago, IL, p. B75
ROURKE, Thomas E., Administrator, Glen Oaks Hospital, Greenville, TX, p. A414
ROUSH, Sharon L., Chief Executive Officer, Tallahassee Community Hospital, Tallahassee, FL, p. A96
ROWAN, Michael Terrance
  President and Chief Executive Officer, St. Elizabeth Health Center, Youngstown, OH, p. A340
  President and Chief Executive Officer, St. Joseph Health Center, Warren, OH, p. A339
ROWE, Gary L., President and Chief Executive Officer, St. John's Regional Medical Center, Joplin, MO, p. A248
ROWE, John W., M.D., President, Mount Sinai–NYU Hospitals/Health System, New York, NY, p. A298
ROWLAND, Phil, Chief Executive Officer, Grandview Medical Center, Jasper, TN, p. A393

ROWLEY, K. Steven, CHE, President and Chief Executive Officer, Wilson N. Jones Medical Center, Sherman, TX, p. A431
ROWTON, William, Chief Executive Officer, Cozby–Germany Hospital, Grand Saline, TX, p. A414
ROYAL, Stephen L., President and Chief Executive Officer, Southwest Florida Regional Medical Center, Fort Myers, FL, p. A85
ROYER, Thomas C., M.D., President, Christus Health, Irving, TX, p. B72
ROYNAN, Joseph, Administrator, Northwestern Institute, Fort Washington, PA, p. A360
ROZEK, Thomas M., President and Chief Executive Officer, Miami Children's Hospital, Miami, FL, p. A90
RUBERTE, Henry, Executive Director, Hospital Metropolitan, San Juan, PR, p. A483
RUBIN, Harold, FACHE, President and Chief Executive Officer, Midland Memorial Hospital, Midland, TX, p. A424
RUCKDESCHEL, John C., M.D., Director and Chief Executive Officer, H. Lee Moffitt Cancer Center and Research Institute, Tampa, FL, p. A96
RUDEGEAIR, Bernard C., President and Chief Executive Officer, Hazleton–St. Joseph Medical Center, Hazleton, PA, p. A361
RUDES, Bryan F.
  Executive Director, Richard H. Hutchings Psychiatric Center, Syracuse, NY, p. A306
  Executive Director, Rochester Psychiatric Center, Rochester, NY, p. A304
RUDES, Sarah F., Executive Director, Mohawk Valley Psychiatric Center, Utica, NY, p. A306
RUELAS, Raul D., M.D., Administrator, Gulf Coast Treatment Center, Fort Walton Beach, FL, p. A85
RUFFIN, Edward W., Administrator, Coliseum Psychiatric Center, Macon, GA, p. A107
RUGGE, John, M.D., Chief Executive Officer, McClellan Health System, Cambridge, NY, p. A289
RUGLE, Kenneth, Interim Director, Central Alabama Veteran Affairs Health Care System, Montgomery, AL, p. A17
RUIZ, Manuel Diaz, President, Mepsi Center, Bayamon, PR, p. A482
RUMLEY, Darrell, Service Unit Director and Chief Executive Officer, U. S. Public Health Service Indian Hospital, Sells, AZ, p. A26
RUMPZ, Mary Renetta, FACHE, President and Chief Executive Officer, St. Mary Hospital, Livonia, MI, p. A218
RUNDIO, Robert A., Executive Director of Hospital Operations, Valley Lutheran Hospital, Mesa, AZ, p. A23
RUPIPER, Allen V., President, Adena Health System, Chillicothe, OH, p. A327
RUPP, William, M.D., President and Chief Executive Officer, Luther Hospital, Eau Claire, WI, p. A468
RUPPERT, James C., Administrator, Alegent Health Mercy Hospital, Corning, IA, p. A149
RUSE, William E., FACHE, President and Chief Executive Officer, Blanchard Valley Health Association System, Findlay, OH, p. A332
RUSH, Domenica, Administrator, Sierra Vista Hospital, Truth or Consequences, NM, p. A286
RUSH, Donald J., Chief Executive Officer, Sidney Health Center, Sidney, MT, p. A259
RUSH, Matthew, President, Hayes–Green–Beach Memorial Hospital, Charlotte, MI, p. A212
RUSHING, R. Lynn, Chief Executive Officer, Brook Lane Health Services, Hagerstown, MD, p. A198
RUSKAN, Jeff, Administrator, HEALTHSOUTH Rehabilitation Hospital of Virginia, Richmond, VA, p. A449
RUSSEL, Kimberly A., President and Chief Executive Officer, Mary Greeley Medical Center, Ames, IA, p. A148
RUSSELL, Daniel F., President and Chief Executive Officer, Catholic Health East, Newtown Square, PA, p. B66
RUSSELL, Gordon H., Administrator, Hi-Plains Hospital, Hale Center, TX, p. A415
RUSSELL, James D. M., Chief Executive Officer, St. Mary's Healthcare Center, Pierre, SD, p. A387
RUSSELL, Linda B., President, The Woman's Hospital of Texas, Houston, TX, p. A418
RUSSELL, Mark R., Chief Executive Officer, Riveredge Hospital, Forest Park, IL, p. A126
RUSSELL, Tim, Administrator, Stillwater Community Hospital, Columbus, MT, p. A257
RUSSELL, Webster T., Chief Executive Officer, South Central Kansas Regional Medical Center, Arkansas City, KS, p. A159
RUSSELL, William, Chief Executive Officer, Riverton Memorial Hospital, Riverton, WY, p. A479
RUTENBERG, Jack, Administrator, Villa Maria Hospital, North Miami, FL, p. A91
RUTHERFORD, James A., President and Chief Executive Officer, St. Clare's Hospital and Health Center, New York, NY, p. A300
RUTLEDGE, Valinda, President, St. Anthony Hospital, Oklahoma City, OK, p. A346
RUYLE, W. Kenneth, Director, Veterans Affairs Medical Center, Tuscaloosa, AL, p. A19
RUZYCKI, Frank C., Executive Director, Roosevelt Warm Springs Institute for Rehabilitation, Warm Springs, GA, p. A111
RYAN, Michael J., Administrator, Nemaha Valley Community Hospital, Seneca, KS, p. A167
RYAN, Patricia, Senior Vice President, Bryn Mawr Rehabilitation Hospital, Malvern, PA, p. A363
RYAN, Thomas E., President, Alamance Regional Medical Center, Burlington, NC, p. A310
RYAN, Mary Jean, President and Chief Executive Officer, SSM Health Care, Saint Louis, MO, p. B136
RYLE, Deborah L., Chief Executive Officer, Round Rock Hospital, Round Rock, TX, p. A427

S

SABA, Francis M., President and Chief Executive Officer, Milford–Whitinsville Regional Hospital, Milford, MA, p. A206
SABIN, Margaret D., Chief Executive Officer, Yampa Valley Medical Center, Steamboat Springs, CO, p. A73
SABIN, Robert H., Director, Aleda E. Lutz Veterans Affairs Medical Center, Saginaw, MI, p. A221
SABO, Michael A., Director, Veterans Affairs Hudson Valley Health Care System–F.D. Roosevelt Hospital, Montrose, NY, p. A294
SABOL, Don J., Chief Executive Officer, Hardin Memorial Hospital, Kenton, OH, p. A333
SACCO, Frank V., FACHE, Chief Executive Officer, Memorial Healthcare System, Los Angeles, FL, p. B110
SACK, Michael V., President and Chief Executive Officer, Union Hospital, Elkton, MD, p. A198
SACKETT, John, Chief Executive Officer, Avista Adventist Hospital, Louisville, CO, p. A72
SACKETT, Walter, Chief Executive Officer, Sunhealth Specialty Hospital for Denver, Thornton, CO, p. A73
SADAU, Ernie W., President and Chief Executive Officer, Hinsdale Hospital, Hinsdale, IL, p. A128
SADLACK, Frank J., Ph.D., Executive Director, La Hacienda Treatment Center, Hunt, TX, p. A419
SADLER, Blair L., President and Chief Executive Officer, Children's Hospital and Health Center, San Diego, CA, p. A58
SADLER, Wanda H., Chief Executive Officer, ValueMark West End Behavioral Healthcare System, Richmond, VA, p. A449
SADVARY, Thomas J., FACHE, Senior Vice President and Chief Operating Officer, Scottsdale Healthcare–Shea, Scottsdale, AZ, p. A25
SAFIAN, Keith F., President and Chief Executive Officer, Phelps Memorial Hospital Center, Sleepy Hollow, NY, p. A305
SAGO, Glenn R., Administrator, Arkansas State Hospital, Little Rock, AR, p. A31
SAHAGIAN, Janine, Administrator and Chief Executive Officer, Wilson Center Psychiatric Facility for Children and Adolescents, Faribault, MN, p. A228
SAIRLS, C. Ronnie, Administrator, St. Vincent Rehabilitation Hospital, Sherwood, AR, p. A33
SAKS, Stephen H., Chief Executive Officer, John F. Kennedy Memorial Hospital, Philadelphia, PA, p. A367
SALA, Jr, Anthony S., Chief Executive Officer, Highland Hospital, Shreveport, LA, p. A188
SALANGER, Matthew J., President and Chief Executive Officer, United Health Services Hospitals–Binghamton, Binghamton, NY, p. A288
SALBER, M. Agnes, Prioress, Missionary Benedictine Sisters American Province, Norfolk, NE, p. B111
SALEAPAGA, Iotamo T., M.D., Director Health, Lyndon B. Johnson Tropical Medical Center, Pago Pago, AS, p. A481
SALLUZZO, Richard, Chief Executive Officer, Conemaugh Memorial Medical Center, Johnstown, PA, p. A362
SALMON, Robert J.
  Administrator, Deuel County Memorial Hospital, Clear Lake, SD, p. A385
  Chief Executive Officer, Sioux Valley Canby Campus, Canby, MN, p. A226
SALTZMAN, M. Joanne, Interim Administrator, Vencor Hospital–Mansfield, Mansfield, TX, p. A423
SAMPSON, Arthur J., President and Chief Executive Officer, Newport Hospital, Newport, RI, p. A376
SANCHEZ, Jose R.
  Executive Director, Lincoln Medical and Mental Health Center, New York, NY, p. A297
  Executive Director, Metropolitan Hospital Center, New York, NY, p. A298
SANDER, Larry J., FACHE, Director, Veterans Affairs Medical Center–Louisville, Louisville, KY, p. A176
SANDERS, David, Administrator, Brooks County Hospital, Quitman, GA, p. A108
SANDERS, John W., Chief Executive Officer, Forest Park Hospital, Saint Louis, MO, p. A253
SANDERS, Larry, FACHE, Chairman and Chief Executive Officer, Columbus Regional Health System, Columbus, GA, p. B73
SANDERS, Steve, Vice President and Chief Executive Officer, Memorial Hermann The Woodlands Hospital, The Woodlands, TX, p. A432
SANDLIN, Keith, Chief Executive Officer, Emory Cartersville Medical Center, Cartersville, GA, p. A102
SANFORD, Edward J., Chief Executive Officer, Cumberland County Hospital, Burkesville, KY, p. A170
SANGER, William A., President and Chief Executive Officer, Cancer Treatment Centers of America, Arlington Heights, IL, p. B63
SANNER, Charlotte K., M.D., Director Health Service, Simpson Infirmary, Wellesley College, Wellesley, MA, p. A209
SANTIAGO, Pedro Juan, Executive Director, Caguas Regional Hospital, Caguas, PR, p. A482
SANTIAGO–VEGA, Francisco, Consultor, Lafayette Hospital, Arroyo, PR, p. A481
SANTILLI, Arthur E., President, Masonic Geriatric Healthcare Center, Wallingford, CT, p. A77
SANTORO, Thomas A., Administrator, Elizabethtown Community Hospital, Elizabethtown, NY, p. A291
SANZONE, Raymond D., Executive Director, Tewksbury Hospital, Tewksbury, MA, p. A209
SARDONE, Frank J.
  President and Chief Executive Officer, Bronson Healthcare Group, Inc., Kalamazoo, MI, p. B63
  President and Chief Executive Officer, Bronson Methodist Hospital, Kalamazoo, MI, p. A218
  President, Bronson Vicksburg Hospital, Vicksburg, MI, p. A223
SARKAR, George A., JD, Executive Director, Manhattan Eye, Ear and Throat Hospital, New York, NY, p. A298
SARKIS, Lucy, M.D., Executive Director, South Beach Psychiatric Center, New York, NY, p. A300
SARLE, C. Richard, President and Chief Executive Officer, Carrier Foundation, Belle Mead, NJ, p. A274
SARNESO, Mark, Chief Executive Officer, Cove Forge Behavioral Health System, Williamsburg, PA, p. A374
SATCHER, Richard H., Chief Executive Officer, Aiken Regional Medical Centers, Aiken, SC, p. A378
SATO, James, Senior Vice President and Chief Executive Officer, Western Arizona Regional Medical Center, Bullhead City, AZ, p. A22
SATZGER, Bruce G., President, Commmunity Hospital of San Bernardino, San Bernardino, CA, p. A58
SAULS, Randy, Administrator, Louis Smith Memorial Hospital, Lakeland, GA, p. A106

Index of Health Care Professionals / Saulters

SAULTERS, W. Dale, Administrator, Winston Medical Center, Louisville, MS, p. A240
SAUNDERS, Donald F., President, Androscoggin Valley Hospital, Berlin, NH, p. A271
SAUNDERS, Linda, Administrator, Guyan Valley Hospital, Logan, WV, p. A462
SCHADER, JoAnne G., R.N., Interim Chief Executive Officer, Sharp Chula Vista Medical Center, Chula Vista, CA, p. A38
SCHADT, Alton M., Executive Director, Warren General Hospital, Warren, PA, p. A373
SCHAEFER, Michele, Chief Executive Officer, Saint Joseph Health Center, Kansas City, MO, p. A248
SCHAENGOLD, Phillip S., JD, Chief Executive Officer, George Washington University Hospital, Washington, DC, p. A79
SCHAETZLE, Daniel J., Administrator, Community Hospital–Lakeview, Eufaula, OK, p. A343
SCHAFER, Michael, Chief Executive Officer, Spooner Health System, Spooner, WI, p. A475
SCHAFFER, Arnold R., President and Chief Executive Officer, Glendale Memorial Hospital and Health Center, Glendale, CA, p. A42
SCHAFFER, Gregory F., President, Johns Hopkins Bayview Medical Center, Baltimore, MD, p. A195
SCHAFFNER, Leroy, Chief Executive Officer, Coon Memorial Hospital and Home, Dalhart, TX, p. A408
SCHANDLER, Jon B., President and Chief Executive Officer, White Plains Hospital Center, White Plains, NY, p. A307
SCHANWALD, Pamela R., Chief Executive Officer, Children's Home of Pittsburgh, Pittsburgh, PA, p. A369
SCHAPER, Robert F., President and Chief Executive Officer, Tomball Regional Hospital, Tomball, TX, p. A432
SCHAPPER, Robert A., Chief Executive Officer, Palm Drive Hospital, Sebastopol, CA, p. A63
SCHATZLEIN, Michael H., M.D., President and Chief Executive Officer, St. Joseph Hospital, Fort Wayne, IN, p. A140
SCHAUER, Charles A., Ph.D., President and Chief Executive Officer, Brooks Rehabilitation Hospital, Jacksonville, FL, p. A86
SCHAUM, James H., President and Chief Executive Officer, Allen Memorial Hospital, Oberlin, OH, p. A336
SCHAUMBURG, John, Administrator, Lanai Community Hospital, Lanai City, HI, p. A113
SCHERR, Morris L., Executive Vice President and Chief Operating Officer, Taylor Manor Hospital, Ellicott City, MD, p. A198
SCHERTZ, David A., Administrator, Saint Anthony Medical Center, Rockford, IL, p. A134
SCHIMPFF, Stephen C., M.D., Chief Executive Officer, University of Maryland Medical Center, Baltimore, MD, p. A196
SCHIMSCHEINER, Mary Joel, Chief Executive Officer, Kenmore Mercy Hospital, Kenmore, NY, p. A293
SCHINDELAR, Carl J., President, Franklin Square Hospital Center, Baltimore, MD, p. A195
SCHINTZ, Conrad W., Senior Vice–President Operations, Penn State Geisinger Wyoming Valley Medical Center, Wilkes-Barre, PA, p. A374
SCHIOP, Judi, Administrator, Harbor Oaks Hospital, New Baltimore, MI, p. A220
SCHIROS, Judy, Administrator, Campbellton Graceville Hospital, Graceville, FL, p. A85
SCHLAUTMAN, Jacolyn M., Executive Vice President and Administrator, St. Joseph's Hospital, Breese, IL, p. A120
SCHLEGELMILCH, Kurt W., CHE, Director, Veterans Affairs Medical Center, Grand Junction, CO, p. A71
SCHLEIF, John V., Administrator, St. Francis Medical Center–West, Ewa Beach, HI, p. A112
SCHMELTER, Robert, President, Community Hospital of Ottawa, Ottawa, IL, p. A132
SCHMIDT, Craig W. C.
President and Chief Executive Officer, Berlin Memorial Hospital, Berlin, WI, p. A467
President and Chief Executive Officer, Wild Rose Community Memorial Hospital, Wild Rose, WI, p. A477
SCHMIDT, Gene E., President, Hutchinson Hospital Corporation, Hutchinson, KS, p. A163

SCHMIDT, Mark, President and Chief Executive Officer, Gettysburg Medical Center, Gettysburg, SD, p. A386
SCHMIDT, Marvy, Administrator, Schick Shadel Hospital, Seattle, WA, p. A456
SCHMIDT, Michael A., President and Chief Executive Officer, Saint Joseph's Hospital, Marshfield, WI, p. A471
SCHMIDT, Richard T., Executive Director, Decatur Hospital, Decatur, GA, p. A103
SCHMIDT, Steve, Chief Executive Officer, Redding Medical Center, Redding, CA, p. A56
SCHMIDT, Timothy E., Chief Executive Officer, Mimbres Memorial Hospital, Deming, NM, p. A284
SCHMIDT , Jr, Richard O.
President and Chief Executive Officer, Kenosha Hospital and Medical Center, Kenosha, WI, p. A469
President and Chief Executive Officer, St. Catherine's Hospital, Kenosha, WI, p. A470
SCHMITT, M. Eileen, M.D., President and Chief Executive Officer, St. Francis Hospital, Wilmington, DE, p. A78
SCHMITT, Thomas, Administrator, Integris Bass Baptist Health Center, Enid, OK, p. A343
SCHNEDLER, Lisa, Administrator, Van Buren County Hospital, Keosauqua, IA, p. A153
SCHNEIDER, Barry S., Chief Executive Officer, Watsonville Community Hospital, Watsonville, CA, p. A67
SCHNEIDER, C. W., President and Chief Executive Officer, Northwest Hospital, Seattle, WA, p. A456
SCHNEIDER, Carol, Chief Executive Officer, Christ Hospital and Medical Center, Oak Lawn, IL, p. A131
SCHNEIDER, Charles F., President, Day Kimball Hospital, Putnam, CT, p. A76
SCHNEIDER, David R., Executive Director, Langlade Memorial Hospital, Antigo, WI, p. A466
SCHNEIDER, Mark E., Chief Executive Officer, Rivendell Behavioral Health Services, Benton, AR, p. A28
SCHNEIDER, Thomas R., Administrator, Shriners Hospitals for Children, Shreveport, Shreveport, LA, p. A189
SCHOCK, Carl, Superintendent, Austin State Hospital, Austin, TX, p. A402
SCHOEN, William J.
Vice President, Allied Services Rehabilitation Hospital, Scranton, PA, p. A371
Chairman and Chief Executive Officer, Health Management Associates, Naples, FL, p. B94
SCHOENHOLTZ, Jack C., M.D., Medical Director, Administrator and President, Rye Hospital Center, Rye, NY, p. A304
SCHON, John, Administrator and Chief Executive Officer, Dickinson County Healthcare System, Iron Mountain, MI, p. A217
SCHRADER, Michael E., President and Chief Executive Officer, Wyoming Medical Center, Casper, WY, p. A478
SCHRAMM, Michael, Administrator, Arlington Municipal Hospital, Arlington, MN, p. A225
SCHRECK, Edward, Chief Executive Officer, USC University Hospital, Los Angeles, CA, p. A50
SCHRECK, Ted, Chief Executive Officer, University of Southern California–Kenneth Norris Jr. Cancer Hospital, Los Angeles, CA, p. A50
SCHREEG, Timothy M., President and Chief Executive Officer, Jasper County Hospital, Rensselaer, IN, p. A145
SCHREIVOGEL, Herman, Administrator and Chief Executive Officer, Lincoln Community Hospital and Nursing Home, Hugo, CO, p. A71
SCHROEDER, Connie L., Chief Executive Officer, Illini Community Hospital, Pittsfield, IL, p. A133
SCHROEDER, Dudley J., Deputy Commander, Bassett Army Community Hospital, Fort Wainwright, AK, p. A20
SCHROTH, Lynn, Dr.PH, Executive Vice President, The Methodist Hospital, Houston, TX, p. A418
SCHRUPP, Richard, President and Chief Executive Officer, Mercy Hospital of Franciscan Sisters, Oelwein, IA, p. A155
SCHUETZ, Charles D., Chief Executive Officer, Kingwood Medical Center, Kingwood, TX, p. A420
SCHULER, G. Wayne, Executive Director, Madison County Medical Center, Canton, MS, p. A237

SCHULER, William J., Chief Executive Officer, Portsmouth Regional Hospital and Pavilion, Portsmouth, NH, p. A273
SCHULLER, David E., M.D., Chief Executive Officer, Arthur G. James Cancer Hospital and Richard J. Solove Research Institute, Columbus, OH, p. A329
SCHULTE, James E., Administrator, Redwood Falls Municipal Hospital, Redwood Falls, MN, p. A232
SCHULTE, Paul A., Chief Executive Officer, Brunswick Community Hospital, Supply, NC, p. A318
SCHULTZ, Michael H., Chief Executive Officer, Feather River Hospital, Paradise, CA, p. A54
SCHULTZ, Steve C., President, Callahan Eye Foundation Hospital, Birmingham, AL, p. A12
SCHULZ, Charles K., Chief Executive Officer, York General Hospital, York, NE, p. A267
SCHULZ, Larry A., President and Chief Executive Officer, St. Gabriel's Hospital, Little Falls, MN, p. A229
SCHURMEIER, L. Jon, President and Chief Executive Officer, Southwest General Health Center, Middleburg Heights, OH, p. A335
SCHURRA, Ronald J., Administrator, Hilo Medical Center, Hilo, HI, p. A112
SCHUSTER, Christine C., Chief Executive Officer, Quincy Medical Center, Quincy, MA, p. A208
SCHUSTER, Emmett C., Chief Executive Officer and Administrator, Choctaw Memorial Hospital, Hugo, OK, p. A344
SCHWAB, Caryn A., Executive Director, The Mount Sinai Hospital of Queens, New York, NY, p. A300
SCHWANKE, Dan, Executive Director, St. Francis Health Care Centre, Green Springs, OH, p. A332
SCHWARM, Tony, President, Clay County Hospital, Flora, IL, p. A126
SCHWARTZ, John N., Chief Executive Officer, Trinity Hospital, Chicago, IL, p. A124
SCHWARTZ, Mark, Administrator, Hartford Memorial Hospital, Hartford, WI, p. A469
SCHWARTZ, Michael J., President and Chief Executive Officer, Prince William Hospital, Manassas, VA, p. A446
SCHWARTZBERG, Gil, President and Chief Executive Officer, City of Hope National Medical Center, Duarte, CA, p. A40
SCHWARZ, Donald E., Administrator, Vencor Hospital–Boston, Boston, MA, p. A203
SCHWEIGERT, Byron, Chief Executive Officer, Long Beach Memorial Medical Center, Long Beach, CA, p. A46
SCHWEIKHART, Douglas P., Administrator, Tyler Healthcare Center/Avera Health, Tyler, MN, p. A234
SCHWEITZER, Alex, Superintendent and Chief Executive Officer, North Dakota State Hospital, Jamestown, ND, p. A323
SCHWEITZER, Robert, Ed.D.
Executive Director, Queens Children's Psychiatric Center, New York, NY, p. A299
Executive Director, Sagamore Children's Psychiatric Center, Huntington Station, NY, p. A293
SCHWEMER, David J., Administrator, Woodrow Wilson Rehabilitation Center, Fishersville, VA, p. A444
SCHWIENTEK, Barbara, Executive Director, Monticello Big Lake Hospital, Monticello, MN, p. A231
SCIOLA, Anthony, President and Chief Executive Officer, Shaughnessy–Kaplan Rehabilitation Hospital, Salem, MA, p. A208
SCOTT, Camille, Administrator, Benewah Community Hospital, Saint Maries, ID, p. A117
SCOTT, Charles F., President and Chief Executive Officer, Doctors Hospital of Sarasota, Sarasota, FL, p. A95
SCOTT, Grady, President and Chief Executive Officer, Copper Basin Medical Center, Copperhill, TN, p. A391
SCOTT, Jerry B., Chief Executive Officer, Northeastern Regional Hospital, Las Vegas, NM, p. A285
SCOTT, John R., Director, St. Lawrence Psychiatric Center, Ogdensburg, NY, p. A302
SCOTT, Mark D., President, Mid–Columbia Medical Center, The Dalles, OR, p. A354
SCOTT, Richard E., President, Hillcrest Baptist Medical Center, Waco, TX, p. A434

SCOTT, Steve, Chief Executive Officer, Pinelands Hospital, Nacogdoches, TX, p. A425
SCOTT, Thomas L., FACHE, President and Chief Executive Officer, Burdette Tomlin Memorial Hospital, Cape May Court House, NJ, p. A275
SEABERG, Lynn, Administrator and Chief Executive Officer, Indian Valley Hospital District, Greenville, CA, p. A43
SEAGRAVE, Richard E., Executive Director and Chief Operating Officer, Phoenixville Hospital of the University of Pennsylvania Health System, Phoenixville, PA, p. A368
SEAL, Ronald, President and Chief Executive Officer, Marion Memorial Hospital, Marion, IL, p. A130
SEALE, Corey A., Chief Executive Officer, Fallbrook Hospital District, Fallbrook, CA, p. A41
SEALE, Paul E., Chief Executive Officer, New Island Hospital, Bethpage, NY, p. A288
SEEL, W. Joseph, Administrator, Edgefield County Hospital, Edgefield, SC, p. A380
SEGLER, Randall K., Chief Executive Officer, Comanche County Memorial Hospital, Lawton, OK, p. A344
SEIBEL, Jacqueline, Administrator, Jacobson Memorial Hospital Care Center, Elgin, ND, p. A322
SEIDEL, Ken, Chief Executive Officer, Claremore Regional Hospital, Claremore, OK, p. A342
SEIDLER, Richard A., FACHE, Chief Executive Officer, Allen Memorial Hospital, Waterloo, IA, p. A157
SEIFERT, David P., President and Chief Executive Officer, St. Anthony's Medical Center, Saint Louis, MO, p. A253
SEILER, Edward H., Director, Veterans Affairs Medical Center, West Palm Beach, FL, p. A98
SEILER, Steven L., Senior Vice President and Chief Executive Officer, Good Samaritan Regional Medical Center, Phoenix, AZ, p. A24
SEIM, Richard L., Senior Vice President, Christ Hospital, Cincinnati, OH, p. A327
SEITTER, IV, Girard, CHE, Administrator, Warm Springs Rehabilitation Hospital, San Antonio, TX, p. A430
SEITZ, Stewart R., Chief Executive Officer, Gladys Spellman Specialty Hospital and Nursing Center, Cheverly, MD, p. A197
SELBERG, Jeffrey D.
President and Chief Executive Officer, Exempla Healthcare, Inc., Denver, CO, p. B84
President and Chief Executive Officer, Exempla Lutheran Medical Center, Wheat Ridge, CO, p. A73
President and Chief Executive Officer, Exempla Saint Joseph Hospital, Denver, CO, p. A69
SELDEN, Thomas A., President and Chief Executive Officer, Parma Community General Hospital, Parma, OH, p. A336
SELL, John, USAF, Administrator, U. S. Air Force Hospital, Cannon AFB, NM, p. A284
SELLARDS, Michael G., Executive Director, Pleasant Valley Hospital, Point Pleasant, WV, p. A463
SELLARS, Thomas V., Superintendent, Memphis Mental Health Institute, Memphis, TN, p. A396
SELTZER, Charlotte, Chief Executive Officer, Creedmoor Psychiatric Center, New York, NY, p. A296
SELZ, Timothy P., President and Chief Executive Officer, Provena Saint Therese Medical Center, Waukegan, IL, p. A136
SENKER, Thomas J., Interim Chief Executive Officer, Logan General Hospital, Logan, WV, p. A462
SENNEFF, Robert G., Chief Executive Officer, DeWitt Community Hospital, De Witt, IA, p. A150
SENSOR, Wayne A., Chief Executive Officer, Christus Schumpert Medical Center, Shreveport, LA, p. A188
SERAPHINE, Jeffrey G., President and Chief Executive Officer, Georgetown Community Hospital, Georgetown, KY, p. A172
SERCY, Dalmer P., Director, William S. Hall Psychiatric Institute, Columbia, SC, p. A380
SERLE, John, Administrator, Clark Fork Valley Hospital, Plains, MT, p. A259
SERNULKA, John M., President and Chief Executive Officer, Carroll County General Hospital, Westminster, MD, p. A200
SERRILL, G. B., President and Chief Executive Officer, Ellis Hospital, Schenectady, NY, p. A304
SEVERANCE, Matt, Administrator, Roper Hospital, Charleston, SC, p. A379

SEWELL, Hybard D., Administrator, Grove Hill Memorial Hospital, Grove Hill, AL, p. A15
SEWELL, Jon, Administrator, North Colorado Medical Center, Greeley, CO, p. A71
SEXTON, Charles F., Chief Executive Officer, Valley Regional Medical Center, Brownsville, TX, p. A405
SEXTON, J. Dennis, President, All Children's Hospital, Saint Petersburg, FL, p. A94
SEXTON, James J., President and Chief Executive Officer, Mercy Medical Center – North Iowa, Mason City, IA, p. A154
SEXTON, Kevin J., President and Chief Executive Officer, Holy Cross Hospital of Silver Spring, Silver Spring, MD, p. A200
SEXTON, William P., Administrator, Franciscan Skemp Healthcare–Sparta Campus, Sparta, WI, p. A475
SEYMOUR, James A., Regional Administrator, Alegent Health Community Memorial Hospital, Missouri Valley, IA, p. A154
SGANGA, Fred S., President and Chief Executive Officer, Bergen Regional Medical Center, Paramus, NJ, p. A279
SHAFER, Ronald J., Chief Executive Officer, Eastern New Mexico Medical Center, Roswell, NM, p. A285
SHAFFER, David D., Chief Executive Officer, Stonewall Jackson Memorial Hospital, Weston, WV, p. A465
SHAFFETT, Donald A., Chief Executive Officer, Clear Lake Regional Medical Center, Webster, TX, p. A434
SHAHEER, Jim, Chief Executive Officer, Charter Savannah Behavioral Health System, Savannah, GA, p. A109
SHANKER, Deo, CPA, Chief Executive Officer, Intracare North Hospital, Houston, TX, p. A417
SHANKS, James A., Administrator, Orlando Regional–Lucerne, Orlando, FL, p. A92
SHAPIRO, Edward R., M.D., Medical Director and Chief Executive Officer, Austen Riggs Center, Stockbridge, MA, p. A208
SHAPIRO, Marcia S., Chief Executive Officer, Chicago Lakeshore Hospital, Chicago, IL, p. A121
SHARFSTEIN, Steven S., M.D., President, Medical Director and Chief Executive Officer, Sheppard and Enoch Pratt Hospital, Baltimore, MD, p. A196
SHARMA, Timothy, M.D., President, Cambridge International, Inc., Houston, TX, p. B63
SHARP, Joseph, Chief Executive Officer, Capital Medical Center, Olympia, WA, p. A455
SHARP, Joseph W., Administrator, Runnells Specialized Hospital of Union County, Berkeley Heights, NJ, p. A274
SHAW, David B., Chief Executive Officer and Administrator, Nor–Lea General Hospital, Lovington, NM, p. A285
SHAW, Douglas A., Administrator, Mad River Community Hospital, Arcata, CA, p. A35
SHAW, Douglas E., President, Jewish Hospital, Louisville, KY, p. A175
SHAW, J. Michael, Administrator, Rusk County Memorial Hospital and Nursing Home, Ladysmith, WI, p. A470
SHAW, Robert C., President and Chief Executive Officer, Los Robles Regional Medical Center, Thousand Oaks, CA, p. A64
SHEAR, Bruce A., President and Chief Executive Officer, Pioneer Behavioral Health, Peabody, MA, p. B119
SHEEDY, Lucille K., Administrator and Chief Executive Officer, Wyoming County Community Hospital, Warsaw, NY, p. A307
SHEEHAN, Daniel F., Administrator, Research Belton Hospital, Belton, MO, p. A244
SHEEHAN, Kevin P., President and Chief Executive Officer, Youth and Family Centered Services, Austin, TX, p. B155
SHEEHAN, Michael J., Administrator, Hastings Regional Center, Hastings, NE, p. A263
SHEEHY, Earl N., Administrator, Mid Dakota Hospital, Chamberlain, SD, p. A385
SHEHORN, Patricia, Chief Executive Officer, Westlake Hospital, Melrose Park, IL, p. A130
SHELBY, Dennis R., Chief Executive Officer, HEALTHSOUTH Rehabilitation Hospital, Fayetteville, AR, p. A29
SHELBY, Marla, Administrator and Chief Executive Officer, South Lincoln Medical Center, Kemmerer, WY, p. A479

SHELDON, Lyle Ernest
President and Chief Executive Officer, Fallston General Hospital, Fallston, MD, p. A198
President and Chief Executive Officer, Harford Memorial Hospital, Havre De Grace, MD, p. A199
President and Chief Executive Officer, Upper Chesapeake Health System, Fallston, MD, p. B150
SHELL, Robert G., Chief Executive Officer, Santa Teresita Hospital, Duarte, CA, p. A40
SHELTON, James D., Chairman and Chief Executive Officer, Triad Hospitals, Inc., Dallas, TX, p. B143
SHELTON, John, President, Montclair Baptist Medical Center, Birmingham, AL, p. A12
SHELTON, II, W. Allen, Administrator and Chief Executive Officer, Eye and Ear Clinic of Charleston, Charleston, WV, p. A460
SHEPARD, Bruce, Administrator, Clinch Memorial Hospital, Homerville, GA, p. A106
SHEPARD, R. Coert, President, Anderson Hospital, Maryville, IL, p. A130
SHERMAN, James F., President and Chief Executive Officer, West Hills Hospital and Medical Center, Los Angeles, CA, p. A50
SHERON, William E., Chief Executive Officer, Wooster Community Hospital, Wooster, OH, p. A339
SHERROD, Rhonda, Administrator, Shands at Live Oak, Live Oak, FL, p. A88
SHERWOOD, John M., FACHE, Chief Executive Officer, Jefferson Memorial Hospital, Ranson, WV, p. A464
SHIELS, Rob, Administrator, Mary Shiels Hospital, Dallas, TX, p. A409
SHIMONO, Jiro R., Director, Delaware Psychiatric Center, New Castle, DE, p. A78
SHIN, Peter, DPM, President and Chairman of the Board, MedLink Hospital and Nursing Center at Capitol Hill, Washington, DC, p. A79
SHIRK, Michael B., President and Senior Executive Officer, Boone Hospital Center, Columbia, MO, p. A245
SHIRTCLIFF, Christine, Executive Vice President, Mary Lane Hospital, Ware, MA, p. A209
SHOCKNEY, Brian T., President and Chief Executive Officer, Memorial Hospital, Logansport, IN, p. A143
SHOOK, Scott E., President, Riverside Mercy Hospital, Toledo, OH, p. A338
SHORE, Muriel M., R.N., Chief Executive Officer, Essex County Hospital Center, Cedar Grove, NJ, p. A275
SHOVELIN, Wayne F., President and Chief Executive Officer, Gaston Memorial Hospital, Gastonia, NC, p. A313
SHUGARMAN, Mark, President, Mercy Hospital, Tiffin, OH, p. A338
SHULER, Priscilla J., Chief Executive Officer, Capitol Medical Center, Richmond, VA, p. A448
SHUTER, Mark H.
President, Grant/Riverside Methodist Hospitals–Grant Campus, Columbus, OH, p. A330
President, Grant/Riverside Methodist Hospitals–Riverside Campus, Columbus, OH, p. A330
SHYAVITZ, Linda, President and Chief Executive Officer, Sturdy Memorial Hospital, Attleboro, MA, p. A201
SICURELLA, John, Chief Executive Officer, Reynolds Memorial Hospital, Glen Dale, WV, p. A461
SIEBER, Thomas L., President and Chief Executive Officer, Genesis HealthCare System, Zanesville, OH, p. A340
SIEGERT, Stasha, Administrator, Throckmorton County Memorial Hospital, Throckmorton, TX, p. A432
SIEMEN–MESSING, Pauline, R.N., President and Chief Executive Officer, Harbor Beach Community Hospital, Harbor Beach, MI, p. A216
SIEMERS, Thomas R., Chief Executive Officer, Rebsamen Medical Center, Jacksonville, AR, p. A30
SIEPMAN, Milton R., Ph.D.
President and Chief Executive Officer, Baton Rouge General Medical Center, Baton Rouge, LA, p. A180
President and Chief Executive Officer, General Health System, Baton Rouge, LA, p. B86
SILBERNAGEL, Gilbert, Chief Executive Officer, Sutter Lakeside Hospital, Lakeport, CA, p. A45
SILVA, William G., Executive Director, Metropolitan State Hospital, Norwalk, CA, p. A53

Index of Health Care Professionals / Silver

SILVER, Jack B., M.P.H., Chief Executive Officer, Arizona State Hospital, Phoenix, AZ, p. A24
SILVER, Richard A., Director, James A. Haley Veterans Hospital, Tampa, FL, p. A96
SILVERMAN, Susan, Chief Executive Officer, Women's and Children's Hospital, Lafayette, LA, p. A184
SILVERNALE, Vern, Administrator, Johnson Memorial Health Services, Dawson, MN, p. A227
SILVIA, Clarence J., President and Chief Executive Officer, Bradley Memorial Hospital and Health Center, Southington, CT, p. A77
SIMMONS, Nancy, Administrator, St. John's Episcopal Hospital–South Shore, New York, NY, p. A300
SIMMONS, Stephen H.
   Senior Administrator, University of South Alabama Hospitals, Mobile, AL, p. B149
   Administrator, University of South Alabama Medical Center, Mobile, AL, p. A16
SIMMONS, Wallace R., Chief Executive Officer, Crawford Memorial Hospital, Robinson, IL, p. A133
SIMMONS, William, President and Chief Executive Officer, San Jacinto Methodist Hospital, Baytown, TX, p. A404
SIMMS, John L., President and Chief Executive Officer, Trinity Community Medical Center of Brenham, Brenham, TX, p. A405
SIMONIN, Steve J., Chief Executive Officer, Community Memorial Hospital, Clarion, IA, p. A149
SIMONIS, Iris, Chief Executive Officer, Bayou City Medical Center, Houston, TX, p. A416
SIMPATICO, Thomas, M.D., Facility Director and Network System Manager, Chicago–Read Mental Health Center, Chicago, IL, p. A121
SIMPSON, Mack N., Administrator, McCone County Medical Assistance Facility, Circle, MT, p. A256
SIMPSON, Tim, Administrator, Vencor–North Florida, Green Cove Springs, FL, p. A85
SIMS, Craig E.
   President and Chief Executive Officer, RHD Memorial Medical Center, Dallas, TX, p. A409
   President, Trinity Medical Center, Carrollton, TX, p. A406
SIMS, Jr, John H., Director, Veterans Affairs Medical Center, Togus, ME, p. A194
SINCLAIR, Mike, Administrator, Kane County Hospital, Kanab, UT, p. A436
SINEK, James J., Chief Executive Officer, Buena Vista County Hospital, Storm Lake, IA, p. A157
SINGLE, John L.
   Chief Executive Officer and Administrator, De Smet Memorial Hospital, De Smet, SD, p. A385
   Chief Executive Officer, Huron Regional Medical Center, Huron, SD, p. A386
SINGLETON, J. Knox, President and Chief Executive Officer, Inova Health System, Falls Church, VA, p. B100
SINGLETON, Thomas W., President and Chief Executive Officer, New American Healthcare Corporation, Brentwood, TN, p. B113
SINNER, James, Chief Executive Officer, Medina Memorial Hospital, Medina, NY, p. A294
SIPES, Don, Chief Executive Officer, Saint Luke's Northland Hospital–Smithville Campus, Smithville, MO, p. A254
SIPKOSKI, Michael, Executive Vice President and Administrator, St. Francis Hospital, Litchfield, IL, p. A129
SISEMORE, Roxanne, Acting Director, Jonathan M. Wainwright Memorial VA Medical Center, Walla Walla, WA, p. A458
SISK, Glenn C., President, Marion Baptist Medical Center, Hamilton, AL, p. A15
SISSON, William G., President, Central Baptist Hospital, Lexington, KY, p. A174
SISTI, Judith L., MS, Administrator, Vineland Developmental Center Hospital, Vineland, NJ, p. A281
SISTO, Dennis, President and Chief Executive Officer, Queen of the Valley Hospital, Napa, CA, p. A52
SKAGGS, Jo Ann, Chief Executive Officer, U. S. Public Health Service Indian Hospital, Mescalero, NM, p. A285
SKALSKY, Susan, M.D., Director, Hurtado Health Center, New Brunswick, NJ, p. A278

SKELLEY, Dennis B., President and Chief Executive Officer, Walton Rehabilitation Hospital, Augusta, GA, p. A101
SKILLINGS, Charles E., President and Chief Executive Officer, Shawnee Regional Hospital, Shawnee, OK, p. A347
SKINNER, Davis D., President, Missouri Baptist Hospital of Sullivan, Sullivan, MO, p. A255
SKINNER, Eileen F., Director, Ochsner Foundation Hospital, New Orleans, LA, p. A187
SKOGSBERGH, James H., President, Iowa Methodist Medical Center, Des Moines, IA, p. A151
SKOMOROCH, Orianna A.
   Regional Chief Executive Officer, Kauai Veterans Memorial Hospital, Waimea, HI, p. A114
   Regional Chief Executive Officer, Samuel Mahelona Memorial Hospital, Kapaa, HI, p. A113
SKORICK, Cynthia, Chief Executive Officer, Fergus Falls Regional Treatment Center, Fergus Falls, MN, p. A228
SKOWLUND, Kathleen, Site Administrator and Chief Nurse Executive, Lakeland Medical Center, Elkhorn, WI, p. A468
SKUBA, Herbert S., President and Chief Executive Officer, Ellwood City Hospital, Ellwood City, PA, p. A359
SKUBIC, Mark, Vice President, Methodist Hospital HealthSystem Minnesota, Saint Louis Park, MN, p. A233
SKVAREK, Joann A., Chief Executive Officer, Edgewater Medical Center, Chicago, IL, p. A121
SLABACH, Brock A., Administrator, Field Memorial Community Hospital, Centreville, MS, p. A237
SLAGTER, Dean G., Administrator, Renville County Hospital, Olivia, MN, p. A231
SLAUBAUGH, D. Ray, President, Graham Hospital, Canton, IL, p. A120
SLIETER, Jr, Richard G., Administrator, Weiner Memorial Medical Center, Marshall, MN, p. A230
SLOAN, Gary
   Chief Executive Officer, Doctors Medical Center–Pinole Campus, Pinole, CA, p. A55
   Chief Executive Officer, Doctors Medical Center–San Pablo Campus, San Pablo, CA, p. A61
SLOAN, Joseph F., CHE, Chief Executive Officer, Plains Memorial Hospital, Dimmitt, TX, p. A410
SLOAN, Robert L., Chief Executive Officer, Sibley Memorial Hospital, Washington, DC, p. A80
SLUNECKA, Fredrick, President and Chief Executive Officer, Avera McKennan Hospital, Sioux Falls, SD, p. A388
SLUSKY, Richard, Administrator, Mt. Ascutney Hospital and Health Center, Windsor, VT, p. A441
SLYTER, Mark, Administrator, Hillcrest Hospital, Simpsonville, SC, p. A383
SMALL, Sandra H.
   Administrator, Kaiser Foundation Hospital, Walnut Creek, CA, p. A67
   Administrator, Kaiser Foundation Hospital and Rehabilitation Center, Vallejo, CA, p. A66
SMART, Rob, Chief Executive Officer, Bourbon Community Hospital, Paris, KY, p. A177
SMART, Robert M., Area Manager and Chief Executive Officer, HEALTHSOUTH Medical Center, Dallas, TX, p. A409
SMEDLEY, Craig M., Administrator, Valley View Medical Center, Cedar City, UT, p. A436
SMILEY, David, Administrator and Chief Executive Officer, Kentfield Rehabilitation Hospital, Kentfield, CA, p. A44
SMILEY, Jon D., Chief Executive Officer, Sunnyside Community Hospital, Sunnyside, WA, p. A458
SMILEY, W. David, Chief Executive Officer, San Joaquin Valley Rehabilitation Hospital, Fresno, CA, p. A42
SMITH, Arthur R., Chief Executive Officer, Artesia General Hospital, Artesia, NM, p. A284
SMITH, Bernadette M., Chief Operating Officer, Seton Medical Center, Daly City, CA, p. A39
SMITH, C. W., President and Chief Executive Officer, Parkview Medical Center, Pueblo, CO, p. A72

SMITH, Charles M., M.D.
   President and Chief Executive Officer, Christiana Care Health System, Wilmington, DE, p. B71
   President and Chief Executive Officer, Christiana Hospital, Newark, DE, p. A78
SMITH, Connie, Chief Executive Officer, The Medical Center at Bowling Green, Bowling Green, KY, p. A170
SMITH, Dennis H.
   Director, Veterans Affairs Maryland Health Care System–Baltimore Division, Baltimore, MD, p. A196
   Director, Veterans Affairs Maryland Health Care System–Fort Howard Division, Fort Howard, MD, p. A198
   Director, Veterans Affairs Maryland Health Care System–Perry Point Division, Perry Point, MD, p. A199
SMITH, F. Curtis, President, Massachusetts Eye and Ear Infirmary, Boston, MA, p. A202
SMITH, Frances T., Administrator, Childress Regional Medical Center, Childress, TX, p. A406
SMITH, Gordon, Administrator and Chief Executive Officer, Merrill Pioneer Community Hospital, Rock Rapids, IA, p. A156
SMITH, Gregory M., Chief Executive Officer, Allentown State Hospital, Allentown, PA, p. A355
SMITH, H. Gerald, President and Chief Executive Officer, St. Francis Medical Center, Monroe, LA, p. A186
SMITH, Harlan J., President and Chief Executive Officer, Franklin Medical Center, Greenfield, MA, p. A205
SMITH, Harley, Chief Executive Officer, Miller County Hospital, Colquitt, GA, p. A102
SMITH, James E., Superintendent, North Texas State Hospital, Wichita Falls Campus, Wichita Falls, TX, p. A435
SMITH, Jeffrey H., Ph.D., Superintendent, Logansport State Hospital, Logansport, IN, p. A143
SMITH, Jim B., President and Chief Executive Officer, Goodall–Witcher Healthcare, Clifton, TX, p. A406
SMITH, Joe E., Administrator and Chief Executive Officer, DeWitt City Hospital, De Witt, AR, p. A29
SMITH, Johnny J., Chief Executive Officer, High Pointe, Oklahoma City, OK, p. A
SMITH, Johnson L., Chief Executive Officer and Administrator, St. Anthony's Healthcare Center, Morrilton, AR, p. A32
SMITH, Jon, Interim Administrator, Pershing General Hospital, Lovelock, NV, p. A269
SMITH, Joseph S., Chief Executive Officer, Boone County Hospital, Boone, IA, p. A148
SMITH, Keith, Chief Executive Officer, Bledsoe Community Medical Center, Pikeville, TN, p. A399
SMITH, Lex, Administrator, Park View Hospital, El Reno, OK, p. A343
SMITH, Lloyd V., President and Chief Executive Officer, Benefis Healthcare, Great Falls, MT, p. A257
SMITH, Louis H., Executive Vice President and Administrator, Cornwall Hospital, Cornwall, NY, p. A290
SMITH, Martin D., Chief Executive Officer, Cleveland Community Hospital, Cleveland, TN, p. A391
SMITH, Meredith H., Administrator, Dodge County Hospital, Eastman, GA, p. A104
SMITH, Michael N., Director Healthcare Services, San Joaquin General Hospital, French Camp, CA, p. A41
SMITH, Randy, Chief Executive Officer, Chilton Medical Center, Clanton, AL, p. A13
SMITH, Raymond N., Chief Executive Officer, Community Hospital of Gardena, Gardena, CA, p. A42
SMITH, Richard
   Administrator, Logan Regional Hospital, Logan, UT, p. A436
   Administrator, Plains Regional Medical Center, Clovis, NM, p. A284
SMITH, Richard G., Chief Executive Officer, Oneida Healthcare Center, Oneida, NY, p. A302
SMITH, Robbie, Administrator, Higgins General Hospital, Bremen, GA, p. A101
SMITH, Robert B., President and Chief Executive Officer, Zale Lipshy University Hospital, Dallas, TX, p. A410
SMITH, Robert L.
   President and Chief Executive Officer, Decatur General Hospital, Decatur, AL, p. A13
   Chief Executive Officer, Paracelsus Healthcare Corporation, Houston, TX, p. B118

SMITH, Rodney R., President and Chief Executive Officer, Central Florida Regional Hospital, Sanford, FL, p. A95
SMITH, Sherry J., Executive Director, Woman's Hospital at River Oaks, Jackson, MS, p. A239
SMITH, Steve, Chief Executive Officer, Carson Tahoe Hospital, Carson City, NV, p. A268
SMITH, Steven L., President and Chief Executive Officer, Memorial Medical Center, Las Cruces, NM, p. A285
SMITH, Stuart, Vice President Clinical Operations and Executive Director, MUSC Medical Center of Medical University of South Carolina, Charleston, SC, p. A379
SMITH, Terry J., Administrator, Bibb Medical Center, Centreville, AL, p. A13
SMITH, Thomas G., Chief Executive Officer, Audubon County Memorial Hospital, Audubon, IA, p. A148
SMITH, Thomas W., President and Chief Executive Officer, Ephraim McDowell Regional Medical Center, Danville, KY, p. A171
SMITH, Tim, President and Chief Executive Officer, Fountain Valley Regional Hospital and Medical Center, Fountain Valley, CA, p. A41
SMITH, Todd A., Chief Executive Officer, Charter Behavioral Health System of Southern California–Charter Oak, Covina, CA, p. A39
SMITH, Tommy J., President and Chief Executive Officer, Baptist Healthcare System, Louisville, KY, p. B58
SMITH, W. David, Director, Veterans Affairs Medical Center, Canandaigua, NY, p. A290
SMITH, Wayne T., President and Chief Executive Officer, Community Health Systems, Inc., Brentwood, TN, p. B73
SMITH, William R., Administrator, Hamilton Hospital, Olney, TX, p. A425
SMITH, II, W. Don, President and Chief Executive Officer, Cabell Huntington Hospital, Huntington, WV, p. A461
SMITH, Jr, P. Paul, Executive Director, Lake Norman Regional Medical Center, Mooresville, NC, p. A316
SMITH, Jr, P. W., Administrator and Chief Executive Officer, Joel Pomerene Memorial Hospital, Millersburg, OH, p. A335
SMITH–BLACKWELL, Olivia, M.P.H., President and Chief Executive Officer, Sheehan Memorial Hospital, Buffalo, NY, p. A289
SMITHERS, Joe, Administrator, Integrated Specialty Hospital, Edmond, OK, p. A343
SMITHMIER, Kenneth L., President and Chief Executive Officer, Decatur Memorial Hospital, Decatur, IL, p. A124
SMOCK, Dennis, Chief Executive Officer, Baptist DeKalb Hospital, Smithville, TN, p. A399
SMOLIK, Chris, Chief Executive Officer, Edinburg Regional Medical Center, Edinburg, TX, p. A411
SMOOT, Steven, Chief Executive Officer, Mineral Community Hospital, Superior, MT, p. A259
SNEAD, Benjamin E., President and Chief Executive Officer, St. Clair Memorial Hospital, Pittsburgh, PA, p. A369
SNEDIGAR, Rudy, Chief Executive Officer, Clarinda Regional Health Center, Clarinda, IA, p. A149
SNIPES, Lucas A., FACHE, Director, Carilion Medical Center, Roanoke, VA, p. A449
SNOW, Mel L., Administrator, West Holt Memorial Hospital, Atkinson, NE, p. A261
SNOWDEN, Raymond W., President and Chief Executive Officer, Memorial Hospital and Health Care Center, Jasper, IN, p. A142
SNYDER, David M., Chief Executive Officer, Bedford County Medical Center, Shelbyville, TN, p. A399
SNYDERMAN, Ralph, M.D., President and Chief Executive Officer, Duke University Health System, Durham, NC, p. B83
SOBEHART, Richard E., President, UPMC St. Margaret, Pittsburgh, PA, p. A370
SOBOTA, Richard E., President and Chief Executive Officer, Pike Community Hospital, Waverly, OH, p. A339
SODERBLOM, Alan, Administrator, Loma Linda University Behavioral Medicine Center, Redlands, CA, p. A56

SODOMKA, Patricia, FACHE, Executive Director, Medical College of Georgia Hospital and Clinics, Augusta, GA, p. A101
SOKOL, Dennis A., President and Chief Executive Officer, Firelands Community Hospital, Sandusky, OH, p. A337
SOKOLOW, Norman J., Chairman and Chief Executive Officer, Cornerstone of Medical Arts Center Hospital, New York, NY, p. A296
SOLARE, Frank A., President and Chief Executive Officer, Thorek Hospital and Medical Center, Chicago, IL, p. A124
SOLBERG, Penny, Administrator, Tweeten Health Services, Spring Grove, MN, p. A233
SOLHEIM, John H., President and Chief Executive Officer, St. Peter's Hospital, Helena, MT, p. A258
SOLVIBILE, Edward R., Chief Executive Officer, Mercy Suburban Hospital, Norristown, PA, p. A365
SOMMERS, Thomas W., President and Chief Executive Officer, Central Kansas Medical Center, Great Bend, KS, p. A161
SONDECKER, James, Director, St. Joseph's Behavioral Health Center, Stockton, CA, p. A64
SONENREICH, Steven, Chief Executive Officer, Cedars Medical Center, Miami, FL, p. A89
SOULE, Frederick L., President and Chief Executive Officer, Caldwell Memorial Hospital, Lenoir, NC, p. A315
SPANG, A. James, Administrator, Shriners Hospitals for Children–Chicago, Chicago, IL, p. A123
SPARKMAN, Dena C., Administrator, McDowell ARH Hospital, McDowell, KY, p. A176
SPARKMAN, Ronald L., Administrator, Randolph County Hospital, Roanoke, AL, p. A18
SPARKS, Gary R., Chief Executive Officer, CrossBridge Community Hospital, Wynne, AR, p. A34
SPARKS, Julian, Board Chairman, Marshall County Health Care Authority, Guntersville, AL, p. B108
SPARKS, Richard G., President, Watauga Medical Center, Boone, NC, p. A310
SPARTZ, Gregory G., Chief Executive Officer, Willmar Regional Treatment Center, Willmar, MN, p. A235
SPARTZ, Jeff, Administrator, Hennepin County Medical Center, Minneapolis, MN, p. A230
SPAUDE, Paul A., President and Chief Executive Officer, Wausau Hospital, Wausau, WI, p. A477
SPAULDING, Don, Administrator and Chief Executive Officer, Fort Duncan Medical Center, Eagle Pass, TX, p. A421
SPAUSTER, Edward, Ph.D., Executive Director, Arms Acres, Carmel, NY, p. A290
SPEED, Marilyn, Administrator, Beacham Memorial Hospital, Magnolia, MS, p. A240
SPELLMAN, Warren K., Administrator, Holy Cross Hospital, Taos, NM, p. A286
SPENCER, Corte J., Chief Executive Officer, Oswego Hospital, Oswego, NY, p. A302
SPENCER, Herman J., Administrator, Northern Inyo Hospital, Bishop, CA, p. A37
SPENCER, Steven H., Chief Executive Officer, Memorial Community Hospital, Edgerton, WI, p. A468
SPICER, John R., President and Chief Executive Officer, Sound Shore Medical Center of Westchester, New Rochelle, NY, p. A295
SPICER, Michael J., President and Chief Executive Officer, St. Joseph's Medical Center, Yonkers, NY, p. A308
SPIELER, John L., FACHE, Executive Director, St. Francis Hospital Cranberry, Cranberry, PA, p. A358
SPIKE, Colleen A., Administrator, Community Hospital and Health Care Center, Saint Peter, MN, p. A233
SPINELLI, Robert J., Administrator and Chief Executive Officer, Bloomsburg Hospital, Bloomsburg, PA, p. A356
SPIVEY, Sue, Administrator, Irwin County Hospital, Ocilla, GA, p. A108
SPIVEY-PAUL, Cathi, Acting Director, Veterans Affairs Medical Center, Danville, IL, p. A124
SPOELMAN, Roger, President and Chief Executive Officer, Mercy General Health Partners, Muskegon, MI, p. A220
SPRAY, William Russell, Chief Executive Officer, Southern Tennessee Medical Center, Winchester, TN, p. A400

SPRENGER, Gordon M., President, Allina Health System, Minneapolis, MN, p. B52
SPRENGER, Jay D., USAF, Commander, U. S. Air Force Academy Hospital, USAF Academy, CO, p. A73
SPROUSE, James P., Associate Administrator for Psychiatric Services, Behavioral Health Care of Cape Fear Valley Health System, Fayetteville, NC, p. A312
SPYHALSKI, Richard A., Chief Executive Officer, Northwest Medical Center, Thief River Falls, MN, p. A234
ST. GEORGE, George H., Chief Executive Officer, Screven County Hospital, Sylvania, GA, p. A110
STAAS, Jr, William E., President and Medical Director, Magee Rehabilitation Hospital, Philadelphia, PA, p. A367
STACEY, Bryan, Administrator, Ashland Health Center, Ashland, KS, p. A159
STACEY, Rulon F., President and Chief Executive Officer, Poudre Valley Hospital, Fort Collins, CO, p. A70
STACK, Edward A., President and Chief Executive Officer, Behavioral Healthcare Corporation, Nashville, TN, p. B59
STAFFORD, J. Scott, Chief Executive Officer and Administrator, St. Helena Parish Hospital, Greensburg, LA, p. A182
STAMBAUGH, Dennis, Director, Missouri Rehabilitation Center, Mount Vernon, MO, p. A250
STAMM, Scott C., Chief Executive Officer, Columbia River Park Hospital, Huntington, WV, p. A462
STAMP, Burl E., Chief Executive Officer, Phoenix Children's Hospital, Phoenix, AZ, p. A24
STAMPOHAR, Jeffry, Chief Executive Officer, Deer River Healthcare Center, Deer River, MN, p. A227
STANDEFFER, Luke, Administrator and Chief Executive Officer, HEALTHSOUTH Medical Center, Birmingham, AL, p. A12
STANKO, J. Richard, President and Chief Executive Officer, St. Joseph Hospital, Omaha, NE, p. A265
STANZIONE, Dominick M., Chief Operating Officer and Executive Vice President, Sisters of Charity Medical Center, New York, NY, p. A300
STAPLES, Nancy, Administrator, Elgin Mental Health Center, Elgin, IL, p. A125
STARK, Charles A., CHE, Administrator, Chief Executive Officer and Regional Vice President, HEALTHSOUTH Medical Center, Richmond, VA, p. A448
STARK, David, Chief Operating Officer, Iowa Lutheran Hospital, Des Moines, IA, p. A151
STARNES, Gregory D., Chief Executive Officer, St. Clare Medical Center, Crawfordsville, IN, p. A138
STARR, Gerald A., Executive Officer, Delano Regional Medical Center, Delano, CA, p. A40
STARR, Jr, Hickory, Administrator, William W. Hastings Indian Hospital, Tahlequah, OK, p. A348
STASIK, Randall, President and Chief Executive Officer, Borgess Medical Center, Kalamazoo, MI, p. A217
STATUTO, Richard, Chief Executive Officer, St. Joseph Health System, Orange, CA, p. B137
STAUDER, Mark S., President and Chief Executive Officer, Mercy Health Center, Laredo, TX, p. A421
STEADHAM, Mark B., President and Chief Executive Officer, St. Catherine Hospital, Garden City, KS, p. A161
STECKLER, Michael J., President and Chief Executive Officer, Jennie M. Melham Memorial Medical Center, Broken Bow, NE, p. A261
STEED, Larry N., Administrator, Tanner Medical Center–Villa Rica, Villa Rica, GA, p. A111
STEED, Robert A., President, Willamette Falls Hospital, Oregon City, OR, p. A352
STEEGE, Armin L., Interim Administrator, Seton Shoal Creek Hospital, Austin, TX, p. A403
STEELE, Barbara, President, The Toledo Hospital, Toledo, OH, p. A338
STEELEY, Hubert, Administrator, Gulf Pines Hospital, Port Saint Joe, FL, p. A93
STEFANIDES, Christine M., CHE, President and Chief Executive Officer, Civista Health, La Plata, MD, p. A199
STEFFEE, Sam L., Executive Director and Chief Executive Officer, Polly Ryon Memorial Hospital, Richmond, TX, p. A427

STEFFEN, Keith E., Administrator, OSF Saint Francis Medical Center, Peoria, IL, p. A132
STEIN, Benjamin M., M.D., President, Brunswick General Hospital, Amityville, NY, p. A287
STEIN, Bob, Executive Director, Vencor Hospital–Houston, Houston, TX, p. A418
STEIN, Dale J., President and Chief Executive Officer, Avera St. Luke's, Aberdeen, SD, p. A385
STEIN, Gary M., President and Chief Executive Officer, Touro Infirmary, New Orleans, LA, p. A187
STEIN, Norman V., President, University Community Hospital, Tampa, FL, p. A96
STEIN, Sheldon J., Chief Operating Officer, Mt. Washington Pediatric Hospital, Baltimore, MD, p. A196
STEINER, Garith W., Chief Executive Officer and Administrator, Vernon Memorial Hospital, Viroqua, WI, p. A476
STEINER, Keith M., Chief Executive Officer, Madison Memorial Hospital, Rexburg, ID, p. A117
STEINHAUER, Bruce W., M.D., President and Chief Executive Officer, Regional Medical Center at Memphis, Memphis, TN, p. A397
STEINHAURER, Gordon L., Chief Executive Officer, BHC Valle Vista Hospital, Greenwood, IN, p. A140
STEINHOFF, Earl J., Administrator and Chief Executive Officer, Prowers Medical Center, Lamar, CO, p. A71
STEINRUCK, Jim, CHE, Administrator and Chief Executive Officer, Vencor Hospital Seattle, Seattle, WA, p. A457
STEITZ, David P., Chief Executive Officer, Frankfort Regional Medical Center, Frankfort, KY, p. A172
STELLE, Walter, Ph.D., Director, Dorothea Dix Hospital, Raleigh, NC, p. A316
STELLER, Tim, Chief Executive Officer, North Central Health Care Facilities, Wausau, WI, p. A476
STELZER, Jr, V. Richard, Chief Administrative Officer, Lakewood Hospital, Lakewood, OH, p. A333
STENBERG, Scott, Chief Executive Officer, Sutter Amador Hospital, Jackson, CA, p. A44
STENGER, Michael J., Executive Vice President and Administrator, St. Nicholas Hospital, Sheboygan, WI, p. A475
STENSAGER, Mark, President and Chief Executive Officer, Guthrie Healthcare System, Sayre, PA, p. B88
STENSON, Richard, President and Chief Executive Officer, Tuality Healthcare, Hillsboro, OR, p. A351
STENSRUD, Kirk, Administrator, Hendricks Community Hospital, Hendricks, MN, p. A229
STENZLER, Mark R., Vice President Administration, North Shore University Hospital at Glen Cove, Glen Cove, NY, p. A291
STEPANIK, Mark J., Interim Chief Executive Officer, Mid–America Rehabilitation Hospital, Overland Park, KS, p. A166
STEPHANS, J. Michael, Administrator, Medical Center Hospital, Odessa, TX, p. A425
STEPHEN, Ron, Executive Vice President and Administrator, Osteopathic Medical Center of Texas, Fort Worth, TX, p. A413
STEPHENS, Michael D., President and Chief Executive Officer, Hoag Memorial Hospital Presbyterian, Newport Beach, CA, p. A53
STEPHENS, Michael R., President, Greene Memorial Hospital, Xenia, OH, p. A340
STEPHENS, Norman F., Chief Executive Officer, Rehabilitation Hospital of Fort Wayne, Fort Wayne, IN, p. A140
STEPHENS, Terry A., Executive Director, Sierra Tucson, Tucson, AZ, p. A27
STEPHENS, Jr, Jack T., President and Chief Executive Officer, Lakeland Regional Medical Center, Lakeland, FL, p. A88
STEPHENSON, Christy, Chief Administrative Officer, Robert Wood Johnson University Hospital at Hamilton, Hamilton, NJ, p. A276
STEPHENSON, David, Administrator, Kearney County Health Services, Minden, NE, p. A264
STEPP, Merle E., President and Chief Executive Officer, Clark Memorial Hospital, Jeffersonville, IN, p. A142
STERN, Ron, Chief Executive Officer, Palmetto General Hospital, Hialeah, FL, p. A86

STEVENS, April A., R.N., Chief Executive Officer, LifeCare Hospital of Pittsburgh, Pittsburgh, PA, p. A369
STEVENS, Diana, Administrator, Garden County Hospital, Oshkosh, NE, p. A266
STEVENS, Essimae, Service Unit Director, U.S. Public Health Service Indian Hospital, Redlake, MN, p. A232
STEVENS, Robert, President and Chief Executive Officer, Ridgeview Medical Center, Waconia, MN, p. A234
STEVENS, Velinda, President and Chief Executive Officer, Kalispell Regional Medical Center, Kalispell, MT, p. A258
STEVENS, Ward W., CHE, Chief Executive Officer, Alleghany Regional Hospital, Low Moor, VA, p. A445
STEVENS, Jr, Vernon R., Administrator, Riverland Medical Center, Ferriday, LA, p. A182
STEVENSON, Jerry L.
President and Chief Executive Officer, Mercy Health System of Kansas, Fort Scott, KS, p. A161
President and Chief Executive Officer, Mercy Health System of Kansas, Independence, KS, p. A163
STEVENSON, Mike, Administrator, Murphy Medical Center, Murphy, NC, p. A316
STEWART, Charles L., Administrator, Northport Medical Center, Northport, AL, p. A17
STEWART, Christine R., President and Chief Executive Officer, Russellville Hospital, Russellville, AL, p. A18
STEWART, Diane Gail, Chief Administrative Officer, Sutter Center for Psychiatry, Sacramento, CA, p. A57
STEWART, Donald L., Chief Executive Officer, Bayshore Medical Center, Pasadena, TX, p. A426
STEWART, Joseph A., Chief Executive Officer, Butler Health System, Butler, PA, p. A357
STEWART, Lawrence C., Director, Veterans Affairs Medical Center, Long Beach, CA, p. A47
STEWART, Paul R., President and Chief Executive Officer, Merle West Medical Center, Klamath Falls, OR, p. A351
STEWART, Shirley A., President and Chief Executive Officer, Tulane University Hospital and Clinic, New Orleans, LA, p. A187
STILLWAGON, Richard A., Superintendent, Torrance State Hospital, Torrance, PA, p. A372
STILLWELL, James M., Director, Impact Drug and Alcohol Treatment Center, Pasadena, CA, p. A55
STINDT, John L., Chief Executive Officer, Standish Community Hospital, Standish, MI, p. A222
STINSON, Karl R., CHE, Chief Executive Officer, Medical Arts Hospital, Lamesa, TX, p. A421
STIPE, Allan, President and Chief Executive Officer, Sunrise Hospital and Medical Center, Las Vegas, NV, p. A268
STITZER, Roxane, Ph.D., Chief Executive Officer, Metropolitan Nashville General Hospital, Nashville, TN, p. A398
STOCK, Greg K., Chief Executive Officer, Thibodaux Regional Medical Center, Thibodaux, LA, p. A189
STOCKTON, Eddy R., Chief Executive Officer, Jane Todd Crawford Hospital, Greensburg, KY, p. A172
STODDARD, Mark R.
President, Central Valley Medical Center, Nephi, UT, p. A437
President, Rural Health Management Corporation, Nephi, UT, p. B129
STOKER, Teresa, Chief Executive Officer, Hillside Hospital, Atlanta, GA, p. A100
STOKES, Barry S., President and Chief Executive Officer, Edward White Hospital, Saint Petersburg, FL, p. A94
STOKES, Gary L., Chief Executive Officer, Gulf Coast Medical Center, Biloxi, MS, p. A236
STOKES, Randell G., Chief Executive Officer, Palestine Regional Medical Center, Palestine, TX, p. A425
STOLL, Lee D., Chief Executive Officer, Saint Louis University Hospital, Saint Louis, MO, p. A253
STOLL, Leona D., Chief Executive Officer, Compton Heights Hospital, Saint Louis, MO, p. A252
STOLZENBERG, Edward A., President and Chief Executive Officer, Westchester Medical Center, Valhalla, NY, p. A306
STONE, James L., Commissioner, New York State Department of Mental Health, Albany, NY, p. B114

STONE, Ken, Administrator, Vencor Hospital – Central Tampa, Tampa, FL, p. A97
STONE, Maxine, Superintendent, Eastern Oregon Psychiatric Center, Pendleton, OR, p. A352
STONE, Robert, President, Blythedale Children's Hospital, Valhalla, NY, p. A306
STONE, Thomas J., Administrator and Chief Executive Officer, St. Tammany Parish Hospital, Covington, LA, p. A181
STORDAHL, Dean R., Chief Executive Officer, Jerry L. Pettis Memorial Veterans Medical Center, Loma Linda, CA, p. A46
STORY, Bettye W., Ph.D., Director, Veterans Affairs Medical Center, Hampton, VA, p. A445
STORY, Lawrence, Administrator, Cypress Creek Hospital, Houston, TX, p. A416
STORY, Jr, James L., M.D., Acting President, John D. Archbold Memorial Hospital, Thomasville, GA, p. A110
STOUT, Dick L., Administrator, North Runnels Hospital, Winters, TX, p. A435
STRANGE, John, President and Chief Executive Officer, St. Luke's Hospital, Duluth, MN, p. A227
STRANKO, Teresa K., Chief Executive Officer, HEALTHSOUTH MountainView Regional Rehabilitation Hospital, Morgantown, WV, p. A463
STRASSHEIM, Dale S., President, BroMenn Healthcare, Normal, IL, p. A131
STRATTON, Terry, Chief Executive Officer, Appling Healthcare System, Baxley, GA, p. A101
STRAUCH, Walter A., Executive Director, Franklin Regional Hospital, Franklin, NH, p. A271
STRAUSS, Thomas J., President and Chief Executive Officer, Summa Health System, Akron, OH, p. A325
STRECK, William F., M.D., President and Chief Executive Officer, Mary Imogene Bassett Hospital, Cooperstown, NY, p. A290
STRECKER, E. Bradley, Chief Executive Officer, Vencor Hospital–Kansas City, Kansas City, MO, p. A249
STREET, Jackie, President, Idaho Falls Recovery Center, Idaho Falls, ID, p. A116
STRIANO, Joseph, Acting Director, Veterans Affairs Medical Center, Bath, NY, p. A288
STRICKER, Sean, Administrator, Liberty–Dayton Hospital, Liberty, TX, p. A421
STRICKLAND, Al, Administrator, Cobb Memorial Hospital, Royston, GA, p. A109
STRICKLAND, Wallace, President and Chief Executive Officer, Rush Health Systems, Meridian, MS, p. B129
STRIEBY, John F., Chief Executive Officer, Nix Health Care System, San Antonio, TX, p. A429
STRINE, Mervin F., President and Chief Executive Officer, Massillon Community Hospital, Massillon, OH, p. A335
STROMAN, W. Neil, President, ViaHealth of Wayne, Newark, NY, p. A301
STROMBERG, Audrey, Administrator, Roosevelt Memorial Medical Center, Culbertson, MT, p. A257
STRUBLE, Lynne M., MSN, Chief Executive Officer, Southwood Psychiatric Hospital, Pittsburgh, PA, p. A369
STRUTHERS, Tony
Vice President Operations and Administrator, St. Joseph Northeast Heights Hospital, Albuquerque, NM, p. A283
Vice President and Administrator, St. Joseph West Mesa Hospital, Albuquerque, NM, p. A284
STRUXNESS, Ronald E., Executive Vice President and Chief Executive Officer, Our Lady of the Resurrection Medical Center, Chicago, IL, p. A122
STRUYK, Douglas A., President and Chief Executive Officer, Christian Health Care Center, Wyckoff, NJ, p. A282
STUART, Philip, Administrator, Tomah Memorial Hospital, Tomah, WI, p. A476
STUART, Wilma D., Administrator, North Baldwin Hospital, Bay Minette, AL, p. A11
STUBBLEFIELD, Alfred G., President, Baptist Health Care Corporation, Pensacola, FL, p. B57
STUBBS, Deborah, Chief Executive Officer, South Barry County Memorial Hospital, Cassville, MO, p. A245
STUBER, Joseph A., Chief Executive Officer, Perry County Memorial Hospital, Tell City, IN, p. A146

STUCKEY, Jane, Interim Chief Executive Officer, Pocono Medical Center, East Stroudsburg, PA, p. A359
STUENKEL, Kurt, FACHE, President and Chief Executive Officer, Floyd Medical Center, Rome, GA, p. A108
STYLES, Jr, John H.
  Administrator, Doctors Hospital Parkway, Houston, TX, p. A416
  Administrator, Doctors Hospital–Tidwell, Houston, TX, p. A416
SUCHOCKI, Celeste L., Chief Executive Officer, Grant Hospital, Chicago, IL, p. A121
SUDDERS, Marylou, Commissioner, Massachusetts Department of Mental Health, Boston, MA, p. B108
SUDDUTH, Tony G., Chief Executive Officer, Dunn Memorial Hospital, Bedford, IN, p. A137
SUEIRO, Edwin, Executive Director, Hospital Doctor Gubern, Fajardo, PR, p. A482
SUGG, William T., President and Chief Executive Officer, Sumner Regional Medical Center, Gallatin, TN, p. A392
SUGIYAMA, Deborah
  President, NorthBay Medical Center, Fairfield, CA, p. A41
  President, VacaValley Hospital, Vacaville, CA, p. A66
SULLIVAN, Charles, President and Chief Executive Officer, Reading Hospital and Medical Center, Reading, PA, p. A371
SULLIVAN, Michael J., Director, Veterans Affairs Medical Center, Philadelphia, PA, p. A368
SULLIVAN, Margaret T., President and Chief Executive Officer, St. Agnes Medical Center, Philadelphia, PA, p. A368
SUMMERS, Stephen M., CHE, Chief Executive Officer, Decatur Community Hospital, Decatur, TX, p. A410
SUMMERS, William L., Executive Director, Patton State Hospital, Patton, CA, p. A55
SUMMERSETT, II, James A., FACHE, President and Chief Executive Officer, Wadley Regional Medical Center, Texarkana, TX, p. A432
SUROWITZ, Dale, Chief Executive Officer, Encino–Tarzana Regional Medical Center Tarzana Campus, Los Angeles, CA, p. A47
SUSI, Jeffrey L., President and Chief Executive Officer, Indian River Memorial Hospital, Vero Beach, FL, p. A97
SUSSMAN, Elliot J., M.D.
  President and Chief Executive Officer, Lehigh Valley Hospital, Allentown, PA, p. A355
  President and Chief Executive Officer, Muhlenberg Hospital Center, Bethlehem, PA, p. A356
SUTTON, Frank, Vice President Hospital Services, Searhc MT. Edgecumbe Hospital, Sitka, AK, p. A21
SUYENAGA, Lee, Chief Executive Officer, Alhambra Hospital Medical Center, Alhambra, CA, p. A35
SWAFFORD, Lea, Acting Director, Alvin C. York Veterans Affairs Medical Center, Murfreesboro, TN, p. A397
SWAN, Allen D., Chief Executive Officer, District Memorial Hospital, Andrews, NC, p. A309
SWARTWOUT, John A., Administrator, Shriners Hospitals for Children, Galveston Burns Hospital, Galveston, TX, p. A413
SWAVELY, Tom, Administrator and Chief Executive Officer, HEALTHSOUTH Nittany Valley Rehabilitation Hospital, Pleasant Gap, PA, p. A370
SWEARINGEN, Lawrence L., President and Chief Executive Officer, Blessing Hospital, Quincy, IL, p. A133
SWEEDEN, Dick, Administrator, Scott and White Memorial Hospital, Temple, TX, p. A432
SWIGART, Russell W., Administrator, Howard County Community Hospital, Saint Paul, NE, p. A266
SWINIARSKI, Wayne A., FACHE, Chief Executive Officer, West Calcasieu Cameron Hospital, Sulphur, LA, p. A189
SWINNEY, Keith, Chief Executive Officer, Southwest General Hospital, San Antonio, TX, p. A429
SWISHER, Charles D., President, St. Francis Hospital–Mooresville, Mooresville, IN, p. A144
SWITZER, Bruce, Administrator, Broken Arrow Medical Center, Broken Arrow, OK, p. A342
SWORD, Russ D., Administrator, Ashley County Medical Center, Crossett, AR, p. A29
SWORD, William L., President and Chief Executive Officer, Texas County Memorial Hospital, Houston, MO, p. A247
SYKES, Jr, Donald K., Chief Executive Officer, BHC Windsor Hospital, Chagrin Falls, OH, p. A327
SYPNIEWSKI, Al, Administrator, Baptist Memorial Hospital–Booneville, Booneville, MS, p. A236
SZABO, Charleen R., FACHE, Chief Executive Officer, Veterans Affairs Medical Center, Lebanon, PA, p. A363

T

TACHOVSKY, Barbara, Senior Vice President, Paoli Memorial Hospital, Paoli, PA, p. A366
TADLOCK, Cindy, Interim Administrator, Leake Memorial Hospital, Carthage, MS, p. A237
TAITANO, Tyrone J., Administrator, Guam Memorial Hospital Authority, Tamuning, GU, p. A481
TALLEY, James J., Administrator, Wheaton Community Hospital, Wheaton, MN, p. A235
TALLY, James E., Ph.D.
  President and Chief Executive Officer, Children's Healthcare of Atlanta, Atlanta, GA, p. B71
  President and Chief Executive Officer, Children's Healthcare of Atlanta at Egleston, Atlanta, GA, p. A99
  President and Chief Executive Officer, Children's Healthcare of Atlanta at Scottish Rite, Atlanta, GA, p. A100
TALMO, Michael S., Chief Executive Officer, Highland Ridge Hospital, Midvale, UT, p. A437
TAMAR, Earl, Chief Operating Officer, Cape Coral Hospital, Cape Coral, FL, p. A82
TAMME, Susan Stout, President, Baptist Hospital East, Louisville, KY, p. A175
TAN–LACHICA, Nieves, M.D., Superintendent, Andrew McFarland Mental Health Center, Springfield, IL, p. A135
TANNER, Anthony J., Executive Vice President, HEALTHSOUTH Corporation, Birmingham, AL, p. B96
TANNER, Gale V., Administrator, Monroe County Hospital, Forsyth, GA, p. A105
TANNER, Laurence A., President and Chief Executive Officer, New Britain General Hospital, New Britain, CT, p. A75
TAPPAN, Hugh C., Chief Executive Officer, Hughston Sports Medicine Hospital, Columbus, GA, p. A102
TARBET, Michele T., R.N., Chief Executive Officer, Grossmont Hospital, La Mesa, CA, p. A45
TARR, Judith, Chief Executive Officer, Miles Memorial Hospital, Damariscotta, ME, p. A192
TARRANT, Jeffrey S., Administrator, Lafayette Regional Health Center, Lexington, MO, p. A250
TASCONE, Deborah, MS
  Executive Director, North Shore University Hospital at Plainview, Plainview, NY, p. A302
  Executive Director, North Shore University Hospital at Syosset, Syosset, NY, p. A305
TASSE, Joseph, Administrator, Oakwood Hospital and Medical Center–Dearborn, Dearborn, MI, p. A213
TATE, Joel W., FACHE, Chief Executive Officer, McAlester Regional Health Center, McAlester, OK, p. A344
TATUM, Stanley D., Chief Executive Officer, Edmond Medical Center, Edmond, OK, p. A343
TAUSSIG, Lynn M., M.D., President and Chief Executive Officer, National Jewish Medical and Research Center, Denver, CO, p. A69
TAVARY, James, Administrator, Prosser Memorial Hospital, Prosser, WA, p. A455
TAVENNER, Marilyn B., Chief Executive Officer, Chippenham Medical Center/Johnston–Willis Hospital, Richmond, VA, p. A448
TAYLOR, Alfred P., Administrator and Chief Executive Officer, Milan General Hospital, Milan, TN, p. A397
TAYLOR, James H., President and Chief Executive Officer, University of Louisville Hospital, Louisville, KY, p. A176
TAYLOR, Kevin, Administrator, Early Memorial Hospital, Blakely, GA, p. A101
TAYLOR, Mark R., President, St. Marys Health Center, Jefferson City, MO, p. A247
TAYLOR, Meredith, Administrator, Vencor Hospital–Sacramento, Folsom, CA, p. A41
TAYLOR, Nancy, Chief Executive Officer, Broadwater Health Center, Townsend, MT, p. A260
TAYLOR, Steven L., Chief Executive Officer, Harrison County Hospital, Corydon, IN, p. A138
TAYLOR, Jr, L. Clark, Ph.D., President and Chief Executive Officer, Memorial Hospital, Chattanooga, TN, p. A391
TEAGUE, Michael E., Chief Executive Officer, Louisiana State Hospitals, New Orleans, LA, p. B106
TEEL, Kenneth R., Administrator, Lake Pointe Medical Center, Rowlett, TX, p. A427
TEIGEN, Bobbe, Administrator, Sauk Prairie Memorial Hospital, Prairie Du Sac, WI, p. A474
TEJIDOR, Roberto, Chief Executive Officer, Pan American Hospital, Miami, FL, p. A90
TEMBREULL, John P., Administrator, Baraga County Memorial Hospital, L'Anse, MI, p. A218
TENAGLIA, Nicholas, M.D., Chief Executive Officer, Progressions Group, Inc., Fort Washington, PA, p. B120
TENNANT, Gail, Director, H. Douglas Singer Mental Health and Developmental Center, Rockford, IL, p. A134
TENNISON, Randal, Chief Executive Officer, Dexter Memorial Hospital, Dexter, MO, p. A246
TERREBONNE, Terry J., Chief Executive Officer, Jennings American Legion Hospital, Jennings, LA, p. A183
TERRILL, John, Administrator, Smith County Memorial Hospital, Smith Center, KS, p. A168
TERRY, Michael I., Chief Executive Officer, Lakeway Regional Hospital, Morristown, TN, p. A397
TESAR, James D., Chief Executive Officer, North Oak Regional Medical Center, Senatobia, MS, p. A242
TEST, Russell A., Administrator and Chief Executive Officer, The Hospital, Sidney, NY, p. A305
TESTERMAN, R. Frank, Administrator, Hawkins County Memorial Hospital, Rogersville, TN, p. A399
THACHER, Frederick J., President and Chief Executive Officer, Charles River Hospital, Wellesley, MA, p. A209
THAW, James G., President and Chief Executive Officer, Lafayette General Medical Center, Lafayette, LA, p. A184
THEBEAU, Robert S., President and Chief Executive Officer, Kishwaukee Health System, De Kalb, IL, p. B104
THEROULT, Thomas N., Administrator, Vencor Hospital–Minneapolis, Golden Valley, MN, p. A228
THIEBEN, William H., Chief Executive Officer, Kewanee Hospital, Kewanee, IL, p. A129
THIER, Samuel O., M.D., President and Chief Executive Officer, Partners HealthCare System, Inc., Boston, MA, p. B119
THOMAS, James R., Chief Executive Officer, Redmond Regional Medical Center, Rome, GA, p. A109
THOMAS, Lacy, Director, Cook County Hospital, Chicago, IL, p. A121
THOMAS, Marcile, Administrator, Providence Medical Center, Wayne, NE, p. A267
THOMAS, Michael P., Administrator, Meade District Hospital, Meade, KS, p. A165
THOMAS, Philip P., Chief Executive Officer, Veterans Affairs Medical Center–West Los Angeles, Los Angeles, CA, p. A50
THOMAS, Richard C., Administrator, Bascom Palmer Eye Institute–Anne Bates Leach Eye Hospital, Miami, FL, p. A89
THOMAS, Richard Lee, Superintendent, Lakeshore Mental Health Institute, Knoxville, TN, p. A395
THOMAS, Richard M., President, Pattie A. Clay Hospital, Richmond, KY, p. A178
THOMAS, Robert, Administrator, Columbus Community Hospital, Columbus, TX, p. A407
THOMAS, Telford W., President and Chief Executive Officer, Washington Hospital, Washington, PA, p. A373
THOMPSON, Bobby G., President and Chief Executive Officer, Mercy Memorial Health Center, Ardmore, OK, p. A341

Index of Health Care Professionals / Thompson

THOMPSON, Charolette, Administrator, Tri-Ward General Hospital, Bernice, LA, p. A181

THOMPSON, Deborah A., Director, Veterans Affairs Medical Center, Iron Mountain, MI, p. A217

THOMPSON, Floyd, Chief Executive Officer, Gallup Indian Medical Center, Gallup, NM, p. A285

THOMPSON, Frederick G., Ph.D., Administrator and Chief Executive Officer, Anson Community Hospital, Wadesboro, NC, p. A319

THOMPSON, Harriet A., Administrator, Hancock County Memorial Hospital, Britt, IA, p. A148

THOMPSON, Jim, Ph.D., Chief Executive Officer, HealthMark Regional Medical Center, De Funiak Springs, FL, p. A83

THOMPSON, John William, Ph.D., President and Chief Executive Officer, Lakeland Regional Hospital, Springfield, MO, p. A254

THOMPSON, Larry
Senior Vice President and Executive Director, Harris Continued Care Hospital, Fort Worth, TX, p. A412
Vice President and Administrator, Harris Methodist Northwest, Azle, TX, p. A403

THOMPSON, Mark E., Chief Executive Officer, Monroe County Medical Center, Tompkinsville, KY, p. A178

THOMPSON, Michael S., Administrator, White County Medical Center, Carmi, IL, p. A120

THOMPSON, Thomas R., Chief Executive Officer, St. Mary's Regional Health Center, Detroit Lakes, MN, p. A227

THOMPSON, Wes, Administrator and Chief Executive Officer, Alta View Hospital, Sandy, UT, p. A439

THOMPSON , Jr, Paul, Interim Senior Vice President, Rehabilitation Institute of Michigan, Detroit, MI, p. A214

THOMS, Maryellen, Warden, Federal Medical Center, Lexington, KY, p. A174

THOMSON, Thomas, Administrator, Delta County Memorial Hospital, Delta, CO, p. A69

THORESON, Scott, Administrator, Springfield Medical Center-Mayo Health System, Springfield, MN, p. A233

THORNHILL, Larry, Chief Executive Officer, Paulding County Hospital, Paulding, OH, p. A336

THORNTON, Dale E., CHE, President and Chief Executive Officer, Mercy Hospital of Willard, Willard, OH, p. A339

THORNTON, William M., Presdent and Chief Executive Officer, Miami Valley Hospital, Dayton, OH, p. A331

THORP, Gretchen, R.N., Administrator, Casa, A Special Hospital, Houston, TX, p. A416

THORSLAND , Jr, Ed, Director, Veterans Affairs Medical Center, Denver, CO, p. A70

THORWARD, S. R., M.D., Chief Operating Officer, OSU& Harding Behavioral Healthcare and Medicine, Worthington, OH, p. A340

THWEATT, James W., Chief Executive Officer, Clinch Valley Medical Center, Richlands, VA, p. A448

TIBBITTS, Tom, President, Trinity Regional Hospital, Fort Dodge, IA, p. A152

TICE, Kirk C., President and Chief Executive Officer, Rahway Hospital, Rahway, NJ, p. A280

TIEDEMANN, Frank, President, St. Paul Medical Center, Dallas, TX, p. A409

TIESI, Mike, Administrator, Alegent Health Bergan Mercy Medical Center, Omaha, NE, p. A265

TILLER, Gary L., Chief Executive Officer, Ninnescah Valley Health System, Kingman, KS, p. A163

TILTON, David P., President and Chief Executive Officer, Atlantic City Medical Center, Atlantic City, NJ, p. A274

TINKER, A. James, President and Chief Executive Officer, Mercy Medical Center, Cedar Rapids, IA, p. A149

TINKER, David E., President and Chief Executive Officer, Samaritan Medical Center, Watertown, NY, p. A307

TINTLE, Keith, Chief Executive Officer, Pioneer Valley Hospital, Salt Lake City, UT, p. A439

TIPPETS, Wayne C., Director, Veterans Affairs Medical Center, Boise, ID, p. A115

TITUS , II, Rexford W., President and Chief Executive Officer, Waukesha Memorial Hospital, Waukesha, WI, p. A476

TOBIN, John H., President and Chief Executive Officer, Waterbury Hospital, Waterbury, CT, p. A77

TOBIN, Timothy C., Chief Executive Officer, Coliseum Medical Centers, Macon, GA, p. A107

TODHUNTER, Neil E., Chief Executive Officer, Northwest Medical Centers, Oil City, PA, p. A365

TOEBBE, Nelson, Chief Executive Officer, Rockdale Hospital and Health System, Conyers, GA, p. A103

TOENBER, Garry A., Ph.D., Director, Colorado Mental Health Institute at Fort Logan, Denver, CO, p. A69

TOERING, Marla, Administrator, Sioux Center Community Hospital and Health Center/Avera Health, Sioux Center, IA, p. A156

TOLL, Sidney A., President, North Country Hospital and Health Center, Newport, VT, p. A440

TOLMAN, Russell K., President and Chief Executive Officer, Cook Children's Medical Center, Fort Worth, TX, p. A412

TOLMIE, John Kerr, President and Chief Executive Officer, St. Joseph Hospital, Lancaster, PA, p. A362

TOLOSKY, Mark R., Chief Executive Officer, Baystate Medical Center, Springfield, MA, p. A208

TOMPKINS, John, Administrator, Baptist Memorial Hospital-Union County, New Albany, MS, p. A241

TOMT, Gene, FACHE, Chief Executive Officer, Bonner General Hospital, Sandpoint, ID, p. A117

TONGATE, Scott, Chief Administrative Officer, Carthage General Hospital, Carthage, TN, p. A390

TONNESON, Ida, Chief Executive Officer, Craig House Center, Beacon, NY, p. A288

TOOMER, Eugene, Chief Operating Officer, Bon Secours-Richmond Community Hospital, Richmond, VA, p. A448

TOOMEY, Joseph F., President and Chief Executive Officer, Resurrection Health Care Corporation, Chicago, IL, p. B128

TOOMEY, Richard Kirk, President and Chief Executive Officer, Nash Health Care Systems, Rocky Mount, NC, p. A317

TOPP , II, Walter, Administrator, Cibola General Hospital, Grants, NM, p. A285

TOPPER, David, Chief Executive Officer, Alta Healthcare System, Santa Monica, CA, p. B52

TORBA, Gerald M., Chief Executive Officer, Callaway Community Hospital, Fulton, MO, p. A247

TORCHIA, Jude, Chief Executive Officer, Deering Hospital, Miami, FL, p. A89

TORRES, Diane D., R.N., Executive Director, Sebastian River Medical Center, Sebastian, FL, p. A95

TORRES, Jorge, Vice President and Chief Executive Officer, First Hospital Panamericano, Cidra, PR, p. A482

TORRES-ZAYAS, Domingo, Executive Director, Hospital Menonita De Cayey, Cayey, PR, p. A482

TORRESCANO, Bob, Administrator, North Florida Reception Center Hospital, Lake Butler, FL, p. A87

TOTH, Cynthia M., Administrator, Shands Rehab Hospital, Gainesville, FL, p. A85

TOURVILLE, James C., Administrator, Douglas County Hospital, Omaha, NE, p. A265

TOUSSAINT, John S., M.D., President and Chief Executive Officer, ThedaCare, Inc., Appleton, WI, p. B143

TOWNSEND, Walden, Service Unit Director, U. S. Public Health Service Owyhee Community Health Facility, Owyhee, NV, p. A269

TOWNSEND , Jr, C. Vincent, Senior Vice President, St. Joseph Medical Center, Albuquerque, NM, p. A283

TOY, Joseph A., President and Chief Executive Officer, Eastern State Hospital, Lexington, KY, p. A174

TRABER, Peter G., M.D.
Chief Executive Officer and Dean, Hospital of the University of Pennsylvania, Philadelphia, PA, p. A367
Chief Executive Officer and Dean, University of Pennsylvania Health System, Philadelphia, PA, p. B149

TRACEY, Robert M., Administrator, Franciscan Skemp Healthcare-Arcadia Campus, Arcadia, WI, p. A466

TRACHTA, Michael D.
Chief Executive Officer, Keokuk County Health Center, Sigourney, IA, p. A156
Administrator, Marengo Memorial Hospital, Marengo, IA, p. A154

TRACY, Tim, Executive Vice President and Chief Operating Officer, John C Lincoln Hospital-Deer Valley, Phoenix, AZ, p. A24

TRACY, Timothy J., Chief Executive Officer, Towner County Medical Center, Cando, ND, p. A321

TRACY, John, Commander, Naval Hospital, Oak Harbor, WA, p. A455

TRAHAN, Alcus, Administrator, Acadia-St. Landry Hospital, Church Point, LA, p. A181

TRAHAN, Daniel M., Administrator, Leonard J. Chabert Medical Center, Houma, LA, p. A183

TRAHAN, Lyman, Chief Executive Officer, Abrom Kaplan Memorial Hospital, Kaplan, LA, p. A183

TRAMP, Francis, President, Burgess Health Center, Onawa, IA, p. A155

TRAUTMAN, Robert J., Administrator, Vencor Hospital-Ontario, Ontario, CA, p. A54

TRAVERSE, Bruce L., President, Carson City Hospital, Carson City, MI, p. A212

TREFRY, Robert J., President and Chief Executive Officer, Bridgeport Hospital, Bridgeport, CT, p. A74

TREMBATH, Douglas R., President and Chief Executive Officer, Audrain Medical Center, Mexico, MO, p. A250

TREXLER, David V., President, Decatur County Memorial Hospital, Greensburg, IN, p. A140

TRIANA, Milton, President and Chief Executive Officer, St. Mary Medical Center, Hobart, IN, p. A141

TRIEBES, David G., Chief Executive Officer, Wood River Township Hospital, Wood River, IL, p. A136

TRIMBLE, Charley O.
President and Chief Executive Officer, Covenant Children's Hospital, Lubbock, TX, p. A422
President and Chief Executive Officer, Covenant Medical Center, Lubbock, TX, p. A422
President and Chief Executive Officer, Covenant Medical Center-Lakeside, Lubbock, TX, p. A422

TRIMBLE, Deborah L., Administrator, Paul B. Hall Regional Medical Center, Paintsville, KY, p. A177

TRIMM, Robert M., President and Chief Executive Officer, Satilla Regional Medical Center, Waycross, GA, p. A111

TRIMMER, Mary R., President and Chief Executive Officer, Mercy Hospital, Port Huron, MI, p. A221

TROTTER, Patrick J., Chief Executive Officer, Two Rivers Community Hospital and Hamilton Memorial Home, Two Rivers, WI, p. A476

TROWER, G. Wil, President and Chief Executive Officer, North Broward Hospital District, Fort Lauderdale, FL, p. B114

TROY, Thomas J., President and Chief Executive Officer, Grays Harbor Community Hospital, Aberdeen, WA, p. A452

TRSTENSKY, Jomary, President, Hospital Sisters Health System, Springfield, IL, p. B99

TRUDELL, Thomas J., President and Chief Executive Officer, Marymount Hospital, Garfield Heights, OH, p. A332

TRUELOVE, Lynn, Administrator, Singing River Hospital, Pascagoula, MS, p. A241

TRUJILLO, Michael, M.P.H., Director, U. S. Public Health Service Indian Health Service, Rockville, MD, p. B145

TRULL, David J., President and Chief Executive Officer, Faulkner Hospital, Boston, MA, p. A202

TRUSKOLOSKI, Roger, Vice President and Chief Executive Officer, Memorial Hermann Rehabilitation Hospital, Houston, TX, p. A417

TRUSLEY , II, James F., Director, Veterans Affairs Medical Center, Dublin, GA, p. A104

TSCHIDER, Richard A., FACHE, Administrator and Chief Executive Officer, St. Alexius Medical Center, Bismarck, ND, p. A321

TSO, Ronald, Chief Executive Officer, Chinle Comprehensive Health Care Facility, Chinle, AZ, p. A22

TUCHSCHMIDT, James, M.D., Chief Executive Officer, Veterans Affairs Medical Center, Portland, OR, p. A353

TUCKER, Edgar L., Director, Veterans Affairs Eastern Kansas Health Care System, Topeka, KS, p. A168

TUCKER, John A., Chief Executive Officer, Memorial Hospital of Center, Center, TX, p. A406

TUCKER, Paul, Administrator, Highline Community Hospital, Seattle, WA, p. A456

TUELL, William J., Director, De Jarnette Center, Staunton, VA, p. A450
TULLMAN, Stephen M.
  Chief Executive Officer, Century City Hospital, Los Angeles, CA, p. A47
  Chief Executive Officer, Midway Hospital Medical Center, Los Angeles, CA, p. A48
TUNGATE, Rex A., Administrator, Westlake Regional Hospital, Columbia, KY, p. A171
TURK, Herbert A., FACHE, Administrator, Sweeny Community Hospital, Sweeny, TX, p. A431
TURK, Jan, Chief Executive Officer, Vencor Hospital - New Orleans, New Orleans, LA, p. A187
TURNBULL, James, Administrator and Chief Executive Officer, Clara Barton Hospital, Hoisington, KS, p. A162
TURNER, Andrew L., Chief Executive Officer and Chairman of the Board, Sun Healthcare Group, Albuquerque, NM, p. B138
TURNER, Howard D., Chief Executive Officer, Heart of the Rockies Regional Medical Center, Salida, CO, p. A72
TURNER, Jeff, President and Chief Executive Officer, University Health System, San Antonio, TX, p. A430
TURNER, John, Chief Executive Officer, Quillen Rehabilitation Hospital, Johnson City, TN, p. A394
TURNER, Joseph F., President, Central Suffolk Hospital, Riverhead, NY, p. A303
TURNER, M. Sue, Administrator, Latimer County General Hospital, Wilburton, OK, p. A349
TURNER, Mark, Chief Executive Officer, Ojai Valley Community Hospital, Ojai, CA, p. A53
TURNER, Robert J., Chief Operating Officer, St. Elizabeth Hospital, Appleton, WI, p. A466
TURNEY, Brian, Chief Executive Officer, Kingman Regional Medical Center, Kingman, AZ, p. A23
TUTEN, E. Allen, Administrator, Lincoln General Hospital, Ruston, LA, p. A188
TWISS, Gayla J., Service Unit Director, U. S. Public Health Service Indian Hospital, Rosebud, SD, p. A387
TYLER, Rosamond, Administrator, Bolivar General Hospital, Bolivar, TN, p. A390
TYRA, Allen, Administrator, Healthsouth Rehabilitation Hospital of Kokomo, Kokomo, IN, p. A142

U

UDAYAKUMAR, Gowdagere, Chief Executive Officer, Lee County Community Hospital, Pennington Gap, VA, p. A447
UFFER, Mark H., Chief Executive Officer, Arrowhead Regional Medical Center, Colton, CA, p. A39
UHLING, Casey, Chief Executive Officer, St. Mary's Hospital, Cottonwood, ID, p. A116
ULAND, Jonas S., Executive Director, Greene County General Hospital, Linton, IN, p. A143
ULBRICHT, William G., Chief Operating Officer, South Florida Baptist Hospital, Plant City, FL, p. A93
ULICNY, Gary R., Ph.D., President and Chief Executive Officer, Shepherd Center, Atlanta, GA, p. A100
ULLIAN, Elaine S., President and Chief Executive Officer, Boston Medical Center, Boston, MA, p. A202
ULMER, Evonne G., JD, Chief Executive Officer, Ionia County Memorial Hospital, Ionia, MI, p. A217
ULMER, Sr, J. L., Commanding Officer, U. S. Naval Hospital, Agana, GU, p. A481
ULSETH, Randy, Administrator, Community Hospital, Cannon Falls, MN, p. A226
UMBDENSTOCK, Richard J., President and Chief Executive Officer, Providence Services, Spokane, WA, p. B121
UNDERKOFLER, Joseph, Director, Veterans Affairs Montana Healthcare System, Fort Harrison, MT, p. A257
UNDERRINER, David T., Operations Administrator, Providence Portland Medical Center, Portland, OR, p. A353
UNDERWOOD, Eugene, Chief Executive Officer, Richwood Area Community Hospital, Richwood, WV, p. A464
UNROE, Larry J., President, Marietta Memorial Hospital, Marietta, OH, p. A334
UNRUH, Greg, Chief Executive Officer, Scott County Hospital, Scott City, KS, p. A167
URCIUOLI, Robert A., President and Chief Executive Officer, Roger Williams Medical Center, Providence, RI, p. A376
UROSEVICH, Steve L., Chief Executive Officer, St. Croix Regional Medical Center, Saint Croix Falls, WI, p. A475
URQUHART, Teresa C., Administrator and Chief Operating Officer, Rio Vista Physical Rehabilitation Hospital, El Paso, TX, p. A411
URSO, Susan, Administrator, Mendota Community Hospital, Mendota, IL, p. A130
URVAND, Leslie O., Administrator, St. Luke's Hospital, Crosby, ND, p. A321
USHIJIMA, Arthur A., President and Chief Executive Officer, Queen's Medical Center, Honolulu, HI, p. A112
UTLEY, Karen, Executive Director, Pathways, Jackson, TN, p. A393

V

VAAGENES, Carl P., Administrator, Pipestone County Medical Center/Avera Health, Pipestone, MN, p. A232
VADELLA, Anthony J., Chief Executive Officer, Poplar Springs Hospital, Petersburg, VA, p. A447
VALENTINE, Billy M., Director, Overton Brooks Veterans Affairs Medical Center, Shreveport, LA, p. A188
VALIANTE, John, Chief Executive Officer, St. John's Hospital and Living Center, Jackson, WY, p. A479
VALLIANT, Robert F., Administrator, Bartlett Regional Hospital, Juneau, AK, p. A21
VAN DORNICK, Jim, Administrator, Community Memorial Hospital, Oconto Falls, WI, p. A473
VAN DRIEL, Allen, Administrator, Harlan County Health System, Alma, NE, p. A261
VAN LITH, Richard
  Chief Executive Officer, Bon Secours Cottage Health Services–Bon Secours Hospital, Grosse Pointe, MI, p. A216
  Chief Executive Officer, Bon Secours Cottage Health Services–Cottage Hospital, Grosse Pointe Farms, MI, p. A216
VAN STRATEN, Elizabeth, President and Chief Executive Officer, St. Bernard Hospital and Health Care Center, Chicago, IL, p. A123
VAN VRANKEN, Ross, Chief Executive Officer, University of Utah Neuropsychiatric Institute, Salt Lake City, UT, p. A438
VANASKIE, William F., President and Chief Executive Officer, Robert Packer Hospital, Sayre, PA, p. A371
VANDENBROEK, Deborah, President and Chief Executive Officer, Mercy Medical Center–Sioux City, Sioux City, IA, p. A156
VANDER DOES, Victor, Administrator, Pioneer Memorial Hospital, Heppner, OR, p. A351
VANDERHOOF, Terry L., President and Chief Executive Officer, River Valley Health System, Ironton, OH, p. A333
VANDERVEER, Robert W., President and Chief Executive Officer, Knapp Medical Center, Weslaco, TX, p. A434
VANDERVORT, Darryl L., President and Chief Executive Officer, Katherine Shaw Bethea Hospital, Dixon, IL, p. A125
VANEK, James, Administrator, Lavaca Medical Center, Hallettsville, TX, p. A415
VANOURNY, Stephen E., M.D., President and Chief Executive Officer, St. Luke's Hospital, Cedar Rapids, IA, p. A149
VARGAS, Laura, Administrator and Chief Executive Officer, BHC Hospital San Juan Capestrano, San Juan, PR, p. A483
VARLAND, Carol A.
  Administrator, Community Memorial Hospital/Avera Health, Burke, SD, p. A385
  Chief Executive Officer, Gregory Community Hospital, Gregory, SD, p. A386
VARMUS, Harold, M.D., President and Chief Executive Officer, Memorial Sloan–Kettering Cancer Center, New York, NY, p. A298
VARNADO, Jerry C., Administrator, Hardeman County Memorial Hospital, Quanah, TX, p. A427
VARNUM, James W., President, Mary Hitchcock Memorial Hospital, Lebanon, NH, p. A272
VARONE, Rick J., President, Staten Island University Hospital, New York, NY, p. A300
VASKELIS, Glenna L., Interim Vice President and Chief Operating Officer, St. Louise Regional Hospital, Gilroy, CA, p. A42
VATTER, Russell K., Superintendent, Moccasin Bend Mental Health Institute, Chattanooga, TN, p. A391
VAUGHAN, Page, Executive Director, Carolina Pines Regional Medical Center, Hartsville, SC, p. A382
VAUGHT, Richard H., Administrator, William Newton Memorial Hospital, Winfield, KS, p. A169
VAZQUEZ, Manuel J., Administrator, Hospital Matilde Brenes, Bayamon, PR, p. A481
VECCHIONE, George A., President, Lifespan Corporation, Providence, RI, p. B105
VEENSTRA, Henry A., President, Zeeland Community Hospital, Zeeland, MI, p. A224
VEITZ, Larry W., Chief Executive Officer, Canton–Inwood Memorial Hospital, Canton, SD, p. A385
VELEZ, Domingo, Administrator, Industrial Hospital, San Juan, PR, p. A484
VELEZ, Pete, Executive Director, Elmhurst Hospital Center, New York, NY, p. A296
VELICK, Stephen H., Chief Executive Officer, Henry Ford Hospital, Detroit, MI, p. A213
VELLINGA, David H., President and Chief Executive Officer, Mercy Medical Center–Des Moines, Des Moines, IA, p. A151
VELTE, Carl J., Chief Executive Officer, Munising Memorial Hospital, Munising, MI, p. A219
VENTURA, N. Lawrence, Superintendent, Bangor Mental Health Institute, Bangor, ME, p. A191
VERK, Chelle, Executive Administrator, Pittsburgh Specialty Hospital, Pittsburgh, PA, p. A369
VERMAELEN, Elizabeth A., President, Sisters of Charity Center, New York, NY, p. B133
VERNEGAARD, Niels P., Chief Executive Officer, Parkridge Medical Center, Chattanooga, TN, p. A391
VERNOR, Robert E., Administrator, Seymour Hospital, Seymour, TX, p. A430
VERNOSKI, Barbara, Commanding Officer, Naval Hospital, Jacksonville, FL, p. A86
VIA, Bob, Chief Executive Officer, Emanuel County Hospital, Swainsboro, GA, p. A110
VIATOR, Kyle J., Chief Executive Officer, Dauterive Hospital, New Iberia, LA, p. A186
VICE, Jon E., President and Chief Executive Officer, Children's Hospital of Wisconsin, Milwaukee, WI, p. A471
VICTORY, Ronald D., Administrator, Penobscot Valley Hospital, Lincoln, ME, p. A193
VILAR, Ramon J., Administrator, Wilma N. Vazquez Medical Center, Vega Baja, PR, p. A484
VILLARREAL, Xavier, Chief Executive Officer, Fairfax Memorial Hospital, Fairfax, OK, p. A343
VINARDI, Gregory B., President and Chief Executive Officer, Western Missouri Medical Center, Warrensburg, MO, p. A255
VINCENT, Rose, President and Chief Executive Officer, St. Elizabeth Medical Center, Utica, NY, p. A306
VINCENZ, Felix T., Ph.D., Chief Executive Officer, Fulton State Hospital, Fulton, MO, p. A247
VINSON, Daniel M., CPA
  Senior Vice President, St. Luke Hospital East, Fort Thomas, KY, p. A172
  Senior Vice President, St. Luke Hospital West, Florence, KY, p. A172
VINSON, Roy S., President, McAllen Heart Hospital, McAllen, TX, p. A423
VINTURELLA, Joseph C., Chief Executive Officer, Southeast Louisiana Hospital, Mandeville, LA, p. A185
VINYARD, II, Roy G., President and Chief Executive Officer, Asante Health System, Medford, OR, p. B53
VIOLI, Ronald L., President and Chief Executive Officer, Children's Hospital of Pittsburgh, Pittsburgh, PA, p. A369
VITO, Christopher A., Chief Executive Officer, Monrovia Community Hospital, Monrovia, CA, p. A51
VIVALDI, Domingo Cruz, Administrator, San Jorge Children's Hospital, San Juan, PR, p. A484

Index of Health Care Professionals / Vlach

VLACH, Karen, Administrator, Oakland Memorial Hospital, Oakland, NE, p. A265
VODENICKER, Johnette L., Administrator, Memorial Hospital–West Volusia, De Land, FL, p. A83
VOGT, Allen J., Administrator, Cook Hospital and Convalescent Nursing Care Unit, Cook, MN, p. A227
VOLCKERS, Alfredo, Executive Director, Hospital Pavia–Santurce, San Juan, PR, p. A483
VOLK, Ronald J., President, St. Aloisius Medical Center, Harvey, ND, p. A322
VOLPE, Michele M., Executive Director, Presbyterian Medical Center of the University of Pennsylvania Health System, Philadelphia, PA, p. A367
VONDERFECHT, Dennis
 President and Chief Executive Officer, Johnson City Medical Center, Johnson City, TN, p. A394
 President and Chief Executive Officer, Mountain States Health Alliance, Johnson City, TN, p. B112
VONDRAK, Darrell E., Administrator, Palo Alto Health System, Emmetsburg, IA, p. A151
VORSETH, Duane R., Chief Executive Officer, SCCI Hospital of Kokomo, Kokomo, IN, p. A142
VOSS, Daryle, Chief Executive Officer, Kingfisher Regional Hospital, Kingfisher, OK, p. A344
VOSS, Wayne M., Chief Executive Officer, Memorial Hermann Memorial City Hospital, Houston, TX, p. A417
VOWELL, John H., Interim Administrator, Sitka Community Hospital, Sitka, AK, p. A21
VOZOS, Frank J., FACS, Executive Director, Monmouth Medical Center, Long Branch, NJ, p. A277
VREELAND, James C., FACHE, President and Chief Executive Officer, UPMC Bedford Memorial, Everett, PA, p. A360
VU, Dac, M.D., Chief Executive Officer, Northside General Hospital, Houston, TX, p. A417
VYVERBERG, Robert W., Ed.D., Director, George A. Zeller Mental Health Center, Peoria, IL, p. A132

W

WADE, Linda, Administrator and Director of Operations, HEALTHSOUTH Rehabilitation Hospital of Montgomery, Montgomery, AL, p. A17
WAGES, N. Gary, President and Chief Executive Officer, Saint Luke's Northland Hospital, Kansas City, MO, p. A248
WAGGENER, Rob S., Chief Executive Officer, Charter Lakeside Behavioral Health System, Memphis, TN, p. A396
WAGNER, Arthur, Chief Operating Officer, North Central Bronx Hospital, New York, NY, p. A299
WAGNER, David S., Vice President and Administrator, Christus Spohn Hospital Beeville, Beeville, TX, p. A404
WAGNER, Henry C., President, Jewish Hospital HealthCare Services, Louisville, KY, p. B102
WAGNER, Janet, Chief Administrative Officer, Sutter Davis Hospital, Davis, CA, p. A39
WAHLMEIER, James, Administrator, Phillips County Hospital, Phillipsburg, KS, p. A166
WAHPEPAH, Frank H., M.P.H., Administrator, Creek Nation Community Hospital, Okemah, OK, p. A345
WAITE, Marguerite, President and Chief Executive Officer, St. Mary's Hospital, Waterbury, CT, p. A77
WAITE , II, Ralph J., Chief Executive Officer, BHC Meadow Wood Hospital, Baton Rouge, LA, p. A180
WAKEFIELD , Jr, Robert D., Chief Executive Officer, Lemuel Shattuck Hospital, Boston, MA, p. A202
WAKEMAN, Daniel, Chief Executive Officer, Chippewa County War Memorial Hospital, Sault Ste. Marie, MI, p. A222
WALB, William R., President and Chief Executive Officer, Hanover Hospital, Hanover, PA, p. A361
WALDBILLIG, Kurt, Chief Executive Officer, Richardton Health Center, Richardton, ND, p. A323
WALDO, Bruce, Chief Executive Officer, Richland Hospital, Mansfield, OH, p. A334
WALDROUP, Gerald E., Administrator, Lawrence County Memorial Hospital, Lawrenceville, IL, p. A129
WALK, Rex D., Chief Executive Officer, Memorial Health Center, Sidney, NE, p. A266

WALKER, Benjamin H., Facility Administrator, Georgia Regional Hospital at Augusta, Augusta, GA, p. A101
WALKER, Bethy W., Chief Executive Officer, Doctors' Hospital of Opelousas, Opelousas, LA, p. A187
WALKER, Gale, Administrator, Avera St. Benedict Health Center, Parkston, SD, p. A387
WALKER, Gregory J., Chief Executive Officer, Wentworth–Douglass Hospital, Dover, NH, p. A271
WALKER, Henry G., President and Chief Executive Officer, Providence Health System, Seattle, WA, p. B120
WALKER, James R., FACHE, President and Chief Executive Officer, North Arundel Hospital, Glen Burnie, MD, p. A198
WALKER, Jerry, Administrator, Leahi Hospital, Honolulu, HI, p. A112
WALKER, John E., Chief Executive Officer, Doctors Hospital of Jefferson, Metairie, LA, p. A185
WALKER, Larry D., Chief Executive Officer, Eunice Community Medical Center, Eunice, LA, p. A182
WALKER, Melvin E., Administrator, Baptist Memorial Hospital–Desoto, Southaven, MS, p. A242
WALKER, Robert J., President, Castle Medical Center, Kailua, HI, p. A113
WALKER, Ronnie D., President, Southwestern Memorial Hospital, Weatherford, OK, p. A349
WALKLEY , Jr, Philip H., Chief Executive Officer, Regional Medical Center of Northeast Arkansas, Jonesboro, AR, p. A31
WALL, Daniel J., President and Chief Executive Officer, Emma Pendleton Bradley Hospital, East Providence, RI, p. A376
WALL, Eldon A., Administrator, Memorial Hospital, Aurora, NE, p. A261
WALL, Joseph C., Chief Executive Officer, Kona Community Hospital, Kealakekua, HI, p. A113
WALLACE, Archie T., Chief Executive Officer, Thomas B. Finan Center, Cumberland, MD, p. A198
WALLACE, David T., President and Chief Executive Officer, Brown County General Hospital, Georgetown, OH, p. A332
WALLACE, James D., Executive Director, Choctaw Health Center, Philadelphia, MS, p. A241
WALLACE, Lloyd E., President and Chief Executive Officer, Valdese General Hospital, Valdese, NC, p. A319
WALLACE, Mark A., Executive Director and Chief Executive Officer, Texas Children's Hospital, Houston, TX, p. A418
WALLACE, Michael S., Chief Executive Officer, Lucas County Health Center, Chariton, IA, p. A149
WALLACE, Patrick L., Administrator, East Texas Medical Center Athens, Athens, TX, p. A402
WALLACE, Samuel T., President, Iowa Health System, Des Moines, IA, p. B101
WALLACE, Thomas M., President and Chief Executive Officer, Granada Hills Community Hospital, Los Angeles, CA, p. A47
WALLER, Richard, Chief Executive Officer, Millinocket Regional Hospital, Millinocket, ME, p. A193
WALLER, Richard E., M.D., Interim Administrator, Quitman County Hospital and Nursing Home, Marks, MS, p. A240
WALLING, John R., President and Chief Executive Officer, Greater Lafayette Health Service, Lafayette, IN, p. A143
WALLIS, Larry D.
 President and Chief Executive Officer, Cox Health System, Springfield, MO, p. B76
 President and Chief Executive Officer, Lester E. Cox Medical Centers, Springfield, MO, p. A254
WALLMAN, Gerald H., Administrator, Doctors Hospital of West Covina, West Covina, CA, p. A67
WALLS, Michael L.
 Chief Executive Officer, Alameda County Medical Center, San Leandro, CA, p. A61
 Chief Executive Officer, Alameda County Medical Center–Highland Campus, Oakland, CA, p. A53
WALMSLEY , II, George J., President and Chief Executive Officer, North Philadelphia Health System, Philadelphia, PA, p. A367
WALSH, Daniel P., President and Chief Executive Officer, Winthrop–University Hospital, Mineola, NY, p. A294

WALSH, Mary Beth, M.D., Chief Executive Officer, Burke Rehabilitation Hospital, White Plains, NY, p. A307
WALSH, Maura, Chief Executive Officer, Mainland Medical Center, Texas City, TX, p. A432
WALSH, Raoul, Chief Executive Officer, Greene County Memorial Hospital, Waynesburg, PA, p. A373
WALSH, William, Executive Director, Coney Island Hospital, New York, NY, p. A296
WALTER, William R., Chief Executive Officer, Maury Regional Hospital, Columbia, TN, p. A391
WALTERS, Farah M.
 President and Chief Executive Officer, University Hospitals Health System, Cleveland, OH, p. B148
 President and Chief Executive Officer, University Hospitals of Cleveland, Cleveland, OH, p. A329
WALTERS, Kevin, Administrator, Southeast Baptist Hospital, San Antonio, TX, p. A429
WALTERS, Norman E., Administrator, R. J. Reynolds–Patrick County Memorial Hospital, Stuart, VA, p. A450
WALTERS, Robert M., Administrator, St. Luke's Hospital, Jacksonville, FL, p. A87
WALTON, Carlyle L. E., President, Takoma Adventist Hospital, Greeneville, TN, p. A393
WALTON, Michael W., Director, Veterans Affairs Medical Center, Chillicothe, OH, p. A327
WALTZ, Ronald D., Chief Executive Officer, Memorial Health Care Systems, Seward, NE, p. A266
WALZ, George, CHE, Chief Executive Officer, Breckinridge Memorial Hospital, Hardinsburg, KY, p. A172
WALZ, Patrick T., Chief Executive Officer, Mesa General Hospital Medical Center, Mesa, AZ, p. A23
WANGENSTEIN, Martha C., Vice President and Site Administrator, Legacy Good Samaritan Hospital and Medical Center, Portland, OR, p. A353
WANGER, David, Chief Executive Officer, White Mountain Regional Medical Center, Springerville, AZ, p. A26
WANGLER, Patricia, Chief Executive Officer, First Care Medical Services, Fosston, MN, p. A228
WARBOYS, Anita, R.N., Administrator, Winslow Memorial Hospital, Winslow, AZ, p. A27
WARD, Sandy, Administrator, Johnson County Healthcare Center, Buffalo, WY, p. A478
WARDELL, Patrick R., President and Chief Executive Officer, St. Joseph's Hospital and Medical Center, Paterson, NJ, p. A279
WARDELL, Scott F., Administrator, U. S. Air Force Hospital, Fairchild AFB, WA, p. A453
WARDEN, Gail L., President and Chief Executive Officer, Henry Ford Health System, Detroit, MI, p. B98
WARMAN , Jr, Harold C., President and Chief Executive Officer, Highlands Regional Medical Center, Prestonsburg, KY, p. A178
WARNER, Donald L., Chief Executive Officer, Arborview Hospital, Warren, MI, p. A223
WARNER , Jr, Gerard H., Chief Executive Officer, Mid–Valley Hospital, Peckville, PA, p. A366
WARREN, Larry, Executive Director, University of Michigan Hospitals and Health Centers, Ann Arbor, MI, p. A211
WARREN, Richard M., Chief Executive Officer, El Camino Hospital, Mountain View, CA, p. A52
WARREN, Roger D., M.D., Administrator, Hanover Hospital, Hanover, KS, p. A162
WASHBURN, Melinda, Chief Operating Officer, Saint Joseph Hospital East, Lexington, KY, p. A174
WASSERMAN, Joseph A., President and Chief Executive Officer, Lakeland Medical Center–St. Joseph, Saint Joseph, MI, p. A222
WASSERMAN, Neil H., Chief Executive Officer, Hawthorn Center, Northville, MI, p. A220
WASSON, Ted D., President and Chief Executive Officer, William Beaumont Hospital Corporation, Royal Oak, MI, p. B155
WATERS, Michael C., FACHE, President, Hendrick Health System, Abilene, TX, p. A401
WATERSTON, Judith C., President and Chief Executive Officer, Schwab Rehabilitation Hospital and Care Network, Chicago, IL, p. A123
WATHEN, James A., Chief Executive Officer, Southern Coos Hospital and Health Center, Bandon, OR, p. A350

Index of Health Care Professionals / White

WATSON, Craig B., Chief Executive Officer, Delta Medical Center, Memphis, TN, p. A396

WATSON, Gary L., FACHE, Senior Executive Officer, Crittenton, Kansas City, MO, p. A248

WATSON, James B., Chief Executive Officer, Ira Davenport Memorial Hospital, Bath, NY, p. A288

WATSON, James R., Administrator, Ashland Community Hospital, Ashland, OR, p. A350

WATSON, T. Gregg
 Administrator, Sheboygan Memorial Medical Center, Sheboygan, WI, p. A475
 Administrator, Valley View Medical Center, Plymouth, WI, p. A474

WATSON, Virgil, Administrator, Sumner County Hospital District One, Caldwell, KS, p. A159

WATTERS, Steve, Chief Executive Officer, Mendota Mental Health Institute, Madison, WI, p. A470

WAUGH, Patrick D., Chief Executive Officer, St. Luke's Behavioral Health Center, Phoenix, AZ, p. A25

WEADICK, James F., Administrator and Chief Executive Officer, Newton General Hospital, Covington, GA, p. A103

WEATHERFORD, Dennis, Interim Administrator, Putnam County Hospital, Greencastle, IN, p. A140

WEATHERLY, Jesse O., President, Cullman Regional Medical Center, Cullman, AL, p. A13

WEAVER, Judy, Administrator, Vencor Hospital–Pittsburgh, Oakdale, PA, p. A365

WEAVER, Thomas H., FACHE, Director, Veterans Affairs Medical Center, Bay Pines, FL, p. A81

WEAVER, William, Administrator, Bradford Health Services at Oak Mountain, Pelham, AL, p. A17

WEBB, Lynn E., Chief Executive Officer and Administrator, Psychiatric Hospital at Vanderbilt, Nashville, TN, p. A398

WEBB, Ronald W., Chief Executive Officer, Our Lady of Lourdes Regional Medical Center, Lafayette, LA, p. A184

WEBBER, Deborah G., Chief Executive Officer, Greater El Monte Community Hospital, South El Monte, CA, p. A63

WEBER, Mark, FACHE, President, St. John's Mercy Medical Center, Saint Louis, MO, p. A253

WEBER, Michael T., President and Chief Executive Officer, Putnam Hospital Center, Carmel, NY, p. A290

WEBER, Peter M., President and Chief Executive Officer, Huguley Memorial Medical Center, Fort Worth, TX, p. A413

WEBER, Jr, Everett P., President and Chief Executive Officer, Grady Memorial Hospital, Delaware, OH, p. A331

WEBSTER, Mark, President, Troy Community Hospital, Troy, PA, p. A373

WEE, Donald J., Executive Director, Pioneer Memorial Hospital, Prineville, OR, p. A353

WEEKS, Donnie J., President and Chief Executive Officer, Kershaw County Medical Center, Camden, SC, p. A378

WEEKS, Steven Douglas
 Senior Vice President and Administrator, Baptist Health Medical Center–Little Rock, Little Rock, AR, p. A31
 Senior Vice President and Administrator, Baptist Health Rehabilitation Institute, Little Rock, AR, p. A31

WEGENER, Kathleen S., Administrator, Kaiser Sunnyside Medical Center, Clackamas, OR, p. A350

WEHMEYER, Kerry, Chief Executive Officer, Springhill Medical Center, Springhill, LA, p. A189

WEIGHTMAN, George, Commander, McDonald Army Community Hospital, Fort Eustis, VA, p. A444

WEILER, Joseph W., President, McKenzie Memorial Hospital, Sandusky, MI, p. A222

WEINBAUM, Barry G., Chief Executive Officer, Alvarado Hospital Medical Center, San Diego, CA, p. A58

WEINBERG, Arnold N., M.D., Director, M. I. T. Medical Department, Cambridge, MA, p. A204

WEINBERG, Barth A., Vice President, Inpatient Rehabilitation, Frazier Rehabilitation Center, Louisville, KY, p. A175

WEINER, David S., Chief Executive Officer, Children's Hospital, Boston, MA, p. A202

WEINER, Jack, President and Chief Executive Officer, St. Joseph's Mercy Hospitals and Health Services, Clinton Township, MI, p. A213

WEINHOLD, Keith J., Interim Director, University Hospitals and Clinics, Columbia, MO, p. A246

WEINSTEIN, Stephen M., President, Michael Reese Hospital and Medical Center, Chicago, IL, p. A122

WEINSTOCK, Dean R., Director, Kingsboro Psychiatric Center, New York, NY, p. A297

WEIR, Silas M., Chief Executive Officer, Centura Special Care Hospital, Denver, CO, p. A69

WEISS, Thomas M., Chief Executive Officer, Crestwood Medical Center, Huntsville, AL, p. A15

WELBORN, Bobby, Administrator, Perry County General Hospital, Richton, MS, p. A242

WELCH, Bill, Administrator, Jefferson Community Health Center, Fairbury, NE, p. A262

WELCH, Nelda K., Administrator, East Texas Medical Center Crockett, Crockett, TX, p. A408

WELLINGER, M. Rosita, President and Chief Executive Officer, St. Francis Health System, Pittsburgh, PA, p. B137

WELLMAN, Roxann A., Chief Executive Officer, Minnewaska District Hospital, Starbuck, MN, p. A234

WELLS, Mary, Administrator, Community Memorial Hospital, Sumner, IA, p. A157

WELLS, Mary Ellen, Administrator, Buffalo Hospital, Buffalo, MN, p. A226

WELLS, Scott, Administrator, Franklin General Hospital, Hampton, IA, p. A152

WELSH, John H., Chief Executive Officer, Rumford Hospital, Rumford, ME, p. A194

WELSH, Jr, J. L., President and Chief Executive Officer, Southeastern Regional Medical Center, Lumberton, NC, p. A315

WELTZIN, Richard, USAF, Administrator, Scott Medical Center, Scott AFB, IL, p. A134

WENDLING, Jeffrey T., President and Chief Executive Officer, Northern Michigan Regional Health System, Petoskey, MI, p. A220

WENTE, James W., CHE, Administrator, Southeast Missouri Hospital, Cape Girardeau, MO, p. A245

WENTWORTH, Philip M., FACHE, President, Presbyterian Hospital of Plano, Plano, TX, p. A426

WENTZ, Robert J., President and Chief Executive Officer, Oroville Hospital, Oroville, CA, p. A54

WERFT, Ron
 Chief Executive Officer, Cottage Health System, Santa Barbara, CA, p. B75
 President and Chief Executive Officer, Santa Barbara Cottage Hospital, Santa Barbara, CA, p. A62
 President and Chief Executive Officer, Santa Ynez Valley Cottage Hospital, Solvang, CA, p. A63

WERNER, Daniel J., Administrator, Owatonna Hospital, Owatonna, MN, p. A231

WERNER, Thomas J., Chief Executive Officer, Richland Hospital, Richland Center, WI, p. A474

WERNER, Thomas L., President, Adventist Health System Sunbelt Health Care Corporation, Winter Park, FL, p. B50

WERNER, Todd S., Senior Executive Officer, La Grange Memorial Hospital, La Grange, IL, p. A129

WERNICK, Joel, President and Chief Executive Officer, Phoebe Putney Memorial Hospital, Albany, GA, p. A99

WERTZ, Randy S., Administrator, Golden Valley Memorial Hospital, Clinton, MO, p. A245

WESOLOWSKI, Jaime A., Chief Executive Officer, Oak Hill Hospital, Spring Hill, FL, p. A95

WESP, James H., Administrator, Vencor Hospital–Louisville, Louisville, KY, p. A176

WESSNER, David, President and Chief Executive Officer, HealthSystem Minnesota, Saint Louis Park, MN, p. B98

WEST, Daniel R., Administrator, Vencor Hospital–Milwaukee, Greenfield, WI, p. A469

WEST, John, Administrator, Jackson Hospital, Marianna, FL, p. A89

WEST, Steven J., Chief Executive Officer, Blackford County Hospital, Hartford City, IN, p. A141

WEST, Warren K., President, Copley Hospital, Morrisville, VT, p. A440

WESTFALL, Bernard G., President and Chief Executive Officer, West Virginia United Health System, Fairmont, WV, p. B154

WESTON, Audrey, Administrator, Hadley Memorial Hospital, Washington, DC, p. A79

WESTON–HALL, Patricia, Executive Director, Glenbeigh Health Sources, Rock Creek, OH, p. A337

WETTA, Jr, Daniel J., Chief Executive Officer, John Randolph Medical Center, Hopewell, VA, p. A445

WHALEN, David, Chief Executive Officer, Twin Cities Hospital, Niceville, FL, p. A91

WHATLEY, David, Director, Veterans Affairs Medical Center, Houston, TX, p. A418

WHATLEY, Gary Lex
 President and Chief Executive Officer, Memorial Health System of East Texas, Lufkin, TX, p. A422
 President and Chief Executive Officer, Memorial Health System of East Texas, Lufkin, TX, p. B110

WHEELER, Michael K., Director, Veterans Affairs Medical Center, Battle Creek, MI, p. A212

WHEELER, Michael D., MSC, Deputy Commander, Administration, Evans U. S. Army Community Hospital, Fort Carson, CO, p. A70

WHEELEY, Barbara, Vice President, Sisters of Mercy of the Americas–Regional Community of Baltimore, Baltimore, MD, p. B134

WHEELOCK, Major W., President, Crotched Mountain Rehabilitation Center, Greenfield, NH, p. A271

WHELAN, Sharon, Administrator, River Falls Area Hospital, River Falls, WI, p. A475

WHELAN, Thomas, Acting Administrator, St. Mary's Hospital, Streator, IL, p. A135

WHIPKEY, Neil, Administrator, Shands at Lake Shore, Lake City, FL, p. A88

WHIPPLE, Ingrid L., Administrator and Chief Executive Officer, BHC Heritage Oaks Hospital, Sacramento, CA, p. A57

WHITAKER, David D., FACHE, President and Chief Executive Officer, Norman Regional Hospital, Norman, OK, p. A345

WHITAKER, E. Berton, President and Chief Executive Officer, Southeast Georgia Regional Medical Center, Brunswick, GA, p. A101

WHITAKER, Harold H., Administrator, Webster Health Services, Eupora, MS, p. A237

WHITAKER, James B., President, Circles of Care, Melbourne, FL, p. A89

WHITBY, Lea, Administrator, Calumet Medical Center, Chilton, WI, p. A467

WHITCOMB, John R., Interim President and Chief Executive Officer, Morgan County Memorial Hospital, Martinsville, IN, p. A143

WHITE, Alvin C., President and Chief Executive Officer, Rome Memorial Hospital, Rome, NY, p. A304

WHITE, Ben, Administrator, Mangum City Hospital, Mangum, OK, p. A344

WHITE, Cindy, Chief Financial Officer, Blackwell Regional Hospital, Blackwell, OK, p. A341

WHITE, Dale A., Chief Executive Officer, Northeast Kansas Center for Health and Wellness, Horton, KS, p. A162

WHITE, Daryl Sue, Chief Executive Officer and Managing Director, River Oaks Hospital, New Orleans, LA, p. A187

WHITE, Doug, Chief Executive Officer, Grand Strand Regional Medical Center, Myrtle Beach, SC, p. A382

WHITE, Dudley R., Administrator, Anson General Hospital, Anson, TX, p. A402

WHITE, Jeffrey L., Chief Executive Officer, Low Country General Hospital, Ridgeland, SC, p. A383

WHITE, John B., President and Chief Executive Officer, Lima Memorial Hospital, Lima, OH, p. A333

WHITE, John R., Chief Executive Officer and Superintendent, Newport Community Hospital, Newport, WA, p. A455

WHITE, Kevin A., CHE, Administrator, Medicine Lodge Memorial Hospital, Medicine Lodge, KS, p. A165

WHITE, Mary M., President and Chief Executive Officer, Swedish Medical Center, Englewood, CO, p. A70

WHITE, Roy E., Administrator, Decatur County Hospital, Leon, IA, p. A154

WHITE, Stephani, Vice President and Site Administrator, Legacy Emanuel Hospital and Health Center, Portland, OR, p. A353

WHITE, Terry R., President and Chief Executive Officer, MetroHealth Medical Center, Cleveland, OH, p. A329

Index of Health Care Professionals / White

WHITE, Thomas, President and Chief Executive Officer, Jameson Hospital, New Castle, PA, p. A365

WHITE, Thomas M., President, Empire Health Services, Spokane, WA, p. B84

WHITE, Jr, Lawrence L., President, St. Patrick Hospital, Missoula, MT, p. A259

WHITEHORN, Jeffrey, Chief Executive Officer, Southern Hills Medical Center, Nashville, TN, p. A398

WHITEHOUSE, Edward J., Chief Executive Office, Atlantic Shores Hospital, Fort Lauderdale, FL, p. A84

WHITFIELD, Gary R., FACHE, Director, Veterans Affairs Sierra Nevada Health Care System, Reno, NV, p. A269

WHITFIELD, Jr, Charles H., President and Chief Executive Officer, Laughlin Memorial Hospital, Greeneville, TN, p. A393

WHITNEY, Harry E., President and Chief Executive Officer, Santa Marta Hospital, Los Angeles, CA, p. A49

WHITTEY, Charlotte, Chief Executive Officer, Mahnomen Health Center, Mahnomen, MN, p. A230

WHITTINGTON, Terry G., Chief Executive Officer and Administrator, Lane Memorial Hospital, Zachary, LA, p. A190

WICK, Timothy J., Chief Executive Officer, Burnett Medical Center, Grantsburg, WI, p. A468

WIDENER, Steve, Chief Executive Officer, Nature Coast Regional Hospital, Williston, FL, p. A98

WIENER, Mark S., Administrator, St. Luke's Medical Center, Milwaukee, WI, p. A472

WIERCINSKI, John P., President and Chief Executive Officer, Shamokin Area Community Hospital, Coal Township, PA, p. A358

WIESNER, Gerald, Administrator, Miami County Medical Center, Paola, KS, p. A166

WIGGINS, Louise, Chief Executive Officer and Administrator, Summit Hospital of Northwest Louisiana, Bossier City, LA, p. A181

WIGGINS, Stephen P., Director, Western State Hospital, Hopkinsville, KY, p. A173

WILBANKS, John F., Administrator, Baptist Medical Center, Jacksonville, FL, p. A86

WILCOX, Sallye M., Ph.D., Executive Director, Mississippi Hospital Restorative Care, Jackson, MS, p. A239

WILCZEK, Joseph W., President and Chief Executive Officer, St. Francis Hospital, Federal Way, WA, p. A453

WILES, Patrick J.
President and Chief Executive Officer, Sisters of Charity Hospital of Buffalo, Buffalo, NY, p. A289
President and Chief Executive Officer, St. Joseph Hospital, Cheektowaga, NY, p. A290

WILES, Paul M., President and Chief Executive Officer, Novant Health, Winston Salem, NC, p. B116

WILEY, Donald J., Senior Vice President and Chief Operating Officer, St. Joseph's Medical Center, Stockton, CA, p. A64

WILEY, Stan, Administrator, Crane Memorial Hospital, Crane, TX, p. A408

WILFORD, Dan S., President and Chief Executive Officer, Memorial Hermann Healthcare System, Houston, TX, p. B110

WILHELM, Mary Eileen, President and Chief Executive Officer, Mercy Medical, Daphne, AL, p. A13

WILHELMSEN, Jr, Thomas E., President and Chief Executive Officer, Southern New Hampshire Medical Center, Nashua, NH, p. A272

WILHOIT, Ellen, President and Chief Administrative Officer, Fort Sanders–Sevier Medical Center, Sevierville, TN, p. A399

WILK, Leonard E., Administrator, Sinai Samaritan Medical Center, Milwaukee, WI, p. A472

WILKERSON, Donald H., Chief Executive Officer, North Austin Medical Center, Austin, TX, p. A403

WILKERSON, Larry D., Chief Executive Officer, Augusta Medical Complex, Augusta, KS, p. A159

WILKINS, Patricia S., Administrator, North Caddo Medical Center, Vivian, LA, p. A189

WILKINS, William W., Chief Executive Officer, OhioHealth, Columbus, OH, p. B117

WILKINSON, Gary L., Director, Veterans Affairs Medical Center, Iowa City, IA, p. A153

WILKINSON, Steven D., President and Chief Executive Officer, Menorah Medical Center, Shawnee Mission, KS, p. A167

WILL, Daniel, Administrator, Zumbrota Health Care, Zumbrota, MN, p. A235

WILLARD, Larry, Administrator, Hocking Valley Community Hospital, Logan, OH, p. A334

WILLAUER, Glenn R., Administrator, U. S. Air Force Hospital, Hampton, VA, p. A444

WILLCOXON, Phil, Chief Executive Officer, Freeman Neosho Hospital, Neosho, MO, p. A251

WILLEKE, Louis R., Administrator, Refugio County Memorial Hospital, Refugio, TX, p. A427

WILLERT, Todd, Administrator, Story County Hospital and Long Term Care Facility, Nevada, IA, p. A155

WILLETT, Richard, Chief Executive Officer, Redington–Fairview General Hospital, Skowhegan, ME, p. A194

WILLHELM, Judene, Administrator, Memorial Hospital, Kermit, TX, p. A420

WILLIAMS, Cindy, FACHE, Administrator, Carraway Methodist Medical Center, Birmingham, AL, p. A12

WILLIAMS, David R., Chief Executive Officer, Montgomery Regional Hospital, Blacksburg, VA, p. A442

WILLIAMS, Denise R., President and Chief Executive Officer, Memorial Hospital of Salem County, Salem, NJ, p. A280

WILLIAMS, Gerald L., Director and Chief Executive Officer, James E. Van Zandt Veterans Affairs Medical Center, Altoona, PA, p. A355

WILLIAMS, John, Chief Executive Officer, Sequoia Hospital, Redwood City, CA, p. A56

WILLIAMS, John G., President and Chief Executive Officer, Seton Medical Center Coastside, Moss Beach, CA, p. A52

WILLIAMS, Oreta, Administrator, Jeff Davis Hospital, Hazlehurst, GA, p. A106

WILLIAMS, Perry E., Administrator, Alliance HealthCare System, Holly Springs, MS, p. A238

WILLIAMS, R. D., Administrator and Chief Executive Officer, Ashe Memorial Hospital, Jefferson, NC, p. A314

WILLIAMS, Richard C., President and Chief Executive Officer, St. Mary's Health System, Knoxville, TN, p. A395

WILLIAMS, Robert B., Administrator, Shands at AGH, Gainesville, FL, p. A85

WILLIAMS, Robert D., Administrator, Mercy Special Care Hospital, Nanticoke, PA, p. A365

WILLIAMS, Roby D., Administrator, Hardin County General Hospital, Rosiclare, IL, p. A134

WILLIAMS, Roger, Chief Executive Officer, Carroll County Hospital, Carrollton, KY, p. A171

WILLIAMS, Scott, Chief Executive Officer, Sycamore Shoals Hospital, Elizabethton, TN, p. A392

WILLIAMS, Stephen A., President, Norton Healthcare, Louisville, KY, p. B115

WILLIAMS, Stuart W., Interim Chief Executive Officer, Madison County Hospital, London, OH, p. A334

WILLIAMS, Timothy B., Director, Veterans Affairs Puget Sound Health Care System, Seattle, WA, p. A457

WILLIAMS, II, Raymond, CHE, President and Chief Executive Officer, Sumner Regional Medical Center, Wellington, KS, p. A169

WILLIAMS, Jr, Elton L., CPA, President, Lake Charles Memorial Hospital, Lake Charles, LA, p. A184

WILLIS, Bill, Chief Executive Officer, Women and Children's Hospital–Lake Charles, Lake Charles, LA, p. A184

WILLIS, Dell, Administrator, Dr. Dan C. Trigg Memorial Hospital, Tucumcari, NM, p. A286

WILLMON, Gary R., Administrator, Grafton City Hospital, Grafton, WV, p. A461

WILLMORE, Perry, Vice President Operations, Baptist Medical Center, San Antonio, TX, p. A428

WILLS, Andrew, Chief Executive Officer, Estes Park Medical Center, Estes Park, CO, p. A70

WILLS, Laura S., R.N., Administrator, Vencor Hospital–Sycamore, Sycamore, IL, p. A135

WILSON, Asa B., Ph.D., Administrator, Community Medical Center, Falls City, NE, p. A262

WILSON, Bill, Chief Executive Officer, Alexander Community Hospital, Taylorsville, NC, p. A319

WILSON, Bill D., Administrator, Wayne County Hospital, Corydon, IA, p. A149

WILSON, Carole, CHE
Administrator, Recovery Inn of Menlo Park, Menlo Park, CA, p. A51
Administrator and Chief Executive Officer, Vencor Hospital–San Leandro, San Leandro, CA, p. A61

WILSON, David C., Chief Executive Officer, Harton Regional Medical Center, Tullahoma, TN, p. A400

WILSON, Hugh D., Chief Executive Officer, Doctors Hospital, Columbus, GA, p. A102

WILSON, James M., President and Chief Executive Officer, St. Catherine of Siena Medical Center, Smithtown, NY, p. A305

WILSON, Jim, President and Chief Executive Officer, Susan B. Allen Memorial Hospital, El Dorado, KS, p. A160

WILSON, John A., President and Chief Executive Officer, The Children's Institute of Pittsburgh, Pittsburgh, PA, p. A370

WILSON, John M., President, San Pedro Peninsula Hospital, Los Angeles, CA, p. A49

WILSON, L. Steven, Administrator, Dixie Regional Medical Center, Saint George, UT, p. A438

WILSON, Larry, President and Chief Executive Officer, Columbia Hospital for Women Medical Center, Washington, DC, p. A79

WILSON, Mark D., Administrator, Barron Medical Center–Mayo Health System, Barron, WI, p. A466

WILSON, Paul J., Administrator, Los Alamos Medical Center, Los Alamos, NM, p. A285

WILSON, Ralph J., Administrator, Red Bay Hospital, Red Bay, AL, p. A18

WILSON, Shala S., R.N., Chief Executive Officer, Mediplex Rehabilitation Hospital, Bowling Green, KY, p. A170

WILSON, William G., President and Chief Executive Officer, Jackson County Memorial Hospital, Altus, OK, p. A341

WILSON, Jr, V. Otis, President, Grace Hospital, Morganton, NC, p. A316

WILTERMOOD, Michael C., Chief Executive Officer, Coulee Community Hospital, Grand Coulee, WA, p. A454

WINDER, Todd, Administrator, Oneida County Hospital, Malad City, ID, p. A116

WINGATE, Jane, Chief Executive Officer, Tustin Hospital and Medical Center, Tustin, CA, p. A65

WINGATE–JONES, Phyllis, President, Prince George's Hospital Center, Cheverly, MD, p. A197

WINKLE, Christian, Chief Executive Officer, Mariner Post–Acute Network, Inc., Atlanta, GA, p. B108

WINKLER, Gordon W., Administrator, Ringgold County Hospital, Mount Ayr, IA, p. A154

WINN, George, Administrator, Sanpete Valley Hospital, Mount Pleasant, UT, p. A437

WINN, Grant M., President, Community Medical Center, Missoula, MT, p. A259

WINN, Roger P., Administrator, Miners Hospital Northern Cambria, Hastings, PA, p. A361

WINTER, William E., Administrative Director, Silverton Hospital, Silverton, OR, p. A354

WINTHROP, Michael K., President, Bellevue Hospital, Bellevue, OH, p. A326

WISE, Brenda, Administrator, Okolona Community Hospital, Okolona, MS, p. A241

WISE, Franklin E., Administrator, Fulton County Hospital, Salem, AR, p. A33

WISE, Jerry R., Administrator, Hart County Hospital, Hartwell, GA, p. A105

WISE, Robert P., President and Chief Executive Officer, Hunterdon Medical Center, Flemington, NJ, p. A276

WISE, Skip, Chief Executive Officer, Washington County Regional Medical Center, Sandersville, GA, p. A109

WISEMAN, John G., Administrator, U. S. Air Force Hospital, Abilene, TX, p. A401

WISSLER, James, President and Chief Executive Officer, Nicholas H. Noyes Memorial Hospital, Dansville, NY, p. A290

WITHERS, Ivan, Chief Executive Officer, Pocahontas Memorial Hospital, Buckeye, WV, p. A460

WITT, Stephen, Chief Executive Officer, College Hospital, Cerritos, CA, p. A38

Index of Health Care Professionals / Zastrow

WOERNER, Steven
Chief Executive Officer, Corpus Christi Medical Center, Corpus Christi, TX, p. A407
Chief Executive Officer, Corpus Christi Medical Center Bay Area, Corpus Christi, TX, p. A407
WOLF, Chris, Chief Executive Officer, Chesterfield General Hospital, Cheraw, SC, p. A379
WOLF, Edward H., President and Chief Executive Officer, Lakeview Medical Center, Rice Lake, WI, p. A474
WOLF, James N., Chief Executive Officer, District One Hospital, Faribault, MN, p. A227
WOLF, Laura J., President, Franciscan Sisters of Christian Charity HealthCare Ministry, Inc, Manitowoc, WI, p. B86
WOLFE, Philip R., President and Chief Executive Officer, Enloe Medical Center, Chico, CA, p. A38
WOLFE, Stephen A., President and Chief Executive Officer, Indiana Hospital, Indiana, PA, p. A362
WOLFF, Ronald V., President and Chief Executive Officer, Bay Medical Center, Panama City, FL, p. A92
WOLFORD, Dennis A., FACHE, Administrator, Macon County General Hospital, Lafayette, TN, p. A395
WOLFRAM, Patricia L., R.N., Chief Executive Officer, San Clemente Hospital and Medical Center, San Clemente, CA, p. A58
WOLIN, Harry, Administrator and Chief Executive Officer, Mason District Hospital, Havana, IL, p. A127
WOLLEN, Nancy L., Executive Director, Community Medical Center, Toms River, NJ, p. A280
WOLTER, Nicholas J., M.D., Chief Executive Officer, Deaconess Billings Clinic, Billings, MT, p. A256
WOLTERS, Erich J., Chief Executive Officer, San Luis Obispo General Hospital, San Luis Obispo, CA, p. A61
WONG, Kate, President and Chief Operating Officer, Rockford Memorial Hospital, Rockford, IL, p. A134
WOOD, Barbara, Administrator, McGehee–Desha County Hospital, McGehee, AR, p. A32
WOOD, Gregory C., Chief Executive Officer, Scotland Memorial Hospital, Laurinburg, NC, p. A315
WOOD, James B., Chief Executive Officer, Fairview Park Hospital, Dublin, GA, p. A104
WOOD, James R., Chairman and Chief Executive Officer, Maryland General Hospital, Baltimore, MD, p. A196
WOOD, Kenneth R., Administrator, Johnson Regional Medical Center, Clarksville, AR, p. A28
WOOD, Kenneth W., Chief Executive Officer, St. Francis Hospital, Evanston, IL, p. A126
WOOD, Michael B., M.D., President and Chief Executive Officer, Mayo Foundation, Rochester, MN, p. B108
WOOD, Michael C., President and Chief Executive Officer, Ukiah Valley Medical Center, Ukiah, CA, p. A65
WOODALL, Jay, Chief Executive Officer, Trinity Hospital, Erin, TN, p. A392
WOODIN, Joseph L., President and Chief Executive Officer, Gifford Medical Center, Randolph, VT, p. A440
WOODLAND, Dave, President, Brim Healthcare, Inc., Brentwood, TN, p. B62
WOODLOCK, David J., Executive Director, Rockland Children's Psychiatric Center, Orangeburg, NY, p. A302
WOODRELL, Frederick, Director, University Hospitals and Clinics, University of Mississippi Medical Center, Jackson, MS, p. A239
WOODS, Daniel J., Executive Vice President and Administrator, St. Anthony's Memorial Hospital, Effingham, IL, p. A125
WOODS, E. Anthony, President, Deaconess Hospital, Cincinnati, OH, p. A327
WOODS, Eugene A., Chief Executive Officer, Roy Lester Schneider Hospital, Saint Thomas, VI, p. A484
WOODS, Kim, Chief Executive Officer, Kimball County Hospital, Kimball, NE, p. A264
WOODSIDE, Jeffrey R., M.D., Executive Director, University of Tennessee Bowld Hospital, Memphis, TN, p. A397
WOODSON, Hank, Administrator, Plateau Medical Center, Oak Hill, WV, p. A463
WOODY, Fred, Chief Executive Officer, Carlsbad Medical Center, Carlsbad, NM, p. A284
WOOTEN, Richard L., President and Chief Executive Officer, Leesburg Regional Medical Center, Leesburg, FL, p. A88
WORDELMAN, Scott, President and Chief Executive Officer, Fairview Red Wing Hospital, Red Wing, MN, p. A232
WORKMAN, John R., Chief Executive Officer, Athens Regional Medical Center, Athens, TN, p. A390
WORLEY, Steve, President and Chief Executive Officer, Children's Hospital, New Orleans, LA, p. A186
WORRELL, James W., Chief Executive Officer, Richmond Eye and Ear Hospital, Richmond, VA, p. A449
WORRICK, Gerald M., President and Chief Executive Officer, Door County Memorial Hospital, Sturgeon Bay, WI, p. A476
WORSHAM, Sharon, Chief Executive Officer, The Brown Schools at Shadow Mountain, Tulsa, OK, p. A349
WOZNIAK, Gregory T., President and Chief Executive Officer, St. Mary Medical Center, Langhorne, PA, p. A363
WRAALSTAD, Kimber, President and Chief Executive Officer, Presentation Medical Center, Rolla, ND, p. A323
WRAY, Christine R., Chief Executive Officer, St. Mary's Hospital, Leonardtown, MD, p. A199
WRIGHT, Betsy T., President and Chief Executive Officer, Woman's Christian Association Hospital, Jamestown, NY, p. A293
WRIGHT, Brandt C., Administrator, Baptist Memorial Hospital–Blytheville, Blytheville, AR, p. A28
WRIGHT, Charles T., Chief Executive, Southern Oregon Service Area, Providence Medford Medical Center, Medford, OR, p. A352
WRIGHT, Joseph, Administrator, Ward Memorial Hospital, Monahans, TX, p. A424
WRIGHT, Rick, CPA, President and Chief Executive Officer, Keweenaw Memorial Medical Center, Laurium, MI, p. A218
WRIGHT, Robert N., President and Chief Operating Officer, Bay Medical Center, Bay City, MI, p. A212
WRIGHT, Roy W., Chief Executive Officer, Siloam Springs Memorial Hospital, Siloam Springs, AR, p. A34
WRIGHT, Skip, Administrator, Vencor Hospital–Atlanta, Atlanta, GA, p. A100
WRIGHT, Stephen F., Chief Executive Officer, Christus St. Frances Cabrini Hospital, Alexandria, LA, p. A180
WRIGHT, Susan L., Administrator, Springbrook Hospital, Brooksville, FL, p. A82
WRIGHT, Margaret, President, Palos Community Hospital, Palos Heights, IL, p. A132
WRIGHT–GRIGGS, Stephanie, Chief Operating Officer, Provident Hospital of Cook County, Chicago, IL, p. A122
WYATT, Leslie G., Administrator, Children's Hospital, Richmond, VA, p. A448
WYNN, Chester A., President and Chief Executive Officer, Passavant Area Hospital, Jacksonville, IL, p. A128
WYSE, LaMar L., President and Chief Executive Officer, Holzer Medical Center, Gallipolis, OH, p. A332

X

XINIS, James J., President and Chief Executive Officer, Calvert Memorial Hospital, Prince Frederick, MD, p. A199

Y

YAGER, Jolene, R.N., Administrator, Lincoln County Hospital, Lincoln, KS, p. A164
YANAI, Christopher, M.D., Warden and Chief Executive Officer, Oakwood Correctional Facility, Lima, OH, p. A333
YARBOROUGH, James, Chief Executive Officer, Alleghany Memorial Hospital, Sparta, NC, p. A318
YARBROUGH, David L., JD, Administrator, Trinity Hospital, Weaverville, CA, p. A67
YARMEL, Jeffrey, Chief Executive Officer, Warminster Hospital, Warminster, PA, p. A373
YCRE, Jr, Louis R., FACHE, President and Chief Executive Officer, Pascack Valley Hospital, Westwood, NJ, p. A281
YEARTY, Patrick, Administrator, Washington County Hospital, Plymouth, NC, p. A316
YEARY, John M., FACHE, Administrator, Eastland Memorial Hospital, Eastland, TX, p. A411
YELLAN, Robert J., President, Huron Valley–Sinai Hospital, Commerce Township, MI, p. A213
YENAWINE, Kelly R., Administrator, Gibson General Hospital, Trenton, TN, p. A400
YIM, Herbert K., Administrator, Kohala Hospital, Kohala, HI, p. A113
YINGST, Thomas E., MSC, Administrator, U. S. Air Force Hospital, Edwards AFB, CA, p. A40
YOCHUM, Richard E., President and Chief Executive Officer, Pomona Valley Hospital Medical Center, Pomona, CA, p. A55
YORKE, Harvey M., President and Chief Executive Officer, Southwestern Vermont Medical Center, Bennington, VT, p. A440
YOSHIOKA, James T.
President, Citrus Valley Medical Center–Queen of the Valley Campus, West Covina, CA, p. A67
President and Chief Executive Officer, Henry Mayo Newhall Memorial Hospital, Valencia, CA, p. A66
YOSKO, Kathleen C., President and Chief Executive Officer, Marianjoy Rehabilitation Hospital, Wheaton, IL, p. A136
YOUNG, Anthony R., Chief Executive Officer, SouthCrest Hospital, Tulsa, OK, p. A348
YOUNG, Charles R., Administrator, Shriners Hospitals for Children–Spokane, Spokane, WA, p. A457
YOUNG, J. Phillip
Chief Executive Officer, Eastmoreland Hospital, Portland, OR, p. A353
Chief Executive Officer, Woodland Park Hospital, Portland, OR, p. A353
YOUNG, John, President and Chief Executive Officer, Cleveland Regional Medical Center, Shelby, NC, p. A318
YOUNG, Mary Ann, R.N., Administrator, Utah Valley Regional Medical Center, Provo, UT, p. A438
YOUNG, Randall A., Administrator, Lamb Healthcare Center, Littlefield, TX, p. A421
YOUNG, Richard T., President, St. John Detroit Riverview Hospital, Detroit, MI, p. A214
YOUNG, Robert C., M.D., President, Fox Chase Cancer Center–American Oncologic Hospital, Philadelphia, PA, p. A366
YOUNG, Susan, Chief Executive Officer, BHC Spirit of St. Louis Hospital, Saint Charles, MO, p. A252
YOUNG, Sylvia, President and Chief Executive Officer, Medical Center of Aurora–South, Aurora, CO, p. A68
YOUNG, James H., Administrator, U. S. Air Force Hospital, Davis–Monthan AFB, AZ, p. A22
YOUNG, Jr, Frederick C., President, Pendleton Memorial Methodist Hospital, New Orleans, LA, p. A187
YOUREE, James H., Interim Chief Executive Officer, Iberia Medical Center, New Iberia, LA, p. A186
YUTZY, LaVern J., Chief Executive Officer, Philhaven, Bahavioral Healthcare Services, Mount Gretna, PA, p. A364

Z

ZACCAGNINO, Joseph A.
President and Chief Executive Officer, Yale New Haven Health System, New Haven, CT, p. B155
President and Chief Executive Officer, Yale–New Haven Hospital, New Haven, CT, p. A76
ZAGER, Joe, Chief Executive Officer, Monroe County Hospital, Monroeville, AL, p. A16
ZALAR, Karl, Administrator, Mercy Memorial Hospital, Urbana, OH, p. A338
ZANFINI, Gaetano, Chief Executive Officer, Brea Community Hospital, Brea, CA, p. A37
ZASTROW, Allan, FACHE, Chief Executive Officer, Keokuk Area Hospital, Keokuk, IA, p. A153

© 2000 AHA Guide

ZAYAS, Domingo Torres, CHE, Executive Director, Mennonite General Hospital, Aibonito, PR, p. A481
ZECHMAN, Jr, Edwin K., President and Chief Executive Officer, Children's National Medical Center, Washington, DC, p. A79
ZEH, Brian R., Administrator, St. Vincent Frankfort Hospital, Frankfort, IN, p. A140
ZEINE, Edward, Administrator and Chief Executive Officer, Cordova Community Medical Center, Cordova, AK, p. A20
ZEITLIN, Alan P., M.D., Chief Executive Officer, Parkway Hospital, New York, NY, p. A299
ZELLERS, Thomas J., Chief Operating Officer, Deaconess Medical Center–Spokane, Spokane, WA, p. A457
ZICHAL, Fran, Chief Executive Officer, Central Community Hospital, Elkader, IA, p. A151
ZIEMAN, Michael A., Administrator, Memorial Behavioral Health, Gulfport, MS, p. A238
ZIMMERMAN, Ann, Acting Administrator, Mohave Valley Hospital and Medical Center, Bullhead City, AZ, p. A22
ZIMMERMAN, Joann
  Administrator, Kaiser Foundation Hospital, Santa Clara, CA, p. A62
  Administrator, Santa Teresa Community Medical Center, San Jose, CA, p. A61
ZIMMERMAN, Joanne, Administrator, Kaiser Foundation Hospital, Redwood City, CA, p. A56
ZIMMERMAN, Nancy, R.N., Administrator, Comanche County Hospital, Coldwater, KS, p. A160
ZIOMEK, Janice, Administrator, Moreno Valley Community Hospital, Moreno Valley, CA, p. A52
ZOLLER, Gregg G., FACHE
  President and Chief Executive Officer, Mercy Hospital of Pittsburgh, Pittsburgh, PA, p. A369
  President and Chief Executive Officer, Mercy Providence Hospital, Pittsburgh, PA, p. A369
ZORNES, Donald H., President and Chief Executive Officer, Columbus Community Hospital, Columbus, NE, p. A262
ZUBER, Eugene, Administrator, Newport Hospital and Clinic, Newport, AR, p. A32
ZUBKOFF, William, Ph.D., Chief Executive Officer, South Shore Hospital and Medical Center, Miami Beach, FL, p. A90
ZUCKERMAN, Gary W., USN, Commanding Officer, Naval Hospital, Beaufort, SC, p. A378
ZULIANI, Michael E., Chief Executive Officer, Angel Medical Center, Franklin, NC, p. A313
ZWICKEY, Tim, Administrator, Clearwater Valley Hospital and Clinics, Orofino, ID, p. A117
ZWIGART, Donna, FACHE, Chief Executive Officer, St. Francis Medical Center, Pittsburgh, PA, p. A369

AHA Membership Categories

The American Hospital Association is primarily an organization of hospitals and related institutions. Its object, according to its bylaws, is "to promote high–quality health care and health services for all the people through leadership in the development of public policy, leadership in the representation and advocacy of hospital and health care organization interests, and leadership in the provision of services to assist hospitals and health care organizations in meeting the health care needs of their communities."

The major source of income for the AHA is its membership dues, which are established by the membership through the House of Delegates. The types of membership are described in the following paragraphs.

Institutional Members

Type I–Hospitals or health services organizations or systems which provide a continuum of integrated, community health resources and which include at least one licensed hospital that is owned, leased, managed or religiously sponsored.

Type I members include hospitals, health care systems, integrated delivery systems, and physician hospital organizations (PHOs) and health maintenance organizations (HMOs) wholly or partially owned by or owning a member hospital or system. A Type I member hospital, health care system or integrated delivery system may, at its decretion and upon approval of a membership application by the Association chief executive officer, extend membership to the health care provider organizations, other than a hospital that it owns, leases, or fully controls.

Type II–Freestanding Health Care Provider Organizations

These are health provider organizations, other than registered hospitals, that provide patient care services, including, but not limited to, ambulatory, preventive, rehabilitative, specialty, post–acute and continuing care, as well as physician groups, health insurance services, and staff and group model health maintenance organizations without a hospital component. Type II members are not owned or controlled by a Type I hospital, health care system or integrated delivery system member. They may, however, be part of an organization eligible for, but not holding, Type I membership.

Type III–Other Organizations

Type III membership includes organizations interested in the objectives of the Association, but not eligible for Type I or Type II membership. Organizations eligible for Type III membership shall include, but not be limited to, associations, societies, foundations, corporations, educational and academic institutions, companies, government agencies, international health providers, and organizations having an interest in and a desire to support the objectives of the Association.

Provisional Members

Hospitals that are in the planning or construction stage and that, on completion, will be eligible for institutional membership type I or type II. Provisional membership may also be granted to applicant institutions that cannot, at present, meet the requirements of type I or type II membership.

Government Institution Group Members

Groups of government hospitals operated by the same unit of government may obtain institutional membership under a group plan. Membership dues are based on a special schedule set forth in the bylaws of the AHA.

Contracting Hospitals

The AHA also provides membership services to certain hospitals that are prevented from holding membership because of legal or other restrictions.

Other Institutional Members

Types IA
Hospitals

U.S. hospitals and hospitals in areas associated with the U.S. that are type IA members of the American Hospital Association are included in the list of hospitals in section A. Canadian types I members of the American Hospital Association are listed below.

Canada

ALBERTA

Edmonton: MISERICORDIA COMMUNITY HEALTH CENTRE, 16940 87th Avenue, Zip T5R 4H5; tel. 780/930-5611; Carl Roy, President

Lamont: LAMONT HEALTH CARE CENTRE, 5216-53rd Street, Zip T0B 2R0; tel. 780/895-2211; Harold James, Chief Executive Officer

MANITOBA

Portage La Prarie: PORTAGE DISTRICT GENERAL HOSPITAL, 524 Fifth Street S.E., Zip R1N 3A8; tel. 204/239-2211; Garry C. Mattin, Executive Director

Winnipeg: RIVERVIEW HEALTH CENTRE, 1 Morley Avenue East, Zip R3L 2P4; tel. 204/452-3411; Norman R. Kasian, President

ONTARIO

Brantford: ST. JOSEPH'S HOSPITAL, 99 Wayne Gretzky Parkway, Zip N3S 6T6; tel. 519/753-8641; Romeo Cercone, President and Chief Executive Officer

London: ST. JOSEPH'S HEALTH CENTRE, P.O. Box 5777, Zip 4V2 4L6; tel. 519/646-6000; Clifford A. Nordal, President and Chief Executive Officer

North York: BAYCREST CENTRE-GERIATRIC CARE, 3560 Bathurst Street, Zip M6A 2E1; tel. 416/789-5131; Stephen W. Herbert, President and Chief Executive Officer

Ottawa: ROYAL OTTAWA HOSPITAL, 1145 Carling Avenue, Zip K1Z 7K4; tel. 613/722-6521; George F. Langill, Executive Director

Parry Sound: WEST PARRY SOUND HEALTH CENTRE, 10 James Street, Zip P2A 1T3; tel. 705/746-9321; Norman Maciver, Chief Executive Officer

Renfrew: RENFREW VICTORIA HOSPITAL, 499 Raglan Street North, Zip K7V 1P6; tel. 613/432-4851; Randy V. Penney, Executive Director

Thornhill: SHOULDICE HOSPITAL, P.O. Box 370, Zip L3T 4A3; tel. 905/889-1125; Alan O'Dell, Administrator

Toronto: MOUNT SINAI HOSPITAL, 600 University Avenue, Zip M5G 1X5; tel. 416/596-4200; Theodore J. Freedman, President and Chief Executive Officer

ST. JOSEPH'S HEALTH CENTRE, 30 the Queensway, Zip M6R 1B5; tel. 416/534-9531; Marilyn Bruner, President and Chief Executive Officer

TORONTO REHABILITATION INSTITUTE, 550 University Avenue, Zip M5G 2A2; tel. 416/597-5111; Mark Rochon, President and Chief Executive Officer

QUEBEC

Montreal: CENTRE HOSPITALIER DE L' UNIVERISITE DE MONTREAL, 3840 Saint Urbain Street, Zip H2W 1T8; tel. 514/843-2794; Cecile Cleroux, Executive Director

MONTREAL CHILDREN'S HOSPITAL, 2300 Tupper Street, Zip H3H 1P3; tel. 514/934-4400; Patricia Sheppard, Director

MOUNT SINAI HOSPITAL CENTER, 5690 Cavendish Cote St-Luc', Zip H4W 1S7; tel. 514/369-2222; Joseph Rothbart, Executive Director

Other Institutional Members / Programs in Health Administration

Associated University Programs in Health Administration

ALABAMA

Birmingham: UNIVERSITY OF ALABAMA AT BIRMINGHAM, 1675 University Boulevard, Zip 35294-3361; tel. 205/934-5661; Charles L. Joiner, Ph.D., Dean

CALIFORNIA

Los Angeles: UCLA SCHOOL OF PUBLIC HEALTH, P.O. Box 951772, Zip 90095-1772; tel. 310/825-2594; Thomas Rice, M.D., Administrator

San Francisco: GOLDEN GATE UNIVERSITY, 536 Mission Street, General Library, Zip 94105; tel. 415/442-0777; Steven Dunlap, Assistant Librarian

DISTRICT OF COLUMBIA

Washington: SCHOOL OF PUBLIC HEALTH AND HEALTH SERVICES, THE GEORGE WASHINGTON UNIVERSITY, 2300 Eye Street N.W., Suite 106H, Zip 20037; tel. 202/994-3139; Richard F. Southby, Ph.D., Associate Dean Health Services and Friesen Professor of International Health School of Public Health and Health Service

GEORGIA

Atlanta: GEORGIA STATE UNIVERSITY, INSTITUTE OF HEALTH ADMINISTRATION, University Plaza, Zip 30303; tel. 404/651-2000; Andrew T. Sumner, Director

ILLINOIS

Carbondale: SOUTHERN ILLINOIS UNIVERSITY, COLLEGE OF APPLIED SCIENCES AND ARTS, Zip 62901; tel. 618/536-6682; Frederic L. Morgan, Ph.D., Chair Health Care Professions

Chicago: UNIVERSITY OF CHICAGO, GRADUATE PROGRAM IN HEALTH ADMINISTRATION AND POLICY, 5841 South Maryland Avenue, Zip 60637; tel. 773/834-3618; Peggy Berndt, Program Administrator

Evanston: HEALTH SERVICE MANAGEMENT PROGRAM, KELLOGG GRADUATE SCHOOL OF MANAGEMENT, NORTHWESTERN UNIVERSITY, 2001 Sheridan Road, Zip 60208; tel. 847/492-5540; Joel Shalowitz, M.D., Professor and Director

University Park: PROGRAM IN HEALTH SERVICE ADMINISTRATION, SCHOOL OF HEALTH PROFESSIONS, GOVERNORS STATE UNIVERSITY, Zip 60466; tel. 847/534-4030; Sang-O Rhee, Chairman

IOWA

Iowa City: DEPARTMENT OF HEALTH MANAGEMENT AND POLICY, UNIVERSITY OF IOWA, 2700 Steindler Building, Zip 52242; tel. 319/335-9814; Douglas Wakefield, Ph.D., Interim Head

MARYLAND

Bethesda: NAVAL SCHOOL OF HEALTH SCIENCES, Naval Medical Command, National Region, Zip 20889-5611; tel. 301/295-1251; Captain Harry Coffey, Commanding Officer

MISSOURI

Saint Louis: WASHINGTON UNIVERSITY, SCHOOL OF MEDICINE, 4547 Clayton Avenue, Zip 63110; tel. 314/362-2477; James O. Hepner, Ph.D., Director Health Administration Program

NEW YORK

Valhalla: NEW YORK MEDICAL COLLEGE, Administration Building, Zip 10595; tel. 914/347-5044; Father Harry C. Barrett, M.P.H., President and Chief Executive Officer

OHIO

Columbus: GRADUATE PROGRAM IN HEALTH SERVICES MANAGEMENT AND POLICY, OHIO STATE UNIVERSITY, 1583 Perry Street, Room 246 Samp, Zip 43210; tel. 614/292-9708; Stephen F. Loebs, Ph.D., Chairman and Associate Professor

PENNSYLVANIA

Philadelphia: TEMPLE UNIVERSITY, DEPARTMENT OF HEALTH ADMINISTRATION, SCHOOL OF BUSINESS ADMINISTRATION, Zip 19122-6083; tel. 215/787-8082; William Aaronson, Professor and Chairman

University Park: PENNSYLVANIA STATE UNIVERSITY, 116 Henderson Building, Zip 16802; tel. 814/863-2859; Diane Brannon, Ph.D., Interim Department Head, Health Policy and Administration

TEXAS

Brooks AFB: U. S. AIR FORCE SCHOOL OF AEROSPACE MEDICINE, USAFSAM-CCE, Zip 78235-5301; tel. 512/536-3342

Fort Sam Houston: ARMY-BAYLOR UNIVERSITY PROGRAM IN HEALTH CARE ADMINISTRATION, Academy of Health Sciences-USA, Zip 78234; tel. 512/221-5009

San Antonio: TRINITY UNIVERSITY, 715 Stadium Drive, Suite 58, Zip 78212-7200; tel. 210/736-8107; Niccie McKay, Ph.D., Chairman

Sheppard AFB: U. S. AIR FORCE SCHOOL OF HEALTH CARE SCIENCES, Building 1900, MSTL/114, Academic Library, Zip 76311; tel. 817/851-2511

PUERTO RICO

San Juan: SCHOOL OF PUBLIC HEALTH, P.O. Box 5067, Zip 00936; tel. 809/767-9626; Orlando Nieves, Dean

Other Institutional Members / Schools of Nursing

Hospital Schools of Nursing

ILLINOIS
Canton: GRAHAM HOSPITAL School of Nursing

MASSACHUSETTS
Brockton: BROCKTON HOSPITAL School of Nursing

NEW JERSEY
Plainfield: MUHLENBERG REGIONAL MEDICAL CENTER School of Nursing

NEW YORK
Elmira: ARNOT–OGDEN MEMORIAL HOSPITAL School of Nursing

OHIO
Canton: AULTMAN HOSPITAL School of Nursing
Cincinnati: GOOD SAMARITAN HOSPITAL School of Nursing

PENNSYLVANIA
Johnstown: CONEMAUGH VALLEY MEMORIAL HOSPITAL School of Nursing
New Castle: JAMESON MEMORIAL HOSPITAL School of Nursing
Philadelphia: METHODIST HOSPITAL School of Nursing
Pittsburgh: ST. FRANCIS MEDICAL CENTER School of Nursing
WESTERN PENNSYLVANIA HOSPITAL School of Nursing
Sewickley: SEWICKLEY VALLEY HOSPITAL School of Nursing

TENNESSEE
Memphis: BAPTIST COLLEGE OF HEALTH SCIENCES
METHODIST HOSPITALS OF MEMPHIS–CENTRAL School of Nursing

TEXAS
Lubbock: METHODIST HOSPITAL School of Nursing

Other Institutional Members / Preacute and Postacute Care Facilities

Nonhospital Preacute and Postacute Care Facilities

ALABAMA
Fort McClellan: NOBLE ARMY HEALTH CLINIC, Zip 36205–5083; tel. 256/848–2232
Montgomery: MAXWELL CLINIC, 330 Kirkpatrick Avenue East, Zip 36112–6219; tel. 334/953–7801; Colonel Mary Ann E. Cardinali, USAF, Commander
Redstone Arsenal: FOX ARMY HEALTH CENTER, Zip 35809–7000; tel. 256/876–4147; Colonel Mark Kirk, Commander

ALASKA
Anchorage: DEPARTMENT OF VETERANS AFFAIRS ALASKA MEDICAL AND REGIONAL OFFICE CENTER, 2925 Debarr Road, Zip 99508–2989; tel. 907/257–6930; Alonzo M. Poteet, , II, Director
SOUTHCENTRAL FOUNDATION, 4501 Diplomacy Drive, Suite 200, Zip 99508; tel. 907/265–4955; Katherine Grosdidier, President and Chief Executive Officer

ARIZONA
Fort Huachuca: RAYMOND W. BLISS ARMY HEALTH CENTER, Zip 85613–7040; tel. 520/533–2350; Major Christopher Hale, Deputy Commander
Phoenix: JESSE OWENS MEMORIAL MEDICAL CENTER, 325 East Baseline Road, Zip 85040; tel. 602/238–3314; Jeffrey K. Norman, Chief Executive Officer
PMH FAMILY HEALTH CENTER–CAMELBACK, P.O. Box 21207, Zip 85036–1207; tel. 602/266–4381; Jeffrey K. Norman, Chief Executive Officer
PMH FAMILY HEALTH CENTER–WEST MCDOWELL, P.O. Box 21207, Zip 85036–1207; tel. 602/2383314; Jeffrey K. Norman, Chief Executive Officer

ARKANSAS
Jacksonville: U. S. AIR FORCE CLINIC LITTLE ROCK, Little Rock AFB, Zip 72099–5057; tel. 501/987–7411; Colonel Rebecca A. Russell, USAF, Commander
Little Rock: CENTRAL ARKANSAS RADIATION THERAPY INSTITUTE, P.O. Box 55050, Zip 72215; tel. 501/664–8573; Janice E. Burford, President and Chief Executive Officer

CALIFORNIA
Beale AFB: U. S. AIR FORCE HOSPITAL, 15301 Warren Shingle Road, Zip 95903–1907; tel. 530/634–4838; Lieutenant Colonel Robert G. Quinn, MSC, USAF, FACHE, Administrator
Long Beach: NAVAL MEDICAL CLINIC, Reeves Avenue, Building 831, Zip 90822–5073; tel. 562/521–4201; Captain J. M. Lamdin, Commanding Officer
Los Angeles: DEPARTMENT OF VETERANS AFFAIRS, OUTPATIENT CLINIC, 351 East Temple Street, Room A–102, Zip 90012; tel. 213/253–5000; Jules Morevec, Ph.D., Director
Pleasant Hill: VETERANS AFFAIRS NORTHERN CALIFORNIA HEALTH SYSTEM, 2300 Contra Costa Boulevard, 440, Zip 94523–3961; tel. 510/372–2047; Janet R. Johnson, Chief Acquisitions and Materials Management
Port Hueneme: NAVAL AMBULATORY CARE CENTER, Zip 93043; tel. 805/982–6301; Captain Fred White, Officer–in–Charge
San Francisco: VETERANS AFFAIRS OUTPATIENT CLINIC, 4150 Clement Street, Zip 94121; tel. 415/221–4810; Lawrence C. Stewart, Director
Sepulveda: VETERANS AFFAIRS MEDICAL CENTER, 16111 Plummer Street, Zip 91343; tel. 818/891–7711; Smith Jenkins, , Jr, Acting Chief Executive Officer

CONNECTICUT
Groton: NAVAL HOSPITAL, 1 Wahoo Drive, Box 600, Zip 06349–5600; tel. 860/694–3261; Captain Kathleen Hiatt, Deputy Commanding Officer
Newington: VETERANS AFFAIRS MEDICAL CENTER–NEWINGTON CAMPUS, 555 Willard Avenue, Zip 06111–2600; tel. 860/666–6951; Paul J. McCool, Director
Stamford: THE REHABILITATION CENTER, 26 Palmer's Hill Road, Zip 06902; tel. 203/325–1544; Kathleen Murphy, President

DELAWARE
Dover: U. S. AIR FORCE HOSPITAL DOVER, 300 Tuskegee Boulevard, Zip 19902–7307; tel. 302/677–2525; Lieutenant Colonel Frederick L. Woods, MSC, USAF, Administrator
New Castle: CHRISTIANA CARE VISITING NURSE ASSOCIATION, One Reads Way, Zip 19720; tel. 302/323–8200; Richard Cherrin, President
SCHWEIZER'S THERAPY AND REHABILITATION, 100 Corporate Commons, Suite 1, Zip 19720
Newark: CHRISTIANA CARE IMAGING CENTER, 4751 Ogletown–Stanton Road, Zip 19718
CHRISTIANA SURGICENTER, 4755 Ogletown–Stanton Road, Zip 19718
HEALTH CARE CENTER AT CHRISTIANA, 200 Hygeia Drive, Zip 19714
Wilmington: EUGENE DUPONT PREVENTIVE MEDICINE AND REHABILITATION INSTITUTE
INFUSION SERVICES OF DELAWARE, 1701 Rockland Road, Suite 102, Zip 19803

FLORIDA
Key West: NAVAL REGIONAL MEDICAL CLINIC, Roosevelt Boulevard, Zip 33040; tel. 305/293–4500; Captain F. L. Anzalone, Officer–in–Charge
Miami: VITAS HEALTHCARE CORPORATION, 100 South Biscayne Boulevard, Zip 33131; tel. 305/374–4143; Hugh Westbrook, Chairman and Chief Executive Officer
Riverview: TAMPA BAY ACADEMY, 12012 Boyette Road, Zip 33569; tel. 813/677–6700; Edward C. Hoefle, Administrator

GEORGIA
Calhoun: ALLIANT HEALTH PLANS, INC., 401 South Wall Street, Suite 201, Zip 30701; tel. 706/629–8848; Louis G. Smith, , Jr, Chief Executive Officer
GEORGIA HEALTH PLUS, 401 South Wall Street, Suite 201, Zip 30701; tel. 706/629–1833; Louis G. Smith, , Jr, Chief Executive Officer
Moody AFB: U. S. AIR FORCE HOSPITAL MOODY, 3278 Mitchell Boulevard, Zip 31699–1500; tel. 912/257–3772; Colonel Anthony Van Goor, Commander
Rome: CENTREX, 420 East Second Avenue, Zip 30161; tel. 706/235–1006; Dee B. Russell, M.D., Chief Executive Officer
COMMUNITY HOSPICECARE, P.O. Box 233, Zip 30162–0233; tel. 706/232–0807; Kurt Stuenkel, FACHE, President and Chief Executive Officer
FLOYD HOME HEALTH AGENCY, P.O. Box 6248, Zip 30162–6248; tel. 706/802–4600; Kurt Stuenkel, FACHE, President and Chief Executive Officer
FLOYD MEDICAL OUTPATIENT SURGERY, P.O. Box 233, Zip 30162–0233; tel. 706/802–2070; Kurt Stuenkel, FACHE, President and Chief Executive Officer
FLOYD REHABILITATION CENTER, P.O. Box 233, Zip 30162–0233; tel. 706/802–2091; Kurt Stuenkel, FACHE, President and Chief Executive Officer

HAWAII
Honolulu: VETERANS AFFAIRS MEDICAL REGIONAL OFFICE, P.O. Box 50188, Zip 96850; tel. 808/541–1582
Pearl Harbor: NAVAL REGIONAL MEDICAL CLINIC, Box 121, Building 1750, Zip 96860–5080; tel. 808/471–3025

IOWA
Eldora: MERCY HEALTH CENTER, 2413 Edgington Avenue, Zip 50627–1541; tel. 515/939–5416; Paul C. Poparad, R.N., Interim Administrator

KANSAS
Fort Leavenworth: MUNSON ARMY HEALTH CENTER, 550 Pope Avenue, Zip 66027–2332; tel. 913/684–6420; Colonel James Dunn, , Jr, Commander
Wichita: U. S. AIR FORCE HOSPITAL, 59570 Leavenworth Street, Suite 6E4, Zip 67221–5300; tel. 316/652–5000; Lieutenant Colonel Charles Wolak, Administrator

LOUISIANA
New Orleans: NAVAL MEDICAL CLINIC, Zip 70142; tel. 504/678–2400; Lieutenant Colonel Deborah Auth, Director, Administration

MAINE
Damariscotta: MILES MEDICAL GROUP, INC., RR 1, Box 4500, Zip 04543; tel. 207/563–1234; Stacey Miller–Friant, Director
Kennebunk: SOUTHERN MAINE HEALTH AND HOME SERVICES, P.O. Box 739, Zip 04043; tel. 207/985–4767; Elaine Brady, R.N., Executive Director

MARYLAND
Annapolis: NAVAL MEDICAL CLINIC, Zip 21402; tel. 410/293–1330
Baltimore: ST. AGNES HEALTH SERVICES, 900 Caton Avenue, Zip 21229; tel. 410/368–2945; Peter Clay, Senior Vice President Managed Care
ST. AGNES HOME CARE AND HOSPICE, 3421 Benson Avenue, Suite G100, Zip 21227; tel. 410/368–2825; Robin Dowell, Director
Fort George G Meade: KIMBROUGH ARMY COMMUNITY HOSPITAL, Zip 20755; tel. 301/677–4171; Colonel David W. Roberts, Commanding Officer
Patuxent River: NAVAL MEDICAL CLINIC, 47149 Buse Road, Zip 20670–5370; tel. 301/342–1418; Captain Ralph A. Puckett, MC, USN, Commanding Officer

MASSACHUSETTS
Falmouth: GOSNOLD ON CAPE COD, P.O. Box 929, Zip 02541; tel. 508/540–6550; Raymond Tamasi, Chief Executive Officer
Springfield: INFUSION AND RESPIRATORY SERVICES, 211 Carando Drive, Zip 01104; tel. 413/794–4663; Maureen Skipper, Senior Vice President Home and Community Based Services
VISITING NURSE ASSOCIATION AND HOSPICE OF WESTERN NEW ENGLAND, INC., 50 Maple Street, Zip 01105; tel. 413/781–5070; Maureen Skipper, President

MICHIGAN
Big Rapids: MECOSTA HEALTH SERVICES, 413 Mecosta, Zip 49307; tel. 717/796–3200; Thomas E. Daugherty, Administrator
Port Huron: TRI–HOSPITAL E.M.S., 309 Grand River Street, Zip 48060; tel. 313/985–7115; Ken Cummings, Chief Executive Officer
WILLOW ENTERPRISES, INC., 1221 Pine Grove Avenue, Zip 48060; tel. 313/989–3737; James B. Bridge, Chief Executive Officer

Other Institutional Members / Preacute and Postacute Care Facilities

Sault Sainte Marie: SAULT SAINTE MARIE TRIBAL HEALTH AND HUMAN SERVICES CENTER, 2864 Ashmun Street, Zip 49783; tel. 906/495-5651; Russell Vizina, Division Director Health

MINNESOTA

Saint Paul: HEALTHEAST CARE, INC., 1690 University Avenue W, Suite 370, Zip 55104-3729; tel. 651/232-5070; Steven N. Burrows, Executive Vice President
HEALTHEAST HOME CARE, INC., 1700 University Avenue, Zip 55104; tel. 651/232-2800; Scott Batulis, Vice President and Administrator
HEALTHEAST MEDICAL RESEARCH INSTITUTE, 559 Capitol Boulevard, Zip 55103; tel. 651/232-2300; Timothy H. Hanson, President and Chief Executive Officer

MISSOURI

Independence: SURGI-CARE CENTER OF INDEPENDENCE, 2311 Redwood Avenue, Zip 64057; tel. 816/373-7995; Michael W. Chappelow, President and Chief Executive Officer
Whiteman AFB: U. S. AIR FORCE CLINIC WHITEMAN, 331 Sijan Avenue, Zip 65305-5001; tel. 660/687-1194; Lieutenant Colonel David Wilmot, USAF, MSC, Administrator

MONTANA

Malmstrom AFB: U. S. AIR FORCE CLINIC, Zip 59402-5300; tel. 406/731-3863
Miles City: VETERANS AFFAIRS MEDICAL CENTER, 210 South Winchester Avenue, Zip 59301-4742; tel. 406/232-3060; Richard J. Stanley, Director

NEBRASKA

Grand Island: GRAND ISLAND DIVISION, 2211 North Broadwell Avenue, Zip 68803-2196; tel. 308/382-3660
North Platte: GREAT PLAINS PHO, INC., P.O. Box 1167, Zip 69103; tel. 308/535-7496; Todd Hlavaty, M.D., Chairman

NEW HAMPSHIRE

Portsmouth: NAVAL MEDICAL CLINIC, Building H-1, Zip 03801; tel. 207/439-1000; Captain F. M. Richardson, Commanding Officer

NEW JERSEY

Fort Monmouth: PATTERSON ARMY HEALTH CLINIC, Zip 07703-5607; tel. 908/532-1266; Colonel Dolores Loew, Commander

NEW YORK

Lake Placid: CAMELOT, 50 Riverside Drive, Zip 12946; tel. 518/523-3605; Father Carlos J. Caguiat, FACHE, Vice President
New York: STATE UNIVERSITY OF NEW YORK, UNIVERSITY OPTOMETRIC CENTER, 100 East 24th Street, Zip 10010; tel. 212/780-4930; Richard C. Weber, Executive Director
Rochester: ROCHESTER REHABILITATION CENTER, 1000 Elmwood Avenue, Zip 14620; tel. 716/271-2520; George H. Gieselman, President
Tuckahoe: HOME NURSING ASSOCIATION OF WESTCHESTER, 69 Main Street, Zip 10707; tel. 919/961-2818; Mary Wehrberger, Director

OHIO

Cleveland: KAISER PERMANENTE, 1001 Lakeside, Zip 44114; tel. 216/362-2000; Jeff Blancett, Vice President
Columbus: OHIOHEALTH GROUP, 300 East Wilson Bridge Road, Zip 43085; tel. 614/566-0123; John Burns, Chief Executive Officer
VETERANS AFFAIRS OUTPATIENT CLINIC, 543 Taylor Avenue, Zip 43203-1278; tel. 614/469-5663
Worthington: HOMEREACH, 404 East Wilson Bridge Road, Suite H., Zip 43085; tel. 614/566-0888; Rebecca Zuccarelli, Vice President Home and Hospice Services

OKLAHOMA

Enid: U. S. AIR FORCE CLINIC, Vance AFB, Building 810, Zip 73705-5000; tel. 405/249-7494; Lieutenant Colonel Andrew F. Love, MSC, USAF, Commander Medical Group
Eufaula: EUFALA INDIAN HEALTH CENTER, 800 Forest Avenue, Zip 74432; tel. 918/689-2547; Shelly Crow, Health System Administrator
Okmulgee: OKMULGEE INDIAN HEALTH SYSTEM, 1313 East 20th, Zip 74447; tel. 918/758-1926; Bert Robinson, Health System Administrator
Sapulpa: SAPULPA INDIAN HEALTH CENTER, 1125 East Clevelend, Zip 74066; tel. 918/224-9310; Judy Aaron, Health System Administrator
Tinker AFB: U. S. AIR FORCE HOSPITAL TINKER, 5700 Arnold Street, Zip 73145; tel. 405/736-2084; Colonel Lloyd A. Reinke, Commander
Tulsa: SURGICARE OF TULSA, 4415 South Harvard, Suite 100, Zip 74135; tel. 918/742-2502; Dirk Foxworthy, Chief Executive Officer

PENNSYLVANIA

Chester: COMMUNITY HOSPITAL, DIVISION OF THE CROZER-CHESTER MEDICAL CENTER, Ninth and Wilson Streets, Zip 19013-2098; tel. 610/494-0700; Joan K. Richards, President
Dallastown: YORK HEALTH SYSTEM MEDICAL GROUP, Zip 17313; tel. 717/851-6515; William R. Richards, Executive Director
Pittsburgh: HEALTH ASSISTANCE PROGRAM FOR PERSONNEL IN INDUSTRY, 4221 Penn Avenue, Zip 15224; tel. 412/622-4994; Eugene Ginchereau, M.D., Director
York: SOUTH CENTRAL PREFERRED, 1803 Mount Rose Avenue, Zip 17403; tel. 717/741-9511; Charles H. Chodroff, M.D., Executive Director
YORK HEALTH CARE SERVICES, 1001 South George Street, Zip 17405; tel. 717/851-2121; Brian A. Gragnolati, Senior Vice President Operations

RHODE ISLAND

Newport: NAVAL HOSPITAL, Zip 02841-1002; tel. 401/841-3915; Captain C. Henderson, , II, MSC, USN, Commanding Officer

TEXAS

Brenham: TRINITY CARE CENTER, 400 East Sayles, Zip 77833; tel. 409/830-2204; DyAnn Lauzon, Executive Director
Bryan: ST. JOSEPH MANOR, 2345 Manor Drive, Zip 77802; tel. 409/821-7590; John Turton, Administrator
Caldwell: BURLESON ST. JOSEPH MANOR, 1022 Presidential Corridor, Zip 77836; tel. 509/567-0920; Harold Cottrell, Administrator
El Paso: VETERANS AFFAIRS HEALTHCARE CENTER, 5001 North Piedras Street, Zip 79930-4211; tel. 915/564-6100; Edward Valenzuela, Director
Houston: GRAMERCY OUTPATIENT SURGERY CENTER. LTD., 2727 Gramercy, Zip 77025; Carol Simons, Administrator
SURGICARE OF TRAVIS CENTER, INC., 6655 Travis, Suite 200, Zip 77030; tel. 713/520-1782; Carol Simons, Administrator
WEST HOUSTON SURGICARE, 970 Campbell Road, Zip 77024; tel. 713/461-3547; Edward Downs, Administrator
Laughlin AFB: U. S. AIR FORCE HOSPITAL, 590 Mitchell Boulevard, Zip 78843-5200; tel. 210/298-6311
San Antonio: U. S. AIR FORCE CLINIC BROOKS, Building 615, Zip 78235-5300; tel. 210/536-2087; Major Edward M. Jenkins, Administrator
Webster: BAY AREA SURGICARE CENTER, P.O. Box 201645, Zip 77216-1445; tel. 281/332-2433; Mary Colombo, Administrator

VIRGINIA

Fort Lee: KENNER ARMY HEALTH CLINIC, 700 24th Street, Zip 23801-1716; tel. 804/734-9256
Quantico: NAVAL REGIONAL MEDICAL CLINIC, Zip 22134; tel. 703/640-2236

WISCONSIN

Green Bay: UNITY HOSPICE, P.O. Box 28345, Zip 54324-8345; tel. 920/494-0225; Donald Seibel, Executive Director

WYOMING

Cheyenne: U. S. AIR FORCE HOSPITAL, 6900 Alden Drive, Zip 82005-3913; tel. 307/773-2045; Major Brenda Bullard, Administrator

Provisional Hospitals

CALIFORNIA

Modesto: STANISLAUS SURGERY CENTER, 1421 Oakdale Road, Zip 95355; tel. 209/572–2700; Michael Lipomi, Chief Executive Officer

NEW MEXICO

Albuquerque: HEART HOSPITAL OF NEW MEXICO, 504 Elm Street, Zip 87102; tel. 505/724–2000; Trudy Land, Chief Executive Officer

OHIO

Dayton: DAYTON HEART HOSPITAL, 707 South Edwin C. Moses Boulevard, Zip 45408; tel. 937/221–8000; Austin B. Cleveland, President and Chief Executive Officer

Associate Members

Ambulatory Centers and Home Care Agencies

United States

FLORIDA

NEMOURS CHILDREN'S CLINIC, 807 Nira Street, Jacksonville, Zip 32207; tel. 904/390–3600; Barry P. Sales, Administrator

NEW HAMPSHIRE

DARTMOUTH COLLEGE HEALTH SERVICE, 7 Rope Ferry Road, Hanover, Zip 03755–1421; tel. 603/650–1400; John Turco, M.D., Director

NEW YORK

WESTFALL SURGERY CENTER, 1065 Senator Keating Boulevard, Rochester, Zip 14618; tel. 716/256–1330; Gary J. Scott, Administrative Director

PENNSYLVANIA

CRAIG HOUSE–TECHNOMA, 751 North Negley Avenue, Pittsburgh, Zip 15206; tel. 412/361–2801; Richard L. Kerchnner, Administrator

WISCONSIN

CURATIVE REHABILITATION SERVICES, 1000 North 92nd Street, Wauwatosa, Zip 53226; tel. 414/259–1414; Robert H. Coons, , Jr, President

Philippines

DEPARTMENT OF VETERANS AFFAIRS, OUTPATIENT CLINIC, Manila, Zip 96440; tel. 632/521–7116

Blue Cross Plans

United States

ARIZONA

BLUE CROSS AND BLUE SHIELD OF ARIZONA, Box 13466, Phoenix, Zip 85002–3466; tel. 602/864–4400; Robert B. Bulla, President and Chief Executive Officer

MICHIGAN

BLUE CROSS AND BLUE SHIELD OF MICHIGAN, 600 East Lafayette, Mail Code 744, Detroit, Zip 48226; tel. 313/225–9101; Mark Johnson, Vice President Provider Contracting and Quality Assessment

NEW YORK

EXCELLUS HEALTH PLAN, INC., 165 Court Street, Rochester, Zip 14647; tel. 716/454–1700; David Mack, Senior Vice President Corporate Relations

OKLAHOMA

BLUE CROSS AND BLUE SHIELD OF OKLAHOMA, Box 3283, Tulsa, Zip 74102; tel. 918/583–0861; Ronald F. King, President and Chief Executive Officer

PENNSYLVANIA

CAPITAL BLUE CROSS, 2500 Elmerton Avenue, Harrisburg, Zip 17110; tel. 717/541–7000; James M. Mead, President

HIGHMARK BLUE CROSS BLUE SHIELD, 120 Fifth Avenue Place, Suite 3014, Pittsburgh, Zip 15222; tel. 412/544–7646; Sandra R. Tomlinson, Senior Vice President, Provider Affairs

INDEPENDENCE BLUE CROSS, 1901 Market Street, Philadelphia, Zip 19103; tel. 215/241–3300; Denise Dodd, Manager

Shared Services Organizations

TEXAS

TEXAS HOSPITAL ASSOCIATION, P.O. Box 15587, Austin, Zip 78761–5587; tel. 512/465–1000; Terry Townsend, FACHE, President and Chief Executive Officer

Other Members

UNITED STATES

Architecture:

BURT HILL KOSAR RITTELMANN ASSOCIATES, 400 Morgan Center, Butler, Pennsylvania Zip 16001-5977;
tel. 412/285-4761; John E. Brock, Principal
EARL SWENSSON ASSOCIATES, INC., 2100 West End Avenue, Suite 1200, Nashville, Tennessee Zip 37203;
tel. 615/329-9445; Richard L. Miller, President
MARSHALL CRAFT ASSOCIATES, INC., 6112 York Road, Baltimore, Maryland Zip 21212; tel. 410/532-3131; Tonia Burnette, Principal
MATTHEI AND COLIN ASSOCIATES, 332 South Michigan Avenue, Suite 614, Chicago, Illinois Zip 60604;
tel. 312/939-4002; Ronald G. Kobold, Managing Partner
SMITHGROUP, 1919 Santa Monica Boulevard, 4th Floor, Santa Monica, California Zip 90404;
tel. 310/586-5425; William Roger, Managing Director
WILLIAM A. BERRY & SON, INC., 100 Conifer Hill Drive, Danvers, Massachusetts Zip 01923;
tel. 978/774-1057; Ronda Paradis, Vice President

Behavioral Health Center:

DEVEREUX–VICTORIA, 120 David Wade Drive, Victoria, Texas Zip 77902-2666; tel. 512/575-8271; L. Gail Atkinson, Executive Director

Consulting Firm:

A.P.M./CSC HEALTHCARE, INC., 1675 Broadway, 18th Floor, New York, New York Zip 10019;
tel. 212/903-9300; Karen Flaherty, Coordinator Marketing
ARTHUR ANDERSEN & COMPANY, 33 West Monroe Street, Chicago, Illinois Zip 60603; tel. 312/580-0033; Edward Giniat, Director
BENEFIT RECOVERY ANALYSTS, INC., 403 West Fisher Avenue, Greensboro, North Carolina Zip 27401;
tel. 336/273-0737; Lisa Holt, Senior Analyst
CAMPBELL WILSON, 9400 Central Expressway, Suite 613, Dallas, Texas Zip 75231; tel. 214/373-7077; Danna J. Wilson, Principal
HAMILTON–KSA, 1355 Peachtree Street N.E., Suite 900, Atlanta, Georgia Zip 30309-0900; tel. 404/892-0321; C. B. Souther, Communication Director
HEALTHCARE FINANCIAL ENTERPRISES, INC., 1475 West Cypress Creek Road, 204, Fort Lauderdale, Florida Zip 33309; tel. 954/772-7878; Peter A. Carvalho, President
HEIDRICK AND STRUGGLES, 233 South Wacker, Suite 7000, Chicago, Illinois Zip 60606; tel. 312/372-8811; Richard P. Gustafson, Partner
MCKESSON HBO, 5995 Windward Parkway, Alpharetta, Georgia Zip 30005; tel. 404/338-3519; Louise Smith, R.N., Manager, Regulatory Assessment and Operations
MMI COMPANIES, INC., 540 Lake Cook Road, Deerfield, Illinois Zip 60015-5290; tel. 847/940-7550; Michelle Cooney, Vice President
PRESS, GANEY ASSOCIATES, INC., 404 Columbia Place, South Bend, Indiana Zip 46601; tel. 219/232-3387; Dennis W. Heck, FACHE, Vice President Corporate Development
RURAL HEALTH CONSULTANTS, 2500 West Sixth, Suite H, Lawrence, Kansas Zip 66049; tel. 785/832-8778; Diann Stogsdill, Senior Consultant
TIBER GROUP, INC., 200 South Wacker Drive, Suite 2620, Chicago, Illinois Zip 60601; tel. 312/609-9935; Davi Hirsch, Chief Operating Officer
TOWERS PERRIN, 100 Summit Lake Drive, Valhalla, New York Zip 10595; tel. 212/309-3400; Leslie Tobias, Information Specialist
VICTOR KRAMER COMPANY, INC., 405 Murray Hill Parkway, Suite 1040, Rutherford, New Jersey Zip 07070;
tel. 201/935-0414; Thomas Mara, President
WEST HUDSON, INC., 5230 Pacific Concourse Drive, Suite 400, Dallas, Texas Zip 75240; tel. 972/982-8700; Angela Carver, Administrative Coordinator

YAFFE AND COMPANY, INC., 409 Washington Avenue, Suite 700, Towson, Maryland Zip 21204;
tel. 410/494-4100; Rian M. Yaffe, President

Educational Services:

CALIFORNIA COLLEGE FOR HEALTH SCIENCES, 222 West 24th Street, National City, California Zip 91950;
tel. 619/477-4800; Dale K. Bean, Program Director

Facilities Management:

JOHNSON CONTROLS, INC., 3354 Perimeter Hill Drive, Suite 105, Franklin, Tennessee Zip 37067;
tel. 615/771-1400; C. Patrick Hardwick, Business Development Manager
SERVICEMASTER COMPANY, One Servicemaster Way, Downers Grove, Illinois Zip 60515; tel. 708/964-1300; C. William Pollard, Chairman

Health Care Alliance:

PREMIER, INC., 3 Westbrook Corporate Center, 9th Floor, San Diego, California Zip 92130; tel. 619/481-2727; Richard A. Norling, Chief Executive Officer
UNIVERSITY HEALTH SYSTEM OF NEW JERSEY, 154 West State Street, Trenton, New Jersey Zip 08608;
tel. 609/656-9600; Thomas E. Terrill, Ph.D., President
UNIVERSITY HEALTHSYSTEM CONSORTIUM, INC., 2001 Spring Road, Suite 700, Oak Brook, Illinois Zip 60523; tel. 630/954-1700; Robert J. Baker, President and Chief Executive Officer
VHA, INC., P.O. Box 140909, Irving, Texas Zip 75014-0909; tel. 972/830-0000; C. Thomas Smith, President and Chief Executive Officer

Information Systems:

3M HEALTH INFORMATION SYSTEMS, P.O. Box 57900, Murray, Utah Zip 84157; tel. 801/265-4400; Scott Slivka, Marketing Manager
CERNER CORPORATION, 2800 Rockcreek Parkway, Kansas City, Missouri Zip 64117; tel. 816/221-1024; Jack Newman, , Jr, Executive Vice President
FIRST COAST SYSTEMS, 6430 Southpoint Parkway, Suite 250, Jacksonville, Florida Zip 32216-0978;
tel. 904/296-4200; Charles R. Gibbs, President
MOTOROLA HEALTHCARE COMMUNICATIONS SOLUTIONS, 1301 East Algonquin Road, Schaumburg, Illinois Zip 60196; tel. 847/576-5000; James R. Hubbard, Director
SUPERIOR CONSULTANT COMPANY, INC., 4000 Town Center, Suite 1100, Southfield, Michigan Zip 48075;
tel. 810/386-8300; Richard D. Helppie, President

Insurance Broker:

AETNA RETIREMENT SERVICES, 151 Farmington Avenue–TS41, Hartford, Connecticut Zip 06156;
tel. 860/273-6053; Lloyd Duggan, , Jr, Market Research Manager
HEALTHCARE UNDERWRITERS MUTUAL INSURANCE COMPANY, 8 British American Boulevard, Latham, New York Zip 12110; tel. 518/786-2700; Gerald J. Cassidy, President and Chief Executive Officer
LOCKTON COMPANIES, 7400 State Line Road, Prairie Village, Kansas Zip 66208; tel. 913/676-9546; Becky Sullivan, Senior Vice President and Unit Manager
PRINCIPAL FINANCIAL GROUP, 711 High Street, Des Moines, Iowa Zip 50392-4620; tel. 515/247-5222; Joan Burns, Technical Senior Consultant

Investment Broker:

STEPHENS, INC., 111 Center Street, Little Rock, Arkansas Zip 72201; tel. 501/377-8125; Nancy Weaver, Research Analyst

Manufacturer/Supplier:

ABBOTT LABORATORIES, One Abbott Park Road, Abbott Park, Illinois Zip 60064; tel. 847/937-4576; William M. Dwyer, Senior Director Strategic Marketing

AMGEN, INC., 1840 Dehavilland Drive, Department 631, Thousand Oaks, California Zip 91320;
tel. 805/447-2106; Philip Villavicencio, Market Segment Director
BAXTER INTERNATIONAL, INC., One Baxter Parkway, Deerfield, Illinois Zip 60015; tel. 847/948-2000; Harry J. Kraemer, Chief Executive Officer
BAXTER PERFUSION SERVICES, 16818 Via Del Campo Court, San Diego, California Zip 92127;
tel. 619/485-5599; Jeffrey C. Crowley, Vice President Clinical Operations
BOSTON SCIENTIFIC CORPORATION, One Boston Scientific Place, Natick, Massachusetts Zip 01760;
tel. 508/650-8427; Susan Simpson, Marketing and Research Assistant
ELI LILLY AND COMPANY, Lilly Corporate Center, Suite 18, Indianapolis, Indiana Zip 46285-4113;
tel. 317/276-8744; Diane C. Waters, Market Analyst
GENERAL ELECTRIC MEDICAL SYSTEMS, P.O. Box 414, Milwaukee, Wisconsin Zip 53201; tel. 414/544-3011; Frank Cheng, Manager Market and Group Analysis
JOHNSON & JOHNSON, 425 Hoes Lane, Piscataway, New Jersey Zip 08855; tel. 732/562-3058; Cathi Brozena, Manager Professional Affairs
MANAGEMENT SCIENCE ASSOCIATES, INC., 4801 Cliff Avenue, Independence, Missouri Zip 64055;
tel. 816/795-1947; Kenneth J. McDonald, President
MEDSTAT GROUP/INFORUM, 424 Church Street, Suite 2600, Nashville, Tennessee Zip 37219;
tel. 800/829-0600; Kelly Tolson, Director Marketing
MERCK U. S. HUMAN HEALTH, WP35-150, West Point, Pennsylvania Zip 19486; tel. 215/652-5000; Phyllis Rausch, Marketing Associate
MILCARE, INC., A. HERMAN MILLER COMPANY, 8500 Byron Road, Zeeland, Michigan Zip 49464;
tel. 616/654-8000; David Reid, Senior Vice President and General Manager
NEMSCHOFF CHAIRS, INC., P.O. Box 129, Sheboygan, Wisconsin Zip 53082-0129; tel. 920/459-1216; David Stinson, Vice President
PFIZER U.S. PHARMACEUTICALS GROUP, 235 East 42nd Street, New York, New York Zip 10017;
tel. 212/573-7877; Daniel J. Coakley, Director Trade Development and Industry Affairs

Metro Health Care Assn:

HEALTHCARE ASSOCIATION OF SOUTHERN CALIFORNIA, 201 North Figueroa Street, 4th Floor, Los Angeles, California Zip 90071-3322; tel. 213/538-0700; James D. Barber, President

Other:

ADVISORY BOARD COMPANY, 600 New Hampshire Avenue N.W., Washington, District of Columbia Zip 20037-2403; tel. 202/672-5600; Scott Fassbach, Director
ALLIED HEALTHCARE PRODUCTS, INC., 1720 Sublette Avenue, Saint Louis, Missouri Zip 63110;
tel. 314/771-2400; Dave Grabowski, Vice President Sales and Marketing
AMERICA'S BLOOD CENTERS, 725 15th Street N.W., Suite 700, Washington, District of Columbia Zip 20005;
tel. 202/393-5725; Jim MacPherson, Executive Director
AMERICAN ASSOCIATION OF NURSE ANESTHETISTS, 222 South Prospect Avenue, Park Ridge, Illinois Zip 60068-4001; tel. 847/692-7050; John F. Garde, Executive Director
AMERICAN BOARD OF MEDICAL SPECIALTIES, 1007 Church Street, Suite 404, Evanston, Illinois Zip 60201-5913; tel. 847/491-9091; Stephen H. Miller, M.D., M.P.H., Executive Vice President
AMERICAN SOCIETY OF HOSPITAL PHARMACISTS, 7272 Wisconsin Avenue, Bethesda, Maryland Zip 20814;
tel. 301/657-3000; Henri R. Manasse, Ph.D., Sc.D., Executive Vice President and Chief Executive Officer
AMERICAN SURGICAL CENTERS, 27550 Schoenherr, Suite 400, Warren, Michigan Zip 48093; tel. 810/498-9440; J. David Posch, President

Associate Members / Other

ARMED FORCES INSTITUTE OF PATHOLOGY, 6825 16th Street N.W., Building 54, Washington, District of Columbia Zip 20306–6000; tel. 202/782–2100; Colonel Michael Dickerson, Director

ARMED FORCES MEDICAL LIBRARY, 5109 Leesburg Pike, Room 670, Falls Church, Virginia Zip 22041–3258; tel. 703/756–8028; D. Zehnpfennig, Administrative Librarian

ASSOCIATION OF UNIVERSITY PROGRAMS IN HEALTH ADMINISTRATION, 1911 North Fort Myer Drive, Suite 503, Washington, District of Columbia Zip 20001–5410; tel. 202/822–8550; Janet Porter, Interim President and Chief Executive Officer

BLUE CROSS AND BLUE SHIELD ASSOCIATION, 225 North Michigan Avenue, Chicago, Illinois Zip 60601–7680; tel. 312/440–6000; Scott Serota, Interim President

BROADCAST MUSIC, INC., 10 Music Square East, Nashville, Tennessee Zip 37203–4399; tel. 615/401–2000; Kathryn D. Crow, Director Industry Development

BUSINESS STRATEGY, INC., 944 520 Fourth Street S.E., Grand Rapids, Michigan Zip 49508; tel. 616/261–2200; Karen Rooney, Marketing Director

CICCORP, INC., 200 Greens Prairie Road, College Station, Texas Zip 77845–9394; tel. 409/690–5200; Rick Loden, Vice President Marketing

CIGNA HEALTHCARE, 1601 Chestnut Street, Suite TL5C, Philadelphia, Pennsylvania Zip 19192; tel. 215/761–1636; Charles Major, Subscription and Publications Manager

CONNECTICUT HOSPITAL ASSOCIATION, Box 90, Wallingford, Connecticut Zip 06492–0090; tel. 203/265–7611; Dennis P. May, President

CRASSOCIATES, INC., 8580 Cinderbed Road, Suite 2400, Newington, Virginia Zip 22122; tel. 703/550–8145; Charles H. Robbins, Chairman and Chief Executive Officer

CURBELL, INC., ELECTRONICS DIVISION, 7 Cobham Drive, Orchard Park, New York Zip 14127–4180; tel. 716/667–3377; Michael P. Donovan, Marketing Manager

DEPARTMENT OF AIR FORCE MEDICAL SERVICE, HQ USAF/SG, Bolling AFB, District of Columbia Zip 20332–6188; tel. 202/545–6700

DEPARTMENT OF THE ARMY, OFFICE OF THE SURGEON GENERAL, 5109 Leesburg Pike, Falls Church, Virginia Zip 22041; tel. 202/690–6467; Rear Admiral Michael Blackwell, Chief of Staff

DEPARTMENT OF THE NAVY, BUREAU OF MEDICINE AND SURGERY, 2300 East Street N.W., Washington, District of Columbia Zip 20372–5300; tel. 202/433–4475

DEPARTMENT OF VETERANS AFFAIRS, 301 Howard Street, Suite 700, San Francisco, California Zip 94105; Linda Pierce, Director, Sierra Pacific Network

DEPARTMENT OF VETERANS AFFAIRS, 810 Vermont Avenue N.W., Washington, District of Columbia Zip 20420; tel. 202/273–5400; Togo West, Secretary

DHHS, PUBLIC HEALTH SERVICE, DIVISION OF INDIAN HEALTH, HEALTH CARE ADMINISTRATION BRANCH, 5600 Fisher Lane, Room 6A–25, Rockville, Maryland Zip 20857; tel. 301/443–1085; Susanne Caviness, M.D., Chief Patient Registration and Quality Management

DIAMOND CRYSTAL SPECIALTY FOODS, INC., 10 Burlington Avenue, Wilmington, Massachusetts Zip 01887–3997; tel. 978/944–3977; Denise C. Kelly, Marketing Manager

DU PONT CORIAN, P.O. Box 80702, Room 1243, Wilmington, Delaware Zip 19880–0702; tel. 302/999–5447; John Burr, Marketing Manager

EMERGENCY CONSULTANTS, INC., 2240 South Airport Road, Traverse City, Michigan Zip 49684; tel. 800/253–1795; James Johnson, M.D., President

EMERGENCY PRACTICE ASSOCIATES, P.O. Box 1260, Waterloo, Iowa Zip 50704; tel. 319/236–3858; Margo Grimm, Chief Executive Officer

EMPACTHEALTH.COM, 3100 West End Avenue, Suite 1230, Nashville, Tennessee Zip 37203; tel. 615/344–5229; Tom Ranseen, Vice President Marketing

GE MEDICAL SYSTEMS HEALTHCARE SOLUTIONS, 10185 Bridgewater Circle, Woodbury, Minnesota Zip 55129; tel. 651/730–9377; Barbara Norman, Vice President Clinical Sales

GRAINGER INDUSTRIAL SUPPLY, 100 Grainger Parkway, Lake Forest, Illinois Zip 60045–0521; tel. 847/535–4532; David Smith, Director Customer Marketing

GUIDANT CORPORATION/CPI, 4100 Hamline Avenue North, Saint Paul, Minnesota Zip 55112; tel. 612/582–4017; Eva R. Shipley, Supervisor, Library Information Center

HAWAII MEDICAL SERVICE ASSOCIATION, P.O. Box 860, Honolulu, Hawaii Zip 96808–0860; tel. 808/948–5482; Waynette Wong-Chu, Manager Facility Reimbursement

HEALTH CARE PROPERTY INVESTORS, INC., 10990 Wilshire Boulevard, Suite 1200, Newport Beach, California Zip 92660–1875; tel. 213/473–1990; Kenneth B. Roath, President and Chief Executive Officer

HEALTHCARE FINANCIAL PARTNERS, 2 Wisconsin Circle, 4th Floor, Chevy Case, Maryland Zip 20815; tel. 301/961–1640; Carolyn Small, Marketing Manager

HEALTHTEK SOLUTIONS, INC., 999 Waterside Drive, Suite 1910, Norfolk, Virginia Zip 23510; tel. 757/625–0800; Anthony Montville, President

HOECHST MARION ROUSSEL, 10236 Marion Park Drive, Kansas City, Missouri Zip 64137–1405; tel. 816/966–4000; Matt Kerr, Market Manager

INTERNATIONAL ASSOCIATION FOR HEALTHCARE SECURITY AND SAFETY, P.O. Box 637, Lombard, Illinois Zip 60148; tel. 630/953–0990; Nancy Felesena, Executive Assistant

J. STEPHENS MAYHUGH AND ASSOCIATES, INC., P.O. Box 3276, Baton Rouge, Louisiana Zip 70821–3276; tel. 800/426–2349; Ron Ellis, Chief Executive Officer

JANZEN, JOHNSTON AND ROCKWELL, EMERGENCY MEDICINE MANAGEMENT SERVICES, INC., 4551 Glencoe Avenue, Suite 260, Marina Del Rey, California Zip 90292; tel. 310/301–2030; Richard W. Sanders, Vice President Marketing

JOBSCIENCE.COM, 1433 Webster Street, Suite 200, Oakland, California Zip 94612; tel. 510/208–5627; Pamela Elliott, Director Development

KEPPLER ASSOCIATES, INC., 4350 North Fairfax Drive, Suite 700, Arlington, Virginia Zip 22203; tel. 703/516–4000; Eric J. Fritz, Associate, Health Division

LEHMAN BROTHERS, 3 World Financial Ctr, 14th Floor, New York, New York Zip 10285; tel. 212/526–5496; Adam Feinstein, Senior Financial Analyst

MALLINCKRODT, P.O. Box 5840, Saint Louis, Missouri Zip 63134; tel. 314/654–8650; Debra L. Cochran, Manager Market Development

MARSH USA, INC., 1255 23rd Street N.W., Suite 400, Washington, District of Columbia Zip 20037; tel. 202/263–7611; Philip A. Balderston, Vice President

MDE/MEDQUIST, INC., 4 Foster Avenue, Suite A., Gibbsboro, New Jersey Zip 08026; tel. 856/784–4300; Joe Durney, Director Client Services

MODERN HEALTHCARE, 740 North Rush Street, Chicago, Illinois Zip 60611; tel. 312/368–6644; Charles S. Lauer, Corporate Vice President

MORRISON HEALTH CARE, INC., 1955 Lake Park Drive, Suite 400, Smyrna, Georgia Zip 30080–8855; tel. 770/437–3300; Glenn Davenport, President and Chief Executive Officer

NATIONAL CENTURY FINANCIAL ENTERPRISES, INC., 6125 Memorial Drive, Dublin, Ohio Zip 43017; tel. 614/764–9944; Dennise Tonn, Marketing Manager

NATIONAL REHAB PARTNERS, INC., 115 East Park Drive, Suite 150, Brentwood, Tennessee Zip 37027; tel. 615/369–2200; John A. Hawes, Chief Executive Officer

NATIONWIDE RETIREMENT SOLUTION, Two Nationwide Plaza, 2nd Floor, Columbus, Ohio Zip 43216; tel. 800/372–0764; Barbara Healy, Vice President Institutional Sales

NAVAL REGIONAL MEDICAL CENTER, PSC 1005, Box 36, FPO, APO/FPO Europe Zip 09593–0136

OLYMPUS AMERICA, INC., 2 Corporte Center Drive, Melville, New York Zip 11747; tel. 516/844–5000; Steven K. Wendt, Senior Manager National Accounts

PPL SPECTRUM, INC., 2 North 9th Street, GEN–GA2, Allentown, Pennsylvania Zip 18101; tel. 610/774–7985; Rick Seibert, Director Marketing

PPO CHECK, P.O. Box 2873, Houston, Texas Zip 77252; tel. 713/651–1533; Ryne Manahan, Chief Operating Officer

PROCTER AND GAMBLE COMPANY, 8700 Mason–Montgomery Road, Box 2071, Mason, Ohio Zip 45040–9462; tel. 513/622–4672; John E. Roney, Associate Director

REHABCARE GROUP, INC., 7733 Forsyth Boulevard, Suite 1700, Saint Louis, Missouri Zip 63105–1817; tel. 314/863–7422; Keith L. Goding, Executive Vice President and Chief Development Officer

SAINT JOSEPH'S REGIONAL MEDICAL CENTER, P.O. Box 1935, South Bend, Indiana Zip 46634; tel. 219/237–7111; Robert L. Beyer, President and Chief Executive Officer

SALICK HEALTH CARE, INC., 8201 Beverly Boulevard, Los Angeles, California Zip 90048; tel. 323/966–3400; Rod Cooley, Vice President Financial Planning

SHARED MEDICAL SYSTEMS, 51 Valley Stream Parkway, Malvern, Pennsylvania Zip 19355; tel. 610/219–3164; Susan B. West, Manager Executive Programs

SPECIALTY LABORATORIES, INC., 2211 Michigan Avenue, Santa Monica, California Zip 90404; tel. 310/828–6543; Susan Bailey, Marketing Manager

STAYWELL COMPANY, 1100 Grundy Lane, San Bruno, California Zip 94066; tel. 650/742–0400; Michelle Simmons, Business Development Manager

T. C. ADVERTISING COMPANY, INC., 450 East Devon Avenue, Suite 155, Itasca, Illinois Zip 60143; tel. 630/773–9855; Roger G. McGregor, Vice President, Sales

TEXAS MEDICAL CENTER, 406 Jesse Jones Library Building, Houston, Texas Zip 77030–3303; tel. 713/791–8805; Rhonda K. Simon, Vice President

THE ASSOCIATES – MUNICIPAL FINANCE DIVISION, P.O. Box 650363, Dallas, Texas Zip 75265–0363; tel. 972/652–2767; Ron L. Klein, Vice President Marketing and Sales

THE TRANE COMPANY, 4831 White Bear Parkway, Saint Paul, Minnesota Zip 55110; tel. 651/407–3822; Peter Berger, Gloval Market Development Manager

TRANSOLUTIONS, INCORPORATED, 18 North Waukegan Road, Suite 100, Lake Bluff, Illinois Zip 60044; tel. 847/234–3461; George Beukema, Director Sales and Marketing

U. S. ARMY MEDICAL COMMAND, 2050 Worth Road, Suite 3, Fort Sam Houston, Texas Zip 78234; tel. 210/221–2212; Lieutenant General Ronald R. Blanck, MS, Commander

UNITED HOSPITAL FUND OF NEW YORK, 350 Fifth Avenue, 23rd Floor, New York, New York Zip 10118; tel. 212/494–0700; James R. Tallon, , Jr, President

URBAN+CARE, 401 North Michigan Avenue, Chicago, Illinois Zip 60611; tel. 312/321–3947; Tena R. Vogt, Vice President Operations

VA HEALTHCARE NETWORK UPSTATE NEW YORK, P.O. Box 8980, Albany, New York Zip 12208–0980; tel. 518/472–1055; Frederick L. Malphurs, Director

VANDERWEIL ENGINEERS, 1055 Maitland Ctr Commons Boulevard, Maitland, Florida Zip 32751; tel. 407/660–0088; Ron Graham, Construction Administrator

VETERANS AFFAIRS CENTRAL REGION OFFICE, P.O. Box 134002, Ann Arbor, Michigan Zip 48113–4002; Linda Belton, Network Director

VETERANS AFFAIRS EASTERN REGION OFFICE, 9600 North Point Road, Fort Howard, Maryland Zip 21052

VETERANS AFFAIRS SOUTHERN REGION, 1600 East Woodrow Wilson Drive, Suite A, 3rd Floor, Jackson, Mississippi Zip 39216; tel. 601/364–7901; Billy M. Valentine, Interim Network Director

VISITING NURSE ASSOCIATION OF BROOKLYN, 138 South Oxford Street, Brooklyn, New York Zip 11217; tel. 718/230–6950; Jane G. Gould, President and Chief Executive Officer

VISN 1 OFFICE, 200 Spring Road, Building 61, Bedford, Massachusetts Zip 01730

VISN 10 OFFICE, 8600 Governor's Hill Road, 115, Cincinnati, Ohio Zip 45259

VISN 12 OFFICE, Fifth Avenue & Roosevelt Road, Hines, Illinois Zip 60141–5000; tel. 708/786–3737; Joan E. Cummings, M.D., Network Director

VISN 13 OFFICE, 54445 Minnehaha Avenue South, 2nd Floor, Minneapolis, Minnesota Zip 55417; tel. 612/727–5967; Robert A. Petzel, M.D., Network Director

VISN 14 OFFICE, 600 South 70th Street, Building 5, Lincoln, Nebraska Zip 68510; tel. 402/484–3202; Vincent Ng, Network Director

VISN 15 OFFICE, 4801 Linwood Boulevard, Kansas City, Missouri Zip 64128

VISN 17 OFFICE, 1901 North Highway 360, Suite 350, Grand Prairie, Texas Zip 75050

VISN 18 OFFICE, 6950 East Williams Field Road, Mesa, Arizona Zip 85212–6033

VISN 19 OFFICE, 4100 East Mississippi Avenue, 510, Glendale, Colorado Zip 80222

VISN 20 OFFICE, P.O. Box 1035, Portland, Oregon Zip 97207

VISN 22 OFFICE, 5901 East Seventh Street, Long Beach, California Zip 90822; tel. 562/494–5963; Smith Jenkins, , Jr, Network Director

VISN 3 OFFICE, 130 West Kingsbridge Road, Building 16, Bronx, New York Zip 10468; James J. Farsetta, FACHE, Network Director

VISN 4 OFFICE, Delafield Road, Pittsburgh, Pennsylvania Zip 15240

Associate Members / Other

VISN 5 OFFICE, 849 International Drive, Suite 275, Linthicum Heights, Maryland Zip 21090
VISN 6 OFFICE, 300 Morgan Street, Suite 1402, Durham, North Carolina Zip 27701
VISN 7 OFFICE, 2200 Century Parkway N.E., Suite 260, Atlanta, Georgia Zip 30345–3203
VISN 8 OFFICE, P.O. Box 5007, Bay Pines, Florida Zip 33744
VISN 9 OFFICE, 1310 24th Avenue South, Nashville, Tennessee Zip 37212–2637
WEB FAMILY VENTURES, INC., 1422 Delgany Street, Suite 40, Denver, Colorado Zip 80302; tel. 720/254–8384; James H. Franklin, Chief Financial Officer

School of Nursing:

ST. JOSEPH HOSPITAL SCHOOL OF NURSING, 200 High Service Avenue, North Providence, Rhode Island Zip 02904; tel. 401/456–3050; Elizabeth H. Decosta, R.N., Director School of Nursing

State Agency for Health:

DEPARTMENT OF HEALTH HOSPITAL AND PATIENT DATA SYSTEMS, CENTER FOR HEALTH STATISTICS, P.O. Box 47811, Olympia, Washington Zip 98504–7811; tel. 360/236–7811; Teresa Jennings, Director

CANADA

Other:

ALBERTA HEALTH–LIBRARY SERVICES BRANCH, P.O. Box 1360, Edmonton, Alberta Zip T5J 2N3; tel. 403/427–8720; Peggy Yeh, Librarian
DARCOR CASTERS, 7 Staffordshire Place, Toronto, Ontario Zip M8W 1T1; tel. 416/255–8563; Cyril J. Muhic, Regional Sales Manager
SHALIT FOODS, INC., 94 Martin Ross Avenue, Toronto, Ontario Zip M3J 2L4; tel. 416/650–9738; Sol Shalit, President
SIGMA ASSISTEL, INC., 1100 Boul Rene–Levesque Quest, Suite 1500, Montreal, Quebec Zip H3B 4N4; tel. 800/465–6390; Louise Des Ormeaux, General Manager
ST. JOSEPH'S HEALTH CARE SYSTEM, P.O. Box 155, LCD 1, Hamilton, Ontario Zip L8L 7V7; tel. 905/528–0138; Brian Guest, Executive Director

FOREIGN

ARGENTINA

Other:

SOCIALMED S.A., Bartolome' Mitre 3565, Buenos Aires, Ramon Cassino, M.D., Chief Executive Officer

AUSTRALIA

Other:

CEDAR COURT REHABILITATION HOSPITAL, 888 Toorak Road, Camberwell, Victoria, Zip 3124; Rodney G. Nissen, General Manager

BAHAMAS

Other:

PRINCESS MARGARET HOSPITAL, P.O. Box N 3730, Nassau, tel. 809/322–2861; Herbert Brown, Administrator

BAHRAIN

Other:

INTERNATIONAL HOSPITAL OF BAHRAIN, P.O. Box 1084, Manama, F. S. Zeerah, M.D., President

BRAZIL

Consulting Firm:

IHC–HOSPITALIUM, Rua dos Pinheiros, 498–cj, 61, San Paulo, Zip 05422–902; Edson Gomez dos Santos, President

Other:

CLINICA SAO VICENTE, Rua Joao Borges 204 – Gavea, Dogue, Zip 22 451–100; Luiz Roberto Londres, President
SANTA MARINA HOSPITAL AND MATERNITY, Avenue Santa Catarina, 2785, Sao Paulo, Zip 04378; Leonardo Santos de Almeida, Supply Manager
SOCIEDADE HOSPITAL SAMARITANO, Rua Conselheiro Brotero, 1486, Sao Paulo, Zip 01232–010; tel. 000/825–1122; Bryan Morgan, Director Superintendente

COLUMBIA

Other:

ASOCIACION COLOMBIANA DE HOSPITALES Y CLINICAS, Carrera 4, No 73–15, Bogota, tel. 091/312–4411; Roberto Esguerra Gutierrez, M.D., President
FUNDACION SANTA FE DE BOGOTA, Calle 116 9–02, Santa Fe De Bogota, Ana Catalina Vesquez Quintero, Manager

ECUADOR

Other:

JUNTA DE BENEFICENCIA DE GUAYAQUIL, P.O. Box 09–01–780, Guayaquil, Lautaro Aspiazu Wright, Director

GREECE

Other:

DIAGNOSTIC AND THERAPEUTIC CENTRE OF ATHENS HYGEIA, S A, 4 Erythrou Stavrou & Kifissiap, Athens, C. Kitsionas, Executive Director
HOSPITAL AFFILIATES INTERNATIONAL, 332 Kifissias Avenue, Halandri, Athens 152 33, A. Philip Chrysafidis, Senior Consultant
IASO S.A. DIAGNOSTIC THERAPEUTIC AND RESEARCH CENTER, OBSTETRICS AND GYNECOLOGY HOSPITAL, 37–39 Kifissias Avenue, Maroussi Athens, Zip 15123

ISRAEL

Other:

HADASSAH MEDICAL ORGANIZATION, Box 12000, Jerusalem, Zip 91120; Avi Israeli, M.D., Director General
S.A.R.E.L. SUPPLIES AND SERVICES FOR MEDICINE LTD., 15 Yehuda & Noah Mozes Street, Tel Aviv, Moshe Modai, Ph.D., Chief Executive Officer

JAPAN

Other:

MEIJI SEIMEI, FSI, 211 Morunouchi, Chiyoda–Ku Tokyo, Yumi Matsubara, Staff Researcher
NAVAL REGIONAL MEDICAL CENTER, FPO, Zip 96362
ST. LUKE'S INTERNATIONAL HOSPITAL, 10–1 Akashi–Cho, Chuo–Ku, Tokyo 104, Shigeaki Hinohara, M.D., Honorary President

LEBANON

Other:

AMERICAN UNIVERSITY OF BEIRUT MEDICAL CENTER, 850 Third Avenue, 18th Floor, New York, Zip 10022; Marina Hajj, M.D., Interim Director
MAKASSED GENERAL HOSPITAL, P.O. Box 6301, Beirut, Moh'd Firikh, Director
SAINT GEORGE HOSPITAL, P.O. Box 166378, Beirut, Ziad Kamel, Assistant Director

MEXICO

Other:

SHRINERS HOSPITAL FOR CHILDREN, Suchil 152, Colonel El Rosario, Mexico City 04380, Araceli Nagore, R.N., Administrator
UNIVERSIDAD AUTONOMA DE GUADALAJARA, Av Patria 1201 Lomas Del Valle, Guadalajara, tel. 210/366–1611; Rosalia Leano, Dean

Other Inpatient Care:

OASIS HOSPITAL, 2247 San Diego Avenue, Suite 235, San Ysidro, Zip 92143; tel. 800/700–1850; Francisco Contreras, Director

PERU

Other:

ASOCIACION BENEFICA ANGLO AMERICANA, Avenue Alfredo Salazar 3 Era, Lima 27, Gonzalo Garrido–Lecca, Director

PHILIPPINES

Other:

ST. LUKE'S MEDICAL CENTER, 279 East Rodriguez Sr Boulevard, Quezon City, Jose F. G. Ledesma, Chief Executive Officer

SAUDI ARABIA

Other:

ABDUL RAHMAN AL MISHARI GENERAL HOSPITAL, Olaya, Riyadh 11564, Abdul Rahman Al Mishari, M.D., President
ELAJ MEDICAL SERVICES COMPANY, LTD., P.O. Box 51141, Jeddah 21463, Mohamed Amin, Medical Director
MUHAMMAD S BASHARAHIL HOSPITAL, P.O. Box 10505, Makkah, Sameer M. Basharahil, Vice President
SAAD MEDICAL CENTER/OASIS RESIDENTIAL RESORT, P.O. Box 3250, Al–Khobar 31952, Hazim A. Khaled, General Manager
SAUDI ARAMCO MEDICAL SERVICES, 9009 West Loop South, MS–549, Houston, Zip 77096; Harris Worchel, Supervisor Information and Image Services

TAIWAN

Other:

CHANG GUNG MEMORIAL HOSPITAL, 199 Tun Hwa North Road, Taipei, Yi–Chou Chuang, Director Administration Center

Associate Members / Other

TURKEY

Other:

ALKAN HOSPITAL, Birlik Mah, 8 Cad 103 Sokak 10, Cankaya, Ankara, Zip 06552; Oguz Engiz, Chief Executive Officer

AMERICAN HOSPITAL OF ISTANBUL, Guzelbaghe SOK 20, Nisantasi, Istanbul, Zip 80020; George D. Roundtree, Chief Executive Officer

BAYINDIR HEALTH CARE SYSTEM, Maslak Pl Buyukdere Cad 69 K. 8, Ayazaga/Istanbul, Zip 80670; Sarper Tanli, M.D., Medical Director

UNITED ARAB EMIRATES

Other:

AMERICAN HOSPITAL–DUBAI, P.O. Box 59, Dubai, Saeed M. Almulla, Chairman

VENEZUELA

Other:

POLICLINICA METROPOLITANA, C.A., P.O. Box 025255, Miami, Zip 33102–5255; Edgar Escalona, M.D., Medical Director

B Networks, Health Care Systems and Alliances

B2 Introduction
3 Networks and their Hospitals
49 Statistics for Multihospital Health Care Systems and their Hospitals
50 Health Care Systems and their Hospitals
156 Headquarters of Health Care Systems, Geographically
163 Alliances

Introduction

This section includes listings for networks, health care systems and alliances.

Networks

The *AHA Guide* shows listings of networks. A network is defined as a group of hospitals, physicians, other providers, insurers and/or community agencies that work together to coordinate and deliver a broad spectrum of services to their community. Organizations listed represent the lead or hub of the network activity. Networks are listed by state, then alphabetically by name including participating partners.

The network identification process has purposely been designed to capture networks of varying organization type. Sources include but are not limited to the following: *AHA Annual Survey,* national, state and metropolitan associations, national news and periodical searches, and the networks and their health care providers themselves. Therefore, networks are included regardless of whether a hospital or healthcare system is the network lead. When an individual hospital does appear in the listing, it is indicative of the role the hospital plays as the network lead. In addition, the network listing is **not** mutually exclusive of the hospital, health care system or alliance listings within this publication.

Networks are very fluid in their composition as goals evolve and partners change. Therefore, some of the networks included in this listing may have dissolved, reformed, or simply been renamed as this section was being produced for publication.

The network identification process is an ongoing and responsive initiative. As more information is collected and validated, it will be made available in other venues, in addition to the *AHA Guide.* For more information concerning the network identification process, please contact Health Forum LLC, an affiliate of the American Hospital Association at 800/821-2039.

Health Care Systems

To reflect the diversity that exists among health care organizations, this publication uses the term health care system to identify both multihospital and diversified single hospital systems.

Multihospital Systems
A multihospital health care system is two or more hospitals owned, leased, sponsored, or contract managed by a central organization.

Single Hospital Systems
Single, freestanding member hospitals may be categorized as health care systems by bringing into membership three or more, and at least 25 percent, of their owned or leased non–hospital preacute and postacute health care organizations. (For purposes of definition, health care delivery is the availability of professional healthcare staff during all hours of the organization's operations). Organizations provide, or provide and finance, diagnostic, therapeutic, and/or consultative patient or client services that normally precede or follow acute, inpatient, hospitalization; or that serve to prevent or substitute for such hospitalization. These services are provided in either a freestanding facility not eligible for licensure as a hospital understate statue or through one that is a subsidiary of a hospital.

The first part of this section is an alphabetical list of multihospital health care systems. Each system listed contains two or more hospitals, which are listed under the system by state. Data for this section were compiled from the 1999 *Annual Survey* and the membership information base as published in section A of the *AHA Guide.*

One of the following codes appears after the name of each system listed to indicate the type of organizational control reported by that system:

CC	Catholic (Roman) church–related system, not–for–profit
CO	Other church–related system, not–for–profit
NP	Other not–for–profit system, including nonfederal, governmental systems
IO	Investor–owned, for profit system
FG	Federal Government

One of the following codes appears after the name of each hospital to indicate how that hospital is related to the system:

O	Owned
L	Leased
S	Sponsored
CM	Contract–managed

Health System Classification System

An identification system for Health Systems was developed jointly by the American Hospital Association's Health Research and Education Trust and Health Forum, and the University of California-Berkeley.[1] A health system is assigned to one of five categories based on how much they differentiate and centeralize their hospital services, physician arrangements, and provider-based insurance products. Differentiation refers to the number of different products or services that the organization offers. Centralization refers to whether decision-making and service delivery emanate from the system level more so than individual hospitals.

The Categories Are:

Centralized Health System: A delivery system in which the system centrally organizes individual hospital service delivery, physician arrangements, and insurance product development. The number of different products/services that are offered across the system is moderate.

Centralized Physician/Insurance Health System: A delivery system with highly centralized physician arrangements and insurance product development. Within this group, hospital services are relatively decentralized with individual hospitals having discretion over the array of services they offer. The number of different products/services that are offered across the system is moderate.

Moderately Centralized Health System: A delivery system that is distinguished by the presence of both centralized and decentralized activity for hospital services, physician arrangements, and insurance product development. For example, a system within this group may have centralized care of expensive, high technology services, such as open heart surgery, but allows individual hospitals to provide an array of other health services based on local needs. The number of different products/services that are offered across the system is moderate.

Decentralized Health System: A delivery system with a high degree of decentralized of hospital services, physician arrangements, and insurance product development. Within this group, systems may lack an overarching structure for coordination. Service and product differentiation is high, which may explain why centralization is hard to achieve. In this group, the system may simply service a role in sharing information and providing administrative support to highly developed local delivery systems centered around hospitals.

Independent Hospital System: A delivery system with limited differentiation in hospital services, physician arrangements, and insurance product development. These systems are largely horizontal affiliations of autonomous hospitals.

No Cluster Assignment: For some systems sufficient data from the Annual Survey were not available to determine a cluster assignment.

The second part of this section lists health care systems indexed geographically by state and city. Every effort has been made to be as inclusive and accurate as possible. However, as in all efforts of this type, there may be omissions. For further information, write to the section for Health Care Systems, American Hospital Association, One North Franklin, Chicago, IL 60606-3401.

Alliances

An alliance is a formal organization, usually owned by shareholders/members, that works on behalf of its individual members in the provision of services and products and in the promotion of activities and ventures. The organization functions under a set of bylaws or other written rules to which each member agrees to abide.

Alliances are listed alphabetically by name. Its members are listed alphabetically by state, city, and then by member name.

---

[1] Bazzoli, CJ; Shortell, SM; Dubbs, N; Chan, C; and Kralovec, P; "A Taxonomy of Health networks and Systems: Bringing Order Out of Chaos" *Health Services Research*, February; 1999

Networks and their Hospitals

ALABAMA

HEALTHGROUP OF ALABAMA
P.O.Box 1246, Madison, AL 35758;
tel. 205/772–4155; Edward D. Boston, Chief Executive Officer

ATHENS–LIMESTONE HOSPITAL, 700 West Market Street, Athens, AL, Zip 35611-2457, Mailing Address: P.O. Box 999, Zip 35612–0999; tel. 256/233–9292; Philip E. Dotson, Chief Executive Officer

ELIZA COFFEE MEMORIAL HOSPITAL, 205 Marengo Street, Florence, AL, Zip 35630–6033, Mailing Address: P.O. Box 818, Zip 35631–0818; tel. 256/768–9191; Richard H. Peck, President and Chief Executive Officer

HUNTSVILLE HOSPITAL, 101 Sivley Road, Huntsville, AL, Zip 35801-4470; tel. 256/517–8020; L. Joe Austin, Chief Executive Officer

ALASKA

KETCHIKAN GENERAL HOSPITAL
3100 Tongass Avenue, Ketchikan, AK 99901; tel. 907/225–5171; Ed Mahn, President

CHARTER NORTH STAR BEHAVIORAL HEALTH SYSTEM, 1650 South Bragaw, Anchorage, AK, Zip 99508-3467; tel. 907/258–7575; Kathleen Cronen, Chief Executive Officer

KETCHIKAN GENERAL HOSPITAL, 3100 Tongass Avenue, Ketchikan, AK, Zip 99901-5746; tel. 907/225–5171; Edward F. Mahn, Chief Executive Officer

NORTON SOUND REGIONAL HOSPITAL
P.O. Box 966, Nome, AK 99762; tel. 907/443–3311; H. Mack, Network Contact

NORTON SOUND REGIONAL HOSPITAL, Bering Straits, Nome, AK, Zip 99762, Mailing Address: P.O. Box 966, Zip 99762-0966; tel. 907/443–3311; Charles Fagerstrom, Vice President

ARIZONA

ARIZONA HEALTHCARE FEDERATION
2701 E. Camelback Road, Suite 510, Phoenix, AZ 85016; tel. 602/468–2070; Saundra Johnson, Chief Operating Officer

ARROWHEAD COMMUNITY HOSPITAL AND MEDICAL CENTER, 18701 North 67th Avenue, Glendale, AZ, Zip 85308-5722; tel. 623/561–1000; Richard S. Alley, Executive Vice President and Chief Executive Officer

CASA GRANDE REGIONAL MEDICAL CENTER, 1800 East Florence Boulevard, Casa Grande, AZ, Zip 85222-5399; tel. 520/426–6300; J. Marty Dernier, President and Chief Executive Officer

CHANDLER REGIONAL HOSPITAL, 475 South Dobson Road, Chandler, AZ, Zip 85224-4230; tel. 480/963–4561; David G. Covert, President and Chief Administrative Officer

FLAGSTAFF MEDICAL CENTER, 1200 North Beaver Street, Flagstaff, AZ, Zip 86001-3198; tel. 520/779–3366; Stephen G. Carlson, President and Chief Operating Officer

LA PAZ REGIONAL HOSPITAL, 1200 Mohave Road, Parker, AZ, Zip 85344-6349; tel. 520/669–9201; William G. Coe, Executive Vice President and Chief Executive Officer

PHOENIX BAPTIST HOSPITAL AND MEDICAL CENTER, 2000 West Bethany Home Road, Phoenix, AZ, Zip 85015-2110; tel. 602/249–0212; Jeffrey K. Norman, Executive Vice President and Chief Executive Officer

UNIVERSITY MEDICAL CENTER, 1501 North Campbell Avenue, Tucson, AZ, Zip 85724-5128; tel. 520/694–6148; Gregory A. Pivirotto, President and Chief Executive Officer

VERDE VALLEY MEDICAL CENTER, 269 South Candy Lane, Cottonwood, AZ, Zip 86326; tel. 520/634–2251; Craig A. Owens, President and Chief Operating Officer

YAVAPAI REGIONAL MEDICAL CENTER, 1003 Willow Creek Road, Prescott, AZ, Zip 86301-1668; tel. 520/445–2700; Timothy Barnett, Chief Executive Officer

YUMA REGIONAL MEDICAL CENTER, 2400 South Avenue A, Yuma, AZ, Zip 85364-7170; tel. 520/344–2000; Robert T. Olsen, CHE, President and Chief Executive Officer

BANNER HEALTH ARIZONA
1441 North 12th Street, Phoenix, AZ 85006; tel. 602/495–4000; Charles H. Welliver, Chief Executive Officer

DESERT SAMARITAN MEDICAL CENTER, 1400 South Dobson Road, Mesa, AZ, Zip 85202-9879; tel. 480/835–3000; Bruce E. Pearson, Senior Vice President and Chief Executive Officer

GOOD SAMARITAN REGIONAL MEDICAL CENTER, 1111 East McDowell Road, Phoenix, AZ, Zip 85006-2666, Mailing Address: P.O. Box 2989, Zip 85062-2989; tel. 602/239–2000; Steven L. Seiler, Senior Vice President and Chief Executive Officer

MESA LUTHERAN HOSPITAL, 525 West Brown Road, Mesa, AZ, Zip 85201-3299; tel. 480/834–1211; James Gingerich, Senior Vice President and Chief Executive Officer

PAGE HOSPITAL, 501 North Navajo Drive, Page, AZ, Zip 86040, Mailing Address: P.O. Box 1447, Zip 86040-1447; tel. 520/645–2424; Richard Polheber, Chief Executive Officer

SAMARITAN BEHAVIORAL HEALTH CENTER–SCOTTSDALE, 7575 East Earll Drive, Scottsdale, AZ, Zip 85251-6998; tel. 480/941–7500; Robert F. Meyer, M.D., Chief Executive Officer

THUNDERBIRD SAMARITAN MEDICAL CENTER, 5555 West Thunderbird Road, Glendale, AZ, Zip 85306-4696; tel. 602/588–5555; Robert H. Curry, Senior Vice President and Chief Executive Officer

CARONDELET HEALTH NETWORK
1601 West Saint Mary's, Tucson, AZ 85745; tel. 602/622–5833; Sister Saint Joan Willert, President & Chief Executive Officer

CARONDELET HOLY CROSS HOSPITAL, 1171 West Target Range Road, Nogales, AZ, Zip 85621-2496; tel. 520/287–2771; Richard Polheber, Interim Vice President and Chief Executive Officer

CARONDELET ST. JOSEPH'S HOSPITAL, 350 North Wilmot Road, Tucson, AZ, Zip 85711-2678; tel. 520/296–3211; Wesley E. Colvin, Senior Vice President and Chief Executive Officer

CARONDELET ST. MARY'S HOSPITAL, 1601 West St. Mary's Road, Tucson, AZ, Zip 85745-2682; tel. 520/622–5833

LUTHERAN HEALTHCARE NETWORK
500 W. 10th Place Suite 237, Mesa, AZ 85201; tel. 602/461–2157; Don Evans, Chief Executive Officer

MESA LUTHERAN HOSPITAL, 525 West Brown Road, Mesa, AZ, Zip 85201-3299; tel. 480/834–1211; James Gingerich, Senior Vice President and Chief Executive Officer

VALLEY LUTHERAN HOSPITAL, 6644 Baywood Avenue, Mesa, AZ, Zip 85206-1797; tel. 480/981–2000; Robert A. Rundio, Executive Director of Hospital Operations

NORTHERN ARIZONA HEALTHCARE
1200 North Beaver Street, Flagstaff, AZ 86001; tel. 520/773–2001; Joseph M. Kortum, President / Chief Executive Officer

FLAGSTAFF MEDICAL CENTER, 1200 North Beaver Street, Flagstaff, AZ, Zip 86001-3198; tel. 520/779–3366; Stephen G. Carlson, President and Chief Operating Officer

VERDE VALLEY MEDICAL CENTER, 269 South Candy Lane, Cottonwood, AZ, Zip 86326; tel. 520/634–2251; Craig A. Owens, President and Chief Operating Officer

SUN HEALTH CORPORATION
13180 N. 103rd Drive, Sun City, AZ 85351; tel. 623/876–5352; Leland W. Peterson, President & Chief Executive Officer

DEL E. WEBB MEMORIAL HOSPITAL, 14502 West Meeker Boulevard, Sun City West, AZ, Zip 85375-5299, Mailing Address: P.O. Box 5169, Sun City, Zip 85375-5169; tel. 623/214–4000; Thomas C. Dickson, Executive Vice President and Chief Operating Officer

WALTER O. BOSWELL MEMORIAL HOSPITAL, 10401 West Thunderbird Boulevard, Sun City, AZ, Zip 85351-3092, Mailing Address: P.O. Box 1690, Zip 85372-1690; tel. 623/977–7211; George Perez, Executive Vice President and Chief Operating Officer

ARKANSAS

BAPTIST HEALTH
9601 Interstate 630, Exit 7, Little Rock, AR 72205; tel. 501/228–0107; Russ Harrington, President

BAPTIST HEALTH BAPTIST MEMORIAL MEDICAL CENTER, 3333 Springhill Drive, North Little Rock, AR, Zip 72117; tel. 501/202–3000; Harrison M. Dean, Senior Vice President and Administrator

BAPTIST HEALTH MEDICAL CENTER–ARKADELPHIA, 3050 Twin Rivers Drive, Arkadelphia, AR, Zip 71923-4299; tel. 870/245–1100; Dan Gathright, Senior Vice President and Administrator

BAPTIST HEALTH MEDICAL CENTER–LITTLE ROCK, 9601 Interstate 630, Exit 7, Little Rock, AR, Zip 72205-7299; tel. 501/202–2000; Steven Douglas Weeks, Senior Vice President and Administrator

BAPTIST HEALTH REHABILITATION INSTITUTE, 9601 Interstate 630, Exit 7, Little Rock, AR, Zip 72205-7249; tel. 501/202–7000; Steven Douglas Weeks, Senior Vice President and Administrator

TENET HEALTHCARE CORP.
12814 Cantrell Rd., Little Rock, AR 72223; tel. 501/219–4260; William Bradley, Senior Vice President

CALIFORNIA

ADVENTIST HEALTH SCIENCES SYSTEM–LOMA LINDA UNIV
11161 Anderson Street, Loma Linda, CA 92350; tel. 909/824–4459; David B. Hinshaw, MD, President

LOMA LINDA UNIVERSITY BEHAVIORAL MEDICINE CENTER, 1710 Barton Road, Redlands, CA, Zip 92373; tel. 909/558–9200; Alan Soderblom, Administrator

LOMA LINDA UNIVERSITY MEDICAL CENTER, 11234 Anderson Street, Loma Linda, CA, Zip 92354-2870, Mailing Address: P.O. Box 2000, Zip 92354-0200; tel. 909/558–4000; B. Lyn Behrens, President and Chief Executive Officer

ADVENTIST HEALTH SOUTHERN CALIFORNIA
1505 Wilson Terrace Suite 220, Glendale, CA 91206; tel. 818/409–8300; Fred Manchur, President & Chief Executive Officer

GLENDALE ADVENTIST MEDICAL CENTER, 1509 Wilson Terrace, Glendale, CA, Zip 91206-4007; tel. 818/409–8000; Fred M. Manchur, President and Chief Executive Officer

SIMI VALLEY HOSPITAL AND HEALTH CARE SERVICES, 2975 North Sycamore Drive, Simi Valley, CA, Zip 93065-1277; tel. 805/955–6000; Alan J. Rice, President

WHITE MEMORIAL MEDICAL CENTER, 1720 Cesar E Chavez Avenue, Los Angeles, CA, Zip 90033-2481; tel. 323/268–5000; Fred M. Manchur, President and Chief Executive Officer

Networks / Catholic Healthcare West

CATHOLIC HEALTHCARE WEST
1700 Montgomery Street, San Francisco, CA 94111; tel. 415/397-9000; Debbie Canta, Director of Corporate Communication

DOMINICAN HOSPITAL, 1555 Soquel Drive, Santa Cruz, CA, Zip 95065; tel. 831/462-7700; Sister Julie Hyer, President and Chief Executive Officer

MARK TWAIN ST. JOSEPH'S HOSPITAL, 768 Mountain Ranch Road, San Andreas, CA, Zip 95249-9710; tel. 209/754-2515; Michael P. Lawson, Administrator

MERCY AMERICAN RIVER/MERCY SAN JUAN HOSPITAL, 6501 Coyle Avenue, Carmichael, CA, Zip 95608, Mailing Address: P.O. Box 479, Zip 95608; tel. 916/537-5000; Michael H. Erne, President and Chief Executive Officer

MERCY GENERAL HOSPITAL, 4001 J Street, Sacramento, CA, Zip 95819; tel. 916/851-2000; Thomas A. Petersen, Vice President and Chief Operating Officer

MERCY HOSPITAL, 2215 Truxtun Avenue, Bakersfield, CA, Zip 93301, Mailing Address: P.O. Box 119, Zip 93302; tel. 661/632-5000; Bernard J. Herman, President and Chief Executive Officer

MERCY HOSPITAL AND HEALTH SERVICES, 2740 M Street, Merced, CA, Zip 95340-2880; tel. 209/384-6444; John Headding, Chief Administrative Officer

MERCY HOSPITAL OF FOLSOM, 1650 Creekside Drive, Folsom, CA, Zip 95630; tel. 916/983-7400; Donald C. Hudson, Vice President and Chief Operating Officer

MERCY MEDICAL CENTER MOUNT SHASTA, 914 Pine Street, Mount Shasta, CA, Zip 96067, Mailing Address: P.O. Box 239, Zip 96067-0239; tel. 530/926-6111; Richard J. Barnett, Executive Vice President and Chief Operating Officer

MERCY MEDICAL CENTER REDDING, 2175 Rosaline Avenue, Redding, CA, Zip 96001, Mailing Address: P.O. Box 496009, Zip 96049-6009; tel. 530/225-6000; John Di Perry, Jr, Executive Vice President and Chief Operating Officer

METHODIST HOSPITAL OF SACRAMENTO, 7500 Hospital Drive, Sacramento, CA, Zip 95823; tel. 916/423-3000; Michael J. Finn, Acting Vice President and Chief Operating Officer

O'CONNOR HOSPITAL, 2105 Forest Avenue, San Jose, CA, Zip 95128; tel. 408/947-2500; Joan A. Bero, Regional Vice President and Chief Operating Officer

ROBERT F. KENNEDY MEDICAL CENTER, 4500 West 116th Street, Hawthorne, CA, Zip 90250; tel. 310/973-1711; Peter P. Aprato, President

SAINT FRANCIS MEMORIAL HOSPITAL, 900 Hyde Street, San Francisco, CA, Zip 94109, Mailing Address: Box 7726, Zip 94120-7726; tel. 415/353-6000; Cheryl A. Fama, Administrator, Vice President and Chief Operating Officer

SEQUOIA HOSPITAL, 170 Alameda De Las Pulgas, Redwood City, CA, Zip 94062; tel. 650/369-5811; John Williams, Chief Executive Officer

SETON MEDICAL CENTER, 1900 Sullivan Avenue, Daly City, CA, Zip 94015; tel. 650/992-4000; Bernadette M. Smith, Chief Operating Officer

SETON MEDICAL CENTER COASTSIDE, Marine Boulevard and Etheldore Street, Moss Beach, CA, Zip 94038; tel. 650/563-7100; John G. Williams, President and Chief Executive Officer

SIERRA NEVADA MEMORIAL HOSPITAL, 155 Glasson Way, Grass Valley, CA, Zip 95945, Mailing Address: P.O. Box 1029, Zip 95945-1029; tel. 530/274-6000; C. Thomas Collier, President and Chief Executive Officer

ST. BERNARDINE MEDICAL CENTER, 2101 North Waterman Avenue, San Bernardino, CA, Zip 92404; tel. 909/883-8711; Steven R. Barron, President

ST. DOMINIC'S HOSPITAL, 1777 West Yosemite Avenue, Manteca, CA, Zip 95337; tel. 209/825-3500; Margaret Hepburn, Chief Administrative Officer and Chief Nurse Executive

ST. ELIZABETH COMMUNITY HOSPITAL, 2550 Sister Mary Columba Drive, Red Bluff, CA, Zip 96080-4397; tel. 530/529-8000; Thomas F. Grimes, II, Executive Vice President and Chief Operating Officer

ST. FRANCIS MEDICAL CENTER, 3630 East Imperial Highway, Lynwood, CA, Zip 90262; tel. 310/603-6000; Gerald T. Kozai, President

ST. JOHN'S PLEASANT VALLEY HOSPITAL, 2309 Antonio Avenue, Camarillo, CA, Zip 93010-1459; tel. 805/389-5800; William J. Clearwater, Vice President and Site Administrator

ST. JOHN'S REGIONAL MEDICAL CENTER, 1600 North Rose Avenue, Oxnard, CA, Zip 93030; tel. 805/988-2500; Charles E. Padilla, Administrator and Chief Operating Officer

ST. JOSEPH'S BEHAVIORAL HEALTH CENTER, 2510 North California Street, Stockton, CA, Zip 95204-5568; tel. 209/948-2100; James Sondecker, Director

ST. JOSEPH'S HOSPITAL AND MEDICAL CENTER, 350 West Thomas Road, Phoenix, AZ, Zip 85013-4496, Mailing Address: P.O. Box 2071, Zip 85001-2071; tel. 602/406-3000; Linda A. Hunt, President and Chief Administrative Officer

ST. JOSEPH'S MEDICAL CENTER, 1800 North California Street, Stockton, CA, Zip 95204, Mailing Address: P.O. Box 213008, Zip 95213-3008; tel. 209/943-2000; Donald J. Wiley, Senior Vice President and Chief Operating Officer

ST. MARY MEDICAL CENTER, 1050 Linden Avenue, Long Beach, CA, Zip 90801, Mailing Address: P.O. Box 887, Zip 90813-0887; tel. 562/491-9000; Thomas G. Hennessy, President and Chief Executive Officer

ST. MARY'S MEDICAL CENTER, 450 Stanyan Street, San Francisco, CA, Zip 94117-1079; tel. 415/668-1000; Rosemary Fox, Vice President and Chief Operating Officer

ST. ROSE DOMINICAN HOSPITAL, 102 Lake Mead Drive, Henderson, NV, Zip 89015-5524; tel. 702/564-2622; Rod A. Davis, President and Chief Executive Officer

ST. VINCENT MEDICAL CENTER, 2131 West Third Street, Los Angeles, CA, Zip 90057-0992, Mailing Address: P.O. Box 57992, Zip 90057; tel. 213/484-7111; William D. Parente, President

WOODLAND HEALTHCARE, 1325 Cottonwood Street, Woodland, CA, Zip 95695-5199; tel. 530/662-3961; Margaret Cleary, Chief Executive Officer

CEDARS SINAI MEDICAL CENTER
8700 Beverly Blvd-Rm2802, Los Angeles, CA 90048; tel. 310/423-5000; Thomas M. Priselac, President/Chief Executive Officer

CEDARS-SINAI MEDICAL CENTER, 8700 Beverly Boulevard, Los Angeles, CA, Zip 90048-1865, Mailing Address: Box 48750, Zip 90048-0750; tel. 310/423-5000; Thomas M. Priselac, President and Chief Executive Officer

EAST BAY MEDICAL NETWORK
2000 Powell Street 9th Flr, Emeryville, CA 94608; tel. 510/450-9850; Belina Rule, Provider Relations

ALAMEDA HOSPITAL, 2070 Clinton Avenue, Alameda, CA, Zip 94501; tel. 510/522-3700; William J. Dal Cielo, Chief Executive Officer

ALTA BATES MEDICAL CENTER-ASHBY CAMPUS, 2450 Ashby Avenue, Berkeley, CA, Zip 94705; tel. 510/204-4444; Warren J. Kirk, President and Chief Administrative Officer

JM/MD HEALTH SYSTEM, 1400 Treat Boulevard, Walnut Creek, CA, Zip 94556; tel. 925/941-2100; J. Kendall Anderson, President and Chief Executive Officer

PATTON STATE HOSPITAL, 3102 East Highland Avenue, Patton, CA, Zip 92369; tel. 909/425-7000; William L. Summers, Executive Director

SAN LEANDRO HOSPITAL, 13855 East 14th Street, San Leandro, CA, Zip 94578-0398; tel. 510/357-6500; Carol B. Freeman, Interim Chief Executive Officer

SUTTER DELTA MEDICAL CENTER, 3901 Lone Tree Way, Antioch, CA, Zip 94509; tel. 925/779-7200; Linda Horn, Chief Executive Officer

WASHINGTON TOWNSHIP HEALTH CARE DISTRICT, 2000 Mowry Avenue, Fremont, CA, Zip 94538-1716; tel. 510/797-1111; Nancy D. Farber, Chief Executive Officer

ESSENTIAL HEALTHCARE NETWORK
525 North Garfield Park, Montery Park, CA 91754; tel. 818/573-2222; A. Schaffer, Acting Executive Director

COMMUNITY HOSPITAL OF HUNTINGTON PARK, 2623 East Slauson Avenue, Huntington Park, CA, Zip 90255; tel. 323/583-1931; Charles Martinez, Ph.D., Chief Executive Officer

GARFIELD MEDICAL CENTER, 525 North Garfield Avenue, Monterey Park, CA, Zip 91754; tel. 626/573-2222; Philip A. Cohen, Chief Executive Officer

GREATER EL MONTE COMMUNITY HOSPITAL, 1701 South Santa Anita Avenue, South El Monte, CA, Zip 91733-9918; tel. 626/579-7777; Deborah G. Webber, Chief Executive Officer

PACIFIC ALLIANCE MEDICAL CENTER, 531 West College Street, Los Angeles, CA, Zip 90012-2385; tel. 213/624-8411; John R. Edwards, Administrator and Chief Executive Officer

QUEEN OF ANGELS-HOLLYWOOD PRESBYTERIAN MEDICAL CENTER, 1300 North Vermont Avenue, Los Angeles, CA, Zip 90027-0069; tel. 323/413-3000; Lou Lazatin, Chief Executive Officer

ROBERT F. KENNEDY MEDICAL CENTER, 4500 West 116th Street, Hawthorne, CA, Zip 90250; tel. 310/973-1711; Peter P. Aprato, President

SANTA MARTA HOSPITAL, 319 North Humphreys Avenue, Los Angeles, CA, Zip 90022-1499; tel. 323/266-6500; Harry E. Whitney, President and Chief Executive Officer

ST. FRANCIS MEDICAL CENTER, 3630 East Imperial Highway, Lynwood, CA, Zip 90262; tel. 310/603-6000; Gerald T. Kozai, President

SUBURBAN MEDICAL CENTER, 16453 South Colorado Avenue, Paramount, CA, Zip 90723; tel. 562/531-3110; Kenneth I. Rivers, Chief Executive Officer

FREMONT-RIDEOUT HEALTH GROUP
989 Plumas Street, Yuba City, CA 95991; tel. 530/751-4046; Deborah Coulter, Community Development

FREMONT MEDICAL CENTER, 970 Plumas Street, Yuba City, CA, Zip 95991; tel. 530/751-4000; Thomas P. Hayes, Chief Executive Officer

RIDEOUT MEMORIAL HOSPITAL, 726 Fourth Street, Marysville, CA, Zip 95901-2128, Mailing Address: 989 Plumas Street, Yuba City, Zip 95991; tel. 530/749-4300; Thomas P. Hayes, Chief Executive Officer

FRIENDLY HILLS HEALTHCARE NETWORK
501 South Idaho Street, LaHabra, CA 90631; tel. 562/905-5204; Dr. Marvin Rice, Chairman & Chief Executive

PLACENTIA LINDA HOSPITAL, 1301 Rose Drive, Placentia, CA, Zip 92870; tel. 714/993-2000; Maxine T. Cooper, Chief Executive Officer

WHITTIER HOSPITAL MEDICAL CENTER, 9080 Colima Road, Whittier, CA, Zip 90605; tel. 562/907-1541; Sandra M. Chester, Chief Executive Officer

HCP/MULLIKEN MEDICAL CENTERS
26000 Altamont Road, Los Altos Hills, CA 94022; tel. 408/947-2866; Patty Raymond, Director-Manged Care

INTERMOUNTAIN HEALTHCARE NETWORK
228 McDowell Street, Alturas, CA 96101; tel. 916/233-5131; Donna Donald, Network Contact

INDIAN VALLEY HOSPITAL DISTRICT, 184 Hot Springs Road, Greenville, CA, Zip 95947; tel. 530/284-7191; Lynn Seaberg, Administrator and Chief Executive Officer

Networks / Sutter Health

* MAYERS MEMORIAL HOSPITAL DISTRICT, Highway 299 East, Fall River Mills, CA, Zip 96028, Mailing Address: Box 459, Zip 96028; tel. 530/336-5511; Judi Beck, Administrator and Chief Executive Officer
MODOC MEDICAL CENTER, 228 McDowell Street, Alturas, CA, Zip 96101; tel. 530/233-5131; Teresa Jacques, Chief Executive Officer
SURPRISE VALLEY COMMUNITY HOSPITAL, Main and Washington Streets, Cedarville, CA, Zip 96104, Mailing Address: P.O. Box 246, Zip 96104-0246; tel. 530/279-6111; Joyce I. Gysin, Administrator

KAISER FOUNDATION HEALTH PLAN OF NORTHERN CALIFORNIA
1 Kaiser Plaza, Oakland, CA 94612; tel. 510/271-2640; Dr. David Lawrence, Chief Executive Officer

KAISER FOUNDATION HOSPITAL, 2425 Geary Boulevard, San Francisco, CA, Zip 94115; tel. 415/202-2000; Julie A. Petrini, Administrator
KAISER FOUNDATION HOSPITAL, 280 West MacArthur Boulevard, Oakland, CA, Zip 94611; tel. 510/987-1000; Bettie L. Coles, R.N., Administrator
KAISER FOUNDATION HOSPITAL, 1425 South Main Street, Walnut Creek, CA, Zip 94596; tel. 925/295-4000; Sandra H. Small, Administrator
KAISER FOUNDATION HOSPITAL, 27400 Hesperian Boulevard, Hayward, CA, Zip 94545-4297; tel. 510/784-4313; Duayna Pucci, Director Operations
KAISER FOUNDATION HOSPITAL, 1150 Veterans Boulevard, Redwood City, CA, Zip 94063-2087; tel. 650/299-2000; Joanne Zimmerman, Administrator
KAISER FOUNDATION HOSPITAL, 6600 Bruceville Road, Sacramento, CA, Zip 95823; tel. 916/688-2430; Edward S. Glavis, Administrator
KAISER FOUNDATION HOSPITAL, 99 Montecillo Road, San Rafael, CA, Zip 94903-3397; tel. 415/444-2000; Julie A. Petrini, Administrator
KAISER FOUNDATION HOSPITAL, 900 Kiely Boulevard, Santa Clara, CA, Zip 95051-5386; tel. 408/236-6400; Joann Zimmerman, Administrator
KAISER FOUNDATION HOSPITAL, 1200 El Camino Real, South San Francisco, CA, Zip 94080-3299; tel. 650/742-2401; Julie A. Petrini, Administrator
KAISER FOUNDATION HOSPITAL AND REHABILITATION CENTER, 975 Sereno Drive, Vallejo, CA, Zip 94589; tel. 707/651-1000; Sandra H. Small, Administrator
REDDING MEDICAL CENTER, 1100 Butte Street, Redding, CA, Zip 96001-0853, Mailing Address: Box 496072, Zip 96049-6072; tel. 530/244-5454; Steve Schmidt, Chief Executive Officer

LITTLE COMPANY OF MARY HEALTH SERVICES
4101 Torrance Boulevard, Torrance, CA 90503; tel. 310/540-7676; Blair Contratto, Chief Executive Officer

LITTLE COMPANY OF MARY HEALTH SERVICES, 4101 Torrance Boulevard, Torrance, CA, Zip 90503-4698; tel. 310/540-7676; Blair Contratto, President and Chief Executive Officer
SAN PEDRO PENINSULA HOSPITAL, 1300 West Seventh Street, San Pedro, CA, Zip 90732; tel. 310/514-5233; John M. Wilson, President

NORTHERN SIERRA RURAL HEALTH
700 Zion Street Suite E., Nevada City, CA 95959; tel. 510/470-9091; Speranza Avram, Executive Director

LASSEN COMMUNITY HOSPITAL, 560 Hospital Lane, Susanville, CA, Zip 96130-4809; tel. 530/257-5325; David S. Anderson, FACHE, Administrator

MAYERS MEMORIAL HOSPITAL DISTRICT, Highway 299 East, Fall River Mills, CA, Zip 96028, Mailing Address: Box 459, Zip 96028; tel. 530/336-5511; Judi Beck, Administrator and Chief Executive Officer
PLUMAS DISTRICT HOSPITAL, 1065 Bucks Lake Road, Quincy, CA, Zip 95971-9599; tel. 530/283-2121; R. Michael Barry, Administrator
SENECA DISTRICT HOSPITAL, 130 Brentwood Drive, Chester, CA, Zip 96020, Mailing Address: Box 737, Zip 96020; tel. 530/258-2151; Bernard G. Hietpas, Chief Executive Officer
SIERRA VALLEY DISTRICT HOSPITAL, 700 Third Street, Loyalton, CA, Zip 96118, Mailing Address: Box 178, Zip 96118; tel. 530/993-1225; Chase Mearian, Administrator
SURPRISE VALLEY COMMUNITY HOSPITAL, Main and Washington Streets, Cedarville, CA, Zip 96104, Mailing Address: P.O. Box 246, Zip 96104-0246; tel. 530/279-6111; Joyce I. Gysin, Administrator

SCRIPPSHEALTH
4275 Campus Point Ct, San Diego, CA 92121; tel. 619/678-6111; Kay Alexander, Executive Assistant

SCRIPPS GREEN HOSPITAL, 10666 North Torrey Pines Road, La Jolla, CA, Zip 92037-1093; tel. 858/455-9100; Thomas C. Gagen, Senior Vice President and Regional Administrator
SCRIPPS MEMORIAL HOSPITAL CHULA VISTA, 435 H Street, Chula Vista, CA, Zip 91912, Mailing Address: P.O. Box 1537, Zip 91910-1537; tel. 619/691-7000; John Grah, Administrator
SCRIPPS MEMORIAL HOSPITAL-ENCINITAS, 354 Santa Fe Drive, Encinitas, CA, Zip 92024, Mailing Address: P.O. Box 230817, Zip 92023; tel. 760/753-6501; Rebecca Ropchan, Administrator
SCRIPPS MEMORIAL HOSPITAL-LA JOLLA, 9888 Genesee Avenue, La Jolla, CA, Zip 92037-1276, Mailing Address: P.O. Box 28, Zip 92038-0028; tel. 858/626-4123; Thomas C. Gagen, Senior Vice President and Regional Administrator
SCRIPPS MERCY HOSPITAL, 4077 Fifth Avenue, San Diego, CA, Zip 92103-2180; tel. 619/294-8111; Thomas A. Gammiere, Senior Vice President and Regional Administrator

SHARP HEALTHCARE
8695 Spectrum Court, San Diego, CA 92123; tel. 858/499-4004; Michael W. Murphy, President & Chief Executive Officer

GROSSMONT HOSPITAL, 5555 Grossmont Center Drive, La Mesa, CA, Zip 91942, Mailing Address: Box 158, Zip 91944-0158; tel. 619/465-0711; Michele T. Tarbet, R.N., Chief Executive Officer
SHARP CABRILLO HOSPITAL, 3475 Kenyon Street, San Diego, CA, Zip 92110-5067; tel. 619/221-3400; Randi Larsson, Vice President
SHARP CHULA VISTA MEDICAL CENTER, 751 Medical Center Court, Chula Vista, CA, Zip 91911, Mailing Address: Box 1297, Zip 91912; tel. 619/482-5800; JoAnne G. Schader, R.N., Interim Chief Executive Officer
SHARP MEMORIAL HOSPITAL, 7901 Frost Street, San Diego, CA, Zip 92123-2788; tel. 858/541-3400; Dan Gross, Chief Executive Officer

SOUTHERN CALIFORNIA HEALTHCARE SYSTEMS
100 W. California Blvd., Pasadena, CA 91105; tel. 626/397-2900; Steve Ralph, President & Chief Executive Officer

HUNTINGTON EAST VALLEY HOSPITAL, 150 West Alosta Avenue, Glendora, CA, Zip 91740-4398; tel. 626/335-0231; James W. Maki, Chief Executive Officer
HUNTINGTON MEMORIAL HOSPITAL, 100 West California Boulevard, Pasadena, CA, Zip 91105, Mailing Address: P.O. Box 7013, Zip 91109-7013; tel. 626/397-5000; Stephen A. Ralph, President and Chief Executive Officer

METHODIST HOSPITAL OF SOUTHERN CALIFORNIA, 300 West Huntington Drive, Arcadia, CA, Zip 91007, Mailing Address: P.O. Box 60016, Zip 91066-6016; tel. 626/445-4441; Dennis M. Lee, President

SUTTER HEALTH
One Capital Mall, Sacramento, CA 95814; tel. 916/733-8800; Van Johnson, President & Chief Executive Officer

ALTA BATES MEDICAL CENTER-ASHBY CAMPUS, 2450 Ashby Avenue, Berkeley, CA, Zip 94705; tel. 510/204-4444; Warren J. Kirk, President and Chief Administrative Officer
CALIFORNIA PACIFIC MEDICAL CENTER, 2333 Buchanan Street, San Francisco, CA, Zip 94115, Mailing Address: P.O. Box 7999, Zip 94120; tel. 415/563-4321; Martin Brotman, M.D., President and Chief Executive Officer
DAMERON HOSPITAL, 525 West Acacia Street, Stockton, CA, Zip 95203; tel. 209/944-5550; Christopher Arismendi, M.D., Administrator
EDEN MEDICAL CENTER, 20103 Lake Chabot Road, Castro Valley, CA, Zip 94546; tel. 510/537-1234; George Bischalaney, President and Chief Executive Officer
MARIN GENERAL HOSPITAL, 250 Bon Air Road, Greenbrae, CA, Zip 94904, Mailing Address: Box 8010, San Rafael, Zip 94912-8010; tel. 415/925-7000; Henry J. Buhrmann, President and Chief Executive Officer
MEMORIAL HOSPITALS ASSOCIATION, Modesto, CA, Mailing Address: P.O. Box 942, Zip 95353-0942; tel. 209/526-4500; David P. Benn, President and Chief Executive Officer
MILLS-PENINSULA HEALTH SERVICES, 1783 El Camino Real, Burlingame, CA, Zip 94010-3205; tel. 650/696-5400; Robert W. Merwin, Chief Executive Officer
NOVATO COMMUNITY HOSPITAL, 1625 Hill Road, Novato, CA, Zip 94947, Mailing Address: P.O. Box 1108, Zip 94948; tel. 415/897-3111; Anne L. Hosfeld, Chief Administrative Officer
SUMMIT MEDICAL CENTER, 350 Hawthorne Avenue, Oakland, CA, Zip 94609; tel. 510/655-4000; Irwin C. Hansen, President and Chief Executive Officer
SUTTER AMADOR HOSPITAL, 200 Mission Boulevard, Jackson, CA, Zip 95642-2379; tel. 209/223-7500; Scott Stenberg, Chief Executive Officer
SUTTER AUBURN FAITH COMMUNITY HOSPITAL, 11815 Education Street, Auburn, CA, Zip 95603; tel. 530/888-4500; Mitch Hanna, Chief Administrative Officer
SUTTER CENTER FOR PSYCHIATRY, 7700 Folsom Boulevard, Sacramento, CA, Zip 95826-2608; tel. 916/386-3000; Diane Gail Stewart, Chief Administrative Officer
SUTTER COAST HOSPITAL, 800 East Washington Boulevard, Crescent City, CA, Zip 95531; tel. 707/464-8511; John E. Menaugh, Chief Executive Officer
SUTTER DAVIS HOSPITAL, 2000 Sutter Place, Davis, CA, Zip 95616, Mailing Address: P.O. Box 1617, Zip 95617; tel. 530/756-6440; Janet Wagner, Chief Administrative Officer
SUTTER DELTA MEDICAL CENTER, 3901 Lone Tree Way, Antioch, CA, Zip 94509; tel. 925/779-7200; Linda Horn, Chief Executive Officer
SUTTER LAKESIDE HOSPITAL, 5176 Hill Road East, Lakeport, CA, Zip 95453-6111; tel. 707/262-5001; Gilbert Silbernagel, Chief Executive Officer
SUTTER MEDICAL CENTER, 5151 F Street, Sacramento, CA, Zip 95819-3295; tel. 916/454-3333; Lawrence A. Maas, Chief Executive Officer
SUTTER MEDICAL CENTER, SANTA ROSA, 3325 Chanate Road, Santa Rosa, CA, Zip 95404; tel. 707/576-4000; Cliff Coates, Chief Executive Officer
SUTTER MERCED MEDICAL CENTER, 301 East 13th Street, Merced, CA, Zip 95340-6211; tel. 209/385-7000; Paul F. Dyer, Administrator

SUTTER ROSEVILLE MEDICAL CENTER, One Medical Plaza, Roseville, CA, Zip 95661–3477; tel. 916/781–1000; Patrick R. Brady, Chief Executive Officer

SUTTER SOLANO MEDICAL CENTER, 300 Hospital Drive, Vallejo, CA, Zip 94589–2517, Mailing Address: P.O. Box 3189, Zip 94589; tel. 707/554–4444; Beverly Gilmore, Chief Executive Officer

SUTTER TRACY COMMUNITY HOSPITAL, 1420 North Tracy Boulevard, Tracy, CA, Zip 95376–3497; tel. 209/835–1500; Gary D. Rapaport, Chief Executive Officer

TENET HEALTHCARE CORP
3820 State Street, Santa Barbara, CA 93105; tel. 805/563–7000; Jeffrey C. Barbakow, Chairman & Chief Executive Officer

ALVARADO HOSPITAL MEDICAL CENTER, 6655 Alvarado Road, San Diego, CA, Zip 92120–5298; tel. 619/287–3270; Barry G. Weinbaum, Chief Executive Officer

CENTURY CITY HOSPITAL, 2070 Century Park East, Los Angeles, CA, Zip 90067; tel. 310/553–6211; Stephen M. Tullman, Chief Executive Officer

COMMUNITY HOSPITAL OF LOS GATOS, 815 Pollard Road, Los Gatos, CA, Zip 95030; tel. 408/378–6131; Daniel P. Doore, Chief Executive Officer

DOCTORS HOSPITAL OF MANTECA, 1205 East North Street, Manteca, CA, Zip 95336; tel. 209/823–3111; Tim A. Joslin, Chief Executive Officer

DOCTORS MEDICAL CENTER, 1441 Florida Avenue, Modesto, CA, Zip 95350–4418, Mailing Address: P.O. Box 4138, Zip 95352–4138; tel. 209/578–1211; Tim A. Joslin, Chief Executive Officer

DOCTORS MEDICAL CENTER–PINOLE CAMPUS, 2151 Appian Way, Pinole, CA, Zip 94564; tel. 510/970–5000; Gary Sloan, Chief Executive Officer

GARDEN GROVE HOSPITAL AND MEDICAL CENTER, 12601 Garden Grove Boulevard, Garden Grove, CA, Zip 92843–1959; tel. 714/537–5160; Mark A. Meyers, President and Chief Executive Officer

GARFIELD MEDICAL CENTER, 525 North Garfield Avenue, Monterey Park, CA, Zip 91754; tel. 626/573–2222; Philip A. Cohen, Chief Executive Officer

IRVINE REGIONAL HOSPITAL AND MEDICAL CENTER, 16200 Sand Canyon Avenue, Irvine, CA, Zip 92618–3714; tel. 949/753–2000; Dan F. Ausman, Chief Executive Officer

JOHN F. KENNEDY MEMORIAL HOSPITAL, 47–111 Monroe Street, Indio, CA, Zip 92201, Mailing Address: P.O. Drawer LLLL, Zip 92202–2558; tel. 760/347–6191; Truman L. Gates, President and Chief Executive Officer

LAKEWOOD REGIONAL MEDICAL CENTER, 3700 East South Street, Lakewood, CA, Zip 90712; tel. 562/531–2550; Kenneth I. Rivers, Chief Executive Officer

LOS ALAMITOS MEDICAL CENTER, 3751 Katella Avenue, Los Alamitos, CA, Zip 90720; tel. 562/598–1311; Michele Finney, Chief Executive Officer

PLACENTIA LINDA HOSPITAL, 1301 Rose Drive, Placentia, CA, Zip 92870; tel. 714/993–2000; Maxine T. Cooper, Chief Executive Officer

REDDING MEDICAL CENTER, 1100 Butte Street, Redding, CA, Zip 96001–0853, Mailing Address: Box 496072, Zip 96049–6072; tel. 530/244–5454; Steve Schmidt, Chief Executive Officer

SAN DIMAS COMMUNITY HOSPITAL, 1350 West Covina Boulevard, San Dimas, CA, Zip 91773–0308; tel. 909/599–6811; Garry M. Olney, R.N., Chief Executive Officer

SAN RAMON REGIONAL MEDICAL CENTER, 6001 Norris Canyon Road, San Ramon, CA, Zip 94583; tel. 925/275–9200; Philip P. Gustafson, Administrator

SIERRA VISTA REGIONAL MEDICAL CENTER, 1010 Murray Street, San Luis Obispo, CA, Zip 93405, Mailing Address: Box 1367, Zip 93406–1367; tel. 805/546–7600; Sean O'Neal, Administrator

TWIN CITIES COMMUNITY HOSPITAL, 1100 Las Tablas Road, Templeton, CA, Zip 93465; tel. 805/434–3500; Harold E. Chilton, Chief Executive Officer

COLORADO

CENTURA PENROSE–ST. FRANCIS
2215 N. Cascade Ave., Colorado Springs, CO 80907; tel. 719/636–8800; Rick O'Connell, Chief Executive Officer

PENROSE–ST. FRANCIS HEALTH SERVICES, Colorado Springs, CO, Rick O'Connell, President and Chief Executive Officer

COLUMBIA – HEALTH ONE, LLC
4643 Ulster Street, Suite 1200, Denver, CO 80237; tel. 303/788–2500; Molly Hagen, Director Planning

MEDICAL CENTER OF AURORA–SOUTH, 1501 South Potomac Street, Aurora, CO, Zip 80012–5499; tel. 303/695–2600; Sylvia Young, President and Chief Executive Officer

NORTH SUBURBAN MEDICAL CENTER, 9191 Grant Street, Thornton, CO, Zip 80229–4341; tel. 303/451–7800; Margaret C. Cain, President and Chief Executive Officer

PRESBYTERIAN–ST. LUKE'S MEDICAL CENTER, 1719 East 19th Avenue, Denver, CO, Zip 80218–1281; tel. 303/839–6000; Madeleine Roberson, President and Chief Executive Officer

ROSE MEDICAL CENTER, 4567 East Ninth Avenue, Denver, CO, Zip 80220–3941; tel. 303/320–2121; Kenneth H. Feiler, President and Chief Executive Officer

SWEDISH MEDICAL CENTER, 501 East Hampden Avenue, Englewood, CO, Zip 80110–0101; tel. 303/788–5000; Mary M. White, President and Chief Executive Officer

COMMUNITY HEALTH PROVIDERS ORGANIZATION
2021 N. 12th Street, Grand Junction, CO 81501; tel. 303/256–6200; Randall Phillips, Chief Executive Officer

COMMUNITY HOSPITAL, 2021 North 12th Street, Grand Junction, CO, Zip 81501–2999; tel. 970/242–0920; Randall M. Phillips, President and Chief Executive Officer

EXEMPLA HEALTHCARE
600 Grant Street, Suite 700, Denver, CO 80203; tel. 303/832–2739; Gary Smith, Member Services

EXEMPLA LUTHERAN MEDICAL CENTER, 8300 West 38th Avenue, Wheat Ridge, CO, Zip 80033–6005; tel. 303/425–4500; Jeffrey D. Selberg, President and Chief Executive Officer

EXEMPLA SAINT JOSEPH HOSPITAL, 1835 Franklin Street, Denver, CO, Zip 80218–1191; tel. 303/837–7111; Jeffrey D. Selberg, President and Chief Executive Officer

SPALDING REHABILITATION HOSPITAL, 900 Potomac Street, Aurora, CO, Zip 80011–6716; tel. 303/367–1166

KIDSMART HEALTH PARTNERS, INC.
600 Grant, Suite 404, Denver, CO 80203; tel. 303/839–1552; Randy Unter, Executive Director

CHILDREN'S HOSPITAL, 1056 East 19th Avenue, Denver, CO, Zip 80218–1088; tel. 303/861–8888; Doris J. Biester, R.N., President and Chief Executive Officer

THE COLORADO NETWORK, INC.
4450 Arapahoe Avenue #200, Boulder, CO 80303; tel. 303/440–5511; John Leavitt, Executive Director

GRAND RIVER HOSPITAL DISTRICT, 701 East Fifth Street, Rifle, CO, Zip 81650–2970, Mailing Address: P.O. Box 912, Zip 81650–0912; tel. 970/625–1510; Patrick Howery, Chief Executive Officer

HEART OF THE ROCKIES REGIONAL MEDICAL CENTER, 448 East First Street, Salida, CO, Zip 81201–0429, Mailing Address: P.O. Box 429, Zip 81201–0429; tel. 719/539–6661; Howard D. Turner, Chief Executive Officer

MEMORIAL HOSPITAL, 785 Russell Street, Craig, CO, Zip 81625–9906; tel. 970/824–9411; M. Randell Phelps, Administrator

MONTROSE MEMORIAL HOSPITAL, 800 South Third Street, Montrose, CO, Zip 81401–4291; tel. 970/249–2211; Kenneth E. S. Platou, Chief Executive Officer

MT. SAN RAFAEL HOSPITAL, 410 Benedicta Avenue, Trinidad, CO, Zip 81082–2093; tel. 719/846–9213; Paul L. Herman, Chief Executive Officer

PARKVIEW MEDICAL CENTER, 400 West 16th Street, Pueblo, CO, Zip 81003–2781; tel. 719/584–4000; C. W. Smith, President and Chief Executive Officer

PIONEERS HOSPITAL OF RIO BLANCO COUNTY, 345 Cleveland Street, Meeker, CO, Zip 81641–0000; tel. 970/878–5047; Thomas E. Lake, Administrator and Chief Executive Officer

PROWERS MEDICAL CENTER, 401 Kendall Drive, Lamar, CO, Zip 81052–3993; tel. 719/336–4343; Earl J. Steinhoff, Administrator and Chief Executive Officer

VALLEY VIEW HOSPITAL, 1906 Blake Avenue, Glenwood Springs, CO, Zip 81601–4259, Mailing Address: P.O. Box 1970, Zip 81602–1970; tel. 970/945–6535; Gary L. Brewer, Chief Executive Officer

THE MEDICAL CENTER OF AURORA
8200 East Belleview Avenue, Suite I200, Englewood, CO 80111; tel. 303/267–8509; Chris Ives, Systems Director

NORTH SUBURBAN MEDICAL CENTER, 9191 Grant Street, Thornton, CO, Zip 80229–4341; tel. 303/451–7800; Margaret C. Cain, President and Chief Executive Officer

PRESBYTERIAN–ST. LUKE'S MEDICAL CENTER, 1719 East 19th Avenue, Denver, CO, Zip 80218–1281; tel. 303/839–6000; Madeleine Roberson, President and Chief Executive Officer

ROSE MEDICAL CENTER, 4567 East Ninth Avenue, Denver, CO, Zip 80220–3941; tel. 303/320–2121; Kenneth H. Feiler, President and Chief Executive Officer

SWEDISH MEDICAL CENTER, 501 East Hampden Avenue, Englewood, CO, Zip 80110–0101; tel. 303/788–5000; Mary M. White, President and Chief Executive Officer

CONNECTICUT

DANBURY HEALTH SYSTEMS
24 Hospital Ave., Danbury, CT 06810; tel. 203/797–7000; Frank J. Kelly, President & Chief Executive Officer

DANBURY HOSPITAL, 24 Hospital Avenue, Danbury, CT, Zip 06810–6099; tel. 203/797–7000; Frank J. Kelly, President and Chief Executive Officer

EASTERN CONNECTICUT HEALTH NETWORK, INC.
71 Haynes Street, Manchester, CT 06040; tel. 860/533–3436; Marc H. Lory, President/Chief Executive Officer

MANCHESTER MEMORIAL HOSPITAL, 71 Haynes Street, Manchester, CT, Zip 06040–4188; tel. 860/646–1222; Marc H. Lory, President and Chief Executive Officer

ROCKVILLE GENERAL HOSPITAL, 31 Union Street, Vernon Rockville, CT, Zip 06066–3160; tel. 860/872–0501; Marc H. Lory, President and Chief Executive Officer

HARTFORD HEALTH CARE CORPORATION
80 Seymour St. P.O. Box 5037, Hartford, CT 06102; tel. 860/545–1490; George M. Kyriacou, Vice President, Network Development

CHARLOTTE HUNGERFORD HOSPITAL, 540 Litchfield Street, Torrington, CT, Zip 06790–0988, Mailing Address: P.O. Box 988, Zip 06790–0988; tel. 860/496–6666; Rosanne U. Griswold, President and Chief Executive Officer

HARTFORD HOSPITAL, 80 Seymour Street, Hartford, CT, Zip 06102–5037, Mailing Address: P.O. Box 5037, Zip 06102–5037; tel. 860/545–5000; John J. Meehan, President and Chief Executive Officer

Networks / Columbia/HCA West Florida Division

HOSPITAL OF SAINT RAPHAEL, 1450 Chapel Street, New Haven, CT, Zip 06511–1450; tel. 203/789–3000; David W. Benfer, FACHE, President and Chief Executive Officer

JOHNSON MEMORIAL HOSPITAL, 201 Chestnut Hill Road, Stafford Springs, CT, Zip 06076–0860, Mailing Address: P.O. Box 860, Zip 06076–0860; tel. 860/684–4251; Alfred A. Lerz, President and Chief Executive Officer

MIDSTATE MEDICAL CENTER, 435 Lewis Avenue, Meriden, CT, Zip 06451–2101; tel. 203/694–8200; Lucille A. Janatka, President and Chief Executive Officer

NATCHAUG HOSPITAL, 189 Storrs Road, Mansfield Center, CT, Zip 06250–1638; tel. 860/456–1311; Stephen W. Larcen, Ph.D., Chief Executive Officer

SHARON HOSPITAL, 50 Hospital Hill Road, Sharon, CT, Zip 06069–0789, Mailing Address: P.O. Box 789, Zip 06069–0789; tel. 860/364–4141; Michael R. Gallacher, President and Chief Executive Officer

ST. VINCENT'S MEDICAL MEDICAL CENTER
2800 Main Street, Bridgeport, CT 06606; tel. 203/576–5131; William J. Riordan, President & Chief Executive Officer

THE GREATER WATERBURY NETWORK
64 Robbins Street, Waterbury, CT 06721; tel. 203/573–7334; John H. Tobin, President

YALE NEW HAVEN HEALTH SYSTEMS
789 Howard Avenue, New Haven, CT 06519; tel. 203/688–4242; Gayle Capozzalo, Executive Vice President, Strategy & System Development

BRIDGEPORT HOSPITAL, 267 Grant Street, Bridgeport, CT, Zip 06610–0120, Mailing Address: P.O. Box 5000, Zip 06610–5000; tel. 203/384–3000; Robert J. Trefry, President and Chief Executive Officer

GREENWICH HOSPITAL, 5 Perryridge Road, Greenwich, CT, Zip 06830–4697; tel. 203/863–3000; Frank A. Corvino, President and Chief Executive Officer

NORWALK HOSPITAL, 34 Maple Street, Norwalk, CT, Zip 06856–5050; tel. 203/852–2000; David W. Osborne, President and Chief Executive Officer

WESTERLY HOSPITAL, 25 Wells Street, Westerly, RI, Zip 02891–2934; tel. 401/596–6000; Michael K. Lally, President and Chief Executive Officer

YALE–NEW HAVEN HOSPITAL, 20 York Street, New Haven, CT, Zip 06504–3202; tel. 203/688–4242; Joseph A. Zaccagnino, President and Chief Executive Officer

DELAWARE

CHRISTIANA CARE
4755 Ogletown – Stanton Rd., Newark, DE 19718; tel. 302/733–1000; James F. Caldas, Executive Vice President/COD

CHRISTIANA HOSPITAL, 4755 Ogletown–Stanton Road, Newark, DE, Zip 19718; tel. 302/733–1000; Charles M. Smith, M.D., President and Chief Executive Officer

DELAWARE NETWORK HEALTH PLAN
801 Middlefield Road, Seaford, DE 19973; tel. 302/629–6611; Edward H. Hancock, President

NANTICOKE MEMORIAL HOSPITAL, 801 Middleford Road, Seaford, DE, Zip 19973–3698; tel. 302/629–6611; Edward H. Hancock, President

FLORIDA

ADVENTIST HEALTH SYSTEM
111 North Orlando Avenue, Winter Park, FL 32789; tel. 497/975–1425; Mardian J. Blair, President

EAST PASCO MEDICAL CENTER, 7050 Gall Boulevard, Zephyrhills, FL, Zip 33541–1399; tel. 813/788–0411; Paul Michael Norman, President

FLORIDA HOSPITAL, 601 East Rollins Street, Orlando, FL, Zip 32803–1489; tel. 407/896–6611; Donald L. Jernigan, President

FLORIDA HOSPITAL HEARTLAND DIVISION, 4200 Sun'n Lake Boulevard, Sebring, FL, Zip 33872, Mailing Address: P.O. Box 9400, Zip 33871–9400; tel. 863/314–4466; John R. Harding, President and Chief Executive Officer

FLORIDA HOSPITAL WATERMAN, 201 North Eustis Street, Eustis, FL, Zip 32726–3488, Mailing Address: P.O. Box B, Zip 32727–0377; tel. 352/589–3333; Kenneth R. Mattison, President and Chief Executive Officer

BAPTIST HEALTH CARE, INC
P.O. Box 17500, Pensacola, FL 32522; tel. 850/469–2338; David Sjoberg, Vice President of Planning

ATMORE COMMUNITY HOSPITAL, 401 Medical Park Drive, Atmore, AL, Zip 36502–3091; tel. 334/368–2500; Robert E. Gowing, Administrator

BAPTIST HOSPITAL, 1000 West Moreno, Pensacola, FL, Zip 32501–2393, Mailing Address: P.O. Box 17500, Zip 32522–7500; tel. 850/469–2313; John R. Heer, Administrator

D. W. MCMILLAN MEMORIAL HOSPITAL, 1301 Belleville Avenue, Brewton, AL, Zip 36426–1306, Mailing Address: P.O. Box 908, Zip 36427–0908; tel. 334/867–8061; Phillip L. Parker, Administrator

GULF BREEZE HOSPITAL, 1110 Gulf Breeze Parkway, Gulf Breeze, FL, Zip 32561, Mailing Address: P.O. Box 159, Zip 32562; tel. 850/934–2000; Richard C. Fulford, Administrator

JAY HOSPITAL, 221 South Alabama Street, Jay, FL, Zip 32565–1070; tel. 850/675–8000; Mark Faulkner, Administrator

COLUMBIA/HCA N & NE FLORIDA DIVISION
1705 Metropolitan, Talahassee, FL 32308; tel. 850/523–0343; Charles Evans, President

FORT WALTON BEACH MEDICAL CENTER, 1000 Mar–Walt Drive, Fort Walton Beach, FL, Zip 32547–6795; tel. 850/862–1111; Wayne Campbell, Chief Executive Officer

GULF COAST MEDICAL CENTER, 449 West 23rd Street, Panama City, FL, Zip 32405–4593, Mailing Address: P.O. Box 15309, Zip 32406–5309; tel. 850/769–8341; Brent A. Marsteller, Chief Executive Officer

MEMORIAL HOSPITAL OF JACKSONVILLE, 3625 University Boulevard South, Jacksonville, FL, Zip 32216–4240, Mailing Address: P.O. Box 16325, Zip 32216–6325; tel. 904/399–6111; H. Rex Etheredge, President and Chief Executive Officer

NORTH FLORIDA REGIONAL MEDICAL CENTER, 6500 Newberry Road, Gainesville, FL, Zip 32605–4392, Mailing Address: P.O. Box 147006, Zip 32614–7006; tel. 352/333–4000; Brian C. Robinson, Chief Executive Officer

OCALA REGIONAL MEDICAL CENTER, 1431 S.W. First Avenue, Ocala, FL, Zip 34474–4058, Mailing Address: P.O. Box 2200, Zip 34478–2200; tel. 352/401–1000; Stephen Mahan, Chief Executive Officer

ORANGE PARK MEDICAL CENTER, 2001 Kingsley Avenue, Orange Park, FL, Zip 32073–5156; tel. 904/276–8500; Robert M. Krieger, Chief Executive Officer

PUTNAM COMMUNITY MEDICAL CENTER, Highway 20 West, Palatka, FL, Zip 32177, Mailing Address: P.O. Box 778, Zip 32178–0778; tel. 904/328–5711; Bland Eng, Interim Chief Executive Officer

SPECIALTY HOSPITAL JACKSONVILLE, 4901 Richard Street, Jacksonville, FL, Zip 32207; tel. 904/737–3120; W. Raymond C. Ford, Chief Executive Officer

TALLAHASSEE COMMUNITY HOSPITAL, 2626 Capital Medical Boulevard, Tallahassee, FL, Zip 32308–4499; tel. 850/656–5000; Sharon L. Roush, Chief Executive Officer

TWIN CITIES HOSPITAL, 2190 Highway 85 North, Niceville, FL, Zip 32578–1045; tel. 850/678–4131; David Whalen, Chief Executive Officer

WEST FLORIDA REGIONAL MEDICAL CENTER, 8383 North Davis Highway, Pensacola, FL, Zip 32514–6088, Mailing Address: P.O. Box 18900, Zip 32523–8900; tel. 850/494–4000; Jerald F. Mitchell, President and Chief Executive Officer

COLUMBIA/HCA S.W. FLORIDA DIVISION
2000 Main Street, Suite 600, Fort Myers, FL 33901; tel. 813/477–3900; Charles Hall, President

DOCTORS HOSPITAL OF SARASOTA, 5731 Bee Ridge Road, Sarasota, FL, Zip 34233–5056; tel. 941/342–1100; Charles F. Scott, President and Chief Executive Officer

EAST POINTE HOSPITAL, 1500 Lee Boulevard, Lehigh Acres, FL, Zip 33936–4897; tel. 941/369–2101; Valerie A. Jackson, Chief Executive Officer

ENGLEWOOD COMMUNITY HOSPITAL, 700 Medical Boulevard, Englewood, FL, Zip 34223–3978; tel. 941/475–6571; Robert C. Meade, Chief Executive Officer

FAWCETT MEMORIAL HOSPITAL, 21298 Olean Boulevard, Port Charlotte, FL, Zip 33952–6765, Mailing Address: P.O. Box 4028, Punta Gorda, Zip 33949–4028; tel. 941/629–1181; Thomas J. Rice, President and Chief Executive Officer

GULF COAST HOSPITAL, 13681 Doctors Way, Fort Myers, FL, Zip 33912–4309; tel. 941/768–5000; Valerie A. Jackson, Chief Executive Officer

SOUTHWEST FLORIDA REGIONAL MEDICAL CENTER, 2727 Winkler Avenue, Fort Myers, FL, Zip 33901–9396; tel. 941/939–1147; Stephen L. Royal, President and Chief Executive Officer

COLUMBIA/HCA WEST FLORIDA DIVISION
26750 U.S. Highway 19 N., Clearwater, FL 33761; tel. 813/286–6000; J. Daniel Miller, President

BLAKE MEDICAL CENTER, 2020 59th Street West, Bradenton, FL, Zip 34209–4669, Mailing Address: P.O. Box 25004, Zip 34206–5004; tel. 941/792–6611; Lindell W. Orr, Chief Executive Officer

BRANDON REGIONAL HOSPITAL, 119 Oakfield Drive, Brandon, FL, Zip 33511–5799; tel. 813/681–5551; Michael M. Fencel, Chief Executive Officer

COMMUNITY HOSPITAL OF NEW PORT RICHEY, 5637 Marine Parkway, New Port Richey, FL, Zip 34652–4331, Mailing Address: P.O. Box 996, Zip 34656–0996; tel. 727/848–1733; Ernie Meier, Administrator

DOCTORS HOSPITAL OF SARASOTA, 5731 Bee Ridge Road, Sarasota, FL, Zip 34233–5056; tel. 941/342–1100; Charles F. Scott, President and Chief Executive Officer

EAST POINTE HOSPITAL, 1500 Lee Boulevard, Lehigh Acres, FL, Zip 33936–4897; tel. 941/369–2101; Valerie A. Jackson, Chief Executive Officer

EDWARD WHITE HOSPITAL, 2323 Ninth Avenue North, Saint Petersburg, FL, Zip 33713–6898, Mailing Address: P.O. Box 12018, Zip 33733–2018; tel. 727/323–1111; Barry S. Stokes, President and Chief Executive Officer

ENGLEWOOD COMMUNITY HOSPITAL, 700 Medical Boulevard, Englewood, FL, Zip 34223–3978; tel. 941/475–6571; Robert C. Meade, Chief Executive Officer

FAWCETT MEMORIAL HOSPITAL, 21298 Olean Boulevard, Port Charlotte, FL, Zip 33952–6765, Mailing Address: P.O. Box 4028, Punta Gorda, Zip 33949–4028; tel. 941/629–1181; Thomas J. Rice, President and Chief Executive Officer

GULF COAST HOSPITAL, 13681 Doctors Way, Fort Myers, FL, Zip 33912–4309; tel. 941/768–5000; Valerie A. Jackson, Chief Executive Officer

LARGO MEDICAL CENTER, 201 14th Street S.W., Largo, FL, Zip 33770–3133, Mailing Address: P.O. Box 2905, Zip 33779–2905; tel. 727/588–5200; Thomas L. Herron, FACHE, President and Chief Executive Officer

Networks / Columbia/HCA West Florida Division

NORTHSIDE HOSPITAL AND HEART INSTITUTE, 6000 49th Street North, Saint Petersburg, FL, Zip 33709-2145; tel. 727/521-4411; Bradley K. Grover, Sr, Ph.D., FACHE, President and Chief Executive Officer

OAK HILL HOSPITAL, 11375 Cortez Boulevard, Spring Hill, FL, Zip 34611, Mailing Address: P.O. Box 5300, Zip 34611-5300; tel. 352/596-6632; Jaime A. Wesolowski, Chief Executive Officer

PASCO COMMUNITY HOSPITAL, 13100 Fort King Road, Dade City, FL, Zip 33525-5294; tel. 352/521-1100; William G. Buck, Chief Executive Officer

REGIONAL MEDICAL CENTER-BAYONET POINT, 14000 Fivay Road, Hudson, FL, Zip 34667-7199; tel. 727/863-2411; Don Griffin, Ph.D., President and Chief Executive Officer

SOUTH BAY HOSPITAL, 4016 State Road 674, Sun City Center, FL, Zip 33573-5298; tel. 813/634-3301; Alan M. Levine, Chief Executive Officer

SOUTHWEST FLORIDA REGIONAL MEDICAL CENTER, 2727 Winkler Avenue, Fort Myers, FL, Zip 33901-9396; tel. 941/939-1147; Stephen L. Royal, President and Chief Executive Officer

ST. PETERSBURG GENERAL HOSPITAL, 6500 38th Avenue North, Saint Petersburg, FL, Zip 33710-1629; tel. 727/384-1414; Daniel J. Friedrich, II, President and Chief Executive Officer

COMMUNITY CARE NETWORK OF INDIAN RIVER
1000 36th Street, Vero Beach, FL 32960; tel. 407/567-4311; Jeffrey L. Susi, President

INDIAN RIVER MEMORIAL HOSPITAL, 1000 36th Street, Vero Beach, FL, Zip 32960-6592; tel. 561/567-4311; Jeffrey L. Susi, President and Chief Executive Officer

FLORIDA HOSPITAL MEDICAL CENTER
601 East Rollins Street, Orlando, FL 32803; tel. 407/896-6611; Thomas L. Werner, President

FLORIDA HOSPITAL, 601 East Rollins Street, Orlando, FL, Zip 32803-1489; tel. 407/896-6611; Donald L. Jernigan, President

FLORIDA HOSPITAL WATERMAN, 201 North Eustis Street, Eustis, FL, Zip 32726-3488, Mailing Address: P.O. Box B, Zip 32727-0377; tel. 352/589-3333; Kenneth R. Mattison, President and Chief Executive Officer

HEARTLAND RURAL HEALTH NETWORK
2010 East Georgia Street, Bartow, FL 33830; tel. 813/533-1111; Valerie Pfister, Executive Director

LAKE OKEECHOBEE RURAL HEALTH NETWORK, INC.
185 U.S. Highway 27 S., South Bay, FL 33493; tel. 561/993-4221; Andrew Behman, Chief Executive Officer

GLADES GENERAL HOSPITAL, 1201 South Main Street, Belle Glade, FL, Zip 33430-4911; tel. 561/996-6571; James E. Purcell, II, Chief Executive Officer

HENDRY REGIONAL MEDICAL CENTER, 500 West Sugarland Highway, Clewiston, FL, Zip 33440-3094; tel. 941/983-9121; Joseph Gonzales, Chief Executive Officer

MEMORIAL HEALTHCARE SYSTEM
3501 Johnson Street, Hollywood, FL 33021; tel. 954/987-2000; Alex Chang, Administrative Resident

MEMORIAL HOSPITAL PEMBROKE, 7800 Sheridan Street, Pembroke Pines, FL, Zip 33024; tel. 954/962-9650; J. E. Piriz, Administrator

MEMORIAL HOSPITAL WEST, 703 North Flamingo Road, Pembroke Pines, FL, Zip 33028; tel. 954/436-5000; Zeff Ross, Administrator

MEMORIAL REGIONAL HOSPITAL, 3501 Johnson Street, Hollywood, FL, Zip 33021-5421; tel. 954/987-2000; C. Kennon Hetlage, Administrator

METHODIST HEALTH SYSTEMS
580 West Eighth Street, Jacksonville, FL 32209; tel. 904/798-8000; Marcus Drewa, President Emeritus

SHANDS JACKSONVILLE MEDICAL CENTER, 655 West Eighth Street, Jacksonville, FL, Zip 32209-6595; tel. 904/549-5000; Robert G. Norton, President and Chief Executive Officer

ORLANDO REGIONAL HEALTHCARE
1414 Kuhl Avenue, Orlando, FL 32806; tel. 407/841-5203; John Hillenmeyer, President & Chief Executive Officer

LEESBURG REGIONAL MEDICAL CENTER, 600 East Dixie Avenue, Leesburg, FL, Zip 34748-5999; tel. 352/323-5000; Richard L. Wooten, President and Chief Executive Officer

ORLANDO REGIONAL MEDICAL CENTER, 1414 Kuhl Avenue, Orlando, FL, Zip 32806-2093; tel. 407/841-5111; Abe Lopman, Executive Director

ORLANDO REGIONAL SOUTH SEMINOLE HOSPITAL, 555 West State Road 434, Longwood, FL, Zip 32750-4999; tel. 407/767-1200; Stephen M. Glazier, Executive Director

ORLANDO REGIONAL-LUCERNE, 818 Main Lane, Orlando, FL, Zip 32801; tel. 407/649-6111; James A. Shanks, Administrator

SOUTH LAKE HOSPITAL, 1099 Citrus Tower Boulevard, Clermont, FL, Zip 34711; tel. 352/394-4071; Leslie Longacre, Executive Director and Chief Executive Officer

ST. CLOUD HOSPITAL, A DIVISION OF ORLANDO REGIONAL HEALTHCARE SYSTEM, 2906 17th Street, Saint Cloud, FL, Zip 34769-6099; tel. 407/892-2135; Jim A. Norris, Executive Director

WINTER HAVEN HOSPITAL
200 Avenue F Northeast, Winter Haven, FL 33881; tel. 941/293-1121; Lance Anastasio, President

WINTER HAVEN HOSPITAL, 200 Avenue F. N.E., Winter Haven, FL, Zip 33881-4193; tel. 941/297-1899; Lance W. Anastasio, President

GEORGIA

COLUMBUS REGIONAL HEALTHCARE SYSTEM
707 Center Street, P.O. Box 790, Columbus, GA 31902; tel. 706/660-6100; Larry Sanders, Fache, Chairman & Chief Executive Officer

PHENIX REGIONAL HOSPITAL, 1707 21st Avenue, Phenix City, AL, Zip 36867-3753, Mailing Address: P.O. Box 190, Zip 36868-0190; tel. 334/291-8502; Lance B. Duke, FACHE, President and Chief Executive Officer

THE MEDICAL CENTER, 710 Center Street, Columbus, GA, Zip 31902, Mailing Address: P.O. Box 951, Zip 31902-0951; tel. 706/571-1000; Lance B. Duke, FACHE, President and Chief Executive Officer

EMORY UNIV SYS OF HEALTHCARE AFFILIATE NETWORK
1365 Clifton Road Northeast, Atlanta, GA 30322; tel. 404/778-3623; Don Wells, Dir of Business Development

FAIRVIEW PARK HOSPITAL, 200 Industrial Boulevard, Dublin, GA, Zip 31021-2997, Mailing Address: P.O. Box 1408, Zip 31040-1408; tel. 912/275-2000; James B. Wood, Chief Executive Officer

HANCOCK MEMORIAL HOSPITAL, 453 Boland Street, Sparta, GA, Zip 31087-1105, Mailing Address: P.O. Box 490, Zip 31087-0490; tel. 706/444-7006; Henry T. Gibbs, Administrator and Chief Executive Officer

TIFT GENERAL HOSPITAL, 901 East 18th Street, Tifton, GA, Zip 31794-3648, Mailing Address: Drawer 747, Zip 31793-0747; tel. 912/382-7120; William T. Richardson, President and Chief Executive Officer

WESLEY WOODS CENTER OF EMORY UNIVERSITY, 1821 Clifton Road N.E., Atlanta, GA, Zip 30329-5102; tel. 404/728-6200; William L. Minnix, Jr, President and Chief Executive Officer

GEORGIA FIRST NETWORK
150 East Ponce de Leon#320, Decatur, GA 30030; tel. 404/778-4939; Russ Toal, President & Chief Executive Officer

APPLING HEALTHCARE SYSTEM, 163 East Tollison Street, Baxley, GA, Zip 31513-2898; tel. 912/367-9841; Terry Stratton, Chief Executive Officer

ATHENS REGIONAL MEDICAL CENTER, 1199 Prince Avenue, Athens, GA, Zip 30606-2793; tel. 706/549-9977; John A. Drew, President and Chief Executive Officer

BROOKS COUNTY HOSPITAL, 903 North Court Street, Quitman, GA, Zip 31643-1315, Mailing Address: P.O. Box 5000, Zip 31643-5000; tel. 912/263-4171; David Sanders, Administrator

CAMDEN MEDICAL CENTER, 2000 Dan Proctor Drive, Saint Marys, GA, Zip 31558; tel. 912/576-6200; Alan E. George, Administrator

CANDLER COUNTY HOSPITAL, Cedar Road, Metter, GA, Zip 30439, Mailing Address: P.O. Box 597, Zip 30439-0597; tel. 912/685-5741; Michael Alexander, President and Chief Executive Officer

CANDLER HOSPITAL, 5353 Reynolds Street, Savannah, GA, Zip 31405-6013; tel. 912/692-6000; Paul P. Hinchey, President and Chief Executive Officer

CHILDREN'S HEALTHCARE OF ATLANTA AT EGLESTON, 1405 Clifton Road N.E., Atlanta, GA, Zip 30322-1101; tel. 404/325-6000; James E. Tally, Ph.D., President and Chief Executive Officer

CRAWFORD LONG HOSPITAL OF EMORY UNIVERSITY, 550 Peachtree Street N.E., Atlanta, GA, Zip 30365-2225; tel. 404/686-4411; John Dunklin Henry, Sr, FACHE, Chief Executive Officer

CRISP REGIONAL HOSPITAL, 902 North Seventh Street, Cordele, GA, Zip 31015-5007; tel. 912/276-3100; D. Wayne Martin, President and Chief Executive Officer

EARLY MEMORIAL HOSPITAL, 630 Columbia Street, Blakely, GA, Zip 31723-1798; tel. 912/723-4241; Kevin Taylor, Administrator

EFFINGHAM HOSPITAL, 459 Highway 119 South, Springfield, GA, Zip 31329-3021, Mailing Address: P.O. Box 386, Zip 31329-0386; tel. 912/754-6451; Terrance R. Frech, Chief Executive Officer

ELBERT MEMORIAL HOSPITAL, 4 Medical Drive, Elberton, GA, Zip 30635-1897; tel. 706/283-3151; Mark LeNeave, Chief Executive Officer

EMORY EASTSIDE MEDICAL CENTER, 1700 Medical Way, Snellville, GA, Zip 30078, Mailing Address: P.O. Box 587, Zip 30078-0587; tel. 770/979-0200; Les Beard, Chief Executive Officer

EMORY UNIVERSITY HOSPITAL, 1364 Clifton Road N.E., Atlanta, GA, Zip 30322-1102; tel. 404/712-7021; John Dunklin Henry, Sr, FACHE, Chief Executive Officer

EMORY-ADVENTIST HOSPITAL, 3949 South Cobb Drive S.E., Smyrna, GA, Zip 30080-6300; tel. 770/434-0710; Dennis Kiley, President

FAIRVIEW PARK HOSPITAL, 200 Industrial Boulevard, Dublin, GA, Zip 31021-2997, Mailing Address: P.O. Box 1408, Zip 31040-1408; tel. 912/275-2000; James B. Wood, Chief Executive Officer

FLOYD MEDICAL CENTER, 304 Turner McCall Boulevard, Rome, GA, Zip 30165-2734, Mailing Address: P.O. Box 233, Zip 30162-0233; tel. 706/802-2000; Kurt Stuenkel, FACHE, President and Chief Executive Officer

GRADY GENERAL HOSPITAL, 1155 Fifth Street S.E., Cairo, GA, Zip 31728-3142, Mailing Address: P.O. Box 360, Zip 31728-0360; tel. 912/377-1150; Glen C. Davis, Administrator

HABERSHAM COUNTY MEDICAL CENTER, Highway 441, Demorest, GA, Zip 30535, Mailing Address: P.O. Box 37, Zip 30535-0037; tel. 706/754-2161; C. Richard Dwozan, President

HIGGINS GENERAL HOSPITAL, 200 Allen Memorial Drive, Bremen, GA, Zip 30110-2012, Mailing Address: P.O. Box 655, Zip 30110-0655; tel. 770/537-5851; Robbie Smith, Administrator

Networks / Southcare Medical Alliance

HOUSTON MEDICAL CENTER, 1601 Watson Boulevard, Warner Robins, GA, Zip 31093–3431, Mailing Address: Box 2886, Zip 31099–2886; tel. 912/922–4281; Arthur P. Christie, Administrator

JOHN D. ARCHBOLD MEMORIAL HOSPITAL, Gordon Avenue at Mimosa Drive, Thomasville, GA, Zip 31792–6113, Mailing Address: P.O. Box 1018, Zip 31799–1018; tel. 912/228–2000; James L. Story, Jr, M.D., Acting President

LIBERTY REGIONAL MEDICAL CENTER, 462 East G. Parkway, Hinesville, GA, Zip 31313, Mailing Address: P.O. Box 919, Zip 31313; tel. 912/369–9438; H. Scott Kroell, Jr, Chief Executive Officer

LOUIS SMITH MEMORIAL HOSPITAL, 852 West Thigpen Avenue, Lakeland, GA, Zip 31635–1099; tel. 912/482–3110; Randy Sauls, Administrator

MEDICAL CENTER OF CENTRAL GEORGIA, 777 Hemlock Street, Macon, GA, Zip 31201–2155, Mailing Address: P.O. Box 6000, Zip 31208–6000; tel. 912/633–1000; A. Donald Faulk, FACHE, President

MEDICAL COLLEGE OF GEORGIA HOSPITAL AND CLINICS, 1120 15th Street, Augusta, GA, Zip 30912–5000; tel. 706/721–0211; Patricia Sodomka, FACHE, Executive Director

MITCHELL COUNTY HOSPITAL, 90 Stephens Street, Camilla, GA, Zip 31730–1899, Mailing Address: P.O. Box 639, Zip 31730–0639; tel. 912/336–5284; Ronald M. Gilliard, FACHE, Administrator

NEWTON GENERAL HOSPITAL, 5126 Hospital Drive, Covington, GA, Zip 30014; tel. 770/786–7053; James F. Weadick, Administrator and Chief Executive Officer

NORTH FULTON REGIONAL HOSPITAL, 3000 Hospital Boulevard, Roswell, GA, Zip 30076–9930; tel. 770/751–2500; John F. Holland, President

NORTHEAST GEORGIA MEDICAL CENTER, 743 Spring Street N.E., Gainesville, GA, Zip 30501–3899; tel. 770/535–3553; Henry Rigdon, Executive Vice President

NORTHSIDE HOSPITAL, 1000 Johnson Ferry Road N.E., Atlanta, GA, Zip 30342–1611; tel. 404/851–8000; Sidney Kirschner, President and Chief Executive Officer

OCONEE REGIONAL MEDICAL CENTER, 821 North Cobb Street, Milledgeville, GA, Zip 31061–2351, Mailing Address: P.O. Box 690, Zip 31061–0690; tel. 912/454–3500; Brian L. Riddle, President and Chief Executive Officer

PALMYRA MEDICAL CENTERS, 2000 Palmyra Road, Albany, GA, Zip 31702–1908, Mailing Address: P.O. Box 1908, Zip 31702–1908; tel. 912/434–2000; Allen Golson, Chief Executive Officer

SOUTH GEORGIA MEDICAL CENTER, 2501 North Patterson Street, Valdosta, GA, Zip 31602–1735, Mailing Address: P.O. Box 1727, Zip 31603–1727; tel. 912/333–1000; James McGahee, Administrator and Chief Executive Officer

SOUTHEAST GEORGIA REGIONAL MEDICAL CENTER, 3100 Kemble Avenue, Brunswick, GA, Zip 31520–4252, Mailing Address: P.O. Box 1518, Zip 31521–1518; tel. 912/466–7000; E. Berton Whitaker, President and Chief Executive Officer

SOUTHERN REGIONAL MEDICAL CENTER, 11 Upper Riverdale Road S.W., Riverdale, GA, Zip 30274–2600; tel. 770/991–8000; Eugene A. Leblond, FACHE, President and Chief Executive Officer

SPALDING REGIONAL HOSPITAL, 601 South Eighth Street, Griffin, GA, Zip 30224–4294, Mailing Address: P.O. Drawer V, Zip 30224–1168; tel. 770/228–2721; Lex A. Guinn, Chief Executive Officer

SUMTER REGIONAL HOSPITAL, 100 Wheatley Drive, Americus, GA, Zip 31709–3799; tel. 912/924–6011; Jerry W. Adams, President

TANNER MEDICAL CENTER, 705 Dixie Street, Carrollton, GA, Zip 30117–3818; tel. 770/836–9666; Loy M. Howard, Chief Executive Officer

TANNER MEDICAL CENTER–VILLA RICA, 601 Dallas Road, Villa Rica, GA, Zip 30180–1202, Mailing Address: P.O. Box 638, Zip 30180–0638; tel. 770/456–3100; Larry N. Steed, Administrator

THE MEDICAL CENTER, 710 Center Street, Columbus, GA, Zip 31902, Mailing Address: P.O. Box 951, Zip 31902–0951; tel. 706/571–1000; Lance B. Duke, FACHE, President and Chief Executive Officer

TIFT GENERAL HOSPITAL, 901 East 18th Street, Tifton, GA, Zip 31794–3648, Mailing Address: Drawer 747, Zip 31793–0747; tel. 912/382–7120; William T. Richardson, President and Chief Executive Officer

UPSON REGIONAL MEDICAL CENTER, 801 West Gordon Street, Thomaston, GA, Zip 30286–2831, Mailing Address: P.O. Box 1059, Zip 30286–1059; tel. 706/647–8111; Samuel S. Gregory, Administrator

WALTON MEDICAL CENTER, 330 Alcovy Street, Monroe, GA, Zip 30655–2140, Mailing Address: P.O. Box 1346, Zip 30655–1346; tel. 770/267–8461; Ronald L. Campbell, Chief Executive Officer

WEST GEORGIA HEALTH SYSTEM, 1514 Vernon Road, La Grange, GA, Zip 30240–4199; tel. 706/882–1411; Charles L. Foster, Jr, FACHE, President and Chief Executive Officer

GRADY HEALTH SYSTEM
80 Butler Street, Atlanta, GA 30335;
tel. 404/616–4307; Edward Renford,
President

GRADY MEMORIAL HOSPITAL, 80 Butler Street S.E., Atlanta, GA, Zip 30335–3801, Mailing Address: P.O. Box 26189, Zip 30335–3801; tel. 404/616–4252; Edward J. Renford, President and Chief Executive Officer

NATIONAL CARDIOVASCULAR NETWORK
6 Concourse Parkway, #2950, Atlanta, GA
30328; tel. 404/551–5018; Michael
Lanzilotta, President

BAPTIST HOSPITAL OF EAST TENNESSEE, 137 Blount Avenue S.E., Knoxville, TN, Zip 37920–1643, Mailing Address: P.O. Box 1788, Zip 37901–1788; tel. 865/632–5011; Jon Foster, Executive Vice President and Administrator

PHOEBE PUTNEY MEMORIAL HOSPITAL, 417 Third Avenue, Albany, GA, Zip 31701–1828, Mailing Address: P.O. Box 1828, Zip 31703–1828; tel. 912/883–1800; Joel Wernick, President and Chief Executive Officer

NW GEORGIA HEALTHCARE PARTNERSHIP
P.O. Box 308, Dalton, GA 30722;
tel. 706/272–6013; Nancy Kennedy,
Executive Director

HAMILTON MEDICAL CENTER, 1200 Memorial Drive, Dalton, GA, Zip 30720–2529, Mailing Address: P.O. Box 1168, Zip 30722–1168; tel. 706/272–6000

MURRAY MEDICAL CENTER, 707 Old Ellijay Road, Chatsworth, GA, Zip 30705–2060, Mailing Address: P.O. Box 1406, Zip 30705–1406; tel. 706/695–4564; Mickey Rabuka, Administrator

SOUTHCARE MEDICAL ALLIANCE
400 North Creek, Suite 300, Atlanta, GA
30327; tel. 404/231–9911; Ken Bryant,
Executive Director

APPLING HEALTHCARE SYSTEM, 163 East Tollison Street, Baxley, GA, Zip 31513–2898; tel. 912/367–9841; Terry Stratton, Chief Executive Officer

ATHENS REGIONAL MEDICAL CENTER, 1114 West Madison Avenue, Athens, TN, Zip 37303–4150, Mailing Address: P.O. Box 250, Zip 37371–0250; tel. 423/745–1411; John R. Workman, Chief Executive Officer

BERRIEN COUNTY HOSPITAL, 1221 East McPherson Street, Nashville, GA, Zip 31639–2326, Mailing Address: P.O. Box 665, Zip 31639–0665; tel. 912/686–7471; James L. Jarrett, Chief Executive Officer

BRADLEY MEMORIAL HOSPITAL, 2305 Chambliss Avenue N.W., Cleveland, TN, Zip 37311, Mailing Address: P.O. Box 3060, Zip 37320–3060; tel. 423/559–6000; John Barnes, Administrator

BULLOCH MEMORIAL HOSPITAL, 500 East Grady Street, Statesboro, GA, Zip 30458–5105, Mailing Address: P.O. Box 1048, Zip 30459–1048; tel. 912/486–1000; C. Scott Campbell, Executive Director

BURKE COUNTY HOSPITAL, 351 Liberty Street, Waynesboro, GA, Zip 30830–9686; tel. 706/554–4435; Michael A. Haddle, CPA, Chief Executive Officer and Chief Financial Officer

CANDLER COUNTY HOSPITAL, Cedar Road, Metter, GA, Zip 30439, Mailing Address: P.O. Box 597, Zip 30439–0597; tel. 912/685–5741; Michael Alexander, President and Chief Executive Officer

CANDLER HOSPITAL, 5353 Reynolds Street, Savannah, GA, Zip 31405–6013; tel. 912/692–6000; Paul P. Hinchey, President and Chief Executive Officer

CHILDREN'S HEALTHCARE OF ATLANTA AT EGLESTON, 1405 Clifton Road N.E., Atlanta, GA, Zip 30322–1101; tel. 404/325–6000; James E. Tally, Ph.D., President and Chief Executive Officer

CHILDREN'S HEALTHCARE OF ATLANTA AT SCOTTISH RITE, 1001 Johnson Ferry Road N.E., Atlanta, GA, Zip 30342–1600; tel. 404/256–5252; James E. Tally, Ph.D., President and Chief Executive Officer

CLEVELAND COMMUNITY HOSPITAL, 2800 Westside Drive N.W., Cleveland, TN, Zip 37312–3599; tel. 423/339–4100; Martin D. Smith, Chief Executive Officer

COBB MEMORIAL HOSPITAL, 577 Franklin Springs Street, Royston, GA, Zip 30662–3909, Mailing Address: P.O. Box 589, Zip 30662–0589; tel. 706/245–5071; Al Strickland, Administrator

COLISEUM MEDICAL CENTERS, 350 Hospital Drive, Macon, GA, Zip 31213; tel. 912/765–7000; Timothy C. Tobin, Chief Executive Officer

DECATUR HOSPITAL, 450 North Candler Street, Decatur, GA, Zip 30030–2671; tel. 404/501–6700; Richard T. Schmidt, Executive Director

DEKALB MEDICAL CENTER, 2701 North Decatur Road, Decatur, GA, Zip 30033–5995; tel. 404/501–1000; John R. Gerlach, Chief Executive Officer and Administrator

DOCTORS HOSPITAL, 616 19th Street, Columbus, GA, Zip 31901–1528, Mailing Address: P.O. Box 2188, Zip 31902–2188; tel. 706/571–4262; Hugh D. Wilson, Chief Executive Officer

DODGE COUNTY HOSPITAL, 715 Griffin Street S.W., Eastman, GA, Zip 31023–2223, Mailing Address: P.O. Box 4309, Zip 31023–4309; tel. 912/374–4000; Meredith H. Smith, Administrator

DOOLY MEDICAL CENTER, 1300 Union Street, Vienna, GA, Zip 31092–7541, Mailing Address: P.O. Box 278, Zip 31092–0278; tel. 912/268–4141; Kenneth D. Rhudy, Chief Executive Officer

EDGEFIELD COUNTY HOSPITAL, 300 Ridge Medical Plaza, Edgefield, SC, Zip 29824; tel. 803/637–3174; W. Joseph Seel, Administrator

EFFINGHAM HOSPITAL, 459 Highway 119 South, Springfield, GA, Zip 31329–3021, Mailing Address: P.O. Box 386, Zip 31329–0386; tel. 912/754–6451; Terrance R. Frech, Chief Executive Officer

EMANUEL COUNTY HOSPITAL, 117 Kite Road, Swainsboro, GA, Zip 30401–3231, Mailing Address: P.O. Box 879, Zip 30401–0879; tel. 912/237–9911; Bob Via, Chief Executive Officer

EMORY CARTERSVILLE MEDICAL CENTER, 960 Joe Frank Harris Parkway, Cartersville, GA, Zip 30120, Mailing Address: P.O. Box 200008, Zip 30120–9001; tel. 770/382–1530; Keith Sandlin, Chief Executive Officer

EMORY PEACHTREE REGIONAL HOSPITAL, 60 Hospital Road, Newnan, GA, Zip 30264, Mailing Address: P.O. Box 2228, Zip 30264–2228; tel. 770/253–1912; Linda Jubinsky, Chief Executive Officer

Networks / Southcare Medical Alliance

FAIRVIEW PARK HOSPITAL, 200 Industrial Boulevard, Dublin, GA, Zip 31021-2997, Mailing Address: P.O. Box 1408, Zip 31040-1408; tel. 912/275-2000; James B. Wood, Chief Executive Officer

FLOYD MEDICAL CENTER, 304 Turner McCall Boulevard, Rome, GA, Zip 30165-2734, Mailing Address: P.O. Box 233, Zip 30162-0233; tel. 706/802-2000; Kurt Stuenkel, FACHE, President and Chief Executive Officer

GORDON HOSPITAL, 1035 Red Bud Road, Calhoun, GA, Zip 30701-2082, Mailing Address: P.O. Box 12938, Zip 30703-7013; tel. 706/629-2895; Carlene Jamerson, President and Chief Executive Officer

GRANDVIEW MEDICAL CENTER, 1000 Highway 28, Jasper, TN, Zip 37347; tel. 423/837-9500; Phil Rowland, Chief Executive Officer

HART COUNTY HOSPITAL, Gibson and Cade Streets, Hartwell, GA, Zip 30643-0280, Mailing Address: P.O. Box 280, Zip 30643-0280; tel. 706/856-6100; Jerry R. Wise, Administrator

HIGGINS GENERAL HOSPITAL, 200 Allen Memorial Drive, Bremen, GA, Zip 30110-2012, Mailing Address: P.O. Box 655, Zip 30110-0655; tel. 770/537-5851; Robbie Smith, Administrator

HILTON HEAD MEDICAL CENTER AND CLINICS, 25 Hospital Center Boulevard, Hilton Head Island, SC, Zip 29926, Mailing Address: P.O. Box 21117, Zip 29925-1117; tel. 843/681-6122; Dennis Ray Bruns, President and Chief Executive Officer

HUTCHESON MEDICAL CENTER, 100 Gross Crescent Circle, Fort Oglethorpe, GA, Zip 30742-3669; tel. 706/858-2000; Robert T. Jones, M.D., President and Chief Executive Officer

JEFFERSON HOSPITAL, 1067 Peachtree Street, Louisville, GA, Zip 30434-1599; tel. 912/625-7000; Rita Culvern, Administrator

LIBERTY REGIONAL MEDICAL CENTER, 462 East G. Parkway, Hinesville, GA, Zip 31313, Mailing Address: P.O. Box 919, Zip 31313; tel. 912/369-9438; H. Scott Kroell, Jr, Chief Executive Officer

LOUIS SMITH MEMORIAL HOSPITAL, 852 West Thigpen Avenue, Lakeland, GA, Zip 31635-1099; tel. 912/482-3110; Randy Sauls, Administrator

MCDUFFIE REGIONAL MEDICAL CENTER, 521 Hill Street S.W., Thomson, GA, Zip 30824-2199; tel. 706/595-1411; Douglas C. Keir, Chief Executive Officer

MEADOWS REGIONAL MEDICAL CENTER, 1703 Meadows Lane, Vidalia, GA, Zip 30474-8915, Mailing Address: P.O. Box 1048, Zip 30474-1048; tel. 912/537-8921; Alan Kent, Interim Chief Executive Officer

MEMORIAL HEALTH, 4700 Waters Avenue, Savannah, GA, Zip 31404-6283, Mailing Address: P.O. Box 23089, Zip 31403-3089; tel. 912/350-8000; Robert A. Colvin, President and Chief Executive Officer

MEMORIAL HOSPITAL, 2525 De Sales Avenue, Chattanooga, TN, Zip 37404-3322; tel. 423/495-2525; L. Clark Taylor, Jr, Ph.D., President and Chief Executive Officer

MEMORIAL HOSPITAL AND MANOR, 1500 East Shotwell Street, Bainbridge, GA, Zip 31717-4294; tel. 912/246-3500; James G. Peak, Chief Executive Officer

NEWTON GENERAL HOSPITAL, 5126 Hospital Drive, Covington, GA, Zip 30014; tel. 770/786-7053; James F. Weadick, Administrator and Chief Executive Officer

NORTH GEORGIA MEDICAL CENTER, 1362 South Main Street, Ellijay, GA, Zip 30540-0346, Mailing Address: P.O. Box 239, Zip 30540-0346; tel. 706/276-4741; Jodi Beauregard, Chief Executive Officer

NORTHEAST GEORGIA MEDICAL CENTER, 743 Spring Street N.E., Gainesville, GA, Zip 30501-3899; tel. 770/535-3553; Henry Rigdon, Executive Vice President

NORTHSIDE HOSPITAL, 1000 Johnson Ferry Road N.E., Atlanta, GA, Zip 30342-1611; tel. 404/851-8000; Sidney Kirschner, President and Chief Executive Officer

NORTHSIDE HOSPITAL – CHEROKEE, 201 Hospital Road, Canton, GA, Zip 30114-2408, Mailing Address: P.O. Box 906, Zip 30114-0906; tel. 770/720-5100; Douglas M. Parker, Chief Executive Officer

OCONEE REGIONAL MEDICAL CENTER, 821 North Cobb Street, Milledgeville, GA, Zip 31061-2351, Mailing Address: P.O. Box 690, Zip 31061-0690; tel. 912/454-3500; Brian L. Riddle, President and Chief Executive Officer

PALMYRA MEDICAL CENTERS, 2000 Palmyra Road, Albany, GA, Zip 31702-1908, Mailing Address: P.O. Box 1908, Zip 31702-1908; tel. 912/434-2000; Allen Golson, Chief Executive Officer

PHENIX REGIONAL HOSPITAL, 1707 21st Avenue, Phenix City, AL, Zip 36867-3753, Mailing Address: P.O. Box 190, Zip 36868-0190; tel. 334/291-8502; Lance B. Duke, FACHE, President and Chief Executive Officer

PIEDMONT HOSPITAL, 1968 Peachtree Road N.W., Atlanta, GA, Zip 30309-1231; tel. 404/605-5000; Richard B. Hubbard, II, President and Chief Executive Officer

PROMINA GWINNETT HOSPITAL SYSTEM, Lawrenceville, GA, Mailing Address: P.O. Box 348, Zip 30246-0348; tel. 770/995-4321; Franklin M. Rinker, President and Chief Executive Officer

PUTNAM GENERAL HOSPITAL, Lake Oconee Parkway, Eatonton, GA, Zip 31024-4330, Mailing Address: Box 4330, Zip 31024-4330; tel. 706/485-2711; Darrell M. Oglesby, Administrator

ROCKDALE HOSPITAL AND HEALTH SYSTEM, 1412 Milstead Avenue N.E., Conyers, GA, Zip 30207-9990; tel. 770/918-3000; Nelson Toebbe, Chief Executive Officer

SATILLA REGIONAL MEDICAL CENTER, 410 Darling Avenue, Waycross, GA, Zip 31501-5246, Mailing Address: P.O. Box 139, Zip 31502-0139; tel. 912/283-3030; Robert M. Trimm, President and Chief Executive Officer

SHEPHERD CENTER, 2020 Peachtree Road N.W., Atlanta, GA, Zip 30309-1465; tel. 404/352-2020; Gary R. Ulicny, Ph.D., President and Chief Executive Officer

SISKIN HOSPITAL FOR PHYSICAL REHABILITATION, One Siskin Plaza, Chattanooga, TN, Zip 37403-1306; tel. 423/634-1200; Robert P. Main, President and Chief Executive Officer

SOUTH FULTON MEDICAL CENTER, 1170 Cleveland Avenue, East Point, GA, Zip 30344; tel. 404/305-3500; H. Neil Copelan, President and Chief Executive Officer

SOUTH GEORGIA MEDICAL CENTER, 2501 North Patterson Street, Valdosta, GA, Zip 31602-1735, Mailing Address: P.O. Box 1727, Zip 31603-1727; tel. 912/333-1000; James McGahee, Administrator and Chief Executive Officer

SOUTHEAST ALABAMA MEDICAL CENTER, 1108 Ross Clark Circle, Dothan, AL, Zip 36301-3024, Mailing Address: P.O. Box 6987, Zip 36302-6987; tel. 334/793-8111; Ronald S. Owen, Chief Executive Officer

SOUTHEAST GEORGIA REGIONAL MEDICAL CENTER, 3100 Kemble Avenue, Brunswick, GA, Zip 31520-4252, Mailing Address: P.O. Box 1518, Zip 31521-1518; tel. 912/466-7000; E. Berton Whitaker, President and Chief Executive Officer

SOUTHERN REGIONAL MEDICAL CENTER, 11 Upper Riverdale Road S.W., Riverdale, GA, Zip 30274-2600; tel. 770/991-8000; Eugene A. Leblond, FACHE, President and Chief Executive Officer

SPALDING REGIONAL HOSPITAL, 601 South Eighth Street, Griffin, GA, Zip 31405-4294, Mailing Address: P.O. Drawer V, Zip 30224-1168; tel. 770/228-2721; Lex A. Guinn, Chief Executive Officer

ST. MARY'S HEALTH CARE SYSTEM, 1230 Baxter Street, Athens, GA, Zip 30606-3791; tel. 706/548-7581; Thomas E. Fitz, Jr FACHE, President and Chief Executive Officer

STEPHENS COUNTY HOSPITAL, 2003 Falls Road, Toccoa, GA, Zip 30577-9700; tel. 706/282-4200; Edward C. Gambrell, Jr, Administrator

SUMTER REGIONAL HOSPITAL, 100 Wheatley Drive, Americus, GA, Zip 31709-3799; tel. 912/924-6011; Jerry W. Adams, President

TANNER MEDICAL CENTER, 705 Dixie Street, Carrollton, GA, Zip 30117-3818; tel. 770/836-9666; Loy M. Howard, Chief Executive Officer

TANNER MEDICAL CENTER–VILLA RICA, 601 Dallas Road, Villa Rica, GA, Zip 30180-1202, Mailing Address: P.O. Box 638, Zip 30180-0638; tel. 770/456-3100; Larry N. Steed, Administrator

TAYLOR REGIONAL HOSPITAL, Macon Highway, Hawkinsville, GA, Zip 31036, Mailing Address: P.O. Box 1297, Zip 31036-1297; tel. 912/783-0200; Dan S. Maddock, President

THE MEDICAL CENTER, 710 Center Street, Columbus, GA, Zip 31902, Mailing Address: P.O. Box 951, Zip 31902-0951; tel. 706/571-1000; Lance B. Duke, FACHE, President and Chief Executive Officer

UNIVERSITY HEALTH CARE SYSTEM, 1350 Walton Way, Augusta, GA, Zip 30901-2629; tel. 706/722-9011; J. Larry Read, President and Chief Executive Officer

UPSON REGIONAL MEDICAL CENTER, 801 West Gordon Street, Thomaston, GA, Zip 30286-2831, Mailing Address: P.O. Box 1059, Zip 30286-1059; tel. 706/647-8111; Samuel S. Gregory, Administrator

VENCOR HOSPITAL–CHATTANOOGA, 709 Walnut Street, Chattanooga, TN, Zip 37402-1961; tel. 423/266-7721; Steven E. McGraw, Administrator

WALTON REHABILITATION HOSPITAL, 1355 Independence Drive, Augusta, GA, Zip 30901-1037; tel. 706/724-7746; Dennis B. Skelley, President and Chief Executive Officer

WASHINGTON COUNTY REGIONAL MEDICAL CENTER, 610 Sparta Highway, Sandersville, GA, Zip 31082-1362, Mailing Address: P.O. Box 636, Zip 31082-0636; tel. 912/240-2000; Skip Wise, Chief Executive Officer

WAYNE MEMORIAL HOSPITAL, 865 South First Street, Jesup, GA, Zip 31598, Mailing Address: P.O. Box 408, Zip 31598-0408; tel. 912/427-6811; Charles R. Morgan, Administrator

WELLSTAR COBB HOSPITAL, 3950 Austell Road, Austell, GA, Zip 30106-1121; tel. 770/732-4000; Thomas E. Hill, Chief Executive Officer

WELLSTAR DOUGLAS HOSPITAL, 8954 Hospital Drive, Douglasville, GA, Zip 30134-2282; tel. 770/949-1500; Thomas E. Hill, Chief Executive Officer

WELLSTAR PAULDING HOSPITAL, 600 West Memorial Drive, Dallas, GA, Zip 30132-1335; tel. 770/445-4411; Thomas E. Hill, Chief Executive Officer

WELLSTAR WINDY HILL HOSPITAL, 2540 Windy Hill Road, Marietta, GA, Zip 30067-8632; tel. 770/644-1000; Thomas E. Hill, Chief Executive Officer

ST. JOSEPH/CANDLER HEALTH SYSTEM
5353 Reynolds Street, Savannah, GA 31412;
tel. 912/692-2018; Paul Hinchey, President

APPLING HEALTHCARE SYSTEM, 163 East Tollison Street, Baxley, GA, Zip 31513-2898; tel. 912/367-9841; Terry Stratton, Chief Executive Officer

CANDLER COUNTY HOSPITAL, Cedar Road, Metter, GA, Zip 30439, Mailing Address: P.O. Box 597, Zip 30439-0597; tel. 912/685-5741; Michael Alexander, President and Chief Executive Officer

CANDLER HOSPITAL, 5353 Reynolds Street, Savannah, GA, Zip 31405-6013; tel. 912/692-6000; Paul P. Hinchey, President and Chief Executive Officer

EFFINGHAM HOSPITAL, 459 Highway 119 South, Springfield, GA, Zip 31329-3021, Mailing Address: P.O. Box 386, Zip 31329-0386; tel. 912/754-6451; Terrance R. Frech, Chief Executive Officer

EMORY UNIVERSITY HOSPITAL, 1364 Clifton Road N.E., Atlanta, GA, Zip 30322–1102; tel. 404/712–7021; John Dunklin Henry, Sr, FACHE, Chief Executive Officer

LIBERTY REGIONAL MEDICAL CENTER, 462 East G. Parkway, Hinesville, GA, Zip 31313, Mailing Address: P.O. Box 919, Zip 31313; tel. 912/369–9438; H. Scott Kroell, Jr, Chief Executive Officer

MEADOWS REGIONAL MEDICAL CENTER, 1703 Meadows Lane, Vidalia, GA, Zip 30474–8915, Mailing Address: P.O. Box 1048, Zip 30474–1048; tel. 912/537–8921; Alan Kent, Interim Chief Executive Officer

WILLINGWAY HOSPITAL, 311 Jones Mill Road, Statesboro, GA, Zip 30458–4765; tel. 912/764–6236; Jimmy Mooney, Chief Executive Officer

UNIVERSITY HEALTH, INC.
1350 Walton Way, Augusta, GA 30901; tel. 706/722–9011; Jim Showman, MSN, RN, Director, Outreach Services

BARNWELL COUNTY HOSPITAL, 811 Reynolds Road, Barnwell, SC, Zip 29812; tel. 803/259–1000; J. Larry Dozier, Jr, FACHE, Chief Executive Officer

BURKE COUNTY HOSPITAL, 351 Liberty Street, Waynesboro, GA, Zip 30830–9686; tel. 706/554–4435; Michael A. Haddle, CPA, Chief Executive Officer and Chief Financial Officer

DORMINY MEDICAL CENTER, Perry House Road, Fitzgerald, GA, Zip 31750, Mailing Address: Drawer 1447, Zip 31750–1447; tel. 912/424–7100; Steve Barber, Administrator

EDGEFIELD COUNTY HOSPITAL, 300 Ridge Medical Plaza, Edgefield, SC, Zip 29824; tel. 803/637–3174; W. Joseph Seel, Administrator

EMANUEL COUNTY HOSPITAL, 117 Kite Road, Swainsboro, GA, Zip 30401–3231, Mailing Address: P.O. Box 879, Zip 30401–0879; tel. 912/237–9911; Bob Via, Chief Executive Officer

JEFFERSON HOSPITAL, 1067 Peachtree Street, Louisville, GA, Zip 30434–1599; tel. 912/625–7000; Rita Culvern, Administrator

JENKINS COUNTY HOSPITAL, 515 East Winthrope Avenue, Millen, GA, Zip 30442–1600; tel. 912/982–4221; Pete Mills, Chief Executive Officer

MCDUFFIE REGIONAL MEDICAL CENTER, 521 Hill Street S.W., Thomson, GA, Zip 30824–2199; tel. 706/595–1411; Douglas C. Keir, Chief Executive Officer

MINNIE G. BOSWELL MEMORIAL HOSPITAL, 1201 Siloam Highway, Greensboro, GA, Zip 30642–2811; tel. 706/453–7331; John M. Herron, Chief Executive Officer

UNIVERSITY HEALTH CARE SYSTEM, 1350 Walton Way, Augusta, GA, Zip 30901–2629; tel. 706/722–9011; J. Larry Read, President and Chief Executive Officer

WALTON REHABILITATION HOSPITAL, 1355 Independence Drive, Augusta, GA, Zip 30901–1037; tel. 706/724–7746; Dennis B. Skelley, President and Chief Executive Officer

WILLS MEMORIAL HOSPITAL, 120 Gordon Street, Washington, GA, Zip 30673–1602, Mailing Address: P.O. Box 370, Zip 30673–0370; tel. 706/678–2151; Tim E. Merritt, Chief Executive Officer

HAWAII

PACIFIC HEALTH CARE
1946 Young Street, Honolulu, HI 96826; tel. 808/547–9712; Gary Kajiwara, President/Chief Executive Officer

KUAKINI MEDICAL CENTER, 347 North Kuakini Street, Honolulu, HI, Zip 96817–2381; tel. 808/536–2236; Gary K. Kajiwara, President and Chief Executive Officer

ST. FRANCIS MEDICAL CENTER, 2230 Liliha Street, Honolulu, HI, Zip 96817–9979, Mailing Address: P.O. Box 30100, Zip 96820–0100; tel. 808/547–6484; Cynthia Okinaka, Administrator

IDAHO

HEALTH NET
1020 N. Washington, Twin Falls, ID 83301; tel. 208/788–9862; Connie Perry, Coordinator

BARNWELL COUNTY HOSPITAL, 811 Reynolds Road, Barnwell, SC, Zip 29812; tel. 803/259–1000; J. Larry Dozier, Jr, FACHE, Chief Executive Officer

EDGEFIELD COUNTY HOSPITAL, 300 Ridge Medical Plaza, Edgefield, SC, Zip 29824; tel. 803/637–3174; W. Joseph Seel, Administrator

GOODING COUNTY MEMORIAL HOSPITAL, 1120 Montana Street, Gooding, ID, Zip 83330–1858; tel. 208/934–4433; Jim Henshaw, President and Chief Executive Officer

MAGIC VALLEY REGIONAL MEDICAL CENTER, 650 Addison Avenue West, Twin Falls, ID, Zip 83301–5444, Mailing Address: P.O. Box 409, Zip 83303–0409; tel. 208/737–2000; Gerald L. Hart, Chief Executive Officer

MINIDOKA MEMORIAL HOSPITAL AND EXTENDED CARE FACILITY, 1224 Eighth Street, Rupert, ID, Zip 83350–1599; tel. 208/436–0481; Carl Hanson, Administrator

ST. BENEDICTS FAMILY MEDICAL CENTER, 709 North Lincoln Avenue, Jerome, ID, Zip 83338–1851, Mailing Address: P.O. Box 586, Zip 83338–0586; tel. 208/324–4301; Lynne M. Mattison, FACHE, Interim Administrator

TWIN FALLS CLINIC AND HOSPITAL, 666 Shoshone Street East, Twin Falls, ID, Zip 83301–6168, Mailing Address: P.O. Box 1233, Zip 83301–1233; tel. 208/733–3700; Michael Arehart, Chief Executive Officer

WOOD RIVER MEDICAL CENTER, Sun Valley Road, Sun Valley, ID, Zip 83353, Mailing Address: P.O. Box 86, Zip 83353–0086; tel. 208/622–3333; Jon Moses, Administrator

NORTH IDAHO HEALTH NETWORK
700 Ironwood Drive, Suite 220, Coeur d'Alene, ID 83814; tel. 208/666–3212; Richard McMaster, Executive Director

ILLINOIS

ADVOCATE HEALTH CARE
2025 Windsor Drive, Oak Brook, IL 60523; tel. 630/572–9393; Richard R. Risk, President & Chief Executive Officer

BETHANY HOSPITAL, 3435 West Van Buren Street, Chicago, IL, Zip 60624–3399; tel. 773/265–7700; Lena Dobbs–Johnson, Chief Executive

CHRIST HOSPITAL AND MEDICAL CENTER, 4440 West 95th Street, Oak Lawn, IL, Zip 60453–2699; tel. 708/425–8000; Carol Schneider, Chief Executive Officer

GOOD SAMARITAN HOSPITAL, 3815 Highland Avenue, Downers Grove, IL, Zip 60515–1590; tel. 630/275–5900; Jonathan R. Bruss, Chief Executive

GOOD SHEPHERD HOSPITAL, 450 West Highway 22, Barrington, IL, Zip 60010–1901; tel. 847/381–9600; Alan Iftiniuk, Chief Executive

LUTHERAN GENERAL HOSPITAL, 1775 Dempster Street, Park Ridge, IL, Zip 60068–1174; tel. 847/723–2210; Kenneth J. Rojek, Chief Executive

RAVENSWOOD HOSPITAL MEDICAL CENTER, 4550 North Winchester Avenue, Chicago, IL, Zip 60640–5205; tel. 773/878–4300; John E. Blair, Chief Executive

SOUTH SUBURBAN HOSPITAL, 17800 South Kedzie Avenue, Hazel Crest, IL, Zip 60429–0989; tel. 708/799–8000; Patricia A. Martin, Chief Executive

TRINITY HOSPITAL, 2320 East 93rd Street, Chicago, IL, Zip 60617–9984; tel. 773/978–2000; John N. Schwartz, Chief Executive Officer

ALEXIAN BROTHERS HEALTH SYSTEMS
600 Alexian Way, Elk Grove Village, IL 60007; tel. 847/640–7550; Br Thomas Keusenkothen, C.F.A., Chief Executive Officer

ALEXIAN BROTHERS BEHAVIORAL HEALTH HOSPITAL, 1650 Moon Lake Boulevard, Hoffman Estates, IL, Zip 60194–5000; tel. 847/882–1600; Mark A. Frey, President and Chief Executive Officer

ALEXIAN BROTHERS MEDICAL CENTER, 800 Biesterfield Road, Elk Grove Village, IL, Zip 60007–3397; tel. 847/437–5500; Nancy R. Hellyer, President and Chief Executive Officer

ST. ALEXIUS MEDICAL CENTER, 1555 Barrington Road, Hoffman Estates, IL, Zip 60194; tel. 847/843–2000; Edward M. Goldberg, President and Chief Executive Officer

CATHOLIC HEALTH PARTNERS
2913 North Commonwealth Ave., Chicago, IL 60657; tel. 773/883–7300; Sister Theresa Peck, President & Chief Executive Officer

COLUMBUS HOSPITAL, 2520 North Lakeview Avenue, Chicago, IL, Zip 60614–1895; tel. 773/388–7300; Arnold Kimmel, Interim President and Chief Executive Officer

SAINT ANTHONY HOSPITAL, 2875 West 19th Street, Chicago, IL, Zip 60623–3596; tel. 773/521–1710; Arnold Kimmel, Interim President and Chief Executive Officer

ST. JOSEPH HOSPITAL, 2900 North Lake Shore Drive, Chicago, IL, Zip 60657–6274; tel. 773/665–3000; Arnold Kimmel, Interim President and Chief Executive Officer

FAMILY HEALTH NETWORK, INC.
910 W. Van Buren–6th, Chicago, IL 60607; tel. 312/491–1956; Phillip C. Bradley, President & Chief Executive Officer

MERCY HOSPITAL AND MEDICAL CENTER, 2525 South Michigan Avenue, Chicago, IL, Zip 60616–2477; tel. 312/567–2000; Dennis Patterson, Interim President and Chief Executive Officer

MOUNT SINAI HOSPITAL MEDICAL CENTER OF CHICAGO, California Avenue and 15th Street, Chicago, IL, Zip 60608–1610; tel. 773/542–2000; Kenneth A. Richmond, President and Chief Executive Officer

NORWEGIAN–AMERICAN HOSPITAL, Chicago, IL, Mailing Address: 1044 North Francisco Avenue, Zip 60622–2794; tel. 773/292–8200; Michael J. O'Grady, Jr, Interim President and Chief Executive Officer

SAINT MARY OF NAZARETH HOSPITAL CENTER, 2233 West Division Street, Chicago, IL, Zip 60622–3086; tel. 312/770–2000; Sister Sally Marie Kiepura, President and Chief Executive Officer

ST. BERNARD HOSPITAL AND HEALTH CARE CENTER, 326 West 64th Street, Chicago, IL, Zip 60621; tel. 773/962–3900; Sister Elizabeth Van Straten, President and Chief Executive Officer

FREEPORT REGIONAL HEALTH ALLIANCE
1006 West Stephenson, Freeport, IL 61032; tel. 815/235–0272; Sshelly Dunham, Director of Managed Care & Employer Services

FREEPORT MEMORIAL HOSPITAL, 1045 West Stephenson Street, Freeport, IL, Zip 61032–4899; tel. 815/599–6000; Dennis L. Hamilton, Chief Executive Officer

MERCER COUNTY HOSPITAL
409 North West Ninth Avenue, Aledo, IL 61231; tel. 309/582–5301; Bruce D. Peterson, Administrator

MERCER COUNTY HOSPITAL, 409 N.W. Ninth Avenue, Aledo, IL, Zip 61231–1296; tel. 309/582–5301; Bruce D. Peterson, Administrator

RUSH SYSTEM FOR HEALTH
820 West Jackson, Chicago, IL 60607; tel. 312/993–4600; Lora Fallon, Assistant Director

HOLY FAMILY MEDICAL CENTER, 100 North River Road, Des Plaines, IL, Zip 60016–1255; tel. 847/297–1800; Sister Patricia Ann Koschalke, President and Chief Executive Officer

OAK PARK HOSPITAL, 520 South Maple Avenue, Oak Park, IL, Zip 60304–1097; tel. 708/383–9300; Bruce M. Elegant, President and Chief Executive Officer

Networks / Rush System For Health

RIVERSIDE MEDICAL CENTER, 350 North Wall Street, Kankakee, IL, Zip 60901-0749; tel. 815/933-1671; Dennis C. Millirons, President and Chief Executive Officer

RUSH NORTH SHORE MEDICAL CENTER, 9600 Gross Point Road, Skokie, IL, Zip 60076-1257; tel. 847/677-9600; John S. Frigo, President

RUSH-COPLEY MEDICAL CENTER, 2000 Ogden Avenue, Aurora, IL, Zip 60504-4206; tel. 630/978-6200; Martin Losoff, President and Chief Executive Officer

RUSH-PRESBYTERIAN-ST. LUKE'S MEDICAL CENTER, 1653 West Congress Parkway, Chicago, IL, Zip 60612-3833; tel. 312/942-5000; Leo M. Henikoff, M.D., President and Chief Executive Officer

SWEDISHAMERICAN HEALTH SYSTEM
1400 Charles Street, Rockford, IL 61104; tel. 815/968-4400; Katherine Hermansen, Manager-Management Engineering

SWEDISHAMERICAN HEALTH SYSTEM, 1313 East State Street, Rockford, IL, Zip 61104; tel. 815/968-4400; Robert B. Klint, M.D., President and Chief Executive Officer

INDIANA

ANCILLA SYSTEMS INC.
1000 S. Lake Park Ave., Hobart, IN 46342; tel. 219/947-8500; Larry Jagrow, Senior Vice President System Services Compliance Officer

COMMUNITY HOSPITAL OF BREMEN, 411 South Whitlock Street, Bremen, IN, Zip 46506, Mailing Address: P.O. Box 8, Zip 46506-0008; tel. 219/546-2211; Scott R. Graybill, Chief Executive Officer and Administrator

ST. CATHERINE HOSPITAL, 4321 Fir Street, East Chicago, IN, Zip 46312-3097; tel. 219/392-7000; JoAnn Birdzell, President and Chief Executive Officer

ST. ELIZABETH'S HOSPITAL, 1431 North Claremont Avenue, Chicago, IL, Zip 60622-1791; tel. 773/278-2000; JoAnn Birdzell, President and Chief Executive Officer

ST. JOSEPH COMMUNITY HOSPITAL, 215 West Fourth Street, Mishawaka, IN, Zip 46544-1999; tel. 219/259-2431; Mary Roos, President and Chief Executive Officer

ST. MARY MEDICAL CENTER, 1500 South Lake Park Avenue, Hobart, IN, Zip 46342-6699; tel. 219/942-0551; Milton Triana, President and Chief Executive Officer

ST. MARY'S HOSPITAL OF EAST ST. LOUIS, 129 North Eighth Street, East St. Louis, IL, Zip 62201-2999; tel. 618/274-1900; Richard J. Mark, President and Chief Executive Officer

CENTRAL INDIANA HEALTH SYSTEM
2001 W. 86th Street, Indianapolis, IN 46260; tel. 317/338-7000; Vincent Caponi, President & Chief Executive Officer

ST. ELIZABETH ANN SETON HOSPITAL, 1116 Millis Avenue, Boonville, IN, Zip 47601, Mailing Address: P.O. Box 290, Zip 47601-0290; tel. 812/897-7440; Reginald P. Gibson, FACHE, Executive Director

ST. JOSEPH HOSPITAL & HEALTH CENTER, 1907 West Sycamore Street, Kokomo, IN, Zip 46904-9010, Mailing Address: P.O. Box 9010, Zip 46904-9010; tel. 765/452-5611; Kathleen M. Korbelak, President

ST. VINCENT CARMEL HOSPITAL, 13500 North Meridian Street, Carmel, IN, Zip 46032; tel. 317/582-7000

ST. VINCENT FRANKFORT HOSPITAL, 1300 South Jackson Street, Frankfort, IN, Zip 46041-3394, Mailing Address: P.O. Box 669, Zip 46041-0669; tel. 765/659-4731; Brian R. Zeh, Administrator

ST. VINCENT HOSPITALS AND HEALTH SERVICES, 2001 West 86th Street, Indianapolis, IN, Zip 46260-1991, Mailing Address: P.O. Box 40970, Zip 46240-0970; tel. 317/338-2345; Marsha N. Casey, President

ST. VINCENT JENNINGS HOSPITAL, 301 Henry Street, North Vernon, IN, Zip 47265-1097; tel. 812/352-4200; Joseph Roche, Administrator

ST. VINCENT MERCY HOSPITAL, 1331 South A Street, Elwood, IN, Zip 46036-1942; tel. 765/552-4600; David Masterson, Administrator

ST. VINCENT RANDOLPH HOSPITAL, 325 South Oak Street, Winchester, IN, Zip 47394-2235, Mailing Address: P.O. Box 407, Zip 47394-0407; tel. 765/584-9001; James M. Full, FACHE, Chief Executive Officer

ST. VINCENT WILLIAMSPORT HOSPITAL, 412 North Monroe Street, Williamsport, IN, Zip 47993-0215; tel. 765/762-4000; Jane Craigin, Chief Executive Officer

CLARIAN HEALTH PARTNERS, INC.
P.O. Box 1367, Indianapolis, IN 46206; tel. 317/929-2000; William J. Loveday, President & Chief Executive Officer

BEDFORD REGIONAL MEDICAL CENTER, 2900 West 16th Street, Bedford, IN, Zip 47421-3583; tel. 812/275-1200; Bradford W. Dykes, President and Chief Executive Officer

HOWARD COMMUNITY HOSPITAL, 3500 South Lafountain Street, Kokomo, IN, Zip 46904-9011; tel. 765/453-0702; James Alender, President and Chief Executive Officer

JOHNSON MEMORIAL HOSPITAL, 1125 West Jefferson Street, Franklin, IN, Zip 46131-2140, Mailing Address: P.O. Box 549, Zip 46131-0549; tel. 317/736-3300; Gregg A. Bechtold, President and Chief Executive Officer

REHABILITATION HOSPITAL OF INDIANA, 4141 Shore Drive, Indianapolis, IN, Zip 46254-2607; tel. 317/329-2000; Denny Armington, Chief Executive Officer

TIPTON COUNTY MEMORIAL HOSPITAL, 1000 South Main Street, Tipton, IN, Zip 46072-9799; tel. 765/675-8500; Alfonso W. Gatmaitan, Chief Executive Officer

UNION HOSPITAL, 1606 North Seventh Street, Terre Haute, IN, Zip 47804-2780; tel. 812/238-7000; David R. Doerr, Chief Executive Officer

WEST CENTRAL COMMUNITY HOSPITAL, 801 South Main Street, Clinton, IN, Zip 47842-0349; tel. 765/832-2451; Marilyn J. Custer-Mitchell, Administrator

WISHARD HEALTH SERVICES, 1001 West 10th Street, Indianapolis, IN, Zip 46202-2879; tel. 317/630-7356; Randall L. Braddom, M.D., Chief Executive Officer and Medical Director

MEMORIAL HEALTH SYSTEM INC
707 North Michigan Street, Suite 100, South Bend, IN 46601; tel. 219/284-3699; David Sage, Executive Vice President & COO

MEMORIAL HOSPITAL OF SOUTH BEND, 615 North Michigan Street, South Bend, IN, Zip 46601-9986; tel. 219/234-9041; Philip A. Newbold, President and Chief Executive Officer

MIDWEST HEALTH NET INC
6407 Constitution Drive, Fort Wayne, IN 46804; tel. 219/436-7879; Thomas C. Henry, President

BEDFORD REGIONAL MEDICAL CENTER, 2900 West 16th Street, Bedford, IN, Zip 47421-3583; tel. 812/275-1200; Bradford W. Dykes, President and Chief Executive Officer

CAMERON MEMORIAL COMMUNITY HOSPITAL, 416 East Maumee Street, Angola, IN, Zip 46703-2015; tel. 219/665-2141; Dennis L. Knapp, President

CAYLOR-NICKEL MEDICAL CENTER, One Caylor-Nickel Square, Bluffton, IN, Zip 46714-2529; tel. 219/824-3500; William F. Brockmann, President and Chief Executive Officer

COMMUNITY HOSPITAL OF NOBLE COUNTY, 951 East Hospital Drive, Kendallville, IN, Zip 46755-2293, Mailing Address: P.O. Box 249, Zip 46755-0249; tel. 219/347-1100; John M. Hatcher, President

DECATUR COUNTY MEMORIAL HOSPITAL, 720 North Lincoln Street, Greensburg, IN, Zip 47240-1398; tel. 812/663-4331; David V. Trexler, President

DEKALB MEMORIAL HOSPITAL, 1316 East Seventh Street, Auburn, IN, Zip 46706-2515, Mailing Address: P.O. Box 542, Zip 46706-0542; tel. 219/925-4600; Jack M. Corey, President

DOCTORS HOSPITAL OF JACKSON, 110 North Elm Avenue, Jackson, MI, Zip 49202-3595; tel. 517/787-1440; Michael J. Falatko, President and Chief Executive Officer

DUKES MEMORIAL HOSPITAL, 275 West 12th Street, Peru, IN, Zip 46970-1698; tel. 765/472-8000; R. Joe Johnston, President and Chief Executive Officer

FISHER-TITUS MEDICAL CENTER, 272 Benedict Avenue, Norwalk, OH, Zip 44857-2374; tel. 419/668-8101; Patrick J. Martin, President and Chief Executive Officer

GREENE COUNTY GENERAL HOSPITAL, Rural Route 1, Box 1000, Linton, IN, Zip 47441-9457; tel. 812/847-2281; Jonas S. Uland, Executive Director

HANCOCK MEMORIAL HOSPITAL AND HEALTH SERVICES, 801 North State Street, Greenfield, IN, Zip 46140-1270, Mailing Address: P.O. Box 827, Zip 46140-0827; tel. 317/462-5544; Robert C. Keen, Ph.D., CHE, President and Chief Executive Officer

HENRY COUNTY HOSPITAL, 11600 State Route 424, Napoleon, OH, Zip 43545-9399; tel. 419/592-4015; Kimberly Bordenkircher, Chief Executive Officer

HENRY COUNTY MEMORIAL HOSPITAL, 1000 North 16th Street, New Castle, IN, Zip 47362-4319, Mailing Address: P.O. Box 490, Zip 47362-0490; tel. 765/521-0890; Jack Basler, President

HOWARD COMMUNITY HOSPITAL, 3500 South Lafountain Street, Kokomo, IN, Zip 46904-9011; tel. 765/453-0702; James Alender, President and Chief Executive Officer

HUNTINGTON MEMORIAL HOSPITAL, 2001 Stults Road, Huntington, IN, Zip 46750-3696; tel. 219/356-3000; L. Kent McCoy, President

JOHNSON MEMORIAL HOSPITAL, 1125 West Jefferson Street, Franklin, IN, Zip 46131-2140, Mailing Address: P.O. Box 549, Zip 46131-0549; tel. 317/736-3300; Gregg A. Bechtold, President and Chief Executive Officer

KOSCIUSKO COMMUNITY HOSPITAL, 2101 East Dubois Drive, Warsaw, IN, Zip 46580-3288; tel. 219/267-3200; Wayne Hendrix, Chief Executive Officer

LIMA MEMORIAL HOSPITAL, 1001 Bellefontaine Avenue, Lima, OH, Zip 45804-2899; tel. 419/228-3335; John B. White, President and Chief Executive Officer

MEDICAL COLLEGE OF OHIO HOSPITALS, 3000 Arlington Avenue, Toledo, OH, Zip 43614-5805; tel. 419/383-4000; Frank S. McCullough, M.D., President

MERCY MEMORIAL HOSPITAL, 740 North Macomb Street, Monroe, MI, Zip 48161-9974, Mailing Address: P.O. Box 67, Zip 48161-0067; tel. 734/241-1700; Richard S. Hiltz, President and Chief Executive Officer

MORGAN COUNTY MEMORIAL HOSPITAL, 2209 John R. Wooden Drive, Martinsville, IN, Zip 46151-1840, Mailing Address: P.O. Box 1717, Zip 46151-1717; tel. 765/342-8441; John R. Whitcomb, Interim President and Chief Executive Officer

PARKVIEW HOSPITAL, 2200 Randallia Drive, Fort Wayne, IN, Zip 46805-4699; tel. 219/484-6636; Frank D. Byrne, M.D., President

PAULDING COUNTY HOSPITAL, 1035 West Wayne Street, Paulding, OH, Zip 45879-9220; tel. 419/399-4080; Larry Thornhill, Chief Executive Officer

RIVERVIEW HOSPITAL, 395 Westfield Road, Noblesville, IN, Zip 46060-1425, Mailing Address: P.O. Box 220, Zip 46061-0220; tel. 317/773-0760; Seward Horner, President

ST. CATHERINE HOSPITAL, 4321 Fir Street, East Chicago, IN, Zip 46312-3097; tel. 219/392-7000; JoAnn Birdzell, President and Chief Executive Officer

Networks / Sagamore Health Network, Inc

ST. ELIZABETH'S HOSPITAL, 1431 North Claremont Avenue, Chicago, IL, Zip 60622–1791; tel. 773/278–2000; JoAnn Birdzell, President and Chief Executive Officer

ST. JOSEPH COMMUNITY HOSPITAL, 215 West Fourth Street, Mishawaka, IN, Zip 46544–1999; tel. 219/259–2431; Mary Roos, President and Chief Executive Officer

ST. JOSEPH HOSPITAL, 700 Broadway, Fort Wayne, IN, Zip 46802–1493; tel. 219/425–3000; Michael H. Schatzlein, M.D., President and Chief Executive Officer

ST. MARY MEDICAL CENTER, 1500 South Lake Park Avenue, Hobart, IN, Zip 46342–6699; tel. 219/942–0551; Milton Triana, President and Chief Executive Officer

ST. MARY'S HOSPITAL OF EAST ST. LOUIS, 129 North Eighth Street, East St. Louis, IL, Zip 62201–2999; tel. 618/274–1900; Richard J. Mark, President and Chief Executive Officer

ST. VINCENT FRANKFORT HOSPITAL, 1300 South Jackson Street, Frankfort, IN, Zip 46041–3394, Mailing Address: P.O. Box 669, Zip 46041–0669; tel. 765/659–4731; Brian R. Zeh, Administrator

ST. VINCENT RANDOLPH HOSPITAL, 325 South Oak Street, Winchester, IN, Zip 47394–2235, Mailing Address: P.O. Box 407, Zip 47394–0407; tel. 765/584–9001; James M. Full, FACHE, Chief Executive Officer

THE TOLEDO HOSPITAL, 2142 North Cove Boulevard, Toledo, OH, Zip 43606–3896; tel. 419/471–4000; Barbara Steele, President

TIPTON COUNTY MEMORIAL HOSPITAL, 1000 South Main Street, Tipton, IN, Zip 46072–9799; tel. 765/675–8500; Alfonso W. Gatmaitan, Chief Executive Officer

VAN WERT COUNTY HOSPITAL, 1250 South Washington Street, Van Wert, OH, Zip 45891–2599; tel. 419/238–2390; Mark J. Minick, President and Chief Executive Officer

WABASH COUNTY HOSPITAL, 710 North East Street, Wabash, IN, Zip 46992–1924, Mailing Address: P.O. Box 548, Zip 46992–0548; tel. 219/563–3131; David C. Hunter, Chief Executive Officer

WELLS COMMUNITY HOSPITAL, 1100 South Main Street, Bluffton, IN, Zip 46714–3697; tel. 219/824–3210; Thomas A. Clark, Chief Executive Officer

WESTVIEW HOSPITAL, 3630 Guion Road, Indianapolis, IN, Zip 46222–1699; tel. 317/924–6661; David C. Dyar, Chief Executive Officer

WHITE COUNTY MEMORIAL HOSPITAL, 1101 O'Connor Boulevard, Monticello, IN, Zip 47960–1698; tel. 219/583–7111; John M. Avers, Chief Executive Officer

WHITLEY MEMORIAL HOSPITAL, 353 North Oak Street, Columbia City, IN, Zip 46725–1623; tel. 219/244–6191; John M. Hatcher, President

WITHAM MEMORIAL HOSPITAL, 1124 North Lebanon Street, Lebanon, IN, Zip 46052–1776, Mailing Address: P.O. Box 1200, Zip 46052–3005; tel. 765/482–2700; Raymond V. Ingham, President and Chief Executive Officer

PARKVIEW HEALTH SYSTEM
2200 Randallia drive, Fort Wayne, IN 46805; tel. 219/484–6636; Charles Mason, President & Chief Executive Officer

HUNTINGTON MEMORIAL HOSPITAL, 2001 Stults Road, Huntington, IN, Zip 46750–3696; tel. 219/356–3000; L. Kent McCoy, President

PARKVIEW HOSPITAL, 2200 Randallia Drive, Fort Wayne, IN, Zip 46805–4699; tel. 219/484–6636; Frank D. Byrne, M.D., President

WHITLEY MEMORIAL HOSPITAL, 353 North Oak Street, Columbia City, IN, Zip 46725–1623; tel. 219/244–6191; John M. Hatcher, President

SAGAMORE HEALTH NETWORK, INC
11555 North Meridian Suite 400, Carmel, IN 46032; tel. 317/573–2903; Greg Yust, President

ADAMS COUNTY MEMORIAL HOSPITAL, 805 High Street, Decatur, IN, Zip 46733–2311, Mailing Address: P.O. Box 151, Zip 46733–0151; tel. 219/724–2145; Marvin L. Baird, Executive Director

BLOOMINGTON HOSPITAL OF ORANGE COUNTY, 642 West Hospital Road, Paoli, IN, Zip 47454–0499, Mailing Address: P.O. Box 499, Zip 47454–0499; tel. 812/723–2811; L. Gene Perry, Chief Executive Officer

CAMERON MEMORIAL COMMUNITY HOSPITAL, 416 East Maumee Street, Angola, IN, Zip 46703–2015; tel. 219/665–2141; Dennis L. Knapp, President

CLAY COUNTY HOSPITAL, 1206 East National Avenue, Brazil, IN, Zip 47834–2797; tel. 812/448–2675; Jay P. Jolly, Administrator and Chief Executive Officer

COMMUNITY HOSPITAL OF BREMEN, 411 South Whitlock Street, Bremen, IN, Zip 46506, Mailing Address: P.O. Box 8, Zip 46506–0008; tel. 219/546–2211; Scott R. Graybill, Chief Executive Officer and Administrator

COMMUNITY HOSPITAL OF NOBLE COUNTY, 951 East Hospital Drive, Kendallville, IN, Zip 46755–2293, Mailing Address: P.O. Box 249, Zip 46755–0249; tel. 219/347–1100; John M. Hatcher, President

COMMUNITY MEMORIAL HOSPITAL, 208 North Columbus Street, Hicksville, OH, Zip 43526–1299; tel. 419/542–6692; Olas A. Hubbs, Chief Executive Officer

DUKES MEMORIAL HOSPITAL, 275 West 12th Street, Peru, IN, Zip 46970–1698; tel. 765/472–8000; R. Joe Johnston, President and Chief Executive Officer

DUNN MEMORIAL HOSPITAL, 1600 23rd Street, Bedford, IN, Zip 47421–4704; tel. 812/275–3331; Tony G. Sudduth, Chief Executive Officer

FAIRBANKS HOSPITAL, 8102 Clearvista Parkway, Indianapolis, IN, Zip 46256–4698; tel. 317/849–8222; Timothy J. Kelly, M.D., President

FLOYD MEMORIAL HOSPITAL AND HEALTH SERVICES, 1850 State Street, New Albany, IN, Zip 47150–4997; tel. 812/949–5500; Bryant R. Hanson, President and Chief Executive Officer

GIBSON GENERAL HOSPITAL, 1808 Sherman Drive, Princeton, IN, Zip 47670–1043; tel. 812/385–3401; Michael J. Budnick, FACHE, Administrator and Chief Executive Officer

GREENE COUNTY GENERAL HOSPITAL, Rural Route 1, Box 1000, Linton, IN, Zip 47441–9457; tel. 812/847–2281; Jonas S. Uland, Executive Director

HANCOCK MEMORIAL HOSPITAL AND HEALTH SERVICES, 801 North State Street, Greenfield, IN, Zip 46140–1270, Mailing Address: P.O. Box 827, Zip 46140–0827; tel. 317/462–5544; Robert C. Keen, Ph.D., CHE, President and Chief Executive Officer

HENDRICKS COMMUNITY HOSPITAL, 1000 East Main Street, Danville, IN, Zip 46122–0409, Mailing Address: P.O. Box 409, Zip 46122–0409; tel. 317/745–4451; Dennis W. Dawes, President

HENRY COUNTY MEMORIAL HOSPITAL, 1000 North 16th Street, New Castle, IN, Zip 47362–4319, Mailing Address: P.O. Box 490, Zip 47362–0490; tel. 765/521–0890; Jack Basler, President

HUNTINGTON MEMORIAL HOSPITAL, 2001 Stults Road, Huntington, IN, Zip 46750–3696; tel. 219/356–3000; L. Kent McCoy, President

JOHNSON MEMORIAL HOSPITAL, 1125 West Jefferson Street, Franklin, IN, Zip 46131–2140, Mailing Address: P.O. Box 549, Zip 46131–0549; tel. 317/736–3300; Gregg A. Bechtold, President and Chief Executive Officer

KOSCIUSKO COMMUNITY HOSPITAL, 2101 East Dubois Drive, Warsaw, IN, Zip 46580–3288; tel. 219/267–3200; Wayne Hendrix, Chief Executive Officer

LA PORTE REGIONAL HEALTH SYSTEM, 1007 Lincolnway, La Porte, IN, Zip 46350, Mailing Address: P.O. Box 250, Zip 46352–0250; tel. 219/326–1234; Jonathan R. Goble, President and Chief Executive Officer

MEDICAL CENTER OF SOUTHERN INDIANA, 2200 Market Street, Charlestown, IN, Zip 47111–0069, Mailing Address: P.O. Box 69, Zip 47111–0069; tel. 812/256–3301; Kevin J. Miller, FACHE, President and Chief Executive Officer

MEMORIAL HOSPITAL, 1101 Michigan Avenue, Logansport, IN, Zip 46947–7013, Mailing Address: P.O. Box 7013, Zip 46947–7013; tel. 219/753–7541; Brian T. Shockney, President and Chief Executive Officer

MORGAN COUNTY MEMORIAL HOSPITAL, 2209 John R. Wooden Drive, Martinsville, IN, Zip 46151–1840, Mailing Address: P.O. Box 1717, Zip 46151–1717; tel. 765/342–8441; John R. Whitcomb, Interim President and Chief Executive Officer

OAKLAWN PSYCHIATRIC CENTER, INC., 330 Lakeview Drive, Goshen, IN, Zip 46528–9365, Mailing Address: P.O. Box 809, Zip 46527–0809; tel. 219/533–1234; Harold C. Loewen, President

PARKVIEW HOSPITAL, 2200 Randallia Drive, Fort Wayne, IN, Zip 46805–4699; tel. 219/484–6636; Frank D. Byrne, M.D., President

PULASKI MEMORIAL HOSPITAL, 616 East 13th Street, Winamac, IN, Zip 46996–1117; tel. 219/946–6131; Richard H. Mynark, Chief Executive Officer

PUTNAM COUNTY HOSPITAL, 1542 Bloomington Street, Greencastle, IN, Zip 46135–2297; tel. 765/653–5121; Dennis Weatherford, Interim Administrator

REHABILITATION HOSPITAL OF INDIANA, 4141 Shore Drive, Indianapolis, IN, Zip 46254–2607; tel. 317/329–2000; Denny Armington, Chief Executive Officer

RIVERVIEW HOSPITAL, 395 Westfield Road, Noblesville, IN, Zip 46060–1425, Mailing Address: P.O. Box 220, Zip 46061–0220; tel. 317/773–0760; Seward Horner, President

RUSH MEMORIAL HOSPITAL, 1300 North Main Street, Rushville, IN, Zip 46173–1198; tel. 765/932–4111; J. Jay Purvis, Interim Chief Executive Officer

SAINT ANTHONY MEMORIAL HEALTH CENTERS, 301 West Homer Street, Michigan City, IN, Zip 46360–4358; tel. 219/879–8511; Bruce E. Rampage, President and Chief Executive Officer

SAINT JOHN'S HEALTH SYSTEM, 2015 Jackson Street, Anderson, IN, Zip 46016–4339; tel. 765/649–2511; Jerry D. Brumitt, President and Chief Executive Officer

SAINT JOSEPH'S REGIONAL MEDICAL CENTER–PLYMOUTH CAMPUS, 1915 Lake Avenue, Plymouth, IN, Zip 46563–9905, Mailing Address: P.O. Box 670, Zip 46563–9905; tel. 219/936–3181; Brian E. Dietz, FACHE, Executive Vice President

SAINT JOSEPH'S REGIONAL MEDICAL CENTER–SOUTH BEND CAMPUS, 801 East LaSalle, South Bend, IN, Zip 46617–2800; tel. 219/237–7111; Robert L. Beyer, President and Chief Executive Officer

SAINT MARGARET MERCY HEALTHCARE CENTERS, 5454 Hohman Avenue, Hammond, IN, Zip 46320–1999; tel. 219/933–2074; Eugene C. Diamond, President and Chief Executive Officer

ST. ANTHONY MEDICAL CENTER, 1201 South Main Street, Crown Point, IN, Zip 46307–8483; tel. 219/738–2100; Stephen O. Leurck, President and Chief Executive Officer

ST. CATHERINE HOSPITAL, 4321 Fir Street, East Chicago, IN, Zip 46312–3097; tel. 219/392–7000; JoAnn Birdzell, President and Chief Executive Officer

ST. FRANCIS HOSPITAL AND HEALTH CENTERS – NORTH CAMPUS, 1600 Albany Street, Beech Grove, IN, Zip 46107–1593; tel. 317/787–3311; Robert J. Brody, President and Chief Executive Officer

ST. FRANCIS HOSPITAL–MOORESVILLE, 1201 Hadley Road N.W., Mooresville, IN, Zip 46158–1789; tel. 317/831–1160; Charles D. Swisher, President

Networks / Sagamore Health Network, Inc

ST. JOSEPH COMMUNITY HOSPITAL, 215 West Fourth Street, Mishawaka, IN, Zip 46544-1999; tel. 219/259-2431; Mary Roos, President and Chief Executive Officer

ST. JOSEPH HOSPITAL, 700 Broadway, Fort Wayne, IN, Zip 46802-1493; tel. 219/425-3000; Michael H. Schatzlein, M.D., President and Chief Executive Officer

ST. MARY MEDICAL CENTER, 1500 South Lake Park Avenue, Hobart, IN, Zip 46342-6699; tel. 219/942-0551; Milton Triana, President and Chief Executive Officer

ST. MARY'S WARRICK, 1116 Millis Avenue, Boonville, IN, Zip 47601-0629, Mailing Address: Box 629, Zip 47601-0629; tel. 812/897-4800; James M. Hayes, Executive Vice President and Administrator

ST. MARY'S MEDICAL CENTER, 3700 Washington Avenue, Evansville, IN, Zip 47750-0002; tel. 812/485-4000; Jay D. Kasey, President

ST. VINCENT FRANKFORT HOSPITAL, 1300 South Jackson Street, Frankfort, IN, Zip 46041-3394, Mailing Address: P.O. Box 669, Zip 46041-0669; tel. 765/659-4731; Brian R. Zeh, Administrator

ST. VINCENT HOSPITALS AND HEALTH SERVICES, 2001 West 86th Street, Indianapolis, IN, Zip 46260-1991, Mailing Address: P.O. Box 40970, Zip 46240-0970; tel. 317/338-2345; Marsha N. Casey, President

ST. VINCENT MERCY HOSPITAL, 1331 South A Street, Elwood, IN, Zip 46036-1942; tel. 765/552-4600; David Masterson, Administrator

ST. VINCENT RANDOLPH HOSPITAL, 325 South Oak Street, Winchester, IN, Zip 47394-2235, Mailing Address: P.O. Box 407, Zip 47394-0407; tel. 765/584-9001; James M. Full, FACHE, Chief Executive Officer

STARKE MEMORIAL HOSPITAL, 102 East Culver Road, Knox, IN, Zip 46534-2299; tel. 219/772-6231; Kathryn J. Norem, Chief Executive Officer

SULLIVAN COUNTY COMMUNITY HOSPITAL, 2200 North Section Street, Sullivan, IN, Zip 47882, Mailing Address: P.O. Box 10, Zip 47882-0010; tel. 812/268-4311; Thomas J. Hudgins, Administrator

TIPTON COUNTY MEMORIAL HOSPITAL, 1000 South Main Street, Tipton, IN, Zip 46072-9799; tel. 765/675-8500; Alfonso W. Gatmaitan, Chief Executive Officer

UNION HOSPITAL, 1606 North Seventh Street, Terre Haute, IN, Zip 47804-2780; tel. 812/238-7000; David R. Doerr, Chief Executive Officer

WABASH COUNTY HOSPITAL, 710 North East Street, Wabash, IN, Zip 46992-1924, Mailing Address: P.O. Box 548, Zip 46992-0548; tel. 219/563-3131; David C. Hunter, Chief Executive Officer

WELLS COMMUNITY HOSPITAL, 1100 South Main Street, Bluffton, IN, Zip 46714-3697; tel. 219/824-3210; Thomas A. Clark, Chief Executive Officer

WESTVIEW HOSPITAL, 3630 Guion Road, Indianapolis, IN, Zip 46222-1699; tel. 317/924-6661; David C. Dyar, Chief Executive Officer

WHITE COUNTY MEMORIAL HOSPITAL, 1101 O'Connor Boulevard, Monticello, IN, Zip 47960-1698; tel. 219/583-7111; John M. Avers, Chief Executive Officer

WHITLEY MEMORIAL HOSPITAL, 353 North Oak Street, Columbia City, IN, Zip 46725-1623; tel. 219/244-6191; John M. Hatcher, President

WITHAM MEMORIAL HOSPITAL, 1124 North Lebanon Street, Lebanon, IN, Zip 46052-1776, Mailing Address: P.O. Box 1200, Zip 46052-3005; tel. 765/482-2700; Raymond V. Ingham, President and Chief Executive Officer

SUBURBAN HEALTH ORGANIZATION
2780 Waterfront Parkway, East Drive, Suite 300, Indianapolis, IN 46214; tel. 317/692-5222; Julie M. Carmichael, President

HANCOCK MEMORIAL HOSPITAL AND HEALTH SERVICES, 801 North State Street, Greenfield, IN, Zip 46140-1270, Mailing Address: P.O. Box 827, Zip 46140-0827; tel. 317/462-5544; Robert C. Keen, Ph.D., CHE, President and Chief Executive Officer

HENDRICKS COMMUNITY HOSPITAL, 1000 East Main Street, Danville, IN, Zip 46122-0409, Mailing Address: P.O. Box 409, Zip 46122-0409; tel. 317/745-4451; Dennis W. Dawes, President

HENRY COUNTY MEMORIAL HOSPITAL, 1000 North 16th Street, New Castle, IN, Zip 47362-4319, Mailing Address: P.O. Box 490, Zip 47362-0490; tel. 765/521-0890; Jack Basler, President

JOHNSON MEMORIAL HOSPITAL, 1125 West Jefferson Street, Franklin, IN, Zip 46131-2140, Mailing Address: P.O. Box 549, Zip 46131-0549; tel. 317/736-3300; Gregg A. Bechtold, President and Chief Executive Officer

MORGAN COUNTY MEMORIAL HOSPITAL, 2209 John R. Wooden Drive, Martinsville, IN, Zip 46151-1840, Mailing Address: P.O. Box 1717, Zip 46151-1717; tel. 765/342-8441; John R. Whitcomb, Interim President and Chief Executive Officer

PUTNAM COUNTY HOSPITAL, 1542 Bloomington Street, Greencastle, IN, Zip 46135-2297; tel. 765/653-5121; Dennis Weatherford, Interim Administrator

RIVERVIEW HOSPITAL, 395 Westfield Road, Noblesville, IN, Zip 46060-1425, Mailing Address: P.O. Box 220, Zip 46061-0220; tel. 317/773-0760; Seward Horner, President

WESTVIEW HOSPITAL, 3630 Guion Road, Indianapolis, IN, Zip 46222-1699; tel. 317/924-6661; David C. Dyar, Chief Executive Officer

WITHAM MEMORIAL HOSPITAL, 1124 North Lebanon Street, Lebanon, IN, Zip 46052-1776, Mailing Address: P.O. Box 1200, Zip 46052-3005; tel. 765/482-2700; Raymond V. Ingham, President and Chief Executive Officer

IOWA

GENESIS HEALTH SYSTEM
1227 East Rusholme Street, Davenport, IA 52803; tel. 319/421-1000; Jill Dobbe, Planning Analyst

DEWITT COMMUNITY HOSPITAL, 1118 11th Street, De Witt, IA, Zip 52742-1296; tel. 319/659-4200; Robert G. Senneff, Chief Executive Officer

GENESIS MEDICAL CENTER, 1227 East Rusholme Street, Davenport, IA, Zip 52803-2498; tel. 319/421-1000; Leo A. Bressanelli, President and Chief Executive Officer

ILLINI HOSPITAL, 801 Hospital Road, Silvis, IL, Zip 61282-1893; tel. 309/792-9363; Gary E. Larson, Chief Executive Officer

HEALTH NETWORK OF IOWA
1200 Pleasant Street, Des Moines, IA 50304; tel. 515/241-6201; Jim Zahnd, Senior Vice President

MERCY MEDICAL CENTER – NORTH IOWA
1000 4th Street, Southwest, Mason City, IA 50401; tel. 515/422-7000; Jim Fitzpatrick, Senior Vice President, Network Development

BELMOND MEDICAL CENTER, 403 First Street S.E., Belmond, IA, Zip 50421-1201, Mailing Address: P.O. Box 326, Zip 50421-0326; tel. 515/444-3223; Kim Price, Administrator

ELLSWORTH MUNICIPAL HOSPITAL, 110 Rocksylvania Avenue, Iowa Falls, IA, Zip 50126-2431; tel. 515/648-4631; John O'Brien, Administrator

FRANKLIN GENERAL HOSPITAL, 1720 Central Avenue East, Hampton, IA, Zip 50441-1859; tel. 515/456-5000; Scott Wells, Administrator

HANCOCK COUNTY MEMORIAL HOSPITAL, 532 First Street N.W., Britt, IA, Zip 50423-0068, Mailing Address: P.O. Box 68, Zip 50423-0068; tel. 515/843-3801; Harriet A. Thompson, Administrator

KOSSUTH REGIONAL HEALTH CENTER, 1515 South Phillips Street, Algona, IA, Zip 50511-3649; tel. 515/295-2451; Scott Curtis, Administrator and Chief Executive Officer

MERCY MEDICAL CENTER – NORTH IOWA, 1000 Fourth Street S.W., Mason City, IA, Zip 50401-2800; tel. 515/422-7000; James J. Sexton, President and Chief Executive Officer

MERCY MEDICAL CENTER–NEW HAMPTON, 308 North Maple Avenue, New Hampton, IA, Zip 50659-1142; tel. 515/394-4121; Carolyn Martin-Shaw, President

MITCHELL COUNTY REGIONAL HEALTH CENTER, 616 North Eighth Street, Osage, IA, Zip 50461-1498; tel. 515/732-6005; Kimberly J. Miller, CHE, Administrator and Chief Executive Officer

PALO ALTO HEALTH SYSTEM, 3201 First Street, Emmetsburg, IA, Zip 50536-2599; tel. 712/852-5500; Darrell E. Vondrak, Administrator

REGIONAL HEALTH SERVICES OF HOWARD COUNTY, 235 Eighth Avenue West, Cresco, IA, Zip 52136-1098; tel. 319/547-2101; Elizabeth A. Doty, President and Chief Executive Officer

MERCY NETWORK
400 University, Des Moines, IA 50309; tel. 515/247-4277; Sara Drobnick, Vice President

ADAIR COUNTY MEMORIAL HOSPITAL, 609 S.E. Kent Street, Greenfield, IA, Zip 50849-9454; tel. 515/743-2123; Myrna Erb-Gundel, Administrator

AUDUBON COUNTY MEMORIAL HOSPITAL, 515 Pacific Street, Audubon, IA, Zip 50025-1099; tel. 712/563-2611; Thomas G. Smith, Chief Executive Officer

DAVIS COUNTY HOSPITAL, 507 North Madison Street, Bloomfield, IA, Zip 52537-1299; tel. 515/664-2145; John E. Monnahan, Administrator

HAMILTON COUNTY PUBLIC HOSPITAL, 800 Ohio Street, Webster City, IA, Zip 50595-2824, Mailing Address: P.O. Box 430, Zip 50595-0430; tel. 515/832-9400; Roger W. Lenz, Administrator

MADISON COUNTY MEMORIAL HOSPITAL, 300 Hutchings Street, Winterset, IA, Zip 50273-2199; tel. 515/462-2373; Jill Kordick, Administrator

MANNING REGIONAL HEALTHCARE CENTER, 410 Main Street, Manning, IA, Zip 51455-1093; tel. 712/653-2072; Michael S. Ketcham, Chief Executive Officer

MERCY MEDICAL CENTER–CENTERVILLE, 1 St. Joseph's Drive, Centerville, IA, Zip 52544; tel. 515/437-4111; William C. Assell, President and Chief Executive Officer

MERCY MEDICAL CENTER–DES MOINES, 1111 6th Avenue, Des Moines, IA, Zip 50314-2611; tel. 515/247-3121; David H. Vellinga, President and Chief Executive Officer

MONROE COUNTY HOSPITAL, 6580 165th Street, Albia, IA, Zip 52531; tel. 515/932-2134; Gregory A. Paris, Administrator

RINGGOLD COUNTY HOSPITAL, 211 Shellway Drive, Mount Ayr, IA, Zip 50854-1299; tel. 515/464-3226; Gordon W. Winkler, Administrator

ST. ANTHONY REGIONAL HOSPITAL, 311 South Clark Street, Carroll, IA, Zip 51401, Mailing Address: P.O. Box 628, Zip 51401-0628; tel. 712/792-8231; Gary P. Riedmann, President and Chief Executive Officer

STORY COUNTY HOSPITAL AND LONG TERM CARE FACILITY, 630 Sixth Street, Nevada, IA, Zip 50201-2266; tel. 515/382-2111; Todd Willert, Administrator

WAYNE COUNTY HOSPITAL, 417 South East Street, Corydon, IA, Zip 50060-1860, Mailing Address: P.O. Box 305, Zip 50060-0305; tel. 515/872-2260; Bill D. Wilson, Administrator

ST LUKES/IOWA HEALTH SYSTEM
P.O. Box 3026, Cedar Rapids, IA 52406; tel. 319/369-7240; Vice President System Development

IOWA METHODIST MEDICAL CENTER, 1200 Pleasant Street, Des Moines, IA, Zip 50309-9976; tel. 515/241-6212; James H. Skogsbergh, President

Networks / Sunflower Health Network

JONES REGIONAL MEDICAL CENTER, 104 Broadway Place, Anamosa, IA, Zip 52205–1100; tel. 319/462–6131; Vickie Asbe, Administrator

KANSAS

COMMUNITY HEALTH ALLIANCE
240 W. 18th Street, Horton, KS 66439;
tel. 816/276-7580; Dale White, Chairman

COMMUNITY MEMORIAL HEALTHCARE, 708 North 18th Street, Marysville, KS, Zip 66508–1338; tel. 785/562–2311; Jay M. Canter, Chief Executive Officer

GEARY COMMUNITY HOSPITAL, 1102 St. Mary's Road, Junction City, KS, Zip 66441, Mailing Address: P.O. Box 490, Zip 66441–0490; tel. 785/238–4131; David K. Bradley, CHE, Chief Executive Officer

HOLTON COMMUNITY HOSPITAL, 1110 Columbine Drive, Holton, KS, Zip 66436–1545; tel. 785/364–2116; Leonard Hernandez, Chief Executive Officer

MERCY HEALTH CENTER OF MANHATTAN, 1823 College Avenue, Manhattan, KS, Zip 66502–3381, Mailing Address: P.O. Box 1289, Zip 66502–1289; tel. 785/776–3322; Richard L. Allen, President and Chief Executive Officer

MORRIS COUNTY HOSPITAL, 600 North Washington Street, Council Grove, KS, Zip 66846–0275, Mailing Address: P.O. Box 275, Zip 66846–0275; tel. 316/767–6811; James H. Reagan, Jr, Ph.D., Chief Executive Officer

NEMAHA VALLEY COMMUNITY HOSPITAL, 1600 Community Drive, Seneca, KS, Zip 66538–9739; tel. 785/336–6181; Michael J. Ryan, Administrator

NORTHEAST KANSAS CENTER FOR HEALTH AND WELLNESS, 240 West 18th Street, Horton, KS, Zip 66439–1245; tel. 785/486–2642; Dale A. White, Chief Executive Officer

GREAT PLAINS HEALTH ALLIANCE
P.O. Box 366, Phillipsburg, KS 67661;
tel. 785/543-2111; Roger John, President

ASHLAND HEALTH CENTER, 709 Oak Street, Ashland, KS, Zip 67831–0188, Mailing Address: P.O. Box 188, Zip 67831–0188; tel. 316/635–2241; Bryan Stacey, Administrator

CHEYENNE COUNTY HOSPITAL, 210 West First Street, Saint Francis, KS, Zip 67756–0547, Mailing Address: P.O. Box 547, Zip 67756–0547; tel. 785/332–2104; Leslie Lacy, Administrator

COMMUNITY MEDICAL CENTER, 2307 Barada Street, Falls City, NE, Zip 68355–1599; tel. 402/245–2428; Asa B. Wilson, Ph.D., Administrator

ELLINWOOD DISTRICT HOSPITAL, 605 North Main Street, Ellinwood, KS, Zip 67526–1440; tel. 316/564–2548; Marge Conell, Administrator

FREDONIA REGIONAL HOSPITAL, 1527 Madison Street, Fredonia, KS, Zip 66736–1751, Mailing Address: P.O. Box 579, Zip 66736–0579; tel. 316/378–2121; Terry Deschaine, Chief Executive Officer

GREELEY COUNTY HOSPITAL, 506 Third Street, Tribune, KS, Zip 67879–0338, Mailing Address: P.O. Box 338, Zip 67879–0338; tel. 316/376–4221; Jerrell J. Horton, Chief Executive Officer

GRISELL MEMORIAL HOSPITAL DISTRICT ONE, 210 South Vermont, Ransom, KS, Zip 67572–0268, Mailing Address: P.O. Box 268, Zip 67572–0268; tel. 785/731–2231; Kristine Ochs, R.N., Administrator

HARLAN COUNTY HEALTH SYSTEM, 717 North Brown Street, Alma, NE, Zip 68920–0836, Mailing Address: P.O. Box 836, Zip 68920–0836; tel. 308/928–2151; Allen Van Driel, Administrator

HILLSBORO COMMUNITY MEDICAL CENTER, 701 South Main Street, Hillsboro, KS, Zip 67063–1595; tel. 316/947–3114; Tom Faulkner, Chief Executive Officer

KIOWA COUNTY MEMORIAL HOSPITAL, 501 South Walnut Street, Greensburg, KS, Zip 67054–1951, Mailing Address: P.O. Box 616, Zip 67054–0616; tel. 316/723–3341; Cecilia Noll, Administrator

LANE COUNTY HOSPITAL, 243 South Second, Dighton, KS, Zip 67839–0969, Mailing Address: P.O. Box 969, Zip 67839–0969; tel. 316/397–5321; Donna McGowan, Administrator

LINCOLN COUNTY HOSPITAL, 624 North Second Street, Lincoln, KS, Zip 67455–1738, Mailing Address: P.O. Box 406, Zip 67455–0406; tel. 785/524–4403; Jolene Yager, R.N., Administrator

MEDICINE LODGE MEMORIAL HOSPITAL, 710 North Walnut Street, Medicine Lodge, KS, Zip 67104–1019, Mailing Address: P.O. Drawer C, Zip 67104; tel. 316/886–3771; Kevin A. White, CHE, Administrator

MINNEOLA DISTRICT HOSPITAL, 212 Main Street, Minneola, KS, Zip 67865–8511, Mailing Address: P.O. Box 127, Zip 67865–0127; tel. 316/885–4264; Ronald D. Baker, Administrator

MITCHELL COUNTY HOSPITAL, 400 West Eighth, Beloit, KS, Zip 67420–1605, Mailing Address: P.O. Box 399, Zip 67420–0399; tel. 785/738–2266; John M. Osse, Administrator

OSBORNE COUNTY MEMORIAL HOSPITAL, 424 West New Hampshire Street, Osborne, KS, Zip 67473–0070, Mailing Address: P.O. Box 70, Zip 67473–0070; tel. 785/346–2121; Patricia Bernard, R.N., Administrator

OTTAWA COUNTY HEALTH CENTER, 215 East Eighth, Minneapolis, KS, Zip 67467–1999, Mailing Address: P.O. Box 290, Zip 67467–0290; tel. 785/392–2122; Joy Reed, R.N., Administrator

PHILLIPS COUNTY HOSPITAL, 1150 State Street, Phillipsburg, KS, Zip 67661–1799, Mailing Address: P.O. Box 607, Zip 67661–0607; tel. 785/543–5226; James Wahlmeier, Administrator

RAWLINS COUNTY HEALTH CENTER, 707 Grant Street, Atwood, KS, Zip 67730–4700, Mailing Address: P.O. Box 47, Zip 67730–4700; tel. 785/626–3211; Donald J. Kessen, Administrator and Chief Executive Officer

REPUBLIC COUNTY HOSPITAL, 2420 G Street, Belleville, KS, Zip 66935–2400; tel. 785/527–2254; Blaine K. Miller, Administrator

SABETHA COMMUNITY HOSPITAL, 14th and Oregon Streets, Sabetha, KS, Zip 66534–0229, Mailing Address: P.O. Box 229, Zip 66534–0229; tel. 785/284–2121; Rita K. Buurman, Chief Executive Officer

SATANTA DISTRICT HOSPITAL, 401 South Cheyenne Street, Satanta, KS, Zip 67870–0159, Mailing Address: P.O. Box 159, Zip 67870–0159; tel. 316/649–2761; T. G. Lee, Administrator

SMITH COUNTY MEMORIAL HOSPITAL, 614 South Main Street, Smith Center, KS, Zip 66967–0349, Mailing Address: P.O. Box 349, Zip 66967–0349; tel. 785/282–6845; John Terrill, Administrator

TREGO COUNTY-LEMKE MEMORIAL HOSPITAL, 320 North 13th Street, Wakeeney, KS, Zip 67672–2099; tel. 785/743–2182; Lisa J. Freeborn, R.N., Administrator

MED-OP
202 Center Avenue, Oakley, KS 67748;
tel. 913/672-3540; Andrew Draper, Executive Director

CITIZENS MEDICAL CENTER, 100 East College Drive, Colby, KS, Zip 67701–3799; tel. 785/462–7511; Michael E. Boyles, Chief Executive Officer

DECATUR COUNTY HOSPITAL AND CEDAR LIVING CENTER, 810 West Columbia Street, Oberlin, KS, Zip 67749–2450, Mailing Address: P.O. Box 268, Zip 67749–0268; tel. 785/475–2208; Lynn Doeden, Administrator

GOODLAND REGIONAL MEDICAL CENTER, 220 West Second Street, Goodland, KS, Zip 67735–1602; tel. 785/899–3625; Jim Chaddic, Chief Executive Officer

GRAHAM COUNTY HOSPITAL, 304 West Prout Street, Hill City, KS, Zip 67642–1435, Mailing Address: P.O. Box 339, Zip 67642–0339; tel. 785/421–2121; Fred J. Meis, Administrator and Chief Executive Officer

HAYS MEDICAL CENTER, 2220 Canterbury Drive, Hays, KS, Zip 67601–2342, Mailing Address: P.O. Box 8100, Zip 67601–8100; tel. 785/623–5000; John H. Jeter, M.D., President and Chief Executive Officer

LOGAN COUNTY HOSPITAL, 211 Cherry Street, Oakley, KS, Zip 67748–0211; tel. 785/672–3211; Rodney Bates, Administrator

NESS COUNTY HOSPITAL, 312 Custer Street, Ness City, KS, Zip 67560–1654; tel. 785/798–2291; Clyde T. McCracken, Administrator

NORTON COUNTY HOSPITAL, 102 East Holme, Norton, KS, Zip 67654–0250, Mailing Address: P.O. Box 250, Zip 67654–0250; tel. 785/877–3351; Richard Miller, Administrator and Chief Executive Officer

PLAINVILLE RURAL HOSPITAL DISTRICT NUMBER ONE, 304 South Colorado Avenue, Plainville, KS, Zip 67663–0389; tel. 785/434–4553; Richard Q. Bergling, Administrator and Chief Executive Officer

SHERIDAN COUNTY HEALTH COMPLEX, 826 18th Street, Hoxie, KS, Zip 67740–0167, Mailing Address: P.O. Box 167, Zip 67740–0167; tel. 785/675–3281; Brian Kirk, Chief Executive Officer

NORTHWEST KANSAS HEALTH ALLIANCE (CAH NETWORK)
2220 Canterbury Drive, Hays, KS 67601;
tel. 785/623-2301; Jodi Schmidt, Network Coordinator

CHEYENNE COUNTY HOSPITAL, 210 West First Street, Saint Francis, KS, Zip 67756–0547, Mailing Address: P.O. Box 547, Zip 67756–0547; tel. 785/332–2104; Leslie Lacy, Administrator

GRISELL MEMORIAL HOSPITAL DISTRICT ONE, 210 South Vermont, Ransom, KS, Zip 67572–0268, Mailing Address: P.O. Box 268, Zip 67572–0268; tel. 785/731–2231; Kristine Ochs, R.N., Administrator

HAYS MEDICAL CENTER, 2220 Canterbury Drive, Hays, KS, Zip 67601–2342, Mailing Address: P.O. Box 8100, Zip 67601–8100; tel. 785/623–5000; John H. Jeter, M.D., President and Chief Executive Officer

PLAINVILLE RURAL HOSPITAL DISTRICT NUMBER ONE, 304 South Colorado Avenue, Plainville, KS, Zip 67663–0389; tel. 785/434–4553; Richard Q. Bergling, Administrator and Chief Executive Officer

RAWLINS COUNTY HEALTH CENTER, 707 Grant Street, Atwood, KS, Zip 67730–4700, Mailing Address: P.O. Box 47, Zip 67730–4700; tel. 785/626–3211; Donald J. Kessen, Administrator and Chief Executive Officer

SATANTA DISTRICT HOSPITAL
P.O. Box 159, Santana, KS 67870;
tel. 316/649-2761; Tom Lee, Administrator

SATANTA DISTRICT HOSPITAL, 401 South Cheyenne Street, Satanta, KS, Zip 67870–0159, Mailing Address: P.O. Box 159, Zip 67870–0159; tel. 316/649–2761; T. G. Lee, Administrator

SUNFLOWER HEALTH NETWORK
139 N. Penn, Salina, KS 67401;
tel. 785/452-6102; Sheryl Dority, Executive Director

CLAY COUNTY MEDICAL CENTER, 617 Liberty Street, Clay Center, KS, Zip 67432–0512, Mailing Address: P.O. Box 512, Zip 67432–0512; tel. 785/632–2144; Ronald Bender, Chief Executive Officer

CLOUD COUNTY HEALTH CENTER, 1100 Highland Drive, Concordia, KS, Zip 66901–3923; tel. 785/243–1234; Daniel R. Bartz, Chief Executive Officer

Networks / Sunflower Health Network

ELLSWORTH COUNTY MEDICAL CENTER, 1604 Aylward Street, Ellsworth, KS, Zip 67439-0087; Mailing Address: P.O. Box 87, Zip 67439-0087; tel. 785/472-3111; Roger W. Pearson, Administrator

HERINGTON MUNICIPAL HOSPITAL, 100 East Helen Street, Herington, KS, Zip 67449-1606; tel. 785/258-2207; William D. Peterson, Administrator

JEWELL COUNTY HOSPITAL, 100 Crestvue Avenue, Mankato, KS, Zip 66956-2407, Mailing Address: P.O. Box 327, Zip 66956-0327; tel. 785/378-3137; Aloha Kier, Administrator

LINCOLN COUNTY HOSPITAL, 624 North Second Street, Lincoln, KS, Zip 67455-1738, Mailing Address: P.O. Box 406, Zip 67455-0406; tel. 785/524-4403; Jolene Yager, R.N., Administrator

LINDSBORG COMMUNITY HOSPITAL, 605 West Lincoln Street, Lindsborg, KS, Zip 67456-2328; tel. 785/227-3308; Greg Lundstrom, Administrator and Chief Executive Officer

MEMORIAL HOSPITAL, 511 N.E. Tenth Street, Abilene, KS, Zip 67410-2100, Mailing Address: P.O. Box 69, Zip 67410-0069; tel. 785/263-2100; Leon J. Boor, Chief Executive Officer and Administrator

MEMORIAL HOSPITAL, 1000 Hospital Drive, McPherson, KS, Zip 67460-2321; tel. 316/241-2250; Stan Regehr, President and Chief Executive Officer

MITCHELL COUNTY HOSPITAL, 400 West Eighth, Beloit, KS, Zip 67420-1605, Mailing Address: P.O. Box 399, Zip 67420-0399; tel. 785/738-2266; John M. Osse, Administrator

OSBORNE COUNTY MEMORIAL HOSPITAL, 424 West New Hampshire Street, Osborne, KS, Zip 67473-0070, Mailing Address: P.O. Box 70, Zip 67473-0070; tel. 785/346-2121; Patricia Bernard, R.N., Administrator

OTTAWA COUNTY HEALTH CENTER, 215 East Eighth, Minneapolis, KS, Zip 67467-1999, Mailing Address: P.O. Box 290, Zip 67467-0290; tel. 785/392-2122; Joy Reed, R.N., Administrator

REPUBLIC COUNTY HOSPITAL, 2420 G Street, Belleville, KS, Zip 66935-2400; tel. 785/527-2254; Blaine K. Miller, Administrator

SALINA REGIONAL HEALTH CENTER, 400 South Santa Fe Avenue, Salina, KS, Zip 67401-4198, Mailing Address: P.O. Box 5080, Zip 67401-5080; tel. 785/452-7000; Randy Peterson, President and Chief Executive Officer

SMITH COUNTY MEMORIAL HOSPITAL, 614 South Main Street, Smith Center, KS, Zip 66967-0349, Mailing Address: P.O. Box 349, Zip 66967-0349; tel. 785/282-6845; John Terrill, Administrator

ST. FRANCIS AT SALINA, 5097 West Cloud Street, Salina, KS, Zip 67401-2348; tel. 785/825-0563; Father Phillip J. Rapp, President and Chief Executive Officer

KENTUCKY

BAPTIST HEALTHCARE SYSTEM
4007 Kresge Way, Louisville, KY 40207; tel. 502/896-5000; Tommy Smith, President & Chief Executive Officer

BAPTIST HOSPITAL EAST, 4000 Kresge Way, Louisville, KY, Zip 40207-4676; tel. 502/897-8100; Susan Stout Tamme, President

BAPTIST REGIONAL MEDICAL CENTER, 1 Trillium Way, Corbin, KY, Zip 40701-8420; tel. 606/528-1212; John S. Henson, President

CENTRAL BAPTIST HOSPITAL, 1740 Nicholasville Road, Lexington, KY, Zip 40503; tel. 859/260-6100; William G. Sisson, President

HARDIN MEMORIAL HOSPITAL, 913 North Dixie Avenue, Elizabethtown, KY, Zip 42701-2599; tel. 270/737-1212; David L. Gray, President

TRI COUNTY BAPTIST HOSPITAL, 1025 New Moody Lane, La Grange, KY, Zip 40031-0559; tel. 502/222-5385; Dennis B. Johnson, Administrator

WESTERN BAPTIST HOSPITAL, 2501 Kentucky Avenue, Paducah, KY, Zip 42003-3200; tel. 270/575-2100; Larry O. Barton, President

BLUE GRASS FAMILY HEALTH PLAN
651 Perimeter Drive, Lexington, KY 40517; tel. 606/264-4475; Jim Fritz, Chief Executive Officer

BAPTIST REGIONAL MEDICAL CENTER, 1 Trillium Way, Corbin, KY, Zip 40701-8420; tel. 606/528-1212; John S. Henson, President

BEREA HOSPITAL, 305 Estill Street, Berea, KY, Zip 40403-1909; tel. 859/986-3151; David E. Burgio, FACHE, President and Chief Executive Officer

BOURBON COMMUNITY HOSPITAL, 9 Linville Drive, Paris, KY, Zip 40361-2196; tel. 606/987-3600; Rob Smart, Chief Executive Officer

CALDWELL COUNTY HOSPITAL, 101 Hospital Drive, Princeton, KY, Zip 42445-0410, Mailing Address: Box 410, Zip 42445-0410; tel. 270/365-0300; William P. Macri, Chief Executive Officer

CARDINAL HILL REHABILITATION HOSPITAL, 2050 Versailles Road, Lexington, KY, Zip 40504-1499; tel. 859/254-5701; Kerry G. Gillihan, FACHE, President and Chief Executive Officer

CENTRAL BAPTIST HOSPITAL, 1740 Nicholasville Road, Lexington, KY, Zip 40503; tel. 859/260-6100; William G. Sisson, President

CLARK REGIONAL MEDICAL CENTER, West Lexington Avenue, Winchester, KY, Zip 40391, Mailing Address: P.O. Box 630, Zip 40392-0630; tel. 606/745-3500; Robert D. Fraraccio, Chief Executive Officer

CRITTENDEN COUNTY HOSPITAL, Highway 60 South, Marion, KY, Zip 42064, Mailing Address: P.O. Box 386, Zip 42064-0386; tel. 270/965-5281; Greg Moore, Chief Executive Officer

FLEMING COUNTY HOSPITAL, 920 Elizaville Avenue, Flemingsburg, KY, Zip 41041, Mailing Address: P.O. Box 388, Zip 41041-0388; tel. 606/849-5000; Luther E. Reeves, Chief Executive Officer

FORT LOGAN HOSPITAL, 124 Portman Avenue, Stanford, KY, Zip 40484-1200; tel. 606/365-2187; Terry C. Powers, Administrator

FRANKFORT REGIONAL MEDICAL CENTER, 299 King's Daughters Drive, Frankfort, KY, Zip 40601-4186; tel. 502/875-5240; David P. Steitz, Chief Executive Officer

GARRARD COUNTY MEMORIAL HOSPITAL, 308 West Maple Avenue, Lancaster, KY, Zip 40444-1098; tel. 859/792-6844; John P. Rigsby, Administrator

GEORGETOWN COMMUNITY HOSPITAL, 1140 Lexington Road, Georgetown, KY, Zip 40324-9362; tel. 502/868-1100; Jeffrey G. Seraphine, President and Chief Executive Officer

HARLAN ARH HOSPITAL, 81 Ball Park Road, Harlan, KY, Zip 40831-1792; tel. 606/573-8201; Daniel Fitzpatrick, Chief Executive Officer

HARRISON MEMORIAL HOSPITAL, Millersburg Road, Cynthiana, KY, Zip 41031-0250, Mailing Address: P.O. Box 250, Zip 41031-0250; tel. 859/234-2300; Darwin E. Root, Administrator

HIGHLANDS REGIONAL MEDICAL CENTER, 5000 Kentucky Route 321, Prestonsburg, KY, Zip 41653, Mailing Address: P.O. Box 668, Zip 41653-0668; tel. 606/886-8511; Harold C. Warman, Jr, President and Chief Executive Officer

JACKSON PURCHASE MEDICAL CENTER, 1099 Medical Center Circle, Mayfield, KY, Zip 42066-1179, Mailing Address: P.O. Box 1099, Zip 42066-1099; tel. 270/251-4100; Mary Jo Lewis, Chief Executive Officer

JANE TODD CRAWFORD HOSPITAL, 202-206 Milby Street, Greensburg, KY, Zip 42743-1100, Mailing Address: P.O. Box 220, Zip 42743-0220; tel. 270/932-4211; Eddy R. Stockton, Chief Executive Officer

KENTUCKY RIVER MEDICAL CENTER, 540 Jett Drive, Jackson, KY, Zip 41339-9620; tel. 606/666-6305; O. David Bevins, Chief Executive Officer

KNOX COUNTY HOSPITAL, 321 High Street, Barbourville, KY, Zip 40906-1317, Mailing Address: P.O. Box 160, Zip 40906-0160; tel. 606/546-4175; Craig Morgan, Administrator

KOSAIR CHILDREN'S HOSPITAL, 231 East Chestnut Street, Louisville, KY, Zip 40202, Mailing Address: P.O. Box 35070, Zip 40232-5070; tel. 502/629-6000; Douglas J. Eighmey, Chief Administrative Officer

MARCUM AND WALLACE MEMORIAL HOSPITAL, 60 Mercy Court, Irvine, KY, Zip 40336-1331, Mailing Address: P.O. Box 928, Zip 40336-0928; tel. 606/723-2115; James F. Heitzenrater, President and Chief Executive Officer

MARYMOUNT MEDICAL CENTER, 310 East Ninth Street, London, KY, Zip 40741-1299; tel. 606/877-3705; Lowell Jones, President and Chief Executive Officer

MEMORIAL HOSPITAL, 401 Memorial Drive, Manchester, KY, Zip 40962-9156; tel. 606/598-5104; Jimm Bunch, President and Chief Executive Officer

MIDDLESBORO APPALACHIAN REGIONAL HOSPITAL, 3600 West Cumberland Avenue, Middlesboro, KY, Zip 40965-2614, Mailing Address: P.O. Box 340, Zip 40965-0340; tel. 606/242-1101; Paul V. Miles, Administrator

MURRAY-CALLOWAY COUNTY HOSPITAL, 803 Poplar Street, Murray, KY, Zip 42071-2432; tel. 270/762-1100; Isaac S. Coe, President

NORTON AUDUBON HOSPITAL, One Audubon Plaza Drive, Louisville, KY, Zip 40217-1397, Mailing Address: P.O. Box 17550, Zip 40217-0550; tel. 502/636-7111; Thomas D. Kmetz, Chief Administrative Officer

NORTON HOSPITAL, 200 East Chestnut Street, Louisville, KY, Zip 40202-1800, Mailing Address: P.O. Box 35070, Zip 40232-5070; tel. 502/629-8000; M. Michelle Hood, Chief Administrative Officer

NORTON SOUTHWEST HOSPITAL, 9820 Third Street Road, Louisville, KY, Zip 40272-9984; tel. 502/933-8100; James W. Pope, Chief Executive Officer

NORTON SUBURBAN HOSPITAL, 4001 Dutchmans Lane, Louisville, KY, Zip 40207-4799; tel. 502/893-1000; John D. Harryman, President and Chief Executive Officer

OUR LADY OF THE WAY HOSPITAL, 11022 Main Street, Martin, KY, Zip 41649-0910; tel. 606/285-5181; Lowell Jones, Chief Executive Officer

OWEN COUNTY MEMORIAL HOSPITAL, 330 Roland Avenue, Owenton, KY, Zip 40359-1502; tel. 502/484-3441; Richard D. McLeod, Administrator

PARKWAY REGIONAL HOSPITAL, 2000 Holiday Lane, Fulton, KY, Zip 42041; tel. 270/472-2522; Michael Patterson, Chief Executive Officer

PATTIE A. CLAY HOSPITAL, EKU By-Pass, Richmond, KY, Zip 40475, Mailing Address: P.O. Box 1600, Zip 40476-2603; tel. 859/623-3131; Richard M. Thomas, President

PAUL B. HALL REGIONAL MEDICAL CENTER, 625 James South Trimble Boulevard, Paintsville, KY, Zip 41240-0000; tel. 606/789-3511; Deborah L. Trimble, Administrator

PINEVILLE COMMUNITY HOSPITAL ASSOCIATION, 850 Riverview Avenue, Pineville, KY, Zip 40977-0850; tel. 606/337-3051; J. Milton Brooks, II, Administrator

SAINT JOSEPH HOSPITAL, One St. Joseph Drive, Lexington, KY, Zip 40504-3754; tel. 606/278-3436; Tom Matherlee, Interim Chief Executive Officer

SAMARITAN HOSPITAL, 310 South Limestone Street, Lexington, KY, Zip 40508-3008; tel. 606/226-7151; Frank Beirne, Chief Executive Officer

THE JAMES B. HAGGIN MEMORIAL HOSPITAL, 464 Linden Avenue, Harrodsburg, KY, Zip 40330-1862; tel. 859/734-5441; Earl James Motzer, Ph.D., FACHE, Chief Executive Officer

Networks / CHA Provider Network, Inc.

UNIVERSITY OF KENTUCKY HOSPITAL, 800 Rose Street, Lexington, KY, Zip 40536-0084; tel. 859/323-5000; Frank Butler, Director

VENCOR HOSPITAL–LOUISVILLE, 1313 St. Anthony Place, Louisville, KY, Zip 40204-1765; tel. 502/587-7001; James H. Wesp, Administrator

WESTLAKE REGIONAL HOSPITAL, Westlake Drive, Columbia, KY, Zip 42728-1149, Mailing Address: P.O. Box 468, Zip 42728-0468; tel. 270/384-4753; Rex A. Tungate, Administrator

CARITAS HEALTH SERVICES
1850 Bluegrass Avenue, Louisville, KY 40215; tel. 502/361-6140; Conrad H. Thorne, Chief of Network Operations

CARITAS MEDICAL CENTER, 1850 Bluegrass Avenue, Louisville, KY, Zip 40215-1199; tel. 502/361-6000; Peter J. Bernard, President and Chief Executive Officer

CARITAS PEACE CENTER, 2020 Newburg Road, Louisville, KY, Zip 40205-1879; tel. 502/451-3330; Peter J. Bernard, President and Chief Executive Officer

CENTER CARE
1225 Fairway Street, Bowling Green, KY 42103; tel. 270/745-1517; Sean McGuinness, Director, Sales & Provider Relations

BAPTIST HOSPITAL, 2000 Church Street, Nashville, TN, Zip 37236-0002; tel. 615/329-5555; Erie Chapman, II, President and Chief Executive Officer

BAPTIST HOSPITAL EAST, 4000 Kresge Way, Louisville, KY, Zip 40207-4676; tel. 502/897-8100; Susan Stout Tamme, President

BAPTIST REGIONAL MEDICAL CENTER, 1 Trillium Way, Corbin, KY, Zip 40701-8420; tel. 606/528-1212; John S. Henson, President

BEDFORD COUNTY MEDICAL CENTER, 845 Union Street, Shelbyville, TN, Zip 37160-9971; tel. 931/685-5433; David M. Snyder, Chief Executive Officer

CAVERNA MEMORIAL HOSPITAL, 1501 South Dixie Street, Horse Cave, KY, Zip 42749-1477; tel. 270/786-2191; Alan B. Alexander, Administrator

CENTRAL BAPTIST HOSPITAL, 1740 Nicholasville Road, Lexington, KY, Zip 40503; tel. 859/260-6100; William G. Sisson, President

CHRIST HOSPITAL, 2139 Auburn Avenue, Cincinnati, OH, Zip 45219-2989; tel. 513/585-2000; Richard L. Seim, Senior Vice President

CLINTON COUNTY HOSPITAL, 723 Burkesville Road, Albany, KY, Zip 42602-1654; tel. 606/387-6421; Randel Flowers, Ph.D., Administrator

COFFEE MEDICAL CENTER, 1001 McArthur Drive, Manchester, TN, Zip 37355-2455, Mailing Address: P.O. Box 1079, Zip 37349-1079; tel. 931/728-3586; James L. Muse, Administrator

COOKEVILLE REGIONAL MEDICAL CENTER, 142 West Fifth Street, Cookeville, TN, Zip 38501-1760, Mailing Address: P.O. Box 340, Zip 38503-0340; tel. 931/528-2541; Tod N. Lambert, Administrator and Chief Executive Officer

CUMBERLAND COUNTY HOSPITAL, Highway 90 West, Burkesville, KY, Zip 42717-0280, Mailing Address: P.O. Box 280, Zip 42717-0280; tel. 270/864-2511; Edward J. Sanford, Chief Executive Officer

DAUTERIVE HOSPITAL, 600 North Lewis Street, New Iberia, LA, Zip 70560, Mailing Address: P.O. Box 11210, Zip 70562-1210; tel. 318/365-7311; Kyle J. Viator, Chief Executive Officer

DOCTORS' HOSPITAL OF OPELOUSAS, 3972 I-49 South Service Road, Opelousas, LA, Zip 70570-8975; tel. 318/948-2100; Bethy W. Walker, Chief Executive Officer

GATEWAY HEALTH SYSTEM, 1771 Madison Street, Clarksville, TN, Zip 37043-4900, Mailing Address: P.O. Box 3160, Zip 37043-3160; tel. 931/552-6622; James Lee Decker, President and Chief Executive Officer

GOOD SAMARITAN HOSPITAL, 375 Dixmyth Avenue, Cincinnati, OH, Zip 45220-2489; tel. 513/872-1400; John S. Prout, President and Chief Executive Officer

HARDIN MEMORIAL HOSPITAL, 913 North Dixie Avenue, Elizabethtown, KY, Zip 42701-2599; tel. 270/737-1212; David L. Gray, President

HARTON REGIONAL MEDICAL CENTER, 1801 North Jackson Street, Tullahoma, TN, Zip 37388-2201, Mailing Address: P.O. Box 460, Zip 37388-0460; tel. 931/393-3000; David C. Wilson, Chief Executive Officer

HEALTHSOUTH REHABILITATION HOSPITAL OF CENTRAL KENTUCKY, 134 Heartland Drive, Elizabethtown, KY, Zip 42701-2778; tel. 270/769-3100; Mark K. Floro, Chief Operating Officer

HENDERSONVILLE HOSPITAL, 355 New Shackle Island Road, Hendersonville, TN, Zip 37075-2393; tel. 615/264-4000; Robert Klein, Chief Executive Officer

JACKSON PURCHASE MEDICAL CENTER, 1099 Medical Center Circle, Mayfield, KY, Zip 42066-1179, Mailing Address: P.O. Box 1099, Zip 42066-1099; tel. 270/251-4100; Mary Jo Lewis, Chief Executive Officer

JEWISH HOSPITAL, 217 East Chestnut Street, Louisville, KY, Zip 40202-1886; tel. 502/587-4011; Douglas E. Shaw, President

LOGAN MEMORIAL HOSPITAL, 1625 South Nashville Road, Russellville, KY, Zip 42276-8834, Mailing Address: P.O. Box 10, Zip 42276-0010; tel. 270/726-4011; Michael Clark, Chief Executive Officer

MACON COUNTY GENERAL HOSPITAL, 204 Medical Drive, Lafayette, TN, Zip 37083-1799, Mailing Address: P.O. Box 378, Zip 37083-0378; tel. 615/666-2147; Dennis A. Wolford, FACHE, Administrator

MEADOWVIEW REGIONAL MEDICAL CENTER, 989 Medical Park Drive, Maysville, KY, Zip 41056-8750; tel. 606/759-5311; Curtis B. Courtney, Chief Executive Officer

MEDICAL CENTER OF MANCHESTER, 481 Interstate Drive, Manchester, TN, Zip 37355-3108, Mailing Address: P.O. Box 1409, Zip 37349-1409; tel. 931/728-6354; Robert C. Couch, Chief Executive Officer

MEDICAL CENTER OF SOUTHWEST LOUISIANA, 2810 Ambassador Caffery Parkway, Lafayette, LA, Zip 70506-5900; tel. 318/981-2949; Stephen K. Jones, Jr, Chief Executive Officer

MONROE COUNTY MEDICAL CENTER, 529 Capp Harlan Road, Tompkinsville, KY, Zip 42167-1840; tel. 270/487-9231; Mark E. Thompson, Chief Executive Officer

MUHLENBERG COMMUNITY HOSPITAL, 440 Hopkinsville Street, Greenville, KY, Zip 42345-1172, Mailing Address: P.O. Box 387, Zip 42345-0387; tel. 270/338-8000; Albert Pilkington, II, Chief Executive Officer

NASHVILLE MEMORIAL HOSPITAL, 612 West Due West Avenue, Madison, TN, Zip 37115-4474; tel. 615/865-3511; Allyn R. Harris, Chief Executive Officer

NORTH OAKS MEDICAL CENTER, 15790 Medical Center Drive, Hammond, LA, Zip 70403-1436, Mailing Address: P.O. Box 2668, Zip 70404-2668; tel. 504/345-2700; James E. Cathey, Jr, Chief Executive Officer

OHIO COUNTY HOSPITAL, 1211 Main Street, Hartford, KY, Zip 42347-1619; tel. 270/298-7411; Blaine Pieper, Administrator

OWENSBORO MERCY HEALTH SYSTEM, 811 East Parrish Avenue, Owensboro, KY, Zip 42303-3268, Mailing Address: P.O. Box 20007, Zip 42303-0007; tel. 270/688-2000; Greg L. Carlson, President and Chief Executive Officer

PIKEVILLE UNITED METHODIST HOSPITAL OF KENTUCKY, 911 South Bypass, Pikeville, KY, Zip 41501-1595; tel. 606/437-3500; Walter E. May, Interim Administrator

SAINT JOSEPH HOSPITAL, One St. Joseph Drive, Lexington, KY, Zip 40504-3754; tel. 606/278-3436; Tom Matherlee, Interim Chief Executive Officer

SOUTHERN TENNESSEE MEDICAL CENTER, 185 Hospital Road, Winchester, TN, Zip 37398-2468; tel. 931/967-8200; William Russell Spray, Chief Executive Officer

ST. ELIZABETH MEDICAL CENTER–GRANT COUNTY, 238 Barnes Road, Williamstown, KY, Zip 41097-9460; tel. 606/824-2400; Chris Carle, Administrator

ST. ELIZABETH MEDICAL CENTER–SOUTH, One Medical Village Drive, Edgewood, KY, Zip 41017; tel. 859/344-2000; Joseph W. Gross, President and Chief Executive Officer

ST. THOMAS HEALTH SERVICES, 4220 Harding Road, Nashville, TN, Zip 37205-2095, Mailing Address: P.O. Box 380, Zip 37202-0380; tel. 615/222-2111; Thomas E. Beeman, President and Chief Executive Officer

SUMNER REGIONAL MEDICAL CENTER, 555 Hartsville Pike, Gallatin, TN, Zip 37066-2449, Mailing Address: P.O. Box 1558, Zip 37066-1558; tel. 615/452-4210; William T. Sugg, President and Chief Executive Officer

T. J. SAMSON COMMUNITY HOSPITAL, 1301 North Race Street, Glasgow, KY, Zip 42141-3483; tel. 270/651-4444; Dwayne Moss, Chief Executive Officer

TAYLOR COUNTY HOSPITAL, 1700 Old Lebanon Road, Campbellsville, KY, Zip 42718-9600; tel. 270/465-3561; David R. Hayes, President

THE JAMES B. HAGGIN MEMORIAL HOSPITAL, 464 Linden Avenue, Harrodsburg, KY, Zip 40330-1862; tel. 859/734-5441; Earl James Motzer, Ph.D., FACHE, Chief Executive Officer

THE MEDICAL CENTER AT BOWLING GREEN, 250 Park Street, Bowling Green, KY, Zip 42101-1795, Mailing Address: P.O. Box 90010, Zip 42102-9010; tel. 270/745-1000; Connie Smith, Chief Executive Officer

THE MEDICAL CENTER AT FRANKLIN, Brookhaven Road, Franklin, KY, Zip 42135-2929, Mailing Address: P.O. Box 2929, Zip 42135-2929; tel. 270/586-3253; Jeffrey L. Durham, Chief Executive Officer

TWIN LAKES REGIONAL MEDICAL CENTER, 910 Wallace Avenue, Leitchfield, KY, Zip 42754-1499; tel. 270/259-9400; Stephen L. Meredith, Chief Executive Officer

UNIVERSITY MEDICAL CENTER/MCFARLAND HOSPITAL, 1411 Baddour Parkway, Lebanon, TN, Zip 37087-2573; tel. 615/444-8262; Larry W. Keller, Chief Executive Officer

WESTLAKE REGIONAL HOSPITAL, Westlake Drive, Columbia, KY, Zip 42728-1149, Mailing Address: P.O. Box 468, Zip 42728-0468; tel. 270/384-4753; Rex A. Tungate, Administrator

WILLIAMSON MEDICAL CENTER, 2021 Carothers Road, Franklin, TN, Zip 37067-5822, Mailing Address: P.O. Box 681600, Zip 37068-1600; tel. 615/791-0500; Ronald G. Joyner, Chief Executive Officer

WOMEN'S AND CHILDREN'S HOSPITAL, 4600 Ambassador Caffery Parkway, Lafayette, LA, Zip 70508-6923, Mailing Address: P.O. Box 88030, Zip 70598-8030; tel. 337/981-9100; Susan Silverman, Chief Executive Officer

CHA PROVIDER NETWORK, INC.
P.O. Box 24647, Lexington, KY 40524; tel. 606/323-0285; Sallie J. Carter, Network Account Manager

ARH REGIONAL MEDICAL CENTER, 100 Medical Center Drive, Hazard, KY, Zip 41701-1000; tel. 606/439-6833; Charles E. Housley, FACHE, Administrator

BAPTIST HOSPITAL, 2000 Church Street, Nashville, TN, Zip 37236-0002; tel. 615/329-5555; Erie Chapman, II, President and Chief Executive Officer

BECKLEY APPALACHIAN REGIONAL HOSPITAL, 306 Stanaford Road, Beckley, WV, Zip 25801-3142; tel. 304/255-3000; David R. Lyon, Administrator

BEREA HOSPITAL, 305 Estill Street, Berea, KY, Zip 40403-1909; tel. 859/986-3151; David E. Burgio, FACHE, President and Chief Executive Officer

Networks / CHA Provider Network, Inc.

BOONE MEMORIAL HOSPITAL, 701 Madison Avenue, Madison, WV, Zip 25130–1699; tel. 304/369–1230; Tommy H. Mullins, Administrator

CABELL HUNTINGTON HOSPITAL, 1340 Hal Greer Boulevard, Huntington, WV, Zip 25701–0195; tel. 304/526–2000; W. Don Smith, II, President and Chief Executive Officer

CARDINAL HILL REHABILITATION HOSPITAL, 2050 Versailles Road, Lexington, KY, Zip 40504–1499; tel. 859/254–5701; Kerry G. Gillihan, FACHE, President and Chief Executive Officer

CAVERNA MEMORIAL HOSPITAL, 1501 South Dixie Street, Horse Cave, KY, Zip 42749–1477; tel. 270/786–2191; Alan B. Alexander, Administrator

CENTRAL BAPTIST HOSPITAL, 1740 Nicholasville Road, Lexington, KY, Zip 40503; tel. 859/260–6100; William G. Sisson, President

CHARTER RIDGE BEHAVIORAL HEALTH SYSTEM, 3050 Rio Dosa Drive, Lexington, KY, Zip 40509–9990; tel. 606/269–2325; Barbara Kitchen, Chief Executive Officer

CHRIST HOSPITAL, 2139 Auburn Avenue, Cincinnati, OH, Zip 45219–2989; tel. 513/585–2000; Richard L. Seim, Senior Vice President

CLAIBORNE COUNTY HOSPITAL, 1850 Old Knoxville Road, Tazewell, TN, Zip 37879–3625, Mailing Address: P.O. Box 219, Zip 37879–0219; tel. 423/626–4211; Michael T. Hutchins, Administrator

CLARK REGIONAL MEDICAL CENTER, West Lexington Avenue, Winchester, KY, Zip 40391, Mailing Address: P.O. Box 630, Zip 40392–0630; tel. 606/745–3500; Robert D. Fraraccio, Chief Executive Officer

CLINTON COUNTY HOSPITAL, 723 Burkesville Road, Albany, KY, Zip 42602–1654; tel. 606/387–6421; Randel Flowers, Ph.D., Administrator

EPHRAIM MCDOWELL REGIONAL MEDICAL CENTER, 217 South Third Street, Danville, KY, Zip 40422–9983; tel. 606/239–1000; Thomas W. Smith, President and Chief Executive Officer

FLEMING COUNTY HOSPITAL, 920 Elizaville Avenue, Flemingsburg, KY, Zip 41041, Mailing Address: P.O. Box 388, Zip 41041–0388; tel. 606/849–5000; Luther E. Reeves, Chief Executive Officer

FORT LOGAN HOSPITAL, 124 Portman Avenue, Stanford, KY, Zip 40484–1200; tel. 606/365–2187; Terry C. Powers, Administrator

FORT SANDERS LOUDON MEDICAL CENTER, 1125 Grove Street, Loudon, TN, Zip 37774–1512, Mailing Address: P.O. Box 217, Zip 37774–0217; tel. 865/458–8222; Martha O'Regan Chill, Administrator

FORT SANDERS REGIONAL MEDICAL CENTER, 1901 Clinch Avenue S.W., Knoxville, TN, Zip 37916–2394; tel. 423/541–1111; Richard Rose, M.D., President and Chief Administrative Officer

FORT SANDERS–PARKWEST MEDICAL CENTER, 9352 Park West Boulevard, Knoxville, TN, Zip 37923–4387, Mailing Address: P.O. Box 22993, Zip 37933–0993; tel. 865/693–5151; Wayne S. Heatherly, President and Chief Administrative Officer

FORT SANDERS–SEVIER MEDICAL CENTER, 709 Middle Creek Road, Sevierville, TN, Zip 37862–5016, Mailing Address: P.O. Box 8005, Zip 37864–8005; tel. 865/429–6100; Ellen Wilhoit, President and Chief Administrative Officer

GARRARD COUNTY MEMORIAL HOSPITAL, 308 West Maple Avenue, Lancaster, KY, Zip 40444–1098; tel. 859/792–6844; John P. Rigsby, Administrator

HARDIN MEMORIAL HOSPITAL, 913 North Dixie Avenue, Elizabethtown, KY, Zip 42701–2599; tel. 270/737–1212; David L. Gray, President

HARLAN ARH HOSPITAL, 81 Ball Park Road, Harlan, KY, Zip 40831–1792; tel. 606/573–8201; Daniel Fitzpatrick, Chief Executive Officer

HARRISON MEMORIAL HOSPITAL, Millersburg Road, Cynthiana, KY, Zip 41031–0250, Mailing Address: P.O. Box 250, Zip 41031–0250; tel. 859/234–2300; Darwin E. Root, Administrator

HEALTHSOUTH HUNTINGTON REHABILITATION HOSPITAL, 6900 West Country Club Drive, Huntington, WV, Zip 25705–2000; tel. 304/733–1060; John Forester, Chief Operating Officer

HEALTHSOUTH REHABILITATION HOSPITAL OF CENTRAL KENTUCKY, 134 Heartland Drive, Elizabethtown, KY, Zip 42701–2778; tel. 270/769–3100; Mark K. Floro, Chief Operating Officer

HIGHLANDS REGIONAL MEDICAL CENTER, 5000 Kentucky Route 321, Prestonsburg, KY, Zip 41653, Mailing Address: P.O. Box 668, Zip 41653–0668; tel. 606/886–8511; Harold C. Warman, Jr, President and Chief Executive Officer

JANE TODD CRAWFORD HOSPITAL, 202–206 Milby Street, Greensburg, KY, Zip 42743–1100, Mailing Address: P.O. Box 220, Zip 42743–0220; tel. 270/932–4211; Eddy R. Stockton, Chief Executive Officer

JENKINS COMMUNITY HOSPITAL, Main Street, Jenkins, KY, Zip 41537–9614, Mailing Address: P.O. Box 472, Zip 41537–0472; tel. 606/832–2171; Sherrie Newcomb, Administrator

JEWISH HOSPITAL, 217 East Chestnut Street, Louisville, KY, Zip 40202–1886; tel. 502/587–4011; Douglas E. Shaw, President

JEWISH HOSPITAL KENWOOD, 4777 East Galbraith Road, Cincinnati, OH, Zip 45236; tel. 513/686–3000; M. Aurora Lambert, Senior Vice President

KENTUCKY RIVER MEDICAL CENTER, 540 Jett Drive, Jackson, KY, Zip 41339–9620; tel. 606/666–6305; O. David Bevins, Chief Executive Officer

KNOX COUNTY HOSPITAL, 321 High Street, Barbourville, KY, Zip 40906–1317, Mailing Address: P.O. Box 160, Zip 40906–0160; tel. 606/546–4175; Craig Morgan, Administrator

LOGAN MEMORIAL HOSPITAL, 1625 South Nashville Road, Russellville, KY, Zip 42276–8834, Mailing Address: P.O. Box 10, Zip 42276–0010; tel. 270/726–4011; Michael Clark, Chief Executive Officer

MAN ARH HOSPITAL, 700 East McDonald Avenue, Man, WV, Zip 25635–1011; tel. 304/583–8421; Erica McDonald, Administrator

MARCUM AND WALLACE MEMORIAL HOSPITAL, 60 Mercy Court, Irvine, KY, Zip 40336–1331, Mailing Address: P.O. Box 928, Zip 40336–0928; tel. 606/723–2115; James F. Heitzenrater, President and Chief Executive Officer

MARY BRECKINRIDGE HOSPITAL, 130 Kate Ireland Drive, Hyden, KY, Zip 41749–0000; tel. 606/672–2901; Mallie S. Noble, Administrator

MARYMOUNT MEDICAL CENTER, 310 East Ninth Street, London, KY, Zip 40741–1299; tel. 606/877–3705; Lowell Jones, President and Chief Executive Officer

MCDOWELL ARH HOSPITAL, Route 122, McDowell, KY, Zip 41647, Mailing Address: P.O. Box 247, Mc Dowell, Zip 41647–0247; tel. 606/377–3400; Dena C. Sparkman, Administrator

MEMORIAL HOSPITAL, 401 Memorial Drive, Manchester, KY, Zip 40962–9156; tel. 606/598–5104; Jimm Bunch, President and Chief Executive Officer

MIDDLESBORO APPALACHIAN REGIONAL HOSPITAL, 3600 West Cumberland Avenue, Middlesboro, KY, Zip 40965–2614, Mailing Address: P.O. Box 340, Zip 40965–0340; tel. 606/242–1101; Paul V. Miles, Administrator

MONROE COUNTY MEDICAL CENTER, 529 Capp Harlan Road, Tompkinsville, KY, Zip 42167–1840; tel. 270/487–9231; Mark E. Thompson, Chief Executive Officer

MORGAN COUNTY APPALACHIAN REGIONAL HOSPITAL, 476 Liberty Road, West Liberty, KY, Zip 41472–2049, Mailing Address: P.O. Box 579, Zip 41472–0579; tel. 606/743–3186; Dennis R. Chaney, Administrator

NASHVILLE MEMORIAL HOSPITAL, 612 West Due West Avenue, Madison, TN, Zip 37115–4474; tel. 615/865–3511; Allyn R. Harris, Chief Executive Officer

NICHOLAS COUNTY HOSPITAL, 2323 Concrete Road, Carlisle, KY, Zip 40311–9721, Mailing Address: P.O. Box 232, Zip 40311–0232; tel. 606/289–7181; Doris Ecton, Administrator and Chief Executive Officer

OUR LADY OF BELLEFONTE HOSPITAL, St. Christopher Drive, Ashland, KY, Zip 41101, Mailing Address: P.O. Box 789, Zip 41105–0789; tel. 606/833–3333; Robert J. Maher, President

OUR LADY OF THE WAY HOSPITAL, 11022 Main Street, Martin, KY, Zip 41649–0910; tel. 606/285–5181; Lowell Jones, Chief Executive Officer

OWEN COUNTY MEMORIAL HOSPITAL, 330 Roland Avenue, Owenton, KY, Zip 40359–1502; tel. 502/484–3441; Richard D. McLeod, Administrator

PATTIE A. CLAY HOSPITAL, EKU By–Pass, Richmond, KY, Zip 40475, Mailing Address: P.O. Box 1600, Zip 40476–2603; tel. 859/623–3131; Richard M. Thomas, President

PAUL B. HALL REGIONAL MEDICAL CENTER, 625 James South Trimble Boulevard, Paintsville, KY, Zip 41240–0000; tel. 606/789–3511; Deborah L. Trimble, Administrator

PENINSULA HOSPITAL, 2347 Jones Bend Road, Louisville, TN, Zip 37777–5213, Mailing Address: P.O. Box 2000, Zip 37777–2000; tel. 423/970–9800; Barbara S. Blevins, President

PINEVILLE COMMUNITY HOSPITAL ASSOCIATION, 850 Riverview Avenue, Pineville, KY, Zip 40977–0850; tel. 606/337–3051; J. Milton Brooks, II, Administrator

ROCKCASTLE HOSPITAL AND RESPIRATORY CARE CENTER, 145 Newcomb Avenue, Mount Vernon, KY, Zip 40456–2733, Mailing Address: P.O. Box 1310, Zip 40456–1310; tel. 606/256–2195; Lee D. Keene, President and Chief Executive Officer

RUSSELL COUNTY HOSPITAL, Dowell Road, Russell Springs, KY, Zip 42642, Mailing Address: P.O. Box 1610, Zip 42642–1610; tel. 270/866–4141; Patricia Ekdahl, President and Chief Executive Officer

ST. CLAIRE MEDICAL CENTER, 222 Medical Circle, Morehead, KY, Zip 40351–1180; tel. 606/783–6500; Mark J. Neff, President and Chief Executive Officer

ST. LUKE HOSPITAL EAST, 85 North Grand Avenue, Fort Thomas, KY, Zip 41075–1796; tel. 869/572–3100; Daniel M. Vinson, CPA, Senior Vice President

ST. LUKE HOSPITAL WEST, 7380 Turfway Road, Florence, KY, Zip 41042–1337; tel. 859/962–5200; Daniel M. Vinson, CPA, Senior Vice President

ST. MARY'S HEALTH SYSTEM, 900 East Oak Hill Avenue, Knoxville, TN, Zip 37917–4556; tel. 865/545–8000; Richard C. Williams, President and Chief Executive Officer

ST. MARY'S HOSPITAL, 2900 First Avenue, Huntington, WV, Zip 25702–1272; tel. 304/526–1234; J. Thomas Jones, Executive Director

ST. THOMAS HEALTH SERVICES, 4220 Harding Road, Nashville, TN, Zip 37205–2095, Mailing Address: P.O. Box 380, Zip 37202–0380; tel. 615/222–2111; Thomas E. Beeman, President and Chief Executive Officer

SUMMERS COUNTY APPALACHIAN REGIONAL HOSPITAL, Terrace Street, Hinton, WV, Zip 25951, Mailing Address: Drawer 940, Zip 25951–0940; tel. 304/466–1000; Rocco K. Massey, Administrator

Networks / Norton Healthcare, Inc.

T. J. SAMSON COMMUNITY HOSPITAL, 1301 North Race Street, Glasgow, KY, Zip 42141–3483; tel. 270/651–4444; Dwayne Moss, Chief Executive Officer

TAYLOR COUNTY HOSPITAL, 1700 Old Lebanon Road, Campbellsville, KY, Zip 42718–9600; tel. 270/465–3561; David R. Hayes, President

TENNESSEE CHRISTIAN MEDICAL CENTER, 500 Hospital Drive, Madison, TN, Zip 37115–5032; tel. 615/865–2373; Clint Kreitner, President and Chief Executive Officer

THE JAMES B. HAGGIN MEMORIAL HOSPITAL, 464 Linden Avenue, Harrodsburg, KY, Zip 40330–1862; tel. 859/734–5441; Earl James Motzer, Ph.D., FACHE, Chief Executive Officer

THE MEDICAL CENTER AT FRANKLIN, Brookhaven Road, Franklin, KY, Zip 42135–2929, Mailing Address: P.O. Box 2929, Zip 42135–2929; tel. 270/586–3253; Jeffrey L. Durham, Chief Executive Officer

THREE RIVERS MEDICAL CENTER, Highway 644, Louisa, KY, Zip 41230, Mailing Address: P.O. Box 769, Zip 41230–0769; tel. 606/638–9451; Greg Kiser, Chief Executive Officer

UNIVERSITY HOSPITAL, 234 Goodman Street, Cincinnati, OH, Zip 45219–2316; tel. 513/584–1000; Elliot G. Cohen, Senior Vice President

UNIVERSITY OF KENTUCKY HOSPITAL, 800 Rose Street, Lexington, KY, Zip 40536–0084; tel. 859/323–5000; Frank Butler, Director

VANDERBILT UNIVERSITY HOSPITAL, 1161 21st Avenue South, Nashville, TN, Zip 37232; tel. 615/322–5000; Mark L. Penkhus, Chief Executive Officer

WELLMONT HOLSTON VALLEY MEDICAL CENTER, West Ravine Street, Kingsport, TN, Zip 37662–0224, Mailing Address: Box 238, Zip 37662–0224; tel. 423/224–4000; Louis H. Bremer, President and Chief Executive Officer

WELLMONT LONESOME PINE HOSPITAL, 1990 Holton Avenue East, Big Stone Gap, VA, Zip 24219–0230; tel. 540/523–3111; Paul A. Bishop, Administrator

WHITESBURG APPALACHIAN REGIONAL HOSPITAL, 240 Hospital Road, Whitesburg, KY, Zip 41858–1254; tel. 606/633–3600; Donald Fields, Administrator

WILLIAMSON ARH HOSPITAL, 260 Hospital Drive, South Williamson, KY, Zip 41503–4072; tel. 606/237–1710; Louis G. Roe, Jr, Administrator

COMMUNITY CARE NETWORK
110 A. Second Street, Henderson, KY 42420; tel. 502/827–7380; Elizabeth Johnson, Director of Marketing

CALDWELL COUNTY HOSPITAL, 101 Hospital Drive, Princeton, KY, Zip 42445–0410, Mailing Address: Box 410, Zip 42445–0410; tel. 270/365–0300; William P. Macri, Chief Executive Officer

CRITTENDEN COUNTY HOSPITAL, Highway 60 South, Marion, KY, Zip 42064, Mailing Address: P.O. Box 386, Zip 42064–0386; tel. 270/965–5281; Greg Moore, Chief Executive Officer

JENNIE STUART MEDICAL CENTER, 320 West 18th Street, Hopkinsville, KY, Zip 42241–2400, Mailing Address: P.O. Box 2400, Zip 42241–2400; tel. 270/887–0100; Lewis T. Peeples, Chief Executive Officer

LIVINGSTON HOSPITAL AND HEALTHCARE SERVICES, 131 Hospital Drive, Salem, KY, Zip 42078; tel. 270/988–2299; Yvonne Maddux, Interim Chief Executive Officer

METHODIST HOSPITAL, 1305 North Elm Street, Henderson, KY, Zip 42420–2775, Mailing Address: P.O. Box 48, Zip 42420–0048; tel. 270/827–7700; Bruce D. Begley, Executive Director

METHODIST HOSPITAL UNION COUNTY, 4604 Highway 60 West, Morganfield, KY, Zip 42437–9570; tel. 270/389–3030; Patrick Donahue, Administrator

MUHLENBERG COMMUNITY HOSPITAL, 440 Hopkinsville Street, Greenville, KY, Zip 42345–1172, Mailing Address: P.O. Box 387, Zip 42345–0387; tel. 270/338–8000; Albert Pilkington, II, Chief Executive Officer

MURRAY-CALLOWAY COUNTY HOSPITAL, 803 Poplar Street, Murray, KY, Zip 42071–2432; tel. 270/762–1100; Isaac S. Coe, President

REGIONAL MEDICAL CENTER OF HOPKINS COUNTY, 900 Hospital Drive, Madisonville, KY, Zip 42431–1694; tel. 270/825–5100; Bobby H. Dampier, Chief Executive Officer

THE MEDICAL CENTER AT FRANKLIN, Brookhaven Road, Franklin, KY, Zip 42135–2929, Mailing Address: P.O. Box 2929, Zip 42135–2929; tel. 270/586–3253; Jeffrey L. Durham, Chief Executive Officer

COMMUNITY HEALTH DELIVERY SYSTEM, INC
2020 Newbrug Road, Louisville, KY 40205; tel. 502/451–3330; Fran Dotson, Network Contact

BAPTIST HOSPITAL EAST, 4000 Kresge Way, Louisville, KY, Zip 40207–4676; tel. 502/897–8100; Susan Stout Tamme, President

BAPTIST REGIONAL MEDICAL CENTER, 1 Trillium Way, Corbin, KY, Zip 40701–8420; tel. 606/528–1212; John S. Henson, President

BRECKINRIDGE MEMORIAL HOSPITAL, 1011 Old Highway 60, Hardinsburg, KY, Zip 40143–2597; tel. 270/756–7000; George Walz, CHE, Chief Executive Officer

CALDWELL COUNTY HOSPITAL, 101 Hospital Drive, Princeton, KY, Zip 42445–0410, Mailing Address: Box 410, Zip 42445–0410; tel. 270/365–0300; William P. Macri, Chief Executive Officer

CARITAS MEDICAL CENTER, 1850 Bluegrass Avenue, Louisville, KY, Zip 40215–1199; tel. 502/361–6000; Peter J. Bernard, President and Chief Executive Officer

CARITAS PEACE CENTER, 2020 Newburg Road, Louisville, KY, Zip 40205–1879; tel. 502/451–3330; Peter J. Bernard, President and Chief Executive Officer

CARROLL COUNTY HOSPITAL, 309 11th Street, Carrollton, KY, Zip 41008–1400; tel. 502/732–4321; Roger Williams, Chief Executive Officer

CAVERNA MEMORIAL HOSPITAL, 1501 South Dixie Street, Horse Cave, KY, Zip 42749–1477; tel. 270/786–2191; Alan B. Alexander, Administrator

CENTRAL BAPTIST HOSPITAL, 1740 Nicholasville Road, Lexington, KY, Zip 40503; tel. 859/260–6100; William G. Sisson, President

FLAGET MEMORIAL HOSPITAL, 201 Cathedral Manor, Bardstown, KY, Zip 40004–1299; tel. 502/348–3923; Suzanne Reasbeck, President and Chief Executive Officer

JANE TODD CRAWFORD HOSPITAL, 202–206 Milby Street, Greensburg, KY, Zip 42743–1100, Mailing Address: P.O. Box 220, Zip 42743–0220; tel. 270/932–4211; Eddy R. Stockton, Chief Executive Officer

MARYMOUNT MEDICAL CENTER, 310 East Ninth Street, London, KY, Zip 40741–1299; tel. 606/877–3705; Lowell Jones, President and Chief Executive Officer

NORTON HOSPITAL, 200 East Chestnut Street, Louisville, KY, Zip 40202–1800, Mailing Address: P.O. Box 35070, Zip 40232–5070; tel. 502/629–8000; M. Michelle Hood, Chief Administrative Officer

SAINT JOSEPH HOSPITAL, One St. Joseph Drive, Lexington, KY, Zip 40504–3754; tel. 606/278–3436; Tom Matherlee, Interim Chief Executive Officer

ST. ELIZABETH MEDICAL CENTER–GRANT COUNTY, 238 Barnes Road, Williamstown, KY, Zip 41097–9460; tel. 606/824–2400; Chris Carle, Administrator

ST. ELIZABETH MEDICAL CENTER–SOUTH, One Medical Village Drive, Edgewood, KY, Zip 41017; tel. 859/344–2000; Joseph W. Gross, President and Chief Executive Officer

TRI COUNTY BAPTIST HOSPITAL, 1025 New Moody Lane, La Grange, KY, Zip 40031–0559; tel. 502/222–5388; Dennis B. Johnson, Administrator

TRIGG COUNTY HOSPITAL, Highway 68 East, Cadiz, KY, Zip 42211, Mailing Address: P.O. Box 312, Zip 42211–0312; tel. 270/522–3215; Richard Chapman, Administrator

TWIN LAKES REGIONAL MEDICAL CENTER, 910 Wallace Avenue, Leitchfield, KY, Zip 42754–1499; tel. 270/259–9400; Stephen L. Meredith, Chief Executive Officer

WESTERN BAPTIST HOSPITAL, 2501 Kentucky Avenue, Paducah, KY, Zip 42003–3200; tel. 270/575–2100; Larry O. Barton, President

JEWISH HOSPITAL HEALTHCARE SERVICES
201 Abraham Flexner Way, Louisville, KY 40202; tel. 502/587–4011; Greg Pugh, Manager Corp. Planning

CLARK MEMORIAL HOSPITAL, 1220 Missouri Avenue, Jeffersonville, IN, Zip 47130–3743, Mailing Address: Box 69, Zip 47131–0069; tel. 812/282–6631; Merle E. Stepp, President and Chief Executive Officer

FRAZIER REHABILITATION CENTER, 220 Abraham Flexner Way, Louisville, KY, Zip 40202–1887; tel. 502/582–7400; Barth A. Weinberg, Vice President, Inpatient Rehabilitation

JEWISH HOSPITAL, 217 East Chestnut Street, Louisville, KY, Zip 40202–1886; tel. 502/587–4011; Douglas E. Shaw, President

JEWISH HOSPITAL–SHELBYVILLE, 727 Hospital Drive, Shelbyville, KY, Zip 40065–1699; tel. 502/647–4000; Timothy L. Jarm, President

PATTIE A. CLAY HOSPITAL, EKU By-Pass, Richmond, KY, Zip 40475, Mailing Address: P.O. Box 1600, Zip 40476–2603; tel. 859/623–3131; Richard M. Thomas, President

SCOTT MEMORIAL HOSPITAL, 1415 North Gardner Street, Scottsburg, IN, Zip 47170–0430, Mailing Address: Box 430, Zip 47170–0430; tel. 812/752–8500; Clifford D. Nay, Executive Director

TAYLOR COUNTY HOSPITAL, 1700 Old Lebanon Road, Campbellsville, KY, Zip 42718–9600; tel. 270/465–3561; David R. Hayes, President

WASHINGTON COUNTY MEMORIAL HOSPITAL, 911 North Shelby Street, Salem, IN, Zip 47167; tel. 812/883–5881; Rodney M. Coats, President and Chief Executive Officer

NORTON HEALTHCARE, INC.
P.O. Box 35070, Louisville, KY 40232; tel. 502/629–8025; Angela Murphy, Research Analyst

BLACKFORD COUNTY HOSPITAL, 503 East Van Cleve Street, Hartford City, IN, Zip 47348–1897; tel. 765/348–0300; Steven J. West, Chief Executive Officer

BRECKINRIDGE MEMORIAL HOSPITAL, 1011 Old Highway 60, Hardinsburg, KY, Zip 40143–2597; tel. 270/756–7000; George Walz, CHE, Chief Executive Officer

CARROLL COUNTY HOSPITAL, 309 11th Street, Carrollton, KY, Zip 41008–1400; tel. 502/732–4321; Roger Williams, Chief Executive Officer

CAVERNA MEMORIAL HOSPITAL, 1501 South Dixie Street, Horse Cave, KY, Zip 42749–1477; tel. 270/786–2191; Alan B. Alexander, Administrator

DECATUR COUNTY MEMORIAL HOSPITAL, 720 North Lincoln Street, Greensburg, IN, Zip 47240–1398; tel. 812/663–4331; David V. Trexler, President

FAIRFIELD MEMORIAL HOSPITAL, 303 N.W. 11th Street, Fairfield, IL, Zip 62837–1203; tel. 618/842–2611

GIBSON GENERAL HOSPITAL, 1808 Sherman Drive, Princeton, IN, Zip 47670–1043; tel. 812/385–3401; Michael J. Budnick, FACHE, Administrator and Chief Executive Officer

HARRISON COUNTY HOSPITAL, 245 Atwood Street, Corydon, IN, Zip 47112–1774; tel. 812/738–4251; Steven L. Taylor, Chief Executive Officer

© 2000 AHA Guide Networks, Health Care Systems and Alliances **B19**

Networks / Norton Healthcare, Inc.

KOSAIR CHILDREN'S HOSPITAL, 231 East Chestnut Street, Louisville, KY, Zip 40202, Mailing Address: P.O. Box 35070, Zip 40232-5070; tel. 502/629-6000; Douglas J. Eighmey, Chief Administrative Officer

NORTON AUDUBON HOSPITAL, One Audubon Plaza Drive, Louisville, KY, Zip 40217-1397, Mailing Address: P.O. Box 17550, Zip 40217-0550; tel. 502/636-7111; Thomas D. Kmetz, Chief Administrative Officer

NORTON HOSPITAL, 200 East Chestnut Street, Louisville, KY, Zip 40202-1800, Mailing Address: P.O. Box 35070, Zip 40232-5070; tel. 502/629-8000; M. Michelle Hood, Chief Administrative Officer

NORTON SOUTHWEST HOSPITAL, 9820 Third Street Road, Louisville, KY, Zip 40272-9984; tel. 502/933-8100; James W. Pope, Chief Executive Officer

NORTON SPRING VIEW HOSPITAL, 320 Loretto Road, Lebanon, KY, Zip 40033-0320; tel. 270/692-3161; Barry A. Papania, Chief Executive Officer

NORTON SUBURBAN HOSPITAL, 4001 Dutchmans Lane, Louisville, KY, Zip 40207-4799; tel. 502/893-1000; John D. Harryman, President and Chief Executive Officer

PARIS COMMUNITY HOSPITAL, 721 East Court Street, Paris, IL, Zip 61944-2420; tel. 217/465-4141; John D. Fajt, FACHE, President and Chief Operating Officer

PERRY COUNTY MEMORIAL HOSPITAL, 1 Hospital Road, Tell City, IN, Zip 47586-0362; tel. 812/547-7011; Joseph A. Stuber, Chief Executive Officer

RUSH MEMORIAL HOSPITAL, 1300 North Main Street, Rushville, IN, Zip 46173-1198; tel. 765/932-4111; J. Jay Purvis, Interim Chief Executive Officer

RUSSELL COUNTY HOSPITAL, Dowell Road, Russell Springs, KY, Zip 42642, Mailing Address: P.O. Box 1610, Zip 42642-1610; tel. 270/866-4141; Patricia Ekdahl, President and Chief Executive Officer

THE JAMES B. HAGGIN MEMORIAL HOSPITAL, 464 Linden Avenue, Harrodsburg, KY, Zip 40330-1862; tel. 859/734-5441; Earl James Motzer, Ph.D., FACHE, Chief Executive Officer

TWIN LAKES REGIONAL MEDICAL CENTER, 910 Wallace Avenue, Leitchfield, KY, Zip 42754-1499; tel. 270/259-9400; Stephen L. Meredith, Chief Executive Officer

WABASH GENERAL HOSPITAL DISTRICT, 1418 College Drive, Mount Carmel, IL, Zip 62863-2638; tel. 618/262-8621; James R. Farris, CHE, Chief Executive Officer

ST ELIZABETH MEDICAL CENTER
1 Medical Village Drive, Edgewood, KY 41017; tel. 606/344-2000; Joseph W. Gross, President & Chief Executive Officer

ST. ELIZABETH MEDICAL CENTER–GRANT COUNTY, 238 Barnes Road, Williamstown, KY, Zip 41097-9460; tel. 606/824-2400; Chris Carle, Administrator

ST. ELIZABETH MEDICAL CENTER–SOUTH, One Medical Village Drive, Edgewood, KY, Zip 41017; tel. 859/344-2000; Joseph W. Gross, President and Chief Executive Officer

VENCOR, INC.
680 S. Forth Street, Louisville, KY 40202; tel. 502/569-7300; Edward Kuntz, Chief Executive Officer

LOUISIANA

FRANCISCAN MISSIONARIES OF OUR LADY
4200 Essen Lane, Baton Rouge, LA 70809; tel. 225/923-2701; John Finan Jr., President & Chief Executive Officer

ABBEVILLE GENERAL HOSPITAL, 118 North Hospital Drive, Abbeville, LA, Zip 70510-4077, Mailing Address: P.O. Box 580, Zip 70511-0580; tel. 318/893-5466; Ray A. Landry, Chief Executive Officer

ABROM KAPLAN MEMORIAL HOSPITAL, 1310 West Seventh Street, Kaplan, LA, Zip 70548-2998; tel. 318/643-8300; Lyman Trahan, Chief Executive Officer

ACADIA–ST. LANDRY HOSPITAL, 810 South Broadway Street, Church Point, LA, Zip 70525-4497; tel. 318/684-5435; Alcus Trahan, Administrator

AMERICAN LEGION HOSPITAL, 1305 Crowley Rayne Highway, Crowley, LA, Zip 70526-9410; tel. 337/783-3222; Terry W. Osborne, Chief Executive Officer

IBERIA MEDICAL CENTER, 2315 East Main Street, New Iberia, LA, Zip 70560-4031, Mailing Address: P.O. Box 13338, Zip 70562-3338; tel. 318/364-0441; James H. Youree, Interim Chief Executive Officer

JENNINGS AMERICAN LEGION HOSPITAL, 1634 Elton Road, Jennings, LA, Zip 70546-3614; tel. 318/824-2490; Terry J. Terrebonne, Chief Executive Officer

OPELOUSAS GENERAL HOSPITAL, 539 East Prudhomme Street, Opelousas, LA, Zip 70570, Mailing Address: P.O. Box 1208, Zip 70571-1208; tel. 318/948-3011; Daryl J. Doise, Administrator

OUR LADY OF LOURDES REGIONAL MEDICAL CENTER, 611 St. Landry Street, Lafayette, LA, Zip 70506-4697, Mailing Address: Box 4027, Zip 70502-4027; tel. 318/289-2000; Ronald W. Webb, Chief Executive Officer

OUR LADY OF THE LAKE REGIONAL MEDICAL CENTER, 5000 Hennessy Boulevard, Baton Rouge, LA, Zip 70808-4350; tel. 225/765-6565; Robert C. Davidge, Chief Executive Officer

ST. FRANCIS MEDICAL CENTER, 309 Jackson Street, Monroe, LA, Zip 71201-7498, Mailing Address: P.O. Box 1901, Zip 71210-1901; tel. 318/327-4000; H. Gerald Smith, President and Chief Executive Officer

LAKEVIEW REGIONAL MEDICAL CENTER
95 East Fairway Drive, Covington, LA 70433; tel. 504/867-3800; Max Lauderdale, Chief Executive Officer

LAKEVIEW REGIONAL MEDICAL CENTER, 95 East Fairway Drive, Covington, LA, Zip 70433-7507; tel. 504/867-3800; Max Lauderdale, Chief Executive Officer

OCHSNER HEALTH PLAN
One Galleria Boulevard, Suite 850, Metairie, LA 70001; tel. 504/836-6600; Leslie Borel, Manager, Marketing Research & Planning

ABBEVILLE GENERAL HOSPITAL, 118 North Hospital Drive, Abbeville, LA, Zip 70510-4077, Mailing Address: P.O. Box 580, Zip 70511-0580; tel. 318/893-5466; Ray A. Landry, Chief Executive Officer

ACADIA–ST. LANDRY HOSPITAL, 810 South Broadway Street, Church Point, LA, Zip 70525-4497; tel. 318/684-5435; Alcus Trahan, Administrator

ALLEN PARISH HOSPITAL, 108 North Sixth Avenue, Kinder, LA, Zip 70648-3519, Mailing Address: P.O. Box 1670, Zip 70648-1670; tel. 318/738-2527; William C. Jeanmard, Chief Executive Officer

BEAUREGARD MEMORIAL HOSPITAL, 600 South Pine Street, De Ridder, LA, Zip 70634-4998, Mailing Address: P.O. Box 730, Zip 70634-0730; tel. 318/462-7100; Theodore J. Badger, Jr, Chief Executive Officer

BUNKIE GENERAL HOSPITAL, 427 Evergreen Highway, Bunkie, LA, Zip 71322, Mailing Address: P.O. Box 380, Zip 71322-0380; tel. 318/346-6681; Donald L. Kannady, Chief Executive Officer

BYRD REGIONAL HOSPITAL, 1020 West Fertitta Boulevard, Leesville, LA, Zip 71446-4697; tel. 318/239-9041; Roger C. LeDoux, Chief Executive Officer

CHRISTUS SCHUMPERT BOSSIER, 2105 Airline Drive, Bossier City, LA, Zip 71111-3190; tel. 318/741-6000; Gary Kerr, Administrator

CHRISTUS SCHUMPERT MEDICAL CENTER, One St. Mary Place, Shreveport, LA, Zip 71101-4399, Mailing Address: P.O. Box 21976, Zip 71120-1076; tel. 318/681-4500; Wayne A. Sensor, Chief Executive Officer

CHRISTUS ST. FRANCES CABRINI HOSPITAL, 3330 Masonic Drive, Alexandria, LA, Zip 71301-3899; tel. 318/487-1122; Stephen F. Wright, Chief Executive Officer

DE SOTO REGIONAL HEALTH SYSTEM, 207 Jefferson Street, Mansfield, LA, Zip 71052-2603, Mailing Address: P.O. Box 1636, Zip 71052-0672; tel. 318/871-3101; William F. Barrow, President and Chief Executive Officer

DEQUINCY MEMORIAL HOSPITAL, 110 West Fourth Street, DeQuincy, LA, Zip 70633-3508, Mailing Address: P.O. Box 1166, Zip 71210-1166; tel. 318/786-1200; John A. Matheson, Administrator

HIGHLAND HOSPITAL, 1453 East Bert Kouns Industrial Loop, Shreveport, LA, Zip 71105-6050; tel. 318/798-4300; Anthony S. Sala, Jr, Chief Executive Officer

HOMER MEMORIAL HOSPITAL, 620 East College Street, Homer, LA, Zip 71040-3202; tel. 318/927-2024; James W. McClung, Acting Administrator

JENNINGS AMERICAN LEGION HOSPITAL, 1634 Elton Road, Jennings, LA, Zip 70546-3614; tel. 318/824-2490; Terry J. Terrebonne, Chief Executive Officer

LADY OF THE SEA GENERAL HOSPITAL, 200 West 134th Place, Cut Off, LA, Zip 70345-4145; tel. 504/632-6401; Lane M. Cheramie, Chief Executive Officer

LAKE CHARLES MEMORIAL HOSPITAL, 1701 Oak Park Boulevard, Lake Charles, LA, Zip 70601-8911, Mailing Address: P.O. Drawer M, Zip 70602; tel. 318/494-3000; Elton L. Williams, Jr, CPA, President

LANE MEMORIAL HOSPITAL, 6300 Main Street, Zachary, LA, Zip 70791-9990; tel. 225/658-4000; Terry G. Whittington, Chief Executive Officer and Administrator

MINDEN MEDICAL CENTER, 1 Medical Plaza, Minden, LA, Zip 71055-3330, Mailing Address: P.O. Box 5003, Zip 71058-5003; tel. 318/377-2321; George E. French, II, Chief Executive Officer

NATCHITOCHES PARISH HOSPITAL, 501 Keyser Avenue, Natchitoches, LA, Zip 71457-6036, Mailing Address: P.O. Box 2009, Zip 71457-2009; tel. 318/214-4200; Mark E. Marley, Chief Executive Officer

OCHSNER FOUNDATION HOSPITAL, 1516 Jefferson Highway, New Orleans, LA, Zip 70121-2484; tel. 504/842-3000; Eileen F. Skinner, Director

OPELOUSAS GENERAL HOSPITAL, 539 East Prudhomme Street, Opelousas, LA, Zip 70570, Mailing Address: P.O. Box 1208, Zip 70571-1208; tel. 318/948-3011; Daryl J. Doise, Administrator

OUR LADY OF LOURDES REGIONAL MEDICAL CENTER, 611 St. Landry Street, Lafayette, LA, Zip 70506-4697, Mailing Address: Box 4027, Zip 70502-4027; tel. 318/289-2000; Ronald W. Webb, Chief Executive Officer

OUR LADY OF THE LAKE REGIONAL MEDICAL CENTER, 5000 Hennessy Boulevard, Baton Rouge, LA, Zip 70808-4350; tel. 225/765-6565; Robert C. Davidge, Chief Executive Officer

PENDLETON MEMORIAL METHODIST HOSPITAL, 5620 Read Boulevard, New Orleans, LA, Zip 70127-3154; tel. 504/244-5100; Frederick C. Young, Jr, President

POINTE COUPEE GENERAL HOSPITAL, 2202 False River Drive, New Roads, LA, Zip 70760-2698; tel. 225/638-6331; Larry J. Ayres, Administrator and Chief Executive Officer

PREVOST MEMORIAL HOSPITAL, 301 Memorial Drive, Donaldsonville, LA, Zip 70346-4376, Mailing Address: P.O. Box 186, Zip 70346-0186; tel. 225/473-7931; Vince A. Cataldo, Administrator

RIVER WEST MEDICAL CENTER, 59355 River West Drive, Plaquemine, LA, Zip 70764-9543; tel. 225/687-9222; Mark Nosacka, Chief Executive Officer

RIVERLAND MEDICAL CENTER, 1700 North E 'E' Wallace Boulevard, Ferriday, LA, Zip 71334, Mailing Address: P.O. Box 111, Zip 71334-0111; tel. 318/757-6551; Vernon R. Stevens, Jr, Administrator

Networks / Berkshire Health System

SABINE MEDICAL CENTER, 240 Highland Drive, Many, LA, Zip 71449–3718; tel. 318/256–5691; Patrick W. Gandy, Chief Executive Officer

ST. ANNE GENERAL HOSPITAL, 4608 Highway 1, Raceland, LA, Zip 70394; tel. 504/537–6841; Milton D. Bourgeois, Jr, Administrator

ST. HELENA PARISH HOSPITAL, Highway 43 North, Greensburg, LA, Zip 70441, Mailing Address: P.O. Box 337, Zip 70441–0337; tel. 225/222–6111; J. Scott Stafford, Chief Executive Officer and Administrator

WEST FELICIANA PARISH HOSPITAL, Saint Francisville, LA, Mailing Address: P.O. Box 368, Zip 70775–0368; tel. 225/635–3811; John H. Green, Administrator

WOMAN'S HOSPITAL, 9050 Airline Highway, Baton Rouge, LA, Zip 70815–4192, Mailing Address: P.O. Box 95009, Zip 70895–9009; tel. 225/927–1300; Teri G. Fontenot, President and Chief Executive Officer

TENET HEALTH SYSTEM
111 Veterans Boulevard, Metarie, LA 70005; tel. 504/833–1495; Reynold Jennings, Senior Vice President

DOCTORS HOSPITAL OF JEFFERSON, 4320 Houma Boulevard, Metairie, LA, Zip 70006–2973; tel. 504/849–4000; John E. Walker, Chief Executive Officer

KENNER REGIONAL MEDICAL CENTER, 180 West Esplanade Avenue, Kenner, LA, Zip 70065–6001; tel. 504/468–8600; Deborah C. Keel, Chief Executive Officer

MEADOWCREST HOSPITAL, 2500 Belle Chase Highway, Gretna, LA, Zip 70056–7196; tel. 504/392–3131; Gerald L. Parton, Chief Executive Officer

MEMORIAL MEDICAL CENTER, New Orleans, LA, Randall L. Hoover, Chief Executive Officer

NORTHSHORE PSYCHIATRIC HOSPITAL, 104 Medical Center Drive, Slidell, LA, Zip 70461–7838; tel. 504/646–5500; George H. Perry, Ph.D., Chief Executive Officer

NORTHSHORE REGIONAL MEDICAL CENTER, 100 Medical Center Drive, Slidell, LA, Zip 70461–8572; tel. 504/649–7070; L. Rene' Goux, Chief Executive Officer

ST. CHARLES GENERAL HOSPITAL, 3700 St. Charles Avenue, New Orleans, LA, Zip 70115–4680; tel. 504/899–7441; L. Rene' Goux, Chief Executive Officer

MAINE

BLUE HILL MEMORIAL HOSPITAL
P.O. Box 823 Water St., Blue Hill, ME 04614; tel. 207/374–2836; Matthew Flynn, CFO

BLUE HILL MEMORIAL HOSPITAL, Water Street, Blue Hill, ME, Zip 04614–0823, Mailing Address: P.O. Box 823, Zip 04614–0823; tel. 207/374–2836; Bruce D. Cummings, Chief Executive Officer

HEALTH NET, INC.
One Merchants Plaza, 5th Floor, Bangor, ME 04401; tel. 207/942–2844; Dale Bradford, Chief Executive Officer (Interim)

ACADIA HOSPITAL, 268 Stillwater Avenue, Bangor, ME, Zip 04401–3945, Mailing Address: P.O. Box 422, Zip 04402–0422; tel. 207/973–6100; Ali A. Elhaj, President and Chief Exectice Officer

AROOSTOOK MEDICAL CENTER, 140 Academy Street, Presque Isle, ME, Zip 04769–3171, Mailing Address: P.O. Box 151, Zip 04769–0151; tel. 207/768–4000; David A. Peterson, President and Chief Executive Officer

BLUE HILL MEMORIAL HOSPITAL, Water Street, Blue Hill, ME, Zip 04614–0823, Mailing Address: P.O. Box 823, Zip 04614–0823; tel. 207/374–2836; Bruce D. Cummings, Chief Executive Officer

CHARLES A. DEAN MEMORIAL HOSPITAL, Pritham Avenue, Greenville, ME, Zip 04441–1395, Mailing Address: P.O. Box 1129, Zip 04441–1129; tel. 207/695–2223; Philomena A. Marshall, R.N., President and Chief Executive Officer

EASTERN MAINE MEDICAL CENTER, 489 State Street, Bangor, ME, Zip 04401–6674, Mailing Address: P.O. Box 404, Zip 04402–0404; tel. 207/973–7000; Norman A. Ledwin, President and Chief Executive Officer

INLAND HOSPITAL, 200 Kennedy Memorial Drive, Waterville, ME, Zip 04901–4595; tel. 207/861–3000; Wilfred J. Addison, President and Chief Executive Officer

MILLINOCKET REGIONAL HOSPITAL, 200 Somerset Street, Millinocket, ME, Zip 04462–1298; tel. 207/723–5161; Richard Waller, Chief Executive Officer

MOUNT DESERT ISLAND HOSPITAL, Wayman Lane, Bar Harbor, ME, Zip 04609–0008, Mailing Address: P.O. Box 8, Zip 04609–0008; tel. 207/288–5081; Arthur Blank, Chief Executive Officer

NORTHERN MAINE MEDICAL CENTER, 143 East Main Street, Fort Kent, ME, Zip 04743–1497; tel. 207/834–3155; Martin B. Bernstein, Chief Executive Officer

SEBASTICOOK VALLEY HOSPITAL, 99 Grove Street, Pittsfield, ME, Zip 04967–1199; tel. 207/487–5141; John C. May, Chief Executive Officer

SYNERNET INC
222 St. John Street, Suite 329, Portland, ME 04102; tel. 207/771–3456; Susan Homer, Office Manager

AUGUSTA MENTAL HEALTH INSTITUTE, Arsenal Street, Augusta, ME, Zip 04330, Mailing Address: P.O. Box 724, Zip 04330–0724; tel. 207/287–7200; Rodney Bouffard, Superintendent

BLUE HILL MEMORIAL HOSPITAL, Water Street, Blue Hill, ME, Zip 04614–0823, Mailing Address: P.O. Box 823, Zip 04614–0823; tel. 207/374–2836; Bruce D. Cummings, Chief Executive Officer

FRANKLIN MEMORIAL HOSPITAL, 129 Hospital Drive, Farmington, ME, Zip 04938–9990; tel. 207/778–6031; Richard A. Batt, President and Chief Executive Officer

HENRIETTA D. GOODALL HOSPITAL, 25 June Street, Sanford, ME, Zip 04073–2645; tel. 207/324–4310; Peter G. Booth, President

INLAND HOSPITAL, 200 Kennedy Memorial Drive, Waterville, ME, Zip 04901–4595; tel. 207/861–3000; Wilfred J. Addison, President and Chief Executive Officer

MERCY HOSPITAL OF PORTLAND, 144 State Street, Portland, ME, Zip 04101–3795; tel. 207/879–3000; Howard R. Buckley, President

MID COAST HOSPITAL, 1356 Washington Street, Bath, ME, Zip 04530–2897; tel. 207/443–5524; Herbert Paris, President

MILES MEMORIAL HOSPITAL, Bristol Road, Damariscotta, ME, Zip 04543, Mailing Address: Rural Route 2, Box 4500, Zip 04543–9767; tel. 207/563–1234; Judith Tarr, Chief Executive Officer

MOUNT DESERT ISLAND HOSPITAL, Wayman Lane, Bar Harbor, ME, Zip 04609–0008, Mailing Address: P.O. Box 8, Zip 04609–0008; tel. 207/288–5081; Arthur Blank, Chief Executive Officer

NORTHERN MAINE MEDICAL CENTER, 143 East Main Street, Fort Kent, ME, Zip 04743–1497; tel. 207/834–3155; Martin B. Bernstein, Chief Executive Officer

PENOBSCOT BAY MEDICAL CENTER, 6 Glen Cove Drive, Rockport, ME, Zip 04856–4241; tel. 207/596–8000; Roy A. Hitchings, Jr, FACHE, President and Chief Executive Officer

REDINGTON–FAIRVIEW GENERAL HOSPITAL, Fairview Avenue, Skowhegan, ME, Zip 04976, Mailing Address: P.O. Box 468, Zip 04976–0468; tel. 207/474–5121; Richard Willett, Chief Executive Officer

SEBASTICOOK VALLEY HOSPITAL, 99 Grove Street, Pittsfield, ME, Zip 04967–1199; tel. 207/487–5141; John C. May, Chief Executive Officer

SOUTHERN MAINE MEDICAL CENTER, One Medical Center Drive, Biddeford, ME, Zip 04005–9496, Mailing Address: P.O. Box 626, Zip 04005–0626; tel. 207/283–7000; Edward J. McGeachey, President and Chief Executive Officer

ST. JOSEPH HOSPITAL, 360 Broadway, Bangor, ME, Zip 04401–3897, Mailing Address: P.O. Box 403, Zip 04402–0403; tel. 207/262–1000; Sister Mary Norberta Malinowski, President

STEPHENS MEMORIAL HOSPITAL, 181 Main Street, Norway, ME, Zip 04268–1297; tel. 207/743–5933; Timothy A. Churchill, President

WALDO COUNTY GENERAL HOSPITAL, Northport Avenue, Belfast, ME, Zip 04915, Mailing Address: P.O. Box 287, Zip 04915–0287; tel. 207/338–2500; Mark A. Biscone, Executive Director

YORK HOSPITAL, 15 Hospital Drive, York, ME, Zip 03909–1099; tel. 207/351–2395; Jud Knox, President

MARYLAND

DIMENSIONS HEALTHCARE SYSTEM
9200 Basil Court, LaRGO, MD 20774; tel. 301/925–7000; Winfield M. Kelly, Jr, President & Chief Executive Officer

LAUREL REGIONAL HOSPITAL, 7300 Van Dusen Road, Laurel, MD, Zip 20707–9266; tel. 301/725–4300; Patrick F. Mutch, President

PRINCE GEORGE'S HOSPITAL CENTER, 3001 Hospital Drive, Cheverly, MD, Zip 20785–1189; tel. 301/618–2000; Phyllis Wingate–Jones, President

MARYLAND HEALTH NETWORK
1508 Woodlawn Drive, Suite 13, Baltimore, MD 21044; tel. 410/594–2401; Peter Clay, President

GREATER BALTIMORE MEDICAL CENTER, 6701 North Charles Street, Baltimore, MD, Zip 21204–6892; tel. 410/828–2000; Laurence M. Merlis, President and Chief Executive Officer

HOLY CROSS HOSPITAL OF SILVER SPRING, 1500 Forest Glen Road, Silver Spring, MD, Zip 20910–1484; tel. 301/754–7000; Kevin J. Sexton, President and Chief Executive Officer

MONTGOMERY GENERAL HOSPITAL, 18101 Prince Philip Drive, Olney, MD, Zip 20832–1512; tel. 301/774–8882; Peter W. Monge, President and Chief Executive Officer

NORTHWEST HOSPITAL CENTER, 5401 Old Court Road, Randallstown, MD, Zip 21133–5185; tel. 410/521–2200; Robert W. Fischer, President

ST. AGNES HEALTHCARE, 900 Caton Avenue, Baltimore, MD, Zip 21229–5299; tel. 410/368–6000; Robert W. Adams, President and Chief Executive Officer

UNIVERSITY OF MARYLAND MEDICAL SYSTEM
42 South Greene Street, Baltimore, MD 21201; tel. 410/328–8667; Morton I. Rapoport, MD, President & Chief Executive Officer

DEATON SPECIALTY HOSPITAL AND HOME, 601 South Charles Street, Baltimore, MD, Zip 21230–3898; tel. 410/547–8500; James E. Ross, FACHE, Chief Executive Officer

JAMES LAWRENCE KERNAN HOSPITAL, 2200 Kernan Drive, Baltimore, MD, Zip 21207–6697; tel. 410/448–2500; James E. Ross, FACHE, Chief Executive Officer

UNIVERSITY OF MARYLAND MEDICAL CENTER, 22 South Greene Street, Baltimore, MD, Zip 21201; tel. 410/328–8667; Stephen C. Schimpff, M.D., Chief Executive Officer

MASSACHUSETTS

BAYSTATE HEALTH SYSTEM
759 Chestnut Street, Springfield, MA 01199; tel. 413/784–0000; Donna Ross, Vice President, Strategic & Program Planning

BERKSHIRE HEALTH SYSTEM
725 North Street, Pittsfield, MA 01201; tel. 413/447–2000; David Phelps, President

Networks / Berkshire Health System

BERKSHIRE MEDICAL CENTER, 725 North Street, Pittsfield, MA, Zip 01201–4124; tel. 413/447–2000; Ruth P. Blodgett, Chief Operating Officer

FAIRVIEW HOSPITAL, 29 Lewis Avenue, Great Barrington, MA, Zip 01230–1713; tel. 413/528–0790; Eugene A. Dellea, Interim President

BETH ISRAEL HEALTHCARE
330 Brookline Avenue, Boston, MA 02215; tel. 617/735–2000; Mitchell T. Rabkin, President

CAPE COD HEALTHCARE, INC.
88 Lewis Bay Road, Hyannis, MA 02601; tel. 508/862–5010; Stephen Abbott, Chief Executive Officer

CAPE COD HOSPITAL, 27 Park Street, Hyannis, MA, Zip 02601; tel. 508/771–1800; Gail M. Frieswick, Ed.D., Executive Vice President

FALMOUTH HOSPITAL, 100 Ter Heun Drive, Falmouth, MA, Zip 02540–2599; tel. 508/548–5300; Robert A. Gunderson, Executive Vice President

CARITAS CHRISTI HEALTH
736 Cambridge Street, Boston, MA 02135; tel. 617/789–2500; Michael F. Collins, M.D., President & Chief Executive

CARITAS GOOD SAMARITAN MEDICAL CENTER, 235 North Pearl Street, Brockton, MA, Zip 02401–1794; tel. 508/427–3000; Peter J. Holden, President

HOLY FAMILY HOSPITAL AND MEDICAL CENTER, 70 East Street, Methuen, MA, Zip 01844–4597; tel. 978/687–0151; William L. Lane, President

SAINT ANNE'S HOSPITAL, 795 Middle Street, Fall River, MA, Zip 02721–1798; tel. 508/674–5741; Michael W. Metzler, President

ST. ELIZABETH'S MEDICAL CENTER OF BOSTON, 736 Cambridge Street, Brighton, MA, Zip 02135–2997; tel. 617/789–3000; Michael F. Collins, M.D., President

CHILDREN'S HOSPITAL
300 Longwood Avenue, Boston, MA 02115; tel. 617/355–8555; David S. Weiner, Vice President of Network Development

CHILDREN'S HOSPITAL, 300 Longwood Avenue, Boston, MA, Zip 02115–5737; tel. 617/355–6000; David S. Weiner, Chief Executive Officer

CONTINUUM OF CARE NETWORK
57 Union Street, Marlborough, MA 01752; tel. 508/481–5000; Cheryl Herberg, Ntwrk Coordinator

LONG ISLAND COLLEGE HOSPITAL, 339 Hicks Street, Brooklyn, NY, Zip 11201–5509; tel. 718/780–1000; Allan Gibofsky, President and Chief Executive Officer

UMASS MARLBOROUGH HOSPITAL, 57 Union Street, Marlborough, MA, Zip 01752–1297; tel. 508/481–5000; Annette B. Leahy, President and Chief Executive Officer

LAHEY NETWORK
41 Mall Road, Burlington, MA 01805; tel. 718/744–8000; David M. Barrett, M.D., Chief Executive Officer

LAHEY CLINIC HOSPITAL, 41 Mall Road, Burlington, MA, Zip 01805; tel. 781/744–8500; David M. Barrett, M.D., Chief Executive Officer

NORTHEAST HEALTH SYSTEMS
85 Herrick Street, Beverly, MA 01915; tel. 978/922–3000; Elisabeth Babcock, Vice President of Network

BEVERLY HOSPITAL, 85 Herrrick Street, Beverly, MA, Zip 01915–1777; tel. 978/922–3000; Robert R. Fanning, Jr, President and Chief Executive Officer

PARTNERS HEALTHCARE SYSYTEM
32 Fruit Street, Boston, MA 02114; tel. 617/732–5500; John McGonagle, Dir–Community Health Services

BRIGHAM AND WOMEN'S HOSPITAL, 75 Francis Street, Boston, MA, Zip 02115–6195; tel. 617/732–5500; Jeffrey Otten, President

MASSACHUSETTS GENERAL HOSPITAL, 55 Fruit Street, Boston, MA, Zip 02114–2696; tel. 617/726–2000; James J. Mongan, M.D., President

SALEM HOSPITAL, 81 Highland Avenue, Salem, MA, Zip 01970–2768; tel. 978/741–1200; Judith Ritchie, President and Chief Executive Officer

SHAUGHNESSY–KAPLAN REHABILITATION HOSPITAL, Dove Avenue, Salem, MA, Zip 01970–2999; tel. 978/745–9000; Anthony Sciola, President and Chief Executive Officer

PATHWAY HEALTH NETWORK
1 Deaconess Road, Boston, MA 02215; tel. 617/632–9967; Susan K. Glazer, Vice President – Planning

BETH ISRAEL DEACONESS MEDICAL CENTER, 330 Brookline Avenue, Boston, MA, Zip 02215–5491; tel. 617/667–2203; James Reinertsen, M.D., Chief Executive Officer

DEACONESS WALTHAM HOSPITAL, Hope Avenue, Waltham, MA, Zip 02453; tel. 781/647–6000; Dana W. Ramish, FACHE, President and Chief Executive Officer

DEACONESS–GLOVER HOSPITAL CORPORATION, 148 Chestnut Street, Needham, MA, Zip 02192–2483; tel. 781/453–3000; John Dalton, President and Chief Executive Officer

DEACONESS–NASHOBA HOSPITAL, 200 Groton Road, Ayer, MA, Zip 01432–3300; tel. 978/784–9000; Jeffrey R. Kelly, President and Chief Executive Officer

MOUNT AUBURN HOSPITAL, 330 Mount Auburn Street, Cambridge, MA, Zip 02138; tel. 617/499–5700; Jeanette G. Clough, President and Chief Executive Officer

NEW ENGLAND BAPTIST HOSPITAL, 125 Parker Hill Avenue, Boston, MA, Zip 02120–3297; tel. 617/754–5800; Alan H. Robbins, M.D., President

SISTERS OF PROVIDENCE HEALTH SYSTEM
85 Spring Street, Springfield, MA 01105; tel. 413/736–5494; Vincent McCorkle, President/Chief Executive Officer

MERCY HOSPITAL, 271 Carew Street, Springfield, MA, Zip 01104–2398, Mailing Address: P.O. Box 9012, Zip 01102–9012; tel. 413/748–9000; Vincent J. McCorkle, President

MICHIGAN

BATTLE CREEK HEALTH SYSTEM
300 North Avenue, Battle Creek, MI 49016; tel. 616/966–8000; Arthur Knueppeal, President

BATTLE CREEK HEALTH SYSTEM, 300 North Avenue, Battle Creek, MI, Zip 49016–3396; tel. 616/966–8000; Patrick R. Garrett, Chief Executive Officer

BORGESS HEALTH ALLIANCE
1521 Gull Rfoad, Kalamazoo, MI 49001; tel. 616/226–7000; Mike Alfred, Executive Director, Business Dev & Public Relation

BORGESS MEDICAL CENTER, 1521 Gull Road, Kalamazoo, MI, Zip 49001–1640; tel. 616/226–4800; Randall Stasik, President and Chief Executive Officer

COMMUNITY HEALTH CENTER OF BRANCH COUNTY, 274 East Chicago Street, Coldwater, MI, Zip 49036–2088; tel. 517/279–5400; Randy DeGroot, Chief Executive Officer

COMMUNITY HOSPITAL, Medical Park Drive, Watervliet, MI, Zip 49098–0158, Mailing Address: P.O. Box 158, Zip 49098–0158; tel. 616/463–3111; David L. McMann, Chief Executive Officer

DOCTORS HOSPITAL OF JACKSON, 110 North Elm Avenue, Jackson, MI, Zip 49202–3595; tel. 517/787–1440; Michael J. Falatko, President and Chief Executive Officer

HILLSDALE COMMUNITY HEALTH CENTER, 168 South Howell Street, Hillsdale, MI, Zip 49242–2081; tel. 517/437–4451; Charles A. Bianchi, President

LEE MEMORIAL HOSPITAL, 420 West High Street, Dowagiac, MI, Zip 49047–1907; tel. 616/782–8681; Fritz Fahrenbacher, President and Chief Executive Officer

METROPOLITAN HOSPITAL, 1919 Boston Street S.E., Grand Rapids, MI, Zip 49506–4199, Mailing Address: P.O. Box 158, Zip 49501–0158; tel. 616/252–7200; Michael D. Faas, President and Chief Executive Officer

THREE RIVERS AREA HOSPITAL, 1111 West Broadway, Three Rivers, MI, Zip 49093–9362; tel. 616/278–1145; Matthew Chambers, Chief Executive Officer

BUTTERWORTH HEALTH SYSTEM
100 Michigan St. S.E., Grand Rapids, MI 49503; tel. 616/776–2008; Carol Sarosik, Regional Vice President

CARSON CITY HOSPITAL, 406 East Elm Street, Carson City, MI, Zip 48811–0879, Mailing Address: P.O. Box 879, Zip 48811–0879; tel. 517/584–0053; Bruce L. Traverse, President

GERBER MEMORIAL HEALTH SERVICES, 212 South Sullivan Street, Fremont, MI, Zip 49412–1596; tel. 231/924–3300; Ned B. Hughes, Jr, President

METROPOLITAN HOSPITAL, 1919 Boston Street S.E., Grand Rapids, MI, Zip 49506–4199, Mailing Address: P.O. Box 158, Zip 49501–0158; tel. 616/252–7200; Michael D. Faas, President and Chief Executive Officer

PINE REST CHRISTIAN MENTAL HEALTH SERVICES, 300 68th Street S.E., Grand Rapids, MI, Zip 49501–0165, Mailing Address: P.O. Box 165, Zip 49501–0165; tel. 616/455–5000; Daniel L. Holwerda, President and Chief Executive Officer

SPECTRUM HEALTH, 1840 Wealthy Street S.E., Grand Rapids, MI, Zip 49506–2921; tel. 616/774–7444; Terrence M. O'Rourke, President

UNITED MEMORIAL HEALTH CENTER, 615 South Bower Street, Greenville, MI, Zip 48838–2628; tel. 616/754–4691; Lorne J. Archer, Chief Executive Officer

ZEELAND COMMUNITY HOSPITAL, 100 South Pine Street, Zeeland, MI, Zip 49464–1619; tel. 616/772–4644; Henry A. Veenstra, President

DETROIT-MACOMB HOSPITAL CORP
11800 East Twelve Mile Road, Warren, MI 48093; tel. 313/573–5000; George P. Karolis, Administrator

ST. JOHN DETROIT RIVERVIEW HOSPITAL, 7733 East Jefferson Avenue, Detroit, MI, Zip 48214–2598; tel. 313/499–4000; Richard T. Young, President

ST. JOHN MACOMB HOSPITAL, 11800 East Twelve Mile Road, Warren, MI, Zip 48093–3494; tel. 810/573–5000; John E. Knox, President

FIRST CHOICE NETWORK
60 Kalamazoo Ave., South Haven, MI 49090; tel. 616/637–1690; John P. Isaia, Executive Director

COMMUNITY HOSPITAL, Medical Park Drive, Watervliet, MI, Zip 49098–0158, Mailing Address: P.O. Box 158, Zip 49098–0158; tel. 616/463–3111; David L. McMann, Chief Executive Officer

LEE MEMORIAL HOSPITAL, 420 West High Street, Dowagiac, MI, Zip 49047–1907; tel. 616/782–8681; Fritz Fahrenbacher, President and Chief Executive Officer

HENRY FORD HEALTH SYSTEM
One Ford Place, Detroit, MI 48220; tel. 313/874–3436; Mehul Patel, Admin. Fellow

BI-COUNTY COMMUNITY HOSPITAL, 13355 East Ten Mile Road, Warren, MI, Zip 48089–2065; tel. 810/759–7300; Gary W. Popiel, Executive Vice President and Chief Executive Officer

BON SECOURS COTTAGE HEALTH SERVICES–COTTAGE HOSPITAL, 159 Kercheval Avenue, Grosse Pointe Farms, MI, Zip 48236–3692; tel. 313/640–1000; Richard Van Lith, Chief Executive Officer

Networks / Fairview Health Services

HENRY FORD HOSPITAL, 2799 West Grand Boulevard, Detroit, MI, Zip 48202–2689; tel. 313/916–2600; Stephen H. Velick, Chief Executive Officer

HENRY FORD KINGSWOOD HOSPITAL, 10300 West Eight Mile Road, Ferndale, MI, Zip 48220–2198; tel. 248/398–3200; Glenn Black, Associate Vice President and Chief Operating Officer

HENRY FORD WYANDOTTE HOSPITAL, 2333 Biddle Avenue, Wyandotte, MI, Zip 48192–4693; tel. 734/246–6000; William R. Alvin, President

RIVERSIDE OSTEOPATHIC HOSPITAL, 150 Truax Street, Trenton, MI, Zip 48183–2151; tel. 734/676–4200; Dennis R. Lemanski, D.O., Vice President and Chief Executive Officer

SAINT JOSEPH MERCY HEALTH SYSTEM, 5301 East Huron River Drive, Ann Arbor, MI, Zip 48106, Mailing Address: P.O. Box 995, Zip 48106–0995; tel. 734/712–3456; Garry C. Faja, President and Chief Executive Officer

ST. JOSEPH MERCY OAKLAND, 900 Woodward Avenue, Pontiac, MI, Zip 48341–2985; tel. 248/858–3000; Thomas L. Feurig, President and Chief Executive Officer

ST. JOSEPH'S MERCY HOSPITALS AND HEALTH SERVICES, Clinton Township, MI, Jack Weiner, President and Chief Executive Officer

HOSPITAL NETWORK, INC.
252 East Lovell Street, Box 42, Kalamazoo, MI 49007; tel. 616/341–8888; George D. Angelidis, President/Chief Executive Officer

ALLEGAN GENERAL HOSPITAL, 555 Linn Street, Allegan, MI, Zip 49010–1594; tel. 616/673–8424; James A. Klun, President

BRONSON METHODIST HOSPITAL, 252 East Lovell Street, Kalamazoo, MI, Zip 49007–5345; tel. 616/341–6000; Frank J. Sardone, President and Chief Executive Officer

BRONSON VICKSBURG HOSPITAL, 13326 North Boulevard, Vicksburg, MI, Zip 49097–1099; tel. 616/649–2321; Frank J. Sardone, President

OAKLAWN HOSPITAL, 200 North Madison Street, Marshall, MI, Zip 49068–1199; tel. 616/781–4271; Rob Covert, President and Chief Executive Officer

PENNOCK HOSPITAL, 1009 West Green Street, Hastings, MI, Zip 49058–1790; tel. 616/945–3451; Daniel Hamilton, Chief Executive Officer

STURGIS HOSPITAL, 916 Myrtle, Sturgis, MI, Zip 49091–2001; tel. 616/651–7824; James N. Browne, Interim Chief Executive Officer

LAKELAND REGIONAL HEALTH SYSTEM
1234 Napier Avenue, St. Joseph, MI 49085; tel. 616/927–5363; Ben Hill, Marketing Department

BRONSON METHODIST HOSPITAL, 252 East Lovell Street, Kalamazoo, MI, Zip 49007–5345; tel. 616/341–6000; Frank J. Sardone, President and Chief Executive Officer

LAKELAND MEDICAL CENTER–ST. JOSEPH, 1234 Napier Avenue, Saint Joseph, MI, Zip 49085–2112; tel. 616/983–8300; Joseph A. Wasserman, President and Chief Executive Officer

SOUTH HAVEN COMMUNITY HOSPITAL, 955 South Bailey Avenue, South Haven, MI, Zip 49090; tel. 616/637–5271; Craig J. Marks, President and Chief Executive Officer

MUNSON HEALTH CARE SYSTEM
1105 Sixth Street, Traverse City, MI 49684; tel. 616/935–6000; John M. Rockwood, President & Chief Executive Officer

KALKASKA MEMORIAL HEALTH CENTER, 419 South Coral Street, Kalkaska, MI, Zip 49646; tel. 231/258–7500; James D. Austin, CHE, Administrator

LEELANAU MEMORIAL HEALTH CENTER, 215 South High Street, Northport, MI, Zip 49670, Mailing Address: P.O. Box 217, Zip 49670–0217; tel. 231/386–0000; Jayne R. Bull, Administrator

MUNSON MEDICAL CENTER, 1105 Sixth Street, Traverse City, MI, Zip 49684–2386; tel. 231/935–5000; Ralph J. Cerny, President and Chief Executive Officer

PAUL OLIVER MEMORIAL HOSPITAL, 224 Park Avenue, Frankfort, MI, Zip 49635; tel. 231/352–9621; James D. Austin, CHE, Administrator

ST. JOHN HEALTH SYSTEM
22101 Moross Road, Detroit, MI 48236; tel. 313/343–4000; Mark J. Brady, Senior Planning Analyst

POH MEDICAL CENTER, 50 North Perry Street, Pontiac, MI, Zip 48342–2253; tel. 248/338–5000; Patrick Lamberti, Chief Executive Officer

PORT HURON HOSPITAL, 1221 Pine Grove Avenue, Port Huron, MI, Zip 48061–5011; tel. 810/987–5000; Donald C. Fletcher, President and Chief Executive Officer

PROVIDENCE HOSPITAL AND MEDICAL CENTERS, 16001 West Nine Mile Road, Southfield, MI, Zip 48075–4854, Mailing Address: Box 2043, Zip 48037–2043; tel. 248/424–3000; Robert F. Casalou, President

ST. JOHN DETROIT RIVERVIEW HOSPITAL, 7733 East Jefferson Avenue, Detroit, MI, Zip 48214–2598; tel. 313/499–4000; Richard T. Young, President

ST. JOHN HOSPITAL AND MEDICAL CENTER, 22101 Moross Road, Detroit, MI, Zip 48236–2172; tel. 313/343–4000; Timothy J. Grajewski, President and Chief Executive Officer

ST. JOHN MACOMB HOSPITAL, 11800 East Twelve Mile Road, Warren, MI, Zip 48093–3494; tel. 810/573–5000; John E. Knox, President

ST. JOHN NORTHEAST COMMUNITY HOSPITAL, 4777 East Outer Drive, Detroit, MI, Zip 48234–0401; tel. 313/369–9100; Michael F. Breen, President

ST. JOHN OAKLAND HOSPITAL, 27351 Dequindre, Madison Heights, MI, Zip 48071–3499; tel. 248/967–7000; Robert Deputat, President

ST. JOHN RIVER DISTRICT HOSPITAL, 4100 River Road, East China, MI, Zip 48054; tel. 810/329–7111; Frank W. Poma, President

WILLIAM BEAUMONT HOSPITAL
3601 W. Thirteen Mile Road, Royal Oak, MI 48073; tel. 248/551–6405; Holli Zwar, Planning Specialist

WILLIAM BEAUMONT HOSPITAL–ROYAL OAK, 3601 West Thirteen Mile Road, Royal Oak, MI, Zip 48073–6769; tel. 248/551–5000; John D. Labriola, Senior Vice President and Hospital Director

WILLIAM BEAUMONT HOSPITAL–TROY, 44201 Dequindre Road, Troy, MI, Zip 48098–1198; tel. 248/828–5100; Eugene F. Michalski, Senior Vice President and Director

MINNESOTA

AFFILIATED COMMUNITY HEALTH NETWORK, INC
101 Wilmar Avenue S.W., Willmar, MN 56201; tel. 612/231–6719; Burnell J. Mellema, MD, President

AVERA MCKENNAN HOSPITAL, 800 East 21st Street, Sioux Falls, SD, Zip 57105–1096, Mailing Address: P.O. Box 5045, Zip 57117–5045; tel. 605/322–8000; Fredrick Slunecka, President and Chief Executive Officer

REDWOOD FALLS MUNICIPAL HOSPITAL, 100 Fallwood Road, Redwood Falls, MN, Zip 56283–1828; tel. 507/637–4500; James E. Schulte, Administrator

RICE MEMORIAL HOSPITAL, 301 Becker Avenue S.W., Willmar, MN, Zip 56201–3395; tel. 320/235–4543; Lawrence J. Massa, Chief Executive Officer

WEINER MEMORIAL MEDICAL CENTER, 300 South Bruce Street, Marshall, MN, Zip 56258–3900; tel. 507/532–9661; Richard G. Slieter, Jr, Administrator

WILLMAR REGIONAL TREATMENT CENTER, North Highway 71, Willmar, MN, Zip 56201–1128, Mailing Address: Box 1128, Zip 56201–1128; tel. 320/231–5905; Gregory G. Spartz, Chief Executive Officer

ALLINA HEALTH SYSTEM
5601 Smetana Drive, Minnetonka, MN 55430; tel. 612/992–3648; Ann Fleischauer, Vice President Physician Communications

ABBOTT NORTHWESTERN HOSPITAL, 800 East 28th Street, Minneapolis, MN, Zip 55407–3799; tel. 612/863–4000; Mark Dixon, Administrator

BUFFALO HOSPITAL, 303 Catlin Street, Buffalo, MN, Zip 55313–1947; tel. 612/682–7180; Mary Ellen Wells, Administrator

CAMBRIDGE MEDICAL CENTER, 701 South Dellwood Street, Cambridge, MN, Zip 55008–1920; tel. 763/689–7700; Dennis J. Doran, Administrator

COMMUNITY HOSPITAL AND HEALTH CARE CENTER, 618 West Broadway Avenue, Saint Peter, MN, Zip 56082–1327; tel. 507/931–2200; Colleen A. Spike, Administrator

GRANITE FALLS MUNICIPAL HOSPITAL AND MANOR, 345 Tenth Avenue, Granite Falls, MN, Zip 56241–1499; tel. 320/564–3111; George Gerlach, Administrator

HUTCHINSON AREA HEALTH CARE, 1095 Highway 15 South, Hutchinson, MN, Zip 55350–3182; tel. 320/234–5000; Philip G. Graves, Administrator

MERCY HOSPITAL, 4050 Coon Rapids Boulevard, Coon Rapids, MN, Zip 55433–2586; tel. 763/421–8888; Marvin L. Dehne, Executive Officer

MILLE LACS HEALTH SYSTEM, 200 North Elm Street, Onamia, MN, Zip 56359–7978; tel. 320/532–3154; Randall A. Farrow, Administrator

NEW ULM MEDICAL CENTER, 1324 Fifth Street North, New Ulm, MN, Zip 56073–1553, Mailing Address: P.O. Box 577, Zip 56073–0577; tel. 507/354–2111; Brian Kief, Administrator

NORTHFIELD HOSPITAL, 801 West First Street, Northfield, MN, Zip 55057–1697; tel. 507/645–6661; Kendall C. Bank, Administrator

OWATONNA HOSPITAL, 903 Oak Street South, Owatonna, MN, Zip 55060–3234; tel. 507/451–3850; Daniel J. Werner, Administrator

PHILLIPS EYE INSTITUTE, 2215 Park Avenue, Minneapolis, MN, Zip 55404–3756; tel. 612/336–6000; Shari E. Levy, Administrator

ST. FRANCIS REGIONAL MEDICAL CENTER, 1455 St. Francis Avenue, Shakopee, MN, Zip 55379–3380; tel. 952/403–3000; Venetia Kudrle, Administrator

STEVENS COMMUNITY MEDICAL CENTER, 400 East First Street, Morris, MN, Zip 56267–1407, Mailing Address: P.O. Box 660, Zip 56267–0660; tel. 320/589–1313; John Rau, Administrator

UNITED HOSPITAL, 333 North Smith Street, Saint Paul, MN, Zip 55102–2389; tel. 651/220–8000; M. Barbara Balik, MSN, Ed.D., Administrator

UNITED HOSPITAL DISTRICT, 515 South Moore Street, Blue Earth, MN, Zip 56013–2158, Mailing Address: P.O. Box 160, Zip 56013–0160; tel. 507/526–3273; Chad Cooper, Administrator

UNITY HOSPITAL, 550 Osborne Road N.E., Fridley, MN, Zip 55432–2799; tel. 763/421–2222

FAIRVIEW HEALTH SERVICES
2450 Riverside Avenue, Minneapolis, MN 55454; tel. 612/672–6000; David Page, Chief Executive Officer

FAIRVIEW NORTHLAND REGIONAL HEALTH CARE, 911 Northland Drive, Princeton, MN, Zip 55371–2173; tel. 612/389–6300; Jeanne Lally, Senior Vice President and Administrator

FAIRVIEW RIDGES HOSPITAL, 201 East Nicollet Boulevard, Burnsville, MN, Zip 55337–5799; tel. 612/892–2000; Mark M. Enger, Senior Vice President and Administrator

FAIRVIEW SOUTHDALE HOSPITAL, 6401 France Avenue South, Minneapolis, MN, Zip 55435–2199; tel. 612/924–5000; Mark M. Enger, Senior Vice President and Administrator

FAIRVIEW–UNIVERSITY MEDICAL CENTER, 2450 Riverside Avenue, Minneapolis, MN, Zip 55454–1400; tel. 612/672–6000; Gordon L. Alexander, M.D., Senior Vice President and Chief Executive Officer

Networks / Healtheast Care System

HEALTHEAST CARE SYSTEM
559 Capitol Blvd., St. Paul, MN 55103; tel. 651/232-2300; Roger Green, V.P. Strategic Planning

BETHESDA REHABILITATION HOSPITAL, 559 Capitol Boulevard, Saint Paul, MN, Zip 55103-2101; tel. 651/232-2000; Scott Batulis, Vice President and Administrator

ST. JOHN'S HOSPITAL, 1575 Beam Avenue, Maplewood, MN, Zip 55109; tel. 651/232-7000; Douglas P. Cropper, Vice President and Administrator

ST. JOSEPH'S HOSPITAL, 69 West Exchange Street, Saint Paul, MN, Zip 55102-1053; tel. 651/232-3000; Douglas P. Cropper, Vice President and Administrator

HEALTHPARTNERS
8100 34th Avenue South, Minneapolis, MN 55440; tel. 612/883-5585; George Halverson, President

REGIONS HOSPITAL, 640 Jackson Street, Saint Paul, MN, Zip 55101-2595; tel. 651/221-3456; Terry S. Finzen, President

I-35 CORRIDOR HEALTH NETWORK
760 West Fourth Street, Rush City, MN 55069; tel. 612/358-4708; Lynn Clayton, Administrator

FAIRVIEW-UNIVERSITY MEDICAL CENTER, 2450 Riverside Avenue, Minneapolis, MN, Zip 55454-1400; tel. 612/672-6000; Gordon L. Alexander, M.D., Senior Vice President and Chief Executive Officer

KANABEC HOSPITAL, 300 Clark Street, Mora, MN, Zip 55051-1590; tel. 320/679-1212; Thomas D. Kaufman, Administrator

MERCY HOSPITAL AND HEALTH CARE CENTER, 710 South Kenwood Avenue, Moose Lake, MN, Zip 55767-9405; tel. 218/485-4481; Dianne Mandernach, Chief Executive Officer

PINE MEDICAL CENTER, 109 Court Avenue South, Sandstone, MN, Zip 55072-5120; tel. 320/245-2212; Michael D. Hedrix, Administrator

ITASCA PARTNERSHIP FOR QUALITY HEALTHCARE
126 S.E. 1st Ave., Grand Rapids, MN 55744; tel. 218/326-7791; Judy Bergh, Consultant/Executive Director

DEER RIVER HEALTHCARE CENTER, 1002 Comstock Drive, Deer River, MN, Zip 56636-9700; tel. 218/246-2900; Jeffry Stampohar, Chief Executive Officer

ITASCA MEDICAL CENTER, 126 First Avenue S.E., Grand Rapids, MN, Zip 55744-3698; tel. 218/326-3401; Gary Kenner, President and Chief Executive Officer

NORTHERN ITASCA HEALTH CARE CENTER, 258 Pine Tree Drive, Bigfork, MN, Zip 56628, Mailing Address: P.O. Box 258, Zip 56628-0258; tel. 218/743-3177; Richard M. Ash, Chief Executive Officer

MAYO FOUNDATION
200 S.W. First Street, Rochester, MN 55905; tel. 507/284-8860; Michael B. Wood, President

ALBERT LEA MEDICAL CENTER, 404 West Fountain Street, Albert Lea, MN, Zip 56007-2473; tel. 507/373-2384; Ronald A. Harmon, M.D., Chief Executive Officer

BARRON MEDICAL CENTER-MAYO HEALTH SYSTEM, 1222 Woodland Avenue, Barron, WI, Zip 54812-1798; tel. 715/537-3186; Mark D. Wilson, Administrator

BLOOMER MEMORIAL MEDICAL CENTER, 1501 Thompson Street, Bloomer, WI, Zip 54724-1299; tel. 715/568-2000; Mary Kerg, Administrator

FRANCISCAN SKEMP HEALTHCARE-ARCADIA CAMPUS, 464 South St. Joseph Avenue, Arcadia, WI, Zip 54612-1401; tel. 608/323-3341; Robert M. Tracey, Administrator

FRANCISCAN SKEMP HEALTHCARE-LA CROSSE CAMPUS, 700 West Avenue South, La Crosse, WI, Zip 54601-4783; tel. 608/785-0940; Glenn Forbes, M.D., President and Chief Executive Officer

FRANCISCAN SKEMP HEALTHCARE-SPARTA CAMPUS, 310 West Main Street, Sparta, WI, Zip 54656-2171; tel. 608/269-2132; William P. Sexton, Administrator

IMMANUEL ST. JOSEPH'S-MAYO HEALTH SYSTEM, 1025 Marsh Street, Mankato, MN, Zip 56002-4700, Mailing Address: P.O. Box 8673, Zip 56002-8673; tel. 507/625-4031; W. Neath Folger, M.D., President and Chief Executive Officer

LAKE CITY MEDICAL CENTER, 904 South Lakeshore Drive, Lake City, MN, Zip 55041-1899; tel. 651/345-3321; Mark Rinehardt, Administrator

LUTHER HOSPITAL, 1221 Whipple Street, Eau Claire, WI, Zip 54702-4105, Mailing Address: P.O. Box 5, Zip 54702-0005; tel. 715/838-3311; William Rupp, M.D., President and Chief Executive Officer

MAYO CLINIC HOSPITAL, 5777 East Mayo Boulevard, Phoenix, AZ, Zip 85054-4502; tel. 480/515-6296; Thomas C. Bour, Administrator

MYRTLE WERTH HOSPITAL-MAYO HEALTH SYSTEM, 2321 Stout Road, Menomonie, WI, Zip 54751-2397; tel. 715/235-5531; Thomas Miller, II, Chief Executive Officer

ROCHESTER METHODIST HOSPITAL, 201 West Center Street, Rochester, MN, Zip 55902-3084; tel. 507/266-7890; John M. Panicek, Administrator

SAINT MARYS HOSPITAL, 1216 Second Street S.W., Rochester, MN, Zip 55902-1970; tel. 507/255-5123; John M. Panicek, Administrator

SPRINGFIELD MEDICAL CENTER-MAYO HEALTH SYSTEM, 625 North Jackson Avenue, Springfield, MN, Zip 56087-1714, Mailing Address: P.O. Box 146, Zip 56087-0146; tel. 507/723-6201; Scott Thoreson, Administrator

ST. LUKE'S HOSPITAL, 4201 Belfort Road, Jacksonville, FL, Zip 32216-5898; tel. 904/296-3700; Robert M. Walters, Administrator

WASECA MEDICAL CENTER, 501 North State Street, Waseca, MN, Zip 56093; tel. 507/835-1210; Michael Milbrath, Administrator

MINNESOTA RURAL HEALTH COOPERATIVE
P.O. Box 104, Willmar, MN 56201; tel. 612/231-3849; Lyle Munneke, MD, President & Chairperson

APPLETON MUNICIPAL HOSPITAL AND NURSING HOME, 30 South Behl Street, Appleton, MN, Zip 56208-1699; tel. 320/289-2422; Mark E. Paulson, Administrator

CHIPPEWA COUNTY MONTEVIDEO HOSPITAL, 824 North 11th Street, Montevideo, MN, Zip 56265-1683; tel. 320/269-8877; Fred Knutson, Administrator

DIVINE PROVIDENCE HEALTH CENTER/AVERA HEALTH, 312 East George Street, Ivanhoe, MN, Zip 56142-0136, Mailing Address: P.O. Box 136, Zip 56142-0136; tel. 507/694-1414; Patrick Branco, Administrator

GRACEVILLE HEALTH CENTER, 115 West Second Street, Graceville, MN, Zip 56240-0157, Mailing Address: P.O. Box 157, Zip 56240-0157; tel. 320/748-7223; Helen Jorve, Chief Executive Officer

GRANITE FALLS MUNICIPAL HOSPITAL AND MANOR, 345 Tenth Avenue, Granite Falls, MN, Zip 56241-1499; tel. 320/564-3111; George Gerlach, Administrator

HENDRICKS COMMUNITY HOSPITAL, 503 East Lincoln Street, Hendricks, MN, Zip 56136-0106; tel. 507/275-3134; Kirk Stensrud, Administrator

JOHNSON MEMORIAL HEALTH SERVICES, 1282 Walnut Street, Dawson, MN, Zip 56232-2333; tel. 320/769-4323; Vern Silvernale, Administrator

MADISON HOSPITAL, 820 Third Avenue, Madison, MN, Zip 56256-1014, Mailing Address: P.O. Box 184, Zip 56256-0184; tel. 320/598-7556; Thomas Richter, Chief Executive Officer

ORTONVILLE AREA HEALTH SERVICES, 750 Eastvold Avenue, Ortonville, MN, Zip 56278-1133; tel. 320/839-2502; Kenneth W. Archer, Administrator

REDWOOD FALLS MUNICIPAL HOSPITAL, 100 Fallwood Road, Redwood Falls, MN, Zip 56283-1828; tel. 507/637-4500; James E. Schulte, Administrator

RENVILLE COUNTY HOSPITAL, 611 East Fairview Avenue, Olivia, MN, Zip 56277-1397; tel. 320/523-1261; Dean G. Slagter, Administrator

RICE MEMORIAL HOSPITAL, 301 Becker Avenue S.W., Willmar, MN, Zip 56201-3395; tel. 320/235-4543; Lawrence J. Massa, Chief Executive Officer

SIOUX VALLEY CANBY CAMPUS, 112 St. Olaf Avenue South, Canby, MN, Zip 56220-1433; tel. 507/223-7277; Robert J. Salmon, Chief Executive Officer

SWIFT COUNTY-BENSON HOSPITAL, 1815 Wisconsin Avenue, Benson, MN, Zip 56215-1653; tel. 320/843-4232; Frank Lawatsch, Chief Executive Officer

TYLER HEALTHCARE CENTER/AVERA HEALTH, 240 Willow Street, Tyler, MN, Zip 56178-0280, Mailing Address: P.O. Box 280, Zip 56178-0280; tel. 507/247-5521; Douglas P. Schweikhart, Administrator

WEINER MEMORIAL MEDICAL CENTER, 300 South Bruce Street, Marshall, MN, Zip 56258-3900; tel. 507/532-9661; Richard G. Slieter, Jr, Administrator

WHEATON COMMUNITY HOSPITAL, 401 12th Street North, Wheaton, MN, Zip 56296-1099; tel. 320/563-8226; James J. Talley, Administrator

NORTHERN LAKES HEALTH CONSORTIUM
600 East Superior Street, Suite 404, Duluth, MN 55802; tel. 218/727-9393; Terry J. Hill, Executive Director

CLOQUET COMMUNITY MEMORIAL HOSPITAL, 512 Skyline Boulevard, Cloquet, MN, Zip 55720-1199; tel. 218/879-4641; James J. Carroll, Administrator

COOK COUNTY NORTH SHORE HOSPITAL, Gunflint Trail, Grand Marais, MN, Zip 55604, Mailing Address: P.O. Box 10, Zip 55604-0010; tel. 218/387-3040; Diane Pearson, Administrator

COOK HOSPITAL AND CONVALESCENT NURSING CARE UNIT, 10 Fifth Street S.E., Cook, MN, Zip 55723-9745; tel. 218/666-5945; Allen J. Vogt, Administrator

CUMBERLAND MEMORIAL HOSPITAL, 1110 Seventh Avenue, Cumberland, WI, Zip 54829; tel. 715/822-2741; Robert Hansen, Chief Executive Officer

CUYUNA REGIONAL MEDICAL CENTER, 320 East Main Street, Crosby, MN, Zip 56441-1690; tel. 218/546-7000; Thomas F. Reek, Chief Executive Officer

DEER RIVER HEALTHCARE CENTER, 1002 Comstock Drive, Deer River, MN, Zip 56636-9700; tel. 218/246-2900; Jeffry Stampohar, Chief Executive Officer

ELY-BLOOMENSON COMMUNITY HOSPITAL, 328 West Conan Street, Ely, MN, Zip 55731-1198; tel. 218/365-3271; John Fossum, Administrator

FALLS MEMORIAL HOSPITAL, 1400 Highway 71, International Falls, MN, Zip 56649-2189; tel. 218/283-4481; Mary Klimp, Administrator and Chief Executive Officer

FLAMBEAU HOSPITAL, 98 Sherry Avenue, Park Falls, WI, Zip 54552-1467, Mailing Address: P.O. Box 310, Zip 54552-0310; tel. 715/762-2484; Curtis A. Johnson, Administrator

GRAND VIEW HOSPITAL, N10561 Grand View Lane, Ironwood, MI, Zip 49938-9359; tel. 906/932-2525; Frederick Geissler, Chief Executive Officer

Networks / Health Midwest

HAYWARD AREA MEMORIAL HOSPITAL AND NURSING HOME, 11040 North State Road 77, Hayward, WI, Zip 54843; tel. 715/634-8911; Barbara A. Peickert, R.N., Chief Executive Officer

ITASCA MEDICAL CENTER, 126 First Avenue S.E., Grand Rapids, MN, Zip 55744-3698; tel. 218/326-3401; Gary Kenner, President and Chief Executive Officer

LAKE VIEW MEMORIAL HOSPITAL, 325 11th Avenue, Two Harbors, MN, Zip 55616-1360; tel. 218/834-7300; Brian J. Carlson, FACHE, President and Chief Executive Officer

LAKEVIEW MEDICAL CENTER, 1100 North Main Street, Rice Lake, WI, Zip 54868-1238; tel. 715/234-1515; Edward H. Wolf, President and Chief Executive Officer

MERCY HOSPITAL AND HEALTH CARE CENTER, 710 South Kenwood Avenue, Moose Lake, MN, Zip 55767-9405; tel. 218/485-4481; Dianne Mandernach, Chief Executive Officer

MILLE LACS HEALTH SYSTEM, 200 North Elm Street, Onamia, MN, Zip 56359-7978; tel. 320/532-3154; Randall A. Farrow, Administrator

MILLER DWAN MEDICAL CENTER, 502 East Second Street, Duluth, MN, Zip 55805-1982; tel. 218/727-8762; William H. Palmer, President

NORTHERN ITASCA HEALTH CARE CENTER, 258 Pine Tree Drive, Bigfork, MN, Zip 56628, Mailing Address: P.O. Box 258, Zip 56628-0258; tel. 218/743-3177; Richard M. Ash, Chief Executive Officer

ONTONAGON MEMORIAL HOSPITAL, 601 Seventh Street, Ontonagon, MI, Zip 49953-1496; tel. 906/884-4134; Fred Nelson, Administrator

PINE MEDICAL CENTER, 109 Court Avenue South, Sandstone, MN, Zip 55072-5120; tel. 320/245-2212; Michael D. Hedrix, Administrator

RIVERWOOD HEALTHCARE CENTER, 301 Minnesota Avenue South, Aitkin, MN, Zip 56431-1697; tel. 218/927-2121; Debra Boardman, Chief Executive Officer

SPOONER HEALTH SYSTEM, 819 Ash Street, Spooner, WI, Zip 54801-1299; tel. 715/635-2111; Michael Schafer, Chief Executive Officer

ST. LUKE'S HOSPITAL, 915 East First Street, Duluth, MN, Zip 55805-2193; tel. 218/726-5555; John Strange, President and Chief Executive Officer

UNIVERSITY MEDICAL CENTER-MESABI, 750 East 34th Street, Hibbing, MN, Zip 55746-4600; tel. 218/262-4881; Richard W. Dinter, M.D., Chief Operating Officer

VIRGINIA REGIONAL MEDICAL CENTER, 901 Ninth Street North, Virginia, MN, Zip 55792-2398; tel. 218/741-3340; Kyle Hopstad, Administrator

WHITE COMMUNITY HOSPITAL, 5211 Highway 110, Aurora, MN, Zip 55705-1599; tel. 218/229-2211; Larry Ravenberg, Administrator

NORTHSTAR HEALTH CONSORTIUM
715 Delmore Drive, Roseau, MN 56751; tel. 218/463-2500; Dave Hagen, Chairman

KITTSON MEMORIAL HEALTHCARE CENTER, 1010 South Birch Street, Hallock, MN, Zip 56728, Mailing Address: P.O. Box 700, Zip 56728-0700; tel. 218/843-3612; Richard J. Failing, Chief Executive Officer

LAKEWOOD HEALTH CENTER, 600 Main Avenue South, Baudette, MN, Zip 56623; tel. 218/634-2120; SharRay Palm, President and Chief Executive Officer

NORTH VALLEY HEALTH CENTER, 109 South Minnesota Street, Warren, MN, Zip 56762-1499; tel. 218/745-4211; Jon Linnell, Administrator

ROSEAU AREA HOSPITAL AND HOMES, 715 Delmore Avenue, Roseau, MN, Zip 56751-1599; tel. 218/463-2500; David F. Hagen, President and Chief Executive Officer

SOUTHWEST MINNESOTA HEALTH ALLIANCE
MN 56156; tel. 612/896-3417

LUVERNE COMMUNITY HOSPITAL, 305 East Luverne Street, Luverne, MN, Zip 56156-2519, Mailing Address: P.O. Box 1019, Zip 56156-1019; tel. 507/283-2321; Gerald E. Carl, Administrator

MURRAY COUNTY MEMORIAL HOSPITAL, 2042 Juniper Avenue, Slayton, MN, Zip 56172-1016; tel. 507/836-6111; Jerry Bobeldyk, Administrator

SIOUX VALLEY CANBY CAMPUS, 112 St. Olaf Avenue South, Canby, MN, Zip 56220-1433; tel. 507/223-7277; Robert J. Salmon, Chief Executive Officer

SIOUX VALLEY HOSPITAL AND UNIVERSITY MEDICAL CENTER, 1100 South Euclid Avenue, Sioux Falls, SD, Zip 57105-0496, Mailing Address: P.O. Box 5039, Zip 57117-5039; tel. 605/333-1000; Becky Nelson, President

TRACY AREA MEDICAL SERVICES, 251 Fifth Street East, Tracy, MN, Zip 56175-1536; tel. 507/629-3200; Dan Reiner, Administrator and Chief Executive Officer

WINDOM AREA HOSPITAL, Highways 60 and 71 North, Windom, MN, Zip 56101, Mailing Address: P.O. Box 339, Zip 56101-0339; tel. 507/831-2400

WORTHINGTON REGIONAL HOSPITAL, 1018 Sixth Avenue, Worthington, MN, Zip 56187-2202, Mailing Address: P.O. Box 997, Zip 56187-0997; tel. 507/372-2941; Melvin J. Platt, Administrator

MISSISSIPPI

NORTH MISSISSIPPI HEALTH SERVICES
830 South Gloster, Tupelo, MS 38801; tel. 662/841-3148; Len Grice, Marketing Director

CLAY COUNTY MEDICAL CENTER, 835 Medical Center Drive, West Point, MS, Zip 39773-9320; tel. 601/495-2300; David M. Reid, Administrator

IUKA HOSPITAL, 1777 Curtis Drive, Iuka, MS, Zip 38852-1001, Mailing Address: P.O. Box 860, Zip 38852-0860; tel. 662/423-6051; Daniel Perryman, Administrator

NORTH MISSISSIPPI MEDICAL CENTER, 830 South Gloster Street, Tupelo, MS, Zip 38801-4934; tel. 601/841-3000; Jeffrey B. Barber, Dr.PH, President and Chief Executive Officer

PONTOTOC HOSPITAL AND EXTENDED CARE FACILITY, 176 South Main Street, Pontotoc, MS, Zip 38863-3311, Mailing Address: P.O. Box 790, Zip 38863-0790; tel. 662/488-7640; Fred B. Hood, Administrator

WEBSTER HEALTH SERVICES, 500 Highway 9 South, Eupora, MS, Zip 39744; tel. 601/258-6221; Harold H. Whitaker, Administrator

MISSOURI

BJC HEALTH SYSTEM
4444 Forest Park Av-S500, St. Louis, MO 63108; tel. 314/286-2085; Patrick N. Lee, Management Assoc

ALTON MEMORIAL HOSPITAL, One Memorial Drive, Alton, IL, Zip 62002-6722; tel. 618/463-7311; Ronald B. McMullen, President

BARNES-JEWISH HOSPITAL, One Barnes-Jewish Hospital Plaza, Saint Louis, MO, Zip 63110-1094; tel. 314/747-3000; Ronald G. Evens, M.D., President

BARNES-JEWISH ST. PETERS HOSPITAL, 10 Hospital Drive, Saint Peters, MO, Zip 63376-1659; tel. 636/916-9000; Carmelo J. Moceri, President

BARNES-JEWISH WEST COUNTY HOSPITAL, 12634 Olive Boulevard, Saint Louis, MO, Zip 63141-6354; tel. 314/996-8000; Ronald G. Evens, M.D., Interim President and Senior Executive Officer

BOONE HOSPITAL CENTER, 1600 East Broadway, Columbia, MO, Zip 65201-5897; tel. 573/815-8000; Michael B. Shirk, President and Senior Executive Officer

CHRISTIAN HOSPITAL NORTHEAST-NORTHWEST, 11133 Dunn Road, Saint Louis, MO, Zip 63136-6192; tel. 314/653-5000; Mark A. Eustis, President

CLAY COUNTY HOSPITAL, 911 Stacy Burk Drive, Flora, IL, Zip 62839-1823, Mailing Address: P.O. Box 280, Zip 62839-0280; tel. 618/662-2131; Tony Schwarm, President

FAYETTE COUNTY HOSPITAL, Seventh and Taylor Streets, Vandalia, IL, Zip 62471-1096; tel. 618/283-1231; Daniel L. Gantz, President

MISSOURI BAPTIST HOSPITAL OF SULLIVAN, 751 Sappington Bridge Road, Sullivan, MO, Zip 63080-2354, Mailing Address: P.O. Box 190, Zip 63080-0190; tel. 573/468-4186; Davis D. Skinner, President

MISSOURI BAPTIST MEDICAL CENTER, 3015 North Ballas Road, Town and Country, MO, Zip 63131-2374; tel. 314/996-5000; Mark A. Eustis, President and Senior Executive Officer

PARKLAND HEALTH CENTER, 1101 West Liberty Street, Farmington, MO, Zip 63640-1997; tel. 573/756-6451; Richard L. Conklin, President

SALEM TOWNSHIP HOSPITAL, 1201 Ricker Drive, Salem, IL, Zip 62881-6250; tel. 618/548-3194; James E. Robertson, Jr, President

ST. LOUIS CHILDREN'S HOSPITAL, One Children's Place, Saint Louis, MO, Zip 63110-1077; tel. 314/454-6000; Ted W. Frey, President and Senior Executive Officer

CARONDELET HEALTH
P.O. Box 8510, Kansas City, MO 64114; tel. 816/943-2673; George A. Zara, Chief Executive Officer

MCCUNE-BROOKS HOSPITAL, 627 West Centennial Avenue, Carthage, MO, Zip 64836-0677; tel. 417/358-8121; Robert Y. Copeland, Jr, Chief Executive Officer

ST. JOHN'S REGIONAL MEDICAL CENTER, 2727 McClelland Boulevard, Joplin, MO, Zip 64804-1694; tel. 417/781-2727; Gary L. Rowe, President and Chief Executive Officer

ST. JOSEPH HEALTH CENTER, 300 First Capitol Drive, Saint Charles, MO, Zip 63301-2835; tel. 636/947-5000; Kevin F. Kast, President, Chief Executive Officer and Market Executive

ST. MARY'S HOSPITAL OF BLUE SPRINGS, 201 West R. D. Mize Road, Blue Springs, MO, Zip 64014; tel. 816/228-5900; Gordon Docking, Chief Executive Officer

FREEMAN HEALTH SYSTEMS
1102 W. 32nd, Joplin, MO 64804; tel. 417/623-2801; Gary Duncan, President/Chief Executive Officer

HEALTH MIDWEST
2306 E. Meyer Blvd., B-11, Kansas city, MO 64232; tel. 816/276-9130; Thomas Cranshaw, Senior Vice President, Strategic Planning

ALLEN COUNTY HOSPITAL, 101 South First Street, Iola, KS, Zip 66749-3505, Mailing Address: P.O. Box 540, Zip 66749-0540; tel. 316/365-1000; Bill May, Chief Executive Officer

BAPTIST MEDICAL CENTER, 6601 Rockhill Road, Kansas City, MO, Zip 64131-1197; tel. 816/276-7000; Darrell W. Moore, President and Chief Executive Officer

CASS MEDICAL CENTER, 1800 East Mechanic Street, Harrisonville, MO, Zip 64701-2099; tel. 816/380-3474; Alan O. Freeman, Chief Executive Officer

HEDRICK MEDICAL CENTER, 100 Central Avenue, Chillicothe, MO, Zip 64601-1599; tel. 660/646-1480; James K. Johnson, Chief Executive Officer

INDEPENDENCE REGIONAL HEALTH CENTER, 1509 West Truman Road, Independence, MO, Zip 64050-3498; tel. 816/836-8100; Michael W. Chappelow, President and Chief Executive Officer

LAFAYETTE REGIONAL HEALTH CENTER, 1500 State Street, Lexington, MO, Zip 64067-1199; tel. 660/259-2203; Jeffrey S. Tarrant, Administrator

LEE'S SUMMIT HOSPITAL, 530 North Murray Road, Lees Summit, MO, Zip 64081-1497; tel. 816/969-6000; John L. Jacobson, President and Chief Executive Officer

© 2000 AHA Guide

Networks / Health Midwest

MEDICAL CENTER OF INDEPENDENCE, 17203 East 23rd Street, Independence, MO, Zip 64057-1899; tel. 816/478-5000; J. Kent Howard, President and Chief Executive Officer

MENORAH MEDICAL CENTER, 5721 West 119th Street, Shawnee Mission, KS, Zip 66209-3722; tel. 913/498-6000; Steven D. Wilkinson, President and Chief Executive Officer

OVERLAND PARK REGIONAL MEDICAL CENTER, 10500 Quivira Road, Shawnee Mission, KS, Zip 66215-2306, Mailing Address: P.O. Box 15959, Zip 66215-5959; tel. 913/541-5000; Kevin J. Hicks, President and Chief Executive Officer

REHABILITATION INSTITUTE, 3011 Baltimore, Kansas City, MO, Zip 64108-3465; tel. 816/751-7900; Ronald L. Herrick, President

RESEARCH BELTON HOSPITAL, 17065 South 71 Highway, Belton, MO, Zip 64012-2165; tel. 816/348-1200; Daniel F. Sheehan, Administrator

RESEARCH MEDICAL CENTER, 2316 East Meyer Boulevard, Kansas City, MO, Zip 64132-1199; tel. 816/276-4000; Steven R. Newton, President and Chief Executive Officer

RESEARCH PSYCHIATRIC CENTER, 2323 East 63rd Street, Kansas City, MO, Zip 64130-3495; tel. 816/444-8161; Todd Krass, Administrator and Chief Executive Officer

TRINITY LUTHERAN HOSPITAL, 3030 Baltimore Avenue, Kansas City, MO, Zip 64108-3404; tel. 816/751-4600; Ronald A. Ommen, President and Chief Executive Officer

HEARTLAND HEALTH SYSTEM
5325 Faraon Street, St. Joseph, MO 64506; tel. 816/271-6012; Curt Kretzinger, Chief Operating Officer

HEARTLAND REGIONAL MEDICAL CENTER, 5325 Faraon Street, Saint Joseph, MO, Zip 64506-3398; tel. 816/271-6000; Lowell C. Kruse, Chief Executive Officer

NORTHWEST MISSOURI HEALTHCARE AGENDA
705 North College Avenue, Albany, MO 64402; tel. 816/726-3941; John Richmond, Chairman

HEARTLAND REGIONAL MEDICAL CENTER, 5325 Faraon Street, Saint Joseph, MO, Zip 64506-3398; tel. 816/271-6000; Lowell C. Kruse, Chief Executive Officer

SAINT LUKES–SHAWNEE MISSIOU HEALTH SYSTEM
10920 Elm Avenue, Kansas City, MO 64134; tel. 816/932-3377; Ruth Coleman, Vice President, Strategic Planning

ANDERSON COUNTY HOSPITAL, 421 South Maple, Garnett, KS, Zip 66032-1334, Mailing Address: P.O. Box 309, Zip 66032-0309; tel. 785/448-3131; Dennis A. Hachenberg, CHE, Chief Executive Officer

CRITTENTON, 10918 Elm Avenue, Kansas City, MO, Zip 64134-4199; tel. 816/765-6600; Gary L. Watson, FACHE, Senior Executive Officer

SAINT LUKE'S HOSPITAL, 4401 Wornall Road, Kansas City, MO, Zip 64111-3238; tel. 816/932-2000; G. Richard Hastings, President and Chief Executive Officer

SAINT LUKE'S NORTHLAND HOSPITAL, 5830 N.W. Barry Road, Kansas City, MO, Zip 64154; tel. 816/891-6000; N. Gary Wages, President and Chief Executive Officer

SAINT LUKE'S NORTHLAND HOSPITAL–SMITHVILLE CAMPUS, 601 South 169 Highway, Smithville, MO, Zip 64089-9334; tel. 816/532-3700; Don Sipes, Chief Executive Officer

SAINT LUKE'S SOUTH HOSPITAL, 12300 Metcalf Avenue, Overland Park, KS, Zip 66213; tel. 913/317-7000; William G. Robertson, Chief Executive Officer

SHAWNEE MISSION MEDICAL CENTER, 9100 West 74th Street, Shawnee Mission, KS, Zip 66204-4004, Mailing Address: Box 2923, Zip 66201-1323; tel. 913/676-2000; William G. Robertson, Chief Executive Officer

ST. LUKE'S HOSPITAL, 232 South Woods Mill Road, Chesterfield, MO, Zip 63017-3480; tel. 314/434-1500; Gary R. Olson, President

WRIGHT MEMORIAL HOSPITAL, 701 East First Street, Trenton, MO, Zip 64683-0648, Mailing Address: P.O. Box 628, Zip 64683-0628; tel. 660/359-5621; Ralph G. Goodrich, Chief Executive Officer

SSM HEALTH CARE–ST LOUIS
1173 Corporate Lake Drive, St. Louis, MO 63132; tel. 314/989-2000; RONALD J. LEVY, President/Chief Executive Officer

CARDINAL GLENNON CHILDREN'S HOSPITAL, 1465 South Grand Boulevard, Saint Louis, MO, Zip 63104-1095; tel. 314/577-5600; Douglas A. Ries, President

DEPAUL HEALTH CENTER, 12303 DePaul Drive, Saint Louis, MO, Zip 63044-2588; tel. 314/344-6000; Robert G. Porter, President

PIKE COUNTY MEMORIAL HOSPITAL, 2305 West Georgia Street, Louisiana, MO, Zip 63353-0020; tel. 573/754-5531; Gregory C. Reed, Administrator

SSM REHAB, 6420 Clayton Road, Suite 600, Saint Louis, MO, Zip 63117-1861; tel. 314/768-5300; Melinda Clark, President

ST. JOSEPH HEALTH CENTER, 300 First Capitol Drive, Saint Charles, MO, Zip 63301-2835; tel. 636/947-5000; Kevin F. Kast, President, Chief Executive Officer and Market Executive

ST. JOSEPH HOSPITAL WEST, 100 Medical Plaza, Lake Saint Louis, MO, Zip 63367-1395; tel. 314/625-5200; Kevin F. Kast, President, Chief Executive Officer and Market Executive

ST. MARY'S HEALTH CENTER, 6420 Clayton Road, Saint Louis, MO, Zip 63117-1811; tel. 314/768-8000; James B. Rigby, Interim President

ST. MARY'S HOSPITAL OF EAST ST. LOUIS, 129 North Eighth Street, East St. Louis, IL, Zip 62201-2999; tel. 618/274-1900; Richard J. Mark, President and Chief Executive Officer

UNITY HEALTH
12409 Powers Court Drive, St. Louis, MO 63131; tel. 314/364-3000; Jim Hobbs, Interim President

ST. ANTHONY'S MEDICAL CENTER, 10010 Kennerly Road, Saint Louis, MO, Zip 63128-2185; tel. 314/525-1000; David P. Seifert, President and Chief Executive Officer

ST. CLEMENT HEALTH SERVICES, One St. Clement Boulevard, Red Bud, IL, Zip 62278-1194; tel. 618/282-3831; Michael T. McManus, Administrator

ST. JOHN'S MERCY MEDICAL CENTER, 615 South New Ballas Road, Saint Louis, MO, Zip 63141-8277; tel. 314/569-6000; Mark Weber, FACHE, President

ST. LUKE'S HOSPITAL, 232 South Woods Mill Road, Chesterfield, MO, Zip 63017-3480; tel. 314/434-1500; Gary R. Olson, President

UNIVERSITY OF MISSOURI HEALTH
1 Hospital Drive, Columbia, MO 65201; tel. 573/882-4141; Robert Churchill, Interim Director

MONTANA

MONTANA HEALTH NETWORK INC
11 S. 7th Street, Suite 160, Miles City, MT 59301; tel. 406/232-1420; Janet Bastian, Chief Executive Officer

BEARTOOTH HOSPITAL AND HEALTH CENTER, 600 West 20th Street, Red Lodge, MT, Zip 59068, Mailing Address: P.O. Box 590, Zip 59068-0590; tel. 406/446-2345; Kelley Evans, Administrator

CENTRAL MONTANA MEDICAL CENTER, 408 Wendell Avenue, Lewistown, MT, Zip 59457-2261; tel. 406/538-7711; David M. Faulkner, Chief Executive Officer

DANIELS MEMORIAL HOSPITAL, 105 Fifth Avenue East, Scobey, MT, Zip 59263, Mailing Address: P.O. Box 400, Zip 59263-0400; tel. 406/487-2296; Glenn Haugo, Administrator

DEACONESS BILLINGS CLINIC, 2800 10th Avenue North, Billings, MT, Zip 59101-0799, Mailing Address: P.O. Box 37000, Zip 59107-7000; tel. 406/657-4000; Nicholas J. Wolter, M.D., Chief Executive Officer

FALLON MEDICAL COMPLEX, 202 South 4th Street West, Baker, MT, Zip 59313-0820, Mailing Address: P.O. Box 820, Zip 59313-0820; tel. 406/778-3331; David Espeland, Chief Executive Officer

FRANCES MAHON DEACONESS HOSPITAL, 621 Third Street South, Glasgow, MT, Zip 59230-2699; tel. 406/228-3500; Randall G. Holom, Chief Executive Officer

GLENDIVE MEDICAL CENTER, 202 Prospect Drive, Glendive, MT, Zip 59330-1999; tel. 406/345-3306

HOLY ROSARY HEALTH CENTER, 2600 Wilson Street, Miles City, MT, Zip 59301-5094; tel. 406/233-2600

MCCONE COUNTY MEDICAL ASSISTANCE FACILITY, Circle, MT, Mailing Address: P.O. Box 48, Zip 59215-0048; tel. 406/485-3381; Mack N. Simpson, Administrator

NORTHEAST MONTANA HEALTH SERVICES, 315 Knapp Street, Wolf Point, MT, Zip 59201-1898; tel. 406/653-2110; Margaret Norgaard, Administrator

PHILLIPS COUNTY MEDICAL CENTER, 417 South Fourth East, Malta, MT, Zip 59538, Mailing Address: P.O. Box 640, Zip 59538-0640; tel. 406/654-1100; Larry E. Putnam, Administrator

ROOSEVELT MEMORIAL MEDICAL CENTER, 818 Second Avenue East, Culbertson, MT, Zip 59218, Mailing Address: P.O. Box 419, Zip 59218-0419; tel. 406/787-6281; Audrey Stromberg, Administrator

ROUNDUP MEMORIAL HOSPITAL, 1202 Third Street West, Roundup, MT, Zip 59072-1816, Mailing Address: P.O. Box 40, Zip 59072-0040; tel. 406/323-2302; Dave McIvor, Administrator

SHERIDAN MEMORIAL HOSPITAL, 440 West Laurel Avenue, Plentywood, MT, Zip 59254-1596; tel. 406/765-1420; Ella Gutzke, Administrator

SIDNEY HEALTH CENTER, 216 14th Avenue S.W., Sidney, MT, Zip 59270-3586; tel. 406/488-2100; Donald J. Rush, Chief Executive Officer

STILLWATER COMMUNITY HOSPITAL, 44 West Fourth Avenue North, Columbus, MT, Zip 59019, Mailing Address: P.O. Box 959, Zip 59019-0959; tel. 406/322-5316; Tim Russell, Administrator

NEBRASKA

ALEGENT HEALTH
1010 North 96th Street, Omaha, NE 68114; tel. 402/255-1661; Robert Azar, President of Public Health

ALEGENT HEALTH COMMUNITY MEMORIAL HOSPITAL, 631 North Eighth Street, Missouri Valley, IA, Zip 51555-1199; tel. 712/642-2784; James A. Seymour, Regional Administrator

ALEGENT HEALTH IMMANUEL MEDICAL CENTER, 6901 North 72nd Street, Omaha, NE, Zip 68122-1799; tel. 402/572-2121; Barbara K. Goodrich, R.N., Administrator

ALEGENT HEALTH MERCY HOSPITAL, 703 Rosary Drive, Corning, IA, Zip 50841, Mailing Address: P.O. Box 368, Zip 50841-0368; tel. 515/322-3121; James C. Ruppert, Administrator

ALEGENT HEALTH MERCY HOSPITAL, 800 Mercy Drive, Council Bluffs, IA, Zip 51503-3128, Mailing Address: P.O. Box 1C, Zip 51502-3001; tel. 712/328-5000; Charles J. Marr, Chief Executive Officer

ALEGENT HEALTH–MEMORIAL HOSPITAL, 104 West 17th Street, Schuyler, NE, Zip 68661-1396; tel. 402/352-2441; Connie Peters, Operations Leader and Regional Administrator

BEHAVIORAL HEALTH SPECIALIST
600 S. 13th St., Norfolk, NE 68701; tel. 402/370-3401; Jackie O'Brien, Referral Specialist

BLUE RIVER VALLEY HEALTH NETWORK
121 S. 13th Suite 700, Lincoln, NE 68508; tel. 402/475-3865; Rick Boucher, Executive Director

Networks / Saint Mary's Health Network

ANNIE JEFFREY MEMORIAL COUNTY HEALTH CENTER, 531 Beebe Street, Osceola, NE, Zip 68651, Mailing Address: P.O. Box 428, Zip 68651-0428; tel. 402/747-2031; Carol E. Jones, Administrator

BUTLER COUNTY HEALTH CARE CENTER, 372 South Ninth Street, David City, NE, Zip 68632-2199; tel. 402/367-3115; Roger Reamer, Administrator

CRETE MUNICIPAL HOSPITAL, 1540 Grove Street, Crete, NE, Zip 68333-0220, Mailing Address: P.O. Box 220, Zip 68333-0220; tel. 402/826-6800; Joseph W. Lohrman, Administrator

FILLMORE COUNTY HOSPITAL, 1325 H Street, Geneva, NE, Zip 68361-1325, Mailing Address: P.O. Box 193, Zip 68361-0193; tel. 402/759-3167; Larry Eichelberger, Chief Executive Officer

HENDERSON HEALTH CARE SERVICES, 1621 Front Street, Henderson, NE, Zip 68371-0217, Mailing Address: P.O. Box 217, Zip 68371-0217; tel. 402/723-4512; Marianna Harris, Administrator

LITZENBERG MEMORIAL COUNTY HOSPITAL, 1715 26th Street, Central City, NE, Zip 68826-9620, Mailing Address: Route 2, Box 1, Zip 68826-0001; tel. 308/946-3015; Michael R. Bowman, Administrator

MEMORIAL HEALTH CARE SYSTEMS, 300 North Columbia Avenue, Seward, NE, Zip 68434-9907; tel. 402/643-2971; Ronald D. Waltz, Chief Executive Officer

MEMORIAL HOSPITAL, 1423 Seventh Street, Aurora, NE, Zip 68818-1197; tel. 402/694-3171; Eldon A. Wall, Administrator

SAUNDERS COUNTY HEALTH SERVICE, 805 West Tenth Street, Wahoo, NE, Zip 68066-1102, Mailing Address: P.O. Box 185, Zip 68066-0185; tel. 402/443-4191; Ed Hackman, Administrator

THAYER COUNTY HEALTH SERVICES, 120 Park Avenue, Hebron, NE, Zip 68370-2019, Mailing Address: P.O. Box 49, Zip 68370-0049; tel. 402/768-6041; Larry E. Leaming, Administrator

WARREN MEMORIAL HOSPITAL, 905 Second Street, Friend, NE, Zip 68359-1198; tel. 402/947-2541; Joseph W. Lohrman, Administrator

YORK GENERAL HOSPITAL, 2222 Lincoln Avenue, York, NE, Zip 68467-1095; tel. 402/362-0445; Charles K. Schulz, Chief Executive Officer

CENTRAL NEBRASKA PRIMARY
1518 J. Street, Ord, NE 68862;
tel. 308/728-3011; Victoria Bauer,
Foundation President

BOONE COUNTY HEALTH CENTER, 723 West Fairview Street, Albion, NE, Zip 68620-1725, Mailing Address: P.O. Box 151, Zip 68620-0151; tel. 402/395-2191; Victor Lee, FACHE, Chief Executive Officer

VALLEY COUNTY HOSPITAL, 217 Westridge Drive, Ord, NE, Zip 68862-1675; tel. 308/728-3211; Colleen Chapp, Interim Chief Executive Officer and Administrator

HEARTLAND HEALTH ALLIANCE
1600 South 48th Street, Lincoln, NE 68506;
tel. 402/481-8831; Kenneth L. Foster,
Executive Director

BEATRICE COMMUNITY HOSPITAL AND HEALTH CENTER, 1110 North Tenth Street, Beatrice, NE, Zip 68310-2039, Mailing Address: P.O. Box 278, Zip 68310-0278; tel. 402/228-3344; Colleen Chapp, Interim Administrator

BOONE COUNTY HEALTH CENTER, 723 West Fairview Street, Albion, NE, Zip 68620-1725, Mailing Address: P.O. Box 151, Zip 68620-0151; tel. 402/395-2191; Victor Lee, FACHE, Chief Executive Officer

BUTLER COUNTY HEALTH CARE CENTER, 372 South Ninth Street, David City, NE, Zip 68632-2199; tel. 402/367-3115; Roger Reamer, Administrator

CHERRY COUNTY HOSPITAL, Highway 12 and Green Street, Valentine, NE, Zip 69201-0410; tel. 402/376-2525; Brent A. Peterson, Administrator

CHILDREN'S HOSPITAL, 8301 Dodge Street, Omaha, NE, Zip 68114-4114; tel. 402/354-5400; Gary A. Perkins, President and Chief Executive Officer

COMMUNITY HOSPITAL, 1301 East H Street, McCook, NE, Zip 69001-1328, Mailing Address: P.O. Box 1328, Zip 69001-1328; tel. 308/345-2650; Gary Bieganski, President

COMMUNITY MEDICAL CENTER, 2307 Barada Street, Falls City, NE, Zip 68355-1599; tel. 402/245-2428; Asa B. Wilson, Ph.D., Administrator

COMMUNITY MEMORIAL HEALTHCARE, 708 North 18th Street, Marysville, KS, Zip 66508-1338; tel. 785/562-2311; Jay M. Canter, Chief Executive Officer

COMMUNITY MEMORIAL HOSPITAL, 1579 Midland Street, Syracuse, NE, Zip 68446-9732, Mailing Address: P.O. Box N, Zip 68446; tel. 402/269-2011; Al Klaasmeyer, Administrator

CRETE MUNICIPAL HOSPITAL, 1540 Grove Street, Crete, NE, Zip 68333-0220, Mailing Address: P.O. Box 220, Zip 68333-0220; tel. 402/826-6800; Joseph W. Lohrman, Administrator

FILLMORE COUNTY HOSPITAL, 1325 H Street, Geneva, NE, Zip 68361-1325, Mailing Address: P.O. Box 193, Zip 68361-0193; tel. 402/759-3167; Larry Eichelberger, Chief Executive Officer

FRANKLIN COUNTY MEMORIAL HOSPITAL, 1406 Q Street, Franklin, NE, Zip 68939-0315, Mailing Address: P.O. Box 315, Zip 68939-0315; tel. 308/425-6221; Jerrell F. Gerdes, Administrator

GOTHENBURG MEMORIAL HOSPITAL, 910 20th Street, Gothenburg, NE, Zip 69138-1237, Mailing Address: P.O. Box 469, Zip 69138-0469; tel. 308/537-3661; John H. Johnson, Chief Executive Officer

GREAT PLAINS REGIONAL MEDICAL CENTER, 601 West Leota Street, North Platte, NE, Zip 69101-6598, Mailing Address: P.O. Box 1167, Zip 69103-1167; tel. 308/534-9310; Lucinda A. Bradley, President

HARLAN COUNTY HEALTH SYSTEM, 717 North Brown Street, Alma, NE, Zip 68920-0836, Mailing Address: P.O. Box 836, Zip 68920-0836; tel. 308/928-2151; Allen Van Driel, Administrator

JEFFERSON COMMUNITY HEALTH CENTER, 2200 H Street, Fairbury, NE, Zip 68352-1119, Mailing Address: P.O. Box 277, Zip 68352-0277; tel. 402/729-3351; Bill Welch, Administrator

JENNIE M. MELHAM MEMORIAL MEDICAL CENTER, 145 Memorial Drive, Broken Bow, NE, Zip 68822-1378, Mailing Address: P.O. Box 250, Zip 68822-0250; tel. 402/872-6891; Michael J. Steckler, President and Chief Executive Officer

JOHNSON COUNTY HOSPITAL, 202 High Street, Tecumseh, NE, Zip 68450-0599, Mailing Address: P.O. Box 599, Zip 68450-0599; tel. 402/335-3361; John E. Keelan, Ph.D., Administrator

MARY LANNING MEMORIAL HOSPITAL, 715 North St. Joseph Avenue, Hastings, NE, Zip 68901-4497; tel. 402/461-5110; W. Michael Kearney, President

MEMORIAL HEALTH CARE SYSTEMS, 300 North Columbia Avenue, Seward, NE, Zip 68434-9907; tel. 402/643-2971; Ronald D. Waltz, Chief Executive Officer

MEMORIAL HOSPITAL, 1423 Seventh Street, Aurora, NE, Zip 68818-1197; tel. 402/694-3171; Eldon A. Wall, Administrator

MEMORIAL NUCKOLLS COUNTY HOSPITAL, 520 East Tenth Street, Superior, NE, Zip 68978-1225, Mailing Address: P.O. Box 187, Zip 68978-0187; tel. 402/879-3281; Michael J. Ellis, Administrator and Chief Executive Officer

RURAL HEALTHCARE NETWORK
821 Morehead Street, Chadron, NE 69337;
tel. 308/432-5586; Harold Krueger, Chief
Executive Officer

CHADRON COMMUNITY HOSPITAL AND HEALTH SERVICES, 821 Morehead Street, Chadron, NE, Zip 69337-2599; tel. 308/432-5586; Harold L. Krueger, Jr, Chief ExecutiveOfficer

CHASE COUNTY COMMUNITY HOSPITAL, 600 West 12th Street, Imperial, NE, Zip 69033-0819, Mailing Address: P.O. Box 819, Zip 69033-0819; tel. 308/882-7111; Ed Hackman, Administrator

GARDEN COUNTY HOSPITAL, 1100 West Second Street, Oshkosh, NE, Zip 69154, Mailing Address: P.O. Box 320, Zip 69154-0320; tel. 308/772-3283; Diana Stevens, Administrator

GORDON MEMORIAL HOSPITAL DISTRICT, 300 East Eighth Street, Gordon, NE, Zip 69343-9990; tel. 308/282-0401; Gladys Phemister, Chief Executive Officer

KIMBALL COUNTY HOSPITAL, 505 South Burg Street, Kimball, NE, Zip 69145-1398; tel. 308/235-3621; Kim Woods, Chief Executive Officer

MEMORIAL HEALTH CENTER, 645 Osage Street, Sidney, NE, Zip 69162-1799; tel. 308/254-5825; Rex D. Walk, Chief Executive Officer

MORRILL COUNTY COMMUNITY HOSPITAL, 1313 S Street, Bridgeport, NE, Zip 69336-0579, Mailing Address: P.O. Box 579, Zip 69336-0579; tel. 308/262-1616; Julia Morrow, Administrator

REGIONAL WEST MEDICAL CENTER, 4021 Avenue B, Scottsbluff, NE, Zip 69361-4695; tel. 308/635-3711; David M. Nitschke, President and Chief Executive Officer

WESTERN PLAINS COMMUNITY HEALTH SERVICES
302 West 27th Street, Scottsbluff, NE 69361;
tel. 308/635-2260; Steve Hetzel, Executive
Vice President

BOX BUTTE GENERAL HOSPITAL, 2101 Box Butte Avenue, Alliance, NE, Zip 69301-0810, Mailing Address: P.O. Box 810, Zip 69301-0810; tel. 308/762-6660; Terrance J. Padden, Administrator

CHADRON COMMUNITY HOSPITAL AND HEALTH SERVICES, 821 Morehead Street, Chadron, NE, Zip 69337-2599; tel. 308/432-5586; Harold L. Krueger, Jr, Chief ExecutiveOfficer

GARDEN COUNTY HOSPITAL, 1100 West Second Street, Oshkosh, NE, Zip 69154, Mailing Address: P.O. Box 320, Zip 69154-0320; tel. 308/772-3283; Diana Stevens, Administrator

GORDON MEMORIAL HOSPITAL DISTRICT, 300 East Eighth Street, Gordon, NE, Zip 69343-9990; tel. 308/282-0401; Gladys Phemister, Chief Executive Officer

KIMBALL COUNTY HOSPITAL, 505 South Burg Street, Kimball, NE, Zip 69145-1398; tel. 308/235-3621; Kim Woods, Chief Executive Officer

MORRILL COUNTY COMMUNITY HOSPITAL, 1313 S Street, Bridgeport, NE, Zip 69336-0579, Mailing Address: P.O. Box 579, Zip 69336-0579; tel. 308/262-1616; Julia Morrow, Administrator

REGIONAL WEST MEDICAL CENTER, 4021 Avenue B, Scottsbluff, NE, Zip 69361-4695; tel. 308/635-3711; David M. Nitschke, President and Chief Executive Officer

NEVADA

SAINT MARY'S HEALTH NETWORK
235 West Sixth Street, Reno, NV 89520;
tel. 775/789-3000; Tamara Bradshaw,
Research Assistant

SAINT MARY'S REGIONAL MEDICAL CENTER, 235 West Sixth Street, Reno, NV, Zip 89520-0108; tel. 775/323-2041; Jeff K. Bills, Chief Executive Officer

Networks / Saint Mary's Health Network

NEW HAMPSHIRE

CARING COMMUNITY NETWORK OF THE TWIN RIVERS
15 Aiken Ave., Franklin, NH 03235;
tel. 603/934-2060; Walter A. Strauch,
Chairman

FRANKLIN REGIONAL HOSPITAL, 15 Aiken Avenue,
Franklin, NH, Zip 03235-1299;
tel. 603/934-2060; Walter A. Strauch,
Executive Director

HEALTHLINK
80 Highland Street, Laconia, NH 03246;
tel. 603/527-2910; Sharon Swanson, Network
Contact

CATHOLIC MEDICAL CENTER, 100 McGregor Street,
Manchester, NH, Zip 03102-3770;
tel. 603/668-3545; Alyson Pitman Giles,
President and Chief Executive Officer

CONCORD HOSPITAL, 250 Pleasant Street, Concord,
NH, Zip 03301-2598; tel. 603/225-2711;
Michael B. Green, President and Chief Executive
Officer

ELLIOT HOSPITAL, One Elliot Way, Manchester, NH,
Zip 03103; tel. 603/669-5300; Douglas F.
Dean, Jr, President and Chief Executive Officer

LAKES REGION GENERAL HOSPITAL, 80 Highland
Street, Laconia, NH, Zip 03246-3298;
tel. 603/524-3211; Thomas Clairmont,
President

MARY HITCHCOCK MEMORIAL HOSPITAL, One Medical
Center Drive, Lebanon, NH, Zip 03756-0001;
tel. 603/650-5000; James W. Varnum,
President

PARTNERS IN HEALTH
243 Elm Street, Claremont, NH 03743;
tel. 603/542-7771; Jane Manning,
Chairperson

VALLEY REGIONAL HOSPITAL, 243 Elm Street,
Claremont, NH, Zip 03743-2099;
tel. 603/542-7771; Claire L. Bowen, Chief
Executive Officer

NEW JERSEY

ATLANTIC HEALTH SYSTEM
325 Columbia Turnpike, Flortham Park, NJ
07932; tel. 973/660-3100; Richard P. Oths,
President & Chief Executive Officer

ATLANTIC HEALTH SYSTEM, 325 Columbia Turnpike,
Florham Park, NJ, Zip 07932-0959, Mailing
Address: P.O. Box 959, Zip 07932-0959;
tel. 973/660-3100; Richard P. Oths, President
and Chief Executive Officer

ATLANTICARE HEALTH SYSTEM
6725 Delilah Road, Egg Harbor Township, NJ
08234; tel. 609/272-6311; Dominic S. Moffa,
Vice President–Administration

ATLANTIC CITY MEDICAL CENTER, 1925 Pacific
Avenue, Atlantic City, NJ, Zip 08401-6713;
tel. 609/345-4000; David P. Tilton, President
and Chief Executive Officer

CAPE SHORE MEDICAL GROUP
Two Stone Habor Boulevard, Court House, NJ
08210; tel. 609/463-2480; Tom Scott,
President & Chief Executive Officer

ALBERT EINSTEIN MEDICAL CENTER, 5501 Old York
Road, Philadelphia, PA, Zip 19141-3098;
tel. 215/456-7890; Martin Goldsmith, President

ALFRED I. DUPONT HOSPITAL FOR CHILDREN, 1600
Rockland Road, Wilmington, DE,
Zip 19803-3616, Mailing Address: Box 269,
Zip 19899-0269; tel. 302/651-4000; Thomas
P. Ferry, Administrator and Chief Executive

BURDETTE TOMLIN MEMORIAL HOSPITAL, 2 Stone
Harbor Boulevard, Cape May Court House, NJ,
Zip 08210-9990; tel. 609/463-2000; Thomas
L. Scott, FACHE, President and Chief Executive
Officer

CHILDREN'S HOSPITAL OF PHILADELPHIA, 34th
Street and Civic Center Boulevard, Philadelphia,
PA, Zip 19104-4399; tel. 215/590-1000;
Steven M. Altschuler, President and Chief
Executive Officer

FOX CHASE CANCER CENTER–AMERICAN
ONCOLOGIC HOSPITAL, 7701 Burholme Avenue,
Philadelphia, PA, Zip 19111-2412;
tel. 215/728-6900; Robert C. Young, M.D.,
President

LANKENAU HOSPITAL, 100 Lancaster Avenue West,
Wynnewood, PA, Zip 19096-3411;
tel. 610/645-2000; C. Barry Dykes, Senior Vice
President

THE COOPER HEALTH SYSTEM, One Cooper Plaza,
Camden, NJ, Zip 08103-1489;
tel. 856/342-2000; Leslie D. Hirsch, President
and Chief Executive Officer

THOMAS JEFFERSON UNIVERSITY HOSPITAL, 111
South 11th Street, Philadelphia, PA,
Zip 19107-5096; tel. 215/955-7022; Thomas
J. Lewis, President and Chief Executive Officer

CLARA MAASS HEALTH SYSTEM
One Franklin Avenue, Belleville, NJ 07109;
tel. 201/450-2000; Robert S. Curtis,
President

CLARA MAASS HEALTH SYSTEM, 1 Clara Maass
Drive, Belleville, NJ, Zip 07109-3557;
tel. 973/450-2000; Thomas A. Biga, Executive
Director

COMMUNITY MEDICAL CENTER
99 Highway 37 W., Toms River, NJ 08755;
tel. 732/557-8051; Nancy L. Wollen,
Executive Director

COMMUNITY MEDICAL CENTER, 99 Route 37 West,
Toms River, NJ, Zip 08755-6423;
tel. 732/557-8000; Nancy L. Wollen, Executive
Director

FIRST OPTION HEALTH PLAN
2 Bridge Street, Red Bank, NJ 07701;
tel. 908/842-5000; John McCarthy, Vice
President Finance

BARNERT HOSPITAL, 680 Broadway Street, Paterson,
NJ, Zip 07514-1472; tel. 973/977-6600;
Stephen M. Patz, President and Chief Executive
Officer

BAYSHORE COMMUNITY HOSPITAL, 727 North Beers
Street, Holmdel, NJ, Zip 07733-1598;
tel. 732/739-5900; Thomas Goldman, President
and Chief Executive Officer

BETH ISRAEL HOSPITAL, 70 Parker Avenue, Passaic,
NJ, Zip 07055-7000; tel. 973/365-5000;
Jeffrey S. Moll, President and Chief Executive
Officer

BURDETTE TOMLIN MEMORIAL HOSPITAL, 2 Stone
Harbor Boulevard, Cape May Court House, NJ,
Zip 08210-9990; tel. 609/463-2000; Thomas
L. Scott, FACHE, President and Chief Executive
Officer

CENTRASTATE HEALTHCARE SYSTEM, 901 West
Main Street, Freehold, NJ, Zip 07728-2549;
tel. 732/431-2000; Thomas H. Litz, FACHE,
President and Chief Executive Officer

CHILTON MEMORIAL HOSPITAL, 97 West Parkway,
Pompton Plains, NJ, Zip 07444-1696;
tel. 973/831-5000; James J. Doyle, Jr,
President and Chief Executive Officer

CHRIST HOSPITAL, 176 Palisade Avenue, Jersey City,
NJ, Zip 07306-1196, Mailing Address: P.O. Box
J-1, Zip 07306-1196; tel. 201/795-8200;
Francis J. Cronin, President and Chief Executive
Officer

CLARA MAASS HEALTH SYSTEM, 1 Clara Maass
Drive, Belleville, NJ, Zip 07109-3557;
tel. 973/450-2000; Thomas A. Biga, Executive
Director

COMMUNITY MEDICAL CENTER, 99 Route 37 West,
Toms River, NJ, Zip 08755-6423;
tel. 732/557-8000; Nancy L. Wollen, Executive
Director

EAST ORANGE GENERAL HOSPITAL, 300 Central
Avenue, East Orange, NJ, Zip 07019-2819;
tel. 973/672-8400; Darlene L. Cox, President
and Chief Executive Officer

ENGLEWOOD HOSPITAL AND MEDICAL CENTER, 350
Engle Street, Englewood, NJ, Zip 07631-1898;
tel. 201/894-3000; Daniel A. Kane, President
and Chief Executive Officer

HACKETTSTOWN COMMUNITY HOSPITAL, 651 Willow
Grove Street, Hackettstown, NJ,
Zip 07840-1798; tel. 908/852-5100; Gene C.
Milton, President and Chief Executive Officer

HOLY NAME HOSPITAL, 718 Teaneck Road, Teaneck,
NJ, Zip 07666-4281; tel. 201/833-3000;
Michael Maron, President and Chief Executive
Officer

HUNTERDON MEDICAL CENTER, 2100 Wescott Drive,
Flemington, NJ, Zip 08822-4604;
tel. 908/788-6100; Robert P. Wise, President
and Chief Executive Officer

IRVINGTON GENERAL HOSPITAL, 832 Chancellor
Avenue, Irvington, NJ, Zip 07111-0709;
tel. 973/399-6000; Amit Mody, M.D., Executive
Director

JFK MEDICAL CENTER, 65 James Street, Edison, NJ,
Zip 08818-3947; tel. 732/321-7000; John P.
McGee, President and Chief Executive Officer

KIMBALL MEDICAL CENTER, 600 River Avenue,
Lakewood, NJ, Zip 08701-5281;
tel. 732/363-1900; Joanne Carrocino,
Executive Director

MEDICAL CENTER AT PRINCETON, 253 Witherspoon
Street, Princeton, NJ, Zip 08540-3213;
tel. 609/497-4000; Dennis W. Doody, President
and Chief Executive Officer

MONMOUTH MEDICAL CENTER, 300 Second Avenue,
Long Branch, NJ, Zip 07740-6303;
tel. 732/222-5200; Frank J. Vozos, M.D.,
FACS, Executive Director

MUHLENBERG REGIONAL MEDICAL CENTER, 1200
Park Avenue, Plainfield, NJ, Zip 07061;
tel. 908/668-2000; John R. Kopicki, President
and Chief Executive Officer

NEWARK BETH ISRAEL MEDICAL CENTER, 201 Lyons
Avenue, Newark, NJ, Zip 07112-2027;
tel. 973/926-7000; Paul A. Mertz, Executive
Director

NEWTON MEMORIAL HOSPITAL, 175 High Street,
Newton, NJ, Zip 07860-1004;
tel. 973/383-2121; Dennis H. Collette,
President and Chief Executive Officer

OUR LADY OF LOURDES MEDICAL CENTER, 1600
Haddon Avenue, Camden, NJ, Zip 08103-3117;
tel. 856/757-3500; Alexander J. Hatala,
President and Chief Executive Officer

PALISADES MEDICAL CENTER, 7600 River Road,
North Bergen, NJ, Zip 07047-6217;
tel. 201/854-5000; Bruce J. Markowitz,
President and Chief Executive Officer

PASCACK VALLEY HOSPITAL, 250 Old Hook Road,
Westwood, NJ, Zip 07675-3181;
tel. 201/358-3000; Louis R. Ycre, Jr, FACHE,
President and Chief Executive Officer

ROBERT WOOD JOHNSON UNIVERSITY HOSPITAL, 1
Robert Wood Johnson Place, New Brunswick, NJ,
Zip 08903-2601; tel. 732/828-3000; Harvey
A. Holzberg, President and Chief Executive
Officer

SAINT BARNABAS MEDICAL CENTER, 94 Old Short
Hills Road, Livingston, NJ, Zip 07039-5668;
tel. 973/322-5000; Vincent D. Joseph,
Executive Director

SHORE MEMORIAL HOSPITAL, 1 East New York
Avenue, Somers Point, NJ, Zip 08244-2387;
tel. 609/653-3500; Richard A. Pitman,
President

SOMERSET MEDICAL CENTER, 110 Rehill Avenue,
Somerville, NJ, Zip 08876-2598;
tel. 908/685-2200; Dennis C. Miller, President
and Chief Executive Officer

SOUTH JERSEY HOSPITAL, 333 Irving Avenue,
Bridgeton, NJ, Zip 08302-2100;
tel. 856/451-6600; Chester B. Kaletkowski,
President and Chief Executive Officer

SOUTHERN OCEAN COUNTY HOSPITAL, 1140 Route
72 West, Manahawkin, NJ, Zip 08050-2499;
tel. 609/978-8900; Joseph P. Coyle, President
and Chief Executive Officer

ST. FRANCIS MEDICAL CENTER, 601 Hamilton
Avenue, Trenton, NJ, Zip 08629-1986;
tel. 609/599-5000; Judith M. Persichilli,
President and Chief Executive Officer

ST. JOSEPH'S HOSPITAL AND MEDICAL CENTER, 703
Main Street, Paterson, NJ, Zip 07503-2691;
tel. 973/754-2000; Patrick R. Wardell,
President and Chief Executive Officer

Networks / University Hospital

ST. PETER'S UNIVERSITY HOSPITAL, 254 Easton Avenue, New Brunswick, NJ, Zip 08901–1780, Mailing Address: P.O. Box 591, Zip 08903–0591; tel. 732/745–8600; John E. Matuska, President and Chief Executive Officer

TRINITAS HOSPITAL, 925 East Jersey Street, Elizabeth, NJ, Zip 07201–2728; tel. 908/289–8600; David A. Fletcher, President and Chief Executive Officer

UNDERWOOD–MEMORIAL HOSPITAL, 509 North Broad Street, Woodbury, NJ, Zip 08096–1697, Mailing Address: P.O. Box 359, Zip 08096–7359; tel. 856/845–0100; Steven W. Jackmuff, President and Chief Executive Officer

UNION HOSPITAL, 1000 Galloping Hill Road, Union, NJ, Zip 07083–1652; tel. 908/687–1900; Kathryn W. Coyne, Executive Director

VALLEY HOSPITAL, 223 North Van Dien Avenue, Ridgewood, NJ, Zip 07450–9982; tel. 201/447–8000; Audrey Meyers, President and Chief Executive Officer

VIRRUA WEST JERSEY HOSPITAL–MARLTON, 90 Brick Road, Marlton, NJ, Zip 08053–9697; tel. 856/355–6000; Leroy J. Rosenberg, Executive Director

VIRTUA MEMORIAL HOSPITAL BURLINGTON COUNTY, 175 Madison Avenue, Mount Holly, NJ, Zip 08060–2099; tel. 609/267–0700; Donald I. Brunn, Executive Vice President

VIRTUA WEST JERSEY HOSPITAL–BERLIN, 100 Townsend Avenue, Berlin, NJ, Zip 08009–9035; tel. 856/322–3100; Ellen Guarnieri, Vice President and Chief Operating Officer

VIRTUA WEST JERSEY HOSPITAL–CAMDEN, 1000 Atlantic Avenue, Camden, NJ, Zip 08104–1595; tel. 856/246–3000; Carolyn M. Ballard, Executive Director

VIRTUA WEST JERSEY HOSPITAL–VOORHEES, 101 Carnie Boulevard, Voorhees, NJ, Zip 08043–1597; tel. 856/325–3000; Joan T. Meyers, R.N., Vice President and Chief Operating Officer

WEST HUDSON HOSPITAL, 206 Bergen Avenue, Kearny, NJ, Zip 07032–3399; tel. 201/955–7051; Carmen Bruce Alecci, Executive Director

WILLIAM B. KESSLER MEMORIAL HOSPITAL, 600 South White Horse Pike, Hammonton, NJ, Zip 08037–2099; tel. 609/561–6700; Warren E. Gager, President and Chief Executive Officer

QUALCARE INC
242 Old Brunswick Road, Piscataway, NJ 08854; tel. 908/562–2800; Jerry Eisenberg, Network Contact

BAYONNE HOSPITAL, 29 East 29th Street, Bayonne, NJ, Zip 07002–4699; tel. 201/858–5000; Michael R. D'Agnes, President and Chief Executive Officer

BETH ISRAEL HOSPITAL, 70 Parker Avenue, Passaic, NJ, Zip 07055–7000; tel. 973/365–5000; Jeffrey S. Moll, President and Chief Executive Officer

CARRIER FOUNDATION, County Route 601, P.O. Box 147, Belle Mead, NJ, Zip 08502–0147; tel. 908/281–1000; C. Richard Sarle, President and Chief Executive Officer

CENTRASTATE HEALTHCARE SYSTEM, 901 West Main Street, Freehold, NJ, Zip 07728–2549; tel. 732/431–2000; Thomas H. Litz, FACHE, President and Chief Executive Officer

CHILDREN'S SPECIALIZED HOSPITAL, 150 New Providence Road, Mountainside, NJ, Zip 07092–2590; tel. 908/233–3720; Richard B. Ahlfeld, President

COLUMBUS HOSPITAL, 495 North 13th Street, Newark, NJ, Zip 07107–1397; tel. 973/268–1400; John G. Magliaro, President and Chief Executive Officer

COMMUNITY MEDICAL CENTER, 99 Route 37 West, Toms River, NJ, Zip 08755–6423; tel. 732/557–8000; Nancy L. Wollen, Executive Director

HACKENSACK UNIVERSITY MEDICAL CENTER, 30 Prospect Avenue, Hackensack, NJ, Zip 07601–1991; tel. 201/996–2000; John P. Ferguson, FACHE, President and Chief Executive Officer

HOLY NAME HOSPITAL, 718 Teaneck Road, Teaneck, NJ, Zip 07666–4281; tel. 201/833–3000; Michael Maron, President and Chief Executive Officer

HOSPITAL CENTER AT ORANGE, 188 South Essex Avenue, Orange, NJ, Zip 07051; tel. 973/266–2200; James E. Romer, President and Chief Executive Officer

HUNTERDON MEDICAL CENTER, 2100 Wescott Drive, Flemington, NJ, Zip 08822–4604; tel. 908/788–6100; Robert P. Wise, President and Chief Executive Officer

IRVINGTON GENERAL HOSPITAL, 832 Chancellor Avenue, Irvington, NJ, Zip 07111–0709; tel. 973/399–6000; Amit Mody, M.D., Executive Director

KESSLER INSTITUTE FOR REHABILITATION, 1199 Pleasant Valley Way, West Orange, NJ, Zip 07052–1419; tel. 973/731–3600; Robert Brehm, President

KIMBALL MEDICAL CENTER, 600 River Avenue, Lakewood, NJ, Zip 08701–5281; tel. 732/363–1900; Joanne Carrocino, Executive Director

MEMORIAL HOSPITAL OF SALEM COUNTY, 310 Woodstown Road, Salem, NJ, Zip 08079–2080; tel. 856/935–1000; Denise R. Williams, President and Chief Executive Officer

MONMOUTH MEDICAL CENTER, 300 Second Avenue, Long Branch, NJ, Zip 07740–6303; tel. 732/222–5200; Frank J. Vozos, M.D., FACS, Executive Director

NEWARK BETH ISRAEL MEDICAL CENTER, 201 Lyons Avenue, Newark, NJ, Zip 07112–2027; tel. 973/926–7000; Paul A. Mertz, Executive Director

PALISADES MEDICAL CENTER, 7600 River Road, North Bergen, NJ, Zip 07047–6217; tel. 201/854–5000; Bruce J. Markowitz, President and Chief Executive Officer

PASCACK VALLEY HOSPITAL, 250 Old Hook Road, Westwood, NJ, Zip 07675–3181; tel. 201/358–3000; Louis R. Ycre, Jr, FACHE, President and Chief Executive Officer

RAHWAY HOSPITAL, 865 Stone Street, Rahway, NJ, Zip 07065–2797; tel. 732/381–4200; Kirk C. Tice, President and Chief Executive Officer

RARITAN BAY MEDICAL CENTER, 530 New Brunswick Avenue, Perth Amboy, NJ, Zip 08861–3685; tel. 732/442–3700; Keith H. McLaughlin, President and Chief Executive Officer

ROBERT WOOD JOHNSON UNIVERSITY HOSPITAL, 1 Robert Wood Johnson Place, New Brunswick, NJ, Zip 08903–2601; tel. 732/828–3000; Harvey A. Holzberg, President and Chief Executive Officer

ROBERT WOOD JOHNSON UNIVERSITY HOSPITAL AT HAMILTON, One Hamilton Health Place, Hamilton, NJ, Zip 08690–3599; tel. 609/586–7900; Christy Stephenson, Chief Administrative Officer

SAINT BARNABAS MEDICAL CENTER, 94 Old Short Hills Road, Livingston, NJ, Zip 07039–5668; tel. 973/322–5000; Vincent D. Joseph, Executive Director

SAINT CLARE'S HEALTH SERVICES, 25 Pocono Road, Denville, NJ, Zip 07834–2995; tel. 973/625–6000; Kathryn J. McDonagh, President and Chief Executive Officer

SHORE MEMORIAL HOSPITAL, 1 East New York Avenue, Somers Point, NJ, Zip 08244–2387; tel. 609/653–3500; Richard A. Pitman, President

SOMERSET MEDICAL CENTER, 110 Rehill Avenue, Somerville, NJ, Zip 08876–2598; tel. 908/685–2200; Dennis C. Miller, President and Chief Executive Officer

SOUTH JERSEY HOSPITAL, 333 Irving Avenue, Bridgeton, NJ, Zip 08302–2100; tel. 856/451–6600; Chester B. Kaletkowski, President and Chief Executive Officer

SOUTHERN OCEAN COUNTY HOSPITAL, 1140 Route 72 West, Manahawkin, NJ, Zip 08050–2499; tel. 609/978–8900; Joseph P. Coyle, President and Chief Executive Officer

ST. FRANCIS HOSPITAL, 25 McWilliams Place, Jersey City, NJ, Zip 07302–1698; tel. 201/418–1000; Robert S. Chaloner, Chief Executive Officer

ST. JOSEPH'S HOSPITAL AND MEDICAL CENTER, 703 Main Street, Paterson, NJ, Zip 07503–2691; tel. 973/754–2000; Patrick R. Wardell, President and Chief Executive Officer

ST. LAWRENCE REHABILITATION CENTER, 2381 Lawrenceville Road, Lawrenceville, NJ, Zip 08648; tel. 609/896–9500; Charles L. Brennan, Chief Executive Officer

ST. MARY HOSPITAL, 308 Willow Avenue, Hoboken, NJ, Zip 07030–3889; tel. 201/418–1000; Robert S. Chaloner, President and Chief Executive Officer

ST. PETER'S UNIVERSITY HOSPITAL, 254 Easton Avenue, New Brunswick, NJ, Zip 08901–1780, Mailing Address: P.O. Box 591, Zip 08903–0591; tel. 732/745–8600; John E. Matuska, President and Chief Executive Officer

THE COOPER HEALTH SYSTEM, One Cooper Plaza, Camden, NJ, Zip 08103–1489; tel. 856/342–2000; Leslie D. Hirsch, President and Chief Executive Officer

TRINITAS HOSPITAL, 925 East Jersey Street, Elizabeth, NJ, Zip 07201–2728; tel. 908/289–8600; David A. Fletcher, President and Chief Executive Officer

UNDERWOOD–MEMORIAL HOSPITAL, 509 North Broad Street, Woodbury, NJ, Zip 08096–1697, Mailing Address: P.O. Box 359, Zip 08096–7359; tel. 856/845–0100; Steven W. Jackmuff, President and Chief Executive Officer

UNION HOSPITAL, 1000 Galloping Hill Road, Union, NJ, Zip 07083–1652; tel. 908/687–1900; Kathryn W. Coyne, Executive Director

UNIVERSITY OF MEDICINE AND DENTISTRY OF NEW JERSEY–UNIVERSITY HOSPITAL, 150 Bergen Street, Newark, NJ, Zip 07103–2406; tel. 973/972–4300; Daniel L. Marcantuono, FACHE, Acting Vice President and Chief Executive Officer

VIRRUA WEST JERSEY HOSPITAL–MARLTON, 90 Brick Road, Marlton, NJ, Zip 08053–9697; tel. 856/355–6000; Leroy J. Rosenberg, Executive Director

VIRTUA MEMORIAL HOSPITAL BURLINGTON COUNTY, 175 Madison Avenue, Mount Holly, NJ, Zip 08060–2099; tel. 609/267–0700; Donald I. Brunn, Executive Vice President

VIRTUA WEST JERSEY HOSPITAL–CAMDEN, 1000 Atlantic Avenue, Camden, NJ, Zip 08104–1595; tel. 856/246–3000; Carolyn M. Ballard, Executive Director

VIRTUA WEST JERSEY HOSPITAL–VOORHEES, 101 Carnie Boulevard, Voorhees, NJ, Zip 08043–1597; tel. 856/325–3000; Joan T. Meyers, R.N., Vice President and Chief Operating Officer

WARREN HOSPITAL, 185 Roseberry Street, Phillipsburg, NJ, Zip 08865–9955; tel. 908/859–6700; Jeffrey C. Goodwin, President and Chief Executive Officer

WAYNE GENERAL HOSPITAL, 224 Hamburg Turnpike, Wayne, NJ, Zip 07470–2100; tel. 973/942–6900; Geraldine Di Risic, Acting Executive Director

SETON HEALTH NETWORK INC
703 Main Street, Paterson, NJ 07503; tel. 913/754–2790; Stephen Schneider, Executive Director

ST. JOSEPH'S HOSPITAL AND MEDICAL CENTER, 703 Main Street, Paterson, NJ, Zip 07503–2691; tel. 973/754–2000; Patrick R. Wardell, President and Chief Executive Officer

NEW MEXICO

LOVELACE
5400 Gibson Boulevard S.E., Albuquerque, NM 87108; tel. 505/262–7000; Martin Hickey, Chief Executive Officer

LOVELACE HEALTH SYSTEM, 5400 Gibson Boulevard S.E., Albuquerque, NM, Zip 87108–4763; tel. 505/262–7000; Martin Hickey, M.D., Chief Executive Officer

UNIVERSITY HOSPITAL
2211 Lomas Boulevard, N.E., Albuquerque, NM 87106; tel. 505/272–2121; Steve McKernan, Chief Executive

© 2000 AHA Guide Networks, Health Care Systems and Alliances

CARRIE TINGLEY HOSPITAL, 1127 University Boulevard N.E., Albuquerque, NM, Zip 87102–1715; tel. 505/272–5200; Barbara Ohm, Interim Administrator

MENTAL HEALTH CENTER, 2600 Marble N.E., Albuquerque, NM, Zip 87131–2600; tel. 505/272–2263; Stephen W. McKernan, Chief Executive Officer

UNIVERSITY HOSPITAL, 2211 Lomas Boulevard N.E., Albuquerque, NM, Zip 87106–2745; tel. 505/272–2121; Stephen W. McKernan, Chief Executive Officer

UNIVERSITY OF NEW MEXICO CHILDREN'S PSYCHIATRIC HOSPITAL, 1001 Yale Boulevard N.E., Albuquerque, NM, Zip 87131–3830; tel. 505/272–2945; Maggie McGowan, Interim Area Director

NEW YORK

ADIRONDACK RURAL HEALTH NETWORK
100 Park Street, Glens Falls, NY 12801; tel. 518/926–1000; David Kruczlnicki, President

GLENS FALLS HOSPITAL, 100 Park Street, Glens Falls, NY, Zip 12801–9898; tel. 518/926–1000; David G. Kruczlnicki, President and Chief Executive Officer

ALLEGANY RURAL HEALTH NETWORK
191 North Main Street, Wellsville, NY 14895; tel. 716/593–1100; William M. DiBeradino, President & Chief Executive Officer

JONES MEMORIAL HOSPITAL, 191 North Main Street, Wellsville, NY, Zip 14895–1197, Mailing Address: P.O. Box 72, Zip 14895–0072; tel. 716/593–1100; William M. DiBerardino, FACHE, President and Chief Executive Officer

BASSETT HEALTHCARE
1 Atwell Road, Cooperstown, NY 13326; tel. 607/547–3100; William F. Streck, MD, President/Chief Executive Officer

BASSETT HOSPITAL OF SCHOHARIE COUNTY, 41 Grandview Drive, Cobleskill, NY, Zip 12043–1331; tel. 518/234–2511; Donald W. Massey, Administrator

MARY IMOGENE BASSETT HOSPITAL, One Atwell Road, Cooperstown, NY, Zip 13326–1394; tel. 607/547–3100; William F. Streck, M.D., President and Chief Executive Officer

BON SECOURS HEALTH SYSTEM
255 Lafayette Ave., Suffern, NY 10901; tel. 914/368–5000; Karl Miller, President & Chief Executive Officer

GOOD SAMARITAN HOSPITAL, 255 Lafayette Avenue, Suffern, NY, Zip 10901–4869; tel. 914/368–5000; James A. Martin, Chief Executive Officer

MERCY COMMUNITY HOSPITAL, 160 East Main Street, Port Jervis, NY, Zip 12771–2245, Mailing Address: P.O. Box 1014, Zip 12771–1014; tel. 914/856–5351; Michael Parmer, M.D., Executive Vice President and Administrator

ST. ANTHONY COMMUNITY HOSPITAL, 15 Maple Avenue, Warwick, NY, Zip 10990–5180; tel. 914/986–2276; James A. Martin, President and Chief Executive Officer

CHEMUNG COUNTY RURAL HEALTH NETWORK
600 Roe Avenue, Elmira, NY 14905; tel. 607/737–4100; Anthony J. Cooper, President & Chief Executive Officer

COLUMBIA–PRES MED CEN HEALTH ALLIANCE
Columbia–Pres Med Cen, New York, NY 10032; tel. 212/305–2500; William T. Speck, President & Chief Executive Officer

CORNWALL HOSPITAL, 19 Laurel Avenue, Cornwall, NY, Zip 12518–1499; tel. 914/534–7711; Louis H. Smith, Executive Vice President and Administrator

HELEN HAYES HOSPITAL, Route 9W, West Haverstraw, NY, Zip 10993–1195; tel. 914/786–4000; Magdalena Ramirez, Chief Executive Officer

HOLY NAME HOSPITAL, 718 Teaneck Road, Teaneck, NJ, Zip 07666–4281; tel. 201/833–3000; Michael Maron, President and Chief Executive Officer

HORTON MEDICAL CENTER, 60 Prospect Avenue, Middletown, NY, Zip 10940–4133; tel. 914/343–2424; Jeffrey D. Hirsch, Executive Vice President and Administrator

LAWRENCE HOSPITAL, 55 Palmer Avenue, Bronxville, NY, Zip 10708–3491; tel. 914/787–1000; Edward M. Dinan, President and Chief Executive Officer

NEW MILFORD HOSPITAL, 21 Elm Street, New Milford, CT, Zip 06776–2993; tel. 860/355–2611; Richard E. Pugh, President and Chief Executive Officer

NYACK HOSPITAL, 160 North Midland Avenue, Nyack, NY, Zip 10960–1998; tel. 914/348–2000; Greger C. Anderson, President and Chief Executive Officer

PALISADES MEDICAL CENTER, 7600 River Road, North Bergen, NJ, Zip 07047–6217; tel. 201/854–5000; Bruce J. Markowitz, President and Chief Executive Officer

ST. FRANCIS HOSPITAL, 100 Port Washington Boulevard, Roslyn, NY, Zip 11576–1348; tel. 516/562–6000; Alan D. Guerci, M.D., President and Chief Executive Officer

ST. LUKE'S HOSPITAL, 70 Dubois Street, Newburgh, NY, Zip 12550–4898, Mailing Address: P.O. Box 631, Zip 12550–0631; tel. 914/561–4400; Laurence E. Kelly, Executive Vice President and Administrator

VALLEY HOSPITAL, 223 North Van Dien Avenue, Ridgewood, NJ, Zip 07450–9982; tel. 201/447–8000; Audrey Meyers, President and Chief Executive Officer

WHITE PLAINS HOSPITAL CENTER, Davis Avenue and Post Road, White Plains, NY, Zip 10601–4699; tel. 914/681–0600; Jon B. Schandler, President and Chief Executive Officer

CONTINUUM HEALTH PARTNERS
555 West 57th Street, New York, NY 10019; tel. 212/523–0390; Kathleen McGovern, Vice President

BETH ISRAEL MEDICAL CENTER, First Avenue and 16th Street, New York, NY, Zip 10003–3803; tel. 212/420–2000; Matthew E. Fink, M.D., President and Chief Executive Officer

LONG ISLAND COLLEGE HOSPITAL, 339 Hicks Street, Brooklyn, NY, Zip 11201–5509; tel. 718/780–1000; Allan Gibofsky, President and Chief Executive Officer

NEW YORK EYE AND EAR INFIRMARY, 310 East 14th Street, New York, NY, Zip 10003–4201; tel. 212/979–4000; Joseph P. Corcoran, President and Chief Executive Officer

ST. LUKE'S–ROOSEVELT HOSPITAL CENTER, 1111 Amsterdam Avenue, New York, NY, Zip 10025; tel. 212/523–4300; Sigurd H. Ackerman, M.D., President and Chief Executive Officer

EPISCOPAL HEALTH SERVICES INC
333 Earle Ovington Boulevard, Uniondale, NY 11787; tel. 516/228–6100; Lorna McBarnette, Executive Director

ST. CATHERINE OF SIENA MEDICAL CENTER, 50 Route 25–A, Smithtown, NY, Zip 11787–1398; tel. 631/862–3000; James M. Wilson, President and Chief Executive Officer

ST. JOHN'S EPISCOPAL HOSPITAL–SOUTH SHORE, 327 Beach 19th Street, Far Rockaway, NY, Zip 11691–4424; tel. 718/869–7000; Nancy Simmons, Administrator

FIRST CHOICE NETWORK, INC
165 EAB Plaza, West Tower 6, Uniondale, NY 11556; tel. 516/474–6000; Dana Metzler, Acting Executive Director

EASTERN LONG ISLAND HOSPITAL, 201 Manor Place, Greenport, NY, Zip 11944–1298; tel. 631/477–1000; Paul J. Connor, II, President and Chief Executive Officer

SOUTHAMPTON HOSPITAL, 240 Meeting House Lane, Southampton, NY, Zip 11968–5090; tel. 516/726–8555; Thomas B. Doolan, Acting President and Chief Executive Officer

SOUTHSIDE HOSPITAL, 301 East Main Street, Bay Shore, NY, Zip 11706–8458; tel. 631/968–3000; Theodore A. Jospe, President

ST. CATHERINE OF SIENA MEDICAL CENTER, 50 Route 25–A, Smithtown, NY, Zip 11787–1398; tel. 631/862–3000; James M. Wilson, President and Chief Executive Officer

ST. CHARLES HOSPITAL AND REHABILITATION CENTER, 200 Belle Terre Road, Port Jefferson, NY, Zip 11777; tel. 631/474–6000; David A. Dibner, FACHE, Interim President and Chief Executive Officer

ST. JOHN'S EPISCOPAL HOSPITAL–SOUTH SHORE, 327 Beach 19th Street, Far Rockaway, NY, Zip 11691–4424; tel. 718/869–7000; Nancy Simmons, Administrator

WINTHROP–UNIVERSITY HOSPITAL, 259 First Street, Mineola, NY, Zip 11501; tel. 516/663–2200; Daniel P. Walsh, President and Chief Executive Officer

FOUR LAKES RURAL HEALTH NETWORK
196 North St., Geneva, NY 14456; tel. 315/787–4000; James J. Dooley, President & Chief Executive Officer

GENEVA GENERAL HOSPITAL, 196 North Street, Geneva, NY, Zip 14456–1694; tel. 315/787–4000; James J. Dooley, President and Chief Executive Officer

SOLDIERS AND SAILORS MEMORIAL HOSPITAL OF YATES COUNTY, 418 North Main Street, Penn Yan, NY, Zip 14527–1085; tel. 315/531–2000; James J. Dooley, President and Chief Executive Officer

HAMILTON–BASSETT–CROUSE RURAL HEALTH NETWORK
150 South Broad Street, Hamilton, NY 13346; tel. 315/598–4735; David Felton, President/Chief Executive Officer

COMMUNITY MEMORIAL HOSPITAL, 150 Broad Street, Hamilton, NY, Zip 13346–9518; tel. 315/824–1100; David Felton, President and Chief Executive Officer

CROUSE HOSPITAL, 736 Irving Avenue, Syracuse, NY, Zip 13210–1690; tel. 315/470–7111; Kent A. Arnold, President and Chief Executive Officer

HEALTH FIRST
25 Broadway, New York, NY 10019; tel. 212/801–1500; Paul Dickstein, Network Contact

BETH ISRAEL MEDICAL CENTER, First Avenue and 16th Street, New York, NY, Zip 10003–3803; tel. 212/420–2000; Matthew E. Fink, M.D., President and Chief Executive Officer

BRONX–LEBANON HOSPITAL CENTER, 1276 Fulton Avenue, Bronx, NY, Zip 10456–3499; tel. 718/590–1800; Miguel A. Fuentes, President and Chief Executive Officer

BROOKLYN HOSPITAL CENTER, 121 DeKalb Avenue, Brooklyn, NY, Zip 11201–5493; tel. 718/250–8005; Frederick D. Alley, President and Chief Executive Officer

BRUNSWICK GENERAL HOSPITAL, 366 Broadway, Amityville, NY, Zip 11701–9820; tel. 631/789–7000; Benjamin M. Stein, M.D., President

INTERFAITH MEDICAL CENTER, 555 Prospect Place, Brooklyn, NY, Zip 11238–4299; tel. 718/935–7000; Corbett A. Price, Chief Executive Officer

JAMAICA HOSPITAL MEDICAL CENTER, 8900 Van Wyck Expressway, Jamaica, NY, Zip 11418–2832; tel. 718/206–6000; David P. Rosen, President

KINGSBROOK JEWISH MEDICAL CENTER, 585 Schenectady Avenue, Brooklyn, NY, Zip 11203–1891; tel. 718/604–5000; Linda Brady, M.D., President and Chief Executive Officer

MAIMONIDES MEDICAL CENTER, 4802 Tenth Avenue, Brooklyn, NY, Zip 11219–2916; tel. 718/283–6000; Stanley Brezenoff, President

MONTEFIORE MEDICAL CENTER, 111 East 210th Street, Bronx, NY, Zip 10467–2490; tel. 718/920–4321; Spencer Foreman, M.D., President

Networks / North Shore–LIJ Health System

MOUNT SINAI–NYU HOSPITALS/HEALTH SYSTEM, One Gustave Levy Place, New York, NY, Zip 10019–6574; tel. 212/241–6500; John W. Rowe, M.D., President

NASSAU COUNTY MEDICAL CENTER, 2201 Hempstead Turnpike, East Meadow, NY, Zip 11554–1854; tel. 516/572–6011; Jerald C. Newman, President and Chief Executive Officer

STATEN ISLAND UNIVERSITY HOSPITAL, 475 Seaview Avenue, Staten Island, NY, Zip 10305–9998; tel. 718/226–9000; Rick J. Varone, President

UNIVERSITY HOSPITAL, State University of New York, Stony Brook, NY, Zip 11794–8410; tel. 631/689–8333; Michael A. Maffetone, Director and Chief Executive Officer

UNIVERSITY HOSPITAL OF BROOKLYN–STATE UNIVERSITY OF NEW YORK HEALTH SCIENCE CENTER AT BROOKLYN, 445 Lenox Road, Brooklyn, NY, Zip 11203–2098; tel. 718/270–2404; John C. LaRosa, M.D., President and Chief Executive Officer

HEALTH STAR NETWORK
1 North Greenwich Road, Armonk, NY 10504; tel. 914/273–2850; Kevin G. Murphy, Vice President & Chief

LAWRENCE HOSPITAL, 55 Palmer Avenue, Bronxville, NY, Zip 10708–3491; tel. 914/787–1000; Edward M. Dinan, President and Chief Executive Officer

NORTHERN WESTCHESTER HOSPITAL CENTER, 400 Main Street, Mount Kisco, NY, Zip 10549–3477; tel. 914/666–1200; Donald W. Davis, President

PHELPS MEMORIAL HOSPITAL CENTER, 701 North Broadway, Sleepy Hollow, NY, Zip 10591–1096; tel. 914/366–3000; Keith F. Safian, President and Chief Executive Officer

WHITE PLAINS HOSPITAL CENTER, Davis Avenue and Post Road, White Plains, NY, Zip 10601–4699; tel. 914/681–0600; Jon B. Schandler, President and Chief Executive Officer

KALEIDA HEALTH
901 Washington Street, Buffalo, NY 14203; tel. 716/843–7500; Carrie Whitcher, Administrative Project Manager

BERTRAND CHAFFEE HOSPITAL, 224 East Main Street, Springville, NY, Zip 14141–1497; tel. 716/592–2871; Steve Krisiak, Chief Executive Officer

BROOKS MEMORIAL HOSPITAL, 529 Central Avenue, Dunkirk, NY, Zip 14048–2599; tel. 716/366–1111; Richard H. Ketcham, President

BUFFALO GENERAL HOSPITAL, 100 High Street, Buffalo, NY, Zip 14203–1154; tel. 716/845–5600; John E. Friedlander, President and Chief Executive Officer

CHILDREN'S HOSPITAL, 219 Bryant Street, Buffalo, NY, Zip 14222–2099; tel. 716/878–7000; Karen Blount, R.N., Chief Operating Officer

DE GRAFF MEMORIAL HOSPITAL, 445 Tremont Street, North Tonawanda, NY, Zip 14120–0750, Mailing Address: P.O. Box 0750, Zip 14120–0750; tel. 716/694–4500; Marcia B. Gutfeld, Vice President and Chief Operating Officer

LAKE SHORE HOSPITAL, 845 Route 5 and 20, Irving, NY, Zip 14081–9716; tel. 716/934–2654; James B. Foster, Chief Executive Officer

LOCKPORT MEMORIAL HOSPITAL, 521 East Avenue, Lockport, NY, Zip 14094–3299; tel. 716/514–5700; Clare A. Haar, Chief Executive Officer

MEDINA MEMORIAL HOSPITAL, 200 Ohio Street, Medina, NY, Zip 14103–1095; tel. 716/798–2000; James Sinner, Chief Executive Officer

MILLARD FILLMORE GATES CIRCLE HOSPITAL, 3 Gates Circle, Buffalo, NY, Zip 14209–9986; tel. 716/887–4600; Joyce Korzen, R.N., Chief Operating Officer

SHEEHAN MEMORIAL HOSPITAL, 425 Michigan Avenue, Buffalo, NY, Zip 14203–2297; tel. 716/848–2000; Olivia Smith-Blackwell, M.D., M.P.H., President and Chief Executive Officer

TRI–COUNTY MEMORIAL HOSPITAL, 100 Memorial Drive, Gowanda, NY, Zip 14070–1194; tel. 716/532–3377; Diane J. Osika, Chief Executive Officer

LAKE ONTARIO RURAL HEALTH NETWORK
200 Ohio Street, Medina, NY 14103; tel. 716/798–2000; Walter S. Becker, Administrator

MEDINA MEMORIAL HOSPITAL, 200 Ohio Street, Medina, NY, Zip 14103–1095; tel. 716/798–2000; James Sinner, Chief Executive Officer

UNITED MEMORIAL MEDICAL CENTER, 127 North Street, Batavia, NY, Zip 14020–2260; tel. 716/343–3131; Charles S. Kinney, Chief Executive Officer

WYOMING COUNTY COMMUNITY HOSPITAL, 400 North Main Street, Warsaw, NY, Zip 14569–1097; tel. 716/786–2233; Lucille K. Sheedy, Administrator and Chief Executive Officer

MOHAWK VALLEY NETWORK, INC
P.O. Box 4308, Utica, NY 13504; tel. 315/798–6386; Fred Asforth, Network Vice President

FAXTON–ST. LUKE'S HEALTHCARE, Utica, NY, Mailing Address: P.O. Box 479, Zip 13503–0479; tel. 315/798–6000; Andrew E. Peterson, President and Chief Executive Officer

LITTLE FALLS HOSPITAL, 140 Burwell Street, Little Falls, NY, Zip 13365–1725; tel. 315/823–1000; David S. Armstrong, Jr, President and Chief Executive Officer

MOUNT SINAI NYU HEALTH NETWORK
P.O. Box 1068, New York, NY 10029; tel. 212/241–6500; John W. Rowe, President

CABRINI MEDICAL CENTER, 227 East 19th Street, New York, NY, Zip 10003–2600; tel. 212/995–6000; Jeffrey Frerichs, President and Chief Executive Officer

ELMHURST HOSPITAL CENTER, 79–01 Broadway, Elmhurst, NY, Zip 11373; tel. 718/334–4000; Pete Velez, Executive Director

ENGLEWOOD HOSPITAL AND MEDICAL CENTER, 350 Engle Street, Englewood, NJ, Zip 07631–1898; tel. 201/894–3000; Daniel A. Kane, President and Chief Executive Officer

GREENVILLE HOSPITAL, 1825 John F. Kennedy Boulevard, Jersey City, NJ, Zip 07305–2198; tel. 201/547–6100; Jonathan M. Metsch, Dr.PH, President and Chief Executive Officer

HOSPITAL FOR JOINT DISEASES ORTHOPAEDIC INSTITUTE, 301 East 17th Street, New York, NY, Zip 10003–3890; tel. 212/598–6000; John N. Kastanis, FACHE, President and Chief Executive Officer

JERSEY CITY MEDICAL CENTER, 50 Baldwin Avenue, Jersey City, NJ, Zip 07304–3199; tel. 201/915–2000; Jonathan M. Metsch, Dr.PH, President and Chief Executive Officer

LONG BEACH MEDICAL CENTER, 455 East Bay Drive, Long Beach, NY, Zip 11561–2300, Mailing Address: P.O. Box 300, Zip 11561–2300; tel. 516/897–1000; Martin F. Nester, Jr, Chief Executive Officer

LUTHERAN MEDICAL CENTER, 150 55th Street, Brooklyn, NY, Zip 11220–2570; tel. 718/630–7000; Dominic J. Lodato, Interim President

MAIMONIDES MEDICAL CENTER, 4802 Tenth Avenue, Brooklyn, NY, Zip 11219–2916; tel. 718/283–6000; Stanley Brezenoff, President

MEADOWLANDS HOSPITAL MEDICAL CENTER, 55 Meadowland Parkway, Secaucus, NJ, Zip 07096–1580; tel. 201/392–3100; Paul V. Cavalli, M.D., President

MOUNT SINAI–NYU HOSPITALS/HEALTH SYSTEM, One Gustave Levy Place, New York, NY, Zip 10019–6574; tel. 212/241–6500; John W. Rowe, M.D., President

NEW YORK UNIVERSITY DOWNTOWN HOSPITAL, 170 William Street, New York, NY, Zip 10038–2649; tel. 212/312–5000; Leonard A. Aubrey, President and Chief Executive Officer

PHELPS MEMORIAL HOSPITAL CENTER, 701 North Broadway, Sleepy Hollow, NY, Zip 10591–1096; tel. 914/366–3000; Keith F. Safian, President and Chief Executive Officer

QUEENS HOSPITAL CENTER, 82–68 164th Street, Jamaica, NY, Zip 11432–1104; tel. 718/883–3000; Antonio D. Martin, Chief Operating Officer

SAINT FRANCIS HOSPITAL, 241 North Road, Poughkeepsie, NY, Zip 12601–1399; tel. 914/483–5000; Sister M. Ann Elizabeth, President

ST. ELIZABETH HOSPITAL, 225 Williamson Street, Elizabeth, NJ, Zip 07202–3600; tel. 908/527–5000; Sister Elizabeth Ann Maloney, President and Chief Executive Officer

ST. JOSEPH'S HOSPITAL AND MEDICAL CENTER, 703 Main Street, Paterson, NJ, Zip 07503–2691; tel. 973/754–2000; Patrick R. Wardell, President and Chief Executive Officer

ST. MARY'S HOSPITAL, 901 45th Street, West Palm Beach, FL, Zip 33407–2495, Mailing Address: P.O. Box 24620, Zip 33416–4620; tel. 561/844–6300; Steven R. Nathan, President and Chief Executive Officer

THE MOUNT SINAI HOSPITAL OF QUEENS, 25–10 30th Avenue, Astoria Station, Long Island City, NY, Zip 11102–2495; tel. 718/932–1000; Caryn A. Schwab, Executive Director

VASSAR BROTHERS HOSPITAL, 45 Reade Place, Poughkeepsie, NY, Zip 12601–3990; tel. 914/454–8500; Ronald T. Mullahey, President

VETERANS AFFAIRS MEDICAL CENTER, 130 West Kingsbridge Road, Bronx, NY, Zip 10468–3992; tel. 718/584–9000; Maryann Musumeci, Director

NEW YORK PRESBYTERIAN HEALTHCARE NETWORK
525 East 68th Street Box 572, New York, NY 10021; tel. 212/746–4030; Jonathan Albert, Director, Admin. Services

GRACIE SQUARE HOSPITAL, 420 East 76th Street, New York, NY, Zip 10021–3104; tel. 212/988–4400; Frank Bruno, Chief Executive Officer

HOSPITAL FOR SPECIAL SURGERY, 535 East 70th Street, New York, NY, Zip 10021–4898; tel. 212/606–1000; John R. Reynolds, President and Chief Executive Officer

NEW YORK COMMUNITY HOSPITAL OF BROOKLYN, 2525 Kings Highway, Brooklyn, NY, Zip 11229–1798; tel. 718/692–5300; Lin H. Mo, President and Chief Executive Officer

NEW YORK METHODIST HOSPITAL, 506 Sixth Street, Brooklyn, NY, Zip 11215–3645; tel. 718/780–3000; Mark J. Mundy, President and Chief Executive Officer

NEW YORK UNITED HOSPITAL MEDICAL CENTER, 406 Boston Post Road, Port Chester, NY, Zip 10573–7300; tel. 914/934–3000; Kevin Dahill, President and Chief Executive Officer

WYCKOFF HEIGHTS MEDICAL CENTER, 374 Stockholm Street, Brooklyn, NY, Zip 11237–4099; tel. 718/963–7102; Dominick J. Gio, President and Chief Executive Officer

NORTH SHORE–LIJ HEALTH SYSTEM
150 Community Drive, Great Neck, NY 11021; tel. 516/465–8000; Jeffrey A. Kraut, Senior Vice President, Planning

FRANKLIN HOSPITAL MEDICAL CENTER, 900 Franklin Avenue, Valley Stream, NY, Zip 11580–2190; tel. 516/256–6000; William Kowalewski, President and Chief Executive Officer

HUNTINGTON HOSPITAL, 270 Park Avenue, Huntington, NY, Zip 11743–2799; tel. 631/351–2200; J. Ronald Gaudreault, President and Chief Executive Officer

LONG ISLAND JEWISH MEDICAL CENTER, 270–05 76th Avenue, New Hyde Park, NY, Zip 11040–1496; tel. 718/470–7000; Paul S. Hochenberg, President

NORTH SHORE UNIVERSITY HOSPITAL, 300 Community Drive, Manhasset, NY, Zip 11030–3876; tel. 516/562–0100; Dennis Dowling, Executive Director

Networks / North Shore–LIJ Health System

NORTH SHORE UNIVERSITY HOSPITAL AT GLEN COVE, 101 St. Andrews Lane, Glen Cove, NY, Zip 11542; tel. 516/674-7300; Mark R. Stenzler, Vice President Administration

NORTH SHORE UNIVERSITY HOSPITAL AT PLAINVIEW, 888 Old Country Road, Plainview, NY, Zip 11803-4978; tel. 516/719-3000; Deborah Tascone, R.N., MS, Executive Director

NORTH SHORE UNIVERSITY HOSPITAL AT SYOSSET, 221 Jericho Turnpike, Syosset, NY, Zip 11791-4567; tel. 516/496-6400; Deborah Tascone, R.N., MS, Executive Director

NORTH SHORE UNIVERSITY HOSPITAL–FOREST HILLS, Forest Hills, NY, Mailing Address: 102-01 66th Road, Zip 11375; tel. 718/830-4000; Andrew J. Mitchell, Executive Director

SOUTHSIDE HOSPITAL, 301 East Main Street, Bay Shore, NY, Zip 11706-8458; tel. 631/968-3000; Theodore A. Jospe, President

STATEN ISLAND UNIVERSITY HOSPITAL, 475 Seaview Avenue, Staten Island, NY, Zip 10305-9998; tel. 718/226-9000; Rick J. Varone, President

NORTHERN NY RURAL HEALTH CARE ALLIANCE
200 Washington Street, Suite 300, Watertown, NY 13601; tel. 315/786-0565; Janice Charles, Chairman

CARTHAGE AREA HOSPITAL, 1001 West Street, Carthage, NY, Zip 13619-9703; tel. 315/493-1000; Walter S. Becker, Chief Executive Officer

E. J. NOBLE HOSPITAL SAMARITAN, 19 Fuller Street, Alexandria Bay, NY, Zip 13607; tel. 315/482-2511; Donna S. MacPherson, Administrator and Chief Operating Officer

SAMARITAN HOSPITAL, 2215 Burdett Avenue, Troy, NY, Zip 12180-2475; tel. 518/271-3300; Paul A. Milton, Chief Operating Officer

NYU HOSPITALS
550 First Avenue, New York, NY 10016; tel. 212/263-5500; John P. Harney, Vice President & COO

HOSPITAL FOR JOINT DISEASES ORTHOPAEDIC INSTITUTE, 301 East 17th Street, New York, NY, Zip 10003-3890; tel. 212/598-6000; John N. Kastanis, FACHE, President and Chief Executive Officer

MOUNT SINAI–NYU HOSPITALS/HEALTH SYSTEM, One Gustave Levy Place, New York, NY, Zip 10019-6574; tel. 212/241-6500; John W. Rowe, M.D., President

NEW YORK UNIVERSITY DOWNTOWN HOSPITAL, 170 William Street, New York, NY, Zip 10038-2649; tel. 212/312-5000; Leonard A. Aubrey, President and Chief Executive Officer

PREFERRED HEALTH NETWORK INC
45 Avenue & Parsons Boulevard, Flushing, NY 11355; tel. 718/963-7102; Charles J. Pandola, President

NEW YORK FLUSHING HOSPITAL MEDICAL CENTER, 45th Avenue at Parsons Boulevard, Flushing, NY, Zip 11355-2100; tel. 718/670-5000; David P. Rosen, President and Chief Executive Officer

WYCKOFF HEIGHTS MEDICAL CENTER, 374 Stockholm Street, Brooklyn, NY, Zip 11237-4099; tel. 718/963-7102; Dominick J. Gio, President and Chief Executive Officer

QUEENS HOSPITAL CENTER
79-01 Broadway, Elmhurst, NY 11373; tel. 718/334-4000; Peter Velez, Network Senior Vice President

ELMHURST HOSPITAL CENTER, 79-01 Broadway, Elmhurst, NY, Zip 11373; tel. 718/334-4000; Pete Velez, Executive Director

RURAL HEALTH NETWORK
70 Bunner Street, Oswego, NY 13126; tel. 315/349-3435; Steven Rose, Chairman

ALBERT LINDLEY LEE MEMORIAL HOSPITAL, 510 South Fourth Street, Fulton, NY, Zip 13069-2994; tel. 315/592-2224; Dennis A. Casey, Executive Director

OSWEGO HOSPITAL, 110 West Sixth Street, Oswego, NY, Zip 13126-9985; tel. 315/349-5511; Corte J. Spencer, Chief Executive Officer

SETON HEALTH SYSTEM
1300 Massachusetts Avenue, Troy, NY 12180; tel. 518/268-5000; Dr. Mark Donavan, President

SETON HEALTH SYSTEM, 1300 Massachusetts Avenue, Troy, NY, Zip 12180-1695; tel. 518/268-5000; Mark A. Donovan, M.D., President and Chief Executive Officer

SHARED HEALTH NETWORK
125 Wolf Road, Suite 404, Albany, NY 12205; tel. 518/458-8607; Eugene Stearns, Executive Director

ELLIS HOSPITAL, 1101 Nott Street, Schenectady, NY, Zip 12308-2487; tel. 518/243-4000; G. B. Serrill, President and Chief Executive Officer

GLENS FALLS HOSPITAL, 100 Park Street, Glens Falls, NY, Zip 12801-9898; tel. 518/926-1000; David G. Kruczlnicki, President and Chief Executive Officer

LITTLE FALLS HOSPITAL, 140 Burwell Street, Little Falls, NY, Zip 13365-1725; tel. 315/823-1000; David S. Armstrong, Jr, President and Chief Executive Officer

MEMORIAL HOSPITAL, 600 Northern Boulevard, Albany, NY, Zip 12204-1083; tel. 518/471-3221; Norman E. Dascher, Jr, Chief Executive Officer

NATHAN LITTAUER HOSPITAL AND NURSING HOME, 99 East State Street, Gloversville, NY, Zip 12078-1293; tel. 518/773-5500; Thomas J. Dowd, President

SAMARITAN HOSPITAL, 2215 Burdett Avenue, Troy, NY, Zip 12180-2475; tel. 518/271-3300; Paul A. Milton, Chief Operating Officer

SARATOGA HOSPITAL, 211 Church Street, Saratoga Springs, NY, Zip 12866-1003; tel. 518/587-3222; David Andersen, President and Chief Executive Officer

SETON HEALTH SYSTEM, 1300 Massachusetts Avenue, Troy, NY, Zip 12180-1695; tel. 518/268-5000; Mark A. Donovan, M.D., President and Chief Executive Officer

ST. CLARE'S HOSPITAL OF SCHENECTADY, 600 McClellan Street, Schenectady, NY, Zip 12304-1090; tel. 518/382-2000; Paul J. Chodkowski, President and Chief Executive Officer

ST. MARY'S HOSPITAL, 427 Guy Park Avenue, Amsterdam, NY, Zip 12010-1095; tel. 518/842-1900; Peter E. Capobianco, President and Chief Executive Officer

ST. PETER'S HOSPITAL, 315 South Manning Boulevard, Albany, NY, Zip 12208-1789; tel. 518/525-1550; Steven P. Boyle, President and Chief Executive Officer

SUNNYVIEW HOSPITAL AND REHABILITATION CENTER, 1270 Belmont Avenue, Schenectady, NY, Zip 12308-2104; tel. 518/382-4500; Robert J. Bylancik, CHE, President and Chief Executive Officer

SISTERS OF CHARITY HEALTHCARE
75 Vanderbilt Ave., Staten Island, NY 10304; tel. 354/718-5080; John J. DePierro, FACHE, President & Chief Executive Officer

SISTERS OF CHARITY MEDICAL CENTER, 355 Bard Avenue, Staten Island, NY, Zip 10310-1699; tel. 718/876-1234; Dominick M. Stanzione, Chief Operating Officer and Executive Vice President

THE BROOKLYN HEALTH NETWORK
121 DeKalb Avenue, Brooklyn, NY 11201; tel. 718/250-8000; Fred Alley, Chief Executive Officer

BROOKLYN HOSPITAL CENTER, 121 DeKalb Avenue, Brooklyn, NY, Zip 11201-5493; tel. 718/250-8005; Frederick D. Alley, President and Chief Executive Officer

INTERFAITH MEDICAL CENTER, 555 Prospect Place, Brooklyn, NY, Zip 11238-4299; tel. 718/935-7000; Corbett A. Price, Chief Executive Officer

KINGSBROOK JEWISH MEDICAL CENTER, 585 Schenectady Avenue, Brooklyn, NY, Zip 11203-1891; tel. 718/604-5000; Linda Brady, M.D., President and Chief Executive Officer

VICTORY MEMORIAL HOSPITAL, 9036 Seventh Avenue, Brooklyn, NY, Zip 11228-3625; tel. 718/567-1234; Krishin L. Bhatia, Administrator

THE NEW YORK HOSPITAL HEALTH PLAN
525 E. 68th Street, New York, NY 10021; tel. 212/297-5510; Robert Chernow, Chief Executive Officer

UNITY HEALTH SYSTEM
89 Genesee Street, Rochester, NY 14611; tel. 716/464-3203; Timothy R. McCormick, President

PARK RIDGE HOSPITAL, 1555 Long Pond Road, Rochester, NY, Zip 14626-4182; tel. 716/723-7000; Martin E. Carlin, President

VIAHEALTH
150 N. Chestnut St., Rochester, NY 14604; tel. 716/922-3000; John R. Kessler, Jr., Vice President Marketing/PL/PR

CLIFTON SPRINGS HOSPITAL AND CLINIC, 2 Coulter Road, Clifton Springs, NY, Zip 14432-1189; tel. 315/462-1311; John P. Galati, President and Chief Executive Officer

GENESEE HOSPITAL, 224 Alexander Street, Rochester, NY, Zip 14607-4055; tel. 716/922-6000; Richard S. Constantino, M.D., President

ROCHESTER GENERAL HOSPITAL, 1425 Portland Avenue, Rochester, NY, Zip 14621-3099; tel. 716/338-4000; Richard S. Constantino, M.D., President

VIAHEALTH OF WAYNE, Driving Park Avenue, Newark, NY, Zip 14513, Mailing Address: P.O. Box 111, Zip 14513-0111; tel. 315/332-2022; W. Neil Stroman, President

NORTH CAROLINA

BLADEN RURAL HEALTH NETWORK
P.O. Box 398, Elizabethtown, NC 28337; tel. 910/862-5178; Leo Petit, Chief Executive Officer

BLADEN COUNTY HOSPITAL, 501 South Poplar Street, Elizabethtown, NC, Zip 28337-0398, Mailing Address: P.O. Box 398, Zip 28337-0398; tel. 910/862-5100; Leo A. Petit, Jr, Chief Executive Officer

DUKE HEALTH NETWORK
3100 Tower Building, Suite 600, Durham, NC 27707; tel. 919/419-5001; Paul Rosenberg, Chief Operating Officer

DUKE UNIVERSITY MEDICAL CENTER, Erwin Road, Durham, NC, Zip 27710, Mailing Address: P.O. Box 3708, Zip 27710-3708; tel. 919/684-8111; Michael D. Israel, Chief Executive Officer and Vice Chancellor

MARIA PARHAM HOSPITAL, 566 Ruin Creek Road, Henderson, NC, Zip 27536-2957; tel. 252/438-4143; Philip S. Lakernick, President and Chief Executive Officer

HOSPITAL ALLIANCE FOR COMMUNITY HEALTH
c/o Peter J. Morris, MD MPH, P.O. Box 46833, Raleigh, NC 27620; tel. 919/250-3813; Peter J. Morris MD MPH, Secretary

RALEIGH COMMUNITY HOSPITAL, 3400 Wake Forest Road, Raleigh, NC, Zip 27609-7373, Mailing Address: P.O. Box 28280, Zip 27611-8280; tel. 919/954-3000; James E. Raynor, Chief Executive Officer

REX HEALTHCARE, 4420 Lake Boone Trail, Raleigh, NC, Zip 27607-6599; tel. 919/784-3100; James W. Albright, President and Chief Executive Officer

WAKE MEDICAL CENTER, 3000 New Bern Avenue, Raleigh, NC, Zip 27610-1295; tel. 919/350-8000; Raymond L. Champ, President

MISSION ST. JOSEPH'S HEALTH SYSTEM
509 Biltmore Avenue, Asheville, NC 28801; tel. 828/213-1144; Robert F. Burgin, President & Chief Executive Officer

Networks / Medcenter One Health Services

MISSION ST. JOSEPH'S HEALTH, 509 Biltmore Avenue, Asheville, NC, Zip 28801-4690; tel. 828/255-4000; Robert F. Burgin, President and Chief Executive Officer

SPRUCE PINE COMMUNITY HOSPITAL, 125 Hospital Drive, Spruce Pine, NC, Zip 28777-3035, Mailing Address: P.O. Drawer 9, Zip 28777-0009; tel. 828/765-4201; Keith S. Holtsclaw, Chief Executive Officer

NORTH CAROLINA HEALTH
P.O. Box 668800, Charlotte, NC 28266; tel. 704/529-3300; Rose Duncan, Interim Director

MOSES CONE HEALTH SYSTEM, 1200 North Elm Street, Greensboro, NC, Zip 27401-1020; tel. 336/832-1000; Dennis R. Barry, President

UNC HEALTH NETWORK
101 Manning Drive, Chapel Hill, NC 27514; tel. 919/966-3709; Carol Straight, Network Development

ALAMANCE REGIONAL MEDICAL CENTER, 1240 Huffman Mill Road, Burlington, NC, Zip 27216-0202, Mailing Address: P.O. Box 202, Zip 27216-0202; tel. 336/538-7000; Thomas E. Ryan, President

CHATHAM HOSPITAL, West Third Street and Ivy Avenue, Siler City, NC, Zip 27344-2343, Mailing Address: P.O. Box 649, Zip 27344; tel. 919/663-2113; Woodrow W. Hathaway, Jr, Chief Executive Officer

COLUMBUS COUNTY HOSPITAL, 500 Jefferson Street, Whiteville, NC, Zip 28472-9987; tel. 910/642-8011; William S. Clark, Chief Executive Officer

FIRSTHEALTH MOORE REGIONAL HOSPITAL, 155 Memorial Drive, Pinehurst, NC, Zip 28374, Mailing Address: P.O. Box 3000, Zip 28374-3000; tel. 910/215-1000; Charles T. Frock, President and Chief Executive Officer

GOOD HOPE HOSPITAL, 410 Denim Drive, Erwin, NC, Zip 28339-0668, Mailing Address: P.O. Box 668, Zip 28339-0668; tel. 910/897-6151; Donald E. Annis, Chief Executive Officer

GRANVILLE MEDICAL CENTER, 1010 College Street, Oxford, NC, Zip 27565-2507, Mailing Address: Box 947, Zip 27565-0947; tel. 919/690-3000; Joe W. Pollard, Jr, Chief Executive Officer

JOHNSTON MEMORIAL HOSPITAL, 509 North Bright Leaf Boulevard, Smithfield, NC, Zip 27577-1376, Mailing Address: P.O. Box 1376, Zip 27577-1376; tel. 919/934-8171; Leland E. Farnell, President

MARIA PARHAM HOSPITAL, 566 Ruin Creek Road, Henderson, NC, Zip 27536-2957; tel. 252/438-4143; Philip S. Lakernick, President and Chief Executive Officer

MOREHEAD MEMORIAL HOSPITAL, 117 East King's Highway, Eden, NC, Zip 27288-5299; tel. 336/623-9711; Robert Enders, President

NORTH CAROLINA BAPTIST HOSPITAL, Medical Center Boulevard, Winston-Salem, NC, Zip 27157; tel. 336/716-2011; Len B. Preslar, Jr, President and Chief Executive Officer

SAMPSON REGIONAL MEDICAL CENTER, 607 Beaman Street, Clinton, NC, Zip 28328-2697, Mailing Address: Drawer 258, Zip 28329-0258; tel. 910/592-8511; Lee Pridgen, Jr, Administrator

SCOTLAND MEMORIAL HOSPITAL, 500 Lauchwood Drive, Laurinburg, NC, Zip 28352-5599; tel. 910/291-7000; Gregory C. Wood, Chief Executive Officer

SOUTHEASTERN REGIONAL MEDICAL CENTER, 300 West 27th Street, Lumberton, NC, Zip 28358-3017, Mailing Address: P.O. Box 1408, Zip 28359-1408; tel. 910/671-5000; J. L. Welsh, Jr, President and Chief Executive Officer

UNIVERSITY OF NORTH CAROLINA HOSPITALS, 101 Manning Drive, Chapel Hill, NC, Zip 27514-4220; tel. 919/966-4131; Eric B. Munson, President and Chief Executive Officer

WAKE MEDICAL CENTER, 3000 New Bern Avenue, Raleigh, NC, Zip 27610-1295; tel. 919/350-8000; Raymond L. Champ, President

WAKE FOREST UNIVERSITY BAPTIST MEDICAL CENTER
Medical Center Boulevard, Winston-Salem, NC 27157; tel. 336/716-7840; G. Douglas Atkinson, Associate Dean/Vice President of Networks

ALEXANDER COMMUNITY HOSPITAL, 326 Third Street S.W., Taylorsville, NC, Zip 28681-3096; tel. 828/632-4282; Bill Wilson, Chief Executive Officer

ALLEGHANY MEMORIAL HOSPITAL, 233 Doctors Street, Sparta, NC, Zip 28675-0009, Mailing Address: P.O. Box 9, Zip 28675-0009; tel. 336/372-5511; James Yarborough, Chief Executive Officer

ANGEL MEDICAL CENTER, Riverview and White Oak Streets, Franklin, NC, Zip 28734, Mailing Address: P.O. Box 1209, Zip 28744; tel. 828/524-8411; Michael E. Zuliani, Chief Executive Officer

ASHE MEMORIAL HOSPITAL, 200 Hospital Avenue, Jefferson, NC, Zip 28640; tel. 336/246-7101; R. D. Williams, Administrator and Chief Executive Officer

BLOWING ROCK HOSPITAL, Chestnut Street, Blowing Rock, NC, Zip 28605-0148, Mailing Address: Box 148, Zip 28605-0148; tel. 828/295-3136; Patricia Gray, Administrator and Chief Executive Officer

CALDWELL MEMORIAL HOSPITAL, 321 Mulberry Street S.W., Lenoir, NC, Zip 28645-5720, Mailing Address: P.O. Box 1890, Zip 28645-1890; tel. 828/757-5100; Frederick L. Soule, President and Chief Executive Officer

CATAWBA MEMORIAL HOSPITAL, 810 Fairgrove Church Road S.E., Hickory, NC, Zip 28602-9643; tel. 828/326-3000; J. Anthony Rose, President and Chief Executive Officer

HOOTS MEMORIAL HOSPITAL, 624 West Main Street, Yadkinville, NC, Zip 27055-7804, Mailing Address: P.O. Box 68, Zip 27055-0068; tel. 336/679-2041; Lance C. Labine, President

HUGH CHATHAM MEMORIAL HOSPITAL, Parkwood Drive, Elkin, NC, Zip 28621-0560, Mailing Address: P.O. Box 560, Zip 28621-0560; tel. 336/527-7000; Richard D. Osmus, Chief Executive Officer

LEXINGTON MEMORIAL HOSPITAL, 250 Hospital Drive, Lexington, NC, Zip 27292, Mailing Address: P.O. Box 1817, Zip 27293-1817; tel. 336/248-5161; John A. Cashion, FACHE, President

MEMORIAL HOSPITAL OF MARTINSVILLE AND HENRY COUNTY, 320 Hospital Drive, Martinsville, VA, Zip 24112-1981, Mailing Address: Box 4788, Zip 24115-4788; tel. 540/666-7200; Joseph Roach, Chief Executive Officer

MOREHEAD MEMORIAL HOSPITAL, 117 East King's Highway, Eden, NC, Zip 27288-5299; tel. 336/623-9711; Robert Enders, President

NORTHERN HOSPITAL OF SURRY COUNTY, 830 Rockford Street, Mount Airy, NC, Zip 27030-5365, Mailing Address: P.O. Box 1101, Zip 27030-1101; tel. 336/719-7000; William B. James, Chief Executive Officer

ROWAN REGIONAL MEDICAL CENTER, 612 Mocksville Avenue, Salisbury, NC, Zip 28144-2799; tel. 704/638-1000; James M. Freeman, Chief Executive Officer

RUTHERFORD HOSPITAL, 288 South Ridgecrest Avenue, Rutherfordton, NC, Zip 28139-3097; tel. 828/286-5000; Robert D. Jones, President

STOKES-REYNOLDS MEMORIAL HOSPITAL, Danbury, NC, Mailing Address: P.O. Box 10, Zip 27016-0010; tel. 336/593-2831; Sandra D. Priddy, President

TWIN COUNTY REGIONAL HOSPITAL, 200 Hospital Drive, Galax, VA, Zip 24333-2283; tel. 540/236-8181; Marcus G. Kuhn, President and Chief Executive Officer

VETERANS AFFAIRS MEDICAL CENTER, 1601 Brenner Avenue, Salisbury, NC, Zip 28144-2559; tel. 704/638-9000; Timothy May, Director

WILKES REGIONAL MEDICAL CENTER, 1370 West D Street, North Wilkesboro, NC, Zip 28659-3506, Mailing Address: P.O. Box 609, Zip 28659-0609; tel. 336/651-8100; David L. Henson, Chief Executive Officer

WESTERN NORTH CAROLINA HEALTH NETWORK
P.O. Box 2295, Asheville, NC 28802; tel. 828/257-2983; Carla Elliott, Projects Manager

ANGEL MEDICAL CENTER, Riverview and White Oak Streets, Franklin, NC, Zip 28734, Mailing Address: P.O. Box 1209, Zip 28744; tel. 828/524-8411; Michael E. Zuliani, Chief Executive Officer

DISTRICT MEMORIAL HOSPITAL, 415 Whitaker Lane, Andrews, NC, Zip 28901-9229; tel. 828/321-1291; Allen D. Swan, Chief Executive Officer

HARRIS REGIONAL HOSPITAL, 68 Hospital Road, Sylva, NC, Zip 28779-2795; tel. 828/586-7000; Mark Leonard, Chief Executive Officer

HAYWOOD REGIONAL MEDICAL CENTER, 262 Leroy George Drive, Clyde, NC, Zip 28721-9434; tel. 828/456-7311; David O. Rice, President

HIGHLANDS-CASHIERS HOSPITAL, Hospital Drive, Highlands, NC, Zip 28741, Mailing Address: P.O. Drawer 190, Zip 28741-0190; tel. 828/526-1200; H. James Graham, Administrator

MARGARET R. PARDEE MEMORIAL HOSPITAL, 715 Fleming Street, Hendersonville, NC, Zip 28791-2563; tel. 828/696-1000; Frank J. Aaron, Jr, Chief Executive Officer

MCDOWELL HOSPITAL, 100 Rankin Drive, Marion, NC, Zip 28752-4989, Mailing Address: P.O. Box 730, Zip 28752-0730; tel. 828/659-5000; Jeffrey M. Judd, President and Chief Executive Officer

MURPHY MEDICAL CENTER, 4130 U.S. Highway 64 East, Murphy, NC, Zip 28906-7917; tel. 828/837-8161; Mike Stevenson, Administrator

PARK RIDGE HOSPITAL, Naples Road, Fletcher, NC, Zip 28732, Mailing Address: P.O. Box 1569, Zip 28732-1569; tel. 828/684-8501; Michael V. Gentry, President

RUTHERFORD HOSPITAL, 288 South Ridgecrest Avenue, Rutherfordton, NC, Zip 28139-3097; tel. 828/286-5000; Robert D. Jones, President

SPRUCE PINE COMMUNITY HOSPITAL, 125 Hospital Drive, Spruce Pine, NC, Zip 28777-3035, Mailing Address: P.O. Drawer 9, Zip 28777-0009; tel. 828/765-4201; Keith S. Holtsclaw, Chief Executive Officer

ST. LUKE'S HOSPITAL, 220 Hospital Drive, Columbus, NC, Zip 28722-9473; tel. 828/894-3311; C. Cameron Highsmith, Jr, President and Chief Executive Officer

SWAIN COUNTY HOSPITAL, 45 Plateau Street, Bryson City, NC, Zip 28713-6784; tel. 828/488-4013; James M. Kirby, Administrator

THOMS REHABILITATION HOSPITAL, 68 Sweeten Creek Road, Asheville, NC, Zip 28803-1599, Mailing Address: P.O. Box 15025, Zip 28813-0025; tel. 828/274-2400; Dennis A. Giles, President

TRANSYLVANIA COMMUNITY HOSPITAL, Hospital Drive, Brevard, NC, Zip 28712-1116, Mailing Address: Box 1116, Zip 28712-1116; tel. 828/884-9111; Robert J. Bednarek, President and Chief Executive Officer

NORTH DAKOTA

HEARTLAND INDEPENDENT PROVIDER NETWORK
1711 S. University Drive, Fargo, ND 58103; tel. 701/461-5782; John Kutch, Executive Director

DAKOTA HEARTLAND HEALTH SYSTEM, 1720 South University Drive, Fargo, ND, Zip 58103-4994; tel. 701/280-4100; Louis Kauffman, President and Chief Executive Officer

MEDCENTER ONE HEALTH SERVICES
300 North 7th St. P.O. Box 5525, Bismarck, ND 58506; tel. 701/323-6000; Terrance G. Brosseau, President/Chief Executive Officer

JACOBSON MEMORIAL HOSPITAL CARE CENTER, 601 East Street North, Elgin, ND, Zip 58533-0376; tel. 701/584-2792; Jacqueline Seibel, Administrator

Networks / Medcenter One Health Services

MCKENZIE COUNTY MEMORIAL HOSPITAL, 516 North Main Street, Watford City, ND, Zip 58854–0548, Mailing Address: P.O. Box 548, Zip 58854–0548; tel. 701/842–3000; Colette Anderson, Administrator

MEDCENTER ONE, 300 North Seventh Street, Bismarck, ND, Zip 58501–4439, Mailing Address: P.O. Box 5525, Zip 58506–5525; tel. 701/323–6000; Terrance G. Brosseau, President and Chief Executive Officer

RICHARDTON HEALTH CENTER, 212 Third Avenue West, Richardton, ND, Zip 58652–7103, Mailing Address: P.O. Box H, Zip 58652; tel. 701/974–3304; Kurt Waldbillig, Chief Executive Officer

ST. LUKE'S TRI-STATE HOSPITAL, 202 Sixth Avenue S.W., Bowman, ND, Zip 58623–0009, Mailing Address: P.O. Drawer C, Zip 58623; tel. 701/523–5265; Darrold Bertsch, Administrator

MERITCARE HEALTH SYSTEM
737 Broadway, Fargo, ND 58123;
tel. 701/234–2621; Angie Heckaman,
Managed Care Analyst

MERITCARE HEALTH SYSTEM, 720 Fourth Street North, Fargo, ND, Zip 58122–0002; tel. 701/234–6000; Roger Gilbertson, M.D., President

UNITED HOSPITAL
1200 South Columbia Road, Grand Forks, ND 58201; tel. 701/780–5000; Rosemary Jacobson, President & Chief Executive

ALTRU HEALTH SYSTEM, 1000 South Columbia Road, Grand Forks, ND, Zip 58201; tel. 701/780–5000

OHIO

BLANCHARD VALLEY HEALTH ASSOCIATION
145 W. Wallace, Findlay, OH 45840;
tel. 419/423–5201; William Ruse, President

BLANCHARD VALLEY HEALTH ASSOCIATION SYSTEM, 145 West Wallace Street, Findlay, OH, Zip 45840–1299; tel. 419/423–4500; William E. Ruse, FACHE, President and Chief Executive Officer

CLEVELAND HEALTH NETWORK
9500 Euclid Avenue H18, Independence, OH 44131; tel. 216/328–7550; Dennis Pijor, Executive Vice–President/COO

ASHTABULA COUNTY MEDICAL CENTER, 2420 Lake Avenue, Ashtabula, OH, Zip 44004–4993; tel. 440/997–2262; R. D. Richardson, President and Chief Executive Officer

BARBERTON CITIZENS HOSPITAL, 155 Fifth Street N.E., Barberton, OH, Zip 44203–3398; tel. 330/745–1611; Ronald J. Elder, Chief Executive Officer

BOSTON MEDICAL CENTER, One Boston Medical Center Place, Boston, MA, Zip 02118–2393; tel. 617/638–8000; Elaine S. Ullian, President and Chief Executive Officer

CHILDREN'S HOSPITAL MEDICAL CENTER OF AKRON, One Perkins Square, Akron, OH, Zip 44308–1062; tel. 330/543–1000; William H. Considine, President

CLEVELAND CLINIC FOUNDATION, 9500 Euclid Avenue, Cleveland, OH, Zip 44195–5108; tel. 216/444–2200; Frank L. Lordeman, Chief Operating Officer

CUYAHOGA FALLS GENERAL HOSPITAL, 1900 23rd Street, Cuyahoga Falls, OH, Zip 44223–1499; tel. 330/971–7000; Fred Anthony, President and Chief Executive Officer

DOCTORS HOSPITAL OF STARK COUNTY, 400 Austin Avenue N.W., Massillon, OH, Zip 44646–3554; tel. 330/837–7200; Thomas E. Cecconi, Chief Executive Officer

EMH AMHERST HOSPITAL, 254 Cleveland Avenue, Amherst, OH, Zip 44001–1699; tel. 440/988–6000; Kevin C. Martin, President and Chief Executive Officer

EMH REGIONAL MEDICAL CENTER, 630 East River Street, Elyria, OH, Zip 44035–5902; tel. 440/329–7500; Kevin C. Martin, President and Chief Executive Officer

EUCLID HOSPITAL, 18901 Lake Shore Boulevard, Euclid, OH, Zip 44119–1090; tel. 216/531–9000; Lauren Rock, Chief Operating Officer

FAIRVIEW HOSPITAL, 18101 Lorain Avenue, Cleveland, OH, Zip 44111–5656; tel. 216/476–7000; Louis P. Caravella, M.D., Chief Executive Officer

FIRELANDS COMMUNITY HOSPITAL, 1101 Decatur Street, Sandusky, OH, Zip 44870–3335; tel. 419/626–7795; Dennis A. Sokol, President and Chief Executive Officer

FISHER–TITUS MEDICAL CENTER, 272 Benedict Avenue, Norwalk, OH, Zip 44857–2374; tel. 419/668–8101; Patrick J. Martin, President and Chief Executive Officer

HAMOT MEDICAL CENTER, 201 State Street, Erie, PA, Zip 16550–0002; tel. 814/877–6000; John T. Malone, President and Chief Executive Officer

LAKEWOOD HOSPITAL, 14519 Detroit Avenue, Lakewood, OH, Zip 44107–4383; tel. 216/521–4200; V. Richard Stelzer, Jr, Chief Administrative Officer

LUTHERAN HOSPITAL, 1730 West 25th Street, Cleveland, OH, Zip 44113; tel. 216/696–4300; John Brocketi, Associate Vice President

MARYMOUNT HOSPITAL, 12300 McCracken Road, Garfield Heights, OH, Zip 44125–2975; tel. 216/581–0500; Thomas J. Trudell, President and Chief Executive Officer

MERIDIA HILLCREST HOSPITAL, 6780 Mayfield Road, Cleveland, OH, Zip 44124–2202; tel. 440/449–4500; Catherine B. Leary, R.N., Chief Operating Officer

MERIDIA HURON HOSPITAL, 13951 Terrace Road, Cleveland, OH, Zip 44112–4399; tel. 216/761–3300; Beverly Lozar, Chief Operating Officer

METROHEALTH MEDICAL CENTER, 2500 MetroHealth Drive, Cleveland, OH, Zip 44109–1998; tel. 216/778–7800; Terry R. White, President and Chief Executive Officer

PARMA COMMUNITY GENERAL HOSPITAL, 7007 Powers Boulevard, Parma, OH, Zip 44129–5495; tel. 440/743–3000; Thomas A. Selden, President and Chief Executive Officer

ST. ELIZABETH HEALTH CENTER, 1044 Belmont Avenue, Youngstown, OH, Zip 44501, Mailing Address: P.O. Box 1790, Zip 44501–1790; tel. 330/746–7211; Michael Terrance Rowan, President and Chief Executive Officer

ST. JOSEPH HEALTH CENTER, 667 Eastland Avenue S.E., Warren, OH, Zip 44484–4531; tel. 330/841–4000; Michael Terrance Rowan, President and Chief Executive Officer

SUMMA HEALTH SYSTEM, Akron, OH, Thomas J. Strauss, President and Chief Executive Officer

WADSWORTH–RITTMAN HOSPITAL, 195 Wadsworth Road, Wadsworth, OH, Zip 44281–9505; tel. 330/334–1504; James W. Brumlow, Jr, President and Chief Executive Officer

COMMUNITY HOSPITALS OF OHIO
1320 West Main Street, Newark, OH 43055;
tel. 614/344–0331; William J. Andrews, President

LICKING MEMORIAL HOSPITAL, 1320 West Main Street, Newark, OH, Zip 43055–3699; tel. 740/348–4000; William J. Andrews, President

COMPREHENSIVE HEALTHCARE OF OHIO, INC
630 East River Street, Elyria, OH 44035;
tel. 440/329–7591; Donald Miller, Vice President–Operations

EMH AMHERST HOSPITAL, 254 Cleveland Avenue, Amherst, OH, Zip 44001–1699; tel. 440/988–6000; Kevin C. Martin, President and Chief Executive Officer

EMH REGIONAL MEDICAL CENTER, 630 East River Street, Elyria, OH, Zip 44035–5902; tel. 440/329–7500; Kevin C. Martin, President and Chief Executive Officer

COUNTY BASED HEALTHCARE NETWORK
2420 Lake Avenue, Ashtabula, OH 44004;
tel. 216/997–2262; Doy Gillespie, Vice President of Business Development

GOOD SAMRITAN HOSPITAL
375 Dixsmyth, Cincinnati, OH 45220;
tel. 513/872–1828; John Prout, President & Chief Executive Officer

BETHESDA NORTH HOSPITAL, 10500 Montgomery Road, Cincinnati, OH, Zip 45242–4415; tel. 513/745–1111; John S. Prout, President and Chief Executive Officer

GOOD SAMARITAN HOSPITAL, 375 Dixmyth Avenue, Cincinnati, OH, Zip 45220–2489; tel. 513/872–1400; John S. Prout, President and Chief Executive Officer

HEALTH CARE ALLIANCE
6001 East Broad Street, Columbus, OH 43213; tel. 614/868–6000; Dale St. Arnold, President

ADENA HEALTH SYSTEM, 272 Hospital Road, Chillicothe, OH, Zip 45601–0708; tel. 740/779–7500; Allen V. Rupiper, President

BERGER HEALTH SYSTEM, 600 North Pickaway Street, Circleville, OH, Zip 43113–1499; tel. 740/420–8231; Brian R. Colfack, CHE, President and Chief Executive Officer

MOUNT CARMEL HEALTH SYSTEM, Columbus, OH, Mailing Address: 793 West State Street, Zip 43222–1551; tel. 614/234–5423; Joseph T. Calvaruso, President and Chief Executive Officer

LAKE ERIE HEALTH ALLIANCE
2142 North Cove Boulevard – Suite 950, Jobst Tower, Toledo, OH 43606; tel. 419/471–3450; John Horn, President

BELLEVUE HOSPITAL, 811 Northwest Street, Bellevue, OH, Zip 44811, Mailing Address: P.O. Box 8004, Zip 44811–8004; tel. 419/483–4040; Michael K. Winthrop, President

BLANCHARD VALLEY HEALTH ASSOCIATION SYSTEM, 145 West Wallace Street, Findlay, OH, Zip 45840–1299; tel. 419/423–4500; William E. Ruse, FACHE, President and Chief Executive Officer

DEFIANCE HOSPITAL, 1206 East Second Street, Defiance, OH, Zip 43512–2495; tel. 419/783–6955; Robert J. Coholich, President

FIRELANDS COMMUNITY HOSPITAL, 1101 Decatur Street, Sandusky, OH, Zip 44870–3335; tel. 419/626–7795; Dennis A. Sokol, President and Chief Executive Officer

FISHER–TITUS MEDICAL CENTER, 272 Benedict Avenue, Norwalk, OH, Zip 44857–2374; tel. 419/668–8101; Patrick J. Martin, President and Chief Executive Officer

FLOWER HOSPITAL, 5200 Harroun Road, Sylvania, OH, Zip 43560–2196; tel. 419/824–1444; Randall Kelley, President

FOSTORIA COMMUNITY HOSPITAL, 501 Van Buren Street, Fostoria, OH, Zip 44830–0907, Mailing Address: P.O. Box 907, Zip 44830–0907; tel. 419/435–7734; Brad A. Higgins, President

FULTON COUNTY HEALTH CENTER, 725 South Shoop Avenue, Wauseon, OH, Zip 43567–1701; tel. 419/335–2015; E. Dean Beck, Administrator

H. B. MAGRUDER MEMORIAL HOSPITAL, 615 Fulton Street, Port Clinton, OH, Zip 43452–2034; tel. 419/734–3131; David R. Norwine, President and Chief Executive Officer

HENRY COUNTY HOSPITAL, 11600 State Route 424, Napoleon, OH, Zip 43545–9399; tel. 419/592–4015; Kimberly Bordenkircher, Chief Executive Officer

LIMA MEMORIAL HOSPITAL, 1001 Bellefontaine Avenue, Lima, OH, Zip 45804–2899; tel. 419/228–3335; John B. White, President and Chief Executive Officer

MEDCENTRAL HEALTH SYSTEM, 335 Glessner Avenue, Mansfield, OH, Zip 44903–2265; tel. 419/526–8000; James E. Meyer, President and Chief Executive Officer

MEDICAL COLLEGE OF OHIO HOSPITALS, 3000 Arlington Avenue, Toledo, OH, Zip 43614–5805; tel. 419/383–4000; Frank S. McCullough, M.D., President

Networks / Integris Health

MEMORIAL HOSPITAL, 715 South Taft Avenue, Fremont, OH, Zip 43420-3200; tel. 419/332-7321; John A. Gorman, Chief Executive Officer

MERCY MEMORIAL HOSPITAL, 740 North Macomb Street, Monroe, MI, Zip 48161-9974, Mailing Address: P.O. Box 67, Zip 48161-0067; tel. 734/241-1700; Richard S. Hiltz, President and Chief Executive Officer

ST. FRANCIS HEALTH CARE CENTRE, 401 North Broadway, Green Springs, OH, Zip 44836-9653; tel. 419/639-2626; Dan Schwanke, Executive Director

THE TOLEDO HOSPITAL, 2142 North Cove Boulevard, Toledo, OH, Zip 43606-3896; tel. 419/471-4000; Barbara Steele, President

WOOD COUNTY HOSPITAL, 950 West Wooster Street, Bowling Green, OH, Zip 43402-2699; tel. 419/354-8900; Michael A. Miesle, Administrator

LAKE HOSPITAL SYSTEM
10 East Washington, Painesville, OH 44077; tel. 216/354-2400; Cynthia Moore-Hardy, President & Chief Executive Officer

LAKE HOSPITAL SYSTEM, 10 East Washington, Painesville, OH, Zip 44077-3472; tel. 440/354-2400; Cynthia Ann Moore-Hardy, President and Chief Executive Officer

MERCY HEALTH PARTNERS - SOUTHWEST OHIO
4340 Glendale-Milford, Cincinnati, OH 45242; tel. 513/483-5270; Julie Hanser, President & Chief Executive Officer

MERCY FRANCISCAN HOSPITAL-MOUNT AIRY, 2446 Kipling Avenue, Cincinnati, OH, Zip 45239-6650; tel. 513/853-5000; Steven Grinnell, President

MERCY HOSPITAL, Hamilton, OH, Mailing Address: P.O. Box 418, Zip 45012-0418; tel. 513/867-6400; David A. Ferrell, President

MERCY HOSPITAL ANDERSON, 7500 State Road, Cincinnati, OH, Zip 45255-2492; tel. 513/624-4500; Fred L. Kolb, President

MERCY HOSPITAL CLERMONT, 3000 Hospital Drive, Batavia, OH, Zip 45103-1998; tel. 513/732-8200; John M. Dawes, Vice President Operations

OHIO STATE HEALTH NETWORK
1375 Perry, Suite 518, Columbus, OH 43201; tel. 614/293-3756; Terry Vanderhoof, Chairman

ARTHUR G. JAMES CANCER HOSPITAL AND RICHARD J. SOLOVE RESEARCH INSTITUTE, 300 West Tenth Avenue, Columbus, OH, Zip 43210-1240; tel. 614/293-5485; David E. Schuller, M.D., Chief Executive Officer

BARNESVILLE HOSPITAL ASSOCIATION, 639 West Main Street, Barnesville, OH, Zip 43713-0309, Mailing Address: P.O. Box 309, Zip 43713-0309; tel. 740/425-3941; Richard L. Doan, Chief Executive Officer

MADISON COUNTY HOSPITAL, 210 North Main Street, London, OH, Zip 43140-1115; tel. 740/852-1372; Stuart W. Williams, Interim Chief Executive Officer

MARY RUTAN HOSPITAL, 205 Palmer Avenue, Bellefontaine, OH, Zip 43311-2298; tel. 937/592-4015; Ewing H. Crawfis, President

OHIO STATE UNIVERSITY MEDICAL CENTER, 410 West 10th Avenue, Columbus, OH, Zip 43210-1240; tel. 614/293-8000; R. Reed Fraley, Vice President for Health Services

PIKE COMMUNITY HOSPITAL, 100 Dawn Lane, Waverly, OH, Zip 45690-9664; tel. 740/947-2186; Richard E. Sobota, President and Chief Executive Officer

RIVER VALLEY HEALTH SYSTEM, 2228 South Ninth Street, Ironton, OH, Zip 45638-2526; tel. 740/532-3231; Terry L. Vanderhoof, President and Chief Executive Officer

WYANDOT MEMORIAL HOSPITAL, 885 North Sandusky Avenue, Upper Sandusky, OH, Zip 43351-1098; tel. 419/294-4991; Joseph A. D'Ettorre, Chief Executive Officer

PHS MOUNT SINAI MEDICAL CENTER
One Mt Sinai Drive, Cleveland, OH 44106; tel. 216/421-4000; Michael Autrey, President & Chief Executive Officer

DEACONESS HOSPITAL OF CLEVELAND, 4229 Pearl Road, Cleveland, OH, Zip 44109-4218; tel. 216/459-6300; Geoffrey D. Moebius, Chief Executive Officer

SAINT MICHAEL HOSPITAL, 5163 Broadway Avenue, Cleveland, OH, Zip 44127-1532; tel. 216/429-8000; Richard J. Frenchie, Chief Executive Officer

PROMEDICA NETWORK
2142 North Cove Boulevard, Toledo, OH 43606; tel. 419/471-4000; Daniel Rissing, Chief Executive Officer

FLOWER HOSPITAL, 5200 Harroun Road, Sylvania, OH, Zip 43560-2196; tel. 419/824-1444; Randall Kelley, President

THE TOLEDO HOSPITAL, 2142 North Cove Boulevard, Toledo, OH, Zip 43606-3896; tel. 419/471-4000; Barbara Steele, President

PROVIDERS SOLUTION
3521 Briarfield Blvd., Maumee, OH 43537; tel. 419/534-2000; Annette Leslie, Director of Marketing

ST. LUKE'S HOSPITAL, 5901 Monclova Road, Maumee, OH, Zip 43537-1899; tel. 419/893-5911; Frank J. Bartell, II, President and Chief Executive Officer

SUMMA HEALTH SYSTEM
525 East Market Street, Akron, OH 44309; tel. 330/375-3101; Gary Robinson, Director, Strategic Planning

AKRON GENERAL MEDICAL CENTER, 400 Wabash Avenue, Akron, OH, Zip 44307-2433; tel. 330/384-6000; Alan J. Bleyer, President

SUMMA HEALTH SYSTEM, Akron, OH, Thomas J. Strauss, President and Chief Executive Officer

SUMMA HEALTH SYSTEM, Akron, OH, Thomas J. Strauss, President and Chief Executive Officer

THE METROHEALTH SYSTEM
2500 MetroHealth Drive, Cleveland, OH 44109; tel. 216/778-7800; Terry White, President & Chief Executive Officer

METROHEALTH MEDICAL CENTER, 2500 MetroHealth Drive, Cleveland, OH, Zip 44109-1998; tel. 216/778-7800; Terry R. White, President and Chief Executive Officer

UNITED HEALTH PARTNERS
2213 Cherry Street, Toledo, OH 43608; tel. 419/321-3232; David Crane, Vice President of Marketing

BELLEVUE HOSPITAL, 811 Northwest Street, Bellevue, OH, Zip 44811, Mailing Address: P.O. Box 8004, Zip 44811-8004; tel. 419/483-4040; Michael K. Winthrop, President

DEFIANCE HOSPITAL, 1206 East Second Street, Defiance, OH, Zip 43512-2495; tel. 419/783-6955; Robert J. Coholich, President

FISHER-TITUS MEDICAL CENTER, 272 Benedict Avenue, Norwalk, OH, Zip 44857-2374; tel. 419/668-8101; Patrick J. Martin, President and Chief Executive Officer

FOSTORIA COMMUNITY HOSPITAL, 501 Van Buren Street, Fostoria, OH, Zip 44830-0907, Mailing Address: P.O. Box 907, Zip 44830-0907; tel. 419/435-7734; Brad A. Higgins, President

FULTON COUNTY HEALTH CENTER, 725 South Shoop Avenue, Wauseon, OH, Zip 43567-1701; tel. 419/335-2015; E. Dean Beck, Administrator

MEMORIAL HOSPITAL, 715 South Taft Avenue, Fremont, OH, Zip 43420-3200; tel. 419/332-7321; John A. Gorman, Chief Executive Officer

MERCY HOSPITAL, 485 West Market Street, Tiffin, OH, Zip 44883-0727; tel. 419/448-3133; Mark Shugarman, President

MERCY HOSPITAL OF WILLARD, 110 East Howard Street, Willard, OH, Zip 44890-1611; tel. 419/964-5000; Dale E. Thornton, M.P.H., CHE, President and Chief Executive Officer

PROVIDENCE HOSPITAL, 1912 Hayes Avenue, Sandusky, OH, Zip 44870-4736; tel. 419/621-7000; Sister Nancy Linenkugel, FACHE, President and Chief Executive Officer

ST. VINCENT MERCY MEDICAL CENTER, 2213 Cherry Street, Toledo, OH, Zip 43608-2691; tel. 419/251-3232; Steven L. Mickus, President and Chief Executive Officer

WOOD COUNTY HOSPITAL, 950 West Wooster Street, Bowling Green, OH, Zip 43402-2699; tel. 419/354-8900; Michael A. Miesle, Administrator

UPPER VALLEY MEDICAL
3130 North Dixie Highway, Troy, OH 45373; tel. 937/492-3775; Michele Elam, Financial Coordinator

UPPER VALLEY MEDICAL CENTER, 3130 North Dixie Highway, Troy, OH, Zip 45373; tel. 937/440-7500; David J. Meckstroth, President and Chief Executive Officer

WEST CENTRAL OHIO REGIONAL HLTHCRE ALLIANCE, LTD.
730 West Market Street, Lima, OH 45801; tel. 419/226-9085; P. Anthony Long, Executive Director

JOINT TOWNSHIP DISTRICT MEMORIAL HOSPITAL, 200 St. Clair Street, Saint Marys, OH, Zip 45885-2400; tel. 419/394-3387; James R. Chick, President

MARY RUTAN HOSPITAL, 205 Palmer Avenue, Bellefontaine, OH, Zip 43311-2298; tel. 937/592-4015; Ewing H. Crawfis, President

MERCER COUNTY JOINT TOWNSHIP COMMUNITY HOSPITAL, 800 West Main Street, Coldwater, OH, Zip 45828-1698; tel. 419/678-2341; James W. Isaacs, Chief Executive Officer

PAULDING COUNTY HOSPITAL, 1035 West Wayne Street, Paulding, OH, Zip 45879-9220; tel. 419/399-4080; Larry Thornhill, Chief Executive Officer

ST. RITA'S MEDICAL CENTER, 730 West Market Street, Lima, OH, Zip 45801-4670; tel. 419/227-3361; James P. Reber, President

VAN WERT COUNTY HOSPITAL, 1250 South Washington Street, Van Wert, OH, Zip 45891-2599; tel. 419/238-2390; Mark J. Minick, President and Chief Executive Officer

OKLAHOMA

EASTERN OKLAHOMA HEALTH NETWORK
110 West 7th Street Ste. 2520, Tulsa, OK 74114; tel. 918/579-7856; Dale Harris, Regional Development

DOCTORS HOSPITAL, 2323 South Harvard Avenue, Tulsa, OK, Zip 74114-3370; tel. 918/744-4000; Kenneth Noteboom, Chief Executive Officer

HILLCREST MEDICAL CENTER, 1120 South Utica, Tulsa, OK, Zip 74104-4090; tel. 918/579-1000; Donald A. Lorack, Jr, President and Chief Executive Officer

WAGONER COMMUNITY HOSPITAL, 1200 West Cherokee, Wagoner, OK, Zip 74467-4681, Mailing Address: Box 407, Zip 74477-0407; tel. 918/485-5514; John W. Crawford, Chief Executive Officer

INTEGRIS HEALTH
3366 N.W. Expressway, Suite 800, Oklahoma City, OK 73112; tel. 405/949-6066; Trevor D. Shipley, Administrative Resident

BLACKWELL REGIONAL HOSPITAL, 710 South 13th Street, Blackwell, OK, Zip 74631-3700; tel. 580/363-2311; Cindy White, Chief Financial Officer

DRUMRIGHT MEMORIAL HOSPITAL, 501 South Lou Allard Drive, Drumright, OK, Zip 74030-4899; tel. 918/352-2525; James L. Clough, Administrator

INTEGRIS BAPTIST MEDICAL CENTER, 3300 N.W. Expressway, Oklahoma City, OK, Zip 73112-4481; tel. 405/949-3011; Thomas R. Rice, FACHE, President and Chief Operating Officer

INTEGRIS BAPTIST REGIONAL HEALTH CENTER, 200 Second Street S.W., Miami, OK, Zip 74354-6830, Mailing Address: P.O. Box 1207, Zip 74355-1207; tel. 918/542-6611; W. Eugene Baxter, Dr.PH, FACHE, Interim Administrator

Networks / Integris Health

INTEGRIS BASS BAPTIST HEALTH CENTER, 600 South Monroe Street, Enid, OK, Zip 73701, Mailing Address: P.O. Box 3168, Zip 73702–3168; tel. 580/233–2300; Thomas Schmitt, Administrator

INTEGRIS GROVE GENERAL HOSPITAL, 1310 South Main Street, Grove, OK, Zip 74344–1310; tel. 918/786–2243; Greg Martin, Administrator and Chief Executive Officer

INTEGRIS MENTAL HEALTH SYSTEM–SPENCER, 2601 North Spencer Road, Spencer, OK, Zip 73084–3699, Mailing Address: P.O. Box 11137, Oklahoma City, Zip 73136–0137; tel. 405/427–2441; Murali Krishna, M.D., President and Chief Operating Officer

INTEGRIS SOUTHWEST MEDICAL CENTER, 4401 South Western, Oklahoma City, OK, Zip 73109–3441; tel. 405/636–7000; Thomas R. Rice, FACHE, President and Chief Operating Officer

INTERGRIS CLINTON REGIONAL HOSPITAL, 100 North 30th Street, Clinton, OK, Zip 73601–3117, Mailing Address: P.O. Box 1569, Zip 73601–1569; tel. 580/323–2363; Jerry Jones, Administrator

MARSHALL MEMORIAL HOSPITAL, 1 Hospital Drive, Madill, OK, Zip 73446, Mailing Address: P.O. Box 827, Zip 73446–0827; tel. 580/795–3384; Norma Howard, Administrator

MAYES COUNTY MEDICAL CENTER, 129 North Kentucky Street, Pryor, OK, Zip 74361–4211, Mailing Address: P.O. Box 278, Zip 74362–0278; tel. 918/825–1600; W. Charles Jordan, Administrator

PAWNEE MUNICIPAL HOSPITAL, 1212 Fourth Street, Pawnee, OK, Zip 74058–4046, Mailing Address: P.O. Box 467, Zip 74058–0467; tel. 918/762–2577; John H. Ketring, Administrator

MERCY HEALTH SYSTEM
4300 West Memorial Road, Oklahoma City, OK 73120; tel. 405/752–3754; Michael Packnett, President & Chief Executive Officer

MERCY HEALTH CENTER, 4300 West Memorial Road, Oklahoma City, OK, Zip 73120–8362; tel. 405/755–1515; Michael J. Packnett, President and Chief Executive Officer

MERCY MEMORIAL HEALTH CENTER, 1011 14th Street N.W., Ardmore, OK, Zip 73401–1889; tel. 580/223–5400; Bobby G. Thompson, President and Chief Executive Officer

ST. MARY'S MERCY HOSPITAL, 305 South Fifth Street, Enid, OK, Zip 73701–5899, Mailing Address: Box 232, Zip 73702–0232; tel. 580/233–6100; Frank Lopez, FACHE, President and Chief Executive Officer

UNIVERSITY HEALTH PARTNERS
6501 North Broadway, Oklahoma City, OK 73116; tel. 405/879–0999; David Dunlap, Chief Executive Officer

EDMOND MEDICAL CENTER, 1 South Bryant Street, Edmond, OK, Zip 73034–4798; tel. 405/341–6100; Stanley D. Tatum, Chief Executive Officer

SEMINOLE MEDICAL CENTER, 2401 Wrangler Boulevard, Seminole, OK, Zip 74868; tel. 405/303–4000; Janet Jackman, Chief Executive Officer

SOUTHWESTERN MEDICAL CENTER, 5602 S.W. Lee Boulevard, Lawton, OK, Zip 73505–9635, Mailing Address: P.O. Box 7290, Zip 73506–7290; tel. 580/531–4700; Thomas L. Rine, President and Chief Executive Officer

UNIVERSITY HEALTH PARTNERS, 6501 North Broadway, Suite 200, Oklahoma City, OK, Zip 73116; tel. 405/879–0900; Jeffrey A. Dorsey, Chief Executive Officer

UNIVERSITY HOSPITALS
P.O. Box 26307, Oklahoma City, OK 73104; tel. 405/271–6165; Gerald Maier, Chief Executive Officer

UNIVERSITY HEALTH PARTNERS, 6501 North Broadway, Suite 200, Oklahoma City, OK, Zip 73116; tel. 405/879–0900; Jeffrey A. Dorsey, Chief Executive Officer

OREGON

HEALTH FUTURE, LLC
825 East Main Street Suite D., Medford, OR 97504; tel. 541/772–3062; Hans G. Wiik, President & Chief Executive Officer

ASHLAND COMMUNITY HOSPITAL, 280 Maple Street, Ashland, OR, Zip 97520, Mailing Address: P.O. Box 98, Zip 97520; tel. 541/482–2441; James R. Watson, Administrator

BAY AREA HOSPITAL, 1775 Thompson Road, Coos Bay, OR, Zip 97420–2198; tel. 541/269–8111; Dale Jessup, President and Chief Executive Officer

COLUMBIA MEMORIAL HOSPITAL, 2111 Exchange Street, Astoria, OR, Zip 97103; tel. 503/325–4321; Terry O. Finklein, Chief Executive Officer

GOOD SHEPHERD MEDICAL CENTER, 610 N.W. 11th Street, Hermiston, OR, Zip 97838–9696; tel. 541/667–3400; Dennis E. Burke, President

GRANDE RONDE HOSPITAL, 900 Sunset Drive, La Grande, OR, Zip 97850, Mailing Address: P.O. Box 3290, Zip 97850; tel. 541/963–8421; James A. Mattes, President

LOWER UMPQUA HOSPITAL DISTRICT, 600 Ranch Road, Reedsport, OR, Zip 97467–1795; tel. 541/271–2171; Sandra Reese, Administrator

MERCY MEDICAL CENTER, 2700 Stewart Parkway, Roseburg, OR, Zip 97470–1297; tel. 541/673–0611; Victor J. Fresolone, FACHE, President and Chief Executive Officer

MERLE WEST MEDICAL CENTER, 2865 Daggett Street, Klamath Falls, OR, Zip 97601–1180; tel. 541/882–6311; Paul R. Stewart, President and Chief Executive Officer

MID–COLUMBIA MEDICAL CENTER, 1700 East 19th Street, The Dalles, OR, Zip 97058–3316; tel. 541/296–1111; Mark D. Scott, President

OHSU HOSPITAL, 3181 S.W. Sam Jackson Park Road, Portland, OR, Zip 97201–3098; tel. 503/494–8311; Timothy M. Goldfarb, Director Health Systems

PIONEER MEMORIAL HOSPITAL, 564 East Pioneer Drive, Heppner, OR, Zip 97836, Mailing Address: P.O. Box 9, Zip 97836; tel. 541/676–9133; Victor Vander Does, Administrator

ROGUE VALLEY MEDICAL CENTER, 2825 East Barnett Road, Medford, OR, Zip 97504–8332; tel. 541/608–4900; Roseanne McLaren, Senior Vice President

SILVERTON HOSPITAL, 342 Fairview Street, Silverton, OR, Zip 97381; tel. 503/873–1500; William E. Winter, Administrative Director

ST. ANTHONY HOSPITAL, 1601 S.E. Court Avenue, Pendleton, OR, Zip 97801–3297; tel. 541/276–5121; Jeffrey S. Drop, President and Chief Executive Officer

ST. CHARLES MEDICAL CENTER, 2500 N.E. Neff Road, Bend, OR, Zip 97701–6015; tel. 541/382–4321; James T. Lussier, President and Chief Executive Officer

WALLOWA MEMORIAL HOSPITAL, 401 East First Street, Enterprise, OR, Zip 97828, Mailing Address: P.O. Box 460, Zip 97828; tel. 541/426–3111; Kim Dahlman, Chief Executive Officer

INTER COMMUNITY HEALTH NETWORK
3600 North Samaritan Drive, Corvallis, OR 97339; tel. 541/757–5377; Larry Mullins, Chairman

ALBANY GENERAL HOSPITAL, 1046 West Sixth Avenue, Albany, OR, Zip 97321–1999; tel. 541/812–4000; Richard J. Delano, President

GOOD SAMARITAN HOSPITAL CORVALLIS, 3600 N.W. Samaritan Drive, Corvallis, OR, Zip 97330, Mailing Address: P.O. Box 1068, Zip 97339; tel. 541/757–5111; Steven W. Jasperson, Executive Vice President Operations

LEBANON COMMUNITY HOSPITAL, 525 North Santiam Highway, Lebanon, OR, Zip 97355, Mailing Address: P.O. Box 739, Zip 97355–0739; tel. 541/258–2101; Steven W. Jasperson, Executive Vice President Operations

LEGACY HEALTH SYSTEM
1919 N.W. Lovejoy Street, Portland, OR 97209; tel. 503/415–5619; Lin Rigutto, Admin Fellow

LEGACY EMANUEL HOSPITAL AND HEALTH CENTER, 2801 North Gantenbein Avenue, Portland, OR, Zip 97227–1674; tel. 503/413–2200; Stephani White, Vice President and Site Administrator

LEGACY GOOD SAMARITAN HOSPITAL AND MEDICAL CENTER, 1015 N.W. 22nd Avenue, Portland, OR, Zip 97210; tel. 503/413–7711; Martha C. Wangenstein, Vice President and Site Administrator

LEGACY MERIDIAN PARK HOSPITAL, 19300 S.W. 65th Avenue, Tualatin, OR, Zip 97062–9741; tel. 503/692–1212; Jeff Cushing, Vice President and Site Administrator

LEGACY MOUNT HOOD MEDICAL CENTER, 24800 S.E. Stark, Gresham, OR, Zip 97030–0154; tel. 503/667–1122; Thomas S. Parker, Site Administrator

PEACE HEALTH
770 E. 11th Avenue, Eugene, OR 97440–1479; tel. 503/686–3660; Sister Monica Heeran, Executive Director

PROVIDENCE HEALTH SYSTEM IN OREGON
1235 N.E. 47fth Ave., Suite 299, Portland, OR 97213; tel. 503/215–4700; Mary Stoneman, Senior Planning Associate

ALBANY GENERAL HOSPITAL, 1046 West Sixth Avenue, Albany, OR, Zip 97321–1999; tel. 541/812–4000; Richard J. Delano, President

ASHLAND COMMUNITY HOSPITAL, 280 Maple Street, Ashland, OR, Zip 97520, Mailing Address: P.O. Box 98, Zip 97520; tel. 541/482–2441; James R. Watson, Administrator

BLUE MOUNTAIN HOSPITAL, 170 Ford Road, John Day, OR, Zip 97845; tel. 541/575–1311; Robert Houser, Chief Executive Officer

CENTRAL OREGON DISTRICT HOSPITAL, 1253 North Canal Boulevard, Redmond, OR, Zip 97756–1395; tel. 541/548–8131; James A. Diegel, CHE, Executive Director

COLUMBIA MEMORIAL HOSPITAL, 2111 Exchange Street, Astoria, OR, Zip 97103; tel. 503/325–4321; Terry O. Finklein, Chief Executive Officer

GOOD SAMARITAN HOSPITAL CORVALLIS, 3600 N.W. Samaritan Drive, Corvallis, OR, Zip 97330, Mailing Address: P.O. Box 1068, Zip 97339; tel. 541/757–5111; Steven W. Jasperson, Executive Vice President Operations

HARNEY DISTRICT HOSPITAL, 557 West Washington Street, Burns, OR, Zip 97720–1497; tel. 541/573–7281; David L. Harman, Administrator

LAKE DISTRICT HOSPITAL, 700 South J Street, Lakeview, OR, Zip 97630–1679; tel. 541/947–2114; Gordon Ensley, Acting Administrator

LEBANON COMMUNITY HOSPITAL, 525 North Santiam Highway, Lebanon, OR, Zip 97355, Mailing Address: P.O. Box 739, Zip 97355–0739; tel. 541/258–2101; Steven W. Jasperson, Executive Vice President Operations

MCKENZIE–WILLAMETTE HOSPITAL, 1460 G Street, Springfield, OR, Zip 97477–4197; tel. 541/726–4400; Roy J. Orr, President and Chief Executive Officer

MOUNTAIN VIEW HOSPITAL DISTRICT, 470 N.E. A Street, Madras, OR, Zip 97741; tel. 541/475–3882; Susan McGough, Administrator

OCEAN BEACH HOSPITAL, First and Fir, Ilwaco, WA, Zip 98624, Mailing Address: P.O. Drawer H, Zip 98624; tel. 360/642–3181; Pamela Ott, R.N., Chief Executive Officer

PEACE HARBOR HOSPITAL, 400 Ninth Street, Florence, OR, Zip 97439, Mailing Address: P.O. Box 580, Zip 97439; tel. 541/997–8412; James Barnhart, Chief Executive Officer

PIONEER MEMORIAL HOSPITAL, 1201 N.E. Elm Street, Prineville, OR, Zip 97754; tel. 541/447–6254; Donald J. Wee, Executive Director

PROVIDENCE HOOD RIVER MEMORIAL HOSPITAL, 13th and May Streets, Hood River, OR, Zip 97031, Mailing Address: P.O. Box 149, Zip 97031; tel. 541/386-3911; Larry Bowe, JD, Chief Executive Officer

PROVIDENCE MEDFORD MEDICAL CENTER, 1111 Crater Lake Avenue, Medford, OR, Zip 97504-6241; tel. 541/732-5000; Charles T. Wright, Chief Executive, Southern Oregon Service Area

PROVIDENCE MILWAUKIE HOSPITAL, 10150 S.E. 32nd Avenue, Milwaukie, OR, Zip 97222-6593; tel. 503/513-8300; Janice Burger, Operations Administrator

PROVIDENCE NEWBERG HOSPITAL, 501 Villa Road, Newberg, OR, Zip 97132; tel. 503/537-1555; Mark W. Meinert, CHE, Chief Executive, Yamhill Service Area

PROVIDENCE PORTLAND MEDICAL CENTER, 4805 N.E. Glisan Street, Portland, OR, Zip 97213-2967; tel. 503/215-1111; David T. Underriner, Operations Administrator

PROVIDENCE SEASIDE HOSPITAL, 725 South Wahanna Road, Seaside, OR, Zip 97138-7735; tel. 503/717-7000; Gail Harper, R.N., Chief Executive

PROVIDENCE ST. VINCENT MEDICAL CENTER, 9205 S.W. Barnes Road, Portland, OR, Zip 97225-6661; tel. 503/216-1234; Donald Elsom, Operations Administrator

SACRED HEART MEDICAL CENTER, 1255 Hilyard Street, Eugene, OR, Zip 97401, Mailing Address: P.O. Box 10905, Zip 97440; tel. 541/686-7300; Judy Hodgson, Administrator

SALEM HOSPITAL, 665 Winter Street S.E., Salem, OR, Zip 97301-3959, Mailing Address: Box 14001, Zip 97309-5014; tel. 503/370-5200; Dennis Noonan, President and Chief Executive Officer

SANTIAM MEMORIAL HOSPITAL, 1401 North 10th Avenue, Stayton, OR, Zip 97383; tel. 503/769-2175; Terry L. Fletchall, Administrator

SILVERTON HOSPITAL, 342 Fairview Street, Silverton, OR, Zip 97381; tel. 503/873-1500; William E. Winter, Administrative Director

SOUTHWEST WASHINGTON MEDICAL CENTER, 400 N.E. Mother Joseph Place, Vancouver, WA, Zip 98664, Mailing Address: P.O. Box 1600, Zip 98668; tel. 360/256-2000; Geoffrey N. Lang, President and Chief Executive Officer

ST. CHARLES MEDICAL CENTER, 2500 N.E. Neff Road, Bend, OR, Zip 97701-6015; tel. 541/382-4321; James T. Lussier, President and Chief Executive Officer

ST. JOHN MEDICAL CENTER, 1615 Delaware Street, Longview, WA, Zip 98632, Mailing Address: P.O. Box 3002, Zip 98632-0302; tel. 360/414-2000; Mark E. McGourty, Regional Chief Executive Officer

THREE RIVERS COMMUNITY HOSPITAL AND HEALTH CENTER, 715 N.W. Dimmick Street, Grants Pass, OR, Zip 97526-1596; tel. 541/476-6831; Paul Janke, Senior Vice President

TUALITY HEALTHCARE, 335 S.E. Eighth Avenue, Hillsboro, OR, Zip 97123; tel. 503/681-1111; Richard Stenson, President and Chief Executive Officer

VALLEY COMMUNITY HOSPITAL, 550 S.E. Clay Street, Dallas, OR, Zip 97338, Mailing Address: P.O. Box 378, Zip 97338; tel. 503/623-8301; Kim Flitcroft, President

WILLAMETTE FALLS HOSPITAL, 1500 Division Street, Oregon City, OR, Zip 97045-1597; tel. 503/656-1631; Robert A. Steed, President

WILLAMETTE VALLEY MEDICAL CENTER, 2700 Three Mile Lane, McMinnville, OR, Zip 97128-6498; tel. 503/472-6131; Rosemari Davis, Chief Executive Officer

PENNSYLVANIA

ALBERT EINSTEIN HEALTH CARE NETWORK
5500 Old York Road, Philadelphia, PA 19141; tel. 215/456-7890; Martin Goldsmith, Chief Executive Officer

ALBERT EINSTEIN MEDICAL CENTER, 5501 Old York Road, Philadelphia, PA, Zip 19141-3098; tel. 215/456-7890; Martin Goldsmith, President

BELMONT CENTER FOR COMPREHENSIVE TREATMENT, 4200 Monument Road, Philadelphia, PA, Zip 19131-1625; tel. 215/877-2000; Jack H. Dembow, General Director and Vice President

CATHOLIC HEALTH EAST
14 Campus Blvd., Suite 300, Newtown Square, PA 19073; tel. 610/355-2000; Sal Foti, V.P. Communications

BAYFRONT MEDICAL CENTER, 701 Sixth Street South, Saint Petersburg, FL, Zip 33701-4891; tel. 727/823-1234; Sue G. Brody, President and Chief Executive Officer

GIRARD MEDICAL CENTER, Girard Avenue at Eighth Street, Philadelphia, PA, Zip 19122; tel. 215/787-2000

GOOD SAMARITAN MEDICAL CENTER, Flagler Drive at Palm Beach Lakes Boulevard, West Palm Beach, FL, Zip 33401-3499; tel. 561/655-5511; Steven R. Nathan, President and Chief Executive Officer

HOLY CROSS HOSPITAL, 4725 North Federal Highway, Fort Lauderdale, FL, Zip 33308-4668, Mailing Address: P.O. Box 23460, Zip 33307-3460; tel. 954/771-8000; John C. Johnson, Chief Executive Officer

KENMORE MERCY HOSPITAL, 2950 Elmwood Avenue, Kenmore, NY, Zip 14217-1390; tel. 716/447-6100; Sister Mary Joel Schimscheiner, Chief Executive Officer

MEASE HOSPITAL DUNEDIN, 601 Main Street, Dunedin, FL, Zip 34698-5891, Mailing Address: P.O. Box 760, Zip 34697-0760; tel. 727/733-1111; James A. Pfeiffer, Chief Operating Officer

MERCY COMMUNITY HOSPITAL, 2000 Old West Chester Pike, Havertown, PA, Zip 19083-2712; tel. 610/853-7000; Mary C. Morrison, R.N., Chief Executive Officer

MERCY HOSPITAL, 271 Carew Street, Springfield, MA, Zip 01104-2398, Mailing Address: P.O. Box 9012, Zip 01102-9012; tel. 413/748-9000; Vincent J. McCorkle, President

MERCY HOSPITAL, 3663 South Miami Avenue, Miami, FL, Zip 33133-4237; tel. 305/854-4400; Edward J. Rosasco, Jr, President and Chief Executive Officer

MERCY HOSPITAL OF PORTLAND, 144 State Street, Portland, ME, Zip 04101-3795; tel. 207/879-3000; Howard R. Buckley, President

MERCY MEDICAL, 101 Villa Drive, Daphne, AL, Zip 36526-4653, Mailing Address: P.O. Box 1090, Zip 36526-1090; tel. 334/626-2694; Sister Mary Eileen Wilhelm, President and Chief Executive Officer

MERCY PROVIDENCE HOSPITAL, 1004 Arch Street, Pittsburgh, PA, Zip 15212-5235; tel. 412/323-5600; Gregg G. Zoller, FACHE, President and Chief Executive Officer

MERCY SUBURBAN HOSPITAL, 2701 DeKalb Pike, Norristown, PA, Zip 19401-1820; tel. 610/278-2000; Edward R. Solvibile, Chief Executive Officer

OUR LADY OF LOURDES MEDICAL CENTER, 1600 Haddon Avenue, Camden, NJ, Zip 08103-3117; tel. 856/757-3500; Alexander J. Hatala, President and Chief Executive Officer

OUR LADY OF VICTORY HOSPITAL, 55 Melroy Road, Lackawanna, NY, Zip 14218-1687; tel. 716/825-8000; John P. Davanzo, President and Chief Executive Officer

RANCOCAS HOSPITAL, 218-A Sunset Road, Willingboro, NJ, Zip 08046-1162; tel. 609/835-2900; Joseph Flamini, Chief Executive Officer

SAINT JOSEPH'S HOSPITAL OF ATLANTA, 5665 Peachtree Dunwoody Road N.E., Atlanta, GA, Zip 30342-1764; tel. 404/851-7001; Brue Chandler, President and Chief Executive Officer

SISTERS OF CHARITY HOSPITAL OF BUFFALO, 2157 Main Street, Buffalo, NY, Zip 14214-2692; tel. 716/862-1000; Patrick J. Wiles, President and Chief Executive Officer

SOUTH FLORIDA BAPTIST HOSPITAL, 301 North Alexander Street, Plant City, FL, Zip 33566-9058, Mailing Address: Drawer H, Zip 33564-9058; tel. 813/757-1200; William G. Ulbricht, Chief Operating Officer

ST. ANTHONY'S HOSPITAL, 1200 Seventh Avenue North, Saint Petersburg, FL, Zip 33705-1388, Mailing Address: P.O. Box 12588, Zip 33733-2588; tel. 727/825-1100; Sue G. Brody, President and Chief Executive Officer

ST. JAMES MERCY HOSPITAL, 411 Canisteo Street, Hornell, NY, Zip 14843-2197; tel. 607/324-8000; William G. Connors, President and Chief Executive Officer

ST. JOSEPH HOSPITAL, 2605 Harlem Road, Cheektowaga, NY, Zip 14225-4097; tel. 716/891-2400; Patrick J. Wiles, President and Chief Executive Officer

ST. JOSEPH'S HOSPITAL, 3001 West Martin Luther King Jr. Boulevard, Tampa, FL, Zip 33607-6387, Mailing Address: P.O. Box 4227, Zip 33677-4227; tel. 813/870-4000; Isaac Mallah, President and Chief Executive Officer

ST. MARY'S HEALTH CARE SYSTEM, 1230 Baxter Street, Athens, GA, Zip 30606-3791; tel. 706/548-7581; Thomas E. Fitz, Jr, FACHE, President and Chief Executive Officer

ST. MARY'S HOSPITAL, 901 45th Street, West Palm Beach, FL, Zip 33407-2495, Mailing Address: P.O. Box 24620, Zip 33416-4620; tel. 561/844-6300; Steven R. Nathan, President and Chief Executive Officer

ST. PETER'S HOSPITAL, 315 South Manning Boulevard, Albany, NY, Zip 12208-1789; tel. 518/525-1550; Steven P. Boyle, President and Chief Executive Officer

COVENANT HOME HEALTH CARE
Fourth & Chew Streets, Allentown, PA 18102; tel. 610/776-4500; Joseph M. Cimerola, FACHE

CROZER-KEYSTONE HEALTH SYSTEM
Healthplex Pavilion II, 100 West Sproul Road, Springfield, PA 19064; tel. 610/338-8203; John C. McMeekin, President & Chief Executive Officer

CROZER-CHESTER MEDICAL CENTER, One Medical Center Boulevard, Upland, PA, Zip 19013-3995; tel. 610/447-2000; Joan K. Richards, President

DELAWARE COUNTY MEMORIAL HOSPITAL, 501 North Lansdowne Avenue, Drexel Hill, PA, Zip 19026-1114; tel. 610/284-8100; Joan K. Richards, President

FOX CHASE NETWORK
8 Huntingdon Pike, 3rd, Rockledge, PA 19046; tel. 215/728-4773; Susan Higman, Vice President

DELAWARE COUNTY MEMORIAL HOSPITAL, 501 North Lansdowne Avenue, Drexel Hill, PA, Zip 19026-1114; tel. 610/284-8100; Joan K. Richards, President

FOX CHASE CANCER CENTER-AMERICAN ONCOLOGIC HOSPITAL, 7701 Burholme Avenue, Philadelphia, PA, Zip 19111-2412; tel. 215/728-6900; Robert C. Young, M.D., President

HUNTERDON MEDICAL CENTER, 2100 Wescott Drive, Flemington, NJ, Zip 08822-4604; tel. 908/788-6100; Robert P. Wise, President and Chief Executive Officer

NORTH PENN HOSPITAL, 100 Medical Campus Drive, Lansdale, PA, Zip 19446-1200; tel. 215/368-2100; Robert H. McKay, President

PAOLI MEMORIAL HOSPITAL, 255 West Lancaster Avenue, Paoli, PA, Zip 19301-1792; tel. 610/648-1000; Barbara Tachovsky, Senior Vice President

PINNACLEHEALTH SYSTEM, 17 South Market Square, Harrisburg, PA, Zip 17101-2003, Mailing Address: P.O. Box 8700, Zip 17105-8700; tel. 717/782-5678; John S. Cramer, FACHE, President and Chief Executive Officer

READING HOSPITAL AND MEDICAL CENTER, Sixth Avenue and Spruce Street, Reading, PA, Zip 19611-1428, Mailing Address: P.O. Box 16052, Zip 19612-6052; tel. 610/988-8000; Charles Sullivan, President and Chief Executive Officer

Networks / Fox Chase Network

ST. FRANCIS MEDICAL CENTER, 601 Hamilton Avenue, Trenton, NJ, Zip 08629–1986; tel. 609/599–5000; Judith M. Persichilli, President and Chief Executive Officer

ST. MARY MEDICAL CENTER, Langhorne–Newtown Road, Langhorne, PA, Zip 19047–1295; tel. 215/750–2000; Gregory T. Wozniak, President and Chief Executive Officer

GREAT LAKES HEALTH NETWORK
201 State Street, Erie, PA 16550; tel. 814/877–7053; Andrew J. Glass, President

ASHTABULA COUNTY MEDICAL CENTER, 2420 Lake Avenue, Ashtabula, OH, Zip 44004–4993; tel. 440/997–2262; R. D. Richardson, President and Chief Executive Officer

BLANCHARD VALLEY HEALTH ASSOCIATION SYSTEM, 145 West Wallace Street, Findlay, OH, Zip 45840–1299; tel. 419/423–4500; William E. Ruse, FACHE, President and Chief Executive Officer

BRADFORD REGIONAL MEDICAL CENTER, 116 Interstate Parkway, Bradford, PA, Zip 16701–0218; tel. 814/368–4143; George E. Leonhardt, President and Chief Executive Officer

CORRY MEMORIAL HOSPITAL, 612 West Smith Street, Corry, PA, Zip 16407–1152; tel. 814/664–4641; Barbara Nichols, Acting President

ELK REGIONAL HEALTH CENTER, 763 Johnsonburg Road, Saint Marys, PA, Zip 15857–3417; tel. 814/781–7500; Paul A. DeSantis, President

HAMOT MEDICAL CENTER, 201 State Street, Erie, PA, Zip 16550–0002; tel. 814/877–6000; John T. Malone, President and Chief Executive Officer

UHHS BROWN MEMORIAL HOSPITAL, 158 West Main Road, Conneaut, OH, Zip 44030–2039, Mailing Address: P.O. Box 648, Zip 44030–0648; tel. 440/593–1131; William P. Lawrence, Chief Executive Officer

WOMAN'S CHRISTIAN ASSOCIATION HOSPITAL, 207 Foote Avenue, Jamestown, NY, Zip 14702–9975, Mailing Address: P.O. Box 840, Zip 14702–0840; tel. 716/487–0141; Betsy T. Wright, President and Chief Executive Officer

JEFFERSON HEALTH SYSTEM
259 Radnor Chester Road, Radnor, PA 190875288; tel. 610/225–6200; Douglas S. Peters, President & Chief Executive Officer

ALBERT EINSTEIN MEDICAL CENTER, 5501 Old York Road, Philadelphia, PA, Zip 19141–3098; tel. 215/456–7890; Martin Goldsmith, President

ALFRED I. DUPONT HOSPITAL FOR CHILDREN, 1600 Rockland Road, Wilmington, DE, Zip 19803–3616, Mailing Address: Box 269, Zip 19899–0269; tel. 302/651–4000; Thomas P. Ferry, Administrator and Chief Executive

BRYN MAWR HOSPITAL, 130 South Bryn Mawr Avenue, Bryn Mawr, PA, Zip 19010–3160; tel. 610/526–3000; Andrea F. Gilbert, Senior Vice President

BRYN MAWR REHABILITATION HOSPITAL, 414 Paoli Pike, Malvern, PA, Zip 19355–3300, Mailing Address: P.O. Box 3007, Zip 19355–3300; tel. 610/251–5400; Patricia Ryan, Senior Vice President

FRANKFORD HOSPITAL OF THE CITY OF PHILADELPHIA, Knights and Red Lion Roads, Philadelphia, PA, Zip 19114–1486; tel. 215/612–4000; Roy A. Powell, President

GERMANTOWN HOSPITAL AND COMMUNITY HEALTH SERVICES, One Penn Boulevard, Philadelphia, PA, Zip 19144–1498; tel. 215/951–8000; Cynthia McGlone, Chief Operating Officer

LANKENAU HOSPITAL, 100 Lancaster Avenue West, Wynnewood, PA, Zip 19096–3411; tel. 610/645–2000; C. Barry Dykes, Senior Vice President

PAOLI MEMORIAL HOSPITAL, 255 West Lancaster Avenue, Paoli, PA, Zip 19301–1792; tel. 610/648–1000; Barbara Tachovsky, Senior Vice President

POTTSTOWN MEMORIAL MEDICAL CENTER, 1600 East High Street, Pottstown, PA, Zip 19464–5008; tel. 610/327–7000; John J. Buckley, President and Chief Executive Officer

THOMAS JEFFERSON UNIVERSITY HOSPITAL, 111 South 11th Street, Philadelphia, PA, Zip 19107–5096; tel. 215/955–7022; Thomas J. Lewis, President and Chief Executive Officer

UNDERWOOD–MEMORIAL HOSPITAL, 509 North Broad Street, Woodbury, NJ, Zip 08096–1697, Mailing Address: P.O. Box 359, Zip 08096–7359; tel. 856/845–0100; Steven W. Jackmuff, President and Chief Executive Officer

WILLS EYE HOSPITAL, 900 Walnut Street, Philadelphia, PA, Zip 19107–5598; tel. 215/928–3000; D. McWilliams Kessler, Executive Director and Chief Executive Officer

LAUREL HEALTH SYSTEM
15 Meade St., Suite U–6, Wellsboro, PA 16901; tel. 570/723–0500; Ron Butler, President & Chief Executive Officer

SOLDIERS AND SAILORS MEMORIAL HOSPITAL, 32–36 Central Avenue, Wellsboro, PA, Zip 16901–1899; tel. 570/724–1631; Jan E. Fisher, R.N., Executive Director

PARTNERSHIP for COMMUNITY HEALTH–LEHIGH VALLEY
P.O. Box 689, Allentown, PA 18105; tel. 610/954–8964; Leo Conners, Chairman

SACRED HEART HOSPITAL, 421 Chew Street, Allentown, PA, Zip 18102–3490; tel. 610/776–4500; Joseph M. Cimerola, FACHE, President and Chief Executive Officer

PARTNERSHIP FOR HEALTHY COMMUNITIES
P.O. Box 447, DuBois, PA 158010447; tel. 814/375–3495; Diane Blasdell, Pub Relations Mgr

DUBOIS REGIONAL MEDICAL CENTER, 100 Hospital Avenue, Du Bois, PA, Zip 15801–1440, Mailing Address: P.O. Box 447, Zip 15801–0447; tel. 814/371–2200; Raymond A. Graeca, President and Chief Executive Officer

PENN STATE GEISINGER HEALTH CARE SYSTEM
2601 Marketplace Commerce Ct Suite 300, Harrisburg, PA 17110; tel. 570/214–2254; Pat Thompson, CIO

GEISINGER MEDICAL CENTER, 100 North Academy Avenue, Danville, PA, Zip 17822–0150; tel. 570/271–6211; Nancy L. Rizzo, Senior Vice President, Operations

PENN STATE GEISINGER WYOMING VALLEY MEDICAL CENTER, 1000 East Mountain Drive, Wilkes–Barre, PA, Zip 18711–0027; tel. 570/826–7300; Conrad W. Schintz, Senior Vice–President Operations

PRIME CARE
2601 North 3rd Street, Harrisburg, PA 17110; tel. 717/230–3434; Alan Davidson, President

PROVIDENCE HEALTH SYSTEM FOUNDATION
1100 Grampian Boulevard, Williamsport, PA 17701; tel. 717/326–8181; Sister Jean Mohl, President

MUNCY VALLEY HOSPITAL, 215 East Water Street, Muncy, PA, Zip 17756–8700; tel. 570/546–8282

SUSQUEHANNA HEALTH SYSTEM, 1001 Grampian Boulevard, Williamsport, PA, Zip 17701–1946; tel. 570/320–7000; Donald R. Creamer, President and Chief Executive Officer

THOMAS JEFFERSON UNIVERSITY HOSPITAL, 111 South 11th Street, Philadelphia, PA, Zip 19107–5096; tel. 215/955–7022; Thomas J. Lewis, President and Chief Executive Officer

SAINT VINCENT HEALTH SYSTEM
232 West 25th Street, Erie, PA 16544; tel. 814/452–5000; Karen Surkala, Planning Associate

SAINT VINCENT HEALTH CENTER, 232 West 25th Street, Erie, PA, Zip 16544–0001; tel. 814/452–5000; Sister Catherine Manning, President and Chief Executive Officer

UNION CITY MEMORIAL HOSPITAL, 130 North Main Street, Union City, PA, Zip 16438–1094, Mailing Address: P.O. Box 111, Zip 16438–0111; tel. 814/438–1000; Thomas McLoughlin, President and Chief Executive Officer

WESTFIELD MEMORIAL HOSPITAL, 189 East Main Street, Westfield, NY, Zip 14787–1195; tel. 716/326–4921; Mary E. LaRowe, President and Chief Executive Officer

ST FRANCIS HEALTH SYSTEM
4401 Penn Avenue, Pittsburgh, PA 15224; tel. 412/622–4214; Sister M. Rosita Wellinger, President & Chief Executive Officer

ST. FRANCIS CENTRAL HOSPITAL, 1200 Centre Avenue, Pittsburgh, PA, Zip 15219–3507; tel. 412/562–3000; Robin Z. Mohr, Chief Executive Officer

ST. FRANCIS HOSPITAL OF NEW CASTLE, 1000 South Mercer Street, New Castle, PA, Zip 16101–4673; tel. 724/658–3511; Sister Patricia Fogle, Chief Executive Officer

UNIVERSITY OF PENNSYLVANIA
21 Penn Tower, 399 S. 34th Street, Philadelphia, PA 19104; tel. 215/898–5181; William N. Kelley, M.D., Chief Executive Officer

HOSPITAL OF THE UNIVERSITY OF PENNSYLVANIA, 3400 Spruce Street, Philadelphia, PA, Zip 19104–4385; tel. 215/662–4000; Peter G. Traber, M.D., Chief Executive Officer and Dean

PRESBYTERIAN MEDICAL CENTER OF THE UNIVERSITY OF PENNSYLVANIA HEALTH SYSTEM, 51 North 39th Street, Philadelphia, PA, Zip 19104–2640; tel. 215/662–8000; Michele M. Volpe, Executive Director

UNIVERSITY OF PITTSBURGH MEDICAL CENTER
3811 O'Hara Street, Pittsburgh, PA 15213; tel. 412/647–3000; Jeffrey Romoff, President

CHILDREN'S HOSPITAL OF PITTSBURGH, 3705 Fifth Avenue at De Soto Street, Pittsburgh, PA, Zip 15213–2583; tel. 412/692–5325; Ronald L. Violi, President and Chief Executive Officer

MAGEE–WOMENS HOSPITAL, 300 Halket Street, Pittsburgh, PA, Zip 15213–3180; tel. 412/641–1000; Irma E. Goertzen, President and Chief Executive Officer

UPMC PRESBYTERIAN, Pittsburgh, PA, Henry A. Mordoh, President

UPMC ST. MARGARET, 815 Freeport Road, Pittsburgh, PA, Zip 15215–3301; tel. 412/784–4000; Richard E. Sobehart, President

WASHINGTON HOSPITAL, 155 Wilson Avenue, Washington, PA, Zip 15301–3398; tel. 724/225–7000; Telford W. Thomas, President and Chief Executive Officer

VANTAGE HEALTH CARE
265 Conneaut Lake Road, Meadville, PA 16335; tel. 814/337–0000; Gerald P. Alonge, Executive Director

MEADVILLE MEDICAL CENTER, 751 Liberty Street, Meadville, PA, Zip 16335–2555; tel. 814/333–5000; Anthony J. DeFail, President and Chief Executive Officer

MILLCREEK COMMUNITY HOSPITAL, 5515 Peach Street, Erie, PA, Zip 16509–2695; tel. 814/864–4031; Mary L. Eckert, President and Chief Executive Officer

NORTHWEST MEDICAL CENTERS, 174 Bissell Avenue, Oil City, PA, Zip 16301–0568; tel. 814/437–7000; Neil E. Todhunter, Chief Executive Officer

SAINT VINCENT HEALTH CENTER, 232 West 25th Street, Erie, PA, Zip 16544–0001; tel. 814/452–5000; Sister Catherine Manning, President and Chief Executive Officer

TITUSVILLE AREA HOSPITAL, 406 West Oak Street, Titusville, PA, Zip 16354–1404; tel. 814/827–1851; Anthony J. Nasralla, FACHE, President and Chief Executive Officer

UPMC HORIZON, Greenville, PA, J. Larry Heinike, President and Chief Executive Officer

WARREN GENERAL HOSPITAL, 2 Crescent Park West, Warren, PA, Zip 16365–2111, Mailing Address: P.O. Box 68, Zip 16365–2111; tel. 814/723–4973; Alton M. Schadt, Executive Director

RHODE ISLAND

CARE NEW ENGLAND HEALTH
45 Willard Avenue, Providence, RI 02905; tel. 401/453–7900; John J. Hynes, Esq., President & Chief Executive

BUTLER HOSPITAL, 345 Blackstone Boulevard, Providence, RI, Zip 02906–4829; tel. 401/455–6200; Patricia R. Recupero, JD, M.D., President and Chief Executive Officer

KENT COUNTY MEMORIAL HOSPITAL, 455 Tollgate Road, Warwick, RI, Zip 02886–2770; tel. 401/737–7000; Robert E. Baute, M.D., President and Chief Executive Officer

WOMEN AND INFANTS HOSPITAL OF RHODE ISLAND, 101 Dudley Street, Providence, RI, Zip 02905–2499; tel. 401/274–1100; Thomas G. Parris, Jr, President

LIFESPAN
167 Point Street, Providence, RI 02903; tel. 401/444–3500; George A. Vecchione, President/Chief Executive Officer

EMMA PENDLETON BRADLEY HOSPITAL, 1011 Veterans Memorial Parkway, East Providence, RI, Zip 02915–5099; tel. 401/432–1000; Daniel J. Wall, President and Chief Executive Officer

MIRIAM HOSPITAL, 164 Summit Avenue, Providence, RI, Zip 02906–2895; tel. 401/793–2500; Kathleen C. Hittner, M.D., President and Chief Executive Officer

NEW ENGLAND MEDICAL CENTER, 750 Washington Street, Boston, MA, Zip 02111–1845; tel. 617/636–5000; Thomas F. O'Donnell, Jr, M.D., FACS, President and Chief Executive Officer

NEWPORT HOSPITAL, 11 Friendship Street, Newport, RI, Zip 02840–2299; tel. 401/846–6400; Arthur J. Sampson, President and Chief Executive Officer

RHODE ISLAND HOSPITAL, 593 Eddy Street, Providence, RI, Zip 02903–4900; tel. 401/444–4000; Joseph E. Amaral, M.D., President and Chief Executive Officer

ST JOSEPH HOSPITAL
200 High Service Avenue, Providence, RI 02904; tel. 401/456–4419; Kathy Monteith, Coordinator

ST. JOSEPH HEALTH SERVICES OF RHODE ISLAND, 200 High Service Avenue, North Providence, RI, Zip 02904–5199; tel. 401/456–3000; H. John Keimig, President and Chief Executive Officer

SOUTH CAROLINA

BON SECOURS ST FRANCIS HEALTH SYSTEM
One St. Francis Drive, Greenville, SC 29601; tel. 803/255–1015; Rebecca Phillips, Plan Coordinator

ST. FRANCIS HEALTH SYSTEM, One St. Francis Drive, Greenville, SC, Zip 29601–3207; tel. 864/255–1000; Richard C. Neugent, Chief Executive Officer

CAROLINA HEALTHCHOICE NETWORK
1718 Saint Julian Place, Columbia, SC 29204; tel. 803/254–0984; Suzanne H. Catalano, Executive Director

CLARENDON MEMORIAL HOSPITAL, 10 Hospital Street, Manning, SC, Zip 29102, Mailing Address: P.O. Box 550, Zip 29102–0550; tel. 803/435–8463; Edward R. Frye, Jr, Administrator

FAIRFIELD MEMORIAL HOSPITAL, 102 U.S. Highway 321 By–Pass North, Winnsboro, SC, Zip 29180, Mailing Address: P.O. Box 620, Zip 29180–0620; tel. 803/635–5548; J. Larry Dozier, Jr, FACHE, Chief Executive Officer

KERSHAW COUNTY MEDICAL CENTER, Haile and Roberts Streets, Camden, SC, Zip 29020–7003, Mailing Address: P.O. Box 7003, Zip 29020–7003; tel. 803/432–4311; Donnie J. Weeks, President and Chief Executive Officer

NEWBERRY COUNTY MEMORIAL HOSPITAL, 2669 Kinard Street, Newberry, SC, Zip 29108–0497, Mailing Address: P.O. Box 497, Zip 29108–0497; tel. 803/276–7570; Lynn W. Beasley, President and Chief Executive Officer

REGIONAL MEDICAL CENTER OF ORANGEBURG AND CALHOUN COUNTIES, 3000 St. Matthews Road, Orangeburg, SC, Zip 29118–1470; tel. 803/533–2200; Thomas C. Dandridge, President

TUOMEY HEALTHCARE SYSTEM, 129 North Washington Street, Sumter, SC, Zip 29150–4983; tel. 803/778–9000; Jay Cox, President and Chief Executive Officer

PREMIER HEALTH SYSTEM, INC
Taylor at Marion Streets, Columbia, SC 29220; tel. 803/988–8999; Frank Riley, President/Chief Executive Officer

ABBEVILLE COUNTY MEMORIAL HOSPITAL, 901 West Greenwood Street, Abbeville, SC, Zip 29620–0887, Mailing Address: P.O. Box 887, Zip 29620–0887; tel. 864/459–5011; Alvin Hoover, CHE, Administrator

ALLEN BENNETT HOSPITAL, 313 Memorial Drive, Greer, SC, Zip 29650–1521; tel. 864/848–8200; Michael W. Massey, Administrator

ALLENDALE COUNTY HOSPITAL, Highway 278 West, Fairfax, SC, Zip 29827–0278, Mailing Address: Box 218, Zip 29827–0218; tel. 803/632–3311; M. K. Hiatt, Administrator

BAMBERG COUNTY MEMORIAL HOSPITAL AND NURSING CENTER, North and McGee Streets, Bamberg, SC, Zip 29003–0507, Mailing Address: P.O. Box 507, Zip 29003–0507; tel. 803/245–4321; Warren E. Hammett, Administrator

BARNWELL COUNTY HOSPITAL, 811 Reynolds Road, Barnwell, SC, Zip 29812; tel. 803/259–1000; J. Larry Dozier, Jr, FACHE, Chief Executive Officer

BON SECOURS–ST. FRANCIS XAVIER HOSPITAL, 2095 Henry Tecklenburg Drive, Charleston, SC, Zip 29414–0001, Mailing Address: P.O. Box 160001, Zip 29414–0001; tel. 843/402–1000; Allen P. Carroll, Chief Executive Officer

CANNON MEMORIAL HOSPITAL, 123 West G. Acker Drive, Pickens, SC, Zip 29671, Mailing Address: P.O. Box 188, Zip 29671–0188; tel. 864/878–4791; Norman G. Rentz, President and Chief Executive Officer

CAROLINAS HOSPITAL SYSTEM–LAKE CITY, 258 North Ron McNair Boulevard, Lake City, SC, Zip 29560–1029, Mailing Address: Box 1029, Zip 29560–1029; tel. 843/394–2036; Clarence W. Bowman, Chief Executive Officer

CHESTER COUNTY HOSPITAL AND NURSING CENTER, 1 Medical Park Drive, Chester, SC, Zip 29706–9799; tel. 803/581–9400; William H. Bundy, Chief Executive Officer

CHESTERFIELD GENERAL HOSPITAL, Highway 9 West, Cheraw, SC, Zip 29520, Mailing Address: P.O. Box 151, Zip 29520–0151; tel. 843/537–7881; Chris Wolf, Chief Executive Officer

CLARENDON MEMORIAL HOSPITAL, 10 Hospital Street, Manning, SC, Zip 29102, Mailing Address: P.O. Box 550, Zip 29102–0550; tel. 803/435–8463; Edward R. Frye, Jr, Administrator

EAST COOPER REGIONAL MEDICAL CENTER, 1200 Johnnie Dodds Boulevard, Mount Pleasant, SC, Zip 29464–3294; tel. 843/881–0100; Jack Dusenbery, President

EDGEFIELD COUNTY HOSPITAL, 300 Ridge Medical Plaza, Edgefield, SC, Zip 29824; tel. 803/637–3174; W. Joseph Seel, Administrator

FAIRFIELD MEMORIAL HOSPITAL, 102 U.S. Highway 321 By–Pass North, Winnsboro, SC, Zip 29180, Mailing Address: P.O. Box 620, Zip 29180–0620; tel. 803/635–5548; J. Larry Dozier, Jr, FACHE, Chief Executive Officer

GEORGETOWN MEMORIAL HOSPITAL, 606 Black River Road, Georgetown, SC, Zip 29440–3368, Mailing Address: Drawer 1718, Zip 29442–1718; tel. 843/527–7000; Paul D. Gatens, Sr, Administrator

GREENVILLE MEMORIAL HOSPITAL, 701 Grove Road, Greenville, SC, Zip 29605–4295; tel. 864/455–7000; J. Bland Burkhardt, Jr, Senior Vice President and Administrator

HEALTHSOUTH REHABILITATION HOSPITAL, 2935 Colonial Drive, Columbia, SC, Zip 29203–6811; tel. 803/254–7777; Debbie W. Johnston, Director Operations

HILLCREST HOSPITAL, 729 S.E. Main Street, Simpsonville, SC, Zip 29681–3280; tel. 864/967–6100; Mark Slyter, Administrator

HILTON HEAD MEDICAL CENTER AND CLINICS, 25 Hospital Center Boulevard, Hilton Head Island, SC, Zip 29926, Mailing Address: P.O. Box 21117, Zip 29925–1117; tel. 843/681–6122; Dennis Ray Bruns, President and Chief Executive Officer

KERSHAW COUNTY MEDICAL CENTER, Haile and Roberts Streets, Camden, SC, Zip 29020–7003, Mailing Address: P.O. Box 7003, Zip 29020–7003; tel. 803/432–4311; Donnie J. Weeks, President and Chief Executive Officer

LAURENS COUNTY HEALTHCARE SYSTEM, Highway 76 West, Clinton, SC, Zip 29325, Mailing Address: P.O. Box 976, Zip 29325–0976; tel. 864/833–9100; Michael A. Kozar, Chief Executive Officer

LEXINGTON MEDICAL CENTER, 2720 Sunset Boulevard, West Columbia, SC, Zip 29169–4816; tel. 803/791–2000; Michael J. Biediger, President

MARLBORO PARK HOSPITAL, 1138 Cheraw Highway, Bennettsville, SC, Zip 29512–0738, Mailing Address: P.O. Box 738, Zip 29512–0738; tel. 843/479–2881; William M. Donohoo, FACHE, Chief Executive Officer

MARY BLACK HEALTH SYSTEM, 1700 Skylyn Drive, Spartanburg, SC, Zip 29307–1061, Mailing Address: P.O. Box 3217, Zip 29304–3217; tel. 864/573–3000; William W. Fox, Chief Executive Officer

NEWBERRY COUNTY MEMORIAL HOSPITAL, 2669 Kinard Street, Newberry, SC, Zip 29108–0497, Mailing Address: P.O. Box 497, Zip 29108–0497; tel. 803/276–7570; Lynn W. Beasley, President and Chief Executive Officer

PALMETTO BAPTIST MEDICAL CENTER EASLEY, 200 Fleetwood Drive, Easley, SC, Zip 29640–2076, Mailing Address: P.O. Box 2129, Zip 29641–2129; tel. 864/855–7200; Roddey E. Gettys, II, Executive Vice President

PALMETTO BAPTIST MEDICAL CENTER/COLUMBIA, Taylor at Marion Streets, Columbia, SC, Zip 29220; tel. 803/296–5010; James M. Bridges, Executive Vice President and Chief Operating Officer

PROVIDENCE HOSPITAL, 2435 Forest Drive, Columbia, SC, Zip 29204–2098; tel. 803/256–5300; Stephen A. Purves, CHE, President and Chief Executive Officer

ROPER HOSPITAL, 316 Calhoun Street, Charleston, SC, Zip 29401–1125; tel. 843/724–2000; Matt Severance, Administrator

SELF MEMORIAL HOSPITAL, 1325 Spring Street, Greenwood, SC, Zip 29646–3860; tel. 864/227–4111; M. John Heydel, President and Chief Executive Officer

ST. JOSEPH'S CANDLER HEALTH SYSTEM, 11705 Mercy Boulevard, Savannah, GA, Zip 31419–1791; tel. 912/925–4100; Paul P. Hinchey, President and Chief Executive Officer

UPSTATE CAROLINA MEDICAL CENTER, 1530 North Limestone Street, Gaffney, SC, Zip 29340–4738; tel. 864/487–4271; Joe D. Howell, Executive Director

WILLINGWAY HOSPITAL, 311 Jones Mill Road, Statesboro, GA, Zip 30458–4765; tel. 912/764–6236; Jimmy Mooney, Chief Executive Officer

RICHLAND COMMUNITY HEALTH PARTNERS
3 Medical Park, Suite 100, Columbia, SC 29203; tel. 803/434–3100; Tom Brown, Director

PALMETTO RICHLAND MEMORIAL HOSPITAL, Five Richland Medical Park Drive, Columbia, SC, Zip 29203, Mailing Address: P.O. Box 2266, Zip 29203–2266; tel. 803/434–7000; B. Daniel Paysinger, M.D., Chief Operating Officer

Networks / Richland Community Health Partners

SOUTH DAKOTA

BLACK HILLS HEALTHCARE
930 10th Street, Spearfish, SD 57783;
tel. 605/642-4641; MaLinda Birkeland,
Coordinator of Marketing Communications

LOOKOUT MEMORIAL HOSPITAL, 1440 North Main Street, Spearfish, SD, Zip 57783-1504; tel. 605/642-2617; Deb J. Krmpotic, R.N., Administrator

STURGIS COMMUNITY HEALTH CARE CENTER, 949 Harmon Street, Sturgis, SD, Zip 57785-2452; tel. 605/347-2536; Roger R. Heidt, Administrator

RAPID CITY REGIONAL HOSPITAL SYSTEM OF CARE
P.O. Box 6000, Rapid City, SD 57709;
tel. 605/341-1000; Carol Helfenstein,
Director of Public Relations/Marketing

CUSTER COMMUNITY HOSPITAL, 1039 Montgomery Street, Custer, SD, Zip 57730-1397; tel. 605/673-2229; Jason Petik, Administrator

FIVE COUNTIES HOSPITAL, 405 Sixth Avenue West, Lemmon, SD, Zip 57638-1318, Mailing Address: P.O. Box 479, Zip 57638-0479; tel. 605/374-3871; James Haeder, Interim Administrator

NORTHERN HILLS GENERAL HOSPITAL, 61 Charles Street, Deadwood, SD, Zip 57732-1303; tel. 605/578-2313; Jack Brinkers, CHE, Interim Chief Executive Officer

RAPID CITY REGIONAL HOSPITAL SYSTEM OF CARE, 353 Fairmont Boulevard, Rapid City, SD, Zip 57701-7393, Mailing Address: P.O. Box 6000, Zip 57709-6000; tel. 605/341-1000; Adil M. Ameer, President and Chief Executive Officer

WESTON COUNTY HEALTH SERVICES, 1124 Washington Street, Newcastle, WY, Zip 82701-2996; tel. 307/746-4491; Greg Nielsen, Administrator

TENNESSEE

CHATTANOOGA HEALTHCARE NETWORK
401 Chestnut Street, Suite 222, Chattanooga, TN 37402; tel. 615/266-5174; Judy Clay, Network Contact

ATHENS REGIONAL MEDICAL CENTER, 1114 West Madison Avenue, Athens, TN, Zip 37303-4150, Mailing Address: P.O. Box 250, Zip 37371-0250; tel. 423/745-1411; John R. Workman, Chief Executive Officer

GRANDVIEW MEDICAL CENTER, 1000 Highway 28, Jasper, TN, Zip 37347; tel. 423/837-9500; Phil Rowland, Chief Executive Officer

COVENANT HEALTH
100 Fort Sanders West Boulevard, Knoxville, TN 37922; tel. 423/531-5555; Max Shell, Senior Vice President, Marketing & Planning

CARTHAGE GENERAL HOSPITAL, 130 Lebanon Highway, Carthage, TN, Zip 37030-2955, Mailing Address: P.O. Box 319, Zip 37030-0319; tel. 615/735-9815; Scott Tongate, Chief Administrative Officer

FORT SANDERS LOUDON MEDICAL CENTER, 1125 Grove Street, Loudon, TN, Zip 37774-1512, Mailing Address: P.O. Box 217, Zip 37774-0217; tel. 865/458-8222; Martha O'Regan Chill, Administrator

FORT SANDERS REGIONAL MEDICAL CENTER, 1901 Clinch Avenue S.W., Knoxville, TN, Zip 37916-2394; tel. 423/541-1111; Richard Rose, M.D., President and Chief Administrative Officer

FORT SANDERS–PARKWEST MEDICAL CENTER, 9352 Park West Boulevard, Knoxville, TN, Zip 37923-4387, Mailing Address: P.O. Box 22993, Zip 37933-0993; tel. 865/693-5151; Wayne S. Heatherly, President and Chief Administrative Officer

FORT SANDERS–SEVIER MEDICAL CENTER, 709 Middle Creek Road, Sevierville, TN, Zip 37862-5016, Mailing Address: P.O. Box 8005, Zip 37864-8005; tel. 865/429-6100; Ellen Wilhoit, President and Chief Administrative Officer

METHODIST MEDICAL CENTER OF OAK RIDGE, 990 Oak Ridge Turnpike, Oak Ridge, TN, Zip 37830-6976, Mailing Address: P.O. Box 2529, Zip 37831-2529; tel. 865/481-1000; George A. Mathews, President and Chief Administrative Officer

PENINSULA HOSPITAL, 2347 Jones Bend Road, Louisville, TN, Zip 37777-5213, Mailing Address: P.O. Box 2000, Zip 37777-2000; tel. 423/970-9800; Barbara S. Blevins, President

HIGHLANDS WELLMONT HEALTH
1 Medical Park Boulevard, Bristol, TN 37621; tel. 423/844-4186; Glynn Hughes, Senior Vice President – Integration Strategies

NORTON COMMUNITY HOSPITAL, 100 15th Street N.W., Norton, VA, Zip 24273-1699; tel. 540/679-9600; Ricky D. Napper, Chief Executive Officer

WELLMONT BRISTOL REGIONAL MEDICAL CENTER, 1 Medical Park Boulevard, Bristol, TN, Zip 37620-7434; tel. 423/844-4200; Randall M. Olson, President

WELLMONT HOLSTON VALLEY MEDICAL CENTER, West Ravine Street, Kingsport, TN, Zip 37662-0224, Mailing Address: Box 238, Zip 37662-0224; tel. 423/224-4000; Louis H. Bremer, President and Chief Executive Officer

WELLMONT LONESOME PINE HOSPITAL, 1990 Holton Avenue East, Big Stone Gap, VA, Zip 24219-0230; tel. 540/523-3111; Paul A. Bishop, Administrator

METHODIST MEDICAL CENTER
1211 Union Avenue Suite 700, Memphis, TN 38104; tel. 901/726-8273; Maurice Elliott, President

METHODIST HEALTHCARE – MCKENZIE, 161 Hospital Drive, McKenzie, TN, Zip 38201-1636; tel. 901/352-5344; Richard M. McCormick, Administrator

METHODIST HEALTHCARE– DYERSBURG HOSPITAL, 400 Tickle Street, Dyersburg, TN, Zip 38024-3182; tel. 901/285-2410; R. Coleman Foss, Chief Executive Officer

METHODIST HEALTHCARE–LEXINGTON HOSPITAL, 200 West Church Street, Lexington, TN, Zip 38351-2014; tel. 901/968-3646; Eugene Ragghianti, Administrator

METHODIST HEALTHCARE–MEMPHIS HOSPITAL, 1265 Union Avenue, Memphis, TN, Zip 38104-3499; tel. 901/726-7000; David L. Ramsey, President

METHODIST HEALTHCARE–SOMERVILLE, 214 Lakeview Drive, Somerville, TN, Zip 38068; tel. 901/465-0532; Michael Blome', Administrator

MOUNTAIN STATES HEALTHCARE NETWORK
400 North State of Franklin Road, Johnson City, TN 37604; tel. 615/461-6810; Richard Kramer, President

CHARLES A. CANNON JR, MEMORIAL HOSPITAL, One Crossnore Drive, Crossnore, NC, Zip 28616, Mailing Address: Drawer 470, Zip 28616; tel. 828/737-7000; Edward C. Greene, Jr, President

CLINCH VALLEY MEDICAL CENTER, 2949 West Front Street, Richlands, VA, Zip 24641-2099; tel. 540/596-6000; James W. Thweatt, Chief Executive Officer

JOHNSON CITY MEDICAL CENTER, 400 North State of Franklin Road, Johnson City, TN, Zip 37604-6094; tel. 423/431-6111; Dennis Vonderfecht, President and Chief Executive Officer

JOHNSTON MEMORIAL HOSPITAL, 351 Court Street N.E., Abingdon, VA, Zip 24210-2921; tel. 540/676-7000; Clark R. Beil, Chief Executive Officer

LAKEWAY REGIONAL HOSPITAL, 726 McFarland Street, Morristown, TN, Zip 37814-3990; tel. 423/586-2302; Michael I. Terry, Chief Executive Officer

LEE COUNTY COMMUNITY HOSPITAL, West Morgan Avenue, Pennington Gap, VA, Zip 24277-0070, Mailing Address: P.O. Box 70, Zip 24277-0070; tel. 540/546-1440; Gowdagere Udayakumar, Chief Executive Officer

MORRISTOWN–HAMBLEN HOSPITAL, 908 West Fourth North Street, Morristown, TN, Zip 37816-1178, Mailing Address: P.O. Box 1178, Zip 37816-1178; tel. 423/586-4231; Richard L. Clark, Administrator and Chief Executive Officer

TAKOMA ADVENTIST HOSPITAL, 401 Takoma Avenue, Greeneville, TN, Zip 37743-4647; tel. 423/639-3151; Carlyle L. E. Walton, President

UNICOI COUNTY MEMORIAL HOSPITAL, 100 Greenway Circle, Erwin, TN, Zip 37650-2196, Mailing Address: P.O. Box 802, Zip 37650-0802; tel. 423/743-3141; Jim S. Pate, Acting Chief Executive Officer

WOODRIDGE HOSPITAL, 403 State of Franklin Road, Johnson City, TN, Zip 37604-6009, Mailing Address: P.O. Box 2226, Zip 37604-2226; tel. 423/928-7111; Donald Larkin, Ph.D., Administrator

NASHVILLE HEALTHCARE PARTNERSHIP
161 Fourth Avenue North, Nashville, TN 37219; tel. 615/259-4786; Joanne F. Pulles, Executive Director

ST. THOMAS HEALTH SERVICES, 4220 Harding Road, Nashville, TN, Zip 37205-2095, Mailing Address: P.O. Box 380, Zip 37202-0380; tel. 615/222-2111; Thomas E. Beeman, President and Chief Executive Officer

TENNESSEE CHRISTIAN MEDICAL CENTER, 500 Hospital Drive, Madison, TN, Zip 37115-5032; tel. 615/865-2373; Clint Kreitner, President and Chief Executive Officer

VANDERBILT UNIVERSITY HOSPITAL, 1161 21st Avenue South, Nashville, TN, Zip 37232; tel. 615/322-5000; Mark L. Penkhus, Chief Executive Officer

ST THOMAS HOSPITAL
P.O. Box 380-4220, Nashville, TN 37205; tel. 615/222-6800; Greg Pope, Executive Director

ST. THOMAS HEALTH SERVICES, 4220 Harding Road, Nashville, TN, Zip 37205-2095, Mailing Address: P.O. Box 380, Zip 37202-0380; tel. 615/222-2111; Thomas E. Beeman, President and Chief Executive Officer

WEST TENNESSEE HEALTHCARE
708 West Forest, Jackson, TN 38301; tel. 901/425-5000; Jim Moss, Chief Executive Officer

BOLIVAR GENERAL HOSPITAL, 650 Nuckolls Road, Bolivar, TN, Zip 38008-1500; tel. 901/658-3100; Rosamond Tyler, Administrator

CAMDEN GENERAL HOSPITAL, 175 Hospital Drive, Camden, TN, Zip 38320-1617; tel. 901/584-6135; John M. Carruth, Administrator

DECATUR COUNTY GENERAL HOSPITAL, 969 Tennessee Avenue South, Parsons, TN, Zip 38363-0250, Mailing Address: Box 250, Zip 38363-0250; tel. 901/847-3031; Larry N. Lindsey, Administrator and Chief Executive Officer

GIBSON GENERAL HOSPITAL, 200 Hospital Drive, Trenton, TN, Zip 38382-3313; tel. 901/855-7900; Kelly R. Yenawine, Administrator

HARDIN COUNTY GENERAL HOSPITAL, 2006 Wayne Road, Savannah, TN, Zip 38372-2294; tel. 901/925-4954; Charlotte Burns, Administrator and Chief Executive Officer

HENRY COUNTY MEDICAL CENTER, 301 Tyson Avenue, Paris, TN, Zip 38242-4544, Mailing Address: Box 1030, Zip 38242-1030; tel. 901/642-1220; Thomas H. Gee, Administrator

HUMBOLDT GENERAL HOSPITAL, 3525 Chere Carol Road, Humboldt, TN, Zip 38343-3699; tel. 901/784-0301; Bill Kail, Administrator

JACKSON–MADISON COUNTY GENERAL HOSPITAL, 708 West Forest Avenue, Jackson, TN, Zip 38301-3855; tel. 901/425-5000; James T. Moss, President and Chief Executive Officer

Networks / Memorial/Sisters of Charity Health Network

MILAN GENERAL HOSPITAL, 4039 South Highland, Milan, TN, Zip 38358; tel. 901/686-1591; Alfred P. Taylor, Administrator and Chief Executive Officer

TEXAS

BAYLOR HEALTH CARE NETWORK
2625 Elm Street, Suite 204, Dallas, TX 75226; tel. 214/820-3425; Bill Cook, President

BAYLOR CENTER FOR RESTORATIVE CARE, 3504 Swiss Avenue, Dallas, TX, Zip 75204-6224; tel. 214/820-9700; Geraldine Brueckner, R.N., Executive Director

BAYLOR MEDICAL CENTER AT GARLAND, 2300 Marie Curie Boulevard, Garland, TX, Zip 75042-5706; tel. 972/487-5000; John B. McWhorter, II, Executive Director

BAYLOR MEDICAL CENTER AT GRAPEVINE, 1650 West College Street, Grapevine, TX, Zip 76051-1650; tel. 817/481-1588; Mark C. Hood, Executive Director

BAYLOR MEDICAL CENTER AT IRVING, 1901 North MacArthur Boulevard, Irving, TX, Zip 75061-2291; tel. 972/579-8100; Michael F. O'Keefe, FACHE, Executive Director

BAYLOR MEDICAL CENTER–ELLIS COUNTY, 1405 West Jefferson Street, Waxahachie, TX, Zip 75165-2275; tel. 972/923-7000; Ronald Hudspeth, Executive Director

BAYLOR UNIVERSITY MEDICAL CENTER, 3500 Gaston Avenue, Dallas, TX, Zip 75246-2088; tel. 214/820-0111; Boone Powell, Jr, President and Chief Executive Officer

BAYLOR/ RICHARDSON MEDICAL CENTER, 401 West Campbell Road, Richardson, TX, Zip 75080-3499; tel. 972/498-4000; Ronald L. Boring, President and Chief Executive Officer

HOPKINS COUNTY MEMORIAL HOSPITAL, 115 Airport Road, Sulphur Springs, TX, Zip 75482-0115; tel. 903/885-7671; Richard L. Goddard, Chief Executive Officer

BRAZO'S VALLEY HEALTH NETWORK
4547 Lake Shore Drive, Waco, TX 76710; tel. 254/202-5320; Don Reeves, Executive Director

CENTRAL TEXAS HOSPITAL, 806 North Crockett Avenue, Cameron, TX, Zip 76520-2599; tel. 254/697-6591; Tariq Mahmood, Chief Executive Officer

GOODALL–WITCHER HEALTHCARE, 101 South Avenue T, Clifton, TX, Zip 76634-1897, Mailing Address: P.O. Box 549, Zip 76634-0549; tel. 254/675-8322; Jim B. Smith, President and Chief Executive Officer

LIMESTONE MEDICAL CENTER, 701 McClintic Street, Groesbeck, TX, Zip 76642-2105; tel. 254/729-3281; Penny Gray, Administrator and Chief Executive Officer

CENTRAL TEXAS RURAL HEALTH NETWORK
503 E. 4th Street, Harrietsville, TX 77964-2824; tel. 512/798-2302; Marcella V. Henke, Executive Director

CENTRAL TEXAS HOSPITAL, 806 North Crockett Avenue, Cameron, TX, Zip 76520-2599; tel. 254/697-6591; Tariq Mahmood, Chief Executive Officer

FALLS COMMUNITY HOSPITAL AND CLINIC, 322 Coleman Street, Marlin, TX, Zip 76661-2358, Mailing Address: Box 60, Zip 76661-0060; tel. 254/803-3561; Willis L. Reese, Administrator

GOODALL–WITCHER HEALTHCARE, 101 South Avenue T, Clifton, TX, Zip 76634-1897, Mailing Address: P.O. Box 549, Zip 76634-0549; tel. 254/675-8322; Jim B. Smith, President and Chief Executive Officer

HAMILTON GENERAL HOSPITAL, 400 North Brown Street, Hamilton, TX, Zip 76531-1598; tel. 254/386-3151; Michael R. Graham, Administrator

HILL REGIONAL HOSPITAL, 101 Circle Drive, Hillsboro, TX, Zip 76645-2670; tel. 254/582-8425; Jan McClure, Chief Executive Officer

HILLCREST MEDICAL CENTER AT WEST, 501 Meadow Drive, West, TX, Zip 76691-1018, Mailing Address: P.O. Box 478, Zip 76691-0478; tel. 254/202-7000; Marilyn K. Lord, Administrator

LAKE WHITNEY MEDICAL CENTER, 200 North San Jacinto Street, Whitney, TX, Zip 76692-2388, Mailing Address: P.O. Box 458, Zip 76692-0458; tel. 254/694-3165; Ruth Ann Crow, Administrator

LIMESTONE MEDICAL CENTER, 701 McClintic Street, Groesbeck, TX, Zip 76642-2105; tel. 254/729-3281; Penny Gray, Administrator and Chief Executive Officer

PARKVIEW REGIONAL HOSPITAL, 312 East Glendale Street, Mexia, TX, Zip 76667-3608; tel. 254/562-5332; Tim Adams, CHE, Administrator and Chief Executive Officer

CHRISTUS SPOHN HEALTH SYSTEM
1702 Santa Fe, Corpus Christi, TX 78404; tel. 361/881-3400; Jake Henry, Jr., President and Chief Executive Officer

CHRISTUS SPOHN HOSPITAL ALICE, 700 North Flournoy Road, Alice, TX Zip 78332; tel. 361/661-8000; Dominic Dominguez, Vice President and Administrator

CHRISTUS SPOHN HOSPITAL BEEVILLE, 1500 East Houston Street, Beeville, TX Zip 78102; tel. 361/354-2000; David S. Wagner, Vice President and Administrator

CHRISTUS SPOHN HOSPITAL KLEBERG, 1311 General Cavazos Boulevard, Kingsville, TX Zip 78363-1197, Mailing Address: P.O. Box 1197, Zip 78363-1197; tel. 361/595-1661; Ernesto G. Flores , Jr, Administrator

CHRISTUS SPOHN HOSPITAL MEMORIAL, 2606 Hospital Boulevard, Corpus Christi, TX Zip 78405-1818, Mailing Address: Box 5280, Zip 78465-5280; tel. 361/902-4000; Thomas G. Neff, Vice President and Administrator

CHRISTUS SPOHN HOSPITAL SHORELINE, 600 Elizabeth Street, Corpus Christi, TX Zip 78404; tel. 361/881-3000; Andrew M. Harris, Vice President and Administrator

CHRISTUS SPOHN HOSPITAL SOUTH, 5950 Saratoga, Corpus Christi, TX Zip 78414; tel. 361/985-5000; Nora Frazier, Vice President and Administrator

GOOD SHEPARD HEALTH NETWORK
700 East Marshall Avenue, Longview, TX 75601; tel. 903/236-2000; Dr. Rebecca Burrow, Executive Director

GOOD SHEPHERD MEDICAL CENTER, 700 East Marshall Avenue, Longview, TX, Zip 75601-5571; tel. 903/236-2000; Jerry D. Adair, President and Chief Executive Officer

HEALTHCARE PARTNERS OF EAST TEXAS, INC
P.O. Box 6340, Tyler, TX 75711; tel. 903/533-0684; Cindy Martinez, Executive Director / President

CHRISTUS ST. MICHAEL HEALTH SYSTEM, 2600 St. Michael Drive, Texarkana, TX, Zip 75503-2372; tel. 903/614-1000; Don A. Beeler, President and Chief Executive Officer

COZBY–GERMANY HOSPITAL, 707 North Waldrip Street, Grand Saline, TX, Zip 75140-1555; tel. 903/962-4242; William Rowton, Chief Executive Officer

DOCTORS MEMORIAL HOSPITAL, 1400 West Southwest Loop 323, Tyler, TX, Zip 75701; tel. 903/561-3771; Olie E. Clem, Chief Executive Officer

EAST TEXAS MEDICAL CENTER ATHENS, 2000 South Palestine Street, Athens, TX, Zip 75751-5610; tel. 903/676-1000; Patrick L. Wallace, Administrator

EAST TEXAS MEDICAL CENTER CARTHAGE, 409 Cottage Road, Carthage, TX, Zip 75633-1466, Mailing Address: P.O. Box 549, Zip 75633-0549; tel. 903/693-3841; Gary Mikeal Hudson, Administrator

EAST TEXAS MEDICAL CENTER FAIRFIELD, 125 Newman Street, Fairfield, TX, Zip 75840-1499; tel. 903/389-2121; Ruth Cook, Administrator

EAST TEXAS MEDICAL CENTER JACKSONVILLE, 501 South Ragsdale Street, Jacksonville, TX, Zip 75766-2413; tel. 903/541-5000; Steve Bowen, President

EAST TEXAS MEDICAL CENTER PITTSBURG, 414 Quitman Street, Pittsburg, TX, Zip 75686-1032; tel. 903/856-6663; W. Perry Henderson, Administrator

EAST TEXAS MEDICAL CENTER–MOUNT VERNON, 500 Highway 37 South, Mount Vernon, TX, Zip 75457, Mailing Address: P.O. Box 477, Zip 75457-0477; tel. 903/537-4552; Perry Henderson, Administrator

EAST TEXAS MEDICAL CENTER–QUITMAN, 117 Winnsboro Street, Quitman, TX, Zip 75783-2144, Mailing Address: P.O. Box 1000, Zip 75783-1000; tel. 903/763-4505; Michael J. McCoy, Administrator

GOOD SHEPHERD MEDICAL CENTER, 700 East Marshall Avenue, Longview, TX, Zip 75601-5571; tel. 903/236-2000; Jerry D. Adair, President and Chief Executive Officer

HENDERSON MEMORIAL HOSPITAL, 300 Wilson Street, Henderson, TX, Zip 75652-5956; tel. 903/657-7541; George T. Roberts, Jr, FACHE, Chief Executive Officer

HUNTSVILLE MEMORIAL HOSPITAL, 485 I-45 South, Huntsville, TX, Zip 77340-4362, Mailing Address: P.O. Box 4001, Zip 77342-4001; tel. 409/291-3411; Ralph E. Beaty, Administrator

LINDEN MUNICIPAL HOSPITAL, 404 North Kaufman Street, Linden, TX, Zip 75563-5235; tel. 903/756-5561; Richard D. Arnold, CHE, Administrator and Chief Executive Officer

MEMORIAL HEALTH SYSTEM OF EAST TEXAS, 1201 West Frank Avenue, Lufkin, TX, Zip 75904-3357, Mailing Address: P.O. Box 1447, Zip 75902-1447; tel. 936/634-8111; Gary Lex Whatley, President and Chief Executive Officer

MEMORIAL HOSPITAL OF CENTER, 602 Hurst Street, Center, TX, Zip 75935-3414, Mailing Address: P.O. Box 1749, Zip 75935-1749; tel. 409/598-2781; John A. Tucker, Chief Executive Officer

MEMORIAL MEDICAL CENTER, 602 East Church Street, Livingston, TX, Zip 77351-1257, Mailing Address: P.O. Box 1257, Zip 77351-1257; tel. 936/327-4381; James C. Dickson, Administrator

NACOGDOCHES MEMORIAL HOSPITAL, 1204 North Mound Street, Nacogdoches, TX, Zip 75961-4061; tel. 409/568-8520; G. W. Jones, Administrator

PINELANDS HOSPITAL, 4632 Northeast Stallings Drive, Nacogdoches, TX, Zip 75961-1617, Mailing Address: P.O. Box 1004, Zip 79563-1004; tel. 409/560-5900; Steve Scott, Chief Executive Officer

PRESBYTERIAN HOSPITAL OF WINNSBORO, 719 West Coke Road, Winnsboro, TX, Zip 75494-3098, Mailing Address: P.O. Box 628, Zip 75494-0628; tel. 903/342-5227; Dan Noteware, Senior Vice President and Executive Director

ROY H. LAIRD MEMORIAL HOSPITAL, 1612 South Henderson Boulevard, Kilgore, TX, Zip 75662-3594; tel. 903/984-3505; Roderick G. La Grone, President and Chief Executive Officer

TITUS REGIONAL MEDICAL CENTER, 2001 North Jefferson Avenue, Mount Pleasant, TX, Zip 75455-2398; tel. 903/577-6000; Steven K. Jacobson, Chief Executive Officer

TRINITY VALLEY MEDICAL CENTER, 2900 South Loop 256, Palestine, TX, Zip 75801-6958; tel. 903/731-1000; Larry C. Bozeman, Chief Executive Officer

MEMORIAL/SISTERS OF CHARITY HEALTH NETWORK
7737 S.W. Freeway Suite 200, Houston, TX 77074; tel. 713/776-6992; Dan Wilford, President

ANGLETON–DANBURY GENERAL HOSPITAL, 132 East Hospital Drive, Angleton, TX, Zip 77515-4197; tel. 409/849-7721; David A. Bleakney, Administrator

© 2000 AHA Guide

Networks, Health Care Systems and Alliances B41

Networks / Memorial/Sisters of Charity Health Network

MEMORIAL HERMANN BEHAVIORAL HEALTH CENTER, 2801 Gessner, Houston, TX, Zip 77080–2599; tel. 713/462–4000; Sue E. Green, Vice President and Chief Executive Officer

MEMORIAL HERMANN MEMORIAL CITY HOSPITAL, 920 Frostwood Drive, Houston, TX, Zip 77024–9173; tel. 713/932–3000; Wayne M. Voss, Chief Executive Officer

MEMORIAL HERMANN SOUTHWEST HOSPITAL, 7600 Beechnut, Houston, TX, Zip 77074–1850; tel. 713/776–5000; Jerel T. Humphrey, Chief Executive Officer

MEMORIAL HERMANN THE WOODLANDS HOSPITAL, 9250 Pinecroft Drive, The Woodlands, TX, Zip 77380–3225; tel. 281/364–2300; Steve Sanders, Vice President and Chief Executive Officer

POLLY RYON MEMORIAL HOSPITAL, 1705 Jackson Street, Richmond, TX, Zip 77469–3289; tel. 281/341–3000; Sam L. Steffee, Executive Director and Chief Executive Officer

TOMBALL REGIONAL HOSPITAL, 605 Holderrieth Street, Tomball, TX, Zip 77375–0889, Mailing Address: Box 889, Zip 77377–0889; tel. 281/351–1623; Robert F. Schaper, President and Chief Executive Officer

METHODIST HEALTH CARE SYSTEM
7550 IH 10 West, Suite 1000, San Antonio, TX 78229; tel. 210/377–1647; John Hornbeak, President

METHODIST CHILDREN'S HOSPITAL OF SOUTH TEXAS, 7700 Floyd Curl Drive, San Antonio, TX, Zip 78229–3383; tel. 210/575–7138; Arthur E. Marlin, M.D., Chief Executive Officer

METHODIST SPECIALTY AND TRANSPLANT HOSPITAL, 8026 Floyd Curl Drive, San Antonio, TX, Zip 78229–3915; tel. 210/575–8110; John E. Hornbeak, Chief Executive Officer

METROPOLITAN METHODIST HOSPITAL, 1310 McCullough Avenue, San Antonio, TX, Zip 78212–2617; tel. 210/208–2200; Mark L. Bernard, Chief Executive Officer

NORTHEAST METHODIST HOSPITAL, 12412 Judson Road, San Antonio, TX, Zip 78233–3272, Mailing Address: P.O. Box 659510, Zip 78265–9510; tel. 210/650–4949; Mark L. Bernard, Chief Executive Officer

SOUTHWEST TEXAS METHODIST HOSPITAL, 7700 Floyd Curl Drive, San Antonio, TX, Zip 78229–3993; tel. 210/575–4000; John E. Hornbeak, Chief Executive Officer

NORTH TEXAS HEALTH NETWORK
5601 MacArthur Suite 300, Irving, TX 75038; tel. 214/751–0047; Charlie Cod, President

BAYLOR CENTER FOR RESTORATIVE CARE, 3504 Swiss Avenue, Dallas, TX, Zip 75204–6224; tel. 214/820–9700; Geraldine Brueckner, R.N., Executive Director

BAYLOR INSTITUTE FOR REHABILITATION, 3505 Gaston Avenue, Dallas, TX, Zip 75246–2018; tel. 214/826–7030; Laura J. Lycan, Executive Director

BAYLOR MEDICAL CENTER AT GARLAND, 2300 Marie Curie Boulevard, Garland, TX, Zip 75042–5706; tel. 972/487–5000; John B. McWhorter, II, Executive Director

BAYLOR MEDICAL CENTER AT GRAPEVINE, 1650 West College Street, Grapevine, TX, Zip 76051–1650; tel. 817/481–1588; Mark C. Hood, Executive Director

BAYLOR UNIVERSITY MEDICAL CENTER, 3500 Gaston Avenue, Dallas, TX, Zip 75246–2088; tel. 214/820–0111; Boone Powell, Jr, President and Chief Executive Officer

MEDICAL CENTER AT TERRELL, 1551 Highway 34 South, Terrell, TX, Zip 75160–4833; tel. 972/563–7611; Ronald J. Ensor, Chief Executive Officer

OUR CHILDREN'S HOUSE AT BAYLOR, 3301 Swiss Avenue, Dallas, TX, Zip 75204–6219; tel. 214/820–9838; Geraldine Brueckner, R.N., Executive Director

PRESBYTERIAN HOSPITAL OF PLANO, 6200 West Parker Road, Plano, TX, Zip 75093–7914; tel. 972/981–8000; Philip M. Wentworth, FACHE, President

PERMIAN BASIN RURAL HEALTH NETWORK
P.O. Box 1648, Fort Stockton, TX 79735; tel. 915/336–2241; George Miller Jr, President

BIG BEND REGIONAL MEDICAL CENTER, 2600 Highway 118 North, Alpine, TX, Zip 79830; tel. 915/837–3447; David Conejo, Chief Executive Officer

BIG SPRING STATE HOSPITAL, Lamesa Highway, Big Spring, TX, Zip 79720, Mailing Address: P.O. Box 231, Zip 79721–0231; tel. 915/267–8216; Edward Moughon, Superintendent

CRANE MEMORIAL HOSPITAL, 1310 South Alford Street, Crane, TX, Zip 79731–3899; tel. 915/558–3555; Stan Wiley, Administrator

MARTIN COUNTY HOSPITAL DISTRICT, 610 North St. Peter Street, Stanton, TX, Zip 79782, Mailing Address: P.O. Box 640, Zip 79782–0640; tel. 915/756–3345; Doris Bergerson, Interim Administrator

MCCAMEY HOSPITAL, Highway 305 South, McCamey, TX, Zip 79752, Mailing Address: P.O. Box 1200, Zip 79752–1200; tel. 915/652–8626; Bill Boswell, Chief Executive Officer

MEDICAL ARTS HOSPITAL, 1600 North Bryan Avenue, Lamesa, TX, Zip 79331; tel. 806/872–2183; Karl R. Stinson, CHE, Chief Executive Officer

MEDICAL CENTER HOSPITAL, 500 West Fourth Street, Odessa, TX, Zip 79761–5059, Mailing Address: P.O. Drawer 7239, Zip 79760–7239; tel. 915/640–4000; J. Michael Stephans, Administrator

MEMORIAL HOSPITAL, 821 Jeffee Drive, Kermit, TX, Zip 79745–4696, Mailing Address: Drawer H, Zip 79745–6008; tel. 915/586–5864; Judene Willhelm, Administrator

MEMORIAL HOSPITAL, 209 N.W. Eighth Street, Seminole, TX, Zip 79360–3447; tel. 915/758–5811; Steve Beck, Chief Executive Officer and Administrator

MIDLAND MEMORIAL HOSPITAL, 2200 West Illinois Avenue, Midland, TX, Zip 79701–6499; tel. 915/685–1111; Harold Rubin, FACHE, President and Chief Executive Officer

PECOS COUNTY GENERAL HOSPITAL, 305 West Fifth Street, Iraan, TX, Zip 79744, Mailing Address: P.O. Box 665, Zip 79744–2057; tel. 915/639–2871; Nicholas R. Blythe, Interim Administrator and Chief Executive Officer

PECOS COUNTY MEMORIAL HOSPITAL, Sanderson Highway, Fort Stockton, TX, Zip 79735, Mailing Address: P.O. Box 1648, Zip 79735–1648; tel. 915/336–2241; Nicholas R. Blythe, Interim Administrator and Chief Executive Officer

PERMIAN GENERAL HOSPITAL, Northeast By–Pass, Andrews, TX, Zip 79714, Mailing Address: P.O. Box 2108, Zip 79714–2108; tel. 915/523–2200; Randy R. Richards, Chief Executive Officer

RANKIN HOSPITAL DISTRICT, 1105 Elizabeth Street, Rankin, TX, Zip 79778, Mailing Address: P.O. Box 327, Zip 79778–0327; tel. 915/693–2443; John Paul Loyless, Administrator

REAGAN MEMORIAL HOSPITAL, 805 North Main Street, Big Lake, TX, Zip 76932–3999; tel. 915/884–2561; Ron Galloway, Administrator

REEVES COUNTY HOSPITAL, 2323 Texas Street, Pecos, TX, Zip 79772–7338; tel. 915/447–3551; Charles N. Butts, Chief Executive Officer

SCENIC MOUNTAIN MEDICAL CENTER, 1601 West 11th Place, Big Spring, TX, Zip 79720–4198; tel. 915/263–1211; Loren F. Chandler, Chief Executive Officer

VETERANS AFFAIRS MEDICAL CENTER, 300 Veterans Boulevard, Big Spring, TX, Zip 79720–5500; tel. 915/263–7361; Cary D. Brown, Director

WARD MEMORIAL HOSPITAL, 406 South Gary Street, Monahans, TX, Zip 79756–4798, Mailing Address: P.O. Box 40, Zip 79756–0040; tel. 915/943–2511; Joseph Wright, Administrator

PRESBYTERIAN HEALTHCARE SYSTEM
8200 Walnut Hill Lane, Dallas, TX 75231; tel. 214/345–8486; Charles Spiler, Adm Resident

HUNT MEMORIAL HOSPITAL DISTRICT, 4215 Joe Ramsey Boulevard, Greenville, TX, Zip 75401–7899, Mailing Address: P.O. Drawer 1059, Zip 75403–1059; tel. 903/408–5000; Richard Carter, Chief Executive Officer

MCCUISTION REGIONAL MEDICAL CENTER, 865 Deshong Drive, Paris, TX, Zip 75462–2097; tel. 903/737–1111; Michael J. McBride, FACHE, President

PRESBYTERIAN HOSPITAL OF DALLAS, 8200 Walnut Hill Lane, Dallas, TX, Zip 75231–4402; tel. 214/345–6789; Mark H. Merrill, President

PRESBYTERIAN HOSPITAL OF KAUFMAN, 850 Highway 243 West, Kaufman, TX, Zip 75142–9998, Mailing Address: P.O. Box 310, Zip 75142–0310; tel. 972/932–7200; Kirk King, Senior Vice President and Executive Director

PRESBYTERIAN HOSPITAL OF PLANO, 6200 West Parker Road, Plano, TX, Zip 75093–7914; tel. 972/981–8000; Philip M. Wentworth, FACHE, President

PRESBYTERIAN HOSPITAL OF WINNSBORO, 719 West Coke Road, Winnsboro, TX, Zip 75494–3098, Mailing Address: P.O. Box 628, Zip 75494–0628; tel. 903/342–5227; Dan Noteware, Senior Vice President and Executive Director

PRIMARY CARE NETWORK OF TEXAS
62443 IH 10 W, Suite 1001, San Antonio, TX 78201; tel. 210/704–4800; Susan Ginnity, Network Contact

CHRISTUS SANTA ROSA HEALTH CARE, 519 West Houston Street, San Antonio, TX, Zip 78207–3108; tel. 210/704–2011; James P. Houser, President and Chief Executive Officer

REGIONAL HEALTHCARE ALLIANCE
800 East Dawson, Tyler, TX 75701; tel. 903/531–4449; John Webb, President

ATLANTA MEMORIAL HOSPITAL, Highway 77 at South William, Atlanta, TX, Zip 75551, Mailing Address: P.O. Box 1049, Zip 75551–1049; tel. 903/799–3000; Tom Crow, Administrator

BAYLOR UNIVERSITY MEDICAL CENTER, 3500 Gaston Avenue, Dallas, TX, Zip 75246–2088; tel. 214/820–0111; Boone Powell, Jr, President and Chief Executive Officer

CHILDREN'S MEDICAL CENTER OF DALLAS, 1935 Motor Street, Dallas, TX, Zip 75235–7794; tel. 214/456–7000; George D. Farr, President and Chief Executive Officer

CHRISTUS SCHUMPERT MEDICAL CENTER, One St. Mary Place, Shreveport, LA, Zip 71101–4399, Mailing Address: P.O. Box 21976, Zip 71120–1076; tel. 318/681–4500; Wayne A. Sensor, Chief Executive Officer

COZBY–GERMANY HOSPITAL, 707 North Waldrip Street, Grand Saline, TX, Zip 75140–1555; tel. 903/962–4242; William Rowton, Chief Executive Officer

EAST TEXAS MEDICAL CENTER CARTHAGE, 409 Cottage Road, Carthage, TX, Zip 75633–1466, Mailing Address: P.O. Box 549, Zip 75633–0549; tel. 903/693–3841; Gary Mikeal Hudson, Administrator

EAST TEXAS MEDICAL CENTER FAIRFIELD, 125 Newman Street, Fairfield, TX, Zip 75840–1499; tel. 903/389–2121; Ruth Cook, Administrator

EAST TEXAS MEDICAL CENTER–QUITMAN, 117 Winnsboro Street, Quitman, TX, Zip 75783–2144, Mailing Address: P.O. Box 1000, Zip 75783–1000; tel. 903/763–4505; Michael J. McCoy, Administrator

GOOD SHEPHERD MEDICAL CENTER, 700 East Marshall Avenue, Longview, TX, Zip 75601–5571; tel. 903/236–2000; Jerry D. Adair, President and Chief Executive Officer

HEALTHSOUTH REHABILITATION HOSPITAL–TYLER, 3131 Troup Highway, Tyler, TX, Zip 75701–8352; tel. 903/510–7000; Sharla Anderson, Interim Chief Executive Officer

HENDERSON MEMORIAL HOSPITAL, 300 Wilson Street, Henderson, TX, Zip 75652–5956; tel. 903/657–7541; George T. Roberts, Jr, FACHE, Chief Executive Officer

Networks / Texoma Health Network

HOPKINS COUNTY MEMORIAL HOSPITAL, 115 Airport Road, Sulphur Springs, TX, Zip 75482-0115; tel. 903/885-7671; Richard L. Goddard, Chief Executive Officer

LINDEN MUNICIPAL HOSPITAL, 404 North Kaufman Street, Linden, TX, Zip 75563-5235; tel. 903/756-5561; Richard D. Arnold, CHE, Administrator and Chief Executive Officer

MARSHALL REGIONAL MEDICAL CENTER, 811 South Washington Avenue, Marshall, TX, Zip 75670-5336, Mailing Address: P.O. Box 1599, Zip 75671-1599; tel. 903/927-6000; James E. Hodges, Chief Operating Officer

NACOGDOCHES MEDICAL CENTER, 4920 N.E. Stallings, Nacogdoches, TX, Zip 75961-1200, Mailing Address: P.O. Box 631604, Zip 75963-1604; tel. 409/568-3380; Glenn A. Robinson, Chief Executive Officer

PINELANDS HOSPITAL, 4632 Northeast Stallings Drive, Nacogdoches, TX, Zip 75961-1617, Mailing Address: P.O. Box 1004, Zip 79563-1004; tel. 409/560-5900; Steve Scott, Chief Executive Officer

PRESBYTERIAN HOSPITAL OF DALLAS, 8200 Walnut Hill Lane, Dallas, TX, Zip 75231-4402; tel. 214/345-6789; Mark H. Merrill, President

PRESBYTERIAN HOSPITAL OF KAUFMAN, 850 Highway 243 West, Kaufman, TX, Zip 75142-9998, Mailing Address: P.O. Box 310, Zip 75142-0310; tel. 972/932-7200; Kirk King, Senior Vice President and Executive Director

PRESBYTERIAN HOSPITAL OF WINNSBORO, 719 West Coke Road, Winnsboro, TX, Zip 75494-3098, Mailing Address: P.O. Box 628, Zip 75494-0628; tel. 903/342-5227; Dan Noteware, Senior Vice President and Executive Director

ROY H. LAIRD MEMORIAL HOSPITAL, 1612 South Henderson Boulevard, Kilgore, TX, Zip 75662-3594; tel. 903/984-3505; Roderick G. La Grone, President and Chief Executive Officer

TITUS REGIONAL MEDICAL CENTER, 2001 North Jefferson Avenue, Mount Pleasant, TX, Zip 75455-2398; tel. 903/577-6000; Steven K. Jacobson, Chief Executive Officer

TRINITY MOTHER FRANCES HEALTH SYSTEM, 910 East Houston, Tyler, TX, Zip 75702; tel. 903/531-4445; J. Lindsey Bradley, Jr, FACHE, President and Chief Administrative Officer

UNIVERSITY OF TEXAS HEALTH CENTER AT TYLER, 11937 Highway 271, Tyler, TX, Zip 75708-3154; tel. 903/877-3451; Ronald F. Garvey, M.D., President

WILLIS–KNIGHTON MEDICAL CENTER, 2600 Greenwood Road, Shreveport, LA, Zip 71103-2600, Mailing Address: P.O. Box 32600, Zip 71130-2600; tel. 318/632-4600; James K. Elrod, President and Chief Executive Officer

SE TEXAS HOSPITAL SYSTEM
233 W. 10th Street, Dallas, TX 75208;
tel. 214/943-3582; Bob McElearney, Interim President

CITIZENS MEDICAL CENTER, 2701 Hospital Drive, Victoria, TX, Zip 77901-5749; tel. 361/573-9181; David P. Brown, Administrator

CUERO COMMUNITY HOSPITAL, 2550 North Esplanade Street, Cuero, TX, Zip 77954-4716; tel. 361/275-6191; James E. Buckner, Jr, Administrator

DRISCOLL CHILDREN'S HOSPITAL, 3533 South Alameda Street, Corpus Christi, TX, Zip 78411-1785, Mailing Address: P.O. Box 6530, Zip 78466-6530; tel. 361/694-5000; Rick W. Merrill, President and Chief Executive Officer

EL CAMPO MEMORIAL HOSPITAL, 303 Sandy Corner Road, El Campo, TX, Zip 77437-9535; tel. 409/543-6251; Steve Gularte, Administrator

JACKSON COUNTY HOSPITAL, 1013 South Wells Street, Edna, TX, Zip 77957-4098; tel. 361/782-5241; Marcella V. Henke, Administrator and Chief Executive Officer

LAVACA MEDICAL CENTER, 1400 North Texana Street, Hallettsville, TX, Zip 77964-2099; tel. 361/798-3671; James Vanek, Administrator

MEMORIAL MEDICAL CENTER, 815 North Virginia Street, Port Lavaca, TX, Zip 77979-3025, Mailing Address: P.O. Box 25, Zip 77979-0025; tel. 361/552-6713; Bob L. Bybee, President and Chief Executive Officer

REFUGIO COUNTY MEMORIAL HOSPITAL, 107 Swift Street, Refugio, TX, Zip 78377-2425; tel. 361/526-2321; Louis R. Willeke, Administrator

REGIONAL MEDICAL CENTER, 101 Medical Drive, Victoria, TX, Zip 77904-3198; tel. 361/573-6100; William R. Blancher, Chief Executive Officer

YOAKUM COMMUNITY HOSPITAL, 1200 Carl Ramert Drive, Yoakum, TX, Zip 77995-4198, Mailing Address: P.O. Box 753, Zip 77995-0753; tel. 361/293-2321; Jeff R. Egbert, Chief Executive Officer

SE TEXAS INTEGRATED COMMUNITY HEALTH NETWORK
2600 North Loop, Houston, TX 77092;
tel. 713/681-8877; Stanley T. Urban, President/Chief Executive Officer

CHRISTUS ST. ELIZABETH HOSPITAL, 2830 Calder Avenue, Beaumont, TX, Zip 77702, Mailing Address: P.O. Box 5405, Zip 77726-5405; tel. 409/892-7171; Edward W. Myers, Chief Executive Officer

CHRISTUS ST. JOHN HOSPITAL, 18300 St. John Drive, Nassau Bay, TX, Zip 77058; tel. 281/333-5503; Thomas Permetti, Chief Executive Officer

CHRISTUS ST. JOSEPH HOSPITAL, 1919 LaBranch Street, Houston, TX, Zip 77002; tel. 713/757-1000; Sally E. Jeffcoat, Chief Executive Officer

CHRISTUS ST. MARY HOSPITAL, 3600 Gates Boulevard, Port Arthur, TX, Zip 77642-3601, Mailing Address: P.O. Box 3696, Zip 77643-3696; tel. 409/985-7431; Alice Baker, Chief Executive Officer

SOUTHWEST TEXAS RURAL HEALTH ALLIANCE
143 East Garza, New Braunfels, TX 78130;
tel. 210/606-9111; Johnny Johnson, President

CENTRAL TEXAS MEDICAL CENTER, 1301 Wonder World Drive, San Marcos, TX, Zip 78666-7544; tel. 512/353-8979; Ken Bacon, President and Chief Executive Officer

DIMMIT COUNTY MEMORIAL HOSPITAL, 704 Hospital Drive, Carrizo Springs, TX, Zip 78834-3836; tel. 830/876-2424; Ernesto G. Flores, Jr, Administrator

FRIO HOSPITAL, 320 Berry Ranch Road, Pearsall, TX, Zip 78061-3998; tel. 830/334-3617; Alan D. Holmes, Chief Executive Officer

GUADALUPE VALLEY HOSPITAL, 1215 East Court Street, Seguin, TX, Zip 78155-5189; tel. 830/379-2411; Don L. Richey, Administrator

HILL COUNTRY MEMORIAL HOSPITAL, 1020 Kerrville Road, Fredericksburg, TX, Zip 78624, Mailing Address: P.O. Box 835, Zip 78624-0835; tel. 830/997-4353; Jeff A. Bourgeois, Chief Executive Officer

KIMBLE HOSPITAL, 2101 Main Street, Junction, TX, Zip 76849-2101; tel. 915/446-3321; Jamie R. Jacoby, Administrator

MCKENNA MEMORIAL HOSPITAL, 600 North Union Avenue, New Braunfels, TX, Zip 78130; tel. 830/606-9111; Tim Brierty, Chief Executive Officer

MEDINA COMMUNITY HOSPITAL, 3100 Avenue East, Hondo, TX, Zip 78861-3599; tel. 830/741-4677; Elwood E. Currier, Jr, CHE, Administrator

MEMORIAL HOSPITAL, Highway 90A By-Pass, Gonzales, TX, Zip 78629, Mailing Address: P.O. Box 587, Zip 78629-0587; tel. 830/672-7581; Douglas Langley, Administrator

OTTO KAISER MEMORIAL HOSPITAL, 3349 South Highway 181, Kenedy, TX, Zip 78119-5240; tel. 830/583-3401; Nancy Kinkler, Administrator

SETON EDGAR B. DAVIS HOSPITAL, 130 Hays Street, Luling, TX, Zip 78648-3207; tel. 830/875-5643; Neal Kelley, Administrator

SID PETERSON MEMORIAL HOSPITAL, 710 Water Street, Kerrville, TX, Zip 78028-5398; tel. 830/896-4200; James Patrick Murray, Chief Executive Officer

SOUTH TEXAS REGIONAL MEDICAL CENTER, 1905 Highway 97 East, Jourdanton, TX, Zip 78026, Mailing Address: P.O. Box 189, Zip 78026-0189; tel. 830/769-3515; Stephen B. Hill, Chief Executive Officer

UVALDE COUNTY HOSPITAL AUTHORITY, 1025 Garner Field Road, Uvalde, TX, Zip 78801-1025; tel. 830/278-6251; Ben M. Durr, Administrator

VAL VERDE REGIONAL MEDICAL CENTER, 801 Bedell Avenue, Del Rio, TX, Zip 78840-4185, Mailing Address: P.O. Box 1527, Zip 78840-1527; tel. 830/775-8566; Patrick J. Jacobus, Chief Executive Officer

WARM SPRINGS REHABILITATION HOSPITAL, Gonzales, TX, Mailing Address: P.O. Box 58, Zip 78629-0058; tel. 830/672-6592; John W. Davis, Administrator

WILSON MEMORIAL HOSPITAL, 1301 Hospital Boulevard, Floresville, TX, Zip 78114-2798; tel. 830/393-3122; Robert Duffield, Administrator

ST DAVID'S HEALTH NETWORK
P.O. Box 49192, Austin, TX 78765;
tel. 512/.40-8700; Sharon J. Alvis, Executive Director

ROUND ROCK HOSPITAL, 2400 Round Rock Avenue, Round Rock, TX, Zip 78681-4097; tel. 512/341-1000; Deborah L. Ryle, Chief Executive Officer

SOUTH AUSTIN HOSPITAL, 901 West Ben White Boulevard, Austin, TX, Zip 78704-6903; tel. 512/447-2211; Richard W. Klusmann, Chief Executive Officer

ST. DAVID'S MEDICAL CENTER, 919 East 32nd Street, Austin, TX, Zip 78705-2709, Mailing Address: P.O. Box 4039, Zip 78765-4039; tel. 512/476-7111; Cole C. Eslyn, Chief Executive Officer

ST. DAVID'S PAVILION, 1025 East 32nd Street, Austin, TX, Zip 78765; tel. 512/867-5800; Cole C. Eslyn, Chief Executive Officer

ST. DAVID'S REHABILITATION CENTER, 1005 East 32nd Street, Austin, TX, Zip 78705-2705, Mailing Address: P.O. Box 4270, Zip 78765-4270; tel. 512/867-5100; Cole C. Eslyn, Chief Executive Officer

TEXOMA HEALTH NETWORK
1600 10th Street, Wichita Falls, TX 76301;
tel. 817/872-1126; Teresa Pontius, Executive Director

BOWIE MEMORIAL HOSPITAL, 705 East Greenwood Avenue, Bowie, TX, Zip 76230-3199; tel. 940/872-1126; Joyce Crumpler, R.N., Administrator

CHILLICOTHE HOSPITAL DISTRICT, 303 Avenue I, Chillicothe, TX, Zip 79225, Mailing Address: P.O. Box 370, Zip 79225-0370; tel. 940/852-5131; Linda Hall, Administrator

CLAY COUNTY MEMORIAL HOSPITAL, 310 West South Street, Henrietta, TX, Zip 76365-3399; tel. 940/538-5621; Jimmy Ben Gill, Chief Executive Officer and Administrator

ELECTRA MEMORIAL HOSPITAL, 1207 South Bailey Street, Electra, TX, Zip 76360-3221, Mailing Address: P.O. Box 1112, Zip 76360-1112; tel. 940/495-3981; Jan A. Reed, CPA, Administrator and Chief Executive Officer

FAITH COMMUNITY HOSPITAL, 717 Magnolia Street, Jacksboro, TX, Zip 76458-1111; tel. 940/567-6633; Don Hopkins, Administrator

HAMILTON HOSPITAL, 903 West Hamilton Street, Olney, TX, Zip 76374-1725, Mailing Address: P.O. Box 158, Zip 76374-0158; tel. 940/564-5521; William R. Smith, Administrator

HARDEMAN COUNTY MEMORIAL HOSPITAL, 402 Mercer Street, Quanah, TX, Zip 79252-4026, Mailing Address: P.O. Box 90, Zip 79252-0090; tel. 940/663-2795; Jerry C. Varnado, Administrator

© 2000 AHA Guide Networks, Health Care Systems and Alliances B43

Networks / Texoma Health Network

NOCONA GENERAL HOSPITAL, 100 Park Street, Nocona, TX, Zip 76255-3616; tel. 940/825-3235; Charles Norris, Administrator

SEYMOUR HOSPITAL, 200 Stadium Drive, Seymour, TX, Zip 76380-2344; tel. 940/888-5572; Robert E. Vernor, Administrator

THROCKMORTON COUNTY MEMORIAL HOSPITAL, 802 North Minter Street, Throckmorton, TX, Zip 76483, Mailing Address: P.O. Box 729, Zip 76483-0729; tel. 940/849-2151; Stasha Siegert, Administrator

UTAH

INTERMOUNTAIN HEALTH CARE
36 South State Street, Suite 2100, Salt Lake City, UT 84102; tel. 801/442-3587; Bill Nelson, President & Chief Executive Officer

ALTA VIEW HOSPITAL, 9660 South 1300 East, Sandy, UT, Zip 84094-3793; tel. 801/501-2600; Wes Thompson, Administrator and Chief Executive Officer

AMERICAN FORK HOSPITAL, 170 North 1100 East, American Fork, UT, Zip 84003-2096; tel. 801/763-3300; Keith N. Alexander, Administrator and Chief Operating Officer

BEAR RIVER VALLEY HOSPITAL, 440 West 600 North, Tremonton, UT, Zip 84337-2497; tel. 435/257-7441; Robert F. Jex, Administrator

CASSIA REGIONAL MEDICAL CENTER, 1501 Hiland Avenue, Burley, ID, Zip 83318-2648; tel. 208/678-4444; Michael R. Olson, Administrator

COTTONWOOD HOSPITAL MEDICAL CENTER, 5770 South 300 East, Murray, UT, Zip 84107-6186, Mailing Address: P.O. Box 57800, Salt Lake City, UT 84107-0800; tel. 801/262-3461; Douglas R. Fonnesbeck, Administrator and Chief Executive Officer

DELTA COMMUNITY MEDICAL CENTER, 126 South White Sage Avenue, Delta, UT, Zip 84624-8928; tel. 435/864-5591; James E. Beckstrand, Administrator

DIXIE REGIONAL MEDICAL CENTER, 544 South 400 East, Saint George, UT, Zip 84770-3799; tel. 435/634-4000; L. Steven Wilson, Administrator

FILLMORE COMMUNITY MEDICAL CENTER, 674 South Highway 99, Fillmore, UT, Zip 84631-9701; tel. 435/743-5591; James E. Beckstrand, Administrator

GARFIELD MEMORIAL HOSPITAL AND CLINICS, 200 North 400 East, Panguitch, UT, Zip 84759, Mailing Address: P.O. Box 389, Zip 84759-0389; tel. 435/676-8811; Eric Packer, Administrator

HEBER VALLEY MEDICAL CENTER, 1485 South Highway 40, Heber City, UT, Zip 84032-3522; tel. 435/654-2500; Randall K. Probst, Administrator

LDS HOSPITAL, Eighth Avenue and C Street, Salt Lake City, UT, Zip 84143-0001; tel. 801/408-1100; Richard M. Cagen, Chief Executive Officer and Administrator

LOGAN REGIONAL HOSPITAL, 1400 North 500 East, Logan, UT, Zip 84341-2499; tel. 435/716-1000; Richard Smith, Administrator

MCKAY-DEE HOSPITAL CENTER, 3939 Harrison Boulevard, Ogden, UT, Zip 84409-0370, Mailing Address: Box 9370, Zip 84409-0370; tel. 801/398-2800; Thomas F. Hanrahan, FACHE, Chief Executive Officer and Regional Vice President

OREM COMMUNITY HOSPITAL, 331 North 400 West, Orem, UT, Zip 84057-1999; tel. 801/224-4080; Kim Nielsen, Administrator and Chief Operating Officer

POCATELLO REGIONAL MEDICAL CENTER, 777 Hospital Way, Pocatello, ID, Zip 83201-2797; tel. 208/234-0777; Tracy J. Farnsworth, Administrator

PRIMARY CHILDREN'S MEDICAL CENTER, 100 North Medical Drive, Salt Lake City, UT, Zip 84113-1100; tel. 801/588-2000; Joseph R. Horton, Chief Executive Officer and Administrator

SANPETE VALLEY HOSPITAL, 1100 South Medical Drive, Mount Pleasant, UT, Zip 84647-2222; tel. 435/462-2441; George Winn, Administrator

SEVIER VALLEY HOSPITAL, 1100 North Main Street, Richfield, UT, Zip 84701-1843; tel. 435/896-8271; Gary E. Beck, Administrator

UTAH VALLEY REGIONAL MEDICAL CENTER, 1034 North 500 West, Provo, UT, Zip 84604-3337; tel. 801/373-7850; Mary Ann Young, R.N., Administrator

VALLEY VIEW MEDICAL CENTER, 595 South 75 East, Cedar City, UT, Zip 84720-3462; tel. 435/586-6587; Craig M. Smedley, Administrator

PARACELSUS HEALTH CARE
2500 South State Street, Salt Lake City, UT 84115; tel. 801/461-6666; David L. Jones, Assistant Vice President

VERMONT

FLETCHER ALLEN HEALTH CARE
111 Colchester Avenue, Burlington, VT 05401; tel. 802/847-0000; William V. Boettcher, Chief Executive Officer

FLETCHER ALLEN HEALTH CARE, 111 Colchester Avenue, Burlington, VT, Zip 05401-1429; tel. 802/847-2345; William V. Boettcher, Chief Executive Officer

VIRGINIA

CARILION HEALTH SYSTEM
1212 Third Street, S.W., Roanoke, VA 24016; tel. 703/981-7900; Randy Edwards, Executive Vice President

CARILION BEDFORD MEMORIAL HOSPITAL, 1613 Oakwood Street, Bedford, VA, Zip 24523-0688, Mailing Address: P.O. Box 688, Zip 24523-0688; tel. 540/586-2441; Howard Ainsley, Vice President and Hospital Director

CARILION FRANKLIN MEMORIAL HOSPITAL, 180 Floyd Avenue, Rocky Mount, VA, Zip 24151-1389; tel. 540/483-5277; Matthew J. Perry, Director

CARILION GILES MEMORIAL HOSPITAL, 1 Taylor Avenue, Pearisburg, VA, Zip 24134-1932; tel. 540/921-6000; Morris D. Reece, Administrator and Chief Executive Officer

CARILION MEDICAL CENTER, Belleview at Jefferson Street, Roanoke, VA, Zip 24014, Mailing Address: P.O. Box 13367, Zip 24033-3367; tel. 540/981-7000; Lucas A. Snipes, FACHE, Director

CARILION NEW RIVER VALLEY MEDICAL CENTER, 2900 Tyler Road, Radford, VA, Zip 24073, Mailing Address: P.O. Box 5, Zip 24141-0005; tel. 540/731-2000; Virginia Ousley, Vice President and Hospital Director

CARILION SAINT ALBANS HOSPITAL, Route 11, Lee Highway, Radford, VA, Zip 24143, Mailing Address: P.O. Box 3608, Zip 24143-3608; tel. 540/639-2481; Janet McKinney Crawford, Vice President and Administrator

CENTRAL VIRGINIA HEALTH NETWORK
8100 Three Chopt-Ste 209, Richmond, VA 23229; tel. 804/359-4500; Michael Matthews, Chief Executive Officer

BON SECOURS ST. MARY'S HOSPITAL, 5801 Bremo Road, Richmond, VA, Zip 23226-1900; tel. 804/285-2011; Ann E. Honeycutt, Executive Vice President and Administrator

BON SECOURS-RICHMOND COMMUNITY HOSPITAL, 1500 North 28th Street, Richmond, VA, Zip 23223-5396, Mailing Address: Box 27184, Zip 23261-7184; tel. 804/225-1700; Eugene Toomer, Chief Operating Officer

BON SECOURS-STUART CIRCLE, 413 Stuart Circle, Richmond, VA, Zip 23220-3799; tel. 804/358-7051; Ann E. Honeycutt, Executive Vice President and Administrator

COMMUNITY MEMORIAL HEALTHCENTER, 125 Buena Vista Circle, South Hill, VA, Zip 23970-0090, Mailing Address: P.O. Box 90, Zip 23970-0090; tel. 804/447-3151; W. Scott Burnette, President

MARY IMMACULATE HOSPITAL, 2 Bernardine Drive, Newport News, VA, Zip 23602-4499; tel. 757/886-6000; Cynthia B. Farrand, Executive Vice President and Administrator

MEMORIAL REGIONAL MEDICAL CENTER, 8260 Atlee Road, Mechanicsville, VA, Zip 23116, Mailing Address: P.O. Box 26783, Richmond, Zip 23261-6783; tel. 804/764-6102; Michael Robinson, Executive Vice President and Administrator

RAPPAHANNOCK GENERAL HOSPITAL, 101 Harris Drive, Kilmarnock, VA, Zip 22482, Mailing Address: P.O. Box 1449, Zip 22482-1449; tel. 804/435-8000; James M. Holmes, President and Chief Executive Officer

SHELTERING ARMS REHABILITATION HOSPITAL, 1311 Palmyra Avenue, Richmond, VA, Zip 23227-4418; tel. 804/342-4100; Jack A. Carroll, Ph.D., President and Chief Executive Officer

SOUTHSIDE REGIONAL MEDICAL CENTER, 801 South Adams Street, Petersburg, VA, Zip 23803-5133; tel. 804/862-5000; David S. Dunham, President

UNIVERSITY OF VIRGINIA MEDICAL CENTER, Jefferson Park Avenue, Charlottesville, VA, Zip 22908, Mailing Address: P.O. Box 800788, Zip 22908-0788; tel. 804/924-0211; William E. Carter, Jr, Senior Associate Vice President for Operations

DEPAUL MEDICAL CENTER GROUP
150 Kingsley Lane, Norfolk, VA 23505; tel. 757/889-5000; David McCombs, President & Chief Executive Officer

BON SECOURS-DEPAUL MEDICAL CENTER, 150 Kingsley Lane, Norfolk, VA, Zip 23505-4650; tel. 757/889-5000; David J. McCombs, Executive Vice President and Administrator

PREFERRED CARE OF RICHMOND
P.O. Box 13739, Richmond, VA 23225; tel. 804/560-4160; Richard Morrow, Network Coordinator

CHIPPENHAM MEDICAL CENTER/JOHNSTON-WILLIS HOSPITAL, 7101 Jahnke Road, Richmond, VA, Zip 23225-4044; tel. 804/320-3911; Marilyn B. Tavenner, Chief Executive Officer

HENRICO DOCTORS' HOSPITAL, 1602 Skipwith Road, Richmond, VA, Zip 23229-5298; tel. 804/289-4500; Patrick W. Farrell, Chief Executive Officer

JOHN RANDOLPH MEDICAL CENTER, 411 West Randolph Road, Hopewell, VA, Zip 23860, Mailing Address: P.O. Box 971, Zip 23860; tel. 804/541-1600; Daniel J. Wetta, Jr, Chief Executive Officer

RETREAT HOSPITAL, 2621 Grove Avenue, Richmond, VA, Zip 23220-4308; tel. 804/254-5100; Paul L. Baldwin, Chief Executive Officer

SENTARA HEALTHCARE
6015 Poplar Hall Dr-Ste306, Norfolk, VA 23502; tel. 757/455-7170; David Bernd, Chief Executive Officer

SENTARA BAYSIDE HOSPITAL, 800 Independence Boulevard, Virginia Beach, VA, Zip 23455-6076; tel. 757/363-6100; Rosemary C. Check, Administrator

SENTARA HAMPTON GENERAL HOSPITAL, 3120 Victoria Boulevard, Hampton, VA, Zip 23661-1585, Mailing Address: Drawer 640, Zip 23669-0640; tel. 757/727-7000; Megan Perry, Administrator

SENTARA LEIGH HOSPITAL, 830 Kempsville Road, Norfolk, VA, Zip 23502-3981; tel. 757/466-6000; Darleen S. Anderson, R.N., MSN, Site Administrator

SENTARA NORFOLK GENERAL HOSPITAL, 600 Gresham Drive, Norfolk, VA, Zip 23507-1999; tel. 757/668-3000; Mark R. Gavens, President

SENTARA VIRGINIA BEACH GENERAL HOSPITAL, 1060 First Colonial Road, Virginia Beach, VA, Zip 23454-9000; tel. 757/395-8000; Robert L. Graves, Administrator

WILLIAMSBURG COMMUNITY HOSPITAL, 301 Monticello Avenue, Williamsburg, VA, Zip 23187-8700, Mailing Address: Box 8700, Zip 23187-8700; tel. 757/259-6000; Les A. Donahue, President and Chief Executive Officer

Networks / Health Parners Network, Iknc.

TIDEWATER HEALTH CARE
1080 First Colonial Road, Virginia Beach, VA 23454; tel. 757/496–6100; Douglas L. Johnson, Ph. D., President/ Chief Executive Officer

SENTARA VIRGINIA BEACH GENERAL HOSPITAL, 1060 First Colonial Road, Virginia Beach, VA, Zip 23454–9000; tel. 757/395–8000; Robert L. Graves, Administrator

VALLEY HEALTH SYSTEM
P.O. Box 3340, Winchester, VA 22604; tel. 703/722–8024; Michael Halseth, Chief Executive Officer

WARREN MEMORIAL HOSPITAL, 1000 Shenandoah Avenue, Front Royal, VA, Zip 22630–3598; tel. 540/636–0300; Charlie M. Horton, President

WINCHESTER MEDICAL CENTER, 1840 Amherst Street, Winchester, VA, Zip 22601–2540, Mailing Address: P.O. Box 3340, Zip 22604–3340; tel. 540/722–8000; George B. Caley, President

VIRGINIA HEALTH NETWORK
7400 Beaufont Springs Drive, Suite 505, Richmond, VA 23225; tel. 804/320–3837; David Keplinger, Marketing Vice President

AUGUSTA HEALTH CARE, 96 Medical Center Drive, Fishersville, VA, Zip 22939, Mailing Address: P.O. Box 1000, Zip 22939–1000; tel. 540/932–4000; Richard H. Graham, President and Chief Executive Officer

BON SECOURS ST. MARY'S HOSPITAL, 5801 Bremo Road, Richmond, VA, Zip 23226–1900; tel. 804/285–2011; Ann E. Honeycutt, Executive Vice President and Administrator

BON SECOURS–DEPAUL MEDICAL CENTER, 150 Kingsley Lane, Norfolk, VA, Zip 23505–4650; tel. 757/889–5000; David J. McCombs, Executive Vice President and Administrator

BON SECOURS–RICHMOND COMMUNITY HOSPITAL, 1500 North 28th Street, Richmond, VA, Zip 23223–5396, Mailing Address: Box 27184, Zip 23261–7184; tel. 804/225–1700; Eugene Toomer, Chief Operating Officer

BON SECOURS–STUART CIRCLE, 413 Stuart Circle, Richmond, VA, Zip 23220–3799; tel. 804/358–7051; Ann E. Honeycutt, Executive Vice President and Administrator

CHARTER BEHAVIORAL HEALTH SYSTEM OF CHARLOTTESVILLE, 2101 Arlington Boulevard, Charlottesville, VA, Zip 22903–1593; tel. 804/977–1120; David Carlini, Chief Executive Officer

CHESAPEAKE GENERAL HOSPITAL, 736 Battlefield Boulevard North, Chesapeake, VA, Zip 23320–4941, Mailing Address: P.O. Box 2028, Zip 23327–2028; tel. 757/312–8121; Donald S. Buckley, FACHE, President

CHILDREN'S HOSPITAL OF THE KING'S DAUGHTERS, 601 Children's Lane, Norfolk, VA, Zip 23507–1971; tel. 757/668–7700; Robert I. Bonar, Jr, President and Chief Executive Officer

COMMUNITY MEMORIAL HEALTHCENTER, 125 Buena Vista Circle, South Hill, VA, Zip 23970–0090, Mailing Address: P.O. Box 90, Zip 23970–0090; tel. 804/447–3151; W. Scott Burnette, President

GREENSVILLE MEMORIAL HOSPITAL, 214 Weaver Avenue, Emporia, VA, Zip 23847–1482; tel. 804/348–2000; Gene Faile, Chief Executive Officer

HEALTHSOUTH REHABILITATION HOSPITAL OF VIRGINIA, 5700 Fitzhugh Avenue, Richmond, VA, Zip 23226–1800; tel. 804/288–5700; Jeff Ruskan, Administrator

LOUISE OBICI MEMORIAL HOSPITAL, 1900 North Main Street, Suffolk, VA, Zip 23434–4323, Mailing Address: P.O. Box 1100, Zip 23439–1100; tel. 757/934–4000; William C. Giermak, President and Chief Executive Officer

MARTHA JEFFERSON HOSPITAL, 459 Locust Avenue, Charlottesville, VA, Zip 22902–9940; tel. 804/982–7000; James E. Haden, President and Chief Executive Officer

MARY IMMACULATE HOSPITAL, 2 Bernardine Drive, Newport News, VA, Zip 23602–4499; tel. 757/886–6000; Cynthia B. Farrand, Executive Vice President and Administrator

MARY WASHINGTON HOSPITAL, 1001 Sam Perry Boulevard, Fredericksburg, VA, Zip 22401–3354; tel. 540/899–1100; Fred M. Rankin, II, President and Chief Executive Officer

MARYVIEW MEDICAL CENTER, 3636 High Street, Portsmouth, VA, Zip 23707–3236; tel. 757/398–2200; Wayne Jones, Executive Vice President and Administrator

MEDICAL COLLEGE OF VIRGINIA HOSPITALS, VIRGINIA COMMONWEALTH UNIVERSITY, 401 North 12th Street, Richmond, VA, Zip 23219, Mailing Address: P.O. Box 980510, Zip 23298–0510; tel. 804/828–9000; Carl R. Fischer, Associate Vice President and Chief Executive Officer

MEMORIAL REGIONAL MEDICAL CENTER, 8260 Atlee Road, Mechanicsville, VA, Zip 23116, Mailing Address: P.O. Box 26783, Richmond, Zip 23261–6783; tel. 804/764–6102; Michael Robinson, Executive Vice President and Administrator

RIVERSIDE REGIONAL MEDICAL CENTER, 500 J. Clyde Morris Boulevard, Newport News, VA, Zip 23601–1976; tel. 757/594–2000; M. Caroline Martin, President

RIVERSIDE TAPPAHANNOCK HOSPITAL, 618 Hospital Road, Tappahannock, VA, Zip 22560; tel. 804/443–3311; Elizabeth J. Martin, Vice President and Administrator

RIVERSIDE WALTER REED HOSPITAL, 7519 Hospital Drive, Gloucester, VA, Zip 23061–4178, Mailing Address: P.O. Box 1130, Zip 23061–1130; tel. 804/693–8800; Grady W. Philips, II, Vice President and Administrator

SENTARA NORFOLK GENERAL HOSPITAL, 600 Gresham Drive, Norfolk, VA, Zip 23507–1999; tel. 757/668–3000; Mark R. Gavens, President

SENTARA VIRGINIA BEACH GENERAL HOSPITAL, 1060 First Colonial Road, Virginia Beach, VA, Zip 23454–9000; tel. 757/395–8000; Robert L. Graves, Administrator

SHELTERING ARMS REHABILITATION HOSPITAL, 1311 Palmyra Avenue, Richmond, VA, Zip 23227–4418; tel. 804/342–4100; Jack A. Carroll, Ph.D., President and Chief Executive Officer

SOUTHAMPTON MEMORIAL HOSPITAL, 100 Fairview Drive, Franklin, VA, Zip 23851–1206, Mailing Address: P.O. Box 817, Zip 23851–0817; tel. 757/569–6100; Gwen S. Eddleman, R.N., Interim Chief Executive Officer

SOUTHSIDE REGIONAL MEDICAL CENTER, 801 South Adams Street, Petersburg, VA, Zip 23803–5133; tel. 804/862–5000; David S. Dunham, President

UNIVERSITY OF VIRGINIA MEDICAL CENTER, Jefferson Park Avenue, Charlottesville, VA, Zip 22908, Mailing Address: P.O. Box 800788, Zip 22908–0788; tel. 804/924–0211; William E. Carter, Jr, Senior Associate Vice President for Operations

WILLIAMSBURG COMMUNITY HOSPITAL, 301 Monticello Avenue, Williamsburg, VA, Zip 23187–8700, Mailing Address: Box 8700, Zip 23187–8700; tel. 757/259–6000; Les A. Donahue, President and Chief Executive Officer

WASHINGTON

GROUP HEALTH COOP OF PUGENT SOUND
521 Wall Street, Seattle, WA 98121; tel. 206/326–3000; Phil Nudelman, PhD, President & Chief Executive Officer

THE EASTSIDE HOSPITAL, 2700 152nd Avenue N.E., Redmond, WA, Zip 98052–5560; tel. 425/883–5151; Patricia Kennedy-Scott, Northern Region Vice President

LINCOLN COUNTY PUBLIC HEALTH
90 Nicholls, Davenport, WA 99122; tel. 509/725–1001; Rand Masteller, Administrator

LINCOLN HOSPITAL, 10 Nichols Street, Davenport, WA, Zip 99122; tel. 509/725–7101; Thomas J. Martin, Administrator

ODESSA MEMORIAL HOSPITAL, 502 East Amende, Odessa, WA, Zip 99159–0368, Mailing Address: P.O. Box 368, Zip 99159–0368; tel. 509/982–2611; Jon R. Davis, Administrator

MULTICARE HEALTH SYSTEM
P.O. Box 5299, Tacoma, WA 98415; tel. 253/403–1000; Diane Cecchettini, President

MARY BRIDGE CHILDREN'S HOSPITAL AND HEALTH CENTER, 317 Martin Luther King Jr. Way, Tacoma, WA, Zip 98405–0299, Mailing Address: Box 5299, Zip 98405–0299; tel. 253/403–1400; Diane Cecchettini, President and Chief Executive Officer

TACOMA GENERAL HOSPITAL, 315 Martin Luther King Jr. Way, Tacoma, WA, Zip 98405–0299, Mailing Address: P.O. Box 5299, Zip 98405–0299; tel. 253/403–1000; Diane Cecchettini, President and Chief Executive Officer

WEST VIRGINIA

CAMDEN–CLARK MEMORIAL HOSPITAL
P.O. Box 718, Parkersburg, WV 26102; tel. 304/424–2111; Iris McCrady, Network Contact

CAMDEN–CLARK MEMORIAL HOSPITAL, 800 Garfield Avenue, Parkersburg, WV, Zip 26101, Mailing Address: P.O. Box 718, Zip 26102–0718; tel. 304/424–2111; Thomas J. Corder, President and Chief Executive Officer

SISTERSVILLE GENERAL HOSPITAL, 314 South Wells Street, Sistersville, WV, Zip 26175–1098; tel. 304/652–2611; F. David Richardson, Ph.D., Chief Executive Officer

EASTERN PANHANDLE INTERGRATED DELIVERY SYSTEM
P.O. Box 758, Martinsburg, WV 25402; tel. 304/262–0201; Joseph Zarbo, Administrator

CITY HOSPITAL, Dry Run Road, Martinsburg, WV, Zip 25401, Mailing Address: P.O. Box 1418, Zip 25402–1418; tel. 304/264–1000; Jon D. Applebaum, Chief Executive Officer

GRANT MEMORIAL HOSPITAL, Route 55 West, Petersburg, WV, Zip 26847, Mailing Address: P.O. Box 1019, Zip 26847–1019; tel. 304/257–1026; Robert L. Harman, Administrator

JEFFERSON MEMORIAL HOSPITAL, 300 South Preston Street, Ranson, WV, Zip 25438–1699; tel. 304/728–1600; John M. Sherwood, FACHE, Chief Executive Officer

MORGAN COUNTY WAR MEMORIAL HOSPITAL, 1124 Fairfax Street, Berkeley Springs, WV, Zip 25411–1718; tel. 304/258–1234; Patrick Nolan, Administrator

HEALTH PARNERS NETWORK, IKNC.
1000 Technology Drive, Suite 2320, Fairmont, WV 26554; tel. 304/368–2740; William G. Maclean, Chief Operating Officer

BROADDUS HOSPITAL, College Hill, Philippi, WV, Zip 26416–1051; tel. 304/457–1760; Susannah Higgins, Chief Executive Officer

CAMDEN–CLARK MEMORIAL HOSPITAL, 800 Garfield Avenue, Parkersburg, WV, Zip 26101, Mailing Address: P.O. Box 718, Zip 26102–0718; tel. 304/424–2111; Thomas J. Corder, President and Chief Executive Officer

DAVIS MEMORIAL HOSPITAL, Gorman Avenue and Reed Street, Elkins, WV, Zip 26241, Mailing Address: P.O. Box 1484, Zip 26241–1484; tel. 304/636–3300; Robert L. Hammer, II, Chief Executive Officer

FAIRMONT GENERAL HOSPITAL, 1325 Locust Avenue, Fairmont, WV, Zip 26554–1435; tel. 304/367–7100; Richard W. Graham, FACHE, President and Chief Executive Officer

GRAFTON CITY HOSPITAL, 500 Market Street, Grafton, WV, Zip 26354–1187; tel. 304/265–0400; Gary R. Willmon, Administrator

HEALTHSOUTH HUNTINGTON REHABILITATION HOSPITAL, 6900 West Country Club Drive, Huntington, WV, Zip 25705–2000; tel. 304/733–1060; John Forester, Chief Operating Officer

Networks / Health Parners Network, Iknc.

HEALTHSOUTH MOUNTAINVIEW REGIONAL REHABILITATION HOSPITAL, 1160 Van Voorhis Road, Morgantown, WV, Zip 26505–3435; tel. 304/598–1100; Teresa K. Stranko, Chief Executive Officer

HEALTHSOUTH WESTERN HILLS REGIONAL REHABILITATION HOSPITAL, 3 Western Hills Drive, Parkersburg, WV, Zip 26101–8122; tel. 304/420–1300; Thomas Heller, Administrator

MINNIE HAMILTON HEALTHCARE CENTER, High Street, Grantsville, WV, Zip 26147, Mailing Address: Route 1, Box 1A, Zip 26147; tel. 304/354–9244; Barbara Lay, Administrator

ST. JOSEPH'S HOSPITAL OF BUCKHANNON, Amalia Drive, Buckhannon, WV, Zip 26201–2222; tel. 304/473–2000; Wayne B. Griffith, FACHE, Chief Executive Officer

STONEWALL JACKSON MEMORIAL HOSPITAL, Weston, WV, Mailing Address: Route 4, Box 10, Zip 26452; tel. 304/269–8000; David D. Shaffer, Chief Executive Officer

UNITED HOSPITAL CENTER, Route 19 South, Clarksburg, WV, Zip 26301, Mailing Address: P.O. Box 1680, Zip 26302–1680; tel. 304/624–2121; Bruce C. Carter, President

WEBSTER COUNTY MEMORIAL HOSPITAL, 324 Miller Mountain Drive, Webster Springs, WV, Zip 26288–1087; tel. 304/847–5682; Stephen M. Gavalchik, Administrator

WEST VIRGINIA UNIVERSITY HOSPITALS, Medical Center Drive, Morgantown, WV, Zip 26506–4749; tel. 304/598–4000; Bruce McClymonds, President

INTEGRATED PROVIDER NETWORK
7000 Hampton Center, Suite F., Morgantown, WV 26505; tel. 304/598–3911; Brad Minton, Network Contact

UNITED HOSPITAL CENTER, Route 19 South, Clarksburg, WV, Zip 26301, Mailing Address: P.O. Box 1680, Zip 26302–1680; tel. 304/624–2121; Bruce C. Carter, President

WEST VIRGINIA UNIVERSITY HOSPITALS, Medical Center Drive, Morgantown, WV, Zip 26506–4749; tel. 304/598–4000; Bruce McClymonds, President

PARTNERS IN HEALTH NETWORK, INC
3411 Virginia Avenue, S.E., Charleston, WV 25304; tel. 304/388–7385; Scot Mitchell, Chief Executive Officer

BOONE MEMORIAL HOSPITAL, 701 Madison Avenue, Madison, WV, Zip 25130–1699; tel. 304/369–1230; Tommy H. Mullins, Administrator

BRAXTON COUNTY MEMORIAL HOSPITAL, 100 Hoylman Drive, Gassaway, WV, Zip 26624–9320; tel. 304/364–5156; Tony E. Atkins, Administrator

CHARLESTON AREA MEDICAL CENTER, 501 Morris Street, Charleston, WV, Zip 25301–1300, Mailing Address: P.O. Box 1547, Zip 25326–1547; tel. 304/348–5432; Phillip H. Goodwin, FACHE, President and Chief Executive Officer

EYE AND EAR CLINIC OF CHARLESTON, 1306 Kanawha Boulevard East, Charleston, WV, Zip 25301, Mailing Address: P.O. Box 2271, Zip 25328–2271; tel. 304/343–4371; W. Allen Shelton, II, Administrator and Chief Executive Officer

JACKSON GENERAL HOSPITAL, Pinnell Street, Ripley, WV, Zip 25271, Mailing Address: P.O. Box 720, Zip 25271–0720; tel. 304/372–2731; Richard L. Rohaley, President and Chief Executive Officer

MINNIE HAMILTON HEALTHCARE CENTER, High Street, Grantsville, WV, Zip 26147, Mailing Address: Route 1, Box 1A, Zip 26147; tel. 304/354–9244; Barbara Lay, Administrator

MONTGOMERY GENERAL HOSPITAL, 401 Sixth Avenue, Montgomery, WV, Zip 25136–0270, Mailing Address: P.O. Box 270, Zip 25136–0270; tel. 304/442–5151; William R. Laird, IV, President and Chief Executive Officer

PLATEAU MEDICAL CENTER, 430 Main Street, Oak Hill, WV, Zip 25901–3455; tel. 304/469–8600; Hank Woodson, Administrator

RICHWOOD AREA COMMUNITY HOSPITAL, Riverside Addition, Richwood, WV, Zip 26261; tel. 304/846–2573; Eugene Underwood, Chief Executive Officer

ROANE GENERAL HOSPITAL, 200 Hospital Drive, Spencer, WV, Zip 25276–1060; tel. 304/927–4444; Lewis Newberry, Chief Executive Officer

SOUTHERN VIRGINIA RURAL
500 A. Cherry Street, Suite 7, Bluefield, WV 24701; tel. 304/324–7123; Jean Henshaw, Network Coordinator

BLUEFIELD REGIONAL MEDICAL CENTER, 500 Cherry Street, Bluefield, WV, Zip 24701–3390; tel. 304/327–1100; Eugene P. Pawlowski, President

PRINCETON COMMUNITY HOSPITAL, 12th Street, Princeton, WV, Zip 24740–1369, Mailing Address: P.O. Box 1369, Zip 24740–1369; tel. 304/487–7000; Daniel C. Dunmyer, Chief Executive Officer

TRI-STATE COMMUNITY CARE
601 Colliers Way, Weirton, WV 26062; tel. 304/797–6413; Cynthia R. Nixon, Chief Financial Officer

WEIRTON MEDICAL CENTER, 601 Colliers Way, Weirton, WV, Zip 26062–5091; tel. 304/797–6000; Donald Muhlenthaler, FACHE, President and Chief Executive Officer

WISCONSIN

AFFINITY HEALTH SYSTEM, INC (CORPORATE OFFICES)
1570 Midway Place, Menash, WI 54954; tel. 920/720–1713; Kevin E. Nolan, Chief Executive Officer

MERCY MEDICAL CENTER, 631 Hazel Street, Oshkosh, WI, Zip 54901–4680, Mailing Address: P.O. Box 1100, Zip 54902–1100; tel. 920/236–2000; Otto L. Cox, President

ST. ELIZABETH HOSPITAL, 1506 South Oneida Street, Appleton, WI, Zip 54915–1397; tel. 920/738–2000; Robert J. Turner, Chief Operating Officer

ALL SAINTS HEALTHCARE SYSTEM
3801 Spring Street, Racine, WI 53405; tel. 414/636–4860; Ed DeMeulenaere, President

ALL SAINT'S HEALTHCARE SYSTEM, 3801 Spring Street, Racine, WI, Zip 53405–1690; tel. 262/636–4011; Kenneth R. Buser, President and Chief Executive Officer

ST. LUKE'S MEMORIAL HOSPITAL, 1320 Wisconsin Avenue, Racine, WI, Zip 53403–1987; tel. 262/636–2011; Kenneth R. Buser, President and Chief Executive Officer

COLUMBIA– ST. MARY'S, INC.
2025 East Newport Avenue, Milwaukee, WI 53211; tel. 414/961–3638; Paul Westrick, Vice President Planning/Marketing

COLUMBIA HOSPITAL, 2025 East Newport Avenue, Milwaukee, WI, Zip 53211–2990; tel. 414/961–3300; Susan Henckel, Executive Vice President and Chief Operating Officer

SACRED HEART REHABILITATION INSTITUTE, 2350 North Lake Drive, Milwaukee, WI, Zip 53211–4507, Mailing Address: P.O. Box 392, Zip 53201–0392; tel. 414/298–6700; Nancy D. Kuelz, Administrator

ST. MARY'S HOSPITAL, 2323 North Lake Drive, Milwaukee, WI, Zip 53211–9682, Mailing Address: P.O. Box 503, Zip 53201–0503; tel. 414/291–1000; Susan Henckel, Chief Operating Officer

ST. MARY'S HOSPITAL OZAUKEE, 13111 North Port Washington Road, Mequon, WI, Zip 53097–2416; tel. 262/243–7300; Therese B. Pandl, Executive Vice President and Chief Operating Officer

COMMUNITY HEALTH CARE, INC
425 Pine Ridge Boulevard, Wausau, WI 54401; tel. 715/847–2118; Paul A. Spaude, Chief Administrative Officer

GOOD SAMARITAN HEALTH CENTER OF MERRILL, 601 Center Avenue South, Merrill, WI, Zip 54452–3404; tel. 715/536–5511; Michael Hammer, President and Chief Executive Officer

LANGLADE MEMORIAL HOSPITAL, 112 East Fifth Avenue, Antigo, WI, Zip 54409–2796; tel. 715/623–2331; David R. Schneider, Executive Director

MEMORIAL HOSPITAL OF TAYLOR COUNTY, 135 South Gibson Street, Medford, WI, Zip 54451–1696; tel. 715/748–8100; Greg Roraff, President and Chief Executive Officer

UNIVERSITY OF WISCONSIN HOSPITAL AND CLINICS, 600 Highland Avenue, Madison, WI, Zip 53792–0002; tel. 608/263–6400; Gordon M. Derzon, Chief Executive Officer

WAUSAU HOSPITAL, 333 Pine Ridge Boulevard, Wausau, WI, Zip 54401–4187, Mailing Address: P.O. Box 1847, Zip 54402–1847; tel. 715/847–2121; Paul A. Spaude, President and Chief Executive Officer

COMMUNITY HEALTH NETWORK, INC
225 Memorial Drive, Berlin, WI 54923; tel. 414/361–5580; Craig W. C. Schmidt, President & Chief Executive Officer

BERLIN MEMORIAL HOSPITAL, 225 Memorial Drive, Berlin, WI, Zip 54923–1295; tel. 920/361–1313; Craig W. C. Schmidt, President and Chief Executive Officer

WILD ROSE COMMUNITY MEMORIAL HOSPITAL, 601 Grove Avenue, Wild Rose, WI, Zip 54984, Mailing Address: P.O. Box 243, Zip 54984–0243; tel. 920/622–3257; Craig W. C. Schmidt, President and Chief Executive Officer

COVENANT HEALTHCARE SYSTEM, INC.
1126 South 70th Street, Suite S306, Milwaukee, WI 53214; tel. 414/456–2300; E. Thomas Sheahan, President & Chief Executive Officer

ELMBROOK MEMORIAL HOSPITAL, 19333 West North Avenue, Brookfield, WI, Zip 53045–4198; tel. 262/785–2000; Kimry A. Johnsrud, President

MARQUETTE GENERAL HEALTH SYSTEM, 580 West College Avenue, Marquette, MI, Zip 49855–2794; tel. 906/228–9440; William Nemacheck, Chief Executive Officer

ST. FRANCIS HOSPITAL, 3237 South 16th Street, Milwaukee, WI, Zip 53215–4592; tel. 414/647–5000; Jerrold A. Maki, President

ST. JOSEPH'S HOSPITAL, 5000 West Chambers Street, Milwaukee, WI, Zip 53210–9988; tel. 414/447–2000; Patricia A. Kaldor, R.N., President

ST. JOSEPH'S HOSPITAL BLUEMOUND, 10010 West Bluemound Road, Wauwatosa, WI, Zip 53226; tel. 414/259–7200; J. E. Race, Administrator and Chief Executive Officer

ST. MICHAEL HOSPITAL, 2400 West Villard Avenue, Milwaukee, WI, Zip 53209–4999; tel. 414/527–8000; Jeffrey K. Jenkins, President

ST. NICHOLAS HOSPITAL, 1601 North Taylor Drive, Sheboygan, WI, Zip 53081–2496; tel. 920/459–8300; Michael J. Stenger, Executive Vice President and Administrator

FELICIAN HEALTH CARE, INC.
3237 South 16th, Milwaukee, WI 53215; tel. 414/647–5622; Sister Mary Clarette, President of Felician Health

ST. FRANCIS HOSPITAL, 3237 South 16th Street, Milwaukee, WI, Zip 53215–4592; tel. 414/647–5000; Jerrold A. Maki, President

ST. MARY'S HOSPITAL, 400 North Pleasant Avenue, Centralia, IL, Zip 62801–3091; tel. 618/532–6731; James W. McDowell, President

FRANCISCAN SKEMP HEALTHCARE
700 West Avenue S., LaCrosse, WI 54601; tel. 608/791–9710; Glenn Forbes, MD, President/Chief Executive Officer

FRANCISCAN SKEMP HEALTHCARE–ARCADIA CAMPUS, 464 South St. Joseph Avenue, Arcadia, WI, Zip 54612–1401; tel. 608/323–3341; Robert M. Tracey, Administrator

Networks / University of Wisconsin Hosp & Clinics

FRANCISCAN SKEMP HEALTHCARE–LA CROSSE CAMPUS, 700 West Avenue South, La Crosse, WI, Zip 54601–4783; tel. 608/785–0940; Glenn Forbes, M.D., President and Chief Executive Officer

FRANCISCAN SKEMP HEALTHCARE–SPARTA CAMPUS, 310 West Main Street, Sparta, WI, Zip 54656–2171; tel. 608/269–2132; William P. Sexton, Administrator

HEALTH CARE NETWORK OF WISCONSIN
250 Bishops Way, Suite 300, Brookfield, WI 53005; tel. 414/784–0223; Jim Wrocklage, President

AGNESIAN HEALTHCARE, 430 East Division Street, Fond Du Lac, WI, Zip 54935–0385, Mailing Address: P.O. Box 385, Zip 54936–0385; tel. 920/929–2300; Robert A. Fale, President and Chief Executive Officer

BURNETT MEDICAL CENTER, 257 West St. George Avenue, Grantsburg, WI, Zip 54840–7827; tel. 715/463–5353; Timothy J. Wick, Chief Executive Officer

CHILDREN'S HOSPITAL OF WISCONSIN, 9000 West Wisconsin Avenue, Milwaukee, WI, Zip 53226–4810, Mailing Address: P.O. Box 1997, Zip 53201–1997; tel. 414/266–2000; Jon E. Vice, President and Chief Executive Officer

COLUMBIA HOSPITAL, 2025 East Newport Avenue, Milwaukee, WI, Zip 53211–2990; tel. 414/961–3300; Susan Henckel, Executive Vice President and Chief Operating Officer

COMMUNITY MEMORIAL HOSPITAL, W180 N8085 Town Hall Road, Menomonee Falls, WI, Zip 53051, Mailing Address: P.O. Box 408, Zip 53052–0408; tel. 262/251–1000; Robert E. Drisner, President and Chief Executive Officer

COMMUNITY MEMORIAL HOSPITAL, 855 South Main Street, Oconto Falls, WI, Zip 54154–1296; tel. 920/846–3444; Jim Van Dornick, Administrator

ELMBROOK MEMORIAL HOSPITAL, 19333 West North Avenue, Brookfield, WI, Zip 53045–4198; tel. 262/785–2000; Kimry A. Johnsrud, President

FROEDTERT MEMORIAL LUTHERAN HOSPITAL, 9200 West Wisconsin Avenue, Milwaukee, WI, Zip 53226–3596, Mailing Address: P.O. Box 26099, Zip 53226–3596; tel. 414/259–3000; William D. Petasnick, President

HARTFORD MEMORIAL HOSPITAL, 1032 East Sumner Street, Hartford, WI, Zip 53027–1698; tel. 262/673–2300; Mark Schwartz, Administrator

HUDSON MEDICAL CENTER, 400 Wisconsin Street, Hudson, WI, Zip 54016–1600; tel. 715/386–9321; Marian M. Furlong, R.N., Chief Executive Officer

MEMORIAL HOSPITAL CORPORATION OF BURLINGTON, 252 McHenry Street, Burlington, WI, Zip 53105–1828; tel. 262/767–6000; Lief Erickson, M.D., President

OCONOMOWOC MEMORIAL HOSPITAL, 791 Summit Avenue, Oconomowoc, WI, Zip 53066–3896; tel. 262/569–9400; Douglas Guy, President and Chief Executive Officer

SHEBOYGAN MEMORIAL MEDICAL CENTER, 2629 North Seventh Street, Sheboygan, WI, Zip 53083–4998; tel. 920/451–5000; T. Gregg Watson, Administrator

SINAI SAMARITAN MEDICAL CENTER, 945 North 12th Street, Milwaukee, WI, Zip 53233–1337, Mailing Address: P.O. Box 342, Zip 53201–0342; tel. 414/219–2000; Leonard E. Wilk, Administrator

ST. CATHERINE'S HOSPITAL, 3556 Seventh Avenue, Kenosha, WI, Zip 53140–2595; tel. 262/656–2011; Richard O. Schmidt, Jr, President and Chief Executive Officer

ST. CLARE HOSPITAL AND HEALTH SERVICES, 707 14th Street, Baraboo, WI, Zip 53913–1597; tel. 608/356–1400; David B. Jordahl, FACHE, President

ST. CROIX REGIONAL MEDICAL CENTER, 204 South Adams Street, Saint Croix Falls, WI, Zip 54024–9400; tel. 715/483–3261; Steve L. Urosevich, Chief Executive Officer

ST. FRANCIS HOSPITAL, 3237 South 16th Street, Milwaukee, WI, Zip 53215–4592; tel. 414/647–5000; Jerrold A. Maki, President

ST. JOSEPH'S COMMUNITY HOSPITAL OF WEST BEND, 551 South Silverbrook Drive, West Bend, WI, Zip 53095–3898; tel. 414/334–5533; Gregory T. Burns, Executive Director

ST. JOSEPH'S HOSPITAL, 5000 West Chambers Street, Milwaukee, WI, Zip 53210–9988; tel. 414/447–2000; Patricia A. Kaldor, R.N., President

ST. LUKE'S MEDICAL CENTER, 2900 West Oklahoma Avenue, Milwaukee, WI, Zip 53215–4330, Mailing Address: P.O. Box 2901, Zip 53201–2901; tel. 414/649–6000; Mark S. Wiener, Administrator

ST. LUKE'S MEMORIAL HOSPITAL, 1320 Wisconsin Avenue, Racine, WI, Zip 53403–1987; tel. 262/636–2011; Kenneth R. Buser, President and Chief Executive Officer

ST. MARY'S HOSPITAL, 2323 North Lake Drive, Milwaukee, WI, Zip 53211–9682, Mailing Address: P.O. Box 503, Zip 53201–0503; tel. 414/291–1000; Susan Henckel, Chief Operating Officer

ST. MARY'S HOSPITAL OF SUPERIOR, 3500 Tower Avenue, Superior, WI, Zip 54880–5395; tel. 715/392–8281; Terry Jacobson, Administrator

ST. MARYS HOSPITAL MEDICAL CENTER, 707 South Mills Street, Madison, WI, Zip 53715–0450; tel. 608/251–6100; Gerald W. Lefert, President

ST. MICHAEL HOSPITAL, 2400 West Villard Avenue, Milwaukee, WI, Zip 53209–4999; tel. 414/527–8000; Jeffrey K. Jenkins, President

VALLEY VIEW MEDICAL CENTER, 901 Reed Street, Plymouth, WI, Zip 53073–2409; tel. 920/893–1771; T. Gregg Watson, Administrator

WAUKESHA MEMORIAL HOSPITAL, 725 American Avenue, Waukesha, WI, Zip 53188–5099; tel. 262/928–1000; Rexford W. Titus, II, President and Chief Executive Officer

WAUPUN MEMORIAL HOSPITAL, 620 West Brown Street, Waupun, WI, Zip 53963–1799; tel. 920/324–5581; James E. Baer, FACHE, President

WEST ALLIS MEMORIAL HOSPITAL, 8901 West Lincoln Avenue, West Allis, WI, Zip 53227–0901, Mailing Address: P.O. Box 27901, Zip 53227–0901; tel. 414/328–6000; Richard A. Kellar, Administrator

HORIZON HEALTHCARE INC
2300 North Mayfair Road Suite 550, Milwaukee, WI 53226; tel. 414/257–3888; Sis. Renee Rose, President & Chief Executive Officer

COLUMBIA HOSPITAL, 2025 East Newport Avenue, Milwaukee, WI, Zip 53211–2990; tel. 414/961–3300; Susan Henckel, Executive Vice President and Chief Operating Officer

COMMUNITY MEMORIAL HOSPITAL, W180 N8085 Town Hall Road, Menomonee Falls, WI, Zip 53051, Mailing Address: P.O. Box 408, Zip 53052–0408; tel. 262/251–1000; Robert E. Drisner, President and Chief Executive Officer

FROEDTERT MEMORIAL LUTHERAN HOSPITAL, 9200 West Wisconsin Avenue, Milwaukee, WI, Zip 53226–3596, Mailing Address: P.O. Box 26099, Zip 53226–3596; tel. 414/259–3000; William D. Petasnick, President

KENOSHA HOSPITAL AND MEDICAL CENTER, 6308 Eighth Avenue, Kenosha, WI, Zip 53143–5082; tel. 262/656–2011; Richard O. Schmidt, Jr, President and Chief Executive Officer

ST. MARY'S HOSPITAL, 2323 North Lake Drive, Milwaukee, WI, Zip 53211–9682, Mailing Address: P.O. Box 503, Zip 53201–0503; tel. 414/291–1000; Susan Henckel, Chief Operating Officer

ST. MARY'S HOSPITAL OZAUKEE, 13111 North Port Washington Road, Mequon, WI, Zip 53097–2416; tel. 262/243–7300; Therese B. Pandl, Executive Vice President and Chief Operating Officer

LUTHER/MIDELFORT/MAYO HEALTH SYSTEM
733 West Clairmont, Eau Claire, WI 54701; tel. 715/838–6732; William C. Rupp, President & Chief Executive Officer

BARRON MEDICAL CENTER–MAYO HEALTH SYSTEM, 1222 Woodland Avenue, Barron, WI, Zip 54812–1798; tel. 715/537–3186; Mark D. Wilson, Administrator

BLOOMER MEMORIAL MEDICAL CENTER, 1501 Thompson Street, Bloomer, WI, Zip 54724–1299; tel. 715/568–2000; Mary Kerg, Administrator

LUTHER HOSPITAL, 1221 Whipple Street, Eau Claire, WI, Zip 54702–4105, Mailing Address: P.O. Box 5, Zip 54702–0005; tel. 715/838–3311; William Rupp, M.D., President and Chief Executive Officer

OSSEO AREA HOSPITAL AND NURSING HOME, 13025 Eighth Street, Osseo, WI, Zip 54758, Mailing Address: P.O. Box 70, Zip 54758–0070; tel. 715/597–3121; Bradley D. Groseth, Administrator

LUTHERAN HEALTH SYSTEM
1910 South Avenue, LaCrosse, WI 54601; tel. 608/785–0530; Phillip Dahlberg, M.D., President

GUNDERSEN LUTHERAN, 1910 South Avenue, La Crosse, WI, Zip 54601–9980; tel. 608/785–0530; Philip J. Dahlberg, M.D., Chief Executive Officer

TRI–COUNTY MEMORIAL HOSPITAL, 18601 Lincoln Street, Whitehall, WI, Zip 54773–0065; tel. 715/538–4361; Ronald B. Fields, President

MARSHFIELD CLINIC
1000 North Oak Avenue, Marshfield, WI 54449; tel. 715/389–4884; Julie Thompson, Division Administrator

FLAMBEAU HOSPITAL, 98 Sherry Avenue, Park Falls, WI, Zip 54552–1467, Mailing Address: P.O. Box 310, Zip 54552–0310; tel. 715/762–2484; Curtis A. Johnson, Administrator

MINISTRY HEALTH CARE
11925 W. Lake Park Drive, Suite 100, Milwaukee, WI 53224; tel. 414/359–1060; Tim Drinan, Assistant Director of Marketing & Communications

PRAIRIE DU CHIEN PARTNERSHIP
705 East Taylor Street, Prairie du Chien, WI 53821; tel. 608/326–2431; Ellen Zwirlein, Network Contact

PRAIRIE DU CHIEN MEMORIAL HOSPITAL, 705 East Taylor Street, Prairie Du Chien, WI, Zip 53821–2196; tel. 608/326–2431; Harold W. Brown, Chief Executive Officer

PROHEALTH CARE, INC.
725 American Avenue, Waukesha, WI 53188; tel. 414/544–2011; Donald Fundingsland, President

OCONOMOWOC MEMORIAL HOSPITAL, 791 Summit Avenue, Oconomowoc, WI, Zip 53066–3896; tel. 262/569–9400; Douglas Guy, President and Chief Executive Officer

WAUKESHA MEMORIAL HOSPITAL, 725 American Avenue, Waukesha, WI, Zip 53188–5099; tel. 262/928–1000; Rexford W. Titus, II, President and Chief Executive Officer

SOUTHERN WISCONSIN HEALTH CARE SYSTEM
1000 Mineral Point Avenue, Janesville, WI 53547; tel. 608/756–6000; Joseph D. Nemeth, Vice President & Chief Executive Officer

MERCY HEALTH SYSTEM, 1000 Mineral Point Avenue, Janesville, WI, Zip 53547–5003, Mailing Address: P.O. Box 5003, Zip 53547–5003; tel. 608/756–6000; Javon R. Bea, President and Chief Executive Officer

UNIVERSITY OF WISCONSIN HOSP & CLINICS
600 Highland Avenue, Madison, WI 53792; tel. 608/263–6400; Donna Sollenberger, Chief Executive Officer

UNIVERSITY OF WISCONSIN HOSPITAL AND CLINICS, 600 Highland Avenue, Madison, WI, Zip 53792–0002; tel. 608/263–6400; Gordon M. Derzon, Chief Executive Officer

Networks / University of Wisconsin Hosp & Clinics

WYOMING

WYOMING INTEGRATED NETWORK
1233 E. 2nd Street, Casper, WY 82601;
tel. 307/577-2153; Dan Hampton, Network Contact

IVINSON MEMORIAL HOSPITAL, 255 North 30th Street, Laramie, WY, Zip 82070-5195; tel. 307/742-2141; Thomas A. Nord, FACHE, Chief Executive Officer

WYOMING MEDICAL CENTER, 1233 East Second Street, Casper, WY, Zip 82601-2988; tel. 307/577-7201; Michael E. Schrader, President and Chief Executive Officer

Statistics for Multihospital Health Care Systems and their Hospitals

The following tables describing multihospital health care systems refer to information in section B of the 2000/2001 *AHA Guide*.

Table 1 shows the number of multihospital health care systems by type of control. Table 2 provides a breakdown of the number of systems that own, lease, sponsor or contract manage hospitals within each control category. Table 3 gives the number of hospitals and beds in each control category as well as total hospitals and beds. Finally, Table 4 shows the percentage of hospitals and beds in each control category.

For more information on multihospital health care systems, please write to the Section for Health Care Systems, One North Franklin, Chicago, Illinois 60606–3401 or call 312/422–3000.

Table 1. Multihospital Health Care Systems, by Type of Organizaton Control

Type of Control	Code	Number of Systems
Catholic (Roman) church–related	CC	44
Other church–related	CO	11
Subtotal, church–related		55
Other not-for-profit	NP	190
Subtotal, not-for-profit		245
Investor Owned	IO	52
Federal Government	FG	5
Total		302

Table 2. Multihospital Health Care Systems, by Type of Ownership and Control

Type of Ownership	Catholic Church–Related (CC)	Other Church–Related (CO)	Total Church–Related (CC + CO)	Other Not-for-Profit (NP)	Total Not-for-Profit (CC, CO, + NP)	Investor–Owned (IO)	Federal Government	All Systems
Systems that only own, lease or sponsor	34	8	42	161	203	44	5	252
Systems that only contract–manage	0	0	0	3	3	2	0	5
Systems that manage, own, lease, or sponsor	10	3	13	26	39	6	0	45
Total	44	11	55	190	245	52	5	302

Table 3. Hospitals and Beds in Multihospital Health Care Systems, by Type of Ownership and Control

Type of Ownership	Catholic Church–Related (CC)		Other Church–Related (CO)		Total Church–Related (CC + CO)		Other Not-for-Profit (NP)		Total Not-for-Profit (CC, CO, + NP)		Investor–Owned (IO)		Federal Government		All Systems	
	H	B	H	B	H	B	H	B	H	B	H	B	H	B	H	B
Owned, leased or sponsored	513	110,579	89	18,022	602	128,601	986	228,352	1,588	356,953	827	116,439	267	57,104	2,682	530,496
Contract–managed	34	2,469	3	476	37	2,945	114	11,479	151	14,424	243	22,671	0	0	394	37,095
Total	547	113,048	92	18,498	639	131,546	1,100	239,831	1,739	371,377	1,070	139,110	267	57,104	3,076	567,591

H = hospitals; B = beds.

Table 4. Hospitals and Beds in Multihospital Health Care Systems, by Type of Ownership and Control as a Percentage of All Systems

Type of Ownership	Catholic Church–Related (CC)		Other Church–Related (CO)		Total Church–Related (CC + CO)		Other Not-for-Profit (NP)		Total Not-for-Profit (CC, CO, + NP)		Investor–Owned (IO)		Federal Government		All Systems	
	H	B	H	B	H	B	H	B	H	B	H	B	H	B	H	B
Owned, leased or sponsored	19.1	20.8	3.3	3.4	22.4	24.2	36.8	43.0	59.2	67.3	30.8	21.9	10.0	10.8	100.0	100.0
Contract–managed	8.6	6.7	0.8	1.3	9.4	7.9	28.9	30.9	38.3	38.9	61.7	61.1	0.0	0.0	100.0	100.0
Total	17.8	19.9	3.0	3.3	20.8	23.2	35.8	42.3	56.5	65.4	34.8	24.5	8.7	10.1	100.0	100.0

H = hospitals; B = beds.
*Please note that figures may not always equal the provided subtotal or total percentages due to rounding.

Health Care Systems and Their Hospitals

0071: ACCORD HEALTH CARE CORPORATION (IO)
3696 Ulmerton Road, Clearwater, FL Zip 33762;
tel. 727/573–1755; Stephen H. Noble, President

GEORGIA: STEWART–WEBSTER HOSPITAL (O, 25 beds) 300 Alston Street, Richland, GA Zip 31825–1406, Mailing Address: P.O. Box 190, Zip 31825–0190; tel. 912/887–3366; Stephen H. Noble, President

WHEELER COUNTY HOSPITAL (O, 40 beds) 111 Third Street, Glenwood, GA Zip 30428, Mailing Address: P.O. Box 398, Zip 30428–0398; tel. 912/523–5113; Brenda Josey, Administrator

Owned, leased, sponsored:	2 hospitals	65 beds
Contract–managed:	0 hospitals	0 beds
Totals:	2 hospitals	65 beds

★**0235: ADVENTIST HEALTH** (CO)
2100 Douglas Boulevard, Roseville, CA Zip 95661–3898, Mailing Address: P.O. Box 619002, Zip 95661–9002; tel. 916/781–2000; Donald R. Ammon, President
(Moderately Centralized Health System)

CALIFORNIA: CENTRAL VALLEY GENERAL HOSPITAL (O, 40 beds) 1025 North Douty Street, Hanford, CA Zip 93230, Mailing Address: Box 480, Zip 93232; tel. 559/583–2100; Kendall R. Fults, Chief Operating Officer
Web address: www.hanfordhealth.org

FEATHER RIVER HOSPITAL (O, 122 beds) 5974 Pentz Road, Paradise, CA Zip 95969–5593; tel. 530/877–9361; Michael H. Schultz, Chief Executive Officer
Web address: www.adventisthealth.org

FRANK R. HOWARD MEMORIAL HOSPITAL (L, 28 beds) 1 Madrone Street, Willits, CA Zip 95490; tel. 707/459–6801; Kevin R. Erich, President
Web address: www.adventisthealth.org

GLENDALE ADVENTIST MEDICAL CENTER (O, 396 beds) 1509 Wilson Terrace, Glendale, CA Zip 91206–4007; tel. 818/409–8000; Fred M. Manchur, President and Chief Executive Officer
Web address: www.glendaleadventist.com

HANFORD COMMUNITY MEDICAL CENTER (O, 59 beds) 450 Greenfield Avenue, Hanford, CA Zip 93230–0240, Mailing Address: Box 240, Zip 93232–0240; tel. 559/582–9000; Darwin R. Remboldt, President and Chief Executive Officer
Web address: www.adventisthealth.org

PARADISE VALLEY HOSPITAL (O, 130 beds) 2400 East Fourth Street, National City, CA Zip 91950; tel. 619/470–4321; David Butler, Chief Executive Officer
Web address: www.adventisthealth.org

REDBUD COMMUNITY HOSPITAL (O, 40 beds) 18th Avenue and Highway 53, Clearlake, CA Zip 95422, Mailing Address: P.O. Box 6720, Zip 95422; tel. 707/994–6486; Richard D. Hathaway, Chief Operating Officer
Web address: www.adventisthealth.org

SAN JOAQUIN COMMUNITY HOSPITAL (O, 178 beds) 2615 Eye Street, Bakersfield, CA Zip 93301, Mailing Address: Box 2615, Zip 93303–2615; tel. 661/395–3000; Douglas L. Lafferty, President and Chief Executive Officer
Web address: www.adventisthealth.org

SELMA COMMUNITY HOSPITAL (C, 57 beds) 1141 Rose Avenue, Selma, CA Zip 93662–3293; tel. 559/891–2201; Richard L. Rawson, President
Web address: www.adventisthealth.org

SIMI VALLEY HOSPITAL AND HEALTH CARE SERVICES (O, 225 beds) 2975 North Sycamore Drive, Simi Valley, CA Zip 93065–1277; tel. 805/955–6000; Alan J. Rice, President
Web address: www.adventisthealth.org

SONORA COMMUNITY HOSPITAL (O, 118 beds) 1 South Forest Road, Sonora, CA Zip 95370; tel. 209/532–3161; Lary Davis, President
Web address: www.sonoracom.com

SOUTH COAST MEDICAL CENTER (O, 155 beds) 31872 Coast Highway, South Laguna, CA Zip 92677; tel. 949/499–1311; T. Michael Murray, President
Web address: www.southcoastmedcenter.com

ST. HELENA HOSPITAL (O, 168 beds) 650 Sanitarium Road, Deer Park, CA Zip 94576, Mailing Address: P.O. Box 250, Zip 94576; tel. 707/963–3611; JoAline Olson, R.N., President and Chief Executive Officer
Web address: www.sthelenahospital.org

UKIAH VALLEY MEDICAL CENTER (O, 85 beds) 275 Hospital Drive, Ukiah, CA Zip 95482; tel. 707/462–3111; Michael C. Wood, President and Chief Executive Officer
Web address: www.adventisthealth.org

WHITE MEMORIAL MEDICAL CENTER (O, 344 beds) 1720 Cesar E Chavez Avenue, Los Angeles, CA Zip 90033–2481; tel. 323/268–5000; Fred M. Manchur, President and Chief Executive Officer
Web address: www.adventisthealth.org

HAWAII: CASTLE MEDICAL CENTER (O, 157 beds) 640 Ulukahiki Street, Kailua, HI Zip 96734–4498; tel. 808/263–5500; Robert J. Walker, President
Web address: www.cmc.ah.org

OREGON: ADVENTIST MEDICAL CENTER (O, 214 beds) 10123 S.E. Market, Portland, OR Zip 97216–2599; tel. 503/257–2500; Deryl L. Jones, President
Web address: www.adventisthealthnw.com

TILLAMOOK COUNTY GENERAL HOSPITAL (L, 33 beds) 1000 Third Street, Tillamook, OR Zip 97141–3430; tel. 503/842–4444; Wendell Hesseltine, President

WASHINGTON: WALLA WALLA GENERAL HOSPITAL (O, 72 beds) 1025 South Second Avenue, Walla Walla, WA Zip 99362–1398, Mailing Address: Box 1398, Zip 99362–1398; tel. 509/525–0480; Morre Dean, President
Web address: www.wwgh.com

Owned, leased, sponsored:	18 hospitals	2564 beds
Contract–managed:	1 hospital	57 beds
Totals:	19 hospitals	2621 beds

★**4165: ADVENTIST HEALTH SYSTEM SUNBELT HEALTH CARE CORPORATION** (CO)
111 North Orlando Avenue, Winter Park, FL Zip 32789–3675;
tel. 407/975–1417; Thomas L. Werner, President
(Decentralized Health System)

FLORIDA: EAST PASCO MEDICAL CENTER (O, 139 beds) 7050 Gall Boulevard, Zephyrhills, FL Zip 33541–1399; tel. 813/788–0411; Paul Michael Norman, President

FLORIDA HOSPITAL (O, 1389 beds) 601 East Rollins Street, Orlando, FL Zip 32803–1489; tel. 407/896–6611; Donald L. Jernigan, President
Web address: www.flhosp.org

FLORIDA HOSPITAL HEARTLAND DIVISION (O, 195 beds) 4200 Sun'n Lake Boulevard, Sebring, FL Zip 33872, Mailing Address: P.O. Box 9400, Zip 33871–9400; tel. 863/314–4466; John R. Harding, President and Chief Executive Officer
Web address: www.flhosp–heartland.org

FLORIDA HOSPITAL WATERMAN (O, 182 beds) 201 North Eustis Street, Eustis, FL Zip 32726–3488, Mailing Address: P.O. Box B, Zip 32727–0377; tel. 352/589–3333; Kenneth R. Mattison, President and Chief Executive Officer
Web address: www.fhwat.org

GEORGIA: EMORY–ADVENTIST HOSPITAL (O, 54 beds) 3949 South Cobb Drive S.E., Smyrna, GA Zip 30080–6300; tel. 770/434–0710; Dennis Kiley, President

GORDON HOSPITAL (O, 54 beds) 1035 Red Bud Road, Calhoun, GA Zip 30701–2082, Mailing Address: P.O. Box 12938, Zip 30703–7013; tel. 706/629–2895; Carlene Jamerson, President and Chief Executive Officer

For explanation of codes following names, see page B2.
★ *Indicates Type III membership in the American Hospital Association.*

Systems / Albert Einstein Healthcare Network

ILLINOIS: GLENOAKS HOSPITAL (O, 116 beds) 701 Winthrop Avenue, Glendale Heights, IL Zip 60139–1403; tel. 630/545–8000; Brinsley Lewis, Senior Executive Officer
Web address: www.glenoaks.org

HINSDALE HOSPITAL (O, 331 beds) 120 North Oak Street, Hinsdale, IL Zip 60521–3890; tel. 630/856–9000; Ernie W. Sadau, President and Chief Executive Officer
Web address: www.keepingyouwell.com

LA GRANGE MEMORIAL HOSPITAL (O, 231 beds) 5101 South Willow Spring Road, La Grange, IL Zip 60525–2680; tel. 708/352–1200; Todd S. Werner, Senior Executive Officer
Web address: www.ahss.org

KENTUCKY: MEMORIAL HOSPITAL (O, 63 beds) 401 Memorial Drive, Manchester, KY Zip 40962–9156; tel. 606/598–5104; Jimm Bunch, President and Chief Executive Officer

NORTH CAROLINA: PARK RIDGE HOSPITAL (O, 96 beds) Naples Road, Fletcher, NC Zip 28732, Mailing Address: P.O. Box 1569, Zip 28732–1569; tel. 828/684–8501; Michael V. Gentry, President
Web address: www.ahss.org

PUERTO RICO: BELLA VISTA HOSPITAL (C, 157 beds) State Road 349, Mayaguez, PR Zip 00680, Mailing Address: P.O. Box 1750, Zip 00681; tel. 787/834–6000; Ruth M. Ortiz, Chief Operating Officer

TENNESSEE: JELLICO COMMUNITY HOSPITAL (L, 54 beds) 188 Hospital Lane, Jellico, TN Zip 37762–4400; tel. 423/784–7252; Jimm Bunch, President and Chief Executive Officer
Web address: www.ahss.org

TAKOMA ADVENTIST HOSPITAL (O, 80 beds) 401 Takoma Avenue, Greeneville, TN Zip 37743–4647; tel. 423/639–3151; Carlyle L. E. Walton, President

TENNESSEE CHRISTIAN MEDICAL CENTER (O, 288 beds) 500 Hospital Drive, Madison, TN Zip 37115–5032; tel. 615/865–2373; Clint Kreitner, President and Chief Executive Officer

TEXAS: CENTRAL TEXAS MEDICAL CENTER (O, 113 beds) 1301 Wonder World Drive, San Marcos, TX Zip 78666–7544; tel. 512/353–8979; Ken Bacon, President and Chief Executive Officer

HUGULEY MEMORIAL MEDICAL CENTER (O, 189 beds) 11801 South Freeway, Fort Worth, TX Zip 76115, Mailing Address: P.O. Box 6337, Zip 76115–6337; tel. 817/293–9110; Peter M. Weber, President and Chief Executive Officer

METROPLEX ADVENTIST HOSPITAL (O, 213 beds) 2201 South Clear Creek Road, Killeen, TX Zip 76542–9305; tel. 254/526–7523; Kenneth A. Finch, Chief Executive Officer

WISCONSIN: CHIPPEWA VALLEY HOSPITAL AND OAKVIEW CARE CENTER (O, 83 beds) 1220 Third Avenue West, Durand, WI Zip 54736–1600, Mailing Address: P.O. Box 224, Zip 54736–0224; tel. 715/672–4211; Douglas R. Peterson, President and Chief Executive Officer

Owned, leased, sponsored:	18 hospitals	3870 beds
Contract–managed:	1 hospital	157 beds
Totals:	19 hospitals	4027 beds

0214: ADVENTIST HEALTHCARE (IO)
1801 Research Boulevard, Rockville, MD Zip 20850; tel. 301/315–3538; Robert Henderschedt, Chief Executive Officer

MARYLAND: SHADY GROVE ADVENTIST HOSPITAL (O, 253 beds) 9901 Medical Center Drive, Rockville, MD Zip 20850–3395; tel. 301/279–6000; Cory Chambers, President and Chief Executive Officer
Web address: www.adventisthealthcare.com

WASHINGTON ADVENTIST HOSPITAL (O, 300 beds) 7600 Carroll Avenue, Takoma Park, MD Zip 20912–6392; tel. 301/891–7600; Kiltie Leach, Chief Operating Officer
Web address: www.adventisthealthcare.com

Owned, leased, sponsored:	2 hospitals	553 beds
Contract–managed:	0 hospitals	0 beds
Totals:	2 hospitals	553 beds

★**0064: ADVOCATE HEALTH CARE** (NP)
2025 Windsor Drive, Oak Brook, IL Zip 60523; tel. 630/990–5010; Richard R. Risk, President and Chief Executive Officer
(Moderately Centralized Health System)

ILLINOIS: BETHANY HOSPITAL (O, 102 beds) 3435 West Van Buren Street, Chicago, IL Zip 60624–3399; tel. 773/265–7700; Lena Dobbs–Johnson, Chief Executive
Web address: www.advocatehealth.com

CHRIST HOSPITAL AND MEDICAL CENTER (O, 620 beds) 4440 West 95th Street, Oak Lawn, IL Zip 60453–2699; tel. 708/425–8000; Carol Schneider, Chief Executive Officer
Web address: www.advocatehealth.com

GOOD SAMARITAN HOSPITAL (O, 258 beds) 3815 Highland Avenue, Downers Grove, IL Zip 60515–1590; tel. 630/275–5900; Jonathan R. Bruss, Chief Executive
Web address: www.advocatehealth.com

GOOD SHEPHERD HOSPITAL (O, 154 beds) 450 West Highway 22, Barrington, IL Zip 60010–1901; tel. 847/381–9600; Alan Iftiniuk, Chief Executive
Web address: www.advocatehealth.com

LUTHERAN GENERAL HOSPITAL (O, 573 beds) 1775 Dempster Street, Park Ridge, IL Zip 60068–1174; tel. 847/723–2210; Kenneth J. Rojek, Chief Executive
Web address: www.advocatehealth.com

RAVENSWOOD HOSPITAL MEDICAL CENTER (O, 324 beds) 4550 North Winchester Avenue, Chicago, IL Zip 60640–5205; tel. 773/878–4300; John E. Blair, Chief Executive
Web address: www.advocatehealth.com

SOUTH SUBURBAN HOSPITAL (O, 235 beds) 17800 South Kedzie Avenue, Hazel Crest, IL Zip 60429–0989; tel. 708/799–8000; Patricia A. Martin, Chief Executive
Web address: www.advocatehealth.com

TRINITY HOSPITAL (O, 217 beds) 2320 East 93rd Street, Chicago, IL Zip 60617–9984; tel. 773/978–2000; John N. Schwartz, Chief Executive Officer
Web address: www.advocatehealth.com

Owned, leased, sponsored:	8 hospitals	2483 beds
Contract–managed:	0 hospitals	0 beds
Totals:	8 hospitals	2483 beds

0225: ALAMEDA COUNTY HEALTH CARE SERVICES AGENCY (NP)
1850 Fairway Drive, San Leandro, CA Zip 94577; tel. 510/351–1367; David J. Kears, Director

CALIFORNIA: ALAMEDA COUNTY MEDICAL CENTER (O, 193 beds) 15400 Foothill Boulevard, San Leandro, CA Zip 94578–1091; tel. 510/437–4800; Michael L. Walls, Chief Executive Officer

ALAMEDA COUNTY MEDICAL CENTER–HIGHLAND CAMPUS (O, 269 beds) 1411 East 31st Street, Oakland, CA Zip 94602; tel. 510/437–4800; Michael L. Walls, Chief Executive Officer

Owned, leased, sponsored:	2 hospitals	462 beds
Contract–managed:	0 hospitals	0 beds
Totals:	2 hospitals	462 beds

1685: ALBERT EINSTEIN HEALTHCARE NETWORK (NP)
5501 Old York Road, Philadelphia, PA Zip 19141–3098; tel. 215/456–7890; Martin Goldsmith, President
(Moderately Centralized Health System)

PENNSYLVANIA: ALBERT EINSTEIN MEDICAL CENTER (O, 701 beds) 5501 Old York Road, Philadelphia, PA Zip 19141–3098; tel. 215/456–7890; Martin Goldsmith, President

BELMONT CENTER FOR COMPREHENSIVE TREATMENT (O, 146 beds) 4200 Monument Road, Philadelphia, PA Zip 19131–1625; tel. 215/877–2000; Jack H. Dembow, General Director and Vice President

---

For explanation of codes following names, see page B2.
★ Indicates Type III membership in the American Hospital Association.

Systems / Albert Einstein Healthcare Network

Owned, leased, sponsored:	2 hospitals	847 beds
Contract-managed:	0 hospitals	0 beds
Totals:	2 hospitals	847 beds

0065: ALEXIAN BROTHERS HEALTH SYSTEM, INC. (CC)
600 Alexian Way, Elk Grove Village, IL Zip 60007-3395;
tel. 847/640-7550; Brother Thomas Keusenkothen, President and Chief Executive Officer
(Centralized Physician/Insurance Health System)

ILLINOIS: ALEXIAN BROTHERS BEHAVIORAL HEALTH HOSPITAL (O, 94 beds) 1650 Moon Lake Boulevard, Hoffman Estates, IL Zip 60194-5000; tel. 847/882-1600; Mark A. Frey, President and Chief Executive Officer

ALEXIAN BROTHERS MEDICAL CENTER (O, 391 beds) 800 Biesterfield Road, Elk Grove Village, IL Zip 60007-3397; tel. 847/437-5500; Nancy R. Hellyer, President and Chief Executive Officer
Web address: www.alexian.org

ST. ALEXIUS MEDICAL CENTER (O, 194 beds) 1555 Barrington Road, Hoffman Estates, IL Zip 60194; tel. 847/843-2000; Edward M. Goldberg, President and Chief Executive Officer
Web address: www.stalexius.org

Owned, leased, sponsored:	3 hospitals	679 beds
Contract-managed:	0 hospitals	0 beds
Totals:	3 hospitals	679 beds

★0041: ALLINA HEALTH SYSTEM (NP)
5601 Smetana Drive, Minneapolis, MN Zip 55343, Mailing Address: P.O. Box 9310, Zip 55440-9310; tel. 612/992-3992; Gordon M. Sprenger, President
(Moderately Centralized Health System)

MINNESOTA: ABBOTT NORTHWESTERN HOSPITAL (O, 642 beds) 800 East 28th Street, Minneapolis, MN Zip 55407-3799; tel. 612/863-4000; Mark Dixon, Administrator
Web address: www.allina.com

BUFFALO HOSPITAL (O, 30 beds) 303 Catlin Street, Buffalo, MN Zip 55313-1947; tel. 612/682-7180; Mary Ellen Wells, Administrator
Web address: www.allina.com

CAMBRIDGE MEDICAL CENTER (O, 81 beds) 701 South Dellwood Street, Cambridge, MN Zip 55008-1920; tel. 763/689-7700; Dennis J. Doran, Administrator

COMMUNITY HOSPITAL AND HEALTH CARE CENTER (C, 118 beds) 618 West Broadway Avenue, Saint Peter, MN Zip 56082-1327; tel. 507/931-2200; Colleen A. Spike, Administrator

GRANITE FALLS MUNICIPAL HOSPITAL AND MANOR (C, 87 beds) 345 Tenth Avenue, Granite Falls, MN Zip 56241-1499; tel. 320/564-3111; George Gerlach, Administrator

HUTCHINSON AREA HEALTH CARE (C, 187 beds) 1095 Highway 15 South, Hutchinson, MN Zip 55350-3182; tel. 320/234-5000; Philip G. Graves, Administrator

MERCY HOSPITAL (O, 198 beds) 4050 Coon Rapids Boulevard, Coon Rapids, MN Zip 55433-2586; tel. 763/421-8888; Marvin L. Dehne, Executive Officer
Web address: www.allina.com

MILLE LACS HEALTH SYSTEM (C, 98 beds) 200 North Elm Street, Onamia, MN Zip 56359-7978; tel. 320/532-3154; Randall A. Farrow, Administrator

NEW ULM MEDICAL CENTER (O, 47 beds) 1324 Fifth Street North, New Ulm, MN Zip 56073-1553, Mailing Address: P.O. Box 577, Zip 56073-0577; tel. 507/354-2111; Brian Kief, Administrator

NORTHFIELD HOSPITAL (C, 67 beds) 801 West First Street, Northfield, MN Zip 55057-1697; tel. 507/645-6661; Kendall C. Bank, Administrator
Web address: www.allina.com

OWATONNA HOSPITAL (O, 44 beds) 903 Oak Street South, Owatonna, MN Zip 55060-3234; tel. 507/451-3850; Daniel J. Werner, Administrator
Web address: www.allina.com

PHILLIPS EYE INSTITUTE (O, 10 beds) 2215 Park Avenue, Minneapolis, MN Zip 55404-3756; tel. 612/336-6000; Shari E. Levy, Administrator
Web address: www.allina.com

ST. FRANCIS REGIONAL MEDICAL CENTER (O, 63 beds) 1455 St. Francis Avenue, Shakopee, MN Zip 55379-3380; tel. 952/403-3000; Venetia Kudrle, Administrator

STEVENS COMMUNITY MEDICAL CENTER (C, 39 beds) 400 East First Street, Morris, MN Zip 56257-1407, Mailing Address: P.O. Box 660, Zip 56267-0660; tel. 320/589-1313; John Rau, Administrator

UNITED HOSPITAL (O, 483 beds) 333 North Smith Street, Saint Paul, MN Zip 55102-2389; tel. 651/220-8000; M. Barbara Balik, MSN, Ed.D., Administrator
Web address: www.allina.com

UNITED HOSPITAL DISTRICT (C, 43 beds) 515 South Moore Street, Blue Earth, MN Zip 56013-2158, Mailing Address: P.O. Box 160, Zip 56013-0160; tel. 507/526-3273; Chad Cooper, Administrator
Web address: www.uhd.org

UNITY HOSPITAL (O, 201 beds) 550 Osborne Road N.E., Fridley, MN Zip 55432-2799; tel. 763/421-2222;
Web address: www.allina.com

WISCONSIN: RIVER FALLS AREA HOSPITAL (O, 31 beds) 1629 East Division Street, River Falls, WI Zip 54022-1571; tel. 715/425-6155; Sharon Whelan, Administrator
Web address: www.allina.com

Owned, leased, sponsored:	11 hospitals	1830 beds
Contract-managed:	7 hospitals	639 beds
Totals:	18 hospitals	2469 beds

0187: ALTA HEALTHCARE SYSTEM (IO)
3000 Ocean Park Boulevard, Santa Monica, CA Zip 90405; tel. 310/399-1349; David Topper, Chief Executive Officer
(Independent Hospital System)

CALIFORNIA: HOLLYWOOD COMMUNITY HOSPITAL OF HOLLYWOOD (O, 160 beds) 6245 De Longpre Avenue, Los Angeles, CA Zip 90028-9001; tel. 323/462-2271; Evan Rayner, Administrator

LOS ANGELES COMMUNITY HOSPITAL (O, 186 beds) 4081 East Olympic Boulevard, Los Angeles, CA Zip 90023-3300; tel. 323/267-0477; Remy Hart, Chief Executive Officer

MONROVIA COMMUNITY HOSPITAL (O, 49 beds) 323 South Heliotrope Avenue, Monrovia, CA Zip 91016, Mailing Address: P.O. Box 707, Zip 91017-0707; tel. 626/359-8341; Christopher A. Vito, Chief Executive Officer

ORANGE COUNTY COMMUNITY HOSPITAL OF BUENA PARK (O, 55 beds) 6850 Lincoln Avenue, Buena Park, CA Zip 90620-5703; tel. 714/827-1161; Michael Kerr, Chief Executive Officer

Owned, leased, sponsored:	4 hospitals	450 beds
Contract-managed:	0 hospitals	0 beds
Totals:	4 hospitals	450 beds

★0135: ANCILLA SYSTEMS INC. (CC)
1000 South Lake Park Avenue, Hobart, IN Zip 46342-5970; tel. 219/947-8500; Elizabeth K. Kaminski, President and Chief Executive Officer
(Moderately Centralized Health System)

ILLINOIS: ST. ELIZABETH'S HOSPITAL (O, 250 beds) 1431 North Claremont Avenue, Chicago, IL Zip 60622-1791; tel. 773/278-2000; JoAnn Birdzell, President and Chief Executive Officer
Web address: www.ancilla.org

ST. MARY'S HOSPITAL OF EAST ST. LOUIS (O, 119 beds) 129 North Eighth Street, East St. Louis, IL Zip 62201-2999; tel. 618/274-1900; Richard J. Mark, President and Chief Executive Officer
Web address: www.ancilla.org

INDIANA: COMMUNITY HOSPITAL OF BREMEN (C, 24 beds) 411 South Whitlock Street, Bremen, IN Zip 46506, Mailing Address: P.O. Box 8, Zip 46506-0008; tel. 219/546-2211; Scott R. Graybill, Chief Executive Officer and Administrator

ST. CATHERINE HOSPITAL (O, 188 beds) 4321 Fir Street, East Chicago, IN Zip 46312-3097; tel. 219/392-7000; JoAnn Birdzell, President and Chief Executive Officer

For explanation of codes following names, see page B2.
★ Indicates Type III membership in the American Hospital Association.

Systems / Ascension Health

ST. JOSEPH COMMUNITY HOSPITAL (O, 100 beds) 215 West Fourth Street, Mishawaka, IN Zip 46544-1999; tel. 219/259-2431; Mary Roos, President and Chief Executive Officer
Web address: www.ancillahealthcare.org

ST. MARY MEDICAL CENTER (O, 146 beds) 1500 South Lake Park Avenue, Hobart, IN Zip 46342-6699; tel. 219/942-0551; Milton Triana, President and Chief Executive Officer
Web address: www.stmary-hobart.com

Owned, leased, sponsored:	5 hospitals	803 beds
Contract-managed:	1 hospital	24 beds
Totals:	6 hospitals	827 beds

0145: APPALACHIAN REGIONAL HEALTHCARE (NP)
1220 Harrodsburg Road, Lexington, KY Zip 40504, Mailing Address: P.O. Box 8086, Zip 40533-8086; tel. 606/226-2440; Stephen C. Hanson, President
(Centralized Physician/Insurance Health System)

KENTUCKY: ARH REGIONAL MEDICAL CENTER (O, 288 beds) 100 Medical Center Drive, Hazard, KY Zip 41701-1000; tel. 606/439-6833; Charles E. Housley, FACHE, Administrator
Web address: www.arh.org

HARLAN ARH HOSPITAL (O, 130 beds) 81 Ball Park Road, Harlan, KY Zip 40831-1792; tel. 606/573-8201; Daniel Fitzpatrick, Chief Executive Officer

MCDOWELL ARH HOSPITAL (O, 40 beds) Route 122, McDowell, KY Zip 41647, Mailing Address: P.O. Box 247, Mc Dowell, Zip 41647-0247; tel. 606/377-3400; Dena C. Sparkman, Administrator
Web address: www.arh.org

MIDDLESBORO APPALACHIAN REGIONAL HOSPITAL (O, 96 beds) 3600 West Cumberland Avenue, Middlesboro, KY Zip 40965-2614, Mailing Address: P.O. Box 340, Zip 40965-0340; tel. 606/242-1101; Paul V. Miles, Administrator

MORGAN COUNTY APPALACHIAN REGIONAL HOSPITAL (L, 45 beds) 476 Liberty Road, West Liberty, KY Zip 41472-2049, Mailing Address: P.O. Box 579, Zip 41472-0579; tel. 606/743-3186; Dennis R. Chaney, Administrator
Web address: www.2.arh.org

WHITESBURG APPALACHIAN REGIONAL HOSPITAL (O, 69 beds) 240 Hospital Road, Whitesburg, KY Zip 41858-1254; tel. 606/633-3600; Donald Fields, Administrator

WILLIAMSON ARH HOSPITAL (O, 148 beds) 260 Hospital Drive, South Williamson, KY Zip 41503-4072; tel. 606/237-1710; Louis G. Roe, Jr, Administrator
Web address: www.arh.org

WEST VIRGINIA: BECKLEY APPALACHIAN REGIONAL HOSPITAL (O, 173 beds) 306 Stanaford Road, Beckley, WV Zip 25801-3142; tel. 304/255-3000; David R. Lyon, Administrator

MAN ARH HOSPITAL (O, 46 beds) 700 East McDonald Avenue, Man, WV Zip 25635-1011; tel. 304/583-8421; Erica McDonald, Administrator
Web address: www.arh.org

SUMMERS COUNTY APPALACHIAN REGIONAL HOSPITAL (L, 50 beds) Terrace Street, Hinton, WV Zip 25951, Mailing Address: Drawer 940, Zip 25951-0940; tel. 304/466-1000; Rocco K. Massey, Administrator
Web address: www.arh.org

Owned, leased, sponsored:	10 hospitals	1085 beds
Contract-managed:	0 hospitals	0 beds
Totals:	10 hospitals	1085 beds

0104: ARCHBOLD MEDICAL CENTER (NP)
910 South Broad Street, Thomasville, GA Zip 31792-6113; tel. 912/228-2739; Ken B. Beverly, President and Chief Executive Officer
(Moderately Centralized Health System)

GEORGIA: BROOKS COUNTY HOSPITAL (L, 35 beds) 903 North Court Street, Quitman, GA Zip 31643-1315, Mailing Address: P.O. Box 5000, Zip 31643-5000; tel. 912/263-4171; David Sanders, Administrator

EARLY MEMORIAL HOSPITAL (L, 159 beds) 630 Columbia Street, Blakely, GA Zip 31723-1798; tel. 912/723-4241; Kevin Taylor, Administrator

GRADY GENERAL HOSPITAL (L, 49 beds) 1155 Fifth Street S.E., Cairo, GA Zip 31728-3142, Mailing Address: P.O. Box 360, Zip 31728-0360; tel. 912/377-1150; Glen C. Davis, Administrator
Web address: www.archbold.org

JOHN D. ARCHBOLD MEMORIAL HOSPITAL (O, 264 beds) Gordon Avenue at Mimosa Drive, Thomasville, GA Zip 31792-6113, Mailing Address: P.O. Box 1018, Zip 31799-1018; tel. 912/228-2000; James L. Story, Jr, M.D., Acting President
Web address: www.archbold.org

MITCHELL COUNTY HOSPITAL (L, 179 beds) 90 Stephens Street, Camilla, GA Zip 31730-1899, Mailing Address: P.O. Box 639, Zip 31730-0639; tel. 912/336-5284; Ronald M. Gilliard, FACHE, Administrator

Owned, leased, sponsored:	5 hospitals	686 beds
Contract-managed:	0 hospitals	0 beds
Totals:	5 hospitals	686 beds

★0094: ASANTE HEALTH SYSTEM (NP)
2650 Siskiyou Boulevard, Suite 218, Medford, OR Zip 97504-8389; tel. 541/608-4100; Roy G. Vinyard, II, President and Chief Executive Officer

OREGON: ROGUE VALLEY MEDICAL CENTER (O, 264 beds) 2825 East Barnett Road, Medford, OR Zip 97504-8332; tel. 541/608-4900; Roseanne McLaren, Senior Vice President

THREE RIVERS COMMUNITY HOSPITAL AND HEALTH CENTER (O, 71 beds) 715 N.W. Dimmick Street, Grants Pass, OR Zip 97526-1596; tel. 541/476-6831; Paul Janke, Senior Vice President

Owned, leased, sponsored:	2 hospitals	335 beds
Contract-managed:	0 hospitals	0 beds
Totals:	2 hospitals	335 beds

★0198: ASCENSION HEALTH (CC)
4600 Edmundson Road, Saint Louis, MO Zip 63134-3806; tel. 314/253-6700; Donald A. Brennan, President and Chief Executive Officer

ALABAMA: PROVIDENCE HOSPITAL (S, 349 beds) 6801 Airport Boulevard, Mobile, AL Zip 36608-3785, Mailing Address: P.O. Box 850429, Zip 36685-0429; tel. 334/633-1000; John R. Roeder, President and Chief Executive Officer
Web address: www.providencehospital.org

ST. VINCENT'S HOSPITAL (S, 255 beds) 810 St. Vincent's Drive, Birmingham, AL Zip 35205-1695, Mailing Address: P.O. Box 12407, Zip 35202-2407; tel. 205/939-7000; Curtis James, President and Chief Executive Officer
Web address: www.stv.org

CONNECTICUT: ST. VINCENT'S MEDICAL CENTER (S, 291 beds) 2800 Main Street, Bridgeport, CT Zip 06606-4292; tel. 203/576-6000; William J. Riordan, President and Chief Executive Officer

DISTRICT OF COLUMBIA: PROVIDENCE HOSPITAL (S, 544 beds) 1150 Varnum Street N.E., Washington, DC Zip 20017-2180; tel. 202/269-7000; Sister Carol Keehan, President and Chief Executive Officer
Web address: www.provhosp.org

FLORIDA: SACRED HEART HEALTH SYSTEM (S, 520 beds) 5151 North Ninth Avenue, Pensacola, FL Zip 32504-8795, Mailing Address: P.O. Box 2700, Zip 32513-2700; tel. 850/416-7000; Patrick J. Madden, President and Chief Executive Officer
Web address: www.sacred-heart.org

ST. VINCENT'S MEDICAL CENTER (S, 756 beds) 1800 Barrs Street, Jacksonville, FL Zip 32204-2982, Mailing Address: P.O. Box 2982, Zip 32203-2982; tel. 904/308-7300; John W. Logue, Executive Vice President and Chief Operating Officer
Web address: www.baptist-stvincents.com

ILLINOIS: HARRISBURG MEDICAL CENTER (S, 80 beds) 100 Hospital Drive, Harrisburg, IL Zip 62946-0017, Mailing Address: P.O. Box 428, Zip 62946-0428; tel. 618/253-7671; Claude Chatterton, Administrator

For explanation of codes following names, see page B2.
★ Indicates Type III membership in the American Hospital Association.

Systems / Ascension Health

INDIANA: ST. ELIZABETH ANN SETON HOSPITAL (O, 25 beds) 1116 Millis Avenue, Boonville, IN Zip 47601, Mailing Address: P.O. Box 290, Zip 47601-0290; tel. 812/897-7440; Reginald P. Gibson, FACHE, Executive Director

ST. JOSEPH HOSPITAL & HEALTH CENTER (S, 167 beds) 1907 West Sycamore Street, Kokomo, IN Zip 46904-9010, Mailing Address: P.O. Box 9010, Zip 46904-9010; tel. 765/452-5611; Kathleen M. Korbelak, President
Web address: www.stjhhc.org

ST. MARY'S WARRICK (S, 28 beds) 1116 Millis Avenue, Boonville, IN Zip 47601-0629, Mailing Address: Box 629, Zip 47601-0629; tel. 812/897-4800; James M. Hayes, Executive Vice President and Administrator
Web address: www.stmarys.org

ST. MARY'S MEDICAL CENTER (S, 787 beds) 3700 Washington Avenue, Evansville, IN Zip 47750-0002; tel. 812/485-4000; Jay D. Kasey, President

ST. VINCENT HOSPITALS AND HEALTH SERVICES (S, 752 beds) 2001 West 86th Street, Indianapolis, IN Zip 46260-1991, Mailing Address: P.O. Box 40970, Zip 46240-0970; tel. 317/338-2345; Marsha N. Casey, President
Web address: www.stvincent.org

ST. VINCENT JENNINGS HOSPITAL (S, 34 beds) 301 Henry Street, North Vernon, IN Zip 47265-1097; tel. 812/352-4200; Joseph Roche, Administrator

ST. VINCENT MERCY HOSPITAL (S, 40 beds) 1331 South A Street, Elwood, IN Zip 46036-1942; tel. 765/552-4600; David Masterson, Administrator
Web address: www.stvincent.org

ST. VINCENT WILLIAMSPORT HOSPITAL (S, 22 beds) 412 North Monroe Street, Williamsport, IN Zip 47993-0215; tel. 765/762-4000; Jane Craigin, Chief Executive Officer
Web address: www.stvincent.org

MARYLAND: MEMORIAL HOSPITAL AND MEDICAL CENTER OF CUMBERLAND (S, 187 beds) 600 Memorial Avenue, Cumberland, MD Zip 21502-3797; tel. 301/723-4000; Thomas C. Dowdell, Executive Director and Senior Vice President
Web address: www.wmhs.com

SACRED HEART HOSPITAL (S, 287 beds) 900 Seton Drive, Cumberland, MD Zip 21502-1874; tel. 301/759-4200; Francis A. Pommett, Jr, Executive Director and Senior Vice President
Web address: www.wmhs.com

ST. AGNES HEALTHCARE (S, 422 beds) 900 Caton Avenue, Baltimore, MD Zip 21229-5299; tel. 410/368-6000; Robert W. Adams, President and Chief Executive Officer
Web address: www.stagnes.org

MICHIGAN: BORGESS MEDICAL CENTER (S, 383 beds) 1521 Gull Road, Kalamazoo, MI Zip 49001-1640; tel. 616/226-4800; Randall Stasik, President and Chief Executive Officer
Web address: www.borgess.com

GENESYS REGIONAL MEDICAL CENTER (S, 379 beds) One Genesys Parkway, Grand Blanc, MI Zip 48439-8066; tel. 810/606-5000; Elliot T. Joseph, President and Chief Executive Officer
Web address: www.genesys.org

LEE MEMORIAL HOSPITAL (S, 40 beds) 420 West High Street, Dowagiac, MI Zip 49047-1907; tel. 616/782-8681; Fritz Fahrenbacher, President and Chief Executive Officer

PROVIDENCE HOSPITAL AND MEDICAL CENTERS (S, 379 beds) 16001 West Nine Mile Road, Southfield, MI Zip 48075-4854, Mailing Address: Box 2043, Zip 48037-2043; tel. 248/424-3000; Robert F. Casalou, President
Web address: www.providence-hospital.org

ST. JOHN DETROIT RIVERVIEW HOSPITAL (S, 230 beds) 7733 East Jefferson Avenue, Detroit, MI Zip 48214-2598; tel. 313/499-4000; Richard T. Young, President

ST. JOHN HOSPITAL AND MEDICAL CENTER (S, 656 beds) 22101 Moross Road, Detroit, MI Zip 48236-2172; tel. 313/343-4000; Timothy J. Grajewski, President and Chief Executive Officer

ST. JOHN MACOMB HOSPITAL (S, 274 beds) 11800 East Twelve Mile Road, Warren, MI Zip 48093-3494; tel. 810/573-5000; John E. Knox, President
Web address: www.stjohn.org

ST. JOHN NORTHEAST COMMUNITY HOSPITAL (S, 222 beds) 4777 East Outer Drive, Detroit, MI Zip 48234-0401; tel. 313/369-9100; Michael F. Breen, President
Web address: www.stjohn.org

ST. JOHN OAKLAND HOSPITAL (S, 196 beds) 27351 Dequindre, Madison Heights, MI Zip 48071-3499; tel. 248/967-7000; Robert Deputat, President

ST. JOHN RIVER DISTRICT HOSPITAL (S, 68 beds) 4100 River Road, East China, MI Zip 48054; tel. 810/329-7111; Frank W. Poma, President

ST. JOSEPH HEALTH SYSTEM (S, 49 beds) 200 Hemlock Street, Tawas City, MI Zip 48763, Mailing Address: P.O. Box 659, Zip 48764-0659; tel. 517/362-3411; Patrick Murtha, President and Chief Executive Officer

ST. MARY'S MEDICAL CENTER (S, 268 beds) 800 South Washington Avenue, Saginaw, MI Zip 48601-2594; tel. 517/776-8000; Frederic L. Fraizer, President and Chief Executive Officer
Web address: www.saintmarys-saginaw.org

NEW YORK: MOUNT ST. MARY'S HOSPITAL AND HEALTH CENTER (S, 179 beds) 5300 Military Road, Lewiston, NY Zip 14092-1997; tel. 716/297-4800; Angelo G. Calbone, President and Chief Executive Officer

OUR LADY OF LOURDES MEMORIAL HOSPITAL (S, 184 beds) 169 Riverside Drive, Binghamton, NY Zip 13905-4198; tel. 607/798-5111; John D. O'Neil, President and Chief Executive Officer
Web address: www.lourdes.com

SETON HEALTH SYSTEM (S, 344 beds) 1300 Massachusetts Avenue, Troy, NY Zip 12180-1695; tel. 518/268-5000; Mark A. Donovan, M.D., President and Chief Executive Officer
Web address: www.setonhealth.org

PENNSYLVANIA: GOOD SAMARITAN REGIONAL MEDICAL CENTER (S, 153 beds) 700 East Norwegian Street, Pottsville, PA Zip 17901-2798; tel. 570/621-4000; Gino J. Pazzaglini, President and Chief Executive Officer
Web address: www.goodsamrmc.com

TENNESSEE: ST. THOMAS HEALTH SERVICES (S, 523 beds) 4220 Harding Road, Nashville, TN Zip 37205-2095, Mailing Address: P.O. Box 380, Zip 37202-0380; tel. 615/222-2111; Thomas E. Beeman, President and Chief Executive Officer

TEXAS: BRACKENRIDGE HOSPITAL (L, 312 beds) 601 East 15th Street, Austin, TX Zip 78701-1996; tel. 512/324-7000; Susan McClernon, Administrator
Web address: www.goodhealth.com

PROVIDENCE HEALTH CENTER (S, 427 beds) 6901 Medical Parkway, Waco, TX Zip 76712-7998, Mailing Address: P.O. Box 2589, Zip 76702-2589; tel. 254/751-4000; Kent A. Keahey, President and Chief Executive Officer
Web address: www.providence-waco.org

SETON EDGAR B. DAVIS HOSPITAL (S, 21 beds) 130 Hays Street, Luling, TX Zip 78648-3207; tel. 830/875-5643; Neal Kelley, Administrator
Web address: www.goodhealth.com

SETON HIGHLAND LAKES (S, 26 beds) Highway 281 South, Burnet, TX Zip 78611, Mailing Address: P.O. Box 1219, Zip 78611-0840; tel. 512/756-6000; Janna Maturo, R.N., Administrator and Vice President Operations
Web address: www.goodhealth.com/fac/highlandlakes.html

SETON MEDICAL CENTER (S, 527 beds) 1201 West 38th Street, Austin, TX Zip 78705-1056; tel. 512/324-1000; Gregory R. Angle, Administrator
Web address: www.goodhealth.com

SETON SHOAL CREEK HOSPITAL (S, 118 beds) 3501 Mills Avenue, Austin, TX Zip 78731-6391; tel. 512/452-0361; Armin L. Steege, Interim Administrator
Web address: www.goodhealth.com

WISCONSIN: SACRED HEART REHABILITATION INSTITUTE (S, 45 beds) 2350 North Lake Drive, Milwaukee, WI Zip 53211-4507, Mailing Address: P.O. Box 392, Zip 53201-0392; tel. 414/298-6700; Nancy D. Kuelz, Administrator
Web address: www.columbia-stmarys.com

ST. MARY'S HOSPITAL (S, 241 beds) 2323 North Lake Drive, Milwaukee, WI Zip 53211-9682, Mailing Address: P.O. Box 503, Zip 53201-0503; tel. 414/291-1000; Susan Henckel, Chief Operating Officer
Web address: www.columbia-stmarys.com

For explanation of codes following names, see page B2.
★ Indicates Type III membership in the American Hospital Association.

Systems / Avera Health

ST. MARY'S HOSPITAL OZAUKEE (S, 82 beds) 13111 North Port Washington Road, Mequon, WI Zip 53097–2416; tel. 262/243–7300; Therese B. Pandl, Executive Vice President and Chief Operating Officer
Web address: www.columbia–stmarys.com

Owned, leased, sponsored:	44 hospitals	11872 beds
Contract–managed:	0 hospitals	0 beds
Totals:	44 hospitals	11872 beds

0202: ASSOCIATES CAPITAL GROUP, LLC (IO)
Birmingham, AL Mailing Address: P.O. Box 380995, Zip 35242; tel. 205/408–9095; Len Bryant, Chief Executive Officer

MISSISSIPPI: NORTH OAK REGIONAL MEDICAL CENTER (O, 52 beds) 401 Getwell Drive, Senatobia, MS Zip 38668–2213, Mailing Address: P.O. Box 648, Zip 38668–0648; tel. 601/562–3100; James D. Tesar, Chief Executive Officer

TENNESSEE: BLEDSOE COMMUNITY MEDICAL CENTER (O, 26 beds) 128 Wheelertown Road, Pikeville, TN Zip 37367, Mailing Address: P.O. Box 699, Zip 37367–0699; tel. 423/447–2112; Keith Smith, Chief Executive Officer

Owned, leased, sponsored:	2 hospitals	78 beds
Contract–managed:	0 hospitals	0 beds
Totals:	2 hospitals	78 beds

★2215: AURORA HEALTH CARE (NP)
3000 West Montana, Milwaukee, WI Zip 53215–3268, Mailing Address: P.O. Box 343910, Zip 53234–3910; tel. 414/647–3000; G. Edwin Howe, President
(Moderately Centralized Health System)

WISCONSIN: HARTFORD MEMORIAL HOSPITAL (O, 71 beds) 1032 East Sumner Street, Hartford, WI Zip 53027–1698; tel. 262/673–2300; Mark Schwartz, Administrator
Web address: www.aurorahealthcare.org

LAKELAND MEDICAL CENTER (O, 78 beds) West 3985 County Road NN, Elkhorn, WI Zip 53121, Mailing Address: P.O. Box 1002, Zip 53121–1002; tel. 262/741–2000; Kathleen Skowlund, Site Administrator and Chief Nurse Executive
Web address: www.aurorahealthcare.org

MEMORIAL HOSPITAL CORPORATION OF BURLINGTON (O, 87 beds) 252 McHenry Street, Burlington, WI Zip 53105–1828; tel. 262/767–6000; Lief Erickson, M.D., President
Web address: www.aurorahealthcare.org

MILWAUKEE PSYCHIATRIC HOSPITAL (O, 75 beds) 1220 Dewey Avenue, Wauwatosa, WI Zip 53213–2598; tel. 414/454–6600; James A. Moore, Chief Operating Officer and Chief Financial Officer
Web address: www.aurorahealthcare.org

SHEBOYGAN MEMORIAL MEDICAL CENTER (O, 217 beds) 2629 North Seventh Street, Sheboygan, WI Zip 53083–4998; tel. 920/451–5000; T. Gregg Watson, Administrator
Web address: www.aurorahealthcare.org

SINAI SAMARITAN MEDICAL CENTER (O, 255 beds) 945 North 12th Street, Milwaukee, WI Zip 53233–1337, Mailing Address: P.O. Box 342, Zip 53201–0342; tel. 414/219–2000; Leonard E. Wilk, Administrator
Web address: www.aurorahealthcare.org

ST. LUKE'S MEDICAL CENTER (O, 747 beds) 2900 West Oklahoma Avenue, Milwaukee, WI Zip 53215–4330, Mailing Address: P.O. Box 2901, Zip 53201–2901; tel. 414/649–6000; Mark S. Wiener, Administrator
Web address: www.aurorahealthcare.org

ST. MARY'S KEWAUNEE AREA MEMORIAL HOSPITAL (O, 18 beds) 810 Lincoln Street, Kewaunee, WI Zip 54216; tel. 920/388–2210; Cathie A. Kocourek, Acting Administrator

TWO RIVERS COMMUNITY HOSPITAL AND HAMILTON MEMORIAL HOME (O, 138 beds) 2500 Garfield Street, Two Rivers, WI Zip 54241–2399; tel. 920/793–1178; Patrick J. Trotter, Chief Executive Officer
Web address: www.aurorahealthcare.org

VALLEY VIEW MEDICAL CENTER (O, 92 beds) 901 Reed Street, Plymouth, WI Zip 53073–2409; tel. 920/893–1771; T. Gregg Watson, Administrator
Web address: www.aurorahealthcare.org

WEST ALLIS MEMORIAL HOSPITAL (O, 147 beds) 8901 West Lincoln Avenue, West Allis, WI Zip 53227–0901, Mailing Address: P.O. Box 27901, Zip 53227–0901; tel. 414/328–6000; Richard A. Kellar, Administrator
Web address: www.aurorahealthcare.org

Owned, leased, sponsored:	11 hospitals	1925 beds
Contract–managed:	0 hospitals	0 beds
Totals:	11 hospitals	1925 beds

★5255: AVERA HEALTH (CC)
610 West 23rd Street, Yankton, SD Zip 57078, Mailing Address: P.O. Box 38, Zip 57078–0038; tel. 605/322–7050; John T. Porter, President and Chief Executive Officer
(Decentralized Health System)

IOWA: AVERA HOLY FAMILY HOSPITAL (O, 35 beds) 826 North Eighth Street, Estherville, IA Zip 51334–1598; tel. 712/362–2631; William Bumgarner, Chief Executive Officer

FLOYD VALLEY HOSPITAL/AVERA HEALTH (C, 44 beds) Highway 3 East, Le Mars, IA Zip 51031–0010, Mailing Address: P.O. Box 10, Zip 51031–0010; tel. 712/546–3398; Michael Donlin, Administrator
Web address: www.floydvalleyhospital.org

HEGG MEMORIAL HEALTH CENTER/AVERA HEALTH (C, 123 beds) 1202 21st Avenue, Rock Valley, IA Zip 51247–1497; tel. 712/476–8000; Vern Carda, Administrator

OSCEOLA COMMUNITY HOSPITAL (C, 32 beds) Ninth Avenue North, Sibley, IA Zip 51249–0258, Mailing Address: P.O. Box 258, Zip 51249–0258; tel. 712/754–2574; Janet Dykstra, Administrator

SIOUX CENTER COMMUNITY HOSPITAL AND HEALTH CENTER/AVERA HEALTH (C, 90 beds) 605 South Main Avenue, Sioux Center, IA Zip 51250–1398; tel. 712/722–1271; Marla Toering, Administrator

MINNESOTA: DIVINE PROVIDENCE HEALTH CENTER/AVERA HEALTH (C, 79 beds) 312 East George Street, Ivanhoe, MN Zip 56142–0136, Mailing Address: P.O. Box 136, Zip 56142–0136; tel. 507/694–1414; Patrick Branco, Administrator

PIPESTONE COUNTY MEDICAL CENTER/AVERA HEALTH (C, 76 beds) 911 Fifth Avenue S.W., Pipestone, MN Zip 56164–0370, Mailing Address: P.O. Box 370, Zip 56164–0370; tel. 507/825–6125; Carl P. Vaagenes, Administrator

TYLER HEALTHCARE CENTER/AVERA HEALTH (C, 63 beds) 240 Willow Street, Tyler, MN Zip 56178–0280, Mailing Address: P.O. Box 280, Zip 56178–0280; tel. 507/247–5521; Douglas P. Schweikhart, Administrator

NEBRASKA: AVERA ST. ANTHONY'S HOSPITAL (C, 29 beds) Second and Adams Streets, O'Neill, NE Zip 68763–1569; tel. 402/336–2611; Ronald J. Cork, President and Chief Executive Officer
Web address: www.avera–sta.org

SOUTH DAKOTA: AVERA MCKENNAN HOSPITAL (O, 521 beds) 800 East 21st Street, Sioux Falls, SD Zip 57105–1096, Mailing Address: P.O. Box 5045, Zip 57117–5045; tel. 605/322–8000; Fredrick Slunecka, President and Chief Executive Officer
Web address: www.mckennan.org

AVERA QUEEN OF PEACE (O, 183 beds) 525 North Foster, Mitchell, SD Zip 57301–2999; tel. 605/995–2000; Ronald L. Jacobson, President and Chief Executive Officer
Web address: www.averaqueenofpeace.org

AVERA SACRED HEART (C, 257 beds) 501 Summit Avenue, Yankton, SD Zip 57078–3899; tel. 605/668–8000; Pamela J. Rezac, President and Chief Executive Officer
Web address: www.shhsservices.com

AVERA ST. BENEDICT HEALTH CENTER (C, 105 beds) Glynn Drive, Parkston, SD Zip 57366, Mailing Address: P.O. Box B, Zip 57366; tel. 605/928–3311; Gale Walker, Administrator
Web address: www.parkston.com

AVERA ST. LUKE'S (O, 224 beds) 305 South State Street, Aberdeen, SD Zip 57402–4450; tel. 605/622–5000; Dale J. Stein, President and Chief Executive Officer
Web address: www.averastlukes.org

COMMUNITY MEMORIAL HOSPITAL/AVERA HEALTH (C, 16 beds) Eighth and Jackson, Burke, SD Zip 57523, Mailing Address: P.O. Box 319, Zip 57523–0319; tel. 605/775–2621; Carol A. Varland, Administrator

For explanation of codes following names, see page B2.
★ Indicates Type III membership in the American Hospital Association.

Systems / Avera Health

EUREKA COMMUNITY HEALTH SERVICES/AVERA HEALTH (C, 6 beds) 410 Ninth Street, Eureka, SD Zip 57437–0517, Mailing Address: P.O. Box 517, Zip 57437–0517; tel. 605/284–2661; Robert A. Dockter, Administrator

FLANDREAU MUNICIPAL HOSPITAL/AVERA HEALTH (C, 18 beds) 214 North Prairie Avenue, Flandreau, SD Zip 57028–1243; tel. 605/997–2433; John E. Barrett, Administrator

HAND COUNTY MEMORIAL HOSPITAL/AVERA HEALTH (C, 43 beds) 300 West Fifth Street, Miller, SD Zip 57362–1238; tel. 605/853–2421; Clarence A. Lee, Administrator

LANDMANN–JUNGMAN MEMORIAL HOSPITAL (C, 19 beds) 600 Billars Street, Scotland, SD Zip 57059–2026; tel. 605/583–2226; Philip Hibnick, Administrator

MARSHALL COUNTY HEALTHCARE CENTER/AVERA HEALTH (C, 20 beds) 413 Ninth Street, Britton, SD Zip 57430–0230, Mailing Address: Box 230, Zip 57430–0230; tel. 605/448–2253; Stephanie Lulewicz, Administrator

PLATTE HEALTH CENTER/AVERA HEALTH (C, 63 beds) 601 East Seventh, Platte, SD Zip 57369–2123, Mailing Address: P.O. Box 200, Zip 57369–0200; tel. 605/337–3364; Mark Burket, Chief Executive Officer

Owned, leased, sponsored:	4 hospitals	963 beds
Contract-managed:	17 hospitals	1083 beds
Totals:	21 hospitals	2046 beds

★**0194: BANNER HEALTH SYSTEM** (NP)
4310 17th Avenue S.W., Fargo, ND Zip 58103; tel. 701/277–7500; Steven R. Orr, Chairman and Chief Executive Officer

ALASKA: FAIRBANKS MEMORIAL HOSPITAL (L, 209 beds) 1650 Cowles Street, Fairbanks, AK Zip 99701; tel. 907/452–8181; Michael K. Powers, Administrator
Web address: www.lhsnet.org

ARIZONA: DESERT SAMARITAN MEDICAL CENTER (O, 551 beds) 1400 South Dobson Road, Mesa, AZ Zip 85202–9879; tel. 480/835–3000; Bruce E. Pearson, Senior Vice President and Chief Executive Officer
Web address: www.samaritan.edu

GOOD SAMARITAN REGIONAL MEDICAL CENTER (O, 687 beds) 1111 East McDowell Road, Phoenix, AZ Zip 85006–2666, Mailing Address: P.O. Box 2989, Zip 85062–2989; tel. 602/239–2000; Steven L. Seiler, Senior Vice President and Chief Executive Officer
Web address: www.samaritan.edu

MESA LUTHERAN HOSPITAL (O, 278 beds) 525 West Brown Road, Mesa, AZ Zip 85201–3299; tel. 480/834–1211; James Gingerich, Senior Vice President and Chief Executive Officer

PAGE HOSPITAL (C, 25 beds) 501 North Navajo Drive, Page, AZ Zip 86040, Mailing Address: P.O. Box 1447, Zip 86040–1447; tel. 520/645–2424; Richard Polheber, Chief Executive Officer

SAMARITAN BEHAVIORAL HEALTH CENTER–SCOTTSDALE (O, 82 beds) 7575 East Earll Drive, Scottsdale, AZ Zip 85251–6998; tel. 480/941–7500; Robert F. Meyer, M.D., Chief Executive Officer

THUNDERBIRD SAMARITAN MEDICAL CENTER (O, 288 beds) 5555 West Thunderbird Road, Glendale, AZ Zip 85306–4696; tel. 602/588–5555; Robert H. Curry, Senior Vice President and Chief Executive Officer
Web address: www.samaritan.edu

VALLEY LUTHERAN HOSPITAL (O, 172 beds) 6644 Baywood Avenue, Mesa, AZ Zip 85206–1797; tel. 480/981–2000; Robert A. Rundio, Executive Director of Hospital Operations

WICKENBURG REGIONAL HOSPITAL (L, 80 beds) 520 Rose Lane, Wickenburg, AZ Zip 85390–1447; tel. 520/684–5421; David Garnas, Administrator

CALIFORNIA: LASSEN COMMUNITY HOSPITAL (O, 59 beds) 560 Hospital Lane, Susanville, CA Zip 96130–4809; tel. 530/257–5325; David S. Anderson, FACHE, Administrator
Web address: www.lshnet.org

COLORADO: EAST MORGAN COUNTY HOSPITAL (L, 25 beds) 2400 West Edison Street, Brush, CO Zip 80723–1640; tel. 970/842–5151; Anne Platt, Administrator
Web address: www.wphn.com

MCKEE MEDICAL CENTER (O, 108 beds) 2000 Boise Avenue, Loveland, CO Zip 80538–4281, Mailing Address: P.O. Box 830, Zip 80539–0830; tel. 970/669–4640; Charles F. Harms, Administrator
Web address: www.wphn.com

NORTH COLORADO MEDICAL CENTER (L, 262 beds) 1801 16th Street, Greeley, CO Zip 80631–5199; tel. 970/352–4121; Jon Sewell, Administrator
Web address: www.ncmcgreeley.com

STERLING REGIONAL MEDCENTER (O, 36 beds) 615 Fairhurst Street, Sterling, CO Zip 80751–0500, Mailing Address: P.O. Box 3500, Zip 80751–0500; tel. 970/522–0122; Michael J. Gillen, Administrator
Web address: www.lhsnet.org

KANSAS: DECATUR COUNTY HOSPITAL AND CEDAR LIVING CENTER (L, 74 beds) 810 West Columbia Street, Oberlin, KS Zip 67749–2450, Mailing Address: P.O. Box 268, Zip 67749–0268; tel. 785/475–2208; Lynn Doeden, Administrator
Web address: www.lhsnet.com

ST. LUKE HOSPITAL AND LIVING CENTER (L, 54 beds) 1014 East Melvin, Marion, KS Zip 66861–1299; tel. 316/382–2179; Craig Hanson, Administrator
Web address: www.lhsnet.com

NEBRASKA: OGALLALA COMMUNITY HOSPITAL (L, 29 beds) 300 East Tenth Street, Ogallala, NE Zip 69153–1509; tel. 308/284–4011; Linda Morris, Administrator

NEVADA: CHURCHILL COMMUNITY HOSPITAL (O, 40 beds) 801 East Williams Avenue, Fallon, NV Zip 89406–3052; tel. 775/423–3151; Jeffrey Feike, Administrator and Chief Executive Officer

PERSHING GENERAL HOSPITAL (C, 34 beds) 855 Sixth Street, Lovelock, NV Zip 89419, Mailing Address: P.O. Box 661, Zip 89419–0661; tel. 775/273–2621; Jon Smith, Interim Administrator

NEW MEXICO: LOS ALAMOS MEDICAL CENTER (O, 47 beds) 3917 West Road, Los Alamos, NM Zip 87544–2293; tel. 505/662–4201; Paul J. Wilson, Administrator

NORTH DAKOTA: LISBON MEDICAL CENTER (O, 70 beds) 905 Main Street, Lisbon, ND Zip 58054–0353, Mailing Address: P.O. Box 353, Zip 58054–0353; tel. 701/683–5241; Michael Matthews, Administrator
Web address: www.lhsnet.com

PEMBINA COUNTY MEMORIAL HOSPITAL AND WEDGEWOOD MANOR (L, 89 beds) 301 Mountain Street East, Cavalier, ND Zip 58220–4015; tel. 701/265–8461; George A. Rohrich, Administrator

OREGON: CENTRAL OREGON DISTRICT HOSPITAL (C, 48 beds) 1253 North Canal Boulevard, Redmond, OR Zip 97756–1395; tel. 541/548–8131; James A. Diegel, CHE, Executive Director
Web address: www.codh.org

PIONEER MEMORIAL HOSPITAL (C, 30 beds) 1201 N.E. Elm Street, Prineville, OR Zip 97754; tel. 541/447–6254; Donald J. Wee, Executive Director
Web address: www.pmhprineville.org

SOUTH DAKOTA: GREGORY COMMUNITY HOSPITAL (O, 84 beds) 400 Park Avenue, Gregory, SD Zip 57533–0400, Mailing Address: P.O. Box 408, Zip 57533–0408; tel. 605/835–8394; Carol A. Varland, Chief Executive Officer

LOOKOUT MEMORIAL HOSPITAL (O, 32 beds) 1440 North Main Street, Spearfish, SD Zip 57783–1504; tel. 605/642–2617; Deb J. Krmpotic, R.N., Administrator

STURGIS COMMUNITY HEALTH CARE CENTER (O, 114 beds) 949 Harmon Street, Sturgis, SD Zip 57785–2452; tel. 605/347–2536; Roger R. Heidt, Administrator

WYOMING: COMMUNITY HOSPITAL (O, 36 beds) 2000 Campbell Drive, Torrington, WY Zip 82240–1597; tel. 307/532–4181; Charles Myers, Administrator

PLATTE COUNTY MEMORIAL HOSPITAL (L, 86 beds) 201 14th Street, Wheatland, WY Zip 82201–3201, Mailing Address: P.O. Box 848, Zip 82201–0848; tel. 307/322–3636; Steve Hannah, Administrator

WASHAKIE MEDICAL CENTER (L, 30 beds) 400 South 15th Street, Worland, WY Zip 82401–3531, Mailing Address: P.O. Box 700, Zip 82401–0700; tel. 307/347–3221; Kent Aland, Interim Administrator

Owned, leased, sponsored:	26 hospitals	3622 beds
Contract-managed:	4 hospitals	137 beds
Totals:	30 hospitals	3759 beds

For explanation of codes following names, see page B2.
★ Indicates Type III membership in the American Hospital Association.

0150: BAPTIST HEALTH (NP)
2105 East South Boulevard, Montgomery, AL Zip 36116–2498; tel. 334/286–2970; Victor D. Butler, Acting President and Chief Executive Officer
(Moderately Centralized Health System)

ALABAMA: BAPTIST MEDICAL CENTER (O, 454 beds) 2105 East South Boulevard, Montgomery, AL Zip 36116–2498, Mailing Address: Box 11010, Zip 36111–0010; tel. 334/288–2100; Victor D. Butler, President and Chief Executive Officer

BAPTIST MEDICAL CENTER EAST (O, 130 beds) 400 Taylor Road, Montgomery, AL Zip 36117–3512, Mailing Address: P.O. Box 241267, Zip 36124–1267; tel. 334/244–8178; John W. Melton, Administrator

CRENSHAW BAPTIST HOSPITAL (O, 52 beds) 101 Baptist Lane, Luverne, AL Zip 36049; tel. 334/335–3374; Moultrie D. Plowden, CHE, Administrator

PRATTVILLE BAPTIST HOSPITAL (O, 54 beds) 124 South Memorial Drive, Prattville, AL Zip 36067–3619, Mailing Address: P.O. Box 681630, Zip 36067–1638; tel. 334/365–0651; William E. Hines, Administrator

SELMA BAPTIST HOSPITAL (O, 130 beds) 1015 Medical Center Parkway, Selma, AL Zip 36701–6352; tel. 334/418–4100; Lee Ashbury, Chief Executive Officer

Owned, leased, sponsored:	5 hospitals	820 beds
Contract–managed:	0 hospitals	0 beds
Totals:	5 hospitals	820 beds

★**0355: BAPTIST HEALTH** (NP)
9601 Interstate 630, Exit 7, Little Rock, AR Zip 72205–7299; tel. 501/202–2000; Russell D. Harrington, Jr, President
(Centralized Physician/Insurance Health System)

ARKANSAS: BAPTIST HEALTH BAPTIST MEMORIAL MEDICAL CENTER (O, 200 beds) 3333 Springhill Drive, North Little Rock, AR Zip 72117; tel. 501/202–3000; Harrison M. Dean, Senior Vice President and Administrator
Web address: www.baptist–health.org

BAPTIST HEALTH MEDICAL CENTER–ARKADELPHIA (L, 57 beds) 3050 Twin Rivers Drive, Arkadelphia, AR Zip 71923–4299; tel. 870/245–1100; Dan Gathright, Senior Vice President and Administrator
Web address: www.baptist–health.org

BAPTIST HEALTH MEDICAL CENTER–HEBER SPRINGS (L, 24 beds) 2319 Highway 110 West, Heber Springs, AR Zip 72543; tel. 501/206–3000; Edward L. Lacy, Administrator

BAPTIST HEALTH MEDICAL CENTER–LITTLE ROCK (O, 620 beds) 9601 Interstate 630, Exit 7, Little Rock, AR Zip 72205–7299; tel. 501/202–2000; Steven Douglas Weeks, Senior Vice President and Administrator
Web address: www.baptist–health.org

BAPTIST HEALTH REHABILITATION INSTITUTE (O, 100 beds) 9601 Interstate 630, Exit 7, Little Rock, AR Zip 72205–7249; tel. 501/202–7000; Steven Douglas Weeks, Senior Vice President and Administrator
Web address: www.baptist–health.org

Owned, leased, sponsored:	5 hospitals	1001 beds
Contract–managed:	0 hospitals	0 beds
Totals:	5 hospitals	1001 beds

0185: BAPTIST HEALTH CARE CORPORATION (NP)
1717 North E Street, Suite 320, Pensacola, FL Zip 32501–6335; tel. 850/469–7643; Alfred G. Stubblefield, President
(Moderately Centralized Health System)

ALABAMA: ATMORE COMMUNITY HOSPITAL (L, 51 beds) 401 Medical Park Drive, Atmore, AL Zip 36502–3091; tel. 334/368–2500; Robert E. Gowing, Administrator

D. W. MCMILLAN MEMORIAL HOSPITAL (L, 67 beds) 1301 Belleville Avenue, Brewton, AL Zip 36426–1306, Mailing Address: P.O. Box 908, Zip 36427–0908; tel. 334/867–8061; Phillip L. Parker, Administrator
Web address: www.bhcpns.org

FLORIDA: BAPTIST HOSPITAL (O, 492 beds) 1000 West Moreno, Pensacola, FL Zip 32501–2393, Mailing Address: P.O. Box 17500, Zip 32522–7500; tel. 850/469–2313; John R. Heer, Administrator
Web address: www.bhcpns.org

GULF BREEZE HOSPITAL (O, 45 beds) 1110 Gulf Breeze Parkway, Gulf Breeze, FL Zip 32561, Mailing Address: P.O. Box 159, Zip 32562; tel. 850/934–2000; Richard C. Fulford, Administrator
Web address: www.bhcpns.org

JAY HOSPITAL (L, 55 beds) 221 South Alabama Street, Jay, FL Zip 32565–1070; tel. 850/675–8000; Mark Faulkner, Administrator
Web address: www.bhcpns.org

THE FRIARY OF BAPTIST HEALTH CENTER (O, 30 beds) 4400 Hickory Shores Boulevard, Gulf Breeze, FL Zip 32561–9113; tel. 850/932–9375; Leo J. Donnelly, Executive Director

Owned, leased, sponsored:	6 hospitals	740 beds
Contract–managed:	0 hospitals	0 beds
Totals:	6 hospitals	740 beds

0265: BAPTIST HEALTH SYSTEM (CO)
200 Concord Plaza, Suite 900, San Antonio, TX Zip 78216; tel. 210/297–1000; Fred R. Mills, President and Chief Executive Officer
(Centralized Physician/Insurance Health System)

TEXAS: BAPTIST MEDICAL CENTER (O, 445 beds) 111 Dallas Street, San Antonio, TX Zip 78205–1230; tel. 210/297–7000; Perry Willmore, Vice President Operations
Web address: www.baptisthealthsystem.org

NORTH CENTRAL BAPTIST HOSPITAL (O, 126 beds) 520 Madison Oak Drive, San Antonio, TX Zip 78258–3912; tel. 210/297–4000; Kim Murphy–Abdouch, Vice President Operations

NORTHEAST BAPTIST HOSPITAL (O, 234 beds) 8811 Village Drive, San Antonio, TX Zip 78217–5440; tel. 210/297–2000; Dan Brown, Vice President Operations
Web address: www.baptisthealthsystem.org

SOUTHEAST BAPTIST HOSPITAL (O, 167 beds) 4214 East Southcross Boulevard, San Antonio, TX Zip 78222–3740; tel. 210/297–3000; Kevin Walters, Administrator
Web address: www.baptisthealthsystem.org

ST. LUKE'S BAPTIST HOSPITAL (O, 195 beds) 7930 Floyd Curl Drive, San Antonio, TX Zip 78229–0100; tel. 210/297–5000; Virginia Dempsey, Vice President Operations
Web address: www.baptisthealthsystem.org

Owned, leased, sponsored:	5 hospitals	1167 beds
Contract–managed:	0 hospitals	0 beds
Totals:	5 hospitals	1167 beds

★**0345: BAPTIST HEALTH SYSTEM** (CO)
Birmingham, AL Mailing Address: P.O. Box 830605, Zip 35283–0605; tel. 205/715–5319; Dennis A. Hall, President
(Centralized Physician/Insurance Health System)

ALABAMA: CHEROKEE BAPTIST MEDICAL CENTER (O, 45 beds) 400 Northwood Drive, Centre, AL Zip 35960–1023; tel. 256/927–5531; Barry S. Cochran, President
Web address: www.bhsala.com

CITIZENS BAPTIST MEDICAL CENTER (O, 97 beds) 604 Stone Avenue, Talladega, AL Zip 35160–2217, Mailing Address: P.O. Box 978, Zip 35161–0978; tel. 256/362–8111; Steven M. Johnson, President
Web address: www.bhsala.com

COOSA VALLEY BAPTIST MEDICAL CENTER (O, 176 beds) 315 West Hickory Street, Sylacauga, AL Zip 35150–2996; tel. 256/249–5000; Steven M. Johnson, President
Web address: www.bhsala.com

CULLMAN REGIONAL MEDICAL CENTER (O, 115 beds) 1912 Alabama Highway 157, Cullman, AL Zip 35055, Mailing Address: P.O. Box 1108, Zip 35056–1108; tel. 256/737–2000; Jesse O. Weatherly, President
Web address: www.crmc–bhs.com

DEKALB BAPTIST MEDICAL CENTER (O, 91 beds) 200 Medical Center Drive, Fort Payne, AL Zip 35968–3415, Mailing Address: P.O. Box 680778,

For explanation of codes following names, see page B2.
★ Indicates Type III membership in the American Hospital Association.

Systems / Baptist Health System

Zip 35968–1608; tel. 256/845–3150; Barry S. Cochran, President
Web address: www.bhsala.com

LAWRENCE BAPTIST MEDICAL CENTER (L, 30 beds) 202 Hospital Street, Moulton, AL Zip 35650–0039, Mailing Address: P.O. Box 39, Zip 35650–0039; tel. 256/974–2200; Steven Honeycutt, Administrator
Web address: www.bhsala.com

MARION BAPTIST MEDICAL CENTER (L, 112 beds) 1256 Military Street South, Hamilton, AL Zip 35570–5001; tel. 205/921–6200; Glenn C. Sisk, President
Web address: www.bhsala.com

MONTCLAIR BAPTIST MEDICAL CENTER (O, 463 beds) 800 Montclair Road, Birmingham, AL Zip 35213–1984; tel. 205/592–1000; John Shelton, President
Web address: www.bhsala.com

PRINCETON BAPTIST MEDICAL CENTER (O, 320 beds) 701 Princeton Avenue S.W., Birmingham, AL Zip 35211–1305; tel. 205/783–3000; Charlie Faulkner, President
Web address: www.bhsala.com

SHELBY BAPTIST MEDICAL CENTER (O, 228 beds) 1000 First Street North, Alabaster, AL Zip 35007–0488; tel. 205/620–8100; Charles C. Colvert, President
Web address: www.bhsala.com

WALKER BAPTIST MEDICAL CENTER (O, 157 beds) 3400 Highway 78 East, Jasper, AL Zip 35501–8956, Mailing Address: P.O. Box 3547, Zip 35502–3547; tel. 205/387–4000; Evan S. Dillard, President
Web address: www.bhsala.com

Owned, leased, sponsored:	11 hospitals	1834 beds
Contract–managed:	0 hospitals	0 beds
Totals:	11 hospitals	1834 beds

0122: BAPTIST HEALTH SYSTEM OF SOUTH FLORIDA (NP)
6855 Red Road, Suite 600, Coral Gables, FL Zip 33143–3632; tel. 305/273–2333; Brian E. Keeley, President and Chief Executive Officer
(Centralized Physician/Insurance Health System)

FLORIDA: BAPTIST HOSPITAL OF MIAMI (O, 392 beds) 8900 North Kendall Drive, Miami, FL Zip 33176–2197; tel. 305/596–1960; Lee S. Huntley, Chief Executive Officer
Web address: www.baptisthealth.net

HOMESTEAD HOSPITAL (O, 100 beds) 160 N.W. 13th Street, Homestead, FL Zip 33030–4299; tel. 305/248–3232; Bo Boulenger, Chief Executive Officer
Web address: www.baptisthealth.net

MARINERS HOSPITAL (S, 42 beds) 91500 Overseas Highway, Tavernier, FL Zip 33070–1582; tel. 305/853–1582; Robert H. Luse, Chief Executive Officer
Web address: www.baptisthealth.net/

SOUTH MIAMI HOSPITAL (O, 397 beds) 6200 S.W. 73rd Street, Miami, FL Zip 33143–9990; tel. 305/661–4611; D. Wayne Brackin, Chief Executive Officer
Web address: www.baptisthealth.net

Owned, leased, sponsored:	4 hospitals	931 beds
Contract–managed:	0 hospitals	0 beds
Totals:	4 hospitals	931 beds

2155: BAPTIST HEALTH SYSTEM OF TENNESSEE (NP)
137 Blount Avenue S.E., Knoxville, TN Zip 37920–1643, Mailing Address: P.O. Box 1788, Zip 37901–1788; tel. 865/532–5011; Dale Collins, President and Chief Executive Officer
(Centralized Physician/Insurance Health System)

TENNESSEE: BAPTIST HOSPITAL OF COCKE COUNTY (O, 109 beds) 435 Second Street, Newport, TN Zip 37821–3799; tel. 423/625–2200; Wayne Buckner, Administrator
Web address: www.baptistoneword.org/

BAPTIST HOSPITAL OF EAST TENNESSEE (O, 316 beds) 137 Blount Avenue S.E., Knoxville, TN Zip 37920–1643, Mailing Address: P.O. Box 1788, Zip 37901–1788; tel. 865/632–5011; Jon Foster, Executive Vice President and Administrator
Web address: www.bhset.org

Owned, leased, sponsored:	2 hospitals	425 beds
Contract–managed:	0 hospitals	0 beds
Totals:	2 hospitals	425 beds

★0315: BAPTIST HEALTHCARE SYSTEM (CO)
4007 Kresge Way, Louisville, KY Zip 40207–4677; tel. 502/896–5000; Tommy J. Smith, President and Chief Executive Officer
(Centralized Physician/Insurance Health System)

KENTUCKY: BAPTIST HOSPITAL EAST (O, 407 beds) 4000 Kresge Way, Louisville, KY Zip 40207–4676; tel. 502/897–8100; Susan Stout Tamme, President
Web address: www.baptisteast.com

BAPTIST REGIONAL MEDICAL CENTER (O, 263 beds) 1 Trillium Way, Corbin, KY Zip 40701–8420; tel. 606/528–1212; John S. Henson, President
Web address: www.bhsi.com

CENTRAL BAPTIST HOSPITAL (O, 355 beds) 1740 Nicholasville Road, Lexington, KY Zip 40503; tel. 859/260–6100; William G. Sisson, President
Web address: www.centralbap.com

HARDIN MEMORIAL HOSPITAL (C, 262 beds) 913 North Dixie Avenue, Elizabethtown, KY Zip 42701–2599; tel. 270/737–1212; David L. Gray, President
Web address: www.hmh.net

TRI COUNTY BAPTIST HOSPITAL (O, 105 beds) 1025 New Moody Lane, La Grange, KY Zip 40031–0559; tel. 502/222–5388; Dennis B. Johnson, Administrator
Web address: www.tri–countybaptist.com

WESTERN BAPTIST HOSPITAL (O, 271 beds) 2501 Kentucky Avenue, Paducah, KY Zip 42003–3200; tel. 270/575–2100; Larry O. Barton, President
Web address: www.bhsi.com

Owned, leased, sponsored:	5 hospitals	1401 beds
Contract–managed:	1 hospital	262 beds
Totals:	6 hospitals	1663 beds

★1625: BAPTIST MEMORIAL HEALTH CARE CORPORATION (NP)
899 Madison Avenue, Memphis, TN Zip 38146–0001; tel. 901/227–5117; Stephen Curtis Reynolds, President and Chief Executive Officer
(Decentralized Health System)

ARKANSAS: BAPTIST MEMORIAL HOSPITAL–BLYTHEVILLE (L, 166 beds) 1520 North Division Street, Blytheville, AR Zip 72315, Mailing Address: P.O. Box 108, Zip 72316–0108; tel. 870/838–7300; Brandt C. Wright, Administrator
Web address: www.bmhcc.org

BAPTIST MEMORIAL HOSPITAL–FORREST CITY (L, 86 beds) 1601 Newcastle Road, Forrest City, AR Zip 72335, Mailing Address: P.O. Box 667, Zip 72336–0667; tel. 870/261–0000; Charles R. Daugherty, Administrator
Web address: www.bmhcc.org

BAPTIST MEMORIAL HOSPITAL–OSCEOLA (L, 59 beds) 611 West Lee Avenue, Osceola, AR Zip 72370–3001, Mailing Address: P.O. Box 607, Zip 72370–0607; tel. 870/563–7000; Joel E. North, Administrator
Web address: www.bmhcc.org

MISSISSIPPI: BAPTIST MEMORIAL HOSPITAL–BOONEVILLE (L, 99 beds) 100 Hospital Street, Booneville, MS Zip 38829–3359; tel. 662/720–5000; Al Sypniewski, Administrator

BAPTIST MEMORIAL HOSPITAL–DESOTO (O, 260 beds) 7601 Southcrest Parkway, Southaven, MS Zip 38671–4742; tel. 662/349–4000; Melvin E. Walker, Administrator
Web address: www.bmhcc.org

BAPTIST MEMORIAL HOSPITAL–GOLDEN TRIANGLE (L, 328 beds) 2520 Fifth Street North, Columbus, MS Zip 39703–2095, Mailing Address: P.O. Box 1307, Zip 39701–1307; tel. 662/244–1000; Dean A. Griffin, Chief Executive Officer
Web address: www.bmhcc.org

For explanation of codes following names, see page B2.
★ Indicates Type III membership in the American Hospital Association.

BAPTIST MEMORIAL HOSPITAL–NORTH MISSISSIPPI (L, 204 beds) 2301 South Lamar Boulevard, Oxford, MS Zip 38655, Mailing Address: P.O. Box 946, Zip 38655–0946; tel. 662/232–8100; James Hahn, Administrator
Web address: www.bmhcc.org

BAPTIST MEMORIAL HOSPITAL–UNION COUNTY (L, 153 beds) 200 Highway 30 West, New Albany, MS Zip 38652–3197; tel. 601/538–7631; John Tompkins, Administrator

TIPPAH COUNTY HOSPITAL (C, 110 beds) 1005 City Avenue North, Ripley, MS Zip 38663–0499; tel. 601/837–9221; Jerry Green, Administrator

TENNESSEE: BAPTIST MEMORIAL HOSPITAL (O, 1054 beds) 899 Madison Avenue, Memphis, TN Zip 38146–0002; tel. 901/227–2727; Stephen Curtis Reynolds, President and Chief Executive Officer
Web address: www.baptistonline.org

BAPTIST MEMORIAL HOSPITAL–HUNTINGDON (O, 70 beds) 631 R. B. Wilson Drive, Huntingdon, TN Zip 38344–1675; tel. 901/986–4461; Susan M. Breeden, Administrator
Web address: www.bmhcc.org

BAPTIST MEMORIAL HOSPITAL–LAUDERDALE (O, 60 beds) 326 Asbury Road, Ripley, TN Zip 38063–9701; tel. 901/221–2200; Zach Chandler, Administrator
Web address: www.baptistonline.org

BAPTIST MEMORIAL HOSPITAL–TIPTON (O, 70 beds) 1995 Highway 51 South, Covington, TN Zip 38019–3635; tel. 901/476–2621; Glenn Baker, Administrator
Web address: www.bmhcc.org

BAPTIST MEMORIAL HOSPITAL–UNION CITY (O, 133 beds) 1201 Bishop Street, Union City, TN Zip 38261–5403, Mailing Address: P.O. Box 310, Zip 38281–0310; tel. 901/884–8601; Mike Perryman, Administrator
Web address: www.bmhcc.org

BAPTIST REHABILITATION–GERMANTOWN (O, 63 beds) 2100 Exeter Road, Germantown, TN Zip 38138; tel. 901/757–1350; Paula Gisler, Administrator
Web address: www.bmhcc.org

Owned, leased, sponsored:	14 hospitals	2805 beds
Contract–managed:	1 hospital	110 beds
Totals:	15 hospitals	2915 beds

★**0095: BAYLOR HEALTH CARE SYSTEM** (CO)
3500 Gaston Avenue, Dallas, TX Zip 75226–2088; tel. 214/820–0111; Joel T. Allison, President and Chief Executive Officer
(Centralized Health System)

TEXAS: BAYLOR CENTER FOR RESTORATIVE CARE (O, 72 beds) 3504 Swiss Avenue, Dallas, TX Zip 75204–6224; tel. 214/820–9700; Geraldine Brueckner, R.N., Executive Director
Web address: www.baylordallas.edu/

BAYLOR INSTITUTE FOR REHABILITATION (O, 92 beds) 3505 Gaston Avenue, Dallas, TX Zip 75246–2018; tel. 214/826–7030; Laura J. Lycan, Executive Director
Web address: www.bhcs.com

BAYLOR MEDICAL CENTER AT GARLAND (O, 195 beds) 2300 Marie Curie Boulevard, Garland, TX Zip 75042–5706; tel. 972/487–5000; John B. McWhorter, II, Executive Director
Web address: www.baylordallas.edu

BAYLOR MEDICAL CENTER AT GRAPEVINE (O, 97 beds) 1650 West College Street, Grapevine, TX Zip 76051–1650; tel. 817/481–1588; Mark C. Hood, Executive Director
Web address: www.bhcs.com

BAYLOR MEDICAL CENTER AT IRVING (L, 235 beds) 1901 North MacArthur Boulevard, Irving, TX Zip 75061–2291; tel. 972/579–8100; Michael F. O'Keefe, FACHE, Executive Director
Web address: www.bhcs.com/irving

BAYLOR MEDICAL CENTER–ELLIS COUNTY (O, 81 beds) 1405 West Jefferson Street, Waxahachie, TX Zip 75165–2275; tel. 972/923–7000; Ronald Hudspeth, Executive Director
Web address: www.baylordallas.edu

BAYLOR UNIVERSITY MEDICAL CENTER (O, 876 beds) 3500 Gaston Avenue, Dallas, TX Zip 75246–2088; tel. 214/820–0111; Boone Powell, Jr, President and Chief Executive Officer
Web address: www.bhcs.com

Owned, leased, sponsored:	7 hospitals	1648 beds
Contract–managed:	0 hospitals	0 beds
Totals:	7 hospitals	1648 beds

★**1095: BAYSTATE HEALTH SYSTEM, INC.** (NP)
759 Chestnut Street, Springfield, MA Zip 01199–0001; tel. 413/794–0000; Michael J. Daly, President
(Centralized Physician/Insurance Health System)

MASSACHUSETTS: BAYSTATE MEDICAL CENTER (O, 564 beds) 759 Chestnut Street, Springfield, MA Zip 01199–0001; tel. 413/794–0000; Mark R. Tolosky, Chief Executive Officer
Web address: www.baystatehealth.com

FRANKLIN MEDICAL CENTER (O, 85 beds) 164 High Street, Greenfield, MA Zip 01301–2613; tel. 413/773–0211; Harlan J. Smith, President and Chief Executive Officer
Web address: www.baystatehealth.com

MARY LANE HOSPITAL (O, 31 beds) 85 South Street, Ware, MA Zip 01082–1697; tel. 413/967–6211; Christine Shirtcliff, Executive Vice President
Web address: www.baystatehealth.com

Owned, leased, sponsored:	3 hospitals	680 beds
Contract–managed:	0 hospitals	0 beds
Totals:	3 hospitals	680 beds

0069: BEHAVIORAL HEALTHCARE CORPORATION (IO)
102 Woodmont Boulevard, Suite 800, Nashville, TN Zip 37205–2287; tel. 615/269–3492; Edward A. Stack, President and Chief Executive Officer
(Independent Hospital System)

ARKANSAS: BHC PINNACLE POINTE HOSPITAL (O, 102 beds) 11501 Financial Center Parkway, Little Rock, AR Zip 72211–3715; tel. 501/223–3322; Lucinda DeBruce, Chief Executive Officer

CALIFORNIA: BHC ALHAMBRA HOSPITAL (O, 98 beds) 4619 North Rosemead Boulevard, Rosemead, CA Zip 91770–1498, Mailing Address: P.O. Box 369, Zip 91770; tel. 626/286–1191; Peggy Minnick, R.N., Chief Executive Officer

BHC CEDAR VISTA HOSPITAL (O, 61 beds) 7171 North Cedar Avenue, Fresno, CA Zip 93720; tel. 559/449–8000; Deborah Quinn, Administrator

BHC FREMONT HOSPITAL (O, 78 beds) 39001 Sundale Drive, Fremont, CA Zip 94538; tel. 510/796–1100; Edward Owen, Chief Executive Officer
Web address: www.fremonthospital.com

BHC HERITAGE OAKS HOSPITAL (O, 76 beds) 4250 Auburn Boulevard, Sacramento, CA Zip 95841; tel. 916/489–3336; Ingrid L. Whipple, Administrator and Chief Executive Officer

BHC ROSS HOSPITAL (O, 56 beds) 1111 Sir Francis Drake Boulevard, Kentfield, CA Zip 94904; tel. 415/258–6900; Judy G. House, Chief Executive Officer

BHC SAN LUIS REY HOSPITAL (O, 122 beds) 335 Saxony Road, Encinitas, CA Zip 92024–2723; tel. 760/753–1245; James S. Plummer, Chief Executive Officer

BHC SIERRA VISTA HOSPITAL (O, 72 beds) 8001 Bruceville Road, Sacramento, CA Zip 95823; tel. 916/423–2000; Tom Pinizzotto, Administrator and Chief Executive Officer

BHC VISTA DEL MAR HOSPITAL (O, 79 beds) 801 Seneca Street, Ventura, CA Zip 93001; tel. 805/653–6434; Diana L. Goulet, Administrator and Chief Executive Officer

BHC WALNUT CREEK HOSPITAL (O, 108 beds) 175 La Casa Via, Walnut Creek, CA Zip 94598; tel. 925/933–7990; Jay R. Kellison, Chief Executive Officer

CANYON RIDGE HOSPITAL (O, 59 beds) 5353 G Street, Chino, CA Zip 91710; tel. 909/590–3700; Diana C. Hanyak, Chief Executive Officer

FLORIDA: BHC FORT LAUDERDALE HOSPITAL (O, 100 beds) 1601 East Las Olas Boulevard, Fort Lauderdale, FL Zip 33301–2393; tel. 954/463–4321; Andrew Fuhrman, Chief Executive Officer

For explanation of codes following names, see page B2.
★ Indicates Type III membership in the American Hospital Association.

Systems / Behavioral Healthcare Corporation

IDAHO: BHC INTERMOUNTAIN HOSPITAL (O, 95 beds) 303 North Allumbaugh Street, Boise, ID Zip 83704-9266; tel. 208/377-8400; Vernon G. Garrett, Chief Executive Officer

ILLINOIS: BHC STREAMWOOD HOSPITAL (O, 100 beds) 1400 East Irving Park Road, Streamwood, IL Zip 60107-3203; tel. 630/837-9000; Jeff Bergren, Chief Executive Officer and Administrator

INDIANA: BHC VALLE VISTA HOSPITAL (O, 96 beds) 898 East Main Street, Greenwood, IN Zip 46143-1400; tel. 317/887-1348; Gordon L. Steinhaurer, Chief Executive Officer

BEHAVIORAL HEALTHCARE OF NORTHERN INDIANA (O, 76 beds) 1800 North Oak Road, Plymouth, IN Zip 46563-3492; tel. 219/936-3784; Wayne T. Miller, Administrator

BEHAVIORAL HEALTHCARE-COLUMBUS (O, 60 beds) 2223 Poshard Drive, Columbus, IN Zip 47203-1844, Mailing Address: P.O. Box 1549, Zip 47203-1844; tel. 812/376-1711; Bryan W. Lett, Chief Executive Officer

LOUISIANA: BHC EAST LAKE HOSPITAL (O, 52 beds) 5650 Read Boulevard, New Orleans, LA Zip 70127-3145; tel. 504/241-0888; Darlene Brennan, Chief Executive Officer

BHC MEADOW WOOD HOSPITAL (O, 55 beds) 9032 Perkins Road, Baton Rouge, LA Zip 70810-1507; tel. 225/766-8553; Ralph J. Waite, II, Chief Executive Officer

MISSISSIPPI: MEMORIAL BEHAVIORAL HEALTH (O, 60 beds) 11150 Highway 49 North, Gulfport, MS Zip 39503-4110; tel. 228/831-1700; Michael A. Zieman, Administrator

MISSOURI: BHC SPIRIT OF ST. LOUIS HOSPITAL (O, 104 beds) 5931 Highway 94 South, Saint Charles, MO Zip 63304-5601; tel. 314/441-7300; Susan Young, Chief Executive Officer

NEVADA: BHC MONTEVISTA HOSPITAL (O, 80 beds) 5900 West Rochelle Avenue, Las Vegas, NV Zip 89103-3327; tel. 702/364-1111; Allan J. Kydd, Chief Executive Officer

BHC WEST HILLS HOSPITAL (O, 95 beds) 1240 East Ninth Street, Reno, NV Zip 89512-2997, Mailing Address: P.O. Box 30012, Zip 89520-0012; tel. 775/323-0478; Alan G. Chapman, Chief Executive Officer
Web address: www.hcahealthcare.com

BHC WILLOW SPRINGS RESIDENTIAL TREATMENT CENTER (O, 68 beds) 690 Edison Way, Reno, NV Zip 89502-4135; tel. 775/858-3303; Nancy N. Dandliker, Executive Director

NEW MEXICO: BHC MESILLA VALLEY HOSPITAL (O, 115 beds) 3751 Del Rey Boulevard, Las Cruces, NM Zip 88012-8526, Mailing Address: P.O. Box 429, Zip 88004-0429; tel. 505/382-3500; Terry G. Johnson, Chief Executive Officer

OHIO: BHC BELMONT PINES HOSPITAL (O, 77 beds) 615 Churchill-Hubbard Road, Youngstown, OH Zip 44505-1379; tel. 330/759-2700; Richard I. Feldman, Chief Executive Officer
Web address: www.belmontpines.com

BHC FOX RUN HOSPITAL (O, 65 beds) 67670 Traco Drive, Saint Clairsville, OH Zip 43950-9375; tel. 740/695-2131; R. Dale Reynolds, Chief Executive Officer

BHC WINDSOR HOSPITAL (O, 50 beds) 115 East Summit Street, Chagrin Falls, OH Zip 44022-2750; tel. 440/247-5300; Donald K. Sykes, Jr, Chief Executive Officer

OREGON: PACIFIC GATEWAY HOSPITAL AND COUNSELING CENTER (O, 66 beds) 1345 S.E. Harney, Portland, OR Zip 97202; tel. 503/234-5353; Karl R. Brady, Chief Executive Officer
Web address: www.pacificgate.com

PUERTO RICO: BHC HOSPITAL SAN JUAN CAPESTRANO (O, 88 beds) San Juan, PR Mailing Address: Rural Route 2, Box 11, Zip 00926; tel. 787/760-0222; Laura Vargas, Administrator and Chief Executive Officer

TEXAS: BHC MILLWOOD HOSPITAL (O, 82 beds) 1011 North Cooper Street, Arlington, TX Zip 76011-5517; tel. 817/261-3121; Wayne Hallford, Chief Executive Officer

WASHINGTON: BHC FAIRFAX HOSPITAL (O, 133 beds) 10200 N.E. 132nd Street, Kirkland, WA Zip 98034; tel. 425/821-2000; Ron Escarda, Chief Executive Officer

Owned, leased, sponsored:	32 hospitals	2628 beds
Contract-managed:	0 hospitals	0 beds
Totals:	32 hospitals	2628 beds

0515: BENEDICTINE HEALTH SYSTEM (CC)
503 East Third Street, Duluth, MN Zip 55805-1964; tel. 218/786-2370; Barry J. Halm, President and Chief Executive Officer
(Moderately Centralized Health System)

IDAHO: CLEARWATER VALLEY HOSPITAL AND CLINICS (L, 23 beds) 301 Cedar, Orofino, ID Zip 83544-9029; tel. 208/476-4555; Tim Zwickey, Administrator
Web address: www.cvh-clrwater.com

ST. MARY'S HOSPITAL (O, 28 beds) Lewiston and North Streets, Cottonwood, ID Zip 83522, Mailing Address: P.O. Box 137, Zip 83522-0137; tel. 208/962-3251; Casey Uhling, Chief Executive Officer

MINNESOTA: ITASCA MEDICAL CENTER (C, 84 beds) 126 First Avenue S.E., Grand Rapids, MN Zip 55744-3698; tel. 218/326-3401; Gary Kenner, President and Chief Executive Officer

PINE MEDICAL CENTER (C, 106 beds) 109 Court Avenue South, Sandstone, MN Zip 55072-5120; tel. 320/245-2212; Michael D. Hedrix, Administrator

ST. JOSEPH'S MEDICAL CENTER (O, 152 beds) 523 North Third Street, Brainerd, MN Zip 56401-3098; tel. 218/829-2861; Thomas K. Prusak, President
Web address: www.stjosephsmedicalctr.com

ST. MARY'S MEDICAL CENTER (S, 288 beds) 407 East Third Street, Duluth, MN Zip 55805-1984; tel. 218/786-4000; Sister Kathleen Hofer, President
Web address: www.smdc.org

ST. MARY'S REGIONAL HEALTH CENTER (O, 163 beds) 1027 Washington Avenue, Detroit Lakes, MN Zip 56501-3598; tel. 218/847-5611; Thomas R. Thompson, Chief Executive Officer
Web address: www.stmaryshealthcenter.com

TRINITY HOSPITAL (O, 85 beds) 3410-213th Street West, Farmington, MN Zip 55024-1197; tel. 651/463-7825; David A. Grundstrom, Chief Executive Officer

WISCONSIN: ST. MARY'S HOSPITAL OF SUPERIOR (S, 42 beds) 3500 Tower Avenue, Superior, WI Zip 54880-5395; tel. 715/392-8281; Terry Jacobson, Administrator
Web address: www.smdc.org

Owned, leased, sponsored:	7 hospitals	781 beds
Contract-managed:	2 hospitals	190 beds
Totals:	9 hospitals	971 beds

0545: BENEDICTINE SISTERS OF THE ANNUNCIATION (CC)
7520 University Drive, Bismarck, ND Zip 58504-9653; tel. 701/255-1520; Sister Susan Berger, Prioress
(Independent Hospital System)

NORTH DAKOTA: GARRISON MEMORIAL HOSPITAL (S, 54 beds) 407 Third Avenue S.E., Garrison, ND Zip 58540-0039; tel. 701/463-2275; Dennis Goebel, Administrator

ST. ALEXIUS MEDICAL CENTER (S, 272 beds) 900 East Broadway, Bismarck, ND Zip 58501-4586, Mailing Address: P.O. Box 5510, Zip 58506-5510; tel. 701/224-7000; Richard A. Tschider, FACHE, Administrator and Chief Executive Officer
Web address: www.st.alexius.org

Owned, leased, sponsored:	2 hospitals	326 beds
Contract-managed:	0 hospitals	0 beds
Totals:	2 hospitals	326 beds

★**2435: BERKSHIRE HEALTH SYSTEMS, INC.** (NP)
725 North Street, Pittsfield, MA Zip 01201-4124; tel. 413/447-2743; David E. Phelps, President and Chief Executive Officer
(Moderately Centralized Health System)

For explanation of codes following names, see page B2.
★ Indicates Type III membership in the American Hospital Association.

Systems / Bon Secours Health System, Inc.

MASSACHUSETTS: BERKSHIRE MEDICAL CENTER (O, 310 beds) 725 North Street, Pittsfield, MA Zip 01201–4124; tel. 413/447–2000; Ruth P. Blodgett, Chief Operating Officer
Web address: www.bhs1.org

FAIRVIEW HOSPITAL (O, 46 beds) 29 Lewis Avenue, Great Barrington, MA Zip 01230–1713; tel. 413/528–0790; Eugene A. Dellea, Interim President
Web address: www.bhs1.org/fairviewhospital.htm

Owned, leased, sponsored:	2 hospitals	356 beds
Contract-managed:	0 hospitals	0 beds
Totals:	2 hospitals	356 beds

★**0051: BJC HEALTH SYSTEM** (NP)
4444 Forest Park Avenue, Saint Louis, MO Zip 63108–2259; tel. 314/286–2000; Steven H. Lipstein, President and Chief Operating Officer
(Centralized Physician/Insurance Health System)

ILLINOIS: ALTON MEMORIAL HOSPITAL (O, 202 beds) One Memorial Drive, Alton, IL Zip 62002–6722; tel. 618/463–7311; Ronald B. McMullen, President
Web address: www.bjc.org

CLAY COUNTY HOSPITAL (C, 31 beds) 911 Stacy Burk Drive, Flora, IL Zip 62839–1823, Mailing Address: P.O. Box 280, Zip 62839–0280; tel. 618/662–2131; Tony Schwarm, President
Web address: www.bjc.org

FAYETTE COUNTY HOSPITAL (L, 142 beds) Seventh and Taylor Streets, Vandalia, IL Zip 62471–1296; tel. 618/283–1231; Daniel L. Gantz, President
Web address: www.provenamercy.com

SALEM TOWNSHIP HOSPITAL (C, 31 beds) 1201 Ricker Drive, Salem, IL Zip 62881–6250; tel. 618/548–3194; James E. Robertson , Jr, President

MISSOURI: BARNES–JEWISH HOSPITAL (O, 941 beds) One Barnes–Jewish Hospital Plaza, Saint Louis, MO Zip 63110–1094; tel. 314/747–3000; Ronald G. Evens, M.D., President
Web address: www.bjc.org/bjh.html

BARNES–JEWISH ST. PETERS HOSPITAL (O, 84 beds) 10 Hospital Drive, Saint Peters, MO Zip 63376–1659; tel. 636/916–9000; Carmelo J. Moceri, President
Web address: www.bjc.org/bjsph.html

BARNES–JEWISH WEST COUNTY HOSPITAL (O, 91 beds) 12634 Olive Boulevard, Saint Louis, MO Zip 63141–6354; tel. 314/996–8000; Ronald G. Evens, M.D., Interim President and Senior Executive Officer
Web address: www.bjc.org/chnenw.html

BOONE HOSPITAL CENTER (L, 335 beds) 1600 East Broadway, Columbia, MO Zip 65201–5897; tel. 573/815–8000; Michael B. Shirk, President and Senior Executive Officer
Web address: www.boone.org

CHRISTIAN HOSPITAL NORTHEAST–NORTHWEST (O, 546 beds) 11133 Dunn Road, Saint Louis, MO Zip 63136–6192; tel. 314/653–5000; Mark A. Eustis, President
Web address: www.bjc.org

MISSOURI BAPTIST HOSPITAL OF SULLIVAN (O, 46 beds) 751 Sappington Bridge Road, Sullivan, MO Zip 63080–2354, Mailing Address: P.O. Box 190, Zip 63080–0190; tel. 573/468–4186; Davis D. Skinner, President
Web address: www.bjc.org/mbhs.html

MISSOURI BAPTIST MEDICAL CENTER (O, 370 beds) 3015 North Ballas Road, Town and Country, MO Zip 63131–2374; tel. 314/996–5000; Mark A. Eustis, President and Senior Executive Officer

PARKLAND HEALTH CENTER (O, 94 beds) 1101 West Liberty Street, Farmington, MO Zip 63640–1997; tel. 573/756–6451; Richard L. Conklin, President
Web address: www.bjc.org/phc.html

ST. LOUIS CHILDREN'S HOSPITAL (O, 235 beds) One Children's Place, Saint Louis, MO Zip 63110–1077; tel. 314/454–6000; Ted W. Frey, President and Senior Executive Officer
Web address: www.STLOUISCHILDRENS.ORG

Owned, leased, sponsored:	11 hospitals	3086 beds
Contract-managed:	2 hospitals	62 beds
Totals:	13 hospitals	3148 beds

● ★**0053: BLUE WATER HEALTH SERVICES CORPORATION** (NP)
1221 Pine Grove Avenue, Port Huron, MI Zip 48060–3568; tel. 810/989–3717; Donald C. Fletcher, President and Chief Executive Officer
(Moderately Centralized Health System)

MICHIGAN: PORT HURON HOSPITAL (O, 173 beds) 1221 Pine Grove Avenue, Port Huron, MI Zip 48061–5011; tel. 810/987–5000; Donald C. Fletcher, President and Chief Executive Officer
Web address: www.porthuronhosp.org

Owned, leased, sponsored:	1 hospital	173 beds
Contract-managed:	0 hospitals	0 beds
Totals:	1 hospital	173 beds

★**5085: BON SECOURS HEALTH SYSTEM, INC.** (CC)
1505 Marriottsville Road, Marriottsville, MD Zip 21104–1399; tel. 410/442–5511; Christopher M. Carney, President and Chief Executive Officer
(Moderately Centralized Health System)

FLORIDA: BON SECOURS–ST. JOSEPH HEALTHCARE GROUP (O, 313 beds) 2500 Harbor Boulevard, Port Charlotte, FL Zip 33952–5396; tel. 941/766–4122; Michael L. Harrington, Chief Executive Officer

BON SECOURS–VENICE HOSPITAL (O, 281 beds) 540 The Rialto, Venice, FL Zip 34285–2900; tel. 941/485–7711; Michael G. Guley, Chief Executive Officer
Web address: www.bonsecours.org/florida/

MARYLAND: BON SECOURS BALTIMORE HEALTH SYSTEM (O, 148 beds) 2000 West Baltimore Street, Baltimore, MD Zip 21223–1597; tel. 410/362–3000; Percy Allen , II, FACHE, Chief Executive Officer
Web address: www.bonsecours.org

MICHIGAN: BON SECOURS COTTAGE HEALTH SERVICES–BON SECOURS HOSPITAL (O, 237 beds) 468 Cadieux Road, Grosse Pointe, MI Zip 48230–1592; tel. 313/343–1000; Richard Van Lith, Chief Executive Officer
Web address: www.bonsecoursmi.com

BON SECOURS COTTAGE HEALTH SERVICES–COTTAGE HOSPITAL (O, 65 beds) 159 Kercheval Avenue, Grosse Pointe Farms, MI Zip 48236–3692; tel. 313/640–1000; Richard Van Lith, Chief Executive Officer

PENNSYLVANIA: BON SECOURS–HOLY FAMILY REGIONAL HEALTH SYSTEM (O, 153 beds) 2500 Seventh Avenue, Altoona, PA Zip 16602–2099; tel. 814/944–1681; Barbara H. Biehner, Chief Executive Officer
Web address: www.mercynet.org

VIRGINIA: BON SECOURS ST. MARY'S HOSPITAL (O, 348 beds) 5801 Bremo Road, Richmond, VA Zip 23226–1900; tel. 804/285–2011; Ann E. Honeycutt, Executive Vice President and Administrator

BON SECOURS–DEPAUL MEDICAL CENTER (O, 293 beds) 150 Kingsley Lane, Norfolk, VA Zip 23505–4650; tel. 757/889–5000; David J. McCombs, Executive Vice President and Administrator

BON SECOURS–RICHMOND COMMUNITY HOSPITAL (O, 88 beds) 1500 North 28th Street, Richmond, VA Zip 23223–5396, Mailing Address: Box 27184, Zip 23261–7184; tel. 804/225–1700; Eugene Toomer, Chief Operating Officer

BON SECOURS–STUART CIRCLE (O, 158 beds) 413 Stuart Circle, Richmond, VA Zip 23220–3799; tel. 804/358–7051; Ann E. Honeycutt, Executive Vice President and Administrator

MARY IMMACULATE HOSPITAL (O, 225 beds) 2 Bernardine Drive, Newport News, VA Zip 23602–4499; tel. 757/886–6000; Cynthia B. Farrand, Executive Vice President and Administrator
Web address: www.mihospital.com

MARYVIEW MEDICAL CENTER (O, 466 beds) 3636 High Street, Portsmouth, VA Zip 23707–3236; tel. 757/398–2200; Wayne Jones, Executive Vice President and Administrator
Web address: www.bonsecours.com

For explanation of codes following names, see page B2.
★ Indicates Type III membership in the American Hospital Association.
● Single hospital health care system

Systems / Bon Secours Health System, Inc.

MEMORIAL REGIONAL MEDICAL CENTER (O, 200 beds) 8260 Atlee Road, Mechanicsville, VA Zip 23116, Mailing Address: P.O. Box 26783, Richmond, Zip 23261–6783; tel. 804/764–6102; Michael Robinson, Executive Vice President and Administrator

Owned, leased, sponsored:	13 hospitals	2975 beds
Contract–managed:	0 hospitals	0 beds
Totals:	13 hospitals	2975 beds

2455: BRADFORD HEALTH SERVICES (IO)
2101 Magnolia Avenue South, Suite 518, Birmingham, AL Zip 35205; tel. 205/251–7753; Jerry W. Crowder, President and Chief Executive Officer
(Independent Hospital System)

ALABAMA: BRADFORD HEALTH SERVICES AT HUNTSVILLE (O, 84 beds) 1600 Browns Ferry Road, Madison, AL Zip 35758–9769, Mailing Address: P.O. Box 176, Zip 35758–0176; tel. 256/461–7272; Bob Hinds, Executive Director

BRADFORD HEALTH SERVICES AT OAK MOUNTAIN (O, 56 beds) 2280 Highway 35, Pelham, AL Zip 35124–6120; tel. 205/664–3480; William Weaver, Administrator
Web address: www.bradfordhealth.com

Owned, leased, sponsored:	2 hospitals	140 beds
Contract–managed:	0 hospitals	0 beds
Totals:	2 hospitals	140 beds

★**0585: BRIM HEALTHCARE, INC.** (IO)
105 Westwood Place, Suite 300, Brentwood, TN Zip 37027; tel. 615/309–6053; Dave Woodland, President
(Decentralized Health System)

ARIZONA: COBRE VALLEY COMMUNITY HOSPITAL (C, 49 beds) 5880 South Hospital Drive, Globe, AZ Zip 85501; tel. 520/425–3261; Charles E. Bill, CHE, Chief Executive Officer

NAVAPACHE REGIONAL MEDICAL CENTER (C, 54 beds) 2200 Show Low Lake Road, Show Low, AZ Zip 85901–7800; tel. 520/537–4375; Leigh Cox, Chief Executive Officer
Web address: www.nrmc.org

NORTHERN COCHISE COMMUNITY HOSPITAL (C, 48 beds) 901 West Rex Allen Drive, Willcox, AZ Zip 85643–1009; tel. 520/384–3541; Chris Cronberg, Chief Executive Officer

CALIFORNIA: CORCORAN DISTRICT HOSPITAL (C, 32 beds) 1310 Hanna Avenue, Corcoran, CA Zip 93212, Mailing Address: Box 758, Zip 93212; tel. 559/992–5051; David R. Green, Chief Executive Officer

HAZEL HAWKINS MEMORIAL HOSPITAL (C, 72 beds) 911 Sunset Drive, Hollister, CA Zip 95023–5695; tel. 831/637–5711; Keith Mesmer, Chief Executive Officer

PIONEERS MEMORIAL HEALTHCARE DISTRICT (C, 99 beds) 207 West Legion Road, Brawley, CA Zip 92227–9699; tel. 760/351–3333; Claire Kuczkowski, Chief Executive Officer
Web address: www.pmhd.org

SAN GORGONIO MEMORIAL HOSPITAL (C, 68 beds) 600 North Highland Springs Avenue, Banning, CA Zip 92220; tel. 909/845–1121; Donald N. Larkin, Chief Executive Officer
Web address: www.sgmhf.org

TEHACHAPI VALLEY HEALTHCARE DISTRICT (C, 28 beds) 115 West E Street, Tehachapi, CA Zip 93561, Mailing Address: P.O. Box 1900, Zip 93581; tel. 661/822–3241; Raymond T. Hino, Chief Executive Officer

COLORADO: RIO GRANDE HOSPITAL (C, 12 beds) 1280 Grande Avenue, Del Norte, CO Zip 81132; tel. 719/657–2510; Rebecca Patterson, Administrator

FLORIDA: JUPITER MEDICAL CENTER (C, 276 beds) 1210 South Old Dixie Highway, Jupiter, FL Zip 33458–7299; tel. 561/747–2234; R. Michael Barry, Chief Executive Officer
Web address: www.jupitermed.com

ILLINOIS: HAMMOND–HENRY HOSPITAL (C, 105 beds) 210 West Elk Street, Geneseo, IL Zip 61254–1099; tel. 309/944–6431; Nathan C. Olson, President and Chief Executive Officer

HILLSBORO AREA HOSPITAL (C, 100 beds) 1200 East Tremont Street, Hillsboro, IL Zip 62049–1900; tel. 217/532–6111; Rex H. Brown, President

WOOD RIVER TOWNSHIP HOSPITAL (C, 60 beds) 101 East Edwardsville Road, Wood River, IL Zip 62095–1332; tel. 618/251–7101; David G. Triebes, Chief Executive Officer
Web address: www.ezl.com/~wrth101/

INDIANA: WIRTH REGIONAL HOSPITAL (C, 20 beds) Highway 64 West, Oakland City, IN Zip 47660–9379, Mailing Address: Rural Route 3, Box 14A, Zip 47660–9379; tel. 812/749–6111; Jeff Probus, Interim Chief Exective Officer

LOUISIANA: IBERIA MEDICAL CENTER (C, 90 beds) 2315 East Main Street, New Iberia, LA Zip 70560–4031, Mailing Address: P.O. Box 13338, Zip 70562–3338; tel. 318/364–0441; James H. Youree, Interim Chief Executive Officer
Web address: www.iberiamedicalcenter.com

LADY OF THE SEA GENERAL HOSPITAL (C, 55 beds) 200 West 134th Place, Cut Off, LA Zip 70345–4145; tel. 504/632–6401; Lane M. Cheramie, Chief Executive Officer

MONTANA: BARRETT MEMORIAL HOSPITAL (C, 23 beds) 1260 South Atlantic Street, Dillon, MT Zip 59725–3597; tel. 406/683–3000; John M. Mootry, Chief Executive Officer
Web address: www.barretthospital.org

BIG HORN COUNTY MEMORIAL HOSPITAL (C, 53 beds) 17 North Miles Avenue, Hardin, MT Zip 59034–0430, Mailing Address: P.O. Box 430, Zip 59034–0430; tel. 406/665–2310; Robert G. Notarianni, Chief Executive Officer
Web address: www.mcn.net/~medlab/

MINERAL COMMUNITY HOSPITAL (C, 30 beds) Roosevelt and Brooklyn, Superior, MT Zip 59872, Mailing Address: P.O. Box 66, Zip 59872–0066; tel. 406/822–4841; Steven Smoot, Chief Executive Officer

NORTHERN MONTANA HOSPITAL (C, 259 beds) 30 13th Street, Havre, MT Zip 59501–5222, Mailing Address: P.O. Box 1231, Zip 59501–1231; tel. 406/265–2211; David Henry, Chief Executive Officer

ROUNDUP MEMORIAL HOSPITAL (C, 48 beds) 1202 Third Street West, Roundup, MT Zip 59072–1816, Mailing Address: P.O. Box 40, Zip 59072–0040; tel. 406/323–2302; Dave McIvor, Administrator

NEBRASKA: TRI–VALLEY HEALTH SYSTEM (C, 65 beds) West Highway 6 and 34, Cambridge, NE Zip 69022–0488, Mailing Address: P.O. Box 488, Zip 69022–0488; tel. 308/697–3329; Arthur H. Frable, Chief Executive Officer

NEW MEXICO: UNION COUNTY GENERAL HOSPITAL (C, 25 beds) 301 Harding Street, Clayton, NM Zip 88415–3321, Mailing Address: P.O. Box 489, Zip 88415–0489; tel. 505/374–2585; W. C. McElhannon, Administrator

NEW YORK: ADIRONDACK MEDICAL CENTER (C, 78 beds) Lake Colby Drive, Saranac Lake, NY Zip 12983, Mailing Address: P.O. Box 471, Zip 12983–0471; tel. 518/891–4141; Chandler M. Ralph, President and Chief Executive Officer
Web address: www.northnet.org/adirondackmedcenter

THE HOSPITAL (C, 87 beds) 43 Pearl Street West, Sidney, NY Zip 13838–1399; tel. 607/561–2153; Russell A. Test, Administrator and Chief Executive Officer
Web address: www.thehospital.org

OHIO: ADAMS COUNTY HOSPITAL (C, 49 beds) 210 North Wilson Drive, West Union, OH Zip 45693–1574; tel. 937/544–5571; Linda Niles, Interim Chief Executive Officer

OREGON: BLUE MOUNTAIN HOSPITAL (C, 73 beds) 170 Ford Road, John Day, OR Zip 97845; tel. 541/575–1311; Robert Houser, Chief Executive Officer

TEXAS: DE LEON HOSPITAL (C, 14 beds) 407 South Texas Street, De Leon, TX Zip 76444–1947; tel. 254/893–2011; Michael K. Hare, Administrator

WASHINGTON: SUNNYSIDE COMMUNITY HOSPITAL (C, 38 beds) 10th and Tacoma Avenue, Sunnyside, WA Zip 98944–0719, Mailing Address: P.O. Box 719, Zip 98944–0719; tel. 509/837–1650; Jon D. Smiley, Chief Executive Officer
Web address: www.televar.com/sch

WISCONSIN: BURNETT MEDICAL CENTER (C, 70 beds) 257 West St. George Avenue, Grantsburg, WI Zip 54840–7827; tel. 715/463–5353; Timothy J. Wick, Chief Executive Officer

For explanation of codes following names, see page B2.
★ Indicates Type III membership in the American Hospital Association.

COMMUNITY MEMORIAL HOSPITAL (C, 27 beds) 855 South Main Street, Oconto Falls, WI Zip 54154–1296; tel. 920/846–3444; Jim Van Dornick, Administrator
Web address: www.cmhospital.org

GRANT REGIONAL HEALTH CENTER (C, 28 beds) 507 South Monroe Street, Lancaster, WI Zip 53813–2099; tel. 608/723–2143; Larry D. Rentfro, FACHE, President and Chief Executive Officer
Web address: www.grantregionalhealthctr.com

MEMORIAL COMMUNITY HOSPITAL (C, 125 beds) 313 Stoughton Road, Edgerton, WI Zip 53534–1198; tel. 608/884–3441; Steven H. Spencer, Chief Executive Officer

RIPON MEDICAL CENTER (C, 29 beds) 933 Newbury Street, Ripon, WI Zip 54971–1798, Mailing Address: P.O. Box 390, Zip 54971–0390; tel. 920/748–3101; Jon W. Baker, Chief Executive Officer
Web address: www.riponmedicalcenter.com

SHAWANO MEDICAL CENTER (C, 46 beds) 309 North Bartlette Street, Shawano, WI Zip 54166–0477; tel. 715/526–2111; John J. Kestly, Administrator
Web address: www.shawanomed.org

SOUTHWEST HEALTH CENTER (C, 143 beds) 250 Camp Street, Platteville, WI Zip 53818–1703; tel. 608/348–2331; Anne K. Klawiter, President and Chief Executive Officer
Web address: www.southwesthealth.org

SPOONER HEALTH SYSTEM (C, 136 beds) 819 Ash Street, Spooner, WI Zip 54801–1299; tel. 715/635–2111; Michael Schafer, Chief Executive Officer

ST. JOSEPH'S COMMUNITY HEALTH SERVICES (C, 80 beds) 400 Water Avenue, Hillsboro, WI Zip 54634–0527, Mailing Address: P.O. Box 527, Zip 54634–0527; tel. 608/489–2211; Billy J. Bruce , Jr, Chief Executive Officer

TOMAH MEMORIAL HOSPITAL (C, 45 beds) 321 Butts Avenue, Tomah, WI Zip 54660–1412; tel. 608/372–2181; Philip Stuart, Administrator

WYOMING: POWELL HOSPITAL (C, 130 beds) 777 Avenue H, Powell, WY Zip 82435–2296; tel. 307/754–2267; Rod Barton, Chief Executive Officer
Web address: www.wir.net/powell–hospital

Owned, leased, sponsored:	0 hospitals	0 beds
Contract–managed:	40 hospitals	2869 beds
Totals:	40 hospitals	2869 beds

★**0595: BRONSON HEALTHCARE GROUP, INC.** (NP)
One Healthcare Plaza, Kalamazoo, MI Zip 49007–5345; tel. 616/341–6000; Frank J. Sardone, President and Chief Executive Officer
(Centralized Physician/Insurance Health System)

MICHIGAN: BRONSON METHODIST HOSPITAL (O, 307 beds) 252 East Lovell Street, Kalamazoo, MI Zip 49007–5345; tel. 616/341–6000; Frank J. Sardone, President and Chief Executive Officer
Web address: www.bronsonhealth.com

BRONSON VICKSBURG HOSPITAL (O, 41 beds) 13326 North Boulevard, Vicksburg, MI Zip 49097–1099; tel. 616/649–2321; Frank J. Sardone, President
Web address: www.bronsonhealth.com

Owned, leased, sponsored:	2 hospitals	348 beds
Contract–managed:	0 hospitals	0 beds
Totals:	2 hospitals	348 beds

0395: BROWN SCHOOLS, INC. (IO)
1407 West Stassney Lane, Austin, TX Zip 78745–2998, Mailing Address: P.O. Box 4088, Zip 78765–4088; tel. 512/464–0200; Thomas Riley, Chief Executive Officer
(Independent Hospital System)

COLORADO: CEDAR SPRINGS BEHAVIORAL HEALTH SYSTEM (O, 114 beds) 2135 Southgate Road, Colorado Springs, CO Zip 80906–2693; tel. 719/633–4114; Connie Mull, Chief Executive Officer
Web address: www.brownschools.com

OKLAHOMA: THE BROWN SCHOOLS AT SHADOW MOUNTAIN (O, 100 beds) 6262 South Sheridan Road, Tulsa, OK Zip 74133–4099; tel. 918/492–8200; Sharon Worsham, Chief Executive Officer

TEXAS: BROWN SCHOOLS REHABILITATION CENTER (O, 30 beds) 1106 West Dittmar, Austin, TX Zip 78745–9990, Mailing Address: P.O. Box 150459, Zip 78715–0459; tel. 512/444–4835; Kay Peck, Chief Executive Officer
Web address: www.brownschools.com

CYPRESS CREEK HOSPITAL (O, 94 beds) 17750 Cali Drive, Houston, TX Zip 77090–2700; tel. 281/586–7600; Lawrence Story, Administrator
Web address: www.brownschools.com

WEST OAKS HOSPITAL (O, 40 beds) 6500 Hornwood Drive, Houston, TX Zip 77074–5095; tel. 713/995–0909; Charlene Arnett, Chief Executive Officer
Web address: www.brownschools.com/services/westoaks.html

VIRGINIA: CUMBERLAND, A BROWN SCHOOLS HOSPITAL FOR CHILDREN AND ADOLESCENTS (O, 84 beds) 9407 Cumberland Road, New Kent, VA Zip 23124–2029; tel. 804/966–2242; Ernest C. Priddy , II, Chief Executive Officer

Owned, leased, sponsored:	6 hospitals	462 beds
Contract–managed:	0 hospitals	0 beds
Totals:	6 hospitals	462 beds

0077: CAMBRIDGE INTERNATIONAL, INC, (IO)
7505 Fannin, Suite 680, Houston, TX Zip 77225; tel. 713/790–1153; Timothy Sharma, M.D., President
(Independent Hospital System)

TEXAS: INTRACARE MEDICAL CENTER HOSPITAL (O, 100 beds) 7601 Fannin Street, Houston, TX Zip 77054–1905; tel. 713/790–0949; Alice Hiniker, Ph.D., Administrator

INTRACARE NORTH HOSPITAL (O, 48 beds) 1120 Cypress Station, Houston, TX Zip 77090–3031; tel. 281/893–7200; Deo Shanker, CPA, Chief Executive Officer

Owned, leased, sponsored:	2 hospitals	148 beds
Contract–managed:	0 hospitals	0 beds
Totals:	2 hospitals	148 beds

★**0955: CAMCARE, INC.** (NP)
501 Morris Street, Charleston, WV Zip 25301–1300, Mailing Address: P.O. Box 1547, Zip 25326–1547; tel. 304/348–5432; Phillip H. Goodwin, FACHE, President and Chief Executive Officer
(Centralized Physician/Insurance Health System)

WEST VIRGINIA: BRAXTON COUNTY MEMORIAL HOSPITAL (O, 25 beds) 100 Hoylman Drive, Gassaway, WV Zip 26624–9320; tel. 304/364–5156; Tony E. Atkins, Administrator
Web address: www.pihn.org

CHARLESTON AREA MEDICAL CENTER (O, 765 beds) 501 Morris Street, Charleston, WV Zip 25301–1300, Mailing Address: P.O. Box 1547, Zip 25326–1547; tel. 304/348–5432; Phillip H. Goodwin, FACHE, President and Chief Executive Officer
Web address: www.camcare.com

PLATEAU MEDICAL CENTER (O, 74 beds) 430 Main Street, Oak Hill, WV Zip 25901–3455; tel. 304/469–8600; Hank Woodson, Administrator

Owned, leased, sponsored:	3 hospitals	864 beds
Contract–managed:	0 hospitals	0 beds
Totals:	3 hospitals	864 beds

0113: CANCER TREATMENT CENTERS OF AMERICA (IO)
3455 West Salt Creek Lane, Arlington Heights, IL Zip 60005–1080; tel. 847/342–7400; William A. Sanger, President and Chief Executive Officer
(Independent Hospital System)

ILLINOIS: MIDWESTERN REGIONAL MEDICAL CENTER (O, 70 beds) 2520 Elisha Avenue, Zion, IL Zip 60099–2587; tel. 847/872–4561; Roger C. Cary, President and Chief Executive Officer
Web address: www.pulbiconline.com/=mrmc

For explanation of codes following names, see page B2.
★ Indicates Type III membership in the American Hospital Association.

Systems / Cancer Treatment Centers Of America

OKLAHOMA: CANCER TREATMENT CENTERS OF AMERICA–TULSA (O, 40 beds) 2408 East 81st Street, Tulsa, OK Zip 74137–4210; tel. 918/496–5000; Joseph A. Gagliardi, President and Chief Executive Officer
Web address: www.cancercenter.com

Owned, leased, sponsored:	2 hospitals	110 beds
Contract–managed:	0 hospitals	0 beds
Totals:	2 hospitals	110 beds

0124: CAPE COD HEALTHCARE, INC. (NP)
88 Lewis Bay Road, Hyannis, MA Zip 02601–5210; tel. 508/862–5000; Stephen L. Abbott, President and Chief Executive Officer

MASSACHUSETTS: CAPE COD HOSPITAL (O, 214 beds) 27 Park Street, Hyannis, MA Zip 02601; tel. 508/771–1800; Gail M. Frieswick, Ed.D., Executive Vice President

FALMOUTH HOSPITAL (O, 83 beds) 100 Ter Heun Drive, Falmouth, MA Zip 02540–2599; tel. 508/548–5300; Robert A. Gunderson, Executive Vice President

Owned, leased, sponsored:	2 hospitals	297 beds
Contract–managed:	0 hospitals	0 beds
Totals:	2 hospitals	297 beds

★0099: CARE NEW ENGLAND HEALTH SYSTEM (NP)
45 Willard Avenue, Providence, RI Zip 02905–3218; tel. 401/453–7900; John J. Hynes, President and Chief Executive Officer
(Centralized Health System)

RHODE ISLAND: BUTLER HOSPITAL (O, 105 beds) 345 Blackstone Boulevard, Providence, RI Zip 02906–4829; tel. 401/455–6200; Patricia R. Recupero, JD, M.D., President and Chief Executive Officer
Web address: www.butler.org

KENT COUNTY MEMORIAL HOSPITAL (O, 339 beds) 455 Tollgate Road, Warwick, RI Zip 02886–2770; tel. 401/737–7000; Robert E. Baute, M.D., President and Chief Executive Officer
Web address: www.kentri.org

WOMEN AND INFANTS HOSPITAL OF RHODE ISLAND (O, 197 beds) 101 Dudley Street, Providence, RI Zip 02905–2499; tel. 401/274–1100; Thomas G. Parris , Jr, President
Web address: www.womenandinfants.com

Owned, leased, sponsored:	3 hospitals	641 beds
Contract–managed:	0 hospitals	0 beds
Totals:	3 hospitals	641 beds

★0096: CAREGROUP (NP)
375 Longwood Avenue, Boston, MA Zip 02215–5395; tel. 617/975–6060; James Reinertsen, M.D., Chief Executive Officer
(Moderately Centralized Health System)

MASSACHUSETTS: BETH ISRAEL DEACONESS MEDICAL CENTER (O, 589 beds) 330 Brookline Avenue, Boston, MA Zip 02215–5491; tel. 617/667–2203; James Reinertsen, M.D., Chief Executive Officer
Web address: www.bidmc.harvard.edu

DEACONESS WALTHAM HOSPITAL (O, 199 beds) Hope Avenue, Waltham, MA Zip 02453; tel. 781/647–6000; Dana W. Ramish, FACHE, President and Chief Executive Officer

DEACONESS–GLOVER HOSPITAL CORPORATION (O, 41 beds) 148 Chestnut Street, Needham, MA Zip 02192–2483; tel. 781/453–3000; John Dalton, President and Chief Executive Officer
Web address: www.glover.caregroup.org/

DEACONESS–NASHOBA HOSPITAL (O, 41 beds) 200 Groton Road, Ayer, MA Zip 01432–3300; tel. 978/784–9000; Jeffrey R. Kelly, President and Chief Executive Officer

MOUNT AUBURN HOSPITAL (O, 172 beds) 330 Mount Auburn Street, Cambridge, MA Zip 02138; tel. 617/499–5700; Jeanette G. Clough, President and Chief Executive Officer
Web address: www.mtauburn.caregroup.org/

NEW ENGLAND BAPTIST HOSPITAL (O, 162 beds) 125 Parker Hill Avenue, Boston, MA Zip 02120–3297; tel. 617/754–5800; Alan H. Robbins, M.D., President
Web address: www.nebh.org

Owned, leased, sponsored:	6 hospitals	1204 beds
Contract–managed:	0 hospitals	0 beds
Totals:	6 hospitals	1204 beds

★0070: CARILION HEALTH SYSTEM (NP)
101 Elm Avenue S.E., Roanoke, VA Zip 24013, Mailing Address: P.O. Box 13727, Zip 24036–3727; tel. 540/981–7347; Thomas L. Robertson, President and Chief Executive Officer
(Centralized Physician/Insurance Health System)

VIRGINIA: CARILION BEDFORD MEMORIAL HOSPITAL (O, 160 beds) 1613 Oakwood Street, Bedford, VA Zip 24523–0688, Mailing Address: P.O. Box 688, Zip 24523–0688; tel. 540/586–2441; Howard Ainsley, Vice President and Hospital Director
Web address: www.carilion.com

CARILION FRANKLIN MEMORIAL HOSPITAL (O, 37 beds) 180 Floyd Avenue, Rocky Mount, VA Zip 24151–1389; tel. 540/483–5277; Matthew J. Perry, Director
Web address: www.carilion.com

CARILION GILES MEMORIAL HOSPITAL (O, 52 beds) 1 Taylor Avenue, Pearisburg, VA Zip 24134–1932; tel. 540/921–6000; Morris D. Reece, Administrator and Chief Executive Officer
Web address: www.carilion.com

CARILION MEDICAL CENTER (O, 740 beds) Belleview at Jefferson Street, Roanoke, VA Zip 24014, Mailing Address: P.O. Box 13367, Zip 24033–3367; tel. 540/981–700C; Lucas A. Snipes, FACHE, Director
Web address: www.carilion.com

CARILION NEW RIVER VALLEY MEDICAL CENTER (O, 97 beds) 2900 Tyler Road, Radford, VA Zip 24073, Mailing Address: P.O. Box 5, Zip 24141–0005; tel. 540/731–2000; Virginia Ousley, Vice President and Hospital Director
Web address: www.carilion.com

CARILION SAINT ALBANS HOSPITAL (O, 60 beds) Route 11, Lee Highway, Radford, VA Zip 24143, Mailing Address: P.O. Box 3608, Zip 24143–3608; tel. 540/639–2481; Janet McKinney Crawford, Vice President and Administrator
Web address: www.carilion.com

SMYTH COUNTY COMMUNITY HOSPITAL (O, 285 beds) 565 Radio Hill Road, Marion, VA Zip 24354–3526, Mailing Address: P.O. Box 880, Zip 24354–0880; tel. 540/782–1234; William Mahone , V, Interim President and Chief Executive Officer

SOUTHSIDE COMMUNITY HOSPITAL (C, 88 beds) 800 Oak Street, Farmville, VA Zip 23901–1199; tel. 804/392–8811; John H. Greer, President

TAZEWELL COMMUNITY HOSPITAL (C, 38 beds) 141 Ben Bolt Avenue, Tazewell, VA Zip 24651–9700; tel. 540/988–2506; Craig B. James, President and Chief Executive Officer
Web address: www.tazecommhospital.org

WYTHE COUNTY COMMUNITY HOSPITAL (O, 90 beds) 600 West Ridge Road, Wytheville, VA Zip 24382–1099; tel. 540/228–0200; Larry H. Chewning , II, Chief Executive Officer
Web address: www.wcch.org

Owned, leased, sponsored:	8 hospitals	1521 beds
Contract–managed:	2 hospitals	126 beds
Totals:	10 hospitals	1647 beds

★0141: CARITAS CHRISTI HEALTH CARE (NP)
736 Cambridge Street, Boston, MA Zip 02135–2997; tel. 617/789–2500; Michael F. Collins, M.D., President
(Moderately Centralized Health System)

For explanation of codes following names, see page B2.
★ Indicates Type III membership in the American Hospital Association.

MASSACHUSETTS: CARITAS GOOD SAMARITAN MEDICAL CENTER (S, 193 beds) 235 North Pearl Street, Brockton, MA Zip 02401–1794; tel. 508/427–3000; Peter J. Holden, President
Web address: www.caritaschristi.org/locations.html

CARITAS NORWOOD HOSPITAL (S, 329 beds) 800 Washington Street, Norwood, MA Zip 02062–3487; tel. 781/278–6001; Delia O'Connor, President

CARNEY HOSPITAL (S, 174 beds) 2100 Dorchester Avenue, Dorchester, MA Zip 02124–5666; tel. 617/296–4000; Joyce A. Murphy, President
Web address: www.caritaschristi.org/locations.html

HOLY FAMILY HOSPITAL AND MEDICAL CENTER (S, 249 beds) 70 East Street, Methuen, MA Zip 01844–4597; tel. 978/687–0151; William L. Lane, President
Web address: www.holyfamilyhosp.org

SAINT ANNE'S HOSPITAL (S, 155 beds) 795 Middle Street, Fall River, MA Zip 02721–1798; tel. 508/674–5741; Michael W. Metzler, President

ST. ELIZABETH'S MEDICAL CENTER OF BOSTON (S, 247 beds) 736 Cambridge Street, Brighton, MA Zip 02135–2997; tel. 617/789–3000; Michael F. Collins, M.D., President
Web address: www.semc.org

Owned, leased, sponsored:	6 hospitals	1347 beds
Contract–managed:	0 hospitals	0 beds
Totals:	6 hospitals	1347 beds

0705: CAROLINAS HEALTHCARE SYSTEM (NP)
1000 Blythe Boulevard, Charlotte, NC Zip 28203–5871, Mailing Address: P.O. Box 32861, Zip 28232–2861; tel. 704/355–2000; Harry A. Nurkin, Ph.D., President
(Moderately Centralized Health System)

NORTH CAROLINA: ANNIE PENN HOSPITAL (C, 129 beds) 618 South Main Street, Reidsville, NC Zip 27320–5094; tel. 336/634–1010; Susan H. Fitzgibbon, President and Chief Executive Officer
Web address: www.anniepenn.org

ANSON COMMUNITY HOSPITAL (O, 125 beds) 500 Morven Road, Wadesboro, NC Zip 28170–2745; tel. 704/694–5131; Frederick G. Thompson, Ph.D., Administrator and Chief Executive Officer
Web address: www.carolinas.org

CAROLINAS MEDICAL CENTER (O, 761 beds) 1000 Blythe Boulevard, Charlotte, NC Zip 28203–5871, Mailing Address: P.O. Box 32861, Zip 28232–2861; tel. 704/355–2000; Paul S. Franz, President
Web address: www.carolinas.org

CHARLOTTE INSTITUTE OF REHABILITATION (O, 118 beds) 1100 Blythe Boulevard, Charlotte, NC Zip 28203–5864; tel. 704/355–4300; Cynthia King, Acting Administrator
Web address: www.carolinas.org

CLEVELAND REGIONAL MEDICAL CENTER (L, 334 beds) 201 Grover Street, Shelby, NC Zip 28150–3940; tel. 704/487–3000; John Young, President and Chief Executive Officer
Web address: www.carolinas.org

CRAWLEY MEMORIAL HOSPITAL (C, 51 beds) 315 West College Avenue, Boiling Springs, NC Zip 28017, Mailing Address: P.O. Box 996, Zip 28017–0996; tel. 704/434–9466; Gail McKillop, President

KINGS MOUNTAIN HOSPITAL (O, 82 beds) 706 West King Street, Kings Mountain, NC Zip 28086–2708, Mailing Address: P.O. Box 339, Zip 28086–0339; tel. 704/739–3601; Hank Neal, Administrator

MERCY HOSPITAL (O, 224 beds) 2001 Vail Avenue, Charlotte, NC Zip 28207–1289; tel. 704/379–5100; C. Curtis Copenhaver, President
Web address: www.carolinas.org

UNION REGIONAL MEDICAL CENTER (L, 223 beds) 600 Hospital Drive, Monroe, NC Zip 28112–6000, Mailing Address: P.O. Box 5003, Zip 28111–5003; tel. 704/283–3100; John W. Roberts, President and Chief Executive Officer
Web address: www.carolinas.org

UNIVERSITY HOSPITAL (O, 122 beds) 8800 North Tryon Street, Charlotte, NC Zip 28262–8415, Mailing Address: P.O. Box 560727, Zip 28256–0727; tel. 704/548–6000; W. Spencer Lilly, Administrator

VALDESE GENERAL HOSPITAL (O, 199 beds) Valdese, NC Mailing Address: P.O. Box 700, Zip 28690–0700; tel. 828/874–2251; Lloyd E. Wallace, President and Chief Executive Officer
Web address: www.carolinas.org

SOUTH CAROLINA: BON SECOURS–ST. FRANCIS XAVIER HOSPITAL (C, 145 beds) 2095 Henry Tecklenburg Drive, Charleston, SC Zip 29414–0001, Mailing Address: P.O. Box 160001, Zip 29414–0001; tel. 843/402–1000; Allen P. Carroll, Chief Executive Officer
Web address: www.sfxhospital.com

ROPER HOSPITAL (C, 375 beds) 316 Calhoun Street, Charleston, SC Zip 29401–1125; tel. 843/724–2000; Matt Severance, Administrator
Web address: www.carealliance.com

ROPER HOSPITAL NORTH (C, 104 beds) 2750 Speissegger Drive, Charleston, SC Zip 29405–8294; tel. 843/745–2800; John C. Hales , Jr, FACHE, President and Chief Executive Officer
Web address: www.carealliance.com

Owned, leased, sponsored:	9 hospitals	2188 beds
Contract–managed:	5 hospitals	804 beds
Totals:	14 hospitals	2992 beds

★5945: CARONDELET HEALTH SYSTEM (CC)
13801 Riverport Drive, Suite 300, Saint Louis, MO Zip 63043–4810; tel. 314/770–0333; Gary Christiansen, President and Chief Executive Officer
(Moderately Centralized Health System)

ARIZONA: CARONDELET HOLY CROSS HOSPITAL (O, 80 beds) 1171 West Target Range Road, Nogales, AZ Zip 85621–2496; tel. 520/287–2771; Richard Polheber, Interim Vice President and Chief Executive Officer

CARONDELET ST. JOSEPH'S HOSPITAL (O, 287 beds) 350 North Wilmot Road, Tucson, AZ Zip 85711–2678; tel. 520/296–3211; Wesley E. Colvin, Senior Vice President and Chief Executive Officer

CARONDELET ST. MARY'S HOSPITAL (O, 345 beds) 1601 West St. Mary's Road, Tucson, AZ Zip 85745–2682; tel. 520/622–5833;
Web address: www.carondelet.org

CALIFORNIA: DANIEL FREEMAN MARINA HOSPITAL (O, 138 beds) 4650 Lincoln Boulevard, Venice, CA Zip 90291–6360; tel. 310/823–8911; Joseph W. Dunn, Ph.D., Chief Executive Officer
Web address: www.danielfreeman.org

DANIEL FREEMAN MEMORIAL HOSPITAL (O, 360 beds) 333 North Prairie Avenue, Inglewood, CA Zip 90301–4514; tel. 310/674–7050; Joseph W. Dunn, Ph.D., President and Chief Executive Officer
Web address: www.danielfreeman.org

SANTA MARTA HOSPITAL (O, 83 beds) 319 North Humphreys Avenue, Los Angeles, CA Zip 90022–1499; tel. 323/266–6500; Harry E. Whitney, President and Chief Executive Officer
Web address: www.santamarta.org

GEORGIA: ST. JOSEPH HOSPITAL (O, 145 beds) 2260 Wrightsboro Road, Augusta, GA Zip 30904–4726; tel. 706/481–7000; J. William Paugh, President and Chief Executive Officer
Web address: www.stjoshosp.org

IDAHO: ST. JOSEPH REGIONAL MEDICAL CENTER (O, 156 beds) 415 Sixth Street, Lewiston, ID Zip 83501–0816; tel. 208/743–2511; Howard A. Hayes, President and Chief Executive Officer
Web address: www.sjrmc.org

MISSOURI: SAINT JOSEPH HEALTH CENTER (O, 267 beds) 1000 Carondelet Drive, Kansas City, MO Zip 64114–4673; tel. 816/942–4400; Michele Schaefer, Chief Executive Officer

ST. MARY'S HOSPITAL OF BLUE SPRINGS (O, 115 beds) 201 West R. D. Mize Road, Blue Springs, MO Zip 64014; tel. 816/228–5900; Gordon Docking, Chief Executive Officer

NEW YORK: ST. JOSEPH'S HOSPITAL (O, 240 beds) 555 East Market Street, Elmira, NY Zip 14902–1512; tel. 607/733–6541; Sister Marie Castagnaro, President and Chief Executive Officer
Web address: www.stjosephs.org

For explanation of codes following names, see page B2.
★ Indicates Type III membership in the American Hospital Association.

Systems / Carondelet Health System

ST. MARY'S HOSPITAL (O, 143 beds) 427 Guy Park Avenue, Amsterdam, NY Zip 12010–1095; tel. 518/842–1900; Peter E. Capobianco, President and Chief Executive Officer
Web address: www.smha.org

WASHINGTON: LOURDES COUNSELING CENTER (O, 32 beds) 1175 Carondelet Drive, Richland, WA Zip 99352–1175; tel. 509/943–9104; James F. Dover, FACHE, Chief Executive Officer
Web address: www.lourdesonline.com

LOURDES MEDICAL CENTER (O, 132 beds) 520 North Fourth Avenue, Pasco, WA Zip 99301–2568, Mailing Address: P.O. Box 2568, Zip 99302–2568; tel. 509/547–7704; James F. Dover, FACHE, Chief Executive Officer
Web address: www.cbvcp.com\healthcenter

Owned, leased, sponsored:	14 hospitals	2523 beds
Contract-managed:	0 hospitals	0 beds
Totals:	14 hospitals	2523 beds

0126: CARRAWAY METHODIST HEALTH SYSTEM (NP)
1600 Carraway Boulevard, Birmingham, AL Zip 35234–1990; tel. 205/502–6000; Robert M. Carraway, M.D., Chairman and Chief Executive Officer
(Moderately Centralized Health System)

ALABAMA: CARRAWAY BURDICK WEST MEDICAL CENTER (O, 99 beds) Highway 195 East, Haleyville, AL Zip 35565–9536, Mailing Address: P.O. Box 780, Zip 35565–0780; tel. 205/486–5213; Donald J. Jones, Administrator
Web address: www.carraway.com

CARRAWAY METHODIST MEDICAL CENTER (O, 383 beds) 1600 Carraway Boulevard, Birmingham, AL Zip 35234–1990; tel. 205/502–6000; Cindy Williams, FACHE, Administrator
Web address: www.carraway.org

CARRAWAY NORTHWEST MEDICAL CENTER (O, 63 beds) Highway 78 West, Winfield, AL Zip 35594, Mailing Address: P.O. Box 130, Zip 35594–0130; tel. 205/487–7000; Robert E. Henger, Administrator
Web address: www.carraway.org

Owned, leased, sponsored:	3 hospitals	545 beds
Contract-managed:	0 hospitals	0 beds
Totals:	3 hospitals	545 beds

6545: CATHEDRAL HEALTHCARE SYSTEM, INC. (CC)
219 Chestnut Street, Newark, NJ Zip 07105–1558; tel. 973/690–3600; Frank L. Fumai, President and Chief Executive Officer
(Moderately Centralized Health System)

NEW JERSEY: COLUMBUS HOSPITAL (O, 206 beds) 495 North 13th Street, Newark, NJ Zip 07107–1397; tel. 973/268–1400; John G. Magliaro, President and Chief Executive Officer

HOSPITAL CENTER AT ORANGE (O, 195 beds) 188 South Essex Avenue, Orange, NJ Zip 07051; tel. 973/266–2200; James E. Romer, President and Chief Executive Officer

SAINT JAMES HOSPITAL OF NEWARK (O, 189 beds) 155 Jefferson Street, Newark, NJ Zip 07105; tel. 973/589–1300; Ceu Cirne-Neves, Administrator

SAINT MICHAEL'S MEDICAL CENTER (O, 270 beds) 268 Dr. Martin Luther King Jr. Boulevard, Newark, NJ Zip 07102–2094; tel. 973/877–5000; Barbara Loughney, Administrator
Web address: www.cathedralhealthcare.org

Owned, leased, sponsored:	4 hospitals	860 beds
Contract-managed:	0 hospitals	0 beds
Totals:	4 hospitals	860 beds

★0136: CATHOLIC HEALTH EAST (CC)
14 Campus Boulevard, Suite 300, Newtown Square, PA Zip 19073–3277; tel. 610/355–2000; Daniel F. Russell, President and Chief Executive Officer
(Decentralized Health System)

ALABAMA: MERCY MEDICAL (O, 162 beds) 101 Villa Drive, Daphne, AL Zip 36526–4653, Mailing Address: P.O. Box 1090, Zip 36526–1090; tel. 334/626–2694; Sister Mary Eileen Wilhelm, President and Chief Executive Officer
Web address: www.mercymedical.com

FLORIDA: BAYFRONT MEDICAL CENTER (O, 268 beds) 701 Sixth Street South, Saint Petersburg, FL Zip 33701–4891; tel. 727/823–1234; Sue G. Brody, President and Chief Executive Officer
Web address: www.bayfront.org

GOOD SAMARITAN MEDICAL CENTER (S, 341 beds) Flagler Drive at Palm Beach Lakes Boulevard, West Palm Beach, FL Zip 33401–3499; tel. 561/655–5511; Steven R. Nathan, President and Chief Executive Officer

HOLY CROSS HOSPITAL (O, 437 beds) 4725 North Federal Highway, Fort Lauderdale, FL Zip 33308–4668, Mailing Address: P.O. Box 23460, Zip 33307–3460; tel. 954/771–8000; John C. Johnson, Chief Executive Officer
Web address: www.holy-cross.com

MERCY HOSPITAL (O, 339 beds) 3663 South Miami Avenue, Miami, FL Zip 33133–4237; tel. 305/854–4400; Edward J. Rosasco, Jr, President and Chief Executive Officer
Web address: www.mercymiami.com

MORTON PLANT MEASE–NORTH BAY HOSPITAL (S, 122 beds) 6600 Madison Street, New Port Richey, FL Zip 34652–1900; tel. 727/842–8468; William M. Jennings, Administrator and Chief Operating Officer

SOUTH FLORIDA BAPTIST HOSPITAL (O, 96 beds) 301 North Alexander Street, Plant City, FL Zip 33566–9058, Mailing Address: Drawer H, Zip 33564–9058; tel. 813/757–1200; William G. Ulbricht, Chief Operating Officer

ST. ANTHONY'S HOSPITAL 1200 Seventh Avenue North, Saint Petersburg, FL Zip 33705–1388, Mailing Address: P.O. Box 12588, Zip 33733–2588; tel. 727/825–1100; Sue G. Brody, President and Chief Executive Officer
Web address: www.stanthonys.org

ST. JOSEPH'S HOSPITAL (S, 883 beds) 3001 West Martin Luther King Jr. Boulevard, Tampa, FL Zip 33607–6387, Mailing Address: P.O. Box 4227, Zip 33677–4227; tel. 813/870–4000; Isaac Mallah, President and Chief Executive Officer

ST. MARY'S HOSPITAL (S, 460 beds) 901 45th Street, West Palm Beach, FL Zip 33407–2495, Mailing Address: P.O. Box 24620, Zip 33416–4620; tel. 561/844–6300; Steven R. Nathan, President and Chief Executive Officer

GEORGIA: SAINT JOSEPH'S HOSPITAL OF ATLANTA (O, 346 beds) 5665 Peachtree Dunwoody Road N.E., Atlanta, GA Zip 30342–1764; tel. 404/851–7001; Brue Chandler, President and Chief Executive Officer
Web address: www.stjosephsatlanta.org

ST. MARY'S HEALTH CARE SYSTEM (O, 292 beds) 1230 Baxter Street, Athens, GA Zip 30606–3791; tel. 706/548–7581; Thomas E. Fitz, Jr, FACHE, President and Chief Executive Officer
Web address: www.stmarysathens.com

MAINE: MERCY HOSPITAL OF PORTLAND (O, 166 beds) 144 State Street, Portland, ME Zip 04101–3795; tel. 207/879–3000; Howard R. Buckley, President
Web address: www.mercyhospital.com

MASSACHUSETTS: MERCY HOSPITAL (O, 311 beds) 271 Carew Street, Springfield, MA Zip 01104–2398, Mailing Address: P.O. Box 9012, Zip 01102–9012; tel. 413/748–9000; Vincent J. McCorkle, President

NEW JERSEY: OUR LADY OF LOURDES MEDICAL CENTER (O, 300 beds) 1600 Haddon Avenue, Camden, NJ Zip 08103–3117; tel. 856/757–3500; Alexander J. Hatala, President and Chief Executive Officer
Web address: www.lourdesnet.org

RANCOCAS HOSPITAL (O, 237 beds) 218–A Sunset Road, Willingboro, NJ Zip 08046–1162; tel. 609/835–2900; Joseph Flamini, Chief Executive Officer

NEW YORK: ST. JAMES MERCY HOSPITAL (O, 256 beds) 411 Canisteo Street, Hornell, NY Zip 14843–2197; tel. 607/324–8000; William G. Connors, President and Chief Executive Officer
Web address: www.sjmh.org

ST. PETER'S HOSPITAL (O, 437 beds) 315 South Manning Boulevard, Albany, NY Zip 12208–1789; tel. 518/525–1550; Steven P. Boyle, President and Chief Executive Officer

---

For explanation of codes following names, see page B2.
★ Indicates Type III membership in the American Hospital Association.

Systems / Catholic Health Initiatives

PENNSYLVANIA: MERCY COMMUNITY HOSPITAL (O, 107 beds) 2000 Old West Chester Pike, Havertown, PA Zip 19083–2712; tel. 610/853–7000; Mary C. Morrison, R.N., Chief Executive Officer

MERCY HEALTH SYSTEM OF SOUTHEASTERN PENNSYLVANIA (O, 536 beds) 1 West Elm Street, Conshohocken, PA Zip 19428–2007; tel. 610/567–6000; Mark T. O'Neil , Jr, President and Chief Executive Officer
Web address: www.mercyhealth.org

MERCY HOSPITAL OF PITTSBURGH (O, 399 beds) 1400 Locust Street, Pittsburgh, PA Zip 15219–5166; tel. 412/232–8111; Gregg G. Zoller, FACHE, President and Chief Executive Officer
Web address: www.mercylink.org

MERCY PROVIDENCE HOSPITAL (O, 146 beds) 1004 Arch Street, Pittsburgh, PA Zip 15212–5235; tel. 412/323–5600; Gregg G. Zoller, FACHE, President and Chief Executive Officer
Web address: www.mercylink.org

MERCY SUBURBAN HOSPITAL (O, 115 beds) 2701 DeKalb Pike, Norristown, PA Zip 19401–1820; tel. 610/278–2000; Edward R. Solvibile, Chief Executive Officer
Web address: www.mercyhealth.org

NORTH PHILADELPHIA HEALTH SYSTEM (C, 315 beds) 16th Street and Girard Avenue, Philadelphia, PA Zip 19130–1615; tel. 215/787–9000; George J. Walmsley , II, President and Chief Executive Officer

Owned, leased, sponsored:	22 hospitals	6756 beds
Contract–managed:	1 hospital	315 beds
Totals:	23 hospitals	7071 beds

★0092: CATHOLIC HEALTH INITIATIVES (CC)
1999 Broadway, Suite 2605, Denver, CO Zip 80202–4004; tel. 303/298–9100; Patricia A. Cahill, President and Chief Executive Officer
(Decentralized Health System)

ARKANSAS: ST. VINCENT DOCTORS HOSPITAL (S, 308 beds) 6101 West Capitol, Little Rock, AR Zip 72205–5331; tel. 501/661–4000; Larry Marr, Senior Vice President and Administrator

ST. VINCENT INFIRMARY MEDICAL CENTER (S, 605 beds) Two St. Vincent Circle, Little Rock, AR Zip 72205–5499; tel. 501/660–3000; William A. McDonald, President and Chief Executive Officer
Web address: www.stvincenthealth.org

ST. VINCENT REHABILITATION HOSPITAL (S, 60 beds) 2201 Wildwood Avenue, Sherwood, AR Zip 72120–5074, Mailing Address: P.O. Box 6930, Zip 72124–6930; tel. 501/834–1800; C. Ronnie Sairls, Administrator

COLORADO: MERCY MEDICAL CENTER (S, 81 beds) 375 East Park Avenue, Durango, CO Zip 81301; tel. 970/247–4311; Kirk Dignum, Ph.D., President and Chief Executive Officer
Web address: www.mercydurango.org

PENROSE–ST. FRANCIS HEALTH SERVICES (S, 384 beds) Colorado Springs, CO Rick O'Connell, President and Chief Executive Officer

ST. ANTHONY CENTRAL HOSPITAL (S, 417 beds) 4231 West 16th Avenue, Denver, CO Zip 80204–4098; tel. 303/629–3511; Matthew S. Fulton, Senior Vice President and Administrator

ST. ANTHONY NORTH HOSPITAL (S, 106 beds) 2551 West 84th Avenue, Westminster, CO Zip 80030–3887; tel. 303/426–2151; Peggy Gustafson, Administrator
Web address: www.centura.org

ST. MARY–CORWIN MEDICAL CENTER (S, 261 beds) 1008 Minnequa Avenue, Pueblo, CO Zip 81004–3798; tel. 719/560–4000; Thomas E. Anderson, Chief Executive Officer
Web address: www.centura.org

ST. THOMAS MORE HOSPITAL AND PROGRESSIVE CARE CENTER (S, 218 beds) 1338 Phay Avenue, Canon City, CO Zip 81212–2221; tel. 719/269–2000; C. Ray Honaker, Chief Executive Officer
Web address: www.centura.org

DELAWARE: ST. FRANCIS HOSPITAL (S, 222 beds) Seventh and Clayton Streets, Wilmington, DE Zip 19805–0500, Mailing Address: P.O. Box 2500, Zip 19805–0500; tel. 302/421–4100; M. Eileen Schmitt, M.D., President and Chief Executive Officer

IDAHO: MERCY MEDICAL CENTER (S, 149 beds) 1512 12th Avenue Road, Nampa, ID Zip 83686–6008; tel. 208/467–1171; Joseph Messmer, President and Chief Executive Officer

IOWA: ALEGENT HEALTH MERCY HOSPITAL (S, 22 beds) 703 Rosary Drive, Corning, IA Zip 50841, Mailing Address: P.O. Box 368, Zip 50841–0368; tel. 515/322–3121; James C. Ruppert, Administrator

ALEGENT HEALTH MERCY HOSPITAL (S, 189 beds) 800 Mercy Drive, Council Bluffs, IA Zip 51503–3128, Mailing Address: P.O. Box 1C, Zip 51502–3001; tel. 712/328–5000; Charles J. Marr, Chief Executive Officer

MERCY MEDICAL CENTER–CENTERVILLE (S, 57 beds) 1 St. Joseph's Drive, Centerville, IA Zip 52544; tel. 515/437–4111; William C. Assell, President and Chief Executive Officer

MERCY MEDICAL CENTER–DES MOINES (S, 591 beds) 1111 6th Avenue, Des Moines, IA Zip 50314–2611; tel. 515/247–3121; David H. Vellinga, President and Chief Executive Officer
Web address: www.mercydesmoines.org

KANSAS: CENTRAL KANSAS MEDICAL CENTER (S, 184 beds) 3515 Broadway Street, Great Bend, KS Zip 67530–3633; tel. 316/792–2511; Thomas W. Sommers, President and Chief Executive Officer

ST. CATHERINE HOSPITAL (S, 93 beds) 410 East Walnut, Garden City, KS Zip 67846–5600; tel. 316/272–2222; Mark B. Steadham, President and Chief Executive Officer
Web address: www.phn.org

KENTUCKY: CARITAS MEDICAL CENTER (S, 213 beds) 1850 Bluegrass Avenue, Louisville, KY Zip 40215–1199; tel. 502/361–6000; Peter J. Bernard, President and Chief Executive Officer
Web address: www.chi-caritas.org

CARITAS PEACE CENTER (S, 225 beds) 2020 Newburg Road, Louisville, KY Zip 40205–1879; tel. 502/451–3330; Peter J. Bernard, President and Chief Executive Officer

FLAGET MEMORIAL HOSPITAL (S, 52 beds) 201 Cathedral Manor, Bardstown, KY Zip 40004–1299; tel. 502/348–3923; Suzanne Reasbeck, President and Chief Executive Officer
Web address: www.flaget.com

MARYMOUNT MEDICAL CENTER (S, 95 beds) 310 East Ninth Street, London, KY Zip 40741–1299; tel. 606/877–3705; Lowell Jones, President and Chief Executive Officer

OUR LADY OF THE WAY HOSPITAL (S, 39 beds) 11022 Main Street, Martin, KY Zip 41649–0910; tel. 606/285–5181; Lowell Jones, Chief Executive Officer
Web address: www.olwh.org

SAINT JOSEPH HOSPITAL (S, 361 beds) One St. Joseph Drive, Lexington, KY Zip 40504–3754; tel. 606/278–3436; Tom Matherlee, Interim Chief Executive Officer
Web address: www.sjhlex.org

SAINT JOSEPH HOSPITAL EAST (S, 119 beds) 150 North Eagle Creek Drive, Lexington, KY Zip 40509–1807; tel. 606/268–4800; Melinda Washburn, Chief Operating Officer

MARYLAND: ST. JOSEPH MEDICAL CENTER (S, 381 beds) 7601 York Road, Towson, MD Zip 21204–7582; tel. 410/337–1000; James J. Cullen, President and Chief Executive Officer
Web address: www.sjmcmd.org

MINNESOTA: ALBANY AREA HOSPITAL AND MEDICAL CENTER (S, 15 beds) 300 Third Avenue, Albany, MN Zip 56307–9363; tel. 320/845–2121; Ben Koppelman, Administrator

LAKEWOOD HEALTH CENTER (S, 64 beds) 600 Main Avenue South, Baudette, MN Zip 56623; tel. 218/634–2120; SharRay Palm, President and Chief Executive Officer

ST. FRANCIS MEDICAL CENTER (S, 171 beds) 415 Oak Street, Breckenridge, MN Zip 56520–1298; tel. 218/643–3000; David A. Nelson, President and Chief Executive Officer

ST. GABRIEL'S HOSPITAL (S, 199 beds) 815 Second Street S.E., Little Falls, MN Zip 56345–3596; tel. 320/632–5441; Larry A. Schulz, President and Chief Executive Officer
Web address: www.stgabriels.com

ST. JOSEPH'S AREA HEALTH SERVICES (S, 39 beds) 600 Pleasant Avenue, Park Rapids, MN Zip 56470–1432; tel. 218/732–3311; Peter Jacobson, President and Chief Executive Officer

---

For explanation of codes following names, see page B2.
★ Indicates Type III membership in the American Hospital Association.

Systems / Catholic Health Initiatives

MISSOURI: ST. JOHN'S REGIONAL MEDICAL CENTER (S, 367 beds) 2727 McClelland Boulevard, Joplin, MO Zip 64804–1694; tel. 417/781–2727; Gary L. Rowe, President and Chief Executive Officer
Web address: www.stj.com

NEBRASKA: ALEGENT HEALTH BERGAN MERCY MEDICAL CENTER (S, 549 beds) 7500 Mercy Road, Omaha, NE Zip 68124; tel. 402/343–4410; Mike Tiesi, Administrator

GOOD SAMARITAN HEALTH SYSTEMS (S, 267 beds) 10 East 31st Street, Kearney, NE Zip 68847–2926, Mailing Address: P.O. Box 1990, Zip 68848–1990; tel. 308/865–7100; William C. Luke, Interim President and Chief Executive Officer

SAINT ELIZABETH REGIONAL MEDICAL CENTER (S, 197 beds) 555 South 70th Street, Lincoln, NE Zip 68510–2494; tel. 402/489–7181; Robert J. Lanik, President and Chief Executive Officer
Web address: www.stez.org

ST. FRANCIS MEDICAL CENTER (S, 198 beds) 2620 West Faidley Avenue, Grand Island, NE Zip 68803–4297, Mailing Address: P.O. Box 9804, Zip 68802–9804; tel. 308/384–4600; Michael R. Gloor, FACHE, President and Chief Executive Officer
Web address: www.sfmc–gi.org

ST. MARY'S HOSPITAL (S, 28 beds) 1314 Third Avenue, Nebraska City, NE Zip 68410–1999; tel. 402/873–3321; Daniel J. Kelly, President and Chief Executive Officer

NEW JERSEY: ST. FRANCIS MEDICAL CENTER (S, 254 beds) 601 Hamilton Avenue, Trenton, NJ Zip 08629–1986; tel. 609/599–5000; Judith M. Persichilli, President and Chief Executive Officer

NEW MEXICO: ST. JOSEPH MEDICAL CENTER (S, 179 beds) 601 Martin Luther King Jr. Drive N.E., Albuquerque, NM Zip 87102, Mailing Address: P.O. Box 25555, Zip 87125–0555; tel. 505/727–8000; C. Vincent Townsend , Jr, Senior Vice President

ST. JOSEPH NORTHEAST HEIGHTS HOSPITAL (S, 78 beds) 4701 Montgomery Boulevard N.E., Albuquerque, NM Zip 87109–1251, Mailing Address: P.O. Box 25555, Zip 87125–0555; tel. 505/727–7800; Tony Struthers, Vice President Operations and Administrator

ST. JOSEPH REHABILITATION HOSPITAL AND OUTPATIENT CENTER (S, 62 beds) 505 Elm Street N.E., Albuquerque, NM Zip 87102–2500, Mailing Address: P.O. Box 25555, Zip 87125–5555; tel. 505/727–4700; Mary Lou Coors, Vice President
Web address: www.sjhs.org

ST. JOSEPH WEST MESA HOSPITAL (S, 74 beds) 10501 Golf Course Road N.W., Albuquerque, NM Zip 87114–5000, Mailing Address: P.O. Box 25555, Zip 87125–0555; tel. 505/727–2000; Tony Struthers, Vice President and Administrator

NORTH DAKOTA: CARRINGTON HEALTH CENTER (S, 70 beds) 800 North Fourth Street, Carrington, ND Zip 58421–1217; tel. 701/652–3141; Brian J. McDermott, President and Chief Executive Officer

MERCY HOSPITAL (S, 35 beds) 1031 Seventh Street, Devils Lake, ND Zip 58301–2798; tel. 701/662–2131; Marlene J. Krein, President and Chief Executive Officer

MERCY HOSPITAL (S, 50 beds) 570 Chautauqua Boulevard, Valley City, ND Zip 58072–3199; tel. 701/845–6400; Jane Bissel, President and Chief Executive Officer

MERCY MEDICAL CENTER (S, 93 beds) 1301 15th Avenue West, Williston, ND Zip 58801–3896; tel. 701/774–7400; M. Thomas Mitchell, President and Chief Executive Officer
Web address: www.dia.net/mercy

OAKES COMMUNITY HOSPITAL (S, 25 beds) 314 South Eighth Street, Oakes, ND Zip 58474–2099; tel. 701/742–3291; Bradley D. Burris, President and Chief Executive Officer

ST. ANSGAR'S HEALTH CENTER (S, 20 beds) 115 Vivian Street, Park River, ND Zip 58270–0708; tel. 701/284–7500; Michael D. Mahrer, President

ST. JOSEPH'S HOSPITAL AND HEALTH CENTER (S, 90 beds) 30 Seventh Street West, Dickinson, ND Zip 58601–4399; tel. 701/225–7200; Greg Hanson, President
Web address: www.stjoeshospital.org

OHIO: GOOD SAMARITAN HOSPITAL (S, 419 beds) 375 Dixmyth Avenue, Cincinnati, OH Zip 45220–2489; tel. 513/872–1400; John S. Prout, President and Chief Executive Officer
Web address: www.trihealth.com

GOOD SAMARITAN HOSPITAL AND HEALTH CENTER (S, 496 beds) 2222 Philadelphia Drive, Dayton, OH Zip 45406–1813; tel. 937/278–2612; K. Douglas Deck, President and Chief Executive Officer

OREGON: HOLY ROSARY MEDICAL CENTER (S, 74 beds) 351 S.W. Ninth Street, Ontario, OR Zip 97914–2693; tel. 541/881–7000; Bruce C. Jensen, President and Chief Executive Officer

MERCY MEDICAL CENTER (S, 114 beds) 2700 Stewart Parkway, Roseburg, OR Zip 97470–1297; tel. 541/673–0611; Victor J. Fresolone, FACHE, President and Chief Executive Officer
Web address: www.mercyrose.org

ST. ANTHONY HOSPITAL (S, 49 beds) 1601 S.E. Court Avenue, Pendleton, OR Zip 97801–3297; tel. 541/276–5121; Jeffrey S. Drop, President and Chief Executive Officer

ST. ELIZABETH HEALTH SERVICES (S, 134 beds) 3325 Pocahontas Road, Baker City, OR Zip 97814; tel. 541/523–6461; John R. Perushek, President and Chief Executive Officer

PENNSYLVANIA: NAZARETH HOSPITAL (S, 236 beds) 2601 Holme Avenue, Philadelphia, PA Zip 19152–2007; tel. 215/335–6000; Patricia B. DeAngelis, President and Chief Operating Officer

ST. AGNES MEDICAL CENTER (S, 172 beds) 1900 South Broad Street, Philadelphia, PA Zip 19145–2304; tel. 215/339–4100; Sister Margaret T. Sullivan, President and Chief Executive Officer
Web address: www.chi–east.org

ST. JOSEPH HOSPITAL (S, 208 beds) 250 College Avenue, Lancaster, PA Zip 17604, Mailing Address: P.O. Box 3509, Zip 17604–3509; tel. 717/291–8211; John Kerr Tolmie, President and Chief Executive Officer
Web address: www.chieast.org

ST. JOSEPH MEDICAL CENTER (S, 269 beds) 215 North 12th Street, Reading, PA Zip 19603–0316, Mailing Address: P.O. Box 316, Zip 19603–0316; tel. 610/378–2000; John R. Morahan, President
Web address: www.chi–east.org/

ST. MARY MEDICAL CENTER (S, 257 beds) Langhorne–Newtown Road, Langhorne, PA Zip 19047–1295; tel. 215/750–2000; Gregory T. Wozniak, President and Chief Executive Officer

SOUTH DAKOTA: GETTYSBURG MEDICAL CENTER (S, 61 beds) 606 East Garfield, Gettysburg, SD Zip 57442–1398; tel. 605/765–2480; Mark Schmidt, President and Chief Executive Officer

ST. MARY'S HEALTHCARE CENTER (S, 191 beds) 800 East Dakota Avenue, Pierre, SD Zip 57501–3313; tel. 605/224–3100; James D. M. Russell, Chief Executive Officer
Web address: www.st–marys.com

TENNESSEE: MEMORIAL HOSPITAL (S, 370 beds) 2525 De Sales Avenue, Chattanooga, TN Zip 37404–3322; tel. 423/495–2525; L. Clark Taylor , Jr, Ph.D., President and Chief Executive Officer

WASHINGTON: ST. CLARE HOSPITAL (S, 60 beds) 11315 Bridgeport Way S.W., Lakewood, WA Zip 98499–0998, Mailing Address: P.O. Box 99998, Zip 98499–0998; tel. 253/588–1711; Syd Bersante, Chief of Operations

ST. FRANCIS HOSPITAL (S, 99 beds) 34515 Ninth Avenue South, Federal Way, WA Zip 98003–9710; tel. 253/927–9700; Joseph W. Wilczek, President and Chief Executive Officer

ST. JOSEPH MEDICAL CENTER (S, 283 beds) 1717 South J Street, Tacoma, WA Zip 98405–3004, Mailing Address: P.O. Box 2197, Zip 98401–2197; tel. 253/627–4101; June C. Bowman, R.N., Chief Operating Officer and Nurse Executive

WISCONSIN: GOOD SAMARITAN HEALTH CENTER OF MERRILL (S, 63 beds) 601 Center Avenue South, Merrill, WI Zip 54452–3404; tel. 715/536–5511; Michael Hammer, President and Chief Executive Officer

Owned, leased, sponsored:	66 hospitals	12111 beds
Contract–managed:	0 hospitals	0 beds
Totals:	66 hospitals	12111 beds

For explanation of codes following names, see page B2.
★ Indicates Type III membership in the American Hospital Association.

Systems / Catholic Healthcare West

0079: CATHOLIC HEALTH PARTNERS (CC)
2913 North Commonwealth, Chicago, IL Zip 60657–6296; tel. 773/665–3757; Arnie Kimmel, President and Chief Executive Officer
(Centralized Health System)

ILLINOIS: COLUMBUS HOSPITAL (S, 128 beds) 2520 North Lakeview Avenue, Chicago, IL Zip 60614–1895; tel. 773/388–7300; Arnold Kimmel, Interim President and Chief Executive Officer
Web address: www.cath–health.org

SAINT ANTHONY HOSPITAL (S, 163 beds) 2875 West 19th Street, Chicago, IL Zip 60623–3596; tel. 773/521–1710; Arnold Kimmel, Interim President and Chief Executive Officer
Web address: www.cath–health.org

ST. JOSEPH HOSPITAL (S, 408 beds) 2900 North Lake Shore Drive, Chicago, IL Zip 60657–6274; tel. 773/665–3000; Arnold Kimmel, Interim President and Chief Executive Officer
Web address: www.cath–health.org

Owned, leased, sponsored:	3 hospitals	699 beds
Contract–managed:	0 hospitals	0 beds
Totals:	3 hospitals	699 beds

5155: CATHOLIC HEALTHCARE PARTNERS (CC)
615 Elsinore Place, Cincinnati, OH Zip 45202; tel. 513/639–2827; Michael D. Connelly, President and Chief Executive Officer
(Moderately Centralized Health System)

KENTUCKY: LOURDES HOSPITAL (S, 290 beds) 1530 Lone Oak Road, Paducah, KY Zip 42003, Mailing Address: P.O. Box 7100, Zip 42002–7100; tel. 270/444–2444; Robert P. Goodwin, President and Chief Executive Officer
Web address: www.lourdes–pad.org

MARCUM AND WALLACE MEMORIAL HOSPITAL (S, 25 beds) 60 Mercy Court, Irvine, KY Zip 40336–1331, Mailing Address: P.O. Box 928, Zip 40336–0928; tel. 606/723–2115; James F. Heitzenrater, President and Chief Executive Officer

ST. ELIZABETH MEDICAL CENTER–GRANT COUNTY (O, 20 beds) 238 Barnes Road, Williamstown, KY Zip 41097–9460; tel. 606/824–2400; Chris Carle, Administrator

ST. ELIZABETH MEDICAL CENTER–SOUTH (O, 397 beds) One Medical Village Drive, Edgewood, KY Zip 41017; tel. 859/344–2000; Joseph W. Gross, President and Chief Executive Officer
Web address: www.stelizabeth.com

OHIO: FRANCISCAN HOSPITAL–WESTERN HILLS (O, 223 beds) 3131 Queen City Avenue, Cincinnati, OH Zip 45238–2396; tel. 513/389–5000; Charles C. Lobeck, President
Web address: www.mercy.health–partners.org

LORAIN COMMUNITY/ST. JOSEPH REGIONAL HEALTH CENTER (S, 282 beds) 3700 Kolbe Road, Lorain, OH Zip 44053–1697; tel. 440/960–3000; Brian C. Lockwood, President and Chief Executive Officer

MERCY FRANCISCAN HOSPITAL–MOUNT AIRY (O, 246 beds) 2446 Kipling Avenue, Cincinnati, OH Zip 45239–6650; tel. 513/853–5000; Steven Grinnell, President
Web address: www.mercy.health–partners.org

MERCY HOSPITAL (S, 205 beds) Hamilton, OH Mailing Address: P.O. Box 418, Zip 45012–0418; tel. 513/867–6400; David A. Ferrell, President
Web address: www.mercy.health–partners.org

MERCY HOSPITAL (S, 66 beds) 485 West Market Street, Tiffin, OH Zip 44883–0727; tel. 419/448–3133; Mark Shugarman, President
Web address: www.mhsnr.org

MERCY HOSPITAL ANDERSON (S, 151 beds) 7500 State Road, Cincinnati, OH Zip 45255–2492; tel. 513/624–4500; Fred L. Kolb, President
Web address: www.mercy.health–partners.org

MERCY HOSPITAL CLERMONT (S, 85 beds) 3000 Hospital Drive, Batavia, OH Zip 45103–1998; tel. 513/732–8200; John M. Dawes, Vice President Operations
Web address: www.mercy.health–partners.org

MERCY HOSPITAL OF WILLARD (S, 30 beds) 110 East Howard Street, Willard, OH Zip 44890–1611; tel. 419/964–5000; Dale E. Thornton, M.P.H., CHE, President and Chief Executive Officer
Web address: www.mhsnr.org

MERCY MEDICAL CENTER (S, 218 beds) 1343 North Fountain Boulevard, Springfield, OH Zip 45501–1380; tel. 937/390–5000; Marian R. Purdue, Senior Vice President and Chief Operating Officer

MERCY MEMORIAL HOSPITAL (S, 20 beds) 904 Scioto Street, Urbana, OH Zip 43078–2200; tel. 937/653–5231; Karl Zalar, Administrator

RIVERSIDE MERCY HOSPITAL (S, 162 beds) 1600 North Superior Street, Toledo, OH Zip 43604–2199; tel. 419/729–6000; Scott E. Shook, President
Web address: www.mhsnr.org

ST. CHARLES MERCY HOSPITAL (S, 309 beds) 2600 Navarre Avenue, Oregon, OH Zip 43616–3297; tel. 419/696–7200; Cathleen K. Nelson, President and Chief Executive Officer
Web address: www.mercyweb.org

ST. ELIZABETH HEALTH CENTER (S, 339 beds) 1044 Belmont Avenue, Youngstown, OH Zip 44501, Mailing Address: P.O. Box 1790, Zip 44501–1790; tel. 330/746–7211; Michael Terrance Rowan, President and Chief Executive Officer
Web address: www.hmhs.org

ST. JOSEPH HEALTH CENTER (S, 136 beds) 667 Eastland Avenue S.E., Warren, OH Zip 44484–4531; tel. 330/841–4000; Michael Terrance Rowan, President and Chief Executive Officer
Web address: www.hmhs.org

ST. RITA'S MEDICAL CENTER (S, 351 beds) 730 West Market Street, Lima, OH Zip 45801–4670; tel. 419/227–3361; James P. Reber, President
Web address: www.mercy.com/srmc

ST. VINCENT MERCY MEDICAL CENTER (S, 459 beds) 2213 Cherry Street, Toledo, OH Zip 43608–2691; tel. 419/251–3232; Steven L. Mickus, President and Chief Executive Officer
Web address: www.mercyweb.org

PENNSYLVANIA: MERCY HOSPITAL OF SCRANTON (S, 265 beds) 746 Jefferson Avenue, Scranton, PA Zip 18501–1624; tel. 570/348–7100; Susan Petula, President
Web address: www.mhs–nepa.com

MERCY HOSPITAL OF WILKES–BARRE (S, 215 beds) 25 Church Street, Wilkes–Barre, PA Zip 18765–0999, Mailing Address: P.O. Box 658, Zip 18765–0658; tel. 570/826–3100; V. Gail Blaum, President
Web address: www.mhs–nepa.com

MERCY SPECIAL CARE HOSPITAL (S, 38 beds) 128 West Washington Street, Nanticoke, PA Zip 18634–3113; tel. 570/735–5000; Robert D. Williams, Administrator

TENNESSEE: JEFFERSON MEMORIAL HOSPITAL (L, 29 beds) 1800 Bishop Avenue, Jefferson City, TN Zip 37760–1992, Mailing Address: P.O. Box 560, Zip 37760–0560; tel. 865/475–2091; Michael C. Hicks, President and Chief Executive Officer
Web address: www.jeffersonhealthinc.com

ST. MARY'S HEALTH SYSTEM (S, 300 beds) 900 East Oak Hill Avenue, Knoxville, TN Zip 37917–4556; tel. 865/545–8000; Richard C. Williams, President and Chief Executive Officer
Web address: www.mercy.com/stmarys

Owned, leased, sponsored:	25 hospitals	4861 beds
Contract–managed:	0 hospitals	0 beds
Totals:	25 hospitals	4861 beds

★5205: CATHOLIC HEALTHCARE WEST (CC)
1700 Montgomery Street, Suite 300, San Francisco, CA Zip 94111–9603; tel. 415/438–5500; Lloyd H. Dean, President and Chief Executive Officer
(Decentralized Health System)

ARIZONA: CHANDLER REGIONAL HOSPITAL (O, 120 beds) 475 South Dobson Road, Chandler, AZ Zip 85224–4230; tel. 480/963–4561; David G. Covert, President and Chief Administrative Officer
Web address: www.evrhs.org

ST. JOSEPH'S HOSPITAL AND MEDICAL CENTER (S, 514 beds) 350 West Thomas Road, Phoenix, AZ Zip 85013–4496, Mailing Address: P.O. Box

For explanation of codes following names, see page B2.
★ Indicates Type III membership in the American Hospital Association.

Systems / Catholic Healthcare West

2071, Zip 85001-2071; tel. 602/406-3000; Linda A. Hunt, President and Chief Administrative Officer
Web address: www.chw.edu

CALIFORNIA: BAKERSFIELD MEMORIAL HOSPITAL (S, 299 beds) 420 34th Street, Bakersfield, CA Zip 93301, Mailing Address: P.O. Box 1888, Zip 93303-1888; tel. 661/327-1792; C. Larry Carr, Regional Executive Vice President and President
Web address: www.chw.edu

CALIFORNIA HOSPITAL MEDICAL CENTER (O, 245 beds) 1401 South Grand Avenue, Los Angeles, CA Zip 90015-3063; tel. 213/748-2411; Melinda D. Beswick, President
Web address: www.chmcla.com

COMMMUNITY HOSPITAL OF SAN BERNARDINO (O, 373 beds) 1805 Medical Center Drive, San Bernardino, CA Zip 92411; tel. 909/887-6333; Bruce G. Satzger, President
Web address: www.chsb.org

DOMINICAN HOSPITAL (S, 275 beds) 1555 Soquel Drive, Santa Cruz, CA Zip 95065; tel. 831/462-7700; Sister Julie Hyer, President and Chief Executive Officer
Web address: www.dominicanhospital.org

GLENDALE MEMORIAL HOSPITAL AND HEALTH CENTER (O, 290 beds) 1420 South Central Avenue, Glendale, CA Zip 91204-2594; tel. 818/502-1900; Arnold R. Schaffer, President and Chief Executive Officer
Web address: www.glendalememorial.com

LONG BEACH COMMUNITY MEDICAL CENTER (O, 278 beds) 1720 Termino Avenue, Long Beach, CA Zip 90804; tel. 562/498-1000; Thomas G. Hennessy, President and Chief Executive Officer
Web address: www.lbcommunty.com

MARIAN MEDICAL CENTER (O, 225 beds) 1400 East Church Street, Santa Maria, CA Zip 93454, Mailing Address: Box 1238, Zip 93456; tel. 805/739-3000; Charles J. Cova, Executive Vice President and Chief Operating Officer
Web address: www.chw.edu

MARK TWAIN ST. JOSEPH'S HOSPITAL (S, 30 beds) 768 Mountain Ranch Road, San Andreas, CA Zip 95249-9710; tel. 209/754-2515; Michael P. Lawson, Administrator
Web address: www.chw.edu

MERCY AMERICAN RIVER/MERCY SAN JUAN HOSPITAL (S, 352 beds) 6501 Coyle Avenue, Carmichael, CA Zip 95608, Mailing Address: P.O. Box 479, Zip 95608; tel. 916/537-5000; Michael H. Erne, President and Chief Executive Officer

MERCY GENERAL HOSPITAL (S, 402 beds) 4001 J Street, Sacramento, CA Zip 95819; tel. 916/851-2000; Thomas A. Petersen, Vice President and Chief Operating Officer
Web address: www.mercysac.org

MERCY HOSPITAL (O, 422 beds) 2215 Truxtun Avenue, Bakersfield, CA Zip 93301, Mailing Address: P.O. Box 119, Zip 93302; tel. 661/632-5000; Bernard J. Herman, President and Chief Executive Officer

MERCY HOSPITAL AND HEALTH SERVICES (S, 101 beds) 2740 M Street, Merced, CA Zip 95340-2880; tel. 209/384-6444; John Headding, Chief Administrative Officer
Web address: www.chw.edu

MERCY HOSPITAL OF FOLSOM (S, 95 beds) 1650 Creekside Drive, Folsom, CA Zip 95630; tel. 916/983-7400; Donald C. Hudson, Vice President and Chief Operating Officer
Web address: www.mercysacramento.org

MERCY MEDICAL CENTER MOUNT SHASTA (S, 80 beds) 914 Pine Street, Mount Shasta, CA Zip 96067, Mailing Address: P.O. Box 239, Zip 96067-0239; tel. 530/926-6111; Richard J. Barnett, Executive Vice President and Chief Operating Officer
Web address: www.mercy.org

MERCY MEDICAL CENTER REDDING (S, 219 beds) 2175 Rosaline Avenue, Redding, CA Zip 96001, Mailing Address: P.O. Box 496009, Zip 96049-6009; tel. 530/225-6000; John Di Perry, Jr, Executive Vice President and Chief Operating Officer
Web address: www.mercy.org

MERCY WESTSIDE HOSPITAL (S, 84 beds) 110 East North Street, Taft, CA Zip 93268; tel. 661/763-4211; Margo Arnold, Administrator

METHODIST HOSPITAL OF SACRAMENTO (S, 325 beds) 7500 Hospital Drive, Sacramento, CA Zip 95823; tel. 916/423-3000; Michael J. Finn, Acting Vice President and Chief Operating Officer
Web address: www.mercysacto.org

NORTHRIDGE HOSPITAL MEDICAL CENTER-ROSCOE BOULEVARD CAMPUS (O, 413 beds) 18300 Roscoe Boulevard, Northridge, CA Zip 91328; tel. 818/885-8500; Richard D. Lyons, Interim President and Chief Executive Officer

NORTHRIDGE HOSPITAL AND MEDICAL CENTER, SHERMAN WAY CAMPUS (O, 195 beds) 14500 Sherman Circle, Van Nuys, CA Zip 91405; tel. 818/997-0101; Richard D. Lyons, Senior Vice President and Chief Operating Officer
Web address: www.chw.edu

O'CONNOR HOSPITAL (S, 283 beds) 2105 Forest Avenue, San Jose, CA Zip 95128; tel. 408/947-2500; Joan A. Bero, Regional Vice President and Chief Operating Officer
Web address: www.chwbay.org

OAK VALLEY DISTRICT HOSPITAL (O, 148 beds) 350 South Oak Street, Oakdale, CA Zip 95361; tel. 209/847-3011; Dev Mahadevan, Chief Executive Officer

ROBERT F. KENNEDY MEDICAL CENTER (S, 195 beds) 4500 West 116th Street, Hawthorne, CA Zip 90250; tel. 310/973-1711; Peter P. Aprato, President
Web address: www.chw.edu

SAINT FRANCIS MEMORIAL HOSPITAL (S, 187 beds) 900 Hyde Street, San Francisco, CA Zip 94109, Mailing Address: Box 7726, Zip 94120-7726; tel. 415/353-6000; Cheryl A. Fama, Administrator, Vice President and Chief Operating Officer
Web address: www.chw.edu

SAN GABRIEL VALLEY MEDICAL CENTER (O, 274 beds) 438 West Las Tunas Drive, San Gabriel, CA Zip 91776, Mailing Address: P.O. Box 1507, Zip 91778-1507; tel. 626/289-5454; Steven A. Fellows, President
Web address: www.sgvmc.org

SEQUOIA HOSPITAL (S, 245 beds) 170 Alameda De Las Pulgas, Redwood City, CA Zip 94062; tel. 650/369-5811; John Williams, Chief Executive Officer
Web address: www.chwbay.org

SETON MEDICAL CENTER (S, 255 beds) 1900 Sullivan Avenue, Daly City, CA Zip 94015; tel. 650/992-4000; Bernadette M. Smith, Chief Operating Officer
Web address: www.chwwestbay.org

SETON MEDICAL CENTER COASTSIDE (S, 121 beds) Marine Boulevard and Etheldore Street, Moss Beach, CA Zip 94038; tel. 650/563-7100; John G. Williams, President and Chief Executive Officer
Web address: www.chw.edu

SIERRA NEVADA MEMORIAL HOSPITAL (S, 61 beds) 155 Glasson Way, Grass Valley, CA Zip 95945, Mailing Address: P.O. Box 1029, Zip 95945-1029; tel. 530/274-6000; C. Thomas Collier, President and Chief Executive Officer
Web address: www.snmh.org

ST. BERNARDINE MEDICAL CENTER (S, 268 beds) 2101 North Waterman Avenue, San Bernardino, CA Zip 92404; tel. 909/883-8711; Steven R. Barron, President

ST. DOMINIC'S HOSPITAL (S, 77 beds) 1777 West Yosemite Avenue, Manteca, CA Zip 95337; tel. 209/825-3500; Margaret Hepburn, Chief Administrative Officer and Chief Nurse Executive
Web address: www.chw.edu

ST. ELIZABETH COMMUNITY HOSPITAL (S, 61 beds) 2550 Sister Mary Columba Drive, Red Bluff, CA Zip 96080-4397; tel. 530/529-8000; Thomas F. Grimes, II, Executive Vice President and Chief Operating Officer
Web address: www.mercy.org

ST. FRANCIS MEDICAL CENTER (S, 414 beds) 3630 East Imperial Highway, Lynwood, CA Zip 90262; tel. 310/603-6000; Gerald T. Kozai, President

ST. FRANCIS MEDICAL CENTER OF SANTA BARBARA (O, 85 beds) 601 East Micheltorena Street, Santa Barbara, CA Zip 93103; tel. 805/568-5705; Ron Biscaro, Administrator and Chief Operating Officer

ST. JOHN'S PLEASANT VALLEY HOSPITAL (S, 180 beds) 2309 Antonio Avenue, Camarillo, CA Zip 93010-1459; tel. 805/389-5800; William J. Clearwater, Vice President and Site Administrator
Web address: www.chw.edu

For explanation of codes following names, see page B2.
★ *Indicates Type III membership in the American Hospital Association.*

ST. JOHN'S REGIONAL MEDICAL CENTER (S, 230 beds) 1600 North Rose Avenue, Oxnard, CA Zip 93030; tel. 805/988–2500; Charles E. Padilla, Administrator and Chief Operating Officer
Web address: www.chw.edu

ST. JOSEPH'S BEHAVIORAL HEALTH CENTER (S, 35 beds) 2510 North California Street, Stockton, CA Zip 95204–5568; tel. 209/948–2100; James Sondecker, Director
Web address: www.sjrhs.org

ST. JOSEPH'S MEDICAL CENTER (S, 291 beds) 1800 North California Street, Stockton, CA Zip 95204, Mailing Address: P.O. Box 213008, Zip 95213–3008; tel. 209/943–2000; Donald J. Wiley, Senior Vice President and Chief Operating Officer
Web address: www.sjrhs.org

ST. MARY MEDICAL CENTER (S, 479 beds) 1050 Linden Avenue, Long Beach, CA Zip 90801, Mailing Address: P.O. Box 887, Zip 90813–0887; tel. 562/491–9000; Thomas G. Hennessy, President and Chief Executive Officer
Web address: www.sc.chw.edu

ST. MARY'S MEDICAL CENTER (S, 280 beds) 450 Stanyan Street, San Francisco, CA Zip 94117–1079; tel. 415/668–1000; Rosemary Fox, Vice President and Chief Operating Officer

ST. VINCENT MEDICAL CENTER (S, 350 beds) 2131 West Third Street, Los Angeles, CA Zip 90057–0992, Mailing Address: P.O. Box 57992, Zip 90057; tel. 213/484–7111; William D. Parente, President
Web address: www.stvincentmedicalcenter.com

WOODLAND HEALTHCARE (S, 103 beds) 1325 Cottonwood Street, Woodland, CA Zip 95695–5199; tel. 530/662–3961; Margaret Cleary, Chief Executive Officer
Web address: www.chw.edu

NEVADA: ST. ROSE DOMINICAN HOSPITAL (S, 143 beds) 102 Lake Mead Drive, Henderson, NV Zip 89015–5524; tel. 702/564–2622; Rod A. Davis, President and Chief Executive Officer
Web address: www.srdh.com

Owned, leased, sponsored:	44 hospitals	10102 beds
Contract–managed:	0 hospitals	0 beds
Totals:	44 hospitals	10102 beds

★**2265: CENTRA HEALTH, INC.** (NP)
1920 Atherholt Road, Lynchburg, VA Zip 24501–1104; tel. 804/947–4700; George W. Dawson, President
(Centralized Health System)

VIRGINIA: LYNCHBURG GENERAL HOSPITAL (O, 350 beds) 1901 Tate Springs Road, Lynchburg, VA Zip 24501–1167; tel. 804/947–3000; L. Darrell Powers, Senior Vice President
Web address: www.centrahealth.com

VIRGINIA BAPTIST HOSPITAL (O, 323 beds) 3300 Rivermont Avenue, Lynchburg, VA Zip 24503–9989; tel. 804/947–4000; Thomas C. Jividen, Senior Vice President
Web address: www.centrahealth.com

Owned, leased, sponsored:	2 hospitals	673 beds
Contract–managed:	0 hospitals	0 beds
Totals:	2 hospitals	673 beds

0184: CENTRACARE (NP)
20 Ninth Street S.E., Long Prairie, MN Zip 56347; tel. 320/732–2141; Clayton R. Peterson, President
(Moderately Centralized Health System)

MINNESOTA: LONG PRAIRIE MEMORIAL HOSPITAL AND HOME (O, 117 beds) 20 Ninth Street S.E., Long Prairie, MN Zip 56347–1404; tel. 320/732–2141; Clayton R. Peterson, President

MELROSE AREA HOSPITAL (O, 87 beds) 11 North Fifth Avenue West, Melrose, MN Zip 56352–1098; tel. 320/256–4231; Joan Jackson, Administrator

ST. CLOUD HOSPITAL (O, 697 beds) 1406 Sixth Avenue North, Saint Cloud, MN Zip 56303–0016; tel. 320/251–2700; John Frobenius, President and Chief Executive Officer
Web address: www.stcloudhospital.com

Owned, leased, sponsored:	3 hospitals	901 beds
Contract–managed:	0 hospitals	0 beds
Totals:	3 hospitals	901 beds

0665: CENTURY HEALTHCARE DEVELOPMENT CORPORATION (IO)
5727 South Lewis, Suite 125, Tulsa, OK Zip 74105–7119; tel. 918/712–7010; William Grey, President and Chief Executive Officer

ARIZONA: WESTBRIDGE TREATMENT CENTER (O, 78 beds) 1830 East Roosevelt Street, Phoenix, AZ Zip 85006–3641; tel. 602/254–0884; Mike Perry, Chief Executive Officer

OKLAHOMA: HIGH POINTE (O, 36 beds) 6501 N.E. 50th Street, Oklahoma City, OK Zip 73141–9613; tel. 405/424–3383; Johnny J. Smith, Chief Executive Officer

Owned, leased, sponsored:	2 hospitals	114 beds
Contract–managed:	0 hospitals	0 beds
Totals:	2 hospitals	114 beds

0114: CHILDREN'S COMPREHENSIVE SERVICES, INC. (IO)
3401 West End Avenue, Suite 500, Nashville, TN Zip 37203–0376; tel. 615/383–0376; William J. Ballard, Chief Executive Officer
(Independent Hospital System)

ARKANSAS: RIVENDELL BEHAVIORAL HEALTH SERVICES (O, 77 beds) 100 Rivendell Drive, Benton, AR Zip 72015–9100; tel. 501/316–1255; Mark E. Schneider, Chief Executive Officer

MICHIGAN: RIVENDELL OF MICHIGAN (O, 31 beds) 101 West Townsend Road, Saint Johns, MI Zip 48879–9200; tel. 517/224–1177; Roger Rohall, Chief Executive Officer

UTAH: COPPER HILLS YOUTH CENTER (O, 98 beds) 5899 West Rivendell Drive, West Jordan, UT Zip 84088–5700; tel. 801/561–3377; David Damshen, Chief Executive Officer

Owned, leased, sponsored:	3 hospitals	206 beds
Contract–managed:	0 hospitals	0 beds
Totals:	3 hospitals	206 beds

0148: CHILDREN'S HEALTHCARE OF ATLANTA (NP)
2200 Century Parkway, Suite 450, Atlanta, GA Zip 30345; tel. 404/250–2211; James E. Tally, Ph.D., President and Chief Executive Officer
(Moderately Centralized Health System)

GEORGIA: CHILDREN'S HEALTHCARE OF ATLANTA AT EGLESTON (O, 206 beds) 1405 Clifton Road N.E., Atlanta, GA Zip 30322–1101; tel. 404/325–6000; James E. Tally, Ph.D., President and Chief Executive Officer

CHILDREN'S HEALTHCARE OF ATLANTA AT SCOTTISH RITE (O, 165 beds) 1001 Johnson Ferry Road N.E., Atlanta, GA Zip 30342–1600; tel. 404/256–5252; James E. Tally, Ph.D., President and Chief Executive Officer
Web address: www.srcmc.org

Owned, leased, sponsored:	2 hospitals	371 beds
Contract–managed:	0 hospitals	0 beds
Totals:	2 hospitals	371 beds

●★**0131: CHRISTIANA CARE HEALTH SYSTEM** (NP)
501 West 14th Street, Wilmington, DE Zip 19899, Mailing Address: P.O. Box 1668, Zip 19899; tel. 302/428–2570; Charles M. Smith, M.D., President and Chief Executive Officer
(Moderately Centralized Health System)

DELAWARE: CHRISTIANA HOSPITAL (O, 866 beds) 4755 Ogletown–Stanton Road, Newark, DE Zip 19718; tel. 302/733–1000; Charles M. Smith, M.D., President and Chief Executive Officer
Web address: www.christianacare.org

For explanation of codes following names, see page B2.
★ Indicates Type III membership in the American Hospital Association.
● Single hospital health care system

Systems / Christiana Care Health System

Owned, leased, sponsored:	1 hospital	866 beds
Contract-managed:	0 hospitals	0 beds
Totals:	1 hospital	866 beds

★0192: **CHRISTUS HEALTH** (CC)
6363 North Highway 161, Suite 450, Irving, TX Zip 75038;
tel. 877/980-0100; Thomas C. Royer, M.D., President

ARKANSAS: MAGNOLIA HOSPITAL (C, 62 beds) 101 Hospital Drive, Magnolia, AR Zip 71753-2416, Mailing Address: Box 629, Zip 71753-0629; tel. 870/235-3000; Kirk Reamey, Chief Executive Officer
Web address: www.magnolia-net.com

LOUISIANA: CHRISTUS COUSHATTA HEALTH CARE CENTER (O, 49 beds) 1635 Marvel Street, Coushatta, LA Zip 71019-9022, Mailing Address: P.O. Box 589, Zip 71019-0589; tel. 318/932-2000; Sister Laureen Painter, Chief Executive Officer

CHRISTUS SCHUMPERT BOSSIER (O, 131 beds) 2105 Airline Drive, Bossier City, LA Zip 71111-3190; tel. 318/741-6000; Gary Kerr, Administrator

CHRISTUS SCHUMPERT MEDICAL CENTER (O, 486 beds) One St. Mary Place, Shreveport, LA Zip 71101-4399, Mailing Address: P.O. Box 21976, Zip 71120-1076; tel. 318/681-4500; Wayne A. Sensor, Chief Executive Officer

CHRISTUS ST. FRANCES CABRINI HOSPITAL (O, 227 beds) 3330 Masonic Drive, Alexandria, LA Zip 71301-3899; tel. 318/487-1122; Stephen F. Wright, Chief Executive Officer

CHRISTUS ST. PATRICK HOSPITAL (O, 359 beds) 524 South Ryan Street, Lake Charles, LA Zip 70601-5799, Mailing Address: P.O. Box 3401, Zip 70602-3401; tel. 318/436-2511; James E. Gardner, Jr, Chief Executive Officer

HIGHLAND HOSPITAL (O, 121 beds) 1453 East Bert Kouns Industrial Loop, Shreveport, LA Zip 71105-6050; tel. 318/798-4300; Anthony S. Sala, Jr, Chief Executive Officer

NATCHITOCHES PARISH HOSPITAL (C, 166 beds) 501 Keyser Avenue, Natchitoches, LA Zip 71457-6036, Mailing Address: P.O. Box 2009, Zip 71457-2009; tel. 318/214-4200; Mark E. Marley, Chief Executive Officer

TEXAS: CHRISTUS JASPER MEMORIAL HOSPITAL (L, 57 beds) 1275 Marvin Hancock Drive, Jasper, TX Zip 75951-4995; tel. 409/384-5461; George N. Miller, Jr, Chief Executive Officer

CHRISTUS SANTA ROSA HEALTH CARE (O, 636 beds) 519 West Houston Street, San Antonio, TX Zip 78207-3108; tel. 210/704-2011; James P. Houser, President and Chief Executive Officer
Web address: www.sch.org

CHRISTUS SPOHN HOSPITAL ALICE (O, 49 beds) 700 North Flournoy Road, Alice, TX Zip 78332; tel. 361/661-8000; Dominic Dominguez, Vice President and Administrator

CHRISTUS SPOHN HOSPITAL BEEVILLE (O, 67 beds) 1500 East Houston Street, Beeville, TX Zip 78102; tel. 361/354-2000; David S. Wagner, Vice President and Administrator
Web address: www.sch.org

CHRISTUS SPOHN HOSPITAL KLEBERG (O, 100 beds) 1311 General Cavazos Boulevard, Kingsville, TX Zip 78363-1197, Mailing Address: P.O. Box 1197, Zip 78363-1197; tel. 361/595-1661; Ernesto G. Flores, Jr, Administrator
Web address: www.sch.org

CHRISTUS SPOHN HOSPITAL MEMORIAL (O, 270 beds) 2606 Hospital Boulevard, Corpus Christi, TX Zip 78405-1818, Mailing Address: Box 5280, Zip 78465-5280; tel. 361/902-4000; Thomas G. Neff, Vice President and Administrator
Web address: www.sch.org

CHRISTUS SPOHN HOSPITAL SHORELINE (O, 377 beds) 600 Elizabeth Street, Corpus Christi, TX Zip 78404; tel. 361/881-3000; Andrew M. Harris, Vice President and Administrator
Web address: www.sch.org

CHRISTUS SPOHN HOSPITAL SOUTH (O, 95 beds) 5950 Saratoga, Corpus Christi, TX Zip 78414; tel. 361/985-5000; Nora Frazier, Vice President and Administrator

CHRISTUS ST. ELIZABETH HOSPITAL (O, 447 beds) 2830 Calder Avenue, Beaumont, TX Zip 77702, Mailing Address: P.O. Box 5405, Zip 77726-5405; tel. 409/892-7171; Edward W. Myers, Chief Executive Officer
Web address: www.sch.org

CHRISTUS ST. JOHN HOSPITAL (O, 135 beds) 18300 St. John Drive, Nassau Bay, TX Zip 77058; tel. 281/333-5503; Thomas Permetti, Chief Executive Officer

CHRISTUS ST. JOSEPH HOSPITAL (O, 424 beds) 1919 LaBranch Street, Houston, TX Zip 77002; tel. 713/757-1000; Sally E. Jeffcoat, Chief Executive Officer
Web address: www.sch.org

CHRISTUS ST. JOSEPH'S HEALTH SYSTEM (O, 175 beds) 820 Clarksville Street, Paris, TX Zip 75460-9070, Mailing Address: P.O. Box 9070, Zip 75461-9070; tel. 903/785-4521; Monty E. McLaurin, President
Web address: www.stjosephhc.com

CHRISTUS ST. MARY HOSPITAL (O, 242 beds) 3600 Gates Boulevard, Port Arthur, TX Zip 77642-3601, Mailing Address: P.O. Box 3696, Zip 77643-3696; tel. 409/985-7431; Alice Baker, Chief Executive Officer
Web address: www.sch.org

CHRISTUS ST. MICHAEL HEALTH SYSTEM (O, 239 beds) 2600 St. Michael Drive, Texarkana, TX Zip 75503-2372; tel. 903/614-1000; Don A. Beeler, President and Chief Executive Officer
Web address: www.smhcc.org

Owned, leased, sponsored:	20 hospitals	4686 beds
Contract-managed:	2 hospitals	228 beds
Totals:	22 hospitals	4914 beds

0101: **CITRUS VALLEY HEALTH PARTNERS** (NP)
210 West San Bernardino Road, Covina, CA Zip 91723; tel. 626/938-7577; Peter E. Makowski, President and Chief Executive Officer
(Centralized Physician/Insurance Health System)

CALIFORNIA: CITRUS VALLEY MEDICAL CENTER INTER-COMMUNITY CAMPUS (O, 252 beds) 210 West San Bernardino Road, Covina, CA Zip 91723-1901, Mailing Address: P.O. Box 6108, Zip 91722-5108; tel. 626/331-7331; Peter E. Makowski, President and Chief Executive Officer

CITRUS VALLEY MEDICAL CENTER-QUEEN OF THE VALLEY CAMPUS (O, 263 beds) 1115 South Sunset Avenue, West Covina, CA Zip 91790, Mailing Address: Box 1980, Zip 91793; tel. 626/962-4011; James T. Yoshioka, President

FOOTHILL PRESBYTERIAN HOSPITAL-MORRIS L. JOHNSTON MEMORIAL (O, 106 beds) 250 South Grand Avenue, Glendora, CA Zip 91741; tel. 626/963-8411; Larry S. Fetters, Administrator and Chief Operating Officer

Owned, leased, sponsored:	3 hospitals	621 beds
Contract-managed:	0 hospitals	0 beds
Totals:	3 hospitals	621 beds

0212: **CLEVELAND CLINIC HEALTH SYSTEM** (NP)
9500 Euclid, Cleveland, OH Zip 44195-5108; tel. 216/444-2200; Fred Loop, M.D., President

OHIO: CLEVELAND CLINIC CHILDREN'S HOSPITAL FOR REHABILITATION (O, 46 beds) Cleveland, OH Mailing Address: 2801 Martin Luther King Jr. Drive, Zip 44104-3865; tel. 216/721-5400; Thomas A. Rathbone, President
Web address: www.clevelandclinic.org/childrensrehab

CLEVELAND CLINIC FOUNDATION (O, 1001 beds) 9500 Euclid Avenue, Cleveland, OH Zip 44195-5108; tel. 216/444-2200; Frank L. Lordeman, Chief Operating Officer
Web address: www.ccf.org

EUCLID HOSPITAL (O, 187 beds) 18901 Lake Shore Boulevard, Euclid, OH Zip 44119-1090; tel. 216/531-9000; Lauren Rock, Chief Operating Officer
Web address: www.meridia.org

FAIRVIEW HOSPITAL (O, 428 beds) 18101 Lorain Avenue, Cleveland, OH Zip 44111-5656; tel. 216/476-7000; Louis P. Caravella, M.D., Chief Executive Officer

For explanation of codes following names, see page B2.
★ Indicates Type III membership in the American Hospital Association.

Systems / Community Health Systems, Inc.

LAKEWOOD HOSPITAL (O, 328 beds) 14519 Detroit Avenue, Lakewood, OH Zip 44107–4383; tel. 216/521–4200; V. Richard Stelzer , Jr, Chief Administrative Officer

LUTHERAN HOSPITAL (O, 219 beds) 1730 West 25th Street, Cleveland, OH Zip 44113; tel. 216/696–4300; John Brocketi, Associate Vice President

MARYMOUNT HOSPITAL (O, 213 beds) 12300 McCracken Road, Garfield Heights, OH Zip 44125–2975; tel. 216/581–0500; Thomas J. Trudell, President and Chief Executive Officer

MERIDIA HILLCREST HOSPITAL (O, 305 beds) 6780 Mayfield Road, Cleveland, OH Zip 44124–2202; tel. 440/449–4500; Catherine B. Leary, R.N., Chief Operating Officer
Web address: www.meridia.org

MERIDIA HURON HOSPITAL (O, 163 beds) 13951 Terrace Road, Cleveland, OH Zip 44112–4399; tel. 216/761–3300; Beverly Lozar, Chief Operating Officer
Web address: www.meridia.org

MERIDIA SOUTH POINTE HOSPITAL (O, 198 beds) 4110 Warrensville Center Road, Warrensville Heights, OH Zip 44122–7099; tel. 216/491–6000; Kathleen A. Rice, Chief Operating Officer
Web address: www.meridia.com

Owned, leased, sponsored:	10 hospitals	3088 beds
Contract–managed:	0 hospitals	0 beds
Totals:	10 hospitals	3088 beds

★**0152: COFFEE HEALTH GROUP** (NP)
205 Marengo Street, Florence, AL Zip 35630–6033; tel. 256/768–9191; Carl W. Bailey, President and Chief Executive Officer
(Independent Hospital System)

ALABAMA: ELIZA COFFEE MEMORIAL HOSPITAL (O, 455 beds) 205 Marengo Street, Florence, AL Zip 35630–6033, Mailing Address: P.O. Box 818, Zip 35631–0818; tel. 256/768–9191; Richard H. Peck, President and Chief Executive Officer

RUSSELLVILLE HOSPITAL (O, 100 beds) 15155 Highway 43, Russellville, AL Zip 35653, Mailing Address: P.O. Box 1089, Zip 35653–1089; tel. 256/332–1611; Christine R. Stewart, President and Chief Executive Officer

SHOALS HOSPITAL (O, 128 beds) 201 Avalon Avenue, Muscle Shoals, AL Zip 35661–2805, Mailing Address: P.O. Box 3359, Zip 35662–3359; tel. 256/386–1600; Connie Hawthorne, Chief Executive Officer

Owned, leased, sponsored:	3 hospitals	683 beds
Contract–managed:	0 hospitals	0 beds
Totals:	3 hospitals	683 beds

0076: COLLEGE HEALTH ENTERPRISES (IO)
17100 Pioneer Boulevard, Suite 300, Downey, CA Zip 90241; tel. 949/642–2734; Dale A. Kirby, President

CALIFORNIA: COLLEGE HOSPITAL (O, 124 beds) 10802 College Place, Cerritos, CA Zip 90703–1579; tel. 562/924–9581; Stephen Witt, Chief Executive Officer

COLLEGE HOSPITAL COSTA MESA (O, 119 beds) 301 Victoria Street, Costa Mesa, CA Zip 92627; tel. 949/574–3322; Dale A. Kirby, Chief Executive Officer

Owned, leased, sponsored:	2 hospitals	243 beds
Contract–managed:	0 hospitals	0 beds
Totals:	2 hospitals	243 beds

★**0161: COLUMBUS REGIONAL HEALTH SYSTEM** (NP)
707 Center Street, Suite 400, Columbus, GA Zip 31901; tel. 706/660–6100; Larry Sanders, FACHE, Chairman and Chief Executive Officer
(Centralized Physician/Insurance Health System)

ALABAMA: PHENIX REGIONAL HOSPITAL (O, 114 beds) 1707 21st Avenue, Phenix City, AL Zip 36867–3753, Mailing Address: P.O. Box 190, Zip 36868–0190; tel. 334/291–8502; Lance B. Duke, FACHE, President and Chief Executive Officer

GEORGIA: THE MEDICAL CENTER (O, 537 beds) 710 Center Street, Columbus, GA Zip 31902, Mailing Address: P.O. Box 951, Zip 31902–0951; tel. 706/571–1000; Lance B. Duke, FACHE, President and Chief Executive Officer
Web address: www.columbusregional.com

Owned, leased, sponsored:	2 hospitals	651 beds
Contract–managed:	0 hospitals	0 beds
Totals:	2 hospitals	651 beds

0080: COMMUNITY HEALTH SYSTEMS, INC. (IO)
155 Franklin Road, Suite 400, Brentwood, TN Zip 37027–4600, Mailing Address: P.O. Box 217, Zip 37024–0217; tel. 615/373–9600; Wayne T. Smith, President and Chief Executive Officer
(Moderately Centralized Health System)

ALABAMA: EDGE REGIONAL MEDICAL CENTER (O, 87 beds) 1330 Highway 231 South, Troy, AL Zip 36081–1224; tel. 334/670–5000; David E. Loving, Chief Executive Officer

HARTSELLE MEDICAL CENTER (O, 50 beds) 201 Pine Street N.W., Hartselle, AL Zip 35640–2309, Mailing Address: P.O. Box 969, Zip 35640–0969; tel. 256/773–6511; Mike H. McNair, Chief Executive Officer

L. V. STABLER MEMORIAL HOSPITAL (O, 74 beds) 29 L. V. Stabler Drive, Greenville, AL Zip 36037; tel. 334/382–2676; Tom R. McDougal , Jr, Chief Executive Officer

PARKWAY MEDICAL CENTER HOSPITAL (O, 94 beds) 1874 Beltline Road S.W., Decatur, AL Zip 35601–5509, Mailing Address: P.O. Box 2211, Zip 35609–2211; tel. 256/350–2211; Danny Crowe, Interim Chief Executive Officer

SOUTH BALDWIN REGIONAL MEDICAL CENTER (O, 82 beds) 1613 North McKenzie Street, Foley, AL Zip 36535–2299; tel. 334/952–3400; Sandy D. McGill, Administrator
Web address: www.southbaldwinrmc.com

WOODLAND MEDICAL CENTER (O, 100 beds) 1910 Cherokee Avenue S.E., Cullman, AL Zip 35055–5599; tel. 256/739–3500; Lowell S. Benton, Executive Director
Web address: www.woodlandmedicalcenter.com

ARIZONA: PAYSON REGIONAL MEDICAL CENTER (O, 66 beds) 807 South Ponderosa Street, Payson, AZ Zip 85541–5599; tel. 520/474–3222; Russell V. Judd, Chief Executive Officer
Web address: www.paysonhospital.com

WESTERN ARIZONA REGIONAL MEDICAL CENTER (O, 182 beds) 2735 Silver Creek Road, Bullhead City, AZ Zip 86442–8303; tel. 520/763–2273; James Sato, Senior Vice President and Chief Executive Officer
Web address: www.baptisthealth.com

ARKANSAS: HARRIS HOSPITAL (O, 88 beds) 1205 McLain Street, Newport, AR Zip 72112–3533; tel. 870/523–8911; David W. Fuller, Chief Executive Officer

RANDOLPH COUNTY MEDICAL CENTER (L, 50 beds) 2801 Medical Center Drive, Pocahontas, AR Zip 72455–9497; tel. 870/892–6000; Michael G. Layfield, Chief Executive Officer

CALIFORNIA: BARSTOW COMMUNITY HOSPITAL (L, 56 beds) 555 South Seventh Street, Barstow, CA Zip 92311; tel. 760/256–1761; George F. Naylor , II, CHE, Chief Executive Officer
Web address: www.barstowhospital.com

WATSONVILLE COMMUNITY HOSPITAL (O, 130 beds) 75 Nielson Street, Watsonville, CA Zip 95076; tel. 831/724–4741; Barry S. Schneider, Chief Executive Officer
Web address: www.watsonville.com\hospital

FLORIDA: DOCTORS MEMORIAL HOSPITAL (L, 34 beds) 401 East Byrd Avenue, Bonifay, FL Zip 32425–3007, Mailing Address: P.O. Box 188, Zip 32425–0188; tel. 850/547–1120; Dale Larson, Chief Executive Officer

NORTH OKALOOSA MEDICAL CENTER (O, 91 beds) 151 Redstone Avenue S.E., Crestview, FL Zip 32539–6026; tel. 850/689–8100; Roger L. Hall, Chief Executive Officer

For explanation of codes following names, see page B2.
★ Indicates Type III membership in the American Hospital Association.

Systems / Community Health Systems, Inc.

GEORGIA: BERRIEN COUNTY HOSPITAL (O, 153 beds) 1221 East McPherson Street, Nashville, GA Zip 31639–2326, Mailing Address: P.O. Box 665, Zip 31639–0665; tel. 912/686–7471; James L. Jarrett, Chief Executive Officer

FANNIN REGIONAL HOSPITAL (O, 32 beds) 2855 Old Highway 5, Blue Ridge, GA Zip 30513; tel. 706/632–3711; Barry L. Mousa, Chief Executive Officer

ILLINOIS: CROSSROADS COMMUNITY HOSPITAL (O, 37 beds) 8 Doctors Park Road, Mount Vernon, IL Zip 62864–6224; tel. 618/244–5500; Ruth McDaniel, Chief Executive Officer

MARION MEMORIAL HOSPITAL (L, 84 beds) 917 West Main Street, Marion, IL Zip 62959–1836; tel. 618/997–5341; Ronald Seal, President and Chief Executive Officer

KENTUCKY: KENTUCKY RIVER MEDICAL CENTER (L, 49 beds) 540 Jett Drive, Jackson, KY Zip 41339–9620; tel. 606/666–6305; O. David Bevins, Chief Executive Officer

PARKWAY REGIONAL HOSPITAL (O, 38 beds) 2000 Holiday Lane, Fulton, KY Zip 42041; tel. 270/472–2522; Michael Patterson, Chief Executive Officer

THREE RIVERS MEDICAL CENTER (O, 90 beds) Highway 644, Louisa, KY Zip 41230, Mailing Address: P.O. Box 769, Zip 41230–0769; tel. 606/638–9451; Greg Kiser, Chief Executive Officer
Web address: www.trmc.net

LOUISIANA: BYRD REGIONAL HOSPITAL (O, 59 beds) 1020 West Fertitta Boulevard, Leesville, LA Zip 71446–4697; tel. 318/239–9041; Roger C. LeDoux, Chief Executive Officer

RIVER WEST MEDICAL CENTER (O, 72 beds) 59355 River West Drive, Plaquemine, LA Zip 70764–9543; tel. 225/687–9222; Mark Nosacka, Chief Executive Officer

SABINE MEDICAL CENTER (O, 48 beds) 240 Highland Drive, Many, LA Zip 71449–3718; tel. 318/256–5691; Patrick W. Gandy, Chief Executive Officer

MISSISSIPPI: KING'S DAUGHTERS HOSPITAL (O, 103 beds) 300 Washington Avenue, Greenville, MS Zip 38701–3614, Mailing Address: P.O. Box 1857, Zip 38702–1857; tel. 601/378–2020; Donald Joe Fisher, Administrator

MISSOURI: MOBERLY REGIONAL MEDICAL CENTER (O, 92 beds) 1515 Union Avenue, Moberly, MO Zip 65270–9449, Mailing Address: P.O. Box 3000, Zip 65270–3000; tel. 660/263–8400; Cathryn A. Hibbs, Chief Executive Officer

NEW MEXICO: EASTERN NEW MEXICO MEDICAL CENTER (O, 168 beds) 405 West Country Club Road, Roswell, NM Zip 88201–9981; tel. 505/622–8170; Ronald J. Shafer, Chief Executive Officer
Web address: www.enmmc.com

MIMBRES MEMORIAL HOSPITAL (O, 119 beds) 900 West Ash Street, Deming, NM Zip 88030–4098, Mailing Address: P.O. Box 710, Zip 88031–0710; tel. 505/546–2761; Timothy E. Schmidt, Chief Executive Officer

NORTH CAROLINA: MARTIN GENERAL HOSPITAL (O, 49 beds) 310 South McCaskey Road, Williamston, NC Zip 27892–2150, Mailing Address: P.O. Box 1128, Zip 27892–1128; tel. 252/809–6121; Scott M. Landrum, Chief Executive Officer

PENNSYLVANIA: BERWICK HOSPITAL CENTER (O, 340 beds) 701 East 16th Street, Berwick, PA Zip 18603–2397; tel. 570/759–5000; Donald Henderson, President and Chief Executive Officer

SOUTH CAROLINA: CHESTERFIELD GENERAL HOSPITAL (O, 58 beds) Highway 9 West, Cheraw, SC Zip 29520, Mailing Address: P.O. Box 151, Zip 29520–0151; tel. 843/537–7881; Chris Wolf, Chief Executive Officer
Web address: www.chs.net/chesterfield.html

MARLBORO PARK HOSPITAL (O, 111 beds) 1138 Cheraw Highway, Bennettsville, SC Zip 29512–0738, Mailing Address: P.O. Box 738, Zip 29512–0738; tel. 843/479–2881; William M. Donohoo, FACHE, Chief Executive Officer

SPRINGS MEMORIAL HOSPITAL (O, 208 beds) 800 West Meeting Street, Lancaster, SC Zip 29720–2298; tel. 803/286–1214; Daniel E. McKay, Chief Executive Officer

TENNESSEE: CLEVELAND COMMUNITY HOSPITAL (O, 70 beds) 2800 Westside Drive N.W., Cleveland, TN Zip 37312–3599; tel. 423/339–4100; Martin D. Smith, Chief Executive Officer

LAKEWAY REGIONAL HOSPITAL (O, 135 beds) 726 McFarland Street, Morristown, TN Zip 37814–3990; tel. 423/586–2302; Michael I. Terry, Chief Executive Officer

SCOTT COUNTY HOSPITAL (L, 77 beds) 18797 Alberta Avenue, Oneida, TN Zip 37841–4939, Mailing Address: P.O. Box 4939, Zip 37841–4939; tel. 423/569–8521; Peter T. Petruzzi, Chief Executive Officer
Web address: www.scottcountyhospital.com

WHITE COUNTY COMMUNITY HOSPITAL (O, 60 beds) 401 Sewell Road, Sparta, TN Zip 38583–1299; tel. 931/738–9211; Mark Cain, Chief Executive Officer

TEXAS: BIG BEND REGIONAL MEDICAL CENTER (O, 36 beds) 2600 Highway 118 North, Alpine, TX Zip 79830; tel. 915/837–3447; David Conejo, Chief Executive Officer
Web address: www.overland.net/bbrmc

CLEVELAND REGIONAL MEDICAL CENTER (O, 115 beds) 300 East Crockett Street, Cleveland, TX Zip 77327–4062, Mailing Address: P.O. Box 1688, Zip 77328–1688; tel. 281/593–1811; Ron J. MacLaren, Chief Executive Officer
Web address: www.crmcr.com

HIGHLAND MEDICAL CENTER (O, 123 beds) 2412 50th Street, Lubbock, TX Zip 79412–2494; tel. 806/788–4060; John D. Brock, Chief Executive Officer

HILL REGIONAL HOSPITAL (O, 80 beds) 101 Circle Drive, Hillsboro, TX Zip 76645–2670; tel. 254/582–8425; Jan McClure, Chief Executive Officer

LAKE GRANBURY MEDICAL CENTER (L, 34 beds) 1310 Paluxy Road, Granbury, TX Zip 76048–5699; tel. 817/573–2683; Mike Pruitt, Chief Executive Officer

NORTHEAST MEDICAL CENTER (O, 39 beds) 504 Lipscomb Boulevard, Bonham, TX Zip 75418–4096, Mailing Address: P.O. Drawer C, Zip 75418–4096; tel. 903/583–8585; Kenneth May, Chief Executive Officer

SCENIC MOUNTAIN MEDICAL CENTER (O, 128 beds) 1601 West 11th Place, Big Spring, TX Zip 79720–4198; tel. 915/263–1211; Loren F. Chandler, Chief Executive Officer
Web address: www.smmccares.com

UTAH: TOOELE VALLEY REGIONAL MEDICAL CENTER (O, 108 beds) 211 South 100 East, Tooele, UT Zip 84074–2794; tel. 435/843–3611; Brent Cope, Chief Executive Officer

VIRGINIA: GREENSVILLE MEMORIAL HOSPITAL (L, 154 beds) 214 Weaver Avenue, Emporia, VA Zip 23847–1482; tel. 804/348–2000; Gene Faile, Chief Executive Officer

RUSSELL COUNTY MEDICAL CENTER (O, 78 beds) Carroll and Tate Streets, Lebanon, VA Zip 24266–4510; tel. 540/889–1224; David L. Brash, Chief Executive Officer
Web address: www.rcmc.net

WYOMING: EVANSTON REGIONAL HOSPITAL (O, 38 beds) 190 Arrowhead Drive, Evanston, WY Zip 82930–9266; tel. 307/789–3636; Robert W. Allen, Chief Executive Officer
Web address: www.ihc.com

Owned, leased, sponsored:	48 hospitals	4369 beds
Contract-managed:	0 hospitals	0 beds
Totals:	48 hospitals	4369 beds

★**1085: COMMUNITY MEDICAL CENTERS** (NP) Fresno and R Streets, Fresno, CA Zip 93721, Mailing Address: P.O. Box 1232, Zip 93715–1232; tel. 559/459–6000; J. Philip Hinton, M.D., President and Chief Executive Officer

CALIFORNIA: COMMUNITY MEDICAL CENTER–CLOVIS (O, 143 beds) 2755 Herndon Avenue, Clovis, CA Zip 93611; tel. 559/324–4000; J. Philip Hinton, M.D., President and Chief Executive Officer
Web address: www.communitymedical.org

COMMUNITY MEDICAL CENTER–FRESNO (O, 375 beds) 2823 Fresno Street, Fresno, CA Zip 93721, Mailing Address: P.O. Box 1232, Zip 93715–1232; tel. 559/459–6000; Marge Beekman, Facility Director
Web address: www.communitymedical.org

UNIVERSITY MEDICAL CENTER (O, 334 beds) 445 South Cedar Avenue, Fresno, CA Zip 93702–2907; tel. 559/459–4000; Andres Fernandez, Director

---

For explanation of codes following names, see page B2.
★ Indicates Type III membership in the American Hospital Association.

Systems / Covenant Health Systems, Inc.

Owned, leased, sponsored:	3 hospitals	852 beds
Contract–managed:	0 hospitals	0 beds
Totals:	3 hospitals	852 beds

0014: CONNECTICUT DEPARTMENT OF MENTAL HEALTH AND ADDICTION SERVICES (NP)
410 Capitol Avenue, Hartford, CT Zip 06134, Mailing Address: P.O. Box 341431, Zip 06134–1431; tel. 860/418–6969; Thomas A. Kirk, Jr, Ph.D., Commissioner
(Independent Hospital System)

CONNECTICUT: CEDARCREST HOSPITAL (O, 131 beds) 525 Russell Road, Newington, CT Zip 06111–1595; tel. 860/666–4613; Peter Mendelson, Superintendent

CONNECTICUT MENTAL HEALTH CENTER (O, 36 beds) 34 Park Street, New Haven, CT Zip 06519–1187, Mailing Address: P.O. Box 1842, Zip 06508–1842; tel. 203/974–7144; Selby Jacobs, M.D., Director

CONNECTICUT VALLEY HOSPITAL (O, 418 beds) Silver Street, Middletown, CT Zip 06457–7023, Mailing Address: P.O. Box 351, Zip 06457–0351; tel. 860/262–5000; Garrell S. Mullaney, Chief Executive Officer

SOUTHWEST CONNECTICUT MENTAL HEALTH SYSTEM (O, 62 beds) 1635 Central Avenue, Bridgeport, CT Zip 06610–2700, Mailing Address: P.O. Box 5117, Zip 06610–5117; tel. 203/551–7444; James M. Pisciotta, Chief Executive Officer

Owned, leased, sponsored:	4 hospitals	647 beds
Contract–managed:	0 hospitals	0 beds
Totals:	4 hospitals	647 beds

★0127: CONTINUUM HEALTH PARTNERS (NP)
555 West 57th Street, New York, NY Zip 10019; tel. 212/523–8390; Robert G. Newman, M.D., President
(Decentralized Health System)

NEW YORK: BETH ISRAEL MEDICAL CENTER (O, 1245 beds) First Avenue and 16th Street, New York, NY Zip 10003–3803; tel. 212/420–2000; Matthew E. Fink, M.D., President and Chief Executive Officer
Web address: www.bethisraelny.org

LONG ISLAND COLLEGE HOSPITAL (O, 388 beds) 339 Hicks Street, Brooklyn, NY Zip 11201–5509; tel. 718/780–1000; Allan Gibofsky, President and Chief Executive Officer
Web address: www.lich.org

NEW YORK EYE AND EAR INFIRMARY (O, 30 beds) 310 East 14th Street, New York, NY Zip 10003–4201; tel. 212/979–4000; Joseph P. Corcoran, President and Chief Executive Officer
Web address: www.nyee.edu

ST. LUKE'S–ROOSEVELT HOSPITAL CENTER (O, 715 beds) 1111 Amsterdam Avenue, New York, NY Zip 10025; tel. 212/523–4300; Sigurd H. Ackerman, M.D., President and Chief Executive Officer
Web address: www.wehealnewyork.org

Owned, leased, sponsored:	4 hospitals	2378 beds
Contract–managed:	0 hospitals	0 beds
Totals:	4 hospitals	2378 beds

0016: COOK COUNTY BUREAU OF HEALTH SERVICES (NP)
1900 West Polk Street, Suite 220, Chicago, IL Zip 60612; tel. 312/633–6820; Ruth M. Rothstein, Chief
(Moderately Centralized Health System)

ILLINOIS: COOK COUNTY HOSPITAL (O, 770 beds) 1835 West Harrison, Chicago, IL Zip 60612–3785; tel. 312/633–6000; Lacy Thomas, Director

OAK FOREST HOSPITAL OF COOK COUNTY (O, 601 beds) 15900 South Cicero Avenue, Oak Forest, IL Zip 60452; tel. 708/687–7200; Cynthia T. Henderson, M.D., M.P.H., Director and Chief Operating Officer

PROVIDENT HOSPITAL OF COOK COUNTY (O, 113 beds) 500 East 51st Street, Chicago, IL Zip 60615–2494; tel. 312/572–2000; Stephanie Wright–Griggs, Chief Operating Officer

Owned, leased, sponsored:	3 hospitals	1484 beds
Contract–managed:	0 hospitals	0 beds
Totals:	3 hospitals	1484 beds

0103: COTTAGE HEALTH SYSTEM (NP)
Pueblo at Bath Streets, Santa Barbara, CA Zip 93102, Mailing Address: P.O. Box 689, Zip 93102; tel. 805/682–7111; Ron Werft, Chief Executive Officer
(Independent Hospital System)

CALIFORNIA: GOLETA VALLEY COTTAGE HOSPITAL (O, 79 beds) 351 South Patterson Avenue, Santa Barbara, CA Zip 93111, Mailing Address: Box 6306, Zip 93160; tel. 805/967–3411; James L. Ash, President and Chief Executive Officer
Web address: www.sbch.org

SANTA BARBARA COTTAGE HOSPITAL (O, 336 beds) Pueblo at Bath Streets, Santa Barbara, CA Zip 93105, Mailing Address: Box 689, Zip 93102; tel. 805/682–7111; Ron Werft, President and Chief Executive Officer
Web address: www.cottagehealthsystem.org

SANTA YNEZ VALLEY COTTAGE HOSPITAL (O, 20 beds) 700 Alamo Pintado Road, Solvang, CA Zip 93463; tel. 805/688–6431; Ron Werft, President and Chief Executive Officer
Web address: www.cottagehealthsystem.org

Owned, leased, sponsored:	3 hospitals	435 beds
Contract–managed:	0 hospitals	0 beds
Totals:	3 hospitals	435 beds

0123: COVENANT HEALTH (NP)
100 Fort Sanders West Boulevard, Knoxville, TN Zip 37922; tel. 423/531–5555; Alan C. Guy, President and Chief Executive Officer
(Centralized Physician/Insurance Health System)

TENNESSEE: FORT SANDERS LOUDON MEDICAL CENTER (O, 50 beds) 1125 Grove Street, Loudon, TN Zip 37774–1512, Mailing Address: P.O. Box 217, Zip 37774–0217; tel. 865/458–8222; Martha O'Regan Chill, Administrator
Web address: www.covenanthealth.com

FORT SANDERS REGIONAL MEDICAL CENTER (O, 422 beds) 1901 Clinch Avenue S.W., Knoxville, TN Zip 37916–2394; tel. 423/541–1111; Richard Rose, M.D., President and Chief Administrative Officer
Web address: www.covenanthealth.com

FORT SANDERS–PARKWEST MEDICAL CENTER (O, 262 beds) 9352 Park West Boulevard, Knoxville, TN Zip 37923–4387, Mailing Address: P.O. Box 22993, Zip 37933–0993; tel. 865/693–5151; Wayne S. Heatherly, President and Chief Administrative Officer
Web address: www.covenanthealth.com

FORT SANDERS–SEVIER MEDICAL CENTER (O, 104 beds) 709 Middle Creek Road, Sevierville, TN Zip 37862–5016, Mailing Address: P.O. Box 8005, Zip 37864–8005; tel. 865/429–6100; Ellen Wilhoit, President and Chief Administrative Officer
Web address: www.covenanthealth.com

METHODIST MEDICAL CENTER OF OAK RIDGE (O, 290 beds) 990 Oak Ridge Turnpike, Oak Ridge, TN Zip 37830–6976, Mailing Address: P.O. Box 2529, Zip 37831–2529; tel. 865/481–1000; George A. Mathews, President and Chief Administrative Officer
Web address: www.mmcoakridge.com

Owned, leased, sponsored:	5 hospitals	1128 beds
Contract–managed:	0 hospitals	0 beds
Totals:	5 hospitals	1128 beds

★5885: COVENANT HEALTH SYSTEMS, INC. (CC)
420 Bedford Street, Lexington, MA Zip 02420–1502; tel. 781/862–1634; David R. Lincoln, President and Chief Executive Officer
(Moderately Centralized Health System)

For explanation of codes following names, see page B2.
★ Indicates Type III membership in the American Hospital Association.

Systems / Covenant Health Systems, Inc.

MAINE: ST. MARY'S REGIONAL MEDICAL CENTER (O, 187 beds) 45 Golder Street, Lewiston, ME Zip 04240–6033, Mailing Address: P.O. Box 291, Zip 04243–0291; tel. 207/777–8100; James E. Cassidy, President and Chief Executive Officer
Web address: www.stmarysmaine.com

MASSACHUSETTS: YOUVILLE LIFECARE (O, 286 beds) 1575 Cambridge Street, Cambridge, MA Zip 02138–4398; tel. 617/876–4344; Daniel P. Leahey, President and Chief Executive Officer

NEW HAMPSHIRE: ST. JOSEPH HOSPITAL (O, 208 beds) 172 Kinsley Street, Nashua, NH Zip 03061; tel. 603/882–3000; Peter B. Davis, President and Chief Executive Officer
Web address: www.nh-healthcare.org

Owned, leased, sponsored:	3 hospitals	681 beds
Contract-managed:	0 hospitals	0 beds
Totals:	3 hospitals	681 beds

0179: COX HEALTH SYSTEM (NP)
1423 North Jefferson Avenue, Springfield, MO Zip 65802–1988; tel. 417/269–3108; Larry D. Wallis, President and Chief Executive Officer
(Centralized Physician/Insurance Health System)

MISSOURI: COX MONETT HOSPITAL (O, 53 beds) 801 Lincoln Avenue, Monett, MO Zip 65708–1698; tel. 417/354–1400; Gregory D. Johnson, Administrator
Web address: www.coxnet.org/whoarewe/hospital_seche.cfm

LESTER E. COX MEDICAL CENTERS (O, 676 beds) 1423 North Jefferson Street, Springfield, MO Zip 65802–1988; tel. 417/269–3000; Larry D. Wallis, President and Chief Executive Officer
Web address: www.coxnet.org/whoarewe/coxsouth.cfm

Owned, leased, sponsored:	2 hospitals	729 beds
Contract-managed:	0 hospitals	0 beds
Totals:	2 hospitals	729 beds

★0008: CROZER–KEYSTONE HEALTH SYSTEM (NP)
100 West Sproul Road, Springfield, PA Zip 19064; tel. 610/338–8200; John C. McMeekin, President and Chief Executive Officer
(Centralized Health System)

PENNSYLVANIA: CROZER–CHESTER MEDICAL CENTER (O, 574 beds) One Medical Center Boulevard, Upland, PA Zip 19013–3995; tel. 610/447–2000; Joan K. Richards, President

DELAWARE COUNTY MEMORIAL HOSPITAL (O, 231 beds) 501 North Lansdowne Avenue, Drexel Hill, PA Zip 19026–1114; tel. 610/284–8100; Joan K. Richards, President

Owned, leased, sponsored:	2 hospitals	805 beds
Contract-managed:	0 hospitals	0 beds
Totals:	2 hospitals	805 beds

★1825: DCH HEALTH SYSTEM (NP)
809 University Boulevard East, Tuscaloosa, AL Zip 35401; tel. 205/759–7111; Bryan N. Kindred, President and Chief Executive Officer
(Centralized Physician/Insurance Health System)

ALABAMA: DCH REGIONAL MEDICAL CENTER (O, 383 beds) 809 University Boulevard East, Tuscaloosa, AL Zip 35401–9961; tel. 205/759–7111; William H. Cassels, Administrator
Web address: www.dchhealthcare.com

FAYETTE MEDICAL CENTER (L, 183 beds) 1653 Temple Avenue North, Fayette, AL Zip 35555–1314, Mailing Address: P.O. Drawer 878, Zip 35555–0878; tel. 205/932–5966; Harold Reed, Administrator

NORTHPORT MEDICAL CENTER (O, 196 beds) 2700 Hospital Drive, Northport, AL Zip 35476–1079, Mailing Address: P.O. Box 1079, Zip 35476–1079; tel. 205/333–4500; Charles L. Stewart, Administrator
Web address: www.dchsystem.com

Owned, leased, sponsored:	3 hospitals	762 beds
Contract-managed:	0 hospitals	0 beds
Totals:	3 hospitals	762 beds

9655: DEPARTMENT OF NAVY (FG)
2300 East Street N.W., Washington, DC Zip 20372–5300; tel. 202/762–3701; Admiral Richard A. Nelson, Surgeon General
(Moderately Centralized Health System)

CALIFORNIA: NAVAL HOSPITAL (O, 25 beds) 930 Franklin Avenue, Lemoore, CA Zip 93246–5000; tel. 559/998–4201; Captain Christine M. Bruzek-Kohler, Commanding Officer
Web address: www.lenhfsa.med.navy.mil

NAVAL HOSPITAL (O, 209 beds) Camp Pendleton, CA Mailing Address: Box 555191, Zip 92055–5191; tel. 760/725–1288; Captain Thomas Burkhard, Commanding Officer

NAVAL HOSPITAL (O, 29 beds) Twentynine Palms, CA Mailing Address: Box 788250, MCAGCC, Zip 92278–8250; tel. 760/830–2190; Captain Joan M. Huber, Commanding Officer
Web address: www.nhtp.med.navy.mil/nhtp

NAVAL MEDICAL CENTER (O, 288 beds) 34800 Bob Wilson Drive, San Diego, CA Zip 92134–5000; tel. 619/532–6400; Rear Admiral Alberto Diaz , Jr, MC, USN, Commander

FLORIDA: NAVAL HOSPITAL (O, 84 beds) 2080 Child Street, Jacksonville, FL Zip 32214–5000; tel. 904/777–7300; Captain Barbara Vernoski, Commanding Officer

NAVAL HOSPITAL (O, 113 beds) 6000 West Highway 98, Pensacola, FL Zip 32512–0003; tel. 850/505–6413; Mark F. Bernier, Director

GUAM: U. S. NAVAL HOSPITAL (O, 55 beds) Agana, GU Mailing Address: PSC 490, Box 7607, FPO, APZip 96538–1600; tel. 671/344–9340; Captain J. L. Ulmer , Sr, Commanding Officer

ILLINOIS: NAVAL HOSPITAL (O, 59 beds) 3001A Sixth Street, Great Lakes, IL Zip 60088–5230; tel. 847/688–4560; Captain Elaine C. Holmes, MC, USN, Commanding Officer
Web address: greatlakes.med.navy.mil

MARYLAND: NATIONAL NAVAL MEDICAL CENTER (O, 135 beds) 8901 Wisconsin Avenue, Bethesda, MD Zip 20889–5600; tel. 301/295–5800; Rear Admiral Bonnie B. Potter, Commander

NORTH CAROLINA: NAVAL HOSPITAL (O, 117 beds) Camp Lejeune, NC Mailing Address: P.O. Box 10100, Zip 28547–0100; tel. 910/450–4300; Captain Thomas R. Collison, Commanding Officer
Web address: lej-www.med.navy.mil

NAVAL HOSPITAL (O, 23 beds) Cherry Point, NC Mailing Address: PSC Box 8023, Zip 28533–0023; tel. 252/466–0266; Captain Joan A. Bold, Commanding Officer

PUERTO RICO: U. S. NAVAL HOSPITAL (O, 35 beds) Roosevelt Roads, PR Mailing Address: P.O. Box 3007, FPO, AAZip 34051–8100; tel. 787/865–5762; Captain G. R. Brown, Commanding Officer

SOUTH CAROLINA: NAVAL HOSPITAL (O, 20 beds) 1 Pinckney Boulevard, Beaufort, SC Zip 29902–6148; tel. 843/525–5301; Captain Gary W. Zuckerman, MSC, USN, Commanding Officer

NAVAL HOSPITAL (O, 15 beds) 3600 Rivers Avenue, North Charleston, SC Zip 29405; tel. 843/743–7000; Captain John M. Mateczun, Commanding Officer
Web address: www.nhchasn.med.navy.mil

TEXAS: NAVAL HOSPITAL (O, 25 beds) 10651 E Street, Corpus Christi, TX Zip 78419–5131; tel. 361/961–2688; Captain Elizabeth R. Barker, Commanding Officer
Web address: www.nhcc.med.navy.mil

VIRGINIA: NAVAL MEDICAL CENTER (O, 330 beds) 620 John Paul Jones Circle, Portsmouth, VA Zip 23708–2197; tel. 757/953–7424; Rear Admiral Marion Balsam, MC, USN, Commander
Web address: www.164.167.49.190/

WASHINGTON: NAVAL HOSPITAL (O, 91 beds) Boone Road, Bremerton, WA Zip 98312–1898; tel. 360/475–4000; Captain Gregg S. Parker, Commanding Officer
Web address: www.nh_bremerton.med.navy.mil

For explanation of codes following names, see page B2.
★ Indicates Type III membership in the American Hospital Association.

Systems / Department of the Army, Office of the Surgeon General

NAVAL HOSPITAL (O, 25 beds) 3475 North Saratoga Street, Oak Harbor, WA Zip 98278–8800; tel. 360/257–9500; Captain John Tracy, Commander

Owned, leased, sponsored:	18 hospitals	1678 beds
Contract–managed:	0 hospitals	0 beds
Totals:	18 hospitals	1678 beds

9495: DEPARTMENT OF THE AIR FORCE (FG)
110 Luke Avenue, Room 400, Bowling AFB, DC Zip 20332–7050; tel. 202/767–5066; Paul Carlton, M.D., Surgeon General
(Moderately Centralized Health System)

ALASKA: U. S. AIR FORCE REGIONAL HOSPITAL (O, 64 beds) 24800 Hospital Drive, Elmendorf AFB, AK Zip 99506–3700; tel. 907/552–4033

ARIZONA: U. S. AIR FORCE HOSPITAL (O, 20 beds) 4175 South Alamo Avenue, Davis–Monthan AFB, AZ Zip 85707–4405; tel. 520/228–2930; Colonel James H. Young, Administrator

U. S. AIR FORCE HOSPITAL LUKE (O, 23 beds) Luke AFB, 7219 Litchfield Road, Glendale, AZ Zip 85309–1525; tel. 623/856–7501; Colonel Michael Lischak, MC, USAF, Commander

CALIFORNIA: DAVID GRANT MEDICAL CENTER (O, 185 beds) 101 Bodin Circle, Travis AFB, CA Zip 94535–1800; tel. 707/423–7300; Lieutenant Colonel David Costa, Administrator

U. S. AIR FORCE HOSPITAL (O, 8 beds) 338 South Dakota Street, Vandenberg AFB, CA Zip 93437–6307; tel. 805/606–1110; Colonel Alan D. Newton, Commander

U. S. AIR FORCE HOSPITAL (O, 10 beds) 30 Hospital Road, Building 5500, Edwards AFB, CA Zip 93524–1730; tel. 661/277–2010; Lieutenant Colonel Thomas E. Yingst, USAF, MSC, Administrator

COLORADO: U. S. AIR FORCE ACADEMY HOSPITAL (O, 30 beds) 4102 Pinion Drive, USAF Academy, CO Zip 80840–4000; tel. 719/333–5102; Colonel Jay D. Sprenger, USAF, Commander

FLORIDA: U. S. AIR FORCE HOSPITAL (O, 25 beds) 340 Magnolia Circle, Tyndall AFB, FL Zip 32403–5612; tel. 850/283–7515; Colonel Michael J. Murphy, Commander

U. S. AIR FORCE HOSPITAL (O, 50 beds) 8415 Bayshore Boulevard, MacDill AFB, FL Zip 33621–1607; tel. 813/828–3258; Colonel Gregory C. Baggerly, MC, USAF, Commander

U. S. AIR FORCE REGIONAL HOSPITAL (O, 85 beds) 307 Boatner Road, Suite 114, Eglin AFB, FL Zip 32542–1282; tel. 850/883–8221; Colonel Monica A. Figun, MSC, USAF, Administrator

GEORGIA: U. S. AIR FORCE HOSPITAL ROBINS (O, 32 beds) 655 Seventh Street, Robins AFB, GA Zip 31098–2227; tel. 912/327–7996; Colonel John A. Lee, USAF, MSC, Commander
Web address: www.robins.af.mil/orgs/abw/78MEDGP/INEX/HTM

IDAHO: U. S. AIR FORCE HOSPITAL MOUNTAIN HOME (O, 29 beds) 90 Hope Drive, Building 600, Mountain Home AFB, ID Zip 83648–5300; tel. 208/828–7600; Colonel Gwenda McClure, USAF, Commanding Officer

ILLINOIS: SCOTT MEDICAL CENTER (O, 25 beds) 310 West Losey Street, Scott AFB, IL Zip 62225–5252; tel. 618/256–7456; Colonel Richard Weltzin, MSC, USAF, Administrator
Web address: www.satx.disa.mil/mtf3751

LOUISIANA: U. S. AIR FORCE HOSPITAL (O, 25 beds) 243 Curtiss Road, Suite 100, Barksdale AFB, LA Zip 71110–5300; tel. 318/456–6004; Colonel Dennis Marquardt, USAF, Commander

MARYLAND: MALCOLM GROW MEDICAL CENTER (O, 55 beds) 1050 West Perimeter, Andrews AFB, MD Zip 20762–6600, Mailing Address: 1050 West Perimeter, Suite A1–19, Zip 20762–6600; tel. 240/857–3000; Colonel Jeffrey L. Butler, Administrator

MISSISSIPPI: U. S. AIR FORCE HOSPITAL (O, 7 beds) 201 Independence, Suite 235, Columbus, MS Zip 39701–5300; tel. 662/434–2297; Lieutenant Colonel Mark L. Allen, MSC, USAF, Administrator

U. S. AIR FORCE MEDICAL CENTER KEESLER (O, 185 beds) 301 Fisher Street, Suite 1A132, Keesler AFB, MS Zip 39534–2519; tel. 228/377–6510; Colonel Randall W. Hartley, Administrator
Web address: www.81mdg06.keesler.af.mil/index.cgi

NEBRASKA: EHRLING BERGQUIST HOSPITAL (O, 45 beds) 2501 Capehart Road, Offutt AFB, NE Zip 68113–2160; tel. 402/294–7312; Colonel Thomas J. Eslick, MSC, USAF, Commander

NEVADA: MIKE O'CALLAGHAN FEDERAL HOSPITAL (O, 94 beds) 4700 Las Vegas Boulevard North, Suite 2419, Nellis AFB, NV Zip 89191–6601; tel. 702/653–2000; Colonel John A. Butler, MSC, Administrator

NEW MEXICO: U. S. AIR FORCE HOSPITAL (O, 7 beds) 280 First Street, Holloman AFB, NM Zip 88330–8273; tel. 505/572–3777; Colonel Marilyn S. Abu–Ghusson, USAF, Commander

U. S. AIR FORCE HOSPITAL (O, 10 beds) 208 West Casablanca Avenue, Cannon AFB, NM Zip 88103–5300; tel. 505/784–6318; Major John Sell, MSC, USAF, Administrator

U. S. AIR FORCE HOSPITAL–KIRTLAND (O, 10 beds) 1951 Second Street S.E., Kirtland AFB, NM Zip 87117–5559; tel. 505/846–3547; Colonel Royetta Marconi–Dooley, Commander

NORTH CAROLINA: U. S. AIR FORCE HOSPITAL SEYMOUR JOHNSON (O, 41 beds) 1050 Curtis Avenue, Seymour Johnson AFB, NC Zip 27531–5300; tel. 919/722–1812; Colonel Bradford Lee, Commanding Officer
Web address: www.med.navy.mil

NORTH DAKOTA: U. S. AIR FORCE HOSPITAL (O, 15 beds) 220 G Street, Grand Forks AFB, ND Zip 58205–6332; tel. 701/747–5391; Lieutenant Colonel Robert J. Rennie, Administrator

U. S. AIR FORCE REGIONAL HOSPITAL (O, 39 beds) 10 Missile Avenue, Minot, ND Zip 58705–5024; tel. 701/723–5103; Colonel David L. Clark, Commander

OHIO: U. S. AIR FORCE MEDICAL CENTER WRIGHT–PATTERSON (O, 65 beds) 4881 Sugar Maple Drive, Wright-Patterson AFB, OH Zip 45433–5529; tel. 937/257–8762; Brigadier General Joseph Kelley, Commander
Web address: www.wpmc1.wpafb.af.mil

OKLAHOMA: U. S. AIR FORCE HOSPITAL ALTUS (O, 14 beds) 301 North First Street, Altus, OK Zip 73523–5005; tel. 580/481–7347; Colonel David L. Clark, USAF, Commander

SOUTH CAROLINA: U. S. AIR FORCE HOSPITAL SHAW (O, 35 beds) 431 Meadowlark Street, Shaw A F B, SC Zip 29152–5019; tel. 803/895–6324; Lieutenant Colonel Daniel P. Dickinson, Administrator
Web address: www.shaw.af.mil

SOUTH DAKOTA: U. S. AIR FORCE HOSPITAL (O, 31 beds) 2900 Doolittle Drive, Ellsworth AFB, SD Zip 57706–4821; tel. 605/385–3201; Colonel Farley Howell, Commanding Officer
Web address: www.elsworth.af.mil/~medge/index.htm

TEXAS: U. S. AIR FORCE HOSPITAL (O, 20 beds) 7th Medical Group, Dyess AFB, Abilene, TX Zip 79607–1367; tel. 915/696–5429; Major John G. Wiseman, Administrator

U. S. AIR FORCE REGIONAL HOSPITAL–SHEPPARD (O, 65 beds) 149 Hart Street, Suite 1, Sheppard AFB, TX Zip 76311–3478; tel. 940/676–2010; Lieutenant Colonel Karen A. Bradway, MSC, USAF, Administrator

WILFORD HALL MEDICAL CENTER (O, 284 beds) 2200 Bergquist Drive, Suite 1, Lackland AFB, TX Zip 78236–5300; tel. 210/292–7353; Colonel Arthur E. Aenchbacher, Jr, Administrator

VIRGINIA: U. S. AIR FORCE HOSPITAL (O, 59 beds) 45 Pine Street, Hampton, VA Zip 23665–2080; tel. 757/764–6969; Colonel Glenn R. Willauer, Administrator

WASHINGTON: U. S. AIR FORCE HOSPITAL (O, 35 beds) 701 Hospital Loop, Suite 102, Fairchild AFB, WA Zip 99011–8701; tel. 509/247–5217; Major Scott F. Wardell, Administrator

Owned, leased, sponsored:	34 hospitals	1727 beds
Contract–managed:	0 hospitals	0 beds
Totals:	34 hospitals	1727 beds

9395: DEPARTMENT OF THE ARMY, OFFICE OF THE SURGEON GENERAL (FG)
5109 Leesburg Pike, Falls Church, VA Zip 22041; tel. 703/681–3114
(Moderately Centralized Health System)

ALABAMA: LYSTER U. S. ARMY COMMUNITY HOSPITAL (O, 37 beds) U.S. Army Aeromedical Center, Fort Rucker, AL Zip 36362–5333; tel. 334/255–7361; Lieutenant Colonel Donald Henderson, Jr, Deputy Commander for Administration

For explanation of codes following names, see page B2.
★ *Indicates Type III membership in the American Hospital Association.*

Systems / Department of the Army, Office of the Surgeon General

ALASKA: BASSETT ARMY COMMUNITY HOSPITAL (O, 43 beds) 1060 Gaffney Road, Box 7400, Fort Wainwright, AK Zip 99703–7400; tel. 907/353–5108; Lieutenant Colonel Dudley J. Schroeder, Deputy Commander

CALIFORNIA: WEED ARMY COMMUNITY HOSPITAL (O, 27 beds) Fort Irwin, CA Zip 92310–5065; tel. 760/380–3108; Colonel Michael McCaffrey, Commander

COLORADO: EVANS U. S. ARMY COMMUNITY HOSPITAL (O, 112 beds) Fort Carson, CO Zip 80913–5101; tel. 719/526–7200; Lieutenant Colonel Michael D. Wheeler, MSC, Deputy Commander, Administration

DISTRICT OF COLUMBIA: WALTER REED ARMY MEDICAL CENTER (O, 474 beds) 6900 Georgia Avenue N.W., Washington, DC Zip 20307–5001; tel. 202/782–3501; Colonel Michael A. Dunn, Commander

GEORGIA: DWIGHT DAVID EISENHOWER ARMY MEDICAL CENTER (O, 313 beds) Hospital Drive, Building 300, Fort Gordon, GA Zip 30905–5650; tel. 706/787–8191; Lieutenant Colonel Julie Martin, Chief Operating Officer
Web address: www.ddeamc.amedd.army.mil

MARTIN ARMY COMMUNITY HOSPITAL (O, 126 beds) Fort Benning, GA Mailing Address: P.O. Box 56100, Building 9200, Zip 31905–6100; tel. 706/544–2516; Lieutenant Colonel Joe W. Butler, Deputy Commander for Administration
Web address: www.martin.amedd.army.mil

WINN ARMY COMMUNITY HOSPITAL (O, 93 beds) 1061 Harmon Avenue, Hinesville, GA Zip 31314–5611; tel. 912/370–6965; Colonel George V. Masi, Commander

HAWAII: TRIPLER ARMY MEDICAL CENTER (O, 256 beds) Honolulu, HI Zip 96859–5000; tel. 808/433–6661; Major General Nancy R. Adams, Commander
Web address: www.tamc.amedd.army.mil

KANSAS: IRWIN ARMY COMMUNITY HOSPITAL (O, 44 beds) 600 Caisson Hill Road, Fort Riley, KS Zip 66442–7037; tel. 785/239–7555; Colonel Dean R. Giulitto, Commander

KENTUCKY: COLONEL FLORENCE A. BLANCHFIELD ARMY COMMUNITY HOSPITAL (O, 107 beds) 650 Joel Drive, Fort Campbell, KY Zip 42223–5349; tel. 270/798–8040; Colonel Virgil T. Deal, Commander
Web address: 198.250.216.210/

IRELAND ARMY COMMUNITY HOSPITAL (O, 76 beds) 851 Ireland Loop, Fort Knox, KY Zip 40121–5520; tel. 502/624–9020; Lieutenant Colonel David Huddleston, Deputy Commander for Administration

LOUISIANA: BAYNE–JONES ARMY COMMUNITY HOSPITAL (O, 58 beds) 1585 Third Street, Fort Polk, LA Zip 71459–5110; tel. 318/531–3928; Lieutenant Colonel Mark D. Moore, Deputy Commander and Administrator

MARSHALL ISLANDS: KWAJALEIN HOSPITAL (O, 14 beds) U.S. Army Kwajalein Atoll, Kwajalein Island, MH Zip 96960, Mailing Address: Box 1702, APO, AP Zip 96555–5000; tel. 805/355–2225; Elaine McMahon, Administrator

MISSOURI: GENERAL LEONARD WOOD ARMY COMMUNITY HOSPITAL (O, 97 beds) 126 Missouri Avenue, Fort Leonard Wood, MO Zip 65473–8952; tel. 573/596–0414; Lieutenant Colonel Mark A. Miller, Deputy Commander for Administration
Web address: glwach.leonardwood.amedd.army.mil

NEW YORK: KELLER ARMY COMMUNITY HOSPITAL (O, 49 beds) U.S. Military Academy, West Point, NY Zip 10996–1197; tel. 914/938–4837; Colonel Gordon Miller, Deputy Commander Clincial Services
Web address: www.wramc.amedd.army.mil/wp

WILCOX ARMY COMMUNITY HOSPITAL (O, 30 beds) Fort Drum, NY Zip 13602–5004

NORTH CAROLINA: WOMACK ARMY MEDICAL CENTER (O, 187 beds) Normandy Drive, Fort Bragg, NC Zip 28307–5000; tel. 910/432–4802; Colonel Daniel F. Perugini, Commander

OKLAHOMA: REYNOLDS ARMY COMMUNITY HOSPITAL (O, 73 beds) 4301 Mow–way Street, Fort Sill, OK Zip 73503–6300; tel. 580/458–3000; Colonel Alice Demarais, Commander

SOUTH CAROLINA: MONCRIEF ARMY COMMUNITY HOSPITAL (O, 91 beds) 4500 Stuart Street, Fort Jackson, SC Zip 29207–5720; tel. 803/751–2284; Colonel Stephen G. Oswald, Commander

TEXAS: BROOKE ARMY MEDICAL CENTER (O, 226 beds) Fort Sam Houston, San Antonio, TX Zip 78234–6200; tel. 210/916–2225; Colonel Martin J. Fisher, MSC, USA, Deputy Commander for Administration

DARNALL ARMY COMMUNITY HOSPITAL (O, 109 beds) 36000 Darnall Loop, Fort Hood, TX Zip 76544–4752; tel. 254/288–8000; Colonel Gerald M. Cross, USA, Commander
Web address: www.hood-meddac.army.mil

WILLIAM BEAUMONT ARMY MEDICAL CENTER (O, 209 beds) 5005 North Piedras Street, El Paso, TX Zip 79920–5001; tel. 915/569–2121; Lieutenant Colonel William Barrett , Jr, Chief of Staff

VIRGINIA: DEWITT ARMY COMMUNITY HOSPITAL (O, 62 beds) 9501 Farrell Road, Fort Belvoir, VA Zip 22060–5901; tel. 703/805–0510; Colonel James W. Martin, Commander
Web address: www.dewitt.wramc.amedd.army.mil

MCDONALD ARMY COMMUNITY HOSPITAL (O, 30 beds) Jefferson Avenue, Fort Eustis, VA Zip 23604–5548; tel. 757/314–7501; Colonel George Weightman, Commander

WASHINGTON: MADIGAN ARMY MEDICAL CENTER (O, 216 beds) Tacoma, WA Zip 98431–5000; tel. 253/968–1110; Brigadier General Mack C. Hill, Commanding General
Web address: www.mamc.amedd.army.mil

Owned, leased, sponsored:	26 hospitals	3159 beds
Contract-managed:	0 hospitals	0 beds
Totals:	26 hospitals	3159 beds

9295: DEPARTMENT OF VETERANS AFFAIRS (FG)
810 Vermont Avenue N.W., Washington, DC Zip 20420; tel. 202/273–5781; Thomas L. Garthwaite, M.D., Acting Undersecretary for Health
(Decentralized Health System)

ALABAMA: CENTRAL ALABAMA VETERAN AFFAIRS HEALTH CARE SYSTEM (O, 355 beds) 215 Perry Hill Road, Montgomery, AL Zip 36109–3798; tel. 334/272–4670; Kenneth Rugle, Interim Director
Web address: www.va.gov/stations97/guide/home.asp?DIVISION=ALL

VETERANS AFFAIRS MEDICAL CENTER (O, 122 beds) 700 South 19th Street, Birmingham, AL Zip 35233–1927; tel. 205/933–8101; Y. C. Parris, Director
Web address: www.va.gov

VETERANS AFFAIRS MEDICAL CENTER (O, 307 beds) 3701 Loop Road, Tuscaloosa, AL Zip 35404–5015; tel. 205/554–2000; W. Kenneth Ruyle, Director
Web address: www.va.gov/stations97/guide/home.asp?DIVISION=ALL

ARIZONA: CARL T. HAYDEN VETERANS AFFAIRS MEDICAL CENTER (O, 285 beds) 650 East Indian School Road, Phoenix, AZ Zip 85012–1892; tel. 602/277–5551; John R. Fears, Director
Web address: www.va.gov

NORTHERN ARIZONA VA HEALTH CARE SYSTEM (O, 287 beds) 500 Highway 89 North, Prescott, AZ Zip 86313–5000; tel. 520/445–4860; Patricia A. McKlem, Chief Executive Officer
Web address: www.va.gov/stations97/guide/home.asp?DIVISION=ALL

SOUTHERN ARIZONA VETERANS AFFAIRS HEALTHCARE SYSTEM (O, 210 beds) 3601 South 6th Avenue, Tucson, AZ Zip 85723–0002; tel. 520/792–1450; Jonathan H. Gardner, Chief Executive Officer
Web address: www.va.gov/stations97/guide/home.asp?DIVISION=ALL

ARKANSAS: CENTRAL ARKANSAS VETERANS AFFAIRS HEALTHCARE SYSTEM (O, 512 beds) 4300 West Seventh Street, Little Rock, AR Zip 72205–5484; tel. 501/257–1000; George H. Gray , Jr, Director
Web address: www.visn16.med.va.gov

VETERANS AFFAIRS MEDICAL CENTER (O, 51 beds) 1100 North College Avenue, Fayetteville, AR Zip 72703–6995; tel. 501/443–4301; Richard F. Robinson, Director
Web address: www.va.gov/stations97/guide/home.asp?DIVISION=ALL

CALIFORNIA: JERRY L. PETTIS MEMORIAL VETERANS MEDICAL CENTER (O, 315 beds) 11201 Benton Street, Loma Linda, CA Zip 92357; tel. 909/825–7084; Dean R. Stordahl, Chief Executive Officer
Web address: www.desertpacific.med.va.gov

VETERANS AFFAIRS MEDICAL CENTER (O, 145 beds) 2615 East Clinton Avenue, Fresno, CA Zip 93703; tel. 559/225–6100; Alan S. Perry, Director
Web address: www.fresno.med.va.gov

For explanation of codes following names, see page B2.
★ Indicates Type III membership in the American Hospital Association.

Systems / Department of Veterans Affairs

VETERANS AFFAIRS MEDICAL CENTER (O, 426 beds) 5901 East Seventh Street, Long Beach, CA Zip 90822–5201; tel. 562/494–5400; Lawrence C. Stewart, Director
Web address: www.long-beach.va.gov

VETERANS AFFAIRS MEDICAL CENTER (O, 232 beds) 3350 LaJolla Village Drive, San Diego, CA Zip 92161; tel. 858/552–8585; Gary J. Rossio, Director and Chief Executive Officer
Web address: www.va.gov/stations97/guide/home.asp?DIVISION=ALL

VETERANS AFFAIRS MEDICAL CENTER (O, 244 beds) 4150 Clement Street, San Francisco, CA Zip 94121–1598; tel. 415/221–4810; Sheila M. Cullen, Director
Web address: www.va.gov/stations97/guide/home.asp?DIVISION=ALL

VETERANS AFFAIRS MEDICAL CENTER–WEST LOS ANGELES (O, 1327 beds) 11301 Wilshire Boulevard, Los Angeles, CA Zip 90073–0275; tel. 310/268–3132; Philip P. Thomas, Chief Executive Officer
Web address: www.va.gov/stations97/guide/home.asp?DIVISION=ALL

VETERANS AFFAIRS PALO ALTO HEALTH CARE SYSTEM (O, 967 beds) 3801 Miranda Avenue, Palo Alto, CA Zip 94304–1207; tel. 650/493–5000; James A. Goff, FACHE, Director
Web address: www.icon.palo-alto.med.va.gov

COLORADO: VETERANS AFFAIRS MEDICAL CENTER (O, 336 beds) 1055 Clermont Street, Denver, CO Zip 80220–3877; tel. 303/399–8020; Ed Thorsland , Jr, Director
Web address: www.va.gov/stations97/guide/home.asp?DIVISION=ALL

VETERANS AFFAIRS MEDICAL CENTER (O, 53 beds) 2121 North Avenue, Grand Junction, CO Zip 81501–6499; tel. 970/242–0731; Kurt W. Schlegelmilch, M.D., CHE, Director
Web address: www.va.gov/stations97/guide/home.asp?DIVISION=ALL

CONNECTICUT: VETERANS AFFAIRS CONNECTICUT HEALTHCARE SYSTEM–WEST HAVEN DIVISION (O, 200 beds) 950 Campbell Avenue, New Haven, CT Zip 06516–2770; tel. 203/932–5711; Paul J. McCool, Director
Web address: www.va.gov/stations97/guide/home.asp?DIVISION=ALL

DELAWARE: VETERANS AFFAIRS MEDICAL CENTER (O, 118 beds) 1601 Kirkwood Highway, Wilmington, DE Zip 19805–4989; tel. 302/633–5201; Dexter D. Dix, Director
Web address: www.va.gov/station

DISTRICT OF COLUMBIA: VETERANS AFFAIRS MEDICAL CENTER (O, 287 beds) 50 Irving Street N.W., Washington, DC Zip 20422–0002; tel. 202/745–8100; Sanford M. Garfunkel, Director
Web address: www.va.gov/station

FLORIDA: JAMES A. HALEY VETERANS HOSPITAL (O, 640 beds) 13000 Bruce B. Downs Boulevard, Tampa, FL Zip 33612–4798; tel. 813/972–2000; Richard A. Silver, Director

MALCOM RANDALL VETERANS AFFAIRS MEDICAL CENTER (O, 594 beds) 1601 S.W. Archer Road, Gainesville, FL Zip 32608–1197; tel. 352/376–1611; Elwood J. Headley, M.D., System Director
Web address: www.va.gov

VETERANS AFFAIRS MEDICAL CENTER (O, 453 beds) Bay Pines & 100 Way, Bay Pines, FL Zip 33744, Mailing Address: P.O. Box 5005, Zip 33744–5005; tel. 727/398–6661; Thomas H. Weaver, FACHE, Director
Web address: www.va.gov/stations97/guide/home.asp?DIVISION=ALL

VETERANS AFFAIRS MEDICAL CENTER (O, 192 beds) 7305 North Military Trail, West Palm Beach, FL Zip 33410–6400; tel. 561/882–8262; Edward H. Seiler, Director
Web address: www.va.gov

VETERANS AFFAIRS MEDICAL CENTER (O, 669 beds) 1201 N.W. 16th Street, Miami, FL Zip 33125–1624; tel. 305/324–4455; Thomas C. Doherty, Medical Director
Web address: www.va.gov/stations97/guide/home.asp?DIVISION=ALL

VETERANS AFFAIRS MEDICAL CENTER (O, 360 beds) 801 South Marion Street, Lake City, FL Zip 32025–5898; tel. 904/755–3016; Marlis Meyer, Division Director
Web address: www.va.gov/stations97/guide/home.asp?DIVISION=ALL

GEORGIA: VETERANS AFFAIRS MEDICAL CENTER (O, 271 beds) 1670 Clairmont Road, Decatur, GA Zip 30033–4004; tel. 404/321–6111; Robert A. Perreault, Director
Web address: www.va.gov/stations97/guide/home.asp?DIVISION=ALL

VETERANS AFFAIRS MEDICAL CENTER (O, 587 beds) 1 Freedom Way, Augusta, GA Zip 30904–6285; tel. 706/733–0188; Ellen DeGeorge–Smith, FACHE, Director
Web address: www.va.gov

VETERANS AFFAIRS MEDICAL CENTER (O, 253 beds) 1826 Veterans Boulevard, Dublin, GA Zip 31021–3620; tel. 912/272–1210; James F. Trusley , II, Director
Web address: www.va.gov/stations97/guide/home.asp?DIVISION=ALL

IDAHO: VETERANS AFFAIRS MEDICAL CENTER (O, 176 beds) 500 West Fort Street, Boise, ID Zip 83702–4598; tel. 208/422–1100; Wayne C. Tippets, Director
Web address: www.va.gov/stations97/guide/home.asp?DIVISION=ALL

ILLINOIS: VETERANS AFFAIRS CHICAGO HEALTH CARE SYSTEM (O, 325 beds) 333 East Huron Street, Chicago, IL Zip 60611–3004; tel. 312/640–2100; Richard S. Citron, Director

VETERANS AFFAIRS EDWARD HINES, JR. HOSPITAL (O, 385 beds) Fifth Avenue & Roosevelt Road, Hines, IL Zip 60141–5000, Mailing Address: P.O. Box 5000, Zip 60141–5000; tel. 708/202–8387; John R. Fears, Acting Director
Web address: www.va.gov/stations97/guide/home.asp?DIVISION=ALL

VETERANS AFFAIRS MEDICAL CENTER (O, 439 beds) 1900 East Main Street, Danville, IL Zip 61832–5198; tel. 217/442–8000; Cathi Spivey–Paul, Acting Director
Web address: www.va.gov/stations97/guide/home.asp?DIVISION=ALL

VETERANS AFFAIRS MEDICAL CENTER (O, 836 beds) 3001 Green Bay Road, North Chicago, IL Zip 60064–3049; tel. 847/688–1900; Alfred S. Pate, Director
Web address: www.va.gov/stations97/guide/home.asp?DIVISION=ALL

VETERANS AFFAIRS MEDICAL CENTER (O, 99 beds) 2401 West Main Street, Marion, IL Zip 62959–1194; tel. 618/997–5311; Earl F. Falast, Director
Web address: www.va.gov/stations97/guide/home.asp?DIVISION=ALL

INDIANA: RICHARD L. ROUDEBUSH VETERANS AFFAIRS MEDICAL CENTER (O, 139 beds) 1481 West Tenth Street, Indianapolis, IN Zip 46202–2884; tel. 317/554–0000; Susan P. Bowers, Acting Director

VETERANS AFFAIRS NORTHERN INDIANA HEALTH CARE SYSTEM (O, 423 beds) 2121 Lake Avenue, Fort Wayne, IN Zip 46805–5347; tel. 219/460–1310; Michael W. Murphy, Ph.D., Director and Chief Executive Officer
Web address: www.va.gov/stations97/guide/home.asp?DIVISION=ALL

IOWA: VETERANS AFFAIRS CENTRAL IOWA HEALTH CARE SYSTEM (O, 327 beds) 3600 30th Street, Des Moines, IA Zip 50310–5774; tel. 515/699–5999; Donald C. Cooper, Director
Web address: www.va.gov/stations97/guide/home.asp?DIVISION=ALL

VETERANS AFFAIRS MEDICAL CENTER (O, 106 beds) 601 Highway 6 West, Iowa City, IA Zip 52246–2208; tel. 319/338–0581; Gary L. Wilkinson, Director
Web address: www.va.gov/stations97/guide/home.asp?DIVISION=ALL

KANSAS: VETERANS AFFAIRS EASTERN KANSAS HEALTH CARE SYSTEM (O, 588 beds) 2200 Gage Boulevard, Topeka, KS Zip 66622–0002; tel. 785/350–3111; Edgar L. Tucker, Director
Web address: www.va.gov/stations97/guide/home.asp?DIVISION=ALL

VETERANS AFFAIRS MEDICAL AND REGIONAL OFFICE CENTER (O, 41 beds) 5500 East Kellogg, Wichita, KS Zip 67218; tel. 316/685–2221; Kent D. Hill, Director
Web address: www.va.gov/stations97/guide/home.asp?DIVISION=ALL

KENTUCKY: VETERANS AFFAIRS MEDICAL CENTER–LEXINGTON (O, 413 beds) 2250 Leestown Pike, Lexington, KY Zip 40511–1093; tel. 606/233–4511; Helen K. Cornish, Director
Web address: www.va.gov/stations97/guide/home.asp?DIVISION=ALL

VETERANS AFFAIRS MEDICAL CENTER–LOUISVILLE (O, 110 beds) 800 Zorn Avenue, Louisville, KY Zip 40206–1499; tel. 502/895–3401; Larry J. Sander, FACHE, Director
Web address: www.va.gov/603louisville

LOUISIANA: OVERTON BROOKS VETERANS AFFAIRS MEDICAL CENTER (O, 100 beds) 510 East Stoner Avenue, Shreveport, LA Zip 71101–4295; tel. 318/221–8411; Billy M. Valentine, Director
Web address: www.va.gov/stations97/guide/home.asp?DIVISION=ALL

For explanation of codes following names, see page B2.
★ Indicates Type III membership in the American Hospital Association.

Systems / Department of Veterans Affairs

VETERANS AFFAIRS MEDICAL CENTER (O, 257 beds) Shreveport Highway, Alexandria, LA Zip 71306-6002; tel. 318/473-0010; Allen J. Colston, Director
Web address: www.va.gov/stations97/guide/home.asp?DIVISION=ALL

VETERANS AFFAIRS MEDICAL CENTER (O, 204 beds) 1601 Perdido Street, New Orleans, LA Zip 70112-1262; tel. 504/568-0811; John D. Church, Jr, Director
Web address: www.va.gov/stations97/guide/home.asp?DIVISION=ALL

MAINE: VETERANS AFFAIRS MEDICAL CENTER (O, 176 beds) 1 VA Center, Togus, ME Zip 04330; tel. 207/623-8411; John H. Sims, Jr, Director
Web address: www.visn1.med.va.gov

MARYLAND: VETERANS AFFAIRS MARYLAND HEALTH CARE SYSTEM–BALTIMORE DIVISION (O, 897 beds) 10 North Greene Street, Baltimore, MD Zip 21201-1524; tel. 410/605-7001; Dennis H. Smith, Director

VETERANS AFFAIRS MARYLAND HEALTH CARE SYSTEM–FORT HOWARD DIVISION (O, 245 beds) 9600 North Point Road, Fort Howard, MD Zip 21052-9989; tel. 410/477-1800; Dennis H. Smith, Director

VETERANS AFFAIRS MARYLAND HEALTH CARE SYSTEM–PERRY POINT DIVISION (O, 526 beds) Circle Drive, Perry Point, MD Zip 21902; tel. 410/642-2411; Dennis H. Smith, Director

MASSACHUSETTS: BROCKTON VETERANS AFFAIRS MEDICAL CENTER (O, 495 beds) 940 Belmont Street, Brockton, MA Zip 02401-5596; tel. 508/583-4500; Roland E. Moore, Director
Web address: www.va.gov/stations97/guide/home.asp?DIVISION=ALL

EDITH NOURSE ROGERS MEMORIAL VETERANS HOSPITAL (O, 411 beds) 200 Springs Road, Bedford, MA Zip 01730-1198; tel. 781/687-2000; William A. Conte, Director
Web address: www.va.gov/stations97/guide/home.asp?DIVISION=ALL

VETERANS AFFAIRS BOSTON HEALTHCARE SYSTEM (O, 188 beds) Boston, MA Mailing Address: 150 South Huntington Avenue, Jamaica Plain Station, Zip 02130-4820; tel. 617/232-9500; Michael E. Lawson, Director
Web address: www.va.gov/stations97/guide/home.asp?DIVISION=ALL

VETERANS AFFAIRS MEDICAL CENTER (O, 197 beds) 421 North Main Street, Leeds, MA Zip 01053-9764; tel. 413/584-4040; Bruce A. Gordon, Director
Web address: www.va.gov/stations97/guide/home.asp?DIVISION=ALL

MICHIGAN: ALEDA E. LUTZ VETERANS AFFAIRS MEDICAL CENTER (O, 114 beds) 1500 Weiss Street, Saginaw, MI Zip 48602-5298; tel. 517/497-2500; Robert H. Sabin, Director

JOHN D. DINGELL VETERANS AFFAIRS MEDICAL CENTER (O, 218 beds) 4646 John R Street, Detroit, MI Zip 48201-1932; tel. 313/576-1000; Carlos B. Lott, Jr, Director
Web address: www.va.gov/stations97/guide/home.asp?DIVISION=ALL

VETERANS AFFAIRS MEDICAL CENTER (O, 162 beds) 2215 Fuller Road, Ann Arbor, MI Zip 48105-2399; tel. 734/769-7100; James W. Roseborough, CHE, Director
Web address: www.va.gov/stations97/guide/home.asp?DIVISION=ALL

VETERANS AFFAIRS MEDICAL CENTER (O, 376 beds) 5500 Armstrong Road, Battle Creek, MI Zip 49016; tel. 616/966-5600; Michael K. Wheeler, Director
Web address: www.va.gov/stations97/guide/home.asp?DIVISION=ALL

VETERANS AFFAIRS MEDICAL CENTER (O, 74 beds) 325 East H Street, Iron Mountain, MI Zip 49801-4792; tel. 906/774-3300; Deborah A. Thompson, Director
Web address: www.va.gov/stations97/guide/home.asp?DIVISION=ALL

MINNESOTA: VETERANS AFFAIRS MEDICAL CENTER (O, 361 beds) One Veterans Drive, Minneapolis, MN Zip 55417-2399; tel. 612/725-2000; Steven Kleinglass, Acting Director

VETERANS AFFAIRS MEDICAL CENTER (O, 382 beds) 4801 Eighth Street North, Saint Cloud, MN Zip 56303-2099; tel. 320/252-1670; Barry I. Bahl, Director

MISSISSIPPI: G.V. MONTGOMERY VETERANS AFFAIRS MEDICAL CENTER (O, 443 beds) 1500 East Woodrow Wilson Drive, Jackson, MS Zip 39216-5199; tel. 601/364-1201; Richard F. Miller, Director
Web address: www.visn16.med.va.gov

VA GULF COAST VETERANS HEALTH CARE SYSTEM (O, 510 beds) 400 Veterans Avenue, Biloxi, MS Zip 39531-2410; tel. 228/523-5000; Julie A. Catellier, Director

MISSOURI: HARRY S. TRUMAN MEMORIAL VETERANS HOSPITAL (O, 104 beds) 800 Hospital Drive, Columbia, MO Zip 65201-5297; tel. 573/814-6300; Gary L. Campbell, Director

JOHN J. PERSHING VETERANS AFFAIRS MEDICAL CENTER (O, 56 beds) 1500 North Westwood Boulevard, Poplar Bluff, MO Zip 63901-3318; tel. 573/686-4151; Nancy Arnold, Director

VETERANS AFFAIRS MEDICAL CENTER (O, 355 beds) 1 Jefferson Barracks Drive, Saint Louis, MO Zip 63125-4199; tel. 314/652-4100; Linda Kurz, CHE, Director

VETERANS AFFAIRS MEDICAL CENTER (O, 126 beds) 4801 Linwood Boulevard, Kansas City, MO Zip 64128-2295; tel. 816/861-4700; Hugh F. Doran, Director

MONTANA: VETERANS AFFAIRS MONTANA HEALTHCARE SYSTEM (O, 45 beds) Highway 12 and William Street, Fort Harrison, MT Zip 59636; tel. 406/442-6410; Joseph Underkofler, Director
Web address: www.va.gov/stations97/guide/home.asp?DIVISION=ALL

NEBRASKA: VETERANS AFFAIRS GREATER NEBRASKA HEALTH CARE SYSTEM (O, 191 beds) 600 South 70th Street, Lincoln, NE Zip 68510-2493; tel. 402/489-3802; David Asper, Director
Web address: www.va.gov/stations97/guide/home.asp?DIVISION=ALL

VETERANS AFFAIRS MEDICAL CENTER (O, 122 beds) 4101 Woolworth Avenue, Omaha, NE Zip 68105-1873; tel. 402/449-0600; John J. Phillips, Director
Web address: www.va.gov/stations97/guide/home.asp?DIVISION=ALL

NEVADA: VETERANS AFFAIRS SIERRA NEVADA HEALTH CARE SYSTEM (O, 126 beds) 1000 Locust Street, Reno, NV Zip 89520-0111; tel. 775/786-7200; Gary R. Whitfield, FACHE, Director

VETERANS AFFAIRS SOUTHERN NEVADA HEALTHCARE SYSTEM (O, 52 beds) 1700 Vegas Drive, Las Vegas, NV Zip 89106; tel. 702/636-3000; Ramon J. Reevey, Director

NEW HAMPSHIRE: VETERANS AFFAIRS MEDICAL CENTER (O, 180 beds) 718 Smyth Road, Manchester, NH Zip 03104-4098; tel. 603/624-4366; Marc Levenson, Administrator
Web address: www.va.gov/stations97/guide/home.asp?DIVISION=ALL

NEW JERSEY: VETERANS AFFAIRS NEW JERSEY HEALTH CARE SYSTEM (O, 934 beds) 385 Tremont Avenue, East Orange, NJ Zip 07018-1095; tel. 973/676-1000; Kenneth H. Mizrach, Director
Web address: www.va.gov/stations97/guide/home.asp?DIVISION=ALL

NEW MEXICO: VETERANS AFFAIRS MEDICAL CENTER (O, 327 beds) 1501 San Pedro S.E., Albuquerque, NM Zip 87108-5138; tel. 505/265-1711; Norman E. Browne, Director
Web address: www.va.gov

NEW YORK: VETERANS ADMINISTRATION NEW YORK HARBOR HEALTHCARE SYSTEM (O, 618 beds) 800 Poly Place, Brooklyn, NY Zip 11209-7104; tel. 718/630-3500; John J. Donnellan, Jr, Director

VETERANS AFFAIRS HUDSON VALLEY HEALTH CARE SYSTEM–F.D. ROOSEVELT HOSPITAL (O, 597 beds) Montrose, NY Mailing Address: P.O. Box 100, Zip 10548-0110; tel. 914/737-4400; Michael A. Sabo, Director

VETERANS AFFAIRS MEDICAL CENTER (O, 298 beds) 113 Holland Avenue, Albany, NY Zip 12208-3473; tel. 518/462-3311; Clyde L. Parkis, Director
Web address: www.va.gov/stations97/guide/home.asp?DIVISION=ALL

VETERANS AFFAIRS MEDICAL CENTER (O, 615 beds) 76 Veterans Avenue, Bath, NY Zip 14810-0842; tel. 607/664-4000; Joseph Striano, Acting Director
Web address: www.va.gov/stations97/guide/home.asp?DIVISION=ALL

VETERANS AFFAIRS MEDICAL CENTER (O, 626 beds) 400 Fort Hill Avenue, Canandaigua, NY Zip 14424-1197; tel. 716/394-2000; W. David Smith, Director
Web address: www.va.gov/visns/visn02/can_nf.html

VETERANS AFFAIRS MEDICAL CENTER (O, 328 beds) 130 West Kingsbridge Road, Bronx, NY Zip 10468-3992; tel. 718/584-9000; Maryann Musumeci, Director
Web address: www.va.gov/stations97/guide/home.asp?DIVISION=ALL

VETERANS AFFAIRS MEDICAL CENTER (O, 699 beds) 79 Middleville Road, Northport, NY Zip 11768-2293; tel. 631/261-4400; Mary A. Dowling, Director
Web address: www.va.gov/stations97/guide/home.asp?DIVISION=ALL

For explanation of codes following names, see page B2.
★ Indicates Type III membership in the American Hospital Association.

Systems / Department of Veterans Affairs

VETERANS AFFAIRS MEDICAL CENTER (O, 175 beds) 800 Irving Avenue, Syracuse, NY Zip 13210–2796; tel. 315/476–7461; James P. Cody, Director
Web address: www.va.gov/stations97/guide/home.asp?DIVISION=ALL

VETERANS AFFAIRS WESTERN NEW YORK HEALTHCARE SYSTEM–BATAVIA DIVISION (O, 158 beds) 222 Richmond Avenue, Batavia, NY Zip 14020–1288; tel. 716/343–7500; Richard S. Droske, Director

VETERANS AFFAIRS WESTERN NEW YORK HEALTHCARE SYSTEM–BUFFALO DIVISION (O, 233 beds) 3495 Bailey Avenue, Buffalo, NY Zip 14215–1129; tel. 716/834–9200; William F. Feeley, Director
Web address: www.va.gov/stations97/guide/home.asp?DIVISION=ALL

NORTH CAROLINA: VETERANS AFFAIRS MEDICAL CENTER (O, 382 beds) 508 Fulton Street, Durham, NC Zip 27705–3897; tel. 919/286–0411; Michael B. Phaup, Director
Web address: www.va.gov/stations97/guide/home.asp?DIVISION=ALL

VETERANS AFFAIRS MEDICAL CENTER (O, 193 beds) 2300 Ramsey Street, Fayetteville, NC Zip 28301–3899; tel. 910/822–7059; Richard J. Baltz, Director
Web address: www.va.gov/stations97/guide/home.asp?DIVISION=ALL

VETERANS AFFAIRS MEDICAL CENTER (O, 389 beds) 1100 Tunnel Road, Asheville, NC Zip 28805–2087; tel. 828/298–7911; James A. Christian, Director
Web address: www.va.gov

VETERANS AFFAIRS MEDICAL CENTER (O, 533 beds) 1601 Brenner Avenue, Salisbury, NC Zip 28144–2559; tel. 704/638–9000; Timothy May, Director
Web address: www.va.gov/stations97/guide/home.asp?DIVISION=ALL

NORTH DAKOTA: VETERANS AFFAIRS MEDICAL AND REGIONAL OFFICE CENTER (O, 109 beds) 2101 Elm Street, Fargo, ND Zip 58102–2498; tel. 701/232–3241; Douglas M. Kenyon, Director

OHIO: VETERANS AFFAIRS MEDICAL CENTER (O, 817 beds) 10701 East Boulevard, Cleveland, OH Zip 44106–1702; tel. 216/791–3800; William D. Montague, Director

VETERANS AFFAIRS MEDICAL CENTER (O, 304 beds) 17273 State Route 104, Chillicothe, OH Zip 45601–0999; tel. 740/773–1141; Michael W. Walton, Director
Web address: www.bright.net/~vachilli

VETERANS AFFAIRS MEDICAL CENTER (O, 240 beds) 3200 Vine Street, Cincinnati, OH Zip 45220–2288; tel. 513/861–3100; Gary N. Nugent, Medical Director
Web address: www.va.gov/stations97/guide/home.asp?DIVISION=ALL

VETERANS AFFAIRS MEDICAL CENTER (O, 835 beds) 4100 West Third Street, Dayton, OH Zip 45428–1002; tel. 937/268–6511; Steven M. Cohen, M.D., Director
Web address: www.va.gov/stations97/guide/home.asp?DIVISION=ALL

OKLAHOMA: VETERANS AFFAIRS MEDICAL CENTER (O, 50 beds) 1011 Honor Heights Drive, Muskogee, OK Zip 74401–1399; tel. 918/683–3261;
Web address: www.visn16.med.va.gov

VETERANS AFFAIRS MEDICAL CENTER (O, 277 beds) 921 N.E. 13th Street, Oklahoma City, OK Zip 73104–5028; tel. 405/270–0501; Steven J. Gentling, Director
Web address: www.va.gov/stations97/guide/home.asp?DIVISION=ALL

OREGON: VETERANS AFFAIRS MEDICAL CENTER (O, 591 beds) 3710 S.W. U.S. Veterans Hospital Road, Portland, OR Zip 97201; tel. 503/220–8262; James Tuchschmidt, M.D., Chief Executive Officer
Web address: www.va.gov/stations97/guide/home.asp?DIVISION=ALL

VETERANS AFFAIRS ROSEBURG HEALTHCARE SYSTEM (O, 132 beds) 913 N.W. Garden Valley Boulevard, Roseburg, OR Zip 97470–6513; tel. 541/440–1000; George Marnell, Director

PENNSYLVANIA: JAMES E. VAN ZANDT VETERANS AFFAIRS MEDICAL CENTER (O, 68 beds) 2907 Pleasant Valley Boulevard, Altoona, PA Zip 16602–4377; tel. 814/943–8164; Gerald L. Williams, Director and Chief Executive Officer
Web address: www.va.gov/stations97/guide/home.asp?DIVISION=ALL

VETERANS AFFAIRS MEDICAL CENTER (O, 170 beds) 325 New Castle Road, Butler, PA Zip 16001–2480; tel. 724/287–4781; Michael E. Moreland, Director
Web address: www.va.gov/station/529–butler

VETERANS AFFAIRS MEDICAL CENTER (O, 607 beds) 1400 Black Horse Hill Road, Coatesville, PA Zip 19320–2097; tel. 610/384–7711; Gary W. Devansky, Chief Executive Officer
Web address: www.coatesville.med.va.gov

VETERANS AFFAIRS MEDICAL CENTER (O, 61 beds) 135 East 38th Street, Erie, PA Zip 16504–1559; tel. 814/860–2576; Stephen M. Lucas, Chief Executive Officer
Web address: www.erie.net/~vamcerie

VETERANS AFFAIRS MEDICAL CENTER (O, 285 beds) 1700 South Lincoln Avenue, Lebanon, PA Zip 17042–7529; tel. 717/272–6621; Charleen R. Szabo, FACHE, Chief Executive Officer
Web address: www.va.gov

VETERANS AFFAIRS MEDICAL CENTER (O, 389 beds) University and Woodland Avenues, Philadelphia, PA Zip 19104–4594; tel. 215/823–5800; Michael J. Sullivan, Director
Web address: www.va.gov/stations97/guide/home.asp?DIVISION=ALL

VETERANS AFFAIRS MEDICAL CENTER (O, 339 beds) 1111 East End Boulevard, Wilkes–Barre, PA Zip 18711–0026; tel. 570/824–3521; Reedes Hurt, Chief Executive Officer
Web address: www.va.gov/stations97/guide/home.asp?DIVISION=ALL

VETERANS AFFAIRS PITTSBURGH HEALTHCARE SYSTEM (O, 809 beds) Delafield Road, Pittsburgh, PA Zip 15240–1001; tel. 412/784–3900; John C. Lowe, Acting Director
Web address: www.pitt.edu

PUERTO RICO: VETERANS AFFAIRS MEDICAL CENTER (O, 693 beds) One Veterans Plaza, San Juan, PR Zip 00936–5800; tel. 787/641–7582; James A. Palmer, Director
Web address: www.va.gov/stations97/guide/home.asp?DIVISION=ALL

RHODE ISLAND: VETERANS AFFAIRS MEDICAL CENTER (O, 66 beds) 830 Chalkstone Avenue, Providence, RI Zip 02908–4799; tel. 401/457–3042; Louise McMahon, Acting Director
Web address: www.va.gov/stations97/guide/home.asp?DIVISION=ALL

SOUTH CAROLINA: RALPH H. JOHNSON VETERANS AFFAIRS MEDICAL CENTER (O, 161 beds) 109 Bee Street, Charleston, SC Zip 29401–5703; tel. 843/577–5011

WM. JENNINGS BRYAN DORN VETERANS AFFAIRS MEDICAL CENTER (O, 280 beds) 6439 Garners Ferry Road, Columbia, SC Zip 29209–1639; tel. 803/776–4000; Brian Heckert, Medical Center Director

SOUTH DAKOTA: ROYAL C. JOHNSON VETERANS MEMORIAL HOSPITAL (O, 84 beds) 2501 West 22nd Street, Sioux Falls, SD Zip 57105–9920, Mailing Address: P.O. Box 5046, Zip 57117–9920; tel. 605/336–3230; Ronald T. Porzio, Chief Operating Officer
Web address: www.va.gov/stations97/guide/home.asp?DIVISION=ALL

VETERANS AFFAIRS BLACK HILLS HEALTH CARE SYSTEM (O, 163 beds) 113 Comanche Road, Fort Meade, SD Zip 57741–1099; tel. 605/347–2511; Peter P. Henry, Director
Web address: www.va.gov/stations97/guide/home.asp?DIVISION=ALL

TENNESSEE: ALVIN C. YORK VETERANS AFFAIRS MEDICAL CENTER (O, 372 beds) 3400 Lebanon Pike, Murfreesboro, TN Zip 37129–1236; tel. 615/867–6100; Lea Swafford, Acting Director
Web address: www.va.gov/murfreesboro.htm

JAMES H. QUILLEN VETERANS AFFAIRS MEDICAL CENTER (O, 390 beds) Mountain Home, TN Zip 37684–4000; tel. 423/926–1171; Carl J. Gerber, M.D., Ph.D., Director

VETERANS AFFAIRS MEDICAL CENTER (O, 293 beds) 1030 Jefferson Avenue, Memphis, TN Zip 38104–2193; tel. 901/523–8990; K. L. Mulholland, Jr, Director
Web address: www.va.gov/stations97/guide/home.asp?DIVISION=ALL

VETERANS AFFAIRS MEDICAL CENTER (O, 137 beds) 1310 24th Avenue South, Nashville, TN Zip 37212–2637; tel. 615/327–4751; William A. Mountcastle, Director
Web address: www.nashville.med.va.gov

TEXAS: CENTRAL TEXAS VETERANS AFFAIRS HEALTHCARE SYSTEM (O, 1852 beds) 1901 South First Street, Temple, TX Zip 76504–7493; tel. 254/778–4811; Dean S. Billik, Director

SOUTH TEXAS VETERANS HEALTH CARE SYSTEM (O, 1112 beds) 7400 Merton Minter Boulevard, San Antonio, TX Zip 78284–5799; tel. 210/617–5140; Jose R. Coronado, FACHE, Director
Web address: www.vasthcs.med.va.gov

For explanation of codes following names, see page B2.
★ Indicates Type III membership in the American Hospital Association.

Systems / Department of Veterans Affairs

VETERANS AFFAIRS MEDICAL CENTER (O, 218 beds) 6010 Amarillo Boulevard West, Amarillo, TX Zip 79106–1992; tel. 806/354–7801; Wallace M. Hopkins, FACHE, Chief Executive Officer

VETERANS AFFAIRS MEDICAL CENTER (O, 189 beds) 300 Veterans Boulevard, Big Spring, TX Zip 79720–5500; tel. 915/263–7361; Cary D. Brown, Director

VETERANS AFFAIRS MEDICAL CENTER (O, 859 beds) 2002 Holcombe Boulevard, Houston, TX Zip 77030–4298; tel. 713/791–1414; David Whatley, Director
Web address: www.va.gov/stations97/guide/home.asp?DIVISION=ALL

VETERANS AFFAIRS NORTH TEXAS HEALTH CARE SYSTEM (O, 1031 beds) 4500 South Lancaster Road, Dallas, TX Zip 75216–7167; tel. 214/742–8387; Alan G. Harper, Director

UTAH: VETERANS AFFAIRS MEDICAL CENTER (O, 121 beds) 500 Foothill Drive, Salt Lake City, UT Zip 84148–0002; tel. 801/582–1565; James R. Floyd, Director
Web address: www.va.gov/stations97/guide/home.asp?DIVISION=ALL

VERMONT: VETERANS AFFAIRS MEDICAL CENTER (O, 60 beds) North Hartland Road, White River Junction, VT Zip 05009–0001; tel. 802/295–9363; Gary M. De Gasta, Center Director
Web address: www.va.gov

VIRGINIA: HUNTER HOLMES MCGUIRE VETERANS AFFAIRS MEDICAL CENTER (O, 616 beds) 1201 Broad Rock Boulevard, Richmond, VA Zip 23249–0002; tel. 804/675–5000; James W. Dudley, Director

VETERANS AFFAIRS MEDICAL CENTER (O, 470 beds) 100 Emancipation Drive, Hampton, VA Zip 23667–0001; tel. 757/722–9961; Bettye W. Story, Ph.D., Director
Web address: www.va.gov

VETERANS AFFAIRS MEDICAL CENTER (O, 268 beds) 1970 Roanoke Boulevard, Salem, VA Zip 24153; tel. 540/982–2463; Stephen L. Lemons, Ed.D., Director
Web address: www.va.gov

WASHINGTON: JONATHAN M. WAINWRIGHT MEMORIAL VA MEDICAL CENTER (O, 76 beds) 77 Wainwright Drive, Walla Walla, WA Zip 99362–3994; tel. 509/525–5200; Roxanne Sisemore, Acting Director
Web address: www.va.gov/stations97/guide/home.asp?DIVISION=ALL

VETERANS AFFAIRS MEDICAL CENTER (O, 86 beds) North 4815 Assembly Street, Spokane, WA Zip 99205–6197; tel. 509/434–7200; Joseph M. Manley, Director
Web address: www.va.gov/stations97/guide/home.asp?DIVISION=ALL

VETERANS AFFAIRS PUGET SOUND HEALTH CARE SYSTEM (O, 557 beds) 1660 South Columbian Way, Seattle, WA Zip 98108–1597; tel. 206/762–1010; Timothy B. Williams, Director

WEST VIRGINIA: LOUIS A. JOHNSON VETERANS AFFAIRS MEDICAL CENTER (O, 160 beds) 1 Medical Center Drive, Clarksburg, WV Zip 26301–4199; tel. 304/623–3461; Michael W. Neusch, FACHE, Director

VETERANS AFFAIRS MEDICAL CENTER (O, 90 beds) 200 Veterans Avenue, Beckley, WV Zip 25801–6499; tel. 304/255–2121; Gerard P. Husson, Director
Web address: www.va.gov/stations97/guide/home.asp?DIVISION=ALL

VETERANS AFFAIRS MEDICAL CENTER (O, 80 beds) 1540 Spring Valley Drive, Huntington, WV Zip 25704–9300; tel. 304/429–6741; David N. Pennington, FACHE, Chief Executive Officer
Web address: www.va.gov

VETERANS AFFAIRS MEDICAL CENTER (O, 370 beds) Charles Town Road, Martinsburg, WV Zip 25401–0205; tel. 304/263–0811; George Moore, Director
Web address: www.va.gov/visn5

WISCONSIN: CLEMENT J. ZABLOCKI VETERANS AFFAIRS MEDICAL CENTER (O, 566 beds) 5000 West National Avenue, Milwaukee, WI Zip 53295; tel. 414/384–2000; Glen W. Grippen, Director

VETERANS AFFAIRS MEDICAL CENTER (O, 569 beds) 500 East Veterans Street, Tomah, WI Zip 54660; tel. 608/372–3971; Stan Johnson, Medical Center Director

WILLIAM S. MIDDLETON MEMORIAL VETERANS HOSPITAL (O, 200 beds) 2500 Overlook Terrace, Madison, WI Zip 53705–2286; tel. 608/256–1901; Nathan L. Geraths, Director

WYOMING: VETERANS AFFAIRS MEDICAL CENTER (O, 71 beds) 2360 East Pershing Boulevard, Cheyenne, WY Zip 82001–5392; tel. 307/778–7550; Richard Fry, Director
Web address: www.va.gov/stations97/guide/home.asp?DIVISION=ALL

VETERANS AFFAIRS MEDICAL CENTER (O, 114 beds) 1898 Fort Road, Sheridan, WY Zip 82801–8320; tel. 307/672–3473; Maureen Humphrys, Director
Web address: www.va.gov/stations97/guide/home.asp?DIVISION=ALL

Owned, leased, sponsored:	139 hospitals	48460 beds
Contract–managed:	0 hospitals	0 beds
Totals:	139 hospitals	48460 beds

★**2145: DETROIT MEDICAL CENTER** (NP)
3663 Woodward Avenue, Suite 200, Detroit, MI Zip 48201–2403; tel. 313/578–2020; Arthur Porter, M.D., President and Chief Executive Officer
(Centralized Physician/Insurance Health System)

MICHIGAN: CHILDREN'S HOSPITAL OF MICHIGAN (O, 218 beds) 3901 Beaubien Street, Detroit, MI Zip 48201–9985; tel. 313/745–0073; Larry Fleischmann, M.D., President
Web address: www.dmc.org/chm

DETROIT RECEIVING HOSPITAL AND UNIVERSITY HEALTH CENTER (O, 258 beds) 4201 St. Antoine Boulevard, Detroit, MI Zip 48201–2194; tel. 313/745–3603; Leslie C. Bowman, Senior Vice President Operations
Web address: www.dmc.org

HARPER HOSPITAL (O, 427 beds) 3990 John R, Detroit, MI Zip 48201–9027; tel. 313/745–8040; Jeff Dankins, Vice President Operations

HURON VALLEY–SINAI HOSPITAL (O, 136 beds) 1 William Carls Drive, Commerce Township, MI Zip 48382–2201; tel. 248/937–3300; Robert J. Yellan, President

HUTZEL HOSPITAL (O, 243 beds) 4707 St. Antoine Boulevard, Detroit, MI Zip 48201–0154; tel. 313/745–7555; Mark McNash, Vice President Operations

REHABILITATION INSTITUTE OF MICHIGAN (O, 94 beds) 261 Mack Boulevard, Detroit, MI Zip 48201–2495; tel. 313/745–1203; Paul Thompson, Jr, Interim Senior Vice President
Web address: www.mdc.org

SINAI/GRACE HOSPITAL (O, 821 beds) 6071 West Outer Drive, Detroit, MI Zip 48235–2679; tel. 313/966–3300; Anne M. Regling, Senior Vice President
Web address: www.dmc.org

Owned, leased, sponsored:	7 hospitals	2197 beds
Contract–managed:	0 hospitals	0 beds
Totals:	7 hospitals	2197 beds

0845: DEVEREUX FOUNDATION (NP)
444 Deveraux Drive, Villanova, PA Zip 19085, Mailing Address: P.O. Box 638, Zip 19333–0638; tel. 610/520–3000; Ronald P. Burd, President and Chief Executive Officer
(Independent Hospital System)

FLORIDA: DEVEREUX HOSPITAL AND CHILDREN'S CENTER OF FLORIDA (O, 100 beds) 8000 Devereux Drive, Melbourne, FL Zip 32940–7907; tel. 407/242–9100; Michael Becker, Executive Director
Web address: www.devereux.org

GEORGIA: DEVEREUX GEORGIA TREATMENT NETWORK (O, 125 beds) 1291 Stanley Road N.W., Kennesaw, GA Zip 30152–4359; tel. 770/422–2135; Elizabeth M. Chadwick, JD, Executive Director
Web address: www.devereux.org

PENNSYLVANIA: DEVEREUX MAPLETON PSYCHIATRIC INSTITUTE–MAPLETON CENTER (O, 13 beds) 655 Sugartown Road, Malvern, PA Zip 19355–0297, Mailing Address: Box 297, Zip 19355–0297; tel. 610/296–6974; James M. Cole, Executive Director

TEXAS: DEVEREUX TEXAS TREATMENT NETWORK (O, 88 beds) 1150 Devereux Drive, League City, TX Zip 77573–2043; tel. 281/335–1000; L. Gail Atkinson, Executive Director
Web address: www.devereux.org

For explanation of codes following names, see page B2.
★ Indicates Type III membership in the American Hospital Association.

Systems / East Texas Medical Center Regional Healthcare System

Owned, leased, sponsored:	4 hospitals	326 beds
Contract-managed:	0 hospitals	0 beds
Totals:	4 hospitals	326 beds

★**0029: DIMENSIONS HEALTH CORPORATION** (NP)
9200 Basil Court, Largo, MD Zip 20774; tel. 301/925-7000;
Winfield M. Kelly, Jr, President and Chief Executive Officer
(Centralized Physician/Insurance Health System)

MARYLAND: LAUREL REGIONAL HOSPITAL (O, 133 beds) 7300 Van Dusen Road, Laurel, MD Zip 20707-9266; tel. 301/725-4300; Patrick F. Mutch, President
Web address: www.laurelregionalhospital.org

PRINCE GEORGE'S HOSPITAL CENTER (O, 370 beds) 3001 Hospital Drive, Cheverly, MD Zip 20785-1189; tel. 301/618-2000; Phyllis Wingate-Jones, President
Web address: www.princegeorgeshospital.org

Owned, leased, sponsored:	2 hospitals	503 beds
Contract-managed:	0 hospitals	0 beds
Totals:	2 hospitals	503 beds

0010: DIVISION OF MENTAL HEALTH SERVICES, DEPARTMENT OF HUMAN SERVICES, STATE OF NEW JERSEY (NP)
Capital Center, P.O. Box 727, Trenton, NJ Zip 08625-0727;
tel. 609/777-0702; Alan G. Kaufman, Director

NEW JERSEY: ANCORA PSYCHIATRIC HOSPITAL (O, 625 beds) 202 Spring Garden Road, Ancora, NJ Zip 08037-9699; tel. 609/561-1700; Gregory P. Roberts, Chief Executive Officer

GREYSTONE PARK PSYCHIATRIC HOSPITAL (O, 605 beds) Central Avenue, Greystone Park, NJ Zip 07950, Mailing Address: P.O. Box A, Zip 07950; tel. 973/538-1800; Michael Greenstein, Chief Executive Officer

SENATOR GARRETT T. W. HAGEDORN GERO PSYCHIATRIC HOSPITAL (O, 181 beds) 200 Sanitorium Road, Glen Gardner, NJ Zip 08826-9752; tel. 908/537-2141; Donald A. Bruckman, Acting Chief Executive Officer

TRENTON PSYCHIATRIC HOSPITAL (O, 395 beds) Sullivan Way, Trenton, NJ Zip 08625, Mailing Address: P.O. Box 7500, West Trenton, Zip 08628-7500; tel. 609/633-1500; Joseph Jupin, Jr, Chief Executive Officer

Owned, leased, sponsored:	4 hospitals	1806 beds
Contract-managed:	0 hospitals	0 beds
Totals:	4 hospitals	1806 beds

0164: DOCTORS COMMUNITY HEALTHCARE CORPORATION (IO)
6730 North Scottsdale Road, Suite 200, Scottsdale, AZ Zip 85253; tel. 602/348-9800; Melvin Redman, President and Chief Operating Officer
(Independent Hospital System)

CALIFORNIA: BREA COMMUNITY HOSPITAL (O, 60 beds) 380 West Central Avenue, Brea, CA Zip 92821; tel. 714/529-0211; Gaetano Zanfini, Chief Executive Officer

PACIFICA HOSPITAL OF THE VALLEY (O, 204 beds) 9449 San Fernando Road, Sun Valley, CA Zip 91352; tel. 818/767-3310; Casey Fatch, Administrator and Chief Operating Officer

PINE GROVE HOSPITAL (O, 80 beds) 7011 Shoup Avenue, Canoga Park, CA Zip 91307; tel. 818/348-0500; Patty Lepe, Administrator

DISTRICT OF COLUMBIA: GREATER SOUTHEAST COMMUNITY HOSPITAL (O, 305 beds) 1310 Southern Avenue S.E., Washington, DC Zip 20032-4699; tel. 202/574-6000; Ana Raley, Chief Executive Officer

HADLEY MEMORIAL HOSPITAL (O, 109 beds) 4601 Martin Luther King Jr. Avenue S.W., Washington, DC Zip 20032-1199; tel. 202/574-5700; Audrey Weston, Administrator
Web address: www.doctorscommunity.com

ILLINOIS: MICHAEL REESE HOSPITAL AND MEDICAL CENTER (O, 523 beds) 2929 South Ellis Avenue, Chicago, IL Zip 60616-3376; tel. 312/791-2000; Stephen M. Weinstein, President

Owned, leased, sponsored:	6 hospitals	1281 beds
Contract-managed:	0 hospitals	0 beds
Totals:	6 hospitals	1281 beds

0190: DUKE UNIVERSITY HEALTH SYSTEM (NP)
Erwin Road, Durham, NC Zip 27710, Mailing Address: P.O. Box 3708, Zip 27710-3708; tel. 919/684-2255; Ralph Snyderman, M.D., President and Chief Executive Officer
(Centralized Physician/Insurance Health System)

NORTH CAROLINA: DUKE UNIVERSITY MEDICAL CENTER (O, 852 beds) Erwin Road, Durham, NC Zip 27710, Mailing Address: P.O. Box 3708, Zip 27710-3708; tel. 919/684-8111; Michael D. Israel, Chief Executive Officer and Vice Chancellor

DURHAM REGIONAL HOSPITAL (O, 213 beds) 3643 North Roxboro Road, Durham, NC Zip 27704-2763; tel. 919/470-4000; Richard L. Myers, President and Chief Executive Officer
Web address: www.drh.duhs.duke.edu

RALEIGH COMMUNITY HOSPITAL (O, 164 beds) 3400 Wake Forest Road, Raleigh, NC Zip 27609-7373, Mailing Address: P.O. Box 28280, Zip 27611-8280; tel. 919/954-3000; James E. Raynor, Chief Executive Officer

Owned, leased, sponsored:	3 hospitals	1229 beds
Contract-managed:	0 hospitals	0 beds
Totals:	3 hospitals	1229 beds

1895: EAST TEXAS MEDICAL CENTER REGIONAL HEALTHCARE SYSTEM (NP)
1000 South Beckham Street, Tyler, TX Zip 75701-1996, Mailing Address: P.O. Box 6400, Zip 75711-6400; tel. 903/535-6211; Elmer G. Ellis, President and Chief Executive Officer
(Centralized Physician/Insurance Health System)

TEXAS: EAST TEXAS MEDICAL CENTER ATHENS (L, 108 beds) 2000 South Palestine Street, Athens, TX Zip 75751-5610; tel. 903/676-1000; Patrick L. Wallace, Administrator

EAST TEXAS MEDICAL CENTER CARTHAGE (L, 30 beds) 409 Cottage Road, Carthage, TX Zip 75633-1466, Mailing Address: P.O. Box 549, Zip 75633-0549; tel. 903/693-3841; Gary Mikeal Hudson, Administrator
Web address: www.etmc.org

EAST TEXAS MEDICAL CENTER CROCKETT (L, 68 beds) 1100 Loop 304 East, Crockett, TX Zip 75835-1810; tel. 936/546-3862; Nelda K. Welch, Administrator

EAST TEXAS MEDICAL CENTER FAIRFIELD (L, 19 beds) 125 Newman Street, Fairfield, TX Zip 75840-1499; tel. 903/389-2121; Ruth Cook, Administrator

EAST TEXAS MEDICAL CENTER JACKSONVILLE (L, 83 beds) 501 South Ragsdale Street, Jacksonville, TX Zip 75766-2413; tel. 903/541-5000; Steve Bowen, President

EAST TEXAS MEDICAL CENTER PITTSBURG (L, 42 beds) 414 Quitman Street, Pittsburg, TX Zip 75686-1032; tel. 903/856-6663; W. Perry Henderson, Administrator
Web address: www.etmc.org

EAST TEXAS MEDICAL CENTER REHABILITATION CENTER (O, 49 beds) 701 Olympic Plaza Circle, Tyler, TX Zip 75701-1996; tel. 903/596-3000; Eddie L. Howard, Vice President and Chief Operating Officer
Web address: www.etmc.org

EAST TEXAS MEDICAL CENTER TRINITY (L, 22 beds) 900 Prospect Drive, Trinity, TX Zip 75862-0471, Mailing Address: P.O. Box 471, Zip 75862-0471; tel. 409/594-3541; Grady Hooper, Chief Executive Officer

EAST TEXAS MEDICAL CENTER TYLER (O, 362 beds) 1000 South Beckham Street, Tyler, TX Zip 75701-1996, Mailing Address: Box 6400, Zip 75711-6400; tel. 903/597-0351; Robert B. Evans, Administrator and Chief Executive Officer
Web address: www.etmc.org

EAST TEXAS MEDICAL CENTER-CLARKSVILLE (L, 36 beds) 3000 Highway 82 West, Clarksville, TX Zip 75426, Mailing Address: P.O. Box 1270, Zip 75426-1270; tel. 903/427-3851; Terry Cutler, Administrator and Chief Operating Officer

For explanation of codes following names, see page B2.
★ Indicates Type III membership in the American Hospital Association.

Systems / East Texas Medical Center Regional Healthcare System

EAST TEXAS MEDICAL CENTER–MOUNT VERNON (L, 30 beds) 500 Highway 37 South, Mount Vernon, TX Zip 75457, Mailing Address: P.O. Box 477, Zip 75457-0477; tel. 903/537-4552; Perry Henderson, Administrator
Web address: www.etmc.org

EAST TEXAS MEDICAL CENTER–QUITMAN (L, 15 beds) 117 Winnsboro Street, Quitman, TX Zip 75783-2144, Mailing Address: P.O. Box 1000, Zip 75783-1000; tel. 903/763-4505; Michael J. McCoy, Administrator
Web address: www.etmc.org

Owned, leased, sponsored:	12 hospitals	864 beds
Contract–managed:	0 hospitals	0 beds
Totals:	12 hospitals	864 beds

★0100: EASTERN HEALTH SYSTEM, INC. (NP)
48 Medical Park East Drive, 450, Birmingham, AL Zip 35235; tel. 205/838-3999; Robert C. Chapman, FACHE, President and Chief Executive Officer
(Centralized Physician/Insurance Health System)

ALABAMA: MEDICAL CENTER BLOUNT (L, 40 beds) 150 Gilbreath, Oneonta, AL Zip 35121-2534, Mailing Address: P.O. Box 1000, Zip 35121-1000; tel. 205/274-3000; Jacki Jennings, Chief Executive Officer

MEDICAL CENTER EAST (O, 257 beds) 50 Medical Park East Drive, Birmingham, AL Zip 35235-9987; tel. 205/838-3000; Gary R. Colberg, CHE, Chief Executive Officer
Web address: www.ehs–inc.com

ST. CLAIR REGIONAL HOSPITAL (C, 51 beds) 2805 Hospital Drive, Pell City, AL Zip 35125-1499; tel. 205/338-3301

Owned, leased, sponsored:	2 hospitals	297 beds
Contract–managed:	1 hospital	51 beds
Totals:	3 hospitals	348 beds

★0555: EASTERN MAINE HEALTHCARE (NP)
489 State Street, Bangor, ME Zip 04401-6674, Mailing Address: P.O. Box 404, Zip 04402-0404; tel. 207/973-7045; Norman A. Ledwin, President and Chief Executive Officer
(Centralized Health System)

MAINE: ACADIA HOSPITAL (O, 91 beds) 268 Stillwater Avenue, Bangor, ME Zip 04401-3945, Mailing Address: P.O. Box 422, Zip 04402-0422; tel. 207/973-6100; Ali A. Elhaj, President and Chief Exective Officer
Web address: www.emh.org

AROOSTOOK MEDICAL CENTER (O, 152 beds) 140 Academy Street, Presque Isle, ME Zip 04769-3171, Mailing Address: P.O. Box 151, Zip 04769-0151; tel. 207/768-4000; David A. Peterson, President and Chief Executive Officer
Web address: www.tamc.org

CHARLES A. DEAN MEMORIAL HOSPITAL (O, 45 beds) Pritham Avenue, Greenville, ME Zip 04441-1395, Mailing Address: P.O. Box 1129, Zip 04441-1129; tel. 207/695-2223; Philomena A. Marshall, R.N., President and Chief Executive Officer
Web address: www.moosehead.net/cadean

EASTERN MAINE MEDICAL CENTER (O, 319 beds) 489 State Street, Bangor, ME Zip 04401-6674, Mailing Address: P.O. Box 404, Zip 04402-0404; tel. 207/973-7000; Norman A. Ledwin, President and Chief Executive Officer
Web address: www.emh.org

INLAND HOSPITAL (O, 120 beds) 200 Kennedy Memorial Drive, Waterville, ME Zip 04901-4595; tel. 207/861-3000; Wilfred J. Addison, President and Chief Executive Officer

Owned, leased, sponsored:	5 hospitals	727 beds
Contract–managed:	0 hospitals	0 beds
Totals:	5 hospitals	727 beds

★0945: EMPIRE HEALTH SERVICES (NP)
West 800 Fifth Avenue, Spokane, WA Zip 99204, Mailing Address: P.O. Box 248, Zip 99210-0248; tel. 509/473-7960; Thomas M. White, President
(Centralized Physician/Insurance Health System)

WASHINGTON: DEACONESS MEDICAL CENTER–SPOKANE (O, 326 beds) 800 West Fifth Avenue, Spokane, WA Zip 99204, Mailing Address: P.O. Box 248, Zip 99210-0248; tel. 509/458-5800; Thomas J. Zellers, Chief Operating Officer
Web address: www.deaconess–spokane.org

VALLEY HOSPITAL AND MEDICAL CENTER (O, 117 beds) 12606 East Mission Avenue, Spokane, WA Zip 99216-1090; tel. 509/924-6650; Michael T. Liepman, Chief Operating Officer

Owned, leased, sponsored:	2 hospitals	443 beds
Contract–managed:	0 hospitals	0 beds
Totals:	2 hospitals	443 beds

★0735: EPISCOPAL HEALTH SERVICES INC. (CO)
700 Hicksville Road, Bethpage, NY Zip 11714; tel. 516/349-6132; Corbett A. Price, Chief Executive Officer

NEW YORK: ST. CATHERINE OF SIENA MEDICAL CENTER (O, 366 beds) 50 Route 25-A, Smithtown, NY Zip 11787-1398; tel. 631/862-3000; James M. Wilson, President and Chief Executive Officer

ST. JOHN'S EPISCOPAL HOSPITAL–SOUTH SHORE (O, 314 beds) 327 Beach 19th Street, Far Rockaway, NY Zip 11691-4424; tel. 718/869-7000; Nancy Simmons, Administrator

Owned, leased, sponsored:	2 hospitals	680 beds
Contract–managed:	0 hospitals	0 beds
Totals:	2 hospitals	680 beds

★0134: EXEMPLA HEALTHCARE, INC. (NP)
600 Grant Street, Suite 700, Denver, CO Zip 80203; tel. 303/813-5000; Jeffrey D. Selberg, President and Chief Executive Officer
(Centralized Physician/Insurance Health System)

COLORADO: EXEMPLA LUTHERAN MEDICAL CENTER (O, 335 beds) 8300 West 38th Avenue, Wheat Ridge, CO Zip 80033-6005; tel. 303/425-4500; Jeffrey D. Selberg, President and Chief Executive Officer
Web address: www.exempla.org

EXEMPLA SAINT JOSEPH HOSPITAL (O, 480 beds) 1835 Franklin Street, Denver, CO Zip 80218-1191; tel. 303/837-7111; Jeffrey D. Selberg, President and Chief Executive Officer

Owned, leased, sponsored:	2 hospitals	815 beds
Contract–managed:	0 hospitals	0 beds
Totals:	2 hospitals	815 beds

★1325: FAIRVIEW HEALTH SERVICES (NP)
2450 Riverside Avenue, Minneapolis, MN Zip 55454-1400; tel. 612/672-6300; David R. Page, President and Chief Executive Officer
(Centralized Physician/Insurance Health System)

MINNESOTA: FAIRVIEW LAKES REGIONAL MEDICAL CENTER (O, 78 beds) 5200 Fairview Boulevard, Wyoming, MN Zip 55092-8013; tel. 651/982-7000; Daniel K. Anderson, Senior Vice President and Administrator
Web address: www.fairview.org

FAIRVIEW NORTHLAND REGIONAL HEALTH CARE (O, 41 beds) 911 Northland Drive, Princeton, MN Zip 55371-2173; tel. 612/389-6300; Jeanne Lally, Senior Vice President and Administrator
Web address: www.fairview.org

FAIRVIEW RED WING HOSPITAL (O, 70 beds) 1407 West Fourth Street, Red Wing, MN Zip 55066-2198; tel. 651/388-6721; Scott Wordelman, President and Chief Executive Officer
Web address: www.fairview.org

FAIRVIEW RIDGES HOSPITAL (O, 127 beds) 201 East Nicollet Boulevard, Burnsville, MN Zip 55337-5799; tel. 612/892-2000; Mark M. Enger, Senior Vice President and Administrator
Web address: www.fairview.org

For explanation of codes following names, see page B2.
★ *Indicates Type III membership in the American Hospital Association.*

FAIRVIEW SOUTHDALE HOSPITAL (O, 348 beds) 6401 France Avenue South, Minneapolis, MN Zip 55435-2199; tel. 612/924-5000; Mark M. Enger, Senior Vice President and Administrator
Web address: www.fairview.org

FAIRVIEW–UNIVERSITY MEDICAL CENTER (O, 1028 beds) 2450 Riverside Avenue, Minneapolis, MN Zip 55454-1400; tel. 612/672-6000; Gordon L. Alexander, M.D., Senior Vice President and Chief Executive Officer
Web address: www.fairview.org

UNIVERSITY MEDICAL CENTER–MESABI (O, 132 beds) 750 East 34th Street, Hibbing, MN Zip 55746-4600; tel. 218/262-4881; Richard W. Dinter, M.D., Chief Operating Officer

Owned, leased, sponsored:	7 hospitals	1824 beds
Contract–managed:	0 hospitals	0 beds
Totals:	7 hospitals	1824 beds

★0166: **FAY–WEST HEALTH SYSTEM** (NP)
508 South Church Street, Mount Pleasant, PA Zip 15666-1790; tel. 724/547-1500; Rodney L. Gunderson, Chief Executive Officer
(Independent Hospital System)

PENNSYLVANIA: FRICK HOSPITAL (O, 171 beds) 508 South Church Street, Mount Pleasant, PA Zip 15666-1790; tel. 724/547-1500; Rodney L. Gunderson, Chief Executive Officer

HIGHLANDS HOSPITAL (O, 87 beds) 401 East Murphy Avenue, Connellsville, PA Zip 15425-2700; tel. 724/628-1500; Michelle Cunningham, Chief Executive Officer

Owned, leased, sponsored:	2 hospitals	258 beds
Contract–managed:	0 hospitals	0 beds
Totals:	2 hospitals	258 beds

● 2635: **FHC HEALTH SYSTEMS** (IO)
240 Corporate Boulevard, Norfolk, VA Zip 23502-4950; tel. 757/459-5100; Ronald I. Dozoretz, M.D., Chairman
(Independent Hospital System)

PUERTO RICO: FIRST HOSPITAL PANAMERICANO (O, 165 beds) State Road 787 KM 1 5, Cidra, PR Zip 00739, Mailing Address: P.O. Box 1398, Zip 00739; tel. 787/739-5555; Jorge Torres, Vice President and Chief Executive Officer

Owned, leased, sponsored:	1 hospital	165 beds
Contract–managed:	0 hospitals	0 beds
Totals:	1 hospital	165 beds

0174: **FORUM HEALTH** (NP)
3530 Belmont Avenue, Suite 7, Youngstown, OH Zip 44505; tel. 330/759-4090; Gary E. Kaatz, Chief Executive Officer
(Centralized Health System)

OHIO: HILLSIDE REHABILITATION HOSPITAL (O, 47 beds) 8747 Squires Lane N.E., Warren, OH Zip 44484-1649; tel. 330/841-3700; Rodney Jones, Chief Operating Officer
Web address: www.forumhealth.org

TRUMBULL MEMORIAL HOSPITAL (O, 284 beds) 1350 East Market Street, Warren, OH Zip 44482-6628; tel. 330/841-9011; N. Kristopher Hoce, Interim President and Chief Executive Officer
Web address: www.forumhealth.org

WESTERN RESERVE CARE SYSTEM (O, 361 beds) 500 Gypsy Lane, Youngstown, OH Zip 44501-0240, Mailing Address: P.O. Box 990, Zip 44501-0990; tel. 330/747-0777; N. Kristopher Hoce, Interim President and Chief Executive Officer
Web address: www.forumhealth.org

Owned, leased, sponsored:	3 hospitals	692 beds
Contract–managed:	0 hospitals	0 beds
Totals:	3 hospitals	692 beds

1485: **FRANCISCAN HEALTH PARTNERSHIP, INC.** (CC)
8 Airport Park Boulevard, Latham, NY Zip 12110; tel. 518/783-5257; James H. Flynn, Jr, President and Chief Executive Officer
(Moderately Centralized Health System)

KENTUCKY: OUR LADY OF BELLEFONTE HOSPITAL (S, 194 beds) St. Christopher Drive, Ashland, KY Zip 41101, Mailing Address: P.O. Box 789, Zip 41105-0789; tel. 606/833-3333; Robert J. Maher, President
Web address: www.olbh.com

NEW JERSEY: ST. FRANCIS HOSPITAL (S, 161 beds) 25 McWilliams Place, Jersey City, NJ Zip 07302-1698; tel. 201/418-1000; Robert S. Chaloner, Chief Executive Officer

ST. MARY HOSPITAL (S, 223 beds) 308 Willow Avenue, Hoboken, NJ Zip 07030-3889; tel. 201/418-1000; Robert S. Chaloner, President and Chief Executive Officer

NEW YORK: GOOD SAMARITAN HOSPITAL (S, 308 beds) 255 Lafayette Avenue, Suffern, NY Zip 10901-4869; tel. 914/368-5000; James A. Martin, Chief Executive Officer

MERCY COMMUNITY HOSPITAL (O, 187 beds) 160 East Main Street, Port Jervis, NY Zip 12771-2245, Mailing Address: P.O. Box 1014, Zip 12771-1014; tel. 914/856-5351; Michael Parmer, M.D., Executive Vice President and Administrator
Web address: www.mercycommunityhospital.org

ST. ANTHONY COMMUNITY HOSPITAL (S, 73 beds) 15 Maple Avenue, Warwick, NY Zip 10990-5180; tel. 914/986-2276; James A. Martin, President and Chief Executive Officer

OHIO: FRANCISCAN MEDICAL CENTER–DAYTON CAMPUS (S, 317 beds) One Franciscan Way, Dayton, OH Zip 45408-1498; tel. 937/229-6000; James E. Grobmyer, Interim Chief Executive Officer

Owned, leased, sponsored:	7 hospitals	1463 beds
Contract–managed:	0 hospitals	0 beds
Totals:	7 hospitals	1463 beds

★1475: **FRANCISCAN MISSIONARIES OF OUR LADY HEALTH SYSTEM, INC.** (CC)
4200 Essen Lane, Baton Rouge, LA Zip 70809; tel. 225/923-2701; John J. Finan, Jr, President and Chief Executive Officer
(Centralized Physician/Insurance Health System)

LOUISIANA: OUR LADY OF LOURDES REGIONAL MEDICAL CENTER (O, 248 beds) 611 St. Landry Street, Lafayette, LA Zip 70506-4697, Mailing Address: Box 4027, Zip 70502-4027; tel. 318/289-2000; Ronald W. Webb, Chief Executive Officer
Web address: www.lourdes.net/

OUR LADY OF THE LAKE REGIONAL MEDICAL CENTER (O, 668 beds) 5000 Hennessy Boulevard, Baton Rouge, LA Zip 70808-4350; tel. 225/765-6565; Robert C. Davidge, Chief Executive Officer
Web address: www.ololrmc.com

ST. FRANCIS MEDICAL CENTER (O, 341 beds) 309 Jackson Street, Monroe, LA Zip 71201-7498, Mailing Address: P.O. Box 1901, Zip 71210-1901; tel. 318/327-4000; H. Gerald Smith, President and Chief Executive Officer
Web address: www.stfran.com

Owned, leased, sponsored:	3 hospitals	1257 beds
Contract–managed:	0 hospitals	0 beds
Totals:	3 hospitals	1257 beds

★5375: **FRANCISCAN SERVICES CORPORATION** (CC)
6832 Convent Boulevard, Sylvania, OH Zip 43560-2897; tel. 419/882-8373; John W. O'Connell, President
(Moderately Centralized Health System)

OHIO: PROVIDENCE HOSPITAL (S, 170 beds) 1912 Hayes Avenue, Sandusky, OH Zip 44870-4736; tel. 419/621-7000; Sister Nancy Linenkugel, FACHE, President and Chief Executive Officer
Web address: www.providencehealth.org

TRINITY HEALTH SYSTEM (S, 355 beds) 380 Summit Avenue, Steubenville, OH Zip 43952-2699; tel. 740/283-7000; Fred B. Brower, President and Chief Executive Officer
Web address: www.trinityhealth.com

For explanation of codes following names, see page B2.
★ Indicates Type III membership in the American Hospital Association.
● Single hospital health care system

Systems / Franciscan Services Corporation

TEXAS: BURLESON ST. JOSEPH HEALTH CENTER (S, 30 beds) 1101 Woodson Drive, Caldwell, TX Zip 77836–1052, Mailing Address: P.O. Drawer 360, Zip 77836–0360; tel. 409/567–3245; Reed Edmundson, Administrator
Web address: www.st-joseph.org/

MADISON ST. JOSEPH HEALTH CENTER (S, 35 beds) 100 West Cross Street, Madisonville, TX Zip 77864–0698, Mailing Address: Box 698, Zip 77864–0698; tel. 409/348–2631; Reed Edmundson, Administrator

ST. JOSEPH REGIONAL HEALTH CENTER (S, 289 beds) 2801 Franciscan Drive, Bryan, TX Zip 77802–2599; tel. 979/776–3777; Daniel L. Buche, Chief Executive Officer
Web address: www.st-joseph.org

TRINITY COMMUNITY MEDICAL CENTER OF BRENHAM (S, 60 beds) 700 Medical Parkway, Brenham, TX Zip 77833–5498; tel. 979/836–6173; John L. Simms, President and Chief Executive Officer
Web address: www.trinitymed.com

Owned, leased, sponsored:	6 hospitals	939 beds
Contract-managed:	0 hospitals	0 beds
Totals:	6 hospitals	939 beds

★1455: FRANCISCAN SISTERS OF CHRISTIAN CHARITY HEALTHCARE MINISTRY, INC (CC)
1415 South Rapids Road, Manitowoc, WI Zip 54220–9302; tel. 920/684–7071; Sister Laura J. Wolf, President
(Moderately Centralized Health System)

NEBRASKA: ST. FRANCIS MEMORIAL HOSPITAL (O, 102 beds) 430 North Monitor Street, West Point, NE Zip 68788–1595; tel. 402/372–2404; Ronald O. Briggs, President

OHIO: GENESIS HEALTHCARE SYSTEM (O, 433 beds) 2951 Maple Avenue, Zanesville, OH Zip 43701–2881; tel. 740/454–5000; Thomas L. Sieber, President and Chief Executive Officer

WISCONSIN: HOLY FAMILY MEMORIAL MEDICAL CENTER (O, 176 beds) 2300 Western Avenue, Manitowoc, WI Zip 54220, Mailing Address: P.O. Box 1450, Zip 54221–1450; tel. 920/684–2011; Daniel B. McGinty, President and Chief Executive Officer
Web address: www.hfmhealth.org

Owned, leased, sponsored:	3 hospitals	711 beds
Contract-managed:	0 hospitals	0 beds
Totals:	3 hospitals	711 beds

★9650: FRANCISCAN SKEMP HEALTHCARE (CC)
700 West Avenue South, La Crosse, WI Zip 54601–4796; tel. 608/791–9710; Glenn Forbes, M.D., President and Chief Executive Officer
(Independent Hospital System)

FRANCISCAN SKEMP HEALTHCARE–ARCADIA CAMPUS (O, 101 beds) 464 South St. Joseph Avenue, Arcadia, WI Zip 54612–1401; tel. 608/323–3341; Robert M. Tracey, Administrator
Web address: www.mayo.edu/fsh

FRANCISCAN SKEMP HEALTHCARE–LA CROSSE CAMPUS (O, 213 beds) 700 West Avenue South, La Crosse, WI Zip 54601–4783; tel. 608/785–0940; Glenn Forbes, M.D., President and Chief Executive Officer
Web address: www.mayo.edu/fsh/

FRANCISCAN SKEMP HEALTHCARE–SPARTA CAMPUS (O, 59 beds) 310 West Main Street, Sparta, WI Zip 54656–2171; tel. 608/269–2132; William P. Sexton, Administrator
Web address: www.mayo.edu/fsh

Owned, leased, sponsored:	3 hospitals	373 beds
Contract-managed:	0 hospitals	0 beds
Totals:	3 hospitals	373 beds

2115: FREMONT–RIDEOUT HEALTH GROUP (NP)
989 Plumas Street, Yuba City, CA Zip 95991; tel. 530/751–4010; Thomas P. Hayes, Chief Executive Officer
(Independent Hospital System)

CALIFORNIA: FREMONT MEDICAL CENTER (O, 90 beds) 970 Plumas Street, Yuba City, CA Zip 95991; tel. 530/751–4000; Thomas P. Hayes, Chief Executive Officer
Web address: www.frhg.org

RIDEOUT MEMORIAL HOSPITAL (O, 89 beds) 726 Fourth Street, Marysville, CA Zip 95901–2128, Mailing Address: 989 Plumas Street, Yuba City, Zip 95991; tel. 530/749–4300; Thomas P. Hayes, Chief Executive Officer
Web address: www.frhg.org

Owned, leased, sponsored:	2 hospitals	179 beds
Contract-managed:	0 hospitals	0 beds
Totals:	2 hospitals	179 beds

★5570: GEISINGER HEALTH SYSTEM (NP)
100 North Academy Avenue, Danville, PA Zip 17822; tel. 570/271–5555; Victor Marks, M.D., Interim President and Chief Executive Officer
(Centralized Physician/Insurance Health System)

PENNSYLVANIA: GEISINGER MEDICAL CENTER (O, 333 beds) 100 North Academy Avenue, Danville, PA Zip 17822–0150; tel. 570/271–6211; Nancy L. Rizzo, Senior Vice President, Operations
Web address: www.ghs.edu

PENN STATE GEISINGER WYOMING VALLEY MEDICAL CENTER (O, 132 beds) 1000 East Mountain Drive, Wilkes–Barre, PA Zip 18711–0027; tel. 570/826–7300; Conrad W. Schintz, Senior Vice–President Operations
Web address: www.psghs.edu

Owned, leased, sponsored:	2 hospitals	465 beds
Contract-managed:	0 hospitals	0 beds
Totals:	2 hospitals	465 beds

★0775: GENERAL HEALTH SYSTEM (NP)
3600 Florida Boulevard, Baton Rouge, LA Zip 70806–3854; tel. 225/237–1603; Milton R. Siepman, Ph.D., President and Chief Executive Officer
(Centralized Physician/Insurance Health System)

LOUISIANA: BATON ROUGE GENERAL MEDICAL CENTER (O, 423 beds) 3600 Florida Street, Baton Rouge, LA Zip 70806–3889, Mailing Address: P.O. Box 2511, Zip 70821–2511; tel. 225/387–7000; Milton R. Siepman, Ph.D., President and Chief Executive Officer

VERMILION HOSPITAL FOR PSYCHIATRIC AND ADDICTIVE MEDICINE (O, 54 beds) 2520 North University Avenue, Lafayette, LA Zip 70507–5306, Mailing Address: P.O. Box 91526, Zip 70509–1526; tel. 318/234–5614; William A. Ferry, Administrator

Owned, leased, sponsored:	2 hospitals	477 beds
Contract-managed:	0 hospitals	0 beds
Totals:	2 hospitals	477 beds

★0138: GEORGIA BAPTIST HEALTH CARE SYSTEM (NP)
100 10th Street, Atlanta, GA Zip 30309; tel. 404/253–3011; David E. Harrell, Chief Executive Officer
(Independent Hospital System)

GEORGIA: BAPTIST HOSPITAL, WORTH COUNTY (O, 49 beds) 807 South Isabella Street, Sylvester, GA Zip 31791–0545, Mailing Address: Box 545, Zip 31791–0545; tel. 912/776–6961; Billy Hayes, Administrator

BAPTIST MEDICAL CENTER (O, 41 beds) 1200 Baptist Medical Center Drive, Cumming, GA Zip 30041; tel. 770/887–2355; Jim Litchford, Administrator

BAPTIST MERIWETHER HOSPITAL (L, 117 beds) 5995 Spring Street, Warm Springs, GA Zip 31830, Mailing Address: P.O. Box 8, Zip 31830–0008; tel. 706/655–3331; Susan Milner, Administrator
Web address: www.gbhcs.org

MINNIE G. BOSWELL MEMORIAL HOSPITAL (C, 55 beds) 1201 Siloam Highway, Greensboro, GA Zip 30642–2811; tel. 706/453–7331; John M. Herron, Chief Executive Officer

---

For explanation of codes following names, see page B2.
★ *Indicates Type III membership in the American Hospital Association.*

Owned, leased, sponsored:	3 hospitals	207 beds
Contract-managed:	1 hospital	55 beds
Totals:	4 hospitals	262 beds

★**1535: GREAT PLAINS HEALTH ALLIANCE, INC.** (NP)
625 Third Street, Phillipsburg, KS Zip 67661-2138, Mailing Address: P.O. Box 366, Zip 67661-0366; tel. 785/543-2111; Roger S. John, President and Chief Executive Officer
(Independent Hospital System)

KANSAS: ASHLAND HEALTH CENTER (C, 48 beds) 709 Oak Street, Ashland, KS Zip 67831-0188, Mailing Address: P.O. Box 188, Zip 67831-0188; tel. 316/635-2241; Bryan Stacey, Administrator
Web address: www.phn.org

CHEYENNE COUNTY HOSPITAL (L, 16 beds) 210 West First Street, Saint Francis, KS Zip 67756-0547, Mailing Address: P.O. Box 547, Zip 67756-0547; tel. 785/332-2104; Leslie Lacy, Administrator
Web address: www.gpha.com

COMANCHE COUNTY HOSPITAL (C, 14 beds) Second and Frisco Streets, Coldwater, KS Zip 67029, Mailing Address: HC 65, Box 8A, Zip 67029; tel. 316/582-2144; Nancy Zimmerman, R.N., Administrator
Web address: www.gpha.com

ELLINWOOD DISTRICT HOSPITAL (L, 12 beds) 605 North Main Street, Ellinwood, KS Zip 67526-1440; tel. 316/564-2548; Marge Conell, Administrator
Web address: www.gpha.com

FREDONIA REGIONAL HOSPITAL (C, 51 beds) 1527 Madison Street, Fredonia, KS Zip 66736-1751, Mailing Address: P.O. Box 579, Zip 66736-0579; tel. 316/378-2121; Terry Deschaine, Chief Executive Officer
Web address: www.gpha.com

GREELEY COUNTY HOSPITAL (L, 48 beds) 506 Third Street, Tribune, KS Zip 67879-0338, Mailing Address: P.O. Box 338, Zip 67879-0338; tel. 316/376-4221; Jerrell J. Horton, Chief Executive Officer
Web address: www.gpha.com

GRISELL MEMORIAL HOSPITAL DISTRICT ONE (C, 46 beds) 210 South Vermont, Ransom, KS Zip 67572-0268, Mailing Address: P.O. Box 268, Zip 67572-0268; tel. 785/731-2231; Kristine Ochs, R.N., Administrator
Web address: www.gpha.com

JEWELL COUNTY HOSPITAL (C, 52 beds) 100 Crestvue Avenue, Mankato, KS Zip 66956-2407, Mailing Address: P.O. Box 327, Zip 66956-0327; tel. 785/378-3137; Aloha Kier, Administrator

KIOWA COUNTY MEMORIAL HOSPITAL (L, 46 beds) 501 South Walnut Street, Greensburg, KS Zip 67054-1951, Mailing Address: P.O. Box 616, Zip 67054-0616; tel. 316/723-3341; Cecilia Noll, Administrator
Web address: www.gpha.com

LANE COUNTY HOSPITAL (C, 31 beds) 243 South Second, Dighton, KS Zip 67839-0969, Mailing Address: P.O. Box 969, Zip 67839-0969; tel. 316/397-5321; Donna McGowan, Administrator
Web address: www.gpha.com

LINCOLN COUNTY HOSPITAL (C, 34 beds) 624 North Second Street, Lincoln, KS Zip 67455-1738, Mailing Address: P.O. Box 406, Zip 67455-0406; tel. 785/524-4403; Jolene Yager, R.N., Administrator
Web address: www.gpha.com

MEDICINE LODGE MEMORIAL HOSPITAL (C, 42 beds) 710 North Walnut Street, Medicine Lodge, KS Zip 67104-1019, Mailing Address: P.O. Drawer C, Zip 67104; tel. 316/886-3771; Kevin A. White, CHE, Administrator

MINNEOLA DISTRICT HOSPITAL (C, 15 beds) 212 Main Street, Minneola, KS Zip 67865-8511, Mailing Address: P.O. Box 127, Zip 67865-0127; tel. 316/885-4264; Ronald D. Baker, Administrator
Web address: www.gpha.com

MITCHELL COUNTY HOSPITAL (L, 89 beds) 400 West Eighth, Beloit, KS Zip 67420-1605, Mailing Address: P.O. Box 399, Zip 67420-0399; tel. 785/738-2266; John M. Osse, Administrator
Web address: www.gpha.com

OSBORNE COUNTY MEMORIAL HOSPITAL (C, 29 beds) 424 West New Hampshire Street, Osborne, KS Zip 67473-0070, Mailing Address: P.O. Box 70, Zip 67473-0070; tel. 785/346-2121; Patricia Bernard, R.N., Administrator
Web address: www.gpha.com

OTTAWA COUNTY HEALTH CENTER (L, 53 beds) 215 East Eighth, Minneapolis, KS Zip 67467-1999, Mailing Address: P.O. Box 290, Zip 67467-0290; tel. 785/392-2122; Joy Reed, R.N., Administrator
Web address: www.gpha.com

PHILLIPS COUNTY HOSPITAL (L, 62 beds) 1150 State Street, Phillipsburg, KS Zip 67661-1799, Mailing Address: P.O. Box 607, Zip 67661-0607; tel. 785/543-5226; James Wahlmeier, Administrator
Web address: www.phillips.hpmin.com/

RAWLINS COUNTY HEALTH CENTER (C, 24 beds) 707 Grant Street, Atwood, KS Zip 67730-4700, Mailing Address: P.O. Box 47, Zip 67730-4700; tel. 785/626-3211; Donald J. Kessen, Administrator and Chief Executive Officer
Web address: www.gpha.com

REPUBLIC COUNTY HOSPITAL (L, 86 beds) 2420 G Street, Belleville, KS Zip 66935-2400; tel. 785/527-2254; Blaine K. Miller, Administrator
Web address: www.gpha.com

SABETHA COMMUNITY HOSPITAL (L, 27 beds) 14th and Oregon Streets, Sabetha, KS Zip 66534-0229, Mailing Address: P.O. Box 229, Zip 66534-0229; tel. 785/284-2121; Rita K. Buurman, Chief Executive Officer
Web address: www.gpha.com

SATANTA DISTRICT HOSPITAL (C, 45 beds) 401 South Cheyenne Street, Satanta, KS Zip 67870-0159, Mailing Address: P.O. Box 159, Zip 67870-0159; tel. 316/649-2761; T. G. Lee, Administrator
Web address: www.gpha.com

SMITH COUNTY MEMORIAL HOSPITAL (L, 54 beds) 614 South Main Street, Smith Center, KS Zip 66967-0349, Mailing Address: P.O. Box 349, Zip 66967-0349; tel. 785/282-6845; John Terrill, Administrator
Web address: www.gpha.com

TREGO COUNTY-LEMKE MEMORIAL HOSPITAL (C, 73 beds) 320 North 13th Street, Wakeeney, KS Zip 67672-2099; tel. 785/743-2182; Lisa J. Freeborn, R.N., Administrator
Web address: www.gpha.com

NEBRASKA: COMMUNITY MEDICAL CENTER (C, 35 beds) 2307 Barada Street, Falls City, NE Zip 68355-1599; tel. 402/245-2428; Asa B. Wilson, Ph.D., Administrator
Web address: www.gpha.com

HARLAN COUNTY HEALTH SYSTEM (C, 25 beds) 717 North Brown Street, Alma, NE Zip 68920-0836, Mailing Address: P.O. Box 836, Zip 68920-0836; tel. 308/928-2151; Allen Van Driel, Administrator
Web address: www.gpha.com

Owned, leased, sponsored:	10 hospitals	493 beds
Contract-managed:	15 hospitals	564 beds
Totals:	25 hospitals	1057 beds

0144: GREATER HUDSON VALLEY HEALTH SYSTEM (NP)
600A Stony Brook Court, Newburgh, NY Zip 12550; tel. 914/568-6050; Val S. Gray, Interim President and Chief Executive Officer
(Moderately Centralized Health System)

NEW YORK: CORNWALL HOSPITAL (O, 125 beds) 19 Laurel Avenue, Cornwall, NY Zip 12518-1499; tel. 914/534-7711; Louis H. Smith, Executive Vice President and Administrator

HORTON MEDICAL CENTER (O, 169 beds) 60 Prospect Avenue, Middletown, NY Zip 10940-4133; tel. 914/343-2424; Jeffrey D. Hirsch, Executive Vice President and Administrator

ST. LUKE'S HOSPITAL (O, 175 beds) 70 Dubois Street, Newburgh, NY Zip 12550-4898, Mailing Address: P.O. Box 631, Zip 12550-0631; tel. 914/561-4400; Laurence E. Kelly, Executive Vice President and Administrator
Web address: www.stlukeshospital.org

For explanation of codes following names, see page B2.
★ Indicates Type III membership in the American Hospital Association.

Systems / Greater Hudson Valley Health System

Owned, leased, sponsored:	3 hospitals	469 beds
Contract-managed:	0 hospitals	0 beds
Totals:	3 hospitals	469 beds

★1555: **GREENVILLE HOSPITAL SYSTEM** (NP)
701 Grove Road, Greenville, SC Zip 29605-4211;
tel. 864/455-7000; Frank D. Pinckney, President
(Centralized Physician/Insurance Health System)

SOUTH CAROLINA: ALLEN BENNETT HOSPITAL (O, 146 beds) 313 Memorial Drive, Greer, SC Zip 29650-1521; tel. 864/848-8200; Michael W. Massey, Administrator
Web address: www.ghs.org

GREENVILLE MEMORIAL HOSPITAL (O, 809 beds) 701 Grove Road, Greenville, SC Zip 29605-4295; tel. 864/455-7000; J. Bland Burkhardt, Jr, Senior Vice President and Administrator
Web address: www.ghs.org

HILLCREST HOSPITAL (O, 46 beds) 729 S.E. Main Street, Simpsonville, SC Zip 29681-3280; tel. 864/967-6100; Mark Slyter, Administrator
Web address: www.ghs.org

Owned, leased, sponsored:	3 hospitals	1001 beds
Contract-managed:	0 hospitals	0 beds
Totals:	3 hospitals	1001 beds

★0675: **GUTHRIE HEALTHCARE SYSTEM** (NP)
Guthrie Square, Sayre, PA Zip 18840; tel. 570/888-6666; Mark Stensager, President and Chief Executive Officer
(Independent Hospital System)

NEW YORK: CORNING HOSPITAL (O, 264 beds) 176 Denison Parkway East, Corning, NY Zip 14830-2899; tel. 607/937-7200; Timothy J. Dentry, President and Chief Executive Officer
Web address: www.corninghospital.com

PENNSYLVANIA: ROBERT PACKER HOSPITAL (O, 252 beds) 1 Guthrie Square, Sayre, PA Zip 18840-1698; tel. 570/888-6666; William F. Vanaskie, President and Chief Executive Officer
Web address: www.guthrie.org

TROY COMMUNITY HOSPITAL (O, 32 beds) 100 John Street, Troy, PA Zip 16947-0036; tel. 570/297-2121; Mark Webster, President
Web address: www.guthrie.org

Owned, leased, sponsored:	3 hospitals	548 beds
Contract-managed:	0 hospitals	0 beds
Totals:	3 hospitals	548 beds

3555: **HAWAII HEALTH SYSTEMS CORPORATION** (NP)
3675 Kilauea Avenue, Honolulu, HI Zip 96816; tel. 808/586-4416; Thomas M. Driskill, Jr, President and Chief Executive Officer
(Independent Hospital System)

HAWAII: HALE HO'OLA HAMAKUA (O, 50 beds) 45-547 Plumeria Street, Honokaa, HI Zip 96727, Mailing Address: P.O. Box 237, Zip 96727-0237; tel. 808/775-7211; Romel Dela Cruz, Administrator

HILO MEDICAL CENTER (O, 164 beds) 1190 Waianuenue Avenue, Hilo, HI Zip 96720-2095; tel. 808/974-4743; Ronald J. Schurra, Administrator

KAU HOSPITAL (O, 21 beds) 1 Kamani Street, Pahala, HI Zip 96777, Mailing Address: P.O. Box 40, Zip 96777-0040; tel. 808/928-8331; Dawn S. Pung, Administrator

KAUAI VETERANS MEMORIAL HOSPITAL (O, 49 beds) Waimea Canyon Road, Waimea, HI Zip 96796, Mailing Address: P.O. Box 337, Zip 96796-0337; tel. 808/338-9431; Orianna A. Skomoroch, Regional Chief Executive Officer

KOHALA HOSPITAL (O, 26 beds) 54-383 Hospital Road, Kohala, HI Zip 96755, Mailing Address: P.O. Box 10, Kapaau, Zip 96755-0010; tel. 808/889-6211; Herbert K. Yim, Administrator

KONA COMMUNITY HOSPITAL (O, 75 beds) Haukapila Street, Kealakekua, HI Zip 96750, Mailing Address: P.O. Box 69, Zip 96750-0069; tel. 808/322-4429; Joseph C. Wall, Chief Executive Officer

KULA HOSPITAL (C, 105 beds) 204 Kula Highway, Kula, HI Zip 96790-9499; tel. 808/878-1221; Alan G. Lee, Administrator

LANAI COMMUNITY HOSPITAL (O, 14 beds) 628 Seventh Street, Lanai City, HI Zip 96763-0650, Mailing Address: P.O. Box 630650, Zip 96763-0650; tel. 808/565-6411; John Schaumburg, Administrator

LEAHI HOSPITAL (O, 192 beds) 3675 Kilauea Avenue, Honolulu, HI Zip 96816; tel. 808/733-8000; Jerry Walker, Administrator

MAUI MEMORIAL MEDICAL CENTER (O, 194 beds) 221 Mahalani Street, Wailuku, HI Zip 96793-2581; tel. 808/244-9056; William B. Kleefisch, Chief Executive Officer

SAMUEL MAHELONA MEMORIAL HOSPITAL (O, 81 beds) 4800 Kawaihau Road, Kapaa, HI Zip 96746-1998; tel. 808/822-4961; Orianna A. Skomoroch, Regional Chief Executive Officer
Web address: www.mahelona.org

Owned, leased, sponsored:	11 hospitals	971 beds
Contract-managed:	0 hospitals	0 beds
Totals:	11 hospitals	971 beds

★0048: **HCA – THE HEALTHCARE COMPANY** (IO)
One Park Plaza, Nashville, TN Zip 37203-1548; tel. 615/344-9551; Jack O. Bovender, Jr, President and Chief Operating Officer
(Decentralized Health System)

ALASKA: ALASKA REGIONAL HOSPITAL (O, 194 beds) 2801 Debarr Road, Anchorage, AK Zip 99508, Mailing Address: P.O. Box 143889, Zip 99514-3889; tel. 907/276-1754; Edward H. Lamb, President and Chief Executive Officer

CALIFORNIA: CHINO VALLEY MEDICAL CENTER (O, 104 beds) 5451 Walnut Avenue, Chino, CA Zip 91710; tel. 909/464-8600; Stephen E. Dixon, Chief Executive Officer
Web address: www.cvmc.com

LAS ENCINAS HOSPITAL (O, 138 beds) 2900 East Del Mar Boulevard, Pasadena, CA Zip 91107-4375; tel. 626/795-9901; Roland Metivier, Chief Executive Officer
Web address: www.hcahealthcare.com

LOS ROBLES REGIONAL MEDICAL CENTER (O, 255 beds) 215 West Janss Road, Thousand Oaks, CA Zip 91360-1899; tel. 805/497-2727; Robert C. Shaw, President and Chief Executive Officer
Web address: www.losrobleshospital.com

REGIONAL MEDICAL CENTER OF SAN JOSE (O, 192 beds) 225 North Jackson Avenue, San Jose, CA Zip 95116-1691; tel. 408/259-5000; Steven R. Barron, President and Chief Executive Officer

RIVERSIDE COMMUNITY HOSPITAL (O, 276 beds) 4445 Magnolia Avenue, Riverside, CA Zip 92501-1669, Mailing Address: P.O. Box 1669, Zip 92502-1669; tel. 909/788-3000; Bryan R. Rogers, President and Chief Executive Officer
Web address: www.pchmc.org

SAN JOSE MEDICAL CENTER (O, 327 beds) 675 East Santa Clara Street, San Jose, CA Zip 95112, Mailing Address: P.O. Box 240003, Zip 95154-2403; tel. 408/998-3212; William L. Gilbert, Chief Executive Officer
Web address: www.hcahealthcare.com

WEST HILLS HOSPITAL AND MEDICAL CENTER (O, 236 beds) 7300 Medical Center Drive, West Hills, CA Zip 91307-9937, Mailing Address: P.O. Box 7937, Zip 91309-9937; tel. 818/676-4000; James F. Sherman, President and Chief Executive Officer
Web address: www.westhillshospital.com

COLORADO: MEDICAL CENTER OF AURORA–SOUTH (O, 334 beds) 1501 South Potomac Street, Aurora, CO Zip 80012-5499; tel. 303/695-2600; Sylvia Young, President and Chief Executive Officer
Web address: www.hcahealthcare.com

NORTH SUBURBAN MEDICAL CENTER (O, 125 beds) 9191 Grant Street, Thornton, CO Zip 80229-4341; tel. 303/451-7800; Margaret C. Cain, President and Chief Executive Officer
Web address: www.hcahealthcare.com

PRESBYTERIAN–ST. LUKE'S MEDICAL CENTER (O, 479 beds) 1719 East 19th Avenue, Denver, CO Zip 80218-1281; tel. 303/839-6000; Madeleine Roberson, President and Chief Executive Officer

Systems / HCA – The Healthcare Company

ROSE MEDICAL CENTER (O, 250 beds) 4567 East Ninth Avenue, Denver, CO Zip 80220–3941; tel. 303/320–2121; Kenneth H. Feiler, President and Chief Executive Officer
Web address: www.rosebabies.com

SPALDING REHABILITATION HOSPITAL (O, 138 beds) 900 Potomac Street, Aurora, CO Zip 80011–6716; tel. 303/367–1166

SWEDISH MEDICAL CENTER (O, 368 beds) 501 East Hampden Avenue, Englewood, CO Zip 80110–0101; tel. 303/788–5000; Mary M. White, President and Chief Executive Officer
Web address: www.swedishhospital.com

FLORIDA: AVENTURA HOSPITAL AND MEDICAL CENTER (O, 407 beds) 20900 Biscayne Boulevard, Miami, FL Zip 33180–1407; tel. 305/682–7100; Davide M. Carbone, Chief Executive Officer
Web address: www.aventurahospital.com

BLAKE MEDICAL CENTER (O, 284 beds) 2020 59th Street West, Bradenton, FL Zip 34209–4669, Mailing Address: P.O. Box 25004, Zip 34206–5004; tel. 941/792–6611; Lindell W. Orr, Chief Executive Officer
Web address: www.hcahealthcare.com

BRANDON REGIONAL HOSPITAL (O, 225 beds) 119 Oakfield Drive, Brandon, FL Zip 33511–5799; tel. 813/681–5551; Michael M. Fencel, Chief Executive Officer
Web address: www.brandonhospital.com

CEDARS MEDICAL CENTER (O, 500 beds) 1400 N.W. 12th Avenue, Miami, FL Zip 33136–1003; tel. 305/325–5511; Steven Sonenreich, Chief Executive Officer
Web address: www.cedarsmed.com

CENTRAL FLORIDA REGIONAL HOSPITAL (O, 226 beds) 1401 West Seminole Boulevard, Sanford, FL Zip 32771–6764; tel. 407/321–4500; Rodney R. Smith, President and Chief Executive Officer
Web address: www.hcahealthcare.com

COLUMBIA HOSPITAL (O, 250 beds) 2201 45th Street, West Palm Beach, FL Zip 33407–2069; tel. 561/842–6141; Eric Goldman, Chief Operating Officer
Web address: www.hcahealthcare.com

COMMUNITY HOSPITAL OF NEW PORT RICHEY (O, 414 beds) 5637 Marine Parkway, New Port Richey, FL Zip 34652–4331, Mailing Address: P.O. Box 996, Zip 34656–0996; tel. 727/848–1733; Ernie Meier, Administrator

DEERING HOSPITAL (O, 233 beds) 9333 S.W. 152nd Street, Miami, FL Zip 33157–1780; tel. 305/256–5100; Jude Torchia, Chief Executive Officer
Web address: www.hcahealthcare.com

DOCTORS HOSPITAL OF SARASOTA (O, 147 beds) 5731 Bee Ridge Road, Sarasota, FL Zip 34233–5056; tel. 941/342–1100; Charles F. Scott, President and Chief Executive Officer
Web address: www.doctorsofsarasota.com

EAST POINTE HOSPITAL (O, 88 beds) 1500 Lee Boulevard, Lehigh Acres, FL Zip 33936–4897; tel. 941/369–2101; Valerie A. Jackson, Chief Executive Officer
Web address: www.hcahealthcare.com

EDWARD WHITE HOSPITAL (O, 134 beds) 2323 Ninth Avenue North, Saint Petersburg, FL Zip 33713–6898, Mailing Address: P.O. Box 12018, Zip 33733–2018; tel. 727/323–1111; Barry S. Stokes, President and Chief Executive Officer
Web address: www.hcahealthcare.com

ENGLEWOOD COMMUNITY HOSPITAL (O, 100 beds) 700 Medical Boulevard, Englewood, FL Zip 34223–3978; tel. 941/475–6571; Robert C. Meade, Chief Executive Officer
Web address: www.hcahealthcare.com

FAWCETT MEMORIAL HOSPITAL (O, 241 beds) 21298 Olean Boulevard, Port Charlotte, FL Zip 33952–6765, Mailing Address: P.O. Box 4028, Punta Gorda, Zip 33949–4028; tel. 941/629–1181; Thomas J. Rice, President and Chief Executive Officer
Web address: www.hcahealthcare.com

FORT WALTON BEACH MEDICAL CENTER (O, 247 beds) 1000 Mar–Walt Drive, Fort Walton Beach, FL Zip 32547–6795; tel. 850/862–1111; Wayne Campbell, Chief Executive Officer
Web address: www.hcahealthcare.com

GULF COAST HOSPITAL (O, 120 beds) 13681 Doctors Way, Fort Myers, FL Zip 33912–4309; tel. 941/768–5000; Valerie A. Jackson, Chief Executive Officer

GULF COAST MEDICAL CENTER (O, 165 beds) 449 West 23rd Street, Panama City, FL Zip 32405–4593, Mailing Address: P.O. Box 15309, Zip 32406–5309; tel. 850/769–8341; Brent A. Marsteller, Chief Executive Officer
Web address: www.hcahealthcare.com

J. F. K. MEDICAL CENTER (O, 363 beds) 5301 South Congress Avenue, Atlantis, FL Zip 33462–1197; tel. 561/965–7300; Phillip D. Robinson, Chief Executive Officer
Web address: www.hcahealthcare.com

KENDALL MEDICAL CENTER (O, 316 beds) 11750 Bird Road, Miami, FL Zip 33175–3530; tel. 305/223–3000; Victor Maya, Chief Executive Officer
Web address: www.kendallmed.com

LAKE CITY MEDICAL CENTER (O, 75 beds) 1050 Commerce Boulevard North, Lake City, FL Zip 32055–3718; tel. 904/719–9000; Todd Gallati, Chief Executive Officer
Web address: www.lakecitymedical.com

LARGO MEDICAL CENTER (O, 243 beds) 201 14th Street S.W., Largo, FL Zip 33770–3133, Mailing Address: P.O. Box 2905, Zip 33779–2905; tel. 727/588–5200; Thomas L. Herron, FACHE, President and Chief Executive Officer
Web address: www.largomedical.com

LAWNWOOD REGIONAL MEDICAL CENTER (O, 375 beds) 1700 South 23rd Street, Fort Pierce, FL Zip 34950–0188; tel. 561/461–4000; Thomas R. Pentz, President and Executive Officer
Web address: www.hcahealthcare.com

MEMORIAL HOSPITAL OF JACKSONVILLE (O, 310 beds) 3625 University Boulevard South, Jacksonville, FL Zip 32216–4240, Mailing Address: P.O. Box 16325, Zip 32216–6325; tel. 904/399–6111; H. Rex Etheredge, President and Chief Executive Officer
Web address: www.hcahealthcare.com

MIAMI HEART INSTITUTE AND MEDICAL CENTER (O, 278 beds) 4701 North Meridian Avenue, Miami, FL Zip 33140–2910; tel. 305/674–3114; Ralph A. Aleman, Chief Executive Officer

NORTH FLORIDA REGIONAL MEDICAL CENTER (O, 266 beds) 6500 Newberry Road, Gainesville, FL Zip 32605–4392, Mailing Address: P.O. Box 147006, Zip 32614–7006; tel. 352/333–4000; Brian C. Robinson, Chief Executive Officer
Web address: www.hcahealthcare.com

NORTHSIDE HOSPITAL AND HEART INSTITUTE (O, 288 beds) 6000 49th Street North, Saint Petersburg, FL Zip 33709–2145; tel. 727/521–4411; Bradley K. Grover , Sr, Ph.D., FACHE, President and Chief Executive Officer
Web address: www.northsidehospital.com

NORTHWEST MEDICAL CENTER (O, 150 beds) 2801 North State Road 7, Pompano Beach, FL Zip 33063–5727, Mailing Address: P.O. Box 639002, Margate, Zip 33063–9002; tel. 954/978–4000; Gina Melby, Chief Executive Officer
Web address: www.hcahealthcare.com

OAK HILL HOSPITAL (O, 204 beds) 11375 Cortez Boulevard, Spring Hill, FL Zip 34611, Mailing Address: P.O. Box 5300, Zip 34611–5300; tel. 352/596–6632; Jaime A. Wesolowski, Chief Executive Officer
Web address: www.hcahealthcare.com

OCALA REGIONAL MEDICAL CENTER (O, 210 beds) 1431 S.W. First Avenue, Ocala, FL Zip 34474–4058, Mailing Address: P.O. Box 2200, Zip 34478–2200; tel. 352/401–1000; Stephen Mahan, Chief Executive Officer

ORANGE PARK MEDICAL CENTER (O, 196 beds) 2001 Kingsley Avenue, Orange Park, FL Zip 32073–5156; tel. 904/276–8500; Robert M. Krieger, Chief Executive Officer

OSCEOLA REGIONAL MEDICAL CENTER (O, 156 beds) 700 West Oak Street, Kissimmee, FL Zip 34741–4996, Mailing Address: P.O. Box 422589, Zip 34742–2589; tel. 407/846–2266; E. Tim Cook, Chief Executive Officer
Web address: www.hcahealthcare.com

PALMS WEST HOSPITAL (O, 117 beds) 13001 Southern Boulevard, Loxahatchee, FL Zip 33470–1150; tel. 561/798–3300; Heather J. Rohan, Chief Executive Officer
Web address: www.hcahealthcare.com

For explanation of codes following names, see page B2.
★ Indicates Type III membership in the American Hospital Association.

Systems / HCA – The Healthcare Company

PASCO COMMUNITY HOSPITAL (O, 120 beds) 13100 Fort King Road, Dade City, FL Zip 33525–5294; tel. 352/521–1100; William G. Buck, Chief Executive Officer
Web address: www.hcahealthcare.com

PLANTATION GENERAL HOSPITAL (O, 264 beds) 401 N.W. 42nd Avenue, Plantation, FL Zip 33317–2882; tel. 954/587–5010; Anthony M. Degina, Jr, Chief Executive Officer
Web address: www.hcahealthcare.com

PUTNAM COMMUNITY MEDICAL CENTER (O, 141 beds) Highway 20 West, Palatka, FL Zip 32177, Mailing Address: P.O. Box 778, Zip 32178–0778; tel. 904/328–5711; Bland Eng, Interim Chief Executive Officer
Web address: www.hcahealthcare.com

RAULERSON HOSPITAL (O, 101 beds) 1796 Highway 441 North, Okeechobee, FL Zip 34972, Mailing Address: P.O. Box 1307, Zip 34973–1307; tel. 941/763–2151; Frank Irby, Chief Executive Officer

REGIONAL MEDICAL CENTER–BAYONET POINT (O, 256 beds) 14000 Fivay Road, Hudson, FL Zip 34667–7199; tel. 727/863–2411; Don Griffin, Ph.D., President and Chief Executive Officer
Web address: www.hcahealthcare.com

SOUTH BAY HOSPITAL (O, 112 beds) 4016 State Road 674, Sun City Center, FL Zip 33573–5298; tel. 813/634–3301; Alan M. Levine, Chief Executive Officer
Web address: www.hcahealthcare.com

SOUTHWEST FLORIDA REGIONAL MEDICAL CENTER (O, 400 beds) 2727 Winkler Avenue, Fort Myers, FL Zip 33901–9396; tel. 941/939–1147; Stephen L. Royal, President and Chief Executive Officer
Web address: www.swfrmc.com

SPECIALTY HOSPITAL JACKSONVILLE (O, 61 beds) 4901 Richard Street, Jacksonville, FL Zip 32207; tel. 904/737–3120; W. Raymond C. Ford, Chief Executive Officer
Web address: www.heartofhealthcare.com

ST. LUCIE MEDICAL CENTER (O, 150 beds) 1800 S.E. Tiffany Avenue, Port St. Lucie, FL Zip 34952–7580; tel. 561/335–4000; Gary Cantrell, President and Chief Executive Officer

ST. PETERSBURG GENERAL HOSPITAL (O, 160 beds) 6500 38th Avenue North, Saint Petersburg, FL Zip 33710–1629; tel. 727/384–1414; Daniel J. Friedrich, II, President and Chief Executive Officer
Web address: www.stpetegeneralhospital.com

TALLAHASSEE COMMUNITY HOSPITAL (O, 180 beds) 2626 Capital Medical Boulevard, Tallahassee, FL Zip 32308–4499; tel. 850/656–5000; Sharon L. Roush, Chief Executive Officer
Web address: www.hcahealthcare.com

TWIN CITIES HOSPITAL (O, 60 beds) 2190 Highway 85 North, Niceville, FL Zip 32578–1045; tel. 850/678–4131; David Whalen, Chief Executive Officer
Web address: www.hcahealthcare.com

UNIVERSITY HOSPITAL AND MEDICAL CENTER (O, 211 beds) 7201 North University Drive, Tamarac, FL Zip 33321–2996; tel. 954/721–2200; James A. Cruickshank, Chief Executive Officer
Web address: www.hcahealthcare.com

WEST FLORIDA REGIONAL MEDICAL CENTER (O, 531 beds) 8383 North Davis Highway, Pensacola, FL Zip 32514–6088, Mailing Address: P.O. Box 18900, Zip 32523–8900; tel. 850/494–4000; Jerald F. Mitchell, President and Chief Executive Officer
Web address: www.hcahealthcare.com

WESTSIDE REGIONAL MEDICAL CENTER (O, 204 beds) 8201 West Broward Boulevard, Plantation, FL Zip 33324–9937; tel. 954/473–6600; Michael G. Joseph, Chief Executive Officer
Web address: www.hcahealthcare.com

WINTER PARK MEMORIAL HOSPITAL (O, 339 beds) 200 North Lakemont Avenue, Winter Park, FL Zip 32792–3273; tel. 407/646–7000; Douglas P. DeGraaf, Chief Executive Officer
Web address: www.hcahealthcare.com

GEORGIA: COLISEUM MEDICAL CENTERS (O, 180 beds) 350 Hospital Drive, Macon, GA Zip 31213; tel. 912/765–7000; Timothy C. Tobin, Chief Executive Officer
Web address: www.hcahealthcare.com

COLISEUM PSYCHIATRIC CENTER (O, 92 beds) 340 Hospital Drive, Macon, GA Zip 31217–8002; tel. 912/741–1355; Edward W. Ruffin, Administrator
Web address: www.hcahealthcare.com

DOCTORS HOSPITAL (O, 216 beds) 3651 Wheeler Road, Augusta, GA Zip 30909–6426; tel. 706/651–3232; Michael K. Kerner, President and Chief Executive Officer
Web address: www.doctors–hospital.net/

DOCTORS HOSPITAL (O, 171 beds) 616 19th Street, Columbus, GA Zip 31901–1528, Mailing Address: P.O. Box 2188, Zip 31902–2188; tel. 706/571–4262; Hugh D. Wilson, Chief Executive Officer
Web address: www.hcahealthcare.com

EMORY CARTERSVILLE MEDICAL CENTER (O, 80 beds) 960 Joe Frank Harris Parkway, Cartersville, GA Zip 30120, Mailing Address: P.O. Box 200008, Zip 30120–9001; tel. 770/382–1530; Keith Sandlin, Chief Executive Officer

EMORY DUNWOODY MEDICAL CENTER (O, 140 beds) 4575 North Shallowford Road, Atlanta, GA Zip 30338–6499; tel. 770/454–2000; Thomas D. Gilbert, President and Chief Executive Officer
Web address: www.hcahealthcare.com

EMORY EASTSIDE MEDICAL CENTER (O, 131 beds) 1700 Medical Way, Snellville, GA Zip 30078, Mailing Address: P.O. Box 587, Zip 30078–0587; tel. 770/979–0200; Les Beard, Chief Executive Officer

EMORY NORTHLAKE REGIONAL MEDICAL CENTER (O, 112 beds) 1455 Montreal Road, Tucker, GA Zip 30084; tel. 770/270–3000; Thomas D. Gilbert, Chief Executive Officer

EMORY PARKWAY MEDICAL CENTER (O, 182 beds) 1000 Thornton Road, Lithia Springs, GA Zip 30122, Mailing Address: P.O. Box 570, Zip 30122–0570; tel. 770/732–7777; John D. Anderson, Chief Executive Officer
Web address: www.hcahealthcare.com/

EMORY PEACHTREE REGIONAL HOSPITAL (O, 144 beds) 60 Hospital Road, Newnan, GA Zip 30264, Mailing Address: P.O. Box 2228, Zip 30264–2228; tel. 770/253–1912; Linda Jubinsky, Chief Executive Officer

FAIRVIEW PARK HOSPITAL (O, 190 beds) 200 Industrial Boulevard, Dublin, GA Zip 31021–2997, Mailing Address: P.O. Box 1408, Zip 31040–1408; tel. 912/275–2000; James B. Wood, Chief Executive Officer
Web address: www.hcahealthcare.com

HUGHSTON SPORTS MEDICINE HOSPITAL (O, 100 beds) 100 First Court, Columbus, GA Zip 31908–7188, Mailing Address: P.O. Box 7188, Zip 31908–7188; tel. 706/576–2101; Hugh C. Tappan, Chief Executive Officer
Web address: www.hughstonsports.com

LANIER PARK HOSPITAL (O, 119 beds) 675 White Sulphur Road, Gainesville, GA Zip 30505, Mailing Address: P.O. Box 1354, Zip 30503–1354; tel. 770/503–3000; Gerald N. Fulks, Chief Executive Officer
Web address: www.lanierpark.com

MACON NORTHSIDE HOSPITAL (O, 103 beds) 400 Charter Boulevard, Macon, GA Zip 31210–4853, Mailing Address: P.O. Box 4627, Zip 31208–4627; tel. 912/757–8200; Bud Costello, Administrator and Chief Executive Officer
Web address: www.hcahealthcare.com

METROPOLITAN HOSPITAL (O, 64 beds) 3223 Howell Mill Road N.W., Atlanta, GA Zip 30327–4135; tel. 404/351–0500; Jean Calhoun, Administrator
Web address: www.hcahealthcare.com

MIDDLE GEORGIA HOSPITAL (O, 119 beds) 888 Pine Street, Macon, GA Zip 31201–2186, Mailing Address: P.O. Box 6278, Zip 31208–6278; tel. 912/751–1111; Richard L. McConahy, Chief Executive Officer
Web address: www.hcahealthcare.com

PALMYRA MEDICAL CENTERS (O, 163 beds) 2000 Palmyra Road, Albany, GA Zip 31702–1908, Mailing Address: P.O. Box 1908, Zip 31702–1908; tel. 912/434–2000; Allen Golson, Chief Executive Officer
Web address: www.palmyramedicalcenters.com

POLK MEDICAL CENTER (O, 40 beds) 424 North Main Street, Cedartown, GA Zip 30125–2698; tel. 770/748–2500; Mark Nichols, Chief Executive Officer

REDMOND REGIONAL MEDICAL CENTER (O, 199 beds) 501 Redmond Road, Rome, GA Zip 30165–7001, Mailing Address: Box 107001, Zip 30164–7001; tel. 706/291–0291; James R. Thomas, Chief Executive Officer
Web address: www.hcahealthcare.com/

IDAHO: EASTERN IDAHO REGIONAL MEDICAL CENTER (O, 289 beds) 3100 Channing Way, Idaho Falls, ID Zip 83404–7533, Mailing Address: P.O. Box 2077, Zip 83403–2077; tel. 208/529–6111; Douglas Crabtree, Chief Executive Officer
Web address: www.eirmc.org

For explanation of codes following names, see page B2.
★ Indicates Type III membership in the American Hospital Association.

Systems / HCA – The Healthcare Company

WEST VALLEY MEDICAL CENTER (O, 122 beds) 1717 Arlington, Caldwell, ID Zip 83605–4864; tel. 208/459–4641; Mark Adams, Chief Executive Officer
Web address: www.westvalleymedctr.com

INDIANA: TERRE HAUTE REGIONAL HOSPITAL (O, 238 beds) 3901 South Seventh Street, Terre Haute, IN Zip 47802–4299; tel. 812/232–0021; Jerry Dooley, Chief Executive Officer
Web address: www.regionalhospital.com

WOMEN'S HOSPITAL–INDIANAPOLIS (O, 102 beds) 8111 Township Line Road, Indianapolis, IN Zip 46260–8043; tel. 317/875–5994; Steven B. Reed, President and Chief Executive Officer
Web address: www.womenshospital.org

KANSAS: WESLEY MEDICAL CENTER (O, 534 beds) 550 North Hillside Avenue, Wichita, KS Zip 67214–4976; tel. 316/688–2000; Carl W. Fitch, Sr, President and Chief Executive Officer
Web address: www.wesleymc.com

KENTUCKY: FRANKFORT REGIONAL MEDICAL CENTER (O, 146 beds) 299 King's Daughters Drive, Frankfort, KY Zip 40601–4186; tel. 502/875–5240; David P. Steitz, Chief Executive Officer
Web address: www.frankfortregional.com

GREENVIEW REGIONAL HOSPITAL (O, 211 beds) 1801 Ashley Circle, Bowling Green, KY Zip 42104–3384, Mailing Address: P.O. Box 90024, Zip 42102–9024; tel. 270/793–1000; Phillip A. Clendenin, Chief Executive Officer
Web address: www.greenviewhospital.com

LOUISIANA: AVOYELLES HOSPITAL (O, 47 beds) 4231 Highway 1192, Marksville, LA Zip 71351, Mailing Address: P.O. Box 249, Zip 71351; tel. 318/253–8611; David M. Mitchel, Chief Executive Officer

DAUTERIVE HOSPITAL (O, 86 beds) 600 North Lewis Street, New Iberia, LA Zip 70560, Mailing Address: P.O. Box 11210, Zip 70562–1210; tel. 318/365–7311; Kyle J. Viator, Chief Executive Officer

LAKELAND MEDICAL CENTER (O, 140 beds) 6000 Bullard Avenue, New Orleans, LA Zip 70128; tel. 504/241–6335; Tracy A. Rogers, Chief Executive Officer
Web address: www.hcahealthcare.com

LAKESIDE HOSPITAL (O, 75 beds) 4700 I–10 Service Road, Metairie, LA Zip 70001–1269; tel. 504/885–3342; Gerald A. Fornoff, Chief Executive Officer

LAKEVIEW REGIONAL MEDICAL CENTER (O, 145 beds) 95 East Fairway Drive, Covington, LA Zip 70433–7507; tel. 504/867–3800; Max Lauderdale, Chief Executive Officer

MEDICAL CENTER OF SOUTHWEST LOUISIANA (O, 138 beds) 2810 Ambassador Caffery Parkway, Lafayette, LA Zip 70506–5900; tel. 318/981–2949; Stephen K. Jones, Jr, Chief Executive Officer
Web address: www.medicalcentersw.com

NORTH MONROE HOSPITAL (O, 210 beds) 3421 Medical Park Drive, Monroe, LA Zip 71203–2399; tel. 318/388–1946; George E. Miller, Chief Executive Officer

OAKDALE COMMUNITY HOSPITAL (O, 54 beds) 130 North Hospital Drive, Oakdale, LA Zip 71463–4004, Mailing Address: P.O. Box 629, Zip 71463–0629; tel. 318/335–3700; Kevin N. Fowler, Chief Executive Officer

RAPIDES REGIONAL MEDICAL CENTER (O, 320 beds) 211 Fourth Street, Alexandria, LA Zip 71301–8421, Mailing Address: Box 30101, Zip 71301–8421; tel. 318/473–3000; A. C. Buchanan, President and Chief Executive Officer
Web address: www.rapidesregional.com

SAVOY MEDICAL CENTER (O, 330 beds) 801 Poinciana Avenue, Mamou, LA Zip 70554–2298; tel. 318/468–5261; J. E. Richardson, Chief Executive Officer

TULANE UNIVERSITY HOSPITAL AND CLINIC (O, 336 beds) 1415 Tulane Avenue, New Orleans, LA Zip 70112–2632; tel. 504/588–5263; Shirley A. Stewart, President and Chief Executive Officer
Web address: www.tuhc.com

WINN PARISH MEDICAL CENTER (O, 103 beds) 301 West Boundary Street, Winnfield, LA Zip 71483–3427, Mailing Address: P.O. Box 152, Zip 71483–0152; tel. 318/628–2721; Bobby Jordan, Chief Executive Officer

WOMEN'S AND CHILDREN'S HOSPITAL (O, 75 beds) 4600 Ambassador Caffery Parkway, Lafayette, LA Zip 70508–6923, Mailing Address: P.O. Box 88030, Zip 70598–8030; tel. 337/981–9100; Susan Silverman, Chief Executive Officer

MISSISSIPPI: COLUMBIA GARDEN PARK HOSPITAL (O, 97 beds) 1520 Broad Avenue, Gulfport, MS Zip 39501, Mailing Address: P.O. Box 1240, Zip 39502–1240; tel. 228/864–4210; William E. Peaks, Chief Executive Officer

NEVADA: MOUNTAINVIEW HOSPITAL (O, 120 beds) 3100 North Tenaya Way, Las Vegas, NV Zip 89128; tel. 702/255–5000; Mark J. Howard, President and Chief Executive Officer
Web address: www.mountainview–hospital.com

SUNRISE HOSPITAL AND MEDICAL CENTER (O, 675 beds) 3186 Maryland Parkway, Las Vegas, NV Zip 89109–2306, Mailing Address: P.O. Box 98530, Zip 89193–8530; tel. 702/731–8000; Allan Stipe, President and Chief Executive Officer
Web address: www.sunrisehospital.com

NEW HAMPSHIRE: PARKLAND MEDICAL CENTER (O, 79 beds) One Parkland Drive, Derry, NH Zip 03038–2750; tel. 603/432–1500; Alex M. Marceline Poirier, President and Chief Executive Officer
Web address: www.parklandmc.com

PORTSMOUTH REGIONAL HOSPITAL AND PAVILION (O, 179 beds) 333 Borthwick Avenue, Portsmouth, NH Zip 03801–7004; tel. 603/436–5110; William J. Schuler, Chief Executive Officer
Web address: www.portsmouthhospital.com

NORTH CAROLINA: BRUNSWICK COMMUNITY HOSPITAL (O, 56 beds) 1 Medical Center Drive, Supply, NC Zip 28462–3350, Mailing Address: P.O. Box 139, Zip 28462–0139; tel. 910/755–8121; Paul A. Schulte, Chief Executive Officer

OKLAHOMA: EDMOND MEDICAL CENTER (O, 84 beds) 1 South Bryant Street, Edmond, OK Zip 73034–4798; tel. 405/341–6100; Stanley D. Tatum, Chief Executive Officer
Web address: www.edmondmedctr.com

SEMINOLE MEDICAL CENTER (O, 39 beds) 2401 Wrangler Boulevard, Seminole, OK Zip 74868; tel. 405/303–4000; Janet Jackman, Chief Executive Officer

SOUTHWESTERN MEDICAL CENTER (O, 158 beds) 5602 S.W. Lee Boulevard, Lawton, OK Zip 73505–9635, Mailing Address: P.O. Box 7290, Zip 73506–7290; tel. 580/531–4700; Thomas L. Rine, President and Chief Executive Officer
Web address: www.hcahealthcare.com

UNIVERSITY HEALTH PARTNERS (O, 621 beds) 6501 North Broadway, Suite 200, Oklahoma City, OK Zip 73116; tel. 405/879–0900; Jeffrey A. Dorsey, Chief Executive Officer

SOUTH CAROLINA: COLLETON MEDICAL CENTER (O, 131 beds) 501 Robertson Boulevard, Walterboro, SC Zip 29488–5714; tel. 843/549–2000; Rebecca T. Brewer, CHE, Chief Executive Officer

GRAND STRAND REGIONAL MEDICAL CENTER (O, 186 beds) 809 82nd Parkway, Myrtle Beach, SC Zip 29572–1413; tel. 803/692–1100; Doug White, Chief Executive Officer
Web address: www.medtropolis.com/medtropolis/fac_right.asp?facility_id=3

SUMMERVILLE MEDICAL CENTER (O, 85 beds) 295 Midland Parkway, Summerville, SC Zip 29485–8104; tel. 843/832–5100; Steven M. Anderson, Chief Executive Officer

TRIDENT MEDICAL CENTER (O, 305 beds) 9330 Medical Plaza Drive, Charleston, SC Zip 29406–9195; tel. 843/797–7000; Michael P. Joyce, President and Chief Executive Officer
Web address: www.tridenthealthsystem.com

TENNESSEE: ATHENS REGIONAL MEDICAL CENTER (O, 91 beds) 1114 West Madison Avenue, Athens, TN Zip 37303–4150, Mailing Address: P.O. Box 250, Zip 37371–0250; tel. 423/745–1411; John R. Workman, Chief Executive Officer
Web address: www.columbiachat.com/athens

CENTENNIAL MEDICAL CENTER AND PARTHENON PAVILION (O, 680 beds) 2300 Patterson Street, Nashville, TN Zip 37203–1528; tel. 615/342–1000; Lawrence Kloess, President
Web address: www.hcahealthcare.com

CHEATHAM MEDICAL CENTER (O, 29 beds) 313 North Main Street, Ashland City, TN Zip 37015–1358; tel. 615/792–3030; Michael W. Garfield, Administrator
Web address: www.hcahealthcare.com

For explanation of codes following names, see page B2.
★ Indicates Type III membership in the American Hospital Association.

Systems / HCA – The Healthcare Company

GRANDVIEW MEDICAL CENTER (O, 50 beds) 1000 Highway 28, Jasper, TN Zip 37347; tel. 423/837–9500; Phil Rowland, Chief Executive Officer
Web address: www.hcahealthcare.com

HENDERSONVILLE HOSPITAL (O, 66 beds) 355 New Shackle Island Road, Hendersonville, TN Zip 37075–2393; tel. 615/264–4000; Robert Klein, Chief Executive Officer
Web address: www.hvillehospital.com

HORIZON MEDICAL CENTER (O, 168 beds) 111 Highway 70 East, Dickson, TN Zip 37055–2033; tel. 615/441–2357; Benjamin J. Everett, Chief Executive Officer
Web address: www.hcahealthcare.com

NASHVILLE MEMORIAL HOSPITAL (O, 250 beds) 612 West Due West Avenue, Madison, TN Zip 37115–4474; tel. 615/865–3511; Allyn R. Harris, Chief Executive Officer
Web address: www.hcahealthcare.com

PARKRIDGE MEDICAL CENTER (O, 517 beds) 2333 McCallie Avenue, Chattanooga, TN Zip 37404–3285; tel. 423/698–6061; Niels P. Vernegaard, Chief Executive Officer
Web address: www.hcahealthcare.com

RIVER PARK HOSPITAL (O, 90 beds) 1559 Sparta Road, McMinnville, TN Zip 37110–1316; tel. 931/815–4000; Terry J. Gunn, Chief Executive Officer
Web address: www.hcahealthcare.com

SOUTHERN HILLS MEDICAL CENTER (O, 140 beds) 391 Wallace Road, Nashville, TN Zip 37211–4859; tel. 615/781–4000; Jeffrey Whitehorn, Chief Executive Officer
Web address: www.hcahealthcare.com

SUMMIT MEDICAL CENTER (O, 204 beds) 5655 Frist Boulevard, Hermitage, TN Zip 37076–2053; tel. 615/316–3000; Bryan K. Dearing, Chief Executive Officer
Web address: www.summitmedctr.com

TEXAS: BAYSHORE MEDICAL CENTER (O, 307 beds) 4000 Spencer Highway, Pasadena, TX Zip 77504–1294; tel. 713/359–2000; Donald L. Stewart, Chief Executive Officer
Web address: www.bayshoremedical.com

BELLAIRE MEDICAL CENTER (O, 209 beds) 5314 Dashwood Street, Houston, TX Zip 77081–4689; tel. 713/512–1200; Walter Leleux, Chief Executive Officer
Web address: www.hcahealthcare.com

CLEAR LAKE REGIONAL MEDICAL CENTER (O, 377 beds) 500 Medical Center Boulevard, Webster, TX Zip 77598–4286; tel. 281/338–3110; Donald A. Shaffett, Chief Executive Officer
Web address: www.hcahealthcare.com

COLUMBIA BEHAVIORAL CENTER (O, 49 beds) 1155 Idaho Street, El Paso, TX Zip 79902–1699; tel. 915/544–4000; Serena Pickman, Director
Web address: www.hcahealthcare.com

COLUMBIA MEDICAL CENTER WEST (O, 228 beds) 1801 North Oregon Street, El Paso, TX Zip 79902–3591; tel. 915/521–1200; Hank Hernandez, Chief Executive Officer
Web address: www.hcahealthcare.com

CONROE REGIONAL MEDICAL CENTER (O, 244 beds) 504 Medical Boulevard, Conroe, TX Zip 77304, Mailing Address: P.O. Box 1538, Zip 77305–1538; tel. 936/539–1111; Russell Meyers, Chief Executive Officer
Web address: www.conroeregional.com

CORPUS CHRISTI MEDICAL CENTER (O, 237 beds) 3315 South Alameda Street, Corpus Christi, TX Zip 78411–1883, Mailing Address: P.O. Box 8991, Zip 78468–8991; tel. 361/857–1400; Steven Woerner, Chief Executive Officer
Web address: www.hcahealthcare.com

CORPUS CHRISTI MEDICAL CENTER BAY AREA (O, 398 beds) 7101 South Padre Island Drive, Corpus Christi, TX Zip 78412–4999; tel. 361/985–1200; Steven Woerner, Chief Executive Officer

DALLAS SOUTHWEST MEDICAL CENTER (O, 107 beds) 2929 South Hampton Road, Dallas, TX Zip 75224–3026; tel. 214/330–4611; Carolyn Caldwell, Chief Executive Officer
Web address: www.hcahealthcare.com

DEL SOL MEDICAL CENTER (O, 299 beds) 10301 Gateway West, El Paso, TX Zip 79925–7798; tel. 915/595–9000; Douglas A. Matney, Chief Executive Officer
Web address: www.hcahealthcare.com

DENTON REGIONAL MEDICAL CENTER (O, 222 beds) 3535 South 1–35 East, Denton, TX Zip 76205; tel. 940/384–3535; Bob Haley, Chief Executive Officer
Web address: www.dentonregional.com

EAST HOUSTON REGIONAL MEDICAL CENTER (O, 121 beds) 13111 East Freeway, Houston, TX Zip 77015; tel. 713/393–2000; Terry Hutton, Chief Executive Officer
Web address: www.hcahealthcare.com

GREEN OAKS HOSPITAL (O, 106 beds) 7808 Clodus Fields Drive, Dallas, TX Zip 75251–2206; tel. 972/991–9504; Thomas M. Collins, Chief Executive Officer
Web address: www.greenoakspsych.com

KINGWOOD MEDICAL CENTER (O, 153 beds) 22999 U.S. Highway 59, Kingwood, TX Zip 77339; tel. 281/359–7500; Charles D. Schuetz, Chief Executive Officer
Web address: www.hcahealthcare.com

LAS COLINAS MEDICAL CENTER (O, 77 beds) 6800 North MacArthur Boulevard, Irving, TX Zip 75039–2422; tel. 972/969–2000; Stan Morton, Chief Executive Officer
Web address: www.lascolinasmedical.com

MAINLAND MEDICAL CENTER (O, 180 beds) 6801 E F Lowry Expressway, Texas City, TX Zip 77591; tel. 409/938–5000; Maura Walsh, Chief Executive Officer
Web address: www.mainlandmedical.com

MEDICAL CENTER AT LANCASTER (O, 79 beds) 2600 West Pleasant Run Road, Lancaster, TX Zip 75146–1199; tel. 972/223–9600; Ernest C. Lynch, II, Chief Executive Officer
Web address: www.hcahealthcare.com

MEDICAL CENTER OF ARLINGTON (O, 188 beds) 3301 Matlock Road, Arlington, TX Zip 76015–2998; tel. 817/465–3241; Michael R. Burroughs, FACHE, President and Chief Executive Officer
Web address: www.medicalcenterarlington.com

MEDICAL CENTER OF LEWISVILLE (O, 116 beds) 500 West Main, Lewisville, TX Zip 75057–3699; tel. 972/420–1000; Raymond M. Dunning, Jr, Chief Executive Officer
Web address: www.lewisvillemedical.com

MEDICAL CENTER OF PLANO (O, 265 beds) 3901 West 15th Street, Plano, TX Zip 75075–7799; tel. 972/596–6800; Harvey L. Fishero, President and Chief Executive Officer
Web address: www.hcahealthcare.com

MEDICAL CITY DALLAS HOSPITAL (O, 530 beds) 7777 Forest Lane, Dallas, TX Zip 75230–2598; tel. 972/566–7000; Britt Berrett, President and Chief Executive Officer
Web address: www.medicalcityhospital.com

METHODIST AMBULATORY SURGERY HOSPITAL (O, 37 beds) 9150 Huebner Road, Suite 100, San Antonio, TX Zip 78240–1545; tel. 210/691–8000; Elaine F. Morris, Administrator
Web address: www.hcahealthcare.com

METHODIST CHILDREN'S HOSPITAL OF SOUTH TEXAS (O, 150 beds) 7700 Floyd Curl Drive, San Antonio, TX Zip 78229–3383; tel. 210/575–7138; Arthur E. Marlin, M.D., Chief Executive Officer
Web address: www.mhshealthcare.com

METHODIST SPECIALTY AND TRANSPLANT HOSPITAL (O, 218 beds) 8026 Floyd Curl Drive, San Antonio, TX Zip 78229–3915; tel. 210/575–8110; John E. Hornbeak, Chief Executive Officer
Web address: www.mhshealthcare.com

METROPOLITAN METHODIST HOSPITAL (O, 228 beds) 1310 McCullough Avenue, San Antonio, TX Zip 78212–2617; tel. 210/208–2200; Mark L. Bernard, Chief Executive Officer
Web address: www.mhshealthcare.com

NORTH AUSTIN MEDICAL CENTER (O, 128 beds) 12221 MoPac Expressway North, Austin, TX Zip 78758–2483; tel. 512/901–1000; Donald H. Wilkerson, Chief Executive Officer
Web address: www.hcahealthcare.com

NORTH BAY HOSPITAL (O, 69 beds) 1711 West Wheeler Avenue, Aransas Pass, TX Zip 78336–4536; tel. 361/758–8585; John Krogness, Chief Executive Officer
Web address: www.hcahealthcare.com

For explanation of codes following names, see page B2.
★ *Indicates Type III membership in the American Hospital Association.*

Systems / HCA – The Healthcare Company

NORTH CENTRAL MEDICAL CENTER (O, 159 beds) 4500 Medical Center Drive, McKinney, TX Zip 75069–3499; tel. 972/547–8000; John F. Adams, Chief Executive Officer
Web address: www.hcahealthcare.com

NORTH HILLS HOSPITAL (O, 129 beds) 4401 Booth Calloway Road, North Richland Hills, TX Zip 76180–7399; tel. 817/255–1000; Randolph Moresi, Chief Executive Officer
Web address: www.northhillshospital.com

NORTHEAST METHODIST HOSPITAL (O, 99 beds) 12412 Judson Road, San Antonio, TX Zip 78233–3272, Mailing Address: P.O. Box 659510, Zip 78265–9510; tel. 210/650–4949; Mark L. Bernard, Chief Executive Officer
Web address: www.mhshealthcare.com

NORTHWEST REGIONAL HOSPITAL (O, 73 beds) 13725 Northwest Boulevard, Corpus Christi, TX Zip 78410–5199; tel. 361/241–4243; Winston Borland, Chief Executive Officer
Web address: www.hcahealthcare.com

PLAZA MEDICAL CENTER OF FORT WORTH (O, 261 beds) 900 Eighth Avenue, Fort Worth, TX Zip 76104–3986; tel. 817/347–5857; Stephen Bernstein, FACHE, Chief Executive Officer
Web address: www.hcahealthcare.com

RIO GRANDE REGIONAL HOSPITAL (O, 230 beds) 101 East Ridge Road, McAllen, TX Zip 78503–1299; tel. 956/632–6000; William A. Burns, Chief Executive Officer
Web address: www.riohealth.com

ROUND ROCK HOSPITAL (O, 103 beds) 2400 Round Rock Avenue, Round Rock, TX Zip 78681–4097; tel. 512/341–1000; Deborah L. Ryle, Chief Executive Officer
Web address: www.hcahealthcare.com

SOUTH AUSTIN HOSPITAL (O, 200 beds) 901 West Ben White Boulevard, Austin, TX Zip 78704–6903; tel. 512/447–2211; Richard W. Klusmann, Chief Executive Officer

SOUTHWEST TEXAS METHODIST HOSPITAL (O, 774 beds) 7700 Floyd Curl Drive, San Antonio, TX Zip 78229–3993; tel. 210/575–4000; John E. Hornbeak, Chief Executive Officer
Web address: www.mhshealthcare.com

SPRING BRANCH MEDICAL CENTER (O, 345 beds) 8850 Long Point Road, Houston, TX Zip 77055–3082; tel. 713/467–6555; Patricia Currie, Chief Executive Officer
Web address: www.hcahealthcare.com

ST. DAVID'S MEDICAL CENTER (O, 298 beds) 919 East 32nd Street, Austin, TX Zip 78705–2709, Mailing Address: P.O. Box 4039, Zip 78765–4039; tel. 512/476–7111; Cole C. Eslyn, Chief Executive Officer
Web address: www.hcahealthcare.com

ST. DAVID'S PAVILION (O, 38 beds) 1025 East 32nd Street, Austin, TX Zip 78765; tel. 512/867–5800; Cole C. Eslyn, Chief Executive Officer
Web address: www.hcahealthcare.com

ST. DAVID'S REHABILITATION CENTER (O, 67 beds) 1005 East 32nd Street, Austin, TX Zip 78705–2705, Mailing Address: P.O. Box 4270, Zip 78765–4270; tel. 512/867–5100; Cole C. Eslyn, Chief Executive Officer
Web address: www.hcahealthcare.com

TEXAS ORTHOPEDIC HOSPITAL (O, 49 beds) 7401 South Main Street, Houston, TX Zip 77030–4509; tel. 713/799–8600; Beryl Ramsey, Chief Executive Officer
Web address: www.hcahealthcare.com

THE WOMAN'S HOSPITAL OF TEXAS (O, 199 beds) 7600 Fannin Street, Houston, TX Zip 77054–1900; tel. 713/790–1234; Linda B. Russell, President
Web address: www.hcahealthcare.com

VALLEY REGIONAL MEDICAL CENTER (O, 177 beds) 100A Alton Gloor Boulevard, Brownsville, TX Zip 78526, Mailing Address: P.O. Box 3710, Zip 78521–3710; tel. 956/350–7101; Charles F. Sexton, Chief Executive Officer
Web address: www.valleyregionalmedicalcenter.com

WEST HOUSTON MEDICAL CENTER (O, 169 beds) 12141 Richmond Avenue, Houston, TX Zip 77082–2499; tel. 281/558–3444; Jeffrey S. Holland, Chief Executive Officer
Web address: www.hcahealthcare.com

UTAH: BRIGHAM CITY COMMUNITY HOSPITAL (O, 49 beds) 950 South Medical Drive, Brigham City, UT Zip 84302; tel. 435/734–9471; Tad A. Morley, Chief Executive Officer
Web address: www.brighamcityhospital.com

LAKEVIEW HOSPITAL (O, 128 beds) 630 East Medical Drive, Bountiful, UT Zip 84010–4996; tel. 801/292–6231; Craig Preston, Chief Executive Officer
Web address: www.hcahealthcare.com

MOUNTAIN VIEW HOSPITAL (O, 126 beds) 1000 East 100 North, Payson, UT Zip 84651–1690; tel. 801/465–9201; Kevin Johnson, Chief Executive Officer
Web address: www.hcahealthcare.com

OGDEN REGIONAL MEDICAL CENTER (O, 179 beds) 5475 South 500 East, Ogden, UT Zip 84405–6978; tel. 801/479–2111; Steven B. Bateman, Chief Executive Officer
Web address: www.hcahealthcare.com

ST. MARK'S HOSPITAL (O, 229 beds) 1200 East 3900 South, Salt Lake City, UT Zip 84124–1390; tel. 801/268–7111; John Hanshaw, Chief Executive Officer
Web address: www.stmarkshospital.com

TIMPANOGOS REGIONAL HOSPITAL (O, 51 beds) 750 West 800 North, Orem, UT Zip 84059; tel. 801/714–6000; Kenneth Armstrong, Chief Executive Officer
Web address: www.hcahealthcare.com

VIRGINIA: ALLEGHANY REGIONAL HOSPITAL (O, 156 beds) One ARH Lane, Low Moor, VA Zip 24457, Mailing Address: P.O. Box 7, Zip 24457–0007; tel. 540/862–6011; Ward W. Stevens, CHE, Chief Executive Officer
Web address: www.hcahealthcare.com

CHIPPENHAM MEDICAL CENTER/JOHNSTON–WILLIS HOSPITAL (O, 748 beds) 7101 Jahnke Road, Richmond, VA Zip 23225–4044; tel. 804/320–3911; Marilyn B. Tavenner, Chief Executive Officer

CLINCH VALLEY MEDICAL CENTER (O, 200 beds) 2949 West Front Street, Richlands, VA Zip 24641–2099; tel. 540/596–6000; James W. Thweatt, Chief Executive Officer
Web address: www.ccvmc.com

DOMINION HOSPITAL (O, 100 beds) 2960 Sleepy Hollow Road, Falls Church, VA Zip 22044–2001; tel. 703/536–2000; Barbara D. S. Hekimian, Chief Executive Officer
Web address: www.dominionhospital.com

HENRICO DOCTORS' HOSPITAL (O, 340 beds) 1602 Skipwith Road, Richmond, VA Zip 23229–5298; tel. 804/289–4500; Patrick W. Farrell, Chief Executive Officer
Web address: www.hcahealthcare.com

JOHN RANDOLPH MEDICAL CENTER (O, 222 beds) 411 West Randolph Road, Hopewell, VA Zip 23860, Mailing Address: P.O. Box 971, Zip 23860; tel. 804/541–1600; Daniel J. Wetta, Jr, Chief Executive Officer
Web address: www.hcahealthcare.com

LEWIS–GALE MEDICAL CENTER (O, 521 beds) 1900 Electric Road, Salem, VA Zip 24153–7494; tel. 540/776–4000; William B. Downey, President and Chief Executive Officer
Web address: www.lewis-gale.com

MONTGOMERY REGIONAL HOSPITAL (O, 115 beds) 3700 South Main Street, Blacksburg, VA Zip 24060–7081, Mailing Address: P.O. Box 90004, Zip 24062–9004; tel. 540/951–1111; David R. Williams, Chief Executive Officer
Web address: www.montreghosp.com

PENINSULA BEHAVIORAL CENTER (O, 115 beds) 2244 Executive Drive, Hampton, VA Zip 23666–2430; tel. 757/827–1001; Steuart A. Kimmeth, Vice President and Administrator
Web address: www.hcahealthcare.com

PULASKI COMMUNITY HOSPITAL (O, 99 beds) 2400 Lee Highway, Pulaski, VA Zip 24301–0759, Mailing Address: P.O. Box 759, Zip 24301–0759; tel. 540/994–8100; Jack Nunley, Chief Executive Officer
Web address: www.pch-va.com

RESTON HOSPITAL CENTER (O, 121 beds) 1850 Town Center Parkway, Reston, VA Zip 20190–3298; tel. 703/689–9000; William A. Adams, President and Chief Executive Officer
Web address: www.restonhospital.net

RETREAT HOSPITAL (O, 100 beds) 2621 Grove Avenue, Richmond, VA Zip 23220–4308; tel. 804/254–5100; Paul L. Baldwin, Chief Executive Officer

For explanation of codes following names, see page B2.
★ Indicates Type III membership in the American Hospital Association.

Systems / HCA – The Healthcare Company

WASHINGTON: CAPITAL MEDICAL CENTER (O, 110 beds) 3900 Capital Mall Drive S.W., Olympia, WA Zip 98502–5026, Mailing Address: P.O. Box 19002, Zip 98507–9002; tel. 360/754–5858; Joseph Sharp, Chief Executive Officer
Web address: www.capitalmedical.com

WEST VIRGINIA: COLUMBIA RIVER PARK HOSPITAL (O, 125 beds) 1230 Sixth Avenue, Huntington, WV Zip 25701–2312, Mailing Address: P.O. Box 1875, Zip 25719–1875; tel. 304/526–9111; Scott C. Stamm, Chief Executive Officer
Web address: www.hcahealthcare.com

PUTNAM GENERAL HOSPITAL (O, 64 beds) 1400 Hospital Drive, Hurricane, WV Zip 25526–9210, Mailing Address: P.O. Box 900, Zip 25526–0900; tel. 304/757–1700; Patsy Hardy, Administrator
Web address: www.hcahealthcare.com

RALEIGH GENERAL HOSPITAL (O, 325 beds) 1710 Harper Road, Beckley, WV Zip 25801–3397; tel. 304/256–4100; David B. Darden, Chief Executive Officer
Web address: www.raleighgeneral.com

SAINT FRANCIS HOSPITAL (O, 151 beds) 333 Laidley Street, Charleston, WV Zip 25301–1628, Mailing Address: P.O. Box 471, Zip 25322–0471; tel. 304/347–6500; Dan Lauffer, Chief Executive Officer

Owned, leased, sponsored:	192 hospitals	38446 beds
Contract-managed:	0 hospitals	0 beds
Totals:	192 hospitals	38446 beds

★0082: HEALTH ALLIANCE OF GREATER CINCINNATI (NP)
3200 Burnet Avenue, Cincinnati, OH Zip 45229; tel. 513/585–6000; Jack M. Cook, President and Chief Executive Officer
(Centralized Health System)

KENTUCKY: ST. LUKE HOSPITAL EAST (O, 211 beds) 85 North Grand Avenue, Fort Thomas, KY Zip 41075–1796; tel. 869/572–3100; Daniel M. Vinson, CPA, Senior Vice President
Web address: www.health-alliance.com

ST. LUKE HOSPITAL WEST (O, 168 beds) 7380 Turfway Road, Florence, KY Zip 41042–1337; tel. 859/962–5200; Daniel M. Vinson, CPA, Senior Vice President
Web address: www.health-alliance.com

OHIO: CHRIST HOSPITAL (O, 431 beds) 2139 Auburn Avenue, Cincinnati, OH Zip 45219–2989; tel. 513/585–2000; Richard L. Seim, Senior Vice President
Web address: www.health-alliance.com

FORT HAMILTON HOSPITAL (O, 181 beds) 630 Eaton Avenue, Hamilton, OH Zip 45013–2770; tel. 513/867–2000; James A. Kingsbury, President and Chief Executive Officer
Web address: www.health-alliance.com

JEWISH HOSPITAL KENWOOD (O, 169 beds) 4777 East Galbraith Road, Cincinnati, OH Zip 45236; tel. 513/686–3000; M. Aurora Lambert, Senior Vice President
Web address: www.health-alliance.com

UNIVERSITY HOSPITAL (O, 429 beds) 234 Goodman Street, Cincinnati, OH Zip 45219–2316; tel. 513/584–1000; Elliot G. Cohen, Senior Vice President
Web address: www.health-alliance.com

Owned, leased, sponsored:	6 hospitals	1589 beds
Contract-managed:	0 hospitals	0 beds
Totals:	6 hospitals	1589 beds

1775: HEALTH MANAGEMENT ASSOCIATES (IO)
5811 Pelican Bay Boulevard, Suite 500, Naples, FL Zip 34108; tel. 941/598–3131; William J. Schoen, Chairman and Chief Executive Officer
(Decentralized Health System)

ALABAMA: RIVERVIEW REGIONAL MEDICAL CENTER (O, 281 beds) 600 South Third Street, Gadsden, AL Zip 35901–5399, Mailing Address: P.O. Box 268, Zip 35999–0268; tel. 256/543–5200; J. David McCormack, Executive Director

STRINGFELLOW MEMORIAL HOSPITAL (L, 125 beds) 301 East 18th Street, Anniston, AL Zip 36207–0038, Mailing Address: P.O. Box 38, Zip 36207–0038; tel. 256/235–8900; Vincent T. Cherry, Jr, Administrator

ARKANSAS: CRAWFORD MEMORIAL HOSPITAL (L, 103 beds) East Main and South 20th Streets, Van Buren, AR Zip 72956, Mailing Address: P.O. Box 409, Zip 72957–0409; tel. 501/474–3401; Richard Boone, Executive Director
Web address: www.noonanrusso.com

SOUTHWEST REGIONAL MEDICAL CENTER (O, 76 beds) 11401 Interstate 30, Little Rock, AR Zip 72209–7056; tel. 501/455–7100; Randall R. Cason, Chief Executive Officer

FLORIDA: BROOKSVILLE REGIONAL HOSPITAL (L, 91 beds) 55 Ponce De Leon Boulevard, Brooksville, FL Zip 34601–0037, Mailing Address: P.O. Box 37, Zip 34605–0037; tel. 352/796–5111; Thomas D. Barb, Executive Director

CHARLOTTE REGIONAL MEDICAL CENTER (O, 148 beds) 809 East Marion Avenue, Punta Gorda, FL Zip 33950–3898, Mailing Address: P.O. Box 51-1328, Zip 33951–1328; tel. 941/639–3131; Joshua S. Putter, Executive Director
Web address: www.charlotteregional.com

FISHERMEN'S HOSPITAL (L, 58 beds) 3301 Overseas Highway, Marathon, FL Zip 33050–0068; tel. 305/743–5533; Alberto J. Aboud, Administrator

HEART OF FLORIDA BEHAVIORAL CENTER (O, 40 beds) 2510 North Florida Avenue, Lakeland, FL Zip 33805–2298; tel. 941/682–6105; David M. Polunas, Administrator and Chief Executive Officer

HEART OF FLORIDA REGIONAL MEDICAL CENTER (O, 51 beds) 1615 U.S. Highway 27N, Davenport, FL Zip 33837, Mailing Address: P.O. Box 67, Haines City, Zip 33844–0067; tel. 863/422–4971; Robert Mahaffey, Administrator

HIGHLANDS REGIONAL MEDICAL CENTER (L, 126 beds) 3600 South Highlands Avenue, Sebring, FL Zip 33870–5495, Mailing Address: Drawer 2066, Zip 33871–2066; tel. 863/471–5800; Michael A. Callahan, Chief Executive Officer

LOWER KEYS MEDICAL CENTER (L, 169 beds) 5900 College Road, Key West, FL Zip 33040–4396, Mailing Address: P.O. Box 9107, Zip 33041–9107; tel. 305/294–5531; Ronald L. Bierman, Chief Executive Officer

SANDYPINES (O, 60 beds) 11301 S.E. Tequesta Terrace, Tequesta, FL Zip 33469–8146; tel. 561/744–0211; Mary S. Bohne', Administrator

SEBASTIAN RIVER MEDICAL CENTER (O, 133 beds) 13695 North U.S. Highway 1, Sebastian, FL Zip 32958–3230, Mailing Address: Box 780838, Zip 32978–0838; tel. 561/589–3186; Diane D. Torres, R.N., Executive Director
Web address: www.srmcenter.com

SPRING HILL REGIONAL HOSPITAL (L, 75 beds) 10461 Quality Drive, Spring Hill, FL Zip 34609; tel. 352/688–8200; Thomas Bard, Chief Executive Officer

UNIVERSITY BEHAVIORAL CENTER (O, 100 beds) 2500 Discovery Drive, Orlando, FL Zip 32826–3711; tel. 407/281–7000; David L. Beardsley, Administrator

GEORGIA: BULLOCH MEMORIAL HOSPITAL (O, 158 beds) 500 East Grady Street, Statesboro, GA Zip 30458–5105, Mailing Address: P.O. Box 1048, Zip 30459–1048; tel. 912/486–1000; C. Scott Campbell, Executive Director

KENTUCKY: PAUL B. HALL REGIONAL MEDICAL CENTER (O, 72 beds) 625 James South Trimble Boulevard, Paintsville, KY Zip 41240–0000; tel. 606/789–3511; Deborah L. Trimble, Administrator

MISSISSIPPI: BILOXI REGIONAL MEDICAL CENTER (L, 153 beds) 150 Reynoir Street, Biloxi, MS Zip 39530–4199, Mailing Address: P.O. Box 128, Zip 39533–0128; tel. 228/432–1571; Keith G. Leblanc, Chief Executive Officer

CENTRAL MISSISSIPPI MEDICAL CENTER (L, 317 beds) 1850 Chadwick Drive, Jackson, MS Zip 39204–3479, Mailing Address: P.O. Box 59001, Zip 39204–9001; tel. 601/376–1000; John R. Finnegan, Chief Executive Officer

NATCHEZ COMMUNITY HOSPITAL (O, 101 beds) 129 Jefferson Davis Boulevard, Natchez, MS Zip 39120–5100, Mailing Address: P.O. Box 1203, Zip 39121–1203; tel. 601/445–6200; Raymond Bane, Executive Director

---

For explanation of codes following names, see page B2.
★ Indicates Type III membership in the American Hospital Association.

Systems / Health Systems America

NORTHWEST MISSISSIPPI REGIONAL MEDICAL CENTER (L, 195 beds) 1970 Hospital Drive, Clarksdale, MS Zip 38614–7204, Mailing Address: P.O. Box 1218, Zip 38614–1218; tel. 601/627–3410; John M. Faulkner, Executive Director

RANKIN MEDICAL CENTER (L, 90 beds) 350 Crossgates Boulevard, Brandon, MS Zip 39042–2698; tel. 601/825–2811; Robert L. Hammond , Jr, Executive Director

RILEY MEMORIAL HOSPITAL (O, 180 beds) 1102 21st Avenue, Meridian, MS Zip 39301–4096, Mailing Address: P.O. Box 1810, Zip 39301–1810; tel. 601/693–2511; Carl J. Etter, Chief Executive Officer

RIVER OAKS HOSPITAL (O, 109 beds) 1030 River Oaks Drive, Jackson, MS Zip 39208–9729, Mailing Address: P.O. Box 5100, Zip 39296–5100; tel. 601/932–1030; John J. Cleary, President and Chief Executive Officer

WOMAN'S HOSPITAL AT RIVER OAKS (O, 76 beds) 1026 North Flowood Drive, Jackson, MS Zip 39208–9599, Mailing Address: P.O. Box 4546, Zip 39296–4546; tel. 601/932–1000; Sherry J. Smith, Executive Director

NORTH CAROLINA: FRANKLIN REGIONAL MEDICAL CENTER (O, 85 beds) 100 Hospital Drive, Louisburg, NC Zip 27549–2256, Mailing Address: P.O. Box 609, Zip 27549–0609; tel. 919/497–8401; Ann Barnhart, Executive Director

LAKE NORMAN REGIONAL MEDICAL CENTER (O, 105 beds) 171 Fairview Road, Mooresville, NC Zip 28117, Mailing Address: P.O. Box 3250, Zip 28117; tel. 704/660–4000; P. Paul Smith , Jr, Executive Director

SANDHILLS REGIONAL MEDICAL CENTER (O, 64 beds) 1000 West Hamlet Avenue, Hamlet, NC Zip 28345, Mailing Address: P.O. Box 1109, Zip 28345–1109; tel. 910/205–8000; John W. McClellan, Executive Director

OKLAHOMA: MEDICAL CENTER OF SOUTHEASTERN OKLAHOMA (O, 103 beds) 1800 University Boulevard, Durant, OK Zip 74701–3006, Mailing Address: P.O. Box 1207, Zip 74702–1207; tel. 580/924–3080; Jacquelyn Harms, R.N., Executive Director

MIDWEST REGIONAL MEDICAL CENTER (L, 247 beds) 2825 Parklawn Drive, Midwest City, OK Zip 73110–4258; tel. 405/610–4411; Tim Parker, Chief Executive Officer

PENNSYLVANIA: COMMUNITY HOSPITAL OF LANCASTER (O, 142 beds) 1100 East Orange Street, Lancaster, PA Zip 17602–3218, Mailing Address: P.O. Box 3002, Zip 17604–3002; tel. 717/397–3711; Maureen Gallo, Administrator
Web address: www.chol.org

SOUTH CAROLINA: CAROLINA PINES REGIONAL MEDICAL CENTER (O, 116 beds) 1304 West BoBo Newsom Highway, Hartsville, SC Zip 29550; tel. 843/339–2100; Page Vaughan, Executive Director
Web address: www.hartsvillesc.com/byerly.html

UPSTATE CAROLINA MEDICAL CENTER (O, 125 beds) 1530 North Limestone Street, Gaffney, SC Zip 29340–4738; tel. 864/487–4271; Joe D. Howell, Executive Director

WEST VIRGINIA: WILLIAMSON MEMORIAL HOSPITAL (O, 76 beds) 859 Alderson Street, Williamson, WV Zip 25661–3215, Mailing Address: P.O. Box 1980, Zip 25661–1980; tel. 304/235–2500; Andrew Knizley, Chief Executive Officer

Owned, leased, sponsored:	34 hospitals	4150 beds
Contract-managed:	0 hospitals	0 beds
Totals:	34 hospitals	4150 beds

★**8815: HEALTH MIDWEST** (NP)
2304 East Meyer Boulevard, Suite A–20, Kansas City, MO Zip 64132–4104; tel. 816/276–9181; Richard W. Brown, President and Chief Executive Officer
(Centralized Health System)

KANSAS: ALLEN COUNTY HOSPITAL (L, 49 beds) 101 South First Street, Iola, KS Zip 66749–3505, Mailing Address: P.O. Box 540, Zip 66749–0540; tel. 316/365–1000; Bill May, Chief Executive Officer

MENORAH MEDICAL CENTER (O, 158 beds) 5721 West 119th Street, Shawnee Mission, KS Zip 66209–3722; tel. 913/498–6000; Steven D. Wilkinson, President and Chief Executive Officer
Web address: www.healthmidwest.org

OVERLAND PARK REGIONAL MEDICAL CENTER (L, 269 beds) 10500 Quivira Road, Shawnee Mission, KS Zip 66215–2306, Mailing Address: P.O. Box 15959, Zip 66215–5959; tel. 913/541–5000; Kevin J. Hicks, President and Chief Executive Officer
Web address: www.healthmidwest.org

MISSOURI: BAPTIST MEDICAL CENTER (O, 265 beds) 6601 Rockhill Road, Kansas City, MO Zip 64131–1197; tel. 816/276–7000; Darrell W. Moore, President and Chief Executive Officer
Web address: www.healthmidwest.org

CASS MEDICAL CENTER (C, 37 beds) 1800 East Mechanic Street, Harrisonville, MO Zip 64701–2099; tel. 816/380–3474; Alan O. Freeman, Chief Executive Officer
Web address: www.healthmidwest.org

HEDRICK MEDICAL CENTER (L, 80 beds) 100 Central Avenue, Chillicothe, MO Zip 64601–1599; tel. 660/646–1480; James K. Johnson, Chief Executive Officer
Web address: www.healthmidwest.org

INDEPENDENCE REGIONAL HEALTH CENTER (L, 329 beds) 1509 West Truman Road, Independence, MO Zip 64050–3498; tel. 816/836–8100; Michael W. Chappelow, President and Chief Executive Officer
Web address: www.healthmidwest.org

LAFAYETTE REGIONAL HEALTH CENTER (L, 37 beds) 1500 State Street, Lexington, MO Zip 64067–1199; tel. 660/259–2203; Jeffrey S. Tarrant, Administrator
Web address: www.healthmidwest.org

LEE'S SUMMIT HOSPITAL (O, 83 beds) 530 North Murray Road, Lees Summit, MO Zip 64081–1497; tel. 816/969–6000; John L. Jacobson, President and Chief Executive Officer
Web address: www.healthmidwest.org

MEDICAL CENTER OF INDEPENDENCE (O, 99 beds) 17203 East 23rd Street, Independence, MO Zip 64057–1899; tel. 816/478–5000; J. Kent Howard, President and Chief Executive Officer
Web address: www.healthmidwest.org

REHABILITATION INSTITUTE (O, 32 beds) 3011 Baltimore, Kansas City, MO Zip 64108–3465; tel. 816/751–7900; Ronald L. Herrick, President
Web address: www.healthmidwest.org

RESEARCH BELTON HOSPITAL (O, 47 beds) 17065 South 71 Highway, Belton, MO Zip 64012–2165; tel. 816/348–1200; Daniel F. Sheehan, Administrator
Web address: www.healthmidwest.org

RESEARCH MEDICAL CENTER (O, 483 beds) 2316 East Meyer Boulevard, Kansas City, MO Zip 64132–1199; tel. 816/276–4000; Steven R. Newton, President and Chief Executive Officer
Web address: www.healthmidwest.org

RESEARCH PSYCHIATRIC CENTER (O, 100 beds) 2323 East 63rd Street, Kansas City, MO Zip 64130–3495; tel. 816/444–8161; Todd Krass, Administrator and Chief Executive Officer
Web address: www.healthmidwest.org

TRINITY LUTHERAN HOSPITAL (O, 334 beds) 3030 Baltimore Avenue, Kansas City, MO Zip 64108–3404; tel. 816/751–4600; Ronald A. Ommen, President and Chief Executive Officer
Web address: www.healthmidwest.org

Owned, leased, sponsored:	14 hospitals	2365 beds
Contract-managed:	1 hospital	37 beds
Totals:	15 hospitals	2402 beds

0204: HEALTH SYSTEMS AMERICA (IO)
555 S.W. 148th Avenue, Sunrise, FL Zip 33325; tel. 954/915–0474; Michael Piercey, M.D., President and Chief Executive Officer

FLORIDA: SUNRISE REGIONAL MEDICAL CENTER (O, 100 beds) 555 S.W. 148th Avenue, Sunrise, FL Zip 33325–3072; tel. 954/370–0200; Humberto J. Munoz, Chief Executive Officer
Web address: www.sunriseregional.com

TEXAS: DESERT SPRINGS MEDICAL CENTER (O, 48 beds) 3300 South FM 1788, Midland, TX Zip 79711–2699, Mailing Address: P.O. Box 60608, Zip 79711–0608; tel. 915/563–1200; Marjorie McLoughlin, Chief Executive Officer

For explanation of codes following names, see page B2.
★ Indicates Type III membership in the American Hospital Association.

Systems / Health Systems America

Owned, leased, sponsored:	2 hospitals	148 beds
Contract-managed:	0 hospitals	0 beds
Totals:	2 hospitals	148 beds

2795: HEALTHCORP OF TENNESSEE, INC. (IO)
735 Broad Street, Chattanooga, TN Zip 37402; tel. 423/267-8406; T. Farrell Hayes, President
(Independent Hospital System)

ALABAMA: LAKESHORE COMMUNITY HOSPITAL (C, 28 beds) 201 Mariarden Road, Dadeville, AL Zip 36853, Mailing Address: P.O. Box 248, Zip 36853-0248; tel. 256/825-7821; Sue Boxx, Administrator

LAKEVIEW COMMUNITY HOSPITAL (C, 74 beds) 820 West Washington Street, Eufaula, AL Zip 36027-1899; tel. 334/687-5761; Carl A. Brown, Administrator

ARKANSAS: DALLAS COUNTY HOSPITAL (O, 32 beds) 201 Clifton Street, Fordyce, AR Zip 71742-3099; tel. 870/352-3155; Greg R. McNeil, Administrator

Owned, leased, sponsored:	1 hospital	32 beds
Contract-managed:	2 hospitals	102 beds
Totals:	3 hospitals	134 beds

★2185: HEALTHEAST (NP)
559 Capitol Boulevard, 6-South, Saint Paul, MN Zip 55103-0000; tel. 651/232-2300; Timothy H. Hanson, President and Chief Executive Officer
(Independent Hospital System)

MINNESOTA: BETHESDA REHABILITATION HOSPITAL (O, 127 beds) 559 Capitol Boulevard, Saint Paul, MN Zip 55103-2101; tel. 651/232-2000; Scott Batulis, Vice President and Administrator
Web address: www.healtheast.org

ST. JOHN'S HOSPITAL (O, 150 beds) 1575 Beam Avenue, Maplewood, MN Zip 55109; tel. 651/232-7000; Douglas P. Cropper, Vice President and Administrator
Web address: www.healtheast.org

ST. JOSEPH'S HOSPITAL (O, 292 beds) 69 West Exchange Street, Saint Paul, MN Zip 55102-1053; tel. 651/232-3000; Douglas P. Cropper, Vice President and Administrator
Web address: www.healtheast.org

Owned, leased, sponsored:	3 hospitals	569 beds
Contract-managed:	0 hospitals	0 beds
Totals:	3 hospitals	569 beds

0023: HEALTHSOUTH CORPORATION (IO)
One Healthsouth Parkway, Birmingham, AL Zip 35243; tel. 205/967-7116; Anthony J. Tanner, Executive Vice President
(Moderately Centralized Health System)

ALABAMA: HEALTHSOUTH LAKESHORE REHABILITATION HOSPITAL (O, 100 beds) 3800 Ridgeway Drive, Birmingham, AL Zip 35209-5599; tel. 205/868-2000; Terry Brown, Administrator and Chief Executive Officer

HEALTHSOUTH MEDICAL CENTER (O, 169 beds) 1201 11th Avenue South, Birmingham, AL Zip 35205-5299; tel. 205/930-7000; Luke Standeffer, Administrator and Chief Executive Officer

HEALTHSOUTH REHABILITATION HOSPITAL OF MONTGOMERY (O, 90 beds) 4465 Narrow Lane Road, Montgomery, AL Zip 36116-2900; tel. 334/284-7700; Linda Wade, Administrator and Director of Operations

HEALTHSOUTH REHABILITATION HOSPITAL OF NORTH ALABAMA (O, 50 beds) 107 Governors Drive S.W., Huntsville, AL Zip 35801-4329; tel. 256/535-2300; Rod Moss, Chief Executive Officer

HEALTHSOUTH METRO WEST HOSPITAL (O, 150 beds) 701 Richard M. Scrushy Parkway, Fairfield, AL Zip 35064; tel. 205/783-5121; Karen Davis, Chief Executive Officer

ARIZONA: HEALTHSOUTH MERIDIAN POINT REHABILITATION HOSPITAL (O, 40 beds) 11250 North 92nd Street, Scottsdale, AZ Zip 85260-6148; tel. 480/860-0671; Elizabeth Lamkin, Administrator

HEALTHSOUTH REHABILITATION INSTITUTE OF TUCSON (O, 80 beds) 2650 North Wyatt Drive, Tucson, AZ Zip 85712-6108; tel. 520/325-1300; Robbee Caseldine, Administrator

HEALTHSOUTH VALLEY OF THE SUN REHABILITATION HOSPITAL (O, 42 beds) 13460 North 67th Avenue, Glendale, AZ Zip 85304-1042; tel. 602/878-8800; Michael J. Oliver, Administrator

ARKANSAS: HEALTHSOUTH REHABILITATION HOSPITAL (O, 60 beds) 153 East Monte Painter Drive, Fayetteville, AR Zip 72703-4002; tel. 501/444-2200; Dennis R. Shelby, Chief Executive Officer
Web address: www.healthsouth.com

HEALTHSOUTH REHABILITATION HOSPITAL OF FORT SMITH (O, 80 beds) 1401 South J Street, Fort Smith, AR Zip 72901-5155; tel. 501/785-3300; Raymond Lenz, Director Operations
Web address: www.healthsouth.com

HEALTHSOUTH REHABILITATION HOSPITAL OF JONESBORO (O, 60 beds) 1201 Fleming Avenue, Jonesboro, AR Zip 72401-4311, Mailing Address: P.O. Box 1680, Zip 72403-1680; tel. 870/932-0440; Brenda Antwine, Administrator
Web address: www.healthsouth.com

CALIFORNIA: HEALTHSOUTH BAKERSFIELD REHABILITATION HOSPITAL (O, 60 beds) 5001 Commerce Drive, Bakersfield, CA Zip 93309; tel. 661/323-5500; Robyn Field, Ph.D., Chief Operating Officer

FLORIDA: HEALTHSOUTH DOCTORS' HOSPITAL (O, 157 beds) 5000 University Drive, Coral Gables, FL Zip 33146-2094; tel. 305/666-2111; Lincoln S. Mendez, Chief Executive Officer
Web address: www.healthsouth.com

HEALTHSOUTH REHABILITATION HOSPITAL (O, 60 beds) 901 North Clearwater-Largo Road, Largo, FL Zip 33770; tel. 727/586-2999; Elaine D. Ebaugh, Chief Executive Officer
Web address: www.healthsouth.com

HEALTHSOUTH REHABILITATION HOSPITAL (O, 45 beds) 20601 Old Cutler Road, Miami, FL Zip 33189-2400; tel. 305/251-3800; Nelson Lazo, Chief Executive Officer
Web address: www.healthsouth.com

HEALTHSOUTH REHABILITATION HOSPITAL OF SARASOTA (O, 60 beds) 3251 Proctor Road, Sarasota, FL Zip 34231-8538; tel. 941/921-8600; Jeff Garber, Administrator and Chief Executive Officer
Web address: www.healthsouth.com

HEALTHSOUTH REHABILITATION HOSPITAL OF TALLAHASSEE (O, 70 beds) 1675 Riggins Road, Tallahassee, FL Zip 32308-5315; tel. 850/656-4800; Armando Colombo, Chief Executive Officer
Web address: www.healthsouth.com

HEALTHSOUTH SEA PINES REHABILITATION HOSPITAL (O, 80 beds) 101 East Florida Avenue, Melbourne, FL Zip 32901-9966; tel. 321/984-4600; Denise B. McGrath, Chief Executive Officer
Web address: www.healthsouth.com

HEALTHSOUTH SUNRISE REHABILITATION HOSPITAL (O, 116 beds) 4399 Nob Hill Road, Fort Lauderdale, FL Zip 33351-5899; tel. 954/749-0300; Kevin R. Conn, Administrator
Web address: www.healthsouth.com

HEALTHSOUTH TREASURE COAST REHABILITATION HOSPITAL (O, 90 beds) 1600 37th Street, Vero Beach, FL Zip 32960-6549; tel. 561/778-2100; Jason N. Roebuck, Chief Executive Officer
Web address: www.healthsouth.com

GEORGIA: HEALTHSOUTH CENTRAL GEORGIA REHABILITATION HOSPITAL (O, 50 beds) 3351 Northside Drive, Macon, GA Zip 31210-2591; tel. 912/471-3536; Elbert T. McQueen, Chief Executive Officer
Web address: www.healthsouth.com

INDIANA: HEALTHSOUTH TRI-STATE REHABILITATION HOSPITAL (O, 80 beds) 4100 Covert Avenue, Evansville, IN Zip 47714-5567, Mailing Address: P.O. Box 5349, Zip 47716-5349; tel. 812/476-9983; Barbara Butler, Administrator and Chief Operating Officer
Web address: www.healthsouth.com

HEALTHSOUTH REHABILITATION HOSPITAL OF KOKOMO (O, 60 beds) 829 North Dixon Road, Kokomo, IN Zip 46901-7709; tel. 765/452-6700; Allen Tyra, Administrator
Web address: www.healthsouth.com

REHABILITATION HOSPITAL OF FORT WAYNE (O, 60 beds) 7970 West Jefferson Boulevard, Fort Wayne, IN Zip 46804-4140; tel. 219/436-2644; Norman F. Stephens, Chief Executive Officer

For explanation of codes following names, see page B2.
★ Indicates Type III membership in the American Hospital Association.

Systems / Healthsouth Corporation

KANSAS: MID-AMERICA REHABILITATION HOSPITAL (O, 80 beds) 5701 West 110th Street, Overland Park, KS Zip 66211; tel. 913/491-2400; Mark J. Stepanik, Interim Chief Executive Officer

WESLEY REHABILITATION HOSPITAL (O, 65 beds) 8338 West 13th Street North, Wichita, KS Zip 67212-2984; tel. 316/729-9999; Robyn Chadwick, Administrator

KENTUCKY: HEALTHSOUTH NORTHERN KENTUCKY REHABILITATION HOSPITAL (O, 40 beds) 201 Medical Village Drive, Covington, KY Zip 41017-3407; tel. 606/341-2044; Timothy W. Mitchell, Chief Executive Officer

HEALTHSOUTH REHABILITATION HOSPITAL OF CENTRAL KENTUCKY (O, 40 beds) 134 Heartland Drive, Elizabethtown, KY Zip 42701-2778; tel. 270/769-3100; Mark K. Floro, Chief Operating Officer

LOUISIANA: HEALTHSOUTH NORTH LOUISIANA REHABILITATION HOSPITAL (O, 90 beds) 1401 Ezell Street, Ruston, LA Zip 71270-7221, Mailing Address: P.O. Box 490, Zip 71273-0490; tel. 318/251-5354; Mark Rice, Chief Executive Officer

HEALTHSOUTH REHABILITATION HOSPITAL OF BATON ROUGE (O, 80 beds) 8595 United Plaza Boulevard, Baton Rouge, LA Zip 70809-2251; tel. 225/927-0567; Michael D. Marshall, Chief Executive Officer

MAINE: NEW ENGLAND REHABILITATION HOSPITAL OF PORTLAND (O, 76 beds) 335 Brighton Avenue, Portland, ME Zip 04102; tel. 207/775-4000; Amy Morse, Chief Executive Officer

MARYLAND: HEALTHSOUTH CHESAPEAKE REHABILITATION HOSPITAL (O, 42 beds) 220 Tilghman Road, Salisbury, MD Zip 21804-1921; tel. 410/546-4600; William Roth, Chief Executive Officer

MASSACHUSETTS: FAIRLAWN REHABILITATION HOSPITAL (O, 110 beds) 189 May Street, Worcester, MA Zip 01602-4399; tel. 508/791-6351; Peter M. Mantegazza, President and Chief Executive Officer

HEALTHSOUTH BRAINTREE REHABILITATION HOSPITAL (O, 187 beds) 250 Pond Street, Braintree, MA Zip 02185-9020; tel. 781/848-5353; Anne M. MacRitchie, Chief Executive Officer

HEALTHSOUTH NEW ENGLAND REHABILITATION HOSPITAL (O, 273 beds) Two Rehabilitation Way, Woburn, MA Zip 01801-6098; tel. 781/935-5050; Mary Moscato, Chief Executive Officer

HEALTHSOUTH REHABILITATION HOSPITAL OF WESTERN MASSACHUSETTS (O, 40 beds) 14 Chestnut Place, Ludlow, MA Zip 01056-3460; tel. 413/589-7581; R. David Richer, Administrator

NEW HAMPSHIRE: HEALTHSOUTH REHABILITATION HOSPITAL (O, 50 beds) 254 Pleasant Street, Concord, NH Zip 03301-2508; tel. 603/226-9800; Lori Manor Underwood, Administrator

NEW JERSEY: HEALTHSOUTH REHABILITATION HOSPITAL OF NEW JERSEY (O, 155 beds) 14 Hospital Drive, Toms River, NJ Zip 08755-6470; tel. 732/244-3100; Patricia Ostaszewski, Chief Executive Officer and Administrator

NEW MEXICO: HEALTHSOUTH REHABILITATION CENTER (O, 60 beds) 7000 Jefferson N.E., Albuquerque, NM Zip 87109-4357; tel. 505/344-9478; Darby Brockette, Chief Executive Officer

OKLAHOMA: HEALTHSOUTH REHABILITATION HOSPITAL (O, 46 beds) 700 N.W. Seventh Street, Oklahoma City, OK Zip 73102-1295; tel. 405/553-1192; Hank Ross, Chief Executive Officer

PENNSYLVANIA: HEALTHSOUTH GREATER PITTSBURGH REHABILITATION HOSPITAL (O, 89 beds) 2380 McGinley Road, Monroeville, PA Zip 15146-4400; tel. 412/856-2400; Faith A. Deigan, Administrator and Chief Executive Officer
Web address: www.healthsouth.com

HEALTHSOUTH HARMARVILLE REHABILITATION HOSPITAL (O, 202 beds) Guys Run Road, Pittsburgh, PA Zip 15238-0460, Mailing Address: Box 11460, Guys Run Road, Zip 15238-0460; tel. 412/781-5700; Faith A. Deigan, Interim Administrator

HEALTHSOUTH LAKE ERIE INSTITUTE OF REHABILITATION (O, 99 beds) 143 East Second Street, Erie, PA Zip 16507-1403; tel. 814/453-5602; Louis M. Condrasky, Chief Executive Officer

HEALTHSOUTH NITTANY VALLEY REHABILITATION HOSPITAL (O, 87 beds) 550 West College Avenue, Pleasant Gap, PA Zip 16823-8808; tel. 814/359-3421; Tom Swavely, Administrator and Chief Executive Officer

HEALTHSOUTH READING REHABILITATION HOSPITAL (O, 76 beds) 1623 Morgantown Road, Reading, PA Zip 19607-9455; tel. 610/796-6000; Tammy L. Ober, Administrator and Chief Executive Officer
Web address: www.healthsouth.com

HEALTHSOUTH REHABILITATION HOSPITAL (O, 25 beds) 303 Camp Meeting Road, Sewickley, PA Zip 15143-8348; tel. 412/741-9500; Kenneth J. Anthony, President and Chief Executive Officer
Web address: www.healthsouth.com

HEALTHSOUTH REHABILITATION HOSPITAL OF ALTOONA (O, 70 beds) 2005 Valley View Boulevard, Altoona, PA Zip 16602-4598; tel. 814/944-3535; Scott Filler, Chief Executive Officer

HEALTHSOUTH REHABILITATION HOSPITAL OF ERIE (O, 108 beds) 143 East Second Street, Erie, PA Zip 16507-1595; tel. 814/878-1200; Louis M. Condrasky, Chief Executive Officer

HEALTHSOUTH REHABILITATION HOSPITAL OF YORK (O, 88 beds) 1850 Normandie Drive, York, PA Zip 17404-1534; tel. 717/767-6941; Cheryl Fleming, Chief Executive Officer

HEALTHSOUTH REHABILITATION OF MECHANICSBURG (O, 103 beds) 175 Lancaster Boulevard, Mechanicsburg, PA Zip 17055-0736, Mailing Address: P.O. Box 2016, Zip 17055-2016; tel. 717/691-3700; Melissa Kutz, Administrator and Chief Executive Officer

SOUTH CAROLINA: HEALTHSOUTH REHABILITATION HOSPITAL (O, 87 beds) 2935 Colonial Drive, Columbia, SC Zip 29203-6811; tel. 803/254-7777; Debbie W. Johnston, Director Operations
Web address: www.healthsouth.com

HEALTHSOUTH REHABILITATION HOSPITAL (O, 88 beds) 900 East Cheves Street, Florence, SC Zip 29506-2704; tel. 843/679-9000; Dennis A. Lofe, FACHE, Chief Executive Officer
Web address: www.healthsouth.com

TENNESSEE: HEALTHSOUTH CHATTANOOGA REHABILITATION HOSPITAL (O, 69 beds) 2412 McCallie Avenue, Chattanooga, TN Zip 37404-3398; tel. 423/698-0221; Donna Bourdon, Chief Operating Officer
Web address: www.healthsouth.com

HEALTHSOUTH REHABILITATION HOSPITAL (O, 50 beds) 113 Cassel Drive, Kingsport, TN Zip 37660-3775; tel. 423/246-7240; Terry R. Maxhimer, Administrator and Chief Executive Officer
Web address: www.healthsouth.com

HEALTHSOUTH REHABILITATION HOSPITAL (O, 80 beds) 1282 Union Avenue, Memphis, TN Zip 38104-3414; tel. 901/722-2000; Jerry Gray, Administrator
Web address: www.healthsouth.com

TEXAS: HEALTHSOUTH HOUSTON REHABILITATION INSTITUTE (O, 79 beds) 17506 Red Oak Drive, Houston, TX Zip 77090-7721, Mailing Address: P.O. Box 73684, Zip 77273-3684; tel. 281/580-1212; Anne R. Leon, Chief Executive Officer
Web address: www.healthsouth.com

HEALTHSOUTH MEDICAL CENTER (O, 86 beds) 2124 Research Row, Dallas, TX Zip 75235-2504; tel. 214/904-6100; Robert M. Smart, Area Manager and Chief Executive Officer
Web address: www.healthsouth.com

HEALTHSOUTH PLANO REHABILITATION HOSPITAL (O, 62 beds) 2800 West 15th Street, Plano, TX Zip 75075-7526; tel. 972/612-9000; Tracey Nixon, Chief Executive Officer
Web address: www.healthsouth.com

HEALTHSOUTH REHABILITATION HOSPITAL (O, 60 beds) 19002 McKay Drive, Humble, TX Zip 77338-5701; tel. 281/446-6148; Darrell L. Pile, Regional Vice President
Web address: www.healthsouth.com

HEALTHSOUTH REHABILITATION HOSPITAL OF ARLINGTON (O, 65 beds) 3200 Matlock Road, Arlington, TX Zip 76015-2911; tel. 817/468-4000; Philip Patterson, Administrator and Chief Operating Officer
Web address: www.healthsouth.com

HEALTHSOUTH REHABILITATION HOSPITAL OF AUSTIN (O, 79 beds) 1215 Red River Street, Austin, TX Zip 78701; tel. 512/474-5700; Laurie Bajich, Chief Executive Officer
Web address: www.healthsouth.com

HEALTHSOUTH REHABILITATION HOSPITAL OF BEAUMONT (O, 61 beds) 3340 Plaza 10 Boulevard, Beaumont, TX Zip 77707; tel. 409/835-0835; Michael Hagen, Administrator
Web address: www.healthsouth.com

For explanation of codes following names, see page B2.
★ *Indicates Type III membership in the American Hospital Association.*

Systems / Healthsouth Corporation

HEALTHSOUTH REHABILITATION HOSPITAL OF FORT WORTH (O, 60 beds) 1212 West Lancaster Avenue, Fort Worth, TX Zip 76102–4510; tel. 817/870–2336; S. Denise Borroni, Administrator and Chief Executive Officer
Web address: www.healthsouth.com

HEALTHSOUTH REHABILITATION HOSPITAL OF TEXARKANA (O, 60 beds) 515 West 12th Street, Texarkana, TX Zip 75501–4416; tel. 903/793–0088; Nate Miller, Chief Executive Officer
Web address: www.healthsouth.com

HEALTHSOUTH REHABILITATION HOSPITAL–CITYVIEW (O, 62 beds) 6701 Oakmont Boulevard, Fort Worth, TX Zip 76132–2957; tel. 817/370–4700; Mark Bennett, Administrator and Chief Executive Officer
Web address: www.healthsouth.com

HEALTHSOUTH REHABILITATION HOSPITAL–TYLER (O, 63 beds) 3131 Troup Highway, Tyler, TX Zip 75701–8352; tel. 903/510–7000; Sharla Anderson, Interim Chief Executive Officer
Web address: www.healthsouth.com

HEALTHSOUTH REHABILITATION HOSPITAL–WICHITA FALLS (O, 63 beds) 3901 Armory Road, Wichita Falls, TX Zip 76302–2204; tel. 940/720–5700; Martin A. Lautner, Chief Executive Officer
Web address: www.healthsouth.com

HEALTHSOUTH REHABILITATION INSTITUTE OF SAN ANTONIO (O, 108 beds) 9119 Cinnamon Hill, San Antonio, TX Zip 78240–5401; tel. 210/691–0737; Diane B. Lampe, Administrator and Chief Executive Officer
Web address: www.healthsouth.com

UTAH: HEALTHSOUTH REHABILITATION HOSPITAL OF UTAH (O, 86 beds) 8074 South 1300 East, Sandy, UT Zip 84094–0743; tel. 801/561–3400; Richard M. Richards, Administrator

VIRGINIA: HEALTHSOUTH MEDICAL CENTER (O, 147 beds) 7700 East Parham Road, Richmond, VA Zip 23294–4301; tel. 804/747–5600; Charles A. Stark, CHE, Administrator, Chief Executive Officer and Regional Vice President
Web address: www.healthsouth-richmond.com

HEALTHSOUTH REHABILITATION HOSPITAL OF VIRGINIA (O, 40 beds) 5700 Fitzhugh Avenue, Richmond, VA Zip 23226–1800; tel. 804/288–5700; Jeff Ruskan, Administrator
Web address: www.healthsouth.com

WEST VIRGINIA: HEALTHSOUTH HUNTINGTON REHABILITATION HOSPITAL (O, 40 beds) 6900 West Country Club Drive, Huntington, WV Zip 25705–2000; tel. 304/733–1060; John Forester, Chief Operating Officer

HEALTHSOUTH MOUNTAINVIEW REGIONAL REHABILITATION HOSPITAL (O, 80 beds) 1160 Van Voorhis Road, Morgantown, WV Zip 26505–3435; tel. 304/598–1100; Teresa K. Stranko, Chief Executive Officer
Web address: www.healthsouth.com

HEALTHSOUTH SOUTHERN HILLS REHABILITATION HOSPITAL (O, 54 beds) 120 Twelfth Street, Princeton, WV Zip 24740–2312; tel. 304/487–8000; Ken Howell, Administrator
Web address: www.healthsouth.com

HEALTHSOUTH WESTERN HILLS REGIONAL REHABILITATION HOSPITAL (O, 40 beds) 3 Western Hills Drive, Parkersburg, WV Zip 26101–8122; tel. 304/420–1300; Thomas Heller, Administrator

Owned, leased, sponsored:	75 hospitals	6059 beds
Contract–managed:	0 hospitals	0 beds
Totals:	75 hospitals	6059 beds

1985: HEALTHSYSTEM MINNESOTA (NP)
6500 Excelsior Boulevard, Saint Louis Park, MN Zip 55426–4702; tel. 612/993–5000; David Wessner, President and Chief Executive Officer
(Centralized Physician/Insurance Health System)

MINNESOTA: GLENCOE REGIONAL HEALTH SERVICES (C, 149 beds) 705 East 18th Street, Glencoe, MN Zip 55336–1499; tel. 320/864–3121; Jon D. Braband, President and Chief Executive Officer
Web address: www.glencoeregionalhealth.org

METHODIST HOSPITAL HEALTHSYSTEM MINNESOTA (O, 376 beds) 6500 Excelsior Boulevard, Saint Louis Park, MN Zip 55426–4702, Mailing Address: P.O. Box 650, Minneapolis, Zip 55440–0650; tel. 952/993–5000; Mark Skubic, Vice President
Web address: www.healthsystemminnesota.com

Owned, leased, sponsored:	1 hospital	376 beds
Contract–managed:	1 hospital	149 beds
Totals:	2 hospitals	525 beds

★9505: HENRY FORD HEALTH SYSTEM (NP)
One Ford Place, Detroit, MI Zip 48202–3067; tel. 313/876–8715; Gail L. Warden, President and Chief Executive Officer
(Centralized Physician/Insurance Health System)

MICHIGAN: BI–COUNTY COMMUNITY HOSPITAL (O, 164 beds) 13355 East Ten Mile Road, Warren, MI Zip 48089–2065; tel. 810/759–7300; Gary W. Popiel, Executive Vice President and Chief Executive Officer

HENRY FORD HOSPITAL (O, 668 beds) 2799 West Grand Boulevard, Detroit, MI Zip 48202–2689; tel. 313/916–2600; Stephen H. Velick, Chief Executive Officer
Web address: www.henryfordhealth.org

HENRY FORD KINGSWOOD HOSPITAL (O, 64 beds) 10300 West Eight Mile Road, Ferndale, MI Zip 48220–2198; tel. 248/398–3200; Glenn Black, Associate Vice President and Chief Operating Officer

HENRY FORD WYANDOTTE HOSPITAL (O, 355 beds) 2333 Biddle Avenue, Wyandotte, MI Zip 48192–4693; tel. 734/246–6000; William R. Alvin, President
Web address: www.henryfordhealth.org

RIVERSIDE OSTEOPATHIC HOSPITAL (O, 138 beds) 150 Truax Street, Trenton, MI Zip 48183–2151; tel. 734/676–4200; Dennis R. Lemanski, D.O., Vice President and Chief Executive Officer
Web address: www.henryfordhealth.org

Owned, leased, sponsored:	5 hospitals	1389 beds
Contract–managed:	0 hospitals	0 beds
Totals:	5 hospitals	1389 beds

★0130: HILLCREST HEALTHCARE SYSTEM (NP)
1120 South Utica, Tulsa, OK Zip 74104–4090; tel. 918/579–1000; Donald A. Lorack, Jr, President and Chief Executive Officer
(Centralized Physician/Insurance Health System)

OKLAHOMA: BRISTOW MEMORIAL HOSPITAL (L, 22 beds) Seventh and Spruce Streets, Bristow, OK Zip 74010, Mailing Address: P.O. Box 780, Zip 74010–0780; tel. 918/367–2215; Ron Cackler, President and Chief Executive Officer

CHILDREN'S MEDICAL CENTER (O, 108 beds) 5300 East Skelly Drive, Tulsa, OK Zip 74135–6599, Mailing Address: P.O. Box 35648, Zip 74153–0648; tel. 918/664–6600; Gerald Rothlein, Chief Executive Officer

CLEVELAND AREA HOSPITAL (L, 19 beds) 1401 West Pawnee Street, Cleveland, OK Zip 74020–3019; tel. 918/358–2501; Thomas Henton, Chief Executive Officer

DOCTORS HOSPITAL (O, 121 beds) 2323 South Harvard Avenue, Tulsa, OK Zip 74114–3370; tel. 918/744–4000; Kenneth Noteboom, Chief Executive Officer
Web address: www.hillcrest.com

EASTERN OKLAHOMA MEDICAL CENTER (L, 72 beds) 105 Wall Street, Poteau, OK Zip 74953, Mailing Address: P.O. Box 1148, Zip 74953–1148; tel. 918/647–8161; L. Gene Matthews, Chief Executive Officer

FAIRFAX MEMORIAL HOSPITAL (L, 15 beds) Taft Avenue and Highway 18, Fairfax, OK Zip 74637, Mailing Address: P.O. Box 219, Zip 74637–0219; tel. 918/642–3291; Xavier Villarreal, Chief Executive Officer

HILLCREST MEDICAL CENTER (O, 421 beds) 1120 South Utica, Tulsa, OK Zip 74104–4090; tel. 918/579–1000; Donald A. Lorack, Jr, President and Chief Executive Officer
Web address: www.hillcrest.com

HILLCREST SPECIALTY HOSPITAL (O, 22 beds) 2408 East 81st Street, 2500, Tulsa, OK Zip 74137–4210; tel. 918/491–2400; Kenneth Noteboom, Chief Executive Officer
Web address: www.hcahealthcare.com

For explanation of codes following names, see page B2.
★ Indicates Type III membership in the American Hospital Association.

Systems / Iasis Healthcare

HURLEY HEALTH CENTER (L, 95 beds) 6 North Covington Street, Coalgate, OK Zip 74538-2002, Mailing Address: P.O. Box 326, Zip 74538; tel. 580/927-2327; Dan A. Clements, Chief Executive Officer

PRAGUE MUNICIPAL HOSPITAL (L, 19 beds) 1322 Klabzuba Avenue, Prague, OK Zip 74864, Mailing Address: P.O. Drawer S, Zip 74864; tel. 405/567-4922; Chris Mattingly, Chief Executive Officer

TULSA REGIONAL MEDICAL CENTER (O, 255 beds) 744 West Ninth Street, Tulsa, OK Zip 74127-9990; tel. 918/599-5900; Steve Dobbs, Chief Executive Officer

WAGONER COMMUNITY HOSPITAL (L, 100 beds) 1200 West Cherokee, Wagoner, OK Zip 74467-4681, Mailing Address: Box 407, Zip 74477-0407; tel. 918/485-5514; John W. Crawford, Chief Executive Officer

Owned, leased, sponsored:	12 hospitals	1269 beds
Contract-managed:	0 hospitals	0 beds
Totals:	12 hospitals	1269 beds

★0027: **HORIZON HEALTHCARE, INC.** (NP)
2300 North Mayfair Road, Suite 550, Milwaukee, WI Zip 53226-1508; tel. 414/257-3888; Sister Renee Rose, President and Chief Executive Officer
(Moderately Centralized Health System)

WISCONSIN: COLUMBIA HOSPITAL (C, 328 beds) 2025 East Newport Avenue, Milwaukee, WI Zip 53211-2990; tel. 414/961-3300; Susan Henckel, Executive Vice President and Chief Operating Officer
Web address: www.columbia-stmarys.com

COMMUNITY MEMORIAL HOSPITAL (C, 142 beds) W180 N8085 Town Hall Road, Menomonee Falls, WI Zip 53051, Mailing Address: P.O. Box 408, Zip 53052-0408; tel. 262/251-1000; Robert E. Drisner, President and Chief Executive Officer
Web address: www.communitymemorial.com

FROEDTERT MEMORIAL LUTHERAN HOSPITAL (C, 472 beds) 9200 West Wisconsin Avenue, Milwaukee, WI Zip 53226-3596, Mailing Address: P.O. Box 26099, Zip 53226-3596; tel. 414/259-3000; William D. Petasnick, President
Web address: www.froedtert.com

KENOSHA HOSPITAL AND MEDICAL CENTER (C, 143 beds) 6308 Eighth Avenue, Kenosha, WI Zip 53143-5082; tel. 262/656-2011; Richard O. Schmidt, Jr, President and Chief Executive Officer

Owned, leased, sponsored:	0 hospitals	0 beds
Contract-managed:	4 hospitals	1085 beds
Totals:	4 hospitals	1085 beds

★5355: **HOSPITAL SISTERS HEALTH SYSTEM** (CC)
Springfield, IL Mailing Address: P.O. Box 19431, Zip 62794-9431; tel. 217/523-4747; Sister Jomary Trstensky, President
(Moderately Centralized Health System)

ILLINOIS: ST. ANTHONY'S MEMORIAL HOSPITAL (O, 146 beds) 503 North Maple Street, Effingham, IL Zip 62401-2099; tel. 217/342-2121; Daniel J. Woods, Executive Vice President and Administrator
Web address: www.stanthonyhospital.org

ST. ELIZABETH'S HOSPITAL (O, 289 beds) 211 South Third Street, Belleville, IL Zip 62220-1998; tel. 618/234-2120; Gerald M. Harman, Executive Vice President and Administrator
Web address: www.steliz.org

ST. FRANCIS HOSPITAL (O, 97 beds) 1215 Franciscan Drive, Litchfield, IL Zip 62056, Mailing Address: P.O. Box 1215, Zip 62056-1215; tel. 217/324-2191; Michael Sipkoski, Executive Vice President and Administrator

ST. JOHN'S HOSPITAL (O, 568 beds) 800 East Carpenter Street, Springfield, IL Zip 62769-0002; tel. 217/544-6464; Allison C. Laabs, Executive Vice President and Administrator
Web address: www.st-johns.org

ST. JOSEPH'S HOSPITAL (O, 57 beds) 9515 Holy Cross Lane, Breese, IL Zip 62230-0099; tel. 618/526-4511; Jacolyn M. Schlautman, Executive Vice President and Administrator

ST. JOSEPH'S HOSPITAL (O, 106 beds) 1515 Main Street, Highland, IL Zip 62249-1656; tel. 618/654-7421; Anthony G. Mastrangelo, Executive Vice President and Administrator
Web address: www.stjosephs-highland.org

ST. MARY'S HOSPITAL (O, 176 beds) 1800 East Lake Shore Drive, Decatur, IL Zip 62521-3883; tel. 217/464-2966; Anthony D. Pfitzer, Executive Vice President and Administrator
Web address: www.stmarys-hospital.com

ST. MARY'S HOSPITAL (O, 170 beds) 111 East Spring Street, Streator, IL Zip 61364-3399; tel. 815/673-2311; Thomas Whelan, Acting Administrator
Web address: www.ortelco.com/~stmaryl

WISCONSIN: SACRED HEART HOSPITAL (O, 179 beds) 900 West Clairemont Avenue, Eau Claire, WI Zip 54701-6122; tel. 715/839-4121; Stephen F. Ronstrom, Executive Vice President and Administrator
Web address: www.sacredhearthospital-ec.org

ST. JOSEPH'S HOSPITAL (O, 127 beds) 2661 County Highway I, Chippewa Falls, WI Zip 54729-1498; tel. 715/723-1811; David B. Fish, Executive Vice President
Web address: www.stjoeschipfalls.com

ST. MARY'S HOSPITAL MEDICAL CENTER (O, 119 beds) 1726 Shawano Avenue, Green Bay, WI Zip 54303-3282; tel. 920/498-4200; James G. Coller, Executive Vice President and Administrator
Web address: www.stmgb.org

ST. NICHOLAS HOSPITAL (O, 185 beds) 1601 North Taylor Drive, Sheboygan, WI Zip 53081-2496; tel. 920/459-8300; Michael J. Stenger, Executive Vice President and Administrator
Web address: www.stnicholashospital.org

ST. VINCENT HOSPITAL (O, 285 beds) 835 South Van Buren Street, Green Bay, WI Zip 54307-3508, Mailing Address: P.O. Box 13508, Zip 54307-3508; tel. 920/433-0111; Joseph J. Neidenbach, Administrator and Chief Executive Officer
Web address: www.stvgb.org

Owned, leased, sponsored:	13 hospitals	2504 beds
Contract-managed:	0 hospitals	0 beds
Totals:	13 hospitals	2504 beds

0201: **IASIS HEALTHCARE** (IO)
104 Woodmont Boulevard, Suite 101, Nashville, TN Zip 37205; tel. 615/844-2747; Wayne Gower, President and Chief Executive Officer

ARIZONA: MESA GENERAL HOSPITAL MEDICAL CENTER (O, 143 beds) 515 North Mesa Drive, Mesa, AZ Zip 85201-5989; tel. 480/969-9111; Patrick T. Walz, Chief Executive Officer

ST. LUKE'S BEHAVIORAL HEALTH CENTER (O, 70 beds) 1800 East Van Buren, Phoenix, AZ Zip 85006-3742; tel. 602/251-8546; Patrick D. Waugh, Chief Executive Officer

ST. LUKE'S MEDICAL CENTER (O, 282 beds) 1800 East Van Buren Street, Phoenix, AZ Zip 85006-3742; tel. 602/251-8100; Robert M. Luther, Chief Executive Officer

TEMPE ST. LUKE'S HOSPITAL (O, 110 beds) 1500 South Mill Avenue, Tempe, AZ Zip 85281-6699; tel. 480/784-5510; Joel F. Engles, Administrator

FLORIDA: MEMORIAL HOSPITAL OF TAMPA (O, 140 beds) 2901 Swann Avenue, Tampa, FL Zip 33609-4057; tel. 813/873-6400; John Mainieri, Interim Chief Executive Officer
Web address: www.tenethealth.com/tampa

PALMS OF PASADENA HOSPITAL (O, 267 beds) 1501 Pasadena Avenue South, Saint Petersburg, FL Zip 33707-3798; tel. 727/381-1000; John D. Bartlett, Chief Executive Officer
Web address: www.tenethealth.com

TOWN AND COUNTRY HOSPITAL (O, 148 beds) 6001 Webb Road, Tampa, FL Zip 33615-3291; tel. 813/885-6666; Phillip J. Mazzuca, Chief Executive Officer
Web address: www.tenethealth.com

TEXAS: MID-JEFFERSON HOSPITAL (O, 138 beds) Highway 365 and 27th Street, Nederland, TX Zip 77627-6288, Mailing Address: P.O. Box 1917, Zip 77627-1917; tel. 409/727-2321; Michael Miller, Chief Executive Officer
Web address: www.tenethealth.com

For explanation of codes following names, see page B2.
★ Indicates Type III membership in the American Hospital Association.

Systems / Iasis Healthcare

ODESSA REGIONAL HOSPITAL (O, 100 beds) 520 East Sixth Street, Odessa, TX Zip 79761-4565, Mailing Address: P.O. Box 4859, Zip 79760-4859; tel. 915/334-8200; Michael S. Potter, FACHE, President and Chief Execfutive Officer
Web address: www.orh.net

PARK PLACE MEDICAL CENTER (O, 219 beds) 3050 39th Street, Port Arthur, TX Zip 77642-5535, Mailing Address: P.O. Box 1648, Zip 77641-1648; tel. 409/983-4951; Michael S. Miller, Chief Executive Officer
Web address: www.tenethealth.com

SOUTHWEST GENERAL HOSPITAL (O, 200 beds) 7400 Barlite Boulevard, San Antonio, TX Zip 78224-1399; tel. 210/921-2000; Keith Swinney, Chief Executive Officer
Web address: www.tenethealth.comswgh

UTAH: DAVIS HOSPITAL AND MEDICAL CENTER (O, 126 beds) 1600 West Antelope Drive, Layton, UT Zip 84041-1142; tel. 801/825-9561; Bruce A. Baldwin, Chief Executive Officer

JORDAN VALLEY HOSPITAL (O, 50 beds) 3580 West 9000 South, West Jordan, UT Zip 84088-8811; tel. 801/561-8888; Jeffrey J. Manley, Chief Executive Officer

PIONEER VALLEY HOSPITAL (O, 127 beds) 3460 South Pioneer Parkway, Salt Lake City, UT Zip 84120-2648; tel. 801/964-3100; Keith Tintle, Chief Executive Officer

SALT LAKE REGIONAL MEDICAL CENTER (O, 138 beds) 1050 East South Temple, Salt Lake City, UT Zip 84102-1599; tel. 801/350-4111; Kay Matsumura, Chief Executive Officer

Owned, leased, sponsored:	15 hospitals	2258 beds
Contract-managed:	0 hospitals	0 beds
Totals:	15 hospitals	2258 beds

2025: INFIRMARY HEALTH SYSTEM, INC. (NP)
3 Mobile Infirmary Circle, Mobile, AL Zip 36607-3520; tel. 334/435-5500; E. Chandler Bramlett , Jr, President and Chief Executive Officer
(Moderately Centralized Health System)

ALABAMA: GROVE HILL MEMORIAL HOSPITAL (C, 34 beds) 295 South Jackson Street, Grove Hill, AL Zip 36451-0935, Mailing Address: P.O. Box 935, Zip 36451-0935; tel. 334/275-3191; Hybard D. Sewell, Administrator

MOBILE INFIRMARY MEDICAL CENTER (O, 502 beds) 5 Mobile Infirmary Drive North, Mobile, AL Zip 36601, Mailing Address: P.O. Box 2144, Zip 36652-2144; tel. 334/435-2400; E. Chandler Bramlett , Jr, President and Chief Executive Officer
Web address: www.mimc.com

THOMASVILLE INFIRMARY (O, 27 beds) 33700 Highway 43, Thomasville, AL Zip 36784; tel. 334/636-4431; Albert Ban , Jr, Administrator

WASHINGTON COUNTY INFIRMARY AND NURSING HOME (C, 94 beds) St. Stephens Avenue, Chatom, AL Zip 36518, Mailing Address: P.O. Box 597, Zip 36518-0597; tel. 334/847-2223; John S. Eads, Administrator

Owned, leased, sponsored:	2 hospitals	529 beds
Contract-managed:	2 hospitals	128 beds
Totals:	4 hospitals	657 beds

★1305: INOVA HEALTH SYSTEM (NP)
8110 Gatehouse Road, Falls Church, VA Zip 22042; tel. 703/289-2069; J. Knox Singleton, President and Chief Executive Officer
(Centralized Health System)

VIRGINIA: INOVA ALEXANDRIA HOSPITAL (O, 311 beds) 4320 Seminary Road, Alexandria, VA Zip 22304-1594; tel. 703/504-3000; Kenneth H. Kozloff, FACHE, Administrator
Web address: www.inova.com

INOVA FAIR OAKS HOSPITAL (O, 151 beds) 3600 Joseph Siewick Drive, Fairfax, VA Zip 22033-1709; tel. 703/391-3600; William A. Brown, CHE, Vice President and Administrator
Web address: www.inova.com

INOVA FAIRFAX HOSPITAL (O, 656 beds) 3300 Gallows Road, Falls Church, VA Zip 22042-3300; tel. 703/698-1110; Steven E. Brown, Administrator
Web address: www.inova.com

INOVA MOUNT VERNON HOSPITAL (O, 229 beds) 2501 Parker's Lane, Alexandria, VA Zip 22306-3209; tel. 703/664-7000; Susan Herbert, Administrator
Web address: www.inova.org

Owned, leased, sponsored:	4 hospitals	1347 beds
Contract-managed:	0 hospitals	0 beds
Totals:	4 hospitals	1347 beds

0182: INTEGRATED HEALTH SERVICES (IO)
910 Rudgebrook Road, Sparks Glencoe, MD Zip 21152; tel. 410/773-1000; Robert Elkins, M.D., Chairman and Chief Exective Officer
(Independent Hospital System)

OKLAHOMA: INTEGRATED SPECIALTY HOSPITAL (O, 43 beds) 1100 East Ninth Street, Edmond, OK Zip 73034-5755; tel. 405/341-8150; Joe Smithers, Administrator

INTEGRATED SPECIALTY HOSPITAL (O, 31 beds) 8210 National Avenue, Midwest City, OK Zip 73110; tel. 405/739-0800; Gayla Campbell, Administrator

TEXAS: IHS HOSPITAL AT SAN ANTONIO (O, 27 beds) 7310 Oak Manor Drive, San Antonio, TX Zip 78229-4509; tel. 210/308-0261; Peggy Cliff, Administrator
Web address: www.ihs-inc.com

IHS HOSPITAL OF LUBBOCK (O, 88 beds) 1409 9th Street, Lubbock, TX Zip 79401-2601; tel. 806/767-9133; Steve Grappe, Administrator
Web address: www.ihs-inc.com

IHS OF AMARILLO (O, 20 beds) 5601 Plum Creek Drive, Amarillo, TX Zip 79124; tel. 806/351-1000; Neal Duncan, Executive Director
Web address: www.ihs-inc.com

Owned, leased, sponsored:	5 hospitals	209 beds
Contract-managed:	0 hospitals	0 beds
Totals:	5 hospitals	209 beds

★0305: INTEGRIS HEALTH (NP)
3366 N.W. Expressway, Suite 800, Oklahoma City, OK Zip 73112-9756; tel. 405/949-6068; Stanley F. Hupfeld, President and Chief Executive Officer
(Moderately Centralized Health System)

OKLAHOMA: BLACKWELL REGIONAL HOSPITAL (L, 34 beds) 710 South 13th Street, Blackwell, OK Zip 74631-3700; tel. 580/363-2311; Cindy White, Chief Financial Officer

DRUMRIGHT MEMORIAL HOSPITAL (L, 15 beds) 501 South Lou Allard Drive, Drumright, OK Zip 74030-4899; tel. 918/352-2525; James L. Clough, Administrator

INTEGRIS BAPTIST MEDICAL CENTER (O, 503 beds) 3300 N.W. Expressway, Oklahoma City, OK Zip 73112-4481; tel. 405/949-3011; Thomas R. Rice, FACHE, President and Chief Operating Officer
Web address: www.integris-health.com

INTEGRIS BAPTIST REGIONAL HEALTH CENTER (O, 113 beds) 200 Second Street S.W., Miami, OK Zip 74354-6830, Mailing Address: P.O. Box 1207, Zip 74355-1207; tel. 918/542-6611; W. Eugene Baxter, Dr.PH, FACHE, Interim Administrator
Web address: www.integris-health.com

INTEGRIS BASS BEHAVIORAL HEALTH SYSTEM (O, 50 beds) 2216 South Van Buren Street, Enid, OK Zip 73703-8299; tel. 580/234-2220; James Hutchison, Director

INTEGRIS BASS BAPTIST HEALTH CENTER (O, 119 beds) 600 South Monroe Street, Enid, OK Zip 73701, Mailing Address: P.O. Box 3168, Zip 73702-3168; tel. 580/233-2300; Thomas Schmitt, Administrator
Web address: www.integris-health.com

For explanation of codes following names, see page B2.
★ Indicates Type III membership in the American Hospital Association.

Systems / Iowa Health System

INTEGRIS GROVE GENERAL HOSPITAL (O, 72 beds) 1310 South Main Street, Grove, OK Zip 74344–1310; tel. 918/786–2243; Greg Martin, Administrator and Chief Executive Officer
Web address: www.integris–health.com

INTEGRIS MENTAL HEALTH SYSTEM–SPENCER (O, 44 beds) 2601 North Spencer Road, Spencer, OK Zip 73084–3699, Mailing Address: P.O. Box 11137, Oklahoma City, Zip 73136–0137; tel. 405/427–2441; Murali Krishna, M.D., President and Chief Operating Officer
Web address: www.integris–health.com

INTEGRIS SOUTHWEST MEDICAL CENTER (O, 325 beds) 4401 South Western, Oklahoma City, OK Zip 73109–3441; tel. 405/636–7000; Thomas R. Rice, FACHE, President and Chief Operating Officer
Web address: www.integris–health.com

INTERGRIS CLINTON REGIONAL HOSPITAL (L, 49 beds) 100 North 30th Street, Clinton, OK Zip 73601–3117, Mailing Address: P.O. Box 1569, Zip 73601–1569; tel. 580/323–2363; Jerry Jones, Administrator
Web address: www.integris–health.com

MARSHALL MEMORIAL HOSPITAL (L, 25 beds) 1 Hospital Drive, Madill, OK Zip 73446, Mailing Address: P.O. Box 827, Zip 73446–0827; tel. 580/795–3384; Norma Howard, Administrator

MAYES COUNTY MEDICAL CENTER (L, 38 beds) 129 North Kentucky Street, Pryor, OK Zip 74361–4211, Mailing Address: P.O. Box 278, Zip 74362–0278; tel. 918/825–1600; W. Charles Jordan, Administrator

PAWNEE MUNICIPAL HOSPITAL (L, 40 beds) 1212 Fourth Street, Pawnee, OK Zip 74058–4046, Mailing Address: P.O. Box 467, Zip 74058–0467; tel. 918/762–2577; John H. Ketring, Administrator

Owned, leased, sponsored:	13 hospitals	1427 beds
Contract–managed:	0 hospitals	0 beds
Totals:	13 hospitals	1427 beds

★**1815: INTERMOUNTAIN HEALTH CARE, INC.** (NP)
36 South State Street, 22nd Floor, Salt Lake City, UT Zip 84111–1453; tel. 801/442–2000; William H. Nelson, President and Chief Executive Officer
(Decentralized Health System)

IDAHO: CASSIA REGIONAL MEDICAL CENTER (O, 87 beds) 1501 Hiland Avenue, Burley, ID Zip 83318–2648; tel. 208/678–4444; Michael R. Olson, Administrator
Web address: www.ihc.com

POCATELLO REGIONAL MEDICAL CENTER (O, 87 beds) 777 Hospital Way, Pocatello, ID Zip 83201–2797; tel. 208/234–0777; Tracy J. Farnsworth, Administrator
Web address: www.ihc.com

UTAH: ALTA VIEW HOSPITAL (O, 72 beds) 9660 South 1300 East, Sandy, UT Zip 84094–3793; tel. 801/501–2600; Wes Thompson, Administrator and Chief Executive Officer
Web address: www.ihc.com

AMERICAN FORK HOSPITAL (O, 66 beds) 170 North 1100 East, American Fork, UT Zip 84003–2096; tel. 801/763–3300; Keith N. Alexander, Administrator and Chief Operating Officer
Web address: www.ihc.com

BEAR RIVER VALLEY HOSPITAL (O, 58 beds) 440 West 600 North, Tremonton, UT Zip 84337–2497; tel. 435/257–7441; Robert F. Jex, Administrator
Web address: www.ihc.com

COTTONWOOD HOSPITAL MEDICAL CENTER (O, 182 beds) 5770 South 300 East, Murray, UT Zip 84107–6186, Mailing Address: P.O. Box 57800, Salt Lake City, Zip 84107–0800; tel. 801/262–3461; Douglas R. Fonnesbeck, Administrator and Chief Executive Officer
Web address: www.ihc.com

DELTA COMMUNITY MEDICAL CENTER (O, 20 beds) 126 South White Sage Avenue, Delta, UT Zip 84624–8928; tel. 435/864–5591; James E. Beckstrand, Administrator
Web address: www.ihc.com

DIXIE REGIONAL MEDICAL CENTER (O, 137 beds) 544 South 400 East, Saint George, UT Zip 84770–3799; tel. 435/634–4000; L. Steven Wilson, Administrator
Web address: www.ihc.com

FILLMORE COMMUNITY MEDICAL CENTER (O, 20 beds) 674 South Highway 99, Fillmore, UT Zip 84631–9701; tel. 435/743–5591; James E. Beckstrand, Administrator
Web address: www.ihc.com

GARFIELD MEMORIAL HOSPITAL AND CLINICS (O, 44 beds) 200 North 400 East, Panguitch, UT Zip 84759, Mailing Address: P.O. Box 389, Zip 84759–0389; tel. 435/676–8811; Eric Packer, Administrator
Web address: www.ihc.com

HEBER VALLEY MEDICAL CENTER (O, 25 beds) 1485 South Highway 40, Heber City, UT Zip 84032–3522; tel. 435/654–2500; Randall K. Probst, Administrator
Web address: www.ihc.com

LDS HOSPITAL (O, 433 beds) Eighth Avenue and C Street, Salt Lake City, UT Zip 84143–0001; tel. 801/408–1100; Richard M. Cagen, Chief Executive Officer and Administrator
Web address: www.ihcweb.co.ihc.com

LOGAN REGIONAL HOSPITAL (O, 112 beds) 1400 North 500 East, Logan, UT Zip 84341–2499; tel. 435/716–1000; Richard Smith, Administrator
Web address: www.ihc.com

MCKAY–DEE HOSPITAL CENTER (O, 293 beds) 3939 Harrison Boulevard, Ogden, UT Zip 84409–0370, Mailing Address: Box 9370, Zip 84409–0370; tel. 801/398–2800; Thomas F. Hanrahan, FACHE, Chief Executive Officer and Regional Vice President
Web address: www.ihc.com

OREM COMMUNITY HOSPITAL (O, 20 beds) 331 North 400 West, Orem, UT Zip 84057–1999; tel. 801/224–4080; Kim Nielsen, Administrator and Chief Operating Officer
Web address: www.ihc.com

PRIMARY CHILDREN'S MEDICAL CENTER (O, 191 beds) 100 North Medical Drive, Salt Lake City, UT Zip 84113–1100; tel. 801/588–2000; Joseph R. Horton, Chief Executive Officer and Administrator
Web address: www.ihc.com

SANPETE VALLEY HOSPITAL (O, 20 beds) 1100 South Medical Drive, Mount Pleasant, UT Zip 84647–2222; tel. 435/462–2441; George Winn, Administrator
Web address: www.ihc.com

SEVIER VALLEY HOSPITAL (O, 26 beds) 1100 North Main Street, Richfield, UT Zip 84701–1843; tel. 435/896–8271; Gary E. Beck, Administrator
Web address: www.ihc.com

UTAH VALLEY REGIONAL MEDICAL CENTER (O, 343 beds) 1034 North 500 West, Provo, UT Zip 84604–3337; tel. 801/373–7850; Mary Ann Young, R.N., Administrator
Web address: www.ihc.com

VALLEY VIEW MEDICAL CENTER (O, 36 beds) 595 South 75 East, Cedar City, UT Zip 84720–3462; tel. 435/586–6587; Craig M. Smedley, Administrator
Web address: www.ihc.com

Owned, leased, sponsored:	20 hospitals	2272 beds
Contract–managed:	0 hospitals	0 beds
Totals:	20 hospitals	2272 beds

★**0061: IOWA HEALTH SYSTEM** (NP)
1200 Pleasant Street, Des Moines, IA Zip 50309–1453; tel. 515/241–6161; Samuel T. Wallace, President
(Moderately Centralized Health System)

ILLINOIS: TRINITY MEDICAL CENTER–WEST CAMPUS (O, 338 beds) 2701 17th Street, Rock Island, IL Zip 61201–5393; tel. 309/779–5000; Eric Crowell, President and Chief Executive Officer
Web address: www.trinityqc.com

IOWA: ALLEN MEMORIAL HOSPITAL (O, 202 beds) 1825 Logan Avenue, Waterloo, IA Zip 50703–1916; tel. 319/235–3987; Richard A. Seidler, FACHE, Chief Executive Officer

BUENA VISTA COUNTY HOSPITAL (C, 30 beds) 1525 West Fifth Street, Storm Lake, IA Zip 50588–0309, Mailing Address: P.O. Box 309, Zip 50588–0309; tel. 712/732–4030; James J. Sinek, Chief Executive Officer

CLARKE COUNTY HOSPITAL (C, 48 beds) 800 South Fillmore Street, Osceola, IA Zip 50213; tel. 515/342–2184; David M. Coates, Ph.D., Chief Executive Officer
Web address: www.clarkehosp.org

For explanation of codes following names, see page B2.
★ Indicates Type III membership in the American Hospital Association.

Systems / Iowa Health System

COMMUNITY MEMORIAL HOSPITAL (C, 33 beds) 1316 South Main Street, Clarion, IA Zip 50525; tel. 515/532-2811; Steve J. Simonin, Chief Executive Officer
Web address: www.trcnet.net

DALLAS COUNTY HOSPITAL (C, 33 beds) 610 10th Street, Perry, IA Zip 50220-2221, Mailing Address: P.O. Box 608, Zip 50220-0608; tel. 515/465-3547; Kari L. Engholm, Administrator and Chief Executive Officer
Web address: www.perryia.org/Healthcare/health.htm

FINLEY HOSPITAL (O, 139 beds) 350 North Grandview Avenue, Dubuque, IA Zip 52001-6392; tel. 319/582-1881; Kevin L. Rogols, President and Chief Executive Officer
Web address: www.finleyhospital.org

GREATER COMMUNITY HOSPITAL (C, 49 beds) 1700 West Townline, Creston, IA Zip 50801-1099; tel. 515/782-7091; Ronald D. Davis, Chief Executive Officer

GRUNDY COUNTY MEMORIAL HOSPITAL (C, 71 beds) 201 East J Avenue, Grundy Center, IA Zip 50638-2096; tel. 319/824-5421; Janice McCart, Chief Executive Officer

GUTTENBERG MUNICIPAL HOSPITAL (C, 20 beds) Second and Main Street, Guttenberg, IA Zip 52052-0550, Mailing Address: P.O. Box 550, Zip 52052-0550; tel. 319/252-1121; Kim Gau, Interim Chief Executive Officer

HUMBOLDT COUNTY MEMORIAL HOSPITAL (C, 49 beds) 1000 North 15th Street, Humboldt, IA Zip 50548-1008; tel. 515/332-4200; Monte Neitzel, Administrator and Chief Executive Officer
Web address: trv1.trvnet.net/~hcmh/

IOWA LUTHERAN HOSPITAL (O, 232 beds) 700 East University Avenue, Des Moines, IA Zip 50316-2392; tel. 515/263-5612; David Stark, Chief Operating Officer
Web address: www.ihsdesmoines.org

IOWA METHODIST MEDICAL CENTER (O, 464 beds) 1200 Pleasant Street, Des Moines, IA Zip 50309-9976; tel. 515/241-6212; James H. Skogsbergh, President
Web address: www.ihsdesmoines.org

JONES REGIONAL MEDICAL CENTER (L, 17 beds) 104 Broadway Place, Anamosa, IA Zip 52205-1100; tel. 319/462-6131; Vickie Asbe, Administrator

LORING HOSPITAL (C, 54 beds) 211 Highland Avenue, Sac City, IA Zip 50583-0217, Mailing Address: P.O. Box 217, Zip 50583-0217; tel. 712/662-7105; Greg Miner, Administrator

POCAHONTAS COMMUNITY HOSPITAL (C, 25 beds) 606 N.W. Seventh, Pocahontas, IA Zip 50574-1099; tel. 712/335-3501

ST. LUKE'S HOSPITAL (O, 384 beds) 1026 A Avenue N.E., Cedar Rapids, IA Zip 52402-3026, Mailing Address: P.O. Box 3026, Zip 52406-3026; tel. 319/369-7211; Stephen E. Vanourny, M.D., President and Chief Executive Officer

ST. LUKE'S REGIONAL MEDICAL CENTER (O, 193 beds) 2720 Stone Park Boulevard, Sioux City, IA Zip 51104-2000; tel. 712/279-3500; John D. Daniels, President and Chief Executive Officer
Web address: www.siouxlan.com/stlukes

TRINITY MEDICAL CENTER-NORTH CAMPUS (O, 105 beds) 1111 West Kimberly Road, Davenport, IA Zip 52806-5913; tel. 319/445-4020; Robert J. Lundin, II, Chief Executive Officer

TRINITY REGIONAL HOSPITAL (O, 161 beds) 802 Kenyon Road, Fort Dodge, IA Zip 50501-5795; tel. 515/573-3101; Tom Tibbitts, President
Web address: www.trh-fd.org

Owned, leased, sponsored:	10 hospitals	2235 beds
Contract-managed:	10 hospitals	412 beds
Totals:	20 hospitals	2647 beds

★7775: **JEFFERSON HEALTH SYSTEM** (NP)
259 Radnor-Chester Road, Suite 290, Wayne, PA Zip 19087-5288; tel. 610/225-6200; Douglas S. Peters, President and Chief Executive Officer
(Centralized Health System)

PENNSYLVANIA: BRYN MAWR HOSPITAL (O, 277 beds) 130 South Bryn Mawr Avenue, Bryn Mawr, PA Zip 19010-3160; tel. 610/526-3000; Andrea F. Gilbert, Senior Vice President
Web address: www.jeffersonhealth.org

BRYN MAWR REHABILITATION HOSPITAL (O, 141 beds) 414 Paoli Pike, Malvern, PA Zip 19355-3300, Mailing Address: P.O. Box 3007, Zip 19355-3300; tel. 610/251-5400; Patricia Ryan, Senior Vice President
Web address: www.jeffersonhealth.org

FRANKFORD HOSPITAL OF THE CITY OF PHILADELPHIA (O, 567 beds) Knights and Red Lion Roads, Philadelphia, PA Zip 19114-1486; tel. 215/612-4000; Roy A. Powell, President
Web address: www.jeffersonhealth.org/frankford/index.html

GERMANTOWN HOSPITAL AND COMMUNITY HEALTH SERVICES (O, 158 beds) One Penn Boulevard, Philadelphia, PA Zip 19144-1498; tel. 215/951-8000; Cynthia McGlone, Chief Operating Officer

LANKENAU HOSPITAL (O, 309 beds) 100 Lancaster Avenue West, Wynnewood, PA Zip 19096-3411; tel. 610/645-2000; C. Barry Dykes, Senior Vice President
Web address: www.jeffersonhealth.org

MAGEE REHABILITATION HOSPITAL (O, 96 beds) Six Franklin Plaza, Philadelphia, PA Zip 19102-1177; tel. 215/587-3099; William E. Staas, Jr, President and Medical Director
Web address: www.mageerehab.org

PAOLI MEMORIAL HOSPITAL (O, 138 beds) 255 West Lancaster Avenue, Paoli, PA Zip 19301-1792; tel. 610/648-1000; Barbara Tachovsky, Senior Vice President
Web address: www.jeffersonhealth.org/paoli/index.html

THOMAS JEFFERSON UNIVERSITY HOSPITAL (O, 981 beds) 111 South 11th Street, Philadelphia, PA Zip 19107-5096; tel. 215/955-7022; Thomas J. Lewis, President and Chief Executive Officer
Web address: www.jeffersonhealth.org

Owned, leased, sponsored:	8 hospitals	2667 beds
Contract-managed:	0 hospitals	0 beds
Totals:	8 hospitals	2667 beds

★0052: **JEWISH HOSPITAL HEALTHCARE SERVICES** (NP)
217 East Chestnut Street, Louisville, KY Zip 40202-1886; tel. 502/587-4011; Henry C. Wagner, President
(Moderately Centralized Health System)

INDIANA: CLARK MEMORIAL HOSPITAL (C, 243 beds) 1220 Missouri Avenue, Jeffersonville, IN Zip 47130-3743, Mailing Address: Box 69, Zip 47131-0069; tel. 812/282-6631; Merle E. Stepp, President and Chief Executive Officer
Web address: www.cmhl.com

SCOTT MEMORIAL HOSPITAL (C, 45 beds) 1415 North Gardner Street, Scottsburg, IN Zip 47170-0430, Mailing Address: Box 430, Zip 47170-0430; tel. 812/752-8500; Clifford D. Nay, Executive Director
Web address: www.scottcounty.hsonline.com

SOUTHERN INDIANA REHABILITATION HOSPITAL (O, 60 beds) 3104 Blackiston Boulevard, New Albany, IN Zip 47150-9579; tel. 812/941-8300; Randy L. Napier, President and Chief Executive Officer

WASHINGTON COUNTY MEMORIAL HOSPITAL (C, 58 beds) 911 North Shelby Street, Salem, IN Zip 47167; tel. 812/883-5881; Rodney M. Coats, President and Chief Executive Officer

KENTUCKY: FRAZIER REHABILITATION CENTER (O, 93 beds) 220 Abraham Flexner Way, Louisville, KY Zip 40202-1887; tel. 502/582-7400; Barth A. Weinberg, Vice President, Inpatient Rehabilitation
Web address: www.jhhs.org

JEWISH HOSPITAL (O, 435 beds) 217 East Chestnut Street, Louisville, KY Zip 40202-1886; tel. 502/587-4011; Douglas E. Shaw, President
Web address: www.jhhs.org

JEWISH HOSPITAL-SHELBYVILLE (O, 58 beds) 727 Hospital Drive, Shelbyville, KY Zip 40065-1699; tel. 502/647-4000; Timothy L. Jarm, President
Web address: www.jhhs.org

PATTIE A. CLAY HOSPITAL (C, 105 beds) EKU By-Pass, Richmond, KY Zip 40475, Mailing Address: P.O. Box 1600, Zip 40476-2603; tel. 859/623-3131; Richard M. Thomas, President

For explanation of codes following names, see page B2.
★ Indicates Type III membership in the American Hospital Association.

Systems / Kaiser Foundation Hospitals

TAYLOR COUNTY HOSPITAL (C, 90 beds) 1700 Old Lebanon Road, Campbellsville, KY Zip 42718–9600; tel. 270/465–3561; David R. Hayes, President

UNIVERSITY OF LOUISVILLE HOSPITAL (C, 271 beds) 530 South Jackson Street, Louisville, KY Zip 40202–3611; tel. 502/562–3000; James H. Taylor, President and Chief Executive Officer
Web address: www.ulh.org

Owned, leased, sponsored:	4 hospitals	646 beds
Contract–managed:	6 hospitals	812 beds
Totals:	10 hospitals	1458 beds

0218: JOHN C LINCOLN HEALTH NETWORK (NP)
250 East Dunlap Avenue, Phoenix, AZ Zip 85020–2446; tel. 602/943–2381; Dan C. Coleman, President and Chief Executive Officer

ARIZONA: JOHN C LINCOLN HOSPITAL–DEER VALLEY (O, 97 beds) 19829 North 27th Avenue, Phoenix, AZ Zip 85027–4002; tel. 623/879–6100; Tim Tracy, Executive Vice President and Chief Operating Officer
Web address: www.jcl.com

JOHN C. LINCOLN HOSPITAL – NORTH MOUNTAIN (O, 239 beds) 250 East Dunlap Avenue, Phoenix, AZ Zip 85020–2446; tel. 602/943–2381; Dan C. Coleman, President and Chief Executive Officer
Web address: www.jcl.com

Owned, leased, sponsored:	2 hospitals	336 beds
Contract–managed:	0 hospitals	0 beds
Totals:	2 hospitals	336 beds

★1015: JOHNS HOPKINS HEALTH SYSTEM (NP)
600 North Wolfe Street, Baltimore, MD Zip 21287–1193; tel. 410/955–5000; Ronald R. Peterson, President
(Centralized Physician/Insurance Health System)

MARYLAND: HOWARD COUNTY GENERAL HOSPITAL (O, 163 beds) 5755 Cedar Lane, Columbia, MD Zip 21044–2912; tel. 410/740–7710; Victor A. Broccolino, President and Chief Executive Officer
Web address: www.hcgh.org

JOHNS HOPKINS BAYVIEW MEDICAL CENTER (O, 658 beds) 4940 Eastern Avenue, Baltimore, MD Zip 21224–2780; tel. 410/550–0100; Gregory F. Schaffer, President
Web address: www.jhbmc.jhu.edu

JOHNS HOPKINS HOSPITAL (O, 844 beds) 600 North Wolfe Street, Baltimore, MD Zip 21287–2182; tel. 410/955–5000; Ronald R. Peterson, President
Web address: www.med.jhu.edu

Owned, leased, sponsored:	3 hospitals	1665 beds
Contract–managed:	0 hospitals	0 beds
Totals:	3 hospitals	1665 beds

★2105: KAISER FOUNDATION HOSPITALS (NP)
One Kaiser Plaza, Oakland, CA Zip 94612–3600; tel. 510/271–5910; David M. Lawrence, M.D., Chairman and Chief Executive Officer
(Moderately Centralized Health System)

CALIFORNIA: KAISER FOUNDATION HOSPITAL (O, 210 beds) 2425 Geary Boulevard, San Francisco, CA Zip 94115; tel. 415/202–2000; Julie A. Petrini, Administrator
Web address: www.kaiserpermanente.org

KAISER FOUNDATION HOSPITAL (O, 103 beds) 401 Bicentennial Way, Santa Rosa, CA Zip 95403; tel. 707/571–4000; Julie A. Petrini, Administrator
Web address: www.ca.kaiserpermanente.org

KAISER FOUNDATION HOSPITAL (O, 384 beds) 4747 Sunset Boulevard, Los Angeles, CA Zip 90027–6072; tel. 323/783–4011; Anthony A. Armada, Senior Vice President and Service Area Manager
Web address: www.lac.usc.org

KAISER FOUNDATION HOSPITAL (O, 121 beds) 7300 North Fresno Street, Fresno, CA Zip 93720; tel. 559/448–4555; Toni Flores, Director Operations
Web address: www.kaiserpermanente.org

KAISER FOUNDATION HOSPITAL (O, 264 beds) 280 West MacArthur Boulevard, Oakland, CA Zip 94611; tel. 510/987–1000; Bettie L. Coles, R.N., Administrator
Web address: www.kaiserpermanente.org

KAISER FOUNDATION HOSPITAL (O, 210 beds) 1425 South Main Street, Walnut Creek, CA Zip 94596; tel. 925/295–4000; Sandra H. Small, Administrator
Web address: www.kaiserpermanente.org

KAISER FOUNDATION HOSPITAL (O, 150 beds) 441 North Lakeview Avenue, Anaheim, CA Zip 92807; tel. 714/279–4100; Janice Head, Administrator
Web address: www.kaiserpermanente.org

KAISER FOUNDATION HOSPITAL (O, 158 beds) 1011 Baldwin Park Boulevard, Baldwin Park, CA Zip 91706; tel. 626/851–1011; Gregory A. Adams, Senior Vice President and Service Area Manager

KAISER FOUNDATION HOSPITAL (O, 299 beds) 9961 Sierra Avenue, Fontana, CA Zip 92335–6794; tel. 909/427–5000; Susan Caulk, Director Operations
Web address: www.kaiserpermanente.org

KAISER FOUNDATION HOSPITAL (O, 189 beds) 25825 South Vermont Avenue, Harbor City, CA Zip 90710; tel. 310/325–5111; Carolyn Orlowski, Director Operations
Web address: www.kaiserpermanente.org

KAISER FOUNDATION HOSPITAL (O, 204 beds) 27400 Hesperian Boulevard, Hayward, CA Zip 94545–4297; tel. 510/784–4313; Duayna Pucci, Director Operations
Web address: www.kaiserpermanente.org

KAISER FOUNDATION HOSPITAL (O, 310 beds) 4647 Zion Avenue, San Diego, CA Zip 92120; tel. 619/528–5000; Terry A. Belmont, Administrator
Web address: www.kaiserpermanente.org

KAISER FOUNDATION HOSPITAL (O, 171 beds) 1150 Veterans Boulevard, Redwood City, CA Zip 94063–2087; tel. 650/299–2000; Joanne Zimmerman, Administrator
Web address: www.kaiserpermanente.org

KAISER FOUNDATION HOSPITAL (O, 304 beds) 2025 Morse Avenue, Sacramento, CA Zip 95825–2115; tel. 916/973–5000; Edward S. Glavis, Administrator
Web address: www.kaiserpermanente.org

KAISER FOUNDATION HOSPITAL (O, 221 beds) 6600 Bruceville Road, Sacramento, CA Zip 95823; tel. 916/688–2430; Edward S. Glavis, Administrator
Web address: www.kaiserpermanente.org

KAISER FOUNDATION HOSPITAL (O, 119 beds) 99 Montecillo Road, San Rafael, CA Zip 94903–3397; tel. 415/444–2000; Julie A. Petrini, Administrator
Web address: www.kaiserpermanente.org

KAISER FOUNDATION HOSPITAL (O, 249 beds) 900 Kiely Boulevard, Santa Clara, CA Zip 95051–5386; tel. 408/236–6400; Joann Zimmerman, Administrator
Web address: www.kaiserpermanente.org

KAISER FOUNDATION HOSPITAL (O, 79 beds) 1200 El Camino Real, South San Francisco, CA Zip 94080–3299; tel. 650/742–2401; Julie A. Petrini, Administrator

KAISER FOUNDATION HOSPITAL (O, 211 beds) 13652 Cantara Street, Panorama City, CA Zip 91402; tel. 818/375–2000; Deborah M. Lee–Eddie, Administrator
Web address: www.kaiserpermanente.org

KAISER FOUNDATION HOSPITAL (O, 140 beds) 5601 DeSoto Avenue, Woodland Hills, CA Zip 91365–4084; tel. 818/719–3808; Deborah M. Lee–Eddie, Administrator
Web address: www.kaiserpermanente.org

KAISER FOUNDATION HOSPITAL AND REHABILITATION CENTER (O, 219 beds) 975 Sereno Drive, Vallejo, CA Zip 94589; tel. 707/651–1000; Sandra H. Small, Administrator
Web address: www.kaiserpermanente.org

KAISER FOUNDATION HOSPITAL–BELLFLOWER (O, 282 beds) 9400 East Rosecrans Avenue, Bellflower, CA Zip 90706–2246; tel. 562/461–3000; Karen K. Ringl, Director Hospital Operations
Web address: www.ca.kaiserpermanente.org

For explanation of codes following names, see page B2.
★ Indicates Type III membership in the American Hospital Association.

Systems / Kaiser Foundation Hospitals

KAISER FOUNDATION HOSPITAL–RIVERSIDE (O, 188 beds) 10800 Magnolia Avenue, Riverside, CA Zip 92505–3000; tel. 909/353–4600; Gerald A. McCall, Chief Executive Officer
Web address: www.kaiserpermanente.org

KAISER FOUNDATION HOSPITAL–WEST LOS ANGELES (O, 180 beds) 6041 Cadillac Avenue, Los Angeles, CA Zip 90034; tel. 323/857–2201; Alice Isani, Acting Administrator
Web address: www.kaiserpermanente.org

SANTA TERESA COMMUNITY MEDICAL CENTER (O, 178 beds) 250 Hospital Parkway, San Jose, CA Zip 95119; tel. 408/972–7000; Joann Zimmerman, Administrator

HAWAII: KAISER FOUNDATION HOSPITAL (O, 190 beds) 3288 Moanalua Road, Honolulu, HI Zip 96819; tel. 808/834–5333; Robert Matsuwaka, Regional Administrator
Web address: www.kaiserhawaii.com

OREGON: KAISER SUNNYSIDE MEDICAL CENTER (O, 178 beds) 10180 S.E. Sunnyside Road, Clackamas, OR Zip 97015–9303; tel. 503/652–2880; Kathleen S. Wegener, Administrator

Owned, leased, sponsored:	27 hospitals	5511 beds
Contract–managed:	0 hospitals	0 beds
Totals:	27 hospitals	5511 beds

0102: KALEIDA HEALTH (NP)
901 Washington Street, Buffalo, NY Zip 14203; tel. 716/843–7500; John E. Friedlander, President and Chief Executive Officer

NEW YORK: BUFFALO GENERAL HOSPITAL (O, 965 beds) 100 High Street, Buffalo, NY Zip 14203–1154; tel. 716/845–5600; John E. Friedlander, President and Chief Executive Officer

CHILDREN'S HOSPITAL (O, 313 beds) 219 Bryant Street, Buffalo, NY Zip 14222–2099; tel. 716/878–7000; Karen Blount, R.N., Chief Operating Officer

DE GRAFF MEMORIAL HOSPITAL (O, 210 beds) 445 Tremont Street, North Tonawanda, NY Zip 14120–0750, Mailing Address: P.O. Box 0750, Zip 14120–0750; tel. 716/694–4500; Marcia B. Gutfeld, Vice President and Chief Operating Officer

MILLARD FILLMORE GATES CIRCLE HOSPITAL (O, 588 beds) 3 Gates Circle, Buffalo, NY Zip 14209–9986; tel. 716/887–4600; Joyce Korzen, R.N., Chief Operating Officer
Web address: www.mfhs.edu

Owned, leased, sponsored:	4 hospitals	2076 beds
Contract–managed:	0 hospitals	0 beds
Totals:	4 hospitals	2076 beds

0149: KISHWAUKEE HEALTH SYSTEM (NP)
626 Bethany Road, De Kalb, IL Zip 60115–4939, Mailing Address: P.O. Box 707, Zip 60115–4939; tel. 815/756–1521; Robert S. Thebeau, President and Chief Executive Officer
(Independent Hospital System)

ILLINOIS: KISHWAUKEE COMMUNITY HOSPITAL (O, 114 beds) 626 Bethany Road, De Kalb, IL Zip 60115–4939, Mailing Address: P.O. Box 707, Zip 60115–0707; tel. 815/756–1521; Brad Copple, Administrator
Web address: www.kishhospital.org

VALLEY WEST COMMUNITY HOSPITAL (O, 35 beds) 11 East Pleasant Avenue, Sandwich, IL Zip 60548–0901; tel. 815/786–8484; Roger L. Holloway, Administrator
Web address: www.uwch.com

Owned, leased, sponsored:	2 hospitals	149 beds
Contract–managed:	0 hospitals	0 beds
Totals:	2 hospitals	149 beds

★2755: LEGACY HEALTH SYSTEM (NP)
1919 N.W. Lovejoy Street, Portland, OR Zip 97209–1503; tel. 503/415–5600; Robert Pallari, President and Chief Executive Officer
(Centralized Health System)

OREGON: LEGACY EMANUEL HOSPITAL AND HEALTH CENTER (O, 356 beds) 2801 North Gantenbein Avenue, Portland, OR Zip 97227–1674; tel. 503/413–2200; Stephani White, Vice President and Site Administrator
Web address: www.legacyhealth.org

LEGACY GOOD SAMARITAN HOSPITAL AND MEDICAL CENTER (O, 279 beds) 1015 N.W. 22nd Avenue, Portland, OR Zip 97210; tel. 503/413–7711; Martha C. Wangenstein, Vice President and Site Administrator
Web address: www.legacyhealth.org

LEGACY MERIDIAN PARK HOSPITAL (O, 117 beds) 19300 S.W. 65th Avenue, Tualatin, OR Zip 97062–9741; tel. 503/692–1212; Jeff Cushing, Vice President and Site Administrator
Web address: www.legacyhealth.org

LEGACY MOUNT HOOD MEDICAL CENTER (O, 58 beds) 24800 S.E. Stark, Gresham, OR Zip 97030–0154; tel. 503/667–1122; Thomas S. Parker, Site Administrator
Web address: www.legacyhealth.org

Owned, leased, sponsored:	4 hospitals	810 beds
Contract–managed:	0 hospitals	0 beds
Totals:	4 hospitals	810 beds

0173: LIBERTY HEALTHCARE SYSTEM (NP)
50 Baldwin Avenue, Jersey City, NJ Zip 07304–3199; tel. 201/915–2000; Jonathan M. Metsch, Dr.PH, President and Chief Executive Officer
(Independent Hospital System)

NEW JERSEY: GREENVILLE HOSPITAL (O, 86 beds) 1825 John F. Kennedy Boulevard, Jersey City, NJ Zip 07305–2198; tel. 201/547–6100; Jonathan M. Metsch, Dr.PH, President and Chief Executive Officer

JERSEY CITY MEDICAL CENTER (O, 487 beds) 50 Baldwin Avenue, Jersey City, NJ Zip 07304–3199; tel. 201/915–2000; Jonathan M. Metsch, Dr.PH, President and Chief Executive Officer

MEADOWLANDS HOSPITAL MEDICAL CENTER (O, 173 beds) 55 Meadowland Parkway, Secaucus, NJ Zip 07096–1580; tel. 201/392–3100; Paul V. Cavalli, M.D., President

Owned, leased, sponsored:	3 hospitals	746 beds
Contract–managed:	0 hospitals	0 beds
Totals:	3 hospitals	746 beds

0206: LIBERTY MANAGEMENT GROUP, INC. (IO)
19 Spear Road, Suite 305, Ramsey, NJ Zip 07446; tel. 201/236–8880; William J. Hartigan, President and Chief Executive Officer

FLORIDA: SAVANNAS HOSPITAL (O, 70 beds) 2550 S.E. Walton Road, Port St. Lucie, FL Zip 34952–7197; tel. 561/335–0400; Patricia W. Brown, Ph.D., Executive Director

NEW YORK: HOLLISWOOD HOSPITAL (C, 100 beds) 87–37 Palermo Street, Holliswood, NY Zip 11423; tel. 718/776–8181; Jeffrey Borenstein, M.D., Chief Executive Officer and Medical Director

OKLAHOMA: ROLLING HILLS HOSPITAL (O, 40 beds) 1000 Rolling Hills Lane, Ada, OK Zip 74820–9415; tel. 580/436–3600; Darnell Powell, Executive Director

Owned, leased, sponsored:	2 hospitals	110 beds
Contract–managed:	1 hospital	100 beds
Totals:	3 hospitals	210 beds

★0158: LIFEBRIDGE HEALTH (NP)
2401 West Belvedere Avenue, Baltimore, MD Zip 21215; tel. 410/601–5134; Warren A. Green, President and Chief Executive Officer
(Independent Hospital System)

MARYLAND: LEVINDALE HEBREW GERIATRIC CENTER AND HOSPITAL (O, 296 beds) 2434 West Belvedere Avenue, Baltimore, MD Zip 21215–5271; tel. 410/466–8700; Ronald Rothstein, President and Chief Executive Officer
Web address: www.sinai–balt.com

For explanation of codes following names, see page B2.
★ Indicates Type III membership in the American Hospital Association.

Systems / Lifespan Corporation

NORTHWEST HOSPITAL CENTER (O, 160 beds) 5401 Old Court Road, Randallstown, MD Zip 21133–5185; tel. 410/521–2200; Robert W. Fischer, President

SINAI HOSPITAL OF BALTIMORE (O, 387 beds) 2401 West Belvedere Avenue, Baltimore, MD Zip 21215–5271; tel. 410/601–9000; Neil M. Meltzer, President and Chief Operating Officer
Web address: www.lifebridgehealth.org

Owned, leased, sponsored:	3 hospitals	843 beds
Contract–managed:	0 hospitals	0 beds
Totals:	3 hospitals	843 beds

0191: LIFECARE MANAGEMENT SERVICES (IO)
6161 Harry Hines Boulevard, Dallas, TX Zip 75235; tel. 214/525–0600; David B. Leblanc, President
(Independent Hospital System)

LOUISIANA: LIFECARE HOSPITALS (O, 65 beds) 9320 Linwood Avenue, Shreveport, LA Zip 71106, Mailing Address: 9320 Lindwood Avenue, Zip 71106; tel. 318/688–8504; Robert A. Loepp, Jr, CHE, Administrator
Web address: www.lifecare–hospitals.com

NEVADA: TAHOE PACIFIC HOSPITAL (O, 27 beds) 2375 East Prater Way, Sparks, NV Zip 89434; tel. 775/331–1044; Clifton Neal Orme, Administrator and Chief Executive Officer

PENNSYLVANIA: LIFECARE HOSPITAL OF PITTSBURGH (O, 152 beds) 225 Penn Avenue, Pittsburgh, PA Zip 15221–2173; tel. 412/247–2424; April A. Stevens, R.N., Chief Executive Officer

Owned, leased, sponsored:	3 hospitals	244 beds
Contract–managed:	0 hospitals	0 beds
Totals:	3 hospitals	244 beds

★**0180: LIFEPOINT HOSPITALS, INC.** (IO)
103 Powell Court, Suite 200, Brentwood, TN Zip 37027; tel. 615/372–8500; James M. Fleetwood, Jr, Chairman, President, Chief Executive Officer and Chief Operating Officer
(Moderately Centralized Health System)

ALABAMA: ANDALUSIA REGIONAL HOSPITAL (O, 101 beds) 849 South Three Notch Street, Andalusia, AL Zip 36420–5325, Mailing Address: P.O. Box 760, Zip 36420–0760; tel. 334/222–8466; Barry L. Keel, Chief Executive Officer

FLORIDA: BARTOW MEMORIAL HOSPITAL (O, 88 beds) 2200 Osprey Boulevard, Bartow, FL Zip 33830, Mailing Address: P.O. Box 1050, Zip 33830–1050; tel. 941/533–8111; Brian P. Baumgardner, Administrator
Web address: www.koala.columbia.net

GEORGIA: BARROW MEDICAL CENTER (O, 56 beds) 316 North Broad Street, Winder, GA Zip 30680–2150, Mailing Address: P.O. Box 768, Zip 30680–0768; tel. 770/867–3400; Randy Mills, Chief Executive Officer
Web address: www.barrowmedical.com

KANSAS: WESTERN PLAINS MEDICAL COMPLEX (O, 99 beds) 3001 Avenue A, Dodge City, KS Zip 67801–6508, Mailing Address: P.O. Box 1478, Zip 67801–1478; tel. 316/225–8400; Ken Hutchenrider, President and Chief Executive Officer

KENTUCKY: BOURBON COMMUNITY HOSPITAL (O, 58 beds) 9 Linville Drive, Paris, KY Zip 40361–2196; tel. 606/987–3600; Rob Smart, Chief Executive Officer

GEORGETOWN COMMUNITY HOSPITAL (O, 58 beds) 1140 Lexington Road, Georgetown, KY Zip 40324–9362; tel. 502/868–1100; Jeffrey G. Seraphine, President and Chief Executive Officer

JACKSON PURCHASE MEDICAL CENTER (O, 106 beds) 1099 Medical Center Circle, Mayfield, KY Zip 42066–1179, Mailing Address: P.O. Box 1099, Zip 42066–1099; tel. 270/251–4100; Mary Jo Lewis, Chief Executive Officer
Web address: www.hcahealthcare.com

LAKE CUMBERLAND REGIONAL HOSPITAL (O, 227 beds) 305 Langdon Street, Somerset, KY Zip 42501, Mailing Address: P.O. Box 620, Zip 42502–2750; tel. 606/679–7441; Jon C. O'Shaughnessy, President and Chief Executive Officer

LOGAN MEMORIAL HOSPITAL (O, 63 beds) 1625 South Nashville Road, Russellville, KY Zip 42276–8834, Mailing Address: P.O. Box 10, Zip 42276–0010; tel. 270/726–4011; Michael Clark, Chief Executive Officer

MEADOWVIEW REGIONAL MEDICAL CENTER (O, 101 beds) 989 Medical Park Drive, Maysville, KY Zip 41056–8750; tel. 606/759–5311; Curtis B. Courtney, Chief Executive Officer

LOUISIANA: RIVERVIEW MEDICAL CENTER (O, 104 beds) 1125 West Louisiana Highway 30, Gonzales, LA Zip 70737; tel. 225/647–5000; Kathy J. Bobbs, Chief Executive Officer

SPRINGHILL MEDICAL CENTER (O, 86 beds) 2001 Doctors Drive, Springhill, LA Zip 71075, Mailing Address: P.O. Box 920, Zip 71075–0920; tel. 318/539–1000; Kerry Wehmeyer, Chief Executive Officer

TENNESSEE: CROCKETT HOSPITAL (O, 98 beds) U.S. Highway 43 South, Lawrenceburg, TN Zip 38464–0847, Mailing Address: P.O. Box 847, Zip 38464–0847; tel. 931/762–6571; Jack S. Buck, Chief Executive Officer
Web address: www.crocketthospital.com

HILLSIDE HOSPITAL (O, 86 beds) 1265 East College Street, Pulaski, TN Zip 38478–4541; tel. 931/363–7531; James H. Edmondson, Chief Executive Officer and Administrator

LIVINGSTON REGIONAL HOSPITAL (O, 85 beds) 315 Oak Street, Livingston, TN Zip 38570, Mailing Address: P.O. Box 550, Zip 38570–0550; tel. 931/823–5611; Timothy W. McGill, Chief Executive Officer

SMITH COUNTY MEMORIAL HOSPITAL (O, 40 beds) 158 Hospital Drive, Carthage, TN Zip 37030–1096; tel. 615/735–1560; Jerry H. Futrell, Chief Executive Officer

SOUTHERN TENNESSEE MEDICAL CENTER (O, 211 beds) 185 Hospital Road, Winchester, TN Zip 37398–2468; tel. 931/967–8200; William Russell Spray, Chief Executive Officer

UTAH: ASHLEY VALLEY MEDICAL CENTER (O, 29 beds) 151 West 200 North, Vernal, UT Zip 84078–1907; tel. 435/789–3342; Ronald J. Perry, Chief Executive Officer
Web address: www.avmc–hospital.com

CASTLEVIEW HOSPITAL (O, 84 beds) 300 North Hospital Drive, Price, UT Zip 84501–4200; tel. 435/637–4800; Jeff Frandsen, Chief Executive Officer

WYOMING: RIVERTON MEMORIAL HOSPITAL (O, 59 beds) 2100 West Sunset Drive, Riverton, WY Zip 82501–2274; tel. 307/856–4161; William Russell, Chief Executive Officer
Web address: www.riverton–hospital.com

Owned, leased, sponsored:	20 hospitals	1839 beds
Contract–managed:	0 hospitals	0 beds
Totals:	20 hospitals	1839 beds

★**0060: LIFESPAN CORPORATION** (NP)
167 Point Street, Providence, RI Zip 02903–4771; tel. 401/444–3500; George A. Vecchione, President
(Moderately Centralized Health System)

MASSACHUSETTS: NEW ENGLAND MEDICAL CENTER (O, 323 beds) 750 Washington Street, Boston, MA Zip 02111–1845; tel. 617/636–5000; Thomas F. O'Donnell, Jr, M.D., FACS, President and Chief Executive Officer
Web address: www.nemc.org/home/

RHODE ISLAND: EMMA PENDLETON BRADLEY HOSPITAL (O, 60 beds) 1011 Veterans Memorial Parkway, East Providence, RI Zip 02915–5099; tel. 401/432–1000; Daniel J. Wall, President and Chief Executive Officer
Web address: www.lifespan.org

MIRIAM HOSPITAL (O, 227 beds) 164 Summit Avenue, Providence, RI Zip 02906–2895; tel. 401/793–2500; Kathleen C. Hittner, M.D., President and Chief Executive Officer
Web address: www.lifespan.org

NEWPORT HOSPITAL (O, 116 beds) 11 Friendship Street, Newport, RI Zip 02840–2299; tel. 401/846–6400; Arthur J. Sampson, President and Chief Executive Officer
Web address: www.lifespan.org

For explanation of codes following names, see page B2.
★ Indicates Type III membership in the American Hospital Association.

Systems / Lifespan Corporation

RHODE ISLAND HOSPITAL (O, 529 beds) 593 Eddy Street, Providence, RI Zip 02903–4900; tel. 401/444–4000; Joseph E. Amaral, M.D., President and Chief Executive Officer
Web address: www.lifespan.org

Owned, leased, sponsored:	5 hospitals	1255 beds
Contract–managed:	0 hospitals	0 beds
Totals:	5 hospitals	1255 beds

2295: LITTLE COMPANY OF MARY SISTERS HEALTHCARE SYSTEM (CC)
9350 South California Avenue, Evergreen Park, IL Zip 60805–2595; tel. 708/229–5491; Sister Carol Pacini, Provincialate Superior
(Moderately Centralized Health System)

CALIFORNIA: LITTLE COMPANY OF MARY HEALTH SERVICES (O, 335 beds) 4101 Torrance Boulevard, Torrance, CA Zip 90503–4698; tel. 310/540–7676; Blair Contratto, President and Chief Executive Officer
Web address: www.lcmhs.org

SAN PEDRO PENINSULA HOSPITAL (O, 309 beds) 1300 West Seventh Street, San Pedro, CA Zip 90732; tel. 310/514–5233; John M. Wilson, President
Web address: www.lchms.org

ILLINOIS: LITTLE COMPANY OF MARY HOSPITAL AND HEALTH CARE CENTERS (O, 306 beds) 2800 West 95th Street, Evergreen Park, IL Zip 60805–2795; tel. 708/422–6200; Sister Kathleen McIntyre, President
Web address: www.lcmh.org

INDIANA: MEMORIAL HOSPITAL AND HEALTH CARE CENTER (O, 124 beds) 800 West Ninth Street, Jasper, IN Zip 47546–2516; tel. 812/482–2345; Raymond W. Snowden, President and Chief Executive Officer
Web address: www.mhhcc.org

Owned, leased, sponsored:	4 hospitals	1074 beds
Contract–managed:	0 hospitals	0 beds
Totals:	4 hospitals	1074 beds

2175: LOMA LINDA UNIVERSITY HEALTH SCIENCES CENTER (NP)
11161 Anderson Street, Loma Linda, CA Zip 92350; tel. 909/824–4540; B. Lyn Behrens, President

CALIFORNIA: LOMA LINDA UNIVERSITY BEHAVIORAL MEDICINE CENTER (O, 89 beds) 1710 Barton Road, Redlands, CA Zip 92373; tel. 909/558–9200; Alan Soderblom, Administrator

LOMA LINDA UNIVERSITY MEDICAL CENTER (O, 653 beds) 11234 Anderson Street, Loma Linda, CA Zip 92354–2870, Mailing Address: P.O. Box 2000, Zip 92354–0200; tel. 909/558–4000; B. Lyn Behrens, President and Chief Executive Officer
Web address: www.llumc.edu

Owned, leased, sponsored:	2 hospitals	742 beds
Contract–managed:	0 hospitals	0 beds
Totals:	2 hospitals	742 beds

5755: LOS ANGELES COUNTY–DEPARTMENT OF HEALTH SERVICES (NP)
313 North Figueroa Street, Room 912, Los Angeles, CA Zip 90012–2691; tel. 213/240–8101; Mark Finucane, Director Health Services
(Centralized Physician/Insurance Health System)

LAC–HARBOR–UNIVERSITY OF CALIFORNIA AT LOS ANGELES MEDICAL CENTER (O, 336 beds) 1000 West Carson Street, Torrance, CA Zip 90509; tel. 310/222–2101; Tecla A. Mickoseff, Administrator

LAC–HIGH DESERT HOSPITAL (O, 82 beds) 44900 North 60th Street West, Lancaster, CA Zip 93536; tel. 661/945–8461; Mel Grussing, Administrator

LAC–KING–DREW MEDICAL CENTER (O, 257 beds) 12021 South Wilmington Avenue, Los Angeles, CA Zip 90059; tel. 310/668–4321; Randall S. Foster, Administrator and Chief Executive Officer

LAC–OLIVE VIEW–UCLA MEDICAL CENTER (O, 213 beds) 14445 Olive View Drive, Sylmar, CA Zip 91342–1495; tel. 818/364–1555; Melinda Anderson, Administrator

LAC–RANCHO LOS AMIGOS NATIONAL REHABILITATION CENTER (O, 207 beds) 7601 East Imperial Highway, Downey, CA Zip 90242; tel. 562/401–7022; Consuelo C. Diaz, Chief Executive Officer
Web address: www.rancho.org

LAC/UNIVERSITY OF SOUTHERN CALIFORNIA MEDICAL CENTER (O, 756 beds) 1200 North State Street, Los Angeles, CA Zip 90033–1084; tel. 323/226–2622; Roberto Rodriguez, Executive Director and Chief Executive Officer
Web address: www.lacusc.org

Owned, leased, sponsored:	6 hospitals	1851 beds
Contract–managed:	0 hospitals	0 beds
Totals:	6 hospitals	1851 beds

0047: LOUISIANA STATE HOSPITALS (NP)
210 State Street, New Orleans, LA Zip 70118–5797; tel. 504/897–3400; Michael E. Teague, Chief Executive Officer
(Independent Hospital System)

LOUISIANA: CENTRAL LOUISIANA STATE HOSPITAL (O, 216 beds) 242 West Shamrock Avenue, Pineville, LA Zip 71361–5031, Mailing Address: P.O. Box 5031, Zip 71361–5031; tel. 318/484–6200; Gary S. Grand, Chief Executive Officer

EAST LOUISIANA STATE HOSPITAL (O, 452 beds) Jackson, LA Mailing Address: P.O. Box 498, Zip 70748–0498; tel. 225/634–0100; Warren T. Price , Jr, Chief Executive Officer

EASTERN LOUISIANA MENTAL HEALTH SYSTEM/GREENWELL SPRING CAMPUS (O, 104 beds) 23260 Greenwell Springs Road, Greenwell Springs, LA Zip 70739–0999, Mailing Address: P.O. Box 549, Zip 70739–0549; tel. 225/261–2730; Lauren Guttzeit, Acting Chief Executive Officer

NEW ORLEANS ADOLESCENT HOSPITAL (O, 95 beds) 210 State Street, New Orleans, LA Zip 70118–5797; tel. 504/897–3400; William J. Malone, M.P.H., Acting Chief Executive Officer

SOUTHEAST LOUISIANA HOSPITAL (O, 231 beds) Mandeville, LA Mailing Address: P.O. Box 3850, Zip 70470–3850; tel. 504/626–6300; Joseph C. Vinturella, Chief Executive Officer

Owned, leased, sponsored:	5 hospitals	1098 beds
Contract–managed:	0 hospitals	0 beds
Totals:	5 hospitals	1098 beds

★0715: LSU MEDICAL CENTER HEALTH CARE SERVICES DIVISION (NP)
8550 United Plaza Boulevard, 4th Floor, Baton Rouge, LA Zip 70809; tel. 225/922–0490; James L. Brexler, President and Chief Executive Officer
(Moderately Centralized Health System)

E. A. CONWAY MEDICAL CENTER (O, 174 beds) 4864 Jackson Street, Monroe, LA Zip 71202–6497, Mailing Address: P.O. Box 1881, Zip 71210–1881; tel. 318/330–7000; Aryon McGuire, Acting Administrator

EARL K. LONG MEDICAL CENTER (O, 204 beds) 5825 Airline Highway, Baton Rouge, LA Zip 70805–2498; tel. 225/358–1000; Jonathan Roberts, Dr.PH, Administrator

HUEY P. LONG MEDICAL CENTER (O, 123 beds) 352 Hospital Boulevard, Pineville, LA Zip 71360, Mailing Address: P.O. Box 5352, Zip 71361–5352; tel. 318/448–0811; James E. Morgan, Administrator

LALLIE KEMP MEDICAL CENTER (O, 68 beds) 52579 Highway 51 South, Independence, LA Zip 70443–2231; tel. 504/878–9421; LeVern S. Meades, Administrator

LEONARD J. CHABERT MEDICAL CENTER (O, 123 beds) 1978 Industrial Boulevard, Houma, LA Zip 70363–7094; tel. 504/873–2200; Daniel M. Trahan, Administrator

MEDICAL CENTER OF LOUISIANA AT NEW ORLEANS (O, 643 beds) 2021 Perdido Street, New Orleans, LA Zip 70112–1396; tel. 504/588–3000; John S. Berault, Chief Executive Officer

UNIVERSITY MEDICAL CENTER (O, 133 beds) 2390 West Congress Street, Lafayette, LA Zip 70506–4298, Mailing Address: P.O. Box 69300, Zip 70596–9300; tel. 337/261–6001; Lawrence T. Dorsey, Administrator
Web address: www.umcip.lsums.edu

For explanation of codes following names, see page B2.
★ Indicates Type III membership in the American Hospital Association.

Systems / Marian Health System

WALTER OLIN MOSS REGIONAL MEDICAL CENTER (O, 74 beds) 1000 Walters Street, Lake Charles, LA Zip 70605; tel. 318/475–8100; Clay Dunaway, Administrator

WASHINGTON–ST. TAMMANY REGIONAL MEDICAL CENTER (O, 50 beds) 400 Memphis Street, Bogalusa, LA Zip 70427–0040, Mailing Address: Box 40, Zip 70427–0040; tel. 504/735–1322; Larry R. King, Administrator

Owned, leased, sponsored:	9 hospitals	1592 beds
Contract–managed:	0 hospitals	0 beds
Totals:	9 hospitals	1592 beds

★0036: LUBBOCK METHODIST HOSPITAL SYSTEM (NP)
3615 19th Street, Lubbock, TX Zip 79410–1201; tel. 806/725–1011; George H. McCleskey, President and Chief Executive Officer
(Independent Hospital System)

NEW MEXICO: NOR–LEA GENERAL HOSPITAL (C, 28 beds) 1600 North Main Avenue, Lovington, NM Zip 88260–2871; tel. 505/396–6611; David B. Shaw, Chief Executive Officer and Administrator
Web address: www.nlgh.org

TEXAS: FISHER COUNTY HOSPITAL DISTRICT (C, 23 beds) Roby Highway, Rotan, TX Zip 79546, Mailing Address: Drawer F, Zip 79546; tel. 915/735–2256; Ella Raye Helms, Administrator

LAMB HEALTHCARE CENTER (C, 41 beds) 1500 South Sunset, Littlefield, TX Zip 79339–4899; tel. 806/385–6411; Randall A. Young, Administrator

MITCHELL COUNTY HOSPITAL (C, 25 beds) 1543 Chestnut Street, Colorado City, TX Zip 79512–3998; tel. 915/728–3431; Roland K. Rickard, Administrator

MULESHOE AREA MEDICAL CENTER (C, 79 beds) 708 South First Street, Muleshoe, TX Zip 79347–3627; tel. 806/272–4524; Jim G. Bone, Interim Administrator

REEVES COUNTY HOSPITAL (C, 44 beds) 2323 Texas Street, Pecos, TX Zip 79772–7338; tel. 915/447–3551; Charles N. Butts, Chief Executive Officer
Web address: www.rchd.org

Owned, leased, sponsored:	0 hospitals	0 beds
Contract–managed:	6 hospitals	240 beds
Totals:	6 hospitals	240 beds

0695: MAGELLAN HEALTH SERVICES (IO)
3414 Peachtree Road N.E., Suite 1400, Atlanta, GA Zip 30326; tel. 404/841–9200; Henry Harbin, M.D., President and Chief Executive Officer
(Independent Hospital System)

ALASKA: CHARTER NORTH STAR BEHAVIORAL HEALTH SYSTEM (O, 34 beds) 1650 South Bragaw, Anchorage, AK Zip 99508–3467; tel. 907/258–7575; Kathleen Cronen, Chief Executive Officer

CHARTER NORTH STAR BEHAVIORAL HEALTH SYSTEM (O, 80 beds) 2530 DeBarr Road, Anchorage, AK Zip 99508; tel. 907/258–7575; Kathleen Cronen, Chief Executive Officer
Web address: www.charterbehavioral.com

ARKANSAS: CHARTER BEHAVIORAL HEALTH SYSTEM OF NORTHWEST ARKANSAS (O, 49 beds) 4253 North Crossover Road, Fayetteville, AR Zip 72703–4596; tel. 501/521–5731; Patrick Kelly, Chief Executive Officer

FLORIDA: CHARTER SPRINGS HOSPITAL (O, 92 beds) 3130 S.W. 27th Avenue, Ocala, FL Zip 34474–4485, Mailing Address: P.O. Box 3338, Zip 34478–3338; tel. 352/237–7293; Marina Cecchini, Chief Executive Officer

GEORGIA: CHARTER ANCHOR HOSPITAL (O, 84 beds) 5454 Yorktowne Drive, Atlanta, GA Zip 30349–5305; tel. 770/991–6044; Matthew Crouch, Chief Executive Officer
Web address: www.talbottcampus.com

CHARTER BEHAVIORAL HEALTH SYSTEM OF ATLANTA (O, 40 beds) 811 Juniper Street N.E., Atlanta, GA Zip 30308–1398; tel. 404/881–5800; John McKenna, Administrator

CHARTER BEHAVIORAL HEALTH SYSTEM OF ATLANTA AT PEACHFORD (O, 224 beds) 2151 Peachford Road, Atlanta, GA Zip 30338–6599; tel. 770/455–3200; Ron Fincher, Chief Executive Officer

CHARTER SAVANNAH BEHAVIORAL HEALTH SYSTEM (O, 112 beds) 1150 Cornell Avenue, Savannah, GA Zip 31406–2797; tel. 912/354–3911; Jim Shaheer, Chief Executive Officer

CHARTER BY–THE–SEA BEHAVIORAL HEALTH SYSTEM (O, 98 beds) 2927 Demere Road, Saint Simons Island, GA Zip 31522–1620; tel. 912/638–1999; Wes Robbins, Chief Executive Officer

INDIANA: CHARTER BEACON (O, 97 beds) 1720 Beacon Street, Fort Wayne, IN Zip 46805–4700; tel. 219/423–3651; Robert Hails, Chief Executive Officer
Web address: www.charterbeacon.com

KENTUCKY: CHARTER RIDGE BEHAVIORAL HEALTH SYSTEM (O, 110 beds) 3050 Rio Dosa Drive, Lexington, KY Zip 40509–9990; tel. 606/269–2325; Barbara Kitchen, Chief Executive Officer

MASSACHUSETTS: PEMBROKE HOSPITAL (O, 80 beds) 199 Oak Street, Pembroke, MA Zip 02359–1953; tel. 781/826–8161; Kenneth A. Davis, Chief Executive Officer

MISSISSIPPI: PARKWOOD BEHAVIORAL HEALTH SYSTEM (O, 66 beds) 8135 Goodman Road, Olive Branch, MS Zip 38654–2199; tel. 662/895–4900; M. Andrew Mayo, Chief Executive Officer

NEW JERSEY: CHARTER BEHAVIORAL HEALTH SYSTEM OF NEW JERSEY–SUMMIT (O, 90 beds) 19 Prospect Street, Summit, NJ Zip 07902–0100; tel. 908/522–7000; Lori Ann Rizzuto, Chief Executive Officer

NORTH CAROLINA: CHARTER BEHAVIORAL HEALTH SYSTEM OF WINSTON–SALEM (O, 99 beds) 3637 Old Vineyard Road, Winston–Salem, NC Zip 27104–4835; tel. 336/768–7710; Marsha Olender, Chief Executive Officer
Web address: www.charterbehavioral.com

HOLLY HILL/ CHARTER BEHAVIORAL HEALTH SYSTEM (O, 108 beds) 3019 Falstaff Road, Raleigh, NC Zip 27610–1812; tel. 919/250–7000; Andy Delbridge, Chief Operating Officer
Web address: www.hcahealthcare.com

PENNSYLVANIA: CHARTER FAIRMOUNT BEHAVIORAL HEALTH SYSTEM (O, 146 beds) 561 Fairthorne Avenue, Philadelphia, PA Zip 19128–2499; tel. 215/487–4000; Diane Kiddy, Chief Executive Officer
Web address: www.charterbehavioral.com

SOUTH CAROLINA: CHARTER CHARLESTON BEHAVIORAL HEALTH SYSTEM (O, 70 beds) 2777 Speissegger Drive, Charleston, SC Zip 29405–8299; tel. 843/747–5830; Anne Battin, Administrator

CHARTER GREENVILLE BEHAVIORAL HEALTH SYSTEM (O, 66 beds) 2700 East Phillips Road, Greer, SC Zip 29650–4816; tel. 864/968–6300; William L. Callison, Chief Executive Officer
Web address: www.charterbehavioral.com/locations/sc_gville.html

CHARTER RIVERS BEHAVIORAL HEALTH SYSTEM (O, 66 beds) 2900 Sunset Boulevard, West Columbia, SC Zip 29169–3422; tel. 803/796–9911; R. Andy Hanner, Chief Executive Officer
Web address: www.charterbehavioral.com

TENNESSEE: CHARTER LAKESIDE BEHAVIORAL HEALTH SYSTEM (O, 174 beds) 2911 Brunswick Road, Memphis, TN Zip 38133–4199, Mailing Address: P.O. Box 341308, Zip 38134–1308; tel. 901/377–4700; Rob S. Waggener, Chief Executive Officer

VIRGINIA: CHARTER BEHAVIORAL HEALTH SYSTEM OF CHARLOTTESVILLE (O, 62 beds) 2101 Arlington Boulevard, Charlottesville, VA Zip 22903–1593; tel. 804/977–1120; David Carlini, Chief Executive Officer

NORFOLK PSYCHIATRIC CENTER (O, 77 beds) 860 Kempsville Road, Norfolk, VA Zip 23502–3980; tel. 757/461–4565; Arlene Manzella, Administrator

Owned, leased, sponsored:	23 hospitals	2124 beds
Contract–managed:	0 hospitals	0 beds
Totals:	23 hospitals	2124 beds

★5305: MARIAN HEALTH SYSTEM (CC)
Tulsa, OK Mailing Address: P.O. Box 4753, Zip 74159–0753; tel. 918/742–9988; Sister M. Therese Gottschalk, President
(Moderately Centralized Health System)

For explanation of codes following names, see page B2.
★ Indicates Type III membership in the American Hospital Association.

Systems / Marian Health System

MINNESOTA: ST. ELIZABETH HOSPITAL (O, 155 beds) 1200 Fifth Grand Boulevard West, Wabasha, MN Zip 55981-1098; tel. 651/565-4531; Thomas Crowley, President
Web address: www.ministryhealthcare.org

NEW JERSEY: SAINT CLARE'S HEALTH SERVICES (O, 662 beds) 25 Pocono Road, Denville, NJ Zip 07834-2995; tel. 973/625-6000; Kathryn J. McDonagh, President and Chief Executive Officer
Web address: www.saintclares.org

OKLAHOMA: ST. JOHN MEDICAL CENTER (O, 556 beds) 1923 South Utica Avenue, Tulsa, OK Zip 74104-5445; tel. 918/744-2345; David Pynn, President and Chief Executive Officer
Web address: www.sjmc.org

ST. JOHN SAPULPA (O, 113 beds) 519 South Division Street, Sapulpa, OK Zip 74066-4501, Mailing Address: P.O. Box 1368, Zip 74067-1368; tel. 918/224-4280; Raymond L. Replogle, President and Chief Executive Officer

WISCONSIN: DOOR COUNTY MEMORIAL HOSPITAL (O, 75 beds) 323 South 18th Avenue, Sturgeon Bay, WI Zip 54235-1495; tel. 920/743-5566; Gerald M. Worrick, President and Chief Executive Officer
Web address: www.doorcounty-wi.com

FLAMBEAU HOSPITAL (O, 42 beds) 98 Sherry Avenue, Park Falls, WI Zip 54552-1467, Mailing Address: P.O. Box 310, Zip 54552-0310; tel. 715/762-2484; Curtis A. Johnson, Administrator
Web address: www.ministryhealth.org/facility/fh.html

SACRED HEART-ST. MARY'S HOSPITALS (O, 53 beds) 1044 Kabel Avenue, Rhinelander, WI Zip 54501-3998; tel. 715/369-6600; Kevin J. O'Donnell, President and Chief Executive Officer
Web address: www.ministryhealth.org

SAINT JOSEPH'S HOSPITAL (O, 524 beds) 611 St. Joseph Avenue, Marshfield, WI Zip 54449-1898; tel. 715/387-1713; Michael A. Schmidt, President and Chief Executive Officer
Web address: www.stjosephs-marshfield.org

SAINT MICHAEL'S HOSPITAL (O, 114 beds) 900 Illinois Avenue, Stevens Point, WI Zip 54481-3196; tel. 715/346-5000; Jeffrey L. Martin, President and Chief Executive Officer
Web address: www.smhosp.org

VICTORY MEDICAL CENTER (O, 111 beds) 230 East Fourth Avenue, Stanley, WI Zip 54768-1298; tel. 715/644-5571; Cynthia Eichman, Chief Executive Officer and Administrator
Web address: www.victorymedicalcenter.org

Owned, leased, sponsored:	10 hospitals	2405 beds
Contract-managed:	0 hospitals	0 beds
Totals:	10 hospitals	2405 beds

0207: MARINER POST-ACUTE NETWORK, INC. (IO)
1 Ravinia Drive, Suite 1500, Atlanta, GA Zip 30346; tel. 678/443-7000; Christian Winkle, Chief Executive Officer

TEXAS: SPECIALTY HOSPITAL OF AUSTIN (O, 133 beds) 4207 Burnet Road, Austin, TX Zip 78756-3396; tel. 512/706-1900; Robert F. Berry, Chief Executive Officer

SPECIALTY HOSPITAL OF HOUSTON (O, 106 beds) 5556 Gasmer Drive, Houston, TX Zip 77035-4598; tel. 713/551-5300; Ronald J. Castagno, FACHE, Chief Executive Officer

Owned, leased, sponsored:	2 hospitals	239 beds
Contract-managed:	0 hospitals	0 beds
Totals:	2 hospitals	239 beds

1975: MARSHALL COUNTY HEALTH CARE AUTHORITY (NP)
8000 Alabama Highway 69, Guntersville, AL Zip 35976; tel. 256/753-8000; Julian Sparks, Board Chairman
(Centralized Physician/Insurance Health System)

ALABAMA: MARSHALL MEDICAL CENTER NORTH (O, 90 beds) 8000 Alabama Highway 69, Guntersville, AL Zip 35976; tel. 256/753-8000; Gary R. Gore, Chief Executive Officer
Web address: www.mmcnorth.com

MARSHALL MEDICAL CENTER SOUTH (O, 102 beds) U.S. Highway 431 North, Boaz, AL Zip 35957-0999, Mailing Address: P.O. Box 758, Zip 35957-0758; tel. 256/593-8310; J. Marlin Hanson, Administrator

Owned, leased, sponsored:	2 hospitals	192 beds
Contract-managed:	0 hospitals	0 beds
Totals:	2 hospitals	192 beds

0013: MASSACHUSETTS DEPARTMENT OF MENTAL HEALTH (NP)
25 Staniford Street, Boston, MA Zip 02114-2575; tel. 617/626-8123; Marylou Sudders, Commissioner
(Independent Hospital System)

MASSACHUSETTS: MEDFIELD STATE HOSPITAL (O, 147 beds) 45 Hospital Road, Medfield, MA Zip 02052-1099; tel. 508/359-7312; Margaret E. LaMontagne, R.N., Chief Operating Officer

TAUNTON STATE HOSPITAL (O, 185 beds) 60 Hodges Avenue Extension, Taunton, MA Zip 02780-3034, Mailing Address: P.O. Box 4007, Zip 02780-4007; tel. 508/977-3000; Katherine Chmiel, R.N., MS, Administrator and Chief Operating Officer

WESTBOROUGH STATE HOSPITAL (O, 220 beds) Lyman Street, Westborough, MA Zip 01581-0288, Mailing Address: P.O. Box 288, Zip 01581-0288; tel. 508/366-4401; Theodore E. Kirousis, Area Director

WORCESTER STATE HOSPITAL (O, 176 beds) 305 Belmont Street, Worcester, MA Zip 01604-1695; tel. 508/368-3300; Raymond Robinson, Chief Operating Officer

Owned, leased, sponsored:	4 hospitals	728 beds
Contract-managed:	0 hospitals	0 beds
Totals:	4 hospitals	728 beds

2505: MATAGORDA COUNTY HOSPITAL DISTRICT (NP)
1115 Avenue G, Bay City, TX Zip 77414-3544; tel. 979/245-6383; Wendell H. Baker, Jr, District Administrator
(Moderately Centralized Health System)

TEXAS: MATAGORDA GENERAL HOSPITAL (O, 67 beds) 1115 Avenue G, Bay City, TX Zip 77414-3544; tel. 979/245-6383; Wendell H. Baker, Jr, Chief Executive Officer

WAGNER GENERAL HOSPITAL (O, 6 beds) 310 Green Street, Palacios, TX Zip 77465-3214, Mailing Address: P.O. Box 859, Zip 77465-0859; tel. 361/972-2511; Kevin Hecht, Director

Owned, leased, sponsored:	2 hospitals	73 beds
Contract-managed:	0 hospitals	0 beds
Totals:	2 hospitals	73 beds

★1875: MAYO FOUNDATION (NP)
200 S.W. First Street, Rochester, MN Zip 55905-0002; tel. 507/284-2511; Michael B. Wood, M.D., President and Chief Executive Officer
(Moderately Centralized Health System)

ARIZONA: MAYO CLINIC HOSPITAL (O, 178 beds) 5777 East Mayo Boulevard, Phoenix, AZ Zip 85054-4502; tel. 480/515-6296; Thomas C. Bour, Administrator

FLORIDA: ST. LUKE'S HOSPITAL (O, 240 beds) 4201 Belfort Road, Jacksonville, FL Zip 32216-5898; tel. 904/296-3700; Robert M. Walters, Administrator

IOWA: FLOYD COUNTY MEMORIAL HOSPITAL (C, 31 beds) 800 Eleventh Street, Charles City, IA Zip 50616-3499; tel. 515/228-6830; Bill D. Faust, Administrator
Web address: www.willowtree.com/~fcmh/

MINNESOTA: ALBERT LEA MEDICAL CENTER (O, 129 beds) 404 West Fountain Street, Albert Lea, MN Zip 56007-2473; tel. 507/373-2384; Ronald A. Harmon, M.D., Chief Executive Officer

For explanation of codes following names, see page B2.
★ Indicates Type III membership in the American Hospital Association.

Systems / Memorial Health System

IMMANUEL ST. JOSEPH'S–MAYO HEALTH SYSTEM (O, 147 beds) 1025 Marsh Street, Mankato, MN Zip 56002–4700, Mailing Address: P.O. Box 8673, Zip 56002–8673; tel. 507/625–4031; W. Neath Folger, M.D., President and Chief Executive Officer
Web address: www.isj–mhs.net/isjmhs.html

ROCHESTER METHODIST HOSPITAL (O, 335 beds) 201 West Center Street, Rochester, MN Zip 55902–3084; tel. 507/266–7890; John M. Panicek, Administrator

SAINT MARYS HOSPITAL (O, 797 beds) 1216 Second Street S.W., Rochester, MN Zip 55902–1970; tel. 507/255–5123; John M. Panicek, Administrator

WISCONSIN: BARRON MEDICAL CENTER–MAYO HEALTH SYSTEM (C, 92 beds) 1222 Woodland Avenue, Barron, WI Zip 54812–1798; tel. 715/537–3186; Mark D. Wilson, Administrator

BLOOMER MEMORIAL MEDICAL CENTER (C, 107 beds) 1501 Thompson Street, Bloomer, WI Zip 54724–1299; tel. 715/568–2000; Mary Kerg, Administrator

LUTHER HOSPITAL (O, 179 beds) 1221 Whipple Street, Eau Claire, WI Zip 54702–4105, Mailing Address: P.O. Box 5, Zip 54702–0005; tel. 715/838–3311; William Rupp, M.D., President and Chief Executive Officer

OSSEO AREA HOSPITAL AND NURSING HOME (C, 77 beds) 13025 Eighth Street, Osseo, WI Zip 54758, Mailing Address: P.O. Box 70, Zip 54758–0070; tel. 715/597–3121; Bradley D. Groseth, Administrator

Owned, leased, sponsored:	7 hospitals	2005 beds
Contract–managed:	4 hospitals	307 beds
Totals:	11 hospitals	2312 beds

0200: MEDCATH, INC. (IO)
7621 Little Avenue, Suite 106, Charlotte, NC Zip 28226; tel. 704/541–3228; Stephen R. Puckett, Chairman, President and Chief Executive Officer

ARIZONA: ARIZONA HEART HOSPITAL (O, 56 beds) 1930 East Thomas Road, Phoenix, AZ Zip 85016; tel. 602/532–1000; John L. Harrington , Jr, FACHE, President

ARKANSAS: ARKANSAS HEART HOSPITAL (O, 84 beds) 1701 South Shackleford Road, Little Rock, AR Zip 72211; tel. 501/219–7000; David Blackburn, President
Web address: www.arheart.com

TEXAS: MCALLEN HEART HOSPITAL (O, 60 beds) 1900 South D. Street, McAllen, TX Zip 78503; tel. 956/994–2000; Roy C. Vinson, President

Owned, leased, sponsored:	3 hospitals	200 beds
Contract–managed:	0 hospitals	0 beds
Totals:	3 hospitals	200 beds

★**0154: MEDSTAR HEALTH** (NP)
5565 Sterrett Place, 5th Floor, Columbia, MD Zip 21044; tel. 410/772–6500; John P. McDaniel, Chief Executive Officer
(Centralized Health System)

DISTRICT OF COLUMBIA: NATIONAL REHABILITATION HOSPITAL (O, 128 beds) 102 Irving Street N.W., Washington, DC Zip 20010–2949; tel. 202/877–1000; Edward A. Eckenhoff, President and Chief Executive Officer
Web address: www.nrhrehab.org/index.htm

WASHINGTON HOSPITAL CENTER (O, 791 beds) 110 Irving Street N.W., Washington, DC Zip 20010–2975; tel. 202/877–7000; Michael H. Covert, FACHE, President
Web address: www.whcenter.org

MARYLAND: FRANKLIN SQUARE HOSPITAL CENTER (O, 405 beds) 9000 Franklin Square Drive, Baltimore, MD Zip 21237–3998; tel. 410/682–7000; Carl J. Schindelar, President
Web address: www.helix.org

GOOD SAMARITAN HOSPITAL OF MARYLAND (O, 254 beds) 5601 Loch Raven Boulevard, Baltimore, MD Zip 21239–2995; tel. 410/532–8000; Lawrence M. Beck, President and Chief Executive Officer
Web address: www.helixhealth.com

HARBOR HOSPITAL CENTER (O, 182 beds) 3001 South Hanover Street, Baltimore, MD Zip 21225–1290; tel. 410/350–3200; L. Barney Johnson, President and Chief Executive Officer
Web address: www.helixhealth.com

UNION MEMORIAL HOSPITAL (O, 318 beds) 201 East University Parkway, Baltimore, MD Zip 21218–2895; tel. 410/554–2000; Harrison J. Rider, II, President
Web address: www.medstarhealth.org

Owned, leased, sponsored:	6 hospitals	2078 beds
Contract–managed:	0 hospitals	0 beds
Totals:	6 hospitals	2078 beds

0084: MEMORIAL HEALTH SERVICES (NP)
2801 Atlantic Avenue, Long Beach, CA Zip 90806, Mailing Address: P.O. Box 1428, Zip 90801–1428; tel. 562/933–9700; Thomas J. Collins, President and Chief Executive Officer
(Independent Hospital System)

CALIFORNIA: ANAHEIM MEMORIAL MEDICAL CENTER (O, 375 beds) 1111 West La Palma Avenue, Anaheim, CA Zip 92801; tel. 714/774–1450; Michael C. Carter, Chief Executive Officer

LONG BEACH MEMORIAL MEDICAL CENTER (O, 726 beds) 2801 Atlantic Avenue, Long Beach, CA Zip 90806, Mailing Address: P.O. Box 1428, Zip 90801–1428; tel. 562/933–2000; Byron Schweigert, Chief Executive Officer
Web address: www.memorialcare.org

ORANGE COAST MEMORIAL MEDICAL CENTER (O, 230 beds) 9920 Talbert Avenue, Fountain Valley, CA Zip 92708; tel. 714/378–7000; Barry S. Arbuckle, Ph.D., Chief Executive Officer
Web address: www.memorialcare.org

SADDLEBACK MEMORIAL MEDICAL CENTER (O, 220 beds) 24451 Health Center Drive, Laguna Hills, CA Zip 92653; tel. 949/837–4500; Barry S. Arbuckle, Ph.D., Chief Executive Officer
Web address: www.memorialcare.org

Owned, leased, sponsored:	4 hospitals	1551 beds
Contract–managed:	0 hospitals	0 beds
Totals:	4 hospitals	1551 beds

2335: MEMORIAL HEALTH SERVICES (IO)
706 North Parrish Avenue, Adel, GA Zip 31620–2064, Mailing Address: P.O. Box 677, Zip 31620–0677; tel. 912/896–2251; Wade E. Keck, Chief Executive Officer
(Independent Hospital System)

GEORGIA: BLECKLEY MEMORIAL HOSPITAL (C, 25 beds) 408 Peacock Street, Cochran, GA Zip 31014–1559, Mailing Address: P.O. Box 536, Zip 31014–0536; tel. 912/934–6211; Cary Martin, Administrator

SMITH HOSPITAL (C, 71 beds) 117 East Main Street, Hahira, GA Zip 31632–1156, Mailing Address: P.O. Box 337, Zip 31632–0337; tel. 912/794–1912; Robert Bauer, Administrator

TELFAIR COUNTY HOSPITAL (C, 52 beds) U.S. 341 South, McRae, GA Zip 31055, Mailing Address: P.O. Box 150, Zip 31055–0150; tel. 912/868–5621; Gail Leggett, Administrator

Owned, leased, sponsored:	0 hospitals	0 beds
Contract–managed:	3 hospitals	148 beds
Totals:	3 hospitals	148 beds

★**0086: MEMORIAL HEALTH SYSTEM** (NP)
701 North First Street, Springfield, IL Zip 62781–0001; tel. 217/788–3000; Robert T. Clarke, President and Chief Executive Officer
(Centralized Physician/Insurance Health System)

ILLINOIS: ABRAHAM LINCOLN MEMORIAL HOSPITAL (O, 60 beds) 315 8th Street, Lincoln, IL Zip 62656–2698; tel. 217/732–2161; Forrest G. Hester, President and Chief Executive Officer
Web address: www.almh.com

For explanation of codes following names, see page B2.
★ Indicates Type III membership in the American Hospital Association.

Systems / Memorial Health System

MEMORIAL MEDICAL CENTER (O, 453 beds) 701 North First Street, Springfield, IL Zip 62781–0001; tel. 217/788–3000; Robert T. Clarke, President and Chief Executive Officer
Web address: www.memorialmedical.com

ST. VINCENT MEMORIAL HOSPITAL (S, 151 beds) 201 East Pleasant Street, Taylorville, IL Zip 62568–1597; tel. 217/824–3331; Daniel J. Raab, President and Chief Executive Officer

Owned, leased, sponsored:	3 hospitals	664 beds
Contract–managed:	0 hospitals	0 beds
Totals:	3 hospitals	664 beds

0176: MEMORIAL HEALTH SYSTEM OF EAST TEXAS (NP)
1201 West Frank Avenue, Lufkin, TX Zip 75904–3357; tel. 409/634–8111; Gary Lex Whatley, President and Chief Executive Officer
(Centralized Physician/Insurance Health System)

TEXAS: MEMORIAL HEALTH SYSTEM OF EAST TEXAS (O, 234 beds) 1201 West Frank Avenue, Lufkin, TX Zip 75904–3357, Mailing Address: P.O. Box 1447, Zip 75902–1447; tel. 936/634–8111; Gary Lex Whatley, President and Chief Executive Officer
Web address: www.memorialhealth.org

MEMORIAL MEDICAL CENTER (O, 31 beds) 602 East Church Street, Livingston, TX Zip 77351–1257, Mailing Address: P.O. Box 1257, Zip 77351–1257; tel. 936/327–4381; James C. Dickson, Administrator

MEMORIAL MEDICAL CENTER OF SAN AUGUSTINE (O, 16 beds) 511 East Hospital Street, San Augustine, TX Zip 75972–2121, Mailing Address: P.O. Box 658, Zip 75972–0658; tel. 409/275–3446; Terry Napper, Administrator
Web address: www.memorialhealth.org

Owned, leased, sponsored:	3 hospitals	281 beds
Contract–managed:	0 hospitals	0 beds
Totals:	3 hospitals	281 beds

★2615: MEMORIAL HEALTH SYSTEMS (NP)
770 West Granada Boulevard, Ormond Beach, FL Zip 32174–5197; tel. 904/615–4100; Richard A. Lind, President and Chief Executive Officer
(Moderately Centralized Health System)

FLORIDA: MEMORIAL HOSPITAL–FLAGLER (O, 81 beds) Moody Boulevard, Bunnell, FL Zip 32110, Mailing Address: HCR1, Box 2, Zip 32110; tel. 904/437–2211; Clark P. Christianson, Senior Vice President and Administrator
Web address: www.memorialhealth.com

MEMORIAL HOSPITAL–ORMOND BEACH (O, 205 beds) 875 Sterthaus Avenue, Ormond Beach, FL Zip 32174–5197; tel. 904/676–6000; Clark P. Christianson, Senior Vice President and Administrator

MEMORIAL HOSPITAL–PENINSULA (O, 119 beds) 264 South Atlantic Avenue, Ormond Beach, FL Zip 32176–8192; tel. 904/672–4161; Clark P. Christianson, Senior Vice President and Administrator

MEMORIAL HOSPITAL–WEST VOLUSIA (L, 156 beds) 701 West Plymouth Avenue, De Land, FL Zip 32720–3291, Mailing Address: P.O. Box 6509, Zip 32721–6509; tel. 904/734–3320; Johnette L. Vodenicker, Administrator

Owned, leased, sponsored:	4 hospitals	561 beds
Contract–managed:	0 hospitals	0 beds
Totals:	4 hospitals	561 beds

★0083: MEMORIAL HEALTHCARE SYSTEM (NP)
3501 Johnson Street, Hollywood, FL Zip 33021–5487; tel. 954/985–5805; Frank V. Sacco, FACHE, Chief Executive Officer
(Centralized Health System)

MEMORIAL HOSPITAL PEMBROKE (L, 301 beds) 7800 Sheridan Street, Pembroke Pines, FL Zip 33024; tel. 954/962–9650; J. E. Piriz, Administrator
Web address: www.mhs-net.com

MEMORIAL HOSPITAL WEST (O, 174 beds) 703 North Flamingo Road, Pembroke Pines, FL Zip 33028; tel. 954/436–5000; Zeff Ross, Administrator
Web address: www.mhs-net.com

MEMORIAL REGIONAL HOSPITAL (O, 672 beds) 3501 Johnson Street, Hollywood, FL Zip 33021–5421; tel. 954/987–2000; C. Kennon Hetlage, Administrator
Web address: www.mhs-net.com

Owned, leased, sponsored:	3 hospitals	1147 beds
Contract–managed:	0 hospitals	0 beds
Totals:	3 hospitals	1147 beds

★2645: MEMORIAL HERMANN HEALTHCARE SYSTEM (NP)
7737 S.W. Freeway, Suite 200, Houston, TX Zip 77074–1800; tel. 713/776–6992; Dan S. Wilford, President and Chief Executive Officer
(Centralized Health System)

TEXAS: HERMANN HOSPITAL (O, 625 beds) 6411 Fannin, Houston, TX Zip 77030–1501; tel. 713/704–4000; James E. Eastham, Senior Vice President and Chief Executive Officer
Web address: www.mhhs.org

KATY MEDICAL CENTER (O, 80 beds) 5602 Medical Center Drive, Katy, TX Zip 77494–6399; tel. 281/392–1111; Brian S. Barbe, Chief Executive Officer

MEMORIAL HERMANN BAPTIST HOSPITAL–EAST CAMPUS (O, 372 beds) 3080 College Street, Beaumont, TX Zip 77701–4689, Mailing Address: P.O. Box 5817, Zip 77726–5817; tel. 409/833–1411; David N. Parmer, President and Chief Executive Officer

MEMORIAL HERMANN BAPTIST HOSPITAL–WEST CAMPUS (O, 184 beds) College and 11th Streets, Beaumont, TX Zip 77701, Mailing Address: Drawer 1591, Zip 77704–1591; tel. 409/835–3781; David N. Parmer, President and Chief Executive Officer

MEMORIAL HERMANN FORT BEND HOSPITAL (O, 65 beds) 3803 FM 1092 at Highway 6, Missouri City, TX Zip 77459; tel. 281/499–4800; Rod Brace, Chief Executive Officer
Web address: www.mhhs.org

MEMORIAL HERMANN MEMORIAL CITY HOSPITAL (L, 324 beds) 920 Frostwood Drive, Houston, TX Zip 77024–9173; tel. 713/932–3000; Wayne M. Voss, Chief Executive Officer
Web address: www.mhhs.org

MEMORIAL HERMANN REHABILITATION HOSPITAL (L, 106 beds) 3043 Gessner Drive, Houston, TX Zip 77080–2597; tel. 713/462–2515; Roger Truskoloski, Vice President and Chief Executive Officer
Web address: www.mhhs.org

MEMORIAL HERMANN SOUTHWEST HOSPITAL (O, 877 beds) 7600 Beechnut, Houston, TX Zip 77074–1850; tel. 713/776–5000; Jerel T. Humphrey, Chief Executive Officer
Web address: www.mhhs.org

MEMORIAL HERMANN THE WOODLANDS HOSPITAL (O, 90 beds) 9250 Pinecroft Drive, The Woodlands, TX Zip 77380–3225; tel. 281/364–2300; Steve Sanders, Vice President and Chief Executive Officer
Web address: www.mhhs.org

Owned, leased, sponsored:	9 hospitals	2723 beds
Contract–managed:	0 hospitals	0 beds
Totals:	9 hospitals	2723 beds

★7235: METHODIST HEALTH CARE SYSTEM (CO)
6565 Fannin Street, D–200, Houston, TX Zip 77030–2707; tel. 713/790–2221; Peter W. Butler, President and Chief Executive Officer
(Centralized Physician/Insurance Health System)

DIAGNOSTIC CENTER HOSPITAL (O, 109 beds) 6447 Main Street, Houston, TX Zip 77030–1595; tel. 713/790–0790; Marc Boom, M.D., Chief Executive Officer
Web address: www.tmh.tmc.edi/

METHODIST HEALTH CENTER–SUGAR LAND (O, 22 beds) 16655 S.W. Freeway, Sugar Land, TX Zip 77479; tel. 281/274–8000; Joan Damon, Administrator
Web address: www.methodisthealth.com

For explanation of codes following names, see page B2.
★ Indicates Type III membership in the American Hospital Association.

Systems / Mississippi State Department of Mental Health

SAN JACINTO METHODIST HOSPITAL (O, 231 beds) 4401 Garth Road, Baytown, TX Zip 77521–3160; tel. 281/420–8600; William Simmons, President and Chief Executive Officer
Web address: www.sanjacintomethodisthospital.com

THE METHODIST HOSPITAL (O, 879 beds) 6565 Fannin Street, Houston, TX Zip 77030–2707; tel. 713/790–3311; Lynn Schroth, Dr.PH, Executive Vice President
Web address: www.methodisthealth.com

Owned, leased, sponsored:	4 hospitals	1241 beds
Contract–managed:	0 hospitals	0 beds
Totals:	4 hospitals	1241 beds

★**9345: METHODIST HEALTHCARE** (CO)
1211 Union Avenue, Suite 700, Memphis, TN Zip 38104–6600; tel. 901/726–2300; Maurice W. Elliott, Chief Executive Officer
(Centralized Physician/Insurance Health System)

TENNESSEE: METHODIST HEALTHCARE – MCKENZIE (O, 29 beds) 161 Hospital Drive, McKenzie, TN Zip 38201–1636; tel. 901/352–5344; Richard M. McCormick, Administrator
Web address: www.methodisthealth.org

METHODIST HEALTHCARE– DYERSBURG HOSPITAL (O, 105 beds) 400 Tickle Street, Dyersburg, TN Zip 38024–3182; tel. 901/285–2410; R. Coleman Foss, Chief Executive Officer
Web address: www.methodisthealth.org

METHODIST HEALTHCARE–BROWNSVILLE (O, 44 beds) 2545 North Washington Avenue, Brownsville, TN Zip 38012–1697; tel. 901/772–4110; Sandra Bailey, Administrator
Web address: www.methodisthealth.org

METHODIST HEALTHCARE–LEXINGTON HOSPITAL (O, 32 beds) 200 West Church Street, Lexington, TN Zip 38351–2014; tel. 901/968–3646; Eugene Ragghianti, Administrator
Web address: www.methodisthealth.org

METHODIST HEALTHCARE–MCNAIRY HOSPITAL (O, 48 beds) 705 East Poplar Avenue, Selmer, TN Zip 38375–1748; tel. 901/645–3221; John R. Borden, Administrator
Web address: www.methodisthealth.org

METHODIST HEALTHCARE–MEMPHIS HOSPITAL (O, 1272 beds) 1265 Union Avenue, Memphis, TN Zip 38104–3499; tel. 901/726–7000; David L. Ramsey, President
Web address: www.methodisthealth.org

METHODIST HEALTHCARE–SOMERVILLE (O, 38 beds) 214 Lakeview Drive, Somerville, TN Zip 38068; tel. 901/465–0532; Michael Blome', Administrator
Web address: www.methodisthealth.org

METHODIST HEALTHCARE–VOLUNTEER HOSPITAL (L, 65 beds) 161 Mount Pelia Road, Martin, TN Zip 38237–0967, Mailing Address: P.O. Box 967, Zip 38237–0967; tel. 901/587–4261; Eugene Ragghianti, Administrator
Web address: www.methodisthealth.org

METHODIST LEBONHEUR HEALTHCARE–JACKSON (L, 120 beds) 367 Hospital Boulevard, Jackson, TN Zip 38305–4518, Mailing Address: P.O. Box 3310, Zip 38303–0310; tel. 901/661–2000; Richard M. McCormick, Administrator
Web address: www.regionalhospital.com

Owned, leased, sponsored:	9 hospitals	1753 beds
Contract–managed:	0 hospitals	0 beds
Totals:	9 hospitals	1753 beds

★**2735: METHODIST HOSPITALS OF DALLAS** (NP)
1441 North Beckley Avenue, Dallas, TX Zip 75203–1201, Mailing Address: P.O. Box 655999, Zip 75265–5999; tel. 214/947–8181; Howard M. Chase, FACHE, President and Chief Executive Officer
(Centralized Physician/Insurance Health System)

TEXAS: CHARLTON METHODIST HOSPITAL (O, 130 beds) 3500 West Wheatland Road, Dallas, TX Zip 75237, Mailing Address: Box 225357, Zip 75222–5357; tel. 214/947–7500; David L. Knocke, CHE, Executive Director
Web address: www.mhd.com

METHODIST MEDICAL CENTER (O, 362 beds) 1441 North Beckley Avenue, Dallas, TX Zip 75203–1201, Mailing Address: Box 655999, Zip 75265–5999; tel. 214/947–8181; Kim N. Hollon, FACHE, Executive Director
Web address: www.mhd.com

Owned, leased, sponsored:	2 hospitals	492 beds
Contract–managed:	0 hospitals	0 beds
Totals:	2 hospitals	492 beds

★**0001: MIDMICHIGAN HEALTH** (NP)
4005 Orchard Drive, Midland, MI Zip 48670–0001; tel. 517/839–3000; Terence F. Moore, President
(Centralized Physician/Insurance Health System)

MICHIGAN: MIDMICHIGAN MEDICAL CENTER–CLARE (O, 64 beds) 104 West Sixth Street, Clare, MI Zip 48617–1409; tel. 517/386–9951; Lawrence F. Barco, President

MIDMICHIGAN MEDICAL CENTER–GLADWIN (O, 42 beds) 515 South Quarter Street, Gladwin, MI Zip 48624–1918; tel. 517/426–9286; Mark E. Bush, Executive Vice President

MIDMICHIGAN MEDICAL CENTER–MIDLAND (O, 250 beds) 4005 Orchard Drive, Midland, MI Zip 48670–3000; tel. 517/839–3000; David A. Reece, President
Web address: www.midmichigan.org

Owned, leased, sponsored:	3 hospitals	356 beds
Contract–managed:	0 hospitals	0 beds
Totals:	3 hospitals	356 beds

2855: MISSIONARY BENEDICTINE SISTERS AMERICAN PROVINCE (CC)
300 North 18th Street, Norfolk, NE Zip 68701–3687; tel. 402/371–3438; Sister M. Agnes Salber, Prioress
(Independent Hospital System)

MINNESOTA: GRACEVILLE HEALTH CENTER (O, 92 beds) 115 West Second Street, Graceville, MN Zip 56240–0157, Mailing Address: P.O. Box 157, Zip 56240–0157; tel. 320/748–7223; Helen Jorve, Chief Executive Officer

NEBRASKA: FAITH REGIONAL HEALTH SERVICES (O, 226 beds) 2700 Norfolk Avenue, Norfolk, NE Zip 68702–0869, Mailing Address: P.O. BOX 869, Zip 68702–0869; tel. 402/644–7201; Robert L. Driewer, Chief Executive Officer
Web address: www.frhs.org

PROVIDENCE MEDICAL CENTER (O, 32 beds) 1200 Providence Road, Wayne, NE Zip 68787–1299; tel. 402/375–3800; Marcile Thomas, Administrator

Owned, leased, sponsored:	3 hospitals	350 beds
Contract–managed:	0 hospitals	0 beds
Totals:	3 hospitals	350 beds

0017: MISSISSIPPI STATE DEPARTMENT OF MENTAL HEALTH (NP)
1101 Robert E Lee Building, Jackson, MS Zip 39201–1101; tel. 601/359–1288; Roger McMurtry, Chief Mental Health Bureau
(Independent Hospital System)

MISSISSIPPI: EAST MISSISSIPPI STATE HOSPITAL (O, 633 beds) 4555 Highland Park Drive, Meridian, MS Zip 39307–5498, Mailing Address: Box 4128, West Station, Zip 39304–4128; tel. 601/482–6186; Ramiro J. Martinez, M.D., Director

MISSISSIPPI STATE HOSPITAL (O, 1297 beds) Whitfield, MS Zip 39193–0157; tel. 601/351–8000; James G. Chastain, Director

Owned, leased, sponsored:	2 hospitals	1930 beds
Contract–managed:	0 hospitals	0 beds
Totals:	2 hospitals	1930 beds

For explanation of codes following names, see page B2.
★ Indicates Type III membership in the American Hospital Association.

Systems / Morton Plant Mease Health Care

1335: MORTON PLANT MEASE HEALTH CARE (NP)
601 Main Street, Dunedin, FL Zip 34698, Mailing Address: P.O. Box 760, Zip 34697-0760; tel. 727/733-1111; Philip K. Beauchamp, FACHE, President and Chief Executive Officer

FLORIDA: MEASE COUNTRYSIDE HOSPITAL (O, 100 beds) 3231 McMullen-Booth Road, Safety Harbor, FL Zip 34695-1098, Mailing Address: P.O. 1098, Zip 34695-1098; tel. 727/725-6111; James A. Pfeiffer, Chief Operating Officer

MEASE HOSPITAL DUNEDIN (O, 258 beds) 601 Main Street, Dunedin, FL Zip 34698-5891, Mailing Address: P.O. Box 760, Zip 34697-0760; tel. 727/733-1111; James A. Pfeiffer, Chief Operating Officer

MORTON PLANT HOSPITAL (S, 742 beds) 323 Jeffords Street, Clearwater, FL Zip 33756, Mailing Address: P.O. Box 210, Zip 34657-0210; tel. 727/462-7000; Philip K. Beauchamp, FACHE, President and Chief Executive Officer

Owned, leased, sponsored:	3 hospitals	1100 beds
Contract-managed:	0 hospitals	0 beds
Totals:	3 hospitals	1100 beds

0167: MOUNTAIN STATES HEALTH ALLIANCE (NP)
400 North State of Franklin, Johnson City, TN Zip 37604; tel. 423/431-6111; Dennis Vonderfecht, President and Chief Executive Officer
(Centralized Health System)

TENNESSEE: INDIAN PATH MEDICAL CENTER (O, 196 beds) 2000 Brookside Drive, Kingsport, TN Zip 37660-4604; tel. 423/392-7000; Randy Cook, Administrator and Chief Executive Officer

JOHNSON CITY MEDICAL CENTER (O, 410 beds) 400 North State of Franklin Road, Johnson City, TN Zip 37604-6094; tel. 423/431-6111; Dennis Vonderfecht, President and Chief Executive Officer
Web address: www.jcmc.com

JOHNSON CITY SPECIALTY HOSPITAL (O, 49 beds) 203 East Watauga Avenue, Johnson City, TN Zip 37601-4651; tel. 423/926-1111; Carolyn Gemmell, Director Operations and Chief Nursing Officer
Web address: www.MSHA.com

QUILLEN REHABILITATION HOSPITAL (O, 60 beds) 2511 Wesley Street, Johnson City, TN Zip 37601-1723; tel. 423/283-0700; John Turner, Chief Executive Officer

SYCAMORE SHOALS HOSPITAL (O, 105 beds) 1501 West Elk Avenue, Elizabethton, TN Zip 37643-1368; tel. 423/542-1300; Scott Williams, Chief Executive Officer

Owned, leased, sponsored:	5 hospitals	820 beds
Contract-managed:	0 hospitals	0 beds
Totals:	5 hospitals	820 beds

6555: MULTICARE HEALTH SYSTEM (NP)
315 Martin Luther King Jr. Way, Tacoma, WA Zip 98415, Mailing Address: P.O. Box 5299, Zip 98415-0299; tel. 253/403-1000; Diane Cecchettini, President and Chief Executive Officer
(Centralized Physician/Insurance Health System)

WASHINGTON: MARY BRIDGE CHILDREN'S HOSPITAL AND HEALTH CENTER (O, 72 beds) 317 Martin Luther King Jr. Way, Tacoma, WA Zip 98405-0299, Mailing Address: Box 5299, Zip 98405-0299; tel. 253/403-1400; Diane Cecchettini, President and Chief Executive Officer
Web address: www.multicare.com

TACOMA GENERAL HOSPITAL (O, 377 beds) 315 Martin Luther King Jr. Way, Tacoma, WA Zip 98405-0299, Mailing Address: P.O. Box 5299, Zip 98405-0299; tel. 253/403-1000; Diane Cecchettini, President and Chief Executive Officer
Web address: www.multicare.org

Owned, leased, sponsored:	2 hospitals	449 beds
Contract-managed:	0 hospitals	0 beds
Totals:	2 hospitals	449 beds

★1465: MUNSON HEALTHCARE (NP)
1105 Sixth Street, Traverse City, MI Zip 49684-2386; tel. 231/935-6502; John M. Rockwood, Jr, President and Chief Executive Officer
(Centralized Physician/Insurance Health System)

MICHIGAN: KALKASKA MEMORIAL HEALTH CENTER (C, 81 beds) 419 South Coral Street, Kalkaska, MI Zip 49646; tel. 231/258-7500; James D. Austin, CHE, Administrator

LEELANAU MEMORIAL HEALTH CENTER (O, 85 beds) 215 South High Street, Northport, MI Zip 49670, Mailing Address: P.O. Box 217, Zip 49670-0217; tel. 231/386-0000; Jayne R. Bull, Administrator

MUNSON MEDICAL CENTER (O, 368 beds) 1105 Sixth Street, Traverse City, MI Zip 49684-2386; tel. 231/935-5000; Ralph J. Cerny, President and Chief Executive Officer
Web address: www.mhc.net

PAUL OLIVER MEMORIAL HOSPITAL (O, 48 beds) 224 Park Avenue, Frankfort, MI Zip 49635; tel. 231/352-9621; James D. Austin, CHE, Administrator
Web address: www.benzie.com

Owned, leased, sponsored:	3 hospitals	501 beds
Contract-managed:	1 hospital	81 beds
Totals:	4 hospitals	582 beds

0116: NETCARE HEALTH SYSTEMS, INC. (IO)
424 Church Street, Suite 2100, Nashville, TN Zip 37219; tel. 615/742-8500; Michael A. Koban, Jr, Chief Executive Officer
(Moderately Centralized Health System)

ALABAMA: CHILTON MEDICAL CENTER (O, 45 beds) 1010 Lay Dam Road, Clanton, AL Zip 35045; tel. 205/755-2500; Randy Smith, Chief Executive Officer

CALIFORNIA: SAN CLEMENTE HOSPITAL AND MEDICAL CENTER (O, 71 beds) 654 Camino De Los Mares, San Clemente, CA Zip 92673; tel. 949/496-1122; Patricia L. Wolfram, R.N., Chief Executive Officer
Web address: www.sanclementehospital.com

GEORGIA: CHESTATEE REGIONAL HOSPITAL (O, 49 beds) 227 Mountain Drive, Dahlonega, GA Zip 30533; tel. 706/864-6136; Charles T. Adams, Chief Executive Officer

NORTH GEORGIA MEDICAL CENTER (O, 150 beds) 1362 South Main Street, Ellijay, GA Zip 30540-0346, Mailing Address: P.O. Box 2239, Zip 30540-0346; tel. 706/276-4741; Jodi Beauregard, Chief Executive Officer

MISSISSIPPI: TRACE REGIONAL HOSPITAL (O, 84 beds) Highway 8 East, Houston, MS Zip 38851, Mailing Address: P.O. Box 626, Zip 38851-0626; tel. 662/456-3700; Charles Nasem, Chief Executive Officer
Web address: www.traceregional.com

MISSOURI: DEXTER MEMORIAL HOSPITAL (O, 48 beds) 1200 North One Mile Road, Dexter, MO Zip 63841-1099; tel. 573/624-5566; Randal Tennison, Chief Executive Officer

NORTH CAROLINA: DAVIS MEDICAL CENTER (O, 132 beds) 218 Old Mocksville Road, Statesville, NC Zip 28625, Mailing Address: P.O. Box 1823, Zip 28687-1823; tel. 704/873-0281; R. Alan Larson, Chief Executive Officer

TEXAS: DENTON COMMUNITY HOSPITAL (O, 122 beds) 207 North Bonnie Brae Street, Denton, TX Zip 76201-3798; tel. 940/898-7000; Timothy Charles, Chief Executive Officer
Web address: www.dentonhospital.com

WEST VIRGINIA: GREENBRIER VALLEY MEDICAL CENTER (O, 122 beds) 202 Maplewood Avenue, Ronceverte, WV Zip 24970-0497, Mailing Address: P.O. Box 497, Zip 24970-0497; tel. 304/647-4411; Stephen Brandt, Interim Chief Executive Officer
Web address: www.gvmc.com

Owned, leased, sponsored:	9 hospitals	823 beds
Contract-managed:	0 hospitals	0 beds
Totals:	9 hospitals	823 beds

For explanation of codes following names, see page B2.
★ Indicates Type III membership in the American Hospital Association.

Systems / New York Presbyterian Healthcare System

0163: NEW AMERICAN HEALTHCARE CORPORATION (IO)
109 Westpark Drive, Suite 440, Brentwood, TN Zip 37027, Mailing Address: P.O. Box 3689, Zip 37024; tel. 615/221–5070; Thomas W. Singleton, President and Chief Executive Officer
(Moderately Centralized Health System)

GEORGIA: MEMORIAL HOSPITAL OF ADEL (O, 155 beds) 706 North Parrish Avenue, Adel, GA Zip 31620–0677, Mailing Address: P.O. Box 677, Zip 31620–0677; tel. 912/896–2251; Greg Griffith, Chief Executive Officer

MISSISSIPPI: CROSBY MEMORIAL HOSPITAL (O, 71 beds) 801 Goodyear Boulevard, Picayune, MS Zip 39466–3221, Mailing Address: P.O. Box 909, Zip 39466–0909; tel. 601/798–4711; Harry Albis, Interim Chief Executive Officer
Web address: www.crosbyhospital.com

MISSOURI: DOCTORS HOSPITAL (O, 94 beds) 500 Medical Drive, Wentzville, MO Zip 63385–0711; tel. 314/327–1000; Joan Phillips, R.N., Interim Chief Executive Officer
Web address: www.healthmidwest.org

OREGON: EASTMORELAND HOSPITAL (O, 77 beds) 2900 S.E. Steele Street, Portland, OR Zip 97202; tel. 503/234–0411; J. Phillip Young, Chief Executive Officer
Web address: www.eastmorelandhospital.net

WOODLAND PARK HOSPITAL (O, 121 beds) 10300 N.E. Hancock, Portland, OR Zip 97220; tel. 503/257–5500; J. Phillip Young, Chief Executive Officer
Web address: www.woodlandparkhospital.net

TEXAS: DOLLY VINSANT MEMORIAL HOSPITAL (O, 33 beds) 400 East U.S. Highway 77, San Benito, TX Zip 78586–5310, Mailing Address: P.O. Box 42, Zip 78586–0042; tel. 956/399–1313; Mark Dooley, Chief Executive Officer
Web address: www.dollyvinsant.nahc.net

MEMORIAL HOSPITAL OF CENTER (O, 46 beds) 602 Hurst Street, Center, TX Zip 75935–3414, Mailing Address: P.O. Box 1749, Zip 75935–1749; tel. 409/598–2781; John A. Tucker, Chief Executive Officer
Web address: www.memorial.nahc.net

WASHINGTON: PUGET SOUND HOSPITAL (O, 146 beds) 215 South 36th Street, Tacoma, WA Zip 98408–6853, Mailing Address: P.O. Box 11412, Zip 98411–0412; tel. 253/474–0561; C. Mark Gregson, Chief Executive Officer
Web address: www.puretsound.nahc.net

WYOMING: LANDER VALLEY MEDICAL CENTER (O, 102 beds) 1320 Bishop Randall Drive, Lander, WY Zip 82520–3996; tel. 307/335–6330; Andrew Gramlich, Chief Executive Officer
Web address: www.landerhospital.com

Owned, leased, sponsored:	9 hospitals	845 beds
Contract–managed:	0 hospitals	0 beds
Totals:	9 hospitals	845 beds

★**0213: NEW HANOVER HEALTH NETWORK** (IO)
2131 South 17th Street, Wilmington, NC Zip 28401–9000; tel. 910/343–7040; William K. Atkinson, II, Ph.D., President and Chief Executive Officer

NORTH CAROLINA: NEW HANOVER REGIONAL MEDICAL CENTER (O, 622 beds) 2131 South 17th Street, Wilmington, NC Zip 28401–7483, Mailing Address: P.O. Box 9000, Zip 28402–9000; tel. 910/343–7000; William K. Atkinson, II, Ph.D., President and Chief Executive Officer
Web address: www.nhrmc.org

PENDER MEMORIAL HOSPITAL (C, 86 beds) 507 Freemont Street, Burgaw, NC Zip 28425; tel. 910/259–5451; Matthew Mendez, Site Administrator

Owned, leased, sponsored:	1 hospital	622 beds
Contract–managed:	1 hospital	86 beds
Totals:	2 hospitals	708 beds

3075: NEW YORK CITY HEALTH AND HOSPITALS CORPORATION (NP)
125 Worth Street, Room 514, New York, NY Zip 10013–4006; tel. 212/788–3321; Luis R. Marcos, M.D., President
(Decentralized Health System)

NEW YORK: BELLEVUE HOSPITAL CENTER (O, 771 beds) 462 First Avenue, New York, NY Zip 10016–9198, Mailing Address: 462 First Avenue, ME–8, Zip 10016–9198; tel. 212/562–4141; Carlos Perez, Executive Director
Web address: www.bellevuehospitalcenter.org/html/core.html

COLER MEMORIAL HOSPITAL (O, 1025 beds) Roosevelt Island, New York, NY Zip 10044; tel. 212/848–6000; Samuel Lehrfeld, Executive Director

CONEY ISLAND HOSPITAL (O, 406 beds) 2601 Ocean Parkway, Brooklyn, NY Zip 11235–7795; tel. 718/616–3000; William Walsh, Executive Director
Web address: www.ci.nyc.ny.us/html/hhc/html/coneyisland.html

ELMHURST HOSPITAL CENTER (O, 506 beds) 79–01 Broadway, Elmhurst, NY Zip 11373; tel. 718/334–4000; Pete Velez, Executive Director

GOLDWATER MEMORIAL HOSPITAL (O, 991 beds) Franklin D. Roosevelt Island, New York, NY Zip 10044; tel. 212/318–8000; Samuel Lehrfeld, Executive Director
Web address: www.coler–goldwater.org

HARLEM HOSPITAL CENTER (O, 297 beds) 506 Lenox Avenue, New York, NY Zip 10037–1894; tel. 212/939–1000; John M. Palmer, Ph.D., Executive Director

JACOBI MEDICAL CENTER (O, 545 beds) Pelham Parkway South and Eastchester Road, Bronx, NY Zip 10461–1197; tel. 718/918–5000; Joseph S. Orlando, Executive Director
Web address: www.ci.nyc.ny.us/html/hhc/html/jacobi.html

KINGS COUNTY HOSPITAL CENTER (O, 686 beds) 451 Clarkson Avenue, Brooklyn, NY Zip 11203–2097; tel. 718/245–3131; Jean G. Leon, R.N., Senior Vice President

LINCOLN MEDICAL AND MENTAL HEALTH CENTER (O, 438 beds) 234 East 149th Street, Bronx, NY Zip 10451–9998; tel. 718/579–5700; Jose R. Sanchez, Executive Director

METROPOLITAN HOSPITAL CENTER (O, 325 beds) 1901 First Avenue, New York, NY Zip 10029–7496; tel. 212/423–6262; Jose R. Sanchez, Executive Director

NORTH CENTRAL BRONX HOSPITAL (O, 255 beds) 3424 Kossuth Avenue, Bronx, NY Zip 10467–2489; tel. 718/519–3500; Arthur Wagner, Chief Operating Officer
Web address: www.ci.nyc.ny.us/html/hhc/html/northcentralbronx.html

QUEENS HOSPITAL CENTER (O, 266 beds) 82–68 164th Street, Jamaica, NY Zip 11432–1104; tel. 718/883–3000; Antonio D. Martin, Chief Operating Officer

WOODHULL MEDICAL AND MENTAL HEALTH CENTER (O, 382 beds) 760 Broadway Street, Brooklyn, NY Zip 11206–5383; tel. 718/963–8000; Cynthia Carrington–Murray, R.N., MS, Senior Vice President

Owned, leased, sponsored:	13 hospitals	6893 beds
Contract–managed:	0 hospitals	0 beds
Totals:	13 hospitals	6893 beds

★**0142: NEW YORK PRESBYTERIAN HEALTHCARE SYSTEM** (NP)
525 East 68th Street, New York, NY Zip 10021–4885; tel. 212/746–4000; Herbert Pardes, M.D., Chief Executive Officer
(Moderately Centralized Health System)

NEW JERSEY: PALISADES MEDICAL CENTER (S, 202 beds) 7600 River Road, North Bergen, NJ Zip 07047–6217; tel. 201/854–5000; Bruce J. Markowitz, President and Chief Executive Officer
Web address: www.palisadesmedical.org

NEW YORK: BROOKLYN HOSPITAL CENTER (S, 653 beds) 121 DeKalb Avenue, Brooklyn, NY Zip 11201–5493; tel. 718/250–8005; Frederick D. Alley, President and Chief Executive Officer

GRACIE SQUARE HOSPITAL (S, 130 beds) 420 East 76th Street, New York, NY Zip 10021–3104; tel. 212/988–4400; Frank Bruno, Chief Executive Officer

HOSPITAL FOR SPECIAL SURGERY (S, 138 beds) 535 East 70th Street, New York, NY Zip 10021–4898; tel. 212/606–1000; John R. Reynolds, President and Chief Executive Officer
Web address: www.hss.edu

For explanation of codes following names, see page B2.
★ Indicates Type III membership in the American Hospital Association.

Systems / New York Presbyterian Healthcare System

NEW YORK COMMUNITY HOSPITAL OF BROOKLYN (S, 125 beds) 2525 Kings Highway, Brooklyn, NY Zip 11229–1798; tel. 718/692–5300; Lin H. Mo, President and Chief Executive Officer

NEW YORK HOSPITAL MEDICAL CENTER OF QUEENS (S, 421 beds) 56–45 Main Street, Flushing, NY Zip 11355–5000; tel. 718/670–1231; Stephen S. Mills, President and Chief Executive Officer
Web address: www.nyhq.org

NEW YORK METHODIST HOSPITAL (S, 560 beds) 506 Sixth Street, Brooklyn, NY Zip 11215–3645; tel. 718/780–3000; Mark J. Mundy, President and Chief Executive Officer
Web address: www.nym.org

NEW YORK UNITED HOSPITAL MEDICAL CENTER (S, 231 beds) 406 Boston Post Road, Port Chester, NY Zip 10573–7300; tel. 914/934–3000; Kevin Dahill, President and Chief Executive Officer
Web address: www.uhmc.com

NEW YORK–PRESBYTERIAN HOSPITAL (O, 2346 beds) 525 East 68th Street, New York, NY Zip 10021–4885; tel. 212/746–5454; Herbert Pardes, M.D., President and Chief Executive Officer
Web address: www.nyp.org

WESTCHESTER SQUARE MEDICAL CENTER (S, 205 beds) 2475 St. Raymond Avenue, Bronx, NY Zip 10461–3198; tel. 718/430–7300; Alan Kopman, President and Chief Executive Officer

WYCKOFF HEIGHTS MEDICAL CENTER (S, 324 beds) 374 Stockholm Street, Brooklyn, NY Zip 11237–4099; tel. 718/963–7102; Dominick J. Gio, President and Chief Executive Officer

Owned, leased, sponsored:	11 hospitals	5335 beds
Contract–managed:	0 hospitals	0 beds
Totals:	11 hospitals	5335 beds

0009: NEW YORK STATE DEPARTMENT OF MENTAL HEALTH (NP)
44 Holland Avenue, Albany, NY Zip 12229–3411; tel. 518/447–9611; James L. Stone, Commissioner
(Independent Hospital System)

BINGHAMTON PSYCHIATRIC CENTER (O, 177 beds) 425 Robinson Street, Binghamton, NY Zip 13901–4198; tel. 607/724–1391; Margaret R. Dugan, Executive Director

BRONX CHILDREN'S PSYCHIATRIC CENTER (O, 75 beds) 1000 Waters Place, Bronx, NY Zip 10461–2799; tel. 718/239–3600; E. Richard Feinberg, M.D., Executive Director

BRONX PSYCHIATRIC CENTER (O, 450 beds) 1500 Waters Place, Bronx, NY Zip 10461–2796; tel. 718/931–0600; LeRoy Carmichael, Executive Director
Web address: www.omh.state.ny.us

BUFFALO PSYCHIATRIC CENTER (O, 240 beds) 400 Forest Avenue, Buffalo, NY Zip 14213–1298; tel. 716/885–2261; George A. Roets, R.N., MS, Executive Director
Web address: www.omh.state.ny.us

CAPITAL DISTRICT PSYCHIATRIC CENTER (O, 200 beds) 75 New Scotland Avenue, Albany, NY Zip 12208–3474; tel. 518/447–9611; Jesse Nixon, Jr, Ph.D., Director

CREEDMOOR PSYCHIATRIC CENTER (O, 494 beds) Jamaica, NY Mailing Address: 80–45 Winchester Boulevard, Queens Village, Zip 11427–2199; tel. 718/264–3300; Charlotte Seltzer, Chief Executive Officer

ELMIRA PSYCHIATRIC CENTER (O, 93 beds) 100 Washington Street, Elmira, NY Zip 14901–2898; tel. 607/737–4739; William Benedict, Executive Director

HUDSON RIVER PSYCHIATRIC CENTER (O, 460 beds) 373 North Road, Poughkeepsie, NY Zip 12601–1197; tel. 914/452–8000; James Regan, Ph.D., Chief Executive Officer

KINGSBORO PSYCHIATRIC CENTER (O, 400 beds) 681 Clarkson Avenue, Brooklyn, NY Zip 11203–2199; tel. 718/221–7395; Dean R. Weinstock, Director

MANHATTAN PSYCHIATRIC CENTER–WARD'S ISLAND (O, 745 beds) 600 East 125th Street, New York, NY Zip 10035–9998; tel. 212/369–0500; Eileen Consilvio, R.N., MS, Executive Director

MIDDLETOWN PSYCHIATRIC CENTER (O, 170 beds) 122 Dorothea Dix Drive, Middletown, NY Zip 10940–6198; tel. 914/342–5511; James H. Bopp, Executive Director

MOHAWK VALLEY PSYCHIATRIC CENTER (O, 614 beds) 1400 Noyes, Utica, NY Zip 13502–3803; tel. 315/797–6800; Sarah F. Rudes, Executive Director

NEW YORK STATE PSYCHIATRIC INSTITUTE (O, 58 beds) 1051 Riverside Drive, New York, NY Zip 10032–2695; tel. 212/543–5000; John M. Oldham, M.D., Director

PILGRIM PSYCHIATRIC CENTER (O, 744 beds) 998 Crooked Hill Road, Brentwood, NY Zip 11717–1087; tel. 631/761–3500; Kathleen Kelly, Chief Executive Officer

QUEENS CHILDREN'S PSYCHIATRIC CENTER (O, 84 beds) 74–03 Commonwealth Boulevard, Jamaica, NY Zip 11426–1890; tel. 718/264–4506; Robert Schweitzer, Ed.D., Executive Director

RICHARD H. HUTCHINGS PSYCHIATRIC CENTER (O, 136 beds) 620 Madison Street, Syracuse, NY Zip 13210–2319; tel. 315/473–4980; Bryan F. Rudes, Executive Director
Web address: www.omh.state.ny.us

ROCHESTER PSYCHIATRIC CENTER (O, 247 beds) 1111 Elmwood Avenue, Rochester, NY Zip 14620–3005; tel. 716/473–3230; Bryan F. Rudes, Executive Director

ROCKLAND CHILDREN'S PSYCHIATRIC CENTER (O, 54 beds) 599 Convent Road, Orangeburg, NY Zip 10962; tel. 914/359–7400; David J. Woodlock, Executive Director

ROCKLAND PSYCHIATRIC CENTER (O, 525 beds) 140 Old Orangeburg Road, Orangeburg, NY Zip 10962–0071; tel. 914/359–1000; James H. Bopp, Executive Director

SAGAMORE CHILDREN'S PSYCHIATRIC CENTER (O, 69 beds) 197 Half Hollow Road, Huntington Station, NY Zip 11746; tel. 516/673–7700; Robert Schweitzer, Ed.D., Executive Director

SOUTH BEACH PSYCHIATRIC CENTER (O, 331 beds) 777 Seaview Avenue, Staten Island, NY Zip 10305–3499; tel. 718/667–2300; Lucy Sarkis, M.D., Executive Director

ST. LAWRENCE PSYCHIATRIC CENTER (O, 114 beds) 1 Chimney Point Drive, Ogdensburg, NY Zip 13669–2291; tel. 315/393–3000; John R. Scott, Director

WESTERN NEW YORK CHILDREN'S PSYCHIATRIC CENTER (O, 46 beds) 1010 East and West Road, Buffalo, NY Zip 14224–3698; tel. 716/674–9730; Jed M. Cohen, Acting Executive Director
Web address: www.omh.state.ny.us

Owned, leased, sponsored:	23 hospitals	6526 beds
Contract–managed:	0 hospitals	0 beds
Totals:	23 hospitals	6526 beds

★3115: NORTH BROWARD HOSPITAL DISTRICT (NP)
303 S.E. 17th Street, Fort Lauderdale, FL Zip 33316–2510; tel. 954/355–5100; G. Wil Trower, President and Chief Executive Officer
(Moderately Centralized Health System)

FLORIDA: BROWARD GENERAL MEDICAL CENTER (O, 545 beds) 1600 South Andrews Avenue, Fort Lauderdale, FL Zip 33316–2510; tel. 954/355–4400; Timothy P. Menton, Administrator

CORAL SPRINGS MEDICAL CENTER (O, 182 beds) 3000 Coral Hills Drive, Coral Springs, FL Zip 33065; tel. 954/344–3000; Deborah Mulvihill, Regional Vice President and Administrator

IMPERIAL POINT MEDICAL CENTER (O, 160 beds) 6401 North Federal Highway, Fort Lauderdale, FL Zip 33308–1495; tel. 954/776–8500; Dorothy J. Mancini, R.N., Regional Vice President Administration

NORTH BROWARD MEDICAL CENTER (O, 334 beds) 201 Sample Road, Pompano Beach, FL Zip 33064–3502; tel. 954/941–8300; James R. Chromik, Regional Vice President, Administration
Web address: www.nbhd.org

Owned, leased, sponsored:	4 hospitals	1221 beds
Contract–managed:	0 hospitals	0 beds
Totals:	4 hospitals	1221 beds

For explanation of codes following names, see page B2.
★ *Indicates Type III membership in the American Hospital Association.*

Systems / Norton Healthcare

0032: NORTH MISSISSIPPI HEALTH SERVICES, INC. (NP)
830 South Gloster Street, Tupelo, MS Zip 38801–4996;
tel. 601/841–3136; Jeffrey B. Barber, Dr.PH, President and Chief Executive Officer
(Centralized Physician/Insurance Health System)

MISSISSIPPI: CLAY COUNTY MEDICAL CENTER (O, 60 beds) 835 Medical Center Drive, West Point, MS Zip 39773–9320; tel. 601/495–2300; David M. Reid, Administrator

IUKA HOSPITAL (O, 48 beds) 1777 Curtis Drive, Iuka, MS Zip 38852–1001, Mailing Address: P.O. Box 860, Zip 38852–0860; tel. 662/423–6051; Daniel Perryman, Administrator

NORTH MISSISSIPPI MEDICAL CENTER (O, 724 beds) 830 South Gloster Street, Tupelo, MS Zip 38801–4934; tel. 601/841–3000; Jeffrey B. Barber, Dr.PH, President and Chief Executive Officer
Web address: www.nmhs.net

PONTOTOC HOSPITAL AND EXTENDED CARE FACILITY (L, 71 beds) 176 South Main Street, Pontotoc, MS Zip 38863–3311, Mailing Address: P.O. Box 790, Zip 38863–0790; tel. 662/488–7640; Fred B. Hood, Administrator

WEBSTER HEALTH SERVICES (L, 76 beds) 500 Highway 9 South, Eupora, MS Zip 39744; tel. 601/258–6221; Harold H. Whitaker, Administrator

Owned, leased, sponsored:	5 hospitals	979 beds
Contract–managed:	0 hospitals	0 beds
Totals:	5 hospitals	979 beds

★0062: NORTH SHORE– LONG ISLAND JEWISH HEALTH SYSTEM (NP)
145 Community Drive, Great Neck, NY Zip 11021;
tel. 516/465–8100; John S. T. Gallagher, Chief Executive Officer
(Centralized Physician/Insurance Health System)

NEW YORK: FRANKLIN HOSPITAL MEDICAL CENTER (C, 310 beds) 900 Franklin Avenue, Valley Stream, NY Zip 11580–2190; tel. 516/256–6000; William Kowalewski, President and Chief Executive Officer
Web address: www.northshorelij.com

HUNTINGTON HOSPITAL (C, 263 beds) 270 Park Avenue, Huntington, NY Zip 11743–2799; tel. 631/351–2200; J. Ronald Gaudreault, President and Chief Executive Officer
Web address: www.hunthosp.org

LONG ISLAND JEWISH MEDICAL CENTER (O, 802 beds) 270–05 76th Avenue, New Hyde Park, NY Zip 11040–1496; tel. 718/470–7000; Paul S. Hochenberg, President
Web address: www.lij.edu

NORTH SHORE UNIVERSITY HOSPITAL (O, 987 beds) 300 Community Drive, Manhasset, NY Zip 11030–3876; tel. 516/562–0100; Dennis Dowling, Executive Director
Web address: www.northshorelij.com

NORTH SHORE UNIVERSITY HOSPITAL AT GLEN COVE (O, 265 beds) 101 St. Andrews Lane, Glen Cove, NY Zip 11542; tel. 516/674–7300; Mark R. Stenzler, Vice President Administration
Web address: www.northshorelij.com

NORTH SHORE UNIVERSITY HOSPITAL AT PLAINVIEW (O, 279 beds) 888 Old Country Road, Plainview, NY Zip 11803–4978; tel. 516/719–3000; Deborah Tascone, R.N., MS, Executive Director
Web address: www.northshorelij.com

NORTH SHORE UNIVERSITY HOSPITAL AT SYOSSET (O, 186 beds) 221 Jericho Turnpike, Syosset, NY Zip 11791–4567; tel. 516/496–6400; Deborah Tascone, R.N., MS, Executive Director
Web address: www.northshorelij.com

NORTH SHORE UNIVERSITY HOSPITAL–FOREST HILLS (O, 231 beds) Forest Hills, NY Mailing Address: 102–01 66th Road, Zip 11375; tel. 718/830–4000; Andrew J. Mitchell, Executive Director
Web address: www.northshorelij.com

SOUTHSIDE HOSPITAL (C, 439 beds) 301 East Main Street, Bay Shore, NY Zip 11706–8458; tel. 631/968–3000; Theodore A. Jospe, President
Web address: www.northshorelij.com

STATEN ISLAND UNIVERSITY HOSPITAL (C, 617 beds) 475 Seaview Avenue, Staten Island, NY Zip 10305–9998; tel. 718/226–9000; Rick J. Varone, President
Web address: www.northshorelij.com

Owned, leased, sponsored:	6 hospitals	2750 beds
Contract–managed:	4 hospitals	1629 beds
Totals:	10 hospitals	4379 beds

★2075: NORTHBAY HEALTHCARE SYSTEM (NP)
1200 B Gale Wilson Boulevard, Fairfield, CA Zip 94533–3587;
tel. 707/429–7809; Gary J. Passama, President and Chief Executive Officer
(Independent Hospital System)

CALIFORNIA: NORTHBAY MEDICAL CENTER (O, 121 beds) 1200 B. Gale Wilson Boulevard, Fairfield, CA Zip 94533–3587; tel. 707/429–3600; Deborah Sugiyama, President
Web address: www.northbay.org

VACAVALLEY HOSPITAL (O, 43 beds) 1000 Nut Tree Road, Vacaville, CA Zip 95687; tel. 707/446–4000; Deborah Sugiyama, President
Web address: www.northbay.org

Owned, leased, sponsored:	2 hospitals	164 beds
Contract–managed:	0 hospitals	0 beds
Totals:	2 hospitals	164 beds

0208: NORTHEAST HEALTH MANAGEMENT, INC. (IO)
104 Log Canoe Circle, Stevensville, MD Zip 21666;
tel. 410/643–3393; Harold A. McBee, President

TEXAS: LIBERTY–DAYTON HOSPITAL (O, 29 beds) 1353 North Travis Street, Liberty, TX Zip 77575–1353; tel. 409/336–7316; Sean Stricker, Administrator

WEST VIRGINIA: HAMPSHIRE MEMORIAL HOSPITAL (O, 47 beds) 549 Center Avenue, Romney, WV Zip 26757–1199; tel. 304/822–4561; Roberta D. McCauley, Chief Executive Officer

POTOMAC VALLEY HOSPITAL (O, 42 beds) 167 South Mineral Street, Keyser, WV Zip 26726–2699; tel. 304/788–3141; Larry Abrams, Administrator

WISCONSIN: INDIANHEAD MEDICAL CENTER (O, 49 beds) 113 Fourth Avenue West, Shell Lake, WI Zip 54871; tel. 715/468–7833; Paul Naglosky, Administrator

Owned, leased, sponsored:	4 hospitals	167 beds
Contract–managed:	0 hospitals	0 beds
Totals:	4 hospitals	167 beds

★2285: NORTON HEALTHCARE (NP)
234 East Gray Street, Suite 225, Louisville, KY Zip 40202, Mailing Address: P.O. Box 35070, Zip 40232–5070; tel. 502/629–8000; Stephen A. Williams, President
(Decentralized Health System)

ILLINOIS: FAIRFIELD MEMORIAL HOSPITAL (C, 185 beds) 303 N.W. 11th Street, Fairfield, IL Zip 62837–1203; tel. 618/842–2611

MASSAC MEMORIAL HOSPITAL (C, 38 beds) 28 Chick Street, Metropolis, IL Zip 62960–2481, Mailing Address: P.O. Box 850, Zip 62960–0850; tel. 618/524–2176; Mark Edwards, Chief Executive Officer

PARIS COMMUNITY HOSPITAL (C, 49 beds) 721 East Court Street, Paris, IL Zip 61944–2420; tel. 217/465–4141; John D. Fajt, FACHE, President and Chief Operating Officer

WABASH GENERAL HOSPITAL DISTRICT (C, 56 beds) 1418 College Drive, Mount Carmel, IL Zip 62863–2638; tel. 618/262–8621; James R. Farris, CHE, Chief Executive Officer

INDIANA: BLACKFORD COUNTY HOSPITAL (C, 25 beds) 503 East Van Cleve Street, Hartford City, IN Zip 47348–1897; tel. 765/348–0300; Steven J. West, Chief Executive Officer

DECATUR COUNTY MEMORIAL HOSPITAL (C, 67 beds) 720 North Lincoln Street, Greensburg, IN Zip 47240–1398; tel. 812/663–4331; David V. Trexler, President

---

For explanation of codes following names, see page B2.
★ Indicates Type III membership in the American Hospital Association.

Systems / Norton Healthcare

GIBSON GENERAL HOSPITAL (C, 109 beds) 1808 Sherman Drive, Princeton, IN Zip 47670-1043; tel. 812/385-3401; Michael J. Budnick, FACHE, Administrator and Chief Executive Officer
Web address: www.gibsongeneral.org

HARRISON COUNTY HOSPITAL (C, 47 beds) 245 Atwood Street, Corydon, IN Zip 47112-1774; tel. 812/738-4251; Steven L. Taylor, Chief Executive Officer

PERRY COUNTY MEMORIAL HOSPITAL (C, 38 beds) 1 Hospital Road, Tell City, IN Zip 47586-0362; tel. 812/547-7011; Joseph A. Stuber, Chief Executive Officer
Web address: www.pchospital.org

RUSH MEMORIAL HOSPITAL (C, 46 beds) 1300 North Main Street, Rushville, IN Zip 46173-1198; tel. 765/932-4111; J. Jay Purvis, Interim Chief Executive Officer
Web address: www.rushmemorial.com

ST. VINCENT RANDOLPH HOSPITAL (C, 25 beds) 325 South Oak Street, Winchester, IN Zip 47394-2235, Mailing Address: P.O. Box 407, Zip 47394-0407; tel. 765/584-9001; James M. Full, FACHE, Chief Executive Officer

KENTUCKY: BRECKINRIDGE MEMORIAL HOSPITAL (C, 45 beds) 1011 Old Highway 60, Hardinsburg, KY Zip 40143-2597; tel. 270/756-7000; George Walz, CHE, Chief Executive Officer
Web address: www.multiplan.com

CARROLL COUNTY HOSPITAL (L, 39 beds) 309 11th Street, Carrollton, KY Zip 41008-1400; tel. 502/732-4321; Roger Williams, Chief Executive Officer
Web address: www.nortonhealthcare.com

CAVERNA MEMORIAL HOSPITAL (C, 28 beds) 1501 South Dixie Street, Horse Cave, KY Zip 42749-1477; tel. 270/786-2191; Alan B. Alexander, Administrator

NORTON AUDUBON HOSPITAL (O, 235 beds) One Audubon Plaza Drive, Louisville, KY Zip 40217-1397, Mailing Address: P.O. Box 17550, Zip 40217-0550; tel. 502/636-7111; Thomas D. Kmetz, Chief Administrative Officer

NORTON HEALTHCARE PAVILION (O, 178 beds) 315 East Broadway, Louisville, KY Zip 40202; tel. 502/629-2000; M. Michelle Hood, Chief Administrative Officer

NORTON HOSPITAL (O, 687 beds) 200 East Chestnut Street, Louisville, KY Zip 40202-1800, Mailing Address: P.O. Box 35070, Zip 40232-5070; tel. 502/629-8000; M. Michelle Hood, Chief Administrative Officer
Web address: www.nortonhealthcare.com

NORTON SOUTHWEST HOSPITAL (O, 108 beds) 9820 Third Street Road, Louisville, KY Zip 40272-9984; tel. 502/933-8100; James W. Pope, Chief Executive Officer
Web address: www.nortonhealthcare.com

NORTON SPRING VIEW HOSPITAL (O, 85 beds) 320 Loretto Road, Lebanon, KY Zip 40033-0320; tel. 270/692-3161; Barry A. Papania, Chief Executive Officer
Web address: www.nortonhealthcare.com

NORTON SUBURBAN HOSPITAL (O, 230 beds) 4001 Dutchmans Lane, Louisville, KY Zip 40207-4799; tel. 502/893-1000; John D. Harryman, President and Chief Executive Officer
Web address: www.nortonhealthcare.com

RUSSELL COUNTY HOSPITAL (C, 45 beds) Dowell Road, Russell Springs, KY Zip 42642, Mailing Address: P.O. Box 1610, Zip 42642-1610; tel. 270/866-4141; Patricia Ekdahl, President and Chief Executive Officer

THE JAMES B. HAGGIN MEMORIAL HOSPITAL (C, 64 beds) 464 Linden Avenue, Harrodsburg, KY Zip 40330-1862; tel. 859/734-5441; Earl James Motzer, Ph.D., FACHE, Chief Executive Officer

TWIN LAKES REGIONAL MEDICAL CENTER (C, 75 beds) 910 Wallace Avenue, Leitchfield, KY Zip 42754-1499; tel. 270/259-9400; Stephen L. Meredith, Chief Executive Officer
Web address: www.tlrmc.com

Owned, leased, sponsored:	7 hospitals	1562 beds
Contract-managed:	16 hospitals	942 beds
Totals:	23 hospitals	2504 beds

★0139: **NOVANT HEALTH** (NP)
3333 Silas Creek Parkway, Winston Salem, NC Zip 27103-3090; tel. 336/718-5000; Paul M. Wiles, President and Chief Executive Officer
(Centralized Physician/Insurance Health System)

NORTH CAROLINA: COMMUNITY GENERAL HOSPITAL OF THOMASVILLE (O, 89 beds) 207 Old Lexington Road, Thomasville, NC Zip 27360, Mailing Address: P.O. Box 789, Zip 27361-0789; tel. 336/472-2000; Lynn Ingram Boggs, President and Chief Executive Officer
Web address: www.cghp.org

DAVIE COUNTY HOSPITAL (L, 30 beds) 223 Hospital Street, Mocksville, NC Zip 27028-2038, Mailing Address: P.O. Box 1209, Zip 27028-1209; tel. 336/751-8100; Mike Kimel, Administrator
Web address: www.novanthealth.org

FORSYTH MEDICAL CENTER (O, 714 beds) 3333 Silas Creek Parkway, Winston-Salem, NC Zip 27103-3090; tel. 336/718-5000; Gregory J. Beier, President
Web address: www.novanthealth.org

MEDICAL PARK HOSPITAL (O, 59 beds) 1950 South Hawthorne Road, Winston-Salem, NC Zip 27103-3993, Mailing Address: P.O. Box 24728, Zip 27114-4728; tel. 336/718-0600; Eduard R. Koehler, Administrator

PRESBYTERIAN HOSPITAL (O, 840 beds) 200 Hawthorne Lane, Charlotte, NC Zip 28204-2528, Mailing Address: P.O. Box 33549, Zip 28233-3549; tel. 704/384-4000; Thomas R. Revels, President and Chief Executive Officer
Web address: www.presbyterian.org

PRESBYTERIAN HOSPITAL-MATTHEWS (O, 82 beds) 1500 Matthews Township Parkway, Matthews, NC Zip 28105, Mailing Address: P.O. Box 3310, Zip 28106-3310; tel. 704/384-6500; Mark R. Farmer, Vice President and Administrator
Web address: www.presbyterian.org

PRESBYTERIAN-ORTHOPAEDIC HOSPITAL (O, 156 beds) 1901 Randolph Road, Charlotte, NC Zip 28207-1195; tel. 704/375-6792; Tom McGraw, Administrator
Web address: www.presbyterian.org

Owned, leased, sponsored:	7 hospitals	1970 beds
Contract-managed:	0 hospitals	0 beds
Totals:	7 hospitals	1970 beds

★1165: **OAKWOOD HEALTHCARE, INC.** (NP)
One Parklane Boulevard, Suite 1000E, Dearborn, MI Zip 48126; tel. 313/253-6050; Gerald D. Fitzgerald, President and Chief Executive Officer
(Centralized Health System)

MICHIGAN: OAKWOOD ANNAPOLIS HOSPITAL (O, 183 beds) 33155 Annapolis Road, Wayne, MI Zip 48184-2493; tel. 734/467-4000; Thomas Kochis, Chief Administrative Officer
Web address: www.oakwood.org

OAKWOOD HERITAGE HOSPITAL (O, 257 beds) 10000 Telegraph Road, Taylor, MI Zip 48180-3349; tel. 313/295-5000; Edward E. Freysinger, Administrator

OAKWOOD HOSPITAL AND MEDICAL CENTER-DEARBORN (O, 585 beds) 18101 Oakwood Boulevard, Dearborn, MI Zip 48124-4093, Mailing Address: P.O. Box 2500, Zip 48123-2500; tel. 313/593-7000; Joseph Tasse, Administrator
Web address: www.oakwood.org

OAKWOOD SEAWAY HOSPITAL (O, 82 beds) 5450 Fort Street, Trenton, MI Zip 48183-4625; tel. 734/671-3800; Brian Peltz, Administrator
Web address: www.oakwood.org

Owned, leased, sponsored:	4 hospitals	1107 beds
Contract-managed:	0 hospitals	0 beds
Totals:	4 hospitals	1107 beds

★3315: **OHIO VALLEY HEALTH SERVICES** (NP)
2000 Eoff Street, Wheeling, WV Zip 26003; tel. 304/234-8383; Thomas P. Galinski, President and Chief Executive Officer

---

For explanation of codes following names, see page B2.
★ Indicates Type III membership in the American Hospital Association.

Systems / OSF Healthcare System

OHIO: EAST OHIO REGIONAL HOSPITAL (O, 165 beds) 90 North Fourth Street, Martins Ferry, OH Zip 43935–1648; tel. 740/633–1100; Brian K. Felici, Vice President and Administrator
Web address: www.wvha.com/web/ovmc/

WEST VIRGINIA: OHIO VALLEY MEDICAL CENTER (O, 363 beds) 2000 Eoff Street, Wheeling, WV Zip 26003–3870; tel. 304/234–0123; Thomas P. Galinski, President and Chief Executive Officer

Owned, leased, sponsored:	2 hospitals	528 beds
Contract–managed:	0 hospitals	0 beds
Totals:	2 hospitals	528 beds

★0162: **OHIOHEALTH** (NP)
3555 Olentangy River Road, 4000, Columbus, OH Zip 43214–3900; tel. 614/566–5424; William W. Wilkins, Chief Executive Officer
(Centralized Physician/Insurance Health System)

OHIO: DOCTORS HOSPITAL (O, 380 beds) 1087 Dennison Avenue, Columbus, OH Zip 43201–3496; tel. 614/297–4000; Dennis J. Freudeman, President
Web address: www.doctorshospital.org

DOCTORS HOSPITAL OF NELSONVILLE (O, 70 beds) 1950 Mount Saint Mary Drive, Nelsonville, OH Zip 45764–1193; tel. 740/753–1931; Joel Kaiser, Chief Executive Officer

GALION COMMUNITY HOSPITAL (C, 108 beds) 269 Portland Way South, Galion, OH Zip 44833–2399; tel. 419/468–4841; Lyndon J. Christman, President and Chief Executive Officer
Web address: www.galionhospital.org

GRANT/RIVERSIDE METHODIST HOSPITALS–GRANT CAMPUS (O, 460 beds) 111 South Grant Avenue, Columbus, OH Zip 43215–1898; tel. 614/566–9000; Mark H. Shuter, President
Web address: www.ohiohealth.com

GRANT/RIVERSIDE METHODIST HOSPITALS–RIVERSIDE CAMPUS (O, 778 beds) 3535 Olentangy Road, Columbus, OH Zip 43214–3998; tel. 614/566–5000; Mark H. Shuter, President
Web address: www.ohiohealth.com

HARDIN MEMORIAL HOSPITAL (O, 51 beds) 921 East Franklin Street, Kenton, OH Zip 43326–2099, Mailing Address: P.O. Box 710, Zip 43326–0710; tel. 419/673–0761; Don J. Sabol, Chief Executive Officer

MARION GENERAL HOSPITAL (O, 188 beds) 1000 McKinley Park Drive, Marion, OH Zip 43302–6397; tel. 740/383–8400; Ronald J. Bachman, Interim President and Chief Executive Officer
Web address: www.mariongeneral.com

MORROW COUNTY HOSPITAL (C, 75 beds) 651 West Marion Road, Mount Gilead, OH Zip 43338–1096; tel. 419/946–5015; Alan C. Pauley, Administrator
Web address: www.mtgilead.com

SOUTHERN OHIO MEDICAL CENTER (O, 205 beds) 1805 27th Street, Portsmouth, OH Zip 45662–2400; tel. 740/354–5000; Randal M. Arnett, President and Chief Executive Officer
Web address: www.somc.org

Owned, leased, sponsored:	7 hospitals	2132 beds
Contract–managed:	2 hospitals	183 beds
Totals:	9 hospitals	2315 beds

0018: **OKLAHOMA STATE DEPARTMENT OF MENTAL HEALTH AND SUBSTANCE ABUSE SERVICES** (NP)
1200 N.E. 13th Street, Oklahoma City, OK Zip 73152, Mailing Address: P.O. Box 53277, Zip 73152–3277; tel. 405/522–3908; Sharron D. Boehler, Commissioner
(Independent Hospital System)

OKLAHOMA: EASTERN STATE HOSPITAL (O, 314 beds) Vinita, OK Mailing Address: P.O. Box 69, Zip 74301–0069; tel. 918/256–7841; William T. Burkett, Chief Executive Officer

GRIFFIN MEMORIAL HOSPITAL (O, 182 beds) 900 East Main Street, Norman, OK Zip 73071–5305, Mailing Address: P.O. Box 151, Zip 73070–0151; tel. 405/321–4880; Don Bowen, Superintendent

WESTERN STATE PSYCHIATRIC CENTER (O, 102 beds) 1222 10th Street, Suite 211, Woodward, OK Zip 73801; tel. 580/571–3233; Steve Norwood, Executive Director

Owned, leased, sponsored:	3 hospitals	598 beds
Contract–managed:	0 hospitals	0 beds
Totals:	3 hospitals	598 beds

3355: **ORLANDO REGIONAL HEALTHCARE** (NP)
1414 Kuhl Avenue, Orlando, FL Zip 32806–2093; tel. 407/841–5111; John Hillenmeyer, President and Chief Executive Officer
(Moderately Centralized Health System)

FLORIDA: LEESBURG REGIONAL MEDICAL CENTER (O, 414 beds) 600 East Dixie Avenue, Leesburg, FL Zip 34748–5999; tel. 352/323–5000; Richard L. Wooten, President and Chief Executive Officer
Web address: www.Leesburgregional.org

ORLANDO REGIONAL MEDICAL CENTER (O, 1226 beds) 1414 Kuhl Avenue, Orlando, FL Zip 32806–2093; tel. 407/841–5111; Abe Lopman, Executive Director
Web address: www.orhs.org

ORLANDO REGIONAL SOUTH SEMINOLE HOSPITAL (O, 206 beds) 555 West State Road 434, Longwood, FL Zip 32750–4999; tel. 407/767–1200; Stephen M. Glazier, Executive Director

ORLANDO REGIONAL–LUCERNE (O, 267 beds) 818 Main Lane, Orlando, FL Zip 32801; tel. 407/649–6111; James A. Shanks, Administrator
Web address: www.cenflhealthcare.com

SOUTH LAKE HOSPITAL (O, 68 beds) 1099 Citrus Tower Boulevard, Clermont, FL Zip 34711; tel. 352/394–4071; Leslie Longacre, Executive Director and Chief Executive Officer

ST. CLOUD HOSPITAL, A DIVISION OF ORLANDO REGIONAL HEALTHCARE SYSTEM (O, 68 beds) 2906 17th Street, Saint Cloud, FL Zip 34769–6099; tel. 407/892–2135; Jim A. Norris, Executive Director

Owned, leased, sponsored:	6 hospitals	2249 beds
Contract–managed:	0 hospitals	0 beds
Totals:	6 hospitals	2249 beds

★5335: **OSF HEALTHCARE SYSTEM** (CC)
800 N.E. Glen Oak Avenue, Peoria, IL Zip 61603–3200; tel. 309/655–2852; Sister Frances Marie Masching, President
(Centralized Physician/Insurance Health System)

ILLINOIS: OSF SAINT FRANCIS MEDICAL CENTER (O, 532 beds) 530 N.E. Glen Oak Avenue, Peoria, IL Zip 61637; tel. 309/655–2000; Keith E. Steffen, Administrator
Web address: www.osfhealthcare.org

OSF SAINT JAMES HOSPITAL (O, 81 beds) 610 East Water Street, Pontiac, IL Zip 61764–2194; tel. 815/842–2828; David T. Ochs, Administrator
Web address: www.osfhealthcare.org

OSF ST. JOSEPH MEDICAL CENTER (O, 154 beds) 2200 East Washington Street, Bloomington, IL Zip 61701–4323; tel. 309/662–3311; Kenneth J. Natzke, Administrator
Web address: www.osfhealthcare.org

OSF ST. MARY MEDICAL CENTER (O, 141 beds) 3333 North Seminary Street, Galesburg, IL Zip 61401–1299; tel. 309/344–3161; Richard S. Kowalski, Administrator and Chief Executive Officer
Web address: www.osfhealthcare.org

SAINT ANTHONY MEDICAL CENTER (O, 221 beds) 5666 East State Street, Rockford, IL Zip 61108–2472; tel. 815/226–2000; David A. Schertz, Administrator
Web address: www.osfhealthcare.org

MICHIGAN: ST. FRANCIS HOSPITAL (O, 66 beds) 3401 Ludington Street, Escanaba, MI Zip 49829–1377; tel. 906/786–3311; Roger M. Burgess, Administrator
Web address: www.osfhealthcare.com

For explanation of codes following names, see page B2.
★ Indicates Type III membership in the American Hospital Association.

Systems / OSF Healthcare System

Owned, leased, sponsored:	6 hospitals	1195 beds
Contract-managed:	0 hospitals	0 beds
Totals:	6 hospitals	1195 beds

0110: OUR LADY OF MERCY HEALTHCARE SYSTEM, INC. (CC)
600 East 233 Street, New York, NY Zip 10466–2697; tel. 718/920–9000; Gary S. Horan, FACHE, President and Chief Executive Officer
(Moderately Centralized Health System)

NEW YORK: OUR LADY OF MERCY MEDICAL CENTER (O, 508 beds) 600 East 233rd Street, Bronx, NY Zip 10466–2697; tel. 718/920–9000; Gary S. Horan, FACHE, President and Chief Executive Officer
Web address: www.ourladyofmercy.com

ST. AGNES HOSPITAL (O, 184 beds) 305 North Street, White Plains, NY Zip 10605–2299; tel. 914/681–4500; Gary S. Horan, FACHE, President and Chief Executive Officer
Web address: www.saintagneshospital.com

Owned, leased, sponsored:	2 hospitals	692 beds
Contract-managed:	0 hospitals	0 beds
Totals:	2 hospitals	692 beds

0435: PACIFIC HEALTH CORPORATION (IO)
14642 Newport Avenue, Tustin, CA Zip 92780; tel. 714/669–2085; Jens Mueller, Chairman

CALIFORNIA: BELLFLOWER MEDICAL CENTER (O, 145 beds) 9542 East Artesia Boulevard, Bellflower, CA Zip 90706; tel. 562/925–8355; Stanley Otake, Administrator and Chief Executive Officer

LOS ANGELES METROPOLITAN MEDICAL CENTER (O, 173 beds) 2231 South Western Avenue, Los Angeles, CA Zip 90018–1399; tel. 323/730–7342; Marc A. Furstman, Chief Executive Officer

Owned, leased, sponsored:	2 hospitals	318 beds
Contract-managed:	0 hospitals	0 beds
Totals:	2 hospitals	318 beds

★4155: PALMETTO HEALTH ALLIANCE (CO)
Columbia, SC Mailing Address: P.O. Box 2266, Zip 29202–2266; tel. 803/296–2000; Charles D. Beaman, Jr, President
(Moderately Centralized Health System)

SOUTH CAROLINA: PALMETTO BAPTIST MEDICAL CENTER EASLEY (O, 106 beds) 200 Fleetwood Drive, Easley, SC Zip 29640–2076, Mailing Address: P.O. Box 2129, Zip 29641–2129; tel. 864/855–7200; Roddey E. Gettys, II, Executive Vice President
Web address: www.palmettohealth.org/

PALMETTO BAPTIST MEDICAL CENTER/COLUMBIA (O, 383 beds) Taylor at Marion Street, Columbia, SC Zip 29220; tel. 803/296–5010; James M. Bridges, Executive Vice President and Chief Operating Officer
Web address: www.palmettohealth.org/

PALMETTO RICHLAND MEMORIAL HOSPITAL (O, 612 beds) Five Richland Medical Park Drive, Columbia, SC Zip 29203, Mailing Address: P.O. Box 2266, Zip 29203–2266; tel. 803/434–7000; B. Daniel Paysinger, M.D., Chief Operating Officer
Web address: www.rmh.edu

Owned, leased, sponsored:	3 hospitals	1101 beds
Contract-managed:	0 hospitals	0 beds
Totals:	3 hospitals	1101 beds

★7555: PALOMAR POMERADO HEALTH SYSTEM (NP)
15255 Innovation Drive, Suite 204, San Diego, CA Zip 92128–3410; tel. 858/675–5100; Norman F. Gruber, President and Chief Executive Officer
(Centralized Physician/Insurance Health System)

CALIFORNIA: PALOMAR MEDICAL CENTER (O, 395 beds) 555 East Valley Parkway, Escondido, CA Zip 92025–3084; tel. 760/739–3000; Gerald E. Bracht, Vice President and Administrator
Web address: www.pphs.org

POMERADO HOSPITAL (O, 258 beds) 15615 Pomerado Road, Poway, CA Zip 92064; tel. 858/485–6511; Marvin C. Levenson, M.D., Administrator and Chief Operating Officer
Web address: www.pphs.org

Owned, leased, sponsored:	2 hospitals	653 beds
Contract-managed:	0 hospitals	0 beds
Totals:	2 hospitals	653 beds

5765: PARACELSUS HEALTHCARE CORPORATION (IO)
515 West Greens Road, Suite 500, Houston, TX Zip 77067–4511; tel. 281/774–5100; Robert L. Smith, Chief Executive Officer
(Moderately Centralized Health System)

LANCASTER COMMUNITY HOSPITAL (O, 123 beds) 43830 North Tenth Street West, Lancaster, CA Zip 93534; tel. 661/948–4781; Michael McAndrew, Chief Executive Officer

FLORIDA: SANTA ROSA MEDICAL CENTER (O, 129 beds) 1450 Berryhill Road, Milton, FL Zip 32570–4028, Mailing Address: P.O. Box 648, Zip 32572–0648; tel. 850/626–7762; M. P. Gandy, Jr, Chief Executive Officer

GEORGIA: FLINT RIVER COMMUNITY HOSPITAL (O, 49 beds) 509 Sumter Street, Montezuma, GA Zip 31063–0770, Mailing Address: P.O. Box 770, Zip 31063–0770; tel. 912/472–3100; Robert V. Deen, Interim Chief Executive Officer

NORTH DAKOTA: DAKOTA HEARTLAND HEALTH SYSTEM (O, 203 beds) 1720 South University Drive, Fargo, ND Zip 58103–4994; tel. 701/280–4100; Louis Kauffman, President and Chief Executive Officer
Web address: www.dakotaheartland.com

TENNESSEE: CUMBERLAND RIVER HOSPITAL (O, 66 beds) 100 Old Jefferson Street, Celina, TN Zip 38551, Mailing Address: P. O. Box 427, Zip 38551–0427; tel. 931/243–3581; Patrick J. Gray, President and Chief Executive Officer

FENTRESS COUNTY GENERAL HOSPITAL (O, 73 beds) Highway 52 West, Jamestown, TN Zip 38556, Mailing Address: P.O. Box 1500, Zip 38556; tel. 931/879–8171; Patrick J. Gray, Chief Executive Officer

TEXAS: BAYCOAST MEDICAL CENTER (O, 191 beds) 1700 James Bowie Drive, Baytown, TX Zip 77520–3386; tel. 281/420–6100; Walter J. Ornsteen, President and Chief Executive Officer

MEDICAL CENTER OF MESQUITE (O, 176 beds) 1011 North Galloway Avenue, Mesquite, TX Zip 75149–2433; tel. 972/320–7000; Terry J. Fontenot, President and Chief Executive Officer

WESTWOOD MEDICAL CENTER (O, 86 beds) 4214 Andrews Highway, Midland, TX Zip 79703–4861; tel. 915/522–2273; Dan Gideon, President and Chief Executive Officer
Web address: www.westwoodmed.com

VIRGINIA: CAPITOL MEDICAL CENTER (O, 135 beds) 701 West Grace Street, Richmond, VA Zip 23220–4191; tel. 804/775–4100; Priscilla J. Shuler, Chief Executive Officer

Owned, leased, sponsored:	10 hospitals	1231 beds
Contract-managed:	0 hospitals	0 beds
Totals:	10 hospitals	1231 beds

0159: PARKVIEW HEALTH SYSTEM (NP)
2200 Randallia Drive, Fort Wayne, IN Zip 46805; tel. 219/470–8200; Charles H. Mason, Jr, President and Chief Executive Officer
(Centralized Physician/Insurance Health System)

INDIANA: HUNTINGTON MEMORIAL HOSPITAL (O, 37 beds) 2001 Stults Road, Huntington, IN Zip 46750–3696; tel. 219/356–3000; L. Kent McCoy, President

For explanation of codes following names, see page B2.
★ Indicates Type III membership in the American Hospital Association.

Systems / Presbyterian Healthcare Services

PARKVIEW HOSPITAL (O, 505 beds) 2200 Randallia Drive, Fort Wayne, IN Zip 46805–4699; tel. 219/484–6636; Frank D. Byrne, M.D., President

WHITLEY MEMORIAL HOSPITAL (O, 122 beds) 353 North Oak Street, Columbia City, IN Zip 46725–1623; tel. 219/244–6191; John M. Hatcher, President

Owned, leased, sponsored:	3 hospitals	664 beds
Contract–managed:	0 hospitals	0 beds
Totals:	3 hospitals	664 beds

★1785: **PARTNERS HEALTHCARE SYSTEM, INC.** (NP)
800 Boylston Street, Suite 1150, Boston, MA Zip 02199–8001; tel. 617/278–1004; Samuel O. Thier, M.D., President and Chief Executive Officer
(Moderately Centralized Health System)

MASSACHUSETTS: BRIGHAM AND WOMEN'S HOSPITAL (O, 694 beds) 75 Francis Street, Boston, MA Zip 02115–6195; tel. 617/732–5500; Jeffrey Otten, President
Web address: www.partners.org

FAULKNER HOSPITAL (O, 125 beds) Boston, MA Mailing Address: 1153 Centre Sreet, Zip 02130–3400; tel. 617/983–7000; David J. Trull, President and Chief Executive Officer
Web address: www.faulknerhospital.org

MASSACHUSETTS GENERAL HOSPITAL (O, 853 beds) 55 Fruit Street, Boston, MA Zip 02114–2696; tel. 617/726–2000; James J. Mongan, M.D., President
Web address: www.mgh.harvard.edu/

MCLEAN HOSPITAL (O, 150 beds) 115 Mill Street, Belmont, MA Zip 02478–9106; tel. 617/855–2000; Bruce M. Cohen, M.D., Ph.D., President and Psychiatrist–in–Chief
Web address: www.mcleanhospital.org

NEWTON–WELLESLEY HOSPITAL (O, 228 beds) 2014 Washington Street, Newton Lower Falls, MA Zip 02462–1699; tel. 617/243–6000; John P. Bihldorff, President and Chief Executive Officer
Web address: www.nwh.org

SALEM HOSPITAL (O, 291 beds) 81 Highland Avenue, Salem, MA Zip 01970–2768; tel. 978/741–1200; Judith Ritchie, President and Chief Executive Officer
Web address: www.nsmc.partners.org

SHAUGHNESSY–KAPLAN REHABILITATION HOSPITAL (O, 160 beds) Dove Avenue, Salem, MA Zip 01970–2999; tel. 978/745–9000; Anthony Sciola, President and Chief Executive Officer
Web address: www.nsmc.partners.org

SPAULDING REHABILITATION HOSPITAL (O, 333 beds) 125 Nashua Street, Boston, MA Zip 02114–1198; tel. 617/573–7000; John E. Cupples, President
Web address: www.spauldingrehab.org

THE UNION HOSPITAL (O, 189 beds) 500 Lynnfield Street, Lynn, MA Zip 01904–1487; tel. 781/581–9200; Judith Ritchie, President and Chief Executive Officer

Owned, leased, sponsored:	9 hospitals	3023 beds
Contract–managed:	0 hospitals	0 beds
Totals:	9 hospitals	3023 beds

★5415: **PEACEHEALTH** (CC)
15325 S.E. 30th Place, Suite 300, Bellevue, WA Zip 98007; tel. 425/747–1711; John Hayward, President and Chief Executive Officer
(Moderately Centralized Health System)

ALASKA: KETCHIKAN GENERAL HOSPITAL (L, 65 beds) 3100 Tongass Avenue, Ketchikan, AK Zip 99901–5746; tel. 907/225–5171; Edward F. Mahn, Chief Executive Officer

OREGON: PEACE HARBOR HOSPITAL (O, 21 beds) 400 Ninth Street, Florence, OR Zip 97439, Mailing Address: P.O. Box 580, Zip 97439; tel. 541/997–8412; James Barnhart, Chief Executive Officer
Web address: www.peacehealth.org

SACRED HEART MEDICAL CENTER (O, 404 beds) 1255 Hilyard Street, Eugene, OR Zip 97401, Mailing Address: P.O. Box 10905, Zip 97440; tel. 541/686–7300; Judy Hodgson, Administrator
Web address: www.peacehealth.com

WASHINGTON: ST. JOHN MEDICAL CENTER (O, 178 beds) 1615 Delaware Street, Longview, WA Zip 98632, Mailing Address: P.O. Box 3002, Zip 98632–0302; tel. 360/414–2000; Mark E. McGourty, Regional Chief Executive Officer
Web address: www.peacehealth.org

ST. JOSEPH HOSPITAL (O, 189 beds) 2901 Squalicum Parkway, Bellingham, WA Zip 98225–1898; tel. 360/734–5400; Nancy J. Bitting, Regional Chief Executive Officer
Web address: www.peacehealth.org

Owned, leased, sponsored:	5 hospitals	857 beds
Contract–managed:	0 hospitals	0 beds
Totals:	5 hospitals	857 beds

0091: **PIONEER BEHAVIORAL HEALTH** (IO)
200 Lake Street, Suite 102, Peabody, MA Zip 01960–4780; tel. 978/536–2777; Bruce A. Shear, President and Chief Executive Officer
(Independent Hospital System)

MICHIGAN: HARBOR OAKS HOSPITAL (O, 64 beds) 35031 23 Mile Road, New Baltimore, MI Zip 48047–2097; tel. 810/725–5777; Judi Schiop, Administrator

UTAH: HIGHLAND RIDGE HOSPITAL (O, 32 beds) 175 West 7200 South, Midvale, UT Zip 84047; tel. 801/569–2153; Michael S. Talmo, Chief Executive Officer

VIRGINIA: MOUNT REGIS CENTER (O, 25 beds) 405 Kimball Avenue, Salem, VA Zip 24153–6299; tel. 540/389–4761; Gail S. Basham, Chief Executive Officer

Owned, leased, sponsored:	3 hospitals	121 beds
Contract–managed:	0 hospitals	0 beds
Totals:	3 hospitals	121 beds

●★0034: **PMH HEALTH RESOURCES, INC.** (NP)
1201 South Seventh Avenue, Phoenix, AZ Zip 85007–3913, Mailing Address: P.O. Box 21207, Zip 85036–1207; tel. 602/824–3321; Reginald M. Ballantyne , II, President
(Centralized Physician/Insurance Health System)

ARIZONA: PHOENIX MEMORIAL HEALTH SYSTEM (O, 195 beds) 1201 South Seventh Avenue, Phoenix, AZ Zip 85007–3995; tel. 602/258–5111; Robert J. Conaway , Jr, Chief Executive Officer
Web address: www.phzmemorialhospital.com

Owned, leased, sponsored:	1 hospital	195 beds
Contract–managed:	0 hospitals	0 beds
Totals:	1 hospital	195 beds

★3505: **PRESBYTERIAN HEALTHCARE SERVICES** (CO)
5901 Harper Drive N.E., Albuquerque, NM Zip 87109–3589, Mailing Address: P.O. Box 26666, Zip 87125–6666; tel. 505/260–6500; James H. Hinton, President and Chief Executive Officer
(Moderately Centralized Health System)

NEW MEXICO: DR. DAN C. TRIGG MEMORIAL HOSPITAL (L; 37 beds) 301 East Miel De Luna Avenue, Tucumcari, NM Zip 88401–3810, Mailing Address: P.O. Box 608, Zip 88401–0608; tel. 505/461–0141; Dell Willis, Administrator

ESPANOLA HOSPITAL (O, 80 beds) 1010 Spruce Street, Espanola, NM Zip 87532–2746; tel. 505/753–7111; Marcella A. Romero, Administrator

LINCOLN COUNTY MEDICAL CENTER (L, 27 beds) 211 Sudderth Drive, Ruidoso, NM Zip 88345–6043, Mailing Address: P.O. Box 8000, Zip 88345–8000; tel. 505/257–7381; James P. Gibson, Administrator

PLAINS REGIONAL MEDICAL CENTER (O, 74 beds) 2100 North Thomas Street, Clovis, NM Zip 88101–9412, Mailing Address: P.O. Box 1688, Zip 88101–1688; tel. 505/769–2141; Richard Smith, Administrator

For explanation of codes following names, see page B2.
★ Indicates Type III membership in the American Hospital Association.
● Single hospital health care system

Systems / Presbyterian Healthcare Services

PRESBYTERIAN HOSPITAL (O, 383 beds) 1100 Central Avenue S.E., Albuquerque, NM Zip 87106–4934, Mailing Address: P.O. Box 26666, Zip 87125–6666; tel. 505/841–1234; Mark W. Reifsteck, Senior Vice President and Chief Operating Officer
Web address: www.phs.org

PRESBYTERIAN KASEMAN HOSPITAL (O, 138 beds) 8300 Constitution Avenue N.E., Albuquerque, NM Zip 87110–7624, Mailing Address: P.O. Box 26666, Zip 87125–6666; tel. 505/291–2000; Robert A. Garcia, Administrative Director

SOCORRO GENERAL HOSPITAL (O, 24 beds) 1202 Highway 60 West, Socorro, NM Zip 87801, Mailing Address: P.O. Box 1009, Zip 87801–1009; tel. 505/835–1140; Jeff Dye, Administrator

Owned, leased, sponsored:	7 hospitals	763 beds
Contract-managed:	0 hospitals	0 beds
Totals:	7 hospitals	763 beds

0209: PROGRESSIONS GROUP, INC. (IO)
450 Bethlehem Pike, Fort Washington, PA Zip 19034; tel. 215/641–5300; Nicholas Tenaglia, M.D., Chief Executive Officer

PENNSYLVANIA: EUGENIA HOSPITAL (O, 126 beds) 660 Thomas Road, Lafayette Hill, PA Zip 19444–1199; tel. 215/836–7700; John P. Ash, FACHE, President and Chief Executive Officer

MALVERN INSTITUTE (O, 40 beds) 940 King Road, Malvern, PA Zip 19355–3167; tel. 610/647–0330; Thomas Cain, Administrator and Chief Executive Officer

NORTHWESTERN INSTITUTE (O, 146 beds) 450 Bethlehem Pike, Fort Washington, PA Zip 19034–0209; tel. 215/641–5300; Joseph Roynan, Administrator

TEXAS: PINELANDS HOSPITAL (O, 38 beds) 4632 Northeast Stallings Drive, Nacogdoches, TX Zip 75961–1617, Mailing Address: P.O. Box 1004, Zip 79563–1004; tel. 409/560–5900; Steve Scott, Chief Executive Officer

Owned, leased, sponsored:	4 hospitals	350 beds
Contract-managed:	0 hospitals	0 beds
Totals:	4 hospitals	350 beds

0153: PROHEALTH CARE (NP)
725 American Avenue, Waukesha, WI Zip 53188; tel. 262/928–2241; Donald W. Fundingsland, Chief Executive Officer
(Moderately Centralized Health System)

WISCONSIN: OCONOMOWOC MEMORIAL HOSPITAL (O, 72 beds) 791 Summit Avenue, Oconomowoc, WI Zip 53066–3896; tel. 262/569–9400; Douglas Guy, President and Chief Executive Officer

WAUKESHA MEMORIAL HOSPITAL (O, 288 beds) 725 American Avenue, Waukesha, WI Zip 53188–5099; tel. 262/928–1000; Rexford W. Titus, II, President and Chief Executive Officer
Web address: www.phci.org

Owned, leased, sponsored:	2 hospitals	360 beds
Contract-managed:	0 hospitals	0 beds
Totals:	2 hospitals	360 beds

★0197: PROMEDICA HEALTH SYSTEM (NP)
2121 Hughes Drive, 4th Floor, Toledo, OH Zip 43606; tel. 419/291–7176; Alan W. Brass, FACHE, President and Chief Executive Officer
(Centralized Physician/Insurance Health System)

MICHIGAN: BIXBY MEDICAL CENTER, LENAWEE HEALTH ALLIANCE (O, 77 beds) 818 Riverside Avenue, Adrian, MI Zip 49221–1496; tel. 517/265–0900; John R. Robertstad, President and Chief Executive Officer
Web address: www.lhanet.org

HERRICK MEMORIAL HOSPITAL, LENAWEE HEALTH ALLIANCE (O, 88 beds) 500 East Pottawatamie Street, Tecumseh, MI Zip 49286–2097; tel. 517/424–3000; John R. Robertstad, President and Chief Executive Officer
Web address: www.lhanet.org

OHIO: DEFIANCE HOSPITAL (O, 80 beds) 1206 East Second Street, Defiance, OH Zip 43512–2495; tel. 419/783–6955; Robert J. Coholich, President
Web address: www.promedica.org

FLOWER HOSPITAL (O, 468 beds) 5200 Harroun Road, Sylvania, OH Zip 43560–2196; tel. 419/824–1444; Randall Kelley, President
Web address: www.promedica.org

FOSTORIA COMMUNITY HOSPITAL (O, 39 beds) 501 Van Buren Street, Fostoria, OH Zip 44830–0907, Mailing Address: P.O. Box 907, Zip 44830–0907; tel. 419/435–7734; Brad A. Higgins, President
Web address: www.fchosp.org

THE TOLEDO HOSPITAL (O, 673 beds) 2142 North Cove Boulevard, Toledo, OH Zip 43606–3896; tel. 419/471–4000; Barbara Steele, President
Web address: www.promedica.org

Owned, leased, sponsored:	6 hospitals	1425 beds
Contract-managed:	0 hospitals	0 beds
Totals:	6 hospitals	1425 beds

★0132: PROVENA HEALTH (NP)
9223 West St. Francis Road, Frankfort, IL Zip 60423–8334; tel. 815/469–4888; Joseph S. Feth, Chief Executive Officer
(Moderately Centralized Health System)

ILLINOIS: PROVENA COVENANT MEDICAL CENTER (O, 258 beds) 1400 West Park Street, Urbana, IL Zip 61801–2396; tel. 217/337–2000; Diane Friedman, R.N., President and Chief Executive Officer
Web address: www.provenacovenant.org

PROVENA MERCY CENTER (O, 180 beds) 1325 North Highland Avenue, Aurora, IL Zip 60506; tel. 630/859–2222; John K. Barto, Jr, Interim President and Chief Executive Officer
Web address: www.provenamercy.com

PROVENA SAINT JOSEPH HOSPITAL (O, 183 beds) 77 North Airlite Street, Elgin, IL Zip 60123–4912; tel. 847/695–3200; Larry Narum, President
Web address: www.provenahealth.com

PROVENA SAINT JOSEPH MEDICAL CENTER (O, 369 beds) 333 North Madison Street, Joliet, IL Zip 60435–6595; tel. 815/725–7133; Thomas A. Reitinger, Chief Executive Officer
Web address: www.provena.org

PROVENA SAINT THERESE MEDICAL CENTER (O, 254 beds) 2615 Washington Street, Waukegan, IL Zip 60085–4988; tel. 847/249–3900; Timothy P. Selz, President and Chief Executive Officer
Web address: www.sainttherese.org

PROVENA ST. MARY'S HOSPITAL (O, 174 beds) 500 West Court Street, Kankakee, IL Zip 60901–3661; tel. 815/937–2180; Paula Jacobi, President and Chief Executive Officer
Web address: www.provena–stmarys.com

PROVENA UNITED SAMARITANS MEDICAL CENTER (O, 308 beds) 812 North Logan, Danville, IL Zip 61832–3788; tel. 217/443–5000; James W. Pope, President and Chief Executive Officer
Web address: www.provenausmc.org

Owned, leased, sponsored:	7 hospitals	1726 beds
Contract-managed:	0 hospitals	0 beds
Totals:	7 hospitals	1726 beds

★5275: PROVIDENCE HEALTH SYSTEM (CC)
506 Second Avenue, Suite 1200, Seattle, WA Zip 98104–2329; tel. 206/464–3355; Henry G. Walker, President and Chief Executive Officer
(Decentralized Health System)

ALASKA: PROVIDENCE ALASKA MEDICAL CENTER (O, 341 beds) 3200 Providence Drive, Anchorage, AK Zip 99508, Mailing Address: P.O. Box 196604, Zip 99519–6604; tel. 907/562–2211; Gene L. O'Hara, Administrator
Web address: www.providence.org

For explanation of codes following names, see page B2.
★ Indicates Type III membership in the American Hospital Association.

Systems / Province Healthcare Corporation

PROVIDENCE KODIAK ISLAND MEDICAL CENTER (L, 44 beds) 1915 East Rezanof Drive, Kodiak, AK Zip 99615; tel. 907/486–3281; Phillip E. Cline, Administrator
Web address: www.providence.org

PROVIDENCE SEWARD MEDICAL CENTER (L, 6 beds) 417 First Avenue, Seward, AK Zip 99664, Mailing Address: P.O. Box 365, Zip 99664–0365; tel. 907/224–5205; Judy Christine Rathje, Administrator
Web address: www.providence.org

CALIFORNIA: PROVIDENCE HOLY CROSS MEDICAL CENTER (O, 255 beds) 15031 Rinaldi Street, Mission Hills, CA Zip 91345–1285; tel. 818/365–8051; Georgianne Jessen, Chief Executive Officer
Web address: www.providence.org

PROVIDENCE SAINT JOSEPH MEDICAL CENTER (O, 448 beds) 501 South Buena Vista Street, Burbank, CA Zip 91505–4866; tel. 818/843–5111; Georgianne Jessen, Chief Executive Officer
Web address: www.providence.org

OREGON: PROVIDENCE HOOD RIVER MEMORIAL HOSPITAL (O, 31 beds) 13th and May Streets, Hood River, OR Zip 97031, Mailing Address: P.O. Box 149, Zip 97031; tel. 541/386–3911; Larry Bowe, JD, Chief Executive Officer
Web address: www.hrmh.org

PROVIDENCE MEDFORD MEDICAL CENTER (O, 121 beds) 1111 Crater Lake Avenue, Medford, OR Zip 97504–6241; tel. 541/732–5000; Charles T. Wright, Chief Executive, Southern Oregon Service Area
Web address: www.providence.org

PROVIDENCE MILWAUKIE HOSPITAL (O, 56 beds) 10150 S.E. 32nd Avenue, Milwaukie, OR Zip 97222–6593; tel. 503/513–8300; Janice Burger, Operations Administrator
Web address: www.providence.org

PROVIDENCE NEWBERG HOSPITAL (O, 35 beds) 501 Villa Road, Newberg, OR Zip 97132; tel. 503/537–1555; Mark W. Meinert, CHE, Chief Executive, Yamhill Service Area
Web address: www.phsor.org

PROVIDENCE PORTLAND MEDICAL CENTER (O, 380 beds) 4805 N.E. Glisan Street, Portland, OR Zip 97213–2967; tel. 503/215–1111; David T. Underriner, Operations Administrator
Web address: www.providence.org

PROVIDENCE SEASIDE HOSPITAL (L, 45 beds) 725 South Wahanna Road, Seaside, OR Zip 97138–7735; tel. 503/717–7000; Gail Harper, R.N., Chief Executive
Web address: www.providence.org

PROVIDENCE ST. VINCENT MEDICAL CENTER (O, 389 beds) 9205 S.W. Barnes Road, Portland, OR Zip 97225–6661; tel. 503/216–1234; Donald Elsom, Operations Administrator
Web address: www.providence.org/portland/hospitals

WASHINGTON: MARK REED HOSPITAL (C, 7 beds) 322 South Birch Street, McCleary, WA Zip 98557; tel. 360/495–3244; Jean E. Roberts, Administrator

MORTON GENERAL HOSPITAL (C, 50 beds) 521 Adams Street, Morton, WA Zip 98356, Mailing Address: Drawer C, Zip 98356–0019; tel. 360/496–5112; Mike Lee, Superintendent

PROVIDENCE CENTRALIA HOSPITAL (O, 142 beds) 914 South Scheuber Road, Centralia, WA Zip 98531; tel. 360/736–2803; Steve Burdick, Administrator
Web address: www.providence.org

PROVIDENCE EVERETT MEDICAL CENTER (O, 283 beds) 1321 Colby Street, Everett, WA Zip 98206, Mailing Address: P.O. Box 1147, Zip 98206–1147; tel. 425/261–2000; Mel Pyne, Administrator
Web address: www.providence.org

PROVIDENCE SEATTLE MEDICAL CENTER (O, 296 beds) 500 17th Avenue, Seattle, WA Zip 98122–1008, Mailing Address: P.O. Box 34008, Zip 98124–1008; tel. 206/320–2000; Craig L. Hendrickson, Chief Operating Officer
Web address: www.providence.org

PROVIDENCE ST. PETER HOSPITAL (O, 314 beds) 413 Lilly Road N.E., Olympia, WA Zip 98506–5116; tel. 360/491–9480; C. Scott Bond, Administrator and Chief Executive Officer
Web address: www.providence.org

PROVIDENCE TOPPENISH HOSPITAL (O, 48 beds) 502 West Fourth Avenue, Toppenish, WA Zip 98948–0672, Mailing Address: P.O. Box 672, Zip 98948–0672; tel. 509/865–3105; Larry Anthony, Administrator
Web address: www.providence.org

PROVIDENCE YAKIMA MEDICAL CENTER (O, 197 beds) 110 South Ninth Avenue, Yakima, WA Zip 98902–3397; tel. 509/575–5000; Andrew S. Robertson, M.D., Chief Executive Officer
Web address: www.providence.org

Owned, leased, sponsored:	18 hospitals	3431 beds
Contract-managed:	2 hospitals	57 beds
Totals:	20 hospitals	3488 beds

★**5265: PROVIDENCE SERVICES** (CC)
9 East Ninth Avenue, Spokane, WA Zip 99202; tel. 509/742–7337; Richard J. Umbdenstock, President and Chief Executive Officer
(Moderately Centralized Health System)

MONTANA: BENEFIS HEALTHCARE (S, 470 beds) 1101 26th Street South, Great Falls, MT Zip 59405; tel. 406/455–5000; Lloyd V. Smith, President and Chief Executive Officer
Web address: www.benefis.org

ST. JOSEPH HOSPITAL (S, 22 beds) Skyline Drive and 14th Avenue, Polson, MT Zip 59860, Mailing Address: P.O. Box 1010, Zip 59860–1010; tel. 406/883–5377; John W. Glueckert, President

ST. PATRICK HOSPITAL (S, 195 beds) 500 West Broadway, Missoula, MT Zip 59802–4096, Mailing Address: Box 4587, Zip 59806–4587; tel. 406/543–7271; Lawrence L. White, Jr, President
Web address: www.saintpatrick.org

WASHINGTON: DEER PARK HOSPITAL (S, 26 beds) East 1015 D Street, Deer Park, WA Zip 99006–0742, Mailing Address: P.O. Box 742, Zip 99006–0742; tel. 509/276–5061; Garvin Olson, Chief Operating Officer

HOLY FAMILY HOSPITAL (S, 190 beds) North 5633 Lidgerwood Avenue, Spokane, WA Zip 99207–2533; tel. 509/482–0111; Thomas Corley, President and Chief Executive Officer
Web address: www.holy-family.org

MOUNT CARMEL HOSPITAL (S, 33 beds) 982 East Columbia Street, Colville, WA Zip 99114–0351, Mailing Address: Box 351, Zip 99114–0351; tel. 509/684–2561; Gloria Cooper, Chief Executive Officer

SACRED HEART MEDICAL CENTER (S, 607 beds) West 101 Eighth Avenue, Spokane, WA Zip 99220–2555, Mailing Address: P.O. Box 2555, Zip 99220–2555; tel. 509/474–3040; Ryland P. Davis, President and Chief Executive Officer
Web address: www.shmc.org

ST. JOSEPH'S HOSPITAL (S, 65 beds) 500 East Webster Street, Chewelah, WA Zip 99109–0197, Mailing Address: P.O. Box 197, Zip 99109–0197; tel. 509/935–8211; Gary V. Peck, Chief Executive Officer

ST. MARY MEDICAL CENTER (S, 107 beds) 401 West Poplar Street, Walla Walla, WA Zip 99362–1477, Mailing Address: Box 1477, Zip 99362–1477; tel. 509/525–3320; John A. Isely, President

Owned, leased, sponsored:	9 hospitals	1715 beds
Contract-managed:	0 hospitals	0 beds
Totals:	9 hospitals	1715 beds

0108: PROVINCE HEALTHCARE CORPORATION (IO)
105 Westwood Place, Suite 400, Brentwood, TN Zip 37027; tel. 615/370–1377; Marty Rash, President and Chief Executive Officer
(Moderately Centralized Health System)

ARIZONA: HAVASU REGIONAL MEDICAL CENTER (O, 118 beds) 101 Civic Center Lane, Lake Havasu City, AZ Zip 86403–5683; tel. 520/855–8185; Kevin P. Poorten, Chief Executive Officer

CALIFORNIA: COLORADO RIVER MEDICAL CENTER (O, 49 beds) 1401 Bailey Avenue, Needles, CA Zip 92363; tel. 760/326–4531; James Arp, Chief Executive Officer

GENERAL HOSPITAL (O, 65 beds) 2200 Harrison Avenue, Eureka, CA Zip 95501; tel. 707/445–5111; Martin Love, Chief Executive Officer

For explanation of codes following names, see page B2.
★ Indicates Type III membership in the American Hospital Association.

Systems / Province Healthcare Corporation

OJAI VALLEY COMMUNITY HOSPITAL (O, 104 beds) 1306 Maricopa Highway, Ojai, CA Zip 93023-3180; tel. 805/646-1401; Mark Turner, Chief Executive Officer

PALO VERDE HOSPITAL (O, 35 beds) 250 North First Street, Blythe, CA Zip 92225; tel. 760/922-4115; M. Victoria Clark, Chief Executive Officer

COLORADO: COLORADO PLAINS MEDICAL CENTER (O, 50 beds) 1000 Lincoln Street, Fort Morgan, CO Zip 80701-3298; tel. 970/867-3391; Solon H. Boggus, Jr, Interim Chief Executive Officer

FLORIDA: GLADES GENERAL HOSPITAL (O, 73 beds) 1201 South Main Street, Belle Glade, FL Zip 33430-4911; tel. 561/996-6571; James E. Purcell, II, Chief Executive Officer

INDIANA: STARKE MEMORIAL HOSPITAL (O, 35 beds) 102 East Culver Road, Knox, IN Zip 46534-2299; tel. 219/772-6231; Kathryn J. Norem, Chief Executive Officer

LOUISIANA: DOCTORS' HOSPITAL OF OPELOUSAS (O, 105 beds) 3972 I-49 South Service Road, Opelousas, LA Zip 70570-8975; tel. 318/948-2100; Bethy W. Walker, Chief Executive Officer

EUNICE COMMUNITY MEDICAL CENTER (O, 62 beds) 400 Moosa Boulevard, Eunice, LA Zip 70535; tel. 318/457-5244; Larry D. Walker, Chief Executive Officer
Web address: www.eunicemedical.com/

MISSISSIPPI: BOLIVAR MEDICAL CENTER (O, 148 beds) 901 Highway 8 East, Cleveland, MS Zip 38732-9722, Mailing Address: P.O. Box 1380, Zip 38732-1380; tel. 662/846-0061; Robert L. Hawley, Jr, Chief Executive Officer

NEVADA: ELKO GENERAL HOSPITAL (O, 50 beds) 1297 College Avenue, Elko, NV Zip 89801-3499; tel. 775/738-5151; Fredrick W. Hodges, Chief Executive Officer
Web address: www.elkogeneral.hbocvan.com

TEXAS: PALESTINE REGIONAL MEDICAL CENTER (O, 97 beds) 4000 South Loop 256, Palestine, TX Zip 75801-8467, Mailing Address: P.O. Box 4070, Zip 75802-4070; tel. 903/731-1000; Randell G. Stokes, Chief Executive Officer
Web address: www.palestineregional.com

PARKVIEW REGIONAL HOSPITAL (O, 44 beds) 312 East Glendale Street, Mexia, TX Zip 76667-3608; tel. 254/562-5332; Tim Adams, CHE, Administrator and Chief Executive Officer
Web address: www.parkviewregional.com

Owned, leased, sponsored:	14 hospitals	1035 beds
Contract-managed:	0 hospitals	0 beds
Totals:	14 hospitals	1035 beds

0011: PUERTO RICO DEPARTMENT OF HEALTH (NP)
Building A – Medical Center, San Juan, PR Zip 00936, Mailing Address: Call Box 70184, Zip 00936; tel. 787/274-7676; Carmen Feliciano De Melecio, M.D., Secretary of Health
(Independent Hospital System)

PUERTO RICO: AGUADILLA GENERAL HOSPITAL (O, 110 beds) Carr Aguadilla San Juan, Aguadilla, PR Zip 00605, Mailing Address: P.O. Box 4036, Zip 00605; tel. 787/891-3534; Marco Reyes, Executive Director

ARECIBO REGIONAL HOSPITAL (O, 188 beds) 129 San Luis Avenue, Arecibo, PR Zip 00612, Mailing Address: P.O. Box 659, Zip 00613; tel. 787/878-7272; Samuel Monroig, Vice President for Administration

CAGUAS REGIONAL HOSPITAL (O, 256 beds) Carretera Caguas A Cidra, Caguas, PR Zip 00725, Mailing Address: Call Box 4964, Zip 00726-4964; tel. 787/744-2500; Pedro Juan Santiago, Executive Director

DR. RAMON E. BETANCES HOSPITAL–MAYAGUEZ MEDICAL CENTER BRANCH (O, 253 beds) 410 Hostos Avenue, Mayaguez, PR Zip 00680; tel. 787/834-8686; Maria Del Pilar Rodriguez, Chief Executive Officer

HOSPITAL SUB-REGIONAL DR. VICTOR R. NUNEZ (O, 83 beds) Avenida Tejas, Expreso Cruz Ortiz Stella, Humacao, PR Zip 00791; tel. 787/852-2727; Ahmed Alvarez Pabon, Executive Director

HOSPITAL UNIVERSITARIO DR. RAMON RUIZ ARNAU (O, 341 beds) Avenue Laurel, Santa Juanita, Bayamon, PR Zip 00956; tel. 787/787-5151; Nilda E. Diaz, Executive Director

PONCE REGIONAL HOSPITAL (O, 324 beds) 917 Tito Castro Avenue, Ponce, PR Zip 00731; tel. 787/844-2080; Julio Andino Rodriguez, Executive Director

STATE PSYCHIATRIC HOSPITAL (O, 425 beds) Monacillos Avenue, San Juan, PR Zip 00936, Mailing Address: Call Box 2100, Caparra Heights Station, Zip 00922-2100; tel. 787/766-4646; Ivette Molena, Administrator

UNIVERSITY HOSPITAL (O, 297 beds) Puerto Rico Medical Center, Rio Piedras Station, San Juan, PR Zip 00920-2116; tel. 787/777-3535; Betty Ocasio, Executive Director

Owned, leased, sponsored:	9 hospitals	2277 beds
Contract-managed:	0 hospitals	0 beds
Totals:	9 hospitals	2277 beds

★0040: QUEEN'S HEALTH SYSTEMS (NP)
1099 Alakea Street, Suite 1100, Honolulu, HI Zip 96813; tel. 808/532-6100; Richard L. Griffith, President and Chief Executive Officer
(Centralized Physician/Insurance Health System)

HAWAII: MOLOKAI GENERAL HOSPITAL (O, 29 beds) Kaunakakai, HI Mailing Address: P.O. Box 408, Zip 96748-0408; tel. 808/553-5331; Calvin M. Ichinose, Administrator
Web address: www.queens.org

QUEEN'S MEDICAL CENTER (O, 451 beds) 1301 Punchbowl Street, Honolulu, HI Zip 96813; tel. 808/538-9011; Arthur A. Ushijima, President and Chief Executive Officer
Web address: www.queens.org

Owned, leased, sponsored:	2 hospitals	480 beds
Contract-managed:	0 hospitals	0 beds
Totals:	2 hospitals	480 beds

★0002: QUORUM HEALTH GROUP (IO)
103 Continental Place, Brentwood, TN Zip 37027; tel. 615/371-7979; James E. Dalton, Jr, President and Chief Executive Officer
(Decentralized Health System)

ALABAMA: FLOWERS HOSPITAL (O, 215 beds) 4370 West Main Street, Dothan, AL Zip 36305, Mailing Address: P.O. Box 6907, Zip 36302-6907; tel. 334/793-5000; Keith Granger, President and Chief Executive Officer

GADSDEN REGIONAL MEDICAL CENTER (O, 257 beds) 1007 Goodyear Avenue, Gadsden, AL Zip 35903-1195; tel. 256/494-4000; James F. O'Loughlin, Chief Executive Officer
Web address: www.gadsdenregional.com

JACKSONVILLE HOSPITAL (O, 56 beds) 1701 Pelham Road South, Jacksonville, AL Zip 36265-3399, Mailing Address: P.O. Box 999, Zip 36265-0999; tel. 256/435-4970; Charles Mitchener, Jr, Chief Executive Officer
Web address: www.jaxhosp.com

MEDICAL CENTER ENTERPRISE (O, 117 beds) 400 North Edwards Street, Enterprise, AL Zip 36330-9981; tel. 334/347-0584; Keith Granger, President and Chief Executive Officer

MONROE COUNTY HOSPITAL (C, 59 beds) 1901 South Alabama Avenue, Monroeville, AL Zip 36460, Mailing Address: P.O. Box 886, Zip 36461-0886; tel. 334/575-3111; Joe Zager, Chief Executive Officer

ALASKA: BARTLETT REGIONAL HOSPITAL (C, 64 beds) 3260 Hospital Drive, Juneau, AK Zip 99801; tel. 907/586-2611; Robert F. Valliant, Administrator
Web address: www.bartletthospital.org

ARIZONA: CASA GRANDE REGIONAL MEDICAL CENTER (C, 244 beds) 1800 East Florence Boulevard, Casa Grande, AZ Zip 85222-5399; tel. 520/426-6300; J. Marty Dernier, President and Chief Executive Officer
Web address: www.casagrandehospital.com

MARICOPA MEDICAL CENTER (C, 481 beds) 2601 East Roosevelt Street, Phoenix, AZ Zip 85008-4956; tel. 602/344-5011; Mark Hillard, Chief Executive Officer
Web address: www.maricopa.gov/medcenter/mmc.html

For explanation of codes following names, see page B2.
★ Indicates Type III membership in the American Hospital Association.

Systems / Quorum Health Group

ARKANSAS: CHICOT MEMORIAL HOSPITAL (C, 52 beds) 2729 Highway 65 and 82 South, Lake Village, AR Zip 71653, Mailing Address: P.O. Box 512, Zip 71653–0512; tel. 870/265–5351; Robert R. Reddish, Administrator and Chief Executive Officer

DE QUEEN REGIONAL MEDICAL CENTER (C, 75 beds) 1306 Collin Raye Drive, De Queen, AR Zip 71832–2198; tel. 870/584–4111; Craig R. Cudworth, Chief Executive Officer
Web address: www.hcahealthcare.com

DELTA MEMORIAL HOSPITAL (C, 20 beds) 300 East Pickens Street, Dumas, AR Zip 71639–2710, Mailing Address: P.O. Box 887, Zip 71639–0887; tel. 870/382–4303; Kurt Meyer, Administrator

HELENA REGIONAL MEDICAL CENTER (C, 145 beds) 1801 Martin Luther King Drive, Helena, AR Zip 72342, Mailing Address: P.O. Box 788, Zip 72342–0788; tel. 870/338–5800; Steve Reeder, Chief Executive Officer

HOWARD MEMORIAL HOSPITAL (C, 50 beds) 800 West Leslie Street, Nashville, AR Zip 71852–0381, Mailing Address: Box 381, Zip 71852–0381; tel. 870/845–4400; Rex Jones, Chief Executive Officer

MENA MEDICAL CENTER (C, 42 beds) 311 North Morrow Street, Mena, AR Zip 71953–2516; tel. 501/394–6100; Travis W. Roderick, Administrator and Chief Executive Officer

NORTHWEST MEDICAL CENTER (O, 222 beds) 609 West Maple Avenue, Springdale, AR Zip 72764–5394, Mailing Address: P.O. Box 47, Zip 72765–0047; tel. 501/751–5711;
Web address: www.northwesthealth.org

REBSAMEN MEDICAL CENTER (C, 113 beds) 1400 West Braden Street, Jacksonville, AR Zip 72076–3788; tel. 501/985–7000; Thomas R. Siemers, Chief Executive Officer

SALINE MEMORIAL HOSPITAL (C, 87 beds) 1 Medical Park Drive, Benton, AR Zip 72015–3354; tel. 501/776–6000; Roger D. Feldt, FACHE, President and Chief Executive Officer
Web address: www.scmc.com

SILOAM SPRINGS MEMORIAL HOSPITAL (C, 52 beds) 205 East Jefferson Street, Siloam Springs, AR Zip 72761–3697; tel. 501/524–4141; Roy W. Wright, Chief Executive Officer

CALIFORNIA: SANTA PAULA MEMORIAL HOSPITAL (C, 34 beds) 825 North Tenth Street, Santa Paula, CA Zip 93060–0270, Mailing Address: P.O. Box 270, Zip 93061–0270; tel. 805/525–7171; William M. Greene, FACHE, President and Chief Executive Officer
Web address: www.santapaulamemorial.org

COLORADO: ARKANSAS VALLEY REGIONAL MEDICAL CENTER (C, 182 beds) 1100 Carson Avenue, La Junta, CO Zip 81050–2799; tel. 719/383–6000; Lynn Crowell, Chief Executive Officer

HEART OF THE ROCKIES REGIONAL MEDICAL CENTER (C, 33 beds) 448 East First Street, Salida, CO Zip 81201–0429, Mailing Address: P.O. Box 429, Zip 81201–0429; tel. 719/539–6661; Howard D. Turner, Chief Executive Officer
Web address: www.hrrmc.com

MEMORIAL HOSPITAL (C, 29 beds) 785 Russell Street, Craig, CO Zip 81625–9906; tel. 970/824–9411; M. Randell Phelps, Administrator

MONTROSE MEMORIAL HOSPITAL (C, 62 beds) 800 South Third Street, Montrose, CO Zip 81401–4291; tel. 970/249–2211; Kenneth E. S. Platou, Chief Executive Officer

MT. SAN RAFAEL HOSPITAL (C, 31 beds) 410 Benedicta Avenue, Trinidad, CO Zip 81082–2093; tel. 719/846–9213; Paul L. Herman, Chief Executive Officer

PARKVIEW MEDICAL CENTER (C, 260 beds) 400 West 16th Street, Pueblo, CO Zip 81003–2781; tel. 719/584–4000; C. W. Smith, President and Chief Executive Officer
Web address: www.parkviewmc.com

PIONEERS HOSPITAL OF RIO BLANCO COUNTY (C, 46 beds) 345 Cleveland Street, Meeker, CO Zip 81641–0000; tel. 970/878–5047; Thomas E. Lake, Administrator and Chief Executive Officer

PROWERS MEDICAL CENTER (C, 40 beds) 401 Kendall Drive, Lamar, CO Zip 81052–3993; tel. 719/336–4343; Earl J. Steinhoff, Administrator and Chief Executive Officer
Web address: www.pmchospital.org

SOUTHWEST MEMORIAL HOSPITAL (C, 42 beds) 1311 North Mildred Road, Cortez, CO Zip 81321–2299; tel. 970/565–6666; Robert M. Peterson, President and Chief Executive Officer

VALLEY VIEW HOSPITAL (C, 63 beds) 1906 Blake Avenue, Glenwood Springs, CO Zip 81601–4259, Mailing Address: P.O. Box 1970, Zip 81602–1970; tel. 970/945–6535; Gary L. Brewer, Chief Executive Officer
Web address: www.vvh.org

FLORIDA: BASCOM PALMER EYE INSTITUTE–ANNE BATES LEACH EYE HOSPITAL (C, 35 beds) 900 N.W. 17th Street, Miami, FL Zip 33136–1199, Mailing Address: Box 016880, Zip 33101–6880; tel. 305/326–6000; Richard C. Thomas, Administrator
Web address: www.bpei.med.miami.edu

DESOTO MEMORIAL HOSPITAL (C, 49 beds) 900 North Robert Avenue, Arcadia, FL Zip 34266–8765, Mailing Address: P.O. Box 2180, Zip 34265–2180; tel. 941/494–3535; Edward J. Hannon, President and Chief Executive Officer

HENDRY REGIONAL MEDICAL CENTER (C, 32 beds) 500 West Sugarland Highway, Clewiston, FL Zip 33440–3094; tel. 941/983–9121; Joseph Gonzales, Chief Executive Officer

JACKSON HOSPITAL (C, 84 beds) 4250 Hospital Drive, Marianna, FL Zip 32446–1939, Mailing Address: P.O. Box 1608, Zip 32447–1608; tel. 850/526–2200; John West, Administrator

UNIVERSITY OF MIAMI HOSPITAL AND CLINICS (C, 40 beds) 1475 N.W. 12th Avenue, Miami, FL Zip 33136–1002; tel. 305/243–6418; John Rossfeld, Administrator

GEORGIA: CAMDEN MEDICAL CENTER (C, 40 beds) 2000 Dan Proctor Drive, Saint Marys, GA Zip 31558; tel. 912/576–6200; Alan E. George, Administrator

ELBERT MEMORIAL HOSPITAL (C, 42 beds) 4 Medical Drive, Elberton, GA Zip 30635–1897; tel. 706/283–3151; Mark LeNeave, Chief Executive Officer

HABERSHAM COUNTY MEDICAL CENTER (C, 159 beds) Highway 441, Demorest, GA Zip 30535, Mailing Address: P.O. Box 37, Zip 30535–0037; tel. 706/754–2161; C. Richard Dwozan, President

HIGGINS GENERAL HOSPITAL (C, 36 beds) 200 Allen Memorial Drive, Bremen, GA Zip 30110–2012, Mailing Address: P.O. Box 655, Zip 30110–0655; tel. 770/537–5851; Robbie Smith, Administrator

MCDUFFIE REGIONAL MEDICAL CENTER (C, 35 beds) 521 Hill Street S.W., Thomson, GA Zip 30824–2199; tel. 706/595–1411; Douglas C. Keir, Chief Executive Officer
Web address: www.mcch.org

MEMORIAL HEALTH (C, 373 beds) 4700 Waters Avenue, Savannah, GA Zip 31404–6283, Mailing Address: P.O. Box 23089, Zip 31403–3089; tel. 912/350–8000; Robert A. Colvin, President and Chief Executive Officer
Web address: www.memorialhealth.org

OCONEE REGIONAL MEDICAL CENTER (C, 147 beds) 821 North Cobb Street, Milledgeville, GA Zip 31061–2351, Mailing Address: P.O. Box 690, Zip 31061–0690; tel. 912/454–3500; Brian L. Riddle, President and Chief Executive Officer

SOUTHEAST GEORGIA REGIONAL MEDICAL CENTER (C, 316 beds) 3100 Kemble Avenue, Brunswick, GA Zip 31520–4252, Mailing Address: P.O. Box 1518, Zip 31521–1518; tel. 912/466–7000; E. Berton Whitaker, President and Chief Executive Officer

TANNER MEDICAL CENTER (C, 176 beds) 705 Dixie Street, Carrollton, GA Zip 30117–3818; tel. 770/836–9666; Loy M. Howard, Chief Executive Officer
Web address: www.tanner.org/

TANNER MEDICAL CENTER–VILLA RICA (C, 36 beds) 601 Dallas Road, Villa Rica, GA Zip 30180–1202, Mailing Address: P.O. Box 638, Zip 30180–0638; tel. 770/456–3100; Larry N. Steed, Administrator
Web address: www.tanner.org

UPSON REGIONAL MEDICAL CENTER (C, 115 beds) 801 West Gordon Street, Thomaston, GA Zip 30286–2831, Mailing Address: P.O. Box 1059, Zip 30286–1059; tel. 706/647–8111; Samuel S. Gregory, Administrator

WALTON MEDICAL CENTER (C, 115 beds) 330 Alcovy Street, Monroe, GA Zip 30655–2140, Mailing Address: P.O. Box 1346, Zip 30655–1346; tel. 770/267–8461; Ronald L. Campbell, Chief Executive Officer

For explanation of codes following names, see page B2.
★ Indicates Type III membership in the American Hospital Association.

Systems / Quorum Health Group

WAYNE MEMORIAL HOSPITAL (C, 110 beds) 865 South First Street, Jesup, GA Zip 31598, Mailing Address: P.O. Box 408, Zip 31598–0408; tel. 912/427–6811; Charles R. Morgan, Administrator
Web address: www.wmhweb.com

HAWAII: WAHIAWA GENERAL HOSPITAL (C, 162 beds) 128 Lehua Street, Wahiawa, HI Zip 96786; tel. 808/621–8411; Tyler A. Erickson, Chief Executive Officer

IDAHO: BINGHAM MEMORIAL HOSPITAL (C, 112 beds) 98 Poplar Street, Blackfoot, ID Zip 83221–1799; tel. 208/785–4100; Louis Kraml, Chief Executive Officer
Web address: www.binghammemorial.org

GRITMAN MEDICAL CENTER (C, 35 beds) 700 South Main Street, Moscow, ID Zip 83843–3047; tel. 208/882–4511;
Web address: www.gritman.org

SHOSHONE MEDICAL CENTER (C, 26 beds) 3 Jacobs Gulch, Kellogg, ID Zip 83837–2096; tel. 208/784–1221; Gary Moore, Chief Executive Officer

ILLINOIS: COMMUNITY MEMORIAL HOSPITAL (C, 44 beds) 400 Caldwell Street, Staunton, IL Zip 62088–1499; tel. 618/635–2200; Patrick B. Heise, Chief Executive Officer

CRAWFORD MEMORIAL HOSPITAL (C, 93 beds) 1000 North Allen Street, Robinson, IL Zip 62454; tel. 618/546–1234; Wallace R. Simmons, Chief Executive Officer

GIBSON AREA HOSPITAL AND HEALTH SERVICES (C, 82 beds) 1120 North Melvin Street, Gibson City, IL Zip 60936–1066, Mailing Address: P.O. Box 429, Zip 60936–0429; tel. 217/784–4251; Craig A. Jesiolowski, Chief Executive Officer

MEMORIAL HOSPITAL (C, 59 beds) South Adams Street, Carthage, IL Zip 62321, Mailing Address: P.O. Box 160, Zip 62321–0160; tel. 217/357–3131; Keith E. Heuser, Chief Executive Officer

INDIANA: CAYLOR–NICKEL MEDICAL CENTER (O, 95 beds) One Caylor–Nickel Square, Bluffton, IN Zip 46714–2529; tel. 219/824–3500; William F. Brockmann, President and Chief Executive Officer
Web address: www.caylornickel.com

DAVIESS COUNTY HOSPITAL (C, 85 beds) 1314 East Walnut Street, Washington, IN Zip 47501–2198, Mailing Address: P.O. Box 760, Zip 47501–0760; tel. 812/254–2760; David G. Fuqua, R.N., Chief Executive Officer
Web address: www.dchosp.org

KOSCIUSKO COMMUNITY HOSPITAL (O, 72 beds) 2101 East Dubois Drive, Warsaw, IN Zip 46580–3288; tel. 219/267–3200; Wayne Hendrix, Chief Executive Officer
Web address: www.kch.com

LUTHERAN HOSPITAL OF INDIANA (O, 377 beds) 7950 West Jefferson Boulevard, Fort Wayne, IN Zip 46804–1677; tel. 219/435–7001; Thomas D. Miller, President and Chief Executive Officer
Web address: www.lutheran–hosp.com

ST. JOSEPH HOSPITAL (O, 194 beds) 700 Broadway, Fort Wayne, IN Zip 46802–1493; tel. 219/425–3000; Michael H. Schatzlein, M.D., President and Chief Executive Officer
Web address: www.stjoehospital.com

SULLIVAN COUNTY COMMUNITY HOSPITAL (C, 37 beds) 2200 North Section Street, Sullivan, IN Zip 47882, Mailing Address: P.O. Box 10, Zip 47882–0010; tel. 812/268–4311; Thomas J. Hudgins, Administrator

IOWA: BOONE COUNTY HOSPITAL (C, 57 beds) 1015 Union Street, Boone, IA Zip 50036–4898; tel. 515/432–3140; Joseph S. Smith, Chief Executive Officer
Web address: www.boonehospital.com

FORT MADISON COMMUNITY HOSPITAL (C, 50 beds) 5445 Avenue O, Fort Madison, IA Zip 52627–0174, Mailing Address: P.O. Box 174, Zip 52627–0174; tel. 319/372–6530; C. James Platt, Chief Executive Officer
Web address: www.fmchcares.com

KNOXVILLE AREA COMMUNITY HOSPITAL (C, 52 beds) 1002 South Lincoln Street, Knoxville, IA Zip 50138–3121; tel. 515/842–2151; Jim Murphy, Chief Executive Officer

WASHINGTON COUNTY HOSPITAL (C, 91 beds) 400 East Polk Street, Washington, IA Zip 52353–0909, Mailing Address: P.O. Box 909, Zip 52353–0909; tel. 319/653–5481; Donald E. Patterson, Chief Executive Officer
Web address: www.wchc.org

KANSAS: BOB WILSON MEMORIAL GRANT COUNTY HOSPITAL (C, 30 beds) 415 North Main Street, Ulysses, KS Zip 67880–2133; tel. 316/356–1266; Steven G. Daniel, Administrator
Web address: www.phn.org

COFFEYVILLE REGIONAL MEDICAL CENTER (C, 116 beds) 1400 West Fourth, Coffeyville, KS Zip 67337–0856; tel. 316/251–1200; Gerald J. Marquette, Jr, Chief Executive Officer

NEOSHO MEMORIAL REGIONAL MEDICAL CENTER (C, 60 beds) 629 South Plummer, Chanute, KS Zip 66720–0426, Mailing Address: P.O. Box 426, Zip 66720–0426; tel. 316/431–4000; Murray L. Brown, Administrator

NEWMAN MEMORIAL COUNTY HOSPITAL (C, 110 beds) 1201 West 12th Avenue, Emporia, KS Zip 66801–2597; tel. 316/343–6800; Terry R. Lambert, CHE, Chief Executive Officer
Web address: www.newmanhospital.org

KENTUCKY: CALDWELL COUNTY HOSPITAL (C, 38 beds) 101 Hospital Drive, Princeton, KY Zip 42445–0410, Mailing Address: Box 410, Zip 42445–0410; tel. 270/365–0300; William P. Macri, Chief Executive Officer

CRITTENDEN COUNTY HOSPITAL (C, 67 beds) Highway 60 South, Marion, KY Zip 42064, Mailing Address: P.O. Box 386, Zip 42064–0386; tel. 270/965–5281; Greg Moore, Chief Executive Officer
Web address: www.crittenden–health.org

CUMBERLAND COUNTY HOSPITAL (C, 31 beds) Highway 90 West, Burkesville, KY Zip 42717–0280, Mailing Address: P.O. Box 280, Zip 42717–0280; tel. 270/864–2511; Edward J. Sanford, Chief Executive Officer

FLEMING COUNTY HOSPITAL (C, 43 beds) 920 Elizaville Avenue, Flemingsburg, KY Zip 41041, Mailing Address: P.O. Box 388, Zip 41041–0388; tel. 606/849–5000; Luther E. Reeves, Chief Executive Officer

JENNIE STUART MEDICAL CENTER (C, 139 beds) 320 West 18th Street, Hopkinsville, KY Zip 42241–2400, Mailing Address: P.O. Box 2400, Zip 42241–2400; tel. 270/887–0100; Lewis T. Peeples, Chief Executive Officer
Web address: www.jsmc.org

MARSHALL COUNTY HOSPITAL (C, 80 beds) 503 George McClain Drive, Benton, KY Zip 42025, Mailing Address: P.O. Box 630, Zip 42025–0630; tel. 270/527–4800; Kathy Long, Chief Executive Officer
Web address: www.healthcareonline.org

MONROE COUNTY MEDICAL CENTER (C, 49 beds) 529 Capp Harlan Road, Tompkinsville, KY Zip 42167–1840; tel. 270/487–9231; Mark E. Thompson, Chief Executive Officer

MUHLENBERG COMMUNITY HOSPITAL (C, 135 beds) 440 Hopkinsville Street, Greenville, KY Zip 42345–1172, Mailing Address: P.O. Box 387, Zip 42345–0387; tel. 270/338–8000; Albert Pilkington, II, Chief Executive Officer

OHIO COUNTY HOSPITAL (C, 49 beds) 1211 Main Street, Hartford, KY Zip 42347–1619; tel. 270/298–7411; Blaine Pieper, Administrator
Web address: www.ohiocountyhospital.com

LOUISIANA: BOGALUSA COMMUNITY MEDICAL CENTER (C, 70 beds) 433 Plaza Street, Bogalusa, LA Zip 70427–3793; tel. 504/732–7122; William R. Hatton, Chief Executive Officer and Administrator

FRANKLIN FOUNDATION HOSPITAL (C, 60 beds) 1501 Hospital Avenue, Franklin, LA Zip 70538–3724, Mailing Address: P.O. Box 577, Zip 70538–0577; tel. 318/828–0760; Patricia Luker, Chief Executive Officer
Web address: www.franklinfoundation.org

LANE MEMORIAL HOSPITAL (C, 137 beds) 6300 Main Street, Zachary, LA Zip 70791–9990; tel. 225/658–4000; Terry G. Whittington, Chief Executive Officer and Administrator
Web address: www.lanehospital.org

For explanation of codes following names, see page B2.
★ Indicates Type III membership in the American Hospital Association.

Systems / Quorum Health Group

NORTH OAKS MEDICAL CENTER (C, 215 beds) 15790 Medical Center Drive, Hammond, LA Zip 70403-1436, Mailing Address: P.O. Box 2668, Zip 70404-2668; tel. 504/345-2700; James E. Cathey, Jr, Chief Executive Officer
Web address: www.northoaks.org

OPELOUSAS GENERAL HOSPITAL (C, 134 beds) 539 East Prudhomme Street, Opelousas, LA Zip 70570, Mailing Address: P.O. Box 1208, Zip 70571-1208; tel. 318/948-3011; Daryl J. Doise, Administrator
Web address: www.opelousasgeneral.com

SUMMIT HOSPITAL (O, 183 beds) 17000 Medical Center Drive, Baton Rouge, LA Zip 70816-3224; tel. 225/755-4800; Steve Grimm, CHE, Chief Executive Officer

THIBODAUX REGIONAL MEDICAL CENTER (C, 140 beds) 602 North Acadia Road, Thibodaux, LA Zip 70301-4847, Mailing Address: P.O. Box 1118, Zip 70302-1118; tel. 504/447-5500; Greg K. Stock, Chief Executive Officer
Web address: www.thibodaux.com

MAINE: CALAIS REGIONAL HOSPITAL (C, 57 beds) 50 Franklin Street, Calais, ME Zip 04619-1398; tel. 207/454-7521; Ray H. Davis, Jr, Chief Executive Officer
Web address: www.calaishospital.com

CARY MEDICAL CENTER (C, 55 beds) 163 Van Buren Road, Suite 1, Caribou, ME Zip 04736-2599; tel. 207/498-3111; Kris Doody-Chabre, Chief Executive Officer
Web address: www.carymed.org

DOWN EAST COMMUNITY HOSPITAL (C, 36 beds) Upper Court Street, Machias, ME Zip 04654, Mailing Address: Rural Route 1, Box 11, Zip 04654-9702; tel. 207/255-3356; Philo D. Hall, Chief Executive Officer
Web address: www.nemaine.com

HOULTON REGIONAL HOSPITAL (C, 75 beds) 20 Hartford Street, Houlton, ME Zip 04730-9998; tel. 207/532-9471; Thomas J. Moakler, Chief Executive Officer
Web address: www.houlton.net/hrh

MAINE COAST MEMORIAL HOSPITAL (C, 48 beds) 50 Union Street, Ellsworth, ME Zip 04605-1599; tel. 207/667-5311; Douglas T. Jones, Chief Executive Officer

MAYO REGIONAL HOSPITAL (C, 46 beds) 75 West Main Street, Dover-Foxcroft, ME Zip 04426-1099; tel. 207/564-8401; Ralph Gabarro, Chief Executive Officer
Web address: www.mayohospital.com

MILLINOCKET REGIONAL HOSPITAL (C, 20 beds) 200 Somerset Street, Millinocket, ME Zip 04462-1298; tel. 207/723-5161; Richard Waller, Chief Executive Officer
Web address: www.millinockethospital.com

PENOBSCOT VALLEY HOSPITAL (C, 42 beds) Transalpine Road, Lincoln, ME Zip 04457-0368, Mailing Address: P.O. Box 368, Zip 04457-0368; tel. 207/794-3321; Ronald D. Victory, Administrator

MASSACHUSETTS: HALE HOSPITAL (C, 129 beds) 140 Lincoln Avenue, Haverhill, MA Zip 01830-6798; tel. 978/374-2000; Robert J. Ingala, Chief Executive Officer

HUBBARD REGIONAL HOSPITAL (C, 47 beds) 340 Thompson Road, Webster, MA Zip 01570-0608; tel. 508/943-2600; Gerald J. Barbini, Administrator and Chief Executive Officer
Web address: www.hubbard-hospital.org

MICHIGAN: ALLEGAN GENERAL HOSPITAL (C, 63 beds) 555 Linn Street, Allegan, MI Zip 49010-1594; tel. 616/673-8424; James A. Klun, President
Web address: www.aghosp.org

COMMUNITY HEALTH CENTER OF BRANCH COUNTY (C, 88 beds) 274 East Chicago Street, Coldwater, MI Zip 49036-2088; tel. 517/279-5400; Randy DeGroot, Chief Executive Officer
Web address: www.chcbc.com

COMMUNITY HOSPITAL (C, 56 beds) Medical Park Drive, Watervliet, MI Zip 49098-0158, Mailing Address: P.O. Box 158, Zip 49098-0158; tel. 616/463-3111; David L. McMann, Chief Executive Officer

HAYES-GREEN-BEACH MEMORIAL HOSPITAL (C, 35 beds) 321 East Harris Street, Charlotte, MI Zip 48813-1697; tel. 517/543-1050; Matthew Rush, President
Web address: www.hgbadmin@voyager.net

LAKEVIEW COMMUNITY HOSPITAL (C, 168 beds) 408 Hazen Street, Paw Paw, MI Zip 49079-1019; tel. 616/657-3141; Sue E. Johnson-Phillippe, Chief Executive Officer

MARLETTE COMMUNITY HOSPITAL (C, 91 beds) 2770 Main Street, Marlette, MI Zip 48453-0307, Mailing Address: P.O. Box 307, Zip 48453-0307; tel. 517/635-4000; David S. McEwen, Chief Executive Officer

MECOSTA COUNTY GENERAL HOSPITAL (C, 50 beds) 405 Winter Avenue, Big Rapids, MI Zip 49307-2099; tel. 231/796-8691; Thomas E. Daugherty, Administrator
Web address: www.mecoscountygeneral.com

STURGIS HOSPITAL (C, 67 beds) 916 Myrtle, Sturgis, MI Zip 49091-2001; tel. 616/651-7824; James N. Browne, Interim Chief Executive Officer

THREE RIVERS AREA HOSPITAL (C, 60 beds) 1111 West Broadway, Three Rivers, MI Zip 49093-9362; tel. 616/278-1145; Matthew Chambers, Chief Executive Officer
Web address: www.trah.org

MINNESOTA: FALLS MEMORIAL HOSPITAL (C, 35 beds) 1400 Highway 71, International Falls, MN Zip 56649-2189; tel. 218/283-4481; Mary Klimp, Administrator and Chief Executive Officer

VIRGINIA REGIONAL MEDICAL CENTER (C, 199 beds) 901 Ninth Street North, Virginia, MN Zip 55792-2398; tel. 218/741-3340; Kyle Hopstad, Administrator
Web address: www.vrmc-mn.com

MISSISSIPPI: DELTA REGIONAL MEDICAL CENTER (C, 160 beds) 1400 East Union Street, Greenville, MS Zip 38703-3246, Mailing Address: P.O. Box 5247, Zip 38704-5247; tel. 662/378-3783; Barton A. Hove, Chief Executive Officer

FIELD MEMORIAL COMMUNITY HOSPITAL (C, 66 beds) 270 West Main Street, Centreville, MS Zip 39631, Mailing Address: P.O. Box 639, Zip 39631-0639; tel. 601/645-5221; Brock A. Slabach, Administrator

H. C. WATKINS MEMORIAL HOSPITAL (C, 45 beds) 605 South Archusa Avenue, Quitman, MS Zip 39355-2398; tel. 601/776-6925; Lawrence H. McAvoy, Interim President and Chief Executive Officer

HANCOCK MEDICAL CENTER (C, 104 beds) 149 Drinkwater Boulevard, Bay Saint Louis, MS Zip 39521-2790, Mailing Address: P.O. Box 2790, Zip 39521-2790; tel. 228/467-8600; Hal W. Leftwich, FACHE, Administrator
Web address: www.hmc.org

KING'S DAUGHTERS MEDICAL CENTER (C, 109 beds) 427 Highway 51 North, Brookhaven, MS Zip 39601-2600, Mailing Address: P.O. Box 948, Zip 39602-0948; tel. 662/833-6011; Phillip L. Grady, Chief Executive Officer
Web address: www.kdmc.org

MAGNOLIA REGIONAL HEALTH CENTER (C, 163 beds) 611 Alcorn Drive, Corinth, MS Zip 38834-9368; tel. 662/293-1000; Douglas Garner, Chief Executive Officer

NATCHEZ REGIONAL MEDICAL CENTER (C, 112 beds) Seargent S Prentiss Drive, Natchez, MS Zip 39120, Mailing Address: P.O. Box 1488, Zip 39121-1488; tel. 601/443-2100; Karen A. Fiducia, Interim Chief Executive Officer

NESHOBA COUNTY GENERAL HOSPITAL (C, 166 beds) 1001 Holland Avenue, Philadelphia, MS Zip 39350-2161, Mailing Address: P.O. Box 648, Zip 39350-0648; tel. 601/663-1200; Lawrence Graeber, Administrator

PARKVIEW REGIONAL MEDICAL CENTER (O, 197 beds) 100 McAuley Drive, Vicksburg, MS Zip 39180-2897, Mailing Address: P.O. Box 590, Zip 39181-0590; tel. 601/631-2131; R. Allan Daugherty, Chief Executive Officer

UNIVERSITY HOSPITALS AND CLINICS, UNIVERSITY OF MISSISSIPPI MEDICAL CENTER (C, 613 beds) 2500 North State Street, Jackson, MS Zip 39216-4505; tel. 601/984-1000; Frederick Woodrell, Director

VICKSBURG MEDICAL CENTER (O, 365 beds) 1111 North Frontage Road, Vicksburg, MS Zip 39180; tel. 601/619-3800; Rob Followell, Chief Operating Officer and Administrator

WESLEY MEDICAL CENTER (O, 211 beds) 5001 Hardy Street, Hattiesburg, MS Zip 39402, Mailing Address: P.O. Box 16509, Zip 39404-6509; tel. 601/268-8000; Dan H. Akin, Interim Chief Executive Officer
Web address: www.wesley.com

For explanation of codes following names, see page B2.
★ Indicates Type III membership in the American Hospital Association.

Systems / Quorum Health Group

MISSOURI: NEVADA REGIONAL MEDICAL CENTER (C, 85 beds) 800 South Ash Street, Nevada, MO Zip 64772–3223; tel. 417/667–3355; Robert B. Ohlen, President and Chief Executive Officer
Web address: www.nrmchealth.com

MONTANA: CENTRAL MONTANA MEDICAL CENTER (C, 124 beds) 408 Wendell Avenue, Lewistown, MT Zip 59457–2261; tel. 406/538–7711; David M. Faulkner, Chief Executive Officer

COMMUNITY HOSPITAL OF ANACONDA (C, 92 beds) 401 West Pennsylvania Street, Anaconda, MT Zip 59711–1999; tel. 406/563–8500; Sam J. Allen, Chief Executive Officer

GLACIER COUNTY MEDICAL CENTER (C, 59 beds) 802 Second Street S.E., Cut Bank, MT Zip 59427–3331; tel. 406/873–2251; Dale E. Polla, Chief Executive Officer

NORTH VALLEY HOSPITAL (C, 99 beds) 6575 Highway 93 South, Whitefish, MT Zip 59937; tel. 406/863–3500; Craig E. Aasved, Chief Executive Officer
Web address: www.nvhosp.org

WHEATLAND MEMORIAL HOSPITAL (C, 54 beds) 530 Third Street North, Harlowton, MT Zip 59036, Mailing Address: P.O. Box 287, Zip 59036–0287; tel. 406/632–4351; Craig E. Aasved, Administrator

NEBRASKA: GREAT PLAINS REGIONAL MEDICAL CENTER (C, 99 beds) 601 West Leota Street, North Platte, NE Zip 69101–6598, Mailing Address: P.O. Box 1167, Zip 69103–1167; tel. 308/534–9310; Lucinda A. Bradley, President

PHELPS MEMORIAL HEALTH CENTER (C, 31 beds) 1220 Miller Street, Holdrege, NE Zip 68949–0828, Mailing Address: P.O. Box 828, Zip 68949–0828; tel. 308/995–2211; Walter W. Brownlee, Interim Chief Executive Officer

NEW HAMPSHIRE: LITTLETON REGIONAL HOSPITAL (C, 49 beds) 262 Cottage Street, Littleton, NH Zip 03561–4101; tel. 603/444–7731; Robert S. Pearson, Administrator
Web address: www.littletonhospital.org

NEW MEXICO: CIBOLA GENERAL HOSPITAL (C, 22 beds) 1212 Bonita Avenue, Grants, NM Zip 87020–2104; tel. 505/287–4446; Walter Topp, II, Administrator

GERALD CHAMPION REGIONAL MEDICAL CENTER (C, 73 beds) 2669 North Scenic Drive, Alamogordo, NM Zip 88310; tel. 505/439–2100; Carl W. Mantey, Administrator

GILA REGIONAL MEDICAL CENTER (C, 67 beds) 1313 East 32nd Street, Silver City, NM Zip 88061; tel. 505/538–4000; Polly Pine, Administrator
Web address: www.grmc.org

HOLY CROSS HOSPITAL (C, 34 beds) 1397 Weimer Road, Taos, NM Zip 87571, Mailing Address: P.O. Box DD, Zip 87571; tel. 505/758–8883; Warren K. Spellman, Administrator
Web address: www.hospital@taoshospital.org

NEW YORK: AMSTERDAM MEMORIAL HOSPITAL (C, 242 beds) 4988 State Highway 30, Amsterdam, NY Zip 12010–1699; tel. 518/842–3100; Cornelio R. Catena, President and Chief Executive Officer

AURELIA OSBORN FOX MEMORIAL HOSPITAL (C, 246 beds) 1 Norton Avenue, Oneonta, NY Zip 13820–2697; tel. 607/432–2000; John R. Remillard, President
Web address: www.foxcarenetwork.com

ELLIS HOSPITAL (C, 351 beds) 1101 Nott Street, Schenectady, NY Zip 12308–2487; tel. 518/243–4000; G. B. Serrill, President and Chief Executive Officer
Web address: www.shine.org

NORTH CAROLINA: ALLEGHANY MEMORIAL HOSPITAL (C, 46 beds) 233 Doctors Street, Sparta, NC Zip 28675–0009, Mailing Address: P.O. Box 9, Zip 28675–0009; tel. 336/372–5511; James Yarborough, Chief Executive Officer

ANGEL MEDICAL CENTER (C, 59 beds) Riverview and White Oak Streets, Franklin, NC Zip 28734, Mailing Address: P.O. Box 1209, Zip 28744; tel. 828/524–8411; Michael E. Zuliani, Chief Executive Officer

ASHE MEMORIAL HOSPITAL (C, 115 beds) 200 Hospital Avenue, Jefferson, NC Zip 28640; tel. 336/246–7101; R. D. Williams, Administrator and Chief Executive Officer
Web address: www.ashememorial.org

CHATHAM HOSPITAL (C, 35 beds) West Third Street and Ivy Avenue, Siler City, NC Zip 27344–2343, Mailing Address: P.O. Box 649, Zip 27344; tel. 919/663–2113; Woodrow W. Hathaway, Jr, Chief Executive Officer

COLUMBUS COUNTY HOSPITAL (C, 117 beds) 500 Jefferson Street, Whiteville, NC Zip 28472–9987; tel. 910/642–8011; William S. Clark, Chief Executive Officer
Web address: www.cchospital.com

DISTRICT MEMORIAL HOSPITAL (C, 25 beds) 415 Whitaker Lane, Andrews, NC Zip 28901–9229; tel. 828/321–1291; Allen D. Swan, Chief Executive Officer

GOOD HOPE HOSPITAL (C, 72 beds) 410 Denim Drive, Erwin, NC Zip 28339–0668, Mailing Address: P.O. Box 668, Zip 28339–0668; tel. 910/897–6151; Donald E. Annis, Chief Executive Officer
Web address: www.goodhopehospital.org

GRANVILLE MEDICAL CENTER (C, 146 beds) 1010 College Street, Oxford, NC Zip 27565–2507, Mailing Address: Box 947, Zip 27565–0947; tel. 919/690–3000; Joe W. Pollard, Jr, Chief Executive Officer

HUGH CHATHAM MEMORIAL HOSPITAL (C, 201 beds) Parkwood Drive, Elkin, NC Zip 28621–0560, Mailing Address: P.O. Box 560, Zip 28621–0560; tel. 336/527–7000; Richard D. Osmus, Chief Executive Officer
Web address: www.hughchatham.org

JOHNSTON MEMORIAL HOSPITAL (C, 127 beds) 509 North Bright Leaf Boulevard, Smithfield, NC Zip 27577–1376, Mailing Address: P.O. Box 1376, Zip 27577–1376; tel. 919/934–8171; Leland E. Farnell, President
Web address: www.vipmedia.com

MOREHEAD MEMORIAL HOSPITAL (C, 236 beds) 117 East King's Highway, Eden, NC Zip 27288–5299; tel. 336/623–9711; Robert Enders, President
Web address: www.morehead.org

NORTHERN HOSPITAL OF SURRY COUNTY (C, 103 beds) 830 Rockford Street, Mount Airy, NC Zip 27030–5365, Mailing Address: P.O. Box 1101, Zip 27030–1101; tel. 336/719–7000; William B. James, Chief Executive Officer
Web address: www.nhsc.org

RUTHERFORD HOSPITAL (C, 261 beds) 288 South Ridgecrest Avenue, Rutherfordton, NC Zip 28139–3097; tel. 828/286–5000; Robert D. Jones, President
Web address: www.rutherfordhosp.org

NORTH DAKOTA: KENMARE COMMUNITY HOSPITAL (O, 42 beds) 317 First Avenue N.W., Kenmare, ND Zip 58746–7104, Mailing Address: P.O. Box 697, Zip 58746–0697; tel. 701/385–4296; Jared Ferguson, Administrator and Chief Executive Officer

UNIMED MEDICAL CENTER (O, 160 beds) 407 3rd Street S.E., Minot, ND Zip 58702–5001; tel. 701/857–2000; Michael L. Mullins, Chief Executive Officer
Web address: www.unimedmedical.com

OHIO: BARBERTON CITIZENS HOSPITAL (O, 255 beds) 155 Fifth Street N.E., Barberton, OH Zip 44203–3398; tel. 330/745–1611; Ronald J. Elder, Chief Executive Officer
Web address: www.barbhosp.com

BROWN COUNTY GENERAL HOSPITAL (C, 53 beds) 425 Home Street, Georgetown, OH Zip 45121–1407; tel. 937/378–6121; David T. Wallace, President and Chief Executive Officer
Web address: www.bcgh.org

DOCTORS HOSPITAL OF STARK COUNTY (O, 110 beds) 400 Austin Avenue N.W., Massillon, OH Zip 44646–3554; tel. 330/837–7200; Thomas E. Cecconi, Chief Executive Officer
Web address: www.drshospital.com

FAYETTE COUNTY MEMORIAL HOSPITAL (C, 35 beds) 1430 Columbus Avenue, Washington Court House, OH Zip 43160–1791; tel. 740/335–1210; Francis G. Albarano, Administrator
Web address: www.fcmh.org

KNOX COMMUNITY HOSPITAL (C, 75 beds) 1330 Coshocton Road, Mount Vernon, OH Zip 43050–1495; tel. 740/393–9000; Robert G. Polahar, Chief Executive Officer

MEMORIAL HOSPITAL (C, 121 beds) 715 South Taft Avenue, Fremont, OH Zip 43420–3200; tel. 419/332–7321; John A. Gorman, Chief Executive Officer
Web address: www.fremontmemorial.org

For explanation of codes following names, see page B2.
★ Indicates Type III membership in the American Hospital Association.

Systems / Quorum Health Group

SELBY GENERAL HOSPITAL (C, 54 beds) 1106 Colegate Drive, Marietta, OH Zip 45750–1323; tel. 740/373–0582; Maryann J. Greenwell, Chief Executive Officer
Web address: www.selby.wscc.edu

WOOSTER COMMUNITY HOSPITAL (C, 90 beds) 1761 Beall Avenue, Wooster, OH Zip 44691–2342; tel. 330/263–8100; William E. Sheron, Chief Executive Officer

OKLAHOMA: CHOCTAW MEMORIAL HOSPITAL (C, 34 beds) 1405 East Kirk Road, Hugo, OK Zip 74743–3603; tel. 580/326–6414; Emmett C. Schuster, Chief Executive Officer and Administrator

CUSHING REGIONAL HOSPITAL (L, 75 beds) 1027 East Cherry Street, Cushing, OK Zip 74023–4101, Mailing Address: P.O. Box 1409, Zip 74023–1409; tel. 918/225–2915; Ron Cackler, President and Chief Executive Officer

HENRYETTA MEDICAL CENTER (L, 28 beds) Dewey Bartlett and Main Streets, Henryetta, OK Zip 74437, Mailing Address: P.O. Box 1269, Zip 74437–1269; tel. 918/652–4463; James P. Bailey, President and Chief Executive Officer

HOLDENVILLE GENERAL HOSPITAL (C, 22 beds) 100 McDougal Drive, Holdenville, OK Zip 74848–9700; tel. 405/379–6631; Shawn Morrow, Chief Executive Officer and Administrator

KINGFISHER REGIONAL HOSPITAL (C, 27 beds) 500 South Ninth Street, Kingfisher, OK Zip 73750–3528, Mailing Address: P.O. Box 59, Zip 73750–0059; tel. 405/375–3141; Daryle Voss, Chief Executive Officer
Web address: www.kingfisherhospital.com

LOGAN HOSPITAL AND MEDICAL CENTER (C, 32 beds) Highway 33 West at Academy Road, Guthrie, OK Zip 73044, Mailing Address: P.O. Box 1017, Zip 73044–1017; tel. 405/282–6700; Judith K. Feuquay, Chief Executive Officer

MCCURTAIN MEMORIAL HOSPITAL (C, 81 beds) 1301 Lincoln Road, Idabel, OK Zip 74745–7341; tel. 580/286–7623; Claude E. Camp , II, Chief Executive Officer

PERRY MEMORIAL HOSPITAL (C, 28 beds) 501 14th Street, Perry, OK Zip 73077–5099; tel. 580/336–3541; Joe Duerr, Chief Executive Officer

PURCELL MUNICIPAL HOSPITAL (C, 22 beds) 1500 North Green Avenue, Purcell, OK Zip 73080–1699, Mailing Address: P.O. Box 511, Zip 73080–0511; tel. 405/527–6524; Curtis R. Pryor, Administrator

SAYRE MEMORIAL HOSPITAL (C, 46 beds) 501 East Washington Street, Sayre, OK Zip 73662, Mailing Address: P.O. Box 680, Zip 73662; tel. 580/928–5541; Larry Anderson, Administrator

SHARE MEDICAL CENTER (C, 117 beds) 800 Share Drive, Alva, OK Zip 73717–3699, Mailing Address: P.O. Box 727, Zip 73717–0727; tel. 580/327–2800; Barbara Oestmann, Chief Executive Officer

WATONGA MUNICIPAL HOSPITAL (C, 24 beds) 500 North Nash Boulevard, Watonga, OK Zip 73772–0370, Mailing Address: Box 370, Zip 73772–0370; tel. 580/623–7211; David R. Jordan, Ph.D., Chief Executive Officer
Web address: www.watongahospital.com

WOODWARD HOSPITAL AND HEALTH CENTER (C, 68 beds) 900 17th Street, Woodward, OK Zip 73801–2423; tel. 580/256–5511; Joel A. Hart, Chief Executive Officer

PENNSYLVANIA: BROWNSVILLE GENERAL HOSPITAL (C, 115 beds) 125 Simpson Road, Brownsville, PA Zip 15417–9699; tel. 724/785–7200; Richard D. Constantine, Chief Executive Officer
Web address: www.bghlink.com

CARLISLE HOSPITAL AND HEALTH SERVICES (C, 110 beds) 246 Parker Street, Carlisle, PA Zip 17013–3618; tel. 717/249–1212; Michael J. Halstead, President and Chief Executive Officer
Web address: www.chhs.org

CLARION HOSPITAL (C, 77 beds) One Hospital Drive, Clarion, PA Zip 16214–8599; tel. 814/226–9500; Donald D. Evans, President and Chief Executive Officer
Web address: www.clarionhospital.org

GREENE COUNTY MEMORIAL HOSPITAL (C, 65 beds) Seventh Street and Bonar Avenue, Waynesburg, PA Zip 15370–1697; tel. 724/627–3101; Raoul Walsh, Chief Executive Officer

J. C. BLAIR MEMORIAL HOSPITAL (C, 104 beds) 1225 Warm Springs Avenue, Huntingdon, PA Zip 16652–2398; tel. 814/643–2290; Richard E. D'Alberto, Chief Executive Officer
Web address: www.JCBlair.Org

JERSEY SHORE HOSPITAL (C, 49 beds) 1020 Thompson Street, Jersey Shore, PA Zip 17740–1794; tel. 570/398–0100; Louis A. Ditzel , Jr, President and Chief Executive Officer

LOCK HAVEN HOSPITAL (C, 195 beds) 24 Cree Drive, Lock Haven, PA Zip 17745–2699; tel. 570/893–5000; Gary R. Rhoads, President and Chief Executive Officer

MEMORIAL HOSPITAL (C, 93 beds) One Hospital Drive, Towanda, PA Zip 18848–9702; tel. 570/265–2191; Gary A. Baker, President
Web address: www.memorialhospital.org

OHIO VALLEY GENERAL HOSPITAL (C, 118 beds) 25 Heckel Road, McKees Rocks, PA Zip 15136–1694; tel. 412/777–6161; William F. Provenzano, President

POTTSVILLE HOSPITAL AND WARNE CLINIC (C, 197 beds) 420 South Jackson Street, Pottsville, PA Zip 17901–3692; tel. 570/621–5000; Donald R. Gintzig, President and Chief Executive Officer
Web address: www.pottsville.com/hospital

TYRONE HOSPITAL (C, 59 beds) One Hospital Drive, Tyrone, PA Zip 16686–1810; tel. 814/684–1255; Thomas G. Bartlett , II, Chief Executive Officer

SOUTH CAROLINA: ABBEVILLE COUNTY MEMORIAL HOSPITAL (C, 60 beds) 901 West Greenwood Street, Abbeville, SC Zip 29620–0887, Mailing Address: P.O. Box 887, Zip 29620–0887; tel. 864/459–5011; Alvin Hoover, CHE, Administrator

CAROLINAS HOSPITAL SYSTEM (O, 320 beds) 805 Pamplico Highway, Florence, SC Zip 29505, Mailing Address: P.O. Box 100550, Zip 29501–0550; tel. 843/674–5000; David A. McClellan, Chief Executive Officer
Web address: www.carolinashospital.com

CAROLINAS HOSPITAL SYSTEM–KINGSTREE (O, 47 beds) 500 Nelson Boulevard, Kingstree, SC Zip 29556–4027, Mailing Address: P.O. Drawer 568, Zip 29556–0568; tel. 843/354–9661; Clarence W. Bowman, Chief Executive Officer
Web address: www.carolinashospital.com

CAROLINAS HOSPITAL SYSTEM–LAKE CITY (O, 40 beds) 258 North Ron McNair Boulevard, Lake City, SC Zip 29560–1029, Mailing Address: P.O. Box 1029, Zip 29560–1029; tel. 843/394–2036; Clarence W. Bowman, Chief Executive Officer

GEORGETOWN MEMORIAL HOSPITAL (C, 141 beds) 606 Black River Road, Georgetown, SC Zip 29440–3368, Mailing Address: Drawer 1718, Zip 29442–1718; tel. 843/527–7000; Paul D. Gatens , Sr, Administrator
Web address: www.gmhsc.com

LAURENS COUNTY HEALTHCARE SYSTEM (C, 85 beds) Highway 76 West, Clinton, SC Zip 29325, Mailing Address: P.O. Box 976, Zip 29325–0976; tel. 864/833–9100; Michael A. Kozar, Chief Executive Officer
Web address: www.lchcs.org

MARY BLACK HEALTH SYSTEM (O, 212 beds) 1700 Skylyn Drive, Spartanburg, SC Zip 29307–1061, Mailing Address: P.O. Box 3217, Zip 29304–3217; tel. 864/573–3000; William W. Fox, Chief Executive Officer

NEWBERRY COUNTY MEMORIAL HOSPITAL (C, 77 beds) 2669 Kinard Street, Newberry, SC Zip 29108–0497, Mailing Address: P.O. Box 497, Zip 29108–0497; tel. 803/276–7570; Lynn W. Beasley, President and Chief Executive Officer

REGIONAL MEDICAL CENTER OF ORANGEBURG AND CALHOUN COUNTIES (C, 295 beds) 3000 St. Matthews Road, Orangeburg, SC Zip 29118–1470; tel. 803/533–2200; Thomas C. Dandridge, President
Web address: www.regmed.com

TUOMEY HEALTHCARE SYSTEM (C, 251 beds) 129 North Washington Street, Sumter, SC Zip 29150–4983; tel. 803/778–9000; Jay Cox, President and Chief Executive Officer
Web address: www.tuomey.com

WALLACE THOMSON HOSPITAL (C, 220 beds) 322 West South Street, Union, SC Zip 29379–2857, Mailing Address: P.O. Box 789, Zip 29379–0789; tel. 864/429–2600; Harrell L. Connelly, Chief Executive Officer
Web address: www.wallacethomson.com/index.htm/default.htm

SOUTH DAKOTA: HURON REGIONAL MEDICAL CENTER (C, 61 beds) 172 Fourth Street S.E., Huron, SD Zip 57350–2590; tel. 605/353–6200; John L. Single, Chief Executive Officer

For explanation of codes following names, see page B2.
★ Indicates Type III membership in the American Hospital Association.

Systems / Quorum Health Group

TENNESSEE: BEDFORD COUNTY MEDICAL CENTER (C, 180 beds) 845 Union Street, Shelbyville, TN Zip 37160–9971; tel. 931/685–5433; David M. Snyder, Chief Executive Officer

LINCOLN COUNTY HEALTH FACILITIES (C, 51 beds) 700 West Maple Street, Fayetteville, TN Zip 37334–3202; tel. 931/438–1111; Gary G. Kendrick, Chief Executive Officer

MACON COUNTY GENERAL HOSPITAL (C, 43 beds) 204 Medical Drive, Lafayette, TN Zip 37083–1799, Mailing Address: P.O. Box 378, Zip 37083–0378; tel. 615/666–2147; Dennis A. Wolford, FACHE, Administrator

RHEA MEDICAL CENTER (C, 131 beds) 7900 Rhea County Highway, Dayton, TN Zip 37321–5912; tel. 423/775–1121; Kennedy L. Croom, Jr, Administrator and Chief Executive Officer

TEXAS: ABILENE REGIONAL MEDICAL CENTER (O, 187 beds) 6250 Highway 83–84 at Antilley Road, Abilene, TX Zip 79606–5299; tel. 915/695–9900; Mary T. Brasseaux, Chief Executive Officer
Web address: www.abilene.com/armc

BRAZOSPORT MEMORIAL HOSPITAL (C, 156 beds) 100 Medical Drive, Lake Jackson, TX Zip 77566–9983; tel. 979/297–4411; Wesley W. Oswald, Chief Executive Officer
Web address: www.brazosportmemorial.com

CAMPBELL HEALTH SYSTEM (C, 67 beds) 713 East Anderson Street, Weatherford, TX Zip 76086–9971; tel. 817/596–8751; John B. Millstead, Chief Executive Officer

DALLAS–FORT WORTH MEDICAL CENTER (C, 147 beds) 2709 Hospital Boulevard, Grand Prairie, TX Zip 75051–1083; tel. 972/641–5000; Robert A. Ficken, Chief Executive Officer
Web address: www.dfwmedicalcenter.com

HENDERSON MEMORIAL HOSPITAL (C, 96 beds) 300 Wilson Street, Henderson, TX Zip 75652–5956; tel. 903/657–7541; George T. Roberts, Jr, FACHE, Chief Executive Officer

HUNTSVILLE MEMORIAL HOSPITAL (C, 104 beds) 485 I–45 South, Huntsville, TX Zip 77340–4362, Mailing Address: P.O. Box 4001, Zip 77342–4001; tel. 409/291–3411; Ralph E. Beaty, Administrator
Web address: www.huntsvillememorial.com

MISSION HOSPITAL (C, 138 beds) 900 South Bryan Road, Mission, TX Zip 78572–6613; tel. 956/580–9000; Paul H. Ballard, Chief Executive Officer
Web address: www.missionhosp.com

TITUS REGIONAL MEDICAL CENTER (C, 165 beds) 2001 North Jefferson Avenue, Mount Pleasant, TX Zip 75455–2398; tel. 903/577–6000; Steven K. Jacobson, Chief Executive Officer

VERMONT: NORTHEASTERN VERMONT REGIONAL HOSPITAL (C, 49 beds) Hospital Drive, Saint Johnsbury, VT Zip 05819–9962, Mailing Address: P.O. Box 905, Zip 05819–9962; tel. 802/748–8141; Paul R. Bengtson, Chief Executive Officer

NORTHWESTERN MEDICAL CENTER (C, 53 beds) 131 Fairfield Street, Saint Albans, VT Zip 05478–1734, Mailing Address: P.O. Box 1370, Zip 05478–1370; tel. 802/524–5911; Peter A. Hofstetter, Chief Executive Officer
Web address: www.nmcinc.org

VIRGINIA: BUCHANAN GENERAL HOSPITAL (C, 144 beds) Grundy, VA Mailing Address: Route 5, Box 20, Zip 24614–9611; tel. 540/935–1000; Randy Brown, Interim Administrator

HALIFAX REGIONAL HEALTH SYSTEM (C, 138 beds) 2204 Wilborn Avenue, South Boston, VA Zip 24592–1638; tel. 804/517–3100; Chris A. Lumsden, Chief Executive Officer
Web address: www.hrhs.org

MEMORIAL HOSPITAL OF MARTINSVILLE AND HENRY COUNTY (C, 152 beds) 320 Hospital Drive, Martinsville, VA Zip 24112–1981, Mailing Address: Box 4788, Zip 24115–4788; tel. 540/666–7200; Joseph Roach, Chief Executive Officer
Web address: www.martinsvillehospital.org

RICHMOND EYE AND EAR HOSPITAL (C, 32 beds) 1001 East Marshall Street, Richmond, VA Zip 23219–1993; tel. 804/775–4500; James W. Worrell, Chief Executive Officer

SOUTHSIDE REGIONAL MEDICAL CENTER (C, 292 beds) 801 South Adams Street, Petersburg, VA Zip 23803–5133; tel. 804/862–5000; David S. Dunham, President
Web address: www.srmconline.com

WASHINGTON: KADLEC MEDICAL CENTER (C, 124 beds) 888 Swift Boulevard, Richland, WA Zip 99352–3542; tel. 509/946–4611; Marcel Loh, President and Chief Executive Officer
Web address: www.kadlecmed.com

WEST VIRGINIA: FAIRMONT GENERAL HOSPITAL (C, 181 beds) 1325 Locust Avenue, Fairmont, WV Zip 26554–1435; tel. 304/367–7100; Richard W. Graham, FACHE, President and Chief Executive Officer
Web address: www.fghi.com

PRESTON MEMORIAL HOSPITAL (C, 56 beds) 300 South Price Street, Kingwood, WV Zip 26537–1495; tel. 304/329–1400; Charles Lonchar, President and Chief Executive Officer

WISCONSIN: AMERY REGIONAL MEDICAL CENTER (C, 15 beds) 225 Scholl Court, Amery, WI Zip 54001–1292; tel. 715/268–8000; Michael Karuschak, Jr, Chief Executive Officer

RIVERSIDE MEDICAL CENTER (C, 32 beds) 800 Riverside Drive, Waupaca, WI Zip 54981–1999; tel. 715/258–1000; Craig A. Kantos, Chief Executive Officer
Web address: www.riversidemedical.org

WYOMING: WEST PARK HOSPITAL (C, 122 beds) 707 Sheridan Avenue, Cody, WY Zip 82414; tel. 307/527–7501; Douglas A. McMillan, Administrator and Chief Executive Officer
Web address: www.westparkhospital.org

Owned, leased, sponsored:	24 hospitals	4037 beds
Contract–managed:	194 hospitals	19178 beds
Totals:	218 hospitals	23215 beds

0405: RAMSAY YOUTH SERVICES (IO)
1 Alhambra Plaza, Suite 750, Coral Gables, FL Zip 33134–5217; tel. 305/569–6993; Bert Cibran, President and Chief Operating Officer
(Independent Hospital System)

ALABAMA: HILL CREST BEHAVIORAL HEALTH SERVICES (O, 119 beds) 6869 Fifth Avenue South, Birmingham, AL Zip 35212–1866; tel. 205/833–9000; Steve McCabe, Chief Executive Officer

FLORIDA: GULF COAST TREATMENT CENTER (O, 79 beds) 1015 Mar–Walt Drive, Fort Walton Beach, FL Zip 32547–6612; tel. 850/863–4160; Raul D. Ruelas, M.D., Administrator

MICHIGAN: HAVENWYCK HOSPITAL (O, 150 beds) 1525 University Drive, Auburn Hills, MI Zip 48326–2675; tel. 248/373–9200; Robert A. Kercorian, Chief Executive Officer

MISSOURI: HEARTLAND BEHAVIORAL HEALTH SERVICES (O, 30 beds) 1500 West Ashland Street, Nevada, MO Zip 64772–1710; tel. 417/667–2666; David Morrison, Chief Executive Officer
Web address: www.hardtoplacekids.com

NORTH CAROLINA: BRYNN MARR BEHAVIORAL HEALTHCARE SYSTEM (O, 76 beds) 192 Village Drive, Jacksonville, NC Zip 28546–7299; tel. 910/577–1400; Dale Armstrong, Chief Executive Officer

TEXAS: MISSION VISTA BEHAVIORAL HEALTH SYSTEM (L, 16 beds) 14747 Jones Maltsberger, San Antonio, TX Zip 78247–3713; tel. 210/490–0000; Holly Minnis, Chief Executive Officer

UTAH: BENCHMARK BEHAVIORAL HEALTH SYSTEMS (O, 68 beds) 592 West 1350 South, Woods Cross, UT Zip 84087–1665; tel. 801/299–5300; Richard O. Hurt, Ph.D., Chief Executive Officer

Owned, leased, sponsored:	7 hospitals	538 beds
Contract–managed:	0 hospitals	0 beds
Totals:	7 hospitals	538 beds

0171: RESURRECTION HEALTH CARE CORPORATION (CC)
7435 West Talcott Avenue, Chicago, IL Zip 60631; tel. 773/792–5150; Joseph F. Toomey, President and Chief Executive Officer
(Moderately Centralized Health System)

For explanation of codes following names, see page B2.
★ Indicates Type III membership in the American Hospital Association.

ILLINOIS: OUR LADY OF THE RESURRECTION MEDICAL CENTER (O, 282 beds) 5645 West Addison Street, Chicago, IL Zip 60634–4455; tel. 773/282–7000; Ronald E. Struxness, Executive Vice President and Chief Executive Officer
Web address: www.reshealthcare.org

RESURRECTION MEDICAL CENTER (O, 667 beds) 7435 West Talcott Avenue, Chicago, IL Zip 60631–3746; tel. 773/774–8000; Sister Donna Marie, Executive Vice President and Chief Executive Officer
Web address: www.reshealthcare.org

ST. FRANCIS HOSPITAL (O, 325 beds) 355 Ridge Avenue, Evanston, IL Zip 60202–3399; tel. 847/316–4000; Kenneth W. Wood, Chief Executive Officer

WESTLAKE HOSPITAL (O, 247 beds) 1225 Lake Street, Melrose Park, IL Zip 60160–4000; tel. 708/681–3000; Patricia Shehorn, Chief Executive Officer

Owned, leased, sponsored:	4 hospitals	1521 beds
Contract–managed:	0 hospitals	0 beds
Totals:	4 hospitals	1521 beds

4810: RIVERSIDE HEALTH SYSTEM (NP)
606 Denbigh Boulevard, Suite 601, Newport News, VA Zip 23608; tel. 757/875–7500; Richard J. Pearce, President and Chief Operating Officer
(Centralized Health System)

VIRGINIA: RIVERSIDE REGIONAL MEDICAL CENTER (O, 360 beds) 500 J. Clyde Morris Boulevard, Newport News, VA Zip 23601–1976; tel. 757/594–2000; M. Caroline Martin, President
Web address: www.riverside–online.com

RIVERSIDE TAPPAHANNOCK HOSPITAL (O, 44 beds) 618 Hospital Road, Tappahannock, VA Zip 22560; tel. 804/443–3311; Elizabeth J. Martin, Vice President and Administrator
Web address: www.riverside–online.com

RIVERSIDE WALTER REED HOSPITAL (O, 71 beds) 7519 Hospital Drive, Gloucester, VA Zip 23061–4178, Mailing Address: P.O. Box 1130, Zip 23061–1130; tel. 804/693–8800; Grady W. Philips , II, Vice President and Administrator
Web address: www.riverside–online.com

Owned, leased, sponsored:	3 hospitals	475 beds
Contract–managed:	0 hospitals	0 beds
Totals:	3 hospitals	475 beds

★0109: RURAL HEALTH MANAGEMENT CORPORATION (NP)
549 North 400 East, Nephi, UT Zip 84648–1226; tel. 435/623–4924; Mark R. Stoddard, President
(Independent Hospital System)

UTAH: ALLEN MEMORIAL HOSPITAL (L, 38 beds) 719 West 400 North Street, Moab, UT Zip 84532–2297, Mailing Address: P.O. Box 998, Zip 84532–0998; tel. 435/259–7191; Charles A. Davis, Administrator and Chief Executive Officer

CENTRAL VALLEY MEDICAL CENTER (L, 20 beds) 549 North 400 East, Nephi, UT Zip 84648–1226; tel. 435/623–1242; Mark R. Stoddard, President

GUNNISON VALLEY HOSPITAL (C, 20 beds) 64 East 100 North, Gunnison, UT Zip 84634, Mailing Address: P.O. Box 759, Zip 84634–0759; tel. 435/528–7246; Greg Rosenvall, Administrator

MILFORD VALLEY MEMORIAL HOSPITAL (C, 34 beds) 451 North Main Street, Milford, UT Zip 84751–0640, Mailing Address: P.O. Box 640, Zip 84751–0640; tel. 435/387–2411; John E. Gledhill, Administrator

Owned, leased, sponsored:	2 hospitals	58 beds
Contract–managed:	2 hospitals	54 beds
Totals:	4 hospitals	112 beds

0220: RUSH HEALTH SYSTEMS (NP)
1314 19th Avenue, Meridian, MS Zip 39301; tel. 601/483–0011; Wallace Strickland, President and Chief Executive Officer

MISSISSIPPI: RUSH FOUNDATION HOSPITAL (O, 195 beds) 1314 19th Avenue, Meridian, MS Zip 39301–4195; tel. 601/483–0011; Dan M. Harrison, Executive Vice President and Administrator

SPECIALTY HOSPITAL OF MERIDIAN (O, 40 beds) 1314 19th Avenue, Meridian, MS Zip 39301; tel. 601/486–4211; Annette V. Drennan, R.N., President

Owned, leased, sponsored:	2 hospitals	235 beds
Contract–managed:	0 hospitals	0 beds
Totals:	2 hospitals	235 beds

★3855: RUSH–PRESBYTERIAN–ST. LUKE'S MEDICAL CENTER (NP)
1653 West Congress Parkway, Chicago, IL Zip 60612–3864; tel. 312/942–5000; Leo M. Henikoff, M.D., President
(Centralized Physician/Insurance Health System)

ILLINOIS: RUSH NORTH SHORE MEDICAL CENTER (O, 226 beds) 9600 Gross Point Road, Skokie, IL Zip 60076–1257; tel. 847/677–9600; John S. Frigo, President
Web address: www.rush.edu

RUSH–COPLEY MEDICAL CENTER (O, 142 beds) 2000 Ogden Avenue, Aurora, IL Zip 60504–4206; tel. 630/978–6200; Martin Losoff, President and Chief Executive Officer
Web address: www.rushcopley.com

RUSH–PRESBYTERIAN–ST. LUKE'S MEDICAL CENTER (O, 713 beds) 1653 West Congress Parkway, Chicago, IL Zip 60612–3833; tel. 312/942–5000; Leo M. Henikoff, M.D., President and Chief Executive Officer
Web address: www.rush.edu

Owned, leased, sponsored:	3 hospitals	1081 beds
Contract–managed:	0 hospitals	0 beds
Totals:	3 hospitals	1081 beds

★0118: SAINT BARNABAS HEALTH CARE SYSTEM (NP)
95 Old Short Hills Road, West Orange, NJ Zip 07052; tel. 973/322–4001; Ronald J. Del Mauro, President and Chief Executive Officer
(Moderately Centralized Health System)

NEW JERSEY: CLARA MAASS HEALTH SYSTEM (O, 644 beds) 1 Clara Maass Drive, Belleville, NJ Zip 07109–3557; tel. 973/450–2000; Thomas A. Biga, Executive Director
Web address: www.sbhcs.com

COMMUNITY MEDICAL CENTER (O, 465 beds) 99 Route 37 West, Toms River, NJ Zip 08755–6423; tel. 732/557–8000; Nancy L. Wollen, Executive Director
Web address: www.sbhcs.com

IRVINGTON GENERAL HOSPITAL (O, 157 beds) 832 Chancellor Avenue, Irvington, NJ Zip 07111–0709; tel. 973/399–6000; Amit Mody, M.D., Executive Director
Web address: www.sbhcs.com

KIMBALL MEDICAL CENTER (O, 300 beds) 600 River Avenue, Lakewood, NJ Zip 08701–5281; tel. 732/363–1900; Joanne Carrocino, Executive Director
Web address: www.sbhcs.com

MONMOUTH MEDICAL CENTER (O, 435 beds) 300 Second Avenue, Long Branch, NJ Zip 07740–6303; tel. 732/222–5200; Frank J. Vozos, M.D., FACS, Executive Director
Web address: www.sbhcs.com

NEWARK BETH ISRAEL MEDICAL CENTER (O, 532 beds) 201 Lyons Avenue, Newark, NJ Zip 07112–2027; tel. 973/926–7000; Paul A. Mertz, Executive Director
Web address: www.saintbarnabas.com

SAINT BARNABAS MEDICAL CENTER (O, 581 beds) 94 Old Short Hills Road, Livingston, NJ Zip 07039–5668; tel. 973/322–5000; Vincent D. Joseph, Executive Director
Web address: www.sbhcs.com

UNION HOSPITAL (O, 148 beds) 1000 Galloping Hill Road, Union, NJ Zip 07083–1652; tel. 908/687–1900; Kathryn W. Coyne, Executive Director
Web address: www.sbhcs.com

For explanation of codes following names, see page B2.
★ Indicates Type III membership in the American Hospital Association.

Systems / Saint Barnabas Health Care System

WAYNE GENERAL HOSPITAL (O, 146 beds) 224 Hamburg Turnpike, Wayne, NJ Zip 07470–2100; tel. 973/942–6900; Geraldine Di Risic, Acting Executive Director
Web address: www.sbhcs.com

WEST HUDSON HOSPITAL (O, 217 beds) 206 Bergen Avenue, Kearny, NJ Zip 07032–3399; tel. 201/955–7051; Carmen Bruce Alecci, Executive Director
Web address: www.sbhcs.com

Owned, leased, sponsored:	10 hospitals	3625 beds
Contract–managed:	0 hospitals	0 beds
Totals:	10 hospitals	3625 beds

0120: SAINT LUKE'S SHAWNEE MISSION HEALTH SYSTEM (NP)
10920 Elm Avenue, Kansas City, MO Zip 64134–4108; tel. 816/932–3377; G. Richard Hastings, President and Chief Executive Officer
(Centralized Health System)

KANSAS: ANDERSON COUNTY HOSPITAL (O, 57 beds) 421 South Maple, Garnett, KS Zip 66032–1334, Mailing Address: P.O. Box 309, Zip 66032–0309; tel. 785/448–3131; Dennis A. Hachenberg, CHE, Chief Executive Officer

SAINT LUKE'S SOUTH HOSPITAL (O, 342 beds) 12300 Metcalf Avenue, Overland Park, KS Zip 66213; tel. 913/317–7000; William G. Robertson, Chief Executive Officer

SHAWNEE MISSION MEDICAL CENTER (O, 333 beds) 9100 West 74th Street, Shawnee Mission, KS Zip 66204–4004, Mailing Address: Box 2923, Zip 66201–1323; tel. 913/676–2000; William G. Robertson, Chief Executive Officer

MISSOURI: CRITTENTON (O, 127 beds) 10918 Elm Avenue, Kansas City, MO Zip 64134–4199; tel. 816/765–6600; Gary L. Watson, FACHE, Senior Executive Officer
Web address: www.saint–lukes.org

SAINT LUKE'S HOSPITAL (O, 510 beds) 4401 Wornall Road, Kansas City, MO Zip 64111–3238; tel. 816/932–2000; G. Richard Hastings, President and Chief Executive Officer
Web address: www.saint–lukes.org

SAINT LUKE'S NORTHLAND HOSPITAL (O, 63 beds) 5830 N.W. Barry Road, Kansas City, MO Zip 64154; tel. 816/891–6000; N. Gary Wages, President and Chief Executive Officer
Web address: www.saint–lukes.org

SAINT LUKE'S NORTHLAND HOSPITAL–SMITHVILLE CAMPUS (O, 59 beds) 601 South 169 Highway, Smithville, MO Zip 64089–9334; tel. 816/532–3700; Don Sipes, Chief Executive Officer
Web address: www.saint–lukes.org

WRIGHT MEMORIAL HOSPITAL (O, 34 beds) 701 East First Street, Trenton, MO Zip 64683–0648, Mailing Address: P.O. Box 628, Zip 64683–0628; tel. 660/359–5621; Ralph G. Goodrich, Chief Executive Officer
Web address: www.saint–lukes.org

Owned, leased, sponsored:	8 hospitals	1525 beds
Contract–managed:	0 hospitals	0 beds
Totals:	8 hospitals	1525 beds

0186: SAMARITAN HEALTH SERVICES (NP)
3600 N.W. Samaritan Drive, Corvallis, OR Zip 97330, Mailing Address: P.O. Box 1068, Zip 97339; tel. 541/757–5111; Larry A. Mullins, President and Chief Executive Officer
(Moderately Centralized Health System)

OREGON: ALBANY GENERAL HOSPITAL (O, 71 beds) 1046 West Sixth Avenue, Albany, OR Zip 97321–1999; tel. 541/812–4000; Richard J. Delano, President

GOOD SAMARITAN HOSPITAL CORVALLIS (O, 124 beds) 3600 N.W. Samaritan Drive, Corvallis, OR Zip 97330, Mailing Address: P.O. Box 1068, Zip 97339; tel. 541/757–5111; Steven W. Jasperson, Executive Vice President Operations
Web address: www.goodsam.com

LEBANON COMMUNITY HOSPITAL (O, 49 beds) 525 North Santiam Highway, Lebanon, OR Zip 97355, Mailing Address: P.O. Box 739, Zip 97355–0739; tel. 541/258–2101; Steven W. Jasperson, Executive Vice President Operations

NORTH LINCOLN HOSPITAL (C, 30 beds) 3043 N.E. 28th Street, Lincoln City, OR Zip 97367–4523, Mailing Address: P.O. Box 767, Zip 97367–0767; tel. 541/994–3661; David C. Bigelow, Chief Executive Officer

Owned, leased, sponsored:	3 hospitals	244 beds
Contract–managed:	1 hospital	30 beds
Totals:	4 hospitals	274 beds

★0037: SCOTTSDALE HEALTHCARE (NP)
3621 Wells Fargo Avenue, Scottsdale, AZ Zip 85251–5607; tel. 480/675–4324; Max Poll, President and Chief Executive Officer
(Moderately Centralized Health System)

ARIZONA: SCOTTSDALE HEALTHCARE–OSBORN (O, 258 beds) 7400 East Osborn Road, Scottsdale, AZ Zip 85251–6403; tel. 480/675–4000; Peggy Reiley, Senior Vice President and Chief Clinical Officer
Web address: www.shc.org

SCOTTSDALE HEALTHCARE–SHEA (O, 251 beds) 9003 East Shea Boulevard, Scottsdale, AZ Zip 85260–6771; tel. 480/860–3000; Thomas J. Sadvary, FACHE, Senior Vice President and Chief Operating Officer
Web address: www.shc.org

Owned, leased, sponsored:	2 hospitals	509 beds
Contract–managed:	0 hospitals	0 beds
Totals:	2 hospitals	509 beds

★1505: SCRIPPS HEALTH (NP)
4275 Campus Point Court, San Diego, CA Zip 92121; tel. 858/678–7200; Stan Pappelbaum, M.D., President and Chief Executive Officer
(Independent Hospital System)

CALIFORNIA: SCRIPPS GREEN HOSPITAL (O, 165 beds) 10666 North Torrey Pines Road, La Jolla, CA Zip 92037–1093; tel. 858/455–9100; Thomas C. Gagen, Senior Vice President and Regional Administrator
Web address: www.chw.edu

SCRIPPS MEMORIAL HOSPITAL CHULA VISTA (O, 183 beds) 435 H Street, Chula Vista, CA Zip 91912, Mailing Address: P.O. Box 1537, Zip 91910–1537; tel. 619/691–7000; John Grah, Administrator
Web address: www.scrippshealth.org

SCRIPPS MEMORIAL HOSPITAL–ENCINITAS (O, 145 beds) 354 Santa Fe Drive, Encinitas, CA Zip 92024, Mailing Address: P.O. Box 230817, Zip 92023; tel. 760/753–6501; Rebecca Ropchan, Administrator

SCRIPPS MEMORIAL HOSPITAL–LA JOLLA (O, 431 beds) 9888 Genesee Avenue, La Jolla, CA Zip 92037–1276, Mailing Address: P.O. Box 28, Zip 92038–0028; tel. 858/626–4123; Thomas C. Gagen, Senior Vice President and Regional Administrator

SCRIPPS MERCY HOSPITAL (O, 447 beds) 4077 Fifth Avenue, San Diego, CA Zip 92103–2180; tel. 619/294–8111; Thomas A. Gammiere, Senior Vice President and Regional Administrator

Owned, leased, sponsored:	5 hospitals	1371 beds
Contract–managed:	0 hospitals	0 beds
Totals:	5 hospitals	1371 beds

0181: SELECT MEDICAL CORPORATION (IO)
4718 Old Gettysburg Road, Mechanicsburg, PA Zip 17055; tel. 717/972–1100; Rocco A. Ortenzio, Chief Executive Officer
(Independent Hospital System)

TEXAS: SELECT SPECIALTY HOSPITAL–DALLAS/FORTH WORTH (O, 36 beds) 10 Medical Parkway, Suite 205, Dallas, TX Zip 75234; tel. 972/488–9167; LouAnn O. Mathews, Administrator

SELECT SPECIALTY HOSPITAL–HOUSTON HEIGHTS (O, 170 beds) 1917 Ashland Street, Houston, TX Zip 77008–3994; tel. 713/861–6161

For explanation of codes following names, see page B2.
★ Indicates Type III membership in the American Hospital Association.

Systems / Shriners Hospitals for Children

SELECT SPECIALTY HOSPITAL–HOUSTON MEDICAL CENTER (O, 34 beds) 6447 Main Street, Houston, TX Zip 77030, Mailing Address: 6500 Fannin Street, Suite 907, Zip 77030; tel. 713/791–9393; Guido J. Cubellis, Chief Executive Officer

Owned, leased, sponsored:	3 hospitals	240 beds
Contract–managed:	0 hospitals	0 beds
Totals:	3 hospitals	240 beds

★2565: **SENTARA HEALTHCARE** (NP)
6015 Poplar Hall Drive, Norfolk, VA Zip 23502–3800; tel. 757/455–7000; David L. Bernd, Chief Executive Officer
(Centralized Health System)

VIRGINIA: SENTARA BAYSIDE HOSPITAL (O, 100 beds) 800 Independence Boulevard, Virginia Beach, VA Zip 23455–6076; tel. 757/363–6100; Rosemary C. Check, Administrator
Web address: www.sentara.com

SENTARA HAMPTON GENERAL HOSPITAL (O, 193 beds) 3120 Victoria Boulevard, Hampton, VA Zip 23661–1585, Mailing Address: Drawer 640, Zip 23669–0640; tel. 757/727–7000; Megan Perry, Administrator
Web address: www.sentara.com

SENTARA LEIGH HOSPITAL (O, 212 beds) 830 Kempsville Road, Norfolk, VA Zip 23502–3981; tel. 757/466–6000; Darleen S. Anderson, R.N., MSN, Site Administrator
Web address: www.sentara.com

SENTARA NORFOLK GENERAL HOSPITAL (O, 478 beds) 600 Gresham Drive, Norfolk, VA Zip 23507–1999; tel. 757/668–3000; Mark R. Gavens, President
Web address: www.sentara.com

SENTARA VIRGINIA BEACH GENERAL HOSPITAL (O, 193 beds) 1060 First Colonial Road, Virginia Beach, VA Zip 23454–9000; tel. 757/395–8000; Robert L. Graves, Administrator
Web address: www.sentara.com

WILLIAMSBURG COMMUNITY HOSPITAL (C, 100 beds) 301 Monticello Avenue, Williamsburg, VA Zip 23187–8700, Mailing Address: Box 8700, Zip 23187–8700; tel. 757/259–6000; Les A. Donahue, President and Chief Executive Officer

Owned, leased, sponsored:	5 hospitals	1176 beds
Contract–managed:	1 hospital	100 beds
Totals:	6 hospitals	1276 beds

★0111: **SHANDS HEALTHCARE** (NP)
1600 S.W. Archer Road, Gainesville, FL Zip 32610–0326; tel. 352/395–0421; J. Richard Gaintner, M.D., Chief Executive Officer
(Centralized Physician/Insurance Health System)

FLORIDA: SHANDS JACKSONVILLE MEDICAL CENTER (O, 678 beds) 655 West Eighth Street, Jacksonville, FL Zip 32209–6595; tel. 904/549–5000; Robert G. Norton, President and Chief Executive Officer

SHANDS REHAB HOSPITAL (O, 40 beds) 8900 N.W. 39th Avenue, Gainesville, FL Zip 32606–5625; tel. 352/338–0091; Cynthia M. Toth, Administrator
Web address: www.shands.org

SHANDS AT AGH (O, 269 beds) 801 S.W. Second Avenue, Gainesville, FL Zip 32601–6289; tel. 352/372–4321; Robert B. Williams, Administrator
Web address: www.shands.org

SHANDS AT LAKE SHORE (L, 83 beds) 560 East Franklin Street, Lake City, FL Zip 32055–3047, Mailing Address: P.O. Box 1989, Zip 32056–1989; tel. 904/754–8000; Neil Whipkey, Administrator
Web address: www.shands.org

SHANDS AT LIVE OAK (O, 16 beds) 1100 S.W. 11th Street, Live Oak, FL Zip 32060–3608, Mailing Address: P.O. Drawer X, Zip 32060; tel. 904/362–1413; Rhonda Sherrod, Administrator
Web address: www.shands.org

SHANDS AT STARKE (O, 30 beds) 922 East Call Street, Starke, FL Zip 32091–3699; tel. 904/368–2300; Jeannie Baker, Administrator
Web address: www.shands.org

SHANDS AT THE UNIVERSITY OF FLORIDA (O, 558 beds) 1600 S.W. Archer Road, Gainesville, FL Zip 32610–0326, Mailing Address: P.O. Box 100326, Zip 32610–0326; tel. 352/395–0111; Jodi J. Mansfield, Executive Vice President and Chief Operating Officer
Web address: www.shands.org

Owned, leased, sponsored:	7 hospitals	1674 beds
Contract–managed:	0 hospitals	0 beds
Totals:	7 hospitals	1674 beds

★2065: **SHARP HEALTHCARE** (NP)
8695 Spectrum Center Court, San Diego, CA Zip 92123–1489; tel. 858/499–4000; Michael Murphy, President and Chief Executive Officer
(Moderately Centralized Health System)

CALIFORNIA: GROSSMONT HOSPITAL (C, 414 beds) 5555 Grossmont Center Drive, La Mesa, CA Zip 91942, Mailing Address: Box 158, Zip 91944–0158; tel. 619/465–0711; Michele T. Tarbet, R.N., Chief Executive Officer
Web address: www.sharp.com

SHARP CABRILLO HOSPITAL (O, 227 beds) 3475 Kenyon Street, San Diego, CA Zip 92110–5067; tel. 619/221–3400; Randi Larsson, Vice President
Web address: www.sharp.com

SHARP CHULA VISTA MEDICAL CENTER (O, 306 beds) 751 Medical Center Court, Chula Vista, CA Zip 91911, Mailing Address: Box 1297, Zip 91912; tel. 619/482–5800; JoAnne G. Schader, R.N., Interim Chief Executive Officer
Web address: www.sharp.com

SHARP CORONADO HOSPITAL (C, 195 beds) 250 Prospect Place, Coronado, CA Zip 92118; tel. 619/522–3600; Marcia K. Hall, Chief Executive Officer
Web address: www.sharp.com

SHARP MEMORIAL HOSPITAL (O, 488 beds) 7901 Frost Street, San Diego, CA Zip 92123–2788; tel. 858/541–3400; Dan Gross, Chief Executive Officer
Web address: www.sharp.com

SHARP MESA VISTA HOSPITAL (O, 166 beds) 7850 Vista Hill Avenue, San Diego, CA Zip 92123–2790; tel. 858/694–8300; Karenlee Robinson, Chief Operating Officer
Web address: www.sharp.com

Owned, leased, sponsored:	4 hospitals	1187 beds
Contract–managed:	2 hospitals	609 beds
Totals:	6 hospitals	1796 beds

4125: **SHRINERS HOSPITALS FOR CHILDREN** (NP)
2900 Rocky Point Drive, Tampa, FL Zip 33607–1435, Mailing Address: Box 31356, Zip 33631–3356; tel. 813/281–0300; Joseph E. Melchiorre, Jr, CHE, Executive Administrator
(Independent Hospital System)

SHRINERS HOSPITALS FOR CHILDREN, LOS ANGELES (O, 50 beds) 3160 Geneva Street, Los Angeles, CA Zip 90020–1199; tel. 213/388–3151; Frank LaBonte, FACHE, Administrator

SHRINERS HOSPITALS FOR CHILDREN, NORTHERN CALIFORNIA (O, 50 beds) 2425 Stockton Boulevard, Sacramento, CA Zip 95817–2215; tel. 916/453–2000; Margaret Bryan, Administrator
Web address: www.shrinershq.org

FLORIDA: SHRINERS HOSPITALS FOR CHILDREN, TAMPA (O, 60 beds) 12502 North Pine Drive, Tampa, FL Zip 33612–9499; tel. 813/972–2250; John Holtz, Administrator

HAWAII: SHRINERS HOSPITALS FOR CHILDREN, HONOLULU (O, 40 beds) 1310 Punahou Street, Honolulu, HI Zip 96826–1099; tel. 808/941–4466; Thomas J. Brotherton, Administrator
Web address: www.shrinershq.org

ILLINOIS: SHRINERS HOSPITALS FOR CHILDREN–CHICAGO (O, 60 beds) 2211 North Oak Park Avenue, Chicago, IL Zip 60707; tel. 773/622–5400; A. James Spang, Administrator
Web address: www.shrinerschicago.org

KENTUCKY: SHRINERS HOSPITALS FOR CHILDREN–LEXINGTON (O, 50 beds) 1900 Richmond Road, Lexington, KY Zip 40502–1298; tel. 606/266–2101; Tony Lewgood, Administrator

For explanation of codes following names, see page B2.
★ Indicates Type III membership in the American Hospital Association.

Systems / Shriners Hospitals for Children

LOUISIANA: SHRINERS HOSPITALS FOR CHILDREN, SHREVEPORT (O, 45 beds) 3100 Samford Avenue, Shreveport, LA Zip 71103–4289; tel. 318/222–5704; Thomas R. Schneider, Administrator

MASSACHUSETTS: SHRINERS HOSPITALS FOR CHILDREN, SHRINERS BURNS HOSPITAL–BOSTON (O, 30 beds) 51 Blossom Street, Boston, MA Zip 02114–2699; tel. 617/722–3000; Robert F. Bories, Jr, FACHE, Administrator
Web address: www.shrinershq.org

SHRINERS HOSPITALS FOR CHILDREN, SPRINGFIELD (O, 40 beds) 516 Carew Street, Springfield, MA Zip 01104–2396; tel. 413/787–2000; Mark L. Niederpruem, Administrator
Web address: www.shrinerspfld.org

MINNESOTA: SHRINERS HOSPITALS FOR CHILDREN, TWIN CITIES (O, 40 beds) 2025 East River Parkway, Minneapolis, MN Zip 55414–3696; tel. 612/596–6100; Laurence E. Johnson, Administrator
Web address: www.shrinershq.org

MISSOURI: SHRINERS HOSPITALS FOR CHILDREN, ST. LOUIS (O, 80 beds) 2001 South Lindbergh Boulevard, Saint Louis, MO Zip 63131–3597; tel. 314/432–3600; Carolyn P. Golden, Administrator

OHIO: SHRINERS HOSPITALS FOR CHILDREN, SHRINERS BURNS HOSPITAL, CINCINNATI (O, 30 beds) 3229 Burnet Avenue, Cincinnati, OH Zip 45229–3095; tel. 513/872–6000; Ronald R. Hitzler, Administrator
Web address: www.shrinershq.org

OREGON: SHRINERS HOSPITALS FOR CHILDREN, PORTLAND (O, 40 beds) 3101 S.W. Sam Jackson Park Road, Portland, OR Zip 97201; tel. 503/241–5090; C. Thomas D'Esmond, Administrator
Web address: www.shcc.org

PENNSYLVANIA: SHRINERS HOSPITALS FOR CHILDREN, ERIE (O, 30 beds) 1645 West 8th Street, Erie, PA Zip 16505–5007; tel. 814/875–8700; Richard W. Brzuz, Administrator

SHRINERS HOSPITALS FOR CHILDREN, PHILADELPHIA (O, 80 beds) 3551 North Broad Street, Philadelphia, PA Zip 19140–4105; tel. 215/430–4000; Sharon J. Rajnic, Administrator

SOUTH CAROLINA: SHRINERS HOSPITALS FOR CHILDREN, GREENVILLE (O, 50 beds) 950 West Faris Road, Greenville, SC Zip 29605–4277; tel. 864/271–3444; Gary F. Fraley, Administrator
Web address: www.shrinershq.org

TEXAS: SHRINERS HOSPITALS FOR CHILDREN, GALVESTON BURNS HOSPITAL (O, 30 beds) 815 Market Street, Galveston, TX Zip 77550–2725; tel. 409/770–6600; John A. Swartwout, Administrator
Web address: www.shrinershq.org

SHRINERS HOSPITALS FOR CHILDREN, HOUSTON (O, 40 beds) 6977 Main Street, Houston, TX Zip 77030–3701; tel. 713/797–1616; Steven B. Reiter, Administrator
Web address: www.shc–houston.org

UTAH: SHRINERS HOSPITALS FOR CHILDREN–INTERMOUNTAIN (O, 40 beds) Fairfax Road and Virginia Street, Salt Lake City, UT Zip 84103–4399; tel. 801/536–3500; J. Craig Patchin, Administrator
Web address: www.shriners.com

WASHINGTON: SHRINERS HOSPITALS FOR CHILDREN–SPOKANE (O, 30 beds) 911 West Fifth Avenue, Spokane, WA Zip 99204–2901, Mailing Address: P.O. Box 2472, Zip 99210–2472; tel. 509/455–7844; Charles R. Young, Administrator
Web address: www.shrinershq.org

Owned, leased, sponsored:	20 hospitals	915 beds
Contract–managed:	0 hospitals	0 beds
Totals:	20 hospitals	915 beds

0067: SINGING RIVER HOSPITAL SYSTEM (NP)
2101 Highway 90, Gautier, MS Zip 39553; tel. 228/497–7907; Chris Anderson, Chief Executive Officer
(Centralized Physician/Insurance Health System)

MISSISSIPPI: OCEAN SPRINGS HOSPITAL (O, 108 beds) 3109 Bienville Boulevard, Ocean Springs, MS Zip 39564–4361; tel. 228/818–1111; Dwight Rimes, Administrator

SINGING RIVER HOSPITAL (O, 273 beds) 2809 Denny Avenue, Pascagoula, MS Zip 39581–5301; tel. 228/809–5000; Lynn Truelove, Administrator
Web address: www.srhshealth.com

Owned, leased, sponsored:	2 hospitals	381 beds
Contract–managed:	0 hospitals	0 beds
Totals:	2 hospitals	381 beds

★0078: SIOUX VALLEY HOSPITALS AND HEALTH SYSTEM (NP)
1100 South Euclid Avenue, Sioux Falls, SD Zip 57105–0496; tel. 605/333–1000; Kelby K. Krabbenhoft, President
(Moderately Centralized Health System)

IOWA: MERRILL PIONEER COMMUNITY HOSPITAL (O, 16 beds) 801 South Greene Street, Rock Rapids, IA Zip 51246–1998; tel. 712/472–2591; Gordon Smith, Administrator and Chief Executive Officer

NORTHWEST IOWA HEALTH CENTER (O, 127 beds) 118 North Seventh Avenue, Sheldon, IA Zip 51201–1235, Mailing Address: P.O. Box 250, Zip 51201–0250; tel. 712/324–5041; Charles R. Miller, Chief Executive Officer

ORANGE CITY HEALTH SYSTEM (C, 113 beds) 400 Central Avenue N.W., Orange City, IA Zip 51041–1398; tel. 712/737–4984; Martin W. Guthmiller, Administrator and Chief Executive Officer

SPENCER MUNICIPAL HOSPITAL (C, 85 beds) 1200 First Avenue East, Spencer, IA Zip 51301–4321; tel. 712/264–6111; John Allen, President and Chief Executive Officer

MINNESOTA: ARNOLD MEMORIAL HEALTH CARE CENTER (O, 50 beds) 601 Louisiana Avenue, Adrian, MN Zip 56110–0279, Mailing Address: P.O. Box 279, Zip 56110–0279; tel. 507/483–2668; Gerald E. Carl, Administrator
Web address: www.siouxvalley.org

JACKSON MEDICAL CENTER (O, 41 beds) 1430 North Highway, Jackson, MN Zip 56143–1098; tel. 507/847–2420; Charlotte Heitkamp, Chief Executive Officer

LUVERNE COMMUNITY HOSPITAL (O, 38 beds) 305 East Luverne Street, Luverne, MN Zip 56156–2519, Mailing Address: P.O. Box 1019, Zip 56156–1019; tel. 507/283–2321; Gerald E. Carl, Administrator
Web address: www.siouxvalley.org

MURRAY COUNTY MEMORIAL HOSPITAL (C, 25 beds) 2042 Juniper Avenue, Slayton, MN Zip 56172–1016; tel. 507/836–6111; Jerry Bobeldyk, Administrator

ORTONVILLE AREA HEALTH SERVICES (C, 105 beds) 750 Eastvold Avenue, Ortonville, MN Zip 56278–1133; tel. 320/839–2502; Kenneth W. Archer, Administrator

SIOUX VALLEY CANBY CAMPUS (O, 94 beds) 112 St. Olaf Avenue South, Canby, MN Zip 56220–1433; tel. 507/223–7277; Robert J. Salmon, Chief Executive Officer
Web address: www.siouxvalley.org

TRACY AREA MEDICAL SERVICES (O, 27 beds) 251 Fifth Street East, Tracy, MN Zip 56175–1536; tel. 507/629–3200; Dan Reiner, Administrator and Chief Executive Officer

WESTBROOK HEALTH CENTER (O, 8 beds) 920 Bell Avenue, Westbrook, MN Zip 56183–0188, Mailing Address: P.O. Box 188, Zip 56183–0188; tel. 507/274–6121; Dan Reiner, Administrator and Chief Executive Officer

WINDOM AREA HOSPITAL (C, 35 beds) Highways 60 and 71 North, Windom, MN Zip 56101, Mailing Address: P.O. Box 339, Zip 56101–0339; tel. 507/831–2400

WORTHINGTON REGIONAL HOSPITAL (C, 66 beds) 1018 Sixth Avenue, Worthington, MN Zip 56187–2202, Mailing Address: P.O. Box 997, Zip 56187–0997; tel. 507/372–2941; Melvin J. Platt, Administrator

SOUTH DAKOTA: CANTON–INWOOD MEMORIAL HOSPITAL (L, 25 beds) 440 North Hiawatha Drive, Canton, SD Zip 57013–9404; tel. 605/987–2621; Larry W. Veitz, Chief Executive Officer

DEUEL COUNTY MEMORIAL HOSPITAL (O, 20 beds) 701 Third Avenue South, Clear Lake, SD Zip 57226–1037, Mailing Address: P.O. Box 1037, Zip 57226–1037; tel. 605/874–2141; Robert J. Salmon, Administrator

LAKE AREA HOSPITAL (O, 26 beds) North First Street, Webster, SD Zip 57274, Mailing Address: P.O. Box 489, Zip 57274–0489; tel. 605/345–3336; Donald J. Finn, Administrator

MID DAKOTA HOSPITAL (L, 36 beds) 300 South Byron Boulevard, Chamberlain, SD Zip 57325–9741; tel. 605/734–5511; Earl N. Sheehy, Administrator

For explanation of codes following names, see page B2.
★ Indicates Type III membership in the American Hospital Association.

Systems / Sisters of Mary of the Presentation Health Corporation

PIONEER MEMORIAL HOSPITAL AND HEALTH SERVICES (C, 64 beds) 315 North Washington Street, Viborg, SD Zip 57070, Mailing Address: P.O. Box 368, Zip 57070–0368; tel. 605/326–5161; Georgia Pokorney, Chief Executive Officer

PRAIRIE LAKES HOSPITAL AND CARE CENTER (C, 119 beds) 400 Tenth Avenue N.W., Watertown, SD Zip 57201–6210, Mailing Address: P.O. Box 1210, Zip 57201–1210; tel. 605/882–7000; Paul A. Hanson, Chief Executive Officer
Web address: www.prairielakes.com

SIOUX VALLEY HOSPITAL AND UNIVERSITY MEDICAL CENTER (O, 496 beds) 1100 South Euclid Avenue, Sioux Falls, SD Zip 57105–0496, Mailing Address: P.O. Box 5039, Zip 57117–5039; tel. 605/333–1000; Becky Nelson, President
Web address: www.siouxvalley.org

SIOUX VALLEY VERMILLION CAMPUS (O, 118 beds) 20 South Plum Street, Vermillion, SD Zip 57069–3346; tel. 605/624–2611; John E. Paulson, Chief Executive Officer
Web address: www.siouxvalley.org

WINNER REGIONAL HEALTHCARE CENTER (C, 116 beds) 745 East Eighth Street, Winner, SD Zip 57580–2677, Mailing Address: P.O. Box 745, Zip 57580–0745; tel. 605/842–7100; Michael M. Penticoff, Administrator

Owned, leased, sponsored:	14 hospitals	1122 beds
Contract-managed:	9 hospitals	728 beds
Totals:	23 hospitals	1850 beds

5995: SISTERS OF CHARITY CENTER (CC)
Mount St. Vincent on Hudson, New York, NY Zip 10471–9930; tel. 718/549–9200; Sister Elizabeth A. Vermaelen, President
(Moderately Centralized Health System)

NEW YORK: SAINT VINCENTS HOSPITAL AND MEDICAL CENTER (S, 978 beds) 170 West 12th Street, New York, NY Zip 10011–8397; tel. 212/604–7000; David J. Campbell, President and Chief Executive Officer
Web address: www.svh.nymc.edu/

ST. JOSEPH'S MEDICAL CENTER (S, 194 beds) 127 South Broadway, Yonkers, NY Zip 10701–4080; tel. 914/378–7000; Michael J. Spicer, President and Chief Executive Officer
Web address: www.stjosephs.org

Owned, leased, sponsored:	2 hospitals	1172 beds
Contract-managed:	0 hospitals	0 beds
Totals:	2 hospitals	1172 beds

★5095: SISTERS OF CHARITY OF LEAVENWORTH HEALTH SERVICES CORPORATION (CC)
4200 South Fourth Street, Leavenworth, KS Zip 66048–5054; tel. 913/682–1338; William M. Murray, President
(Moderately Centralized Health System)

CALIFORNIA: SAINT JOHN'S HOSPITAL AND HEALTH CENTER (O, 234 beds) 1328 22nd Street, Santa Monica, CA Zip 90404–2032; tel. 310/829–5511; Bruce Lamoureux, Chief Executive Officer
Web address: www.stjohns.org

COLORADO: ST. MARY'S HOSPITAL AND MEDICAL CENTER (O, 281 beds) 2635 North 7th Street, Grand Junction, CO Zip 81501–8204, Mailing Address: P.O. Box 1628, Zip 81502–1628; tel. 970/244–2273; Robert W. Ladenburger, President and Chief Executive Officer

KANSAS: BETHANY MEDICAL CENTER (O, 251 beds) 51 North 12th Street, Kansas City, KS Zip 66102–5161; tel. 913/281–8400; Keith R. Poisson, President and Chief Executive Officer

PROVIDENCE MEDICAL CENTER (O, 219 beds) 8929 Parallel Parkway, Kansas City, KS Zip 66112–1636; tel. 913/596–4000; Francis V. Creeden, Jr, Senior Executive Officer
Web address: www.pmc-sjh.org

SAINT JOHN HOSPITAL (O, 36 beds) 3500 South Fourth Street, Leavenworth, KS Zip 66048–5043; tel. 913/680–6000; Mark J. Jaeger, CHE, President and Chief Executive Officer
Web address: www.pmc-sjh.org

ST. FRANCIS HOSPITAL AND MEDICAL CENTER (O, 269 beds) 1700 West Seventh Street, Topeka, KS Zip 66606–1690; tel. 785/295–8000; Sister Loretto Marie Colwell, President and Chief Executive Officer
Web address: www.stfrancistopeka.org

MONTANA: HOLY ROSARY HEALTH CENTER (O, 151 beds) 2600 Wilson Street, Miles City, MT Zip 59301–5094; tel. 406/233–2600;
Web address: www.svhhc.org

SAINT VINCENT HOSPITAL AND HEALTH CENTER (O, 249 beds) 1233 North 30th Street, Billings, MT Zip 59101–0165, Mailing Address: P.O. Box 35200, Zip 59107–5200; tel. 406/237–7000; Patrick M. Hermanson, Senior Executive Officer
Web address: www.svhhc.org

ST. JAMES COMMUNITY HOSPITAL (O, 100 beds) 400 South Clark Street, Butte, MT Zip 59701–2328, Mailing Address: P.O. Box 3300, Zip 59702–3300; tel. 406/723–2500; Robert Rodgers, Administrator and Senior Executive Officer
Web address: www.svhhc.org

Owned, leased, sponsored:	9 hospitals	1790 beds
Contract-managed:	0 hospitals	0 beds
Totals:	9 hospitals	1790 beds

●5125: SISTERS OF CHARITY OF ST. AUGUSTINE HEALTH SYSTEM (CC)
2351 East 22nd Street, Cleveland, OH Zip 44115–3197; tel. 216/696–5560; Sister Judith Ann Karam, President and Chief Executive Officer
(Moderately Centralized Health System)

SOUTH CAROLINA: PROVIDENCE HOSPITAL (S, 228 beds) 2435 Forest Drive, Columbia, SC Zip 29204–2098; tel. 803/256–5300; Stephen A. Purves, CHE, President and Chief Executive Officer
Web address: www.provhosp.com

Owned, leased, sponsored:	1 hospital	228 beds
Contract-managed:	0 hospitals	0 beds
Totals:	1 hospital	228 beds

5805: SISTERS OF MARY OF THE PRESENTATION HEALTH CORPORATION (CC)
1102 Page Drive S.W., Fargo, ND Zip 58106–0007, Mailing Address: P.O. Box 10007, Zip 58106–0007; tel. 701/237–9290; Aaron Alton, President
(Moderately Centralized Health System)

ILLINOIS: ST. MARGARET'S HOSPITAL (O, 123 beds) 600 East First Street, Spring Valley, IL Zip 61362–2034; tel. 815/664–5311; Tim Muntz, President
Web address: www.st.margarets.com

IOWA: VAN BUREN COUNTY HOSPITAL (C, 40 beds) Highway 1 North, Keosauqua, IA Zip 52565, Mailing Address: P.O. Box 70, Zip 52565–0070; tel. 319/293–3171; Lisa Schnedler, Administrator
Web address: www.netins.net/showcase/forhealth/

NORTH DAKOTA: PRESENTATION MEDICAL CENTER (O, 102 beds) 213 Second Avenue N.E., Rolla, ND Zip 58367–7153, Mailing Address: P.O. Box 759, Zip 58367–0759; tel. 701/477–3161; Kimber Wraalstad, President and Chief Executive Officer

ST. ALOISIUS MEDICAL CENTER (O, 141 beds) 325 East Brewster Street, Harvey, ND Zip 58341–1605; tel. 701/324–4651; Ronald J. Volk, President

ST. ANDREW'S HEALTH CENTER (O, 67 beds) 316 Ohmer Street, Bottineau, ND Zip 58318–1018; tel. 701/228–2255; Keith Korman, President

Owned, leased, sponsored:	4 hospitals	433 beds
Contract-managed:	1 hospital	40 beds
Totals:	5 hospitals	473 beds

For explanation of codes following names, see page B2.
★ Indicates Type III membership in the American Hospital Association.
● Single hospital health care system

Systems / Sisters of Mercy Health System–St. Louis

★5185: SISTERS OF MERCY HEALTH SYSTEM–ST. LOUIS (CC)
2039 North Geyer Road, Saint Louis, MO Zip 63131–0902, Mailing Address: P.O. Box 31902, Zip 63131–0902; tel. 314/965–6100; Ronald B. Ashworth, Chief Executive Officer
(Decentralized Health System)

ARKANSAS: CARROLL REGIONAL MEDICAL CENTER (O, 31 beds) 214 Carter Street, Berryville, AR Zip 72616–4303; tel. 870/423–3355; Rudy Darling, President and Chief Executive Officer
Web address: www.carrollregional.com

H.S.C. MEDICAL CENTER (O, 92 beds) 1001 Schneider Drive, Malvern, AR Zip 72104–4828; tel. 501/337–4911; Jeff Curtis, President and Chief Executive Officer

HARBOR VIEW MERCY HOSPITAL (O, 80 beds) 10301 Mayo Road, Fort Smith, AR Zip 72903–1631, Mailing Address: P.O. Box 17000, Zip 72917–7000; tel. 501/484–5550; Richard Cameron, M.D., Administrator

MERCY HOSPITAL OF SCOTT COUNTY (O, 127 beds) Highways 71 and 80, Waldron, AR Zip 72958–9984, Mailing Address: P.O. Box 2230, Zip 72958–2230; tel. 501/637–4135; Jim L. Maddox, Administrator

MERCY HOSPITAL–TURNER MEMORIAL (O, 39 beds) 801 West River Street, Ozark, AR Zip 72949–3000; tel. 501/667–4138; Jim L. Maddox, Regional Administrator

NORTH LOGAN MERCY HOSPITAL (O, 16 beds) 500 East Academy, Paris, AR Zip 72855–4099; tel. 501/963–6101

ST. EDWARD MERCY MEDICAL CENTER (O, 343 beds) 7301 Rogers Avenue, Fort Smith, AR Zip 72903–4189, Mailing Address: P.O. Box 17000, Zip 72917–7000; tel. 501/484–6000; Michael L. Morgan, President and Chief Executive Officer

ST. JOSEPH'S REGIONAL HEALTH CENTER (O, 248 beds) 300 Werner Street, Hot Springs National Park, AR Zip 71913–9937, Mailing Address: P.O. Box 29001, Zip 71913–9001; tel. 501/622–1000; Randall J. Fale, FACHE, President and Chief Executive Officer
Web address: www.saintjosephs.com

ST. MARY–ROGERS MEMORIAL HOSPITAL (O, 92 beds) 1200 West Walnut Street, Rogers, AR Zip 72756–3599; tel. 501/636–0200; Susan Barrett, President and Chief Executive Officer
Web address: www.mercyhealthnwa.smhs.com

ILLINOIS: ST. CLEMENT HEALTH SERVICES (O, 75 beds) One St. Clement Boulevard, Red Bud, IL Zip 62278–1194; tel. 618/282–3831; Michael T. McManus, Administrator

KANSAS: MERCY HEALTH SYSTEM OF KANSAS (O, 94 beds) 821 Burke Street, Fort Scott, KS Zip 66701–2409; tel. 316/223–2200; Jerry L. Stevenson, President and Chief Executive Officer

MERCY HEALTH SYSTEM OF KANSAS (O, 58 beds) 800 West Myrtle Street, Independence, KS Zip 67301–9980, Mailing Address: P.O. Box 388, Zip 67301–0388; tel. 316/331–2200; Jerry L. Stevenson, President and Chief Executive Officer

MISSOURI: BREECH REGIONAL MEDICAL CENTER (O, 41 beds) 100 Hospital Drive, Lebanon, MO Zip 65536–2317; tel. 417/533–6100; Gary W. Pulsipher, President

ST. FRANCIS HOSPITAL (O, 17 beds) Highway 60, Mountain View, MO Zip 65548, Mailing Address: P.O. Box 82, Zip 65548–0082; tel. 417/934–2246; Gary W. Jordan, President and Chief Executive Officer
Web address: www.stfran@socket.net

ST. JOHN'S MERCY MEDICAL CENTER (O, 898 beds) 615 South New Ballas Road, Saint Louis, MO Zip 63141–8277; tel. 314/569–6000; Mark Weber, FACHE, President

ST. JOHN'S REGIONAL HEALTH CENTER (O, 743 beds) 1235 East Cherokee Street, Springfield, MO Zip 65804–2263; tel. 417/885–2000; Robert T. Brodhead, President

ST. LUKE'S HOSPITAL (O, 369 beds) 232 South Woods Mill Road, Chesterfield, MO Zip 63017–3480; tel. 314/434–1500; Gary R. Olson, President

OKLAHOMA: MERCY HEALTH CENTER (O, 363 beds) 4300 West Memorial Road, Oklahoma City, OK Zip 73120–8362; tel. 405/755–1515; Michael J. Packnett, President and Chief Executive Officer
Web address: www.mercyok.com

MERCY MEMORIAL HEALTH CENTER (O, 199 beds) 1011 14th Street N.W., Ardmore, OK Zip 73401–1889; tel. 580/223–5400; Bobby G. Thompson, President and Chief Executive Officer
Web address: www.mercyok.com

TEXAS: MERCY HEALTH CENTER (O, 320 beds) 1700 East Saunders Avenue, Laredo, TX Zip 78041, Mailing Address: Drawer 2068, Zip 78044–2068; tel. 956/718–6222; Mark S. Stauder, President and Chief Executive Officer
Web address: www.mhst.smhs.com

Owned, leased, sponsored:	20 hospitals	4245 beds
Contract–managed:	0 hospitals	0 beds
Totals:	20 hospitals	4245 beds

6015: SISTERS OF MERCY OF THE AMERICAS–REGIONAL COMMUNITY OF BALTIMORE (CC)
1300 Northern Parkway, Baltimore, MD Zip 21239, Mailing Address: P.O. Box 11448, Zip 21239; tel. 410/435–4400; Sister Barbara Wheeley, Vice President
(Independent Hospital System)

GEORGIA: ST. JOSEPH'S CANDLER HEALTH SYSTEM (S, 216 beds) 11705 Mercy Boulevard, Savannah, GA Zip 31419–1791; tel. 912/925–4100; Paul P. Hinchey, President and Chief Executive Officer

MARYLAND: MERCY MEDICAL CENTER (O, 200 beds) 301 St. Paul Place, Baltimore, MD Zip 21202–2165; tel. 410/332–9000; Thomas R. Mullen, President and Chief Executive Officer
Web address: www.mercymed.com

Owned, leased, sponsored:	2 hospitals	416 beds
Contract–managed:	0 hospitals	0 beds
Totals:	2 hospitals	416 beds

★5345: SISTERS OF ST. FRANCIS HEALTH SERVICES, INC. (CC)
1515 Dragoon Trail, Mishawaka, IN Zip 46546–1290, Mailing Address: P.O. Box 1290, Zip 46546–1290; tel. 219/256–3935; Kevin D. Leahy, President and Chief Executive Officer
(Moderately Centralized Health System)

ILLINOIS: ST. JAMES HOSPITAL AND HEALTH CENTERS – CHICAGO HEIGHTS CAMPUS (O, 332 beds) 1423 Chicago Road, Chicago Heights, IL Zip 60411–3483; tel. 708/756–1000; Peter J. Murphy, President and Chief Executive Officer
Web address: www.st jameshhc.org

ST. JAMES HOSPITALS AND HEALTH CENTERS – OLYMPIA FIELDS CAMPUS (O, 164 beds) 20201 South Crawford Avenue, Olympia Fields, IL Zip 60461–1080; tel. 708/747–4000; David Scott Koenig, Chief Executive Officer

INDIANA: SAINT ANTHONY MEMORIAL HEALTH CENTERS (O, 207 beds) 301 West Homer Street, Michigan City, IN Zip 46360–4358; tel. 219/879–8511; Bruce E. Rampage, President and Chief Executive Officer
Web address: www.sahhc.org

SAINT MARGARET MERCY HEALTHCARE CENTERS (O, 624 beds) 5454 Hohman Avenue, Hammond, IN Zip 46320–1999; tel. 219/933–2074; Eugene C. Diamond, President and Chief Executive Officer
Web address: www.smmhc.com

ST. ANTHONY MEDICAL CENTER (O, 228 beds) 1201 South Main Street, Crown Point, IN Zip 46307–8483; tel. 219/738–2100; Stephen O. Leurck, President and Chief Executive Officer

ST. CLARE MEDICAL CENTER (O, 89 beds) 1710 Lafayette Road, Crawfordsville, IN Zip 47933–1099; tel. 765/362–2800; Gregory D. Starnes, Chief Executive Officer

ST. FRANCIS HOSPITAL AND HEALTH CENTERS – NORTH CAMPUS (O, 402 beds) 1600 Albany Street, Beech Grove, IN Zip 46107–1593; tel. 317/787–3311; Robert J. Brody, President and Chief Executive Officer
Web address: www.stfrancis–indy.org

ST. FRANCIS HOSPITAL–MOORESVILLE (O, 60 beds) 1201 Hadley Road N.W., Mooresville, IN Zip 46158–1789; tel. 317/831–1160; Charles D. Swisher, President

For explanation of codes following names, see page B2.
★ Indicates Type III membership in the American Hospital Association.

Owned, leased, sponsored:	8 hospitals	2106 beds
Contract–managed:	0 hospitals	0 beds
Totals:	8 hospitals	2106 beds

5955: SISTERS OF THE 3RD FRANCISCAN ORDER (CC)
2500 Grant Boulevard, Syracuse, NY Zip 13208–1713;
tel. 315/425–0115; Sister Marion Kikukawa, General Minister
(Moderately Centralized Health System)

HAWAII: ST. FRANCIS MEDICAL CENTER (S, 249 beds) 2230 Liliha Street, Honolulu, HI Zip 96817–9979, Mailing Address: P.O. Box 30100, Zip 96820–0100; tel. 808/547–6484; Cynthia Okinaka, Administrator
Web address: www.stfrancishawaii.org

ST. FRANCIS MEDICAL CENTER–WEST (S, 102 beds) 91–2141 Fort Weaver Road, Ewa Beach, HI Zip 96706; tel. 808/678–7000; John V. Schleif, Administrator
Web address: www.sfhs–hi.org

NEW YORK: ST. ELIZABETH MEDICAL CENTER (S, 172 beds) 2209 Genesee Street, Utica, NY Zip 13501–5999; tel. 315/798–8100; Sister Rose Vincent, President and Chief Executive Officer
Web address: www.stemc.org

ST. JOSEPH'S HOSPITAL HEALTH CENTER (S, 431 beds) 301 Prospect Avenue, Syracuse, NY Zip 13203–1895; tel. 315/448–5111; Theodore M. Pasinski, President
Web address: www.SJHSYR.ORG

Owned, leased, sponsored:	4 hospitals	954 beds
Contract–managed:	0 hospitals	0 beds
Totals:	4 hospitals	954 beds

5575: SISTERS OF THE HOLY FAMILY OF NAZARETH–SACRED HEART PROVINCE (CC)
310 North River Road, Des Plaines, IL Zip 60016–1211;
tel. 847/298–6760; Sister Marie Kielanowicz, Provincial Superior
(Moderately Centralized Health System)

ILLINOIS: HOLY FAMILY MEDICAL CENTER (O, 183 beds) 100 North River Road, Des Plaines, IL Zip 60016–1255; tel. 847/297–1800; Sister Patricia Ann Koschalke, President and Chief Executive Officer

SAINT MARY OF NAZARETH HOSPITAL CENTER (O, 325 beds) 2233 West Division Street, Chicago, IL Zip 60622–3086; tel. 312/770–2000; Sister Sally Marie Kiepura, President and Chief Executive Officer
Web address: www.stmaryofnazareth.org

Owned, leased, sponsored:	2 hospitals	508 beds
Contract–managed:	0 hospitals	0 beds
Totals:	2 hospitals	508 beds

★8855: SOLARIS HEALTH SYSTEM (NP)
80 James Street, 2nd Floor, Edison, NJ Zip 08820–3998;
tel. 732/632–1500; John P. McGee, President and Chief Executive Officer

NEW JERSEY: JFK JOHNSON REHABILITATION INSTITUTE (O, 92 beds) 65 James Street, Edison, NJ Zip 08818–3059; tel. 732/321–7050; Scott Gebhard, Senior Vice President Operations
Web address: www.solarishs.org

JFK MEDICAL CENTER (O, 380 beds) 65 James Street, Edison, NJ Zip 08818–3947; tel. 732/321–7000; John P. McGee, President and Chief Executive Officer
Web address: jfkmc.org/index.htm

MUHLENBERG REGIONAL MEDICAL CENTER (O, 261 beds) 1200 Park Avenue, Plainfield, NJ Zip 07061; tel. 908/668–2000; John R. Kopicki, President and Chief Executive Officer
Web address: www.solarishs.org/

Owned, leased, sponsored:	3 hospitals	733 beds
Contract–managed:	0 hospitals	0 beds
Totals:	3 hospitals	733 beds

★0068: SOUTH CENTRAL COMMUNITY HEALTH (NP)
1001 South George Street, York, PA Zip 17405–3645;
tel. 717/851–2345; Bruce M. Bartels, President
(Centralized Physician/Insurance Health System)

PENNSYLVANIA: GETTYSBURG HOSPITAL (O, 99 beds) 147 Gettys Street, Gettysburg, PA Zip 17325–0786; tel. 717/334–2121; Steven W. Renner, CPA, President and Chief Executive Officer
Web address: www.gettysburghosp.org

YORK HOSPITAL (O, 437 beds) 1001 South George Street, York, PA Zip 17405–3645; tel. 717/851–2345; Brian A. Gragnolati, President
Web address: www.yorkhealth.org

Owned, leased, sponsored:	2 hospitals	536 beds
Contract–managed:	0 hospitals	0 beds
Totals:	2 hospitals	536 beds

0151: SOUTH JERSEY HEALTH SYSTEM (NP)
333 Irving Avenue, Bridgeton, NJ Zip 08302–2100;
tel. 856/451–6600; Paul S. Cooper, Chief Executive Officer
(Independent Hospital System)

NEW JERSEY: SOUTH JERSEY HOSPITAL (O, 340 beds) 333 Irving Avenue, Bridgeton, NJ Zip 08302–2100; tel. 856/451–6600; Chester B. Kaletkowski, President and Chief Executive Officer
Web address: www.sjhs.com

SOUTH JERSEY HOSPITAL–NEWCOMB (O, 139 beds) 65 South State Street, Vineland, NJ Zip 08360–4893; tel. 856/507–8500; Chester B. Kaletkowski, President and Chief Executive Officer

Owned, leased, sponsored:	2 hospitals	479 beds
Contract–managed:	0 hospitals	0 beds
Totals:	2 hospitals	479 beds

★0106: SOUTHERN CALIFORNIA HEALTHCARE SYSTEMS (NP)
100 West California Boulevard, Pasadena, CA Zip 91105;
tel. 626/397–5555; Stephen A. Ralph, President and Chief Executive Officer
(Moderately Centralized Health System)

CALIFORNIA: HUNTINGTON EAST VALLEY HOSPITAL (O, 128 beds) 150 West Alosta Avenue, Glendora, CA Zip 91740–4398; tel. 626/335–0231; James W. Maki, Chief Executive Officer
Web address: www.schs.com

HUNTINGTON MEMORIAL HOSPITAL (O, 525 beds) 100 West California Boulevard, Pasadena, CA Zip 91105, Mailing Address: P.O. Box 7013, Zip 91109–7013; tel. 626/397–5000; Stephen A. Ralph, President and Chief Executive Officer
Web address: www.schs.com

METHODIST HOSPITAL OF SOUTHERN CALIFORNIA (O, 304 beds) 300 West Huntington Drive, Arcadia, CA Zip 91007, Mailing Address: P.O. Box 60016, Zip 91066–6016; tel. 626/445–4441; Dennis M. Lee, President

Owned, leased, sponsored:	3 hospitals	957 beds
Contract–managed:	0 hospitals	0 beds
Totals:	3 hospitals	957 beds

★4175: SOUTHERN ILLINOIS HOSPITAL SERVICES (NP)
1239 East Main Street, Carbondale, IL Zip 62901, Mailing Address: P.O. Box 3988, Zip 62902–3988; tel. 618/457–5200; John J. Buckley, Jr, President
(Moderately Centralized Health System)

ILLINOIS: FERRELL HOSPITAL (O, 36 beds) 1201 Pine Street, Eldorado, IL Zip 62930–1634; tel. 618/273–3361; William Hartley, Administrator
Web address: www.sih.net

FRANKLIN HOSPITAL AND SKILLED NURSING CARE UNIT (L, 117 beds) 201 Bailey Lane, Benton, IL Zip 62812–1999; tel. 618/439–3161; Becky Ashton, Administrator
Web address: www.sih.net

For explanation of codes following names, see page B2.
★ Indicates Type III membership in the American Hospital Association.

Systems / Southern Illinois Hospital Services

HERRIN HOSPITAL (O, 92 beds) 201 South 14th Street, Herrin, IL Zip 62948-3631; tel. 618/942-2171; Virgil Hannig, Senior Vice President and Administrator
Web address: www.sih.net

MEMORIAL HOSPITAL OF CARBONDALE (O, 132 beds) 405 West Jackson Street, Carbondale, IL Zip 62901-1467, Mailing Address: P.O. Box 10000, Zip 62902-9000; tel. 618/549-0721; George Maroney, Senior Vice President and Administrator
Web address: www.sih.net

ST. JOSEPH MEMORIAL HOSPITAL (O, 40 beds) 2 South Hospital Drive, Murphysboro, IL Zip 62966-3333; tel. 618/687-3157; Betty Gaffney, Senior Vice President and Administrator
Web address: www.sih.net

UNITED MINE WORKERS OF AMERICA UNION HOSPITAL (O, 20 beds) 507 West St. Louis Street, West Frankfort, IL Zip 62896-1999; tel. 618/932-2155; Becky Ashton, Senior Vice President and Administrator
Web address: www.sih.net

Owned, leased, sponsored:	6 hospitals	437 beds
Contract-managed:	0 hospitals	0 beds
Totals:	6 hospitals	437 beds

★4195: SPARTANBURG REGIONAL HEALTHCARE SYSTEM (NP)
101 East Wood Street, Spartanburg, SC Zip 29303-3016; tel. 864/560-6000; Joseph Michael Oddis, President
(Moderately Centralized Health System)

SOUTH CAROLINA: B.J. WORKMAN MEMORIAL HOSPITAL (O, 43 beds) 751 East Georgia Street, Woodruff, SC Zip 29388, Mailing Address: P.O. Box 699, Zip 29388-0699; tel. 864/476-8122; Alan Caldwell, Administrator
Web address: www.srhs.com

SPARTANBURG HOSPITAL FOR RESTORATIVE CARE (O, 63 beds) 389 Serpentine Drive, Spartanburg, SC Zip 29303; tel. 864/560-3280; Anita M. Butler, Chief Executive Officer
Web address: www.srhs.com

SPARTANBURG REGIONAL MEDICAL CENTER (O, 408 beds) 101 East Wood Street, Spartanburg, SC Zip 29303-3016; tel. 864/560-6000; Joseph Michael Oddis, President
Web address: www.srhs.com

Owned, leased, sponsored:	3 hospitals	514 beds
Contract-managed:	0 hospitals	0 beds
Totals:	3 hospitals	514 beds

0905: SPECIALTY HOSPITAL GROUP (IO)
5 Concourse Parkway, Suite 800, Atlanta, GA Zip 30328-6111; tel. 770/392-1454; Bill Cook, President and Chief Executive Officer
(Independent Hospital System)

LOUISIANA: SUMMIT HOSPITAL OF NORTHWEST LOUISIANA (O, 54 beds) 4900 Medical Drive, Bossier City, LA Zip 71112-4596; tel. 318/747-9500; Louise Wiggins, Chief Executive Officer and Administrator

WEST CALCASIEU CAMERON HOSPITAL (O, 85 beds) 701 East Cypress Street, Sulphur, LA Zip 70663-5000, Mailing Address: P.O. Box 2509, Zip 70664-2509; tel. 337/527-4240; Wayne A. Swiniarski, FACHE, Chief Executive Officer

Owned, leased, sponsored:	2 hospitals	139 beds
Contract-managed:	0 hospitals	0 beds
Totals:	2 hospitals	139 beds

0177: SPECTRUM HEALTH (NP)
100 Michigan Street N.E., Grand Rapids, MI Zip 49503-2551; tel. 616/391-1174; Terrence M. O'Rourke, Interim Chief Executive Officer
(Moderately Centralized Health System)

MICHIGAN: SPECTRUM HEALTH (O, 857 beds) 1840 Wealthy Street S.E., Grand Rapids, MI Zip 49506-2921; tel. 616/774-7444; Terrence M. O'Rourke, President
Web address: www.spectrum-health.org

SPECTRUM HEALTH-KENT COMMUNITY CAMPUS (C, 356 beds) 750 Fuller Avenue N.E., Grand Rapids, MI Zip 49503-1995; tel. 616/336-3300; Lori Portfleet, Chief Executive Officer

SPECTRUM HEALTH-REED CITY CAMPUS (O, 85 beds) 300 North Patterson Road, Reed City, MI Zip 49677-0075; tel. 231/832-3271; Gary L. Petersen, President and Chief Executive Officer

Owned, leased, sponsored:	2 hospitals	942 beds
Contract-managed:	1 hospital	356 beds
Totals:	3 hospitals	1298 beds

★5455: SSM HEALTH CARE (CC)
477 North Lindbergh Boulevard, Saint Louis, MO Zip 63141-7813; tel. 314/994-7800; Sister Mary Jean Ryan, President and Chief Executive Officer
(Moderately Centralized Health System)

ILLINOIS: GOOD SAMARITAN REGIONAL HEALTH CENTER (O, 141 beds) 605 North 12th Street, Mount Vernon, IL Zip 62864-2899; tel. 618/242-4600; Leo F. Childers, Jr, FACHE, President
Web address: www.stmarys-goodsamaritan.com

SAINT FRANCIS HOSPITAL AND HEALTH CENTER (O, 256 beds) 12935 South Gregory Street, Blue Island, IL Zip 60406-2470; tel. 708/597-2000; Jay E. Kreuzer, FACHE, President
Web address: www.stfrancisblueisland.com

ST. MARY'S HOSPITAL (C, 276 beds) 400 North Pleasant Avenue, Centralia, IL Zip 62801-3091; tel. 618/532-6731; James W. McDowell, President

MISSOURI: CARDINAL GLENNON CHILDREN'S HOSPITAL (O, 172 beds) 1465 South Grand Boulevard, Saint Louis, MO Zip 63104-1095; tel. 314/577-5600; Douglas A. Ries, President
Web address: www.cardinalglennon.com/internet/net10hom.nsf/?Open

DEPAUL HEALTH CENTER (O, 375 beds) 12303 DePaul Drive, Saint Louis, MO Zip 63044-2588; tel. 314/344-6000; Robert G. Porter, President

PIKE COUNTY MEMORIAL HOSPITAL (C, 31 beds) 2305 West Georgia Street, Louisiana, MO Zip 63353-0020; tel. 573/754-5531; Gregory C. Reed, Administrator

SSM REHAB (O, 78 beds) 6420 Clayton Road, Suite 600, Saint Louis, MO Zip 63117-1861; tel. 314/768-5300; Melinda Clark, President

ST. FRANCIS HOSPITAL AND HEALTH SERVICES (O, 53 beds) 2016 South Main Street, Maryville, MO Zip 64468-2693; tel. 660/562-2600; Michael Baumgartner, President

ST. JOSEPH HEALTH CENTER (O, 273 beds) 300 First Capitol Drive, Saint Charles, MO Zip 63301-2835; tel. 636/947-5000; Kevin F. Kast, President, Chief Executive Officer and Market Executive

ST. JOSEPH HOSPITAL WEST (O, 58 beds) 100 Medical Plaza, Lake Saint Louis, MO Zip 63367-1395; tel. 314/625-5200; Kevin F. Kast, President, Chief Executive Officer and Market Executive

ST. JOSEPH HOSPITAL OF KIRKWOOD (O, 213 beds) 525 Couch Avenue, Saint Louis, MO Zip 63122-5594; tel. 314/966-1500; Carla S. Baum, President
Web address: www.stjosephkirkwood.com/internet/home/stjokirk.nsf

ST. MARY'S HEALTH CENTER (O, 460 beds) 6420 Clayton Road, Saint Louis, MO Zip 63117-1811; tel. 314/768-8000; James B. Rigby, Interim President

ST. MARYS HEALTH CENTER (O, 167 beds) 100 St. Marys Medical Plaza, Jefferson City, MO Zip 65101-1601; tel. 573/761-7000; Mark R. Taylor, President
Web address: www.stmarys-jeffcity.com/internet/home/stmaryjeff.nsf

OKLAHOMA: BONE AND JOINT HOSPITAL (O, 89 beds) 1111 North Dewey Avenue, Oklahoma City, OK Zip 73103-2615; tel. 405/552-9100; James A. Hyde, Administrator

HILLCREST HEALTH CENTER (O, 181 beds) 2129 S.W. 59th Street, Oklahoma City, OK Zip 73119-7001; tel. 405/685-6671; Ray Brazier, President

---

For explanation of codes following names, see page B2.
★ Indicates Type III membership in the American Hospital Association.

MISSION HILL MEMORIAL HOSPITAL (L, 49 beds) 1900 Gordon Cooper Drive, Shawnee, OK Zip 74801-8600; tel. 405/273-2240; Gray Cox, President

ST. ANTHONY HOSPITAL (O, 362 beds) 1000 North Lee Street, Oklahoma City, OK Zip 73102-1080, Mailing Address: P.O. Box 205, Zip 73101-0205; tel. 405/272-7000; Valinda Rutledge, President

WISCONSIN: ST. CLARE HOSPITAL AND HEALTH SERVICES (O, 82 beds) 707 14th Street, Baraboo, WI Zip 53913-1597; tel. 608/356-1400; David B. Jordahl, FACHE, President
Web address: www.stclare.com

ST. MARYS HOSPITAL MEDICAL CENTER (O, 287 beds) 707 South Mills Street, Madison, WI Zip 53715-0450; tel. 608/251-6100; Gerald W. Lefert, President
Web address: www.stmarysmadison.com

Owned, leased, sponsored:	17 hospitals	3296 beds
Contract-managed:	2 hospitals	307 beds
Totals:	19 hospitals	3603 beds

★**2255: ST. FRANCIS HEALTH SYSTEM** (NP)
4401 Penn Avenue, Pittsburgh, PA Zip 15224-1334; tel. 412/622-4214; Sister M. Rosita Wellinger, President and Chief Executive Officer
(Moderately Centralized Health System)

PENNSYLVANIA: ST. FRANCIS CENTRAL HOSPITAL (O, 136 beds) 1200 Centre Avenue, Pittsburgh, PA Zip 15219-3507; tel. 412/562-3000; Robin Z. Mohr, Chief Executive Officer
Web address: www.sfhs.edu

ST. FRANCIS HOSPITAL CRANBERRY (O, 185 beds) One St. Francis Way, Cranberry, PA Zip 16066; tel. 724/772-5300; John L. Spieler, Dr.PH, FACHE, Executive Director

ST. FRANCIS HOSPITAL OF NEW CASTLE (O, 193 beds) 1000 South Mercer Street, New Castle, PA Zip 16101-4673; tel. 724/658-3511; Sister Patricia Fogle, Chief Executive Officer
Web address: www.sfhs.edu

ST. FRANCIS MEDICAL CENTER (O, 715 beds) 400 45th Street, Pittsburgh, PA Zip 15201-1198; tel. 412/622-4343; Sister Donna Zwigart, FACHE, Chief Executive Officer
Web address: www.sfhs.edu

Owned, leased, sponsored:	4 hospitals	1229 beds
Contract-managed:	0 hospitals	0 beds
Totals:	4 hospitals	1229 beds

★**5425: ST. JOSEPH HEALTH SYSTEM** (CC)
440 South Batavia Street, Orange, CA Zip 92868-3995, Mailing Address: P.O. Box 14132, Zip 92613-1532; tel. 714/997-7690; Richard Statuto, Chief Executive Officer
(Decentralized Health System)

CALIFORNIA: MISSION HOSPITAL REGIONAL MEDICAL CENTER (O, 208 beds) 27700 Medical Center Road, Mission Viejo, CA Zip 92691; tel. 949/364-1400; Peter F. Bastone, President and Chief Executive Officer
Web address: www.mhrmc.com

NORTH COAST HEALTH CARE CENTERS (O, 119 beds) 1287 Fulton Road, Santa Rosa, CA Zip 95401; tel. 707/543-2400; Jeffrey Flocken, Interim President and Chief Executive Officer

PETALUMA VALLEY HOSPITAL (L, 82 beds) 400 North McDowell Boulevard, Petaluma, CA Zip 94954-2339; tel. 707/778-1111; Ramona Faith, R.N., MS, Site Administrator and Chief Nurse Executive

QUEEN OF THE VALLEY HOSPITAL (O, 166 beds) 1000 Trancas Street, Napa, CA Zip 94558, Mailing Address: Box 2340, Zip 94558; tel. 707/252-4411; Dennis Sisto, President and Chief Executive Officer
Web address: www.thequeen.org

REDWOOD MEMORIAL HOSPITAL (O, 35 beds) 3300 Renner Drive, Fortuna, CA Zip 95540; tel. 707/725-3361; Michael L. Purvis, President and Chief Executive Officer

SAINT JOSEPH HOSPITAL (O, 96 beds) 2700 Dolbeer Street, Eureka, CA Zip 95501; tel. 707/445-8121; Michael L. Purvis, President and Chief Executive Officer

SAINT MARY REGIONAL MEDICAL CENTER (O, 137 beds) 18300 Highway 18, Apple Valley, CA Zip 92307-0725, Mailing Address: P.O. Box 7025, Zip 92307-0725; tel. 760/242-2311; Catherine M. Pelley, President and Chief Executive Officer

SANTA ROSA MEMORIAL HOSPITAL (O, 225 beds) 1165 Montgomery Drive, Santa Rosa, CA Zip 95405, Mailing Address: P.O. Box 522, Zip 95402; tel. 707/546-3210; David J. Ameen, President and Chief Executive Officer

ST. JOSEPH HOSPITAL (O, 324 beds) 1100 West Stewart Drive, Orange, CA Zip 92668, Mailing Address: P.O. Box 5600, Zip 92613-5600; tel. 714/633-9111; Larry K. Ainsworth, President and Chief Executive Officer
Web address: www.sjo.stjoe.org

ST. JUDE MEDICAL CENTER (O, 347 beds) 101 East Valencia Mesa Drive, Fullerton, CA Zip 92835; tel. 714/992-3000; Robert J. Fraschetti, President and Chief Executive Officer
Web address: www.mhrmc.com

TEXAS: COVENANT CHILDREN'S HOSPITAL (O, 65 beds) 3610 21st Street, Lubbock, TX Zip 79410-1218; tel. 806/725-1011; Charley O. Trimble, President and Chief Executive Officer
Web address: www.covenanthealth.org

COVENANT HOSPITAL PLAINVIEW (O, 36 beds) 2601 Dimmitt Road, Plainview, TX Zip 79072-1833; tel. 806/296-5531; Joe S. Langford, Chief Executive Officer

COVENANT HOSPITAL-LEVELLAND (O, 49 beds) 1900 South College Avenue, Levelland, TX Zip 79336-6508; tel. 806/894-4963; Jerry Osburn, Administrator

COVENANT MEDICAL CENTER (O, 520 beds) 3615 19th Street, Lubbock, TX Zip 79410-1201, Mailing Address: P.O. Box 1201, Zip 79408-1201; tel. 806/725-1011; Charley O. Trimble, President and Chief Executive Officer
Web address: www.covenanthealth.org

COVENANT MEDICAL CENTER-LAKESIDE (O, 410 beds) 4000 24th Street, Lubbock, TX Zip 79410-1894; tel. 806/725-6000; Charley O. Trimble, President and Chief Executive Officer

CROSBYTON CLINIC HOSPITAL (C, 30 beds) 710 West Main Street, Crosbyton, TX Zip 79322-2143; tel. 806/675-2382; Jeffrey Madison, Administrator and Chief Executive Officer

D. M. COGDELL MEMORIAL HOSPITAL (C, 64 beds) 1700 Cogdell Boulevard, Snyder, TX Zip 79549-6198; tel. 915/573-6374; Jeff Reecer, Chief Executive Officer

SWISHER MEMORIAL HOSPITAL DISTRICT (C, 26 beds) 539 Southeast Second, Tulia, TX Zip 79088-2403, Mailing Address: P.O. Box 808, Zip 79088-0808; tel. 806/995-8200; Steve S. Holmes, Chief Executive Officer

YOAKUM COUNTY HOSPITAL (C, 21 beds) 412 Mustang Avenue, Denver City, TX Zip 79323-2750, Mailing Address: P.O. Drawer 1130, Zip 79323-1130; tel. 806/592-5484; Edward Rodgers, Chief Executive Officer

Owned, leased, sponsored:	15 hospitals	2819 beds
Contract-managed:	4 hospitals	141 beds
Totals:	19 hospitals	2960 beds

★**0156: STANFORD HEALTH CARE** (NP)
5 Thomas Mellon Circle, 305, San Francisco, CA Zip 94134; tel. 415/353-4500; David Hunter, Interim President and Chief Executive Officer
(Moderately Centralized Health System)

CALIFORNIA: LUCILE SALTER PACKARD CHILDREN'S HOSPITAL AT STANFORD (O, 214 beds) 725 Welch Road, Palo Alto, CA Zip 94304; tel. 650/497-8000; Christopher G. Dawes, President

STANFORD HOSPITAL AND CLINICS (O, 417 beds) 300 Pasteur Drive, Stanford, CA Zip 94305-5584; tel. 650/723-4000; Malinda S. Mitchell, President and Chief Executive Officer
Web address: www.med.stanford.edu/sumc/

Owned, leased, sponsored:	2 hospitals	631 beds
Contract-managed:	0 hospitals	0 beds
Totals:	2 hospitals	631 beds

For explanation of codes following names, see page B2.
★ Indicates Type III membership in the American Hospital Association.

Systems / Summit Health

0189: SUMMIT HEALTH (NP)
112 North Seventh Street, Chambersburg, PA Zip 17201;
tel. 717/267-7138; Norman B. Epstein, President
(Centralized Physician/Insurance Health System)

PENNSYLVANIA: CHAMBERSBURG HOSPITAL (O, 223 beds) 112 North Seventh Street, Chambersburg, PA Zip 17201-6005, Mailing Address: P.O. Box 6005, Zip 17201-6005; tel. 717/267-3000; Norman B. Epstein, President
Web address: www.summithealth.org

WAYNESBORO HOSPITAL (O, 62 beds) 501 East Main Street, Waynesboro, PA Zip 17268-2394; tel. 717/765-4000; Rita C. Brizzee, Chief Operating Officer
Web address: www.summithealth.org

Owned, leased, sponsored:	2 hospitals	285 beds
Contract-managed:	0 hospitals	0 beds
Totals:	2 hospitals	285 beds

★**0030: SUN HEALTH CORPORATION** (NP)
13180 North 103rd Drive, Sun City, AZ Zip 85351-3038, Mailing Address: P.O. Box 1278, Zip 85372-1278; tel. 623/876-5301; Leland W. Peterson, President and Chief Executive Officer
(Centralized Health System)

ARIZONA: DEL E. WEBB MEMORIAL HOSPITAL (O, 188 beds) 14502 West Meeker Boulevard, Sun City West, AZ Zip 85375-5299, Mailing Address: P.O. Box 5169, Sun City, Zip 85375-5169; tel. 623/214-4000; Thomas C. Dickson, Executive Vice President and Chief Operating Officer
Web address: www.sunhealth.org

WALTER O. BOSWELL MEMORIAL HOSPITAL (O, 313 beds) 10401 West Thunderbird Boulevard, Sun City, AZ Zip 85351-3092, Mailing Address: P.O. Box 1690, Zip 85372-1690; tel. 623/977-7211; George Perez, Executive Vice President and Chief Operating Officer
Web address: www.sunhealth.org

Owned, leased, sponsored:	2 hospitals	501 beds
Contract-managed:	0 hospitals	0 beds
Totals:	2 hospitals	501 beds

●**0210: SUN HEALTHCARE GROUP** (IO)
101 Sun Avenue Northeast, Albuquerque, NM Zip 87109;
tel. 505/821-3355; Andrew L. Turner, Chief Executive Officer and Chairman of the Board

KENTUCKY: MEDIPLEX REHABILITATION HOSPITAL (O, 60 beds) 1300 Campbell Lane, Bowling Green, KY Zip 42104-4162; tel. 270/782-6900; Shala S. Wilson, R.N., Chief Executive Officer
Web address: www.sunh.com

Owned, leased, sponsored:	1 hospital	60 beds
Contract-managed:	0 hospitals	0 beds
Totals:	1 hospital	60 beds

★**8795: SUTTER HEALTH** (NP)
One Capitol Mall, Sacramento, CA Zip 95814, Mailing Address: P.O. Box 160727, Zip 95816-0727; tel. 916/733-8800; Van R. Johnson, President and Chief Executive Officer
(Moderately Centralized Health System)

CALIFORNIA: ALTA BATES MEDICAL CENTER-ASHBY CAMPUS (O, 468 beds) 2450 Ashby Avenue, Berkeley, CA Zip 94705; tel. 510/204-4444; Warren J. Kirk, President and Chief Administrative Officer
Web address: www.ahabates.com

CALIFORNIA PACIFIC MEDICAL CENTER (C, 520 beds) 2333 Buchanan Street, San Francisco, CA Zip 94115, Mailing Address: P.O. Box 7999, Zip 94120; tel. 415/563-4321; Martin Brotman, M.D., President and Chief Executive Officer
Web address: www.cpmc.org

DAMERON HOSPITAL (O, 211 beds) 525 West Acacia Street, Stockton, CA Zip 95203; tel. 209/944-5550; Christopher Arismendi, M.D., Administrator
Web address: www.sutterhealth.org

EDEN MEDICAL CENTER (O, 258 beds) 20103 Lake Chabot Road, Castro Valley, CA Zip 94546; tel. 510/537-1234; George Bischalaney, President and Chief Executive Officer
Web address: www.edenmedcenter.org

MARIN GENERAL HOSPITAL (O, 165 beds) 250 Bon Air Road, Greenbrae, CA Zip 94904, Mailing Address: Box 8010, San Rafael, Zip 94912-8010; tel. 415/925-7000; Henry J. Buhrmann, President and Chief Executive Officer
Web address: www.maringeneral.com

MEMORIAL HOSPITALS ASSOCIATION (O, 296 beds) Modesto, CA Mailing Address: P.O. Box 942, Zip 95353-0942; tel. 209/526-4500; David P. Benn, President and Chief Executive Officer
Web address: www.sutterhealth.org

MILLS-PENINSULA HEALTH SERVICES (O, 358 beds) 1783 El Camino Real, Burlingame, CA Zip 94010-3205; tel. 650/696-5400; Robert W. Merwin, Chief Executive Officer
Web address: www.mphs.org

NOVATO COMMUNITY HOSPITAL (O, 33 beds) 1625 Hill Road, Novato, CA Zip 94947, Mailing Address: P.O. Box 1108, Zip 94948; tel. 415/897-3111; Anne L. Hosfeld, Chief Administrative Officer
Web address: www.novatocommunity.com

SUMMIT MEDICAL CENTER (O, 420 beds) 350 Hawthorne Avenue, Oakland, CA Zip 94609; tel. 510/655-4000; Irwin C. Hansen, President and Chief Executive Officer

SUTTER AMADOR HOSPITAL (O, 85 beds) 200 Mission Boulevard, Jackson, CA Zip 95642-2379; tel. 209/223-7500; Scott Stenberg, Chief Executive Officer
Web address: www.sutterhealth.org

SUTTER AUBURN FAITH COMMUNITY HOSPITAL (O, 105 beds) 11815 Education Street, Auburn, CA Zip 95603; tel. 530/888-4500; Mitch Hanna, Chief Administrative Officer
Web address: www.sutterhealth.org

SUTTER CENTER FOR PSYCHIATRY (O, 69 beds) 7700 Folsom Boulevard, Sacramento, CA Zip 95826-2608; tel. 916/386-3000; Diane Gail Stewart, Chief Administrative Officer
Web address: www.sutterhealth.org

SUTTER COAST HOSPITAL (O, 59 beds) 800 East Washington Boulevard, Crescent City, CA Zip 95531; tel. 707/464-8511; John E. Menaugh, Chief Executive Officer
Web address: www.sutterhealth.org

SUTTER DAVIS HOSPITAL (O, 48 beds) 2000 Sutter Place, Davis, CA Zip 95616, Mailing Address: P.O. Box 1617, Zip 95617; tel. 530/756-6440; Janet Wagner, Chief Administrative Officer
Web address: www.sutterhealth.org

SUTTER DELTA MEDICAL CENTER (O, 111 beds) 3901 Lone Tree Way, Antioch, CA Zip 94509; tel. 925/779-7200; Linda Horn, Chief Executive Officer
Web address: www.sutterhealth.org

SUTTER LAKESIDE HOSPITAL (O, 54 beds) 5176 Hill Road East, Lakeport, CA Zip 95453-6111; tel. 707/262-5001; Gilbert Silbernagel, Chief Executive Officer
Web address: www.sutterlake.org

SUTTER MATERNITY AND SURGERY CENTER OF SANTA CRUZ (O, 30 beds) 2900 Chanticleer Avenue, Santa Cruz, CA Zip 95065-1816;
tel. 831/477-2200; David T. Hughes, FACHE, Chief Executive Officer
Web address: www.sutterhealth.org

SUTTER MEDICAL CENTER (O, 469 beds) 5151 F Street, Sacramento, CA Zip 95819-3295; tel. 916/454-3333; Lawrence A. Maas, Chief Executive Officer
Web address: www.sutterhealth.org

SUTTER MEDICAL CENTER, SANTA ROSA (O, 128 beds) 3325 Chanate Road, Santa Rosa, CA Zip 95404; tel. 707/576-4000; Cliff Coates, Chief Executive Officer
Web address: www.sutterhealth.org

SUTTER MERCED MEDICAL CENTER (O, 158 beds) 301 East 13th Street, Merced, CA Zip 95340-6211; tel. 209/385-7000; Paul F. Dyer, Administrator
Web address: www.sutterhealth.org

For explanation of codes following names, see page B2.
★ Indicates Type III membership in the American Hospital Association.
● Single hospital health care system

Systems / Tenet Healthcare Corporation

SUTTER ROSEVILLE MEDICAL CENTER (O, 183 beds) One Medical Plaza, Roseville, CA Zip 95661-3477; tel. 916/781-1000; Patrick R. Brady, Chief Executive Officer
Web address: www.sutterhealth.org

SUTTER SOLANO MEDICAL CENTER (O, 111 beds) 300 Hospital Drive, Vallejo, CA Zip 94589-2517, Mailing Address: P.O. Box 3189, Zip 94589; tel. 707/554-4444; Beverly Gilmore, Chief Executive Officer
Web address: www.sutterhealth.org

SUTTER TRACY COMMUNITY HOSPITAL (O, 71 beds) 1420 North Tracy Boulevard, Tracy, CA Zip 95376-3497; tel. 209/835-1500; Gary D. Rapaport, Chief Executive Officer
Web address: www.suttertracy.org

HAWAII: KAHI MOHALA (O, 88 beds) 91-2301 Fort Weaver Road, Ewa Beach, HI Zip 96706; tel. 808/671-8511; Margi Drue, Administrator
Web address: www.kahi.org

Owned, leased, sponsored:	23 hospitals	3978 beds
Contract-managed:	1 hospital	520 beds
Totals:	24 hospitals	4498 beds

0039: TARRANT COUNTY HOSPITAL DISTRICT (NP)
1500 South Main Street, Fort Worth, TX Zip 76104-4941; tel. 817/927-1230; Anthony J. Alcini, President and Chief Executive Officer
(Independent Hospital System)

TEXAS: JPS HEALTH NETWORK (O, 293 beds) 1500 South Main Street, Fort Worth, TX Zip 76104-4941; tel. 817/921-3431; Anthony J. Alcini, President and Chief Executive Officer
Web address: www.jpshealthnet.org

TRINITY SPRINGS PAVILION (O, 34 beds) 1500 South Main Street, Fort Worth, TX Zip 76104-4917; tel. 817/927-3636; Robert N. Bourassa, Executive Director

Owned, leased, sponsored:	2 hospitals	327 beds
Contract-managed:	0 hospitals	0 beds
Totals:	2 hospitals	327 beds

0169: TEMPLE UNIVERSITY HEALTH SYSTEM (NP)
3401 North Broad Street, 1st Floor, Philadelphia, PA Zip 19140; tel. 215/707-8000; Leon S. Malmud, M.D., President
(Moderately Centralized Health System)

PENNSYLVANIA: EPISCOPAL HOSPITAL (O, 218 beds) 100 East Lehigh Avenue, Philadelphia, PA Zip 19125-1098; tel. 215/427-7000; Kathleen Barron, Executive Director

JEANES HOSPITAL (O, 188 beds) 7600 Central Avenue, Philadelphia, PA Zip 19111-2499; tel. 215/728-2000; G. Roger Martin, President and Chief Executive Officer
Web address: www.jeanes.com

LOWER BUCKS HOSPITAL (O, 166 beds) 501 Bath Road, Bristol, PA Zip 19007-3190; tel. 215/785-9200; Nathan Bosk, FACHE, Chief Executive Officer

NORTHEASTERN HOSPITAL OF PHILADELPHIA (O, 166 beds) 2301 East Allegheny Avenue, Philadelphia, PA Zip 19134-4497; tel. 215/291-3000; Lynn Holder, Executive Director

TEMPLE EAST, NEUMANN MEDICAL CENTER (O, 166 beds) 1741 Frankford Avenue, Philadelphia, PA Zip 19125-2495; tel. 215/291-2000; Robert P. Perry, Executive Director and Chief Executive Officer
Web address: www.neumann.org

TEMPLE UNIVERSITY HOSPITAL (O, 439 beds) Broad and Ontario Streets, Philadelphia, PA Zip 19140-5192; tel. 215/707-2000; Paul Boehringer, Executive Director
Web address: www.allcet.com/tuhs/index.htm

Owned, leased, sponsored:	6 hospitals	1343 beds
Contract-managed:	0 hospitals	0 beds
Totals:	6 hospitals	1343 beds

★0063: TENET HEALTHCARE CORPORATION (IO)
3820 State Street, Santa Barbara, CA Zip 93105, Mailing Address: P.O. Box 31907, Zip 93130; tel. 805/563-7000; Jeffrey Barbakow, Chairman and Chief Executive Officer
(Decentralized Health System)

ALABAMA: BROOKWOOD MEDICAL CENTER (O, 497 beds) 2010 Brookwood Medical Center Drive, Birmingham, AL Zip 35209; tel. 205/877-1000; John R. Nickens, II, Chief Executive Officer
Web address: www.brookwood-medical.com

ARKANSAS: CENTRAL ARKANSAS HOSPITAL (O, 148 beds) 1200 South Main Street, Searcy, AR Zip 72143-7397; tel. 501/278-3131; David C. Laffoon, CHE, Chief Executive Officer
Web address: www.tenethealth.com

NATIONAL PARK MEDICAL CENTER (O, 166 beds) 1910 Malvern Avenue, Hot Springs, AR Zip 71901-7799; tel. 501/321-1000; Jerry D. Mabry, Executive Director
Web address: www.tenethealth.com

REGIONAL MEDICAL CENTER OF NORTHEAST ARKANSAS (O, 104 beds) 3024 Stadium Boulevard, Jonesboro, AR Zip 72401-7493; tel. 870/972-7000; Philip H. Walkley, Jr, Chief Executive Officer
Web address: www.tenethealth.com/jonesboro

SAINT MARY'S REGIONAL MEDICAL CENTER (O, 150 beds) 1808 West Main Street, Russellville, AR Zip 72801-2724; tel. 501/968-2841; Mike McCoy, Chief Executive Officer
Web address: www.tenethealth.com/saintmarys

CALIFORNIA: ALVARADO HOSPITAL MEDICAL CENTER (O, 144 beds) 6655 Alvarado Road, San Diego, CA Zip 92120-5298; tel. 619/287-3270; Barry G. Weinbaum, Chief Executive Officer
Web address: www.tenethealh.com

BROTMAN MEDICAL CENTER (O, 244 beds) 3828 Delmas Terrace, Culver City, CA Zip 90231-2459, Mailing Address: Box 2459, Zip 90231-2459; tel. 310/836-7000; Sonja Hagel, Chief Executive Officer
Web address: www.tenethealth.com

CENTINELA HOSPITAL MEDICAL CENTER (O, 377 beds) 555 East Hardy Street, Inglewood, CA Zip 90301-4073, Mailing Address: Box 720, Zip 90307-0720; tel. 310/673-4660; Michael A. Rembis, FACHE, Chief Executive Officer
Web address: www.tenethealth.com

CENTURY CITY HOSPITAL (L, 156 beds) 2070 Century Park East, Los Angeles, CA Zip 90067; tel. 310/553-6211; Stephen M. Tullman, Chief Executive Officer
Web address: www.tenethealth.com

CHAPMAN MEDICAL CENTER (L, 40 beds) 2601 East Chapman Avenue, Orange, CA Zip 92869; tel. 714/633-0011; Maxine T. Cooper, Chief Executive Officer
Web address: www.tenethealth.com

COASTAL COMMUNITIES HOSPITAL (O, 178 beds) 2701 South Bristol Street, Santa Ana, CA Zip 92704-9911; tel. 714/754-5454; Robert C. Caldwell, Chief Executive Officer
Web address: www.tenethealth.com

COMMUNITY HOSPITAL OF HUNTINGTON PARK (L, 226 beds) 2623 East Slauson Avenue, Huntington Park, CA Zip 90255; tel. 323/583-1931; Charles Martinez, Ph.D., Chief Executive Officer
Web address: www.tenethealh.com

COMMUNITY HOSPITAL OF LOS GATOS (L, 153 beds) 815 Pollard Road, Los Gatos, CA Zip 95030; tel. 408/378-6131; Daniel P. Doore, Chief Executive Officer

DESERT REGIONAL MEDICAL CENTER (L, 348 beds) 1150 North Indian Canyon Drive, Palm Springs, CA Zip 92262, Mailing Address: Box 2739, Zip 92263; tel. 760/323-6511; Truman L. Gates, President and Chief Executive Officer
Web address: www.tenethealh.com

DOCTORS HOSPITAL OF MANTECA (O, 73 beds) 1205 East North Street, Manteca, CA Zip 95336; tel. 209/823-3111; Tim A. Joslin, Chief Executive Officer

DOCTORS MEDICAL CENTER (O, 392 beds) 1441 Florida Avenue, Modesto, CA Zip 95350-4418, Mailing Address: P.O. Box 4138, Zip 95352-4138; tel. 209/578-1211; Tim A. Joslin, Chief Executive Officer

---

For explanation of codes following names, see page B2.
★ Indicates Type III membership in the American Hospital Association.

Systems / Tenet Healthcare Corporation

DOCTORS MEDICAL CENTER–PINOLE CAMPUS (L, 137 beds) 2151 Appian Way, Pinole, CA Zip 94564; tel. 510/970–5000; Gary Sloan, Chief Executive Officer
Web address: www.tenethealth.com

DOCTORS MEDICAL CENTER–SAN PABLO CAMPUS (L, 286 beds) 2000 Vale Road, San Pablo, CA Zip 94806; tel. 510/970–5102; Gary Sloan, Chief Executive Officer

ENCINO–TARZANA REGIONAL MEDICAL CENTER ENCINO CAMPUS (L, 151 beds) 16237 Ventura Boulevard, Encino, CA Zip 91436–2201; tel. 818/995–5000

ENCINO–TARZANA REGIONAL MEDICAL CENTER TARZANA CAMPUS (L, 232 beds) 18321 Clark Street, Tarzana, CA Zip 91356; tel. 818/881–0800; Dale Surowitz, Chief Executive Officer
Web address: www.tenethealh.com

FOUNTAIN VALLEY REGIONAL HOSPITAL AND MEDICAL CENTER (O, 396 beds) 17100 Euclid at Warner, Fountain Valley, CA Zip 92708; tel. 714/966–7200; Tim Smith, President and Chief Executive Officer
Web address: www.tenethealh.com

GARDEN GROVE HOSPITAL AND MEDICAL CENTER (O, 167 beds) 12601 Garden Grove Boulevard, Garden Grove, CA Zip 92843–1959; tel. 714/537–5160; Mark A. Meyers, President and Chief Executive Officer
Web address: www.tenethealh.com

GARFIELD MEDICAL CENTER (O, 211 beds) 525 North Garfield Avenue, Monterey Park, CA Zip 91754; tel. 626/573–2222; Philip A. Cohen, Chief Executive Officer
Web address: www.tenethealh.com

GREATER EL MONTE COMMUNITY HOSPITAL (O, 115 beds) 1701 South Santa Anita Avenue, South El Monte, CA Zip 91733–9918; tel. 626/579–7777; Deborah G. Webber, Chief Executive Officer
Web address: www.tenethealh.com

IRVINE REGIONAL HOSPITAL AND MEDICAL CENTER (L, 176 beds) 16200 Sand Canyon Avenue, Irvine, CA Zip 92618–3714; tel. 949/753–2000; Dan F. Ausman, Chief Executive Officer
Web address: www.tenethealh.com

JOHN F. KENNEDY MEMORIAL HOSPITAL (O, 130 beds) 47–111 Monroe Street, Indio, CA Zip 92201, Mailing Address: P.O. Drawer LLLL, Zip 92202–2558; tel. 760/347–6191; Truman L. Gates, President and Chief Executive Officer
Web address: www.tenethealh.com

LAKEWOOD REGIONAL MEDICAL CENTER (O, 148 beds) 3700 East South Street, Lakewood, CA Zip 90712; tel. 562/531–2550; Kenneth I. Rivers, Chief Executive Officer
Web address: www.tenethealh.com

LOS ALAMITOS MEDICAL CENTER (O, 173 beds) 3751 Katella Avenue, Los Alamitos, CA Zip 90720; tel. 562/598–1311; Michele Finney, Chief Executive Officer
Web address: www.tenethealh.com

MIDWAY HOSPITAL MEDICAL CENTER (O, 150 beds) 5925 San Vicente Boulevard, Los Angeles, CA Zip 90019–6696; tel. 323/938–3161; Stephen M. Tullman, Chief Executive Officer
Web address: www.tenethealh.com

MONTEREY PARK HOSPITAL (O, 95 beds) 900 South Atlantic Boulevard, Monterey Park, CA Zip 91754; tel. 626/570–9000; Philip A. Cohen, Chief Executive Officer
Web address: www.tenethealh.com

PLACENTIA LINDA HOSPITAL (O, 114 beds) 1301 Rose Drive, Placentia, CA Zip 92870; tel. 714/993–2000; Maxine T. Cooper, Chief Executive Officer
Web address: www.tenethealth.com/placentialinda

QUEEN OF ANGELS–HOLLYWOOD PRESBYTERIAN MEDICAL CENTER (O, 409 beds) 1300 North Vermont Avenue, Los Angeles, CA Zip 90027–0069; tel. 323/413–3000; Lou Lazatin, Chief Executive Officer
Web address: www.tenethealh.com

RANCHO SPRINGS MEDICAL CENTER (O, 99 beds) 25500 Medical Center Drive, Murrieta, CA Zip 92562–5966; tel. 909/696–6000; Harris Koenig, Chief Executive Officer
Web address: www.tenethealh.com

REDDING MEDICAL CENTER (O, 188 beds) 1100 Butte Street, Redding, CA Zip 96001–0853, Mailing Address: Box 496072, Zip 96049–6072; tel. 530/244–5454; Steve Schmidt, Chief Executive Officer

SAN DIMAS COMMUNITY HOSPITAL (O, 93 beds) 1350 West Covina Boulevard, San Dimas, CA Zip 91773–0308; tel. 909/599–6811; Garry M. Olney, R.N., Chief Executive Officer
Web address: www.tenethealth.com

SAN RAMON REGIONAL MEDICAL CENTER (O, 95 beds) 6001 Norris Canyon Road, San Ramon, CA Zip 94583; tel. 925/275–9200; Philip P. Gustafson, Administrator
Web address: www.sanramonmedctr.com

SANTA ANA HOSPITAL MEDICAL CENTER (L, 90 beds) 1901 North Fairview Street, Santa Ana, CA Zip 92706; tel. 714/554–1653; Robert C. Caldwell, Chief Executive Officer
Web address: www.tenethealth.com

SIERRA VISTA REGIONAL MEDICAL CENTER (O, 117 beds) 1010 Murray Street, San Luis Obispo, CA Zip 93405, Mailing Address: Box 1367, Zip 93406–1367; tel. 805/546–7600; Sean O'Neal, Administrator
Web address: www.tenethealth.com

ST. LUKE MEDICAL CENTER (O, 148 beds) 2632 East Washington Boulevard, Pasadena, CA Zip 91107–1994; tel. 626/797–1141; Phyllis Bushart, R.N., Chief Executive Officer
Web address: www.tenethealh.com

SUBURBAN MEDICAL CENTER (L, 130 beds) 16453 South Colorado Avenue, Paramount, CA Zip 90723; tel. 562/531–3110; Kenneth I. Rivers, Chief Executive Officer
Web address: www.tenethealth.com/suburban

TWIN CITIES COMMUNITY HOSPITAL (O, 72 beds) 1100 Las Tablas Road, Templeton, CA Zip 93465; tel. 805/434–3500; Harold E. Chilton, Chief Executive Officer
Web address: www.tenethealth.com

USC UNIVERSITY HOSPITAL (L, 285 beds) 1500 San Pablo Street, Los Angeles, CA Zip 90033–4585; tel. 323/442–8500; Edward Schreck, Chief Executive Officer
Web address: www.uscuh.com

UNIVERSITY OF SOUTHERN CALIFORNIA–KENNETH NORRIS JR. CANCER HOSPITAL (O, 60 beds) 1441 Eastlake Avenue, Los Angeles, CA Zip 90033–1085, Mailing Address: P.O. Box 33804, Zip 90033–3804; tel. 323/865–3000; Ted Schreck, Chief Executive Officer
Web address: www.uscnorris.com

WESTERN MEDICAL CENTER HOSPITAL ANAHEIM (O, 183 beds) 1025 South Anaheim Boulevard, Anaheim, CA Zip 92805; tel. 714/533–6220; Mark A. Meyers, President and Chief Executive Officer
Web address: www.tenethealth.com

WESTERN MEDICAL CENTER–SANTA ANA (O, 296 beds) 1001 North Tustin Avenue, Santa Ana, CA Zip 92705–3502; tel. 714/835–3555; Daniel Brothman, Chief Executive Officer
Web address: www.tenethealth.com/westermedical

WHITTIER HOSPITAL MEDICAL CENTER (O, 181 beds) 9080 Colima Road, Whittier, CA Zip 90605; tel. 562/907–1541; Sandra M. Chester, Chief Executive Officer
Web address: www.tenethealth.com

FLORIDA: CORAL GABLES HOSPITAL (O, 150 beds) 3100 Douglas Road, Coral Gables, FL Zip 33134–6990; tel. 305/445–8461; Martha Garcia, Chief Executive Officer
Web address: www.tenethealth.com/coralgables

DELRAY MEDICAL CENTER (O, 313 beds) 5352 Linton Boulevard, Delray Beach, FL Zip 33484–6580; tel. 561/498–4440; Mitchell S. Feldman, Chief Executive Officer

FLORIDA MEDICAL CENTER (O, 459 beds) 5000 West Oakland Park Boulevard, Fort Lauderdale, FL Zip 33313–1585; tel. 954/735–6000; Joel Bergenfeld, Chief Executive Officer
Web address: www.tenethealth.com

HIALEAH HOSPITAL (O, 411 beds) 651 East 25th Street, Hialeah, FL Zip 33013–3878; tel. 305/693–6100; Aurelio Fernandez, Chief Executive Officer
Web address: www.tenethealth.com

HOLLYWOOD MEDICAL CENTER (O, 238 beds) 3600 Washington Street, Hollywood, FL Zip 33021–8216; tel. 954/966–4500; Steven MacLauchlan, Chief Executive Officer
Web address: www.tenethealth.com

For explanation of codes following names, see page B2.
★ Indicates Type III membership in the American Hospital Association.

Systems / Tenet Healthcare Corporation

NORTH RIDGE MEDICAL CENTER (O, 391 beds) 5757 North Dixie Highway, Fort Lauderdale, FL Zip 33334–4182, Mailing Address: P.O. Box 23160, Zip 33307; tel. 954/776–6000; Clifford J. Bauer, Chief Executive Officer
Web address: www.tenethealth/northridge.com

NORTH SHORE MEDICAL CENTER (O, 286 beds) 1100 N.W. 95th Street, Miami, FL Zip 33150–2098; tel. 305/835–6000; Allan E. Atzrott, President and Chief Executive Officer
Web address: www.northshoremedical.com/

PALM BEACH GARDENS MEDICAL CENTER (L, 204 beds) 3360 Burns Road, Palm Beach Gardens, FL Zip 33410–4304; tel. 561/622–1411; Clint Matthews, Chief Executive Officer
Web address: www.tenethealth.com

PALMETTO GENERAL HOSPITAL (O, 360 beds) 2001 West 68th Street, Hialeah, FL Zip 33016–1898; tel. 305/823–5000; Ron Stern, Chief Executive Officer
Web address: www.tenethealth.com

PARKWAY REGIONAL MEDICAL CENTER (O, 392 beds) 160 N.W. 170th Street, North Miami Beach, FL Zip 33169–5576; tel. 305/654–5050; Peter A. Marmerstein, Chief Executive Officer
Web address: www.tenethealth.com

PINECREST REHABILITATION HOSPITAL (O, 90 beds) 5360 Linton Boulevard, Delray Beach, FL Zip 33484–6538; tel. 561/495–0400; Paul D. Echelard, Administrator
Web address: www.tenethealth.com

SEVEN RIVERS COMMUNITY HOSPITAL (O, 128 beds) 6201 North Suncoast Boulevard, Crystal River, FL Zip 34428–6712; tel. 352/795–6560; Donald McKenna, Chief Executive Officer
Web address: www.sevenrivershospital.com/

WEST BOCA MEDICAL CENTER (O, 150 beds) 21644 State Road 7, Boca Raton, FL Zip 33428–1899; tel. 561/488–8000; Richard Gold, Chief Executive Officer
Web address: www.tenethealth.com

GEORGIA: ATLANTA MEDICAL CENTER (O, 450 beds) 303 Parkway Drive N.E., Atlanta, GA Zip 30312–1212; tel. 404/265–4000; Bruce F. Buchanan, FACHE, President and Chief Executive Officer
Web address: www.atlantamedcenter.com

NORTH FULTON REGIONAL HOSPITAL (L, 167 beds) 3000 Hospital Boulevard, Roswell, GA Zip 30076–9930; tel. 770/751–2500; John F. Holland, President
Web address: www.northfultonregional.com/

SPALDING REGIONAL HOSPITAL (O, 160 beds) 601 South Eighth Street, Griffin, GA Zip 30224–4294, Mailing Address: P.O. Drawer V, Zip 30224–1168; tel. 770/228–2721; Lex A. Guinn, Chief Executive Officer

SYLVAN GROVE HOSPITAL (L, 28 beds) 1050 McDonough Road, Jackson, GA Zip 30233–1599; tel. 770/775–7861; Jean Dodson, Administrator
Web address: www.tenethealth.com

INDIANA: WINONA MEMORIAL HOSPITAL (O, 169 beds) 3232 North Meridian Street, Indianapolis, IN Zip 46208–4693; tel. 317/924–3392; David L. Callecod, CHE, Chief Executive Officer
Web address: www.tenethealth.com

LOUISIANA: DOCTORS HOSPITAL OF JEFFERSON (L, 130 beds) 4320 Houma Boulevard, Metairie, LA Zip 70006–2973; tel. 504/849–4000; John E. Walker, Chief Executive Officer
Web address: www.tenethealth.com

KENNER REGIONAL MEDICAL CENTER (O, 213 beds) 180 West Esplanade Avenue, Kenner, LA Zip 70065–6001; tel. 504/468–8600; Deborah C. Keel, Chief Executive Officer
Web address: www.tenethealh.com

MEADOWCREST HOSPITAL (O, 181 beds) 2500 Belle Chase Highway, Gretna, LA Zip 70056–7196; tel. 504/392–3131; Gerald L. Parton, Chief Executive Officer
Web address: www.tenethealth.com

MEMORIAL MEDICAL CENTER (O, 389 beds) New Orleans, LA Randall L. Hoover, Chief Executive Officer

NORTHSHORE PSYCHIATRIC HOSPITAL (O, 58 beds) 104 Medical Center Drive, Slidell, LA Zip 70461–7838; tel. 504/646–5500; George H. Perry, Ph.D., Chief Executive Officer
Web address: www.tenethealth.com

NORTHSHORE REGIONAL MEDICAL CENTER (L, 147 beds) 100 Medical Center Drive, Slidell, LA Zip 70461–8572; tel. 504/649–7070; L. Rene' Goux, Chief Executive Officer
Web address: www.tenethealth.com

ST. CHARLES GENERAL HOSPITAL (O, 137 beds) 3700 St. Charles Avenue, New Orleans, LA Zip 70115–4680; tel. 504/899–7441; L. Rene' Goux, Chief Executive Officer
Web address: www.tenethealth.com

MASSACHUSETTS: METROWEST MEDICAL CENTER (O, 398 beds) 115 Lincoln Street, Framingham, MA Zip 01702; tel. 508/383–1000; Mary Jo Gregory, Chief Executive Officer
Web address: www.mwmc.com

SAINT VINCENT HOSPITAL (O, 369 beds) 25 Winthrop Street, Worcester, MA Zip 01604–4593; tel. 508/798–1234; Robert E. Maher, Jr, President and Chief Executive Officer
Web address: www.svh–worc.com

MISSISSIPPI: GULF COAST MEDICAL CENTER (O, 189 beds) 180–A Debuys Road, Biloxi, MS Zip 39531–4405; tel. 228/388–6711; Gary L. Stokes, Chief Executive Officer

MISSOURI: COMPTON HEIGHTS HOSPITAL (O, 192 beds) 3545 Lafayette Avenue, Saint Louis, MO Zip 63104–9984; tel. 314/865–6500; Leona D. Stoll, Chief Executive Officer
Web address: www.tenethealth.com

DES PERES HOSPITAL (O, 93 beds) 2345 Dougherty Ferry Road, Saint Louis, MO Zip 63122–3313; tel. 314/768–3000; Michele C. Meyer, Chief Executive Officer
Web address: www.tenethealth.com

FOREST PARK HOSPITAL (O, 288 beds) 6150 Oakland Avenue, Saint Louis, MO Zip 63139–3297; tel. 314/768–3000; John W. Sanders, Chief Executive Officer
Web address: www.tenethealth.com

LUCY LEE HOSPITAL (L, 173 beds) 2620 North Westwood Boulevard, Poplar Bluff, MO Zip 63901–2341, Mailing Address: P.O. Box 88, Zip 63901–2341; tel. 573/785–7721; Timothy F. Brady, FACHE, Chief Executive Officer
Web address: www.tenethealth.com

SAINT LOUIS UNIVERSITY HOSPITAL (O, 303 beds) 3635 Vista at Grand Boulevard, Saint Louis, MO Zip 63110–0250, Mailing Address: P.O. Box 15250, Zip 63110–0250; tel. 314/577–8000; Lee D. Stoll, Chief Executive Officer
Web address: www.stlucare.edu

SOUTHPOINTE HOSPITAL (O, 249 beds) 2639 Miami Street, Saint Louis, MO Zip 63118–3999; tel. 314/772–1456; Doug Doris, Chief Executive Officer
Web address: www.tenethealth.com

TWIN RIVERS REGIONAL MEDICAL CENTER (O, 116 beds) 1301 First Street, Kennett, MO Zip 63857–2508; tel. 573/888–4522; Dale R. Mulder, Chief Executive Officer
Web address: www.tenethealth.com

NEBRASKA: ST. JOSEPH HOSPITAL (O, 278 beds) 601 North 30th Street, Omaha, NE Zip 68131–2197; tel. 402/449–5021; J. Richard Stanko, President and Chief Executive Officer

NEVADA: LAKE MEAD HOSPITAL MEDICAL CENTER (O, 184 beds) 1409 East Lake Mead Boulevard, North Las Vegas, NV Zip 89030–7197; tel. 702/649–7711; William P. Moore, Chief Executive Officer
Web address: www.tenethealth.com

NORTH CAROLINA: CENTRAL CAROLINA HOSPITAL (O, 137 beds) 1135 Carthage Street, Sanford, NC Zip 27330; tel. 919/774–2100; L. Glenn Davis, Executive Director
Web address: www.centralcarolinahosp.com/

FRYE REGIONAL MEDICAL CENTER (L, 355 beds) 420 North Center Street, Hickory, NC Zip 28601–5049; tel. 828/322–6070; Dennis J. Phillips, Chief Executive Officer

PENNSYLVANIA: ELKINS PARK HOSPITAL (O, 158 beds) 60 East Township Line Road, Elkins Park, PA Zip 19027–2220; tel. 215/663–6000; Richard Centafont, Chief Executive Officer
Web address: www.auhs.edu

GRADUATE HOSPITAL (O, 198 beds) One Graduate Plaza, Philadelphia, PA Zip 19146–1407; tel. 215/893–2000; Christopher DiCicco, Chief Executive Officer

For explanation of codes following names, see page B2.
★ Indicates Type III membership in the American Hospital Association.

Systems / Tenet Healthcare Corporation

HAHNEMANN UNIVERSITY HOSPITAL (O, 540 beds) Broad and Vine Streets, Philadelphia, PA Zip 19102–1192; tel. 215/762–7000; Michael P. Halter, Chief Executive Officer
Web address: www.auhs.edu

MEDICAL COLLEGE OF PENNSYLVANIA HOSPITAL (O, 369 beds) 3300 Henry Avenue, Philadelphia, PA Zip 19129–1121; tel. 215/842–6000; Richard S. Freeman, Chief Executive Officer

PARKVIEW HOSPITAL (O, 165 beds) 1331 East Wyoming Avenue, Philadelphia, PA Zip 19124–3808; tel. 215/537–7400; David J. Fikse, Chief Executive Officer

ST. CHRISTOPHER'S HOSPITAL FOR CHILDREN (O, 178 beds) Erie Avenue at Front Street, Philadelphia, PA Zip 19134–1095; tel. 215/427–5000; Jeffrey Green, Chief Executive Officer

WARMINSTER HOSPITAL (O, 132 beds) 225 Newtown Road, Warminster, PA Zip 18974–5221; tel. 215/441–6600; Jeffrey Yarmel, Chief Executive Officer
Web address: www.warminsterhospital.com

SOUTH CAROLINA: EAST COOPER REGIONAL MEDICAL CENTER (O, 112 beds) 1200 Johnnie Dodds Boulevard, Mount Pleasant, SC Zip 29464–3294; tel. 843/881–0100; Jack Dusenbery, President
Web address: www.tenethealth.com

HILTON HEAD MEDICAL CENTER AND CLINICS (O, 79 beds) 25 Hospital Center Boulevard, Hilton Head Island, SC Zip 29926, Mailing Address: P.O. Box 21117, Zip 29925–1117; tel. 843/681–6122; Dennis Ray Bruns, President and Chief Executive Officer
Web address: www.tenethealth.com

PIEDMONT HEALTHCARE SYSTEM (O, 276 beds) 222 Herlong Avenue, Rock Hill, SC Zip 29732–1952; tel. 803/329–1234; Charles F. Miller, President and Chief Executive Officer
Web address: www.tenethealth.com

TENNESSEE: HARTON REGIONAL MEDICAL CENTER (O, 137 beds) 1801 North Jackson Street, Tullahoma, TN Zip 37388–2201, Mailing Address: P.O. Box 460, Zip 37388–0460; tel. 931/393–3000; David C. Wilson, Chief Executive Officer
Web address: www.tenethealth.com\harton\

MEDICAL CENTER OF MANCHESTER (L, 49 beds) 481 Interstate Drive, Manchester, TN Zip 37355–3108, Mailing Address: P.O. Box 1409, Zip 37349–1409; tel. 931/728–6354; Robert C. Couch, Chief Executive Officer

SAINT FRANCIS HOSPITAL (O, 503 beds) 5959 Park Avenue, Memphis, TN Zip 38119–5198, Mailing Address: P.O. Box 171808, Zip 38187–1808; tel. 901/765–1000; David L. Archer, Chief Executive Officer
Web address: www.tenethealth.com/saintfrancis

UNIVERSITY MEDICAL CENTER/MCFARLAND HOSPITAL (O, 225 beds) 1411 Baddour Parkway, Lebanon, TN Zip 37087–2573; tel. 615/444–8262; Larry W. Keller, Chief Executive Officer

TEXAS: BAYOU CITY MEDICAL CENTER (O, 356 beds) 4200 Portsmouth Street, Houston, TX Zip 77027–6899; tel. 713/623–2500; Iris Simonis, Chief Executive Officer

BROWNSVILLE MEDICAL CENTER (O, 219 beds) 1040 West Jefferson Street, Brownsville, TX Zip 78520–5829, Mailing Address: P.O. Box 3590, Zip 78523–3590; tel. 956/544–1400; John M. Chubb, Chief Executive Officer
Web address: www.tenethealth.com

CYPRESS FAIRBANKS MEDICAL CENTER (O, 140 beds) 10655 Steepletop Drive, Houston, TX Zip 77065–4297; tel. 281/890–4285; Elizabeth A. Primeaux, Chief Executive Officer
Web address: www.tenethealth.com/cypressfairbanks

DOCTORS HOSPITAL OF DALLAS (O, 198 beds) 9440 Poppy Drive, Dallas, TX Zip 75218–3694; tel. 214/324–6100; Robert S. Freymuller, Chief Executive Officer
Web address: www.tenethealth.com/

GARLAND COMMUNITY HOSPITAL (O, 113 beds) 2696 West Walnut Street, Garland, TX Zip 75042–6499; tel. 972/276–7116; Gene Miller, Chief Executive Officer
Web address: www.tenethealh.com

HOUSTON NORTHWEST MEDICAL CENTER (O, 386 beds) 710 FM 1960 West, Houston, TX Zip 77090–3496; tel. 281/440–1000; James Kelly, Chief Executive Officer
Web address: www.hnmc.com/home/home.cfm

LAKE POINTE MEDICAL CENTER (O, 97 beds) 6800 Scenic Drive, Rowlett, TX Zip 75088, Mailing Address: P.O. Box 1550, Zip 75030–1550; tel. 972/412–2273; Kenneth R. Teel, Administrator
Web address: www.lakepointemedical.com

NACOGDOCHES MEDICAL CENTER (O, 124 beds) 4920 N.E. Stallings, Nacogdoches, TX Zip 75961–1200, Mailing Address: P.O. Box 631604, Zip 75963–1604; tel. 409/568–3380; Glenn A. Robinson, Chief Executive Officer
Web address: www.tenethealth.com/nacogdoches

PARK PLAZA HOSPITAL (O, 299 beds) 1313 Hermann Drive, Houston, TX Zip 77004–7092; tel. 713/527–5000; Robert L. Quist, Chief Executive Officer
Web address: www.parkplazahospital.com

PROVIDENCE MEMORIAL HOSPITAL (O, 392 beds) 2001 North Oregon Street, El Paso, TX Zip 79902–3368; tel. 915/577–6011; Thomas E. Casaday, President and Chief Executive Officer
Web address: www.tenethealh.com

RHD MEMORIAL MEDICAL CENTER (L, 141 beds) Seven Medical Parkway, Dallas, TX Zip 75381, Mailing Address: P.O. Box 819094, Zip 75381–9094; tel. 972/247–1000; Craig E. Sims, President and Chief Executive Officer
Web address: www.tenethealth.com

RIO VISTA PHYSICAL REHABILITATION HOSPITAL (O, 100 beds) 1740 Curie Drive, El Paso, TX Zip 79902–2900; tel. 915/544–3399; Teresa C. Urquhart, Administrator and Chief Operating Officer
Web address: www.tenethealth.com

SIERRA MEDICAL CENTER (O, 328 beds) 1625 Medical Center Drive, El Paso, TX Zip 79902–5044; tel. 915/747–4000; Thomas E. Casaday, President and Chief Executive Officer
Web address: www.tenethealth.com

TRINITY MEDICAL CENTER (L, 137 beds) 4343 North Josey Lane, Carrollton, TX Zip 75010–4691; tel. 972/492–1010; Craig E. Sims, President
Web address: www.tenethealth.com

Owned, leased, sponsored:	113 hospitals	23799 beds
Contract–managed:	0 hospitals	0 beds
Totals:	113 hospitals	23799 beds

0020: TEXAS DEPARTMENT OF HEALTH (NP)
1100 West 49th Street, Austin, TX Zip 78756–3199; tel. 512/458–7111; William R. Archer, II, M.D., Commissioner
(Independent Hospital System)

SOUTH TEXAS HOSPITAL (O, 60 beds) 1301 Rangerville Road, Harlingen, TX Zip 78552–7609, Mailing Address: P.O. Box 592, Zip 78551–0592; tel. 956/423–3420; Mary Diaz, R.N., Ed.D., Director
Web address: www.tdh.texas.gov

TEXAS CENTER FOR INFECTIOUS DISEASE (O, 109 beds) 2303 S.E. Military Drive, San Antonio, TX Zip 78223–3597; tel. 210/534–8857; James N. Elkins, FACHE, Director
Web address: www.tdh.state.tx.us

Owned, leased, sponsored:	2 hospitals	169 beds
Contract–managed:	0 hospitals	0 beds
Totals:	2 hospitals	169 beds

★**0129: TEXAS HEALTH RESOURCES** (NP)
600 East Las Colinas Boulevard, Suite 1550, Irving, TX Zip 75039, Mailing Address: 600 East Las Colinas Boulevard, 1550, Zip 75039; tel. 214/818–4500; Douglas D. Hawthorne, President and Chief Executive Officer
(Centralized Physician/Insurance Health System)

ARLINGTON MEMORIAL HOSPITAL (O, 339 beds) 800 West Randol Mill Road, Arlington, TX Zip 76012–2503; tel. 817/548–6100; Wayne N. Clark, President and Chief Executive Officer

HARRIS CONTINUED CARE HOSPITAL (O, 10 beds) 1301 Pennsylvania Avenue, 4th Floor, Fort Worth, TX Zip 76104–2190, Mailing Address: P.O. Box 3471, Zip 76113–3471; tel. 817/878–5500; Larry Thompson, Senior Vice President and Executive Director
Web address: www.hmhs.com

For explanation of codes following names, see page B2.
★ Indicates Type III membership in the American Hospital Association.

Systems / Triad Hospitals, Inc.

HARRIS METHODIST FORT WORTH (O, 518 beds) 1301 Pennsylvania Avenue, Fort Worth, TX Zip 76104–2895; tel. 817/882-2000; Barclay E. Berdan, President
Web address: www.texashealth.org

HARRIS METHODIST NORTHWEST (O, 36 beds) 108 Denver Trail, Azle, TX Zip 76020–3697; tel. 817/444-8600; Larry Thompson, Vice President and Administrator
Web address: www.hmhs.com

HARRIS METHODIST SOUTHWEST (O, 83 beds) 6100 Harris Parkway, Fort Worth, TX Zip 76132–4199; tel. 817/346-5050; Stansel Harvey, Senior Executive Vice President, Executive Director/Administrator
Web address: www.hmhs.com

HARRIS METHODIST–ERATH COUNTY (O, 75 beds) 411 North Belknap Street, Stephenville, TX Zip 76401–3415, Mailing Address: P.O. Box 1399, Zip 76401–1399; tel. 254/965-1500; Ronald E. Dorris, Senior Vice President and Executive Director
Web address: www.hmhs.com

HARRIS METHODIST–HEB (O, 180 beds) 1600 Hospital Parkway, Bedford, TX Zip 76022–6913, Mailing Address: P.O. Box 669, Zip 76095–0669; tel. 817/685-4000; Jack McCabe, President and Chief Executive Officer
Web address: www.hmhs.com

MCCUISTION REGIONAL MEDICAL CENTER (O, 152 beds) 865 Deshong Drive, Paris, TX Zip 75462–2097; tel. 903/737-1111; Michael J. McBride, FACHE, President
Web address: www.texashealth.com

PRESBYTERIAN HOSPITAL OF DALLAS (O, 656 beds) 8200 Walnut Hill Lane, Dallas, TX Zip 75231–4402; tel. 214/345-6789; Mark H. Merrill, President
Web address: www.texashealth.org

PRESBYTERIAN HOSPITAL OF KAUFMAN (O, 62 beds) 850 Highway 243 West, Kaufman, TX Zip 75142–9998, Mailing Address: P.O. Box 310, Zip 75142–0310; tel. 972/932-7200; Kirk King, Senior Vice President and Executive Director
Web address: www.phscare.org

PRESBYTERIAN HOSPITAL OF PLANO (O, 155 beds) 6200 West Parker Road, Plano, TX Zip 75093–7914; tel. 972/981-8000; Philip M. Wentworth, FACHE, President
Web address: www.texashealth.org

PRESBYTERIAN HOSPITAL OF WINNSBORO (O, 46 beds) 719 West Coke Road, Winnsboro, TX Zip 75494–3098, Mailing Address: P.O. Box 628, Zip 75494–0628; tel. 903/342-5227; Dan Noteware, Senior Vice President and Executive Director
Web address: www.phscare.org

ST. PAUL MEDICAL CENTER (O, 339 beds) 5909 Harry Hines Boulevard, Dallas, TX Zip 75235–6285; tel. 214/879-1000; Frank Tiedemann, President
Web address: www.texashealth.com

WALLS REGIONAL HOSPITAL (O, 137 beds) 201 Walls Drive, Cleburne, TX Zip 76031–1008; tel. 817/641-2551; Brent D. Magers, FACHE, President
Web address: www.hmhs.com

Owned, leased, sponsored:	14 hospitals	2788 beds
Contract-managed:	0 hospitals	0 beds
Totals:	14 hospitals	2788 beds

★0058: **THE UNIVERSITY OF CHICAGO HOSPITALS AND HEALTH SYSTEM** (NP)
322 South Green Street, Suite 500, Chicago, IL Zip 60637; tel. 773/702-6240; Ralph W. Muller, President and Chief Executive Officer

ILLINOIS: LOUIS A. WEISS MEMORIAL HOSPITAL (O, 200 beds) 4646 North Marine Drive, Chicago, IL Zip 60640–1501; tel. 773/564-5000; Edward A. Cucci, President
Web address: www.weisshospital.org

UNIVERSITY OF CHICAGO HOSPITALS (O, 533 beds) 5841 South Maryland Avenue, Chicago, IL Zip 60637–1470; tel. 773/702-1000; Ralph W. Muller, President and Chief Executive Officer

Owned, leased, sponsored:	2 hospitals	733 beds
Contract-managed:	0 hospitals	0 beds
Totals:	2 hospitals	733 beds

★2445: **THEDACARE, INC.** (NP)
Five Innovation Court, Appleton, WI Zip 54914–1663, Mailing Address: P.O. Box 8025, Zip 54912; tel. 920/831-6706; John S. Toussaint, M.D., President and Chief Executive Officer
(Centralized Physician/Insurance Health System)

WISCONSIN: APPLETON MEDICAL CENTER (O, 146 beds) 1818 North Meade Street, Appleton, WI Zip 54911–3496; tel. 920/731-4101; Robert H. Malte, Senior Vice President
Web address: www.thedacare.org

THEDA CLARK MEDICAL CENTER (O, 216 beds) 130 Second Street, Neenah, WI Zip 54956–2883, Mailing Address: P.O. Box 2021, Zip 54957–2021; tel. 920/729-3100; Robert H. Malte, Senior Vice President
Web address: www.thedacare.org

Owned, leased, sponsored:	2 hospitals	362 beds
Contract-managed:	0 hospitals	0 beds
Totals:	2 hospitals	362 beds

★0178: **TRIAD HOSPITALS, INC.** (IO)
13455 Noel Road, 20th Floor, Dallas, TX Zip 75240; tel. 972/789-2700; James D. Shelton, Chairman and Chief Executive Officer
(Decentralized Health System)

ALABAMA: CRESTWOOD MEDICAL CENTER (O, 120 beds) One Hospital Drive, Huntsville, AL Zip 35801–3403; tel. 256/882-3100; Thomas M. Weiss, Chief Executive Officer

ARIZONA: EL DORADO HOSPITAL (O, 166 beds) 1400 North Wilmot Road, Tucson, AZ Zip 85712–4498, Mailing Address: P.O. Box 13070, Zip 85732–3070; tel. 520/886-6361; Rhonda Dean, Chief Executive Officer
Web address: www.eldoradohospital.com

NORTHWEST MEDICAL CENTER (O, 134 beds) 6200 North La Cholla Boulevard, Tucson, AZ Zip 85741–3599; tel. 520/742-9000; W. Jefferson Comer, FACHE, Chief Executive Officer
Web address: www.northwestmedicalcenter.com

PARADISE VALLEY HOSPITAL (O, 140 beds) 3929 East Bell Road, Phoenix, AZ Zip 85032–2196; tel. 602/867-1881; Rebecca C. Kuhn, Chief Executive Officer

ARKANSAS: MEDICAL CENTER OF SOUTH ARKANSAS (O, 162 beds) 700 West Grove Street, El Dorado, AR Zip 71730–4416, Mailing Address: P.O. Box 1998, Zip 71731–1998; tel. 870/864-3200; Luther J. Lewis, Chief Executive Officer
Web address: www.mcsaeldo.com

MEDICAL PARK HOSPITAL (O, 71 beds) 2001 South Main Street, Hope, AR Zip 71801–8194; tel. 870/777-2323; Jimmy Leopard, Chief Executive Officer

CALIFORNIA: MISSION BAY HOSPITAL (O, 91 beds) 3030 Bunker Hill Street, San Diego, CA Zip 92109–5780; tel. 619/274-7721; Deborah Brehe, Chief Executive Officer
Web address: www.mbhosp.com

SAN LEANDRO HOSPITAL (O, 136 beds) 13855 East 14th Street, San Leandro, CA Zip 94578–0398; tel. 510/357-6500; Carol B. Freeman, Interim Chief Executive Officer

LOUISIANA: WOMEN AND CHILDREN'S HOSPITAL–LAKE CHARLES (O, 80 beds) 4200 Nelson Road, Lake Charles, LA Zip 70605–4118; tel. 318/474-6370; Bill Willis, Chief Executive Officer
Web address: www.women–childrens.com

NEW MEXICO: CARLSBAD MEDICAL CENTER (O, 110 beds) 2430 West Pierce Street, Carlsbad, NM Zip 88220–3597; tel. 505/887-4100; Fred Woody, Chief Executive Officer
Web address: www.hcahealthcare.com

LEA REGIONAL MEDICAL CENTER (O, 250 beds) 5419 North Lovington Highway, Hobbs, NM Zip 88240–9125, Mailing Address: P.O. Box 3000, Zip 88240–3000; tel. 505/392-6581; William J. Gresco, Chief Executive Officer

OKLAHOMA: CLAREMORE REGIONAL HOSPITAL (O, 68 beds) 1202 North Muskogee Place, Claremore, OK Zip 74017–3036; tel. 918/341-2556; Ken Seidel, Chief Executive Officer

For explanation of codes following names, see page B2.
★ Indicates Type III membership in the American Hospital Association.

Systems / Triad Hospitals, Inc.

SOUTHCREST HOSPITAL (O, 119 beds) 8801 South 101st East Avenue, Tulsa, OK Zip 74133; tel. 918/294-4000; Anthony R. Young, Chief Executive Officer
Web address: www.southcresthospital.com

OREGON: WILLAMETTE VALLEY MEDICAL CENTER (O, 67 beds) 2700 Three Mile Lane, McMinnville, OR Zip 97128-6498; tel. 503/472-6131; Rosemari Davis, Chief Executive Officer
Web address: www.hcahealthcare.com

TEXAS: ALICE REGIONAL HOSPITAL (O, 112 beds) 2500 East Main Street, Alice, TX Zip 78332-4794; tel. 361/664-4376; Bradley E. Jones, Chief Executive Officer

BROWNWOOD REGIONAL MEDICAL CENTER (O, 163 beds) 1501 Burnet Drive, Brownwood, TX Zip 76801-5933, Mailing Address: P.O. Box 760, Zip 76804-0760; tel. 915/646-8541; Tim Lancaster, Chief Executive Officer
Web address: www.brmc-cares.com

COLLEGE STATION MEDICAL CENTER (O, 119 beds) 1604 Rock Prairie Road, College Station, TX 77845-8345, Mailing Address: P.O. Box 10000, Zip 77842-3500; tel. 979/764-5100; Thomas W. Jackson, Chief Executive Officer
Web address: www.csmedcenter.com

COMMUNITY MEDICAL CENTER SHERMAN (O, 128 beds) 1111 Gallagher Road, Sherman, TX Zip 75090-1798; tel. 903/870-7000; William A. Keaton, Chief Executive Officer
Web address: www.hcahealthcare.com

DETAR HOSPITAL (O, 211 beds) 506 East San Antonio Street, Victoria, TX Zip 77901-6060, Mailing Address: Box 2089, Zip 77902-2089; tel. 361/575-7441; William R. Blanchard, Chief Executive Officer
Web address: www.detar.com

GULF COAST MEDICAL CENTER (O, 161 beds) 1400 Highway 59, Wharton, TX Zip 77488-3004, Mailing Address: P.O. Box 3004, Zip 77488-3004; tel. 409/532-2500; Michael D. Murphy, Chief Executive Officer
Web address: www.gulfcoastmedical.com

LONGVIEW REGIONAL MEDICAL CENTER (O, 164 beds) 2901 North Fourth Street, Longview, TX Zip 75605-5191, Mailing Address: P.O. Box 14000, Zip 75607-4000; tel. 903/758-1818; Vicki L. Romero, Chief Executive Officer
Web address: www.longviewregional.com

MEDICAL CENTER AT TERRELL (O, 130 beds) 1551 Highway 34 South, Terrell, TX Zip 75160-4833; tel. 972/563-7611; Ronald J. Ensor, Chief Executive Officer

NAVARRO REGIONAL HOSPITAL (O, 144 beds) 3201 West State Highway 22, Corsicana, TX Zip 75110; tel. 903/654-6800; Nancy A. Byrnes, Chief Executive Officer
Web address: www.hcahealthcare.com

PAMPA REGIONAL MEDICAL CENTER (O, 107 beds) One Medical Plaza, Pampa, TX Zip 79065; tel. 806/665-3721; Mike Munnerlyn, Chief Executive Officer
Web address: www.cmcp.com

REGIONAL MEDICAL CENTER (O, 108 beds) 101 Medical Drive, Victoria, TX Zip 77904-3198; tel. 361/573-6100; William R. Blancher, Chief Executive Officer
Web address: www.detar.com

SAN ANGELO COMMUNITY MEDICAL CENTER (O, 136 beds) 3501 Knickerbocker Road, San Angelo, TX Zip 76904-7698; tel. 915/949-9511; Samuel G. Feazell, Chief Executive Officer

WOODLAND HEIGHTS MEDICAL CENTER (O, 138 beds) 505 South John Redditt Drive, Lufkin, TX Zip 75904, Mailing Address: P.O. Box 150610, Zip 75915-0610; tel. 936/634-8311; Don H. McBride, Chief Executive Officer

Owned, leased, sponsored:	27 hospitals	3535 beds
Contract-managed:	0 hospitals	0 beds
Totals:	27 hospitals	3535 beds

★**0219: TRINITY HEALTH** (CC)
Novi, MI Mailing Address: P.O. Box 8001, Zip 48376-8001; tel. 248/489-6000; Judith Pelham, President and Chief Executive Officer

CALIFORNIA: SAINT AGNES MEDICAL CENTER (O, 326 beds) 1303 East Herndon Avenue, Fresno, CA Zip 93720-3309; tel. 559/449-3000; Sister Ruth Marie Nickerson, President and Chief Executive Officer
Web address: www.samc.com

IDAHO: CASCADE MEDICAL CENTER (O, 10 beds) 402 Old State Highway, Cascade, ID Zip 83611, Mailing Address: P.O. Box 151, Zip 83611-0151; tel. 208/382-4242; Frank Clark, Chief Executive Officer

ELMORE MEDICAL CENTER (O, 78 beds) 895 North Sixth East Street, Mountain Home, ID Zip 83647, Mailing Address: P.O. Box 1270, Zip 83647-1270; tel. 208/587-8401; Gregory L. Maurer, Administrator

MCCALL MEMORIAL HOSPITAL (O, 15 beds) 1000 State Street, McCall, ID Zip 83638; tel. 208/634-2221; Karen J. Kellie, President

SAINT ALPHONSUS REGIONAL MEDICAL CENTER (O, 281 beds) 1055 North Curtis Road, Boise, ID Zip 83706-1370; tel. 208/378-2121; Sandra B. Bruce, President and Chief Executive Officer
Web address: www.saintalphonsus.org

ST. BENEDICTS FAMILY MEDICAL CENTER (O, 60 beds) 709 North Lincoln Avenue, Jerome, ID Zip 83338-1851, Mailing Address: P.O. Box 586, Zip 83338-0586; tel. 208/324-4301; Lynne M. Mattison, FACHE, Interim Administrator

ILLINOIS: MORRISON COMMUNITY HOSPITAL (C, 60 beds) 303 North Jackson Street, Morrison, IL Zip 61270-3042; tel. 815/772-4003; Mark F. Fedyk, Administrator

INDIANA: SAINT JOHN'S HEALTH SYSTEM (O, 205 beds) 2015 Jackson Street, Anderson, IN Zip 46016-4339; tel. 765/649-2511; Jerry D. Brumitt, President and Chief Executive Officer
Web address: www.stjohnshealthsystem.org

SAINT JOSEPH'S REGIONAL MEDICAL CENTER–PLYMOUTH CAMPUS (O, 36 beds) 1915 Lake Avenue, Plymouth, IN Zip 46563-9905, Mailing Address: P.O. Box 670, Zip 46563-9905; tel. 219/936-3181; Brian E. Dietz, FACHE, Executive Vice President
Web address: www.sjmed.com

SAINT JOSEPH'S REGIONAL MEDICAL CENTER–SOUTH BEND CAMPUS (O, 310 beds) 801 East LaSalle, South Bend, IN Zip 46617-2800; tel. 219/237-7111; Robert L. Beyer, President and Chief Executive Officer
Web address: www.sjmed.com

IOWA: BAUM HARMON MERCY HOSPITAL (O, 16 beds) 255 North Welch Avenue, Primghar, IA Zip 51245-1034, Mailing Address: P.O. Box 528, Zip 51245-0528; tel. 712/757-2300; Trudy Pfeiffer, Administrator

BELMOND MEDICAL CENTER (O, 22 beds) 403 First Street S.E., Belmond, IA Zip 50421-1201, Mailing Address: P.O. Box 326, Zip 50421-0326; tel. 515/444-3223; Kim Price, Administrator

CENTRAL COMMUNITY HOSPITAL (O, 16 beds) 901 Davidson Street N.W., Elkader, IA Zip 52043; tel. 319/245-7000; Fran Zichal, Chief Executive Officer

ELLSWORTH MUNICIPAL HOSPITAL (O, 40 beds) 110 Rocksylvania Avenue, Iowa Falls, IA Zip 50126-2431; tel. 515/648-4631; John O'Brien, Administrator

FRANKLIN GENERAL HOSPITAL (O, 82 beds) 1720 Central Avenue East, Hampton, IA Zip 50441-1859; tel. 515/456-5000; Scott Wells, Administrator
Web address: www.franklingeneral.com

HANCOCK COUNTY MEMORIAL HOSPITAL (O, 26 beds) 532 First Street N.W., Britt, IA Zip 50423-0068, Mailing Address: P.O. Box 68, Zip 50423-0068; tel. 515/843-3801; Harriet A. Thompson, Administrator

HAWARDEN COMMUNITY HOSPITAL (O, 17 beds) 1111 11th Street, Hawarden, IA Zip 51023-1999; tel. 712/551-3100; Stuart A. Katz, FACHE, Chief Executive Officer
Web address: www.acsnet.com/~commhosp/

KOSSUTH REGIONAL HEALTH CENTER (C, 24 beds) 1515 South Phillips Street, Algona, IA Zip 50511-3649; tel. 515/295-2451; Scott Curtis, Administrator and Chief Executive Officer

MERCY MEDICAL CENTER – NORTH IOWA (O, 255 beds) 1000 Fourth Street S.W., Mason City, IA Zip 50401-2800; tel. 515/422-7000; James J. Sexton, President and Chief Executive Officer
Web address: www.mercynorthiowa.com

For explanation of codes following names, see page B2.
★ Indicates Type III membership in the American Hospital Association.

Systems / U. S. Public Health Service Indian Health Service

MERCY MEDICAL CENTER–CLINTON (O, 364 beds) 1410 North Fourth Street, Clinton, IA Zip 52732–2999; tel. 319/244–5555; Thomas J. Hesselmann, President and Chief Executive Officer
Web address: www.samhealth.com

MERCY MEDICAL CENTER–DUBUQUE (O, 385 beds) 250 Mercy Drive, Dubuque, IA Zip 52001–7360; tel. 319/589–8000; Russell M. Knight, President and Chief Executive Officer
Web address: www.mercyhealth.com

MERCY MEDICAL CENTER–NEW HAMPTON (O, 58 beds) 308 North Maple Avenue, New Hampton, IA Zip 50659–1142; tel. 515/394–4121; Carolyn Martin–Shaw, President
Web address: www.mercynewhampton.com

MERCY MEDICAL CENTER–SIOUX CITY (O, 284 beds) 801 Fifth Street, Sioux City, IA Zip 51102, Mailing Address: P.O. Box 3168, Zip 51102–3168; tel. 712/279–2010; Deborah VandenBroek, President and Chief Executive Officer
Web address: www.mercysiouxcity.com

MITCHELL COUNTY REGIONAL HEALTH CENTER (O, 28 beds) 616 North Eighth Street, Osage, IA Zip 50461–1498; tel. 515/732–6005; Kimberly J. Miller, CHE, Administrator and Chief Executive Officer

PALO ALTO HEALTH SYSTEM (O, 54 beds) 3201 First Street, Emmetsburg, IA Zip 50536–2599; tel. 712/852–5500; Darrell E. Vondrak, Administrator
Web address: www.northiowamercy.com

REGIONAL HEALTH SERVICES OF HOWARD COUNTY (O, 32 beds) 235 Eighth Avenue West, Cresco, IA Zip 52136–1098; tel. 319/547–2101; Elizabeth A. Doty, President and Chief Executive Officer
Web address: www.rhshc.com

MARYLAND: HOLY CROSS HOSPITAL OF SILVER SPRING (O, 460 beds) 1500 Forest Glen Road, Silver Spring, MD Zip 20910–1484; tel. 301/754–7000; Kevin J. Sexton, President and Chief Executive Officer

MICHIGAN: BATTLE CREEK HEALTH SYSTEM (O, 378 beds) 300 North Avenue, Battle Creek, MI Zip 49016–3396; tel. 616/966–8000; Patrick R. Garrett, Chief Executive Officer
Web address: www.bchealth.com

DECKERVILLE COMMUNITY HOSPITAL (O, 17 beds) 3559 Pine Street, Deckerville, MI 48427–0126, Mailing Address: P.O. Box 126, Zip 48427–0126; tel. 810/376–2835; Edward L. Gamache, Administrator

MCPHERSON HOSPITAL (O, 45 beds) 620 Byron Road, Howell, MI Zip 48843–1093; tel. 517/545–6000; Patricia Claffey, Executive Director
Web address: www.sjmh.com

MERCY GENERAL HEALTH PARTNERS (O, 191 beds) 1500 East Sherman Boulevard, Muskegon, MI Zip 49443; tel. 231/739–9341; Roger Spoelman, President and Chief Executive Officer

MERCY HEALTH SERVICES NORTH–GRAYLING (O, 74 beds) 1100 East Michigan Avenue, Grayling, MI Zip 49738–1398; tel. 517/348–5461; Stephanie J. Riemer–Matuzak, Chief Executive Officer
Web address: www.mercyhealth.com/north

MERCY HOSPITAL (O, 89 beds) 400 Hobart Street, Cadillac, MI Zip 49601–9596; tel. 231/876–7131; John L. MacLeod, Chief Executive Officer
Web address: www.mercyhealth.com

MERCY HOSPITAL (O, 119 beds) 2601 Electric Avenue, Port Huron, MI Zip 48060; tel. 810/985–1510; Mary R. Trimmer, President and Chief Executive Officer
Web address: www.mercyporthuron.com

SAINT JOSEPH MERCY HEALTH SYSTEM (O, 467 beds) 5301 East Huron River Drive, Ann Arbor, MI Zip 48106, Mailing Address: P.O. Box 995, Zip 48106–0995; tel. 734/712–3456; Garry C. Faja, President and Chief Executive Officer
Web address: www.sjmh.com

SAINT MARY'S MERCY MEDICAL CENTER (O, 287 beds) 200 Jefferson Avenue S.E., Grand Rapids, MI Zip 49503–4598; tel. 616/752–6090; Joyce A. Helms, Interim President and Chief Executive Officer
Web address: www.trinity-health.org/

SALINE COMMUNITY HOSPITAL (O, 39 beds) 400 West Russell Street, Saline, MI Zip 48176–1101; tel. 734/429–1500; Garry C. Faja, President and Chief Executive Officer
Web address: www.sjmh.com

ST. JOSEPH MERCY OAKLAND (O, 428 beds) 900 Woodward Avenue, Pontiac, MI Zip 48341–2985; tel. 248/858–3000; Thomas L. Feurig, President and Chief Executive Officer
Web address: www.mercyhealth.com/oakland

ST. JOSEPH'S MERCY HOSPITALS AND HEALTH SERVICES (O, 462 beds) Clinton Township, MI Jack Weiner, President and Chief Executive Officer
Web address: www.stjoe–macomb.com

NEBRASKA: PENDER COMMUNITY HOSPITAL (O, 30 beds) 603 Earl Street, Pender, NE Zip 68047–0100, Mailing Address: P.O. Box 100, Zip 68047–0100; tel. 402/385–3083; Roger Mazour, Administrator

OHIO: MOUNT CARMEL HEALTH SYSTEM (O, 929 beds) Columbus, OH Mailing Address: 793 West State Street, Zip 43222–1551; tel. 614/234–5423; Joseph T. Calvaruso, President and Chief Executive Officer
Web address: www.mchs.com

Owned, leased, sponsored:	39 hospitals	7015 beds
Contract–managed:	2 hospitals	84 beds
Totals:	41 hospitals	7099 beds

★**9255: TRUMAN HEALTH SYSTEM** (NP)
2301 Holmes Street, Kansas City, MO Zip 64108–2677; tel. 816/556–3000; John W. Bluford, Executive Director and Chief Executive Officer
(Moderately Centralized Health System)

MISSOURI: TRUMAN MEDICAL CENTER–EAST (C, 302 beds) 7900 Lee's Summit Road, Kansas City, MO Zip 64139–1241; tel. 816/373–4415; James R. Kelly, Chief Operating Officer

TRUMAN MEDICAL CENTER–HOSPITAL HILL (C, 227 beds) 2301 Holmes Street, Kansas City, MO Zip 64108–2677; tel. 816/556–3000; Catherine D. Disch, Chief Operating Officer

Owned, leased, sponsored:	0 hospitals	0 beds
Contract–managed:	2 hospitals	529 beds
Totals:	2 hospitals	529 beds

9195: U. S. PUBLIC HEALTH SERVICE INDIAN HEALTH SERVICE (FG)
5600 Fishers Lane, Rockville, MD Zip 20857; tel. 301/443–1083; Michael Trujillo, M.D., M.P.H., Director
(Moderately Centralized Health System)

ALASKA: ALASKA NATIVE MEDICAL CENTER (O, 140 beds) 4315 Diplomacy Drive, Anchorage, AK Zip 99508; tel. 907/563–2662; Richard Mandsager, M.D., Administrator

KANAKANAK HOSPITAL (O, 16 beds) Dillingham, AK Mailing Address: P.O. Box 130, Zip 99576; tel. 907/842–5201; Darrel C. Richardson, Chief Operating Officer

MANIILAQ HEALTH CENTER (O, 17 beds) Kotzebue, AK Zip 99752–0043; tel. 907/442–3321; Tim J. Gilbert, Administrator
Web address: www.maniilaq.org

NORTON SOUND REGIONAL HOSPITAL (O, 34 beds) Bering Straits, Nome, AK Zip 99762, Mailing Address: P.O. Box 966, Zip 99762–0966; tel. 907/443–3311; Charles Fagerstrom, Vice President
Web address: www.nshcorp.org

SAMUEL SIMMONDS MEMORIAL HOSPITAL (O, 15 beds) 1296 Agvik Street, Barrow, AK Zip 99723, Mailing Address: P.O. Box 29, Zip 99723; tel. 907/852–4611; Michael S. Herring, Administrator

SEARHC MT. EDGECUMBE HOSPITAL (O, 60 beds) 222 Tongass Drive, Sitka, AK Zip 99835–9416; tel. 907/966–2411; Frank Sutton, Vice President Hospital Services
Web address: www.searhc.org

YUKON–KUSKOKWIM DELTA REGIONAL HOSPITAL (O, 50 beds) Bethel, AK Mailing Address: P.O. Box 528, Zip 99559–3000; tel. 907/543–6300; Edwin L. Hansen, Vice President

ARIZONA: CHINLE COMPREHENSIVE HEALTH CARE FACILITY (O, 46 beds) Highway 191, Chinle, AZ Zip 86503, Mailing Address: P.O. Drawer PH, Zip 86503; tel. 520/674–7011; Ronald Tso, Chief Executive Officer

---

For explanation of codes following names, see page B2.
★ Indicates Type III membership in the American Hospital Association.

Systems / U. S. Public Health Service Indian Health Service

FORT DEFIANCE INDIAN HEALTH SERVICE HOSPITAL (O, 49 beds) Fort Defiance, AZ Mailing Address: P.O. Box 649, Zip 86504–0649; tel. 520/729–5741; Franklin Freeland, Ed.D., Chief Executive Officer

HUHUKAM MEMORIAL HOSPITAL (O, 10 beds) Seed Farm and Skill Center Road, Sacaton, AZ Zip 85247–0038, Mailing Address: P.O. Box 38, Zip 85247–0038; tel. 602/528–1200; Viola L. Johnson, M.P.H., Chief Executive Officer

TUBA CITY INDIAN MEDICAL CENTER (O, 69 beds) 167 Main Street, Tuba City, AZ Zip 86045–0611, Mailing Address: P.O. Box 600, Zip 86045–0600; tel. 520/283–2501; Susie John, M.D., Chief Executive Officer

U. S. PUBLIC HEALTH SERVICE INDIAN HOSPITAL (O, 18 beds) Parker, AZ Mailing Address: Route 1, Box 12, Zip 85344; tel. 520/669–2137; Gary Davis, Service Unit Director

U. S. PUBLIC HEALTH SERVICE INDIAN HOSPITAL (O, 34 beds) Sells, AZ Mailing Address: P.O. Box 548, Zip 85634–0548; tel. 520/383–7251; Darrell Rumley, Service Unit Director and Chief Executive Officer

U. S. PUBLIC HEALTH SERVICE INDIAN HOSPITAL (O, 28 beds) San Carlos, AZ Mailing Address: P.O. Box 208, Zip 85550–0208; tel. 520/475–2371; Nella Ben, Chief Executive Officer

U. S. PUBLIC HEALTH SERVICE INDIAN HOSPITAL (O, 45 beds) State Route 73, Box 860, Whiteriver, AZ Zip 85941–0860; tel. 520/338–4911; Carla Alchesay-Nachu, Service Unit Director

U. S. PUBLIC HEALTH SERVICE PHOENIX INDIAN MEDICAL CENTER (O, 137 beds) 4212 North 16th Street, Phoenix, AZ Zip 85016–5389; tel. 602/263–1200; Anna Albert, Chief Executive Officer

U. S. PUBLIC HEALTH SERVICES INDIAN HOSPITAL (O, 17 beds) Keams Canyon, AZ Mailing Address: P.O. Box 98, Zip 86034–0098; tel. 520/738–2211; Anthony Marshall, Service Unit Director

CALIFORNIA: U. S. PUBLIC HEALTH SERVICE INDIAN HOSPITAL (O, 34 beds) Winterhaven, CA Mailing Address: P.O. Box 1368, Yuma, AZZip 85366–1368; tel. 760/572–0217; Hortense Miguel, R.N., Service Unit Director

MARYLAND: WARREN G. MAGNUSON CLINICAL CENTER, NATIONAL INSTITUTES OF HEALTH (O, 290 beds) 9000 Rockville Pike, Bethesda, MD Zip 20892–1504; tel. 301/496–4114; John I. Gallin, M.D., Director
Web address: www.cc.nih.gov

MINNESOTA: U. S. PUBLIC HEALTH SERVICE INDIAN HOSPITAL (O, 13 beds) 7th Street and Grant Utley Avenue N.W., Cass Lake, MN Zip 56633, Mailing Address: Rural Route 3, Box 211, Zip 56633; tel. 218/335–2293; Luella Brown, Service Unit Director

U.S. PUBLIC HEALTH SERVICE INDIAN HOSPITAL (O, 23 beds) Highway 1, Redlake, MN Zip 56671; tel. 218/679–3912; Essimae Stevens, Service Unit Director

MISSISSIPPI: CHOCTAW HEALTH CENTER (O, 35 beds) Highway 16 West, Philadelphia, MS Zip 39350, Mailing Address: Route 7, Box R–50, Zip 39350; tel. 601/656–2211; James D. Wallace, Executive Director

MONTANA: U. S. PUBLIC HEALTH SERVICE BLACKFEET COMMUNITY HOSPITAL (O, 25 beds) Browning, MT Mailing Address: P.O. Box 760, Zip 59417–0760; tel. 406/338–6100; Reis Fisher, Service Unit Director

U. S. PUBLIC HEALTH SERVICE INDIAN HOSPITAL (O, 24 beds) Crow Agency, MT Mailing Address: P.O. Box 9, Zip 59022–0009; tel. 406/638–2626; Tennyson Doney, Service Unit Director

U. S. PUBLIC HEALTH SERVICE INDIAN HOSPITAL (O, 12 beds) Rural Route 1, Box 67, Harlem, MT Zip 59526; tel. 406/353–3100; Charles D. Plumage, Director

NEBRASKA: U. S. PUBLIC HEALTH SERVICE INDIAN HOSPITAL (O, 30 beds) Highway 7577, Winnebago, NE Zip 68071; tel. 402/878–2231; Donald Lee, Service Unit Director

NEVADA: U. S. PUBLIC HEALTH SERVICE OWYHEE COMMUNITY HEALTH FACILITY (O, 15 beds) Owyhee, NV Mailing Address: P.O. Box 130, Zip 89832–0130; tel. 775/757–2415; Walden Townsend, Service Unit Director

NEW MEXICO: ACOMA–CANONCITO–LAGUNA HOSPITAL (O, 15 beds) San Fidel, NM Mailing Address: P.O. Box 130, Zip 87049–0130; tel. 505/552–5300; R. C. Begay, Chief Executive Officer

GALLUP INDIAN MEDICAL CENTER (O, 79 beds) 516 East Nizhoni Boulevard, Gallup, NM Zip 87301–5748, Mailing Address: P.O. Box 1337, Zip 87305–1337; tel. 505/722–1000; Floyd Thompson, Chief Executive Officer

NORTHERN NAVAJO MEDICAL CENTER (O, 59 beds) Shiprock, NM Mailing Address: P.O. Box 160, Zip 87420–0160; tel. 505/368–6001; Dee Hutchison, Chief Executive Officer

PHS SANTA FE INDIAN HOSPITAL (O, 39 beds) 1700 Cerrillos Road, Santa Fe, NM Zip 87505–3554; tel. 505/988–9821; Lawrence A. Jordan, Director

PUBLIC HEALTH SERVICE INDIAN HOSPITAL (O, 28 beds) 801 Vassar Drive N.E., Albuquerque, NM Zip 87106–2799; tel. 505/248–4000; Cheri Lyon, Service Unit Director

U. S. PUBLIC HEALTH SERVICE INDIAN HOSPITAL (O, 32 beds) Crownpoint, NM Mailing Address: P.O. Box 358, Zip 87313–0358; tel. 505/786–5291; Anita Muneta, Chief Executive Officer

U. S. PUBLIC HEALTH SERVICE INDIAN HOSPITAL (O, 13 beds) Mescalero, NM Mailing Address: Box 210, Zip 88340–0210; tel. 505/671–4441; Jo Ann Skaggs, Chief Executive Officer

U. S. PUBLIC HEALTH SERVICE INDIAN HOSPITAL (O, 25 beds) Zuni, NM Mailing Address: P.O. Box 467, Zip 87327–0467; tel. 505/782–4431; Jean Othole, Service Unit Director

NORTH CAROLINA: U. S. PUBLIC HEALTH SERVICE INDIAN HOSPITAL (O, 30 beds) Hospital Road, Cherokee, NC Zip 28719, Mailing Address: Caller Box C–26, Zip 28719; tel. 828/497–9163; Edwin McLemore, Administrator

NORTH DAKOTA: U. S. PUBLIC HEALTH SERVICE INDIAN HOSPITAL (O, 42 beds) Belcourt, ND Mailing Address: P.O. Box 160, Zip 58316–0160; tel. 701/477–6111; Ray Grandbois, M.P.H., Service Unit Director

U. S. PUBLIC HEALTH SERVICE INDIAN HOSPITAL (O, 14 beds) N 10 North River Road, Fort Yates, ND Zip 58538, Mailing Address: P.O. Box J, Zip 58538; tel. 701/854–3831; Terry Pourier, Services Unit Director

OKLAHOMA: CARL ALBERT INDIAN HEALTH FACILITY (O, 28 beds) 1001 North Country Club Road, Ada, OK Zip 74820–2847; tel. 580/436–3980; Bruce A. Bennett, Administrator

CHOCTAW NATION HEALTH CARE CENTER (O, 37 beds) One Choctaw Way, Talihina, OK Zip 74571–9517; tel. 918/567–7000; Robert W. Blum, FACHE, Administrator
Web address: www.choctawnation.com

CREEK NATION COMMUNITY HOSPITAL (O, 34 beds) 309 North 14th Street, Okemah, OK Zip 74859–2099; tel. 918/623–1424; Frank H. Wahpepah, M.P.H., Administrator

U. S. PUBLIC HEALTH SERVICE COMPREHENSIVE INDIAN HEALTH FACILITY (O, 46 beds) 101 South Moore Avenue, Claremore, OK Zip 74017–5091; tel. 918/342–6434; John Daugherty , Jr, Service Unit Director

U. S. PUBLIC HEALTH SERVICE INDIAN HOSPITAL (O, 11 beds) Clinton, OK Mailing Address: Route 1, Box 3060, Zip 73601–9303; tel. 580/323–2884; Thedis V. Mitchell, Director

U. S. PUBLIC HEALTH SERVICE INDIAN HOSPITAL (O, 44 beds) 1515 Lawrie Tatum Road, Lawton, OK Zip 73507–3099; tel. 580/353–0350

WILLIAM W. HASTINGS INDIAN HOSPITAL (O, 60 beds) 100 South Bliss Avenue, Tahlequah, OK Zip 74464–3399; tel. 918/458–3100; Hickory Starr , Jr, Administrator

SOUTH DAKOTA: INDIAN HEALTH SERVICE HOSPITAL (O, 32 beds) 3200 Canyon Lake Drive, Rapid City, SD Zip 57702–8197; tel. 605/355–2280; Michelle Leach, Director

U. S. PUBLIC HEALTH SERVICE INDIAN HOSPITAL (O, 27 beds) Eagle Butte, SD Mailing Address: P.O. Box 1012, Zip 57625–1012; tel. 605/964–3001; Donald D. Annis, Service Unit Director

U. S. PUBLIC HEALTH SERVICE INDIAN HOSPITAL (O, 46 beds) Pine Ridge, SD Mailing Address: P.O. Box 1201, Zip 57770–1201; tel. 605/867–5131; Vern F. Donnell, Service Unit Director

U. S. PUBLIC HEALTH SERVICE INDIAN HOSPITAL (O, 35 beds) Highway 18, Soldier Creek Road, Rosebud, SD Zip 57570; tel. 605/747–2231; Gayla J. Twiss, Service Unit Director

U. S. PUBLIC HEALTH SERVICE INDIAN HOSPITAL (O, 18 beds) Chestnut Street, Sisseton, SD Zip 57262, Mailing Address: P.O. Box 189, Zip 57262–0189; tel. 605/698–7606; Richard Huff, Administrator
Web address: www.home.aberdeen.his.gov

For explanation of codes following names, see page B2.
★ *Indicates Type III membership in the American Hospital Association.*

Systems / Universal Health Services, Inc.

Owned, leased, sponsored:	50 hospitals	2080 beds
Contract-managed:	0 hospitals	0 beds
Totals:	50 hospitals	2080 beds

1765: UNITED HOSPITAL CORPORATION (IO)
6189 East Shelby Drive, Memphis, TN Zip 38115; James C. Henson, President

ALABAMA: FLORALA MEMORIAL HOSPITAL (O, 23 beds) 515 East Fifth Avenue, Florala, AL Zip 36442–0189, Mailing Address: P.O. Box 189, Zip 36442–0189; tel. 334/858–3287; Blair W. Henson, Administrator

ARKANSAS: OZARK HEALTH MEDICAL CENTER (C, 144 beds) Highway 65 South, Clinton, AR Zip 72031, Mailing Address: P.O. Box 206, Zip 72031–0206; tel. 501/745–7000; George S. Fray, Administrator

Owned, leased, sponsored:	1 hospital	23 beds
Contract-managed:	1 hospital	144 beds
Totals:	2 hospitals	167 beds

9605: UNITED MEDICAL CORPORATION (IO)
603 Main Street, Windermere, FL Zip 34786–3548, Mailing Address: P.O. Box 1100, Zip 34786–1100; tel. 407/876–2200; Donald R. Dizney, Chairman
(Independent Hospital System)

FLORIDA: TEN BROECK HOSPITAL JACKSONVILLE (O, 60 beds) 6300 Beach Boulevard, Jacksonville, FL Zip 32216–2782; tel. 904/724–9202; Patrick Hammer, Chief Executive Officer

KENTUCKY: TEN BROECK HOSPITAL (O, 94 beds) 8521 Old LaGrange Road, Louisville, KY Zip 40242–3800; tel. 502/426–6380; Pat Hammer, Chief Executive Officer

LOUISIANA: ST. CLAUDE MEDICAL CENTER (O, 136 beds) 3419 St. Claude Avenue, New Orleans, LA Zip 70117–6198; tel. 504/948–8200; Gwendolyn M. McInnis, R.N., Chief Executive Officer

PUERTO RICO: HOSPITAL DOCTOR GUBERN (O, 51 beds) 110 Antonio R. Barcelo, Fajardo, PR Zip 00738, Mailing Address: P.O. Box 846, Zip 00738–0846; tel. 787/863–0669; Edwin Sueiro, Executive Director

HOSPITAL PAVIA–HATO REY (O, 105 beds) San Juan, PR Mailing Address: 435 Ponce De Leon, Hato Rey, Zip 00917; tel. 787/754–0909; Alfredo Bolchers, Executive Vice President

HOSPITAL PAVIA–SANTURCE (O, 183 beds) 1462 Asia Street, San Juan, PR Zip 00909, Mailing Address: Box 11137, Santurce Station, Zip 00910; tel. 787/727–6060; Alfredo Volckers, Executive Director

HOSPITAL PEREA (O, 82 beds) 15 Basora Street, Mayaguez, PR Zip 00681, Mailing Address: P.O. Box 170, Zip 00681; tel. 787/834–0101; Ramon Lopez, Administrator

SAN JORGE CHILDREN'S HOSPITAL (O, 85 beds) 258 San Jorge Avenue, San Juan, PR Zip 00912; tel. 787/727–1000; Domingo Cruz Vivaldi, Administrator

Owned, leased, sponsored:	8 hospitals	796 beds
Contract-managed:	0 hospitals	0 beds
Totals:	8 hospitals	796 beds

9555: UNIVERSAL HEALTH SERVICES, INC. (IO)
367 South Gulph Road, King of Prussia, PA Zip 19406–0958; tel. 610/768–3300; Alan B. Miller, President and Chief Executive Officer
(Decentralized Health System)

ARKANSAS: BRIDGEWAY (L, 70 beds) 21 Bridgeway Road, North Little Rock, AR Zip 72113; tel. 501/771–1500; Barry Pipkin, Chief Executive Officer and Managing Director

CALIFORNIA: DEL AMO HOSPITAL (O, 166 beds) 23700 Camino Del Sol, Torrance, CA Zip 90505; tel. 310/530–1151; Lisa K. Montes, Administrator and Chief Executive Officer

INLAND VALLEY REGIONAL MEDICAL CENTER (L, 80 beds) 36485 Inland Valley Drive, Wildomar, CA Zip 92595; tel. 909/677–1111; Christopher L. Boyd, Chief Executive Officer and Managing Director

DISTRICT OF COLUMBIA: GEORGE WASHINGTON UNIVERSITY HOSPITAL (O, 277 beds) 901 23rd Street N.W., Washington, DC Zip 20037–2377; tel. 202/715–4000; Phillip S. Schaengold, JD, Chief Executive Officer
Web address: www.gwumc.edu

FLORIDA: MANATEE MEMORIAL HOSPITAL (O, 512 beds) 206 Second Street East, Bradenton, FL Zip 34208–1000; tel. 941/746–5111; Michael Marquez, Chief Executive Officer

WELLINGTON REGIONAL MEDICAL CENTER (L, 93 beds) 10101 Forest Hill Boulevard, West Palm Beach, FL Zip 33414–6199; tel. 561/798–8500; Gregory E. Boyer, Chief Executive Officer
Web address: www.wrmhospital@icanect.net

GEORGIA: TURNING POINT HOSPITAL (O, 59 beds) 319 East By–Pass, Moultrie, GA Zip 31768, Mailing Address: P.O. Box 1177, Zip 31776–1177; tel. 912/985–4815; Ben Marion, Chief Executive Officer

ILLINOIS: HARTGROVE HOSPITAL (O, 128 beds) 520 North Ridgeway Avenue, Chicago, IL Zip 60624–1299; tel. 773/722–3113; Suzanne Barry, Administrator and Chief Operating Officer

THE PAVILION (O, 46 beds) 809 West Church Street, Champaign, IL Zip 61820; tel. 217/373–1700; Nina W. Eisner, Chief Executive Officer

LOUISIANA: CHALMETTE MEDICAL CENTER (L, 196 beds) 9001 Patricia Street, Chalmette, LA Zip 70043–1727; tel. 504/620–6000; Larry M. Graham, Chief Executive Officer

DOCTORS' HOSPITAL OF SHREVEPORT (L, 118 beds) 1130 Louisiana Avenue, Shreveport, LA Zip 71101–3998, Mailing Address: P.O. Box 1526, Zip 71165–1526; tel. 318/227–1211; Charles E. Boyd, Chief Executive Officer and Managing Director

RIVER OAKS HOSPITAL (O, 94 beds) 1525 River Oaks Road West, New Orleans, LA Zip 70123–2199; tel. 504/734–1740; Daryl Sue White, Chief Executive Officer and Managing Director
Web address: www.riveroakshospital.com

RIVER PARISHES HOSPITAL (O, 106 beds) 500 Rue De Sante, La Place, LA Zip 70068–5420; tel. 504/652–7000; B. Ann Kuss, Chief Executive Officer and Managing Director

MASSACHUSETTS: ARBOUR H. R. I. HOSPITAL (O, 51 beds) 227 Babcock Street, Brookline, MA Zip 02146; tel. 617/731–3200; Roy A. Ettlinger, Chief Executive Officer
Web address: www.arbourhealth.com

ARBOUR HOSPITAL (O, 118 beds) 49 Robinwood Avenue, Boston, MA Zip 02130–2156, Mailing Address: P.O. Box 9, Zip 02130; tel. 617/522–4400; Roy A. Ettlinger, Chief Executive Officer

ARBOUR–FULLER HOSPITAL (O, 46 beds) 200 May Street, Attleboro, MA Zip 02703–5515; tel. 508/761–8500; Gary M. Gilberti, Chief Executive Officer

MICHIGAN: FOREST VIEW HOSPITAL (O, 62 beds) 1055 Medical Park Drive S.E., Grand Rapids, MI Zip 49546–3671; tel. 616/942–9610; John F. Kuhn, Chief Executive Officer
Web address: www.forestview.com

MISSOURI: TWO RIVERS PSYCHIATRIC HOSPITAL (O, 80 beds) 5121 Raytown Road, Kansas City, MO Zip 64133–2141; tel. 816/356–5688; Linda Berridge, Chief Executive Officer
Web address: www.tworivershospital.com

NEVADA: DESERT SPRINGS HOSPITAL (O, 225 beds) 2075 East Flamingo Road, Las Vegas, NV Zip 89119–5121, Mailing Address: P.O. Box 19204, Zip 89132–9204; tel. 702/733–8800; John Lloyd Hummer, Chief Executive Officer

NORTHERN NEVADA MEDICAL CENTER (O, 100 beds) 2375 East Prater Way, Sparks, NV Zip 89434–9900; tel. 775/331–7000; James R. Pagels, Chief Executive Officer and Managing Director
Web address: www.nnmc.com

VALLEY HOSPITAL MEDICAL CENTER (O, 365 beds) 620 Shadow Lane, Las Vegas, NV Zip 89106–4119; tel. 702/388–4000; Roger Collins, Chief Executive Officer and Managing Director

PENNSYLVANIA: CLARION PSYCHIATRIC CENTER (O, 52 beds) 2 Hospital Drive, Clarion, PA Zip 16214–9424; tel. 814/226–9545; Michael R. Keefer, CHE, Chief Executive Officer and Managing Director

HORSHAM CLINIC (O, 138 beds) 722 East Butler Pike, Ambler, PA Zip 19002–2398; tel. 215/643–7800; David A. Baron, D.O., Medical Director

For explanation of codes following names, see page B2.
★ Indicates Type III membership in the American Hospital Association.

Systems / Universal Health Services, Inc.

KEYSTONE CENTER (O, 84 beds) 2001 Providence Avenue, Chester, PA Zip 19013-5504; tel. 610/876-9000; Jimmy Patton, Chief Executive Officer and Managing Director

MEADOWS PSYCHIATRIC CENTER (O, 101 beds) 132 The Meadows Drive, Centre Hall, PA Zip 16828-9798; tel. 814/364-2161; Joseph Barszczewski, Chief Executive Officer and Managing Director

PUERTO RICO: HOSPITAL SAN FRANCISCO (O, 160 beds) 371 Avenida De Diego, Rio Piedras, PR Zip 00923, Mailing Address: P.O. Box 29025, San Juan, Zip 00929-0025; tel. 787/767-2528; Eric Grafals, Executive Director
Web address: www.sanpablo.com

HOSPITAL SAN PABLO (O, 364 beds) Calle Santa Cruz 70, Bayamon, PR Zip 00961, Mailing Address: P.O. Box 236, Zip 00960; tel. 787/740-4747; Jorge Matta, Associate Administrator
Web address: www.sanpablo.com

HOSPITAL SAN PABLO DEL ESTE (O, 107 beds) Avenida General Valero, 404, Fajardo, PR Zip 00738, Mailing Address: P.O. Box 1028, Zip 00738-1028; tel. 787/863-0505; Maria Elena Rodriguez, Executive Administrator
Web address: www.sanpablo.com

SOUTH CAROLINA: AIKEN REGIONAL MEDICAL CENTERS (O, 269 beds) 302 University Parkway, Aiken, SC Zip 29801-2757, Mailing Address: P.O. Box 1117, Zip 29802-1117; tel. 803/641-5000; Richard H. Satcher, Chief Executive Officer

TEXAS: DOCTORS HOSPITAL OF LAREDO (O, 114 beds) 500 East Mann Road, Laredo, TX Zip 78041-2699; tel. 956/723-1131; Abraham Martinez, Chief Executive Officer
Web address: www.hcahealthcare.com

EDINBURG REGIONAL MEDICAL CENTER (O, 163 beds) 1102 West Trenton Road, Edinburg, TX Zip 78539-6199; tel. 956/388-6000; Chris Smolik, Chief Executive Officer
Web address: www.uhsermc.com

GLEN OAKS HOSPITAL (O, 54 beds) 301 East Division, Greenville, TX Zip 75402; tel. 903/454-6000; Thomas E. Rourke, Administrator

MCALLEN MEDICAL CENTER (L, 467 beds) 301 West Expressway 83, McAllen, TX Zip 78503; tel. 956/632-4000; Daniel P. McLean, Executive Director
Web address: www.uhsmmc.com

MERIDELL ACHIEVEMENT CENTER (L, 78 beds) 12550 West Highway 29, Liberty Hill, TX Zip 78642, Mailing Address: P.O. Box 87, Zip 78642-0087; tel. 800/366-8656; Trish Mitchell, Chief Executive Officer

NORTHWEST TEXAS HEALTHCARE SYSTEM (O, 353 beds) 1501 South Coulter Avenue, Amarillo, TX Zip 79106-1790, Mailing Address: P.O. Box 1110, Zip 79175-1110; tel. 806/354-1000; Moody L. Chisholm, Chief Executive Officer and Managing Director
Web address: www.nwths.com

RIVER CREST HOSPITAL (O, 80 beds) 1636 Hunters Glen Road, San Angelo, TX Zip 76901-5016; tel. 915/949-5722; Larry Grimes, Managing Director

TIMBERLAWN MENTAL HEALTH SYSTEM (O, 92 beds) 4600 Samuell Boulevard, Dallas, TX Zip 75228-6800; tel. 214/381-7181; Craig Nuckles, Group Director
Web address: www.timberlawn.com

WASHINGTON: AUBURN REGIONAL MEDICAL CENTER (O, 100 beds) 202 North Division, Plaza One, Auburn, WA Zip 98001-4908; tel. 253/833-7711; Michael M. Gherardini, Chief Executive Officer and Managing Director

Owned, leased, sponsored:	38 hospitals	5768 beds
Contract-managed:	0 hospitals	0 beds
Totals:	38 hospitals	5768 beds

0217: UNIVERSITY HEALTH SYSTEMS OF EASTERN CAROLINA (NP)
2100 Srantonsburg Road, Greenville, NC Zip 27835, Mailing Address: P.O. Box 6028, Zip 27835-6028; tel. 252/816-4100; Dave C. McRae, President and Chief Executive Officer

NORTH CAROLINA: BERTIE MEMORIAL HOSPITAL (O, 15 beds) 401 Sterlingworth Street, Windsor, NC Zip 27983-1726, Mailing Address: P.O. Box 40, Zip 27983-1726; tel. 252/794-3141; Anthony F. Mullen, Administrator
Web address: www.bertie.uhseast.com

CHOWAN HOSPITAL (O, 111 beds) 211 Virginia Road, Edenton, NC Zip 27932-0629, Mailing Address: P.O. Box 629, Zip 27932-0629; tel. 252/482-8451; Barbara R. Cale, President
Web address: www.uhseast.com

HERITAGE HOSPITAL (O, 127 beds) 111 Hospital Drive, Tarboro, NC Zip 27886-2011; tel. 252/641-7700; Janet Mullaney, President
Web address: www.uhseast.com

PITT COUNTY MEMORIAL HOSPITAL–UNIVERSITY HEALTH SYSTEMS OF EASTERN CAROLINA (O, 695 beds) 2100 Stantonsburg Road, Greenville, NC Zip 27835-6028, Mailing Address: Box 6028, Zip 27835-6028; tel. 252/816-4451; Dave C. McRae, President and Chief Executive Officer
Web address: www.pcmh.com

ROANOKE–CHOWAN HOSPITAL (O, 118 beds) 500 South Academy Street, Ahoskie, NC Zip 27910, Mailing Address: P.O. Box 1385, Zip 27910-1385; tel. 252/209-3000; Susan S. Lassiter, President and Chief Executive Officer
Web address: www.rch.uhseast.com

Owned, leased, sponsored:	5 hospitals	1066 beds
Contract-managed:	0 hospitals	0 beds
Totals:	5 hospitals	1066 beds

0112: UNIVERSITY HOSPITALS HEALTH SYSTEM (NP)
11100 Euclid Avenue, Cleveland, OH Zip 44106-5000; tel. 216/844-1000; Farah M. Walters, President and Chief Executive Officer

(Centralized Physician/Insurance Health System)

OHIO: MERCY MEDICAL CENTER (S, 374 beds) 1320 Mercy Drive N.W., Canton, OH Zip 44708-2641; tel. 330/489-1000; Christopher M. Dadlez, President and Chief Executive Officer

SAINT MICHAEL HOSPITAL (O, 199 beds) 5163 Broadway Avenue, Cleveland, OH Zip 44127-1532; tel. 216/429-8000; Richard J. Frenchie, Chief Executive Officer

ST. JOHN WEST SHORE HOSPITAL (S, 183 beds) 29000 Center Ridge Road, Cleveland, OH Zip 44145-5219; tel. 440/835-8000; Fred M. DeGrandis, President

ST. VINCENT CHARITY HOSPITAL (S, 471 beds) 2351 East 22nd Street, Cleveland, OH Zip 44115-3111; tel. 216/861-6200; Alan H. Channing, Chief Executive Officer

UHHS BEDFORD MEDICAL CENTER (O, 99 beds) 44 Blaine Avenue, Bedford, OH Zip 44146-2799; tel. 440/439-2000; Arlene A. Rak, President

UHHS BROWN MEMORIAL HOSPITAL (O, 51 beds) 158 West Main Road, Conneaut, OH Zip 44030-2039, Mailing Address: P.O. Box 648, Zip 44030-0648; tel. 440/593-1131; William P. Lawrence, Chief Executive Officer

UHHS GEAUGA REGIONAL HOSPITAL (O, 142 beds) 13207 Ravenna Road, Chardon, OH Zip 44024-9012; tel. 440/269-6000; Richard J. Frenchie, President and Chief Executive Officer
Web address: www.uhhs.com/uhhs/geauga/index.html

UHHS LAURELWOOD HOSPITAL (O, 120 beds) 35900 Euclid Avenue, Willoughby, OH Zip 44094-4648; tel. 440/953-3000; Farshid Afsarifard, Ph.D., President
Web address: www.laurelwoodhospital.com

UHHS RICHMOND HEIGHTS HOSPITAL (O, 98 beds) 27100 Chardon Road, Richmond Heights, OH Zip 44143-1198; tel. 440/585-6500; William P. Lawrence, President and Chief Executive Officer

UHHS–MEMORIAL HOSPITAL OF GENEVA (O, 40 beds) 870 West Main Street, Geneva, OH Zip 44041-1295; tel. 440/466-1141; William P. Lawrence, President and Chief Executive Officer
Web address: www.uhhs.com

UNIVERSITY HOSPITALS OF CLEVELAND (O, 752 beds) 11100 Euclid Avenue, Cleveland, OH Zip 44106-2602; tel. 216/844-1000; Farah M. Walters, President and Chief Executive Officer
Web address: www.uhhs.com/uhhs/

For explanation of codes following names, see page B2.
★ Indicates Type III membership in the American Hospital Association.

Systems / University of South Alabama Hospitals

Owned, leased, sponsored:	11 hospitals	2529 beds
Contract-managed:	0 hospitals	0 beds
Totals:	11 hospitals	2529 beds

9105: UNIVERSITY OF ALABAMA SYSTEM (NP)
619 South 19th Street, Birmingham, AL Zip 35233;
tel. 205/975–7545; David J. Fine, Chief Executive Officer

ALABAMA: CALLAHAN EYE FOUNDATION HOSPITAL (O, 20 beds) 1720 University Boulevard, Birmingham, AL Zip 35233–1816;
tel. 205/325–8100; Steve C. Schultz, President
Web address: www.health.uab.edu/eyes

UNIVERSITY OF ALABAMA HOSPITAL (O, 870 beds) 619 South 19th Street, Birmingham, AL Zip 35233–6505; tel. 205/934–4011; Martin Nowak, Interim Executive Director
Web address: www.uab.edu

Owned, leased, sponsored:	2 hospitals	890 beds
Contract-managed:	0 hospitals	0 beds
Totals:	2 hospitals	890 beds

6405: UNIVERSITY OF CALIFORNIA–SYSTEMWIDE ADMINISTRATION (NP)
300 Lakeside Drive, 18th Floor, Oakland, CA Zip 94612–3550;
tel. 510/987–9701; Cornelius L. Hopper, M.D., Vice President Health Affairs
(Moderately Centralized Health System)

CALIFORNIA: SANTA MONICA–UCLA MEDICAL CENTER (O, 221 beds) 1250 16th Street, Santa Monica, CA Zip 90404–1200; tel. 310/319–4000; Ellen Pollack, R.N., Interim Chief Operating Officer and Director Nursing

UNIVERSITY OF CALIFORNIA LOS ANGELES MEDICAL CENTER (L, 650 beds) 10833 Le Conte Avenue, Los Angeles, CA Zip 90095–1730;
tel. 310/825–9111; Michael Karpf, M.D., Vice Provost Hospital System and Director Medical Center
Web address: www.medctr.ucla.edu

UNIVERSITY OF CALIFORNIA LOS ANGELES NEUROPSYCHIATRIC HOSPITAL (O, 117 beds) 760 Westwood Plaza, Los Angeles, CA Zip 90095;
tel. 310/825–0511; Fawzy I. Fawzy, M.D., Medical Director
Web address: www.npi.ucla.edu

UNIVERSITY OF CALIFORNIA SAN DIEGO MEDICAL CENTER (O, 468 beds) 200 West Arbor Drive, San Diego, CA Zip 92103–8970; tel. 619/543–6222; Sumiyo E. Kastelic, Director

UNIVERSITY OF CALIFORNIA SAN FRANCISCO MEDICAL CENTER (O, 661 beds) 500 Parnassus, San Francisco, CA Zip 94143–0296;
tel. 415/476–1000; Mark R. Laret, Chief Executive Officer
Web address: www.ucsfstanford.org

UNIVERSITY OF CALIFORNIA, DAVIS MEDICAL CENTER (O, 464 beds) 2315 Stockton Boulevard, Sacramento, CA Zip 95817–2282; tel. 916/734–2011; Martha H. Marsh, Director

UNIVERSITY OF CALIFORNIA, IRVINE MEDICAL CENTER (O, 383 beds) 101 The City Drive, Orange, CA Zip 92868–3298; tel. 714/456–6011; Ralph Cygan, M.D., Interim Director
Web address: www.ucihealth.com

Owned, leased, sponsored:	7 hospitals	2964 beds
Contract-managed:	0 hospitals	0 beds
Totals:	7 hospitals	2964 beds

★0216: UNIVERSITY OF MARYLAND MEDICAL SYSTEM (NP)
22 South Green Street, Baltimore, MD Zip 21201–1595;
tel. 410/328–8667; Morton I. Rapoport, M.D., President and Chief Executive Officer

MARYLAND: DEATON SPECIALTY HOSPITAL AND HOME (O, 277 beds) 601 South Charles Street, Baltimore, MD Zip 21230–3898;
tel. 410/547–8500; James E. Ross, FACHE, Chief Executive Officer

JAMES LAWRENCE KERNAN HOSPITAL (O, 152 beds) 2200 Kernan Drive, Baltimore, MD Zip 21207–6697; tel. 410/448–2500; James E. Ross, FACHE, Chief Executive Officer

MARYLAND GENERAL HOSPITAL (O, 225 beds) 827 Linden Avenue, Baltimore, MD Zip 21201–4681; tel. 410/225–8000; James R. Wood, Chairman and Chief Executive Officer

UNIVERSITY OF MARYLAND MEDICAL CENTER (O, 606 beds) 22 South Greene Street, Baltimore, MD Zip 21201; tel. 410/328–8667; Stephen C. Schimpff, M.D., Chief Executive Officer
Web address: www.umm.edu

Owned, leased, sponsored:	4 hospitals	1260 beds
Contract-managed:	0 hospitals	0 beds
Totals:	4 hospitals	1260 beds

0021: UNIVERSITY OF NEW MEXICO (NP)
915 Camino De Salud, Albuquerque, NM Zip 87131–0001;
tel. 505/272–5849; R. Philip Eaton, M.D., Vice President Health Scences
(Moderately Centralized Health System)

NEW MEXICO: CARRIE TINGLEY HOSPITAL (O, 18 beds) 1127 University Boulevard N.E., Albuquerque, NM Zip 87102–1715; tel. 505/272–5200; Barbara Ohm, Interim Administrator

MENTAL HEALTH CENTER (O, 60 beds) 2600 Marble N.E., Albuquerque, NM Zip 87131–2600; tel. 505/272–2263; Stephen W. McKernan, Chief Executive Officer
Web address: www.mhc.unm.edu

UNIVERSITY HOSPITAL (O, 261 beds) 2211 Lomas Boulevard N.E., Albuquerque, NM Zip 87106–2745; tel. 505/272–2121; Stephen W. McKernan, Chief Executive Officer
Web address: www.unm.edu

UNIVERSITY OF NEW MEXICO CHILDREN'S PSYCHIATRIC HOSPITAL (O, 53 beds) 1001 Yale Boulevard N.E., Albuquerque, NM Zip 87131–3830;
tel. 505/272–2945; Maggie McGowan, Interim Area Director
Web address: www.cph.unm.edu

Owned, leased, sponsored:	4 hospitals	392 beds
Contract-managed:	0 hospitals	0 beds
Totals:	4 hospitals	392 beds

0168: UNIVERSITY OF PENNSYLVANIA HEALTH SYSTEM (NP)
399 South 34th Street, 21st Floor, Philadelphia, PA
Zip 19104–4385; tel. 215/898–5181; Peter G. Traber, M.D., Chief Executive Officer and Dean
(Centralized Health System)

PENNSYLVANIA: HOSPITAL OF THE UNIVERSITY OF PENNSYLVANIA (O, 659 beds) 3400 Spruce Street, Philadelphia, PA Zip 19104–4385;
tel. 215/662–4000; Peter G. Traber, M.D., Chief Executive Officer and Dean
Web address: www.med.upenn.edu

PENNSYLVANIA HOSPITAL (O, 414 beds) 800 Spruce Street, Philadelphia, PA Zip 19107–6192; tel. 215/829–3000; Timothy O. Morgan, Executive Director
Web address: www.pahosp.com

PHOENIXVILLE HOSPITAL OF THE UNIVERSITY OF PENNSYLVANIA HEALTH SYSTEM (O, 126 beds) 140 Nutt Road, Phoenixville, PA Zip 19460–0809, Mailing Address: P.O. Box 809, Zip 19460–0809; tel. 610/983–1000; Richard E. Seagrave, Executive Director and Chief Operating Officer
Web address: www.med.upenn.edu/health/ms.html

PRESBYTERIAN MEDICAL CENTER OF THE UNIVERSITY OF PENNSYLVANIA HEALTH SYSTEM (O, 325 beds) 51 North 39th Street, Philadelphia, PA Zip 19104–2640; tel. 215/662–8000; Michele M. Volpe, Executive Director
Web address: www.health.upenn.edu/pmc

Owned, leased, sponsored:	4 hospitals	1524 beds
Contract-managed:	0 hospitals	0 beds
Totals:	4 hospitals	1524 beds

0057: UNIVERSITY OF SOUTH ALABAMA HOSPITALS (NP)
2451 Fillingim Street, Mobile, AL Zip 36617–2293;
tel. 334/471–7000; Stephen H. Simmons, Senior Administrator

For explanation of codes following names, see page B2.
★ Indicates Type III membership in the American Hospital Association.

Systems / University of South Alabama Hospitals

ALABAMA: USA CHILDREN'S AND WOMEN'S HOSPITAL (O, 152 beds) 1700 Center Street, Mobile, AL Zip 36604–3391; tel. 334/415–1000; Stanley K. Hammack, Administrator

UNIVERSITY OF SOUTH ALABAMA KNOLLWOOD PARK HOSPITAL (O, 150 beds) 5600 Girby Road, Mobile, AL Zip 36693–3398; tel. 334/660–5120; Thomas J. Gibson, Administrator

UNIVERSITY OF SOUTH ALABAMA MEDICAL CENTER (O, 316 beds) 2451 Fillingim Street, Mobile, AL Zip 36617–2293; tel. 334/471–7000; Stephen H. Simmons, Administrator

Owned, leased, sponsored:	3 hospitals	618 beds
Contract-managed:	0 hospitals	0 beds
Totals:	3 hospitals	618 beds

0033: UNIVERSITY OF TEXAS SYSTEM (NP)
601 Colorado Street, Austin, TX Zip 78701–2982; tel. 512/499–4224; Charles B. Mullins, M.D., Executive Vice Chancellor
(Moderately Centralized Health System)

TEXAS: HARRIS COUNTY PSYCHIATRIC CENTER (O, 193 beds) 2800 South MacGregor Way, Houston, TX Zip 77021–1000, Mailing Address: P.O. Box 20249, Zip 77225–0249; tel. 713/741–5000; Robert W. Guynn, M.D., Executive Director
Web address: www.uth.tmc.edu

UNIVERSITY OF TEXAS HEALTH CENTER AT TYLER (O, 117 beds) 11937 Highway 271, Tyler, TX Zip 75708–3154; tel. 903/877–3451; Ronald F. Garvey, M.D., President
Web address: www.uthct.edu

UNIVERSITY OF TEXAS M. D. ANDERSON CANCER CENTER (O, 437 beds) 1515 Holcombe Boulevard, Box 91, Houston, TX Zip 77030–4095; tel. 713/792–6000; John Mendelsohn, M.D., President and Chief Executive Officer
Web address: www.mdanderson.org

UNIVERSITY OF TEXAS MEDICAL BRANCH HOSPITALS (O, 776 beds) 301 University Boulevard, Galveston, TX Zip 77555–0138; tel. 409/772–1011; David S. Lopez, FACHE, Senior Executive Director
Web address: www.utmb.edu

Owned, leased, sponsored:	4 hospitals	1523 beds
Contract-managed:	0 hospitals	0 beds
Totals:	4 hospitals	1523 beds

★0137: UPMC HEALTH SYSTEM (NP)
200 Lothrop, Pittsburgh, PA Zip 15213; tel. 412/647–2345; Jeffrey A. Romoff, President
(Moderately Centralized Health System)

PENNSYLVANIA: MAGEE–WOMENS HOSPITAL (O, 263 beds) 300 Halket Street, Pittsburgh, PA Zip 15213–3180; tel. 412/641–1000; Irma E. Goertzen, President and Chief Executive Officer
Web address: www.magee.edu

UPMC BEAVER VALLEY (O, 112 beds) 2500 Hospital Drive, Aliquippa, PA Zip 15001–2123; tel. 724/857–1212; Susan Dachille, Interim President
Web address: www.upmc.edu

UPMC BEDFORD MEMORIAL (O, 27 beds) 10455 Lincoln Highway, Everett, PA Zip 15537–7046; tel. 814/623–6161; James C. Vreeland, FACHE, President and Chief Executive Officer
Web address: www.bedford.org

UPMC BRADDOCK (O, 148 beds) 400 Holland Avenue, Braddock, PA Zip 15104–1599; tel. 412/636–5000; Margaret Priselac, R.N., Chief Executive Officer
Web address: www.upmc.edu

UPMC HORIZON (O, 243 beds) Greenville, PA J. Larry Heinike, President and Chief Executive Officer
Web address: www.hhs.org

UPMC LEE REGIONAL (O, 217 beds) 320 Main Street, Johnstown, PA Zip 15901–1694; tel. 814/533–0123; David R. Davis, President and Chief Executive Officer
Web address: www.upmc.edu/lee/

UPMC MCKEESPORT (O, 320 beds) 1500 Fifth Avenue, McKeesport, PA Zip 15132–2482; tel. 412/664–2000; Ronald H. Ott, President and Chief Executive Officer
Web address: www.upmc.edu/mckeesport

UPMC PASSAVANT (O, 199 beds) 9100 Babcock Boulevard, Pittsburgh, PA Zip 15237–5815; tel. 412/367–6700; Raymond J. Beck, President and Chief Executive Officer
Web address: www.upmc.edu/passavant

UPMC PRESBYTERIAN (O, 752 beds) Pittsburgh, PA Henry A. Mordoh, President
Web address: www.upmc.edu

UPMC SHADYSIDE (O, 502 beds) 5230 Centre Avenue, Pittsburgh, PA Zip 15232–1304; tel. 412/623–2121; Henry A. Mordoh, President
Web address: www.upmc.edu

UPMC SOUTH SIDE (O, 136 beds) 2000 Mary Street, Pittsburgh, PA Zip 15203–2095; tel. 412/488–5550; Marcie S. Caplan, Chief Executive Officer
Web address: www.upmc.edu/southside/

UPMC ST. MARGARET (O, 223 beds) 815 Freeport Road, Pittsburgh, PA Zip 15215–3301; tel. 412/784–4000; Richard E. Sobehart, President
Web address: www.upmc.edu

Owned, leased, sponsored:	12 hospitals	3142 beds
Contract-managed:	0 hospitals	0 beds
Totals:	12 hospitals	3142 beds

★0038: UPPER CHESAPEAKE HEALTH SYSTEM (NP)
1916 Belair Road, Fallston, MD Zip 21047–2797; tel. 410/893–0322; Lyle Ernest Sheldon, President and Chief Executive Officer
(Independent Hospital System)

MARYLAND: FALLSTON GENERAL HOSPITAL (O, 113 beds) 200 Milton Avenue, Fallston, MD Zip 21047–2777; tel. 410/877–3700; Lyle Ernest Sheldon, President and Chief Executive Officer

HARFORD MEMORIAL HOSPITAL (O, 157 beds) 501 South Union Avenue, Havre De Grace, MD Zip 21078–3493; tel. 410/939–2400; Lyle Ernest Sheldon, President and Chief Executive Officer

Owned, leased, sponsored:	2 hospitals	270 beds
Contract-managed:	0 hospitals	0 beds
Totals:	2 hospitals	270 beds

★0043: VALLEY HEALTH SYSTEM (NP)
1117 East Devonshire Avenue, Hemet, CA Zip 92543; tel. 909/652–2811; John P. Lauri, Chief Executive Officer
(Independent Hospital System)

CALIFORNIA: HEMET VALLEY MEDICAL CENTER (O, 285 beds) 1117 East Devonshire Avenue, Hemet, CA Zip 92543; tel. 909/652–2811; Jack A. Burrows, Administrator

MENIFEE VALLEY MEDICAL CENTER (O, 84 beds) 28400 McCall Boulevard, Sun City, CA Zip 92585–9537; tel. 909/679–8888; Susan Ballard, Administrator

MORENO VALLEY COMMUNITY HOSPITAL (O, 66 beds) 27300 Iris Avenue, Moreno Valley, CA Zip 92555; tel. 909/243–0811; Janice Ziomek, Administrator

Owned, leased, sponsored:	3 hospitals	435 beds
Contract-managed:	0 hospitals	0 beds
Totals:	3 hospitals	435 beds

0128: VALLEY HEALTH SYSTEM (IO)
1840 Amherst Street, Winchester, VA Zip 22601, Mailing Address: P.O. Box 3340, Zip 22604–1334; tel. 540/722–8024; Michael J. Halseth, President and Chief Executive Officer
(Centralized Physician/Insurance Health System)

For explanation of codes following names, see page B2.
★ Indicates Type III membership in the American Hospital Association.

Systems / Vencor, Incorporated

VIRGINIA: WARREN MEMORIAL HOSPITAL (O, 91 beds) 1000 Shenandoah Avenue, Front Royal, VA Zip 22630–3598; tel. 540/636–0300; Charlie M. Horton, President
Web address: www.valleyhealthlink.com

WINCHESTER MEDICAL CENTER (O, 387 beds) 1840 Amherst Street, Winchester, VA Zip 22601–2540, Mailing Address: P.O. Box 3340, Zip 22604–3340; tel. 540/722–8000; George B. Caley, President
Web address: www.valleyhealthlink.com

WEST VIRGINIA: MORGAN COUNTY WAR MEMORIAL HOSPITAL (C, 44 beds) 1124 Fairfax Street, Berkeley Springs, WV Zip 25411–1718; tel. 304/258–1234; Patrick Nolan, Administrator
Web address: www.valleyhealthlink.com

Owned, leased, sponsored:	2 hospitals	478 beds
Contract–managed:	1 hospital	44 beds
Totals:	3 hospitals	522 beds

0097: VALLEYCARE HEALTH SYSTEM (NP)
5575 West Las Positas Boulevard, 300, Pleasanton, CA Zip 94588; tel. 925/447–7000; Marcy L. Feit, Chief Executive Officer

CALIFORNIA: VALLEYCARE MEDICAL CENTER (O, 68 beds) 5555 West Positas Boulevard, Pleasanton, CA Zip 94588, Mailing Address: 555 West Los Positas Boulevard, Zip 94588; tel. 925/847–3000; Marcy L. Feit, Chief Executive Officer

VALLEYCARE MEMORIAL HOSPITAL (O, 110 beds) 1111 East Stanley Boulevard, Livermore, CA Zip 94550; tel. 925/447–7000; Marcy L. Feit, Chief Executive Officer
Web address: www.valleycare.com

Owned, leased, sponsored:	2 hospitals	178 beds
Contract–managed:	0 hospitals	0 beds
Totals:	2 hospitals	178 beds

0081: VALUEMARK HEALTHCARE SYSTEMS, INC. (IO)
300 Galleria Parkway, Suite 650, Atlanta, GA Zip 30339; tel. 770/933–5500; James T. McAfee, Jr, Chairman, President and Chief Executive Officer
(Independent Hospital System)

MISSOURI: HALLMARK YOUTHCARE OF KANSAS CITY (O, 97 beds) 4800 N.W. 88th Street, Kansas City, MO Zip 64154–2757; tel. 816/436–3900; James R. Laws, Chief Executive Officer

VIRGINIA: VALUEMARK WEST END BEHAVIORAL HEALTHCARE SYSTEM (O, 84 beds) 12800 West Creek Parkway, Richmond, VA Zip 23238–1116; tel. 804/784–2200; Wanda H. Sadler, Chief Executive Officer

Owned, leased, sponsored:	2 hospitals	181 beds
Contract–managed:	0 hospitals	0 beds
Totals:	2 hospitals	181 beds

0193: VANGUARD HEALTH SYSTEM (IO)
20 Burton Hills Boulevard, Suite 10, Nashville, TN Zip 37210; tel. 615/665–6000; Charles N. Martin, Jr, President and Chief Executive Officer

ARIZONA: ARROWHEAD COMMUNITY HOSPITAL AND MEDICAL CENTER (O, 115 beds) 18701 North 67th Avenue, Glendale, AZ Zip 85308–5722; tel. 623/561–1000; Richard S. Alley, Executive Vice President and Chief Executive Officer
Web address: www.baptisthealth.com

MARYVALE HOSPITAL MEDICAL CENTER (O, 171 beds) 5102 West Campbell Avenue, Phoenix, AZ Zip 85031–1799; tel. 623/848–5000; Art Layne, Chief Executive Officer

PHOENIX BAPTIST HOSPITAL AND MEDICAL CENTER (O, 201 beds) 2000 West Bethany Home Road, Phoenix, AZ Zip 85015–2110; tel. 602/249–0212; Jeffrey K. Norman, Executive Vice President and Chief Executive Officer
Web address: www.baptisthealth.com

CALIFORNIA: HUNTINGTON BEACH HOSPITAL (O, 116 beds) 17772 Beach Boulevard, Huntington Beach, CA Zip 92647–9932; tel. 714/842–1473; David K. Culberson, Chief Executive Officer

LA PALMA INTERCOMMUNITY HOSPITAL (O, 139 beds) 7901 Walker Street, La Palma, CA Zip 90623–5850, Mailing Address: P.O. Box 5850, Buena Park, Zip 90622; tel. 714/670–7400; David K. Culberson, Chief Executive Officer
Web address: www.unihealth.org

WEST ANAHEIM MEDICAL CENTER (O, 219 beds) 3033 West Orange Avenue, Anaheim, CA Zip 92804–3184; tel. 714/827–3000; David K. Culberson, Chief Executive Officer

ILLINOIS: MACNEAL HOSPITAL (O, 315 beds) 3249 South Oak Park Avenue, Berwyn, IL Zip 60402–0715; tel. 708/783–9100; Brian J. Lemon, President
Web address: www.macneal.com

Owned, leased, sponsored:	7 hospitals	1276 beds
Contract–managed:	0 hospitals	0 beds
Totals:	7 hospitals	1276 beds

0026: VENCOR, INCORPORATED (IO)
1 Vencor Place, 680 S. 4th Avenue, Louisville, KY Zip 40202–2412; tel. 502/596–7300; Edward L. Kuntz, Board Chairman, President and Chief Executive Officer
(Independent Hospital System)

ARIZONA: VENCOR HOSPITAL – TUCSON (O, 51 beds) 355 North Wilmot Road, Tucson, AZ Zip 85711–2635; tel. 520/747–8200; Kevin Christiansen, Administrator

VENCOR HOSPITAL–PHOENIX (O, 58 beds) 40 East Indianola Avenue, Phoenix, AZ Zip 85012–2059; tel. 602/280–7000

CALIFORNIA: RECOVERY INN OF MENLO PARK (O, 16 beds) 570 Willow Road, Menlo Park, CA Zip 94025; tel. 650/324–8500; Carole Wilson, MSN, CHE, Administrator

VENCOR HOSPITAL–BREA (O, 48 beds) 875 North Brea Boulevard, Brea, CA Zip 92821; tel. 714/529–6842; Virgis Narbutas, Executive Director

VENCOR HOSPITAL–LOS ANGELES (O, 81 beds) 5525 West Slauson Avenue, Los Angeles, CA Zip 90056; tel. 310/642–0325; Judith McCurdy, Administrator and Chief Executive Officer

VENCOR HOSPITAL–ONTARIO (O, 100 beds) 550 North Monterey, Ontario, CA Zip 91764; tel. 909/391–0333; Robert J. Trautman, Administrator

VENCOR HOSPITAL–SACRAMENTO (O, 32 beds) 223 Fargo Way, Folsom, CA Zip 95630; tel. 916/351–9151; Meredith Taylor, Administrator

VENCOR HOSPITAL–SAN DIEGO (O, 70 beds) 1940 El Cajon Boulevard, San Diego, CA Zip 92104; tel. 619/543–4500; William Mitchell, Administrator

VENCOR HOSPITAL–SAN LEANDRO (O, 42 beds) 2800 Benedict Drive, San Leandro, CA Zip 94577; tel. 510/357–8300; Carole Wilson, MSN, CHE, Administrator and Chief Executive Officer

FLORIDA: VENCOR HOSPITAL – CENTRAL TAMPA (O, 73 beds) 4801 North Howard Avenue, Tampa, FL Zip 33603–1484; tel. 813/874–7575; Ken Stone, Administrator
Web address: www.vencor.com

VENCOR HOSPITAL–CORAL GABLES (O, 53 beds) 5190 S.W. Eighth Street, Coral Gables, FL Zip 33134–2495; tel. 305/445–1364; Jane Jackson, Chief Executive Officer
Web address: www.vencor.com

VENCOR HOSPITAL–FORT LAUDERDALE (O, 64 beds) 1516 East Las Olas Boulevard, Fort Lauderdale, FL Zip 33301–2399; tel. 954/764–8900; Lewis A. Ransdell, Administrator
Web address: www.vencor.com

VENCOR HOSPITAL–ST PETERSBURG (O, 60 beds) 3030 Sixth Street South, Saint Petersburg, FL Zip 33705–3720; tel. 727/894–8719; Pamela M. Riter, R.N., Administrator
Web address: www.vencor.com

VENCOR HOSPITAL–TAMPA (O, 73 beds) 4555 South Manhattan Avenue, Tampa, FL Zip 33611–2397; tel. 813/839–6341; Theresa Hunkins, Administrator
Web address: www.vencor.com

VENCOR–NORTH FLORIDA (O, 60 beds) 801 Oak Street, Green Cove Springs, FL Zip 32043–4317; tel. 904/284–9230; Tim Simpson, Administrator
Web address: www.vencor.com

For explanation of codes following names, see page B2.
★ Indicates Type III membership in the American Hospital Association.

Systems / Vencor, Incorporated

GEORGIA: VENCOR HOSPITAL–ATLANTA (O, 66 beds) 705 Juniper Street N.E., Atlanta, GA Zip 30365–2500; tel. 404/873–2871; Skip Wright, Administrator

ILLINOIS: VENCOR HOSPITAL–CHICAGO CENTRAL (O, 81 beds) 4058 West Melrose Street, Chicago, IL Zip 60641–4797; tel. 773/736–7000; Richard Cerceo, Administrator
Web address: www.vencor.com

VENCOR HOSPITAL–CHICAGO NORTH (O, 164 beds) 2544 West Montrose Avenue, Chicago, IL Zip 60618–1589; tel. 773/267–2622; Susan Legg, Administrator
Web address: www.vencor.com

VENCOR HOSPITAL–SYCAMORE (O, 50 beds) 225 Edward Street, Sycamore, IL Zip 60178–2197; tel. 815/895–2144; Laura S. Wills, R.N., Administrator
Web address: www.vencor.com

INDIANA: VENCOR HOSPITAL–LAGRANGE (O, 57 beds) 207 North Townline Road, LaGrange, IN Zip 46761–1325; tel. 219/463–2143; Shelleye Hicks, Administrator
Web address: www.vencor.com

KENTUCKY: VENCOR HOSPITAL–LOUISVILLE (O, 156 beds) 1313 St. Anthony Place, Louisville, KY Zip 40204–1765; tel. 502/587–7001; James H. Wesp, Administrator

LOUISIANA: VENCOR HOSPITAL – NEW ORLEANS (O, 78 beds) 3601 Coliseum Street, New Orleans, LA Zip 70115–3606; tel. 504/899–1555; Jan Turk, Chief Executive Officer

MASSACHUSETTS: VENCOR HOSPITAL NORTH SHORE (O, 50 beds) 15 King Street, Peabody, MA Zip 01960–4268; tel. 978/531–2900; Steven E. Levitsky, Administrator
Web address: www.vencor.com

VENCOR HOSPITAL–BOSTON (O, 59 beds) 1515 Commonwealth Avenue, Boston, MA Zip 02135–3696; tel. 617/254–1100; Donald E. Schwarz, Administrator

MICHIGAN: VENCOR HOSPITAL–METRO DETROIT (O, 112 beds) 2700 Martin Luther King Boulevard, Detroit, MI Zip 48208; tel. 313/361–8000; Daniel A. Eppley, FACHE, Executive Director
Web address: www.vencor.com

MINNESOTA: VENCOR HOSPITAL–MINNEAPOLIS (O, 111 beds) 4101 Golden Valley Road, Golden Valley, MN Zip 55422; tel. 612/588–2750; Thomas N. Theroult, Administrator

MISSOURI: VENCOR HOSPITAL–KANSAS CITY (O, 100 beds) 8701 Troost Avenue, Kansas City, MO Zip 64131–3495; tel. 816/995–2000; E. Bradley Strecker, Chief Executive Officer

NEVADA: VENCOR HOSPITAL–LAS VEGAS (O, 52 beds) 5100 West Sahara Avenue, Las Vegas, NV Zip 89102–3436; tel. 702/871–1418; Linn P. Billingsley, Administrator

NEW MEXICO: VENCOR HOSPITAL – ALBUQUERQUE (O, 56 beds) 700 High Street N.E., Albuquerque, NM Zip 87102–2565; tel. 505/242–4444; Jeanne Koester, Chief Executive Officer

NORTH CAROLINA: VENCOR HOSPITAL–GREENSBORO (O, 124 beds) 2401 Southside Boulevard, Greensboro, NC Zip 27406–3311; tel. 336/271–2800; Leanne Fiorentino, Chief Executive Officer

PENNSYLVANIA: VENCOR HOSPITAL–PHILADELPHIA (O, 52 beds) 6129 Palmetto Street, Philadelphia, PA Zip 19111–5729; tel. 215/722–8555; Garrett Arneson, Administrator
Web address: www.vencor.com

VENCOR HOSPITAL–PITTSBURGH (O, 63 beds) 7777 Steubenville Pike, Oakdale, PA Zip 15071–3409; tel. 412/494–5500; Judy Weaver, Administrator
Web address: www.vencor.com

TENNESSEE: VENCOR HOSPITAL–CHATTANOOGA (O, 44 beds) 709 Walnut Street, Chattanooga, TN Zip 37402–1961; tel. 423/266–7721; Steven E. McGraw, Administrator
Web address: www.vencor.com

TEXAS: VENCOR ARLINGTON, TEXAS (O, 63 beds) 1000 North Cooper Street, Arlington, TX Zip 76011–5540; tel. 817/543–0200; Joy Dier, Administrator

VENCOR HOSPITAL – DALLAS (O, 125 beds) 9525 Greenville Avenue, Dallas, TX Zip 75243–4116; tel. 214/355–2600; Dorothy J. Elford, Executive Director and Administrator

VENCOR HOSPITAL–FORT WORTH SOUTHWEST (O, 41 beds) 7800 Oakmont Boulevard, Fort Worth, TX Zip 76132–4299; tel. 817/346–0094; Robert L. McNew, Administrator

VENCOR HOSPITAL–HOUSTON (O, 110 beds) 6441 Main Street, Houston, TX Zip 77030–1596; tel. 713/790–0500; Bob Stein, Executive Director
Web address: www.vencor.com

VENCOR HOSPITAL–MANSFIELD (O, 122 beds) 1802 Highway 157 North, Mansfield, TX Zip 76063–9555; tel. 817/473–6101; M. Joanne Saltzman, Interim Administrator

VIRGINIA: NORTHERN VIRGINIA COMMUNITY HOSPITAL (O, 96 beds) 601 South Carlin Springs Road, Arlington, VA Zip 22204–1096; tel. 703/671–1200; Mark Aanonson, Administrator
Web address: www.nvchospital.com

WASHINGTON: VENCOR HOSPITAL SEATTLE (O, 42 beds) 10560 Fifth Avenue N.E., Seattle, WA Zip 98125–0977; tel. 206/364–2050; Jim Steinruck, CHE, Administrator and Chief Executive Officer
Web address: www.vencor.com

WISCONSIN: VENCOR HOSPITAL–MILWAUKEE (O, 34 beds) 5017 South 110th Street, Greenfield, WI Zip 53228; tel. 414/427–8282; Daniel R. West, Administrator
Web address: www.vencor.com

VENCOR HOSPITAL–MILWAUKEE (O, 60 beds) 5700 West Layton Avenue, Milwaukee, WI 53202; tel. 414/427–8282; E. Kay Gray, Interim Administrator

Owned, leased, sponsored:	42 hospitals	3049 beds
Contract–managed:	0 hospitals	0 beds
Totals:	42 hospitals	3049 beds

5435: VIA CHRISTI HEALTH SYSTEM (CC)
818 North Emporia, Wichita, KS Zip 67214–3725; tel. 316/268–5000; LeRoy E. Rheault, President and Chief Executive Officer
(Centralized Physician/Insurance Health System)

CALIFORNIA: ST. ROSE HOSPITAL (O, 175 beds) 27200 Calaroga Avenue, Hayward, CA Zip 94545–4383; tel. 510/264–4000; Michael P. Mahoney, President and Chief Executive Officer
Web address: www.strosehospital.org

KANSAS: MERCY HEALTH CENTER OF MANHATTAN (O, 114 beds) 1823 College Avenue, Manhattan, KS Zip 66502–3381, Mailing Address: P.O. Box 1289, Zip 66502–1289; tel. 785/776–3322; Richard L. Allen, President and Chief Executive Officer

MOUNT CARMEL MEDICAL CENTER (O, 126 beds) 1102 East Centennial Drive, Pittsburg, KS Zip 66762–6643; tel. 316/231–6100; John Daniel Lingor, President and Chief Executive Officer

VIA CHRISTI REGIONAL MEDICAL CENTER (O, 942 beds) 929 North St. Francis Street, Wichita, KS Zip 67214–3882; tel. 316/268–5000; Randall G. Nyp, President and Chief Executive Officer
Web address: www.via-christi.org

OKLAHOMA: ST. JOSEPH REGIONAL MEDICAL CENTER OF NORTHERN OKLAHOMA (O, 100 beds) 14th Street and Hartford Avenue, Ponca City, OK Zip 74601–2035, Mailing Address: Box 1270, Zip 74602–1270; tel. 580/765–3321; Garry L. England, President and Chief Executive Officer
Web address: www.sjrmcpc.com

Owned, leased, sponsored:	5 hospitals	1457 beds
Contract–managed:	0 hospitals	0 beds
Totals:	5 hospitals	1457 beds

★**0046: VIA HEALTH** (NP)
150 North Chestnut, Rochester, NY Zip 14604; tel. 716/922–3000; Fritz Leibert, Interim Chief Executive Officer
(Moderately Centralized Health System)

For explanation of codes following names, see page B2.
★ Indicates Type III membership in the American Hospital Association.

Systems / Wellstar Health System

NEW YORK: GENESEE HOSPITAL (O, 269 beds) 224 Alexander Street, Rochester, NY Zip 14607–4055; tel. 716/922–6000; Richard S. Constantino, M.D., President

ROCHESTER GENERAL HOSPITAL (O, 476 beds) 1425 Portland Avenue, Rochester, NY Zip 14621–3099; tel. 716/338–4000; Richard S. Constantino, M.D., President
Web address: www.viahealth.org/

VIAHEALTH OF WAYNE (O, 255 beds) Driving Park Avenue, Newark, NY Zip 14513, Mailing Address: P.O. Box 111, Zip 14513–0111; tel. 315/332–2022; W. Neil Stroman, President
Web address: www.viahealth.org

Owned, leased, sponsored:	3 hospitals	1000 beds
Contract–managed:	0 hospitals	0 beds
Totals:	3 hospitals	1000 beds

0012: VIRGINIA DEPARTMENT OF MENTAL HEALTH (NP)
1220 Bank Street, Richmond, VA Zip 23219–3623, Mailing Address: P.O. Box 1797, Zip 23218–1797; tel. 804/786–3921; Richard E. Kellogg, Commissioner
(Independent Hospital System)

VIRGINIA: CATAWBA HOSPITAL (O, 171 beds) 5525 Catawba Hospital Drive, Catawba, VA Zip 24070, Mailing Address: P.O. Box 200, Zip 24070–0200; tel. 540/375–4200; James S. Reinhard, M.D., Director

CENTRAL STATE HOSPITAL (O, 366 beds) 26317 West Washington Street, Petersburg, VA Zip 23803, Mailing Address: P.O. Box 4030, Zip 23803–4030; tel. 804/524–7000; Larry L. Latham, Director
Web address: www.csh.state.va.us

CENTRAL VIRGINIA TRAINING CENTER (O, 1112 beds) 210 East Colony Road, Madison Heights, VA Zip 24572–2005, Mailing Address: P.O. Box 1098, Lynchburg, Zip 24505–1098; tel. 804/947–6326; Judy Dudley, Director

DE JARNETTE CENTER (O, 60 beds) 1355 Richmond Road, Staunton, VA Zip 24401–1091, Mailing Address: Box 2309, Zip 24402–2309; tel. 540/332–2100; William J. Tuell, Director

EASTERN STATE HOSPITAL (O, 581 beds) 4601 Ironbound Road, Williamsburg, VA Zip 23187–8791, Mailing Address: P.O. Box 8791, Zip 23187–8791; tel. 757/253–5161; John M. Favret, Director
Web address: www.easternstatehospital.org

NORTHERN VIRGINIA MENTAL HEALTH INSTITUTE (O, 137 beds) 3302 Gallows Road, Falls Church, VA Zip 22042–3398; tel. 703/207–7110; Mohamed El-Sabaawi, M.D., Acting Facility Director

PIEDMONT GERIATRIC HOSPITAL (O, 210 beds) 900 East Patrick Henry, Burkeville, VA Zip 23922–0427, Mailing Address: P.O. Box 427, Zip 23922–0427; tel. 804/767–4401; Willard R. Pierce , Jr, Director

SOUTHERN VIRGINIA MENTAL HEALTH INSTITUTE (O, 96 beds) 382 Taylor Drive, Danville, VA Zip 24541–4023; tel. 804/799–6220; Constance N. Fletcher, Ph.D., Director

SOUTHWESTERN VIRGINIA MENTAL HEALTH INSTITUTE (O, 266 beds) 340 Bagley Circle, Marion, VA Zip 24354–3390; tel. 540/783–1200; Gerald E. Deans, Director

WESTERN STATE HOSPITAL (O, 488 beds) 1301 Richmond Avenue, Staunton, VA Zip 24401–9146, Mailing Address: P.O. Box 2500, Zip 24402–2500; tel. 540/332–8000; Jack W. Barber, M.D., Director
Web address: www.wsh.state.va.us

Owned, leased, sponsored:	10 hospitals	3487 beds
Contract–managed:	0 hospitals	0 beds
Totals:	10 hospitals	3487 beds

★6725: VIRTUA HEALTH (NP)
94 Brick Road, Suite 200, Marlton, NJ Zip 08053; tel. 856/355–0005; Richard P. Miller, President and Chief Executive Officer
(Moderately Centralized Health System)

NEW JERSEY: VIRRUA WEST JERSEY HOSPITAL–MARLTON (O, 167 beds) 90 Brick Road, Marlton, NJ Zip 08053–9697; tel. 856/355–6000; Leroy J. Rosenberg, Executive Director
Web address: www.wjhs.org

VIRTUA MEMORIAL HOSPITAL BURLINGTON COUNTY (O, 413 beds) 175 Madison Avenue, Mount Holly, NJ Zip 08060–2099; tel. 609/267–0700; Donald I. Brunn, Executive Vice President
Web address: www.virtua.org

VIRTUA WEST JERSEY HOSPITAL–BERLIN (O, 79 beds) 100 Townsend Avenue, Berlin, NJ Zip 08009–9035; tel. 856/322–3100; Ellen Guarnieri, Vice President and Chief Operating Officer
Web address: www.virtua.org

VIRTUA WEST JERSEY HOSPITAL–CAMDEN (O, 117 beds) 1000 Atlantic Avenue, Camden, NJ Zip 08104–1595; tel. 856/246–3000; Carolyn M. Ballard, Executive Director
Web address: www.wjhs.org

VIRTUA WEST JERSEY HOSPITAL–VOORHEES (O, 253 beds) 101 Carnie Boulevard, Voorhees, NJ Zip 08043–1597; tel. 856/325–3000; Joan T. Meyers, R.N., Vice President and Chief Operating Officer
Web address: www.virtua.org

Owned, leased, sponsored:	5 hospitals	1029 beds
Contract–managed:	0 hospitals	0 beds
Totals:	5 hospitals	1029 beds

0188: WELLMONT HEALTH SYSTEM (NP)
1905 American Way, Kingsport, TN Zip 37662–0224; tel. 423/224–3000; Eddie A. George, President and Chief Executive Officer
(Centralized Physician/Insurance Health System)

TENNESSEE: WELLMONT BRISTOL REGIONAL MEDICAL CENTER (O, 348 beds) 1 Medical Park Boulevard, Bristol, TN Zip 37620–7434; tel. 423/844–4200; Randall M. Olson, President
Web address: www.wellmont.com

WELLMONT HOLSTON VALLEY MEDICAL CENTER (O, 375 beds) West Ravine Street, Kingsport, TN Zip 37662–0224, Mailing Address: Box 238, Zip 37662–0224; tel. 423/224–4000; Louis H. Bremer, President and Chief Executive Officer
Web address: www.wellmont.org

VIRGINIA: WELLMONT LONESOME PINE HOSPITAL (O, 49 beds) 1990 Holton Avenue East, Big Stone Gap, VA Zip 24219–0230; tel. 540/523–3111; Paul A. Bishop, Administrator

Owned, leased, sponsored:	3 hospitals	772 beds
Contract–managed:	0 hospitals	0 beds
Totals:	3 hospitals	772 beds

★0995: WELLSTAR HEALTH SYSTEM (NP)
805 Sandy Plains Road, Marietta, GA Zip 30066; tel. 770/792–5012; Thomas E. Hill, Chief Executive Officer
(Moderately Centralized Health System)

GEORGIA: WELLSTAR COBB HOSPITAL (O, 311 beds) 3950 Austell Road, Austell, GA Zip 30106–1121; tel. 770/732–4000; Thomas E. Hill, Chief Executive Officer
Web address: www.promina.org

WELLSTAR DOUGLAS HOSPITAL (O, 98 beds) 8954 Hospital Drive, Douglasville, GA Zip 30134–2282; tel. 770/949–1500; Thomas E. Hill, Chief Executive Officer
Web address: www.wellstar.org

WELLSTAR KENNESTONE HOSPITAL (O, 439 beds) 677 Church Street, Marietta, GA Zip 30060–1148; tel. 770/793–5000; Thomas E. Hill, Chief Executive Officer

WELLSTAR PAULDING HOSPITAL (O, 208 beds) 600 West Memorial Drive, Dallas, GA Zip 30132–1335; tel. 770/445–4411; Thomas E. Hill, Chief Executive Officer

WELLSTAR WINDY HILL HOSPITAL (O, 100 beds) 2540 Windy Hill Road, Marietta, GA Zip 30067–8632; tel. 770/644–1000; Thomas E. Hill, Chief Executive Officer

Owned, leased, sponsored:	5 hospitals	1156 beds
Contract–managed:	0 hospitals	0 beds
Totals:	5 hospitals	1156 beds

For explanation of codes following names, see page B2.
★ Indicates Type III membership in the American Hospital Association.

Systems / West Penn Allegheny Health System

★**0199: WEST PENN ALLEGHENY HEALTH SYSTEM** (NP)
320 East North Avenue, Pittsburgh, PA Zip 15221–2173;
tel. 412/359–3010; Charles M. O'Brien, Jr, President and Chief Executive Officer

PENNSYLVANIA: ALLEGHENY UNIVERSITY HOSPITALS, ALLEGHENY GENERAL (O, 492 beds) 320 East North Avenue, Pittsburgh, PA Zip 15212–4756; tel. 412/359–3131; Connie M. Cibrone, President and Chief Executive Officer
Web address: www.allhealth.edu

ALLEGHENY UNIVERSITY HOSPITALS, ALLEGHENY VALLEY (O, 258 beds) 1301 Carlisle Street, Natrona Heights, PA Zip 15065–1192; tel. 724/224–5100; Joseph Calig, President and Chief Executive Officer

ALLEGHENY UNIVERSITY HOSPITALS, FORBES REGIONAL (O, 335 beds) 2570 Haymaker Road, Monroeville, PA Zip 15146–3592; tel. 412/858–2000; Barry H. Roth, President and Chief Executive Officer

CANONSBURG GENERAL HOSPITAL (O, 120 beds) 100 Medical Boulevard, Canonsburg, PA Zip 15317–9762; tel. 724/745–6100; Barbara A. Bensaia, Chief Executive Officer

SUBURBAN GENERAL HOSPITAL (O, 144 beds) 100 South Jackson Avenue, Pittsburgh, PA Zip 15202–3428; tel. 412/734–6000; Frank G. DeLisi, II, CHE, President and Chief Executive Officer
Web address: www.wphs.org/westpennhospital.htm

WESTERN PENNSYLVANIA HOSPITAL (O, 462 beds) 4800 Friendship Avenue, Pittsburgh, PA Zip 15224–1722; tel. 412/578–5000; James M. Collins, President and Chief Executive Officer
Web address: www.westpennhospital.org

Owned, leased, sponsored:	6 hospitals	1811 beds
Contract–managed:	0 hospitals	0 beds
Totals:	6 hospitals	1811 beds

★**0004: WEST TENNESSEE HEALTHCARE** (NP)
708 West Forest Avenue, Jackson, TN Zip 38301–3901;
tel. 901/425–5000; James T. Moss, President
(Independent Hospital System)

TENNESSEE: BOLIVAR GENERAL HOSPITAL (O, 47 beds) 650 Nuckolls Road, Bolivar, TN Zip 38008–1500; tel. 901/658–3100; Rosamond Tyler, Administrator
Web address: www.wth.net

CAMDEN GENERAL HOSPITAL (O, 40 beds) 175 Hospital Drive, Camden, TN Zip 38320–1617; tel. 901/584–6135; John M. Carruth, Administrator
Web address: www.wth.net

GIBSON GENERAL HOSPITAL (O, 42 beds) 200 Hospital Drive, Trenton, TN Zip 38382–3313; tel. 901/855–7900; Kelly R. Yenawine, Administrator
Web address: www.wth.net

HUMBOLDT GENERAL HOSPITAL (O, 42 beds) 3525 Chere Carol Road, Humboldt, TN Zip 38343–3699; tel. 901/784–0301; Bill Kail, Administrator
Web address: www.wth.net

JACKSON–MADISON COUNTY GENERAL HOSPITAL (O, 567 beds) 708 West Forest Avenue, Jackson, TN Zip 38301–3855; tel. 901/425–5000; James T. Moss, President and Chief Executive Officer
Web address: www.wth.net

MILAN GENERAL HOSPITAL (O, 62 beds) 4039 South Highland, Milan, TN Zip 38358; tel. 901/686–1591; Alfred P. Taylor, Administrator and Chief Executive Officer
Web address: www.wth.net

PATHWAYS (O, 25 beds) 238 Summar Drive, Jackson, TN Zip 38301–3982; tel. 901/935–8200; Karen Utley, Executive Director

Owned, leased, sponsored:	7 hospitals	825 beds
Contract–managed:	0 hospitals	0 beds
Totals:	7 hospitals	825 beds

0119: WEST VIRGINIA UNITED HEALTH SYSTEM (NP)
1000 Technology Drive, Suite 2320, Fairmont, WV Zip 26554;
tel. 304/368–2700; Bernard G. Westfall, President and Chief Executive Officer
(Centralized Physician/Insurance Health System)

WEST VIRGINIA: BROADDUS HOSPITAL (O, 72 beds) College Hill, Philippi, WV Zip 26416–1051; tel. 304/457–1760; Susannah Higgins, Chief Executive Officer

DAVIS MEMORIAL HOSPITAL (O, 115 beds) Gorman Avenue and Reed Street, Elkins, WV Zip 26241, Mailing Address: P.O. Box 1484, Zip 26241–1484; tel. 304/636–3300; Robert L. Hammer, II, Chief Executive Officer
Web address: www.davishealthcare.com

UNITED HOSPITAL CENTER (O, 367 beds) Route 19 South, Clarksburg, WV Zip 26301, Mailing Address: P.O. Box 1680, Zip 26302–1680; tel. 304/624–2121; Bruce C. Carter, President
Web address: www.uhcwv.org

WEST VIRGINIA UNIVERSITY HOSPITALS (O, 401 beds) Medical Center Drive, Morgantown, WV Zip 26506–4749; tel. 304/598–4000; Bruce McClymonds, President
Web address: www.wvhealth.wvu.edu

Owned, leased, sponsored:	4 hospitals	955 beds
Contract–managed:	0 hospitals	0 beds
Totals:	4 hospitals	955 beds

★**6745: WHEATON FRANCISCAN SERVICES, INC.** (CC)
26W171 Roosevelt Road, Wheaton, IL Zip 60189–0667, Mailing Address: P.O. Box 667, Zip 60189–0667; tel. 630/462–9271; Wilfred F. Loebig, Jr, President and Chief Executive Officer
(Decentralized Health System)

ILLINOIS: MARIANJOY REHABILITATION HOSPITAL (O, 116 beds) 26 West 171 Roosevelt Road, Wheaton, IL Zip 60187–0795, Mailing Address: P.O. Box 795, Zip 60189–0795; tel. 630/462–4000; Kathleen C. Yosko, President and Chief Executive Officer
Web address: www.marianjoy.org

OAK PARK HOSPITAL (O, 176 beds) 520 South Maple Avenue, Oak Park, IL Zip 60304–1097; tel. 708/383–9300; Bruce M. Elegant, President and Chief Executive Officer

IOWA: COVENANT MEDICAL CENTER (O, 283 beds) 3421 West Ninth Street, Waterloo, IA Zip 50702–5499; tel. 319/272–8000; Raymond F. Burfeind, President
Web address: www.covhealth.com

MERCY HOSPITAL OF FRANCISCAN SISTERS (O, 64 beds) 201 Eighth Avenue S.E., Oelwein, IA Zip 50662–2447; tel. 319/283–6000; Richard Schrupp, President and Chief Executive Officer

SARTORI MEMORIAL HOSPITAL (O, 62 beds) 515 College Street, Cedar Falls, IA Zip 50613–2599; tel. 319/268–3000

WISCONSIN: ALL SAINT'S HEALTHCARE SYSTEM (O, 215 beds) 3801 Spring Street, Racine, WI Zip 53405–1690; tel. 262/636–4011; Kenneth R. Buser, President and Chief Executive Officer

ELMBROOK MEMORIAL HOSPITAL (O, 136 beds) 19333 West North Avenue, Brookfield, WI Zip 53045–4198; tel. 262/785–2000; Kimry A. Johnsrud, President
Web address: www.covhealth.org

ST. CATHERINE'S HOSPITAL (O, 114 beds) 3556 Seventh Avenue, Kenosha, WI Zip 53140–2595; tel. 262/656–2011; Richard O. Schmidt, Jr, President and Chief Executive Officer
Web address: www.acronet.net/~stcath

ST. ELIZABETH HOSPITAL (S, 166 beds) 1506 South Oneida Street, Appleton, WI Zip 54915–1397; tel. 920/738–2000; Robert J. Turner, Chief Operating Officer

ST. FRANCIS HOSPITAL (S, 212 beds) 3237 South 16th Street, Milwaukee, WI Zip 53215–4592; tel. 414/647–5000; Jerrold A. Maki, President
Web address: www.covhealth.org

ST. JOSEPH'S HOSPITAL (O, 473 beds) 5000 West Chambers Street, Milwaukee, WI Zip 53210–9988; tel. 414/447–2000; Patricia A. Kaldor, R.N., President
Web address: www.covhealth.org

ST. LUKE'S MEMORIAL HOSPITAL (O, 151 beds) 1320 Wisconsin Avenue, Racine, WI Zip 53403–1987; tel. 262/636–2011; Kenneth R. Buser, President and Chief Executive Officer

ST. MICHAEL HOSPITAL (O, 179 beds) 2400 West Villard Avenue, Milwaukee, WI Zip 53209–4999; tel. 414/527–8000; Jeffrey K. Jenkins, President
Web address: www.covhealth.org

For explanation of codes following names, see page B2.
★ Indicates Type III membership in the American Hospital Association.

Systems / Youth and Family Centered Services

Owned, leased, sponsored:	13 hospitals	2347 beds
Contract-managed:	0 hospitals	0 beds
Totals:	13 hospitals	2347 beds

★9575: **WILLIAM BEAUMONT HOSPITAL CORPORATION** (NP)
3601 West Thirteen Mile Road, Royal Oak, MI Zip 48073–6769;
tel. 248/551–5000; Ted D. Wasson, President and Chief Executive Officer
(Centralized Health System)

MICHIGAN: WILLIAM BEAUMONT HOSPITAL–ROYAL OAK (O, 899 beds) 3601 West Thirteen Mile Road, Royal Oak, MI Zip 48073–6769; tel. 248/551–5000; John D. Labriola, Senior Vice President and Hospital Director
Web address: www.beaumont.edu

WILLIAM BEAUMONT HOSPITAL–TROY (O, 189 beds) 44201 Dequindre Road, Troy, MI Zip 48098–1198; tel. 248/828–5100; Eugene F. Michalski, Senior Vice President and Director
Web address: www.beaumont.edu

Owned, leased, sponsored:	2 hospitals	1088 beds
Contract-managed:	0 hospitals	0 beds
Totals:	2 hospitals	1088 beds

★0157: **YALE NEW HAVEN HEALTH SYSTEM** (NP)
789 Howard Avenue, New Haven, CT Zip 06519;
tel. 203/688–2608; Joseph A. Zaccagnino, President and Chief Executive Officer
(Centralized Physician/Insurance Health System)

CONNECTICUT: BRIDGEPORT HOSPITAL (O, 334 beds) 267 Grant Street, Bridgeport, CT Zip 06610–0120, Mailing Address: P.O. Box 5000, Zip 06610–5000; tel. 203/384–3000; Robert J. Trefry, President and Chief Executive Officer
Web address: www.bridgeporthospital.com

GREENWICH HOSPITAL (O, 160 beds) 5 Perryridge Road, Greenwich, CT Zip 06830–4697; tel. 203/863–3000; Frank A. Corvino, President and Chief Executive Officer
Web address: www.greenhosp.chime.org

YALE–NEW HAVEN HOSPITAL (O, 722 beds) 20 York Street, New Haven, CT Zip 06504–3202; tel. 203/688–4242; Joseph A. Zaccagnino, President and Chief Executive Officer
Web address: www.ynhh.org

Owned, leased, sponsored:	3 hospitals	1216 beds
Contract-managed:	0 hospitals	0 beds
Totals:	3 hospitals	1216 beds

0211: **YOUTH AND FAMILY CENTERED SERVICES** (IO)
1705 Capital of TX Highway South, Austin, TX Zip 78746;
tel. 512/327–1119; Kevin P. Sheehan, President and Chief Executive Officer

MISSOURI: LAKELAND REGIONAL HOSPITAL (O, 78 beds) 440 South Market Street, Springfield, MO Zip 65806–2090; tel. 417/865–5581; John William Thompson, Ph.D., President and Chief Executive Officer

NEW MEXICO: DESERT HILLS HOSPITAL (O, 35 beds) 5310 Sequoia Road N.W., Albuquerque, NM Zip 87120–1249; tel. 505/836–7330; Carol Bickelman, President and Chief Executive Officer

PENNSYLVANIA: SOUTHWOOD PSYCHIATRIC HOSPITAL (O, 50 beds) 2575 Boyce Plaza Road, Pittsburgh, PA Zip 15241–3925; tel. 412/257–2290; Lynne M. Struble, MSN, Chief Executive Officer

Owned, leased, sponsored:	3 hospitals	163 beds
Contract-managed:	0 hospitals	0 beds
Totals:	3 hospitals	163 beds

Headquarters of Health Care Systems

Geographically

United States

ALABAMA

Birmingham: 0202 ASSOCIATES CAPITAL GROUP, LLC Mailing Address: P.O. Box 380995, Zip 35242; tel. 205/408–9095; Len Bryant, Chief Executive Officer, p. B55

0345 ★ BAPTIST HEALTH SYSTEM Mailing Address: P.O. Box 830605, Zip 35283–0605; tel. 205/715–5319; Dennis A. Hall, President, p. B57

2455 BRADFORD HEALTH SERVICES 2101 Magnolia Avenue South, Suite 518, Zip 35205; tel. 205/251–7753; Jerry W. Crowder, President and Chief Executive Officer, p. B62

0126 CARRAWAY METHODIST HEALTH SYSTEM 1600 Carraway Boulevard, Zip 35234–1990; tel. 205/502–6000; Robert M. Carraway, M.D., Chairman and Chief Executive Officer, p. B66

0100 ★ EASTERN HEALTH SYSTEM, INC. 48 Medical Park East Drive, 450, Zip 35235; tel. 205/838–3999; Robert C. Chapman, FACHE, President and Chief Executive Officer, p. B84

0023 HEALTHSOUTH CORPORATION One Healthsouth Parkway, Zip 35243; tel. 205/967–7116; Anthony J. Tanner, Executive Vice President, p. B96

9105 UNIVERSITY OF ALABAMA SYSTEM 619 South 19th Street, Zip 35233; tel. 205/975–7545; David J. Fine, Chief Executive Officer, p. B149

Florence: 0152 ★ COFFEE HEALTH GROUP 205 Marengo Street, Zip 35630–6033; tel. 256/768–9191; Carl W. Bailey, President and Chief Executive Officer, p. B73

Guntersville: 1975 MARSHALL COUNTY HEALTH CARE AUTHORITY 8000 Alabama Highway 69, Zip 35976; tel. 256/753–8000; Julian Sparks, Board Chairman, p. B108

Mobile: 2025 INFIRMARY HEALTH SYSTEM, INC. 3 Mobile Infirmary Circle, Zip 36607–3520; tel. 334/435–5500; E. Chandler Bramlett, Jr, President and Chief Executive Officer, p. B100

0057 UNIVERSITY OF SOUTH ALABAMA HOSPITALS 2451 Fillingim Street, Zip 36617–2293; tel. 334/471–7000; Stephen H. Simmons, Senior Administrator, p. B149

Montgomery: 0150 BAPTIST HEALTH 2105 East South Boulevard, Zip 36116–2498; tel. 334/286–2970; Victor D. Butler, Acting President and Chief Executive Officer, p. B57

Tuscaloosa: 1825 ★ DCH HEALTH SYSTEM 809 University Boulevard East, Zip 35401; tel. 205/759–7111; Bryan N. Kindred, President and Chief Executive Officer, p. B76

ARIZONA

Phoenix: 0218 JOHN C LINCOLN HEALTH NETWORK 250 East Dunlap Avenue, Zip 85020–2446; tel. 602/943–2381; Dan C. Coleman, President and Chief Executive Officer, p. B103

0034 ★ PMH HEALTH RESOURCES, INC. 1201 South Seventh Avenue, Zip 85007–3913, Mailing Address: P.O. Box 21207, Zip 85036–1207; tel. 602/824–3321; Reginald M. Ballantyne, II, President, p. B119

Scottsdale: 0164 DOCTORS COMMUNITY HEALTHCARE CORPORATION 6730 North Scottsdale Road, Suite 200, Zip 85253; tel. 602/348–9800; Melvin Redman, President and Chief Operating Officer, p. B83

0037 ★ SCOTTSDALE HEALTHCARE 3621 Wells Fargo Avenue, Zip 85251–5607; tel. 480/675–4324; Max Poll, President and Chief Executive Officer, p. B130

Sun City: 0030 ★ SUN HEALTH CORPORATION 13180 North 103rd Drive, Zip 85351–3038, Mailing Address: P.O. Box 1278, Zip 85372–1278; tel. 623/876–5301; Leland W. Peterson, President and Chief Executive Officer, p. B138

ARKANSAS

Little Rock: 0355 ★ BAPTIST HEALTH 9601 Interstate 630, Exit 7, Zip 72205–7299; tel. 501/202–2000; Russell D. Harrington, Jr, President, p. B57

CALIFORNIA

Covina: 0101 CITRUS VALLEY HEALTH PARTNERS 210 West San Bernardino Road, Zip 91723; tel. 626/938–7577; Peter E. Makowski, President and Chief Executive Officer, p. B72

Downey: 0076 COLLEGE HEALTH ENTERPRISES 17100 Pioneer Boulevard, Suite 300, Zip 90241; tel. 949/642–2734; Dale A. Kirby, President, p. B73

Fairfield: 2075 ★ NORTHBAY HEALTHCARE SYSTEM 1200 B Gale Wilson Boulevard, Zip 94533–3587; tel. 707/429–7809; Gary J. Passama, President and Chief Executive Officer, p. B115

Fresno: 1085 ★ COMMUNITY MEDICAL CENTERS Fresno and R Streets, Zip 93721, Mailing Address: P.O. Box 1232, Zip 93715–1232; tel. 559/459–6000; J. Philip Hinton, M.D., President and Chief Executive Officer, p. B74

Hemet: 0043 ★ VALLEY HEALTH SYSTEM 1117 East Devonshire Avenue, Zip 92543; tel. 909/652–2811; John P. Lauri, Chief Executive Officer, p. B150

Loma Linda: 2175 LOMA LINDA UNIVERSITY HEALTH SCIENCES CENTER 11161 Anderson Street, Zip 92350; tel. 909/824–4540; B. Lyn Behrens, President, p. B106

Long Beach: 0084 MEMORIAL HEALTH SERVICES 2801 Atlantic Avenue, Zip 90806, Mailing Address: P.O. Box 1428, Zip 90801–1428; tel. 562/933–9700; Thomas J. Collins, President and Chief Executive Officer, p. B109

Los Angeles: 5755 LOS ANGELES COUNTY–DEPARTMENT OF HEALTH SERVICES 313 North Figueroa Street, Room 912, Zip 90012–2691; tel. 213/240–8101; Mark Finucane, Director Health Services, p. B106

Oakland: 2105 ★ KAISER FOUNDATION HOSPITALS One Kaiser Plaza, Zip 94612–3600; tel. 510/271–5910; David M. Lawrence, M.D., Chairman and Chief Executive Officer, p. B103

6405 UNIVERSITY OF CALIFORNIA–SYSTEMWIDE ADMINISTRATION 300 Lakeside Drive, 18th Floor, Zip 94612–3550; tel. 510/987–9701; Cornelius L. Hopper, M.D., Vice President Health Affairs, p. B149

Orange: 5425 ★ ST. JOSEPH HEALTH SYSTEM 440 South Batavia Street, Zip 92868–3995, Mailing Address: P.O. Box 14132, Zip 92613–1532; tel. 714/997–7690; Richard Statuto, Chief Executive Officer, p. B137

Pasadena: 0106 ★ SOUTHERN CALIFORNIA HEALTHCARE SYSTEMS 100 West California Boulevard, Zip 91105; tel. 626/397–5555; Stephen A. Ralph, President and Chief Executive Officer, p. B135

Pleasanton: 0097 VALLEYCARE HEALTH SYSTEM 5575 West Las Positas Boulevard, 300, Zip 94588; tel. 925/447–7000; Marcy L. Feit, Chief Executive Officer, p. B151

Roseville: 0235 ★ ADVENTIST HEALTH 2100 Douglas Boulevard, Zip 95661–3898, Mailing Address: P.O. Box 619002, Zip 95661–9002; tel. 916/781–2000; Donald R. Ammon, President, p. B50

Sacramento: 8795 ★ SUTTER HEALTH One Capitol Mall, Zip 95814, Mailing Address: P.O. Box 160727, Zip 95816–0727; tel. 916/733–8800; Van R. Johnson, President and Chief Executive Officer, p. B138

San Diego: 7555 ★ PALOMAR POMERADO HEALTH SYSTEM 15255 Innovation Drive, Suite 204, Zip 92128–3410; tel. 858/675–5100; Norman F. Gruber, President and Chief Executive Officer, p. B118

1505 ★ SCRIPPS HEALTH 4275 Campus Point Court, Zip 92121; tel. 858/678–7200; Stan Pappelbaum, M.D., President and Chief Executive Officer, p. B130

2065 ★ SHARP HEALTHCARE 8695 Spectrum Center Court, Zip 92123–1489; tel. 858/499–4000; Michael Murphy, President and Chief Executive Officer, p. B131

San Francisco: 5205 ★ CATHOLIC HEALTHCARE WEST 1700 Montgomery Street, Suite 300, Zip 94111–9603; tel. 415/438–5500; Lloyd H. Dean, President and Chief Executive Officer, p. B69

0156 ★ UCSF STANFORD HEALTH CARE 5 Thomas Mellon Circle, 305, Zip 94134; tel. 415/353–4500; David Hunter, Interim President and Chief Executive Officer, p. B137

Headquarters of Health Care Systems / Geographically

San Leandro: 0225 ALAMEDA COUNTY HEALTH CARE SERVICES AGENCY 1850 Fairway Drive, Zip 94577; tel. 510/351–1367; David J. Kears, Director, p. B51

Santa Barbara: 0103 COTTAGE HEALTH SYSTEM Pueblo at Bath Streets, Zip 93102, Mailing Address: P.O. Box 689, Zip 93102; tel. 805/682–7111; Ron Werft, Chief Executive Officer, p. B75

0063 ★ TENET HEALTHCARE CORPORATION 3820 State Street, Zip 93105, Mailing Address: P.O. Box 31907, Zip 93130; tel. 805/563–7000; Jeffrey Barbakow, Chairman and Chief Executive Officer, p. B139

Santa Monica: 0187 ALTA HEALTHCARE SYSTEM 3000 Ocean Park Boulevard, Zip 90405; tel. 310/399–1349; David Topper, Chief Executive Officer, p. B52

Tustin: 0435 PACIFIC HEALTH CORPORATION 14642 Newport Avenue, Zip 92780; tel. 714/669–2085; Jens Mueller, Chairman, p. B118

Yuba City: 2115 FREMONT–RIDEOUT HEALTH GROUP 989 Plumas Street, Zip 95991; tel. 530/751–4010; Thomas P. Hayes, Chief Executive Officer, p. B86

COLORADO

Denver: 0092 ★ CATHOLIC HEALTH INITIATIVES 1999 Broadway, Suite 2605, Zip 80202–4004; tel. 303/298–9100; Patricia A. Cahill, President and Chief Executive Officer, p. B67

0134 ★ EXEMPLA HEALTHCARE, INC. 600 Grant Street, Suite 700, Zip 80203; tel. 303/813–5000; Jeffrey D. Selberg, President and Chief Executive Officer, p. B84

CONNECTICUT

Hartford: 0014 CONNECTICUT DEPARTMENT OF MENTAL HEALTH AND ADDICTION SERVICES 410 Capitol Avenue, Zip 06134, Mailing Address: P.O. Box 341431, Zip 06134–1431; tel. 860/418–6969; Thomas A. Kirk, Jr, Ph.D., Commissioner, p. B75

New Haven: 0157 ★ YALE NEW HAVEN HEALTH SYSTEM 789 Howard Avenue, Zip 06519; tel. 203/688–2608; Joseph A. Zaccagnino, President and Chief Executive Officer, p. B155

DELAWARE

Wilmington: 0131 ★ CHRISTIANA CARE HEALTH SYSTEM 501 West 14th Street, Zip 19899, Mailing Address: P.O. Box 1668, Zip 19899; tel. 302/428–2570; Charles M. Smith, M.D., President and Chief Executive Officer, p. B71

DISTRICT OF COLUMBIA

Bowling AFB: 9495 DEPARTMENT OF THE AIR FORCE 110 Luke Avenue, Room 400, Zip 20332–7050; tel. 202/767–5066; Paul Carlton, M.D., Surgeon General, p. B77

Washington: 9655 DEPARTMENT OF NAVY 2300 East Street N.W., Zip 20372–5300; tel. 202/762–3701; Admiral Richard A. Nelson, Surgeon General, p. B76

9295 DEPARTMENT OF VETERANS AFFAIRS 810 Vermont Avenue N.W., Zip 20420; tel. 202/273–5781; Thomas L. Garthwaite, M.D., Acting Undersecretary for Health, p. B78

FLORIDA

Clearwater: 0071 ACCORD HEALTH CARE CORPORATION 3696 Ulmerton Road, Zip 33762; tel. 727/573–1755; Stephen H. Noble, President, p. B50

Coral Gables: 0122 BAPTIST HEALTH SYSTEM OF SOUTH FLORIDA 6855 Red Road, Suite 600, Zip 33143–3632; tel. 305/273–2333; Brian E. Keeley, President and Chief Executive Officer, p. B58

0405 RAMSAY YOUTH SERVICES 1 Alhambra Plaza, Suite 750, Zip 33134–5217; tel. 305/569–6993; Bert Cibran, President and Chief Operating Officer, p. B128

Dunedin: 1335 MORTON PLANT MEASE HEALTH CARE 601 Main Street, Zip 34698, Mailing Address: P.O. Box 760, Zip 34697–0760; tel. 727/733–1111; Philip K. Beauchamp, FACHE, President and Chief Executive Officer, p. B112

Fort Lauderdale: 3115 ★ NORTH BROWARD HOSPITAL DISTRICT 303 S.E. 17th Street, Zip 33316–2510; tel. 954/355–5100; G. Wil Trower, President and Chief Executive Officer, p. B114

Gainesville: 0111 ★ SHANDS HEALTHCARE 1600 S.W. Archer Road, Zip 32610–0326; tel. 352/395–0421; J. Richard Gaintner, M.D., Chief Executive Officer, p. B131

Hollywood: 0083 ★ MEMORIAL HEALTHCARE SYSTEM 3501 Johnson Street, Zip 33021–5487; tel. 954/985–5805; Frank V. Sacco, FACHE, Chief Executive Officer, p. B110

Naples: 1775 HEALTH MANAGEMENT ASSOCIATES 5811 Pelican Bay Boulevard, Suite 500, Zip 34108; tel. 941/598–3131; William J. Schoen, Chairman and Chief Executive Officer, p. B94

Orlando: 3355 ORLANDO REGIONAL HEALTHCARE 1414 Kuhl Avenue, Zip 32806–2093; tel. 407/841–5111; John Hillenmeyer, President and Chief Executive Officer, p. B117

Ormond Beach: 2615 ★ MEMORIAL HEALTH SYSTEMS 770 West Granada Boulevard, Zip 32174–5197; tel. 904/615–4100; Richard A. Lind, President and Chief Executive Officer, p. B110

Pensacola: 0185 BAPTIST HEALTH CARE CORPORATION 1717 North E Street, Suite 320, Zip 32501–6335; tel. 850/469–7643; Alfred G. Stubblefield, President, p. B57

Sunrise: 0204 HEALTH SYSTEMS AMERICA 555 S.W. 148th Avenue, Zip 33325; tel. 954/915–0474; Michael Piercey, M.D., President and Chief Executive Officer, p. B95

Tampa: 4125 SHRINERS HOSPITALS FOR CHILDREN 2900 Rocky Point Drive, Zip 33607–1435, Mailing Address: Box 31356, Zip 33631–3356; tel. 813/281–0300; Joseph E. Melchiorre, Jr, CHE, Executive Administrator, p. B131

Windermere: 9605 UNITED MEDICAL CORPORATION 603 Main Street, Zip 34786–3548, Mailing Address: P.O. Box 1100, Zip 34786–1100; tel. 407/876–2200; Donald R. Dizney, Chairman, p. B147

Winter Park: 4165 ★ ADVENTIST HEALTH SYSTEM SUNBELT HEALTH CARE CORPORATION 111 North Orlando Avenue, Zip 32789–3675; tel. 407/975–1417; Thomas L. Werner, President, p. B50

GEORGIA

Adel: 2335 MEMORIAL HEALTH SERVICES 706 North Parrish Avenue, Zip 31620–2064, Mailing Address: P.O. Box 677, Zip 31620–0677; tel. 912/896–2251; Wade E. Keck, Chief Executive Officer, p. B109

Atlanta: 0148 CHILDREN'S HEALTHCARE OF ATLANTA 2200 Century Parkway, Suite 450, Zip 30345; tel. 404/250–2211; James E. Tally, Ph.D., President and Chief Executive Officer, p. B71

0138 ★ GEORGIA BAPTIST HEALTH CARE SYSTEM 100 10th Street, Zip 30309; tel. 404/253–3011; David E. Harrell, Chief Executive Officer, p. B86

0695 MAGELLAN HEALTH SERVICES 3414 Peachtree Road N.E., Suite 1400, Zip 30326; tel. 404/841–9200; Henry Harbin, M.D., President and Chief Executive Officer, p. B107

0207 MARINER POST–ACUTE NETWORK, INC. 1 Ravinia Drive, Suite 1500, Zip 30346; tel. 678/443–7000; Christian Winkle, Chief Executive Officer, p. B108

0905 SPECIALTY HOSPITAL GROUP 5 Concourse Parkway, Suite 800, Zip 30328–6111; tel. 770/392–1454; Bill Cook, President and Chief Executive Officer, p. B136

0081 VALUEMARK HEALTHCARE SYSTEMS, INC. 300 Galleria Parkway, Suite 650, Zip 30339; tel. 770/933–5500; James T. McAfee, Jr, Chairman, President and Chief Executive Officer, p. B151

Columbus: 0161 ★ COLUMBUS REGIONAL HEALTH SYSTEM 707 Center Street, Suite 400, Zip 31901; tel. 706/660–6100; Larry Sanders, FACHE, Chairman and Chief Executive Officer, p. B73

Marietta: 0995 ★ WELLSTAR HEALTH SYSTEM 805 Sandy Plains Road, Zip 30066; tel. 770/792–5012; Thomas E. Hill, Chief Executive Officer, p. B153

Thomasville: 0104 ARCHBOLD MEDICAL CENTER 910 South Broad Street, Zip 31792–6113; tel. 912/228–2739; Ken B. Beverly, President and Chief Executive Officer, p. B53

HAWAII

Honolulu: 3555 HAWAII HEALTH SYSTEMS CORPORATION 3675 Kilauea Avenue, Zip 96816; tel. 808/586–4416; Thomas M. Driskill, Jr, President and Chief Executive Officer, p. B88

0040 ★ QUEEN'S HEALTH SYSTEMS 1099 Alakea Street, Suite 1100, Zip 96813; tel. 808/532–6100; Richard L. Griffith, President and Chief Executive Officer, p. B122

ILLINOIS

Arlington Heights: 0113 CANCER TREATMENT CENTERS OF AMERICA 3455 West Salt Creek Lane, Zip 60005–1080; tel. 847/342–7400; William A. Sanger, President and Chief Executive Officer, p. B63

Carbondale: 4175 ★ SOUTHERN ILLINOIS HOSPITAL SERVICES 1239 East Main Street, Zip 62901, Mailing Address: P.O. Box 3988, Zip 62902–3988; tel. 618/457–5200; John J. Buckley, Jr, President, p. B135

Chicago: 0079 CATHOLIC HEALTH PARTNERS 2913 North Commonwealth, Zip 60657–6296; tel. 773/665–3757; Arnie Kimmel, President and Chief Executive Officer, p. B69

0016 COOK COUNTY BUREAU OF HEALTH SERVICES 1900 West Polk Street, Suite 220, Zip 60612; tel. 312/633–6820; Ruth M. Rothstein, Chief, p. B75

0171 RESURRECTION HEALTH CARE CORPORATION 7435 West Talcott Avenue, Zip 60631; tel. 773/792–5150; Joseph F. Toomey, President and Chief Executive Officer, p. B128

Headquarters of Health Care Systems / Geographically

3855 ★ RUSH–PRESBYTERIAN–ST. LUKE'S MEDICAL CENTER 1653 West Congress Parkway, Zip 60612–3864; tel. 312/942–5000; Leo M. Henikoff, M.D., President, p. B129

0058 ★ THE UNIVERSITY OF CHICAGO HOSPITALS AND HEALTH SYSTEM 322 South Green Street, Suite 500, Zip 60637; tel. 773/702–6240; Ralph W. Muller, President and Chief Executive Officer, p. B143

De Kalb: 0149 KISHWAUKEE HEALTH SYSTEM 626 Bethany Road, Zip 60115–4939, Mailing Address: P.O. Box 707, Zip 60115–4939; tel. 815/756–1521; Robert S. Thebeau, President and Chief Executive Officer, p. B104

Des Plaines: 5575 SISTERS OF THE HOLY FAMILY OF NAZARETH–SACRED HEART PROVINCE 310 North River Road, Zip 60016–1211; tel. 847/298–6760; Sister Marie Kielanowicz, Provincial Superior, p. B135

Elk Grove Village: 0065 ALEXIAN BROTHERS HEALTH SYSTEM, INC. 600 Alexian Way, Zip 60007–3395; tel. 847/640–7550; Brother Thomas Keusenkothen, President and Chief Executive Officer, p. B52

Evergreen Park: 2295 LITTLE COMPANY OF MARY SISTERS HEALTHCARE SYSTEM 9350 South California Avenue, Zip 60805–2595; tel. 708/229–5491; Sister Carol Pacini, Provincialate Superior, p. B106

Frankfort: 0132 ★ PROVENA HEALTH 9223 West St. Francis Road, Zip 60423–8334; tel. 815/469–4888; Joseph S. Feth, Chief Executive Officer, p. B120

Oak Brook: 0064 ★ ADVOCATE HEALTH CARE 2025 Windsor Drive, Zip 60523; tel. 630/990–5010; Richard R. Risk, President and Chief Executive Officer, p. B51

Peoria: 5335 ★ OSF HEALTHCARE SYSTEM 800 N.E. Glen Oak Avenue, Zip 61603–3200; tel. 309/655–2852; Sister Frances Marie Masching, President, p. B117

Springfield: 5355 ★ HOSPITAL SISTERS HEALTH SYSTEM Mailing Address: P.O. Box 19431, Zip 62794–9431; tel. 217/523–4747; Sister Jomary Trstensky, President, p. B99

0086 ★ MEMORIAL HEALTH SYSTEM 701 North First Street, Zip 62781–0001; tel. 217/788–3000; Robert T. Clarke, President and Chief Executive Officer, p. B109

Wheaton: 6745 ★ WHEATON FRANCISCAN SERVICES, INC. 26W171 Roosevelt Road, Zip 60189–0667, Mailing Address: P.O. Box 667, Zip 60189–0667; tel. 630/462–9271; Wilfred F. Loebig, Jr, President and Chief Executive Officer, p. B154

INDIANA

Fort Wayne: 0159 PARKVIEW HEALTH SYSTEM 2200 Randallia Drive, Zip 46805; tel. 219/470–8200; Charles H. Mason, Jr, President and Chief Executive Officer, p. B118

Hobart: 0135 ★ ANCILLA SYSTEMS INC. 1000 South Lake Park Avenue, Zip 46342–5970; tel. 219/947–8500; Elizabeth K. Kaminski, President and Chief Executive Officer, p. B52

Mishawaka: 5345 ★ SISTERS OF ST. FRANCIS HEALTH SERVICES, INC. 1515 Dragoon Trail, Zip 46546–1290, Mailing Address: P.O. Box 1290, Zip 46546–1290; tel. 219/256–3935; Kevin D. Leahy, President and Chief Executive Officer, p. B134

IOWA

Des Moines: 0061 ★ IOWA HEALTH SYSTEM 1200 Pleasant Street, Zip 50309–1453; tel. 515/241–6161; Samuel T. Wallace, President, p. B101

KANSAS

Leavenworth: 5095 ★ SISTERS OF CHARITY OF LEAVENWORTH HEALTH SERVICES CORPORATION 4200 South Fourth Street, Zip 66048–5054; tel. 913/682–1338; William M. Murray, President, p. B133

Phillipsburg: 1535 ★ GREAT PLAINS HEALTH ALLIANCE, INC. 625 Third Street, Zip 67661–2138, Mailing Address: P.O. Box 366, Zip 67661–0366; tel. 785/543–2111; Roger S. John, President and Chief Executive Officer, p. B87

Wichita: 5435 VIA CHRISTI HEALTH SYSTEM 818 North Emporia, Zip 67214–3725; tel. 316/268–5000; LeRoy E. Rheault, President and Chief Executive Officer, p. B152

KENTUCKY

Lexington: 0145 APPALACHIAN REGIONAL HEALTHCARE 1220 Harrodsburg Road, Zip 40504, Mailing Address: P.O. Box 8086, Zip 40533–8086; tel. 606/226–2440; Stephen C. Hanson, President, p. B53

Louisville: 0315 ★ BAPTIST HEALTHCARE SYSTEM 4007 Kresge Way, Zip 40207–4677; tel. 502/896–5000; Tommy J. Smith, President and Chief Executive Officer, p. B58

0052 ★ JEWISH HOSPITAL HEALTHCARE SERVICES 217 East Chestnut Street, Zip 40202–1886; tel. 502/587–4011; Henry C. Wagner, President, p. B102

2285 ★ NORTON HEALTHCARE 234 East Gray Street, Suite 225, Zip 40202, Mailing Address: P.O. Box 35070, Zip 40232–5070; tel. 502/629–8000; Stephen A. Williams, President, p. B115

0026 VENCOR, INCORPORATED 1 Vencor Place, 680 S. 4th Avenue, Zip 40202–2412; tel. 502/596–7300; Edward L. Kuntz, Board Chairman, President and Chief Executive Officer, p. B151

LOUISIANA

Baton Rouge: 1475 ★ FRANCISCAN MISSIONARIES OF OUR LADY HEALTH SYSTEM, INC. 4200 Essen Lane, Zip 70809; tel. 225/923–2701; John J. Finan, Jr, President and Chief Executive Officer, p. B85

0775 ★ GENERAL HEALTH SYSTEM 3600 Florida Boulevard, Zip 70806–3854; tel. 225/237–1603; Milton R. Siepman, Ph.D., President and Chief Executive Officer, p. B86

0715 ★ LSU MEDICAL CENTER HEALTH CARE SERVICES DIVISION 8550 United Plaza Boulevard, 4th Floor, Zip 70809; tel. 225/922–0490; James L. Brexler, President and Chief Executive Officer, p. B106

New Orleans: 0047 LOUISIANA STATE HOSPITALS 210 State Street, Zip 70118–5797; tel. 504/897–3400; Michael E. Teague, Chief Executive Officer, p. B106

MAINE

Bangor: 0555 ★ EASTERN MAINE HEALTHCARE 489 State Street, Zip 04401–6674, Mailing Address: P.O. Box 404, Zip 04402–0404; tel. 207/973–7045; Norman A. Ledwin, President and Chief Executive Officer, p. B84

MARYLAND

Baltimore: 1015 ★ JOHNS HOPKINS HEALTH SYSTEM 600 North Wolfe Street, Zip 21287–1193; tel. 410/955–5000; Ronald R. Peterson, President, p. B103

0158 ★ LIFEBRIDGE HEALTH 2401 West Belvedere Avenue, Zip 21215; tel. 410/601–5134; Warren A. Green, President and Chief Executive Officer, p. B104

6015 SISTERS OF MERCY OF THE AMERICAS–REGIONAL COMMUNITY OF BALTIMORE 1300 Northern Parkway, Zip 21239, Mailing Address: P.O. Box 11448, Zip 21239; tel. 410/435–4400; Sister Barbara Wheeley, Vice President, p. B134

0216 ★ UNIVERSITY OF MARYLAND MEDICAL SYSTEM 22 South Green Street, Zip 21201–1595; tel. 410/328–8667; Morton I. Rapoport, M.D., President and Chief Executive Officer, p. B149

Columbia: 0154 ★ MEDSTAR HEALTH 5565 Sterrett Place, 5th Floor, Zip 21044; tel. 410/772–6500; John P. McDaniel, Chief Executive Officer, p. B109

Fallston: 0038 ★ UPPER CHESAPEAKE HEALTH SYSTEM 1916 Belair Road, Zip 21047–2797; tel. 410/893–0322; Lyle Ernest Sheldon, President and Chief Executive Officer, p. B150

Largo: 0029 ★ DIMENSIONS HEALTH CORPORATION 9200 Basil Court, Zip 20774; tel. 301/925–7000; Winfield M. Kelly, Jr, President and Chief Executive Officer, p. B83

Marriottsville: 5085 ★ BON SECOURS HEALTH SYSTEM, INC. 1505 Marriottsville Road, Zip 21104–1399; tel. 410/442–5511; Christopher M. Carney, President and Chief Executive Officer, p. B61

Rockville: 0214 ADVENTIST HEALTHCARE 1801 Research Boulevard, Zip 20850; tel. 301/315–3538; Robert Henderschedt, Chief Executive Officer, p. B51

9195 U. S. PUBLIC HEALTH SERVICE INDIAN HEALTH SERVICE 5600 Fishers Lane, Zip 20857; tel. 301/443–1083; Michael Trujillo, M.D., M.P.H., Director, p. B145

Sparks Glencoe: 0182 INTEGRATED HEALTH SERVICES 910 Rudgebrook Road, Zip 21152; tel. 410/773–1000; Robert Elkins, M.D., Chairman and Chief Exective Officer, p. B100

Stevensville: 0208 NORTHEAST HEALTH MANAGEMENT, INC. 104 Log Canoe Circle, Zip 21666; tel. 410/643–3393; Harold A. McBee, President, p. B115

MASSACHUSETTS

Boston: 0096 ★ CAREGROUP 375 Longwood Avenue, Zip 02215–5395; tel. 617/975–6060; James Reinertsen, M.D., Chief Executive Officer, p. B64

0141 ★ CARITAS CHRISTI HEALTH CARE 736 Cambridge Street, Zip 02135–2997; tel. 617/789–2500; Michael F. Collins, M.D., President, p. B64

0013 MASSACHUSETTS DEPARTMENT OF MENTAL HEALTH 25 Staniford Street, Zip 02114–2575; tel. 617/626–8123; Marylou Sudders, Commissioner, p. B108

1785 ★ PARTNERS HEALTHCARE SYSTEM, INC. 800 Boylston Street, Suite 1150, Zip 02199–8001; tel. 617/278–1004; Samuel O. Thier, M.D., President and Chief Executive Officer, p. B119

Headquarters of Health Care Systems / Geographically

Hyannis: 0124 CAPE COD HEALTHCARE, INC. 88 Lewis Bay Road, Zip 02601–5210; tel. 508/862–5000; Stephen L. Abbott, President and Chief Executive Officer, p. B64

Lexington: 5885 ★ COVENANT HEALTH SYSTEMS, INC. 420 Bedford Street, Zip 02420–1502; tel. 781/862–1634; David R. Lincoln, President and Chief Executive Officer, p. B75

Peabody: 0091 PIONEER BEHAVIORAL HEALTH 200 Lake Street, Suite 102, Zip 01960–4780; tel. 978/536–2777; Bruce A. Shear, President and Chief Executive Officer, p. B119

Pittsfield: 2435 ★ BERKSHIRE HEALTH SYSTEMS, INC. 725 North Street, Zip 01201–4124; tel. 413/447–2743; David E. Phelps, President and Chief Executive Officer, p. B60

Springfield: 1095 ★ BAYSTATE HEALTH SYSTEM, INC. 759 Chestnut Street, Zip 01199–0001; tel. 413/794–0000; Michael J. Daly, President, p. B59

MICHIGAN

Dearborn: 1165 ★ OAKWOOD HEALTHCARE, INC. One Parklane Boulevard, Suite 1000E, Zip 48126; tel. 313/253–6050; Gerald D. Fitzgerald, President and Chief Executive Officer, p. B116

Detroit: 2145 ★ DETROIT MEDICAL CENTER 3663 Woodward Avenue, Suite 200, Zip 48201–2403; tel. 313/578–2020; Arthur Porter, M.D., President and Chief Executive Officer, p. B82

9505 ★ HENRY FORD HEALTH SYSTEM One Ford Place, Zip 48202–3067; tel. 313/876–8715; Gail L. Warden, President and Chief Executive Officer, p. B98

Grand Rapids: 0177 SPECTRUM HEALTH 100 Michigan Street N.E., Zip 49503–2551; tel. 616/391–1174; Terrence M. O'Rourke, Interim Chief Executive Officer, p. B136

Kalamazoo: 0595 ★ BRONSON HEALTHCARE GROUP, INC. One Healthcare Plaza, Zip 49007–5345; tel. 616/341–6000; Frank J. Sardone, President and Chief Executive Officer, p. B63

Midland: 0001 ★ MIDMICHIGAN HEALTH 4005 Orchard Drive, Zip 48670–0001; tel. 517/839–3000; Terence F. Moore, President, p. B111

Novi: 0219 ★ TRINITY HEALTH Mailing Address: P.O. Box 8001, Zip 48376–8001; tel. 248/489–6000; Judith Pelham, President and Chief Executive Officer, p. B144

Port Huron: 0053 ★ BLUE WATER HEALTH SERVICES CORPORATION 1221 Pine Grove Avenue, Zip 48060–3568; tel. 810/989–3717; Donald C. Fletcher, President and Chief Executive Officer, p. B61

Royal Oak: 9575 ★ WILLIAM BEAUMONT HOSPITAL CORPORATION 3601 West Thirteen Mile Road, Zip 48073–6769; tel. 248/551–5000; Ted D. Wasson, President and Chief Executive Officer, p. B155

Traverse City: 1465 ★ MUNSON HEALTHCARE 1105 Sixth Street, Zip 49684–2386; tel. 231/935–6502; John M. Rockwood, Jr, President and Chief Executive Officer, p. B112

MINNESOTA

Duluth: 0515 BENEDICTINE HEALTH SYSTEM 503 East Third Street, Zip 55805–1964; tel. 218/786–2370; Barry J. Halm, President and Chief Executive Officer, p. B60

Long Prairie: 0184 CENTRACARE 20 Ninth Street S.E., Zip 56347; tel. 320/732–2141; Clayton R. Peterson, President, p. B71

Minneapolis: 0041 ★ ALLINA HEALTH SYSTEM 5601 Smetana Drive, Zip 55343, Mailing Address: P.O. Box 9310, Zip 55440–9310; tel. 612/992–3992; Gordon M. Sprenger, President, p. B52

1325 ★ FAIRVIEW HEALTH SERVICES 2450 Riverside Avenue, Zip 55454–1400; tel. 612/672–6300; David R. Page, President and Chief Executive Officer, p. B84

Rochester: 1875 ★ MAYO FOUNDATION 200 S.W. First Street, Zip 55905–0002; tel. 507/284–2511; Michael B. Wood, M.D., President and Chief Executive Officer, p. B108

Saint Louis Park: 1985 HEALTHSYSTEM MINNESOTA 6500 Excelsior Boulevard, Zip 55426–4702; tel. 612/993–5000; David Wessner, President and Chief Executive Officer, p. B98

Saint Paul: 2185 ★ HEALTHEAST 559 Capitol Boulevard, 6–South, Zip 55103–0000; tel. 651/232–2300; Timothy H. Hanson, President and Chief Executive Officer, p. B96

MISSISSIPPI

Gautier: 0067 SINGING RIVER HOSPITAL SYSTEM 2101 Highway 90, Zip 39553; tel. 228/497–7907; Chris Anderson, Chief Executive Officer, p. B132

Jackson: 0017 MISSISSIPPI STATE DEPARTMENT OF MENTAL HEALTH 1101 Robert E Lee Building, Zip 39201–1101; tel. 601/359–1288; Roger McMurtry, Chief Mental Health Bureau, p. B111

Meridian: 0220 RUSH HEALTH SYSTEMS 1314 19th Avenue, Zip 39301; tel. 601/483–0011; Wallace Strickland, President and Chief Executive Officer, p. B129

Tupelo: 0032 NORTH MISSISSIPPI HEALTH SERVICES, INC. 830 South Gloster Street, Zip 38801–4996; tel. 601/841–3136; Jeffrey B. Barber, Dr.PH, President and Chief Executive Officer, p. B115

MISSOURI

Kansas City: 8815 ★ HEALTH MIDWEST 2304 East Meyer Boulevard, Suite A–20, Zip 64132–4104; tel. 816/276–9181; Richard W. Brown, President and Chief Executive Officer, p. B95

0120 SAINT LUKE'S SHAWNEE MISSION HEALTH SYSTEM 10920 Elm Avenue, Zip 64134–4108; tel. 816/932–3377; G. Richard Hastings, President and Chief Executive Officer, p. B130

9255 ★ TRUMAN HEALTH SYSTEM 2301 Holmes Street, Zip 64108–2677; tel. 816/556–3000; John W. Bluford, Executive Director and Chief Executive Officer, p. B145

Saint Louis: 0198 ★ ASCENSION HEALTH 4600 Edmundson Road, Zip 63134–3806; tel. 314/253–6700; Donald A. Brennan, President and Chief Executive Officer, p. B53

0051 ★ BJC HEALTH SYSTEM 4444 Forest Park Avenue, Zip 63108–2259; tel. 314/286–2000; Steven H. Lipstein, President and Chief Operating Officer, p. B61

5945 ★ CARONDELET HEALTH SYSTEM 13801 Riverport Drive, Suite 300, Zip 63043–4810; tel. 314/770–0333; Gary Christiansen, President and Chief Executive Officer, p. B65

5185 ★ SISTERS OF MERCY HEALTH SYSTEM–ST. LOUIS 2039 North Geyer Road, Zip 63131–0902, Mailing Address: P.O. Box 31902, Zip 63131–0902; tel. 314/965–6100; Ronald B. Ashworth, Chief Executive Officer, p. B134

5455 ★ SSM HEALTH CARE 477 North Lindbergh Boulevard, Zip 63141–7813; tel. 314/994–7800; Sister Mary Jean Ryan, President and Chief Executive Officer, p. B136

Springfield: 0179 COX HEALTH SYSTEM 1423 North Jefferson Avenue, Zip 65802–1988; tel. 417/269–3108; Larry D. Wallis, President and Chief Executive Officer, p. B76

NEBRASKA

Norfolk: 2855 MISSIONARY BENEDICTINE SISTERS AMERICAN PROVINCE 300 North 18th Street, Zip 68701–3687; tel. 402/371–3438; Sister M. Agnes Salber, Prioress, p. B111

NEW JERSEY

Bridgeton: 0151 SOUTH JERSEY HEALTH SYSTEM 333 Irving Avenue, Zip 08302–2100; tel. 856/451–6600; Paul S. Cooper, Chief Executive Officer, p. B135

Edison: 8855 ★ SOLARIS HEALTH SYSTEM 80 James Street, 2nd Floor, Zip 08820–3998; tel. 732/632–1500; John P. McGee, President and Chief Executive Officer, p. B135

Jersey City: 0173 LIBERTY HEALTHCARE SYSTEM 50 Baldwin Avenue, Zip 07304–3199; tel. 201/915–2000; Jonathan M. Metsch, Dr.PH, President and Chief Executive Officer, p. B104

Marlton: 6725 ★ VIRTUA HEALTH 94 Brick Road, Suite 200, Zip 08053; tel. 856/355–0005; Richard P. Miller, President and Chief Executive Officer, p. B153

Newark: 6545 CATHEDRAL HEALTHCARE SYSTEM, INC. 219 Chestnut Street, Zip 07105–1558; tel. 973/690–3600; Frank L. Fumai, President and Chief Executive Officer, p. B66

Ramsey: 0206 LIBERTY MANAGEMENT GROUP, INC. 19 Spear Road, Suite 305, Zip 07446; tel. 201/236–8880; William J. Hartigan, President and Chief Executive Officer, p. B104

Trenton: 0010 DIVISION OF MENTAL HEALTH SERVICES, DEPARTMENT OF HUMAN SERVICES, STATE OF NEW JERSEY Capital Center, P.O. Box 727, Zip 08625–0727; tel. 609/777–0702; Alan G. Kaufman, Director, p. B83

West Orange: 0118 ★ SAINT BARNABAS HEALTH CARE SYSTEM 95 Old Short Hills Road, Zip 07052; tel. 973/322–4001; Ronald J. Del Mauro, President and Chief Executive Officer, p. B129

NEW MEXICO

Albuquerque: 3505 ★ PRESBYTERIAN HEALTHCARE SERVICES 5901 Harper Drive N.E., Zip 87109–3589, Mailing Address: P.O. Box 26666, Zip 87125–6666; tel. 505/260–6500; James H. Hinton, President and Chief Executive Officer, p. B119

0210 SUN HEALTHCARE GROUP 101 Sun Avenue Northeast, Zip 87109; tel. 505/821–3355; Andrew L. Turner, Chief Executive Officer and Chairman of the Board, p. B138

0021 UNIVERSITY OF NEW MEXICO 915 Camino De Salud, Zip 87131–0001; tel. 505/272–5849; R. Philip Eaton, M.D., Vice President Health Scences, p. B149

Headquarters of Health Care Systems / Geographically

NEW YORK

Albany: 0009 NEW YORK STATE DEPARTMENT OF MENTAL HEALTH 44 Holland Avenue, Zip 12229–3411; tel. 518/447–9611; James L. Stone, Commissioner, p. B114

Bethpage: 0735 ★ EPISCOPAL HEALTH SERVICES INC. 700 Hicksville Road, Zip 11714; tel. 516/349–6132; Corbett A. Price, Chief Executive Officer, p. B84

Buffalo: 0102 KALEIDA HEALTH 901 Washington Street, Zip 14203; tel. 716/843–7500; John E. Friedlander, President and Chief Executive Officer, p. B104

Great Neck: 0062 ★ NORTH SHORE– LONG ISLAND JEWISH HEALTH SYSTEM 145 Community Drive, Zip 11021; tel. 516/465–8100; John S. T. Gallagher, Chief Executive Officer, p. B115

Latham: 1485 FRANCISCAN HEALTH PARTNERSHIP, INC. 8 Airport Park Boulevard, Zip 12110; tel. 518/783–5257; James H. Flynn, Jr, President and Chief Executive Officer, p. B85

New York: 0127 ★ CONTINUUM HEALTH PARTNERS 555 West 57th Street, Zip 10019; tel. 212/523–8390; Robert G. Newman, M.D., President, p. B75

3075 NEW YORK CITY HEALTH AND HOSPITALS CORPORATION 125 Worth Street, Room 514, Zip 10013–4006; tel. 212/788–3321; Luis R. Marcos, M.D., President, p. B113

0142 ★ NEW YORK PRESBYTERIAN HEALTHCARE SYSTEM 525 East 68th Street, Zip 10021–4885; tel. 212/746–4000; Herbert Pardes, M.D., Chief Executive Officer, p. B113

0110 OUR LADY OF MERCY HEALTHCARE SYSTEM, INC. 600 East 233 Street, Zip 10466–2697; tel. 718/920–9000; Gary S. Horan, FACHE, President and Chief Executive Officer, p. B118

5995 SISTERS OF CHARITY CENTER Mount St. Vincent on Hudson, Zip 10471–9930; tel. 718/549–9200; Sister Elizabeth A. Vermaelen, President, p. B133

Newburgh: 0144 GREATER HUDSON VALLEY HEALTH SYSTEM 600A Stony Brook Court, Zip 12550; tel. 914/568–6050; Val S. Gray, Interim President and Chief Executive Officer, p. B87

Rochester: 0046 ★ VIA HEALTH 150 North Chestnut, Zip 14604; tel. 716/922–3000; Fritz Leibert, Interim Chief Executive Officer, p. B152

Syracuse: 5955 SISTERS OF THE 3RD FRANCISCAN ORDER 2500 Grant Boulevard, Zip 13208–1713; tel. 315/425–0115; Sister Marion Kikukawa, General Minister, p. B135

NORTH CAROLINA

Charlotte: 0705 CAROLINAS HEALTHCARE SYSTEM 1000 Blythe Boulevard, Zip 28203–5871, Mailing Address: P.O. Box 32861, Zip 28232–2861; tel. 704/355–2000; Harry A. Nurkin, Ph.D., President, p. B65

0200 MEDCATH, INC. 7621 Little Avenue, Suite 106, Zip 28226; tel. 704/541–3228; Stephen R. Puckett, Chairman, President and Chief Executive Officer, p. B109

Durham: 0190 DUKE UNIVERSITY HEALTH SYSTEM Erwin Road, Zip 27710, Mailing Address: P.O. Box 3708, Zip 27710–3708; tel. 919/684–2255; Ralph Snyderman, M.D., President and Chief Executive Officer, p. B83

Greenville: 0217 UNIVERSITY HEALTH SYSTEMS OF EASTERN CAROLINA 2100 Srantonsburg Road, Zip 27835, Mailing Address: P.O. Box 6028, Zip 27835–6028; tel. 252/816–4100; Dave C. McRae, President and Chief Executive Officer, p. B148

Wilmington: 0213 ★ NEW HANOVER HEALTH NETWORK 2131 South 17th Street, Zip 28401–9000; tel. 910/343–7040; William K. Atkinson, II, Ph.D., President and Chief Executive Officer, p. B113

Winston Salem: 0139 ★ NOVANT HEALTH 3333 Silas Creek Parkway, Zip 27103–3090; tel. 336/718–5000; Paul M. Wiles, President and Chief Executive Officer, p. B116

NORTH DAKOTA

Bismarck: 0545 BENEDICTINE SISTERS OF THE ANNUNCIATION 7520 University Drive, Zip 58504–9653; tel. 701/255–1520; Sister Susan Berger, Prioress, p. B60

Fargo: 0194 ★ BANNER HEALTH SYSTEM 4310 17th Avenue S.W., Zip 58103; tel. 701/277–7500; Steven R. Orr, Chairman and Chief Executive Officer, p. B56

5805 SISTERS OF MARY OF THE PRESENTATION HEALTH CORPORATION 1102 Page Drive S.W., Zip 58106–0007, Mailing Address: P.O. Box 10007, Zip 58106–0007; tel. 701/237–9290; Aaron Alton, President, p. B133

OHIO

Cincinnati: 5155 CATHOLIC HEALTHCARE PARTNERS 615 Elsinore Place, Zip 45202; tel. 513/639–2827; Michael D. Connelly, President and Chief Executive Officer, p. B69

0082 ★ HEALTH ALLIANCE OF GREATER CINCINNATI 3200 Burnet Avenue, Zip 45229; tel. 513/585–6000; Jack M. Cook, President and Chief Executive Officer, p. B94

Cleveland: 0212 CLEVELAND CLINIC HEALTH SYSTEM 9500 Euclid, Zip 44195–5108; tel. 216/444–2200; Fred Loop, M.D., President, p. B72

5125 SISTERS OF CHARITY OF ST. AUGUSTINE HEALTH SYSTEM 2351 East 22nd Street, Zip 44115–3197; tel. 216/696–5560; Sister Judith Ann Karam, President and Chief Executive Officer, p. B133

0112 UNIVERSITY HOSPITALS HEALTH SYSTEM 11100 Euclid Avenue, Zip 44106–5000; tel. 216/844–1000; Farah M. Walters, President and Chief Executive Officer, p. B148

Columbus: 0162 ★ OHIOHEALTH 3555 Olentangy River Road, 4000, Zip 43214–3900; tel. 614/566–5424; William W. Wilkins, Chief Executive Officer, p. B117

Sylvania: 5375 ★ FRANCISCAN SERVICES CORPORATION 6832 Convent Boulevard, Zip 43560–2897; tel. 419/882–8373; John W. O'Connell, President, p. B85

Toledo: 0197 ★ PROMEDICA HEALTH SYSTEM 2121 Hughes Drive, 4th Floor, Zip 43606; tel. 419/291–7176; Alan W. Brass, FACHE, President and Chief Executive Officer, p. B120

Youngstown: 0174 FORUM HEALTH 3530 Belmont Avenue, Suite 7, Zip 44505; tel. 330/759–4090; Gary E. Kaatz, Chief Executive Officer, p. B85

OKLAHOMA

Oklahoma City: 0305 ★ INTEGRIS HEALTH 3366 N.W. Expressway, Suite 800, Zip 73112–9756; tel. 405/949–6068; Stanley F. Hupfeld, President and Chief Executive Officer, p. B100

0018 OKLAHOMA STATE DEPARTMENT OF MENTAL HEALTH AND SUBSTANCE ABUSE SERVICES 1200 N.E. 13th Street, Zip 73152, Mailing Address: P.O. Box 53277, Zip 73152–3277; tel. 405/522–3908; Sharron D. Boehler, Commissioner, p. B117

Tulsa: 0665 CENTURY HEALTHCARE DEVELOPMENT CORPORATION 5727 South Lewis, Suite 125, Zip 74105–7119; tel. 918/712–7010; William Grey, President and Chief Executive Officer, p. B71

0130 ★ HILLCREST HEALTHCARE SYSTEM 1120 South Utica, Zip 74104–4090; tel. 918/579–1000; Donald A. Lorack, Jr, President and Chief Executive Officer, p. B98

5305 ★ MARIAN HEALTH SYSTEM Mailing Address: P.O. Box 4753, Zip 74159–0753; tel. 918/742–9988; Sister M. Therese Gottschalk, President, p. B107

OREGON

Corvallis: 0186 SAMARITAN HEALTH SERVICES 3600 N.W. Samaritan Drive, Zip 97330, Mailing Address: P.O. Box 1068, Zip 97339; tel. 541/757–5111; Larry A. Mullins, President and Chief Executive Officer, p. B130

Medford: 0094 ★ ASANTE HEALTH SYSTEM 2650 Siskiyou Boulevard, Suite 218, Zip 97504–8389; tel. 541/608–4100; Roy G. Vinyard, II, President and Chief Executive Officer, p. B53

Portland: 2755 ★ LEGACY HEALTH SYSTEM 1919 N.W. Lovejoy Street, Zip 97209–1503; tel. 503/415–5600; Robert Pallari, President and Chief Executive Officer, p. B104

PENNSYLVANIA

Chambersburg: 0189 SUMMIT HEALTH 112 North Seventh Street, Zip 17201; tel. 717/267–7138; Norman B. Epstein, President, p. B138

Danville: 5570 ★ GEISINGER HEALTH SYSTEM 100 North Academy Avenue, Zip 17822; tel. 570/271–5555; Victor Marks, M.D., Interim President and Chief Executive Officer, p. B86

Fort Washington: 0209 PROGRESSIONS GROUP, INC. 450 Bethlehem Pike, Zip 19034; tel. 215/641–5300; Nicholas Tenaglia, M.D., Chief Executive Officer, p. B120

King of Prussia: 9555 UNIVERSAL HEALTH SERVICES, INC. 367 South Gulph Road, Zip 19406–0958; tel. 610/768–3300; Alan B. Miller, President and Chief Executive Officer, p. B147

Mechanicsburg: 0181 SELECT MEDICAL CORPORATION 4718 Old Gettysburg Road, Zip 17055; tel. 717/972–1100; Rocco A. Ortenzio, Chief Executive Officer, p. B130

Mount Pleasant: 0166 ★ FAY–WEST HEALTH SYSTEM 508 South Church Street, Zip 15666–1790; tel. 724/547–1500; Rodney L. Gunderson, Chief Executive Officer, p. B85

Newtown Square: 0136 ★ CATHOLIC HEALTH EAST 14 Campus Boulevard, Suite 300, Zip 19073–3277; tel. 610/355–2000; Daniel F. Russell, President and Chief Executive Officer, p. B66

Philadelphia: 1685 ALBERT EINSTEIN HEALTHCARE NETWORK 5501 Old York Road, Zip 19141–3098; tel. 215/456–7890; Martin Goldsmith, President, p. B51

0169 TEMPLE UNIVERSITY HEALTH SYSTEM 3401 North Broad Street, 1st Floor, Zip 19140; tel. 215/707–8000; Leon S. Malmud, M.D., President, p. B139

0168 UNIVERSITY OF PENNSYLVANIA HEALTH SYSTEM 399 South 34th Street, 21st Floor, Zip 19104–4385; tel. 215/898–5181; Peter G. Traber, M.D., Chief Executive Officer and Dean, p. B149

Pittsburgh: 2255 ★ ST. FRANCIS HEALTH SYSTEM 4401 Penn Avenue, Zip 15224–1334; tel. 412/622–4214; Sister M. Rosita Wellinger, President and Chief Executive Officer, p. B137

0137 ★ UPMC HEALTH SYSTEM 200 Lothrop, Zip 15213; tel. 412/647–2345; Jeffrey A. Romoff, President, p. B150

0199 ★ WEST PENN ALLEGHENY HEALTH SYSTEM 320 East North Avenue, Zip 15221–2173; tel. 412/359–3010; Charles M. O'Brien, Jr, President and Chief Executive Officer, p. B154

Sayre: 0675 ★ GUTHRIE HEALTHCARE SYSTEM Guthrie Square, Zip 18840; tel. 570/888–6666; Mark Stensager, President and Chief Executive Officer, p. B88

Springfield: 0008 ★ CROZER–KEYSTONE HEALTH SYSTEM 100 West Sproul Road, Zip 19064; tel. 610/338–8200; John C. McMeekin, President and Chief Executive Officer, p. B76

Villanova: 0845 DEVEREUX FOUNDATION 444 Deveraux Drive, Zip 19085, Mailing Address: P.O. Box 638, Zip 19333–0638; tel. 610/520–3000; Ronald P. Burd, President and Chief Executive Officer, p. B82

Wayne: 7775 ★ JEFFERSON HEALTH SYSTEM 259 Radnor–Chester Road, Suite 290, Zip 19087–5288; tel. 610/225–6200; Douglas S. Peters, President and Chief Executive Officer, p. B102

York: 0068 ★ SOUTH CENTRAL COMMUNITY HEALTH 1001 South George Street, Zip 17405–3645; tel. 717/851–2345; Bruce M. Bartels, President, p. B135

PUERTO RICO

San Juan: 0011 PUERTO RICO DEPARTMENT OF HEALTH Building A – Medical Center, Zip 00936, Mailing Address: Call Box 70184, Zip 00936; tel. 787/274–7676; Carmen Feliciano De Melecio, M.D., Secretary of Health, p. B122

RHODE ISLAND

Providence: 0099 ★ CARE NEW ENGLAND HEALTH SYSTEM 45 Willard Avenue, Zip 02905–3218; tel. 401/453–7900; John J. Hynes, President and Chief Executive Officer, p. B64

0060 ★ LIFESPAN CORPORATION 167 Point Street, Zip 02903–4771; tel. 401/444–3500; George A. Vecchione, President, p. B105

SOUTH CAROLINA

Columbia: 4155 ★ PALMETTO HEALTH ALLIANCE Mailing Address: P.O. Box 2266, Zip 29202–2266; tel. 803/296–2000; Charles D. Beaman, Jr, President, p. B118

Greenville: 1555 ★ GREENVILLE HOSPITAL SYSTEM 701 Grove Road, Zip 29605–4211; tel. 864/455–7000; Frank D. Pinckney, President, p. B88

Spartanburg: 4195 ★ SPARTANBURG REGIONAL HEALTHCARE SYSTEM 101 East Wood Street, Zip 29303–3016; tel. 864/560–6000; Joseph Michael Oddis, President, p. B136

SOUTH DAKOTA

Sioux Falls: 0078 ★ SIOUX VALLEY HOSPITALS AND HEALTH SYSTEM 1100 South Euclid Avenue, Zip 57105–0496; tel. 605/333–1000; Kelby K. Krabbenhoft, President, p. B132

Yankton: 5255 ★ AVERA HEALTH 610 West 23rd Street, Zip 57078, Mailing Address: P.O. Box 38, Zip 57078–0038; tel. 605/322–7050; John T. Porter, President and Chief Executive Officer, p. B55

TENNESSEE

Brentwood: 0585 ★ BRIM HEALTHCARE, INC. 105 Westwood Place, Suite 300, Zip 37027; tel. 615/309–6053; Dave Woodland, President, p. B62

0080 COMMUNITY HEALTH SYSTEMS, INC. 155 Franklin Road, Suite 400, Zip 37027–4600, Mailing Address: P.O. Box 217, Zip 37024–0217; tel. 615/373–9600; Wayne T. Smith, President and Chief Executive Officer, p. B73

0180 ★ LIFEPOINT HOSPITALS, INC. 103 Powell Court, Suite 200, Zip 37027; tel. 615/372–8500; James M. Fleetwood, Jr, Chairman, President, Chief Executive Officer and Chief Operating Officer, p. B105

0163 NEW AMERICAN HEALTHCARE CORPORATION 109 Westpark Drive, Suite 440, Zip 37027, Mailing Address: P.O. Box 3689, Zip 37024; tel. 615/221–5070; Thomas W. Singleton, President and Chief Executive Officer, p. B113

0108 PROVINCE HEALTHCARE CORPORATION 105 Westwood Place, Suite 400, Zip 37027; tel. 615/370–1377; Marty Rash, President and Chief Executive Officer, p. B121

0002 ★ QUORUM HEALTH GROUP 103 Continental Place, Zip 37027; tel. 615/371–7979; James E. Dalton, Jr, President and Chief Executive Officer, p. B122

Chattanooga: 2795 HEALTHCORP OF TENNESSEE, INC. 735 Broad Street, Zip 37402; tel. 423/267–8406; T. Farrell Hayes, President, p. B96

Jackson: 0004 ★ WEST TENNESSEE HEALTHCARE 708 West Forest Avenue, Zip 38301–3901; tel. 901/425–5000; James T. Moss, President, p. B154

Johnson City: 0167 MOUNTAIN STATES HEALTH ALLIANCE 400 North State of Franklin, Zip 37604; tel. 423/431–6111; Dennis Vonderfecht, President and Chief Executive Officer, p. B112

Kingsport: 0188 WELLMONT HEALTH SYSTEM 1905 American Way, Zip 37662–0224; tel. 423/224–3000; Eddie A. George, President and Chief Executive Officer, p. B153

Knoxville: 2155 BAPTIST HEALTH SYSTEM OF TENNESSEE 137 Blount Avenue S.E., Zip 37920–1643, Mailing Address: P.O. Box 1788, Zip 37901–1788; tel. 865/532–5011; Dale Collins, President and Chief Executive Officer, p. B58

0123 COVENANT HEALTH 100 Fort Sanders West Boulevard, Zip 37922; tel. 423/531–5555; Alan C. Guy, President and Chief Executive Officer, p. B75

Memphis: 1625 ★ BAPTIST MEMORIAL HEALTH CARE CORPORATION 899 Madison Avenue, Zip 38146–0001; tel. 901/227–5117; Stephen Curtis Reynolds, President and Chief Executive Officer, p. B58

9345 ★ METHODIST HEALTHCARE 1211 Union Avenue, Suite 700, Zip 38104–6600; tel. 901/726–2300; Maurice W. Elliott, Chief Executive Officer, p. B111

1765 UNITED HOSPITAL CORPORATION 6189 East Shelby Drive, Zip 38115; James C. Henson, President, p. B147

Nashville: 0069 BEHAVIORAL HEALTHCARE CORPORATION 102 Woodmont Boulevard, Suite 800, Zip 37205–2287; tel. 615/269–3492; Edward A. Stack, President and Chief Executive Officer, p. B59

0114 CHILDREN'S COMPREHENSIVE SERVICES, INC. 3401 West End Avenue, Suite 500, Zip 37203–0376; tel. 615/383–0376; William J. Ballard, Chief Executive Officer, p. B71

0048 ★ HCA – THE HEALTHCARE COMPANY One Park Plaza, Zip 37203–1548; tel. 615/344–9551; Jack O. Bovender, Jr, President and Chief Operating Officer, p. B88

0201 IASIS HEALTHCARE 104 Woodmont Boulevard, Suite 101, Zip 37205; tel. 615/844–2747; Wayne Gower, President and Chief Executive Officer, p. B99

0116 NETCARE HEALTH SYSTEMS, INC. 424 Church Street, Suite 2100, Zip 37219; tel. 615/742–8500; Michael A. Koban, Jr, Chief Executive Officer, p. B112

0193 VANGUARD HEALTH SYSTEM 20 Burton Hills Boulevard, Suite 10, Zip 37210; tel. 615/665–6000; Charles N. Martin, Jr, President and Chief Executive Officer, p. B151

TEXAS

Austin: 0395 BROWN SCHOOLS, INC. 1407 West Stassney Lane, Zip 78745–2998, Mailing Address: P.O. Box 4088, Zip 78765–4088; tel. 512/464–0200; Thomas Riley, Chief Executive Officer, p. B63

0020 TEXAS DEPARTMENT OF HEALTH 1100 West 49th Street, Zip 78756–3199; tel. 512/458–7111; William R. Archer, II, M.D., Commissioner, p. B142

0033 UNIVERSITY OF TEXAS SYSTEM 601 Colorado Street, Zip 78701–2982; tel. 512/499–4224; Charles B. Mullins, M.D., Executive Vice Chancellor, p. B150

0211 YOUTH AND FAMILY CENTERED SERVICES 1705 Capital of TX Highway South, Zip 78746; tel. 512/327–1119; Kevin P. Sheehan, President and Chief Executive Officer, p. B155

Bay City: 2505 MATAGORDA COUNTY HOSPITAL DISTRICT 1115 Avenue G, Zip 77414–3544; tel. 979/245–6383; Wendell H. Baker, Jr, District Administrator, p. B108

Dallas: 0095 ★ BAYLOR HEALTH CARE SYSTEM 3500 Gaston Avenue, Zip 75226–2088; tel. 214/820–0111; Joel T. Allison, President and Chief Executive Officer, p. B59

0191 LIFECARE MANAGEMENT SERVICES 6161 Harry Hines Boulevard, Zip 75235; tel. 214/525–0600; David B. Leblanc, President, p. B105

2735 ★ METHODIST HOSPITALS OF DALLAS 1441 North Beckley Avenue, Zip 75203–1201, Mailing Address: P.O. Box 655999, Zip 75265–5999; tel. 214/947–8181; Howard M. Chase, FACHE, President and Chief Executive Officer, p. B111

Headquarters of Health Care Systems / Geographically

0178 ★ TRIAD HOSPITALS, INC. 13455 Noel Road, 20th Floor, Zip 75240; tel. 972/789-2700; James D. Shelton, Chairman and Chief Executive Officer, p. B143

Fort Worth: 0039 TARRANT COUNTY HOSPITAL DISTRICT 1500 South Main Street, Zip 76104-4941; tel. 817/927-1230; Anthony J. Alcini, President and Chief Executive Officer, p. B139

Houston: 0077 CAMBRIDGE INTERNATIONAL, INC, 7505 Fannin, Suite 680, Zip 77225; tel. 713/790-1153; Timothy Sharma, M.D., President, p. B63

2645 ★ MEMORIAL HERMANN HEALTHCARE SYSTEM 7737 S.W. Freeway, Suite 200, Zip 77074-1800; tel. 713/776-6992; Dan S. Wilford, President and Chief Executive Officer, p. B110

7235 ★ METHODIST HEALTH CARE SYSTEM 6565 Fannin Street, D-200, Zip 77030-2707; tel. 713/790-2221; Peter W. Butler, President and Chief Executive Officer, p. B110

5765 PARACELSUS HEALTHCARE CORPORATION 515 West Greens Road, Suite 500, Zip 77067-4511; tel. 281/774-5100; Robert L. Smith, Chief Executive Officer, p. B118

Irving: 0192 ★ CHRISTUS HEALTH 6363 North Highway 161, Suite 450, Zip 75038; tel. 877/980-0100; Thomas C. Royer, M.D., President, p. B72

0129 ★ TEXAS HEALTH RESOURCES 600 East Las Colinas Boulevard, Suite 1550, Zip 75039, Mailing Address: 600 East Las Colinas Boulevard, 1550, Zip 75039; tel. 214/818-4500; Douglas D. Hawthorne, President and Chief Executive Officer, p. B142

Lubbock: 0036 ★ LUBBOCK METHODIST HOSPITAL SYSTEM 3615 19th Street, Zip 79410-1201; tel. 806/725-1011; George H. McCleskey, President and Chief Executive Officer, p. B107

Lufkin: 0176 MEMORIAL HEALTH SYSTEM OF EAST TEXAS 1201 West Frank Avenue, Zip 75904-3357; tel. 409/634-8111; Gary Lex Whatley, President and Chief Executive Officer, p. B110

San Antonio: 0265 BAPTIST HEALTH SYSTEM 200 Concord Plaza, Suite 900, Zip 78216; tel. 210/297-1000; Fred R. Mills, President and Chief Executive Officer, p. B57

Tyler: 1895 EAST TEXAS MEDICAL CENTER REGIONAL HEALTHCARE SYSTEM 1000 South Beckham Street, Zip 75701-1996, Mailing Address: P.O. Box 6400, Zip 75711-6400; tel. 903/535-6211; Elmer G. Ellis, President and Chief Executive Officer, p. B83

UTAH

Nephi: 0109 ★ RURAL HEALTH MANAGEMENT CORPORATION 549 North 400 East, Zip 84648-1226; tel. 435/623-4924; Mark R. Stoddard, President, p. B129

Salt Lake City: 1815 ★ INTERMOUNTAIN HEALTH CARE, INC. 36 South State Street, 22nd Floor, Zip 84111-1453; tel. 801/442-2000; William H. Nelson, President and Chief Executive Officer, p. B101

VIRGINIA

Falls Church: 9395 DEPARTMENT OF THE ARMY, OFFICE OF THE SURGEON GENERAL 5109 Leesburg Pike, Zip 22041; tel. 703/681-3114, p. B77

1305 ★ INOVA HEALTH SYSTEM 8110 Gatehouse Road, Zip 22042; tel. 703/289-2069; J. Knox Singleton, President and Chief Executive Officer, p. B100

Lynchburg: 2265 ★ CENTRA HEALTH, INC. 1920 Atherholt Road, Zip 24501-1104; tel. 804/947-4700; George W. Dawson, President, p. B71

Newport News: 4810 RIVERSIDE HEALTH SYSTEM 606 Denbigh Boulevard, Suite 601, Zip 23608; tel. 757/875-7500; Richard J. Pearce, President and Chief Operating Officer, p. B129

Norfolk: 2635 FHC HEALTH SYSTEMS 240 Corporate Boulevard, Zip 23502-4950; tel. 757/459-5100; Ronald I. Dozoretz, M.D., Chairman, p. B85

2565 ★ SENTARA HEALTHCARE 6015 Poplar Hall Drive, Zip 23502-3800; tel. 757/455-7000; David L. Bernd, Chief Executive Officer, p. B131

Richmond: 0012 VIRGINIA DEPARTMENT OF MENTAL HEALTH 1220 Bank Street, Zip 23219-3623, Mailing Address: P.O. Box 1797, Zip 23218-1797; tel. 804/786-3921; Richard E. Kellogg, Commissioner, p. B153

Roanoke: 0070 ★ CARILION HEALTH SYSTEM 101 Elm Avenue S.E., Zip 24013, Mailing Address: P.O. Box 13727, Zip 24036-3727; tel. 540/981-7347; Thomas L. Robertson, President and Chief Executive Officer, p. B64

Winchester: 0128 VALLEY HEALTH SYSTEM 1840 Amherst Street, Zip 22601, Mailing Address: P.O. Box 3340, Zip 22604-1334; tel. 540/722-8024; Michael J. Halseth, President and Chief Executive Officer, p. B150

WASHINGTON

Bellevue: 5415 ★ PEACEHEALTH 15325 S.E. 30th Place, Suite 300, Zip 98007; tel. 425/747-1711; John Hayward, President and Chief Executive Officer, p. B119

Seattle: 5275 ★ PROVIDENCE HEALTH SYSTEM 506 Second Avenue, Suite 1200, Zip 98104-2329; tel. 206/464-3355; Henry G. Walker, President and Chief Executive Officer, p. B120

Spokane: 0945 EMPIRE HEALTH SERVICES West 800 Fifth Avenue, Zip 99204, Mailing Address: P.O. Box 248, Zip 99210-0248; tel. 509/473-7960; Thomas M. White, President, p. B84

5265 ★ PROVIDENCE SERVICES 9 East Ninth Avenue, Zip 99202; tel. 509/742-7337; Richard J. Umbdenstock, President and Chief Executive Officer, p. B121

Tacoma: 6555 MULTICARE HEALTH SYSTEM 315 Martin Luther King Jr. Way, Zip 98415, Mailing Address: P.O. Box 5299, Zip 98415-0299; tel. 253/403-1000; Diane Cecchettini, President and Chief Executive Officer, p. B112

WEST VIRGINIA

Charleston: 0955 ★ CAMCARE, INC. 501 Morris Street, Zip 25301-1300, Mailing Address: P.O. Box 1547, Zip 25326-1547; tel. 304/348-5432; Phillip H. Goodwin, FACHE, President and Chief Executive Officer, p. B63

Fairmont: 0119 WEST VIRGINIA UNITED HEALTH SYSTEM 1000 Technology Drive, Suite 2320, Zip 26554; tel. 304/368-2700; Bernard G. Westfall, President and Chief Executive Officer, p. B154

Wheeling: 3315 ★ OHIO VALLEY HEALTH SERVICES 2000 Eoff Street, Zip 26003; tel. 304/234-8383; Thomas P. Galinski, President and Chief Executive Officer, p. B116

WISCONSIN

Appleton: 2445 ★ THEDACARE, INC. Five Innovation Court, Zip 54914-1663, Mailing Address: P.O. Box 8025, Zip 54912; tel. 920/831-6706; John S. Toussaint, M.D., President and Chief Executive Officer, p. B143

La Crosse: 9650 ★ FRANCISCAN SKEMP HEALTHCARE 700 West Avenue South, Zip 54601-4796; tel. 608/791-9710; Glenn Forbes, M.D., President and Chief Executive Officer, p. B86

Manitowoc: 1455 ★ FRANCISCAN SISTERS OF CHRISTIAN CHARITY HEALTHCARE MINISTRY, INC 1415 South Rapids Road, Zip 54220-9302; tel. 920/684-7071; Sister Laura J. Wolf, President, p. B86

Milwaukee: 2215 ★ AURORA HEALTH CARE 3000 West Montana, Zip 53215-3268, Mailing Address: P.O. Box 343910, Zip 53234-3910; tel. 414/647-3000; G. Edwin Howe, President, p. B55

0027 ★ HORIZON HEALTHCARE, INC. 2300 North Mayfair Road, Suite 550, Zip 53226-1508; tel. 414/257-3888; Sister Renee Rose, President and Chief Executive Officer, p. B99

Waukesha: 0153 PROHEALTH CARE 725 American Avenue, Zip 53188; tel. 262/928-2241; Donald W. Fundingsland, Chief Executive Officer, p. B120

Alliances

ALLIANCE OF INDEPENDENT ACADEMIC MEDICAL CENTERS
435 N Michigan Ave, Ste 2700, Chicago, IL Zip 60611; tel. 312/923–9770; Ms Nancie Noie, Managing Director

ARIZONA
Phoenix
Member
  Good Samaritan Regional Medical Center
  Maricopa Medical Center
  St. Joseph's Hospital and Medical Center

CALIFORNIA
Long Beach
Member
  Long Beach Memorial Medical Center

Los Angeles
Member
  Cedars–Sinai Medical Center

Oakland
Member
  Kaiser Foundation Hospital

San Francisco
Member
  California Pacific Medical Center

CONNECTICUT
Hartford
Member
  Saint Francis Hospital and Medical Center

DELAWARE
Wilmington
Member
  Christiana Care Health System

DISTRICT OF COLUMBIA
Washington
Member
  Washington Hospital Center

FLORIDA
Miami Beach
Member
  Mount Sinai Medical Center

Orlando
Member
  Orlando Regional Medical Center

ILLINOIS
Berwyn
Member
  MacNeal Hospital

Chicago
Shareholder
  Illinois Masonic Medical Center

Park Ridge
Member
  Lutheran General Hospital

INDIANA
Indianapolis
  St. Vincent Hospitals and Health Services

LOUISIANA
Baton Rouge
  Baton Rouge General Medical Center

New Orleans
Member
  Ochsner Foundation Hospital

MAINE
Portland
Member
  Maine Medical Center

MARYLAND
Columbia
Member
  MedStar Health

MASSACHUSETTS
Springfield
Member
  Baystate Medical Center

MICHIGAN
Detroit
Member
  Henry Ford Health System

Royal Oak
Member
  William Beaumont Hospital–Royal Oak

MISSOURI
Kansas City
Member
  Children's Mercy Hospital
  Saint Luke's Hospital

Saint Louis
  St. John's Mercy Medical Center

NEW JERSEY
Florham Park
Member
  Atlantic Health System

Livingston
Member
  Saint Barnabas Medical Center

Long Branch
Partner
  Monmouth Medical Center

Paterson
Member
  St. Joseph's Hospital and Medical Center

NEW YORK
Bronx
Member
  Bronx–Lebanon Hospital Center

Brooklyn
Member
  Maimonides Medical Center

Mineola
Member
  Winthrop–University Hospital

New Hyde Park
Member
  Long Island Jewish Medical Center

New York
Member
  Lenox Hill Hospital

NORTH CAROLINA
Charlotte
Member
  Carolinas Medical Center

OHIO
Akron
Member
  Akron General Medical Center

Columbus
Member
  Grant/Riverside Methodist Hospitals–Riverside Campus

PENNSYLVANIA
Allentown
Member
  Lehigh Valley Hospital

Jersey Shore
Member
  Jersey Shore Hospital

Philadelphia
Member
  Albert Einstein Medical Center

Pittsburgh
Member
  Mercy Hospital of Pittsburgh
  Western Pennsylvania Hospital

SOUTH CAROLINA
Columbia
Member
  Palmetto Richland Memorial Hospital

Greenville
Member
  Greenville Hospital System

TEXAS
Dallas
Member
  Baylor University Medical Center

VIRGINIA
Falls Church
Member
  Inova Fairfax Hospital

ASSOCIATION OF INDEPENDENT HOSPITALS
8300 Troost, Kansas City, MO Zip 64131; tel. 816/276–7580; Mr Jeff Tindle, President and Chief Executive Officer

KANSAS
Council Grove
Member
  Morris County Hospital

Garnett
Member
  Anderson County Hospital

Girard
Member
  Crawford County Hospital District One

Holton
Member
  Holton Community Hospital

Horton
Member
  Northeast Kansas Center for Health and Wellness

Iola
Member
  Allen County Hospital

Junction City
Member
  Geary Community Hospital

Kansas City
Member
  University of Kansas Medical Center

Lawrence
Member
  Lawrence Memorial Hospital

Manhattan
Member
  Mercy Health Center of Manhattan

Marysville
Member
  Community Memorial Healthcare

Onaga
Member
  Community Hospital Onaga

Ottawa
Member
  Ransom Memorial Hospital

Pittsburg
Member
  Mount Carmel Medical Center

Seneca
Member
  Nemaha Valley Community Hospital

Shawnee Mission
Member
  Menorah Medical Center
  Overland Park Regional Medical Center

Alliances

Topeka
Member
St. Francis Hospital and Medical Center

Wamego
Member
Wamego City Hospital

MISSOURI

Albany
Member
Gentry County Memorial Hospital

Belton
Member
Research Belton Hospital

Bethany
Member
Harrison County Community Hospital

Boonville
Member
Cooper County Memorial Hospital

Brookfield
Member
General John J. Pershing Memorial Hospital

Carrollton
Member
Carroll County Memorial Hospital

Carthage
Member
McCune–Brooks Hospital

Chillicothe
Member
Hedrick Medical Center

Clinton
Member
Golden Valley Memorial Hospital

Columbia
Member
University Hospitals and Clinics

Excelsior Springs
Member
Excelsior Springs Medical Center

Fairfax
Member
Community Hospital Association

Farmington
Member
Mineral Area Regional Medical Center

Fulton
Affiliate
Callaway Community Hospital

Hannibal
Member
Hannibal Regional Hospital

Harrisonville
Member
Cass Medical Center

Hermann
Member
Hermann Area District Hospital

Independence
Member
Independence Regional Health Center
Medical Center of Independence

Jefferson City
Member
Capital Region Medical Center

Joplin
Member
St. John's Regional Medical Center

Kansas City
Member
Baptist Medical Center
Research Medical Center
Trinity Lutheran Hospital

Kirksville
Affiliate
Northeast Regional Medical Center–Jefferson Campus

Lees Summit
Member
Lee's Summit Hospital

Lexington
Member
Lafayette Regional Health Center

Macon
Affiliate
Samaritan Memorial Hospital

Memphis
Affiliate
Scotland County Memorial Hospital

Mexico
Member
Audrain Medical Center

Milan
Affiliate
Sullivan County Memorial Hospital

Nevada
Member
Nevada Regional Medical Center

North Kansas City
Member
North Kansas City Hospital

Osceola
Member
Sac–Osage Hospital

Richmond
Affiliate
Ray County Memorial Hospital

Saint Joseph
Member
Heartland Regional Medical Center

Warrensburg
Member
Western Missouri Medical Center

CHILD HEALTH CORPORATION OF AMERICA
6803 West 64th Street, Ste 208, Shawnee Mission, KS Zip 66202; tel. 913/262–1436; Mr Don C Black, President and Chief Executive Officer

ALABAMA

Birmingham
Member
Children's Hospital of Alabama

ARIZONA

Phoenix
Member
Phoenix Children's Hospital

ARKANSAS

Little Rock
Member
Arkansas Children's Hospital

CALIFORNIA

Los Angeles
Member
Childrens Hospital of Los Angeles

Madera
Member
Valley Children's Hospital

Oakland
Member
Children's Hospital Oakland

Orange
Member
Children's Hospital of Orange County

Palo Alto
Member
Lucile Salter Packard Children's Hospital at Stanford

San Diego
Member
Children's Hospital and Health Center

COLORADO

Denver
Member
Children's Hospital

DISTRICT OF COLUMBIA

Washington
Member
Children's National Medical Center

FLORIDA

Miami
Member
Miami Children's Hospital

Saint Petersburg
Member
All Children's Hospital

GEORGIA

Atlanta
Member
Children's Healthcare of Atlanta at Egleston

ILLINOIS

Chicago
Member
Children's Memorial Hospital

LOUISIANA

New Orleans
Member
Children's Hospital

MASSACHUSETTS

Boston
Member
Children's Hospital

MICHIGAN

Detroit
Member
Children's Hospital of Michigan

MINNESOTA

Minneapolis
Member
Children's Hospitals and Clinics, Minneapolis

MISSOURI

Kansas City
Member
Children's Mercy Hospital

Saint Louis
Member
St. Louis Children's Hospital

NEBRASKA

Omaha
Member
Children's Hospital

NEW YORK

Buffalo
Member
Children's Hospital

OHIO

Akron
Member
Children's Hospital Medical Center of Akron

Cincinnati
Member
Children's Hospital Medical Center

Columbus
Member
Children's Hospital

Dayton
Member
Children's Medical Center

PENNSYLVANIA

Philadelphia
Member
Children's Hospital of Philadelphia

Pittsburgh
Member
Children's Hospital of Pittsburgh

TENNESSEE

Memphis
Member
Le Bonheur Children's Medical Center

TEXAS
Corpus Christi
Member
  Driscoll Children's Hospital

Dallas
Member
  Children's Medical Center of Dallas

Fort Worth
Member
  Cook Children's Medical Center

Houston
Member
  Texas Children's Hospital

VIRGINIA
Norfolk
Member
  Children's Hospital of The King's Daughters

WASHINGTON
Seattle
Member
  Children's Hospital and Regional Medical Center

WISCONSIN
Milwaukee
Member
  Children's Hospital of Wisconsin

CONSOLIDATED CATHOLIC HEALTH CARE
1301 W 22nd Street, Suite 202, Oak Brook, IL Zip 60523; tel. 630/990-2242; Mr Roger N Butler, Executive Director

CALIFORNIA
Orange
Member
  St. Joseph Health System

San Francisco
Member
  Catholic Healthcare West

COLORADO
Denver
Member
  Catholic Health Initiatives

ILLINOIS
Frankfort
Member
  Provena Health

Wheaton
Member
  Wheaton Franciscan Services, Inc.

INDIANA
Mishawaka
Member
  Sisters of St. Francis Health Services, Inc.

KANSAS
Leavenworth
Shareholder
  Sisters of Charity of Leavenworth Health Services Corporation

Wichita
Member
  Via Christi Health System

MARYLAND
Marriottsville
Member
  Bon Secours Health System, Inc.

MISSOURI
Saint Louis
Member
  Carondelet Health System

NEW YORK
Latham
Member
  Franciscan Health Partnership, Inc.

OHIO
Cincinnati
Member
  Catholic Healthcare Partners

Sylvania
Member
  Franciscan Services Corporation

PENNSYLVANIA
Newtown Square
Member
  Catholic Health East

SOUTH DAKOTA
Yankton
Member
  Avera Health

WASHINGTON
Seattle
Member
  Providence Health System

HOSPITAL NETWORK, INC.
One Healthcare Plaza, Kalamazoo, MI Zip 49007; tel. 616/341-8888; Mr George Angelidis, President and Chief Executive Officer

MICHIGAN
Allegan
Member
  Allegan General Hospital

Hastings
Member
  Pennock Hospital

Kalamazoo
Member
  Bronson Healthcare Group, Inc.
  Bronson Methodist Hospital

Marshall
Member
  Oaklawn Hospital

Sturgis
Member
  Sturgis Hospital

Vicksburg
Member
  Bronson Vicksburg Hospital

INTERHEALTH
2550 University Ave W, Ste 233, Saint Paul, MN Zip 55114; tel. 612/646-5574; Mr Benjamin Aune, President and Chief Executive Officer

ALABAMA
Birmingham
Member
  Baptist Health System

ILLINOIS
Normal
Member
  BroMenn Healthcare

Oak Brook
Member
  Advocate Health Care

Rock Island
Member
  Trinity Medical Center–West Campus

LOUISIANA
New Orleans
Member
  Southern Baptist Health System

MICHIGAN
Bay City
Member
  Bay Health Systems

MINNESOTA
Duluth
Member
  Benedictine Health System

Saint Paul
Member
  HealthEast

MISSOURI
Saint Louis
Member
  Forest Park Hospital

OHIO
Kettering
Member
  Kettering Medical Center–Network

TEXAS
Houston
Member
  Memorial Hermann Healthcare System

JORDAN HOSPITAL
275 Sandwich Street, Plymouth, MA Zip 02360-2196; tel. 508/746-2001; Mr Alan D Knight, President and Chief Executive Officer

MASSACHUSETTS
Andover
Affiliate
  Yankee Alliance

PHOENIX CHILDREN'S HOSPITAL
1111 East McDowell Road, Phoenix, AZ Zip 85006-2666; tel. 602/239-5960; Mr Burl E Stamp, Chief Executive Officer

KANSAS
Shawnee Mission
Member
  Child Health Corporation of America

PREMIER, INC.
3 Westbrook Corporate Center, 9th Floor, San Diego, CA Zip 92130; tel. 619/481-2727; Mr Richard A Norling, Chief Executive Officer

ALABAMA
Birmingham
Member
  Callahan Eye Foundation Hospital
  Children's Hospital of Alabama

Dadeville
Member
  Lakeshore Community Hospital

Daphne
Member
  Mercy Medical

Dothan
Member
  Flowers Hospital
  Southeast Alabama Medical Center

Enterprise
Member
  Medical Center Enterprise

Gadsden
Member
  Gadsden Regional Medical Center

Geneva
Member
  Wiregrass Medical Center

Jacksonville
Member
  Jacksonville Hospital

Monroeville
Member
  Monroe County Hospital

Opelika
Member
  East Alabama Medical Center

Valley
Member
  Lanier Health Services

ALASKA
Anchorage
Member
  Providence Alaska Medical Center

Alliances

Cordova
Affiliate
 Cordova Community Medical Center

Fairbanks
Member
 Fairbanks Memorial Hospital

Homer
Member
 South Peninsula Hospital

Juneau
Member
 Bartlett Regional Hospital

Ketchikan
Member
 Ketchikan General Hospital

Kodiak
Member
 Providence Kodiak Island Medical Center

Palmer
Member
 Valley Hospital

Seward
Affiliate
 Providence Seward Medical Center

Soldotna
Member
 Central Peninsula General Hospital

Valdez
Member
 Valdez Community Hospital

ARIZONA

Bullhead City
Member
 Western Arizona Regional Medical Center

Casa Grande
Member
 Casa Grande Regional Medical Center

Ganado
Member
 Sage Memorial Hospital

Glendale
Member
 Arrowhead Community Hospital and Medical Center

Mesa
Member
 Mesa Lutheran Hospital
 Valley Lutheran Hospital

Phoenix
Member
 Maricopa Medical Center
 Phoenix Baptist Hospital and Medical Center

Prescott
Member
 Yavapai Regional Medical Center

ARKANSAS

Ashdown
Member
 Little River Memorial Hospital

Batesville
Shareholder
 White River Medical Center

Benton
Member
 Saline Memorial Hospital

Camden
Member
 Ouachita Medical Center

Crossett
Shareholder
 Ashley County Medical Center

Danville
Shareholder
 Chambers Memorial Hospital

Dardanelle
Shareholder
 Dardanelle Hospital

De Witt
Shareholder
 DeWitt City Hospital

Dumas
Member
 Delta Memorial Hospital

Gravette
Shareholder
 Gravette Medical Center Hospital

Harrison
Shareholder
 North Arkansas Regional Medical Center

Hot Springs National Park
Shareholder
 Levi Hospital

Jacksonville
Member
 Rebsamen Medical Center

Lake Village
Member
 Chicot Memorial Hospital

Little Rock
Shareholder
 Arkansas Children's Hospital

Magnolia
Shareholder
 Magnolia Hospital

McGehee
Shareholder
 McGehee–Desha County Hospital

Mena
Member
 Mena Medical Center

Monticello
Shareholder
 Drew Memorial Hospital

Nashville
Member
 Howard Memorial Hospital

Paragould
Shareholder
 Arkansas Methodist Hospital

Pine Bluff
Shareholder
 Jefferson Regional Medical Center

Siloam Springs
Member
 Siloam Springs Memorial Hospital

Springdale
Shareholder
 Northwest Medical Center

Warren
Shareholder
 Bradley County Medical Center

West Memphis
Shareholder
 Crittenden Memorial Hospital

CALIFORNIA

Alhambra
Member
 Alhambra Hospital Medical Center

Apple Valley
Member
 Saint Mary Regional Medical Center

Arroyo Grande
Member
 Arroyo Grande Community Hospital

Bakersfield
Member
 Kern Medical Center
 San Joaquin Community Hospital

Burbank
Member
 Providence Saint Joseph Medical Center

Chula Vista
Member
 Sharp Chula Vista Medical Center

Clearlake
Member
 Redbud Community Hospital

Corona
Member
 Corona Regional Medical Center

Coronado
Member
 Sharp Coronado Hospital

Deer Park
Member
 St. Helena Hospital

Delano
Member
 Delano Regional Medical Center

Escondido
Member
 Palomar Medical Center

Eureka
Member
 Saint Joseph Hospital

Fortuna
Member
 Redwood Memorial Hospital

Fullerton
Member
 St. Jude Medical Center

Glendale
Member
 Glendale Adventist Medical Center
 Glendale Memorial Hospital and Health Center

Hanford
Member
 Hanford Community Medical Center

La Mesa
Member
 Grossmont Hospital

La Palma
Member
 La Palma Intercommunity Hospital

Lompoc
Member
 Lompoc Healthcare District

Long Beach
Member
 Long Beach Community Medical Center

Los Angeles
Member
 California Hospital Medical Center
 Childrens Hospital of Los Angeles
 White Memorial Medical Center

Madera
Member
 Valley Children's Hospital

Mission Hills
Member
 Providence Holy Cross Medical Center

Mission Viejo
Member
 Mission Hospital Regional Medical Center

Murrieta
Member
 Rancho Springs Medical Center

Napa
Member
 Queen of the Valley Hospital

National City
Member
 Paradise Valley Hospital

Northridge
Member
 Northridge Hospital Medical Center–Roscoe Boulevard Campus

Oakland
Member
 Children's Hospital Oakland
 Summit Medical Center

Orange
Affiliate
 Children's Hospital of Orange County
Member
 St. Joseph Health System
 St. Joseph Hospital

Alliances

Palo Alto
Member
 Lucile Salter Packard Children's Hospital at Stanford
Paradise
Member
 Feather River Hospital
Petaluma
Member
 Petaluma Valley Hospital
Poway
Member
 Pomerado Hospital
Rancho Mirage
Member
 Eisenhower Memorial Hospital and Betty Ford Center at Eisenhower
Roseville
Member
 Adventist Health
San Diego
Member
 Children's Hospital and Health Center
 Palomar Pomerado Health System
 Sharp Cabrillo Hospital
 Sharp Healthcare
 Sharp Memorial Hospital
 Sharp Mesa Vista Hospital
San Gabriel
Member
 San Gabriel Valley Medical Center
San Luis Obispo
Member
 French Hospital Medical Center
San Pedro
Member
 San Pedro Peninsula Hospital
Santa Paula
Member
 Santa Paula Memorial Hospital
Santa Rosa
Member
 Santa Rosa Memorial Hospital
Selma
Member
 Selma Community Hospital
Simi Valley
Member
 Simi Valley Hospital and Health Care Services
Sonora
Member
 Sonora Community Hospital
South Laguna
Member
 South Coast Medical Center
Susanville
Member
 Lassen Community Hospital
Torrance
Affiliate
 Little Company of Mary Health Services
Ukiah
Member
 Ukiah Valley Medical Center
Vallejo
Member
 California Specialty Hospital
Van Nuys
Member
 Northridge Hospital and Medical Center, Sherman Way Campus
Victorville
Member
 Victor Valley Community Hospital
Willits
Member
 Frank R. Howard Memorial Hospital

COLORADO
Brush
Member
 East Morgan County Hospital
Cortez
Member
 Southwest Memorial Hospital
Craig
Member
 Memorial Hospital
Delta
Member
 Delta County Memorial Hospital
Denver
Member
 Children's Hospital
Glenwood Springs
Member
 Valley View Hospital
Greeley
Member
 North Colorado Medical Center
Holyoke
Member
 Melissa Memorial Hospital
Lamar
Member
 Prowers Medical Center
Loveland
Member
 McKee Medical Center
Meeker
Member
 Pioneers Hospital of Rio Blanco County
Montrose
Member
 Montrose Memorial Hospital
Pueblo
Member
 Parkview Medical Center
Rifle
Member
 Grand River Hospital District
Salida
Member
 Heart of the Rockies Regional Medical Center
Sterling
Member
 Sterling Regional MedCenter
Trinidad
Member
 Mt. San Rafael Hospital
Yuma
Affiliate
 Yuma District Hospital

CONNECTICUT
Bristol
Member
 Bristol Hospital
Hartford
Member
 Saint Francis Hospital and Medical Center
New Haven
Member
 Hospital of Saint Raphael
Stafford Springs
Member
 Johnson Memorial Hospital

DELAWARE
Dover
Affiliate
 Bayhealth Medical Center
Lewes
Member
 Beebe Medical Center
Newark
Affiliate
 Christiana Hospital
Seaford
Member
 Nanticoke Memorial Hospital
Wilmington
Member
 Alfred I. duPont Hospital for Children
 Christiana Care Health System
 Eugene Dupont Preventive Medicine and Rehabilitation Institute

DISTRICT OF COLUMBIA
Washington
Member
 Children's National Medical Center
 Columbia Hospital for Women Medical Center
 George Washington University Hospital
 Greater Southeast Community Hospital
 Sibley Memorial Hospital

FLORIDA
Altamonte Springs
Member
 Florida Hospital–Altamonte
Apopka
Member
 Florida Hospital–Apopka
Arcadia
Member
 DeSoto Memorial Hospital
Belle Glade
Member
 Glades General Hospital
Brooksville
Member
 Brooksville Regional Hospital
Bunnell
Member
 Memorial Hospital–Flagler
Clearwater
Member
 Accord Health Care Corporation
Clewiston
Member
 Hendry Regional Medical Center
Coral Springs
Member
 Coral Springs Medical Center
De Land
Member
 Memorial Hospital–West Volusia
Dunedin
Member
 Mease Hospital Dunedin
 Morton Plant Mease Health Care
Eustis
Member
 Florida Hospital Waterman
Fernandina Beach
Member
 Baptist Medical Center–Nassau
Fort Lauderdale
Member
 Broward General Medical Center
 Cleveland Clinic Hospital
 Holy Cross Hospital
 Imperial Point Medical Center
 North Broward Hospital District
Gainesville
Member
 AvMed–Santa Fe
Hollywood
Member
 Memorial Regional Hospital
Homestead
Member
 Homestead Hospital
Jacksonville
Member
 St. Vincent's Medical Center
Jacksonville Beach
Member
 Baptist Medical Center–Beaches
Jupiter
Member
 Jupiter Medical Center

Alliances

Kissimmee
Member
 Florida Hospital Kissimmee

Largo
Member
 Sun Coast Hospital

Marianna
Member
 Jackson Hospital

Miami
Member
 Baptist Hospital of Miami
 Bascom Palmer Eye Institute–Anne Bates Leach Eye Hospital
 Miami Children's Hospital
 Pan American Hospital
 South Miami Hospital

Miami Beach
Member
 Mount Sinai Medical Center

Naples
Member
 Naples Community Hospital

New Port Richey
Member
 Morton Plant Mease–North Bay Hospital

New Smyrna Beach
Member
 Bert Fish Medical Center

Orange City
Member
 Florida Hospital Fish Memorial

Orlando
Member
 Florida Hospital

Ormond Beach
Member
 Memorial Health Systems
 Memorial Hospital–Ormond Beach

Pembroke Pines
Member
 Memorial Hospital Pembroke
 Memorial Hospital West

Plant City
Member
 South Florida Baptist Hospital

Pompano Beach
Member
 North Broward Medical Center

Port Charlotte
Member
 Bon Secours–St. Joseph Healthcare Group

Rockledge
Member
 Wuesthoff Health System

Safety Harbor
Member
 Mease Countryside Hospital

Saint Petersburg
Member
 All Children's Hospital
 Bayfront Medical Center
 St. Anthony's Hospital

Sebring
Member
 Florida Hospital Heartland Division

Spring Hill
Member
 Spring Hill Regional Hospital

Tampa
Member
 H. Lee Moffitt Cancer Center and Research Institute
 St. Joseph's Hospital
 Tampa Children's Hospital at St. Joseph's, St. Joseph's Women's Hospital – Tampa

Tarpon Springs
Member
 Helen Ellis Memorial Hospital

Tavernier
Member
 Mariners Hospital

Titusville
Member
 Parrish Medical Center

Venice
Member
 Bon Secours–Venice Hospital

Vero Beach
Member
 Indian River Memorial Hospital

Winter Haven
Member
 Winter Haven Hospital

Winter Park
Member
 Adventist Health System Sunbelt Health Care Corporation

Zephyrhills
Member
 East Pasco Medical Center

GEORGIA

Athens
Member
 St. Mary's Health Care System

Atlanta
Member
 Children's Healthcare of Atlanta at Egleston
 Northside Hospital
 Saint Joseph's Hospital of Atlanta

Augusta
Member
 University Health Care System
 Walton Rehabilitation Hospital

Blairsville
Member
 Union General Hospital

Bremen
Member
 Higgins General Hospital

Brunswick
Member
 Southeast Georgia Regional Medical Center

Calhoun
Member
 Gordon Hospital

Carrollton
Member
 Tanner Medical Center

Columbus
Member
 St. Francis Hospital

Cumming
Member
 Baptist Medical Center

Demorest
Member
 Habersham County Medical Center

Elberton
Member
 Elbert Memorial Hospital

Fort Oglethorpe
Member
 Hutcheson Medical Center

Glenwood
Member
 Wheeler County Hospital

Greensboro
Member
 Minnie G. Boswell Memorial Hospital

Jesup
Member
 Wayne Memorial Hospital

La Grange
Member
 West Georgia Health System

Macon
Member
 Macon Northside Hospital
 Middle Georgia Hospital

Milledgeville
Member
 Oconee Regional Medical Center

Monroe
Member
 Walton Medical Center

Richland
Member
 Stewart–Webster Hospital

Saint Marys
Member
 Camden Medical Center

Savannah
Member
 Candler Hospital
 Memorial Health
 St. Joseph's Candler Health System

Smyrna
Member
 Emory–Adventist Hospital

Sparta
Member
 Hancock Memorial Hospital

Sylvania
Member
 Screven County Hospital

Sylvester
Member
 Baptist Hospital, Worth County

Thomaston
Member
 Upson Regional Medical Center

Thomson
Member
 McDuffie Regional Medical Center

Tifton
Member
 Tift General Hospital

Vienna
Member
 Dooly Medical Center

Villa Rica
Member
 Tanner Medical Center–Villa Rica

Warm Springs
Member
 Baptist Meriwether Hospital

Washington
Member
 Wills Memorial Hospital

IDAHO

Blackfoot
Member
 Bingham Memorial Hospital

Moscow
Member
 Gritman Medical Center

ILLINOIS

Aurora
Member
 Provena Mercy Center

Barrington
Member
 Good Shepherd Hospital

Blue Island
Member
 Saint Francis Hospital and Health Center

Canton
Member
 Graham Hospital

Carmi
Member
 White County Medical Center

Carrollton
Member
 Thomas H. Boyd Memorial Hospital

Carthage
Member
 Memorial Hospital

Alliances

Centralia
Member
St. Mary's Hospital

Chicago
Member
Children's Memorial Hospital
Mercy Hospital and Medical Center
Mount Sinai Hospital Medical Center of Chicago
Our Lady of the Resurrection Medical Center
Ravenswood Hospital Medical Center
Resurrection Medical Center
Thorek Hospital and Medical Center
Trinity Hospital

Downers Grove
Member
Good Samaritan Hospital

Elk Grove Village
Member
Alexian Brothers Medical Center

Galesburg
Member
Galesburg Cottage Hospital

Geneva
Member
Delnor-Community Hospital

Gibson City
Member
Gibson Area Hospital and Health Services

Hazel Crest
Member
South Suburban Hospital

Hinsdale
Member
Hinsdale Hospital

Hoopeston
Member
Hoopeston Community Memorial Hospital

Melrose Park
Member
Gottlieb Memorial Hospital

Metropolis
Member
Massac Memorial Hospital

Morrison
Member
Morrison Community Hospital

Mount Carmel
Member
Wabash General Hospital District

Mount Vernon
Member
Good Samaritan Regional Health Center

Nashville
Member
Washington County Hospital

Oak Brook
Member
Advocate Health Care

Oak Lawn
Member
Christ Hospital and Medical Center

Ottawa
Member
Community Hospital of Ottawa

Paris
Member
Paris Community Hospital

Park Ridge
Member
Lutheran General Hospital

Peoria
Member
Methodist Health Services Corporation
Methodist Medical Center of Illinois

Pinckneyville
Member
Pinckneyville Community Hospital

Pittsfield
Member
Illini Community Hospital

Robinson
Member
Crawford Memorial Hospital

Staunton
Member
Community Memorial Hospital

Urbana
Member
Carle Foundation Hospital

Winfield
Member
Central DuPage Hospital

INDIANA

Brazil
Member
Clay County Hospital

Charlestown
Member
Medical Center of Southern Indiana

Frankfort
Member
St. Vincent Frankfort Hospital

Gary
Member
Methodist Hospitals

Greensburg
Member
Decatur County Memorial Hospital

Hartford City
Member
Blackford County Hospital

Jeffersonville
Member
Clark Memorial Hospital

Princeton
Member
Gibson General Hospital

Rushville
Member
Rush Memorial Hospital

Salem
Member
Washington County Memorial Hospital

Scottsburg
Member
Scott Memorial Hospital

Sullivan
Member
Sullivan County Community Hospital

Tell City
Member
Perry County Memorial Hospital

Wabash
Member
Wabash County Hospital

Washington
Member
Daviess County Hospital

Winchester
Member
St. Vincent Randolph Hospital

IOWA

Algona
Member
Kossuth Regional Health Center

Ames
Member
Mary Greeley Medical Center

Anamosa
Member
Jones Regional Medical Center

Belmond
Member
Belmond Medical Center

Boone
Member
Boone County Hospital

Britt
Member
Hancock County Memorial Hospital

Cedar Rapids
Member
Mercy Medical Center
St. Luke's Hospital

Chariton
Member
Lucas County Health Center

Charles City
Member
Floyd County Memorial Hospital

Clarion
Member
Community Memorial Hospital

Clinton
Member
Mercy Medical Center-Clinton

Corning
Member
Alegent Health Mercy Hospital

Council Bluffs
Member
Alegent Health Mercy Hospital

Cresco
Member
Regional Health Services of Howard County

Davenport
Member
Genesis Medical Center

De Witt
Member
DeWitt Community Hospital

Des Moines
Member
Harrison Treat and Rehabilitation Center
Iowa Lutheran Hospital
Iowa Methodist Medical Center
Owner
Iowa Health System

Dubuque
Member
Finley Hospital
Mercy Medical Center-Dubuque

Dyersville
Member
Mercy Medical Center-Dyersville

Eldora
Member
Mercy Health Center

Elkader
Member
Central Community Hospital

Emmetsburg
Member
Palo Alto Health System

Estherville
Member
Avera Holy Family Hospital

Fairfield
Member
Jefferson County Hospital

Fort Dodge
Member
Trinity Regional Hospital

Fort Madison
Member
Fort Madison Community Hospital

Grinnell
Member
Grinnell Regional Medical Center

Hampton
Member
Franklin General Hospital

Hawarden
Member
Hawarden Community Hospital

Alliances

Humboldt
Member
  Humboldt County Memorial Hospital

Iowa City
Member
  Mercy Hospital

Iowa Falls
Member
  Ellsworth Municipal Hospital

Knoxville
Member
  Knoxville Area Community Hospital

Manchester
Member
  Regional Medical Center of Northeast Iowa and Delaware County

Maquoketa
Member
  Jackson County Public Hospital

Marengo
Member
  Marengo Memorial Hospital

Marshalltown
Member
  Marshalltown Medical and Surgical Center

Mason City
Member
  Mercy Medical Center – North Iowa

Missouri Valley
Member
  Alegent Health Community Memorial Hospital

New Hampton
Member
  Mercy Medical Center–New Hampton

Newton
Member
  Skiff Medical Center

Osage
Member
  Mitchell County Regional Health Center

Osceola
Member
  Clarke County Hospital

Oskaloosa
Member
  Mahaska County Hospital

Ottumwa
Member
  Ottumwa Regional Health Center

Pella
Member
  Pella Regional Health Center

Pocahontas
Member
  Pocahontas Community Hospital

Primghar
Member
  Baum Harmon Mercy Hospital

Rock Valley
Member
  Hegg Memorial Health Center/Avera Health

Sac City
Member
  Loring Hospital

Shenandoah
Member
  Shenandoah Medical Center

Sibley
Member
  Osceola Community Hospital

Sioux City
Member
  Mercy Medical Center–Sioux City
  St. Luke's Regional Medical Center

Spencer
Member
  Spencer Municipal Hospital

Storm Lake
Member
  Buena Vista County Hospital

Washington
Member
  Washington County Hospital

Waterloo
Member
  Allen Memorial Hospital

West Burlington
Member
  Great River Medical Center

Winterset
Member
  Madison County Memorial Hospital

KANSAS

Chanute
Member
  Neosho Memorial Regional Medical Center

Coffeyville
Member
  Coffeyville Regional Medical Center

Emporia
Member
  Newman Memorial County Hospital

Eureka
Member
  Greenwood County Hospital

Iola
Member
  Allen County Hospital

Lawrence
Member
  Lawrence Memorial Hospital

Marion
Member
  St. Luke Hospital and Living Center

Neodesha
Member
  Wilson County Hospital

Oberlin
Member
  Decatur County Hospital and Cedar Living Center

Shawnee Mission
Member
  Menorah Medical Center

Ulysses
Member
  Bob Wilson Memorial Grant County Hospital

KENTUCKY

Benton
Member
  Marshall County Hospital

Berea
Member
  Berea Hospital

Bowling Green
Member
  The Medical Center at Bowling Green

Burkesville
Member
  Cumberland County Hospital

Cadiz
Member
  Trigg County Hospital

Campbellsville
Member
  Taylor County Hospital

Carrollton
Member
  Carroll County Hospital

Corbin
Member
  Baptist Regional Medical Center

Elizabethtown
Member
  Hardin Memorial Hospital

Flemingsburg
Member
  Fleming County Hospital

Franklin
Member
  The Medical Center at Franklin

Glasgow
Member
  T. J. Samson Community Hospital

Greensburg
Member
  Jane Todd Crawford Hospital

Greenville
Member
  Muhlenberg Community Hospital

Hardinsburg
Member
  Breckinridge Memorial Hospital

Harrodsburg
Member
  The James B. Haggin Memorial Hospital

Hartford
Member
  Ohio County Hospital

Henderson
Member
  Methodist Hospital

Hopkinsville
Member
  Jennie Stuart Medical Center

Horse Cave
Member
  Caverna Memorial Hospital

Irvine
Member
  Marcum and Wallace Memorial Hospital

La Grange
Member
  Tri County Baptist Hospital

Lancaster
Member
  Garrard County Memorial Hospital

Leitchfield
Member
  Twin Lakes Regional Medical Center

Lexington
Member
  Central Baptist Hospital
  Saint Joseph Hospital East

Louisville
Member
  Baptist Healthcare System
  Baptist Hospital East
  Frazier Rehabilitation Center
  Jewish Hospital
  Kosair Children's Hospital
  Norton Healthcare
  Norton Hospital
  University of Louisville Hospital

Manchester
Member
  Memorial Hospital

Marion
Member
  Crittenden County Hospital

Morganfield
Member
  Methodist Hospital Union County

Mount Sterling
Member
  Gateway Regional Health System
  Mary Chiles Hospital Extended Care Facility

Mount Vernon
Member
  Rockcastle Hospital and Respiratory Care Center

Murray
Member
  Murray–Calloway County Hospital

Alliances

Paducah
Member
  Lourdes Hospital
  Western Baptist Hospital

Pikeville
Member
  Pikeville United Methodist Hospital of Kentucky

Pineville
Member
  Pineville Community Hospital Association

Princeton
Member
  Caldwell County Hospital

Richmond
Member
  Pattie A. Clay Hospital

Russell Springs
Member
  Russell County Hospital

Salem
Member
  Livingston Hospital and Healthcare Services

Shelbyville
Member
  Jewish Hospital–Shelbyville

Tompkinsville
Member
  Monroe County Medical Center

Winchester
Member
  Clark Regional Medical Center

LOUISIANA

Alexandria
Member
  Christus St. Frances Cabrini Hospital

Baton Rouge
  Baton Rouge General Medical Center
Member
  General Health System
  Woman's Hospital

Bogalusa
  Bogalusa Community Medical Center

Bossier City
Member
  Christus Schumpert Bossier

Breaux Bridge
Affiliate
  Gary Memorial Hospital

Farmerville
Member
  Union General Hospital

Franklin
Member
  Franklin Foundation Hospital

Hammond
Member
  North Oaks Medical Center

Homer
Member
  Homer Memorial Hospital

Houma
Member
  Terrebonne General Medical Center

Jena
Member
  LaSalle General Hospital

Kaplan
Member
  Abrom Kaplan Memorial Hospital

Lafayette
Member
  Lafayette General Medical Center

Lake Charles
Member
  Christus St. Patrick Hospital
  Dubuis Hospital for Continuing Care

Lutcher
Member
  St. James Parish Hospital

Marrero
Member
  West Jefferson Medical Center

Morgan City
Member
  Lakewood Medical Center

Natchitoches
Member
  Natchitoches Parish Hospital

New Orleans
Member
  Children's Hospital
  Touro Infirmary

Opelousas
Member
  Opelousas General Hospital

Raceland
Member
  St. Anne General Hospital

Shreveport
Member
  Christus Schumpert Medical Center

Tallulah
Member
  Madison Parish Hospital

Thibodaux
Member
  Thibodaux Regional Medical Center

Ville Platte
Member
  Ville Platte Medical Center

West Monroe
Member
  Glenwood Regional Medical Center

Zachary
  Lane Memorial Hospital

MAINE

Blue Hill
Member
  Blue Hill Memorial Hospital

Brunswick
Member
  Parkview Hospital

Calais
Member
  Calais Regional Hospital

Caribou
Member
  Cary Medical Center

Dover–Foxcroft
Member
  Mayo Regional Hospital

Ellsworth
Member
  Maine Coast Memorial Hospital

Houlton
Member
  Houlton Regional Hospital

Lewiston
Member
  St. Mary's Regional Medical Center

Lincoln
Member
  Penobscot Valley Hospital

Machias
Member
  Down East Community Hospital

Millinocket
Member
  Millinocket Regional Hospital

Portland
Member
  Mercy Hospital of Portland

MARYLAND

Annapolis
Member
  Anne Arundel Medical Center

Baltimore
Member
  Bon Secours Baltimore Health System
  Franklin Square Hospital Center
  Good Samaritan Hospital of Maryland
  Harbor Hospital Center
  Mercy Medical Center
  Mt. Washington Pediatric Hospital
  Sinai Hospital of Baltimore
  Union Memorial Hospital

Berlin
Member
  Atlantic General Hospital

Bethesda
Member
  Suburban Hospital

Cheverly
Member
  Prince George's Hospital Center

Columbia
Member
  Howard County General Hospital
  MedStar Health

Cumberland
Member
  Memorial Hospital and Medical Center of Cumberland
  Sacred Heart Hospital

Elkton
Member
  Union Hospital

Fort Washington
Member
  Fort Washington Hospital

Frederick
Member
  Frederick Memorial Hospital

Glen Burnie
Member
  North Arundel Hospital

Hagerstown
Member
  Washington County Health System

Lanham
Member
  Doctors Community Hospital

Laurel
Member
  Laurel Regional Hospital

Marriottsville
Member
  Bon Secours Health System, Inc.

Olney
Member
  Montgomery General Hospital

Randallstown
Member
  Northwest Hospital Center

Rockville
Member
  Shady Grove Adventist Hospital

Salisbury
Member
  Peninsula Regional Health System

Takoma Park
Member
  Washington Adventist Hospital

Westminster
Member
  Carroll County General Hospital

MASSACHUSETTS

Attleboro
Member
  Sturdy Memorial Hospital

Ayer
Member
  Deaconess–Nashoba Hospital

Boston
Member
  Beth Israel Deaconess Medical Center
  Boston Medical Center
  Children's Hospital
  New England Baptist Hospital

Alliances

Braintree
Member
  Massachusetts Respiratory Hospital

Brockton
Member
  Brockton Hospital
  Caritas Good Samaritan Medical Center

Cambridge
Member
  Youville Lifecare

Fall River
Member
  Southcoast Hospitals Group

Great Barrington
Member
  Fairview Hospital

Greenfield
Member
  Franklin Medical Center

Haverhill
Member
  Hale Hospital

Lexington
Member
  Covenant Health Systems, Inc.

Lowell
Member
  Saints Memorial Medical Center

Needham
Member
  Deaconess–Glover Hospital Corporation

Palmer
Member
  Wing Memorial Hospital and Medical Centers

Pittsfield
Member
  Berkshire Medical Center

Plymouth
Member
  Jordan Hospital

Quincy
Member
  Quincy Medical Center

Springfield
Member
  Baystate Health System, Inc.
  Baystate Medical Center

Waltham
Member
  Deaconess Waltham Hospital

Ware
Member
  Mary Lane Hospital

Webster
Member
  Hubbard Regional Hospital

Winchester
Member
  Winchester Hospital

Worcester
Member
  UMass Memorial Health Care

MICHIGAN

Allegan
Member
  Allegan General Hospital

Alma
Member
  Gratiot Community Hospital

Ann Arbor
Member
  Saint Joseph Mercy Health System

Battle Creek
Member
  Battle Creek Health System

Big Rapids
Member
  Mecosta County General Hospital

Cadillac
Member
  Mercy Hospital

Carson City
Member
  Carson City Hospital

Chelsea
Member
  Chelsea Community Hospital

Clinton Township
Member
  St. Joseph's Mercy Hospitals and Health Services

Commerce Township
Member
  Huron Valley–Sinai Hospital

Detroit
Member
  Detroit Medical Center
  Detroit Receiving Hospital and University Health Center
  Harper Hospital
  Henry Ford Health System
  Henry Ford Hospital
  Hutzel Hospital
  Sinai/Grace Hospital
  St. John Detroit Riverview Hospital

Dowagiac
Member
  Lee Memorial Hospital

Farmington Hills
Member
  Botsford General Hospital

Flint
Member
  McLaren Regional Medical Center

Frankfort
Member
  Paul Oliver Memorial Hospital

Garden City
Member
  Garden City Hospital

Grand Rapids
  Spectrum Health
Member
  Metropolitan Hospital
  Saint Mary's Mercy Medical Center

Grayling
Member
  Mercy Health Services North–Grayling

Grosse Pointe
Member
  Bon Secours Cottage Health Services–Bon Secours Hospital

Grosse Pointe Farms
Member
  Bon Secours Cottage Health Services–Cottage Hospital

Hillsdale
Member
  Hillsdale Community Health Center

Jackson
Member
  Doctors Hospital of Jackson
  W. A. Foote Memorial Hospital

Kalamazoo
Member
  Borgess Medical Center

Kalkaska
Member
  Kalkaska Memorial Health Center

Lansing
Member
  Ingham Regional Medical Center
  Sparrow Health System

Lapeer
Member
  Lapeer Regional Hospital

Madison Heights
Member
  Madison Community Hospital
  St. John Oakland Hospital

Marlette
Member
  Marlette Community Hospital

Mount Clemens
Member
  Mount Clemens General Hospital

Mount Pleasant
Member
  Central Michigan Community Hospital

Muskegon
Member
  Mercy General Health Partners

Northport
Member
  Leelanau Memorial Health Center

Paw Paw
Member
  LakeView Community Hospital

Pontiac
Member
  POH Medical Center
  St. Joseph Mercy Oakland

Port Huron
Member
  Mercy Hospital

Rochester
Member
  Crittenton Hospital

Romeo
Member
  St. Joseph's Mercy–North

Saginaw
Member
  HealthSource Saginaw

Saint Johns
Member
  Clinton Memorial Hospital

Saline
Member
  Saline Community Hospital

Southfield
Member
  Straith Hospital for Special Surgery

Sturgis
Member
  Sturgis Hospital

Tecumseh
Member
  Herrick Memorial Hospital, Lenawee Health Alliance

Three Rivers
Member
  Three Rivers Area Hospital

Traverse City
Member
  Munson Medical Center

Trenton
Member
  Riverside Osteopathic Hospital

Warren
Member
  Bi-County Community Hospital
  St. John Macomb Hospital

Watervliet
Member
  Community Hospital

Wyandotte
Member
  Henry Ford Wyandotte Hospital

MINNESOTA

Aitkin
Member
  Riverwood HealthCare Center

Alexandria
Member
  Douglas County Hospital

Austin
Member
  Austin Medical Center

Alliances

Burnsville
Member
  Fairview Ridges Hospital

Cloquet
Member
  Cloquet Community Memorial Hospital

Cook
Member
  Cook Hospital and Convalescent Nursing Care Unit

Crosby
Member
  Cuyuna Regional Medical Center

Duluth
Member
  Miller Dwan Medical Center

Ely
Member
  Ely–Bloomenson Community Hospital

Fairmont
Member
  Fairmont Community Hospital

Glencoe
Member
  Glencoe Regional health Services

Hibbing
Member
  University Medical Center–Mesabi

International Falls
Member
  Falls Memorial Hospital

Litchfield
Member
  Meeker County Memorial Hospital

Minneapolis
Member
  Fairview Health Services
  Fairview Southdale Hospital
  Fairview–University Medical Center

Monticello
Member
  Monticello Big Lake Hospital

Moose Lake
Member
  Mercy Hospital and Health Care Center

Mora
Member
  Kanabec Hospital

New Prague
Member
  Queen of Peace Hospital

Northfield
Member
  Northfield Hospital

Ortonville
Member
  Ortonville Area Health Services

Pipestone
Member
  Pipestone County Medical Center/Avera Health

Princeton
Member
  Fairview Northland Regional Health Care

Red Wing
Member
  Fairview Red Wing Hospital

Robbinsdale
Member
  North Memorial Health Care

Rochester
Member
  Olmsted Medical Center

Saint Louis Park
Member
  HealthSystem Minnesota

Sandstone
Member
  Pine Medical Center

Staples
Member
  Lakewood Health System

Stillwater
Member
  Lakeview Hospital

Tyler
Member
  Tyler Healthcare Center/Avera Health

Virginia
Member
  Virginia Regional Medical Center

Wadena
Member
  Tri–County Hospital

Winona
Member
  Winona Community Memorial Hospital

Wyoming
Member
  Fairview Lakes Regional Medical Center

MISSISSIPPI

Amory
Member
  Gilmore Memorial Hospital

Bay Saint Louis
Member
  Hancock Medical Center

Bay Springs
Member
  Jasper General Hospital

Brookhaven
Member
  King's Daughters Medical Center

Centreville
Member
  Field Memorial Community Hospital

Cleveland
Member
  Bolivar Medical Center

Columbia
Member
  Marion General Hospital

Corinth
Member
  Magnolia Regional Health Center

Durant
Member
  University Hospitals and Clinics of Holmes County–Durant

Greenville
Member
  Delta Regional Medical Center
  King's Daughters Hospital

Grenada
Member
  Grenada Lake Medical Center

Hattiesburg
Member
  Wesley Medical Center

Jackson
Member
  Central Mississippi Medical Center
  Mississippi Baptist Health Systems
  University Hospitals and Clinics, University of Mississippi Medical Center

Laurel
Member
  South Central Regional Medical Center

Lexington
Member
  University Hospitals and Clinics – Holmes County

Louisville
Member
  Winston Medical Center

Magee
Member
  Magee General Hospital

Meridian
Member
  Rush Foundation Hospital

Natchez
Member
  Natchez Regional Medical Center

Philadelphia
Member
  Neshoba County General Hospital

Picayune
Member
  Crosby Memorial Hospital

Prentiss
Member
  Prentiss Regional Hospital and Extended Care Facilities

Quitman
Member
  H. C. Watkins Memorial Hospital

Union
Member
  Laird Hospital

Vicksburg
Member
  Parkview Regional Medical Center

Yazoo City
Member
  King's Daughters Hospital

MISSOURI

Albany
Member
  Gentry County Memorial Hospital

Belton
Member
  Research Belton Hospital

Bethany
Member
  Harrison County Community Hospital

Bridgeton
Member
  DePaul Hospital

Carrollton
Member
  Carroll County Memorial Hospital

Fairfax
Member
  Community Hospital Association

Farmington
Member
  Mineral Area Regional Medical Center

Harrisonville
Member
  Cass Medical Center

Independence
Member
  Medical Center of Independence

Jefferson City
Member
  St. Marys Health Center

Kansas City
Member
  Baptist Medical Center
  Children's Mercy Hospital
  Health Midwest
  Research Medical Center
  Trinity Lutheran Hospital

Lake Saint Louis
Member
  St. Joseph Hospital West

Lees Summit
Member
  Lee's Summit Hospital

Lexington
Member
  Lafayette Regional Health Center

Louisiana
Member
  Pike County Memorial Hospital

Alliances

Maryville
Member
St. Francis Hospital and Health Services

Mexico
Member
Audrain Medical Center

Nevada
Member
Nevada Regional Medical Center

Rolla
Member
Phelps County Regional Medical Center

Saint Charles
Member
St. Joseph Health Center

Saint Joseph
Member
Heartland Regional Medical Center

Saint Louis
Member
Cardinal Glennon Children's Hospital
SSM Health Care
St. Joseph Hospital of Kirkwood
St. Mary's Health Center

West Plains
Member
Ozarks Medical Center

MONTANA

Anaconda
Member
Community Hospital of Anaconda

Cut Bank
Member
Glacier County Medical Center

Great Falls
Member
Benefis Health Care–West Campus
Benefis Healthcare

Harlowton
Member
Wheatland Memorial Hospital

Lewistown
Member
Central Montana Medical Center

Missoula
Member
St. Patrick Hospital

Plains
Member
Clark Fork Valley Hospital

Polson
Member
St. Joseph Hospital

Whitefish
Member
North Valley Hospital

NEBRASKA

Ainsworth
Member
Brown County Hospital

Albion
Member
Boone County Health Center

Atkinson
Member
West Holt Memorial Hospital

Auburn
Member
Nemaha County Hospital

Aurora
Member
Memorial Hospital

Bassett
Member
Rock County Hospital

Central City
Member
Litzenberg Memorial County Hospital

Chadron
Member
Chadron Community Hospital and Health Services

Cozad
Member
Cozad Community Hospital

Creighton
Member
Creighton Area Health Services

Fairbury
Member
Jefferson Community Health Center

Fremont
Member
Fremont Area Medical Center

Geneva
Member
Fillmore County Hospital

Genoa
Member
Genoa Community Hospital

Gordon
Member
Gordon Memorial Hospital District

Gothenburg
Member
Gothenburg Memorial Hospital

Hebron
Member
Thayer County Health Services

Henderson
Member
Henderson Health Care Services

Holdrege
Member
Phelps Memorial Health Center

Imperial
Member
Chase County Community Hospital

Lynch
Member
Niobrara Valley Hospital

North Platte
Member
Great Plains Regional Medical Center

O'Neill
Member
Avera St. Anthony's Hospital

Oakland
Member
Oakland Memorial Hospital

Ogallala
Member
Ogallala Community Hospital

Omaha
Member
Alegent Health Bergan Mercy Medical Center
Alegent Health Immanuel Medical Center
Boys Town National Research Hospital

Ord
Member
Valley County Hospital

Osceola
Member
Annie Jeffrey Memorial County Health Center

Papillion
Member
Alegent-Health Midlands Community Hospital

Pawnee City
Member
Pawnee County Memorial Hospital

Pender
Member
Pender Community Hospital

Red Cloud
Member
Webster County Community Hospital

Saint Paul
Member
Howard County Community Hospital

Schuyler
Member
Alegent Health–Memorial Hospital

Seward
Member
Memorial Health Care Systems

Superior
Member
Memorial Nuckolls County Hospital

Syracuse
Member
Community Memorial Hospital

Tecumseh
Member
Johnson County Hospital

Valentine
Member
Cherry County Hospital

Wahoo
Member
Saunders County Health Service

Wayne
Member
Providence Medical Center

West Point
Member
St. Francis Memorial Hospital

NEVADA

Fallon
Member
Churchill Community Hospital

Las Vegas
Member
Desert Springs Hospital

Lovelock
Member
Pershing General Hospital

NEW HAMPSHIRE

Exeter
Member
Exeter Hospital

Littleton
Member
Littleton Regional Hospital

Manchester
Member
Catholic Medical Center
Elliot Hospital

Nashua
Member
St. Joseph Hospital

NEW JERSEY

Belleville
Member
Clara Maass Health System

Edison
Member
JFK Medical Center
Solaris Health System

Englewood
Member
Englewood Hospital and Medical Center

Freehold
Member
CentraState Healthcare System

Hackensack
Member
Hackensack University Medical Center

Hackettstown
Member
Hackettstown Community Hospital

Holmdel
Member
Bayshore Community Hospital

Alliances

Irvington
Member
  Irvington General Hospital
Jersey City
Member
  Greenville Hospital
  Jersey City Medical Center
Kearny
Member
  West Hudson Hospital
Lakewood
Member
  Kimball Medical Center
Livingston
Member
  Saint Barnabas Medical Center
Long Branch
Member
  Monmouth Medical Center
Manahawkin
Member
  Southern Ocean County Hospital
Newark
Member
  Newark Beth Israel Medical Center
Passaic
Member
  Beth Israel Hospital
Paterson
Member
  Barnert Hospital
  St. Joseph's Hospital and Medical Center
Salem
Member
  Memorial Hospital of Salem County
Secaucus
Member
  Meadowlands Hospital Medical Center
Toms River
Member
  Community Medical Center
Union
Member
  Union Hospital
Wayne
Member
  Wayne General Hospital
West Orange
Member
  Saint Barnabas Health Care System

NEW MEXICO
Alamogordo
Member
  Gerald Champion Regional Medical Center
Albuquerque
Member
  Presbyterian Healthcare Services
  Presbyterian Hospital
  Presbyterian Kaseman Hospital
Artesia
Member
  Artesia General Hospital
Clovis
Member
  Plains Regional Medical Center
Espanola
Member
  Espanola Hospital
Grants
Member
  Cibola General Hospital
Los Alamos
Member
  Los Alamos Medical Center
Ruidoso
Member
  Lincoln County Medical Center
Silver City
Member
  Gila Regional Medical Center

Socorro
Member
  Socorro General Hospital
Taos
Member
  Holy Cross Hospital
Truth or Consequences
Member
  Sierra Vista Hospital
Tucumcari
Member
  Dr. Dan C. Trigg Memorial Hospital

NEW YORK
Albany
Member
  Albany Medical Center
  St. Peter's Hospital
Amityville
Affiliate
  South Oaks Hospital
Amsterdam
Member
  Amsterdam Memorial Hospital
Batavia
Member
  United Memorial Medical Center
Bath
Member
  Ira Davenport Memorial Hospital
Bayside
Member
  St. Mary's Hospital for Children
Beacon
Member
  Saint Francis Hospital–Beacon
Bethpage
Member
  Episcopal Health Services Inc.
  New Island Hospital
Brockport
Member
  Lakeside Memorial Hospital
Bronx
  St Barnabas Hospital
Member
  Bronx–Lebanon Hospital Center
  Calvary Hospital
  Fulton Division
  Jewish Home and Hospital for Aged
  Montefiore Medical Center
  Our Lady of Mercy Healthcare System, Inc.
  Our Lady of Mercy Medical Center
Brooklyn
Member
  Brookdale Hospital Medical Center
  Interfaith Medical Center
  Kingsbrook Jewish Medical Center
  Long Island College Hospital
  Lutheran Medical Center
  Maimonides Medical Center
  New York Methodist Hospital
  St. Mary's Hospital of Brooklyn
  University Hospital of Brooklyn–State University of
    New York Health Science Center at Brooklyn
  Victory Memorial Hospital
Buffalo
Member
  Brylin Hospitals
  Children's Hospital
  Mercy Hospital
  Millard Fillmore Gates Circle Hospital
  Sheehan Memorial Hospital
Canandaigua
Member
  F. F. Thompson Health System
Cheektowaga
Member
  St. Joseph Hospital
Clifton Springs
Member
  Clifton Springs Hospital and Clinic

Corning
Member
  Corning Hospital
Cortlandt Manor
Member
  Hudson Valley Hospital Center
Dansville
Member
  Nicholas H. Noyes Memorial Hospital
Dobbs Ferry
Member
  Community Hospital at Dobbs Ferry
Elizabethtown
Member
  Elizabethtown Community Hospital
Elmira
Member
  Arnot Ogden Medical Center
  St. Joseph's Hospital
Far Rockaway
  Peninsula Hospital Center
  St. John's Episcopal Hospital–South Shore
Flushing
Member
  Parkway Hospital
  St. John's Queens Hospital
  St. Joseph's Hospital
Glen Oaks
Member
  Hillside Hospital
Glens Falls
Member
  Glens Falls Hospital
Hornell
Member
  St. James Mercy Hospital
Irving
Member
  Lake Shore Hospital
Jamaica
Member
  Catholic Medical Centers
  Jamaica Hospital Medical Center
Kenmore
Member
  Kenmore Mercy Hospital
Lackawanna
Member
  Our Lady of Victory Hospital
Long Beach
Member
  Long Beach Medical Center
Long Island City
Member
  The Mount Sinai Hospital of Queens
Medina
Member
  Medina Memorial Hospital
Mineola
Member
  Winthrop–University Hospital
Montour Falls
Member
  Schuyler Hospital
Mount Vernon
Member
  Mount Vernon Hospital
New Hyde Park
Member
  Long Island Jewish Medical Center
  Schneider Children's Hospital
New York
Member
  Cabrini Medical Center
  Hospital for Special Surgery
  Lenox Hill Hospital
  Manhattan Eye, Ear and Throat Hospital
  Mount Sinai–NYU Hospitals/Health System
  New York Eye and Ear Infirmary
  North General Hospital
  Saint Vincents Hospital and Medical Center
  St. Clare's Hospital and Health Center
  St. Luke's–Roosevelt Hospital Center

Alliances

Newfane
Member
  Inter-Community Memorial Hospital

Oceanside
Member
  South Nassau Communities Hospital

Oneonta
Member
  Aurelia Osborn Fox Memorial Hospital

Patchogue
Member
  Brookhaven Memorial Hospital Medical Center

Penn Yan
Member
  Soldiers and Sailors Memorial Hospital of Yates County

Plattsburgh
Member
  Champlain Valley Physicians Hospital Medical Center

Port Jefferson
Member
  John T. Mather Memorial Hospital
  St. Charles Hospital and Rehabilitation Center

Poughkeepsie
Member
  Saint Francis Hospital
  Vassar Brothers Hospital

Rochester
Member
  Genesee Hospital
  Monroe Community Hospital
  Rochester General Hospital

Rockville Centre
Member
  Mercy Medical Center

Roslyn
Member
  St. Francis Hospital

Schenectady
Member
  Ellis Hospital

Seaford
Member
  Massapequa General Hospital

Smithtown
Member
  St. Catherine of Siena Medical Center

Staten Island
Member
  Doctors' Hospital of Staten Island
  Sisters of Charity Healthcare
  Sisters of Charity Medical Center
  Staten Island University Hospital

Syracuse
Member
  University Hospital-SUNY Health Science Center at Syracuse

Troy
Member
  Samaritan Hospital

Valhalla
Member
  Blythedale Children's Hospital
  Westchester Medical Center

Warsaw
Member
  Wyoming County Community Hospital

West Islip
Member
  Good Samaritan Hospital Medical Center

Westfield
Member
  Westfield Memorial Hospital

White Plains
Member
  St. Agnes Hospital

Williamsville
Member
  Millard Fillmore Suburban Hospital

Yonkers
Member
  St. John's Riverside Hospital
  Yonkers General Hospital

NORTH CAROLINA

Albemarle
Member
  Stanly Memorial Hospital

Andrews
Member
  District Memorial Hospital

Asheboro
Member
  Randolph Hospital

Asheville
Member
  Mission St. Joseph's Health
  Thoms Rehabilitation Hospital

Blowing Rock
Member
  Blowing Rock Hospital

Boiling Springs
Member
  Crawley Memorial Hospital

Boone
Member
  Watauga Medical Center

Brevard
Member
  Transylvania Community Hospital

Bryson City
Member
  Swain County Hospital

Burgaw
Member
  Pender Memorial Hospital

Burlington
Member
  Alamance Regional Medical Center

Clinton
Member
  Sampson Regional Medical Center

Clyde
Member
  Haywood Regional Medical Center

Columbus
Member
  St. Luke's Hospital

Danbury
Member
  Stokes-Reynolds Memorial Hospital

Durham
Member
  Durham Regional Hospital

Eden
Member
  Morehead Memorial Hospital

Edenton
Member
  Chowan Hospital

Elizabethtown
Member
  Bladen County Hospital

Elkin
Member
  Hugh Chatham Memorial Hospital

Erwin
Member
  Good Hope Hospital

Fayetteville
Member
  Behavioral Health Care of Cape Fear Valley Health System
  Cape Fear Valley Health System

Fletcher
Member
  Park Ridge Hospital

Franklin
Member
  Angel Medical Center

Gastonia
Member
  Gaston Memorial Hospital

Goldsboro
Member
  Wayne Memorial Hospital

Henderson
Member
  Maria Parham Hospital

Hendersonville
Member
  Margaret R. Pardee Memorial Hospital

Hickory
Member
  Catawba Memorial Hospital

Jefferson
Member
  Ashe Memorial Hospital

Kenansville
Member
  Duplin General Hospital

Kinston
Member
  Lenoir Memorial Hospital

Laurinburg
Member
  Scotland Memorial Hospital

Lenoir
Member
  Caldwell Memorial Hospital

Lexington
Member
  Lexington Memorial Hospital

Lumberton
Member
  Southeastern Regional Medical Center

Marion
Member
  McDowell Hospital

Matthews
Member
  Presbyterian Hospital-Matthews

Morganton
Member
  Grace Hospital

Mount Airy
Member
  Northern Hospital of Surry County

Murphy
Member
  Murphy Medical Center

North Wilkesboro
Member
  Wilkes Regional Medical Center

Oxford
Member
  Granville Medical Center

Pinehurst
Member
  FirstHealth Moore Regional Hospital

Plymouth
Member
  Washington County Hospital

Raleigh
Member
  Rex Healthcare

Roanoke Rapids
Member
  Halifax Regional Medical Center

Roxboro
Member
  Person Memorial Hospital

Rutherfordton
Member
  Rutherford Hospital

Shelby
Member
  Cleveland Regional Medical Center

Alliances

Siler City
Member
  Chatham Hospital

Smithfield
Member
  Johnston Memorial Hospital

Sparta
Member
  Alleghany Memorial Hospital

Spruce Pine
Member
  Spruce Pine Community Hospital

Statesville
Member
  Iredell Memorial Hospital

Sylva
Member
  Harris Regional Hospital

Taylorsville
Member
  Alexander Community Hospital

Troy
Member
  FirstHealth Montgomery Memorial Hospital

Whiteville
Member
  Columbus County Hospital

Williamston
Member
  Martin General Hospital

Wilmington
Member
  New Hanover Regional Medical Center

Wilson
Member
  Wilson Memorial Hospital

Winston–Salem
Member
  North Carolina Baptist Hospital

Yadkinville
Member
  Hoots Memorial Hospital

NORTH DAKOTA

Cavalier
Member
  Pembina County Memorial Hospital and Wedgewood Manor

Kenmare
Member
  Kenmare Community Hospital

Lisbon
Member
  Lisbon Medical Center

Minot
Member
  UniMed Medical Center

OHIO

Akron
Member
  Akron City Hospital
  Children's Hospital Medical Center of Akron
  Edwin Shaw Hospital for Rehabilitation
  Saint Thomas Hospital
  Summa Health System

Alliance
Member
  Alliance Community Hospital

Amherst
Member
  EMH Amherst Hospital

Ashtabula
Member
  Ashtabula County Medical Center

Barberton
Member
  Barberton Citizens Hospital

Batavia
Member
  Mercy Hospital Clermont

Cincinnati
Member
  Bethesda North Hospital
  Catholic Healthcare Partners
  Children's Hospital Medical Center
  Mercy Hospital Anderson

Cleveland
Member
  Cleveland Clinic Children's Hospital for Rehabilitation
  Cleveland Clinic Foundation
  Fairview Hospital
  Grace Hospital
  Lutheran Hospital
  Meridia Hillcrest Hospital
  Meridia Huron Hospital
  MetroHealth Medical Center

Columbus
Member
  Children's Hospital
  Ohio State University Hospital East

Dayton
Member
  Children's Medical Center
  Good Samaritan Hospital and Health Center

Defiance
Member
  Defiance Hospital

Dennison
Member
  Twin City Hospital

East Liverpool
Member
  East Liverpool City Hospital

Elyria
Member
  EMH Regional Medical Center

Euclid
Member
  Euclid Hospital

Fremont
Member
  Memorial Hospital

Garfield Heights
Member
  Marymount Hospital

Georgetown
Member
  Brown County General Hospital

Green Springs
Member
  St. Francis Health Care Centre

Greenfield
Member
  Greenfield Area Medical Center

Hamilton
Member
  Mercy Hospital

Kettering
Member
  Kettering Medical Center–Network

Lakewood
Member
  Lakewood Hospital

Lima
Member
  St. Rita's Medical Center

Lodi
Member
  Lodi Community Hospital

Lorain
Member
  Lorain Community/St. Joseph Regional Health Center

Marietta
Member
  Selby General Hospital

Marysville
Member
  Memorial Hospital

Massillon
Member
  Doctors Hospital of Stark County
  Massillon Community Hospital

Middleburg Heights
Member
  Southwest General Health Center

Mount Vernon
Member
  Knox Community Hospital

Oberlin
Member
  Allen Memorial Hospital

Oregon
Member
  St. Charles Mercy Hospital

Parma
Member
  Parma Community General Hospital

Paulding
Member
  Paulding County Hospital

Sandusky
Member
  Providence Hospital

Springfield
Member
  Mercy Medical Center

Tiffin
Member
  Mercy Hospital

Toledo
Member
  Riverside Mercy Hospital
  St. Vincent Mercy Medical Center

Urbana
Member
  Mercy Memorial Hospital

Van Wert
Member
  Van Wert County Hospital

Wadsworth
Member
  Wadsworth–Rittman Hospital

Warren
Member
  Hillside Rehabilitation Hospital
  St. Joseph Health Center

Warrensville Heights
Member
  Meridia South Pointe Hospital

Washington Court House
Member
  Fayette County Memorial Hospital

Willard
Member
  Mercy Hospital of Willard

Wooster
Member
  Wooster Community Hospital

Youngstown
Member
  St. Elizabeth Health Center
  Youngstown Osteopathic Hospital

OKLAHOMA

Alva
Member
  Share Medical Center

Atoka
Member
  Atoka Memorial Hospital

Cordell
Member
  Cordell Memorial Hospital

Cushing
Member
  Cushing Regional Hospital

Frederick
Member
  Memorial Hospital

Alliances

Guthrie
Member
  Logan Hospital and Medical Center

Henryetta
Member
  Henryetta Medical Center

Holdenville
Member
  Holdenville General Hospital

Idabel
Member
  McCurtain Memorial Hospital

Kingfisher
Member
  Kingfisher Regional Hospital

Lawton
Member
  Comanche County Memorial Hospital

Mangum
Member
  Mangum City Hospital

Oklahoma City
Member
  Bone and Joint Hospital
  Hillcrest Health Center
  St. Anthony Hospital

Okmulgee
Affiliate
  Okmulgee Memorial Hospital
Member
  Okmulgee Memorial Hospital Authority

Perry
Member
  Perry Memorial Hospital

Purcell
Member
  Purcell Municipal Hospital

Sayre
Member
  Sayre Memorial Hospital

Seiling
Member
  Seiling Hospital

Seminole
Member
  Seminole Medical Center

Tahlequah
Member
  Tahlequah City Hospital

Tulsa
Member
  Laureate Psychiatric Clinic and Hospital
  Saint Francis Hospital

Watonga
Member
  Watonga Municipal Hospital

Woodward
Member
  Woodward Hospital and Health Center

OREGON

Dallas
Member
  Valley Community Hospital

Eugene
Member
  Sacred Heart Medical Center

Florence
Member
  Peace Harbor Hospital

Gold Beach
Member
  Curry General Hospital

Gresham
Member
  Legacy Mount Hood Medical Center

Heppner
Member
  Pioneer Memorial Hospital

Lakeview
Member
  Lake District Hospital

Lebanon
Member
  Lebanon Community Hospital

Lincoln City
Member
  North Lincoln Hospital

Medford
  Providence Medford Medical Center

Milwaukie
Member
  Providence Milwaukie Hospital

Newberg
Member
  Providence Newberg Hospital

Newport
Member
  Pacific Communities Health District

Portland
Member
  Adventist Medical Center
  Colonial Manor Sanitarium
  Legacy Good Samaritan Hospital and Medical Center
  Legacy Health System
  Providence St. Vincent Medical Center

Prineville
Member
  Pioneer Memorial Hospital

Salem
Member
  Salem Hospital

Seaside
Member
  Providence Seaside Hospital

Springfield
Member
  McKenzie–Willamette Hospital

Stayton
Member
  Santiam Memorial Hospital

Tillamook
Member
  Tillamook County General Hospital

Tualatin
Member
  Legacy Meridian Park Hospital

PENNSYLVANIA

Altoona
Member
  Bon Secours–Holy Family Regional Health System

Berwick
Member
  Berwick Hospital Center

Bethlehem
Member
  St. Luke's Hospital and Health Network

Brownsville
Member
  Brownsville General Hospital

Bryn Mawr
Member
  Bryn Mawr Hospital
  Bryn Mawr Hospital

Carlisle
Member
  Carlisle Hospital and Health Services

Clarion
Member
  Clarion Hospital

Coaldale
Member
  Miner's Memorial Medical Center

Corry
Member
  Corry Memorial Hospital

Danville
Member
  Geisinger Health System
  Geisinger Medical Center

Darby
Member
  Mercy Fitzgerald Hospital

East Stroudsburg
Member
  Pocono Medical Center

Easton
Member
  Easton Hospital

Erie
Member
  Millcreek Community Hospital
  Saint Vincent Health Center

Hastings
Member
  Miners Hospital Northern Cambria

Havertown
Member
  Mercy Community Hospital

Hazleton
Member
  Hazleton–St. Joseph Medical Center

Hershey
Member
  Penn State Geisinger Health System–Milton S. Hershey Medical Center

Huntingdon
Member
  J. C. Blair Memorial Hospital

Jersey Shore
Member
  Jersey Shore Hospital

Kane
Member
  Kane Community Hospital

Lock Haven
Member
  Lock Haven Hospital

Malvern
Member
  Bryn Mawr Rehabilitation Hospital

McKees Rocks
Member
  Ohio Valley General Hospital

Meadville
Member
  Meadville Medical Center

Media
Member
  Riddle Memorial Hospital

Monroeville
Member
  Allegheny University Hospitals, Forbes Regional

Nanticoke
Member
  Mercy Special Care Hospital

Newtown Square
Member
  Catholic Health East

Palmerton
Member
  Palmerton Hospital

Paoli
Member
  Paoli Memorial Hospital

Philadelphia
Member
  Albert Einstein Healthcare Network
  Albert Einstein Medical Center
  Belmont Center for Comprehensive Treatment
  Children's Hospital of Philadelphia
  Germantown Hospital and Community Health Services
  Mercy Hospital of Philadelphia
  Methodist Hospital
  Thomas Jefferson University Hospital
  Wills Eye Hospital

Alliances

Pittsburgh
Member
  Children's Hospital of Pittsburgh
  LifeCare Hospital of Pittsburgh
  Mercy Hospital of Pittsburgh
  Mercy Providence Hospital
  Suburban General Hospital
  Western Pennsylvania Hospital

Pottsville
Member
  Pottsville Hospital and Warne Clinic

Ridley Park
Member
  Taylor Hospital

Scranton
Member
  Mercy Hospital of Scranton

Titusville
Member
  Titusville Area Hospital

Towanda
Member
  Memorial Hospital

Tyrone
Member
  Tyrone Hospital

Union City
Member
  Union City Memorial Hospital

Warren
Member
  Warren General Hospital

Wayne
Member
  Jefferson Health System

Waynesburg
Member
  Greene County Memorial Hospital

West Grove
Member
  Southern Chester County Medical Center

Wilkes–Barre
Member
  Mercy Hospital of Wilkes–Barre
  Penn State Geisinger Wyoming Valley Medical Center

Wynnewood
Member
  Lankenau Hospital

York
Member
  Memorial Hospital

PUERTO RICO

Mayaguez
Member
  Bella Vista Hospital

Ponce
Member
  Hospital De Damas

RHODE ISLAND

Providence
Member
  Roger Williams Medical Center

SOUTH CAROLINA

Abbeville
Member
  Abbeville County Memorial Hospital

Anderson
Member
  Anderson Area Medical Center

Beaufort
Member
  Beaufort Memorial Hospital

Camden
Member
  Kershaw County Medical Center

Charleston
Member
  Bon Secours–St. Francis Xavier Hospital
  Roper Hospital
  Roper Hospital North

Clinton
Member
  Laurens County Healthcare System

Columbia
Member
  Palmetto Richland Memorial Hospital

Conway
Member
  Conway Hospital

Dillon
Member
  Saint Eugene Medical Center

Edgefield
Member
  Edgefield County Hospital

Florence
Member
  Carolinas Hospital System
  McLeod Regional Medical Center

Greenville
Member
  Greenville Hospital System
  Greenville Memorial Hospital
  Shriners Hospitals for Children, Greenville

Greenwood
Member
  Self Memorial Hospital

Greer
Member
  Allen Bennett Hospital

Kingstree
Member
  Carolinas Hospital System–Kingstree

Lake City
Member
  Carolinas Hospital System–Lake City

Lexington
Member
  Keisler Nursing Home

Loris
Member
  Loris Community Hospital

Newberry
Member
  Newberry County Memorial Hospital

Orangeburg
Member
  Regional Medical Center of Orangeburg and Calhoun Counties

Pickens
Member
  Cannon Memorial Hospital

Ridgeland
Member
  Low Country General Hospital

Simpsonville
Member
  Hillcrest Hospital

Spartanburg
Member
  Mary Black Health System
  Spartanburg Regional Medical Center

Sumter
Member
  Tuomey Healthcare System

Union
Member
  Wallace Thomson Hospital

West Columbia
Member
  Lexington Medical Center

Winnsboro
Member
  Fairfield Memorial Hospital

Woodruff
Member
  B.J. Workman Memorial Hospital

SOUTH DAKOTA

Aberdeen
Member
  Avera St. Luke's

Armour
Member
  Douglas County Memorial Hospital

Britton
Member
  Marshall County Healthcare Center/Avera Health

Burke
Member
  Community Memorial Hospital/Avera Health

Custer
Member
  Custer Community Hospital

Deadwood
Member
  Northern Hills General Hospital

Dell Rapids
Member
  Dells Area Health Center

Eureka
Member
  Eureka Community Health Services/Avera Health

Faulkton
Member
  Faulk County Memorial Hospital

Flandreau
Member
  Flandreau Municipal Hospital/Avera Health

Gregory
Member
  Gregory Community Hospital

Hoven
Member
  Holy Infant Hospital

Huron
Member
  Huron Regional Medical Center

Martin
Member
  Bennett County Healthcare Center

Milbank
Member
  St. Bernard's Providence Hospital

Miller
Member
  Hand County Memorial Hospital/Avera Health

Mitchell
Member
  Avera Queen of Peace

Parkston
Member
  Avera St. Benedict Health Center

Platte
Member
  Platte Health Center/Avera Health

Rapid City
Member
  Rapid City Regional Hospital System of Care

Redfield
Member
  Community Memorial Hospital

Scotland
Member
  Landmann–Jungman Memorial Hospital

Sioux Falls
Member
  Avera McKennan Hospital

Spearfish
Member
  Lookout Memorial Hospital

Sturgis
Member
  Sturgis Community Health Care Center

Tyndall
Member
  St. Michael's Hospital

Alliances

Wagner
Member
  Wagner Community Memorial Hospital
Watertown
Member
  Prairie Lakes Hospital and Care Center
Wessington Springs
Member
  Weskota Memorial Medical Center
Yankton
Member
  Avera Health
  Avera Sacred Heart

TENNESSEE
Bristol
Member
  Wellmont Bristol Regional Medical Center
Brownsville
Member
  Haywood County Memorial Hospital
Chattanooga
Member
  Siskin Hospital for Physical Rehabilitation
Cleveland
Member
  Bradley Memorial Hospital
Copperhill
Member
  Copper Basin Medical Center
Crossville
Member
  Cumberland Medical Center
Dayton
Member
  Rhea Medical Center
Dyersburg
Member
  Methodist Healthcare– Dyersburg Hospital
Erwin
Member
  Unicoi County Memorial Hospital
Etowah
Member
  Woods Memorial Hospital District
Fayetteville
Member
  Lincoln County Health Facilities
Gallatin
Member
  Sumner Regional Medical Center
Greeneville
Member
  Takoma Adventist Hospital
Jackson
Member
  Jackson–Madison County General Hospital
Jefferson City
Member
  Jefferson Memorial Hospital
Jellico
Member
  Jellico Community Hospital
Johnson City
Member
  Johnson City Medical Center
Kingsport
Member
  Wellmont Holston Valley Medical Center
Knoxville
Member
  Baptist Hospital of East Tennessee
  St. Mary's Health System
La Follette
Member
  La Follette Medical Center
Lafayette
Member
  Macon County General Hospital
Lexington
Member
  Methodist Healthcare–Lexington Hospital
Madison
Member
  Tennessee Christian Medical Center
Maryville
Member
  Blount Memorial Hospital
McKenzie
Member
  Methodist Healthcare – McKenzie
Memphis
Member
  Extendicare of Memphis
  Methodist Healthcare
  Methodist Healthcare–Memphis Hospital
  Regional Medical Center at Memphis
  St. Jude Children's Research Hospital
Morristown
Member
  Morristown–Hamblen Hospital
Nashville
Member
  Vanderbilt University Hospital
Newport
Member
  Baptist Hospital of Cocke County
Rockwood
Member
  Baptist Urgent Care
Rogersville
Member
  Hawkins County Memorial Hospital
Somerville
Member
  Methodist Healthcare–Somerville
Sweetwater
Member
  Sweetwater Hospital
Tazewell
Member
  Claiborne County Hospital

TEXAS
Abilene
Member
  Abilene Regional Medical Center
  Hendrick Health System
Anahuac
Member
  Bayside Community Hospital
Anson
Member
  Anson General Hospital
Aspermont
Member
  Stonewall Memorial Hospital
Azle
Member
  Harris Methodist Northwest
Ballinger
Member
  Ballinger Memorial Hospital
Bay City
Member
  Matagorda General Hospital
Beaumont
Member
  Christus St. Elizabeth Hospital
Bedford
Member
  Harris Methodist–HEB
Big Lake
Member
  Reagan Memorial Hospital
Bowie
Member
  Bowie Memorial Hospital
Brady
Member
  Heart of Texas Memorial Hospital
Breckenridge
Member
  Stephens Memorial Hospital
Brenham
Member
  Trinity Community Medical Center of Brenham
Bryan
Member
  St. Joseph Regional Health Center
Burnet
Member
  Seton Highland Lakes
Caldwell
Member
  Burleson St. Joseph Health Center
Canadian
Member
  Hemphill County Hospital
Carrizo Springs
Member
  Dimmit County Memorial Hospital
Childress
Member
  Childress Regional Medical Center
Chillicothe
Member
  Chillicothe Hospital District
Cleburne
Member
  Walls Regional Hospital
Clifton
Member
  Goodall–Witcher Healthcare
Coleman
Member
  Coleman County Medical Center
Columbus
Member
  Columbus Community Hospital
Comanche
Member
  Comanche Community Hospital
Commerce
Member
  Presbyterian Hospital of Commerce
Corpus Christi
Member
  Driscoll Children's Hospital
Crane
Member
  Crane Memorial Hospital
Crosbyton
Member
  Crosbyton Clinic Hospital
Dallas
Member
  Charlton Methodist Hospital
  Children's Medical Center of Dallas
  Methodist Hospitals of Dallas
  Methodist Medical Center
  Presbyterian Hospital of Dallas
  St. Paul Medical Center
Decatur
Member
  Decatur Community Hospital
Denison
Member
  Texoma Medical Center Restorative Care Hospital
Denver City
Member
  Yoakum County Hospital
Dimmitt
Member
  Plains Memorial Hospital
Eagle Lake
Member
  Rice Medical Center

Alliances

Eagle Pass
Member
  Fort Duncan Medical Center
Eastland
Member
  Eastland Memorial Hospital
Eden
Member
  Concho County Hospital
Edna
Member
  Jackson County Hospital
El Campo
Member
  El Campo Memorial Hospital
El Paso
Member
  R. E. Thomason General Hospital
Eldorado
Member
  Schleicher County Medical Center
Fort Stockton
Member
  Pecos County Memorial Hospital
Fort Worth
Member
  Cook Children's Medical Center
  Harris Methodist Fort Worth
  Harris Methodist Health System
  Harris Methodist Southwest
  Huguley Memorial Medical Center
  Osteopathic Medical Center of Texas
Fredericksburg
Member
  Hill Country Memorial Hospital
Friona
Member
  Parmer County Community Hospital
Galveston
Member
  University of Texas Medical Branch Hospitals
Graham
Member
  Graham Regional Medical Center
Grand Prairie
Member
  Dallas–Fort Worth Medical Center
Greenville
Member
  Presbyterian Hospital of Greenville
Groves
Member
  Doctors Hospital
Hale Center
Member
  Hi–Plains Hospital
Hallettsville
Member
  Lavaca Medical Center
Hamilton
Member
  Hamilton General Hospital
Hamlin
Member
  Hamlin Memorial Hospital
Haskell
Member
  Haskell Memorial Hospital
Henderson
Member
  Henderson Memorial Hospital
Hondo
Member
  Medina Community Hospital
Houston
Member
  Christus St. Joseph Hospital
  Methodist Health Care System
  St. Luke's Episcopal Health System
  Texas Children's Hospital
  The Methodist Hospital
  University of Texas M. D. Anderson Cancer Center

Irving
Member
  Texas Health Resources
Jasper
Member
  Christus Jasper Memorial Hospital
Junction
Member
  Kimble Hospital
Kaufman
Member
  Presbyterian Hospital of Kaufman
Kenedy
Member
  Otto Kaiser Memorial Hospital
Kermit
Member
  Memorial Hospital
Killeen
Member
  Metroplex Adventist Hospital
Knox City
Member
  Knox County Hospital
Lake Jackson
Member
  Brazosport Memorial Hospital
Lamesa
Member
  Medical Arts Hospital
Livingston
Member
  Memorial Medical Center
Lockney
Member
  W. J. Mangold Memorial Hospital
Lubbock
Member
  Covenant Medical Center–Lakeside
  University Medical Center
Lufkin
Member
  Memorial Health System of East Texas
Luling
Member
  Seton Edgar B. Davis Hospital
Madisonville
Member
  Madison St. Joseph Health Center
McAllen
Member
  McAllen Medical Center
Midland
Member
  Westwood Medical Center
Mineral Wells
Member
  Palo Pinto General Hospital
Mission
Member
  Mission Hospital
Monahans
Member
  Ward Memorial Hospital
Morton
Member
  Cochran Memorial Hospital
Mount Pleasant
Member
  Titus Regional Medical Center
Muleshoe
Member
  Muleshoe Area Medical Center
Nacogdoches
Member
  Nacogdoches Memorial Hospital
Nassau Bay
Member
  Christus St. John Hospital

Navasota
Member
  Grimes St. Joseph Health Center
Nocona
Member
  Nocona General Hospital
Olney
Member
  Hamilton Hospital
Paris
Member
  McCuistion Regional Medical Center
Pecos
Member
  Reeves County Hospital
Plano
Member
  Presbyterian Hospital of Plano
Port Arthur
Member
  Christus St. Mary Hospital
Quanah
Member
  Hardeman County Memorial Hospital
Rockdale
Member
  Richards Memorial Hospital
Rotan
Member
  Fisher County Hospital District
San Augustine
Member
  Memorial Medical Center of San Augustine
San Marcos
Member
  Central Texas Medical Center
Seminole
Member
  Memorial Hospital
Seymour
Member
  Seymour Hospital
Shamrock
Member
  Shamrock General Hospital
Snyder
Member
  D. M. Cogdell Memorial Hospital
Sonora
Member
  Lillian M. Hudspeth Memorial Hospital
Spearman
Member
  Hansford Hospital
Stamford
Member
  Stamford Memorial Hospital
Stanton
Member
  Martin County Hospital District
Stephenville
Member
  Harris Methodist–Erath County
Sweetwater
Member
  Rolling Plains Memorial Hospital
Tahoka
Member
  Lynn County Hospital District
Texarkana
Member
  Christus St. Michael Health System
Throckmorton
Member
  Throckmorton County Memorial Hospital
Tulia
Member
  Swisher Memorial Hospital District

Alliances

Van Horn
Member
  Culberson Hospital District

Weatherford
Member
  Campbell Health System

Wellington
Member
  Collingsworth General Hospital

Weslaco
Member
  Knapp Medical Center

Whitney
Member
  Lake Whitney Medical Center

Winnie
Member
  Medical Center of Winnie

Winnsboro
Member
  Presbyterian Hospital of Winnsboro

Winters
Member
  North Runnels Hospital

UTAH

Monticello
Member
  San Juan Hospital

VERMONT

Saint Albans
Member
  Northwestern Medical Center

Saint Johnsbury
Member
  Northeastern Vermont Regional Hospital

VIRGINIA

Abingdon
Member
  Johnston Memorial Hospital

Alexandria
Member
  Inova Alexandria Hospital
  Inova Mount Vernon Hospital

Bedford
Member
  Carilion Bedford Memorial Hospital

Big Stone Gap
Member
  Wellmont Lonesome Pine Hospital

Chesapeake
Member
  Chesapeake General Hospital

Culpeper
Member
  Culpeper Regional Hospital

Danville
Member
  Danville Regional Medical Center

Emporia
Member
  Greensville Memorial Hospital

Fairfax
Member
  Inova Fair Oaks Hospital

Falls Church
Member
  Inova Fairfax Hospital
  Inova Health System

Farmville
Member
  Southside Community Hospital

Front Royal
Member
  Warren Memorial Hospital

Galax
Member
  Twin County Regional Hospital

Gloucester
Member
  Riverside Walter Reed Hospital

Grundy
Member
  Buchanan General Hospital

Kilmarnock
Member
  Rappahannock General Hospital

Leesburg
Member
  Loudoun Hospital Center

Lexington
Member
  Stonewall Jackson Hospital

Luray
Member
  Page Memorial Hospital

Manassas
Member
  Prince William Hospital

Marion
Member
  Smyth County Community Hospital

Martinsville
Member
  Memorial Hospital of Martinsville and Henry County

Mechanicsville
Member
  Memorial Regional Medical Center

Nassawadox
Member
  Shore Memorial Hospital

Newport News
Member
  Mary Immaculate Hospital
  Riverside Health System
  Riverside Regional Medical Center
  Riverside Rehabilitation Institute

Norfolk
Member
  Bon Secours–DePaul Medical Center
  Children's Hospital of The King's Daughters

Norton
Member
  Norton Community Hospital

Pearisburg
Member
  Carilion Giles Memorial Hospital

Pennington Gap
Member
  Lee County Community Hospital

Petersburg
Member
  Southside Regional Medical Center

Portsmouth
Member
  Maryview Medical Center

Radford
Member
  Carilion New River Valley Medical Center

Richmond
Member
  Bon Secours St. Mary's Hospital
  Bon Secours–Richmond Community Hospital
  Bon Secours–Stuart Circle
  Children's Hospital
  Richmond Eye and Ear Hospital

Roanoke
Member
  Carilion Health System
  Carilion Medical Center

Rocky Mount
Member
  Carilion Franklin Memorial Hospital

South Boston
Member
  Halifax Regional Health System

South Hill
Member
  Community Memorial Healthcenter

Stuart
Member
  R. J. Reynolds–Patrick County Memorial Hospital

Suffolk
Member
  Louise Obici Memorial Hospital

Tappahannock
Member
  Riverside Tappahannock Hospital

Tazewell
Member
  Tazewell Community Hospital

Virginia Beach
Member
  Sentara Virginia Beach General Hospital
  Tidewater Health Care, Inc.

Warrenton
Member
  Fauquier Hospital

Winchester
Member
  Valley Health System
  Winchester Medical Center

Woodbridge
Member
  Potomac Hospital

Woodstock
Member
  Shenandoah Memorial Hospital

Wytheville
Member
  Wythe County Community Hospital

WASHINGTON

Aberdeen
Member
  Grays Harbor Community Hospital

Bellevue
Member
  Overlake Hospital Medical Center
  PeaceHealth

Bellingham
Member
  St. Joseph Hospital

Brewster
Member
  Okanogan–Douglas County Hospital

Centralia
Member
  Providence Centralia Hospital

Chelan
Member
  Lake Chelan Community Hospital

Chewelah
Member
  St. Joseph's Hospital

Clarkston
Member
  Tri-State Memorial Hospital

Colfax
Member
  Whitman Hospital and Medical Center

Colville
Member
  Mount Carmel Hospital

Coupeville
Member
  Whidbey General Hospital

Davenport
Member
  Lincoln Hospital

Deer Park
Member
  Deer Park Hospital

Edmonds
Member
  Stevens Healthcare

Ephrata
Member
  Columbia Basin Hospital

Alliances

Everett
Member
  Providence Everett Medical Center
Grand Coulee
Member
  Coulee Community Hospital
Kirkland
Member
  Evergreen Community Health Center
Longview
Member
  St. John Medical Center
Morton
Member
  Morton General Hospital
Moses Lake
Member
  Samaritan Healthcare
Newport
Member
  Newport Community Hospital
Odessa
Member
  Odessa Memorial Hospital
Olympia
Member
  Providence St. Peter Hospital
Omak
Member
  Mid–Valley Hospital
Othello
Member
  Othello Community Hospital
Prosser
Member
  Prosser Memorial Hospital
Pullman
Member
  Pullman Memorial Hospital
Puyallup
Member
  Good Samaritan Community Healthcare
Quincy
Member
  Quincy Valley Medical Center
Redmond
Member
  The Eastside Hospital
Renton
Member
  Valley Medical Center
Republic
Member
  Ferry County Memorial Hospital
Richland
Member
  Kadlec Medical Center
Ritzville
Member
  East Adams Rural Hospital
Seattle
Member
  Children's Hospital and Regional Medical Center
  Highline Community Hospital
  Northwest Hospital
  Providence Health System
  Providence Seattle Medical Center
  Regional Hospital for Respiratory and Complex Care
Shelton
Member
  Mason General Hospital
Spokane
Member
  Deaconess Medical Center–Spokane
  Empire Health Services
  Holy Family Hospital
  Providence Services
  Sacred Heart Medical Center
  Shriners Hospitals for Children–Spokane
  St. Lukes Rehabilitation Institute
  Valley Hospital and Medical Center

Tonasket
Member
  North Valley Hospital
Toppenish
Member
  Providence Toppenish Hospital
Vancouver
Member
  Southwest Washington Medical Center
  Woodside Hospital
Walla Walla
Member
  St. Mary Medical Center
  Walla Walla General Hospital
Wenatchee
Member
  Central Washington Hospital
Yakima
Member
  Providence Yakima Medical Center

WEST VIRGINIA
Berkeley Springs
Member
  Morgan County War Memorial Hospital
Bluefield
Member
  Bluefield Regional Medical Center
Buckhannon
Member
  St. Joseph's Hospital of Buckhannon
Clarksburg
Member
  United Hospital Center
Elkins
Member
  Davis Memorial Hospital
Fairmont
Member
  Fairmont General Hospital
Huntington
Member
  St. Mary's Hospital
Keyser
Member
  Potomac Valley Hospital
Kingwood
Member
  Preston Memorial Hospital
Martinsburg
Member
  City Hospital
Morgantown
Member
  Monongalia General Hospital
Parkersburg
Member
  Camden–Clark Memorial Hospital
Petersburg
Member
  Grant Memorial Hospital
Philippi
Member
  Broaddus Hospital
Point Pleasant
Member
  Pleasant Valley Hospital
Ranson
Member
  Jefferson Memorial Hospital
Romney
Member
  Hampshire Memorial Hospital
Sistersville
Member
  Sistersville General Hospital
South Charleston
Member
  Thomas Memorial Hospital

Summersville
Member
  Summersville Memorial Hospital
Weirton
Member
  Weirton Medical Center
Weston
Member
  Stonewall Jackson Memorial Hospital

WISCONSIN
Amery
Member
  Amery Regional Medical Center
Baldwin
Member
  Baldwin Area Medical Center
Baraboo
Member
  St. Clare Hospital and Health Services
Barron
Member
  Barron Medical Center–Mayo Health System
Berlin
Member
  Berlin Memorial Hospital
Burlington
Member
  Memorial Hospital Corporation of Burlington
Cumberland
Member
  Cumberland Memorial Hospital
Durand
Member
  Chippewa Valley Hospital and Oakview Care Center
Elkhorn
Member
  Lakeland Medical Center
Green Bay
Member
  Bellin Hospital
Hartford
Member
  Hartford Memorial Hospital
Janesville
Member
  Mercy Health System
Kewaunee
Member
  St. Mary's Kewaunee Area Memorial Hospital
Madison
Member
  St. Marys Hospital Medical Center
Marinette
Member
  Bay Area Medical Center
Milwaukee
Member
  Children's Hospital of Wisconsin
  Sinai Samaritan Medical Center
  St. Luke's Medical Center
Monroe
Member
  The Monroe Clinic
Osceola
Member
  Osceola Medical Center
Plymouth
Member
  Valley View Medical Center
Sheboygan
Member
  Sheboygan Memorial Medical Center
Two Rivers
Member
  Two Rivers Community Hospital and Hamilton Memorial Home
Viroqua
Member
  Vernon County Hospital

Alliances

Waupaca
Member
  Riverside Medical Center

West Allis
Member
  West Allis Memorial Hospital

WYOMING

Buffalo
Member
  Johnson County Healthcare Center

Cody
Member
  West Park Hospital

Gillette
Member
  Campbell County Memorial Hospital

Jackson
Member
  St. John's Hospital and Living Center

Newcastle
Member
  Weston County Health Services

Sundance
Member
  Crook County Medical Services District

Torrington
Member
  Community Hospital

Wheatland
Member
  Platte County Memorial Hospital Nursing Home

Worland
Member
  Washakie Medical Center

SYNERNET, INC.
222 St John Street, Portland, ME Zip 04102; tel. 207/775–6081; Mr Paul I Davis, II, President

MAINE

Bangor
Member
  St. Joseph Hospital

Bar Harbor
Member
  Mount Desert Island Hospital

Bath
Member
  Mid Coast Hospital

Belfast
Member
  Waldo County General Hospital

Biddeford
Member
  Southern Maine Medical Center

Blue Hill
Member
  Blue Hill Memorial Hospital

Bridgton
Member
  Bridgton Hospital

Damariscotta
Member
  Miles Memorial Hospital

Farmington
Member
  Franklin Memorial Hospital

Fort Kent
Member
  Northern Maine Medical Center

Lewiston
Member
  St. Mary's Regional Medical Center

Norway
Member
  Stephens Memorial Hospital

Pittsfield
Member
  Sebasticook Valley Hospital

Portland
Member
  Mercy Hospital of Portland

Rockport
Member
  Penobscot Bay Medical Center

Rumford
Member
  Rumford Hospital

Sanford
Member
  Henrietta D. Goodall Hospital

Skowhegan
Member
  Redington–Fairview General Hospital

Waterville
Member
  Inland Hospital

York
Member
  York Hospital

UNIVERSITY HEALTH SYSTEM OF NEW JERSEY
154 West State Street, Trenton, NJ Zip 08608; tel. 609/656–9600; Dr Thomas E Terrill, Ph.D., President

NEW JERSEY

Camden
Member
  The Cooper Health System

Flemington
Member
  Hunterdon Medical Center

Florham Park
Member
  Atlantic Health System

Hackensack
Member
  Hackensack University Medical Center

Hamilton
Member
  Robert Wood Johnson University Hospital at Hamilton

New Brunswick
Member
  Robert Wood Johnson University Hospital

Newark
Member
  University of Medicine and Dentistry of New Jersey–University Hospital

Phillipsburg
Member
  Warren Hospital

Somerville
Member
  Somerset Medical Center

Trenton
Member
  Capital Health System at Mercer

West Orange
Member
  Kessler Institute for Rehabilitation

UNIVERSITY HEALTHSYSTEM CONSORTIUM, INC.
2001 Spring Road, Suite 700, Oak Brook, IL Zip 60523; tel. 630/954–1700; Mr Robert J Baker, President and Chief Executive Officer

ALABAMA

Birmingham
Member
  University of Alabama Hospital

Mobile
Affiliate
  University of South Alabama Knollwood Park Hospital
Member
  University of South Alabama Medical Center

ARIZONA

Tucson
Member
  University Medical Center

ARKANSAS

Little Rock
Member
  University Hospital of Arkansas

CALIFORNIA

Downey
Affiliate
  LAC–Rancho Los Amigos National Rehabilitation Center

Lancaster
Affiliate
  LAC–High Desert Hospital

Los Angeles
Member
  LAC–King–Drew Medical Center
  LAC/University of Southern California Medical Center
  University of California Los Angeles Medical Center

Martinez
Affiliate
  Contra Costa Regional Medical Center

Moreno Valley
Affiliate
  Riverside County Regional Medical Center

Orange
Member
  University of California, Irvine Medical Center

Sacramento
Member
  University of California, Davis Medical Center

San Diego
Member
  University of California San Diego Medical Center

San Francisco
Affiliate
  University of California–San Francisco Mount Zion Medical Center
Member
  San Francisco General Hospital Medical Center

San Jose
Affiliate
  Santa Clara Valley Medical Center

San Leandro
Affiliate
  Alameda County Medical Center

Santa Monica
Affiliate
  Santa Monica–UCLA Medical Center

Stanford
Member
  Stanford Hospital and Clinics

Sylmar
Affiliate
  LAC–Olive View–UCLA Medical Center

Torrance
Member
  LAC–Harbor–University of California at Los Angeles Medical Center

Valencia
Affiliate
  Henry Mayo Newhall Memorial Hospital

COLORADO

Denver
Affiliate
  National Jewish Medical and Research Center
Member
  Denver Health Medical Center
  University of Colorado Hospital

CONNECTICUT

Farmington
Member
  University of Connecticut Health Center, John Dempsey Hospital

Alliances

New Haven
Member
  Yale–New Haven Hospital

DISTRICT OF COLUMBIA
Washington
Member
  Georgetown University Hospital
  Howard University Hospital

FLORIDA
Gainesville
Affiliate
  Shands at AGH
Member
  Shands at the University of Florida

Lake City
Affiliate
  Shands at Lake Shore

Live Oak
Affiliate
  Shands at Live Oak

Starke
Affiliate
  Shands at Starke

Tampa
Member
  Tampa General Healthcare

GEORGIA
Atlanta
Member
  Crawford Long Hospital of Emory University
  Emory University Hospital

Augusta
Member
  Medical College of Georgia Hospital and Clinics

ILLINOIS
Chicago
Affiliate
  Cook County Hospital
  Louis A. Weiss Memorial Hospital
Member
  University of Chicago Hospitals
  University of Illinois at Chicago Medical Center

Maywood
Member
  Loyola University Medical Center

INDIANA
Indianapolis
Member
  Clarian Health Partners
  Wishard Health Services

IOWA
Iowa City
Member
  University of Iowa Hospitals and Clinics

KANSAS
Kansas City
Member
  University of Kansas Medical Center

KENTUCKY
Lexington
Member
  University of Kentucky Hospital

LOUISIANA
Shreveport
Member
  LSU Medical Center–University Hospital

MARYLAND
Baltimore
Affiliate
  James Lawrence Kernan Hospital
Member
  University of Maryland Medical Center

MASSACHUSETTS
Boston
Member
  Brigham and Women's Hospital
  Massachusetts General Hospital

Clinton
Affiliate
  Clinton Hospital

Marlborough
Affiliate
  UMass Marlborough Hospital

MICHIGAN
Ann Arbor
Member
  University of Michigan Hospitals and Health Centers

MINNESOTA
Minneapolis
Affiliate
  Hennepin County Medical Center

MISSOURI
Columbia
Member
  University Hospitals and Clinics

NEBRASKA
Omaha
Member
  Nebraska Health System

NEVADA
Las Vegas
Affiliate
  University Medical Center

NEW JERSEY
New Brunswick
Member
  Robert Wood Johnson University Hospital

Newark
Member
  University of Medicine and Dentistry of New Jersey–University Hospital

NEW YORK
Albany
Member
  Albany Medical Center

Brooklyn
Member
  University Hospital of Brooklyn–State University of New York Health Science Center at Brooklyn

Stony Brook
Member
  University Hospital

Syracuse
Member
  University Hospital–SUNY Health Science Center at Syracuse

NORTH CAROLINA
Ahoskie
Affiliate
  Roanoke–Chowan Hospital

Chapel Hill
Member
  University of North Carolina Hospitals

Greenville
Member
  Pitt County Memorial Hospital–University Health Systems of Eastern Carolina

Windsor
Affiliate
  Bertie Memorial Hospital

Winston–Salem
Member
  North Carolina Baptist Hospital

OHIO
Bedford
Affiliate
  UHHS Bedford Medical Center

Chardon
Affiliate
  UHHS Geauga Regional Hospital

Cincinnati
Member
  University Hospital

Cleveland
Member
  University Hospitals of Cleveland

Columbus
Member
  Ohio State University Medical Center

Conneaut
Affiliate
  UHHS Brown Memorial Hospital

Geneva
Affiliate
  UHHS–Memorial Hospital of Geneva

Ironton
Affiliate
  River Valley Health System

Toledo
Member
  Medical College of Ohio Hospitals

Waverly
Affiliate
  Pike Community Hospital

Willoughby
Affiliate
  UHHS Laurelwood Hospital

OREGON
Portland
Member
  OHSU Hospital

PENNSYLVANIA
Philadelphia
Affiliate
  Friends Hospital
  Presbyterian Medical Center of the University of Pennsylvania Health System
  Thomas Jefferson University Hospital
Member
  Hospital of the University of Pennsylvania

Phoenixville
Affiliate
  Phoenixville Hospital of the University of Pennsylvania Health System

Pittsburgh
Member
  UPMC Presbyterian

SOUTH CAROLINA
Charleston
Affiliate
  Charleston Memorial Hospital
Member
  MUSC Medical Center of Medical University of South Carolina

TENNESSEE
Knoxville
Member
  University of Tennessee Memorial Hospital

Memphis
Member
  University of Tennessee Bowld Hospital

TEXAS
Dallas
Member
  Zale Lipshy University Hospital

Galveston
Member
  University of Texas Medical Branch Hospitals

Houston
Member
  Hermann Hospital

Tyler
Affiliate
  University of Texas Health Center at Tyler

UTAH
Salt Lake City
Member
  University of Utah Hospitals and Clinics

VIRGINIA
Charlottesville
Member
  University of Virginia Medical Center

Alliances

Richmond
Member
  Medical College of Virginia Hospitals, Virginia Commonwealth University

WASHINGTON
Seattle
Member
  Harborview Medical Center
  University of Washington Medical Center

WISCONSIN
Antigo
Affiliate
  Langlade Memorial Hospital

Madison
Member
  University of Wisconsin Hospital and Clinics

Medford
Affiliate
  Memorial Hospital of Taylor County

Merrill
Affiliate
  Good Samaritan Health Center of Merrill

Milwaukee
Member
  Froedtert Memorial Lutheran Hospital

Wausau
Affiliate
  Wausau Hospital

VHA, INC.
220 East Las Colinas Boulevard, Irving, TX Zip 75039-5500; tel. 972/830-0000; Mr C Thomas Smith, President and Chief Executive Officer

ALABAMA
Anniston
Partner
  Northeast Alabama Regional Medical Center

Athens
Partner
  Athens–Limestone Hospital

Birmingham
Shareholder
  Baptist Health System

Cullman
Partner
  Cullman Regional Medical Center

Decatur
  Decatur General Hospital

Florence
Partner
  Eliza Coffee Memorial Hospital

Guntersville
Partner
  Marshall County Health Care Authority

Jackson
Partner
  Jackson Medical Center

Mobile
Shareholder
  Infirmary Health System, Inc.

Montgomery
Shareholder
  Baptist Medical Center

Scottsboro
Partner
  Jackson County Hospital

Tuscaloosa
Partner
  DCH Health System

ARIZONA
Tucson
Shareholder
  Health Partners of Southern Arizona

ARKANSAS
Fayetteville
Partner
  Washington Regional Medical Center

Fort Smith
Shareholder
  Sparks Regional Medical Center

Jonesboro
Partner
  St. Bernards Regional Medical Center

Little Rock
Shareholder
  Baptist Health

CALIFORNIA
Anaheim
Partner
  Anaheim Memorial Medical Center

Covina
Partner
  Citrus Valley Health Partners

Fresno
Shareholder
  Community Medical Centers

La Jolla
Shareholder
  Scripps Memorial Hospital–La Jolla

Lancaster
Partner
  Antelope Valley Hospital

Long Beach
Shareholder
  Memorial Health Services

Los Angeles
Shareholder
  Cedars–Sinai Medical Center

Modesto
Partner
  Memorial Hospitals Association

Newport Beach
Shareholder
  Hoag Memorial Hospital Presbyterian

Pasadena
Partner
  Southern California Healthcare Systems

Pomona
Partner
  Pomona Valley Hospital Medical Center

Riverside
Partner
  Riverside Community Hospital

Sacramento
Shareholder
  Sutter Health

San Francisco
Shareholder
  California Pacific Medical Center

Santa Barbara
Partner
  Santa Barbara Cottage Hospital

Stockton
Partner
  St. Joseph's Regional Health System

Torrance
Partner
  Torrance Memorial Medical Center

Turlock
Partner
  Emanuel Medical Center

Valencia
Partner
  Santa Clarita Health Care Association

Van Nuys
Partner
  Valley Presbyterian Hospital

Whittier
Partner
  Presbyterian Intercommunity Hospital

COLORADO
Alamosa
Partner
  San Luis Valley Regional Medical Center

Aspen
Partner
  Aspen Valley Hospital District

Boulder
Partner
  Boulder Community Hospital

Colorado Springs
Partner
  Memorial Hospital

Englewood
Shareholder
  HealthONE Healthcare System

Grand Junction
Partner
  Community Hospital

La Junta
Partner
  Arkansas Valley Regional Medical Center

Longmont
Partner
  Longmont United Hospital

Steamboat Springs
Partner
  Yampa Valley Medical Center

Vail
Shareholder
  Vail Valley Medical Center

Wheat Ridge
Shareholder
  Exempla Lutheran Medical Center

CONNECTICUT
Danbury
Partner
  Danbury Hospital

Greenwich
Partner
  Greenwich Hospital

Hartford
Shareholder
  Hartford Hospital

Meriden
Partner
  MidState Medical Center

Middletown
Partner
  Middlesex Hospital

Stamford
Partner
  Stamford Health System

Torrington
Partner
  Charlotte Hungerford Hospital

FLORIDA
Boca Raton
Partner
  Boca Raton Community Hospital

Boynton Beach
Partner
  Bethesda Memorial Hospital

Daytona Beach
Shareholder
  Halifax Medical Center

Fort Myers
Partner
  Lee Memorial Health System

Inverness
Partner
  Citrus Memorial Hospital

Jacksonville
Partner
  St. Luke's Hospital

Lakeland
Shareholder
  Lakeland Regional Medical Center

Melbourne
Shareholder
  Holmes Regional Medical Center

Alliances

Miami
Partner
  South Miami Hospital
Ocala
Partner
  Munroe Regional Medical Center
Orlando
Shareholder
  Orlando Regional Healthcare
Panama City
Partner
  Bay Medical Center
Pensacola
Shareholder
  Baptist Health Care Corporation
Saint Petersburg
Partner
  Bayfront Medical Center
Sarasota
Partner
  Sarasota Memorial Hospital
Stuart
Partner
  Martin Memorial Health Systems
Tallahassee
Shareholder
  Tallahassee Memorial HealthCare
Tampa
Partner
  University Community Hospital
West Palm Beach
Partner
  Good Samaritan Medical Center

GEORGIA
Albany
Partner
  Phoebe Putney Memorial Hospital
Athens
Partner
  Athens Regional Medical Center
Atlanta
Partner
  Northside Hospital
Shareholder
  Piedmont Hospital
Columbus
Partner
  Columbus Regional Health Care System, Inc
Dalton
Partner
  Hamilton Medical Center
Decatur
Partner
  DeKalb Medical Center
East Point
Partner
  South Fulton Medical Center
Gainesville
Partner
  Northeast Georgia Health Services
Lawrenceville
Partner
  Promina Gwinnett Hospital System
Macon
Partner
  Medical Center of Central Georgia
Marietta
Partner
  WellStar Kennestone Hospital
Riverdale
Partner
  Southern Regional Medical Center
Rome
Partner
  Floyd Medical Center
Royston
Partner
  Cobb Memorial Hospital

Savannah
Partner
  Candler Hospital
Thomasville
Partner
  Archbold Medical Center
  John D. Archbold Memorial Hospital
Valdosta
Partner
  South Georgia Medical Center

HAWAII
Honolulu
Shareholder
  Queen's Medical Center

IDAHO
Boise
Shareholder
  St. Luke's Regional Medical Center
Coeur D'Alene
Partner
  Kootenai Medical Center
Pocatello
Partner
  Bannock Regional Medical Center
Twin Falls
Partner
  Magic Valley Regional Medical Center

ILLINOIS
Arlington Heights
Partner
  Northwest Community Healthcare
Berwyn
Partner
  MacNeal Hospital
Carbondale
Partner
  Southern Illinois Hospital Services
Chicago
Shareholder
  Northwestern Memorial Hospital
  Rush–Presbyterian–St. Luke's Medical Center
De Kalb
Partner
  Kishwaukee Community Hospital
Decatur
Shareholder
  Decatur Memorial Hospital
Dixon
Partner
  Katherine Shaw Bethea Hospital
Elgin
Partner
  Sherman Hospital
Elmhurst
Partner
  Elmhurst Memorial Hospital
Evanston
  Evanston Northwestern Healthcare Corporation
Evergreen Park
Partner
  Little Company of Mary Hospital and Health Care Centers
Freeport
Partner
  Freeport Memorial Hospital
Harvey
Shareholder
  Ingalls Health System
  Ingalls Hospital
Jacksonville
Partner
  Passavant Area Hospital
Joliet
Partner
  Silver Cross Hospital
Kankakee
Partner
  Riverside Medical Center

Macomb
Partner
  McDonough District Hospital
Maryville
Partner
  Anderson Hospital
Mattoon
Partner
  Sarah Bush Lincoln Health Center
Normal
Partner
  BroMenn Healthcare
Oak Brook
Shareholder
  Advocate Health Care
Quincy
Partner
  Blessing Hospital
Rock Island
Partner
  Trinity Medical Center–West Campus
Rockford
Partner
  Rockford Memorial Hospital
Springfield
Shareholder
  Memorial Medical Center
  Memorial Medical Center System

INDIANA
Bloomington
Partner
  Bloomington Hospital
Columbus
Partner
  Columbus Regional Hospital
Danville
Partner
  Hendricks Community Hospital
Elkhart
Partner
  Elkhart General Hospital
Evansville
Shareholder
  Deaconess Hospital
Fort Wayne
Partner
  Parkview Hospital
Indianapolis
Shareholder
  Clarian Health Partners
  Community Hospitals Indianapolis
La Porte
Partner
  La Porte Regional Health System
Madison
Partner
  King's Daughters' Hospital and Health Services
Marion
Partner
  Marion General Hospital
Muncie
Shareholder
  Ball Memorial Hospital
New Albany
Partner
  Floyd Memorial Hospital and Health Services
Noblesville
Partner
  Riverview Hospital
Richmond
Partner
  Reid Hospital and Health Care Services
South Bend
Shareholder
  Memorial Health System, Inc.
Terre Haute
Partner
  Union Hospital

Alliances

Valparaiso
Partner
  Porter Memorial Hospital

Vincennes
Partner
  Good Samaritan Hospital

IOWA

Atlantic
Shareholder
  Cass County Memorial Hospital

Council Bluffs
Shareholder
  Jennie Edmundson Memorial Hospital

Keokuk
Shareholder
  Keokuk Area Hospital

Red Oak
Shareholder
  Montgomery County Memorial Hospital

Sioux City
Shareholder
  St. Luke's Regional Medical Center

KANSAS

Atchison
Shareholder
  Atchison Hospital

Colby
Shareholder
  Citizens Medical Center

Hays
Shareholder
  Hays Medical Center

Hutchinson
Shareholder
  Hutchinson Hospital Corporation

Kansas City
Shareholder
  Bethany Medical Center

Liberal
Shareholder
  Southwest Medical Center

Phillipsburg
Shareholder
  Great Plains Health Alliance, Inc.

Pratt
Shareholder
  Pratt Regional Medical Center

Salina
Partner
  Salina Regional Health Center

Shawnee Mission
Shareholder
  Shawnee Mission Medical Center

Topeka
Partner
  St. Francis Hospital and Medical Center
Shareholder
  Stormont–Vail HealthCare

Wichita
Partner
  Via Christi Health System

KENTUCKY

Fort Thomas
Partner
  St. Luke Hospital East

Madisonville
Partner
  Regional Medical Center of Hopkins County

LOUISIANA

Baton Rouge
Member
  Our Lady of the Lake Regional Medical Center
Partner
  Woman's Hospital

Crowley
Partner
  American Legion Hospital

De Ridder
Partner
  Beauregard Memorial Hospital

Lafayette
Partner
  Our Lady of Lourdes Regional Medical Center

Lake Charles
Partner
  Lake Charles Memorial Hospital

Monroe
Partner
  St. Francis Medical Center

New Orleans
Partner
  Pendleton Memorial Methodist Hospital
Shareholder
  Ochsner Foundation Hospital

Ruston
Partner
  Lincoln General Hospital

Shreveport
Shareholder
  Willis–Knighton Medical Center

MAINE

Bangor
Partner
  Eastern Maine Healthcare

Biddeford
Shareholder
  Southern Maine Medical Center

Lewiston
Shareholder
  Central Maine Medical Center

Portland
Shareholder
  Maine Medical Center

Waterville
Shareholder
  MaineGeneral Medical Center–Waterville Campus

MARYLAND

Easton
Partner
  Memorial Hospital at Easton Maryland

Fallston
Partner
  Upper Chesapeake Health System

MASSACHUSETTS

Beverly
Partner
  Beverly Hospital

Boston
Partner
  Massachusetts Eye and Ear Infirmary
Shareholder
  New England Medical Center
  Partners HealthCare System, Inc.

Cambridge
Partner
  Mount Auburn Hospital

Concord
Partner
  Emerson Hospital

Fall River
Member
  Southcoast Hospitals Group

Hyannis
Partner
  Cape Cod Hospital

Lawrence
Owner
  Lawrence General Hospital

Leominster
Partner
  Health Alliance Hospitals

Lowell
Partner
  Lowell General Hospital

Melrose
Partner
  Melrose–Wakefield Hospital

Newton
Partner
  Newell Home Health Service

South Weymouth
Partner
  South Shore Health & Education Corporation

Southbridge
Partner
  Harrington Memorial Hospital

Worcester
Partner
  Saint Vincent Hospital

MICHIGAN

Bay City
Partner
  Bay Medical Center

Dearborn
Member
  Oakwood Healthcare, Inc.

Detroit
Partner
  St. John Hospital and Medical Center

Flint
Partner
  Genesys Health System

Holland
Partner
  Holland Community Hospital

Kalamazoo
Partner
  Bronson Healthcare Group, Inc.

Lansing
Partner
  Michigan Capital Healthcare

Monroe
Partner
  Mercy Memorial Hospital

Petoskey
Partner
  Healthshare Group

Port Huron
Partner
  Blue Water Health Services Corporation

Royal Oak
Shareholder
  William Beaumont Hospital–Royal Oak

MINNESOTA

Bemidji
Partner
  North Country Regional Hospital

Duluth
Partner
  St. Luke's Hospital

Fergus Falls
Partner
  Lake Region Healthcare Corporation

Mankato
Partner
  Immanuel St. Joseph's–Mayo Health System

Minneapolis
Shareholder
  Allina Health System

Saint Cloud
Partner
  St. Cloud Hospital

Saint Paul
Shareholder
  HealthEast

Waconia
Partner
  Ridgeview Medical Center

Willmar
Partner
  Rice Memorial Hospital

Alliances

MISSISSIPPI
Gautier
Partner
  Singing River Hospital System
Greenwood
Partner
  Greenwood Leflore Hospital
Gulfport
Partner
  Memorial Hospital at Gulfport
Hattiesburg
Partner
  Forrest General Hospital
Jackson
Partner
  St. Dominic–Jackson Memorial Hospital
McComb
Partner
  Southwest Mississippi Regional Medical Center
Meridian
Partner
  Jeff Anderson Regional Medical Center
Tupelo
Shareholder
  North Mississippi Health Services, Inc.

MISSOURI
Bolivar
Partner
  Citizens Memorial Hospital
Branson
Partner
  Skaggs Community Health Center
Cameron
Partner
  Cameron Community Hospital
Cape Girardeau
Partner
  Saint Francis Medical Center
  Southeast Missouri Hospital
Carthage
Partner
  McCune–Brooks Hospital
Joplin
Partner
  Freeman Health System
  Freeman Hospital West
Kansas City
Shareholder
  Saint Luke's Hospital
  Saint Luke's Shawnee Mission Health System
Liberty
Partner
  Liberty Hospital
Saint Louis
Shareholder
  BJC Health System
Springfield
Shareholder
  Cox Health Systems
West Plains
Partner
  Ozarks Medical Center

MONTANA
Billings
Partner
  Deaconess Billings Clinic
Bozeman
Partner
  Bozeman Deaconess Hospital
Great Falls
Partner
  Benefis Health Care–East Campus
Helena
Partner
  St. Peter's Hospital

NEBRASKA
Aurora
Partner
  Memorial Hospital
Beatrice
Partner
  Beatrice Community Hospital and Health Center
Columbus
Partner
  Columbus Community Hospital
Hastings
Partner
  Mary Lanning Memorial Hospital
Norfolk
Partner
  Faith Regional Health Services
Omaha
Partner
  Children's Hospital
Shareholder
  Nebraska Methodist Hospital
Scottsbluff
Partner
  Regional West Medical Center

NEW HAMPSHIRE
Concord
Partner
  Capital Region Family Health Center
Dover
Partner
  Wentworth–Douglass Hospital
Keene
Partner
  Cheshire Medical Center
Nashua
Partner
  Southern New Hampshire Medical Center
Rochester
Partner
  Frisbie Memorial Hospital

NEW JERSEY
Belleville
Shareholder
  Clara Maass Health System
Camden
Partner
  Our Lady of Lourdes Medical Center
Elizabeth
Partner
  Trinitas Hospital
Flemington
Partner
  Hunterdon Medical Center
Florham Park
Shareholder
  Atlantic Health System
Hackettstown
Partner
  Hackettstown Community Hospital
Hammonton
Partner
  William B. Kessler Memorial Hospital
Jersey City
Partner
  Christ Hospital
Mount Holly
Shareholder
  Virtua Memorial Hospital Burlington County
Newton
Partner
  Newton Memorial Hospital
Phillipsburg
Partner
  Warren Hospital
Plainfield
Partner
  Muhlenberg Regional Medical Center
Pompton Plains
Partner
  Chilton Memorial Hospital
Rahway
Partner
  Rahway Hospital
Somers Point
Partner
  Shore Memorial Hospital
Toms River
Shareholder
  Community Medical Center
Trenton
Partner
  Capital Health System
Woodbury
Partner
  Underwood–Memorial Hospital

NEW MEXICO
Albuquerque
Partner
  University Hospital
Farmington
Partner
  San Juan Regional Medical Center
Gallup
Partner
  Rehoboth McKinley Christian Hospital
Las Cruces
Partner
  Memorial Medical Center
Roswell
Partner
  Eastern New Mexico Medical Center

NEW YORK
Binghamton
Shareholder
  United Health Services Hospitals–Binghamton
Brooklyn
Partner
  Brooklyn Hospital Center
Cobleskill
Partner
  Bassett Hospital of Schoharie County
Geneva
Partner
  Geneva General Hospital
Great Neck
Partner
  North Shore– Long Island Jewish Health System
Ithaca
Partner
  Cayuga Medical Center at Ithaca
Jamestown
Partner
  Woman's Christian Association Hospital
Mount Kisco
Partner
  Northern Westchester Hospital Center
New Rochelle
Partner
  Sound Shore Medical Center of Westchester
New York
Partner
  Lenox Hill Hospital
  St. Luke's–Roosevelt Hospital Center
North Tonawanda
Partner
  De Graff Memorial Hospital
Plattsburgh
Partner
  Champlain Valley Physicians Hospital Medical Center
Rochester
Partner
  Highland Hospital of Rochester
  Park Ridge Health System
Rockville Centre
Partner
  Mercy Medical Center
Southampton
Partner
  Southampton Hospital
Suffern
Partner
  Good Samaritan Hospital

Alliances

Syracuse
Partner
  Crouse Hospital

Troy
Partner
  Samaritan Hospital

Utica
Partner
  Mohawk Valley Psychiatric Center

White Plains
Partner
  White Plains Hospital Center

Yonkers
Partner
  St. John's Riverside Hospital

NORTH CAROLINA

Charlotte
Shareholder
  Carolinas HealthCare System

Raleigh
Partner
  Wake Medical Center

Rocky Mount
Partner
  Nash Health Care Systems

Thomasville
Partner
  Community General Hospital of Thomasville

Winston–Salem
Shareholder
  Carolina Medicorp, Inc.

NORTH DAKOTA

Bismarck
Partner
  MedCenter One

Fargo
Shareholder
  MeritCare Health System

Grand Forks
Partner
  Altru Health System

Jamestown
Partner
  Jamestown Hospital

Minot
Partner
  Trinity Health

OHIO

Akron
Shareholder
  Akron General Medical Center

Ashtabula
Partner
  Ashtabula County Medical Center

Cincinnati
Partner
  Bethesda Corporate Health Services
Shareholder
  Christ Hospital

Columbus
Member
  OhioHealth

Dover
Partner
  Union Hospital

Elyria
Partner
  EMH Regional Medical Center

Fremont
Partner
  Memorial Hospital

Garfield Heights
Partner
  Marymount Hospital

Hamilton
Partner
  Fort Hamilton Hospital

Lima
Partner
  Lima Memorial Hospital

Mansfield
Partner
  Mansfield Hospital

Maumee
Partner
  St. Luke's Hospital

Middletown
Partner
  Middletown Regional Hospital

Painesville
Partner
  Lake Hospital System

Springfield
Partner
  Community Hospital

Steubenville
Partner
  Trinity Health System

Toledo
Shareholder
  The Toledo Hospital

Troy
Partner
  Upper Valley Medical Center

Xenia
Partner
  Greene Memorial Hospital

Zanesville
Partner
  Genesis HealthCare System

OKLAHOMA

Ada
Partner
  Valley View Regional Hospital

Altus
Partner
  Jackson County Memorial Hospital

Ardmore
Partner
  Mercy Memorial Health Center

Chickasha
Partner
  Grady Memorial Hospital

Duncan
Partner
  Duncan Regional Hospital

McAlester
Partner
  McAlester Regional Health Center

Midwest City
Partner
  Midwest Regional Medical Center

Muskogee
Partner
  Muskogee Regional Medical Center

Norman
Partner
  Norman Regional Hospital

Oklahoma City
Partner
  Deaconess Hospital
Shareholder
  Oklahoma Health System

Poteau
Partner
  Eastern Oklahoma Medical Center

Stillwater
Partner
  Stillwater Medical Center

Tulsa
Shareholder
  Hillcrest Medical Center

OREGON

Hillsboro
Partner
  Tuality Healthcare

PENNSYLVANIA

Allentown
Shareholder
  Lehigh Valley Hospital

Altoona
Partner
  Altoona Hospital

Bristol
Partner
  Lower Bucks Hospital

Butler
Partner
  Butler Health System

Erie
Shareholder
  Hamot Health Systems

Johnstown
Partner
  Conemaugh Valley Memorial Hospital

Kingston
Partner
  Wyoming Valley Health Care System

Lancaster
Partner
  Lancaster General Hospital

Latrobe
Partner
  Latrobe Area Hospital

Natrona Heights
Partner
  Allegheny University Hospitals, Allegheny Valley

Norristown
Partner
  Montgomery Hospital

Philadelphia
Partner
  Chestnut Hill HealthCare
  Episcopal Hospital
  Frankford Hospital of the City of Philadelphia
  Jeanes Health System
Shareholder
  Pennsylvania Hospital

Pittsburgh
Partner
  St. Clair Memorial Hospital
  UPMC Shadyside
  UPMC St. Margaret

Pottstown
Partner
  Pottstown Memorial Medical Center

Reading
Partner
  Reading Hospital and Medical Center

Sayre
Shareholder
  Guthrie Healthcare System

Scranton
Partner
  Community Medical Center

Sellersville
Partner
  Grand View Hospital

Sewickley
Partner
  Valley Medical Facilities

Springfield
Shareholder
  Crozer–Keystone Health System

Uniontown
Partner
  Uniontown Hospital

Washington
Partner
  Washington Hospital

West Chester
Partner
  Chester County Hospital

Williamsport
Partner
  Susquehanna Health System

Alliances

York
Partner
  South Central Community Health

RHODE ISLAND
Providence
Shareholder
  Lifespan Corporation
  Rhode Island Hospital

SOUTH CAROLINA
Columbia
Shareholder
  Palmetto Health Alliance

SOUTH DAKOTA
Sioux Falls
Shareholder
  Sioux Valley Hospital and University Medical Center

TENNESSEE
Jackson
Shareholder
  West Tennessee Healthcare

Knoxville
Shareholder
  Fort Sanders Alliance

Memphis
Shareholder
  Baptist Memorial Hospital

Nashville
Shareholder
  Baptist Hospital

Oak Ridge
Partner
  Methodist Medical Center of Oak Ridge

TEXAS
Amarillo
Partner
  Baptist St. Anthony Health System

Arlington
Partner
  Arlington Memorial Hospital

Austin
Partner
  St. David's Medical Center

Beaumont
Partner
  Memorial Hermann Baptist Hospital–West Campus

Dallas
Shareholder
  Baylor Health Care System

El Paso
Partner
  Providence Memorial Hospital

Fort Worth
Shareholder
  All Saints Episcopal Hospital of Fort Worth

Grapevine
Partner
  Baylor Medical Center at Grapevine

Harlingen
Partner
  Valley Baptist Medical Center

Houston
Shareholder
  Memorial Hermann Southwest Hospital

Irving
Partner
  Baylor Medical Center at Irving

Lubbock
Shareholder
  Lubbock Methodist Hospital System

Marshall
Partner
  Marshall Regional Medical Center

Midland
Partner
  Midland Memorial Hospital

San Antonio
Partner
  Baptist Health System

Sherman
Partner
  Wilson N. Jones Medical Center

Temple
Partner
  King's Daughters Hospital

Texarkana
Partner
  Wadley Regional Medical Center

Waco
Partner
  Hillcrest Baptist Medical Center

Wichita Falls
Partner
  United Regional Health Care System

VERMONT
Barre
Partner
  Central Vermont Medical Center

Burlington
Shareholder
  Fletcher Allen Health Care

Rutland
Partner
  Rutland Regional Medical Center

VIRGINIA
Alexandria
Partner
  Inova Alexandria Hospital

Charlottesville
Partner
  Martha Jefferson Hospital

Franklin
Partner
  Southampton Memorial Hospital

Fredericksburg
Partner
  MWH Medicorp

Harrisonburg
Partner
  Rockingham Memorial Hospital

Lynchburg
Partner
  Centra Health, Inc.

Norfolk
Shareholder
  Sentara Healthcare

Richmond
Partner
  Children's Hospital

Warrenton
Partner
  Fauquier Hospital

WASHINGTON
Tacoma
Shareholder
  MultiCare Health System

WEST VIRGINIA
Charleston
Shareholder
  Camcare, Inc.

Glen Dale
Partner
  Reynolds Memorial Hospital

Huntington
Partner
  Cabell Huntington Hospital

Morgantown
Partner
  West Virginia University Hospitals

Parkersburg
Owner
  St. Joseph's Hospital

Princeton
Partner
  Princeton Community Hospital

Wheeling
Partner
  Wheeling Hospital

WISCONSIN
Appleton
Shareholder
  ThedaCare, Inc.

Beaver Dam
Partner
  Beaver Dam Community Hospitals

Eau Claire
Partner
  Luther Hospital

Green Bay
Partner
  Bellin Hospital

Kenosha
Partner
  Kenosha Hospital and Medical Center

La Crosse
Shareholder
  Gundersen Lutheran

Madison
Shareholder
  Meriter Hospital

Menomonee Falls
Partner
  Community Memorial Hospital

Milwaukee
Partner
  Columbia Hospital
  Froedtert Memorial Lutheran Hospital
  Horizon Healthcare, Inc.

Rice Lake
Partner
  Lakeview Medical Center

Watertown
Partner
  Watertown Memorial Hospital

Waukesha
Partner
  Waukesha Health System, Inc.

West Bend
Owner
  St. Joseph's Community Hospital of West Bend

WYOMING
Casper
Partner
  Wyoming Medical Center

Cheyenne
Partner
  United Medical Center

Laramie
Partner
  Ivinson Memorial Hospital

Sheridan
Partner
  Memorial Hospital of Sheridan County

VANTAGE HEALTH GROUP
265 Conneaut Lake Road, Meadville, PA Zip 16335; tel. 814/337-0000; Mr David C Petno, Vice President Business Development

PENNSYLVANIA
Erie
Member
  Millcreek Community Hospital
  Saint Vincent Health Center

Greenville
Member
  UPMC Horizon

Meadville
Member
  Meadville Medical Center

Oil City
Member
  Northwest Medical Centers

Alliances

Titusville
Member
 Titusville Area Hospital

Warren
Member
 Warren General Hospital

YANKEE ALLIANCE
300 Brickstone Square, 5th Floor, Andover, MA Zip 01810–1429; tel. 978/475–2000; Mr R Paul O'Neill, President

CONNECTICUT
New Haven
Member
 Hospital of Saint Raphael

MAINE
Blue Hill
Affiliate
 Blue Hill Memorial Hospital

Lewiston
Member
 St. Mary's Regional Medical Center

MASSACHUSETTS
Attleboro
Affiliate
 Sturdy Memorial Hospital

Boston
Member
 Boston Medical Center

Cambridge
Member
 Youville Lifecare

Fall River
Member
 Southcoast Hospitals Group

Great Barrington
Member
 Fairview Hospital

Lexington
Member
 Covenant Health Systems, Inc.

Lowell
Member
 Saints Memorial Medical Center

North Adams
Affiliate
 North Adams Regional Hospital

Pittsfield
Member
 Berkshire Health Systems, Inc.
 Berkshire Medical Center

Winchester
Member
 Winchester Hospital

NEW HAMPSHIRE
Manchester
Affiliate
 Catholic Medical Center
 Elliot Hospital

Nashua
Member
 St. Joseph Hospital

NEW YORK
Albany
Member
 Albany Medical Center

Elizabethtown
Affiliate
 Elizabethtown Community Hospital

Glens Falls
Member
 Glens Falls Hospital

Plattsburgh
Affiliate
 Champlain Valley Physicians Hospital Medical Center

Troy
Member
 Samaritan Hospital

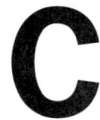

Health Organizations, Agencies, and Providers

C2	Description of Lists
3	National Organizations
12	Healthfinder
29	International Organizations
31	U.S. Government Agencies
	State and Local Organizations and Agencies
32	*Blue Cross and Blue Shield Plans*
34	*Health Systems Agencies*
35	*Hospital Associations*
37	*Hospital Licensure Agencies*
39	*Medical and Nursing Licensure Agencies*
42	*Peer Review Organizations*
43	*State Health Planning and Development Agencies*
44	*State and Provincial Government Agencies*
	Health Care Providers
57	*Health Maintenance Organizations*
69	*State Government Agencies for Health Maintenance Organizations*
71	*Freestanding Ambulatory Surgery Centers*
98	*State Government Agencies for Freestanding Ambulatory Surgery Centers*
100	*Freestanding Hospices*
120	*State Government Agencies for Freestanding Hospices*
122	*JCAHO Accredited Freestanding Long—Term Care Organizations†*
146	*JCAHO Accredited Freestanding Mental Health Care Organizations†*
156	*JCAHO Accredited Freestanding Substance Abuse Organizations†*

†List supplied by the Joint Commission on Accreditation of Healthcare Organizations

Description of Lists

This section was compiled to provide a directory of information useful to the health care field.

National and International Organizations

The national and international lists include many types of voluntary organizations concerned with matters of interest to the health care field. The organizational information includes address, telephone number, FAX number, and the contact person. For organizations that maintain permanent offices, office addresses and telephone numbers are given. For organizations not maintaining offices, the addresses and telephone numbers given are those of their corresponding secretaries. The information was obtained directly from the organizations.

National Organizations are listed alphabetically by their full names. International Organizations are grouped alphabetically by country.

Also included is the Healthfinder listings. The Healthfinder is composed of two listing types: toll–free numbers for health information and federal health information centers and clearinghouses. Organizations are listed alphabetically by topic area.

We present this list simply as a convenient directory. Inclusion or omission of any organization's name indicates neither approval nor disapproval by Health Forum LLC, an American Hospital Association company.

United States Government Agencies

National agencies concerned with health–related matters are listed by the major department of government under which the different functions fall.

State and Local Organizations and Agencies

The lists of organizations in states, associated areas, and provinces include Blue Cross and Blue Shield plans, health systems agencies, hospital associations and councils, hospital licensure agencies, medical and nursing licensure agencies, peer review organizations, state health planning and development agencies, and statewide health coordinating councils.

There are many active local organizations that do not fall within these categories. Contact the hospital association of the state or province for information about such additional groups. The hospital association and councils listed have offices with full-time executives.

The selected state and provincial government agencies include those within state departments of health and welfare, and other agencies, such as comprehensive health planning, crippled children's services, maternal and child health, mental health, and vocational rehabilitation.

Health Care Providers

Lists of JCAHO Accredited Freestanding Long–Term Care Organizations, Health Maintenance Organizations, Freestanding Ambulatory Surgery Centers, Freestanding Hospices, JCAHO Accredited Freestanding Substance Abuse Organizations, JCAHO Accredited Freestanding Mental Health Care Organizations are provided in this section. The lists were developed from information supplied by the providers themselves.

As with the lists of National and International Organizations, these lists are provided simply as a convenient directory. Inclusion or omission of any organization's name indicates neither approval nor disapproval by Health Forum LLC.

National Organizations

A

Academy for Implants and Transplants, P.O. Box 223, Springfield, VA 22150; tel. 703/451-0001; FAX. 703/451-0004; Anthony J. Viscido, D.D.S., Secretary-Treasurer

Academy of Dentistry for Persons with Disabilities, 211 East Chicago Avenue, 5th Floor, Chicago, IL 60611; tel. 312/440-2660; FAX. 312/440-2824; James J. Balija, CAE, Executive Director

Academy of General Dentistry, 211 East Chicago Avenue, Suite 900, Chicago, IL 60611-2670; tel. 312/440-4300; FAX. 312/440-0559; Harold E. Donnell, Jr., Executive Director

Academy of Oral Dynamics, 1590 West Street Road, Warminster, PA 18974; tel. 215/957-0700; FAX. 215/957-0703; Dr. William J. Crielly, Treasurer

Academy of Oral Dynamics, 8919 Sudley Road, Manassas, VA 20110-5016; tel. 703/365-2616; FAX. 703/331-0356; Dr. E. Paul Byrne, Secretary

Accreditation Association for Ambulatory Health Care, 9933 Lawler Avenue, Skokie, IL 60077-3708; tel. 847/676-9610; FAX. 847/676-9628; John E. Burke, Ph. D., Executive Director

Acute Long Term Hospital Association, 1055 North Fairfax Street, Suite 201, Alexandria, VA 22314; tel. 703/299-5571; FAX. 703/299-5574; Brad Traverse, Executive Director, ALTHA

ADARA: Professionals Networking for Excellence in Service Delivery, Individuals Who are Deaf or Hard of Hearing, P.O. Box 6956, San Mateo, CA 94403-6956; tel. 650/372-0620; FAX. 650/372-0661; Elizabeth Charlson, Ph.D.

Aerospace Medical Association, 320 South Henry Street, Alexandria, VA 22314-3579; tel. 703/739-2240; FAX. 703/739-9652; Russell B. Rayman, M.D., Executive Director

Alexander Graham Bell Association for the Deaf, Inc., 3417 Volta Place, N.W., Washington, DC 20007; tel. 202/337-5220; FAX. 202/337-8314; Elissa M. Brooks, Development/PR

Allergy Associates, 2004 Grand Avenue, Baldwin, NY 11510; tel. 516/223-7656; FAX. 516/223-0583; Joseph d'amour, M.D.

Alliance for Children & Families, 11700 West Lake Park Drive, Milwaukee, WI 53224; tel. 414/359-1040; FAX. 414/359-1074; Peter B. Goldberg, President and CEO

Alliance of Cardiovascular Professionals, 910 Charles Street, Fredericksburg, VA 22408; tel. 540/370-0102; FAX. 540/370-0015; Peggy McElgunn, Executive Director

Alzheimer's Association, (Alzheimer's Disease and Related Disorders Association, Inc.), 919 North Michigan Avenue, Suite 1000, Chicago, IL 60611; tel. 312/335-8700; FAX. 312/335-1110; Stephen McConnell, VP, Public Policy Programs and Services

Ambulatory Pediatric Association, 6728 Old McLean Village Drive, McLean, VA 22101; tel. 703/556-9222; FAX. 703/556-8729; Marge Degnon, Executive Director

America's Blood Centers, 725 15th Street, N.W., Suite 700, Washington, DC 20005-2109; tel. 202/393-5725; FAX. 202/393-1282; Jim MacPherson, Executive Director

American Academy for Cerebral Palsy and Developmental Medicine, 6300 North River Road, Suite 727, Rosemont, IL 60018-4226; tel. 847/698-1635; FAX. 847/823-0536; Sheril King, Executive Director

American Academy of Allergy, Asthma and Immunology, 611 East Wells Street, Milwaukee, WI 53202; tel. 414/272-6071; FAX. 414/272-6070; Rick Iber, Executive Vice President

American Academy of Child and Adolescent Psychiatry, 3615 Wisconsin Avenue, N.W., Washington, DC 20016; tel. 202/966-7300; FAX. 202/966-2891; Virginia Q. Anthony, Executive Director

American Academy of Dental Electrosurgery, Planetarium Station, P.O. Box 374, New York, NY 10024; tel. 212/595-1925; Maurice J. Oringer, D.D.S., Executive Secretary

American Academy of Dental Practice Administration, 1063 Whippoorwill Lane, Palatine, IL 60067; tel. 847/934-4404; Kathleen Uebel, Executive Director

American Academy of Dermatology, P.O. Box 40141, Schaumburg, IL 60168-4014; tel. 847/330-0230; FAX. 847/330-0050; Bradford W. Claxton, Executive Director

American Academy of Family Physicians, 11400 Tomahawk Creek Parkway, Leawood, MO 66211; tel. 913/906-6000; FAX. 913/906-6083; Robert Graham, M.D., Executive Vice President

American Academy of Insurance Medicine, P.O. Box 59811, Potomac, MD 20859-9811; tel. 301/365-3572; FAX. 301/365-7705; Russell E. Barker, C.A.E., Executive Vice President

American Academy of Medical Administrators, 701 Lee Street, Suite 600, DesPlaines, IL 60016; tel. 847-759-8601; FAX. 847/759-8602; Renee Schleicher, CAE, President and CEO

American Academy of Neurology, 1080 Montreal Avenue, St. Paul, MN 55116-2325; tel. 612/695-1940; FAX. 612/695-2791; Catherine Rydell, Executive Director

American Academy of Ophthalmology, 655 Beach Street, P.O. Box 7424, San Francisco, CA 94120; tel. 415/561-8500; FAX. 415/561-8533; H. Dunbar Hoskins, Jr., M.D., Executive Vice President

American Academy of Optometry, 6110 Executive Boulevard, Suite 506, Rockville, MD 20852; tel. 301/984-1441; FAX. 301/984-4737; Lois Schoenbrun, CAE, Executive Director

American Academy of Oral Medicine, 2910 Lightfoot Drive, Baltimore, MD 21209-1452; tel. 410/602-8585; Mrs. Joyce Caplan, Executive Secretary

American Academy of Orthopaedic Surgeons, 6300 North River Road, Rosemont, IL 60018-4262; tel. 847/823-7186; FAX. 847/823-8125; William W. Tipton, Jr., M.D., Executive Vice President

American Academy of Otolaryngic Allergy, 8455 Colesville Road, Suite 745, Silver Spring, MD 20910-9998; tel. 301/588-1800; FAX. 301/588-2454; Jami Lucas, Executive Director

American Academy of Otolaryngology-Head and Neck Surgery, Inc., One Prince Street, Alexandria, VA 22314; tel. 703/836-4444; FAX. 703/683-5100; G. Richard Holt, M.D., MPH

American Academy of Pain Management, 13947 Mono Way, Suite A, Sonora, CA 95370-2807; tel. 209/533-9744; FAX. 209/533-9750; Richard S. Weiner, Ph.D., Executive Director

American Academy of Pediatrics, 141 Northwest Point Boulevard, Elk Grove Village, IL 60007; tel. 847/228-5005; FAX. 847/228-5027; Joe M. Sanders, Jr., M.D., Executive Director

American Academy of Physical Medicine and Rehabilitation, One IBM Plaza, Suite 2500, Chicago, IL 60611-3604; tel. 312/464-9700; FAX. 312/464-0227; Ronald A. Henrichs, CAE, Executive Director

American Academy of Physician Assistants, 950 North Washington Street, Alexandria, VA 22314; tel. 703/836-2272; FAX. 703/684-1924; Stephen C. Crane, Ph.D., MPH, Executive Vice President

American Academy of Psychoanalysis, 47 East 19th Street, Sixth Floor, New York, NY 10003; tel. 212/475-7980; FAX. 212/475-8101; Dianne Gabriele, Executive Director

American Academy of Restorative Dentistry, Mid-Continental Tower, Suite 1800, 401 South Boston Avenue, Tulsa, OK 74103; tel. 918-582-3877; FAX. 918/582-3879; James C. Kessler, DDS, Secretary-Treasurer

American Aging Association, The Sally Balin Medical Center, 110 Chesley Drive, Media, PA 19063; tel. 610/627-2626; FAX. 610/565-9747; Arthur K. Balin, M.D., Ph.D., Executive Director

American Alliance for Health, Physical Education, Recreation & Dance, 1900 Association Drive, Reston, VA 20191; tel. 703/476-3400; FAX. 703/476-9527; Michael G. Davis, Executive Vice President

American Ambulance Association, 1255 23rd Street, NW, Washington, DC 20037; tel. 202/452-8888; FAX. 202/452-0005; Steve Haracznak, Executive Vice President

American Art Therapy Association, 1202 Allanson Road, Mundelein, IL 60060; tel. 847/949-6064; FAX. 847/566-4580; Edward J. Stygar, Jr., Executive Director

American Assembly for Men in Nursing, NYSNA, 11 Cornel Road, Latham, NY 12110-1499; tel. 518/782-9400; FAX. 518/782-9530; David Sprouse, President

American Association for Adult and Continuing Education, 1200 19th Street, N.W., Suite 300, Washington, DC 20036; tel. 202/429-5131; FAX. 202/223-4579; Anna Darin, Association Manager

American Association for Clinical Chemistry, Inc., 2101 L Street, N.W., Suite 202, Washington, DC 20037; tel. 202/857-0717; FAX. 202/887-5093; Richard Flaherty, Executive Vice President

American Association for Dental Research, 1619 Duke Street, Alexandria, VA 22314-3406; tel. 703/548-0066; FAX. 703/548-1883; Eli Schwarz, DDS, MPH, Ph.D., Executive Director

American Association for Laboratory Animal Science, 9190 Crestwyn Hills Drive, Memphis, TN 38125; tel. 901/754-8620; FAX. 901/753-0046; Michael R. Sondag, Executive Director

American Association for Respiratory Care, 11030 Ables Lane, Dallas, TX 75229; tel. 972/243-2272; FAX. 972/484-2720; Sam P. Giordano, Executive Director

American Association for the Advancement of Science, 1200 New York Avenue, N.W., Washington, DC 20005; tel. 202/326-6400; FAX. 202/321-5526; Richard S. Nicholson, Executive Officer

American Association for the Surgery of Trauma, Department of Surgery, UCLA Medical Center, Room 72-178 CHS, Los Angeles, CA 90095; tel. 310/794-4210; FAX. 310/794-4251; H. Gill Cryer, M.D., Secretary-Treasurer

American Association of Anatomists, Department of Anatomy, Tulane Medical School, New Orleans, LA 70112; FAX. 504/584-1687; Robert Yates, Secretary-Treasurer

American Association of Bioanalysts, 917 Locust Street, Suite 1100, St. Louis, MO 63101-1419; tel. 314/241-1445; FAX. 314/241-1449; Mark S. Birenbaum, Ph.D., Administrator

American Association of Certified Orthoptists, St. Louis Children's Hospital, Eye Center, 2 South 89, St.. Louis, MO 63110; tel. 314/454-6026; FAX. 314/454-2368; Kyle Arnold, President

American Association of Colleges of Nursing, One Dupont Circle, N.W., Suite 530, Washington, DC 20036; tel. 202/463-6930; FAX. 202/785-8320; Geraldine Bednash, Ph.D., RN, FAAN, Executive Director

American Association of Colleges of Pharmacy, 1426 Prince Street, Alexandria, VA 22314-2841; tel. 703/739-2330; FAX. 703/836-8982; Richard P. Penna, Pharm.D., Executive Vice President

American Association of Colleges of Podiatric Medicine, 1350 Piccard Drive, Suite 322, Rockville, MD 20850-4307; tel. 301/990-7400; FAX. 301/990-2807; Anthony J. McNevin, CAE, President

American Association of Critical-Care Nurses, 101 Columbia, Suite 200, Aliso Viejo, CA 92656-1491; tel. 949/362-2000; FAX. 949/362-2020; Wanda L. Johanson, RN, MN, CEO

American Association of Dental Consultants, Inc., P.O. Box 3345, Lawrence, KS 66046; tel. 785/749-2727; FAX. 785/749-1140; Ed Schooley, D.D.S., Secretary-Treasurer

Organizations / National Organizations

American Association of Dental Schools, 1625 Massachusetts Avenue, N.W., Suite 600, Washington, DC 20036; tel. 202/667–9433; FAX. 202/667–0642; Richard W. Valachonic, D.M.D., Executive Director

American Association of Endodontists, 211 East Chicago Avenue, Suite 1100, Chicago, IL 60611; tel. 312/266–7255; FAX. 312/266–9867; Irma S. Kudo, Executive Director

American Association of Fund–Raising Counsel, Inc., 37 east 28th Street, Suite 902, New York, NY 10016; tel. 212/354–5799; FAX. 212/768–1795; Ann Kaplan, Research Director

American Association of Health Plans, (AAHP), 1129 20th Street, N.W., Suite 600, Washington, DC 20036–3421; tel. 202/778–3200; FAX. 202/778–8486; Charles W. Stellar, Executive Vice President

American Association of Healthcare Administrative Management, (Formerly The American Guild of Patient Account Management), 1200 19th Street, N.W., Suite 300, Washington, DC 20036; tel. 202/857–1179; FAX. 202/223–4579; Dennis E. Smeage, Executive Director

American Association of Healthcare Consultants, 11208 Waples Mill Road, Suite 109, Fairfax, VA 22030; tel. 800/362–4674; FAX. 703/691–2247; Vaughan A. Smith, President and CEO

American Association of Homes and Services for the Aging, 901 E Street, N.W., Suite 500, Washington, DC 20004–2011; tel. 202/783–2242; FAX. 202/783–2255; Len Fishman, President

American Association of Hospital Dentists, Inc., 211 East Chicago Avenue, 5th Floor, Chicago, IL 60611; tel. 312/440–2661; FAX. 312/440–2824; James J. Balija, CAE, Executive Director

American Association of Kidney Patients, 100 South Ashley Drive, Suite 280, Tampa, FL 33602; tel. 800/749–2257; FAX. 813/223–0001; Kris Robinson, Executive Director

American Association of Medical Assistants, 20 North Wacker Drive, Suite 1575, Chicago, IL 60606–2968; tel. 312/899–1500; FAX. 312/899–1259; Donald A. Balasa, J.D., M.B.A., Executive Director, Legal Counsel

American Association of Neuroscience Nurses, 4700 West Lake Avenue, Glenview, IL 60025–1485; tel. 847/375–4733; FAX. 847/375–6333; Diane K. Burghar, Executive Director

American Association of Nurse Anesthetists, 222 South Prospect Avenue, Park Ridge, IL 60068–4001; tel. 847/692–7050; FAX. 847/692–6968; John F. Garde, CRNA, M.S., FAAN, Executive Director

American Association of Nutritional Consultants, 870 Canarios Court, Chula Vista, CA 91910; tel. 619/482–8533; FAX. 619/482–4485; Lenda Summerfield, Administrator

American Association of Occupational Health Nurses, Inc., 2920 Brandywine Road, Suite 100, Atlanta, GA 30341–4146; tel. 770/455–7757; FAX. 770/455–7271; Ann R. Cox, CAE, Executive Director

American Association of Oral and Maxillofacial Surgeons, 9700 West Bryn Mawr Avenue, Rosemont, IL 60018–5701; tel. 847/678–6200; FAX. 847/678–6286; Robert C. Rinadi, Ph.D., Executive Director

American Association of Orthodontists, 401 North Lindbergh Boulevard, St. Louis, MO 63141–7816; tel. 314/993–1700; FAX. 314/997–1745; Ronald S. Moen, Executive Director

American Association of Pastoral Counselors, 9504A Lee Highway, Fairfax, VA 22031–2303; tel. 703/385–6967; FAX. 703/352–7725; C. Roy Woodruff, Ph.D., Executive Director

American Association of Physicists in Medicine, One Physics Ellipse, College Park, MD 20740–3846; tel. 301/209–3350; FAX. 301/209–0862; Salvatore Trofi, Jr., Executive Director

American Association of Plastic Surgeons, 4900 B South 31st Street, Arlington, VA 22206; tel. 703/820–7400; FAX. 703–931–4520; Thomas F. Fise, Executive Secretary

American Association of Poison Control Centers, 3201 New Mexico Avenue, N.W., Suite 310, Washington, DC 20016; tel. 202/362–7217; Rose Ann Soloway, RN, MSED, ABAT

American Association of Psychiatric Technicians, Inc., A.A.P.T., 336 Johnson Road, Suite 2, Michigan, IN 46360; tel. 800/391–7589; George Blake, Ph.D., Director

American Association of Public Health Dentistry, A.A.P.H.D. National Office, 3760 SW Lyle Court, Portland, OR 97221; tel. 503/242–0712; FAX. 503–242–0721; James Toothaker, D.D.S., M.D., Executive Director

American Association of Public Health Physicians, 515 North State Street, 14th Floor, Chicago, IL 60610; tel. 312/464–4299; FAX. 312/464–5993; David Cloud, Executive Manager

American Association on Mental Retardation, 444 North Capitol Street, N.W., Suite 846, Washington, DC 20001–1512; tel. 202/387–1968; FAX. 202/387–2193; M. Doreen Croser, Executive Director

American Baptist Homes and Hospitals Association, P.O. Box 851, Valley Forge, PA 19482–0851; tel. 610/768–2411; FAX. 610/768–2453; Rosalie Norman–McNaney, Director

American Board of Allergy and Immunology, A Conjoint Board of the American Board of Internal Medicine, 510 Walnut Street, Suite 1701, Philadelphia, PA 19106–3699; tel. 215/592–9466; FAX. 215/592–9411; John W. Yunginger, M.D., Executive Secretary

American Board of Anesthesiology, 4101 Lake Boone Trail, Suite 510, Raleigh, NC 27607–7506; tel. 919/881–2570; FAX. 919/881–2575; M. Jane Matjasko, M.D., Secretary

American Board of Cardiovascular Perfusion, 207 North 25th Avenue, Hattiesburg, MS 39401; tel. 601/582–2227; FAX. 601/582–2271; Beth A. Richmond, Ph.D., Mark G. Richmond, Ed.D.

American Board of Colon and Rectal Surgery, 20600 Eureka Road, Suite 713, Taylor, MI 48180; tel. 734/282–9400; FAX. 734/282–9402; Herand Abcarian, M.D., Executive Director

American Board of Dermatology, Inc., Henry Ford Hospital, One Ford Place, Detroit, MI 48202–3450; tel. 313/874–1088; FAX. 313/872–3221; Harry J. Hurley, M.D., Executive Director

American Board of Emergency Medicine, 3000 Coolidge Road, East Lansing, MI 48823; tel. 517/332–4800; FAX. 517/332–2234; Mary Ann Reinhart, Ph.D., Acting Executive Director

American Board of Family Practice, Inc., 2228 Young Drive, Lexington, KY 40505; tel. 606/269–5626; FAX. 606/335–7501; Robert F. Avant, M.D., Executive Director

American Board of Internal Medicine, 510 Walnut Street, Suite 1700, Philadelphia, PA 19106–3699; tel. 215/446–3500; FAX. 215/446–3473; Harry R. Kimball, M.D., President

American Board of Medical Management, 4890 West Kennedy Boulevard, Suite 200, Tampa, FL 33609–2575; tel. 813/287–2815; FAX. 813/287–8993; Roger S. Schenke, Executive Vice President

American Board of Medical Specialties, 1007 Church Street, Suite 404, Evanston, IL 60201–5913; tel. 847/491–9091; FAX. 847/328–3596; Stephen H. Miller, M.D., MPH, Executive Vice–President

American Board of Neurological Surgery, 6550 Fanning Street, Suite 2139, Houston, TX 77030; tel. 713/790–6015; FAX. 713/794–0207; Mary Louise Sanderson, Administrator

American Board of Nuclear Medicine, 900 Veteran Avenue, Los Angeles, CA 90024; tel. 310/825–6787; FAX. 310/825–9433; Joseph F. Ross, M.D., President

American Board of Ophthalmology, 111 Presidential Boulevard, Suite 241, Bala Cynwyd, PA 19004; tel. 610/664–1175; FAX. 610/664–6503; Denis M. O'Day, M.D., Executive Director

American Board of Oral and Maxillofacial Surgery, 625 North Michigan Avenue, Suite 1820, Chicago, IL 60611; tel. 312/642–0070; FAX. 312/642–8584; Cheryl E. Mounts, Executive Secretary

American Board of Orthopedic Surgery, Inc., 400 Silver Cedar Court, Chapel Hill, NC 27514; tel. 919/929–7103; FAX. 919/942–8988; G. Paul De Rosa, M.D., Executive Director

American Board of Otolaryngology, 2211 Norfolk, Suite 800, Houston, TX 77098; tel. 713/528–6200; FAX. 713/528–1171; Robert W. Cantrell, M.D., Executive Vice President

American Board of Pathology, One Urban Centre, 4830 West Kennedy Boulevard, Tampa, FL 33622–5915; tel. 813/286–2444; FAX. 813/289–5279; William H. Hartmann, M.D., Executive Vice President

American Board of Pediatric Dentistry, 1193 Woodgate Drive, Carmel, IN 46033–9232; tel. 317/573–0877; FAX. 317/846–7235; James R. Roche, D.D.S., Executive Secretary–Treasurer

American Board of Pediatrics, Inc., 111 Silver Cedar Court, Chapel Hill, NC 27514; tel. 919/929–0461; FAX. 919/929–9255; James A. Stockman, III, M.D., President

American Board of Physical Medicine and Rehabilitation, Norwest Center, Suite 674, 21 First Street, S.W., Rochester, MN 55902; tel. 507/282–1776; FAX. 507/282–9242; Anthony Tarvestad, JD, Executive Director

American Board of Podiatric Surgery, 3330 Mission Street, San Francisco, CA 94110–5009; tel. 415/826–3200; FAX. 415/826–4640; James A. Lamb, Executive Director

American Board of Preventive Medicine, Inc., 9950 West Lawrence Avenue, Suite 106, Schiller Park, IL 60176; tel. 847/671–1750; FAX. 847/671–1751; James M. Vanderploeg, M.D., MPH

American Board of Prosthodontics, P.O. Box 8437, Atlanta, GA 31106; tel. 404/876–2625; FAX. 404/872–8804; William D. Culpepper, D.D.S., M.S.D., Executive Director

American Board of Psychiatry and Neurology, Inc., 500 Lake Cook Road, Suite 335, Deerfield, IL 60015; tel. 847/945–7900; FAX. 847/945–1146; Stephen C. Scheiber, M.D., Executive Vice President

American Board of Quality Assurance and Utilization Review, 2120 Range Road, Clearwater, FL 33765; tel. 727/298–8777; FAX. 727/449–0555; H.E. Hartsell, Chief Operating Officer

American Board of Radiology, 5255 East Williams Circle, Suite 3200, Tucson, AZ 85711; tel. 520/790–2900; FAX. 520/790–3200; M. Paul Capp, M.D., Executive Director

American Board of Surgery, Inc., 1617 John F. Kennedy Boulevard, Suite 860, Philadelphia, PA 19103; tel. 215/568–4000; FAX. 215/563–5718; Wallace P. Ritchie, Jr., M.D., Executive Director

American Board of Thoracic Surgery, One Rotary Center, Suite 803, Evanston, IL 60201; tel. 847/475–1520; FAX. 847/475–6240; Richard J. Cleveland, M.D., Secretary–Treasurer

American Broncho–Esophagological Association, Vanderbilt University Medical Center, Department of Otolaryngology, S–2100, Nashville, TN 37232–2559; tel. 615/322–7267; FAX. 615/343–7604; James A. Duncavage, M.D., Secretary

American Burn Association, 625 North Michigan Avenue, Suite 1530, Chicago, IL 60611; tel. 312/642–9260; FAX. 312/642–9130; John Krichbaum, J.D., Executive Director

American Cancer Society, 1599 Clifton Road, N.E., Atlanta, GA 30329; tel. 404/320–3333; Gerald P. Murphy, M.D., Senior Vice President

American Center for the Alexander Technique, Inc., 39 W. 14th Street, #507, New York, NY 10011; tel. 212/633–2229; Jane Tomkiewiez, Executive Director

American Chiropractic Association, 1701 Clarendon Boulevard, Arlington, VA 22209; tel. 703/276–8800; FAX. 703/243–2593; Garrett F. Cuneo, Executive Vice President

American Cleft Palate–Craniofacial Association, 104 S. Estes Drive, Suite 204, Chapel Hill, NC 27514; tel. 919/933–9044; FAX. 919/933–9604; Nancy C. Smythe, Executive Director

American Clinical Neurophysiology Society, (formerly the American Electroencephalographic Society), One Regency Drive, P.O. Box 30, Bloomfield, CT 06002; tel. 203/243–3977; FAX. 203/286–0787; Jacquelyn T. Coleman, Executive Director

Organizations / National Organizations

American College Health Association, P.O. Box 28937, Baltimore, MD 21240–8937; tel. 410/859–1500; FAX. 410/859–1510; Doyle E. Randol, MS, Executive Director

American College of Allergy, Asthma and Immunology, 85 West Algonquin Road, Suite 550, Arlington Heights, IL 60005; tel. 847/427–1200; FAX. 847/427–1294; James R. Slawny, Executive Director

American College of Apothecaries, P.O. Box 341266, Bartlett, TN 38184; tel. 901/383–8119; FAX. 901/383–8882; D. C. Huffman, Jr., Ph.D., Executive Vice President

American College of Cardiology, 9111 Old Georgetown Road, Bethesda, MD 20814; tel. 800/253–4636; FAX. 301/897–9745; Christine McEntee, Executive Vice President

American College of Cardiovascular Nursing, 11219 Rice Creek Road, Riverview, FL 33569; tel. 813/671–8912; FAX. 813/671–8912; Jonni Cooper, Chief Executive Officer

American College of Chest Physicians, 3300 Dundee Road, Northbrook, IL 60062–2348; tel. 847/498–1400; FAX. 847/498–5460; Alvin Lever, Executive Vice President and CEO

American College of Dentists, 839 Quince Orchard Boulevard, Suite J, Gaithersburg, MD 20878–1614; tel. 301/977–3223; FAX. 301/977–3330; Stephen A. Ralls, D.D.S.

American College of Emergency Physicians, P.O. Box 619911, Dallas, TX 75261–9911; tel. 972/550–0911; FAX. 972/580–2816; Colin C. Rorrie, Jr., Ph.D., CAE, Executive Director

American College of Foot and Ankle Surgeons, 515 Busse Highway, Park Ridge, IL 60068–3150; tel. 847/292–2237; FAX. 847/292–2022; Thomas R. Schedler, CAE, Executive Director

American College of Health Care Administrators, 1800 Diagonal Road, Suite 355, Alexandria, VA 22314; tel. 703/739–7900; FAX. 703/739–7901; Karen S. Tucker, CAE, President and CEO

American College of Healthcare Executives, One North Franklin, Suite 1700, Chicago, IL 60606–3491; tel. 312/424–2800; FAX. 312/424–0023; Thomas C. Dolan, Ph.D., FACHE, CAE, President and CEO

American College of Legal Medicine, 611 East Wells Street, Milwaukee, WI 53202; tel. 414/276–1881; FAX. 414/276–3349; Janet Haynes, Executive Director

American College of Medical Staff Development, 6855 Jimmy Carter Blvd., Suite 2100, Norcross, GA 30071; tel. 770/734–9904; FAX. 770/734–9709; Jan McElroy, Director of Education

American College of MOHS Micrographic Surgery and Cutaneous On, 930 North Meacham, Schaumburg, IL 60173–4965; tel. 847/330–9830; FAX. 847/330–1135; Sherrie Traficano, Executive Director

American College of Nurse–Midwives, 818 Connecticut Avenue, N.W., Suite 900, Washington, DC 20006; tel. 202/728–9860; FAX. 202/728–9897; Deanne Williams, Executive Director

American College of Obstetricians and Gynecologists, 409 12th Street, S.W., Washington, DC 20024–2188; tel. 202/638–5577; FAX. 202/484–5107; Ralph W. Hale, M.D., Executive Vice President

American College of Occupational and Environmental Medicine, (Includes ACOEM Research and Education Fund, and Occupational, 1114 N. Arlington Heights Road, Arlington Heights, IL 60004; tel. 847/818–1800; FAX. 847/818–9289; E. Eugene Handley, Ph.D., Executive Director

American College of Physician Executives, 4890 West Kennedy Boulevard, Suite 200, Tampa, FL 33609–2575; tel. 813/287–2000; FAX. 813/287–8993; Roger S. Schenke, Executive Vice President

American College of Physicians, American Society of Internal Medicine, 190 North Independence Mall West, Philadelphia, PA 19106–1572; tel. 215/351–2800; FAX. 215/351–2829; Walter J. McDonald, M.D., F.A.C.P., Executive Vice President

American College of Preventive Medicine, 1660 L Street, N.W., Washington, DC 20036; tel. 202/466–2044; FAX. 202/466–2662; Jordan H. Richland, MPH, Executive Director

American College of Radiology, 1891 Preston White Drive, Reston, VA 20191–4397; tel. 703/648–8900; FAX. 703/648–9176; John J. Curry, Executive Director

American College of Rheumatology, 1800 Century Place, Suite 150, Atlanta, GA 30345; tel. 404/633–3777; FAX. 404/633–1870; Lynn Bonfiglio, Director, Membership

American College of Sports Medicine, P.O. Box 1440, Indianapolis, IN 46206–1440; tel. 317/637–9200; FAX. 317/634–7817; James R. Whitehead, Executive Vice President

American College of Surgeons, 633 N. Saint Clair Street, Chicago, IL 60611; tel. 312/202–5000; FAX. 312/202–5001; Thomas R. Russell, M.D., Executive Director

American Congress of Rehabilitation Medicine, 5987 E. 71st Street, Suite 111, Indianapolis, IN 46220; tel. 317/915–2250; FAX. 317/915–2245; Carllyn L. Braddom, Ed.D., Executive Director

American Council on Pharmaceutical Education, Inc., 311 West Superior Street, Suite 512, Chicago, IL 60610; tel. 312/664–3575; FAX. 312/664–4652; Daniel A. Nona, Ph.D., Executive Director

American Dental Assistants Association, 203 North LaSalle, Suite 1320, Chicago, IL 60601; tel. 312/541–1550; FAX. 312/541–1496; Lawrence H. Sepin, Executive Director

American Dental Association, 211 East Chicago Avenue, Chicago, IL 60611; tel. 312/440–2500; FAX. 312/440–7494; John S. Zapp, D.D.S., Executive Director

American Dental Society of Anesthesiology, Inc., 211 East Chicago Avenue, Suite 780, Chicago, IL 60611; tel. 312/664–8270; FAX. 312/642–9713; R. Knight Charlton, Executive Secretary

American Diabetes Association, Inc., 1701 N. Beauregard Street, Alexandria, VA 22311; tel. 703/549–1500; FAX. 703/836–7439; John H. Graham IV, Chief Executive Officer

American Dietetic Association, 216 West Jackson Boulevard, Suite 800, Chicago, IL 60606–6995; tel. 312/899–0040; FAX. 312/899–1758; Connie L. Rivera, Chief Executive Officer

American Federation for Medical Research, 1200 19th Street, N.W., Suite 300, Washington, DC 20036–2422; tel. 202/429–5161; FAX. 202/223–4579; Antinette Turner, Director of Programs & Services

American Foundation for Aging Research, North Carolina State University, Biochemistry Department, Raleigh, NC 27695–7622; tel. 919/515–5679; FAX. 919/515–2047; Paul F. Agris, President

American Foundation for AIDS Research, 120 Wall Street, 13th Floor, New York, NY 10005; tel. 212/860/1600; FAX. Mathilde Krim, Ph.D., Founding Co–Chair and Chairman

American Foundation for the Blind, Inc., 11 Penn Plaza, Suite 300, New York, NY 10001; tel. 212/502–7600; FAX. 212/502–7770; Liz Greco, Vice President, Communications

American Fracture Association, Rural Route 6, Box 8, Bloomington, IL 61704; tel. 309/828–2815; FAX. 309/828–1499; Sarah Olson, Executive Secretary

American Geriatrics Society, 770 Lexington Avenue, Suite 300, New York, NY 10021; tel. 212/308–1414; FAX. 212/832–8646; Linda Hiddemen Baroness, Executive Vice President

American Group Psychotherapy Association, Inc., 25 East 21st Street, Sixth Floor, New York, NY 10010; tel. 212/477–2677; FAX. 212/979–6627; Marsha S. Block, CAE, Chief Executive Officer

American Head and Neck Society, 203 Lothrop Street, Suite 519, Pittsburgh, PA 15213; tel. 414/647–2227; FAX. 412/647–8944; Jonas T. Johnson, M.D., Secretary

American Headache Society, 19 Mantua Road, Mt. Royal, NJ 08061; tel. 856/423–0043; FAX. 856/423–0082; Linda McGillicuddy, Executive Director

American Health Care Association, 1201 L Street, N.W., Washington, DC 20005; tel. 202/842–4444; FAX. 202/842–3860; Charles H. Roadman, II, M.D., President and CEO

American Health Foundation, One Dana Road, Valhalla, NY 10595; tel. 914/789–7122; FAX. 212/687–2339; Daniel W. Nixon, M.D., President

American Health Information Management Association, 233 North Michigan Avenue, Suite 2150, Chicago, IL 60611; tel. 312/233–1100; FAX. 312/233–1090; Linda Kloss, R.H.I.A., Executive Vice President and CEO

American Health Lawyers Association, 1025 Connecticut Avenue, N.W., Suite 600, Washington, DC 20036; tel. 202/833–1100; FAX. 202/833–1105; Peter M. Leibold, Esq, Executive Vice President and CEO

American Health Planning Association, 7245 Arlington Boulevard, Suite 300, Falls Church, VA 22042; tel. 703/573–3103; FAX. 703/573–1276; Dean Montgomery

American Healthcare Radiology Administrators, P.O. Box 334, Sudbury, MA 01776; tel. 978/443–7591; FAX. 978/443–8046; Mary Reitter, Executive Director

American Heart Association, Inc., Office of Scientific Affairs, 7272 Greenville Avenue, Dallas, TX 75231; tel. 214/706–1446; FAX. 214/373–9818; Rodman D. Starke, M.D., Executive Vice President

American Hospital Association, One North Franklin, Chicago, Chicago, IL 60606–3491; tel. 312/422–3000; Richard J. Davidson, President

American Hospital Association, 325 Seventh Street, N.W., Washington, DC 20004; tel. 202/626–2363; FAX. 202/626–2303; Richard J. Davidson, President

American Hospital Association, 5412 Idylwild Trail, Suite 108, Boulder, CO 80301; tel. 303/516–9709; FAX. 303/516–9710; Marcia Desmond, Regional Executive

American Hospital Association, Washington Office, 325 Seventh Street, N.W., Suite 700, Washington, DC 20004; tel. 202/638–1100; FAX. 202/626–2345; Richard Pollack, Executive Vice President, Government Public Affairs

American Juvenile Arthritis Organization, Council, Arthritis Foundation, 1330 West Peachtree Street, Atlanta, GA 30309; tel. 404/872–7100; FAX. 404/872–9559; Janet S. Austin, Ph.D., Vice President

American Laryngological Association, Department of Otolaryngology, S–2100 Medical Center North, Nashville, TN 37232–2559; tel. 615/322–7267; FAX. 615/343–7604; R.H. Ossoff, DMD, M.D., Secretary

American Library Association, 50 East Huron Street, Chicago, IL 60611; tel. 312/280–5044; FAX. 312/944–8520; Debra Davis, PR Specialist

American Lung Association, 1740 Broadway, New York, NY 10019–4374; tel. 212/315–8700; FAX. 212/765–7876; John R. Garrison, Managing Director

American Lung Association of Ohio, Dayton Office, 7560 McEwen Road, Dayton, OH 45459; tel. 937/291–0451; FAX. 937/291–0453; Roberta M. Taylor, Director

American Medical Association, 515 North State Street, Chicago, IL 60610; tel. 312/464–5000; FAX. 312/464–4184; E. Ratcliffe Anderson, Jr., M.D., Executive V.P. and CEO

American Medical Association Alliance, 515 North State Street, Chicago, IL 60610; tel. 312/464–4470; FAX. 312/464–5020; Hazel J. Lewis, Executive Director

American Medical Group Association, Inc., 1422 Duke Street, Alexandria, VA 22314–3430; tel. 703/838–0033; FAX. 703/548–1890; Donald W. Fisher, Ph.D., Chief Executive Officer

American Medical Student Association/Foundation, 1902 Association Drive, Reston, VA 22091; tel. 703/620–6600; FAX. 703/620–5873; Paul R. Wright, Executive Director

American Medical Technologists, 710 Higgins Road, Park Ridge, IL 60068; tel. 847/823–5169; FAX. 847/823–0458; Gerard P. Boe, Ph.D., Executive Director

American Medical Women's Association, Inc., 800 North Fairfax Street, Suite 400, Alexandria, VA 22314; tel. 703/838–0500; FAX. 703/549–3864; Eileen McGrath, J.D., CAE, Executive Director

© 2000 AHA Guide — Health Organizations, Agencies, and Providers

Organizations / National Organizations

American Medical Writers Association, 40 West Gude Drive #101, Rockville, MD 20850-1192; tel. 301/294-5303; FAX. 301/294-9006; Lillian Sablack, Executive Director

American Music Therapy Association, (Formerly The National Association for Music Therapy), 8455 Colesville Road, Suite 1000, Silver Spring, MD 20910; tel. 301/589-3300; FAX. 301/589-5175; Andrea Farbman, Ed.D., Executive Director

American National Standards Institute, 11 West 42nd Street, New York, NY 10036; tel. 212/642-4900; FAX. 212/398-0023; Sergio Mazza, President

American Nephrology Nurses' Association, East Holly Avenue, P.O. Box 56, Pitman, NJ 08071; tel. 609/256-2320; FAX. 609/589-7463

American Neurological Association, 5841 Cedar Lake Road, Suite 204, Minneapolis, MN 55416; tel. 612/545-6284; FAX. 612/545-6073; Linda Wilkerson, Executive Director

American Nurses' Association, 600 Maryland Avenue, S.W., Suite 100 W, Washington, DC 20024-2571; tel. 202/651-7000; FAX. 202/651-7001; David Hennage, Ph.D., M.B.A.

American Occupational Therapy Association, Inc., 4720 Montgomery Lane, P.O. Box 31220, Bethesda, MD 20824-1220; tel. 301/652-2682; FAX. 301/652-7711; Chris Bluhm, CMA, CPA, Interim Executive Director

American Ontological Society, Inc., Loyola University Medical Center, 2160 South First Avenue, Building 105, Number 1870, Maywood, IL 60153; tel. 708/216-8526; FAX. 708/216-4834; Gregory J. Matz, M.D., Secretary-Treasurer

American Ophthalmological Society, P.O. Box 193940, San Francisco, CA 94119-3940; tel. 415/561-8578; FAX. 415/561-8531; Charles P. Wilkinson, M.D., Secretary-Treasurer

American Optometric Association, 243 North Lindbergh Boulevard, St. Louis, MO 63141; tel. 314/991-4100; FAX. 314/991-4101; Michael D. Jones, O.D., Executive Director

American Organization of Nurse Executives (AONE), One North Franklin, 34th Floor, Chicago, IL 60606; tel. 312/422-2800; FAX. 312/422-4503; Marjorie Beyers, RN, Ph.D., FAAN

American Orthopsychiatric Association, 330 Seventh Avenue, 18th Floor, New York, NY 10001; tel. 212/564-5930; FAX. 212/564-6180; Gale Siegel, M.S.W., Executive Director

American Orthoptic Council, 3914 Nakoma Road, Madison, WI 53711; tel. 608/233-5383; FAX. 608/263-4247; Leslie France, Administrator

American Osteopathic Association, 142 East Ontario Street, Chicago, IL 60611; tel. 312/202-8000; FAX. 312/202-8212; John B. Crosby, J.D., Executive Director

American Parkinson Disease Association, Inc., 1250 Hylan Boulevard, Suite 4B, Staten Island, NY 10305; tel. 800/223-2732; FAX. 718/981-4399; G. Maestrone, D.V.M., Scientific and Medical Affairs Director

American Pediatric Society, Inc., 3400 Research Forest Drive, Suite B7, The Woodlands, TX 77381; tel. 281/419-0052; FAX. 281/419-0082; Kathy Cannon, Associate Executive Director

American Pharmaceutical Association, 2215 Constitution Avenue, N.W., Washington, DC 20037; tel. 202/628-4410; FAX. 202/783-2351; John A. Gans, Pharm.D., Executive Vice President

American Physical Therapy Association, 1111 North Fairfax Street, Alexandria, VA 22314; tel. 703/684-2782; FAX. 703/684-7343; Francis J. Mallon, Esq., Chief Executive Officer

American Physiological Society, 9650 Rockville Pike, Bethesda, MD 20814-3991; tel. 301/530-7164; FAX. 301/571-8305; Martin Frank, Ph.D., Executive Director

American Podiatric Medical Association, 9312 Old Georgetown Road, Bethesda, MD 20814-1698; tel. 301/571-9200; FAX. 301/530-2752; Glenn B. Gastwirth, DPM, Executive Director

American Psychiatric Association, 1400 K Street, N.W., Washington, DC 20005; tel. 202/682-6000; FAX. 202/682-6114; Steven M. Mirin, M.D., Medical Director

American Psychoanalytic Association, 309 East 49th Street, New York, NY 10017; tel. 212/752-0450; FAX. 212/593-0571; Ellen B. Fertig, Administrative Director

American Psychological Association, 750 First Street, N.E., Washington, DC 20002-4242; tel. 202/336-5500; FAX. 202/336-5797; Russ Newman, Ph.D., J.D., Executive Director,

American Psychosomatic Society, 6728 Old McLean Village Drive, McLean, VA 22101; tel. 703/556-9222; George K. Degnon, Executive Director

American Public Health Association, 800 I. Street, NW, Washington, DC 20001-3710; tel. 202/777-APHA; FAX. 202/777-2534; Mohammed N. Akhter, M.D., MPH, Executive Vice President

American Public Welfare Association, 810 First Street, N.E., Suite 500, Washington, DC 20002; tel. 202/682-0100; FAX. 202/289-6555; Sidney Johnson, III, Executive Director

American Red Cross, National Headquarters, 8111 Gatehouse Road, Falls Church, VA 22042; tel. 703/206-7764; FAX. 703/206-7765; Susan M. Livingstone, Vice President, Health and Safety

American Registry of Medical Assistants, 69 Southwick Road, Suite A, Westfield, MA 01085-4729; tel. 800/527-2762; FAX. 413/562-9021; Annette H. Heyman, R.M.A., Director

American Registry of Radiologic Technologists, 1255 Northland Drive, St. Paul, MN 55120; tel. 651/687-0048; Jerry B. Reid, Ph.D., Executive Director

American Rhinologic Society, Department of Otolaryngology/Head and Neck Surgery, LSU Health Services Center, Shreveport, LA 71130; tel. 888/520-9585; FAX. 318/675-6260; Fred J. Stucker, M.D., Secretary

American Roentgen Ray Society, 44211 Slate Stone Court, Leesburg, VA 20176; tel. 703/648-8992; FAX. 703/264-8863; Paul R. Fullagar, Executive Director

American School Health Association, 7263 S.R. 43, P.O. Box 708, Kent, OH 44240-0708; tel. 330/678-1601; FAX. 330/678-4526; Susan Wooley, Ph.D., CHES, Executive Director

American Society for Adolescent Psychiatry, 4340 East West Highway, Suite 401, Bethesda, MD 20814; tel. 301/718-6502; FAX. 301/656-0989; Ann T. Loew, Ed.M.

American Society for Biochemistry and Molecular Biology, Inc., 9650 Rockville Pike, Bethesda, MD 20814-3996; tel. 301/530-7145; FAX. 301/571-1824; Charles C. Hancock, Executive Officer

American Society for Clinical Laboratory Science, 7910 Woodmont Avenue, Suite 530, Bethesda, MD 20814; tel. 301/657-2768; FAX. 301/657-2909; Elissa Passiment, Executive Director

American Society for Clinical Pharmacology and Therapeutics, 528 North Washington Street, Alexandria, VA 22314; tel. 703/836-6981; FAX. 703/836-5223; Sharon J. Swans, CAE, Executive Director

American Society for Cytotechnology, 4101 Lake Boone Trail, Suite 2A, Raleigh, NC 27607; tel. 919/787-5181; FAX. 919/787-4916; Kathleen Norris, Executive Director

American Society for Healthcare Central Service Professionals , One North Franklin, 31st Floor, Chicago, IL 60606; tel. 312/422-3570; FAX. 312/422-4573; Patti Costello, Director of Educational Product Development and Programs

American Society for Healthcare Engineering (ASHE), One North Franklin, Chicago, IL 60606; tel. 312/422-3800; FAX. 312/422-4571; Jacqueline Croteau, Interim Executive Director

American Society for Healthcare Food Service Administrators (AHA), One North Franklin, Chicago, IL 60606; tel. 312/422-3870; FAX. 312/422-4581; Patricia Burton, Executive Director

American Society for Healthcare Human Resources Administration, One North Franklin, 31st Floor, Chicago, IL 60606; tel. 312/422-3720; FAX. 312/422-4579; Mary Anne Kelly, Executive Director

American Society for Healthcare Risk Management (AHA), One North Franklin, Chicago, IL 60606; tel. 312/422-3980; FAX. 312/422-4580; David Strickland, Executive Director

American Society for Investigative Pathology, 9650 Rockville Pike, Bethesda, MD 20814-3993; tel. 301/530-7130; FAX. 301/571-1879; Frances A. Pitlick, Ph.D., Executive Officer

American Society for Laser Medicine and Surgery, Inc., 2404 Stewart Square, Wausau, WI 54401; tel. 715/845-9283; FAX. 715/848-2493; Richard O. Gregory, M.D., Secretary

American Society for Microbiology, 1752 North Street, NW, Washington, DC 20036; tel. 202/924-9265; FAX. 202/942-9333; Michael I. Goldberg, Ph.D., Executive Director

American Society for Pharmacology and Experimental Therapeutic, 9650 Rockville Pike, Bethesda, MD 20814-3995; tel. 301/530-7060; FAX. 301/530-7061; Christine K. Carrico, Ph. D., Executive Officer

American Society for Public Administration, 1120 G Street, N.W., Suite 700, Washington, DC 20005; tel. 202/393-7878; FAX. 202/638-4952; Mary Hamilton, Executive Director

American Society for Reproductive Medicine, (formerly The American Fertility Society), 1209 Montgomery Highway, Birmingham, AL 35216-2809; tel. 205/978-5000; FAX. 205/978-5005; Benjamin Younger, M.D., Executive Director

American Society for the Advancement of Anesthesia in Dentistry, Six East Union Avenue, P.O. Box 551, Bound Brook, NJ 08805; tel. 732/469-9050; FAX. 732/271-1985; David Crystal, D.D.S., Executive Secretary

American Society for Therapeutic Radiology and Oncology, 12500 Fair Lakes Circle, Suite 375, Fairfax, VA 22033-3882; tel. 703/502-1550; FAX. 703/502-7852; Frank Malouff, Executive Director

American Society of Anesthesiologists, 520 North Northwest Highway, Park Ridge, IL 60068; tel. 847/825-5586; FAX. 847/825-1692; Glenn W. Johnson, Executive Director

American Society of Clinical Pathologists., (Includes Board of Registry), 2100 West Harrison Street, Chicago, IL 60612-3798; tel. 312/738-1336; FAX. 312/738-9798; Robert C. Rock, M.D., Executive Vice President

American Society of Colon and Rectal Surgeons, 85 West Algonquin Road, Suite 550, Arlington Heights, IL 60005; tel. 847/290-9184; FAX. 847/290-9203; James Slawny, Executive Director

American Society of Consultant Pharmacists, 1321 Duke Street, Alexandria, VA 22314-3563; tel. 703/739-1300; FAX. 703/739-1321; R. Timothy Webster, Executive Director

American Society of Contemporary Medicine and Surgery, 820 N. Orleans, Suite 208, Chicago, IL 60610; tel. 800/621-4002; FAX. 312/440-0580; Randall T. Bellows, M.D., Director

American Society of Contemporary Ophthalmology, 4711 Golf Road, Suite 408, Skokie, IL 60076; tel. 800/621-4002; FAX. 847/568-1527; Randall T. Bellows, M.D., Director

American Society of Cytopathology, 400 West Ninth Street, Suite 201, Wilmington, DE 19801; tel. 302/429-8802; FAX. 302/429-8807; Joseph L. Eckrich, Executive Director

American Society of Dentistry for Children, John Hancock Center, 875 North Michigan Avenue, Suite 4040, Chicago, IL 60611; tel. 312/943-1244; FAX. 312/943-5341; Dr. Peter Fos, Interim Executive Director

American Society of Directors of Volunteer Services (AHA), One North Franklin, Chicago, IL 60606; tel. 312/422-3938; FAX. 312/422-4575; Nancy A. Brown, Executive Director

American Society of Electroneurodiagnostic Technologists, Inc., 204 West Seventh Street, Carroll, IA 51401-2317; tel. 712/792-2978; FAX. 712/792-6962; M. Fran Pedelty, Executive Director

American Society of Group Psychodrama and Psychotherapy, 6728 Old McLean Village Drive, McLean, VA 22101; tel. 703/556-9222; George K. Degnon, Executive Director

Organizations / National Organizations

American Society of Health-System Pharmacists, 7272 Wisconsin Avenue, Bethesda, MD 20814; tel. 301/657-3000; FAX. 301/664-8872; Henri R. Manasse, Jr., Executive VP and CEO

American Society of Internal Medicine, 2011 Pennsylvania Avenue, N.W., Suite 800, Washington, DC 20006-1808; tel. 202/835-2746; FAX. 202/835-0443; Alan R. Nelson, M.D., Executive Vice President

American Society of Law, Medicine & Ethics, 765 Commonwealth Avenue, 16th Floor, Boston, MA 02215; tel. 617/262-4990; FAX. 617/437-7596; Benjamin W. Moulton, JD, MPH, Executive Director

American Society of Maxillofacial Surgeons, 444 East Algonquin Road, Arlington Heights, IL 60005; tel. 847/228-8375; FAX. 847/228-6509; Gina Cappellania, Administrative Coordinator

American Society of Neuroimaging, 5841 Cedar Lake Road, Suite 204, Minneapolis, MN 55416; tel. 612/545-6291; FAX. 612/545-6073; Theresa Gutoski, Society Manager

American Society of Plastic Surgeons, 444 East Algonquin Road, Arlington Heights, IL 60005; tel. 847/228-9900; FAX. 847/228-9517; Thomas C. Adams, CAE, Executive Director

American Society of Radiologic Technologists, 15000 Central Avenue, S.E., Albuquerque, NM 87123-3917; tel. 505/298-4500; FAX. 505/298-5063; Joan L. Parsons, Executive Vice President, Operations

American Speech-Language-Hearing Association, 10801 Rockville Pike, Rockville, MD 20852; tel. 301/897-5700; FAX. 301/571-0457; Frederick T. Spahr, Ph.D., Executive Director

American Surgical Association, 13 Elm Street, Manchester, MA 01944; tel. 978/526-8330; FAX. 978/526-4018; Carlos A. Pellegrini, M.D., Secretary

American Thoracic Society, 1740 Broadway, New York, NY 10019-4374; tel. 212/315-8700; FAX. 212/315-6498; Carl C. Booberg, Executive Director

American Thyroid Association, Inc., Townhouse Office Park, 55 Old Nyack turnpike – Suite 611, Nanuet, NY 10954; tel. 914/623-1800; FAX. 914/623-3736; Diane P. Miller, Administrator

American Trauma Society, 8903 Presidential Parkway, Suite 512, Upper Marlboro, MD 20772-2656; tel. 800/556-7890; FAX. 301/420-0617; Harry Teter, Executive Director

American Urological Association, Inc., 1120 North Charles Street, Baltimore, MD 21201; tel. 410/727-1100; FAX. 410/223-4370; G. James Gallagher, Executive Director

AORN, Association of Operating Room Nurses, Inc., 2170 South Parker Road, Suite 300, Denver, CO 80231-5711; tel. 303/755-6300; FAX. 303/750-2927; Pat Palmer, RN, M.S., CAE, MNM, Executive Director

Arthritis Foundation, 1330 West Peachtree Street, Atlanta, GA 30309; tel. 404/872-7100; FAX. 404/872-3458; Don L. Riggin, President and CEO

Association for Applied Psychophysiology and Biofeedback, 10200 West 44th Avenue, Suite 304, Wheat Ridge, CO 80033; tel. 303/422-8436; FAX. 303/422-8894; Francine Butler, Ph.D., Executive Director

Association for Clinical Pastoral Education, Inc., 1549 Clairmont Road, Suite 103, Decatur, GA 30033; tel. 404/320-1472; FAX. 404/320-0849; Teresa E. Snorton, Executive Director

Association for Healthcare Philanthropy, 313 Park Avenue, Suite 400, Falls Church, VA 22046; tel. 703/532-6243; FAX. 703/532-7170; Dr. William C. McGinly, CAE, President and CEO

Association for Healthcare Resource Materials Management (AHA), One North Franklin, Chicago, IL 60606-3491; tel. 312/422-3840; FAX. 312/422-4573; Albert J. Sunseri, Ph.D., Executive Director

Association for Hospital Medical Education, 1200 19th Street, N.W., Suite 300, Washington, DC 20036-2422; tel. 202/857-1196; FAX. 202/223-4579; Dennis Smeage, Executive Director

Association for Professionals in Infection Control and Epidemiology, 1275 K Street. NW, Suite 1000, Washington, DC 20005; tel. 202/789-1890; FAX. 202/789-1899; Christopher E. Laxton, Executive Director

Association for Quality HealthCare, Inc., P.O. Box 670, Columbus, GA 31902; tel. 404/571-2122; FAX. 404/571-2650; L. B. Skip Teaster, Executive Director

Association for the Advancement of Automotive Medicine, 2340 DesPlaines Avenue, Suite 106, Des Plaines, IL 60018; tel. 847/390-8927; FAX. 847/390-9962; Elaine Petrucelli, Executive Director

Association for the Advancement of Medical Instrumentation, 3330 Washington Boulevard, Suite 400, Arlington, VA 22201-4598; tel. 703/525-4890; FAX. 703/276-0793; Maureen Malinowski, Director for Educational Activities

Association of American Medical Colleges, 2450 N Street, N.W., Washington, DC 20037-1127; tel. 202/828-0400; FAX. 202/828-1125; Jordan J. Cohen, M.D., President

Association of American Physicians, Krannert Institute of Cardiology, Indiana University School of Medicine, Indianapolis, IN 46202-4800; tel. 317/630-7712; FAX. 317/274-9697; David R. Hathaway, M.D., Secretary

Association of American Physicians and Surgeons, Inc., 1601 North Tucson Boulevard, Suite Nine, Tucson, AZ 85716; tel. 520/327-4885; FAX. 520/325-4230; Jane M. Orient, M.D., Executive Director

Association of Birth Defect Children, 930 Woodcock Road, Suite 270, Orlando, FL 32803; tel. 407/245-7035; FAX. 407/245-7087; Betty Mekdeci, Executive Director

Association of Community Cancer Centers, 11600 Nebel Street, Suite 201, Rockville, MD 20852-2587; tel. 301/984-9496; FAX. 301/770-1949; Lee E. Mortenson, DPA, Executive Director

Association of Mental Health Administrators, 60 Revere Drive, Suite 500, Northbrook, IL 60062; tel. 847/480-9626; FAX. 847/480-9282; Alison C. Brown, Executive Director

Association of Professional Chaplains, 1701 East Woodfield Road, Suite 311, Schaumburg, IL 60173-5191; tel. 847/240-1014; FAX. 847/240-1015; Jo Schrader, Executive Administrator

Association of Schools of Allied Health Professions, 1730 M Street, N.W., Suite 500, Washington, DC 20036; tel. 202/293-4848; FAX. 202/293-4852; Thomas W. Elwood, Dr. P.H., Executive Director

Association of Schools of Public Health, Inc., 1660 L Street, N.W., Suite 204, Washington, DC 20036; tel. 202/296-1099; FAX. 202/296-1252; Michael K. Gemmell, CAE, Executive Director

Association of Specialized and Cooperative Library Agencies A Division of the American Library Ass., 50 East Huron Street, Chicago, IL 60611; tel. 312/280-4399; FAX. 312/944-8085; Cathleen Bourdon, ASCLA, Executive Director

Association of State and Territorial Health Officials, 1275 K Street, NW, Suite 800, Washington, DC 20005-4006; tel. 202/371-9090; FAX. 202/371-9797; Cheryl A. Beversdorf, RN, M.H.S., CAE, Executive Vice President

Association of Surgical Technologists, Inc., 7108–C South Alton Way, Englewood, CO 80112-2106; tel. 303/694-9130; FAX. 303/694-9169; William J. Teutsch, Executive Director

Association of University Anesthesiologists, 2150 N. 107th Street, Suite 205, Seattle, WA 98133-9009; tel. 206/367-8704; FAX. 206/367-8777; Shirley Bishop

Association of University Programs in Health Administration, 1110 Vermont Avenue, NW, Suite 220, Washington, DC 20005-3500; tel. 202/822-8550; FAX. 202/822-8555; Janet Porter, Ph.D., Interim President and CEO

Asthma and Allergy Foundation of America, 1233 20th Street,NW, Suite 402, Washington, DC 20036; tel. 202/466-7643; FAX. 202/466-8940; Mary E. Worstell, MPH, Executive Director

Asthma Foundation of Southern Arizona, P.O. Box 30069, Tucson, AZ 85751-0069; tel. 602/323-6046; FAX. 602/324-1137; Lynn Krust, Executive Director

B

Banner Health System, Box 6200, 4310 17th Avenue, S.W., Fargo, ND 58106-6200; tel. 701/277-7500; FAX. 701/277-7636; Steven R. Orr, Chairman and CEO

BCS Financial Corporation, 676 North St. Clair, Chicago, IL 60611; tel. 312/951-7700; FAX. 312/951-7777; Edward J. Baran, Chairman and CEO

Bereavement Services, Gundersen Lutheran Medical Center, 1910 South Avenue, La Crosse, WI 54601; tel. 800/362-9567; FAX. 608/791-5137; Fran Rybarik, Director

Biological Photographic Association, Inc., 1819 Peachtree Road, N.E., Suite 620, Atlanta, GA 30309; tel. 404/351-6300; FAX. 404/351-3348; William Just, Executive Director

Biological Stain Commission, Inc., University of Rochester, Department Pathology, Rochester, NY 14642-0001; tel. 716/275-6335; FAX. 716/442-8993; David P. Penney, Ph.D., Treasurer

Blinded Veterans Association, 477 H Street, N.W., Washington, DC 20001; tel. 800/669-7079; FAX. 202/371-8258; Thomas H. Miller, Executive Director

Blue Cross and Blue Shield Association, 225 N. Michigan Avenue, Chicago, IL 60601; tel. 312/297-6010; FAX. 312/297-6120; Ray McCaskey, President and CEO

C

Catholic Health Association of the United States, 4455 Woodson Road, St. Louis, MO 63134-3797; tel. 314/427-2500; FAX. 314/427-0029; Rev. Michael D. Place, STD, President and CEO

Catholic Medical Association, 850 Elm Grove Road, Elm Grove, WI 53122; tel. 414/784-3435; FAX. 414/782-8788; Michael J. Herzog, Executive Director

Center for Health Administration Studies, University of Chicago, 969 East 60th Street, Chicago, IL 60637; tel. 773/702-7104; FAX. 773/702-7222; Kristiana Raube, Ph.D., Acting Director

Central Neuropsychiatric Association, 128 East Milltown Road, Wooster, OH 44691; tel. 330/345-6555; FAX. 330/345-6648; Dennis O. Helmuth, M.D., Secretary-Treasurer

Central Surgical Association, Loyola University Medical Center, Department of Surgery, 2160 South First Avenue, Maywood, IL 60153; tel. 708/327-2685; FAX. 708/327-2810; William H. Baker, M.D., Secretary-CSA

Children's Rights Council (CRC), formerly National Council for Children's Rights, 300 Eye Street, N.E., Suite 401, Washington, DC 20002; tel. 202/547-6227; FAX. 202/546-4272; David E. Levy, Esq., President & Chief Executive Officer

Christian Record Services, Inc., 4444 South 52nd Street, Lincoln, NE 68516; tel. 402/488-0981; FAX. 402/488-7582; Ron Bowes, Public Relations Director

College of American Pathologists, 325 Waukegan Road, Northfield, IL 60093-2750; tel. 847/832-7000; FAX. 847/832-8151; Lee VanBremen, Ph.D., Executive Vice President

Commission on Accreditation of Rehabilitation Facilities, 4891 East Grant Road, Tucson, AZ 85712; tel. 520/325-1044; FAX. 520/318-1129; Donald E. Galvin, Ph.D., President & Chief Executive Officer

Committee of Interns and Residents, 386 Park Avenue, S., New York, NY 10016; tel. 212/725-5500; FAX. 212/779-2413; John Ronches, Executive Director

Cooley's Anemia Foundation, Inc., 129-09 26th Avenue, Suite 203, Flushing, NY 11354; tel. 800/522-7222; FAX. 718/321-3340; Gina Cioffi, Esq. National Executive Director

Organizations / National Organizations

Corporate Angel Network, Inc., CAN (Arranges Free Air Transportation for Cancer Patients, Westchester County Airport, One Loop Road, White Plains, NY 10604; tel. 914/328-1313; FAX. 914/328-4226; Liz Lockwood, Director of Volunteers

Council of Jewish Federations, Inc., 730 Broadway, New York, NY 10003; tel. 212/475-5000; FAX. 212/529-5842; Martin S. Kraar, Executive Vice President

Council of Medical Specialty Societies, 51 Sherwood Terrace, Suite M, Lake Bluff, IL 60044; tel. 847/295-3456; FAX. 847/295-3759; Rebecca R. Gschwend, M.A., M.B.A., Executive Vice President

Council of State Administrators of Vocational Rehabilitation, P.O. Box 3776, Washington, DC 20007; tel. 202/638-4634; Jack G. Duncan, General Counsel, Rehabilitation Policy

Council on Education for Public Health, 1015 Fifteenth Street, N.W., Washington, DC 20005; tel. 202/789-1050; FAX. 202/789-1895; Patricia P. Evans, Executive Director

Council on Social Work Education, 1600 Duke Street, Alexandria, VA 22314; tel. 703/683-8080; FAX. 703/683-8099; Donald W. Beless, Ph.D., Executive Director

Crohn's and Colitis Foundation of America, Inc., 386 Park Avenue, S., 17th Floor, New York, NY 10016-8804; tel. 800/932-2423; FAX. 212/779-4098; James V. Romano, Ph. D., President and CEO

Cystic Fibrosis Foundation, 6931 Arlington Road, Bethesda, MD 20814; tel. 301/951-4422; FAX. 301/951-6378; Robert J. Beally, Ph.D., President and CEO

D

Damien Dutton Society for Leprosy Aid, Inc., 616 Bedford Avenue, Bellmore, NY 11710; tel. 516/221-5829; FAX. 516/221-5909; Howard E. Crouch, President

Delta Dental Plans Association, 211 East Chicago Avenue, Suite 800, Chicago, IL 60611; tel. 312/337-4707; FAX. 312/337-7991; James Bonk, President

Dermatology Foundation, 1560 Sherman Avenue, Evanston, IL 60201-4802; tel. 847/328-2256; FAX. 847/328-0509; Sandra Rahn Goldman, Executive Director

Dietary Managers Association, 406 Surrey Woods Drive, St. Charles, IL 60174; tel. 630/587-6336; FAX. 630/587-6308; William St. John, President

Dysautonomia Foundation, Inc., 20 East 46th Street, Suite 302, New York, NY 10017; tel. 212/949-6644; FAX. 212/682-7625; Lenore F. Roseman, Executive Director

E

Easter Seals, Inc., 230 West Monroe Street, Suite 1800, Chicago, IL 60606-4802; tel. 312/726-6200; FAX. 312/726-1494; James E. Williams, Jr., President and CEO

Eastern Orthopaedic Association, Inc., Pier Five North, Suite 5D, Seven North Columbus Boulevard, Philadelphia, PA 19106-1486; tel. 215/351-4110; FAX. 215/351-1825; Elizabeth F. Capella, Executive Director

ECRI, 5200 Butler Pike, Plymouth Meet, PA 19462; tel. 610/825-6000; FAX. 610/834-1275; Joel J. Nobel, M.D., President

Educational Commission for Foreign Medical Graduates, 3624 Market Street, Philadelphia, PA 19104-2685; tel. 215/386-5900; FAX. 215/387-9963; Nancy E. Gary, M.D., President and CEO

Ehlers-Danlos National Foundation, P.O. Box 13157, Richmond, VA 23225; tel. 804/320-8192; FAX. 804/320-8192; Susan L. Stephenson, Vice President, Patient Advocate

Emergency Nurses Association, 216 Higgins Road, Park Ridge, IL 60068-5736; tel. 847/698-9400; FAX. 847/698-9406; Executive Office

Epilepsy Foundation of America, 4351 Garden City Drive, Landover, MD 20785-2267; tel. 301/459-3700; FAX. 301/577-2684; Eric Hargis, Chief Executive Officer

Epilepsy Foundation of Connecticut, 1800 Silas Deane Highway, Suite 168, Rocky Hill, CT 06067; tel. 860/721-9226; Linda Wallace

F

Federation of American Health Systems, 1111 19th Street, N.W., Suite 402, Washington, DC 20036; tel. 202/833-3090; FAX. 202/861-0063; Thomas A. Scully, President & Chief Executive Officer

Federation of State Medical Boards of the United States, Inc., 400 Fuller Wiser Road, Suite 300, Euless, TX 76039-3855; tel. 817/868-4000; FAX. 817/868-4099; James R. Winn, M.D., Executive Vice President

Financial Accounting Standards Board, 401 Merritt 7, P.O. Box 5116, Norwalk, CT 06856-5116; tel. 203/847-0700; FAX. 203/849-9714; Timothy S. Lucas, Director, Research, Technical Activities

Foundation for Chiropractic Education and Research, 1330 Beacon Street, Suite 315, Brookline, MA 02146-3202; tel. 617/734-3397; FAX. 617/734-0989; Anthony L. Rosner, Ph.D., Director of Research and Education

G

Gerontological Society of America, 1030 15 Street, NW, suite 250, Washington, DC 20005-1503; tel. 202/842-1275; FAX. 202/842-1150; Carol A. Schutz, Executive Director

Great Plains Health Alliance, Inc., 625 Third Street, Box 366, Phillipsburg, KS 67661; tel. 785/543-2111; FAX. 785/543-5098; Roger S. John, President and CEO

Guide Dog Users, Inc., 57 Grandview Avenue, Watertown, MA 02472; tel. 617/926-9198; FAX. 617-923-0004; Kim Charlson, Editor

H

Health Industry Distributors Association, 66 Canal Center Plaza, Suite 520, Alexandria, VA 22314-1591; tel. 703/549-4432; FAX. 703/549-6495; S. Wayne Kay, President & Chief Executive Officer

Health Industry Manufacturers Association, 1200 G Street, N.W., Suite 400, Washington, DC 20005; tel. 202/783-8700; FAX. 202/783-8750; Alan H. Magazine, President

Health Research and Educational Trust, One North Franklin, Chicago, IL 60606; tel. 312/422-2624; FAX. 312/422-4568; Deborah Bohr, Vice President

Healthcare Council of MidMichigan, 3927 Beecher Road, Flint, MI 48532; tel. 810/766-8898; FAX. 810/762-4108; Marlene Soderstrom, President

Healthcare Financial Management Association, Two Westbrook Corporate Center, Suite 700, Westchester, IL 60154; tel. 708/531-9600; FAX. 708/531-0032; Richard L. Clarke, F.H.F.M.A., President

Healthcare Information and Management Systems Society (HIMSS), 230 East Ohio Street, Suite 500, Chicago, IL 60611-3201; tel. 312/664-4467; FAX. 312/664-6143; John A. Page, Executive Director

HEAR Center, 301 East Del Mar Boulevard, Pasadena, CA 91101; tel. 626/796-2016; FAX. 626/796-2320; Josephine Wilson, Executive Director

Hispanic American Geriatrics Society, One Cutts Road, Durham, NH 03824-3102; tel. 603/868-5757; Eugene E. Tillock, Ed.D., President

Histochemical Society, Inc., Department of Neurology, University of Washington, Seattle, WA 98195; tel. 206/764-2088; FAX. 206/764-2164

Huntington's Disease Society of America, Inc., 158 West 29th Street, 7th Floor, New York, NY 10001-5300; tel. 800/345-HDSA; FAX. 212/243-2443; Barbara T. Boyle, National Executive Director/CEO

I

Institutes for the Achievement of Human Potential, 8801 Stenton Avenue, Wyndmoor, PA 19038; tel. 215/233-2050; FAX. 215/233-3940; Coralee Thompson, M.D.

InterHealth, P.O. Box 10624, White Bear Lake, MN 55110; tel. 612/407-7075; FAX. 612/407-7077; Thomas LaMotte, Chairman of the Board

International Childbirth Education Association, Inc., P.O. Box 20048, Minneapolis, MN 55420-0048; tel. 612/854-8660; FAX. 612/854-8772; Doris Olson, Administrator

International College of Surgeons/United States Section, 1516 North Lake Shore Drive, Chicago, IL 60610-1694; tel. 312/787-6274; FAX. 312/787-9289; Susan Zelner, Director, Meeting and Publications

International Council for Health, Physical Education, Recreation, Sport and Dance, 1900 Association Drive, Reston, VA 20191; tel. 703/476-3486; FAX. 703/476-9527; Dr. Dong Ja Yang, Secretary General

Intravenous Nurses Society, Inc., Fresh Pond Square, 10 Fawcett Street, Cambridge, MA 02138; tel. 617/441-3008; FAX. 617/576-5452; Mary Alexander, Chief Executive Officer

J

John Milton Society for the Blind, 475 Riverside Drive, Suite 455, New York, NY 10115; tel. 212/870-3335; FAX. 212/870-3229; Darcy Quigley, Executive Director

Joint Commission on Accreditation of Healthcare Organizations, One Renaissance Boulevard, Oakbrook Terr, IL 60181; tel. 630/792-5000; FAX. 630/792-5005; Dennis S. O'Leary, M.D., President

L

Lamaze International, Inc., (formerly ASPO/LAMAZE), 1200 19th Street, N.W., Suite 300, Washington, DC 20036; tel. 800/368-4404; FAX. 202/828-6051; Linda L. Harmon, Executive Director

Lupus Foundation of America, Inc., 1300 Piccard Drive, Suite 200, Rockville, MD 20850; tel. 301/670-9292; FAX. 301/670-9486; Anne Rapoza, Health Educator

M

March of Dimes Birth Defects Foundation, 1275 Mamaroneck Avenue, White Plains, NY 10605; tel. 914/428-7100; FAX. 914/428-8203; Jennifer L. Howse, Ph.D., President

Medical Group Management Association, 104 Inverness Terrace, E., Englewood, CO 80112-5306; tel. 888/608-5601; FAX. 303/643-4427; Thomas L. Adams, CAE, Chief Executive Officer

Medical Library Association, 65 East Wacker Drive, Suite 1900, Chicago, IL 60601-7298; tel. 312/419-9094; FAX. 312/419-8950; Carla J. Funk, Executive Director

MedicAlert Foundation, 2323 Colorado Avenue, Turlock, CA 95382; tel. 800/825-3785; FAX. 209/669-2495; David Roth, Public Relations

Mended Hearts, Inc., 7272 Greenville Avenue, Dallas, TX 75231; tel. 214/706-1442; FAX. 214/706-5231; Darla Bonham, Executive Director

Muscular Dystrophy Association, 3300 East Sunrise Drive, Tucson, AZ 85718; tel. 520/529-2000; FAX. 520/529-5400; Robert Ross, Senior VP and Executive Director

N

National Academy of Sciences, National Research Council/Commission on Life Sciences, 2101 Constitution Avenue, N.W., NAS 343, Washington, DC 20418; tel. 202/334-2500; FAX. 202/334-1639; Paul Gilman, Ph.D., Executive Director

National Accreditation Council for Agencies Serving the Blind, 260 Northland Blvd., Suite 233, Cincinnati, OH 45246; tel. 513/772-8449; FAX. 513/772-8854; Dr. Gerald W. Mundy, Executive Director

National Accrediting Agency for Clinical Laboratory Sciences, 8410 West Bryn Mawr, Suite 670, Chicago, IL 60631-3415; tel. 773/714-8880; FAX. 773/714-8886; Olive M. Kimball, Executive Director

National Alliance for the Mentally Ill, Colonial Place Three, 2107 Wilson Blvd, Suite 300, Arlington, VA 22203-3754; tel. 703/524-7600; FAX. 703/524-9094; Laurie Flynn, Executive Director

National Assembly on School Based Health Care, 666 11th Street, NW, Suite 735, Washington, DC 20005; tel. 202/638-5872; FAX. 202/638-5879; John Schlitt, Executive Director

National Association for Home Care, 228 Seventh Street, S.E., Washington, DC 20003; tel. 202/547-7424; FAX. 202/547-3540; Val J. Halamandaris, President

National Association for Medical Equipment Services (NAMES), 625 Slaters Lane, Suite 200, Alexandria, VA 22314-1171; tel. 703/836-6263; FAX. 703/836-6730; William D. Coughlan, CAE, President and CEO

National Association for Practical Nurse Education and Service, 1400 Spring Street, Suite 330, Silver Spring, MD 20910; tel. 301/588-2491; FAX. 301/588-2839; John H. Word, LPN, Executive Director

National Association Medical Staff Services, 631 East Butterfield, Suite 311, Lombard, IL 60148; tel. 630/271-9814; FAX. 630/271-0295; Robert A. Dengler, CAE, CMP, Executive Director

National Association of Boards of Pharmacy, 700 Busse Highway, Park Ridge, IL 60068; tel. 847/698-6227; FAX. 847/698-0124; Carmen A. Catizone, R.Ph., M.S., Executive Director/Secretary

National Association of Children's Hospitals and Related Institutes, 401 Wythe Street, Alexandria, VA 22314; tel. 703/684-1355; FAX. 703/684-1589; Lawrence A. McAndrews, President and CEO

National Association of Childrens Hospitals, 401 Wythe Street, Alexandria, VA 22314; tel. 703/684-1355; FAX. 703/684-1589; Lawrence A. McAndrews, President and CEO

National Association of Dental Assistants, 900 South Washington, Suite G13, Falls Church, VA 22046; tel. 703/237-8616; S. Young, Director

National Association of Dental Laboratories, (Includes National Board for Certification in Dental Laboratory Technology), 8201 Greensboro Drive, Suite 300, McLean, VA 22102; tel. 800/950-1150; FAX. 703/610-9005; Nattily Dang, Office Administrator

National Association of Health Services Executives, 8630 Fenton Street, Suite 126, Silver Spring, MD 20910; tel. 202/628-3953; FAX. 301/588-0011; Ozzie Jenkins, CMP, Executive Director

National Association of Hospital Hospitality Houses, Inc., 4915 Auburn Avenue, Suite 303, Bethesda, MD 20814; tel. 800/542-9730; FAX. 301/961-3094; Martha J. Lockwood, CAE, APR, Executive Director

National Association of Institutional Laundry Managers, 781 Twin Oaks Avenue, Chula Vista, CA 92010; tel. 619/420-1396; FAX. 619/420-1396; Betty Conard, Executive Secretary

National Association of Psychiatric Health Systems, 325 Seventh Street, NW, Suite 625, Washington, DC 20004-2802; tel. 202/393-6700; FAX. 202/783-6041; Mark J. Covall, Executive Director

National Association of Social Workers, Inc., 750 First Street, N.E., Suite 700, Washington, DC 20002; tel. 202/408-8600; FAX. 202/336-8311; Senior Staff Associate, Health, Mental

National Association of State Mental Health Program Directors, 66 Canal Center Plaza, Suite 302, Alexandria, VA 22314; tel. 703/739-9333; FAX. 703/548-9517; Robert W. Glover, Ph.D., Executive Director

National Board for Respiratory Care, 8310 Nieman Road, Lenexa, KS 66214; tel. 913/599-4200; FAX. 913/541-0156; Steven K. Bryant, Executive Director

National Board of Anesthesiology, Inc, 308 Maine Street, Lawrence, KS 66044; tel. 785/842-7067; FAX. 785/842-7088; Thomas Nique, M.D., D.D.S., President

National Board of Medical Examiners, 3750 Market Street, Philadelphia, PA 19104; tel. 215/590-9500; FAX. 215/590-9755; L. Thompson Bowles, M.D., Ph.D., President

National Children's Eye Care Foundation, P.O. Box 795069, Dallas, TX 75379-5069; tel. 972/407-0404; FAX. 972/407-0616; Suzanne C. Beauchamp, Administrator

National Council on Alcoholism and Drug Dependence, Inc., 12 West 21st Street, New York, NY 10010; tel. 212/206-6770; FAX. 212/645-1690; Jeffrey Hon, Director, Public Information

National Council on Radiation Protection and Measurements, 7910 Woodmont Avenue, Suite 800, Bethesda, MD 20814; tel. 301/657-2652; FAX. 301/907-8768; William M. Beckner, Executive Director

National Council on the Aging, Inc., 409 Third Street, S.W., Suite 200, Washington, DC 20024; tel. 202/479-1200; FAX. 202/479-0735; James Firman, President

National Dental Association, 5506 Connecticut Avenue, N.W., Suite 24-25, Washington, DC 20015; tel. 202/244-7555; FAX. 202/244-5992; Robert S. Johns, Executive Director

National Depressive and Manic-Depressive Association, 730 North Franklin Street, Suite 501, Chicago, IL 60610; tel. 312/642-0049; FAX. 312/642-7243; Lydia Lewis, Executive Director

National Environmental Health Association, 720 South Colorado Boulevard, South Tower, Suite, Denver, CO 80222; tel. 303/756-9090; FAX. 303/691-9490; Nelson Fabian, Executive Director

National Federation of Licensed Practical Nurses, 893 Highway, 70 West, Suite 202, Garner, NC 27529; tel. 919/779-0046; FAX. 919/779-5642; Charlene Barbour, Executive Director

National Fire Protection Association, P.O. Box 9101, One Batterymarck Park, Quincy, MA 02269-9101; tel. 617/770-3000; FAX. 617/770-7110; Craig H. Kampmier, Sr Fire Protection Specialist

National Gaucher Foundation, 11140 Rockville Pike, Suite 350, Rockville, MD 20852; tel. 301/816-1515; FAX. 301/816-1516; Rhonda Buyers, Executive Director

National Headache Foundation, 428 West St. James Place, Second Floor, Chicago, IL 60614-2750; tel. 888/NHF-5552; FAX. 773/525-7357; Suzanne Simons, Executive Director

National Health Council, Inc., 1730 M Street, N.W., Suite 500, Washington, DC 20036; tel. 202/785-3910; FAX. 202/785-5923; Myrl Weinberg, CAE, President

National Hemophilia Foundation, 116 West 32nd Street, 11th Floor, New York, NY 10001; tel. 212/328-3700; FAX. 212/328-9247; Stephen E. Bajard, Executive Director

National Institute for Jewish Hospice, Central Telephone Network, P.O. Box 48025, Los Angeles, CA 90048; tel. 800/446-4448; Levana Lev, Executive Director

National Kidney Foundation, 30 East 33rd Street, New York, NY 10016; tel. 800/622-9010; FAX. 212/779-0068; John Davis, Chief Executive Officer

National Medical Association, 1012 10th Street, N.W., Washington, DC 20001; tel. 202/347-1895; FAX. 202/842-3293; Lorraine Cole, Ph.D., Executive Director

National Mental Health Association, 1021 Prince Street, Alexandria, VA 22314-2971; tel. 703/684-7722; FAX. 703/684-5968; Michael M. Faenza, President and CEO

National Multiple Sclerosis Society, 733 Third Avenue, New York, NY 10017; tel. 212/986-3240; FAX. 212/986-7981; Dwayne Howell, Executive Vice President

National Parkinson Foundation, Inc., 1501 Northwest Ninth Avenue, Miami, FL 33136-1494; tel. 305/547-6666; FAX. 305/548-4403; Brian Morton, Controller

National Perinatal Association, 3500 East Fletcher Avenue, Suite 209, Tampa, FL 33613-4712; tel. 813/971-1008; FAX. 813/971-9306; Sheila S. Sorkin, Executive Director

National Recreation and Park Association, 22377 Belmont Ridge Road, Ashburn, VA 20148; tel. 703/858-0784; FAX. 703/858-0794; R. Dean Tice, Executive Director

National Registry of Certified Chemists, 815 15th Street, N.W., Suite 508, Washington, DC 20005; tel. 202/393-7140; FAX. 202/393-4059; Gilbert E. Smith, Ph.D., Executive Director

National Registry of Emergency Medical Technicians, 6610 Busch Boulevard, P.O. Box 29233, Columbus, OH 43229; tel. 614/888-4484; William E. Brown, Jr., Executive Director

National Rehabilitation Association, (Includes Nine National Associations and 58 Affiliate Chapters), 633 South Washington Street, Alexandria, VA 22314; tel. 703/836-0850; FAX. 703/836-0848; Michelle A. Vaughan, Executive Director

National Resident Matching Program, 2450 N Street, N.W., Suite 201, Washington, DC 20037-1141; tel. 202/828-0676; FAX. 202/828-1121; Robert L. Beran, Ph. D., Deputy Executive Director

National Rural Health Association, 1320 19th Street, N.W., Suite 350, Washington, DC 20036-1610; tel. 202/232-6200; FAX. 202/232-1133; Darin E. Johnson, Vice President for Policy and Public Affairs

National Safety Council, P.O. Box 558, Itasca, IL 60143-0558; tel. 800/621-7619; FAX. 630/285-0797; Customer Service Department

National Student Nurses' Association, Inc., 555 West 57th Street, Suite 1327, New York, NY 10019; tel. 212/581-2211; FAX. 212/581-2368; Diane J. Mancino, Ed.D., RN, CAE, Executive Director

National Tay-Sachs and Allied Diseases Association, 2001 Beacon Street, Suite 204, Brighton, MA 02135; tel. 800/90-NTSAD; FAX. 617/277-0134; Jayne C. Gershkowitz, Executive Director

New England Gerontological Association, One Cutts Road, Durham, NH 03824-3102; tel. 603/868-5757; Eugene E. Tillock, Ed.D., Executive Director

Organizations / National Organizations

NSF International, 789 Dixboro Road, P.O. Box 130140, Ann Arbor, MI 48113–0140; tel. 313/769–8010; FAX. 313/769–0109; Dennis R. Mangino, Ph. D., President and CEO

O

Osteogenesis Imperfecta Foundation, Inc., 804 West Diamond Avenue, Suite 210, Gaithersburg, MD 20878; tel. 301/947–0083; FAX. 301/947–0456; Heller An Shapiro, Executive Director

P

Pan American Health Organization, 525 23rd Street, N.W., Washington, DC 20037; tel. 202/974–3000; Daniel Lopez Acuna, Director, HSP

Parkinson's Disease Foundation, Inc, (Formerly United Parkinson Foundation), 833 West Washington Boulevard, Chicago, IL 60607; tel. 312/733–1893; FAX. 312/733–1896; Jeanne Lee – Rosner, Manager

Physician Executive Management Center, 3403 West Fletcher Avenue, Tampa, FL 33618–2813; tel. 813/963–1800; FAX. 813/264–2207; David R. Kirschman, President

Pilot Dogs, Inc., 625 West Town Street, Columbus, OH 43215; tel. 614/221–6367; FAX. 614/221–1577; J. Jay Gray, Executive Director

Prevent Blindness America, 500 East Remington Road, Schaumburg, IL 60173–4557; tel. 800/331–2020; FAX. 847/843–8458; Richard T. Hellner, President and CEO

Public Relations Society of America, 33 Irving Place, New York, NY 10003–2376; tel. 212/995–2230; FAX. 212/995–0757; Ray Gaulke, President and COO

R

Radiological Society of North America, Inc., 820 Jorie Boulevard, Oak Brook, IL 60523; tel. 630/571–2670; FAX. 630/571–7837; Joe Taylor, Marketing Communications

Recording for the Blind and Dyslexic, 20 Roszel Road, Princeton, NJ 08540; tel. 609/452–0606; FAX. 609/520–7990; Richard O. Scribner, President

Renal Physicians Association, 2011 Pennsylvania Avenue, N.W., Suite 800, Washington, DC 20006–1808; tel. 202/835–0436; FAX. 202/835–0443; Dale Singer, MHA, Executive Director

Robert Wood Johnson Foundation, P.O. Box 2316, Route One and College Road East, Princeton, NJ 08543–2316; tel. 609/452–8701; FAX. 609/987–8845; Richard J. Toth, Director, Office of Proposal Management

S

Shriners Hospitals for Children, P.O. Box 31356, Tampa, FL 33631–3356; tel. 813/281–0300; FAX. 813/281–8113; Melody Lewis, Executive Secretary

Sickle Cell Disease Foundation of Greater New York, 127 West 127th Street, Suite 421, New York, NY 10027; tel. 212/865–1500; FAX. 212/865–0917; Beryl Murray, Executive Director

Society for Academic Emergency Medicine, 901 North Washington Avenue, Lansing, MI 48906; tel. 517/485–5484; FAX. 517/485–0801; Mary Ann Schropp, Executive Director

Society for Adolescent Medicine, Inc., 1916 Northwest Copper Oaks Circle, Blue Springs, MO 64015; tel. 816/224–8010; FAX. 816/224–8009; Edie Moore, Administrative Director

Society for Healthcare Consumer Advocacy, One North Franklin, Chicago, IL 60606; tel. 312/422–3774; FAX. 312/422–4580; Eleanore Kirsch, Executive Director

Society for Healthcare Strategy and Market Development, of the American Hospital Association, One North Franklin, 31st Floor, Chicago, IL 60606; tel. 312/422–3888; FAX. 312/422–4579; Lauren A. Barnett, Executive Director

Society for Occupational and Environmental Health, 6728 Old McLean Village Drive, McLean, VA 22101; tel. 703/556–9222; FAX. 703/556–8729; Robin Turner, Account Manager

Society for Pediatric Pathology, 6728 Old McLean Village Drive, McLean, VA 22101; tel. 703/556–9222; FAX. 703/556–8729; Kathryn Kelley, Associate Director

Society for Social Work Administrators in Health Care, One North Franklin, Chicago, IL 60606–3401; tel. 312/422–3774; FAX. 312/422–4580; Eleanore Kirsch, Executive Director

Society of Critical Care Medicine, 8101 East Kaiser Boulevard, Anaheim, CA 92808–2214; tel. 714/282–6000; FAX. 714/282–6050; Steven Seekins, Chief Executive Officer

Society of Neurological Surgeons, New England Medical Center, Department of Neurosurgery, Boston, MA 02111; tel. 617/636–5858; William Shucart, M.D., Secretary

Society of Nuclear Medicine, 1850 Samuel Morse Drive, Reston, VA 22090; tel. 703/708–9000; FAX. 703/708–9015; c/o Administrator

Society of University Otolaryngologists–Head and Neck Surgeons, USC School of Medicine, Department of Otolaryngology, Los Angeles, CA 90083; tel. 323/226–7315; FAX. 323/226–2780; Donna Hoffman, M.A., Executive Director

Southeastern Healthcare Association, 1345 Carmichael Way, P.O. Box 11126, Montgomery, AL 36111–0126; tel. 334/260–8600; FAX. 205/260–0023; Tommy R. McDougal, FACHE, President

T

Technologist Section, Society of Nuclear Medicine, 1850 Samuel Morse Drive, Reston, VA 22090; tel. 703/708–9000; FAX. 703/708–9015; Virginia M. Pappas, Deputy Executive Director

The Alliance For Healthcare Strategy And Marketing, 11 South LaSalle, Suite 2300, Suite 2300, Chicago, IL 60603; tel. 312/704–9700; FAX. 312/704–9709; Carla Windhorst, President

The American Association of Immunologists, 9650 Rockville Pike, Bethesda, MD 20814; tel. 301/530–7178; FAX. 301/571–1816; M. Michele Hogan, Ph.D., Executive Director

The American Board of Obstetrics and Gynecology, Inc., 2915 Vine Street, Dallas, TX 75204; tel. 214/871–1619; FAX. 214/871–1943; Dr. Norman F. Gant, Executive Director

The American Board of Plastic Surgery, Inc., Seven Penn Center, Suite 400, 1635 Market Street, Philadelphia, PA 19103–2204; tel. 215/587–9322; FAX. 215/587–9622; Terry M. Cullison, RN, MSN, Administrator

The American Board of Professional Disability Consultants, 1350 Beverly Road, Suite 115–327, McLean, VA 22101; tel. 703/790–8644; Taras J. Cerkevitch, Ph.D., Director, Operations

The American Board of Urology, Inc., 2216 Ivy Road, Suite 210, Charlottesville, VA 22903; tel. 804/979–0059; FAX. 804/979–0266; Stuart S. Howards, M.D., Executive Secretary

The American Institute of Architects, Academy of Architecture for Health, 1735 New York Avenue, N.W., Washington, DC 20006; tel. 202/626–7429; FAX. 206/626–7518; Gail B. Dym, Director

The American Orthopaedic Association, 6300 North River Road, Suite 300, Rosemont, IL 60018–4263; tel. 847/318–7330; FAX. 847/318–7339; Hildegard A. Weiler, Executive Director

The Arc of the United States, Formerly Association for Retarded Citizens, 500 East Border Street, Suite 300, Arlington, TX 76011; tel. 817/640–0204; FAX. 817/277–3491; Alan Abeson, Ed.D., Executive Director

The Association for Research in Vision and Ophthalmology, 9650 Rockville Pike, Suite 1500, Bethesda, MD 20814–3998; tel. 301/571–1844; FAX. 301/571–8311; Joanne G. Angle, Executive Director

The Association of Medical Illustrators, 1819 Peachtree Street, N.E., Suite 712, Atlanta, GA 30309; tel. 404/350–7900; FAX. 404/351–3348; William H. Just, Executive Director

The Association of Military Surgeons of the United States, 9320 Old Georgetown Road, Bethesda, MD 20814; tel. 301/897–8800; FAX. 301/530–5446; RADM Frederic G. Sanford, MC, USN Ret.

The Association of Women's Health, Obstetric, and Neonatal Nurses, 2000 L. Street, NW, Suite 740, Washington, DC 20036; tel. 202/261–2400; FAX. 201/728–0575; Gail G. Kincaide, Executive Director

The Duke Endowment, 100 North Tryon Street, Suite 3500, Charlotte, NC 28202; tel. 704/376–0291; FAX. 704/376–9336; Elizabeth H. Locke, President

The Endocrine Society, 4350 East West Highway, Suite 500, Bethesda, MD 20814–4410; tel. 301/941–0200; FAX. 301/941–0259; Susan Koppi, Director, Public Affairs

The Foundation Fighting Blindness, Executive Plaza I, Suite 800, 11350 McCormick Road, Hunt Valley, MD 21031–1014; tel. 800/683–5555; FAX. 410/771–9470; Robert M. Gray, Chief Executive Officer

The Foundation for Ichthyosis and Related Skin Types, Inc., (F.I.R.S.T.), 650 N. Cannon Avenue, Suie 17, Lansdale, PA 19446; tel. 215/631–1411; FAX. 215/631–1413; Jean Pickford, Executive Director

The Institute for Rehabilitation and Research, 1333 Moursound, Houston, TX 77030; tel. 713/799–5000; FAX. 713/799–7095; Louisa Adelung, President and CEO

The International Dyslexia Association, (Formerly The Orton Dyslexia Society), Chester Building, Suite 382, 8600 LaSalle Road, Baltimore, MD 21286; tel. 410/296–0232; FAX. 410/321–5069; Judith Dudek, Director, Marketing and Membership

The Leukemia and Lymphoma Society, 600 Third Avenue, New York, NY 10016; tel. 212/573–8484; FAX. 212/856–9686; Dwayne Howell, President and CEO

The Points of Light Foundation, 1737 H Street, N.W., Washington, DC 20006; tel. 202/223–9186; FAX. 202/223–9256; Yael Israel, Customer Information Coordinator

The Salvation Army National Corporation, 615 Slaters Lane, P.O. Box 269, Alexandria, VA 22313; tel. 703/684–5500; FAX. 703/684–3478; Commissioner John Busby, National Commander

The Seeing Eye, Inc., Washington Valley Road, Box 375, Morristown, NJ 07963–0375; tel. 973/539–4425; FAX. 973/539–0922; Kenneth Rosenthal, President

The Southwestern Surgical Congress, 401 North Michigan Avenue, Chicago, IL 60611–4267; tel. 312/527–6667; FAX. 312/321–6869; Thomas E. Stautzenbach, Executive Director

U

UCLA Medical Center, Surgery/Neurosurgery, Box 957039, Room 18–228 NPI, Los Angeles, CA 90095–7039; tel. 310/825–3998; FAX. 310/794–5836; Donald P. Becker, M.D.

Organizations / National Organizations

United Cerebral Palsy Associations, Inc., 1660 L Street, N.W., Suite 700, Washington, DC 20036; tel. 800/872-5827; Kirsten A. Nyrop, Executive Director

United Methodist Association of Health and Welfare Ministries, 601 West Riverview Avenue, Dayton, OH 45406-5543; tel. 937/227-9494; FAX. 937/222-7364; Dean W. Pulliam, President and CEO

United Ostomy Association, Inc., 19772 MacArthur Boulevard, Suite 200, Irvine, CA 92613; tel. 800/826-0826; FAX. 714/660-9262; Darlene A. Smith, Executive Director

United Way of America, 701 North Fairfax Street, Alexandria, VA 22314-2045; tel. 703/836-7100; FAX. 703/683-7840; Betty Stanley Beene, President

USP, 12601 Twinbrook Parkway, Rockville, MD 20852; tel. 301/881-0666; FAX. 301/816-8299; Roger L. Williams, Executive Vice President, Chief Executive Officer

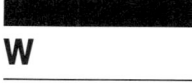

W

Western Orthopaedic Association, 1834 First Street, Suite 3, Napa, CA 94559-2353; tel. 707/259-9481; FAX. 707/259-9486; Susan Hanf, Executive Director

Western Surgical Association, Mayo Clinic, 200 First Street, S.W., Rochester, MN 55905; Jon A. VanHeerden, M.D., Secretary

Healthfinder

Healthfinder® is composed of two listing types: toll–free numbers for health information and federal health information centers and clearinghouses. Toll–free numbers are listed first, followed by the federal numbers.

This file was released for 2000. This document is revised annually.

This Federal document is in the public domain, but is distributed subject to two conditions: 1) Any person or organization posting and/or distributing this document in electronic or paper form MUST respect the integrity of the document and post or distribute it ONLY in its entirety, including this paragraph, and without any change whatsoever; and 2) Any person or organization either posting or distributing this document MUST agree to post and/or distribute future editions of the document in the same manner as this edition to ensure that the most current information is made available to those parties who received the earlier version.

If you would like more information, contact the U.S. Department of Health and Human Services, or visit the internet site at www.healthfinder.net.

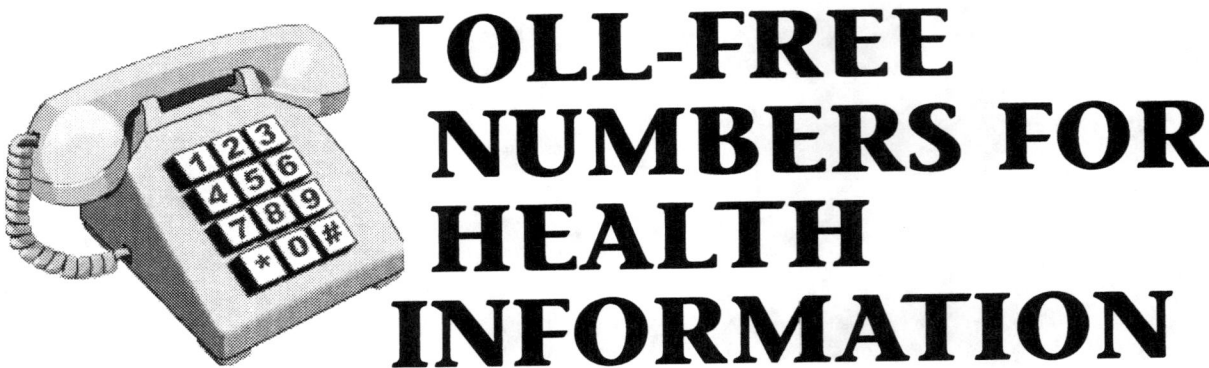

TOLL-FREE NUMBERS FOR HEALTH INFORMATION

These selected toll-free numbers for organizations provide health-related information, education, and support. These organizations do NOT diagnose or recommend treatment for any disease. Some of the organizations use recorded messages; others provide personalized counseling and referrals. Most offer educational materials; some charge handling fees.

Organizations that provide crisis assistance are listed under the heading, *Crisis Intervention*. The *Rare Disorders* category includes diseases and disorders that affect less than 1 percent of the population at any given time. Groups in the *Professional Organizations* section offer consumer information.

Unless otherwise stated, numbers can be reached within the continental United States 24 hours a day, 7 days a week.

Inclusion of an information source in this publication does not imply endorsement by the U.S. Department of Health and Human Services.

This information is in the public domain. Duplication is encouraged.

TOLL-FREE NUMBERS FOR HEALTH INFORMATION 2000

ADOPTION

Bethany Christian Services
(800)238–4269
8 a.m.–12 p.m.

National Adoption Center
(800)TO–ADOPT
9 a.m.–5 p.m.

AGING

American Health Assistance Foundation
(800)437–2423
9 a.m.–5 p.m.

Eldercare Locator
(800)677–1116
9 a.m.–8 p.m.

National Institute on Aging Information Center
(800)222–2225: (800)222–4225 (TTY)
8:30 a.m.–5 p.m.

AIDS/HIV

AIDS Clinical Trials Information Service
(800)874–2572
9 a.m.–7 p.m.

CDC National HIV/AIDS Hotline
(800)342–2437 (English) (24 hours)
(800)344–7432 (Spanish)
(800)243–7889 (TTY)
10 a.m.–10 p.m.

CDC National Prevention Information Network (NPIN)
(800)458–5231; (800)243–7012 (TTY)
(888)282–7681 (Fax)
info@cdcnac.org (E-Mail)
9 a.m.–6 p.m.

HIV/AIDS Treatment Information Service
(800)HIV–0440
9 a.m.–7 p.m. All calls are confidential.

Project Inform National HIV/ AIDS Treatment Hotline
(800)822–7422
9 a.m.–5 p.m., Monday-Friday
10 a.m. - 4:00 p.m. (Pacific) Saturday

ALCOHOL ABUSE

See also DRUG ABUSE

ADCARE Hospital Helpline
(800)ALCOHOL

Al-Anon Family Group Headquarters
(800)356–9996
8 a.m.–6 p.m.

Alcohol and Drug Helpline
(800)821–4357

American Council on Alcoholism
(800)527–5344
9 a.m.–5 p.m.

Calix Society
(800)398-0524
9 a.m.–3 p.m.

Children of Alcoholics Foundation
(800)359-COAF

National Clearinghouse for Alcohol and Drug Information
(800)729–6686; (800)487–4889 (TTY/TDD)
8 a.m.–7 p.m.

National Council on Alcoholism and Drug Dependence, Inc.
(800)622–2255
9 a.m.–5 p.m.

National Woman's Christian Temperance Union
(800)755-1321
9 a.m.–5 p.m. (Central)

ALLERGY/ASTHMA

See LUNG DISEASE/ASTHMA/ALLERGY

The Food Allergy Network
(800)929-4040
9 a.m.–5 p.m.

ALZHEIMER'S DISEASE

See also AGING

Alzheimer's Association
(800)272–3900
The information and referral line is available 24 hours; operators staff the line 8 a.m.–5 p.m. (Central).
Leave message after hours.

Alzheimer's Disease Education and Referral Center
(800)438–4380
adear@alzheimers.org (E-mail)
8:30 a.m.–5 p.m.

ARTHRITIS

American Juvenile Arthritis Organization
(800)283-7800
8:30 a.m.–4:30 p.m.

U.S. DEPARTMENT OF HEALTH AND HUMAN SERVICES, OFFICE OF PUBLIC HEALTH AND SCIENCE

Arthritis Foundation Information Line
(800)283–7800

Lyme Disease Foundation, Inc.
(800)886–5963

AUDIOVISUALS

See LIBRARY SERVICES

AUTISM

See CHILD DEVELOPMENT/PARENTING

AUTOIMMUNE DISEASES

American Autoimmune Related Diseases Association, Inc.
(800)598-4668
9:30 a.m.–5 p.m.

BONE MARROW

See CANCER

BONE DISEASE

Osteoporosis and Related Bone Diseases National Resource Center
(800)624-BONE [(800)624-2663]

BRAIN TUMORS

American Brain Tumor Association
(800)886-2282
8:30 a.m.–5 p.m. (Central)

The Brain Tumor Society
(800)770-TBTS
8:30 a.m.–5:30 p.m.

National Brain Tumor Foundation
(800)934-CURE
9 a.m.–5 p.m. (Pacific)

CANCER

ACS, National Cancer Information Center
(800)227–2345 (Voice/TDD/TT)

Cancer Information Service
(800)422–6237
9 a.m.–4:30 p.m.

Cancer Hope Network
(877)HOPENET
9 a.m.–5:30 p.m.

Candlelighters Childhood Cancer Foundation
(800)366-2223
10 a.m.–4 p.m.

Organizations / Healthfinder

TOLL-FREE NUMBERS FOR HEALTH INFORMATION 2000

Komen Breast Cancer Foundation
(800)462–9273
9 a.m.–4:30 p.m. (Central)

National Alliance of Breast Cancer Organizations
(800)719-9154

National Bone Marrow Transplant Link
(800)546-5268

National Kidney Cancer Association
(800)850-9132
8 a.m.–5 p.m. (Central)

National Marrow Donor Program®
(800)627–7692
Professional staff answer questions from 8 a.m.–6 p.m. (Central); recorded message at all other times.

Reach to Recovery Program
(800)227-2345

Us Too International
(800)808-7866
8:30 a.m.–4:30 p.m. (Central)

Y-Me National Breast Cancer Organization
(800)221–2141 (English)
(800)986–9505 (Spanish)
9 a.m.–5 p.m. (Central)

CEREBRAL PALSY

See RARE DISORDERS

CHEMICAL PRODUCTS/ PESTICIDES

See also HOUSING

Chemtrec Non-Emergency Services Hotline
(800)262–8200
9 a.m.–5 p.m.

National Pesticide Telecommunications Network
(800)858–7378-TDD capability
6:30 a.m.–4:30 p.m. (Pacific)
Voice mail provided for off-hours calls.

CHILD ABUSE/MISSING CHILDREN/MENTAL HEALTH

Boys Town National Hotline
(800)448–3000; (800)448–1833 (TDD)
Spanish-speaking operators available; TDD capability.

Child Find of America, Inc.
(800)426–5678 (I–AM–LOST)
9 a.m.–5 p.m.

A–WAY–OUT
(800)292–9688
9 a.m.–5 p.m.

CHILDHELP/IOF Foresters
National Child Abuse Hotline
(800)422–4453; (800)222–4453 (TDD)

Covenant House Nineline
(800)999–9999

National Center for Missing and Exploited Children
(800)843–5678; (800)826–7653 (TDD)
Ability to serve callers in over 140 languages.

National Child Safety Council Childwatch
(800)222–1464
7 a.m.–3:30 p.m.

National Clearinghouse on Child Abuse and Neglect Information
(800)394–3366
nccanch@calibcom (E-mail)
8:30 a.m.–5:30 p.m.

National Runaway Switchboard
(800)621–4000; (800)621–0394 (TDD)
Has access to AT&T Language Line

National Youth Crisis Hotline
(800)448–4663

CHILD DEVELOPMENT/ PARENTING

Association for the Care of Children's Health
(800)808-2224 x327
9 a.m.–5 p.m.

Association of Birth Defect Children
(800)313–2232

Autism Society of America
(800)328–3476

The MAGIC Foundation for Children's Growth
(800)362–4423
9 a.m.–5 p.m. (Central)

National Association for the Education of Young Children
(800)424–2460
9 a.m.–5 p.m.

National Institute of Child Health and Human Development, Public Information and Communications Branch
(800)505-2742 (SIDS Information Line)
8 a.m.–8 p.m.

National Lekotek Center
(800)366-7529
(800)573-4446 (Voice and TTY)
9 a.m.–5 p.m. (Central)

National Organization on Fetal Alcohol Syndrome
(800)666–6327

Pediatric Projects, Inc.
(800)947-0947

Starlight Children's Foundation
(800)274-7827
9 a.m.–5 p.m. (Pacific)

Zero to Three: National Center for Infants, Toddlers and Families
(800)899-4301
9 a.m.–5 p.m.

U.S. DEPARTMENT OF HEALTH AND HUMAN SERVICES, OFFICE OF PUBLIC HEALTH AND SCIENCE

**TOLL-FREE NUMBERS
FOR HEALTH INFORMATION
2000**

CRISIS INTERVENTION

All operate 24 hours.

Boys Town National Hotline
(800)448–3000
(800)448–1833 (TDD)
Provides short-term intervention and counseling and refers callers to local community resources. Counsels on parent-child conflicts, family issues, suicide, pregnancy, runaway youth, physical and sexual abuse, and other issues that impact children and families. Spanish-speaking operators are available. TDD capability.

A–WAY–OUT
(800)292–9688
Provides unique crisis mediation program for parents contemplating abduction of their children, or who have already abducted their children and want to use Child Find Volunteer Family Mediators to resolve their custody dispute.

**CHILDHELP/IOF Foresters
National Child Abuse Hotline**
(800)422–4453
(800)222–4453 (TDD)
Provides multilingual crisis intervention and professional counseling on child abuse and domestic violence issues. Gives referrals to local agencies offering counseling and other services related to child abuse, adult survivor issues, and domestic violence. Provides literature on child abuse in English and Spanish.

Covenant House Nineline
(800)999–9999
Crisis line for youth, teens, and families. Locally based referrals throughout the United States. Help for youth and parents regarding drugs, abuse, homelessness, runaway children, and message relays.

National Center for Missing and Exploited Children
(800)843–5678
(800)826–7653 (TDD)
Operates a hotline for reporting missing children and sightings of missing children. Offers assistance and training to law enforcement agents. Takes reports of sexually exploited children. Serves as the National Child Porn TipLine. Provides books and other publications on prevention and issues related to missing and sexually exploited children. Ability to serve callers in over 140 languages.

National Runaway Switchboard
(800)621–4000
(800)621–0394 (TDD)
Provides crisis intervention and travel assistance information to runaways. Gives referrals to shelters nationwide. Also relays messages to, or sets up conference calls with, parents at the request of the child. Has access to AT&T Language Line.

National Youth Crisis Hotline
(800)448–4663
Provides counseling and referrals to local drug treatment centers, shelters, and counseling services. Responds to youth dealing with pregnancy, molestation, suicide, and child abuse.

Rape, Abuse, and Incest National Network
(800)656–4673
Connects caller to the nearest counseling center which provides counseling for rape, abuse, and incest victims.

CYSTIC FIBROSIS

See RARE DISORDERS

DIABETES/DIGESTIVE DISEASES

American Association of Diabetes Educators
(800)832–6874

American Diabetes Association
(800)232–3472
(800)ADA–ORDER (Fax, Order Fulfillment)
8:30 a.m.–5 p.m.

Crohn's and Colitis Foundation of America, Inc.
(800)932–2423
(800)343–3637 (Warehouse)
9 a.m.–5 p.m. Recording after hours.
Warehouse is open 8 a.m.–5 p.m.

Juvenile Diabetes Foundation International Hotline
(800)223–1138
9 a.m.–5 p.m.

DISABLING CONDITIONS/DISABILITIES ACCESS

Americans with Disabilities Act Hotline
(800)514–0301; (800)514–0383 (TTY)
ADA Specialists available 10 a.m.–6 p.m. on Monday, Tuesday, Wednesday, and Friday and 1 p.m.–6 p.m. on Thursday.

U.S. DEPARTMENT OF HEALTH AND HUMAN SERVICES, OFFICE OF PUBLIC HEALTH AND SCIENCE

ADA Technical Assistance Hotline
(800)466–4232
9 a.m.–5 p.m. (Pacific)

Children's Craniofacial Association
(800)535-3643

FACES: The National Craniofacial Association
(800)332-2373
9 a.m.–5 p.m.

Families of Spinal Muscular Atrophy
(800)886-1762

Job Accommodation Network
(800)232–9675 (Voice/TDD)
(800)526–7234 (Voice/TDD)
(800)526–2262 (in Canada)
Services available in English, Spanish, and French.
8 a.m.–8 p.m., Monday–Thursday;
8 a.m.–7 p.m., Friday

National Center for Chronic Disease Prevention and Health Promotion, CDC
(877)CDC–DIAB; (877)232–3422

National Easter Seal Society
(800)221–6827
8:30 a.m.–5 p.m. (Central)

National Information Center for Children and Youth with Disabilities
(800)695–0285 (Voice/TT)
nichcy@aed.org
9:30 a.m.–6:30 p.m., or leave recorded message after hours.

National Rehabilitation Information Center (NARIC)
(800)346–2742 (Voice/TDD)
Spanish-speaking operators available.
9 a.m.–5 p.m.

Scoliosis Association
(800)800–0669
1 p.m.–5:30 p.m.

DOWN SYNDROME

See RARE DISORDERS

DRINKING WATER SAFETY

Safe Drinking Water Hotline
(800)426–4791
sdwa@epamail.epa.gov (E-mail)
Information provided in English, Spanish, French, Lebanese, and Persian.
9 a.m.–5:30 p.m., weekdays, except Federal holidays.

Organizations / Healthfinder

TOLL-FREE NUMBERS FOR HEALTH INFORMATION 2000

Water Quality Association
(800)749-0234 (Consumer Information)

DRUG ABUSE

See also ALCOHOL ABUSE and SUBSTANCE ABUSE

Drug Help
(800)378-4435; (800)202-2463

Housing and Urban Development Drug Information and Strategy Clearinghouse
(800)955-2232
9 a.m.–6 p.m.

National Parents Resource Institute for Drug Education
(800)279-6361
(800)853-7867
9 a.m.–5 p.m.

DWARFISM

Human Growth Foundation
(800)451-6434
8:30 a.m.–5 p.m.

Little People of America
(888)LPA-2001

DYSLEXIA

See LEARNING DISORDERS

ENDOMETRIOSIS

See WOMEN

ENVIRONMENT

Indoor Air Quality Information Clearinghouse
(800)438-4318
9 a.m.–5 p.m.

U.S. Environmental Protection Agency, Environmental Justice
(800)962-6215
8 a.m. to 5:30 p.m.

EPILEPSY

See RARE DISORDERS

ETHICS

Joseph and Rose Kennedy Institute of Ethics, National Reference Center for Bioethics Literature
(800)633-3849
medethx@gunet.georgetown.edu (E-mail)
9 a.m.–5 p.m., Monday, Wednesday, Thursday, Friday; 9 a.m.–8 p.m., Tuesday; 10 a.m.–3 p.m., Saturday, except summers and holidays.

FIRE PREVENTION

National Fire Protection Association
(800)344-3555 (Customer Service)
8:30 a.m.–8 p.m.

FITNESS

Aerobics and Fitness Foundation of America
(800)446-2322 (For Professionals)
(800)968-7263 (Consumer Hotline)
7:00 a.m.–6:00 p.m. (Pacific)

American Running and Fitness Association
(800)776-2732
9 a.m.–6:30 p.m.

Consumer Fitness Hotline
(800)529-8227 (Recording)
8 a.m. 5 p.m. (Pacific)

The Weight Control Information Network, NIDDK
(800)WIN-8098 (Recording)

TOPS Club, Inc.
(800)932-8677
8 a.m.–4:30 p.m. (Central)

YMCA of the USA
(800)872-9622
8:30 a.m.–5 p.m. (Central)

FOOD SAFETY

Food Labeling Hotline Meat and Poultry Hotline
(888)535-4555
10 a.m.–4 p.m.

Seafood Hotline
(888)SAFEFOOD
12 p.m.–4 p.m.

GENERAL HEALTH

Agency for Health Care Policy and Research Clearinghouse
(800)358-9295
9 a.m.–5 p.m.

Air Lifeline
(800)446-1231
7:30 - 4:30 (Pacific)

American Chiropractic Association
(800)986-4636
8:30 a.m.–5:30 p.m.

American Podiatric Medical Association, Inc.
(800)366-8227 (Recording)

American Osteopathic Association
(800)621-1773
8:30 a.m.–4:30 p.m. (Central)

MedicAlert Foundation
(800)432-5378; (800)344-3226

Mercy Medical Airlift
(800)296-1191 (Recording)

National Health Service Corps
(800)221-9393 (Recruitment/Loans)
(800)638-0824 (Medical Scholarship Programs)
8:30 a.m.–5:30 p.m. (Central)

National Health Information Center
(800)336-4797
nhicinfo@health.org (E-Mail)
9 a.m.–5 p.m.

National Center for Complementary and Alternative Medicine Clearinghouse
(888)644-6226 (Voice and TTY)
(800)531-1794 (Fax-back)
8:30 a.m. to 5:00 p.m.

Office for Civil Rights
(800)368-1019 (Recording)
(800)527-7697 (TDD)

Office of Consumer Affairs, FDA
(800)332-1088 (Medwatch)
(800)532-4440 (Consumer Inquiries)

People's Medical Society
(800)624-8773
9 a.m.–5 p.m.

Well Spouse Foundation
(800)838-0879
10 a.m.–4 p.m.

U.S. DEPARTMENT OF HEALTH AND HUMAN SERVICES, OFFICE OF PUBLIC HEALTH AND SCIENCE

Organizations / Healthfinder

**TOLL-FREE NUMBERS
FOR HEALTH INFORMATION
2000**

HEADACHE/HEAD INJURY

American Council for Headache Education
(800)255-ACHE

Brain Injury Association, Inc.
(800)444-6443 (Family Helpline)
9 a.m.–5 p.m.

National Headache Foundation
(888)NHF-5552
8 a.m.–6 p.m. (Central)

HEARING AND SPEECH

American Society for Deaf Children
(800)942-2732

American Speech-Language-Hearing Association
(800)638-8255
8:30 a.m.–5 p.m.

**DB-Link
(National Clearinghouse on Children Who Are Deaf-Blind)**
(800)438-9376
(800)854-7013 (TTY)
8:30 a.m.–5 p.m.

Deafness Research Foundation
(800)535-3323
9 a.m.–5 p.m.

Dial A Hearing Screening Test
(800)222-3277 (Voice/TDD)
9 a.m.–5 p.m.

The Ear Foundation at Baptist Hospital
(800)545-4327
8:30 a.m.–4:30 p.m. (Central), or leave recorded message after hours.

Hear Now
(800)648-4327 (Voice/TDD)
9 a.m.–4 p.m. (Mountain)

John Tracy Clinic
(800)522-4582 (Voice/TTY)
8 a.m.–4 p.m. (Pacific)
Leave recorded message after hours.

International Hearing Society
(800)521-5247 (Recording)
10 a.m.–4 p.m.

National Family Association for Deaf-Blind
(800)255-0411, ext. 275
9 a.m.–5 p.m.

National Institute on Deafness and Other Communication Disorders Information Clearinghouse
(800)241-1044; (800)241-1055 (TT)
8:30 a.m.–5 p.m.

LEAD LINE
(800)352-8888 (Voice/TDD in the U.S.)
(800)287-4763
blincoln@hci.org (E-Mail)
8 a.m.–5 p.m. (Pacific), or leave recorded message after hours.

Vestibular Disorders Association
(800)837-8428

HEART DISEASE

American Heart Association
(800)242-8721
9 a.m.–5 p.m.

The Coronary Club, Inc.
(800)478-4255

Heart Information Service
(800)292-2221
7 a.m.–6 p.m. (Central), or leave a recorded message after hours.

National Heart, Lung, and Blood Institute Information Center
(800)575-9355 (High Blood Pressure and Cholesterol Info. Hotline)
24-hour recording of information on high blood pressure and high blood cholesterol in English and Spanish.

HISTIOCYTOSIS

See RARE DISORDERS

HOMELESSNESS

National Resource Center on Homelessness and Mental Illness
(800)444-7415
8 a.m.–5 p.m.

HORMONAL DISORDERS

Thyroid Foundation of America, Inc.
(800)832-8321
8:30 a.m.–4 p.m.

The Thyroid Society for Education and Research
(800)849-7643
8 a.m.–4 p.m. (Central)

U.S. DEPARTMENT OF HEALTH AND
HUMAN SERVICES, OFFICE OF PUBLIC
HEALTH AND SCIENCE

HOSPITAL/HOSPICE CARE

Children's Hospice International
(800)242-4453
9:00 a.m.–5:00 p.m.

Hill-Burton Hospital Free Care
(800)638-0742; (800)492-0359 (in MD)
9:30 a.m.–5:30 p.m., or leave a recorded message after hours.

Hospice Education Institute "Hospice Link"
(800)331-1620
9 a.m.–4 p.m.

National Association of Hospitality Houses, Inc.
(800)542-9730

National Hospice Organization
(800)658-8898

Shriners Hospital Referral Line
(800)237-5055
8 a.m.–5 p.m.

HOUSING

See also CHEMICAL PRODUCTS/PESTICIDES and LEAD

Housing and Urban Development User
(800)245-2691; (800)483-2209 (TDD)
8:30 a.m.–5:15 p.m.

HUNTINGTON'S DISEASE

See RARE DISORDERS

IMMUNIZATION

CDC Immunization Hotline
(800)232-7468
8 a.m.–11 p.m.

IMPOTENCE

Impotence Information Center
(800)843-4315; (800)543-9632
8:30 a.m.–5 p.m. (Central), or leave a recorded message after hours.

INSURANCE/MEDICARE/MEDICAID

DHHS Inspector General's Hotline
(800)447-8477
8 a.m.–5 p.m.

Medicare Issues Hotline
(800)638-6833; (800)820-1202 (TDD/TTY)
8 a.m.–8 p.m.

Organizations / Healthfinder

TOLL-FREE NUMBERS FOR HEALTH INFORMATION 2000

Health Insurance Association of America Consumer Helpline
(800)942–4242
7 a.m.–7 p.m. (Mountain)

Pension Benefit Guaranty Corporation
(800)400-7242
8 a.m.–5 p.m.

Social Security Administration
(800)772–1213
7 a.m.–7 p.m.

JUSTICE

National Criminal Justice Reference Service (NCJRS)
(800)851–3420
8:30 a.m.–7 p.m. Leave recorded message after hours.

KIDNEY DISEASE

See UROLOGICAL DISORDERS

LEAD

See also HOUSING

National Lead Information Center
(800)532–3394(Hotline)
(800)424–5323 (Clearinghouse)
nlic@optimus.corp.com (E-mail)
8:30 a.m.–6 p.m.

LEARNING DISORDERS

Children and Adults with Attention Deficit Disorders (CH.A.D.D.)
(800)233–4050
8:30 a.m.–5 p.m.

The Orton Dyslexia Society
(800)222–3123 (Recording and mail box)

LIBRARY SERVICES

Captioned Films/Videos Programs, The National Association of the Deaf
(800)237–6213 (Voice/TTY)
(800)538–5636 (Fax)
8:30 a.m.–5 p.m.

National Library Service for the Blind and Physically Handicapped
(800)424–8567
8 a.m.–4:30 p.m.

Recording for the Blind and Dyslexic
(800)221–4792
8:30 a.m.–4:30 p.m.

LIVER DISEASES

American Liver Foundation
(800)223–0179
9 a.m.–5 p.m.

Hepatitis Foundation International
(800)891–0707
8:30 a.m.–5 p.m.

LUNG DISEASE/ASTHMA/ALLERGY

American Lung Association
(800)586–4872
8:30 a.m.–4:30 p.m.

Asthma and Allergy Foundation of America
(800)7–ASTHMA (727–8462)
7 a.m.–Midnight. Provides recording when not in operation.

Asthma Information Line
(800)822–2762

Lung Line National Jewish Medical and Research Center
(800)222–5864
(800)552–LUNG (LUNG FACTS)
8 a.m.–5 p.m. (Mountain)
LUNG FACTS, a companion to LUNG LINE, is a 24-hour, 7-days-a-week automated information service.

MATERNAL AND INFANT HEALTH

Alliance of Genetic Support Groups
(800)336-4363
9 a.m.–5:30 p.m.

La Leche League International
(800)525–3243
9 a.m.–3 p.m. (Central)

National Fragile X Foundation
(800)688-8765

National Life Center/Pregnancy Hotline
(800)848-5683

Prenatal Care Hotline
(800)311-2229 (English)
(800)504-7081 (Spanish)
8:30 a.m.–5 p.m.

MEDICARE/MEDICAID

See INSURANCE/MEDICARE/MEDICAID

U.S. DEPARTMENT OF HEALTH AND HUMAN SERVICES, OFFICE OF PUBLIC HEALTH AND SCIENCE

MENTAL HEALTH

See also CHILD ABUSE/MISSING CHILDREN/MENTAL HEALTH

American Academy of Child and Adolescent Psychiatry
(800)333–7636
8:30 a.m.–5 p.m.

Anxiety Disorders Information, NIMH
(888)826–9438
9 a.m.–5 p.m.

Depression Awareness, Recognition, and Treatment (D/ART)
(800)421–4211

National Alliance for the Mentally Ill
(800)950-6264

National Clearinghouse on Family Support and Children's Mental Health
(800)628–1696 (Recording)

National Council on Problem Gambling
(800)522-4700

National Foundation for Depressive Illness
(800)248–4344 (Recording)
NAFDI@pipeline.com (E-mail)

National Gaucher Foundation
(800)925-8885

National Institute for Mental Health Information Line
(800)647–2642

National Mental Health Association
(800)969–6642
9 a.m.–5 p.m.

National Mental Health Services, Knowledge Exchange Network
(800)789-2647; (800)790-2647
8:30 a.m.–5 p.m.

The Arc of the United States
(800)433–5255
8:30 a.m.–5:30 p.m. (Central)

MINORITY HEALTH

Office of Minority Health Resource Center
(800)444–6472
8:30 a.m.–5 p.m.

Organizations / Healthfinder

**TOLL-FREE NUMBERS
FOR HEALTH INFORMATION
2000**

NUTRITION

American Dietetic Association's Consumer Nutrition Hotline
(800)366–1655
8:30 a.m.–4:45 p.m. (Central)
TDD available.

American Institute for Cancer Research
(800)843–8114
8:30 a.m.–9:30 p.m.

National Dairy Council
(800)426–8271
8:30 a.m.–5 p.m. (Central)

ORAL HEALTH

American Dental Association
(800)947–4746
8:30 a.m.–5 p.m. (Central)

ORGAN DONATION

See also VISION and UROLOGICAL DISORDERS

The Living Bank
(800)528–2971
7:30 a.m.–4:30 p.m. (Central)

National Marrow Donor Program®
(800)627–7692

United Network for Organ Sharing
(800)243–6667

PARALYSIS AND SPINAL CORD INJURY

See also STROKE

Christopher Reeve Paralysis Association
(800)225–0292
9 a.m.–5 p.m.

National Rehabilitation Information Center
(800)346–2742 (Voice/TDD)
9 a.m.–5 p.m.

National Spinal Cord Injury Association
(800)962–9629
(Members and individuals with spinal cord injuries; no vendors)
9 a.m.–noon, 1 p.m.–4 p.m.

National Spinal Cord Injury Hotline
(800)526–3456
9 a.m.–5 p.m.
24-hour answering service will page for emergency.

National Stroke Association
(800)787–6537
7 a.m.–4:30 p.m. (Mountain)

Paralyzed Veterans of America
(800)424–8200; (800)795–4327 (TDD)

PARKINSON'S DISEASE

American Parkinson's Disease Association
(800)223–2732
9 a.m.–5 p.m.
Leave recorded message after hours.

National Parkinson Foundation, Inc.
(800)327–4545
8 a.m.–5 p.m., Monday–Friday; recorded messages at all other times.

Parkinson's Disease Foundation
(800)457-6676
9 a.m.–5 p.m.

PESTICIDES

See CHEMICAL PRODUCTS/PESTICIDES

PRACTITIONER REPORTING

USP Practitioners Reporting Network
(800)487–7776
(800)233–7767 (Medication error)
Recording operates 24 hours a day; staff available 9 a.m.–4:30 p.m., Monday–Friday. Medication error telephone number records information 24 hours a day.

PREGNANCY/MISCARRIAGE

Bradley Method of Natural Childbirth
(800)422–4784
9 a.m.–5 p.m. (Pacific).
Leave recorded message after hours.

Lamaze International
(800)368–4404
lamaze@dc.sba.com (E-mail)
9 a.m.–5 p.m.

DES Action USA
(800)337-9288
10 a.m.–4 p.m. (Pacific)

U.S. DEPARTMENT OF HEALTH AND HUMAN SERVICES, OFFICE OF PUBLIC HEALTH AND SCIENCE

International Childbirth Education Association
(800)624–4934 (Book Center orders)
8 a.m.–4:30 p.m. (Central)
Summers: 8 a.m.–1 p.m., Fridays

Liberty Godparent Home
(800)542–4453

National Abortion Federation
(800)772-9100
9 a.m.–7 p.m.

PROFESSIONALS

Alopecia Areata Research Foundation
(800)941-4223

American Academy of Allergy, Asthma and Immunology
(800)822-2762 (Central)

American Academy of Ophthalmology
(800)222–3937
8 a.m.-4 p.m. (Pacific)

American Alliance for Health, Recreation, Physical Education, and Dance
(800)213-7193
8 a.m.–4:30 p.m.

American Association of Critical Care Nurses
(800)899-2226
7:30 a.m.–5:30 p.m. (Pacific)

American Council for the Blind
(800)424-8666
9 a.m.–5 p.m.

American Counseling Association
(800)347-6647
8 a.m.–6 p.m.

American Nurses Association
(800)274-4ANA
9 a.m. - 5 p.m.

American Occupational Therapy Association
(800)377-8555

American School Food Service Association
(800)877-8822
8:30 a.m.-5:30 p.m.

Aplastic Anemia Foundation of America
(800)747-2820
9 a.m.-5 p.m.

Organizations / Healthfinder

**TOLL-FREE NUMBERS
FOR HEALTH INFORMATION
2000**

Arthritis National Research Foundation
(800)588–2873
8:30 a.m.-5 p.m. (Pacific)

Association for Applied Psychophysiology and Biofeedback
(800)477-8892
8 a.m.-5 p.m. (Mountain)

Association of American Physicians and Surgeons
(800)635-1196
8 a.m.-6 p.m. (Mountain)

Association of Operating Room Nurses
(800)755–2676
8 a.m.-4:30 p.m. (Mountain)

Center for Substance Abuse Treatment, SAMHSA
(800)662-4357

College of American Pathologists
(800)323-4040
8:30 a.m.-5 p.m. (Central)

Dystonia Medical Research Foundation
(800)377-3978
9 a.m.-5 p.m. (Central)

For Kids Sake, Inc.
(800)898-4543
9 a.m.–5 p.m. (Central)

Federal Emergency Management Agency
(800)879-6076
8 a.m.-4:30 p.m.

Federal Information Center, GSA
(800)688-9889
9 a.m.-8 p.m.

Glaucoma Research Foundation
(800)826-6693
8:30 a.m.-4:30 p.m. (Pacific)

Immune Deficiency Foundation
(800)296-4433
9 a.m.-5 p.m.

International Childbirth Education Association
(800)624-4934
8:30 a.m.-4:30 p.m. (Central)

International Chiropractors Association
(800)423-4690
9 a.m.-5:30 p.m.

Leukemia Society Of America
(800)955-4572
4 a.m.-6 p.m.

Lighthouse National Center for Vision and Aging
(800)829-0500
8:30 a.m.-5 p.m.

Medical Institute for Sexual Health
(800)892–9484
8 a.m.-5:00 p.m. (Central)

National Center for Disability Services
(800)949-4232
8:30 a.m.-5 p.m.

National Child Care Information Center, ACF
(800)516-2242; (800)616-2242 (TTY)
8:30 a.m.-5:30 p.m.,
Wednesdays, 8:30 a.m.-8 p.m.

National Clearinghouse of Rehabilitation Training Materials
(800)223-5219
8 a.m.-5 p.m. (Central)

National Information Prevention Network
(800)458-5231
9 a.m.-6 p.m.

National Jewish Medical and Research Association
(800)552-5864
8 a.m.-5 p.m. (Mountain)

National Pediculosis Association
(800)446-4672
8:30 a.m.–4:30 p.m., 24-hour voice mail

National Resource Center on Domestic Violence
(800)537-2238; (800)553-2508 (TTY)
8 a.m.-5 p.m., 24-hour voice mail

National Sexually Transmitted Disease Hotline (CDC)
(800)227-8922
8 a.m.-11 p.m.

National Technical Information Service
(800)553-6847
8 a.m.-6 p.m.

NIOSH, CDC
(800)356-4674
9 a.m.–4 p.m.

U.S. DEPARTMENT OF HEALTH AND
HUMAN SERVICES, OFFICE OF PUBLIC
HEALTH AND SCIENCE

Office of the National Drug Control Policy
(800)666-3332
8:30 a.m.-5 :15 p.m.

Prevent Child Abuse America
(800)556-2722 (Recording)

Research to Prevent Blindness
(800)621-0026
9 a.m.-5 p.m.

The Alliance for Aging Research
(800)639-2421
9 a.m.-5 p.m., 24-hour voice mail

RADIATION

National Association of Radiation Survivors
(800)798-5102
9 a.m.–5 p.m. (Pacific)

RARE DISORDERS*

*A rare disorder is defined as a disorder that affects less than 1 percent of the population at any given time.

American Behcet's Disease Association
(800)723-4238
9 a.m.–5 p.m. (Pacific)

American Cleft Palate-Craniofacial Association/Cleft Palate Foundation
(800)242-5338
CLEFTLINE operates 24 hours.
Spanish-speaking operators available.
8:30 a.m.–4:30 p.m.

American Leprosy Missions (Hansen's Disease)
(800)543–3135
8 a.m.–5:30 p.m. Monday-Thursday
8 a.m.–noon Friday

American SIDS Institute
(800)232–7437; (800)847–7437 (in GA)
9 a.m.–5 p.m. Leave recorded message after hours (staff on call).

Amyotrophic Lateral Sclerosis Association (ALS, Lou Gehrig's Disease)
(800)782–4747
7:30 a.m.–4:30 p.m. (Pacific)
Leave a recorded message after hours.

Batten's Disease Support and Research Association
(800)448–4570
8 a.m.–5 p.m. 24-hour recording

Organizations / Healthfinder

**TOLL-FREE NUMBERS
FOR HEALTH INFORMATION
2000**

Charcot-Marie-Tooth Association
(800)606-2682
8:30 a.m.–5 p.m.

Cooley's Anemia Foundation
(800)522-7222
9 a.m.–5 p.m.

Cornelia de Lange Syndrome Foundation, Inc.
(800)223-8355
(800)753-2357 (U.S. and Canada)
9 a.m.–5:00 p.m.
Leave a recorded message after hours.

Cystic Fibrosis Foundation
(800)344-4823
8:30 a.m.–5:30 p.m.

Epilepsy Foundation of America
(800)332-1000
(800)213-5821 (Publications)
9 a.m.–5 p.m. Monday-Thursday
9 a.m.–3 p.m. Friday

Epilepsy Information Service
(800)642-0500
8 a.m.–5 p.m.

Fibromyalgia Network
(800)853-2929
8 a.m.–4 p.m. (Mountain) Monday-Thursday

Gillis W. Long Hansen's Disease Center
(800)642-2477
8 a.m.–4:30 p.m. (Central)

Histiocytosis Association
(800)548-2758
9:00 a.m.–4:30 p.m.
Voice mail after hours.

Huntington's Disease Society of America, Inc.
(800)345-4372
9 a.m.–5 p.m.

International Rett Syndrome Association
(800)818-7388
9 a.m.–5 p.m.

Les Turner Amyotrophic Lateral Sclerosis Foundation, Ltd.
(888)ALS-1107
8:30 a.m.–4:30 p.m. (Central)

Multiple Sclerosis Association of America
(800)532-7667
8 a.m.–6 p.m., Monday–Thursday

Multiple Sclerosis Foundation
(800)441-7055
9 a.m.–5 p.m.

Muscular Dystrophy Association
(800)572-1717
9 a.m.–5 p.m. (Mountain)

Myasthenia Gravis Foundation
(800)541-5454
8:45 a.m.–4:45 p.m. (Central)

National Down Syndrome Congress
(800)232-6372
9 a.m.–5:30 p.m. Recording after hours.

National Down Syndrome Society Hotline
(800)221-4602
9 a.m.–5 p.m.

National Hemophilia Foundation
(888)463-6643
9 a.m.–5 p.m.
Summer: 9 a.m.–5:30 p.m. Monday-Thursday, 9 a.m.–3 p.m. Friday

National Lymphedema Network
(800)541-3259
9:30 a.m.–5:30 p.m. (Pacific)
Leave recorded message.

National Marfan Foundation
(800)862-7326
8 a.m.–3:30 p.m.

National Multiple Sclerosis Society
(800)344-4867
11 a.m.–5 p.m.

National Neurofibromatosis Foundation
(800)323-7938
9 a.m.–5 p.m.

National Organization for Albinism and Hypopigmentation
(800)473-2310

National Organization for Rare Disorders
(800)999-6673
9 a.m.–5 p.m.
Leave recorded message after hours.

National Reye's Syndrome Foundation
(800)233-7393
8 a.m.–5 p.m.
Leave recorded message after hours.

National Sjogren's Syndrome Association
(800)395-6772

National Spasmodic Torticollis Association
(800)487-8385
9 a.m.–5:30 p.m. (Pacific)

National Tuberous Sclerosis Association
(800)225-6872
8:30 a.m.–5 p.m.

Neurofibromatosis, Inc.
(800)942-6825, 24-hour message line

Office of Orphan Products Development, Food and Drug Administration
(800)300-7469
8 a.m.–4:30 p.m.

Osteogenesis Imperfecta Foundation
(800)981-2663
9 a.m.–5 p.m.

The Paget Foundation for Paget's Disease of Bone and Related Disorders
(800)237-2438
9 a.m.–5 p.m.

Prader-Willi Syndrome Association
(800)926-4797
9 a.m.–7 p.m.

Scleroderma Foundation
(800)722-4673
8:30 a.m.–5:00 p.m.

Sickle Cell Disease Association of America, Inc.
(800)421-8453
8:30 a.m.–5 p.m. (Pacific)
Recording after hours.

SIDS Alliance
(800)221-7437
9 a.m.–5 p.m.

Sjogren's Syndrome Foundation, Inc.
(800)475-6473
9 a.m.–5 p.m.

Spina Bifida Association of America
(800)621-3141
9 a.m.–5 p.m.

Spondylitis Association of America
(800)777-8189
8 a.m.–5 p.m. (Pacific)
Leave recorded message after hours.

U.S. DEPARTMENT OF HEALTH AND HUMAN SERVICES, OFFICE OF PUBLIC HEALTH AND SCIENCE

Organizations / Healthfinder

**TOLL-FREE NUMBERS
FOR HEALTH INFORMATION
2000**

Sturge-Weber Foundation
(800)627–5482
9 a.m.–3 p.m.

Sudden Infant Death Syndrome Network
(800)560-1454

Support Organization for Trisomy 18, 13 and Related Disorders
(800)716-7638
Leave recorded message.

Tourette Syndrome Association, Inc.
(800)237–0717
9 a.m.–5 p.m.

Treacher Collins Foundation
(800)823-2055

Turner's Syndrome Society of the United States
(800)365-9944

United Cerebral Palsy Association
(800)872–5827
9 a.m.–5 p.m.

United Leukodystrophy Foundation
(800)728-5483
8:30 a.m.–8:30 p.m., 7days (Central)

Wegener's Granulomatosis Support Group, Inc.
(800)277-9474
8:00 a.m.–5:00 p.m. (Central)

Wilson's Disease Association
(800)399-0266

REHABILITATION

See also DISABLING CONDITIONS and PARALYSIS AND SPINAL CORD INJURY

ABLEDATA
(800)227-0216
8:00 a.m. to 5:30 p.m.

National Institute for Rehabilitation Engineering
(800)736-2216
9 a.m.–5 p.m.

Phoenix Society for Burn Survivors
(800)888-2876
9 a.m.–5 p.m.

United Ostomy Association
(800)826-0826
6:30 a.m.–4:30 p.m., Monday - Thursday
6:30 a.m.–3:30 p.m., Friday (Pacific)

RURAL

Rural Information Center Health Service (RICHS)
(800)633-7701
ric@nalusda.gov (E-mail)
8 a.m.–4:30 p.m.

SAFETY

See also CHEMICAL PRODUCTS/PESTICIDES

Clearinghouse for Occupational Safety and Health Information, National Institute for Occupational Safety and Health
(800)356-4674
9 a.m.–4 p.m.

The Danny Foundation
(800)83-DANNY (Recording)

National Child Safety Council Childwatch
(800)222-1464
7 a.m.–4:30 p.m.

National Highway Traffic Safety Administration Auto Safety Hotline
(800)424–9393 (Recording)
(800)424–9153 (TTY)
8 a.m.–10 p.m.

National Program for Playground Safety
(800)554-7529
7:30 a.m.–4:30 p.m.

National Safety Council
(800)621-7615
(800)767-7236 (National Radon Hotline)
8:30 a.m.–4:45 p.m.

Office of Navigation Safety and Waterway Services, U.S. Coast Guard Customer Infoline
(800)368–5647; (800)689–0816 (TDD/TT)
8 a.m.–4 p.m.

Safe Sitter
(800)255-4089
8 a.m.–5:30 p.m.

U.S. Consumer Product Safety Commission Hotline
(800)638–2772; (800)638–8270 (TDD)
info@cpsc.gov
24-hour messages

U.S. DEPARTMENT OF HEALTH AND HUMAN SERVICES, OFFICE OF PUBLIC HEALTH AND SCIENCE

SEXUAL EDUCATION

Planned Parenthood Federation of America, Inc.
(800)669–0156
(800)230–7526 (Recording)

SEXUALLY TRANSMITTED DISEASES

See also AIDS/HIV

Centers for Disease Control and Prevention National STD Hotline
(800)227–8922
8 a.m.–11 p.m.

Herpes Resource Center
(800)230–6039
9 a.m.–3:30 p.m.

Skin Disease

Foundation for Ichthyosis and Related Skin Types, Inc.
(800)545-3286
9 a.m.–5 p.m.

National Psoriasis Foundation
(800)723-9166
8 a.m.–5 p.m. (Pacific)

SPINAL CORD INJURY

See PARALYSIS AND SPINAL CORD INJURY

SMOKING

Office on Smoking and Health
(800)232-1311 (Recording)

STROKE

See also PARALYSIS AND SPINAL CORD INJURY

American Heart Association Stroke Connection
(800)553–6321
7:30 a.m.–7 p.m. (Central)

National Institute of Neurological Disorders and Stroke
(800)352-9424
8:30 a.m.–5 p.m.

STUTTERING

National Center for Stuttering
(800)221–2483
10 a.m.–5 p.m.

Stuttering Foundation of America
(800)992–9392
9 a.m.–5 p.m.

**TOLL-FREE NUMBERS
FOR HEALTH INFORMATION
2000**

SUBSTANCE ABUSE

See also ALCOHOL ABUSE and DRUG ABUSE

National Inhalant Prevention Coalition
(800)269–4237 (Recording)
8 a.m.–7 p.m. (Central)

SUDDEN INFANT DEATH SYNDROME

See RARE DISORDERS

SURGERY/FACIAL PLASTIC SURGERY

American Society for Dermatologic Surgery, Inc.
(800)441–2737 (Recording)
8:30 a.m.–5 p.m. (Central)

American Society of Plastic and Reconstructive Surgeons, Inc.
(800)635–0635
8:30 a.m.–4:30 p.m. (Central).
Leave recorded message after hours.

Facial Plastic Surgery Information Service
(800)332–3223
8 a.m.–6 p.m.

TRAUMA

American Trauma Society (ATS)
(800)556–7890
8:30 a.m.–4:30 p.m.

UROLOGICAL DISORDERS

American Association of Kidney Patients
(800)749–2257
8:30 a.m.–5 p.m.

American Foundation for Urologic Disease
(800)242–2383 (Recording)

American Kidney Fund
(800)638–8299
8:30 a.m.–5 p.m.

Incontinence Information Center
(800)843–4315; (800)543–9632
8:00 a.m.–4 p.m. (Central), or leave recorded message after hours

National Association for Continence
(800)252-3337
8 a.m.–5 p.m.

National Kidney Foundation
(800)622–9010
8:30 a.m.–5:30 p.m.

Polycystic Kidney Research Foundation
(800)753-2873
8 a.m.–5 p.m. (Central)

The Simon Foundation for Continence
(800)237–4666

VENEREAL DISEASES

See SEXUALLY TRANSMITTED DISEASES

VETERANS

Persian Gulf Veterans Information Helpline
(800)749-8387
8 a.m.–4 p.m. (Central)

Vietnam Veterans Agent Orange Victims
(800)521-0198
9 a.m.–4 p.m.

VISION

See also LIBRARY SERVICES and HEARING AND SPEECH

American Council of the Blind
(800)424–8666
hcraff@ACCESS.DIGEX.NET (E-mail)
3p.m.–5:30 p.m.

American Foundation for the Blind
(800)232–5163

Better Vision Institute
(800)424-8422
9 a.m.–5 p.m.

Braille Institute
(800)272-4553
8 a.m.–5 p.m. (Pacific)

Blind Children's Center
(800)222–3566 ; (800)222–3567
ncrabb@acb.org (E-mail)
9 a.m.–5 p.m. (Pacific).

DB-Link
(800)438-9376
8:30 a.m.–5 p.m.

The Foundation Fighting Blindness
(800)683–5555; (800)683–5551 (TDD)
8:30 a.m.–5 p.m.

Guide Dog Foundation for the Blind, Inc.
(800)548–4337
8 a.m.–5 p.m.

Guide Dogs for the Blind
(800)295-4050
8 a.m.–5 p.m. (Pacific)

The Lighthouse National Center for Education
(800)334–5497

Louisiana Center for the Blind
(800)234–4166
8 a.m.–5 p.m. (Central)

National Alliance of Blind Students
(800)424-8666
9 a.m.–5:30 p.m.

National Association for Parents of the Visually Impaired
(800)562–6265 (Recording)
9 a.m.–5 p.m.

National Eye Care Project Helpline
(800)222–EYES (3937)
8 a.m.–4 p.m. (Pacific)

National Eye Research Foundation
(800)621–2258
8:30 a.m.–5 p.m. (Central)
Leave recorded message after hours.

National Family Association for Deaf-Blind
(800)255–0411, ext. 275
9 a.m.–5 p.m.

Prevent Blindness Center for Sight
(800)331–2020
8 a.m.–5 p.m. (Central)

U.S. DEPARTMENT OF HEALTH AND HUMAN SERVICES, OFFICE OF PUBLIC HEALTH AND SCIENCE

Organizations / Healthfinder

**TOLL-FREE NUMBERS
FOR HEALTH INFORMATION
2000**

VIOLENCE

National Domestic Violence Hotline
(800)787-3224 (TDD); (800)799-7233

National Organization for Victim Assistance
(800)879-6682

Rape, Abuse, and Incest National Network
(800)656–4673

WOMEN

Endometriosis Association
(800)992–3636 (Recording)

National Osteoporosis Foundation
(800)223–9994

National Women's Health Information Center
(800)994–9662; (888)220-5446 (TDD)
9 a.m.-6 p.m.

PMS Access
(800)222–4767 (Recording)
7:30 a.m.–5:30 p.m. (Central)

Women's Health America Group
(800)558-7046 (Recording)

Women's Sports Foundation
(800)227–3988
9: a.m.–5 p.m.

**U.S. DEPARTMENT OF HEALTH AND
HUMAN SERVICES, OFFICE OF PUBLIC
HEALTH AND SCIENCE**

TOLL-FREE NUMBERS FOR HEALTH INFORMATION•DIAL 1-800
(UNLESS 888 IS SPECIFIED)

ABLEDATA, 227-0216

ACS, National Cancer Information Center, 227–2345 (Voice /TDD/TT)

ADA Technical Assistance Hotline, 466-4232

ADCARE Hospital Helpline, 252–6465

Aerobics and Fitness Foundation of America, 968–7263 (Consumers); 446–2322 (Professionals)

Alliance of Genetic Support Groups, 336-4363

Agency for Health Care Policy and Research Clearinghouse, 358–9295

AIDS Clinical Trials Information Service, 874–2572

Al-Anon Family Group Headquarters, 356–9996

Alcohol and Drug Helpline, 821–4357

Alzheimer's Association, 272–3900

Alzheimer's Disease Education and Referral Center, 438–4380

American Academy of Child and Adolescent Psychiatry, 333–7636

American Alliance for Health, Recreation, Physical Education, and Dance, 213–7193

American Association of Diabetes Educators, 832–6874

American Association of Kidney Patients, 749–2257

American Autoimmune Related Diseases Association, Inc., 598-4668

American Behcet's Disease Association, 723-4238

American Brain Tumor Association, 886-2282

American Chiropractic Association, 986-4636

American Cleft Palate-Craniofacial Association/Cleft Palate Foundation, 242-5338

American Council for Headache Education, 255-ACHE

American Council on Alcoholism, 527–5344

American Council of the Blind, 424–8666

American Dental Association, 947–4746

American Diabetes Association, 232–3472, 232–6733 (Fax Order Fulfillment)

American Dietetic Association's Consumer Nutrition Hotline, 366–1655

American Foundation for the Blind, 232–5163

American Foundation for Urologic Disease, 242–2383

American Health Assistance Foundation, 437-2423

American Heart Association, 242–8721

American Heart Association Stroke Connection, 553–6321

American Institute for Cancer Research, 843–8114

American Juvenile Arthritis Organization, 283-7800

American Kidney Fund, 638–8299

American Leprosy Missions (Hansen's Disease), 543–3135

American Liver Foundation, 223–0179

American Lung Association, 586–4872; 528–2971 (Living Bank)

American Osteopathic Association, 621–1773

American Parkinson's Disease Association, 223–2732

American Podiatric Medical Association, Inc., 366–8227

American Running and Fitness Association, 776-2732

American School Food Service Association, 877–8822

American SIDS Institute, 232–7437; 847–7437

American Society for Deaf Children, 942-2732

American Society for Dermatologic Surgery, Inc., 441–2737

American Society of Plastic and Reconstructive Surgeons, Inc. 635–0635

American Speech-Language-Hearing Association, 638–8255

American Trauma Society, 556–7890

Americans with Disabilities Act Hotline, 514–0301; 514–0383 (TTY)

Amyotrophic Lateral Sclerosis Association, 782–4747

Anxiety Disorders Information, NIMH, (888)8-ANXIETY

ARC of the United States, 433–5255

Arthritis Foundation Information Hotline, 283–7800

Association for the Care of Children's Health, 808-2224 x327

Association of Birth Defect Children, 313-2232

Association of Operating Room Nurses, 755–2676

Asthma and Allergy Foundation of America, 727–8462

Asthma Information Line, 822–2762

Autism Society of America, 328–8476

A WAY OUT, 292–4688

Batten's Disease Support and Research Association, 448–4570

Bethany Christian Services, 238–4269

Better Vision Institute, 424-8422

Blind Children's Center, 222–3566; 222–3567 (California only)

Boys Town National Hotline, 448–3000; 448–1833 (TDD)

Bradley Method of Natural Childbirth, 422–4784

Braille Institute, 272-4553

Brain Injury Association, 444–6443

Brain Tumor Society, The, 770-TBTS

Calix Society, 398-0524

Captioned Films/Videos Programs, the National Association of the Deaf, 237–6213 (Voice/TTY)

Cancer Hope Network, (877)HOPENET

Cancer Information Service, 422–6237

Candlelighters Childhood Cancer Foundation, 366-2223

CDC Immunization Hotline, 232–7468

CDC National HIV/AIDS Hotline, 342–2437 (English); 344–7432 (Spanish); 243–7889 (TDD)

CDC National Prevention Information Network (NPIN), 458–5231; 243–7012 (TTY); (888)282–7681 (Fax)

Centers for Disease Control National STD Hotline, 227–8922

Charcot-Marie-Tooth Association, 606-2682

Chemtrec Non-Emergency Services Hotline, 262–8200

Child Find of America, Inc., 426–5678; 292–9688

U.S. DEPARTMENT OF HEALTH AND HUMAN SERVICES, OFFICE OF PUBLIC HEALTH AND SCIENCE

Organizations / Healthfinder

**TOLL-FREE NUMBERS
FOR HEALTH INFORMATION
2000**

CHILDHELP/IOF Foresters National Child Abuse Hotline, 422–4453; 222–4453 (TDD)
Children and Adults with Attention Deficit Disorder, 233–4050
Children of Alcoholics Foundation, 359-COAF
Children's Craniofacial Association, 535-3643
Children's Hospice International, 242–4453
Christopher Reeve Paralysis Association, 225–0292
Clearinghouse for Occupational Safety and Health Information, National Institute for Occupational Safety and Health, 356–4674
Consumer Fitness Hotline, 529–8227
Cooley's Anemia Foundation, 522–7222
Cornelia de Lange Syndrome Foundation, 223–8355; 753–2357
Coronary Club, Inc., The, 478-4255
Covenant House Nineline, 999–9999
Crohn's and Colitis Foundation of America, Inc., 932–2423
Cystic Fibrosis Foundation, 344–4823
Danny Foundation, The, 83-DANNY
DB-Link, 438-9376; 854–7013 (TTY)
Deafness Research Foundation, 535–3323
Depression Awareness, Recognition, and Treatment (D/ART), 421–4211
DES Action USA, DES-9288
DHHS Inspector General's Hotline, 447–8477
Dial A Hearing Screening Test, 222–3277 (Voice/TDD)
Drug Help, 378–4435; 202–2463
Ear Foundation at Baptist Hospital, The, 545–4327
Eldercare Locator, 677–1116
Endometriosis Association, 992–3636
Epilepsy Foundation of America, 332–1000; 213–5821 (Publications)
Epilepsy Information Service, 642–0500
FACES: The National Craniofacial Association, 332-2373
Facial Plastic Surgery Information Service, 332–3223
Families of Spinal Muscular Atrophy, 886-1762
Fibromyalgia Network, 853–2929
Food Allergy Network, The, 929-4040
Food Labeling Hotline, Meat and Poultry Hotline, 535–4555

For Kids Sake, Inc, 898–4543
Foundation Fighting Blindness, The, 683–5555; 683–5551 (TDD)
Foundation for Ichthyosis and Related Skin Types, Inc., 545-3286
Gillis W. Long Hansen's Disease Center, 642-2477
Guide Dog Foundation for the Blind, Inc., 548–4337
Guide Dogs for the Blind, 295-4050
Health Insurance Association of America Consumer Hotline, 942–4242
Hear Now, 648–4327 (Voice/TDD)
Heart Information Service, 292-2221
Hepatitis Foundation International, 891–0707
Herpes Resource Center, 230–6039
Hill-Burton Hospital Free Care, 638–0742; 492–0359 (in MD)
Histiocytosis Association, 548–2758
HIV/AIDS Treatment Information Service, 448–0440
Hospice Education Institute "Hospice Link," 331–1620
Housing and Urban Development Drug Information and Strategy Clearinghouse, 955–2232
Housing and Urban Development User, 245–2691; 483–2209 (TDD)
Human Growth Foundation, 451–6434
Huntington's Disease Society of America, 345–4372
Impotence Information Center, 843–4315; 543–9632
Incontinence Information Center, 843–4315; 543–9632
Indoor Air Quality Information Clearinghouse, 438–4318
International Childbirth Education Association, 624–4934 (orders only)
International Hearing Society, 521–5247
International Rett Syndrome Association, 818-7388
Job Accommodation Network, 232–9675 (Voice/TDD); 526–7234 (Voice/TDD); 526–2262 (in Canada)
John Tracy Clinic, 522–4582 (Voice/TTY)
Joseph and Rose Kennedy Institute of Ethics, 633–3849
Juvenile Diabetes Foundation International Hotline, 223–1138
La Leche League International, 525–3243

U.S. DEPARTMENT OF HEALTH AND HUMAN SERVICES, OFFICE OF PUBLIC HEALTH AND SCIENCE

Lamaze International, 368–4404
LEAD LINE, 352–8888 (Voice/TDD); 287–4763
Les Turner Amyotrophic Lateral Sclerosis Foundation, Ltd., (888)ALS-1107
Liberty Godparent Home, 542–4453
Lighthouse National Center for Education, The, 334–5497
Lighthouse National Center for Vision and Aging, 829–0500
Little People of America, (888)LPA–2001
Living Bank, The, 528–2971
Louisiana Center for the Blind, 234–4166
Lung Line National Jewish Medical and Research Center, 222–5864; 552–5864 (LUNG FACTS)
Lupus Foundation of America, 558–0121 (English); 558–0231 (Spanish)
Lyme Disease Foundation, Inc., 886–5963
MAGIC Foundation for Children's Growth, The, 3-MAGIC-3
MedicAlert Foundation, 432–5378; 344–3226
Medical Institute for Sexual Dysfunction, 892–9484
Medicare Issues Hotline, 638–6833; 820–1202 (TDD/TTY)
Mercy Medical Airlift, 296-1191
Multiple Sclerosis Association of America, LEARN-MS
Multiple Sclerosis Foundation, 441-7055
Muscular Dystrophy Association, 572–1717
Myasthenia Gravis Foundation, 541–5454
National Abortion Federation, 772-9100
National Adoption Center, 862–3678
National Alliance for the Mentally Ill, 950-6264
National Alliance of Blind Students, 424-8666
National Alliance of Breast Cancer Organizations, 719-9154
National Association for Continence, 252-3337
National Association for the Education of Young Children, 424–2460
National Association for Parents of the Visually Impaired, 562–6265

Organizations / Healthfinder

TOLL-FREE NUMBERS FOR HEALTH INFORMATION 2000

National Association of Hospitality Houses, Inc., 542-9730

National Association of Radiation Survivors, 798-5102

National Bone Marrow Transplant Link, LINK-BMT

National Brain Tumor Foundation, 934-CURE

National Center for Chronic Disease Prevention and Health Promotion, (877)CDC–DIAB; (877)232–3422

National Center for Complementary and Alternative Medicine Clearinghouse, (888)644-6226 (Voice and TTY); (800)531-1794 (Fax-back)

National Center for Missing and Exploited Children, 843-5678; 826-7653 (TDD)

National Center for Stuttering, 221-2483

National Child Safety Council Childwatch, 222-1464

National Clearinghouse for Alcohol and Drug Information, 729-6686; 487-4889 (TTY/TDD)

National Clearinghouse on Child Abuse and Neglect Information, 394-3366

National Clearinghouse on Family Support and Children's Mental Health, 628-1696

National Council on Problem Gambling, 522-4700

National Council on Alcoholism and Drug Dependence, Inc., 622-2255

National Criminal Justice Reference Service, 851-3420

National Dairy Council, 426-8271; 974-6455 (Fax)

National Down Syndrome Congress, 232-6372

National Domestic Violence Hotline, 787-3224 (TDD); 799-SAFE

National Down Syndrome Society Hotline, 221-4602

National Easter Seal Society, 221-6827

National Eye Care Project Helpline, 222-3937

National Eye Research Foundation, 621-2258

National Eye Research Foundation's Memorial Eye Clinic, The, 621-2258

National Family Association for Deaf-Blind, 255-0411, ext. 275

National Fire Protection Association, 344-3555

National Foundation for Depressive Illness, 248-4344

National Fragile X Foundation, 688-8765

National Gaucher Foundation, 925-8885

National Headache Foundation, (888)NHF–5552

National Health Information Center, 336-4797

National Health Service Corps, 221-9393 (Recruitment/Loans); 638-0824 (Medical Scholarship Programs)

National Heart, Lung, and Blood Institute's Information Center, 575–WELL (High Blood Pressure and Cholesterol Information Hotline)

National Hemophilia Foundation, (888)INFO-NHF

National Highway Traffic Safety Administration Auto Safety Hotline, 424-9393; 424-9153 (TTY)

National Hospice Organization, 658-8898

National Information Center for Children and Youth With Disabilities, 695–0285 (Voice/TT)

National Information Prevention Network, 458-5231

National Inhalant Prevention Coalition, 269-4237

National Institute for Mental Health Information Line, 647-2642

National Institute for Rehabilitation Engineering, 736-2216

National Institute of Child Health and Human Development, Public Information & Communications Branch, 505-CRIB (SIDS Information Line)

National Institute of Neurological Disorders and Stroke, 352-9424

National Institute on Aging Information Center, 222-2225; 222-4225 (TTY)

National Institute on Deafness and Other Communication Disorders Information Clearinghouse, 241-1044;241-1055 (TT)

National Insurance Consumer Helpline, 942-4242

National Kidney Cancer Association, 850-9132

National Kidney Foundation, 622-9010

U.S. DEPARTMENT OF HEALTH AND HUMAN SERVICES, OFFICE OF PUBLIC HEALTH AND SCIENCE

National Lead Information Hotline, LEAD–FYI (Hotline); 424–LEAD (Clearinghouse); 526–5456 (TDD)

National Leigh's Disease Foundation, 819-2551

National Lekotek Center, 366-PLAY; 573-4446 (Voice and TTY)

National Library of Medicine, 272-4787

National Library Service for the Blind and Physically Handicapped, 424–8567

National Life Center, 848-5683

National Lymphedema Network, 541-3259

National Marfan Foundation, 8-MARFAN

National Marrow Donor Program®, MARROW-2

National Mental Health Association, 969-6642

National Mental Health Services, Knowledge Exchange Network, 789-2647; 790-2647

National Multiple Sclerosis Society, 344-4867

National Neurofibromatosis Foundation, 323-7938

National Organization for Albinism and Hypopigmentation; 473-2310

National Organization for Rare Disorders, 999-6673

National Organization for Victim Assistance, TRY-NOVA

National Organization on Fetal Alcohol Syndrome, 66-NOFAS

National Osteoporosis Foundation, 464-6700

National Parents Resource Institute for Drug Education, 279-6361; 853-7867 (Taped Drug Information)

National Parkinson Foundation, Inc., 327-4545

National Pesticide Telecommunications Network, 858-7378

National Program for Playground Safety, 554-PLAY

National Psoriasis Foundation, 723-9166

National Rehabilitation Information Center, 346-2742 (Voice/TDD)

National Resource Center on Homelessness and Mental Illness, 444-7415

National Reye's Syndrome Foundation, 233-7393

Organizations / Healthfinder

TOLL-FREE NUMBERS FOR HEALTH INFORMATION 2000

National Runaway Switchboard, 621–4000; 621–0394 (TDD)
National Safety Council, 621–7615
National Sexually Transmitted Disease Hotline (CDC) 227–8922
National Sjogren's Syndrome Association, 395-6772
National Spasmodic Torticollis Association, 487-8385
National Spinal Cord Injury Association, 962–9629
National Spinal Cord Injury Hotline, 526–3456
National Stroke Association, STROKES
National Tuberous Sclerosis Association, 225–6872
National Woman's Christian Temperance Union, 755-1321
National Women's Health Information Center, 994–9662
National Youth Crisis Hotline, 448–4663
Neurofibromatosis, Inc., 942-6825
Office for Civil Rights, 368-1019; 527-7697 (TDD)
Office of Consumer Affairs, FDA, 332-1088 (Medwatch); 532-4440 (Consumer Inquiries)
Office of Minority Health Resource Center, 444–6472
Office of Navigation Safety and Waterway Services, U.S. Coast Guard Customer InfoLine, 368–5647, 689–0816 (TDD/TT)
Office of Orphan Products Development, Food and Drug Administration, 300–7469
Office on Smoking and Health, CDC-1311
Orton Dyslexia Society, The, 222–3123
Osteogenesis Imperfecta Foundation, 981-BONE
Osteoporosis and Related Bone Diseases National Resource Center, 624-BONE
Paget Foundation for Paget's Disease of Bone and Related Disorders, 237–2438
Paralyzed Veterans of America, 424–8200; 416–7622 (TDD)
Parkinson's Disease Foundation, 457-6676
Pediatric Projects, Inc., 947-0947
Pension Benefit Guaranty Corporation, 400-PBGC

People's Medical Society, 624-8773
Persian Gulf Veterans Information Helpline, PGW-VETS
Phoenix Society for Burn Survivors, 888-2876
Planned Parenthood, 230–7526; 669–0156
PMS Access, 222–4767
Polycystic Kidney Research Foundation, 753-2873
Prader-Willi Syndrome Association, 926-4797
Prenatal Care Hotline, 311-BABY (English); 504-7081 (Spanish)
Prevent Blindness Center for Sight, 331–2020
Prevent Child Abuse America, 556–2722
Project Inform HIV/AIDS Treatment Hotline, 822–7422
Rape, Abuse, and Incest National Network, 656–4673
Reach to Recovery Program, 227-2345
Recording for the Blind and Dyslexic, 221–4792
Rural Information Center Health Service, 633–7701
Safe Drinking Water Hotline, 426–4791
Safe Sitter, 255-4089
Scleroderma Foundation, 722–4673
Scoliosis Association, 800–0669
Seafood Hotline, (888)SAFEFOOD
Shriners Hospital Referral Line, 237–5055
Sickle Cell Disease Association of America, Inc., 421–8453
SIDS Alliance, 221–7437
Simon Foundation for Continence, The, 237–4666
Sjogren's Syndrome Foundation, Inc., 475-6473
Social Security Administration, 772–1213
Spina Bifida Association of America, 621–3141
Spondylitis Association of America, 777–8189
Starlight Children's Foundation, 274-7827
Sturge-Weber Foundation, 627–5482
Stuttering Foundation of America, 992–9392

U.S. DEPARTMENT OF HEALTH AND HUMAN SERVICES, OFFICE OF PUBLIC HEALTH AND SCIENCE

Sudden Infant Death Syndrome Network, 560-1454
Support Organization for Trisomy 18, 13 and Related Disorders, 716-SOFT
Susan G. Komen Breast Cancer Foundation, 462–9273
Thyroid Foundation of America, Inc., 832–8321
Thyroid Society for Education and Research, The, THYROID
TOPS Club, Inc., 932-8677
Tourette Syndrome Association, Inc., 237–0717
Treacher Collins Foundation, TCF-2055
Turner's Syndrome Society of the United States, (800)365-9944
United Cerebral Palsy Association, 872–5827
United Leukodystrophy Foundation, 728-5483
United Network for Organ Sharing, 243–6667
United Ostomy Association, 826-0826
U.S. Consumer Product Safety Commission Hotline, 638–2772; 638–8270 (TDD)
U.S. Environmental Protection Agency, 962-6215
USP Practitioners Reporting Network, 487–7776; 233–7767 (Medication Error)
Us Too International, 808-7866
Vestibular Disorders Association, 837-8428
Vietnam Veterans Agent Orange Victims, 521-0198
Water Quality Association, 749-0234 (Consumer Information)
Wegener's Granulomatosis Support Group, Inc., 277-9474
Weight Control Information Network, NIDDK, The, WIN-8098
Well Spouse Foundation, 838-0879
Wilson's Disease Association, 399-0266
Women's Health America Group, 558-7046
Women's Sports Foundation, 227–3988
YMCA of the USA, 872–9622
Y-ME National Organization for Breast Cancer Information Support Program, 221–2141 (English), 986–9505 (Spanish)
Zero to Three: National Center for Infants, Toddlers and Families, 899-4301

International Organizations

ARGENTINA
Argentinan Association of Dermatology (AAD), Asociacion Argentina De Dermatologia, Mexico 1720, 1100 Buenos Aires; tel. 114/381-2737; FAX. 114/381-2737; Dra. Lidia Ester Valle, Chairman

Camara Argentina De Empresas De Salud, (Argentina Hospital Association), Tucuman 1668, 2 Piso, C.P. 1050 Buenos Aires

AUSTRALIA
Australian Healthcare Association, P.O. Box 54, Deakin West, 2600; tel. +612 628-5148; FAX. +612 6282239; Tracey Turner, Office Manager

BELGIUM
International Federation of Oto–Rhino–Laryngological Societies, IFOS–MISA–NKO Oosterveldlaan 24, 2610 WILRIJK; tel. 3 4433611; Ms. Gadeyne, Administrator, Publication Manager

Verbond der Verzorgingsinstellingen V.Z.W., 1, Guimardstraat, Brussels 1040; tel. 2 5118008; FAX. 2 5135269; Mrs. C. Boonen, M.D., General Manager

BRAZIL
Fraternidade Crista De Doentes E Deficientes, Cap. Correa Pacheco 134, Americana, SP; tel. 0 194 619754; Celso Zoppi

CANADA
Association des Medecins de langue francaise du Canada, 8355 St. Laurent Boulevard, Montreal, PQ H2P 2Z6; tel. 514/388-2228; FAX. 514/388-5335; Andre' de Seve, General Director

Canadian Anesthesiologists' Society, One Eglinton Avenue East, Suite 208, Toronto, ON M4P 3A1; tel. 416/480-0602; FAX. 416/480-0320; Angela Fritsch, Director

Canadian Association of Pathologists, Office of the Secretariat, 774 Echo Drive, Ottawa, ON K1S 5N8; tel. 613-730-6230; FAX. 613/730-0260; Dr. Roger Amy, Secretary–Treasurer

Canadian Association of Social Workers, 383 Parkdale Avenue, Suite 402, Ottawa, ON K1Y 4R4; tel. 613/729-6668; FAX. 613/729-9608; Eugenia Repetur Moreno, Executive Director

Canadian Cancer Society, 10 Alcorn Avenue, Suite 200, Toronto, ON M4V 3B1; tel. 416/961-7223; FAX. 416/961-4189; Maaika Asselbergo, Executive Director

Canadian Cardiovascular Society, 222 Queen Street, Suite 1403, Ottawa, On K1P SV9; tel. 613/569-3407; FAX. 613/569-6574; Charles Shields, Jr., Executive Director

Canadian College of Health Record Administrators, Canadian Health Record Association, 1090 Don Mills Road, Suite 501, Don Mills, ON M3C 3G8; tel. 416/447-4900; FAX. 416/447-4598; Deborah Del Duca, Executive Director

Canadian Council of the Blind, 396 Cooper Street, Suite 405, Ottawa, ON K2P 2H7; tel. 613/567-0311; FAX. 613/567-2728; Sharon E. Davis, Executive Assistant – National

Canadian Council on Social Development, 441 Maclaren, Fourth Floor, Ottawa, ON K2P 2H3; tel. 613/236-8977; FAX. 613/236-2750; Nancy Perkins, Communications Coordinator

Canadian Dental Association, 1815 Alta Vista Drive, Ottawa, ON K1G 3Y6; tel. 613/523-1770; FAX. 613/523-7736; Jardine Neilson, Executive Director

Canadian Healthcare Association, Association Canadian des soins de sante, 17 York Street, Suite 100, Ottawa, ON K1N 9J6; tel. 613/241-8005; FAX. 613/241-5055; Sharon Sholzberg–Gray, President

Canadian Medical Engineering Consultants, 594 Bush Street, Belfountain, ON L0N 1B0; tel. 519/927-3286; FAX. 519/927-9440; A. M. Dolan, President

Canadian Mental Health Association, 2160 Yonge Street, Toronto, ON M4S 2Z3; tel. 416/484-7750; FAX. 416/484-4617; Edward J. Pennington, General Director

Canadian National Institute for the Blind, 320 McLeod Street, Ottawa, ON K2P1A3; tel. 613/563-4021; FAX. 416/480-7677; Angelo Nikias, National Director, Gov't Relations and

Canadian Nurses Association, 50 Driveway, Ottawa, ON K2P 1E2; tel. 613/237-2133; FAX. 613/237-3520; Mary Ellen Jeans, RN, Ph.D., Executive Director

Canadian Orthopaedic Association, 1440 Ste. Catherine Street, W., Suite 320, Montreal, PQ H3G 1R8; tel. 514/874-9003; FAX. 514/874-0464; Dr. David Petrie, President

Canadian Pharmacists Association, 1785 Alta Vista Drive, Ottawa, ON K1G 3Y6; tel. 613/523-7877; FAX. 613/523-0445; Jeff Poston, Executive Director

Canadian Physiotherapy Association, National Office, 2345 Yonge Street, Suite 410, Toronto, ON M4P 2E5; tel. 416/932-1888; FAX. 416/932-9708; Dan Stapleton, Chief Executive Officer

Canadian Psychiatric Association, 441 MacLaren Street, Suite 260, Ottawa, ON K2P2H3; tel. 613/234-2815; FAX. 613/234-9857; Alex Saunders, Chief Executive Officer

Canadian Public Health Association, 1565 Carling Avenue, Suite 400, Ottawa, ON K1Z 8R1; tel. 613/725-3769; FAX. 613/725-9826; Gerald H. Dafoe, M.H.A., Chief Executive Officer

Canadian Rehabilitation Council for the Disabled, 45 Sheppard Avenue, E., Suite 801, Toronto, ON M2N 5W9; tel. 416/250-7490; FAX. 416/229-1371; Henry Botchford, National Executive Director

Canadian Society for Medical Laboratory Science, Box 2830, LCD 1, Hamilton, ON L8N 3N8; tel. 905/528-8642; FAX. 905/528-4968; Kurt H. Davis, Executive Director

Canadian Society of Hospital Pharmacists, 1145 Hunt Club Road, Suite 350, Ottawa, ON K1V 0Y3; tel. 613/736-9733; FAX. 613/736-5660; Bill Leslie, Executive Director

Catholic Health Association of Canada, 1247 Kilborn Place, Ottawa, ON K1H 6K9; tel. 613/731-7148; FAX. 613/731-7797; Richard Haughian, President

College des medecins du Quebec, 2170, boul. Rene-Levesque Quest, Montreal, PQ H3H 2T8; tel. 514/933-4441; FAX. 514/993-3112; Joelle Lescop, M.D., Secretary General

College of Family Physicians of Canada, 2630 Skymark Avenue, Mississauga, ON L4W 5A4; tel. 905/629-0900; FAX. 905/629-0893; Dr. Claude A. Renaud, Director, Professional Affairs

Dietitians of Canada/Les dietetistes du Canada, 480 University Avenue, Suite 604, Toronto, ON M5G 1V2; tel. 416/596-0857; FAX. 416/596-0603; Marsha Sharp, Chief Executive Officer

National Cancer Institute of Canada, 10 Alcorn Avenue, Suite 200, Toronto, ON M4V 3B1; tel. 416/961-7223; FAX. 416/961-4189; Robert A. Phillips, Ph. D., Executive Director

The Canadian Hearing Society, 271 Spadina Road, Toronto, ON M5R 2V3; tel. 416/964-9595; FAX. 416/928-2506; David Allen, Executive Director

The Canadian Medical Association, Box 8650, Ottawa, ON K1G 0G8; tel. 613/731-9331; FAX. 613/731-7314; Leo-Paul Landry, M.D., Secretary General

The Canadian Red Cross Society, National Office, 1800 Alta Vista Drive, Ottawa, ON K1G 4J5; tel. 613/739-2220; FAX. 613/739-2505; Claude Houde, National Director, Blood Services

The College of Physicians and Surgeons of New Brunswick, One Hampton Road, Suite 300, Rothesay, NB E2E 5K8; tel. 506/849-5050; FAX. 506/849-5069; Ed Schollenberg, M.D., Registrar

The Royal College of Physicians and Surgeons of Canada, 774 Echo Drive, Ottawa, ON K1S 5N8; tel. 613/730-6201; FAX. 613/730-2410; Mrs. Pierrette Leonard, APR, Manager Communications Group

World Federation of Hemophilia, 1425 Rene devesque Blvd. West, Suite 1010, Montreal, PQ; tel. 5148757944; FAX. 514/8758916; Mrs. Line Robillard, Executive Director

COLOMBIA
Associacion Colombiana De Hospitales, (Colombia Hospital Association), Calle 98 no. 17 A, 34 Oficina 205-3, Santafe, de Bogota, Colombia

COSTA RICA
Associacion Coctarricense De Hospitales, (Costa Rica Hospital Association), Aparatado 267, 1005 San Jose; tel. 506/255-0363; FAX. 506/221-4919; Carlos Enrique Fuentes Bolanos

DENMARK
Amtsradsforeningen, Dampfaergevej 22, Postboks 2593, Copenhagen; tel. +45 35 29 81; FAX. +45 35 29 83; Ida Sofie Jensen, Assistant Director

Association of County Councils in Denmark, (Denmark Hospital Association), Dampfaergevi 22, P.O. Box 2593; tel. +4535298100; FAX. +4535298300

Danish Dental Association, Amaliegade 17, Postboks 143, Copenhagen; tel. 45 33157711; FAX. 45 33151637; Karsten Thuen, Chief Executive Director

National Committee for Danish Hospitals, Amtsradsforeningen, Dampfaergevej 22, Postboks 2593; tel. 45 35298196; FAX. 45 35298337; Peder Ring, Assistant Director

ENGLAND
British Medical Association, B.M.A. House Tavistock Square, London, WCH1 9JP; tel. 0207/387-4499; FAX. 0207/388-6400; Dr. E.M. Armstrong, BSC., FRCP Ed Glas.,FRCCP

European Association of Poisons/Centres and Clinical Toxicology, City Hospital, Birmingham, B187QH; tel. (44) 121 507; FAX. (44) 121 507; Dr. Allister Vale, President

Institute of Healthcare Management, 7–10 Chandos Street, London,WIM,9DE; tel. 0171/460-765; FAX. 0171/460-765; Suzanne Tyler, Deputy Director

International Hospital Federation, Hospital Federation, 46 Grosvenor Gardens, London, SW1WOEB, UK; tel. 44/207881922; FAX. 44/207881922; Professor Per–Gunnar Svensson, Director General

King's Fund, 11–13 Cavendish Square, London, W1M 0AN; tel. 0171/3072400; FAX. 0171/3072801; Rabbi Julia Neuberger, Chief Executive

Nuffield Trust, 59 New Cavendish Street, London W1 7RD; tel. 0207/631-8450; FAX. 0207/631-8451; John Wyn Owen, Secretary

FINLAND
National Research and Development Centre for Welfare and Health, (Finland Hospital Association), Siltasaarenkatu 18A, P.O. Box 220, 00531 Helsinki

FRANCE
Federation hospitaliere De France, (France Hospital Association), Avenue d'Italie 33, Paris 75013

World Medical Association, 13 Chemin du Levant, B.P. 63; tel. 450 407575; FAX. 450 405937; Dr. Delon Human, Secretary General

GERMANY
Deutsche Krankenhausgesellschaft, (German Hospital Association), Tersteegenstrasse 9, D40474, Dusseldorf; tel. 211 454730; FAX. 211 4547361; Jorg Robbers, Director General

International Academy of Cytology, Burgunderstr. 1, 79104 Freiburg; tel. 49 761 292 3801; FAX. 49 761 292 3802; Volker Schneider, M.D., FIAC, Office of Secretary General

HUNGARY
Magyar Korhazszovetseg, (Hungary Hospital Association), Fogaskereku U.4-6., 1125 Budapest; tel. 36–121451118; FAX. 36–12149715; Dr. Zoltan Ajkay, President

INDIA
Indian Hospital Association, B–401 Sarita Vihar, New Delhi, India, 110044

INDONESIA
Indonesian Hospital Association (PERSI), Jl. Danau Sunter Utara, Blok J 12/68, Sunter Podomoro, Jakarta, Utara, 14350; tel. 6221 6510962; FAX. 6221 6514531; A.W. Boediarso, M.D., SKM, MBA

IRELAND
Comhairle na nOspideal (Ireland Hospital Council), Corrigan House, Fenian Street, Dublin 2; tel. 003531676347; FAX. 003531676143; Thomas Martin, Chief Officer

ITALY
Federazione Italiana delle Aziende Sanitarie e Ospedaliere (FIASO), (Italy Hospital Association), Azienda Ospedaliera S Orsola Malpoghi Via Albertoni 15, 40138 Bologna

Organizations / International Organizations

KOREA
Korean Hospital Association, (Mapo Hyun Dai Building), 35–1 Mapo–don; tel. 2 7187521; FAX. 2 7187522; Ho Uk Ha, Ph.D., Vice President

MANGOLIA
Mongolian Hospital Association, P.O. Box 48/146, MHSW Olympic Street

MEXICO
Asociacion Mexicana De Hospitales AC, (Mexico Hospital Association), Queretaro 210, Col Roma Mexico DF, 06700
Federacion Latinoamericana de Hospitales, Apartado Postal 107–076, C.P. 06741; tel. 5 482650; Dr. Guillermo Fajardo, Representative

NORWAY
Norsk Sykehus Helsetjenesten, (Norway Hospital Association), Nedre Slottsgt 7, 0157 Oslo, Norske Kommuners sentralforbund, Vika Oslo 1

PANAMA
Asociacion Panamena De Hospitales Privados, (Panama Hospital Association), Apartado 7503, Panama City 5

PERU
Peruvian Hospital Association, Av. Dos De Mayo 8502 Of. 203, San Isidro, L; tel. 14 419546; Arturo Vasi Paez, President

PHILIPPINES
Philippine Hospital Association, 14 Kamias Road, Quezon City–1; tel. 2 9227674/75; Thelma Navarrete–Clemente, M.D., M.H.A., President

SOUTH AFRICA
Provincial Administration, Health Services Branch, P.O. Box 517; tel. 051/4055818; FAX. 051/304958; Dr. J. H. Kotze
South African Hospital Federation, Department of Health, Facilities Planning and Hospital, Private Bag X828, Pretoria 0001

SWEDEN
Federation of Swedish County Councils, Box 70491, S–10726 Stockholm

SWITZERLAND
H+ Die Spitaler der Schweiz, (Swiss Hospital Association), Rain 32, Aarau; tel. 62 824 1222; FAX. 62 822 33 35; Mr. Christof Haudenschild, Director
World Health Organization, Avenue Appia 20, 1211 Geneva 27; tel. +41 22 791 2111; FAX. +41 22 791 3111; Hiroshi Nakajima, M.D., Ph.D., Director–General

TAIWAN
Hospital Association of Taiwan, 4f, No 5 Chung Cheng Road, Section 2, Shihlin, Taipei; tel. 88 622 833 8829; FAX. 88 622 832 3571; Grace Y. L. Hsu, Head of Department

UNITED STATES
American College of Gastroenterology, 4900B South 31st Street, Arlington, VA 22206; tel. 703/820–7400; FAX. 703/931–4520; Thomas F. Fise, Executive Director
American Society for Testing and Materials, 100 Barr Harbor Drive, West Conshoho, PA 19428–2959; tel. 610/832–9672; FAX. 610/832–9666; Kenneth C. Pearson, Vice President
Association for Assessment and Accreditation of Laboratory Animal, Care International, 11300 Rockville Pike, Suite 1211, Rockville, MD 20852–3035; tel. 301/231–5353; FAX. 301/231–8282; Dr. John G. Miller, Executive Director
Association for Volunteer Administration, P.O. Box 32092, Richmond, VA 23294; tel. 804/346–2266; FAX. 804/346–3318; Katherine H. Campbell, Executive Director
International Academy of Podiatric Medicine (IAPM), 4603 Highway 95 South, P.O. Box 39, Cocolalla, ID 83813–0039; tel. 208/683–3900; FAX. 208/683–3700; Judith A. Baerg, Executive Director
International Aid, 17011 West Hickory, Spring Lake, MI 49456–9712; tel. 616/846–7490; FAX. 616/846–3842; Warren L. Prelesnik, FACHE, Director of Hospital Management
International Association for Dental Research, 1619 Duke Street, Alexandria, VA 22314–3406; tel. 703/548–0066; FAX. 703/548–1883; Eli Schwarz, DDS, MPH, Ph.D., Executive Director
International Association of Ocular Surgeons, 820 North Orleans, Suite 208, Chicago, IL 60610; tel. 312/440–0699; FAX. 312/440–0580; Randall T. Bellows, M.D., Director
International Association of Pediatric Laboratory Medicine, 6728 Old McLean Village Drive, McLean, VA 22101; tel. 703/556–9222; FAX. 703/556–8729; Merrill Ferber, Executive Director
International Executive Housekeepers Association, Inc., 1001 Eastwind Drive, Suite 301, Westerville, OH 43081–3361; tel. 800/200–6342; FAX. 614/895–1248; Beth Risinger, CEO/ Executive Director
International Tremor Foundation, 7046 W. 105th Street, Overland Park, KS 66212–1803; tel. 888/387–3667; FAX. 913/341–1296; Catherine S. Rice, Executive Director
Rehabilitation International, 25 East 21st Street, New York, NY 10010; tel. 212/420–1500; FAX. 212/505–0871; Arthur O'Reilly, President
Sigma Theta Tau International Honor Society of Nursing, 550 West North Street, Indianapolis, IN 46202; tel. 317/634–8171; FAX. 317/634–8188; Nancy A. Dickenson–Hazard, Executive Officer
U.S. Council on International Social Welfare, 750 First Street, N.E., Washington, DC 20002; tel. 202/336–8274; FAX. 202/336–8311; Helen Whetzel, Secretary
World Federation of Public Health Associations, c/o APHA, 1015 15th Street, N., Washington, DC 20005; tel. 202/789–5696; FAX. 202/789–5681; Allen K. Jones, Ph.D., Executive Secretary

VENEZUELA
Latin American Association for the Study of the Liver (LAASL), P.O. Box 51890, Sabana Grande; tel. 58–2–9799380; FAX. 58–2–9799380; Dr. Miguel A. Garassini, President

U. S. GOVERNMENT AGENCIES

The following information is based on data available as of April 2000. For more information about U.S. government agencies, consult the U.S. Government Manual, *available from the Office of the* Federal Register, *National Archives and Records Service, Washington, DC 20408. A telephone directory of the U.S. Department of Health and Human Services is available from the Superintendent of Documents, Government Printing Office, Washington, DC 20402. Additional assistance may be obtained by contacting the American Hospital Association's Washington office, 325 Seventh Street, N.W., Washington, DC 20004.*

Executive Office of the President
tel. 202/456-1414
Counsel to the President: Charles Ruff; 202/456–2632
Chief of Staff: Erskine Bowles; 202/456–6797
Assistant to the President for Economic Policy: Gene B. Sperling; 202/456–5808
Assistant to the President for Domestic Policy: Bruce Reed; 202/456–2216
Assistant to the President and Director of Public Liaison: Minyon Moore; 202/456–2930

COUNCIL OF ECONOMIC ADVISORS
Chairman: Martin N. Baily

OFFICE OF MANAGEMENT AND BUDGET
Director: Jacob J. Lew

Department of Agriculture
tel. 202/720-8732
Secretary: Dan Glickman; 202/720–3631

Department of Commerce
tel. 202/482-2000
Secretary: William M. Daley; 202/482–2112
BUREAU OF ECONOMIC ANALYSIS
Director: Steven Landefeld; 202/606–2600
ECONOMIC DEVELOPMENT ADMINISTRATION
Acting Assistant Secretary: Chester J. Straub, Jr.
NATIONAL INSTITUTE OF STANDARDS AND TECHNOLOGY
Director: Raymond Krammer; 301/975–3058

Department of Defense
tel. 703/545-6700
Secretary: William S. Cohen; 703/695–5261
Assistant Secretary of Defense (Health Affairs): Sue Bailey; 703/545-6700
UNIFORMED SERVICES UNIVERSITY OF THE HEALTH SCIENCES
President: James A. Zimble; 301/295–3030
DEPARTMENT OF THE AIR FORCE
Lt. Gen. Paul K. Carlton, Jr.
DEPARTMENT OF THE ARMY
Surgeon General: Lt. Gen. Ronald R. Blanck; 703/681–3000
DEPARTMENT OF THE NAVY
Vice Adm. R. A. Nelson

Department of Education
tel. 202/401-2000
Secretary: Richard W. Riley; 202/401–3000

Department of Health and Human Services
tel. 202/619-0257
Secretary: Donna E. Shalala; 202/690–7000
General Counsel: Harriet Rabb; 202/690–7741

MANAGEMENT AND BUDGET
Assistant Secretary: John J. Callahan, Ph.D.; 202/690–6396

HEALTH
Assistant Secretary: James O'Hara; 202/690–7694

ADMINISTRATION FOR CHILDREN AND FAMILIES
Assistant Secretary: Olivia A. Golden; 202/401–2337

LEGISLATION
Assistant Secretary/Designate: Richard J. Tarplin; 202/690–7627

PLANNING AND EVALUATION
Margaret A. Hamburg, M.D.

PUBLIC AFFAIRS
Assistant Secretary: Melissa Skolfield; 202/690–7850

PUBLIC HEALTH SERVICE
Surgeon General: David Satcher, M.D.; 301/443–4000

Centers for Disease Control, Atlanta 30333
Administrator: Jeffrey P. Koplan

Food and Drug Administration, Rockville, MD 20857
Jane E. Henney

Health Resources and Services Administration, Rockville, MD 20857
Administrator: Claude E. Fox, M.D.

National Institutes of Health, Bethesda, MD 20892
Ruth Kirschstein, M.D.

Substance Abuse and Mental Health Services Administration, Rockville, MD
Administrator: Nelba Chavez, Ph.D.; 301/443–4795

HEALTH CARE FINANCING ADMINISTRATION
Administrator: Nancy-Ann Min De Parle; 202/690–6726

SOCIAL SECURITY ADMINISTRATION: Baltimore, MD 21235
Commissioner: Kenneth S. Apfel; 410/965–7700
Regional Commissioners telephone: 800/772-1213
(1) Boston
Manuel J. Vaz
(2) New York
Beatrice M. Disman
(3) Philadelphia
Larry G. Massanari
(4) Atlanta
Myrtle S. Habersham
(5) Chicago
Jeff F. Martin
(6) Dallas
Horace L. Dickerson
(7) Kansas City
Michael Grochowski
(8) Denver
Richard J. Gonzalez
(9) San Francisco
Linda S. McMahon
(10) Seattle
Carmen Maria Keller

Department of Housing and Urban Development
tel. 202/708-1112
Secretary: Andrew Cuomo; 202/708–0417

Department of Justice
tel. 202/514-2000
Attorney General: Janet Reno; 202/514–2000

DRUG ENFORCEMENT ADMINISTRATION
Administrator: Thomas A. Constantine; 202/307–8000

Department of Labor
tel. 202/219-5000
Secretary: Alexis M. Herman; 202/219–8271

BUREAU OF LABOR STATISTICS
Commissioner: Katharine G. Abraham; 202/606–7800

EMPLOYMENT AND TRAINING ADMINISTRATION
Assistant Secretary: Raymond L. Brammucci; 202/219–6050

OCCUPATIONAL SAFETY AND HEALTH ADMINISTRATION
Acting Assistant Secretary: Charles Jeffress; 202/219–7162

Department of State
tel. 202/647-4000
Secretary: Madeleine Albright; 202/647–6575

AGENCY FOR INTERNATIONAL DEVELOPMENT
Administrator: J. Brian Atwood; 202/647–9620

Independent Agencies
U.S. COMMISSION ON CIVIL RIGHTS
Chairperson: Mary Frances Berry; 202/376–7572

CONSUMER PRODUCT SAFETY COMMISSION
Chairperson: Ann Brown; 301/504–0213

ENVIRONMENTAL PROTECTION AGENCY
Administrator: Carol M. Browner; 202/260–4700

EQUAL EMPLOYMENT OPPORTUNITY COMMISSION
Chairwoman: Ida L. Castro

FEDERAL EMERGENCY MANAGEMENT AGENCY
Director: James Lee Witt; 202/646–3923

Government-Related Groups
Federally aided corporations and quasi–official agencies, such as American Red Cross, National Academy of Sciences and World Health Organization, are listed with International, National, and Regional Organizations beginning on page C3.

State and Local Organizations and Agencies

Blue Cross–Blue Shield Plans

The following listing is based on information provided by the agencies themselves. Inclusion or omission of any organization's name indicates neither approval nor disapproval by Health Forum LLC, an American Hospital Association Company.

United States

ALABAMA: Blue Cross and Blue Shield of Alabama, 450 Riverchase Parkway, E., Birmingham, AL 35244; tel. 205/988–2200; FAX. 205/444–6555; H.L. Jones, Chief Executive Officer

ARIZONA: Blue Cross and Blue Shield Arizona, 2444 West Las Palmaritas Drive, Phoenix, AZ 85021; tel. 6028644444; FAX. 602/864–4184; Robert B. Bulla, Chief Executive Officer

ARKANSAS: Arkansas Blue Cross and Blue Shield, a Mutual Insurance Company, 601 Gaines Street, Little Rock, AR 72201; tel. 501/378–2010; FAX. 501/378–2037; Robert L. Shoptaw, Chief Executive Officer

CALIFORNIA: Blue Cross of California, 21555 Oxnard Street, Woodland Hills, CA 91367; tel. 805/557–6000; Leonard D. Schaeffer, Chief Executive Officer

Blue Shield of California, California Physicians' Service Corporation, 50 Beale Street, San Francisco, CA 94105; tel. 415/229–5000; FAX. 415/229–5056; Wayne R. Moon, Chief Executive Officer

COLORADO: Blue Cross and Blue Shield Colorado, Rocky Mountain Hospital and Medical Service, 700 Broadway, Denver, CO 80273; tel. 303/831–2131; FAX. 303/830–0887; C. David Kikumoto, Chief Executive Officer

CONNECTICUT: Anthem Insurance Companies of Connecticut, Anthem Insurance Companies, Inc., 370 Bassett Road, North Haven, CT 06473; tel. 317/488–6493; Larry G. Glasscock, Chief Executive Officer

DELAWARE: Blue Cross and Blue Shield Delaware, Blue Cross and Blue Shield Delaware, CareFirst Inc., One Brandywine Gateway, Wilmington, DE 19899; tel. 302/421–3210; FAX. 302/421–2089; Paul C. King, Jr., Chief Executive Officer

DISTRICT OF COLUMBIA: CareFirst Blue Cross and Blue Shield, 550 12th Street, S.W., Washington, DC 21117; tel. 410/998–5252; William L. Jews, Chief Executive Officer

FLORIDA: Blue Cross and Blue Shield Florida, Inc., 4800 Deerwood Campus Parkway, Jacksonville, FL 32246; tel. 904/905–6115; FAX. 904/905–6638; Michael Cascone, Jr., Chief Executive Officer

GEORGIA: Blue Cross and Blue Shield Georgia, Cerulean Companies, Inc., 3350 Peachtree Road, N.E., Atlanta, GA 30326; tel. 404/842–8410; FAX. 404/842–8010; Richard D. Shirk, Chief Executive Officer

HAWAII: Blue Cross and Blue Shield Hawaii, Hawaii Medical Service Association, 818 Keeaumoku Street, Honolulu, HI 96804; tel. 808/948–5517; FAX. 808/948–5999; Robert P. Hiam, Chief Executive Officer

IDAHO: Blue Cross of Idaho Health Services, 3000 East Pine Avenue, Meridian, ID 83642; tel. 208/331–7333; FAX. 208/331–7311; David L. Barnett, Chief Executive Officer

Regence BlueShield of Idaho, 1602 21st Avenue, Lewiston, ID 83501; tel. 208/798–2169; John Ruch, Chief Executive Officer

ILLINOIS: Blue Cross and Blue Shield Illinois, 300 East Randolph Street, Chicago, IL 60601; tel. 312/653–6746; FAX. 312/819–1220; Raymond F. McCaskey, Chief Executive Officer

INDIANA: Anthem Blue Cross and Blue Shield, Anthem Insurance Companies, Inc., 120 Monument Circle, Indianapolis, IN 46204; tel. 317/488–6057; FAX. 317/488–6477; L. Ben Lytle, Chief Executive Officer

IOWA: Wellmark Blue Cross and Blue Shield of Iowa, Wellmark, Inc., 636 Grand Avenue, Des Moines, IA 50309; tel. 515/245–4545; FAX. 515/245–5090; John D. Forsyth, Chief Executive Officer

KANSAS: Blue Cross and Blue Shield Kansas, 1133 Topeka Boulevard, Topeka, KS 66629; tel. 785/291–8700; John W. Knack, Chief Executive Officer

LOUISIANA: Blue Cross and Blue Shield Louisiana, Louisiana Health Service and Indemnity Company, 5525 Reitz Avenue, Baton Rouge, LA 708093802; tel. 225/295–2266; Kathryn Sullivan, Chief Executive Officer

MAINE: Blue Cross and Blue Shield Maine, Associated Hospital Service of Maine, 2 Gannett Drive, South Portland, ME 04106-6911; tel. 207/822–7000; FAX. 207/822–7350; Keith W. Vangeison, Chief Executive Officer

MARYLAND: CareFirst Blue Cross and Blue Shield, 10455 Mill Run Circle, Owings Mills, MD 21117; tel. 410/998–5252; FAX. 410/998–5576; William L. Jews, Chief Executive Officer

MASSACHUSETTS: Blue Cross and Blue Shield Massachusetts, 100 Summer Street, Boston, MA 02110; tel. 617/832–3300; FAX. 617/832–3353; William C. Van Faasen, Chief Executive Officer

MICHIGAN: Blue Cross and Blue Shield Michigan, 600 Lafayette East, Detroit, MI 48226-2998; tel. 313/225–9000; FAX. 313/225–6239; Richard E. Whitmer, Chief Executive Officer

MINNESOTA: Blue Cross and Blue Shield Minnesota, Aware Integrated, Inc., 3535 Blue Cross Road, St. Paul, MN 55122; tel. 651/662–8438; FAX. 651/662–7767; Mark W. Banks, M.D., Chief Executive Officer

MISSISSIPPI: Blue Cross and Blue Shield Mississippi, Blue Cross and Blue Shield of Mississippi, a Mutual Insurance Co., 3545 Lakeland Drive, Jackson, MS 392089799; tel. 601/664–4200; FAX. 601/939–7035; Richard J. Hale, Chief Executive Officer

MISSOURI: Blue Cross and Blue Shield Kansas City, 2301 Main Street, Kansas City, MO 64108; tel. 816/395–2222; FAX. 816/395–2035; John Mascotte, Chief Executive Officer

Blue Cross and Blue Shield Missouri, 1831 Chestnut Street, St. Louis, MO 63103-2275; tel. 314/923–4444; FAX. 314/923–4809; John A. O'Rourke, Chief Executive Officer

MONTANA: Blue Cross and Blue Shield Montana, 560 North Park Avenue, Helena, MT 59601; tel. 406/444–8200; FAX. 406/442–6946; Terry Screnar, Chief Executive Officer

NEBRASKA: Blue Cross and Blue Shield Nebraska, 7261 Mercy Road, Omaha, NE 68180-0001; tel. 402/390–1800; FAX. 402/392–2141; Richard L. Guffey, Chief Executive Officer

NEVADA: Blue Cross and Blue Shield Nevada, Anthem Insurance Companies, Inc., 5250 South Virginia Street, Reno, NV 89520; tel. 303/831–3234; C. David Kikumoto, Chief Executive Officer

NEW HAMPSHIRE: Blue Cross and Blue Shield New Hampshire, Anthem Insurance Companies, Inc., 3000 Goffs Falls Road, Manchester, NH 03111-0001; tel. 603/695–7000; FAX. 603/695–7304; David A. Jensen, Chief Executive Officer

NEW JERSEY: Horizon Blue Cross and Blue Shield of New Jersey, Inc., Horizon Healthcare Services, Inc., 3 Penn Plaza East, Newark, NJ 07105; tel. 973/466–8300; FAX. 973/466–8762; William J. Marino, Chief Executive Officer

NEW MEXICO: Blue Cross and Blue Shield New Mexico, 12800 Indian School Road, N.E., Albuquerque, NM 87112; tel. 505/271–4463; Norman P. Becker, Chief Executive Officer

NEW YORK: Blue Cross and Blue Shield Central New York, Excellus, Inc., 344 South Warren Street, Syracuse, NY 13202; tel. 315/448–3700; FAX. 315/448–4922; Howard F. Beacham, III, Chief Executive Officer

Blue Cross and Blue Shield of the Rochester Area, Excellus, Inc., 165 Court Street, Rochester, NY 14647; tel. 716/238–4351; FAX. 716/238–4400; Howard J. Berman, Chief Executive Officer

Blue Cross and Blue Shield Utica-Watertown, Excellus, Inc., 12 Rhoads Drive, Utica, NY 13502-6398; tel. 315/798–4200; FAX. 315/797–4288; Christopher D. Perna, Chief Executive Officer

Blue Cross and Blue Shield Western New York, 1901 Main Street, Buffalo, NY 14240-0080; tel. 716/887–6949; FAX. 716/887–8981; Thomas P. Hartnett, Ph.D., Chief Executive Officer

Empire Blue Cross and Blue Shield, One World Trade Center, New York, NY 10048-0682; tel. 212/476–7623; Michael A. Stocker, M.D., Chief Executive Officer

NORTH CAROLINA: Blue Cross and Blue Shield North Carolina, 5901 Chapel Hill Road, Durham, NC 27707; tel. 919/765–2400; FAX. 919/765–7105; Kenneth C. Otis, II, Chief Executive Officer

NORTH DAKOTA: Blue Cross and Blue Shield North Dakota, Noridian Mutual Insurance Company, 4510 13th Avenue, S.W., Fargo, ND 58121-0001; tel. 701/282–1327; FAX. 701/282–1866; Michael B. Unhjem, Chief Executive Officer

OHIO: Anthem Blue Cross and Blue Shield, Anthem Insurance Companies, Inc., 4361 Irwin Simpson Road, Mason, OH 45040; tel. 317/488–6577; Keith R. Faller, Chief Executive Officer

OKLAHOMA: Blue Cross and Blue Shield Oklahoma, 1215 South Boulder Avenue, Tulsa, OK 741192800; tel. 918/560–3500; FAX. 918/560–2095; Ronald F. King, Chief Executive Officer

OREGON: Regence Blue Cross and Blue Shield Oregon, The Regence Group, 100 S.W. Market Street, Portland, OR 97201; tel. 503/225–5206; FAX. 503/225–5232; Donald P. Sacco, Chief Executive Officer

PENNSYLVANIA: Blue Cross Northeastern Pennsylvania, Hospital Service Association of Northeastern Pennsylvania, 70 North Main Street, Wilkes-Barre, PA 18711; tel. 570/829–8801; FAX. 570/829–8420; Denise S. Cesare, Chief Executive Officer

Capital Blue Cross, 2500 Elmerton Avenue, Harrisburg, PA 17110; tel. 717/541–7000; FAX. 717/541–7405; James M. Mead, Chief Executive Officer

Independence Blue Cross, 1901 Market Street, Philadelphia, PA 19103; tel. 215/241–2422; FAX. 215/241–3824; G. Fred DiBona, Jr., Esq., Chief Executive Officer

Pennsylvania Blue Shield, Highmark, Inc., 1800 Center Street, Camp Hill, PA 17089; tel. 412/544–8208; John S. Brouse, Chief Executive Officer

Pennsylvania Blue Shield, Highmark, Inc., 120 Fifth Avenue, Pittsburgh, PA 15222-3099; tel. 412/544–8202; John S. Brouse, Chief Executive Officer

RHODE ISLAND: Blue Cross and Blue Shield Rhode Island, 444 Westminster Street, Providence, RI 02903-3279; tel. 401/459–1200; FAX. 401/459–1290; Ronald A. Battista, Chief Executive Officer

SOUTH CAROLINA: Blue Cross and Blue Shield South Carolina, I-20 East at Alpine Road, Columbia, SC 29219; tel. 803/788–3860; FAX. 803/736–3420; M. Edward Sellers, Chief Executive Officer

SOUTH DAKOTA: Wellmark Blue Cross and Blue Shield South Dakota, Wellmark, Inc., 1601 West Madison Street, Sioux Falls, SD 57104; tel. 515/245–4545; John D. Forsyth, Chief Executive Officer

TENNESSEE: Blue Cross and Blue Shield Tennessee, 801 Pine Street, Chattanooga, TN 37402; tel. 423/755–5620; FAX. 423/755–2178; Thomas Kinser, Chief Executive Officer

TEXAS: Blue Cross and Blue Shield Texas, 901 South Central Expressway, Richardson, TX 75080; tel. 972/766–6900; FAX. 972/766–8586; Roger K. Coleman, M.D., Chief Executive Officer

Organizations / BlueCross BlueShield Association

UTAH: Regence Blue Cross and Blue Shield Utah, 2890 E. Cottonwood Parkway, Salt Lake City, UT 84130; tel. 802/371-3770; Jed H. Pitcher, Chief Executive Officer

VERMONT: Blue Cross and Blue Shield Vermont, 445 Industrial Lane, Berlin, VT 05602; tel. 802/223-6131; FAX. 802/229-0511; William R. Milnes, Jr., Chief Executive Officer

VIRGINIA: Trigon Blue Cross and Blue Shield, Trigon Healthcare, Inc., 2015 Staples Mill Road, Richmond, VA 23230; tel. 804/354-7173; FAX. 804/354-7044; Thomas Snead, Chief Executive Officer

WASHINGTON: Blue Cross and Blue Shield Alaska, Premera Blue Cross, P.O Box 327, Seattle, WA 98111-0327; tel. 425/670-5780; FAX. 425/670-4900; Betty Woods, Chief Executive Officer

Northwest Washington Medical Bureau, 1100 South Second Street, Mount Vernon, WA 98273; tel. 360/336-9660; Karen J. Larson, Chief Executive Officer

Regence Blue Shield, The Regence Group, 1800 Ninth Avenue, Seattle, WA 981011322; tel. 206/464-3600; FAX. 206/389-6778; Rich D. Nelson, Chief Executive Officer

WEST VIRGINIA: Mountain State Blue Cross and Blue Shield, 700 Market Square, P.O. Box 1948, Parkersburg, WV 26101; tel. 304/424-7732; FAX. 304/424-7789; Gregory K. Smith, Chief Executive Officer

WISCONSIN: Blue Cross and Blue Shield United of Wisconsin, 401 West Michigan Street, Milwaukee, WI 53203; tel. 414/226-6295; FAX. 414/226-5488; Thomas R. Hefty, Chief Executive Officer

WYOMING: Blue Cross and Blue Shield Wyoming, 4000 House Avenue, Cheyenne, WY 820012266; tel. 307/634-1393; Tim J. Crilly, Chief Executive Officer

U.S. Associated Areas

PUERTO RICO: La Cruz Azul de Puerto Rico, Independence Blue Cross, Carr. 1 Km 17.3, Rio Piedras, PR 00927; tel. 787/272-7800; Rafael Santos Del Valle, Esq., Chief Executive Officer

Triple-S, Inc., Triple-S Management Corporation, 1441 F. D. Roosevelt Avenue, Caparra, PR 00920; tel. 809/749-4114; Miguel A. Vazquez Deynes, Chief Executive Officer

Canada

ALBERTA: Alberta Blue Cross Plan, 10009-108th Street, Edmonton, AB T5J 3C5; tel. 780/498-8297; FAX. 780/498-8383; V. George Ward, President and CEO

MANITOBA: Manitoba Blue Cross, United Health Services Corporation, 100A Polo Park Centre, 1485 Portage Avenue, Winnipeg, MB R3G 0W, Winnipeg, MB R3C 2X7; tel. 204/775-0161; FAX. 204/774-1761; Kerry V. Bittner, President

NEW BRUNSWICK: Blue Cross in Ontario, (Moncton Office), 644 Main Street, Moncton, NB E1C 1E2, P.O. Box 220, Moncton, NB E1C 8L3; tel. 506/853-1811; FAX. 506/867-4646; Leon R. Furlong, President and CEO

Blue Cross of Atlantic Canada, 644 Main Street, Moncton, NB E1C 1E2, P.O. Box 220, Moncton, NB E1C 8L3; tel. 506/853-1811; FAX. 506/853-4651; Leon R. Furlong, President and CEO

ONTARIO: Blue Cross in Ontario, (Ontario Office), 185 The West Mall, Suite 600, Etobicoke, ON M9C 5P1; tel. 416/626-1688; FAX. 416/626-0997; Claude Bovin, President

QUEBEC: Quebec Blue Cross Quebec Hospital Service Association, 550 Sherbrooke Street, W., Suite B-9, Montreal, PQ H3A 1B9; tel. 514/286-8482; FAX. 514/286-8475; Claude Bolvin, CA, President and CEO

SASKATCHEWAN: Saskatchewan Blue Cross, 516 Second Avenue, N., Saskatoon, SK S7K 2C5, P.O. Box 4030, Saskatoon, SK S7K 3T2; tel. 306/244-1192; FAX. 306/664-1945; Terry R. Brash, President and CEO

Health Systems Agencies

The following list is based on information provided by the agencies themselves. For information about other local agencies and organizations that fulfill similar functions, contact the state or metropolitan hospital associations; see also the list of State Health Planning and Development Agencies in section C.

United States

FLORIDA: Broward Regional Health Planning Council (District 10), 915 Middle River Drive, Suite 521, Fort Lauderdale, FL 33304; tel. 954/561–9681; FAX. 954/561–9685; John H. Werner, Chief Executive Officer

Health Council of South Florida, Inc., 5757 Blue Lagoon Drive, Suite 170, Miami, FL 33126; tel. 305/263–9020; FAX. 305/262–9905; Sonya Albury, Executive Director

Health Planning Council of Northeast Florida, Inc., 900 University Blvd. N, Suite 202, Jacksonville, FL 32211; tel. 904/745–3050; FAX. 904/745–3054; Lori A. Bilello, Executive Director

Health Planning Council of Southwest Florida, Inc., 9250 College Parkway, Suite Three, Fort Myers, FL 33919; tel. 941/433–4600; FAX. 941/433–6703; Ron Burris, Executive Director

North Central Florida Health Planning Council, 18 N.W. 33rd Court, Gainesville, FL 32607; tel. 352/955–2264; FAX. 352/955–3109; Edith M. Orsini, Executive Director

Suncoast Health Council, Inc. (District Five), 9800 4th Street North, Suite 206, St. Petersburg, FL 33702-2451; tel. 727/217–7070; FAX. 727/570–3033; Elizabeth Rugg, Executive Director

The Local Health Council of East Central Florida Inc., 1155 South Semoran Boulevard, Suite 1, Winter Park, FL 32792-5505; tel. 407/671–2005; Dieter Carlton, Chief Executive Officer

Treasure Coast Health Council, Inc. (District Nine), 4152 W. Blue Heron Blvd, Suite 229, Riviera Beach, FL 33404; tel. 561/844–4220; FAX. 516/844–3310; Barbara H. Jacobowitz, Executive Director

MARYLAND: Chesapeake Health Planning System, Inc., P.O. Box 773, Cambridge, MD 21613; tel. 410/221–0907; FAX. 410/221–2605; John Bennett, President

MINNESOTA: Region 1 (Northwest MN) and Region II (Northeast MN), Regional Coordinating Boards, Minnesota Department of Health, P.O. Box 64975, St. Paul, MN 55164-0975; tel. 612/282–5644; FAX. 612/282–5628; Michele Holten

NEW JERSEY: Health Visions, Inc., 6981 North Park Drive, East Building, Suite 309, Pennsauken, NJ 08109; tel. 609/662–2050; FAX. 609/662–2261; Charles Steinmetz, Senior Vice President, CPAC

NEW YORK: Central New York Health Systems Agency, Inc., 701 Erie Boulevard West, Syracuse, NY 13204; tel. 315/472–8099; FAX. 315/472–8033; Timothy J. Bobo, Executive Director

Finger Lakes Health Systems Agency, 1150 University Avenue, Rochester, NY 14607; tel. 716/461–3520; FAX. 716/461–0997; Martha P. Bond, Executive Director

New York State Public Health Association, Pine West Plaza, One United Way, Albany, NY 12205-5558; tel. 518/452–3300; FAX. 518/452–3305; Robert Guerrin, Ph.D., President

NY Penn Health Systems Agency, 84 Court Street, Suite 300, Binghamton, NY 13901; tel. 607/772–0336; FAX. 607/772–0158; Denise Murray, President

OHIO: Health Planning and Resource Development Association of Central, Ohio River Valley, 35 East Seventh Street, Suite 311, Cincinnati, OH 45202; tel. 513/621–2434; FAX. 513/621–4307; James F. Sandmann, President

Health Systems Agency, 415 Bulkley Building, 2910 Euclid Avenue, Cleveland, OH 44115; tel. 216/771–6814; FAX. 216/771–2939; Nancy J. Roth, Executive Director

Lake to River Health Care Coalition, 280 N. Park Avenue, Park Pointer Building 3rd Floor, Warren, OH 44481-1123; tel. 330/306–0827; FAX. 330/306–0829; Jack Roberts, Executive Director

Miami Valley Health Improvement Council, 2076 B. North Broad Street, Fairborn, OH 45324; tel. 937/754–9520; FAX. 937/754–9750; Rudolph P. Arnold, M.D., President and CEO

Northwest Ohio Health Planning, Inc., 635 North Erie Street, Toledo, OH 43624; tel. 419/255–1190; FAX. 419/255–2900; David G. Pollick, Executive Director

Scioto Valley Health Systems Agency (SVHSA), 600 West Spring Street, Rear, Columbus, OH 43215-2327; tel. 614/645–7438; FAX. 614/645–5531; Franklin Hirsch, Executive Director

VIRGINIA: Central Virginia Health Planning Agency, Inc., P.O. Box 24287, Richmond, VA 23224; tel. 804/233–6206; FAX. 804/233–8834; Karen L. Cameron, Chief Executive Officer

Eastern Virginia Health Systems Agency, Inc., The Koger Center, Suite 232, Norfolk, VA 23502; tel. 757/461–4834; FAX. 757/461–3255; Paul M. Boynton, Executive Director

Health Systems Agency of Northern Virginia, 7245 Arlington Boulevard, Suite 300, Falls Church, VA 22042; tel. 703/573–3100; FAX. 703/573–1276; Dean Montgomery, Executive Director

Northwestern Virginia Health Systems Agency, 1924 Arlington Boulevard, Suite 211, Charlottesville, VA 22903; tel. 804/977–6010; FAX. 804/977–0748; Margaret P. King, Executive Director

Southwest Virginia Health Systems Agency, Inc., Health Planning Agency of Southwest Virginia, Inc., 3100-A Peters Creek Road, N.W., Roanoke, VA 24019; tel. 540/362–9528; FAX. 540/362–9676; Pamela P. Clark, MPA, Executive Director

Hospital Associations

The following list of state and metropolitan hospital associations is derived from the American Hospital Association.

United States

ALABAMA: Alabama Hospital Association, 500 North East Boulevard, P.O. Box 210759, Montgomery, AL 36121-0759; tel. 334/272-8781; FAX. 334/270-9527; J. Michael Horsley, President and CEO

ALASKA: Alaska State Hospital and Nursing Home Association, 426 Main Street, Juneau, AK 99801; tel. 907/586-1790; FAX. 907/463-3573; Laraine Derr, President and CEO

ARIZONA: Arizona Hospital and Healthcare Association, 1501 W. Fountainhead Parkway, Suite 650, Tempe, AZ 85282; tel. 480/968-1083; FAX. 480/967-2029; John R. Rivers, President and CEO

ARKANSAS: Arkansas Hospital Association, 419 Natural Resources Drive, Little Rock, AR 72205-1539; tel. 501/224-7878; FAX. 501/224-0519; James R. Teeter, President and CEO

CALIFORNIA: California Healthcare Association, 1201 K. Street, Suite 800, Sacramento, CA 95814-1100; tel. 916/443-7401; FAX. 916/552-7596; C. Duane Dauner, President

Healthcare Association of San Diego and Imperial Counties, 402 West Broadway, 22nd Floor, San Diego, CA 92101-3542; tel. 619/544-0777; FAX. 619/544-0888; Gary R. Stephany, President and CEO

Healthcare Association of Southern California, 515 South Figueroa Street, Suite 1300, Los Angeles, CA 90071-3322; tel. 213/538-0700; FAX. 213/629-4272; James D. Barber, President and CEO

Hospital Council of Northern and Central California, 1215 K. Street, Suite 730, Sacramento, CA 95814; tel. 916/552-7608; FAX. 916/552-2618; Gregg Schnepple, President and CEO

COLORADO: Colorado Health and Hospital Association, 7335 East Orchard Road, Suite 100, Englewood, CO 80111; tel. 720/489-1630; FAX. 720/489-9400; Larry Wall, President

CONNECTICUT: Connecticut Hospital Association, 110 Barnes Road, P.O. Box 90, Wallingford, CT 06492-0090; tel. 203/265-7611; FAX. 203/284-9318; Dennis P. May, President

DELAWARE: Delaware Healthcare Association, 1280 South Governors Avenue, Dover, DE 19904-4802; tel. 302/674-2853; FAX. 302/734-2731; Joseph M. Letnaunchyn, President

DISTRICT OF COLUMBIA: District of Columbia Hospital Association, 1250 Eye Street, N.W., Suite 700, Washington, DC 20005-3930; tel. 202/682-1581; FAX. 202/371-8151; Robert A. Malson, President

FLORIDA: Florida Hospital Association, 307 Park Lake Circle, P.O. Box 531107, Orlando, FL 32853-1107; tel. 407/841-6230; FAX. 407/422-5948; Charles F. Pierce, Jr., President

South Florida Hospital and Healthcare Association, Inc, 6363 Taft Street, Suite 200, Hollywood, FL 33024; tel. 954/964-1660; FAX. 954/962-1260; Linda S. Quick, President

GEORGIA: GHA: An Association of Hospitals and Health Systems, 1675 Terrell Mill Road, Marietta, GA 30067; tel. 770/955-0324; FAX. 770/955-5801; Joseph A. Parker, President

HAWAII: Healthcare Association of Hawaii, 932 Ward Avenue, Suite 430, Honolulu, HI 96814-2126; tel. 808/521-8961; FAX. 808/599-2879; Richard E. Meiers, President and CEO

IDAHO: Idaho Hospital Association, 802 West Bannock Street, Suite 500, Boise, ID 83701-1278; tel. 208/338-5100; FAX. 208/338-7800; Steven A. Millard, President

ILLINOIS: Illinois Hospital and HealthSystems Association, 1151 East Warrenville Road, P.O. Box 3015, Naperville, IL 60566-7015; tel. 630/505-7777; FAX. 630/505-9457; Kenneth C. Robbins, President

Metropolitan Chicago Healthcare Council, 222 South Riverside Plaza, 19th Floor, Chicago, IL 60606; tel. 312/906-6000; FAX. 312/993-0779; Earl C. Bird, President

INDIANA: Indiana Hospital & Health Association, One American Square, P.O. Box 82063, Indianapolis, IN 46282; tel. 317/633-4870; FAX. 317/633-4875; Kenneth G. Stella, President

IOWA: Iowa Hospital Association, 100 East Grand Avenue, Suite 100, Des Moines, IA 50309; tel. 515/288-1955; FAX. 515/283-9366; Stephen F. Brenton, President

KANSAS: Kansas Hospital Association, 215 SE 8th Street, Topeka, KS 66603; tel. 785/233-7436; FAX. 785/233-6955; Donald A. Wilson, President

KENTUCKY: KHA: An Association of Kentucky Hospitals and Health Systems, 2501 Nelson Miller Parkway, P.O. Box 436629, Louisville, KY 40253-6629; tel. 502/426-6220; FAX. 502/426-6226; Michael T. Rust, President

LOUISIANA: Louisiana Hospital Association, 9521 Brookline Avenue, Baton Rouge, LA 70809-1431; tel. 225/928-0026; FAX. 225/923-1004; Lynn B. Nicholas, FACHE, President and CEO

Metropolitan Hospital Council of New Orleans, 2450 Severn Avenue, Suite 210, Metairie, LA 70001; tel. 504/837-1171; FAX. 504/837-1174; John J. Finn, Ph.D., President

MAINE: Maine Hospital Association, 150 Capitol Street, Augusta, ME 04330; tel. 207/622-4794; FAX. 207/622-3073; Steven R. Michaud, President

MARYLAND: Healthcare Council of the National Capital Area, 8201 Corporate Drive, Suite 410, Landover, MD 20785-2229; tel. 301/731-4700; FAX. 301/731-8286; Joseph P. Burns, President and CEO

MHA: The Association of Maryland Hospitals & Health Systems, 6820 Deerpath Road, Elkridge, MD 21075-6234; tel. 410/379-6200; FAX. 410/379-8239; Calvin M. Pierson, President

MASSACHUSETTS: Massachusetts Hospital Association, Five New England Executive Park, Burlington, MA 01803; tel. 781/272-8000; FAX. 781/272-0466; Ronald M. Hollander, President

MICHIGAN: Healthcare Council of MidMichigan, 3927 Beecher Road, Flint, MI 48532-3803; tel. 810/766-6898; FAX. 810/762-4108; Marlene Soderstrom, President

Hospital Council of East Central Michigan, 141 Harrow Lane, Suite 11, Saginaw, MI 48603; tel. 517/792-1725; FAX. 517/792-3099; John C. Halstead, Acting President

Michigan Health & Hospital Association, 6215 West St. Joseph Highway, Lansing, MI 48917; tel. 517/323-3443; FAX. 517/323-0946; Spencer C. Johnson, President

North Central Council of MHA, 114 North Court Street, Gaylord, MI 49735; tel. 517/732-7002; FAX. 517/732-3059; Elizabeth Gertz, Executive Director

Southeast Michigan Health and Hospital Council, 24725 West Twelve Mile Road, Suite 104A, Southfield, MI 48034; tel. 248/358-2950; FAX. 248/358-1098; Donald P. Potter, President

Southwestern Michigan Hospital Council, 6215 West St. Joseph Highway, Lansing, MI 48917; tel. 517/323-3443; FAX. 517/323-0946; Clark R. Ballard, President

MINNESOTA: Minnesota Hospital and Healthcare Partnership, 2550 University Avenue, W., Suite 350S, St. Paul, MN 55114-1900; tel. 651/641-1121; FAX. 651/659-1477; Bruce J. Rueben, President

MISSISSIPPI: Mississippi Hospital Association, 6425 Lakeover Road, P.O. Box 16444, Jackson, MS 392366444; tel. 800/289-8884; FAX. 601/368-3200; Sam W. Cameron, President and CEO

MISSOURI: Missouri Hospital Association, P.O. Box 60, Jefferson City, MO 65102-0060; tel. 573/893-3700; FAX. 573/893-2809; Marc D. Smith, President

The Health Alliance of MidAmerica, 10401 Holmes Road, Suite 280, Kansas City, MO 64131-3368; tel. 816/941-3800; FAX. 816/941-0818; Michael R. Dunaway, Senior Vice President

MONTANA: MHA... An Association of Montana Health Care Providers, 1720 Ninth Avenue, P.O. Box 5119, Helena, MT 59604; tel. 406/442-1911; FAX. 406/443-3894; James F. Ahrens, President

NEBRASKA: Nebraska Association of Hospitals and Health Systems, 1640 L Street, Suite D, Lincoln, NE 68508; tel. 402/458-4900; FAX. 402/475-4091; Laura J. Redoutey, CHE, President

NEVADA: Nevada Hospital Association, 4600 Kietzke Lane, Suite A-106, Reno, NV 89502; tel. 775/827-0184; FAX. 775/827-0190; Bill M. Welch, President and CEO

NEW HAMPSHIRE: New Hampshire Hospital Association, 125 Airport Road, Concord, NH 03301-5388; tel. 603/225-0900; FAX. 603/225-4346; Michael J. Hill, President

NEW JERSEY: New Jersey Hospital Association, P.O. Box One, 760 Alexander Road, CN-1, Princeton, NJ 08543-0001; tel. 609/275-4000; FAX. 609/275-4100; Gary S. Carter, FACHE, President and CEO

NEW MEXICO: New Mexico Hospitals and Health Systems Association, 2121 Osuna Road, N.E., Albuquerque, NM 87113; tel. 505/343-0010; FAX. 505/343-0012; Maureen L. Boshier, President and CEO

NEW YORK: Greater New York Hospital Association, Subsidiaries, and Affiliates, 555 West 57 Street, 15th Floor, New York, NY 10019; tel. 212/246-7100; FAX. 212/262-6350; Kenneth E. Raske, President

Healthcare Association of New York State, One Empire Drive, Rensselaer, NY 12144; tel. 518/431-7600; FAX. 518/431-7915; Daniel Sisto, President

Iroquois Healthcare Alliance, 17 Halfmoon Executive Park Drive, Clifton Park, NY 12065; tel. 518/383-5060; FAX. 518/383-2616; Gary J. Fitzgerald, President

Nassau-Suffolk Hospital Council, Inc, 3001 Expressway Drive North, Suite 300, Islandia, NY 11749-5308; tel. 631/435-3000; FAX. 631/435-2343; Peter M. Sullivan, Executive President and CEO

Northern Metropolitan Hospital Association, 400 Stony Brook Court, Newburgh, NY 12550; tel. 914/562-7520; FAX. 914/562-0187; Arthur E. Weintraub, President

Rochester Regional Healthcare Association, 3445 Winton Place, Rochester, NY 14623; tel. 716/273-8180; FAX. 716/273-8189; Robert M. Swinnerton, President and CEO

Western New York Healthcare Association, 1876 Niagara Falls Boulevard, Tonawanda, NY 14150-6439; tel. 716/695-0843; FAX. 716/695-0073; William D. Pike, President

NORTH CAROLINA: NCHA, An Association of Hospitals and Health Networks, P.O. Box 4449, Cary, NC 27519-4449; tel. 919/677-2400; FAX. 919/677-4200; William A. Pully, President

NORTH DAKOTA: North Dakota Healthcare Association, 1121 N. 13th Street, Suite 1, Bismarck, ND 58501; tel. 701/224-9732; FAX. 701/224-9529; Arnold R. Thomas, President

OHIO: Akron Regional Hospital Association, 190 Montrose West Ave., Suite 201, Akron, OH 44321-2786; tel. 330/668-6180; FAX. 330/668-2013; Marianne G. Lorini, President

Greater Cincinnati Health Council, 2100 Sherman Avenue, Suite 100, Cincinnati, OH 45212-2775; tel. 513/531-0200; FAX. 513/531-0278; Lynn R. Olman, President

Greater Dayton Area Hospital Association, 32 North Main Street, Suite 1441, Dayton, OH 45402; tel. 937/228-1000; FAX. 937/228-1035; Joseph M. Krella, President

Hospital Council of Northwest Ohio, 3231 Central Park West Drive, Suite 200, Toledo, OH 43614; tel. 419/842-0800; FAX. 419/843-8889; W. Scott Fry, President and CEO

Organizations / Hospital Associations

OHA: The Association for Hospitals and Health Systems, 155 East Broad Street, Columbus, OH 43215; tel. 614/221-7614; FAX. 614/221-4771; James R. Castle, President and CEO

The Center for Health Affairs, 1226 Huron Road, Cleveland, OH 44115; tel. 216/696-6900; FAX. 216/696-1837; C. Wayne Rice, Ph.D., President and CEO

OKLAHOMA: Greater Oklahoma City Hospital Council, 4000 Lincoln Boulevard, Oklahoma City, OK 73105; tel. 405/359-5530; FAX. 405/359-5500; Stanley Tatum, Chairman

Oklahoma Hospital Association, 4000 Lincoln Boulevard, Oklahoma City, OK 73105; tel. 405/359-5530; FAX. 405/359-5500; Craig W. Jones, President

OREGON: Oregon Association of Hospitals and Health Systems, 4000 Kruse Way Place, Building 2, Suite 100, Lake Oswego, OR 97035-2543; tel. 503/636-2204; FAX. 503/636-8310; Kenneth M. Rutledge, President

PENNSYLVANIA: Hospital Council of Western Pennsylvania, 500 Commonwealth Drive, Warrendale, PA 15086; tel. 724/776-6400; FAX. 724/776-6969; Ian G. Rawson, Ph.D., President

The Delaware Valley Healthcare Council of HAP, 121 South Broad Street, 20th Floor, Philadelphia, PA 19107; tel. 215/735-9695; FAX. 215/790-1267; Andrew B. Wigglesworth, President

The Hospital & Healthsystem Association of Pennsylvania, 4750 Lindle Road, P.O. Box 8600, Harrisburg, PA 17105-8600; tel. 717/564-9200; FAX. 717/561-5334; Carolyn F. Scanlan, President and CEO

RHODE ISLAND: Hospital Association of Rhode Island, 880 Butler Drive, Suite One, Providence, RI 02906; tel. 401/274-4274; FAX. 401/274-1838; Edward Quinlan, President

SOUTH CAROLINA: South Carolina Health Alliance, 101 Medical Circle, P.O. Box 6009, West Columbia, SC 29171-6009; tel. 803/796-3080; FAX. 803/796-2938; Ken A. Shull, FACHE, President

SOUTH DAKOTA: South Dakota Association of Healthcare Organizations, 3708 Brooks Place, Sioux Falls, SD 57106; tel. 605/361-2281; FAX. 605/361-5175; David R. Hewett, President and CEO

TENNESSEE: THA: An Association of Hospitals and Health Systems, 500 Interstate Boulevard, South, Nashville, TN 37210; tel. 615/256-8240; FAX. 615/242-4803; Craig A. Becker, President

TEXAS: Dallas-Forth Worth Hospital Council, 250 Decker Drive, Irving, TX 75062; tel. 972/719-4900; FAX. 972/719-4009; John C. Gavras, President

Greater San Antonio Hospital Council, 8620 North New Braunfels, Suite 420, San Antonio, TX 78217; tel. 210/820-3500; FAX. 210/820-3888; William Dean Rasco, FACHE, President and CEO

Texas Hospital Association, 6225 U.S. Highway 290, E, P.O. Box 15587, Austin, TX 78761-5587; tel. 512/465-1000; FAX. 512/465-1090; Terry Townsend, FACHE, CAE, President and CEO

UTAH: UHA: Utah Hospital and Health Systems Association, 2180 South 1300 East, Suite 440, Salt Lake City, UT 84106-2843; tel. 801/486-9915; FAX. 801/486-0882; Richard B. Kinnersley, President

VERMONT: Vermont Association of Hospitals and Health Systems, 148 Main Street, Montpelier, VT 05602; tel. 802/223-3461; FAX. 802/223-0364; Norman E. Wright, President

VIRGINIA: Virginia Hospital & Healthcare Association, 4200 Inslake Drive, P.O. Box 31394, Richmond, VA 23294; tel. 804/747-8600; FAX. 804/965-0475; Laurens Sartoris, President

WASHINGTON: Washington State Hospital Association, 300 Elliott Avenue, West, Suite 300, Seattle, WA 98119-4118; tel. 206/281-7211; FAX. 206/283-6122; Leo F. Greenawalt, President and CEO

WEST VIRGINIA: West Virginia Hospital Association, 100 Association Drive, Charleston, WV 25311-1571; tel. 304/344-9744; FAX. 304/344-9745; Steven J. Summer, President

WISCONSIN: Wisconsin Health and Hospital Association, 5721 Odana Road, Madison, WI 53719-1289; tel. 608/274-1820; FAX. 608/274-8554; Robert C. Taylor, President and CEO

WYOMING: Wyoming Hospital Association, P.O. Box 249, Cheyenne, WY 82003; tel. 307/632-9344; FAX. 307/632-9347; Robert C. Kidd, II, President

U.S. Associated Areas

PUERTO RICO: Puerto Rico Hospital Association, Officina 101-103, Villa Navarez Professional Center, Centro Commercial Villa Navarez, San Juan, PR 00927; tel. 787/764-0290; FAX. 787/753-9748; Juan Rivera, Executive Vice President

Canada

ALBERTA: Provincial Health Authorities of Alberta, 44 Capital Boulevard, 200-10044-108 Street, NW, Edmonton, AB AB T5J 3S7; tel. 403/424-4309; FAX. 403/424-4309; E. Michael Higgins, Executive Director

NEW BRUNSWICK: New Brunswick Healthcare Association, 861 Woodstock Road, Fredericton, NB E3B 7R7; tel. 506/451-0750; FAX. 506/451-0760; Michel J. Poirier, Executive Director

NEWFOUNDLAND: NFLD & Lab Health Boards Association, P.O. Box 8234, St. John's, NF A1B-3N5; tel. 709/364-7701; FAX. 709/364-6460; John F. Peddle, Executive Director

NORTHWEST TERRITORIES: Northwest Territories Health Care Association, P.O. Box 1709, Yellowknife, NT X1A-2P3; tel. 867/873-9253; FAX. 867/873-9254; Sharon Ehaloak, Executive Director

NOVA SCOTIA: Nova Scotia Association of Health Organizations, Bedford Professional Centre, 2 Dartmouth Road, Bedford, NS B4A-2K7; tel. 902/832-8500; FAX. 902/832-8505; Robert A. Cook, President and CEO

ONTARIO: Catholic Health Association of Canada, 1247 Kilborn Place, Ottawa, ON K1H-6K9; tel. 613/731-7148; FAX. 613/731-7797; Richard Haughian, D.Th., President

Ontario Hospital Association, 200 Front Street, W, Suite 2000, Toronto, ON M5V-3L1; tel. 416/205-1300; FAX. 416/205-1310; David MacKinnon, President

PRINCE EDWARD ISLAND: Health Association of PEI, Inc., 10 Pownal Street, Charlottetown, PEI C1A-3V6; tel. 902/368-3901; FAX. 902/368-3231; Ken Ezeard, President

QUEBEC: Quebec Hospital Association, 505 boulevard de Maisonneuve, W, Suite 400, Montreal, PQ H3-3C2; tel. 514/842-4861; FAX. 514/282-4271; Daniel Adam, Executive Vice President

SASKATCHEWAN: Saskatchewan Association of Health Organizations, 1445 Park Street, Regina, SK S4N-4C5; tel. 306/347-5500; FAX. 306/347-5500; Arliss Wright, President and CEO

Hospital Licensure Agencies

Information for the following list of state hospital licensure agencies was obtained directly from the agencies.

United States

ALABAMA: Alabama Department of Public Health, Division of Health Care Facilities, The RSA Tower, P.O. Box 303017, Montgomery, AL 36130-3017; tel. 334/206-5075; FAX. 334/206-5088; Elva Goldman, Director

Alabama Department of Public Health, Division of Provider Services, The RSA Tower, P.O. Box 303017, Montgomery, AL 36130-3017; tel. 334/206-5079; FAX. 334/206-5219; Jimmy D. Prince, Director

ALASKA: Health Facilities Licensing and Certification, 4730 Business Park Boulevard, Building H, Anchorage, AK 99503-7137; tel. 907/561-8081; FAX. 907/561-3011; Shelbert Larsen, Administrator

ARIZONA: Arizona Department of Health Services Office of Health Care, Office of Health Care Licensing /Medical Facilities Section, 1647 East Morten Avenue, Suite 160, Phoenix, AZ 85020; tel. 602/674-9750; FAX. 602/395-8913; Mary Madden, Program Manager

ARKANSAS: Division of Health Facility Services, Arkansas Department of Health, 5800 West 10th Street, Suite 400, Little Rock, AR 72204-9916; tel. 501/661-2201; FAX. 501/661-2468; Renee Mallory, Director

CALIFORNIA: Licensing and Certification, Department of Health Services, 1800 Third Street, Suite 210,, P.O. Box 942732, Sacramento, CA 94234-7320; tel. 916/445-2070; FAX. 916/445-6979; Brenda Klutz, Deputy Director

COLORADO: Health Facilities Division, Colorado Department of Public Health and Environment, 4300 Cherry Creek Drive, S., Denver, CO 80246-1530; tel. 303/692-2800; FAX. 303/782-4883; Paul Daraghy, Director

CONNECTICUT: Department of Public Health, Division of Health Systems Regulation, 410 Capitol Avenue, Hartford, CT 06134-0308; tel. 860/509-7400; FAX. 860/509-7543; Kathleen Zarrella, R.N., Director

DELAWARE: Office of Health Facilities Licensing and Certification, Department of Health and Social Services, 2055 Limestone Road, Suite 200, Wilmington, DE 19808; tel. 302/995-8521; FAX. 302/995-8529; Mary E. Peterson, Director

DISTRICT OF COLUMBIA: Licensing Regulation Administration, 614 H Street, N.W., Suite 1003, Washington, DC 20001; tel. 202/727-7190; FAX. 202/727-7780; Geraldine K. Sykes

FLORIDA: Division of Health Quality Assurance, Hospital and Outpatient , Agency for Health Care Administration, 2727 Mahan Drive, Tallahassee, FL 32308; tel. 850/487-2717; FAX. 850/487-6240; Mary Loepp, Unit Manager

GEORGIA: Health Care Section, Office of Regulatory Services, Georgia Department of Human Resources, Two Peachtree Street, N.W., Room 33-250, Atlanta, GA 30303-3142; tel. 404/657-5550; FAX. 404/657-8934; Susie M. Woods, Director

HAWAII: Hawaii Department of Health, Office of Health Care Assurance, P.O. Box 3378, Honolulu, HI 96801; tel. 808/586-4080; FAX. 808/586-4747; Helen K. Yoshimi, B.S.N., MPH, Chief, OHCA

IDAHO: Bureau of Facility Standards, Department of Health and Welfare, P.O. Box 83720, Boise, ID 83720-0036; tel. 208/334-6626; FAX. 208/364-1888; Sylvia Creswell, Supervisor, Non-Long Term Care

ILLINOIS: Division of Health Care Facilities and Programs, Illinois Department of Public Health, 525 West Jefferson Street, Springfield, IL 62761; tel. 217/782-7412; FAX. 217/782-0382; Enrique J. Unanue, AIA, Chief

INDIANA: Division of Acute Care, Indiana State Department of Health, Two North Meridian Street, Indianapolis, IN 46204; tel. 317/233-7472; FAX. 317/233-7157; Mary Azbill, Director

IOWA: Division of Health Facilities, Iowa State Department of Inspections and Appeals, Lucas State Office Building, 321 East 12th Street, Des Moines, IA 50319; tel. 515/281-4115; FAX. 515/242-5022; David Werning, Public Information Officer

KANSAS: Kansas Department of Health and Environment, Bureau of Health Facilities, 900 Southwest Jackson, Suite 1001, Topeka, KS 66612-1290; tel. 785/296-0131; FAX. 785/296-1266; Beth Vaurhees, Director of Medical Facilites and Support

KENTUCKY: Division of Licensing and Regulation, Cabinet for Health Services, 275 East Main Street, 4E-A, Frankfort, KY 40621; tel. 502/564-2800; FAX. 502/564-6546; Rebecca J. Cecil, R.Ph., Director

LOUISIANA: Health Standards Section, Louisiana Department of Health and Hospitals, P.O. Box 3767, Baton Rouge, LA 70821; tel. 504/342-0415; FAX. 504/342-5292; Lisa Deaton, RN, Manager

MAINE: Division of Licensing and Certification, Department of Human Services, State House, Station 11, Augusta, ME 04333; tel. 207/624-5443; FAX. 207/624-5378; Louis Dorogi, Director

MARYLAND: Department of Health and Mental Hygiene, Office of Health Care Quality, 55 Wade Avenue - SGHC, Catonsville, MD 21228; tel. 410/402-8007; FAX. 410/402-8211; Joseph I. Berman, Medical Director

MASSACHUSETTS: Massachusetts Department of Public Health, Division of Health Care Quality, 10 West Street, Fifth Floor, Boston, MA 02111; tel. 617/753-8000; FAX. 617/753-8125; Paul I. Dreyer, Ph.D., Director

MICHIGAN: Bureau of Health Systems, Michigan Department of Consumer and Industry Service, 525 West Ottawa, P.O. Box 30664, Lansing, MI 48909; tel. 517/241-4160; FAX. 517/241-2635; Gladys M. Thomas, Ph. D., Division Director

MINNESOTA: Facility and Provider Compliance Division, Minnesota Department of Health, 85 East Seventh Place, P.O. Box 64900, St. Paul, MN 55164-0900; tel. 651/215-8700; FAX. 651/215-8710; Linda G. Sutherland, Director

MISSISSIPPI: Division of Health Facilities Licensure and Certification, Mississippi State Department of Health, P.O. Box 1700, Jackson, MS 39215; tel. 601/576-7300; FAX. 601/354-7230; Vanessa Phipps, Director

MISSOURI: Bureau of Health Facility Regulation, Missouri Department of Health, P.O. Box 570, Jefferson City, MO 65102; tel. 573/751-6303; FAX. 573/526-3621; Calvin L. Badding, Administrator

MONTANA: Division of Quality Assurance, Department of Public Health and Human Services, 2401 Colonial Drive, P.O. Box 202953, Helena, MT 59620-2953; tel. 406/444-2037; FAX. 406/444-1742; Denzel Davis, Administrator

NEBRASKA: Nebraska Department of Regulation and Licensure, Credentialing Division, 301 Centennial Mall, S., P.O. Box 95007, Lincoln, NE 68509-5007; tel. 402/471-2946; FAX. 402/471-0555; Nancy Brown, Program Administrator

NEVADA: Bureau of Licensure and Certification, Nevada Health Division, 1550 East College Parkway, Suite 158, Carson City, NV 89706-7921; tel. 775/687-4475; FAX. 775/687-6588; Richard J. Panelli, Chief

NEW HAMPSHIRE: Bureau of Health Facilities Administration, Office of Program Support, Licensure and Regulation, 129 Pleasant Street, Brown Building, Concord, NH 03301; tel. 603/271-4966; FAX. 603/271-4968; Raymond Rusin, Bureau Chief

NEW JERSEY: Certificate of Need and Acute Care Licensing, N.J. Department of Health and Senior Services, P.O. Box 360, Trenton, NJ 08625-0360; tel. 609/292-8773; FAX. 609/292-3780; John Calabria, Director

NEW MEXICO: Department of Health, Health Facility Licensing & Certification Bureau, 525 Camino de los Marquez, Suite Two, Santa Fe, NM 87501; tel. 505/827-4200; FAX. 505/827-4203; Wilma Hammar, Bureau Chief

NEW YORK: New York State Department of Health, Bureau of Hospital and Primary Care Services, Hedley Park Place, Suite 303, 433 River Street, Troy, NY 12180-2299; tel. 518/402-1003; FAX. 518/402-1010; Frederick J. Heigel, Director

NORTH CAROLINA: Division of Facility Services, Department of Human Resources, 2715 Mail Service Center, Raleigh, NC 27699-2715; tel. 919/733-1610; FAX. 919/733-3207; Steve White, Section Chief

NORTH DAKOTA: Health Resources Section, State Department of Health, 600 East Boulevard Avenue, Bismarck, ND 58505-0200; tel. 701/328-2352; FAX. 701/328-1890; Darleen Bartz, Chief Health Resources Section

OHIO: Bureau of Quality Assessment and Improvement, Department of Health, P.O. Box 118, Columbus, OH 43266-0118; tel. 614/644-7230; FAX. 614/644-8661; Louis Pomerantz, Chief, Bureau of Quality Assessment a

OKLAHOMA: State Department of Health, 1000 Northeast 10th, Oklahoma City, OK 73117; tel. 405/271-4200; FAX. 405/271-3431; Jerry R. Nida, M.D., Commissioner

OREGON: Health Care Licensure and Certification, Oregon Health Division, P.O. Box 14450, Portland, OR 97293-0450; tel. 503/731-4013; FAX. 503/731-4080; Kathleen Smail, Manager

PENNSYLVANIA: Division of Acute and Ambulatory Care Facilities, Pennsylvania Department of Health, Division of Acute and Ambulatory Care, P.O. Box 90, Harrisburg, PA 17100; tel. 717/783-8980; FAX. 717/772-2163; Elaine Gibble, Director

RHODE ISLAND: Rhode Island Department of Health, Division of Facilities Regulation, Three Capitol Hill, Providence, RI 02908-5097; tel. 401/222-2566; FAX. 401/222-3999; Wayne I. Farrington, Division Chief, Facilities Regulator

SOUTH CAROLINA: Department of Health and Environmental Control, Division of Health Licensing, 2600 Bull Street, Columbia, SC 29201; tel. 803/737-7370; FAX. 803/737-7212; Jerry Paul, Director

SOUTH DAKOTA: Office of Health Care Facilities Licensure and Certification, State Department of Health, Health Lab, 615 E. 4th Street, Pierre, SD 57501-1700; tel. 605/773-3356; FAX. 605/773-6667; Joan Bachman, Administrator

TENNESSEE: Tennessee Department of Health, Division of Health Care Facilities, 425 5th Avenue North, Cordell Hull, 1st Floor, Nashville, TN 37247-0508; tel. 615/741-7294; FAX. 615/741-7051; Ken Murray, Director

TEXAS: Health Facility Compliance Division, Texas Department of Health, 1100 West 49th Street, Austin, TX 78756-3199; tel. 512/834-6650; FAX. 512/834-6653; Nance Stearman, RN, M.S.N., Director

UTAH: Utah State Department of Health, Bureau of Licensing, Box 142003, Salt Lake City, UT 84114-2003; tel. 801/538-6152; FAX. 801/538-6325; Debra Wynkoop, Director

Organizations / Hospital Licensure Agencies

VERMONT: Health Improvement, Vermont Department of Health, 108 Cherry Street, P.O. Box 70, Burlington, VT 05402; tel. 802/863–7606; FAX. 802/651–1634; Ellen B. Thompson, Planning Chief

VIRGINIA: Center for Quality Health Care Services and Consumer Protection, Virginia Department of Health, 3600 Centre, Suite 216, Richmond, VA 23230; tel. 804/367–2102; FAX. 804/367–2149; Nancy R. Hofheimer, Director

WASHINGTON: Acute Care and In-Home Services, Washington Department of Health, Target Plaza, Suite 500, 2725 Harrison Avenue, Olympia, WA 98504-7852; tel. 360/705–6612; FAX. 360/705–6654; Byron Plan, Acute Care Manager

WEST VIRGINIA: Office of Health Facility Licensure and Certification, West Virginia Division of Health, 350 Capitol Street, Room 206, Charleston, WV 25301-3715; tel. 304/558–0050; FAX. 304/558–2515; John Wilkinson, Director

WISCONSIN: Bureau of Quality Assurance, Division of Supportive Living, Department of Health and Family Services, One West Wilson Street, P.O. Box 2969, Madison, WI 53701-2969; tel. 608/267–7185; FAX. 608/266–8481; Susan Schroeder, Director

WYOMING: Office of Health Quality, Health Facilities Licensing, 2020 Carey Avenue, Eighth Floor, Cheyenne, WY 82002; tel. 307/777–7123; FAX. 307/777–7127; K. Wagner, Nurse Administrator

Medical and Nursing Licensure Agencies

The following information is based on information provided by state government entities and the agencies themselves.

United States

ALABAMA
- **Alabama State Board of Medical Examiners**, 848 Washington Avenue, Zip 36104, P.O. Box 946, Montgomery, AL 36101-0946; tel. 334/242-4116; FAX. 334/242-4155; Larry D. Dixon, Executive Director

ALASKA
- **Alaska Board of Nursing, Division of Occupational Licensing**, 3601 C Street, Suite 722, Anchorage, AK 99503; tel. 907/269-8161; FAX. 907/269-8156; Dorothy Fulton, Executive Administrator
- **Alaska State Medical Board, Division of Occupational Licensing**, 3601 C Street, Suite 722, Anchorage, AK 99503; tel. 907/269-8163; FAX. 907/269-8196; Leslie G. Abel, Executive Administrator

ARIZONA
- **Arizona Board of Osteopathic Examiners in Medicine and Surgery**, 9535 E. Doubletree Ranch Road, Scottsdale, AZ 85258; tel. 602/657-7703; FAX. 602/657-7715; Ann Marie Berger, Executive Director
- **Arizona State Board of Medical Examiners**, 1651 East Morton, Suite 210, Phoenix, AZ 85020; tel. 602/255-3751; FAX. 602/255-1848; Claudia Fontz, Executive Director
- **Arizona State Board of Nursing**, 1651 East Morten, Suite 150, Phoenix, AZ 85020; tel. 602/331-8111; FAX. 602/906-9365; Joey Ridenour, RN, M.S.N., Executive Director

ARKANSAS
- **Arkansas State Board of Nursing**, University Tower Building, Suite 800, 1123 South University Avenue, Little Rock, AR 72204; tel. 501/686-2700; FAX. 501/686-2714; Faith A. Fields, M.S.N., RN, Executive Director
- **Arkansas State Medical Board**, 2100 Riverfront Drive, Suite 200, Little Rock, AR 72202; tel. 501/296-1802; FAX. 501/296-1805; Peggy Pryor, Executive Secretary

CALIFORNIA
- **California Board of Registered Nursing**, 400 R Street, Suite 4030, Sacramento, CA 94244-2100; tel. 800/838-6828; FAX. 916/327-4402; Ruth Ann Terry, MPH, RN, Executive Officer
- **Medical Board of California**, 1426 Howe Avenue, Suite 54, Sacramento, CA 95825; tel. 916/263-2344; FAX. 916/263-2487; Ron Joseph, Executive Director

COLORADO
- **Colorado State Board of Medical Examiners**, 1560 Broadway, Suite 1300, Denver, CO 80202-5140; tel. 303/894-7690; FAX. 303/894-7692; Susan Miller, Program Administrator
- **Colorado State Board of Nursing**, 1560 Broadway, Suite 880, Denver, CO 80202; tel. 303/894-2430; FAX. 303/894-2821; Patricia Uris, RN, Ph.D., Program Administrator

CONNECTICUT
- **Connecticut Board of Examiners for Nursing, Department of Public Health**, 410 Capitol Avenue, MS #12 HSR, P.O. Box 340308, Hartford, CT 06134-0308; tel. 860/509-7624; FAX. 860/509-7286; Wendy H. Furniss, RNC., M.S., Public Health Services Manager
- **Connecticut Department of Public Health**, 410 Capitol Avenue, MS #12 APP, P.O. Box 340308, Hartford, CT 06134-0308; tel. 860/509-7563; FAX. 860/509-8457; Jennifer Filippone, Health Program Supervisor

DELAWARE
- **Delaware Board of Medical Practice**, Cannon Building, 861 Silver Lake Boulevard, Suite 203, Dover, DE 19901; tel. 302/739-4522; FAX. 302/739-2711; Doug Reed, Executive Director
- **Delaware Board of Nursing**, Cannon Building, Suite 203, 861 Silver Lake Boulevard, Suite 203, Dover, DE 19904; tel. 302/739-4522; FAX. 302/739-2711; Iva J. Boardman, RN, M.S.N., Executive Director

DISTRICT OF COLUMBIA
- **District of Columbia Board of Medicine**, 825 North Capital Street, NE, Room 2224, Washington, DC 20002; tel. 202/442-9200; FAX. 202/442-9431; James R. Granger, Jr., Executive Director
- **District of Columbia Board of Nursing**, 614 H Street, N.W., Washington, DC 20001; tel. 202/727-7461; FAX. 202/727-8030; Barbara Hatcher, Chairperson

FLORIDA
- **Florida Board of Medicine**, 2020 Capital Circle S.E., Bin #C03, Tallahassee, FL 32399-3253; tel. 850/488-3622; FAX. 850/922-3040; Tanya Williams, Board Director
- **Florida Board of Osteopathic Medicine**, 2020 Capital Circle, SE, Bin #6, Tallahassee, FL 32399-3256; tel. 850/488-0595; FAX. 850/487-9874; Christy Robinson, RSI
- **Florida State Board of Nursing**, 4080 Woodcock Drive, Suite 202, Jacksonville, FL 32207; tel. 904/858-6940; FAX. 904/858-6964; Ruth R. Stiehl, Ph.D.,RN, Executive Director

GEORGIA
- **Georgia Board of Nursing**, 237 Coliseum Drive, Macon, GA 31217; tel. 912/207-1640; FAX. 912/207-1660; Shirley A. Camp, RN, J.D., Executive Director
- **Georgia Composite State Board of Medical Examiners**, 2 Peachtree Street, 6th Floor, Atlanta, GA 30303; tel. 404/656-3913; FAX. 404/656-9723; Karen Mason, Director

HAWAII
- **Hawaii Board of Medical Examiners, Department of Commerce and Consumer Affairs**, 1010 Richards Street, Zip 96813, P.O. Box 3469, Honolulu, HI 96801; tel. 808/586-3000; Constance Cabral-Makanani, Executive Officer
- **Hawaii Board of Nursing**, P.O. Box 3469, Honolulu, HI 96801; tel. 808/586-3000; FAX. 808/586-2689; Kathy Yokouchi, Executive Officer

IDAHO
- **Idaho State Board of Medicine**, 1755 Westgate Drive, Suite 140, Boise, ID 83720-0058; tel. 208/334-2822; FAX. 203/334-2801; Darleene Thorsted, Executive Director
- **Idaho State Board of Nursing**, 280 North 8th Street, P.O. Box 83720, Boise, ID 83720-0061; tel. 208/327-7000; FAX. 208/327-7005; Sandra Evans, Executive Director

ILLINOIS
- **Illinois Department of Professional Regulation**, 320 West Washington Street, Springfield, IL 62786; tel. 217/782-0458; FAX. 217/557-8073; Tony Sanders, Public Information Officer
- **Illinois Department of Professional Regulation**, James R. Thompson Center, 100 West Randolph Street, Suite 9-300, Chicago, IL 60601; tel. 312/814-4500; FAX. 312/814-1837; Leonard A. Sherman, Director

INDIANA
- **Indiana Health Professions Bureau, Medical Licensing Board of Indiana**, 402 West Washington, Suite 041, Indianapolis, IN 46204; tel. 317/233-4401; FAX. 317/233-4236; Laura Langford, Executive Director
- **Indiana State Board of Nursing, Health Professions Bureau**, 402 West Washington, Suite 041, Indianapolis, IN 46204; tel. 317/233-4405; FAX. 317/233-4236; Gina Voorhies, Board Administrator

IOWA
- **Iowa Board of Nursing**, Riverpoint Business Park, 400 S.W. 8th Street, Des Moines, IA 50309-4685; tel. 515/281-3255; FAX. 515/281-4825; Lorinda K. Inman, RN, M.S.N., Executive Director
- **Iowa State Board of Medical Examiners**, 400 S.W. 8th Street, Suite C, Des Moines, IA 50309-4686; tel. 515/281-5171; FAX. 515/242-5908; Ann E. Mowery, Ph.D., Executive Director

KANSAS
- **Kansas State Board of Healing Arts**, 235 Southwest Topeka Boulevard, Topeka, KS 66603-3068; tel. 913/296-7413; FAX. 913/296-0852; Lawrence T. Buening, Jr., J.D., Executive Director
- **Kansas State Board of Nursing**, Landon State Office Building, 900 Southwest, Topeka, KS 66612-1230; tel. 785/296-4929; FAX. 785/296-3929; Mary Blubaugh RN, Executive Administrator

KENTUCKY
- **Kentucky Board of Medical Licensure**, The Hurstbourne Office Park, 310 Whittington Parkway, Suite 1B, Louisville, KY 40222; tel. 502/429-8046; FAX. 502/429-9923; C. William Schmidt, Executive Director
- **Kentucky Board of Nursing**, 312 Whittington Parkway, Suite 300, Louisville, KY 40222; tel. 502/329-7000; FAX. 502/329-7011; Sharon M. Weisenbeck, M.S., RN, Executive Director

LOUISIANA
- **Louisiana State Board of Medical Examiners**, P.O. Box 30250, New Orleans, LA 70190-0250; tel. 504/524-6763; FAX. 504/568-8893; Mrs. Delmar Rorison, Executive Director
- **Louisiana State Board of Nursing**, 912 Pere Marquette Building, New Orleans, LA 70112; tel. 504/568-5467; FAX. 504/568-5464; Barbara L. Morvant, RN, M.S.N., Executive Director

MAINE
- **Maine Board of Licensure in Medicine**, Two Bangor Street, 137 State House Station, Augusta, ME 04333-0137; tel. 207/287-3601; FAX. 207/287-6590; Randal C. Manning, Executive Director
- **Maine Board of Osteopathic Licensure**, 142 State House Station, Two Bangor Street, Augusta, ME 04333-0142; tel. 207/287-2480; FAX. 207/287-2480; Susan E. Stout, Executive Secretary
- **Maine State Board of Nursing**, 24 Stone Street, 158 State House Station, Augusta, ME 04333; tel. 207/287-1133; FAX. 207/287-1149; Myra A. Broadway, J.D., MS, RN, Executive Director

MARYLAND
- **Maryland Board of Nursing**, 4140 Patterson Avenue, Baltimore, MD 21215; tel. 410/585-1900; FAX. 410/358-3530; Donna M. Dorsey, RN, M.S., Executive Director
- **Maryland Board of Physician Quality Assurance**, 4201 Patterson Avenue, Third Floor, P.O. Box 2571, Baltimore, MD 21215-0095; tel. 800/492-6836; FAX. 410/358-2252; J. Michael Compton, Executive Director

MASSACHUSETTS
- **Massachusetts Board of Registration in Medicine**, 10 West Street, Third Floor, Boston, MA 02111; tel. 617/727-3086; FAX. 617/451-9568; Nancy Achin Sullivan, Executive Director
- **Massachusetts Board of Registration in Nursing**, 100 Cambridge Street, Suite 1519, Boston, MA 02202; tel. 617/727-9961; FAX. 617/727-1630; Theresa M. Bonanno, M.S.N., RN, Executive Director

MICHIGAN
- **Michigan Board of Medicine**, 611 West Ottawa Street, First Floor, P.O. Box 30670, Lansing, MI 48909; tel. 517/373-6873; FAX. 517/373-2179
- **Michigan Board of Nursing, Department of Consumer and Industry Service**, 611 West Ottawa Street, P.O. Box 30670, Lansing, MI 48909; tel. 517/335-0918; FAX. 517/373-2179; Doris Foley, Licensing Administrator
- **Michigan Board of Osteopathic Medicine and Surgery**, 611 West Ottawa Street, First Floor, P.O. Box 30670, Lansing, MI 48909; tel. 517/335-0918; FAX. 517/373-2179; Doris Foley, Licensing Administrator

Organizations / Medical and Nursing Licensure Agencies

MINNESOTA
Minnesota Board of Medical Practice, 2829 University Avenue, S.E., Suite 400, Minneapolis, MN 55414-3246; tel. 612/617-2130; FAX. 612/617-2166; Robert A. Leach, Executive Director
Minnesota Board of Nursing, 2829 University Avenue, S.E., Suite 500, Minneapolis, MN 55414-3253; tel. 612/617-2270; FAX. 612/617-2190; Joyce M. Schowalter, Executive Director

MISSISSIPPI
Mississippi Board of Nursing, 1935 Lakeland Drive, Suite B, Jackson, MS 39216-5014; tel. 601/987-4188; FAX. 601/364-2352; Marcia M. Rachel, Ph.D., RN, Executive Director
Mississippi State Board of Medical Licensure, 2600 Insurance Center Drive, Suite 200-B, Jackson, MS 39216; tel. 601/987-3079; FAX. 601/987-4159; W. Joseph Burnett, M.D., Executive Director

MISSOURI
Missouri State Board of Nursing, 3605 Missouri Boulevard, P.O. Box 656, Jefferson City, MO 65102; tel. 573/751-0681; FAX. 573/751-0075; Calvina Thomas, Executive Director

MONTANA
Montana Board of Medical Examiners, 111 North Jackson, P.O. Box 200513, Helena, MT 59620-0513; tel. 406/444-4284; FAX. 406/444-9396; Charlene Norris, J.D., Acting Executive Secretary
Montana State Board of Nursing, 111 North Jackson-4C, P.O. Box 200513, Helena, MT 59620-0513; tel. 406/444-2071; FAX. 406/444-7759; Joan Bowers, Administrative Assistant

NEBRASKA
Nebraska State Board of Examiners in Medicine and Surgery, 301 Centennial Mall, S., P.O. Box 94986, Lincoln, NE 68509-4986; tel. 402/471-2118; FAX. 402/471-3577; Becky Wisell, Executive Secretary

NEVADA
Nevada State Board of Medical Examiners, 1105 Terminal Way, Suite 301, Zip 89502, P.O. Box 7238, Reno, NV 89510; tel. 702/688-2559; FAX. 702/688-2321; Larry D. Lessly, Executive Director
Nevada State Board of Nursing, 4330 S. Valley View, Suite 106, Las Vegas, NV 89103; tel. 775/688-2620; FAX. 775/688-2628; Kathy Apple, Executive Director
Nevada State Board of Osteopathic Medicine, 2950 East Flamingo Road, Suite E-3, Las Vegas, NV 89121; tel. 702/732-2147; FAX. 702/732-2079; Larry J. Tarno, D.O., Executive Director

NEW HAMPSHIRE
New Hampshire Board of Medicine, Two Industrial Park Drive, Suite Eight, Concord, NH 03301; tel. 603/271-1203; FAX. 603/271-6702; Penny Taylcr, Acting Administrator
New Hampshire State Board of Nursing, 78 Regional Drive, P.O. Box 3898, Concord, NH 03302-3898; tel. 603/271-2323; FAX. 603/271-6605; Doris G. Nuttelman, RN, Ed.D., Executive Director

NEW JERSEY
New Jersey Board of Nursing, P.O. Box 45010, Newark, NJ 07101; tel. 973/504-6430; FAX. 973/648-3481; Patricia A. Polansky, Executive Director
New Jersey State Board of Medical Examiners, 140 East Front Street, Second Floor, P.O. Box 183, Trenton, NJ 08625-0183; tel. 609/826-7100; FAX. 609/984-3930; Judith I. Gleason, Executive Director

NEW MEXICO
New Mexico Board of Osteopathic Medical Examiners, 2055 S. Pacheco, P.O. Box 25101, Santa Fe, NM 87504; tel. 505/476-7120; FAX. 505/476-7095; Liz Z. Montoya
New Mexico State Board of Medical Examiners, 491 Old Santa Fe Trail, Lamy Building, Second Floor, Santa Fe, NM 87501; tel. 505/827-5022; FAX. 505/827-7377; Kristen A. Hedrick, Executive Director
State of New Mexico Board of Nursing, 4206 Louisiana, N.E., Suite A, Albuquerque, NM 87109; tel. 505/841-8340; FAX. 505/841-8347; Nancy L. Twigg, Executive Director

NEW YORK
New York Board for Professional Medical Conduct, State Department of Health, 433 River Street, Suite 303, Troy, NY 12180-2299; tel. 800/663-6114; FAX. 518/402-0866; Anne F. Saile, Director
New York State Board for Nursing, State Education Department, The Cultural Center, Suite 3023, Albany, NY 12230; tel. 518/474-3845; FAX. 518/474-3706; Milene A. Sowers, Ph.D., RN, Executive Secretary
New York State Division of Professional Licensing Services, Cultural Education Center, Suite 3000, Empire State Plaza, Albany, NY 12230; tel. 518/474-3817; FAX. 518/473-0578; Robert G. Bentley, Director, Professional Licensing

NORTH CAROLINA
North Carolina Board of Nursing, P.O. Box 2129, Raleigh, NC 27602-2129; tel. 919/782-3211; FAX. 919/781-9461; Mary P. Johnson, RN, MSN, Executive Director
North Carolina Medical Board, P.O. Box 20007, Raleigh, NC 27619; tel. 919/326-1100; FAX. 919/326-1130; Andrew W. Watry, Executive Director

NORTH DAKOTA
North Dakota Board of Nursing, 919 South Seventh Street, Suite 504, Bismarck, ND 58504-5881; tel. 701/328-9777; FAX. 701/328-9785; Constance Kalanek, Ph D., RN, Executive Director
North Dakota State Board of Medical Examiners, City Center Plaza, Suite 12, 418 East Broadway Avenue, Bismarck, ND 58501; tel. 701/328-6500; FAX. 701/328-6505; Rolf P. Sletten, Executive Secretary-Treasurer

OHIO
Ohio Board of Nursing, 17 South Highstreet, Suite 400, Columbus, OH 43215-3413; tel. 614/466-3947; FAX. 614/466-0388; Dorothy Fiorino, RN, Executive Director
State Medical Board of Ohio, 77 South High Street, 17th Floor, Columbus, OH 43266-0315; tel. 614/466-3934; FAX. 614/728-5946; Tom Dilling, Executive Director

OKLAHOMA
Oklahoma Board of Nursing, 2915 North Classen Boulevard, Suite 524, Oklahoma City, OK 73106; tel. 405/962-1800; FAX. 405/962-1821; Norma Wallace, Executive Secretary
Oklahoma Board of Osteopathic Examiners, 4848 North Lincoln Boulevard, Suite 100, Oklahoma City, OK 73105-3321; tel. 405/528-8625; FAX. 405/557-0653; Gary R. Clark, Executive Director
Oklahoma State Board of Medical Licensure and Supervision, 5104 North Francis, Suite C, Oklahoma City, OK 73118, Oklahoma City, OK 73154-0256; tel. 405/848-6841; FAX. 405/848-8240; Lyle Kelsey, Executive Director

OREGON
Oregon Board of Medical Examiners, 620 Crown Plaza, Portland, OR 97201-5826; tel. 503/229-5770; FAX. 503/229-6543; Kathleen Haley, J.D., Executive Director
Oregon State Board of Nursing, 800 Northeast Oregon Street, Suite 465, Portland, OR 97232-2162; tel. 503/731-4745; FAX. 503/731-4755; Joan C. Bouchard, Executive Director

PENNSYLVANIA
Pennsylvania State Board of Medicine, P.O. Box 2649, Harrisburg, PA 17105-2649; tel. 717/783-1400; FAX. 717/787-7769; Cindy L. Warner, Administrative Officer
Pennsylvania State Board of Nursing, Department of State, P.O. Box 2649, Harrisburg, PA 17105-2649; tel. 717/783-7142; FAX. 717/783-0822; Board Administrator
Pennsylvania State Board of Osteopathic Medicine, P.O. Box 2649, Harrisburg, PA 17105-2649; tel. 717/783-4858; FAX. 717/787-7769; Gina Bittner, Administrative Assistant

RHODE ISLAND
Board of Nursing Education and Nurse Registration, Three Capitol Hill, Room 104, Providence, RI 02908-5097; tel. 401/222-1827; FAX. 401/222-1272; Charles R. Alexandre, RN, M.S.N., Director
Rhode Island Board of Medical Licensure and Discipline, Rhode Island Department of Health, Room 205, 3 Capitol Hill, Providence, RI 02908-5097; tel. 401/222-3855; FAX. 401/222-2158; Milton W. Hamolsky, M.D., Chief Administrative Officer

SOUTH CAROLINA
Department of Labor, Licensing and Regulation, State Board of Nursing for South Carolina, 110 Centerview Drive, Columbia, SC 29211; tel. 803/896-4550; FAX. 803/896-4525; Dorothy Buchanan, Board of Administrative Assistant
South Carolina Department of Labor, Licensing and Regulation, Board of Medical Examiners, 110 Centerview Drive, Suite 202, Columbia, S.C. 29210, Columbia, SC 29211-1289; tel. 803/896-4500; FAX. 803/896-4515; John D. Volmer, Board Administrator

SOUTH DAKOTA
South Dakota Board of Nursing, 4300 South Louise Avenue, Sioux Falls, SD 57106; tel. 605/362-2760; FAX. 605/362-2768; Diana Vander Woude, Executive Secretary
South Dakota State Board of Medical and Osteopathic Examiners, 1323 South Minnesota Avenue, Sioux Falls, SD 57105; tel. 605/336-1965; FAX. 605/336-0270; L. Hall Jensen, Executive Secretary

TENNESSEE
Tennessee Board of Medical Examiners, Cordell Hull Building, 1st Floor, 425 Fifth Avenue, N, Nashville, TN 37247-1010; tel. 888/310-4650; FAX. 615/253-4484; Yarnell Beatty, Director
Tennessee Board of Nursing, Cordell Hull Building, 1st Floor, 425 Fifth avenue, N, Nashville, TN 37247; tel. 888/310-4650; FAX. 615/741-7899; Elizabeth J. Lund, RN, Executive Director
Tennessee State Board of Osteopathic Examination, First Floor, Cordell Hull Building, 425 Fifth Avenue, N., Nashville, TN 37247-1010; tel. 888/310-4650; FAX. 615/253-4484; Vickie Pentecost, Administrator

TEXAS
Texas State Board of Medical Examiners, 333 Guadalupe, Tower Three, Suite 610, P.O. Box 2018, Austin, TX 78768-2018; tel. 512/305-7010; FAX. 512/305-7008; Bruce A. Levy, M.D., J.D., Executive Director

UTAH
Utah Physicians Licensing Board, Division of Occupational and Professional Licensure, Heber M. Wells Building, Fourth Floor, 160 East 300 South, Salt Lake City, UT 84114-6741; tel. 801/530-6628; FAX. 801/530-6511; Laura Poe, Bureau Manager
Utah State Board of Nursing, 160 East 300 South, Box 146741, Salt Lake City, UT 84114-6741; tel. 801/530-6628; FAX. 801/530-6511; Laura Poe, Executive Administrator

VERMONT
Vermont Board of Medical Practice, 109 State Street, Montpelier, VT 05609-1106; tel. 802/828-2673; FAX. 802/828-5450; Barbara Neuman, J.D., Executive Director
Vermont Board of Nursing Licensure and Regulation Division, 81 River Street, Montpelier, VT 05609-1106; tel. 802/828-2396; FAX. 802/828-2484; Anita Ristau, RN, M.S., Executive Director
Vermont Board of Osteopathic Physicians and Surgeons, 26 Terrace Street, Drawer 09, Montpelier, VT 05609-1106; tel. 802/828-2373; FAX. 802/828-2465; Peggy Atkins, Staff Assistant

VIRGINIA
Virginia Board of Medicine, 6606 West Broad Street, Fourth Floor, Richmond, VA 23230-1717; tel. 804/662-9908; FAX. 804/662-9517; William L. Harp, M.D., Executive Director
Virginia Board of Nursing, 6606 West Broad Street, Fourth Floor, Richmond, VA 23230; tel. 804/662-9909; FAX. 804/662-9512; Nancy K. Durrett, RN, Executive Director

WASHINGTON
Washington State Board of Osteopathic Medicine and Surgery, Department of Health, 1300 Southeast Quince Street, P.O. Box 47870, Olympia, WA 98504-7870; tel. 360/236-4943; FAX. 360/586-0745; Karen T. Maasjo, Administrative Assistant
Washington State Medical Quality Assurance Commission, 1300 Southeast Quince Street, P.O. Box 47866, Olympia, WA 98504-7866; tel. 360/236-4800; FAX. 360/586-4573; Bonnie L. King, Executive Director
Washington State Nursing Care Quality Assurance Commission, Department of Health, 1300 Southeast Quince Street, P.O. Box 47864, Olympia, WA 98504-7864; tel. 360/236-4713; FAX. 360/586-5935; Paula Meyer, RN, M.S.N., Executive Director

Organizations / Medical and Nursing Licensure Agencies

WEST VIRGINIA
West Virginia Board of Examiners for Registered Professional Nurses, 101 Dee Drive, Charleston, WV 25311-1620; tel. 304/558-3596; FAX. 304/558-3666; Laura S. Rhodes, RN, M.S.N., Executive Secretary
West Virginia Board of Medicine, 101 Dee Drive, Charleston, WV 25311; tel. 304/558-2921; FAX. 304/558-2084; Ronald D. Walton, Executive Director
West Virginia Board of Osteopathy, 334 Penco Road, Weirton, WV 26062; tel. 304/723-4638; FAX. 304/723-6723; Cheryl D. Schreiber, Executive Secretary

WISCONSIN
Division of Health Professions and Services Licensing, 1400 East Washington Avenue, Room 178, P.O. Box 8935, Madison, WI 53708-8935; tel. 608/266-2911; FAX. 608/266-0145; Patrick D. Braatr, Division Director
Wisconsin Medical Examining Board, 1400 East Washington Avenue, Zip 53702, P.O. Box 8935, Madison, WI 53708; tel. 608/266-2811; FAX. 608/261-7083; Patrick D. Braatz, Administrator

WYOMING
Wyoming Board of Medicine, The Colony Building, 211 West 19th Street, Cheyenne, WY 82002; tel. 307/778-7053; FAX. 307/778-2069; Carole Shotwell, Executive Secretary
Wyoming State Board of Nursing, 2020 Carey Avenue, Suite 110, Cheyenne, WY 82002; tel. 307/777-7601; FAX. 307/777-3519; Cheryl Koski, MN, RN, Executive Director

U.S. Associated Areas

GUAM
Guam Board of Medical Examiners, 1304 East Sunset Boulevard, Barrigada, GU 96913; tel. 671/475-0251; FAX. 671/477-4733; Teofila P. Cruz, Administrator
Guam Board of Nurse Examiners, Department of Public Health and Social Serv, 1304 East Sunset Boulevard, P.O. Box 2816, Agana, GU 96910; tel. 671/475-0251; FAX. 671/477-4733; Teofila P. Cruz, RN, M.S., Administrator

PUERTO RICO
Council on Higher Education of Puerto Rico, UPR Station, P.O. Box 23305, San Juan, PR 00931-3305; tel. 809/758-3356; Madeline Quilichini Paz, Director, Office of Licensing
Puerto Rico Board of Medical Examiners, Kennedy Avenue, ILA Building, Hogar del Obrero Portuario, Piso 8, Puert Nuevo, San Juan, PR 00908; tel. 787/782-8989; FAX. 787/782-8733; Ivonne M. Fernandez, Executive Director

Canada

ALBERTA
College of Physicians and Surgeons of Alberta, 900 Manulife Place, 10180-101 Street, Edmonton, AB T5J 4P8; tel. 780/423-4764; FAX. 780/420-0651; Dr. L.R. Ohlhauser, Registrar

MANITOBA
College of Physicians and Surgeons of Manitoba, 494 St. James Street, Winnipeg, MB R3G 3J4; tel. 204/774-4344; FAX. 204/774-0750; William D.B. Pope, M.D., Registrar

NEW BRUNSWICK
College of Physicians and Surgeons of New Brunswick, One Hampton Road, Rothesay, NB E2E 5K8; tel. 506/849-5050; FAX. 506/849-5069; Dr. Ed Schollenberg, Registrar

NOVA SCOTIA
College of Physicians and Surgeons of Nova Scotia, Office of the Registrar, 5248 Morris Street, Halifax, NS B3J 1B4; tel. 902/422-5823; FAX. 902/422-5035; Dr. Cameron Little, Registrar

PRINCE EDWARD ISLAND
College of Physicians and Surgeons of Prince Edward Island, 199 Grafton Street, Charlottetown, PE C1A 1L2; tel. 902/566-3861; FAX. 902/566-3861; C.A. Moyse, M.D., Registrar

QUEBEC
College des medecins du Quebec, 2170, boul. Rene-Levesque Quest, Montreal, PQ H3H 2T8; tel. 514/933-4441; FAX. 514/933-3112; Joelle Lescop, M.D., Secretary General

SASKATCHEWAN
College of Physicians and Surgeons of Saskatchewan, 211 Fourth Avenue, S., Saskatoon, SK S7K 1N1; tel. 306/244-7355; FAX. 306/244-0090; D. A. Kendel, M.D., Registrar

Peer Review Organizations

The following list of PROs was obtained from the Office of Medical Review, Division of Program Operation, HCFA.

United States

ALABAMA: Alabama Quality Assurance Foundation, One Perimeter Park, S., Suite 200 North, Birmingham, AL 35243-2354; tel. 205/970-1600; FAX. 205/970-1616; H. Terrell Lindsey, President and CEO

ALASKA: PRO-West, 721 Sesame Street, Suite 1A, Anchorage, AK 98133; tel. 907/562-2252; FAX. 907/562-5659; Jonathan Sugarman, M.D., MPH

ARIZONA: Health Services Advisory Group, Inc., 301 East Bethany Home Road, Suite B-1, Phoenix, AZ 85012; tel. 602/264-6382; FAX. 602/241-0757; Lawrence J. Shapiro, M.D., President and CEO

ARKANSAS: Arkansas Foundation for Medical Care, Inc., 2201 Brooken Hill Drive, P.O. Box 180001, Fort Smith, AR 72918-0001; tel. 501/649-8501; FAX. 501/649-8180; Russell G. Brasher, Ph.D., Chief Executive Officer

CALIFORNIA: CMRI (California Medical Review, Inc)., One Sansome Street, Suite 600, San Francisco, CA 94104; tel. 415/677-2000; FAX. 415/677-2195; Jo Ellen H. Ross, President and CEO

COLORADO: Colorado Foundation for Medical Care, 2851 South Parker Road, Suite 200, Aurora, CO 80014-2713; tel. 303/695-3300; FAX. 303/695-3350; Arja P. Adair, Jr., President and CEO

CONNECTICUT: Connecticut Peer Review Organization, Inc., d.b.a Qualidigm, 100 Roscommon Drive, Suite 200, Middletown, CT 06457; tel. 860/632-2008; FAX. 860/632-5865; Marcia K. Petrillo, Chief Executive Officer

DELAWARE: Quality Insights of Delaware, Plaza III, 1847 marsh Road, Wilmington, DE 19810; tel. 302/475-8100; FAX. 302/475-7317; John Wiesendanger, CEO

DISTRICT OF COLUMBIA: Delmarva Foundation for Medical Care, Inc., 1620 L Street, NW, Suite 1275, Washington, DC 20036; tel. 410/822-0697; FAX. 410/822-7971; Thomas Schaefer, M.D., CEO

FLORIDA: Florida Medical Quality Assurance, Inc., 4350 West Cypress Street, Suite 900, Tampa, FL 33607; tel. 813/354-9111; FAX. 813/354-0737; LaNona Robinson, Acting President and CEO

GEORGIA: Georgia Medical Care Foundation, 57 Executive Park, S., Suite 200, Atlanta, GA 30329; tel. 404/982-0411; FAX. 404/982-7584; Tom W. Williams, Chief Executive Officer

HAWAII: Mountain-Pacific Quality Health Foundation, 1360 South Beretania Street, Suite 501, Honolulu, HI 96814; tel. 808/545-2550; FAX. 808/440-6030; Dee Dee Nelson, Director of Hawaii Office

IDAHO: PRO-West/Idaho, 720 Park Boulevard, Suite 120, Boise, ID 83712-7756; tel. 208/343-4617; FAX. 208/343-4705; Jonathan Sugarman, M.D., MPH

INDIANA: Health Care Excel, Incorporated, 2901 Ohio Boulevard, P.O. Box 3713, Terre Haute, IN 47803; tel. 812/234-1499; FAX. 812/232-6167; Philip L. Morphew, Chief Executive Officer

IOWA: Iowa Foundation for Medical Care, The Sunderbruch Corporation, 6000 Westown Parkway, Suite 350E, West Des Moines, IA 50266; tel. 515/233-2900; FAX. 402/474-7410; Fred Ferree, Executive Vice President

Iowa Foundation for Medical Care/The Sunderbruch Corporation/, Illinois Foundation for Quality Health, 6000 Westown Parkway, Suite 350E, West Des Moines, IA 50266-7771; tel. 515/223-2900; FAX. 515/222-2407; Fred A. Ferree, Executive Vice President

KANSAS: The Kansas Foundation for Medical Care, Inc., 2947 Southwest Wanamaker Drive, Topeka, KS 66614; tel. 785/273-2552; FAX. 785/273-5130; Larry Pitman, President and CEO

KENTUCKY: Health Care Excel, Incorporated, 9300 Shelbyville Road, The Hurstburg Place, Suite 600, Louisville, KY 40222; tel. 502/339-7442; FAX. 502/339-8641; Philip L. Morphew, Chief Executive Officer

LOUISIANA: Louisiana Health Care Review, Inc., 8591 United Plaza Boulevard, Suite 270, Baton Rouge, LA 70809; tel. 504/926-6353; FAX. 504/923-0957; Leo Stanley, Chief Executive Officer

MARYLAND: Delmarva Foundation for Medical Care, Inc., 9240 Centreville Road, Easton, MD 21601; tel. 410/822-0697; FAX. 410/822-9572; Thomas J. Schaefer, Chief Executive Officer

MASSACHUSETTS: Massachusetts Peer Review Organization, Inc., 235 Wyman Street, Waltham, MA 02154-1231; tel. 781/890-0011; FAX. 781/487-0083; Kathleen E. McCarthy, President and CEO

MICHIGAN: Michigan Peer Review Organization, 40600 Ann Arbor Road, Suite 200, Plymouth, MI 48170-4495; tel. 734/459-0900; FAX. 734/454-7301; Sheryl L. Stogis, Dr Ph, Chief Executive Officer

MINNESOTA: Stratis Health, 2901 Metro Drive, Suite 400, Bloomington, MN 55425; tel. 612/854-3306; FAX. 612/853-8503; Patricia Riley, Chief Executive Officer

MISSISSIPPI: I.Q.H., Information & Quality Healthcare, 385 Highland Colony Parkway, Suite 120, Ridgeland, MS 39157; tel. 601/957-1575; FAX. 601/956-1173; James McIlwain, M.D., President

MISSOURI: Missouri Patient Care Review Foundation, 505 Hobbs Road, Suite 100, Jefferson City, MO 65109; tel. 573/893-7900; FAX. 573/893-5827; Sarah A. Grim, MHA, CHE, Chief Executive Officer

MONTANA: Mountain Pacific Quality Health Foundation, 3404 Cooney Drive, Helena, MT 59602; tel. 406/443-4020; FAX. 406/443-4585; Steve Wallace, M.D., President

Mountain-Pacific Quality Health Foundation, 3404 Cooney Drive, Helena, MT 59602; tel. 406/443-4020; FAX. 406/443-4585; Janice Connors, Executive Director

NEW HAMPSHIRE: Northeast Health Care Quality Foundaiton, 15 Old Rollinsford Road, Suite 302, Dover, NH 03820; tel. 603/749-1641; FAX. 603/749-1195; Robert A. Aurilio, CEO

Northeast Health Care Quality Foundation, 15 Old Rollinsford Road, Suite 302, Dover, NH 03820-2830; tel. 603/749-1641; FAX. 603/749-1195; Robert A. Aurilio, Chief Executive Officer

NEW JERSEY: The Peer Review Organization of New Jersey, Inc., 557 Cranbury Road, Suite 21, East Brunswick, NJ 08816; tel. 732/238-5570; FAX. 732/238-7766; Martin P. Margolies, Chief Executive Officer

NEW MEXICO: NMMRA, (New Mexico Medical Review Association), 2340 Menaul Blvd., NE, Suite 300, P.O. Box 3200, Albuquerque, NM 87190-3200; tel. 505/998-9898; FAX. 505/998-9899; Gary Horvat, Chief Executive Officer

NEW YORK: IPRO, 1979 Marcus Avenue, First Floor, Lake Success, NY 11042-1002; tel. 516/326-7767; FAX. 516/328-2310; Theodore O. Will, Executive Vice President

NORTH CAROLINA: Medical Review of North Carolina, Inc., 5625 Dillard Drive, Suite 203, Cary, NC 27511-9227; tel. 919/851-2955; FAX. 919/851-8457; Charles Riddick, Executive Director

NORTH DAKOTA: North Dakota Health Care Review Inc., 800 31st Avenue S.W., Minot, ND 58701; tel. 701/852-4231; FAX. 701/838-6009; David Remillard, Chief Executive Officer

OHIO: Peer Review Systems, Inc., 757 Brooksedge Plaza Drive, Westerville, OH 43081-4913; tel. 614/895-9900; FAX. 614/895-6784; Gregory J. Dykes, Chief Executive Officer

OKLAHOMA: Oklahoma Foundation for Medical Quality, Inc., The Paragon Building, 5801 Broadway Extension, Suite 400, Oklahoma City, OK 73118-7489; tel. 405/840-2891; FAX. 405/840-1343; Jim L. Williams, President and CEO

OREGON: Oregon Medical Professional Review Organization, 2020 S.W. 4th Avenue, Suite 520, Portland, OR 97201-4960; tel. 503/279-0100; FAX. 503/279-0190; Robert S. Kinoshita, President

PENNSYLVANIA: Keystone Peer Review Organization, Inc., 777 East Park Drive, P.O. Box 8310, Harrisburg, PA 17105-8310; tel. 717/564-8288; FAX. 717/564-4188; John DiNardi, III, Executive Director

RHODE ISLAND: Rhode Island Quality Partners, Inc., 9 Hayes Street, Providence, RI 02908; tel. 860/632-2008; FAX. 860/632-5865; Marcia K. Petrillo, Executive Director

SOUTH CAROLINA: Carolina Medical Review, 250 Berryhill Road, Suite 101, Columbia, SC 29210; tel. 803/731-8225; FAX. 803/731-8229; Diana M. Zona, Communications Manager

SOUTH DAKOTA: South Dakota Foundation for Medical Care, 1323 South Minnesota Avenue, Sioux Falls, SD 57105; tel. 605/336-3505; FAX. 605/336-0270; Mark Hoven, Chief Executive Officer

TENNESSEE: Mid-South Foundation for Medical Care, Inc., 6401 Poplar Avenue, Suite 400, Memphis, TN 38119; tel. 901/682-0381; FAX. 901/761-3786; Logan Malone, Chief Executive Officer

TEXAS: Texas Medical Foundation, Barton Oaks Plaza Two, Suite 200, 901 Mopac Expressway, S., Austin, TX 78746-5799; tel. 512/329-6610; FAX. 512/327-7159; Phillip K. Dunne, Chief Executive Officer

UTAH: HealthInsight, 348 E. 4500 South, Suite 300, Salt Lake City, UT 84107; tel. 702/826-1996; FAX. 702/826-5865; David Buchanan, President/CEO

HealthInsight, 348 East 4500 South, Suite 300, Salt Lake City, UT 84107; tel. 801/892-0155; FAX. 801/892-0160; E. David Buchanan, President and CEO

VIRGINIA: Virginia Health Quality Center, 1604 Santa Rosa Road, Suite 200, Richmond, VA 23288-0070; tel. 804/289-5320; FAX. 804/289-5324; Joy Hogan Rozman, Executive Director

WASHINGTON: PRO-WEST, 10700 Meridian Avenue, N., Suite 100, Seattle, WA 98133-9075; tel. 206/364-9700; FAX. 206/368-2427; Jonathan Sugarman, Interim Chief Executive Officer

WEST VIRGINIA: West Virginia Medical Institute, Inc., 3001 Chesterfield Place, Charleston, WV 25304; tel. 304/346-9864; FAX. 304/346-9863; Mabel M. Stevenson, M.D., President

WISCONSIN: Meta Star, 2909 Landmark Place, Madison, WI 53713; tel. 608/274-1940; FAX. 608/274-5008; Greg E. Simmons, President and CEO

U.S. Associated Areas

PUERTO RICO: Quality Improvement Professional Research Organization, Mercantile Plaza Building, Suite 605, Hato Rey, PR 00918; tel. 787/753-6705; FAX. 787/753-6885; Jose Robles, Chief Executive Officer

VIRGIN ISLANDS: Virgin Islands Medical Institute, Inc., 1AD Estate Diamond Ruby, P.O. Box 5989, St. Croix, VI 00823-5989; tel. 340/712-2400; FAX. 340-712-2449; Patrick Peterson, Chief Executive Officer

State Health Planning and Development Agencies

The following is a list of state health planning and development agencies. The information was obtained from the agencies themselves. For information about other state agencies and organizations that fulfill many of the same functions, contact the state or metropolitan hospital associations.

United States

ALABAMA: State Health Planning and Development Agency, 100 North Union Street, Suite 870, Montgomery, AL 36104; tel. 334/242–4103; FAX. 334/242–4113; Alva Lambert, Executive Director

ALASKA: Facilities and Planning Section, Department of Health and Social Services, P.O. Box 110650, Juneau, AK 99811-0650; tel. 907/465–3015; FAX. 907/465–2499; Larry J. Streuber, Section Chief

ARIZONA: Office of Health Planning, Evaluation and Statistics, 2700 North 3rd Street, Suite 4075, Phoenix, AZ 85007; tel. 602/542–1216; FAX. 602/542–1244; Ross Barchner, Chief

CALIFORNIA: Office of Statewide Health Planning and Development, 1600 Ninth Street, Suite 440, Sacramento, CA 95814; tel. 916/654–2087; FAX. 916/654–3138; Priscilla Gonzalez-Leiva, RN, Deputy Director

COLORADO: Colorado Department of Public Health and Environment, Rural and Primary Health Program, 4300 Cherry Creek Drive, S., Denver, CO 80246-1530; tel. 303/692–2470; FAX. 303/782–5576; Susan Rehak, Program Director

CONNECTICUT: Connecticut Department of Public Health, Office of Policy, Planning and Evaluation, 410 Capitol Avenue, MS# 13PPE, Hartford, CT 06134-0308; tel. 860/509–7123; FAX. 860/509–7160; Michael Hoffman, Ph.D., Director

DELAWARE: Bureau of Health Planning and Resources Management, Department of Health and Social Services, P.O. Box 637, Dover, DE 19903; tel. 302/739–4776; FAX. 302/739–4784; Robert I. Welch, Director

DISTRICT OF COLUMBIA: Plan Development and Implementation Division, 825 North Capital Street, N.E., Third Floor, Washington, DC 20002; tel. 202/442–5875; FAX. 202/442–5894; Virginia Knox Woods, Director

GEORGIA: State Health Planning Agency, Planning and Implementation Division, 2 Peach Tree Street, Room 34262, Atlanta, GA 30303-3142; tel. 404/656–0654; FAX. 404/656–0655; Vallery Hepburn, Director, Planning and Data Management

HAWAII: Hawaii State Health Planning and Development Agency, 1177 Alakea Street, Suite 402, Honolulu, HI 96813; tel. 808/587–0788; FAX. 808/587–0783; Marilyn A. Matsunaga, Administrator

IDAHO: Center for Vital Statistics and Health Policy, Division of Health, Idaho Department of Health and Welfare, 450 West State Street, First Floor, P.O. Box 83720, Boise, ID 83720-0036; tel. 208/334–5976; FAX. 208/334–0685; Jane Smith, Chief

ILLINOIS: Illinois Department of Public Health, Division of Health Policy, 525 West Jefferson, Springfield, IL 62761; tel. 217/782–6235; FAX. 217/785–4308; Patti Kimmel, Actintg Chief

INDIANA: Indiana State Department of Health, Local Liaison Office, Two North Meridian Street, Suite Eight-B, Indianapolis, IN 46204-3003; tel. 317/233–7846; FAX. 317/233–7761; Raymond Guest, Office of Primary Health Manager

IOWA: Department of Public Health, Division of Substance Abuse and Health Promotion, Lucas State Office Building, Des Moines, IA 50319; tel. 515/281–5914; FAX. 515/281–4535; Ronald Eckoff, Medical Director

KANSAS: Health Care Commission, 900 Southwest Jackson, Ninth Floor, Landon State Office B, Topeka, KS 66612; tel. 785/296–7488; FAX. 785/368–7180; Steve Ashley

MAINE: Office of Health Data and Program Management, Bureau of Health, 35 Anthony Ave., SHS #11, Augusta, ME 04330-0011; tel. 207/624–5424; FAX. 207/624–5431; Sophie Glidden, Primary Care Director

MARYLAND: Maryland Health Care Commission, 4201 Patterson Avenue, Baltimore, MD 21215-2299; tel. 410/764–3460; FAX. 410/358–1311; John M. Colmars, Executive Director

MINNESOTA: Division of Community Health Services, Bureau of Family and Community Health, Metro Square Building, Suite 460, St.Paul, MN 55164-0975; tel. 651/296–9720; FAX. 651/296–9362; Ryan Church, Director

MISSISSIPPI: Mississippi State Department of Health, Health Planning and Resource Development Division, 2423 North State Street, P.O. Box 1700, Jackson, MS 39215-1700; tel. 601/576–7874; FAX. 601/576–7530; Harold B. Armstrong, Chief

MISSOURI: Missouri Department of Health, 920 Wildwood, P.O. Box 570, Jefferson City, MO 65102; tel. 573/751–6001; FAX. 573/751–6041; Maureen Dempsey, M.D., Director

MONTANA: Health Policy and Services Division, Department of Public Health and Human Services, Cogswell Building, P.O. Box 202951, Helena, MT 59620-2951; tel. 406/444–4540; FAX. 406/444–1861; Nancy Ellery, Administrator

NEBRASKA: Nebraska Health and Human Services, Finance and Support, Research and Performance Measure, Nebraska State Office Building-5th Floor, 301 Centennial Mall South, Lincoln, NE 68509; tel. 402/471–8941; FAX. 402/471–7049; Paula Hartig, Administrator

NEVADA: State Health Division, Bureau of Health Planning and Statistics, 505 East King Street, Suite 102, Carson City, NV 89701-4749; tel. 775/684–4218; FAX. 775/684–4156; Emil DeJan, Chief

NEW HAMPSHIRE: Office of Health Services Planning and Review, Six Hazen Drive, Concord, NH 03301-6527; tel. 603/271–4606; FAX. 603/271–4141; Paula M. Minnehan, Administrator

NEW JERSEY: Certificate of Need and Acute Care Licensure Program, New Jersey Department of Health and Senior Services, CN 360, John Fitch Plaza, Trenton, NJ 08625-0360; tel. 609/292–8773; FAX. 609/292–3780; John A. Calabria, Director

NEW MEXICO: New Mexico Health Policy Commission, 2055 S. Pacheco Street, Suite 200, Santa Fe, NM 87505; tel. 505/424–3200; FAX. 505/424–3222; Katherine Ganz, M.D., Director

NEW YORK: New York State Department of Health, Division of Planning, Policy and Resource Development, Corning Tower, Suite 1495, Empire State Plaza, Albany, NY 12237; tel. 518/474–0180; FAX. 518/474–5450; Judith Arnold, Deputy Commissioner

NORTH CAROLINA: Medical Facilities Planning Section, P.O. Box 29530, Raleigh, NC 27626-0530; tel. 919/733–2342; FAX. 919/733–2757; Bonnie M. Cramer, Assistant Director, Division of Facility Services

NORTH DAKOTA: North Dakota Department of Health, Office of Community Assistance, 600 East Boulevard Avenue, Bismarck, ND 58505-0200; tel. 701/328–2894; FAX. 701/328–1890; Gary Garland, Director

OKLAHOMA: Oklahoma State Department of Health, Healthcare Information, 1000 Northeast 10th Street, Oklahoma City, OK 73117-1299; tel. 405/271–1110; FAX. 405/271–1225; Sue Mallonee, Director of Healthcare Information

PENNSYLVANIA: Bureau of Health Planning, Pennsylvania Department of Health, Health and Welfare Building, Room 833, P.O. Box 90, Harrisburg, PA 17108; tel. 717/772–5298; FAX. 717/705–6525; Joseph B. May, Director

RHODE ISLAND: Rhode Island Department of Health, Cannon Building, Three Capitol Hill, Suite 401, Providence, RI 02908; tel. 401/277–2231; FAX. 401/277–6548; William J. Waters, Jr., Ph.D., Deputy Director

SOUTH CAROLINA: DHEC, Division of Planning and Certificate of Need, 2600 Bull Street, Columbia, SC 29201; tel. 803/737–7200; FAX. 803/737–7579; Albert Whiteside, Director

SOUTH DAKOTA: South Dakota Department of Health, Division of Administration, 600 East Capitol Avenue, Pierre, SD 57501-3185; tel. 605/773–3361; FAX. 605/773–5683; Jerry Hofer, Director, Division of Administration

TENNESSEE: Assessment and Planning, Tennessee Department of Health, Cordell Hull Building, Sixth Floor, Nashville, TN 37247-5261; tel. 615/741–0244; FAX. 615/253–1688; Arthur Mader, Health Planner

TEXAS: Office of Policy and Planning, Texas Department of Health, 1100 West 49th Street, Austin, TX 78756; tel. 512/458–7261; FAX. 512/458–7344; Rick A. Danko, Planning Director

VERMONT: Division of Health Care Administration, Department of Banking Insurance, Securities, and Health Care Administration, 89 Main Street, Drawer 20, Montpelier, VT 05620-3601; tel. 802/828–2900; FAX. 802/828–2949; Stan Lane, Policy Analyst

VIRGINIA: Virginia Department of Health, Division of Certificate of Public Need, 3600 West Broad Street, Suite 216, Richmond, VA 23220; tel. 804/367–2126; FAX. 804/367–2206; Eric O'Bodeen, III, Acting Director

WASHINGTON: Washington State Board of Health, 1102 SE Quince Street, P.O. Box 47990, Olympia, WA 98504-7990; tel. 360/236–4100; FAX. 360/236–4088; Don Sloma, MPH, Executive Director

WEST VIRGINIA: West Virginia Health Care Authority, 100 Dee Drive, Charleston, WV 25311; tel. 304/558–7000; FAX. 304/558–7001; D. Parker Haddix

WYOMING: Department of Health, Health Planning & Implementation Division, 2020 Carey Avenue, 8th Floor, Cheyenne, WY 82002; tel. 307/777–7123; FAX. 307/777–7127; Douglas Thiede, Manager

State and Provincial Government Agencies

The following list includes state departments of health and welfare, and their subagencies as well as such independent agencies as those for children's services, maternal and child health, mental health, and vocational rehabilitation. The information was obtained directly from the agencies.

United States

ALABAMA
The Honorable Don Seigelman, Governor, 334/242-7100

Health
- **Alabama Department of Public Health, Bureau of Family Health Services,** The RSA Tower, P.O. Box 303017, Montgomery, AL 36130-3017; tel. 334/206-2940; FAX. 334/206-2950; Thomas M. Miller, M.D., MPH, Director
- **Alabama Department of Public Health, Division of Licensure and Certification,** The RSA Tower, P.O. Box 303017, Montgomery, AL 36130-3017; tel. 334/206-2940; FAX. 334/206-2950; Thomas M. Miller, M.D., MPH, Director
- **Department of Public Health,** 201 Monroe Street, P.O. Box 303017, Montgomery, AL 36130-3017; tel. 334/206-5200; FAX. 334/206-2008; Donald E. Williamson, M.D., State Health Officer

Insurance
- **Department of Insurance,** 201 Monroe Street, Suite 1700, Montgomery, AL 36130; tel. 334/241-4101; FAX. 334/241-4192; David Parsors, Acting Commissioner

Licensing
- **Alabama Board of Nursing, RSA Plaza,** 770 Washirgton Avenue, Suite 250, Montgomery, AL 36130; tel. 334/242-4060; FAX. 334/242-4360; N. Genell Lee, RN, M.S.N. JD, Executive Officer

Social Services
- **Alabama Medicaid Agency,** 501 Dexter Avenue, P.O. Box 5624, Montgomery, AL 36103-5624; tel. 334/242-5010; FAX. 334/242-5097; W. Dale Walley, Acting Commissioner
- **Department of Human Resources,** Gordon Persons Building, 50 Ripley Street, Montgomery, AL 36130; tel. 334/242-1160; FAX. 334/242-0198; Tony Petelos, Commissioner
- **Department of Rehabilitation Services,** 2129 East South Boulevard, Montgomery, AL 36116; tel. 800/441-7607; FAX. 334/281-1973; Steve Shivers, Commissioner
- **State Department of Mental Health and Mental Retardation,** RSA Union, 100 North Union Street, Montgomery, AL 36130-1410; tel. 334/242-3107; FAX. 334/242-0684; Kathy E. Sowers, Commissioner

Other
- **State Department of Education,** Gordon Persons Building, P.O. Box 302101, Montgomery, AL 36130-2101; tel. 334/242-9700; FAX. 334/242-9708; Ed Richardson, Superintendent

ALASKA
The Honorable Tony Knowles, Governor, 907/465-3500

Health
- **Health Facilities Licensing and Certification,** 4730 Business Park Boulevard, Suite 18, Anchorage, AK 99503-7137; tel. 907/561-8081; FAX. 907/561-3011; Shelbert Larsen, Administrator
- **Division of Mental Health and Developmental Disabilities,** P.O. Box 110620, Juneau, AK 99811-0620; tel. 907/465-3370; FAX. 907/465-2668; Karl Brimner, Director

Licensing
- **Alaska Board of Nursing,** 3601 C Street, Suite 722, Anchorage, AK 99503; tel. 907/269-8160; FAX. 907/269-8156; Dorothy P. Fulton, RN, M.A., Executive Administrator
- **Department of Communitye and Economic Development, Division of Occupational Licensing, State Medical Board,** 3601 C Street, Suite 722, Anchorage, AK 99503; tel. 907/269-8160; FAX. 907/269-8156; Leslie G. Abel, Executive Administrator

Social Services
- **Department Health and Social Services, Division Alcoholism and Drug Abuse,** 240 Main Street, Suite 701, P.O. Box 110607, Juneau, AK 99811-0607; tel. 907/465-2071; FAX. 907/465-2185; Ernie Turner, Director
- **Department of Health and Social Services,** 350 Main Street, Room 229, P.O. Box 110601, Juneau, AK 99811-0601; tel. 907/465-3030; FAX. 907/465-3068; Karen Perdue, Commissioner
- **Division of Administrative Services, Department of Health and Social Services,** P.O. Box 110650, Juneau, AK 99811-0650; tel. 907/465-3082; FAX. 907/465-2499; Janet E. Clarke, Director
- **Division of Family and Youth Services,** P.O. Box 110630, Juneau, AK 99811; tel. 907/465-3191; FAX. 907/465-3397; Theresa Tanoury, Director
- **Division of Medical Assistance,** P.O. Box 110660, Juneau, AK 99811-0660; tel. 907/465-3355; FAX. 907/465-2204; Bob Labbe, Director
- **Division of Vocational Rehabilitation,** 801 West 10th Street, Suite A, Juneau, AK 99801-1894; tel. 907/465-2814; FAX. 907/465-2856; Duane M. French, Director
- **State of Alaska, Division of Medical Assistance,** P.O. 110660, Juneau, AK 99811-0640; tel. 907/465-3355; FAX. 907/465-2204; Bob Labbe, Director
- **State of Alaska, Department of Health and Social Services,** 350 Main Street, Room 229, P.O. Box 110601, Juneau, AK 99811-0601; tel. 907/465-3030; FAX. 907/465-3068; Jay A. Livey, Deputy Commissioner

Other
- **Department of Education and Early Development,** 801 West 10th Street, Suite 200, Juneau, AK 99801-1894; tel. 907/465-2887; FAX. 907/465-2713; Beth Shober, Health Promotion Specialist

ARIZONA
The Honorable Jane Dee Hull, Governor, 602/542-4331

Health
- **Arizona Department of Health Services,** 1740 West Adams Street, Suite 407, Phoenix, AZ 85007; tel. 602/542-1025; FAX. 602/542-1062; James R. Schamadan, M.D.
- **Arizona Department of Health Services, Division of Health and Child Care Review Services, Office,** 1647 East Morten, Phoenix, AZ 85020; tel. 602/255-1197; FAX. 602/255-1135; John Zemaitis, Assistant Director
- **Arizona Department of Health Services, Division of Public Health, Bureau of Epidemiology and Disease Control Services,** 3815 North Black Canyon Highway, Phoenix, AZ 85015; tel. 602/230-5808; FAX. 602/230-5959; Lee A. Bland, Bureau Chief

Licensing
- **Arizona Board of Medical Examiners,** 1651 East Morten, Suite 210, Phoenix, AZ 85020; tel. 602/255-3751; FAX. 602/255-1848; Claudia Fontz, Executive Director
- **Arizona State Board of Nursing,** 1651 East Morten, Suite 150, Phoenix, AZ 85020; tel. 602/331-8111; FAX. 602/906-9365

Social Services
- **Community and Family Health Services,** 1740 West Adams Street, Suite 307, Phoenix, AZ 85007; tel. 602/542-1223; FAX. 602/542-1265; Elsie E. Eyer, M.S., Bureau Chief
- **Division of Behavioral Health Services, Arizona Department of Health Services,** 2122 East Highland, Suite 100, Phoenix, AZ 85016; tel. 602/381-8999; FAX. 602/553-9140; Ronald Smith, Assistant Director
- **Office for Children with Special Health Care Needs,** Administrative Offices, 1740 West Adams Street, Phoenix, AZ 85007; tel. 602/542-1860; FAX. 602/542-2589; Susan Burke, Chief
- **Rehabilitation Services Administration (930A),** 1789 West Jefferson, Second Floor Northwest, Phoenix, AZ 85007; tel. 602/542-3332; FAX. 602/542-3778; Skip Bingham, Administrator

Other
- **Arizona Department of Environmental Quality,** 3033 North Central Avenue, Phoenix, AZ 85012; tel. 602/207-2300; FAX. 602/207-2218; Jacqueine E. Schaffer, Director
- **Department of Economic Security,** Site Code 010A, P.O. Box 6123, Phoenix, AZ 85005; tel. 602/542-5678; FAX. 602/542-5339; John L. Clayton, Director

ARKANSAS
The Honorable Mike Huckabee, Governor, 501/682-2345

Health
- **Arkansas Department of Health,** 4815 West Markham Street, Slot 39, Little Rock, AR 72205-3867; tel. 501/661-2000; FAX. 501/671-1450; Fay W. Boozman, III, M.D.
- **Arkansas Department of Health, Bureau of Community Health Services,** 4815 West Markham Street, Slot 2, Little Rock, AR 72205-3867; tel. 501/661-2167; FAX. 501/661-2601; Jim Mills, Director
- **Arkansas Department of Health, Public Health,** 4815 West Markham, Slot 55, Little Rock, AR 72205; tel. 501/661-2238; FAX. 501/661-2414; Gail Gannaway, Director
- **Bureau of Administrative Support,** State Health Building, Little Rock, AR 72205-3867; tel. 501/661-2252; Tom Butler, Director
- **Bureau of Health Resources, Arkansas Department of Health,** 4815 West Markham Street, Slot 21, Little Rock, AR 72205-3867; tel. 501/661-2268; FAX. 501/661-2544; Henry C. Robinson, Acting Director
- **Children's Medical Service,** Donaghey Plaza South, Seventh and Main Streets, Little Rock, AR 72203; tel. 501/682-8202; FAX. 501/682-8247; G. A. Buchanan, M.D., Medical Director
- **Division of Health Facility Services, Department of Health,** 5800 West 10th Street, Suite 400, Little Rock, AR 72204; tel. 501/661-2201; FAX. 501/661-2165; Renee Mallory, Director, Health Facility Service
- **Division of Medical Services,** Donaghey Building – 11th Floor, 103 E. Seventh Street, Little Rock, AR 72203-1437; tel. 501/682-8292; FAX. 501/682-1197; Ray Hanley, Director

Insurance
- **Arkansas Insurance Department,** 1200 W. 3rd Street, Little Rock, AR 72201; tel. 501/371-2600; FAX. 501/371-2626; Mike Pickens, Insurance Commissioner

Licensing
- **Arkansas State Board of Nursing,** University Tower Building, Suite 800, 1123 South University Avenue, Little Rock, AR 72204; tel. 501/686-2700; FAX. 501/686-2714; Faith A. Fields, M.S.N., RN, Executive Director

Social Services
- **Arkansas Department of Human Services,** P.O. Box 1437, Little Rock, AR 72203-1437; tel. 501/682-8650; FAX. 501/682-6836; Kurk Knickrehm
- **Arkansas Division of Mental Health Services, Arkansas State Hospital,** 4313 West Markham, Little Rock, AR 72205-4096; tel. 501/686-9000; FAX. 501/686-9182; Richard Hill, Director
- **Arkansas Rehabilitation Services,** 1616 Brookwood, P.O. Box 3781, Little Rock, AR 72203; tel. 501/296-1616; FAX. 501/296-1675; Bobby C. Simpson, Commissioner
- **Bureau of Alcohol & Drug Abuse Prevention,** Freeway Medical Center, Suite 907, 5800 West 10th Street, Little Rock, AR 72204; tel. 501/280-4501; FAX. 501/280-4532; Joe M. Hill, Director

Organizations / State and Provincial Government Agencies

Bureau of Public Health Programs, Arkansas Department of Health, 4815 West Markham Street, Slot 41, Little Rock, AR 72205–3867; tel. 501/661–2243; FAX. 501/661–2055; Martha Hiett, Director

Division of Aging and Adult Services, P.O. Box 1437, Slot 1412, Little Rock, AR 72203–1437; tel. 501/682–2441; FAX. 501/682–8155; Herb Sanderson, Director

Office of Long–Term Care, Lafayette Building, Sixth and Louisiana Streets, Little Rock, AR 72203–8059; tel. 501/682–8487; FAX. 501/682–6955; Carol Shockley, Interim Director

CALIFORNIA
The Honorable Gray Davis, Governor, 916/445–2841

Health
Department of Developmental Services, 1600 Ninth Street, Suite 240, Sacramento, CA 95814; tel. 916/654–1897; FAX. 916/654–2167; Cliff Allenby, Director

Department of Health Services, 714 P Street, Suite 1253, Sacramento, CA 95814; tel. 916/657–1425; FAX. 916/657–5183; Diana M. Bonta, RN, DrPH, Director

Licensing
Board of Registered Nursing, 400 R Street, Suite 4030, P.O. Box 944210, Sacramento, CA 94244–2100; tel. 916/322–3350; FAX. 916/327–4402; Ruth Ann Terry, MPH, RN, Executive Officer

Board of Vocational Nursing and Psychiatric Technicians, 2535 Capitol Oaks Drive, Suite 205, Sacramento, CA 95833; tel. 916/263–7800; FAX. 916/263–7859; Teresa Bello–Jones, J.D., M.S.N., RN, Executive Officer

Medical Board of California, 1426 Howe Avenue, Suite 54, Sacramento, CA 95825–3236; tel. 916/263–2389; FAX. 916/263–2387; Ron Joseph, Executive Director

Social Services
Community Resources Development Section, California Department of Rehabilitation, 2000 Evergreen Street, Sacramento, CA 95815; tel. 916/263–7374; FAX. 916/263–7456; Sig Brivkalns, Chief

Department of Alcohol and Drug Programs, 1700 K Street, Sacramento, CA 95814; tel. 916/445–1943; FAX. 916/323–5873; Position vacant at this time

Department of Mental Health, 1600 Ninth Street, Room 151, Sacramento, CA 95814; tel. 916/654–2309; FAX. 916/654–3198; Stephen W. Mayberg, Ph.D., Director

Department of Social Services, 744 P Street, Sacramento, CA 95814; tel. 916/657–3661; FAX. 916/654–2049; Rita Saenz, Director

Human Services Agency, Office of the Secretary, 1600 Ninth Street, Suite 460, Sacramento, CA 95814; tel. 916/654–3454; FAX. 916/654–3343; Sandy Stiles, Manager, Administrative Services

Other
Department of Corporations, Health Care Division, 3700 Wilshire Boulevard, Suite 600, Los Angeles, CA 90010–3001; tel. 213/736–2776; Gary G. Hagen, Assistant Commissioner

COLORADO
The Honorable Bill Owens, Governor, 303/866–2471

Health
Colorado Department of Public Health and Environment, 4300 Cherry Creek Drive, S., Denver, CO 80222–1530; tel. 303/692–2000; FAX. 303/782–0095; Jane E. Norton, Executive Director

Colorado Department of Public Health and Environment, Health Facilities Division, 4300 Cherry Creek Drive S., Denver, CO 80246–1530; tel. 303/692–2100; FAX. 303/691–7702; Patti Shwayder, Executive Director

State Department of Health Care Policy and Financing, 1575 Sherman Street, 10th Floor, Denver, CO 80203–1714; tel. 303/866–2993; FAX. 303/866–4411; James T. Rizzuto, Executive Director

Insurance
Division of Insurance, 1560 Broadway, Suite 850, Denver, CO 80202; tel. 303/894–7499; FAX. 303/894–7455; Jack Ehnes, Commissioner

Licensing
Colorado Board of Medical Examiners, 1560 Broadway, Suite 1300, Denver, CO 80202–5140; tel. 303/894–7690; FAX. 303/894–7692; Susan Miller, Program Administrator

Department of Regulatory Agencies, 1560 Broadway, Suite 1550, Denver, CO 80202; tel. 303/894–7855; FAX. 303/894–7885; M. Michael Cooke, Executive Director

Social Services
Alcohol and Drug Abuse Division, Colorado Department of Human Services, 4300 Cherry Creek Drive South, Denver, CO 80222; tel. 303/692–2930; FAX. 303/753–9775; Robert Aukerman, Director

Department of Human Services, 1575 Sherman Street, Eighth Floor, Denver, CO 80203; tel. 303/866–5096; FAX. 303/866–4740; Marva Livingston Hammons, Executive Director

Division of Aging and Adult Services, Colorado Department of Human Services, 110 16th Street, Second Floor, Denver, CO 80202; tel. 303/620–4127; FAX. 303/620–4191; Rita A. Barreras, Director

Family and Community Health Services Division, Colorado Department of Public Health and Environment, 4300 Cherry Creek Drive South, Denver, CO 80246–1530; tel. 303/692–2310; FAX. 303/753–9249; Merril Stern, Director

Mental Health Services, 3824 West Princeton Circle, Denver, CO 80236; tel. 303/366–7400; FAX. 303/866–7428; Thomas J. Barrett, Ph.D., Director

CONNECTICUT
The Honorable John G. Rowland, Governor, 800/406–1527

Health
Department of Health Services, 150 Washington Street, Hartford, CT 06106; tel. 203/566–2038; Frederick G. Adams, D.D.S., MPH, Commissioner

Department of Public Health, 410 Capitol Avenue, Mail Stop 12APP, Hartford, CT 06134–0308; tel. 860/509–7579; FAX. 860/509–8457; Cynthia Denne, Director

Department of Public Health, 410 Capitol Avenue, P.O. Box 340308, Hartford, CT 06134–0308; tel. 860/509–7101; FAX. 860/509–7111; Joxel Garcia, M.D., Commissioner

Department of Public Health, Division of Health Systems Regulation, 410 Capitol Avenue, Mail Stop HSR, Hartford, CT 06134–0308; tel. 860/509–7407; FAX. 860/509–7539; Kathleenn Zarrella, RN, BS, Director

Insurance
Department of Insurance, P.O. Box 816, Hartford, CT 06142–0816; tel. 860/297–3862; FAX. 860/297–3941; Mary Ellen Breault, Director, Life and Health Division

Licensing
Connecticut Board of Examiners for Nursing, Department of Public Health – MS#13ADJ, 410 Capital Avenue, P.O. Box 340308, Hartford, CT 06134–0308; tel. 860/509–7624; FAX. 860/509–7286; Wendy H. Furniss, RNC, MS, Public Health Services Manager

Social Services
Department of Social Services, 25 Sigourney Street, Hartford, CT 06106; tel. 860/424–5008; FAX. 860/424–5129; Patricia A. Wilson–Coker, JD, MSW, Commissioner

Department of Social Services, Bureau of Rehabilitation Service, Division of Organizational Support, 10 Griffin Road, N., Windsor, CT 06095; tel. 203/298–2032; FAX. 203/298–9590; John J. Galiette, Chief

Elderly Services Division, Department of Social Services, 25 Sigourney Street, Hartford, CT 06106–5033; tel. 203/424–5277; FAX. 203/424–4966; Christine M. Lewis, Director

State Department of Mental Health and Addiction Services, 410 Capitol Avenue, P.O. Box 341431, Hartford, CT 6134; tel. 860/418–7000; FAX. 860/418–6691; Albert J. Solnit, M.D., Commissioner

Other
Department of Education, 165 Capitol Avenue, Hartford, CT 06145; tel. 203/566–5061; FAX. 203/566–8964

DELAWARE
The Honorable Thomas R. Carper, Governor, 302/739–4101

Health
Community Health Care Access Section, Jesse Cooper Building, Dover, DE 19903; tel. 302/739–4785; FAX. 302/739–6653; Prudence Kobasa, Public Health Nursing Director

Delaware Office of Emergency Medical Services, Blue Hen Corporate Center, 655 South Bay Road, Dover, DE 19901; tel. 302/739–4710; FAX. 302/739–2352; Bill Stevenson, EMS Director

Delaware Public Health Laboratory, 30 Sunnyside Road, P.O. Box 1047, Smyrna, DE 19977–1047; tel. 302/653–2870; FAX. 302/653–2877; Christopher K. Zimmerman, M.A., Acting Director

Division of Public Health, P.O. Box 637, Dover, DE 19903; tel. 302/739–4700; FAX. 302/739–6659; Steven F. Boedigheimer, Deputy Director

Division of Public Health, Community Health Care Access Section, Jesse S. Cooper Building, Federal Street, Dover, DE 19903; tel. 302/739–4785; FAX. 302/739–6653

Licensing
Delaware Board of Medical Practice, Cannon Building, Suite 203, 861 Silver Lake Boulevard, Dover, DE 19901; tel. 302/739–4522; FAX. 302/739–2711; Brenda D. Petty-Ball, Executive Director

Delaware Board of Nursing, Cannon Building, Suite 203, 861 Silver Lake Boulevard, Dover, DE 19904; tel. 302/739–4522; FAX. 302/739–2711; Iva J. Boardman, RN, M.S.N., Executive Director

Office of Health Facilities Licensing and Certification, Department of Health and Social Services, Three Mill Road, Suite 308, Wilmington, DE 19806; tel. 302/577–6666; FAX. 302/577–6672; Ellen Reap, Director

Social Services
Delaware Psychiatric Center, Division of Alcoholism, Drug Abuse and Mental Health, 1901 North DuPont Highway, New Castle, DE 19720; tel. 302/577–4000; FAX. 302/577–4359; Jiro R. Shimond, AGSW, Hospital Director

Department of Health and Social Services, 1901 North DuPont Highway, Main Administration Building, New Castle, DE 19720; tel. 302/577–4500; FAX. 302/577–4510

Department of Labor, Division of Vocational Rehabilitation, 4425 North Market Street, Wilmington, DE 19802; tel. 302/761–8275; FAX. 302/761–6611; Michelle P. Pointer, Director

Division of Services for Aging and Adults with Physical Disabilities, 1901 North DuPont Highway, 2nd Floor Annex, New Castle, DE 19720; tel. 302/577–4791; FAX. 302/577–4793; Eleanor L. Cain, Director

Division of Social Services, P.O. Box 906, New Castle, DE 19720; tel. 302/577–4400; FAX. 302/577–4405; Elaine Archangelo, Director

Family Health Services, Division of Public Health, P.O. Box 637, Dover, DE 19903; tel. 302/739–4785; FAX. 302/739–6653; Joan Powell, MPA, Director

DISTRICT OF COLUMBIA
Governor Swithboard, 202/727–1000

Health
Commission on Mental Health Services, Office of the Receiver, 4301 Conn. Avenue, N.W., Washington, DC 20008; tel. 202/364–3422; FAX. 202/364–4886; Dr. Scott H. Nelson, Receiver

D.C. Department of Public Health, 800 Ninth Street, S.W., Washington, DC 20024; tel. 202/645–5556; FAX. 202/645–0526; Allan S. Noonan, M.D., MPH

Department of Health, 800 9th Street, S.E., 3rd Floor, Washington, DC 20024; tel. 202/645–5556; FAX. 202/645–0627; Allan S. Noonan, M.D., MPH

Department of Health, Preventive Health Services Administration, 800 Ninth Street, S.W., Second Floor, Washington, DC 20024; tel. 202/645–5550; FAX. 202/645–0454; Administrator, PHSA

Licensing
Department of Consumer and Regulatory Affairs, 614 H Street, N.W., Suite 1120, Washington, DC 20001; tel. 202/727–7120; FAX. 202/727–8073; Lloyd J. Jordan, Director

Department of Consumer and Regulatory Affairs, Licensing Regulation Administration, 614 H Street, N.W., Suite 1003, Washington, DC 20001; tel. 202/727–7190; FAX. 202/727–7780; Geraldine K. Sykes, Administrator

Organizations / State and Provincial Government Agencies

Occupational and Professional Licensing Administration, Department of Consumer and Regulatory Affairs, 614 H Street, N.W., Suite 903, Washington, DC 20001; tel. 202/727-7480; FAX. 202/727-7662; Winnie R. Huston, Administrator

Social Services
Alcohol and Drug Abuse Services Administration, 1300 1st Street, N.E., Washington, DC 20002; tel. 202/727-1762; FAX. 202/535-2028

Bureau of Maternal and Child Health Services, Dept. of Health, Office of Maternal and Child Health, 800 Ninth Street, S.W., 3rd Floor, Washington, DC 20024; tel. 202/645-5653; Michelle S. Davis, M.S.P.H., Interim Chief

Commission on Social Services, 609 H Street, N.E., F fth Floor, Washington, DC 20002; tel. 202/727-5930; FAX. 202/727-6529; A. Sue Brown, Acting Commissioner of Social Services

Rehabilitation Services Administration, 810 First Street, N.E., 10th Floor, Washington, DC 20024; tel. 202/442-8663; FAX. 202/442-8742; Monique C. Brown, Secretary

FLORIDA
The Honorable Jeb Bush, Governor, 850/488-2272

Health
Children's Medical Services, 2020 Capital Circle, SE, Bir A-06, Tallahassee, FL 32399-1700; tel. 850/245-4200; FAX. 904/488-3813; Eric G. Handler, M.D., MPH, Director, CMS

Department of Health, Secretary's Office, 2020 Capital Circle, SE, Bin #A00, Tallahassee, FL 32399-1700; tel. 850/245-4443; FAX. 904/487-3729; Robert G. Brooks, M.D., Secretary

Department of Health, Secretary's Office, 1317 Winewood Boulevard, Building Six, Tallahassee, FL 32399-0700; tel. 904/487-2945; FAX. 904/487-3729; James T. Howell, M.D., MPH, Secretary

Insurance
Department of Insurance, Bureau of Specialty Insurers, 200 East Gaines Street, Tallahassee, FL 32399; tel. 904/488-6766; FAX. 904/488-0313; Al Willis, Chief

Licensing
Division of Health Quality Assurance, 2727 Mahan Drive, Tallahassee, FL 32308; tel. 850/487-2528; FAX. 850/487-6240; Pete J. Buigas, Director

Florida Board of Medicine, 2020 Capital Circle S.E., Bin # C03, Tallahassee, FL 32399-3253; tel. 850/488-3622; FAX. 850/488-9325; Tanya Williams, Board Director

Social Services
Adult Services, 1317 Winewood Boulevard, Building 8, Room 327, Tallahassee, FL 32399-0700; tel. 904/488-8922; Ms. Nancy Fulton, Director, Adult Services

Certificate of Need/Financial Analysis, Agency for Health Care Administration, 2727 Mahan Drive, Tallahassee, FL 32308; tel. 904/488-8673; FAX. 904/922-6964; Jeff Gregg, Chief

Department of Health and Rehabilitative Services, Alcohol, Drug Abuse and Mental Health Program Office, 1317 Winewood Boulevard, Tallahassee, FL 32399-0700; tel. 904/488-8304; FAX. 904/487-2239

Department of Labor and Employment Security, 2012 Capital Circle, S.E., 303 Hartman Building, Tallahassee, FL 32399-2152; tel. 904/922-7021; FAX. 904/488-8930; Mary B. Hooks, Secretary

Division of Vocational Rehabilitation, 2002 Old St. Augustine Road, Building A, Tallahassee, FL 32399-0696; tel. 850/488-6210; FAX. 850/921-7215; Michael Moore, Acting Director

GEORGIA
The Honorable Roy Barnes, Governor, 404/656-1776

Health
Division of Public Health, Two Peachtree Street, NW, Suite 715-470-300, Atlanta, GA 30303-3682; tel. 404/657-2700; FAX. 404/657-6709; Kathleen E. Toomay, M.D., MPH, Director

Insurance
Office of Commissioner of Insurance, Two Martin Luther King, Jr. Drive, Seventh Floor, West Tower, Floyd Build, Atlanta, GA 30334; tel. 404/656-2056; FAX. 404/656-4030; John W. Oxendine, Commissioner of Insurance

Licensing
Child Care Licensing Section, Two Peachtree Street, N.W., 32-458, Atlanta, GA 30303; tel. 404/657-5562; FAX. 404/657-8936; Jo Cato, Director

Composite State Board of Medical Examiners, 166 Pryor Street, S.W., Atlanta, GA 30303; tel. 404/656-3913; FAX. 404/656-9723; Gregg W. Scheder, Acting Executive Director

Diagnostic Services Unit, Health Care Section, Office of Regulatory Services, Two Peachtree Street, N.W., 33rd Floor, Room 250, Atlanta, GA 30303-3142; tel. 404/657-5447; FAX. 404/657-8934; Betty J. Logan, Regional Director, Diagnostic Services

Georgia Board of Nursing, 166 Pryor Street, S.W., Atlanta, GA 30303; tel. 404/656-3943; FAX. 404/657-7489; Shirley A. Camp, Executive Director

Social Services
Department of Human Resources, Two Peachtree N.W., Suite 29.250, Atlanta, GA 30303; tel. 404/656-5680; FAX. 404/651-8669; Audrey W. Horne, Commissioner

Department of Human Resources, Office of Regulatory Services, Health Care Section, Two Peachtree Street, N.W., Suite 33.250, Atlanta, GA 30303-3167; tel. 404/657-5550; FAX. 404/657-8934; Susie M. Woods, Director of the HCS

Division of Mental Health, Mental Retardation and Substance Abuse, Two Peachtree Street, NW., 22-205, Atlanta, GA 30303; tel. 404/657-2252; FAX. 404/657-1137; Carl E. Roland, Jr., Director

Division of Rehabilitation Services, Two Peachtree Street, N.W., 35th Floor, Atlanta, GA 30303-3142; tel. 404/657-3000; FAX. 404/657-3079; Peggy Rosser, Director

Office of Regulatory Services, Georgia Department of Human Resources, Two Peachtree Street, N.W., Room 32-415, Atlanta, GA 30303-3142; tel. 404/657-5700; FAX. 404/657-5708; Martin J. Rotter, Director

Personal Care Home Program, Office of Regulatory Services, Two Peachtree Street, 31st Floor, Atlanta, GA 30303-3167; tel. 404/657-4076; FAX. 404/657-3655; Victoria L. Flynn, Director

HAWAII
The Honorable Benjamin J. Cayetano, Governor, 808/586-0034

Health
Adult Mental Health Division, P.O. Box 3378, Honolulu, HI 96801-3378; tel. 808/586-4677; FAX. 808/586-4745; Linda Fox, Ph.D.

Communicable Disease Division, P.O. Box 3378, Honolulu, HI 96801; tel. 808/586-4580; FAX. 808/586-4595; Richard L. Vogt, M.D., State Epidemiologist

Dental Health Division, 1700 Lanakila Avenue, Suite 203, Honolulu, HI 96817-2199; tel. 808/832-5700; FAX. 808/832-5722; Mark H.K. Greer, D.M.D., MPH, Chief

Hawaii Department of Health, P.O. Box 3378, Honolulu, HI 96801; tel. 808/586-4410; FAX. 808/586-4444; Bruce S. Anderson, Ph.D., MPH, Director

State Health Planning and Development Agency, 335 Merchant Street, Suite 214 E, Honolulu, HI 96813; tel. 808/587-0788; FAX. 808/587-0783; Patrick J. Boland, Administrator

Licensing
Department of Commerce and Consumer Affairs, Board of Medical Examiners, P.O. Box 3469, Honolulu, HI 96801; tel. 808/586-2708; Constance Cabral-Makanani, Executive Officer

Department of Health/Office of Health Care Assurance, Licensing and Certification, P.O. Box 3378, Honolulu, HI 96801; tel. 808/586-4080; FAX. 808/586-5844; Helen K. Yoshimi, B.S.N., MPH, Chief, OHCA

Social Services
Alcohol and Drug Abuse Division, Department of Health, State of Hawaii, 601 Kamokila Blvd., Room 360, Kapolei, HI 96707; tel. 808/692-7506; FAX. 808/692-7521; Elaine Wilson, Chief

Department of Human Services, Med-QUEST Division, 601 Kamokila Boulevard, Room 518, Box 339, Honolulu, HI 96809; tel. 808/692-8050; FAX. 808/692-8173; Charles C. Duarte, Med-QUEST Administrator

Department of Labor and Industrial Relations, Disability Compensation Division, P.O. Box 3769, Honolulu, HI 96812; tel. 808/586-9151; FAX. 808/586-9219; Gary S. Hamada, Administrator

Family Health Services Division, Hawaii State Department of Health, 1250 Punchbowl Street, Room 216, Honolulu, HI 96813; tel. 808/586-4122; FAX. 808/586-9303; Loretta J. Fuddy, A.C.S.W., M.P.H

Vocational Rehabilitation, 601 Kamokila Blvd, Room 515, Kapolei, HI 96707; tel. 808/692-7715; FAX. 808/692-7727; Neil Shim, Administrator

Other
Environmental Management Division, 919 Ala Mona Boulevard, Room 300, Honolulu, HI 96814; tel. 808/586-4304; FAX. 808/586-4352; Thomas E. Aritumi, Chief Environmental

IDAHO
The Honorable Dirk Kempthorne, Governor, 208/334-2100

Health
Bureau of Emergency Medical Services, P.O. Box 83720, Boise, ID 83720-0036; tel. 208/334-4000; FAX. 208/334-4015; Dia Gainor, Bureau Chief

Center for Vital Statistics and Health Policy, 450 West State, First Floor, P.O. Box 83720, Boise, ID 83720-0036; tel. 208/334-5976; FAX. 208/332-7260; Jane S. Smith, State Registrar, Chief

Insurance
Department of Insurance, 700 West State Street, Third Floor, P.O. Box 83720, Boise, ID 83720-0043; tel. 208/334-4250; FAX. 208/334-4398; Mary L. Hartung, Director

Licensing
Bureau of Facility Standards, Department of Health and Welfare, P.O. Box 83720, Boise, ID 83720-0036; tel. 208/334-6626; FAX. 208/364-1888; Sylvia Creswell, Supervisor-Non LTC

Idaho State Board of Medicine, 280 North Eighth Street, Suite 202, P.O. Box 83720, Boise, ID 83720-0058; tel. 208/334-2822; FAX. 208/334-2801; Darlene Thorsted, Executive Director

Idaho State Board of Nursing, 280 North Eighth Street, Suite 210, Boise, ID 83720-0061; tel. 208/334-3110; FAX. 208/334-3262; Sandra Evans, MA.,Ed., RN, Executive Director

Social Services
Bureau of Clinical and Preventive Services, P.O. Box 83720, Boise, ID 83720-0036; tel. 208/334-5930; FAX. 208/332-7307; Roger Perotto, Chief

Department of Health and Welfare, Division of Health, 450 West State, Fourth Floor, P.O. Box 83720, Boise, ID 83720-0036; tel. 208/334-5945; FAX. 208/334-6581; Richard H. Schultz, Administrator

Division of Family and Community Services, Bureau of Mental Health and Substance Abuse, P.O. Box 83720, Boise, ID 83720-0036; tel. 208/334-5935; FAX. 208/334-6664; Tina Klamt, Substance Abuse Project Manager

Vocational Rehabilitation, 650 West State, P.O. Box 83720, Boise, ID 83720-0096; tel. 208/334-3390; FAX. 208/334-5305; F. Pat Young, Interim Administrator

Other
Bureau of Laboratories, 2220 Old Penitentiary Road, Boise, ID 83712; tel. 208/334-2235; FAX. 208/334-2382; Richard F. Hudson, Ph.D., Chief

ILLINOIS
The Honorable George H. Ryan, Governor, 217/782-0244

Health
Illinois Department of Public Health, 535 West Jefferson Street, Springfield, IL 62761; tel. 217/782-4977; FAX. 217/782-3987; John R. Lumpkin, M.D., MPH, Director

Illinois Department of Public Health, Office of Epidemiology & Health Systems Development, 525 West Jefferson Street, Springfield, IL 62761; tel. 217/785-2040; FAX. 217/785-4308; Laura B. Landrum, Deputy Director

Illinois Department of Public Health, Office of Health Care Regulation, 525 West Jefferson Street, 5th floor, Springfield, IL 62761; tel. 217/782-2913; FAX. 217/524-6292; William A. Bell, Deputy Director

Organizations / State and Provincial Government Agencies

Illinois Department of Public Health, Office of Health Protection, 525 West Jefferson Street, Springfield, IL 62761; tel. 217/782-3984; FAX. 217/524-0802; Dave King, Deputy Director

Illinois Department of Public Health Laboratories, 825 North Rutledge Street, P.O. Box 19435, Springfield, IL 62794-9435; tel. 217/782-6562; FAX. 217/524-7924; Bernard T. Johnson, Acting, State Laboratory Director

Illinois Department of Public Health, Office of Health Care Resources, Bureau of Hospitals and Ambulatory Services, 525 West Jefferson Street, Fourth Floor, Springfield, IL 62761; tel. 217/782-7412; FAX. 217/782-0382; Catherine M. Stokes, Assistant Deputy Director

Insurance

Department of Insurance, 320 West Washington Street, Fourth Floor, Springfield, IL 62767; tel. 217/782-4515; FAX. 217/782-5020; Nathaniel S. Sharp, Director

Licensing

Illinois Department of Professional Regulation, James R. Thompson Center, 100 West Randolph, Chicago, IL 60601; tel. 312/814-4500; FAX. 312/814-1837; Leonard A. Sherman, Director

Social Services

Department of Public Aid, 201 South Grand Avenue, E., Springfield, IL 62763; tel. 217/782-1200; FAX. 217/524-7979; Ann Patla, Director

Division of Specialized Care for Children, University of Illinois, (Illinois' Title V Program for Children with Special Health Care Needs), 2815 West Washington, Suite 300, Springfield, IL 62794-9481; tel. 217/793-2350; FAX. 217/793-0773; Charles N. Onufer, M.D., Director

Illinois Department of Human Services, 100 South Grand Avenue East, Springfield, IL 62762; tel. 217/557-1601; FAX. 217/557-1647; Howard A. Peters, III, Secretary

Illinois Department of Human Services, 100 S. Grand Avenue, East, Springfield, IL 62762; tel. 217/557-2109; FAX. 217/557-2112; Linda Renee Baker, Secretary

Illinois Department of Human Services, Office of Rehabilitation Services Home Services Program, 623 East Adams Street, P.O. Box 19509, Springfield, IL 62794-9509; tel. 217/782-2722; FAX. 217/557-0142; Rob Kilbury, Assistant Bureau Chief, Home Service Program

Office of Finance and Administration, 535 West Jefferson Street, Springfield, IL 62761; tel. 217/785-2033; FAX. 217/782-3987; Gary Robinson, Deputy Director

INDIANA
The Honorable Frank O'Bannon, Governor, 317/232-4567

Health

Children's Special Health Care Services, Indiana State Department of Health, Two North Meridian Street, Section 7B, Indianapolis, IN 46204; tel. 317/233-5578; FAX. 317/233-5609; Wendy S. Gettelfinger, Director

Indiana State Department of Health, Division of Acute Care, Two North Meridian Street, Indianapolis, IN 46204; tel. 317/233-7474; FAX. 317/233-7157; Mary Azbill, Director

Insurance

Department of Insurance, 311 West Washington Street, Suite 300, Indianapolis, IN 46204; tel. 317/232-2387; FAX. 317/232-5251; Liz Carroll, Chief Deputy Commissioner

Licensing

Indiana State Board of Nursing, Health Professions Bureau, 402 West Washington Street, Room 041, Indianapolis, IN 46204; tel. 317/232-1105; FAX. 317/233-4236; Barbara Powers, Director

Medical Licensing Board of Indiana, Health Professions Bureau, 402 West Washington, Suite 041, Indianapolis, IN 46204; tel. 317/232-2960; FAX. 317/233-4236

Social Services

Division of Long Term Care, Two North Meridian Street, Fourth Floor, Indianapolis, IN 46204; tel. 317/233-7442; FAX. 317/233-7322; Suzanne Hornstein, Director

Indiana Family and Social Services Administration, 402 West Washington Street, P.O. Box 7083, Indianapolis, IN 46207-7083; tel. 317/233-4454; FAX. 317/233-4693; Venita J. Moore, Interim Secretary

Indiana Family and Social Services Administration, Division of Mental Health, Indiana Government Center-South, W353, 402 West Washington Street, Indianapolis, IN 46204; tel. 317/232-7800; FAX. 317/233-3472; Patrick Sullivan, Ph.D., Director

Indiana Family and Social Services Administration, Office of Medicaid Policy and Planning, Indiana Government Center-South, 402 West Washington, Room W 382, Indianapolis, IN 46204-2739; tel. 317/233-4455; FAX. 317/232-7382; Kathleen D. Gifford, Assistant Secretary

Maternal and Child Health Services, Indiana State Department of Health, Two North Meridian Street, Suite 700, Indianapolis, IN 46204; tel. 317/233-1262; FAX. 317/233-1299; Judith A. Ganser, M.D., MPH, Medical Director

IOWA
The Honorable Thomas Vilsack, Governor, 515/281-5211

Health

Center for Health Policy, Iowa Department of Public Health, Lucas State Office Building, Fourth Floor, Des Moines, IA 50319; tel. 515/281-4346; FAX. 515/281-4958; Gerd Clabaugh, Director

Department of Public Health, Lucas State Office Building, Des Moines, IA 50319-0075; tel. 515/281-5605; FAX. 515/281-4958; Stephen C. Gleason, DO, Director

Division of Family and Community Health, Iowa Department of Public Health, Lucas State Office Building, Fifth Floor, Des Moines, IA 50319; tel. 515-281-7785; FAX. 515/281-4529; Mary Weaver

Insurance

Division of Insurance, 330 E. Maple, Des Moines, IA 50319-0065; tel. 515/281-5705; FAX. 515/281-3059; Therese M. Vaughan, Commissioner

Licensing

Department of Inspection and Appeals, Division of Health Facilities, Lucas State Office Building, Des Moines, IA 50319; tel. 515/281-4115; FAX. 515/242-5022; Marvin Toman, Administrator

Iowa Board of Medical Examiners, 400 S.W. 8th Street, Suite C, Des Moines, IA 50309-4686; tel. 515/281-5171; FAX. 515/242-5908; Ann E. Mowery, PhD, Executive Director

Iowa Board of Nursing, 400 S.W. 8th Street, Suite B, Des Moines, IA 50309-4685; tel. 515/281-3255; FAX. 515/281-4825; Lorinda K. Inman, RN, M.S.N., Executive Director

Social Services

Child Health Specialty Clinics, 247 Hospital School, Iowa City, IA 52242-1011; tel. 319/356-1469; FAX. 319/356-3715; Jeffrey G. Lobas, M.D., Director

Department of Human Services, Hoover State Office Building, Des Moines, IA 50319; tel. 515/281-5452; FAX. 515-281-4980; Jessie K. Rasmussen, Director

Division of Mental Health/Developmental Disabilities, Hoover State Office Building, Des Moines, IA 50319-0114; tel. 515/281-5874; FAX. 515/281-4597; Division Administrator

Division of Substance Abuse and Health Promotion, Iowa Department of Public Health, Lucas State Office Building, 321 East 12th Street, Des Moines, IA 50319-0075; tel. 515/281-3641; FAX. 515/281-4535; Janet Zwick, Director

Governor's Alliance on Substance Abuse, Lucas State Office Building, Des Moines, IA 50319; tel. 515/281-4518; FAX. 515/242-6390; Dale Woolery, Associate Coordinator

Iowa Department of Elder Affairs, 200 – 10th, 3rd Floor, Des Moines, IA 50309-3609; tel. 515/281-5187; FAX. 515/281-4036; Judith A. Conlin, M.D., Executive Director

Other

Department of Education, Division of Vocational Rehabilitation Services, 510 East 12th Street, Des Moines, IA 50319; tel. 515/281-4211; FAX. 515/281-4703; Dwight R. Carlson, Administrator

KANSAS
The Honorable Bill Graves, Governor, 913/296-6240

Health

Kansas Department of Health and Environment, Capital Tower, 400 S.W. 8th Street, Topeka, KS 66603; tel. 913/296-0461; FAX. 913/368-6368; Clyde Graeber, Secretary, Kansas Health and Environment

Insurance

Kansas Insurance Department, 420 Southwest Ninth, Topeka, KS 66612; tel. 913/296-3071; FAX. 913/296-2283; Kathleen Sebelius, Commissioner, Insurance

Kansas Insurance Department, Accident and Health Division, 420 Southwest Ninth, Topeka, KS 66612; tel. 913/296-7850; FAX. 913/296-2283; Thomas C. Foley, Director of Accident and Health

Licensing

Kansas State Board of Healing Arts, 235 South Topeka Boulevard, Topeka, KS 66603-3068; tel. 913/296-7413; FAX. 913/296-0852; Lawrence T. Buening, Jr., Executive Director

Kansas State Board of Nursing, Landon State Office Building, 900 Southwest Jackson, Topeka, KS 66612-1230; tel. 785/296-4929; FAX. 785/296-3929; Mary Blubaugh, MSN, RN, Executive Administrator

Social Services

Division of Health Care Policy, Docking State Office Building, Fifth Floor-N, Topeka, KS 66612; tel. 913/296-3773; FAX. 913/296-6142; J. Lyn Entrikin Goering, Assistant Secretary

Health Care Policy/Medicaid, Docking State Office Building, 915 Southwest Harrison, Topeka, KS 66612; tel. 913/296-3981; FAX. 913/296-4813; Robert Day, Director

Kansas Department of Health and Bureau of Health Facilities, Bureau of Health Facilities, 900 Southwest Jackson, Suite 1001, Topeka, KS 66612-1290; tel. 913/296-1240; FAX. 913/296-1266; Beth Voorhees, Director of Medical Facilities and Support

Rehabilitation Services, 3640 SW Topeka Blvd., Suite 150, Topeka, KS 66611-2373; tel. 785/267-5301; FAX. 785-267-0263; Dennis D. Rogers, Director

State Department of Social and Rehabilitation Services, Economic & Employment Support, Docking State Office Building, Suite 681-W, Topeka, KS 66612; tel. 913/296-6750; FAX. 913/296-6960; Sandra C. Hazlett, Director

KENTUCKY
The Honorable Paul E. Patton, Governor, 502/564-2611

Health

Commission for Children with Special Health Care Needs, 982 Eastern Parkway, Louisville, KY 40217; tel. 502/595-4459; FAX. 502/595-4673; Ann Marks, Executive Director

Department For Mental Health/Mental Retardation Services, 100 Fair Oaks Lane, Frankfort, KY 40621-0001; tel. 502/564-4527; FAX. 502/564-5478; Margaret A. Pennington, MSSW, Commissioner

Department for Public Health, Cabinet for Health Services, 275 East Main Street, Frankfort, KY 40621; tel. 502/564-3970; FAX. 502/564-6533; Rice C. Leach, M.D., MSHSA, Commissioner

Office of Certificate of Need, 275 East Main Street, Frankfort, KY 40621; tel. 502/564-9589; FAX. 502/564-0302; John H. Gray, Director

Surveillance and Health Date Branch, 275 East Main Street, HSIE-C, Frankfort, KY 40621; tel. 502/564-2757; FAX. 502/564-6533; George Robertson, Manager

Insurance

Department of Insurance, Division of Health Policy and Managed Care, 215 West Main Street, P.O. Box 517, Frankfort, KY 40602; tel. 502/564-6088; FAX. 502/564-2728; Carrie Banahan, Branch Manager

Licensing

Division of Licensing and Regulation, Office of Inspector General, C.H.R. Building, Fourth Floor, E., 275 East Main Street – 4ES, Frankfort, KY 40621; tel. 502/564-2800; FAX. 502/565-6546; Rebecca J. Cecil, R.Ph., Director

Kentucky Board of Nursing, 312 Whittington Parkway, Suite 300, Louisville, KY 40222-5172; tel. 502/329-7000; FAX. 502/329-7011; Sharon M. Weisenbeck, M.S., RN, Executive Director

Social Services

Department for Community Based Services, 3rd Floor West, 275 East Main Street, Frankfort, KY 40621; tel. 502/564-3703; FAX. 502/564-6907; Dietra Paris, Commissioner

Department for Medicaid Services, 275 East Main Street, Frankfort, KY 40621; tel. 502/564-4321; FAX. 502/564-6917; John Morse, Commissioner

Organizations / State and Provincial Government Agencies

Department of Vocational Rehabilitation, 209 St. Clair Street, Frankfort, KY 40601; tel. 502/564–4440; FAX. 502/564–6745; Sam Serraglio, Commissioner

LOUISIANA
The Honorable Murphy Foster, Jr., Governor, 225/342–7015

Health
Department of Health and Hospitals, Bureau of Health Services, Health Standards Section, Box 3767, Baton Rouge, LA 70821; tel. 504/342–0138; FAX. 504/342–5292; Lily W. McAlister, RN, Manager, Health Standards Section

Louisiana Department of Health and Hospitals, P.O. Box 629 Bin 2, Baton Rouge, LA 70821; tel. 504/342–9509; FAX. 504/342–9508; Rose V. Forrest, Secretary

Louisiana State University Health Sciences Center, Health Care Services Division–Medical Center of LA at New Orleans, 2021 Perdido Street, New Orleans, LA 70112–1352; tel. 504/588–3332; FAX. 504/588–3580; John S. Berault, MSPH, Chief Executive Officer

Louisiana State University Medical Center, Health Care Services Division, 8550 United Plaza Boulevard, Fourth Floor, Baton Rouge, LA 70809; tel. 504/922–0490; FAX. 504/922–2259; Cary M. Dougherty, Jr., Chief Operating Officer

Insurance
Department of Insurance, P.O. Box 94214, Baton Rouge, LA 70804; tel. 225/342–1355; FAX. 225/342–5711; James H. Brown, Commissioner

Licensing
Louisiana State Board of Medical Examiners, P.O. Box 30250, New Orleans, LA 70190–0250; tel. 504/524–6763; FAX. 504/568–8893; Virginia Gerace Benoist, Executive Director

Louisiana State Board of Nursing, 150 Baronne Street, New Orleans, LA 70112; tel. 504/568–5464; Barbara L. Movant, RN, M.S.N.

Louisiana State Board of Practical Nurse Examiners, 3421 North Causeway Boulevard, Suite 203, Metairie, LA 70002; tel. 504/838–5791; FAX. 504/838–5279; Dennis S. Mann, Esq., Executive Director

Social Services
Office for Addictive Disorders, P.O. Box 2790, Baton Rouge, LA 70821–2790; tel. 504/342–6717; FAX. 504/342–3875; Alton E. Hadley, Assistant Secretary

Office of Community Services, P.O. Box 3318, Baton Rouge, LA 70821; tel. 504/342–2297; FAX. 504/342–2268; Carmen Weisner, Assistant Secretary

Office of Family Support, P.O. Box 94065, Baton Rouge, LA 70804–9065; tel. 225/342–3950; FAX. 225/342–4252; Vera W. Blakes, Assistant Secretary

Other
Office of The Secretary, P.O. Box 629, Baton Rouge, LA 70821; tel. 225/342–9500; FAX. 225/342–5568; David W. Hood, Secretary

MAINE
The Honorable Angus S. King, Jr., Governor, 207/287–3531

Health
Bureau of Health, Department of Human Services, 11 State House Station, Augusta, ME 04333; tel. 207/287–8016; FAX. 207/287–9058; Dora Anne Mills, M.D., MPH, Director

Division of Community and Family Health, 151 Capitol Street, 11 State House Station, Augusta, ME 04333–0011; tel. 207/287–3311; FAX. 207/287–4631; Valerie Ricker, MSN, MS, NP

Insurance
Bureau of Insurance, Department of Professional and Financial Regulation, 34 State House Station, Augusta, ME 04333; tel. 207/624–8475; FAX. 207/624–8599; David Stetson, Supervisor, Life and Health Division

Licensing
Board of Licensure in Medicine, Two Bangor Street, 137 State House Station, Augusta, ME 04333; tel. 207/287–3601; FAX. 207/287–6590; Randal C. Manning, Executive Director

Department of Professional and Financial Regulation, 35 State House Station, Augusta, ME 04333; tel. 207/624–8511; FAX. 207/624–8595; S. Catherine Longley, Commissioner

Division of Licensing and Certification, Department of Human Services, 35 Anthony Avenue, Station 11, Augusta, ME 04333; tel. 207/624–5443; FAX. 207/624–5378; Louis Dorogi, Director

Maine State Board of Nursing, 24 Stone Street, 158 State House Station, Augusta, ME 04333; tel. 207/287–1133; FAX. 207/287–1149; Myra A. Broadway, J.D., RN, Executive Director

Social Services
Bureau of Elder and Adult Services, 35 Anthony Avenue, Station 11, Augusta, ME 04333; tel. 207/624–5335; FAX. 207/624–5361; Christine Gianopoulos, Director

Bureau of Rehabilitation Services, 150 State House Station, Augusta, ME 04333–0150; tel. 207/287–5145; FAX. 207/287–5166; John Shattuck, Director

Bureau of Rehabilitation Services, Division of Deafness, 150 State House Station, Augusta, ME 04333–0150; tel. 207/287–5145; FAX. 207/287–5166; Jan DeVinney, Director

Department of Human Services, Bureau of Medical Services, State House, Station 11, Augusta, ME 04333; tel. 207/287–2674; FAX. 207/287–2675; Francis T. Finnegan, Jr., Director

Department of Mental Health, Mental Retardation and Substance, State House Station 40, Augusta, ME 04333; tel. 207/287–4220; FAX. 207/287–4268; Susan Wygal, Commissioner, Programs

Department of Mental Health, Mental Retardation and Substance, Abuse Services, 40 State House Station, Augusta, ME 04333–0040; tel. 207/287–4223; FAX. 207/287–4268; Melodie J. Peet, Commissioner

Division for the Blind and Visually Impaired, 150 State House Station, Augusta, ME 04333–0150; tel. 207/287–5256; FAX. 207/287–5166; Harold Lewis, Director

Maine Department of Human Services, State House, Station 11, Augusta, ME 04333; tel. 207/287–2736; FAX. 207/287–3005; Kevin W. Concannon, Commissioner

MARYLAND
The Honorable Parris N. Glendening, Governor, 410/974–3901

Health
Community and Public Health Administration, 201 West Preston Street, Baltimore, MD 21201; tel. 410/225–5300; FAX. 410/333–7106; Dr. Carlossia Hussein, Director

Department of Health and Mental Hygiene, 201 West Preston Street, Room 500, Baltimore, MD 21201; tel. 410/767–6500; FAX. 410/767–6489; Georges C. Benjamin, M.D., Secretary

Insurance
Maryland Insurance Administration, 525 St. Paul Place, Baltimore, MD 21202; tel. 410/468–2000; FAX. 410/468–2020; Steven B. Larsen, Insurance Commissioner

Licensing
Board of Physician Quality Assurance, 4201 Patterson Avenue, Baltimore, MD 21215; tel. 800/492–6836; FAX. 410/358–2252; J. Michael Compton, Executive Director

Maryland Board of Nursing, 4140 Patterson Avenue, Baltimore, MD 21215–2254; tel. 410/585–1900; FAX. 410/358–3530; Donna M. Dorsey, RN, M.S., Executive Director

Office of Health Care Quality, Bland Bryant Building, Spring Grove Center, 55 Wade Avenue, Catonsville, MD 21228; tel. 410/402–8018; FAX. 410/402–8211; Carol Benner, Director

Social Services
Alcohol and Drug Abuse Administration, 201 West Preston Street, Baltimore, MD 21201; tel. 410/767–6925; FAX. 410/333–7206; Thomas Davis, Director

Community and Public Health Administration, 201 West Preston Street, Baltimore, MD 21201; tel. 410/767–5300; FAX. 410/333–7106; Carlessia A. Hussein, Dr.P.H., Director

Developmental Disabilities Administration, 201 West Preston Street, Baltimore, MD 21201; tel. 410/767–5600; FAX. 410/767–5850; Diane K. Coughlin, Director

Division of Rehabilitation Services, 2301 Argonne Drive, Baltimore, MD 21218–1696; tel. 410/554–9385; FAX. 410/554–9412; Robert A. Burns, Assistant State Superintendent

Mental Hygiene Administration, 201 West Preston Street, Baltimore, MD 21201; tel. 410/767–6655; FAX. 410/333–5402; Oscar L. Morgan, Director

Social Services Administration, 311 West Saratoga Street, Fifth Floor, Baltimore, MD 21201; tel. 410/767–7216; FAX. 410/333–0127; Linda E. Mouzon, Executive Director

Other
Laboratories Administration, 201 West Preston Street, Baltimore, MD 21201; tel. 410/767–6100; FAX. 410/333–5403; J. Mehsen Joseph, Ph.D., Director

Maryland Department of the Environment, Office of Environmental Health Coordination, 2500 Broening Highway, Baltimore, MD 21224; tel. 410/631–3851; FAX. 410/631–4112; Tom Allen, Director

Maryland State Department of Education, 200 West Baltimore Street, Baltimore, MD 21201–1595; tel. 410/767–0100; FAX. 410/333–6033; Nancy S. Grasmick, State Superintendent of Schools

Office of Planning and Capital Financing, 201 West Preston Street, Baltimore, MD 21201; tel. 410/767–6816; FAX. 410/333–7525; Elizabeth G. Barnard, Director

MASSACHUSETTS
The Honorable Argeo Paul Cellucci, Governor, 617/727–3600

Health
Bureau of Environmental Health Assessment, 250 Washington Street, Seventh Floor, Boston, MA 02108; tel. 617/624–5757; FAX. 617/624–5777; Suzanne K. Condon, Director

Bureau of Health Quality Management, Massachusetts Department of Public Health, 250 Washington Street, Boston, MA 02108–4619; tel. 617/624–5280; FAX. 617/624–5046; Nancy Ridley, Assistant Commissioner

Bureau of Health Statistics, Research and Evaluation, Massachusetts Department of Public Health, 250 Washington Street, Sixth Floor, Boston, MA 02108–4619; tel. 617/624–5613; FAX. 617/624–5698; Daniel J. Friedman, Ph.D., Assistant Commissioner

Department of Transitional Assistance, 600 Washington Street, Boston, MA 02111; tel. 617/348–8402; FAX. 617/348–8575; Claire McIntire, Commissioner

Office of Emergency Medical Services, 470 Atlantic Avenue, Second Floor, Boston, MA 02210–2208; tel. 617/753–8300; FAX. 617/753–8350; Louise Goyette, Director

Insurance
Division of Insurance, Boston, MA 02110–2208; tel. 617/521–7794; FAX. 617/521–7773; Linda Ruthardt, Commissioner

Licensing
Board of Registration in Medicine, Commonwealth of Massachusetts, Boston, MA 02111; tel. 617/727–3086; FAX. 617/451–9568; Alexander F. Fleming, Executive Director

Division of Health Care Quality, 10 West Street, Fifth Floor, Boston, MA 02111; tel. 617/753–8100; FAX. 617/753–8125; Paul I. Dreyer, Ph.D., Director

Massachusetts Board of Registration in Nursing, 100 Cambridge Street, Suite 1519, Boston, MA 02202; tel. 617/727–9961; FAX. 617/727–1630; Theresa M. Bonanno, M.S.N., RN, Executive Director

Social Services
Commission for the Blind, 88 Kingston Street, Boston, MA 02111; tel. 617/727–5550; FAX. 617/727–5960; David Govostes, Commissioner

Massachusetts Department of Mental Health, Central Office, 25 Stanford Street, Boston, MA 02114; tel. 617/626–8123; FAX. 617/626–8131; Marylou Sudders, Commissioner

Massachusetts Department of Public Health, Bureau of Substance Abuse, 250 Washington Street, Third Floor, Boston, MA 02108–4619; tel. 617/624–5111; FAX. 617/624–5185; Mayra Rodriguez–Howard, Director

Massachusetts Rehabilitation Commission, Fort Point Place, 27–43 Wormwood Street, Boston, MA 02210–1606; tel. 617/204–3600; FAX. 617/727–1354; Elmer C. Bartels, Commissioner

MICHIGAN
The Honorable John Engler, Governor, 517/335–3400

Organizations / State and Provincial Government Agencies

Health

Bureau of Health Systems, Michigan Department of Consumer and Industry Services, 525 West Ottawa, P.O. Box 30664, Lansing, MI 48909; tel. 517/241-2626; FAX. 517/241-2635; Walter S. Wheeler, III, Director

Division of Chronic Disease and Injury Control, Michigan Department of Community Health, 3423 North Martin Luther King, Jr. Boulevard, P.O. Box 30195, Lansing, MI 48909; tel. 517/335-8368; FAX. 517/335-8593; Jean Chabut, Director

Medical Services Administration, 400 South Pine, P.O. Box 30037, Lansing, MI 48909; tel. 517/373-6561; FAX. 517/335-5007; Robert M. Smedes, Deputy Director

Licensing

Department of Consumer and Industry Services, Michigan Insurance Bureau, 611 West Ottawa, Second Floor, P.O. Box 30220, Lansing, MI 48909-7720; tel. 877/999-6442; FAX. 517/335-4978; Frank M. Fitzgerald, Commissioner

Division of Licensing and Certification, 3500 North Logan Street, Lansing, MI 48909; tel. 517/335-8505; Nancy Graham, Supervisor

Managed Care Quality Assessment and Improvement Division, Michigan Department of Community Health, P.O. Box 30195, Lansing, MI 48909; tel. 517/241-8551; FAX. 517/241-9953; Julia Harris Griffith, Director

Michigan Board of Medicine, 611 West Ottawa Street, Box 30670, Lansing, MI 48909; tel. 517/373-6873; FAX. 517/373-2179; Carole Hakala Engle, Director, Licensing

Michigan Board of Nursing, 611 West Ottawa Street, Box 30670, Lansing, MI 48909; tel. 517/335-0918; FAX. 517/373-2179; Doris Foley, Licensing Administrator

Social Services

Bureau of Rehabilitation and Disability Determination, Box 30010, Lansing, MI 48909; tel. 517/373-3390; Ivan L. Cotman, Associate Superintendent

Bureau of Substance Abuse Services, Michigan Department of Community Health, 320 S. Walnut Street, Lewis Cass Building, Lansing, MI 48913; tel. 517/335-0278; FAX. 517/241-2611; Deborah J. Hollis, Acting Director

Michigan Department of Community Health, Lewis Cass Building, Lansing, MI 48913; tel. 517/373-3500; FAX. 517/335-3090; James K. Haveman, Jr., Director

Michigan Department of Community Health, Community Public Health Agency, 3423 North Martin Luther King, Jr. Boulevard, Lansing, MI 48909; tel. 517/335-0267; FAX. 517/335-3090; James K. Haveman, Jr., Director, MDCH

Michigan Department of Community Health, Health Legislation and Policy Development, 320 S. Walnut Street, Lewis Cass Building, 6th Floor, Lansing, MI 48913; tel. 517/373-2559; FAX. 517/241-1200; Carol L. Isaacs, Deputy Director

Office of Health and Human Services, Michigan Department of Management and Budget, Lewis Cass Building, Box 30026, Lansing, MI 48909; tel. 517/373-1076; FAX. 517/373-3624; Paul Reinhart, Director

Office of Services to the Aging, P.O. Box 30026, Lansing, MI 48909; tel. 517/373-8230; FAX. 517/373-4092; Carol Parr, Acting Director

Other

Department of Education, Box 30008, Lansing, MI 48909; tel. 517/373-7247; FAX. 517/373-1233; Patricia Nichols, Supervisor, School Health Programs U

Michigan Department of Consumer and Industry Services, Office of Health Services, Box 30670, Lansing, MI 48909; tel. 517/373-8068; FAX. 517/241-3082; Thomas C. Lindsay, II, Director

Michigan Department of Consumer and Industry Services, Laboratories, Laboratory Improvement Section, P.O. Box 30664, Lansing, MI 48909; tel. 517/241-2640; FAX. 517/241-2635; Richard J. Benson, Chief

Michigan Department of Environmental Quality, Drinking Water and Radiological Protection Division, Medical Waste Regulatory Program, 3423 North Martin Luther King, Jr. Boulevard, P.O. Box 30630, Lansing, MI 48909; tel. 517/335-8637; FAX. 517/335-9033; John N. Gohlke, R.S., M.S.A., Program Chief

Michigan Family Independence Agency, 235 South Grand Avenue, P.O. Box 30037, Lansing, MI 48909; tel. 517/373-2035; FAX. 517/335-6236; Mark Jasonowicz – Interim Director

Office of Health Services, Department of Consumer and Industry Services, P.O. Box 30670, Lansing, MI 48909; tel. 517/373-8068; FAX. 517/373-2179; Thomas C. Lindsay, II, Director

MINNESOTA

The Honorable Jesse Ventura, Governor, 651/296-3391

Health

Division of Environmental Health, 121 East Seventh Place, P.O. Box 64975, St. Paul, MN 55164-0975; tel. 651/215-0700; FAX. 651/215-0979; Patricia A. Bloomgren, Director

Minnesota Department of Health, 85 East 7th Place, Suite 400, St. Paul, MN 55164-0882; tel. 651/215-5806; FAX. 651/215-5801; Jan K. Malcolm, Commissioner

Minnesota Department of Health, Division of Finance and Administration, 121 East 7th Place, P.O. Box 64975, St. Paul, MN 55164-0975; tel. 651/282-2999; FAX. 651/282-3832; David Johnson, Assistant Commissioner

Minnesota Department of Health, Office of Regulatory Reform, 121 East Seventh Place, P.O. Box 64975, St. Paul, MN 55164-0975; tel. 612/282-5627; FAX. 612/282-3839; Nanette M. Schroeder, Director

Public Health Laboratory Division, 717 Southeast Delaware Street, P.O. Box 9441, Minneapolis, MN 55440; tel. 612/676-5331; FAX. 612/676-5514; Norman Crouch, PhD, Director

Licensing

Facility and Provider Compliance Division, Minnesota Department of Health, 393 North Dunlap Street, P.O. Box 64900, St. Paul, MN 55164-0900; tel. 612/643-2100; FAX. 612/643-2593; Linda G. Sutherland, Director

Licensing and Certification, 393 North Dunlap Street, P.O. Box 64900, St. Paul, MN 55164-0900; tel. 612/643-2130; FAX. 612/643-3534; Carol Hirschfeld, Supervisor, Program Assurance Unit

Minnesota Board of Medical Practice, 2829 University Avenue, S.E., Suite 400, Minneapolis, MN 55414-3246; tel. 612/617-2130; FAX. 612/617-2166; Robert A. Leach, Executive Director

Minnesota Board of Nursing, 2829 University Avenue, S.E., Suite 500, Minneapolis, MN 55414-3253; tel. 612/617-2270; FAX. 612/617-2190; Shirley A. Brekken, Executive Director

Social Services

Minnesota Department of Health, Division of Community Health Services, Metro Square Building, Suite 460, 121 East Seventh Place, Zip 55101, St. Paul, MN 55164-0975; tel. 651/296-9720; FAX. 651/296-9362; Ryan Church, Director

Minnesota Department of Health, Division of Disease Prevention and Control, 717 Southeast Delaware Street, P.O. Box 9441, Minneapolis, MN 55440-9441; tel. 612/676-5363; FAX. 612/676-5666; Martin Laventure, Acting Director

Minnesota Department of Health, Division of Family Health, 717 Southeast Delaware Street, P.O. Box 9441, Minneapolis, MN 55440; tel. 612/623-5167; FAX. 612/623-5442; Norbert Hirschhorn, M.D., Director

Minnesota Department of Human Services, 444 Lafayette Road, N., St. Paul, MN 55155; tel. 651/296-6117; FAX. 651/296-6244; Michael O'Keefe, Commissioner

Rehabilitation Services Branch, 390 North Robert Street, Fifth Floor, St. Paul, MN 55101; tel. 612/296-7510; FAX. 612/296-0994; Howard E. Grad, Assistant Commissioner

Other

Department of Commerce, 133 East Seventh Street, St. Paul, MN 55101; tel. 612/296-4026; FAX. 612/296-4328; David B. Gruenes

MISSISSIPPI

The Honorable David Renold Musgrove, Governor, 601/737-9540

Health

Bureau of Environmental Health, Mississippi State Department of Health, Felix J. Underwood State Board of Health Building, P.O. Box 1700, Jackson, MS 32915-1700; tel. 601/576-7680; FAX. 601/576-7800; Rick Harrington, Director

Bureau of Health Services, Felix J. Underwood State Board of Health Building An, P.O. Box 1700, Jackson, MS 32915; tel. 601/960-7472; FAX. 601/960-7480; Michael J. Gandy, Ed.D., Bureau Director, Deputy

Department of Health, Felix J. Underwood State Board of Health Building, P.O. Box 1700, Jackson, MS 32915-1700; tel. 601/576-7634; FAX. 601/576-7931; F.E. Thompson, Jr., M.D., MPH, State Health Officer

Health Planning and Resources Development Division, Mississippi State Department of Health, Felix J. Underwood State Board of Health Building, 2423 North State Street, Jackson, MS 39215-1700; tel. 601/576-7874; FAX. 601/576-7530; Harold B. Armstrong, Chief

Mississippi State Department of Health, Felix J. Underwood State Board of Health Building, P.O. Box 1700, Jackson, MS 32915-1700; tel. 601/960-7634; Betty Jane Phillips, Dr. P.H. Deputy State Health Officer

Public Health Statistics, Mississippi State Department of Health, Bureau of Health Statistics, Box 1700, Jackson, MS 39215-1700; tel. 601/576-7960; FAX. 601/576-7505; Nita C. Gunter, Director

Licensing

Division of Health Facilities Licensure and Certification, P.O. Box 1700, Jackson, MS 39215; tel. 601/354-7300; FAX. 601/354-7230; Vanessa Phipps, Director

Mississippi Board of Nursing, 1935 Lakeland Drive, Suite B, Jackson, MS 39216-5014; tel. 601/987-4188; FAX. 601/364-2352; Marcia M. Rachel, Ph.D., RN, M.S.N., Executive Director

Social Services

Children's Medical Program, 421 Stadium Circle, P.O. Box 1700, Jackson, MS 39215-1700; tel. 601/987-3965; FAX. 601/987-5560; Mike Gallarno, Director

Department of Mental Health, 1101 Robert E. Lee Building, Jackson, MS 39201; tel. 601/359-1288; FAX. 601/359-6295; Randy Hendrix, Ph.D., Director

Mississippi Department of Human Services, P.O. Box 352, Jackson, MS 39205-0352; tel. 601/359-4480; FAX. 601/359-4477; Bettye W. Fletcher, Executive Director

State Department of Rehabilitation Services, P.O. Box 1698, Jackson, MS 39215-1698; tel. 601/853-5100; FAX. 601/853-5205; H.S. McMillian, Executive Director

Other

State Epidemiologist, Underwood Annex, P.O Box 1700, Jackson, MS 32915-1700; tel. 601/960-7725; FAX. 601/354-6061; Mary Currier, M.D., MPH

MISSOURI

The Honorable Mel Carnahan, Governor, 573/751-3222

Health

Center for Health Information Management and Epidemiology (CHIME), Box 570, Jefferson City, MO 65102; tel. 573/751-6272; FAX. 573/526-4102; Garland H. Land, Director

Department of Health, P.O. Box 570, Jefferson City, MO 65102; tel. 314/751-6001; FAX. 314/751-6041; Maureen E. Dempsey, M.D., Director

Missouri Department of Health – Bureau of Special Health Care Needs, 930 Wildwood Drive, P.O. Box 570, Jefferson City, MO 65109; tel. 314/751-6246; FAX. 314/751-6237; Richard Brown, Chief

Insurance

Department of Insurance, P.O. Box 690, Jefferson City, MO 65102; tel. 314/751-4126; FAX. 314/751-1165; Keith Wenzel, Director

Licensing

Bureau of Hospital Licensing and Certification, Missouri Department of Health, Box 570, Jefferson City, MO 65102; tel. 314/751-6302; FAX. 314/526-3621; Darrell Hendrickson, Administrator

Organizations / State and Provincial Government Agencies

Missouri State Board of Registration for the Healing Arts, 3605 Missouri Boulevard, Zip 65109, P.O. Box 4, Jefferson City, MO 65102; tel. 314/751-0098; FAX. 314/751-3166; Tina Steinman, Executive Director

Social Services
Department of Mental Health, 1706 East Elm Street, P.O. Box 687, Jefferson City, MO 65102; tel. 573/751-4122; FAX. 573/751-8224; Roy C. Wilson, M.D., Director

Life and Health Section, Missouri Department of Insurance, P.O. Box 690, Jefferson City, MO 65102; tel. 573/751-4363; FAX. 573/526-6075; James W. Casey, Supervisor

Missouri Division of Vocational Rehabilitation, 3024 West Truman Boulevard, Jefferson City, MO 65109-0525; tel. 573/751-3251; FAX. 314/751-1441; Ronald W. Vessell, Assistant Commissioner

Other
Department of Elementary and Secondary Education, 205 Jefferson, P.O. Box 480, Jefferson City, MO 65102; tel. 573/751-4446; FAX. 573/751-1179; Dr. Robert E. Bartman, Commissioner of Education

Division of Nutritional Health and Services, 930 Wildwood Drive, P.O. Box 570, Jefferson City, MO 65109; tel. 573/526-5520; FAX. 573/526-5348; Gretchen C. Wartman, Director

MONTANA
The Honorable Marc Racicot, Governor, 406/444-3111

Health
Health Policy and Services Division, Montana Department of Public Health and Human Services, 1400 Broadway, P.O. Box 202951, Helena, MT 59620-2951; tel. 406/444-4540; FAX. 406/444-1861; Nancy Ellery, Administrator

Licensing
Quality Assurance Division, Department of Public Health and Human Services, Certification Bureau, Cogswell Building, 1400 Broadway, Helena, MT 59620-2951; tel. 406/444-2099; FAX. 406/444-3456; Linda Sandman, Chief

Social Services
Aging Services, Senior and Long Term Care Division, Department of Public Health and Human Services, 111 Sanders, P.O. Box 4210, Helena, MT 59604; tel. 406/444-7785; FAX. 406/444-7743; Robin Homan, State Long Term Care Ombudsman

Child and Family Services Division, P.O. Box 8005, Helena, MT 59604-8005; tel. 406/444-5902; FAX. 406/444-5956; Hank Hudson, Administrator

Department of Public Health and Human Services, 111 North Sanders Street, Box 4210, Helena, MT 59604-4210; tel. 406/444-5622; FAX. 406/444-1970; Laurie Ekanger, Director

Disability Services Division, P.O. Box 4210, Helena, MT 59604; tel. 406/444-2590; FAX. 406/444-3632; Joe A. Mathews, Administrator

Family/Maternal and Child Health Services Bureau, W. F. Cogswell Building, Helena, MT 5962C; tel. 406/444-4740; FAX. 406/444-2606; JoAnn Walsh Dotson, RN MSN, Bureau Chief

Montana Department of Public Health and Human Services, 111 North Sanders, P.O. Box 4210, Helena, MT 59604; tel. 406/444-5622; FAX. 406/444-1970; Laurie Ekanger, Director

Other
Department of Commerce, Montana State Board of Nursing, Arcade Building – 4-C, 111 North Jackson, Helena, MT 59620-0513; tel. 406/444-2071; FAX. 406/444-7759; Joan Bowers, Administrative Assistant

NEBRASKA
The Honorable Mike Johanns, Governor, 402/471-2244

Insurance
Department of Insurance, 941 O Street, Suite 400, Lincoln, NE 68508; tel. 402/471-2201; FAX. 402/471-4610; L. Tim Wagner, Director

Licensing
Division of Health Policy and Planning, 301 Centennial Mall, S., P.O. Box 95007, Lincoln, NE 68509; tel. 402/471-0146; FAX. 402/471-7783; David Palm, Ph.D., Director

HHS R&L Credentialing Division, 301 Centennial Mall, S., Box 94986, Lincoln, NE 68509-4986; tel. 402/471-2115; FAX. 402/471-3577; Helen L. Meeks, Director

Nebraska Department of Regulation and Licensure, Credentialing Division, 301 Centennial Mall, S., P.O. Box 94986, Lincoln, NE 68509-4986; tel. 402/471-2115; FAX. 402/471-3557; Helen L. Meeks, Administrator

Social Services
Department of Health and Human Services – Regulation, Certificate of Need Program and Licensure, P.O. Box 95007, Lincoln, NE 68509-5007; tel. 402/471-2105; FAX. 402/471-0555; Don Smith, Fiscal Analyst

Division of Family Health, Nebraska Department of Health and Human Services, 301 Centennial Mall South, P.O. Box 95044, Lincoln, NE 68509-5044; tel. 402/471-3980; FAX. 402/471-7049; Paula Eurek, R.D., Division Administrator

Nebraska Department of Health & Human Services, Regulation & Licensure, 301 Centennial Mall South, P.O. Box 951007, Lincoln, NE 68509-5007; tel. 402/471-2133; FAX. 402/471-9449; Richard P. Nelson, Director

Nebraska Department of Health and Human Services, Services, 301 Centennial Mall, S., P.O. Box 95044, Lincoln, NE 68509; tel. 402/471-0191; FAX. 402/471-8259; Sue Medinger, Administrator

Nebraska Department of Health and Human Services, Special Services for Children and Adults, 301 Centennial Mall, S., P.O. Box 95044, Lincoln, NE 68509-5044; tel. 402/471-9345; FAX. 402/471-9455; Mary Jo Iwan, Administrator

Nebraska Health and Human Services, Finance and Support Medicaid Division Medical Services Division, 301 Centennial Mall, S., P.O. Box 95026, Lincoln, NE 68509; tel. 402/471-9147; FAX. 402/471-9092; Cec Brady, Administrator

Nebraska Health and Human Services System, 301 Centennial Mall, South., P.O. Box 95026, Lincoln, NE 68509-5026; tel. 402/471-9433; FAX. 401/471-9449; Chris Peterson, Policy Secretary

Other
Department of Education, Vocational Rehabilitation, 301 Centennial Mall, S., P.O. Box 94987, Lincoln, NE 68509; tel. 402/471-3644; Frank Lloyd, Assistant Commissioner

Nebraska Department of Health, Division of Radiological Health, 301 Centennial Mall, S., P.O. Box 95007, Lincoln, NE 68509; tel. 402/471-2168; FAX. 402/471-0169; Harold Borchert, Director

NEVADA
The Honorable Kenny C. Guinn, Governor, 702/684-5670

Health
Bureau of Health Planning and Statistics, Nevada State Health Division, 505 East King Street, Room 102, Carson City, NV 89701-4749; tel. 775/684-4218; FAX. 775/684-4156; Emil DeJan, Chief

Children With Special Health Care Needs Program, Nevada State Health Division, Kinkead Building, 505 East King, Suite 205, Carson City, NV 89710; tel. 775/684-4243; FAX. 775/684-4245; Gloria Deyhle, MCH Nurse Consultant

Division of Mental Health and Developmental Services, Kinkead Building, Suite 602, 505 East King Street, Carson City, NV 89701-3790; tel. 775/684-5943; FAX. 775/684-5966; Carlos Brandenburg, Ph.D., Administrator

Nevada Division of Health, Kinkead Building, 505 East King Street, Room 201, Carson City, NV 89701-4761; tel. 775/684-4200; FAX. 775/684-4211; Yvonne Sylva, Administrator

Nevada State Health Division, Bureau of Community Health Services, 3656 Research Way, Suite 32, Carson City, NV 89706; tel. 775/687-6944; FAX. 775/687-7693; Mary D. Sassi, Bureau Chief

Nevada State Health Laboratory, 1660 North Virginia Street, Reno, NV 89503; tel. 702/688-1335; FAX. 702/688-1460; Arthur F. DiSalvo, M.D., Director

Insurance
Division of Insurance, 788 Fairview Drive, Suite 300, Carson City, NV 89701; tel. 775/687-4270; FAX. 775/687-3937; Alice A. Molasky-Arman, Commissioner

Licensing
Bureau of Licensure and Certification, Nevada Health Division, 1550 College Parkway, Capitol Complex, Suite 158, Carson City, NV 89706-7921; tel. 775/687-4475; FAX. 775/687-6588; Richard J. Panelli, Chief

Nevada State Board of Medical Examiners, 1105 Terminal Way, Suite 301, Zip 89502, P.O. Box 7238, Reno, NV 89510; tel. 702/688-2559; FAX. 702/688-2321; Larry D. Lessly, Executive Director

Nevada State Board of Nursing, 1755 East Plumb Lane, Suite 260, Reno, NV 89502; tel. 775/688-2620; FAX. 775/688-2628; Kathy Apple, M.S., RN, Executive Director

Social Services
Department of Human Resources, Kinkead Building, Carson City, NV 89710; tel. 775/684-4000; FAX. 775/684-4010; Charlotte Crawford, Director

Division of Health Care Financing & Policy, 1100 East William Street, Carson City, NV 89710; tel. 702/684-4176; FAX. 702/684-8792; Janice Wright, Administrator

Division of Health Care Financing and Policy–Medicaid, 2527 North Carson Street, Carson City, NV 84706-0113; tel. 775/687-4775; FAX. 775/687-8724; Mary Wherry, MS, CS, RN, Deputy Administrator

Rehabilitation Division, Kinkead Building, 505 East King, Room 502, Carson City, NV 89710; tel. 75/684-4040; FAX. 775/684-4184; Maynard R. Yasmer, Administrator

Other
Nevada Department of Business and Industry, Director's Office, 555 East Washington, Suite 4900, Las Vegas, NV 89101; tel. 702/486-2750; FAX. 702/486-2758; Sydney H. Wickliffe, Director

NEW HAMPSHIRE
The Honorable Jeanne Shaheen, Governor, 603/271-2121

Health
Department of Health and Human Services, Six Hazen Drive, Concord, NH 03301-6527; tel. 603/271-4372; FAX. 603/271-4827; William J. Kassler, M.D., MPH, State Medical Director

Department of Health and Human Services, Office of Health Management, Six Hazen Drive, Concord, NH 03301-6527; tel. 603/271-4726; FAX. 603/271-4827; William J. Kassler, M.D., MPH, State Medical Director

Department of Health and Human Services, Office of The Commissioner, 129 Pleasant Street, Brown Building, Concord, NH 03301; tel. 603/271-4602; FAX. 603/271-4912; Kathleen G. Sgambati, Deputy Commissioner

Division of Public Health Services, Office of Family and Community Health, Health and Welfare Building, Six Hazen Drive, Concord, NH 03301; tel. 603/271-4726; FAX. 603/271-4779; Roger Taillefer, Assistant Director

Insurance
Department of Insurance, 169 Manchester Street, Concord, NH 03301; tel. 603/271-2661; FAX. 603/271-1406; Sylvio L. Dupuis, O.D., Commissioner

State of New Hampshire, Insurance Department, Examination Division, 56 Old Suncook Road, Concord, NH 03301-5151; tel. 603/271-2241; FAX. 603/271-1406; Thomas S. Burke, Director

Licensing
New Hampshire Board of Medicine, Board of Medicine, Two Industrial Park Drive, Concord, NH 03301; tel. 603/271-1203; FAX. 603/271-6702; Allen Hall, Administrator

New Hampshire Board of Nursing, 78 Regional Drive, P.O. Box 3898, Concord, NH 03302-3898; tel. 603/271-2323; FAX. 603/271-6605; Doris G. Nuttelman, RN, Ed.D., Executive Director

Office of Program Support, Licensing and Regulation, Health Facilities Administration, 129 Pleasant Street, Concord, NH 03301; tel. 603/271-4966; FAX. 603/271-5590; Raymond Rusin, Chief

Social Services
Department of Health and Human Services, Office of Family Services, 129 Pleasant Street, Concord, NH 03301-3857; tel. 603/271-4321; FAX. 603/271-4727; Richard A. Chevrefils, Assistant Commissioner

Organizations / State and Provincial Government Agencies

New Hampshire Department of Health and Human Services, Office of Community and Public Health, Six Hazen Drive, Concord, NH 03301; tel. 603/271–4496; FAX. 603/271–4933; Kathy Dunn, Director

Office of Community Supports and Long Term Care, State Office Park, S., 105 Pleasant Street, Concord, NH 03301; tel. 603/271–5007; FAX. 603/271–5058; Paul G. Gorman, Ed.D., Director

Vocational Rehabilitation Division, 78 Regional Drive, Concord, NH 03301; tel. 603/271–3471; Bruce A. Archambault, Director

Other

Department of Environmental Services, Six Hazen Drive, Concord, NH 03301; tel. 603/271–3503; FAX. 603/271–2867; Robert W. Varney, Commissioner

State Department of Education, 101 Pleasant Street, State Office Park, S., Concord, NH 03301; tel. 603/271–3494; FAX. 603/271–1953; Elizabeth M. Twomey, Commissioner

NEW JERSEY
The Honorable Christine T. Whitman, Governor, 609/292–6000

Health

Division of Health Care Systems Analysis, CN–360, Trenton, NJ 08625; tel. 609/292–8772; FAX. 609/984–3165; Maria Morgan, Assistant Commissioner

New Jersey Department of Health and Senior Services, Certificate of Need and Acute Care Licensing, P.O. Box 360, Trenton, NJ 08625–0360; tel. 609/292–8773; FAX. 609/292–3780; John A. Calabria, Director

Office of Managed Care, New Jersey State Department of Health, P.O. Box 360, Trenton, NJ 08625; tel. 609/633–0660; FAX. 609/633–0807; Edwin V. Kelleher, Chief

Licensing

Division of Consumer Affairs, 124 Halsey Street, P.O. Box 45027, Newark, NJ 07101; tel. 201/504–6534; FAX. 201/648–3538; Mark S. Herr, Director

New Jersey Board of Nursing, P.O. Box 45010, Newark, NJ 07101; tel. 973/504–6430; FAX. 973/648–3481; Patricia Polansky, Executive Director

State Board of Medical Examiners, 140 East Front Street, Second Floor, Trenton, NJ 08608; tel. 609/826–7100; FAX. 609/984–3930; Kevin B. Earle, Executive Director

Social Services

Department of Law and Public Safety, P.O. Box 080, 25 Market Street, Trenton, NJ 08625; tel. 609/292–8740; FAX. 609/292–3508; John J. Farmer, Jr., Attorney General

Division of Family Development, P.O. Box 716, Trenton, NJ 08625–0716; tel. 609/588–2401; FAX. 609/584–4404; David C. Heins, Director

Division of Family Health Services, 50 East State Street, P.O. Box 364, Trenton, NJ 08625; tel. 609/292–4043; FAX. 609/292–9599; Celeste Andviot–Wood

Maternal, Child and Community Health, New Jersey Department of Health and Senior Services, 50 East State Street, CN 364, P.O. Box 364, Trenton, NJ 08625–0364; tel. 609/984–1384; FAX. 609/292–3580; Len Massey, Acting Director

N.J. Department of Health and Senior Services, Office of the Commissioner, CN–360, Trenton, NJ 08625; tel. 609/292–7874; FAX. 609/292–0053; William Conroy, RN, Ph.D., Deputy Commissioner

New Jersey Department of Health and Senior Services, Office of the Commissioner, P.O. Box 360, Trenton, NJ 08625–0360; tel. 609/292–7837; FAX. 609/292–0053; Christine Grant, State Commissioner of Health and Senior Services

Other

Health Facilities Construction Service, CN–367, 300 Whitehead Road, Trenton, NJ 08625; tel. 609/588–7731; FAX. 609/588–7823; Kenneth A. Hess, Director

NEW MEXICO
The Honorable Gary E. Johnson, Governor, 505/827–3000

Health

Department of Health, P.O. Box 26110, Santa Fe, NM 87502–6110; tel. 505/827–2613; FAX. 505/827–2530; J. Alex Valdez, Secretary

Public Health Division, Department of Health, P.O. Box 26110, Santa Fe, NM 87502–6110; tel. 505/827–2389; FAX. 505/827–2329; Barak Wolff, Interim Director

Insurance

New Mexico Department of Insurance, P.O. Drawer 1269, Santa Fe, NM 87504–1269; tel. 505/827–4601; FAX. 505/827–4734; Helen Hordes, Manager, Life and Health Forms Division

State Corporation Commission, P.O. Drawer 1269, Santa Fe, NM 87504; tel. 505/827–4529; Eric P. Serna, Chairman

Licensing

Health Facility Licensing and Certification Bureau, Long Term Care Program, 525 Camino de los Marquez, Suite Two, Santa Fe, NM 87501; tel. 505/827–4200; FAX. 505/827–4203; Matthew M. Gervase, Bureau Chief

New Mexico Board of Medical Examiners, 491 Old Santa Fe Trail, Lamy Building, Second Floor, Santa Fe, NM 87501; tel. 505/827–5022; FAX. 505/827–7377; Kristen A. Hedrick, Executive Secretary

State of New Mexico, Board of Nursing, 4206 Louisiana, N.E., Suite A, Albuquerque, NM 87109; tel. 505/841–8340; FAX. 505/841–8340; Debra Brady, Executive Director

Social Services

Division of Vocational Rehabilitation, 435 St. Michaels Drive, Building D, Santa Fe, NM 87505; tel. 505/954–8511; FAX. 505/954–8562; Terry Brigance, Director

Human Services Department, P.O. Box 2348, Santa Fe, NM 87504–2348; tel. 505/827–7750; FAX. 505/827–6286; Duke Rodriguez, Secretary

Income Support Division, P.O. Box 2348, Santa Fe, NM 87504–2348; tel. 505/827–7252; FAX. 505/827–7203; Linda Chaug, Administrator

Protective Services Division, P.O. Box 5160, Santa Fe, NM 87502–5160; tel. 505/827–8400; FAX. 505/827–8480; Janet M. Escuedero, Acting Director

Other

State Department of Education, Education Building, 300 Don Gaspar, Santa Fe, NM 87501–2786; tel. 505/827–6516; FAX. 505/827–6696; Michael J. Davis, State Superintendent of Public Instruction

NEW YORK
The Honorable George E. Pataki, Governor, 518/474–8390

Health

Bureau of Home Health Care Services, New York State Department of Health, Freer Building, 2 Third Street, Troy, NY 12180; tel. 518/271–2741; FAX. 518/271–2771; Dr. Nancy Barhydt, Director

New York State Department of Health, Tower Building, Empire State Plaza, Room 1417, Albany, NY 12237; tel. 518/473–1124; FAX. 518/473–9674

New York State Department of Health, Empire State Plaza, Corning Tower, Room 1466, Albany, NY 12237; tel. 518/486–4803; FAX. 518/486–6852; Kathryn Kuhmerker, Deputy Commissioner – Office of Medicaid Management

New York State Department of Health, Office of Managed Care, Bureau of Managed Care Certification and Surveillance, Room 1911 Corning Tower Building, Empire State Plaza, Albany, NY 12237; tel. 518/473–4842; FAX. 518/473–3583; Vallencia Lloyd, Director

State Department of Health, Tower Building, Empire State Plaza, Albany, NY 12237; tel. 518/474–2011; FAX. 518/474–5450; Barbara A. DeBuono, M.D., MPH, Commissioner

Licensing

New York State Board for Medicine, Cultural Education Center, Albany, NY 12230; tel. 518/474–3841; FAX. 518/486–4846; Thomas J. Monahan, Executive Secretary

State Board for Nursing, New York State Education Department, Cultural Education Center, Room 3023, Albany, NY 12230; tel. 518/474–3843; FAX. 518/474–3706; Milene A. Sower, Ph.D., RN, Executive Secretary

Social Services

New York State Education Department, Vocational and Educational Services for Individuals with Disabilities, One Commerce Plaza, Suite 1606, Albany, NY 12234; tel. 518/474–2714; Lawrence C. Gloeckler, Deputy Commissioner

New York State Office of Alcoholism and Substance Abuse Services, 1450 Western Avenue, Albany, NY 12203; tel. 518/457–2061; FAX. 518/457–5474; Jean Somers Miller, Commissioner

New York State Office of Mental Health, 44 Holland Avenue, Albany, NY 12229; tel. 518/474–4403; FAX. 518/474–2149; James L. Stone, M.S.W., CSW Commissioner

Office of Mental Retardation and Developmental Disabilities, 44 Holland Avenue, Albany, NY 12229; tel. 518/473–1997; FAX. 518/473–1271; Thomas A. Maul, Commissioner

Other

Bureau of Project Management, New York State Department of Health, 433 River Street, Suite 303, Troy, NY 12180–2299; tel. 518/402–0911; FAX. 518/402–0975; Dominick F. Testo, Director

New York State Education Department, Main Education Building, Room 111, Albany, NY 12234; tel. 518/474–5844; FAX. 518/473–4909

Office of Health Systems Management, Tower Building, Empire State Plaza, Room 1441, Albany, NY 12237–0701; tel. 518/474–7028; FAX. 518/486–2564

Wadsworth Center for Laboratories and Research, Clinical Lab Evaluation, P.O. Box 509, Empire State Plaza, Albany, NY 12201–0509; tel. 518/474–7592; FAX. 518/474–3439; Lawrence S. Sturman, M.D., Ph.D., Director

NORTH CAROLINA
The Honorable James B. Hunt, Jr., Governor, 919/733–4240

Health

Department of Health and Human Services, P.O. Box 29526, Raleigh, NC 27626–0526; tel. 919/733–4534; FAX. 919/715–4645; Ronald H. Levine, M.D., MPH, Deputy Secretary

Department of Health and Human Services, 2001 Mail Service Center, Raleigh, NC 27626; tel. 919/733–4534; FAX. 919/715–4645; H. David Bruton, M.D., Secretary

Department of Health and Human Services, Division of Facility Services, 701 Barbour Drive, Raleigh, NC 27603; tel. 919/733–2342; FAX. 919/733–2757; Lynda D. McDaniel, Director

Insurance

Department of Insurance, P.O. Box 26387, Raleigh, NC 27611; tel. 919/733–7343; FAX. 919/733–6495; James E. Long, Commissioner

Licensing

North Carolina Board of Nursing, P.O. Box 2129, Raleigh, NC 27602; tel. 919/782–3211; FAX. 919/781–9461; Mary P. Johnson, RN, MSN, Executive Director

North Carolina Medical Board, P.O. Box 20007, Raleigh, NC 27619; tel. 919/326–1100; FAX. 919/326–1130; Andrew W. Watry, Executive Director

Social Services

Division of Medical Assistance, 2517 Mail Service Center, Raleigh, NC 27699–2517; tel. 919/857–4011; FAX. 919/733–6608; Paul R. Perruzzi, Director

Division of Mental Health, Developmental Disabilities and Substance Abuse Services, 325 North Salisbury Street, Raleigh, NC 27603; tel. 919/733–7011; FAX. 919/733–9455; J. Iverson Riddle, M.D.

Division of Vocational Rehabilitation Services, 2801 Math Services Center, Raleigh, NC 27609–2801; tel. 919/733–3364; FAX. 919/733–7968; Bob H. Philbeck, Director

NORTH DAKOTA
The Honorable Edward T. Schafer, Governor, 701/328–2200

Health

Children's Special Health Services, Department of Human Services, State Capitol, 600 East Boulevard Avenue, Dept 325, Bismarck, ND 58505–0269; tel. 701/328–2436; FAX. 701/328–2359; Robert W. Nelson, Director

Division of Health Facilities, North Dakota Department of Health, 600 East Boulevard Avenue, Bismarck, ND 58505–0200; tel. 701/328–2352; FAX. 701/328–1890; Darleen Bartz, Director

Health Resources Section, North Dakota Department of Health, 600 East Boulevard Avenue, Bismarck, ND 58505–0200; tel. 701/328–2352; FAX. 701/328–1890; Daeleen Bartz, Chief, Health Resources Section

Organizations / State and Provincial Government Agencies

Medical Services Division, North Dakota Department of Human Services, 600 East Boulevard Avenue, Dept 325, Bismarck, ND 58505-0261; tel. 701/328-2321; FAX. 701/328-1544; David J. Zentner, Director

State Department of Health, 600 East Boulevard Avenue, Bismarck, ND 58505-0200; tel. 701/328-2372; FAX. 701/328-4727; Londa Rodahl, Administrative Assistant

Insurance
North Dakota Department of Insurance, State Capitol, 600 East Boulevard, 5th Floor, Bismarck, ND 58505-0320; tel. 701/328-2440; FAX. 701/328-4880; Glenn Pomeroy, Commissioner

Licensing
North Dakota Board of Nursing, 919 South Seventh Street, Suite 504, Bismarck, ND 58504-5881; tel. 701/328-9777; FAX. 701/328-9785; Constance Kalanek, Ph.D, RN, Executive Director

North Dakota State Board of Medical Examiners, City Center Plaza, Suite 12, Bismarck, ND 58501; tel. 701/328-6500; FAX. 701/328-6505; Rolf P. Sletten, Executive Secretary, Treasurer

Social Services
Developmental Disabilities Unit, Disability Services Division, Department of Human Services, 600 South Second Street, Suite 1A, Bismarck, ND 58504-5729; tel. 701/328-8930; FAX. 701/328-8969; Gene Hysjulien, Director

Division of Alcoholism and Drug Abuse, 600 South Second Street, Suite 1E, Bismarck, ND 58504-5729; tel. 701/328-8920; FAX. 701/328-8969; Karen Larson, Director

Division of Maternal and Child Health, North Dakota Department of Health, State Capitol, 600 East Boulevard Avenue, Bismarck, ND 58505-0200; tel. 701/328-2493; FAX. 701/328-1412; Sandra Anseth, Director

Division of Mental Health and Substance Abuse Services, 600 S. 2nd Street, Suite 1D, Bismarck, ND 58504-5729; tel. 701/328-8940; FAX. 701/328-8969; Mark Kolling, Director

Office of Economic Assistance, North Dakota Department of Human Services, 600 East Boulevard Avenue Dept 325, Bismarck, ND 58505-0250; tel. 701/328-2332; FAX. 701/328-2359; Carol K. Olson, Executive Director

Office of Vocational Rehabilitation, Department of Human Services, 400 East Broadway Avenue, Suite 303, Bismarck, ND 58501-4038; tel. 701/328-3999; FAX. 701/328-3976; Gene Hysjulien, Director

Other
Facility Management Division, Office of Management and Budget, 600 East Boulevard, Ave, Dept 130, State Capitol, Bismarck, ND 58505-0130; tel. 701/328-2471; FAX. 701/328-3230; Curt Zimmerman, Director, Facility Management

Program and Policy, State Capitol, 600 East Boulevard Avenue Dept 325, Bismarck, ND 58505-0265; tel. 701/328-2310; FAX. 701/328-2359; Carol K. Olson, Executive Director

OHIO
The Honorable Bob Taft, Governor, 614/466-3555

Health
Managed Care Division, 2100 Stella Court, Columbus, OH 43215-1067; tel. 614/644-2661; FAX. 614/728-5238; Teresa Reedus, Senior Contract Analyst

Ohio Department of Health, 246 North High Street, Columbus, OH 43266-0588; tel. 614/466-3543; FAX. 614/644-0085; J.Nick Baird, M.D., Director

Ohio Department of Health, Bureau of Diagnostics Safety and Personnel Certification, 246 North High Street, P.O. Box 118, Columbus, OH 43266-0118; tel. 614/644-7230; FAX. 614/752-4157; Christine Kenney, Health Services Policy Specialist

Ohio Department of Health, Bureau of Local Services, 246 North High Street, Columbus, OH 43266-0118; tel. 614/466-0666; FAX. 614/644-4556; John Wanchick, M.P.A., R.S., Chief

Insurance
Department of Insurance, 2100 Stella Court, Columbus, OH 43215-1067; tel. 614/644-2658; FAX. 614/644-3743; J. Lee Covington, III, Director

Licensing
Division of Quality Assurance, Ohio Department of Health, 246 North High Street, Columbus, OH 43266-0588; tel. 614/466-7857; FAX. 614/644-0208; Rebecca S. Maust, Chief

Ohio Board of Nursing, 17 South High Street, Suite 400, Columbus, OH 43215-0413; tel. 614/466-3947; FAX. 614/466-0388; Dorothy Fiorino, RN, M.S., Executive Director

State Medical Board of Ohio, 77 South High Street, 17th Floor, Columbus, OH 43266-0315; tel. 614/466-3934; FAX. 614/728-5946; Ray Q. Bumgarner, Executive Director

Social Services
Bureau of Disability Determination, P.O. Box 359001, Columbus, OH 43235-9001; tel. 614/438-1500; FAX. 614/438-1504; Kathleen Johnson, Director

Department of Mental Health, 30 East Broad Street, Eighth Floor, Columbus, OH 43266-0414; tel. 614/466-2596; FAX. 614/752-9453; Michael F. Hogan, Ph.D., Director

Department of Mental Retardation and Developmental Disability, 30 East Broad Street, Columbus, OH 43266-0415; tel. 614/466-5214; FAX. 614/644-5013; Kenneth Ritchey, Director

Division of Family and Community Health Services, 246 North High Street, P.O. Box 118, Columbus, OH 43266-0118; tel. 614/466-3263; FAX. 614/728-3616; Kathryn K. Peppe, RN, M.S., Chief

Ohio Department of Alcohol and Drug Addiction Services, Two Nationwide Plaza, 280 North High Street, 12th Floor, Columbus, OH 43215-2537; tel. 614/466-3445; FAX. 614/752-8645; Luceille Fleming, Director

Ohio Department of Human Services, 30 East Broad Street, 32nd Floor, Columbus, OH 43266-0423; tel. 614/466-6282; FAX. 614/466-2815; Wayne W. Sholes, Director

Ohio Department of Human Services, Office of Medicaid, 30 East Broad Street, 31st Floor, Columbus, OH 43266-0423; tel. 614/644-0140; FAX. 614/752-3986; Barbara Coulter Edwards, Deputy Director

Ohio Rehabilitation Services Commission, Bureau of Services for the Visually Impaired, 400 East Campus View Boulevard, Columbus, OH 43235-4604; tel. 614/438-1255; FAX. 614/438-1257; William A. Casto, II, Director

Ohio Rehabilitation Services Commission, Bureau of Vocational Rehabilitation, 400 East Campus View Boulevard (SW3), Columbus, OH 43235-4604; tel. 614/438-1250; FAX. 614/438-1257; June K. Gutterman, Ed.D., Director

Other
Bureau of Plan Operations, 30 East Broad Street, 31st Floor, Columbus, OH 43266-0423; tel. 614/466-2365; FAX. 614/752-7701; Martha Lang, Acting Director

OKLAHOMA
The Honorable Frank Keating, Governor, 405/521-2342

Health
Oklahoma Health Care Authority, 4545 North Lincoln, Suite 124, Oklahoma City, OK 73105; tel. 405/530-3439; FAX. 405/530-4787; Garth L. Splinter, M.D., M.B.A., Chief Executive Officer

Oklahoma Health Care Authority, 4545 North Lincoln Boulevard, Suite 124, Oklahoma City, OK 73105; tel. 405/530-3373; FAX. 405/530-3478; Mike Fogarty, State Medicaid Director

Oklahoma Health Care Authority, Medical Authorization Unit, 4545 North Lincoln Boulevard, Suite 124, Oklahoma City, OK 73105; tel. 405/530-3439; FAX. 405/530-3215; Mike Fogarty, Medicaid Operations

Public Health Laboratory Services, 1000 Northeast 10th, Oklahoma City, OK 73117-1299; tel. 405/271-5070; FAX. 405/271-4850; Garry McKee, Ph.D., Chief

Special Health Services, 1000 Northeast 10th, Oklahoma City, OK 73117-1299; tel. 405/271-6576; FAX. 405/271-1308; Gary Glover, Chief, Medical Facilities

State Department of Health, 1000 Northeast 10th, Oklahoma City, OK 73117-1299; tel. 405/271-4200; FAX. 405/271-3431; Jerry R. Nida, M.D., Commissioner of Health

State Department of Health, Dental Services, 1000 Northeast 10th Street, Oklahoma City, OK 73117-1299; tel. 405/271-5502; FAX. 405/271-6199; Michael L. Morgan, D.D.S., Chief

State Department of Health, Nursing Service, 1000 Northeast 10th Street, Oklahoma City, OK 73117-1299; tel. 405/271-5183; FAX. 405/271-1897; Toni Frioux, M.S., RN, C.N.S.

State Department of Health, Special Health Services, 1000 Northeast 10th, Oklahoma City, OK 73117-1299; tel. 405/271-4200; FAX. 405/271-2632; Brent E. VanMeter, Deputy Commissioner

Licensing
Oklahoma Board of Nursing, 2915 North Classen Boulevard, Suite 524, Oklahoma City, OK 73106; tel. 405/962-1800; FAX. 405/962-1821; Kim Glazier, RN, M.Ed., Executive Director

Oklahoma State Board of Medical Licensure and Supervision, P.O. Box 18256, Oklahoma City, OK 73154-0256; tel. 405/848-6841; FAX. 405/848-8240; Lyle Kelsey, Executive Director

Social Services
Aging Services Division, Oklahoma Department of Human Services, 312 Northeast 28th, Oklahoma City, OK 73105; tel. 405/521-2327; FAX. 405/521-2086; Roy R. Keen, Division Administrator

Department of Mental Health and Substance Abuse Services, P.O. Box 53277, Oklahoma City, OK 73152; tel. 405/522-3877; FAX. 405/522-0637; David V. Statton, Interim Commissioner

Maternal and Child Health Service, 1000 Northeast 10th Street, Oklahoma City, OK 73117-1299; tel. 405/271-4470; FAX. 405/271-2944; Edd D. Rhoades, M.D., MPH, Chief

Rehabilitation Services, 3535 Northwest 58th Street, Suite 500, Oklahoma City, OK 73112-4815; tel. 405/951-3400; FAX. 405/951-3529; Linda Parker, Director

OREGON
The Honorable John A. Kitzhaber, Governor, 503/378-3111

Health
Oregon Health Division, 800 Oregon Street, Suite 925, Portland, OR 97232; tel. 503/731-4000; FAX. 503/731-4078; Elinor Hall, MPH, Administrator

Licensing
Department of Consumer and Business Services/Oregon, Insurance Division, 350 Winter Street, N.E., Salem, OR 97301-3883; tel. 503/947-7270; FAX. 503/378-4351; Joel Ario

Oregon Health Division, Health Care Licensure and Certification, P.O. Box 14450, Portland, OR 97214-0450; tel. 503/731-4013; FAX. 503/731-4080; Kathleen Smail, Manager

Oregon State Board of Nursing, 800 Northeast Oregon Street, Suite 465, Portland, OR 97232-2162; tel. 503/731-4745; FAX. 503/731-4755; Joan C. Bouchard, RN, M.S.N., Executive Director

Social Services
Adult and Family Services Division, 500 Summer Street, N.E., Salem, OR 97310-1013; tel. 503/945-5601; Sandie Hoback, Administrator

Child Development and Rehabilitation Center, Oregon Health Sciences University, Box 574, Portland, OR 97207; tel. 503/494-8362; FAX. 503/494-6868; Clifford J. Sells, M.D., Director

Mental Health and Developmental Disability Services Division, 2575 Bittern Street, N.E., P.O. Box 14250, Salem, OR 97309-0740; tel. 503/945-9499; FAX. 503/378-3796; Barry S. Kast, M.S.W., Administrator

Office of Alcohol and Drug Abuse Programs, 500 Summer Street, N.E., Salem, OR 97310-1016; tel. 503/945-5763; FAX. 503/378-8467

Vocational Rehabilitation Division, Human Services Building, 500 Summer Street N.E., Salem, OR 97310-1018; tel. 503/945-5880; FAX. 503/378-3318; Bobby C. Simpson, Administrator

Other
Oregon State Public Health Laboratory, P.O. Box 275, Portland, OR 97207-0275; tel. 503/229-5882; FAX. 503/229-5682; Michael R. Skeels, Ph.D., MPH

PENNSYLVANIA
The Honorable Tom Ridge, Governor, 717/787-2500

Health
Bureau of Health Planning, 709 Health and Welfare Building, Harrisburg, PA 17120; tel. 717/772-5298; Joseph B. May, Director

Organizations / State and Provincial Government Agencies

Department of Health, Bureau of Laboratories, P.O. Box 500, Exton, PA 19341-0500; tel. 610/363-8500; FAX. 610/436-3346; Dr. Bruce Kleger, Director

Division of Acute and Ambulatory Care, Health and Welfare Building, Room 532, Harrisburg, PA 17120; tel. 717/783-8980; FAX. 717/772-2163; Elaine Gibble, MPA, RHIA, CTR, Director

Pennsylvania Department of Health, Health and Welfare Building, Suite 802, Harrisburg, PA 17120; tel. 717/787-6436; FAX. 717/787-0191; Daniel F. Hoffmann, Secretary

Pennsylvania Department of Health, Health and Welfare Building, Suite 806, Harrisburg, PA 17120; tel. 717/783-8770; FAX. 717/772-6959

Pennsylvania Department of Health, Division Home Health, 132 Kline Plaza, Suite A, Harrisburg, PA 17104; tel. 717/783-1379; FAX. 717/787-3188; Jan Staloski, Director

Pennsylvania Department of Health, Public Health Programs, 809 Health and Welfare Building, Harrisburg, PA 17120; tel. 717/787-9857; FAX. 717/772-6959; Gary Giofian, Deputy Secretary fpr Public Health Program

Insurance
Department of Insurance, 1326 Strawberry Square, Harrisburg, PA 17120; tel. 717/783-0442; FAX. 717/772-1969; M. Diane Koken, Insurance Commissioner

Pennsylvania Insurance Department, Office of Rate and Policy Regulation, 1311 Strawberry Square, Harrisburg, PA 17120; tel. 717/783-5079; FAX. 717/787-8555; Gregory Martino, Deputy Insurance Commissioner

Licensing
Bureau of Facility Licensure and Certification, Health and Welfare Building, Room 930, Harrisburg, PA 17120; tel. 717/787-8015; FAX. 717/787-1491

Pennsylvania Department of Health, Quality Assurance, Health and Welfare Building, Room 805, P.O. Box 90, Harrisburg, PA 17108; tel. 717/783-1078; FAX. 717/772-6959; Richard H. Lee, Deputy Secretary

Pennsylvania State Board of Nursing, Department of State, P.O. Box 2649, Harrisburg, PA 17105-2649; tel. 717/783-7142; FAX. 717/783-0822; Miriam H. Limo, Executive Secretary

State Board of Medicine, P.O. Box 2649, Harrisburg, PA 17105-2649; tel. 717/783-1400; FAX. 717/787-7769; Cindy L. Warner, Administrative Officer

Social Services
Mental Health and Substance Abuse Services, Health and Welfare Building, Room 502, P.O. Box 2675, Harrisburg, PA 17120; tel. 717/787-6443; FAX. 717/787-5394; Charles G. Curie, Deputy Secretary, Mental Health

Office of Children, Youth, and Families, Department of Public Welfare, P.O. Box 2675, Harrisburg, PA 17105-2675; tel. 717/787-4756; FAX. 717/787-0414; Jo Ann R. Lawer, Deputy Secretary

Office of Income Maintenance, Health and Welfare Building, Room 432, Harrisburg, P, P.O. Box 2675, Harrisburg, PA 17105; tel. 717/783-3063; FAX. 717/787-6765; Sherri Z. Heller, Deputy Secretary

Office of Vocational Rehabilitation, Labor and Industry Building, 909 Green Street, Harrisburg, PA 17120; tel. 717/787-5244; FAX. 717/783-5221; Susan L. Aldrete, Executive Director

Pennsylvania Department of Health, Bureau of Drug and Alcohol Programs, 933 Health and Welfare Building, P.O. Box 90, Harrisburg, PA 17108; tel. 717/783-8200; FAX. 717/787-6285; Gene R. Boyle, Director

Pennsylvania Department of Public Welfare, Office of Medical Assistance Programs, Health and Welfare Building, Room 515, Harrisburg, PA 17120; tel. 717/787-1870; FAX. 717/787-4639; Peg J. Dierkers, Ph.D., Deputy Secretary

Other
Division of Laboratory Improvement, Bureau of Laboratories, 110 Pickering Way, Lionville, PA 19353; tel. 610/280-3464; FAX. 610/436-3346; Joseph W. Gasiewski, Director

RHODE ISLAND
The Honorable Lincoln Almond, Governor, 401/222-2080

Health
Department of Health, Three Capitol Hill, Providence, RI 02908-5097; tel. 401/277-2231; FAX. 401/277-6548; Barbara A. DeBuono, M.D., MPH, Director, Health

Division of Medical Services, 600 New London Avenue, Cranston, RI 02920; tel. 401/464-5274; John Young, Associate Director

Rhode Island Department of Health, Three Capitol Hill, Room 401, Providence, RI 02908-5097; tel. 401/222-2231; FAX. 401/222-6548; William J. Waters, Jr., Ph.D., Deputy Director

Rhode Island Department of Health, Division of Family Health, Three Capitol Hill, Room 302, Providence, RI 02908-5097; tel. 401/222-2312; FAX. 401/222-1442; William H. Hollinshead, M.D., MPH, Medical Director

Rhode Island Department of Health, Office of Health Systems Development, Three Capitol Hill, Providence, RI 02908-5097; tel. 401/222-2788; FAX. 401/273-4350; John X. Donahue, Chief

Insurance
Division of Insurance, 233 Richmond Street, Suite 233, Providence, RI 02903-4233; tel. 401/277-2223; FAX. 401/751-4887; Charles P. Kwolek, Jr., CPA, Associate Director, Supervisor

Licensing
Division of Professional Regulation, Rhode Island Department of Health, Three Capitol Hill, Suite 104, Providence, RI 02908-5097; tel. 401/222-2827; FAX. 401/222-1272; Russell J. Spaight, Administrator

Social Services
Department of Human Services, 600 New London Avenue, Cranston, RI 02920; tel. 401/464-3575; FAX. 401/464-2174; John Young, Associate Director, Division of Medical Services

Office of Rehabilitation Services, 40 Fountain Street, Providence, RI 02903; tel. 401/421-7005; FAX. 401/421-9259; Raymond A. Carroll, Administrator

Rhode Island Department of Health, Division of Facilities Regulation, Three Capitol Hill, Providence, RI 02908-5097; tel. 401/222-2566; FAX. 401/222-3999; Wayne I. Farrington, Chief

Rhode Island Department of Mental Health, Retardation and Hospitalization, Barry Hall, 14 Harrington Road, Cranston, RI 02920; tel. 401/462-3201; FAX. 401/462-3204; A. Kathryn Power, Director

Other
Department of Business Regulation, 233 Richmond Street, Suite 237, Providence, RI 02903-4237; tel. 401/222-2246; FAX. 401/222-6098; Barry G. Hittner, Director

SOUTH CAROLINA
The Honorable James Hodges, Governor, 803/734-9400

Health
Bureau of Environmental Health, 2600 Bull Street, Columbia, SC 29201; tel. 803/896-0646; FAX. 803/896-0645; Richard L. Hatfield, Chief

Bureau of Maternal and Child Health, South Carolina Department of Health, Robert Mills Complex, P.O. Box 101106, Columbia, SC 29211; tel. 803/898-0789; FAX. 803/734-4442; Linda Price, Acting Director

Department of Health and Environmental Control, 2600 Bull Street, Columbia, SC 29201; tel. 803/898-3300; FAX. 803/898-3323; Douglas E. Bryant, Commissioner

Department of Health and Human Services, 1801 Main Street, P.O. Box 8206, Columbia, SC 29202-8206; tel. 803/898-2500; FAX. 803/898-4515; J. Samuel Griswold, Director

Division of Preventive and Personal Health, South Carolina Department of Health and Environmental Control, 2600 Bull Street, Columbia, SC 29201; tel. 803/737-4040; FAX. 803/737-4036; Mick Henry, Division Chief

Licensing
Department of Health and Environmental Control, Division of Health Licensing, 2600 Bull Street, Columbia, SC 29201; tel. 803/737-7370; FAX. 803/737-7212; Jerry Paul, Director

South Carolina Department of Labor, Licensing and Regulation, Board of Medical Examiners, 110 Centerview Drive, Suite 202, Columbia, SC, 29210; P.O. Box 11289, Columbia, SC 29211-1289; tel. 803/896-4500; FAX. 803/896-4515; Aaron Kozloski, Board Administrator

Social Services
Bureau of Drug Control, South Carolina Department of Health and Environmental Control, 2600 Bull Street, Columbia, SC 29201; tel. 803/896-063; FAX. 803/896-0638; Wilbur L. Harling, Director

LLR Board of Nursing, 110 Centerview Drive, Columbia, SC 29210; tel. 803/896-4550; FAX. 803/896-4525; Debbie Herman, Administrator

South Carolina Commission for the Blind, P.O. Box 79, Columbia, SC 29202-0079; tel. 803/898-8822; FAX. 803/898-8824; Joan Barker Miller, Commissioner

South Carolina Department of Alcohol and Other Drug Abuse Services, 3700 Forest Drive, Suite 300, Columbia, SC 29204; tel. 803/734-9520; FAX. 803/734-9663; Rick C. Wade, Director

South Carolina Department of Disabilities and Special Needs, 3440 Harden Street Extension, P.O. Box 4706, Columbia, SC 29240; tel. 803/737-6444; FAX. 803/737-6323; Philip S. Massey, Ph.D, State Director

South Carolina Department of Health and Environmental Control, Bureau of Home Health Services and Long Term Care, 2600 Bull Street, Columbia, SC 29201; tel. 803/898-0559; FAX. 803/898-0350; Michael Byrd, Program Manager

South Carolina Department of Health and Human Services, Office of Seniority and Long Term Care Services, 1801 Main Street, P.O. Box 8206, Columbia, SC 29202-8206; tel. 803/898-2500; FAX. 803/898-4565; Elizabeth M. Fuller, Deputy Director – Officer

South Carolina Department of Social Services, P.O. Box 1520, Columbia, SC 29202; tel. 803/898-7360; FAX. 803/898-7277; Elizabeth G. Patterson. J.D., State Director

State Department of Mental Health, 2414 Bull Street, P.O. Box 485, Columbia, SC 29202; tel. 803/898-8319; FAX. 803/898-8586; Stephen M. Soltys, M.D., State Director

Vocational Rehabilitation Department, 1410 Boston Avenue, P.O. Box 15, West Columbia, SC 29171-0015; tel. 803/896-6500; P. Charles LaRosa, Jr., Commissioner

Other
Bureau of Laboratories, P.O. Box 2202, Columbia, SC 29202; tel. 803/935-7045; FAX. 803/935-7357; Sarah J. Robinson, Acting Chief

SOUTH DAKOTA
The Honorable William T. Janklow, Governor, 605/773-3212

Health
Division of Developmental Disabilities, Hillsview Plaza, E. Highway 34, c/o 500 East Capitol, Pierre, SD 57501-5070; tel. 605/773-3438; FAX. 605/773-5483; Kim Malsam-Rysdon, Director

Division of Health and Medical Services, 615 East Fourth Street, Pierre, SD 57501; tel. 605/773-3737; FAX. 605/773-5509; Laurie Gill, Administrator

Division of Health Systems Development and Regulation, South Dakota Department of Health, Health Building, 600 East Capitol, Pierre, SD 57501; tel. 605/773-3364; FAX. 605/773-5904; Kevin Forsch, Division Director

South Dakota Department of Health, 600 East Capitol, Pierre, SD 57501-2536; tel. 605/773-3361; FAX. 605/773-5683; Doneen B. Hollingsworth, Secretary of Health

Licensing
Office of Health Care Facilities Licensure and Certification, State Department of Health, 615 E. Fourth Street, Pierre, SD 57501; tel. 605/773-3356; FAX. 605/773-6667; Joan Bachman, Administrator

State Board of Medical and Osteopathic Examiners, 1323 South Minnesota Avenue, Sioux Falls, SD 57105; tel. 605/336-1965; FAX. 605/336-0270; Robert D. Johnson, Executive Secretary

Social Services
Department of Human Services, East Highway 34, Hillsview Plaza, c/o 500 East Capitol, Pierre, SD 57501; tel. 605/773-5990; FAX. 605/773-5483; John N. Jones, Secretary

Department of Social Services, 700 Governors Drive, Pierre, SD 57501-2291; tel. 605/773-3165; FAX. 605/773-4855; James W. Ellenbecker, Secretary

Organizations / State and Provincial Government Agencies

Division of Alcohol and Drug Abuse, 3800 East Highway 34, Hillsview Plaza, Pierre, SD 57501; tel. 605/773-3123; FAX. 605/773-7076; Gilbert Sudbeck, Director

Office of Medical Services, 700 Governor's Drive, Pierre, SD 57501-2291; tel. 605/773-3495; FAX. 605/773-5246; David Christensen, Administrator

TENNESSEE
The Honorable Don Sundquist, Governor, 615/741-2001

Health
Department of Health, Cordell Hull Building, 425 Fifth Avenue, N., Nashville, TN 37247-0101; tel. 615/741-3111; FAX. 615/741-2491; Fredia Wadley, State Health Officer

Tennessee Department of Health, Commissioner's Office, Cordell Hull Building, 425 Fifth Avenue,N., Nashville, TN 37247-0101; tel. 615/741-3111; FAX. 615/741-2491; Tammy Barton, Executive Administrative Assistant

Licensing
Board for Licensing Health Care Facilities, Cordell Hull Building, 425 Fifth Avenue, N., Nashville, TN 37247-0530; tel. 615/741-7221; FAX. 615/741-7051; Katy Gammon, Director

Department of Health, Office of Health Licensure and Regulation, Cordell Hull Building, 425 Fifth Avenue, N., Nashville, TN 37247-0501; tel. 615/741-8402; FAX. 615/741-5542; Judy Eads, Assistant Commissioner

Tennessee Board of Medical Examiners, Cordell Hull Building, First Floor, 425 Fifth Avenue, North, Nashville, TN 37247-1010; tel. 800/310-4650; FAX. 615/253-4484; Yarnell Beatty, Director

Tennessee Board of Nursing, Cordell Hull Building, 1st Floor, 425 Fifth Avenue, N., Nashville, TN 37247-1010; tel. 888/310-4650; FAX. 615/741-7899; Elizabeth J. Lund, RN, Executive Director

Tennessee Medical Laboratory Board, Cordell Hull Building, 425 Fifth Avenue, N., Nashville, TN 37247-1010; tel. 615/532-5128; FAX. 615/532-5369; Lynda England, BSMT(ASCP), Administrator/Consultant

Social Services
Bureau of Alcohol and Drug Abuse Services – TN Dept. of Health, Cordell Hull Building, 425 Fifth Avenue, Nashville, TN 37247-4401; tel. 615/741-1921; FAX. 615/532-2419; Stephanie W. Perry, M.D., Assistant Commissioner

Department of Children's Services, Program Operations which includes Departmental Services, Cordell Hull Building, 436 Sixth Avenue, N., Nashville, TN 37243-1290; tel. 615/532-1102; FAX. 615/532-6495; Cathy Rogers Smith, Assistant Commissioner, Department

Division of Health Care Facilities, Cordell Hull Building, 426 Fifth Avenue N., 1st Floor, Nashville, TN 37247-0508; tel. 615/741-7221; FAX. 615/741-7051; Kennard Murray, Director

Division of Rehabilitation Services, Citizens Plaza State Office Building, 15th Floor, Nashville, TN 37248-0060; tel. 615/313-4714; FAX. 615/741-4165; Carl Brown, Assistant Commissioner

Family Assistance, 400 Deaderick Street, Nashville, TN 37248-0070; tel. 615/313-4712; FAX. 615/741-4165; Michael O'Hara, Assistant Commissioner

Medicaid/TennCare, 729 Church Street, Nashville, TN 37247-6501; tel. 615/741-0213; FAX. 615/741-0882; John F. Tighe, Deputy Commissioner

Tennessee Commission on Aging, 500 Deaderick Street, Ninth Floor, Nashville, TN 37243-0860; tel. 615/741-2056; FAX. 615/741-3309; James S. Whaley, Executive Director

Tennessee Department of Human Services, 400 Deaderick Street, Nashville, TN 37248; tel. 615/741-3241; FAX. 615/741-4165; Robert A. Grunow, Commissioner

Tennessee Department of Mental Health and Mental Retardation, Cordell Hull Building, 425 Fifth Avenue, N, Nashville, TN 37243-0675; tel. 615/532-6500; FAX. 615/532-6514; Elizabeth Rukeyser, Commissioner

Tennessee Rehabilitation Center, 460 Ninth Avenue, Smyrna, TN 37167; tel. 615/741-4921; FAX. 615/355-1373; David Holmes, Superintendent

Other
Bureau of Environment, L & C Tower–21st Floor, 401 Church Street, Nashville, TN 37243-1530; tel. 615/532-0220; FAX. 615/532-0120; John M. Leonard, Assistant Commissioner

Office of Budget and Finance, Tennessee Department of Health, Andrew Johnson Tower, Tenth Floor, Nashville, TN 37247-0301; tel. 615/741-3824; FAX. 615/253-1998; Donna Dickens, Director

TEXAS
The Honorable George W. Bush, Governor, 512/463-2000

Health
Bureau of Children's Health, (Texas Department of Health), 1100 West 49th Street, Austin, TX 78756; tel. 512/458-7700; FAX. 512/458-7203; Mike Montgomery, Chief

Texas Department of Health, 1100 West 49th Street, Austin, TX 78756; tel. 512/458-7375; FAX. 512/458-7477; William R. Archer, III, M.D., Commissioner

Texas Department of Health, 1100 West 49th Street, Austin, TX 78756-3167; tel. 512/338-6501; FAX. 512/338-6945; Randy P. Washington, Deputy Commissioner, Health Care

Texas Department of Health, Community Health and Prevention, 1100 West 49th Street, Suite M543, Austin, TX 78756; tel. 512/458-7555; FAX. 512/458-7713; John E. Evans, Deputy Commissioner

Texas Department of Health, Health Facility Licensing and Compliance Division, 1100 West 49th Street, Austin, TX 78756; tel. 512/834-6650; FAX. 512/834-6653; Nancy Stearman, RN, M.S.N., Director

Texas Department of Health, Office of Policy and Planning, 1100 West 49th Street, Austin, TX 78756; tel. 512/458-7261; FAX. 512/458-7344; Ann Henry, Assistant Director

Texas Department of Mental Health and Mental Retardation, 909 West 45th Street, P.O. Box 12668, Capitol Station, Austin, TX 78751; tel. 512/454-3761; FAX. 512/206-4560; Tex Killion, Deputy Medical Director for Administration

Insurance
Texas Department of Insurance, P.O. Box 149104, Mail Code 106-1A, Austin, TX 78714-9104; tel. 512/322-3401; FAX. 512/322-3552; Ana M. Smith-Daley, Deputy Commissioner, Life/Health Division

Licensing
Board of Nurse Examiners for the State of Texas, P.O. Box 430, Austin, TX 78767-0430; tel. 512/305-7400; FAX. 512/305-7401; Katherine A. Thomas, M.S.N., RN, Executive Director

Board of Vocational Nurse Examiners, William P. Hobby Building, 333 Guadalupe Street, Austin, TX 78701; tel. 512/305-8100; FAX. 512/305-8101; Mary M. Strange, Executive Director

Bureau of Licensing and Certification, Texas Department of Health, 1100 West 49th Street, Austin, TX 78756-3199; tel. 512/834-6645; FAX. 512/834-6653; Maurice B. Shaw, Chief

UTAH
The Honorable Michael O. Leavitt, Governor, 801/538-1000

Health
Utah Department of Health, P.O. Box 14100, Salt Lake City, UT 84114-1000; tel. 801/538-6111; FAX. 801/538-6306; Rod L. Betit, Executive Director

Utah Department of Health, Bureau of Licensing, Box 142003, Salt Lake City, UT 84114-2003; tel. 801/538-6152; FAX. 801/538-6325; Debra Wynkoop, Director

Utah Department of Health, Bureau of Primary Care and Rural Health Systems, P.O. Box 142050, Salt Lake City, UT 84114-2005; tel. 801/538-6113; FAX. 801/538-6387; Marilyn Haynes-Brokopp, Bureau Director

Utah Department of Health, Community and Family Health Services Division, P.O. Box 142001, Salt Lake City, UT 84114-2001; tel. 801/538-6901; FAX. 801/538-6510; George Delavan, M.D., Director

Utah Department of Health, Division of Epidemiology and Laboratories, 46 North Medical Drive, Salt Lake City, UT 84113; tel. 801/584-8400; FAX. 801/584-8486; Charles D. Brokopp, Dr.P.H., Director

Insurance
Insurance Department, State Office Building, Suite 3110, Salt Lake City, UT 84114; tel. 801/538-3800; FAX. 801/538-3829; Merwin U. Stewart, Insurance Commissioner

Licensing
Division of Occupational and Professional Licensing, Heber M. Wells Building, 160 East 300 South, Salt Lake City, UT 84114-6741; tel. 801/530-6628; FAX. 801/530-6511; A. Gary Bowen, Division Director

Office of The Medical Examiners, State of Utah, 48 North Medical Drive, Salt Lake City, UT 84113; tel. 801/584-8410; FAX. 801/584-8435; Todd C. Grey, M.D., Director

Social Services
Department of Human Services, 120 North 200 West, P.O. Box 45500, Salt Lake City, UT 84145-0500; tel. 801/538-4001; FAX. 801/538-4016; Robin Arnold-Williams, Executive Director

Division of Aging and Adult Services, 120 North 200 West, Room 325, Salt Lake City, UT 84103; tel. 801/538-3910; FAX. 801/538-4395; Helen Goddard, Director

Division of Child and Family Services, 120 North. 200 W., Suite 225, Salt Lake City, UT 84103; tel. 801/538-4100; FAX. 801/538-3993; Ken Patterson, Director

Division of Health Care Financing (Utah Medicaid), P.O. Box 143101, Salt Lake City, UT 84114-3101; tel. 801/538-6406; FAX. 801/538-6099; Michael J. Deily, Director

Division of Services for People With Disabilities, 120 North 200 West, Suite 411, Salt Lake City, UT 84103; tel. 801/538-4200; FAX. 801/538-4279; Sue Geary, Ph.D., Director

Mental Health, P.O. Box 45500, Salt Lake City, UT 84145-0500; tel. 801/538-4270; Paul Thorpe, Director

Utah Division of Substance Abuse, 120 North 200 West, Room 201, Salt Lake City, UT 84103; tel. 801/538-3939; FAX. 801/538-4696; Patrick Fleming, Associate Director

Utah State Office of Rehabilitation, 250 East 500 South, Salt Lake City, UT 84111; tel. 801/538-7530; FAX. 801/538-7522; Blaine Petersen, Ed.D., Executive Director

Youth Corrections, P.O. Box 45500, Salt Lake City, UT 84145-0500; tel. 801/538-4330; FAX. 801/538-4334; Gary K. Dalton, Director

Other
Department of Environmental Quality, 168 No 1950 West, Salt Lake City, UT 84116; tel. 801/536-4404; FAX. 801/538-6016; Dianne R. Nielson, Ph.D., Executive Director

State Office of Education, 250 East 500 South, Salt Lake City, UT 84111; tel. 801/538-7500; FAX. 801/538-7521; Steven O. Laing, State Superintendent

VERMONT
The Honorable Howard Dean, M.D., Governor, 802/828-3333

Health
Department of Developmental and Mental Health Services, Weeks Building, 103 South Main Street, Waterbury, VT 05671-1601; tel. 802/241-2610; FAX. 802/241-1129; Rodney E. Copeland, Ph.D., Commissioner

Environmental Health Division, 108 Cherry Street, P.O. Box 70, Burlington, VT 05402; tel. 802/863-7220; FAX. 802/863-7425; William C. Bress, Ph. D., Director

Vermont Department of Health, 108 Cherry Street, P.O. Box 70, Burlington, VT 05402; tel. 802/863-7280; FAX. 802/863-7425; Jan K. Carney, M.D., MPH, Commissioner

Vermont Department of Health, Division of Community Public Health, 108 Cherry Street, P.O. Box 70, Burlington, VT 05402-0070; tel. 802/863-7347; FAX. 802/863-7229; Patricia Berry, Director

Vermont Department of Health, Division of Health Surveillance, Public Health Statistics, 108 Cherry Street, P.O. Box 70, Burlington, VT 05402-0070; tel. 802/863-7300; FAX. 802/865-7701; Jeanetters Voas, Health Surveillance Biostatistician

Vermont Department of Health Infectious Disease Epidemiology, 108 Cherry Street, P.O. Box 70, Burlington, VT 05402; tel. 802/863-7240; FAX. 802/865-7701; Peter Galbraith, State Epidemiologist

Organizations / State and Provincial Government Agencies

Vermont Department of Health Laboratory, 195 Colchester Avenue, P.O. Box 1125, Burlington, VT 05402–1125; tel. 802/863–7335; FAX. 802/863–7632; Burton W. Wilcke, Jr., Ph.D., Director, Division of Health

Insurance
Deparment of Banking, Insurance, Securities & Health Care Adm., 89 Main Street, Drawer 20, Montpelier, VT 05620–3101; tel. 802/828–3301; FAX. 802/828–3306; Elizabeth R. Costle, Commissioner

Licensing
Licensing and Protection, Ladd Hall, 103 South Main Street, Waterbury, VT 05671–2306; tel. 802/241–2345; FAX. 802/241–2358; Laine Lucenti, Director

Vermont Department of Aging and Disabilities, Division of Licensing and Protection, Ladd Hall, 103 South Main Street, Waterbury, VT 05671–2306; tel. 802/241–2345; FAX. 802/241–2358; Loune Lucenti, RN, Director

Vermont State Board of Nursing, 81 River Street, Montpelier, VT 05609–1106; tel. 802/828–2396; FAX. 802/828–2484; Anita Ristau, RN, M.S., Executive Director

Social Services
Agency of Human Services, 103 South Main Street, Waterbury, VT 05676; tel. 802/241–2220; FAX. 802/241–2979; Cornelius Hogan, Secretary

Department of Social and Rehabilitation Services, 103 South Main Street, Waterbury, VT 05671–2401; tel. 802/241–2100; FAX. 802/241–2980; William M. Young, Commissioner

Department of Social Welfare, 103 South Main Street, Waterbury, VT 05671–1201; tel. 802/241–2853; FAX. 802/241–2830; M. Jane Kitchel, Commissioner

Office of Alcohol and Drug Abuse Programs, 108 Cherry Street, Burlington, VT 05401; tel. 802/651–1550; FAX. 802/651–1573; Thomas E. Perras, Director

Office of Vermont Health Access/Medicaid, 103 South Main Street, Waterbury, VT 05671–1201; tel. 802/241–2880; FAX. 802/241–2974; Paul Wallace–Brodeur, Director

Vocational Rehabilitation Division, 103 South Main Street, Waterbury, VT 05671–2303; tel. 802/241–2186; FAX. 802/241–3359; Diane P. Dalmasse, Director

VIRGINIA
The Honorable James S. Gillmore, III, Governor, 804/786–2211

Health
State Department of Health, Main Street Station, P.O. Box 2448, Richmond, VA 23218; tel. 804/786–3561; FAX. 804/786–4616; E. Anne Peterson, M.D., MPH, State Health Commissioner

Insurance
Bureau of Insurance, Virginia State Corporation Commission, P.O. Box 1157, Richmond, VA 23218; tel. 804/371–9691; FAX. 804/371–9944; Life and Health Consumer Services Section

State Corporation Commission Bureau of Insurance, Company Licensing and Regulatory Compliance Section, P.O. Box 1157, Richmond, VA 23209; tel. 904/371–9636; FAX. 904/371–9396; Andy Delbridge, Supervisor

State Corporation Commission–Bureau of Insurance, P.O. Box 1157, Richmond, VA 23218; tel. 804/371–9869; FAX. 804/371–9511; Douglas C. Stolte, Deputy Insurance Commissioner

Licensing
Center for Quality Health Care Services and Consumer Protection, Virginia Department of Health, 3600 Centre, Suite 216, 3600 West Broad Street, Richmond, VA 23230; tel. 804/367–2102; FAX. 804/367–2149; Nancy R. Hofheimer, Director

Virginia State Board of Medicine, 6606 West Board Street, Fourth Floor, Richmond, VA 23230–1717; tel. 804/662–9908; FAX. 804/662–9943; Warren W. Koontz, Jr., M.D., Executive Director

Social Services
Department for the Aging, 1600 Forest Avenue, Suite 102, Richmond, VA 23229; tel. 804/662–9333; FAX. 804/662–9354; Dr. Ann Y McGee, Commissioner

Department of Medical Assistance Services, 600 East Broad Street, Suite 1300, Richmond, VA 23219; tel. 804/786–8099; FAX. 804/371–4981; Dennis G. Smith, Director

Department of Mental Health, Mental Retardation and Substance Abuse Services, P.O. Box 1797, Richmond, VA 23214; tel. 804/786–3921; FAX. 804/371–6638; Richard E. Kellogg, Commissioner

Department of Rehabilitative Services, 8004 Franklin Farms Drive, P.O. Box K–300, Richmond, VA 23288–0300; tel. 804/662–7010; FAX. 804/662–9532; H. Gray Broughton, Commissioner

Division of Child and Adolescent Health, Virginia Department of Health, P.O. Box 2448, Room 13B, Richmond, VA 23218; tel. 804/786–3691; FAX. 804/225–3307; Nancy R. Bullock, RN, MPH, Director

Division of Women's and Infants' Health, 1500 East Main Street, Suite 135, P.O. Box 2448, Richmond, VA 23218–2448; tel. 804/786–5916; FAX. 804/371–6032; Joan Corder-Mabe, RNC, M.S., OGNP, Acting Director

Virginia Department of Social Services, 730 East Broad Street, Richmond, VA 23219–1949; tel. 804/692–1900; FAX. 804/692–1849; Sonia Rivera, Acting Commissioner

WASHINGTON
The Honorable Gary Locke, Governor, 360/902–4111

Health
Department of Health, Facilities and Services Licensing, P.O. Box 47852, Olympia, WA 98504–7852; tel. 206/705–6652; FAX. 206/705–6654; Kathy Stout, Director

Department of Health, Office of Emergency Medical and Trauma Prevention, P.O. Box 47853, Olympia, WA 98504–7853; tel. 360/705–6700; FAX. 360/705–6706; Janet Griffith, Director

Washington State Department of Health, P.O. Box 47812, Mail Stop 7812, Olympia, WA 98504–7812; tel. 206/705–6060; FAX. 206/705–6043; Dan Rubin, Director, Special Projects Office

Insurance
Office of the Insurance Commissioner, Insurance Building, P.O. Box 40255, Olympia, WA 98504–0255; tel. 206/753–7300; FAX. 206/586–3535; Deborah Senn, Insurance Commissioner

Licensing
Health Systems Quality Assurance, Department of Health, 1112 Quince, Mail Stop 7850, Olympia, WA 98504–7851; tel. 360/236–4600; FAX. 360/236–4626; Ron Weaver, Assistant Secretary

Social Services
Division of Alcohol and Substance Abuse, P.O. Box 45330, Mail Stop 5330, Olympia, WA 98504–5330; tel. 206/438–8200; FAX. 206/438–8078; Ken Stark, Director

Division of Vocational Rehabilitation, P.O. Box 45340, Olympia, WA 98504–5340; tel. 206/438–8000; FAX. 206/438–8007; Jeanne Munro, Director

Medical Assistance Administration, P.O. Box 45080, Olympia, WA 98504–5080; tel. 360/902–7807; FAX. 360/902–7855; Tom Bedell, Acting Assistant Secretary

Medical Assistance Administration, P.O. Box 45500, Olympia, WA 98504–5500; tel. 360/725–1500; FAX. 360/586–7498; David R. Cundiff, M.D., MPH

State Department of Social and Health Services, P.O. Box 45080, Olympia, WA 98504–5080; tel. 360/902–7807; FAX. 360/902–7855; Tom Bedell, Acting Assistant Secretary, Medical Assistance Administration

Other
Washington State Nursing Care Quality Assurance Commission, 1300 Southeast Quince Street, P.O. Box 47864, Olympia, WA 98504–7864; tel. 360/236–4713; FAX. 360/236–4738; Paula R. Meyer, MSN, Executive Director

WEST VIRGINIA
The Honorable Cecil H. Underwood, Governor, 304/558–2000

Health
Bureau for Public Health, 350 Capital Street, Room 702, Charleston, WV 25301; tel. 304/558–2971; FAX. 304/558–1035; Henry G. Taylor, M.D., MPH, Commissioner

Bureau of Medical Services, 350 Capitol Street, Room 251, Charleston, WV 25301–3706; tel. 304/558–7055; FAX. 304/558–2866; Janet E. Lucas, Director

Children's Specialty Care, 350 Capitol Street, Room 427, Charleston, WV 25301; tel. 304/558–3071; FAX. 304/558–2866; Patricia Kent, M.S.W., Administrative Director

Department of Health and Human Resources, Capitol Complex, Building Three, Room 206, Charleston, WV 25305; tel. 304/558–0684; FAX. 304/558–1130; Joan E. Ohl, Secretary

Office of Community and Rural Health Services, Bureau for Public Health, 350 Capitol Street, Room 515, Charleston, WV 25301–3013; tel. 304/558–3210; FAX. 504/558–1437

Office of Environmental Health Services, Morrison Building, 815 Quarrier Street, Suite 418, Charleston, WV 25301–2616; tel. 304/558–2981; FAX. 304/558–1291; C. Russell Rader, P.E., Director

West Virginia Department of Health and Human Resources, Division of Primary Care, 350 Capitol Street, Room 515, Charleston, WV 25301–3716; tel. 304/558–4007; FAX. 304/558–1437; Frances L. Jackson, Director

Insurance
Insurance Commissioners Office, P.O. Box 50540, Charleston, WV 25305–0540; tel. 304/558–3354; FAX. 304/558–0412; Hanley C. Clark, Commissioner

Office of the West Virginia Insurance Commissioner, 1124 Smith Street, Charleston, WV 25301; tel. 304/558–2100; FAX. 304/558–1365; Jeffrey W. VanGilder, Director, Chief Examiner

Licensing
Office of Chief Medical Examiner, State of West Virginia, 701 Jefferson Road, South Charles, WV 25309; tel. 304/558–3920; FAX. 304/558–7886; James A. Kaplan, M.D., Chief Medical Examiner

Office of Health Facility Licensure and Certification, West Virginia Division of Health, Capitol Complex, 1900 Kanawha Boulevard., Charleston, WV 25305; tel. 304/558–0050; FAX. 304/558–2515; John Wilkinson, Director

West Virginia Board of Examiners, for Registered Professional Nurses, 101 Dee Drive, Charleston, WV 25311–1620; tel. 304/558–3596; FAX. 304/558–3666; Laura S. Rhodes, M.S.N., RN, Executive Secretary

West Virginia Board of Medicine, 101 Dee Drive, Charleston, WV 25311; tel. 304/558–2921; FAX. 304/558–2084; Ronald D. Walton, Executive Director

Social Services
Division of Rehabilitation Services, P.O. Box 50890, State Capitol Complex, Charleston, WV 25305–0890; tel. 304/766–4601; FAX. 304/766–4905; James S. Jeffers, Director

Division on Alcoholism and Drug Abuse, Capitol Complex, Building Six, Room B–738, Charleston, WV 25305; tel. 304/558–2276; FAX. 304/558–1008; DeDe Serverino, Acting Director

Other
West Virginia Department of Education, Division of Technical and Adult Education Services, 1900 Kanawha Boulevard, Bldg. 6 Room B221, Charleston, WV 25305–0330; tel. 304/558–2346; FAX. 304/558–3946; Adam Sponaugle, Assistant State Superintendent

WISCONSIN
The Honorable Tommy G. Thompson, Governor, 608/266–1212

Health
Bureau of Health Services, P.O. Box 7925, Madison, WI 53707–7925; tel. 608/267–1720; FAX. 608/261–7103; Sharon Zunker, Director

Center for Health Statistics, P.O. Box 309, Madison, WI 53701–0309; tel. 608/266–1334; FAX. 608/261–6380; James John Vaura, Director

Division of Public Health, P.O. Box 2659, Madison, WI 53701–2659; tel. 608/266–1251; FAX. 608/267–2832; John Chapin, Administrator and Kenneth Baldwin, Deputy Administrator

Insurance
Office of the Commissioner of Insurance, 121 East Wilson Street, P.O. Box 7873, Madison, WI 53707–7873; tel. 608/266–3585; FAX. 608/266–9935; Kyle Richmond, Public Information Officer

Licensing
Bureau of Quality Assurance, Division of Supportive Living, Department of Health and F, P.O. Box 2969, Madison, WI 53701–0309; tel. 608/266–8481; FAX. 608/267–0352; Susan Schroeder, Director, Bureau of Quality Assurance

Organizations / State and Provincial Government Agencies

Department of Regulation and Licensing, 1400 East Washington Avenue, Room 173, P.O. Box 8935, Madison, WI 53708–8935; tel. 608/265–8609; FAX. 608/267–0644; Grace Schwingel, Secretary

State of Wisconsin, Department of Regulation and Licensing, 1400 East Washington Avenue, Suite 173, P.O. Box 8935, Madison, WI 53708–8935; tel. 608/266–8609; FAX. 608/267–0644; Marlene A. Cummings, Secretary

Wisconsin Medical Examining Board, 1400 East Washington Avenue, P.O. Box 8935, Madison, WI 53708; tel. 608/266–2811; FAX. 608/261–7083; Patrick D. Braatz, Administrator

Social Services

Department of Health and Family Services, P.O. Box 7850, Madison, WI 53707–7850; tel. 608/266–9622; FAX. 608/266–7882; Joe Leean, Secretary

Division for Learning Support: Equity and Advocacy, Department of Public Instruction, 125 South Webster Street, P.O. Box 7841, Madison, WI 53707–7841; tel. 608/266–8960; FAX. 608/267–3746; Michael J. Thompson, Director Student Services, Prevention and Wellness

Division of Health Care Financing (Wisconsin Medicaid), One West Wilson Street, Room 350, P.O. Box 309, Madison, WI 53701–0309; tel. 608/266–8922; FAX. 608/266–1096; Peggy L. Bartels, Administrator

Division of Vocational Rehabilitation, P.O. Box 7852, Madison, WI 53707–7852; tel. 608/243–5600; FAX. 608/243–5680; Thomas E. Dixon, Jr., Administrator

Other

State Department of Public Instruction, 125 South Webster Street, P.O. Box 7841, Madison, WI 53707–7841; tel. 608/266–1771; FAX. 608/267–1052; Juanita Pawlisch, Assistant Superintendent

WYOMING

The Honorable Jim Geringer, Governor, 307/777–7434

Health

Children's Health Service, Department of Health, Hathaway Building, Fourth Floor, Cheyenne, WY 82002; tel. 307/777–7941; FAX. 307/777–7215; Dorothy Ailes, Program Manager

Department of Health, 117 Hathaway Building, Cheyenne, WY 82002; tel. 307/777–7656; FAX. 307/777–7439

Division of Behavioral Health, 6101 Yellowstone Road, Room 259B, Cheyenne, WY 82002–0480; tel. 307/777–7094; FAX. 307/777–5580; Pablo Hernandez, M.D., Administrator

Wyoming Department of Health, Division of Public Health, Hathaway Building, Room 478, Cheyenne, WY 82002; tel. 307/777–6004; FAX. 307/777–3617

Licensing

Health Facilities Licensing, Department of Health, Metropolitan Bank Building, Eighth Floor, Cheyenne, WY 82002; tel. 307/777–7123; FAX. 307/777–5970; Charlie Simineo, Program Manager

Wyoming Board of Medicine, The Colony Building, Second Floor, 211 West 19th Street, Cheyenne, WY 82002; tel. 307/778–7053; FAX. 307/778–2069; Carole Shotwell, Executive Secretary

Wyoming State Board of Nursing, 2020 Carey Avenue, Suite 110, Cheyenne, WY 82002; tel. 307/777–7601; FAX. 307/777–3519; Toma A. Nisbet, RN, M.S., Executive Director

Social Services

Department of Family Services, Hathaway Building, Third Floor, 2300 Capitol Avenue, Cheyenne, WY 82002–0490; tel. 307/777–7561; FAX. 307/777–7747; Shirley R. Carson, Director

Division of Vocational Rehabilitation, Herschler Building, Room 1100, Cheyenne, WY 82002; tel. 307/777–7386; FAX. 307/777–5939; Gary W. Child, Administrator

Health Care Access and Resources Division, 154 Hathaway Building, Room 259B, Cheyenne, WY 82002; tel. 307/777–7531; FAX. 307/777–6964; Daniel G. Stackis, Administrator

Wyoming Department of Health, Division on Aging, 6101 Yellowstone Road 259B, Cheyenne, WY 82002; tel. 800/442–2766; FAX. 307/777–5340; Wayne A. Milton, Administrator

U.S. Associated Areas

GUAM

Health

Guam Health Planning and Development Agency, P.O. Box 2950, Agana, GU 96910; tel. 671/477–3920; FAX. 671/477–3956; Helen B. Ripple, Director

Social Services

Department of Public Health and Social Services, P.O. Box 2816, Hagatna, GU 96932; tel. 671/735–7102; FAX. 671/734–5910; Dennis G. Rodriguez, Director

Division of Public Welfare, Box 2816, Agana, GU 96910; tel. 671/735–7274; FAX. 671/734–7015; Adoracion A. Solidum, Acting Chief Human Services Administration

PUERTO RICO

Health

Dental Health, Building A–Medical Center, Call Box 70184, San Juan, PR 00936; tel. 809/751–4750; FAX. 809/765–5675; Wanda Urbiztondo, D.M.D., Oral Health Coordinator

Department of Health, Secretaryship for Preventive Medicine and Family Health, Building E–Medical Center, Call Box 70184, San Juan, PR 00936; tel. 809/765–0482; FAX. 809/765–5675; Dr. Raul G. Castellanos Bran, Director, Division of FAA

Environmental Health, Department of Health, Building A, Psiq Hospital, Box 70184, San Juan, PR 00936–0184; tel. 787/274–7798; FAX. 787/758–6285; Herman Horta, Assistant Secretary, Environmental Health

Government of Puerto Rico, Department of Health, P.O. Box 70184, San Juan, PR 00936–8184; tel. 787/274–7601; FAX. 787/250–6547; Carmen A. Feliciano–De–Melecio, Secretary of Health

Mental Health and Anti Addiction Services, P.O. Box 21414, San Juan, PR 00928–1414; tel. 787/764–3795; FAX. 787/765–5895; Dr. Jose Acevedo, Administrator

Social Services

Department of Family, Call Box 11398, San Juan, PR 00910; tel. 809/721–4624; FAX. 809/723–1223; Carmen L. Rodriguez de Rivera, Secretary

Vocational Rehabilitation Program, Department of Social Services, Apartado 191118, San Juan, PR 00919–1118; tel. 809/725–1792; FAX. 809/721–6286; Sr. Francisco Vallejo, Assistant Secretary

Other

Administration, Building A–Medical Center, Call Box 70184, San Juan, PR 00936; tel. 809/765–1616; FAX. 809/250–6547; Antonia Pizarrro Lago, Assistant Secretary for Administrator

Legal Services, Building A–Medical Center, Call Box 70184, San Juan, PR 00936; tel. 809/766–1616; FAX. 809/766–2240; J. Gerardo Cruz–Arroyo, Esq. General Counsel

VIRGIN ISLANDS

Health

Department of Health, Division of Financial Services, Knud Hansen Complex, St. Thomas, VI 00802; tel. 809/774–3171; FAX. 809/777–5120; Alphonse J. Stalliard, Deputy Commissioner

Division of Environmental Health, John Moorehead Complex, Charlotte Amalie, St. Thomas, VI 00802; tel. 809/774–9000; FAX. 809/776–7899; Ethyle T. Joseph

Division of Hospitals and Medical Services, Roy Lester Schneider Hospital, 9048 Sugar Estate, St. Thomas, VI 00802; tel. 809/776–3687; FAX. 809/777–8421; Bruce Goldman, Chief Executive Officer

Prevention, Health, Promotion and Protection, Department of Health, Charles Harwood Hospital, 3500 Richmond Christiansted, St. Croix, VI 00820–4300; tel. 809/773–1311; FAX. 809/772–5895; Olaf G. Hendricks, M.D., Assistant Commissioner

Virgin Islands Department of Health, St. Thomas Hospital, St. Thomas, VI 00802; tel. 809/774–0117; FAX. 809/777–4001; Ralph A. de Chabert, M.D., Acting Commissioner

Social Services

Disabilities and Rehabilitation Services, Department of Human Services, Knud Hansen Complex–Building A, 1303 Hospital Ground, St. Thomas, VI 00802; tel. 809/774–0930; FAX. 809/774–3466; Sedonie Halbert, Administrator

Division of Maternal and Child Health Services, Virgin Islands Department of Health, #2C Contant, AQ Building, 2nd Floor, St. Thomas, VI 00802; tel. 809/776–3580; FAX. 809/774–8633; Dr. Mavis Matthew, Director

Division of Mental Health, Department of Health, Barbel Plaza South, 2nd Floor, St. Thomas, VI 00802; tel. 340/774–4888; FAX. 340/774–4701; Derek V. Spencer, M.D., MPH

Virgin Islands Department of Human Services, Knud Hansen Complex, Building A, St. Thomas, VI 00802; tel. 340/774–1166; FAX. 340/774–3466; Sedonie Halbert, Commissioner

Canada

ALBERTA

Social Services

Department of Family and Social Services, 109 Street and 97 Avenue, Edmonton, AB T5K 2B6; tel. 403/427–2606; FAX. 403/427–0954; Dr. Lyle Oberg, Minister

BRITISH COLUMBIA

Health

Ministry of Health, Parliament Building, Room 306, Victoria, BC V8V 1X4; tel. 604/387–5394; FAX. 604/387–3696; The Honorable Joy K. MacPhail

MANITOBA

Health

Department of Health, 302 Legislative Building, Winnipeg, MB R3C 0V8; tel. 204/945–3731; FAX. 204/945–0441; The Honorable Erie Stefanson, Minister

Social Services

Department of Manitoba Family Services Housing, 450 Broadway, Winnipeg, MB R3C 0V8; tel. 204/945–4173; FAX. 204/945–5149; The Honorable Tim Sale, Minister

NEWFOUNDLAND

Health

Department of Health and Community Services, Confederation Building, P.O. Box 8700, St. John's, NF A1B 4J6; tel. 709/729–3124; FAX. 709/729–0121; Roger D. Grimes, Minister, Health and Community Services

NOVA SCOTIA

Health

Department of Health, P.O. Box 488, Halifax, NS B3J 2R8; tel. 902/424–5818; FAX. 902/424–0559; The Honorable Jamie Muir, M.D.

PRINCE EDWARD ISLAND

Social Services

Department of Health and Social Services, Sullivan Building, Second Floor, P.O. Box 2000, Charlottetown, PE C1A 7N8; tel. 902/368–4930; FAX. 902/368–4969; The Honorable Walter A. McEwen, Q.C./Minister

QUEBEC

Social Services

Ministry of Health and Social Services, Ministere de la Sante et des Services Sociaux, Quebec, PQ G1S 2M1; tel. 418/643–3160; FAX. 418/644–4534; Jean Rochon, Minister

SASKATCHEWAN

Health

Department of Health, 3475 Albert Street, Third Floor, Regina, SK S4S 6X6; tel. 306/787–3168; FAX. 306/787–8677; The Honorable, Clay Serby, Minister

Health Care Providers

Health Maintenance Organizations

The following is a list of Health Maintenance Organizations developed with the assistance of state government agencies and the individual facilities listed.

We present this list simply as a convenient directory. Inclusion or omission of any organization indicates neither approval nor disapproval by Health Forum LLC.

United States

ALABAMA

Apex Healthcare of Alabama, Inc., 104 Inverness Center Parkway, Suite 230, Birmingham, AL 35243; tel. 334/279-5000; Stan Sherlin, Executive Director

Apex Healthcare of Mississippi, Inc, P.O. Box 381173, Birmingham, AL 35238-1173; tel. 800/856-3877; FAX. 800/491-2557

Apex Healthcare, Inc., 104 Inverness Center Parkway, Suite 320, Birmingham, AL 35242; tel. 205/991-3233

CACH HMO, Inc., 1600 7th Avenue South, Birmingham, AL 35233; tel. 205/939-6905; Mike Burgess, CEO

CIGNA Healthcare of Alabama, 10 Inverness Center Parkway, Suite 230, Birmingham, AL 35242; tel. 205/991-1005; FAX. 205/995-8511; Dave Manuso, Executive Director

DirectCare, Inc., 629 Interstate Park Drive, Montgomery, AL 36109; tel. 334/277-6670; FAX. 334/279-8875; T. David Lewis, President & CEO

Foundation Health Plan, 1900 International Park Drive, Suite 200, Birmingham, AL 35243; tel. 205/298-0679; Michael Newman, Acting Executive Director

Health Advantage Plans, Inc., 140 Riverchase Parkway, E., Birmingham, AL 35244; tel. 205/982-8400; FAX. 205/982-8411; James Denman, Chief Executive Officer

Health Maintenance Group of Birmingham, 936 19th Street South, Birmingham, AL 35205; tel. 205/988-2537; Joe Bolen, Director

Health Partners of Alabama, Inc., Two Perimeter Park South, Suite 200W, Birmingham, AL 35243; tel. 205/968-1000; Carl Sather, President & CEO

MedPartners Provider Network, 3000 Gallery Tower, Suite 1700, Birmingham, AL 35244; tel. 205/982-4291; FAX. 205/733-1984; Brad Karro, President and Chief Operating Officer

Primehealth of Alabama, Inc., 1400 South University Boulevard, Suite M, Mobile, AL 36609; tel. 334/342-0022; FAX. 334/342-1176; Becky S. Holliman, President

United Healthcare of Alabama, Inc., 3700 Colonnade Parkway, Birmingham, AL 35243; tel. 205/977-6300; Charles Pitts, President & CEO

Viva Health, Inc., 1401 South 21st Street, Birmingham, AL 35205; tel. 205/939-1718; John Davis, Interim President

ARIZONA

Aetna Health Plan of Arizona, Inc., 7878 North 16th Street, Suite 210, Phoenix, AZ 85020; tel. 602/395-8800; FAX. 602/395-8813; James W. Jones, Acting Vice President, Market Manager

CIGNA HealthCare of Arizona, Inc., 11001 North Black Canyon Highway, Suite 400, Phoenix, AZ 85029; tel. 602/942-4462; FAX. 602/371-2625; Clyde Wright, M.D., President, General Manager

FHP Inc., 410 North 44th Street, P.O. Box 52078, Phoenix, AZ 85072-2078; tel. 602/440-8200; FAX. 602/681-7680; Clifford Klima, President, Arizona Region

Humana Healthcare Plan, Inc., 2710 E. camelback Road, Phoenix, AZ 85016; tel. 602/381-4300; FAX. 602/381-4381; Elizabeth Kelly, Associate Executive Director

Premier Healthcare, Inc., d/b/a Premier Healthcare of Arizona, 100 East Clarendon, Suite 400, Phoenix, AZ 85013; tel. 602/248-0404; FAX. 602/248-7771; David K. Stewart, Vice President, Marketing, Sales

Sun Health Medisun, Inc., 10448 West Coggins Drive, Sun City, AZ 85351; tel. 602/933-1344; FAX. 602/933-5819; Glenn D. Jones, Administrative Director

United Healthcare of Arizona, (formerly Health Partners Health Plan Inc.), 3141 N. Third Avenue, Phoenix, AZ 85013; tel. 888/290-4747

University Physicians Health Maintenance Organization, Inc., 575 East River Road, Tucson, AZ 85704-5822; tel. 520/795-3500

ARKANSAS

American Dental Providers, Inc., 614 Center Street, P.O. Box 34045, Little Rock, AR 72203-4045; tel. 501/376-0544; FAX. 501/371-3820; Robert E. Iriana

Healthsource Arkansas, Inc., 333 Executive Court, Little Rock, AR 72205-4548; tel. 501/227-7222; Donald T. Jack

QCA Health Plan, Inc., 10800 Financial Centre Parkway, Suite 540, Little Rock, AR 72211; tel. 501/954-9595; FAX. 501/228-0135; Tim Brown, President and CEO

United HealthCare of Arkansas, Inc., 415 North McKinley Street, Plaza West Building, Suite 820, Little Rock, AR 72205; tel. 501/664-7700; FAX. 501/664-7768; V. Rob Herndon, III

CALIFORNIA

Access Dental Plan, Inc., 555 University Avenue, Suite 182, Sacramento, CA 95825; tel. 916/922-5000; FAX. 916/646-9000; Reza Abbaszadeh, D.D.S., Chief Executive Officer

Aetna US Healthcare Dental Plan of California, Inc., 2303 Camino Ramon, Suite 100, San Ramon, CA 94583; tel. 925/543-9503; FAX. 925/543-9513; Dr. Robert B. Ouelette, President

Alameda Alliance for Health, 1850 Fairway Drive, San Leandro, CA 94577; tel. 510/895-4532; FAX. 510/483-0536; Irene M. Ibarra, CEO

Alternative Dental Care of California, Inc., 21700 Oxnard Street, Suite 500, Woodland Hill, CA 91367; tel. 818/710-9400; FAX. 818/704-9817; Sargis Khaziran, Chief Finance Officer

American Speciality Health Plans, Inc., 8989 Rio San Diego Drive, Suite 250, San Diego, CA 92108; tel. 619/297-8100; FAX. 619/209-6233; Peggy Kilpatrick, Sales Manager

Ameritas Managed Dental Plan, 151 Kalmus Drive, Suite B-250, Costa Mesa, CA 92626; tel. 714/437-5966; FAX. 714/437-5967; Karin Truxillo, President

Baycare Health Plan, 122 Saratoga Avenue, Suite B, Santa Clara, CA 95051; tel. 408/441-9340; Tracy K. Heeter, D.D.S., President

Brown and Toland Medical Group, 100 Van Ness Avenue, 28th Floor, Suite 2800, San Francisco, CA 94102; tel. 415/553-6567; FAX. 415/553-6791; Michael Abel, M.D., President and CEO

California Dental Health Plan, 14471 Chambers Road, 92680, P.O. Box 899, Tustin, CA 92681-0899; tel. 714/731-4751; FAX. 714/731-2049; James R. Lindsey, President

California Physicians' Service, Blue Shield of California, 50 Beale Street, 22nd Floor, San Francisco, CA 94105; tel. 415/229-5195; FAX. 415/229-5343; Patricia Ernsberger, Associate General Counsel

Care 1st Health Plan, 1000 S. Fremont Avenue, Suite 11100, Alhambra, CA 91803; tel. 626/299-4299; FAX. 626/458-0415; John Edwards, Chief Executive Officer

CareAmerica, 6300 Canoga Avenue, Woodland Hill, CA 91367; tel. 818/228-2207; FAX. 818/228-5117; Robert P. White, President and CEO

Chinese Community Health Plan, 170 Columbus Avenue, Suite 210, San Francisco, CA 94133; tel. 415/397-3190; FAX. 415/397-6140; K.C. Wong, Administrator

ChrioSave, Inc., 3833 Atlantic Avenue, Long Beach, CA 90807; tel. 562/595-8164; FAX. 562/426-5352; J. Rodney Shelley, D.C., President and CEO

Cigna Dental Health of California, Inc., 5990 Sepulveda Blvd., Suite 500, Van Nuys, CA 91411; tel. 954/423-5674; Ann Fulks, Director of Compliance

Cohen Medical Corporation, d/b/a Tower Health Service, 200 Ocean Gate, Sixth Floor, Long Beach, CA 90802; tel. 562/435-2676; FAX. 562/432-3477; Robert Cohen, M.D., President

Community Dental Services, Smilecare, 3501 West Sunflower Ave, Suite 110, Santa Ana, CA 92715; tel. 714/850-3333; M. E. Hardin, President and CEO

Community Health Group, 740 Bay Boulevard, Chula Vista, CA 91910; tel. 619/422-0422; FAX. 619/422-5930; Gabriel Arce, Chief Executive Officer

Contra Costa Health Plan, 595 Center Avenue, Suite 100, Martinez, CA 94553; tel. 925/313-6000; FAX. 925/313-6580; Milton Camhi, Chief Executive Officer

County of Los Angeles, Department of Health Services, d/b/a Community Health Plan, 313 North Figueroa Street – Room 904, Los Angeles, CA 90012; tel. 213/240-7775; FAX. 213/202-5989; Donald R. Oxley, Director

County of Ventura, Ventura County Health Care Plan, 2323 Knoll Drive, Ventura, CA 93003; tel. 805/677-8787; FAX. 805/677-5177; Patricia S. Neumann, Insurance Administrator

Dedicated Dental Systems, Inc., 3990 Ming Avenue, Bakersfield, CA 93309; tel. 661/397-5513; FAX. 661/397-2888; Vicki Garcia, Membership Services Manager

Delta Dental Plan of California, 100 First Street, San Francisco, CA 94105; tel. 415/972-8463; Carl W. Ludwig, Director, Northern California Sales

Dental Benefit Providers of California, Inc., 311 California Street, Suite 550, San Francisco, CA 94104; tel. 415/391-1211; Jill Schultze Evans, Acting COO

Dental Health Services, 3833 Atlantic Avenue, Long Beach, CA 90807-3505; tel. 310/595-6000; FAX. 310/424-0150; Godfrey Pernell, D.D.S., President, Chief Executive Officer

DentiCare of California, Inc., 125 Technology Drive, Suite 100, Irvine, CA 92618; tel. 949/790-3400; FAX. 949/790-3455; Ed Eberhard, President

Dr. Leventhal's Vision Care Centers of America, 3680 Rosecrans Street, Zip 92110, P.O. Box 87808, San Diego, CA 92138; tel. 619/223-5656; FAX. 619/223-2318; Debra Brant, Chief Operating Officer

Eyecare Service Plan, Inc., 100 Corporate Point, Suite 285, Cover City, CA 90230; tel. 310/271-0145; FAX. 310/271-0784; Paige Roben, President

Eyexam 2000 of California, Inc., 170 Newport Center Drive, Suite 130, Newport Beach, CA 92661; tel. 949/583-6373; Keith Borders, Attorney

For Eyes Vision Plan, Inc., 2104 Shattuck Avenue, Berkeley, CA 94704; tel. 510/843-0787; Robert Schoen, President

Foundation Health Psychcare Services, Inc., d/b/a Occupational Health Services (OHS), 1600 Los Gamos Drive, Suite 300, San Rafael, CA 94903; tel. 415/491-7232; Nancy B. Diamond, Director of Admin, Reg. Compliance.

Foundation Health Vision Services, Vision Plans, 125 Technology, PO Box 57074, Irvine, CA 92619-7074; tel. 800/999-2848; Ed Eberhard, President

Golden West Dental and Vision Plan, 888 West Ventura Boulevard, Camarillo, CA 93010; tel. 800/995-4124; FAX. 805/384-9412; Chris R. Kamen, DDS and CEO

Greater California Dental Plan, Smilesaver, Signature Dental Plan, 22144 Clarendon Street, First Floor, P.O. Box 4281, Woodland Hill, CA 91365-4281; tel. 818/348-1500; FAX. 818/348-2942; Mark Johnson, President

Health & Human Resource Center, 9370 Sky Park Court, Suite 140, San Diego, CA 92123; tel. 619/571-1698; FAX. 619/571-1868; Stephen H. Heidel, M.D., President & CEO

Providers / Health Maintenance Organizations

Health and Human Resource Center, 9370 Sky Park Court, Suite 140, San Diego, CA 92123; tel. 858/571-1698; FAX. 858/571-1868; Stephen H. Heidel, M.D., President and CEO

Health Net, 155 Grand Avenue, Oakland, CA 94612; tel. 510/287-4586; FAX. 510/287-4654; Marshall Bentley, Vice President and Counsel

Health Net, 21600 Oxnard Street, Woodland Hills, CA 91367, P.O. Box 9103, Van Nuys, CA 91409-9103; tel. 818/719-6800; FAX. 818/719-5450; Arthur Southam, M.D., Chief Executive Officer

Health Plan of the Redwoods, 3033 Cleveland Avenue, Santa Rosa, CA 95403; tel. 707/525-4231; FAX. 707/547-4101; John W. Baxter, Chief Executive Officer

Healthdent of California, Inc., 2848 Arden Way, Suite 100, Sacramento, CA 95825; tel. 916/486-0749; FAX. 916/486-3642; Edward L. Cruchley, D.D.S., President

HMO California, 17922 Fitch, Irvine, CA 92614; tel. 949/756-5555; FAX. 949/756-5550; Raja Takhar, Chief Operating Officer

Holman Professional Counseling Centers, 21050 Vanowen Street, Canoga Park, CA 91303; tel. 818/704-1444; FAX. 818/704-9339; Ron Holman, Ph.D., President

Human Affairs International of California, 300 North Continental Boulevard, Suite 200, El Segundo, CA 90245; tel. 310/414-0066; FAX. 310/414-9282; Jonathan Wormhoudt, Ph.D., Chief Executive Officer

Ideal Dental Health Plan, Inc, 18911 Portola Drive, Suite C, Salinas, CA 93908; tel. 831/455-3400; FAX. 831/455-3409; Stanley Watkinson, President

Inland Empire Health Plan, 303 East Vanderbilt Way, Suite 400, San Bernardino, CA 92408; tel. 909/890-2000; FAX. 909/890-2003; Richard Bruno, Chief Executive Officer

Inter Valley Health Plan, 300 South Park Avenue, Suite 300, Pomona, CA 91766; tel. 909/623-6333; FAX. 909/622-2907; Mark C. Covington, President and CEO

Kaiser Foundation Health Plan, Inc., 1800 Harrison Street, 3th Floor, Oakland, CA 94612; tel. 510/987-2146; Renee Kullick, Director, H.P. Licensing

Kern Health Systems, 1600 Norris Road, Bakersfield, CA 93308; tel. 661/391-4000; FAX. 661/391-4097; Carol L. Sorrell, RN, Chief Executive Officer

Key Health Plan, Inc., 5959 South Mooney Boulevard, Visalia, CA 93277-9329; tel. 209/730-4100; Sheri A. Shannon, Chief Executive Officer

L.A. Care Health Plan, 3530 Wilshire Blvd., Suite 900, Los Angeles, CA 90010; tel. 213/251-8300; FAX. 213/637-3026; Anthony D. Rodgers, CEO

Landmark Healthplan of California, Inc., 1750 Howe Avenue, Suite 300, Sacramento, CA 95825-3369; tel. 800/638-4557; Sean Allen, Director HMO Sales

Laurel Dental Plan, Inc., 5451 Laurel Canyon Boulevard, Suite 204, North Hollywood, CA 91607; tel. 818/980-0929; FAX. 818/980-4668; Patrick Brooks, President

Lifeguard. Inc., 2840 Junction Avenue, San Jose, CA 95134; tel. 408/943-9400; FAX. 408/383-4259; Mark G. Hyde, President and CEO

Lifeguard. Inc., 1851 McCarthy Blvd., Milpatis, CA 95035; tel. 408/432-3608; Holly McCann, VP and General Counsel

Managed Dental Care of California, 6200 Canoga Avenue, Suite 100, Woodland Hill, CA 91367; tel. 800/273-3330; FAX. 818/347-7302; Candee Bolyog, President

Managed Health Network, Inc., 5100 West Goldleaf Circle, Suite 300, Los Angeles, CA 90056; tel. 213/299-0999; FAX. 213/298-2765; Alethea Caldwell, President

Managed Health Network, Inc., d/b/a California Wellness plan, 5100 W. Goldleaf Circle, Suite 300, Los Angeles, CA 90056; tel. 916/631-6039; Joseph K. Klinger, VP & Counsel

Maxicare, 1149 South Broadway Street, Suite 819, Los Angeles, CA 90015; tel. 213/365-3451; FAX. 213/365-3499; Warren D. Foon, Vice President, General Manager

MCC Behavioral Care of California, Inc., 801 North Brand Blvd., #1150, Glendale, CA 91203; tel. 800/433-5768; Susan Speltz Feltus, VP, Counsel

Merit Behavioral Care of California, Inc., 400 Oyster Point Boulevard, Suite 306, South San Francisco, CA 94080; tel. 415/742-0980; FAX. 415/742-0988; Douglas Studebaker, President

Molina Medical Centers, One Golden Shore, Long Beach, CA 90802; tel. 562/435-3666; John Molina, J.D., Vice President

Monarch Plan, Inc., 201 North Salsipuedes, Suite 206, Santa Barbara, CA 93103-3256; tel. 805/963-0566; FAX. 805/564-4167; Peter J. Leeson, D.O., Chief Executive Officer

National Health Plans, 1005 West Orangeburg Avenue, Suite B, Modesto, CA 95350-4163; tel. 209/527-3350; FAX. 209/527-6773; Mike Sheley, President & Chief Executive Officer

Newport Dental Plan, 3540 Howard Way, Costa Mesa, CA 92626; tel. 714/668-1300; FAX. 714/668-9015; Dennis Fratt, Chief Operating Officer

Omni Healthcare, 2450 Venture Oaks Way, Suite 300, Sacramento, CA 95833-3292; tel. 916/921-4000; FAX. 916/921-4100; Robert L. Fahlman, Chief Executive Officer

One Health Plan of California, Inc., 1740 Technology Drive, Suite 320, San Jose, CA 95110; tel. 408/437-4100; FAX. 408/437-0253; Jackie L. James, President

Oral Health Services, Inc., Mida Dental Plan, 21700 Oxnard Street, Suite 500, Woodland Hill, CA 91367; tel. 818/710-9400; FAX. 818/710-9400; Sargis Khaziran, Chief Financial Officer

Pacific Dental Benefits, Inc., 1390 Willow Pass Road, Suite 800, Concord, CA 94521; tel. 925/363-6000; FAX. 925/363-6098; Lee Schneider, Vice President, Sales

PacifiCare Behavioral Health of California, 23046 Avenida de la Carlota, Suite 700, Laguna Hills, CA 92653; tel. 714/859-7971; William Thomas, Manager Account Services

PacifiCare of California, Secure Horizons, 5995 Plaza Drive, P.O. Box 6006, Cypress, CA 90630-6006; tel. 714/236-5674; FAX. 714/236-7887; Nancy J. Monk, Regulatory Affairs, VP

Pearle Vision Care, Inc., 6727 Flanders Drive, Suite 104, San Diego, CA 92121; tel. 619/625-9173; FAX. 619/625-9781; Debbie Hyde-Duby, President

Preferred Dental Plan, Inc., 3636 Birch Street, Suite 250, Newport Beach, CA 92660; tel. 949/223-0007; FAX. 949/297-0317; Joan Contratti, Secretary/Treasurer

Preventive Dental Systems, Inc., 801 Broadway, Sacramento, CA 95818; tel. 916/448-2994; FAX. 916/448-2997; Gregory Thomas, Interim CEO

Priority Health Services, P.O. Box 25790, Fresno, CA 93729-5790; tel. 559/435-8366; FAX. 559/435-7693; Vreeland O. Jones, President and CEO

Private Medical–Care, Inc., PMI, 12898 Towne Center Drive, Cerritos, CA 90701; tel. 310/924-8311; FAX. 310/924-8039; Robert B. Elliott, President

Prudential Health Care Plan of California, Inc., 5800 Canoga Avenue, Woodland Hill, CA 91367; tel. 818/712-5002; FAX. 818/992-2474; Susan Hallett, President

Regents of the University of California, d/b/a UCSD Health Plan, 1899 McKee Street, San Diego, CA 92101; tel. 619/294-3743; FAX. 619/294-2460; Nancy White, RN, MPH, Director, UCSD Health Plan

Safeguard Health Plans, 505 North Euclid Street, P.O. Box 3210, Anaheim, CA 92803-3210; tel. 714/778-1005; FAX. 714/778-4383; Ronald I. Brendzel, Senior Vice President

San Francisco Health Plan, 568 Howard Street, Fifth Floor, San Francisco, CA 94105; tel. 415/547-7800; FAX. 415/547-7824; Shahnaz Nikpay, Ph.D., Chief Executive Officer

San Joaquin County Health Commission, d/b/a The Health Plan of San Joaquin, 1550 West Fremont Street, Suite 200, Stockton, CA 95203-2643; tel. 209/939-3500; FAX. 209/939-3535; Mr. Terry G. Mack, Chief Executive Officer

Santa Clara Family Health Plan, 4050 Moorpark Avenue, San Jose, CA 95117; tel. 408/260-4490; FAX. 408/260-2016; Leona M. Butler, Chief Executive Officer

Santa Clara Valley Medical Center, Valley Health Plan, 750 South Bascom Avenue, San Jose, CA 95128; tel. 408/885-5704; FAX. 408/885-4050; Roger Wells, Executive Director

SCAN, 3780 Kilroy Airport Way, Suite 600, P.O. Box 22616, Zip 90801-5616, Long Beach, CA 90806-2460; tel. 562/989-5100; FAX. 562/989-5200; Sam L. Ervin, President and CEO

Sharp Health Plan, 9325 Sky Park Court, Suite 300, San Diego, CA 92123; tel. 619/637-6530; FAX. 619/637-6504; Kathlyn Mead, President and CEO

U.S. Behavioral Health Plan, California, 425 Market Street, 27th Floor, San Francisco, CA 94105-2426; tel. 415/547-5294; FAX. 415/547-5512; Kathryn Emery Dougherty, Executive Director

UDC Dental California, Inc., (formerly The Dental Advantage/National Dental Health), 3111 Camino Del Rio North, Suite 1000, San Diego, CA 92108; tel. 800/288-9992; FAX. 619/283-9437; Keith C. Macumber, Senior Vice President, Western Region

United Healthcare of California, Inc., 180 E. Ocloa Boulevard, Suite 500, Long Beach, CA 90802-4708; tel. 562/951-6400; FAX. 562/951-6870; C. Emery Dameron, Chief Executive Officer

Universal Care, 1600 East Hill Street, Signal Hill, CA 90806; tel. 562/424-6200; FAX. 562/427-4634; Jay Davis, Vice President

Value Options of California, Inc, (formerly Value Behavioral Health of California, Inc), 340 Golden Shore, Long Beach, CA 90802; tel. 562/590-9004; FAX. 562/951-6130; Tim Kotas, Acting Executive Director

Vision First Eye care, Inc., 1937–A Tully Road, San Jose, CA 95122; tel. 408/923-0400; James K. Eu, O.D., Ph.D., President

Vision Plan of America, 3255 Wilshire Blvd, suite 1610, Los Angeles, CA 90010; tel. 213/384-2600; FAX. 213/384-0084; Dr. Stuart Needleman

Vision Service Plan, 3333 Quality Drive, Rancho Cordov, CA 95670; tel. 800/852-7600; Al Schubert, Vice President, Managed Care

Visioncare of California, d/b/a Sterling Visioncare, 6540 Lusk Boulevard, Suite 234, San Diego, CA 92121; tel. 619/458-9983; Abb B. Prickett, CFO

Vista Behavioral Health Plans, 2355 Northside Drive, 3rd floor, San Diego, CA 92108; tel. 619/521-4440; FAX. 619/497-5244; Erik Bradbury, Chief Executive Officer

VivaHealth, Inc., d/b/a BPS HMO, 888 South Figueroa Street, Suite 1400, Los Angeles, CA 90017; tel. 213/489-2694; Barbara E. Rodin, Ph.D., President and CEO

Watts Health Foundation, Inc., UHP Healthcare, 3405 W. Imperial Highway, Inglewood, CA 90303; tel. 310/412-3569; FAX. 310/412-7782; Alma Graham, VP and General Counsel

Wellpoint Dental Plan, 21555 Oxnard Street, Woodland Hill, CA 91367; tel. 818/703-2412; Thomas C. Geiser, Senior Vice President, General Counsel

Wellpoint Health Networks, Inc., 21555 Oxnard Street, Woodland Hill, CA 91367; tel. 818/703-2412; FAX. 818/703-4406; Thomas Geiser, Executive Vice President, General Counsel

Wellpoint Pharmacy Plan, 27001 Agoura Road, Suite 325, Calabasas Hill, CA 91301-5339; tel. 818/878-2675; FAX. 818/880-4981; Richard C. Bleil, General Manager

Western Dental Services, Inc., Western Dental Plan, 300 Plaza Alicante, Suite 800, Garden Grove, CA 92640; tel. 714/938-1600; FAX. 714/938-1611; Robert C. Schur, President

Western Health Advantage, 1331 Garden Highway, Suite 100, Sacramento, CA 95833; tel. 916/563-3180; FAX. 916/563-3182; Garry Maisel, Chief Executive Officer

COLORADO

Antero Healthplans, 600 Grant Street, Suite 900, Denver, CO 80203; tel. 303/830-3150; FAX. 303/830-2392; Charlie Stark, President and CEO

Blue Cross/ Blue Shield of Colorado, P.O. Box 1668, Fort Collins, CO 80522; tel. 970/482-8403; FAX. 970/482-8911; Karen Morgan, VP, Group and Member Service

CIGNA HealthCare of Colorado, Inc., 3900 East Mexico Avenue, Suite 1100, Denver, CO 80210-3946; tel. 303/782-1500; FAX. 303/782-1577; Dennis Mouras, General Manager

Colorado Access, 501 South Cherry Street, Suite 700, Denver, CO 80222; tel. 303/355-6707; FAX. 303/355-6779; Donald Hall, CEO

Community Health Plan of the Rockies, Inc., 400 South Colorado Boulevard, Suite 300, Denver, CO 80246; tel. 303/355-3220; FAX. 303/355-3224; Fawn Anderson, Human Resources

Denver Health Medical Plan, Inc., 777 Bannock Street, Mail Code 0278, Denver, CO 80204-4507; tel. 303/436-7253; FAX. 303/436-5714

FHP of Colorado, Inc., 6455 South Yosemite Street, Englewood, CO 80111; tel. 303/220-5800; FAX. 303/714-3999; James J. Swayze, Vice President, Sales and Marketing

Providers / Health Maintenance Organizations

Health Network of Colorado Springs, Inc., 1115 Tejon, Suite 400, Colorado Springs, CO 80903; tel. 719/227-3450; FAX. 719/227-3451; Janet Pogar, Chief Operating Officer
HMO Colorado, Inc., d/b/a HMO Blue, 700 Broadway, Suite 612, Denver, CO 80273; tel. 303/831-2131; FAX. 303/830-0887; Caz Matthews, COO
HMO Health Plans, Inc., d/b/a San Luis Valley HMO, Inc., 95 West First Avenue, Monte Vista, CO 81144; tel. 719/852-4055; FAX. 719/852-3481; Barbara J. Howard, Chief Administrative Officer
Kaiser Foundation Health Plan of Colorado, 2500 S. Havana Street, Aurora, CO 80014-1622; tel. 303/338-3000; Kathryn A. Paul, President
One Health Plan of Colorado, Inc., 8505 East Orchard Road, Englewood, CO 80111; tel. 303/804-6800
Prudential Health Care Plan, Inc., d/b/a Prudential HealthCare HMO, 4643 South Ulster Street, Suite 1000, Denver, CO 80237; tel. 303/796-6161; FAX. 303/796-6183; Denise Saabye, Communication Manager
Qual-Med Plans for Health of Colorado, Inc., P.O. Box 1986, Pueblo, CO 81002-1986; tel. 719/542-0500; FAX. 719/542-4921; Malik Hasan, M.D., Chairman, President
Rocky Mountain Health Maintenance Organization, d/b/a Rocky Mountain HMO, P.O. Box 10600, Grand Junction, CO 81502-5500; tel. 303/244-7760; FAX. 303/244-7880; Michael J. Weber, Executive Director
Sloans Lake Health Plan, Inc., 1355 South Colorado Boulevard, Suite 902, Denver, CO 80222; tel. 303/691-2200
United Healthcare of Colorado, Inc., 6251 Greenwood Plaza Boulevard, Englewood, CO 80111; tel. 303/694-9336; FAX. 303/267-3599

CONNECTICUT
Anthem BCBS of Connecticut, 370 Bassett Road, North Haven, CT 06473; tel. 203/239-8483; FAX. 203/985-4258; Robert Scalettar, M.D., MPH, VP Medical Policy CMO
CIGNA HealthCare of Connecticut, Inc., 900 Cottage Grove Road, A-118, Hartford, CT 06152-1118; tel. 860/769-2300; FAX. 860/769-2399; Donald S. Grossman, M.D., Medical Director
ConnectiCare of Massachusetts, Inc., P.O. Box 522, Farmington, CT 06032-0522; tel. 800/474-1466
ConnectiCare, Inc., 30 Batterson Park Road, Farmington, CT 06032; tel. 860/674-5700; FAX. 860/674-5728; Marcel Gamache, President and CEO
Health Choice of Connecticut Preferred One, 23 Maiden Lane, North Haven, CT 06473; tel. 203/239-7444; FAX. 203/239-5308; Sylvia B. Kelly, Vice President and Executive Director Medicaid
Oxford Health Plans, 800 Connecticut Avenue, Norwalk, CT 06854; tel. 800/444-6222; Julie Summers, Marketing Associate
Oxford Health Plans, Inc., 800 Connecticut Avenue, Norwalk, CT 06854; tel. 800/889-7546; Norman Payson, Chief Executive Officer
Physicians Health Services (PHS), One Far Mill Crossing, P.O. Box 904, Shelton, CT 06484-0944; tel. 800/772-5869; FAX. 203/407-2899; Caryn Coughlin, President
Prudential Health Care of Connecticut, Inc., 101 Merritt Seven, Norwalk, CT 06851; tel. 203/849-1800; FAX. 203/849-8387; Lewis E. Devendorf, Executive Director
Suburban Health Plan, Inc., 680 Bridgeport Avenue, Shelton, CT 06484; tel. 203/926-8882; FAX. 203/925-1202; Tim Pusch, Manager, Sales, Marketing

DELAWARE
Amerihealth HMO, Inc., 919 North Market Street, Suite 1200, Wilmington, DE 19801-3021; Alfred F. Meyer, Executive Director
CareLink Community Health Partners, Georgetown Professional Park, 600 N. Dupont Highway, Georgetown, DE 19947; tel. 302/856-3100; FAX. 302/856-3999; Don Clark, Vice President, Corporate Development
Cigna Health Plan of Pennsylvania, Inc., One Beaver Valley Road, Suite CHP, Wilmington, DE 19803; tel. 302/477-3700
CIGNA Health Plan of Southern New Jersey, CIGNA HealthCare of PA, NJ & DE, One Beaver Valley Road, Suite CHP, Wilmington, DE 19803; tel. 302/477-3700; FAX. 302/477-3707; Norman Scott, M.D.
CIGNA HealthCare of Pennsylvania, New Jersey and Delaware, One Beaver Valley Road, Suite CHP, Wilmington, DE 19803; tel. 302/477-3000; FAX. 302/477-3707; Norman Scott, M.D., Medical Director
Delaware Network Health Plan, 121 South Front Street, Seaford, DE 19973; tel. 302/629-6611; Donald Pinner, Vice President
Total Health, Inc., One Brandywine Gateway, P.O. Box 8792, Wilmington, DE 19899; tel. 302/421-3034; FAX. 302/421-2577; Robert C. Cole, Jr., President

DISTRICT OF COLUMBIA
Capital Care, Inc., 550 12th Street, S.W., Washington, DC 20065; tel. 410/528-7024; FAX. 410/528-7013; Eric R. Baugh, M.D., President
CapitalCare, Inc., 550 12th Street, S.W., Washington, DC 20065-0001; tel. 202/479-3678; FAX. 202/479-3660; M. Bruce Edwards, President
D.C. Chartered Health Plan, Inc., 820 First Street, N.E., Suite LL100, Washington, DC 20002-4205; tel. 202/408-4710; FAX. 202/408-4730; Robert L. Bowles, Jr., DBA, Chairman, President and CEO
United Mine Workers of America, 4455 Connecticut Avenue, N.W., Washington, DC 20008; tel. 202/895-3960; Robert Condra

FLORIDA
AHL Select HMO, Inc., 1776 American Heritage Life Drive, Jacksonville, FL 32224; tel. 904/992-2529; FAX. 904/992-2658; James H. Baum, Administrator
American Medical Healthcare, 1900 Summit Tower Boulevard, Suite 700, Orlando, FL 32810; tel. 407/660-1611; FAX. 407/660-0203; Sandra K. Johnson, President and CEO
AmeriHealth of Florida, Inc., 10151 Deerwood Park Blvd., Bldg. 200, Suite 400, Jacksonville, FL 32256; tel. 904/998-6700; FAX. 904/998-5403; Paul G. Jennings, VP & General Manager
AvMed Health Plan, P.O. Box 749, Gainesville, FL 32606-0749; tel. 352/372-8400; FAX. 352/337-8726; Edward C. Peddie, President and CEO
Beacon Health Plans, Inc., 2511 Ponce de Leon Boulevard, Coral Gables, FL 33134; tel. 305/930-8181; FAX. 305/774-2617; Ana M. Berengver, Vice President
Capital Group Health Services of Florida, Inc., 2140 Centerville Place, P.O. Box 13267, Tallahassee, FL 32317; tel. 904/386-3161; FAX. 904/385-3193; John Hogan, Administrator
CIGNA Dental Health of North Carolina, Inc., P.O. Box 189060, Plantation, FL 33318-9060; tel. 954/423-5800; FAX. 954/423-5491; Randee H. Lehrer, President
CIGNA HealthCare of Florida, Inc., 5404 Cypress Center Drive, P.O. Box 24203, Tampa, FL 33623; tel. 813/281-1000; FAX. 813/282-0356; Joseph C. Gregor, President and General Manager
Community Health Care Systems, Inc., 2301 Lucien Way, Suite 400, Maitland, FL 32751; tel. 800/635-4345; FAX. 407/481-7190; Eric Scott, Director of Sales
DentiCare, Inc., 8130 Baymeadows Way West, Suite 200, Jacksonville, FL 32256; tel. 904/731-1870; Glenn Kollen
Florida Health Care Plan, 1340 Ridgewood Avenue, Holly Hill, FL 32117; tel. 904/676-7193; FAX. 904/676-7196; Edward F. Simpson, Jr., President, Chief Executive Off
Florida 1st Health Plans, Inc., 3425 Lake Alfred Road, P.O. Box 9126, Winter Haven, FL 33883-9126; tel. 863/293-0785; FAX. 863/297-9095; Frank Willis, President and CEO
Foundation Health, a Florida Health Plan, Inc., 1340 Concord Terrace, Sunrise, FL 33323; tel. 954/858-3000; FAX. 954/846-0331; Steven Griffin, Administrator
Foundation Health, a South Florida Health Plan, Inc., 7950 Northwest 53rd Street, Miami, FL 33166; tel. 305/591-3311
Health First Health Plans, Inc., 8247 Devereux Drive, Suite 103, Melbourne, FL 32940-7955; tel. 321/434-5600; FAX. 321/752-1129; Jerry Senne, President and CEO
Health Options, Inc., 532 Riverside Avenue, P.O. Box 60729, Jacksonville, FL 32202; tel. 800/457-4713; FAX. 904/791-6054; Robert I. Lufrano, Administrator
Healthcare USA, Inc., 8705 Perimeter Park Boulevard, Suite Three, Jacksonville, FL 32216; tel. 904/565-2950; FAX. 904/646-9238; Christopher Fey, President and CEO
Healthplan Southeast, Inc., 3520 Thomasville Road, Suite 200, Tallahassee, FL 32308; tel. 800/833-2169; FAX. 850/668-3133; Robert A. Wychulis, Chief Operating Officer
Healthplans of America, Inc., 2605 Maitland Center Parkway, Suite 300, Maitland, FL 32751; tel. 800/882-3054; FAX. 407/875-9581; Robert Flanagan, Administrator
Healthy Palm Beaches, Inc., 324 Datura Street, Suite 401, West Palm Beach, FL 33401; tel. 561/659-1270; FAX. 561/833-9786; Dwight Chenette, Administrator
HIP Health Plan of Florida, Inc., 200 South Park Road, Hollywood, FL 33021; tel. 954/962-3008; FAX. 954/985-4379; David S. Abernathy, Executive Director
Humana Medical Plan, Inc., 3400 Lakeside Drive, Miramar, FL 33027; tel. 305/626-5619; FAX. 305/626-5297; Joe Berding, Vice President, South Florida Market Operations
JMA Health Plans, 1801 Northwest 9th Avenue, Suite 700, Miami, FL 33136; tel. 305/575-3700; FAX. 305/545-5212; Joseph Rogers, Administrator
John Alden Nevadaplus Health Plan, 7300 Corporate Center Drive, Miami, FL 33126
Mayo Health Plans, Inc., 4168 Southpoint Parkway, Suite 102, Jacksonville, FL 32216; tel. 888/279-2646; FAX. 904/279-9777; Patrick Healy, Administrator
Neighborhood Health Partnership, Inc., 7600 Corporate Center Drive, Miami, FL 33126; tel. 800/354-0222; FAX. 305/715-4306; Joseph R. Papa, President and CEO
PCA Family Health Plan, Inc., d/b/a Century Medical Health Plan, Inc., 5959 Blue Lagoon Drive, Miami, FL 33126; tel. 800/562-9262; FAX. 605/267-6290; Elias Hourani, Administrator
Preferred Choice, HMO of Florida Health Choice, Inc., 5300 West Atlantic Avenue, Suite 500, Delray Beach, FL 33484-8190; tel. 800/233-0505; FAX. 407/496-0513; Jeff Keiser, Administrator/Compliance Officer
Preferred Medical Plan, Inc., 4950 SW 8th Street, Coral Gables, FL 33134; tel. 305/669-1501; FAX. 305/667-3957; Sylvia Urlich, President
Principal Health Care of Florida, Inc., 1200 Riverplace Boulevard, Suite 500, Jacksonville, FL 32207; tel. 800/358-6205; FAX. 301/231-1033; Kenneth S. Bryant, Administrator
Principal Health Care of Florida, Inc., 7282 Plantation Road, Suite 200, Pensacola, FL 32504; tel. 904/484-4000; Rebecca McQueen, Executive Director
Prudential Health Care Plan, Inc., d/b/a PruCare, 2301 Lucien Way, Suite 230, Maitland, FL 32751-7086; tel. 800/628-3801; FAX. 201/716-2193; Andrew Crooks, Administrator
Riscorp Health Plan, Inc., 1390 Main Street, Zip 34236, P.O. Box 1598, Sarasota, FL 34230-1598; tel. 800/226-9899; FAX. 813/954-4611; Rich Fogle, Administrator
St. Augustine Health Care, Inc., 1511 N. Westshore Blvd., 7th floor, Tampa, FL 33607; tel. 813/288-7600; FAX. 813/288-7664; Dennis Mihale, M.D., Administrator
Tampa General Healthplan, Inc., 100 South Ashley Drive, Suite 300, Tampa, FL 33602; tel. 813/276-5047; FAX. 813/276-5030; Thelma Czeczotca, Plan Administrator
Total Health Choice, Inc., formerly: PacifiCare of Florida, One Alhambra Plaza, Suite 1000, Coral Gables, FL 33134; tel. 800/887-6888; FAX. 305/443-5445; Kenneth G. Rimmer, Administrator
United Healthcare of Florida, Inc., 800 N. Magnolia Avenue, Orlando, FL 32803; tel. 800/543-3145; FAX. 305/447-3292; Gary L. Scultz, President

GEORGIA
AETNA Health Plans of Georgia, Inc., 11675 Great Oaks Way, Alpharetta, GA 30022; tel. 404/814-4300; FAX. 404/814-4294; Joseph Wild, General Manager
American Dental Plan of North Carolina, Inc., 100 Mansell Court East, Suite 400, Roswell, GA 30076; tel. 770/998-8936; John Gasiorowski
Athens Area Health Plan Select, Inc., 295 West Clayton Street, Athens, GA 30601; tel. 706/549-0549; FAX. 706/549-8004; Richard Tanzella, Executive Director
CIGNA Healthcare of Georgia, Inc., 100 Peachtree Street, N.E., Suite 700, Equitable Building, Atlanta, GA 30301; tel. 404/681-7100; FAX. 404/681-7135; Jack Towsley, President and GM
Complete Health of Georgia, Inc., 2970 Clairmont Road, N.E., Atlanta, GA 30329; tel. 404/698-8600; Gail Smallridge, Executive Director

Providers / Health Maintenance Organizations

FamilyPlus Health Plans of Georgia, Inc., Two Decatur Town Center, 125 Clairemont Road, Decatur, GA 30030; tel. 404/235-1010; FAX. 404/248-3858; Michael Brohm, President

Grady Healthcare, Inc., 100 Edgewood Avenue, Suite 1317, Atlanta, GA 30303; tel. 404/616-5829; FAX. 404/616-8408; Alma Roberts, Executive Director

HMO Georgia, Inc., 3350 Peachtree Road, N.E., P.O. Box 3417, Atlanta, GA 30326; tel. 404/842-8422; FAX. 404/842-8451; John Harris, President

Humana Employers Health Plan of Georgia, Inc., 115 Perimeter Center Place, N.E., Suite 540, Atlanta, GA 30346; tel. 770/399-5916; Gregory H. Wolf, Executive Director

Kaiser Foundation Health Plan of Georgia, Inc., 3495 Piedmont Road, N.E., Building Nine, Atlanta, GA 30305-1736; tel. 404/364-7000; FAX. 404/364-4963; Carolyn Kenny, President

Master Health Plan, Inc., 3652 J. Dewey Gray Circle, Augusta, GA 30909; tel. 706/863-5955; Libby Young, Executive Director

Principal Health Care of Georgia, Inc., 3715 Northside Parkway, 400 Northcreek, Atlanta, GA 30327; tel. 404/231-9911; Kenneth J. Linde, President

Promina Managed Care Organization, 2000 South Park Place, Suite 200, Atlanta, GA 30339-2049; tel. 770/956-6944; FAX. 770/937-4159; Bonnie Phipps, President and CEO

United Healthcare of Georgia, Inc., 2970 Clairmont Road, Atlanta, GA 30329; tel. 404/364-8800; FAX. 404/364-8818; A. Kelly Atkinson, Executive Director

HAWAII

Health Plan Hawaii, 818 Keeaumoku Street, P.O. Box 860, Honolulu, HI 96808; tel. 808/948-5408; FAX. 808/948-5999; Robert C. Nickel, President and CEO

Kaiser Foundation Health Plan, Inc., 3283 Moanaleau Road, Honolulu, HI 96819; tel. 808/834-5333; FAX. 808/834-3944; Bruce Behnke, President

Queens Health Care Plan, Two Waterfront Plaza, Suite 200, 500 Ala Moana Boulevard, Honolulu, HI 96813; tel. 808/532-4114; FAX. 808/532-7996; Nate Nygaard, President

Straub Plan, 888 South King Street, Honolulu, HI 96813; tel. 808/522-4540; FAX. 808/522-4544; Karen Lennox, Executive Director

IDAHO

HealthSense, 1602 21st Avenue, Lewiston, ID 83501; tel. 208/746-2671; FAX. 208/798-2060; Carolyn Steinbrecher-Loera, Assistant Vice President

Primary Health Network, Inc., 800 Park Boulevard, Suite 760, Boise, ID 83712; tel. 208/344-1811; FAX. 208/344-4262; Elden Mitchell, President and CEO

ILLINOIS

Aetna Health Plans of Illinois, Inc., d/b/a Aetna Health Plans of the Midwest, 100 North Riverside Plaza, Chicago, IL 60606; tel. 312/441-3000

Aetna U.S. Healthcare of Illinois, Inc., 100 North Riverside Plaza, 20th Floor, Chicago, IL 60606; tel. 312/928-3000; FAX. 312/928-3202; Robert Mendoza, General Manager

American Health Care Providers, Inc., 142 Towncenter Road, Matteson, IL 60443; tel. 708/503-5000; FAX. 708/503-5001; Asif A. Sayeed, President

BCI HMO, Inc., 300 East Randolph Street, 21st floor, Chicago, IL 60601-5090; tel. 312/653-6699; Eileen Holderbaum, Executive Director

BCI HMO, Inc., (formerly HMO Illinois, Inc.), 233 North Michigan Avenue, Chicago, IL 60601; tel. 312/938-6347; FAX. 312/819-1220; Simeon Martin Hickman, President

Benchmark Health Insurance Company, 2550 Charles Street, Rockford, IL 61108; tel. 815/391-7000; FAX. 815/966-2089; Michael J. Gallagher

CIGNA HealthCare of Illinois, Inc., 525 West Monroe, Suite 1800, Chicago, IL 60661; tel. 312/648-2460; FAX. 312/648-3617; Donna DeFrank, President

Community Health Choice, 650 South Clark, Suite 400, Chicago, IL 60605; tel. 312/922-4501; FAX. 312/922-6358; Nasser Wasim, VP Government Sales

Community Health Plan of Sarah Bush Lincoln, 1000 Health Center Drive, P.O. Box 372, Mattoon, IL 61938-0372; tel. 217/258-2572; FAX. 217/258-2111; Gary L. Barnett, President and CEO

Country Medical Plans, Inc., d/b/a Country Care HMO, PO Box 2000, Bloomington, IL 61702-2000; tel. 309/821-2477; FAX. 309/821-5198; Lori Reel, HMO Administator

Dreyer Health Plans, 1877 West Downer Place, Aurora, IL 60506; tel. 630/859-1100; FAX. 630/906-5100; Richard A. Lutz, President

FHP of Illinois, Inc., One Lincoln Centre, Suite 700, Oakbrook Terr, IL 60181-4260; tel. 630/916-8400; FAX. 630/916-4275; Gary M. Cole, President

First Commonwealth, Inc., 444 North Wells, Suite 600, Chicago, IL 60610; tel. 312/644-1800; FAX. 312/644-1822; Mark R. Lundberg, Vice President, Sales

Harmony Health Plan of Illinois, Inc., 125 South Wacker Drive, Suite 2900, Chicago, IL 60606; tel. 312/630-2025; Kathleen Laspina, Director

Health Alliance Medical Plans, Inc., d/b/a Health Alliance HMO, 102 East Main, Urbana, IL 61801; tel. 217/337-8010; FAX. 217/337-8093; Jeffrey Ingram, CEO

Health Alliance Midwest, Inc., 102 East Main Street, Suite 200, Urbana, IL 61801; tel. 217/337-8000; Robert C. Parker, M.D., President

Heritage National Healthplan, 1300 River Drive, Suite 200, Moline, IL 61265; tel. 309/765-1200; G. Michael Hammes, President

Heritage National Healthplan, Inc., 1515 Fifth Avenue, Suite 200, Moline, IL 61265-1368; tel. 309/765-1200; G. Michael Hammes, President

HMO Illinois a product of Health Care Services Corporation, 300 East Randolph Street, Chicago, IL 60601-5099; tel. 312/653-6000; Ray McCaskey, President

Humana Dental, 222 North LaSalle, Suite 700, Chicago, IL 60601; tel. 312/201-1260; Polly Reese, D.D.S., Dental Director

Humana Health Plan, Inc., 30 South Wacker Drive, Suite 3100, Chicago, IL 60606; tel. 312/441-5350; Barry Averill, Vice President

Illinois Healthcare Insurance Co., 303 E. Washington, Bloomington, IL 61701; tel. 309/829-1061; Thomas J. Pliura, M.D., J.D., President

Illinois Masonic Community Health Plan, 836 West Wellington, Room 1710, Chicago, IL 60657; tel. 773/296-7014; FAX. 773/296-7352; Dana Gilbert, Administrative Director

John Deere Healthplan, 1300 River Drive, Moline, IL 61265-1368; tel. 309/765-1200; FAX. 309/765-1322; Dan O'Keeffe, Manager-Corporate Communications

John Deere Health Care Insurancenc., 3800 23rd Avenue, Suite 200, Moline, IL 61265; tel. 800/330-9205; Dean Anderson, Executive Director

Maxicare Health Plans of the Midwest, Inc., 111 East Wacker Drive, Suite 1500, Chicago, IL 60601; tel. 312/616-4700; FAX. 312/616-4998; Mark Hanrahan, Vice President, General Manager

MetraHealth Care Plan of Illinois, Inc., 1900 East Golf Road, Suite 501, Schaumburg, IL 60173; tel. 708/619-2222

One Health Plan of Illinois, Inc., 6250 River Road, Suite 3030, Rosemont, IL 60018; tel. 847/518-0490; Patricia Ann Moldovan, President

OSF Healthplans, Inc., 7915 N. Hale, Suite D, Peoria, IL 61615-2088; tel. 309/677-8200; FAX. 309/677-8330; Kevin D. Schoeplein, President

Oxford Health Plans, Inc., 9801 West Higgins, Suite 720, Rosemont, IL 60018-4701; tel. 847/685-2273; Aldo Giacchio, President

Personal Care Insurance of Illinois, Inc., 2110 Fox Drive, Champaign, IL 61820; tel. 217/366-1226; FAX. 217/366-5571; Randolph C. Hoffman, President and CEO

Principal Health Care of Illinois, Inc., One Lincoln Center, Suite 1040, Oakbrook Terrace, IL 60181-4267; tel. 630/916-6622; FAX. 630/916-9595; Lee Green, Executive Director

Rockford Health Plans, 3401 North Perryville Road, Rockford, IL 61114; tel. 815/654-3600; FAX. 815/654-5186; John W. Zilavy, Executive Director

Rush Prudential Health Plans, 233 South Wacker Drive, Suite 3900, Chicago, IL 60605-6309; tel. 312/234-7000; FAX. 312/986-4859; Scott Serota, President and CEO

UIHMO, Inc., 2023 West Ogden Avenue, Suite 205, M/C 692, Chicago, IL 60612-3741; tel. 312/996-3553; FAX. 312/996-0035; Diane S. Eng, VP for University Programs

Union Health Service, 1634 West Polk, Chicago, IL 60612; tel. 312/829-4224; FAX. 312/829-8241; W. Joe Garrett, Executive Director

United HealthCare of Illinois, Inc., d/b/a Chicago HMO, Ltd., One South Wacker Drive, P.O. Box 909714, Chicago, IL 60609-9714; tel. 312/424-4605; FAX. 312/424-4914; Marshall Rozzi, President and CEO

Universal Health Services, Inc., 403 West 14th Street, Chicago Heights, IL 60411-2498; tel. 708/755-2462; Ralph R. Crescenzo, President

Wellmark Health Plan of Northern Illinois, Inc., 1420 Kensington Road, Suite 203, Oak Brook, IL 60521-2106; tel. 800/345-7848

INDIANA

Anthem Health Plan, d/b/a Key Health Plan, 120 Monument Circle, Indianapolis, IN 46204; tel. 317/488-6000; FAX. 317/290-5695; Dijuana Lewis, Vice President, Health Care Management

Arnett HMO, Inc., 415 N. 26th Street, Suite 101, Lafayette, IN 47905; tel. 765/448-7440; FAX. 765/448-7700; James A. Brunnemer, Executive Director

Coordinated Care Corporation Indiana, Inc., d/b/a Managed Health Services, 8688 Broadway, Merrillville, IN 46410; tel. 219/756-7134

Health Resources, Inc., 314 Southeast Riverside Drive, P.O. Box 3607, Evansville, IN 47735-3607; tel. 812/424-1444; FAX. 812/424-2096; Edward L. Fritz, D.S., President

Healthpoint, LLC, 8900 Keystone Crossing, Suite 500, Indianapolis, IN 46240; tel. 317/574-8181; FAX. 317/574-8182; L. Denise Smith, Administrative Assistant

IU Health Plan, Inc., 3901 West 86th Street, Suite 230, Indianapolis, IN 46268; tel. 317/872-2202; FAX. 317/871-8833; Sarah Blackman, Sales Coordinator

M Plan, Inc., 8802 North Meridian Street, Suite 100, Indianapolis, IN 46260; tel. 317/571-5300; FAX. 317/571-5306; Alex Slabosky, President

Maxicare Indiana, Inc., 9480 Priority Way, West Drive, Indianapolis, IN 46240-3899; tel. 317/844-5775; FAX. 317/574-0713; Kenneth Kubistu, Vice President, General Manager

Partners National Health Plans of Indiana, Inc., One Michigan Square, 100 East Wayne, Suite 502, South Bend, IN 46601; tel. 219/233-4899; FAX. 219/234-7484; Richard C. Born, Senior Vice President Finance, Operations

Physicians Health Plan of Northern Indiana, Inc., 8101 West Jefferson Boulevard, Fort Wayne, IN 46804-4163; tel. 800/982-6257; FAX. 219/432-0493; Jay M. Gilbert, President and CEO

Principal Health Care of Indiana, Inc., One North Pennsylvania, Suite 1100, Indianapolis, IN 46204; tel. 317/263-0920; FAX. 317/263-9139; Douglas Stratton, Executive Director

Sagamore Health Network, Inc., 11555 North Meridian, Suite 400, Carmel, IN 46032; tel. 317/573-2836; FAX. 317/580-8009; C. Randall Abner, Vice President, Marketing

Southeastern Indiana Health Organization, Inc. (SIHO), 432 Washington Street, P.O. Box 1787, Columbus, IN 47202-1787; tel. 812/378-7000; FAX. 812/348-4592; David S. Barker, President and CEO

SpecialMed of Indiana, Inc., 120 Monument Circle, Indianapolis, IN 46204-4903; tel. 317/488-6128; Mike Hostetter, M.D., President

United Dental Care of Indiana, Inc., 50 South Meridian, Suite 700, Indianapolis, IN 46204-3542; tel. 800/262-5388

Vision Service Plan, 201 N. Illinois Street, Suite 2075, Indianapolis, IN 46204; tel. 317/686-1066; FAX. 317/686-1140

Welborn Clinic/Welborn HMO, Welborn Health Options, 421 Chestnut Street, Evansville, IN 47713; tel. 812/425-3939; James Krueger, M.D., Medical Director

IOWA

Care Choices HMO, 600 Fourth Street, Terra Centre, Suite 401, Sioux City, IA 51101; tel. 712/252-2344; FAX. 712/233-3684; Bill Windsor, Executive Director

Health Alliance Midwest, Inc., 3510 Lincolnway, Ames, IA 50014; tel. 515/296-1656; Jeffrey Ingram, CEO

Medical Associates Health Plan, Inc., 700 Locust Street, PO Box 5002, Dubuque, IA 52004-5002; tel. 319/556-8070; FAX. 319/556-5134; Cynthia C. Thumser, Executive Director

Mercy Health Plans HMO – IA, (d/b/a Care Choices), 522 Fourth Street, Suite 250, Sioux City, IA 51101-1744; tel. 712/252-2344; FAX. 712/294-7018; Marsha Watts, Iowa Site Manager

Providers / Health Maintenance Organizations

Nevada Care, d/b/a Iowa Health Solutions, 300 N. W. Bank Tower, Spruce Hills Drive at Middle Road, Bettendorf, IA 52722; tel. 319/359-8999; FAX. 319/359-8999; Paul C. Carter, Vice President
Principal Health Care of Iowa, Inc., 4600 Westown Parkway, Suite 200, West Des Moines, IA 50266-1099; tel. 515/225-1234; FAX. 515/223-0097; Louis Garcia, CEO
Wellmark Health Plan of Iowa, 636 Grand Avenue, Des Moines, IA 50309; tel. 800/355-2031; Thomas E. Press, President

KANSAS
CIGNA HealthCare of Ohio, Inc.,, dba CIGNA HealthCare of Kansas/Missouri, 7400 West 110th Street, Suite 600, Overland Park, KS 66210; tel. 913/339-4700; FAX. 913/451-0974; James A. Young, President, General Manager
HealthCare American Plans, Inc., P.O. Box 780467, Wichita, KS 67278-0467
HMO Kansas, Inc., 419 West 29th Street, Topeka, KS 66601-0110; tel. 913/291-7000; John W. Knack, Jr., President
Horizon Health Plan, Inc., 623 Southwest 10th Avenue, Suite 300, Topeka, KS 66612-1627; tel. 913/235-0402; Bruce M. Gosser, President
Kaiser Foundation Health Plan of Kansas City, Inc., 10561 Barkley, Suite 200, Overland Park, KS 66212-1886; tel. 913/967-4638; FAX. 913/967-4647; Gerard Grimaldi, Director External Affairs
MetraHealth Care Plan of Kansas City, Inc., (a wholly owned subsidiary of United HealthCare of the Midwest, Inc.), 9300 West 110th Street, Suite 350A, Overland Park, KS 66210; tel. 913/451-5656; FAX. 913/451-0492; Robert S. Bonney, Vice President
Preferred Plus of Kansas, Inc., 8535 E. 21st. N, Wichita, KS 67206; tel. 316/609-2345; FAX. 316/609-2346; Marlon Dauner, President
Premier Health, Inc., d/b/a Premier Blue, 1133 Topeka Avenue, Topeka, KS 66629-0001; tel. 913/291-7000; John W. Knack, Jr., President

KENTUCKY
Advantage Care, Inc., 120 Prosperous Place, Suite 300, Lexington, KY 40509; tel. 606/264-4600; Peter M. Ebner, President and CEO
Alternative Health Delivery Systems, Inc., 1901 Campus Place, Louisville, KY 40299; tel. 502/261-2176; FAX. 502/261-2255; Carol H. Muldoon, Vice President and COO
Anthem Blue Cross and Blue Shield, 9901 Linn Station Road, Louisville, KY 40223; tel. 502/423-2373; FAX. 502/423-6974; George L. Walker, Chief Operating Officer
Anthem Blue Cross Blue Shield, 9901 Linn Station Road, Louisville, KY 40223; tel. 502/423-2277; FAX. 502/423-2729; Robert McIntire, Vice President
Anthem Health Plans of Ky, Inc., 9901 Linn Station Road, Louisville, KY 40223; tel. 502/423-2308; FAX. 502/4213-272; Mike Lorch, Vice President
Bluegrass Family Health, Inc., 651 Perimeter Drive, Suite 300, Lexington, KY 40517; tel. 606/269-4475; FAX. 606/335-3720; James S. Fritz, President and CEO
CHA Health, 300 West Vine Street, 16th Floor, Lexington, KY 40522; tel. 606/271-5055; Mark Birdwhistell, Chief Executive Officer
CompDent Corporation, 1930 Bishop Lane, 16th Floor, Louisville, KY 40218; tel. 800/456-5500; FAX. 502/456-2772; Allan Brockway Morris, President and CEO
Healthsource Kentucky, Inc., 100 Mallard Creek Road, Suite 300, Louisville, KY 40207; tel. 502/899-7500; Paul E. Stamp, Interim Executive Director
Healthwise of Kentucky, Ltd., 2409 Harodsburg Road, Lexington, KY 40504; tel. 606/296-6100; FAX. 606/255-9134; Harold Bischoff, Executive Director
HMO Kentucky, Inc., 9901 Linn Station Road, Louisville, KY 40223; tel. 502/423-2282; FAX. 502/423-6979; G. Douglas Sutherland, President
HMPK, 500 West Main Street, P.O. Box 1438, Louisville, KY 40201-1438; tel. 502/580-1854; FAX. 502/580-5044; Heidi Margulis, Director, Government Programs
HPLAN, Inc., 500 West Main Street, P.O. Box 1438, Louisville, KY 40201-1438; tel. 502/580-1854; Heidi Margulis, Director, Government Programs
Humana Health Plan of Louisiana, Inc., 500 West Main Road, P.O. Box 740036, Louisville, KY 40201-7436; tel. 502/580-1000; James E. Murray, Vice President, Finance
Humana Health Plan of Utah, Inc., 500 West Main Street, 20th Floor, Louisville, KY 40201; tel. 502/580-1000
Humana Health Plan of Washington, Inc., P.O. Box 1438, Louisville, KY 40201-1438; tel. 502/580-3620; FAX. 502/580-3942; Sandra Lewis, Director, Government Compliance
Humana Health Plan, Inc., 500 West Main Street, Louisville, KY 40202; tel. 502/580-1860; FAX. 502/580-3127; Dick Brown, Director, Corporate Communications
United Health Care of Kentucky, 2409 Harrodsburg Road, Lexington, KY 40504; tel. 606/296-6000; Budd Fisher, Chief Executive Officer

LOUISIANA
Advantage Health Plan, Inc., 829 St. Charles Avenue, New Orleans, LA 70130; tel. 504/568-9009; FAX. 504/568-0301; Jane Cooper, President and CEO
Aetna Health Plans of Louisiana, Inc., 3900 North Causeway Boulevard, Suite 410, Metairie, LA 70002-7283; tel. 504/830-5600; FAX. 504/837-6571; Michael L. Rogers, President
AmCare Health Plans of Louisiana, 5353 Essen Lane, Suite 450, Baton Rouge, LA 70809; tel. 504/763-5300; Scott Westbrook, Vice President/Director of Operations
Capitol Health Network, Inc., 4700 Wichers Drive, Suite 300, Marrero, LA 70072; tel. 504/347-4515; John Sudderth, Chief Executive Officer
CIGNA HealthCare of Louisiana, Inc., 4354 South Sherwood Forest Boulevard, Suite 240, Baton Rouge, LA 70816; tel. 225/295-2800; FAX. 225/295-2888; Linda Gage-White, M.D., Executive Director
Gulf South Health Plans, Inc., 5615 Corporate Boulevard, Suite Three, P.O. Box 80339, Baton Rouge, LA 70898-0339; tel. 504/237-1700; FAX. 504/237-1939; Jack W. Walker, President
Health Plus of Louisiana, Inc., 2600 Greenwood Road, Shreveport, LA 71103; tel. 318/632-4590; FAX. 318/632-4463; Peter J. Babin, President
HMO of Louisiana, Inc., P.O. Box 98029, Baton Rouge, LA 70898-8024; tel. 504/295-2383; FAX. 504/295-2491; Michael A. Hayes, Executive Director
NYLCare Health Plans of Louisiana, Inc., 2014 West Pinhook Road, Suite 200, Lafayette, LA 70508; tel. 800/825-0568; FAX. 318/237-1703; Burley J. Pellerin, II, Director, Operations
Ochsner Health Plan, Inc. (HMO), One Galleria Boulevard, Suite 1224, Metairie, LA 70001; tel. 504/836-6600; FAX. 504/836-6566; R. Lyle Luman, President and CEO
Principal Health Care of Louisiana, Inc, 2424 Edenborn Ave, Suite 600, Metairie, LA 70001; tel. 504/834-0840; FAX. 504/834-2694; Keith G. Benoit, Sr., Chief Executive Officer
SMA Health Plan, 111 Veteran's Memorial Boulevard, Heritage Plaza, Suite 500, Metairie, LA 70005; tel. 504/837-7374; FAX. 504/837-7366; Robert Ritchey
Vantage Health Plan, 909 North 18th Street, Suite 201, Monroe, LA 71201; tel. 318/323-2269; Angela Olden, Executive Director

MAINE
Blue Cross and Blue Shield of Maine, Two Gannett Drive, South Portland, ME 04106; tel. 207/822-7000; Nancy Hutchings, Director, Customer Service
CIGNA Healthsource Maine, Two Stonewood Drive, P.O. Box 447, Freeport, ME 04032-0447; tel. 207/865-5000; FAX. 207/865-5632; Richard White, Chief Executive Officer
NYLCare of Maine Health Plans, Inc., One Monument Square, Portland, ME 04102; tel. 207/791-7916; Charlotte Pease, Manager
PMC Medical Management, Inc., 202 US Route One, P.O. Box 165, Falmouth, ME 04105; tel. 207/781-9890; FAX. 207/781-6675; Jeffrey W. Kirby, Controller

MARYLAND
CIGNA HealthCare Mid-Atlantic, Inc., 9700 Patuxent Woods Drive, Columbia, MD 21046; tel. 410/720-5800; Linda Hacker
CIGNA Healthplan of the MidAtlantic, Inc., 9700 Patent Woods Drive, Columbia, MD 21046; tel. 410/720-5800; FAX. 410/720-5860
Columbia Medical Plan, Inc., Two Knoll North Drive, Columbia, MD 21045; tel. 410/997-8500; FAX. 410/964-4563; Marilyn M. Levinson, Director, Patient Services
Delmarva Health Care Plan, 106 Marlboro Road, P.O. Box 2410, Easton, MD 21601; tel. 410/822-7223; FAX. 410/822-8152; Richard Moore, President
Free State Health Plan, Inc., 100 South Charles Street, Tower II, Baltimore, MD 21201; tel. 410/528-7000
George Washington University Health Plan, Inc., 4550 Montgomery Avenue, Suite 800, Bethesda, MD 20814; tel. 301/941-2000; FAX. 301/941-2005; Dr. John E. Ott, Executive Director, Chief Executive Officer
George Washington University Health Plan, Inc., 4550 Montgomery Avenue, Suite 800, Bethesda, MD 20814; tel. 301/941-2000; FAX. 301/941-200; Stanley Aronoritch, President and CEO
Healthcare Corporation of Mid-Atlantic, 100 South Charles Street, Baltimore, MD 21201; tel. 301/828-7000; David D. Wolf, Chief Executive Officer
Healthcare Corporation of the Potomac, Inc., Care First-Free State Potomac, Equitable Bank Center's Tower-II, 100 South Charles Street, Baltimore, MD 21201; tel. 410/528-7025; FAX. 410/528-7013; David Wolf, President
HealthPlus, Inc., NYLCare Health Plans of the Mid-Atlantic, Inc., 7601 Ora Glen Drive, Suite 200, Greenbelt, MD 20770-3641; tel. 301/441-1600; FAX. 301/489-5282; Jeff D. Emerson, President and CEO
Kaiser Foundation Health Plan of the Mid-Atlantic States, 2101 East Jefferson Street, Box 6611, Rockville, MD 20849-6611; tel. 301/468-6000; FAX. 301/816-2424; James Novell, President
M.D. Individual Practice Association, Inc., Four Taft Court, Rockville, MD 20850; tel. 800/544-2853; Susan Goff, President
MAMSI, Four Taft Court, Rockville, MD 20850; tel. 301/294-5100; FAX. 301/309-1709; Thomas P. Barbera, President and CEO
MD Individual Practice Association, Inc, MDIPA/Optimum, Four Taft Court, Rockville, MD 20850; tel. 301/762-8205; FAX. 301/738-1230; Mark D. Groban, M.D., President and CEO
MD-Individual Practice Association, Inc., Four Taft Court, Rockville, MD 20850; tel. 301/294-5100; FAX. 301/309-1709; Susan Goff, President
NYL Care Health Plans of the Mid-Atlantic, Inc., 7601 Ora Glen Drive, Suite 200, Greenbelt, MD 20770; tel. 301/982-0098; FAX. 301/489-5282; Jeff D. Emerson, President and CEO
NYLCare Health Plans of Mid-Atlantic, Inc., 7601 Ora Glen Drive, Suite 200, Greenbelt, MD 20770; tel. 301/982-0098; FAX. 301/489-5282; Jeff D. Emerson, President and CEO
Optimum Choice Inc., Four Taft Court, Rockville, MD 20850; tel. 301/762-8205; Judy Graham, VP, Human Resources
Optimum Choice, Inc., Four Taft Court, Rockville, MD 20850; tel. 301/762-8205
PrimeHealth Corporation, 9602 C Martin Luther King, Jr. Highway, Lanham, MD 20706; Edward L. Mosley, Jr., President
Prudential Health Care Plan, Inc., Seton Court, 2800 North Charles Street, Baltimore, MD 21218; tel. 410/554-7000; FAX. 410/554-7077
Spectera Dental Services, Inc., (formerly United Dental Services), 2811 Lord Baltimore Drive, Baltimore, MD 21244-2644; tel. 410/265-6033; Oscar B. Camp, President
Spectera, Inc., 2811 Lord Baltimore Drive, Baltimore, MD 21244; tel. 410/265-6033; FAX. 410/944-5903; Sue Cox, Vice President, Marketing
Total Health Care, Inc., 2305 North Charles Street, Baltimore, MD 21218; tel. 410/383-8300; FAX. 410/554-9012; Edwin R. Golden, President

MASSACHUSETTS
Central Massachusetts Health Care, Mechanics Tower, 100 Front Street, Suite 300, Worcester, MA 01608; tel. 508/798-8667; FAX. 508/798-4197; Brian D. Wells, Chief Executive Officer
CIGNA HealthCare of Massachusetts, Inc., Three Newton Executive Park, 2223 Washington Street, Newton, MA 02162; tel. 800/345-9458
Fallon Community Health Plan, One Chestnut Place, 10 Chestnut Street, Worcester, MA 01608; tel. 508/799-2100; FAX. 508/831-0921; Gary J. Zelch, Executive Director
Harvard Community Health Plan, Inc., 10 Brookline Place West, Brookline, MA 02146; tel. 617/421-6400; Laura Peabody, Assistant General Counsel

Providers / Health Maintenance Organizations

Harvard Pilgrim Health Care, Inc., 10 Brookline Place West, Brookline, MA 02445; tel. 617/730-4612; FAX. 617/730-4765; Allan Greenberg, President and CEO
Health New England, One Monarch Place, Springfield, MA 01144; tel. 413/787-4000; FAX. 413/734-3356; Phil M. Pin, Interim President
Healthsource Massachusetts, Inc., (d/b/a Healthsource CMHC), 100 Front Street, Worcester, MA 01608-1449; tel. 800/922-8380
HMO Blue, 100 Summer Street, Boston, MA 02110; tel. 617/832-7808; FAX. 617/832-7758; Alan Rosenberg, Vice President, Marketing
Neighborhood Health Plan, 253 Summer Street, Boston, MA 02210; tel. 617/772-5500; FAX. 617/772-5513; James Hooley, President & CEO
One Health Plan of Massachusetts, Inc., One University Office Park, 29 Sawyer Road, 3rd Floor, Waltham, MA 02453; tel. 800/725-0748; FAX. 781/788-9366; Melinda Caggiano, Administrative Assistant
Pilgrim Health Care Inc., 1200 Crown Colony Drive, Quincy, MA 02169; tel. 800/742-8326
Tufts Associated Health Maintenance Organization, Inc., 333 Wyman Street, P.O. Box 9112, Waltham, MA 02254-9112; tel. 617/466-9400
Tufts Health Plan, 333 Wyman Street, P.O. Box 9112, Waltham, MA 02454; tel. 617/466-9400; FAX. 617/466-9430; Harris A. Berman, M.D., CEO
Tufts Health Plan of New England, Inc., 333 Wyman Street, Waltham, MA 02254-9112; tel. 617/466-9055; Theresa Gallinaro, Manager
Tufts Health Plan of New England, Inc., 333 Wyman Street, P.O. Box 9112, Waltham, MA 02254-9112; tel. 800/442-0422

MICHIGAN
Blue Care Network of East Michigan, 4200 Fashion Square Boulevard, Saginaw, MI 48603; tel. 517/249-3200; FAX. 517/249-3730; Arnold C. DuFort, President and CEO
Blue Care Network of Southeast Michigan, 25925 Telegraph, P.O. Box 5043, Southfield, MI 48086-5043; tel. 313/354-7450; FAX. 313/799-6970; David H. Smith, President and CEO
Blue Care Network–Great Lakes, 1769 South Garfield Avenue, Suite B, Traverse City, MI 49684; tel. 616/941-6000; FAX. 616/941-6012; Sharon Carlin, Regional Director
Blue Care Network–Great Lakes, 3624 South Westnedge, Kalamazoo, MI 49008; tel. 616/388-9500; FAX. 616/388-5156; Marcia Lallaman, Regional Manager
Blue Care Network–Great Lakes, 611 Cascade West Parkway, S.E., Grand Rapids, MI 49546; tel. 616/957-5057; FAX. 616/956-5866; Sharon Carlin, President and CEO
Blue Care Network–Health Central, 1403 South Creyts Road, Lansing, MI 48917; tel. 517/322-8000; FAX. 517/322-8015; Arnold C. DuFort, President and CEO
Care Choices HMO, 34605 Twelve Mile Road, Farmington Hi, MI 48331; tel. 810/489-6200
Care Choices–Grand Rapids, 1500 East Beltline S.E., Suite 300, Grand Rapids, MI 49506; tel. 616/285-3801; FAX. 616/285-3810; Janie Begeman, Site Manager
Care Choices–Muskegon, 1560 East Sherman, 145, Muskegon, MI 49444; tel. 231/733-6734; FAX. 231/733-6739; Elyse Winter, Executive Director
Family Health Plan of Michigan, 901 North Macomb, Monroe, MI 48162-3048; tel. 313/457-5370; FAX. 313/457-5506; Robert Campbell, Executive Vice President
Grand Valley Health Plan, 829 Forest Hill Avenue, S.E., Grand Rapids, MI 49546; tel. 616/949-2410; FAX. 616/949-4978; Roland Palmer, President
Great Lakes Health Plan, Inc., 17117 West Nine Mile Road, Suite 1600, Southfield, MI 48075; tel. 810/559-5656; FAX. 810/559-4640; Donald A. Zinner, President
Health Alliance Plan, 2850 West Grand Boulevard, Detroit, MI 48202; tel. 313/664-8354; FAX. 313/664-8433; Joseph E. Schmitt, Chief Financial Officer
HealthPlus of Michigan, 2050 South Linden Road, P.O. Box 1700, Flint, MI 48501-1700; tel. 810/230-2000; FAX. 810/230-2208; Paul A. Fuhs, Ph.D., President and CEO
M–Care, 2301 Commonwealth Boulevard, Ann Arbor, MI 48105-1573; tel. 313/747-8700; FAX. 313/747-7152; Peter W. Roberts, President
Mercy Health Plans, 34605 W. 12 Mile Road, Farmington Hills, MI 48311; tel. 313/971-7667; FAX. 313/971-7455; Dennis Angellis, M.D., Chief Medical Director
MIDA Dental Plans, Inc., 2000 Town Center, Suite 2200, Southfield, MI 48075; tel. 810/353-6410; Walter Knysz, Jr., D.D.S., President
NorthMed HMO, 109 East Front Street, Suite 204, Traverse City, MI 49684; tel. 616/935-0500; FAX. 616/935-0505; Walter J. Hooper, III, President
OmniCare Health Plan, 1155 Brewery Park Boulevard, Suite 250, Detroit, MI 48207-2602; tel. 313/259-4000; FAX. 313/393-7944; Gregory H. Moses, Jr., President and CEO
Paramount Care of Michigan, Inc., 1339 North Telegraph Road, Monroe, MI 48162; tel. 313/241-5604; FAX. 313/241-5998; Robert J. Kolodgy, Vice President, Finance
PHP-Kalamazoo, 106 Farmers Alley, P.O. Box 50271, Kalamazoo, MI 49005; tel. 616/349-6692; FAX. 616/349-1476; Michael Koehler, Executive Director
Physicians Health Plan, P.O. Box 30377, Lansing, MI 48909-7877; tel. 517/349-2101; FAX. 517/347-9460; John G. Ruther, President and CEO
Physicians Health Plan of South Michigan, One Jackson Square, 8th Floor, Jackson, MI 49201; tel. 517/782-7154; FAX. 517/782-4512; Susan K. Sharkey, Chief Executive Officer
Physicians Health Plan–Muskegon, Terrace Plaza, 250 Morris Avenue, Suite 550, Muskegon, MI 49440-1143; tel. 616/728-3900; FAX. 616/728-5189; Ronald Franzese, Chief Executive Officer
Priority Health, 1231 East Beltline, Suite 300, Grand Rapids, MI 49505; tel. 616/942-0954; FAX. 616/942-0145; Olga Dazzo, President and CEO
Priority Health Managed Benefits, Inc., 1231 East Beltline, N.E., Grand Rapids, MI 49546; tel. 800/942-0954; FAX. 616/942-5651; Kimberly K. Horn, President and CEO
SelectCare HMO, Inc., 2401 West Big Beaver Road, Suite 700, Troy, MI 48084; tel. 248/637-5300; FAX. 248/637-6710; Roman T. Kulich, President and CEO
The Wellness Plan, 1060 West Norton Avenue, Suite Four B, Muskegon, MI 49442; tel. 616/780-4722; FAX. 616/780-3557; Evangeline Zimmerman, Health Systems Manager
The Wellness Plan, One East First Street, Genesse Tower, Suite 1620, Flint, MI 48502; tel. 810/767-7400; FAX. 810/767-6338; Sharon P. Matthews, Regional Administrator
The Wellness Plan, 320 North Washington Square, Lansing, MI 48933; tel. 517/484-1400; FAX. 517/484-8801; Mary Anne Sesti, Health Systems Manager
Total Health Care, Inc., 1600 Fisher Building, Detroit, MI 48202; tel. 313/871-2000; FAX. 313/871-6400; Kenneth G. Rimmer, Executive Director

MINNESOTA
Allina Health System, 5601 Smetana Drive, Minneapolis, MN 55440-9310; tel. 612/992-3840; FAX. 612/992-3990; James Ehlen, M.D., President
Blue Plus, P.O. Box 64179, St. Paul, MN 55164; tel. 651/662-2795; FAX. 651/662-6798; Colleen Reitan, President and CEO
First Plan HMO, 1010 Fourth Street, Two Harbors, MN 55616; tel. 218/834-7210; John Bjorum, Executive Director
HealthPartners, 8100-34th Avenue South, P.O. Box 1309, Minneapolis, MN 55440-1309; tel. 612/883-5382; FAX. 612/883-5120; George Halvorson, President, Chief Executive Director
Mayo Health Plan, 21 First Street S.W., Suite 401, Rochester, MN 55902; tel. 507/284-2919; FAX. 507/284-5811; Paula E. Mankosky, Executive Director
Medica Health Plans of Wisconsin, Inc., 5901 Smetana Drive, P.O. Box 9310, Minneapolis, MN 55440-9310; tel. 612/992-2000
Metropolitan Health Plan, 822 South Third Street, Suite 140, Minneapolis, MN 55415; tel. 612/347-8557; FAX. 612/904-4264; David R. Johnson, Chief Operating Officer
UCARE Minnesota, P.O. Box 52, Minneapolis, MN 55440-0052; tel. 612/676-6500; FAX. 612/676-6501; Nancy Feldman, Chief Executive Officer

MISSISSIPPI
American Medical Plans of Mississippi, Inc., 633 North State Street, Suite 211, Jackson, MS 39202; tel. 601/968-9000; FAX. 601/973-2015; Rissa P. Richardson, Director, Provider Relations
Canton Management Group, Inc., 3330 South Liberty Street, Suite 300, Canton, MS 39046; tel. 601/859-4450
Exchange HMO, Inc, 6425 Lakeover Road, Jackson, MS 39213; tel. 601/368-3230; FAX. 601/368-3200
Family Healthcare Plus, 4635 Highway 80 East, P.O. Box 54268, Pearl, MS 39288-4268; tel. 601/825-7280; FAX. 601/825-8130; Margaret A. Gray, DPA, President and CEO
Health Link, Inc., 830 South Gloster Street, Tupelo, MS 38801; tel. 800/453-7536; FAX. 800/453-0648; Pamela J. Hansen, Director
HMO of Mississippi, Inc., 3545 Lakeland Drive, Jackson, MS 39208; tel. 601/932-3704; FAX. 601/664-5084; Thomas C. Fenter, M.D., Executive Director
Integrity Health Plan of Mississippi, Inc., 6360 I-55 North, Suite 460, Suite 160, Jackson, MS 39211; tel. 601/977-0010; FAX. 601/977-1119; Robert S. Parenteau, Director, Marketing
Mississippi Managed Care Network, Inc., 713 South Pear Orchard Road, Suite B-102, Suite B 102, Ridgeland, MS 39157; tel. 601/977-9834; FAX. 601/977-9553; Jesse Buie, President
Mississippi Select Health Care, LLC, 14110 Airport Road, Suite 100, Gulfport, MS 39503; tel. 228/865-0514; FAX. 228/865-0550
Phoenix Healthcare of Mississippi, Inc., 795 Woodlands Parkway, Suite 200, Ridgeland, MS 39157; tel. 601/956-2706; FAX. 601/957-0847; Stephen G. Braden, Executive Director
PhysiciansPlus Baptist & St. Dominic, Inc, 969 Lakeland Drive, Jackson, MS 39216; tel. 601/364-6843; FAX. 601/364-6854; Frank A. Quiricon, Treasurer
United HealthCare of Mississippi, Inc., 795 Woodlands Parkway, Suite 101, Ridgeland, MS 39157; tel. 601/956-8030; FAX. 601/957-0847

MISSOURI
Alliance for Community Health, Inc., d/b/a Community CarePlans, 5615 Pershing, Suite 29, St. Louis, MO 63112; tel. 314/454-0055; FAX. 314/454-9595; Jerry Linder, Chief Executive Officer
Blue-Care, Inc., 2301 Main, Zip 64108-2428, P.O. Box 413163, Kansas City, MO 64141-6163; tel. 816/395-2222; Larry K. Chastain, President
BMA SelectCare, Inc., One Penn Valley Park, P.O. Box 419458, Kansas City, MO 64141; tel. 816/751-5336; FAX. 816/751-5571; Sara L. Adams, Vice President
Children's Mercy Family Plan, 2401 Gilham Road, Kansas City, MO 64108; tel. 816/234-3420; Judy Brooksher
Cigna HealthCare of St. Louis, Inc., 8182 Maryland Avenue, Suite 900, St. Louis, MO 63105; tel. 314/726-7841; FAX. 314/726-7819; James A. Young, General Manager
Citizens Advantage, P.O. Box 479, 1500 North Oakland, Bolivar, MO 65613; tel. 417/777-6000
Community Health Plan, 801 Faraon, St. Joseph, MO 64501; tel. 816/271-1247; FAX. 816/271-1248; Randa Anderson-Stice, Plan Administrator
Cox–Freeman HealthPlans, Inc., 1443 North Robberson, #800, Springfield, MO 65802; tel. 800/205-7665; FAX. 417/269-2925; Gary Jacobs, President
Family Health Partners, 215 West Pershing, 6th Floor, Kansas City, MO 64141; tel. 800/347-9363; FAX. 816/842-2326; Joseph R. Cecil, Executive Director
FirstGuard Health Plan, Inc., 3801 Blue Parkway, Kansas City, MO 64130; tel. 816/922-7250; FAX. 816/922-7205; Joy Wheeler, Executive Director and COO
Gencare Health Systems, Inc., P.O. Box 419079, St. Louis, MO 63141-9079; tel. 314/434-6114
Good Health HMO, Inc., d/b/a Blue–Care, Inc., One Pershing Square, 2301 Main Street, Kansas City, MO 64108; tel. 816/395-2222; FAX. 816/395-3811; Larry K. Chastain, President and COO
Group Health Plan, Inc., 940 West Port Plaza, Suite 300, St. Louis, MO 63146; tel. 314/453-1700; FAX. 314/453-0375; Richard H. Jones, President and CEO
Health Partners of the Midwest, 120 S. Central, Suite 900, St. Louis, MO 63105; tel. 314/505-5000; FAX. 314/725-4251; Dennis Matheis, President
Healthcare USA of Missouri LLC, 100 South Fourth Street, Suite 1100, St. Louis, MO 63102; tel. 800/213-7792; FAX. 314/241-8010; Claudia Bjerre, President and CEO
HealthFirst Health Management Organization, 1102 West 32nd Street, Joplin, MO 64804-3599

Providers / Health Maintenance Organizations

Healthlink HMO, Inc., 777 Craig Road, PO Box 410289, St. Louis, MO 63141; tel. 314/569-7200; FAX. 314/569-3268; Dennis McCart, Executive Director

HealthNet, Inc., 2300 Main Street, Suite 700, Kansas City, MO 64108-2415; tel. 816/221-8400; FAX. 816/221-7709; Beth Johnson, Executive Assistant

HMO Missouri (Bluechoice), 1831 Chestnut Street, P.O. Box 66828, St. Louis, MO 63166-6828; tel. 314/923-4444; FAX. 314/923-6618; John O'Rowrke, President and Chairman

Humana Health Plan, Inc., 10450 Holmes, Suite 200, Kansas City, MO 64131-3471; tel. 800/715-4862

Humana Kansas City, Inc., 10450 Holmes Road, Kansas City, MO 64131-3471; tel. 816/941-8900; FAX. 816/941-3910; David W. Fields, Executive Director

Medical Center Health Plan, d/b/a Partners HMO, 2 City Place Drive, Suite 330, St. Louis, MO 63141; tel. 314/567-6660; FAX. 314/567-3627; Robert Schering, General Manager

Mercy Health Plans of Missouri, Inc., 425 S. Woods Mill Road, Suite 100, Chesterfield, MO 63017-3441; tel. 314/214-8100; FAX. 314/214-8101; Thomas L. Kelly, President and CEO

Missouri Advantage LLC, 428 East Capital Avenue, 3rd Floor, Jefferson City, MO 65101; tel. 573/659-5200; FAX. 573/659-5222; Kevin G. McRoberts, Executive Director

Missouri Care, 2404 Forum Blvd., Columbia, MO 65203; tel. 573/441-2100; Donna Checkett

Physicians Health Plan of Greater St. Louis, Inc., 77 West Port Plaza, Suite 500, St. Louis, MO 63146; tel. 314/275-7000; FAX. 314/542-1155; Thomas Zorumski, President and CEO

Principal Health Care of Kansas City, Inc., 1001 East 101st Terrace, Suite 230, Kansas City, MO 64131; tel. 816/941-3030; FAX. 816/941-8516; Kenneth J. Linde, President

Principal Health Care of St. Louis, Inc., 12312 Olive Boulevard, Suite 150, St. Louis, MO 63141; tel. 314/434-6990; FAX. 314/434-7540; Barbara C. Buenemann, Executive Director

Prudential Health Care Plan, Inc., 4600 Madison Avenue, Suite 300, Kansas City, MO 64112; tel. 816/756-5588; FAX. 816/756-5667; David W. Dingley, Executive Director

Prudential Health Care Plan, Inc., 12312 Olive Boulevard, Suite 500, St. Louis, MO 63141; tel. 314/579-7718; Gary C. Hawkins, Vice President

TriSource HealthCare, Inc., d/b/a Blue Advantage, 2301 Main Street, P.O. Box 419130, Kansas City, MO 64141-6130; tel. 816/395-3636; FAX. 816/395-3811; Larry K. Chastain, President and CEO

Trucare, Inc., 2301 Holmes, Kansas City, MO 64108; tel. 816/556-3186; Joseph Cecil, President

Truman Medical Center, Inc., 2301 Holmes Street, Kansas City, MO 64108; tel. 816/556-3094; James J. Morgan, M.D., Executive Director

United Healthcare of the Midwest, 13655 Riverport Drive, Maryland Heights, MO 63043; tel. 314/434-6114; FAX. 314/592-7157; Vic Turvey, President and CEO

UnitedHealthcare of the Midwest, Inc, 13655 Riverport Drive, Maryland Heights, MO 63043; tel. 800/627-0687; FAX. 314/592-7560; Mary Nowotny, Director Corporate Communications

MONTANA

HMO Montana, 560 North Park, Helena, MT 59604; tel. 406/444-8540; FAX. 406/447-3570; Paul Pedersen, Manager

Yellowstone Community Health, 1233 North 30th Street #200, Billings, MT 59101; tel. 406/238-6868; FAX. 406/238-6898; Jennifer A. Parise, Marketing Director

NEBRASKA

Exclusive Healthcare, Inc., Mutual of Omaha Plaza, 10250 Regency Circle, Omaha, NE 68124-7012; tel. 402/255-1629; FAX. 402/255-1665; Grete Vaught, Chief Operating Officer

Exclusive Healthcare, Inc., Mutual of Omaha Plaza, Omaha, NE 68175; tel. 402/978-2869; FAX. 402/978-2999; Kurt Irlbeck, Administrative Services Coordinator

Exclusive Healthcare, Inc., Mutual of Omaha of South Dakota and Community Health Plus, HMO, Inc., 10250 Regency Circle, Omaha, NE 68124-7012; tel. 402/255-1662; FAX. 402/255-1665; Jacque Alt, Executive Director

Mutual of Omaha Health Plans of Lincoln, Inc., 220 South 17th Street, Lincoln, NE 68508; tel. 402/475-7000; FAX. 402/475-6005; Steve Burnham, Chief Operating Officer

Principal Health Care of Nebraska, Inc., 330 North 117th Street, Omaha, NE 68154-2595; tel. 402/333-1720; FAX. 402/333-1116; John Klaasmeyer, Executive Director

United Healthcare of Midlands, Inc., 2717 North 118th Circle, Omaha, NE 68164; tel. 402/445-5000; FAX. 402/445-5575; Pat Krueger, Marketing Coordinator

NEVADA

Amil International of Nevada, 1050 East Flamingo Road, Suite E-120, Las Vegas, NV 89119; tel. 702/693-5250; FAX. 702/693-5399; Jeff Allen, Director, Provider Relations Director

Health Plan of Nevada, Inc., 3016 W. Charleston, #100, Mailing Address: P.O. Box 15645, Las Vegas, NV 89102; tel. 702/242-7300; Donald J. Giancursio, VP, Sales and Marketing

HMO Colorado, Inc., d/b/a HMO Nevada, 6900 Westcliff Drive, Suite 600, Las Vegas, NV 89145; tel. 702/228-2583; FAX. 702/228-1259; Kevin R. Clark, Vice President, Sales and Marketing

Hometown Health Plan, Inc., 400 South Wells Avenue, Reno, NV 89502; tel. 702/325-3000; FAX. 702/325-3220; Ed Holme, Executive Director

St. Mary's HealthFirst, 5290 Neil Road, Reno, NV 89502; tel. 702/829-6000; FAX. 702/829-6010; Lin Howland, Executive Director

NEW HAMPSHIRE

CIGNA HealthCare/Healthsource New Hampshire, Two College Drive, P.O. Box 2041, Hooksett, NH 03106; tel. 603/268-7000; FAX. 603/268-7907; Brian D. Wells, Chief Executive Officer

Healthsource New Hampshire, Donovan Street Extension, P.O. Box 2041, Concord, NH 03302; tel. 603/225-5077; FAX. 603/225-7621; Susan Berry, Director, Marketing

HMO Blue, c/o Blue Cross Blue Shield of New Hampshire, 3000 Goffs Falls Road, Manchester, NH 03111-0001; tel. 800/621-3724

Matthew Thornton Health Plan, 3000 Goffs Falls Road, Manchester, NH 03111-0001; tel. 603/695-7000; FAX. 603/695-7304; David a Jensen, President and CEO

Matthew Thorton Health Plan, Inc., 43 Constitution Drive, Bedford, NH 03110; tel. 800/874-7122

Oxford Health Plans, 10 Tara Boulevard, Nashua, NH 03062; tel. 603/891-7000; FAX. 603/891-7015; Craig Tobin, Regional Chief Executive Officer

NEW JERSEY

Aetna Health Plans of New Jersey, 8000 Midlantic Drive, Suite 100 North, Mount Laurel, NJ 08054; tel. 609/866-7880; Dennis Allen, Medical Director

AltantiCare Health Plans, 6727 Delilah Road, Egg Harbor To, NJ 08234; tel. 609/272-6330; FAX. 609/407-7770; Patricia Koelling, Chief Executive Officer

American Preferred Provider Plan, Inc., 810 Broad Street, Newark, NJ 07102; tel. 201/799-0900; FAX. 201/799-0911; Harold E. Smith, President and CEO

Amerihealth Insurance Company, 8000 Midlantic Drive, Suite 333, Mount Laurel, NJ 08054; tel. 856/778-6500; FAX. 856/802-3110; Richard J. Gilfillan, M.D., General Manager

Community Healthcare Plan, 309 Market Street, Camden, NJ 08102; tel. 609/541-7526; FAX. 609/635-9328; Mark R. Bryant, President

First Option Health Plan, The Galleria, Two Bridge Avenue, Building Six, Second Floor, Red Bank, NJ 07701-1106; tel. 908/842-5000; Donald Paris, Senior Vice President, Secretary, General

Garden State Health Plan, CN-712, Trenton, NJ 08625-0712; tel. 800/525-0047; FAX. 609/588-4643; Beverly Blacher, EIDG, Chief Executive Officer

HIP Health Plan of New Jersey, One HIP Plaza, North Brunswig, NJ 08902; tel. 908/937-7600; FAX. 908/937-7870; Victoria A. Wicks, President and CEO

HMO New Jersey, U.S. HealthCare, 55 Lane Road, Fairfield, NJ 07004; tel. 201/575-5600; Andrew Schuyler, M.D., Medical Director

Horizon HMO, Three Penn Plaza East, Newark, NJ 07105-2000; tel. 973/466-4000; FAX. 973/466-8288; Christy W. Bell, SVP, HCM

Liberty Health Plan, 115 Christopher Columbus Drive, Jersey City, NJ 07302; tel. 201/946-6800; FAX. 201/946-1740; Donald L. Picuri, Senior Vice President and COO

Managed Health Care Systems of New Jersey, Inc., Two Gateway Center, Newark, NJ 07102; tel. 973/297-5500; Thelma Duggin, CEO

One Health Plan of New Jersey, Inc, One Centennial Avenue, Piscataway, NJ 08855; tel. 732/980-8570; Daniel Dragalin, M.D., CEO

Physician Health Services of New Jersey, Inc., Mack Centre IV, South 61 Paramus Road, Paramus, NJ 07652; tel. 201/291-9300; Ronald L. Helm, Executive Director

PruCare of New Jersey, (Northern Division), 200 Wood Avenue, S., Iselin, NJ 08830; tel. 908/632-7333; FAX. 908/494-8207; Paul Conlin, Vice President, Group Operations

Qualcare, 242 Old New Brunswick Road, Piscataway, NJ 08854; Annette Catino, CEO

University Health Plan, Inc, 60 Park Place, 15th Floor, Newark, NJ 07102; tel. 973/623-8700; FAX. 973/623-3635; Alexander McLean, President and CEO

NEW MEXICO

HMO New Mexico, 12800 Indian School Road, N.E., Zip 87112, P.O. Box 11968, Albuquerque, NM 87192; tel. 505/271-4441; FAX. 505/237-5324; Blair Christensen, President

Lovelace, Inc., P.O. Box 27107, Albuquerque, NM 87125-7107; tel. 505/262-7363; Derick Pasternak, M.D., President

Presbyterian Health Plan, d/b/a FHP of El Paso, 2501 Buena Vista Drive, SE, Albuquerque, NM 87100; tel. 505/881-7900; FAX. 505/923-5585; Mark Zobel, Regional Compliance Officer

Qual-Med, Inc.-New Mexico Health Plan, 6100 Uptown Boulevard, N.E., Suite 400, Albuquerque, NM 87110; tel. 505/889-8800; FAX. 505/889-8819; Michael J. Mayer, President

NEW YORK

ABC Health Plan, Inc., 16 East 16th Street, New York, NY 10003; tel. 212/633-0815; FAX. 212/627-2958; Audrey Brahamsha, Executive Director

Aetna Health Plans of New York, Inc., 2700 Westchester Avenue, Purchase, NY 10577; tel. 914/251-0600; FAX. 914/251-0260; Paula Adderson, President

Better Health Plan, Inc., 120 Pineview Drive, Amherst, NY 14228; tel. 518/482-1200; Daniel Tillotson, Chief Executive Officer

Blue Cross and Blue Shield of Western New York, Community Blue, 1901 Main Street, P.O. Box 159, Buffalo, NY 14240-0159; tel. 716/887-8874; FAX. 716/887-7911; Nora K. McGuire, Executive Director

Capital Area Community Health Plan, Inc., 1201 Troy-Schenectady Road, Latham, NY 12110; tel. 518/783-1864; FAX. 518/783-0234; John Baackes, President and CEO

Capital District Physicians Health Plan, 17 Columbia Circle, Albany, NY 12203; tel. 518/862-3700; FAX. 516/218-6396; Richard A. Kramer, Director, Accounting

Capital District Physicians' Health Plan, Inc., 17 Columbia Circle, Albany, NY 12203; tel. 518/862-3700; FAX. 518/452-0003; Diane E. Bergman, President and CEO

CenterCare, Inc., 555 West 57th Street, 18th Floor, New York, NY 10019-2925; tel. 212/293-9200; FAX. 212/293-9298; Julio Bellber, President and Chief Operating Officer

CIGNA HealthCare of New York, Inc., 195 Broadway, Eighth Floor, New York, NY 10007; tel. 212/618-4200; FAX. 212/618-4258; Tom Garvey, Assistant Vice President, Network Management

Community Choice Health Plan of Westchester, Inc., 35 East Grassy Sprain Road, Suite 300, Yonkers, NY 10710; tel. 914/337-6908; FAX. 914/337-6919; Lynda G. Gray, Chief Executive Officer

Community Health Plan (CHP), 1201 Troy-Schenectady Road, Latham, NY 12110; tel. 518/783-1864; FAX. 518/783-0234; John Baackes, President and CEO

Community Premier Plus, Inc., 534 W. 135th Street, New York, NY 10031; tel. 212/491-2333; FAX. 212/491-2315; Harris Lampert, M.D., President and CEO

Elderplan, Inc., 6323 Seventh Avenue, Brooklyn, NY 11220; tel. 718/921-7990; FAX. 718/921-7962; Eli S. Feldman, President and CEO

Empire Health Choice, Inc., One World Trade Center, New York, NY 10017-0682; tel. 800/453-0113; Michael Stocker, M.D., Chief Executive Officer

Providers / Health Maintenance Organizations

Finger Lakes Blue Cross/Blue Shield, Blue Choice, 150 East Main Street, Rochester, NY 14647; tel. 716/454–1700; FAX. 716/238–4526; Richard D. Dent, M.D., Senior Vice President, Managed Care
GENESIS Healthplan, Inc., One Executive Boulevard, Second Floor, Yonkers, NY 10701; tel. 914/476–6000; FAX. 914/476–0762; Maura Bluestone, President and CEO
Health Insurance Plan of Greater New York (HIP), Seven West 34th Street, New York, NY 10001; tel. 212/630–3440; FAX. 212/630–8290; Daniel T. McGowan, President and COO
Health Services Medical Corporation of Central New York, Inc., a/k/a Prepaid Health Plan (PHP) in Syracuse, NY, PHP/SDMN, 8278 Willett Parkway, Baldwinsville, NY 13027; tel. 315/638–2133; FAX. 315/638–0985; Frederick F. Yanni, Jr., President and CEO
HealthFirst PHSP, Inc., 25 Broadway, Ninth Floor, New York, NY 10004; tel. 212/801–6000; FAX. 212/801–1799; Paul Dickstein, Chief Executive Officer
HealthPlus, Inc., 5800 Third Avenue, Brooklyn, NY 11220; tel. 718/745–0030; FAX. 718–745–1180; Thomas Early, Chief Executive Officer
HMO–CNY, Inc., 344 South Warren Street, P.O. Box 4809, Syracuse, NY 13221; tel. 315/448–4931; FAX. 315/448–6802; Ralph Carelli, Jr., Senior Vice President
Independent Health, 511 Farber Lakes Drive, Buffalo, NY 14221; tel. 716/631–3001; FAX. 716/635–3838; Frank Colantuono, President and CEO
Kaiser Foundation Health Plan of New York, 210 Westchester Avenue, White Plains, NY 10604; tel. 914/682–6401; FAX. 914/682–6403; Maura Carley, New York Area Operations Manager
MagnaHealth, 100 Garden City Plaza, Garden City, NY 11530; tel. 516/294–0700; Anthony Bacchi, Chief Executive Officer
Managed Healthcare Systems of New York, Inc., Seven Hanover Square, Fifth Floor, New York, NY 10004; tel. 212/509–5999; FAX. 212/509–1929; Karen Clark, Chief Executive Officer
MDNY Healthcare, 1 Huntington Quadrangle, Suite 4C01, Melville, NY 11747; tel. 516/454–1900; FAX. 516/396–8169; Richard Radoccia, Chief Executive Officer
Metrahealth Care Plan of Upstate New York, Two Penn Plaza, Suite 700, New York, NY 10121; tel. 212/216–6591; James T. Kerr, Chief Executive Officer
Metroplus Health Plan, 11 West 42nd Street, Second Floor, New York, NY 10036; tel. 212/597–8600; FAX. 212/597–8666; Denice F. Davis, J.D., Executive Director
Mohawk Valley Physicians Health Plan, 111 Liberty Street, Schenectady, NY 12305; tel. 518/370–4793; David Oliker, Chief Executive Officer
MVP Health Plan, 111 Liberty Street, P.O. Box 2207, Schenectady, NY 12301–2207; tel. 518/370–4793; David W. Oliker, President
Neighborhood Health Providers, 521 5th Avenue, 3rd Floor, New York, NY 10017; tel. 212/808–4775; FAX. 212/808–4772; Steven Bory, President and CEO
New York Hospital Community Health Plan, 333 East 38th Street, New York, NY 10016; tel. 212/297–5547; FAX. 212/297–5923; Rosaire McDonald, Chief Executive Officer
North Medical Community Health Plan, Inc., 5112 West Taft Road, Suite R, Liverpool, NY 13088; tel. 315/452–2500; James Butler, Chief Executive Officer
Physicians Health Services of New York, Inc., Crosswest Office Center, 399 Knollwood Road, Suite 220, White Plains, NY 10603; tel. 914/682–8006; FAX. 914/682–5692; Ronald L. Helm, Executive Director
Prudential HealthCare, Prudential Healthcare Building, Suite 300, Suffern, NY 10901; tel. 914/368–4497; Dennis Ashley, Site Manager
Rochester Area HMO, Inc., d/b/a Preferred Care, 259 Monroe Avenue, Suite A, Rochester, NY 14607; tel. 716/325–3920; FAX. 716/325–3122; John Urban, President
SCHC Total Care, Inc., 819 South Salina Street, Syracuse, NY 13202; tel. 315/476–7921; FAX. 315/475–4713; Ruben Cowart, D.D.S., Chief Executive Officer
Signa Healthcare of New York, Inc., P.O. Box 1498, Syracuse, NY 13201–1498; tel. 315/449–1100; FAX. 315/449–2200; Ron Harms, Chief Executive Officer

St. Barnabas Community Health Plan, d/b/a Partners in Health, 2595 Webster Avenue, Bronx, NY 10458; tel. 718/960–9476; FAX. 718/960–3652; Arlene Ortiz–Allende, Associate Executive Director
Suffolk Health Plan, 225 Rabro Drive, E., Happauge, NY 11788–4290; tel. 877/747–6789; Clare B. Bradley, M.D., MPH, Chief Executive Officer
The Bronx Health Plan, One Fordham Plaza, Bronx, NY 10458; tel. 718/817–6670; FAX. 718/817–6893; Maura Bluestone, Chief Executive Officer
U.S. Healthcare, Inc., Nassau Omni West, 333 Earle Ovington Boulevard, Uniondale, NY 11553; tel. 516/794–6565; Michael A. Stocker, M.D., President
United Healthcare of Upstate NY, 5015 CampusWood Drive, Suite 303, East Syracuse, NY 13057; tel. 315/433–5700; FAX. 315/433–5826; Jay Fischer, Director
United HealthCare Plan of NY, Inc., United HealthCare Plan of NJ, Two Penn Plaza, Suite 700, New York, NY 10121; tel. 212/216–6401; FAX. 212/216–6595
Univera Healthcare, Guaranty Building, 28 Church Street, Room 100, Buffalo, NY 14202; tel. 716/847–1480; FAX. 716/847–1817; Arthur R. Goshin, M.D., Plan President and CEO
Utica–Watertown Health Insurance Co., Inc., The Utica Business Park, 12 Rhoads Drive, Utica, NY 13502; tel. 315/798–4358; FAX. 315/797–4298; Thomas Flannery, M.D.
Vytra Health Plans, Corporate Center, 395 North Service Road, Melville, NY 11747–3127; tel. 516/694–4000; FAX. 516/694–5780; David S. Reynolds, Ph.D., President
WellCare of New York, Inc., P.O. Box 4800, Park West/Hurley Avenue Ext., Kingston, NY 12402; tel. 914/334–7185; FAX. 914/338–0566; Darcy Shepard, Vice President
Westchester Prepaid Health Services Plan, Inc., d/b/a HealthSource and Hudson Health Plan, 303 South Broadway, Suite 321, Tarrytown, NY 10591; tel. 914/631–1611; FAX. 914/631–1615; Georganne Chapin, Chief Executive Officer

NORTH CAROLINA
Aetna U.S. Healthcare of the Carolinas, Inc., 201 S. College Street, Suite 1010, Charlotte, NC 28244–0002; tel. 704/559–7250; Michael J. Cardillo, President
Association of Eye Care Centers Total Vision Health Plan, Inc., P.O. Box 7185, 110 Zebulon Court, Rocky Mount, NC 27804; tel. 919/937–6650; FAX. 919/451–2182; Samuel B. Petteway, Jr., President
Blue Cross Blue Shield of North Carolina, P.O. Box 2291, Durham, NC 27702; tel. 919/765–2400; Ken Otis, II, President
Carolina Summit Healthcare, Inc., 2100 Stantonsburg Rd., Greenville, NC 27835; tel. 919/816–6751; William Bull
CIGNA Health Plan of North Carolina, Inc., P.O. Box 470068, Charlotte, NC 28247; tel. 704/544–4350; FAX. 704/544–4375; Joseph L. Murgo
CIGNA Healthcare of North Carolina, 701 Corporate Center Dr., Raleigh, NC 27604; tel. 919/460–1610; Barry Martins
Community Choice of North Carolina, Inc., 100 North Green Street, Greensboro, NC 27401; tel. 910/691–3001; Randolph Ferguson
Coventry Health Care of the Carolinas, Inc., Six Coliseum Center, 2815 Coliseum Cintre Drive, Suite 550, Charlotte, NC 28217; tel. 704/357–1421; FAX. 704/357–3164; Stephen H. Nolte, CEO
Doctors Health Plan of North Carolina, Inc., 2828 Croasdaile Drive, Box 15309, Durham, NC 27704; tel. 919/383–4175; FAX. 919/383–3286; Bertram E. Walls, M.D., President and CEO
Generations Family Health Plan, Inc., 6330 Quadrangle Dr., Suite 100, Chapel Hill, NC 27514; tel. 919/490–0102; FAX. 919/490–1790; John C. Hays, President and CEO
Healthsource North Carolina, Inc., 701 Corporate Center Drive, Raleigh, NC 27607; tel. 919/854–7000; FAX. 919/854–7102; Steve White, GM and President
Kanawha HealthCare, Inc., 4609 Old Course Drive, Charlotte, NC 28277; tel. 704/333–8810; James L. Tillotson
Maxicare North Carolina, Inc., 5550 77 Center Drive, Suite 380, Charlotte, NC 28217–0700; tel. 704/525–0880; FAX. 704/529–0382; Peter J. Ratican

Optimum Choice of the Carolinas, Inc., 4600 Marriott Drive, Suite 300, Raleigh, NC 27612; tel. 800/469–8470; FAX. 919/788–1486; Jim Bendel, Regional Vice–President
Partners National Health Plans of NC, Inc., 2085 Frontis Plaza Boulevard, Winston–Salem, NC 27103; tel. 336/760–4822; FAX. 336/760–6218; Cosby M. Davis, III, Chief Financial Officer
PARTNERS National Health Plans of North Carolina, Inc., 2085 Frontis Plaza Boulevard, P.O. Box 24907, Winston–Salem, NC 27114–4907; tel. 336–760–4822; FAX. 336–760–3198; John W. Jones, President
Personal Care Plan of North Carolina, Inc., P.O. Box 2291, Durham, NC 27702; tel. 919/489–7431; Kenneth C. Otis, II
Principal Health Care of the Carolinas, Inc., 2300 Yorkmont Road, Suite 710, Charlotte, NC 28217; tel. 704/357–1421; Kenneth J. Linde, President
Prudential Health Care Plan, Inc., 2701 Coltsgate Road, Suite 300, Charlotte, NC 28211; tel. 704/365–6070; FAX. 704/365–9959; Tracey Baker, Executive Director
QualChoice of North Carolina, Inc., P.O. Box 340, Winston–Salem, NC 27102–0340; tel. 336/716–0900; FAX. 336/716–1090; David Patterson, President and CEO
The Wellness Plan of North Carolina, Inc., P.O. Box 12980, Charlotte, NC 28220–2980; tel. 704/944–3700; FAX. 704/944–3900; Timothy O'Brien, Chief Executive Officer
UnitedHealthcare of North Carolina, Northwestern Plaza, 2307 West Cone Boulevard, Greensboro, NC 27408; tel. 336/282–0900; FAX. 336/545–5099; Frank R. Mascia, President and CEO
WellPath Select, Inc., 6330 Quadrangle Drive, Suite 500, Chapel Hill, NC 27514; tel. 919/493–1210; FAX. 919/419–3872; Anna M. Lore, President and CEO

NORTH DAKOTA
Altru Health Plan, 1000 South Columbia Road, Grand Forks, ND 58201; tel. 701/780–1600; FAX. 701/780–1683; Raymond Kuntz
Heart of America HMO, 800 South Main, Rugby, ND 58368; tel. 701/776–5848; FAX. 701/776–5425; Ingvald Teigen, Executive Director

OHIO
Aetna U.S. Healthcare, Inc., 4059 Kinross Lakes Parkway, Richfield, OH 44286–5009; tel. 800/233–9747; FAX. 330/659–8035; Sheldon Orkin, General Manager
Aultcare HMO, 2600 Sixth Street, S.W., Canton, OH 44710; tel. 330/438–6388; FAX. 330/438–2911; Brenda Lehmiller, Vice President, Managed Care
Bethesda Managed Care, Inc., 619 Oak Street, Cincinnati, OH 45206; tel. 513/569–6597; FAX. 513/569–6233; Richard Smith, M.D., Medical Director
ChoiceCare, 655 Eden Park Drive, Cincinnati, OH 45202; tel. 513/784–5200; FAX. 513/784–5300; Robert W. Quirk, Dir. of Legislative & Regulatory Affairs
ChoiceCare Health Plans, Inc., 655 Eden Park Drive, Cincinnati, OH 45202; tel. 513/784–5200; FAX. 513/784–5300; Daniel A. Gregorie, M.D., Chief Executive Officer
CIGNA HealthCare of Ohio, Inc., 3700 Corporate Drive, Suite 200, Business Campus N.E. # Five, Columbus, OH 43231; tel. 614/823–7500; FAX. 614/823–7519; Elmond A. Kenyon, President
Community Health Plan of Ohio, 1915 Tamarack Road, Newark, OH 43055–1841; tel. 614/348–1400; FAX. 614/348–1500; Robert R. Kamps, M.D., President and CEO
Day-Med Health Maintenance Plan, 9797 Springboro Pike, Suite 200, Miamisburg, OH 45342; tel. 937/847–5646; FAX. 937/847–5620; Jeanette Prear, President and CEO
Dayton Area Health Plan, One Dayton Centre, One South Main Street, Dayton, OH 45402–9794; tel. 937/224–3300; FAX. 937/224–3388; Pamela B. Morris, President and CEO
Dental Care Plus, Inc., 4500 Lake Forest Drive, Suite 512, Cincinnati, OH 45242; tel. 513/554–1100; FAX. 513/554–3187; John W. O'Neil, President and Chief Operating Officer
Emerald HMO, Inc., Diamond Building, 100 Superior Avenue, 16th Floor, Cleveland, OH 44114–2591; tel. 216/479–2030; FAX. 216/241–4158; Susan M. Simpson, President
Family Health Plan, Inc., 2200 Jefferson Ave., 6th Floor, Toledo, OH 43624; tel. 419/241–6501; FAX. 419/241–5441; Thomas Beaty, Jr., President and CEO

Providers / Health Maintenance Organizations

Genesis Health Plan of Ohio, Inc., Two Summit Park Drive, Suite 340, Cleveland, OH 44131; tel. 216/642-3344; FAX. 216/901-4856; James Hayden, Executive Director

Health Guard, d/b/a Advantage Health Plan, 3000 Guernsey Street, Bellaire, OH 43906-1598; tel. 614/676-4623; Daniel Splain, President

Health Power HMO, Inc., 560 East Town Street, Columbus, OH 43215-0346; tel. 614/461-9900; FAX. 614/461-0960; Thomas Beaty, Jr., President

HealthFirst, 278 Barks Road West, Marion, OH 43301-1820; tel. 740/387-6355; FAX. 740/383-3840; N. Robert Jones, President and CEO

HealthPledge, a product of OhioHealth Group HMO, Inc., 300 East Wilson Bridge Road, Suite 200, Worthington, OH 43085-2339; tel. 614/566-0111; FAX. 614/566-0403; Colleen M. Tincher, Vice President of Operations

HMO Health Ohio, 2060 East Ninth Street, Cleveland, OH 44115-1355; tel. 216/687-6514; FAX. 216/687-7632; Paula Sauer, R.N., MBA, Care Management

HomeTown Health Plan, 100 Lillian Gish Boulevard, Suite 301, Massillon, OH 44647; tel. 330/837-6880; FAX. 330/837-6869; William C. Epling, Vice President, Chief Operating Officer

John Alden Health Systems, Inc., 5500 Glendon Court, Dublin, OH 43017; tel. 614/798-2930; William F. Sterling, Vice President, Senior Associate

Kaiser Permanente, North Point Tower, 1001 Lakeside Avenue, Suite 1200, Cleveland, OH 44114-1153; tel. 216/479-5251; FAX. 216/623-8776; Jeffrey Werner, Vice President, Marketing

Medical Value Plan, 405 Madison Avenue, P.O. Box 2147, Toledo, OH 43604; tel. 419/245-5165; Hal A. White, M.D., Medical Director

Medohio Health Plan, 445 E. Dublin-Granville Road, Building R, Worthington, OH 43085; tel. 614/293-6336; FAX. 614/293-9360; L.Kelley Millikin, Jr., President

Mount Carmel Health Plan, Inc., 495 Cooper Road, Suite 300, Westerville, OH 43081; tel. 614/898-8750; FAX. 614/898-8960; Mark Richardson, President

Nationwide Health Plans, Inc., 5525 Parkcenter Circle, Dublin, OH 43017-3584; tel. 800/940-3553; FAX. 614/854-3376; Mike Medwid, Sales Manager

OhioHealth Group HMO, Inc., 300 East Wilson Bridge Road, Suite 200, Worthington, OH 43085-2339; tel. 614/566-0111; FAX. 614/566-0400; John Laird, Chief Operating Officer

PacifiCare of Ohio, Inc., 11260 Chester Road, Suite 800, Cincinnati, OH 45246; tel. 513/772-7325; FAX. 513/772-1466; Brenda A. Pettit, Supervisor, Compliance

PacifiCare/FHP of Ohio, Spectrum Office Tower, 11260 Chester Road, Cincinnati, OH 45246-9928; tel. 513/772-7325; FAX. 513/772-1466; Thomas D. Anthony, President and CEO

Paramount Health Care, P.O. Box 928, Toledo, OH 43697-0928; tel. 419/887-2500; FAX. 419/887-2530; John C. Randolph, President

PrimeTime Health Plan, 2600 6th St. SW, Canton, OH 44710; tel. 330/438-6360; Chad Kibler

Prudential HealthCare, 312 Elm Street, Suite 1400, Cincinnati, OH 45202; tel. 513/784-7795; FAX. 513/784-7020; Kim Ballard, Executive Director

QualChoice HMO, 6000 Parkland Boulevard, Cleveland, OH 44124; tel. 440/460-4010; FAX. 440/460-4000; Gerard C. Bradford, Senior Vice President

SummaCare, Inc., 400 West Market Street, P.O. Box 3620, Akron, OH 44309-3620; tel. 330/996-8410; FAX. 330/996-8454; Martin P. Hauser, President

SuperMed HMO, 2060 East Ninth Street, Cleveland, OH 44115; tel. 216/6871951; FAX. 216/687-2622; Michael P. Walker, Director Contracting –Northern Region

The Health Plan, 52160 National Road, East, St. Clarksville, OH 43950-9365; tel. 614/695-3585; FAX. 740/695-5297; Philip D. Wright, President and COO

Total Health Care Plan, Inc., 12800 Shaker Boulevard, Cleveland, OH 44120; tel. 216/991-3000; FAX. 216/991-3011; Donald E. Butler, Acting Chief Executive Officer

United Healthcare of Ohio, Inc., 3650 Olentangy River Road, Columbus, OH 43216-1138; tel. 614/442-7160; Linda Cullen, Manager, Product Administration

United HealthCare of Ohio, Inc., 9200 Worthington Road, Westerfield, OH 43082-8823; tel. 614/410-1011; FAX. 614/410-7599; Robert J. Sheehy, President

VH Foundation, 1100 Dennison Avenue, Columbus, OH 43201; tel. 614/297-4870; Richard A. Mitchell, President

OKLAHOMA

DentiCare of Arkansas, Inc., Regional Administration Office, 7112 South Mingo, Suite 108, Tulsa, OK 74133; tel. 918/254-9055; FAX. 918/254-9076; John K. Wright, Secretary

GHS Health Maintenance Organization, Inc., d/b/a BlueLincs HMO, 1400 South Boston, Tulsa, OK 74119-3630; tel. 918/592-9414; FAX. 918/592-0611; Lyndle R. Ellis, Group Vice President

HealthCare Oklahoma, Inc., 3030 Northwest Expressway, Suite 140, Oklahoma City, OK 73112-4481; tel. 405/951-4700; FAX. 405/951-4701; Jon H. Friesen, President and CEO

PacifiCare of Oklahoma, 7666 East 61st Street, Tulsa, OK 74133-1112; tel. 918/459-1100; FAX. 918/459-1451; Laura Morrow, Vice President, Network Management

Prudential Health Care Plan, Inc., d/b/a Prudential Health Care HMO, 7912 East 31st Court, Tulsa, OK 74145; tel. 918/624-4600; FAX. 918/627-9759; Ann Paul, Executive Director

Prudential HealthCare Plan, Inc., 4005 Northwest Expressway, Suite 300, Oklahoma City, OK 73116; tel. 405/879-1780; James K. McNaughton, Executive Director

OREGON

Health Masters of Oregon, Inc., 201 High Street, S.E., Salem, OR 97301; tel. 503/225-6980; FAX. 503/779-3238; Judd Holtey, Chief Operating Officer, Southern Regional

HMO Oregon, Inc., P.O. Box 1271, Portland, OR 97207; tel. 503/364-4868; FAX. 503/588-4350; Donald P. Secco, President and CEO

Kaiser Foundation Health Plan of the Northwest, d/b/a Kaiser Permente, 500 Northeast Multnomah, Suite 100, Suite 100, Portland, OR 97232-2099; tel. 503/813-2800; FAX. 503/813-2283; Denise L. Honzel, Vice President

PACC, P.O. Box 286, Clackamas, OR 97015-0286; tel. 503/659-4212; FAX. 503/794-3409; Martin A. Preizler, President and CEO

PACC, d/b/a PACC Health Plans of Washington, 12901 Southeast 97th Avenue, P.O. Box 286, Clackamas, OR 97015-0286; tel. 503/659-4212; FAX. 503/786-5319; Ron Morgan

Pacificare of Oregon, Inc., Five Centerpointe Drive, Suite 600, Lake Oswego, OR 97035-8650; tel. 503/620-9324; FAX. 503/603-7377; Mary O. McWilliams, President

Providence Health Plans, l235 Northeast 47th Avenue, Suite 220, Portland, OR 97213; tel. 503/215-2981; FAX. 503/215-7655; Jack Friedman, Executive Director

Regence HMO Oregon, Inc, 200 SW Market Street, Portland, OR 97201; tel. 503/225-6980

PENNSYLVANIA

Aetna Health Plans of Central and Eastern Pennsylvania, Inc., 955 Chesterbrook Boulevard, Suite 200, Wayne, PA 19087; tel. 610/644-3800; FAX. 610/251-6441; Anthony Buividas, Chief Executive Officer

Alliance Health Network, 1700 Peach Street, Suite 244, Erie, PA 16501; tel. 814/878-1700; FAX. 814/878-1811; Steven H. Beloff, President and CEO

Central Medical Health Plan, d/b/a Advantage Health, 121 Seventh Avenue, Suite 500, Pittsburgh, PA 15222-3408; tel. 412/391-9300; FAX. 412/391-0457; Elizabeth Stolkowski, Executive Vice President, Chief

Geisinger Health Plan, Geisinger Office Building, 100 North Academy Avenue, Danville, PA 17822-3020; tel. 570/271-8777; FAX. 570/271-5268; Howard G. Hughes, M.D., Senior Vice President Health Plans

Health Partners of Philadelphia, 833 Chestnute Street, Suite 900, Philadelphia, PA 19107; tel. 215/849-9606; FAX. 215/991-4130; Vicki L. Sessoms, Vice President, Human Resources

HealthAmerica of Pennsylvania, Inc., Five Gateway Center, Pittsburgh, PA 15222; tel. 412/553-7300; FAX. 412/553-7384; Mike Blackwood, Chief Executive Officer

Healthcentral, Inc., 2605 Interstate Drive, Suite 140, Harrisburg, PA 17110; tel. 717/540-0033; FAX. 717/651-9165; Robert J. Dondes, President and CEO

HealthGuard of Lancaster, Inc., 280 Granite Run Drive, Suite 105, Lancaster, PA 17601-6810; tel. 717/560-9049; FAX. 717/581-4580; James R. Godfrey, President

HIP of Pennsylvania, d/b/a HIP Health Plan of Pennsylvania, Six Neshaminy Interplex, Suite 600, Trevose, PA 19053; tel. 215/633-7780; FAX. 215/633-8240

HMO of Northeastern Pennsylvania, d/b/a First Priority Health, 70 North Main Street, Wilkes-Barre, PA 18711; tel. 717/829-6035; FAX. 717/830-6176; Gerry Snyder, Public Relations Manager

Horizon Healthcare, 1700 Market Street, Suite 1050, Philadelphia, PA 19103; tel. 215/575-0530; FAX. 215-575-0537

Keystone Health Plan Central, Inc., 300 Corporate Center Drive, P.O. Box 898812, Camp Hill, PA 17089-8812; tel. 717/763-3458; FAX. 717/975-6895; Joseph M. Pfister, President and CEO

Keystone Health Plan East, Inc., 1901 Market Street, Philadelphia, PA 19101-7516; tel. 215/241-2001; John Daddis, Executive Vice President, COO

Keystone Health Plan West, Inc., Fifth Avenue Place, 120 Fifth Avenue, Suite 3116, Pittsburgh, PA 15222; tel. 412/255-7245; FAX. 412/255-7583; Kenneth R. Melani, M.D., President

NYLCare Health Plans of New Jersey, Inc., 530 East Swedesford Road, Suite 201, Wayne, PA 19087; tel. 610/971-0404; FAX. 610/971-0159; Peter Linder, Executive Director

Optimum Choice, Inc. of Pennsylvania, 1755 Oregon Pike, First Floor, Lancaster, PA 17601; tel. 800/474-6647; FAX. 717/581-3525; J. Steven Dufresne, President

Oxford Health Plans, The Curtis Center, 601 Walnut Street, Suite 900E, Philadelphia, PA 19106; tel. 215/625-8800; FAX. 215/625-5601; Michael C. Gaffney, Chief Executive Officer

Philcare Health Systems, Inc., 2005 Market Street, Suite 500, Philadelphia, PA 19103; tel. 800/371-6664; FAX. 215/564-4204; Mr. Gregory Moses, President

Prudential Health Care Plan, Inc., Prudential HealthCare, 220 Gibraltar Road, Suite 200, P.O. Box 901, Horsham, PA 19044-0901; tel. 215/672-1944; FAX. 215/442-2946; Brian J. Keane, Senior Director, Network Management, O

QualMed Plans for Health, Inc., 1835 Market Street, Ninth Floor, Philadelphia, PA 19103; tel. 215/209-6703; FAX. 215/209-6708; Francis A. Woodward, Director, Legal and Regulatory Affairs

Three Rivers Health Plans, Inc., 300 Oxford Drive, Monroeville, PA 15146; tel. 412/858-4000; FAX. 412/858-4060; Warren Carmichael, Chairman and CEO

U. S. Healthcare, Inc., 980 Jolly Road, P.O. Box 1109, Blue Bell, PA 19422; tel. 215/283-6656; Timothy Nolan, President

U.S. Healthcare, 980 Jolly Road, Blue Bell, PA 19422; tel. 215/628-4800; FAX. 215/283-6858

RHODE ISLAND

Blue Cross & Blue Shield of Rhode Island, 444 Westminster Street, Providence, RI 02903; tel. 401/459-1000; Ronald A. Battista, President

Coordinated Health Partners, Inc., d/b/a Blue Chip/Coordinated Health Partners, Inc., 15 LaSalle Square, Providence, RI 02903; tel. 800/528-4141; FAX. 401/459-5586; James Joy, Chief Financial Officer

Harvard Pilgrim Health Care of New England, One Hoppin Street, Providence, RI 02903-4199; tel. 401/331-3000; FAX. 401/331-0496; Stephen Schoenbaum, M.D., President

United Health Plans of NE, Inc., 475 Kilvert Street, Warwick, RI 02886-1392; tel. 800/447-1245; FAX. 401/732-7208; Robert K. Winston, Director, Corporate Communications

United Health Plans of New England, Inc., 475 Kilvert Street, Suite 310, Warwick, RI 02886-1392; tel. 401/737-6900; FAX. 401/737-6957; Max Powell, Chief Executive Officer

SOUTH CAROLINA

Carolina Care Health Plan, Inc., 111 Stonemark Lane, Suite 202, Columbia, SC 29210; tel. 803/551-5585; FAX. 813/265-6213; Laurie Burrell, Chief Operating Officer

Companion HealthCare Corporation, 200 Arbor Lake Drive, Suite 200, Columbia, SC 29223; tel. 803/786-8466; FAX. 803/754-0300; Harvey L. Galloway, Executive VP and COO

Providers / Health Maintenance Organizations

HealthFirst, Inc., Brookfield Corporate Center, 1041 E. Butler Road, Suite 2400, Greenville, SC 29607-5725; tel. 864/289-3080; FAX. 864/289-3100; Steve Meeker, Chief Financial Officer

Physicians Health Plan of South Carolina, Inc., 201 Executive Center Drive, Suite 300, Columbia, SC 29210-8438; tel. 803/750-7400; FAX. 803/750-7476; Ronald H. Haems, Chief Executive Officer

Preferred Health Systems, Inc., I-20 at Alpine Road, Columbus, SC 29219; tel. 803/788-0222; FAX. 803/736-2851; Gail Bragg, Senior Director

Select Health of South Carolina, Inc., 7410 Northside Drive, Suite 208, North Charles, SC 29420; tel. 803/569-1759; FAX. 803/569-0702; Michael Jernigan, President and CEO

SOUTH DAKOTA

Avera Health Plans, 610 West 23rd Suite 1, P.O. Box 38, Yankton, SD 57078; tel. 605/322-7050; FAX. 605/322-7054; Jean Reed

Mutual of Omaha of South Dakota and Community Health Plus HMO,, 3904 Technology Circle, Sioux Falls, SD 57106; tel. 605/361-9591; FAX. 605/361-9593; William P. Jetter, Executive Director

Sioux Valley Health Plan, 1200 North West Avenue, Sioux Falls, SD 57104; tel. 605/357-6868; FAX. 605/357-6811; Ryan Bohy, Director of Provider Services

South Dakota State Medical Holding Company, Inc., d/b/a Dakota Care, 1323 South Minnesota Avenue, Sioux Falls, SD 57105; tel. 605/334-4000; FAX. 605/336-0270; Robert D. Johnson Chief Executive Officer

Western Services HMO, 353 Fairmont Blvd, Rapid City, SD 57701; tel. 605/341-8302; FAX. 605/341-8053; Rick G. Stracqualursi, CEO

TENNESSEE

Aetna Health Plans of Tennessee, 1801 West End Avenue, Suite 500, Nashville, TN 37203; tel. 615/322-1600; FAX. 615/322-1217; David R. Field, President

Cigna Healthcare of Tennessee, Inc., 6555 Quince Road, Suite 215, Memphis, TN 38119; tel. 901/755-7411; David O. Hollis, M.D., Medical Director

Community Health Plan of Chattanooga, Inc., d/b/a Wellport Health Plan, Franklin Building, Suite 101, Chattanooga, TN 37411; tel. 423/490-1120; Brian E. Dalbey, President

Health 123, Inc., 210 Westwood Place, Suite 200, Brentwood, TN 37203; tel. 615/782-7800; FAX. 615/782-7812; Michael Bailey, Executive VP and COO

HealthNet HMO, Inc., 44 Vantage Way, Suite 300, Nashville, TN 37228; tel. 800/881-9466; John D. Davis, Chief Executive Officer

Healthsource Tennessee, Inc., 5409 Maryland Way, Suite 300, Brentwood, TN 37027; tel. 615/373-6995; FAX. 615/370-9396; Steve White, Chief Executive Officer

Phoenix Healthcare of Tennessee, Inc., 3401 West End Avenue, Suite 470, Nashville, TN 37203; tel. 615/298-3666; FAX. 615/297-2036; Samuel H. Howard, Chairman

PHP Companies, Inc., 1420 Centerpoint Boulevard, Knoxville, TN 37932; tel. 423/470-7470; Lance Hunsinger, Chief Financial Officer

Southern Health Plan, Inc., 600 Jefferson, Memphis, TN 38105; tel. 901/544-2336; FAX. 901/544-2220; Bill Graham, Executive Director

Tennessee Health Care Network, Inc., P.O. Box 1407, Chattanooga, TN 37401-1407; tel. 423/755-2033; FAX. 615/755-5630; Robert M. Fox, President

TriPoint Health Plan, Inc., 706 Church Street, Suite 500, Nashville, TN 37203-3511; tel. 800/557-4874; Barbara Bennett, General Counsel

Vanderbilt Health Plans, Inc., 706 Church Street Building, Suite 500, Nashville, TN 37203; tel. 615/343-2670; FAX. 615/343-2823; Randal B. Farr, Executive Vice President

TEXAS

AECC Total Vision Health Plan of Texas, Inc., 3010 LBJ Freeway, Suite 240, Dallas, TX 75234; tel. 800/268-8847; FAX. 927/620-9484; Bill Henderson, Chief Executive Officer

Aetna Dental Care of Texas, Inc., 2777 Stemmons Freeway, Suite 300, Dallas, TX 75207; tel. 214/470-7990; Jackie Eveslage, Chief Operating Officer

Aetna Health Plans of Texas, Inc., 2900 North Loop West, Suite 200, Houston, TX 77092; tel. 713/683-7500; FAX. 713/683-5819; Joseph T. Blanford, III, General Manager

Aetna U.S. Healthcare of North Texas, Inc., P.O. Box 569440, 2777 Stemmons Freeway, Dallas, TX 75356-9440; tel. 214/401-8610; John Coyle, President

Alpha Dental Programs, Inc., d/b/a Delta Care, 1431 Greenway Drive, Suite 520, Irving, TX 75038; tel. 972/580-1616; FAX. 972/580-1333; Robert Budd, Vice President, Marketing, Western Region

Americaid Texas, Inc., d/b/a Americaid Community Care, 617 Seventh Avenue, Second Floor, Fort Worth, TX 76104; tel. 817/870-1281; James Donovan, Jr., President

Anthem Health Plan of Texas, Inc., 5055 Keller Springs Road, Dallas, TX 75243; tel. 972/732-2000; FAX. 972/732-2043; Joseph W. Hrbek, President

Block Vision of Texas, Inc., 14228 Midway Road, Suite 213, Dallas, TX 75244; tel. 800/914-9795; FAX. 972/991-4704; Andrew Alcorn, President

Certus Healthcare, L.L.C., 1300 North 10th Street, Suite 450, McAllen, TX 78501; tel. 210/630-1956; FAX. 210/630-1957; David Rodriguez, President

CIGNA Dental Health of Texas, Inc., d/b/a CIGNA Dental Health, 600 East Las Colinas Boulevard, Suite 1100, Irving, TX 75039; tel. 800/367-1037; Brent Martin, D.D.S., M.B.A., Chief Executive Officer,

CIGNA HealthCare of Texas, Inc., d/b/a CIGNA HealthCare for Seniors, 600 East Las Colinas Boulevard, Suite 1100, Irving, TX 75039; tel. 214/401-5200; FAX. 214/401-5263; Paul Carter, Associate Vice President of Government Programs

Community Health Choice, Inc., 2525 Holly Hall, Houston, TX 77054; tel. 713/746-6999; FAX. 713/746-4365; Wayne Colson, VP of Finance

Comprehensive Health Services of Texas, Inc., 100 Northeast Loop 410, Suite 675, San Antonio, TX 78217; tel. 210/321-4050; Thomas C. Jackson, Chief Executive Officer

Dental Benefits, Inc., d/b/a Bluecare Dental HMO, 12170 Abrams Road, Dallas, TX 75243; tel. 972/766-6129; FAX. 972/766-6129; Richard A. Clissold

DentiCare, Inc., d/b/a CompDent, 2929 Briarpark Drive, Suite 314, Houston, TX 77042-3709; tel. 713/784-7011; Henry New, President

ECCA Managed Vision Care, Inc., 11103 West Avenue, San Antonio, TX 78213-1392; tel. 800/340-0129; FAX. 210/524-6587; Mark O. Jolly, Senior Vice President of Sales

First American Dental Benefits, Inc., 14800 Landmark Boulevard, Suite 700, Dallas, TX 75240; tel. 214/661-5848; Jim Davenport, President, Acting Chief Executive Officer

Foundation Health A Texas Plan, 5525 N. Macarthur Blvd #850, Irving, TX 78746; tel. 972/756-5000; Penny Zagroba, Operations Manager

Harris Methodist Texas Health Plan, Inc., d/b/a Harris Methodist Health Plan, 611 Ryan Plaza Drive, Suite 900, Arlington, TX 76011-4009; tel. 817/462-7000; FAX. 817/462-6903; Patrick Spehrs, President

Healthplan of Texas, Inc., 110 North College Ave., Suite 900, Tyler, TX 75702; tel. 903/531-4447; Paul Christian, M.D., Chief Executive Officer

HMO Texas, L.C., P.O. Box 42416, Houston, TX 77242-2416; tel. 713/952-6868; FAX. 713/974-1650; John Micale, President

Humana Health Plan of Texas, Inc., d/b/a Humana Health Plan of Dallas, 8431 Fredericksburg Road, San Antonio, TX 78229; tel. 512/617-1000; Brenda Luckett, Executive Director

Humana Health Plan of Texas, Inc., d/b/a Humana Health Plan of San Antonio, 8431 Fredericksburg Road, Suite 570, San Antonio, TX 78229; tel. 210/617-1000; FAX. 210/617-1704; Michael A. Seltzer, Director, Texas Operations

Humana Health Plans of Texas, Inc, 8431 Fredericksburg Road, Suite 570, San Antonio, TX 78229; tel. 210/617-1708; FAX. 210/617-1704; Michael A. Seltzer, Vice President West Region

Kaiser Foundation Health Plan of Texas, 12720 Hillcrest Road, Suite 600, Dallas, TX 75230; tel. 214/479-0332; Sharon Flaherty, President

Memorial Sisters of Charity HMO, LLC, d/b/a MSCH HMO, 9494 Southwest Freeway, Suite 300, Houston, TX 77074; tel. 713/430-1617; FAX. 713/778-2375; Richard Todd, President and CEO

Mercy Health Plans of Missouri, Inc., 5901 McPherson, Suites 1 & 2B, Laredo, TX 78041; tel. 956/723-2144; FAX. 956/723-8246; Ernesto Segura, Executive Director

MethodistCare, Two Greenway Plaza, Suite 500, Houston, TX 77046; tel. 713/479-4100; FAX. 713/479-4263; James Henderson, President and CEO

Metrowest Health Plan, Inc., 1500 South Main Street, 3rd Floor, Fort Worth, TX 76104; tel. 817/927-3999; FAX. 817/927-3996; Robert G. O'Donnell, President

Mid-Con Health Plans, L.C., d/b/a HMO Blue, Southwest Texas, 500 Chestnut Street, Suite 1699, Abilene, TX 79602; tel. 915/738-3518; FAX. 915/738-3519; M. Ted Haynes, President and CEO

NYLCare Dental Plan of the Southwest, Inc., 4500 Fuller Drive, Irving, TX 75038; tel. 972/650-5500; FAX. 972/650-5707; Steve Yerxa, Chief Executive Officer, Executive Direct

NYLCare Health Plans of the Gulf Coast, 2425 West Loop South, Suite 1000, Houston, TX 77027; tel. 713/624-5000; FAX. 713/963-9417; Thomas S. Lucksinger, President and CEO

One Health Plan of Texas, Inc., 10000 North Central Expressway, Suite 900, Dallas, TX 75231; tel. 800/866-3136; Jim White, President

Orthopedic Healthcare of Texas, Inc., 729 Bedford-Euless Road, W., Suite 100, Hurst, TX 76053; tel. 817/282-6905; Edward William Smith, D.O., President

PacifiCare of Texas, Inc., San Antonio Region, 8200 I.H. 10 West, San Antonio, TX 78230; tel. 210/524-9800; Patrick Feyen, President

Parkland Community Health Plan, Inc., 7920 Elmbrook, Suite 120, Dallas, TX 75247; tel. 214/590-2800; Ron J. Anderson, President

Parliament Dental Plans, Inc., 2909 Hillcroft, Suite 515, Houston, TX 77057; tel. 713/784-6262; FAX. 713/784-0488; Paul H. Michael, President

Physicians Care HMO, Inc., 2777 Stemmons Freeway, Suite 957B, Stemmons Place, Dallas, TX 75207; tel. 214/631-0221; FAX. 214/688-7044; Amanullah Khan, President

Principal Health Care of Texas, Inc., 555 North Caracahua, Suite 500, Corpus Christ, TX 78478; tel. 512/887-0101; Diana Tchida, Executive Director

Prudential Dental Maintenance Organization, Inc., Stop 206, One Prudential Circle, Sugar Land, TX 77478-3833; tel. 713/494-6000; FAX. 713/276-3752; Royce Rosemond, Executive Director

Prudential Health Care Plan, Inc., Stop 204, One Prudential Circle, Sugar Land, TX 77478; tel. 713/276-3850; FAX. 713/276-8254; Dennis Edmonds, Executive Director

Prudential Health Care Plan, Inc., PruCare, 24 Greenway Plaza, Suite 500, Houston, TX 77046; tel. 201/716-8174

Rio Grande HMO, Inc., d/b/a HMO Blue, 4150 Pinnacle, Suite 203, El Paso, TX 79902; tel. 800/831-0576; Anne McDow, Vice President, Operations

Safeguard Health Plans, Inc., 14800 Landmark Blvd., 7th Floor, Dallas, TX 75240; tel. 214/265-7041; FAX. 214/265-7702; David Branstetter, Executive Director

Scott & White Health Plan, 2401 South 31st Street, Temple, TX 76508; tel. 254/292-3003; FAX. 254/298-3011; C. Dave Morehead, M.D., President

Seton Health Plan, Inc., 1201 West 38th Street, Austin, TX 78705; tel. 800/749-7404; FAX. 512/323-1952; John H. Evler, III, President and COO

Sha, L.L.C., d/b/a Firstcare, 12940 Research Boulevard, Austin, TX 78750; tel. 806/356-5151; Dale Bowerman, President and CEO

Spectera Dental, Inc., (formerly United Healthcare Dental, Inc.), 1445 North Loop West, Suite 1000, Houston, TX 77008; tel. 713/861-3231; Arlene Sheldon, Executive Director

Superior Healthplan, L.P., 816 Congress Ave., Suite 1100, Austin, TX 78701; tel. 512/480-2206; Jose Comacho, Executive Director

Texas Children's Health Plan, Inc., 1919 South Braeswood Boulevard, P.O. Box 301011, Houston, TX 77230-1011; tel. 713/770-2600; FAX. 713/770-2686; Christopher Born, President

Texas Universities Health Plan, Inc., d/b/a TUHP, 700 University Blvd., Galveston, TX 77550; tel. 409/747-5430

Providers / Health Maintenance Organizations

Unicare of Texas Health Plans, Inc., (formerly **Affiliated Health Plans, Inc.**), 11200 Westheimer, Suite 700, Houston, TX 77042; tel. 713/782-4555; Sam John Nicholson, II, President

United Healthcare of Texas, Inc., (formerly **Metrahealth Care Plan of Texas, Inc.**), 1250 Capital of Texas, Highway South, Austin, TX 78746; tel. 800/424-6480; FAX. 512/338-6812; Karen England, Director, Network Operations

United Healthcare of Texas, Inc., Dallas/Fort Worth Division, 4835 LBJ Freeway, Suite 1100, Dallas, TX 75244; tel. 214/866-6000; FAX. 214/866-6018; Richard Cook, Chief Executive Officer

Universal HealthPlan, Inc., 2900 Elgin, Houston, TX 77004; tel. 713/526-2441

USABLE HMO, Inc., d/b/a **USABLE Health Advantage**, 1406 College Drive, Suite A, Texarkana, TX 75503; tel. 800/844-6047

VHP Dental, Inc., P.O. Box 15800, 7801 North IH 35, Austin, TX 78761; tel. 512/433-1000

Vista Health Plan, Inc., (formerly **The Wellness Health Plan of Texas, Inc.**), 7801 North IH-35, Austin, TX 78753; tel. 512/433-1000; Paul Tovar, President

West Texas Health Plans, d/b/a HMO Blue, West Texas, Sentry Plaza II, 5225 South Loop 289, Lubbock, TX 79424; tel. 806/798-6362; Michael A. Huesman, President

UTAH

Altrus Health Plans, 1041 S. Jordan Gateway #400, South Jordan, UT 84095; tel. 801/355-1234; FAX. 801/323-6400; Larry Hancock, President and COO

American Family Care of Utah, Inc., 2120 S. 1300 E, Suite 303, Salt Lake City, UT 84106; tel. 801/486-1664; Jose Fernandez, President

Benchoice, Inc., 310 East 4500 South, Suite 550, Murray, UT 84157-0906; tel. 801/262-2999; Talmage Pond, President

CIGNA Health Plan of Utah, Inc., 5295 South 320 West, Suite 280, Salt Lake City, UT 84107; tel. 801/265-2777; FAX. 801/261-5349; Robert Immitt, President

Delta Care Dental Plan, Inc., 257 East 200 South, Suite 375, Salt Lake City, UT 84111; tel. 801/575-5168

Educators Health Care, 852 East Arrowhead Lane, Murray, UT 84107-5298; tel. 801/262-7476; FAX. 801/269-9734; Andy I. Galano, Ph.D., President and CEO

HealthWise, 2890 East Cottonwood Parkway, P.O. Box 30270, Salt Lake City, UT 84130-0270; tel. 801/333-2320; Jed H. Pitcher, Chairman

IHC Care, Inc., 36 South State Street, 15th Floor, Salt Lake City, UT 84111; tel. 801/442-5000; FAX. 801/538-5003; Sid Paulson, Chief Operating Officer

Intergroup Utah, Inc, 127 South 500 East, Suite 510, Salt Lake City, UT 84102; tel. 801/532-7665; FAX. 801/297-4585; Elden Mitchell, President

U. S. Dental Plan, Inc., 4001 South 700 East, Suite 300, Salt Lake City, UT 84107; tel. 801/263-8884; Christopher A. Jehle, President

United HealthCare of Utah, 7910 South 3500 East, Salt Lake City, UT 84121; tel. 801/942-6200; FAX. 801/944-0940; Colin Gardner, Chief Executive Officer

Utah Community Health Plan, 36 South State Street, Suite 1020, Salt Lake City, UT 84111-1418; tel. 801/442-3780; FAX. 801/442-3791; William K. Wilson, Executive Director

VIRGINIA

Aetna Health Plans of the Mid-Atlantic, Inc., 7600 A Leesburg Pike, Falls Church, VA 22043; tel. 703/903-7100; Jon Glaudemans, Vice President, Health Services

Amerigroup Corporation, Americaid Community Care, 4425 Corporation Lane, Suite 100, Virginia Beach, VA 23462; tel. 757/490-6900; FAX. 757/473-2738; Ted M. Willie, JR., Chief Operating Officer

CIGNA HealthCare of Virginia, Inc., 4050 Innslake Drive, Glen Allen, VA 23060; tel. 804/273-1100; John E. Sharp, Vice President and Executive Director

Health First, Inc., 621 Lynnhaven Parkway, Suite 450, Virginia Beach, VA 23452-7330; tel. 804/431-5298; Russell F. Mohawk, President

HealthKeepers, Inc., 2220 Edward Holland Drive, P.O. Box 26623, Richmond, VA 23230; tel. 804/354-7961; FAX. 804/354-3554; Sam Weidman, Vice President, Finance

HMO Virginia, Inc., Health Keepers, 2220 Edward Holland Drive, Richmond, VA 23230; tel. 804/354-7961; FAX. 804/354-3554; Sam Weidman, Vice President, Finance

National Capital Health Plan, Inc., 5850 Versar Center, Suite 420, Springfield, VA 22151; tel. 703/914-5650

Optimum Choice, 3025 Hamaker Court, Suite 301, Fairfax, VA 22031; tel. 703/207-6570; Susan Hrubes, Senior Director

Peninsula Health Care, Inc., 606 Denbigh Boulevard, Suite 500, Newport News, VA 23608; tel. 757/875-5760; FAX. 757/875-5785; C. Burke King, President

Physicians Health Plan, Inc., Health Keepers, 2220 Edward Holland Drive, Richmond, VA 23230; tel. 804/354-7961; FAX. 804/354-3554; Sam Weidman, Vice President, Finance

Priority Health Plan, Inc., 621 Lynnhaven Parkway, Suite 450, Virginia Beach, VA 23452-7330; tel. 804/463-4600; Russell F. Mohawk, President

Prudential Health Care Plan, Inc., d/b/a **PruCare and Prudential Health Care Plan of the Mid-**, 1000 Boulders Parkway, Richmond, VA 23225; tel. 804/323-0900; William Patrick Link, President

QualChoice of VA Health Plan, Inc., 1807 Seminole Trail, Charlottesville, VA 22901; tel. 804/975-1212; FAX. 804/975-1414; Martha D' Erasmo, President and CEO

Sentara Health Management, 4417 Corporation Lane, Virginia Beach, VA 23462; tel. 804/552-7400; FAX. 804/552-7396; Michael M. Dudley, President

Sentara Health Plans, Inc., d/b/a Sentara Health Plan, 4417 Corporation Lane, Virginia Beach, VA 23462; tel. 804/552-7100; FAX. 804/552-7396; John E. McNamara, III, President

Southern Health Services, 9881 Mayland Drive, P.O. Box 85603, Richmond, VA 23285-5603; tel. 804/747-3700; FAX. 804/747-8723; James L. Gore, President

WASHINGTON

Group Health Cooperative of Puget Sound, Administration and Conference Center, 521 Wall Street, Seattle, WA 98121-1535; tel. 206/448-6460; FAX. 206/448-6080; Phil Nudelman, Ph.D., President and CEO

Group Health Northwest, 5615 West Sunset Highway, Spokane, WA 99204; tel. 509/838-9100; FAX. 509/838-3823; Henry S. Berman, M.D., President and CEO

HealthFirst Partners, Inc., 601 Union Street, Suite 700, Seattle, WA 98101; tel. 206/667-8070; FAX. 206/667-8060; Eileen Duncan

QualMed Washington Health Plan, Inc, d/b/a Molina Healthcare of Washington, 2331 130th Avenue, N.E., Suite 200, Zip 98009, P.O. Box 3387, Bellevue, WA 98009-3387; tel. 206/869-3500; FAX. 206/869-3568; Mark Rattray, M.D., CEO

QualMed Washington Health Plan, Inc., West 508 Sixth Avenue, Suite 700, P.O. Box 2470, Spokane, WA 99210-2470; tel. 509/459-6690; FAX. 509/458-2705; Nicolette Bryant, Director of Operations

Regence Care, 1800 Ninth Avenue, P.O. Box 2088, Seattle, WA 98111-2088; tel. 206/389-6721; FAX. 206/389-6719; Mary McWilliams, Executive Director

Virginia Mason Health Plan, Inc., Metropolitan Park West, 1100 Olive Way, Suite 1580, Seattle, WA 98101-1828; tel. 206/223-8844; FAX. 206/223-7506; John Clarke, Director, Operations

WEST VIRGINIA

Advantage Health Plan, Adv. Health/QualMed, 137 Waddles Run Road, Wheeling, WV 26003; tel. 304/243-1489

Anthem Health Plan of West Virginia, Inc., d/b/a PrimeONE, 500 Virginia Street East, Suite 400, Charleston, WV 25301; tel. 304/340-6944; FAX. 304/304/6943; A. Paul Holdren, President and CEO

Carelink Health Plans, 141 Summers Square, Charleston, WV 25326-1711; tel. 304/348-2040; FAX. 304/348-2948; Kevin Fulner, Director of Provider Relations

WISCONSIN

Atrium Health Plan, Inc., 2215 Vine Street, Suite E, Hudson, WI 54016-5802; tel. 800/535-4041; FAX. 715/386-8326; Michael L. Christensen, Director of Operations

Compcare Health Services Insurance Corp., 225 South Executive Drive, Brookfield, WI 53005; tel. 262/814-3600; FAX. 262/814-3603; Mary Traver, President and COO

Dean Health Plan, Inc., P.O. Box 56099, Madison, WI 53705-9399; tel. 608/836-1301; FAX. 608/836-9620; John A. Turcott, President and CEO

Dean Health Plan, Inc., 1277 Deming Way, Madison, WI 53717; tel. 608/836-1400; John A. Turcott, President and CEO

Emphesys Wisconsin Insurance Company, 1100 Employers Boulevard, DePere, WI 54115; tel. 800/558-4444; Mark R. Minsloff, Executive Director

Family Health Plan Cooperative, P.O. Box 44260, Milwaukee, WI 53214-7260; tel. 414/256-0006; FAX. 414/256-5681; David Bradford, President

Greater La Crosse Health Plans, Inc., 1285 Rudy Street, Onalaska, WI 54650; tel. 608/782-2638; FAX. 608/781-8862; Steven M. Kunes, Plan Administrator

Group Health Cooperative of Eau Claire, P.O. Box 3217, Eau Claire, WI 54702-3217; tel. 715/552-4300; FAX. 715/836-7683; Peter Farrow, General Manager and CEO

Group Health Cooperative of South Central Wisconsin, 8202 Excelsior Drive, P.O. Box 44971, Madison, WI 53744-4971; tel. 608/251-4156; FAX. 608/257-3842; Lawrence Zanoni, Executive Director

Gundersen Lutheran Health Maintenance Plan, 1836 South Avenue, LaCrosse, WI 54601; tel. 608/775-8000; FAX. 608/791-8042; Patrick Killeen, Executive Director

Humana Wisconsin Health Organization Insurance Corporation, 111 West Pleasant Street, P.O. Box 12359, Milwaukee, WI 53212-0359; tel. 414/223-3300; FAX. 414/223-7777; William L. Carr, Executive Director

Managed Health Services, 2040 W. Wisconsin Ave #452, Milwaukee, WI 53227; tel. 414/345-4600; FAX. 414/345-4624; Michael F. Neidorff, President and CEO

MercyCare Insurance Company, 3430 Palmer Drive, P.O. Box 2770, Janesville, WI 53547-2770; tel. 608/752-3431; FAX. 608/752-3751; Bradley J. Mucek, Executive Vice President

Network Health Plan of Wisconsin, Inc., 1165 Appleton Road, P.O. Box 120, Menasha, WI 54952-0120; tel. 414/727-0100; FAX. 414/727-5634; Michael D. Wolff, President and CEO

North Central Health Protection Plan, 2000 Westwood Drive, Zip 54401, P.O. Box 969, Wausau, WI 54402-0969; tel. 715/842-6730; Larry A. Baker, Administrator

Physicians Plus Insurance Corporation, 340 West Washington Avenue, P.O. Box 2078, Madison, WI 53703; tel. 608/282-8900; FAX. 608/282-8944; Thomas R. Sobocinski, President and CEO

PrimeCare Health Plan, Inc., 10701 West Research Drive, Milwaukee, WI 53226-0649; tel. 800/879-0071; FAX. 414/443-4750; James Schultz, Administrator

Security Health Plan of Wisconsin, Inc., 1515 Saint Joseph Avenue, P.O. Box 8000, Marshfield, WI 54449-8000; tel. 715/221-9678; FAX. 715/221-9500; John C. Smylie, CEO

United Health of Wisconsin Insurance Company, Inc., P.O. Box 507, Appleton, WI 54912-0507; tel. 414/735-6440; FAX. 414/731-7232; Jay Fulkerson, Chief Executive Officer

Unity Health Plans Insurance Corp., 840 Carolina Street, Sauk City, WI 53583; tel. 800/362-3308; FAX. 608/643-2564; Nicholas J. Reiland, III, CEO

Valley Health Plan, 2270 East Ridge Center, P.O. Box 3128, Eau Claire, WI 54702-3128; tel. 715/832-3235; FAX. 715/836-1298; Kathryn R. Teeters, Director

WYOMING

WinHealth Partners, 2515 Warren Avenue, Suite 504, Cheyenne, WY 82001; tel. 307/638-7700; FAX. 307/638-7701; Beth Wasson, Executive Director

U.S. Associated Areas

GUAM

F.H.P., Inc., P.O. Box 6578, Tamunig, GU 96911; tel. 671/646-5824; FAX. 671/646-6923; Edward English, Associate Regional Vice President

Guam Memorial Health Plan, 177 Achalan Pasaheru, Tamunig, GU 96911; tel. 671/646–4647; FAX. 671/647–5048; James W. Gillan, Chief Operating Officer

PUERTO RICO

First Medical Comprehensive Health Care, Inc., (Antes Plan Comprehensive de Salud, Inc.), Apartado 40954, Estacion Minillas, Santurce, PR 00940; tel. 809/723–6016; FAX. 809/723–6014; J. A. Soler, President

Golden Cross HMO Health Plan Corporation, Antes HMO Medical System Corporation, Apartado 9021727, Estacion Viejo San Juan, San Juan, PR 00902–1727; tel. 809/721–0427; FAX. 809/721–5464; Lic Luis F. Hernandez Velez

Humana Puerto Rico, Humana Puerto Rico, Box 192059, San Juan, PR 00919–2059; tel. 787/282–7900; FAX. 787/282–6290; Victor S. Gutierrez, M.D., President

Mennonite General Hospital, Inc., Calle Jose C. Vazquez, Apartado 1379, Aibonito, PR 00705; tel. 809/735–8001; FAX. 809/735–8073; Domingo Torres Zayas, Chief Executive Officer

Plan de Salud de la Federacion de Maestros, de Puerto Rico, Inc., P.O. Box 71336, San Juan, PR 00936–8436; tel. 787/758–5610; FAX. 787/281–7392; Eugenio Aponte, Executive Director

Plan de Salud Hospital de la Concepcion, Inc., Calle Dr. Veve #102, Apartado 39, San German, PR 00683; tel. 787/892–1860; FAX. 787/892–2176; Ivonne Montaluo, Executive Director

Plan de Salud U.I.A., Inc., Calle Mayaguez #49, San Juan, PR 00917; tel. 787/763–4004; FAX. 787/763–7095; Jose E. Sanchez, Consultant

Plan Medico U.T.I. de Puerto Rico, Inc., Apartado 23316–Estacion U.P.R., Rio Piedras, PR 00924; tel. 809/758–1500; FAX. 787/758–3210; David Munoz, President

Ryder Health Plan, Inc., Call Box 859, Humacao, PR 00792; tel. 809/852–0846; FAX. 809/850–4863; Juan L. De Le Rosa, Director

Service Medical, Inc., Avenida Munoz Rivera 402, Parada 31, Hato Rey, PR 00917; tel. 809/758–5555; FAX. 809/250–1425; Lexie Gomez

Servicios de Salud Bella Vista, Inc., Bella Vista Gardens Numero 43, Carr. 349–Cerro Las Mesas, Mayaguez, PR 00680; tel. 787/833–8070; FAX. 787/832–5400; Edson Lugo, President

United Healthcare Plans of Puerto Rico, Inc., (Antes Group Sales and Service of Puerto Rico, Inc.), Rexco Office Park, Apartado 364864, San Juan, PR 00936–4864; tel. 809/782–7005; FAX. 809/782–5269; Luis A. Salgado Munoz, Executive Vice President

State Government Agencies for HMO's

Information for the following list was obtained directly from the agencies.

United States

ALABAMA: Department of Insurance, 201 Monroe Street, Suite 1700, Montgomery, AL 36104; tel. 334/269-3550; FAX. 334/241-4192; David Parsons, Acting Commissioner

ALASKA: Alaska Division of Insurance, P.O. Box 110805, Juneau, AK 99811-0805; tel. 907/465-2596; FAX. 907/465-3422; Marianne K. Burke, Director

ARIZONA: Department of Insurance, 2910 North 44th Street, Suite 210, Phoenix, AZ 85018; tel. 602/912-8443; FAX. 602/912-8453; Mary Butterfield, Assistant Director, Life and Health

ARKANSAS: Arkansas Insurance Department, 1200 West Third Street, Little Rock, AR 72201-1904; tel. 501/371-2600; FAX. 501/371-2618; Mike Pickens, Insurance Commissioner

CALIFORNIA: Department of Corporations, Health Care Service Plan Division, 3200 West 4th Street, Suite 750, Los Angeles, CA 90010; tel. 213/736-2776; FAX. 213/576-7660; Gary G. Hagen, Assistant Commissioner

COLORADO: Department of Regulatory Agencies, Colorado Division of Insurance, 1560 Broadway, Suite 850, Denver, CO 80202; tel. 303/894-7499; FAX. 303/894-7455; Janet Byrne, Corporate Affairs

CONNECTICUT: Department of Insurance, P.O. Box 816, Hartford, CT 06142-0816; tel. 860/297-3800; FAX. 860/566-7410; Mary Ellen Breault, Director, Life and Health Division

DELAWARE: Office of Health Facilities Licensure and Certification, 2055 Limestone Road, Suite 200, Wilmington, DE 19808; tel. 302/577-6666; FAX. 302/577-6672; Ellen T. Reap, Director

DISTRICT OF COLUMBIA: District of Columbia Department of Insurance and Securities Re, 810 1st Street NE, Room 701, Washington, DC 20002; tel. 202/727-8000; FAX. 202/535-1196; Herman Hunter, Chief Consumer Services Branch

FLORIDA: Florida Department of Insurance, Bureau of Life and Health Insurer Solvency and Market Con, 200 East Gaines, Tallahassee, FL 32399-0327; tel. 850/922-3153; FAX. 850/413-9019; Beth Vecchioli, Administrator

GEORGIA: Department of Insurance, 6th West Tower, Floyd Building, Two Martin Luther King, Jr. Drive, Atlanta, GA 30334; tel. 404/656-2074; FAX. 404/657-7743; John Oxendine, Commissioner

HAWAII: State of Hawaii Department of Labor and Industrial Relations, Disability Compensation Division, P.O. Box 3769, Honolulu, HI 96812; tel. 808/586-9151; FAX. 808/586-9219; Gary S. Hamada, Administrator

IDAHO: Department of Insurance, 700 West State Street, Third Floor, P.O. Box 83720, Boise, ID 83720-0043; tel. 208/334-4250; FAX. 208/334-4398; Joan Krosch, Health Insurance Coordinator

ILLINOIS: Department of Insurance, 320 West Washington Street, Fourth Floor, Springfield, IL 62767-0001; tel. 217/782-6369; FAX. 217/524-2122; David E. Grant, Health Care Coordinator

INDIANA: Department of Insurance, 311 West Washington Street, Suite 300, Indianapolis, IN 46204; tel. 317/232-5695; FAX. 317/232-5251; Jim Fuller, Health Deputy

IOWA: Iowa Department of Commerce, Division of Insurance, 330 Maple, Des Moines, IA 50319-0065; tel. 515/281-5705; FAX. 515/281-3059; Therese M. Vaughan, Commissioner

KANSAS: Kansas Insurance Department, 420 Southwest Ninth Street, Topeka, KS 66612; tel. 785/296-3071; FAX. 785/296-2283; Kathleen Sebelius, Commissioner

KENTUCKY: Department of Insurance, Life and Health Division, 215 West Main Street, P.O. Box 517, Frankfort, KY 40602; tel. 502/564-6088; FAX. 502/564-2728; Gale Pearce, Director

LOUISIANA: Department of Insurance, Attn: Company Licensing Division, P.O. Box 94214, Baton Rouge, LA 70804; tel. 504/342-1216; FAX. 504/342-3078; Mike Boutwell, Company Licensing Coordinator

MAINE: Department of Professional and Financial Regulation, Bureau of Insurance, 34 State House Station, Augusta, ME 04333; tel. 207/624-8416; FAX. 207/624-8599; Michael F. McGonigle, Senior Insurance Analyst

MARYLAND: Department of Health and Mental Hygiene, Insurance Division, 201 West Preston Street, Baltimore, MD 21201-2399; tel. 410/767-6860; FAX. 410/767-6489; George C. Benjamin, M.D., Secretary

MASSACHUSETTS: Division of Insurance, 1 South State, Boston, MA 02210-2223; tel. 617/521-7794; FAX. 617/521-7770; Robert Dynan, Company Licensing

MICHIGAN: Department of Community Health, Managed Care Quality Assessment and Improvement Division, P.O. Box 30479, 400 S. Pine, Lansing, MI 48909-7979; tel. 517/241-9809; FAX. 517/241-9953; Janet Olszewski, Director

MINNESOTA: Minnesota Health Technology Advisory Committee (HTAC), 121 East Seventh Place, Suite 400, P.O. Box 64975, St. Paul, MN 55164-0975; tel. 651/282-5600; FAX. 651/282-5628; Brenda Holden, Director

MISSISSIPPI: Mississippi Department of Insurance, P.O. Box 79, Jackson, MS 39205; tel. 601/359-3577; FAX. 601/359-2474; J. Mark Haire, Special Assistant Attorney General

MISSOURI: Department of Insurance, Division of Market Regulation, Managed Care Section, P.O. Box 690, Jefferson City, MO 65102; tel. 573/751-2641; FAX. 573/526-6075; Molly White, Research Anaylst 3

MONTANA: Montana State Auditor, Insurance Department, Mitchell Building, Room 270, 126 North Sanders, Helena, MT 59604-4009; tel. 406/444-4372; FAX. 406/444-3497; James Borchardt, Chief Examiner

NEBRASKA: Department of Insurance, 941 O Street, Suite 400, Lincoln, NE 68508; tel. 402/471-2201; FAX. 402/471-4610; L Tim Wagner, Director

NEVADA: Nevada Division of Insurance, Capitol Complex, 1665 Hot Springs Road, Suite 152, Carson City, NV 89710; tel. 775/687-4270; FAX. 775/687-3937; Alice A. Molasky-Arman, Esq., Commissioner

NEW HAMPSHIRE: Department of Health and Human Services, Office of Community and Public Health, Medicaid Administration Bureau, 6 Hazen Drive, Concord, NH 03301-6521; tel. 603/271-4365; FAX. 603/271-4376; Diane Kemp, Administrator

NEW JERSEY: Department of Health, Office of Managed Care, P.O. Box 360, Trenton, NJ 08625; tel. 609/588-2510; FAX. 609/633-0807; Edwin V. Kelleher, Supervisor Regulatory Compliance

NEW MEXICO: Public Regulation Commission, Insurance Division, P.O. Box 1269, Santa Fe, NM 87504; tel. 505/827-4601; FAX. 505/827-4734; Life and Health Forms Filing Bureau

NEW YORK: The Bureau of Managed Care Certification and Surveillance, Empire State Plaza, Corning Tower, Room 1911, Albany, NY 12237; tel. 518/474-5515; FAX. 518/473-3583; Vallencia Lloyd, Director

NORTH CAROLINA: Department of Insurance, Financial Evaluation Division, P.O. Box 26387, Raleigh, NC 27611; tel. 919/733-5633; FAX. 919/715-6811; Jackie Obusek, Financial Analyst

NORTH DAKOTA: North Dakota Department of Insurance, State Capitol, 600 East Boulevard, 5th Boulevard, Bismarck, ND 58505-0320; tel. 701/328-2440; FAX. 701/328-4880; Glenn Pomeroy, Commissioner

OHIO: Department of Insurance, Managed Care Division, 2100 Stella Court, Columbus, OH 43215-1067; tel. 614/644-3311; FAX. 614/644-2658; Lee Covington, Director

OKLAHOMA: Oklahoma State Department of Health, 1000 Northeast 10th Street, Oklahoma City, OK 73117-1299; tel. 405/271-6868; FAX. 405/271-5600; Lajuana Wire, Director of Managed Care Systems

OREGON: Department of Consumer and Business Services, Insurance Division, 350 Winter St. NE #440, Salem, OR 97301-3883; tel. 503/947-7980; FAX. 503/378-4351; Michael Greenfield, Insurance Commissioner

PENNSYLVANIA: Pennsylvania Insurance Department, Company Licensing Division, 1345 Strawberry Square, Harrisburg, PA 17120; tel. 717/787-2735; FAX. 717/787-8557; Robert E. Brackbill, Chief of Company Licensing Division

RHODE ISLAND: Department of Business Regulation, Division of Insurance, 233 Richmond Street, Suite 233, Providence, RI 02903-4233; tel. 401/222-2223; FAX. 401/222-5475; Alfonso E. Mastrostefano, Associate Director

SOUTH CAROLINA: Office of Insurer Licensing and Solvency Services, 1612 Marion Street, Columbia, SC 29201; tel. 803/737-6221; FAX. 803/737-6232; Timothy W. Campbell, Chief Financial Analyst

SOUTH DAKOTA: Division of Administration, South Dakota Department of Health, 600 East Capitol Avenue, Pierre, SD 57501-2536; tel. 605/773-3361; FAX. 605/773-5683; Doneen Hollingworth, Secretary of Health

TENNESSEE: Department of Commerce and Insurance, 500 James Robertson Parkway, Nashville, TN 37243-1135; tel. 615/741-0472; FAX. 615/532-2788; Don Spann, Chief Financial Executive

TEXAS: Texas Department of Insurance, Mail Code 103-6A, P.O. Box 149104, Austin, TX 78714-9104; tel. 512/322-4266; FAX. 512/322-4260; Blake Brodersen, Deputy Commissioner, HMO/URA/QA

UTAH: Utah Insurance Department, State Office Building, Room 3110, Salt Lake City, UT 84114; tel. 801/538-3800; FAX. 801/538-3829; Jilane Whitby, Information Specialist

VERMONT: Department of Banking, Insurance and Securities, Division of Healthcare Administration, 89 Main Street, Drawer 20, Montpelier, VT 05620-2946; tel. 802/828-2900; FAX. 802/828-2949; Susan Gretkowski, Deputy Commissioner

VIRGINIA: State Corporation Commission, Bureau of Insurance, P.O. Box 1157, Richmond, VA 23218; tel. 804/371-9901; FAX. 804/371-9511; Laura Lee Viergever, Senior Financial Analyst

WASHINGTON: Office of the Insurance Commissioner, Insurance Building, P.O. Box 40255, Olympia, WA 98504-0255; tel. 360/664-8002; FAX. 360/586-3535; Donna Dorris, Manager, Health Care

WEST VIRGINIA: Insurance Commissioner's Office, Financial Conditions Division, 1124 Smith Street, Charleston, WV 25301; tel. 304/558-2100; FAX. 304/558-1365; Jeffrey W. Van Gilder, Director, Chief Examiner

WISCONSIN: Office of the Commissioner of Insurance, P.O. Box 7873, Madison, WI 53707-7873; tel. 608/266-3585; FAX. 608/266-9935; Connie L. O'Connell, Commissioner

Providers / State Government Agencies for HMO's

WYOMING: Department of Insurance, Herschler Building, Third Floor East, Cheyenne, WY 82002; tel. 307/777-7401; FAX. 307/777-5895; Lloyd Wilder, Business Systems Specialist

U.S. Associated Areas

GUAM: Department of Public Health and Social Services, Government of Guam, P.O. Box 2816, Agana, GU 96932; tel. 671/735-7102; FAX. 671/734-5910; Dennis G. Rodriguez, Director

PUERTO RICO: Aurea Lopez, Chief Examiner, Office of the Commissioner of Insurance, P.O. Box 8330, Fernandez Juncos Station, Santurce, PR 00910-8330; tel. 787/722-8686; FAX. 809/722-4400; Aurea Lopez, Chief Examiner

Freestanding Ambulatory Surgery Centers

The following list of freestanding ambulatory surgery centers was developed with the assistance of state government agencies and the individual facilities listed.

The AHA Guide contains two types of ambulatory surgery center listings; those that are hospital based and those that are freestanding. Hospital based ambulatory surgery centers are listed in section A of the AHA Guide and are identified by Facility Code F48. Please refer to that section for information on the over 5,000 hospital based ambulatory surgery centers.

We present this list simply as a convenient directory. Inclusion or omission of any organization's name indicates neither approval nor disapproval by Health Forum LLC, an American Hospital Association company.

United States

ALABAMA

American Surgery Centers of Alabama, d/b/a American Surgery Center, 2802 Ross Clark Circle, S.W., Dothan, AL 36301; tel. 334/793-3411; FAX. 334/712-0227; Carlotta McCallister, Administrator

Baptist Surgery Center, 2035 East South Boulevard, Montgomery, AL 36111-0000; tel. 334/286-3180; FAX. 334/286-3381; Kay Catliffe, Nurse Manager

Birmingham Endoscopy Center, Inc., 2621 19th Street, South, Homewood, AL 35209; tel. 205/271-8200; Norah Hollis, RN Director of Nursing

Birmingham Outpatient Surgery Center, Ltd., d/b/a HealthSouth Outpatient Center, 2720 University Boulevard, Birmingham, AL 35233; tel. 205/933-0050; FAX. 205/933-8212; Jackie Harrison, RN, Administrator

Columbia Surgicare of Mobile, 2890 Dauphin Street, Mobile, AL 36606; tel. 334/473-2020; FAX. 334/478-6737; Sandy Bunch, Administrator

Dauphin West Surgery Center, 3701 Dauphin Street, Mobile, AL 36608; tel. 334/341-3405; FAX. 334/341-3404; James L. Spires, Executive Director

Decatur Ambulatory Surgery Center, 2828 Highway 31, S., Decatur, AL 35603; tel. 256/340-1212; FAX. 256/340-0252; Andrew Hetrick, Administrator

Dothan Surgery Center, 1450 Ross Clark Circle, S.E.Suite 4, Dothan, AL 36301; tel. 334/793-3442; FAX. 334/793-3318; Denise Harrington, Clinic Administrator

Gadsden Surgery Center, 418 South Fifth Street, Gadsden, AL 35901; tel. 205/543-1253; FAX. 205/543-1260; Bobo Martin, RN, Administrator

HealthSouth Florence Surgery Center, 103 Helton Court, Florence, AL 35630; tel. 256/760-0672; FAX. 256/766-4547; Pam Watson, Administrator

HealthSouth Surgical Center of Tuscaloosa, 1400 McFarland Boulevard, N., Tuscaloosa, AL 35406; tel. 205/345-5500; Jeff Hayes, Administrator

Huntsville Endoscopy Center, Inc., 119 Longwood Drive, Huntsville, AL 35801; tel. 205/533-6488; FAX. 205/533-6495; Michael W. Brown, M.D.

Medplex Outpatient Medical Centers, Inc., 4511 Southlake Parkway, Birmingham, AL 35422; tel. 205/985-4398; FAX. 205/985-4486; Dawn Ousley, RN, Administrator

Mobile Surgery Center, 1721 Springhill Avenue, Mobile, AL 36608; tel. 334/438-3614; Julie Saucier, RN, B.S.N., Facility Administrator

Montgomery Eye Surgery Center, 2752 Zelda Road, Montgomery, AL 36106; tel. 334/270-9677; FAX. 334/213-0622; Chris Green, Center Director

Montgomery Surgical Center, 855 East South Boulevard, Montgomery, AL 36116; tel. 334/284-9600; FAX. 334/284-4233; Susan N. Lamar, Administrator

Outpatient Services East, Inc., 52 Medical Park Drive, E., Suite 401, Birmingham, AL 35235; tel. 205/838-3888; FAX. 205/838-6181; James E. Stidham, President and CEO

The Kirklin Clinic, 2000 Sixth Avenue, S., Birmingham, AL 35233; tel. 205/801-8000; Steven C. Schultz, Executive Vice President

The Surgery Center of Huntsville, 721 Madison Street, Huntsville, AL 35801; tel. 205/533-4888; FAX. 205/532-9510; William Sammons, Chief Executive Officer

Tuscaloosa Endoscopy Center, 100 Rice Mine Road, N.E, Suite E, Tuscaloosa, AL 35406; tel. 205/345-0010; FAX. 205/752-1175; A. B. Reddy, M.D., Medical Director

ALASKA

Alaska Surgery Center, 4001 Laurel Street, Anchorage, AK 99508; tel. 907/563-3327; FAX. 907/562-7042; Kim M. Pickerel, Administrator

Alaska Women's Health Services, Inc., 4115 Lake Otis Parkway, Anchorage, AK 99508; tel. 907/563-7228; FAX. 907/563-6278; Ellen Cowgill, Administrator

Geneva Woods Surgical Center, 3730 Rhone Circle, Suite 100, Anchorage, AK 99508; tel. 907/562-4764; FAX. 907/561-8519; Heidi Muckey, Administrator

Pacific Cataract & Laser Institute, 1600 'A' Street, Suite 200, Anchorage, AK 99501; tel. 907/272-2423; FAX. 907/272-2428

Susitna Surgery Center, 950 East Bogard Road, Wasilla, AK 99645, Palmer, AK 99645; tel. 907/746-8729; Lynn Wagoner, RN, Vice President, Clinical Services

ARIZONA

32nd Street Outpatient Surgery Center, 2501 North 32nd Street, Phoenix, AZ 85008; tel. 602/957-6799; FAX. 602/957-0172; Gary W. Hall, M.D., President

A.I.M.S. Outpatient Surgery, 3636 Stockton Hill Road, Kingman, AZ 86401; tel. 602/757-3636; FAX. 602/757-7224; Bill Margita

Adobe Plastic Surgery, 2585 North Wyatt Drive, Tucson, AZ 85712; tel. 602/322-5295; FAX. 602/325-7763; Lucricia Banks, Administrator

Aesthetic Reconstructive Associates, P.C., 4222 East Camelback, Suite H-150, Phoenix, AZ 85018; tel. 602/952-8100; FAX. 602/952-9519; Martin L. Johnson, M.D.

Ambulatory Surgicenter, Inc., 1940 East Southern Avenue, Tempe, AZ 85282; tel. 602/820-7101; FAX. 602/820-9291; H. William Reese, D.P.M., Medical Director

Arizona Diagnostic and Surgical Center, 545 North Mesa Drive, Mesa, AZ 85201; tel. 602/461-4407; FAX. 602/461-4401; Lynnette King, RN, Administrator

Arizona Foot Institute, P.C., 1901 West Glendale Avenue, Phoenix, AZ 85021; tel. 602/246-0816; FAX. 602/433-2257; Barry Kaplan

Arizona Medical Clinic, Ltd., 13640 North Plaza Del Rio Boulevard, Peoria, AZ 85381; tel. 602/876-3800; Jan Kaplan, Director, Operations

Arizona Surgical Arts, Inc., 1245 North Wilmot Road, Tucson, AZ 85712; tel. 520/296-7550; Kelly M. Gordon, Administrator

Barnet Dulaney Eye Center, 4800 N. 22nd Street, Phoenix, AZ 85018; tel. 602/955-1000; FAX. 602/957-9202; Ronald W. Barnet, M.D.

Barnet Dulaney Eye Center, 825 20th Avenue, Safford, AZ 85546; tel. 602/428-6930; FAX. 602/428-7272; Beth Curtis, RN

Barnet Dulaney Eye Center, 1375 West 16th Street, Yuma, AZ 85364; tel. 602/955-1000; FAX. 602/508-4700; Imelda Kelly, Director of Nursing

Barnet Eye Center-Mesa, 6335 East Main Street, Mesa, AZ 85205; tel. 602/981-1000; FAX. 602/981-0467; Carolyn Miller, Administrator

Boswell Eye Institute, 10541 West Thunderbird Boulevard, Sun City, AZ 85351; tel. 602/933-3402; FAX. 602/972-5014; Jan Zellmann, Administrator

Carriker Eye Center, 6425 North 16th Street, Phoenix, AZ 85016; tel. 602/274-1703; FAX. 602/274-3216; Richard G. Carriker, M.D.

Casa Blanca Medical Group, 4001 East Baseline Road, Gilbert, AZ 85234; tel. 602/926-6276; FAX. 602/926-5177; Cathy Romano, Executive Director

Cataract Surgery Clinic, 215 South Power Road, Suite 112, Mesa, AZ 85206; tel. 602/981-1345; Robert P. Gervais, M.D., President

CIGNA Healthplan of Arizona, Outpatient Surgery, 755 East McDowell Road, Phoenix, AZ 85006; tel. 602/271/5207; Karen A. Miller, Administrator

Cochise Eye and Laser, PC, 2445 East Wilcox Drive, Sierra Vista, AZ 85635; tel. 520/458-8131; FAX. 520/458-0422; Sheree H. Christian, Administrator

Cottonwood Day Surgery Center, Inc., 55 South Sixth Street, Cottonwood, AZ 86326; tel. 602/634-8330; FAX. 520/634-8522; Linda Davis, Administrator

Desert Mountain Surgicenter, Ltd., 7776 Pointe Parkway West, Suite 135, Phoenix, AZ 85044; tel. 602/431-8500; FAX. 602/431-1677; David M. Creech, M.D.

Desert Samaritan Surgicenter, 1500 South Dobson Road, Suite 101, Mesa, AZ 85202; tel. 602/835-3590; FAX. 480/835-8774; Brenda Mastopietro, Administrator

Dooley Outpatient Surgery Center, 151 Riviera Drive, Lake Havasu C, AZ 86403; tel. 602/855-9477; FAX. 602/855-2983; William J. Dooley, Jr., M.D., Medical Director

East Valley Surgical Associates, Ltd., 6424 East Broadway Road, Suite 102, Mesa, AZ 85206; tel. 602/833-2216; Manuel J. Chee

Fifty-Ninth Avenue Surgical Facility, Ltd., 8608 North 59th Avenue, Glendale, AZ 85302; tel. 623/934/3211; FAX. 623/930-1891; Mark Gorman, Administrator

Fishkind and Bakewell Eye Care and Surgery Center, 5599 North Oracle Road, Tucson, AZ 85704; tel. 602/293-6740; FAX. 602/293-6771; Kathleen A. Brown, Surgery Center Supervisor

Flagstaff Outpatient Surgery Center, 77 West Forest Avenue, Suite 306, Flagstaff, AZ 86001; tel. 520/773-2597; FAX. 520/773-2327; Jackie Mosier, RN, Administrator

Footcare Surgi Center, 10249 West Thunderbird, Suite 100, Sun City, AZ 85351; tel. 602/979-4466; FAX. 602/933-8354; Gary N. Friedlander, D.P.M.

Footcare Surgi Center of Northern Arizona, 10 West Columbus Avenue, Flagstaff, AZ 86001; tel. 520/774-4191; Dr. Edward L. Wiebe

Glendale Surgicenter, 5757 West Thunderbird Road, Suite E-150, Glendale, AZ 85306; tel. 602/843-1900; FAX. 602/843-5607; Douglas G. Merrill, M.D., Medical Director

Good Samaritan Surgicenter, 1111 B East McDowell Road, Phoenix, AZ 85006; tel. 602/239-2776; FAX. 602/239-5352; Brenda Mastopietro, Administrator

Greenbaum Outpatient Surgery and Recovery Care Center, 3624 Wells Fargo Avenue, Scottsdale, AZ 85251; tel. 602/481-4958; Craig Stout, Administrator

Grimm Eye Clinic and Cataract Institute, P.C., 1502 North Tucson Boulevard, Tucson, AZ 85716; tel. 602/326-4321; Stephen F. Grimm, M.D.

Havasu Arthritis and Sports Medicine Institute, 1840 Mesquite Avenue, Suite G, Lake Havasu, AZ 86403; tel. 602/453-2663; Marc H. Zimmerman, M.D., Administrator

Havasu Foot and Ankle Surgi-Center, 90 Riviera Drive, Lake Havasu, AZ 86403; tel. 520/855-7800; FAX. 520/855-5392; Robert Novack, D.P.M., Director

HealthSouth Surgery Center of Tucson, 310 North Wilmot Road, Suite 309, Tucson, AZ 85711; tel. 520/296-7080; FAX. 520/886-6518; Aaron Chatterson, Administrator

Kokopelli Eye Care, P.C., 2820 North Glassford Hill Road, Suite 106, Prescott Vall, AZ 86314; tel. 520/775-5606; FAX. 520/772-4999; Nina M. Corriere

Lear Surgery Clinic-Sun City, 10615 West Thunderbird, Suite A-100, Sun City, AZ 85351; tel. 602/974-9375; FAX. 602/977-2598; David E. Marine, Executive Director

© 2000 AHA Guide Health Organizations, Agencies, and Providers **C71**

Providers / Freestanding Ambulatory Surgery Centers

Mayo Clinic Scottsdale Ambulatory Surgery Center, 13400 East Shea Boulevard, Scottsdale, AZ 85259 tel. 602/342-2419; FAX. 602/342-2414; Karen A. Biel, Administrator

McCready Eye Surgery Center, 310 North Wilmot Road, Suite 106, Tucson, AZ 85711; tel. 520/885-6783; FAX. 520/885-5366; Joseph L. McCready, M.D., Administrator

Metro Ambulatory Surgery, Inc., a/k/a Metro Recovery Care Center, 3131 West Peoria Avenue, Phoenix, AZ 85029; tel. 602/375-1083; FAX. 602/789-6833; Carole A. Crevier, Administrator

Mohave Surgery Center, Inc., 1919 Florence Avenue, Kingman, AZ 86401; tel. 520/753-5454; FAX. 520/753-7790; Frank Brown, Administrator

Moon Valley Surgery Center, Inc., 14045 North Seventh Street, Suite Two, Phoenix, AZ 85022; tel. 602/942-3966; Andrew E. Lowy

Nogales Medical Clinic Outpatient Surgery, 480 North Morley Avenue, Nogales, AZ 85621; tel. 520/287-2726; Imogene A. Bell, Administrator

Osborn Ambulatory Surgical Center, 3330 North Second Street, Suite 300, Phoenix, AZ 85012; tel. 602/265-0113; FAX. 602/277-8580; Gudrun Anderson, RN, Administrator

Outpatient Surgical Care, Ltd., 1530 West Glendale, Suite 105, Phoenix, AZ 85021; tel. 602/995-3395; FAX. 602/995-1853; James Kennedy, M.D., Medical Director

Outpatient Surgical Center, 456 North Mesa Drive, Mesa, AZ 85201; tel. 602/464-8000; FAX. 602/969-7107; Maddie Dauernheim, Administrator

Phoenix Eye Surgical Center, A.C., 5133 North Central Avenue, Suite 100, Phoenix, AZ 85012; tel. 602/279-2434; FAX. 602/279-6475; Beth Hurley, RN Nursing/Business Administrator

Porter, Michael, D.P.M., 3620 East Campbell, Suite B, Phoenix, AZ 85018; tel. 602/954-6224; Michael Porter

Prescott Outpatient Surgery Center, Inc., 815 Ainsworth Drive, Prescott, AZ 86301; tel. 602/778-9770; Gail Reidhead, Administrative Director

Prescott Urocenter, Ltd., 811 Ainsworth, Suite 101, Prescott, AZ 86301; tel. 520/771-5282; FAX. 520/771-5283; Gregory Oldani

Santa Cruz Ambulatory Surgical Center, 699 West Ajo Way, Tucson, AZ 85713; tel. 602/746-1711; Richard Edward Quint, Administrator

Scottsdale Eye Surgery Center, P.C., 3320 North Miller Road, Scottsdale, AZ 85251; tel. 602/949-1208; FAX. 602/994-3316; Beth Hurley, RN Nursing/Business Administrator

Southwestern Eye Center, 1055 S. Stapley, Mesa, AZ 85204; tel. 480/833/9100; John M. Lewis, M.D.

Southwestern Eye Center-Casa Grande, 1919 North Trekell Road, Casa Grande, AZ 85222; tel. 520/426-9224; FAX. 520/426-1554; Lothaire Bluth, Administrator

Southwestern Eye Center-Yuma, 2179 West 24th Street, Yuma, AZ 85364; tel. 520/726-4120; FAX. 520/341-0315; Lance K. Wozniak, M.D.

Southwestern Eye Surgi Center-Falcon Field, 4760 Falcon Drive, Mesa, AZ 85205; tel. 602/985-7400; Pat Bray, RN, CRNO, Director

Southwestern Eye Surgicenter-Nogales, 1815 North Mastick Way, Nogales, AZ 85621; tel. 520/761/3533; Pat Bray, Administrator

Sun City Endoscopy Center, Inc., 13203 North 103rd Avenue, Suite C 3, Sun City, AZ 85351; tel. 623/972-2116; Jagdish Patel, M.D.

Surgery Center of Peoria, 13260 North 94th Drive, Suite 300, Peoria, AZ 85381; tel. 623/933-2900; FAX. 623/933-2900; Gayle Stockin, Administrator

Surgi-Care, 5115 North Central Avenue, Suite B, Phoenix, AZ 85012; tel. 602/264-1818; FAX. 602/264-2172; Ellison F. Herro, M.D., Administrator

SurgiCenter, 1040 East McDowell Road, Phoenix, AZ 85006; tel. 602/258-1521; FAX. 602/340-0889; Sharon Shafer, RN, Administrator

Surginet of Arizona, Ltd., 7725 North 43rd Avenue, Suite 100, Phoenix, AZ 85051; tel. 623/931-9400; FAX. 623/930-9884; Jan Haffley, Administrator

Swagel Wootton Eye Center, 220 South 63rd Street, Mesa, AZ 85206; tel. 602/641-3937; FAX. 602/924-5096; S. Joyce Graham

T.A.S.I. Surgery Center, 5585 North Oracle Road, Suite B, Tucson, AZ 85704; tel. 602/293-4730; John A. Pierce, M.D., Medical Director

Tempe Surgical Center, Inc., 2000 East Southern Avenue, Suite 106, Tempe, AZ 85282; tel. 602/838-9313; Richard F. Pavese, M.D.

Thunderbird Samaritan Surgicenter, 5555 B West Thunderbird Road, Glendale, AZ 85306-4622; tel. 602/588-5475; FAX. 602/588-5472; Diane Elmore, RN, Administrator

Valley Outpatient Surgery Center, 160 West University Drive, Mesa, AZ 85201; tel. 602/835-7373; FAX. 602/969-7981; Craig R. Cassidy, D.O., President

Vital Sight ASC, dba Eye Institute of Southern Arizona, 5632 East Fifth Street, Tucson, AZ 85711; tel. 520/790-8888; FAX. 520/790-1427; Clara Dupnik

Warner Medical Park Outpatient Surgery, Inc., 604 West Warner Road, Building A, Chandler, AZ 85225; tel. 480/899-2571; FAX. 480/899-4263; Robert Thunberg

White Mountain Ambulatory Surgery Center, 2650 East Show Low Lake Road, Suite Two, Show Low, AZ 85901; tel. 602/537-4240; William J. Waldo

Yuma Outpatient Surgery Center, L.P., 2475 Avenue A, Suite B, Yuma, AZ 85364; tel. 520/726-6910; FAX. 520/726-7423; Stephen Renfro, Facility Administrator

ARKANSAS

Arkansas Endoscopy Center, P.A., 9501 Lile Drive, Suite 100, Little Rock, AR 72205; tel. 501/224-9100; FAX. 501/224-0420; Ronald D. Hardin, M.D.

Arkansas Otolaryngology Ambulatory Surgery Center, 1200 Medical Towers Building, 9601 Lile Drive, Little Rock, AR 72205; tel. 501/227-5050; Joseph R. Phillips, RN, Administrator

Arkansas Surgery and Endoscopy Center, 4800 Hazel Street, Pine Bluff, AR 71603; tel. 870/536-4800; FAX. 870/536-1609; Syed Samad, M.D., FACP, FACG President

Arkansas Surgery Center, 10 Hospital Circle, Batesville, AR 72501; tel. 870/793-4040; FAX. 870/793-5649; Ronald L. Lowery, M.D., Administrator

Arkansas Surgery Center of Fayetteville, 3873 North Parkview Drive, Suite One, Fayetteville, AR 72703; tel. 501/582-3200; FAX. 501/582-1338; Debra Sexton, Administrator

BEC Surgery Center, One Mercy Lane, Suite 201, P.O. Box 6409, Hot Springs, AR 71902; tel. 501/623-0755; Terry D. Brown

Boozman–Hof Eye Surgery and Laser Center, LLC, 3737 West Walnut Street, P.O. Box 1353, Rogers, AR 72757-1353; tel. 501/636-7506; Donna R. Acord, Director

Cooper Clinic Ambulatory Surgery Center, 6801 Rogers Avenue, P.O. Box 3528, Fort Smith, AR 72903; tel. 501/452-2077; FAX. 501/631-2702; Jerry Stewart, M.D. Administrator

Dempsey–McKee, Inc., d/b/a McKee Outpatient Surgery Center, 601 East Matthews, Jonesboro, AR 72401; tel. 501/935-6396; FAX. 501/935-4063; Terry V. DePriest, Administrator

Doctors Surgery Center, 303 West Polk Street, Suite B, West Memphis, AR 72301; tel. 501/732-2100; Doris Davis, Administrator

Endoscopy Center of Hot Springs, 151 McGowan Court, Hot Springs, AR 71913; tel. 501/623-4101; FAX. 501/623-0103; Rebecca Bates, Administrator

H. Lewis Pearson Eye Institute, 3211 Surger Hill Road, Texarkana, AR 71854-9265; tel. 501/772-4440; FAX. 501/772-7190; James Loomis, Comptroller

Hot Springs Outpatient Surgery, 100 Ridgeway Boulevard, Suite Seven, Hot Springs, AR 71901; tel. 501/624-4464; FAX. 501/623-7748; Robert V. Borg, M.D., Administrator

James Trice, M.D., P.A., d/b/a Digestive Disease Center, 7005 South Hazel Street, Pine Bluff, AR 71603; tel. 870/536-3070; FAX. 870/536-3171; Louis Trice, Administrator

Little Rock Diagnostic Clinic ASC, 10001 Lile Drive, Little Rock, AR 72205; tel. 501/227-8000; Roger J. St. Onge, Administrator

Little Rock Pain Clinic, Two Lile Court, Suite 100, Little Rock, AR 72205; tel. 501/224-7246; FAX. 501/224-7644; Virginia Johnson, Administrator

Little Rock Surgery Center, 8820 Knoedl Court, Little Rock, AR 72205; tel. 501/224-6767; FAX. 501/224-8203; Jerri Herron, Administrator

Lowery Medical/Surgical Eye Center, P.A., 105 Central Avenue, Searcy, AR 72143; tel. 501/268-7154; FAX. 501/268-9071; Benjamin R. Lowery, M.D., Administrator

North Hills Gastroenterology Endoscopy Center, Inc., 3344 North Futrall Drive, Fayetteville, AR 72703; tel. 501/582-7280; FAX. 510/582-7279; William C. Martin, M.D.

Northeast Arkansas Surgery Center, Inc., 505 East Matthews, Suite 103, Jonesboro, AR 72401; tel. 501/972-1723; FAX. 501/972-5941; Teresa D. Brown, Administrator

Ozark Eye Center, 360 Highway Five North, Mountain Home, AR 72653; tel. 501/425-2277; Rick Galkoski, Administrator

Physicians Day Surgery Center, 3805 West 28th, Pine Bluff, AR 71603; tel. 501/536-4100; FAX. 501/536-3100; Joan Fletcher, Administrator

Russellville Surgery Center, L.L.C., 2205 West Main Street, P.O. Box 2654, Russellville, AR 72801; tel. 501/890-2654; FAX. 501/890-5101; James Kennedy, Administrator

South Arkansas Surgery Center, 4310 South Mulberry, Pine Bluff, AR 71603; tel. 501/535-5719; Tammy L. Studdard, Administrator

Sparks Medical Plaza, 1500 Dodson Avenue, Fort Smith, AR 72901; tel. 501/788-4000; FAX. 501/441-5420; Harold H. Mings, M.D., Chief Executive Officer

The Center for Day Surgery, 4200 Jenny Lind, Suite A, Fort Smith, AR 72901; tel. 501/648-9496; Monte Wilson, Administrator

The Gastro-Intestinal Center, 405 North University, Little Rock, AR 72205; tel. 501/663-1074; James G. Dunlap, Administrator

The Physicians Surgery Center of Arkansas, Inc., d/b/a Physicians Surgery Center, 1024 North University Avenue, Little Rock, AR 72207; tel. 501/663-0158; FAX. 501/663-4652; Martha Plant, Administrator

CALIFORNIA

Advanced Surgery Center, 5771 North Fresno Street, Suite 101, Fresno, CA 93710; tel. 559/448-9900; FAX. 559/448-9546; B. David, Administrator

Aesthetic Facial Surgery Center of Menlo Park, 2200 Sand Hill Road, Suite 130, Menlo Park, CA 94025; tel. 415/854-6444; Dr. Mary Lynn Maron

Aestheticare Outpatient Surgery Center, 30260 Rancho Viejo Road, San Juan Capital, CA 92675; tel. 949/661-1700; FAX. 949/661-4321; Ronald E. Moser, M.D.

Ambulatory Surgical Center of Chico, 1950 East 20th Street, Suite 102, Chico, CA 95928; tel. 916/343-1674; Robert G. Basinger, D.P.M.

Ambulatory Surgical Center of Southern California, Gastroenterology Diagnostic Center, 880 South Atlantic Boulevard G-10, Monterey Park, CA 91754; tel. 213/483-9080; Zelman Weingaren, M.D.

Ambulatory Surgical Center of the Zeiter Eye, 117 North San Joaquin Street, Stockton, CA 95202; tel. 209/466-5566; FAX. 209/466-0535; Donna M. Tschirky

Ambulatory Surgical Center, Inc., 14400 Bear Valley Road, Suite 201, Victorville, CA 92392; tel. 760/951-5162; FAX. 818/985-0055; Garey L. Weber, D.P.M., Administrator

Ambulatory Surgical Centers, Inc., 18952 Mac Arthur Boulevard, Suite 102, Irvine, CA 92612; tel. 949/833-3406; FAX. 949/985-0055; Garey L. Weber, D.P.M., Administrator

Anaheim Surgical Center, 1324 South Euclid Street, Anaheim, CA 92802; tel. 714/533-9880; FAX. 714/533-1802; Debra Berntsen, RN, Charge Nurse

Antelope Valley Surgery Center, 44301 North Lorimer Avenue, Lancaster, CA 93534; tel. 805/940-1112; FAX. 805/940-6856; Yolanda Gomez

Apple Valley Surgery Center, 18122 Outer Highway 18, Apple Valley, CA 92307; tel. 760/946-1170; FAX. 760/946-2646; Virginia Budington, Administrator

Arlington Podiatry Surgery Center, 7310 Magnolia Avenue, Riverside, CA 92504; tel. 909/354-8787; FAX. 909/354-0350; James A. De Silva, Administrator

Aspen Outpatient Center, 2750 North Sycamore Drive, Simi Valley, CA 93065; tel. 805/955-8100; FAX. 805/583-1084; Bob Ericson, Administrative Director, Ambulatory Care

Associates Outpatient Surgery Center, 2128 Eureka Way, Redding, CA 96001; tel. 916/246-9737; FAX. 916/246-4052; Jesse M. Kramer, M.D., Administrator

Atherton Plastic Surgery Center, 3351 El Camino Real, Suite 201, Atherton, CA 94027; tel. 415/363-0300; FAX. 415/363-0302; David Apfelberg

Bakersfield Endoscopy Center, 1902 B Street, Bakersfield, CA 93301; tel. 805/327-4455; Ramesh Gupta, M.D., Medical Director

Providers / Freestanding Ambulatory Surgery Centers

Bakersfield Surgery Center, 2120 19th Street, Bakersfield, CA 93301; tel. 661/323-2020; FAX. 661/323-6552; Shirley Skelton, Administrator

Beverly Hills Ambulatory Surgery Center, Inc., 9201 Sunset Boulevard, Suite 405, Los Angeles, CA 90069; tel. 310/887-1730; Sandra Cericola, Administrator

Beverly Hills Outpatient Surgery Center, 250 North Robertson Boulevard, Suite 104, Los Angeles, CA 90211; tel. 310/273-9255; FAX. 310/273-6167; Peter Golden, M.D., Medical Director

Beverly Surgical Center, 105 West Beverly Boulevard, Montebello, CA 90640-4375; tel. 213/728-5400; FAX. 213/887-0058; James G. Ovieda, Administrator

Blackhawk Surgery Center, Inc., 4165 Blackhawk Plaza Circle, Suite 195, Danville, CA 94506; tel. 510/736-7881; Molly Healy, Administrator

Bolsa Out-Patient Surgery Center, 10362 Bolsa Avenue, Suite 100, Westminster, CA 92683; tel. 714/775-5690; FAX. 714/775-7405; CO D. L. PHAM, FACOG, M.D., Medical Director

Bonaventure Surgery Center, 221 North Jackson Avenue, San Jose, CA 95116; tel. 408/729-2848; FAX. 408/729-2880; Virginia Field, RN, M.B.A., Director

Brawley Endoscopy and Surgery Center, 205 West Legion Road, Brawley, CA 92227; tel. 619/351-3655; FAX. 619/351-3675; Mahomed Suliman, M.D., Administrator

Brockton Surgical Center, 5905 Brockton Avenue, Suite B, Riverside, CA 92506; tel. 909/686-5373; FAX. 909/778-9064; Michael N. Durrant, D.P.M., MPH

Bruce A. Kaplan, M.D., 39000 Bob Hope Drive, Wright Building, Suite 209, Rancho Mirage, CA 92270; tel. 619/346-5603; FAX. 619/346-5604; Jessie Schumaker

California Eye Clinic, 3747 Sunset Lane, Suite A, Antioch, CA 94509; tel. 510/754-2300; Jean Kemp, Administrator

Camden Surgery Center of Beverly Hills, 414 North Camden Drive, Suite 800, Beverly Hills, CA 90210; tel. 310/859-3991; FAX. 310/859-7126; Yasmin Sibulo, Administrator

Capistrano Surgicenter, Inc., 30280 Rancho Viejo Road, San Juan Capital, CA 92675; tel. 714/248-5757; FAX. 714/248-9339; Jeffrey A. Klein, President

Cardiac Surgery Mercy Medical Center, 2626 Edith Avenue # D, Redding, CA 96001; tel. 530/243-2626; Edward W. Pottmeyer, M.D.

Center for Ambulatory Medicine and Surgery, 111 East Noble Avenue, Visalia, CA 93277; tel. 209/739-8383; FAX. 209/739-7929; Janice M. Weaver, Business Coordinator

Central Coast Surgery Center, 1941 Johnson Avenue, Suite 103, San Luis Obis, CA 93406; tel. 805/546-9999; FAX. 804/546-8904; Helen Swanagon, Nurse Administrator

Channel Islands Surgicenter, 2300 Wankel Way, Oxnard, CA 93030; tel. 805/485-1908; FAX. 805/485-5767; Mary K. Fish, Administrator

Children's Surgery Center, 744 Fifty-Second Street, Oakland, CA 94609; tel. 510/428-3133; FAX. 510/450-5606; Terry Hawes, Administrator

Columbia Los Gatos Surgical Center, 15195 National Avenue, Los Gatos, CA 95032; tel. 408/356-0454; FAX. 408/358-3924; Martha Ponce, Administrator

Columbia Southwest Surgical Clinic, Inc., 4201 Torrance Boulevard, Suite 240, Torrance, CA 90503; tel. 310/540-7803; FAX. 310/316-3903; Otto Munchow, M.D., Director

Columbia Surgicenter of South Bay, 23500 Madison Street, Torrance, CA 90505; tel. 310/539-5120; Debra Saxton

Columbia West Hills Surgical Center, 7240 Medical Center Drive, West Hills, CA 91307; tel. 818/226-9151; FAX. 818/226-6171; Christine Sherman, Administrator

Columbia/Woodward Park Surgicenter, 7055 North Fresno Street, Suite 100, Fresno, CA 93720; tel. 209/449-9977; FAX. 209/449-9350; Lori Ruffner, RN, Administrator

Community Surgery Centre, 17190 Bernado Center Drive, Suite 100, San Diego, CA 92128; tel. 619/675-3270; FAX. 619/675-3260; Regina S. Boore, B.S.N., M.S.

Crown Valley Surgicenter, 26921 Crown Valley Parkway, Suite 110, Mission Viejo, CA 92691; tel. 949/348-7252; FAX. 949/348-7246; Maurice Chammas, M.D., Administrator

Cypress Outpatient Surgical Center, Inc., 1665 Dominican Way, Suite 120, Santa Cruz, CA 95065; tel. 831/476-6943; FAX. 831/476-1473; Sandra Warren, Administrator

Cypress Surgery Center, 842 South Akers Road, Visalia, CA 93277; tel. 209/740-4094; FAX. 209/740-4100; Jack K. Waller

Del Rey Surgery Center, 4640 Admiralty Way, Suite 1020, Marina Del Re, CA 90292; tel. 310/305-7570; Lee Estes, Administrator

Desert Surgery Center, 1180 North Palm Canyon, Palm Springs, CA 92262; tel. 760/320-7600; FAX. 760/320-1694; Rosemary Combs, Executive Director

Digestive Disease Center, 24411 Health Center Drive, Suite 450, Laguna Hills, CA 92653; tel. 714/586-9386; FAX. 714/586-0864; Crisynda Buss, RN

Doctors Surgery Center of Whittier, 8135 South Painter Avenue, Suite 103, Whittier, CA 90602; tel. 310/945-8961; FAX. 310/698-3578; Veronica Coughenour, RN

Doctors Surgical Center, Inc., 9461 Grindlay Street, Suite 102, Cypress, CA 90630; tel. 714/995-3001; R. Wayne Ives, Administrator

Doctors' Surgery Center, 1441 Liberty Street, Suite 104, Redding, CA 96001; tel. 916/244-6300; FAX. 916/246-2051; Joy Schultz, Director

Downey Surgery Center, 8555 East Florence Avenue, Downey, CA 90240; tel. 310/923-9784; Marisol Magana, Administrator

E. N. T. Facial Surgery Center, 1351 East Spruce, Fresno, CA 93720; tel. 209/432-3724; FAX. 209/432-8579; JoAnn LoForti, RN, Division of Nursing

East Bay Medical Surgical Center, 20998 Redwood Road, Castro Valley, CA 94546; tel. 510/538-2828; FAX. 510/538-2508; Yoshitsugu Teramoto, M.D., Administrator

El Camino Surgery Center, 2480 Grant Road, Mountain View, CA 94040-4300; tel. 650/961-1200; FAX. 650/960-7041; Nancy Kessler

El Mirador Surgical Center, 1180 North Indian Canyon Drive, Palm Springs, CA 92262; tel. 760/416-4600; FAX. 760/416-4668; Marilyn M. Perkins, Nurse Administrator

Endoscopy Center of Chula Vista, 681 Third Avenue, Suite B, Chula Vista, CA 91910; tel. 619/425-2150; Robert Penner, M.D., Administrator

Endoscopy Center of Southern California, 2336 Santa Monica Boulevard, Suite 204, Santa Monica, CA 90404; tel. 310/453-4477; FAX. 310/453-4811; Parviz D. Afshani

Endoscopy Center of the Central Coast, 77 Casa Street, Suite 106, San Luis Obis, CA 93405; tel. 805/541-1021; FAX. 805/541-3142; Penny Chamousis, Administrator

Escondido Surgery Center, 343 East Second Avenue, Escondido, CA 92025; tel. 619/480-6606; FAX. 619/480-6671; Marvin W. Levenson, M.D., Managing Medical Director

Eye Center of Northern California Surgicenter, 6500 Fairmount Avenue, Suite Two, El Cerrito, CA 94530; tel. 510/525-2600; FAX. 510/524-1887; William Ellis

Eye Life Institute, 6283 Clark Road, Suite Seven, Paradise, CA 95969; tel. 916/877-2020; FAX. 916/877-4641; Almary Hivale, RN, Administrator

Eye Surgery Center of Southern California, Inc./Med. Group, 2023 West Vista Way, Suite E, Vista, CA 92083; tel. 619/941-8152; FAX. 619/726-4822; Regg V. Antle, M.D., Medical Director

Eye Surgery Center of the Desert, 39700 Bob Hope Drive, Suite 111, Rancho Mirage, CA 92270; tel. 760/340-3937; FAX. 760/340-1940; Timothy T. Milauskas, Administrator

Feather River Surgery Center, 370 Del Norte Avenue, Yuba City, CA 95991; tel. 916/751-4800; FAX. 916/751-4884; Elizabeth LaBouyer, RN, CNOR, Perioperative Coordinator

Fig Garden Surgi-Med Center, 1332 West Herndon Avenue # 101, Fresno, CA 93711-0431; tel. 559/439-2040

Foothill Ambulatory Surgery Center, 1030 East Foothill Boulevard, Suite 101B, Upland, CA 91786; tel. 909/981-5859; FAX. 909/981-8293; Montra M. Kanok, M.D.

Fort Sutter Surgery Center, 2801 K Street, Suite 525, Sacramento, CA 95816; tel. 916/733-5017; FAX. 916/733-8738; Bill Davis, Administrator

Four Thirty-Six North Bedford Surgicenter, 436 North Bedford, Suite 101, Beverly Hills, CA 90210; tel. 310/278-0188; FAX. 310/278-1791; Kay Zacharski, RN, Director of Nursing

Fremont Surgery Center, 2675 Stevenson Boulevard, Fremont, CA 94538; tel. 510/793-4987; FAX. 510/793-5084; Debbie Mack, Director of Nursing

Fritch Eye Care Medical Center, 2525 Eye Street, Suite A and B, Bakersfield, CA 93301; tel. 805/327-8511; FAX. 805/327-9809; Charles D. Fritch, M.D.

Frost Street Outpatient Surgical Center, LP, 8008 Frost Street, Suite 200, San Diego, CA 92123; tel. 619/576-8320; FAX. 619/576-8568; John Cashman, Administrator

GastroDiagnostics, A Medical Group, 1140 West La Veta, Suite 550, Orange, CA 92868; tel. 714/835-5100; FAX. 714/835-5567; Stephanie Quinn, Administrator

Glendale Eye Surgery Center, 607 North Central, Suite 103, Glendale, CA 91203; tel. 818/956-1010; FAX. 818/543-6083; Stephen S. Chang, M.D.

Glenwood Surgical Center, L.P., 8945 Magnolia Avenue, Suite 200, Riverside, CA 92503; tel. 909/688-7270; Calvin Nash

Golden Triangle Surgicenter, 25405 Hancock Avenue, Suite 103, Murrieta, CA 92562; tel. 909/698-4670; FAX. 909/698-4675; Ella Stockstill, Administrator

Golden West Pain Therapy Center, 25405 Hancock Avenue, Suite 110, Murrieta, CA 92562-5964; tel. 909/698-4710; FAX. 909/698-4715; Richard Harris, Administrator

Greater Long Beach Endoscopy Center, 2880 Atlantic Avenue, Suite 180, Long Beach, CA 90806; tel. 562/426-2606; FAX. 562/426-5866; Andrea Campbell, Business Office Manager

Greater Sacramento Surgery Center, 2288 Auburn Boulevard, Suite 201, Sacramento, CA 95821; tel. 916/929-7229; FAX. 916/929-2590; Susan Brunone, MHS, Administrator

Grossmont Plaza Surgery Center, 5525 Grossmont Center Drive, La Mesa, CA 91942; tel. 619/644-4561; Lois Hoke, Administrator

Halcyon Laser and Surgery Center, Inc., 303 South Halcyon Road, Arroyo Grande, CA 93420; tel. 805/489-8254; FAX. 805/474-1997; Sara Pazell, Administrator Michael Bolumberg,M.D.,Medical Director

Harbor-UCLA Medical Foundation, Inc., Ambulatory Surgery Center, 21840 South Normandie Avenue, Suite 700, Torrance, CA 90502; tel. 310/222-5189; Lee Scher, RN, Administrator

Health South Surgery, Center of Ventura, 3525 Loma Vista Road, Ventura, CA 93003; tel. 805/641-6434; FAX. 805/641-6437; Chris Behm, Administrator

HealthSouth Arcadia Outpatient Surgery, Inc., 614 West Duarte Road, Arcadia, CA 91007; tel. 818/445-4714; FAX. 626/445-1701; Susan P. Nunnery, Administrator

HealthSouth Center for Surgery of Encinitas, 477 North El Camino Real, Suite C-100, Encinitas, CA 92024; tel. 760/942-8800; FAX. 760/942-0106; Christine Ree, Administrator

HealthSouth Forest Surgery Center, 2110 Forest Avenue, San Jose, CA 95128; tel. 408/297-3432; FAX. 408/298-3338; Helen Maloney, RN, Administrator

HealthSouth Grossmont Surgery Center, 8881 Fletcher Parkway, Suite 100, La Mesa, CA 91942; tel. 619/698-0930; FAX. 619/698-3093; Administrator

HealthSouth In-Valley Surgery Center, 4487 Stoneridge Drive, Pleasanton, CA 94588; tel. 510/484-3100; FAX. 510/484-3113; Karen Stevens, RN, CNOR, Administrator

HealthSouth North Coast Surgery Center, 3903 Waring Road, Oceanside, CA 92056; tel. 760/940-0997; FAX. 760/940-0407; Donna Danley, Administrator

HealthSouth South Bay Ambulatory Surgical Center, 251 Landis Street, Chula Vista, CA 91910; tel. 619/585-1020; FAX. 619/585-0247; Arthur E. Casey, Administrator

HealthSouth Surgery Center of Auburn, 3123 Professional Drive, Suite 100, Auburn, CA 95603; tel. 530/888-8899; FAX. 530/888-1464; Fran Thompson, Area Administrator

HealthSouth Surgery Center of San Luis Obispo, 1304-C Ella Street, San Luis Obis, CA 93401; tel. 805/544-7874; FAX. 805/544-6057; Kim Heath, RN, B.S.N., MBA

Healthsouth Surgery Center-Alhambra, 1201 Alhambra Boulevard, Sacramento, CA 95816; tel. 916/733-8222; FAX. 916/733-8224; Rita Bowen, Administrator

Providers / Freestanding Ambulatory Surgery Centers

HealthSouth Surgery Center-J Street, 3810 J Street, Sacramento, CA 95816; tel. 916/929-9431; FAX. 916/929-0132; Charlene Nakayama, Administrator

HealthSouth Surgery Center-Scripps, 75 Scripps Drive, Sacramento, CA 95825; tel. 916/929-9431; FAX. 916/929-0132; Charlene Nakayama, Administrator

HealthSouth Surgery Center-Solano, 991 Nut Tree Road, Suite 100, Vacaville, CA 95687; tel. 707/447-5400; FAX. 707/447-2356; Bill Davis, Administrator

Heart Institute of the Desert an The Heart Hospital, 39-600 Bob Hope Drive, Rancho Mirage, CA 92270; tel. 760/324-3278; FAX. 760/346-1867; Jack J. Sternlieb, Administrator

Hemet Cataract Surgery Clinic, 162 North Santa Fe, Hemet, CA 92343; tel. 909/929-3200; FAX. 909/929-8124; Stephen K. Schaller, M.D., Administrator

Hemet Endoscopy Center, 2390 East Florida Avenue, Suite 101, Hemet, CA 92544; tel. 909/652-2252; FAX. 909/925-9252; Milan S. Chakrabarty, M.D.

Hemet Healthcare Surgicenter, 301 North San Jacinto Avenue, Hemet, CA 92543; tel. 909/765-1717; FAX. 909/765-1716; Jodi Freitas

Hesperia Podiatry Surgery Center, 14661 Main Street, Hesperia, CA 92345; tel. 619/244-0222; FAX. 619/244-1242; William S. Beal

Hi-Desert Surgery Center, 18002 Outer Highway 18, Apple Valley, CA 92307; tel. 619/242-5505; FAX. 619/242-3502; Venkat R. Vangala, M.D.

High Desert Endoscopy, 18523 Corwin Road, Suite H2, Apple Valley, CA 92307; tel. 760/242-3000; FAX. 760/242-1802; Raman S. Poola, M.D., Administrator

Hope Square Surgical Center, 39700 Bob Hope Drive, Suite 301, Rancho Mirage, CA 92270; tel. 760/346-7696; FAX. 760/776-1069; Marilee Kyler, Administrator

Huntington Outpatient Surgery Center, 797 South Fair Oaks Avenue, Pasadena, CA 91105; tel. 626/535-2434; FAX. 626/535-2430; Sandra Bidlack, Administrator

Imperial Valley Surgery Center, 608 G Street, Brawley, CA 92227; tel. 619/344-1101; FAX. 619/344-4985; Vida C. Baron, M.D., Administrator

Inland Endoscopy Center, Inc., d/b/a Mountain View Surgery Center, 10408 Industrial Circle, Redlands, CA 92374; tel. 909/796-7803; FAX. 909/796-0614; Khushal Stanisai

Inland Surgery Center, 1620 Laurel Avenue, Redlands, CA 92373; tel. 909/793-4701; FAX. 909/792-6397; Tina Gaac, Facility Administrator

Inland Surgery Center, 361 North San Jacinto, Hemet, CA 92543; tel. 909/652-4343; R. Michael Duffin, M.D., Medical Director

Irvine Multi-Specialty Surgical Care, 4900 Barranca Parkway, Suite 104, Irvine, CA 92604-8603; tel. 714/726-0677; FAX. 714/726-0678; Carol R. Stevenson, RN, Administrator

John Muir/Mt. Diablo HealthCare System, Inc., d/b/a Diablo Valley Surgery Center, 2222 East Street, Suite 200, Concord, CA 94520; tel. 510/671-2222; FAX. 510/671-2672; Virginia Goodrich, Administrator

Kaiser Ambulatory Surgical Center, 2025 Morse Avenue, Sacramento, CA 95825; tel. 916/973-7675; FAX. 916/973-7786; Richard R. Stading, RN, MSHA, A.S.C. Manager

Kaiser Ambulatory Surgical Center, 10725 International Drive, Rancho Cordov, CA 95670; tel. 916/631-2000; FAX. 916/631-2013; Steven Metzger, RN, Manager

Kaiser Permanente Medical Facility-Stockton, 7373 West Lane, Stockton, CA 95210; tel. 209/476-3300; Jose R. Rivera, Administrator

La Jolla Gastroenterology Medical Group, Inc., Endoscopy Center, 9850 Genesee Avenue, Suite 980, La Jolla, CA 92037; tel. 619/453-5200; FAX. 619/453-5753; Otto T. Nebel, M.D., Medical Director

La Veta Surgical Center, 725 West La Veta, Suite 270, Orange, CA 92868; tel. 714/744-0900; FAX. 714/744-0283; Joyce Hall, Administrator

Laser and Skin Surgery Center of La Jolla, 9850 Genesee Avenue, Suite 480, La Jolla, CA 92037; tel. 858/455-7714; FAX. 858/455-9340; Angela Richberg, RN

Laser Surgery Center, LTD., 2021 Ygnacio Valley Road, Building H-102, Walnut Creek, CA 94598; tel. 925/949-9400; FAX. 925/947-2160; Lori Fried, Administrator

Lassen Surgery Center, 103 Fair Drive, P.O. Box 1150, Susanville, CA 96130; tel. 530/257-7772; FAX. 530/257-2939; Shannon Viersla, Medical Staff Secretary

Lodi Outpatient Surgical Center, 521 South Ham Lane, Suite F, Lodi, CA 95242; tel. 209/333-0905; FAX. 209/333-0219; Marklin E. Brown, Administrator

Loma Linda Foot and Ankle Center, Ambulatory Surgical Center, 11332 Mountain View Avenue, Suite A, Loma Linda, CA 92354; tel. 909/796-3707; FAX. 909/796-3709; Sheldon Collis, D.P.M., Administrator

Los Robles Surgicenter, 2190 Lynn Road, Suite 100, Thousand Oaks, CA 91360; tel. 805/497-3737; FAX. 805/373-8878; Le Anne Schai, Administrative Director

M/S Surgery Center, 3510 Martin Luther King Boulevard, Lynwood, CA 90262; tel. 310/635-7550; FAX. 310/603-8749; John H. Shammas, M.D., Medical Director

Madera Ambulatory Endoscopy Center, 1015 West Yosemite Avenue, Suite 101, Madera, CA 93637; tel. 209/673-4000; FAX. 209/673-1430; Naeem M. Akhtar, M.D.

Madison Park Surgery and Laser Center, 3445 Pacific Coast Highway, Suite 250, Torrance, CA 90505; tel. 310/530-2900; FAX. 310/891-0367; R. Reed

Magnolia Outpatient Surgery Center, 14571 Magnolia Street, Suite 107, Westminster, CA 92683; tel. 714/898-6448; FAX. 714/893-1681; Bob Caldwell, Chief Executive Officer

Magnolia Plastic Surgery Center, 10694 Magnolia Avenue, Riverside, CA 92505; tel. 909/358-1445; FAX. 909/688-2803; Alexander Carli

Marin Ophthalmic Surgery Center, 901 E Street, Suite 270, San Rafael, CA 94901; tel. 415/454-2112; FAX. 415/454-6542; Audrey M. DeMars, Administrator

Mariners Bay Surgical Medical Center, 318 South Lincoln Boulevard, Suite 100, Venice, CA 90291; tel. 310/314-2191; FAX. 310/392-8020; Gregory Panos, II, Administrator

Martel Eye Surgical Center, 11216 Trinity River, Rancho Cordov, CA 95670; tel. 916/635-6161; FAX. 916/635-5145; Joseph Martel, M.D.

McHenry Surgery Center, 1524 McHenry Street, Suite 240, Modesto, CA 95350; tel. 209/576-2900; FAX. 209/575-5815; Syd Fuentes, RN, Director

Medical Arts Ambulatory Surgery Center, 205 South West Street, Suite B, Visalia, CA 93291; tel. 209/625-9601; FAX. 209/625-3124; Thomas F. Mitts, M.D., Administrator

Medical Plaza Orthopedic Surgery Center, 1301 20th Street, Suite 140, Santa Monica, CA 90404; tel. 310/315-0333; FAX. 310/315-0341; Carolyn A. Hankinson, RN, Director, Nursing

Merced Ambulatory Endoscopy Center, 750 West Olive Avenue, Suite 107A, Merced, CA 95348; tel. 209/384-3116; FAX. 209/384-0878; Monika Grasley, Administrator

Mercy Surgical and Diagnostic Center, 3303 North M Street, Merced, CA 95348; tel. 209/384-3533; FAX. 209/383-5047; Lynda Pitts, Administrator

Mission Ambulatory Surgicenter, Ltd., 26730 Crown Valley Parkway, First Floor, Mission Viejo, CA 92691; tel. 714/364-2201; FAX. 714/364-5372; Thomas H. Catlett, Administrator

Mission Valley Surgery Center, 39263 Mission Boulevard, Fremont, CA 94539; tel. 510/796-4500; FAX. 510/796-4573; Sarb S. Hundal, M.D.

Mittleman/Moran Asthetiz Facial Surgery CenterReconstructive Surgery, 2200 Sandhill Road, Suite 130, Menlo Park, CA 94025; tel. 415/854-6444; Mary Lynn Moran, M.D., Administrator

Modesto Surgery Center, Inc., 400 East Orangeburg Avenue, Suite One, Modesto, CA 95350; tel. 209/526-3000; FAX. 209/526-3133; Dr. Greg Tesluk, Administrator

Monterey Bay Endoscopy Center, 833 Cass Street, Suite B, Monterey, CA 93940; tel. 408/375-3598; FAX. 408/375-1478; James Farrow, Administrator

Monterey Peninsula Surgery Center, LLC., 966 Cass Street, Suite 210, Monterey, CA 93940; tel. 408/372-2169; FAX. 408/372-6323; J.R. LeBlanc, Administrator

Moreno Valley Ambulatory Surgery Center, 24384 Sunnymead Boulevard, Moreno Valley, CA 92388; tel. 714/247-8080; FAX. 714/247-9381; John E. Bohn, Administrator

Napa Surgery Center, 3444 Valle Verde Drive, Napa, CA 94558; tel. 707/252-9660; Eric Grigsby, M.D., Medical Director

Newport Beach Orange Coast Endoscopy Center, 1525 Superior Avenue, Suite 114, Newport Beach, CA 92663; tel. 949/646-6999; FAX. 949/646-9699; Donald Abraham

Newport Beach Surgery Center, 361 Hospital Road, Suite 124, Newport Beach, CA 92663; tel. 714/631-0988; FAX. 714/631-2036; Eric Reints, Administrator

Newport Surgery Institute, 360 San Miguel Drive, Suite 406, Newport Beach, CA 92660; tel. 714/759-0995; Linda Shelman, Office Manager

North Anaheim Surgicenter, 1154 North Euclid, Anaheim, CA 92801; tel. 714/635-6272; FAX. 714/635-0943; Monica Briton, Administrator

North County Outpatient Surgery Center, 1101 Las Tablas Road, P.O. Box 147, Templeton, CA 93465; tel. 805/434-1333; FAX. 805/434-3171; Carolyn Lash, RN, Administrator

Northern California Kidney Stone Center, 15195 National Avenue, Suite 204, Los Gatos, CA 95032; tel. 408/358-2111; FAX. 408/356-2359; John Kersten Kraft, Medical Director

Northridge Maxillofacial Surgery Center, 18546 Roscoe Boulevard, Suite 125, Northridge, CA 91324; tel. 818/349-8890; FAX. 818/349-1532; Robert G. Hale, D.D.S., Administrator

Northridge Surgery Center, 8327 Reseda Boulevard, Northridge, CA 91324; tel. 818/993-3131; FAX. 818/993-3347; Robert Vassey, Administrator

Optima Ophthalmic Medical Associates, Inc., 1237 B Street, Hayward, CA 94541-2977; tel. 510/886-3937; FAX. 510/886-4465; Nora J. McQuinn, Administrative Director

Orange County Institute of Gastroenterology and Endoscopy, 26732 Crown Valley Parkway, Suite 241, Mission Viejo, CA 92691; tel. 949/364-2611; FAX. 949/364-0226; Ahmad M. Shaban, M.D., Medical Director

Orange County Litho Center, Inc., 12555 Garden Grove Boulevard, Suite 200, Garden Grove, CA 92843; tel. 714/530-6000; FAX. 714/534-7061; Guy A. Biagiotti, M.D.

Orange Surgical Services, 302 West La Veta Avenue, Suite 100, Orange, CA 92866; tel. 714/771-3432; FAX. 714/741-7606; Elizabeth E. Grant, RN, M.S.

Out-Patient Surgery Center, 17752 Beach Boulevard, Huntington Beach, CA 92647; tel. 714/842-1426; FAX. 714/847-1503; Madelyn Tinkler, Administrator

Outpatient Care Surgery Center South, 5225 Kearny Villa Way, Suite 110, San Diego, CA 92123; tel. 619/278-1611; FAX. 619/278-5853; Ronald Gertsch, M.D.

Pacific Dental Surgery Center, 820 34th Street, Suite 201, Bakersfield, CA 93301; tel. 805/327-7878; Charles Nicholson, III, Administrator

Pacific Eye Institute, 555 North 13th Avenue, Upland, CA 91786; tel. 909/982-8846; FAX. 909/949-3967; Robert Fabricant, M.D., FACS, Medical Director

Pacific Hills Surgery Center, Inc., 24022 Calle De La Plata, Suite 180, Laguna Hills, CA 92653; tel. 714/951-9470; FAX. 714/951-9478; Norman D. Peterson, M.D., Medical Director

Pacific Surgicenter, Inc., 1301 20th Street, Suite 470, Santa Monica, CA 90404; tel. 310/315-0222; FAX. 310/828-8852; Jocelyne Rosenthal, RN, Administrator

Palm Desert Ambulatory Surgery Center, 73-345 Highway 111, Palm Desert, CA 92260; tel. 619/346-4780; FAX. 619/340-4650; S. C. Shah, M.D., Administrator

Paul L. Archambeau, M.D., Inc., Ambulatory Surgery Center, 380 Tesconi Court, Santa Rosa, CA 95401; tel. 707/544-3375; FAX. 707/544-0808; Paul L. Archambeau, M.D., Administrator

Petaluma Surgicenter, 1400 Professional Drive, Suite 102, Petaluma, CA 94954; tel. 707/763-9325; FAX. 707/769-0751; Ronald M. La Vigna, D.P.M.

Physician's Surgery Center, 901 Campus Drive, Suite 102, Daly City, CA 94015; tel. 415/991-2000; FAX. 415/755-8638; Kathleen O'Riordan

Physicians Plaza Surgical Center, 6000 Physicians Boulevard, Bakersfield, CA 93301; tel. 805/322-4744; FAX. 805/322-2938; Michael G. Clark, Administrator

Providers / Freestanding Ambulatory Surgery Centers

Physicians Resource Group, d/b/a Barr Eye Surgery Center, 1805 North California Street, Stockton, CA 95204; tel. 209/948-3241; FAX. 209/948-9321; Susan Ford, Administrator

Plastic and Reconstructive Surgery Center, 1387 Santa Rita Road, Pleasanton, CA 94566; tel. 510/462-3700; FAX. 510/462-4681; Ronald Iverson, Administrator

Plastic Surgery Center, 1515 El Camino Real, Palo Alto, CA 94304; tel. 650/322-2723; FAX. 650/322-3260; Grace Bazan, Business MGR.

Plaza Surgical Center, Inc., 168 North Brent Street, Suite 403B, Ventura, CA 93003; tel. 805/643-5438; FAX. 805/643-1625; Dale P. Armstrong, M.D.

Podiatric Surgery Center, 255 North Gilbert, Suite B, Hemet, CA 92543; tel. 909/925-2186; FAX. 909/925-4947; Robert Drake, D.P.M., Administrator

Point Loma Surgical Center, 3434 Midway Drive, Suite 1006, San Diego, CA 92110; tel. 619/223-0910; FAX. 619/221-4456; David M. Kupfer, M.D., Medical Director

Porterville Surgical Center, 577 West Putnam Avenue, Porterville, CA 93257; tel. 209/788-6400; Lucy Lara, Administrator

Premier Endoscopy Center of the Desert, 1100 North Palm Canyon Drive, Suite 209, Palm Springs, CA 92262; tel. 760/416-6322; FAX. 760/416-0483; Phillip R. Roy, Administrator

Premiere Surgery Center, Inc., 700 West El Norte Parkway, Escondido, CA 92026; tel. 760/738-7830; FAX. 760/738-7841; R. K. Massengill, M.D., Medical Director

Providence Ambulatory Surgical Center, 1310 West Stewart Drive, Suite 310, Orange, CA 92668; tel. 714/771-6363; FAX. 714/771-0754; Harrell E. Robinson, M.D., President

Providence Holy Cross Surgery Center, 11550 Indian Hills Road, Suite 160, Mission Hills, CA 91345; tel. 818/898-1061; FAX. 818/898-3866; Laura Moore, Administrator

Pueblo Nuevo Aesthetic and Reconstructive Surgery, 1334 Nelson Avenue, Modesto, CA 95350; tel. 209/524-9904; FAX. 209/524-4101; Diane Payne, Administrator

Redlands Dental Surgery Center, 1180 Nevada Street, Suite 100, Redlands, CA 92374; tel. 909/335-0474; Russell O. Seheult, D.D.S.

Richburg Valley Eye Institute Ambulatory Surgical Center, 1680 East Herndon Avenue, Fresno, CA 93720; tel. 209/432-4200; FAX. 209/432-0147; Frederick Richburg, M.D., Administrator

Riverside Community Surgi-Center, 3980 14th Street, Riverside, CA 92501; tel. 909/787-0580; FAX. 909/787-8201; Pat Finley, Administrator

Riverside Eye, Ear, Nose and Throat Institute Surgery Center, 4500 Brockton Avenue, Suite 105, Riverside, CA 92501; tel. 714/788-2788; FAX. 909/788-4374; B. G. Smith, M.D., Medical Director

Riverside Medical Clinic Surgery Center, 7160 Brockton Avenue, Riverside, CA 92506; tel. 714/782-3801; FAX. 909/782-3861; Geraldine Newell, Surgery Center Manager

Rose Eye Laser Center, 3325 North Broadway, Los Angeles, CA 90031; tel. 323/221-6121; FAX. 323/221-6120; Michael R. Rose, Administrator

Sacramento Eye Surgicenter, 3150 J Street, Sacramento, CA 95816; tel. 916/444-7052; FAX. 916/446-1145; Kim Russell, ASC Director

Sacramento Midtown Endoscopy Center, 3941 J Street, Suite 460, Sacramento, CA 95819; tel. 916/733-6940; FAX. 916/733-6934; Tommy Poirier, M.D.

Saddleback Eye Center, 23161 Moulton Parkway, Laguna Hills, CA 92653; tel. 714/951-4641; FAX. 714/951-4601; Linda Riley, Administrator

Saddleback Valley Outpatient Surgery, 24302 Paseo De Valencia, Laguna Hills, CA 92653; tel. 714/472-0244; FAX. 714/472-0380; Brian Fitzgerald, Administrator

Salinas Surgery Center, 955-A Blanco Circle, Salinas, CA 93901; tel. 408/753-5800; FAX. 408/753-5808; Christine Gallagher, Executive Director

Samaritan Pain Management Center, 2520 Samaritan Drive, San Jose, CA 95124; tel. 408/356-2731; FAX. 408/356-6366; Ilka E. McAlister, Administrator

San Diego Endoscopy Center, A Partnership, 4033 Third Avenue, Suite 106, San Diego, CA 92103; tel. 619/291-6064; FAX. 619/291-3078; John D. Goodman, M.D.

San Diego Outpatient Surgical Center, 770 Washington Street, Suite 101, San Diego, CA 92103; tel. 619/299-9530; FAX. 619/296-5386; Carla G. Ramirez, Administrator

San Francisco Surgi Center, 1635 Divisidero Street, Suite 200, San Francisco, CA 94115; tel. 415/346-1218; FAX. 415/346-2930; Jessie Scott, Administrator

San Gabriel Valley Surgical Center, 1250 South Sunset Avenue, Suite 100, West Covina, CA 91790; tel. 626/960-6623; FAX. 626/962-4341; Susan Raub, Administrator

San Jose Eye Ambulatory Surgicenter, Inc., 4585 Stevens Creek Boulevard, Suite 500, Santa Clara, CA 95051; tel. 408/247-2706; FAX. 408/296-2020; Lolita Ancheta, Clinical Coordinator

San Leandro Surgery Center, 15035 East 14th Street, San Leandro, CA 94578; tel. 510/276-2800; FAX. 510/276-2890; Sheila L. Cook, Executive Director

Sani Eye Surgery Center, 1315 Las Tablas Road, Templeton, CA 93465; tel. 805/434-2533; FAX. 805/434-3037; Javad N. Sani, M.D., Director

Santa Cruz Surgery Center, 3003 Paul Sweet Road, Santa Cruz, CA 95065; tel. 408/462-5512; FAX. 408/462-2451; Mary Ann Dunlap, RN

Santa Monica Surgery and Laser Center, 2001 Santa Monica Boulevard, Suite 1288W, Santa Monica, CA 90404; tel. 310/829-2005; FAX. 310/453-9201; Cindy Schlaak, RN, Administrator

Scoffield Foot Care Center, 3796 North Fresno Street, Suite 103, Fresno, CA 93726; tel. 209/228-1475; Mark H. Scoffield, Administrator

Sebastopol Ambulatory Surgery Center, 6880 Palm Avenue, Sebastopol, CA 95472; tel. 707/823-7628; FAX. 707/823-1521; Edward J. Boland, Administrator

Sequoia Endoscopy Center, 2900 Whipple Avenue, Suite 100, Redwood City, CA 94062; tel. 415/363-5200; FAX. 415/369-4609; Stuart Weisman, Administrator

Shepard Eye Center Medical Group, 1414 East Main Street, Santa Maria, CA 93454-4806; tel. 805/925-2637; FAX. 809/928-2067; Dennis D. Shepard, M.D.

Sierra Plastic Surgery Center, 6153 North Thesta, Fresno, CA 93710; tel. 209/432-5156; FAX. 209/432-2247; Terry A. Gillian, M.D., Medical Director

Sierra Vista Medical Pavilion Ambulatory Surgery, 77 Casa Street, Suite 203, San Luis Obis, CA 93405; tel. 805/544-6471; FAX. 805/544-6471; James W. Thornton, M.D., Administrator

Simi Health Center, 1350 Los Angeles Avenue, Simi Valley, CA 93065; tel. 805/522-3782; FAX. 805/522-1283; Lorna Holland, Administrator

Solis Surgical Arts Center, 4940 Van Nuys Boulevard, Suite 105, Sherman Oaks, CA 91403; tel. 818/787-1144; Dr. H. William Gottschalk, Administrator

Sonora Eye Surgery Center, 940 Sylva Lane, Suite G, Sonora, CA 95370; tel. 209/532-2020; FAX. 209/532-1687; Loretta Monfort

South Bay Endoscopy Center, 256 Landis Avenue, Suite 100, Chula Vista, CA 91910; tel. 619/420-6864; FAX. 619/420-0477; Janet Lemon, Director

South Coast Laser Center, 3420 Bristol Street, Suite 701, Costa Mesa, CA 92626; tel. 714/957-0272; FAX. 714/641-2020; Michael R. Rose, M.D., Medical Director

Southern California Surgery Center, 7305 Pacific Boulevard, Huntington Pa, CA 90255; tel. 213/584-8222; Amgad A. Awad, Administrator

Southland Endoscopy Center, 949 East Calhoun Place, Suite B, Hemet, CA 92543; tel. 909/929-1177; FAX. 909/765-9111; Sreenivasa R. Nakka, M.D., F.A.C.P.

Southwest Surgical Center, 201 New Stine Road, Suite 130, Bakersfield, CA 93309; tel. 661/396-8900; FAX. 661/397-2929; Shirley Skelton, Administrator

St. Joseph Surgery and Laser Center, Inc., 436 South Glassell Street, Orange, CA 92866; tel. 714/633-9566; FAX. 714/633-5193

Stanislaus Surgery Center, 1421 Oakdale Road, Modesto, CA 95355; tel. 209/572-2700; Michael Lipomi, Chief Executive Officer

Stockton Eye Surgery Center, 36 West Yokuts Avenue, Suite 3, Stockton, CA 95207; tel. 209/473-2940; FAX. 209/474-1168; Kathy Barton, Administrator

Surgecenter of Palo Alto, 795 El Camino Road, Palo Alto, CA 94301; tel. 415/324-1832; FAX. 650/330-4520; Rose Parkes, Chief Executive Officer

Surgery Center, 1111 Sonoma Avenue, Lower Level, Santa Rosa, CA 95405; tel. 707/578-4100; Ken Alban, Administrator

Surgery Center of Corona, 1124 South Main Street, Suite 102, Corona, CA 91720; tel. 909/737-9091; FAX. 909/737-9093; Melanie Dastrup, Executive Director

Surgery Center of Northern California, 950 Butte Street, Redding, CA 96001; tel. 916/241-4044; FAX. 916/241-1408; Sarah E. Galewick, RN, B.S.N., Director

Surgery Center of Santa Monica, 2121 Wilshire Boulevard, Santa Monica, CA 90403; tel. 310/264-7300; Ruth F. Andrews

Surgical Eye Care Center, 655 Laguna Drive, Carlsbad, CA 92008; tel. 760/729-7101; FAX. 760/729-7106; Lisa Barron, Administrator

Surgitek Outpatient Center, Inc., 460 North Greenfield Avenue, Suite Eight, Hanford, CA 93230; tel. 209/582-0238; Wiley Elick, Owner, Administrator

Sutter North Procedure Center, 550 B Street, Yuba City, CA 95991; tel. 530/749-3653; FAX. 530/749-3493; Deborah Smith, Ancillary Services Director

The Beverly Hills Center for Special Surgery, 1125 South Beverly Drive, Suite 505, Los Angeles, CA 90035; tel. 310/277-6780; Alina Pnini, Administrator

The Center for Endoscopy, 3921 Waring Road, Suite B, Oceanside, CA 92056; tel. 760/940-6300; FAX. 760/940-8074; Barbara Bockover, RN, Administrator

The Centre for Plastic Surgery, 401 East Highland Avenue, Suite 352, San Bernardino, CA 92404; tel. 909/883-8686; FAX. 909/881-6537; Dennis K. Anderson, Administrator

The Darr Eye Clinic Surgical Medical Group, Inc., 44139 Monterey Avenue, Suite A, Palm Desert, CA 92260; tel. 619/773-3099; FAX. 619/341-6863; Joseph L. Darr, M.D., Administrator

The Endoscopy Center, 870 Shasta Street, Suite 100, Yuba City, CA 95991; tel. 530/671-3636; FAX. 530/671-4099; Floyd V. Burton, M.D.

The Endoscopy Center of the South Bay, 23560 Madison Street, Suite 109, Torrance, CA 90505; tel. 310/325-6331; FAX. 310/325-6335; Norman M. Panitch, M.D., Medical Director

The Eye Surgery Center (Colton), 1900 East Washington, Colton, CA 92324; tel. 909/825-8002; FAX. 909/422-8930; Sally Chalk, RN, Operating Room Manager

The Eye Surgery Center of Northern California, 5959 Greenback Lane, Citrus Height, CA 95621; tel. 916/723-7400; FAX. 916/723-4449; Georgia McDonald, Office Manager

The Eye Surgery Center of Riverside, Inc., 8990 Garfield, Suite One, Riverside, CA 92503; tel. 909/785-5421; FAX. 909/785-0130

The Montebello Surgery Center, 229 East Beverly Boulevard, Montebello, CA 90640; tel. 213/728-7998; Clifton M. Baker, Administrator

The Palos Verdes Ambulatory Surgery Medical Center, 3400 West Lomita Boulevard, Suite 307A, Torrance, CA 90505; tel. 310/517-8689; FAX. 310/517-9916; Christine Petti, M.D., Medical Director

The Plastic Surgery Center Medical Group, Inc., 95 Scripps Drive, Sacramento, CA 95825; tel. 916/929-1833; FAX. 916/929-6730; Mark L. Ross, Administrator

The Sinskey Eye Institute, 2232 Santa Monica Boulevard, Santa Monica, CA 90411; tel. 310/453-8911; FAX. 310/453-2519; Sherry Bennett, Administrator

The Specialists Surgery Center, 2450 Martin Road, Fairfield, CA 94533; tel. 707/429-6060; FAX. 707/429-6088; Ann Karg, Operations Manager

The Surgery Center, 6840 Sepulveda Boulevard, Van Nuys, CA 91405-4401; tel. 818/785-6840; FAX. 818/785-3931; Grace Sussman, RN, Nurse Manager

The Surgery Center, A HealthSouth Surgery Center, 3875 Telegraph Avenue, Oakland, CA 94609; tel. 510/547-2244; FAX. 510/547-6637; Ann Banchero, Administrator

The Valley Endoscopy Center, 18425 Burbank Boulevard, Suite 525, Tarzana, CA 91356; tel. 818/708-6050; FAX. 818/708-6009; Betty Asato, RN, Clinical Director

Third Street Surgery Center, 420 East Third Street, Suite 604, Los Angeles, CA 90013; tel. 213/617-9194; FAX. 213/617-0605; Yukiko Hattori, Director of Nursing

Providers / Freestanding Ambulatory Surgery Centers

Thousand Oaks Endoscopy Center, 227 West Janss Road, Suite 240, Thousand Oaks, CA 91360; tel. 805/371-0455; FAX. 805/371-0459; Hector Caballero, M.D., Administrator

Time Surgical Facility, 720 North Tustin Avenue, Suite 202, Santa Ana, CA 92705; tel. 714/972-1811; Denise Reale, Administrator

Torrance Surgicenter, 22410 Hawthorne Boulevard, Suite Three, Torrance, CA 90505; tel. 310/373-2238; FAX. 310/373-8238; Lindon KenKawahara, M.D., Medical Director

Truxtun Surgery Center, Inc., 4260 Truxtun Avenue, Suite 120, Bakersfield, CA 93309; tel. 805/327-3636; Velma Reed, Administrator

Twin Cities Surgicenter, Inc., 812 Fourth Street, Suite A, Marysville, CA 95901; tel. 916/741-3937; FAX. 916/743-0427; Karen Morasch, Administrator

University Surgi-Center Medical Group, 23961 Calle De La Magdalena, Suite 430, Laguna Hills, CA 92653; tel. 714/830-5500; Bernard Berry, M.D., Administrator

Upland Outpatient Surgical Center, Inc., 1330 San Bernardino Road, Upland, CA 91786; tel. 909/981-8755; FAX. 909/981-9462; Roger E. Murken, M.D., President

UTC Surgicenter, 8929 University Center Lane, Suite 103, San Diego, CA 92122; tel. 619/554-0220; FAX. 619/554-0458; Dawn Ainsworth, RN, Administrator

Valencia Outpatient Surgical Center, L.P., d/b/a Valencia Surgical Center, 24355 Lyons Avenue, Suite 120, Santa Clarita, CA 91321; tel. 661/255-6644; FAX. 661/255-6717; Nina Turner, Administrative Director

Valley Surgical Center, 5555 West Las Positas Boulevard, Pleasanton, CA 94566; tel. 510/734-3360; FAX. 510/734-3358; Beth Combs, RN, Director, Nursing

Ventura Out-Patient Surgery, Inc., 3555 Loma Vista Road, Suite 204, Ventura, CA 93003; tel. 805/653-6765; FAX. 805/653-1470; Brian D. Brantner, M.D.

Victorville Ambulatory Surgery Center, 15030 Seventh Street, Victorville, CA 92392; tel. 619/241-2273; FAX. 619/245-6798; John D. Amar, M.D., Medical Director

Vision Care Surgery Center, 1045 S Street, Fresno, CA 93721; tel. 559/486-2000; Lynn Horton, Chief Executive Officer

Walnut Creek Ambulatory Surgery Center, 112 La Casa Via, Suite 300, Walnut Creek, CA 94598; tel. 925/933-0290; FAX. 925/933-7034; Allison Isaacs, Administrator

Wardlow Surgery Center, 200 West Wardlow Road, Long Beach, CA 90806; tel. 310/424-3574; FAX. 310/490-0329; Marisol Magana, Administrator

Washington Outpatient Surgery Center, 2299 Mowry Avenue, First Floor, Fremont, CA 94538; tel. 510/791-5374; FAX. 510/790-8916; Gerald G. Pousho, M.D.

West Olympic Surgery Center and Laser Institute, 11570 West Olympic Boulevard, Los Angeles, CA 90064; tel. 310/479-4211; FAX. 310/473-6069; Chris Klimaszewski, Operating Room Supervisor

West Valley Surgery Center, 3803 South Bascom Avenue, Suite 106, Campbell, CA 95008; tel. 408/559-4886; FAX. 408/559-4908; Annette Wunderlich, RN, Administrator

Westlake Eye Surgery Center, 2900 Townsgate Road, Suite 201, Westlake Village, CA 91361; tel. 805/496-6789; FAX. 805/494-8392; John Darin, M.D., Medical Director

Westwood Surgery Center, 11819 Wilshire Boulevard, Suite 214, Los Angeles, CA 90025; tel. 310/575-1616; FAX. 310/575-1622; Thomas Cloud, M.D., Administrator

Women's Health Care and Cosmetic Surgical Center, 15306 Devonshire Street, Mission Hills, CA 91311; tel. 818/892-0274; FAX. 818/895-0663; Martha P. Nazemi, Administrator

Woodland Surgery Center, 1321 Cottonwood Street, Woodland, CA 95695; tel. 916/662-9112; FAX. 916/668-5783; Donna Kanas, Manager

COLORADO

Aurora Outpatient Surgery, 2900 South Peoria Street, Suite D, Aurora, CO 80014; tel. 303/752-2496; FAX. 303/752-2577; L. F. Peede, Jr., M.D., Administrator

Aurora Surgery Center LTD, 13701 E. Mississippi, #200, Aurora, CO 80012; tel. 303/363-8646; Beverly Kirchner, RN, Administrator

Aurora Surgery Center, Ltd., 13701 Mississippi Avenue, Suite 200, Aurora, CO 80012; tel. 303/363-8646; FAX. 303/363-8689; Beverly Kirchner, RN, Administrator

Avista Surgery Center, 2525 Fourth Street, Lower Level, Boulder, CO 80304; tel. 303/443-3672; John Sackett, Administrator

Boulder Medical Center, P C, 2750 Broadway, Boulder, CO 80304; tel. 303/440-3000; Mr. Bradford McKane, Administrator

Boulder Medical Center, P.C., 2750 Broadway, Boulder, CO 80304; tel. 303/440-3000; Bradford B. McKane

Centennial Healthcare Plaza, a Division of Healthone/Columbia, 14200 East Arapahoe Road, Englewood, CO 80112; tel. 303/699-3000; FAX. 303/699-3182; Ginger McNally, Administrator

Center for Reproductive Surgery, 799 East Hampden Avenue, Suite 300, Englewood, CO 80110; tel. 303/788-8300; FAX. 303/788-8310; Dr. William Schoolcraft, Administrator

Centrum Surgical Center, 8200 East Belleview, Suite 300, East Tower, Englewood, CO 80111; tel. 303/290-0600; FAX. 303/290-6359; David Parrott, Administrator

Centura Health-Summit Surgery Center, Highway Nine at School Road, P.O. Box 4460, Frisco, CO 80443; tel. 303/668-1458; FAX. 970/668-1703; Carol Turrin, Administrator

Cherry Creek Eye Surgery Center, (Rose Medical Center), 4999 East Kentucky Avenue, Denver, CO 80222; tel. 303/692-0903; Jeffrey Dorsey, Administrator

Colorado Outpatient Eye Surgical Center, 2480 South Downing, Suite G-20, Denver, CO 80210; tel. 303/777-3882; FAX. 303/778-0738; Thomas P. Larkin, M.D.

Colorado Outpatient Eye Surgical Center, 2480 S. Downing, Denver, CO 80210; tel. 303/777-3882; FAX. 303/778-0738; Thomas Larkin, Administrator

Colorado Springs Eye Surgery Center, 2920 North Cascade Avenue, Colorado Springs, CO 80907; tel. 719/636-5054; FAX. 719/520-3576; Dr. Robert Foerster, Medical Director

Colorado Springs Health Partners Ambulatory Surgery Unit, 209 South Nevada Avenue, Colorado Springs, CO 80903; tel. 719/475-7700; FAX. 719/538-2999; Ms. Joan Compton, VP Operations

Denver Eye Surgery Center, Inc., 13772 Denver West Parkway, Building 55, Golden, CO 80401; tel. 303/273-8770; Larry W. Kreider, M.D., Administrator

Denver Midtown Surgery Center, 1919 East 18th Avenue, Denver, CO 80206; tel. 303/322-3993; FAX. 303/322-7329; Lisa Cross, Administrator

Durango Surgicenter, 316 Sawyer Drive, Durango, CO 81301; tel. 970/259-3818; FAX. 970/259-9553; D.J. Winder, M.D., Administrator

ENT Surgicenter, Inc., 1032 Luke, Fort Collins, CO 80524; tel. 970/484-8686; FAX. 970/484-1064; Debbie Brown, Manager

Eye Center of Northern Colorado Surgery Center, 1725 E. Prospect Ave., Fort Collins, CO 80525; tel. 970/221-2222; FAX. 970/221-4286; Carol Wittmer, Administrator

Eye Surgery Center of Colorado, 8403 Bryant Street, Westminster, CO 80030; tel. 303/426-4810; FAX. 303/426-8708; William G. Self, Jr., M.D., Administrator

Foot Surgery Center of Northern Colorado, 1355 Riverside Ave., #B, Fort Collins, CO 80524; tel. 970/484-4620; Connie Nelson, RN

HealthSouth Denver West Surgery Center, 13952 Denver West Parkway, Building 53, Suite 100, Golden, CO 80401; tel. 303/271-1112; FAX. 303/271-1117; Ms. Susan Byers, Administrator

HealthSouth Pueblo Surgery Center, 25 Montebello Road, Pueblo, CO 81001; tel. 719/544-1600; FAX. 719/544-2599; Jennifer Arellano, Administrator

HealthSouth Surgery Center of Colorado Springs, 1615 Medical Center Point, Colorado Springs, CO 80907; tel. 719/635-7740; FAX. 719/635-7750; Melodie Gurrobo, Administrator

HealthSouth Surgery Center of Fort Collins, 1100 East Prospect Road, Fort Collins, CO 80525; tel. 970/493-7200; FAX. 970/493-2380; Alice Fischer, Administrator

Kaiser Permanente Ambulatory Surgery Center, 2045 Franklin Street, Denver, CO 80205; tel. 303/764-4444; Rosemarie Polemi, Director

Lakewood Surgical Center, 2201 Wadsworth Boulevard, Lakewood, CO 80215; tel. 303/234-0445; FAX. 303/232-7182; Connie Holtz, Administrator

Laser Institute of the Rockies, 8400 East Prentice Avenue, Suite 1200, Englewood, CO 80111; tel. 303/793-3000; Jon Dishler, M.D., President

Littleton Day Surgery Center, 8381 South Park Lane, Littleton, CO 80120; tel. 303/795-2244; FAX. 303/795-5965; Judy Rich, Administrator

Mountain View Surgery Center, 1850 N. Boise Ave., P.O. Box 887, Loveland, CO 80538; tel. 970/622-1999; Charles Harms, Administrator

North Denver Surgery Center., 10001 North Washington, Thornton, CO 80229; tel. 303/252-0083; FAX. 303/252-9095; Craig J. Bakken, Administrator

Orthopedic Center of the Rockies Ambulatory Surgery Center, 2500 East Prospect Road, Fort Collins, CO 80525; tel. 303/493-4010; FAX. 303/493-0521; Scott M. Thomas, Executive Director

Pain Management Center, 455 E. Pikes Peak Ave., #201, Colorado Springs, CO 80903; tel. 719/442-0777; FAX. 719/442-0888; Sue Hayes Golden, Administrator

Park Meadows Outpatient Surgery, 7430 Park Meadows Drive, Lonetree, CO 80124; tel. 303/752-2496; Randolph Robinson, Administrator

Pikes Peak Endoscopy & Surgery Center, 1699 Medical Center Pt., #100, Colorado Springs, CO 80907; tel. 719/632-7101; Karen Parks, Administrator

South Denver Endoscopy Center, Inc., 499 East Hampden Avenue, Suite 430, Englewood, CO 80110; tel. 303/788-8888; Dr. Pete Baker, Administrator

Southern Colorado Center for Endoscopy and Surgery, 2002 Lake Avenue, Pueblo, CO 81004; tel. 719/560-7111; FAX. 719/564-0122; Dr. Andrew Perry, Administrator

Spring Creek Surgery Center, Spring Creek Medical Park, 2001 South Shields Street, Building H, Su, Fort Collins, CO 80526; tel. 970/221-9363; FAX. 970/221-9636; Natalie Coubrough, Facility Administrator

Springs Pain Research & Surgery Facility, 1625 Medical Center Point, #240, Colorado Spire, CO 80907; tel. 719/577-9063; FAX. 719/577-9124; Charles Ripp, M.D. Medical Director

Sterling Eye Surgery Center, 1410 S. 7th Ave., P.O. Box 951, Sterling, CO 80751; tel. 970/522-1833; FAX. 970/522-3677; Rashell Fritzler, Administrator

Surgicenter of the San Luis Valley Medical, P.C., 2115 Stuart, Alamosa, CO 81101; tel. 719/589-8010; FAX. 719/589-8112; Lauriann Blakeman, RN, Supervisor

Western Rockies Surgery Center, Inc., 1000 Wellington Avenue, Grand Junction, CO 81501; tel. 970/243-9000; FAX. 970/245-4936; Marilyn M. Smith, RN, Surgery Center Administrator

Western Rockies Surgery Center, Inc., 1000 Wellington Ave., Grand Junction, CO 81501; tel. 970/243-9000; Marilyn Smith, Administrator

CONNECTICUT

Bridgeport Surgical Center, 4920 Main Street, Bridgeport, CT 06606; tel. 203/374-1515; FAX. 203/374-4702; Anthony German, Administrative Director

Connecticut Foot Surgery Center, 318 New Haven Avenue, Milford, CT 06460; tel. 203/882-0065; Martin Pressman, D.P.M., Administrator

Connecticut Surgical Center, 81 Gillett Street, Hartford, CT 06105; tel. 203/247-5555; FAX. 203/249-5860; Margaret Rubino, President

Danbury Surgical Center, 73 Sandpit Road, Suite 101, Danbury, CT 06810; tel. 203/743-2400; Bernard A. Kershner, President

Hartford Surgical Center, 100 Retreat Avenue, Hartford, CT 06106; tel. 860/549-7970; FAX. 860/247-4121; Christine M. Quallen, Administrative Director

Johnson Surgery Center, 148 Hazard Avenue, P.O. Box 909, Enfield, CT 06083; tel. 860/763-7650; FAX. 860/763-7675; Anthony T. Valente, Vice President, Vice President

Middlesex Surgical Center, 530 Saybrook Road, Middletown, CT 06457; tel. 203/343-0400; FAX. 203/343-0396; Louise DeChesser, RN, CNOR, M.S.

Naugatuck Valley Surgical Center, Ltd., 160 Robbins Street, Waterbury, CT 06708; tel. 203/755-6663; FAX. 203/756-9645; Bernard A. Kershner, President

Stamford Surgical Center, 1290 Summer Street, Stamford, CT 06905; tel. 203/961-1345; FAX. 213/324-1470; James Bowden, Administrative Director

Waterbury Outpatient Surgical Center, 87 Grandview Avenue, Waterbury, CT 06708; tel. 203/574-2020; Nancy Noll, Administrator

Providers / Freestanding Ambulatory Surgery Centers

Woman's Surgical Center, 40 Temple Street, New Haven, CT 06510; tel. 203/624–3080; Bruce I. Fisher, Administrator

Yale–New Haven Ambulatory Services Corporation, d/b/a Temple Surgical Center, 60 Temple Street, New Haven, CT 06510; tel. 203/624–6008; Alvin D. Greenberg, M.D., Administrator

DELAWARE

Bayview Endoscopy Center, Inc., 1539 Savannah Road, Lewes, DE 19958; tel. 302/644–0455; FAX. 302/645–5214; Harry J. Anagnostakos, D.O., President

Central Delaware Endoscopy Unit, 644 South Queen Street, Suite 105, Dover, DE 19904; tel. 302/672–1617; William M. Kaplan, M.D., Medical Director

Central Delaware Surgery Center, 100 Scull Terrace, Dover, DE 19901; tel. 302/735–8290; Paul Francisco, Administrator

Endoscopy Center of Delaware, Inc., 1090 Old Churchman's Road, Newark, DE 19713; tel. 302/892–2710; FAX. 302/892–2715; Jean–Marie M. Taylor, Administrator

Eye Care of Delaware Cataract and Laser Center, 4102 Ogletown Road, Suite 1, Newark, DE 19713; tel. 302/454–8802; FAX. 302/454–8801; Jane Baker, Officer Manager

Glasgow Medical Center, L.L.C., 2400 Summit Bridge Road, Newark, DE 19702–4777; tel. 302/536–8350; Joseph M. Rule, Ph.D., Administrator

Limestone Medical Center, Inc., 1941 Limestone Road, Suite 113, Wilmington, DE 19808; tel. 302/633–9873; FAX. 302/992–0563; Thomas E. Mulhern, Executive Director

DISTRICT OF COLUMBIA

Hillcrest Northwest, 7603 Georgia Avenue, N.W., Washington, DC 20012; tel. 202/829–5620; FAX. 202/882–8387; Alice Harper, Administrator

Hillcrest Women's Surgi–Center, 3233 Pennsylvania Avenue, S.E., Washington, DC 20020; tel. 202/584–6500; Ms. Caridad V. Wright, Administrator

Medlantic Center for Ambulatory Surgery, Inc., 1145 19th Street, N.W., Suite 850, Washington, DC 20036; tel. 202/223–9040; FAX. 202/223–9047; William Heron, M.D., Medical Director

New Summit Medical Center II, Inc., 1630 Euclid Street, N.W., Suite 130; Washington, DC 20037; tel. 202/337–7200; Johnette Anderson, RNC, Administrator

Planned Parenthood of Metropolitan Washington, D.C., Schumacher Center, 1108 16th Street, N.W., Washington, DC 20036; tel. 202/347–8512; FAX. 202/347–0281; Lorraine D. White, Center Manager

Premier Surgery Center of D.C., 6323 Georgia Avenue, N.W., Suite 200, Washington, DC 20011; tel. 202/291–0126; FAX. 202/291–0126; Lenora Hollaway, RN, Administrative Director

The Endoscopy Center of Washington, DC, L.P., 2021 K Street, N.W., Suite T-115, Washington, DC 20006; tel. 202/775–8692; FAX. 202/463–1165; Roberta Fernandez–Rojo, RN, Center Director

Washington Surgi–Clinic, 1018 22nd Street, N.W., Washington, DC 20037; tel. 202/659–9403; FAX. 202/467–0056; Maria Barrera, Administrator

FLORIDA

Aesthetic Cosmetic Surgery Center, Inc, 598 Sterthaus Avenue, Ormond Beach, FL 32174; tel. 904/673–2262; FAX. 904/677–3808; Bonnie Dantoni, R.N., D.D.N.

Aker–Kasten Cataract and Laser Institute, 1445 Northwest Boca Raton Boulevard, Boca Raton, FL 33432; tel. 407/338–7722; FAX. 407/338–7785; Kim Harrington, Administrator

Alpha Ambulatory Surgery, Inc., 2160 Capital Circle, N.E., Tallahassee, FL 32308; tel. 904/385–0033; FAX. 904/422–0201; Gloria Jeter, Office Manager

Ambulatory Ankle and Foot Center of Florida, 1509 South Orange Avenue, P.O. Box 536951, Orlando, FL 32853; tel. 407/895–2432; Gregory J. Renton, Administrator

Ambulatory Surgery Center, 4500 East Fletcher Avenue, Tampa, FL 33613; tel. 813/977–8550; FAX. 813/977–7941; Carole Cornell, Administrator

Ambulatory Surgery Center of Brevard, 719 East New Haven Avenue, Melbourne, FL 32901; tel. 407/726–4106; Norm Gagnon, General Manager

Ambulatory Surgery Center of Naples, 1351 Pine Street, Naples, FL 34104; tel. 941/793–0664; FAX. 941/793–4318; Christian Mogelvang, M.D., Medical Director

Ambulatory Surgery Center/Bradenton, 5817 21st Avenue, W., Bradenton, FL 34209; tel. 813/794–0379; J. Leikensohn, M.D., Medical Director

Ambulatory Surgical Care, 1045 North Courtenay Parkway, Merritt Island, FL 32953; tel. 407/452–4448; FAX. 407/452–4533; Melanie Peavler, RN, DON

Ambulatory Surgical Center of Central Florida, Inc., 801 North Stone Street, Deland, FL 32720; tel. 904/734–4431; FAX. 904/738–1045; Albert C. Neumann, M.D., Medical Director

Ambulatory Surgical Center of Lake County, Inc., 803 East Dixie Avenue, Leesburg, FL 32748; tel. 904/787–6656; FAX. 904/787–9008; Patricia R. Hux, RN, Business Manager, Administrator

Ambulatory Surgical Centre, 8700 North Kendall Drive, Suite 100, Miami, FL 33176; tel. 305/595–9511; FAX. 305/271–0383; Gail Tauriello, Administrator

Ambulatory Surgical Facility of South Florida, LTD-East, 4470 Sheridan Street, Hollywood, FL 33021; tel. 305/962–3210; FAX. 305/962–3466; Carl T. Waskiewicz, Executive Director and Administrator

American Surgery Center of Coral Gables, Inc., 10975 W. Le Jeune Road, Miami, FL 33134; tel. 305/461–1300; Laura Lilburn, RN, Nurse Manager

Atlantic Surgery Center, 541 Health Boulevard, Daytona Beach, FL 32114; tel. 904/239–0021

Atlantic Surgery Center, A HealthSouth Facility, 1707 South 25th Street, Fort Pierce, FL 34947; tel. 561/464–8900; FAX. 561/464–1104; Lisa L. Kodya, CMM, Business Office Coordinator

Atlantic Surgical Center, 150 Southwest 12th Avenue, Suite 450, Pompano Beach, FL 33069; tel. 305/941–3369; Ruben Paradela, Chief Executive Officer

Ayers Surgery Center, 720 Southwest Second Avenue, Suite 101, Gainesville, FL 32601; tel. 904/338–7100; FAX. 904/338–7102; Barbara Hyder, RN, Nurse Manager

Barkley Surgicenter, 63 Barkley Circle, Suite 104, Fort Myers, FL 33907; tel. 941/275–8452; Kerri Gantt BS,CMM, Administrative Director

Bay Med Surgery, 1936 Jenks Avenue, Panama City, FL 32405; tel. 904/763–6700; FAX. 904/763–5779; Stan Hicks, CRNA, Manager

Bayfront Medical Plaza Same Day Surgery, 603 Seventh Street South, St. Petersburg, FL 33701; tel. 813/553–7906; FAX. 813/553–7992; Gail A. Cook, RN, Nurse Manager

Beraja Clinics Laser and Surgery Center, 2550 Douglas Road, Suite 301, Coral Gables, FL 33134

Bethesda Health City Same Day Surgery, 10301 Hagen Ranch Road, Boynton Beach, FL 33437; tel. 561/374–5400; FAX. 561/374–5405; Denver Gray, RN, CNOR, Clinical Manager

Boca Raton Outpatient Surgery and Laser Center, 501 Glades Road, Boca Raton, FL 33432; tel. 561/362–4400; FAX. 561/362–4440; Karen Raiano, Administrator

Bon Secours–Venice HealthPark Surgery Center, 1283 Jacaranda Boulevard, Venice, FL 34292; tel. 941/497–5660; FAX. 941/492–3942; Kermit Knight, Administrator

Brevard Surgery Center, 665 Apollo Boulevard, Melbourne, FL 32901; tel. 407/984–0300; FAX. 407/984–0032; Narda Cotman, Surgical Director

Cape Coral Endoscopy and Surgery Center, 1413 Viscaya Parkway, Cape Coral, FL 33990; tel. 941/772–0404; Nancy Rhodes, Administrator

Cape Surgery Center, 1941 Waldemere Street, Sarasota, FL 34239–3555; tel. 941/917–1900; FAX. 941/917–2356; Sharon Tolhurst, RN, M.B.A., Director

Capital Eye Surgery Center, 2535 Capital Medical Boulevard, Tallahassee, FL 32308; tel. 904/942–3937; FAX. 904/942–6279; Renee Harina, Business Manager

Center for Advanced Eye Surgery, L.P., 3920 Bee Ridge Road Building F, Suite C, Sarasota, FL 34233; tel. 941/925–0000; FAX. 941/927–2726; Darice Downs, RN, LHRM, Nurse Manager

Center for Digestive Health and Pain Management, 12700 Creekside Lane, Suite 202, P.O. Box 60045, Fort Myers, FL 33919; tel. 941/489–4454; FAX. 941/489–2114; Vivian DiCarlo, RN, Nursing Director

Central Florida Eye Institute, 3133 Southwest 32nd Avenue, Ocala, FL 34474; tel. 904/237–8400; Thomas L. Croley, M.D.

Clearwater Endoscopy Center, 401 Corbett Street, Suite 220, Clearwater, FL 33756; tel. 727/443–0100; FAX. 727/461–4893; Lori Parrinello, RN Clinical Director

Cleveland Clinic Florida, 3000 West Cypress Creek Road, Fort Lauderdale, FL 33309

Columbia Belleair Surgery Center, 1130 Ponce de Leon Boulevard, Clearwater, FL 34616; tel. 813/581–4800; FAX. 813/585–0319; Margie Maddock, Administrator

Columbia Brandon Surgery Center, 711 South Parsons, Brandon, FL 33511; tel. 813/654–7771; FAX. 813/654–3347; Charlene Harrell, RN, Administrator

Columbia Cape Coral Surgery Center, 2721 Del Prado Boulevard, S., Suite 100, Cape Coral, FL 33904; tel. 941/458–9000; Carol Carr, Administrator

Columbia Center for Special Surgery, 4650 Fourth Street, N., St. Petersburg, FL 33703; tel. 727/527–1919; FAX. 727/527–0714; Paula Russo, RN, CNOR, Administrator

Columbia DeLand Surgery Center, 651 West Plymouth Avenue, Deland, FL 32720; tel. 904/738–6811; FAX. 904/822–4316; Jay Hutcherson, Administrator

Columbia Florida Surgery Center, 180 Boston Avenue, Altamonte Springs, FL 32701; tel. 407/830–0573; FAX. 407/830–4373; Paige L. Adams, Administrator

Columbia North County Surgicenter, 4000 Burns Road, Palm Beach, FL 33410; tel. 407/626–6446; FAX. 561/626–7244; Jennifer Rime, Business Manager

Columbia Outpatient Surgical Services, Ltd., 301 Northwest 82nd Avenue, Plantation, FL 33324; tel. 954/424–1766; FAX. 954/424–1966; Debbie Haga–Cofer, Administrator

Columbia Surgery Center, 3901 University Boulevard #111, Jacksonville, FL 32216; tel. 904/448–1948; Debbie Overton–Raines, Administrator

Columbia Surgery Center at Coral Springs, 967 University Drive, Coral Springs, FL 33071; tel. 954/975–4166; FAX. 954/344–7054

Columbia Surgery Center Merritt Island, 220 North Sykes Creek Parkway, Suite 101, Merritt Island, FL 32953; tel. 321/459–0015; FAX. 321/459–2291; Cynthia Johnson, Administrator

Coral View Surgery Center, 8390 West Flager, Suite 216, Miami, FL 33144; tel. 305/226–5574; Victor Suarez, M.D., President

Cordova Ambulatory Surgical Center, 545 Brent Lane, Pensacola, FL 32503; tel. 904/477–5437; Cynthia Blake, Assistant Administrator

Cortez Foot Surgery Center, PA, 1800 Cortez Road, W., Suite B, Bradenton, FL 34207; tel. 941/758–4608; FAX. 941/755–2901; Margaret Provencher, Administrator

Countryside Surgery Center, 3291 North McMullen Booth Road, Clearwater, FL 33761; tel. 727/725–5800; FAX. 727/797–4002; Karen Nelson, Administrator

Day Surgery, Inc., 1715 Southeast Tiffany Avenue, Port St. Luci, FL 34952; tel. 407/335–7005; Mary Holobaugh, RN, Administrator

Dermatologic and Cosmetic Surgery Center, L.C., 2668 Swamp Cabbage Court, Fort Myers, FL 33901; tel. 813/275–7546; FAX. 813/275–5074; Charles Eby, M.D.

Diagnostic Clinic Center for Outpatient Surgery, 1401 West Bay Drive, Largo, FL 34640; tel. 813/581–8767; FAX. 813/584–1938; Robert R. Dippong, Administrator and CEO

Doctors Surgery Center, 921 North Main Street, Kissimmee, FL 34744; tel. 407/933–7800; FAX. 407/933–0564; Sue Velez, Administrator

Endoscopy Associates of Citrus, 6412 West Gulf to Lake Highway, Crystal River, FL 34429

Endoscopy Center of Ocala, Inc., 1160 Southeast 18th Place, Ocala, FL 34471; tel. 352/732–8679; FAX. 352/732–2440; Lynn Gano, RN, Nurse Manager

Endoscopy Center of Sarasota, 1435 Osprey Avenue, Suite 100, Sarasota, FL 34239; tel. 941/366–4475; FAX. 941/366–4390; Susan M. Brongel, RN, Administrator

Eye Care and Surgery Center of Ft. Lauderdale, 2540 Northeast Ninth Street, Ft. Lauderdale, FL 33304; tel. 954/561–3533; FAX. 954/565–9706; Jane M. Beatly, Administrator

Eye Surgery and Laser Center, 4120 Del Prado Boulevard, Cape Coral, FL 33904; tel. 941/542–2020; FAX. 941/542–0704; Deboras Hughes, RN,BSN, Surgery Director

Eye Surgery and Laser Center of Mid–Florida, Inc., 409 Avenue K, S.E., Winter Haven, FL 33880; tel. 863/299–8574; FAX. 941/294–8305; Jane Dempsey, ASC Supervisor

Providers / Freestanding Ambulatory Surgery Centers

Eye Surgery Facility, P.A., 2808 West Martin Luther King Boulevard, Tampa, FL 33607; tel. 813/876-1331; FAX. 813/872-0647; Phyllis S. Chisholm, RN, M.A., Executive Director

Eye Surgicenter, 2521 Northwest 41st Street, Gainesville, FL 32606; tel. 352/377-7733; FAX. 352/377-9577; William A. Newsome, M.D.

Faculty Clinic, Inc., 653 West Eighth Street, Jacksonville, FL 32209; tel. 904/350-6708

Family Medical Center, 100 Commercial Drive, Keystone Heights, FL 32656; tel. 352/473-6595; FAX. 352/473-6597; Sue Russell, Office Manager

Florida Eye Clinic Ambulatory Surgical Center, 160 Boston Avenue, Altamonte Springs, FL 32701; tel. 407/834-7776; FAX. 407/831-8607; Genevieve Parm, Chief Executive Officer

Florida Eye Institute Surgicenter, Inc., 2750 Indian River Boulevard, Vero Beach, FL 32960; tel. 407/569-9500; FAX. 407/569-9507; Mary Lynne Schlitt, Administrator

Florida Medical Clinic Special Procedures Center, 38135 Market Square, Zephyrhills, FL 33540; tel. 813/780-8266; FAX. 813/715-4150

Forest Oaks Ambulatory Surgical Center, Inc., 7320 Forest Oaks Boulevard, Spring Hill, FL 34606. tel. 904/683-5666; Thomas D. Stelnicki, D.P.M.

Foundation for Advanced Eye Care, 3737 Pine Island Road, Sunrise, FL 33351; tel. 305/572-5888; FAX. 305/572-5994; Andrea B. Lettman, Administrator

Gaskins Eye Care and Surgery Center, 2335 Ninth Street, N., Suite 304, Naples, FL 34103; tel. 941/263-7750; FAX. 941/263-1754; Cindy Gaskins, RN, M.S.N., R.M.

Gulf Coast Endoscopy Center, Inc., 665 Del Prado Boulevard, Cape Coral, FL 33990; tel. 813/772-3800; FAX. 813/772-5073; Randi Gonzalez

Gulf Coast Surgery Center, 411 Second Street, E., Bradenton, FL 34208; tel. 941/746-1121; FAX. 941/746-7816; Carlene Bailey, RN, Administrator

Gulfcoast Surgery Center, 12132 Cortez Boulevard, Brooksville, FL 34613; tel. 352/596-0744; Fawzi Soliman, M.D.

Gulfshore Endoscopy Center, 1064 Goodletter Road, Naples, FL 33940

Harborside Surgery Center, 610 East Olympia Avenue, Punta Gorda, FL 33950; tel. 941/637-0065

HealthSouth Central Florida Outpatient Surgery Center, 11140 West Colonial Drive, Suite Three, Ocoee, FL 34761; tel. 407/656-2700; FAX. 407/877-9432; Antonio Caos, M.D., Medical Director

HealthSouth Citrus Surgery Center, 110 North Lecanto Highway, Lecanto, FL 34461; tel. 352/527-1825; FAX. 352/527-1827; Douglas Vybiral, Facility Administrator

HealthSouth Collier Surgery Center, 800 Goodlette Road, N., Suite 120, Naples, FL 34104; tel. 813/262-5757; FAX. 813/262-6073; Barbara L. Messmer

HealthSouth Emerald Coast Surgery Center, 995 Northwest Mar Walt Drive, Fort Walton B, FL 32547; tel. 904/863-7887; FAX. 904/863-4955; Annah Carethers, Facility Administrator

HealthSouth Indian River Surgery Center, 1200 37th Street, Vero Beach, FL 32960; tel. 407/770-5600; FAX. 407/770-1793; Regina Ludicke, Clinical Administrator

HealthSouth Melbourne Surgery Center, 1340 Medical Park Drive, Suite 101, Melbourne, FL 32901; tel. 407/729-9493; FAX. 407/768-6043; Robert C. Miner, Administrator/CEO

HealthSouth Orlando Center for Outpatient Surgery, 1405 South Orange Avenue, Suite 400, Orlando, FL 32806; tel. 407/426-8331; FAX. 407/425-9582

HealthSouth St. Petersburg Surgery Center, 539 Pasadena Avenue, S., St. Petersburg, FL 33707; tel. 813/345-8337; FAX. 813/347-4675; Patty Grover, Administrator

Hialeah Ambulatory Care Center, 445 East 25th Street, Hialeah, FL 33176; tel. 305/691-4450; FAX. 305/693-0823; Jose Kone, Administrative Director

Holiday Surgery Center, 1109 U.S. Highway 19, Suite B, Holiday, FL 34691; tel. 813/934-5705; Laverne Peyton, Administrator

Institute for Plastic and Reconstructive Surgery, 820 Arthur Godfrey Road, Third Floor, Miami Beach, FL 33140; tel. 305/673-6164; FAX. 305/534-9759; Lawrence B. Robbins, M.D.

Jacksonville Surgery Center, 4253 Salisbury Road, Jacksonville, FL 32216; tel. 904/281-0021; FAX. 904/281-0988; Katherine Anderson, RN, B.S.N., Center Director

Johnson Eye Institute Surgery Center, Inc., 5923 Seventh Street, Zephyrhills, FL 33539; tel. 813/788-7656; FAX. 813/788-6011; Jane Dempsey, RN, Surgery Services Coordinator

Kimmel Outpatient Surgical Center, 903 45th Street, West Palm Beach, FL 33407; tel. 407/845-8343; FAX. 407/840-8970; Susan Glendon, Administrator

Kissimmee Surgery Center, 2275 North Central Avenue, Kissimmee, FL 34741; tel. 407/870-0573; FAX. 407/870-1859; Lou Warmijak, Administrator

Lake Surgery and Endoscopy Center, 8100 CR 44A, Leesburg, FL 34788; tel. 352/323-1995; Pam Campbell, Assistant Administrator

Laser & Surgical Center of FL., L.C., 1717-1799 Woolbright Road, Boynton Beach, FL 33426; tel. 561/737-5500; FAX. 561/737-7055; Lily Lee, Administrator

Lee County Center for Foot and Ankle Surgery, Inc., 12734 Kenwood Lane, Suite 44, Fort Myers, FL 33907; tel. 941/936-2454; FAX. 941/936-1974; Steve Ostendorf, D.P.M.

Leesburg Regional Day Surgery Center, 601 East Dixie Avenue, Plaza 501, Leesburg, FL 34748; tel. 904/365-0700; FAX. 904/365-0758; Renae Vaughn, RN, B.S.N., CNOR, Clinical Director

Lowrey Eye Clinic, 1840 North Highland Avenue, Clearwater, FL 34615-1915; tel. 813/442-4147; FAX. 813/446-9297; Miquel E. Mulet, Jr., M.D.

Manatee Endoscopy Center, Inc., 6010 Pointe West Boulevard, Bradenton, FL 34209; tel. 813/792-4239

Martin Memorial SurgiCenter, 509 Riverside Drive, Suite 100, Stuart, FL 34994; tel. 407/223-5920; FAX. 407/288-5820

Martin Memorial Surgicenter at St. Lucie West, 1095 Northwest St. Lucie West Boulevard, Port St. Luci, FL 34986; tel. 561/223-5945; FAX. 561/223-6862; Charles S. Immordino, RN, Director, Clinical Operation

Mayo Clinic Jacksonville Ambulatory Surgery Center for G.I., 4500 San Pablo Road, Jacksonville, FL 32224; tel. 904/223-2000; Evelyn Leddy, ASC for GI Coordinator

Mayo Outpatient Surgery Center, 4500 San Pablo Road, Jacksonville, FL 32224; tel. 904/953-0100; FAX. 904/953-0019; Debbie Thornblom, Manager

Mease Countryside Surgery Care Center, 1880 Mease Drive, Safety Harbor, FL 34695; tel. 727/725-6373; Nancy Wheeling, Director

Medical Development Corporation of Pasco County, 7315 Hudson Avenue, Hudson, FL 34667; tel. 813/868-9563; FAX. 813/869-6918; Dawn M. Ernst, Director, Nursing

Medical Partners Surgery Center, 4545 Emerson Expressway, Jacksonville, FL 32207; tel. 904/399-2600; Kim Chitty, Director

Medivision of Northern Palm Beach County, 2889 10th Avenue, N., Suite 201, Lake Worth, FL 33461; tel. 407/969-0139; FAX. 407/642-1167; Denise Brower, Administrator

Miami Eye Center, 619 Northwest 12th Avenue, Miami, FL 33136; tel. 305/326-0260; FAX. 305/326-1907; Edward C. Gelber, M.D., F.A.C.S.

Mid Florida Surgery Center, 17564 West Highway 441, Mt. Dora, FL 32757; tel. 352/735-4100; FAX. 352/735-2444; Patsy Lentz, RN, Administrative Director

Montgomery Eye Center, 700 Neapolitan Way, Naples, FL 34103; tel. 941/261-8383; FAX. 941/261-8443; Jay E. Montgomery, Administrator

Mullis Eye Institute, Inc., 1600 Jenks Avenue, Panama City, FL 32405; tel. 904/763-6666; FAX. 904/763-6665; O. Lee Mullis, M.D., Administrator

Naples Day Surgery, 790 Fourth Avenue, N., Naples, FL 33940; tel. 813/263-3863; FAX. 813/263-7429; Sara May McCallum, Executive Director

Naples Day Surgery North, 11161 Health Park Boulevard, Naples, FL 34110; tel. 813/598-3111; FAX. 813/598-1707; Sara May McCallum, Executive Director

New Port Richey Surgery Center, 5415 Gulf Drive, New Port Rich, FL 34652; tel. 727/848-0446; FAX. 727/842-3166; Sandra McFarland, RN, Administrator

New Smyrna Beach Ambulatory Care Center, Inc., 612 Palmetto Street, New Smyrna Beach, FL 32168; tel. 904/423-5500

Newgate Surgery Center, Inc., 5200 Tamiami Trail, Suite 202, Naples, FL 34103; tel. 941/263-6766; FAX. 941/263-3320; Dr. R. Crane

North Florida Eye Clinic Surgicenter, 590 Dundas Drive, Jacksonville, FL 32218; tel. 904/751-3600; FAX. 904/757-8922; Mary Miller, RN, Director Surgical Services

North Florida Surgery Center, 4600 North Davis, Pensacola, FL 32503; tel. 904/494-0048; FAX. 904/494-0065; D. M. Whitehead, Administrator and CEO

North Florida Surgery Center, 2745 South First Street, Lake City, FL 32025; tel. 904/758-8937; Angela Kohlepp, Administrator

North Florida Surgical Pavilion, 6705 Northwest 10th Place, Gainesville, FL 32605; tel. 352/333-4555; FAX. 352/333-4569; Susan Roland, Administrative Director

North Ridge Surgery Center, 4650 North Dixie Highway, Fort Lauderdale, FL 33334; tel. 305/772-7995

Northwest Florida Gastroenterology Center, Inc., 202 Doctors Drive, Panama City, FL 32405; tel. 904/769-7599; FAX. 904/769-7389

Northwest Florida Surgery Center, 767 Airport Road, Panama City, FL 32405; tel. 850/747-0400; FAX. 850/913-9744; Ron Samuelian, Chief Executive Officer

Oak Hill Ambulatory Surgery, 11377 Cortez Boulevard, Brooksville, FL 32806; tel. 352/597-3060

Oak Hill Ambulatory Surgery and Endoscopy Center, 11377 Cortez Boulevard, Spring Hill, FL 34611; tel. 352/597-3060; FAX. 352/597-3077; Kelly Rhineberger, Administrative Director

Oakwater Surgical Center, inc., 3885 Oakwater Circle, Suite B, Orlando, FL 32806; tel. 407/438-9533; FAX. 407/438-9542; Sheila Angove, RN (Administrator)

Orange Park Surgery Center, 2050 Professional Center Drive, Orange Park, FL 32073; tel. 904/272-2550; FAX. 904/272-7911; Michele K. Cook, RN, Administrator, Nursing Director

Orlando Surgery Center, LTD., 2000 North Orange Avenue, Orlando, FL 32804; tel. 407/894-5808; FAX. 407/894-7802; Rodney C. Hollis, Administrator

Ormond Eye Surgi Center, 26 North Beach Street, Suite A, Ormond Beach, FL 32174; tel. 904/673-3344; FAX. 904/672-1854; Karen S. LaMotte, RN, Assistant Administrator

Pal-Med Same Day Surgery, 6950 West 20th Avenue, Hialeah, FL 33016; tel. 305/821-0079; FAX. 305/558-7494; Mario Machado, RN, Director

Palm Beach Endoscopy Center, Inc., 2015 North Flagler Drive, West Palm Beach, FL 33407; tel. 561/659-6543; FAX. 561/659-3533; Eva K. HasenHuttl, Admin. Director

Palm Beach Eye Clinic, 130 Butler Street, West Palm Beach, FL 33407; tel. 561/832-6113; FAX. 561/833-3003; Andre J. Golino, M.D.

Palm Beach Lakes Surgery Center, 2047 Palm Beach Lakes Boulevard, West Palm Beach, FL 33409; tel. 561/684-1375; FAX. 561/683-0332; Marjorie F. Konigsberg, Administrator

Parkside Surgery Center, 2731 Park Street, Jacksonville, FL 32205; tel. 904/389-1077; FAX. 904/389-9959; Chris Edmond, Administrator

Physician's Surgical Care Center, 2056 Aloma Avenue, Winter Park, FL 32792; tel. 407/647-5100; FAX. 407/647-1966

Physicians Ambulatory Surgery Center, 300 Clyde Morris Boulevard, Suite B, Ormond Beach, FL 32174; tel. 904/672-1080; FAX. 904/672-8628; Joel M. Wilder, RN, Administrator

Physicians Surgery Center, Ltd., DBA Lee Island Coast Surgery Center, 4035 Evans Avenue, Fort Myers, FL 33901; tel. 941/939-7375; FAX. 941/275-5248; Judi Schroeder, Administrator

Premier Surgery Center of Zephyrhills, 37834 Medical Arts Court, Zephyrhills, FL 33541; tel. 813/782-8778; FAX. 813/782-2811; Debra Fortenberry, RN, Director, Nursing

Presidential Surgicenter, Inc., 1501 Presidential Way, Suite Nine, West Palm Beach, FL 33401; tel. 407/689-7255; FAX. 407/683-7342; Steve S. Spector, M.D.

Rand Surgical Pavilion Corp., Five West Sample Road, Pompano Beach, FL 33064; tel. 800/782-1711; FAX. 954/782-7490; Deborah Rand, Administrator

Reed Centre for Ambulatory Urological Surgery, 1111 Kane Concourse, Suite 311, Bay Harbor, FL 33154; tel. 305/865-2000

Providers / Freestanding Ambulatory Surgery Centers

Riverside Park Surgicenter, 2001 College Street, Jacksonville, FL 32204; tel. 904/355-9800; Janice Carter, RN, Director, Nursing

Same-Day Surgicenter of Orlando, Ltd., 88 West Kaley Street, Orlando, FL 32806; tel. 407/423-0573; FAX. 407/841-7317; Sandy Moorhead, Administrator

Samuel Wells Surgicenter, Inc., 3599 University Boulevard, S., Suite 604, Jacksonville, FL 32216; tel. 904/399-0905; FAX. 904/346-0757; Faye T. Evans, Administrator

San Pablo Surgery Center, 14444 Beach Boulevard, Suite 50, Jacksonville, FL 32250; tel. 904/223-7800; FAX. 904/223-0081; Katie Anderson

Santa Lucia Surgical Center Inc., 2441 Southwest 37th Avenue, Miami, FL 33145; tel. 305/442-0066; FAX. 305/445-6896

Sarasota Surgery Center, 983 South Beneva Road, Sarasota, FL 34232; tel. 941/365-5355; FAX. 941/953-7080; Administrator

Seven Springs Surgery Center, Inc., 2024 Seven Springs Boulevard, New Port Richey, FL 34655; tel. 813/376-7000; Barbara Perich, Administrator

Southwest Florida Endoscopy Center, 5050 Mason Corbin Court, Ft. Myers, FL 33907; tel. 813/275-6678; FAX. 813/275-1785; Connie Byrd, Administrator

Southwest Florida Institute of Ambulatory Surgery, 3700 Central Avenue, Suite Two, Ft. Myers, FL 33901; tel. 941/275-0665; Susan Hanzevack, Executive Director

St. Augustine Endoscopy Center, 212 South Park Circle, E., St. Augustine, FL 32086; tel. 904/824-6108; FAX. 904/823-9613; Michael D. Schiff, M.D., President

St. John's Surgery Center, Inc., 8901 Conference Drive, Fort Myers, FL 33919; tel. 941/481-8833; FAX. 941/481-7898; Linda Pavletich, RN, Administrator

St. Joseph's Same Day Surgery Center, 3003 West Martin Luther King Boulevard, Tampa, FL 33607; tel. 813/870-4711; FAX. 813/870-4907; Paula McGuiness, Executive Director

St. Lucy's Outpatient Surgery Center, 21275 Olean Boulevard, Port Charlotte, FL 33952; tel. 941/625-1325; FAX. 941/625-6482; Anthony Limoncelli, M.D.

St. Luke's Surgical Center, 43309 U.S. Highway 19, N., P.O. Box 5000, Tarpon Spring, FL 34688-5000; tel. 813/938-2020; FAX. 813/938-5606; Glenn S. Wolfson, M.D., Medical Director

St. Petersburg Medical Group, Ambulatory Surgery and Endoscopy Center, 1099 Fifth Avenue, N., St. Petersburg, FL 33705-1419; tel. 813/821-1221; FAX. 813/892-8770; Iverson Pace, RN, Facility Manager, Director of Nursing

Suburban Medical Ambulatory Surgical Center, 17615 Southwest 97th Avenue, Miami, FL 33157; tel. 305/255-3950; FAX. 305/233-2503; Jules G. Minkes, D.O., Administrator

Suncoast Endoscopy Center, 601 Seventh Street, S., St. Petersburg, FL 33701; tel. 727/824-8337; FAX. 727/824-7177; Ivey Pace, RN, Director, Nursing

Suncoast Eye Center, Eye Surgery Institute, 14003 Lakeshore Boulevard, Hudson, FL 34667; tel. 727/868-9442; FAX. 727/862-6210; Lawrence A. Seigel, M.D., P.A., Medical Director

Suncoast Skin Surgery Clinic, 4519 U.S. Highway 19, New Port Richey, FL 34652; tel. 813/849-8922; FAX. 813/841-7553; Bethany Carvallo, Administrator

Suncoast Surgery Center of Hernando, Inc., 5060 Commercial Way, Spring Hill, FL 34606; tel. 904/596-3696; FAX. 904/596-2707; Bethany Carvallo, Administrator

Sunrise Surgical Center, 110 Yorktowne Drive, Daytona Beach, FL 32119; tel. 904/788-6696; FAX. 904/788-2219; Carolyn Teal

Surgery Center at St. Andrews, Inc., 1350 East Venice Avenue, Venice, FL 34292; tel. 941/488-2030; FAX. 941/484-2010; Lori Chase, Business Office Manager

Surgery Center of Jupiter, Inc., 102 Coastal Way, Jupiter, FL 33477; tel. 561/747-1111; FAX. 560/747-4151; Monroe N. Benaim, M.D., Medical Director

Surgery Center of North Florida, Inc., 6520 Northwest Ninth Boulevard, Gainsville, FL 32615; tel. 352/331-7987; FAX. 352/331-2787; Joy Ingram, Administrator

Surgery Center of Ocala, 3241 Southwest 34th Avenue, Ocala, FL 34474; tel. 352/237-5906; FAX. 352/237-5785; Verla Heffrin, Administrator

Surgery Center of Stuart, 2096 Southeast Ocean Boulevard, Stuart, FL 34996; tel. 561/223-0174; FAX. 561/223-0946; Jill Logan, Administrator

Surgical Center of Central Florida, 3601 South Highlands Avenue, Sebring, FL 33870; tel. 863/382-7500; FAX. 863/385-7132; Sharon Keiber, RN, Administrator

Surgical Licensed Ward, 110 West Underwood Street, Suite B, Orlando, FL 32806; tel. 407/648-9151; FAX. 407/426-7017; Cheryl Modica, RN, Administrator

Surgical Park Center, Ltd., 9100 Southwest 87th Avenue, Miami, FL 33176; tel. 305/271-9100; FAX. 305/270-8527; Rena Coady, Administrator

Surgicare Center, 4101 Evans Avenue, Ft. Myers, FL 33901; tel. 941/939-3456; FAX. 941/936-8776; Robin Fox, Director of Reimbursement

Surgicare Center of Venice, 950 Cooper Street, Venice, FL 34285; tel. 813/485-4868; FAX. 813/484-4084; Jean Matz, RN, CNOR, Director of Nursing

Tallahassee Endoscopy Center, 2400 Miccosukee Road, Tallahassee, FL 32308; tel. 904/877-2105; FAX. 904/942-1761; Noel Withers, Administrator

Tallahassee Outpatient Surgery Center, Inc., 3334 Capital Medical Boulevard, Suite 500, Tallahassee, FL 32308; tel. 904/877-4688; FAX. 904/877-0368; Martin Shipman, Administrator

Tallahassee Single Day Surgery, 1661 Phillips Road, Tallahassee, FL 32308; tel. 850/878-5165; FAX. 850/942-5545; Stacey Dye, Director of Administration

Tampa Bay Surgery Center, Inc., 11811 North Dale Mabry, Tampa, FL 33618; tel. 813/961-8500; FAX. 813/968-6818; Jay L. Rosen, M.D., Executive Director

Tampa Eye Surgery Center, 4302 North Gomez, Tampa, FL 33607; tel. 813/870-6330; FAX. 813/871-3956; Beverly Martin, Administrator

Tampa Outpatient Surgical Facility, 5013 North Armenia Avenue, Tampa, FL 33603; tel. 813/875-0562; FAX. 813/875-1983; Lawrence J. Cyment, Administrator

The Aesthetic Plastic Surgery Center, 135 San Marco Drive, Venice, FL 34285; tel. 941/484-6836; Claudell Crowe, Administrative Director

The Endoscopy Center, 4810 North Davis Highway, Pensacola, FL 32503; tel. 850/474-8988; FAX. 850/478-9903; Alice Cartee, Administrator

The Endoscopy Center of Naples, 150 Tamiami Trail, N., Suite One, Naples, FL 34102; tel. 941/262-8306; FAX. 941/262-3179; Marjorie Rogers, Billing Office Manager

The Endoscopy Center, Inc., 5101 Southwest Eighth Street, Miami, FL 33134; Susan Bobeman, Center Director

The Eye Associates Surgery Center, 6002 Pointe West Boulevard, Bradenton, FL 34209; tel. 941/792-2020; FAX. 941/792-2832; Linda Colson, RN, Director

The Gastrointestinal Center of Hialeah, 135 West 49th Street, Hialeah, FL 33012; tel. 305/825-0500; FAX. 305/826-6910; Annette Decastro, RN

The Ocala Eye Surgery Center, 3330 Southwest 33rd Street, Ocala, FL 34474; tel. 352/873-9311; FAX. 352/873-9652; Carol Hiatt, RN, Nurse Administrator

The Sheridan Surgery Center, 95 Bulldog Boulevard, Melbourne, FL 32901; tel. 407/952-9800; FAX. 407/952-7889; Patrice Curtis, RN, Clinical Director

The Treasure Coast Cosmetic Surgery Center, 1901 Port St. Lucie Boulevard, Port St. Lucie, FL 34952; tel. 407/335-3954; Donato A. Viggiano, M.D.

Total Surgery Center, 130 Tamiami Trail, Suite 210, Naples, FL 33940; tel. 941/434-4118; FAX. 941/434-6343; Elizabeth Ross, Administrator

Treasure Coast Center for Surgery, 1411 East Ocean Boulevard, Stuart, FL 34996; tel. 561/286-8028; FAX. 561/283-6628; Andrea Scoville, Business Office Manager

Trinity Outpatient Center, 2101 Trinity Oaks Boulevard, New Port Richey, FL 34655; tel. 727/372-4000; FAX. 727/372-4065; Nancy Burden, Director

University Surgical Center, 7251 University Boulevard, Suite 100, Winter Park, FL 32792; tel. 407/677-0066; FAX. 407/670-4199; Laura Hoffman, RRA, Director, Operations

Urological Ambulatory Surgery Center, Inc., 1812 North Mills Avenue, Orlando, FL 32803; tel. 407/897-5499; FAX. 407/896-9454; Susan A. Wuerz, Administrator

Urology Center of Florida, Inc., 3201 Southwest 34th Street, Ocala, FL 34474; tel. 352/237-8100; FAX. 352/237-5684; Randy Warellow, Administrator

Urology Health Center, 5652 Meadow Lane, New Port Rich, FL 34652; tel. 813/842-9561; FAX. 813/848-7270; Greg Toney, Administrator

Venture Ambulatory Surgery Center, 16853 Northeast Second Avenue, Suite 400, North Miami Beach, FL 33162; tel. 305/652-2999; FAX. 305/652-8156; Lali Perez, RN, B.S.N., Center Director

Vero Eye Center, 70 Royal Palm Boulevard, Vero Beach, FL 32960; tel. 407/569-6600

Volusia Endoscopy & Surgery Center, Inc., 550 Memorial Circle, Suite G, Ormond Beach, FL 32174; tel. 904/672-0017; FAX. 904/676-0506

Winter Park Ambulatory Surgical Center, 1000 South Orlando Avenue, Winter Park, FL 32789; tel. 407/629-1500; FAX. 407/629-1741; Linda Dingman, Administrator

GEORGIA

Advanced Aesthetics Plastic Surgery Center, 499 Arrowhead Boulevard, Jonesboro, GA 30236; tel. 770/603-6000; FAX. 770/603-7064; Paul D. Feldman, President

Advanced Surgery Center of Georgia, 220 Hospital Road, Canton, GA 30114; tel. 770/479-2202; FAX. 770/479-6666; Debbie Moore, Administrator

Aesthetic Laser & Surgery Facility, 416 Gordon Ave., Thomasville, GA 31792-6644; tel. 912/228-7200; Judy Warmack, Administrator

Aesthetica Surgicenter, P.C., 975 Johnson Ferry Road, Suite 160, Atlanta, GA 30342; tel. 404/531-9995; FAX. 404/531-0649; Sharon A. Pessalanto, Director

Affinity Outpatient Services, 2224 US Highway 41 North, Tifton, GA 31794; tel. 912/391-4299; FAX. 912/391-4291; Barry L. Cutts, Administrator

Albany Ambulatory Surgery Center, 531 Seventh Avenue, Albany, GA 31701; tel. 912/883-3535; FAX. 912/888-1079; J. Kenneth Durham, Medical Director

Ambulatory Foot and Leg Surgical Center, 1650 Mulkey Road, Austell, GA 30001; tel. 770/941-3633; Alan Shaw, D.P.M., Chief Executive Officer

Ambulatory Laser and Surgery Center, 425 Forest Parkway, Suite 103, Forest Park, GA 30297-2135; tel. 404/363-1087; FAX. 404/363-9951; Dr. Paul A. Colon, Medical Director

Athens Plastic Surgery Center, 2325 Prince Avenue, Athens, GA 30606; tel. 706/546-0280; FAX. 404/548-0258; James C. Moore, M.D., Administrator

Atlanta Aesthetic Surgery Center, Inc., 4200 Northside Parkway, Building Eight, Atlanta, GA 30327; tel. 404/233-3833; Debbie Clotfelter, Administrator

Atlanta Endoscopy Center, LTD, 2665 North Decatur Road, Suite 545, Decatur, GA 30033; tel. 404/297-5000; FAX. 404/296-9890; Jennifer Merowchek, RN, Clinical Coordinator

Atlanta Eye Surgery Center, P.C., 3200 Downwood Circle, NW, Suite 200, Atlanta, GA 30327; tel. 404/355-8721; Walter G. Elliott, Administrator

Atlanta Outpatient Peachtree Dunwoody Center, 5505 Peachtree-Dunwoody Road, Suite 150, Atlanta, GA 30342; tel. 404/847-0893; FAX. 404/843-8664; Janie Ellison, Administrator

Atlanta Outpatient Surgery Center, 993 Johnson Ferry Road, Suite 300, Atlanta, GA 30342; tel. 404/252-3074; FAX. 404/843-2089; Marjane Ellison, Administrator

Atlanta Surgi-Center, Inc., 1113 Spring Street, Atlanta, GA 30309; tel. 404/892-8685; FAX. 404/892-8143; Toni P. Hawkins, Administrator

Atlanta Women's Medical Center, Inc., 235 West Wieuca Road, Atlanta, GA 30342; tel. 404/257-0057; FAX. 404/257-1245; Ann Garzia, Administrator

Augusta Plastic Surgery Center, Inc., 811 13th Street, Suite 28, Richmond, GA 30901-2772; tel. 706/724-5611; FAX. 706/724-5435; Betsy Sharp, Office Manager

Augusta Surgical Center, 915 Russell Street, Augusta, GA 30904-4115; tel. 404/738-4925; Beryl Barrett, Administrator

Brunswick Endoscopy Center, 3217 4th Street, Brunswick, GA 31520-3759; tel. 912/267-1802; FAX. 912/267-0061; Rita Warren, Administrator

Center for Plastic Surgery, Inc., 365 East Paces Ferry Road, Atlanta, GA 30305; tel. 404/814-1100; FAX. 404/814-0015; Dr. Vincent Zubowicz, Medical Director

Providers / Freestanding Ambulatory Surgery Centers

Center for Reconstructive Surgery, 5335 Old National Highway, College Park, GA 30349; tel. 404/768-3668; FAX. 404/763-2929; Gregory Alvarez, D.P.M.

Clayton Outpatient Surgical Center, Inc., 6911 Tara Boulevard, Jonesboro, GA 30236; tel. 770/477-9535; FAX. 770/471-7826; Yvonne Guettler, Operating Room Supervisor

Cobb Foot and Leg Surgery Center, 792 Church Street Suite Two, Marietta, GA 30060; tel. 770/422-9864; FAX. 770/984/0303; Glyn Lewis, Administrator

Coliseum Same Day Surgery, 340 Hospital Drive, P.O. Box 6154, Macon, GA 31208; tel. 912/742-1403; FAX. 912/742-1671; Lenore Sell, Administrator

Columbia Augusta Surgical Center, 915 Russell Street, Augusta, GA 30904; tel. 706/738-4925; FAX. 706/738-7224; Beryl Barrett, RN, Administrator

Columbus Ambulatory Surgery Center, 725-22nd Street, Columbus, GA 31904-8845; tel. 706/322-6335; Freda R. Stewart, Administrator

Columbus Women's Health Organization, Inc., 3850 Rosemont Drive, Columbus, GA 31901; tel. 706/323-8363

Decatur Urological Clinic–Ambulatory Surgery Center, Inc., 428 Winn Court, Decatur, GA 30030; tel. 404/298-0217; FAX. 404/298-0218; Denise Ethridge, Office Manager

DeKalb Endoscopy Center, 2675 North Decatur Road, Suite 506, Decatur, GA 30033; tel. 404/299-1679; FAX. 404/501-7558; Peter Leff, M.D.

Dennis Surgery Center, Inc., 3193 Howell Mill Road, Suite 215, Atlanta, GA 30327; tel. 404/355-1312; Valerie Garrett, Administrator

Doctors Hospital Surgery Center, 635 Washington West, Evans, GA 30809; tel. 706/868-3110; Jeff Simless, Assistant Vice President, Finance

Dunwoody Outpatient Surgicenter, Inc., 4553 North Shallowford Road, Suite 60C, Atlanta, GA 30338; tel. 770/455-1198; FAX. 770/457-2823; Janet Davies, Administrator

Endoscopy Center of Columbus, Inc, 1041 Talbotton Road, Columbus, GA 31904-8745; tel. 706/327-0700; Jean Patterson, RN, Administrator

Endoscopy Center of Southeast Georgia, Inc., 200 Maple Drive, P.O. Box 1367, Vidalia, GA 30475; tel. 912/537-9851; Dixie Calhoun, RN, Administrator

Feminist Women's Health Center, 580 14th Street, N.W., Atlanta, GA 30318; tel. 404/874-7551; FAX. 404/875-7644; Jan Lockridge, Administrator

G.I. Endoscopy Center, 6555 Professional Place, Suite B, Riverdale, GA 30274; tel. 404/996-8830; FAX. 404/991-1596; Aruna Jaya Prakash, Administrator

Gainesville Surgery Center, 1945 Beverly Road, Gainesville, GA 30501-2034; tel. 770/287-1500; Mary W. Hoffman, Administrator

Gastrointestinal Endoscopy of Gwinnett, 600 Professional Drive, Suite 130, Lawrenceville, GA 30245; tel. 770/995-7989; FAX. 770/339-8646; Donna Ash, Practice Manager

Georgia Lithotripsy Center, 120 Trinity Place, Athens, GA 30607; tel. 404/543-2718; David C. Allen, M.D., Administrator

Georgia Surgical Centers – South, 541 Forest Parkway, Suite 14, Forest Park, GA 30297-6110; tel. 404/366-5652; Trudy Hunley, Administrator

Golden Isles Surgical Center, Inc., 2916 Glynn Avenue, Brunswick, GA 31530; tel. 912/265-3210; FAX. 912/265-1481; J. Brooker, Office Manager

Gwinnet Endoscopy Center, 575 Professional Drive, Suite 150, Lawrenceville, GA 30245; tel. 770/687-7220; FAX. 770/822-5548; Kerry H. King, M.D., President

HealthSouth Surgery Center of Atlanta, 1140 Hammond Drive, Building F, Suite 6100, Atlanta, GA 30328; tel. 770/551-9944; FAX. 770/551-8826; Nichole Busch, Administrator

HealthSouth Surgery Center of Gwinnett, 2131 Fountain Drive, Snellville, GA 30278; tel. 770/979-8200; FAX. 770/979-1327; Dianne Barrow, RN, Administrator

Hollis Eye Surgery Center, Inc., 7351 Old Moon Road, Columbus, GA 31909; tel. 706/323-8127; Kenneth Hopkins, Administrator

Marietta Surgical Center, Ambulatory Surgery Division, Columbia Healthcare Corporate, 796 Church Street, Marietta, GA 30060; tel. 770/422-1579; FAX. 770/422-1057; Charlotte Bellantoni, Administrator

Medical Eye Associates, Inc., 1429 Oglethorpe Street, Macon, GA 31201; tel. 912/743-7061; FAX. 912/743-6296; Linda Henderson, Office Manager

Midtown Urology Surgical Center, 128 North Avenue, N.E., Suite 100, Atlanta, GA 30308; tel. 404/881-0966; FAX. 404/874-5902; Jenelle E. Foote, M.D., Administrator

North Atlanta Endoscopy Center, 5555 Peachtree–Dunwoody Road, Suite G70, Atlanta, GA 30342-1703; tel. 404/843-0500; Phyllis Pritchett, Administrator

North Atlanta Head and Neck Surgery Center, 980 Johnson Ferry Road, Northside Doctors Building, Atlanta, GA 30342; tel. 404/256-5428; FAX. 404/250-1881; Ramon S. Franco, M.D.

North Fulton Diagnostic Gastrointestinal, 2500 Hospital Boulevard, Suite 480, Roswell, GA 30076; tel. 770/475-3085; David A. Atefi, M.D.

North Georgia Endoscopy Center, Inc., 320 Hospital Road, Canton, GA 30114; tel. 770/479-5535; FAX. 770/479-8821; Kevin W. Kellogg, Administrator

North Georgia Outpatient Surgery Center, 795 Red Bud Road, Calhoun, GA 30701; tel. 706/629-1852; FAX. 706/629-8004; Herbert E. Kosmahl, President

North Oak Ambulatory Surgical Center, 2718 North Oak Street, Valdosta, GA 31602; tel. 912/242-3668; FAX. 912/253-8666; T.E. Pitts, D.P.M.

Northeast Georgia Plastic Surgery Center, 1296 Sims Street, Gainesville, GA 30501; tel. 770/534-1856; FAX. 404/531-0355; Sam Richwine, Medical Director

Northlake Ambulatory Surgical Center, 2193 Northlake Parkway, Building 12, Suite 114, Tucker, GA 30084-4113; tel. 770/938-4860; Winfield Butlin, Administrator

Northlake Endoscopy Center, 1459 Montreal Road, Suite 204, Tucker, GA 30084; tel. 770/939-4721; FAX. 770/939-1187; Gayle Carter, Administrator

Northside Foot and Ankle Outpatient Surgical Center, 3415 Holcomb Bridge Road, Norcross, GA 30092; tel. 770/449-1122; FAX. 770/242-8709; Steven T. Arminio, DPM, Administrator

Northside Hospital Outpatient Surgical Center, 3400-A State Bridge Road, Suite 240, Alpharetta, GA 30202; tel. 404/667-4060; Sidney Kirscher, Administrator

Northside Surgery Center, Inc., 5505 Peachtree–Dunwoody Road, Suite 115, Atlanta, GA 30358-2091; tel. 404/256-0948; FAX. 404/843-1008; Irving Miller, Administrator

Northside Women's Clinic, Inc., 3543 Chamblee–Dunwoody Road, Atlanta, GA 30341; tel. 404/455-4210; FAX. 404/451-9529; James W. Gay, M.D., Administrator

Outpatient Center for Foot Surgery, Inc., 730 South Eighth Street, Suite B, Griffin, GA 30224; tel. 770/228-6644; FAX. 770/228-5769; Pam Roberts, RN

Paces Plastic Surgery Center, Inc., 3200 Downwood Circle, Suite 640, Atlanta, GA 30327; tel. 404/351-0051; FAX. 404/351-0632; Cathy Wood, Administrator

Parkwood Ambulatory Surgical Center, 2605 Parkwood Drive, Brunswick, GA 31520; tel. 912/265-4766; FAX. 912/267-9857; Betty Bauer, RN

Piedmont Surgery Center, 4660 Riverside Park Boulevard, Macon, GA 31210; tel. 912/471-6300; Mikell Peed, Administrator

Planned Parenthood of Reproductive Health Services, 1289 Broad Street, Augusta, GA 30911; tel. 706/724-5557; FAX. 706/724-5293; Karen Gates-Bonnet

Podiatric Surgi Center, 215 Clairemont Avenue, Decatur, GA 30030; tel. 404/373-2529; FAX. 404/370-1688; Jerald N. Kramer, President

Pulliam Ambulatory Surgical Center, 4167 Hospital Drive, Covington, GA 30209, P.O. Box 469, Covington, GA 30210; tel. 404/786-1234; M.M. Pulliam, P.C., Medical Director

Resurgens Surgical Center, 5671 Peachtree Dunwoody Road, Suite 800, Atlanta, GA 30342; tel. 404/847-9999; Kay F. Elliott, RN

Roswell Ambulatory Surgery Center, 1240 Upper Hembree Road, Roswell, GA 30076; tel. 770/663-8011

Savannah Medical Clinic, 120 East 34th Street, Savannah, GA 31401; tel. 912/236-1603; FAX. 912/236-1605; William Knorr, M.D., Administrator

Savannah Outpatient Foot Surgery Center, 310 Eisenhower Drive, Suite Seven, Savannah, GA 31406; tel. 912/355-6503; FAX. 912/355-9837; Dr. Kalman Baruch, President

Savannah Plastic Surgicenter, 4750 Waters Avenue, Suite 505, Savannah, GA 31404; tel. 912/351-5050; FAX. 912/351-5051; F. Christopher Pettigrew, M.D.

Southeastern Fertility Institute Surgical Associates, 5505 Peachtree Dunwood Road, Suite 400, Atlanta, GA 30342; tel. 404/257-1900; FAX. 404/256-1528; Ron Davidson, Administrator

Southlake Ambulatory Surgery Center, 4000 Corporate Center Drive, Suite 100, Morrow, GA 30260-1407; tel. 770/960-2701; FAX. 770/960-2702; Linda Simmons, Administrator

Statesboro Ambulatory Surgery Center, 95 Bel-Air Drive, Statesboro, GA 30461-6879; tel. 912/489-6519; FAX. 912/764-7882; Marie Autry, Office Manager

Surgery Center of Rome, 16 John Maddox Drive, Rome, GA 30165; tel. 706/234-0315; Neal Jochimsen, Director

The Cosmetic and Plastic Surgicenter of South Atlanta, 6524 Professional Place, Riverdale, GA 30274; tel. 770/991-1733; FAX. 770/997-7204; Nabil Elsahy, M.D.

The Emory Clinic Ambulatory Surgery Center, 1365 Clifton Road, N.E., Atlanta, GA 30322; tel. 404/778-5000; W. Mike Mason, Administrator

The Foot Surgery Center, 2520 Windy Hill Road, Suite 105, Marietta, GA 30067; tel. 770/952-0868; L. Susan Rothstein, Administrator

The Rome Surgery Center, 16 John Maddox Drive, Rome, GA 30165; tel. 706/234-0315; FAX. 706/234-1940; Neal Jochimsen, Administrator

Tifton Endoscopy Center, Inc., 1111 E. 20th Street, Tifton, GA 31794-3668; tel. 912/382-9338; FAX. 912/382-4282; Glenda Whittle, Administrator

HAWAII

Aloha Surgical Center, 239 Hoohana Street, Kahului, HI 96732; tel. 808/877-3984; FAX. 808/871-6498; Russell T. Stodd, M.D., Medical Director

Cataract and Retina Center of Hawaii, 1712 Liliha Street, Suite 400, Honolulu, HI 96817; tel. 808/524-1010; FAX. 808/531-1030; Worldster Lee, M.D., Director

Hawaiian Eye Surgicenter, 606 Kilani Avenue, Wahiawa, HI 96786; tel. 808/621-8448; FAX. 808/621-2082; Christopher M. Tortora, M.D., Surgeon, Director

Kaiser Honolulu Clinic, 1010 Pensacola Street, Honolulu, HI 96814; tel. 808/545-2950; FAX. 808/597-2249; Jonathan Ganz, Administrator

Kaiser Wailuku Clinic, 80 Mahalani Street, Wailuku, HI 96793; tel. 808/528-2511; FAX. 808/243-6009; Eileen Payton, Facility Manager

Surgicare of Hawaii, Inc., 550 South Beretania Street, Honolulu, HI 96813; tel. 808/528-2511; FAX. 808/526-0651; Eileen M. Peyton, Facility Manager

The Endoscopy Center, 134 Pu'uhou Way, Hilo, HI 96720; tel. 808/969-3979; FAX. 808/935-7657; Jody Montell, Administrator

The Surgical Suites, LLC, 1100 Ward Avenue, Suite 1001, Honolulu, HI 96814; tel. 808/531-0127; FAX. 808/531-0455; Carlos Omphroy, M.D., President

IDAHO

Addison Surgery Center, 191 Addison Avenue, Twin Falls, ID 83301; tel. 208/734-5993; David A. Blackmer, D.P.M., President

Boise Center for Foot Surgery, 1400 West Bannock, Boise, ID 83702; tel. 208/381-0262; FAX. 2/8429-8575; Marshall D. Odgen, D.P.M., Administrator

Boise Gastroenterology Associates, P.A., Idaho Endoscopy Center, 5680 West Gage, Boise, ID 83706; tel. 208/367-2894; FAX. 208/375-5286; Ike D. Tanabe, M.D., President

Coeur D'Alene Foot and Ankle Surgery Center, 101 Ironwood Drive, Suite 131, Coeur D'Alene, ID 83814; tel. 208/666-0814; Stephen A. Isham, D.P.M., Chairman, Board of Directors

Coeur D'Alene Surgery Center, 2121 Ironwood Center Drive, Coeur D'Alene, ID 83814; tel. 208/765-9059; FAX. 208/664-9998; Peter C. Jones, M.D., President

Emerald Surgical Center, 811 North Liberty, Boise, ID 83704; tel. 208/323-4522; FAX. 208/376-5258; Connie Alexander, Administrator

Idaho Ambucare Center, Inc., 211 West Iowa, Nampa, ID 83686; tel. 208/463-5160; FAX. 208/463-5178; Gary Botimer, Administrator

Providers / Freestanding Ambulatory Surgery Centers

Idaho Eye Surgicenter, 2025 East 17th Street, Idaho Falls, ID 83404; tel. 208/524-2025; FAX. 208/529-1924; Kenneth W. Turley, M.D., Medical Director

Idaho Falls Surgical Center, 1945 East 17th Street, Idaho Falls, ID 83404; tel. 208/529-1945; James A. Haney, M.D., Medical Director

Idaho Foot Surgery Center, 782 South Woodruff, Idaho Falls, ID 83401; tel. 208/529-8393; FAX. 208/529-8078; Bruce G. Tolman, D.P.M., Facility Director

Jefferson Day Surgery Center, 220 West Jefferson, Boise, ID 83702; tel. 208/343-3802; FAX. 208/343-9161; William Stano, President

North Idaho Cataract and Laser Center, Inc., 1814 Lincoln Way, Coeur D'Alene, ID 83814; tel. 208/667-2531; Paul Wail, Administrator

Pacific Cataract and Laser Institute, 250 Bobwhite Court, Suite 100, Boise, ID 83706-3983; tel. 208/385-7576; FAX. 208/385-0050; Sherri Mellville, Site Coordinator

Rock Creek Endoscopy Center, 284 Martin Street, Suite Two, Twin Falls, ID 83301; tel. 208/734-1266; FAX. 208/736-0390; Arlene Hansen, Administrator

Surgicare Center of Idaho, L.C., 360 East Mallard Drive, Suite 125, Boise, ID 83706; tel. 208/336-8700; W. Andrew Lyle, M.D., Medical Director

The Surgery Center, 115 Falls Avenue, W., P.O. Box 1864, Twin Falls, ID 83303-1864; tel. 208/733-1662; FAX. 208/734-3632; Larry Maxwell, M.D., Administrator

ILLINOIS

25 East Same Day Surgery, 25 East Washington, Chicago, IL 60602; tel. 312/726-3329; FAX. 312/726-3823; Pat Wansley, Administrator

A.C.T. Medical Center, 5714 West Division Street, Chicago, IL 60651; tel. 312/921-4300; Anthony Centrachio, Administrator

A.C.U. Health Center, LTD., 736 York Road, Hinsdale, IL 60521; tel. 630/794-0645; FAX. 630/794-0169; Lisa Shyne, Administrator

Able Health Center, Ltd., 1640 Arlington Heights Road, Suite 110, Arlington Heights, IL 60004; tel. 847/255-7400; FAX. 847/398-4585

Access Health Center, Ltd., 1700 75th Street, Downers Grove, IL 60516; tel. 630/964-0000; FAX. 630/964-0047; Diane L. Duddles, RN, Administrator

Advantage Health Care, LTD., 203 E. Irving Park Road, Wood Dale, IL 60191; tel. 630/595-1515; FAX. 630/595-9097; Lynn Pfingsten, Administrator

Albany Medical Surgical Center, 5086 North Elston, Chicago, IL 60630; tel. 312/725-0200; FAX. 312/725-6152; Diana Lammon, Administrator

Ambulatory Surgicenter of Downers Grove, Ltd., 4333 Main Street, Downers Grove, IL 60515; tel. 630/332-9451; Inga Ferdkoff, M.D., Administrator

American Women's Medical Center, 2744 North Western, Chicago, IL 60647; tel. 773/772-7726; FAX. 773/772-3696; Jan Barton, M.D., Administrator

AmSurg/Columbia HCA, 330 North Madison Street, Joliet, IL 60435; tel. 815/744-3000; FAX. 815/744-7916; Anne M. Cole, Administrator

Arlington Health Center, Ltd., 1640 Arlington Heights Road, Suite 210, Arlington Heights, IL 60004; tel. 847/255-7474

Bel–Clair Ambulatory Surgical Treatment Center, 325 West Lincoln, Belleville, IL 62220; tel. 618/235-2299; FAX. 618/235-2556; David Horace, Administrator

Carbondale Clinic Ambulatory Surgical Treatment Center, 2601 West Main Street, Carbondale, IL 62901; tel. 618/549-5361; FAX. 618/549-5128

Carle Surgicenter, 1702 South Mattis Avenue, Champaign, IL 61821; tel. 217/326-2030; Julie Root, RN, Administrator

Center for Reconstructive Surgery, 6311 West 95th Street, Oak Lawn, IL 60453; tel. 708/499-3355; FAX. 708/423-2305; Lori Brown, Administrator

Chang's Medical Arts Surgicenter (DBA), Apple Tree Health Care, Ltd., 2809 North Center Street, Maryville, IL 62062; tel. 618/288-1882; FAX. 618/288-3575; Jackie Nemsky, RN

Children's Pediatric Specialty Services In Westchester, 2301 Enterprise Drive, Westchester, IL 60154; tel. 708/836-4800; FAX. 708/836-4805; Jell Keats, Director,Satallite Services

CMP Surgicenter, Ltd, 3412 West Fullerton Avenue, Chicago, IL 60647; tel. 773/235-8000; FAX. 773/235-7018; Carlos G. Baldoceda, M.D., Medical Director

Columbia Surgicare–North Michigan Avenue, L.P., 60 East Delaware, 15th Floor, Chicago, IL 60611; tel. 312/440-5100; FAX. 312/440-5114; Barbara Villa, Administrator

Columbia–Northwest Surgicare, 1100 West Central Road, Arlington Heights, IL 60005; tel. 847/259-3080; FAX. 847/259-3190; Barbara Cerwin, RN, Administrator

Community Health and Emergency Services, R.R. 1, P.O. Box 233, Cairo, IL 62914; tel. 618/734-4400; FAX. 618/734-2884; Frederick L. Bernstein, Executive Director

Concord Medical Center, 17 West Grand, Chicago, IL 60610; tel. 312/467-6555; FAX. 312/467-9683; Elizabeth Reiker, Administrator

Concord West Medical Center, Ltd., 530 North Cass Avenue, Westmont, IL 60559; tel. 630/963-2500; Faramarz Farahati, Managing Director

Day SurgiCenters, Inc., 18 South Michigan Avenue, Suite 700, Chicago, IL 60603; tel. 312/726-2000; FAX. 312/726-3921; Andy Andrikos, Regional Vice President

Dimensions Medical Center, Ltd., 1455 East Golf Road, Suite 108, Des Plaines, IL 60016; tel. 847/390-9300; FAX. 847/390-0035; Vera Schmidt, Administrator

Dreyer Ambulatory Surgery Center, 1221 North Highland Avenue, Aurora, IL 60506; tel. 630/264-8400; FAX. 630/264-8402; James Kuyper, RN, Administrator

Eastland Medical Plaza SurgiCenter, 1505 Eastland Drive, Bloomington, IL 61701; tel. 309/662-2500; FAX. 309/662-7143; Marsha Reeves, Director

Edwardsville Ambulatory Surgical Center, LLC, 12, Ginger Creek Parkway, Glen Carbon, IL 62034; tel. 618/656-8200; FAX. 618/656-8204; Maxine Johnson, Administrator

Effingham Ambulatory Surgical Treatment Center, LTD., 904 West Temple Street, Effingham, IL 62401; tel. 217/342-1234; FAX. 217/342-1230; Leanne Fish, RN, CNOR, Administrator

Elmwood Park Same Day Surgery Center, 1614 North Harlem Avenue, Elmwood Park, IL 60635; tel. 708/452-6102; FAX. 708/452-1614; Ronald W. Hugar, DPM, Administrator

Foot and Ankle Surgical Center, Ltd., 1455 Golf Road, Suite 134, Des Plaines, IL 60016; tel. 847/390-7666; Lowell S. Weil, DPM, FACFS, Administrator

Golf Surgical Center, 8901 Golf Road, Des Plaines, IL 60016; tel. 847/299-2273; FAX. 847/299-2297; Bernard Abrams, M.D., Administrator

Hauser–Ross Surgicenter, Inc., Kishwaukee Community Hospital., 2240 Gateway Drive, Sycamore, IL 60178; tel. 815/756-8571; FAX. 815/756-1226; Barbara Lauger, Administrator

Health South Surgery Center of Southern Illinois, 806 North TreasTreas, P.O. Box 1729, Marion, IL 62959; tel. 618/993-2113; FAX. 618/993-2041; Linda Bickers, RN, Administrator

HealthSouth Surgery Center of Hawthorn, 1900 Hollister Drive, Suite 100, Libertyville, IL 60048; tel. 847/367-8100; FAX. 847/367-8335; Dr. Gary Rippberger, Administrator

HealthSouth Surgical Center, 1800 McDonough Road, Hoffman Estates, IL 60192; tel. 847/742-7272; FAX. 847/697-3210; Diane Newquist, Area Manager

Hinsdale Surgical Center, Inc., 908 North Elm Street, Suite 401, Hinsdale, IL 60521; tel. 630/325-5035; FAX. 630/325-5134; Shirley E. Zemansky, RN, Executive Director

Hope Clinic for Women, Ltd., 1602 21st Street, Granite City, IL 62040; tel. 800/844-3130; FAX. 615/451-9092; Sally Burgess, MBA, Executive Director

Horizons Ambulatory Surgery Center, 630 Locust Street, Carthage, IL 62321; tel. 217/357-2173; James E. Coeur, M.D., Administrator

Illinois Eye Surgeons Cataract Surgery, 3990 North Illinois Street, Belleville, IL 62221; tel. 618/235-3101; Cathy Vieluf, Administrator

Ingalls Same Day Surgery, 6701 West 159th Street, Tinley Park, IL 60477; tel. 708/429-0222; FAX. 708/429-0293; John Czech, Administrator

Lakeshore Physicians and Surgery Center, 7200 North Western Avenue, Chicago, IL 60645; tel. 773/743-6700; FAX. 773/761-9226; Phyllis J. Allen, RN, Administrator

Loyola Ambulatory Surgery Center at Oakbrook, One South 224 Summit Avenue, Suite 201, Oakbrook Terr, IL 60181; tel. 630/916-7008; Geoff Abbott, Administrator

LP Central Community Halth Centre, 355 East Fifth Ave., P.O. Box 68, Clifton, IL 60927; tel. 815/694-2392; Steve Wilder, Administrator

Magna Surgical Center, 9831 South Western Avenue, Chicago, IL 60643; tel. 312/445-9696; FAX. 312/445-9590; Yadira Martell, Administrator

Midwest Center for Day Surgery, 3811 Highland Avenue, Downers Grove, IL 60515; tel. 630/852-9300; FAX. 630/852-7773; Ronald P. Ladniak, Administrator

Midwest Eye Center, S.C., 1700 East West Road, Calumet City, IL 60409; tel. 708/891-3330; FAX. 708/891-0904; Afzal Ahmad, M.D., Administrator

Midwest Medical Center, 7340 West College Drive, Palos Heights, IL 60463; tel. 708/361-3233; FAX. 708/361-4876; Paul P. Skowron

Naperville Surgical Centre, 1263 Rickert Drive, Naperville, IL 60540; tel. 630/305-3300; FAX. 630/305-3301; Ronald P. Ladniak

North Shore Endoscopy Center, 101 South Waukegan Road, Suite 980, Lake Bluff, IL 60044; tel. 847/604-8700; FAX. 847/604-8711; Everett P. Kirch, M.D., Administrator

North Shore Same Day Surgicenter, 815 Howard Street, Evanston, IL 60202; tel. 847/869-8500; FAX. 847/869-0028; Edward Atkins, M.D., Medical Director

Northern Illinois Surgery Center, 1620 Sauk Road, Dixon, IL 61021; tel. 815/288-7722; FAX. 815/288-7720; Darryl Wahler, CEO

Northern Illinois Women's Center, Ltd., 1400 Broadway Street, Suite 201, Rockford, IL 61104; tel. 815/963-4101; FAX. 815/963-6122; Deborah D. Demars, Administrator

Northwest Community Day Surgery Center, 675 West Kirchoff Road, Arlington Heights, IL 60005; tel. 874/618-7075; FAX. 874/618-7069; Meaghan Reshoft, Administrator

Notre Dame Hills Surgical Center, 28 North 64th Street, Belleville, IL 62223; tel. 618/398-5705; FAX. 618/398-5764; Kathleen Claunch, RN, Administrator

Nova Med Eye Surgery Center of Maryville, L.L.C., 12 Maryville Professional Park Drive, Maryville, IL 62062; tel. 618/288-7483; Adrienne Forsythe, Administrator

NovaMed Eye Surgery Center River Forest, 7427 Lake Street, River Forest, IL 60305; tel. 708/771-3334; FAX. 708/771-0841; Karen Hyman, Administrator

Oak Brook Surgical Centre, Inc., 2425 West 22nd Street, Oak Brook, IL 60521; tel. 630/990-2212; FAX. 630/990-3130; George H. Olsen, Administrator

Oak Park Eye Center, S.C., 7055-61 West North Avenue, Oak Park, IL 60302; tel. 708/848-1182; FAX. 708/848-5033; James L. McCarthy, M.D., Administrator

One Day Surgery Center, 4211 North Cicero Avenue, Chicago, IL 60641-1699; tel. 773/794-1000; FAX. 773/794-9575; Ronald P.Ladniak

Orthopedic and Sports Medicine Clinic, P.C., 4411 Alby, P.O. Box 3195, Alton, IL 62002; tel. 618/474-8052; FAX. 618/474-8054; Bruce T. Vest, Jr., M.D., Director, Surgery

Orthopedic Institute of Illinois Ambulatory Surgery Center, 303 North Kumpf Boulevard, Peoria, IL 61605; tel. 309/676-5559; FAX. 309/676-5045; Donna Adair, Administrator

Peoria Ambulatory Surgery Center, 4909 North Glen Park Place, Peoria, IL 61614; tel. 309/691-9069; FAX. 309/691-9286; Cynthia J. Simpson, MBA, Administrator

Peoria Day Surgery Center, 7309 North Knoxville, Peoria, IL 61614; tel. 309/692-9210; FAX. 309/693-6472; Wanda Spacht, RN, Nursing Administrator

Physicians' Surgical Center, Ltd., 311 West Lincoln, Suite 300, Belleville, IL 62220; tel. 618/233-7077; FAX. 618/234-5650; Cynthia Chapman, RN, Administrator

Planned Parenthood of East Central Illinois, 302 East Stoughton Street, Champaign, IL 61820; tel. 217/359-8022; FAX. 217/359-2683; Robin Beach, Director of Client Services

Quad City Ambulatory Surgery Center, 520 Valley View Drive, Moline, IL 61265; tel. 309/762-1952; FAX. 309/762-3642; Vicki Sullivan, RN, CNOR, BS, Administrative Director

Quad City Endoscopy, 2525 24th Street, Rock Island, IL 61201; tel. 309/788-5624; FAX. 309/788-5668; Najwa Bayrakdar, Administrator

Regional Surgicenter, Ltd., 545 Valley View Drive, Moline, IL 61265; tel. 309/762-5560; FAX. 309/762-7351; Kay Wynn, Administrator

Providers / Freestanding Ambulatory Surgery Centers

Resurrection Health Care Surgery Center, 3101 North Harlem Avenue, Chicago, IL 60634; tel. 773/889–2000; FAX. 773/745–5522; Sandra Ankebrant, Executive Director

River North Same Day Surgery, One East Erie, Suite 115, Chicago, IL 60611; tel. 312/649–3939; FAX. 312/649–5747; Patricia Wamsley, Administrator

Rockford Ambulatory Surgery Center, 1016 Featherstone Drive, Rockford, IL 61107; tel. 815/226–3300; FAX. 815/226–9990; Dr. Steven Gunderson, Administrator/Medical Director

Rockford Endoscopy Center, 401 Roxbury Road, Rockford, IL 61107; tel. 815/397–7340; FAX. 815/397–7388; Nancy Norman, Administrator

Rogers Park One Day Surgery Center, 7616 North Paulina, Chicago, IL 60626; tel. 773/761–0500; FAX. 773/761–0500; Jerry Ruffino, RN Nurse Administrator

South Shore Surgicenter, Inc., 8300 South Brandon Avenue, Chicago, IL 60617; tel. 773/721–6000; FAX. 773/721–9861; Lucy Morales, RN, Administrator

Spiritus Dei Eye Surgery Center, 7600 West College Drive, Palos Heights, IL 60463; tel. 708/361–0010; Audrey Schmidt–Annerino, Administrator

Springfield Clinic Ambulatory Surgical Treatment Center, Inc., 1025 South Seventh Street, Springfield, IL 62794–9248; tel. 217/528–7541; Michae Maynard

Suburban Otolaryngology SurgiCenter, 3340 South Oak Park Avenue, Berwyn, IL 60402; tel. 708/749–3070; FAX. 708/749–3410; Edward A. Razim, M.D., Administrator

SureVision Surgery & Laser Center–Northshore, 3034 West Peterson Avenue, Chicago, IL 60659; tel. 773/973–7432; FAX. 773/973–1119; Dawn Laskey, Administrator

Surgicare Center, Inc., 333 Dixie Highway, Chicago Heights, IL 60411; tel. 708/754–4890; FAX. 708/756–1149; Paul Kats, Administrator

Surgicore, Inc., 10547 South Ewing Avenue, Chicago, IL 60617; tel. 773/221–1690; William Wood, DPM, Medical Director

The Center for Orthopedic Medicine, LLC, 2502–B East Empire, Bloomington, IL 61704; tel. 309/662–6120; FAX. 309/663–8972; Tracy J. Silver, RN, Administrator

The Center for Surgery, 475 East Diehl Road, Naperville, IL 60563–1253; tel. 630/505–7733; FAX. 630/505–0656; Eric Myers, Administrator

The Surgery Center of Centrailia, 1045 Martin Luther King, Jr. Drive, Centralia, IL 62801; tel. 618/532–3110; FAX. 618/532–7226; Rajendra Shroff, M.D., Medical Director

Valley Ambulatory Surgery Center, 2210 Dean Street, St. Charles, IL 60175; tel. 630/584–9800; FAX. 630/584–9805; Mark Mayo, Facility Director

Watertower Surgicenter Corp., 845 North Michigan Avenue, Suite 994–W, Chicago, IL 60611; tel. 312/944–2929; FAX. 312/944–7769; John M. Sevcik, President and CEO

Women's Aid Clinic, 4751 West Touhy Avenue, Lincolnwood, IL 60712–2212; tel. 847/676–2428; Iris Schneider

INDIANA

Aesthetic Surgery Center, 13590 N. Meridian, Carmel, IN 46032; tel. 317/846–0846; FAX. 317/846–0722; William H. Beeson, M.D., Medical Director

Akin Medical Center, 2019 State Street, New Albany, IN 47150–4963; tel. 812/945–3557; FAX. 812/949–3469; Karyn Cureton, RN, Director, Surgery

Broadwest Surgical Center, 315 W. 89th Ave., Merrillville, IN 46410–2904; tel. 219/757–5275; FAX. 219/757–5290; Lisa M. Goranovich, Administrator

Calumet Surgery Center, 7847 Calumet Avenue, Munster, IN 46321–1296; tel. 219/836–5102; FAX. 219/836–4493; Gloria J. Portney, RN, Chief Administrative Officer

Central Indiana Surgery Center, 9002 North Meridian, Lower Level, Indianapolis, IN 46260; tel. 317/846–9906; FAX. 317/846–9949; William E. Whitson, M.D., Medical Director

Columbia Physiciancare Outpatient Surgery Center, L.L.P., 7460 North Shadeland, Indianapolis, IN 46250; tel. 317/577–7450; FAX. 317/577–7462; Maureen Chernoff, RN, Administrator

Columbus Surgery Center, 940 North Marr Road, Suite B, Columbus, IN 47201; tel. 812/372–1370; Colleen M. North, Executive Director

Digestive Health Center, 1120 AAA Way, Suite A, Carmel, IN 46032–3210; tel. 317/848–5494; FAX. 317/575–0392; Daniel J. Stout, M.D., President

Dupont Ambulatory Surgery Center, 2510 East Dupont Road, Suite 130, Fort Wayne, IN 46825; tel. 219/489–8785; FAX. 219/489–2148; Rick C. Trego, Administrator

Evansville Surgery Center, 1212 Lincoln Ave., Evansville, IN 47714–1076; tel. 812/428–0810; FAX. 812/421–6070; Cathy Head, RN, Facility Manager

Foot and Ankle Surgery Center, Inc., 1950 West 86th Street, Suite 105, Indianapolis, IN 46260; tel. 317/334–0232; FAX. 317/334–0268; Anthony E. Miller, D.P.M., Administrator

Fort Wayne Cardiology Outpatient Catheterization Laboratory, 1819 Carew Street, Fort Wayne, IN 46805; tel. 219/481–4896; FAX. 219/481–4814; Douglas W. Martin, RN, M.B.A., Director of Clinical Operations

Fort Wayne Ophthalmic Surgical Center, 321 East Wayne Street, Ft. Wayne, IN 46802–2713; tel. 219/422–5976; FAX. 219/424–4511; J. Rex Parent, M.D., Chief Executive Officer

Fort Wayne Orthopaedics LLC Surgicenter, 7601 West Jefferson Boulevard, P.O. Box 2526, Fort Wayne, IN 46801–2526; tel. 219/436–8383; FAX. 219/436–8477; David H. Fischer, Executive Director

Gastrointestinal Endoscopy Center, 801 St. Mary's Drive, Suite 110 West, Evansville, IN 47714; tel. 812/477–6103; FAX. 812/477–4897; Butch Moors, CPA, Administrator

Grand Park Surgical Center, 1479 East 84th Place, Merrillville, IN 46410; tel. 219/738–2828; FAX. 219/756–3349; Chris Macarthy, Administrator

Grossnickle Eye Surgery Center, Inc., 2251 DuBois Drive, Warsaw, IN 46580–3292; tel. 219/269–3777; FAX. 219/269–9828; Shirley Rhodes, RN, Administrative Director

Illiana Surgery Center, 701 Superior Avenue, Munster, IN 46321; tel. 219/924–1300; FAX. 219/922–4856; Virgil Villaflor, Executive Director

IMA Endoscopy Surgicenter, P.C., 8895 Broadway, Merrillville, IN 46411; tel. 219/736–4660; FAX. 219/736–4663; Dawn Graham, Administrator

Indiana Eye Clinic, 30 North Emerson Avenue, Greenwood, IN 46143–9760; tel. 317/881–3931; FAX. 317/887–4008; Charles O. McComnick, M.D., Administrator

Indiana Surgery Center, 8040 Clearvista Parkway, Indianapolis, IN 46256–1695; tel. 317/841–2000; FAX. 317/841–2005; Amy Glover, Administrator

Indiana Surgery Center, 1550 East County Line Road, Suite 100, Indianapolis, IN 46227; tel. 317/887–7600; FAX. 317/887–7606; Peggy Davidson, Administrator

Indiana Surgery Center – North Campus, 8040 Clearvista Parkway, Indianapolis, IN 46256; tel. 317/841–2000; FAX. 317/841–2005; Amy D. Glover, RN, B.S.N., Administrator

Indianapolis Endoscopy Center, 7353 East 21st Street, Indianapolis, IN 46219; tel. 317/353–2232; FAX. 317/353–2522; David Hollander, M.D.

Lafayette Ambulatory Surgery Center, 3733 Rome Drive, Box 6477, Lafayette, IN 47903; tel. 765/449–5272; FAX. 765/447–1276; Dale T. Krynak, Executive Director

Meridian Endoscopy Center, 1801 North Senate, Suite 400, Indianapolis, IN 46202; tel. 317/929–5660; FAX. 317/929–2346; Robert J. Whitmore, Executive Director

Meridian Plastic Surgery Center, 170 West 106th Street, Indianapolis, IN 46290–1004; tel. 317/575–0110; FAX. 317/571–8667; Ken Dyar, RN, Director

MHC Surgical Center Associates, Inc., d/b/a Broadwest Surgical Center, 315 West 89th Avenue, Merrillville, IN 46410–2904; tel. 219/757–5275; FAX. 219/757–5290; Melvin Lichtenfeld, P.D., Administrator

Michigan Endoscopy Center, LLC, 53830 Generation Drive, South Bend, IN 46635; tel. 219/271–0893; FAX. 219/271–1285; John G. Mathis, M.D., CEO

Midwest Surgery Centers, Inc., 650 Surgery Center Drive, Terre Haute, IN 47802; tel. 812/232–8325; FAX. 812/234–8385; Terry Havens, RN, Administrator

Muncie Ambulatory Surgicenter, LLC, 200 North Tillotson Avenue, Muncie, IN 47304–3988; tel. 765/286–8888; FAX. 765/747–7962; Jeffrey S. Rapkin, M.D., Medical Director

Munster Same Day Surgery Center, 761 Forty Fifth Avenue, Suite 116, Munster, IN 46321; tel. 219/924–3090; FAX. 219/924–2161; Edward Atkins, President

Nasser Smith and Pinkerton Cardiac Cath Lab, 8333 Naab Road, Suite 400, Indianapolis, IN 46260; tel. 317/338–6094; FAX. 317/338–6066; Stephen A. McAdams, M.D., CEO

North Indianapolis Surgery Center, 8651 North Township Line Road, Indianapolis, IN 46260–1578; tel. 317/876–2090; FAX. 317/876–2097; Dean E. Lehmkuhler, Facility Administrator

North Meridian Surgery Center, 10601 North Meridian Street, Suite 100, Indianapolis, IN 46290; tel. 317/574–5400; FAX. 317/575–0173; Susan Matouk, Director

Northeast Indiana Endoscopy Center, 7900 West Jefferson Boulevard, Fort Wayne, IN 46804; tel. 219/436–6213; FAX. 219/432–6388; Jerry Steele, Administrator

Northside Cardiac Cath Lab, 8333 Naab Road, Suite 180, Indianapolis, IN 46260; tel. 317/338–9001; FAX. 317/338–9045; Beth Higgins, RN, MSN, Clinical Director

NovaMed Eyecare Management, L.L.C., 8514 Broadway, Merrillville, IN 46410; tel. 219/756–5010; FAX. 219/736–2222; Joan Klug, Administrator

NovaMed Eyecare Management, L.L.C., d/b/a NovaMed Eye Surgery Center–Hammond, 6836 Hohman Avenue, Hammond, IN 46324; tel. 219/937–5063; FAX. 219/937–5068; Renee Peters, Administrator

Oakview Surgical Center, Inc., 120 E. 18th St., Rochester, IN 66975; tel. 219/224–7500; FAX. 219/223–3057; Laurence C. Rogers, D.P.M., Administrator

Outpatient Surgery Center of Indiana, LLP, 711 Gardner Drive, Marion, IN 46952; tel. 317/664–2000; FAX. 317/668–6797; Dixie Hewitt, RN, Director

Richmond Surgery Center, 1900 Chester Boulevard, Richmond, IN 47374; tel. 765/966–1776; FAX. 765/962–1191; Lynn Greene, Director

Riverpointe Surgery Center, 500 Arcade Avenue, Suite 100, Elkhart, IN 46514–2459; tel. 219/522–9505; Robert Scheller, Administrator

Sagamore Surgical Services, Inc., 2320 Concord Road, Suite B, Lafayette, IN 47909; tel. 317/474–7838; Carol Blanar, Administrator

South Bend Clinic Surgicenter, 211 North Eddy Street, P.O. Box 4061, South Bend, IN 46634–4061; tel. 219/237–9366; FAX. 219/237–9363; Paul J. Meyer, Executive Director

Southern Indiana Surgery Center, 2800 Rex Grossman Boulevard, Bloomington, IN 47403; tel. 812/333–8969; FAX. 812/335–2309; Miriam Malone, RN, B.S.N., Executive Director

Surgery Center of Eye Specialists, 1901 North Meridian Street, Indianapolis, IN 46202; tel. 317/925–2200; FAX. 317/921–6614; Dan Bradford, Administrator

Surgery Center of Fort Wayne, L. P., d/b/a HealthSouth Premier Surgery Center, 1333 Maycrest Drive, Fort Wayne, IN 46805–5478; tel. 219/423–3339; FAX. 219/423–6344; Mary Schafer, Administrator

Surgery Center of Southeastern Indiana, Inc., 999 N. Michigan Ave., Greensburg, IN 47240; tel. 812/663–3222; FAX. 812/663–3622; Deanna Borgman, R.N., DON Administrator

Surgery Center Plus, 7430 North Shadeland Avenue, Suite 100, Indianapolis, IN 46250–2025; tel. 317/841–8005; FAX. 317/577–7538; James Hansen, Administrator

Surgery One, 5052 North Clinton, Fort Wayne, IN 46825–5822; tel. 219/482–5194; FAX. 219/482–5686; Julia Ellert, Director

Surgical Care Center, Inc., 8103 Clearvista Parkway, Indianapolis, IN 46256–4600; tel. 317/842–5173; FAX. 317/570–7429; Brian Smith, Executive Director

Surgical Center of New Albany, 2201 Green Valley Road, New Albany, IN 47150–4648; tel. 812/949–1223; FAX. 812/945–4765; Tamara E. Jones, B.S.N., Administrator

Surgicare, 2907 McIntire Drive, Suite C, Bloomington, IN 47403; tel. 812/339–8000; FAX. 812/339–2524; Sonya M. Zeller, Administrator

Surgicare of Jeffersonville, 1305 Wall Street, Suite 101, Jeffersonville, IN 47130–3898; tel. 812/288–9674; FAX. 812/283–6955; Marsha Parker, Administrator

Providers / Freestanding Ambulatory Surgery Centers

The Ambulatory Care Center d/b/a, Surgicare–Outpatient Surgical Center, 1125 Professional Boulevard, Evansville, IN 47714; tel. 812/475-1000; FAX. 812/475-1001; Diana McDaniel, Facility Administrator

The Center for Specialty Surgery of Fort Wayne, Inc., 2730 East State Boulevard, Fort Wayne, IN 46805-4731; tel. 219/483-2540; FAX. 219/483-3097; Andrea Kelley, RN, Director, Nursing

The Endoscopy Center, 8051 South Emerson, Suite 150, Indianapolis, IN 46237; tel. 317/865-2950; FAX. 317/865-2952; Robert Intress, Ph.D., Administrator

The Heart Group Outpatient Cath Lab, 415 West Columbia Street, Evansville, IN 47710; tel. 812/464-0545; FAX. 812/464-0560; Sue Krieg, RN, Clinical Manager

The Indiana Hand Surgery Center, 8501 Harcourt Road, P.O. Box 80434, Indianapolis, IN 46260-0434; tel. 317/875-9105; FAX. 317/471-4382; Valeria M. Wareham, Chief Operating Officer

Unity Surgery Center, 1011 West Second Street, Bloomington, IN 47403-2216; tel. 812/334-1213; FAX. 812/333-5039; Michael D. Bishop, M.D., CEO

Valley Cataract and Laser Institute, Inc., 220 East Virginia, Evansville, IN 47711; tel. 812/435-1600; FAX. 812/435-1603; Lisa J. Gossman-Werner, Facility Administrator

Valparaiso Physician and Surgery Center, 1700 Pointe Drive, Valparaiso, IN 46383; tel. 219/531-5000; FAX. 219/531-5010; Lilly Veljovic, RN, Manager

Welborn Clinic Surgery Center, 421 Chestnut Street, Evansville, IN 47713; tel. 812/426-9412; Claudia R. Earnest, Administrator

Zollman Surgery Center, Inc., 7439 Woodland Drive, Indianapolis, IN 46268; tel. 317/328-7000; FAX. 317/328-6948; Jackie Kersey, RN, Administrator

IOWA

Ambulatory Surgery Center, 931 13th Avenue, N., P.O. Box 608, Clinton, IA 52733-0608; tel. 319/242-3937; FAX. 319/242-3845; Renelda Ebensberger, Supervisor

Iowa Endoscopy Center, 2600 Grand Avenue, Suite 418, Des Moines, IA 50312; tel. 515/288-3342; Loraine Hansne, B.S.N., Administrator

Iowa Eye Institute, 1721 West 18th Street, Spencer, IA 51301; tel. 712/262-8878; FAX. 712/262-8807; Dennis D. Gordy, M.D., Administrator

Jones Eye Clinic, 4405 Hamilton Boulevard, Sioux City, IA 51104; tel. 712/239-3937; Charles E. Jones, M.D., Medical Director

Mississippi Valley Surgery Center, L.C., 3400 Dexter Court, Suite 200, Davenport, IA 52807; tel. 319/344-6600; FAX. 319/344-6699; John B. Dooley, Administrator

Spring Park Surgery Center, LLC, 3319 Spring Street, Suite 202–A, Davenport, IA 52807; tel. 319/355-6236; FAX. 319/359-6347; Paul Rohlf, M.D., Administrator

Surgery Center of Des Moines, 1301 Penn Avenue, Suite 100, Des Moines, IA 50312; tel. 515/266-3140; FAX. 515/266-3073; Kathleen Supplee, RN, Administrator

KANSAS

College Park Family Care Center, 11725 West 112th Street, Overland Park, KS 66210-2761; tel. 913/469-5579; Chuck Chambers, Administrator

Columbia Mt. Oread Surgery Centre, 3500 Clinton Parkway Place, Lawrence, KS 66047-1985; tel. 913/843-9300; FAX. 913/843-9301; Nancy Sturgeon, Administrator

Comprehensive Health for Women, 4401 West 109th Street, Overland Park, KS 66211-1303; tel. 913/345-1400; Sheila Kostas, Director, Human Resources

Cotton–O'Neil Clinic Endoscopy Center, 823 Southwest Mulvane Street, Suite 375, Topeka, KS 66606-1679; tel. 785/354-0538; FAX. 785/368-0735; Irene Hasenbank, RN,Director

Emporia Ambulatory Surgery Center, 2528 West 15th Avenue, Emporia, KS 66801-6102; tel. 316/343-2233; J. E. Bosiljevac, M.D., Administrator

Endoscopic Services, P.A., 1431 South Bluffview Street, Suite 215, Wichita, KS 67218-3000; tel. 316/687-0234; FAX. 316/687-0360; Jace Hyder, M.D.

Endoscopy and Surgery Center of Topeka, L.P., 2200 Southwest Sixth Avenue, Suite 103, Topeka, KS 66606-1707; tel. 913/354-1254; FAX. 913/354-1255; Ashraf M. Sufi, M.D., Medical Director

EyeSurg of Kansas City, 5520 College Boulevard, Overland Park, KS 66211-1600; tel. 913/491-3757; FAX. 913/469-6686; Phillip Hoopes, M.D., Medical Administrator

Hutchinson Clinic Ambulatory Surgery Center, 2101 North Waldron, Hutchinson, KS 67502; tel. 316/669-2500; Murray Holcomb, Administrator

Laser Center, 1518A East Iron Avenue, Salina, KS 67401-3236; tel. 913/825-6016; Brian E. Conner, M.D., Administrator

Laser Center–Russell, 222 South Kansas, Suite A, Russell, KS 67665-3029; tel. 913/825-6016; Brian Conner, Administrator

Newton Surgery Centre, 215 South Pine Street, Newton, KS 67114-3761; tel. 316/283-4400; Sondra L. Leatherman, Administrator

Ochsner Eye Medical/Associated Eye Surgical Center, 1100 North Topeka Street, Wichita, KS 67214-2810; tel. 316/263-6273; FAX. 316/263-5568; Bruce B. Ochsner, Medical Director

South Pointe Surgery Center, 151 West 151st Street, Suite 200, Olathe, KS 66061-5351; tel. 913/782-3631; FAX. 913/782-2606; Katherine Thon, RN, Administrator

Surgery Center of Kansas, Inc., 1507 West 21st Street, Wichita, KS 67203-2449; tel. 316/838-8388; FAX. 316/838-2999; Karen Gabbert, RN, B.S.N., Administrator

Surgicare of Wichita, Inc., 810 North Lorraine, Wichita, KS 67214-4841; tel. 316/685-2207; FAX. 316/685-2861; Carolyn J. Exley, Administrator

Surgicenter of Johnson County, 8800 Ballentine Street, Overland Park, KS 66214-1985; tel. 913/894-4050; FAX. 913/894-0384; Rose Weintraub, Administrator

Team Vision Surgery Center East, 6100 East Central Street, Suite Six, Wichita, KS 67208-4237; tel. 316/684-8013; Linda S. Buettner, Vice President

Team Vision Surgery Center West, 834 North Socora, Suite One, Wichita, KS 67212-3238; tel. 316/681-2020; Linda Buettner, Administrator

The Center for Same Day Surgery, 818 North Emporia Street, Suite 108, Wichita, KS 67214-3725; tel. 316/262-7263; FAX. 316/262-6253; Michele LeGate, RN, B.S., Administrator

The Headache and Pain Center, 11111 Nall Avenue, Suite 222, Leawood, KS 66211-1625; tel. 913/491-3999; FAX. 913/491-6453; Steven D. Waldman, Administrator

Topeka Single Day Surgery, 823 Southwest Mulvane Street, Suite 101, Topeka, KS 66606-1679; tel. 913/354-8737; FAX. 913/354-1440; Linda Daniel, Executive Director

Wichita Clinic DaySurgery, 3311 East Murdock Street, Wichita, KS 67208-3054; tel. 316/689-9596; Janelle Oliver, RN, Manager

KENTUCKY

Ambulatory Surgery Center, 2831 Lone Oak Road, Paducah, KY 42003; tel. 502/554-8373; FAX. 502/554-8987; Laxmaiah Manchikanti, M.D.

Caritas Surgical Center, 4414 Churchman Avenue, Louisville, KY 40215; tel. 502/366-9525; Danny Cain

Center For Surgical Care, 7575 U.S. 42, Florence, KY 41042; tel. 606/283-9100; FAX. 606/283-6046; Thomas Mayer, M.D., Medical Director

Columbia Owensboro Surgery Center, 1100 Walnut Street, Suite 13, Owensboro, KY 42301; tel. 502/683-2751; FAX. 502/926-1618; Donna R. Norton, Administrator

Cumberland Valley Surgical Center, P.O. Box 580, 2737 North U.S. Highway 25, East Bernstad, KY 40729; tel. 606/843-6100; FAX. 606/843-6115; John Lanning, Administrator

Downing –McPeak Surgery Center, 1507 Bravo Boulevard, Glasgow, KY 42141; tel. 502/651-2181; FAX. 502/651-2183; Sheila Dishman, Administrator

Dupont Surgery Center, 4004 Dupont Circle, Louisville, KY 40207; tel. 502/896-6428; FAX. 502/893-5270; Sherry Oeswein, Administrator

E.M.W. Women's Surgical Center, 138 West Market Street, Louisville, KY 40202; tel. 502/589-2124; FAX. 502/589-1588; Dona F. Wells, Administrator

HealthSouth Surge Center of Louisville, 4005 DuPont Circle, Louisville, KY 40207; tel. 502/897-7401; FAX. 502/897-5652; Sheila S. Boros, Administrator

HealthSouth Surgical Center of Elizabethtown, 708 Westport Road, Elizabethtown, KY 42701; tel. 270/737-5200; FAX. 270/765-5362

Louisville Surgery Center, 614 East Chestnut Street, Louisville, KY 40202; tel. 502/589-9488; FAX. 502/589-9928; Vanessa McDermott, Administrator

Medical Heights Surgery Center, 2374 Nicholasville Road, Lexington, KY 40503; tel. 606/278-1460; FAX. 606/278-0115; John Johnson, Facility Director

Outpatient Care Center at Jewish Hospital, 225 Abraham Flexner Way, Louisville, KY 40202; tel. 502/587-4709; FAX. 502/587-4323; Kim Tharp-Barrie, Administrator

Pikeville United Methodist Hospital of Kentucky, Inc., 911 South By-Pass Road, Pikeville, KY 41501; tel. 606/437-3500; FAX. 606/437-4996; Joann Anderson, Chief Operating Officer

Somerset Surgery Center, 353 Bogle Street, Suite 101, Somerset, KY 42501; tel. 606/679-9322; FAX. 606/678-2666; Kathy Turner, Administrator

Stone Road Surgery Center, 280 Pasadena Drive, Lexington, KY 40503; tel. 606/278-1316; FAX. 606/276-3847; Ballard Wright, President

The Eye Surgery Center of Paducah, 100 Medical Center Drive, P.O. Box 8269, Paducah, KY 42002-8269; tel. 502/442-1024; FAX. 502/442-1001; Kelly Harris, RN, Administrator

Tri-State Digestive Disorder Center Ambulatory Surgery Center, 196 Barnwood Drive, Edgewood, KY 41017; tel. 606/341-3575; Stephen W. Hiltz, M.D.

LOUISIANA

Acadiana Endoscopy Center, 113 St. Louis Street, Lafayette, LA 70506; tel. 318/269-1126; FAX. 318/269-0553; Stephen M. Person, M.D., Administrator

Acadiana Surgery Center, Inc., 1100 Andre Street, Suite 300, New Iberia, LA 70560; tel. 318/364-9680; FAX. 318/364-9689

Alexandria Laser and Surgery Center, 4100 Parliament Drive, Alexandria, LA 71303; tel. 318/487-8342; FAX. 318/487-9942; M. L. Revelett, Administrator

Ambulatory Eye Surgery Center of Louisiana, 3900 Veterans Boulevard, Suite 100, Metairie, LA 70002; tel. 504/455-1550; FAX. 504/455-2011; Mark Brown, Administrator

Baton Rouge Ambulatory Surgicare Services, 5328 Didesse Drive, Baton Rouge, LA 70808; tel. 504/766-1718; FAX. 504/767-3034; Laura B. Cronin, Administrator

Broussard Surgery Institute, 1250 Pecanland Road, Suite E-1, Monroe, LA 71203; tel. 318/387-2015; FAX. 318/387-2097; Gerald Broussard, M.D., Administrator

Browne-McHardy Outpatient Surgery Center, 4315 Houma Boulevard, Metairie, LA 70006-2981; tel. 504/889-5218; FAX. 504/889-5224; Robert L. Goldstein, Chief Administrative Officer

Central Louisiana Ambulatory Surgical Center, 720 Madison Street, P.O. Box 8646, Alexandria, LA 71301; tel. 318/443-3511; FAX. 318/443-5628; Louise Barker, RN, Administrator

Colonnade Surgery, 555 South Ryan Street, Lake Charles, LA 70601; tel. 337/439-6226; FAX. 337/436-6223; Nellie Rideaux, Administrative Assistant

Columbia Greater New Orleans Surgery Center, 3434 Houma Boulevard, Metairie, LA 70006; tel. 504/888-7100; Claire G. Manuel, RN, Administrator

Columbia Surgicare of Lake Charles, 214 South Ryan Street, Lake Charles, LA 70601; tel. 318/436-6941; FAX. 318/439-3384; Debbie Boudreaux, Administrator

Eye Care and Surgery Center, 10423 Old Hammond Highway, Baton Rouge, LA 70816; tel. 504/923-0960; FAX. 504/923-2419; M. Brian Roper

Foot Surgery Center of Shreveport, 9308 Mansfield Road, Suite 300, Shreveport, LA 71118; tel. 318/686-9622; Richard Havens, D.P.M., Administrator

Gamble Ambulatory Surgery Center, 2601 Line Avenue, Suite B, Shreveport, LA 71104; tel. 318/424-3291; Michael Drews, D.P.M., Administrator

Green Clinic Surgery Center, 1200 South Farmerville Street, Ruston, LA 71270; tel. 318/255-3690; FAX. 318/251-6116; Glenn Scott, Executive Director

HealthSouth Surgi-Center of Baton Rouge, 5222 Brittany Drive, Baton Rouge, LA 70808; tel. 225/767-5636; FAX. 225/215-3477; Denise T. Fortenberry, Administrator

Providers / Freestanding Ambulatory Surgery Centers

Hedgewood Surgical Center, 2427 St. Charles Avenue, New Orleans, LA 70130; tel. 504/895-7642; FAX. 504/895-0728; Sally Carpenter, RN

Houma Outpatient Surgery Center, Ltd., 3800 Houma Boulevard, Suite 250, Metairie, LA 70006; tel. 504/456-1515; FAX. 504/454-3810; Jay Weil, III, President and CEO

Houma Surgi Center, Inc., 1020 School Street, Houma, LA 70360; tel. 504/868-4320; FAX. 504/868-3617; Robert M. Alexander, M.D., Administrator

LaHaye Center for Advanced Care, 201 Rue Iberville, Lafayette, LA 70508; tel. 318/235-2149; Darryl Wagley

LaHaye Eye and Ambulatory Surgical Center, 4313 I-49 S. Service Rd., Opelousas, LA 70570; tel. 337/942-2024; FAX. 337/948-8869; Douglas C. Mankin, Administrator

Lake Forest Surgical Center, 10545 Lake Forest Boulevard, New Orleans, LA 70127; tel. 504/244-3000; FAX. 504/246-2600; Karan Prieto, Facility Manager

Lakeview Surgery and Diagnostic Center, Inc., 800 Heavens Drive, Mandeville, LA 70471; tel. 504/845-7100; FAX. 504/845-7596; Glenda P. Escudero-Dobson, Administrator

Laser and Surgery Center of Acadiana, 514 St. Landry Street, Lafayette, LA 70506; tel. 318/234-2020; FAX. 318/234-8230; Barbara L. Azar, Administrator

Laser and Surgery Center of the South, 1101 Audubon Avenue, Suite S-Four, Thibodaux, LA 70301; tel. 504/447-7258; FAX. 504/446-7614; Nate Graff, Administrator

Louisiana Endoscopy Center, Inc., 8150 Jefferson Highway, Baton Rouge, LA 70809; tel. 504/927-0970; FAX. 504/927-0989; Albert Hart, IV, Administrator

Louisville Plaza Surgery Center, 3101 Kilpatrick Boulevard, Suite B, Monroe, LA 71201; tel. 318/322-5916; FAX. 318/322-5916; Beckie Gab, MHA, Manager

LSU Eye Surgery Center, 2020 Gravier Street, Suite B, New Orleans, LA 70112; tel. 504/568-6700; W. L. Blackwell, Chief Executive Officer

Magnolia Surgical Facility, 3939 Houma Boulevard, Suite 216, Metairie, LA 70006; tel. 504/455-7771; FAX. 504/885-5063; Melissa Johnson, Administrator, Medical Director

Marrero SurgiCenter, Inc., 4511 Westbank Expressway, Suite B, Marrero, LA 70072; tel. 504/340-1993; John Schiro, M.D., Administrator

MGA GI Diagnostic and Therapeutic Center, 1111 Medical Center Boulevard, Suite 310, Marrero, LA 70072; tel. 504/349-6401; FAX. 504/349-6444; Thomas D. McCaffery, Jr., President

MGA GI Diagnostic and Therapeutic Center, 2633 Napoleon Avenue, Suite 707, New Orleans, LA 70115; tel. 504/349-6401; FAX. 504/349-6444; Thomas D. McCaffery, Jr., Administrator

Ochsner Clinic–Center for Cosmetic Surgery, 1514 Jefferson Highway, Fifth Floor, New Orleans, LA 70121; tel. 504/842-3950; FAX. 504/842-5003; Rachel Franz, RN, B.S.N., Manager

Omega Ambulatory Surgical Institute, 2525 Severn Avenue, Metairie, LA 70001; tel. 504/832-4200; Rene Rosenson, Administrator

Outpatient Eye Surgery Center, 4324 Veterans Boulevard, Metairie, LA 70006; tel. 504/455-4046; FAX. 504/455-9890; Cheryl Crouse, RN, Administrator

Outpatient Surgery Center for Sight, 550 Connell's Park Lane, Baton Rouge, LA 70809; tel. 504/924-2020; Alan DeCorte, Administrator

P & S Surgery Center, LLC, 312 Grammont Street, P.O. Box 3187, Monroe, LA 71201-3187; tel. 318/388-4040; FAX. 318/388-4099; Terri Hicks, Business Office, Mgr.

Physicians Surgery Center, 218 Corporate Drive, Houma, LA 70360; tel. 504/853-1390; FAX. 504/853-1470; Connie K. Martin, Administrator

Prytania Surgery, Inc., 3525 Prytania Street, New Orleans, LA 70115; tel. 504/897-8880; Jay Weil, III, Administrator

Saints Streets ASC Endoscopy Center, Inc., 201 St. Patrick Street, Suite 202, Lafayette, LA 70506; tel. 337/232-6697; FAX. 337/233-8065; Stephen G. Abshire, M.D., Administrator

Shreveport Endoscopy Center, A.M.C., 3217 Mabel Street, P.O. Box 37045, Shreveport, LA 71133-7045; tel. 318/631-0072; FAX. 318/631-9688; Linda Ray, Administrator

Shreveport Surgery Center, 745 Olive Street, Suite 100, Shreveport, LA 71104; tel. 318/227-1163; FAX. 318/227-0413; Mary Jones, Administrator

Surgery Center, Inc., 1101 South College Road, Suite 100, Lafayette, LA 70503; tel. 337/233-8603; FAX. 337/234-0341; Russell J. Arceneaux, Administrator

Surginet Outpatient Surgery, LLC, 101 La Rue France, Suite 400, Lafayette, LA 70508; tel. 318/269-9828; FAX. 318/269-9823; Millissa R. Coco, Administrator

Surgiunit, Inc., 4204 Teuton Street, Metairie, LA 70006; tel. 504/888-3836; Gustavo A. Colon, M.D., Administrator

The Endoscopy Center of Monroe, 316 South Sixth Street, Monroe, LA 71201; tel. 318/325-2649; FAX. 318/325-0717; Andy W. Waldo, Administrator

The Endoscopy Clinic of Lake Charles Medical and Surgical Clinic, 501 South Ryan, Lake Charles, LA 70601; tel. 318/433-8400; Robert Oates, Administrator

The Outpatient Surgery Center of Baton Rouge, 505 East Airport Drive, Baton Rouge, LA 70806; tel. 504/925-2031; FAX. 504/924-2809; Lorraine Caraway, Administrator

The Plastic Surgery Center, Inc., 4224 Houma Boulevard, Suite 430, Metairie, LA 70006; tel. 504/456-5150; FAX. 504/456-5055; James B. Johnson, M.D., Administrator

The Surgery Suite, 103 Medical Center Drive, Slidell, LA 70461; tel. 504/646-4466; FAX. 504/646-4485; Allison F. Maestro, RN, Administrator

Urology Specialty and Surgery Center, 234 South Ryan Street, Lake Charles, LA 70601; tel. 318/433-5282; FAX. 318/433-1159; Charles Enright, Administrator

West Monroe Endoscopy Center, 102 Thomas Road, Suite 506, West Monroe, LA 71291; tel. 318/388-8878; FAX. 318/388-8870; C.B. Dunn, Jr. M.D.

Westbank Medical Clinic Surgical Facility, Inc., 4700 Wichers Drive, Suite 200, Marrero, LA 70072; tel. 504/347-2297; FAX. 504/347-2299; Robert L. Sudderth, Administrator

Young Eye Surgery Center, Inc., 204 North Magdalen Square, Abbeville, LA 70510; tel. 318/893-4452; FAX. 318/893-7870; Virginia Y. Hebert, Administrator

MAINE

Acadia Medical Arts Ambulatory Surgical Suite, 404 State Street, Bangor, ME 04401; tel. 207/990-0928; Jordan J. Shubert, M.D., President

Aroostook County Regional Ophthalmology Center, 148 Academy Street, Presque Isle, ME 04769; tel. 207/764-0376; FAX. 207/764-7612; Craig W. Young, M.D., Director

Eye Care and Surgery Center of Maine, P.A., 53 Sewall Street, Portland, ME 04102; tel. 207/773-6336; FAX. 207/773-7034; William S. Holt, M.D., President

Maine Cataract and Eye Center, 386 Bridgeton Road, Route 302, Westbrook, ME 04092; tel. 207/797-9214; FAX. 207/797-8236; Elliot Schweid, D.O., Director

Maine Eye Center, P.A., 15 Lowell Street, Portland, ME 04102; tel. 207/774-8277; FAX. 207/871-1415; Frank Read, M.D., Director

Northern Maine Ambulatory Endoscopy Center, 11 Martin Street, P.O. Box 748, Presque Isle, ME 04769-0151; tel. 207/764-2482; FAX. 207/764-1569; Shelley Kenney, RN, Nurse Manager

Orthopedic Surgery Center, 33 Sewall Street, Portland, ME 04102; tel. 207/828-2130; FAX. 207/828-2190; Linda M. Ruterbories, Medical Director

Portland Endoscopy Center, 131 Chadwick Street, Portland, ME 04102-3266; tel. 207/773-7964; FAX. 207/773-9073; Newell Augur M.D., President

Western Avenue Day Surgery Center, a/k/a Plastic and Hand Surgical Associates, P.A., 244 Western Avenue, South Portland, ME 04106; tel. 207/775-3446; FAX. 207/879-1646; Jean J. Labelle, M.D., President

MARYLAND

Albert Shoumer, D.P.M., Dundalk Professional Center, 40 South Dundalk Avenue, Dundalk, MD 21222; tel. 410/282-6434; FAX. 410/284-4636; Darleen Grupp, Office Manager

Albert Shoumer, D.P.M., 1645 Liberty Road, Eldersburg, MD 21784; tel. 310/795-2889

Amber Meadows Ambulatory Care Center, Inc., 198 Thomas Johnson Drive, Suite Three, Frederick, MD 21702; tel. 301/695-9669; FAX. 301/695-0346

Amber Ridge Operating Room Center, 1475 Taney Avenue, Suite 101, Frederick, MD 21702; tel. 301/694-5656; FAX. 301/846-4117; Lorin F. Busselberg, M.D., Director

Ambulatory Foot Surgery Center of Burtonsville, Inc., 15300 Spencerville Court, Suite 101, Burtonsville, MD 20866; tel. 301/421-4286; Dr. Kressin, President

Ambulatory Plastic Surgery Associates, CHTD, 9715 Medical Center Drive, Suite 315, Rockville, MD 20850; tel. 301/948-5670; FAX. 301/948-5598; Page Curtis, OR Manager

American Podiatric Surgery, 10236 River Road, Potomac, MD 20854; tel. 301/983-9873; FAX. 301/299-3985; Amy Meehan, Administrator

Annapolis Plastic Surgery Center, 1300 Ritchie Highway, Arnold, MD 21012; tel. 410/544-0707; FAX. 410/544-0724; Jack Frost, M.D., President

Anne Arundel Gastroenterology Ambulatory Surgery Center, 703 Giddings Avenue, Suite M, Annapolis, MD 21401; tel. 410/224-2116; Gary M. Evans, Practice Administrator

Armiger, William G., M.D., P.A., d/b/a Chesapeake Plastic Surgery Associates, 1421 South Caton Avenue, Suite 203, Baltimore, MD 21227; tel. 410/646-3226; FAX. 410/644-2134; Sandra Pappas, Administrator

Arundel Ambulatory Center for Endoscopy, 621 Ridgely Avenue, Suite 101, Annapolis, MD 21401; tel. 410/224-3636; FAX. 410/224-6971; Jeff Hazel, Practice Administrator

Baltimore Ambulatory Center for Endoscopy, 19 Fontana Lane, Suite 104, Baltimore, MD 21237; tel. 410/574-7776; FAX. 410/574-9038; Dr. V. Sivan, Medical Director

Baltimore County Out-Patient Plastic Surgery Center, 1205 York Road, Suite 36, Lutherville, MD 21093; tel. 410/828-9570; FAX. 410/583-9120; Bernard McGibbon, M.D.

Baltimore Podiatry Group, 5205 East Drive, Suite I, Arbutus, MD 21227; tel. 410/247-5333; Neil Scheffler, D.P.M., President

Baltimore Washington Eye Center, 200 Hospital Drive, Suite 600, Glen Burnie, MD 21061; tel. 410/766-3937; FAX. 410/761-4386; Cheryl Norwood, ASC Coordinator

Bayside Foot and Ankle Center, 8023 Ritchie Highway, Pasadena, MD 21122; tel. 410/761-4190; FAX. 410/761/0265; Sheila Freeze, Office Manager

Beitler, Samuel D., D.P.M. Ambulatory Surgery Center, Glen Burnie Podiatric Surgery Center, 795 Aquahart Road, Suite 125, Glen Burnie, MD 21061; tel. 410/768-0702; FAX. 410/768-0649; Samuel D. Beitler, D.P.M.

Bel Air Ambulatory Surgical Center, LLC, 2007 Rock Spring Road, Lower Level, Forest Hill, MD 21050; tel. 410/879-2474; FAX. 410/879-8194; Cindy Banaszak, Clinical Manager

Bethesda Ambulatory Surgical Center, 5620 Shields Dr., Bethesda, MD 20817; tel. 301/530-4181; FAX. 301/530-4373; John Lydon, D.P.M., Administrator

Bowie Health Center, 15001 Health Center Drive, Bowie, MD 20716; tel. 301/262-5511; FAX. 301/464-3572

Carroll Medicine, d/b/a Steven Shaffer, M.D., 211 Hanover Pike, Hampstead, MD 21074; tel. 410/239-7073

Center for Eye Surgery P.C., 5550 Friendship Boulevard, Suite 270, Chevy Chase, MD 20815; tel. 301/215-7347; FAX. 301/215-7345; Leila Cabrera-Reid, RN, Administrator

Center for Oral & Maxillofacial Surgery, 1212 York Road, Suite A201, Lutherville, MD 21093; tel. 410/337-7755; FAX. 410/337-7922; Laurie Kolmer, Office Manager

Center for Plastic Surgery, 5550 Friendship Boulevard, Suite 130, Chevy Chase, MD 20815; tel. 301/652-7700; Jean, Administrator

Chesapeake Ambulatory Surgery Center, 8028 Governor Ritchie Highway, Suite 100, Pasadena, MD 21122; tel. 410/768-5800; FAX. 410/768-5806; Ira J. Gottlieb, D.P.M., Owner, Administrator

Chesapeake Surgery Center, 145 East Carroll Street, Salisbury, MD 21801; tel. 410/548-1108; FAX. 410/548-2607; Joseph G. Walters, PA-C Administrative Director

Clinical Associates, 515 Fairmont Avenue, Suite 500, Towson, MD 21286; tel. 410/494-1335

De Leonibus and Palmer, L.L.C., A.S.C., MedSurg Foot Center, 2086 Generals Highway, Suite 101, Annapolis, MD 21401; tel. 410/266-7666; FAX. 410/266-7703; Courtney Palmer, DPM

Providers / Freestanding Ambulatory Surgery Centers

Digestive Disease Consultant of Frederick, 915 Toll House Avenue, Suite 201, Frederick, MD 21701; tel. 301/662-7822; James A. Frizzell, M.D.

Dr. Alan W. Hopson, P.A., 560 Riverside Drive, Suite A-101, Salisbury, MD 21801; tel. 410/749-0121; FAX. 410/749-6807; Pat Timmons, Office Manager

Dr. Gary Lieberman, P.A., A.S.C., d/b/a Four Corners Ambulatory Surgical Center, 10101 Lorain Avenue, Silver Spring, MD 20901; tel. 301/681-8400; Ms. Gayle Rickert

Dr. Michael K. Schwartz, D.D.S., P.A., 723 South Charles Street, Baltimore, MD 21230; tel. 410/727-4886

Drs. Smith and Schwartz, D.D.S., P.A., 10 Warren Road, Suite 330, Cockeysville, MD 21030; tel. 410/666-5225; FAX. 410/666-7220; Mary Thompson, Office Manager

Dulaney Eye Institute, 901 Dulaney Valley Road, Towson, MD 21204; tel. 410/583-1000; Andrea Hyatt, Administrator

Dundalk Ambulatory Surgery Center, 1123 Merritt Boulevard, Baltimore, MD 21222; tel. 410/282-6666

Easton Foot Center, 8579 Commerce Drive, Suite 100A, Easton, MD 21061; tel. 410/822-0645

Eye Surgery Center at Greenspring Station of Ophthalmology Ass, 10755 Falls Road, Suite 110B, Lutherville, MD 21093; tel. 410/583-2810; FAX. 410/583-2807; (vacant) Operations Manager

Eye Surgical Center Associates of Baltimore, 1122 Kenilworth Drive, Suite 18, Towson, MD 21204; tel. 410/321-4400; FAX. 410/321-4909; Terry Lewis, Administrator

Facial Plastic Surgicenter, Ltd., 21 Crossroads Drive, Suite 310, Owings Mills, MD 21117; tel. 410/356-1100; FAX. 410/356-1110; Ira D. Papel, M.D., President

Family Foot Health Specialists, P.C., 339 East Antietam Street, Hagerstown, MD 21740; tel. 301/797-7272; Judy Cline, Office Manager

Flaum, Martin/Rockville Podiatry Center, 50 West Edmonston Drive, Suite 306, Rockville, MD 20852; tel. 301/340-8666; FAX. 301/340-7448; Martin C. Flaum, Owner

Foot and Ankle Surgical Center, Kensington Surgery Center, 10901 Connecticut Avenue, Suite 200, Kensington, MD 20895; tel. 301/949-2000; Dr. Gene Mirkin

Foot Care Associates Ambulatory Care Center at Hamilton Foot C, 5508 Harford Road, Baltimore, MD 21214; tel. 410/426-5508

Foot Care Associates Ambulatory Care Center at Joppa Foot Care, 2316 East Joppa Road, Baltimore, MD 21234; tel. 410/882-5100

Footer, Ronald, D.P.M., P.A., 16220 Frederick Avenue, Suite 200, Gaithersburg, MD 20877; tel. 301/948-2995; FAX. 301/948-6056; Maryrose Hanks, Office Manager

Frederick Surgical Center, 915 Toll House Avenue, Suite 103, Frederick, MD 21701; tel. 301/694-3400; FAX. 301/694-3620; Barbara Smith, Administrator

Gastrointestinal Diagnostic Center, 4660 Wilkens Avenue, Suite 302, Baltimore, MD 21229; tel. 410/242-3636; FAX. 410/242-4404; Mary C. Harrison, Business Manager

Gehris, Heroy and Associates of Lutherville, 1212 York Road, Suite 201B, Lutherville, MD 21093; tel. 410/821-6130; James H. Heroy, III, Administrator

Giardina and Glubo, 4660 Wilkens Avenue, Baltimore, MD 21229; tel. 410/242-7066; FAX. 410/242-4126; Eileen Giardina, RN

Gynemed Surgi-Center, 17 Fontana Lane, Suite 201, Baltimore, MD 21237; tel. 410/686-8220; FAX. 410/391-0943; David O'Neil, M.D.

Harford County Ambulatory Surgery Center, 1952-A Pulaski Highway, Edgewood, MD 21040; tel. 410/538-7000; FAX. 410/671-7162; Ms. Linda A. Terzigui, RN, BSN, CNOR, Nurse Administrator

Harford Endoscopy Center, LLC, Two North Avenue, Suite 102, Belair, MD 21014; tel. 410/838-6345; FAX. 410/838-1595; Janet Day, Nurse Manager

HealthSouth Central Maryland Surgery, 1500 John Avenue, Baltimore, MD 21227; tel. 410/536-0012; FAX. 410/536-0016; Thelma Hoerl, RN, Facility Manager

HealthSouth St. Agnes Surgery Center of Ellicott City, 2850 North Ridge Road, Ellicott City, MD 21043; tel. 410/461-1600; FAX. 410/750-7615; Donna Broccolino, Faculty Administrator

Johns Hopkins Plastic Surgery Associates, JHOC 8, 601 North Caroline Street, Baltimore, MD 21287; tel. 410/955-6897; FAX. 410/614-1296

Kaiser-Permanente-Kensington, 10810 Connecticut Avenue, Kensington, MD 20895; tel. 301/929-7100; FAX. 301/929-7577; Wanda McCulley, RN, Supervisor

Kenneth Margolis, M.D., P.A., Ambulatory Endoscopy Surgical Center, 9101 Franklin Square Drive, Suite 213, Baltimore, MD 21237; tel. 410/687-0202; FAX. 410/687-0985; Jo Ann Smith, Office Manager

Klatsky Plastic Surgery Facility, 122 Slade Avenue, Pikesville, MD 21208; tel. 410/484-0400; FAX. 410/484-2993; Stanley A. Klatsky, M.D., Director

Lake Forest Ambulatory Surgical Center, 702 Russell Avenue, Gaithersburg, MD 20877; tel. 301/948-3668; FAX. 301/926-7787

Laser Surgery Center, Inc., 484A Ritchie Highway, Severna Park, MD 21146; tel. 410/544-4600; Dottie Scholes, Office Manager

Laurel Foot and Ankle Center, 14440 Cherry Lane Court, Suite 104, Laurel, MD 20707; tel. 301/953-3668; Dr. Frank Smith, Administrator

Maclean, Kishel, Applestein, M.D., A.S.C., 11085 Little Patuxent Parkway, Columbia, MD 21044; tel. 410/997-1930

Maple Springs Ambulatory Surgery Center, 10810 Darnstown Road, Suite 101, Gaithersburg, MD 20878; tel. 301/762-3338; FAX. 301/762-1585

Maryland Digestive Disease Center, 7350 Van Ducen Road, Suite 230, Laurel, MD 20707; tel. 301/498-5500

Maryland Ear, Nose and Throat Group, P.A., 2112 Bell Air Road, Suite Three, Fallston, MD 21047; tel. 410/879-7049; Barbara Huckeba, Corporate Secretary

Maryland Endoscopy Center, L.L.C., 100 West Road, Suite 115, Towson, MD 21204; tel. 410/494-0144; FAX. 410/494-0147; Gretchen Caron, RN, Administrator

Maryland Kidney Stone Center/AKSM, 6115 Falls Road,LL-a, Baltimore, MD 21209; tel. 410/377-2622; FAX. 410/377-4410; Walter Weinstein, Regional Manager

Maryland Outpatient Foot Surgery Center, Dennis M. Weber D.P.M., 4701 Randolph Road, Suite 115, Rockville, MD 20852; tel. 301/770-5741; FAX. 301/468-1093; Dennis M. Weber, D.P.M., Director

Maryland Urology Surgicenters, LLC, 6830 Hospital Drive, Suite 204, Baltimore, MD 21237; tel. 410/391-6131; FAX. 410/391-6144; Anthony O. Sclama, M.D., President

McCone, Jonathan, Jr., M.D., 6196 Oxon Hill Road, Suite 640, Oxon Hill, MD 20745; tel. 301/567-2400

Metropolitan Ambulatory Urologic Institute Inc., 7753 Belle Point Drive, Greenbelt, MD 20770; tel. 301/474-5583; FAX. 301/474-5742; Mary Moore-Administrator

Michetti, Michael, Dr. of District Heights, 6400 Marlboro Pike, District Heights., MD 20747; tel. 301/736-6900

Mid Shore Surgical Eye Center, 8420 Ocean Gateway, Suite One, Easton, MD 21601; tel. 410/822-0424; FAX. 410/822-2283; Adrienne Welch, RN

Mid-Atlantic Surgery Center, 1120 Professional Court, Hagerstown, MD 21740; tel. 301/739-7900

Montgomery Endoscopy Center P.A., Montgomery Gastroenterology P.A., 12012 Veirs Mill Road, Wheaton, MD 20906; tel. 301/942-3550; FAX. 301/933-3621; Howard Goldberg, M.D., A.S.C Director

Montgomery Surgical Center, 46 West Gude Drive, Rockville, MD 20850; tel. 301/424-6901; FAX. 301/294-7847; Jeannie M. Lohmeyer, RN, CNOR, Administrative Director

Moulsdale, Murphy, Siegelbaum and Lerner, 7505 Osler Drive, Suite 508, Towson, MD 21204; tel. 410/296-0166; FAX. 410/828-7275

Neil J. Napora, D.P.M., 7809 Wise Avenue, Baltimore, MD 21222; tel. 410/285-0310; FAX. 410/288-1569; Neil J. Napora, D.P.M.

North Arundel Plastic Surgery Specialists, 203 Hospital Drive, Suite 308, Glen Burnie, MD 21061; tel. 410/841-5355; FAX. 410/841-6589; Ajia S. Layman, Administrator

Parris-Castro Eye Association, Six North Boulton Street, Bel Air, MD 21014; tel. 410/836-7010; Michael Grasham, Administrator

Peninsula Obstetrics and Gynecology, 314 West Carroll Street, Salisbury, MD 21801; tel. 410/546-3125; FAX. 410/546-3128; J. Cutchin, M.D., Director

Plastic Surgery Specialists, 2448 Holly Avenue, Suite 400, Annapolis, MD 21401; tel. 410/841-5355; FAX. 410/841-6589; Ajia S. Layman, Administrator

Plaza Ambulatory Surgical Center, 6568 Reisterstown Road, Suite 501, Baltimore, MD 21215; tel. 410/764-7044; Brian Kashan, Administrator

Podiatry Associates of Hagerstown, A.S.C, 12821 Oak Hill Avenue, Hagerstown, MD 21742; tel. 301/739-1575; FAX. 301/739-1578; Crystal Shankle, Office Manager

Podiatry Associates, P.A., 9712 Bel Air Road, Baltimore, MD 21236; tel. 410/574-6060; FAX. 410/256-2727; Stanley Book

Podiatry Associates, P.A., One North Main Street, Bel Air, MD 21014; tel. 410/879-1212; FAX. 410/893-1081

Podiatry Associates, P.A., 10840 Little Patuxent Parkway, Columbia, MD 21044; tel. 410/730-0970; FAX. 410/730-0161; Dr. Cappello, Podiatrist

Podiatry Associates, P.A., 6569 North Charles Street, Suite 702, Towson, MD 21204; tel. 410/828-5420; Nancy L. Patterson, Billing Manager

Podiatry Associates, P.A., 9101 Franklin Square Drive, Baltimore, MD 21237; tel. 410/574-3900; FAX. 410/574-3902; Vincent J. Martorana, D.P.M.

Podiatry Group, P.A. of Annapolis, 139 Old Solomons Island Road, Suite C, Annapolis, MD 21401; tel. 410/224-4448; FAX. 410/841-5200; Kate Pearson, Administrator

Podiatry Group, P.A. of Laurel, Ambulatory Surgery Center, 14333 Laurel-Bowie Road, Suite 205, Laurel, MD 20708; tel. 301/725-5650; FAX. 301/953-0365; Bruce A. Wenzel, Administrator

Prince George's Ambulatory Care Center/Endoscopy Suites, Inc., 6001 Landover Road, Suite One, Cheverly, MD 20785; tel. 301/773-3900; FAX. 301/773-7869; Jeannette Figueroa, Administrator

Prince George's Multi-Specialty Surgery Centre, Inc., 8700 Central Avenue, Suite 106, Landover, MD 20785; tel. 301/808-9298; FAX. 301/499-1266; Douglas Hallgren, Administrator

Professional Village Surgical Center, 356 Mill Street, Hagerstown, MD 21740; tel. 301/791-1800

Queen Anne Plastic, L.L.C., 2110 Red Apple Plaza, Chester, MD 2161; tel. 410/643-7207; FAX. 410/643-6945

Queen Anne Surgery Center, 2108 DiDonato Drive, Chester, MD 21619; tel. 410/643-7207; FAX. 410/643-9274; Lisa Parks, Administrator

River Reach Outpatient Surgery Center, 790 Governor Ritchie Highway, Suite E-35, Severna Park, MD 21146; tel. 410/544-2487; FAX. 410/544-1872

Rivertowne Surgery Center, 6196 Oxon Hill Road, Suite 650, Oxon Hill, MD 20745; tel. 301/839-7499; FAX. 301/839-8726; Aimee Gaum, Business Manager

Robinwood Surgery Center, LLC, 11110 Medical Campus Road, Suite 200, Hagerstown, MD 21742; tel. 301/714-4300; FAX. 301/714-4324; Sarah Ann DeBaugh, Office Manager

Roger J. Oldham, M.D., Ambulatory Surgery Center, 10215 Fernwood Road, Suite 412, Bethesda, MD 20817; tel. 301/530-6100; Raquel Lynskey

Rotunda Ambulatory Surgery Center, 711 West 40th Street, Suite 410, Baltimore, MD 21211; tel. 410/889-4885

Sagoskin and Levy, M.D., 9707 Medical Center Drive, Suite 230, Rockville, MD 20850; tel. 301/340-1188; Arthur Sagoskin, M.D., Administrator

Saint Mary's Multispecialty Surgery Center, Inc., Route 235 and Chancellors Run Road, Suite 15, P.O. Box 1310, California, MD 20619; tel. 301/862-3984; FAX. 301/862-3335; Douglas H. Hallgren, Administrator

Siegel and Langer (Drs.), P.A., Ambulatory Surgery Center, 1001 Pine Heights Avenue, Suite 104, Baltimore, MD 21229; tel. 410/644-0929; Narang Ashok, Administrator

Silver Spring Ambulatory Surgical Center, Inc., 1104 Spring Street, Suite T110, Silver Spring, MD 20910; tel. 301/589-7664; FAX. 301/589-3410; Todd A. Nitkin, D.P.M., President

Silverman, David H., M.D., 6490 Landover Road, Suite D, Cleverly, MD 20785; tel. 301/322-5885

Providers / Freestanding Ambulatory Surgery Centers

Smith, Schwartz and Hyatt, D.D.S., P.A. of Owings Mills, 25 Crossroads Drive, Suite 147, Owings Mills, MD 21117; tel. 410/363-7780; FAX. 410/581-9724; Michael K. Schwartz, D.D.S., Administrator

Spector, Adam, D.P.M., Ambulatory Surgery Center, 1111 Spring Street, Silver Spring, MD 20910; tel. 301/589-8886; FAX. 301/589-8889; Adam Spector, D.P.M., Administrator

Suburban Endoscopy Center, L.L.C., 10215 Fernwood Road, Suite 206, Bethesda, MD 20817; tel. 301/530-2800; Maryanne Reimer, RN, Manager of Clinical Services

Sugar, Mark, D.P.M., A.S.C., 6505 Belcrest Road, Suite One, Hyattsville, MD 20782; tel. 301/699-5900; FAX. 301/699-9297; Mark H. Sugar, D.P.M., Director

Suhayl Kalash, Ambulatory Surgery Center, 3455 Wilkens Avenue, Suite 203, Baltimore, MD 21229; tel. 410/646-0330; Bridget Vracar, Accounts Coordinator

Surgical Center of Greater Annapolis, Inc., 83 Church Road, Arnold, MD 21012; tel. 410/757-5018; FAX. 410/757-0632; Denise Adams, RN, Administrator

The Ambulatory Urosurgical Center, 401 East Jefferson Street, Suite 105, Rockville, MD 20850; tel. 301/309-8219; FAX. 301/309-9370; Jacqueline Hillman, RN, B.S.N. M.S., Director of Nursing

The Endoscopy Center, 7402 York Road, Suite 101, Towson, MD 21204; tel. 410/494-0156; FAX. 410/828-1706; Barry Gendaston, General Manager

The SurgiCenter of Baltimore, 23 Crossroads Drive, Suite 100, Owings Mills, MD 21117; tel. 410/356-0300; FAX. 410/356-7507; Jerry W. Henderson, Executive Director

Total Foot Care Surgery Center, Inc., 7525 Greenway Center Drive, Suite 112, Greenbelt, MD 20770; tel. 301/345-4087; FAX. 301/345-0482; Dale Scoville, Office Manager

Tri County Endoscopy, Charlotte Hall, Route Five, Charlotte Hal, MD 20622; tel. 301/884-7322; Dr. Shah, M.D.

United Foot Care Center, 420 South Crain Highway, Glen Burnie, MD 21061; tel. 410/766-7500; Steven Brownstein, Administrator

Vahos Aesthetic Plastic Surgery Institute, 1001 Pine Heights Avenue, Suite 100, Baltimore, MD 21229; tel. 410/644-4877; FAX. 410/525-1346; Mario Vahos, M.D., Director

Waldorf Endoscopy Center, 11340 Pembroke Square, Suite 202, Waldorf, MD 20603; tel. 310/638-5354; FAX. 301/843-5184; Mary Lou Champney, Office Manager

Washington Surgi Center, 6228 Oxon Hill Road, Oxon Hill, MD 20745; tel. 301/839-0770; FAX. 301/839-1350

Western Maryland Eye Surgical Center, 1003 West Seventh Street, Suite 400, Frederick, MD 21701; tel. 301/662-3721; FAX. 301/698-8164

MASSACHUSETTS

Advanced Pain Management Center, Three Woodland Road, Suite 206, Stoneham, MA 02180; tel. 617/662-2243; FAX. 617/662-4878

Andover Surgical Day Care Clinic, 138 Haverhill Street, Andover, MA 01810; tel. 508/475-2880; FAX. 508/475-9562; Edward G. George, Administrator

Boston Center for Ambulatory Surgery, Inc., 170 Commonwealth Avenue, Boston, MA 02116; tel. 617/267-7171; FAX. 617/236-8704; Philip J. Gaven, MBA, Administrator

Boston Eye Surgery & Laser Center, P.C., 50 Stanford Street, Boston, MA 02114; tel. 617/723-2015; FAX. 617/723-7787; Sheila M. Harney, Business Manager

Boston University Eye Assoc., Inc., 90 New State Highway, Raynham, MA 02767; tel. 508/822-8839; FAX. 508/880-3616; Jeanne H. Tierney Chief Operating Officers

Cataract and Laser Center West, P.C., 171 Interstate Drive, West Springfield, MA 01089; tel. 413/732-2333; FAX. 413/732-3514; John Dunne, Administrator

Cataract and Laser Center, Inc., 333 Elm Street, Dedham, MA 02026; tel. 781/326-3800; FAX. 728/326-2120; John Dunne, Administrator

Cosmetic Surgery Center, 68 Camp Street, Hyannis, MA 02601; tel. 508/775-7026; FAX. 508/771-0499; Laura Norkatis, Office Manager

Eye Institute of the Merrimack Valley, 280 Haverhill Street, Lawrence, MA 01840; tel. 508/685-3366

Goddard Medical Association Outpatient Surgery, One Pearl Street, Caputo Building First Floor, Brockton, MA 02401; tel. 508/586-3600

Greater New Bedford Surgicare, Inc., 540 Hawthorne Street, North Dartmouth, MA 02747; tel. 508/997-1271; FAX. 508/992-7701; George A. Picord, Administrator

HealthSouth Maple Surgery Center, 298 Carew Street, Springfield, MA 01104; tel. 413/739-9668; FAX. 413/781-3652; Kathleen S. Loomis, RN, Facility Administrator

McGowan Eye Care Center, 297 Union Avenue, Framingham, MA 01701; tel. 800/873-4590; FAX. 508/872-0038; Bernard L. McGowan, M.D., Director

New England Eye Surgery Center, 696 Main Street, Weymouth, MA 02190; tel. 617/331-3820; FAX. 617/331-1076; Kenneth Camerota

New England Surgicare, One Brookline Place, Suite 201, Brookline, MA 02146; tel. 617/730-9650; Gratia S. Chase, RN, Administrator

Plymouth Laser and Surgical Center, 40 Industrial Park Road, Plymouth, MA 02360; tel. 508/746-8600; FAX. 508/747-0824; Kathleen Murphy, Administrator

Same Day SurgiClinic, 272 Stanley Street, Fall River, MA 02720; tel. 508/672-2290; FAX. 508/679-3766; John Harries, M.D., Chief Executive Officer

Surgery Center of Waltham, 40 Second Avenue, Suite 200, Waltham, MA 02154

Worcester Surgical Center, Inc., 300 Grove Street, Worcester, MA 01650; tel. 508/754-0700; FAX. 508/831-9989; Andy H. Poritz, M.D., Professional Services Director

MICHIGAN

Balian Eye Center, 432 West University Drive, Rochester, MI 48307; tel. 313/651-6122; John V. Balian, M.D.

Birth Control Center, Inc., 2783 Fourteen Mile Road, Sterling Heights, MI 48310; tel. 810/939-4000; Armen Vartanian, Administrator

Borgess at Woodbridge Hills Outpatient Surgery, 7901 Angling Road, Portage, MI 49024; tel. 616/324-8406; FAX. 616/324-8476; Renee Langeland, M.S.N., R.N., Administrator

Castleman Surgery Center, 14050 Dix-Toledo Road, Southgate, MI 48195; tel. 734/283-0500; FAX. 734/283-2720; Linda Phillips, R.N., Administrator

Center for Specialty Care Clinics, 19900 Haggerty Road, Livonia, MI 48152; tel. 313/462-1888; FAX. 313/462-1944; Pamela Cittan, Administrator

Centre for Plastic Surgery, 426 Michigan Street, N.E., Suite 300, Grand Rapids, MI 49503; tel. 616/454-1256; FAX. 616/454-0308; Daniel Reeder, Administrator

Community Surgical Center, 30671 Stephenson Highway, Madison Height, MI 48071; tel. 810/588-8000; FAX. 810/588-9140; C. J. Yanos, Administrator

Detroit Medical Center Surgery Center, 27207 Lahser Road, Suite 100, Southfield, MI 48034; tel. 810/357-0800; FAX. 810/357-1738; Patrick Voight, Administrative Manager

East Michigan Eye Surgery Center, 701 South Ballenger, Flint, MI 48532; tel. 810/238-3603; FAX. 810/767-5194; Bridget Charlesworth, Administrator

Eastside Endoscopy Center, 28963 Little Mack, Suite 103, St. Clair Shores, MI 48081; tel. 810/447-5110; FAX. 810/774-6091; Beth Miller Administrator

Feminine Health Care Clinic of Flint, 2032 South Saginaw Street, Flint, MI 48503; tel. 800/323-6205; FAX. 313/232-8071; Dawn LoRec, Director

Glascco Ambulatory Surgery Center, 1707 West Lake Lansing Road, Lansing, MI 48912; tel. 517/267-0033; FAX. 517/267-0430; Jane Beshore, Administrator

Health Midwest Surgery Center, 125 West Walnut, Kalamazoo, MI 49007; tel. 616/343-1381; Greg Orblix, M.D., Medical Director

Hemorrhoid Clinics of America, 22000 Greenfield Road, Oak Park, MI 48237; tel. 248/967-4140; FAX. 248/967-0745; Max Ali, M.D., President

Henry Ford Hospital Fairlane Center, 19401 Hubbard Drive, Dearborn, MI 48126; tel. 313/593-8100; Jay Zerwekh, Administrator

Henry Ford Medical Center–Ambulatory Surgery, 6777 West Maple Road, West Bloomfield, MI 48322; tel. 248/661-4100; FAX. 248/661-6494; Mary Vidaurri, Ph.D., Regional Administrator

Henry Ford Medical Center–Lakeside Ambulatory Surgery, 14500 Hall Road, Sterling Heights, MI 48313; tel. 810/247-2680; FAX. 810/247-2682; Mary Vidaurri, Ph.D., Regional Administrator

Holland Eye Clinic, 999 South Washington, Holland, MI 49423; tel. 616/396-2316; FAX. 616/396-0085; Kristine Curtis, Assistant Administrator

Hutzel Health Center, 4050 East 12 Mile Road, Warren, MI 48092; tel. 810/573-3140

John Michael Garrett, P.C., 1301 Carpenter Avenue, Iron Mountain, MI 49801; tel. 906/774-1404; FAX. 906/774-8132; Cathy Hartwig, RN, Supervisor

M.D. Surgicenter, 375 Barclay Circle, Rochester Hill, MI 48307; tel. 810/852-3636; FAX. 810/852-3631; Robert Swartz, Administrator

Metropolitan Eye Center, 21711 Greater Mack, St. Clair Shores, MI 48080; tel. 810/774-6820; FAX. 810/777-2214; Richard C. Mertz, Jr., M.D., Director

Michigan Center for Outpatient Ocular Surgery, 33080 Utica Road, P.O. Box 26010, Fraser, MI 48026; tel. 810/296-7250; FAX. 810/296-0276; Norbert P. Czajkowski, M.D., Director

Midwest Health Center, 5050 Schaefer Avenue, Dearborn, MI 48126; tel. 313/581-2600; FAX. 313/581-6013; Mark B. Saffer, M.D., President and CEO

Oakland Surgi Center, Inc., 2820 Crooks Road, Suite 200, Rochester Hill, MI 48309; tel. 248/852-7484; FAX. 248/852-4279; Beverly Huffman, CMM, Administrator

Oakwood Healthcare Center–Dearborn, 10151 Michigan Avenue, Dearborn, MI 48126; tel. 313/624-0855; FAX. 313/624-0857; Patricia Glosser, Nursing Supervisor

Park Eye and Surgicenter, 5014 Villa Linde Parkway, Flint, MI 48532

Planned Parenthood League, Inc., 25932 Dequindre, Warren, MI 48091; tel. 810/758-2100; FAX. 810/758-2104; Carrie Haneckow, Administrator

Planned Parenthood of Mid-Michigan, 3100 Professional Drive, P.O. Box 3673, Ann Arbor, MI 48106-3673; tel. 313/973-0710; FAX. 313/973-0595; Peg Hill-Callahan

Planned Parenthood of South Central Michigan, 4201 West Michigan Avenue, Kalamazoo, MI 49006-5833; tel. 616/372-1205; FAX. 616/372-1279; Rev. Mark Pawlowski, Executive Director, Chief Executive Officer

Providence Hospital Ambulatory Surgery Center, 47601 Grand River, Novi, MI 48374; tel. 810/380-4170; Brian Connolly, Administrator

Providence Surgical Center, 29877 Telegraph Road, Suite 200, Southfield, MI 48034

Sinai Surgery Center, 28500 Orchard Lake Road, Farmington Hi, MI 48334; tel. 810/851-9215; FAX. 810/851-2077; Michael K. Rosenberg, M.D., Medical Director

Somerset Surgery Center, P.C., 1565 West Big Beaver Road, Building F, Troy, MI 48084; tel. 248/649-7343; FAX. 248/643-0999; Frank A. Nesi, M.D., Medical Director

Spectrum Health Surgical Center, Merger of Blodgett & Butterworth, 1000 East Paris S.E., Suite 100, Grand Rapids, MI 49546; tel. 616/285-1822; FAX. 616/285-1820; Deb Williams, Clinical Site Manager

St. John Surgery Center, 21000 12 Mile Road, St. Clair Shores, MI 48081; tel. 810/447-5015; FAX. 810/447-5012; Cheri Dendy, Administrator

St. Mary's Ambulatory Care Center, 4599 Towne Centre, Saginaw, MI 48604; tel. 517/797-3000; FAX. 517/797-3010; Donna Juhala, Director

Superior Endoscopy Center/U P Digestive Disease Associates, P., 1414 West Fair Avenue, Suite 135, Marquette, MI 49855; tel. 906/226-6025; FAX. 906/226-5366; Kristine Garsalitz, R.N., Director of Nursing

Surgery Center of Michigan, 44650 Delco Boulevard, Sterling Heights, MI 48313; tel. 810/254-3391; FAX. 810/254-3344; Jay Novetsky, Administrator

Surgical Care Center of Michigan, 750 East Beltline, N.E., Grand Rapids, MI 49525; tel. 616/940-3600; FAX. 616/954-0216; Kris Kilgore, RN, B.S.N, Administrative Director

Upper Peninsula Surgery Center, 1414 West Fair Avenue, Suite 232, Marquette, MI 49855; tel. 906/225-7547; FAX. 906/225-7548; Sally J. Achatz, RN, Administrator

Waterford Ambulatory Surgi-Center, 1305 North Oakland Boulevard, Waterford, MI 48327; tel. 248/666-5546; FAX. 248/666-5550; Penny Sherwood, Manager/Elaine Lamb, Supervisor

Providers / Freestanding Ambulatory Surgery Centers

MINNESOTA
Centennial Lakes Same Day Surgery Center, 7373 France Avenue, S., Suite 404, Edina, MN 55435; tel. 612/921-0100; FAX. 612/921-0999; Kathleen L. Whatley, Administrator
Children's West, 6050 Clearwater Drive, Minnetonka, MN 55343; tel. 612/930-8600; FAX. 612/930-8650; Jane Price, Director
Columbia St. Cloud Surgical Center, 1526 Northway Drive, St. Cloud, MN 56303; tel. 320/251-8385; FAX. 320/251-1267; Jeanette I. Stack, Administrator
Dakota Clinic, Ltd., 125 East Frazee Street, 312, Detroit Lakes, MN 56501; tel. 218/847-3181; FAX. 218/847-2795; Linda L. Walz, Division Manager
First Eye Care Center, Inc., 9117 Lyndale Avenue, S., Bloomington, MN 55420; tel. 612/884-7568; FAX. 612/884-2656; Barbara McGovern, Administrator
Healtheast St. Paul Endoscopy Center, 17 West Exchange Street, Suite 215, St. Paul, MN 55102; tel. 612/224-9677; FAX. 612/223-5683; Glenda Tims, RN, Clinical Manager
Landmark Surgical Center, 17 West Exchange Street, Suite 307, St. Paul, MN 55102; tel. 612/223-7400; FAX. 651/842-5491; Lesley Nace, R.N., Director
Maplewood Surgery Center, 1655 Beam Ave., Maplewood, MN 55109; tel. 612/232-7780; Sandra Todd, Administrator
Midwest Surgicenter, d/b/a Midwest Eye and Ear Institute, 393 North Dunlap Street, Suite 900, St. Paul, MN 55104; tel. 651/642-1106; FAX. 651/645-3346; H. Joseph Drannen, Administrator
Park Nicollet Clinic Health System Minnesota, 3800 Park Nicollet Boulevard, St. Louis Park, MN 55416; tel. 612/993-1953; FAX. 612/993-9250; Kathy Beckman, RN, Manager
WestHealth, Inc., 2855 Campus Drive, Plymouth, MN 55441; tel. 612/577-7120; FAX. 612/577-7130; Paula Green, Administrator
Willmar Surgery Center, 1320 South First Street, Willmar, MN 56201; tel. 320/235-6506; FAX. 320/235-7069; John Seifert, Medical Director

MISSISSIPPI
Ambu-Care Outpatient Surgery Center, 6204 North State Street, Jackson, MS 39213; tel. 601/956-3251; FAX. 601/957-8456; Frank McCune, M.D., Administrator
Better Living Clinic Endoscopy Center, 3000 Halls Ferry Road, Vicksburg, MS 39180; tel. 601/638-9800; FAX. 601/638-9808; Barbara Neal, Office Manager
Biloxi Outpatient Surgery and Endoscopy Center, Inc., 111 Lameuse Street, Suite 104, Biloxi, MS 39530; tel. 228/374-2130; FAX. 228/374-9308; Michael T. Gossman, Administrator
Columbia Mississippi Surgical Center, 1421 North State Street, Jackson, MS 39202; tel. 601/353-8000; Virginia Brown, Administrator
ENT and Facial Plastic Surgery, 107 Millsaps Drive, P.O. Box 17829, Hattiesburg, MS 39402; tel. 601/268-5131; FAX. 601/268-5138; Pam Carter, Office Manager
Gulf South Outpatient Center, 1206 31st Avenue, P.O. Box 1778, Gulfport, MS 39501; tel. 601/864-0008; FAX. 601/863-1747; Jason V. Smith, M.D., President
Gulfport Outpatient Surgical Center, 1240 Broad Avenue, Gulfport, MS 39501; tel. 601/868-1120; William Peaks, Administrator
Lowery A. Woodall Outpatient Surgery Facility, 105 South 28th Avenue, Hattiesburg, MS 39401; tel. 601/288-1072; FAX. 601/288-3132; Marshall H. Tucker, FACHE, Administrator
North Mississippi Surgery Center, 500 West Eason Boulevard, Tupelo, MS 38801; tel. 601/841-4700; FAX. 601/841-3101; Beth Taylor, RN, Director
Southern Eye Center of Excellence, 1420 South 28th Avenue, Hattiesburg, MS 39402; tel. 601/264-3937; Lynn McMahan, M.D., Medical Director
Southwest Mississippi Ambulatory Surgery Center, 215 Marion Avenue, McComb, MS 39648; tel. 601/249-1477; FAX. 601/249-1375; Norman M. Price, Administrator
Surgicare of Jackson, 766 Lakeland Drive, Jackson, MS 39216; tel. 601/362-8700; FAX. 601/362-6459; Sheila Grillis, RN, Administrator

MISSOURI
Arnold Eye Surgery Center, Inc., 1265 East Primrose, Springfield, MO 65804; tel. 417/886-3937; FAX. 417/886-1285; Stephen C. Sheppard, Administrator
Associated Plastic Surgeons Ambulatory Surgical Center, 6420 Prospect, Suite 115, Kansas City, MO 64132; tel. 816/333-5524; Joni Reist, RN
BarnesCare, 401 Pine Street, St. Louis, MO 63102; tel. 314/331-3000; FAX. 314/331-3012; Gary Payne, Vice President, BJC Corporate Health
Cape Girardeau Outpatient Surgery Center, 1429 Mount Auburn Road, Cape Girardeau, MO 63701; tel. 573/335-9175; FAX. 573/335-2392; Stephanie J. Husted, RN, CNOR, Administrator
Cataract and Glaucoma Outpatient Surgicenter, 7220 Watson Road, St. Louis, MO 63119; tel. 314/352-5515; Stanley C. Becker, M.D.
Cataract Surgery Center of St. Louis, Inc., 900 North Highway 67 (Lindbergh), Florissant, MO 63031; tel. 314/838-0321; FAX. 314/838-4682; Karen E. Wilson, RN, Nurse Manager
Cataract Surgery Center of Young Eye Clinic, Inc., 3201 Ashland Avenue, St. Joseph, MO 64506; tel. 816/279-0079; FAX. 816/364-1100; Judy Watowa, RN, B.S.N., Administrator
Center for Eye Surgery, 6650 Troost, Suite 305, Kansas City, MO 64131; tel. 816/276-7757; FAX. 816/926-2231; Connie B. Watson, Administrator
CMMP Surgical Center, 1705 Christy Drive, Jefferson City, MO 65101; tel. 573/635-7022; FAX. 573/635-7029; Angela R. Sumner-Hahn, Asst. Director
Creekwood Surgery Center, 211 Northeast 54th Street, Suite 100, Kansas City, MO 64118; tel. 816/455-4214; FAX. 816/455-4216; Diana Carr, Administrator
Creve Coeur Surgery Center, 633 Emerson, Creve Coeur, MO 63141; tel. 314/872-7100; Marla Stone, Administrator
Doctors' Park Surgery, Inc., 30 Doctors' Park, Cape Girardeau, MO 63703; tel. 573/334-9606; FAX. 573/334-9608; Ronald G. Wittmer, President
ENT/Urology Surgical Care, Inc., 5301 Faraon Street, St. Joseph, MO 64506; tel. 816/364-2772; Sidney G. Christiansen, M.D.
Eye Surgery Center–The Cliffs, 4801 Cliff Avenue, Suite 101, Independence, MO 64055; tel. 816/478-4400; FAX. 816/478-8240; Jacki Wyrick, R.N., B.S.N., Direct of Nursing
G.I. Diagnostics, Inc., 4321 Washington, Suite 5700, Kansas City, MO 64111; tel. 816/561-2000; FAX. 816/931-7559; Craig B. Reeves, Administrator
HealthSouth Surgery Center of Cape Girardeau, 300 South Mount Auburn Road, Suite 200, Cape Girardea, MO 63701; tel. 573/339-7575; FAX. 573/332-1065; Cinda Silver, Business Office Manager
HealthSouth Surgery Center of West County, 1130 Town and Country Commons, Chesterfield, MO 63017; tel. 314/394-0698; FAX. 314/394-7493; Sandi Baber R.N., Administrator
Hunkeler Eye Surgery Center, Inc., 4321 Washington, Suite 6000, Kansas City, MO 64111; tel. 816/753-6511; FAX. 816/931-9498; Practice Administrator
Kansas City Surgicenter, Ltd., 1800 East Meyer Boulevard, Kansas City, MO 64132; tel. 816/523-0100; FAX. 816/523-6241; Barbara Klein, RN, Administrator
Laser Surgery Center North, 7700 South Florissant Road, St. Louis, MO 63122; tel. 314/261-2020; FAX. 314/821-4080; Irvin C. Hoffman, Administrator
Laser Surgery Center West, 1028 South Kirkwood, St. Louis, MO 63122; tel. 314/984-0080; FAX. 314/821-4080; Irvin C. Hoffman, Administrator
North County Surgery Center, One Village Square, Hazelwood, MO 63042; tel. 314/895-4001; FAX. 314/895-1791; Connie Moore, Administrator
Outpatient Surgery Center, 450 North New Ballas Road, Suite 103, St. Louis, MO 63141; tel. 314/991-0776; FAX. 314/991-3076; Karen Barrow, Administrator
Regional Surgery Center, P.C., 1531 West 32nd Street, Suite 107, Joplin, MO 64804; tel. 417/781-9595; FAX. 417/781-9814; Cynthia Shofner, Administrator
South County Outpatient Surgery Center, 13303 Tesson Ferry Road, St. Louis, MO 63128; tel. 314/842-3200; Gloria Lamb, Administrator
St. Charles County Surgery Center, Inc., 4203 South Cloverleaf Drive, St. Peters, MO 63376; tel. 314/928-0087; FAX. 314/928-1242; Sandi Baber, Administrator
St. Louis University Eye Institute, 5139 Mattis Road, St. Louis, MO 63128; tel. 314/849-8400; FAX. 314/849-5922
Surgery Center of Springfield, L.P., 1350 East Woodhurst Drive, Springfield, MO 65804; tel. 417/887-5243; FAX. 417/887-6507; Joyce Gillespie, Administrator
Surgi-Care Center of Independence, 2311 Redwood Avenue, Independence, MO 64057; tel. 816/373-7995; FAX. 816/373-8580; Dolores Sabia, Administrator
The Ambulatory Head and Neck Surgical Center, 1965 South Fremont, Suite 1940, Springfield, MO 65804; tel. 417/887-5750; FAX. 417/887-6612; Charles R. Taylor, Administrator
The Endoscopy Center, 3800 South Whitney, Independence, MO 64055; tel. 816/478-6868
The Endoscopy Center II, 5330 North Oak Trafficway, Suite 100, Kansas City, MO 64118; tel. 816/478-7144; FAX. 816/478-7129; Jean Thompson, Public Relations, Marketing
The Surgery Center, 802 North Riverside Road, Suite 115, St. Joseph, MO 64507; tel. 816/364-5030; FAX. 816/364-5810; Mari S. May, Administrator
The Tobin Eye Institute, 3902 Sherman Avenue, St. Joseph, MO 64506; tel. 816/279-1363; FAX. 816/233-8936; Linda S. Wildhagen, Administrator
Tri County Surgery Center, 1111 East Sixth Street, Washington, MO 63090; tel. 314/239-1766; FAX. 314/239-2964; Sharry Mohr, RN, Administrator

MONTANA
Billings Cataract and Laser Surgicenter, 1221 North 26th Street, Billings, MT 59101; tel. 406/252-5681; FAX. 406/252-5058
Flathead Outpatient Surgical Center, 66 Claremont Street, Kalispell, MT 59901; tel. 406/752-8484; FAX. 406/756-8008; Victoria L. Johnson, RN, Executive Director
HealthSouth Surgery Center of Billings, 940 North 30th Street, Billings, MT 59101; tel. 406/248-7186; FAX. 406/248-6889; Sharon McLeod, RN, OR Supervisor
Montana Surgical Center, Inc., 840 South Montana, Butte, MT 59701; tel. 406/782-2391; Charles Harris, Manager
Rocky Mountain Eye Surgery Center, 700 West Kent, Missoula, MT 59801; tel. 406/543-8179; Darlene Timmerhoff, Administrator
Same Day Surgery Center, Inc., 300 North Wilson, Suite 600F, Bozeman, MT 59715; tel. 406/586-1956; Ann Guenther, Supervisor
The Eye Surgicenter, 2475 Village Lane, Billings, MT 59102; tel. 406/252-6608; FAX. 406/252-6600; Sara Coleman, Supervisor

NEBRASKA
Aesthetic Surgical Images, P.C., 8900 West Dodge Road, Omaha, NE 68114; tel. 402/390-0100; FAX. 402/390-2711; Rita Petersen, Administrator
Anis Eye Institute, P.C., d/b/a The Nebraska Eye Surgical Center, 1500 South 48th Street, Suite 612, Lincoln, NE 68506; tel. 402/483-7991; FAX. 402/483-4750; Dr. Aziz Y. Anis
Bergan Mercy Surgical Center, 11704 West Center Road, Omaha, NE 68124; tel. 402/333-3111; Richard A. Hachten, III
Clarkson Hospital Outpatient Surgery, 4353 Dodge Street, Omaha, NE 68131; tel. 402/552-6065; Dr. Louis Burgher, Administrator
Clarkson West Medical Center, 2727 S. 144th Street, Omaha, NE 68144; tel. 402/778-5300; FAX. 402/778-5310; Cindy Alloway, Vice President
Jones Eye Clinic, 825 North 90th Street, Omaha, NE 68114; tel. 402/397-2010; Craig Borsdorf, Administrator
Lincoln Surgery Center, 1710 South 70th, Suite 200, Lincoln, NE 68506; tel. 402/483-1550; FAX. 402/483-0476; Robin Linnafelter, Administrator
Omaha Surgical Center, 8051 West Center Road, Omaha, NE 68124; tel. 402/391-3333; James Quinn, M.D., Administrator
The Nebraska Eye Surgical Center, 1500 S. 48th Street, Suite 612, Lincoln, NE 68506; tel. 402/483-7991; FAX. 402/483-4750; Aziz Anis, M.D., Administrator
The Omaha Eye Institute Surgery Center, 11606 Nicholas Street, Suite 200, Omaha, NE 68154; tel. 402/493-2020; FAX. 402/493-8987; Dr. Robert S. Vandervort, Administrator
The Urology Center, P.C., 111 1/2 South 90th Street, Omaha, NE 68114; tel. 402/397-9800; Laura Forehead, Administrator
Tobin Eye Institute, 4151 E Street, Omaha, NE 68107; tel. 402/731-1363; Patricia Moffatt, RN, Administrator

Providers / Freestanding Ambulatory Surgery Centers

NEVADA

Aesthetic Associates Day Surgery Center, 1580 East Desert Inn Road, Las Vegas, NV 89109; tel. 702/735-6755; FAX. 702/733-8221; Charles A. Vinnik, M.D., Administrator

Ambulatory Surgery Center of Nevada, 4631 E. Charleston Blvd., Las Vegas, NV 89104; tel. 702/438-8417; Neal A. Marek, Administrator

American Surgery Center of Las Vegas, 2575 Lindell Road, Las Vegas, NV 89102; tel. 702/362-3937; FAX. 702/362-7935; Fay dela Cruz, Center Director

Carson Ambulatory Surgery Center, Inc., 1299 Mountain Street, Carson City, NV 89703; tel. 775/883-1700; FAX. 775/883-8905; Joan P. Lapham, MHA, Executive Director

Carson Endoscopy Center, 707 North Minnesota, Carson City, NV 89703; tel. 775/884-8818; FAX. 775/884-4569; Jay M. Coller, Executive Director

Carson Valley Ambulatory Surgery Center, 1107 Highway 395, Gardnerville, NV 89410; tel. 775/782-1595; FAX. 775/782-1592; Laura D. Strong, Director

Center for Outpatient Surgery, 343 Elm Street, Suite 100, Reno, NV 89503; tel. 702/770-6500; FAX. 702/770-6535; Christine Balascoe, Executive Director

Columbia Sunrise Flamingo Surgery Center, 2565 East Flamingo Road, Las Vegas, NV 89121; tel. 702/697-7900; FAX. 702/697-5383; Carolyn C. Weaver, Administrator

Columbia Sunrise Surgical Center–Sahara, 2401 Paseo Del Prado, Las Vegas, NV 89102; tel. 702/362-7874; FAX. 702/362-3567; Stephanie Finkelstein, Administrator

Digestive Disease Center, 2136 East Desert Inn Road, Suite B, Las Vegas, NV 89109; tel. 702/734-0075; Osama Haikal, M.D., Administrator

Digestive Health Center, 5250 Kietzke Lane, Reno, NV 89511; tel. 702/829-8855; FAX. 702/829-3757; Jim LaBorde, Administrator

Endoscopic Institute of Nevada, 3777 Pecos–McLeod, Suite 102, Las Vegas, NV 89121; tel. 702/433-5686; Rebecca Duty, Administrator

Endoscopy Center of Nevada, LTD, 700 Shadow Lane, Suite 165B, Las Vegas, NV 89106; tel. 702/382-8101; Dipak K. Desai, Administrator

Eye Surgery Center of Nevada, 3839 North Carson Street, Carson City, NV 89706; tel. 702/882-3950; FAX. 708/882-1726; Michael J. Fischer, M.D., Administrator

Foot Surgery Center of Northern Nevada, 1300 East Plumb Lane, Suite A, Reno, NV 89502; tel. 702/829-8066; FAX. 702/829-8069; Dr. Frank M. Davis, Jr., Administrator

Ford Center for Foot Surgery, 2321 Pyramid Way, Sparks, NV 89431; tel. 702/331-1919; FAX. 702/331-2008; Dr. L. Bruce Ford, Administrator

Gastrointestinal Diagnostic Clinic, 3196 South Maryland Parkway, Suite 207, Las Vegas, NV 89109; tel. 702/369-3400; Nourollah Ghahreman, MD, Administrator

Goldring Surgical Center, 2020 Goldring, Suite 300, Las Vegas, NV 89106; tel. 702/477-7000; Texas Gustavson, Administrator

HealthSouth Reno Medical Plaza, 2005 Silverada Boulevard, Suite 100, Reno, NV 89512; tel. 775/359-0212; FAX. 775/359-0645; Maggie Summerfelt, Administrator

La Tourette Surgical Center, 2300 South Rancho Drive, Suite 216, Las Vegas, NV 89102; tel. 702/386-6979; FAX. 702/386-8700; Gary J. La Tourette, Administrator

Las Vegas Surgicare, Ltd., 870 South Rancho Drive, Las Vegas, NV 89106; tel. 702/870-2090; FAX. 702/870-5468; Kathy King, Administrator

Nevada Surgery Center, 4187 Pecos Road, Las Vegas, NV 89121; tel. 702/458-2522; Lyndell Kewley, Administrator

Northern Nevada Plastic Surgery Associates, 932 Ryland Street, Reno, NV 89502; tel. 702/322-3446; FAX. 702/322-4529; Averill M. Moser, RN, Administrator

Reno Endoscopy Center, LLC, 753 Ryland Street, Reno, NV 89502; tel. 775/329-1009; FAX. 775/329-4992; Jay M. Collier, Executive Director

Reno Outpatient Surgery Center, LTD., 350 West Sixth Street, Reno, NV 89503; tel. 702/334-4888; Sandra Walker–Wright, Administrator

Shepherd Eye Surgicenter, 3575 Pecos McLeod, Las Vegas, NV 89121; tel. 702/731-2088; FAX. 702/734-7836; Christina Kennelley, Administrator

Sierra Center for Foot Surgery, 1801 North Carson, Suite B, Carson City, NV 89701; tel. 702/382-1441; FAX. 702/882-6844; H. Kim Bean, D.P.M., Administrator

SMA Surgery Center, 2450 West Charleston, Las Vegas, NV 89106; tel. 702/877-8660; FAX. 702/877-5180; Steve Evans, M.D., Medical Director

Valley View Surgery Center, 1330 Valley View Boulevard, Las Vegas, NV 89102; tel. 702/870-7101; FAX. 702/870-7118; Michael B. Harkness, Administrator

NEW HAMPSHIRE

Ambulatory Surgery Center, 100 Hitchcock Way, Manchester, NH 03104; tel. 603/695-2500; FAX. 603/629-1730; Cheryl Laferriere, Supervisor–ASC

Bedford Ambulatory Surgical Center, 11 Washington Place, Bedford, NH 03110; tel. 603/622-3670; FAX. 603/626-9750; Laurie T. Raderiques, R.N., CNOR

Clinic Surgery Center (The), 253 Pleasant Street, Concord, NH 03301; tel. 603/226-2200; Kevin Appleton, Administrator

Day Surgery, 590 Court Street, Keene, NH 03431; tel. 603/357-3411; Michael Chelstowski, Director

Dunning Street Ambulatory Care Center, Seven Dunning Street, Claremont, NH 03743; tel. 603/543-3501; July Bradley, Administrator

Elliot One Day Surgery Center, 445 Cypress Street, Manchester, NH 03103; tel. 603/627-4889; FAX. 603/626-4300; Donna Quinn, RN, B.S.N., M.B.A., Director

Nashua Eye Surgery Center, Inc., Five Coliseum Avenue, Nashua, NH 03063; tel. 603/882-9800; FAX. 603/882-0556; Paul O'Leary, Administrator

Northeast Pain Consultation and Management PC, Pinewood Medical Center, 255 State Route 16, Somersworth, NH 03878; tel. 603/692-3166; FAX. 603/692-3168; Michael J. O'Connell, M.D., M.H.A., CEO

Nutfield Surgicenter, Inc., 44 Birch Street, Suite 304, Derry, NH 03038; tel. 603/898-3610; Cynthia Fortune, Administrator

Orthopeadic Surgery Center, 264 Pleasant Street, Concord, NH 03301; tel. 603/228-7211; FAX. 603/228-7192; Gail McNulty, Administrator

Salem Surgery Center, 32 Stiles Road, Salem, NH 03079; tel. 603/898-3610; FAX. 603/890-3313; Cynthia C. Fortune, Director

The Clinic Surgery Center, 253 Pleasant Street, Concord, NH 03301; tel. 603/226-2200; Kevin Appleton, Administrator

NEW JERSEY

A Center for Advanced Surgery, Three Winslow Place, Paramus, NJ 07652; tel. 201/843-9390; FAX. 201/843-0591; Marc L. Reichman, Director of Administration

Affiliated Ambulatory Surgery PA, 182 South Street, Suite One, Morristown, NJ 07960; tel. 973/267-0300; FAX. 973/984-2670; Sylvia Wexler, Administrator

Allan H. Schoenfeld, M.D., PA, 501 Lakehurst Road, Toms River, NJ 08753

Arthur W. Perry, M.D., FACS Plastic Surgery Center, 3055 Route 27, Franklin Park, NJ 08823; tel. 908/422-9600; FAX. 908/422-9606; Arthur W. Perry, M.D., Director

Associated Surgeon of Northern New Jersey, 25 Rockwood Place, Englewood, NJ 07631; tel. 201/567-3999; FAX. 201/567-9288

Atlantic Surgery Center, LLC, 279 Third Avenue,, Suite 105, Long Branch, NJ 07740; tel. 732/222-7373; FAX. 732/229-1556; Daniel B. Goldberg, M.D., President

Atrium Surgery Center, Inc., 195 Route 46, Suite 202, Mine Hill, NJ 07803; tel. 201/989-5185; FAX. 201/328-4097; Jennifer Rand, RN, CNOR, President

Bergen Gastroenterology, 466 Old Hook Road, Suite One, Emerson, NJ 07630; tel. 201/967-8221; FAX. 201/967-0340; Robert Ein, M.D., President

Bergen Surgical Center, Outpatient Surgical Services, One West Ridgewood Avenue, Suite 301, Paramus, NJ 07652; tel. 201/444-7666; FAX. 201/444-5862; Ralph Perricelli, Administrator

Burlington County Internal Medicine, 651 John F Kennedy Way, Willingboro, NJ 08046; tel. 609/871-7070; FAX. 609/835-4510; Toni McNei, Administrator

Campus Eye Group, 1700 Whitehorse Hamilton Square Road, Suite A, Hamilton Square, NJ 08690; tel. 609/587-2020; FAX. 609/588-9545; Denise Agness, O.D., Office Manager

Cataract and Laser Institute, PA, 101 Prospect Street, Suite 102, Lakewood, NJ 08701; tel. 908/367-0699; FAX. 908/367-0937

Cataract Surgery and Laser Center, Inc., 19 21 Fair Lawn Avenue, Fair Lawn, NJ 07410

Center for Special Surgery, 104 Lincoln Avenue, Hawthorne, NJ 07506; tel. 973/427-6800; FAX. 973/427-9602; John Tauber, Business Administrator

Clifton Surgery Center, 1117 Route 46 East Suite 303, Clifton, NJ 07013; tel. 973/779-7210; FAX. 973/779-7387; Ramon Silen, M.D., President and Medical Director

Drs. Scherl Scherl Chessler and Zingler, P.A., 1555 Center Avenue, Fort Lee, NJ 07024; tel. 201/945-6564; FAX. 201/461-9038; Lynn A. Sculley, Practice Administrator

Endo–Surgi Center, 1201 Morris Avenue, Union, NJ 07083; tel. 908/686-0066; Sharon DeMato, Executive Director

Endo/Surgical Center of New Jersey, 925 Clifton Avenue, Clifton, NJ 07013; tel. 201/777-3938; FAX. 201/777-6738; Pauline Perrino, RN, CGRN, Director of Nursing

Englewood Endoscopic Associates, 420 Grand Avenue, Englewood, NJ 07631; tel. 201/569-7044; FAX. 201/569-1999

Enrico Monti and Murphy, PA, 715 Broadway, Second Floor, Paterson, NJ 07514

Essex Eye Surgery and Laser Center, 1460 Broad Street, Bloomfield, NJ 07003; tel. 201/338-5566; FAX. 201/338-0753; Lin Lee, Director Support Services

Eye Institute of Essex Surgeye Center, 50 Newark Avenue, Belleville, NJ 07109; tel. 201/751-6060; FAX. 201/450-1464; Eileen Beltramba, Administrator

Eye Physician of Sussex County Surgical Center, 183 High Street, Newton, NJ 07860; tel. 973/383-6345; FAX. 973/383-0032; Patricia Fowler, RN

Eye Surgery Princeton, 419 North Harrison Street, Princeton, NJ 08540; tel. 609/921-9437; FAX. 609/921-0277; Richard H. Wong, M.D., Medical Director

Freehold Ent, d/b/a Face to Face, Patriots Park, 222 Schanck Road, Freehold, NJ 07728; tel. 908/431-1666; FAX. 908/431-1665

Garden State Ambulatory Surgical Center, One Plaza Drive, Suite 20–21, Toms River, NJ 08757; tel. 732/341-7010; FAX. 732/341-5066; Moshe Rothkopf, M.D., FACS

Gastroenterology Diagnosis Northern New Jersey, 205 Browertown Road, Suite 102, West Paterson, NJ 07424; tel. 973/890-4780; FAX. 973/890-1097; Barbara Wattenberg, Administrative Director

Hand Surgery and Rehabilitation Center of New Jersey, P.A., 5000 Sagemore Drive, Suite 103, Marlton, NJ 08053; tel. 609/983-4263; FAX. 609/983-9362; John D. Wingate, Administrator

HealthSouth Surgical Center of South Jersey, 130 Gaither Drive, Suite 160, Mount Laurel, NJ 08054; tel. 609/722-7000; FAX. 609/722-8962; Eleanor O. Peschko, Administrator

Horizon Laser and Eye Surgery Center, 9701 Ventnor Avenue, Suite 301, Margate City, NJ 08402; tel. 609/822-7171; FAX. 609/822-3211; Suzanne D. Bruno, Administrator

Hunterdon Center for Surgery, LLC T/A Surgery Today, 121 Highway 31, Suite 1300, Flemington, NJ 08822; tel. 908/806-7017; FAX. 908/806-2838; Saleha Faruqi, M.D., Medical Director

James Street Surgical Suite, 261 James Street, Morristown, NJ 07960

Mediplex Surgery Center, 98 James Street, Suite 108, Edison, NJ 08820-3998; tel. 908/632-1600; FAX. 908/632-1678; Ruth Mosher, Administrator

Metropolitan Surgical Association, 40 Eagle Street, Englewood, NJ 07631

Mid Atlantic Eye Center, 70 East Front Street, Red Bank, NJ 07701; tel. 732/741-0858; FAX. 732/219-0180; Walter J. Kahn, M.D.

Middlesex Same Day Surgical Center, 561 Cranbury Road, East Brunswick, NJ 08816; tel. 908/390-4300; FAX. 908/390-4405; Evelyn Tornquist, Office Manager

Newark Mini-Surgi Site, Inc., 145 Roseville Avenue, Newark, NJ 07107; tel. 201/485-3300; FAX. 201/485-2404; Monica Chomsky

North Jersey Center for Surgery, 39 Newton Sparta Road, Newton, NJ 07860; tel. 973/383-0153; FAX. 973/300-9002; Bruno J. Casatelli, D.P.M., Administrator

North Jersey Women's Medical Center, Inc., 6000 Kennedy Boulevard, West New York, NJ 07093; tel. 201/869-9293; Saul Luchs, M.D.

Providers / Freestanding Ambulatory Surgery Centers

Northern New Jersey Eye Institute, 71 Second Street, South Orange, NJ 07079; tel. 973/763-2203; FAX. 973/763-5207; Shirley Vitale, Administrative Director

Northwest Jersey Ambulatory Surgery Center, 350 Sparta Avenue, Building A, Sparta, NJ 07871; tel. 973/729-8580; FAX. 973/729-2344; Sharon L. Marquardt, RN, Operating Room Coordinator

Ocean County Eye Associates, P.C., 18 Mule Road, Toms River, NJ 08755

Ocean Surgical Pavilion, Inc., 1907 Highway 35, Suite Nine, Oakhurst, NJ 07755; tel. 908/517-8885; FAX. 908/517-8589; Valerie Plaska, Practice Mgr.

Ophthalmic Physicians of Monmouth, 733 North Beers Street, Holmdel, NJ 07733; tel. 908/739-0707; FAX. 908/739-6722; Beverly Savlov, Office Manager

Pavonia Surgery Center, Inc., 600 Pavonia Avenue, Fourth Floor, Jersey City, NJ 07306; tel. 201/216-1700; FAX. 201/216-1800; William H. Constad, M.D., President

Princeton Ambulatory Surgery Center, Inc., 281 Witherspoon Street, Third Floor, Princeton, NJ 08542; tel. 609/497-4380; FAX. 609/497-4986; Joseph Bonanno, Director

Princeton Orthopaedic Associates, P.A., 727 State Road, Princeton, NJ 08540; tel. 609/924-8131; FAX. 609/924-8532; William G. Hyncik, Jr., Executive Director

Retina Consultants Surgery Center, 39 Sycamore Avenue, Little Silver, NJ 07739; tel. 732/530-7730; FAX. 732/530-3837

Ridgedale Surgery Center, 14 Ridgedale Avenue, Suite 120, Cedar Knolls, NJ 07927; tel. 201/605-5151; FAX. 201/605-1208; Enza Guagenti, Administrator

Ridgewood Ambulatory Surgery Center, 1200 Ridgewood Avenue, Ridgewood, NJ 07450; tel. 201/444-4499; FAX. 201/612-8114

Roseland Surgery Center, 556 Eagle Rock Avenue, Roseland, NJ 07068; tel. 201/226-1717; FAX. 201/403-9034; Joseph Brandspiegel, Executive Director

Saddle Brook Surgicenter, Inc., 289 Market Street, Saddle Brook, NJ 07663; tel. 201/843-4444; FAX. 201/368-2817; Dr. Ronald Sollitto, President and CEO

Seashore Ambulatory Surgery Center, 1907 New Road, Northfield, NJ 08225; tel. 609/646-2323; FAX. 609/645-9780; Carol A. Leszczynski, Administrator

Shore Surgicenter, Inc., 142 Route 35, Eatontown, NJ 07724; tel. 908/542-9666; FAX. 908/542-9393; Simone Bendary, Manager

Somerset Eye Institute, P.C., 562 Easton Avenue, Somerset, NJ 08873

Somerset Surgical Center, P.A., 1081 Route 22 West, Bridgewater, NJ 08807

South Jersey Endoscopy Center, 17 West Red Bank Avenue, Suite 302, Woodbury, NJ 08096; tel. 856/848-4464; FAX. 856/848-8706; Sue Lampman, Billing Manager

South Jersey Surgicenter, 2835 South Delsea Drive, Vineland, NJ 08360; tel. 856/696-0020; FAX. 856/205-1721; Catherine C. Retzbach, R.N., B.S.N., Administrator

Springfield Eye Surgery Laser Center, 105 Morris Avenue, Springfield, NJ 07081; tel. 201/376-3113; FAX. 201/376-1378; Dr. Christine Zolli

Summit Eye Group T/A Suburban Eye Institute, 369 Springfield Avenue, Berkeley Heights, NJ 07922; tel. 908/464-4600; FAX. 908/464-4737; Patricia K. Ketcham, RN, Administrator

Summit Surgical Center, 110 Carnie Boulevard, Voorhees, NJ 08043; tel. 856/325-5813; FAX. 856/325-5858; Elizabeth Jaques, Administrator Director

Surgery Center of Cherry Hill, 408 Route 70 East, Cherry Hill, NJ 08034; tel. 609/354-1600; FAX. 609/429-7555; Nancy Diflavis, Director of Nursing

Surgicare of Central Jersey, Inc., 40 Stirling Road, Watchung, NJ 07060; tel. 908/769-8000; FAX. 908/668-3139; Marion Jenkins, Executive Director

Surgicare Surgical Associates, PC, 15 01 Broadway, Route 4 West, Suite One and Three, Fairlawn, NJ 07410; tel. 201/791-6585; John H. Haffar, M.D., Medical Director

Teaneck Gastroenterology and Endoscopy Center, 1086 Teaneck Road, Suite Three B, Teaneck, NJ 07666; tel. 201/837-9636; FAX. 201/837-9544

The Endoscopy Center of Red Bank, 365 Broad Street, Red Bank, NJ 07701; tel. 732/842-4294; FAX. 732/842-3854; Elizabeth Boyle, Provider Relations or Marie Scoles, R.N., Office Manager

The Endoscopy Center of South Jersey, 2791 South Delsea Drive, South Vinelan, NJ 08360; tel. 609/691-1400; FAX. 609/691-7117; Richard Wagar, Assistant Director

The Eye Care Center, 500 West Main Street, Freehold, NJ 07728; tel. 908/462-8707; FAX. 908/462-1296; Dale A. Ingram, Administrator

The Hernia Center, 222 Schanck Road, Suite 100, Freehold, NJ 07728; tel. 908/462-2999; FAX. 908/462-7760; Jackie Porter, RN

The New Jersey Eye Center, 21 West Main Street, Bergenfield, NJ 07621; tel. 201/384-7333; FAX. 201/385-3881; Steve Meneve, Director

The Peck Center Incorporated, 1200 Route 46, Clifton, NJ 07013; tel. 201/471-3906; FAX. 201/471-7048; George C. Peck, Jr., M.D.

The Surgical Center at South Jersey Eye Physicians, P.A., 509 South Lenola Road, Building 11, Moorestown, NJ 08057; tel. 609/727-9333; FAX. 609/727-0064; Janet Daniels, RN, ASC Nurse Manager

Trocki Plastic Surgery Center, PA, 635 Tilton Road, Northfield, NJ 08225

NEW MEXICO

Alamogordo Eye Clinic and Surgical Center, 1124 10th Street, Alamogordo, NM 88310; tel. 505/434-1200; FAX. 505/437-3947; Donald J. Ham, Administrator

Eastern New Mexico Eye Clinic, 1820 West 21st Street, Clovis, NM 88101; tel. 505/762-2207; Dik S. Cheung, M.D.

Eye Care Surgery, 110 North Coronado Avenue, Espanola, NM 87532; tel. 505/753-7391; FAX. 505/753-2749; Dr. Gary Puro

HealthSouth Albuquerque Surgery Center, 1720 Wyoming Boulevard, N.E., Albuquerque, NM 87112; tel. 505/292-9200; FAX. 505/292-1398; D'Ann Rohde, Administrator

Lazaro Eye Surgical Center, 1131 Mall Drive, Las Cruces, NM 88011; tel. 505/522-7676; Corine B. Lazaro, M.D., Administrator

Northside Presbyterian, P.O. Box 26666, 5901 Harper Drive, NE, Albuquerque, NM 87125; tel. 505/291-2114; FAX. 505/291-2983; Robert Garcia, Administrator

The Endoscopy Center of Santa Fe, 1650 Hospital Drive, Suite 900, Santa Fe, NM 87505; tel. 505/988-3373; FAX. 505/984-1858; Jim Howlett, Administrator

NEW YORK

Ambulatory Surgery Center of Brooklyn, 313 43rd Street, Brooklyn, NY 11232; tel. 718/369-1900; FAX. 718/965-4157; Michael M. Levi, M.D., Ph.D., Governing Authority

Ambulatory Surgery Center of Greater New York, Inc., 1101 Pelham Parkway, N., Bronx, NY 10469; tel. 718/515-3500; FAX. 718/655-1795; Joanne McLaughlin, Administrator

Brook Plaza Ambulatory Surgical Center, 1901 Utica Avenue, Brooklyn, NY 11234; tel. 718/629-5590; FAX. 718/629-2833; David Doretsky, Administrator

Brooklyn Eye Surgery Center, LLC, 1301-1311 Avenue J, Brooklyn, NY 11230; tel. 718/645-0600; FAX. 718/692-4456; Rosalind A. Kochman, Chief Executive Officer

Buffalo Ambulatory Surgery Center, 3095 Harlem Road, Cheektowaga, NY 14225; tel. 716/896-3815; FAX. 716/896-3015; Dorothy L. Zimdahl, R.N., B.S., CNOR, Administrator

Central New York Eye Center, 22 Green Street, Poughkeepsie, NY 12601; tel. 914/471-3720; Marie Schneider, R.N.

Day-Op Center of Long Island, Inc., 110 Willis Avenue, Mineola, NY 11501; tel. 516/294-0030; FAX. 516/294-0228; Robin Fishman, Executive Director

Fifth Avenue Surgery Center, 1049 Fifth Avenue, New York, NY 10028; tel. 212/772-6667; Francois Simon, Vice President

Harrison Center Outpatient Surgery, Inc., 550 Harrison Street, Suite 230, Syracuse, NY 13202; tel. 315/472-4424; FAX. 315/475-8056; Margaret M. Alteri, Administrator and CEO

Hurley Avenue Surgical Center, Inc., 40 Hurley Avenue, Kingston, NY 12401; tel. 914/338-4777; FAX. 914/339-7339; Steven L. Kelley, CHE, Administrator and CEO

Lattimore Community Surgicenter, 125 Lattimore Road, Rochester, NY 14620; tel. 716/473-9000; FAX. 716/473-9018; John J. Goehle, CPA, Administrator

Long Island Eye Surgery Center, 601 Suffolk Avenue, Brentwood, NY 11717; tel. 631/231-4455; FAX. 631/434-1728; Robert Nelson, RPA-C/Director of Operations and Clinical Services

Long Island Surgi-Center, 1895 Walt Whitman Road, Melville, NY 11747; tel. 516/293-9700; FAX. 516/293-1018; Howard Leemon, D.D.S.

Millard Fillmore Ambulatory Surgery Center, 215 Klein Road, Williamsville, NY 14221; tel. 716/568-6100; FAX. 716/568-6166; Joel C. Farwell, Business Manager

Nassau Center for Ambulatory Surgery, Inc., dba Garden City SurgiCenter, 400 Endo Boulevard, Garden City, NY 11530; tel. 516/832-8504; FAX. 516/832-1085; Charles J. Raab, Chief Executive/Financial Officer

New York Institute for Same Day Surgery, Inc., 99 Dutch Hill Plaza, Orangeburg, NY 10962; tel. 914/359-9000; FAX. 914/359-1495; Richard Sherman, CPA, Director of Finance and Business

North Shore Surgi Center, Inc., 989 Jericho Turnpike, Smithtown, NY 11787; tel. 516/864-7100; FAX. 516/864-7129; Gerald Mazzola, Administrator

Our Lady of Victory Surgery Center, 6300 Powers Road, Orchard Park, NY 14127; tel. 716/667-3222; FAX. 716/667-3120; Dana M. Mata, Administrative Director

Queens Surgi-Center, 83-40 Woodhaven Boulevard, Glendale, NY 11385; tel. 718/849-8700; FAX. 718/849-6523; Stanley H. Kornhauser, Ph.D., Chief Operating Officer

Queens Surgical Community Center, 46-04 31st Avenue, Long Island C, NY 11103; tel. 718/545-5050; FAX. 718/721-8709; Mr. Misk, Partner

Same Day Surgery of Latham, Inc., Seven Century Hill Drive, Latham, NY 12110; tel. 518/785-5741; FAX. 518/785-5741; Judith A. Grady, RN, Administrator

The Mackool Eye Institute, 31-27 41st Street. Astoria, NY 11103; tel. 718/728-3400; FAX. 718/721-7562; Jeanne Mackool, Administrator

Westfall Surgery Center, LLP, 1065 Senator Keating Boulevard, Rochester, NY 14618; tel. 716/256-1330; FAX. 716/256-3823; Gary J. Scott, Administrative Director

NORTH CAROLINA

Asheboro Endoscopy Center, 700 Sunset Avenue, P.O. Box 4830, Asheboro, NC 27203; tel. 910/626-4328; FAX. 910/625-9941; Vickie Whitaker, R.N., Clinical Director

Asheville Hand Ambulatory Surgery Center, 34 Granby Street, P.O. Box 1980, Asheville, NC 28802; tel. 704/258-0847; FAX. 704/258-0374; E. Brown Crosby, M.D., Executive Officer

Blue Ridge Day Surgery Center, 2308 Wesvill Court, Raleigh, NC 27607; tel. 919/781-4311; FAX. 919/781-0625; Susan S. Swift, Facility Manager

Carteret Surgery Center, 3714 Guardian Avenue, Morehead City, NC 28557; tel. 252/247-2101; FAX. 252/247-2031; Frances Meyer, Administrator

Chapel Hill Surgical Center, 109 Conner Drive, Suite 1201, Chapel Hill, NC 27514; tel. 919/968-0611; FAX. 919/967-8637; Gary S. Berger, M.D., President

Charlotte Surgery and Laser Center, 2825 Randolph Road, Charlotte, NC 28211; tel. 704/377-1647; FAX. 704/358-8267; Margaret Slattery, Manager

Christenbury Ambulatory Surgical Center, 449 North Wendover Road Park Place, Charlotte, NC 28211; tel. 704/332-9365; FAX. 704/364-7384; Jama Hammond, R.N., CNOR, Director

Cleveland Ambulatory Services, 1100 North Lafayette Street, Shelby, NC 28150; tel. 704/482-1331; FAX. 704/482-4833; Thomas D. Bailey, M.D., Medical Director

Columbia Medivision Inc., 2200 East Seventh Street, Charlotte, NC 28204; tel. 704/334-4317; FAX. 704/377-1830; Diane H. Matthews, Administrator

Craven Surgery Center, 630 McCarthy Blvd, P.O. Box 12446, New Bern, NC 28561; tel. 252/633-2000; FAX. 252/633-0096; Lila Cotten, Business Manager

Davis Ambulatory Surgical Center, 120 Carver Street, P.O. Box 15727, Durham, NC 27704; tel. 919/477-9677; FAX. 919/479-6755; Susan R. Hollander, Administrator

Eye Surgery and Laser Clinic, 500 Lake Concord Road, N.E., Concord, NC 28025; tel. 704/782-1127; FAX. 704/782-1207; Steven Grubb, Administrator

Providers / Freestanding Ambulatory Surgery Centers

Eye Surgery Center of Shelby, 1622 East Marion Street, Shelby, NC 28150; tel. 704/482-2020; FAX. 704/482-7707; Frank T. Hannah, M.D., Medical Director

Fayetteville Ambulatory Surgery Center, 1781 Metromedical Drive, Fayetteville, NC 28304; tel. 910/323-1647; FAX. 910/323-4142; John T. Henley Jr., M.D., Medical Director

FemCare, 62 Orange Street, Asheville, NC 28801; tel. 828/255-8400; Lorraine M. Cummings M.D., Medical Director

Gaston Ambulatory Surgery, 2545 Court Drive, Gastonia, NC 28054; tel. 704/834-2086; FAX. 704/834-2085; Elizabeth Kohli, Director

Goldsboro Endoscopy Center, Inc., 2705 Medical Office Place, Goldsboro, NC 27534; tel. 919/530-9111; FAX. 919/580-0988; Venkata C. Motaparthy, M.D., Chief Executive Officer

Greensboro Center for Digestive Diseases, 520 North Elam Avenue, P.O. Box 10829, Greensboro, NC 27403; tel. 910/547-1718; FAX. 910/547-1711; Jeannette Perez, Director

Greensboro Specialty Surgical Center, 522 North Elam Avenue, Greensboro, NC 27403; tel. 336/294-1833; FAX. 336/294-8831; Cathy Bryant, Administrator

Hawthorne Surgical Center, 1999 South Hawthorne Road, Winston-Salem, NC 27103; tel. 910/718-6800; FAX. 910/718-6847; Teresa L. Carter, Facility Director

HealthSouth Surgecenter of Wilson, 1709 Medical Park Drive, Wilson, NC 27893; tel. 919/237-5649; Phyllis S. Renfrow, Administrator

HealthSouth Surgery Center of Charlotte, 2825 Randolph Rd., Charlotte, NC 28211; tel. 704/377-1647; Margaret L. Slattery, Administrator

HealthSouth Surgery Center of Greensboro, L.P., 3312 Battleground Avenue, Greensboro, NC 27410; tel. 336/282-8330; FAX. 336/282-2625; Paige Fowler, Administrator

HealthSouth Surgery Center of Hickory, L.P., 27 13th Avenue, N.E., Hickory, NC 28601; tel. 704/328-1493; FAX. 704/322-6097; Kevin Deal, R.N., Administrator

High Point Endoscopy Center, Inc., 624 Quaker Lane, Suite C-106, High Point, NC 27262; tel. 336/885-1400; Lester E. Hurrelbrink, Administrator

High Point Surgery Center, 600 Lindsay Street, P.O. Box 2476, High Point, NC 27261; tel. 336/884-6068; FAX. 336/888-6111; Joan D. Gayle, Administrator

Iredell Head, Neck and Ear Ambulatory Surgery Center, 707 Bryant Street, Statesville, NC 28677; tel. 704/873-5224; FAX. 704/873-5984; Scott Seagle, Administrator

Iredell Surgical Center, 1720 Davie Avenue, Statesville, NC 28677; tel. 704/871-0081; FAX. 704/871-0086; Debra C. Hartman, Administrator

Medivision, 2170 Midland Road, P.O. Box 1938. Southern Pine, NC 28387; tel. 910/295-1221; FAX. 910/295-0512; Kathy Stout, RN, Administrator

Piedmont Gastroenterology Center, Inc., 1901 South Hawthorne Road, Suite 308, Winston-Salem, NC 27103; tel. 910/760-4340; FAX. 919/765-2869; Charles H. Hauser, Administrator

Plastic Surgery Center of North Carolina, Inc., 2901 Maplewood Avenue, Winston-Salem, NC 27103; tel. 336/768-6210; FAX. 336/768-6236; Melba Edwards, Administrator

Quandrangle Endoscopy Center, 620 South Memorial Drive, Greenville, NC 27834; tel. 919/752-6101; Mark Dellasega

Raleigh Endoscopy Center, 3320 Wake Forest Road, Raleigh, NC 27609; tel. 919/878-1151; Robert N. Harper, M.D., Medical Director

Raleigh Plastic Surgery Center, Inc., 1112 Dresser Court, Raleigh, NC 27609; tel. 919/872-2616; FAX. 919/782-2771; Kelly Hodges, Administrator

Raleigh Women's Health Organization, Inc., 3613 Haworth Drive, Raleigh, NC 27609; tel. 919/783-0444; FAX. 919/781-8432; Susan Hill, Vice President

Regional Medical Services Surgery Center, 5200 North Croatan Highway, Kitty Hawk, NC 27949; tel. 919/261-9009; FAX. 919/261-4329; Trish Blackmon, Executive Director

SameDay Surgery Center at Presbyterian, 1800 East Fourth Street, P.O. Box 34425, Charlotte, NC 28234; tel. 704/384-4200; Chip Day, Administrator

Southern Eye Associates, P.A., Ophthalmic Surgery Center, 2801 Blue Ridge Road, Suite 200, Raleigh, NC 27607; tel. 919/571-0081; Brian Klaasmeyer, Administrator

Surgery Center of Morganton Eye Physicians, P.A., 335 East Parker Road, Morganton, NC 28655; tel. 704/433-6225; L. A. Raynor, M.D., Medical Director

Surgical Center of Greensboro, Inc., 1211 Virginia Street, P.O. Box 29347, Greensboro, NC 27429; tel. 919/272-0012; FAX. 919/272-4063; Ken Overbey, Administrator

SurgiCenter of Wilson, 209 Richards Street, Wilson, NC 27893; tel. 919/237-5649; FAX. 919/237-4977; Phyllis Renfrow, President

Surgicenter Services of Pitt, Inc., 102 Bethesda Drive, Greenville, NC 27834; tel. 919/816-7700; FAX. 919/816-7733; Anna M. Weaver, President

The Endoscopy Center, 191 Biltmore Avenue, Asheville, NC 28801; tel. 704/254-0881; Michael Grier, M.D.

The Surgery Center, 166 Memorial Court, Jacksonville, NC 28546; tel. 910/353-9565; FAX. 919/353-5497; Takey Crist, M.D., President

WHA Medical Clinic, PLLC, 1202 Medical Center Drive, Wilmington, NC 28401; tel. 910/341-3433; Diane A. Atkinson, Executive Director

Wilmington SurgCare, 1801 South 17th Street, Wilmington, NC 28401; tel. 910/763-4555; FAX. 910/763-9044; David Gross, Facility Administrator

Wilson OB-GYN, 2500 Horton Boulevard, Zip 27893, P.O. Box 7639, Wilson, NC 27895; tel. 919/206-1000; FAX. 919/237-0704; Daniel P. Michalak, M.D., Administrator

Woman Care and Carolina Birth Center, 712 North Elm Street, High Point, NC 27262; tel. 910/889-3646; Robert C. Crawford, M.D., Chief Executive Officer

NORTH DAKOTA

Bismarck Surgical Associates, 600 N. 9th Street, Bismarck, ND 58501; tel. 701/221-2299; FAX. 701/221-3239; Tim Loch, Administrator

Centennial Medical Center, 1500 24th Avenue, S.W., Minot, ND 58702; tel. 701/852-0777; Dr. Manuel Neto, Administrator

Dakota Clinic Ltd Endoscopy, 1702 S. University Drive, Fargo, ND 58108; tel. 701/280-8900; Larry G. Solberg, Administrator

Dakota Day Surgery, 1717 South University Drive, P.O. Box 6014, Fargo, ND 58103; tel. 701/280-4700; FAX. 701/280-4747; Pauline Fischer, Patient Account Coordinator

Dakota Surgery & Laser Center, 430 E. Sweet Avenue, Bismarck, ND 58504; tel. 701/222-4900; Charles R. Volk, Administrator

Day Surgery-Wahpeton, 275 South 11th Street, Wahpeton, ND 58075; tel. 701/642-2000; FAX. 701/671-4153; Lynn R. Wold, Administrator

Grand Forks Clinic Ltd., ASC, 1000 South Columbia Road, Grand Forks, ND 58201; tel. 701/780-6000; Wayne K. Larson, Associate Administrator

Great Plains Clinic Surgery Center, 33 Ninth Street W., Dickinson, ND 58601; tel. 701/225-6017; FAX. 701/225-5018; Jim LeBrun, Administrator

Institute for Special Surgery, 2301 25th Street, Fargo, ND 58103; tel. 702/271-1045; FAX. 702/271-1044; Timothy Haugen, Administrator

Medical Arts, ASC, Inc., 400 East Burdick Expressway, Minot, ND 58702; tel. 701/857-7000; Doug Eberhard, Exec. Director

North Dakota Surgery Center, 3035 Demers Ave., Grand Forks, ND 58201; tel. 701/775-3151; FAX. 701/775-3153; Ross J. Gonitzke, Administrator

St. Alexius Same Day Surgery Center, 810 East Rosser, Bismarck, ND 58501; tel. 701/530-5000; Sandy Berreth, Director

TMC Western Dakota Medical Group, 1102 Main, Williston, ND 58801; tel. 701/572-7711; Mary Banta, Administrator

Trinity Community Clinic-Western Dakota, 1102 Main, Williston, ND 58801; tel. 701/572-7711; FAX. 701/572-2283; Mary E. Banta, Administrator

OHIO

Advanced Cosmetic and Laser Surgery Center, Inc., 2200 Philadelphia Drive, Suite 651, Dayton, OH 45406; tel. 937/278-0809; FAX. 937/278-3590

Amend Center for Eye Surgery, 5939 Colerain Avenue, Cincinnati, OH 45239; tel. 513/923-3900; FAX. 513/923-3012

Austintown Ambulatory Healthcare Center, 45 North Canfield-Niles Road, Youngstown, OH 44515; tel. 216/792-2722; FAX. 216/793-4883; James M. Conti, President and CEO

Bloomberg Eye Center, 1651 West Main Street, Newark, OH 43055; tel. 614/522-3937; FAX. 614/522-6766; John E. Reid, Executive Director

Carnegie Surgery Center, 10681 Carnegie Avenue, Cleveland, OH 44106; tel. 216/231-5566; FAX. 216/231-1441; K. L. Rosacco, RN, CNOR, Nurse Administrator

Cincinnati Eye Institute and Outpatient Eye Surgery Center, 10494 Montgomery Road, Cincinnati, OH 45242; tel. 513/984-5133; FAX. 513/984-4240; Doris Holton, Administrator

Cincinnati Foot Clinic, Inc., 9600 Colerain Avenue, Suite 400, Cincinnati, OH 45239; tel. 513/385-6946; Robert Hayman, M.D., President

Columbia The Surgery Center, 19250 East Bagley Road, Middleburg Heights, OH 44130; tel. 440/826-3240; FAX. 440/826-3250

Columbus Eye Surgery Center, 5965 East Broad Street, Suite 460, Columbus, OH 43213; tel. 614/751-4080; FAX. 614/751-4092; Toni Van Horn, Executive Director

Consultants in Gastroenterology, Inc., 29001 Cedar Road, Suite 110, Lyndhurst, OH 44124; tel. 216/461-2550; FAX. 216/461-5319; Karen Wahl, Manager

Crystal Clinic Surgery Center, 3975 Embassy Parkway, Akron, OH 44313; tel. 216/668-4085; Katherine L. McNeal, RN, Administrator

Dayton Ear, Nose and Throat Surgeons, Inc., 7076 Corporate Way, Centerville, OH 45459; tel. 937/434-0555; FAX. 937/434-7413; Jana Hilgeman, Administrator

Digestivecare Endoscopy Unit, 75 Sylvania Drive, Beavercreek, OH 45440; tel. 937/325-5065; FAX. 937/325-5060; Patty Mannix, RN, CGRN Endoscopy Coordinator

Endoscopy Center of Dayton LTD, 4200 Indian Ripple Road, Beavercreek, OH 45440; tel. 937/427-1680; FAX. 937/427-9081; Christy L. McBride, Office Manager

Endoscopy Center West, 3654 Werk Road, Cincinnati, OH 45248; tel. 513/451-6001; FAX. 513/451-7310

Eye Care Center of Cincinnati, 5300 Cornell Road, Cincinnati, OH 45242; tel. 513/489-6161; FAX. 513/489-6442; Amy D. Riegler, Coordinator

Eye Institute of Northwestern Ohio, Inc., 5555 Airport Highway, Suite 110, Toledo, OH 43615; tel. 419/865-3866; FAX. 419/865-3451; Carol R. Kollarits, M.D., President

Eye Surgery Center of Wooster, 3519 Friendsville Road, Wooster, OH 44691; tel. 330/345-6371; FAX. 330/345-8029; Michelle Morrison, Director

Facial Surgery Center, 1130 Congress Avenue, Glendale, OH 45246; tel. 513/772-2442; FAX. 513/772-2844; Joseph J. Moravec, M.D., Medical Director

Firas Atassi, M.D. Outpatient Surgery Center, 34500 Center Ridge Road, North Ridgeville, OH 33039; tel. 216/327-2414

Gastroenterology Associates of Cleveland, 6801 Mayfield Road, Suite 142, Mayfield Heights, OH 44124; tel. 440/461-8800; FAX. 440/646-8594; James Andrassy, Administrator

Gastroenterology Associates, Inc., 4665 Belpar Street, NW, P.O. Box 36329, Canton, OH 44735; tel. 216/493-1480; FAX. 216/493-6805

Gastroenterology Specialists, Inc., 2732 Fulton Drive, N.W., Canton, OH 44718; tel. 330/455-5011; FAX. 330/588-7127; Melissa Smith, RN, C.G.C.

Halpin-Poweleit Eye Surgery Center, (Division of Tri-State Eye Care), 8044 Montgomery Road, Suite 155, Cincinnati, OH 45236; tel. 513/791-3937; FAX. 513/791-1473

HealthSouth Western Reserve Surgery Center, LP, 1930 State Route 59, Kent, OH 44240; tel. 216/677-3292; FAX. 330/677-3624; Laurie Simon, Office Manager

Heritage Surgical Associates of Cincinnati, d/b/a Healthsouth Surgery Center of Cincinnati, 2925 Vernon Place, Suite 101, Cincinnati, OH 45219; tel. 513/872-4541; FAX. 513/872-4558; Patti Murphy, RN, Director

Kahn and Diehl Center for Progressive Eye Care, 2740 Navarre Avenue, Oregon, OH 43616; tel. 419/697-3658; FAX. 419/697-2149; Karen R. Hess, RN, C.O.T., O.R. Supervisor

Kunesh Eye Surgery Center, 2601 Far Hills Avenue, Dayton, OH 45419-1665; tel. 937/298-1093; FAX. 937/298-6344; Lucy Helmers, Administrator

Mercy Ambulatory Surgery Center, 2990 Mack Road, Fairfield, OH 45014; tel. 513/874-6440; FAX. 513/682-3906; Lori Vernon, Administrator

Mid-Ohio Outpatient Surgery Center, 245 Taylor Station Road, Columbus, OH 43213; tel. 614/861-0448; FAX. 614/861-7717; Dr. Grace Z. Kim, Director

Providers / Freestanding Ambulatory Surgery Centers

Midwest Eye Center, 119 West Kemper Road, Cincinnati, OH 45246; tel. 513/671–6112; FAX. 513/671–6386; Lorrie Walters, Business Office Supervisor

North Coast Endoscopy, Inc., 9500 Mentor Avenue, Suite 380, Mentor, OH 44060; tel. 216/352–9400; FAX. 216/352–9407; Ahmad Ascha, M.D.

Northshore Endoscopy Center, 850 Columbia Road, Suite 201, Westlake, OH 44145; tel. 216/808–1212

Ohio Eye Associates Eye Surgery Center, 466 South Trimble Road, Mansfield, OH 44906; tel. 419/756–8000; FAX. 419/756–7100; John L. Marquardt, M.D.

Ohio Gastroenterology Group, Inc., Endoscopy Center, 777 West State Street, Suite 402, Columbus, OH 43222; tel. 614/221–7431; FAX. 614/341–2401; Jean Yarletts, RN, B.S.N.

Parkside Women's Center, Inc., 1011 Boardman–Canfield Road, Boardman, OH 44512; tel. 216/758–0975; FAX. 216/758–8453

Parkway Urology Center, Inc., 3500 Executive Parkway, Toledo, OH 43606; tel. 419/531–8349; FAX. 419/534–5337; Gregory K. Emmert, Sr., M.D., Chief Executive Officer

Ram Bandi M.D. A.S.C., 1037 North Main Street, Suite B, Akron, OH 44310; tel. 330/923–0094; FAX. 330/923–2609; Ann Marie Faber, RN

Restorative Vision Center, 4452 Eastgate Boulevard, Suite 305, Cincinnati, OH 45245; tel. 513/752–5700; FAX. 513/752–5716; Holly Schwab, RN, Surgery Manager

Richfield Surgery Center, Inc., 3030 Streetsboro Road, Richfield, OH 44286; tel. 216/659–4790; FAX. 216/659–3355; Carol A. Westfall, Vice President

Ross Park Surgical Services, One Ross Park, Steubenville, OH 43952; tel. 614/282–4790; Kathy Lemasters, RN, Manager

Sandusky Surgeons, Inc., 1221 Hayes Avenue, Sandusky, OH 44870; tel. 419/625–1374; Donald Lenhart, M.D., President

Sidney Foot and Ankle Surgical Center, 1000 Michigan, Sidney, OH 45365; tel. 513/492–1211; FAX. 513/492–6557; Micki Heater, Administrative Director

South Dayton Urological Associates, Inc., 10 Southmoor Circle, N.W., Kettering, OH 45429; tel. 937/294–1489; Donald Bailey, Practice Administrator

Stoneridge Endoscopy Center, 3900 Stoneridge Lane, Dublin, OH 43017; tel. 614/889–5001; FAX. 614/889–5913; Cheryl Miller, Clinic Manager

Surgery Alliance Ltd., 975 Sawburg Avenue, Alliance, OH 44601; tel. 330/821–7997; FAX. 330/821–7295; Hazel Thomas, Administrator

Surgery Center At Southwoods, 7525 California Avenue, Youngstown, OH 44513; tel. 330/758–1954

Surgery Center West, 850 Columbia Road, Westlake, OH 44145; tel. 216/808–4000; FAX. 216/808–4010; Michelle Padden, RN, Administrator

Surgiplex, 950 Clague Road, Westlake, OH 44145; tel. 216/333–1020; FAX. 216/333–3278

Taylor Station Surgery Center, 275 Taylor Station Road, Columbus, OH 43213; tel. 614/751–4466; FAX. 614/751–4475; Bridget A. Huston, Manager

The Endoscopy Center, 3439 Granite Circle, Toledo, OH 43617; tel. 419/843–7993; FAX. 419/841–7789; Alice Horner, R.N. Nurse Manager

The LCA Center for Surgery, 7840 Montgomery Road, Cincinnati, OH 45236; tel. 513/792–9099; FAX. 513/792–5634; Rene Fischer, President and CEO

The Surgical Center of East Liverpool, 16480 St. Clair Avenue, P.O. Box 2640, East Liverpool, OH 43920; tel. 216/386–9000; FAX. 216/386–1255; Robin Menchen, Chief Executive Officer

The Zeeba Clinic, A Meridia Outpatient and Laser Surgery Center, 29017 Cedar Road, Lyndhurst, OH 44124; tel. 216/461–7774; FAX. 216/461–5401; Sharon Luke, RN, B.S.N., Clinical Manager

Tippecanoe Endoscopy, Inc., 1210 Boardman Canfield Road, Youngstown, OH 44512; tel. 330/726–0132; FAX. 330/726–0571; Mary Amorn, RN, Administrator

Toledo Clinic, Inc., 4235 Secor Road, Toledo, OH 43623; tel. 419/473–3561; FAX. 419/472–0838; David J. Sobczak, Senior Vice President, Chief Finance

Toledo Community Lithotripter Center, 3158 West Central Avenue, Toledo, OH 43606; tel. 419/531–3538

University Suburban Health Center, 1611 South Green Road, Suite 124, South Euclid, OH 44121; tel. 216/382–1868; Barbara McCann, Director of Marketing and Communication

Vision America of Ohio, 210 Sharon Road, Suite B, Circleville, OH 43113; tel. 740/477–7200; FAX. 740/477–8349; Teresa Meadows, OR Coordinator

Wedgewood Surgery Center, 10330 Sawmill Parkway, Powell, OH 43065; tel. 614/234–0500; FAX. 614/234–0540; Kim Heimlich, RN, Director

OKLAHOMA

Ambulatory Surgery Associates, 6160 South Yale Avenue, Tulsa, OK 74136; tel. 918/495–2625; FAX. 918/495–2601; Jacquelyn S. Moore, RN, Director

Central Oklahoma Ambulatory Surgical Center, Inc., 3301 Northwest 63rd Street, Oklahoma City, OK 73116; tel. 405/842–9732; FAX. 405/842–9771; Paul Silverstein, M.D., Administrator

Columbia Surgicare of Tulsa, 4415 South Harvard Avenue, Suite 100, Tulsa, OK 74135; tel. 918/742–2502; FAX. 918/745–9750; Dirk Foxworthy, Administrator

Columbia Surgicare–Midtown, 1000 North Lincoln, Suite 150, Oklahoma City, OK 73104; tel. 405/232–8696; FAX. 405/232–6002; Connie M. Belding, RN, Administrator

Digestive Disease Specialists, Inc., 3366 Northwest Expressway, Suite 400, P.O. Box 99521, Oklahoma City, OK 73199; tel. 405/943–2001; FAX. 405/947–1966; Larry A. Bookman, M.D.

Eastern Oklahoma Surgery Center, L. L. C., 5020 East 68th Street, Tulsa, OK 74136; tel. 918/492–1539; FAX. 918/494–8683; Bobbie Huff, RN, Administrator

Grisham Eye Associates, P.O. Box 1437, Bartlesville, OK 74005; tel. 918/333–1990; Dennis McKinley

Heritage Eye Surgicenter of Oklahoma, Heritage Building, 6922 South Western, Oklahoma City, OK 73139; tel. 405/636–1508; Edward D. Glinski, D.O., Administrator

Medical Plaza Endoscopy Unit, 1125 North Porter, Suite 304, Norman, OK 73071; tel. 405/360–2799; FAX. 405/447–0321; Philip C. Bird, M.D.

Oklahoma Ambulatory Surgery Center, 6908–B East Reno, Midwest City, OK 73110; tel. 405/737–6900; FAX. 405/732–0885; A.C. Vyas, M.D., Administrator

Oklahoma City Clinic, 701 Northwest 10th Street, Oklahoma City, OK 73104; tel. 405/280–5700; FAX. 405/280–5200; Mike Klein, Executive Director

Oklahoma Surgicare, 4317 W. Memorial Road, Oklahoma City, OK 73134; tel. 405/755–6240; FAX. 405/752–1819; Linda Slater, Administrator

Orthopedic Associates Ambulatory Surgery Center, Inc., 3301 Northwest 50th Street, P.O. Box 57027, Oklahoma City, OK 73157–7027; tel. 405/947–5610; FAX. 405/947–1341; Thomas H. Flesher, President

Outpatient Surgical Center of Ponca City, 400 Fairview, Ponca City, OK 74601; tel. 405/762–0695; FAX. 405/765–9406; Peggy Maples, RN, Executive Director

Physicians Surgical Center, 805 East Robinson, Norman, OK 73071–6610; tel. 405/364–9789; FAX. 405/366–8081; Ruth Beller, RN, Director

Southern Oklahoma Surgical Center, Inc., 2412 North Commerce, Ardmore, OK 73401; tel. 405/226–5000; Ann Willis, RN, Administrator

Southern Plains Ambulatory Surgery Center, 2222 Iowa Avenue, P.O. Box 1069, Chickasha, OK 73023; tel. 405/224–8111; FAX. 405/222–9557; H. Wayne Delony, Executive Director

Southwest Ambulatory Surgery Center, LLC, 8125 South Walker Avenue, Oklahoma City, OK 73139; tel. 405/631–1014; FAX. 405/631–4964; Anthony L. Cruse, D.O., President

Surgery Center of Edmond, 1700 South State Street, Edmon, OK 73013; tel. 405/330–1003; FAX. 405/330–1087; Timothy A. Gee, Administrator

Surgery Center of Midwest City, 8121 National Avenue, Suite 108, Midwest City, OK 73110; tel. 405/732–7905; FAX. 405/732–3561; Jackie Reed, Administrator

Surgery Center of Oklahoma, 815 Northwest 12th Street, Oklahoma City, OK 73106; tel. 405/235–4525; Olivia Dick, RN, Administrator

Surgery Center of South Oklahoma City, 100 Southeast 59th Street, Oklahoma City, OK 73109; tel. 405/634–9300; FAX. 405/634–8300; Larry Smith, Administrator

The Cataract Center of Lawton, 4214 Southwest Lee Boulevard, Lawton, OK 73505; tel. 405/353–5860; Stephen W. Gilkeson, Executive Administrator

Three Rivers Surgery Center, 3800 West Okmulgee, Muskogee, OK 74401; tel. 918/682–9899; FAX. 918/687–0786; Doug Blessen, Chief Executive Officer

Tower Day Surgery, 1044 Southwest 44th Street, Suite 100, Oklahoma City, OK 73109; tel. 405/636–1701; FAX. 405/636–4314; Marie Smith, RN, Director

Triad Eye Medical Clinic and Cataract Institute, 6140 South Memorial, Tulsa, OK 74133; tel. 918/252–2020; FAX. 918/252–7466; Marc L. Abel, D.O., Medical Director

Wilson Surgery Center, 5404 West Lee Boulevard, Lawton, OK 73505; tel. 405/357–2020; Gary Wilson, M.D., Administrator

OREGON

Aesthetic Breast Care Center, 10201 Southeast Main, Suite 20, Portland, OR 97216; tel. 503/253–3458; FAX. 503/253–0856; Mary K. Barnhart, M.D., Administrator

Center for Cosmetic and Plastic Surgery, 1353 East McAndrews Road, Medford, OR 97504; tel. 541/770–6776; FAX. 541/770–5791; Robert M. Jensen, M.D., Administrator

Eye Surgery Center, 2925 Siskiyou Boulevard, Medford, OR 97504; tel. 541/779–2020; FAX. 541/770–6838; Loren R. Barrus, M.D., Administrator

Eye Surgery Institute, The, 813 S.W. Highland Ave., Redmond, OR 97756; tel. 541/548–7170; FAX. 541/548–3842; Kathleen Peterson, RN, Administrator

Futures Outpatient Surgical Center, Inc., 1849 Northwest Kearney, Suite 302, Portland, OR 97209; tel. 503/224–0723; FAX. 503/224–0722; Bryce E. Potter, M.D.

GI Endoscopy Center, 2560 N.W. Medical Park Drive, Roseburg, OR 97470; tel. 541/673–2046; FAX. 541/673–0454; Ruth E. Harpole, RN, Administrator

Lawrence W. O'Dell, d/b/a Northwest Eye Center, 9975 Southwest Nimbus Avenue, Beaverton, OR 97005; tel. 503/646–7644; Jim Heath, Administrator

Lovejoy Surgicenter, Inc., 933 Northwest 25th Avenue, Portland, OR 97210; tel. 503/221–1870; FAX. 503/221–1488; Allene M. Klass, Administrator

McKenzie Surgery Center, 940 Country Club Road, Eugene, OR 97401; tel. 541/344–2600; FAX. 541/344–3317; Lynn M. Staples, RN, Administrator

Medford Clinic, P.C., 555 Black Oak Drive, Medford, OR 97504; tel. 541/734–3520; FAX. 541/734–3597; Jon D. Ness, Chief Executive Officer

Medford Plastic Surgeons, 1690 East McAndrews Road, Medford, OR 97504; tel. 541/779–5655; FAX. 541/770–6943; R. Kenneth Pons, M.D., Administrator

North Bend Medical Center, Inc., 1900 Woodland Drive, Coos Bay, OR 97420; tel. 503/267–5151; FAX. 503/269–0797; J. Peter Johnson, Administrator

Northbank Surgical Center, 700 Bellevue Street, S., Suite 300, Salem, OR 97301; tel. 503/364–3704; Peggy Seidler, Administrator

Ontario Surgery Center, 251 S.W. 19th Street, Ontario, OR 97914; tel. 541/889–3198; FAX. 541/881–9106; Jeffrey C. Pitts, M.D., Administrator

Oregon Cataract and Laser Institute, 2700 Southeast 14th Avenue, Albany, OR 97321; tel. 503/928–1666; Darrell Genstler, M.D., Administrator

Oregon Eye Surgery Center, Inc., 1550 Oak Street, Eugene, OR 97401; tel. 541/683–8771; FAX. 541/484–4898; Virginia Pecora, RN, Administrator

Roseburg Surgicenter, LTD, 631 West Stanton, Roseburg, OR 97470; tel. 541/440–6311; FAX. 541/440–6784; Bruce Piper, CEO

The Gastroenterology Endoscopy Center, Inc., 6464 Southwest Borland Road, Suite D–4, Tualatin, OR 97062; tel. 503/692–4537; FAX. 503/691–2324; Gale R. Dupek, M.B.A., Administrator

The Oregon Clinic Gastroenterology Division Gresham Office, 24900 Southeast Stark, Suite 205, Gresham, OR 97030; tel. 503/661–2000; FAX. 503/661–2001; Jeffrey S. Albaugh, M.D., Administrator

Providers / Freestanding Ambulatory Surgery Centers

The Portland Clinic Surgical Center, 800 Southwest 13th Avenue, Portland, OR 97205; tel. 503/221-0161; FAX. 503/221-4451; J. Michael Schwab, Administrator
Tigard Surgery Center, 13240 Southwest Pacific Highway, Suite 200, Tigard, OR 97223; tel. 503/639-6571; FAX. 503/624-6037; Ivan L. Bakos, M.D., Administrator
Willamette Valley Eye SurgiCenter, 2001 Commercial Street, S.E., Salem, OR 97302; tel. 503/363-1500; FAX. 503/588-2028; Gordon Miller, M.D., Administrator

PENNSYLVANIA

Abington Surgical Center, 2701 Blair Mill Road, Suite 35, Willow Grove, PA 19090; tel. 215/443-8505; FAX. 215/957-0565; Stanley E. Grissinger, MBA, CHE, Executive Director
Aestique Ambulatory Surgical Center, One Aesthetic Way, Greensburg, PA 15601; tel. 412/832-7555; FAX. 412/832-7568; Theodore A. Lazzaro, M.D., Medical Director
Apple Hill Surgical Center, 25 Monument Road, Suite 270, York, PA 17403; tel. 717/741-8250; FAX. 717/741-8254; Gwendolyn J. Grothouse, RN, Administrative Director
Delaware Valley Laser Surgery Institute, Two Bala Plaza, Pl 33, Bala Cynwd, PA 19004; tel. 215/668-2847; FAX. 215/668-1509; Herbert J. Nevyas, M.D., Medical Director
Dermatologic Surgery Center, P.C., 6415 Bustleton Avenue, Philadelphia, PA 19149
Dermatologic SurgiCenter, 1200 Locust Street, Philadelphia, PA 19107; tel. 215/546-3666; FAX. 215/546-6060; Anthony V. Benedetto, D.O., FACP, Medical Director
Dermatologic SurgiCenter, 2221 Garrett Road, Drexel Hill, PA 19026; tel. 610/623-5885; FAX. 610/623-7276; Anthony V. Benedetto, D.O. Medical Director
Digestive Disease Institute, 899 Poplar Church Road, Camp Hill, PA 17011; tel. 717/763-1239; FAX. 717/763-9854; Iris Garman, Administrator
Eye Clinic Ambulatory Surgical Center, Inc., 601 Wyoming Avenue, Kingston, PA 18704; tel. 717/288-7405; Mark Kelly, Administrator
Fairgrounds Surgical Center, 400 North 17th Street, Suite 300, Allentown, PA 18104; tel. 610/821-2020; FAX. 610/821-2016; Darlene G. Hinkle/ Debi Baker, Co-Administrative Directors
Fort Washington Surgery Center, 467 Pennsylvania Avenue, Fort Washington, PA 19034; tel. 215/628-4300; FAX. 215/628-4253; Charles Pappas, M. D.
Grandview Surgery & Laser Center, 205 Grandview Avenue, Camp Hill, PA 17011; tel. 717/731-5444; FAX. 717/731-0415; Mary Turnbaugh, Administrator
Hanover Surgicenter, 3130 Grandview Road, Building B, Hanover, PA 17331; tel. 717/633-1600; FAX. 717/633-6556; Melvin L. Brooks, Jr., CRNA, Administrator
Healthsouth Mt. Pleasant Surgery Center, 200 Bessemer Road, Mt. Pleasant, PA 15666; tel. 412/547-5432; FAX. 412/547-2435; Brian Kowleczny, Administrative Director
HealthSouth Scranton Surgery and Laser Center, 425 Adams Street, Scranton, PA 18510; tel. 717/348-1114; FAX. 717/347-4351; Nancy A. Nealcn, RN, B.S.N., Administrative Director
HealthSouth Surgery Center of Lancaster, 217 Harrisburg Avenue, Suite 103, Lancaster, PA 17603; tel. 717/295-2500; FAX. 717/295-4898; Mary Turnbaugh, Administrator
Jefferson Surgery Center, Coal Valley Road, P.O. Box 18420, Pittsburgh, PA 15236; tel. 412/469-6060; FAX. 412/469-7322; Sheran Sullivan, Manager
John A. Zitelli, M.D., P.C., Ambulatory Surgery Facility, 5200 Centre Avenue, Suite 303, Pittsburgh, PA 15232; tel. 412/681-9400; FAX. 412/681-5240; John A. Zitelli, M.D.
Kremer Laser Eye Center, 200 Mall Boulevard, King of Pruss, PA 19406; tel. 610/337-1580; FAX. 610/337-1815; Tara Hopewell, RN
Lebanon Outpatient Surgical Center, L.P., 830 Tuck Street, Lebanon, PA 17042; tel. 717/228-1620; FAX. 717/228-1642; Anita Gingrich Fuhrman, R.N., B.S., Director
Lowry SurgiCenter, 1115 Lowry Avenue, Jeannette, PA 15644; tel. 412/527-2885; FAX. 412/527-6885; K. Diddle, M.D., Medical Director
Mt. Lebanon Surgical Center, Professional Office Building, 1050 Bower Hill Road, Suite 102, Pittsburgh, PA 15243; tel. 412/563-6808; FAX. 412/563-6857; Patricia Strosnider, Director, Nursing

N.E.I. Ambulatory Surgery, Inc., 204 Mifflin Avenue, Scranton, PA 18503; tel. 717/342-3145; FAX. 717/342-3136
North Shore Surgi-Center, Two Allegheny Center, Suite 530, Pittsburgh, PA 15212-5493; tel. 412/231-0200; FAX. 412/231-0613; Jack Demos, M.D., FACS
Northwood Surgery Center, 3729 Easton-Nazareth Highway, Easton, PA 18045; tel. 610/559-7110; FAX. 610/559-7317; Chitu Patel, Administrator
Ophthalmology Laser and Surgery Center, Inc., 92 Tuscarora Street, Harrisburg, PA 17104; tel. 717/233-2020; FAX. 717/232-3294; Jeanne Megella, RN,CNOR, Director, Nursing
Paoli Surgery Center, One Industrial Boulevard, Paoli, PA 19301; tel. 610/408-0822; FAX. 610/408-9933; Marcia L. Collymore, Facility Manager
Pennsylvania Eye Surgery Center, 4100 Linglestown Road, Harrisburg, PA 17112; tel. 717/657-2020; FAX. 717/657-2071; Sandra Benner, RN, Director, Surgical Services
Pocono Ambulatory Surgery Center, One Veterans Place, Stroudsburg, PA 18360; tel. 570/421-4978; Mary P. Hayden RN, B.S., Administrative Director
Ridgeway Esper Medical Center Ambulatory Surgical Center, 5050 West Ridge Road, Erie, PA 16506-1298; tel. 814/833-8800; FAX. 814/833-2079; Deborah Hartmann, RN, Director, Nursing
Sewickley Surgical Center at Edgeworth Commons, 301 Ohio River Boulevard, Edgeworth, Suite 100, Sewickley, PA 15143; tel. 412/741-5866; FAX. 412/741-5884; Carol Figas, RN, CNOR, Supervisor
Shadyside Surgi-Center, Inc., 5727 Centre Avenue, Pittsburgh, PA 15206; tel. 412/363-6626; FAX. 412/363-7008; Susan M. Katch, RN, Director
Southwestern Ambulatory Surgery Center, 500 Lewis Run Road, Pittsburgh, PA 15236; tel. 412/469-6964; FAX. 412/469-6948; Pamela Wroblenski, CRNA, M.P.M., Director
Southwestern Pennsylvania Eye Center, 750 East Beau Street, Washington, PA 15301; tel. 412/228-7477; FAX. 412/228-6271; Mary Roth, R.N., Clinical Director
St. Francis Surgery Center North, One St. Francis Way, Cranberry Tow, PA 16066; tel. 412/772-5360; FAX. 412/772-4644; Gerry Matt, RN, M.Ed., Director
Surgery Center of Bucks County, 401 North York Road, Warminster, PA 18974; tel. 215/443-3022; FAX. 215/443-5859; JoAnn Quinn, Director, Nursing
Surgical Center of York, 1750 Fifth Avenue, P.O. Box 290, York, PA 17405; tel. 717/843-7613; FAX. 717/849-5662; Thomas R. Harlow, Administrative Director
Surgical Eye Institute of Western Pennsylvania, 618 Monongahela Avenue, Glassport, PA 15045; tel. 412/664-7874; FAX. 412/673-5720; Shirley A. Smith, RN
The Surgery Center of Chester County, 460 Creamery Way, Oaklands Corporate Center, Exton, PA 19341-2500; tel. 610/594-8900; FAX. 610/594-8907; Stephen P. Barainyak, Executive Director
The SurgiCenter at Ligonier, 221 West Main Street, Ligonier, PA 15658; tel. 724/238-9573; FAX. 724/238-9474; Kim Kenney-Ciarimboli, Manager
UPMC Monroeville Surgery Center, 125 Daugherty Drive, Monroeville, PA 15146-2749; tel. 412/374-9385; FAX. 412/374-9490; Carol Fiske Boumbouras, CMSC, Administrative Assistant, Medical Staff Mgr.
West Shore Endoscopy Center, 423 North 21st Street, Camp Hill, PA 17011; tel. 717/975-2430; FAX. 717/730-2150; Marilee Ball, RN, Director
Wills Eye Surgery Center of the Northeast, 1815 Cottman Avenue, Philadelphia, PA 19111; tel. 215/722-2505; FAX. 215/742-6386; Lawrence S. Schaffzin, M.D., Medical Director
Wyoming Valley Surgery Center, 1130 Highway 315, Wilkes-Barre, PA 18702; tel. 717/821-2830; FAX. 717/825-7962; David N. Culp, Chief Executive Officer

RHODE ISLAND

Bayside Endoscopy Center, 120 Dudley Street, Suite 103, Providence, RI 02905; tel. 401/274-1810; FAX. 401/273-9689; Nicholas Califano, M.D., Administrator
Blackstone Valley Surgicare, Inc., 333 School Street, Pawtucket, RI 02860; tel. 401/728-3800; FAX. 401/723-2440; Ann Dugan, Administrator

Koch Eye Surgi Center, Inc., 566 Tollgate Road, Warwick, RI 02886; tel. 401/738-4800; FAX. 401/738-8153; Paul S. Koch, M.D., Administrator
Ocean State Endoscopy, 100 Highland Avenue, Providence, RI 02906; tel. 401/421-6306; Joel Spellun, M.D.
Planned Parenthood of Rhode Island, 111 Point Street, Providence, RI 02903; tel. 401/421-9620; FAX. 401/621-6250; Miriam Inocencio, President and CEO
Wayland Square Surgicare, 17 Seekonk Street, Providence, RI 02906; tel. 401/453-3311; FAX. 401/351-1280; Ann Dugan, Administrator
Women's Medical Center, 1725 Broad Street, Cranston, RI 02905; tel. 401/467-9111; FAX. 401/461-1390; Nancy Ganem, Administrator

SOUTH CAROLINA

Ambulatory Eye Surgery and Laser Center, Inc., 9297 Medical Plaza Drive, Charleston, SC 29406; tel. 803/572-2888; Margaret A. Thompson
Bay Microsurgical Unit, Inc., 400 Marina Drive, P.O. 2800, Georgetown, SC 29442; tel. 803/546-8421; FAX. 803/546-1173; Janet Spring, Administrator and Director of Nursing
Bearwood Ambulatory Surgery Center, 3031 Highway 81, N., Anderson, SC 29621; tel. 864/226-0837; FAX. 864/226-8367; Patricia P. Smith, Administrator
Carolina Eye Ambulatory Surgery Center, 410 University Parkway, Suite 1500 B, Aiken, SC 29801; tel. 803/649-3953; FAX. 803/641-3801; Stephen K. Vanderbilt, M.D.
Carolina Regional Surgery Center, Ltd., 944 Medical Circle, Myrtle Beach, SC 29572; tel. 803/449-7885; FAX. 803/497-5137; Mary Garvey, RN, Administrator
Carolina Surgical Center, 198 South Herlong Avenue, Rock Hill, SC 29732; tel. 803/327-4664; Gary Fillers, Administrator
Charleston Plastic Surgery Center, Inc., 261 Calhoun St., Ste. 200, Charleston, SC 29401; tel. 843/722-1985; FAX. 843/722-4840; Anna Lambert, Office Manager
Columbia Eye Surgery Center, Inc., 1920 Pickens Street, P.O. Box 1754, Columbia, SC 29202; tel. 803/254-7732; FAX. 803/748-7199; Kenneth W. Gibbons, Administrator
Columbia Gastrointestinal Endoscopy Center, 2739 Laurel Street, Suite One-B, Columbia, SC 29240; tel. 803/254-9588; FAX. 803/252-0052; Cindy Sease, R.N.-CGRN, Center Director
Columbia Surgery Center, Inc., 338 Harbison Boulevard, Columbia, SC 29212; tel. 803/732-6655; FAX. 803/732-6644; Vickie H. Ott, Administrator
Cross Creek Surgery Center of Greenville Hospital System, Nine Doctors Drive, Crosscreek Medical Park, Greenville, SC 29605; tel. 803/455-8400; Barbara Callahan, Administrator
Greenville Endoscopy Center, Inc., 317 St. Francis Drive, Suite 150, Greenville, SC 29601; tel. 864/232-7338; FAX. 864/240-8140; Rebecca K. Swoyer, Administrator
HealthSouth Surgery Center of Charleston, 2690 Lake Park Drive, North Charles, SC 29406; tel. 803/764-0992; FAX. 803/764-3187; Donna Padgette, RN, M.S.N., Facility Manager
Healthsouth Surgery Center of Greenville, Five Memorial Medical Court, Greenville, SC 29605; tel. 864/295-3067; FAX. 864/295-3096; Cathy Rudisill, Facility Manager
Medicus Surgery Center, Inc., 107 Professional Court, P.O. Box 1886, Anderson, SC 29622-1886; tel. 864/225-1933; FAX. 864/716-7965; Ann Geier, R.N., M.S., CNOR, Chief Operating Officer
Outpatient Surgery Center of Lexington Medical Center in Irmo, 7035 Saint Andrews Road, Columbia, SC 29212; tel. 803/749-0924; Barbara Williams, Administrator
Pee Dee Ambulatory Surgery Center, 602 Cheves, P.O. Box F-17, Florence, SC 29506; tel. 803/669-3822; Joseph J. McEvoy, Administrator
Roper West Ashley Surgery Center, 18 Farmfield Avenue, Charleston, SC 29407; tel. 803/763-3763; FAX. 803/763-3881; Maria I. Sample, Administrator
Same Day Surgery East, 10 Enterprise Boulevard, Suite 104, Greenville, SC 29615; tel. 803/458-7141; FAX. 803/676-9116; Mary Jane Knottek, RN, B.S.N., CNOR, Clinical Nurse
Spartanburg Urology Surgicenter, Inc., 391 Serpentine Drive, Suite 330, Spartanburg, SC 29303; tel. 864/585-2002; FAX. 864/585-3300; Mary Alford, RN, OR Director

Providers / Freestanding Ambulatory Surgery Centers

The Greenwood Endoscopy Center, 103 Liner Drive, Greenwood, SC 29646; tel. 803/227-3838; FAX. 803/227-6116; A. A. Ramage, M.D., Administrator

Trident Surgery Center, 9313 Medical Plaza Drive, Suite 102, Charleston, SC 29406; tel. 803/797-8992; FAX. 803/797-4094; Leah J. Dawson, Administrator

SOUTH DAKOTA

Aberdeen Surgical Center, 1200 South Main, Box 1150, Aberdeen, SD 57401-1150; tel. 605/225-2466; Scott H. Berry, M.D., Administrator

Black Hills Regional Eye Surgery Center, 2800 Third Street, Rapid City, SD 57701-7394; tel. 605/341-2000; FAX. 605/341-0278; Richard B. Hanafin, Executive Director

Jones Eye Clinic, 3801 South Elmwood Avenue, Sioux Falls, SD 57105-6565; tel. 605/336-3142; FAX. 605/334-0737; Charles E. Jones, M.D.

Mallard Pointe Surgical Center, 1201 Mickelson Drive, Watertown, SD 57201-7100; tel. 605/882-4743; FAX. 605/882-6064; Mary Petersen, Administrative Director

Medical Associates Surgi Center, 772 East Dakota, Pierre, SD 57501-3399; tel. 605/224-5901; Michael Pfeifer, Administrator

Sioux Falls Surgical Center, 910 East 20th Street, Sioux Falls, SD 57105-1012; tel. 605/334-6730; Donald A. Schellpfeffer, M.D., Ph.D., Medical Director

Spearfish Surgery Center, Inc., 1316 10th Street, Spearfish, SD 57783-1530; tel. 605/642-3113; FAX. 605/642-3117; Linda Redding, Administrator

SurgiClinic, 1010 Ninth Street, Rapid City, SD 57701-3599; tel. 605/348-7607; FAX. 605/342-1359; Ray G. Burnett, M.D., Medical Director

Women's Health Clinic, 909 South Miller, Mitchell, SD 57301; tel. 605/995-5560; Sheri Trudeau, CWP, Clinic Director

TENNESSEE

Appalachian Ambulatory Surgical Center, Medical Arts Building, 106 Rogosin Drive, Elizabethton, TN 37643; tel. 615/543-5888

Atrium Memorial Surgical Center, 1949 Gunbarrel Road, Suite 290, Chattanooga, TN 37421; tel. 615/495-3550; FAX. 615/495-3580; Sandy Proctor, Administrator

Baptist Physicians Pavilion Surgery Center, 360 Wallace Road, Nashville, TN 37211; tel. 615/781-9020; FAX. 615/781-9944

Bristol Surgery Center, 350 Blountville Highway, Suite 108, Bristol, TN 37620; tel. 423/844-6120; FAX. 423/844-6126; Jim Hodge, Administrator

Cataract Surgery Center, 5406 Knight Arnold Road, Memphis, TN 38115; tel. 901/360-8081; FAX. 901/368-3822

Centennial Surgery Center, 340 23rd Avenue, N., Nashville, TN 37203; tel. 615/327-1123; FAX. 615/327-0261; Cynthia S. Duvall, RN, B.S., Administrator

Chattanooga Surgery Center, 400 North Holtzclaw Avenue, Chattanooga, TN 37404; tel. 615/698-6871; Becky Myers, Administrator

Clarksville Endoscopy Center, 132 Hillcrest Drive, Clarksville, TN 37043; tel. 931/552-0180; FAX. 931/572-0915

Cleveland Surgery Center, L.P., 137 25th Street, N.E., Cleveland, TN 37311; tel. 423/472-7874; R. Scott Peterson, Executive Director

Columbia Endoscopy Center, Inc., 1510 1/2 Hatcher Lane, Columbia, TN 38401; tel. 615/381-7818; FAX. 615/381-5625; Dianne Roberts, RN, Head Nurse

Columbia Outpatient Surgery, Inc., 1405 Hatcher Lane, Columbia, TN 38401; tel. 615/381-3700; Judy Griffin, Administrator

Columbia Sullins Surgery Center, 2761 Sullins Street, Knoxville, TN 37919; tel. 423/522-2949; FAX. 423/637-3259; Tina Shelby-Kahl, Assistant Administrator

D D C Surgery Center, Nine Physicians Drive, Jackson, TN 38305; tel. 901/661-0086; Vicki Hale, Administrator

Digestive Disease Endoscopy Center, 22nd Avenue, North, Nashville, TN 37203; tel. 615/340-4625; FAX. 615/340-4628

East Memphis Surgery Center, 80 Humphreys Center Drive, Suite 101, Memphis, TN 38120; tel. 901/747-3233; FAX. 901/747-3230

Endoscopy Center of Kingsport, 2204 Pavilion Drive, Kingsport, TN 37660; tel. 423/392-6100; FAX. 423/392-6159; Penny Loyd, Administrator

Endoscopy Center of Northeast Tennessee, 310 State of Franklin Road, Suite 202, Johnson City, TN 37604; tel. 615/929-7111

Eye Surgery Center of East Tennessee, 1124 Weisgarber Road, Suite 110, Knoxville, TN 37909; tel. 423/588-1037; FAX. 423/909-9104; Pat Puller, RN

Eye Surgery Center of Middle Tennessee, Parkview Tower, Suite 900, 210 25th Avenue, N., Nashville, TN 37203; tel. 615/327-2244; FAX. 615/327-9254; Sharon Reesor, Surgery Center Administrator

Fort Sanders West Outpatient Surgery Center, Ltd., 210 Fort Sanders West Boulevard, Knoxville, TN 37922; tel. 615/531-5222; FAX. 615/531-5043; Leslie Irwin, Administrator

Franklin Surgery Center at MedCore, 2105 Edward Curd Lane, Franklin, TN 37067; tel. 615/794-7320

G. Baker Hubbard Ambulatory Surgery Center, 616 West Forest Avenue, Jackson, TN 38301; tel. 901/422-0330

G. I. Diagnostic and Therapeutic Center, 1068 Cresthaven Road, Suite 300, Memphis, TN 38119; tel. 901/682-6700; FAX. 901/683-3046; Randolph M. McCloy, M.D., Medical Director

Germantown Ambulatory Surgical Center, Inc., 7499 Old Poplar Pike, Germantown, TN 38138; tel. 901/755-6465; FAX. 901/757-5543; Carol Harper, Facility Manager

Health South Surgery Center of Clarksville, 121 Hillcrest Drive, Clarksville, TN 37043; tel. 615/552-9992

HealthSouth Nashville Surgery Center, 1717 Patterson Street, Nashville, TN 37203; tel. 615/329-1888; FAX. 615/329-0179; Patricia Middleton, Facility Manager

HealthSouth Surgery Center of Chattanooga, 924 Spring Creek Road, Chattanooga, TN 37412; tel. 423/899-1600; FAX. 423/899-2171; Melissa Powers, Administrator

Kingsport Bronchoscopy Center, Inc., 135 West Ravine Road, Suite Eight-A, Kingsport, TN 37660; tel. 615/247-5197; FAX. 615/247-5254; Shirley Hawkins, Administrator

Kingsport Endoscopy Corporation, 135 West Ravine Street, Suite 7A, Kingsport, TN 37660; tel. 423/246-6777; Bettye Reed, Administrator

Knoxville Center for Reproductive Health, 1547 West Clinch Avenue, Knoxville, TN 37916; tel. 423/637-3861; FAX. 865/637-0222; Bernadette McNabb, Executive Director

Knoxville Surgery Center, 9300 Park West Boulevard, Knoxville, TN 37923; tel. 615/691-2725; FAX. 615/691-3090; Ranae Thompson, RN, Facility Administrator

Lebanon Surgery Center, Inc., 1414 Baddour Parkway, P.O. Box 549, Lebanon, TN 37088; tel. 615/444-8944; Sheena Sloan, Administrator

LeBonheur East Surgery Center, L.P., 786 Estate Place, Memphis, TN 38120; tel. 901/681-4100; FAX. 901/681-4140; Sarah Wainscott, Director

Maternity Center of East Tennessee, 1925-B Ailor Avenue, Knoxville, TN 37921; tel. 615/524-4422

Mays & Schnapp Pain Clinic and Rehabilitation Center, 55 Humphreys Center Drive, Suite 200, Memphis, TN 38120; tel. 901/747-0040; FAX. 901/747-3424; Lori Parris, RN, Administrator

Medical Center Endoscopy Group, 930 Madison, Suite 870, Memphis, TN 38103; tel. 901/578-2538; FAX. 901/578-2572; John W. Flowers, Business Manager

Memphis Area Medical Center for Women, 29 South Bellevue Boulevard, Memphis, TN 38104; tel. 901/722-8050

Memphis Center for Reproductive Health, 1462 Poplar Avenue, Memphis, TN 38104; tel. 901/274-3550

Memphis Eye and Cataract Ambulatory Surgery Center, 6485 Poplar Avenue, Memphis, TN 38119; tel. 901/767-3937

Memphis Gastroenterology Group, 80 Humphrey's Blvd., Suite 220, Memphis, TN 38120; tel. 901/747-3630; FAX. 901/747-0039; Sylvia Hawkins, RN, Nurse Manager

Memphis Planned Parenthood, Inc., 1407 Union Avenue, Third Floor, Memphis, TN 38104; tel. 901/725-1717

Memphis Regional Gamma Knife Center, 1265 Union Avenue, Memphis, TN 38104; tel. 901/726-6444

Memphis Surgery Center, 1044 Cresthaven Road, Memphis, TN 38119; tel. 901/682-1516; FAX. 901/682-1545; Jane Almon R.N., CNOR, Facility Administrator

Mid-State Endoscopy Center, 2010 Church Street, Suite 420, Nashville, TN 37203; tel. 615/329-2141; FAX. 615/321-0522; Allan H. Bailey, M.D., Medical Director

Nashville Endoscopy Center, 300 20th N., Eighth Floor, Nashville, TN 37203; tel. 615/284-1335; FAX. 615/284-1316; Margaret Sullivan, RN

Nashville Gastrointestinal Endoscopy Center, 4230 Harding Road, Suite 309, Nashville, TN 37205; tel. 615/383-0165; FAX. 615/292-4657; Ron E. Pruitt, M.D.

Ophthalmic Ambulatory Surgery Center, P.C., 342 22nd Street, Nashville, TN 37203; tel. 615/327-2001; FAX. 615/327-2069; Alec Dryden, Administrator

Oral Facial Surgery Center, 322 22nd Avenue, N., Nashville, TN 37203; tel. 615/321-6160; FAX. 615/327-9612; Dawn R. Shirley, C.P.A., Administrator

Physicians Surgery Center, 207 Stonebridge, Jackson, TN 38305; tel. 901/661-6340; FAX. 901/661-6363; Judy Haskins, RN, Manager

Planned Parenthood Association of Nashville, 412 D.B. Todd Boulevard, Nashville, TN 37203; tel. 615/321-7216

Ridge Lake Ambulatory Surgery Center, 825 Ridge Lake Boulevard, Memphis, TN 38119; tel. 901/685-0777

Rivergate Surgery Center, 647 Myatt Drive, Madison, TN 37115; tel. 615/868-8942; FAX. 615/860-3820; Brenda Cruse, Director

Shea Clinic, 6133 Poplar Pike, Memphis, TN 38119; tel. 901/761-9720; FAX. 901/683-8440

Southern Endoscopy Center, 397 Wallace Road, Suite 407, Nashville, TN 37211; tel. 615/832-5530; FAX. 615/832-5713; Robert W. Herring, Jr., M.D., Medical Director

St. Thomas Medical Group Endoscopy Center, 4230 Harding Road, Suite 400, Nashville, TN 37205; tel. 615/297-2700; Deborah MacDonald, R.N.

Surgical Services, P.C., 604 South Main Street, Sweetwater, TN 37874; tel. 423/337-4508; FAX. 423/337-4588

Surgicenter Of Murfreesboro Medical Clinic, P.A., 1004 North Highland Avenue, Murfreesboro, TN 37130; tel. 615/893-4480; FAX. 615/876-7876; Barbara Norton, R.N., Coordinator

Tennessee Endoscopy Center, 1706 East Lamar Alexander Parkway, Maryville, TN 37804; tel. 615/983-0073; FAX. 615/984-1731; Craig Jarvis, M.D., Administrator

The Cookeville Surgery Center, 100 West Fourth Street, Suite 100, Cookeville, TN 38501; tel. 615/528-6115; FAX. 615/526-2962; Diana Welch, RN, Administrator

The Endoscopy Center, 801 Weisgarber Road, Suite 100, Knoxville, TN 37909, Knoxville, TN 37950-9002; tel. 615/588-5121; Gayle Mahan, Office Manager

The Endoscopy Center of Centennial, L.P., 2400 Patterson Street, Suite 515, Nashville, TN 37203; tel. 615/327-2111; FAX. 615/327-9292; Donna Corn, RN, B.S., Endoscopy Administrator

The Eye Surgery Center Oak Ridge, 90 Vermont Avenue, Oak Ridge, TN 37830; tel. 423/482-8894; Sally Jones

Tullahoma Outpatient Surgery Center, 1918 North Jackson, Tullahoma, TN 37388; tel. 615/455-2006

Urology Surgery Center, Inc., 2011 Church Street, Sixth Floor, Nashville, TN 37203; tel. 615/284-4488; David Hill, Chairman

Van Dyke Ambulatory Surgery Center, 1024 Kelley Drive, Paris, TN 38242; tel. 901/642-5003; FAX. 901/642-8756; John T. VanDyck, III, M.D., Owner

Volunteer Medical Clinic, 313 Concord Street, Knoxville, TN 37919; tel. 423/522-5173; FAX. 423/522-9907; Lisa Thomas, Clinical Director

Wesberry Surgery Center, 2900 South Perkins Road, Memphis, TN 38118-3237; tel. 901/362-3100; FAX. 901/362-3372; Jesse Wesberry, Jr., M.D., President

Wesley Ophthalmic Plastic Surgery Center, 250 25th Avenue North, Suite 213, Nashville, TN 37203; tel. 615/329-3624; Janie Stucker, R.N., Director

Women's Wellness and Maternity Center, Inc., 3459 Highway 68, Madisonville, TN 37354; tel. 423/442-6624; FAX. 423/442-5746; Betti Wilson, Administrator

TEXAS

Abilene Cataract and Refractive Surgery Center, 2120 Antilley Road, Abilene, TX 79606; tel. 915/695-1999; FAX. 915/695-2326; Robert W. Cameron, M.D., Medical Director

Abilene Endoscopy Center, 1249 Ambler Avenue, Abilene, TX 79601; tel. 915/695-2020; Gary Roark, M.D., Medical Director

Providers / Freestanding Ambulatory Surgery Centers

Amarillo Cataract and Eye Surgery Center, Inc., 7310 Fleming Avenue, Amarillo, TX 79106; tel. 806/354-8891; FAX. 806/354-2591; Carol A. Pearson, Director

Ambulatory Urological Surgery Center, Inc., 1149 Ambler, Abilene, TX 79601; tel. 915/676-3557; FAX. 915/673-2143; Angela X. Young, RN, Manager

American Surgery Centers of South Texas, LTD, 7810 Louis Pasteur, Suite 101, San Antonio, TX 78229; tel. 210/692-0218; Britt F. Mitchell, C.O.T., Director, Operations

Bailey Square Surgical Center, Ltd., 1111 West 34th Street, Austin, TX 78705; tel. 512/454-6753; FAX. 512/454-4314; Donna Hutto, R.N., CNOR, Director of Nursing Services Operation

Barbara Jean Bartlett Memorial Surgery Center, 4200 Andrews Highway, Midland, TX 79703; tel. 915/520-5888; FAX. 915/520-9801; Sylvan Bartlett, M.D., Administrator

Bay Area Endoscopy Center, 444 FM 1959, Houston, TX 77034; tel. 281/481-9400; FAX. 281/481-9490; N.S. Bala, Medical Director

Bay Area Surgery, 7101 South Padre Island Drive, Corpus Christi, TX 78412; tel. 361/761-3500; FAX. 361/761-3754; Gene Hybner, Administrator

Bay Area Surgicare Center, 502 Medical Center Boulevard, P.O. Box 57767, Webster, TX 77598; tel. 281/332-2433; FAX. 281/332-0619; Carol Simons, Administrator

Baylor SurgiCare, 3920 Worth Street, Dallas, TX 75246; tel. 214/820-2581; FAX. 214/820-7484; Robin Shaw, Administrative Director

Bellaire Surgicare, Inc., 6699 Chimney Rock, Suite 200, Houston, TX 77081; tel. 713/665-1406; FAX. 713/665-8262; Sheila M. Liccketto, Administrator

Brazosport Eye Institute, 103 Parking Way, P.O. Box 369, Lake Jackson, TX 77566; tel. 409/297-2961; FAX. 409/297-2395; Frank J. Grady, M.D., Ph.D., FACS, Director

Brownsville Surgicare, 1024 Los Ebanos Boulevard, Brownsville, TX 78520; tel. 210/548-0101; FAX. 210/541-3752; Norberto J. Sanchez, Administrator

Central Texas Day Surgery Center, L.P., 1817 Southwest Dodgen, Loop, Temple, TX 76502; tel. 817/773-7785; FAX. 817/773-9333; Debby Meyer, Director

Coastal Bend Ambulatory Surgical Center, 900 Morgan, Corpus Christi, TX 78404; tel. 512/888-4288; FAX. 512/888-4786; Barbara VanderBout

Columbia Physicians DaySurgery Center, 3930 Crutcher Street, Dallas, TX 75246; tel. 214/827-0760; FAX. 214/827-0944; Vickie Roberts, RN, Administrator

Columbia Surgery Center of Las Colinas, 4255 North Macarthur Boulevard, Irving, TX 75038; tel. 214/257-0144; FAX. 214/258-0436; Bill Beaman, Administrator

Columbia Surgery Center of Sherman, 3400 North Calais Drive, Sherman, TX 75090; tel. 903/813-3377; FAX. 903/870-7617

Columbia Surgical Center, 2800 East 29th Street, P.O. Box 2700, Bryan, TX 77805; tel. 409/776-4300; FAX. 409/774-7149; Bob Lemay R.N., Director

Columbia Surgical Center of Southeast Texas, 3127 College Street, Beaumont, TX 77701; tel. 409/835-2607; Jim Hoeks, Administrator

Columbia West Houston Surgicare, 970 Campbell Road, Houston, TX 77024-2804; tel. 713/461-3547; FAX. 713/722-8921; Edward Downs, Administrator

Covenant Surgicenter, Ltd., 2301 Quaker Avenue, Lubbock, TX 79410; tel. 806/793-8801; David S. Weil, Executive Director

Crystal Outpatient Surgery Center, Inc., 215 Oak Drive, S., Suite J, Lake Jackson, TX 77566; tel. 409/299-6118; FAX. 409/299-1007; R. Scott Yarish, M.D., Administrator

Cy-Fair Surgery Center, 11250 Fallbrook Drive, Houston, TX 77065; tel. 713/955-7194; FAX. 713/890-0895; Scott Washko, Administrator

Dallas Day Surgery Center, Inc., 411 North Washington, Suite 5400, Dallas, TX 75246; tel. 214/821-8613; Henry S. Byrd, President

Dallas Ophthalmology Center, Inc., 4633 North Central Expressway, Suite 310, Dallas, TX 75205; tel. 214/520-7600; FAX. 214/528-6522; Jean Vining, RN, Administrator

Dallas Surgi Center, 8230 Walnut Hill Lane, Suite 808, Dallas, TX 75231; tel. 214/696-8828; FAX. 214/696-1444

DeHaven Surgical Center, Inc., 1424 East Front Street, Tyler, TX 75702; tel. 903/595-4168; FAX. 903/595-6821; Barbara Shamburger, RN, Administrator

Diagnostic Clinic of San Antonio Ambulatory Surgical Center, 4647 Medical Drive, P.O. Box 29249, San Antonio, TX 78224-3100; tel. 210/692-3382; FAX. 512/692-3397; Nancy Nixon, RN, ASC Supervisor

Doctors Surgery Center, Inc., 5300 North Street, Nacogdoches, TX 75961; tel. 409/569-8278; FAX. 409/569-0275; Robert P. Lehmann, M.D., Director

East El Paso Surgery Center, 7835 Corral Drive, El Paso, TX 79915; tel. 915/595-3353; FAX. 915/595-6796; Connie Ortiz, Administrator

East Side Surgery Center, Inc., 10918 East Freeway, Houston, TX 77029; tel. 713/451-4299; FAX. 713/451-4383; John Bennett, Administrator

East Texas Eye Associates Surgery Center, 1306 Frank Avenue, Lufkin, TX 75904; tel. 409/634-8381; Jo Ann O'Neill, C.O.T., Administrator

El Paso Institute of Eye Surgery, Inc., 1717 North Brown Street, Building Three, El Paso, TX 79902; tel. 915/544-0526; FAX. 915/544-2877; Esthern A. Calderon, Administrator

Elm Place Ambulatory Surgical Center, 2217 South Danville Drive, Abilene, TX 79605; tel. 915/695-0600; FAX. 915/695-3908; Susan King, RN, Director

Endoscopy Center of Dallas, Ambulatory Endoscopy Clinic of Dallas, 6390 LBJ Freeway, Suite 200, Dallas, TX 75240; tel. 972/934-3691; FAX. 972/934-3644; Jeane Suggs, Administrator

Facial Plastic and Cosmetic Surgical Center, 6300 Humana Plaza, Suite 475, Abilene, TX 79606; tel. 915/695-3630; FAX. 915/695-3633; Howard A. Tobin, M.D., FACS, Medical Director

Forest Park Surgery Pavilion, 5920 Forest Park Road, Suite 700, Dallas, TX 75235; tel. 214/350-2400; FAX. 214/352-3853; Mark Turner, Administrator

Fort Worth Endoscopy Center, 1201 Summit Avenue, Suite 400, Fort Worth, TX 76102; tel. 817/332-6500; Donna Drerup, RN, M.S.N., Administrator

Foundation Surgery Center of Dickinson, 3810 Hughes Court, Dickinson, TX 77539; tel. 713/337-7001; FAX. 713/337-7091; Sara Bledsoe, Administrator

Garland Surgery Center L.P., 777 Walter Reed Boulevard, Suite 105, Garland, TX 75042; tel. 214/494-2400; FAX. 214/494-3873; Dan Nicholson, President

Gastroenterology Consultants Outpatient Surgical Center, 8214 Wurzbach, San Antonio, TX 78229; tel. 210/614-1234; FAX. 210/614-7749; Bonnie Draude, B.S.N., RN, C.G.RN, Clinical Manager

Gastrointestinal Endoscopy Center Number Two, LTD, 1600 Coit Road, Suite 401A, Plano, TX 75075; tel. 214/867-0019; Brian Cooley, M.D., Administrator

Gonzaba Surgical Center, 720 Pleasanton Road, San Antonio, TX 78214; tel. 210/921-3826; FAX. 210/923-3825; William Gonzaba, M.D., Chief Executive Officer

Gramercy Outpatient Surgery Center, LTD, 2727 Gramercy, Houston, TX 77025; tel. 713/660-6900; FAX. 713/660-0704; Kimberly Evans, R.N., B.S.N., Clinical Director

Healthsouth Arlington Day Surgery, 918 North Davis Street, Arlington, TX 76012; tel. 817/860-9933; FAX. 817/860-2314; Diane Wood, RN, Administrator

HealthSouth Northeast Surgery Center, 18929 Highway 59, Humble, TX 77338; tel. 713/446-4053; Holly Reems, R.N.

Healthsouth Outpatient Surgery Center, 7515 South Main Street, Suite 800, Houston, TX 77030; tel. 713/796-9666; FAX. 713/796-9660; Joan M. Culberson, RN, Administrator

HealthSouth Surgery Center of Beaumont, 3050 Liberty, Beaumont, TX 77702; tel. 409/835-3535; FAX. 409/835-6005; Tammie Clodfelter, Administrator

HealthSouth Surgery Center of Conroe, 233 Interstate 45 N., P.O. Box 3091, Conroe, TX 77304; tel. 409/760-3443; FAX. 409/760-1322; Kathy Schutz, RN, B.S.N., Facility Administrator

HealthSouth Surgery Center of Dallas, 7150 Greenville Avenue, Suite 200, Dallas, TX 75231; tel. 214/891-0466; FAX. 214/739-4702; Vicki V. Schultz, RN, Administrator

HealthSouth Surgery Center of Southwest Houston, 8111 Southwest Freeway, Houston, TX 77074; tel. 713/988-7600; FAX. 713/988-4070; Karen Whigham, Administrator

HealthSouth Surgery Center or Dunkanville, 1018 East Wheatland Road, Duncanville, TX 75116; tel. 972/296-6912; FAX. 972/296-6912; Dewayne Hodges, Administrator

HealthSouth Waco Surgery Center, 2911 Herring, Waco, TX 76708; tel. 817/755-4430; FAX. 817/755-4590; Kay H. O'Leary, RN, Administrator

Heart of Texas Outpatient Cataract Center, 100 South Park Drive, Brownwood, TX 76801; tel. 915/643-3561; FAX. 915/646-0670; Larry Smith, CRNA, Administrator

Heritage Surgery Center, 1501 Redbud, McKinney, TX 75069; tel. 214/548-0771; FAX. 214/562-2300; Rudolf Churner, M.D., Administrator

Howerton Eye and Laser Surgical Center, 2610 I.H. 35 South, Austin, TX 78704-5703; tel. 512/443-9715; FAX. 512/443-9845; Ernest E. Howerton, M.D., Administrator

Key Whitman Surgery Center, 2801 Lemmon Avenue, Suite 400, Dallas, TX 75204; tel. 214/754-0000; FAX. 214/754-0079; Jeffrey Whitman, M.D.

Longview Ambulatory Surgical Center, 703 East Marshall Avenue, Suite 2000, Longview, TX 75601-5563; tel. 903/236-2111; FAX. 903/236-2479; Jerry D. Adair, President and CEO

Lufkin Endoscopy Center, 317 Gaslight Boulevard, Lufkin, TX 75901; tel. 409/634-3713; FAX. 409/634-8136; Bhagvan R. Malladi, M.D., Administrator

Maddox Outpatient Eye Surgery Center, 1755 Curie Drive, El Paso, TX 79902; tel. 915/544-9597; FAX. 915/533-3460; Robert M. Maddox, M.D., Administrator

Mann Berkeley Eye Center, 1200 Binz, Suite 1000, Houston, TX 77004; tel. 713/526-1600; FAX. 713/529-5254; Darcy Falbey, Director of Nursing

Mann Cataract Surgery Center, 18850 South Memorial Boulevard, Humble, TX 77338; tel. 713/446-9164; Elpidio Fahel, Administrator

Medical City Dallas Ambulatory Surgery Center, 7777 Forest Lane, Suite C-150, Dallas, TX 75220; tel. 214/661-7000; FAX. 214/788-6181; Sheila Everly, Chief Nursing Executive

Medical Mall Surgery Center, Inc., 1665 Antilley Road, Suite 170, Abilene, TX 79606; tel. 915/692-6694; FAX. 915/691-1568; Melissa Boyd, RN

Memorial Herman Subar Land Health-Center, 1211 Highway Six, Suite One, Sugarland, TX 77478; tel. 713/242-7200; Richelle Webb, Administrator

Methodist Ambulatory Surgery Center-Central San Antonio, 1008 Brooklyn Avenue, San Antonio, TX 78215-1600; tel. 210/225-0496; FAX. 210/225-8462; Carl J. Collazo, Administrator

Methodist Malone and Hogan-Texas Surgery, 1501 West 11th Place, Big Spring, TX 79720-4199; tel. 915/267-1623; FAX. 915/267-1137; Penny Phillips, Administrator

Metroplex Ambulatory Surgical Center, 2717 Osler Drive, Suite 102, Grand Prairie, TX 75051; tel. 214/647-6272; FAX. 972/660-1822; Glenda Daniels, RN, Director

Metroplex Surgicare, 1600 Central Drive, Suite 180, Bedford, TX 76022; tel. 817/571-1999; FAX. 817/571-1220; Julie Walker, Administrator

Mid-Town Surgical Center, Inc., 2105 Jackson Street, Suite 200, Houston, TX 77003; tel. 713/659-3050; FAX. 713/659-8359; Sylvia Nunez Reyes, R.N.

North Carrier Surgicenter, 517 North Carrier Parkway, Suite A, Grand Prairie, TX 75050-5494; tel. 214/264-0533; FAX. 214/262-5974; Abraham F. Syrquin, M.D., Medical Director

North Dallas Surgicare, 375 Municipal Drive, Suite 214, Richardson, TX 75080; tel. 214/918-9400; FAX. 214/918-9749; Bill MacKnight, Administrator

North Texas Surgi-Center, 917 Midwestern Parkway, E., Wichita Falls, TX 76302; tel. 817/767-7273; FAX. 817/723-9059; Barbara Dawson, Administrator

Northeast Texas Surgical Center, 1801 Galleria Oaks Drive, Texarkana, TX 75503; tel. 903/792-2108; FAX. 903/792-0606; Ruby Bearden, Business Manager

Northwest Ambulatory Surgery Center, 2833 Babcock Road, San Antonio, TX 78229; tel. 210/705-5100; FAX. 210/705-5025; R. Edwards, R.N., Manager

Providers / Freestanding Ambulatory Surgery Centers

Outpatient Surgical Center, 2507 Medical Row, Suite 101, Grand Prairie, TX 75051; tel. 214/647-8520; Jack Gray, Administrator

Outpatient Surgisite, 401-A East Pinecrest Drive, Marshall, TX 75670; tel. 903/938-3110; Carol C. Hall

Park Central Surgical Center, 12200 Park Central Drive, Third Floor, Dallas, TX 75251; tel. 972/661-0505; FAX. 972/661-0505; Molly Paulose, Administrator

Piney Point Ambulatory Surgery Center, 2500 Fondren, Suite 350, Houston, TX 77063; tel. 713/782-8279; FAX. 713/782-3139

Plano Ambulatory Surgery Associates, L.P., d/b/a Columbia Surgery Center of Plano, 1620 Coit Road, Plano, TX 75075-7799; tel. 972/519-1100; Dolores Holland

Plastic and Reconstructive Surgery Centre of the SW, 461 WestPark Way, Euless, TX 76040; tel. 817/540-1755; Catherine Lugger, Director

Plaza Day Surgery, 909 Ninth Avenue, Fort Worth, TX 76104-3986; tel. 817/336-6060; FAX. 817/339-2329; Deborah Pelton R.N., CNOR, Administrator

Port Arthur Day Surgery Center, 3449 Gates Boulevard, Port Arthur, TX 77642; tel. 409/983-6144; Vicki Clark, Administrative Director

Premier Ambulatory Surgery of Austin, 4207 James Casey, Suite 203, Austin, TX 78745; tel. 512/440-7894; FAX. 512/440-1932; Patricia Philbin, Executive Director

Regional Eye Surgery Center, 107 West 30th Street, Pampa, TX 79065; tel. 806/665-0051; FAX. 806/665-0640; George R. Walters, M.D., President

Rio Grande Surgery Center, 1809 South Cynthia, McAllen, TX 78503; tel. 956/618-4402; FAX. 956/618-4174; Janet R. West, Administrator

San Antonio Digestive Disease Endoscopy Center, 1804 Northeast Loop 410, Suite 101, San Antonio, TX 78217; tel. 210/828-8400; FAX. 210/828-8648

San Antonio Eye Surgicenter, 800 McCullough, San Antonio, TX 78215; tel. 210/226-6169; FAX. 210/226-6383; Carol Harris, Administrator

San Antonio Gastroenterology Endoscopy Center, 520 Euclid Avenue, San Antonio, TX 78212; tel. 210/271-0606; FAX. 210/271-0180; Ernesto Guerra, M.D.

San Antonio Surgery Center, Inc., 5290 Medical Drive, San Antonio, TX 78229; tel. 210/614-0187; FAX. 210/692-7757; Ann Mueller, RN, Facility Administrator

Santa Rose Diagnostic and Surgical Center, 315 North San Saba, San Antonio, TX 78207; tel. 210/704-4000; FAX. 210/704-4014; Julie Meador, Clinical Manager

South Plains Endoscopy Center, 3610 24th Street, Lubbock, TX 79410; tel. 806/797-1015; Pat S. Wheeler, Administrator

South Texas Eye Surgicenter, Inc., 4406 North Laurent, Victoria, TX 77901; tel. 800/352-5928; Robert T. McMahon, M.D., Chief Executive Officer

South Texas Outpatient Surgical Center, Inc., 4025 East Southcross Boulevard, Building Three, Suit, San Antonio, TX 78222; tel. 210/333-0633; FAX. 210/333-0671; Michael P. Lewis, Administrator

South West Surgery Center, 1717 Precinct Line Road, Suite 101, Hurst, TX 76054; tel. 817/788-1881; FAX. 817/656-1490; Caressa Walls, Administrator

Southwest Endoscopy Center, 11803 South Freeway, Suite 115, Fort Worth, TX 76115; tel. 817/293-9292; FAX. 817/551-0616; Pamela Payne, RN

Surgery Center of Fort Worth, 2001 West Rosedale, Fort Worth, TX 76104; tel. 817/877-4777; Debra Delain, RN, Administrator

Surgery Center Southwest, 8230 Walnut Hill Lane, Suite 102, Dallas, TX 75231; tel. 214/345-4076; FAX. 214/345-4055; Tom Blair, Director, PHS

SurgEyeCare, Inc., 5421 La Sierra Drive, Dallas, TX 75231; tel. 214/361-1443; FAX. 214/691-3299; Sandra J. Yankee, Administrator

Surgi-Care Center of Midland, Inc., 3001 West Illinois, Suite Five-A, Midland, TX 79701; tel. 915/697-1067; FAX. 915/697-8802; Brenda Braun, R.N., Director

Surgical and Diagnostic Center, Inc., 729 Bedford Euless Road West 100, Hurst, TX 76053; tel. 817/282-6905; FAX. 817/285-8114; Edward William Smith, D.O., Medical Director

Surgical Center of El Paso, 1815 North Stanton, El Paso, TX 79902; tel. 915/533-8412; FAX. 915/542-0367; Thomas Reynolds, Managing Director

Surgicare of Travis Centre, Inc., 6655 Travis, Suite 200, Houston, TX 77030; tel. 713/526-5100; Carol Simons, Administrator

Surgicare, Ltd., 3534 Vista, Pasadena, TX 77504; tel. 713/947-0330; Evelyn Grimes, Administrator

Surgicenter of San Antonio, L.P., 5290 Medical Drive, San Antonio, TX 78229; tel. 210/614-0187; FAX. 210/692-7757; Ann Mueller, Executive Director

SurgiSystems, Inc., 427 West 20th Street, Houston, TX 77008; tel. 713/868-3641; FAX. 713/865-5460; Jo McBeth, RN

Texarkana Surgery Center, 5404 Summerhill Road, Texarkana, TX 75503; tel. 903/792-7151; Karen Stephens, Director

Texas Ambulatory Surgical Center, Inc., 2505 North Shepherd, Houston, TX 77008; tel. 713/880-3940; FAX. 713/880-1923; Kwang S. Park, Administrator

Texas Institute of Surgery, 12700 North Featherwood Drive, Suite 100, Houston, TX 77034; tel. 713/481-9303; FAX. 713/481-4263; Glenn Rodriguez, Administrator

Texoma Outpatient Surgery Center, Inc., 1712 Eleventh Street, Wichita Falls, TX 76301; tel. 940/723-1274; Tracy Youngblood, Administrator

The Birth Center of Southeast Texas, Inc., 2400 Highway 96 S., Lumberton, TX 77656; tel. 409/755-0252; Dennis D. Riston, M.D., Administrator

The Cataract Center of East Texas, P.A., 802 Turtle Creek Drive, Tyler, TX 75701; tel. 903/595-4333; FAX. 903/535-9845; Nancy G. Grimes, Administrator

The Center for Sight, P.A., Two Medical Center Boulevard, Lufkin, TX 75904-3175; tel. 409/634-8434; FAX. 409/639-2581; Richard J. Ruckman, M.D.

The Endoscopy Center of Southeast Texas, 950 North 11th Street, Beaumont, TX 77702; tel. 409/833-5555; FAX. 409/833-9911; Royce D. Harrell

The Eye Surgery Center of the Rio Grande Valley, 1402 East Sixth Street, Weslaco, TX 78596; tel. 210/968-6155; FAX. 210/968-8291; Linda Funston, Administrator

The Ocular Surgery Center, Inc., 1100 North Main Avenue, San Antonio, TX 78212; tel. 210/222-2154; FAX. 512/222-0706; Jane Wilson, Administrator

The Surgery Center of Mesquite, 2690 North Galloway Avenue, Mesquite, TX 75150; tel. 972/279-8100; FAX. 972/279-3300; Jeffrey S. Houston, Administrator

The Surgery Center of Texas, 155 East Loop 338, Suite 500, Odessa, TX 79762; tel. 915/367-3906; FAX. 915/367-3895; Marsha Smith, Administrator

The Surgery Center of the Woodlands, 1441 Woodstead Court, Suite 100, The Woodlands, TX 77380; tel. 281/363-0058; FAX. 281/363-0450; Kathy Budd, Administrator

Thorstenson Eye Clinic Surgery Center, 3302 Northeast Stallings Drive, Nacogdoches, TX 75963-2020; tel. 409/564-2411; FAX. 409/564-1280; Lyle S. Thorstenson, M.D., FACS, Administrator

University Surgery Center, Inc., 311 University Drive, Fort Worth, TX 76107; tel. 817/877-1002; FAX. 817/877-1006; Lori Schooler, Administrator

Urological Surgery Center of Fort Worth, 418 South Henderson, Fort Worth, TX 76104; tel. 817/338-4637; Charles Bamberger, M.D.

Valley Endoscopy Center, LLP, 3101 South Sunshine Strip, Harlingen, TX 78550; tel. 956/412-2324; FAX. 956/428-2561; Noel B. Searle, M.D.

Valley Eye Surgery Center, 1515 North Ed Carey Drive, Harlingen, TX 78550; tel. 210/423-2773; FAX. 210/423-5618; Michael D. Laney, Administrator

Valley View Surgery Center, 5744 LBJ Freeway, Suite 200, Dallas, TX 75240; tel. 972/490-4333; FAX. 972/490-2494; Ronald W. Disney, Chief Executive Officer

Vista Healthcare, Inc., 4301 Vista, Pasadena, TX 77504; tel. 713/947-0891; FAX. 713/947-1377; Chiu M. Chan, Administrator

WestPark Surgery Center, 130 South Central Expressway, McKinney, TX 75070; tel. 214/542-9382; FAX. 214/548-5303; Debbie Taylor

Westside Surgery Center, Ltd., 16100 Cairnway, Houston, TX 77084; tel. 713/550-5556; FAX. 713/577-7888; Harold F. Taylor, President and CEO

Wilson Surgicenter, 4315 28th Street, Lubbock, TX 79410; tel. 806/792-2104; Bill W. Wilson, M.D., Chief Executive Officer

UTAH

Central Utah Surgical Center, 1067 North 500 West, Provo, UT 84604; tel. 801/374-0354; FAX. 801/374-3210; Jill Andrews, RN, BSN, CNOR, Administrator

HealthSouth Provo Surgical Center, 585 North 500 West, Provo, UT 84601; tel. 801/375-0983; Francis Gibson, Administrator

Institute of Facial and Cosmetic Surgery, 5929 Fashion Boulevard, Salt Lake City, UT 84107; tel. 801/261-3637; FAX. 801/261-4096; Dr. Brent D. Kennedy, Administrator

Intermountain Surgical Center, 359 Eighth Avenue, Salt Lake City, UT 84103; tel. 801/321-3200; FAX. 801/321-3035; Joan W. Lelis, Administrative Director

McKay-Dee Surgical Center, 3903 Harrison Boulevard, Suite 100, Ogden, UT 84403; tel. 801/398-2809; FAX. 801/398-5938; Suzanne Richins, Administrator

Salt Lake Endoscopy Center, 24 South 1100 East, Salt Lake City, UT 84102; tel. 801/355-2987; FAX. 801/531-9704; Pam Bloomquist, Business Manager

Salt Lake Surgical Center, 617 East 3900 South, Salt Lake City, UT 84107; tel. 801/261-3141; FAX. 801/268-2599; Jay T. Lighthall, Administrator

St. George Surgical Center, 676 South Bluff Street, St. George, UT 84770; tel. 435/673-8080; FAX. 435/673-0096; Terrill Dick, Administrator

St. Mark's Outpatient Surgery Center, 1250 East 3900 South, Suite 100, Salt Lake City, UT 84124; tel. 801/262-0358; FAX. 801/262-0901; Marjorie Kimes, Administrator

The SurgiCare Center of Utah, 755 East 3900 South, Salt Lake City, UT 84107; tel. 801/266-2283; FAX. 801/268-6151; Andrew Lyle, M.D., Administrator

Wasatch Endoscopy, 1220 East 3900 South, Suite 1B, Salt Lake City, UT 84124; tel. 801/281-3657; Marjorie Kimes, RN, Administrator

Wasatch Surgery Center, 555 South Foothill Boulevard, Salt Lake City, UT 84112; tel. 801/581-7782; FAX. 801/581-8962; Mark Holyoak, Administrator, Manager

Western Surgery Center, Inc., 850 East 1200 North, Logan, UT 84341; tel. 801/797-3670; FAX. 801/797-3848; Barbara Smehland, Administrator

VERMONT

David S. Chase, M.D., Ambulatory Surgical Center, 183 St. Paul Street, Burlington, VT 05401; tel. 802/864-0381; David S. Chase, M.D., Administrator

VIRGINIA

Ambulatory Surgery Center, 844 Kempsville Road, Norfolk, VA 23502; tel. 757/466-6900; FAX. 757/466-6313; Darleen S. Anderson, Site Administrator

Cataract and Refractive Surgery Center, 2010 Bremo Road, Suite 128, Richmond, VA 23226; tel. 804/285-0680; FAX. 804/282-6365; Jeffry A. Staples, Administrator

Columbia Fairfax Surgical Center, 10730 Main Street, Fairfax, VA 22030; tel. 703/691-0670; Sharon B. Johnson, Chief Executive Officer

CountrySide Ambulatory Surgery Center, Four Pidgeon Hill Drive, Sterling, VA 20165; tel. 703/444-6060; FAX. 703/444-2278; Deborah F. Arminio, RN, Director

Fredericksburg Ambulatory Surgery Center, 2216 Princess Anne Street, Fredericksburg, VA 22401; tel. 540/899-3403; FAX. 540/899-6893; Jeane Bullock, Administrator

Hanover Outpatient Center, 7016 Lee Park Road, Mechanicsville, VA 23111; tel. 804/730-9000; FAX. 804/730-1460; Valene G. Rice, RN, Director

Kaiser Permanente Falls Church Medical Center Ambulatory Surge, 201 North Washington Street, Falls Church, VA 22046; tel. 703/237-4046; FAX. 703/536-1400; Debbie Bland, Director, Surgical Services

Lakeview Medical Center, Inc., 2000 Meade Parkway, Suffolk, VA 23424; tel. 804/539-0251; FAX. 804/934-2620; Michael B. Stout, Executive Director

Lewis-Gale Clinic, Same Day Surgery, 1802 Braeburn Drive, Salem, VA 24153; tel. 540/772-3673; FAX. 540/725-5016; Kay Walker, RN, Director

Providers / Freestanding Ambulatory Surgery Centers

Piedmont Day Surgery Center, Inc., 1040 Main Street, P.O. Box 1360, Danville, VA 24543-1360; tel. 804/792-1433; FAX. 804/797-1398; Aaron Lieberman, Chief Operating Officer

Riverside Surgery Center-Warwick, 12420 Warwick Boulevard, Building 3, Newport News, VA 23606; tel. 804/594-2796; FAX. 804/594-3911; M. Caroline Martin, Executive Vice President

Sentara Care Plex, 3000 Coliseum Drive, Hampton, VA 23666; tel. 804/827-2000; FAX. 804/827-6748; Jeri Eastridge, Director

Surgi Center of Central Virginia, Inc., 12 White Oak Road, Fredericksburg, VA 22405; tel. 703/371-5349; FAX. 703/373-1745; Janet P. O'Keefe, Facility Administrator

Surgi–Center of Winchester, Inc., 1860 Amherst Street, P.O. Box 2660, Winchester, VA 22604; tel. 540/722-8934; FAX. 540/722-8936; Nelson N. Eisenhower, M.D., Administrator

Tuckahoe Surgery Center, Inc., 8919 Three Chopt Road, Richmond, VA 23229; tel. 804/285-4763; FAX. 804/288-2850; Charles A. Stark, CHE, Administrator

Urosurgical Center of Richmond–North, 8228 Meadowbridge Road, Mechanicsville, VA 23111; tel. 804/730-5023; FAX. 804/746-4015; Terry W. Coffey, Administrator

Urosurgical Center of Richmond–South, Urosurgical Center of Richmond, 5224 Monument Avenue, Richmond, VA 23226; tel. 804/288-4137; FAX. 804/282-9874; Terry W. Coffey, Administrator

Virginia Ambulatory Surgery Center, 337-15th Street, S.W., Charlottesville, VA 22903; tel. 804/295-4800; FAX. 804/977-0544; Gerry Dobrasz, Administrator

Virginia Beach Ambulatory Surgery Center, 1700 Will-o-Wisp Drive, Virginia Beach, VA 23454; tel. 804/496-6400; FAX. 804/496-3137; Brian Murray, M.D., Medical Director

Virginia Eye Institute/Eye Surgeons of Richmond, Inc., 400 Westhampton Station, Richmond, VA 23226; tel. 804/282-3931; FAX. 804/287-4210; Michelle Carley, Marketing Director

Virginia Heart Institute, LTD., 205 North Hamilton Street, Richmond, VA 23221; tel. 804/359-9265; Charles L. Baird, Jr., M.D., Director

Woodburn Surgery Center, 3289 Woodburn Road, Suite 100, Annandale, VA 22003; tel. 703/207-7520; Jolene Tornabeni, Senior Vice President, Administrator

WASHINGTON

Aesteem Outpatient Surgery Center, 1200 North Northgate Way, Seattle, WA 98133-8916; tel. 206/522-0200; FAX. 206/522-7019; Peter R. N. Chatard, Jr., M.D., Medical Director

Aesthetic Eye Associates, P.S., 1810 116th Avenue, N.E., Suite B, Bellevue, WA 98004-3020; tel. 426/462-0400; FAX. 425/454-1085; Janet Jordan, Business Manager

Bel–Red Ambulatory Surgical Facility, 1370 116th Avenue, N.E., Suite 209, Bellevue, WA 98004-3825; tel. 625/455-7225; FAX. 425/455-0045; Jah Zewplenyi, M.D., Director

Bellingham Surgery Center, 2980 Squalicum Parkway, Bellingham, WA 98225; tel. 206/671-6933; Richard Brumenschenkel, Managing Agent

Cascade Ambulatory Surgery Center, 407 Northeast 87th Street, Vancouver, WA 98664; tel. 360/253-9201; Joseph R. McFarland, Director

Central Washington Cataract Surgery, 1450 North 16th Avenue, Building J, Yakima, WA 98902; tel. 509/457-5000; FAX. 509/457-6498; Paul Almeida, CRNA

Central Washington Surgicare, 307 South 12th Avenue, Suite Nine, Yakima, WA 98902; tel. 509/248-4900; FAX. 509/248-0609

Covington Day Surgery Center, 17700 Southeast 272nd Street, Kent, WA 98042; tel. 206/639-8302; FAX. 206/639-8301; Victoria Fitzpatrick, B.S.N., Director

Ear, Nose, Throat and Plastic Surgery Center, 101 Second Street, N.E., Auburn, WA 98002; tel. 253/833-6241; FAX. 253/833-4113; William Portuese, M.D., Medical Director

Eastside Podiatry Ambulatory Surgery Center, 15617 Bel–Red Road, Bellevue, WA 98008; tel. 425/881-5592; G. Curda, D.P.M.

Edmonds Surgery Center, 21229 84th Avenue W., Edmonds, WA 98026; tel. 206/775-1505; FAX. 206/775-9078; Mark A. Kuzel, D.P.M., F.A.C.F.S

Everett Surgical Center, Inc., 3025 Rucker Avenue, Everett, WA 98201; tel. 425/339-2464; FAX. 425/252-4700; Rita Sweeney, RNFA, CNOR, Administrator

Evergreen Endoscopy Center, 13030 121st Way, N.E., Suite 101, Kirkland, WA 98034; tel. 206/899-4500; FAX. 425/899-4510; Lynn Bookkeeper

Evergreen Eye Surgery Center, 34719 Sixth Avenue South, Federal Way, WA 98003; tel. 253/874-3969; FAX. 253/661-7383; Richard A. Boudreau, Administrator

Evergreen Surgical Center, 12034 Northeast 130th Lane, Kirkland, WA 98034; tel. 206/821-3131; Ronald E. Abrams, M.D.

Good Samaritan Surgery Center, 1322 Third Street S.E., Suite 100, Puyallup, WA 98372; tel. 206/840-2200; FAX. 206/840-2352; Roger D. Robinett, M.D., Medical Director

Health South, Green River Surgical Center, 126 Auburn Avenue, Suite 200, Auburn, WA 98002; tel. 253/735-0500; FAX. 253/939-8526; Lori McMann, Administrator

Hernia Treatment Center, NW, 205 Lilly Road, NE, Suite D, Olympia, WA 98506; tel. 360/491-8667; Robert Kugel, M.D., Director

Inland Eye Center, South 842 Cowley, Spokane, WA 99202; tel. 509/624-5300; FAX. 509/747-1348; Michael H. Cunningham, M.D., President

Kruger Clinic Day Surgery, 21600 Highway 99, Suite 150, Edmonds, WA 98026; tel. 425/774-2636; FAX. 425/774-2688

Lomas Surgery Center, 17800 Talbot Road, S., Renton, WA 98055; tel. 425/255-0986; FAX. 425/271-5703; Inese A. Lomas, Administrator

Madrona Medical Group, ASC, 4545 Cordata Parkway, Bellingham, WA 98226; tel. 360/676-1712

McIntyre Eye Clinic & Surgical Center, 1920 116th Avenue, N.E., Bellevue, WA 98004; tel. 425/454-3937; FAX. 425/646-5914; David McIntyre, M.D., FACS

Minor & James Medical, PLLC, 515 Minor Avenue, Suite 200, Seattle, WA 98104; tel. 206/386-9500; FAX. 206/386-9605; Sylvia Croy, RN, ASC Coordinator

Monroe Foot Care Associates Ambulatory Surgery Center, 14692 179th Avenue, S.E., Suite 300, Monroe, WA 98272; tel. 206/794-1266; Dr. Brunsman, Medical Director

Moses Lake Surgery Center, 840 East Hill Avenue, Moses Lake, WA 98837; tel. 509/765-0216; John Rodriguez, ASC Manager

North Cascade ENT and Facial Plastic Surgery, 111 South 13th Street, Mount Vernon, WA 98273; tel. 206/336-2178

North Cascade ENT Facial Plastic Surgery, 20302 77th Avenue, N.E., Arlington, WA 98223; tel. 360/435-6300; FAX. 360/435-8381; Alex O'Dell

North Kitsap Ambulatory Surgical Center, 20696 Bond Road, N.E., Poulsbo, WA 98370; tel. 360/779-6527; FAX. 360/697-2743; Susan Simons, R.N., Director of Surgical Services

Northwest Center for Plastic and Reconstructive Surgery, 16259 Sylvester Road, S.W., Suite 302, Seattle, WA 98166; tel. 206/241-5400; FAX. 206/241-8591; Sindi Miller, Office Manager

Northwest Eye Surgery, P.C., 1120 N. Pines Road, Spokane, WA 99206; tel. 509/927-0700

Northwest Gastroenterology, d/b/a Northwest Endoscopy, 3149 Ellis, Suite 301, Bellingham, WA 98225; tel. 360/734-1420; FAX. 360/734-8748; Kathy Burns, Manager

Northwest Nasal Sinus Center, 10330 Meridan Avenue, N., Suite 240, Seattle, WA 98133; tel. 206/525-2525; FAX. 206/525-0346

Northwest Surgery Center, 1920 100th Street, S.E., Everett, WA 98208; tel. 425/316-3700; FAX. 425/316-6881; Chris Vance, President

Northwest Surgery Center, Inc., West 123 Francis, Spokane, WA 99205; tel. 509/483-9363; FAX. 509/483-0355; Douglas P. Romney

NW Aesthetic Surgery Center, 550 16th Avenue, Suite 404, Seattle, WA 98122; tel. 206/328-2250; Jo Olson, Administrator

NW Center for Corrective Jaw Surgery, 550 16th Avenue, Suite 303, Seattle, WA 98122; tel. 206/324-6570; FAX. 206/324-9936; Dotti Miller, Practice Manager

Olympic Ambulatory Surgery Center, Inc., 2601 Cherry Avenue, Suite 115, Bremerton, WA 98310; tel. 206/479-5990; FAX. 360/377-5731; Audrey E. Harris, RN

Olympic Plastic Surgery Suite, 2600 Cherry Avenue Suite 201, Bremerton, WA 98310; tel. 360/415-0762; Suzanne Fletcher, Administrator

Pacific Cataract and Laser Institute, 2517 Northeast Kresky, Chehalis, WA 98532; tel. 206/748-8632; Debbie Eldredge, Vice President and COO

Pacific Cataract and Laser Institute, 10500 Northeast Eighth Street, Suite 1650, Bellevue, WA 98004-4332; tel. 206/462-7664; FAX. 206/462-6429; Maynard Pohl, O.D., Clinical Director

Pacific Cataract and Laser Institute, 8200 West Grandridge, Kennewick, WA 99336; tel. 206/748-8632; Debbie Eldredge, Vice President and COO

Pacific Medical Center, 1200 12th Avenue, S., Seventh Floor, Seattle, WA 98144; tel. 206/326-4000; Carolyn Bodeen, RN, Clinic Director

Pacific NW Facial Plastic Ambulatory Surgery Center, 600 Broadway, Suite 280, Seattle, WA 98122; tel. 206/386-3550; FAX. 206/386-3553

Parkway Surgical Center, 2940 Squalicum Parkway, Suite 204, Bellingham, WA 98225; tel. 206/676-8350; FAX. 206/676-8351; Orville Vandergriend, M.D., Administrator

Physicians Eye Surgical Center, 3930 Hoyt Avenue, Everett, WA 98201; tel. 206/259-2020; Carol Schoenfelder, Administrator

Plastic and Reconstructive Surgeons, 17930 Talbot Road, S., Renton, WA 98055; tel. 206/228-3187; Mack D. Richey, M.D.

Plastic Surgery Center, 1017 South 40th Avenue, Yakima, WA 98904; tel. 509/966-6000; FAX. 509/966-6565; Julie Marquis, RN, Quality Assurance Manager

Plastic Surgicenter of Olympia, 400 Lilly Road, N.E., Building Four, Olympia, WA 98506; tel. 360/456-4400; FAX. 360/491-7619; Wayne L. Dickason, M.D.

Professional Surgical Specialists, 1609 Meridian South, Puyallup, WA 98371; tel. 253/841-1222; FAX. 253/770-0360; Doreen Healy, Office Manager

Redmond Foot Care Associates, ASC, 16146 Cleveland Street, Redmond, WA 98052; tel. 206/885-7004

Rockwood Clinic, d/b/a Gastrointestinal Endoscopy Unit, Sacred Heart Building, West 105 Eighth Avenue, Spokane, WA 99204; tel. 509/838-2531; FAX. 509/455-8828; Stephen Burgert, M.D., Administrator

Rockwood Clinic, PS, East 400 Fifth Avenue, Spokane, WA 99202; tel. 509/838-2531; FAX. 509/455-5315; William R. Poppy, Chief Executive Officer

Seattle Endoscopy Center, 11027 Meridian Avenue, N., Suite 100, Seattle, WA 98133; tel. 206/365-4492; FAX. 206/348-3456; Patty Carroll, CGRN, Manager

Seattle Hand Surgery Group, P.C., 600 Broadway, Suite 440, Seattle, WA 98122; tel. 206/292-6252; FAX. 206/292-7893; Tamiko Gandy, Administrator

Seattle Head and Neck Office Surgery, 515 Minor Avenue, Suite 130, Seattle, WA 98104; tel. 206/682-6103; FAX. 206/682-3012; Debbie Perdue, Director

Seattle Microsurgical Eyecare Center, 5300 17th Avenue, N.W., Seattle, WA 98107; tel. 206/783-3929; Jack C. Bunn, M.D., Medical Director

Seattle Plastic Surgery Center, 600 Broadway, Suite 320, Seattle, WA 98122; tel. 206/324-1120; FAX. 206/720-0800; Diane Wallaia

Seattle Surgery Center, Columbus Pavilion, 900 Terry Avenue, Fourth Floor, Seattle, WA 98104-1240; tel. 206/382-1021; FAX. 206/382-1026; Naya Kehayes, MPH, Administrator

Sequim Same Day Surgery, 777 North Fifth Avenue, Sequim, WA 98382; tel. 360/681-0358; FAX. 360/683-0170; Tammy Paolini, Surgical Technician

South Hill Ambulatory Surgical Center, South 3028 Grand Boulevard, Spokane, WA 99203; tel. 509/747-0279; FAX. 509/747-3220

Southwest Washington Ambulatory Surgery Center, Inc., 102 West Fourth Plain Boulevard, Vancouver, WA 98666; tel. 360/696-4400; FAX. 360/696-4287; Denice Nolan, Office Manager

Spokane Digestive Disease Center, 105 West Eighth Avenue, Suite 6010, Spokane, WA 99204-2318; tel. 509/838-5950; FAX. 509/838-5961; Margie Troske–Johnson, RN, B.S.N., Director

Spokane Eye Surgery Center, West 208 Fifth Street, Spokane, WA 99204; tel. 509/456-8150; FAX. 509/455-9887; Donald Ellingsen, M.D.

Spokane Foot and Ankle Surgery Center, 9405 East Sprague Avenue, Spokane, WA 99206; tel. 509/922-3199; Rita Kinney, RN

Spokane Surgery Center, North 1120 Pines Road, Spokane, WA 99206; tel. 509/924-3235; FAX. 509/928-1990; Stewart P. Brim, D.P.M.

Providers / Freestanding Ambulatory Surgery Centers

St. Mark's Micro Surgical Center, Inc., 502 South M Street, Tacoma, WA 98405; tel. 206/627–8266; Roy Baker, Chief Executive Officer
Stanley M. Jackson, M.D., Plastic and Reconstructive Surgery, 105 27th Avenue, S.E., Puyallup, WA 98374; tel. 206/848–8110; FAX. 206/845–3561; Karen Smith, RN
Sutcliffe Facial And Laser Center, 1229 Madison Street, Suite 1190, Seattle, WA 98104; tel. 206/621–0800; FAX. 206/621–7023; R. Toby Sutcliffe, M.D.
Tacoma Ambulatory Surgery Center, 1112 Sixth Avenue, Suite 100, Tacoma, WA 98405; tel. 206/272–3916; FAX. 206/627–1713; Joan Hoover, Administrator
Tacoma Endoscopy Center, 1112 Sixth Avenue, Suite 200, Tacoma, WA 98405; tel. 253/272–8664; FAX. 253/627–7880; Richard Baerg, M.D., Medical Director
Tacoma Speciality ASU, 209 Martin Luther King, Jr. Way, Tacoma, WA 98405; tel. 206/596–3590; Linda Bradley, Manager
The Eastside Endoscopy Center, P.L.L.C., 1700 116th Avenue, N.E., Suite 100, Bellevue, WA 98004–3049; tel. 425/451–7335; FAX. 425/451–1226; Michelle Steele, CGRN, Clinical Nurse Manager
The Plastic SurgiCentre, Inc., 535 South Pine Street, Spokane, WA 99202; tel. 509/623–2160; FAX. 509/623–1135; Pamala Silvers, RN, Manager
The Polyclinic, Inc., 1145 Broadway, Seattle, WA 98122; tel. 206/329–1760; Lloyd David, Chief Executive Officer
TLC Northwest Eye, Inc., 10330 Meridian Avenue N., Suite 370, Seattle, WA 98133–9451; tel. 206/528–6000; FAX. 206/528–0014; Wendy R. Williams, Marketing Director
Valley Outpatient Surgery Center, North 1414 Houk Road, Suite 204, Spokane, WA 99216; tel. 509/922–0362; FAX. 509/927–8316; Joel San Nicholas, Administrator
Valley Surgi Centre, Five South 14th Avenue, Yakima, WA 98902; tel. 509/248–6813; FAX. 509/457–9691; Liz Hanks, Office Manager
Virginia Mason Federal Way, 33501 First Way South, Federal Way, WA 98003; tel. 253/874–1635; FAX. 253/874–1732; Steven Alley
Virginia Mason–Issaquah, 100 Northeast Gilman Boulevard, Issaquah, WA 98027; tel. 206/557–8000; Bobbie Eatmon, Manager
Washington Centre for Reproductive Medicine, 1370 116th Avenue, N.E., Suite 100, Bellevue, WA 98004; tel. 206/462–6100
Washington Orthopaedic Center, Inc., PS, 1900 Cooks Hill Road, Centralia, WA 98531; tel. 360/736–2889; JoAnn Wilkey, Director
Wenatchee Valley Clinic/Cascade Surgery Center, 820 North Chelan, Wenatchee, WA 98801; tel. 509/663–8711; FAX. 509/665–2309; Dr. Don Paugh, Chief, Cascade Surgery Center
Westlake Surgical Center, 509 Olive Way, Third Floor, Seattle, WA 98101; tel. 206/623–4755; Maria T. Burrows, Administrative Assistant
Whidbey SurgiCare, 31775–SR 20, Suite A Two, Oak Harbor, WA 98277–2334; tel. 360/679–3117; FAX. 360/679–3118; Stephen T. Miller, DPM, Medical Director
Whitehorse Surgical Center, 875 Wesley Street, Suite 160, Arlington, WA 98223; tel. 360/435–6969; FAX. 360/435–1068

WEST VIRGINIA
Anwar Eye Center, 1500 Lafayette Avenue, Moundsville, WV 26041; tel. 304/845–0908; M. F. Anwar, M.D.
Cabell Huntington Surgery Center, 1201 Hal Greer Boulevard, Huntington, WV 25701; tel. 304/523–1885; FAX. 304/523–8942; John Stone, Facility Administrator
Cook Eye Surgery Center, 1300 Third Avenue, Huntington, WV 25701; tel. 304/522–1802; FAX. 304/529–6752; David W. Cook, M.D., President
Jerry N. Black, M.D., Surgical Suite, 10 Amalia Drive, Buckhannon, WV 26201; tel. 304/472–2100; FAX. 304/472–2118; Jerry N. Black, M.D., Medical Director
Kanawha Valley Surgi–Center, 4803 MacCorkle Avenue, S.E., Charleston, WV 25304; tel. 304/925–6390; FAX. 304/925–7931; Gorli Harish, M.D., Medical Director
Lee's Surgi–Center, 415 Morris Street, Suite 200, Charleston, WV 25301; tel. 304/342–1113; FAX. 304/346–2271; Hans Lee, M.D., President
SurgiCare, 3200 MacCorkle Avenue, S.E., Charleston, WV 25304; tel. 304/348–9556; Robert L. Savage, President
West Virginia Surgery Center, Inc., 425 Greenway Avenue, South Charles, WV 25309; tel. 304/768–7310; FAX. 304/768–8211; Nancy Jo Vinson, Administrator

WISCONSIN
Aurora Health Center, 10400 75th Street, Kenosha, WI 53142; tel. 414/697–6907; FAX. 414/697–3022; Thomas M. Warsocki, Administrator
Bay Lake Surgery Outpatient Surgery Center, Inc., 1843 Michigan Street, P.O. Box 678, Sturgeon Bay, WI 54235; tel. 414/746–1070; FAX. 414/746–1072; Michael Herlache, Administrator
Baycare Surgery Center, 2253 West Mason, P.O. Box 33227, Green Bay, WI 54303–0102; tel. 414/592–9100; FAX. 414/497–6830; Jeff Mason, Administrator
Center for Digestive Health, 2801 West Kinnickinnic River Parkway, Suite 560, Milwaukee, WI 53215; tel. 414/649–3522; FAX. 414/649–5454; Roger L. Daris, Administrator
Davis Duehr Day Surgery, 1025 Regent Street, Madison, WI 53715; tel. 608/282–2050; Rodney Sturm, M.D., President
Dean St. Mary's Surgery Center, 800 South Brooks Street, Madison, WI 53715; tel. 608/259–3510; FAX. 608/255–1272; Patricia Klitzman, Director
Eau Claire Surgery Center, 950 West Clairemont Avenue, Eau Claire, WI 54701; tel. 715/839–9339; FAX. 715/839–9033; Kathryn Hentz, RN, Facility Manager
Green Bay Surgical Center, Ltd., 704 South Webster Avenue, Green Bay, WI 54301; tel. 920/432–7433; FAX. 920/432–6003; Herbert F. Sandmire, M.D., Medical Director, Administrator
HealthSouth Surgery Center of Wausau, 2809 Westhill Drive, Wausau, WI 54401; tel. 715/842–4490; FAX. 715/842–4645; Sharon Schwartz, RN, Facility Administrator
LaSalle Surgery Center, 1550 Midway Place, Menasha, WI 54952; tel. 920/727–8200; FAX. 920/727–8203; Laura Ruys, Manager
Marshfield Clinic Ambulatory Surgery Center, 1000 North Oak Avenue, Marshfield, WI 54449; tel. 715/387–5315; FAX. 715/387–5240; Robert J. DeVita, Executive Director
Menomonee Falls Ambulatory Surgery Center, W180 N8045 Town Hall Road, Menomonee Falls, WI 53051; tel. 414/250–0950; FAX. 414/250–0955; Dianne Wallace, Executive Director
Mercy Walworth, ASC, N2950 State Road 67, Lake Geneva, WI 53147; tel. 414/245–0535; Deb Saylor, RN, Team Leader
North Shore Surgical Center, 7007 North Range Line Road, Milwaukee, WI 53209; tel. 414/352–3341; FAX. 414/352–3218; Robert Lonergan, Executive Director
Northlake Surgery Center, 2110 Medical Drive, Box 636, Menomonee, WI 54751; tel. 715/235–8884; Douglas Carson
Northwest Surgery Center, 2300 North Mayfair Road, Wauwatosa, WI 53226; tel. 414/257–3322; Nancy Jones, Administrator
Oshkosh Surgery Center, 1925 Surgery Center Drive, Oshkosh, WI 54901; tel. 920/233–1233; FAX. 920/233–2101; Jean Cox, Administrator
Riverview Surgery Center, 616 North Washington Street, Janesville, WI 53545; tel. 608/758–7300; FAX. 608/758–1050; Lynn Jenkins, Director
Surgery Center of Wisconsin, 10401 West Lincoln Avenue, Suite 201, West Allis, WI 53227; tel. 414/321–7850; FAX. 414/328–5899; Daniel R. Hellman, M.D., Facility Administrator
Surgicenter of Greater Milwaukee, 3223 South 103rd Street, Milwaukee, WI 53227; tel. 414/328–5800; FAX. 414/328–5805; Denise Augustin, President
Surgicenter of Racine, Ltd., 5802 Washington Avenue, Racine, WI 53406; tel. 262/886–9100; FAX. 262/886–9130; Dennis J. Kontra, Administrator
Wauwatosa Surgery Center, d/b/a HealthSouth Surgery Center of Wauwatosa, 10900 West Potter Road, Wauwatosa, WI 53226–3424; tel. 414/774–9227; FAX. 414/774–0957; Kathleen Miller, R.N., M.S.N., Administrator

WYOMING
Casper Endoscopy Center, 167 South Conwell, Suite Seven, Casper, WY 82601; tel. 307/262–3896; Robert A. Schlidt, M.D., Administrator
Gem City Bone and Joint Surgery Center, 1909 Vista Drive, Laramie, WY 82070; tel. 307/745–8851; FAX. 307/742–8851; Trent Kaufman, Admin. Director
Wyoming Endoscopy Center, 1200 East 20th Street, Cheyenne, WY 82001; tel. 307/635–5439; Tracie Brandt, MBA, Administrator
Wyoming Outpatient Services, 5050 Powderhouse Road, Cheyenne, WY 82009; tel. 307/634–1311; FAX. 307/638–6820; Robin Brown, Director
Yellowstone Surgery Center, Ltd., 5201 Yellowstone Road, Cheyenne, WY 82009; tel. 307/635–7070; FAX. 307/632–9920; Linnea McNair, RN, B.S.N., Director

U.S. Associated Areas

PUERTO RICO
ASC Espanola Clinic, Box 490, La Quinta, Mayaguez, PR 00681; tel. 787/832–2094
ASC Hato Rey Comm., 435 Ponce de Leon Avenue, Hato Rey, PR 00919; tel. 787/754–0909; FAX. 787/753–1625
ASC Mimiya, P.O. Box 41245, 303 De Diego Avenue, Santurce, PR 00940; tel. 809/721–2590; Efrain Pinero, MHSA
Cirugia Ambulatoria y Centro de Diagnostico y Tratamiento de S, Box 486, San Sebastian, PR 00755; tel. 809/896–1850
Clinica de Cirugia Ambulatoria de Puerto Rico, Box 3748, Marina Station, Mayaguez, PR 00681; tel. 787/833–4400; FAX. 787/265–6621; Roberto Ruiz, Asencio, Administrator
Clinica del Turabo, P.O. Box 1900, Caguas, PR 00726; tel. 787/746–8899; FAX. 787/258–1776; Jamie L. Olivera, BSIE, MBA, MHSA
Instituto Cirugia Plastica Del Oeste, Plastica Del Oeste, 165 Este Mendez Virgo Street, Mayaguez, PR 00680; tel. 787/833–3248; FAX. 787/831–4400; Oscar Vargas, M.D., Medical Director
Instituto de Ojos y Piel, Carr Three, KM 12.3, Carolina, PR 00985; tel. 809/769–2477
Instituto Quirurgico De Un Dia – Dr. Pila, P.O. Box 1910, Ponce, PR 00733; tel. 809/844–5600
OJOS, Inc., Calle Hipodromo, Esquina Las Palmas, Santurce, PR 00908; tel. 787/721–8330; FAX. 787/722–3222; Maria Delos A. Tirado, Administrator
Southern SurgiCenter, Edificio Parra Office 201, Ponce, PR 00731; tel. 787/841–0303; FAX. 787/841–0387; Mr. Roberto Rentas, MHSA
The New San Juan Health Centre, 150 De Diego Avenue, Esquina Baldorioty, San Juan, PR 00911; tel. 809/725–0202; FAX. 809/725–3060

State Government Agencies for FASC's

Information for the following list was obtained directly from the agencies.

United States

ALABAMA
Alabama Department of Public Health, Division of Licensure and Certification, 434 Monroe Street, Montgomery, AL 36130-1701; tel. 334/240-3503; FAX. 334/240-3147; L. O'Neal Green, Director

ARIZONA
Arizona Department of Health Services, Health and Child Care Review Services, 1647 East Morten, Suite 220, Phoenix, AZ 85020; tel. 602/542-1100; FAX. 602/861-0645; Mary Wiley, Assistant Director

ARKANSAS
Department of Health, Division of Health Facility Services, 5800 West 10th Street, Suite 400, Little Rock, AR 72204-9916; tel. 501/661-2201; FAX. 501/661-2165; Henry Robinson, Director

CALIFORNIA
Department of Health Services, Licensing and Certification Program, 1800 Third Street, Suite 210, P.O. Box 942732, Sacramento, CA 94234-7320; tel. 916/445-2070; FAX. 916/327-4355; Diane L. Ford, Branch Chief

COLORADO
Department of Health, Division of Health Facilities, 4300 Cherry Creek Drive South, Denver, CO 80220; tel. 303/692-2800; FAX. 303/782-4883; Diane Carter, Deputy, Director

CONNECTICUT
Public Health Division of Health Systems Regulation, 410 Capital Avenue, Hartford, CT 06134-0308; tel. 860/509-7400; FAX. 860/509-7538; Cynthia Denne, RN, MPA., Bureau Chief Regulatory Services

DELAWARE
Department of Health and Social Services, Licensing and Certification, Office of Health Facilities, 2055 Limestone Road, Suite 200, Wilmington, DE 19808; tel. 302/995-8521; FAX. 302/995-8524; Mary Peterson, Director

DISTRICT OF COLUMBIA
Department of Health, Licensing Regulation Administration, 614 H Street, N.W., Suite 1003, Washington, DC 20001; tel. 202/727-7190; FAX. 202/727-7780; Geraldine K. Sykes

FLORIDA
Division of Health Quality Assurance, Agency for Health Care Administration, Fort Knox Executive Office Center, 2727 Mahan Drive, Suite 214, Tallahassee, FL 32308-5407; tel. 850/487-2527; Peter J. Euigas, Director

GEORGIA
Health Care Section - Georgia Dept. of Human Resources, Office of Regulatory Services, Two Peachtree Street, N.W., Room 33-250, Atlanta, GA 30303-3142; tel. 404/657-5550; FAX. 404/657-8934; Susie M. Woods, Director

HAWAII
Hawaii Department of Health, Office of Health Care Assurance, P.O. Box 3378, Honolulu, HI 96801; tel. 808/586-4080; FAX. 808/586-4747; Helen K. Yoshimi, B.S.N., MPH, Chief, HMFB

IDAHO
Bureau of Facility Standards, Department of Health and Welfare, P.O. Box 83720, Boise, ID 83720-0036; tel. 208/334-6626; FAX. 208/364-1888; Sylvia Creswell, Supervisor-Non Long Term Care

ILLINOIS
Department of Public Health, Division of Health Care Facilities and Programs, 525 West Jefferson Street, Springfield, IL 62761; tel. 217/782-7412; FAX. 217/782-0382; Enrique Unanue, Acting Division Chief

INDIANA
Indiana State Department of Health, Division of Acute Care, Two North Meridian Street, 4/A, Indianapolis, IN 46204; tel. 317/233-7474; FAX. 317/233-7157; Mary Azbill, MT (ASCP)

IOWA
Department of Inspection and Appeals, Division of Health Facilities, Lucas State Office Building, Des Moines, IA 50319; tel. 515/281-4115; FAX. 515/242-5022; Nancy M. Ruzicka, Bureau Chief

KANSAS
Kansas Department of Health and Environment, Bureau of Adult and Child Care, 900 Southwest Jackson, Suite 1001, Topeka, KS 66612-1290; tel. 785/296-1280; FAX. 785/296-1266; George A. Dugger, Medical Facilities Certification Administrator

KENTUCKY
Cabinet for Health Services, Division of Licensing and Regulation, 275 East Main, 4th Floor, Frankfort, KY 40621; tel. 502/564-2800; FAX. 502/564-6546; Rebecca J. Cecil, R.Ph., Director

LOUISIANA
Department of Health and Hospitals, Bureau of Health Services Financing-Health Standards Section, P.O. Box 3767, Baton Rouge, LA 70821; tel. 504/342-0415; FAX. 504/342-5292; Lisa Deaton, RN, Manager

MAINE
Division of Licensing and Certification, Department of Human Services, 35 Anthony Avenue, Station 11, Augusta, ME 04333; tel. 207/624-5443; FAX. 207/624-5378; Louis Dorogi, Director

MARYLAND
Department of Health and Mental Hygiene, Licensing and Certification, 4201 Patterson Avenue, Baltimore, MD 21215; tel. 410/402-8025; FAX. 410/358-0750; James Ralls, Assistant Director

MASSACHUSETTS
Department of Public Health, Division of Health Care Quality, 80 Boylston Street, Suite 1100, Boston, MA 02116; tel. 617/727-5860; Irene McManus, Director

MICHIGAN
Department of Consumer and Industry Services, Division of Licensing and Certification, P.O. Box 30664, Lansing, MI 48909; tel. 517/241-2626; FAX. 517/241-2635; Pauline DeRose

MINNESOTA
Department of Health, Facility and Provider Compliance Division, Licensing and Certification Program, 85 East Seventh Place, Suite 300, St. Paul, MN 55164-0900; tel. 651/215-8719; FAX. 651/215-8709; Carol Hirschfeld, Program Assurance Unit

MISSISSIPPI
Department of Health, Division of Health Facilities Licensure and Certification, P.O. Box 1700, Jackson, MS 39215; tel. 601/354-7300; FAX. 601/354-7230; Vanessa Phipps, Director

MISSOURI
Missouri Department of Health, Bureau of Hospital Licensing and Certification, 920 Wildwood Drive, P.O. Box 570, Jefferson City, MO 65102; tel. 573/751-6302; FAX. 573/526-3621; Calvin Bidding, Acting Administrator

MONTANA
Quality Assurance Division, Department of Public Health and Human Services, 2401 Colonial Drive, 2nd Floor, P.O. Box 202953, Helena, MT 59620-2953; tel. 406/444-2099; FAX. 406/444-3456; Denzel Davis, Division Administrator

NEBRASKA
Credentialing Division, Nebraska Department of Health and Human Services Regulation & Licensure, 301 Centennial Mall, S., P.O. Box 94986, Lincoln, NE 68509-4986; tel. 402/471-2116; FAX. 402/471-3577; Helen L. Meeks, Director

NEVADA
Bureau of Licensure & Certification, Nevada Health Division, 1550 E. College Parkway, Suite 158, Carson City, NV 89706-7921; tel. 775/687-4475; FAX. 775/687-6588; Richard J. Panelli, Chief

NEW HAMPSHIRE
Office of Program Support, Licensing and Regulation - Health Facilities, 129 Pleasant Street, Concord, NH 03301; tel. 603/271-4592; FAX. 603/271-4968; Raymond Rusin, Chief

NEW JERSEY
Division of Health Systems Analysis, Certificate of Need and Acute Care Licensing, P.O. Box 360, Trenton, NJ 08625-0360; tel. 609/292-5960; FAX. 609/292-3780; John A. Calabria, Director

NEW MEXICO
Department of Health and Environment, Health Facility Licensing and Certification Bureau, 525 Camino de los Marquez, Suite Two, Santa Fe, NM 87501; tel. 505/827-4200; FAX. 505/827-4203; Wilma Hammer, Bureau Chief

NEW YORK
Health Education Services, P.O. Box 7126, Albany, NY 12224; tel. 518/439-7286; FAX. 518/439-7200

NORTH CAROLINA
Department of Human Resources, Division of Facility Services, 701 Barbour Drive, P.O. Box 29530, Raleigh, NC 27626-0530; tel. 919/733-7461; FAX. 919/733-8274; Steve White, Chief, Licensure and Certification

NORTH DAKOTA
North Dakota Department of Health, Health Resources Section, 600 East Boulevard Avenue, Bismarck, ND 58505-0200; tel. 701/328-2352; FAX. 701/328-1890; Darleen Bartz, Director

OHIO
Division of Quality Assurance, Ohio Department of Health, 246 North High Street, Columbus, OH 43266-0588; tel. 614/466-7857; FAX. 614/644-0208; Rebecca Maust, Division Chief

OKLAHOMA
Department of Health, Special Health Services, 1000 Northeast 10th Street, Oklahoma City, OK 73117; tel. 405/271-6576; FAX. 405/271-1308; Gary Glover, Chief, Medical Facilities

OREGON
Health Care Licensure and Certification, Oregon Health Division, 800 Northeast Oregon Street, Suite 640, # 21, P.O. Box 14450, Portland, OR 97293-0450; tel. 503/731-4013; FAX. 503/731-4080; Kathleen Smail, Manager

PENNSYLVANIA
Bureau of Quality Assurance, Division of Acute and Ambulatory Care Facilities, Health and Welfare Building, Room 532, Harrisburg, PA 17120; tel. 717/783-8980; FAX. 717/705-6663; Elaine Gibble, Director

RHODE ISLAND
Rhode Island Department of Health, Division of Facilities Regulation, Three Capitol Hill, Providence, RI 02908-5097; tel. 401/222-2566; FAX. 401/222-3999; Wayne I. Farrington, Chief

SOUTH CAROLINA
Department of Health and Environmental Control, Division of Health Licensing, 2600 Bull Street, Columbia, SC 29201; tel. 803/737-7202; FAX. 803/737-7212; Jerry Paul, Director

SOUTH DAKOTA
Department of Health, Office of Health Care Facilities Licensure and Certification, 615 East 4th Street, Pierre, SD 57501; tel. 605/773-3356; FAX. 605/773-6667; Joan Bachman, Administrator

Providers / State Government Agencies for FASC's

TENNESSEE
Department of Health, Division of Health Care Facilities, Cordell Hull Building, First Floor, 425 Fifth Avenue, N., Nashville, TN 37247-0508; tel. 615/741–7221; FAX. 615/741–7051; Ken Murray, Director

TEXAS
Texas Department of Health, Health Facility Compliance Division, 1100 West 49th Street, Austin, TX 78756; tel. 512/834–6650; FAX. 512/834–6653; Nance Stearman, RN, M.S.N., Director

UTAH
Utah Department of Health, Bureau of Licensing, P.O. Box 142003, Salt Lake City, UT 84114-2003; tel. 801/538–6152; FAX. 801/538–6325; Debra Wynkoop-Green, Director

VERMONT
Department of Aging and Disabilities, 103 South Main Street, Waterbury, VT 05671; tel. 802/241–2400; FAX. 802/241–2325; Patrick Flood, Commissioner

VIRGINIA
Virginia Department of Health, Center for Quality Health Care Services and Consumer Protection, 3600 Centre, Suite 216, 3600 West Broad Street, Richmond, VA 23230; tel. 804/367–2102; FAX. 804/367–2149; Nancy R. Hofheimer, Director

WASHINGTON
Washington Department of Health, Facilities and Services Licensing, Target Plaza, Suite 500, 2725 Harrison Avenue N.W., Olympia, WA 98504-7852; tel. 360/705–6652; FAX. 360/705–6654; Byron R. Plan, Manager

WEST VIRGINIA
Office of Health Facility Licensure and Certification, West Virginia Division of Health, 350 Capital Street, Room 206, Charleston, WV 25301-3718; tel. 304/558–0050; FAX. 304/588–2515; Bonnie Brauner, Program Manager

WISCONSIN
Bureau of Quality Assurance, Division of Supportive Living, Department of Health and Family Services, P.O. Box 2969, Madison, WI 53701-0309; tel. 608/267–7185; FAX. 608/267–0352; Susan Schroder, Director, Bureau of Quality Assurance

WYOMING
Wyoming Department of Health, Health Facilities Licensing, U.S. Bank Building, Eighth Floor, Cheyenne, WY 82001; tel. 307/777–7123; FAX. 307/777–7127; Jerry Bronnenberg, Administrator

U.S. Associated Areas

PUERTO RICO
Department of Health, P. O. Box 70184, San Juan, PR 00936; tel. 809/766–1616; FAX. 809/766–2240; Carmen Feliciano de Melecio, M.D., Secretary of Health

Freestanding Hospices

The following list of freestanding hospices was developed with the assistance of state government agencies and the individual facilities listed. For a complete list of hospital based hospice programs please refer to Section A. In Section A, hospice programs are identified by Facility Code F37.

We present this list simply as a convenient directory. Inclusion or omission of any organization's name indicates neither approval nor disapproval by Health Forum LLC, an American Hospital Association company.

United States

ALABAMA

Baptist Hospice Walker County, 302 Blackwall Dairy Road, Jasper, AL 35504; tel. 205/387-9339; FAX. 205/387-8226; Ray Whittaker, RN, LBSW, Patient Care Coordinator

Birmingham Area Hospice, 1400 Sixth Avenue, S., P.O. Box 2648, Birmingham, AL 35233; tel. 205/930-1330; FAX. 205/930-1390; Flora Y. Blackledge, Director

Brookwood Hospice, 2010 Brookwood Medical Center Drive, Birmingham, AL 35209; tel. 205/877-2140; FAX. 205/823-0364; Barbara Ballard, Administrator

Caring Hands Hospice, Inc., 225 University Blvd., E., Suite 203, Tuscaloosa, AL 35401; tel. 205/349-3065; FAX. 205/349-3295; Toni D. Welbourne, Executive Director

Chattahoochee Hospice, Inc., #6 Medical Park, North, Valley, AL 36854; tel. 334/756-8043; FAX. 334/756-8059; Kaye Maxwell, RN, Administrator

Community Hospice of Baldwin County, 1113B North McKenzie Street, Foley, AL 36535; tel. 334/943-5015; FAX. 334/943-3986; Diana L. Cline, RN, Administrator

Community Hospice of Escambia County, 1023 Douglas Avenue, Suite 106, Brewton, AL 36426; tel. 334/867-6993; FAX. 334/867-7271; Daniel M. Scarbrough, M.D., Administrator

Countryside Hospice, 1826 E. 3 Notch Street, Andalusia, AL 36420; tel. 334/222-7048; FAX. 334/427-7246; Lisa K. Teel

Hospice Family Care, 2225 Drake Avenue, S.W., Suite 8, Huntsville, AL 35805; tel. 256/650-1212; FAX. 256/880-2929; Sue Morgan, Executive Director

Hospice of Blount County, Inc., 204 Washington Avenue, E., Oneonta, AL 35121; tel. 205/274-0549; FAX. 205/274-0550; Debbie Hyde

Hospice of Cullman County, Inc., 402 Fourth Avenue, N.E., P.O. Box 1227, Cullman, AL 35055; tel. 205/739-5185; Roger Hood, Administrator

Hospice of EAMC, 665 Opelika Road, Auburn, AL 36830; tel. 334/826-1899; FAX. 334/826-1899; Nancy A. Penaskovic

Hospice of Limestone County, 405 South Marion Street, P.O. Box 626, Athens, AL 35612; tel. 205/232-5017; FAX. 205/230-0085; Patricia P. Jackson, Administrator

Hospice of Marshall County, 8787 U.S. Highway 431, Albertville, AL 35950; tel. 256/891-7724; FAX. 256/891-7754; Rhonda Osborne, RN, B.S.N., CRNH, Executive Director

Hospice of Montgomery, 1111 Holloway Park, Montgomery, AL 36117; tel. 334/279-6677; FAX. 334/277-2223; Clare W. Lacey, Executive Director

Hospice of Northeast Alabama, a Member of the Baptist Health System, 112 College Street, P.O. Box 981, Scottsboro, AL 35768; tel. 205/574-4622; FAX. 205/259-3772; Virginia Stone, Director

Hospice of Northwest Alabama, 170 Bankhead Highway, Suite A, P.O. Box 1216, Winfield, AL 35594; tel. 205/487-8140; FAX. 205/487-8740; Linda Martin Sewell, Executive Director

Hospice of the Shoals, Inc., 1108 Bradshaw Drive, P.O. Box 307, Florence, AL 35630-0000; tel. 256/767-6699; FAX. 256/767-3116; Blake Edwards, Executive Director

Hospice of the Valley, Inc., 216 Johnston Street, S.E., P.O. Box 2745, Decatur, AL 35602; tel. 256/350-5585; FAX. 256/350-5567; Carolyn Dobson, Executive Director

Hospice of West Alabama, 1800 McFarland Boulevard, N., Suite 310, Tuscaloosa, AL 35406; tel. 205/345-0067; FAX. 205/345-9806; Julie Sittason, Executive Director

Hospice South, Inc., 501 Hargrove Road, Suite 4D, Tuscaloosa, AL 35401; tel. 205/366-9681; FAX. 205/366-9665; Dr. Bobby T. Williams, Chief Executive Officer

Hospice South, Inc., Of Livingston, 112 Lafayette Street, Livingston, AL 35470; tel. 205/652-2451; David Looney, Administrator

Infirmary Hospice Care, Inc., 2601-B Emorgene Street, Mobile, AL 36606; tel. 334/450-3280; FAX. 334/450-3289; David Price, Administrator

Lakeside Hospice, Inc, 17 Lake Plaza, P.O. Box 544, Pell City, AL 35125; tel. 205/884-1111; FAX. 205/884-1114; Nancy Odom, Director

Lakeview Hospice, 820 West Washington Street, Eufaula, AL 36027; tel. 334/687-1073; Rhonda Cotton, RN, Assistant Administrator

Mercy Medical, 101 Villa Drive, P.O. Box 1090, Daphne, AL 36526; tel. 334/626-2694; FAX. 334/626-0315; Sister Mary Eileen Wilhelm

Providence Hospice, 1141 Montlimar Drive, Mobile, AL 36609; tel. 334/344-2234; FAX. 334/344-4642; Frances Glenn, Administrator

Saad's Hospice Services, Inc., 3725 Airport Boulevard, Suite 180, Mobile, AL 36608; tel. 334/343-9600; FAX. 334/380-3328; Barbara S. Fulgham

Unity Hospice Biham Montclair, Princeton & St. Vincent's Hospice, 2145 Highland Ave., Suite 110, Birmingham, AL 35205; tel. 205/939-8797; FAX. 205/939-1682; Debbie Cox, CRNH, Patient Care Manager

Wiregrass Hospice, Inc., 1211 West Main Street, Dothan, AL 36301; tel. 334/792-1101; FAX. 334/792-0009; Ray L. Shrout, Administrator

Wiregrass Hospice, Inc., 2740 Headland Avenue, Dothan, AL 36303; tel. 334/792-1100; FAX. 334/794-0009; Ray L. Shrout, President and CEO

ALASKA

Alaska Home Health Care Agency, Inc., 1200 Airport Heights, Suite 170, Anchorage, AK 99508; tel. 907/272-0018; FAX. 907/272-0014; Lawrence Smith, Title Company President

Hospice of Anchorage, 500 W. International Airport Road #C, Anchorage, AK 99518; tel. 907/561-5322; FAX. 907/561-0334; Julia Thersness, Executive Director

Hospice of Mat-Su, 3051 E. Palmer Wasilla Hwy, Wasilla, AK 99654; tel. 907/352-4800; FAX. 907/352-4801; Kimm Gibson, RN, Director

ARIZONA

Community Hospice, 4330 North Campbell Avenue, Suite 256, Tucson, AZ 85718; tel. 520/544-2273; FAX. 520/577-8862; Bonnie Lindstrom

Dignita Hospice Care, 202 East Earl Drive, Suite 320, Phoenix, AZ 85012; tel. 602/279-0677; FAX. 602/279-1085; Gary Polsky

Hospice Family Care Inpatient Unit, 5037 East Broadway Road, Mesa, AZ 85206; tel. 602/807-2655; FAX. 602/807-2660; Rhonda Huffman, RN, General Manager

Hospice Family Care Inpatient Unit–Santa Rita, 150 North La Canada Drive, Green Valley, AZ 85614; tel. 520/648-3099; Nancy Smith

Hospice Family Care, Inc., 1550 S. Alma School Road, Suite 102, Mesa, AZ 85210; tel. 480/461-3144; FAX. 480/844-9711; Rhonda Huffman, RN, General Manager

Hospice Family Care, Inc. Green Valley Program, 210 West Continental Road, Suite 134, Green Valley, AZ 85614; tel. 520/648-6166; FAX. 520/648-6165; Karen Hoefle

Hospice of Arizona, 2222 W. Northern Avenue, Suite A-100, Phoenix, AZ 85021; tel. 602/678-1313; FAX. 602/242-2178; Jerene Maierle, Administrator

Hospice of Havasu, Inc., 2277 Swanson Ave, Suite A, Lake Havasu C, AZ 86403; tel. 520/453-2111; FAX. 520/453-2353; Nancy Iannone, Administrator

Hospice of the Valley, 1510 East Flower Street, Phoenix, AZ 85014; tel. 602/530-6900; FAX. 602/530-6901; Susan Goldwater, Executive Director

Hospice of the Valley, 2222 South Dobson Road, Suite 401, Mesa, AZ 85202; tel. 602/835-0711; FAX. 602/730-6078; Donna O'Brien

Hospice of the Valley Gardiner Hospice Home, 1522 West Myrtle Avenue, Phoenix, AZ 85021; tel. 602/995-9323; Susan Goldwater, Executive Director

Hospice of Yuma, 1824 South Eighth Avenue, Yuma, AZ 85364; tel. 602/343-2222; FAX. 602/343-0688; Maggie Welsh, RN, BSN, Executive Director

Jacob C. Fruchthendler Jewish Community Hospice, 5100 East Grant Road, P.O. Box 13090, Tucson, AZ 85732-3090; tel. 520/881-5300; FAX. 520/322-3620; Jo Turnbull, RN, B.S.

Mt. Graham Community Hospital–Hospice Services, 1600 20th Avenue, Building E, Safford, AZ 85546; tel. 520/348-4045; FAX. 520/428-3868; Lana Sanderson, Clinical Coordinator

Northland Hospice, 1609 S. Plaza Way, P.O. Box 997, Flagstaff, AZ 86002; tel. 520/779-1227; FAX. 520/779-5884; Marilyn J. Pate, Executive Director

RTA Hospice, 107 East Frontier, Payson, AZ 85541; tel. 602/472-6340; FAX. 602/472-6464; Vicki Dietz, RN, B.S.N., Executive Director

RTA Hospice, Inc., 177 West Cottonwood Lane, Suite 10, Casa Grande, AZ 85222; tel. 520/421-7143; FAX. 520/421-7315; Cindy McCarville, Patient Care Administrator

Sun Health Hospice Care Services & Residence, 12740 N. Plaza del rio blvd, Peoria, AZ 85381; tel. 800/858-9428; FAX. 602/974-7894; Marlene Stolz, Acting Director

Vista Hospice Care, Inc., 6991 East Camelback Road, Suite C-250, Scottsdale, AZ 85251; tel. 602/945-2200; Roseanne Berry

ARKANSAS

Area Agency on Aging Hospice of West Central Arkansas, 103 West Parkway Drive, Suite Two A, Russellville, AR 72801; tel. 501/967-9300; FAX. 501/967-2401; Oren Yates, Program Administrator

Area Agency on Aging Hospice of Western Arkansas, 524 Garrison Avenue, P.O. Box 1724, Fort Smith, AR 72902; tel. 501/783-4500; FAX. 501/783-0029; Jim Medley, Executive Director, CEO

Area Agency on Aging of Southeast Arkansas Hospice Two, 529 West Trotter, P.O. Box 722, Monticello, AR 71655; tel. 501/367-9873; Betty Bradshaw, Administrator

Area Agency on Aging of Southeast Arkansas, Inc. Hospice, 709 East Eighth Avenue, P.O. Box 8569, Pine Bluff, AR 71611; tel. 501/534-3268; Betty Bradshaw, President and CEO

Area Agency on Aging of Western Arkansas, Inc., d/b/a Visiting Nurses Agency of Western Arkansas, Inc., 398 School Street, Winslow, AR 72959; tel. 501/634-3812; FAX. 501/634-3912; Jim Medley, Executive Director

Area Agency on Aging of Western Arkansas, Inc., Mena Hospice, 600 Seventh Street, Mena, AR 71953; tel. 501/394-5458; FAX. 501/394-7675; Mary Keith, RNC, Vice President

Arkansas Department of Health Hospice 10, 40 Allen Chapel Road, P.O. Box 4267, Batesville, AR 72503; tel. 870/251-2848; FAX. 870/251-3449; Susan Coleman, Hospice Specialist

Arkansas Department of Health Hospice Five, Miller County Health Unit, 503 Walnut, Texarkana, AR 71852; tel. 870/773-2108; Mary Johnson, Administrator

Arkansas Department of Health Hospice Nine West, Monroe County Health Unit, 306 West King Drive, Brinkley, AR 72021; tel. 501/734-1461; FAX. 501/734-1024; John Selig, Administrator

Arkansas Department of Health Hospice Six, Area Six Office, Highway 167 South, Hampton, AR 71744; tel. 870/798-3113; Nealia Neal, Administrator

Providers / Freestanding Hospices

Arkansas Department of Health Hospice, Area III, 1708 West 'C' Place, Russellville, AR 72801; tel. 501/968–4177; FAX. 501/890–7211; Vickie Dunn, Coordinator

Arkansas Department of Health–Hospice Area Nine, Crittenden County Health Unit, 901 North Seventh, West Memphis, AR 72301; tel. 501/735–4334; FAX. 501/735–1393; John Selig, Administrator

Baptist Health, d/b/a Baptist Hospice, 11900 Colonel Glenn Road, Suite 2300, Little Rock, AR 72210; tel. 800/900–7474; FAX. 501/202–7793; Becky Pryor, Administrator

Baptist Memorial Regional Home Health Care, d/b/a Arkansas Home Health and Hospice, 824 North Washington, P.O. Box 90, Forrest City, AR 72335; tel. 501/633–6184; Gary Hughes, Administrator

Baptist Memorial Regional Home Health Care, Inc., d/b/a Arkansas Home Health and Hospice–West Memphis, 310 Mid–Continent Building, Suite 400, P.O. Box 2013, West Memphis, AR 72303; tel. 870/735–0363; FAX. 870/735–7156; Gary Hughes, Administrator

Best Care Hospice Services, 1125 East 35th Street, Texarkana, AR 71854; tel. 870/773–4671; Ed Braddock, RN, BSN

CareNetwork, Inc., d/b/a CareNetwork Hospice of Fort Smith, Central Mall, Suite 600, Fort Smith, AR 72903; tel. 501/484–7273; Barny Solomon, Administrator

CareNetwork, Inc., d/b/a CareNetwork of Hot Springs Hospice, 2212 Malvern, Suite 3, Hot Springs, AR 71901; tel. 501/623–5656; Cheryl Drake, Director, Hospice Services

Central Arkansas Area Agency on Aging, d/b/a Hospice of central Arkansas, 706 West Fourth Street, P.O. Box 5988, North Little Rock, AR 72119; tel. 501/372–5300; FAX. 501/688–7443; Beth Landon, Administrator

Country Medical Services of Arkansas, Inc, d/b/a Eastern Ozarks Home Health & Hospice, 120 South Allegheny, Box 7, Cherokee Village, AR 72549; tel. 870/257–4141; Cindy Hall, RN, Administrator

County Medical Services of Arkansas, Inc, d/b/a Eastern Ozarks Home Health and Hospice, 120 Hospital Drive Box 7, Cherokee Village, AR 72529; tel. 870/257–4141; FAX. 870/257–5232; Debra Windham, RN, Director

Crossroads Hospice of Arkansas, LLC, 10816 Executive Center Drive, Suite 203, Little Rock, AR 72211; tel. 501/312–9540; FAX. 501/312–9546; Eva Combee, Executive Director

Eureka Regional Health, d/b/a Eureka Springs Hospital Home Health & Hospice, 24 Norris Street, Eureka Springs, AR 72632; tel. 501/253–5554; FAX. 501/253–9428; Mary Bland, Director

Hospice Care for Southeast Arkansas, Inc., d/b/a Hospice Care Services, 2214 South Blake, Pine Bluff, AR 71603; tel. 870/534–4847; FAX. 870/534–4884; Dianna Millenbaugh, Administrator

Hospice Care Foundation, Inc, P.O Box 410, McGehee, AR 71654; tel. 870/222–5989; FAX. 870/222–5990; Tiffany Walker, Coordinator

Hospice Foundation of Arkansas, d/b/a The Arkansas Hospice, 2200 Fort Roots Drive, North Little Rock, AR 72114–1709; tel. 501/275–3400; FAX. 501/257–3400; Michael V. Aureli, Executive Director

Hospice Home Care, Inc of Pine Bluff, 3067 W. 28th Street, P.O Box 5046, Pine Bluff, AR 71603; tel. 870/540–0727; FAX. 870/534–6300; Cecilia Troppoli, Administrator

Hospice Home Care, Inc., Prospect Building, 1501 North University Avenue, Little Rock, AR 72207; tel. 501/666–9697; FAX. 501/666–4616; Cecilia Troppoli, Administrator

Hospice Home, Inc. of Monticello, 450 West Gaines, Monticello, AR 71657; tel. 870/367–9008; Cecilia Troppoli, Administrator

Hospice of St. Michael Health Care Center, 300 East Fifth Street, Texarkana, AR 75502; tel. 501/779–2720; Steven F. Wright, Administrator

Hospice of Texarkana, Inc., d/b/a Hospice of Hope, 102 East 16th Street, Hope, AR 71801; tel. 870/722–5887; Cynthia L. Marsh, Administrator

Hospice Preferred Choice, Inc., d/b/a Hospice Preferred Choice – Fort Smith, 2910 Jenny Lind, #6 Boston Square, Fort Smith, AR 72903; tel. 501/494–0100; Sheila Brown, Executive Director

Jonesboro Health Services, LLC, d/b/a Regional Hospice of NEA, 2200 Fowler Avenue, Jonesboro, AR 72401; tel. 888/310–1214; Linda A. Fulton, Administrator

Leo N. Levi National Arthritis Hospital Hospice, 300 Prospect Avenue, Hot Springs, AR 71902; tel. 501/624–1281; FAX. 501/622–3500; Patrick G. McCabe, Jr., Administrator

Medical Center of Calico Rock, Home Health Hospice, 103 Grasse Street, P.O. Box 438, Calico Rock, AR 72519; tel. 870/297–3738; FAX. 870/297–3739; Terry L. Amstutz, Administrator

Medshares, Inc of Arkansas, d/b/a Medshares Hospice of Western Arkansas, Inc., 210 South Maple, Nashville, AR 71852; tel. 870/832–4834; Kay Dunn, Administrator

North Arkansas regional Center Hospice, d/b/a Hospice of the Hills, 825 North High Spring, P.O. Box 1927, Harrison, AR 72602–1927; tel. 870/365–2100; FAX. 870/365–2461; Tim Hill, Administrator

Ozarks Regions Health Systems, Inc, d/b/a Hospice Care of Carroll Regional Medical Center, 214 Carter Street, Berryville, AR 72616; tel. 870/423–3355; James Darling, President and CEO

Saline County Medical Center, d/b/a Home Health & Hospice Services of Saline, 1 Medical Park Drive, Benton, AR 72015; tel. 501/776–6250; Roger D. Feldt, President and CEO

Share Foundation, d/b/a Community Hospice, 516 West Faulkner, El Dorado, AR 71730; tel. 501/862–0337; FAX. 501/862–0727; Linda D. Swart, Director

Texarkana Memorial Hospital, Inc., d/b/a Wadley Care Source Hospice, 718 East Fifth Street, Texarkana, AR 71854; tel. 903/798–7660; FAX. 903/798–7667; Hugh R. Hallgren, President and CEO

Visiting Nurses Agency of Western Arkansas, Inc., 207 College Avenue, Clarksville, AR 72830; tel. 501/754–8280; Lois Phillips, RNC, Regional Nursing Supervisor

Washington Regional Medical Center Hospice, 4241 Gable Drive, Fayetteville, AR 72703; tel. 888/611–1094; FAX. 501/444–7120; Kathy Kandar, Patient Care Coordinator

CALIFORNIA

All Nations Hospice, Inc., 3325 Wilshire Boulevard, Los Angeles, CA 90010; tel. 213/738–9741; Ugochi Obuge, Chief Executive Officer

American Home Health Hospice, 1950 E. 17th Street, Second Floor, Santa Ana, CA 92705; tel. 714/550–0800; FAX. 714/550–0521; Marylyn A. Hagerty, Ph.D., Chief Executive Officer

Assisted Home Hospice, 16909 Parthenia Street, Suite 201, North Hills, CA 91343; tel. 818/894–8117; FAX. 818/894–8707; Sherry Netherland, M.A., Executive Director, Hospice

Carl Bean House, 2146 West Adams Boulevard, Los Angeles, CA 90018; tel. 213/766–2326; FAX. 213/730–8244; Don Bustle, D.O.N.,RN

Children's Homecare, 3020 Children's Way, Mail Code 5036, San Diego, CA 92123; tel. 619/495–4941; FAX. 619/495–4956; Michelle Deitz, Director

Citrus Valley Hospice, d/b/a Citrus Valley Home Health, 820 North Phillips Avenue, West Covina, CA 91791; tel. 818/859–2263; FAX. 818/859–2272; Nancy Gillete, RN, Hospice Coordinator

Community Home Care Services/Hospice, 1925 East Dakota, Suite 208, Fresno, CA 93726; tel. 559/459–1615; FAX. 559/459–1009; Debra Henry, RN, DPCS

Community Hospice of the Bay Area, d/b/a Hospice by the Bay, 1540 Market Street, Suite 350, San Francisco, CA 94102–6035; tel. 415/626–5900; FAX. 415/626–7800; Constance L. Borden, Executive Director

Community Hospice, Inc., 601 McHenry Avenue, Modesto, CA 95350; tel. 209/577–0615; FAX. 209/577–0738; Harold A. Peterson, III, Chief Executive Officer

Companion Hospice, 12072 Trask Avenue, Suite 100, Garden Grove, CA 92643; tel. 714/741–0953; FAX. 714/534–0998; Michael Uranga, Administrator

Covina Health Care Center, 233 E. Rowland Street #B, Covina, CA 91723; tel. 626/339–9460; FAX. 626/331–5688; Rajinder Kutty

Crossroads Home Health Care and Hospice, Inc., 1109 Vincen, Suite 104, San Francisco, CA 94110; tel. 415/682–2111; Virginia A. Kahn

Elizabeth Hospice, 150 W. Crest Street, Escondido, CA 92025; tel. 760/737–2050; FAX. 760/796–3875; Laura Miller, Executive Director

Fremont–Rideout Home Health Valley Hospice, 16911 Willow Glen Road, Brownsville, CA 95919; tel. 916/692–1410; Cindy White, RN, Supervisor, Patient Care Coordinator

Garden Grove Hospice, 12882 Shackelford Lane, Garden Grove, CA 92841; tel. 714/638–9470; Rosa Valdivia

Hinds Hospice, 115 North P Street, P.O. Box 1325, Madera, CA 93639; tel. 559/674–0407; FAX. 559/674–3459; Nancy Hinds, Administrator

Hinds Hospice, 1450 E. 27th Street, P.O. Box 763, Merced, CA 95341; tel. 209/383–3123; FAX. 209/383–5308; Nancy Hinds, RN, Administrator

Hinds Hospice Services, 1616 West Shaw Avenue, Suite B–Six, Fresno, CA 93711; tel. 209/226–5683; FAX. 209/226–1028; Nancy Hinds, Administrator, Director of Nursing

Home Health Plus, 2511 Garden Road, Suite B–200, Monterey, CA 93940; tel. 408/373–8442; Anne Mason

Home Health Plus, 1003 Willow Pass Road, Suite 220, Concord, CA 94520; tel. 800/828–0698; FAX. 925/825–6010; Penny Barnes, Hospice Director

Home Health Plus, 2950 Merced Street, Suite 101, San Leandro, CA 94577; tel. 510/357–5852; FAX. 510/357–5969; Betsy Neel, Manager of Patient Care Services

Home Health Plus–Hospice, 825 Sonoma Avenue, Suite B, Santa Rosa, CA 95404; tel. 707/523–0111; FAX. 707/623–1034; Penelope J. Hunt, RN, Manager of Clinical Services

Home Health Plus–NCA, 2005 De La Cruz Boulevard, Suite 221, Santa Clara, CA 95050; tel. 408/986–1801; Mike Geraughty, Regional Hospice Director

Home Health Plus/Hospice, 3120 Chicago Avenue, Suite 190, Riverside, CA 92507; tel. 909/369–8054; Judith K. Kafantaris

Hope Hospice, 6500 Dublin Boulevard, Suite 100, Dublin, CA 94568–3151; tel. 925/829–8770; FAX. 925/829–0868; Teresa Drake, BSN, Executive Director

Horizon Hospice, 12709 Poway Road, Suite E–Two, Poway, CA 92064; tel. 619/748–3030; Thomas Dusmu–Johnson

Hospice and Palliative Care of Contra Costa, 2051 Harrison Street, Concord, CA 94520; tel. 925/609–1830; FAX. 925/609–1841; Cindy Siljestrom, Chief Executive Officer

Hospice by the Sea, 312 South Cedros Street, Suite 250, Solana Beach, CA 92075; tel. 858/794–0195; FAX. 858/794–0147; Kathie Jackson, Administrator

Hospice Cheer, 4032 Wilshire Boulevard, Suite 305, Los Angeles, CA 90010; tel. 213/383–9905; FAX. 213/383–9908; Vivian Graue–Allen, RN

Hospice of Amador, 839 North Highway 49/88, Suite F, Jackson, CA 95642; tel. 209/223–5500; FAX. 209/223–4964; Hazel Joyce, Executive Director

Hospice of Humboldt, Inc., 2010 Myrtle Avenue, Eureka, CA 95501; tel. 707/445–8443; FAX. 707/445–2209; Paul Mueller, Executive Director

Hospice of Marin, 150 Nellen Avenue, P.O. Box 763, Corte Madera, CA 94925; tel. 415/927–2273; FAX. 415/927–2284; Mary Tavema, President

Hospice of Napa Valley, 3299 Claremont Way, Napa, CA 94558; tel. 707/258–9080; FAX. 707/258–9088; Sarah Gorodezdy, Executive Director

Hospice of San Joaquin, 2609 East Hammer Lane, Stockton, CA 95210; tel. 209/957–3888; FAX. 209/957–3986; Barbara Tognoli, Administrator

Hospice of the Central Coast/Adobe Home Health, 100 Barnet Segal Lane, Monterey, CA 93940; tel. 408/648–7744; FAX. 408/648–7746; Patricia Cincone

Hospice of the Sierra, P.O. Box 4805, Sonora, CA 95370; tel. 209/533–6800; FAX. 209/532–6982; Judy Villalobos, Executive Director

Hospice of the Valley, 1150 South Bascom Avenue, Suite Seven A, San Jose, CA 95128; tel. 408/947–1233; FAX. 408/288–4172; Jessica Klinghoffer, Executive Director

Hospice of Tulare County, Inc., 332 North Johnson, Visalia, CA 93291; tel. 209/733–0642; FAX. 209/733–0658; Debbie Westfall

Hospice Preferred Choice, Inc., d/b/a HPC–Concord, 1470 Enea Circle, Suite 1710, Concord, CA 94520; tel. 510/798–1014; Victoria Condon, Executive Director

Hospice Services of Lake County, 1717 South Main Street, Lakeport, CA 95453; tel. 707/263–6222; FAX. 707/263–4045; Michael Brooks

Hospice Services of Santa Barbara, a Division of the Santa Barbara Visiting Nurse Association, 222 East Canon Perdido, Santa Barbara, CA 93101; tel. 805/963–6794; James S. Rivera, President and CEO

Providers / Freestanding Hospices

Hospital Home Health Care–Hospice, 2601 Airport Drive, Suite 110, Torrance, CA 90505; tel. 310/530-3800; FAX. 310/534-1754; Kaye Daniels President

Inland Valley Hospice, 3770 Myers Street, Riverside, CA 92503; tel. 909/360-5848; FAX. 909/360-0811; Katherine L. Allen, Administrator

Livingston Memorial VNA and Hospice, 1996 Eastman Avenue, Suite 101, Ventura, CA 93003; tel. 805/642-0239; FAX. 805/642-2320; Deborah Roberts, RN, B.S.N., President

Madrone Hospice, Inc., 255 Collier Circle, Yreka, CA 96097; tel. 530/842-3160; FAX. 530/842-6412; Audrey Flower, Executive Director

Marian Hospital Homecare and Hospice, 1300 East Cypress, Suite G, Santa Maria, CA 93454; tel. 805/922-9609; FAX. 805/349-9229; Marie Whitford, Vice President, Alternate Care Service

Medshares Home Care and Hospice of Coastal California, 2421 Mendocino Avenue, Suite 150, Santa Rosa, CA 95403; tel. 707/528-4663; FAX. 707/528-2301; Karen Emge, RN, Clinical Manager

Midpeninsula HomeCare and Hospice Services, Inc., 201 San Antonio Circle, Suite 135, Mountain View, CA 94040; tel. 650/949-3029; FAX. 650/949-4317; Barbara Burgess, Executive Director

Mission Hospice, Inc. of San Mateo County, 151 West 20th Avenue, San Mateo, CA 94403; tel. 650/554-1000; FAX. 650/554-1001; Carol L. Gray, RN, Administrator

Mountain Home Health Services, Inc., 35680 Wish-i-ah Road, Auberry, CA 93602; tel. 209/855-2200; FAX. 209/855-2284; Lori M. Harshman

Nations Healthcare, Inc.–Hospice, 9823 Pacific Heights Boulevard, Suite N, San Diego, CA 92121; tel. 619/546-3834; FAX. 619/546-0701; David Golman, Administrator

Odyssey Hospice, 7077 Orangewood Avenue, Suite 201, Garden Grove, CA 92841; tel. 800/797-2686; FAX. 714/934-4515; Jean M. Hunn, General Manager

Orangegrove Hospice, 12332 Garden Grove Boulevard, Garden Grove, CA 92843; tel. 714/534-1041; FAX. 714/534-7921; Maria Aguilar, Director, Hospice Services

Pathways to Care, Hospice, 1650 Iowa Avenue, Suite 220, Riverside, CA 92507; tel. 909/320-7070; FAX. 909/320-7060; Ed Gardner, President

Providence Home Hospice, 3413 Pacific Avenue, Burbank, CA 91505; tel. 818/953-4461; Elo Tanielian, Operations Director

Ramona Care Center Hospice, 11900 Ramona Boulevard, El Monte, CA 91732; tel. 626/442-5721; FAX. 626/444-9884

San Diego Hospice Corporation, 4311 Third Avenue, San Diego, CA 92103; tel. 619/688-1600; FAX. 619/688-9665; Jan Cetti, President and CEO

Self–Help HomeCare and Hospice, 407 Sansome Street, Suite 300, San Francisco, CA 94111; tel. 415/982-9171; FAX. 415/398-5903; Intake RN

St. Ambrose Hospice Care, 15022 Pacific Street, Suite #A, Midway City, CA 92655; tel. 714/379-6738; FAX. 714/379-6740; Mike Peiton, Director, Operations

St. Joseph Health System Home Care Services–Hospice, 1845 West Orangewood Avenue, Suite 100 A, Orange, CA 92868; tel. 714/712-9559; FAX. 714/712-9529; Junith Coyle, Hospice Director

Tri–City Hospice, 2095 West Vista Way, Suite 101, Vista, CA 92083; tel. 760/940-5801; FAX. 760/940-5823; Arthur A. Gonzalez, President and CEO

Tri–Med Hospice, 534 West Manchester Boulevard, Inglewood, CA 90301; tel. 310/419-4836; Margaret R. Lanam

Visiting Nurse Association and Hospice of Northern California, 1900 Powell Street, Suite 300, Emeryville, CA 94608; tel. 510/450-8596; FAX. 510/450-8532; Patricia Murphy, Director

Visiting Nurse Association and Hospice of Pomona/San Bernardin, 150 West First Street, P.O. Box 908, Claremont, CA 91711; tel. 714/624-3574; FAX. 714/624-8904; Marsha Fox, President

Visiting Nurse Service Hospice, Serving Santa Barbara County and San Luis Obispo County, 521 East Chapel Street, P.O. Box 1029, Santa Maria, CA 93454; tel. 805/925-8694; FAX. 805/925-1387; John W. Puryear, Executive Director

Vitas Healthcare, 333 South Anita Drive, Suite 950, Orange, CA 92668; tel. 714/921-2273; FAX. 714/712-5168; Brian Landberg, Director of Admissions

Vitas Healthcare Corporation, 8880 Rio San Diego Drive, Suite 950, San Diego, CA 92108; tel. 619/280-2273; Judy Piazza, RN, Director of Admissions

VNA and Home Hospice, 1110 North Dutton Avenue, Santa Rosa, CA 95401-4606; tel. 707/542-5045; FAX. 707/542-5742; Phyllis L. Cimino, Hospice Clinial Supervisor

VNA Foundation, 101 S. First Street, Suite 407, Burbank, CA 91502; tel. 818/526-1780; FAX. 818/526-1788; June Simmons, Chief Executive Officer

West Healthcare Hospice Services, 180 Otay Lakes Road, Suite 100, Bonita, CA 91902; tel. 619/472-7500; FAX. 619/472-1534; Suzanne L. Purdy

COLORADO

Angel of Shavano Hospice, Department of Health of the Regional Medical Center, 543 East First Street, Salida, CO 81201; tel. 719/539-7638; FAX. 719/539-3699; Diane Rogers, RN

Arkansas Valley Hospice, 118 West Fourth Street, Box 1067, LaJunta, CO 81050; tel. 719/384-8827; FAX. 719/384-2045; Erma J. Isaac, Executive Director

Baca County Hospice, 204 East 10th Avenue, Springfield, CO 81073; tel. 719/523-4851; FAX. 719/523-4513; Shirley Close, Director

Banner Hospice, 615 Fairhurst Street, P.O. Box 3500, Sterling, CO 80751; tel. 970/521-3126; FAX. 970/521-3255; Mike Gillen, Administrator

Boulder County Hospice, Inc., 2825 Marine Street, Boulder, CO 80303; tel. 303/449-7740; FAX. 303/449-6961; Constance Holden, Executive Director

Bristlecone Home Care and Hospice, Inc., 615 Walsen Avenue, Walsenburg, CO 81089; tel. 970/668-5604; FAX. 970/668-3189; Ms. Grace Rome-Kuhn, Administrator

Caring Unlimited Hospice Services, Inc., 615 Walsen Avenue, Walsenburg, CO 81019; tel. 719/738-1929; FAX. 719/738-2113; Karen Clouse, RN

Exempla Homecare and Hospice, 3964 Youngfield, Wheat Ridge, CO 80033; tel. 303/467-4700; FAX. 303/424-5260; Ms. Kim Hegemann, Administrator

Grand Valley Hospice, d/b/a Hospice of the Grand Valley, 2754 Compass Drive, Suite 377, Grand Junction, CO 81506; tel. 970/241-2212; FAX. 970/257-2400; Christy Whitney, President and CEO

Hospice Associates of America, 2223 S. Monaco, #A–Z, Denver, CO 80222; tel. 303/753-0421; Mr. Edward Lowe, Administrator

Hospice Del Valle, Inc., 617 6th Street, P.O. Box 1554, Alamosa, CO 81101; tel. 719/589-9019; FAX. 719/589-5094; Judy M. Lamb, RN, MBA

Hospice of Estes Valley, 555 Prospect, P.O. Box 2740, Estes Park, CO 80517-2740; tel. 970/586-2273; FAX. 970/586-3895; Susan J. Mock, Director

Hospice of Larimer County, 7604 Colland Drive, Fort Collins, CO 80525; tel. 970/663-3500; FAX. 970/663-1180; Brian Hoag, Executive Director

Hospice of Metro Denver, Inc., 425 South Cherry Street, Suite 700, Denver, CO 80246-1234; tel. 303/321-2828; FAX. 303/321-7171; Ber Sloan, President and CEO

Hospice of Northern Colorado, 2726 11th Street Road, Greeley, CO 80631; tel. 970/352-8487; FAX. 970/352-6685; Jane M. Schnell, RN, Executive Director

Hospice of Peace, 1601 A Lowell Boulevard, Denver, CO 80204-1545; tel. 303/575-8393; FAX. 303/575-8390; Ann Luke, Executive Director

Hospice of St. John, 1320 Everett Court, Lakewood, CO 80215; tel. 303/232-7900; FAX. 303/232-3614; Ms. Cindy Morrison, Administrator

Hospice of the Comforter of Colorado, 2345 N. Academy Place, Suite 213, Colorado Springs, CO 80909; tel. 719/573-4166; FAX. 719/573-4164; Mary McGreevy, RN, Executive Administrator

Hospice of the Gunnison Valley, 1500 West Tomichi Avenue, Gunnison, CO 81230; tel. 970/641-0704; FAX. 970/641-5593; Robert Patterson, Administrator

Hospice of the Plains, Inc., 125 W. 5th Street, P.O. Box 365, Wray, CO 80758; tel. 970/332-4116; FAX. 970/332-4102; Donna Roberts, Administrator

Hospice Services of Northwest Colorado, 135 Sixth Street, P.O. Box 775816, Steamboat Springs, CO 80477; tel. 970/879-9218; FAX. 970/870-1326; Janet Fritz, Executive Director

Lamar Area Hospice Association, Inc., 1001 South Main, P.O. Box 843, Lamar, CO 81052; tel. 719/336-2100; Denise Koechner, RN, Executive Director

Life Source Services, Inc., 245 S. Benton Street, Suite 205, Lakewood, CO 80226; tel. 303/237-4673; FAX. 303/237-2773; Candee Wells, Executive Director

Mount Evans Hospice, 3721 Evergreen Parkway, P.O. Box 2770, Evergreen, CO 80439; tel. 303/674-6400; Louisa B. Walthers, Executive Director

Pikes Peak Hospice and Palliative Care, 825 E. Pikes Peak Avenue, Suite 600, Colorado Springs, CO 80903; tel. 719/633-3400; FAX. 719/633-1150; Martha Barton, RN, President and CEO

Porter Hospice, 2420 W. 26th Ave, Suite 200D, Denver, CO 80211; tel. 303/561-5100; FAX. 303/561-5199; Terri Walter, Director

Prospect Home Care Hospice, Inc., 321 West Henrietta Avenue, Suite E, P.O. Box 6278, Woodland Park, CO 80866; tel. 719/687-0549; FAX. 719/687-8558; Joleen Bailey, Executive Director

Sangre de Cristo Hospice, 704 Elmhurst Place, Pueblo, CO 81004; tel. 719/542-0032; FAX. 719/542-1413; Joni Fair, President and CEO

Trinity Hospice, LLC, 6795 East Tennessee, Suite 250, Denver, CO 80224; tel. 303/355-5890; FAX. 303/355-5976; Kevin Webb, Administrator

CONNECTICUT

Bristol Hospital Home Care Agency, Seven North Washington Street, Plainville, CT 06062; tel. 860/585-4752; FAX. 860/747-6719; Linda St. Pierre, RN, Director

East Hartford Visiting Nurse Association, Inc., 111 Founders Plaza, Suite 200, East Hartford, CT 06108-3213; tel. 860/528-2273; FAX. 860/290-6777; Louise Leita, Hospice Director

Foothills Visiting Nurse & Home Care, Inc., 32 Union Street, Winsted, CT 06098; tel. 860/379-8561; FAX. 860/738-7479; Jeannette Jakubiak, RN, Executive Director

Home and Community Health Services, Inc., The Nirenberg Medical Center, 140 Hazard Avenue, P.O. Box 1199, Enfield, CT 06083; tel. 860/763-7603; FAX. 860/763-7613; Kathryn D. Roby, RN, B.S.N., Administrator

Hospice & Palliative Care of Eastern Connecticut, a Program at VNA East, Inc, 34 Ledgebrook Drive, P.O. Box 716, Mansfield Center, CT 06250; tel. 860/456-7288; FAX. 860/456-4267; Claudia M. Marcinczyk, CEO

Hospice at Home, A program of Visiting Nurse Services of Connecticut, Inc, 765 Fairfield Avenue, Bridgeport, CT 06606; tel. 203/366-3821; FAX. 203/334-0543; Lois Ravage – Mass, RN, M.S.N, Hospice Director

Hospice of Northeastern Connecticut, 320 Pomfret Street, Putnam, CT 06260; tel. 860/928-0422; FAX. 860/963-2259; Carol Emmerthal, Hospice Program Director

Hospice of Southeastern Connecticut, Inc., 179 Gallivan Lane, P.O. Box 902, Uncasville, CT 06382-0902; tel. 860/848-5699; FAX. 860/848-6898; Carol Shaber, Executive Director

McLean Visiting Nursing and Community Services, 75 Great Pond Road, Simsbury, CT 06070; tel. 860/658-3950; FAX. 860/408-1319; Nancy E. Ryan, RN, Administrator

Middlesex Visiting Nurse and Home Health Services, Inc., 51 Broad Street, Middletown, CT 06457; tel. 860/704-5600; Janine Fay, Administrator

Project Care, Inc., Home and Hospice Services, 51 Depot Street, Suite 203, Watertown, CT 06795; tel. 860/274-9239; FAX. 860/945-3625; Joel Schlank, Administrator

Regional Hospice of Western Connecticut, Inc., 30 West Street, Danbury, CT 06810; tel. 203/797-1685; Patricia Coyle, RN, Administrator, Supervisor

Salisbury Visiting Nurse Association, Inc., 30 Salmon Kill Road, Salisbury, CT 06068; tel. 860/435-0816; Marilyn Joseph, RN, Administrator/Supervisor

Southington Visiting Nurse Association, Inc., 80 Meriden Avenue, Southington, CT 06489; tel. 203/621-0157; Mary Jane Corn, RN, Administrator

The Connecticut Hospice, Inc., 61 Burban Drive, Branford, CT 06405; tel. 203/481-6231; FAX. 203/483-9539; Rosemary J. Hurzeler, President and CEO

Providers / Freestanding Hospices

The Greater Bristol VNA, Inc., 10 Maltby Street, P.O. Box 2826, Bristol, CT 06011–2826; tel. 860/583–1644; FAX. 860/584–2100; Anita Baldwin, Hospice Coordinator

Visiting Nurse and Health Services of Connecticut, Eight Keynote Drive, Vernon, CT 06066; tel. 860/872-9163; FAX. 860/872-3030; William Pearl, Administrator

Visiting Nurse and Homecare, Inc, 103 Woodland Street, Hartford, CT 06105; tel. 860/525–7001; FAX. 860/278–0581; Donna Boehm, Program Manager

Visiting Nurse Association and Hospice, of Pioneer Valley, Inc., 701 Enfield Street, Enfield, CT 06082; tel. 203/253–5316; Kimberly A. Barbaro, RN, M.B.A., Administrator

Visiting Nurse Association of Central Connecticut, Inc., 205 West Main Street, P.O. Box 1327, New Britain, CT 06050; tel. 860/224–7131; FAX. 860/224–8303; Mary Jane Corn, B.S.N., RN, President and CEO

VNA Health at Home, Inc., 27 Princeton Road, Watertown, CT 06795; tel. 860/274-7531; FAX. 860/274-8492; W. Rennard Wieland, President

VNA Valley Care, Inc., Eight Old Mill Lane, Simsbury, CT 06070–1932; tel. 860/651–3539; FAX. 860/651–5082; Incy Severance, RN, M.P.A., Executive Director

DELAWARE

Compassionate Care Hospice of Delaware, 623 W. Newport Pike, Wilmington, DE 19804; tel. 302/454–7002; FAX. 302/454–7003; Cathy Stauffer Kimble, MPH, Regional Director

Delaware Hospice – Northern Division, 100 Clayton Building, 3515 Silverside Road, Wilmington, DE 19810; tel. 302/478–5707; FAX. 302/479–2586; Susan D. Lloyd, RN, M.S.N., Executive Director

Delaware Hospice, Inc.–Southern Division, 600 DuPont Highway, Suite 107, Georgetown Professional Park, Georgetown, DE 19947; tel. 302/856–7717; Susan D. Lloyd, RN, M.S.N., Executive Director

Delaware Hospice–Central Division, Lotus Plaza, 911 South DuPont Highway, Dover, DE 19901; tel. 302/734–4700; FAX. 302/678–4451; Susan D. Lloyd, RN, M.S.N., Executive Director

First State Hospice, 5193 West Woodmill Drive, Suite 28, Wilmington, DE 19808; tel. 302/995–2273; FAX. 302/995–2280; Terry L. Hastings, RN, Executive Director

DISTRICT OF COLUMBIA

Children's Hospice Services, 111 Michigan Avenue, N.W., Washington, DC 20010; tel. 202/884–4663; FAX. 202/884–6950

Home Care Partners, 1234 Massachusetts Avenue, N.W., Washington, DC 20005; tel. 202/638–2382; FAX. 202/628–3169; Marla Lahat, CEO

Hospice Care of the District of Columbia, 1331 H. Street, NW, Suite 600, Washington, DC 20005; tel. 202/347–1700; FAX. 202/347–3505; Ann Burden, Executive Director

Hospice of Washington, 3720 Upton Street, N.W., Washington, DC 20016; tel. 202/966–3720; FAX. 202/895–0177; Mary Ann Griffin, Vice President Hospice

Inova Health Care–District of Columbia Branch, 1331 Pennsylvania Avenue, N.W., S–500, Washington, DC 20005; tel. 202/638–5828; Regina Silver

Medstar Health VNA Hospice Services, 6000 New Hampshire Ave, NE, Washington, DC 20011; tel. 202/538–8600; FAX. 202/538–8681; Susan Walker, Hospice Director

Urgent Home Health Care, 1535 P Street, N.W., Washington, DC 20005; tel. 202/483–3355; Pauline NGO Bapack

FLORIDA

Big Bend Hospice, Inc., 1723 Mahan Center Boulevard, Tallahassee, FL 32308–5428; tel. 850/878–5310; FAX. 850/309–1638; Elaine C. Bartelt, M.S., President and CEO

Catholic Hospice, Inc., 14100 Palmetto Frontage Road, Suite 370, Miami, FL 33016; tel. 305/822–2380; FAX. 305/824–0665; Janet L. Jones, President and COO

Good Shepherd Hospice of Mid–Florida, 105 Arneson Avenue, Auburndale, FL 33823; tel. 813/297–1880; FAX. 813/965–5601; Mary Ellen Poe, Administrator

Good Shepherd Hospice of Mid–Florida, Inc., 2121 S.E. Lakeview Drive, Sebring, FL 33870; tel. 863/471–3700; FAX. 863/471–9452; Isaac Durance, RN, Director

Hernando–Pasco Hospice, Inc., 12107 Majestic Boulevard, Hudson, FL 34667; tel. 813/863–7971; FAX. 813/868–9261; Rodney Taylor, Executive Director

Hope Hospice of Lee County, Inc., 9470 Health Park Circle, Ft. Myers, FL 33908; tel. 941/482–4673; FAX. 941/482–2488; Samira K. Beckwith, President and CEO

Hospice Care of Broward County, Inc., 309 Southeast 18th Street, Ft. Lauderdale, FL 33316; tel. 954/467–7423; FAX. 954/476–3353; Susan G. Telli, Executive Director

Hospice Care of South Florida, 7270 Northwest 12th Street, Penthouse Six, Miami, FL 33126; tel. 305/591–1606; FAX. 305/591–1618; Rose Marie R. Marty, Administrator, CEO

Hospice of Citrus County, Inc., 3350 West Audubon Park Path, Lecanto, FL 34461–8450; tel. 352/527–2020; FAX. 352/527–0386; Marjorie Budd, RN, Executive Director

Hospice of Health First, Inc, 1900 Dairy Road, West Melbourne, FL 32904; tel. 407/952–0494; FAX. 407/952–0382; Roberta Van Dusen, Director

Hospice of Lake and Sumter, Inc., 12300 Lane Park Road, Taveres, FL 32778–9660; tel. 352/343–1341; FAX. 352/343–6115; Patricia Lehorsky, Chief Executive Officer

Hospice of Naples, Inc., 1095 Whippoorwill Lane, Naples, FL 34105; tel. 941/261–4404; FAX. 941/261–3278; Diane S. Cox, President and CEO

Hospice of Northeast Florida, Inc., 4266 Sunbeam Road, The Earl Hadlow Center for Caring, Jacksonville, FL 32257; tel. 904/268–5200; FAX. 904/596–6036; Susan Ponder-Stansel, President and CEO

Hospice of Northwest Florida, Inc., 2001 North Palafox Street, Pensacola, FL 32501; tel. 904/433–2155; FAX. 904/433–7212; Dale O. Knee, President and CEO

Hospice of Okeechobee, Inc., 411 Southeast Fourth Street, Okeechobee, FL 34973; tel. 813/467–2321; FAX. 813/467–8330; Richard S. Green, Executive Director

Hospice of Palm Beach County, Inc., 5300 East Avenue, West Palm Bea, FL 33407; tel. 561/848–5200; FAX. 561/863–2955; David Fielding, President and CEO

Hospice of Pasco, Inc., 6224–6230 Lafayette Street, New Port Rich, FL 34652–2626; tel. 813/845–5707; FAX. 813/846–8661; Katherine Hirst, Executive Director

Hospice of St. Francis, Inc., 2395 South U.S. Highway 1, P.O. Box 5563, Titusville, FL 32783–5563; tel. 321/269–4240; FAX. 321/269–5428; Bruce Wolters, Executive Director

Hospice of the Comforter, 595 Montgomery Road, Altamonte Springs, FL 32714; tel. 407/682–0808; FAX. 407/682–5737; Robert G. Wilson, President and Director

Hospice of the Florida Keys, 1319 William Street, Key West, FL 33040; tel. 305/294–8812; FAX. 305/294–9348; Liz Kern, President and CEO

Hospice of the Gold Coast H.H.S., 911 East Atlantic Boulevard, Suite 200, Pompano Beach, FL 33060; tel. 305/785–2990; FAX. 305/785–2993; Lynda Friedman, Administrator

Hospice of the Treasure Cost, Inc., 805 Virginia Avenue, Suite 15, Ft. Pierce, FL 34982; tel. 561/465–0504; FAX. 561/465–6309; Sharon A. Rivers, President and CEO

Hospice of Volusia and Flagler, 3800 Woodbriar Trail, Port Orange, FL 32119; tel. 904/322–4701; FAX. 904/324–4702; Debbie Harley, Director

Life Path Hospice, Inc, 3010 West Azeele Street, Tampa, FL 33609–3139; tel. 813/877–2200; FAX. 813/872–7037; Susan E. Lang, Director of Marketing

The Hospice of Martin & St. Lucie, Inc., 2030 Southeast Ocean Boulevard, Stuart, FL 34996; tel. 561/287–7860; FAX. 561/287–7982; Mary C. Knox, Executive Director

The Hospice of North Central Florida, 4200 Northwest 90th Blvd., Gainesville, FL 32606; tel. 352/378–2121; FAX. 352/378–4111; Tim Bowen, Executive Director, CEO

The Hospice of the Florida Suncoast, Inc., 300 East Bay Drive, Largo, FL 33770; tel. 813/586–4432; FAX. 813/581–5846; Mary Labyak, M.S.S.W., L.C.S.W., President

VITAS Healthcare Corporation of Central Florida, Inc., 5151 Adamson Street, Orlando, FL 32804; tel. 407/875–0028; FAX. 407/875–2074; Clark Taylor, General Manager

VNA Hospice of Indian River County, 1111 36th Street, Vero Beach, FL 32960; tel. 407/567–5551; FAX. 407/567–9308; Sharon L. Kennedy, President and CEO

GEORGIA

American HospiceCare, 340 Eisenhower Drive, Building 1400, Suite A, Savannah, GA 31406; tel. 912/356–9090; FAX. 912/356–1155; Mr. Neil Bennett, Administrator

Avondale Hospice Services, Inc., 3500 Kensington Road, Decatus, GA 30032–1328; tel. 404/299–6111; Rachel Waldemar, Administrator

Blue–Gray Community Hospice, Perry House Road, P.O. Box 1349, Fitzgerald, GA 31750–1447; tel. 912/424–7152; Lenora Kirby, RN, Executive Director

Columbus Hospice, Inc., 1315 Delauney Ave., Suite 104, Columbus, GA 31901; tel. 706/327–5153; Mike Smajd, Executive Director

Georgia Mountain Hospice, Inc., 1476 East Church Street, P.O. Box 881, Jasper, GA 30143; tel. 706/692–3491; FAX. 706/692–4300; Lynn Corliss, Executive Director

Hamilton Medical Center–Hospice, P.O. Box 1168, 1200 Memorial Drive, Dalton, GA 30720–1168; tel. 706/278–2848; FAX. 706/272–6417; Judy Hannah, Administrator

Hand In Hand Hospice, 2150 Limestone Parkway, Gainesville, GA 30501; tel. 404/536–0497; FAX. 404/536–0157; Teresa J. Warren, Administrator

Haven House Hospice, Inc., 5411 Northland Drive, Atlanta, GA 30342; tel. 404/874–8313; FAX. 404/875–4363; Clyde W. Johnson, Jr., Vice President and CFO

Healthfield Hospice Services, Inc., 2045 Peachtree Road, N.E., Suite 210, Atlanta, GA 30309–1414; tel. 404/355–3134; Richard Stroder, RN Director

Hospice Atlanta, 1244 Park Vista Drive, Atlanta, GA 30319; tel. 404/869–3000; FAX. 404/869–3099; Patricia Szucs, Administrator

Hospice Care of Carroll County, Inc., P.O. Box 1136, Carrolton, GA 30117; tel. 770/214–2355; FAX. 770/214–8301; Pat Alfrey, Administrator

Hospice Care, Inc., 1310 13th Avenue, Suite 200, Columbus, GA 31901; tel. 706/660–8899; FAX. 706/660–8899; Mr. Adeleye Tokes, Ph.D., Administrator

Hospice of Americus and Sumter County, 119 Brannan Street, P.O. Box 1434, Americus, GA 31709; tel. 912/928–7940; FAX. 912/928–1322; Anne F. Speer, Executive Director

Hospice of Baldwin, Inc., 811 North Cobb Street, Milledgeville, GA 31061; tel. 912/453–8432; FAX. 912/453–8432; Jeannie Sweeney, Administrator

Hospice of Central Georgia, P.O. Box 6533, Macon, GA 31208; tel. 912/781–3340; FAX. 912/781–3349; Sharon Compton, Executive Director

Hospice of Georgia, Inc., 3450 New High Shoals Road, P.O. Box 10, High Shoals, GA 30645; tel. 706/769–8835; FAX. 706/769–5944; Fran Keisel, Administrator

Hospice of Houston Co., Inc., The Heart of Georgia Hospice, 2066 Watson Boulevard, Warner Robins, GA 31093; tel. 912/922–1777; FAX. 912/922–9433; Art Holtz, Executive Director

Hospice of Laurens County, 1103 Bellevue Avenue, P.O. Box 1344, Dublin, GA 31021; tel. 912/272–8333; FAX. 912/272–1695; Kaye Bracewell, Executive Director

Hospice of Northeast Georgia, Inc., Highway 76 West, Clayton, GA 30525; tel. 706/782–7505; FAX. 404/782–3343; Julie Ferguson, RN, Patient Care Coordinator

Hospice of Southeast Georgia, Inc., 333 South Ashley Street, P.O. Box 1077, Kingsland, GA 31548; tel. 912/673–7000; Chuck Chapman, President

Hospice of Southwest Georgia, 818 Gordon Avenue, Thomasville, GA 31792; tel. 912/227–5520; FAX. 912/227–5526; Sheila D. Warren, RN, MSN, Director

Hospice of the Golden Isles, Inc., 1692 Glynco Parkway, Brunswick, GA 31525; tel. 912/265–4735; FAX. 912/265–6100; Cheryl Johns, RN, Executive Director

Hospice of Wilkinson County, Inc., 1046 Mission Farm Road, P.O. Box 920, Gordon, GA 31031; tel. 912/628–5655; Edwin Lavender, Administrator

Hospice Savannah, Inc., 1352 Eisenhower Drive, P.O. Box 13190, Savannah, GA 31406; tel. 912/355–2289; FAX. 912/355–2376; Judith B. Brunger, Executive Director

Providers / Freestanding Hospices

Northside Hospice, 5825 Glenridge Drive, Building Four, Atlanta, GA 30328-5544; tel. 404/851-6300; FAX. 404/252-7708; Cristi Campbell, RN, CCM, Hospice Manager
Ogeechee Area Hospice, 5 West Altman Street, P.O. Box 531, Statesboro, GA 30458; tel. 912/764-8441; FAX. 912/489-8247; Nancy Bryant, RN
Peachtree Hospice, 3600 DeKalb Technology Parkway, P.O. 942029, Atlanta, GA 30340; tel. 404/451-1903; Curtis Stubblefield, Executive Director
Portsbridge, Inc., 4598 Barclay Drive, Dunwoody, GA 30338-5883; tel. 404/936-9546; FAX. 770/936-9547; T.M. Mahone, Administrator
Shepherd's Gate Hospice, Inc., 2149 Pace Street, Covington, GA 30014-6652; tel. 770/784-9200; FAX. 770/784-7650; John J. McBride, Executive Director
Southwest Christian Hospice, 7225 Lester Road, Union City, GA 30291; tel. 404/969-8354; FAX. 404/969-1940; Mike Sorrow, Executive Director
United Hospice of Calhoun, 1195 Curtis Parkway, Calhoun, GA 30701; tel. 706/602-9546; FAX. 706/602-0765; Judy Walters, Administrator
United Hospice of Macon, Inc., 2484 Ingleside Avenue, Building B, Macon, GA 31204; tel. 912/745-9204; FAX. 912/745-9321; Juliette Simpson, Regional Director
United Hospice, Inc., 3945 Lawrenceville Highway, Lilburn, GA 30047; tel. 800/544-4788; FAX. 770/925-4619; Matt Annis, Executive Director
Vencare Hospice-Atlanta, 1190 Winchester Parkway, Suite 200, Smyrna, GA 30080-6544; tel. 770/803-0881; Douglas J. Thompson, Administrator
Vencare Hospice-Columbus, 3646 Edgewood Road, Columbus, GA 31907; tel. 706/569-0200; Margarita Jara, Administrator
VistaCare Hospice-Macon, 750 Baconsfield Drive, Suite 115, Macon, GA 31211; tel. 912/750-9777; FAX. 912/750-0033; Lynda Geddis, Administrator
WellStar Community Hospice, 4040 Hospital West Drive, Suite 340, Austell, GA 30106-8117; tel. 770/732-6710; FAX. 770/732-6732; Cam Drinkwater, Admissions Coordinator
West Georgia Hospice, 1510 Vernon Road, Lagrange, GA 30240-4130; tel. 706/845-3905; FAX. 706/812-2650; Charles Foster, President and CEO
Wiregrass Hospice, Inc., 432 E. Shotwell Street, Bainbridge, GA 31717-4058; tel. 912/246-6330; Ray L. Shrout, Administrator

HAWAII
Hospice Hawaii, Inc, 860 Iwilei Road, Honolulu, HI 96817; tel. 808/924-9255; FAX. 808/922-9161; Stephen A. Kula, Ph.D., President, Chief Professional Officer
Hospice Maui, 400 Mahalani Street, Wailuku, HI 96793; tel. 808/244-5555; FAX. 808/244-5557; Dr. Gregory LaGoy, Executive Director
Hospice of Hilo, 1011 Waianuenue Avenue, Hilo, HI 96720; tel. 808/969-1733; FAX. 808/969-4863; Brenda Ho, Executive Director
Hospice of Kona, Inc., 74-5094 Palani Road, Kailua-Kona, HI 96740; tel. 808/334-0334; FAX. 808/334-0365; David Kula, Administrator
Kauai Hospice, 3175 Elua Street, P.O. Box 3286, Lihue, HI 96766; tel. 808/245-7277; FAX. 808/245-5006; Kathleen Boyle
North Hawaii Hospice, Inc., P.O. Box 1236, Kamuela, HI 96743; tel. 808/885-7547; FAX. 808/885-5592; Nancy Bouvet, Executive Director
St. Francis Hospice, 24 Puiwa Road, Honolulu, HI 96817; tel. 808/595-7566; FAX. 808/595-6996; Sister Francine Gries, Administrator

IDAHO
Blackfoot Medical Clinic, Home Care & Hospice, Inc., 625 West Pacific, Blackfoot, ID 83221; tel. 208/785-2600; James Marriott, Administrator
Good Samaritan Community Hospice, 840 East Elva, Idaho Falls, ID 83401; tel. 208/529-8326; FAX. 208/524-1518; H. Ray Belk, RNC, Director
Hospice of North Idaho, West 280 Prairie Avenue, Coeur D'Alene, ID 83815; tel. 208/772-7994; Dan Kuetemeyer, Director of Finance
Hospice of the Palouse, P.O. Box 9461, Moscow, ID 83843; tel. 208/882-1228; FAX. 208/883-6519; Leslie Park, RN, Director
Hospice of the Palouse, 700 South Main Street, Moscow, ID 83843-0119; tel. 208/882-1228; FAX. 208/883-2239; Julie Nelson, Administrator
Hospice Visions, Inc., 1300 Kimberly Road, Suite 11, Twin Falls, ID 83301; tel. 208/735-0121; FAX. 208/735-0661; Tamala Slatter, Director
Latah Health Home Care & Hospice, 510 West Palouse River Drive, Moscow, ID 83843; tel. 208/882-4802; FAX. 208/882-1819; Irma Laskowski, RNC, Hospice Director
Life's Doors Hospice, Inc., 1111 South Orchard, Suite 400, P.O. Box 5754, Boise, ID 83705; tel. 208/344-6500; FAX. 208/344-6590; Mary L. Langenfeld, Chief Executive Officer
Magic Valley Staffing Service, Inc., 200 Second Avenue, N., Twin Falls, ID 83301; tel. 208/734-0600; FAX. 208/736-9149; Debbie Osborn, Administrator
MSTI - Hospice of Boise, 151 East Bannock, Boise, ID 83712; tel. 208/386-2711; Nan Hart, Administrator
Southeastern District Hospice, 1901 Alvin Ricken Drive, Pocatello, ID 83201; tel. 208/239-5240; FAX. 208/478-6306; Judy Moyer, Administrator
XL Hospice, Inc., 1401 North Whitley Drive, Suite 16, Fruitland, ID 83619; tel. 208/452-5911; FAX. 208/452-4090; Dwight E. Olson, President

ILLINOIS
Advocate Hospice, 1441 Branding Avenue, Suite 240, Downers Grove, IL 60515; tel. 630/963-6800; FAX. 630/963-6877; Leslie A. Williams, Administrative Director
All Care, Inc., 900 Jorie Blvd., Suite 220, Oak Brook, IL 60523; tel. 630/346-2575; Robert M. Wesolowski
Beacon of Hope Hospice, Inc., 615 35th Ave., Moline, IL 61265; tel. 309/757-0579; Diane Lang
Beloit Regional Hospice, Inc., 5512 Elevator Road, Roscoe, IL 61073; tel. 608/365-7421; FAX. 608/363-7426; Virginia Burton, Administrator
Brave Heart Support Services, 78 Cherry Street, Park Forest, IL 60466; tel. 708/481-2104; Susie Zavodnyik, Executive Director
Bureau Valley Area Hospice, 526 Bureau Valley Parkway, Suite B, Princeton, IL 61356; tel. 815/875-7723; FAX. 815/875-4112; Geraldine Devert, RN, MS, Administrator
Carle Hospice, 2011 Round Barn Road, Champagne, IL 61821; tel. 217/383-3151; Sheryl Imlay, Administrator
Cass-Schuyler Area Hospice, 331 South Main Street, Virginia, IL 62691; tel. 217/452-3057; FAX. 217/452-7245; Jan Anderson, RN, Coordinator
CNS Hospice, 690 East North Avenue, Carol Stream, IL 60188; tel. 630/665-7000; FAX. 630/690-9064; Constance O'Neill, RN, Director
Community Hospices of America Northwest Illinois, 256 South Soangetaha Road, Suite 103, Galesburg, IL 61401-5586; tel. 309/342-3007; FAX. 309/342-6973; Sue Myer, Program Director
Covenant Hospice Care Program, 1400 West Park, Urbana, IL 61801; tel. 217/337-2470; Ruth Madewick
DeKalb County Hospice, 2727 Sycamore Road, Suite 1B, DeKalb, IL 60115; tel. 815/756-3000; FAX. 815/758-0962; Karen Hagen, RN, M.S., Executive Director
ENH Hospice, 5215 Old Orchard, Suite200, Skokie, IL 60077; tel. 847/581-1717; FAX. 847/581-1919; Janet Sullivan, Executive Director
Family Hospice of Belleville Area, 11B Park Place, Professional Center, Swansea, IL 62226; tel. 618/277-1800; FAX. 618/277-1074; Diane Smith, Administrator
Fox Valley Hospice, 200 Whitfield Drive, P.O. Box 707, Geneva, IL 60134; tel. 630/232-2233; FAX. 630/232-0023; M.E. Walsh, Executive Director
Grundy Community Hospice, 1802 North Division Street, Suite 307, Morris, IL 60450; tel. 815/942-8525; FAX. 815/942-4934; Joan Sereno, Executive Director
Harbor Light Hospice, 800 Roosevelt Road, Building C, Glen Ellyn, IL 60137; tel. 800/419-0542; FAX. 630/942-0118; Tracr Deleo, Administrator
Home Health Plus Hospice Program, 2215 Enterprise Drive, Suite 1512, Westchester, IL 60154; tel. 708/531-9339; FAX. 708/531-9680; Peggy Janka, Administrator
Home Health Plus Hospice Program, 333 Salem Place, Suite 165, Fairview Heights, IL 62208; tel. 618/632-0304; FAX. 314/453-0290; Robin Carnett, Administrator
Horizon Hospice, Inc., 833 West Chicago Avenue, Chicago, IL 60622; tel. 312/733-2233; FAX. 312/226-8173; Michael Preodor, M.D., President
Hospice Care, 319 East Madison, Suite Three J, Springfield, IL 62701; tel. 217/789-6506; FAX. 217/789-6113; Kathleen Sgro
Hospice Care of Illinois, Visiting Nurse Association of Central Illinois, 720 North Bond Street, Springfield, IL 62702; tel. 217/523-4113; FAX. 217/757-7322; Sue Ellen Billington, Manager
Hospice of Bond County, 305 West Harris, Greenville, IL 62246; tel. 618/664-9701; Elnora Hamel, Administrator
Hospice of Dubuque, 50 Sinsinawa, P.O. Box 236, East Dubuque, IL 61025; tel. 815/747-3622; Barbara Zoeller, Administrator
Hospice of Kankakee Valley, Inc., 1015 North Fifth Avenue, Suite Five, Kankakee, IL 60901; tel. 815/939-4141; FAX. 815/939-1501; Dorothea MacDonald-Lagesse, Executive Director
Hospice of Northeastern Illinois, Inc., 410 South Hager Avenue, Barrington, IL 60010; tel. 847/381-5599; FAX. 847/381-5713; Jane Bilyeu, Executive Director
Hospice of Northwest Illinois, Inc., 155 West Front Street, P.O. Box 185, Stockton, IL 61085-0185; tel. 815/947-3260; FAX. 815/947-4594; Deann Anderson, Administrator
Hospice of Southern Illinois, Inc., 305 South Illinois Street, Belleville, IL 62220; tel. 618/235-1703; FAX. 618/235-3130; Rebecca J. Wisdon, President and CEO
Hospice of the Calumet Area, Inc., 3224 Ridge Road, Suite 202 and 203, Lansing, IL 60438; tel. 708/895-8332; FAX. 708/922-1947; Adrianne May, Administrator
Hospice of the Good Samaritan, 605 N. 12th Street, Mt. Vernon, IL 62864; tel. 618/242-4600; Christina Adams, Administrator
Hospice of the North Shore, A Division of Palliative CareCenter of the North Shore, 2821 Central Street, Evanston, IL 60201; tel. 847/467-7423; FAX. 847/866-6023; Dorothy L. Pitner, RN, BSN., MM, President and CEO
Hospice of the Rock River Valley, 264 Illinois, Route 2, Dixon, IL 61021; tel. 815/288-9573; FAX. 815/288-1181; Donna McCoy, Executive Director
Ingalls Home Hospice, One Ingalls Drive, Harvey, IL 60426; tel. 708/331-1360; FAX. 708/915-2749; Jean Laroche, Administrator
Joliet Area Community Hospice, Inc., 335 West Jefferson Street, Joliet, IL 60435; tel. 815/740-4104; FAX. 815/740-4107; Duane A. Krieger, Executive Director
Lourdes Hospice, 600 Market Street, Metropolis, IL 62960; tel. 618/524-3647; FAX. 618/524-3920; Donna Stewart, Director
Northern Illinois Hospice Association, 4215 Newburg Road, Rockford, IL 61108; tel. 815/398-0500; FAX. 815/398-0588; Carol Couper, Acting Executive Director
Ogle County Hospice Association, 421 Pines Road, P.O. Box 462, Oregon, IL 61061; tel. 815/732-2499; Lorrie Barrows, RN, Executive Director
Provena Hospice - Waukegan, 2615 Washington Street, Waukegan, IL 60085; tel. 847/360-2220; Nancy Delaney, Administrator
QV Hospice, 322 South Green Street, Suite 300, Chicago, IL 60607-3599; tel. 312/738-8622; FAX. 312/738-1238; Dan Woods, President
Rainbow Hospice, Inc., 444 North Northwest Highway, Suite 145, Park Ridge, IL 60068-1427; tel. 847/699-2000; FAX. 847/685-6390; Patricia Ahern, President
Rockford VNA, 4223 East State Street, Rockford, IL 61108; tel. 815/971-3550; FAX. 815/971-3500; Susan Schreier, Administrator
Rush Hospice Partners, 1035 Madison Street, Oak Park, IL 60302; tel. 708/386-9191; FAX. 708/386-9933; Kathleen Nash
Saint Francis Hospice, 355 Ridge Ave., Evanston, IL 60202; tel. 847/316-7114; Virginia G. Niemann, Administrator
Seasons Hospice, 1600 W. Dempster, Park Ridge, IL 60068; tel. 847/759-9449; FAX. 847/759-9448; Marcia Norman, Executive Director
St. Thomas Hospice, Inc., Seven Salt Creek Lane, Suite 101, Hinsdale, IL 60521; tel. 630/850-3990; FAX. 630/850-3969; Marilyn Retter, Administrator
Vitas Corporation, 580 Wateredge, Suite 100, Lombard, IL 60148; tel. 630/495-8484; Nancy Blattler, Administrator
VNA Hospice Care of Central Illinois, 720 North Bond Street, Springfield, IL 62702; tel. 217/523-4113; FAX. 217/757-7322; SueEllen Billington, Mgr
VNA Lincolnland, Inc., 5837 W. Park Drive, Charleston, IL 61920; tel. 217/234-4044; FAX. 217/345-1098; Carol Browning - Whiteside, Administrator

Providers / Freestanding Hospices

VNA of Fox Valley Hospice, 1245 Corporate Boulevard, Aurora, IL 60504; tel. 630/978-2532; FAX. 630/978-1129; Linnea Windel, President and CEO

VNA of Illinois Hospice, 102 Springfield Court, O'Fallon, IL 62269; tel. 618/624-8639; FAX. 618/624-8371; Vivian Carter, Hospice Director

Woodhaven Hospice and Special Support Services, 800 Hoagland Boulevard, Jacksonville, IL 62650; tel. 217/245-0838; Bette Jackson, Administrator

INDIANA

Americare Home Health and Hospice Services, 49 East Monroe, Franklin, IN 46131; tel. 317/736-6005; Kim Weddle, Administrator

Cameron Home Health Care & Hospice, 416 East Maumee Street, Angola, IN 46703; tel. 219/665-2141; Pat Grosenbacher, Administrator

Care at Home Hospice Services, 1721 South Main Street, Goshen, IN 46527; tel. 219/535-2700; FAX. 219/535-2815; Nancy Buss

Clarian Hospice, Clarian Health Partners, Inc., 2039 North Capitol Avenue, Indianapolis, IN 46202; tel. 317/929-4663; FAX. 317/929-3815; William Loveday, Administrator

Comprecare Home Health and Hospice, 1607 East Dowling Street, P.O. Box 517, Kendallville, IN 46755-0517; tel. 800/824-5860; Marilyn Alligood, Administrator

Deaconess Ohio Valley Hospice, 600 Mary Street, Evansville, IN 47747; tel. 812/850-3832; FAX. 812/450-4665; Kim Mans, Director of Home Services

DeKalb Memorial Hospice, 221 N. Main Street, Auburn, IN 46706; tel. 219/927-1640; Annette Vincent, Administrator

Elkhart Community Hospice, Inc., 2020 Industrial Parkway, Elkhart, IN 46516; tel. 219/523-3135; FAX. 219/294-3866; Janice M. Yoder, Administrator

Family Hospice of Northeast Indiana, 1521 W. Main Street, Berne, IN 46711; tel. 219/589-8598; FAX. 219/589-8065; Bernhard P. Wiebe, Medical Director

Good Samaritan Lincoln Trail, 520 South Seventh Street, Vincennes, IN 47591; tel. 812/885-8035; FAX. 812/885-8048; Vonetta Vories, Administrator

Grancare Hospice Services, 1521 E. Tipton Street, Suite 386, Seymour, IN 47274; tel. 812/523-8200; FAX. 812/522-8200; Kathy Dougald, Administrator

Hancock Memorial Hospice, 801 North State Street, Greenfield, IN 46140; tel. 317/468-4522; FAX. 317/468-4217; Darlene Albertson, Homecare and Hospice Administrator

Harbor Light Hospice, 500 West Lincoln Highway, Suite F, Merrillville, IN 46410; tel. 219/793-1200; FAX. 219/793-9292; Stephanie Mayercik, Director

Heartland Hospice, 1315 Directors Row, Suite 206, Fort Wayne, IN 46808; tel. 219/484-7622; FAX. 219/484-5662; Angie Vandeventer, Administrator

Home Hospital Home Health Care, 1415 Salem Street, Lafayette, IN 47904; tel. 765/449-5046; FAX. 765/449-5192; Cheryl Ransom, Administrator

Hoosier Uplands Hospice, 1500 West Main Street, P.O. Box Nine, Mitchell, IN 47446; tel. 812/849-4447; FAX. 812/849-3068; Edna Jackson, B.S.N., RN, Director

Hope Hospice of Fulton County, 100 West 9th Street, Suite 306, P.O. Box 306, Rochester, IN 46975-0621; tel. 219/224-4673; FAX. 219/224-4444; Rev. Ronald C. Purkey, Executive Director

Hospice of Margaret Mary Community, 321 Mitchell Avenue, Batesville, IN 47006; tel. 812/933-5125; FAX. 812/933-5108; Diane C. Helcher, Administrator

Hospice of South Central Indiana, Inc., 2400 East 17th Street, Columbus, IN 47201-5351; tel. 812/376-5813; FAX. 812/376-5929; Sandra Carmichael, Executive Director

Hospice of Southern Indiana, 624 East Market Street, P.O. Box 17, New Albany, IN 47150-4621; tel. 812/945-4596; FAX. 812/945-4735; Susan Miller, Director

Hospice of St. Joseph County, Inc., 111 Sunnybrook Court, South Bend, IN 46637; tel. 219/243-3100; FAX. 219/243-3134; Mark Murray, President, CEO

Hospice of the Calumet Area, Inc., 600 Superior Avenue, Munster, IN 46321-4032; tel. 219/922-2732; FAX. 219/922-1947; Adrianne May, Executive Director

Hospice of Wabash Valley, 600 South 1st Street, Terre Haute, IN 47807; tel. 812/234-2515; FAX. 812/232-2047; Jacquelyn Fox, Administrator

Hospice Preferred Choice, 3905 Vincennes Road, Suite 504, Indianapolis, IN 46268; tel. 317/871-8500; FAX. 317/871-8510; Ferne Squiers, Executive Director

HospiceCare, Inc., 11555 North Meridian, Suite 190, Carmel, IN 46032; tel. 317/580-9336; FAX. 317/580-9346; Jill Ashcraft, Vice President of Hospice Operations

Koseivsko Home Care and Hospice, 902 Provident Drive, Warsaw, IN 46580; tel. 219/372-3401; FAX. 219/372-3414; Jennifer Buhiet, Hospice Director

Oakwood Hospice, 1000 N. 16th Street, New Castle, IN 47362; tel. 765/521-1420; Colleen Fedders, Administrator

Odyssey HealthCare of Central Indiana, Inc., 8765 Guion Road, Indianapolis, IN 46268; tel. 317/334-9302; Joseph D. Lingengelter

Parkview Home Health and Hospice, 105 N. Madison, Columbia City, IN 46725; tel. 219/244-6191; Bridget Dolohanty-Johns

Parkview Home Health and Hospice, 2270 Lake Ave., Suite 200, Fort Wayne, IN 46805; tel. 219/484-6636; Sally Boak, Executive Director

Parkview Home Heath & Hospice, 240 South Jefferson Street, Huntington, IN 46750; tel. 219/356-3000; FAX. 219/358-5272; Tim Miller, Director

Premier Hospice, Inc., 6111 Harrison Street, Merrillville, IN 46410; tel. 219/985-0160; FAX. 219/985-0163; Donna S. Huddleston, Administrator

Saint Joseph at Home Hospice Services, 400 North Main, Kokomo, IN 46903; tel. 317/452-6066; FAX. 317/457-4817; Pam Franklin, RN, Director

The Community VNA Hospice, 1354 South B Street, Elwood, IN 46036; tel. 317/552-3393; FAX. 317/552-3994; Jessie A. Westlund

Vencare Hospice of Indiana, 2601 Fortune Circle East Drive, Suite 105B, Indianapolis, IN 46241; tel. 317/484-9400; FAX. 317/484-9500; Marita Barthuly, Administrator

Visiting Nurse Association Hospice, 610 East Walnut Street, P.O. Box 3487, Evansville, IN 47734-3487; tel. 800/326-4862; FAX. 812/463-4300; Intake and Referral Department

Visiting Nurse Association of Northwest Indiana, Inc., 201 West 89th Avenue, Merrillville, IN 46410-6283; tel. 219/769-3644; FAX. 219/756-7372; Susan Rehrer, Executive Director

Visiting Nurse Service and Hospice, Inc., 3015 South Wayne Avenue, Fort Wayne, IN 46807; tel. 219/456-9888; FAX. 219/456-8883; Sharon Staller, RN, Hospital Phone Nurse

Visiting Nurse Service Hospice of Central Indiana, 4701 North Keystone Avenue, Indianapolis, IN 46205; tel. 317/722-8200; FAX. 317/722-8240; Nancy Utz, Director

VNA Home Care Services Hospice, Inc., 901 South Woodland Avenue, Michigan City, IN 46360-5672; tel. 219/877-2070; FAX. 219/877-2089; Mary Craymer, Chief Executive Officer

VNA Homecare, Hospice and Family Support Services, 901 South Woodland Avenue, Michigan City, IN 46360-5672; tel. 219/877-2070; FAX. 219/877-2089; Mary Craymer, Chief Executive Officer

VNA Hospice Home Care and Hospice Center, 501 Marquette Street, Valparaiso, IN 46383-2058; tel. 219/462-5195; FAX. 219/462-6020; Laura Harting, Executive Director

VNA Hospice of Southeastern Indiana, 1806 East 10th Street, Jeffersonville, IN 47130; tel. 812/288-2700; FAX. 812/285-8111; Nanci Brill, Hospice Director

IOWA

Beacon of Hope Hospice Inc., 3906 Lillie, Suite Six, Davenport, IA 52806; tel. 319/391-6933; FAX. 319/391-5104; Diane Land, Executive Director

Bremer-Butler Hospice, 406 West Bremer Avenue, Suites C and D, Waverly, IA 50677; tel. 319/352-1274; FAX. 319/352-9001; Rod Meyer, Administrator

Calhoun County HHA/Hospice, 501 Court Street, Rockwell City, IA 50579; tel. 712/297-8323; FAX. 712/297-7530; Jane E. Condon, Administrator

Cedar Valley Hospice, 2101 Kimball Avenue, Suite 401, Waterloo, IA 50702; tel. 319/272-2002; FAX. 319/272-2071; Cheryl A. Hoerner, Executive Director

Grinnell Regional Hospice, 106 Fourth Avenue, Grinnell, IA 50112; tel. 515/236-2418; FAX. 515/236-2956; Sandra Bond, Director

Hamilton County PHNS-Hospice Division, 821 Seneca Street, Webster City, IA 50595; tel. 515/832-9565; FAX. 515/832-9554; Jacqueline Butler, Administrator

Home Care Select, 160 South Hayes Avenue, Primghar, IA 51245; tel. 712/757-0060; FAX. 712/757-0060; Jennifer Marco, Hospice Director

Hospice of Cass County, 1501 East Tenth Street, Atlantic, IA 50022; tel. 712/243-3250; Patricia A. Markham, Administrator

Hospice of Central Iowa, 401 Railroad Place, West Des Moines, IA 50265; tel. 515/274-3400; FAX. 515/274-1137; William P. Havekost, President and CEO

Hospice of Comfort, 709 West Main Street, P.O. Box 359, Manchester, IA 52057; tel. 319/927-7303; FAX. 319/927-7444; John Kerns, Operations Manager

Hospice of Compassion, 406 Court, P.O. Box 1034, Williamsburg, IA 52361-1034; tel. 319/668-2262; FAX. 319/668-1656; Carole Moore, Executive Director

Hospice of Dubuque, 2255 John F. Kennedy Road, Asbury Square, Dubuque, IA 52002; tel. 319/582-1220; FAX. 319/582-8089; Barbara Zoeller, Director

Hospice of Lee County, Lee County Health Department-Community Nursing, 2218 Avenue H – Suite A, Fort Madison, IA 52627; tel. 319/372-5225; FAX. 319/372-4374; M. Therese O'Brien, Administrator

Hospice of North Iowa, 232 Second Street, S.E., Mason City, IA 50401; tel. 515/423-3508; FAX. 515/423-5250; Ann MacGregor, Administrator

Hospice of Northwest Iowa, 1200 First Avenue East, Spencer, IA 51301; tel. 515/422-6200; FAX. 515/422-6253; Frances Hoffman, Executive Director

Hospice of Pella, 414 Jefferson Street, Pella, IA 50219; tel. 515/628-6644; FAX. 515/628-6664; Louan Hietbrink, Hospice Manager

Hospice of Siouxland, 224 Fourth Street, Sioux City, IA 51101; tel. 712/233-1298; FAX. 712/233-1123; Linda Todd, Hospice Director

Hospice of the Midlands, 800 Mercy Drive, Council Bluff, IA 51502; tel. 515/328-5106; Denise McNitt, Administrator

Hospice of VNA, 242 North Bluff Boulevard, Clinton, IA 52732; tel. 319/242-7165; FAX. 319/242-7197; Denise Schrader, Administrator

Hospice of Wapello County, 312 East Alta Vista, Ottumwa, IA 52501; tel. 515/682-0684; FAX. 515/684-9209; Cindy Donohue, RN, B.S.N., Director

Hospice Preferred Choice, 508 East Broadway, Council Bluff, IA 51503; tel. 800/591-2273; FAX. 712/325-1895; Lillian Jeppesen, Administrator

Iowa City Hospice, Inc., 613 Bloomington Street, Iowa City, IA 52245; tel. 319/351-5665; FAX. 319/351-5729; Maggie Elliott, Executive Director

Iowa River Hospice, Inc., 206 West Church Street, Marshalltown, IA 50158; tel. 515/753-7704; FAX. 515/753-0379; Brent D. Blackwell, Executive Director

Lyon County Hospice, 803 South Greene Street, Rock Rapids, IA 51246; tel. 712/472-3618; FAX. 712/472-3616; Marge Smith, RN

KANSAS

Central Homecare and Hospice, Inc., 427 S.E. Second, P.O. Box 645, Newton, KS 67114; tel. 316/283-8220; FAX. 316/283-8576; Robert E. Carlton, Executive Director

Community Hospice of Kansas, 1650 South Georgetown, Suite 160, Wichita, KS 67218; tel. 316/686-5999; FAX. 316/686-5634; Karen Everhart, M.Ed., Director

Homecare and Hospice, Inc., 323 Poyntz Avenue, Suite A, Manhattan, KS 66502; tel. 785/537-0688; FAX. 785/537-1309; Jessica Dederer, Executive Director

Hospice Care in Douglas County, 200 Maine, Suite D, Lawrence, KS 66044; tel. 785/843-3738; FAX. 913/843-0757; Patricia Turmes, Clinical Director

Hospice Inc., 313 South Market, P.O. Box 3267, Wichita, KS 67202-3267; tel. 800/835-1043; FAX. 316/265-6066; John G. Carney, President

Hospice of Jefferson County, 1212 Walnut, Highway 59, P.O. Box 324, Oskaloosa, KS 66066-0275; tel. 913/863-2447; FAX. 913/863-2652; Marilyn Zieg, RN, Hospice Coordinator

Hospice of Leavenworth, 218 Choctaw, Leavenworth, KS 66048; tel. 913/684-1305; Charles L. Rogers

Hospice of NE Kansas Multi-County, 326 East Ninth Street, Holton, KS 66436; tel. 913/364-4921; FAX. 913/364-3001; Patricia Scott, RN

Providers / Freestanding Hospices

Hospice of Reno County, Inc., Three Compound Drive, Hutchinson, KS 67502; tel. 316/665-2473; FAX. 316/669-5959; Carolyn Carter, RN, M.S.N., Executive Director

Hospice of Salina, Inc., 333 South Santa Fe, P.O. Box 2238, Salina, KS 67402-2238; tel. 785/825-1717; FAX. 785/825-4949; Kim Fair, President, CEO

Hospice of the Prairie, Inc., 2010 First Avenue, P.O. Box 1294, Dodge City, KS 67801-2623; tel. 316/227-1294; FAX. 316/227-7429; Stan Brown, Executive Director

Hospice Services, Inc., 424 Eighth Street, P.O. Box 116, Phillipsburg, KS 67661; tel. 785/543-2900; FAX. 785/543-5688; Sandy Kuhlman

Midland Hospice Care, Inc., 200 Southwest Frazier Circle, Topeka, KS 66606-2800; tel. 913/232-2044; FAX. 913/232-5567; Karren Weichert, Executive Director

Ottawa County Home Health/Hospice Agency, 307 North Concord, Suite 200, Minneapolis, KS 67467; tel. 913/392-2822; June Clark, RN

SCCS Home Health and Hospice, P.A., 1410 North Woodlawn, Suite D, Derby, KS 67037; tel. 316/788-7626; FAX. 316/788-7072; Cheryl Pelaccic, RN, Administrator

South Wind Hospice, Inc., 920 East 1st Street, P.O. Box 862, Pratt, KS 67124; tel. 316/672-7553; FAX. 316/672-7554; Diane L. Johnson, Director

Southwest Homecare and Hospice, 103 East 11th Street, Liberal, KS 67901; tel. 316/629-2456; FAX. 315/629-2453; Ida Rodkey, Administrator

KENTUCKY

Community Hospice, 1538 Carter Avenue, Ashland, KY 41101; tel. 606/329-1890; FAX. 606/329-0018; Susan Hunt, Administrator

Cumberland Valley District Health Department Hospice, P.O. Box 890, Hwy# 421S, Manchester, KY 40962; tel. 606/287-8437; Lois Powell, Program Director

Heritage Hospice, 337 West Broadway, P.O. Box 1213, Danville, KY 40422; tel. 606/236-2425; FAX. 606/236-6152; Janelle Lane, Executive Director

Hospice and Palliative Care of Louisville, 3532 Ephraim McDowell Drive, Louisville, KY 40205-3224; tel. 502/456-6200; FAX. 502/456-6655; Helen Donaldson, President and CEO

Hospice Care Plus, 210 St. George Street, Richmond, KY 40475-2376; tel. 606/624-8820; FAX. 606/624-9230; Gail McGillis, M.S.N., Chief Executive Officer

Hospice East, 24 West Lexington Avenue, P.O. Box 115, Winchester, KY 40392; tel. 606/744-9866; FAX. 606/744-1971; Carol Richardson, Director

Hospice of Central Kentucky, 105 Diecks Drive, P.O. Box 2149, Elizabethtown, KY 42701-2444; tel. 502/737-6300; FAX. 502/737-4053; Gary Bohannon, Director

Hospice of Hope, One West McDonald Parkway, Maysville, KY 41056; tel. 606/564-4848; FAX. 606/564-7615; Kavin Cartmell, Executive Director

Hospice of Lake Cumberland, 108 College Street, P.O. Box 651, Somerset, KY 42502; tel. 606/679-4389; FAX. 606/678-0191; Jeanne Travis, Executive Director

Hospice of Pike County, 229 College Street, Pikeville, KY 41501; tel. 606/432-2112; FAX. 606/432-4631; Sharon Branham, President and CEO

Hospice of Southern Kentucky, Inc., 1027 Broadway, Bowling Green, KY 42104; tel. 270/782-3402; FAX. 270/782-3496; Betty Preece – Biggerstaff, Executive Director

Hospice of the Bluegrass, 2312 Alexandria Drive, Lexington, KY 40504; tel. 606/276-5344; FAX. 606/223-0490; Gretchen M. Brown, President and CEO

Jessamine County Hospice, 109 Shannon Parkway, P.O. Box 873, Nicholasville, KY 40356; tel. 606/887-2696; FAX. 606/885-1474; Susan G. Swinford, M.S.W., Executive Director

Lourdes Hospice, 2855 Jackson Street, Paducah, KY 42001; tel. 502/444-2262; FAX. 502/444-2380; Donna Stewart, Administrator

Mountain Community Hospice, 3115 North Main Street, Hazard, KY 41701; tel. 606/439-2111; FAX. 606/439-4198; Gene Rice, M.S.W., Director

Mountain Heritage Hospice, Inc., 68 Belkway, Village Center, Building Two, P.O. Box 189, Harlan, KY 40831-0189; tel. 606/573-6111; FAX. 606/573-7964; Bernice Reynolds, Administrator

Pennyroyal Hospice, Inc., 1821 East Ninth Street, Suite 1, Hopkinsville, KY 42240; tel. 502/885-6428; FAX. 502/889-5005; Hanna Sabel, Executive Director

St. Anthony's Hospice, Inc., 2410 South Green Street, P.O. Box 351, Henderson, KY 42420; tel. 502/826-2326; FAX. 502/831-2169; Paula Yeviney, Executive Director

Tri County Hospice, P.O. Box 395, London, KY 40741; tel. 606/877-3950; Ed Valentine

LOUISIANA

Good Shepherd in Hospice, Inc., 327 North Canal Boulevard, P.O. Box 1223, Thibodaux, LA 70302-1223; tel. 504/448-2200; Barbara Lofton

Hospice Care Foundation, 810 Julia Street P.O. Box 278, Rayville, LA 71269; Tiffany Walker, Coordinator

Hospice Care Foundation, Inc., P.O. Box 278, Rayville, LA 71269; tel. 318/728-3060; FAX. 318/728-3080; Kathleen Garley, RN, Patient Care Coordinator

Hospice of Acadiana, Inc., 2600 Johnson Street, Suite 200, Lafayette, LA 70503; tel. 318/232-1234; FAX. 318/232-1297; Nelson Waguespack, Jr., Executive Director

Hospice of Greater Baton Rouge, 8322 One Calais Avenue, Suite A, Baton Rouge, LA 70809-3412; tel. 225/767-4673; FAX. 225/769-8113; Kathryn Grigsby, Executive Director

Hospice of Greater New Orleans, 3616 South I-10 Service Road, Suite 109, New Orleans, LA 70001; tel. 504/838-8944; FAX. 504/838-9034; Jo-Ann Mueller, Chief Executive Officer

Hospice of Jefferson, 3715 Williams Blvd., Suite 240, Kenner, LA 70062; tel. 504/464-7357; FAX. 504/466-9482; Tracy McCann, Administrator

Hospice of South Louisiana, 210 Mystic Boulevard, Houma, LA 70360; tel. 504/851-4273; FAX. 504/872-6543; Dottie Landry, RN, Administration

Hospice of St. Jude, 615 Baronne Street, Suite 300 A, New Orleans, LA 70113; tel. 504/522-7108; Charles C. Harding

Hospice of St. Luke, 237 North Second Street, Eunice, LA 70535; tel. 800/869-2067; Willadean McWhorter, Administrator

Hospice of the Delta, 104 Smart Place, Slidell, LA 70458; tel. 504/641-7373; FAX. 504/641-7374; Winnie Rispoli, Director of Operations

Odyssey Healthcare, Inc, 3340 Severn Avenue, Suite 215, Metairie, LA 70002; tel. 504/887-8128; FAX. 504/887-8206; Kathleen Schellhaas, General Manager

Peoples Hospice, 1743 Stumpf Boulevard, Gretna, LA 70056; tel. 504/364-1494; FAX. 504/362-1056; Sheila A. Osburn, RN, BSN, Administrator

Red River Hospice, Inc., 5501 John Eskew Drive, Alexandria, LA 71303; tel. 318/443-5694; E. W. Parker, Administrator

Samaritan Care Hospice of Louisiana, 411 Meadowview Drive, Munden, LA 71105; tel. 800/238-7628; FAX. 318/869-2744; Toni Camp, Administrator

Trinity Hospice of Louisiana, LLC, 5647 Superior Drive, Baton Rouge, LA 70816; tel. 225/293-1948; FAX. 225/292-1502; Linda Leach, Program Director

MAINE

Androscoggin Home Health Services, 15 Strawberry Avenue, P.O. Box 819, Lewiston, ME 04243-0819; tel. 207/777-7740; Richard C. Stephenson, M.D., Medical Director

Community Health And Nursing Services, d/b/a CHANS Hospice Care, 50 Baribeau Drive, Brunswick, ME 04011; tel. 207/729-6782; FAX. 207/725-5640; Juliana L'Heureux, Executive Director

Community Health Services, Inc., 901 Washington Avenue, Suite 104, Portland, ME 04103; tel. 207/775-7231; FAX. 207/775-5520; Robert P. Liversidge, Jr., President, and CEO

HealthReach Hospice, Eight Highwood Street, P.O. Box 0829, Waterville, ME 04903-1568; tel. 207/873-1127; FAX. 207/873-2059; Rebecca K. Colwell, Vice President, Home Care & Hospice

Hospice of Aroostook, 14 Carroll Street, P.O. Box 688, Caribou, ME 04736; tel. 207/498-2578; FAX. 207/493-3111; Saundra Scott-Adams, Executive Director

Hospice of Hancock County, 14 McKenzie Avenue, P.O. Box 224, Ellsworth, ME 04605; tel. 207/667-2531; FAX. 207/667-9406; Barbara Clark, Director

Hospice of Maine, 693 Congress Street, Rear, Portland, ME 04102-3303; tel. 207/774-4417; Terence Cronin, Executive Director

Hospice of Mid Coast Maine, P.O. Box 741, 331 Maine Street, Suite 14, Brunswick, ME 04011-0741; tel. 207/729-3602; FAX. 207/729-2721; Gary Araujo, Executive Director

Hospice Volunteers of Kennebec Valley, Maine General Medical Center, 150 Dresden Avenue, Gardiner, ME 04345; tel. 207/626-1779; FAX. 207/582-6819; Barbara Bell, Director

Hospice Volunteers of Waldo County, 118 Northport Avenue, P.O. Box 772, Belfast, ME 04915; tel. 207/338-2268; FAX. 207/338-2367; Alelia Hilt, RN, BSN, Volunteer Coordinator

Hospice Volunteers of Waterville Area, 76 Silver Street, Waterville, ME 04901; tel. 207/873-3615; FAX. 207/873-5094; Bonnie Lantz, Executive Director

Kno-Wal-Lin Coastal Family Hospice, 170 Pleasant Street, Rockland, ME 04841; tel. 207/594-9561; FAX. 207/594-2527; Linda Laweryson, Clinical Manager Hospice

Miles Home Health Hospice Division, R.R. 2, P.O. Box 4500, Damariscotta, ME 04543-8903; tel. 207/563-4592; FAX. 207/563-8652; Carol Knipping, Executive Director

New Hope Hospice, Inc., 1344 Main Road, P.O. Box 757 Holden ME 04429, Eddington, ME 04428; tel. 207/843-7521; FAX. 207/843-6645; Nancy S. Burgess, Director

Pine Tree Hospice, 65 West Main Street, Dover-Foxcroft, ME 04426; tel. 207/564-4346; Theresa Boettner, Program Coordinator

Southern Maine Health and Homecare Services, Route One South, P.O. Box 739, Kennebunk, ME 04043; tel. 207/985-4767; FAX. 207/985-6715; Linda Sentner, RN, Hospice Program Director

Visiting Nurse Service, 15 Industrial Park Road, Saco, ME 04072; tel. 207/284-4566; FAX. 207/282-4148; Maryanna Arsenault, Chief Executive Officer

MARYLAND

Calvert Hospice, 238 Merrimac Court, P.O. Box 838, Prince Freder, MD 20678; tel. 410/535-0892; FAX. 301/855-1226; Lynn Bonde, Executive Director

Caroline County Home Health/Hospice, 601 North Sixth Street, P.O. Box 10, Denton, MD 21629; tel. 410/479-3500; FAX. 410/479-3425; L. Carol Smith, Administrator

Carroll Hospice, 95 Carroll Street, Westminster, MD 21157; tel. 410/871-8000; FAX. 410/871-7242; Marie Bossie, Executive Director

Coastal Hospice, Inc., 2604 Old Ocean City Road, P.O. Box 1733, Salisbury, MD 21802-1733; tel. 410/742-8732; FAX. 410/548-5669; Marion F. Keenan, President

Dorchester County Home Health Hospice, 751 Woods Road, Cambridge, MD 21613; tel. 410/228-5860; FAX. 410/228-4475; Joyce T. Hyde, RN, M.S., Director

Holy Cross Home Care and Hospice, 9805 Dameron Drive, Silver Spring, MD 20902; tel. 301/754-7740; FAX. 301/754-7743; Margaret Hadley, Director

Hospice Caring, Inc., Volunteer Hospice, 707 Conservation Lane, Suite 100, Gaithersburg, MD 20878; tel. 301/869-4673; FAX. 301/869-2924; Lisa McKillop, Executive Director

Hospice of Baltimore, Gilchrist Center for Hospice Care, 6601 North Charles Street, Baltimore, MD 21204; tel. 410/512-8200; FAX. 410/512-8284; Regina Bodnar, Director, Clinical Services

Hospice of Charles County, 105 La Grange Avenue, P.O. Box 1703, LaPlata, MD 20646; tel. 888/934-1268; FAX. 301/934-6437; Geri Firosz, President

Hospice of Frederick County, 516 Trail Avenue, Frederick, MD 21702; tel. 301/698-3030; FAX. 301/694-9012; Laurel A. Cucchi, Executive Director

Hospice of Garrett County, 69 Wolf Acres Drive, P.O. Box 271, Oakland, MD 21550; tel. 301/334-5151; FAX. 301/334-5800; Brenda Butscher, Executive Director

Hospice of Prince George's County, 96 Harry Truman Drive, Largo, MD 20774; tel. 301/499-0550; FAX. 301/350-7844; Cheri Sanford, Director, Nursing Services

Hospice of Queen Anne's, Inc., 300 Del Rhodes Avenue, Queenstown, MD 21658; tel. 410/827-0426; FAX. 410/827-4678; Mildred H. Barrette, Executive Director

Hospice of the Chesapeake, Inc., 8424 Veterans Highway, Millersville, MD 21108; tel. 410/987-2003; FAX. 410/729-5263; Erwin E. Abrams, President

Providers / Freestanding Hospices

Hospice of Washington County, 101 East Baltimore Street, Hagerstown, MD 21740; tel. 301/791–6360; FAX. 301/791–6579; Robert Rauch, Executive Director
Jewish Social Service Agency, 6123 Montrose Road, Rockville, MD 20852; tel. 301/881–3700; Ronnie Tobin, Division Director
Joseph Richey Hospice, 828 North Eutaw Street, Baltimore, MD 21201; tel. 410/523–2150; FAX. 410/523–1146; Catherine Hawtin, Coordinator, Admissions
Kent Hospice Foundation, Inc., 103 Dixon Drive, Chestertown, MD 21620; tel. 410/778–7058; FAX. 410/778–7903; Nancy R. Morris, Executive Director
Mid–Atlantic Hospice Care, 4805 Benson Avenue, Baltimore, MD 21227; tel. 410/247–2900; FAX. 410/247–2581; Darlene Armacost
Montgomery Hospice, 1450 Research Boulevard, Suite 310, Rockville, MD 20850; tel. 301/279–2566; FAX. 301/309–8791; Ann Mitchell, Executive Director
Potomac Home Health Care, 6001 Montrose Road, Suite 307, Rockville, MD 20852; tel. 301/896–6999; FAX. 301/896–6275; Lauren Simpson, Executive Director and CEO
Stella Maris Hospice Care Program, 2300 Dulaney Valley Road, Timonim, MD 21204; tel. 410/252–4500; FAX. 410/560–9675; Sister Karen McNally, R.S.M., Chief Administrative Officer
Talbot Hospice Foundation, 586 Cynwood Drive, Easton, MD 21601; tel. 410/822–6681; FAX. 410/822–5576; Liz Freedlander, Executive Director
VNA Hospice of Maryland L.L.C., 7008 Security Blvd, Baltimore, MD 21244–2504; tel. 410/594–9100; FAX. 410/277–4251; Cynthia Corbin, CRNP, RN, Clinical Manager

MASSACHUSETTS
Athol Memorial Home Health & Hospice, 423 Main Street, Athol, MA 01331; tel. 978/249–5366; FAX. 978/249–8993; Cynthia M. Rode, Director
Cura VNA & Cranberry Hospice, 89 Court Street, Plymouth, MA 02360; tel. 508/830–2720; FAX. 508/830–2703; Paul Montgomery, Hospice Manager
Diversified VNA Hospice, 316 Nichols Road, Fitchburg, MA 01420; tel. 978/342–6013; FAX. 978/343–5629; Karen Diamond, Executive Director
Good Samaritan Hospice, Inc., 310 Allston Street, Brighton, MA 02146; tel. 617/566–6242; FAX. 617/566–3055; Leo P. Smith, Executive Director
HealthCare Dimensions, 254 South Street, Waltham, MA 02154–2707; tel. 617/894–1100; FAX. 617/736–0908; Patricia A. Field, Executive Director
Hospice Care of Greater Taunton, One Taunton Green, Taunton, MA 02780; tel. 508/822–1447; Joanne Smith, Vice President, Clinical Services
Hospice Care, Inc., 41 Montvale Avenue, Stoneham, MA 02180; tel. 781/279–4100; FAX. 781/279–4677; Kathleen Colburn, Executive Director
Hospice Community Care, 495 Pleasant Street, Winthrop, MA 02152
Hospice of Boston and Hospice of Greater Brockton, 500 Belmont Street, Suite 215, Brockton, MA 02401; tel. 508/583–0383; FAX. 508/583–1193; Ruth Capernaros, Executive Director
Hospice of Cape Cod, Inc., 923 Route 6A, Yarmouthport, MA 02675; tel. 508/362–1103; FAX. 508/375–0103; Marilyn Hannus, RN, Director, COO
Hospice of Central Massachusetts, Inc., 120 Thomas Street, Worcester, MA 01608; tel. 508/756–7176
Hospice of Community Nurse Association, 40 Centre Street, P.O. Box 831, Fairhaven, MA 02719; tel. 508/999–3400; FAX. 508/999–6401; Brenda M. Van Laarhoven, RN, Coordinator
Hospice of Community Visiting Nurse Agency, 141 Park Street, Attleboro, MA 02703; tel. 508/222–0118; FAX. 508/226–8939; Kathleen M. Trier, Executive Director
Hospice of Greater Milford, 12 Hastings Street, P.O. Box 328, Mendon, MA 01756; tel. 508/634–8382; FAX. 508/634–8738; Renee Merolli, RN, M.A., Director
Hospice of the Good Shepherd, 2042 Beacon Street, Newton, MA 02468; tel. 617/969–6130; FAX. 617/928–1450; Ellen Rudikoff, Ph.D., Psy. D., Executive Director
Hospice of the North Shore, Inc., 10 Elm Street, Danvers, MA 01923; tel. 508/774–7566; FAX. 508/774–4389; Diane Stringer, Executive Director

Hospice of the South Shore, P.O. Box 334, 100 Bay State Drive, Braintree, MA 02184; tel. 781/843–0947; Elaine Coughlan, RN, Program Manager
HospiceCare in the Berkshires, Inc., 369 South Street, Pittsfield, MA 01201; tel. 413/443–2994; FAX. 413/433–7814; Anne Kissel, Executive Director
Merrimack Valley Hospice, Inc., 360 Merrimack Street, Building 9, Lawrence, MA 01843; tel. 978/552–4599; FAX. 978/552–4543; Diane Bergeron, Administrator
Neponset Valley Hospice, Inc., Three Edgewater Drive, Norwood, MA 02062; tel. 617/769–8282; FAX. 617/762–0718; Susan DiBona, Hospice Manager
Noble Visiting Nurse and Hospice Services, Inc., 77 Mill Street, Suite 207, Westfield, MA 01085–3602; tel. 413/562–7049; FAX. 413/568–9434; Kimberly A. Andrews, Executive Director
Old Colony Hospice, Inc., 14 Page Terrace, Stoughton, MA 02072; tel. 781/341–4145; FAX. 781/297–7345; Marjorie Levy, Executive Director
Staff Builders Hospice Program, 529 Main Street, Suite 1M07, Boston, MA 02129; tel. 617/242–4872; FAX. 617/241–2880; Victoria Gunfolino, Director
Visiting Nurse Association and Hospice of Western New England, Inc, 50 Maple Street, P.O. Box 9058, Springfield, MA 01102–9058; tel. 413/781–5070; FAX. 413/739–1423; Maureen Skipper, President
Visiting Nurse Association of Greater Lowell Hospice, 336 Central Street, P.O. Box 1965, Lowell, MA 01853–1965; tel. 978/459–9343; FAX. 978/459–0981; Nancy L. Pettinelli, Executive Director
Visiting Nurse Association of Middlesex–East and Visiting Nurse Hospices, 12 Beacon Street, Stoneham, MA 02180; tel. 617/438–3770; FAX. 617/438–7994; Jacquelyn Galluzzi, Chief Executive Officer
VNA Care Choices, Inc., a VNA care Network, Inc, 186 Alewife Brook Parkway, Suite 206, Cambridge, MA 02138; tel. 800/728–1862; FAX. 617/890–8444; Denise King, Clinical Services Manager
VNA Hospice Alliance, d/b/a Hampshire County Hospice, Inc., 168 Industrial Drive, Northampton, MA 01061; tel. 413/584–1060; FAX. 413/586–3912; Joan Keochakian, Executive Director
VNA of Greater Gardner Hospice, 34 Pearly Lane, Gardner, MA 01440; tel. 508/632–1230; FAX. 508/632–4513; Cynthia M. Roche, Director
Wayside Hospice/Parmenter VNA& Community Care, 266 Cochituate Road, Wayland, MA 01778; tel. 508/358–3000; FAX. 508/358–3005; Marilyn Bonkovsky, Clinical Manager

MICHIGAN
Andy Scholett Memorial, 12426 State Street, P.O. Box 587, Atlanta, MI 49709–0587; tel. 517/785–3134; FAX. 517/785–2834; Shirley Burnham, Executive Director
Angela Hospice Home Care, Inc. and Care Center, 14100 Newburgh Road, Livonia, MI 48154–5010; tel. 313/464–7810; FAX. 313/464–6930; Mary Giovanni, Administrator
Arbor Hospice, 7445 Allen Road, Allen, MI 41801; tel. 313/383–8800; FAX. 313/383–0115; Beverly Spicknall
Arbor Hospice, 2366 Oak Valley Drive, Ann Arbor, MI 48103; tel. 734/662–5999; FAX. 734/662–2330; Bev Spicknall
Arbor Hospice, Home Care and Care–ousel, 7445 Allen Road, Suite 230, Allen Park, MI 48101; tel. 313/383–8800; FAX. 313/383–0115; Karen Basile, RN, Branch Director
Baraga County Hospice, Inc., 913 Meador Street, L'Anse, MI 49946; tel. 906/524–5168
Barry Community Hospice, A Division of Good Samaritan Hospice Care, Inc., 450 Meadow Run Drive, Suite 200, P.O. Box 308, Hastings, MI 49058; tel. 616/948–8452; FAX. 616/948–9545; Barbara VanDyken, Manager
Barry–Eaton District Health Department – Hospice Program, 528 Beech Street, Charlotte, MI 48813; tel. 517/543–2900; FAX. 517/541–2612; Penny Pierce, RN, Director
Blue Water Hospices, Inc., 1422 Lyon Street, Port Huron, MI 48060; tel. 313/982–8809; FAX. 313/984–1612; Carol M. Nichols, Vice President, Operations
Branch–Hillside–St. Joseph DHD, 600 South Lakeview, Sturgis, MI 49091; tel. 616/659–4013; Duke Anderson

Cass Branch Hospice Program, 201 M–62 North, Cassopolis, MI 49031; tel. 616/445–2296; Jill Eldred
Charlevoix County Hospice, 601 Bridge Street, East Jordan, MI 49727; tel. 231/536–2842; FAX. 231/547–1164; Margaret Lasater, Executive Director
Community Home Health & Hospice, G–5095 West Bristol Road, Flint, MI 48507; tel. 810/733–7250; FAX. 810/733–8424; Donna Lloyd, Executive Director
Community Hospice Services, Inc., 32932 Warren Road, Suite 100, Westland, MI 48185; tel. 313/522–4244; FAX. 313/522–2099; Maureen Butrico, Executive Director
Cranbrook Hospice Care, 281 Enterprise Court, Suite 300, Bloomfield, MI 48302–0313; tel. 248/334–6700; FAX. 248/334–7064; Brian Hansen, Director
Dickinson–Iron DHD, 601 Washington Avenue, P.O. Box 516, Stambaugh, MI 49964; tel. 906/265–9913; FAX. 906/265–2950; Marsha Ackerman, RN
Downriver Hospice, Inc., 1545 Kingsway Court, Trenton, MI 48183; tel. 313/671–6343
Genesys Hospice, 7280 South State Road, Goodrich, MI 48438; tel. 810/636–5000; FAX. 810/636–5019; LaVeme A. McCombs, Administrator
Good Samaritan Hospice Care, Inc., 166 East Goodale Avenue, Battle Creek, MI 49017–2728; tel. 561/666–0360; Mary Cunningham, Executive Director
Grand Traverse Area Hospice, 1105 Sixth Street, Traverse City, MI 49684; tel. 616/935–6520; FAX. 616/935–7270; Kay Benisek, Manager
Gratiot Area Hospice, 302 1/2 East Main, Stanton, MI 48888; tel. 517/831–5045; Carol Goffnett
Heartland Hospice, 814 Adams, Suite 109, Bay City, MI 48708; tel. 517/892–0355; FAX. 517/892–0896; Christine Satkowiak, RN, Administrator
Heartland Hospice, 700 West Ash Street, Suite Three–A, Mason, MI 48854; tel. 517/676–6469; FAX. 517/676–7022; Michael Freytag, Administrator
Heartland Hospice, 6504 28th Street, S.E., Suite T, Grand Rapids, MI 49546; tel. 616/942–7733
Henry Ford Hospice–West Bloomfield, 6020 West Maple Road, Suite 500, West Bloomfield, MI 48322; tel. 810/539–0660; FAX. 810/539–8868; Laura Zeile, RN, B.S.N., Manager
Home Health Plus (Homecare & Hospice), 26211 Central Park Boulevard, Suite 110, Southfield, MI 48076; tel. 248/357–3650; FAX. 248/357–1486; Marilyn M. Chirilut, RN, BSN., Director, Operations
Hospice at Home, Inc., 2626 West John Beers Road, P.O. Box 297, Stevensville, MI 49127; tel. 616/429–7100; FAX. 616/428–3499; Cathy Paradise, Clinical Services Director
Hospice Care of Southwest Michigan, 301 West Cedar Street, Kalamazoo, MI 49007–5106; tel. 616/345–0273; FAX. 616/345–8522; Jean Maile, Administrator
Hospice of Bay Area, 1460 West Center Avenue, Essexville, MI 48732; tel. 517/895–4750; FAX. 517/895–4701; Christine Chesny
Hospice of Chippewa County/Chippewa County Health Department, 508 Ashmun Street, Suite 120, Sault Sainte Marie, MI 49783; tel. 906/635–1568; FAX. 906/635–1701; Rosemary Blashill, Administrator
Hospice of Gladwin Area, Inc., 1312 N. State Street, P.O. Box 557, Gladwin, MI 48624; tel. 517/426–4464; FAX. 517/426–3057; Georgann Schuster, Executive Director
Hospice of Helping Hands, Inc., 335 East Houghton Avenue, West Branch, MI 48661; tel. 517/345–4700; FAX. 517/345–2991; Debbie Bills, RN, Clinical Program Director
Hospice of Hillsdale County, 111 South Howell Street, Suite B, Hillsdale, MI 49242; tel. 517/437–5252; FAX. 517/437–5253; Kathryn Aemisegger, Administrator
Hospice of Holland Home, 2100 Raybrook, S.E., Grand Rapids, MI 49546; tel. 616/235–5100; FAX. 616/235–5111; Joanne E. Kellogg, Administrator
Hospice of Holland, Inc., 270 Hoover Boulevard, Holland, MI 49423; tel. 616/396–2972; FAX. 616/396–2808; Judith A. Zylman, RN, Executive Director
Hospice of Integrated Health Services, 24445 Northwestern Highway, Suite 105, Southfield, MI 48075; tel. 800/397–9360; FAX. 248/355–5705; Susan Gadlage, Area Administration

Providers / Freestanding Hospices

Hospice of Ionia, 117 North Depot Street, Ionia, MI 48846; tel. 616/527-0681; Bernice Falsetta

Hospice of Jackson, 915 Airport Road, Jackson, MI 49202; tel. 517/783-2648; FAX. 517/783-2674; Kenneth O. Drees, FACHE, Executive Director

Hospice of Lansing, Inc., 6035 Executive Drive, Suite 103, Lansing, MI 48911; tel. 517/882-4500; FAX. 517/882-3010; Barbara A. Kowalski, M.P.A., Executive Director

Hospice of Lenawee, 415 Mill Road, Adrian, MI 49221; tel. 517/263-2323; FAX. 517/263-1279; Ann Gehoski, Administrator

Hospice of Little Traverse Bay, 416 Connable Avenue, Petoskey, MI 49770; tel. 231/487-4825; FAX. 231/487-4228; Lori Schiller, Clinical Manager

Hospice of Michigan, 16250 Northland Drive, Suite 212, Southfield, MI 48075-5200; tel. 248/559-9209; FAX. 248/559-4037; Dorothy Defemo, President and CEO

Hospice of Michigan – Alpena, 112 West Chisholm, Alpena, MI 49707; tel. 517/354-5258; FAX. 517/356-6931; Annette Miller, Program Director

Hospice of Michigan – Big Rapids, 400 Perry, Big Rapids, MI 49307; tel. 231/796-7371; FAX. 231/796-4841; Heather Stueber, Program Director

Hospice of Michigan – Cadillac, 932 North Mitchell Street, Cadillac, MI 49601; tel. 231/779-9570; FAX. 231/779-0717; Heather Stueber, Program Director

Hospice of Michigan – Chesterfield, 27322 Twenty-three Mile Road, Suite 3, Chesterfield, MI 48051; tel. 810/949-2800; FAX. 810/949-6475; Susan Testa, Program Director

Hospice of Michigan – Detroit, 2990 West Grand Boulevard, Suite 402, Detroit, MI 48202; tel. 313/874-2000; FAX. 313/872-0212; Pamela Joy, Program Director

Hospice of Michigan – Farmington Hills Hospice Home, 25911 Middlebelt, Farmington Hills, MI 48336; tel. 248/426-4000; FAX. 248/426-4092; Cheryl Nicklay, Program Director

Hospice of Michigan – Gaylord, 810 South Otsego, Bavarian Office Center, Suite 111, Gaylord, MI 49735; tel. 517/732-2151; FAX. 517/731-2897; Annette Miller, Program Director

Hospice of Michigan – Grand Rapids, 1260 Ekhart, N.E., Grand Rapids, MI 49503; tel. 616/454-1426; FAX. 616/454-9413; Jean Obermiller, Program Director

Hospice of Michigan – Ludington, 10 Atkinson Drive, Suite 3, Ludington, MI 49431; tel. 616/845-0321; FAX. 616/845-1802; Heather Stueber, Program Director

Hospice of Michigan – Milford, 120 South Main Street, Suite A, Milford, MI 43841; tel. 248/685-1333; FAX. 248/684-5586; Pamela Joy, Program Director

Hospice of Michigan – Pontiac, 530 West Huron, Pontiac, MI 48341; tel. 810/253-2580; FAX. 248/253-2599; Susan Testa, Program Director

Hospice of Michigan – Southfield, 16250 Northland Drive, Suite 212, Southfield, MI 48075; tel. 248/559-3195; FAX. 248/569-3306; Shannon O Neill-Shoberg, Program Director

Hospice of Michigan – Taylor, 9333 Telegraph Road, Taylor, MI 48180; tel. 313/291-9700; FAX. 313/295-0852; Shannon O'Neill-Shoberg, Program Director

Hospice of Michigan –St. Clair Shores, 22811 Greater Mack Avenue, Suite 203, St. Clair Shores, M 48080; tel. 810/445-6855; FAX. 810/445-6855; Susan Testa, Program Director

Hospice of Michigan, Inc., Newaygo County/Freemont, 819 West Main Street, Fremont, MI 49412; tel. 616/924-6123; FAX. 616/924-8028; Marie Malone, RN, B.S.N., Hospice Director

Hospice of Michigan–Roscommon, 709 Lake Street, Suite 102, P.O. Box 532, Roscommon, MI 48653; tel. 517/275-8967; FAX. 517/275-6130; Annette Miller, Program Director

Hospice of Monroe, 502 West Elm Street, Monroe, MI 48161; tel. 313/457-3220; FAX. 313/457-5060; Paul Doerfler, Administrator

Hospice of Muskegon-Oceana, 1095 Third Street, Suite 209, Muskegon, MI 49441; tel. 231/728-3442; FAX. 231/722-0708; Mary Anne Gorman, Executive Director

Hospice of North Ottawa Community, Inc., 1515 South Despelder, Grand Haven, MI 49417; tel. 616/846-2015; FAX. 616/846-7227; Carolyn K. Howes, Executive Director

Hospice of Sturgis, 600 South Lakeview Avenue, Sturgis, MI 49091; Pamela Pope

Hospice of the Straits/Vital Care, 722 South Street, Cheboygan, MI 49721; tel. 616/627-4774; FAX. 616/627-4416; Laura Daniel, Regional Manager

Hospice of Washtenaw, 806 Airport Boulevard, Ann Arbor, MI 48108; tel. 734/327-3400; FAX. 734/327-3273; Teri Turner, Administrator

Hospice's of Henry Ford Health System, 23000 Mack Avenue, Suite 500, St. Clair Shore, MI 48080; tel. 810/774-4141; FAX. 810/774-0515; Sondra Seely, Administrator

Individualized Hospice, 3003 Washtenaw Avenue, Suite Two, Ann Arbor, MI 48104; tel. 313/971-0444; FAX. 313/971-1980; Ingrid Deininga, Administrator

International Pediatric Hospice, 2300 Bull Building, Detroit, MI 48226; tel. 313/965-6100; Paul Manion

Kaleidoscope Kids, 1 Ford Place, 2–A, Detroit, MI 48202; tel. 313/972-1980; Sondra Seely

Karmanos Cancer Institute–Hospice Program, 24601 Northwestern Highway, Southfield, MI 48075; tel. 810/827-1592; FAX. 810/827-0972; Shelia A. Sperti, M.S.N., RN, Administrator

Keweenaw Home Nursing and Hospice, 311 Sixth Street, Calumet, MI 49913; tel. 906/337-5700; FAX. 906/337-9929; Wanda Kolb, Administrator

LMAS DHD Hospice, 200 Hamilton Lake Road, Newberry, MI 49868; tel. 906/293-5107; FAX. 906/293-5453; Rosemary Blashill, Administrator

LMAS DHD Hospice/St. Ignace, 749 Hombach Street, St. Ignace, MI 49781; tel. 906/643-7700; FAX. 906/643-7719; Judy Misner, Home Health Nursing Supervisor

Manistee Area Volunteer Hospice, Inc., P.O. Box 293, Manistee, MI 49660; tel. 616/723-6064; Barbara Hansen, President

Marquette General Home Health and Hospice, Doctors Park, Suite 105, Escanaba, MI 49829; tel. 906/789-1305; FAX. 906/789-9144; Linda S. Lewandowski, Director, Hospice

McLaren HomeCare and Hospice, 237 Davis Lake Road, Lapeer, MI 48446; tel. 810/667-0042; FAX. 810/667-0060; Nancy Griffiths, Manager

Memorial Hospice, 1320 South Carpenter Street, Iron Mountain, MI 48901; tel. 906/774-5589

Mid Michigan VNA Hospice/Clare, 1438 North McEwan, Clare, MI 48617; tel. 517/539-5320; FAX. 517/839-1773; Sandra Simmons, Administrator

MidMichigan Visiting Nurses Association and Hospice, 3007 North Saginaw Road, Midland, MI 48640; tel. 517/839-1770; FAX. 517/839-1749; Sherry Hockstra, Hospice Manager

North County Hospice, Inc., 301 South Cedar, Kalkaska, MI 49646; tel. 616/258-5286; Eleen R. Bubble, Co-Volunteer Director

North Woods Home Nursing and Hospice, 226 South Cedar, P.O. Box 307, Manistique, MI 49854; tel. 906/341-6963; FAX. 906/341-2490; Susan Bjorne, Administrator

Northwest Michigan Community Health Agency, 220 West Garfield Street, Charleviox, MI 49720; tel. 231/547-6523; FAX. 231/547-1164; Nancy Bottomley, Director

South Haven Area Hospice, 05055 Blue Star Highway, P.O. Box 990, South Haven, MI 49090-0990; tel. 616/637-3825; FAX. 616/637-6777; Barbara Reicherts, Executive Director

Sparrow Hospice Services, 304 Brush Street, St. Johns, MI 48879; tel. 517/224-5650; FAX. 517/224-1501; Michelle Wiseman, Director

St. Joseph Huron Home Health and Hospice, Inc., 516 Oak Street, Tawas City, MI 48763; tel. 517/362-4611; FAX. 517/362-8771; Ann Balfour, Administrator

St. Joseph's Hospice/Affiliate of Henry Ford Cottage Hospice, 43411 Garfield Boulevard, Building Two, Clinton Towns, MI 48038; tel. 810/263-2840; FAX. 810/263-2895; Patti Ciechanovski, CRNH, Manager

United Home Hospice, Inc., 2401 20th Street, Detroit, MI 48216; tel. 313/964-1133; Alice Okwu, Director, Nursing

United Hospice Service, Six Eastgate Plaza, Sandusky, MI 48471; tel. 800/635-7490

Upper Peninsula Home Health and Hospice, 1414 West Fair, Suite 44, Marquette, MI 49855; tel. 906/225-4545; FAX. 906/225-7543; Cynthia A. Nyquist, RN, B.S.N., Executive Director, CEO

Visiting Nurse Hospice Services, 348 North Burdick Street, Kalamazoo, MI 49007-3843; tel. 616/343-1396; FAX. 616/382-8686; Jill Eldred

Visiting Nurse Service of Western Michigan Hospice Program, 1401 Cedar, N.E., Grand Rapids, MI 49503; tel. 616/774-2702; FAX. 616/774-7017; Laurie Sefton, RN, M.S.N., Hospice Program Director

VNA of Southwest Michigan Hospice, County Road #681, Suite D, Hartford, MI 49057; tel. 616/621-3154; Jill Eldred

VNA/Hospice Partners in Caring, Division of VNA of Saginaw, 500 South Hamilton, Saginaw, MI 48602; tel. 517/799-6020; FAX. 517/799-6062; S. J. Schultz, B.S.N., M.S., Director

West Bloomfield Hospice, 6020 West Maple Road, Suite 500, West Bloomfield, MI 48322; tel. 810/884-8600; Sondra Seely

Wings of Hope Hospice, Inc. of Allegan County, 663 North 10th Street, Plainwell, MI 49080; tel. 616/685-1645; FAX. 616/685-2105; Nancy Whitley, Executive Director

MINNESOTA

Crossroads Community Hospice, 404 Fountain Street, Albert Lea, MN 56007; tel. 507/377-6385; Shelley Doran, Administrator

Douglas County PHNS Hospice, 725 Elm Street, Suite 1200, Alexandria, MN 56308; tel. 320/763-6018; FAX. 320/763-4127; Mark Lundin, RN

Fairbault Area Hospice, 631 Southeast First Street, Faribault, MN 55021; tel. 507/332-4835; FAX. 507/332-4829; Jeanne Schoenbauer, Manager

Fairview Hospice, 2450 26th Avenue South, Minneapolis, MN 55406; tel. 612/728-2380; Mark Enger

First Care Hospice, 900 Hilligoss Blvd, Southeast, Fosston, MN 56542; tel. 218/435-1133; David S. Hubbard, Administrator

Healtheast Hospice, 69 West Exchange Street, St. Paul, MN 55102; tel. 612/232-3312; Kathleen M. Lucas, Administrator

HealthSpan Home Care and Hospice, 2750 Arthur Street, Roseville, MN 55113; tel. 612/628-4200; FAX. 612/628-9074; Cletis Hoffer, Acting Administrator

HomeCaring and Hospice, 11725 Stinson Avenue, Chisago City, MN 55013; tel. 651/257-8850; FAX. 651/257-8852; Karen Brohaugh, Manager

HomeHealth Partnership, 320 E. Main Street, Crosby, MN 56441; tel. 218/546-2311; Thomas F. Reek, Administrator

Hospice of Luverne Community Hospital, 305 East Luverne Street, P.O. Box 1019, Luverne, MN 56156; tel. 507/283-1805; Linda Reisdorferf, RN, Clinical Director

Hospice of Murray County, 2129 Broadway, Slayton, MN 56172; tel. 507/836-8114; Holly Miller, Administrator

Hospice of the Lakes, 8100 34th Avenue, S., P.O. Box 1309, Minneapolis, MN 55440-1309; tel. 612/883-6877; FAX. 612/883-6883; Becky Eck, Supervisor

Hospice of the Twin Cities, Inc., 7100 Northland Circle, Suite 205, Minneapolis, MN 55428; tel. 800/364-2478; FAX. 612/531-2422; Lisa Abicht Swensen, Executive Director

Hospice Partners, Inc., 6750 France Ave. South, Suite 290, Edina, MN 55435; tel. 612/920-0035; Roberta S. Cline, President and CEO

Immanuel St. Joseph's Hospice, 501 Holly Lane, Suite 10, Mankato, MN 56002; tel. 507/345-2618; W. Neath Folger, M.D., President

Lake City Area Hospice, 904 South Lakeshore Drive, Lake City, MN 55041; tel. 612/345-3321; Mark Rinehardt, Administrator

Lakeland Hospice, Inc., 715 S. Pebble Lake Road, P.O. Box 824, Fergus Falls, MN 56538; tel. 218/736-7885; FAX. 218/736-2231; Phyllis Schmid, Administrator

Lakeview Hospice, 927 West Churchill Street, Stillwater, MN 55082; tel. 612/430-3320; Geri Wagner

Litchfield Area Hospice, 218 N. Holcombe, Litchfield, MN 55355; tel. 320/693-7367; Lores Rogers, Director of Patient Services

Long Prairie Memorial Hospice, 20 Ninth Street Southeast, Long Prairie, MN 56347; tel. 320/732-7287; Rona Bless, Administrator

Mayo Hospice Program, 200 First Street, S.W., Rochester, MN 55905; tel. 507/284-4002; FAX. 507/284-0161; Ann Bartlett, RN, Coordinator

Northern Communities Hospice, 715 Delmore Drive, Roseau, MN 56751; tel. 218/463-3211; David Hagen, Administrator

Owatonna Area Hospice, 903 South Oak Ave., Owatonna, MN 55060; tel. 507/455-7628; Marlene H. Breckner, Administrator

Providers / Freestanding Hospices

Pine to Prairie Hospice Inc., 201 Hillestad Avenue North, Fosston, MN 56542; tel. 218/435–2017; FAX. 218/435–6909; Bev Leier, Administrator
Pope County Hospice, 10 Fourth Avenue, Southeast, Glenwood, MN 56334; tel. 320/634–4521; FAX. 320/634–2253; Douglas Reker, Administrator
Prairie Home Hospice, 300 South Bruce, Marshall, MN 56258; tel. 507/537–9247; FAX. 507/537–9258; Denise Brewers, Administrator
Prairie Home Hospice, Inc., 300 South Bruce, Marshall, MN 56258; tel. 507/537–9247; FAX. 507/537–9258; Lynn Yueill, Administrative Director
Red Wing Hospice, 434 West Fourth Street, Suite 200, Red Wing, MN 55066; tel. 651/385–3410; FAX. 651/385–3414; Bonnie Sheridan, Director
Renville County Hospice, 611 East Fairview Ave., Olivia, MN 56277; tel. 320/523–3427; Dean Slagter, Administrator
Rice Hospice Program, 301 Becker Ave., SW, Willmar, MN 56201; tel. 320/231–4450; Margaret Sietsema, Administrator
Ridgeview Hospice, 240 Willow Street, Tyler, MN 56178; tel. 507/247–5521; Douglas P. Schweikhart, CHE
Riverview Community Hospice, 323 South Minnesota, Crookston, MN 56716; tel. 218/281–9478; Victoria Korynta, Director
Seasons Hospice, 5650 Weatherhill Rd, SW, Rochester, MN 55902; tel. 507/281–3029; Pamela Schaid, Administrator
St. Joseph's Home Care and Hospice, 303 Kingwood Street, Brainerd, MN 56401; tel. 218/828–7444; FAX. 218/828–7579; Barb Anderson, Director
St. Luke's Hospice Duluth, 915 East First Street, Duluth, MN 55805; tel. 218/722–6220; Lynette Rauscher, Administrator
St. Mary's Medical Center Hospice, 407 East Third Street, Duluth, MN 55805; tel. 218/786–4020; FAX. 218/786–7249; Margaret Wolters, Hospice Nurse Manager
St. Mary's Medical Center Hospice, 404 East Fourth Street, Duluth, MN 55805; tel. 218/726–4020; Joanne Hagen, Administrator
St. Michael's Hospice, 425 North Elm Street, Sauk Centre, MN 56378; tel. 320/352–2221; FAX. 320/352–2899; Monica Blaske
The Hospice of Morrison County, 815 Southeast Second Street, Little Falls, MN 56345; tel. 320/632–1144; Dianne Jackson, Administrator
United Hands Hospice, 519 S. Galbraith St., Box 160, Blue Earth, MN 56013; tel. 507/526–3273; FAX. 507/526–3285; Marcia Smith, RN, Nurse Manager
Waseca Area Hospice, Inc., 204 Second Street, N.W., P.O. Box 94, Waseca, MN 56093; tel. 507/835–8983; FAX. 507/835–8737; Linda Grant, Director
Winona Area Hospice Services, 825 Mankato Avenue, Suite 111, Winona, MN 55987; tel. 507/457–4468; Charles R. Haugh, Administrator

MISSISSIPPI
Appletree Hospice, Inc., 521 Main Street, Suite U–Four, Natchez, MS 39121; tel. 601/446–8000; Linda L. Carlton, Administrator
Baptist Home Care and Hospice, 703A North Lamar, Oxford, MS 38655; tel. 601/234–8553; FAX. 601/236–1459; Sharon Johnson, RN, Director
Baptist Memorial Regional Home Health Care, Inc., Magnolia Health Services and Hospice North, 396 Southcrest Court Five, Southhaven, MS 38671; tel. 601/349–1394; Bill Caldwell, Administrator
Delta Area Hospice Care, Ltd., 522 Arnold Avenue, P.O. Box 5915, Greenville, MS 38704–5915; tel. 601/335–7040; FAX. 601/335–7048; Gloria Blakely, Administrator
Friendship Hospice of Natchez, Inc., 133 Jeff Davis Boulevard, Natchez, MS 39120; tel. 601/445–0307; Cynthia Paul, Administrator
Hospice Care Foundation, P.O. Box 351, Crystal Springs, MS 39059; tel. 601/892–3324; FAX. 601/892–3350; Kathy Welch, RN, Patient Care Coordinator
Hospice Care Foundation, P.O. Box 378, Edwards, MS 39066; tel. 601/852–4818; FAX. 601/852–4899; Dora Harris, RN, Patient Care Coordinator
Hospice Care Foundation, 4795 McWillie Drive, Suite 245, Jackson, MS 39216; tel. 601/713–3077; FAX. 601/713–3075; Leslie Scott, Social Worker
Hospice Care Foundation, P.O. Box 727, Magee, MS 39111; tel. 601/849–3025; FAX. 601/849–3074; Karen Walker, RN, Patient Care Coordinator

Hospice Care Foundation, P.O. Box 18427, Natchez, MS 39120; tel. 601/442–3070; FAX. 601/442–3074; Kathy Renfrow, RN, Patient Care Coordinator
Hospice Care Foundation, P.O. Box 119, Philadelphia, MS 39350; tel. 601/389–2006; FAX. 601/389–2202; Brenda Thrash, RN, Patient Care Coordinator
Hospice Care Foundation, P.O. Box 2056, Vicksburg, MS 39180; tel. 601/638–3070; FAX. 601/634–6010; Tiffany Walker, RN, Patient Care Coordinator
Hospice Care Foundation, P.O. Box 1152, Yazoo City, MS ; tel. 601/746–8481; FAX. 601/746–8497; Helen Hanna, RN, Patient Care Coordinator
Hospice Care Foundation, Inc., P.O. Box 2056, Vicksburg, MS 39181; tel. 601/638–3070; FAX. 601/634–6010; Tiffany Walker, RN, Coordinator
Hospice Care Foundation, Inc., 317–B Highland Avenue, Natchez, MS 39120; tel. 601/442–3070; Janie Calloway, Office Manager
Hospice Ministries, 450 Towne Center Blvd., Ridgeland, MS 39157; tel. 601/898–1053; FAX. 601/898–4320; John Fletcher, Executive Director
Hospice Ministries, 450 Towne Center Boulevard, Ridgeland, MS 39157; tel. 601/898–1053; FAX. 601/898–4320; Ronda Marks, Market – Development Director
Hospice of Light, 4341 Gautier & Vancleave Road, Suite Four, Gautier, MS 39553; tel. 228/497–2400; FAX. 228/497–9035; Laurie H. Grady, Nurse Coordinator
Hospice of North Mississippi, Inc., 619 East Lee Street, Sardis, MS 38666; tel. 601/487–1827; FAX. 601/487–1060; Renee Wright, Administrator
Hospice South, 202 South Washington Avenue, Greenville, MS 38701; tel. 601/335–4298; FAX. 601/335–4292; Wendy James, Executive Director
Hospice–North Mississippi Medical Center, 600 West Main, Tupelo, MS 38801; tel. 601/841–3612; Laura Kelley, Administrator
HospiceCare, 187 Stateline Road, Suite 10, P.O. Box 744, Southaven, MS 38671; tel. 601/280–8200; FAX. 601/280–8202; Linda Crum, Administrator
Quality Hospice of Gulf Coast, Inc., P.O. Box 549, Biloxi, MS 39533; tel. 228/374–4434; FAX. 228/436–3679; Patricia Hiers, Administrator
Rush Hospital Hospice, Highway 15, Route Nine, Box 28, Philadelphia, MS 39350; tel. 601/656–8388; Ken Boyette, Patient Care Coordinator, Supervisor
Sta–Home Hospice, 105 North Van Buren, Carthage, MS 39051; tel. 800/898–1159; Claudette Hathcock, Administrator
Sta–Home Hospice, 1620 24th Avenue, Meridan, MS 39305; tel. 601/485–8489; FAX. 601/693–7457; Debbie Emerson, RN, Patient Care Coordinator
Trinity Hospice, LLC, d/b/a Gulf Coast, 15101 LeMoyne Boulevard, D'Iberville, MS 39532; tel. 228/396–5750; FAX. 228/396–5751; JoAnne Swanzy, Intake Coordinator

MISSOURI
American Heartland Hospice, 7555 South Lindbergh Boulevard, St. Louis, MO 63125; tel. 314/894–8189; FAX. 314/894–7334; Susan O'Kane, Administrator
BLC Home Care Services, Inc, 9890 Clayton Road, St. Louis, MO 63124; tel. 314/953–1840; FAX. 314/953–1812; Ruth N. Castellano, Director Operations Administration
Community Hospice of America–Central, 3600 I–70 Drive, S.E., Suite H, Columbia, MO 65201; tel. 573/443–8360; FAX. 573/499–4601; Jean Yokley, RN, Patient Care Supervisor
Community Hospice of America–South Central, 101 East Second Street, Mountain Grove, MO 65711; tel. 417/926–4146; FAX. 417/926–6123; Jo Moody, Administrator
Community Hospice of America–Tri Lakes, 1756 Bee Creek Road, Suite G, Branson, MO 65616; tel. 417/335–2004; FAX. 417/335–2012; Janet Gard, Program Director
Comprehealth, Inc., Hospice Services Division, 2001 South Hanley Road, Suite 105, St. Louis, MO 63144; tel. 314/781–2800; FAX. 314/781–4844; Carolynn Ingerson–Hoffman, Interim Administrator
Hands of Hope Hospice, 801 Faraon Street, St. Joseph, MO 64501; tel. 816/271–7190; FAX. 816/271–7672; Jim Pierce, Resource Specialist
Harrison County Hospice, Highway 136 West, P.O. Box 425, Bethany, MO 64424; tel. 816/425–6324; FAX. 816/425–7642; Nola Martz, RN, B.S.N., Administrator

Heart of America Hospice, L.C., 9229 Ward Parkway, Suite 350, Kansas City, MO 64114; tel. 816/333–1980; FAX. 816/333–2421; Jacquelyn Tuohig, Executive Director
HomeCare of Mid–Missouri Hospice, 102 West Reed Street, Moberly, MO 65270; tel. 660/263–1517; FAX. 660/263–8033; Cherie Aird, LCSW, Hospice Director
Hospice of Integrated Health Services, 10910 Kennerly Road, St. Louis, MO 63128; tel. 314/849–3324; FAX. 314/842–9077; Gay Carlstrom, Administrator
Hospice of Southwest Missouri, 1465 E. Primrose, Suite A, Springfield, MO 65804; tel. 417/882–0453; FAX. 417/882–1245; Richard Williams, President and CEO
HospiceCare, Inc., P.O Box 1000, Mineral Area College, Park Hills, MO 63601; tel. 573/431–0162; FAX. 573/431–6304; Fred McDaniel, Administrator
Howard County Home Health and Hospice, 600 W. Morrison, Suite 10, Fayette, MO 65248; tel. 660/248–2100; FAX. 660/248–3347; Serese M. Wiehardt, Administrator
Kansas City Hospice, 1625 West 92nd Street, Kansas City, MO 64114; tel. 816/363–2600; FAX. 816/523–0068; Elaine McIntosh, President
Lake Ozark Area Home Health and Hospice, A Department of Pulaski County Health Department, 602 Commercial Street, P.O. Box 498, Crocker, MO 65452; tel. 314/736–2219; FAX. 314/736–5847; Beth Hutton, Administrator
Missouri River Hospice, 1440 Aaron Court, Jefferson City, MO 65101; tel. 314/635–5643; FAX. 314/635–6552; Roxanne Reed–Johnson, Director
NorthCare Hospice and Palliative Care, 6501 East Commerce Avenue, Suite 205, Kansas City, MO 64120; tel. 816/241–1994; FAX. 816/471–2434; Linda Ault, Administrator
Pike County Home Health Agency and Hospice, 19 North Main Cross, Bowling Green, MO 63334; tel. 573/324–2111; FAX. 573/324–5517; Lisa Pitzer, RN, Patient Care Coordinator
PRHS, Inc., 1202 Homelife Drive, Rolla, MO 65401; tel. 314/364–2425; FAX. 314/364–1575
Saint Luke's Shawnee Mission Hospice, 3100 Broadway, Suite 300, Kansas City, MO 64111–2415; tel. 816/756–1160; FAX. 816/756–3275; Deanette Sisson, Director
St. Clair County Hospice, 101 Hospital Drive, Osceola, MO 64776; tel. 417/646–8157; FAX. 417/646–8159; Candice J. Baker, Administrator
St. John's HospiceCare, 1235 East Cherokee, Springfield, MO 65804; tel. 417/888–7750; FAX. 417/888–7426; Suzanne Dollar, Administrator
Twin Lakes Hospice, Inc., 725 East Ohio, P.O. Box 502, Clinton, MO 64735; tel. 660/890–2018; FAX. 660/890–2018; Roy Wheeler, Administrator
Unity Health Hospice, 4191 Crescent Drive, Suite A, St. Louis, MO 63129; tel. 314/894–1000; FAX. 314/894–8389; Dawn Counts, Executive Director
Visiting Nurse Association Hospice Care, 9450 Manchester Road, Suite 206, St. Louis, MO 63119; tel. 314/918–7171; Susan Pettit, Administrator
VNA of Southeast Missouri Hospice, 100 East Harrison, Kennett, MO 63857; tel. 573/888–5892; FAX. 573/888–0538; Teresa McCulloch, Administrator

MONTANA
Anaconda Pintler Hospice of Community Hospital of Anaconda, 200 Main Street, P.O. Box 596, Anaconda, MT 59711; tel. 406/563–5422; FAX. 406/563–4245; Alice Cortright, Director
Big Sky Hospice, 3021 Sixth Avenue, N., Suite 205, Billings, MT 59103–1049; tel. 406/248–7442; FAX. 406/248–2572; Bernice Bjertness, RN, M.S.N., Director
Big Sky Hospice Stillwater Team, 350 West Pike Avenue, P.O. Box 1109, Columbus, MT 59019; tel. 406/322–5100; FAX. 406/322–5737; Donna McClure, RN
Highlands Hospice, 507 Centennial Avenue, Butte, MT 59701; tel. 406/723–5780; FAX. 406/723–9595; Virginia Mick, Director
Hospice of Powell County, 310 Milwaukee Avenue, P.O. Box 808, Deer Lodge, MT 59722; tel. 406/846–3975; Nora E. Meier, Office Manager
Kootenai Volunteer Hospice, P.O. Box 781, Libby, MT 59923; tel. 406/293–3923; Theresa Schneider, Director
Lake County Home Health Hospice, 107 6th Ave SW, Ronan, MT 59864; tel. 406/676–7300; FAX. 406/676–5243

Providers / Freestanding Hospices

Partners in Home Care Home Health & Hospice, Inc., 500 North Higgins, Suite 201, Missoula, MT 59801; tel. 406/728-8848; Kate Bratches, RN, Hospice Manager
Pondera Hospice, 300 North Virginia, Suite 305, Conrad, MT 59425; tel. 406/278-5566; FAX. 406/278-5569
Westmont Home Health Services Inc Hospice, 2525 Colonial Drive, P.O. Box 5059, Helena, MT 59601; tel. 406/443-4140; FAX. 406/447-3144; Bridget McGregor, Vice President, Clinical Services

NEBRASKA
Alegent Health Home Care & Hospice, 7070 Spring Street, Omaha, NE 68106-3519; tel. 402/898-8000; Denise McNitt, Operations Director
Central Plains Hospice, 300 E. 12th Street, P.O. Box 108, Cozad, NE 69130; tel. 308/784-4630; FAX. 308/784-4691; Rita Johnson, RN, Administrator
Chadron Community Hospital Hospice, 821 Morehead Street, Chadron, NE 69337; tel. 308/432-5586; FAX. 308/432-2737; Harold Krueger, Jr., Administrator
Fremont Area Medical Center Hospice, 450 East 23rd, Fremont, NE 68025; tel. 402/727-3373; D. Michael Leibert, President and CEO
Hospice Care of Nebraska LLC, 1600 South 70th Street, Suite 201, Lincoln, NE 68506; tel. 402/488-1363; FAX. 402/488-5976; Marcia Cederdahl, RN, CRNH, B.S. Ed.
Hospice of Tabitha, 4720 Randolph Street, Lincoln, NE 68510; tel. 402/483-7671; Roberta Daugherty, RN, Administrator
Hospice Preferred Choice, 407 South 27th Ave., Suite 200, Omaha, NE 68131; tel. 402/346-2273; Barbara Coppa, Administrator
Mary Lanning Hospice, 715 North St. Joseph Ave., Hastings, NE 68901; tel. 402/460-5868; FAX. 402/460-5869; Marcia Donley, Hospice Coordinator
Memorial Health Center Hospice, 1103 Illinois, Sidney, NE 69162; tel. 308/256-5825; Susan Peters, Administrator
St. Francis Hospice, 430 N. Monitor Street, West Point, NE 68788-1595; tel. 402/372-2404; FAX. 402/372-2360; Ronald Briggs, Administrator
St. Joe Ville Homecare and Hospice, 3035 South 72 Street, Omaha, NE 68124; tel. 402/926-4444; FAX. 402/393-8230; Judy M. Larsen, MA, RN, Director
Syracuse Hospice, 1579 Midland Street, Syracuse, NE 68446; tel. 402/269-2011; FAX. 402/269-2795; Al Klaasmeyer, Administrator
VNA Homecare and Hospice of Nebraska, 1941 S. 42nd, Suite 225, Omaha, NE 68127; tel. 402/342-5566; FAX. 402/342-5587; Janice Treml, Administrator

NEVADA
Family Home Hospice, 1701 West Charleston, Suite 201, P.O. Box 15645, Las Vegas, NV 89114-5645; tel. 702/383-0887; FAX. 702/383-9826; Nan Johnson, PSD
Hospice of Integrated Health Service, 5670 West Flamingo, Suite D, Las Vegas, NV 89103; tel. 702/361-6801; Karen Maxfield, Administrator
Nathan Adelson Hospice, 4141 Swenson Street, Las Vegas, NV 89119; tel. 702/733-0320; FAX. 702/796-3195; Richard L. Kilburn, Interim Chief Executive Officer
St. Mary's Hospice of Northern Nevada, 3605 Grant Drive, Reno, NV 89509; tel. 775/770-3081; FAX. 775/325-8320; James Summerfelt, Executive Director
Washoe Home Care Connection, 780 Kuenzli, Suite 200, Reno, NV 89502; tel. 775/982-5860; FAX. 775/982-5795; Michael Girard, Administrator

NEW HAMPSHIRE
Community Health and Hospice, Inc., 780 North Main Street, P.O. Box 578, Laconia, NH 03247-0578; tel. 603/524-8444; FAX. 603/524-8217; Polly Clough, Administrator
Concord Regional VNA–Hospice, 250 Pleasant Street, P.O. Box 1797, Concord, NH 03302; tel. 603/224-4093; FAX. 603/228-7359; Mary B. DeVeau, President and CEO
Connecticut Valley Home Care Inc., 958 John Stark Highway, Newport, NH 03773; tel. 603/543-0164; Lynn Holland, RN
Elliot Home Care and Hospice, 1815 Elmstreet, Manchester, NH 03103; tel. 603/628-4430; FAX. 603/622-4800; Diane LaBossiere, M.S.W.

HCS – Home Healthcare, Hospice and Community Services, Inc., 69L Island Street, P.O. Box 564, Keene, NH 03431; tel. 603/352-2253; FAX. 603/358-3904; Lois Hopkins, Hospice Program Coordinator
Home Health and Hospice, 22 Prospect Street, Nashua, NH 03060; tel. 603/882-2941; FAX. 603/883-1515; Gail Spera, Administrator
Hospice America of New Hampshire, 169 Daniel Webster Highway, Suite 14, Meredith, NH 03253; tel. 603/279-4700; FAX. 603/279-1370; Linda Roberts, Administrator
Hospice America of New Hampshire, Inc., 169 D W Highway, Suite 14, Meredith, NH 03253; tel. 603/279-4700; FAX. 603/279-1370; Linda Roberts, Administrator
Hospice at HCS, 69L Island Street, P.O. Box 564, Keene, NH 03431; tel. 603/352-2253; Lois Hopkins, Administrator
Lake Sunapee Home Care and Hospice, 290 County Road, P.O. Box 2209, New London, NH 03257; tel. 603/526-4077; FAX. 603/526-4272; Barbara Boulton, RN, Hospice Patient Care Coordinator
North Country Home Health Agency, 536 Cottage Street, Littleton, NH 03561; tel. 603/444-5317; FAX. 603/444-0980; Cheryl Guinan, Administrator
Optima Health Visiting Nurse Services, VNA Hospice, 1850 Elm Street, Manchester, NH 03104; tel. 603/622-3781; FAX. 603/641-4074; Jane Clough, Director, Hospice
Pemi–Baker Home Health Agency, 258 Highland Street, Plymouth, NH 03264; tel. 603/536-2232; Elaine Vieira, Administrator
Portsmouth Regional Visiting Nurses Association and Hospice, 127 Parrott Avenue, Portsmouth, NH 03801; tel. 603/436-0815; FAX. 603/431-5457; Joan P. Nickell, President
Rochester Visiting Nurse Association, Inc., 89 Charles Street, Rochester, NH 03867; tel. 603/332-1133; FAX. 603/332-9223; Marianne Gagne, Hospice Coordinator
Rockingham VNA and Hospice, 137 Epping Road, Exeter, NH 03833; tel. 603/772-2981; FAX. 603/772-0931; Ann Blair, RN, Hospice Director
Rural District VNA Inc., 36 Charles Street, Farmington, NH 03835; tel. 603/755-2202; FAX. 603/755-3760; Sue Houle, Director
Seacoast Hospice, 10 Hampton Road, Exeter, NH 03833; tel. 603/778-7391; FAX. 603/772-7692; Susan Cole, Administrator
Souhegan Nursing Association Inc., 24 North River Road, Milford, NH 03055; tel. 603/673-3460; FAX. 603/673-0159; Liane Schubring, Executive Director
Squamscott Visiting Nurse and Hospice Care, 113 New Rochester Rd., Suite 4, Dover, NH 03820; tel. 603/742-7921; FAX. 603/742-3835; Mary Jo Sceggell, Administrator
Tri-Area Visiting Nurse Association, Inc., 301 High Street, Somersworth, NH 03878-1800; tel. 603/692-2112; FAX. 603/692-9940; Susan Karmeris, President and CEO
Tri-Area VNA Hospice, 301 High Street, Somersworth, NH 03878; tel. 603/692-2112; FAX. 603/692-9940; Maxine Lacy, Clinical Services Coordinator
Visiting Nurse and Hospice Care of Northern Carroll County, Route 16, P.O. Box 432, North Conway, NH 03818; tel. 603/447-6766; FAX. 603/447-6370; Kathleen T. Sheehan, Administrator
VNA – Hospice of Southern Carroll County and Vicinity, South Main Street, Wolfeboro, NH 03894; tel. 603/569-2729; FAX. 603/569-2409; Carol C. Tubman, RN, CRNH

NEW JERSEY
Atlantic City Medical Center Hospice, P.O. Box 1626, Pleasantville, NJ 08232; tel. 609/272-2424; FAX. 609/272-2414; Diana Ciurczak, Director
Atlantic Home Care and Hospice, 33 Bleeker Street, Millburn, NJ 07041; tel. 973/379-8440; FAX. 973/379-8412; Mary White, RN, Clinical Coordinator
Center for Hope Hospice & Palliative Care, 176 Hussar Street, Linden, NJ 07036; tel. 908/486-0700; FAX. 908/486-2450; Margaret J. Coloney, President
Community VNA/Community Care Hospice, 586 East Main Street, Bridgewater, NJ 08807; tel. 908/725-9355; FAX. 908/725-1033; Doreen Flanagan, RN, Hospice Manager
Compassionate Care Hospice, 1373 Broad Street, Suite 304, Clifton, NJ 07013; tel. 201/916-1400; FAX. 201/916-0066; Judith Grey, MPH, RNC, Regional Director of New Jersey

Garden State Hospice, 27 Daniel Road West, Fairfield, NJ 07932; tel. 973/882-6100; FAX. 973/882-5599; Nora Nicolosi, RN, Administrator
Holy Redeemer Hospice, 1801 Route Nine North, P.O. Box 280A, Swainton, NJ 08210; tel. 609/465-2082; FAX. 609/465-6185; Arleen Moffitt, ACSW
Hospice at Bergen Community Health Care, 400 Old Hook Road, Westwood, NJ 07675-3131; tel. 201/358-2900; FAX. 201/358-0836; Patricia Hutzelman, RN, Hospice Coordinator
Hospice of New Jersey, 400 Broadacres Drive, Fourth Floor, Bloomfield, NJ 07003; tel. 973/893-0818; FAX. 973/893-0828; Michelle Stefanelli, Administrator, CEO
Hospice of VNA of Northern New Jersey, 38 Elm Street, Morristown, NJ 07960; tel. 973/539-1216; FAX. 973/539-3352; Marcia Lutschewitz, Hospice Patient Care Manager
Hospice Program of Bayonne VNA, 325 Broadway, Bayonne, NJ 07002; tel. 201/339-2500; FAX. 201/339-1255; Barbara Halosz, RN, B.S.N., Coordinator
HospiceCare of South Jersey, Inc., 2848 South Delsea Drive, Vineland, NJ 08360; tel. 856/794-1515; FAX. 856/691-7660; Yvonne Crouch, Executive Director
Jerseycare Hospice, 50 Newark Avenue, Suite 101, Belleville, NJ 07109
Karen Ann Quinlan Hospice, 99 Sparta Avenue, Newton, NJ 07860; tel. 973/383-0115; FAX. 973/383-6889; Mary Guler, Executive Director
Lighthouse Hospice, A Division of Alternative Healthcare System, 4 Executive Campus, 771 Cuthbert Blvd, Cherry Hill, NJ 08002; tel. 856/661-5600; FAX. 856/661-5650; Susan Curry, Director
Meridian Hospice, 615 Hope Road, Building Four, 2nd Floor, Eatontown, NJ 07724; tel. 908/935-1797; Kerri A. Johnston, Hospice Administrator
Passaic Valley Hospice, VHS of New Jersey, Inc., 783 Riverview Drive, Totowa, NJ 07511; tel. 973/256-4636; FAX. 973/256-6778; Elizabeth Geoghegan
The Center for Hospice Care, Inc., An affiliate of the Saint Barnabas Health Care System, 187 Millburn Avenue, Millburn, NJ 07041; tel. 973/379-2200; FAX. 973/322-0248; Lorraine M. Sciara, Executive Director
Trinity Hospice, 150 Ninth Avenue, Runnemede, NJ 08078; tel. 609/939-9000; FAX. 609/939-9010; Eileen D'Amico, Director
Trinity Hospice, Formerly Greater Monmouth VNA Hospice, 111 Union Avenue, Long Branch, NJ 07740; tel. 908/229-0816; FAX. 908/229-0561; Debra Cox, RN, CRNH, Hospice Supervisor
Unity Hospice, 17 Academy Street, Newark, NJ 07102; tel. 201/596-9661; FAX. 201/596-9664; Terry M. Copeland, Administrator
Visiting Nurse and Health Services Hospice, 354 Union Avenue, P.O. Box 170, Elizabeth, NJ 07208; tel. 908/352-5694; FAX. 908/352-9216; Shirley Altman, Hospice Administrator
Visiting Nurse Association Somerset Hills Hospice, 12 Olcott Avenue, Bernardsville, NJ 07924; tel. 908/766-0180; FAX. 908/766-2268; Suzanne VanLoon, Hospice Coordinator
VNA of Central Jersey Hospice, 1100 Wayside Road, Asbury Park, NJ 07712; tel. 732/493-2220; Patricia Vigilante, Director of Hospice
West Essex Hospice, 799 Bloomfield Avenue, Verona, NJ 07044; tel. 973/857-7300; FAX. 973/857-3433; Thomas Koester, President and CEO

NEW MEXICO
Alamogordo Home Care–Hospice, 505 11th Street, Alamogordo, NM 88310; tel. 800/617-3555; FAX. 505/437-2399; Pat Raub, Administrator
Alternative Home Health Care Hospice, 1118 National Avenue, Las Vegas, NM 87701; tel. 800/296-1538; FAX. 505/425-7682; Maxine E. Gonzales, Administrator
Carlsbad Hospice, Inc., 1003 West Riverside Drive, P.O. Drawer PP, Carlsbad, NM 88220; tel. 505/885-8257; Nancy Flanagan, Administrator
Esperanza Home Health Care Hospice, Inc., Highway 518 Buena Vista, P.O. Box 270, Mora, NM 87732; tel. 505/387-2215; Josephine P. Garcia
Helping Hand Hospice, 615 South Second, Tucumcari, NM 88401; tel. 800/662-8840; Diana Beck, Administrator
Hospice of Artesia, 702 North 13th, Artesia, NM 88210; tel. 505/748-3333; FAX. 505/746-8918; Beverly Morehead, RN, Director

Providers / Freestanding Hospices

Hospice Services, Inc., 901 East Bender, P.O. Box 249, Hobbs, NM 88241; tel. 800/658-6844; FAX. 505/393-3985; Brenda Chambers
Los Alamos Visiting Nurse Service Hospice, 901 18th Street, Suite 203, Los Alamos, NM 87544; tel. 505/662-2525; FAX. 505/662-7093; Deborah Simon, Director
Mesilla Valley Hospice, Inc., 299 East Montana Avenue, Las Cruces, NM 88005; tel. 505/523-4700; FAX. 505/527-2204; Margaret Connealy, Executive Director
Mountain Home Health Hospice, 630 Paseo del Pueblo Sur, Suite 180, Taos, NM 87571; tel. 505/758-4786; Patricia Heinen, Administrator
Northwest New Mexico Hospice, 608 Reilly Avenue, P.O. Box 3336, Farmington, NM 87499; tel. 505/327-0301; FAX. 505/325-2477; Debra Lowe, Administrator
Presbyterian Hospice, P.O. Box 26666, Albuquerque, NM 87125; tel. 505/291-5656; FAX. 505/291-2055; Jane Bergquist, RN
Quality Continuum Hospice, 2625 Pennsylvania NE, Suite 225, Albuquerque, NM 87110; tel. 505/881-3937; FAX. 505/881-4319; Sheila D. Nipper, Administrator
Sandia Hospice, 4725 Indianschool N.E., Suite 100, Albuquerque, NM 87100; tel. 505/888-0095; FAX. 505/888-2025; Catherine A. Esterheld, Executive Director
St. Anthony's Hospice, 1008 Douglas Avenue, P.O. Box 1170, Las Vegas, NM 87701; tel. 505/425-3353; Beatrice R. Velasquez, Administrator
Staff Builders Services, Inc., 826 Camino De Monte Rey, P.O. Box 23448, Santa Fe, NM 87502; tel. 505/983-5408; Pamela Brunsell, RN, Administrator
The Hospice Center, 1422 Paseo De Peralta, Santa Fe, NM 87501; tel. 505/988-2211; FAX. 505/986-1833; Barbara Elder Owas, RN, Executive Director
Victory Home Health Hospice, 2810 Hotsprings Boulevard, Las Vegas, NM 87701; tel. 505/454-0499; FAX. 505/425-9105; Maria Luisa Padilla, Administrator
VistaCare Family Hospice, 8804 Washington NE, Suite C, Albuquerque, NM 87113; tel. 505/821-5404; FAX. 505/821-5449; Kathy Garcia, RN, Program Director
VNS Health Services, Inc., 706 La Joya, N.E., Espanola, NM 87532; tel. 505/753-2284; FAX. 505/756-2179; Beatrice Sceery, Manager, Home Health, Hospice

NEW YORK
Caring Community Hospice of Cortland, 4281 North Homer Avenue, Cortland, NY 13045; tel. 607/753-9105; FAX. 607/758-7668; Mary Beach, Director
Catskill Area Hospice Palliative Care, Inc., 542 Main Street, Oneonta, NY 13820; tel. 607/432-6773; FAX. 607/432-7741; Lesley Deleski, Executive Director
Christian Nursing Hospice, Inc., d/b/a Little House Residence, 110 Lake Avenue South, Suite 33, Nesconset, NY 11767; tel. 516/265-5300; FAX. 516/265-5789; Camille Harlow, Executive Director
Comstock Hospice Care Network, 1225 West State Street, Olean, NY 14760; tel. 716/372-2106; FAX. 716/372-4635; Kathleen Mack, Hospice Director
East End Hospice, Inc., 1111 Riverhead Road, P.O. Box 1048, Westhampton B, NY 11978; tel. 516/288-8400; FAX. 512/288-8492; Priscilla Ruffin, Executive Director
Herkimer County Hospice, 301 N. Washington Street, Suite 2343, Herkimer, NY 13350-2908; tel. 315/867-1317; FAX. 315/867-1371; Sue Campagna, Administrator
High Peaks Hospice, Inc., P.O. Box 840, Trudeau Road, Saranac Lake, NY 12983; tel. 518/891-0606; FAX. 518/891-0657; Maureen Sayles, Executive Director
Hospicare of Tompkins County, Inc., 172 East King Road, Ithaca, NY 14850; tel. 607/272-0212; FAX. 607/272-0237; Nina K. Miller, Executive Director
Hospice Buffalo, Inc., 225 Como Park Boulevard, Cheektowaga, NY 14227-1480; tel. 716/686-1900; FAX. 716/686-8181; J. Donald Schumacher, Psy.D., President and CEO
Hospice Care in Westchester and Putnam, an Affiliate of VNA of Hudson Valley, 100 South Bedford Road, Mount Kisco, NY 10549; tel. 914/666-4228; FAX. 914/666-0378; Cornelia Schimert, Director
Hospice Care Network, Merchants Concourse, Westbury, NY 11590; tel. 516/832-7100; FAX. 516/832-7160; Maureen Hinkleman, Chief Executive Officer

Hospice Care, Inc., 4277 Middlesettlement Road, New Hartford, NY 13413; tel. 315/735-6484; FAX. 315/735-8545; Wes Case, Executive Director
Hospice Family Care, 550 East Main Street, Batavia, NY 14020; tel. 716/343-7596; FAX. 716/343-7629; Deborah Schafer, Operating Director
Hospice of Central New York, 990 7th North Street, Liverpool, NY 13088; tel. 315/634-1100; FAX. 315/634-1111; Peter Sarver, President and CEO
Hospice of Chenango County, Inc., 21 Hayes Street, Norwich, NY 13815; tel. 607/334-3556; FAX. 607/334-3688; Laurie Vogel, Executive Director
Hospice of Greater New York, 6323 Seventh Avenue, Brooklyn, NY 11220; tel. 718/921-7900; FAX. 718/921-0752; Abby Gordon, Administrator
Hospice of Jefferson County, Inc., 425 Washington Street, Watertown, NY 13601; tel. 315/788-7323; FAX. 315/785-9932; Judith H. Boros, Executive Director
Hospice of North Country, 386 Rugar Street, Plattsburgh, NY 12901-2306; tel. 518/561-8465; FAX. 518/561-3182; Sarah Anderson, Executive Director
Hospice of Orleans County, 13996 Route 31 West, Albion, NY 14411; tel. 716/589-0809; Mary Ann Fisher, Executive Director
Hospice of Rochester and Hospice of Wayne and Seneca Counties, 70 Metro Park, Rochester, NY 14623; tel. 716/214-1400; FAX. 716/214-1207; Barbara Quinlan, RN, BSN, Director of Palliative Care Services
Hospice of St. Lawrence Valley, Inc., 6439 State Highway 56, Potsdam, NY 13676; tel. 315/265-3105; FAX. 315/265-0323; Brian Gardam, Executive Director
Hospice of the Finger Lakes, 25 William Street, Auburn, NY 13021; tel. 315/255-2733; FAX. 315/252-9080; Theresa Kenny Kline, Executive Director
Hospice Serving Dutchess and Ulster Counties Inc., 362 Violet Avenue, Poughkeepsie, NY 12601; tel. 914/485-2273; Benjamin Wallace, Jr., Chief Executive Officer
Hospice VNSW/WPHC, Inc., d/b/a Hospice of Westchester, 95 South Broadway, 4th Floor, The Esplanade, White Plains, NY 10601; tel. 914/682-1484; FAX. 914/682-9425; George Battern, Executive Director
Jansen Memorial Hospice/Home Nursing Association of Westchester, 69 Main Street, Tuckahoe, NY 10707; tel. 914/961-2818; FAX. 914/961-8654; Lucille D. Winton, Director
Livingston County Hospice, 2 Livingston County Campus, Mount Morris, NY 14510; tel. 716/243-7290; FAX. 716/243-7287; Cheryl Pletcher, Administrator
Mercy Hospice, St. Pius X Service Center, 1220 Front Street, Uniondale, NY 11553; tel. 516/485-3060; FAX. 516/485-1007; Edith Miozzi, Executive Director
Mountain Valley Hospice, 73 North Main Street, Gloversville, NY 12078; tel. 518/725-4545; FAX. 518/725-8066; Nancy Dowd, Executive Director
Niagara Hospice, Inc., 4675 Sunset Drive, Lockport, NY 14094; tel. 716/439-4417; FAX. 716/439-6035; Carol E. Gettings, M.S., Executive Director
Ontario-Yates Hospice, A Program of Finger Lakes VNS, 756 Pre-Emption Road, Geneva, NY 14456; tel. 315/781-0071; FAX. 315/789-7042; Bonnie Hollenbeck, Administrator
Oswego County Hospice, Oswego County Health Department, 70 Bunner Street, Oswego, NY 13126; tel. 315/349-8259; FAX. 315/349-8269; Judith S. Watson, Director
Pax Christi Hospice, 355 Bard Avenue, Staten Island, NY 10310; tel. 718/876-1022; Patricia Farrington, Executive Director
Southern Tier Hospice, Inc., 244 West Water Street, Elmira, NY 14901; tel. 607/734-1570; FAX. 607/734-1902; Mary Ann Starbuck, Executive Director
The Community Hospice, Inc, 295 Valley View Boulevard, Rensselaer, NY 12144; tel. 518/285-8150; FAX. 518/285-8151; Philip G. Di Sorbo, Executive Director
United Hospice of Rockland, 18 Thiells-Mount Ivy Road, Pomona, NY 10970; tel. 914/354-5100; FAX. 914/354-2128; Amy Stern, Executive Director
Visiting Nurse Hospice, 2180 Empire Boulevard, Webster, NY 14580; tel. 716/787-8315; FAX. 716/787-9726; Dorothy Chilton, Administrator

VNS Hospice of Suffolk, 505 Main Street, Northport, NY 11768; tel. 516/261-7200; FAX. 516/261-1985; Joyce Palmier, RN, BSN, Director, Patient Services
VNSNY Hospice Care, 1250 Broadway, New York, NY 10001; tel. 212/290-3888; FAX. 212/290-3933; Renee Martinez, Administrator

NORTH CAROLINA
3HC Home Health and Hospice Care, Inc, 1614 Harbour Drive, Wilmington, NC 28401; tel. 910/799-0018; FAX. 910/452-3198
3HC Home Health and Hospice Care, Inc, 1023 Beaman Street, Clinton, NC 28323-2343; tel. 910/592-1421; FAX. 910/592-7392
3HC Home Health and Hospice Care, Inc, 100 Westlake Road, Fayetteville, NC 28302; tel. 910/860-7858; FAX. 910/860-8279
3HC Home Health and Hospice Care, Inc, 2402 Wayne Memorial Drive, P.O. Box 88, Goldsboro, NC 27533; tel. 919/753-1386; FAX. 919/731-4985
3HC Home Health and Hospice Care, Inc, 503 Bowman Gray Drive Suite C, Greensville, NC 27834; tel. 252/758-8212; FAX. 252/758-1384; Edith H. Farmer, RN, Director of Clinical Services
3HC Home Health and Hospice Care, Inc, 744 Airport Road, P.O. Box 1396, Kinston, NC 28503; tel. 252/527-9561; FAX. 252/527-6617
3HC Home Health and Hospice Care, Inc, 1004 Jenkins Avenue, P.O. Box 190, Maysville, NC 28555-0190; tel. 910/743-2800; FAX. 910/743-2321
3HC Home Health and Hospice Care, Inc, 8208 Brownleigh Drive, P.O. Box 31804, Raleigh, NC 27622-1804; tel. 919/789-4241; FAX. 919/789-4245
3HC Home Health and Hospice Care, Inc, 15 Noble Street, P.O. Box 1524, Smithfield, NC 27577-9300; tel. 919/934-0664; FAX. 919/934-9046
Albemarle Home Care, 103 Charles Street, P.O. Box 189, Hertford, NC 27907; tel. 919/426-5488; Paula Vanhorn, Administrator
Albemarle Home Care, Highway 168, P.O. Box 189, Currituck, NC 27907; tel. 919/232-2026; Victoria Rentrop, Administrator
Albemarle Hospice, 400 S. Road Street, P.O. Box 189, Elizabeth City, NC 27907-0189; tel. 252/338-4066; FAX. 252/338-3767; Ronda Wentz, Director
Angel Home Health and Hospice, 170 Church Street, Franklin, NC 28713; tel. 828/369-4206; FAX. 828/369-4400; Sandy Smith, RN, MPH, Director
Beverly HomeCare – Hospice, 4051 South Memorial Drive, Suite #2, Greenville, NC 27835; tel. 252/353-3326; FAX. 252/353-3331; Barbara Walter, Executive Director
Caldwell County Hospice, Inc., 902 Kirkwood Street, N.W., Lenoir, NC 28645; tel. 828/754-0101; FAX. 828/757-3335; Cathy S. Simmons, Executive Director
Cape Fear Valley Home Health and Hospice, 3418 Village Drive, Fayetteville, NC 28304; tel. 910/609-6740; FAX. 910/609-6573; Pat Pruitt, M.S.N., Director
Cashiers Home Health, Highway 107 South, 59 Hospital Road, Sylva, NC 28779; tel. 704/586-7410
Center of Living Home Health and Hospice, d/b/a Center of Living Homecare, 416 Vision Drive, P.O. Box 9, Asheboro, NC 27204-0009; tel. 336/672-9300; FAX. 336/672-0868; Billie Vuncannon, President and CEO
Community Home Care and Hospice, 5301 Morgantan Road, Fayetteville, NC 28314; tel. 910/323-9816; FAX. 910/484-6724; Robert Reed, Chief Executive Officer
Comprehensive Home Health Care, 3840 Henderson Drive, Jacksonville, NC 28456; tel. 910/346-4800; Linda Powers, Patient Care Manager
Comprehensive Home Health Care, 819 Jefferson Street, P.O. Box 366, Whiteville, NC 28472; tel. 910/642-5808; FAX. 910/640-1374; Sheila Faulk, Director
Comprehensive Home Health Care, 1120 Ocean Highway W, P.O. Box 200, Supply, NC 28462; tel. 910/754-8133; FAX. 910/754-2096; Crystal Floyd, RN, Director
Comprehensive Home Health Care and Comprehensive Hospice, Inc., 101 South Craig Street, P.O. Drawer 2540, Elizabethtown, NC 28337; tel. 910/862-8538; Sherry Hester, Director, Office Operations

Providers / Freestanding Hospices

Comprehensive Home Health Care/Comprehensive Hospice, 1800 Skibo Road, Suite 228, Fayetteville, NC 28303; tel. 910/864–8411; Gwendolyn Harrell, Regional Director

Craven County Home Health–Hospice Agency, 2818 Neuse Boulevard, P.O. Drawer 12610, New Bern, NC 28561; tel. 919/636–4930; FAX. 919/636-5301

Davie County Health Department and Home Health Agency, Hospice of Davie, 210 Hospital Street, P.O. Box 848, Mocksville, NC 27028; tel. 336/751–8770; FAX. 336/751–0335; Joseph B. Bass, Jr., M.S.W., Health Director

Duplin Home Care and Hospice Inc., 234 Smith Chapel Road, Kenansville, NC 28349; tel. 910/296–0819; FAX. 910/296–0482; Rhonda Lucus, RN, Hospice Coordinator

Duplin Home Care and Hospice, Inc., 101 East Main Street, Wallace, NC 28466; tel. 910/285–1100; FAX. 910/285–1172; Glenda Kenan, RN, Home Health Coordinator

Duplin Home Care and Hospice, Inc., P.O. Box 887, Kenansville, NC 28349; tel. 910/296–0819; FAX. 910/296-0482

Edgecombe County HomeCare and Hospice, 2213 St. Andrew Street, Tarboro, NC 27886; tel. 919/641-7558; FAX. 919/641-7004; Jessie Worthington, Hospice Program Director

FirstHealth Hospice, 5 Aviemore Drive, Pinehurst, NC 28374; tel. 910/215–6000; FAX. 910/215–6032; Carole White, Director

Four Seasons Hospice HomeCare (Elizabeth's House), 1825 Asheville Highway, P.O. Box 2395, Hendersonville, NC 28739; tel. 828/692–6178; FAX. 828/692–2365; Mark Miller, Executive Director

Good Shepherd Home Health and Hospice Agency, Inc., P.O. Box 465, Hayesville, NC 28904; tel. 704/389-6311; FAX. 704/389-9584; Ernie Zapetis, Hospice Manager

Home Health and Hospice Care, Inc., 1004 Jenkins Avenue, P.O. Box 190, Maysville, NC 28555; tel. 919/743-2800; Janet Haddow-Green, Administrator

Home Health and Hospice Care, Inc., 1023 Beaman Street, P.O. Box 852, Clinton, NC 28328; tel. 800/695-4442; FAX. 910/592-7392; Richard Stone, Administrator

Home Health and Hospice Care, Inc., 2305 Wellington Drive, Suite G, P.O. Box 3673, Wilson, NC 27895–3673; tel. 252/291–4400; FAX. 252/237-4396; Carolyn Yowell, Marketing Director

Home Health and Hospice Care, Inc., 15 Noble Street, P.O. Box 1524, Smithfield, NC 27577–9300; tel. 919/934–0664; FAX. 919/934-9046; Phil Adams Administrator

Home Health and Hospice Care, Inc., 2419 East Ash Street, Suite Four and Five, Goldsboro, NC 27532; tel. 919/735–1386; FAX. 919/731–4985; Jim Wall, Administrator

Home Health and Hospice Care, Inc., 907A Southeast Second Street, Snow Hill, NC 28580

Home Health and Hospice Care, Inc., d/b/a Kitty Askins Hospice Center, 107 Handley Park Court, Goldsboro, NC 27534; tel. 919/735–5887; FAX. 919/735-5948; Marie K. Abrams, RN, GNP

Home Health and Hospice of Halifax, 1229 Julian R. Allsbrock Road, Roanoke Rapids, NC 27870; tel. 252/308-0700; FAX. 252/537-1872; Sheila Alford, RN, Home Care Director

Home Health and Hospice of Person County, 325 South Morgan Street, Roxboro, NC 27573; tel. 336/597-2542; FAX. 336/597-3367; Joyce Franke, Administrator

Home Health of NC, Inc., 120 Providence Road, Suite 200, Chapel Hill, NC 27514; tel. 919/401-3000; FAX. 919/402-1952; Linda Sutherin, Executive Director

HomeHealth and Hospice Care Inc., 744 Airport Road, P.O. Box 1396, Kinston, NC 28503; tel. 919/527-9561; Ann Harrison, Clinical Director

Hospice at Charlotte, Inc., 1420 East Seventh Street, Charlotte, NC 28204; tel. 704/375–0100; FAX. 704/375-8623; Janet Fortner, President

Hospice at Greensboro–Beacon Place, 2502 Summit Avenue, Greensboro, NC 27405; tel. 336/621–5301; FAX. 336/375–2348; Pat Gibbons, BSN, Nurse Manager

Hospice Home, 918 Chapel Hill Road, Burlington, NC 27215; tel. 336/513–4460; FAX. 336/513–4471; Judy Bowman, Manager

Hospice of Alamance–Caswell, 730 Hermitage Road, P.O. Box 2122, Burlington, NC 27216; tel. 336/538-8040; FAX. 336/538-8049; Jim Higgins, Executive Director

Hospice of Alexander County, Inc., 50 Lucy Echerd Lane, Taylorsville, NC 28681; tel. 704/632–5026; FAX. 704/632-3707; Ruth Jarrell, Executive Director

Hospice of Alleghany, P.O. Box 1278, Sparta, NC 28675; tel. 910/373–8018; Wanda Branch, Administrator

Hospice of Ashe, 392 Highway 16–88 South, Jefferson, NC 28640; tel. 336/246–6443; FAX. 336/246-8504; Trinja Merit, Clinical Director

Hospice of Avery County, Inc., 351 West Mitchell Street, P.O. Box 1357, Newland, NC 28657; tel. 704/733-0663; FAX. 704/733-0375; Melissa Gragg, RN, Patient Care Coordinator

Hospice of Burke County, Inc., 1721 Eron Road, Valdese, NC 28690; tel. 704/879–1601; FAX. 704/879-3500; Marlene Jernigan, Business Manager

Hospice of Cabarrus County, Inc., 1060 Diploma Place, S.W., P.O. Box 1235, Concord, NC 28026–1235; tel. 704/788–9434; FAX. 704/788-6013; Shirley McDowell, Executive Director

Hospice of Carteret County, Inc., P.O. Drawer 1619, Morehead City, NC 28557; tel. 252/ 247–1390; FAX. 252/247-1379; Claudia Lewis, Administrator

Hospice of Catawba Valley, Inc., 3975 Robinson Road, Newton, NC 28658; tel. 828/466–0466; FAX. 828/466-8862; David B. Clarke, Executive Director

Hospice of Chatham County, Inc., 200 East Street, P.O. Box 1077, Pittsboro, NC 27312; tel. 919/542–5545; FAX. 919/542–6232; Susan H. Balfour, RN, Executive Director

Hospice of Cleveland County, Inc., 951 Wendover Heights Drive, Shelby, NC 28150; tel. 704/487–4677; FAX. 704/481–8050; Myra McGinnis Hamrick, Executive Director

Hospice of Cumberland County, 235 N. McPherson Church Road, Suite 210, Fayetteville, NC 28303-4403; tel. 910/860–7178; FAX. 910/860-1660; Stacy Pendarvis, M.S.W., Hospice Coordinator

Hospice of Davidson County, Inc., 524 South State Street, P.O. Box 1941, Lexington, NC 27293-1941; tel. 336/248–6185; FAX. 336/248-4574; Gary Drake, Executive Director

Hospice of Gaston County, Inc., d/b/a Gaston Hospice, 258 East Garrison Boulevard, P.O. Box 3984, Gastonia, NC 28054; tel. 704/861–8405; FAX. 704/865-0590; Lee Bucci, Executive Director

Hospice of Harnett County, Inc., 111A North Ellis Avenue, Dunn, NC 28339; tel. 910/892–1213; FAX. 910/892-1229; Grace E. Tart, Administrator

Hospice of Iredell County, Inc., 403 East Statesville Avenue, Suite One, Mooresville, NC 28115; tel. 704/663-0051; FAX. 704/872–1810; Judy Snowden, Executive Director

Hospice of Lee County, Inc., P.O. Box 1181, Sanford, NC 27331–1181; tel. 919/774–4169; FAX. 919/774-6348; Janet MacLaren Scovil, Executive Director

Hospice of Lincoln County, Inc., 107 North Cedar Street, Lincolnton, NC 28093–1526; tel. 704/732-6146; FAX. 704/736-0264; Leslie Barlowe, RN, Branch Director

Hospice of Macon County, Inc., 208 Roller Mill Road, P.O. Box 1594, Franklin, NC 28734; tel. 828/369-6641; FAX. 828/349-4161; Sandra L. Deke, Executive Director

Hospice of McDowell County, Inc., 116 North Logan Street, Marion, NC 28752; tel. 828/652–1318; FAX. 828/659-1631; Deanna MacLaren, RN, BSN, PCC

Hospice of Mitchell County, P.O. Box 38, 284 Hospital Drive, Spruce Pine, NC 28777; tel. 828/765-5677; FAX. 828/765–5680; Clarice Turner, Executive Director

Hospice of Pamlico County, Inc., 13628 North Carolina Highway 55, Alliance, NC 28509; tel. 919/745-5171; Diane McDaniel, Executive Director

Hospice of Polk County, Inc., 421 North Trade Street, Tryon, NC 28782; tel. 828/859–2270; FAX. 828/859-2731; Jean H. Eckert, Administrator

Hospice of Rockingham County, Inc., 2150 North Carolina 65, P.O. Box 281, Wentworth, NC 27375; tel. 336/427-9022; FAX. 336/427-9030; Rowera P. Sewell, Director

Hospice of Rutherford County, Inc., 374 Hudlow Road, P.O. Box 336, Forest City, NC 28043; tel. 828/245-0095; FAX. 828/248–1035; Rita Burch, Executive Director

Hospice of Scotland County, 610 Lauchwood Drive, P.O. Box 1033, Laurinburg, NC 28353; tel. 910/276–7176; FAX. 910/277–1941; Linda McQueen, RN, Executive Director

Hospice of Stanly County, Inc., 960 North First Street, Albermarle, NC 28001–3350; tel. 704/983–4216; FAX. 704/983–6662; Elvin T. Henry, Executive Director

Hospice of the Carolina Foothills, Inc., 421 North Tryon Street, Tryon, NC 28782; tel. 828/859-2270; FAX. 828/859-2731; Jean H. Eckert, Executive Director

Hospice of the Piedmont/Care Connection, 1801 Westchester Drive, High Point, NC 27262; tel. 910/889-8446; FAX. 910/889-3450; Leslie Kalinowski, President

Hospice of Union County, Inc., 700 West Roosevelt Boulevard, Monroe, NC 28110; tel. 704/292-2100; FAX. 704/292-2190; Charlene C. Broome, Executive Director

Hospice of Wake County, Inc., 1300 St. Mary's Street, 4th Floor, Raleigh, NC 27605; tel. 919/828-1998; Karolyn H. Kaye, Executive Director

Hospice of Watauga, 136 Furman Road, Suite #4, Boone, NC 28607; tel. 828/265–3926; FAX. 828/264-2125; Trinja Merit, Administrator

Hospice of Winston–Salem/Forsyth County, Inc., 1100 –C South Stratford Road, Winston-Salem, NC 27103-3212; tel. 910/768–3972; FAX. 910/659-0461; JoAnn Davis, Chief Executive Officer

Hospice of Yancey County, Inc., 314 West Main Street, P.O. Box 471, Burnsville, NC 28714; tel. 828/682-9675; FAX. 828/682-4713; Donna Messenger, Executive Director

Liberty Hospice, 3045 Henderson Drive, Suite 308, Jacksonville, NC 28546; tel. 910/937–6648; FAX. 910/346-3855; Debra Nixion Jones, Patient Case Manager

Lower Cape Fear Hospice, Inc., 725 – A Wellington Avenue, Wilmington, NC 28401; tel. 910/772-5444; FAX. 910/762-9146; Lauren Myles, Interim Executive Director

Lower Cape Fear Hospice, Inc., 121 West Main Street, P.O. Box 636, Whiteville, NC 28472; tel. 919/642-9051; FAX. 910–642-0223; Mary McNear, RN, BSN, Patient Care Coordinator

Lower Cape Fear Hospice, Inc., 112 Pine Street, P.O. Box 1926, Shallotte, NC 28459; tel. 910/754-5356; FAX. 910/754–5351; Jeff Hickey, Director, Operations

Lower Cape Fear Hospice, Inc., 103 North Morehead Street, Elizabethtown, NC 28337; tel. 910/862-3111; FAX. 910/862-3129; Anita Graber, Community Relations Specialist

Madison Home Care and Hospice, P.O. Box 909, 170 Carl Eller Road, Mars Hill, NC 28754; tel. 704/689-3491; FAX. 704/689-3496; John H. Estes, Executive Director

Mountain Area Hospice, Inc., 85 Zillicoa Street, P.O. Box 16, 28802, Asheville, NC 28801; tel. 828/ 255-0231; FAX. 828/255-2880; Kit Cosgrove, Director of Operations

Northern Hospital Home Care and Hospice, 933 Old Rockford Street, P.O. Box 1605, Mount Airy, NC 27030; tel. 336/719–7434; FAX. 336/719-7435; Kitty Horton, Executive Director

Onslow County Home Health and Hospice, 2013 LeJeune Boulevard, Jacksonville, NC 28546; tel. 910/577-6660; FAX. 910/577-6636; Jeanne Sleiertin, RN, Director

Pemberton Hospice, 106 North Main Street, P.O. Box 3069, Pembroke, NC 28372; tel. 910/521-5550; FAX. 910/521–3335; RD Locklear, II, Administrator

Richmond County Hospice, Inc., 230 South Lawrence Street, P.O. Box 2136, Rockingham, NC 28380; tel. 910/997–4464; FAX. 910/997-4484; Lydia P. Talbert, CRNH, Patient Care Coordinator

Roanoke Home Care, 115 West Boulevard, Williamston, NC 27892; tel. 919/792–5899; FAX. 252-799-3069; Barbara Owens, Nursing Director

Roanoke Home Care–Hospice, 408 Bridge Street, P.O. Box 238, Columbia, NC 27925; tel. 919/796-2681; FAX. 919/796–0818; Barbara Owens, RN, Director, Nursing

Roanoke Home Care–Hospice, 198 North Carolina Highway 45 North, Plymouth, NC 27962; tel. 800/842-8275; FAX. 252/791-3158; Phyllis McCombs, Referrals and Intake

Roanoke–Chowan Hospice, Inc., 521 Myers Street, P.O. Box 272, Ahoskie, NC 27910; tel. 919/332-3392; FAX. 919/332–5705; Brenda Hoggard, Director

Providers / Freestanding Hospices

St. Joseph of the Pines Home Health Agency, 117 Wortham Street, P.O. Box 974, Wadesboro, NC 28170; tel. 704/694-5992; Kathy Appenzeller, Director, Daily Operations

St. Joseph of the Pines Home Health Agency, 404 North Main Street, Troy, NC 27371; tel. 910/572-4962; FAX. 910/572-5010; Barbara Smith, CRNH Coordinator

St. Joseph of the Pines Home Health Agency, 336 South Main Street, Raeford, NC 28376; tel. 910/875-8198; FAX. 910/875-8862; Ronda Pickler, Administrator

Staff Builders, 112 Broad Street, Oxford, NC 27565

Staff Builders/MedVisit Home Health and Hospice, 1937NC Highway 39, Louisburg, NC 27549; tel. 800/377-5827; FAX. 919/496-7052; Sherry Watson, Administrator

Triangle Hospice, 1804 Martin Luther King, Jr. Parkway, Suite 112, Durham, NC 27707; tel. 919/490-8480; FAX. 919/493-0242; Lucy Worth, Executive Director

Triangle Hospice at the Meadowlands, 1001 Corporate Drive, Hillsborough, NC 27278; tel. 919/644-0764; FAX. 919/644-0932; Robin Hill, Manager

Wendover, 953 Wendover Heights Drive, Shelby, NC 28150; tel. 704/487-7018; FAX. 704/487-7028; Myra McGinnis Hamrick, Executive Director

Wilson Home Care, Inc., d/b/a Hometown Hospice, 1705 South Tarboro Street, Wilson, NC 27893; tel. 252/237-4333; FAX. 252/237-1125; Gail Brewer, RN, MPH, Home Care Manager

Yadkin County Home Health/Hospice Agency, 217 East Willow Street, P.O. Box 457, Yadkinville, NC 27055; tel. 910/679-4207; FAX. 910/679-6358; Jackie Harrell, Nursing Supervisor

NORTH DAKOTA

Heart of America Hospice, 800 S. Main, Rugby, ND 58368; tel. 701/776-5261; FAX. 701/776-5448; Dana Johnson, RN

Heartland Hospice, 30 W. 7th Street, Dickinson, ND 58601; tel. 701/264-4251; FAX. 701/264-4809; Peggy Steed, RN, Unit Supervisor

Hospice of the Red River Valley, 702 28th Avenue, N., Fargo, ND 58102; tel. 701/237-4629; FAX. 701/280-9069; Susan J. Fuglie, Executive Director

Mercy Hospice, 1031 7th Street, Devils Lake, ND 58301; tel. 701/662-2131; FAX. 701/662-4862; Marlene Krein, President, CEO

Riveredge Hospice of St. Francis, 415 Oak Street, Breckenridge, ND 56520; tel. 218/643-7594; FAX. 218/643-7506; Cindy Splichal, Director

St. Alexius Hospice, 1120 E. Main Street, Bismarck, ND 58501; tel. 701/224-7888; FAX. 701/224-7811; Barbara Schweitzer, Administrator

Trinity Hospice, 1015 South Broadway, Minot, ND 58701; tel. 701/857-5083; FAX. 701/857-5079; Marilyn Bader, Administrator

United Community Hospice, 407 3rd Street NE, Minot, ND 58701; tel. 701/857-2499; FAX. 701/857-2565; Mary O'Clair, Hospice Care Nurse

OHIO

Allen Hospice, 5700 Southwyck Boulevard, Suite 111, Toledo, OH 43614; tel. 419/867-4655; FAX. 419/865-1601; Jane Wilcox, RN, Executive Director

Appalachian Community Hospice, 280 East State Street, P.O. Box 768, Athens, OH 45701; tel. 614/592-3493; FAX. 614/594-5591; Nancy Pitre', Clinical Director

Aultman Hospice Program, 4510 Dressler Road, N.W., Canton, OH 44718; tel. 330/493-3344; FAX. 330/493-8637; Rebecca Crowl, RN, Program Director

Bridge Home Health and Hospice, 425 Frazier Street, Findlay, OH 45840; tel. 419/423-5351; FAX. 419/423-8967; Karen Mallett, Vice President, Home Care Services

Columbia Mercy Medical Center Hospice, 1445 Harrison Avenue, N.W., Suite 201, Canton, OH 44708; tel. 330/489-6855; FAX. 330/489-6868; Ken Wasiniak, L.I.S.W., Hospice Manager

Community Hospice, 18200 Loraine Road, Cleveland, OH 44111; tel. 216/363-2397; FAX. 216/363-2284; Cheryl Carrino, Program Manager

Community Hospice Care, 182 St. Francis Avenue, Rear Suite, Tiffin, OH 44883; tel. 419/447-4040; FAX. 419/447-4657; Rebecca S. Shank, Executive Director

Geauga County Visiting Nurse Service and Hospice, 13221 Ravenna Road, Chardon, OH 44024; tel. 216/286-9461; Patricia Huels, RN, Director, Patient Services

HomeCare Matters Home Health & Hospice, 352 South Street, P.O. Box 327, Galion, OH 44833; tel. 419/468-7985; FAX. 419/468-9211; Bert Maglott, RN, Executive Director

Hospice and Health Services of Fairfield County, 1111 East Main Street, Lancaster, OH 43130; tel. 740/654-7077; FAX. 740/654-6321; Paul D. Longenecker, RN, MBA, Executive Director

Hospice of Alliance VNA, 885 South Sawburg, Suite 100, Alliance, OH 44601; tel. 330/821-7055; FAX. 330/821-1955; Lin Sever, M.S.N., Executive Director

Hospice of Care Corporation, 831 South Street, Chardon, OH 44024; tel. 440/286-2273; FAX. 440/286-7662; Elizabeth A. Petersen, RN, Vice President, Operations

Hospice of Cincinnati, Inc., 4310 Cooper Road, Cincinnati, OH 45242; tel. 513/891-7700; FAX. 513/792-6980; Leigh Gerdsen, RN, Director

Hospice of Columbus, 181 South Washington Boulevard, Columbus, OH 43215; tel. 614/645-6471; FAX. 614/645-5895; Larry L. Miracle, Director

Hospice of Coshocton County, Inc., 230 South Fourth, P.O. Box 1284, Coshocton, OH 43812; tel. 740/622-7311; FAX. 740/622-7310; Barbara Brooks-Emmons, Director

Hospice of Darke County, Inc., 122 West Martz Street, Greenville, OH 45331; tel. 937/548-2999; FAX. 937/548-7144; Katie Wehri, Executive Director

Hospice of Dayton, Inc., 324 Wilmington Avenue, Dayton, OH 45420; tel. 937/256-4490; FAX. 937/256-5951; Linda Koeppen, President and CEO

Hospice of Guernsey, Inc., 1401 Campbell Avenue, P.O. Box 1165, Cambridge, OH 43725; tel. 740/432-7440; FAX. 740/432-7424; Patricia Howell-Vaughn, RN, Administrator

Hospice of Henry County, 104 East Washington, Suite 302, Napoleon, OH 43545; tel. 419/599-5545; FAX. 419/599-1714; Janelle Cline, RN, Hospice Coordinator

Hospice of Knox County, 302 East High Street, Mount Vernon, OH 43050; tel. 740/397-5188; FAX. 740/397-5189; Melanie Richardson, Executive Director

Hospice of Medina County, 797 North Court Street, Medina, OH 44256; tel. 330/722-4771; FAX. 330/722-5266; Patricia M. Stropko-O'Leary, Executive Director

Hospice of Miami County, Inc., P.O. Box 502, Troy, OH 45373; tel. 937/335-5191; FAX. 937/335-8841; Sidney J. Pinkus, Chief Executive Officer

Hospice of Morrow County, P.O. Box 86, 851 West Marion Road, Mount Gilead, OH 43338; tel. 419/946-9822; FAX. 419/946-9971; Deb Roszman, RN, Executive Director

Hospice of North Central Ohio, Inc., 1605 County Road 1095, Ashland, OH 44805; tel. 419/281-7107; FAX. 419/281-8427; Ruth A. Lindsey, Executive Director

Hospice of Northwest Ohio, 30000 East River Road, Perrysburg, OH 44551; tel. 419/661-4001; FAX. 419/661-4015; Virginia Clifford, Executive Director

Hospice of Pickaway County, 702 Pickaway Street, Circleville, OH 43113; tel. 740/474-3525; FAX. 740/474-1832; Franklin Christmas, Business Manager

Hospice of the Valley, Inc., 5190 Market Street, Youngstown, OH 44512; tel. 330/788-1992; FAX. 330/788-1998; Kenneth O. Drees, Executive Director

Hospice of the Western Reserve, Hospice House, 300 East 185th Street, Cleveland, OH 44119; tel. 216/383-2222; FAX. 216/383-3750; David A. Simpson, Executive Director

Hospice of Tuscarawas County, Inc., 201 West Third Street, Dover, OH 44622; tel. 330/343-7605; FAX. 330/343-3542; Janie Jones, Administrator

Hospice of V.N.A., 1159 Westwood Drive, Van Wert, OH 45891; tel. 419/238-9223; FAX. 419/238-9391; Donna Grimm, President and CEO

Hospice of Visiting Nurse Service, 3358 Ridgewood Road, Akron, OH 44333; tel. 800/335-1455; FAX. 216/668-4680; Patricia Waickman, M.S.N., RN, Vice President, Hospice

Hospice of Wyandot County, 320 West Maple Street, Suite C, Upper Sandusky, OH 43351; tel. 419/294-5787; FAX. 419/294-4721; Susan Barth, RN, Executive Director

Hospice Service of Licking County, Inc., d/b/a Hospice of Central Ohio, Homecare of Central Ohio, 1435 B West Main Street, Newark, OH 43055; tel. 740/344-0311; FAX. 740/344-6577; Michele McMahon, Chief Executive Officer

Hospice, The Caring Way of Defiance County, 197-C Island Park Avenue, Defiance, OH 43512; tel. 419/784-3818; FAX. 419/782-4979; Ruthann Czartoski, Hospice Coordinator

Loving Care Hospice, Inc., 25 W. 5th Street, P.O. Box 445, London, OH 43140; tel. 740/852-7755; FAX. 740/852-7762; Patty Boerger, Board Chair

M J Nursing Registry, 2534 Victory Parkway, Cincinnati, OH 45206; tel. 513/961-1000; FAX. 513/872-7550; Sharon Rachford, RN, Hospice Patient Care Coordinator

Madison County Home Health Hospice Inc., 212 North Main Street, London, OH 43140; tel. 614/852-3915; FAX. 614/852-5125; Kathy Gill, RNCS, Director

Mercy Hospice, 7010 Rowan Hill Drive, Cincinnati, OH 45227; tel. 513/271-1440; FAX. 513/271-2405

Mount Carmel Hospice, 1144 Dublin Road, Columbus, OH 43215; tel. 614/234-0200; FAX. 614/234-0201; Mary Ann Gill, Director of Hospice & Palliative Care Medicine

New Life-Choices in LifeCare, 5255 North Abbe Road, Elyria, OH 44035; tel. 216/934-1458; FAX. 216/934-1567; Micki M. Tubbs, President and CEO

Stein Hospice Services, Inc., 1200 Sycamore Line, Sandusky, OH 44870; tel. 800/625-5269; FAX. 419/625-5761; Jan Bucholz, Executive Director

The Hospice of Staff Builders, 6100 Rockside Woods Boulevard, Suite 100, Independence, OH 44131; tel. 216/642-0202; FAX. 216/642-3273; Marion Keathley, Intake Coordinator

Tri County Hospice, One Park Centre, Suite 20, Wadsworth, OH 44281; tel. 330/336-6595; FAX. 330/334-9925; Kris Lawson, Director

Tricare Hospice, 701 Park Road, Bellefontaine, OH 43311; tel. 800/886-5936; FAX. 513/593-6355; Mary L. Mayer, Director

Valley Hospice, 380 Summit Avenue, Steubenville, OH 43952; tel. 614/264-7161; Karen Nichols, Executive Director

Valley Hospice, Inc., 380 Summit Avenue, Steubenville, OH 43952; tel. 614/283-7487; FAX. 614/283-7507; Karen Nichols, RN, B.S.N., Executive Director

Visiting Nurse Hospice and Health Care, 383 West Dussel Drive, Maumee, OH 43537; tel. 419/897-2803; FAX. 419/897-2810; Nancy Host, Executive Director

VistaCare Hospice, 8135 Beachmont Avenue, Cincinnati, OH 45255; tel. 513/474-2550; FAX. 513/241-4012; Mike Doddy, RN, Administrator

VistaCare Hospice, 92 Northwoods Boulevard, #A, Columbus, OH 43235; tel. 614/781-1444; FAX. 614/781-1450; Danielle Antonares, RN, Patient Care Manager

VNA of Cleveland Hospice, 2500 East 22nd Street, Cleveland, OH 44115; tel. 216/931-1450; FAX. 216/694-6355; Roberta Laurie, Executive Director, Hospice

OKLAHOMA

Blaine County Hospice, 401 North Clarence Nash, P.O. Box 567, Watonga, OK 73772; tel. 405/623-7414; FAX. 405/623-7412; Lisa Watson, RN

Carter Healthcare & Hospice, 4301 Will Rogers Parkway, Suite 900, Oklahoma City, OK 73108; tel. 888/951-1112; FAX. 405/947-7300; Kathi Egan, Director of Hospice

Carter Hospice Care, 828 North Porter, Norman, OK 73069; tel. 888/951-1112; Stanley F. Carter, Administrator

Carter Hospice Care, Inc., 1 West 36 Street, North, Suite 1, Tulsa, OK 74106; tel. 918/425-4000; FAX. 918/428-0780; Stanley F. Carter, Administrator

Columbia Hospice Oklahoma, 7508 North Broadway Extension, Suite 110, Oklahoma City, OK 73116; tel. 800/243-7776; FAX. 405/848-5135; Sharon Collins, RN, CRNH, Hospice Director

Crossroads Hospice of Oklahoma, L.L.C., 9916-B East 43rd Street, Tulsa, OK 74146; tel. 918/663-3234; FAX. 918/663-3334; G. Perry Farmer, Jr., Executive Director

Eastern Oklahoma Hospice, 1301 Reynolds, Poteau, OK 74953; tel. 918/647-8235; Jody L. Shepherd, RN, Agency Director

Four Square Hospice, 223 Plaza, P.O. Box 827, Madill, OK 73446; tel. 405/795-3384; Norma Howard

Providers / Freestanding Hospices

Good Shepherd Hospice, 4411 Highline Boulevard, Oklahoma City, OK 73108; tel. 405/943-0903; FAX. 405/943-0950; Steve Moore, Executive Director
Hospice Circle of Love, 529 N. Grand, Enid, OK 73701; tel. 405/234-2273; FAX. 405/234-1990; Cathy Graber, Director
Hospice of Central Oklahoma, 4549 Northwest 36th Street, Oklahoma City, OK 73122; tel. 405/491-0828; Aaron Barnes, President and CEO
Hospice of Green Country, Inc., 3010 South Harvard, Suite 110, Tulsa, OK 74114-6136; tel. 918/747-2273; FAX. 918/747-2573; Betty Holman, RN, MBA, Executive Director
Hospice of Lawton Area, Inc., 1930 Northwest Ferris Avenue, Suite 105, Lawton, OK 73505; tel. 405/248-5885; FAX. 405/355-2446; Jeff Henderson, Executive Director
Hospice of McAlester, 801 E. Wyandotte, P.O. Box 1333, McAlester, OK 74501; tel. 918/423-3911; FAX. 918/423-4241; Rhonda Kurvink, Executive Director
Hospice of Oklahoma County, Inc., 4334 Northwest Expressway, Suite 106, Oklahoma City, OK 73116-1515; tel. 405/848-8884; FAX. 405/841-4899; Terry Gonsoulin, RN, Executive Director
Hospice of Ponca City, 1904 North Union, Suite 103, Ponca City, OK 74601; tel. 580/762-9102; FAX. 580/762-9111; Melody Lahann, Director
Judith Karman Hospice, Inc., 824 South Main Street, P.O. Box 818, Stillwater, OK 74076; tel. 405/377-8012; FAX. 405/624-9007; Mary Lee Warren, Executive Director
Mid-Lakes Hospice Care, 500 East Main Street, P.O. Box 728, Stigler, OK 74462; tel. 918/967-8499; FAX. 918/967-2584; John C. Neal, Administrator
Mission Hospice, LLC, 7301 North Broadway, Suite 225, Suite 210, Oklahoma City, OK 73116; tel. 405/848-3779; FAX. 405/848-8481; Jerilyn Barthel, Program Director
Russell–Murray Hospice, Inc., 221 South Bickford, P.O. Box 1423, El Reno, OK 73036; tel. 405/262-3088; FAX. 405/262-3082; Cathie Sales, Administrator
The Hospice, 1303 West Broadway, Muskogee, OK 74401; tel. 918/683-1192; FAX. 918/687-0750; Jamie Bridgewater, Executive Director
Trinity Hospice LLC, Lawton, 4645 West Gore Boulevard, Lawton, OK 73505; tel. 800/422-8015; FAX. 405/250-0489; Jerry Darnell, Program Director
Trinity Hospice, LLC, 2327 E. 13th Street, Tulsa, OK 74104; tel. 918/582-8163; FAX. 918/582-8310; Kerri Ellis, Administrator
Visiting Nurses Agency of Eastern Oklahoma Hospice, 220 South Main Street, Spiro, OK 74959; tel. 918/962-9491; Jim Medley, Chief Executive Officer
Visiting Nurses Agency of Eastern Oklahoma, Inc., Four Eastern Heights Shopping Center, P.O. Box 1647, Muldrow, OK 74948; tel. 918/427-1010; FAX. 918/427-7805; Janice Myers, RN, Vice-President
VistaCare Family Hospice, 4900 Richmond Square, Suite 203, Oklahoma City, OK 73118; tel. 405/843-4097; FAX. 405/843-5629; Deborah Brazeal, Executive Director
VistaCare Family Hospice, 4325 E. 51st Street, Suite 103, Tulsa, OK 74135; tel. 918/488-9477; FAX. 918/488-9506; Jo Brewer, Professional Relation Director

OREGON

Benton Hospice Service, Inc., P.O. Box 100, Corvallis, OR 97333; tel. 541/757-9616; FAX. 541/757-1760; Judy List, Executive Director
Curry County Home/Health Hospice, 29984 Ellensburg, P.O. Box 746, Gold Beach, OR 97444; tel. 541/247-7084; FAX. 541/247-2117; Lori Kent, RN
Harney County Home Health/Hospice, 420 North Fairview, Burns, OR 97720; tel. 541/573-8360; FAX. 541/573-8389; Cheryl Keniston, Director
Hospice of Bend, 1303 Northwest Galveston, Bend, OR 97701; tel. 541/383-3910; FAX. 541/388-4221
Hospice of Redmond and Sisters, P.O. Box 1092, Redmond, OR 97756; tel. 541/548-7483; FAX. 541/548-1507; Ellen Garcia, Executive Director
Hospice of the Gorge, Inc., 13th and May Street, P.O. Box 36, Hood River, OR 97031; tel. 503/387-6449; FAX. 503/386-6700; Ina Holman, Executive Director
Kaiser Permanente, Home Health/Hospice, 2701 Northwest Vaughn Street, Suite 140, Portland, OR 97210; tel. 503/499-5200; FAX. 503/499-5200; Linda Van Buren, RN, Administrator
Klamath Hospice, Inc., 437 Main Street, Klamath Falls, OR 97601; tel. 541/882-2902; FAX. 541/883-1992; Teresa C. Pastorius
Legacy VNA Hospice, 2701 Northwest Vaughn, Suite 720, P.O. Box 3426, Portland, OR 97208; tel. 503/225-6370; FAX. 503/225-6398; Patti Berrier, Director
Lower Umpqua Hospice, 600 Ranch Road, Reedsport, OR 97467; tel. 541/271-2171; FAX. 541/271-1108; Sylvia Tommasino, RN, Manager
Mt. Hood Hospice, 17275 Strauss, P.O. Box 1269, Sandy, OR 97055; tel. 503/668-5545; FAX. 503/668-7951; Lindy Blaesing, Executive Director
Pathway Hospice, Inc., 323 West Idaho Avenue, Ontario, OR 97914; tel. 541/889-0847; FAX. 541/889-0849; Betty Cooper, RN
Providence Home Services Hospice, 1235 Northeast 47th, Suite 215, 4805 Northeast Glisan (Mailing Address), Portland, OR 97213; tel. 503/331-4601; FAX. 503/215-4624; Karen Bell, Director
South Coast Hospice, 1620 Thompson Road, Coos Bay, OR 97420; tel. 541/269-2986; FAX. 541/267-0458; Linda J. Furman Grile, Administrator
Washington County Hospice, Inc., 427 Southeast Eighth Avenue, Hillsboro, OR 97123-4519; tel. 503/648-9565; FAX. 503/648-1282; Christine Larch, Administrator

PENNSYLVANIA

Abington Memorial Hospital Home Care Hospice Program, 2510 Maryland Road, Suite 250, Willow Grove, PA 19090-0520; tel. 215/481-5800; FAX. 215/481-5850; Elissa Della Monica, MSN, RN, Executive Director
Albert Gallatin Hospice Program, 20 Highland Park Drive, Suite 203, Uniontown, PA 15401; tel. 412/438-6660; FAX. 412/438-4468; Chris Constantine, RN, Administrator
All Care Hospice, 472 1/2 South Poplar Street, Hazelton, PA 18201; tel. 717/459-2004; Mary Ann Barletta, RN, Administrator
Berks Visiting Nurse Association, Inc., 1170 Berkshire Boulevard, Wyomissing, PA 19610; tel. 610/378-0481; FAX. 610/378-9762; Lucille D. Gough, RN, President and CEO
Brookline Home Care & Hospice, 3901 South Atherton Street, State College, PA 16801; tel. 814-466-4800; FAX. 814-466-4806; Diane Good, Administrator
Centre Hospice, A Program of Centre HomeCare, Inc., 221 West High Street, Bellefonte, PA 16823-1385; tel. 814/355-2273; FAX. 814/353-9292; Linda Scholl, Hospice Manager
Chandler Hall Hospice, 99 Barclay Street, Newtown, PA 18940; tel. 215/860-4000; FAX. 215/860-3458; Jane W. Fox, Executive Director
Clarion Forest VNA Hospice, P.O. Box 668, Knox, PA 16232; tel. 814/797-1492; FAX. 814/797-2698; Deborah J. Kelly, Director of Hospice
Columbia–Montour Home Hospice, Locust Court, 599 East Seventh Street, Bloomsburg, PA 17815; tel. 717/784-1723; FAX. 717/784-8512; Jane Gittler, Chief Executive Officer
Comfort Care Hospice, 205 Grandview Corporate Place, Camp Hill, PA 17011; tel. 800/255-3300; FAX. 717/766-5037; Linda L. Smith, Director
Community Nurses Professional Health Services/Hospice, 99 Erie Avenue, St. Mary's, PA 15857; tel. 814/781-1415; FAX. 814/781-6987; Elizabeth A. Roberts, RN, Executive Director
Family Home Hospice of the VNA of Greater Philadelphia and the VNS of New Jersey, One Winding Way, Monroe Office Center, Philadelphia, PA 19131; tel. 215/581-2046; FAX. 215/473-5047; Rev. Anne G. Huey, Hospice Director
Family Hospice, 250 Mount Lebanon Blvd., Suite 203, Pittsburgh, PA 15234; tel. 412/572-8800; FAX. 412/572-8827; Judy Talbert, Executive Director
Family Hospice of Indiana County, a division of the V.N.A. of Indiana County, 119 Professional Center, 1265 Wayne Avenue, Indiana, PA 15701; tel. 724/463-8711; FAX. 724/463-8907; Linda E. Bettinazzi, BSN, RN, Director, Hospice and Special Care Services
Forbes Hospice–Allegheny VNI Hospitals, 6655 Frankstown Avenue, Pittsburgh, PA 15206; tel. 412/665-3301; FAX. 412/665-3238; Maryanne Fello, RN, Manager
General Care Services, d/b/a Hospice of Warren County, Two Crescent Park, W., P.O. Box 68, Warren, PA 16365; tel. 814/723-2455; FAX. 814/723-1177; Elsa L. Redding, Director
Great Lakes Hospice, Northgate Commons, Suite 107, Erie, PA 16501; tel. 814/877-6120; Debbie Burbules, Director
Guthrie Hospice, R.R. One, P.O. Box 154, Towanda, PA 18848; tel. 800/598-6155; FAX. 717/265-3570; Staci Covey, Administrator
HealthReach Home Care and Hospice, 409 South Second Street, Harrisburg, PA 17104; tel. 717/231-6363; Janet T. Foreman, RN
Holy Family Home Health and Hospice Care, 900 West Market Street, Owigsburg, PA 17961; tel. 717/366-0990; FAX. 717/366-3735; Arlene L. Mongrain, RN, B.S., Executive Director
Holy Redeemer, Nazarath and St. Home Health Services, 12265 Townsend Road, Philadelphia, PA 19154; tel. 215/671-9200; FAX. 215/671-1950; Jerold S. Cohen, President
Home Hospice Agency of St. Francis, 131 Columbus Innerbelt, New Castle, PA 16101; tel. 412/652-8847; FAX. 412/656-0876; Susan N. Ludu, Executive Director
Home Nursing Agency/VNA Hospice Program, 201 Chestnut Avenue, P.O. Box 352, Altoona, PA 16603-0352; tel. 814/946-5411; FAX. 814-941-1648; Robert R. Packer, Chief Executive Officer
Hospice Community Care, Inc., 385 Wyoming Avenue, Kingston, PA 18704; tel. 717/288-2288; FAX. 717/288-7424; Philip Decker, President
Hospice of Central Pennsylvania, 98 South Enola Drive, P.O. Box 266, Enola, PA 17025-0266; tel. 717/732-1000; FAX. 717/732-5348; Karen M. Paris, Chief Executive Officer
Hospice of Crawford County, Inc., 448 Pine Street, Meadville, PA 16335; tel. 814/333-5403; FAX. 814/333-5407; Sister Mary Ellen Dwyer, Director
Hospice of Lancaster County, 685 Good Drive, P.O. Box 4125, Lancaster, PA 17604-4125; tel. 717/295-3900; FAX. 717/391-9582; Mary Graner, President
Hospice of North Penn Visiting Nurse Association, 51 Medical Campus Drive, Lansdale, PA 19446; tel. 215/855-8297; FAX. 215/855-1305; Patty Lengel, Hospice Coordinator
Hospice of the Delaware Valley, 527 Plymouth Road, Suite 417, Plymouth Meet, PA 19462; tel. 610/941-6700; FAX. 610/941-6440; Marcia M. Cook, Administrator
Hospice of the Visiting Nurse Association of Eastern Pennsylvania, 1510 Valley Center Parkway, Suite 200, Bethlehem, PA 18017; tel. 610/691-1100; FAX. 610/691-2271; Halyna Stigura, RN, M.S.N., Chief Executive Officer
Hospice Preferred Choice, Inc., 2400 Ardmore Boulevard, Suite 302, Pittsburgh, PA 15221; tel. 412/271-2273; FAX. 412/271-3361; Christean Dugan, Administrator
Hospice Program/VNA of Hanover and Spring Grove, 440 North Madison Street, Hanover, PA 17331; tel. 717/637-1227; FAX. 717/637-9772; Sandra L. Wojtkowiak, RN, M.S.N., Administrator
Hospice Services of the VNA of York County, 218 East Market Street, York, PA 17403; tel. 717/846-9900; FAX. 717/846-1933; Marie V. Fraser, President and CEO
Hospice–The Bridge, Lewistown Hospital, 1126 West Fourth Street, Lewistown, PA 17044-1909; tel. 717/242-5000; FAX. 717/242-7099; Ruth Anne Sieber, RN, CRNH, Clinical Supervisor
HospiceCare of Pittsburgh, 11 Parkway Center, Suite 275, Pittsburgh, PA 15220; tel. 412/937-8088; FAX. 412/922-9609; Fran Romito, RN, Administrator
In Home Health, Inc., 750 Holiday Drive, Foster Plaza Nine, Pittsburgh, PA 15220; tel. 412/928-2126; FAX. 412/928-2127; Margaret Timm, Director, Operations
Jefferson Hospice–Main Line, Gerhard Building, 130 South Bryn Mawr Avenue, Bryn Mawr, PA 19018; tel. 610/526-4770; Timothy P. Cousounis, Executive Director
Lee Regional Hospice, 1425 Scalp Avenue, Johnstown, PA 15904; tel. 888/553-5503; FAX. 814/262-9616; Donna L. Russian, Executive Director
Lehigh Valley Hospice, 2166 South 12th Street, Allentown, PA 18103; tel. 610/402-7400; FAX. 610/402-7382; Bonnie Kosman, M.S.N., RN, CS, Administrator

Providers / Freestanding Hospices

Lutheran Home Health Care Services, Hospice of the Good Shepherd, 2700 Luther Drive, Chambersburg, PA 17201; tel. 717/264–8178; FAX. 717/264–6347; Diane M. Howell, Executive Director

McKean County VNA Hospice, 20 School Street, P.O. Box 465, Bradford, PA 16701–0465; tel. 814/362–7466; FAX. 814/362–2916; Elizabeth M. Costello, Administrator

Montgomery Hospital Hospice Program, 25 West Fornance Street, Norristown, PA 19401; tel. 610/272–1080; Elise N. Lamarra, B.S.N.

Neighborhood Visiting Nurse Association, 795 East Marshall Street, West Chester, PA 19380; tel. 610/696–6511; FAX. 610/344–7064; Heide Owen, Director of Hospice

North Penn HH Agency/Hospice Program, 520 Ruah Street, P.O. Box Eight, Blossburg, PA 16912; tel. 717/638–2141; FAX. 717/638–2163; Wilma Hall, Program Director

Northeast Health and Hospice Care, Inc., 38 North Main Street, Pittston, PA 18640; tel. 717/654–0220; FAX. 717/654–0360; Stephan Hannon, Administrator

Odyssey Health Care of Pennsylvania, Park West One, Suite 500, Pittsburgh, PA 15275; tel. 412/494–0870; FAX. 412/494–0879; Robert S. Holder, General Manager

Olsten Kimberly QualityCare Hospice, 749 Northern Boulevard, Clarks Summit, PA 18411; tel. 800/870–0085; Peggy Durkin, Administrator

Penn Care at Home, 51 North 39th Street, Philadelphia, PA 19104; tel. 215/662–8996; Rita P. Rebman, RN, M.S.N.

Pinnacle Health Hospice, 3705 Elmwood Drive, Harrisburg, PA 17110; tel. 717/671–3700; FAX. 717/671–3713; Denise K. Harris, M.S.W., Director

Ridgway Community Nurse Service, Inc., Hospice, 20 North Broad Street, Ridgway, PA 15853; tel. 814/773–5705; FAX. 814/776–6246; Catherine M. Grove, RN, Executive Director

Samaritan Care Hospice of Pennsylvania, 6198 Butler Pike, Suite 275, Blue Bell, PA 19422; tel. 215/653–7310; FAX. 215/653–7340; Joan Holcome, DCS

Sivitz Jewish Hospice, 901 West Street, Pittsburgh, PA 15221; tel. 412/422–5700; FAX. 412/247–5626; Deborah Shtulman, Executive Director

SUN Home Health Services, Inc, 61 Duke Street, Northumberland, PA 17857; tel. 888/478–6227; FAX. 570/473–3070; Karen Adams, Hospice Coordinator

Susquehanna Regional Home Health Services and Hospice, 1101 Grampian Boulevard, 4th Floor, Williamsport, PA 17701–1967; tel. 570/320–7690; FAX. 570/323–0716; Patricia L. Smith, RN, Director of Hospice

Three Rivers Family Hospice, Inc., 3029 Jacks Run Road, White Oak, PA 15131; tel. 412/672–6737; FAX. 412/672–5823; Martha Howell, RN, CRNH, Executive Director

Ultimate Home Health and Hospice Care, 212 North Second Street, Girardville, PA 17935; tel. 717/276–1148; Barbara McDonald, Administrator

Upper Bucks Hospice, a Division of Life Quest Home Care, 2075 Quaker Pointe Drive, Quakertown, PA 18951; tel. 215/529–6100; FAX. 215/529–6253; Beth Gotwals, RN, M.S.N., Hospice Manager

Visiting Nurses Association of the Lehigh Valley, Inc., 1710 Union Boulevard, Allentown, PA 18103; tel. 610/434–6134; FAX. 610/821–1982; Patricia Frenduto, President and CEO

VNA Health Care Services, 1789 South Braddock Avenue, Pittsburgh, PA 15218; tel. 412/256–6800; Andrew R. Peacock

VNA Health System, 21 West Independence Street, Shamokin, PA 17872; tel. 800/732–2486; FAX. 570/648–9590; Joseph L. Scopelliti, Jr., Chief Executive Officer

VNA Hospice Services of Erie County, 1305 Peach Street, Erie, PA 16501; tel. 814/454–2831; FAX. 814/453–5357; James J. Jarvszwicz, Administrator

VNA Hospice, Western Pennsylvania, 154 Hindman Road, Butler, PA 16001; tel. 724/282–6806; FAX. 724/282–7517; Liz Powell, RN, M.S.N., CRNP, Vice President

VNA of Central PA, Hospice, 3315 Derry Street, Harrisburg, PA 17111; tel. 717/233–1035; FAX. 717/233–2759; Thomas Tarasewich, Chief Executive Officer

VNA of Easton Hospice, 3421 Nightingale Drive, Easton, PA 18045; tel. 215/258–7189; Theresa P. Onorata

VNA of Pottstown and Vicinity Comprehensive Hospice Program, 1963 East High Street, Pottstown, PA 19464; tel. 610/327–5700; FAX. 610/327–5701; Sandra Levengood, Executive Director

VNA/Hospice of Monroe County, Inc., 502 Independence Boulevard, East Strouds, PA 18301; tel. 570/421–5390; FAX. 570/421–7423; Mark Hodgson, Administrator

White Rose Hospice, 2870 Eastern Boulevard, York, PA 17402; tel. 717/849–5642; FAX. 717/849–5630; Lisa Hanne, RN, Team Leader

Wissahickon Hospice, 8835 Germantown Avenue, Philadelphia, PA 19118; tel. 215/247–0277; FAX. 215/248–3253; Priscilla D. Kissick, RN, M.S.N., Executive Director

RHODE ISLAND

Hospice Care of Rhode Island, 169 George Street, Pawtucket, RI 02860–3868; tel. 401/444–9070; FAX. 401/444–9090; Analee Wulfkuhle, President and CEO

Hospice of Nursing Placement, 339 Angel Street, P.O. Box 603337, Providence, RI 02906; tel. 401/453–4544; Marcia Bigney, Administrator

Kent County Visiting Nurse Association Hospice, 51 Health Lane, Warwick, RI 02886; tel. 401/737–6050; FAX. 401/738–0247; Nancy Roberts, RN, M.S.N., Chief Executive Officer

Northwest Home Care (Hospice), 185 Putnam Pike, P.O. Box 423, Harmony, RI 02829; tel. 401/949–2600; FAX. 401/949–5115; Beverly McGuire, President

Visiting Nurse Services Hospice, 1184 East Main Road, P.O. Box 690, Portsmouth, RI 02871; tel. 401/682–2100; FAX. 401/682–2112; Jean Anderson, RN, M.S., Chief Executive Officer

VNA of Rhode Island, 157 Waterman Avenue, Providence, RI 02906; tel. 401/444–9400; FAX. 401/444–9430; Sandra L. Hooper, RN, M.B.A., CNAA, Director, Adult Services

SOUTH CAROLINA

Hitchcock Rehabilitation Center Home Health and Hospice, 690 Medical Park Drive, Aiken, SC 29801; tel. 803/643–0001; FAX. 803/649–0490; Theresa Altman, Director, Home Health Hospice

Hospice Care of the Low Country, Hospice Care of the Low Country Home Health, 20 Palmetto Parkway, Suite 104, Hilton Head, SC 29926; tel. 803/681–7814; FAX. 803/681–7821; Laura Frieden, Executive Director

Hospice Care of the Piedmont, 303 West Alexander Street, Greenwood, SC 29646; tel. 864/227–9393; FAX. 864/227–9377; Nancy B. Corley, Director

Hospice Care of Tri–County, 111 Executive Pointe Boulevard, Columbia, SC 29212; tel. 803/750–8697; FAX. 803/750–8695; Edna McClain, RN, M.S.N., Administrator

Hospice Community Care, (Serving York, Chester, Lancaster, Cherokee and Union), 325 South Oakland Avenue, Rock Hill, SC 29730; tel. 803/329–4663; FAX. 803/329–5935; Jane Armstrong, Executive Director

Hospice Health Services, One Carriage Lane, Suite F1, Charleston, SC 29407; tel. 843/852–2177; FAX. 843/769–0148; Sylvia Barnes Gailliard, RN, Executive Director

Hospice of Charleston, Inc., 3896 Leeds Avenue, Charleston, SC 29405; tel. 843/529–3100; FAX. 843/529–3111; Carol Younker, Executive Director

Hospice of Chesterfield County, Inc., 140 South Page Street, P.O. Box 293, Chesterfield, SC 29709; tel. 800/572–9322; FAX. 843/623–3833; Monnie W. Bittle, Executive Director

Hospice of Colleton County, Inc., 214 Wichman Street, Walterboro, SC 29488; tel. 803/549–5948; FAX. 803/549–1451; Alfred S. Givens, Administrator

Hospice of Georgetown County, Inc., 2591 North Fraser Street, P.O. Box 1436, Georgetown, SC 29440; tel. 843/546–3410; FAX. 843/527–6964; Brenda Stroup, RN, Executive Director

Hospice of Laurens County, Inc., 16 Peachtree Street, P.O. Box 178, Clinton, SC 29325; tel. 864/833–6287; FAX. 864/833–0556; Amanda Reeves, Executive Director

Hospice of Marlboro County, Inc., P.O. Box 474, Bennettsville, SC 29512; tel. 843/479–5979; FAX. 843/479–3711; Kevin Long, Executive Director

Hospice of the Upstate, Inc., Callie & John Rainey Hospice House, 1835 Rogers Road, Anderson, SC 29621; tel. 864/224–3358; FAX. 864/224–9971; Nancy Garrett–Boyle, Administrator

Interim HealthCare Hospice, 775 Spartan Boulevard, Spartanburg, SC 29301; tel. 864/587–9798; FAX. 864/587–2855; Nancy A. Dereng, Director

Island Hospice, 460 Wilhinton Parkway, Suite D, Hilton Head I, SC 29926; tel. 803/681–7035; FAX. 803/681–8506; Elisha Jones, Administrator

Lutheran Hospice Ministry, Lowman Home–Bolick Building, P.O. Box 444, White Rock, SC 29177; tel. 803/732–8756; Jean Tilley, Administrator

Mercy Hospice of Horry County, Columbus Plaza, Myrtle Beach, SC 29578; tel. 803/347–2282; FAX. 803/236–4306; Connie Fahey, FSM, Executive Director

United Hospice, Inc., 6300 St. Andrews Road, Columbia, SC 29212; tel. 803/798–6605; FAX. 803/798–3001; Debbie Graham

SOUTH DAKOTA

Ellen Stephen Hospice, P.O. Box 1805, Pine Ridge, SD 57770; tel. 605/455–1217; FAX. 605/455–1218; Linda Howell, RN

TENNESSEE

Advanced Home Care and Hospice, Inc., 117 Edenway Drive, P.O. Box 1099, White House, TN 37188; tel. 615/384–0962; FAX. 615/672–7398; Gloria Keen, Administrator

Alive Hospice, Inc., 1718 Patterson Street, Nashville, TN 37203; tel. 615/327–1085; FAX. 615/321–8902; Janet L. Jones, President and CEO

Amedisys Home Health, 446 Highway 46 South, Dickson, TN 37055; tel. 615/441–1365; FAX. 615/446–8109; Glenda Pace, Acting Administrator

Baptist Community Home Care and Hospice, 139 East Swan Street, Centerville, TN 37033; tel. 615/729–4500; FAX. 615/729–9000

Baptist Hospice, 433 Sevier Avenue, Knoxville, TN 37920; tel. 865/632–5718; FAX. 865/549–2065; Debbie Watson, Office Manager

Baptist Trinity Hospice, 1049 Cresthaven Road, Memphis, TN 38119; tel. 901/767–6767; FAX. 901/767–4627; Nancy Averwater, BSN, RN, Executive Director

Buckeye Quality HHA, Inc. Hospice, Highway 52W, P.O. Box 697, Jamestown, TN 38556; tel. 615/879–9928; Sandra Hall, RN, Director, Patient Services

Comprehensive HHC Hospice Services, Inc., P.O. Box 574, Patterson Crossroads, Harrogate, TN 37752; tel. 426/869–5111; FAX. 423/869–5916; Sherri Rowe, Coordinator

Friendship Hospice of Nashville, Inc., 1326 Eighth Avenue, N., Nashville, TN 37203; tel. 615/327–3950; Andre L. Lee, DPA, Chairman of the Board

Home Health Care of East Tennessee, Inc., 1796 Mount Vernon Drive, N.W., Cleveland, TN 37311; tel. 423/479–4581; FAX. 423/479–5422; Annette Green, DOPC

Home–Bound Medical Care, 4355 Highway 58, Suite 101, Chattanooga, TN 37416; tel. 423/855–9128

Home–Bound Medical Care, Inc., 2165 Spicer Cove, Suite One, Memphis, TN 38134; tel. 901/386–5061

Homecare Hospice Services, 115 Vicksburg Avenue, Camden, TN 38320; tel. 901/584–1927; FAX. 901/584–0401

Hospice of Chattanooga, Inc., 165 Hamm Road, Chattanooga, TN 37405; tel. 423/267–6828; FAX. 423/756–4765; Ben Johnston, Executive Director

Hospice of Cumberland County, Inc., 140 North Main, Suite 2, Crossville, TN 38555; tel. 931/484–4748; FAX. 931/456–5096; Ann Marie McFarland, Executive Director

Hospice of Murfreesboro, 417 North University Street, Murfreesboro, TN 37130; tel. 615/896–4663

Hospice of West Tennessee, 1804 Highway 45 Bypass, West Tennessee Healthcare, Jackson, TN 38305; tel. 901/664–4220; FAX. 901/664–4231; Donna Scott, RN, Director

House Call Hospice, Inc., Executive Business Park, 6025 Lee Highway, Chattanooga, TN 37421; tel. 615/892–2561; Caroline McBrayer

Housecall Hospice, 100 Rogosin Drive, Suite B, Elizabethton, TN 37643; tel. 615/547–0852; FAX. 615/543–6449; Rachel Vollman, Hospice Administrator

Housecall Hospice, 1708 Morriah Woods Boulevard, Suite 1, Memphis, TN 38117; tel. 901/685–5300; FAX. 901/761–4321; Lynn Thomasson, Hospice Administrator

Housecall Hospice, 3343 Perimeter Hill Drive, Suite 102, Nashville, TN 37211; tel. 615/333–3995; FAX. 615/333–7953; Andy Baker, Administrator

Lazarus House Hospice, Inc., 260 West Fifth Street, Cookeville, TN 38501; tel. 921/528–5133; FAX. 931/372–0249; J. Steve Mathias, Executive Director

Providers / Freestanding Hospices

Methodist Home Care Services, 1716 Parr Avenue, Dyersburg, TN 38024; tel. 901/287-2307; FAX. 901/287-2174
Procare Support Services, Inc., 1210 Stonebridge Square, Jackson, TN 38305; tel. 800/982-2273; FAX. 901/668-9498; Betty Peeryhouse, Administrator
Smoky Mountain Home Health & Hospice, Inc, 222 Heritage Boulevard, Newport, TN 37821; tel. 423/623-0233; FAX. 423/623-8311; Cynthia Finch, M.S.W., Hospice Administrator
Sumner Hospice, 316 East Main Street, Gallatin, TN 37066; tel. 615/451-6690; FAX. 615/230-6889; Shirlene Campbell, Manager
Tennessee Nursing Services of Morristown, Coldwell Bank Building, 415 North Fairmont, Morristown, TN 37816; tel. 423/581-7690; FAX. 423/581-8164; Glena Duffield, Director, Hospice
TLC Hospice, 1200 Mountain Creek Road, Suite 440, Chattanooga, TN 37405; tel. 423/877-0983; FAX. 423/877-4944; Gloria J. Dodds, RN, B.S.N., Administrator
Tri County Quality Homecare and Hospice, 20 Lee Avenue, Box 308, McKenzie, TN 38201; tel. 901/352-2240; FAX. 901/352-0320; Kay Taylor, RN, Patient Care Coordinator
University Home Health and Hospice, Inc., 135 Kennedy Drive, Martin, TN 38237; tel. 901/587-2996; FAX. 800/627-3228; Kellie Sims, B.S.W., Hospice Director
Willowbrook Hospice, Inc., 145 Southesast Parkway, Suite 100, Franklin, TN 37064; tel. 800/790-8499; June Baldini, RN, Director

TEXAS

Abacus Home Health Care, Inc., 8035 E.R.L. Thornton, Suite 322, Dallas, TX 75228; tel. 214/319-7480; FAX. 214/319-2453; Kathy Russell, M.S.W., Administrator
AIM Hospice, 703 East Concho, P.O. Box 2300, Rockport, TX 78381-2300; tel. 512/729-0507; FAX. 512/790-0243; Judith Johnson, RN, Ph.D., Administrator
American Home Health and Hospice, 315 South Oak, Pecos, TX 79772
Ann's Haven/VNA, 216 West Mulberry Street, Denton, TX 76201; tel. 817/566-6550; FAX. 817/383-4000; Karen Pemberton, RN, B.S.N.
Baptist Saint Anthony's Hospice, 600 North Tyler, P.O. Box 950, Amarillo, TX 79176-0001; tel. 806/212-8777; FAX. 806/212-8290; Sharon Hutchison, RN, Director
BSA Hospice, 800 North Sumner, Pampa, TX 79065; tel. 806/665-6677; FAX. 806/665-8423; Sharon Hutchinson, RN, Executive Director
Burton Hospice Care, Inc., 6640 Eastex Freeway, Suite 140, Beaumont, TX 77708; tel. 409/892-7476; FAX. 409/892-7740; Vergie A. Burton, Administrator
Casual Peak Hospice, 901 North Galloway Avenue, Suite 101, Mesquite, TX 75149; tel. 972/285-3713; FAX. 972/285-3699; Julie Francis, Director
Central Texas Medical Center Hospice, 1345 S Thorpe Lane, San Marcos, TX 78666; tel. 512/753-3584; FAX. 512/392-8489; Brenda L. Bloch, RN, Administrator
Circle of Hope Hospice of VNA, 2211 East Missouri, Suite 220, El Paso, TX 79923; tel. 915/543-6201; Tom Meagher, Vice President, Hospice
Community Care Services, Inc., dba CCS Hospice, 118 E. Live Oak, Suite 104, Dublin, TX 76446; tel. 254/445-4675; FAX. 254/445-2972; Beth Martini, Administrator
Community Hospice of St. Joseph, 1000 Summit, Fort Worth, TX 76102
Crown of Texas Hospice, 1000 South Jefferson, Amarillo, TX 79101; tel. 806/372-7696; FAX. 806/372-2825; Sharla Valdez, B.S.N., CRNH, RN, President
Crown of Texas Hospice, 100 I-45 North, Suite 240, Box 103, Conroe, TX 77301; tel. 409/788-7707; FAX. 409/788-7708; Marsha J. Irwin, RN, Ph.D., Director
Cypress Basin Hospice, Inc., 1805 North Jefferson, P.O. Box 544, Mount Pleasant, TX 75455; tel. 903/577-1510; FAX. 903/577-9377; Edd C. Hess, Executive Director
DNS Hospice, 2101 Kemp Boulevard, Wichita Falls, TX 76309; tel. 817/723-2771; FAX. 817/322-1754; Helen Dipprey, Chief Operating Officer
East Harris County Hospice Services, Inc., Holland Avenue Medical Center, 1313 Holland Avenue, Houston, TX 77029; tel. 713/450-4500; FAX. 281/450-4006; Ipe Mathai, Executive Director

Family Hospice of Dallas, 1140 Empire Central, Suite 235, Dallas, TX 75247; tel. 214/631-7273; FAX. 214/630-4032; Jim Grant, RN, B.S.N., M.S., Executive Director
Family Hospice, Inc., 819 South Fifth Street, Temple, TX 76504; tel. 800/643-3139; FAX. 817/742-2023; Carrie Carson, Administrator
First Community Homecare, 9323 Garland Road, Suite 308, Dallas, TX 75218
Golden Acres Hospice, 2525 Centerville Road, Dallas, TX 75228-2693; tel. 214/327-4503; FAX. 214/319-5974; Robert J. Watson, Executive Director
Heart of the Valley Hospice, 189 S. Fannin, San Benito, TX 78586; tel. 800/333-6131; FAX. 210/399-3553; Rebecca Hernandez, RN, Administrator
Hendrick Hospice Care, 1682 Hickory, Abilene, TX 79602; tel. 915/677-8516; FAX. 915/675-5031; David Stephenson, Executive Director
Hillcrest Community Hospice, 3215 Pine Avenue, Waco, TX 76708; tel. 254/202-5150; FAX. 254/752-3072; Richard E. Scott, President
Home Health Services of Dallas, Inc., 2929 Carlisle Street, Suite 375, Dallas, TX 75204-1050
Home Health Specialists, Inc., 813 South Palestine, Athens, TX 75751; tel. 800/801-8126; FAX. 903/657-9513; Rhonda Crabtree, RN, Administrator
Home Hospice, 516 N. Texas, Odessa, TX 79761; tel. 915/580-9990; FAX. 915/580-9989; Hilton Chancellor, Director
Home Hospice, Grayson County Office, 505 West Center Street, P.O. Box 2306, Sherman, TX 75091; tel. 903/868-9315; FAX. 903/893-2772; Marty Barr, Executive Director
HomeHealth, Inc., 17629 El Camino Real, Suite 400, Houston, TX 77058; tel. 281/990-7000; FAX. 281/990-7672; Suzanne Denson, Administrator
Hospice Care Team, Inc., 1708 Auburn Road, Suite C, Texas City, TX 77591; tel. 409/938-0070; FAX. 409/938-1509; Sue Mistretta, Executive Director
Hospice Home Care, 10221 Desert Sands, Suite 301, San Antonio, TX 78216; tel. 210/377-1033; FAX. 210/377-2560; Al Hafer, Business Administrator
Hospice in the Pines, 116 South Raguet, Lufkin, TX 75904; tel. 800/324-8557; FAX. 409/632-1352; Holly Randall, LSW, Social Services
Hospice New Braunfels, 613 North Walnut, New Braunfels, TX 78130; tel. 830/625-7500; FAX. 830/606-1388; Joyce Fox, Administrator
Hospice of Cedar Lake, 101 E. Market Street, Mabank, TX 75147-8614; tel. 903/887-3772; FAX. 903/887-3700; Lila Shumante, RN
Hospice of East Texas, 3800 Paluxy, Suite 560, Tyler, TX 75703; tel. 903/581-5585; FAX. 903/581-5293; Michael C. Couch, Executive Director
Hospice of El Paso, Inc., 3901 North Mesa, Suite 400, El Paso, TX 79902; tel. 915/532-5699; FAX. 915/532-7822; Charles E. Roark, Ed.D. FACHE
Hospice of HIS, 9535 Forest Lane, Suite 211, Dallas, TX 75243; tel. 972/690-6632; FAX. 972/690-0834; Tim Gellegos, National Director, Hospice Operation
Hospice of Lubbock, Inc., 1102 Slide Road, Suite 3, P.O. Box 53276, Lubbock, TX 79453; tel. 806/795-2751; FAX. 806/795-8464; Linda McMurry, RN, B.S.N.
Hospice of Midland, Inc., 911 West Texas, Midland, TX 79701; tel. 915/682-2855; FAX. 915/682-2989; Carol Armstrong, Executive Director
Hospice of Northeast Texas, 51 North Side Square, Cooper, TX 75432; tel. 903/395-2811; FAX. 903/395-2766; Nicki J. Beeler, Administrator
Hospice of San Angelo, Inc., 36 East Beauregard, Suite 1100, San Angelo, TX 76902; tel. 915/658-6524; FAX. 915/658-8895; David McBride, Executive Director
Hospice of South Texas, 2004 Fagan Circle, Victoria, TX 77901; tel. 361/572-4300; FAX. 361/572-4532; Doug Eaves, Executive Director
Hospice of St. Michael Hospital of Texarkana, 1400 College Drive, Texarkana, TX 75501; tel. 903/794-1206; FAX. 903/735-5390; Tommy McGee, Administrator
Hospice of Texarkana, Inc., 803 Spruce Street, Texarkana, TX 75501; tel. 903/794-4263; FAX. 870/774-1108; Cynthia L. Marsh, Administrator
Hospice of the Big Country, Inc., 3113 Oldham Lane, Abilene, TX 79602; tel. 915/677-1191; FAX. 915/677-1808; Danna L. Clouse, Administrator

Hospice of the Heart, 218 S. San Jacinto, Whitney, TX 76962; tel. 817/694-6009; FAX. 817/694-9926; Mary Flournoy, Executive Director
Hospice of the Plains, Inc., 7109 Olton Road, Plainview, TX 79072; tel. 806/293-5127; FAX. 806/293-5902; Roxey Williams, Executive Director
Hospice of the Three Rivers, 51 North 11th Street, Beaumont, TX 77702-2224; tel. 800/946-7742; Andi Whitmer, Administrator
Hospice of V.N.A., 2905 Sackett, Houston, TX 77098; tel. 713/630-5521; FAX. 713/630-5529; Paula Wehrman, RN, MHA, Chief Executive Officer
Hospice of Wichita Falls, 4909 Johnson Road, Wichita Falls, TX 76310; tel. 940/691-0982; FAX. 940/691-1608; Jan Banta, Executive Director
Hospice Preferred Choice, 427 West 20th, Suite 603, Houston, TX 77008; tel. 713/864-2626; FAX. 713/864-9476; Linda Dumoit Administrator
Houston Hospice, 8811 Gaylord, Suite 100, Houston, TX 77024; tel. 713/468-2441; FAX. 713/468-0879; Margaret Caddy, RN, Executive Director
Houston Hospice – Hospice Support Care, 1102 North Mechanic, El Campo, TX 77437; tel. 409/578-0314; FAX. 409/578-0242; Ruth Kainer, RN, Administrator
Huguley Hospice Care, 11801 South Freeway, Ft. Worth, TX 76115; tel. 817/551-2545; FAX. 817/568-3294; Donna Reddell, RN, Director
La Mariposa Hospice, 2001 North Oregon, El Paso, TX 79902; tel. 915/452-6802; Frances Witt, Director
Lakes Area Hospice, 254 Ethel Street, Jasper, TX 75951; tel. 409/384-5995; FAX. 409/384-9655; Jeanette Coffield, Executive Director
Lone Star Hospice, 1212 Palm Valley Boulevard, Round Rock, TX 78664; tel. 512/467-7423; FAX. 512/218-9288; Cecilia Bunker, RN, CRNH
Managed Home Health Care, 2211 Calder Avenue, Beaumont, TX 77707; tel. 409/832-4164; FAX. 409/832-4182; Charles Bray, CEO
Nurses In Touch Community Hospice, 7410 Blanco Road, Suite 100, San Antonio, TX 78216; tel. 210/979-9771; FAX. 210/979-6644; Mary Helen Tieken, RN, B.S.N., Administrator
Odyssey Center for Hospice Care, 1 Price Street, Suite 200, Baytown, TX 77520; tel. 281/422-8879; FAX. 281/422-8789
Odyssey HealthCare, 5440 Harvert Hill Road, Dallas, TX 75230; tel. 888/285-8081; FAX. 972/720-0115; Judy Kremers, General Manager
Personal Touch Hospice of Texas, Inc., 8200 Brookriver Drive, Suite N109, Dallas, TX 75247; tel. 214/638-0357; FAX. 214/905-8687; Roy W. Terry, RN, Director
Robinson Creek Home Care, Inc., 1000 Westbank Drive, Suite 6B201, Austin, TX 78746; tel. 512/328-7606; Vanessa Nunnelly, Administrator
Rural Hospice, Inc., 501 South Alford, Crane, TX 79731; tel. 888/558-2300; FAX. 915/558-2335; Pam Ross, RN, Director
San Juan Home Health and Hospice, 300 North Nebraska Avenue, San Juan, TX 78589; tel. 210/782-0333; FAX. 210/782-0335; Tony Cortez, Director
Spohn Hospice, 600 Elizabeth Street, Corpus Christi, TX 78404; tel. 512/881-3159; FAX. 512/888-7405; Rita Mueller, RN, Director
St. Joseph Hospice Houston, 1404 Calhoun Cullen Family Building, Houston, TX 77002; tel. 713/757-7488; FAX. 713/756-5127; Maresa Henry, Associate Director
St. Paul Hospice, 7920 Elmbrook Drive, Suite 112, Dallas, TX 75247; tel. 214/637-7474; FAX. 214/637-7474; Debbie Weir, Director
Stephen's Hospice, 925 A North Graham, Stephenville, TX 76401-4216; tel. 817/965-7119; FAX. 817/965-3228; Kim Davis, Administrator
Texas Health Staffing Services, Inc., 1115 Chihuahua Street, Suite B, Laredo, TX 78040; tel. 210/791-3012; Maria Elena Montemayor, Administrator
Texoma Community Hospice, 3821 Wilbarger Street, Vernon, TX 76384; tel. 800/658-6330; FAX. 817/552-2305; Jean Tucker, Administrator
The Hospice at the Texas Medical Center, 1905 Holcombe Boulevard, Houston, TX 77030; tel. 713/467-7423; FAX. 713/677-7177; Brandy R. Hicok, RN, BSN, Vice President for Patient Services
The Southeast Texas Hospice, Inc., 912 West Cherry, P.O. Box 2385, Orange, TX 77630; tel. 409/886-0622; FAX. 409/886-0623; Mary McKenna, Executive Director

Providers / Freestanding Hospices

Thee Hospice, POB 6548, Huntsville, TX 77342-6548; tel. 409/291-8439; FAX. 409/295-8582; Patricia Lee, RN, Patient Care Coordinator

Tomlinson Health Services, Hospice Program, 1300 West Mockingbird, Suite 160, Dallas, TX 75247; tel. 214/630-8847; FAX. 817/573-3160; Reba Tomlinson, Chief Executive Officer

Tyler Hospice, 423 South Beckham Avenue, Tyler, TX 75701; tel. 903/592-9703; FAX. 903/593-0639; Sandra L. Bunch, Administrator

Ultra Home Health Care, Inc., 8303 Southwest Freeway, Suite 410, Houston, TX 77074; tel. 713/988-5872; FAX. 713/271-1002; Noel L Carino, Administrator

Visiting Nurse Association Hospice, 212 Brown Street, Brownwood, TX 76801-2915; tel. 915/646-6500; FAX. 915/646-6412; Mary Suther, President and CEO

Visiting Nurse Association of Texas Hospice, 1440 West Mockingbird Lane, Suite 500, Dallas, TX 75247-4929; tel. 214/689-0000; FAX. 214/689-0010; Judith Bigler

Vista Care Family Hospice, 8701 Shoal Creek Boulevard, Suite 104, Austin, TX 78757; tel. 800/444-2405; FAX. 512/453-4165; Susan Smith – Willeh, Program Director

VistaCare Family Hospice of San Antonio, 5815 Callaghan Road, Suite 102, San Antonio, TX 78228; tel. 210/738-8141; FAX. 210/738-3507; Sharon Sheets, Program Director

Vitas Healthcare Corporation, 5001 LBJ Freeway, Suite 1050, Dallas, TX 75244; tel. 972/661-2004; FAX. 972/448-6542; Cindy Kastler, General Manager

Vitas Healthcare Corporation, 4828 Loop Central Drive, Suite 890, Houston, TX 77081; tel. 713/663-7777; FAX. 713/663-4990; Joi Bodine, General Manager

Vitas Healthcare Corporation Hospice, 211 East Parkwood, Suite 211, Friendswood, TX 77546; tel. 713/996-4400; Joi Bodine, General Manager

VNA and Hospice of South Texas, 8721 Botts, San Antonio, TX 78217; tel. 210/804-5200; FAX. 210/826-5987; Mike Mazzocco, Executive Director

VNA and Hospice of the Texas Gulf Coast, P.O. Box 1777, Angleton, TX 77516-1777; tel. 409/849-6476; FAX. 409/849-0343; Jenny Carswell, Administrator

UTAH

CNS Community Hospice, 6949 South Hitech Drive, Salt Lake City, UT 84007-3757; tel. 801/233-6100; FAX. 801/486-2193; Grant C. Howarth, President and CEO

Creative Health Services, Inc. Hospice Care, 6777 South 1560 East, Salt Lake City, UT 84121; tel. 801/943-8374; FAX. 801/942-2949; Joyce L. Smith, Administrator

Creekside Hospice Care, 1935 East Vine Street, Suite 350, Salt Lake City, UT 84121; tel. 801/272-8617; FAX. 801/277-3790; Maryann Pales, Administrator

Dixie Regional Home Health Hospice, 354 East 600 South, Suite 304, St. George, UT 84770; tel. 801/634-4567; FAX. 801/634-4564; Kathy Andrus, RN, Administrator

Family Hospice Care, 404 East 5600 South, Murray, UT 84107; tel. 801/268-8083; FAX. 801/268-8096; Pat Burns, Director, Home Care Services

Hospice of Cache Valley, 1400 North 500 East, Logan, UT 84341; tel. 801/750-5477; FAX. 801/750-5361; Neil C. Perkes, RN, M.B.A., Administrator

IHC Hospice, 2250 South 1300 West, Suite A, Salt Lake City, UT 84119; tel. 801/977-9900; FAX. 801/977-9956; Shauna Einerson, Administrator

Premier Hospice Care, 4885 South 900 East, Suite 207, Salt Lake City, UT 84117; tel. 801/288-1619; David West, RN, Administrator

Rocky Mountain Hospice, 315 East 400 South, Bountiful, UT 84010; tel. 801/397-4900; Patricia Kruger, Administrator

Uintah Basin Hospice, 26 West 200 North 78-15, Roosevelt, UT 84066; tel. 435/722-2418; FAX. 435/722-6187; Lloyd Neilsen, RNC, BSN, Director

Vista Care, 1093 South Orem Boulevard, Orem, UT 84058; tel. 801/224-2999; Alan Green, Administrator

VERMONT

Brattleboro Area Hospice, 191 Canal Street, P.O. Box 1053, Brattleboro, VT 05302-1053; tel. 802/257-0775; Susan Parris, Executive Director

Caledonia Home Health Care–Hospice, Sherman Drive, P.O. Box 383, St. Johnsbury, VT 05819; tel. 802/748-8116; FAX. 802/748-4628; Brenda B. Smith, Hospice Care Director

Central Vermont Home Health and Hospice, Inc., R.R. 3, Barre, VT 05641; tel. 802/223-1878; FAX. 802/223-6835; Diana Peirce, RN, CRNH, Director, Hospice Services

Franklin County Home Health and Hospice, Three Home Health Circle, St. Albans, VT 05478; tel. 802/527-7531; FAX. 802/527-7533; Janet McCarthy, Executive Director

Hospice of Bennington County, Inc., P.O. Box 1231, Bennington, VT 05201; tel. 802/447-0307; Amy Barber-Thomas, Executive Director

Hospice of Champlain Valley, 1110 Prim Road, Suite 1, Colchester, VT 05446; tel. 802/860-4410; FAX. 802/860-6149; Annette Blanchard, RN, Program Director

Hospice of VNH, 20 South Main Street, White River Junction, VT 05001; tel. 802/295-2604; FAX. 802/295-3163; Marie Kirn, Executive Director

Hospice Volunteer Sucs, P.O. Box 772, Middlebury, VT 05753; tel. 802/388-4111; Catherine Studley, Executive Director

Lamoille Home Health and Hospice, 54 Farr Avenue, Morrisville, VT 05661; tel. 802/888-4651; FAX. 802/888-7822; Ann Mallett, Director

Orleans Essex VNA and Hospice, Inc., 46 Lakemont Road, Newport, VT 05855-1550; tel. 802/334-5213; FAX. 802/334-8822; Diana Hamilton, RN, Director of Hospice Services

Randolph Area Hospice, 36 South Main Street, Randolph, VT 05060; tel. 802/728-6100; Susan O'Malley, Area Chairperson

Rutland Area Visiting Nurse Association, Seven Albert Cree Drive, Rutland, VT 05701; tel. 802/775-0568; FAX. 802/775-2304; Sally Tobin, Associate Director, Community Health Program

Southern Vermont Home Health Agency, 1 Holstein Place, Suite 311, Brattleboro, VT 05301; tel. 802/257-4390; FAX. 802/257-2188; Kathy Anderson

Springfield Area Hospice, Inc., 366 River Street, Springfield, VT 05156; tel. 802/886-2525; Marisa Bolognese, Volunteer Coordinator

Visiting Nurse Alliance of Vermont and New Hampshire, Hospice of Vermont and New Hampshire, 46 South Main Street, Old Court House, White River J, VT 05001; tel. 802/295-2604; FAX. 802/295-3163; Marie Kirn, Executive Director

VIRGINIA

Blue Ridge Hospice, Inc., 333 West Cork Street, Winchester, VA 22601; tel. 540/665-5210; FAX. 540/678-0584; Ernest J. Carnevale, Jr., CEO

Community Hospices of America, Inc., 540 West Main Street, Wytheville, VA 24382; tel. 703/228-5424; FAX. 703/228-9225; Rita C. Cobbs, Program Director

Crater Community Hospice, Inc., 840 W. Roslyn Road, Suite E, Colonial Heights, VA 23834; tel. 804/526-4300; FAX. 804/526-4337; Brenda D. Mitchell, RN

First Choice Home Services, Inc., 915 Central Avenue, P.O. Box 1146, Harrisonburg, VA 22801; tel. 703/434-3916; Diana Berkshire, Administrator

Gentle Shepherd Hospice, Inc., 4040 Franklin Road, S.W., Roanoke, VA 24014; tel. 540/989-6265; FAX. 540/989-1547; Donald A. Eckenroth, III, Administrator

Good Samaritan Hospice, Inc., 3525 Electric Road, Suite A, Roanoke, VA 24018; tel. 540/776-0198; FAX. 540/776-0841; Sue Moore, President

Hospice of Central Virginia, 5540 Falmouth Street, Suite 307, Richmond, VA 23230; tel. 804/281-0541; FAX. 804/281-0954; Jane Isbell, Administrator

Hospice of Northern Virginia, 9540 Center Street, Suite 300, Manassas, VA 20110; tel. 703/392-6707; FAX. 703/392-5116; Mary Simpson, Clinical Manager

Hospice of Northern Virginia, Inc., 6400 Arlington Boulevard, Suite 1000, Falls Church, VA 22042; tel. 703/534-7070; FAX. 703/538-2163; David J. English, President and CEO

Hospice of Northern Virginia, Inc., 885 Harrison Street, S.E., Leesburg, VA 21075; tel. 703/777-7866; FAX. 703/771-8904; Jackie Wright, Regional Vice President

Hospice of the Piedmont, Inc., 1490 Pantops Mountain Place, Suite 200, Charlottesville, VA 22911; tel. 804/975-5500; FAX. 804/975-4040; Roberta White, Executive Director

Hospice of the Rapidan, Inc., 1200 Sunset Lane, Suite 2320, Culpeper, VA 22701; tel. 703/825-4840; FAX. 703/825-7752; Patricia Tuffy, Executive Director

Housecall Hospice, Two Main Street, P.O. Box 850, Jonesville, VA 24263; tel. 703/346-1095; Ethel Combs, Administrator

Housecall Hospice, 2167 Apperson Drive, Salem, VA 24153; tel. 540/776-3213; FAX. 540/776-1849; Peggy Mental, RN, Administrator

Housecall Hospice, 294 C Commonwealth Boulevard, Box 335, Martinsville, VA 24112; tel. 540/632-9611; FAX. 540/632-4414; Pat Coleman, Administrator

In Home Health, 5040 Corporate Woods Drive, Virginia Beach, VA 23462; tel. 757/490-9323; FAX. 757/490-8711; Phyllis Moran, Director of Operations

In Home Health and Hospice, 408 W. Washington, Suffolk, VA 23434; tel. 757/934-7935; FAX. 757/934-7940; Phyllis J. Moran, Director Operations

Jewish Family Service, 7300 Newport Avenue, P.O. Box 9503, Norfolk, VA 23505; tel. 757/489-3111; FAX. 757/451-1796; Harry Graber, Executive Director

Medshares Hospice of Middle Virginia, 9200 Arboretum Parkway, Suite 120, Richmond, VA 23236; tel. 804/327-4445; FAX. 804/327-4467; Michelle G. Nichols, RN, Director

Mountain Regional Hospice, 525 Main Street, P.O. Box 637, Clifton Forge, VA 24422; tel. 540/862-8820; FAX. 540/862-8822; Glenn Perry, Executive Director

New River Valley Hospice, Inc., 111 West Main Street, Christiansburg, VA 24073; tel. 703/381-5001; FAX. 703/381-5008; Bhanu Iyengar, Executive Director

Rockbridge Area Hospice, Inc., 129 South Randolph Street, P.O. Box 948, Lexington, VA 24450; tel. 540/463-1848; FAX. 540/463-5219; Susan Hogg, Executive Director

Sentara Hospice, Eight Koger Executive Building, Suite 210, Norfolk, VA 23502; tel. 804/628-3602; Dorothy Weeks, Manager

Twin County Hospice, 605 Glendale Road, Galaxy, VA 24333; tel. 540/236-7935; Patty S. Cooke, Administrator

WASHINGTON

Associated Health Services, P.O. Box 5200, Tacoma, WA 98415-0200; tel. 206/552-1825; FAX. 206/552-1838; Beverly Hatter, Director Grief, Loss and Transitional

Assured Home Health and Hospice, 576–B Main Street, Chehalis, WA 98532; tel. 360/748-0151; FAX. 360/748-0518; Wilma Wayson, RN, B.S.N., Director

Central Basin Home Health and Hospice, 715 West Third Avenue, Moses Lake, WA 98837; tel. 509/765-1856; FAX. 509/765-3323; Beth S. Laszlo, Executive Director

Community Home Health and Hospice, 1035 11th Avenue, P.O. Box 2067, Longview, WA 98632-8189; tel. 360/425-8510; FAX. 360/425-4667; Angie Armstrong, Executive Director

Evergreen Community Hospice, 12822 – 124th Lane, N.E., Kirkland, WA 98034; tel. 206/899-1040; FAX. 206/899-1099; Mary VanItoomissioin, RN, Director

Group Health Cooperative Hospice Program, 83 South King Street, Suite 515, Seattle, WA 98104-2848; tel. 425/882-2022; FAX. 425/881-7147; Barbara Boyd, Administrator, Home and Community Service

Harbors Home Health and Hospice, 201 Seventh Street, Hoquiam, WA 98550; tel. 360/532-5454; FAX. 360/533-0999; DeLila Thorp, Administrator

Highline Home Care Services, 2801 South 128th, Tukwila, WA 98168; tel. 206/439-9095; FAX. 206/433-1031

Hospice of Snohomish County, 2731 Wetmore Avenue, Suite 520, Everett, WA 98201-3581; tel. 425/261-4800; FAX. 425/258-1097; Mary L. Brueggeman, Executive Director

Hospice of Spokane, West 1325 First Avenue, Suite 200, P.O. Box 2215, Spokane, WA 99210; tel. 888/459-0438; FAX. 509/458-0359; Anne Koepsell, Executive Director

Lower Valley Hospice, 3920 Outlook Road, Sunnyside, WA 98944; tel. 509/837-1676; FAX. 509/837-2878; Vicki Meyer, Executive Director

Providers / Freestanding Hospices

Okanogan Regional Home Health Care Agency, 217 Second Avenue, S., P.O. Box 1248, Okanogan, WA 98840; tel. 509/422-6721; FAX. 509/422-1835; Jeanette Weyrich, Executive Director

Swedish Home Health and Hospice and Infusion, 5701 Sixth Avenue, S., Suite 504, Seattle, WA 98108-2522; tel. 206/386-6602; FAX. 206/385-6613; Marla Mallatt, RN, Acting Director

Tri-Cities Chaplaincy/Hospice and Counseling, 2108 West Entail Avenue, Kennewick, WA 99336; tel. 509/783-7416; FAX. 509/735-7850; Thomas H. Halazon, Executive Director

Walla Community Hospice, P.O. Box 2026, 37 Jade Ave – Suite B, Walla, WA 99362; tel. 509/525-5561; FAX. 509/525-3517; Karyl Ball, Administrator

Whatcom Hospice, 600 Birchwood Avenue, Bellingham, WA 98225; tel. 360/733-5877; FAX. 360/734-9621; Marsha J. Johnson

WEST VIRGINIA

Albert Gallatin Hospice, 3280 University Avenue, Morgantown, WV 25605; tel. 304/598-0226; Christine Constantine, Administrator

Community Home Care and Hospice, 1209 Warwood Avenue, Wheeling, WV 26003; tel. 304/277-1500; FAX. 304/277-1507; Ruth Prosser, M.S.N., RN, Administrator

Community Hospices of America – The Virginias, P.O. Box 6364, Blue Prince Road, Bluefield, WV 24701; tel. 304/325-7220; FAX. 304/325-9384; Rich Bezjak, Program Director

Dignity Hospice of Southern West Virginia, Inc, P.O. Box 4304, Chapmanville, WV 25508; tel. 304/855-1132; FAX. 304/855-1129; Sabrina C. Conley, Director

Hospice Care Corporation, P.O. Box 229, Kingwood, WV 26537; tel. 304/329-1161; FAX. 304/329-3285; Malene J. Davis, RN, Executive Director

Hospice of Huntington, 1101 Sixth Avenue, P.O. Box 464, Huntington, WV 25709; tel. 304/529-4217; FAX. 304/523-6051; Charlene Farrell, Executive Director

Hospice of South West Virginia, 105 South Eisenhower Drive, P.O. Box 1472, Beckley, WV 25802; tel. 304/255-6404; FAX. 304/255-6494; Thomas A. Williams, Executive Director

Hospice of the Panhandle, Inc., 2015 Boyd Orchard Court, Martinsburg, WV 25401; tel. 304/264-0406; FAX. 304/264-0409; Margaret Cogswell, RN, Executive Director

Journey Hospice, 314 South Wells Street, Sisterville, WV 26175; tel. 304/652-2611; FAX. 304/652-3190; Kathy J. Powell, RN, Program Director

Kanawha Hospice Care, Inc., 1143 Dunbar Avenue, Dunbar, WV 25064; tel. 304/768-8523; FAX. 304/768-8627; Shirley Hyatt, Director of Patient Services

Lewis County Home Health and Hospice Care, P.O. Box 1750, Weston, WV 26452; tel. 304/269-6432; FAX. 304/269-8220; Nancy Hosey, RN, Patient Care Coordinator

Monongalia County Health Department Hospice, 453 Van Voorhis Road, Morgantown, WV 26505-3408; tel. 304/598-5151; FAX. 304/598-5167; George Liston, RN, BSN, Hospice Supervisor, Patient Care Coordinator

Morgantown Hospice, 989 Maple Drive, P.O. Box 4222, Morgantown, WV 26504; tel. 304/285-2777; FAX. 304/285-1456; Sharon Weimer, Executive Director

Mountain Hospice, Inc., 1040 Crim Avenue, Belington, WV 26250; tel. 304/823-3922; FAX. 304/823-3926; Debra Goodman, Director

MVA Hospice of Marion County, P.O. Box 1112, 1322 Locust Avenue, Fairmont, WV 26555-1112; tel. 304/366-0700; FAX. 304/366-9529; Bedelia Lienbach, Nurse Coordinator

People's Hospice, United Hospital Center, P.O. Box 1680, Clarksburg, WV 26302-1680; tel. 304/623-0524; FAX. 304/623-3399; Janice Chapman, Director

St. Joseph's Hospice, 92 West Main Street, Buckannon, WV 26201; tel. 304/472-6846; Sandra Knotts, Director

WISCONSIN

Beloit Regional Hospice, Inc., 2958 Prairie Avenue, Beloit, WI 53511; tel. 608/363-7421; FAX. 608/363-7426; Virginia Burton, Administrator

Colland Nelson Crossroads Hospice, 1020 James Drive, Hartland, WI 53029; tel. 262/928-7444; FAX. 262/928-7446; Anne Friedman, Hospice Coordinator

Community Hospice–VNA, 811 Monitor Street, Suite 101, LaCrosse, WI 54603; tel. 608/796-1666; Margaret Mossholder

Covenant Home Health and Hospice, 1055 Prarie Drive, P.O. Box 4045, Racine, WI 53406; tel. 414/884-2980; FAX. 414/884-2999; Sharon Pheiffer, Administrator

Dr. Kate Hospice House, P.O. Box 770, Woodruff, WI 54568; tel. 715/356-8805; FAX. 715/356-8875; Helen Mozuch, RN, Director, Operations

Franciscan Skemp Healthcare Hospice, 212 South 11th Street, LaCrosse, WI 54601; tel. 608/791-9790; FAX. 608/791-9548; Deanna Dickinson, Administrator

Grant County Hospice, 125 S. Monroe Street, Lancaster, WI 53813; tel. 608/723-6416; FAX. 608/723-6501; Linda S. Adrian, Director, Health Officer

Heartland Hospice, 455 Davis Street, P.O. Box 487, Hammond, WI 54015; tel. 715/796-2223; Mary Troftgruben, Director

Hillside Homecare/Hospice, 709 South University Avenue, Beaver Dam, WI 53916; tel. 414/887-4050; FAX. 414/887-6815; Lisa White, Director

Home Health United Hospice, 520 South Boulevard, P.O. Box 527, Baraboo, WI 53913; tel. 608/242-1516; FAX. 608/242-1613; Thomas H. Brown, President

Hope Hospice, Inc., 709 McComb Avenue, P.O. Box 237, Rib Lake, WI 54470; tel. 715/427-3532; FAX. 715/427-3537; Barbara Meyer, Director

Hospice Alliance, Inc., 600 – 52nd Street, Kenosha, WI 53140; tel. 262/652-4440; FAX. 262/652-4628; Connie Matler, Executive Director, Clinical Services

Hospice Preferred Choice, 3118 South 27th Street, Milwaukee, WI 53215; tel. 414/649-8302; FAX. 414/649-8441; Joanne M. Klinko, Executive Director

Hospice Program of Waupaca County, 811 Harding Street, Waupaca, WI 54981; tel. 715/258-6323; Susan Enz, B.S.N., Coordinator

HospiceCare, Inc., 5835 E. Cheryl Parkway, Madison, WI 53713-4521; tel. 608/276-4660; FAX. 608/276-4672; Susan Phillips, Executive Director

Jefferson Home Health and Hospice, 1007 Washington Street, P.O. Box 117, Baraboo, WI 53913; tel. 608/356-7570; FAX. 608/356-2629; William J. Hamilton, Jr., Managing Director

Manitowoc County Community Hospice, 1004 Washington Street, Manitowoc, WI 54220; tel. 920/684-7155; FAX. 920/684-8653; Lynn Seidl-Babcock, RN, B.S.N., Administrator

Mercy Assisted Care, Home Health, Hospice, DME, 901 Mineral Point Avenue, Janesville, WI 53545; tel. 608/754-2201; FAX. 608/754-1147; Caryn Oleston, Executive Director

Monroe Clinic Hospice, 515 22nd Avenue, Monroe, WI 52566; tel. 800/367-8406; FAX. 608/324-1302; Carla Stadel, Administrator

Northwest Wisconsin HomeCare/Hospice, 2321 East Clairemont Parkway, P.O. Box 2060, Eau Claire, WI 54702-2060; tel. 715/831-0100; FAX. 715/831-0108; Jill Hurlburt, RN, B.S.N., Director, Clinical Services

Rainbow Hospice Care, LLC, 147 West Rockwell Street, Jefferson, WI 53549; tel. 920/674-6255; FAX. 920/674-5288; Keni Christiansen, Director of Clinical Services

Regional Hospice, 2101 Beaser Avenue, Ashland, WI 54806; tel. 715/682-8677; FAX. 715/682-6404; Dianne Zaiser, Director of Clinical Services

Rolland Nelson Crossroads Hospice, 1020 James Drive, Hartland, WI 53029; tel. 414/928-7444; FAX. 414/928-7446; Anne Friedman, CHPN, Hospice Coordinator

The Daycare at Home, P.O. Box 469, Neerah, WI 54957-0469; tel. 920/969-0919; FAX. 920/969-0020; Susan Kostka, Homecare/Hospice Supervisor

Unity Hospice, P.O. Box 22395, Green Bay, WI 54305-2395; tel. 414/433-7470; FAX. 414/437-1934; Donald W. Seibel, Director

UPC Health Network–Hospice Services, 3724 West Wisconsin Avenue, Milwaukee, WI 53208; tel. 414/342-9292; FAX. 414/342-8721; Walter Orzechowski, National Director, Hospice Service

Visiting Nurse Association of Wisconsin Hospice, 2314 Kohler Memorial Drive, Sheboygan, WI 53081; tel. 920/458-4314; Robert Walters, VP of Regional Operations

Vitas Healthcare, 450 North Sunny Slope Road, Suite 60, Brookfield, WI 53005; tel. 414/821-6500; FAX. 414/821-6533; Suzanne Weltzien, General Manager

VNA of Wisconsin Hospice, 11333 West National Avenue, Milwaukee, WI 53227; tel. 414/327-2295; FAX. 414/328-4567; Mary Runge, Hospice Director

WYOMING

Central Wyoming Hospice Program, 319 South Wilson Street, Casper, WY 82601; tel. 307/577-4832; FAX. 307/577-4841; Janace Chapman, RN, Director

Hospice of Laramie, 1262 N. 22nd Street, Unit A, Laramie, WY 82072; tel. 307/745-9254; FAX. 307/742-5967; Connie M. Coca, M.S.W., Director

Hospice of Sweetwater County, 809 Thompson, Suite D, Rock Springs, WY 82901; tel. 307/362-1990; FAX. 307/352-6769; Pamela L. Jelaca, Executive Director

Hospice of the Tetons, 555 East Broadway, P.O. Box 428, Jackson, WY 83001; tel. 307/739-7465; FAX. 307/739-7645; Catherine Hadden, Director

Northeast Wyoming Hospice, 400 S. Kendrick #301, P.O. Box 3259, Gillette, WY 82717-3259; tel. 307/682-6570; FAX. 307/682-2781; Donna Suchan, RN, Administrator

Spirit Mountain Hospice, 707 Sheridan Ave., Cody, WY 82414; tel. 307/578-2413; FAX. 307/578-2294; Fred Whitmore, Administrator

Susie Bowling Lawrence Hospice, 497 West Lott, Buffalo, WY 82834; tel. 307/684-5521; FAX. 307/684-5385; Kent Ward, Administrator

U.S. Associated Areas

PUERTO RICO

Caribbean Hospice, 153 Winston Churchill Avenue, Rio Piedras, PR 00926; tel. 787/764-6565; FAX. 787/758-3035; Adalberto Sandoval

Condado Hospice Program, P.O. Box 5417, Station Hato, PR 00919-5417; tel. 809/758-2325; Manuel de Leon

Condado Hospice Program, Inc., Avenue Laurel 2 U-6 2U-6, Bayamon, PR 00956; tel. 787/780-7045; FAX. 787/269-0175; Carmen L. Rosa, Administrator

Corporacioon de Servicios de Salud de Adjuntas, Rodulfo Gonzalez #46, P.O. Box 993, Adjuntas, PR 00601; tel. 787/829-2953; FAX. 787/829-1093; Abraham Gonzalez, Executive Director

Guaynabo Hospice, Nine Jose Julian Acosta Street, Guaynabo, PR 00969; tel. 809/789-7878; Ricardo Larin, President

Hospicio Atencion Medica en el Hogar, Carr. #1, Rm. 34.9 Bo. Bairoa, P.O. Box 5742, Caguas, PR 00726; tel. 787/258-1628; FAX. 787/746-1066; Sandra Torres, Administrator

Hospicio de Esperanza, Avenue General Valero 267, Fajardo, PR 00738; tel. 809/863-0924; Luis Vazquez

Hospicio El Nuevo Amanecer, Calle Garcia De La, Noceda 38, Rio Grande, PR 00745; tel. 809/888-8885; Melvin Acosta Roman

Hospicio Fe y Esperanza, P.O. Box 1834, Manati, PR 00674-1834; tel. 787/854-4971; FAX. 787/884-3757; Eduardo Alvarez, Administrator

Hospicio La Caridad, Calle Cipres El, Villa Turabo, Caguas, PR 00725; tel. 787/286-8745; FAX. 787/746-5750; Glorivette Seneriz

Hospicio La Montana, Road 152 Km 12.4, Cedro Arriba P.O. Box 515, Naranjito, PR 00719; tel. 787/869-9500; FAX. 787/869-4483; Antonia Fortis Santiago

Hospicio La Paz, Calle Jose Rodriguez, Irizarry 152, Arecibo, PR 00612; tel. 809/879-4733; Luis Monrouzeau

Hospicio Luzamor, P.O. Box 1312, Calle Patron, #11, Morovis, PR 00687; tel. 809/862-0608; Ms. Brunilda Otero Declet, Executive Director

Hospicio Nuestra Sra. de la Guadalupe, P.O. Box 7699, Ponce, PR 00732; tel. 787/259-8210; FAX. 787/259-0206; Lucy Gonzalez, Administrator

Hospicio Santa Rita, La Paz Street, Box 1143, Aguada, PR 00602; tel. 787/868-2945; FAX. 787/868-0010; Licedia Rosado

Hospital Sin Paredes, P.O. Box 2015, Hato Rey, PR 00919; tel. 809/767-8959; Luis Serrano

Providers / Freestanding Hospices

La Piedad Hospice, 626 Escorial Hospice, San Juan, PR 00920; tel. 787/792–2411; FAX. 787/781–1643; Antonio Bisono

La Providencia Hospice, 1206 Munoz Rivera Avenue, P.O. Box 10447, Ponce, PR 00717–0689; tel. 787/843–2364; FAX. 787/841–2940; Eyleen Rodriguez Lugo, Executive Director

Monserrate Hospice Care, Inc., P.O. Box 366148, San Juan, PR 00936–6148; tel. 809/754–0449; Luis Class

San Francisco Asis Hospice, P.O. Box 877, Aguada, PR 00602; tel. 787/868–2920; FAX. 787/252–0211; Dilia Dajer, Executive Director

Santa Rita Hospice, Inc., Condominio Medical Center Plaza, Box 1143, Aguada, PR 00602; tel. 787/831–7225; Licedia Rosado

Sendero de Luz Hospice, Inc., 9 Georgett Street, P.O. Box 875, Comerio, PR 00782; tel. 787/875–5701; FAX. 787/875–0887; Juan C. Santiago, Executive Director

St. Lukes Home Care and Hospice Program, 291 Calle Monterrey, Ponce, PR 00717–1376; tel. 787/843–4185; FAX. 787/843–4076; Luz N. Rodriguez, Executive Director

Un Toque de Amor Hospice, Marginal A–2 Urb, San Salvador, Manati, PR 00674; tel. 809/884–3326; Jenny Olivo

Information for the following list was obtained directly from the agencies.

State Government Agencies for Freestanding Hospices

United States

ALABAMA
Alabama Department of Public Health, Division of Licensure and Certification, 434 Monroe Street, Montgomery, AL 36130-1701; tel. 334/240-3503; FAX. 334/240-3147; Rick Harris, Director

ALASKA
Division of Medical Assistance, Health Facilities Licensing and Certification Section, 4730 Business Park Blvd., Suite 18, Anchorage, AK 99503; tel. 907/561-8081; FAX. 907/561-3011; Shelbert Larsen, Administrator

ARIZONA
Arizona Department of Health Services, Health Care Facilities, 1647 East Morten, Phoenix, AZ 85020; tel. 602/542-1100; FAX. 602/861-0645; Mary Wiley, Assistant Director

ARKANSAS
Department of Health, Division of Health Facility Services, 5800 West 10th, Suite 400, Little Rock, AR 72204-9916; tel. 501/661-2201; FAX. 501/661-2165; Henry Robinson, Director

CALIFORNIA
Department of Health Services, Licensing and Certification Program, 1800 Third Street, Suite 210, P.O. Box 942732, Sacramento, CA 94234-7320; tel. 916/324-8628; FAX. 916/445-6979; Marilyn Pearman, Chief, Policy Section

COLORADO
Colorado Department of Public Health and Environment, Health Facilities Division A-Two, 4300 Cherry Creek Drive., Denver, CO 80222-1530; tel. 303/692-2800; FAX. 303/782-4883; Priscilla Ezell, RN, Program Administrator

CONNECTICUT
Department of Public Health Division of Health Systems Regulation, 410 Capital Avenue, Hartforc, CT 06134-0308; tel. 860/509-7400; FAX. 860/509-7538; Cynthia Denne, RN, MPA., Bureau Chief Regulatory Services

DELAWARE
Department of Health and Social Services, Office of Health Facilities Licensing and Certification, 2055 Limestone Road, Suite 200, Wilmington, DE 19808; tel. 302/995-8521; FAX. 302/577-8524; Mary Peterson, Director

DISTRICT OF COLUMBIA
Department of Health Licensing and Regulation, 825 North Capital, NE, Washington, DC 20001; tel. 202/442-5888; FAX. 202/727-7780; Geraldine Sykes, Administrator

FLORIDA
Agency for HealthCare Administration, Division of Health Quality Assurance, Long Term Care Unit, Fort Knox Executive Center, 2727 Mahan Drive, Tallahassee, FL 32308-5407; tel. 850/922-8540; FAX. 850/487-6240; Patricia Hall, Unit Manager

GEORGIA
Health Care Section - Georgia Dept. of Human Resources, Office of Regulatory Services, Two Peachtree Street, N.W., Room 33-250, Atlanta, GA 30303-3142; tel. 404/657-5550; FAX. 404/657-8934; Susie M. Woods, Director

HAWAII
Department of Health, Licensing and Certification, Office Health Care Assurance, P.O. Box 3378, Honolulu, HI 96801; tel. 808/586-4080; FAX. 808/586-4444; Helen K. Yoshimi, B.S.N., MPH, HMF, Branch Chief

IDAHO
Bureau of Facility Standards, Department of Health and Welfare, P.O. Box 83720, Boise, ID 83720-0036; tel. 208/334-6626; FAX. 208/364-1888; Sylvia Cresell, Supervisor

ILLINOIS
Department of Public Health, Office of Health Care Regulation, Bureau of Hospitals and Ambulatory Services, 525 West Jefferson Street, Fourth Floor, Springfield, IL 62761; tel. 217/782-7412; FAX. 217/782-0382; Catherine M. Stokes, Assistant Deputy Director

INDIANA
Indiana State Department of Health, Division of Acute Care, Two North Meridian Street, Indianapolis, IN 46204; tel. 317/233-7474; FAX. 317/233-7157; Mary Azbill, MT (ASCP)

IOWA
Department of Inspection and Appeals, Division of Health Facilities, Lucas State Office Building, Des Moines, IA 50319; tel. 515/281-3765; FAX. 515/242-5022; Nancy M. Ruzicka, Bureau Chief

KANSAS
Department of Health and Environment, Bureau of Health Facility Regulation, 900 Southwest Jackson, Suite 1001, Topeka, KS 66612-0001; tel. 785/296-1280; FAX. 785/296-1266; George A. Dugger, Medical Facilities Certification Administrator

KENTUCKY
Cabinet for Human Resources, Division of Licensing and Regulation, C.H.R. Building, 275 East Main Street, Fourth Floor, East, Frankfort, KY 40621; tel. 502/564-2800; FAX. 502/564-6546; Rebecca J. Cecil, Director

LOUISIANA
Department of Health and Hospitals, Bureau of Health Services, Health Standards Section Licensing Unit, P.O. Box 3767, Baton Rouge, LA 70821; tel. 504/342-0138; FAX. 504/342-5292; Lisa Deaton, RN, Manager

MAINE
Division of Licensing and Certification, Department of Human Services, State House, Station 11, Augusta, ME 04333; tel. 207/624-5443; FAX. 207/624-5378; Louis Dorogi, Director

MARYLAND
Department of Health and Mental Hygiene, Licensing and Certification Administration, 4201 Patterson Avenue, Baltimore, MD 21215; tel. 410/764-4980; FAX. 410/358-0750; James Ralls, Assistant Director

MASSACHUSETTS
Massachusetts Department of Public Health, Division of Health Care Quality, 10 West Street, 5th Floor, Boston, MA 02111; tel. 617/727-5860; Dr. Howard Kyongju Koh New, Commissioner

MICHIGAN
Department of Consumer and Industry Services, Division of Licensing and Certification, G. Mennen Williams Building, 525 W. Ottawa, Lansing, MI 48909; tel. 517/241-2626; Dr. Gladys Thomas, Director

MINNESOTA
Department of Health, Facility and Provider Compliance Division, Licensing and Certification, 85 East Seventh Place, Suite 300, St. Paul, MN 55164-0900; tel. 651/215-8719; FAX. 651/215-8709; Carol Hirschfeld, Supervisor, Program Assurance Unit

MISSISSIPPI
Department of Health, Division of Health Facilities, Licensure and Certification, P.O. Box 1700, Jackson, MS 39215; tel. 601/354-7300; FAX. 601/354-7230; Vanessa Phipps, Director

MISSOURI
Department of Health, Bureau of Home Health Licensing and Certification, P.O. Box 570, Jefferson City, MO 65102; tel. 573/751-6336; FAX. 573/751-6315; Carol Gourd, RN, Administrator

MONTANA
Department of Public Health and Human Services, Quality Assurance Division, Licensure Bureau, Cogswell Building, 1400 Broadway, Helena, MT 59620-2951; tel. 406/444-2676; FAX. 406/444-1742; Roy P. Kemp, Chief

NEBRASKA
Nebraska Department of Health, Health Facility Licensure and Inspection Section, 301 Centennial Mall, South, 3rd Floor., P.O. Box 94986, Lincoln, NE 68509-4980; tel. 402/471-2946; FAX. 402/471-0555; Helen Meeks, Director

NEVADA
Nevada State Health Division, Bureau of Licensure and Certification, 1550 East College Parkway, Suite 158, Carson City, NV 89706-7921; tel. 775/687-4475; FAX. 775/687-6588; Richard J. Panelli, Chief

NEW HAMPSHIRE
Department of Health and Human Services, Licensing and Regulation, Six Hazen Drive, 2nd Floor, West Wing, Concord, NH 03301; tel. 603/271-4592; FAX. 603/271-4968; Raymond Rusin, Bureau Chief

NEW JERSEY
New Jersey Department of Health and Senior Services, Division , Certificate of Need and Acute Care Licensure, Inspections, John Fitchway, Market and Warren Streets, Trenton, NJ 08625-0360; tel. 609/292-8773; FAX. 609/984-3165; John Caiabira, Director

NEW MEXICO
Department of Health, Health Facility Licensing and Certification Bureau, 525 Camino de los Marquez, Suite Two, Santa Fe, NM 87501; tel. 505/827-4200; FAX. 505/827-4222; Wilma Hammer, Bureau Chief

NEW YORK
Bureau of Surveillance and Quality Assurance, 161 Delaware Avenue, Delmar, NY 12054; tel. 518/478-1133; FAX. 518/478-1134; Anna D. Colello, Director

NORTH CAROLINA
Department of Human Resources, Division of Facility Services, 701 Barbour Drive, Raleigh, NC 27626-0530; tel. 919/733-7461; FAX. 919/733-8274; Steve White, Chief, Licensure and Certification

NORTH DAKOTA
Department of Health, Health Resources Section, 600 East Boulevard Avenue, Bismarck, ND 58505; tel. 701/328-2352; FAX. 701/328-4727; Darleen Bartz, Director of Health Facilities

OHIO
Division of Quality Assurance, Ohio Department of Health, 246 North High Street, Columbus, OH 43266-0588; tel. 614/466-7857; FAX. 614/644-0208; Rebecca Maust, Division Chief

OKLAHOMA
Department of Health, Special Health Services, 1000 Northeast 10th Street, Oklahoma City, OK 73117; tel. 405/271-6576; FAX. 405/271-1308; Gary Glover, Chief, Medical Facilities

OREGON
Health Care Licensing and Certification, Oregon Health Division, 800 Northeast Oregon Street, # 21, Suite 640, P.O. Box 14450, Portland, OR 97293-0450; tel. 503/731-4013; FAX. 503/731-4080; Kathleen Smail, Manager

PENNSYLVANIA
Department of Health, Division of Primary Care and Home Health, 132 Kline Plaza, Suite A, Harrisburg, PA 17104; tel. 717/783-1379; FAX. 717/787-3188; Aralene Trostle, Acting Director

Providers / State Government Agencies for Freestanding Hospices

RHODE ISLAND
Rhode Island Department of Health, Division of Facilities Regulation, Three Capitol Hill, Providence, RI 02908-5097; tel. 401/222–2566; FAX. 401/222–3999; Wayne I. Farrington, Chief

SOUTH CAROLINA
Department of Health and Environmental Control, Division of Certification, 2600 Bull Street, Columbia, SC 29201; tel. 803/737–7205; FAX. 803/737–7292; Arthur I. Starnes, Division Director

SOUTH DAKOTA
Department of Health, Office of Health Care Facilities Licensure and Certification, 615 East 4th Street, Pierre, SD 57501-1700; tel. 605/773–3356; FAX. 605/773–6667; Joan Bachman, Administrator

TENNESSEE
Department of Health, Division of Health Care Facilities, Cordell Hull Building, 425 5th Ave. North, 1st Floor, Nashville, TN 37247-0508; tel. 615/741–7603; FAX. 615/367–6397; Carol Brown

TEXAS
Texas Department of Health, Health Facility Compliance Division, 1100 West 49th Street, Austin, TX 78756; tel. 512/834–6650; FAX. 512/834–6653; Nance Stearman, RN, M.S.N., Director

UTAH
Utah Department of Health, Bureau of Health Facility Licensure, Box 142003, Salt Lake City, UT 84114-2003; tel. 801/538–6152; FAX. 801/538–6325; Debra Wynkoop-Green, Director

VERMONT
Hospice Council of Vermont, 10 Maine Street, Montpelier, VT 05602; tel. 802/229–0579; FAX. 802/232–6218; Virginia L. Fry, Director

VIRGINIA
Virginia Department of Health, Center for Quality Health Care Services and Consumer Protection, 3600 Centre, Suite 216, Richmond, VA 23230; tel. 804/367–2102; FAX. 804/367–2149; Nancy R. Hofheimer, Director

WASHINGTON
Washington Department of Health, Facilities and Services Licensing, Target Plaza, Suite 500, 2725 Harrison Avenue, N.W., Olympia, WA 98504-7852; tel. 360/705–6611; FAX. 360/705–6654; Byron Plan, Manager

WEST VIRGINIA
Office of Health Facility Licensure and Certification, West Virginia Division of Health, 350 Capital Street, Room 206, Charleston, WV 25301-3718; tel. 304/558–0050; FAX. 304/558–2515; Bonnie K. Brauner, RN, BSN, Program Manager

WISCONSIN
Bureau of Quality Assurance, Division of Supportive Living, P.O. Box 2969, Madison, WI 53701-2969; tel. 608/267–7185; FAX. 608/267–0352; Susan Schroder, Director, Bureau of Quality Assurance

WYOMING
Department of Health, Office of Health Quality, 2020 Carey Avenue, 8th Floor, Cheyenne, WY 82002; tel. 307/777–7123; FAX. 307/777–7127; Gerald E. Bronnenberg, Administrator

U.S. Associated Areas

PUERTO RICO
Puerto Rico Department of Health, PO Box 70184, San Juan, PR 00936-8184; tel. 787/274–7601; FAX. 787/250–6547; Carmen Feliciano de Melecio, M.D., Secretary of Health

JCAHO Accredited Freestanding Long-Term Care Organizations

The accredited freestanding long-term care organizations listed have been accredited as of March, 2000 by the Joint Commission on Accreditation of Healthcare Organizations by decision of the Accreditation Committee of the Board of Commissioners.

The organizations listed here have been found to be in compliance with the Joint Commission standards for long-term care organizations, as found in the Comprehensive Accreditation Manual for the Long-Term Care Organizations.

Please refer to section A of the AHA Guide for information on hospitals with Long-Term Care services. These hospitals are identified by Facility Code 69. In section A, those hospitals identified by Approval Code 1 are JCAHO accredited.

We present this list simply as a convenient directory. Inclusion or omission of any organization's name indicates neither approval nor disapproval by Health Forum LLC, an American Hospital Association company.

United States

ALABAMA

Cedar Crest, 4490 Virginia Loop Road, Montgomery, AL 36116; tel. 334/281-6826; Mr. James G Griffin

Integrated Health Services at Hanover, 39 Hanover Circle, Birmingham, AL 35205; tel. 205/933-1828; Ms. Vicki Worley

South Haven Manor, 1300 East South Boulevard, Montgomery, AL 36116; tel. 334/288-0122; Ms. Diane G Sorey

Warren Manor Living Center, Number 11 Bell Road, Selma, AL 36701; tel. 334/874-7425; Mr. John B White

ARIZONA

Chris Ridge Village Health Center, 6246 North 19th Avenue, Phoenix, AZ 85015; tel. 602/433-6300; Mr. Gerald L Wissink

Citadel Care Center, 5121 East Broadway Road, Mesa, AZ 85206; tel. 602/832-5555; Mrs. Patricia A Phillips

Desert Cove Nursing Center, 1750 West Frye Road, Chandler, AZ 85224; tel. 602/899-0641; Ms. Melanie S Seamans

Desert Sky Health and Rehabilitation Center, 5125 North 58th Avenue, Glendale, AZ 85301; tel. 602/931-5800; Ms. Virginia Rafferty

East Valley Health Care Center, 420 West 10th Place, Mesa, AZ 85201; tel. 602/833-4226; Ms. Dayna Steenberg

Glendale Care Center, 4704 West Diana Avenue, Glendale, AZ 85302; tel. 623/247-3949; Mr. Daniel E Summers

GranCare Health Care Center, 16640 North 38th Street, Phoenix, AZ 85032; tel. 602/482-6671; Mr. David Gibson

Hacienda Rehabilitation and Care Center, 660 Coronaco Drive, Sierra Vista, AZ 85635; tel. 520/459-4900; Ms. Maria A Ritter

Hearthstone of Mesa, 215 South Power Road, Mesa, AZ 85206; tel. 602/985-6992; Mr. Laura C Niffenegger

Hearthstone of Sun City, 13818 N Thunderbird Boulevard, Sun City, AZ 85351; tel. 623/977-1325; Mr. Steven Flynt

Heritage Health Care Center, PO Box 391, Globe, AZ 85502; tel. 520/425-3118; Mr. Greg LeChemnant

Kachina Point Health Care and Rehabilitation Center, 505 Jacks Canyon Road, Sedona, AZ 86351; tel. 520/284-1000; Ms. Christine Walker

La Canada Care Center, 7970 North La Canada Drive, Tucson, AZ 85704; tel. 520/797-1191; Mr. John P O'Brien, Jr.

La Mesa Rehabilitation and Care Center, 2470 South Arizona Avenue, Yuma, AZ 85364; tel. 520/344-8441; Mr. Scott M Little

Life Care Center at South Mountain, 8008 South Jesse Owens Parkway, Phoenix, AZ 85040; tel. 602/243-2780; Mr. Ricardo P Villa

Life Care Center of North Glendale, 13620 North 55th Avenue, Glendale, AZ 85304; tel. 602/843-8433; Mr. Gary Davis

Life Care Center of Paradise Valley, 4065 East Bell Road, Phoenix, AZ 85032; tel. 602/867-0212; Terry Granger

Life Care Center of Scottsdale, 9494 East Becker Lane, Scottsdale, AZ 85260; tel. 480/860-6396; Ms. Linda L Villa

Life Care Center of Tucson, 6211 West LaCholla Boulevard, Tucson, AZ 85741; tel. 520/575-0900; Mr. Thomas Hines

Life Care Center of Yuma, 2450 South 19th Avenue, Yuma, AZ 85364; tel. 520/344-0425; Mr. Robert Frechette

Mi Casa Nursing Center, 330 South Pinnule Circle, Mesa, AZ 85206; tel. 480/981-0687; Ms. Rosemary Anderson

Payson Care Center, 107 East Lone Pine Drive, Payson, AZ 85541; tel. 520/474-6896; Mr. Todd L Corless

Pecos Nursing and Rehabilitation Center, 1980 West Pecos Road, Chandler, AZ 85224; tel. 602/821-1268; Mr. Vernon Thacker

Phoenix Living Center, 1314 East McDowell Road, Phoenix, AZ 85006; tel. 602/252-5212; Ms. Virginia Rafferty, MBA

Scottsdale Heritage Court, 3339 N Civic Center Boulevard, Scottsdale, AZ 85251; tel. 602/949-5400; Mr. David R Starret

Scottsdale Village Square, 2620 North 68th Street, Scottsdale, AZ 85257; tel. 602/946-6571; Ms. Colleen H Sweet

Silver Ridge Village, 2812 Silver Creek Road, Bullhead City, AZ 86442; tel. 520/763-1404; Ms. Carol Schmoyer

Sonoran Rehabilitation and Care Center, 4202 North 20th Avenue, Phoenix, AZ 85015; tel. 602/264-3824; Mr. David Brown

Sun Grove Village Care Center, 20625 N. Lake Pleasant Drive, Peoria, AZ 85382; tel. 602/566-0642; Ms. Susan Davis

Sun Health Care Center, 10601 West Santa Fe Drive, Sun City, AZ 85351; tel. 602/974-7000; Ms. Genny Rose

Village Green HealthCare Center, 2932 North 14th Street, Phoenix, AZ 85014; tel. 602/264-5274; Mr. David W DeRushia

CALIFORNIA

Akin's Post Acute Rehabilitation Hospital, 2750 Atlantic Avenue, Long Beach, CA 90806; tel. 562/424-8101; Mr. Ronald M Akin

Alamitos Belmont Rehabilitation Hospital, 3901 East Fourth Street, Long Beach, CA 90814; tel. 562/434-8421; Mr. Alan Anderson

Almaden Health and Rehab Center, 2065 Los Gatos Almaden Road, San Jose, CA 95124; tel. 408/377-9275; Ms. Debbie Cota

Anaheim Terrace Care Center, 141 South Knott Avenue, Anaheim, CA 92804; tel. 714/821-7310; Ms. Mona L Fisk

Auburn Gardens Care Center, 260 Racetrack Street, Auburn, CA 95603; tel. 530/885-7051; Mr. Clayton L Green

Autumn Hills Health Care Center, 430 North Glendale Avenue, Glendale, CA 91206; tel. 818/246-5677; Ms. Jenik Akopian

Bay Crest Care Center, 3750 Garnet Street, Torrance, CA 90503; tel. 310/371-2431; Ms. Elaine Kau

Beverly Healthcare, 6700 Sepulveda Boulevard, Van Nuys, CA 91411; tel. 818/988-2501; Mrs. Marcia Weldon

Beverly Manor Nursing and Rehabilitation Center, 1041 South Main Street, Burbank, CA 91506; tel. 818/843-2330; Jennifer Rose

Bixby Knolls Towers Health Care and Rehabilitation Center, 3747 Atlantic Avenue, Long Beach, CA 90807; tel. 562/426-6123; Mr. Buck L Perkins

Brier Oak Terrace Care Center, 5154 Sunset Boulevard, Los Angeles, CA 90027; tel. 213/663-3951; Ms. Sheila Snukal

Brookside Skilled Nursing Hospital, 2620 Flores Street, San Mateo, CA 94403; tel. 650/349-2161; Mr. Carl Braginsky

California Nursing and Rehabilitation Center, 2299 North Indian Canyon, Palm Springs, CA 92262; tel. 760/325-2937; Ms. Linda Jackson

California Special Care Center, Inc., 8787 Center Drive, La Mesa, CA 91942; tel. 619/460-4444; Mr. John Jimenez

Calistoga Care – Nursing and Rehab Center, 1715 Washington Street, Calistoga, CA 94515; tel. 707/942-6253; Ms. Cindy Reed

Carehouse, 1800 Old Tustin Road, Santa Ana, CA 92705; tel. 714/835-4900; Mr. Robert Snukal

Casa Palmera Care Center, Inc., 14750 El Camino Real, Del Mar, CA 92014; tel. 619/481-4411; Mr. Lee A Johnson

Chapman Harbor Skilled Nursing Facility, 12232 West Chapman Avenue, Garden Grove, CA 92840; tel. 714/971-5517; Ms. Patricia A Smith

Clear View Sanitarium and Convalescent Center, 15823 South Western Avenue, Gardena, CA 90247; tel. 310/538-2323; Mr. W. Lee Towns

Colonial Care Center, 1913 East 5th Street, Long Beach, CA 90802; tel. 562/432-5751; Mr. James Preimesderger

Colony Park Nursing and Rehabilitation Center, 159 East Orangeburg Avenue, Modesto, CA 95350; tel. 209/526-2811; Mr. David Yarbrough

Country Villa Belmont Heights, 1730 Grand Avenue, Long Beach, CA 90804; tel. 562/597-8817; Ms. Janice Connelley

Country Villa Los Feliz Nursing Center, 3002 Rowena Avenue, Los Angeles, CA 90039; tel. 323/666-1544; Mr. Stephen E Reissman

Country Villa Nursing and Rehabilitation Center, 340 South Alvarado Street, Los Angeles, CA 90057; tel. 213/484-9730; Mr. Stephen E Reissman

Country Villa Oxnard Manor Healthcare Center, 1400 West Gonzales Road, Oxnard, CA 93030; tel. 805/983-0324; Mr. Stephen E Reissman

Country Villa Pavilion, 5916 West Pico Boulevard, Los Angeles, CA 90035; tel. 323/939-3184; Mr. Stephen E Reissman

Country Villa Plaza Nursing Center, 1209 West Hemlock Way, Santa Ana, CA 92707; tel. 714/546-1966; Mr. Stephen E Reissman

Country Villa Sheraton Nursing and Rehabilitation Center, 9655 Sepulveda Boulevard, North Hills, CA 91343; tel. 818/892-8665; Mr. Steve Reissman

Country Villa South, 3515 Overland Avenue, Los Angeles, CA 90034; tel. 310/839-5201; Mr. Stephen Reissman

Country Villa Westwood Nursing Center, 12121 Santa Monica Boulevard, Los Angeles, CA 90025; tel. 310/826-0821; Mr. Stephen E Reissman

Country Villa Wilshire, 855 North Fairfax Avenue, Los Angeles, CA 90046; tel. 323/653-1521; Mr. Stephen E Reissman

Country Villa Woodman Health Care Center, 13524 Sherman Way, Van Nuys, CA 91405; tel. 818/786-3470; Mr. Geovany Fino

Creekside HealthCare Center, 1900 Church Lane, San Pablo, CA 94806; tel. 510/235-5514; K. J Page

Delta Nursing and Rehabilitation Hospital, 514 North Bridge Street, Visalia, CA 93291; tel. 209/732-8614; Mr. Mark A Fisher

Devonshire Care Center, 1350 East Devonshire Avenue, Hemet, CA 92544; tel. 909/925-2571; Mr. Raymond Villaluz

Diamond Ridge HealthCare Center, 2351 Loveridge Road, Pittsburg, CA 94565; tel. 510/427-4444; Ms. Carol Shields-Wallace

Driftwood Health Care Center, 4109 Emerald Street, Torrance, CA 90503; tel. 310/371-4628; Mr. Gary Yoshida

Providers / JCAHO Accredited Freestanding Long-Term Care Care Organizations

Driftwood Health Care Center, 19700 Hesperian Boulevard, Hayward, CA 94541; tel. 510/785-2880; Mrs. Helen Anderson
Driftwood Healthcare Center, 675 24th Avenue, Santa Cruz, CA 95062; tel. 408/475-6323; Ms. Elizabeth P Byrne
Earlwood Care Center, 20820 Earl Street, Torrance, CA 90503; tel. 310/371-1228; Mr. Robert Snokal
Eastwood Convalescent Hospital, 4029 East Anaheim Street, Long Beach, CA 90804; tel. 562/494-4421; Mr. Ronald M Akin, Jr.
Edgewater Convalescent Hospital, 2625 East 4th Street, Long Beach, CA 90814; tel. 562/434-0974; Ms. Debbie Kremel
El Encanto Healthcare and Habilitation Center, 555 South El Encanto Road, City Of Industry, CA 91745; tel. 626/336-1274; Mr. Steve Blackwell
El Rancho Vista Healthcare Center, 8925 Mines Avenue, Pico Rivera, CA 90660; tel. 562/542-7019; Ms. Shirley B Schouleman
Elmcrest Convalescent Hospital, 3111 Santa Anita Avenue, El Monte, CA 91733; tel. 818/443-0218; Mr. Robert Snukal
Empress Rehabilitation Center, 1020 Termino Avenue, Long Beach, CA 90804; tel. 562/433-6791; Ms. Kini McDonald
English Oaks Convalescent and Rehabilitation Hospital, 2633 West Rumble Road, Modesto, CA 95350; tel. 209/577-1001; Mr. Jerry Holloway
Eskaton Manzanita Manor, 5318 Manzanita Avenue, Carmichael, CA 95608; tel. 916/331-8513; Mr. John Breaux
Eskaton Village, 3939 Walnut Avenue, Carmichael, CA 95608; tel. 916/974-2000; Mr. John Breaux
Evergreen Rehabilitation Care Center, 2030 Evergreen Avenue, Modesto, CA 95350; tel. 209/577-1055; Mr. Benedict V Cipponeri, Jr.
Flagship Healthcare Center, 466 Flagship Road, Newport Beach, CA 92663; tel. 714/642-8044; Mr. Joseph Munoz
Florin Health Care Center, 7400 24th Street, Sacramento, CA 95822; tel. 916/422-4825; Mr. Greg Urban
Fountain Care Center, 1835 West La Veta Avenue, Orange, CA 92868; tel. 714/978-6800; Mr. Henry Kim
Fountain View Convalescent Hospital, 5310 Fountain Avenue, Los Angeles, CA 90029; tel. 213/461-9961; Mr. Robert Snukal
Fremont Health Center, 39022 Presidio Way, Fremont, CA 94538; tel. 510/792-3743; Ms. Lisa Chestnut
Fruitvale Health Care Center, 3020 East 15th Street, Oakland, CA 94601; tel. 510/261-5613; Mrs. Remedios B Tibayan
Grand Terrace Convalescent Hospital, 12000 Mt. Vernon Avenue, Grand Terrace, CA 92313; tel. 909/825-5221; Ms. Diane Machain
Greenhaven Country Place, 455 Florin Road, Sacramento, CA 95831; tel. 916/393-2550; Mr. John Breaux
Guardian Ygnacio, 1449 Ygnacio Valley Road, Walnut Creek, CA 94598; tel. 925/939-5820; Mr. Robert G Peirce
Hancock Park Convalescent Rehabilitation Center, 505 North LaBrea Avenue, Los Angeles, CA 90036; tel. 323/937-4860; Mr. Robert Snukal
Hanford Nursing and Rehabilitation Hospital, 1007 West Lacey Boulevard, Hanford, CA 93230-0911; tel. 209/582-2871; Mr. Mike Mayfield
Hayward Hills Health Care Center, 1768 B Street, Hayward, CA 94541; tel. 510/538-4424; Mr. Bill Curto
Heritage of Stockton, A Convalescent and Rehab Center, 9109 North Davis Road, Stockton, CA 95209; tel. 209/478-6488; Mr. Richard K Matros
Hillside Care Center, 81 Professional Center Parkway, San Rafael, CA 94903; tel. 415/479-5161; Mr. Richard Isaacs
Huntington Beach Convalescent Hospital, 18811 Florida Street, Huntington Beach, CA 92648; tel. 714/847-3515; Mr. Rod Mittchum
Huntington Drive Health and Rehabilitation Center, 400 West Huntington Drive, Arcadia, CA 91007; tel. 626/445-2421; Ms. Melissa L Nelson
Imperial Convalescent Center, 11926 S La Mirada Boulevard, La Mirada, CA 90638; tel. 562/943-7156; Ms. Judith S Gonzalez
Inglewood Healthcare Center, 100 South Hillcrest Boulevard, Inglewood, CA 90301; tel. 310/677-9114; Ms. Shirley B Schouleman
Integrated Health Services at Orange Hills, 5017 East Chapman Avenue, Orange, CA 92669; tel. 714/997-7090; Dr. Charles Kellerman
John Douglas French Center for Alzheimer's Disease, 3951 Katella Avenue, Los Alamitos, CA 90720; tel. 562/493-1555; Ms. Ferri F Kidane
Julia Healthcare Center, 276 Sierra Vista Avenue, Mountain View, CA 94043; tel. 650/967-5714; Mrs. Terry Campbell
La Mariposa Nursing and Rehabilitation Center, 1244 Travis Boulevard, Fairfield, CA 94533; tel. 707/422-7750; Ms. Lisa E Churches
La Salette Health and Rehabilitation Center, 538 East Fulton Street, Stockton, CA 95204; tel. 209/466-2066; Ms. Janey Hargreaves
Lancaster Health Care Center, 1642 West Avenue J, Lancaster, CA 93534; tel. 661/942-8463; Ms. Randy Herzig
LaSierra Care Center, 2424 M Street, Merced, CA 95340; tel. 209/723-4224; Mr. Keith G Braley
Laurelwood Health Care Center, 13000 Victory Boulevard, North Hollywood, CA 91606; tel. 818/985-5990; Mr. Scott Herzig
Leisure Court Nursing Center, 1135 North Leisure Court, Anaheim, CA 92801; tel. 714/772-1353; Ms. Patricia Smith
Live Oak Rehabilitation Center, 537 West Live Oak, San Gabriel, CA 91776; tel. 818/289-3763; Ms. Carol Scanlon
Lytton Gardens, 437 Webster Street, Palo Alto, CA 94301; tel. 650/617-7360; Ms. Vera T Goupille
Madera Rehabilitation and Convalescent Center, 517 South A Street, Madera, CA 93638; tel. 559/673-9228; Mr. Michael Giardullo
Magnolia Gardens Care Center, 1609 Trousdale Drive, Burlingame, CA 94010; tel. 650/697-1865; Ms. Barbara Dabney
Magnolia Special Care Center, 635 South Magnolia, El Cajon, CA 92020; tel. 619/442-8826; Ms. Harriet Haugen
ManorCare Health Services, Inc, 11680 Warner Avenue, Fountain Valley, CA 92708; tel. 714/241-9800; Mr. Anthony Glenn Padama
Marlora Post Acute Rehabilitation Hospital, 3801 East Anaheim Street, Long Beach, CA 90804; tel. 562/494-3311; Ms. Marilyn A Hauser
Merced Living Care Center, 510 West 26th Street, Merced, CA 95340; tel. 209/723-2911; Ms. Arden Bennett
Mission Terrace Convalescent Hospital, 623 West Junipero Street, Santa Barbara, CA 93105; tel. 805/682-7443; Mrs. Evelina Murphy
Nob Hill Healthcare Center, 1359 Pine Street, San Francisco, CA 94109; tel. 415/673-8405; Mr. Paul D Tunnell
Orinda Rehabilitation and Convalescent Hospital, 11 Altarinda Road, Orinda, CA 94563; tel. 925/254-6500; Mr. Charles H Speers
Pacific Coast Manor, 1935 Wharf Road, Capitola, CA 95010; tel. 408/476-0770; Mr. Charles H Bruffey
Pacific Hills Manor, 370 Noble Court, Morgan Hill, CA 95037; tel. 408/779-7346; Ms. Laurie L Behrend
Pacific Regency / Bakersfield, 6212 Tudor Way, Bakersfield, CA 93306; tel. 805/871-3133; Ms. Deana Shannon
Pacifica Nursing and Rehabilitation Center, 385 Esplanade Avenue, Pacifica, CA 94044; tel. 650/993-5576; Mr. William Connell
Palm Grove Care Center, 13075 Blackbird Street, Garden Grove, CA 92843; tel. 714/530-6322; Mr. Tony Ricci
Park Anaheim Healthcare Center, 3435 West Ball Road, Anaheim, CA 92804; tel. 714/827-5880; Mr. Kevin Burkin
Park Tustin Rehabilitation and Healthcare Center, 2210 East First Street, Santa Ana, CA 92705; tel. 714/547-7091; Mr. Mark Schroepfer
Parkmont Rehabilitation and Nursing Care Center, 2400 Parkside Drive, Fremont, CA 94536; tel. 510/793-7222; Ms. Jan Beresford
Parkview Health Care Center, 27350 Tampa Avenue, Hayward, CA 94544-4429; tel. 510/783-8150; Mr. Jeff Lambkin
Petaluma Care and Rehabilitation, 1115 B Street, Petaluma, CA 94952; tel. 707/765-3030; Mr. John Jones
Reche Canyon Rehabilitation and Health Care Center, 1350 Reche Canyon Road, Colton, CA 92324; tel. 909/370-4411; Mr. Fred B Frank
Scripps Oceanview Convalescent Hospital, 900 Santa Fe Drive, Encinitas, CA 92024; tel. 760/753-6423; Ms. Carol J Carroll
Scripps Torrey Pines Convalescent Hospital, 2552 Torrey Pines Road, La Jolla, CA 92037; tel. 858/453-5810; Ms. Sheeri Rockler
Sharon Heights Care & Rehab, 1185 Monte Rosa Drive, Menlo Park, CA 94025-6795; tel. 650/854-3300; Ms. Leslee J Fennell
Skyline Convalescent Hospital, 2065 Forest Avenue, San Jose, CA 95128; tel. 408/298-3950; Mr. W. M. Nicholson, Jr.
Studio City Convalescent, 11429 Ventura Boulevard, Studio City, CA 91604; tel. 818/766-9551; Mr. Mark Donahoe
Subacute Saratoga Hospital, 13425 Sousa Lane, Saratoga, CA 95070; tel. 408/378-8875; Mr. Alton King
Sun Rise Care Center – Park Central, 2100 Parkside Drive, Fremont, CA 94536; tel. 510/797-5300; Ms. Kathleen Voll
Sunbridge Care Center – Huntington Valley, 8382 Newman Avenue, Huntington Beach, CA 92647; tel. 714/842-5551; Peggy Larsen
Sunrise Brittany Care Center, 3900 Garfield Avenue, Carmichael, CA 95608; tel. 916/481-6455; Mrs. Joan B Martellucci
Sunrise Care & Rehabilitation for Glendora, 435 East Gladstone Street, Glendora, CA 91740; tel. 626/963-5955; Ms. Barbara Dube
SunRise Care & Rehabilitation for Hayward, 26660 Patrick Avenue, Hayward, CA 94544; tel. 510/782-1845; Ms. Breda B Conroy
Sunrise Care and Rehab Center for Kentfield, 1251 South Eliseo Drive, Kentfield, CA 94904; tel. 415/461-1900; Mr. Dan Daly
Sunrise Care and Rehab Center for Monteca, 410 Eastwood Avenue, Manteca, CA 95336; tel. 209/239-1222; Mr. Mike Blaufus
SunRise Care Center for San Dimas, 1033 East Arrow Highway, Glendora, CA 91740; tel. 818/963-7531; Ms. Sandra Fahey
Sunrise Care Center for Santa Monica – 17th Street, 1330 17th Street, Santa Monica, CA 90404; tel. 310/829-5411; Ms. Sherri Silverberg
SunRise Care Center for Escondido–West, 201 North Fig Street, Escondido, CA 92025; tel. 619/746-0303; Mr. William Adams
Sunrise Care Center for Santa Monica – Franklin St, 1321 Franklin Street, Santa Monica, CA 90404; tel. 310/828-5596; Mr. Dale Zulauf
Tarzana Health and Rehabilitation Center, 5650 Reseda Boulevard, Tarzana, CA 91356; tel. 818/881-4261; Mr. Pete Stong
The Cloisters of La Jolla, 7160 Fay Avenue, La Jolla, CA 92037; tel. 619/459-4361; Ms. Cheryl M Thompson
The Cloisters of Mission Hills, 3680 Reynard Way, San Diego, CA 92103; tel. 619/297-4484; Mr. Scott M Harmon
The Homestead of Fair Oaks, 11300 Fair Oaks Boulevard, Fair Oaks, CA 95628-5172; tel. 916/965-4663; Mr. John Breaux
Thousand Oaks Health Care Center, 93 West Avenida de Los Arboles, Thousand Oaks, CA 91360; tel. 805/492-2444; Ms. Sherri Silverberg
Totally Kids Specialty Healthcare, 1720 Mountain View Avenue, Loma Linda, CA 92354; tel. 909/796-6915; Mr. Doug Padgett
Tulare Nursing and Rehabilitation Hospital, 680 East Merritt Avenue, Tulare, CA 93274; tel. 209/686-8581; Mr. Mark A Fisher
Vacaville Convalescent and Rehabilitation Center, 585 Nut Tree Court, Vacaville, CA 95687; tel. 707/449-8000; Mr. Michael T Kelly
Vale HealthCare Center, 13484 San Pablo Avenue, San Pablo, CA 94806; tel. 510/232-5945; Ms. Mary Thrower
Valley Manor Rehabilitation Center, 3806 Clayton Road, Concord, CA 94521; tel. 510/689-2266; Dr. Robert Elkin
Verdugo Vista Health Care Center, 3050 Montrose Avenue, La Crescenta, CA 91214; tel. 818/984-0850; Ms. Carole M Lillis
Villa Maria Care Center, 425 East Barcellus Avenue, Santa Maria, CA 93454; tel. 805/922-3558; Ms. Caryn Lisnek
Village Square Nursing and Rehabilitation Center, 1586 West San Marcos Boulevard, San Marcos, CA 92069; tel. 760/471-2986; Ms. Gail Brockway
Vista Knoll, 2000 Westwood Road, Vista, CA 92083; tel. 619/630-2273; Ms. Cheryl Carter
Woodland Care Center, 7120 Corbin Avenue, Reseda, CA 91335; tel. 818/881-4540; Ms. Nancy Spaeth

COLORADO

Alpine Living Center, 501 East Thornton Parkway, Thornton, CO 80229; tel. 303/452-6101; Ms. Marlyan Martinez
Applewood Living Center, 1800 Stroh Place, Longmont, CO 80501; tel. 303/776-6081; Mr. Daniel Balli
Arvada Health Center, 6121 West 60th Avenue, Arvada, CO 80003; tel. 303/420-4550; Ms. Holly Raymer

Providers / JCAHO Accredited Freestanding Long-Term Care Care Organizations

Bethany Healthplex, 5301 West First Avenue, Lakewood, CO 80226; tel. 303/238–8333; Mr. Warren Yule
Bonell Good Samaritan Center, PO Box 1508, Greeley, CO 80632–1508; tel. 970/352–6082; Mr. Art H Hess
Boulder Manor Living Center, 4685 East Baseline Road, Boulder, CO 80303; tel. 303/494–0535; Mr. Butch Cash
Camellia Health Care Center, 500 Geneva Street, Aurora, CO 80010–4305; tel. 303/364–9311; Ms. Patsy M Bagully
Castle Garden Care Center, 401 Malley Drive, Northglenn, CO 80233; tel. 303/452–4700; Ms. Rene Bebout
Cedars Health Care Center, 1599 Ingalls Street, Lakewood, CO 80214; tel. 303/232–3551; Ms. Terrance M Sharron
Cherrelyn Health Care Center, 5555 South Elati Street, Littleton, CO 80120; tel. 303/798–8686; Mr. Mark Bedinger
Cherry Hills Health Care Center, 3575 South Washington Street, Englewood, CO 80110; tel. 303/789–2265; Mr. Bruce Busby
Fort Collins Good Samaritan Village, 508 West Trilby Road, Fort Collins, CO 80525; tel. 970/226–4909; Ms. Sherry L Friesen
Garden Terrace Alzheimer's Center of Excellence, 1600 South Potomac Street, Aurora, CO 80012; tel. 303/750–8418; Jean Sommer
Hallmark Nursing Center, 3701 West Radcliff Avenue, Denver, CO 80236; tel. 303/794–6484; Mr. Kevin Fletcher
IHS of Colorado at Cherry Creek, 14699 East Hampden Avenue, Aurora, CO 80014; tel. 303/693–0111; Ms. Ann Kokish
Integrated Health Services of Canon City, 515 Fairview, Canon City, CO 81212; tel. 719/275–0665; Mr. Larry Lavelle
Integrated Health Services of Parkmoor Village, 3625 Parkmoor Village Drive, Colorado Springs, CO 80917; tel. 719/550–0200; Mr. Robert Crook
Julia Temple Center, 3401 South Lafayette Street, Englewood, CO 80110; tel. 303/761–0075; Ms. Nancy K Schwalm
Kenton Manor, 850 27th Avenue, Greeley, CO 80631; tel. 970/353–1018; Ms. Nancy L Jones
Life Care Center of Aurora, 14101 East Evans Avenue, Aurora, CO 80014; tel. 303/751–2000; Ms. Tiffany M Geist
Life Care Center of Evergreen, 2987 Evergreen Parkway, Evergreen, CO 80439; tel. 303/674–4500; Ms. Anne Deines
Life Care Center of Pueblo, 2118 Chatelat Lane, Pueblo, CO 81005; tel. 719/564–2000; Ms. Terrie Stanton–Nance
Life Care Center of Westminster, 7751 Zenobia Court, Westminster, CO 80030; tel. 303/412–9121; Mr. Gary W Walker
Manor Care Nursing and Rehabilitation Center, 2800 Palo Parkway, Boulder, CO 80301; tel. 303/440–9100; Ms. Marybeth Leavell
Mariner Health of Denver, 895 South Monaco Parkway, Denver, CO 80224; tel. 303/321–3110; Ms. Gloria Jones
Mariner Health of Greenwood Village, 6005 South Holly Street, Littleton, CO 80121; tel. 303/773–1000; Ms. Mary Fisher–Guy
Red Rocks HealthCare Center, 4450 East Jewell, Denver, CO 80222; tel. 303/757–7438; Mr. Todd R Amo
Spring Creek HealthCare Center, 1000 East Stuart Street, Fort Collins, CO 80525; tel. 970/482–5712; Mr. Dan Wellman
Sunbridge Bear Creek Care and Rehabilitation of Morrison, PO Box 117, Morrison, CO 80465; tel. 303/697–8181; Mr. Andrew Turner
Terrace Gardens Health Care Center, 2438 East Fountain Boulevard, Colorado Springs, CO 80910; tel. 719/473–8000; Mr. Gerry LaFont
University Park Care Center, 945 Desert Flower Boulevard, Pueblo, CO 81001; tel. 719/545–5321; Ms. Barbara Strombeck
Vista Grande Rehabilitation and Care Center, PO Box 1718, Cortez, CO 81321; tel. 970/564–2600; Ms. Jo Ann Aldrich

CONNECTICUT
3030 Park Fairfield Health Center, Inc., 118 Jefferson Street, Fairfield, CT 06432; tel. 203/372–4501; Ms. Alice Pisani
Aaron Manor Nursing and Rehabilitation Center, 3 South Wig Hill Road, Chester, CT 06412; tel. 860/526–5316; Mr. Martin Sbriglio
Abbott Terrace Health Center, 44 Abbott Terrace, Waterbury, CT 06702; tel. 203/755–4870; Mrs. Diane MacSweeney
Adams House Healthcare, 80 Fern Drive, Torrington, CT 06790; tel. 860/482–7668; Mr. William Viola
Alexandria Manor, 55 Tunxis Avenue, Bloomfield, CT 06002; tel. 860/242–0703; Ms. Michael Lawless
Ashlar of Newtown, PO Box 5505, Newtown, CT 06470; tel. 203/426–5847; Mr. Thomas M Gutner
Astoria Park, 725 Park Avenue, Bridgeport, CT 06604; tel. 203/366–3653; Mr. Donald L Franco
Avery Heights, 705 New Britain Avenue, Hartford, CT 06106; tel. 860/527–9126; Dr. Mariam Parker
Avon Health Center, 652 West Avon Road, Avon, CT 06001–2999; tel. 860/673–2521; Ms. Laura L Nelson
Bayview Health Care Center, 301 Rope Ferry Road, Waterford, CT 06385; tel. 860/444–1175; Ms. Patricia J Lincoln
Beacon Brook Health Center, 89 Weid Drive, Naugatuck, CT 06770; tel. 203/729–9889; Ms. Marion Najamy
Beechwood Rehabilitation and Nursing Center, P.O Box 308, New London, CT 06320; tel. 860/442–4363; Mr. William G White
Bel-Air Manor Nursing and Rehabilitation Center, 256 New Britain Avenue, Newington, CT 06111; tel. 860/666–5689; Mr. Martin Sbriglio
Bentley Gardens Health Care Center, 310 Terrace Avenue, West Haven, CT 06516–2698; tel. 203/932–2247; Mr. Jack Friedler
Bethel Health and Rehabilitation Center, LLC, 13 Parklawn Drive, Bethel, CT 06801; tel. 203/830–4180; Mrs. Grace Flight
Bickford Health Care Center, Fourteen Main Street, Windsor Locks, CT 06096; tel. 860/623–4351; Ms. Michele Carney
Bishop Wicke Health and Rehabilitation Center, Inc, 584 Long Hill Avenue, Shelton, CT 06484; tel. 203/929–5321; Mr. Robert Clapp
Blair Manor, 612 Hazard Avenue, Enfield, CT 06082; tel. 860/749–8388; Ms. Doris Gordon
Bloomfield Health Care Center, 355 Park Avenue, Bloomfield, CT 06002; tel. 860/242–8595; Mr. Lewis Abrmason
Branford Hills Health Care Center, 189 Alps Road, Branford, CT 06405; tel. 203/481–6221; Mr. Stephen J Shelton
Bridgeport Health Care Center, 600 Bond Street, Bridgeport, CT 06610; tel. 203/384–6400; Miss Rachel Blass
Bridgeport Manor, 540 Bond Street, Bridgeport, CT 06610; tel. 203/384–6500; Ms. Rachel Blass
Brightview of Avon, 220 Scoville Road, Avon, CT 06001; tel. 860/673–3265; Mr. Gregory J Hamley
Brittany Farms Health Center, 400 Brittany Farms Road, New Britain, CT 06053; tel. 860/224–3111; Mr. Thomas M V Tolisano
Brook Hollow Health Care Center, LLC, 55 Kondracki Lane, Wallingford, CT 06492; tel. 203/265–6771; Ms. Elizabeth J Schmeizl
Brookview Health Care Facility, 130 Loomis Drive, West Hartford, CT 06107; tel. 860/521–8700; Mr. Clifton P Mix
Caleb Hitchcock Health Center, 40 Loeffler Road, Bloomfield, CT 06002; tel. 860/726–2000; Mr. Waiter Stroly
Cambridge Manor, 2428 Easton Turnpike, Fairfield, CT 06432; tel. 203/372–0313; Ms. Sandy Podany
Carolton Chronic and Convalescent Hospital, 400 Mill Plain Road, Fairfield, CT 06430; tel. 203/255–3573; Ms. Carmen A Tortora
Cedar Lane Rehabilitation and Health Care Center, 128 Cedar Avenue, Waterbury, CT 06705; tel. 203/592–9271; Ms. Joan P Lyke
Center for Optimum Care – Summit, 97 Preston Road, Griswold, CT 06351–2516; tel. 860/376–4438; Mr. Jim Bates
Cherry Brook Health Care Center, 102 Dyer Avenue, Collinsville, CT 06022; tel. 860/693–7777; Ms. Susan J Wilson
Cheshire Convalescent Center, 745 Highland Avenue, Cheshire, CT 06410; tel. 203/272–7285; Ms. Dawn Kolenda
Cheshire House Health Care and Rehabilitation Center, 3396 East Main Street, Waterbury, CT 06705; tel. 203/754–2161; Ms. Marlene L Faust
Chestelm Health & Rehabilitation Center, PO Box 719, Moodus, CT 06469; tel. 860/873–1455; Ms. Brenda E Marinan
Chesterfields Health Care Center, 132 Main Street, Chester, CT 06412; tel. 860/526–5363; Cathleen A O'Connor
Clifton House Rehabilitation Center, 181 Clifton Street, New Haven, CT 06513; tel. 203/467–1666; Mr. Joel Carmichael
Coccomo Memorial Health Care Center, 33 Cone Avenue, Meriden, CT 06450; tel. 203/238–1606; Mr. Brian Foley
Cook Willow Health Center, 81 Hillside Avenue, Plymouth, CT 06782; tel. 860/283–8208; Mr. Henry Lemoi
Country Manor Health Care Center, PO Box 7060, Prospect, CT 06712; tel. 203/758–4431; Mr. Jack Friedler
Countryside Manor, 1660 Stafford Avenue, Bristol, CT 06010; tel. 860/583–8483; Mr. Charles Hallgren
Crescent Manor, 1243 West Main Street, Waterbury, CT 06708–3101; tel. 203/757–0561; Mr. George Giblin
Crestfield Rehabilitation Center and Fenwood Manor, 565 Vernon Street, Manchester, CT 06040; tel. 860/643–5151; Mr. Rolland Castleman
Cromwell Crest Convalescent Home, PO Box 208, Cromwell, CT 06416; tel. 860/635–5613; Mr. Patrick Keaveny
Ellis Manor, 210 George Street, Hartford, CT 06114; tel. 860/296–9166; Mr. Eric M Dana
Elm Hill Nursing Center, 45 Elm Street, Rocky Hill, CT 06067; tel. 860/529–8661; Ms. Lizbeth A Evans
Essex Meadows, 30 Bokum Road, Essex, CT 06426; tel. 860/767–7201; Ms. Jennifer Rannestad
Evergreen Health Care Center, 205 Chestnut Hill Care Center P.O. Box 549, Stafford Springs, CT 06076; tel. 860/684–6341; Mr. David T Panteleakos
Fairview, PO Box 7218, Groton, CT 06340; tel. 860/445–7478; Mr. Jack V Verdeghem
Filosa Convalescent Home, Inc. Hancock Hall, 13 Hakim Street, Danbury, CT 06810; tel. 203/744–3366; Dr. Frank D Malone
Fowler Nursing Center, Inc., 10 Boston Post Road, Guilford, CT 06437; tel. 203/453–3725; Ms. Gail A Jewiss
Gardner Heights, 172 Rocky Rest Road, Shelton, CT 06484; tel. 203/929–1481; Ms. Margaret Bucknall
Geer Nursing and Rehabilitation Center, PO Box 819, Canaan, CT 06018–0819; tel. 860/824–5137; Mr. Anthony J Nania
Gladeview Health Care Center, 60 Boston Post Road, Old Saybrook, CT 06475; tel. 860/388–6696; Ms. Yvette Dobruck
Glastonbury Health Care Center, 1175 Hebron Avenue, Glastonbury, CT 06033; tel. 860/659–1905; Mr. Thomas C Gaccione
Glen Hill Convalescent Center, One Glen Hill Road, Danbury, CT 06811; tel. 203/744–2840; Mr. John Hooker
Golden Heights Health Center, 62 Coleman Street, Bridgeport, CT 06604; tel. 203/367–8444; Mr. Louis P Affinito
Grant Street Health and Rehabilitation Center, 425 Grant Street, Bridgeport, CT 06610; tel. 203/366–5255; Ms. Donna M Deitch
Greenery Rehabilitation Center at Waterbury, 177 Whitewood Road, Waterbury, CT 06708; tel. 203/757–9491; Mr. Earle Hollings
Greentree Healthcare and Rehabilitation Center, 4 Greentree Drive, Waterford, CT 06385; tel. 860/442–0647; Mr. Kenneth S Kopchik
Greenwood Health Care Center, 5 Greenwood Street, Hartford, CT 06106; tel. 860/236–2901; Ms. Veronica Cretella
Groton Regency Nursing and Rehabilitation Center, 1145 Poquonnock Road, Groton, CT 06340; tel. 860/446–9960; Mr. Richard Howard
Grove Manor Nursing Home, Inc., 145 Grove Street, Waterbury, CT 06710; tel. 860/753–7205; Ms. Rose J Schaefer
Hamilton Rehabilitation and Healthcare Center, 50 Palmer Street, Norwich, CT 06360; tel. 860/889–8358; Mr. Phillip A KrakowiakSr.
Harbor Hill Care Center, Inc., 111 Church Street, Middletown, CT 06457; tel. 860/347–7286; Mr. William Thompson
Harbor View Manor, 308 Savin Avenue, West Haven, CT 06516; tel. 203/932–6411; Ms. Betsy Greenwald
Harborside Healthcare – Willows, 225 Amity Road, Woodbridge, CT 06525; tel. 203/387–0076; Terrence M Brennan
Harborside Healthcare – The Reservoir, One Emily Way, West Hartford, CT 06107; tel. 860/561–7022; Mr. Raymond Talamona
Harborside Healthcare Arden House, 850 Mix Avenue, Hamden, CT 06514; tel. 203/281–3500; Ms. Joanne Scafati
Harborside Healthcare Madison House, 34 Wildwood Avenue, Madison, CT 06443; tel. 203/245–8008; Ms. Kathleen Z Dess
Harrington Court, 59 Harrington Court, Colchester, CT 06415; tel. 860/537–2339; Mr. Charles R Carito

Providers / JCAHO Accredited Freestanding Long-Term Care Care Organizations

Hebrew Home and Hospital, Inc., One Abrahms Boulevard, West Hartford, CT 06117-1525; tel. 860/523-3800; Ms. Bonnie Gautier
Heritage Heights Care Center, 22 Hospital Avenue, Danbury, CT 06810; tel. 203/744-3700; Ms. Susan L Jodoin
High View Health Care Center, 600 Highland Avenue, Middletown, CT 06457; tel. 860/347-3315; Mr. Frank Fiore
HillCrest Health Care Center, 5 Richard Brown Drive, Uncasville, CT 06382; tel. 860/848-8466; Mr. Greg Alston
Honey Hill Care Center, 34 Midrocks Drive, Norwalk, CT 06851; tel. 203/847-9686; Ms. Betty A Karkut
Hughes Health and Rehabilitation, Inc., 29 Highland Street, West Hartford, CT 06119; tel. 860/236-5623; Dr. Eugene R Flaxman
Ingraham Manor, 400 North Main Street, Bristol, CT 06010; tel. 860/584-3400; Ms. Linda A Urbanski
Jerome Home, 975 Corbin Avenue, New Britain, CT 06052; tel. 860/229-3707; Mr. John A Kelly
Jewish Home for the Aged, Inc., 169 Davenport Avenue, New Haven, CT 06519; tel. 203/789-1650; Mrs. Maureen Kolacenko
Jewish Home for the Elderly of Fairfield County, Inc., 175 Jefferson Street, Fairfield, CT 06432; tel. 203/365-6400; Mr. Dennis J Magid
Kettle Brook Care Center, LLC, 96 Prospect Hill Road, East Windsor, CT 06088; tel. 860/623-9846; Mr. Bruce Wood
Kimberly Hall South, One Emerson Drive, Windsor, CT 06095; tel. 860/688-6443; Mr. Allan DeBlasio
Laurel Woods, Inc., 451 North High Street, East Haven, CT 06512; tel. 203/466-6850; Mr. Robert M Mislow
Laurelwood Rehabilitation and Skilled Nursing Center, 642 Danbury Road, Ridgefield, CT 06877; tel. 203/438-8226; Ms. Polly F Schnell
Ledgecrest Health Care Center, Inc., PO Box 453, Kensington, CT 06037; tel. 860/828-0583; Mr. Jarrett McClurg
Liberty Specialty Care Center, Inc., 36 Broadway, Colchester, CT 06415; tel. 860/537-4606; Ms. Mary Filloramo
Litchfield Woods Health Care Center, 255 Roberts Street, Torrington, CT 06790; tel. 860/489-5801; Ms. Ilene Epstine
Lord Chamberlain Nursing and Rehabilitation Center, 7003 Main Street, Stratford, CT 06497; tel. 203/375-5894; Mr. Martin Sbriglio
Maefair Health Care Center, 21 Maefair Court, Trumbull, CT 06611; tel. 203/459-5152; Mrs. Janet Hansen
Manchester Manor, 385 West Center Street, Manchester, CT 06040; tel. 860/646-0129; Mr. Stephen T Surprenant
Mansfield Center for Nursing and Rehabilitation, 100 Warren Circle, Mansfield, CT 06268; tel. 860/487-2300; Ms. Kathleen Sutherland
Maple View Manor, Inc., 856 Maple Street, Rocky Hill, CT 06067; tel. 860/563-2861; Mr. Thomas E Harris
Mariner Health at Pendleton, 44 Maritime Drive, Mystic, CT 06355; tel. 860/572-1700; Ms. Susan D Peglow
Mariner Health Care at Bride Brook, 23 Liberty Way, Niantic, CT 06357; tel. 860/739-4007; Ms. Dianne Caristo
Mariner Health of Southern Connecticut, 126 Ford Street, Ansonia, CT 06401; tel. 203/736-1100; Ms. Heidi Gil
Marlborough Health Care Center, Inc., 85 Stage Harbor Road, Marlborough, CT 06447; tel. 860/295-9531; Mr. Marvin J Ostreicher
Mary Elizabeth Nursing Center, PO Box 98, Mystic, CT 06355; tel. 860/536-9655; Ms. Lisa A Ferreri
McLean Home, 75 Great Pond Road, Simsbury, CT 06070; tel. 860/658-3700; Mr. David R Bailey
MeadowBrook of Granby, 350 Salmon Brook Street, Granby, CT 06035; tel. 860/653-9888; Ms. Lisa Menapace
Mediplex of Danbury, 107 Osborne Street, Danbury, CT 06810; tel. 203/792-8102; Mr. John Kolanda
Mediplex of Darien, 599 Boston Post Road, Darien, CT 06820; tel. 203/655-7727; Ms. Dorothy Feigin
Mediplex of Greater Hartford, 160 Coventry Street, Bloomfield, CT 06002; tel. 860/243-2995; Mr. Albert Saunders
Mediplex of Newington, 240 Church Street, Newington, CT 06111; tel. 860/667-2256; Ms. Jolene M Trombetta
Mediplex of Southbury, 162 South Britain Road, Southbury, CT 06488; tel. 203/264-9600; Ms. Ann M Rogers

Mediplex of Stamford, 710 Long Ridge Road, Stamford, CT 06902; tel. 203/329-4026; Mr. Andrew Turner
Mediplex of Westport, One Burr Road, Westport, CT 06880; tel. 203/226-4201; Mr. R. John Ramano
Mediplex of Wethersfield, 341 Jordan Lane, Wethersfield, CT 06109; tel. 860/563-0101; Mr. J. Kevin Prisco
Mediplex Rehab and Skilled Nursing Center of Central CT, 261 Summit Street, Plantsville, CT 06479; tel. 860/628-0364; Ms. Lisa Jaser
Mediplex Rehabilitation and Skilled Nursing Ctr of Sthn CT, 2028 Bridgeport Avenue, Milford, CT 06460; tel. 203/877-0371; Ms. Mary J Grabell
MercyKnoll, Inc., 243 Steele Road, W Hartford, CT 06117; tel. 860/236-3503; Irene Holowesko
Meridan Center, 845 Paddock Avenue, Meriden, CT 06450; tel. 203/238-2645; Ms. Marie Lanzillotti
Meridian Manor Corporation, 1132 Meriden Road, Waterbury, CT 06705; tel. 203/757-1228; Mr. James E Cleary
Middlesex Convalescent Center, Inc., 100 Randolph Road, Middletown, CT 06457; tel. 860/344-0353; Mr. Robert M Shepard
Milford Health Care Center, Inc., 195 Platt Street, Milford, CT 06460; tel. 203/878-5958; Mr. Paul E Ulatowski
Miller Memorial Community, 360 Broad Street, Meriden, CT 06450; tel. 860/237-8815; Sister Ann Noonan
Monsignor Bojnowski Manor, 50 Pulaski Street, New Britain, CT 06053; tel. 860/229-0336; Sister M. Deborah Blados
Montowese Health and Rehabilitation Center, Inc., 163 Quinnipiac Avenue, North Haven, CT 06473; tel. 203/624-3303; Ms. Eileen M Khan
New London Rehabilitation and Care Center, 88 Clark Lane, Waterford, CT 06385; tel. 860/442-0471; Mr. Denis Twig
Noble Horizons, 17 Cobble Road, Salisbury, CT 06068; tel. 860/435-9851; Mr. Norman E Harper
Northbridge Health Care Center, 2875 Main Street, Bridgeport, CT 06606; tel. 203/336-0232; Ms. Kathy Pajor
Norwichtown Rehabilitation and Care Center, 93 West Town Street, Norwichtown, CT 06360; tel. 860/889-2614; Ms. Rosemary Clark
Notre Dame Convalescent Home, Inc., 76 West Rocks Road, Norwalk, CT 06851; tel. 203/847-5893; Kenneth B Hugo
Oakcliff Convalescent Home, Inc., 71 Plaza Avenue, Waterbury, CT 06710; tel. 203/753-0060; Mr. Raymond T Cruess
Olympus Healthcare Center, 20 Scott Swamp Road, Farmington, CT 06032; tel. 860/677-7707; Ms. Peggy Coburn
Parkway Pavilion Healthcare, 1157 Enfield Street, Enfield, CT 06082; tel. 860/745-1641; Mr. Terrance Kuzman
Pierce Memorial Baptist Home, Inc., PO Box 326, Brooklyn, CT 06234; tel. 860/774-9050; Mr. Leonard Goldberg
Plainville Health Care Center, Inc., 269 Farmington Avenue, Plainville, CT 06062; tel. 860/747-1637; Ms. katie Coburn
Pomperaug Woods Health Center, 80 Heritage Road, Southbury, CT 06488; tel. 203/262-6555; Ms. Sherri Rhodes
Pope John Paul II Center for Health Care, 33 Lincoln Avenue, Danbury, CT 06810; tel. 203/797-9300; Ms. Diane A Pimentel
Portland Care and Rehabilitation Centre, Inc, 333 Main Street, Portland, CT 06480; tel. 860/342-0370; Mr. Gregory A Yuska
Regency House of Wallingford, 181 East Main Street, Wallingford, CT 06492; tel. 203/265-1661; Mr. Marvin Ostreicher
Rehabilitation and Healthcare Center of Litchfield Hills, 225 Wyoming Avenue, Torrington, CT 06790; tel. 860/482-8563; Christine Marek
Ridgeview Health Care Center, 156 Berlin Road, Cromwell, CT 06416; tel. 860/635-1010; Mr. Ken Lewis
Ridgewood Health Care Facility, Inc., 582 Meriden Avenue, Southington, CT 06489; tel. 860/628-0388; Marcel Leveille
Riverside Health and Rehabilitation Center, Inc, 745 Main Street, East Hartford, CT 06108; tel. 860/289-2791; Ms. Karen H Chadderton
Rose Haven, Ltd., PO Box 157, Litchfield, CT 06759; tel. 860/567-9475; Ms. Linda D Klauber
Saint Christopher's Health Center, 60 Crouch Avenue, Norwich, CT 06360; tel. 860/889-2631; Ms. Lizbeth Evans

Saint Mary Home, Incorporated, 2021 Albany Avenue, West Hartford, CT 06117; tel. 860/570-8200; Mr. Richard Kisher
Saint Regis Health Center, 1354 Chapel Street, New Haven, CT 06511; tel. 203/867-8300; Mr. Robert Hellrigel
Salmon Brook Center, 72 Salmon Brook Drive, Glastonbury, CT 06033; tel. 860/633-5244; Mr. Scott Ziskin
Seabury Retirement Community, 200 Seabury Drive, Bloomfield, CT 06002; tel. 860/286-0243; Mr. John S Mobley
Shady Knoll Health Center, 41 Skokorat Street, Seymour, CT 06483; tel. 203/881-2555; Mr. Robert F Fritz
Sharon Health Care Center, PO Box 1268, Sharon, CT 06069; tel. 860/364-1002; Mr. Peter J Belval
Shelton Lakes Residence and Health Care Center, Inc., 5 Lake Road, Shelton, CT 06484; tel. 203/924-2635; Mr. David Bordonaro
Sheriden Woods Health Care Center, 321 Stonecrest Drive, Bristol, CT 06010; tel. 860/583-1827; Mr. Gene Heavens
Skyview Center Rehabilitation Center, Inc., 35 Marc Drive, Wallingford, CT 06492; tel. 203/265-0981; Mr. Robert Guastella
Sound View Nursing Center, One Care Lane, West Haven, CT 06516; tel. 203/934-7955; Ms. Donna Deitch
Southington Care Center, 45 Meriden Avenue, Southington, CT 06489; tel. 860/621-9559; Ms. Patricia M Walden
Southport Manor Convalescent Center, Inc., 930 Mill Hill Terrace, Southport, CT 06490; tel. 203/259-7894; Mr. Gery P Alexander
St. Elizabeth Health Center, 51 Applegate Lane, East Hartford, CT 06118; tel. 860/568-7520; Mr. Robert Guastella
St. Joseph Living Center, 14 Club Road, Windham, CT 06280; tel. 860/456-1107; Ms. Patricia M Hamill
St. Joseph's Manor, 6448 Main Street, Trumbull, CT 06611-2075; tel. 203/268-6204; Sister Michelle Anne Reho
Sterling Manor, Inc., 870 Burnside Avenue, East Hartford, CT 06108; tel. 860/289-9571; Mr. Thomas Blonski
Subacute Center of Bristol, 23 Fair Street, Forestville, CT 06010; tel. 860/589-2923; Ms. Linda Bradigo
The Center for Optimum Care – Elm City, 50 Mead Street, New Haven, CT 06511; tel. 203/777-3491; Ms. Giovanna Griffin
The Center for Optimum Care – New Haven, 915 Ella T Grasso Boulevard, New Haven, CT 06519; tel. 203/865-5155; Mr. Denis Twig
The Center for Optimum Care – Windham, 595 Valley Street, Willimantic, CT 06226; tel. 860/423-2597; Ms. Anne R Manning
The Center for Optimum Care of Danielson, 111 Westcott Road, Danielson, CT 06239; tel. 860/774-9540; Ms. Judy-Ann Johnson
The Center for Optimum Care Waterford, 171 Rope Ferry Road, Waterford, CT 06385; tel. 860/443-8357; Mr. Garry Preble
The Curtis Home, 380 Crown Street, Meriden, CT 06450; tel. 203/237-4338; Mr. Steven M Jackson
The Elim Park Health Care Center, 140 Cook Hill Road, Cheshire, CT 06410; tel. 203/272-3547; Mr. David MacNeill
The Flora and Mary Hewitt Memorial Hospital, Inc., 45 Maltby Street, Shelton, CT 06484; tel. 203/924-4671; Mr. David Sheehan
The Glendale Center, 4 Hazel Avenue, Naugatuck, CT 06770; tel. 203/723-1456; Ms. Patricia Johnson
The Health Center at Evergreen Woods, 88 Notch Hill Road, North Branford, CT 06471; tel. 203/488-8000; Ms. Jeanne P Kinnard
The Kent, PO Box 340, Kent, CT 06757; tel. 860/927-5368; Ms. Judy Begley
The Lutheran Home of Southbury, 990 Main Street North, Southbury, CT 06488; tel. 203/264-9135; Ms. Linda Garcia
The Mary Wade Home, Incorporated, 118 Clinton Avenue, New Haven, CT 06513; tel. 203/562-7222; Mr. David V Hunter
The Suffield House, One Canal Road, Suffield, CT 06078; tel. 860/668-6111; Mr. Harold J Moffie
The William and Sally Tandet Center for Continuing Care, 146 West Broad Street, Stamford, CT 06902; tel. 203/964-8501; Mr. Daniel Katz
Valerie Manor, 1360 Torringford Street, Torrington, CT 06790; tel. 860/489-1008; Mr. Duncan M Hunter

Providers / JCAHO Accredited Freestanding Long-Term Care Care Organizations

Vernon Manor Health Care Center, 180 Regan Rd, Vernon, CT 06066-2818; tel. 860/871-0385; Ms. Pamela B Klapproth
Victorian Heights Health Care Center, 341 Bidwell Street, Manchester, CT 06040; tel. 860/647-9191; Ms. Linda Odaynik
Village Manor Health Care, 16 Windsor Avenue, Plainfield, CT 06374; tel. 860/564-4081; Mr. Stanley Rodowicz, Jr.
Wadsworth Glen Health Care and Rehabilitation Center, 30 Boston Road, Middletown, CT 06457; tel. 860/346-9299; Ms. Elaine Madden
Walnut Hill Care Center, 55 Grand Street, New Britain, CT 06052; tel. 860/223-3617; Mr. Donald J Griggs
Waterbury Extended Care Facility, 35 Bunker Hill Road, Watertown, CT 06795; tel. 860/274-5428; Mr. John Sweeney
Watrous Nursing Center, 9 Neck Road, Madison, CT 06443; tel. 203/245-9483; Ms. Sharon G Craft
Waveny Care Center, 3 Farm Road, New Canaan, CT 06840; tel. 203/966-8725; Mr. Jeremy M Vickers
Westfield Care and Rehabilitation Center, 65 Westfield Road, Meriden, CT 06450; tel. 203/238-1291; Mr. Scott Duell
Wintonbury Healthcare Center, LLC, 140 Park Avenue, Bloomfield, CT 06002; tel. 860/243-9591; Mr. Robert Salazar
Wolcott Hall Nursing Center, Inc., 215 Forest Street, Torrington, CT 06790; tel. 860/482-8554; Mr. Stephen R Barrett
Wolcott View Manor, Inc., PO Box 6192, Wolcott, CT 06716; tel. 203/879-8066; Mr. Dennis H Cleary
Woodlake at Tolland, 26 Shenipsit Lake Road, Tolland, CT 06084; tel. 860/872-2999; Mr. Marc Lory

DELAWARE
Arbors at New Castle Subacute and Rehabilitation Center, 32 Buena Vista Drive, New Castle, DE 19720; tel. 302/328-2580; Mr. Ronald Y Inglis, Jr.
Harbor Healthcare and Rehabilitation Center, 301 Oceanview Boulevard, Lewes, DE 19958; tel. 302/645-4664; Ms. Christine Evans
Harrison House of Georgetown, 110 West North Street, Georgetown, DE 19947; tel. 302/856-4574; Ms. Carole Daniels
Kentmere Nursing Care Center, 1900 Lovering Avenue, Wilmington, DE 19806; tel. 302/652-3311; Ms. Eileen Mahler
Manor Care Health Services, 5651 Limestone Road, Wilmington, DE 19808; tel. 302/239-8583; Ms. Ruth G Marinelli
Methodist Country House, 4830 Kennett Pike, Wilmington, DE 19807; tel. 302/654-5101; Ms. Susan A Weaver
Parkview Nursing and Rehabilitation Center, 2801 West 6th Street, Wilmington, DE 19805; tel. 302/655-6135; Mr. Steve Silver
Seaford Center Genesis Eldercare Network, 1100 Norman Eskridge Highway, Seaford, DE 19973; tel. 305/629-3575; Mr. Lon Kieffer
Silver Lake Center – Genesis Health Care Network, 1080 Silver Lake Boulevard, Dover, DE 19904; tel. 302/734-5990; Ms. Vickie Cox
St. Francis Care Center at Brackenville, 100 St. Claire Drive, Hockessin, DE 19707; tel. 302/234-5420; Ms. Ruth G Marinelli

DISTRICT OF COLUMBIA
Benjamin King Health Center US Soldiers' and Airmen's Home, 3700 North Capitol Street, NW, Washington, DC 20317-9998; tel. 202/722-3323; Dr. Paul D Gleason
Center For Aging's Health Care Institute, 1380 Southern Avenue Southeast, Washington, DC 20032; tel. 202/279-5880; Mrs. Joyce D Jones
Grant Park Care Center, 5000 Nannie Helen Burroughs Avenue, Northeast, Washington, DC 20019; tel. 202/399-7504; Ms. Rosalind L Wright
The Washington Home and Hospice, 3720 Upton Street, Northwest, Washington, DC 20016-2299; tel. 202/895-0107; Mrs. Lynn C O'Connor
Washington Nursing Facility, 2425 25th Street Southeast, Washington, DC 20020; tel. 202/889-3600; Ms. Gail L Jernigan

FLORIDA
Arbor at Jacksonville, 4101 Southpoint Drive East, Jacksonville, FL 32216; tel. 614/791-2920; Terry Carpenter
Arbors at Baynnet Point, 8132 Hudson Ave, Hudson, FL 34667; tel. 727/863-3100; Mr. Stephen Jones
Arbors at Brandon, 701 Victoria Street, Brandon, FL 33510; tel. 813/681-4220; Ms. Marianne Segel
Arbors at Lakeland, 2020 West Lake Parker Drive, Lakeland, FL 33805; tel. 941/682-7580; Mr. Clark Buurma
Arbors at Orange Park, 1215 Kingsley Avenue, Orange Park, FL 32073; tel. 904/269-8922; Mr. Gary Cook
Arbors at Orlando Subacute and Rehabilitation Center, 1099 West Town Parkway, Altamonte Springs, FL 32714; tel. 407/865-8000; Mr. Wes Carter
Arbors at Pensacola, 235 West Airport Boulevard, Pensacola, FL 32505; tel. 904/857-5200; Mr. Daniel W Healy
Arbors at Safety Harbor, 1410 4th Street North, Safety Harbor, FL 34695; tel. 727/726-1181; Ms. Elizabeth K Barton
Arbors at St. Petersburg, 9393 Park Boulevard, Seminole, FL 34642; tel. 614/791-2920; Mr. Greg Roberts
Arbors at Tallahassee, 1650 Phillips Road, Tallahassee, FL 32308; tel. 850/942-9868; Mr. Allan Davis
Arbors at Tampa, 2811 Campus Hill Drive, Tampa, FL 33612; tel. 614/791-2920; Mr. Rich Kase
Baptist Manor, Inc., 10095 Hillview Road, Pensacola, FL 32514; tel. 850/479-4000; Mr. Edward Ranelli
Bay Pointe Nursing Pavilion, 4201 31st Street South, Saint Petersburg, FL 33712-4051; tel. 727/867-1104; Mr. Kenneth D Hawkins
BayShore Convalescent Center, 16650 West Dixie Highway, North Miami Beach, FL 33160; tel. 305/945-7447; Louis Manzo
Beverly Health and Rehab Center – Port St. Lucie, 1655 Southeast Walton Road, Port Saint Lucie, FL 34952; tel. 561/337-1333; Ms. Emma Dial
Beverly Health and Rehab Center of Brandon, 1465 Oakfield Drive, Brandon, FL 33511; tel. 813/655-0404; Ms. Gwenn San Marco
Beverly Health and Rehab Services – Tarpon Springs, 501 South Walton Avenue, Tarpon Springs, FL 34689; tel. 727/938-2814; Ms. Rose Rager
Beverly Health/Rehabilitation Center – Englewood, 1111 Drury Lane, Englewood, FL 34224; tel. 941/474-9371; Ms. Debra Wurz
Boca Raton Rehabilitation Center, 755 Meadows Road, Boca Raton, FL 33486; tel. 561/391-5200; Mr. Brian Tenney
Bon Secours Maria Manor Nursing Care Center, Inc., 10300 4th Street North, Saint Petersburg, FL 33716; tel. 813/576-1025; Mr. Michael Ward
Boulevard Manor, 2839 South Seacrest Boulevard, Boynton Beach, FL 33435; tel. 561/732-2464; Mr. Loren Braner, Jr.
Brandywyne Lakeside Center, 1801 North Lake Mariam Drive, Winter Haven, FL 33884; tel. 941/293-1989; Mr. Richard W Ebersole
Colonial Care Center, 6300 46th Avenue North, Saint Petersburg, FL 33709; tel. 813/544-1444; Ms. Lynn Fecso
Coquina Center, 170 North Center Street, Ormond Beach, FL 32174; tel. 904/672-7113; Mr. Daniel Charpentier
Countryside Health Care Center, 3825 Countryside Boulevard, Palm Harbor, FL 34684; tel. 813/784-2848; Ms. Frances Cady
Cross Creek Health Care Center, 10040 Hillview Road, Pensacola, FL 32514; tel. 904/474-0570; Mr. Mark Daniels
Darcy Hall of Life Care, 2170 Palm Beach Lakes Blvd, West Palm Beach, FL 33409; tel. 561/683-3333; Ms. Patricia Allard
Deltona Healthcare Rehabilitation Center, 1851 Elkcam Boulevard, Deltona, FL 32725; tel. 904/789-3769; Ms. Renee Rizzuti
Drew Village Rehabilitation, 401 Fairwood Avenue, Clearwater, FL 34619; tel. 813/797-6313; Mr. Richard D Richardson
Edgewater of Waterman Village, 300 Brookfield Avenue, Mount Dora, FL 32757; tel. 352/383-0051; Dale Lind
Egret Cove Center, 550 62nd Street South, Saint Petersburg, FL 33707; tel. 727/347-6151; Ms. Mary Huss
Fairway Oaks Center – Genesis ElderCare, 13806 North 46th Street, Tampa, FL 33613; tel. 813/977-4214; Mr. Robert C Murphy
First Coast Health and Rehabilitation Center, 7723 Jasper Avenue, Jacksonville, FL 32211; tel. 904/725-8044; Ms. Hanna Cook
Florida Club Care Center, 220 Sierra Drive, North Miami Beach, FL 33179; tel. 305/653-8427; Mr. Sid L Schiff
Franco Nursing and Rehabilitation Center, 800 Northwest 95th Street, Miami, FL 33150; tel. 305/836-1550; Mr. Paul A Harris
Gramercy Park Nursing Center, 17475 South Dixie Highway, Miami, FL 33157; tel. 305/255-1045; Emma F Dial
Greenbriar Rehabilitation and Nursing Center, 210 21st Avenue West, Bradenton, FL 34205; tel. 941/747-3786; Ms. Nancy Thurman
Greenbrook Nursing and Rehabilitation Center, 1000 24th Street North, Saint Petersburg, FL 33713; tel. 727/323-4711; Ms. Sandra Ryczek
Greynolds Park Manor Rehabilitation Center, 17400 West Dixie Highway, North Miami Beach, FL 33160; tel. 305/944-2361; Mr. Martin E Casper
Hallandale Rehabilitation Center, 2400 E Hallandale Beach Blvd, Hallandale, FL 33009; tel. 954/457-9717; Ms. Beverly T Eliahu
Harborside – Pinebrook, 1240 Pinebrook Road, Venice, FL 34292; tel. 941/488-6733; Ms. Connie S Tolley
Harborside Healthcare of Palm Harbor, 2600 Highlands Boulevard, N, Palm Harbor, FL 34684; tel. 727/785-5671; Mr. Timothy J Selleck
Harborside Healthcare – Brevard, 1775 Huntington Lane, Rockledge, FL 32955; tel. 407/632-7341; Mr. Stephen Guillard
Harborside Healthcare – Clearwater, 1980 Sunset Point Road, Clearwater, FL 34625; tel. 813/443-1588; Marie L Seger
Harborside Healthcare – Gulf Coast, 4927 Voorhees Road, New Port Richey, FL 34653; tel. 727/848-3578; Mr. James M Kobrick
Harborside Healthcare – Ocala, 1501 Southeast 24th Road, Ocala, FL 34471; tel. 352/629-8900; Mr. Steve Watson
Harborside Healthcare – Sarasota, 4602 Northgate Court, Sarasota, FL 34234; tel. 941/355-2913; Mr. Anthony Brunicardi
Harborside Healthcare – Tampa Bay, 3865 Tampa Road, Oldsmar, FL 34677; tel. 813/855-4661; Ms. Michele Forney
Harborside Healthcare of Naples, 2900 12th Street, North, Naples, FL 34103; tel. 941/261-2554; Mr. Brad Evans
HCR/ManorCare, 375 Northwest 51st Street, Boca Raton, FL 33431; tel. 561/997-8111; Ms. Dieudegrace Achille
Heartland Health Care and Rehabilitation Center, 7225 Boca Del Mar Drive, Boca Raton, FL 33433-5517; tel. 561/362-9644; Mr. R. Kevin Mcfeely
Heartland Health Care and Rehabilitation Center, 5401 Sawyer Drive, Sarasota, FL 34233; tel. 941/925-3427; Ms. Teresa Martin
Heartland Health Care and Rehabilitation Center/Sunrise, 9711 W Oakland Park Boulevard, Sunrise, FL 33351; tel. 954/572-4000; Ms. Joylin Nation
Heartland Health Care Center – Fort Myers, 1600 Matthew Drive, Fort Myers, FL 33907; tel. 941/275-6067; Ms. Nancy Zant
Heartland Health Care Center – Jacksonville, 8495 Normandy Boulevard, Jacksonville, FL 32221; tel. 904/783-3749; Ms. Jan Davis
Heartland Health Care Center Miami Lakes, 5725 Northwest 186th Street, Hialeah, FL 33015; tel. 305/625-9857; Mr. Bill Tippins
Heartland Health Care Center of Kendall, 9400 Southwest 137th Avenue, Kendall, FL 33186; tel. 305/385-8290; Mr. David Chamberlain
Heartland Healthcare Center – Boynton Beach, 3600 Old Boynton Road, Boynton Beach, FL 33436; tel. 561/736-9992; Mr. James Lawless
Heartland Healthcare Center – Prosperity Oaks, 11375 Prosperity Farms Road, Palm Beach Gardens, FL 33410; tel. 561/626-9702; Mrs. Sally Gates
Heartland of Brooksville, 575 Lamar Avenue, Brooksville, FL 34601; tel. 352/799-2226; Ms. Linda Howard
Heartland of Tamarac, 5901 Northwest 79th Avenue, Tamarac, FL 33321; tel. 954/722-7001; Mrs. Pamela Green–Allison
Heartland of Zephyrhills, 38220 Henry Drive, Zephyrhills, FL 33540; tel. 813/788-7114; Ms. Susan Shoffstall
Heritage Health Care Center, 1815 Ginger Drive, Tallahassee, FL 32308; tel. 904/877-2177; Mr. Chuck Cascio
Highlands Lake Center, 4240 Lakeland Highlands Road, Lakeland, FL 33813; tel. 941/646-8699; Ms. Dawn Jones
Holmes Regional Nursing Center, 606 East Sheridan Road, Melbourne, FL 32901; tel. 407/727-7990; Ms. Mary Peebles
Horizon Specialty and Rehabilitation Center, 221 Park Place Boulevard, Kissimmee, FL 34741; tel. 407/935-0200; Mr. Stephen C Brown
Human Resources Health Center, 2500 Northwest 22nd Avenue, Miami, FL 33142; tel. 305/638-6661; Ira C Clark

Providers / JCAHO Accredited Freestanding Long-Term Care Care Organizations

IHS at Greenbriar, 9820 North Kendall Drive, Miami, FL 33176; tel. 305/271-6311; Mr. Gary Duncanson

IHS of Florida NO. 8, Inc., 200 16th Avenue Southeast, Largo, FL 33771; tel. 727/585-9377; Ms. Mary Bladen

Indian River Center - Genesis ElderCare, 7201 Greenboro Drive, West Melbourne, FL 32904; tel. 407/727-0990; Ms. Kathryn Kondolf-Harmer

Integrated Health Services at Brandon, 702 South Kings Avenue, Brandon, FL 33511; tel. 813/651-1818; Mr. Bernardo J Carotenuto

Integrated Health Services at Gainesville, 4000 Southwest 20th Avenue, Gainesville, FL 32607; tel. 357/377-1981; Ms. Terrye Dubberly

Integrated Health Services of Florida at Clearwater, 2055 Palmetto Street, Clearwater, FL 34625; tel. 813/461-6613; Ms. Anne Dougherty

Integrated Health Services of Florida at Lake Worth, 1201 12th Avenue South, Lake Worth, FL 33460; tel. 561/586-7404; Adela Baldo

Integrated Health Services of Fort Myers, 13755 Golf Club Parkway, Fort Myers, FL 33919; tel. 941/482-2848; Mr. Walter R Grabda

Integrated Health Services of Jacksonville, 1650 Fouraker Road, Jacksonville, FL 32221; tel. 904/786-8668; Mr. Christopher J Warrick

Integrated Health Services of Palm Bay, 1515 Port Malabar Boulevard, Palm Bay, FL 32905; tel. 407/723-1235; Mr. Gregory Roberts

Integrated Health Services of Pinellas Park, 8701 49th Street North, Pinellas Park, FL 33782; tel. 727/546-4661; Mr. Patrick Dauchot

Laurels Nursing & Rehabilitation Center, 550 9th Avenue South, Saint Petersburg, FL 33701; tel. 813/898-4105; Ms. Laurel J Chadwick

Manor Care Boynton Beach, 3001 South Congress Avenue, Boynton Beach, FL 33426; tel. 561/737-5600; Mr. R Kevin McFeely

ManorCare Health Services, 6931 West Sunrise Boulevard, Plantation, FL 33313; tel. 954/583-6200; Ms. Gilda Anderson

ManorCare Health Services, 870 Patricia Avenue, Dunedin, FL 34698; tel. 727/734-8861; Ms. Carrie Lund

ManorCare Health Services - Carrollwood, 3030 West Bearss Avenue, Tampa, FL 33618; tel. 813/968-8777; Ms. Carmen Telot

Mariner Health of Atlantic Shores, 4251 Stack Boulevard, Melbourne, FL 32901; tel. 407/953-2219; Mr. Gary L Krulewitz

Mariner Health of Belleair, 1150 Ponce de Leon Boulevard, Clearwater, FL 33756; tel. 727/585-5491; Mr. Patrick Neil Heird

Mariner Health of Clearwater, 4470 East Bay Drive, Clearwater, FL 33764; tel. 727/530-7100; Ms. Christina M Johnson

Mariner Health of Deland, 1200 North Stone Street, Deland, FL 32720; tel. 904/734-6200; Mr. Merle W Zinck

Mariner Health of Palm City, 2505 Southwest Martin Highway, Palm City, FL 34990; tel. 561/288-0060; Mr. Don Cochran

Mariner Health of Palmetto, 926 Haben Boulevard, Palmetto, FL 34221; tel. 941/722-0553; Mr. Joseph Keenan

Mariner Health of Port Orange, 5600 Victoria Gardens Blvd, Port Orange, FL 32127; tel. 904/760-7773; Mr. Jon Marc Creighton

Mariner Health of Port St. Lucie, 1800 Southeast Hillmoor Drive, Port Saint Lucie, FL 34952; tel. 561/337-3565; Mrs. Carol Resetco

Mariner Health of St. Augustine, 200 Mariner Health Way, Saint Augustine, FL 32086; tel. 904/797-1800; Mr. Brian M Ferguson

Mariner Health of Tuskawilla, 1024 Willa Springs Drive, Winter Springs, FL 32708; tel. 407/699-5506; Mr. Gary Beaulieu

Marion House Health Care Center, 3930 E Silver Springs Blvd, Ocala, FL 34470; tel. 352/236-2626; Ms. Debbie Wesch

Medicana Nursing Center, 1710 Lake Worth Road, Lake Worth, FL 33460; tel. 561/582-5331; Ms. Maraleita K Jackson

Mediplex Rehab - Bradenton, 5627 Ninth Street East, Bradenton, FL 34203; tel. 941/753-8941; Ms. Anita Faulmann

Menorah Manor, Inc., 255 59th Street North, Saint Petersburg, FL 33710; tel. 727/345-2775; Mr. Marshall Seiden

Miami Jewish Home & Hospital for the Aged, 5200 Northeast 2nd Avenue, Miami, FL 33137; tel. 305/751-8626; Mr. Terry Goodman

Moody Manor, Inc., 7150 Holatee Trail, Fort Lauderdale, FL 33330; tel. 954/434-2016; Mrs. Patricia A Moody

New Horizon Rehabilitation Center, 635 Southeast 17th Street, Ocala, FL 34471; tel. 352/629-7921; Ms. Susan N Chancellor

NHC HealthCare - Hudson, PO Box 5487, Hudson, FL 34667; tel. 727/863-1521; Mr. David Cross

North Florida Rehabilitation and Specialty Care Center, 6700 Northwest 10th Place, Gainesville, FL 32605; tel. 352/331-3111; Mr. George Hamilton

Oak Manor Nursing Center, 3500 Oak Manor Lane, Largo, FL 33774; tel. 813/581-9427; Mr. Robert E Rice

Oakwood Terrace Skilled Nursing & Rehabilitation Cntr, 18905 Northeast 25th Avenue, Aventura, FL 33180; tel. 305/932-6360; Mr. Jon C Aaron

Ormond in the Pines, 103 N Clyde Morris Boulevard, Ormond Beach, FL 32174; tel. 904/673-0450; Ms. Ross Baird

Palm Court Nursing and Rehabilitation Center, 2675 North Andrews Avenue, Fort Lauderdale, FL 33311; tel. 954/563-5711; Ms. Susan Compton

Palm Garden - Jacksonville, 5725 Spring Park Road, Jacksonville, FL 32216; tel. 904/733-6954; Mr. James McCarver

Palm Garden - Orlando, 654 Econlockhatchee Trail, Orlando, FL 32825; tel. 407/273-6158; Mrs. Eloise Abrahams

Palm Garden of Clearwater, 3480 McMullen Booth Road, Clearwater, FL 34621; tel. 727/786-6697; Mr. Roy Meredith

Palm Garden of Gainesville, 227 Southwest 62nd Boulevard, Gainesville, FL 32607; tel. 352/331-0601; Mr. Dwight D Osteen

Palm Garden of Lake City, 920 McFarlane Avenue, Lake City, FL 32025; tel. 904/758-4777; Ms. Sharon Tervola

Palm Garden of Largo, 10500 Starkey Road, Largo, FL 33777; tel. 813/397-8166; Mr. David W Cross

Palm Garden of Ocala, 3400 Southwest 27th Avenue, Ocala, FL 34474; tel. 352/854-6262; Ms. Jennifer Seall

Palm Garden of Tampa, 3612 East 138th Avenue, Tampa, FL 33613; tel. 813/972-8775; Mr. Richard G Moss

Palm Garden of West Palm Beach, 300 Executive Center Drive, West Palm Beach, FL 33401; tel. 561/471-5566; Ms. Peggy Booth

Palmetto Health Center, 6750 West 22nd Court, Hialeah, FL 33016-3918; tel. 305/823-3119; Ms. Rosemary Wedderspoon NHA,BHSA

Perdue Medical Center, 19590 Old Cutler Road, Miami, FL 33157; tel. 305/233-8931; Mr. Ira C Clark

Regents Park of Boca Raton, 6363 Verde Trail, Boca Raton, FL 33433; tel. 561/483-9282; Mr. Stanley H Sternefeld, Jr.

Regents Park of Jacksonville, 7130 Southside Boulevard, Jacksonville, FL 32256; tel. 904/642-7300; Ms. Patricia Hammond

Regents Park of Winter Park, 558 North Semoran Boulevard, Winter Park, FL 32792; tel. 407/679-1515; Ms. Linda Karling

Renova Health Care Center, 750 Bayberry Drive, Lake Park, FL 33403; tel. 561/844-4396; Mr. Richard D Richardson

River Garden Hebrew Home for the Aged, 11401 Old Saint Augustine Road, Jacksonville, FL 32258; tel. 904/260-1818; Mr. Elliott Palevsky

Sabal Palms Health Care Center, 499 Alternate Keene Road, Largo, FL 33771; tel. 813/586-4211; Ms. Susan Hunter

Shore Acres Rehabilitation and Nursing Center, 4500 Indianapolis Street NE, Saint Petersburg, FL 33703; tel. 813/527-5801; Ms. April Doherty

Southern Pines Nursing Center, 6140 Congress Street, New Port Richey, FL 34653; tel. 813/842-8402; Ms. Rebecca Miller

Spanish Gardens Nursing Center, 1061 Virginia Street, Dunedin, FL 34698; tel. 727/733-4189; Mr. Robert A Delimon

St. Anne's Nursing Center, 11855 Quail Roost Drive, Miami, FL 33177; tel. 305/252-4000; Ms. Cynthia Palermo

St. Catherine Labouré' Manor, 1750 Stockton Street, Jacksonville, FL 32204; tel. 904/308-4700; Ms. Maureen F Gartland

Sun Health of the Palm Beaches, 6414 13th Road South, West Palm Beach, FL 33415; tel. 561/478-9900; Mr. Robert Beebee

Sunrise Health and Rehabilitation Center, 4800 Nob Hill Road, Sunrise, FL 33351; tel. 954/748-3400; Mr. John Corrado

Sutton Place Center, 4405 Lakewood Road, Lake Worth, FL 33461; tel. 561/969-1400; Mr. Garland W Cline

Swanholm Nursing and Rehabilitation Center, 6200 Central Avenue, Saint Petersburg, FL 33707; tel. 727/347-5196; Mr. Paul F Jeannotte, Jr.

Tandem Healthcare of Melbourne, 3033 Serno Road, Melbourne, FL 32934; tel. 321/791-2920; Mr. Lawerence Deering

The Fountains Nursing Home, 3800 North Federal Highway, Boca Raton, FL 33431; tel. 561/395-7510; Ms. Helen Kots

The Riverwood Center - Genesis ElderCare Network, 2802 Parental Home Road, Jacksonville, FL 32216; tel. 904/721-0088; Mr. Larry A Montroy

Tierra Pines Center, 7380 Ulmerton Road, Largo, FL 33771; tel. 727/535-9833; Ms. Carol Sweetland

TimberRidge Nursing and Rehabilitation Center, 9848 Southwest 110th Street, Ocala, FL 34481; tel. 352/854-8200; Ms. Caroline Smith

University Village Health Center, 12250 North 22nd Street, Tampa, FL 33612; tel. 813/975-5001; Ms. Patrice E Pelletier-Sanders

Washington Manor Nursing and Rehabilitation Center, 4200 Washington Street, Hollywood, FL 33021; tel. 954/981-6300; John J Wall, Jr.

Water's Edge Extended Care, 1500 Southwest Capri Street, Palm City, FL 34990; tel. 561/283-7775; Mr. Jon P Tagatz

Whitehall Boca Raton, 7300 Del Prado South, Boca Raton, FL 33433; tel. 561/392-3000; Mr. P. Steven Mulder

GEORGIA

American Transitional Care - Northside, 5470 Meridian Mark Road, Atlanta, GA 30342; tel. 404/256-5131; Ms. Jeanine Braaten

Ashton Woods Rehabilitation Center, 3535 Ashton Woods Drive NE, Atlanta, GA 30319; tel. 770/451-0236; Bobby Stigler

Azalea Trace Nursing Center, 910 Talbotton Road, Columbus, GA 31904; tel. 706/323-9513; Barbara Mitchell

Beverly Health and Rehabilitation Center, 2650 Highway 138 SE, Jonesboro, GA 30236; tel. 770/473-4436; Ms. JoEllen Rogers

Brian Center Nursing Center / Powder Springs, 3460 Powder Springs Road, Powder Springs, GA 30073; tel. 770/439-9199; Ms. Susan J McKinley

Budd Terrace, 1833 Clifton Road Northeast, Atlanta, GA 30329; tel. 404/728-4975; Mr. Larry Minnix

Dogwood Health and Rehabilitation, 7560 Butner Road, Fairburn, GA 30213; tel. 770/306-7878; Ms. Kay Beckworth

Dublinair Health Care and Rehabilitation Center, PO Box 1243, Dublin, GA 31040; tel. 912/272-7437; Ms. Janet N Munday

Family Life Enrichment Centers, Inc., PO Box 10, High Shoals, GA 30645; tel. 706/769-7738; Ms. Magda D Bennett

Georgia War Veterans Nursing Home, 1101 15th Street, Augusta, GA 30901; tel. 706/721-2531; Mr. Charles Esposito

Green Acres Nursing Home, 313 Allen Memorial Drive SW, Milledgeville, GA 31061; tel. 912/453-9437; Ms. Jay Nelson

Harvest Heights Nursing Home, 3200 Panthersville Road, Decatur, GA 30034; tel. 404/212-3400; Mr. David Harrell

IHS of Atlanta at Shoreham, 811 Kennesaw Avenue, Marietta, GA 30060; tel. 770/422-2451; Mr. Scott Herndon

Integrated Health Services of Atlanta at Briarcliff Haven, 1000 Briarcliff Road Northeast, Atlanta, GA 30306; tel. 404/875-6456; Mr. Richard Kennedy

Integrated Health Services of Atlanta at Buckhead, 54 Peachtree Park Drive, Atlanta, GA 30309; tel. 404/351-6041; Mr. Herbert L Patton, Jr.

Life Care Center of Gwinnett, 3850 Safehaven Drive, Lawrenceville, GA 30244; tel. 770/923-0005; Mrs. Cheri Underwood

Lilburn Geriatric Center, 788 Indian Trail Road, Lilburn, GA 30047; tel. 770/923-2020; Mr. Melvin Moses

Magnolia Manor Nursing Center, 2001 South Lee Street, Americus, GA 31709; tel. 912/924-9352; Mr. Tom Cronemeyer

Mariner Health of Northeast Atlanta, 1500 South Johnson Ferry Road, Atlanta, GA 30319; tel. 404/252-2002; Ms. Marrianne Wiesen

Marion Memorial Nursing Home, PO Box 197, Buena Vista, GA 31803; tel. 912/649-2331; Ms. Faye Lane

Montezuma Health Care Center, PO Box 639, Montezuma, GA 31063; tel. 912/472-8168; Mrs. Merle Baggett

Providers / JCAHO Accredited Freestanding Long-Term Care Care Organizations

Oak Manor Nursing Home, Inc. / Pine Manor Nursing Home, Inc., PO Box 8828, Columbus, GA 31908-8828; tel. 706/324-0387; Mr. James S Wilson

Quinton Memorial Health Care and Rehabilitation Center, 1114 Burleyson Road, Dalton, GA 30720; tel. 706/226-4642; Ms. Patricia W Haynes

Riverside Nursing Center / Thomaston, 101 Old Talbotton Road, Thomaston, GA 30286; tel. 706/647-8161; Ms. Sue G Estes

Southland Nursing Home, Inc., PO Box 2747, Peachtree City, GA 30269; tel. 770/631-9000; Mr. Gary Massengale

Starcrest of Lithonia, PO Box 855, Lithonia, GA 30058; tel. 770/482-2961; Mr. Tony Eatherly

Windermere, 3618 J Dewey Gray Circle, Augusta, GA 30909; tel. 706/860-7572; Mr. Tom Turner

Winthrop Manor Nursing Center, 12 Chateau Drive, Rome, GA 30161; tel. 706/235-1422; Mr. Bruce Behner

HAWAII

Life Care Center of Hilo, 944 West Kawailani Street, Hilo, HI 96720; tel. 808/959-9151; Mr. Fred Horwitz

IDAHO

Life Care Center of Boise, 808 North Curtis Road, Boise, ID 83706; tel. 208/376-5273; Ms. Ann Swenson

Rexburg Nursing Center, 660 South 200 West, Rexburg, ID 83440; tel. 208/356-0220; Mr. Kent Kellersberger

ILLINOIS

Advocate Transitional Care Center, 10124 South Kedzie Avenue, Evergreen Park, IL 60642; tel. 708/636-9200; Ms. Joanne Jurkovic

Alden Estates of Evanston, 2520 Gross Point Road, Evanston, IL 60201; tel. 847/328-6000; Mr. Floyd A Schlossberg

Alden Poplar Creek - Rehabilitation & Hlth Care Ctr, 1545 Barrington Road, Hoffman Estates, IL 60194; tel. 847/884-0011; Mr. Floyd A Schlossberg

Alden Rehabilitation and Health Care Center - Heather, 15600 South Honore, Harvey, IL 60426; tel. 708/333-9550; Ms. Tonya Hackney

Alden Rehabilitation and Health Care Center - Lakeland, 820 West Lawrence Avenue, Chicago, IL 60640; tel. 773/769-2570; Mr. Floyd A Schlosserg

Alden Rehabilitation and Health Care Center - Morrow, 5001 South Michigan, Chicago, IL 60615; tel. 773/924-9292; Mr. Floyd A Schlossberg

Alden Rehabilitation and Health Care Center - Northmoor, 5831 North Northwest Highway, Chicago, IL 60631; tel. 773/775-8080; Mr. Floyd A Schlossberg

Alden Rehabilitation and Health Care Center - Princeton, 255 West 69th Street, Chicago, IL 60621; tel. 773/224-5900; Mr. Floyd A Schlossberg

Alden Rehabilitation and Health Care Center - Wentworth, 201 West 69th Street, Chicago, IL 60621; tel. 773/487-1200; Mr. Floyd A Schlossberg

Alden Rehabilitation and Health Care Center-Lincoln Pk, 504 West Wellington Avenue, Chicago, IL 60657; tel. 773/281-6200; Mr. Floyd A Schlossberg

Alden Rehabilitation and Health Care Center/Long Grove, Box 2308 RFD, Hickes Road, Long Grove, IL 60047; tel. 847/438-8275; Mr. Floyd A Schlossberg

Alden Rehabilitation and Health Care Center/Naperville, 1525 Oxford Lane, Naperville, IL 60565; tel. 630/983-0500; Mr. Floyd A Schlossberg

Alden Rehabilitation and Health Care Center/Orland Park, 16450 South 97th Avenue, Orland Park, IL 60462; tel. 708/403-6500; Mr. Floyd A Schlossberg

Alden Rehabilitation and Health Care Center/Town Manor, 6120 West Ogden Avenue, Cicero, IL 60804; tel. 708/863-0500; Mr. Floyd A Schlossberg

Alden Rehabilitation and Health Care Cnter-Valley Ridge, 275 Army Trail Road, Bloomingdale, IL 60108; tel. 630/893-9616; Mr. Floyd A Schlossberg

Alden Terrace of McHenry, 803 Royal Drive, Mc Henry, IL 60050; tel. 815/344-2600; Mr. Floyd A Schlossberg

Alma Nelson Manor, Inc., 550 South Mulford Road, Rockford, IL 61108; tel. 815/399-4914; Vickie M Zimmerman

Anchorage of Beecher, 1201 Dixie Highway, Beecher, IL 60401; tel. 708/946-2600; Ms. Marcia Quale

Applewood Nursing and Rehabilitation Center, 21020 Kostner Avenue, Matteson, IL 60443; tel. 708/747-1300; Ms. Heidi Smith

ASTA Care Center of Bloomington, 1509 North Calhoun Street, Bloomington, IL 61701; tel. 309/827-6046; Ms. Patricia A Grady

ASTA Care Center of Elgin, 134 North McLean Boulevard, Elgin, IL 60123; tel. 847/742-8822; Ms. Karen E Kemp

ASTA Care Center of Rockford, 707 West Riverside Boulevard, Rockford, IL 61103; tel. 815/877-5752; Mr. Micheal Gillman

ASTA Care Center of Toluca, Rural Route 1, Box 205, Toluca, IL 61369; tel. 815/452-2367; Ms. Terri Taylor

Barton W. Stone Christian Home, 873 Grove Street, Jacksonville, IL 62650; tel. 217/479-3400; Mrs. Barbara L Hannel

Bethany Terrace Nursing Centre, 8425 North Waukegan Road, Morton Grove, IL 60053; tel. 847/965-8100; Mr. Kenneth Kolich

Bethesda Home and Retirement Center, 2833 North Nordica Avenue, Chicago, IL 60634; tel. 773/622-6144; Ms. Carol Page Beecher

Brentwood North, 3705 Deerfield Road, Riverwoods, IL 60015; tel. 847/459-1200; Mr. Jerome J Aniolowski

Brightview Care Center, 4538 North Beacon Street, Chicago, IL 60640; tel. 773/275-7200; Ms. Ahuva Weinreb

California Gardens Nursing and Rehabilitation Center, 2829 S California Boulevard, Chicago, IL 60608; tel. 773/847-8061; Farhat Sharif

Care Centre of Champaign, 1915 South Mattis, Champaign, IL 61821; tel. 217/352-0516; Ms. Jane Flewelling

Care Centre of Urbana, 907 North Lincoln Avenue, Urbana, IL 61801; tel. 217/367-8421; Ms. Jess Coles

Care Centre of Wauconda, 176 Thomas Court, Wauconda, IL 60084; tel. 847/526-5551; Shael Bellows

Carrington Care Center, 759 Kane Street, South Elgin, IL 60177; tel. 847/697-3310; Mr. Steven Goldstein

Chateau Village Nursing and Rehabilitation Center, 7050 Madison Street, Willowbrook, IL 60521; tel. 630/323-6380; Mr. Alford Grayson

Chevy Chase Nursing and Rehabilitation Center, 3400 South Indiana Avenue, Chicago, IL 60616; tel. 312/842-5000; Mr. Barry Carr

Clark Manor Convalescent Center, 7433 North Clark, Chicago, IL 60626; tel. 773/338-8778; Mr. Mark Schlicting

Colonial Hall Center, 515 Bureau Valley Parkway, Princeton, IL 61356; tel. 815/875-3347; Mr. Robert D Yearian

Community HealthCare Centers, 1136 North Mill Street, Naperville, IL 60563-2580; tel. 630/355-3300; Mr. Norm Gross

Continental Care Center, 5336 North Western Avenue, Chicago, IL 60625; tel. 773/271-5600; Ms. Monica L Ramirez

Council for Jewish Elderly - Lieberman Geriatric Health Ctr, 9700 Gross Point Road, Skokie, IL 60076; tel. 847/674-7210; Mr. Ronald Weismehl

Countryside Care Centre, 2330 West Galena Boulevard, Aurora, IL 60506; tel. 630/896-4686; Shael Bellows

Crestwood Care Centre, 14255 South Cicero Avenue, Crestwood, IL 60445; tel. 708/371-0400; Ms. Jeanette Fox

Danville Care Center, 1701 North Bowman Avenue, Danville, IL 61832; tel. 217/443-2955; Mrs. Cathie Bailey

Deerbrook Care Centre, 306 North Larkin Avenue, Joliet, IL 60435; tel. 815/744-5560; Shael Bellows

Dolton Health Care and Rehabilitation Centre, 14325 South Blackstone Avenue, Dolton, IL 60419; tel. 708/849-5000; Ms. Roxane Goad

Douglas Healthcare Center, PO Box 978, Mattoon, IL 61938; tel. 217/234-6401; Ms. Teresa L Dunsbergen

DuPage Convalescent Center, PO Box 708, Wheaton, IL 60187; tel. 630/665-6400; Mr. Ronald R Reinecke

Elmhurst Extended Care Center, Inc., 200 East Lake Street, Elmhurst, IL 60126; tel. 630/834-4337; Mr. John Massard

Elmwood Center, 1017 West Galena Boulevard, Aurora, IL 60506; tel. 630/897-3100; Ms. Kathryn DyHouse

Fairmont Care Centre, 5061 North Pulaski Road, Chicago, IL 60630; tel. 773/604-8112; Ms. Theresa J Smelser

Farmington Center, PO Box 109, Farmington, IL 61531; tel. 309/245-2407; Ms. Vicki S Hoke

Flora HealthCare Center, 120 Frontage Road, Flora, IL 62839; tel. 618/662-8381; Ms. Jane Melton

Flora Pavilion Nursing Home Center, Inc., 701 Shadwell Avenue, Flora, IL 62839-0309; tel. 618/662-8361; Mr. Bradley Alter

Forest Villa Nursing Center, 6840 West Touhy Avenue, Niles, IL 60714; tel. 847/647-8994; Mr. Michael Kaplan

Garden View Nursing and Rehabilitation Center, 6450 North Ridge Avenue, Chicago, IL 60626; tel. 773/743-8700; Andre' A Matlock

Geneseo Good Samaritan Village, 704 South Illinois Street, Geneseo, IL 61254; tel. 309/944-6424; Michael J Olsen

Genesis Lemont Center, 12450 Walker Road, Lemont, IL 60439; tel. 630/243-0400; Ms. Sara J Szumski

Glen Elston Nursing and Rehabilitation Centre, Ltd, 4340 North Keystone Avenue, Chicago, IL 60641; tel. 773/545-8700; Mr. Steven Schayer

Glen Oaks Nursing and Rehabilitation Centre, Ltd, 270 Skokie Boulevard, Northbrook, IL 60062; tel. 847/498-9320; Mr. Simcha Dachs

GlenBridge Nursing and Rehabilitation Center, Ltd, 8333 West Golf Road, Niles, IL 60714; tel. 847/966-9190; Mr. Jeffrey Garkinkel

Glencrest Nursing and Rehabilitation Centre, 2451 West Touhy Avenue, Chicago, IL 60645; tel. 773/338-6800; Mr. Joshua Ray

GlenShire Nursing and Rehabilitation Centre, Ltd., 22660 South Cicero Avenue, Richton Park, IL 60471; tel. 708/747-6120; Ms. Sherry L Bengtson

Glenview Terrace Nursing Center, 1511 Greenwood Road, Glenview, IL 60025; tel. 847/729-9090; Mr. Mark Hollander

Glenwood Heaalthcare and Rehab, 19330 Cottage Grove, Glenwood, IL 60425; tel. 708/758-6200; Ms. Irene Glass

Halsted Terrace Nursing Centre, 10935 South Halsted, Chicago, IL 60628; tel. 773/928-2000; Mr. Mark Hollander

Hampton Plaza Health Care Center, 9777 Greenwood, Niles, IL 60714; tel. 847/967-7000; Mr. Burton Behr

Harmony Nursing and Rehabilitation Center, 3919 West Foster Avenue, Chicago, IL 60625; tel. 773/588-9500; Mr. Mark Hollander

HCR ManorCare, 600 West Ogden Avenue, Hinsdale, IL 60521; tel. 630/325-9630; Mr. John F Vrba

Heartland Health Care Center, 833 16th Avenue, Moline, IL 61265; tel. 309/764-6744; Ms. Vickie J Toomsen

Heartland Health Care Center - Galesburg, 280 East Losey Street, Galesburg, IL 61401; tel. 309/343-2166; Ms. Kathy Karr

Heartland Health Care Center - Henry, PO Box 215, Henry, IL 61537; tel. 309/364-3905; Ms. Susan M Legner

Heartland Health Care Center - Homewood, 940 Maple Avenue, Homewood, IL 60430; tel. 708/799-0244; Mr. K.P. Henricks

Heartland Health Care Center - Macomb, 8 Doctors Lane, Macomb, IL 61455; tel. 309/833-5555; Ms. Christie Butler

Heartland Health Care Center - Paxton, 1001 East Pells Street, Paxton, IL 60957; tel. 217/379-4361; Mrs. Cindy Sharp

Heartland Health Care Center of Canton, 2081 North Main Street, Canton, IL 61520; tel. 309/647-6135; Mr. Gail McGinnis

Holy Family Health Center, 2380 East Dempster Street, Des Plaines, IL 60016-4898; tel. 847/296-3335; Sister Mary Elizabeth

IHS Chicago at Governors Park, 1420 South Barrington Road, Barrington, IL 60010; tel. 847/382-6664; Ms. Lori Schuetz

Illini Restorative Care Center, 1455 Hospital Road, Silvis, IL 61282; tel. 309/792-7614; Ms. Barbara Mask

Integrated Health Services at Brentwood, 5400 West 87th Street, Burbank, IL 60459; tel. 708/423-1200; Mr. Kam McGavock

Jackson Square Nursing and Rehabilitation Center, 5130 West Jackson Boulevard, Chicago, IL 60644; tel. 773/921-8000; Mr. Barry Carr

Lake Shore HealthCare and Rehabilitation Centre, 7200 North Sheridan Road, Chicago, IL 60626; tel. 773/973-7200; Mr. James R Farlee

Providers / JCAHO Accredited Freestanding Long-Term Care Care Organizations

Lutheran Home and Services, 800 West Oakton Street, Arlington Heights, IL 60004; tel. 847/253-3710; Mr. Roger W Paulsberg
Manor Care Health Services, 6300 West 95th Street, Oak Lawn, IL 60453; tel. 708/599-8800; Ms. Regina Weidner
Manor HealthCare Corp., 200 West Martin Avenue, Naperville, IL 60540; tel. 630/355-4111; Mr. John Vrba
ManorCare Health Services, 9401 South Kostner Avenue, Oak Lawn, IL 60453; tel. 708/423-7882; Mr. John Anderson
ManorCare Health Services, 512 East Ogden Avenue, Westmont, IL 60559; tel. 630/323-4400; Ms. Jeanne P Hansen
ManorCare Health Services – Skokie, 4660 Old Orchard Road, Skokie, IL 60076; tel. 847/676-4800; Mr. Jamie Weibeler
ManorCare Health Services of Arlington Heights, 715 West Central Road, Arlington Heights, IL 60005; tel. 847/392-2020; Ms. Denise Clements
Mariner Health of Westchester, 2901 South Wolf Road, Westchester, IL 60154; tel. 708/531-1441; Ms. Joanna Castro
Maryhaven, 1700 East Lake Avenue, Glenview, IL 60025; tel. 847/729-1300; Ms. Judy Pitzele
Mason City Area Nursing Home, 520 North Price Avenue, Mason City, IL 62664; tel. 217/482-5022; Ms. Joyce Conrady
Mayfield Care Center, 5905 West Washington Boulevard, Chicago, IL 60644; tel. 773/261-7074; Mr. Eli Tropper
Mid-America Care Center, 4920 North Kenmore Avenue, Chicago, IL 60640; tel. 773/769-2700; Mr. Josh Davis
Monroe Pavilion Health and Treatment Center, 1400 West Monroe, Chicago, IL 60607; tel. 312/666-4090; Mr. Barry Carr
Morton Terrace, 191 East Queenwood Road, Morton, IL 61550; tel. 309/266-5331; Ms. Patricia A Chism
Norridge Healthcare and Rehabilitation Centre, 7001 West Cullom Avenue, Norridge, IL 60634; tel. 708/457-0700; Ms. Sandra Bernett
Northwoods Care Centre, 2250 Pearl Street, Belvidere, IL 61008; tel. 815/544-0358; Ms. Susan K Mead
O.S.F. Saint Clare Home, 5533 N Galena Rd, Peoria Heights, IL 61614; tel. 309/682-5428; Mr. Peter J Bolt, III
Oak Brook Healthcare Centre, 2013 Midwest Road, Oak Brook, IL 60521; tel. 630/495-0220; Ms. Paula Park
Oakton Pavilion, Inc., 1660 Oakton Place, Des Plaines, IL 60018; tel. 847/299-5588; Mr. Jay Lewkowitz
Odd Fellow–Rebekah Home, 201 Lafayette Avenue East, Mattoon, IL 61938; tel. 217/235-5449; Ms. Lualyce C Brown
Odin Healthcare Center, 300 Green Street, Odin, IL 62870; tel. 618/775-6444; Ms. Stacy Nies
P. A. Peterson Center for Health, 1311 Parkview Avenue, Rockford, IL 61107; tel. 815/399-9832; Mr. Frederick Aigner
Pavilion of Waukegan, Il, Inc., 2217 Washington Street, Waukegan, IL 60085; tel. 847/244-4100; Mr. Aaron Shpayher
Piatt County Nursing Home, 1111 North State Street, Monticello, IL 61856; tel. 217/762-7332; Ms. Marilyn E Benedino
Pine Acres Care Center, 1212 South Second Street, De Kalb, IL 60115; tel. 815/758-8151; Mr. James Formal
Plaza Terrace, 3249 West 147th Street, Midlothian, IL 60445; tel. 708/389-3141; Mr. Avigdor (Victor) Horowitz
Prairie Manor Health Care Center, 345 Dixie Highway, Chicago Heights, IL 60411; tel. 708/754-7601; Ms. Candace Zanon
Prairie View Care Center of Lewistown, 175 Sycamore Drive, Lewistown, IL 61542; tel. 309/547-2267; Ms. Julia Smith
Red Oaks of Highland Park, 2773 Skokie Valley Road, Highland Park, IL 60035; tel. 847/266-9266; Mr. Richard Haskell, Jr.
Regency Nursing Centre, 6631 North Milwaukee Avenue, Niles, IL 60714; tel. 847/647-7444; Ms. Barbara A Hecht
Renaissance at Hillside, 4600 North Frontage Road, Hillside, IL 60162; tel. 708/544-9933; Mr. Patrick Finn
Renaissance Care Center, 1675 East Ash, Canton, IL 61520; tel. 309/647-5631; Ms. Jennifer L Wilder

Rest Haven Illiana Chrisitan Convalescent Home, 13259 South Central Avenue, Palos Heights, IL 60463; tel. 708/597-1000; Mr. Peter J Klein
Rest Haven South Nursing Home, 16300 South Wausau Avenue, South Holland, IL 60473; tel. 708/225-6160; Ms. Nancy Van Drunen
Rest Haven West, 3450 Saratoga Avenue, Downers Grove, IL 60515; tel. 630/969-2900; Ms. Jacquelyn L Terpstra
Resurrection Nursing and Rehabilitation Center, 1001 North Greenwood Avenue, Park Ridge, IL 60068; tel. 847/692-5600; Ms. Norma Wilson
Ridgeland Center, 12550 South Ridgeland Avenue, Palos Heights, IL 60463; tel. 708/597-9300; Ms. Diane L Androvich
Rivershores Center, 573 West Commercial Street, Marseilles, IL 61341; tel. 815/795-5121; Carolyn Mills
Rosewood Care Center of Alton, Inc., 3490 Humbert Road, Alton, IL 62002; tel. 618/465-2626; Mr. Ken Kabureck
Rosewood Care Center of Northbrook, Inc., 4101 Lake Cook Road, Northbrook, IL 60062; tel. 847/562-1770; Ms. Mary Burnell
Sheridan Health Care Center, 2534 Elim Avenue, Zion, IL 60099; tel. 847/746-8435; Ms. Nanjean Painter
Sherman West Court, 1950 Larkin Avenue, Elgin, IL 60123; tel. 847/742-7070; Ms. Anne Huang
Skokie Meadows Nursing Center – No. 1, 9615 North Knox Avenue, Skokie, IL 60076; tel. 847/679-4161; Ms. Lucy C Lariosa
St. Andrew Home, 7000 North Newark Avenue, Niles, IL 60714; tel. 847/647-8332; Mr. James Kouzios
St. Benedict Home, 6930 West Touhy Avenue, Niles, IL 60714; tel. 847/647-0003; Mr. Peter Goshey
St. Pauls House and Health Care Center, 3800 North California Avenue, Chicago, IL 60618; tel. 773/478-4222; Mr. Lawrence D Carlson
SunBridge Hillside Care & Rehabilitation, 1308 Game Farm Road, Yorkville, IL 60560; tel. 630/553-5811; Ms. Nancy Tettemer
The Abington of Glenview, 3901 Glenview Road, Glenview, IL 60025; tel. 847/729-0000; Mr. Phillip DeLeon, Jr.
The Carlton at the Lake, Inc., 725 West Montrose Avenue, Chicago, IL 60613; tel. 773/929-1700; Ms. Rose Marie Betz
The Claremont Rehab and Living Center, 150 North Weiland Road, Buffalo Grove, IL 60089; tel. 847/465-0200; Ms. Karen Fogel
The Fountains at Crystal Lake, 1000 Brighton Lane, Crystal Lake, IL 60012; tel. 815/477-6400; Mr. Mel Trafford
The Imperial Convalescent and Geriatric Center, 1366 West Fullerton Avenue, Chicago, IL 60614; tel. 773/248-9300; Mr. Michael E Toral
The Neighbors, Inc., 811 West Second Street, Byron, IL 61010; tel. 815/234-2511; Mr. Grant Bullock
The Renaissance at 87th Street, 2940 West 87th Street, Chicago, IL 60652; tel. 773/434-8787; Mr. Ray Dolan
The Willow of Carbondale, Inc., 120 North Tower Road, Carbondale, IL 62901; tel. 618/549-3355; Ms. Debbie Dillion
Villa Scalabrini, 480 North Wolf Road, Northlake, IL 60164; tel. 708/562-0040; Ms. Mary L Grondin
Wagner Health Center, 820 Foster Street, Evanston, IL 60201; tel. 847/492-7700; Mr. Edward F Otto
Walnut Ridge Rehabilitation and Healthcare Center, 555 West Carpenter, Springfield, IL 62702; tel. 217/525-1880; Mr. Fred Aaron
Westmont Convalescent Center, 6501 South Cass Avenue, Westmont, IL 60559; tel. 630/960-2026; Ms. Nancy M Geraci
Whitehall North, 300 Waukegan Road, Deerfield, IL 60015-4988; tel. 847/945-4600; Ms. Barbara Harms
York Convalescent Center, 127 West Diversey Avenue, Elmhurst, IL 60126; tel. 630/530-5225; Ms. Rani Srinivas-Rao

INDIANA
American Transitional Care – Brookview, 7145 East 21st Street, Indianapolis, IN 46219; tel. 317/356-0977; Mr. Greg Limeberry
Arbors at Fort Wayne, 2827 Northgate Blvd., Fort Wayne, IN 46835; tel. 219/485-9691; Ms. Carol Simmons
Covington Manor Health Care Center, 1600 East Liberty Street, Covington, IN 47932; tel. 765/793-4818; Mr. Christopher T Cook
Danville Regional Rehabilitation Center, 255 Meadow Drive, Danville, IN 46122; tel. 317/745-5451; Ms. Melissa Haxton

Harborside Healthcare – Decatur, 4851 Tincher Road, Indianapolis, IN 46221; tel. 317/856-4851; Mr. Stephen Harris
Harborside Healthcare – Indianapolis, 8201 West Washington Street, Indianapolis, IN 46231; tel. 317/244-6848; Mr. Stephen L Guillard
Harborside Healthcare – New Haven, 1201 Daly Drive, New Haven, IN 46774; tel. 219/749-0413; Ms. Judy Privett
Harborside Healthcare – Terre Haute, 1001 East Springhill Drive, Terre Haute, IN 47802; tel. 812/238-2441; Ms. Karen F Rumple
Harrison Healthcare Corporation, 2026 East 54th Street, Indianapolis, IN 46220; tel. 317/253-6950; Ms. Ginger L Fitzpatrick
Healthwin Specialized Care Facility, 20531 Darden Road, South Bend, IN 46637; tel. 219/272-0100; Mr. Grant Shumway
Heartland Health Care Center – Prestwick, 445 South County Road 525E, Avon, IN 46123; tel. 317/745-2522; Mr. Michael Thompson
Heritage Healthcare, 3401 Soldiers Home Road, West Lafayette, IN 47906; tel. 317/463-1541; Shirley Lake
Heritage House Rehabilitation and HealthCare Center, 281 S County Road, 200 East, Connersville, IN 47331; tel. 317/825-2148; Ms. Linda C Lacey
Holiday Care Center, 1201 West Buena Vista Road, Evansville, IN 47710; tel. 812/429-0700; Ms. Kathy Knapp
Holy Cross Care and Rehabilitation Center, 17475 Dugdale Drive, South Bend, IN 46635; tel. 219/271-3990; Mr. Joseph M Doran
Integrated Health Services of Indianapolis at Cambridge, 8530 Township Line Road, Indianapolis, IN 46260; tel. 317/876-9955; Mr. Marc A Hurst
Ironwood Health and Rehabilitation Center, 1950 Ridgedale Avenue, South Bend, IN 46614; tel. 219/291-6722; Mr. Glenn Wagner
Kingston Care Center, 1010 W Washington Center Road, Fort Wayne, IN 46825; tel. 219/489-2552; Ms. Rebecca A Housman
Miller's Merry Manor, PO Box 480, Logansport, IN 46947; tel. 219/722-4006; Ms. Nan Albright
Munster Med–Inn, 7935 Calumet Avenue, Munster, IN 46321; tel. 219/836-8300; Mr. Julian D Robinson
Northwest Manor Health Care Center, 6440 West 34th Street, Indianapolis, IN 46224; tel. 317/293-4930; Ms. Jennifer A Knoll
Paoli Convalescent Center, PO Box 299, Paoli, IN 47454; tel. 812/723-2595; Ms. Donna R Martin
Rensselaer Care Center, 1309 East Grace Street, Rensselaer, IN 47978; tel. 219/866-4181; Ms. Barbara A Slosson
Robin Run Village, 6370 Robin Run West Drive, Indianapolis, IN 46268; tel. 317/298-6255; Mr. Kent Kirkwood
Southlake Nursing and Rehabilitation Center, 8800 Virginia Place, Merrillville, IN 46410; tel. 219/736-1310; Ms. Linda O'Neill
St. Vincent Children's Specialty Hospital, PO Box 40407, Indianapolis, IN 46240-0407; tel. 317/415-5500; Mr. David Carter
The Altenheim Community, 3525 East Hanna Avenue, Indianapolis, IN 46237; tel. 317/788-4261; Mr. Brian Allen
Transitional Health Services of Clark County, 203 Sparks Avenue, Jeffersonville, IN 47130; tel. 812/283-7918; Ms. Julie Hartlage
Vermillion Convalescent and Rehabilitation Center, 1705 South Main Street, Clinton, IN 47842; tel. 317/832-3573; Ms. Melissa Gum
Woodlands Convalescent Center, PO Box 400, Newburgh, IN 47630; tel. 812/853-9567; Mr. John V Foster

IOWA
Anamosa Care Center, PO Box 229, Anamosa, IA 52205; tel. 319/462-4356; Randall Christy
Cedar Falls Lutheran Home, 7511 University Avenue, Cedar Falls, IA 50613; tel. 319/268-0401; Pat Welton
Danville Care Center, PO Box 248, Danville, IA 52623; tel. 319/392-4259; Barbara Howell
Edgewood Convalescent Home, PO Box 39, Edgewood, IA 52042; tel. 319/928-6461; Ms. Ruth Stephens
Elkader Care Center, BOX 519, Elkader, IA 52043; tel. 319/245-1620; Ms. Kristi L Mitchell
Great River Care Center, PO Box 370, McGregor, IA 52157; tel. 319/873-3527; Ms. Raletta Thomas
Iowa Veterans Home, 1301 Summit Street, Marshalltown, IA 50158; tel. 515/752-1501; Mr. Jack J Dack

Providers / JCAHO Accredited Freestanding Long-Term Care Care Organizations

Lone Tree Health Care Center, Inc., 501 East Pioneer Road, Lone Tree, IA 52755; tel. 319/629-4255; Ms. Roberta Shirkey
Manor Care Nursing and Rehabilitation Center, 815 East Locust, Davenport, IA 52803; tel. 319/324-3276; Mr. Glen W Roebuck
Mill Valley Care Center, 1201 Park Avenue, Bellevue, IA 52031; tel. 319/872-5521; Mr. Lyman D Bailey
Montezuma Nursing and Rehabilitation Center, PO Box 790, Montezuma, IA 50171; tel. 515/623-5497; Mr. Todd Kollbaum
New Hampton Nursing and Rehabilitation Center, PO Box 428, New Hampton, IA 50659; tel. 515/394-4153; Mr. Gregg Hanson
St. Luke's Living Center West, 1050 Fourth Avenue Southeast, Cedar Rapids, IA 52403; tel. 319/366-8714; Mr. Fred Brumm
St. Lukes Living Center East, 1220 Fifth Avenue Southeast, Cedar Rapids, IA 52403-4073; tel. 319/366-8701; Mr. Scott L Marnin
State Center Manor, 702 Third Street, State Center, IA 50247; tel. 515/483-2812; Mr. Donald Nicholls
The Monticello Nursing and Rehabilitation Center, 500 Pinehaven Drive, Monticello, IA 52310; tel. 319/465-5415; Sister Donna Venteicher
Wheatland Manor, PO Box 368, Wheatland, IA 52777-0368; tel. 319/374-1295; Mr. Jack McIntosh

KANSAS
ManorCare Health Services, 5211 West 103rd Street, Overland Park, KS 66207; tel. 913/383-2569; Ms. Ann Say
Wilson Nursing Center, PO Box 160, Wilson, KS 67490; tel. 785/658-2505; Mr. Monty Warren

KENTUCKY
Christopher East Health Care Center, PO Box 20909, Louisville, KY 40220; tel. 502/459-8900; Mr. William Johnson
Florence Park Care Center, 6975 Burlington Pike, Florence, KY 41042; tel. 606/525-0007; Ms. Patricia A Feldman
Harrodsburg Health Care Center, 853 Lexington Road, Harrodsburg, KY 40330; tel. 606/734-7791; Ms. Vicki Trump
Hermitage Nursing and Rehabilitation Center, 1614 West Parrish Avenue, Owensboro, KY 42301; tel. 502/684-4559; Ms. Kathy Skaggs
Highlands of Ft. Thomas, 960 Highland Avenue, Fort Thomas, KY 41075; tel. 606/572-0660; Mr. Barry N Bortz
Hillcreek Manor Rehabilitation and Nursing Center, 3116 Breckenridge Lane, Louisville, KY 40220; tel. 502/459-9120; Mr. Bert Sedoris
Hurstbourne Care Centre, 2200 Stony Brook Drive, Louisville, KY 40220; tel. 502/495-6240; Mr. David Grady
Parkview Nursing and Rehabilitation Center, 544 Lone Oak Road, Paducah, KY 42003; tel. 502/443-6543; Ms. Marilyn Ingram
Rosewood Health Care Center, 550 High Street, Bowling Green, KY 42101; tel. 502/843-3296; Ms. Donna Brown
Salyersville Health Care Center, PO Box 819, Salyersville, KY 41465; tel. 606/349-6181; Mr. Thomas E Hummer

LOUISIANA
Chateau Living Center, 716 Village Road, Kenner, LA 70065; tel. 504/464-0604; Mr. Harry Franatovich
IHS of Slidell Rehab Center, 1400 Lindberg Drive, Slidell, LA 70458; tel. 504/641-4985; Dr. James L McEwen
Lafon Nursing Facility of the Holy Family, 6900 Chef Menteur Highway, New Orleans, LA 70126; tel. 504-246-1100; Sr. Augustine McDaniel
Martin de Porres Nursing Home, Inc., PO Box 1294, Lake Charles, LA 70602; tel. 318/439-5761; Ms. Juannie Miller
Meadowcrest Living Center, 535 Commerce Street, Gretna, LA 70056; tel. 504/393-9595; Ms. Jane Fockler
Metairie Healthcare Center, 6401 Riverside Drive, Metairie, LA 70003; tel. 504/885-8611; Mr. Reggie McCue
National Hansen's Disease Programs, 1770 Physicians Park Drive, Baton Rouge, LA 70816; tel. 225/756-3517; Mr. Charles D Stanley
Waldon Healthcare Center, 2401 Idaho Street, Kenner, LA 70062; tel. 504/466-0222; Mr. David Hargrave

MAINE
Brewer Rehabilitation and Living Center, 74 Parkway South, Brewer, ME 04412; tel. 207/989-7300; Mr. Michael Beal
Cedar Ridge Center for Health Care and Rehabilitation, Rural Route 1, Box 1283, Skowhegan, ME 04976; tel. 207/474-9686; Mr. Stephen A Marsden
Courtland Living Center, 38 Court Street, Ellsworth, ME 04605; tel. 207/667-9036; Ms. Alice F Endre
Eastside Rehabilitation and Living Center, 516 Mt. Hope Avenue, Bangor, ME 04401; tel. 207/947-6131; Mr. Marc S Plourde
Maplecrest Rehabilitation and Living Center, 174 Main Street, Madison, ME 04950; tel. 207/696-8225; Mr. Michael J McDougall
Marshwood Center for Healthcare and Rehabilitation, 33 Roger Street, Lewiston, ME 04240; tel. 207/784-0108; Ms. Susanne Heeschen
Montello Manor, 540 College Street, Lewiston, ME 04240; tel. 207/783-2039; Mr. Peter A Davison
Oak Grove Rehabilitation and Living Center, 27 Cool Street, Waterville, ME 04901; tel. 207/873-0721; Ms. Sara J Sylvester
Orono Commons, 117 Bennoch Road, Orono, ME 04473; tel. 207/866-4914; Mr. Gary B Currier
Pine Point Center for Health Care and Rehabilitation, 67 Pine Point Road, Scarborough, ME 04074; tel. 207/883-2468; Ms. Barbara Rentz-Champagne
RiverRidge, 79 Cat Mousam Road, Kennebunk, ME 04043; tel. 207/985-3030; Mr. Irving Faunce
Ross Manor Associates, 758 Broadway, Bangor, ME 04401-3224; tel. 207/941-8400; Ms. Ruth Tozier
Sandy River Center for Nursing and Rehabilitation, RFD 4, Box 5121, Farmington, ME 04938; tel. 207/778-6591; Ms. Geri Bryant
Seaside Rehabilitation and Health Care Center, 850 Baxter Boulevard, Portland, ME 04103; tel. 207/774-7878; Mr. Pierre Morneault
Southridge Rehabilitation and Living Center, PO Box 4138, Biddeford, ME 04005; tel. 207/282-4138; Mr. Philip Jean
Springbrook Center for Healthcare and Rehabilitation, 300 Spring Street, Westbrook, ME 04092; tel. 207/856-1230; Ms. Anne Herrick
St. Marguerite d'Youville Pavilion, 102 Campus Avenue, Lewiston, ME 04240; tel. 207/777-4200; Mr. James Cassidy
Stillwater Health Care, 335 Stillwater Avenue, Bangor, ME 04401; tel. 207/947-1111; Ms. Hope Richards
Westgate Manor, 750 Union Street, Bangor, ME 04401; tel. 207/942-7336; Mr. T. Michael Skirven
Windward Gardens, 105 Mechanic Street, Camden, ME 04843; tel. 207/236-4197; Mr. William F Chase
Woodlawn Rehabilitation and Nursing Center, 91 West Front Street, Skowhegan, ME 04976; tel. 207/474-9300; Mr. Rodney McIntyre

MARYLAND
Adventist HealthCare Sligo Creek Nursing and Rehab Center, 7525 Carroll Avenue, Takoma Park, MD 20912; tel. 301/270-4200; Mr. Ron Wisby
Bradford Oaks Nursing and Rehabilitation Center, 7520 Surratts Road, Clinton, MD 20735; tel. 301/856-1660; Ms. Lori Lusby-Hamilton
Canton Harbor Healthcare, 1300 South Elwood Avenue, Baltimore, MD 21224; tel. 410/342-6644; Mr. Brian H Klausmeyer
Caroline Nursing Home, Inc., 520 Kerr Avenue, Denton, MD 21629; tel. 410/479-2130; Ms. Karen Potter
Carriage Hill Bethesda, Inc., 5215 West Cedar Lane, Bethesda, MD 20814; tel. 301/897-5500; Mr. Joseph R Vucich
Carroll Lutheran Village, Inc., 300 St. Luke Circle, Westminster, MD 21158; tel. 410/848-0090; Geary Milliken
College View Center, 700 Toll House Avenue, Frederick, MD 21701; tel. 301/663-5181; Ms. Jeannine Blomquist
Copper Ridge, Inc., 710 Obrecht Road, Sykesville, MD 21784; tel. 410/795-8808; Ms. Carmel Roques
Cromwell Center - Genesis ElderCare, 8710 Emge Road, Baltimore, MD 21234; tel. 410/661-5955; Mr. Richard Kincaid
Cumberland Villa Nursing Center, PO Box 869, Cumberland, MD 21501-0869; tel. 301/724-6066; Ms. Shirley E Paulus
Fairland Adventist Nursing and Rehabilitation Center, 2101 Fairland Road, Silver Spring, MD 20904; tel. 301/384-6161; Ms. Sheila R Jones
Forest Glen Skilled Nursing and Rehabilitation Center, 2700 Barker Street, Silver Spring, MD 20910; tel. 301/565-0300; Ms. Jane Blum
Fox Chase Rehabilitation and Nursing Center, 2015 East West Highway, Silver Spring, MD 20910; tel. 301/587-2400; Ms. G. Mary Clinton
Franklin Woods Center - Genesis Eldercare Network, 9200 Franklin Square Drive, Baltimore, MD 21237; tel. 410/391-2600; Mr. Robert Harris
Frostburg Village of Allegany County, One Kaylor Circle, Frostburg, MD 21532-2099; tel. 301/689-2425; Ms. Anita L Blauch
Future Care - Pineview, 9106 Pineview Lane, Clinton, MD 20735; tel. 301/856-2930; Ms. Vanessa L Mattox
FutureCare Sandtown - Winchester, 1000 North Gilmor Street, Baltimore, MD 21217; tel. 410/669-2759; Mr. John A Darden
FutureCare Homewood, 2700 North Charles Street, Baltimore, MD 21218; tel. 410/554-6300; Mrs. Elissa Heck
FutureCare Old Court, 5412 Old Court Road, Randallstown, MD 21133-5196; tel. 410/922-3200; Ms. Lorrie J Custodio
FutureCare-CherryWood, 12020 Reisterstown Road, Reisterstown, MD 21136; tel. 410/833-3801; Leslie D Goldschmidt
FutureCare-Chesapeake, 305 College Parkway, Arnold, MD 21012; tel. 410/647-0015; Ms. Carolynne Adams
Genesis ElderCare - Heritage Center, 7232 German Hill Road, Baltimore, MD 21222; tel. 410/282-6310; Mr. Michael E Morin
Genesis ElderCare - Randallstown Center, 9109 Liberty Road, Randallstown, MD 21133; tel. 410/655-7373; Ms. Sharon K Schulz
Genesis ElderCare - Severna Park Center, 24 Truckhouse Road, Severna Park, MD 21146; tel. 410/544-4220; Ms. Joanne M Bonfardeci
Glade Valley Nursing and Rehabilitation Center, 56 West Frederick Street, Walkersville, MD 21793; tel. 301/898-4300; Ms. Ellen Reap
Glen Meadows Retirement Community, 11630 Glen Arm Road, Glen Arm, MD 21057; tel. 410/592-5310; Mr. Charles F Brown
Harborside Healthcare - Larkin Chase, 15005 Health Center Drive, Bowie, MD 20716; tel. 301/805-6070; Mr. Stephen Guillard
Heartland Health Care Center - Adelphi, 1801 Metzerott Road, Adelphi, MD 20783; tel. 301/434-0500; Mr. Brian E Karstetter
Heartland Health Care Center - Hyattsville, 6500 Riggs Road, Hyattsville, MD 20783; tel. 301/559-0300; Mr. Matthew Neiswanger
Hebrew Home of Greater Washington, 6121 Montrose Road, Rockville, MD 20852; tel. 301/770-8310; Mr. Warren R Slavin
Herman Wilson Health Care Cntr Asbury Methodist Village, Inc, 301 Russell Avenue, Gaithersburg, MD 20877; tel. 301/216-4220; Ms. Kathryn J McAlevy
Irvington Knolls Care Center II, Inc., 30 South Athol Avenue, Baltimore, MD 21229; tel. 410/947-3052; Mr. Bruce Goodman
Irvington Knolls Care Center, Inc., 22 South Athol Avenue, Baltimore, MD 21229; tel. 410/947-3052; Ms. Shirley Grandison
Ivy Hall Geriatric and Rehabilitation Center, 1300 Windlass Drive, Baltimore, MD 21220; tel. 410/687-1383; Ms. Yolanda V Walton
Keswick Multi-Care Center, 700 West 40th Street, Baltimore, MD 21211; tel. 410/662-4200; Ms. Elizabeth Bowerman
La Plata Center, 1 Magnolia Drive, La Plata, MD 20646; tel. 301/934-4001; Ms. Margaret McGovern
Layhill Center - Genesis ElderCare Network, 3227 Bel Pre Road, Silver Spring, MD 20906; tel. 301/871-2000; Ms. Martha E Leeson
Levindale Hebrew Geriatric Center and Hospital, Inc., 2434 West Belvedere Avenue, Baltimore, MD 21215; tel. 410/466-8700; Mr. Ronald Rothstein
Magnolia Center, 8200 Good Luck Road, Lanham, MD 20706; tel. 301/552-2000; Ms. Carla Shipley
ManorCare Health Services - Wheaton, 11901 Georgia Avenue, Wheaton, MD 20902; tel. 301/942-2500; Ms. Patricia Megary
ManorCare Health Services of Potomac, 10714 Potomac Tennis Lane, Potomac, MD 20854; tel. 301/299-2273; Mr. Stewart Bainum, Jr.
Mariner Health at Circle Manor, 10231 Carroll Place, Kensington, MD 20895; tel. 301/949-0230; Ms. Jennifer Rosenberg
Mariner Health of Bethesda, 5721 Grosvenor Lane, Bethesda, MD 20814; tel. 301/530-1600; Ms. Barbara Wells
Mariner Health of Greater Laurel, 14200 Laurel Park Drive, Laurel, MD 20707; tel. 410/792-4717; Mr. Gary Czapski

Providers / JCAHO Accredited Freestanding Long-Term Care Care Organizations

Mariner Health of Silver Spring, 901 Arcola Avenue, Silver Spring, MD 20902; tel. 301/649-2400; Ms. Michelle F Kraus

Mariner Health of Southern Maryland, 9211 Stuart Lane, Clinton, MD 20735; tel. 301/868-3600; Ms. Barbara McKenna

Mariner Post Acute Network of Kensington, 3000 McComas Avenue, Kensington, MD 20895; tel. 301/933-0060; Ms. Deborah K Toth

Multi-Medical Center – Genesis ElderCare Network, 7700 York Road, Towson, MD 21204; tel. 410/821-5500; Ms. Margaret A Leonard

Ravenwood Lutheran Village, 1183 Luther Drive, Hagerstown, MD 21740; tel. 301/790-1000; Mr. Garret Falcone, NHA

Salisbury Center: Genesis Eldercare Network, 200 Civic Avenue, Salisbury, MD 21804; tel. 410/749-1466; Bruce R Levin

Shady Grove Adventist Nursing and Rehabilitation Center, 9701 Medical Center Drive, Rockville, MD 20850; tel. 301/424-6400; Ms. Michelle Mahn

Spa Creek Center Genesis ElderCare, 35 Milkshake Lane, Annapolis, MD 21403; tel. 410/269-5100; Renee Verrier

Springbrook Adventist Nursing and Rehabilitation Center, 12325 New Hampshire Avenue, Silver Spring, MD 20904; tel. 301/622-4600; Mr. Richard Balogh

St. Agnes Nursing and Rehabilitation Center, 3000 North Ridge Road, Ellicott City, MD 21043; tel. 410/461-7577; Mrs. Barbara A Gustke

St. Elizabeth Rehabilitation and Nursing Center, 3320 Benson Avenue, Baltimore, MD 21227; tel. 410/644-7100; Ms. Christine L Mour

St. Thomas More Nursing and Rehabilitation Center, 4922 LaSalle Road, Hyattsville, MD 20782; tel. 301/864-2333; Mr. Owen Schwartz

Stella Maris, Inc., 2300 Dulaney Valley Road, Timonium, MD 21093; tel. 410/252-4500; Sister Karen McNally

SunBridge Care for Elkton, One Price Drive, Elkton, MD 21921; tel. 410/398-6474; Ms. Mary Guttendorf

The Pines, 610 Dutchmans Lane, Easton, MD 21601; tel. 410/822-4000; Ms. Stacey E Radcliffe

Transitional Care at Mercy, 301 St. Paul Place, Baltimore, MD 21202-2165; tel. 410/332-9091; Ms. Nancy G Lawerence

Woodside Center – Genesis Eldercare Network, 9101 Second Avenue, Silver Spring, MD 20910; tel. 301/588-5544; Ms. Maureen A Otero

MASSACHUSETTS

Abbott House, 28 Essex Street, Lynn, MA 01902; tel. 781/595-5500; Mr. Richard C Bane

Aberjona Nursing Center, Inc., PO Box 490, Winchester, MA 01890; tel. 781/729-9370; Mr. Robert F Salter

Alden Court Nursing Care and Rehabilitation Center, 389 Alden Road, Fairhaven, MA 02719; tel. 508/991-8600; Mr. David B Manahan

Anchorage Nursing Home, 904 Mohawk Trail, Shelburne, MA 01370; tel. 413/625-2305; Ms. Susan M Page

Apple Valley Nursing and Rehabilitation Center, 400 Groton Road, Ayer, MA 01432; tel. 978/772-1704; Ms. Joyce Sears

Avery Manor, 100 West Street, Needham, MA 02194; tel. 781/433-0202; Mr. Paul O'Connell

Baldwinville Nursing Home, PO Box 24, Baldwinville, MA 01436; tel. 978/939-2196; Mr. Roger E Myers

Bay Path at Duxbury Rehabilitation and Nursing Ctr, 308 Kingstown Way, Duxbury, MA 02332; tel. 781/585-5561; Ms. Marianne Welch-Martinez

Baypointe Rehabilitation and Skilled Care Center, 50 Christy Place, Brockton, MA 02401; tel. 508/580-6800; Ms. Kimberly Sciacca

Bear Hill Nursing Center, 11 North Street, Stoneham, MA 02180; tel. 781/438-8515; Mr. William E Ring, Jr.

Beaumont Rehabilitation and Skilled Nursing Center, PO Box 935, Northbridge, MA 01534-0935; tel. 508/234-9771; Mr. Daniel J Salmon, Jr.

Beaumont Rehabilitation and Skilled Nursing Center, 1 Lyman Street, Westborough, MA 01581; tel. 508/366-9933; Mr. Michael T Murphy

Beaumont Rehabilitation and Skilled Nursing Center, 3 Vision Drive, Route 9 West, Natick, MA 01760; tel. 508/655-3344; Mr. William McGinley

Belmont Manor Nursing Home, Inc., 34 Agassiz Avenue, Belmont, MA 02178; tel. 617/489-1200; Mr. Stewart A Karger

Beverly Health Care East Village, 840 Emerson Gardens Road, Lexington, MA 02173; tel. 781/861-8630; Mr. Mark Carroll

Beverly Healthcare – Dexter House, 120 Main Street, Malden, MA 02148; tel. 781/324-5600; Mr. Scott Dickenson

Beverly Healthcare – Hermitage, 383 Mill Street, Worcester, MA 01602; tel. 508/791-8131; Ms. Mary L Davis

Beverly Healthcare Birchwood Care Center, 1199 John Fitch Highway, Fitchburg, MA 01420; tel. 978/345-0146; Mr. Mark L Moyer

Beverly Healthcare Emerald Court, 460 Washington Street, Norwood, MA 02062; tel. 781/769-2200; Lionel Bergeron

Beverly Healthcare-Melrose, 40 Martin Street, Melrose, MA 02176; tel. 781/665-7050; Mr. Michael Takesian

Beverly Manor of Plymouth Nursing Home, 19 Obery Street, Plymouth, MA 02360; tel. 508/747-4790; Ms. Linda R Valenzano

Beverly Nursing and Rehabilitation Center, 40 Heather Street, Beverly, MA 01915; tel. 978/927-6220; Mr. Eugene Belle

Blaire House Long Term Care Facility of New Bedford, 397 County Street, New Bedford, MA 02740; tel. 508/997-9396; Ms. Marcia MacInnis

Blaire House of Milford, 20 Claflin Street, Milford, MA 01757; tel. 508/473-1272; Mr. John Gerety

Blaire House of Tewksbury, 10 Erlin Terrace, Tewksbury, MA 01876; tel. 978/640-8600; Mr. Frank C Romano

Blue Hills Alzheimer's Care Center, 1044 Park Street, Stoughton, MA 02072; tel. 781/344-7300; Mr. Steven Goold

Blueberry Hill Healthcare, 75 Brimbal Avenue, Beverly, MA 01915; tel. 978/927-2020; Mr. Daniel Micherone

Bolton Manor, 400 Bolton Street, Marlborough, MA 01752; tel. 508/481-6123; Mr. Scott Bullock

Bostonian Nursing Care and Rehabilitation Center, 337 Neponset Avenue, Dorchester, MA 02122; tel. 617/265-2350; Mr. Wayne Pultman

Bourne Manor Extended Care Facility, 146 MacArthur Boulevard, Bourne, MA 02532; tel. 508/759-8880; Mr. William C Jones

Braemoor Rehabilitation and Nursing Center, Inc., 34 North Pearl Street, Brockton, MA 02301; tel. 508/586-3696; Mr. Michael J Roland

Brandon Woods of Dartmouth, 567 Dartmouth Street, South Dartmouth, MA 02748; tel. 508/997-7787; Ms. Deborah Klock

Brewster Senior Care Center, 873 Harwich Road, Brewster, MA 02631; tel. 508/896-7046; Mr. Scott Schuster

Briarwood Continuing Care Retirement Community, 70 Briarwood Circle, Worcester, MA 01606; tel. 508/852-2670; Mr. Kenneth L Hooge

Briarwood Healthcare, 150 Lincoln Street, Needham, MA 02192; tel. 781/449-4040; Mrs. Amy Baxter-McKenzie

Brook Farm Rehabilitation and Nursing Centre, 1190 VFW Parkway, West Roxbury, MA 02132; tel. 617/325-1688; Ms. Kimberly Brailsford

Cape Cod Nursing and Rehabilitation Center, 8 Lewis Point, Buzzards Bay, MA 02532; tel. 508/759-5767; Mr. Jeffrey Aframe

Cape Heritage Rehabilitation and Nursing Center, 37 Route 6A, Sandwich, MA 02563; tel. 508/888-8222; Ms. Steven Garfinkle

Cape Regency Rehabilitation and Nursing Center, 120 South Main Street, Centerville, MA 02632; tel. 508/778-1835; Danette Manzi

CareMatrix of Dedham, 10 CareMatrix Drive, Dedham, MA 02026; tel. 781/461-9663; Ms. Nene A Pallera

Carlyle Nursing Home, Inc., PO Box 2495, Framingham, MA 01701; tel. 508/879-6100; Mr. Dennis Morgan

Catholic Memorial Home, Inc., 2446 Highland Avenue, Fall River, MA 02720-4599; tel. 508/679-0011; Sister Nina Amaral

Center for Extended Care at Amherst, 150 University Drive, Amherst, MA 01002; tel. 413/256-8185; Ms. Sharon E Meyers

Center for Optimum Care Berkshire, 360 West Housatonic Street, Pittsfield, MA 01201; tel. 413/442-4841; Robert Willis

Center for Rehabilitation and Nursing Care, 217 Westfield Street, West Springfield, MA 01089; tel. 413/746-0390; Mr. David J Ianacone

Chamberlain Nursing Home, 123 Gardner Road, Brookline, MA 02146; tel. 617/277-0225; Ms. Barbara A Smith

Charlene Manor Extended Care Facility, 130 Colrain Road, Greenfield, MA 01301; tel. 413/774-3724; Mr. William C Jones, Jr.

Charlwell House, 305 Walpole Street, Norwood, MA 020623098; tel. 781/762-7700; Mr. Donald C Baker

Chestnut Hill Rehabilitation and Nursing Center, 32 Chestnut Street, East Longmeadow, MA 01028; tel. 413/525-1893; Ms. Nancy J Packham

Chetwynde Health and Rehabilitation Center, 1650 Washington Street, West Newton, MA 02165; tel. 617/244-5407; Mr. Jonathan Shadowitz

Christopher House of Worcester, Inc., 10 Mary Scano Drive, Worcester, MA 01605; tel. 508/754-3800; Mr. Arthur S Tirella

Clark House Nursing Center at Fox Hill Village, 30 Longwood Drive, Westwood, MA 02090; tel. 781/326-5652; Ms. Andrea Sklencar

Clifton Rehabilitative Nursing Center, 500 Wilbur Avenue, Somerset, MA 02725-2051; tel. 508/675-7589; Mr. Clifton O Greenwood

Cohasset Knoll Skilled Nursing and Rehabilitation Facility, 1 Chief Justice Cushing Hwy, Cohasset, MA 02025; tel. 781/383-9060; Mr. David Banks

Colonial Rehabilitation & Nursing Center, 125 Broad Street, Weymouth, MA 02188; tel. 781/337-3121; Mr. Richard M Welch

Colony House Nursing and Rehabilitation Center, 277 Washington Street, Abington, MA 02351-0556; tel. 781/871-0200; Ms. Shari Krivyanik

Coolidge House Nursing Care Center, 30 Webster Street, Brookline, MA 02146; tel. 617/734-2300; Mr. Matt Weinstock

Copley at Stoughton Nursing Care Center, 380 Sumner Street, Stoughton, MA 02072; tel. 617/341-2300; Miss Marc Presutti

Country Estates Nursing and Rehabilitation Center, 1200 Suffield Street, Agawam, MA 01001; tel. 413/789-2200; Mr. M. William Sibley

Country Gardens Skilled Nursing and Rehabilitation Ctr, 2045 Grand Army Highway, Swansea, MA 02777; tel. 508/379-9700; Mr. Scott M Sanborn

Country Haven, Inc., 184 Mansfield Avenue, Norton, MA 02766; tel. 508/285-7745; Mr. Jeffrey C Harsfield

Country Manor Rehabilitation and Nursing Center, 180 Low Street, Newburyport, MA 01950; tel. 978/465-5361; Ms. Heidi Paek

Courtyard Nursing Care Center, 200 Governors Avenue, Medford, MA 02155; tel. 781/391-5400; Ms. Joanne Mukerjee

Coyne Healthcare Center, 56 Webster Street, Rockland, MA 02370; tel. 781/871-0555; Ms. Martha Daneault

Cranberry Pointe Rehab and Skilled Care Center, 111 Headwaters Drive, Harwich, MA 02645-1726; tel. 508/430-1717; Cheryl Ferguson

Crawford Skilled Nursing and Rehabilitation Center, 273 Oak Grove Avenue, Fall River, MA 02723; tel. 508/679-4866; Ms. Karen Wadlow

Crestview Healthcare Facility, Inc., 86 Greenleaf Street, Quincy, MA 02169; tel. 617/479-2978; Mr. Joel K Logan

D'Youville Senior Care, Inc., 981 Varnum Avenue, Lowell, MA 01854; tel. 978/454-5681; Mr. Steve Johnson

Den-Mar Rehabilitation and Nursing Center, 44 South Street, Rockport, MA 01966; tel. 978/546-6311; Mr. Stanley T Trocki, Jr.

Deutsches Altenheim, Inc., 2222 Centre Street, West Roxbury, MA 02132; tel. 617/325-1230; Mr. W. Bruce Glass

Devereux House Nursing Home, 39 Lafayette Street, Marblehead, MA 01945-1997; tel. 781/631-6120; Mr. Kenneth D Bane

Don Orione Nursing Home, 111 Orient Avenue, East Boston, MA 02128; tel. 617/569-2100; Rev. Lawrence Tosatto

Eagle Pond Rehabilitation and Living Center, PO Box 208, South Dennis, MA 02660; tel. 508/385-6200; Mr. Scott E Stone

East Longmeadow Skilled Nursing Center, 305 Maple Street, East Longmeadow, MA 01028; tel. 413/525-6361; Mr. William C Jones, Jr.

Easton Lincoln Rehabilitation and Nursing Center, 184 Lincoln Street, North Easton, MA 02356; tel. 508/238-7053; Mr. Steven Garfinkle

Eastpointe Rehabilitation and Skilled Care Center, 255 Central Avenue, Chelsea, MA 02150; tel. 617/884-5700; Mr. Richard Sciacca

Eastwood Care Center, 1007 East Street, Dedham, MA 02026; tel. 781/329-1520; Mr. David Butler

Edgar P. Benjamin Healthcare Center, 120 Fisher Avenue, Boston, MA 02120; tel. 617/738-1500; Ms. Myrna E Wynn

Elihu White Nursing and Rehabilitation Center, 95 Commercial Street, Braintree, MA 02184; tel. 781/848-3678; Ms. Florence E Logan

Providers / JCAHO Accredited Freestanding Long-Term Care Care Organizations

Elizabeth Seton Residence, Inc, 125 Oakland Street, Wellesley Hills, MA 02481; tel. 781/237-2161; Sister Blanche LaRose

Embassy House Skilled Nursing and Rehabilitation Center, 2 Beaumont Avenue, Brockton, MA 02402; tel. 617/588-8550; Mr. Vincent Bettes

Emerson Convalescent Home, 59 Coolidge Hill Road, Watertown, MA 02172-2884; tel. 617/924-1130; Mr. Steven P Duffy

Evanswood Center for Older Adults/Bethesda at Evanswood, 17 Chipman Way, Kingston, MA 02364; tel. 781/585-4100; Mr. Matthew J Muratore

Fairhaven Nursing Home, Inc., 476 Varnum Avenue, Lowell, MA 01854; tel. 508/458-3388; Ms. Lita I Noel

Fairlawn Nursing Home, Inc., 370 West Street, Leominster, MA 01453; tel. 978/537-0771; Mr. Stephen A Trudeau

Fall River Jewish Home, Inc., 538 Robeson Street, Fall River, MA 02720; tel. 508/679-6172; Ms. Christine M Vitale

Farren Care Center, Inc., 340 Montague City Road, Turners Falls, MA 01376; tel. 413/774-3111; Mr. William E Casper

Forestview Nursing Home of Wareham, Inc., 50 Indian Neck Road, Wareham, MA 02571; tel. 508/295-6264; Mr. Edward Turcotte-Shamski

Franklin Skilled Nursing and Rehabilitation Center, 130 Chestnut Street, Franklin, MA 02038; tel. 508/528-4600; Mr. Victor O Emodi

Franvale Nursing and Rehabilitation Center, 20 Pond Street, Braintree, MA 02184; tel. 781/356-6399; Mr. Bruce A Shear

Geriatric Authority of Holyoke, 45 Lower Westfield Road, Holyoke, MA 01040; tel. 413/536-8110; Ms. Sheryl Y Quinn

Geriatric Authority of Milford Nursing and Rehabilitation Ct, 1 Countryside Drive, Milford, MA 01757; tel. 508/473-0435; Mr. James Tracy

Glen Ridge Nursing Care Center, Hospital Road, Malden, MA 02148; tel. 781/391-0800; Mr. Robert F Driscoll

Goddard House, 201 South Huntington Avenue, Jamaica Plain, MA 02130; tel. 617/522-3080; Mr. Barry Chiler

Governor's Center, 66 Broad Street, Westfield, MA 01085; tel. 413/562-5464; Mr. Jeffrey N Heinz

Great Barrington Rehabilitation and Nursing Ctr, 148 Maple Avenue, Great Barrington, MA 01230-1998; tel. 413/528-3320; Mr. Francis Q Meyer

Greenery Extended Care Center at Danvers, 56 Liberty Street, Danvers, MA 01923-3398; tel. 978/777-2700; Mr. Edward J Stewart

Greenery Extended Care Center at North Andover, 75 Park Street, North Andover, MA 01845; tel. 978/685-3372; Mr. James Sullivan

Greenery Rehabilitation and Skilled Nursing Center, PO Box 1330, Middleboro, MA 02346; tel. 508/947-9295; Mr. Paul E Corcoran

Greenery Rehabilitation and Skilled Nursing Center, 89 Lewis Bay Road, Hyannis, MA 02601; tel. 508/775-7601; Mr. Emmanuel P Freddura

Greenery Rehabilitation Center, 99 Chestnut Hill Avenue, Boston, MA 02135; tel. 617/787-3390; Mr. Brian King

Greycliff at Cape Ann, 272 Washington Street, Gloucester, MA 01930; tel. 978/281-0333; Mr. Douglas Fiero

Grosvenor Park Nursing Center, Inc., 7 Loring Hills Avenue, Salem, MA 01970; tel. 978/741-5700; Ms. Naomi Pendergast

Hallmark Nursing and Rehabilitation Center, 1123 Rockdale Avenue, New Bedford, MA 02740-2998; tel. 508/997-7448; Mr. Albert E Crabtree, Jr.

Hancock Park Rehabilitation and Nursing Center, 164 Parkingway, Quincy, MA 02169; tel. 617/773-4222; Ms. Elizabeth Flynn

Hannah Duston Healthcare Center, 126 Monument Street, Haverhill, MA 01832; tel. 978/373-1747; Mr. Edmund Taglieri, Jr.

Harbor House Rehabilitation and Nursing Center, 11 Condito Road, Hingham, MA 02043; tel. 781/749-4774; Mr. Richard Johnson

Harborside Healthcare Danvers Twin Oaks Rehab/Nursing Center, 63 Locust Street, Danvers, MA 01923; tel. 978/777-0011; Mr. Justin D Verge

Harborside Healthcare Northshore, 266 Lincoln Avenue, Saugus, MA 01906; tel. 781/233-6830; Mr. Philip S Sher

Harrington House Nursing and Rehabilitation Center, 160 Main Street, Walpole, MA 02081; tel. 508/660-3080; Mr. Anthony D Lacke

Hathaway Manor, ECF, 863 Hathaway Road, New Bedford, MA 02740; tel. 508/996-6763; Mr. Ken Persinko

Henry C. Nevins Home, Inc., Ten Ingalls Court, Methuen, MA 01844; tel. 978/682-7611; Mr. Felix F Albano, Jr.

Heritage Hall East Nursing and Rehabilitation Center, 464 Main Street, Agawam, MA 01001-2588; tel. 413/786-8000; Mr. Ira M Schoenberger

Heritage Hall West Genesis Eldercare Network, 61 Cooper Street, Agawam, MA 01001; tel. 413/786-8000; Mr. Bill Stafford

Heritage Nursing Care Center, 841 Merrimack Street, Lowell, MA 01854; tel. 978/459-0546; Mr. Michael Lehrman

Hollywell, 975 North Main Street, Randolph, MA 02368; tel. 781/963-8800; Mr. Donald M Gresh

Holy Trinity Nursing and Rehabilitation Center, 300 Barber Avenue, Worcester, MA 01606-2476; tel. 508/852-1000; Ms. Karen Laganelli

Hunt Nursing and Retirement Home, 90 Lindall Street, Danvers, MA 01923; tel. 978/777-3740; Mr. Burt Isaacs

IHS of Greater Boston at Medford, 300 Winthrop Street, Medford, MA 02155; tel. 781/396-4400; Mr. John Heller

Integrated Health Services of Greater Worcester, 215 Mill Street, Worcester, MA 01602; tel. 508/791-3168; Mr. Richard C Corey

Jesmond Nursing Home, 271 Nahant Road, Nahant, MA 01908; tel. 781/581-0420; Mr. Thomas P Costin, Jr.

Jewish Healthcare Center, Inc., 629 Salisbury Street, Worcester, MA 01609; tel. 508/798-8653; Mr. Steven Willens

Jewish Nursing Home of Western Massachusetts, Inc., 770 Converse Street, Longmeadow, MA 01106; tel. 413/567-6211; Ms. Linda Donoghue

JML Care Center, Inc., 184 Ter Heun Drive, Falmouth, MA 02540-2503; tel. 508/457-4621; Mr. Charles A Peterman, Jr.

John Scott House Rehabilita- tion and Nursing Center, 233 Middle Street, Braintree, MA 02184; tel. 781/843-1860; Mr. Thomas D Nolan

Kathleen Daniel Nursing and Rehabilitation Center, 485 Franklin Street, Framingham, MA 01702; tel. 508/872-8801; Mr. Timothy Brainerd

Kenoza Manor Convalescent Home, 190 North Avenue, Haverhill, MA 01830; tel. 978/372-7700; Mr. Richard M Augeri

Keystone Center – Genesis ElderCare, 44 Keystone Drive, Leominster, MA 01453; tel. 978/537-9327; Ms. Donna Trespas

Kimwell Rehabilitation and Nursing Center, 495 New Boston Road, Fall River, MA 02720; tel. 508/679-0106; Mr. Arthur C Taylor

Lakeview House Nursing Home, PO Box 1598, Haverhill, MA 01831-1598; tel. 978/372-1081; Mr. Jon Guarino

Laurel Lake Center for Health and Rehabilitation, 620 Laurel Street, Lee, MA 01238; tel. 413/243-2010; Ms. Jennifer Gay

Laurel Ridge Rehabilitation and Nursing Center, 174 Forest Hills Street, Jamaica Plain, MA 02130; tel. 617/522-1550; Mr. Brad A Truini

Ledgewood Rehabilitation and Skilled Nursing Center, 87 Herrick Street, Beverly, MA 01915; tel. 978/921-1392; Rev. Laurie A Roberto

Leo P. LaChance Center for Rehabilitation and Nursing, 59 Eastwood Circle, Gardner, MA 01440; tel. 978/632-8776; Mr. Dennis Lopata

Liberty Commons of Chatham, 390 Orleans Road, North Chatham, MA 02650; tel. 508/945-4611; Mr. William A Dobson

Life Care Center of Attleboro, 969 Park Street, Attleboro, MA 02703; tel. 508/222-4182; Patrick O'Connor

Life Care Center of Auburn, 14 Masonic Circle, Auburn, MA 01501; tel. 508/832-4800; Mr. James A Nugent

Life Care Center of Merrimack Valley, 80 Boston Road, North Billerica, MA 01862; tel. 978/667-2166; Ms. Colleen Lovering

Life Care Center of Nashoba Valley, 191 Foster Street, Littleton, MA 01460; tel. 978/486-3512; Ms. Ellen Levinson

Life Care Center of Plymouth, 94 Obery Street, Plymouth, MA 02360; tel. 508/747-9800; Mr. Joseph A Veno

Life Care Center of Raynham, 546 South Street East, Raynham, MA 02767; tel. 508/821-5700; Ms. Christine A Schmottlach

Life Care Center of Stoneham, 25 Woodland Road, Stoneham, MA 02180; tel. 781/662-2545; Ms. Carolyn E Lassiter

Life Care Center of the North Shore, 111 Birch Street, Lynn, MA 01902; tel. 781/592-9667; Mr. Joseph Deveau

Life Care Center of the South Shore, PO Box 830, Scituate, MA 02066; tel. 781/545-1370; Mr. Kevin Morris

Life Care Center of West Bridgewater, 765 West Center Street, West Bridgewater, MA 02379; tel. 508/580-4400; Mr. Alan J Richman

Life Care Center of Wilbraham, 2399 Boston Road, Wilbraham, MA 01095; tel. 413/596-3111; Mr. Ronald L Cherubin

Lighthouse Nursing Care Center, 204 Proctor Avenue, Revere, MA 02151; tel. 781/286-3100; Mr. Roger Marks

Lincoln Center, 299 Lincoln Street, Worcester, MA 01605; tel. 508/852-2000; Ms. Patricia Lobb

Linda Manor Extended Care Facility, 349 Haydenville Road, Leeds, MA 01053; tel. 413/586-7700; Mr. William C Jones, Jr.

Logan Nursing & Rehabiltation Center, 175 Grove Street, Braintree, MA 02184; tel. 781/848-2050; Mr. Joel K Logan

Loomis Nursing Center, 298 Jarvis Avenue, Holyoke, MA 01040; tel. 413/538-7551; Ms. Carol C Katz

Lutheran Home of Worcester, 26 Harvard Street, Worcester, MA 01609; tel. 508/754-8877; Ms. Ann M Nadreau

Madonna Manor, Inc., 85 North Washington Street, North Attleboro, MA 02760; tel. 508/699-2740; Rev. Edmund J Fitzgerald

Marian Manor, Inc., 33 Summer Street, Taunton, MA 02780; tel. 508/822-4885; Rev. Edmund J Fitzgerald

Mariner Health at Longwood, 53 Parker Hill Avenue, Boston, MA 02120; tel. 617/278-3700; Mr. Stewart R Goff

Mariner Health Care of Southeastern Massachusetts, 4586 Acushnet Avenue, New Bedford, MA 02745; tel. 508/998-1188; Ms. Marjorie Austin

Mariner Health of Methuen, 480 Jackson Street, Methuen, MA 01844; tel. 508/686-3906; Mr. Kevin Comick

Maristhill Nursing Home & Rehabilitation Center, 66 Newton Street, Waltham, MA 02453; tel. 781/893-0240; Ms. Janet Murphy

Mary Ann Morse Nursing and Rehabilitation Center, 45 Union Street, Natick, MA 01760; tel. 508/650-9003; Ms. Karen Wilkinson

Mary Lyon Nursing Home, 34 Main Street, Hampden, MA 01036; tel. 413/566-5511; Mr. Patrick Laskey

Masconomet Healthcare Center, 123 High Streeet, Topsfield, MA 01983-1926; tel. 978/887-7002; Mr. David Lewis

Masonic Home, Inc., PO Box 1000, Charlton, MA 01507-1000; tel. 508/248-7344; Mr. David C Turner

Mayflower Nursing and Rehabilitation Center, 123 South Street, Plymouth, MA 02360; tel. 508/746-4343; Mr. John H Keeney

Mayflower Place Nursing and Rehabilitation Center, 579 Buck Island Road, W Yarmouth, MA 02673; tel. 508/790-0200; Mr. Sidney Insoft

Meadow Green Nursing and Rehabilitation Center, 45 Woburn Street, Waltham, MA 02452; tel. 781/899-8600; Mr. David L Bell

Meadowbrook Nursing Home, Inc, One Meadowbrook Way, Canton, MA 02021; tel. 781/961-5600; Mr. David D Kurzman

Mediplex of Newton, 2101 Washington Street, Newton, MA 02162; tel. 617/696-4660; Ms. Donna Steirmann

Mediplex Rehabilitation and Skilled Nursing Center, 70 Granite Street, Lynn, MA 01904; tel. 781/581-2400; Mr. John A Holt

Medway Country Manor Skilled Nursing and Rehabilitation, PO Box 106, Medway, MA 02053; tel. 508/533-6634; Mr. John Peters

MI Nursing/Restorative Center, Inc., 172 Lawrence Street, Lawrence, MA 01841; tel. 978/685-6321; Ms. Barbara E Grant

Milton Health Care, 1200 Brush Hill Road, Milton, MA 02186; tel. 617/333-0600; Ms. Elizabeth Wood

Mont Marie Health Care Center, Inc., 34 Lower Westfield Road, Holyoke, MA 01040-2739; tel. 413/536-0853; Ms. Elizabeth T Sullivan

Mount St. Vincent Nursing Home, 35 Holy Family Road, Holyoke, MA 01040-2758; tel. 413/532-3246; Mr. Dennis K McKenna

Mt. Greylock Extended Care Facility, 1000 North Street, Pittsfield, MA 01201; tel. 413/499-7186; Ms. Joyce E Brewer

Providers / JCAHO Accredited Freestanding Long-Term Care Care Organizations

New England Pediatric Care, Inc., 78 Boston Road, North Billerica, MA 01862; tel. 978/667-5123; Ms. Ellen J O'Gorman

Newton & Wellesley Alzheimer Center, 694 Worcester Street, Wellesley, MA 02482; tel. 781/237-6400; Mr. Steven J Tyer

Normandy Senior Care Center, 15 Green Street, Melrose, MA 02176-2811; tel. 781/665-3950; Mr. Laurence Gerber

North End Community Nursing Home, 70 Fulton Street, Boston, MA 02109; tel. 617/367-3750; Ms. Audrey J DiBendetto

Northboro Senior Care Center, 238-1/2 West Main Street, Northboro, MA 01532; tel. 508/393-2368; Mr. Laurence Gerber

Northbridge Nursing and Rehabilitation Center, 2356 Providence Road, Northbridge, MA 01534; tel. 508/234-4641; Mr. Larry Bonds

Northwood Rehabilitation and Nursing Center, 1010 Varnum Avenue, Lowell, MA 01854; tel. 978/458-8773; Mr. Steven Garfinkle

Norwell Knoll Nursing Home, 329 Washington Street, Norwell, MA 02061; tel. 781/659-4901; Mr. Brian G Geany

Norwood Health and Rehabilitation Center, 767 Washington Street, Norwood, MA 02062; tel. 617/769-3704; Lori Peters

Notre Dame Long Term Care Center, 559 Plantation Street, Worcester, MA 01605; tel. 508/852-3011; Ms. Katherine Lemay

Nursing Care Center at Kimball Farms, 235 Walker Street, Lenox, MA 01240; tel. 413/637-4684; Mr. William C Jones, Jr.

Oak Hill Nursing and Rehabilitation Center, 76 North Street, Middleboro, MA 02346; tel. 508/947-4774; Mr. Mark S Nussman

Oak Island Skilled Nursing Facility Limited Partnership, 400 Revere Beach Boulevard, Revere, MA 02151; tel. 781/284-1958; Mr. Marc S Shpritzer

Oak Knoll Health Care Center, 9 Arbetter Drive, Framingham, MA 01701; tel. 508/877-3300; Mr. Norman Michard

Oakdale Rehabilitation and Skilled Nursing Center, 76 North Main Street, West Boylston, MA 01583; tel. 508/835-6076; Mr. David Oriol

Oakwood Rehabilitation and Nursing Center, 11 Pontiac Avenue, Webster, MA 01570; tel. 508/943-3889; Mr. Daniel O'Neil

Odd Fellows Home of Massachusetts, 104 Randolph Road, Worcester, MA 01606; tel. 508/853-6687; Mr. Jeffrey Gangi

Olympus Healthcare Center-Lanessa, 751 School Street, Webster, MA 01570; tel. 508/949-1334; Mr. Robert D Whitkin

Olympus Healthcare Center – Braintree, 1102 Washington Street, Braintree, MA 02184; tel. 781/848-3100; Mr. J. Michael Rose

Olympus Healthcare Center – Hollingsworth, 1120 Washington Street, Braintree, MA 02184; tel. 781/848-4710; Mr. Michael Rose

Olympus Healthcare Center – Webster, 745 School Street, Webster, MA 01570; tel. 508/949-0644; Ms. Ellen Saltarella

On Broadway Nursing and Rehabilitation Center, 932-934 Broadway, Chelsea, MA 02150; tel. 617/889-2250; Ms. Marjorie Minichello

Our Lady's Haven of Fairhaven, Inc., 71 Center Street, Fairhaven, MA 02719; tel. 508/999-4561; Rev. Edmund J Fitzgerald

Palm Manor Nursing Home, 40 Parkhurst Road, Chelmsford, MA 01824; tel. 978/256-3131; Mr. Thomas J Wheatley

Park Avenue Nursing, & Rehabilitation Center, 146 Park Avenue, Arlington, MA 02476; tel. 781/648-9530; Mr. John J Alessandroni

Parkwell Rehabilitation and Nursing Center, 745 Truman Highway, Hyde Park, MA 02136; tel. 617/361-8300; Ms. Mary Kilcommons

Peabody Glen Nursing Center, 199 Andover Street, Peabody, MA 01960; tel. 978/531-0772; Ms. Carmella M Mancini

Pilgrim Manor Skilled Nursing and Rehabilitation Center, 60 Stafford Street, Plymouth, MA 02360; tel. 508/746-7016; Ms. Virginia Roper

Pilgrim Rehabilitation and Skilled Nursing Center, 96 Forest Street, Peabody, MA 01960-3907; tel. 978/532-0303; Mr. Frank P Miller

Pleasant Bay Nursing and Rehabilitation Center, 383 South Orleans Road, Rte 39, Brewster, MA 02631; tel. 508/240-3500; Mr. Joshua L Zuckerman

Pleasant Manor Nursing Home, 193-195 Pleasant Street, Attleboro, MA 02703; tel. 508/222-4950; Ms. Joyce Pinto

Pond Meadow Nursing and Rehabilitation Center, 188 Summer Street, Weymouth, MA 02188; tel. 781/337-6900; Ms. Paul B Mahoney, Jr.

Port Healthcare Center, 113 Low Street, Newburyport, MA 01950; tel. 978/462-7373; Dr. Alfred L Arcidi

Prescott House Nursing Home, 140 Prescott Street, North Andover, MA 01845; tel. 978/685-8086; Ms. Judith E Blinn

Presentation Nursing and Rehabilitation Center, Ten Bellamy Street, Brighton, MA 02135; tel. 617/782-8113; Mr. Mark Jessup

Presidential Rehabilitation and Nursing Center, 43 Old Colony Avenue, Quincy, MA 02170; tel. 617/471-0155; Ms. Valerie Gingras

Quabbin Valley Healthcare, 821 Daniel Shays Highway, Athol, MA 01331; tel. 978/249-3717; Mr. Mark Ailinger

Quaboag on the Common, PO Box 386, West Brookfield, MA 01585; tel. 508/867-7716; Mrs. Loren Salvietti

Queen Anne Nursing Home, Inc., 50 Recreation Park Drive, Hingham, MA 02043; tel. 781/749-4982; Mr. Peter H Starr

Quincy Rehabilitation and Nursing Center, 11 McGrath Highway, Quincy, MA 02169-5311; tel. 617/479-2820; Mr. John Kuo

Renaissance Manor of Westfield, 37 Feeding Hills Road, Westfield, MA 01085; tel. 413/568-2341; Ms. Bonnie J Davis

Reservoir Nursing Home, 1841 Trapelo Road, Waltham, MA 02451; tel. 781/890-5000; Ms. Fran Herr

Ring Health Care Centers/East, PO Box 478, Springfield, MA 01118; tel. 413/734-1133; Ms. Matthew J Leahey

River Terrace, 1675 Main Street, Lancaster, MA 01523; tel. 978/365-4537; Ms. Laura Sansone

Rivercrest Long Term Care Facility, 80 Deaconess Road, Concord, MA 01742; tel. 978/369-5151; Mr. Willis H Brucker

Riverdale Gardens Rehabilitation and Nursing Ctr, 42 Prospect Avenue, West Springfield, MA 01089; tel. 413/733-3151; Sarah M Voss

Rosewood Nursing and Rehabilitation Center, 22 Johnson Street, Peabody, MA 01960; tel. 978/535-8700; Mr. Robert Nolan

Royal Nursing and Alzheimer's Center, 545 Main Street, Falmouth, MA 02540; tel. 508/548-3800; Mr. Thomas Dresser

Sachem Skilled Nursing and Rehabilitation Center, 66 Central Street, East Bridgewater, MA 02333; tel. 508/378-7227; Mr. Stephen Kelly

Sacred Heart Nursing Home, 359 Summer Street, New Bedford, MA 02740-5599; tel. 508/996-6751; Ms. Jean Golitz

Saint Francis Home, 101 Plantation Street, Worcester, MA 01604-3025; tel. 508/755-8605; Sister Jacquelyn Alix, PFM

Sancta Maria Nursing Facility, 799 Concord Avenue, Cambridge, MA 02138-1077; tel. 617/868-2200; Sister Mary M Pizzotti

Sarah S. Brayton Nursing Care Center, 4901 North Main Street, Fall River, MA 02720; tel. 508/675-1001; Mr. Antonio Sousa

Seacoast Nursing and Rehabilitation Center, 292 Washington Street, Gloucester, MA 01930; tel. 978/283-0300; Mr. George Gougian

Sharon Senior Care Center, 259 Norwood Street, Sharon, MA 02067; tel. 781/784-6781; Ms. Linda M Marsh

Sherrill House, Inc., 135 South Huntington Avenue, Boston, MA 02130; tel. 617/731-2400; Mr. Donald M Powell

Sippican Healthcare Center, 15 Mill Street, Marion, MA 02738; tel. 508/748-3830; Ms. Ruth Vital-Hebert

Southpointe Rehabilitation and Skilled Care Center, 100 Amity Street, Fall River, MA 02721; tel. 508/675-2500; Jim Cobbs

Southwood at Norwell Nursing Center, 501 Cordwainer Drive, Norwell, MA 02061; tel. 781/982-7450; Mr. Richard H Starr

SPEC Center, 642 Boston Post Road, Sudbury, MA 01776; tel. 978/443-4646; Ms. Roberta C Henderson

St. Joseph Manor Health Care, Inc., 215 Thatcher Street, Brockton, MA 02402; tel. 508/583-5834; Mr. Thomas J Brown

Stephen Caldwell Memorial Convalescent Home, Inc., 16 Green Street, Ipswich, MA 01938; tel. 978/356-2526; Mr. Lawrence J Pszenny

Suburban Manor Rehabilitation Nursing Center, One Great Road, Acton, MA 01720; tel. 978/263-9101; Mr. Carl H Anderson

SunBridge Care & Rehab for E. Longmeadow, 135 Benton Drive, East Longmeadow, MA 01028; tel. 413/525-3336; Mr. George Mercier

SunBridge Care & Rehabilitation for Beverly, 265 Essex Street, Beverly, MA 01915; tel. 978/927-3260; Diane C Tessier-Efstathin

Sunbridge Care and Rehab for East Boston, 910 Saratoga Street, East Boston, MA 02128; tel. 617/569-1157; Ms. Anne L Brennan

SunBridge Care and Rehabilitation for Brookline, 99 Park Street, Brookline, MA 02446; tel. 617/731-1050; Ms. Christine Baldini

SunBridge Care and Rehabilitation for Lexington, 178 Lowell Street, Lexington, MA 02420; tel. 781/862-7400; Mr. Stephen Davis

SunBridge Care and Rehabilitation for Lowell, 19 Varnum Street, Lowell, MA 01850; tel. 978/454-5644; Mr. Edward Hunt

SunBridge Care and Rehabilitation for Milford, 10 Veterans Memorial Drive, Milford, MA 01757; tel. 508/473-6414; Mr. Donald Perkins

SunBridge Care and Rehabilitation for New Bedford, 221 Fitzgerald Drive, New Bedford, MA 02745; tel. 508/996-4600; Ms. Susan M Gauthier

SunBridge Care and Rehabilitation for Northampton, 548 Elm Street, Northampton, MA 01060; tel. 413/586-3150; Mr. Christopher Durr

SunBridge Care and Rehabilitation for Weymouth, 64 Performance Drive, Weymouth, MA 02189; tel. 781/340-9800; Mr. J. Michael Rose

Sunbridge Care and Rehabilitation for Wilmington, 750 Woburn Street, Wilmington, MA 01887; tel. 978/988-0888; Mr. Delbert Downing

SunBridge for Holyoke, 260 EastHampton Road, Holyoke, MA 01040; tel. 413/538-9733; Mr. Darrell Carlson

Sunbridge for Millbury, 312 Millbury Avenue, Millbury, MA 01527; tel. 508/793-0088; Mr. Joseph Yalmokas

SunBridgeCare & Rehabilitation for Hadley @ Elaine Manor, Box 720, Hadley, MA 01035; tel. 413/584-5057; Ms. Agnes S Mauro

Sunny Acres Nursing Home, Inc., 254 Billerica Road, Chelmsford, MA 01824-4184; tel. 978/256-1616; Ms. Shirley Freitas

SunRise Care and Rehabilitation for Concord, 57 Old Road to Nine Acre Corner, Concord, MA 01742; tel. 978/371-3400; Mr. James A Nugent

Sutton Hill Center, 1801 Turnpike Street, North Andover, MA 01845; tel. 978/688-1212; Ms. LuAnn Kuder

Sweet Brook Care Centers, Inc., 1561 Cold Spring Road, Williamstown, MA 01267; tel. 413/458-8120; Mr. John F Warren

Taber Street Nursing Home, 19 Taber Street, New Bedford, MA 02740; tel. 508/997-0791; Ms. Kathleen Ferranti

The Boston Center For Rehabilitative & Subacute Care, 1245 Centre Street, Roslindale, MA 02131; tel. 617/325-5400; Mr. Michael Walker

The Buckley Center for Nursing and Rehabilitation, 282 Cabot Street, Holyoke, MA 01040; tel. 413/538-7470; Mr. Patrick Laskey

The Center for Optimum Care – Falmouth, 359 Jones Road, Falmouth, MA 02540; tel. 508/457-9000; Mr. Thomas Sullivan

The Center for Optimum Care – Mashpee, 161 Falmouth Road – Route 28, Mashpee, MA 02649; tel. 508/477-2490; Mr. Michael Gallagher

The Center for Optimum Care – Wakefield, Bathol Street, Wakefield, MA 01880; tel. 781/245-7600; Mr. John Brennan

The Center for Optimum Care – Westfield, 60 East Silver Street, Westfield, MA 01085; tel. 413/562-5121; Ms. Audrey Cushing

The Ellis Nursing and Rehabilitation Center, 135 Ellis Avenue, Norwood, MA 02062; tel. 781/762-6880; Mr. George W Seabrook

The Goddard Center, 909 Sumner Street, Stoughton, MA 02072; tel. 781/297-8203; Ms. Barbara Hendricks

The Greenery Extended Care Center, 59 Acton Street, Worcester, MA 01604; tel. 508/791-3147; Ms. Sandra Brunelle

The Guardian Center, 888 North Main Street, Brockton, MA 02401; tel. 508/587-6556; Mr. Dennis Sullivan

The Hellenic Nursing Home for the Aged, 601 Sherman Street, Canton, MA 02021-2025; tel. 781/828-7450; Mr. David Cavalier

The Highlands, 335 Nichols Road, Fitchburg, MA 01420; tel. 978/343-4411; Ms. JoAnn Piedrafite

The Lafayette Convalescent Home, 25 Lafayette Street, Marblehead, MA 01945; tel. 781/631-4535; Mr. William Mantzoukas

Providers / JCAHO Accredited Freestanding Long-Term Care Care Organizations

The Meadows Skilled Nursing and Rehabilitation Center, 111 Huntoon Memorial Highway, Rochdale, MA 01542; tel. 508/892-4858; Ms. Jill Zucco
The Oaks, 4525 Acushnet Avenue, New Bedford, MA 02745; tel. 508/998-7807; Mr. Robert G Noonan
The Oxford, 689 Main Street, Haverhill, MA 01830; tel. 978/373-1131; Mr. John G Albert
Town & Country Nursing Center, 259 Baldwin Street, Lowell, MA 01851; tel. 978/454-5438; Mr. James S Mamary
University Commons Nursing Care Center, 378 Plantation Street, Worcester, MA 01605-4311; tel. 508/755-7300; Mr. Mark S Berman
Wachusett Extended Care Facility, 56 Boyden Road, Holden, MA 01520-2593; tel. 508/829-7383; Mr. James M Oliver
Walden Rehabilitation and Nursing Center, 785 Main Street, Concord, MA 01742; tel. 978/369-6889; Mr. Robert M Hayes
Wedgemere Rehabilitation and Nursing Center, 146 Dean Street, Taunton, MA 02780; tel. 508/823-C767; Mr. William C Moloney, Jr.
Wellesley Health and Rehabilitation Center, 878 Worcester Road, Wellesley, MA 02181; tel. 781/235-6699; George Elkins
West Acres Nursing Home and Rehabilitation Center, 804 Pleasant Street, Brockton, MA 02401-3099; tel. 508/583-6000; Mr. John G Soule
Westborough Nursing Center, 5 Colonial Drive, Westborough, MA 01581; tel. 508/366-9131; Mr. Joel R Stevens
Westford Nursing and Rehabilitation Center, 3 Park Drive, Westford, MA 01886; tel. 978/392-1144; Ms. Wendy D LaBate
Weston Manor Nursing and Rehabilitation Center, 75 Norumbega Road, Weston, MA 02193; tel. 781/891-6100; Ms. Evelyn Insoft
Willow Manor, 30 Princeton Boulevard, Lowell, MA 01851; tel. 978/454-8086; Mr. David A Lewis
Willowood Health Care Center of North Adams, 175 Franklin Street, North Adams, MA 01247; tel. 413/664-4041; Mr. Michael Stroetzel
Willowood Nursing and Retirement Facility, 151 Christian Hill Road, Great Barrington, MA 01230; tel. 413/528-4560; Ms. Deborah Richardson
Willowood of Pittsfield Health Care Center, 169 Valentine Road, Pittsfield, MA 01201; tel. 413/445-2300; Mr. Leo Attella
Willowood of Williamstown, 25 Adams Road, Williamstown, MA 01267; tel. 413/458-2111; Mr. Ron T Cerow
Winchester Nursing Center, Inc, PO Box 490, Winchester, MA 01890; tel. 781/729-9595; Mr. Richard H Salter
Windsor Skilled Nursing and Rehabilitation Center, 265 North Main Street, South Yarmouth, MA 02664; tel. 508/394-3514; Garrett O Driscoll
Wingate at Andover, 80 Andover Street, Andover, MA 01810; tel. 978/470-3434; Mr. John T Kain
Wingate at Brighton Rehabilitative/Skilled Nursing, 100 North Beacon Street, Boston, MA 02134; tel. 617/787-2300; Mr. Paul Dixon
Wingate at Needham, 589 Highland Avenue, Needham, MA 02194; tel. 781/455-9090; Mr. Richard Herrick
Wingate at Reading, 1364 Main Street, Reading, MA 01867; tel. 781/942-1210; Ms. Catherine M Congo
Wingate at Sudbury, Inc., 136 Boston Post Road, Sudbury, MA 01776; tel. 978/443-2722; Mr. Gerald Schuster
Wingate at Wilbraham, 9 Maple Street, Wilbraham, MA 01095; tel. 413/596-2411; Ms. Marcia B Zimmer
Woburn Nursing Center, 18 Frances Street, Woburn, MA 01801; tel. 781/933-8175; Ms. Barbara Wilkins
Woodbriar of Wilmington Rehab and Skilled Nursing Center, 90 West Street, Wilmington, MA 01887; tel. 978/658-2700; Mr. Dennis S Sargent
Woodford of Ayer, 15 Winthrop Avenue, Ayer, MA 01432; tel. 978/772-0409; Mr. Todd McDonagh

MICHIGAN
Bay County Medical Care Facility, 564 West Hampton Road, Essexville, MI 48732; tel. 517/892-3591; Mr. William P Mahoney
Boulder Park Terrace, 14676 West Upright, Charlevoix, MI 49720; tel. 616/547-1005; Ms. Deborah Saur
Brookcrest Christian Nursing Home, 3400 Wilson Avenue, Grandville, MI 49418; tel. 616/534-5487; Mr. Richard Freerksen
Calhoun County Medical Care Facility, 1150 East Michigan Avenue, Battle Creek, MI 49014; tel. 616/962-5458; Ms. Joanne J Konkle
Charter House of Farmington Hills, 21017 Middlebelt Road, Farmington Hills, MI 48336; tel. 248/476-8300; Ms. Lisa Berthold
Christian Rest Home Association, 1000 Edison Ave. N.W., Grand Rapids, MI 49504-3999; tel. 616/453-2475; Mr. Todd Nyeholt
Crestmont HealthCare Center, 111 Trealout Drive, Fenton, MI 48430; tel. 810/629-4105; Ms. Lisa Anetrini
Evangelical Home – Port Huron, 5635 Lakeshore Road, Fort Gratiot, MI 48059; tel. 810/385-7447; Ms. Denise Rabidoux
Farmington Health Care, 34225 Grand River Avenue, Farmington, MI 48335; tel. 248/477-7373; Mr. Neal Elliott
Fraser Villa – A Mercy Living Center, 33300 Utica Road, Fraser, MI 48026; tel. 810/293-3300; Ms. Julie C Kaslly
Genesys Convalescent Center – Grand Blanc, Inc., 8481 Holly Road, Grand Blanc, MI 48439; tel. 810/694-1711; Mr. Robert K Stevens
Haven Park Christian Nursing Home, 285 North State Street, Zeeland, MI 49464; tel. 616/772-4641; Mr. Steve Zuiderveen
Heartland Health Care Center – Allen Park, 9150 Allen Road, Allen Park, MI 48101; tel. 313/386-2150; Mr. Richard Shook
Heartland Health Care Center – Briarwood, 3011 North Center Road, Flint, MI 48506; tel. 810/736-0600; Shawn Coughlin
Heartland Health Care Center – Dearborn Heights, 26001 Ford Road, Dearborn Heights, MI 48127; tel. 313/274-4600; Ms. Leslie Shanlian
Heartland Health Care Center – Dorvin, 29270 Morlock Street, Livonia, MI 48152; tel. 810/476-0555; Mr. Benjamin Duckworth
Heartland Health Care Center – Georgian Bloomfield, 2975 North Adams Road, Bloomfield Hills, MI 48304; tel. 248/645-2900; Ms. Julie Musiol
Heartland Health Care Center – Georgian East, 21401 Mack Avenue, Grosse Pointe, MI 48236; tel. 810/778-0800; Ms. Monte Schloss
Heartland Health Care Center – Kalamazoo, 3625 West Michigan Avenue, Kalamazoo, MI 49006; tel. 616/375-4550; Ms. Mary Ann Bremmer
Heartland Health Care Center – Knollview, 1061 West Hackley Avenue, Muskegon, MI 49441; tel. 616/755-2255; Ms. Nancy Wisner
Heartland Health Care Center – Plymouth Court, 105 Haggerty Road, Plymouth, MI 48170; tel. 313/455-0510; Mr. Michael Perry
Heartland Health Care Center – University, 28550 Five Mile Road, Livonia, MI 48154; tel. 734/427-8270; Ms. Roslind Ferrone
Heartland Healthcare Center – Ann Arbor, 4701 East Huron River Drive, Ann Arbor, MI 48105; tel. 734/975-2600; Ms. Betsy J Perry
Holland Health Care Center, 493 West 32nd Street, Holland, MI 49423; tel. 616/396-1438; Mr. Denis Hill
Holland Home – Breton Manor, 2589 44th Street Southeast, Kentwood, MI 49512; tel. 616/235-5003; Mr. H. David Claus
Holland Home – Fulton Manor, 1450 East Fulton Avenue, Grand Rapids, MI 49503; tel. 616/235-5001; H. David Claus
Holland Home – Raybrook Manor, 2121 Raybrook, Southeast, Grand Rapids, MI 49546; tel. 616/235-5002; David Claus
IHS of Michigan @ Clarkston, 4800 Clintonville Road, Clarkston, MI 48346; tel. 248/674-0903; Ms. Margaret Canny
IHS of Michigan at Howell, 3003 West Grand River, Howell, MI 48843; tel. 517/546-4210; Mr. Todd Funk
Integrated Health Services of Michigan at Riverbend, 11941 Belsay Road, Grand Blanc, MI 48439; tel. 810/694-1970; Mr. Lee Karson
Isabella County Medical Care Facility, 1222 North Drive, Mount Pleasant, MI 48858; tel. 517/772-2957; Ms. Vickie S Block
Martha T. Berry Memorial Medical Care Facility, 43533 Elizabeth Road, Mount Clemens, MI 48043; tel. 810/469-5265; Ms. Josephine Savalle-Dunn
Mercy Pavilion, 80 North 20th Street, Battle Creek, MI 49015; tel. 616/964-5400; Mr. Stephen Abbott
Mercy Services for Aging, 875 Avon Road, Rochester Hills, MI 48307; tel. 248/656-3239; Ms. Karen Struve
Metron of Greenville, 828 East Washington Street, Greenville, MI 48838; tel. 616/754-7186; Mr. Mark Pierpsma
North Ottawa Care Center, 1615 South Despelder, Grand Haven, MI 49417-2633; tel. 616/842-0770; Ms. Susan Pawlak
Oakland County Medical Care Facility, 1200 North Telegraph Road, Pontiac, MI 48341-0469; tel. 248/858-1415; Ms. Shirla F Kugler
Orchard Hills, A Mercy Living Center, 532 Orchard Lake Road, Pontiac, MI 48341; tel. 248/338-7151; Ms. Robyn Gabbard
Porter Hills Health and Rehab Center, 3600 East Fulton Street, Grand Rapids, MI 49546-1395; tel. 616/949-4971; Mr. Jeff Huegli
Rivergate Convalescent Center, 14041 Pennsylvania Road, Riverview, MI 48192; tel. 734/284-7200; Ms. Elizabeth Edenstrom
Rivergate Terrace, 14141 Pennsylvania Road, Riverview, MI 48192; tel. 734/284-8000; Mr. John Polturanus
Shore Haven, A Mercy Living Center, 900 South Beacon Boulevard, Grand Haven, MI 49417; tel. 616/846-1850; Ms. Nancy J Ritchie
Special Tree NeuroCare Center, 39000 Chase Road, Romulus, MI 48174; tel. 734/941-1142; Ms. Cathy A Blevins
The Laurels of Hudsonville, 3650 Van Buren Street, Hudsonville, MI 49426; tel. 616/669-1520; Mr. Dennis G Sherman
The Marvin and Betty Danto Health Care Center, 6800 West Maple, West Bloomfield, MI 48322; tel. 810/788-5300; Mr. Larry Lester
University Park Living Center, 570 South Harvey Street, Muskegon, MI 49442; tel. 231/773-9121; Dr. Ronald D Rop

MINNESOTA
Bloomington Health Care & Rehabilitation, 9200 Nicollet Avenue South, Bloomington, MN 55420; tel. 612/881-8676; Mr. Joseph G Gubbels
Chateau Healthcare Center, 2106 2nd Avenue South, Minneapolis, MN 55404; tel. 612/874-1603; Ms. Phyllis C Winters
Ebenezer Hall and Luther Hall, 2636 Park Avenue South, Minneapolis, MN 55407; tel. 612/879-2286; Ms. Joanne Gilbertson
Ebenezer Ridges Care Center, 13820 Community Drive, Burnsville, MN 55337; tel. 612/435-8116; Ms. Sharon Klefsaas
Greeley Healthcare Center, 313 South Greeley Street, Stillwater, MN 55082; tel. 651/439-5775; Ms. Jean Cole
La Crescent Healthcare Center, 701 Main Street, La Crescent, MN 55947; tel. 507/895-4445; Ms. Gale Bruessel
Lexington Health and Rehabilitation Center, 375 North Lexington Parkway, Saint Paul, MN 55104; tel. 612/645-0577; Ms. Mary Brun
Moorhead Healthcare Center, 2810 2nd Avenue North, Moorhead, MN 56560; tel. 218/233-7578; Mr. David W Erickson
Olivia Healthcare Center, PO Box 229, Olivia, MN 56277; tel. 320/523-1652; Mr. Scott D Spates
Park Health and Rehabilitation Center, 4415 West 36 1/2 Street, Saint Louis Park, MN 55416; tel. 612/927-9717; Ms. Vivian Booker
St. Louis Park Plaza Health Care Center, 3201 Virginia Avenue South, Saint Louis Park, MN 55426; tel. 612/935-0333; Ms. Judi Woloszczyk
Trevilla of Golden Valley, 7505 Country Club Drive, Golden Valley, MN 55427; tel. 612/545-0416; Mr. Larry Vander Poel
Trevilla of New Brighton, 825 First Avenue Northwest, New Brighton, MN 55112; tel. 612/633-7875; Ms. JoAnn Buytendorp
Twin Rivers Care Center, 305 Fremont Street, Anoka, MN 55303; tel. 612/421-5660; Ms. Amy Mackenzie
University Good Samaritan Center, 22 – 27th Avenue Southeast, Minneapolis, MN 55414; tel. 612/332-4262; Mr. Jonathan E Lundberg

MISSISSIPPI
Beverly Healthcare – Eupora, PO Box 918, Eupora, MS 39744-2029; tel. 601/258-8293; Mr. Gerald Gary
Lakeland Health Care Center, 3680 Lakeland Lane, Jackson, MS 39216; tel. 601/982-5505; Ms. Debbie Spence
Ruleville Health Care Center, 800 Stansel Drive, Ruleville, MS 38771; tel. 601/756-4361; Ms. Kathy Hopkins
United States Naval Home, 1800 Beach Drive, Gulfport, MS 39507-1597; tel. 228/897-4003; Capt Jesse H Vasquez

MISSOURI
Alexian Brothers Lansdowne Village, 4624 Lansdowne, Saint Louis, MO 63116; tel. 314/351-6888; Ms. Kim Woodsmall
Balanced Care Hermitage, PO Box 325, Hermitage, MO 65668; tel. 417/745-2111; Mr. Stephen G Marcus

Providers / JCAHO Accredited Freestanding Long-Term Care Care Organizations

Balanced Care Lebanon North, PO Box K, Lebanon, MO 65536; tel. 417/532-9173; Mr. Brad Hollinger
Balanced Care Lebanon South, 514 West Fremont Road, Lebanon, MO 65536; tel. 417/532-5351; Mr. Al Lovitz
BCC at Republic Park Care Center, Inc., PO Box 755, Republic, MO 65738; tel. 417/732-1822; Mr. Stephen G Marcus
Harry S. Truman Restorative Center, 5700 Arsenal Street, St. Louis, MO 63139; tel. 314/768-6600; Mr. Edward M Peters
Integrated Health Services of Kansas City at Alpine North, 4700 Cliff View Drive, Kansas City, MO 64150; tel. 816/741-5105; Ms. Karen Leverich
Integrated Health Services of St. Louis at Gravois, 10954 Kennerly Road, St. Louis, MO 63128; tel. 314/843-8282; Dr. Robert Elkins
John Knox Village Care Center, 600 NW Pryor Road, Lees Summit, MO 64081; tel. 816/246-4343; Mr. Gary Holmes
Life Care Center of Saint Louis, 3520 Chouteau Avenue, Saint Louis, MO 63103; tel. 314/771-2100; Mr. Bill Maggard
ManorCare Health Services, 1200 Graham Road, Florissant, MO 63031; tel. 314/838-6555; Ms. Anita Martinez
Village North Health Center, 11160 Village North Drive, St. Louis, MO 63136; tel. 314/355-8010; Ms. Maureen Dunn
Village North Manor, 6768 North Highway 67, Florissant, MO 63034; tel. 314/741-9101; Ms. Elaine B Piper
Woodbine Healthcare and Rehabilitation Centre, 2900 Kendallwood Parkway, Kansas City, MO 64119; tel. 816/453-1222; Mr. Rick Oros

NEBRASKA
Beverly Healthcare - Scottsbluff, 111 West 36th Street, Scottsbluff, NE 69361; tel. 308/635-2019; Ms. Pamela A Cover
Columbus Manor, PO Box 625, Columbus, NE 68601; tel. 402/564-8014; Mr. Alexander Willford
Good Samaritan Village, PO Box 2149, Hastings, NE 68902-2149; tel. 402/463-3181; Ms. Mary F Kraus
Hallmark Care Center, 5505 Grover Street, Omaha, NE 68106; tel. 402/558-0225; Mr. Kurt Luth
Millard Good Samaritan Center, 12856 Deauville Drive, Omaha, NE 68137; tel. 402/895-2266; Mr. Ronald Fechner
Montclair Nursing and Rehab Center, 2525 South 135th Avenue, Omaha, NE 68144; tel. 402/333-2304; Mr. David Lading
Park Place Health Care and Rehabilitation Center, 610 North Darr, Grand Island, NE 68803; tel. 308/382-2635; Mr. Tim Groshans
Plattsmouth Manor and Rehabilitation Center, 602 South 18th Street, Plattsmouth, NE 68048; tel. 402/296-2800; Mr. William R Gerken
The Ambassador Lincoln, 4405 Normal Boulevard, Lincoln, NE 68506; tel. 402/488-2355; Mr. Michael D Ryan
Valhaven Nursing Center, PO Box 357, Valley, NE 68064; tel. 402/359-2533; Ms. Tammy Sealer

NEW HAMPSHIRE
Dover Rehabilitation and Living Center, 307 Plaza Drive, Dover, NH 03820; tel. 603/742-2676; Ms. Mary Lou Asbell
Genesis ElderCare Network - Keene Center, 677 Court Street, Keene, NH 03431; tel. 603/357-3800; Mr. James C Harrison
Golden View Health Care Center, 19 New Hampshire Route 104, Meredith, NH 03253; tel. 603/279-8111; Ms. Jeanne Sanders
Good Shepherd Nursing Home, 20 Plantation Drive, Jaffrey, NH 03452; tel. 603/532-8762; Ms. Judith A LeBlanc
Greenbriar Terrace Healthcare, 55 Harris Road, Nashua, NH 03062; tel. 603/888-1573; Mr. David Stordy
Hanover Hill Health Care Center, 700 Hanover Street, Manchester, NH 03104; tel. 603/627-3826; Mr. Theodore J Lee
Hanover Terrace Healthcare, 53 Lyme Road, Hanover, NH 03755; tel. 603/643-2854; Mr. Carl Hausler
Harborside Healthcare - Applewood, 8 Snow Road, Winchester, NH 03470; tel. 603/239-6355; Ms. Lorraine Comi
Harborside Healthcare - Crestwood Rehab and Nursing, 40 Crosby Road, Milford, NH 03055; tel. 603/673-7061; Ms. Linda Brooks
Harborside Healthcare - Northwood, 30 Colby Court, Bedford, NH 03110; tel. 603/625-6462; Mr. David Ross
Harborside Healthcare - Pheasant Wood, 100 Pheasant Road, Peterborough, NH 03458; tel. 603/924-7267; Mr. Bruce C Moorhead
Integrated Health Services of New Hampshire at Claremont, RFD 3, Box 47, Hanover Street Extension, Claremont, NH 03743; tel. 603/542-2606; Mr. Sean Stevenson
Integrated Health Services of Derry, 8 Peabody Road, Derry, NH 03038; tel. 603/434-1566; Sean Stevenson
Integrated Health Services of New Hampshire at Manchester, 191 Hackett Hill Road, Manchester, NH 03102; tel. 603/668-8161; Mr. Charles E Bernard
Maple Leaf Health Care Center, 198 Pearl Street, Manchester, NH 03104; tel. 603/669-1660; Ms. Rita Miville
Mount Carmel Nursing Home, 235 Myrtle Street, Manchester, NH 03104; tel. 603/627-3811; Mr. Stephen V Fulchino
Ridgewood Center, 25 Ridgewood Road, Bedford, NH 03110; tel. 603/623-8805; Ms. Bonnie Kisielewski
Rochester Manor, 40 Whitehall Road, Rochester, NH 03867; tel. 603/332-7711; Mr. Mark Finkelstein
Saint Ann Home, 195 Dover Point Road, Dover, NH 03820; tel. 603/742-2612; Sr. Karen J Painter
Saint Vincent de Paul Nursing Home, 29 Providence Avenue, Berlin, NH 03570; tel. 603/752-1820; Mr. Steven E Woods
Seacoast Health Center, 22 Tuck Road, Hampton, NH 03842; tel. 603/926-4551; Mr. Daniel P Trahan
St. Francis Home, 406 Court Street, Laconia, NH 03246; tel. 603/524-0466; Ms. Julieann R Fay
St. Teresa's Manor, 519 Bridge Street, Manchester, NH 03104; tel. 603/668-2373; Mr. Patrick F McManus
The Edgewood Centre, 928 South Street, Portsmouth, NH 03801; tel. 603/436-0099; Ms. Patricia Cummings
Villa Crest Nursing and Retirement Center, 1276 Hanover Street, Manchester, NH 03104; tel. 603/622-3262; Mr. Ron Lusk

NEW JERSEY
Absecon Manor Nursing and Rehabilitation Center, 1020 Pitney Road, Absecon, NJ 08201; tel. 609/646-5400; Ms. Marlene Dziaba
Arbor Glen Center / Genesis ElderCare, Pompton Avenue/E Lindsley Road, Cedar Grove, NJ 07009; tel. 973/256-7220; Mr. Micheal S Ewing
Arnold Walter Nursing Home, 622 Laurel Avenue, Hazlet, NJ 07730; tel. 732/787-6300; Mr. Benezion Schachter
Ashbrook Nursing and Rehabilitation Center, 1610 Raritan Road, Scotch Plains, NJ 07076; tel. 908/889-5500; Carmen Alecci
Atlantic Coast Rehabilitation and Health Care Center, 485 River Avenue, Lakewood, NJ 08701; tel. 732/364-7100; Mr. Melvin Feigenbaum
Barn Hill Care Center, 249 High Street, Newton, NJ 07860; tel. 973/383-5600; Ms. Janice Brown
Barnegat Nursing Center, 859 West Bay Avenue, Barnegat, NJ 08005; tel. 609/698-1400; Karen Scienski
Bartley Healthcare Nursing and Rehabilitation, 175 Bartley Road, Jackson, NJ 08527; tel. 732/370-4700; Mrs. Mary Jane Eicke
Berkeley Heights Convalescent Center, 35 Cottage Street, Berkeley Heights, NJ 07922; tel. 908/464-0048; Mr. Michael Handsman
Bey Lea Village, 1351 Old Freehold Road, Toms River, NJ 08753; tel. 732/240-0090; Ms. Christine Lapid
Brakeley Park Center - Genesis ElderCare Network, 290 Red School Lane, Phillipsburg, NJ 08865; tel. 908/859-2800; Ms. Mary D Tucker
Cedar Oaks Care Center, 1311 Durham Avenue, South Plainfield, NJ 07080; tel. 732/287-9555; Mr. Morris Wiesel
Chestnut Hill Convalescent and Rehabilitation Center, 360 Chestnut Street, Passaic, NJ 07055; tel. 973/777-7800; Mr. Michael G Mazzola
Cinniminson Nursing and Rehabilitation Center, 1700 Wynwood Drive, Cinnaminson, NJ 08077; tel. 609/829-9000; Mr. Ronald Waterman
Clark Nursing and Rehabilitation Center, 1213 Westfield Avenue, Clark, NJ 07066; tel. 732/396-7100; Ms. Joanne Ryan
Cornell Hall, 234 Chestnut Street, Union, NJ 07083; tel. 908/687-7800; Carmen Alecci
Courthouse Convalescent Center, 144 Magnolia Drive, Cape May Court House, NJ 08210; tel. 609/465-7171; Mr. Benjamin Miller
Cranbury Nursing and Rehabilitation Center, 292 Applegarth Road, Cranbury, NJ 08512; tel. 609/860-2500; Mr. J P Cronin
Crestwood Nursing and Rehabilitation Center, 101 Whippany Road, Whippany, NJ 07981; tel. 973/887-0311; Ms. Carol Shepard
Daughters of Israel Geriatric Center, 1155 Pleasant Valley Way, West Orange, NJ 07052; tel. 973/731-5100; Mr. Lawerence Gelfand
Daughters of Miriam / The Gallen Institute, 155 Hazel Street, Clifton, NJ 07015; tel. 973/253-5210; Mr. Jay S Solomon
Delaire Nursing and Convalescent Center, 400 West Stimpson Avenue, Linden, NJ 07036; tel. 908/862-3399; Ms. Barbara Andrews
Dunroven Health Care Center, 221 County Road, Cresskill, NJ 07626; tel. 201/567-9310; Ms. Stefanie Mair
Eastern Shore Nursing and Rehabilitation Center, 1419 Route 9 North, Cape May Court House, NJ 08210; tel. 609/465-2260; Mr. Benjamin Miller
Forrestal Nursing and Rehabilitation Center, 5000 Windrow Drive, Princeton, NJ 08540; tel. 609/987-1221; Ms. Linda Berger
Franklin Convalescent Center, 3371 Route 27, Franklin Park, NJ 08823; tel. 732/821-8000; Mr. Robert Kovacs
Gateway Care Center, 139 Grant Avenue, Eatontown, NJ 07724; tel. 732/542-4700; Mr. Steven Goldberg
Glenside Nursing Center, 144 Gales Drive, New Providence, NJ 07974; tel. 908/464-8600; Ms. Joan Lepore
Green Acres Manor, 1931 Lakewood Road, Route 9, Toms River, NJ 08755; tel. 732/286-2323; Mr. Robert Michael Lapid
Greenbrook Manor, 303 Rock Avenue, Green Brook, NJ 08812; tel. 732/968-5500; Carmen B Alecci
Hamilton Park Health Care Center, 525-535 Monmouth Street, Jersey City, NJ 07302; tel. 201/653-8800; Ms. Natalie Zanetich-Fatigati
Hamilton Plaza Nursing and Rehabilitation Center, 56 Hamilton Avenue, Passaic, NJ 07055; tel. 973/773-7070; Ms. Lynda Solomon
Harborside Healthcare - Woods Edge, 875 Route 202/206 North, Bridgewater, NJ 08807; tel. 908/526-8600; Mr. Alain Bernard
Harrogate, Inc., 400 Locust Street, Lakewood, NJ 08701; tel. 732/905-7070; Mr. Donald A Johansen
Heath Village Retirement Community, Schooley's Mountain Road, Hackettstown, NJ 07840; tel. 908/852-4801; Mr. Patrick E Brady
Inglemoor Care Center, 311 South Livingston Avenue, Livingston, NJ 07039; tel. 973/994-0221; Mr. Daniel Moles
Integrated Health Services of New Jersey at Somerset Valley, 1621 Route 22 West, Bound Brook, NJ 08805; tel. 732/469-2000; Ms. Carolyn Allen
Jackson Center - Genesis ElderCare, 11 History Lane, Jackson, NJ 08527; tel. 732/367-6600; Mr. Chris Vogt
JFK Hartwyck at Cedar Brook, 1340 Park Avenue, Plainfield, NJ 07060; tel. 908/754-3100; Mr. Thomas Lankey
JFK Hartwyck at Edison Estates, 465 Plainfield Avenue, Edison, NJ 08817; tel. 732/985-1500; Mr. Thomas Lankey
JFK Hartwyck at Oak Tree Nrsg, Convalescent, & Rehab Center, 2048 Oak Tree Road, Edison, NJ 08820; tel. 732/906-2100; Mr. Thomas Lankey
Lakeview Subacute Care Center, 130 Terhune Drive, Wayne, NJ 07470; tel. 973/839-4500; Ms. Margaret Nolan
Laurelton Village, 475 Jack Martin Boulevard, Brick, NJ 08724; tel. 732/458-6600; Ms. Sue Jones
Lincoln Park Subacute and Rehab Center Inc., One, 521 Pine Brook Road, Lincoln Park, NJ 07035; tel. 201/696-3300; Ms. Carla Turco-Kipiani
Linwood Convalescent Center, Route 9 and Central Avenue, Linwood, NJ 08221; tel. 609/927-6131; Ms. Ellie Kinsey-Skroski
Llanfair House, 1140 Black Oak Ridge Road, Wayne, NJ 07470; tel. 973/835-7443; Carmen B Alecci
Logan Manor Care Center, 23 Schoolhouse Road, Whiting, NJ 08759; tel. 732/849-4300; Ms. Rita Berardo
Mainland Manor Nursing and Rehabilitation Center, PO Box 1309, Pleasantville, NJ 08232; tel. 609/646-6900; Ms. Margaret Gannon
Manchester Manor Associates, 101 State Highway 70, Lakehurst, NJ 08733; tel. 732/657-1800; Ms. Shawne R Mimna

Providers / JCAHO Accredited Freestanding Long-Term Care Care Organizations

ManorCare Health Services, 1180 Route 22 West, Mountainside, NJ 07092; tel. 908/654-0020; Mr. Jeffrey Floyd

ManorCare Health Services, 1412 Marlton Pike, Cherry Hill, NJ 08034; tel. 856/428-6100; Ms. Marie G Voelicek

ManorCare Health Services, 550 Jessup Road, West Deptford, NJ 08066; tel. 609/848-9551; Mr. Tony Stinson

Marcella Center–Genesis Eldercare, 2305 Rancocas Road, Burlington Township, NJ 08016; tel. 609/387-9300; Mr. Ben Arccadi

Margaret McLaughlin McCarrick Care Center, 15 Dellwood Lane, Somerset, NJ 08873; tel. 732/545-4200; Mr. James F Caron

Meadow View Nursing and Respiratory Care Center, 1328 South Black Horse Pike, Williamstown, NJ 08094; tel. 856/875-0100; Ms. Cass Salema

Medford Care Center, 185 Tuckerton Road, Medford, NJ 08055; tel. 856/983-8500; Mr. Richard Pineles

Medicenter/Neptune City, 2050 Sixth Avenue, Neptune City, NJ 07753-6197; tel. 732/774-8300; Ms. Mary Lou Browning

Millhouse, 325 Jersey Street, Trenton, NJ 08611; tel. 609/394-3400; Mr. Michael D Gentile

Morris Hills Genesis Eldercare Center, 77 Madison Avenue, Morristown, NJ 07960; tel. 973/540-9800; Ms. Ceil Weisbauer

Morris View Nursing Home, PO Box 437, Morris Plains, NJ 07950; tel. 973/285-2820; Mr. Joaquin Deniz

Mt. Laurel Nursing and Rehabilitation Center, 3706 Church Road, Mount Laurel, NJ 08054; tel. 609/235-7100; Mr. Michael Veloric

Neptune ConvaCenter, 101 Walnut Street, Neptune, NJ 07753; tel. 732/774-3550; Mr. George Michals

Oak Ridge Rehabilitation and Nursing Center, 261 Terhune Drive, Wayne, NJ 07470; tel. 973/835-3871; Mr. Robert Valentine

Old Bridge Manor, 6989 Route 18 South, Old Bridge, NJ 08857; tel. 732/360-2277; Ms. Dana McWilliams

Parkway Manor Health Center, 480 Parkway Drive, East Orange, NJ 07017; tel. 973/674-2700; Ms. Ellen Alibrando

Pine Rest Health Care Center, West 90 Ridgewood Avenue, Paramus, NJ 07652; tel. 201/652-1950; Ms. Dorothy Franklin

Regent Care Center, 50 Polifly Road, Hackensack, NJ 07601; tel. 201/646-1166; Mr. Steven Schilsky

Riverview Extended Care Residence, 55 West Front Street, Red Bank, NJ 07701; tel. 908/842-3800; Mr. Laurence C Gumina

Seacrest Village Nursing and Rehabilitation Center, PO Box 1480, Little Egg Harbor Twp, NJ 08087; tel. 609/296-9292; Mr. Brian T Holloway

Silver Care Center, 1423 Brace Road, Cherry Hill, NJ 08034; tel. 856/795-3131; Mr. Marc I Silver

South Mountain Healthcare and Rehabilitation Center, 2385 Springfield Avenue, Vauxhall, NJ 07088-1046; tel. 908/688-3400; Mr. Jacob Frommer

Southern Ocean Nursing and Rehabilitation Center, 1361 Route 72 West, Manahawkin, NJ 08050; tel. 609/978-0600; Mr. Robert E Stark

Sunbridge Care and Rehabilitation for Oradell, 600 Kinderkamack Road, Oradell, NJ 07649; tel. 201/967-0002; Ms. Rebecca Resh

SunRise Care and Rehabilitation for Southern NJ, 2 Cooper Plaza, Camden, NJ 08103; tel. 609/342-7600; Mr. Christopher Gillies

The Health Center at Bloomingdale, 255 Union Avenue, Bloomingdale, NJ 07403; tel. 973/283-1700; Ms. Nancy Cougahlin

The Manor, 689 West Main Street, Freehold, NJ 07728-2511; tel. 732/431-5200; Mr. Thomas H Litz

The Pope John Paul II Pavilion at Saint Mary's Life Center, 135 South Center Street, Orange, NJ 07050; tel. 973/266-3000; Mr. Michael Shipley

Troy Hills Center, 200 Reynolds Avenue, Parsippany, NJ 07054; tel. 973/887-8080; Ms. Laura Sansone

Valley Health Care Center, 300 Old Hook Road, Westwood, NJ 07675; tel. 201/664-8888; Ms. Christine Asmann-Finch

Voorhees Center – Genesis ElderCare Network, 3001 Evesham Road, Voorhees, NJ 08043; tel. 856/751-1600; Mr. Dwight Roche

Voorhees Pediatric Facility, 1304 Laurel Oak Road, Voorhees, NJ 08043-4392; tel. 609/346-3300; Mr. Carl W Underland

Wanaque Operating Company, LP, 1433 Ringwood Avenue, Haskell, NJ 07420; tel. 201/839-2119; Mr. Sidney Schiff

Wayne View Convalescent Center, 2020 Route 23 North, Wayne, NJ 07470; tel. 973/305-8400; Mr. Elliot Baruch

Wellington Hall Care Center, 301 Union Street, Hackensack, NJ 07601; tel. 201/487-4900; Ms. Charlotte Catrillo-Sodora

West Caldwell Care Center, 165 Fairfield Avenue, West Caldwell, NJ 07006; tel. 973/364-0723; Mr. Michael P Duffy

Westfield Center – Genesis ElderCare Network, 1515 Lamberts Mill Road, Westfield, NJ 07090; tel. 908/233-9700; Mr. Joseph Brandspiegel

Whiting Healthcare Center, 3000 Hilltop Road, Whiting, NJ 08759; tel. 908/849-4400; Mr. Thomas Miller

Willow Creek Rehabilitation and Care Center, 1165 Easton Avenue, Somerset, NJ 08873; tel. 732/246-4100; Ms. Allyson Brown

Woodcrest Center, 800 River Road, New Milford, NJ 07646; tel. 201/967-1700; Mr. David Repoli

NEW MEXICO

Casa Arena Blanca Nursing Center, 205 Moonglow, Alamogordo, NM 88310; tel. 505/434-4510; Ms. Cynthia A Myers

La Residencia Nursing Center, 820 Paseo de Peralta, Santa Fe, NM 87501; tel. 505/983-2273; Mr. Jim Riebsomer

Las Palomas Nursing and Rehabilitation Center, 8100 Palomas, NE, Albuquerque, NM 87109; tel. 505/821-4200; Ms. Joan D Earl

NEW YORK

Arbor Hill Care Center, 1175 Monroe Avenue, Rochester, NY 14620-1697; tel. 716/442-0450; Mr. Timothy C Chrzan

Arbor Park Health Care Center, Inc., 2806 George Street, Eden, NY 14057; tel. 716/992-3987; Ms. Lisa A Hennessy

Aurora Park Health Care Center, Inc., 292 Main Street, East Aurora, NY 14052; tel. 716/652-1560; Ms. Lisa L Harr

Autumn View Health Care Facility, 4650 Southwestern Boulevard, Hamburg, NY 14075; tel. 716/648-2450; Mr. David Eaton

Bainbridge Nursing and Rehabilitation Center, 3518 Bainbridge Avenue, Bronx, NY 10467; tel. 718/655-1991; Mr. Matis Weinstock

Beechwood Residence / Beechwood Nursing Home, 2235 Millersport Highway, Getzville, NY 14068; tel. 716/688-8822; Mr. Robert R Meiss

Beth Abraham Health Services, 612 Allerton Avenue, Bronx, NY 10467; tel. 718/519-4001; Ms. Henriette Kole

Birchwood Health Care Center, Inc., 4800 Bear Road, Liverpool, NY 13088; tel. 315/457-9946; Mr. Patrick Deptula

Birchwood Health Center, 78 Birchwood Drive, Huntington Station, NY 11746; tel. 516/423-3673; Mr. Timothy P Steffens, II

Brandywine Nursing Home, 620 Sleepy Hollow Road, Briarcliff Manor, NY 10510; tel. 914/941-5100; Mr. Paul S Roth

Briody Health Care Facility, 909 Lincoln Avenue, Lockport, NY 14094; tel. 716/434-6361; Ms. Ann Briody-Petock

Brooklyn Queens Nursing Home, Inc., 2749 Linden Boulevard, Brooklyn, NY 11208; tel. 718/227-5100; Dr. Anthony A Summers

Center for Nursing and Rehabilitation, 520 Prospect Place, Brooklyn, NY 11238; tel. 718/636-1000; Ms. Clari Gilbert

Central Island Healthcare, 825 Old Country Road, Plainview, NY 11803; tel. 516/433-0600; Ms. Martha Sweet

Clearview Nursing Home, 157-15 19th Avenue, Whitestone, NY 11357; tel. 718/746-0400; Ms. Diane Gariti

Clove Lakes Health Care and Rehabilitation Center, Inc, 25 Fanning Street, Staten Island, NY 10314; tel. 718/289-7900; Ms. Helene A Demisay

Cobble Hill Health Center, Inc, 380 Henry Street, Brooklyn, NY 11201; tel. 718/855-6789; Ms. Olga Lipschitz

College Park Health Care Center, Inc., 9876 Luckey Drive, Houghton, NY 14744; tel. 716/567-2207; Harlie D Clark

Concourse Rehabilitation and Nursing Center, Inc., 1072 Grand Concourse, Bronx, NY 10456; tel. 718/681-4000; Ms. Helen Neiman

Cortland Care Center, 193 Clinton Avenue, Cortland, NY 13045; tel. 607/756-9921; Mr. Anthony Salerno

Crown Nursing & Rehabilitation Center, 3457 Nostrand Avenue, Brooklyn, NY 11229; tel. 718/615-1100; Ms. Diane Carducci

Daughters of Jacob Nursing Home Company, Inc., 1160 Teller Avenue, Bronx, NY 10456; tel. 718/293-1500; Mr. Gilbert Preira

DeWitt Nursing Home, 211 East 79th Street, New York, NY 10021; tel. 212/879-1600; Mr. Saunders Ted Preiss

Dr. Susan Smith McKinney Nursing/Rehabilitation Center, 594 Albany Avenue, Brooklyn, NY 11203; tel. 718/245-7170; Ms. Ruth R Ogieste

Dr. William O. Benenson Rehabilitation Pavilion, 36-17 Parsons Boulevard, Flushing, NY 11354; tel. 718/961-4300; Dr. Esther Benenson

Dumont Masonic Home, 676 Pelham Road, New Rochelle, NY 10805; tel. 914/632-9600; Ms. Beth E Goldstein

East Haven Nursing and Rehab Center, 2323 Eastchester Road, Bronx, NY 10469; tel. 718/655-2848; Mr. Joseph Brachfeld

Eddy Heritage House Nursing Center, 2920 Tibbits Avenue, Troy, NY 12180; tel. 518/274-4125; Mr. Andrew Cruikshank

Eddy-Ford Nursing Home, 421 W. Columbia Street, Cohoes, NY 12047; tel. 518/237-5630; Ms. Albert Pasinella

Eger Health Care and Rehabilitation Center, 140 Meisner Avenue, Staten Island, NY 10306-1200; tel. 718/979-1800; Ms. Adeline M Conroy

Father Baker Manor, 6400 Powers Road, Orchard Park, NY 14127; tel. 716/667-0001; Mr. John R Durno

Florence Nightingale Health Center, 1760 Third Avenue, New York, NY 10029; tel. 212/410-8760; Mr. William J Pascocello

Flushing Manor Care Center, Inc., 139-66 35th Avenue, Flushing, NY 11354; tel. 718/961-5300; Mr. Herb Eisen

Flushing Manor Nursing Home, Inc., 35-15 Parsons Boulevard, Flushing, NY 11354; tel. 718/961-3500; Esther Benenson

Franklin Center for Rehabilitation and Nursing, 142-27 Franklin Avenue, Flushing, NY 11355; tel. 718/670-3400; Mr. Jack Friedman

Glengariff Health Care Center, Dosoris Lane, Glen Cove, NY 11542; tel. 516/676-1100; Mr. Michael D Miness

Golden Gate Health Care Center, Inc., 191 Bradley Avenue, Staten Island, NY 10314; tel. 718/698-8800; Mr. Manny Chopp

Gouverneur Nursing Facility, 227 Madison Street, New York, NY 10002; tel. 212/238-7000; Mr. Samuel Lehrfeld

Grace Plaza of Great Neck, Inc, 15 St. Paul's Place, Great Neck, NY 11021; tel. 516/466-3001; Ms. Celia Strow

Grandell Rehabilitation and Nursing Center, Inc., 645 West Broadway, Long Beach, NY 11561-2902; tel. 516/889-1100; Mr. Sidney Greenberger

Greater Harlem Nursing Home, 30 West 138th Street, New York, NY 10037; tel. 212/690-7400; Ms. Reita Fuller

Gurwin Jewish Geriatric Center, 68 Hauppauge Road, Commack, NY 11725; tel. 516/715-2600; Mr. Herbert H Friedman

Haven Manor Health Care Center, 1441 Gateway Boulevard, Far Rockaway, NY 11691; tel. 718/471-1500; Mr. Aron Cytryn

Hempstead Park Nursing Home, 800 Front Street, Hempstead, NY 11550; tel. 516/560-1422; Mr. Alexander Sajdak

Highgate Manor of Cortland, Inc., PO Box 5510, Cortland, NY 13045-5510; tel. 607/753-9631; Ms. Karen Harvatin

Highgate Manor of Rensselaer, Inc., 100 New Turnpike Road, Troy, NY 12182; tel. 518/235-1410; Ms. Daniel Leahey

Highland Healthcare Center, 160 Seneca Street, Wellsville, NY 14895; tel. 716/593-3750; Mr. James Fuller

Hillcrest Nursing and Rehabilitation Center, 661 North Main Street, Spring Valley, NY 10977; tel. 914/356-0567; Mr. Michael N Rosenblut

Hillside Manor Rehabilitation and Extended Care Center, 182-15 Hillside Avenue, Jamaica Est, NY 11432; tel. 718/291-8200; Ms. Judith Dicker

Hilltop Manor of Niskayuna, 1805 Providence Avenue, Niskayuna, NY 12309; tel. 518/374-2212; Mr. Christopher Alexander

Horizon Care Center, 64-11 Beach Channel Drive, Arverne, NY 11692; tel. 718/945-0700; Mr. Morris Tenenbaum

Providers / JCAHO Accredited Freestanding Long-Term Care Care Organizations

Hudson Valley Rehabilitative and Extended Care Center, 260 Vineyard Avenue, Highland, NY 12528; tel. 914/691-7201; Ms. Judith Dicker
Indian River Rehabilitation and Health Care Center, Inc, 17 Madison Street, Granville, NY 12832; tel. 518/642-2710; Ms. Renee M Groesbeck
Isabella Geriatric Center, 515 Audubon Avenue, New York, NY 10040; tel. 212/342-9300; Mr. Mark Kator
James A. Eddy Memorial Geriatric Center, 2256 Burdett Avenue, Troy, NY 12180; tel. 518/274-9890; Mr. Peter G Young
Kateri Residence, 150 Riverside Drive, New York, NY 10024; tel. 212/769-0744; Mr. Lascelles L Bond
Kings Harbor Multicare Center, 2000 East Gun Hill Road, Bronx, NY 10469; tel. 718/320-0400; Mr. Alexander Stern
Laconia Nursing Home, Inc., 1050 East 230th Street, Bronx, NY 10466; tel. 718/654-5875; Mr. John N Okwodu
Lakewood Health Care Center, Inc., 5775 Maelou Drive, Hamburg, NY 14075; tel. 716/648-2820; Mr. Michael J Murphy
Lawrence Nursing Care Center, Inc., 350 Beach 54th Street, Arverne, NY 11692; tel. 718/945-0400; Ms. Barbara Young
Little Neck Nursing Home, 260-19 Nassau Boulevard, Little Neck, NY 11362; tel. 718/423-6400; Ms. Sue Zimet
Long Island Care Center, 144-61 38th Avenue, Flushing, NY 11354; tel. 718/939-7500; Mr. Paul Konstam
Lyden Nursing Home, 27-37 27th Street, Astoria, NY 11102; tel. 718/932-4613; Chaim Sieger
M.J.G. Nursing Home Company, Inc., 4915 Tenth Avenue, Brooklyn, NY 11219; tel. 718/851-3700; Mr. Eli S Feldman
Manhattanville Health Care Center, 311 West 231st Street, Bronx, NY 10463; tel. 718/601-8400; Mr. Leonard J Wiener
Maplewood Nursing Home, Inc., 100 Daniel Drive, Webster, NY 14580-2983; tel. 716/872-1800; Mr. Gregory J Chambery
Margaret Tietz Center for Nursing Care, 164-11 Chapin Parkway, Jamaica, NY 11432; tel. 718/523-6400; Mr. Kenneth M Brown
Meadowbrook Healthcare, 154 Prospect Avenue, Plattsburgh, NY 12901; tel. 518/563-5440; Mr. Hobbie E Hyatt
Morningside House Nursing Home Company, Inc., 1000 Pelham Parkway South, Bronx, NY 10461; tel. 718/824-4243; Dr. William T Smith
Morris Park Nursing Home, 1235 Pelham Parkway North, Bronx, NY 10469; tel. 718/231-4300; Mr. Morris Berkowitz
Mosholu Parkway Nursing and Rehabilitation Center, 3356 Perry Avenue, Bronx, NY 10467; tel. 718/655-3568; Mr. Alexander Hartman
Nassau Extended Care Center, One Greenwich Street, Hempstead, NY 11550; tel. 516/565-4800; Mr. Kurt Mohr
No Shore Univ Hosp Center for Extended Care & Rehabilitation, 330 Community Drive, Manhasset, NY 11030; tel. 516/562-8070; Mr. Dennis Connors
Northern Manhattan Nursing Home, Inc., 116 East 125th Street, New York, NY 10035; tel. 212/426-1284; Ms. Verna Fitzpatrick
Oakwood Health Care Center, Inc., 200 Bassett Road, Williamsville, NY 14221; tel. 716/689-6681; Mr. Robert Chur
Oceanview Nursing Home, PO Box 628, Far Rockaway, NY 11691; tel. 718/471-6000; Mr. Louis Wolcowitz
Oneonta Nursing and Rehabilitation Center, 330 Chestnut Street, Oneonta, NY 13820; tel. 607/432-8500; Ms. Kristin Russell
Orchard Park Health Care Center, Inc., 6060 Armor Road, Orchard Park, NY 14127; tel. 716/662-4433; Albert C Parton
Palm Gardens Nursing Home, 615 Avenue C, Brooklyn, NY 11218; tel. 718/633-3300; Mr. Israel Lefkowitz
Park Shore Health Care Center, Inc., 447 Lake Shore Drive West, Dunkirk, NY 14048; tel. 716/366-6710; Ms. Lisa A Hennessy
Parker Jewish Institute for Health Care and Rehabilitation, 271-11 76th Avenue, New Hyde Park, NY 11040-1433; tel. 718/289-2100; Mr. David Glaser
Promenade Rehabilitation and Health Care Center, 140 Beach 114th Street, Rockaway Park, NY 11694; tel. 718/945-4600; Mr. Stanley Spector

Prospect Park Care Center Inc, 1455 Coney Island Avenue, Brooklyn, NY 11230; tel. 718/252-9800; Ms. Shirley Kurzman
Providence Rest, 3304 Waterbury Avenue, Bronx, NY 10465; tel. 718/931-3000; Sister Seline Mary Flores
Ramapo Manor Nursing Center, Inc., PO Box 248, Suffern, NY 10901; tel. 914/357-1230; Ms. Marsha Z Squires
Regency Extended Care Center, 65 Ashburton Avenue, Yonkers, NY 10701; tel. 914/963-4000; Mr. Alexander D Sajdak
Resort Nursing Home, 430 Beach 68th Street, Arverne, NY 11692; tel. 718/474-5200; Mr. Michael Tenenbaum
River Park Health Care Center, Inc., 5th and Maple Avenue, Allegany, NY 14706; tel. 716/373-2238; Ms. Charlene Lehman
Riverdale Nursing Home, 641 West 230th Street, Bronx, NY 10463; tel. 718/796-4800; Mr. Eric Paneth
Rivington House – The Nicholas A. Rango Health Care Facility, 45 Rivington Street, New York, NY 10002; tel. 212/539-6200; Mr. Arthur Y Webb
Rome Nursing Home, 950 Floyd Avenue, Rome, NY 13440; tel. 315/336-5400; Mr. Michael Svendsen
Rosewood Gardens Convalescent Home, Inc., 284 Troy Road, Rensselaer, NY 12144-9474; tel. 518/286-1621; Ms. Beverly R Benno
Saint Cabrini Nursing Home, Inc., 115 Broadway, Dobbs Ferry, NY 10522; tel. 914/693-6800; Ms. Patricia A Krasnausky
Sands Point Center for Health and Rehabilitation, 1440 Port Washington Boulevard, Port Washington, NY 11050; tel. 516/719-9400; Mr. David Moskowitz
Sarah Neuman Center for Heathcare and Rehabilitation, 845 Palmer Avenue, Mamaroneck, NY 10543; tel. 914/777-6100; Alvan Small
Schervier Pavilion, 22 Van Duzer Place, Warwick, NY 10990; tel. 914/987-5710; Ms. Adele L Coates
Sea Crest Health Care Center, 3035 West 24th Street, Brooklyn, NY 11224; tel. 718/372-4500; Ms. Evelyn Jones
Sea View Hospital Rehabilitation Center and Home, 460 Brielle Avenue, Staten Island, NY 10314; tel. 718/317-3000; Ms. Violet K Huie
Shore View Nursing Home, 2865 Brighton 3rd Street, Brooklyn, NY 11235; tel. 718/891-4400; Mr. Howard Small
Shorefront Jewish Geriatric Center, 3015 West 29th Street, Brooklyn, NY 11224; tel. 718/266-5700; Ms. Marilyn Reiter
Silvercrest Extended Care Facility, 144-45 87th Avenue, Briarwood, NY 11435; tel. 718/480-4026; Mr. Kenneth A Carter
South Shore Healthcare, 275 West Merrick Road, Freeport, NY 11520; tel. 516/623-4000; Ms. Cathie L Geraghty
St. Ann's Community – St. Ann's Home For The Aged, 1500 Portland Avenue, Rochester, NY 14621; tel. 716/544-6000; Ms. Elizabeth Mullin
St. Elizabeth Ann's Health Care and Rehabilitation Center, 91 Tompkins Avenue, Staten Island, NY 10304; tel. 718/876-4560; Mr. Paul Rosenfield
St. Francis Home of Williamsville, 147 Reist Street, Williamsville, NY 14221; tel. 716/633-5400; Dr. James A Walsh
St. James Healthcare Center, 275 Moriches Road, St James, NY 11780; tel. 516/862-8000; Mr. William J St. George
St. Mary's Hospital for Children, 29-01 216th Street, Bayside, NY 11360; tel. 718/281-8800; Dr. Burton Grebin
Sullivan Park Health Care Center, Inc., 301 Nantucket Drive, Endicott, NY 13760; tel. 607/754-2705; Mr. Mark R Foreman
Sunharbor Manor, 255 Warner Avenue, Roslyn Heights, NY 11577; tel. 516/621-5400; Mr. Clifford R Osinoff
The Arden Hill Life Care Center, 6 Harriman Drive, Goshen, NY 10924; tel. 914/291-3700; Ms. Donna G Case
The Guild Home for Aged Blind, 75 Stratton Street South, Yonkers, NY 10701; tel. 914/963-4661; Mr. Alan R Morse
The Jewish Home and Hospital – Manhattan Division, 120 West 106th Street, New York, NY 10025; tel. 212/870-4902; Mr. Sheldon Goldberg
The Nathan Miller Center for Nursing Care, Inc., 220 West Post Road, White Plains, NY 10606; tel. 914/686-8880; Ms. Lorraine Goldman
The Port Jefferson Health Care Facility, Dark Hollow Road, Port Jefferson, NY 11777; tel. 516/473-5400; Ms. Leslie Saren

The Wartburg, Wartburg Place, Mt Vernon, NY 10552; tel. 914/513-5189; Dr. Dale G Gatz
The Wesley Group, 630 East Avenue, Rochester, NY 14607-2194; tel. 716/241-2101; Mr. Jon R Zemans
Three Rivers Health Care Center, Inc., 101 Creekside Drive, Painted Post, NY 14870; tel. 607/936-4108; Mr. Mark R Foreman
Throgs Neck Extended Care Facility, 707 Throgs Neck Expressway, Bronx, NY 10465; tel. 718/430-0003; Mr. George P Stops
TownHouse Extended Care Center, 755 Hempstead Turnpike, Uniondale, NY 11553; tel. 516/565-1900; Mrs. Caryl Benjamin
Vestal Nursing Center, 860 Old Vestal Road, Vestal, NY 13850; tel. 607/754-4105; Ms. Denise B Johnson
Victory Lake Nursing Center, PO Box 2008, Hyde Park, NY 12538; tel. 914/229-9177; Ms. Patricia Walsh
Village Nursing Home, 607 Hudson Street, New York, NY 10014; tel. 212/255-3003; Mr. Arthur Y Webb
Village Park Health Care Center, Inc., 4540 Lincoln Drive, Gasport, NY 14067; tel. 716/772-2631; Mr. Robert C Travis
Waterfront Health Care Center, Inc., 200 Seventh Street, Buffalo, NY 14201; tel. 716/847-2500; Mr. Lawrence Piselli
Waterview Nursing Care Center, 119-15 27th Avenue, Flushing, NY 11354; tel. 718/461-5000; Mr. Larry I Slatky
Wayne Nursing Home, 3530 Wayne Avenue, Bronx, NY 10467; tel. 718/655-1700; Mr. Howard Wolf
Wedgewood Care Center, 199 Community Drive, Great Neck, NY 11021; tel. 516/365-9229; Mr. Israel Sherman
West Lawrence Care Center, 1410 Seagirt Boulevard, Far Rockaway, NY 11691; tel. 718/471-7000; Mr. Maurice H Radzik
Westfield Health Care Center, Inc., 26 Cass Street, Westfield, NY 14787; tel. 716/326-4646; Mr. Ivan Tarnopoll
Wingate at Dutchess Rehabilitative/Skilled Nursing, 3 Summit Court, Fishkill, NY 12524; tel. 914/896-1500; Mr. Richard Herrick
Wingate at Ulster, One Wingate Way, Highland, NY 12528; tel. 914/691-6800; Mr. Richard Herrick
Woodbury Center for HealthCare, 8533 Jericho Turnpike, Woodbury, NY 11797; tel. 516/692-4100; Mr. Frederick E White

NORTH CAROLINA
Alamance Health Care Center, 1987 Hilton Road, Burlington, NC 27217; tel. 336/226-0848; Mr. Howard Staples
Asheboro Health and Rehabilitation Center, PO Box 4218, Asheboro, NC 27203; tel. 910/629-1447; Mr. Gary L Plasschaert
Asheville Health Care Center, 1270 Highway 70, Swannanoa, NC 28778; tel. 828/298-2214; Ms. Lillian Silvers
Aston Park Health Care Center, Inc., 380 Brevard Road, Asheville, NC 28806; tel. 828/253-4437; Ms. Marsha W Kaufman
Belaire Health Care Center, 2065 Lyon Street, Gastonia, NC 28052; tel. 704/867-7300; Ms. Kathy F Putnam
Beverly Health Care Center, 1000 Western Boulevard, Tarboro, NC 27886-7008; tel. 252/823-0401; Ms. Effie E Webb
Brian Center – Shamrock, 2727 Shamrock Drive, Charlotte, NC 28205; tel. 704/563-0886; Ms. Laura Fitzpatrick
Brian Center Cabarrus, 250 Bishop Lane, Concord, NC 28025; tel. 704/788-6400; Mr. John Klaver
Brian Center Health and Rehabilitation – Brevard, PO Box 1096, Brevard, NC 28712; tel. 828/884-2031; Ms. Debbie Drohan
Brian Center Health and Rehabilitation – Eden, 226 North Oakland Avenue, Eden, NC 27288; tel. 336/623-1750; Ms. Helen S Myers
Brian Center Health and Rehabilitation – Gastonia, 969 Cox Road, Gastonia, NC 28054; tel. 704/866-8596; Ms. Julie D Goforth
Brian Center Health and Rehabilitation – Hertford, 200 River Drive, Hertford, NC 27944; tel. 252/426-5391; Mr. Joseph G France
Brian Center Health and Rehabilitation – Hickory East, 3031 Tate Boulevard Southeast, Hickory, NC 28602; tel. 828/322-3343; Ms. Mary Starnes
Brian Center Health and Rehabilitation – Salisbury, 635 Statesville Boulevard, Salisbury, NC 28144; tel. 704/633-7390; Ms. Deborah Mathis
Brian Center Health and Rehabilitation – Spruce Pine, 218 Laurel Creek Court, Spruce Pine, NC 28777; tel. 704/765-7312; Mr. Walt Cross

Providers / JCAHO Accredited Freestanding Long-Term Care Care Organizations

Brian Center Health and Rehabilitation – Wallace, PO Box 966, Wallace, NC 28466; tel. 910/285-6646; Ms. Bonnie Davis

Brian Center Health and Rehabilitation – Windsor, 1306 South King Street, Windsor, NC 27983; tel. 919/794-5146; Ms. Mary J Tibbs

Brian Center Health and Rehabilitation / Goldsboro, 1700 Wayne Memorial Drive, Goldsboro, NC 27534; tel. 919/731-2805; Ms. Catherine T Hollowell

Brian Center Health and Rehabilitation/Durham, 6000 Fayettville Road, Durham, NC 27713; tel. 919/544-9021; Mr. Keith Lombardi

Brian Center Health and Rehabilitation/Hendersonville, 1870 Pisgah Drive, Hendersonville, NC 28739; tel. 704/693-9796; Mr. Paul Shogren

Brian Center Health and Rehabilitation/Raleigh, 3000 Holston Lane, Raleigh, NC 27610; tel. 919/231-6045; Ms. Melissa McKinney

Brian Center Health and Rehabilitation/Weaverville, 78 Weaver Boulevard, Weaverville, NC 28787; tel. 704/645-4297; Ms. Carol L Prater

Brian Center Health and Rehabilitation/Wilson, PO Box 3566, Wilson, NC 27895-3566; tel. 252/237-5300; Mr. Dan R Cotten

Brian Center Health and Retirement, 4911 Brian Center Lane, Winston Salem, NC 27106-6423; tel. 336/744-5674; Mr. Charles Lentz

Brian Center Health and Retirement – Clayton, 204 Dairy Road, Clayton, NC 27520; tel. 919/553-8232; Mr. Dennis Redmond

Brian Center Health and Retirement – Monroe, 204 Old Highway 74 East, Monroe, NC 28112; tel. 704/283-3066; Mr. Dwight Jessup

Brian Center Health and Retirement – Mooresville, 752 East Center Avenue, Mooresville, NC 28115; tel. 704/663-3448; Mr. Dennis V Reese

Brian Center Hickory/Viewmont, 220 13th Ave Place Northwest, Hickory, NC 28601; tel. 828/328-5646; Ms. Teddie Simmons

Cary Health and Rehabilitation Center, 6590 Tryon Roac, Cary, NC 27511; tel. 919/851-8000; Ms. Deborah Crane

Charlotte Health Care Center, 1735 Toddville Road, Charlotte, NC 28214; tel. 704/394-4001; Mrs. Paula Phillips

Courtland Terrace Nursing Center, 2300 Aberdeen Boulevard, Gastonia, NC 28054; tel. 704/834-4806; Mr. Wayne F Shovelin

Cypress Pointe Rehabilitation and Health Care Centre, 2006 South 16th Street, Wilmington, NC 28401; tel. 910/763-6271; Ms. Faye M Kennedy

Genesis ElderCare – Mooresville Center, 550 Glenwood Drive, Mooresville, NC 28115; tel. 704/664-7494; Ms. Anne Ennis

GreenTree Ridge + The Summit, 70 Sweeten Creek Road, Asheville, NC 28803; tel. 828/274-7646; Ms. Margaret Abbott

Guilford Health Care Center, 2041 Willow Road, Greensboro, NC 27406; tel. 336/272-9700; Ms. Laura W Lucas

Horizon Rehabilitation Center, 3100 Erwin Road, Durham, NC 27705; tel. 919/383-1545; Ms. Sharon Kochanovich

Hunter Woods Nursing and Rehabilitation Center, 620 Tom Hunter Road, Charlotte, NC 28213; tel. 704/598-5136; Mr. James Krob

Integrated Health Services of Charlotte, 333 Hawthorne Lane, Charlotte, NC 28204; tel. 704/372-1270; Mr. Darryl Ehlers

Lexington Health Care Center, 17 Cornelia Drive, Lexington, NC 27292; tel. 336/242-1349; Ms. Linda K Morrison

Lutheran Nursing Home – Albemarle, PO Box 308, Albemarle, NC 28002; tel. 704/982-8191; Ms. Priscilla Vint

Lutheran Nursing Home at Trinity Oaks, PO Box 1310, Salisbury, NC 28144; tel. 704/637-3784; Ms. Lynn A Lancaster

Lutheran Nursing Home, Inc. – Hickory Unit, 1265 21st Street Northeast, Hickory, NC 28601; tel. 828/328-2006; Mr. Ted Goins

Mariner Health of Wilmington, 820 Wellington Avenue, Wilmington, NC 28401; tel. 910/343-0425; Mr. John W Strawcutter

Meadowbrook Manor of Siler City, 900 West Dolphin Street, Siler City, NC 27344; tel. 919/663-3431; Mr. John Edmonds

Mecklenburg Health Care Center, 2415 Sandy Porter Road, Charlotte, NC 28273; tel. 704/583-0430; Ms. Kristi Anthony

North Carolina Special Care Center, 4761 Ward Boulevard, Wilson, NC 27893; tel. 252/399-2112; Mr. William R Benton, Jr.

Salisbury Center/Genesis Elder Care, 710 Julian Road, Salisbury, NC 28147; tel. 704/636-5812; Mr. Patrick Foley

St. Joseph of the Pines, Health Center, 95 Aviemore Drive, Pinehurst, NC 28374; tel. 910/692-1644; Mr. George Kecatos

The Nursing Center at Oak Summit, 5680 Windy Hill Drive, Winston Salem, NC 27105; tel. 336/744-1188; Ms. Ruth Lowe

Transitional Health Services of Kannapolis, 1810 Concord Lake Road, Kannapolis, NC 28083; tel. 704/933-3781; Mr. Paul J Minton, Jr.

Wilora Lake Healthcare Center, 6001 Wilora Lake Road, Charlotte, NC 28212; tel. 704/563-2922; Ms. Bethany Mercer

OHIO

Altercare of Alliance, 11750 Klinger Avenue Northeast, Alliance, OH 44601; tel. 330/823-8263; Mr. Rob Aneshansel

Altercare of Mentor, 9901 Johnnycake Ridge Road, Mentor, OH 44060; tel. 440/357-7900; Mr. Barry Lieberman

Altercare of Navarre, 517 Park Street, Navarre, OH 44662; tel. 330/879-2765; Ms. May Jean Flossie

Americare Marion Nursing and Rehabilitation Center, 524 James Way, Marion, OH 43302-5890; tel. 740/389-6306; Ms. Nita L Hunt

Anna Maria of Aurora, Inc., 889 North Aurora Road, Aurora, OH 44202; tel. 330/562-6171; Mr. George J Norton

Arbors at Canton, 2714 13th Street Northwest, Canton, OH 44708-9970; tel. 216/456-2842; Mr. Rick Kesic

Arbors at Delaware, 2270 Warrensburg Road, Delaware, OH 43015; tel. 740/369-9614; Ms. Suzanne T Johns

Arbors at Fairlawn, 575 S. Cleveland Massillon Rd., Fairlawn, OH 44333; tel. 614/791-2920; Ms. Kimberly Joye

Arbors at Hilliard, 5471 Scioto Darby Road, Hilliard, OH 43026; tel. 614/876-7356; Mr. Michael Lacey

Arbors at London, 218 Elm Street, London, OH 43140; tel. 740/852-3100; Mr. Sam Ullum

Arbors at Marietta, 400 Seventh Street, Marietta, OH 45750; tel. 740/373-3597; Mr. Aaron Loney

Arbors at Milford, 5900 Meadowcreek Drive, Milford, OH 45150; tel. 513/248-1655; Ms. Deonne Schenk

Arbors at Sylvania, 7120 Port Sylvania Drive, Toledo, OH 43617; tel. 419/841-2200; Mr. Martin Jan

Arbors at Toledo, 2920 Cherry Street, Toledo, OH 43608; tel. 419/242-7458; Mr. Franklin E Swinehart

Arbors at Waterville, 555 Anthony Wayne Trail, Waterville, OH 43566; tel. 419/878-3901; Ms. Jennifer Bombrys

Arbors East Skilled and Rehabilitation Center, 5500 East Broad Street, Columbus, OH 43213; tel. 614/575-9003; Ms. Joan W Rankin

Arbors West, 375 West Main Street, West Jefferson, OH 43162; tel. 614/791-2920; Mr. Mike Lacey

Aristocrat Berea Healthcare Center, 255 Front Street, Berea, OH 44017; tel. 440/243-4000; Mr. Robert M Coury

Arlington Court Nursing and Rehabilitation Center, 1605 NW Professional Plaza, Columbus, OH 43220; tel. 614/451-5677; Ms. Linda S Vrable

Aurora Manor Special Care Centre, 101 Bissell Road, Aurora, OH 44202; tel. 330/562-5000; Ms. Christa L Lavigna-Mayes

Batavia Nursing and Convalescent Inn, 4000 Golden Age Drive, Batavia, OH 45103; tel. 513/732-6500; Mr. Glydon Powell

Bethany Lutheran Village, 6451 Far Hills Avenue, Centerville, OH 45459; tel. 937/433-2110; Mr. Willis O Serr, II

BridgePark Centre for Rehabilitation & Nursing Svcs, 145 Olive Street, Akron, OH 44310; tel. 330/762-0901; Mr. Edward Husbands

Broadview Health Care Center, 5151 North Hamilton Road, Columbus, OH 43230; tel. 614/337-1066; Mr. Edward J Powell

Broadview Multi-Care Center, 5520 Broadview Road, Parma, OH 44134; tel. 216/749-4010; Mr. Harold Shachter

Brookwood Retirement Community, 12100 Reed Hartman Highway, Cincinnati, OH 45241; tel. 513/605-2000; Mr. Steven Boymel

Calcutta Health Care Center, 48444 Bell School Road, Calcutta, OH 43920; tel. 330/385-7100; Mr. Thomas D Nordquist

Cambridge Health and Rehabilitation Center, 1471 Wills Creek Valley Drive, Cambridge, OH 43725; tel. 740/439-4437; Ms. Judy Dennis

Carriage Inn of Steubenville, 3102 St. Charles Drive, Steubenville, OH 43952; tel. 740/264-7161; Mr. Peter P Merritt

Chapel Hill Community, 12200 Strausser Road, Canal Fulton, OH 44614; tel. 330/854-4177; Mr. Jason E Miller

Christel Manor of Miamisburg, 1120 South Dunaway, Miamisburg, OH 45342; tel. 937/866-9089; Ms. Patsy VanDyke

Clermont Nursing and Convalescent Center, 934 State Route 28, Milford, OH 45150; tel. 513/831-1770; Mr. Robert D Lehman

College Park Nursing and Rehabilitation Center, 3201 CR 16, Coshocton, OH 43812; tel. 740/622-2074; Mr. Kevin Case

Columbus Alzheimer Care Center, 700 Jasonway Avenue, Columbus, OH 43214; tel. 614/459-7050; Mr. Tim Johnson

Columbus Center, 4301 Clime Road North, Columbus, OH 43228; tel. 614/276-4400; Ms. Karen Mitchell

Columbus Rehabilitation and Subacute Institute, 44 Souder Avenue, Columbus, OH 43222; tel. 614/228-5900; Mr. Bob Brooks

CommuniCare of Clifton, 625 Probasco Street, Cincinnati, OH 45220; tel. 513/281-2464; Mr. David Lucid

Community Care Center, 145 East College Street, Alliance, OH 44601; tel. 330/829-4000; Mr. Stan Jonas, Jr.

Community Healthcare Center, 175 Community Drive, Marion, OH 43302; tel. 740/387-7537; Mr. Roger Drake

Community Multicare Center, PO Box 18669, Fairfield, OH 45018-0669; tel. 513/868-6500; Mr. Aaron Handler

Copley Health Center, 155 Heritage Woods Drive, Akron, OH 44321-1398; tel. 330/666-0980; Mr. Gregory L Ryan

Cortland Center, 369 North High Street, Cortland, OH 44410; tel. 330/638-4015; Mr. Robert Aroesty

Crestview Manor, 4381 Tonawanda Trail, Dayton, OH 45430; tel. 937/426-5033; Mr. James W Unverferth

Cuyahoga Falls Country Place, 2728 Bailey Road, Cuyahoga Falls, OH 44221; tel. 330/929-4231; Mr. Barry Schimer

Darlington House, 2735 Darlington Road, Toledo, OH 436063206; tel. 419/531-4465; Mr. Charles S Weiden

DaySpring Health Care Center and Rehabilitation, 8001 Dayton-Springfield Road, Fairborn, OH 45324; tel. 937/864-5800; Mr. John B Hoenemeyer

East Galbraith Health Care Community, 3889 East Galbraith Road, Cincinnati, OH 45236; tel. 513/793-5222; Mr. Thomas Zemboch

Eastgate Health Care Center and Rehabilitation, 4400 Glen Este Withamsville Rd, Cincinnati, OH 45245; tel. 513/752-3710; Mr. Barry N Bortz

Evergreen Rehabilitation and Specialty Care Center, 555 Springbrook Drive, Medina, OH 44256; tel. 330/725-3393; Ms. Deborah J Lougheed

Fairhaven Community, 850 Marseilles Avenue, Upper Sandusky, OH 433511; tel. 419/294-4973; Mr. Dan Miller

Franklin Plaza Extended Care, 3600 Franklin Boulevard, Cleveland, OH 44113; tel. 216/651-1600; Ms. Tara Coy

Gables Care Center, 350 Lahm Drive, Hopedale, OH 43976; tel. 740/937-2900; Ms. Darlene Woods

Gateway Health Care Center, Three Gateway Drive, Euclid, OH 44119; tel. 216/486-4949; Ms. Linda Bliss

Gibsonburg Health Care Center, 355 Windsor Lane, Gibsonburg, OH 43431; tel. 419/-637-2104; Mr. Larry Tebeau

Grande Pointe Healthcare Community, 3 Merit Drive, Richmond Heights, OH 44143; tel. 216/261-9600; Mr. Barry Braunstein

Greenbriar Quality Care of Boardman, 8064 South Avenue, Boardman, OH 44512; tel. 330/726-3700; Ms. Diane Reese

Harborside Healthcare – Beachwood, 3800 Park East Drive, Beachwood, OH 44122; tel. 216/831-4303; Mr. Don Puteet

Harborside Healthcare – Broadview Heights, 2801 East Royalton Road, Broadview Heights, OH 44147; tel. 440/526-4770; Ms. Anne Marie Johnson

Harborside Healthcare – Defiance, 395 Harding Street, Defiance, OH 43512; tel. 419/784-1450; Ms. Katie Hitchcock

Harborside Healthcare – Northwestern Ohio, 1104 Wesley Avenue, Bryan, OH 43506; tel. 419/636-5071; Ms. Randi M Kiphen

Providers / JCAHO Accredited Freestanding Long-Term Care Care Organizations

Harborside Healthcare – Perrysburg, 28546 Starbright Boulevard, Perrysburg, OH 43551; tel. 419/666-0935; Mrs. Michelle L Dobson
Harborside Healthcare – Swanton, 401 West Airport Highway, Swanton, OH 43558; tel. 419/825-1111; Ms. Michelle L Dobson
Harborside Healthcare – Troy, 512 Crescent Drive, Troy, OH 45373; tel. 937/335-7161; Roger W Walker
Harborside Healthcare – Westlake I, 27601 Westchester Parkway, Westlake, OH 44145; tel. 440/871-5900; Ms. Cathy Henderson
Heartland of Beavercreek, 1974 North Fairfield Road, Dayton, OH 45432; tel. 937/429-1106; Mrs. Jennifer Woodward
Heartland of Browning, 8885 Browning Drive, Waterville, OH 43566; tel. 419/878-8523; Mr. Gregory Nijak
Heartland of Centerburg, PO Box 720, Centerburg, OH 43011; tel. 740/625-5774; Ms. Laurie Zinn
Heartland of Holly Glen, 4293 Monroe Street, Toledo, OH 43606; tel. 419/474-6021; Mr. Doug Mack
Heartland of Kettering, 3313 Wilmington Pike, Kettering, OH 45429; tel. 937/298-8084; Mrs. Jennifer Woodward
Heartland of Marysville, 755 South Plum Street, Marysville, OH 43040; tel. 937/644-8836; Mr. Charles George
Heartland of Mentor, 8200 Mentor Hills Drive, Mentor, OH 44060; tel. 440/256-1496; Ms. Elizabeth Schupp
Heartland of Oak Ridge, 450 Oak Ridge Boulevard, Miamisburg, OH 45342; tel. 937/866-8885; Ms. Jennifer Miller
Heartland of Perrysburg, 10540 Fremont Pike, Perrysburg, OH 43551; tel. 419/874-3578; Mr. James P Berger
Heartland of Piqua, 275 Kienie Drive, Piqua, OH 45356; tel. 937/773-9346; Ms. Myrtle Hickman
Heartland of Springfield, 2615 Derr Road, Springfield, OH 45503; tel. 937/390-0005; Mr. Thomas Cunningham
Heartland of Wauseon, 303 West Leggett Street, Wauseon, OH 43567; tel. 419/337-3050; Mr. Roger E Wyman
Heather Hill Hospital, Health and Care Center, 12340 Bass Lake Road, Chardon, OH 44024; tel. 440/285-4040; Mr. Robert G Harr
Heatherdowns Rehabilitation and Residential Care Center, 2401 Cass Road, Toledo, OH 43614; tel. 419/382-5050; Mr. David A Myrice
Heritage Care, 24579 Broadway Avenue, Oakwood Village, OH 44146; tel. 440/439-7976; Mr. James Baraona
Hickory Creek Nursing Center, 3421 Pinnacle Road, Dayton, OH 45418; tel. 937/268-3488; Ms. Staci Lehmkuhl
Hickory Creek of Athens, 51 East 4th Street, The Plains, OH 45780; tel. 740/797-4561; Mr. Matthew LHNA, Glass
Hillebrand Nursing Center, 4320 Bridgetown Road, Cincinnati, OH 45211; tel. 513/574-4550; Ms. Michelle Glass Schneider
Horizon Village Nursing and Rehabilitation Center, 2473 North Road, Northeast, Warren, OH 44483; tel. 330/372-2251; Mr. David L Burnham
Hospitality Homes, 1301 North Monroe Drive, Xenia, OH 45385; tel. 937/372-4495; Mr. William C Jones, Jr.
IHS at Carriage-by-the-Lake, 1957 North Lakeman Drive, Bellbrook, OH 45305; tel. 937/848-8421; Ms. Melissa S Bennett
IHS of New London at Firelands, 204 West Main Street, New London, OH 44851; tel. 419/929-1563; Ms. Melanie A Bair
IHS of West Carrollton at Elm Creek, 115 Elmwood Circle, Dayton, OH 45449; tel. 937/866-3814; Ms. Patricia A Walter
Integrated Health Services at Waterford Commons, 955 Garden Lake Parkway, Toledo, OH 43614; tel. 419/382-2200; Ms. Vivian Kiraly
Integrated Health Services of Huber Heights at Spring Creek, 5440 Charlesgate Road, Huber Heights, OH 45424; tel. 937/236-6707; Mr. Dennis J Swartzbaugh
Ivy Woods Health Care and Rehabilitation Center, 2025 Wyoming Avenue, Cincinnati, OH 45205; tel. 513/251-2557; Ms. Michelle Schneider
Kent Center– Genesis ElderCare Network, 1290 Fairchild Avenue, Kent, OH 44240; tel. 330/678-4912; Mr. Joseph M Bestic
Kethley House at Benjamin Rose Place, 11900 Fairhill Road, Cleveland, OH 44120; tel. 216/795-5450; Mr. Jerome M Weissfeld

Kettering Convalescent Center, 1150 West Dorothy Lane, Kettering, OH 45409; tel. 937/293-1152; Mr. Timothy Shackleford
Kingston of Ashland, Post Office Box 347, Ashland, OH 44805; tel. 419/289-3859; Mr. Timothy K Callahan
Kingston of Vermilion, 4210 Telegraph Lane, Vermilion, OH 44089; tel. 440/967-1800; Ms. Nicole L Howard
Laurie Ann Nursing Home and Laurie Ann Home Health Care, 2200 Milton Boulevard, Newton Falls, OH 44444; tel. 330/872-1990; Ms. Doris Hooberry
Lebanon Country Manor, 700 Monroe Road, Lebanon, OH 45036; tel. 513/932-0105; Mr. Russell M Holtz
Lebanon Health Care Center, PO Box 376, Lebanon, OH 45036-0376; tel. 513/932-1121; Mr. W. E Ullum
Leisure Oaks Convalescent Center, 214 Harding Street, Defiance, OH 43512; tel. 419/784-1014; Ms. Ellie Stough
Life Care Center of Medina, 2400 Columbia Road, Medina, OH 44256; tel. 330/483-3131; Mr. Jon Rarick
Llanfair Retirement Community, 1701 Llanfair Avenue, Cincinnati, OH 45224; tel. 513/681-4230; Ms. Mariellen Sutton
Magnolia Care and Rehabilitation Center, 365 Johnson Road, Wadsworth, OH 44281; tel. 330/335-1558; Ms. Patricia A Paler
Manor Care at Sycamore Glen, 2175 Leiter Road, Miamisburg, OH 45342; tel. 937/866-5700; Mr. Elliott Fortner
Manor Care Health Services, 23225 Lorain Road, North Olmsted, OH 44070; tel. 216/779-6900; Mr. BJ Centa
ManorCare Health Services, 4102 Rocky River Drive, Cleveland, OH 44135; tel. 216/251-3300; Mr. Jason Gigliotti
ManorCare Health Services, 3801 Woodridge Boulevard, Fairfield, OH 45014; tel. 513/874-9933; Ms. Lori A Saidleman-Yoh
ManorCare Health Services, 5970 Kenwood Road, Madeira, OH 45243; tel. 513/561-4111; Ms. Virginia Uehlin
ManorCare Health Services – Mayfield Heights, 6757 Mayfield Road, Mayfield Heights, OH 44124; tel. 440/473-0090; Ms. Arlene Manross
ManorCare Health Services – Willoughby, 37603 Euclid Avenue, Willoughby, OH 44094; tel. 440/951-5551; Ms. Patricia Tyler
ManorCare Health Services of Akron, 1211 West Market Street, Akron, OH 44313; tel. 330/867-8530; Mr. Gerald L Thomas
Maple Knoll Village, 11100 Springfield Pike, Cincinnati, OH 45246; tel. 513/782-2400; Mr. Jerry D Smart
Mariner Health of Toledo, 1011 North Byrne Road, Toledo, OH 43607; tel. 419/531-5321; Mrs. Mary E McConnell
Mayfair Village Nursing Care Center, 3000 Bethel Road, Columbus, OH 43220; tel. 614/889-6320; Ms. Cheryl Guyman
McCrea Manor Nursing and Rehabilitation Center, 2040 McCrea Street, Alliance, OH 44601; tel. 330/823-9005; Mr. Jim Egli
Menorah Park Center for the Aging, 27100 Cedar Road, Beachwood, OH 44122-1156; tel. 216/831-6500; Mr. Steven Raichilson
Mercy Franciscan at Schroder, 1300 Millville Avenue, Hamilton, OH 45013; tel. 513/867-1300; Ms. Julie Hanser
Mercy Franciscan at West Park, 2950 West Park Drive, Cincinnati, OH 45238; tel. 513/451-8900; Ms. Julie Hanser
Mercy St. Theresa Center, 7010 Rowan Hills Drive, Mariemont, OH 45227; tel. 513/271-7010; Ms. Nancy Hamann
Mill Run Care Center, 3399 Mill Run Drive, Hilliard, OH 43026; tel. 614/527-3000; Ms. Melissa Ray
Monterey Care Center, 3929 Hoover Road, Grove City, OH 43123; tel. 614/875-7700; Ms. Lisa Fair
New Albany Care Center, 5691 Thompson Road, Columbus, OH 43230; tel. 614/855-8866; Ms. Wendy Harbarger
Newark Healthcare Centre, 75 McMillen Drive, Newark, OH 43055; tel. 740/344-0357; Mr. Mark Johnson
Northcrest Nursing and Rehabilitation Center, 240 Northcrest Drive, Napoleon, OH 43545; tel. 419/599-4070; Ms. Carolyn Snedeker
Northland Terrace Medical Center, 5700 Karl Road, Columbus, OH 43229; tel. 614/846-5420; Mr. Gregory Turner

Oak Creek Terrace, 2316 Springmill Road, Kettering, OH 45440; tel. 937/439-1454; Mr. Barry A Kohn
Oak Grove Manor, 1670 Crider Road, Mansfield, OH 44903; tel. 419/589-6222; Mr. David Sink
Oak Grove Quality Care, 620 East Water Street, Deshler, OH 43516; tel. 419/278-6921; Mr. Glenn T Adrian
Ohio Extended Care Center, 3364 Kolbe Road, Lorain, OH 44053; tel. 440/282-2244; Mr. Barry Braunstein
Ohio Valley Manor, 5280 Routes 62 and 68, Ripley, OH 45167-9774; tel. 937/392-4318; Mr. George W Balz
Olmsted Manor Nursing Center, 27500 Mill Road, North Olmsted, OH 44070; tel. 440/777-8444; Mr. James M Eberly
Orchard Villa, 2841 Munding Drive, Oregon, OH 43616; tel. 419/697-4100; Mr. Rey Nevarez
Oregon Nursing and Rehabilitation Center, 904 Isaac Streets Drive, Oregon, OH 43616; tel. 419/691-2483; Ms. Shawnna Hearing
Parkvue Health Care Center, 3800 Boardwalk Boulevard, Sandusky, OH 44870; tel. 419/621-1900; Mr. Kenneth Keller
Pataskala Oaks Care Center, 144 East Broad Street, Pataskala, OH 43062; tel. 740/927-9888; Ms. Kathy Isbister
Pebble Creek Convalescent Center, 670 Jarvis Road, Akron, OH 44319; tel. 330/645-0200; Mr. Barry Braunstein
Pickaway Manor Care Center, 391 Clark Drive, Circleville, OH 43113; tel. 740/474-6036; Mr. John Dunn
Pine Valley Care Center, 4360 Brecksville Road, Richfield, OH 44286; tel. 330/659-6166; Mr. Barry Braunstein
Pleasant Lake Villa, 7260 Ridge Road, Parma, OH 44129; tel. 440/842-2273; Mr. Michael L Milbrandt
Rae-Ann Center, 4650 Rocky River Drive, Cleveland, OH 44135; tel. 216/267-5445; Mr. Kenneth J DiPippo
Ridge Crest Care Center, 1926 Ridge Avenue, Warren, OH 44484; tel. 330/369-4672; Ms. Debra Radecky
Ridgewood Manor, 3231 Manley Road, Maumee, OH 43537; tel. 419/865-1248; Mr. Patrick Kriner
Rittman Nursing and Rehabilitation Center, 275 East Sunset Drive, Rittman, OH 44270; tel. 330/927-2060; Ms. Sandra Zigmont
Riverview Community, 5999 Bender Road, Cincinnati, OH 45233; tel. 513/922-1440; Leigh Deaton
Rockmill Rehabilitation Centre, 3680 Dolson Court Northwest, Carroll, OH 43112; tel. 740/654-0641; Mr. Mark Forman
S.E.M. Haven Health Care Center, 225 Cleveland Avenue, Milford, OH 45150; tel. 513/248-1270; Ms. Barbara Wolf
Scenic Hills, 311 Buckridge Road, Bidwell, OH 45614; tel. 740/446-7150; Mr. David Conaway
Shepherd of the Valley Lutheran Retirement Services, 1500 McKinley Avenue, Niles, OH 44446; tel. 330/544-0771; Mr. Donald Kacmar
Somerset Quality Care Nursing and Rehabilitation Center, 411 South Columbus Street, Somerset, OH 43783; tel. 740/743-2924; Ms. Sheila A Stouder
Southern Hills Health and Rehabilitation Center, 19530 Bagley Road, Middleburg Heights, OH 44130; tel. 216/816-7500; Ms. Stephanie L Morley
St. Augustine Manor, Inc., 7801 Detroit Avenue, Cleveland, OH 44102-2895; tel. 216/634-7400; Mr. K. Patrick Gareau
Sunset View/Castle Nursing Homes, Inc., PO Box 5001, Millersburg, OH 44654; tel. 330/674-0015; Ms. Theda J Hostetler
The Convalarium at Indian Run, 6430 Post Road, Dublin, OH 43016; tel. 614/761-1188; Ms. Chenessa Marbrey
The Corinthian Skilled Nursing and Rehab Center, 320 North Wayne Street, Kenton, OH 43326; tel. 419/673-1295; Mr. Harry Hooyenga
The Corinthian, Inc., 4000 Crocker Road, Westlake, OH 44145; tel. 440/892-2100; Ms. Doula Gaitanaros
The Franciscan at St. Clare, 100 Compton Avenue, Cincinnati, OH 45215; tel. 513/761-9036; Ms. Julie Hanser
The Franciscan at St. Leonard, 8100 Clyo Road, Dayton, OH 45458; tel. 937/439-7119; Ms. Elizabeth Hartman
The LakeMed Nursing and Rehabilitation Center, 70 Normandy Drive, Painesville, OH 44077; tel. 216/357-1311; Mr. Sean Riley

Providers / JCAHO Accredited Freestanding Long-Term Care Care Organizations

The Maria-Joseph Center, 4830 Salem Avenue, Dayton, OH 45416-; tel. 937/278-2692; Ms. Bonnie G Langdon

The Northwestern Quality Care Skilled Nursing/Rehab Center, 570 North Rocky River Drive, Berea, OH 44017; tel. 440/243-2122; Ms. Danielle Mullally

The Oakridge Home, 26520 Center Ridge Road, Westlake, OH 44145; tel. 440/871-3030; Mr. Douglas Dickey

The Patrician Skilled Nursing Center, 9001 West 130th Street, North Royalton, OH 44133; tel. 440/237-3104; Ms. Doula Gaitanaros

The Village at St. Edward Nursing Care, 3131 Smith Road, Fairlawn, OH 44333-2697; tel. 330/666-1183; Mr. John J Hennelly

The Village of Westerville Nursing Center, 1060 Eastwind Drive, Westerville, OH 43081; tel. 614/895-1038; Ms. Susan Emmons

The Whetstone Gardens and Care Center, 3710 Olentangy River Road, Columbus, OH 43214; tel. 614/457-1100; Ms. Michele Engelbach

Trinity Community of Beavercreek, 3218 Indian Ripple Road, Dayton, OH 45440; tel. 937/426-8481; Mr. Brian Allen

Walnut Creek Nursing Center, 5070 Lamme Road, Kettering, OH 45439; tel. 937/293-7703; Mr. Paul DePalma

Walton Manor Health Care Centre, 19859 Alexander Road, Walton Hills, OH 44146; tel. 440/439-4433; Mrs. Wendy Repchick

West Chester Health Care, 9117 Cincinnati-Columbus Road, West Chester, OH 45069; tel. 513/777-6164; Ms. Wilma H Willard

Western Hills Retirement Village, 6210 Cleves Warsaw Pike, Cincinnati, OH 45233; tel. 513/941-0099; Mr. Barry A Kohn

Wickliffe Country Place, 1919 Bishop Road, Wickliffe, OH 44092; tel. 440/944-9400; Mr. Lisa M Mansour

Willard Center, Genesis Eldercare Network, 725 Wessor Avenue, Willard, OH 44890; tel. 419/935-6511; Mr. Roger L Blair

Windsong Care Center at Chambrel, 120 Brookmont Road, Akron, OH 44333; tel. 330/666-7373; Ms. Deborah A Haueter

Woodsfield Nursing and Rehabilitation Center, 37930 Airport Road, Woodsfield, OH 43793; tel. 614/472-1678; Mr. Dick Huffer

OKLAHOMA

ManorCare Health Services - Midwest City, 2900 Parklawn Drive, Midwest City, OK 73110; tel. 405/737-6601; Ms. Chiquita Henderson

Saint Simeon's Episcopal Home, Inc., 3701 North Cincinnati Ave., Tulsa, OK 74106; tel. 918/425-3583; Mrs. Marian P Matthews

OREGON

Cascade Terrace Nursing Center, 5601 Southeast 122nd Avenue, Portland, OR 97236; tel. 503/761-3181; Ms. Beth M Biggs

Meadow Park Health and Specialty Care Center, 75 Shore Drive, St Helens, OR 97051; tel. 503/397-2713; Mr. Michael McCoy

PENNSYLVANIA

Abington Manor, 100 Edella Road, Clarks Summit, PA 18411; tel. 717/586-1002; Ms. Ellen Craven

Adams Manor, 824 Adams Avenue, Scranton, PA 18510; tel. 717/346-5704; Mrs. Romaine Campenni

Altoona Hospital Care Center, 1020 Green Avenue, Altoona, PA 16601; tel. 814/946-2700; Mr. Felix J Mariani

Artman Lutheran Home, 250 North Bethlehem Pike, Ambler, PA 19002-3597; tel. 215/643-6333; Ms. Katrina Kane Wise

Attleboro Nursing and Rehabilitation Center, 300 East Winchester Avenue, Langhorne, PA 19047; tel. 215/757-3739; Mr. James McInerney

Baldock Health Care Center, 8850 Barnes Lake Road, North Huntingdon, PA 15642; tel. 724/864-7190; Mr. Bryan Evans

Baldwin Health Center, 1717 Skyline Drive, Pittsburgh, PA 15227; tel. 412/885-8400; Ms. Shirley Hornfeck

Ball Pavilion, Inc., 5416 East Lake Road, Erie, PA 16511; tel. 814/899-8600; Mr. George Hunter

Baptist Home of Philadelphia, 8301 Roosevelt Boulevard, Philadelphia, PA 19152; tel. 215/624-7575; Mr. David A Smiley

Barclay Friends, 700 North Franklin Street, West Chester, PA 19380; tel. 610/696-5211; Ms. J Carol Hanson

Beacon Manor, Senior Choice, Inc., 1515 Wayne Avenue, Indiana, PA 15701; tel. 724/349-5300; Ms. Kelly Pidgeon

Belvedere Center, 2507 Chestnut Street, Chester, PA 19013; tel. 610/872-5373; Mr. Gerald Miller

Berkshire Manor Nursing and Rehabilitation Center, 5501 Perkiomen Avenue, Reading, PA 19606; tel. 610/779-0600; Mr. William H Timm, Jr.

Bethany Village Retirement Center, 325 Wesley Drive, Mechanicsburg, PA 17055; tel. 717/766-0279; Ms. Bonnie S Mauldin

Beverly Health Care, 129 Franklin Avenue, Uniontown, PA 15401; tel. 724/439-5700; Mr. James A Filippone

Beverly Health Care – Murrysville, 3300 Logans Ferry Road, Murrysville, PA 15668; tel. 724/325-1500; Ms. Mary E Sauer

Beverly Healthcare – Erie, 2686 Peach Street, Erie, PA 16504; tel. 814/453-6641; Ms. Marguerite Jones

Beverly Healthcare – Kinzua valley, 205 Water Street, Warren, PA 16365; tel. 814/726-0820; Ms. Patricia A Auerbeck

Beverly Healthcare – Oakmont, 26 Ann Street, Oakmont, PA 15139; tel. 412/828-7300; Mr. Brad W Nowlen

Beverly Healthcare – Shippenville, 512 South Paint Boulevard, Shippenville, PA 16254; tel. 814/226-5660; Mr. Eric L Funk

Beverly Healthcare – South Hills, 201 Village Drive, Canonsburg, PA 15317; tel. 724/746-1300; Ms. Jennifer Firestone

Beverly Healthcare – Warren, 121 Central Avenue, Warren, PA 16365; tel. 814/726-1420; Mr. Chad Evans

Beverly Healthcare Monroeville, 4142 Monroeville Boulevard, Monroeville, PA 15146; tel. 412/856-7570; Ms. Renee Rosner

Beverly Healthcare– Western Reserve, 1521 West 54th Street, Erie, PA 16509; tel. 814/864-0671; Mrs. Connie L Farabaugh

Beverly Healthcare – William Penn, 163 Summit Drive, Lewistown, PA 17044; tel. 717/248-3941; Ms. Wanda Page

Beverly Healthcare–Meyersdale, 201 Hospital Drive, Meyersdale, PA 15552; tel. 814/634-5966; Mr. George Dayoob

Beverly Healthcare–Richland, 349 Vo-Tech Drive, Johnstown, PA 15904; tel. 814/266-9702; Mr. John Poltrack

Beverly Healthcare–Titusville, 81 Dillon Drive, Titusville, PA 16354; tel. 814/827-2727; Mrs. Dana Paszek

Blue Ridge Haven Convalescent Center – East, 3625 North Progress Avenue, Harrisburg, PA 17110; tel. 717/652-2345; Ms. Virginia Swank

Brethren Village, PO Box 5093, Lancaster, PA 17606-5093; tel. 717/569-2657; Mr. Gary Clouser

Brinton Manor, 549 Baltimore Pike, Glen Mills, PA 19342; tel. 610/358-6005; Ms. Janice Brown

Broomall Presbyterian Home, 146 Marple Road, Broomall, PA 19008-2099; tel. 610/356-0100; Mr. Robert Morrow

Buckingham Valley Rehabilitation and Nursing Ctr, PO Box 447, Buckingham, PA 18912; tel. 215/598-7181; Ms. Mary Elena Shaw

Buffalo Valley Lutheran Village, 211 Fairground Road, Lewisburg, PA 17837; tel. 570/524-2221; Ms. Kathy J Herter

Caledonia Manor, 3301 Lincoln Way East, Fayetteville, PA 17222; tel. 717/352-2101; Ms. Kristine Lowther

Camp Hill Care Center, 46 Erford Road, Camp Hill, PA 17011; tel. 717/763-7361; Ms. Kristine Lowther

Carpenter Care Center, 30 Virginia Drive, Tunkhannock, PA 18657; tel. 717/836-5166; Mr. Joseph A Traino

Cathedral Village, 600 East Cathedral Road, Philadelphia, PA 19128; tel. 215/487-1300; Mr. J. William Owens

Centre Crest, 502 East Howard Street, Bellefonte, PA 16823-2199; tel. 814/355-6777; Ms. Barbara Jackson

Chandler Hall Friends Nursing Home/Hospice Home Health, 99 Barclay Street, Newtown, PA 18940; tel. 215/860-4000; Ms. Jane Fox

Chester Care Center, 15th Street and Shaw Terrace, Chester, PA 19013; tel. 610/499-8800; Ms. Marian Ardinger

Concordia Lutheran Ministries, 615 North Pike Road, Cabot, PA 16023-2299; tel. 724/352-1571; Mr. Keith E Frndak

Conestoga View Nursing Home, 900 East King Street, Lancaster, PA 17602; tel. 717/299-7850; Ms. Carol A Knisely

Dowden Nursing and Rehabilitation Center, 3503 Rhoads Avenue, Newtown Square, PA 19073; tel. 610/359-0300; Ms. Rosemary T Stewart

Doylestown Manor, 432 Maple Avenue, Doylestown, PA 18901; tel. 215/345-1452; Mr. Thomas Scarborough

Dresher Hill Health and Rehabilitation Center, 1390 Camp Hill Road, Dresher, PA 19025; tel. 215/641-1710; Ms. Patricia Keyes

Dunwoody Village, 3500 West Chester Pike, Newtown Square, PA 19073-4168; tel. 610/359-4454; Mr. Robert Domagalski

East Mountain Manor, 101 East Mountain Boulevard, Wilkes Barre, PA 18702-7993; tel. 717/825-5892; Mr. William C Soldrich

Elkins Crest Health and Rehabilitation Center, 265 East Township Line Road, Elkins Park, PA 19027; tel. 215/379-2700; Ms. Jennifer Rittier

Elm Terrace Gardens, 660 North Broad Street, Lansdale, PA 19446; tel. 215/361-5600; Mr. Robert F Lovelace

Ephrata Manor, 99 Bethany Road, Ephrata, PA 17522; tel. 717/738-4940; Mr. John F Esbenshade

Epworth Manor, 951 Washington Avenue, Tyrone, PA 16686; tel. 814/684-0320; Ms. Jeanette B Schroeder

Evangelical Manor, 8401 Roosevelt Boulevard, Philadelphia, PA 19152; tel. 215/624-5800; Mr. J. Edward Burleigh

Fellowship Manor, 3000 Fellowship Drive, Whitehall, PA 18052; tel. 610/799-3000; Mr. Robert H Zentz

Forest Park Health Center, 700 Walnut Bottom Road, Carlisle, PA 17013; tel. 717/243-1032; Ms. Donna J Martin

Fox Subacute Center, 2644 Bristol Road, Warrington, PA 18976; tel. 215/343-2700; Mr. James M Foulke

Frederick Mennonite Community, Box 498, Frederick, PA 19435-0498; tel. 610/754-7878; Mr. Keith Hummel, Jr.

Frey Village Retirement Center, 1020 North Union Street, Middletown, PA 17057; tel. 717/944-0451; Mr. Steve Lindsey

Gettysburg Lutheran Home, 1075 Old Harrisburg Road, Gettysburg, PA 17325; tel. 717/334-6204; Ms. Christina M Ransier

Golden Slipper Club Uptown Home for the Aged, 7800 Bustleton Avenue, Philadelphia, PA 19152; tel. 215/722-2300; Mr. Lee M Davidson

Good Samaritan Nursing Care Center, 1017 Franklin Street, Johnstown, PA 15905; tel. 814/533-1934; Lois I Chapman

Green Acres Rehabilitation and Nursing Center, 1401 Ivy Hill Road, Philadelphia, PA 19150; tel. 215/233-5605; Ms. Elizabeth L Dempsey

Gwynedd Square Center for Nursing and Convalescent Care, 773 Sumneytown Pike, Lansdale, PA 19446; tel. 215/699-5000; Mr. Morris J Kaplan

HAIDA Manor, PO Box 603, Hastings, PA 16646; tel. 814/247-6578; Mrs. Pauline Formeck

Hanover Hall, 267 Frederick Street, Hanover, PA 17331; tel. 717/637-8937; Mr. George R Lorah

Harlee Manor Nursing and Rehabilitation Center, 463 West Sproul Road, Springfield, PA 19064; tel. 610/544-2200; Mr. J. Gregory Cauterucci

HarmarVillage Care Center, 715 Freeport Road, Cheswick, PA 15024; tel. 724/274-3773; Ms. Garnetta Simmons

Harmon House Care Center, 601 South Church Street, Mount Pleasant, PA 15666; tel. 724/547-1890; Mr. Dennis J Murphy

Harrison House of Christiana, 41 Newport Avenue, Christiana, PA 17509; tel. 610/593-6901; Mr. Bruce Kimball

Haverford Nursing and Rehabilitation Center, 2050 Old West Chester Pike, Havertown, PA 19083; tel. 610/449-8600; Mr. John Hadgkiss

HCR - ManorCare at Mercy Fitzgerald, 600 South Wycombe Avenue, Yeadon, PA 19050; tel. 610/626-8065; Mr. Thomas P Garvin

Heartland Health Care Center - Pittsburgh, 550 South Negley Avenue, Pittsburgh, PA 15232; tel. 412/665-2400; Ms. Deborah Koch

Heritage Towers, 200 Veterans Lane, Doylestown, PA 18901; tel. 215/345-4300; Mr. Bruce L Lenich

Hickory House Nursing Home, 3120 Horseshoe Pike, Honey Brook, PA 19344; tel. 610/273-2915; Ms. Mary E Magner

Highland Manor Nursing Home, 750 Schooley Avenue, Exeter, PA 18643; tel. 717/655-3791; Mr. Richard D Lee

Hillview Health and Rehabilitation Center, 700 South Cayuga Avenue, Altoona, PA 16602; tel. 814/946-0471; Mr. James W Wutrich

Providers / JCAHO Accredited Freestanding Long-Term Care Care Organizations

Homestead Center, 1113 North Easton Road, Willow Grove, PA 19090; tel. 215/659-3060; Ms. Nancy Deutsch

IHS at Mt. View, RD #7 Box 249, Sand Hill Road, Greensburg, PA 15601; tel. 724/837-6499; Ms. Kris Duvall

IHS at the Clara Burke Community, 251 Stenton Avenue, Plymouth Meeting, PA 19462; tel. 610/828-2272; Mr. Paul Goldenberg

IHS Greenery of Canonsburg, 2200 Hill Church - Houston Rd, Canonsburg, PA 15317; tel. 724/745-8000; Ms. Kathy D Carter

IHS of Erie at Bayside, 4114 Schaper Avenue, Erie, PA 16508; tel. 818/868-0831; Mr. Gary L Plasschaert

IHS of Greater Pittsburgh, 890 Weatherwood Lane, Greensburg, PA 15601; tel. 724/837-8076; Mr. James A Palmer

Indian Creek Nursing Center, 222 West Edison Avenue, New Castle, PA 16101; tel. 724/652-6340; Mr. Daniel Kenyon

Inglis House, 2600 Belmont Avenue, Philadelphia, PA 19131-2799; tel. 215/581-0733; Mr. John Frederick

Integrated Health Services of Chestnut Hill, 8833 Stenton Avenue, Wyndmoor, PA 19038; tel. 215/836-2100; Ms. Karen A Pulini

Integrated Health Services of Pennsylvania at Plymouth, 900 East Germantown Pike, Norristown, PA 19401; tel. 610/279-7300; Mrs. Kathleen L Glendening

Jameson Care Center, 3349 Wilmington Road, New Castle, PA 16105-1038; tel. 724/598-3300; Mr. Troy Snyder

Jefferson Manor Health Centers, RR 5, Box 42, Brookville, PA 15825; tel. 814/849-8026; Ms. Karen Wilshire

Jewish Home of Greater Harrisburg, 4000 Linglestown Road, Harrisburg, PA 17112; tel. 717/657-0700; Ms. JoAnn Ellenberger

Kittanning Care Center, RD 1, Box 27C, Kittanning, PA 16201; tel. 724/545-2273; Mr. Richard R Adams

Lancashire Hall Nursing and Rehabilitation Center, 2829 Lititz Pike, Lancaster, PA 17601; tel. 717/569-3211; Mr. Ronald E Myers

Langhorne Gardens Rehabilitation & Nursing Ctr, 350 Manor Avenue, Langhorne, PA 19047; tel. 215/757-7667; Ms. Ellen Chabin

LAS/Passavant Retirement Community, 401 South Main Street, Zelienople, PA 16063; tel. 724/452-5400; Mr. Thomas G Chase

LAS/St. John Specialty Care Center, PO Box 928, Mars, PA 16046; tel. 724/625-1571; Mr. Theodore Gillgrist

Laurel Center, 125 Holly Road, Hamburg, PA 19526; tel. 610/562-2284; Ms. Maria A Wagner

Laurel Wood Care Center, 100 Woodmont Road, Johnstown, PA 15905; tel. 814/255-1488; Mr. James E Neely

LGAR Health and Rehabilitation Center, 800 Elsie Street, Turtle Creek, PA 15145; tel. 412/825-9000; Ms. Sandra S O'Toole

Liberty Nursing and Rehab Center, 17th and Allen Streets, Allentown, PA 18104; tel. 610/432-4351; Ms. Marionlee Specter

LifeQuest Nursing Center, 2450 John Fries Highway, Quakertown, PA 18951; tel. 215/536-0770; Ms. April DelPinto

Locust Grove Retirement Village, HCR 67, Box 7, Mifflin, PA 17058; tel. 717/436-8921; Mr. Homer P Smith

Luther Acres Manor, 400 Saint Luke Drive, Lititz, PA 17543; tel. 717/626-6884; Mr. Dennis A Bruce

Luther Crest Nursing Facility, 800 Hausman Road, Allentown, PA 18104; tel. 610/391-8226; Ms. Judee Bavaria

Luther Woods Convalescent Center, 313 West County Line Road, Hatboro, PA 19040; tel. 215/675-5005; Ms. Lynn S McLaughlin

Main Line Nursing and Rehabilitation Center, 283 East Lancaster Avenue, Malvern, PA 19355; tel. 610/296-4170; Mr. John Hadgkiss

Majestic Oaks, 333 Newtown Road, Warminster, PA 18974; tel. 215/672-9082; Mr. Robert A Purdy

Manchester House Nursing and Convalescent Center, 411 Manchester Avenue, Media, PA 19063; tel. 610/565-1800; Ms. Margaret (Meg) Brockett

Manor Care Health Services - Lansdale, 640 Bethlehem Pike, Montgomeryville, PA 18936; tel. 215/368-4350; Mr. Jeffrey Brown

ManorCare Health Services, 1848 Greentree Road, Pittsburgh, PA 15220; tel. 412/344-7744; Ms. Linda Keith

ManorCare Health Services, 1105 Perry Highway, Pittsburgh, PA 15237; tel. 412/369-9955; Mr. Martin Russell

ManorCare Health Services, 113 West McMurray Road, Mc Murray, PA 15317-2427; tel. 412/941-3080; Mr. John M Walsh

ManorCare Health Services, 800 King Russ Road, Harrisburg, PA 17109; tel. 717/657-1520; Mrs. Kathryn Weachock

ManorCare Health Services, 1480 Oxford Valley Road, Yardley, PA 19067; tel. 215/321-3921; Mr. Scott E Miller

ManorCare Health Services - Laurelda1e, 2125 Elizabeth Avenue, Laureldale, PA 19605; tel. 610/921-9292; Ms. Linda Vignati

ManorCare Health Services - Bethlehem, 2029 Westgate Drive, Bethlehem, PA 18017; tel. 610/861-0100; Ms. Mary Reagan

ManorCare Health Services - Carlisle, 940 Walnut Bottom Road, Carlisle, PA 17013; tel. 717/249-0085; Mr. Thomas Wright

ManorCare Health Services - Kingston, 200 Second Avenue, Kingston, PA 18704; tel. 717/288-9315; Mr. Raymond Benkoski

ManorCare Health Services - Lancaster, 100 Abbeyville Road, Lancaster, PA 17603; tel. 717/397-4261; Ms. Teresa Long

ManorCare Health Services - Pottstown, 724 North Charlotte Street, Pottstown, PA 19464; tel. 610/323-1837; Mr. Mark Edquid

ManorCare Health Services - Pottsville, Leader and Pulaski Drives, Pottsville, PA 17901; tel. 717/622-9582; Ms. Mary Cumers

ManorCare Health Services - Williamsport North, 300 Leader Drive, Williamsport, PA 17701; tel. 717/323-8627; Ms. Anne E Holladay, NHA

ManorCare Health Services - York, 1770 Barley Road, York, PA 17404; tel. 717/767-6530; Mr. Craig Thureson

Mansion Nursing Home, 1040 Market Street, Sunbury, PA 17801; tel. 717/286-6922; Ms. Julia Starr

Mariner Health of North Hills, 194 Swinderman Road, Wexford, PA 15090; tel. 724/935-3781; Ms. Nancy Flenner

Mariner Health of West Hills, 951 Brodhead Road, Coraopolis, PA 15108; tel. 412/269-1101; Mr. Bryan Sturgeon

Mary J. Drexel Home, 238 Belmont Avenue, Bala Cynwyd, PA 19004; tel. 610/664-5967; Ms. Rosann Banback

Masonic Homes, One Masonic Drive, Elizabethtown, PA 17022-2199; tel. 717/367-1121; Mr. Joseph E Murphy

Mountain Laurel Nursing and Rehabilitation Center, 700 Leonard Street, Clearfield, PA 16830; tel. 814/765-7546; Ms. Julie A LaBree

Mt. Lebanon Manor, 350 Old Gilkeson Road, Pittsburgh, PA 15228; tel. 412/257-4444; Mr. Anthony J Molinaro, NHA

Normandie Ridge, 1700 Normandie Drive, York, PA 17404; tel. 717/764-6262; Ms. Carol McKinley

North Penn Convalescent Center, 25 West 5th Street, Lansdale, PA 19446; tel. 215/855-9765; Mr. Thomas E Howells

Ohesson Manor, 276 Green Avenue Extended, Lewistown, PA 17044; tel. 717/242-1416; Mr. Harold E Leiter, Jr.

Pembrooke Health and Rehabilitation Residence, 1130 West Chester Pike, West Chester, PA 19382; tel. 610/692-3636; Ms. Cammi Lubking

Penn Lutheran Village, 800 Broad Street, Selinsgrove, PA 17870; tel. 717/374-8181; Mr. Donald S Pote

Pennknoll Village, 208 Pennknoll Road, Everett, PA 15537-6940; tel. 814/623-9018; Ms. Linda N Frederick

Pennsylvania Memorial Home, 51 Euclid Avenue, Brookville, PA 15825; tel. 814/849-3615; Mr. Rob Buzzell

Perry Village, Inc., 213 East Main Street, New Bloomfield, PA 17068; tel. 717/582-4346; Ms. Judith Kauffman

Philadelphia Protestant Home, 6500 Tabor Road, Philadelphia, PA 19111; tel. 215/697-8006; Mr. Ronald Dyson

Phoebe Berks Health Center, 1 Heidelberg Drive, Wernersville, PA 19565; tel. 610/678-4002; Rev. Kenneth V Daniel

Phoebe Home, Inc., 1925 Turner Street, Allentown, PA 18102; tel. 610/435-9037; Mr. Joseph J Hess

Pickering Manor Home, 226 North Lincoln Avenue, Newtown, PA 18940; tel. 215/968-3878; Mr. William Wills

Presbyterian Medical Center of Oakmont, Inc., 1215 Hulton Road, Oakmont, PA 15139; tel. 412/828-5600; Mr. Paul M Winkler

Prospect Park Health and Rehabilitation Residence, 815 Chester Pike, Prospect Park, PA 19076; tel. 610/586-6262; Ms. Marjorie Tomes

Providence Care Center, PO Box 140, Beaver Falls, PA 15010; tel. 412/846-8504; Mr. Richard A Graciano, Jr.

Quakertown Center, 1020 South Main Street, Quakertown, PA 18951-1592; tel. 215/536-9300; Ms. Susan L Ulmer

Redstone Highlands Health Care Center, 6 Garden Center Drive, Greensburg, PA 15601-1397; tel. 724/832-8400; Mr. Ronald G Barrett

Rest Haven-York, 1050 South George Street, York, PA 17403; tel. 717/843-9866; Margaret Evans

Richboro Care Center, 253 Twining Ford Road, Richboro, PA 18954; tel. 215/357-2032; Ms. Susan Fetterolf

Ridge Crest Nursing and Rehabilitation Center, 1730 Buck Road, North, Feasterville, PA 19053; tel. 215/355-3131; Mr. Stanley J Segal

River's Edge Nursing and Rehabilitation Center, 9501 State Road, Philadelphia, PA 19114; tel. 215/632-5700; Ms. Paula Notarfrancisco

Riverside Care Center, 100 Eighth Avenue, Mc Keesport, PA 15132; tel. 412/664-8860; Ms. T. M Graciano

Riverstreet Manor, 440 North River Street, Wilkes Barre, PA 18702; tel. 717/825-5611; Mr. Jeff Rentner

RiverWoods, One River Road, Lewisburg, PA 17837; tel. 717/524-2271; Mr. Douglas Leidig

Rochester Manor, 174 Virginia Avenue, Rochester, PA 15074; tel. 724/775-6400; Ms. Kathryn D Kopsack

Rockhill Mennonite Community, 3250 State Road, Sellersville, PA 18960-1699; tel. 215/257-2751; Mrs. Ellen Livingston

Rosemont Manor, 35 Rosemont Avenue, Rosemont, PA 19010; tel. 610/525-1500; Ms. Carol S Cara

RoseView Center, 1201 Rural Avenue, Williamsport, PA 17701; tel. 717/323-4340; Ms. Janet Kovalich

Roslyn Nursing and Rehabilitation Center, 2630 Woodland Road, Roslyn, PA 19001; tel. 215/884-6776; Ms. Carole S Kramer

Rouse Home, 701 Rouse Avenue, Youngsville, PA 16371; tel. 814/563-7565; Mr. David A Metcalf

Rydal Park of Philadelphia Presbytery Homes, Inc., 1515 the Fairway, Rydal, PA 19046; tel. 215/885-6800; Mr. Peter Heck

Sacred Heart Manor, 6445 Germantown Avenue, Philadelphia, PA 19119-2345; tel. 215/951-0713; Sister M.Patricia Michael Sweeney

Saint John Neumann Nursing Home, 10400 Roosevelt Boulevard, Philadelphia, PA 19116; tel. 215/698-5600; Ms. Michelle Bieszczad

Saint Joseph Villa, 110 West Wissahickon Avenue, Flourtown, PA 19031-1898; tel. 215/836-4179; Sister Marie Rudegeair

Saint Luke Pavilion, 1000 Stacie Drive, Hazleton, PA 18201; tel. 717/455-7578; Mr. Mark Pile

Saint Martha Manor, 470 Manor Avenue, Downingtown, PA 19335; tel. 610/873-8490; Ms. Colleen F Frankenfield

Saint Mary Manor, 701 Lansdale Avenue, Lansdale, PA 19446-2994; tel. 215/368-0900; Ms. Maureen K Heckler

Saunders House, 100 Lancaster Avenue, Wynnewood, PA 19096-3494; tel. 610/658-5100; Mr. William J Grim

Sherwood Oaks, 100 Norman Drive, Cranberry Twp, PA 16066; tel. 412/776-8100; Ms. Cherly Metrick

Shrewsbury Lutheran Retirement Village, 200 Luther Road, Shrewsbury, PA 17361; tel. 717/235-6895; Ms. Brenda J Ferree

Sidney Square Care Center, 2112 Sidney Street, Pittsburgh, PA 15203; tel. 412/481-5566; Ms. Meriann Ritacco

Silver Lake Center - Genesis ElderCare, 905 Tower Road, Bristol, PA 19007; tel. 215/785-3201; Ms. Carol S McQuillan

Simpson House, Inc., 2101 Belmont Avenue, Philadelphia, PA 19131-1628; tel. 215/878-3600; Mr. David W Powell

Slate Belt Nursing and Rehabilitation Center, 701 Slate Belt Boulevard, Bangor, PA 18013; tel. 610/588-6161; Ms. Marie T DeFranco

Somerset Patriot Manor, 495 West Patriot Street, Somerset, PA 15501; tel. 814/445-4549; Ms. Sandra J Wright

South Mountain Restoration Center, 10058 South Mountain Road, South Mountain, PA 17261-0999; tel. 717/749-4000; Mr. Thomas A Buckus

Providers / JCAHO Accredited Freestanding Long-Term Care Care Organizations

Spang Crest Manor, 945 Duke Street, Lebanon, PA 17042; tel. 717/274-1495; Mr. Dennis Bruce
St. Andrew's Village/Julia Wilson Pounds Health Care Ctr., 1155 Indian Springs Road, Indiana, PA 15701; tel. 724/349-4870; Mr. James Bender
St. Anne's Home, 3952 Columbia Avenue, Columbia, PA 17512; tel. 717/285-5443; Sister M. Carmela Guito
Statesman Health and Rehabilitation Center, 2629 Trenton Road, Levittown, PA 19056; tel. 215/943-7777; Mr. Johnathon R Eigen
Stroud Manor, 221 East Brown Street, East Stroudsburg, PA 18301; tel. 717/421-6200; Ms. Mary Lou Shannon
Suburban General Extended Care Center, Inc., 2751 DeKalb Pike, Norristown, PA 19401; tel. 610/278-2700; Mr. Geoffrey L Henry
Summit Health Care Center, 50 North Pennsylvania Avenue, Wilkes Barre, PA 18702; tel. 717/825-3488; Ms. Suzanne Bernatovich
Susque-View Home, Inc., 22 Cree Drive, Lock Haven, PA 17745; tel. 717/748-9377; Ms. Mary V McKerrow
Susquehanna Lutheran Village, 990 Medical Road, Millersburg, PA 17061-1235; tel. 717/692-4751; Mr. Joseph G Mraz
Swaim Health Center at Green Ridge Village, 210 Big Spring Road, Newville, PA 17241; tel. 717/776-3192; Mr. Merle S Arnold
Sycamore Manor Health Center, 1445 Sycamore Road, Montoursville, PA 17754; tel. 570/326-2037; Ms. Diane Burfeindt
Tel Hai Nursing Center, Inc., PO Box 190, Honey Brook, PA 19344; tel. 610/273-9333; Mr. Keith Stuckey
The Bishop Nursing Home, 318 South Orange Street, Media, PA 19063; tel. 610/566-1400; Mrs. Roxann Vance
The Brethren Home Community, PO Box 128, New Oxford, PA 17350-0128; tel. 717/624-2161; Ms. Judith C Wallace
The Fairways at Brookline Village, 1950 Cliffside Drive, State College, PA 16801; tel. 814/238-3139; Mr. Clifford R Coldren
The Healthcare Campus at Colonial Manor, 970 Colonial Avenue, York, PA 17403; tel. 717/845-2661; Ms. Amy M Young
The Lebanon Valley Home, 550 East Main Street, Annville, PA 17003; tel. 717/867-4467; Mrs. Susan J Harley
The Lutheran Home at Hollidaysburg, 916 Hickory Street, Hollidaysburg, PA 16648; tel. 814/696-3501; Ms. Patricia Savage
The Lutheran Home at Johnstown, 807 Goucher Street, Johnstown, PA 15905; tel. 814/255-6844; Ms. Patricia W Savage
The Lutheran Home at Topton (Henry Health Care Center), One South Home Avenue, Topton, PA 19562; tel. 610/682-2145; Ms. Judee Bavaria
The Masonic Home of Pennsylvania, 801 Ridge Pike, Lafayette Hill, PA 19444; tel. 610/825-6100; Mr. Kenneth R Mills
The Presbyterian Medical Center of Washington, PA Inc., 835 South Main Street, Washington, PA 15301; tel. 724/222-4300; Ms. Elaine Bloskis
Thornwald Home, 442 Walnut Bottom Road, Carlisle, PA 17013; tel. 717/249-4118; Ms. Fay Y Henry
Twinbrook Medical Center, 3805 Field Street, Erie, PA 16511; tel. 814/898-5600; Ms. Tamara J Montell
Valley Manor Nursing and Rehabilitation Center, 7650 Route 309, Coopersburg, PA 18036; tel. 610/282-1919; Ms. Audrey Eames
Wallingford Nursing and Rehabilitation Center, 115 South Providence Road, Wallingford, PA 19086; tel. 610/565-3232; Mrs. Andrea Cantymaglia
Warren Manor, 682 Pleasant Drive, Warren, PA 16365; tel. 814/723-7060; Mr. John D McCracken
Waverly Heights, Ltd, 1400 Waverly Road, Gladwyne, PA 19035; tel. 610/645-8600; Mr. William Maguire
Wayne Center, 30 West Avenue, Wayne, PA 19087; tel. 610/688-3635; Ms. Dale Jacobs
West Shore Health and Rehabilitation Center, 770 Poplar Church Road, Camp Hill, PA 17011; tel. 717/763-7070; Ms. Deborah Slemons
Westminster Village, 803 North Wahneta Street, Allentown, PA 18103; tel. 610/434-6245; Ms. Lisa Quimbey
White Billet Nursing And Rehabilitation Center, 412 South York Road, Hatboro, PA 19040; tel. 215/675-2828; Ms. Marguerite D Everly
Wightman Health Center, 2025 Wightman Street, Pittsburgh, PA 15217; tel. 412/421-8443; Ms. Maureen McKinnon-Coyne
Willow Ridge Center, 3485 Davisville Road, Hatboro, PA 19040; tel. 215/830-0400; Ms. Carol E.L. Perfect
Woodhaven Care Center, 2400 McGinley Road, Monroeville, PA 15146; tel. 412/856-4770; Ms. Rebecca D Jobe
York Lutheran Home, 1801 Folkemer Circle, York, PA 17404-1771; tel. 717/767-5404; Rev. John M Brndjar, D.D.
York Terrace, 2401 West Market Street, Pottsville, PA 17901-1833; tel. 570/622-3982; Ms. Arlene S Postupak
Zohlman Nursing Home, PO Box 39, Richlandtown, PA 18955-0039; tel. 215/536-2252; Ms. Debora M Bartsch

RHODE ISLAND

Cedar Crest Nursing Centre, 125 Scituate Avenue, Cranston, RI 02921; tel. 401/944-8500; Ms. Susan K Whipple
Cherry Hill Manor, 2 Cherry Hill Road, Johnston, RI 02919; tel. 401/231-3102; Mr. Hugh J Hall
Elmhurst Extended Care Facility, 50 Maude Street, Providence, RI 02908; tel. 401/456-2623; Mr. Hugh J Hall
Evergreen House Health Center, One Evergreen Drive, East Providence, RI 02914; tel. 401/438-3250; Mr. Brian D Brown
Forest Farm Health Care Centre, Inc., 193 Forest Avenue, Middletown, RI 02842; tel. 401/847-2777; Mr. Karl H Lyon, Jr.
Golden Crest Nursing Centre, 100 Smithfield Road, North Providence, RI 02904; tel. 401/353-1710; Mr. Paul Pezzelli
Heatherwood Nursing and Subacute Center, Inc, 398 Bellevue Avenue, Newport, RI 02840; tel. 401/849-6600; Ms. Jennifer W Fairbanks
Kent Nursing and Rehabilitation Center, Inc, 660 Commonwealth Avenue, Warwick, RI 02886; tel. 401/739-4241; Mr. David R Velander
Metacom Manor Health Center, One Dawn Hill Road, Bristol, RI 02809; tel. 401/253-2300; Ms. Elizabeth Russell
Morgan Health Center, 80 Morgan Avenue, Johnston, RI 02919; tel. 401/944-7800; Mr. David Ryan
Oak Hill Nursing and Rehabilitation Center, 544 Pleasant Street, Pawtucket, RI 02860; tel. 401/725-8888; Mr. Richard E Gamache
Oakland Grove Health Care Center, 560 Cumberland Hill Road, Woonsocket, RI 02895; tel. 401/769-0800; Ms. Susan L LaNinfa
Saint Elizabeth Home, 109 Melrose Street, Providence, RI 02907-1898; tel. 401/941-0200; Mr. Steven J Horowitz
Slater Health Center, Inc., 70 Gill Avenue, Pawtucket, RI 02861; tel. 401/722-7900; Ms. Jo-Ann Melchert
South County Nursing and Subacute Center, 740 Oak Hill Road, North Kingstown, RI 02852; tel. 401/294-4545; Ms. Jennifer W Fairbank
St. Antoine Residence, 400 Mendon Road, North Smithfield, RI 02896-6999; tel. 401/767-3500; Ms. Mary Ann Altrui
Steere House Inc., 100 Borden Street, Providence, RI 02903; tel. 401/454-7970; Mr. Steven J Farrow
The Clipper Home, Inc., 161 Post Road, Westerly, RI 02891; tel. 401/322-8081; Ms. Linda Tucker
The St. Clare Home, 309 Spring Street, Newport, RI 02840; tel. 401/849-3204; Ms. Mary Beth Daigneault
Watch Hill Manor, Ltd., 79 Watch Hill Road, Westerly, RI 02891; tel. 401/596-2664; Ms. Linda A Tucker
Westerly Health Center, 280 High Street, Westerly, RI 02891; tel. 401/348-0020; Ms. Melissa M Prevey
Woonsocket Health and Rehabilitation Center, 262 Poplar Street, Woonsocket, RI 02895; tel. 401/765-2100; Ms. Norma Pezzelli

SOUTH CAROLINA

C. M. Tucker, Jr. / Dowdy Gardner Nursing Care Center, 2200 Harden Street, Columbia, SC 29203; tel. 803/737-5301; Ms. Shielda D Friendly
Heartland Health Care Center - Charleston, 1800 Eagle Landing Boulevard, Hanahan, SC 29406; tel. 803/553-0656; Mr. Paul Cercone
Life Care Center of Charleston, 2600 Elms Plantation Boulevard, Charleston, SC 29406; tel. 843/764-3500; Ms. Beth A Cliett
Life Care Center of Columbia, 2514 Faraway Drive, Columbia, SC 29223; tel. 803/865-1999; Ms. Carol D Cordan
Manor Care - Columbia, 2601 Forest Drive, Columbia, SC 29204; tel. 803/256-4983; Ms. Jeaneane Tam
National HealthCare Center Greenville, 1305 Boiling Springs Road, Greer, SC 29650; tel. 864/458-7566; Mr. William D Bishop
Roper Nursing Center, 2230 Ashley Crossing Drive, Charleston, SC 29417; tel. 803/852-2273; Mr. John Driggers
Springdale HealthCare Center, 146 Battleship Road, Camden, SC 29020; tel. 803/432-3741; Ms. Timothy A Osment

SOUTH DAKOTA

Beverly Healthcare, 1103 South 2nd Street, Milbank, SD 57252; tel. 605/432-4556; Ms. Katherine Holland
Beverly Healthcare Covington Heights, 3900 South Cathy Avenue, Sioux Falls, SD 57106; tel. 605/361-8822; Ms. Carol Ulmer
Colonial Manor Health and Rehabilitation, PO Box 620, Salem, SD 57058; tel. 605/425-2203; Joan Raap
Rapid City Care Center, 916 Mountain View, Rapid City, SD 57702; tel. 605/343-8577; Mr. Bruce Glanzer

TENNESSEE

Allen Morgan Health Center, 177 North Highland, Memphis, TN 38111; tel. 901/325-4003; Mr. James A Brooks
American Transitional Rehab and Specialty Care, 6733 Quince Road, Memphis, TN 38119; tel. 901/755-3860; Mr. Rob Rollans
Fairpark Healthcare Center, PO Box 5477, Maryville, TN 37802; tel. 423/983-0261; Mr. Harold Walker
Farragut Health Care Center, 12823 Kingston Pike, Knoxville, TN 37922; tel. 423/966-0600; Mr. George S Oeakins
Greystone Health Care Center, PO Box 1133, TCAS, Blountville, TN 37617; tel. 423/323-7112; Ms. Judy C Dexter
Life Care Center of Athens, PO Box 786, Athens, TN 37371-0786; tel. 423/754-8181; Mr. Kirk Rogers
Life Care Center of Collegedale, PO Box 658, Collegedale, TN 37315; tel. 423/396-2182; Mr. Richard Mountz
Life Care Center of East Ridge, 1500 Fincher Avenue, East Ridge, TN 37412; tel. 423/894-1254; Ms. Martha A Johnson
Life Care Center of Jefferson City, 336 West Old A.J. Highway, Jefferson City, TN 37760; tel. 423/475-6097; Mr. Keith L Boyce
Life Care Center of Morristown, PO Box 1899, Morristown, TN 37814; tel. 423/581-5435; Mr. Marvin Frey
Life Care Center of Tullahoma, 1715 North Jackson Street, Tullahoma, TN 37388; tel. 931/455-8557; Ms. Dawn R Visscher
Mariner Health of Nashville, 3939 Hillsboro Circle, Nashville, TN 37215; tel. 615/297-2100; Ms. Paula Glover
Maryville Healthcare and Rehabilitation Center, 1012 Jamestown Way, Maryville, TN 37803; tel. 423/984-7400; Mr. J. Joe Maples
McKendree Village, Inc., 4343-47 Lebanon Road, Hermitage, TN 37076; tel. 615/871-8232; Dr. Robert F Willner
Mountainview Rehabilitation and Nursing Center, 1360 Bypass Road, Winchester, TN 37398; tel. 931/967-7082; Mr. Royce J Earp
National HealthCare - Murfreesboro, 100 Vine Street, Murfreesboro, TN 37130; tel. 615/890-2020; Mr. Greg Bidwell
NHC HealthCare, 2120 Highland Ave, Knoxville, TN 37916; tel. 423/525-4131; Mr. Douglas S Ford
NHC Healthcare - Nashville, 2215 Patterson Street, Nashville, TN 37203; tel. 615/327-3011; Ms. Joann Maze
Ridgeview Terrace of Life Care, PO Box 26, Rutledge, TN 37861; tel. 423/828-5295; Mr. Greg Mitchell

TEXAS

Alameda Oaks Nursing Center, 1101 South Alameda, Corpus Christi, TX 78404; tel. 512/882-2711; Mrs. Marta Wellesley
Alamo Heights Health and Rehabilitation Center, 8223 Broadway, San Antonio, TX 78209; tel. 210/828-0606; Mr. J. Randy Baronet
Allenbrook Health Care Center, 4109 Allenbrook Drive, Baytown, TX 77521; tel. 713/422-3546; Mr. Barry Goldstein
Autumn Years Lodge, 424 South Adams, Fort Worth, TX 76104; tel. 817/335-5781; Ms. Patricia Sanders
Bay Villa Health Care Center, 1800 - 13th Street, Bay City, TX 77414; tel. 409/245-6327; Mr. Joshua H Nieto

Providers / JCAHO Accredited Freestanding Long-Term Care Care Organizations

Beacon Health, Ltd., 9182 Six Pines Drive, The Woodlands, TX 77380; tel. 281/364-0317; Ms. Kathy Roberts
Bivins Memorial Nursing Home, 1001 Wallace Boulevard, Amarillo, TX 79106-1736; tel. 806/355-7453; Mr. John Paul Athanasiou
Brazos Valley Geriatric Center, 1115 Anderson Street, College Station, TX 77840; tel. 409/693-1515; Mr. Darryl Thomas
Brookhaven Nursing Center, 1855 Cheyenne Dr., Carrollton, TX 75008; tel. 972/394-7141; Mr. Stephen Powell
CASA, A Special Hospital, 1803 Old Spanish Trail, Houston, TX 77054; tel. 713/796-2272; Ms. Gretchen Thorp
Christian Care Center, 1000 Wiggins Parkway, Mesquite, TX 75150; tel. 972/686-3000; Mr. Russ Chambers
Colonial Manor - Tyler, 930 South Baxter, Tyler, TX 75701; tel. 903/597-2068; Ms. Matt Moore
Coronado Nursing Center, 1751 North 15th Street, Abilene, TX 79603; tel. 915/673-8892; Ms. Cyd Lane
Elizabeth Jane Bivins Home for the Aged, 3115 Tee Anchor Boulevard, Amarillo, TX 79104; tel. 806/373-7671; Ms. Jimmie Sue Chisum
Fort Worth Nursing and Rehabilitation Center, 1000 6th Avenue, Fort Worth, TX 76104; tel. 817/336-2586; Mr. Mark Johnston
Green Acres Convalescent Center, 93 Isaacks Road, Humble, TX 77338; tel. 281/446-7159; Ms. Eddie J Doerre
Green Acres Parkdale, 11025 Old Voth Road, Beaumont, TX 77713; tel. 409/892-9722; Ms. Darline D Rouse
Heart of Texas Health Care & Rehab. Center-Changing Seasons, 545 Denver Street, Vidor, TX 77662; tel. 409/769-4542; Mr. Frances Dupuy
Heart of Texas Health Care & Rehab Center-Colonial Park, 104 Enterprise, Devine, TX 78016; tel. 830/663-4451; Ms. Cathy Peeler
Heart of Texas Health Care & Rehabilitation Center- Del Mar, 4130 Santa Elena, Corpus Christi, TX 78405; tel. 512/882-3655; Mr. Jim Miller
Heart of Texas Health Care & Rehabilitation-Poteet, 329 School Drive, Poteet, TX 78065; tel. 830/742-3525; Ms. Kristy Luna
Hearthstone Nursing and Rehabilitation Center, 401 Oakwood Boulevard, Round Rock, TX 78681; tel. 512/388-7494; Ms. Stacy Adams
Heartland Health Care Center - Austin, 11406 Rustic Rock Drive, Austin, TX 78750; tel. 512/335-5028; Ms. Ann Rayner
Heartland Health Care Center - Bedford, 2001 Forest Ridge Drive, Bedford, TX 76021; tel. 817/571-6804; Mr. Mack Baldridge
Heartland Health Care Center of West Houston, 2939 Woodland Park Drive, Houston, TX 77082; tel. 281/870-9100; Ms. Terri D Humes
Heartland of Corpus Christi, 202 Fortune Drive, Corpus Christi, TX 78405; tel. 512/289-0889; Ms. Marvena Jones
Heartland of San Antonio, One Heartland Drive, San Antonio, TX 78247; tel. 210/653-1219; Mr. Guy Bowles
Heritage Manor, 1621 Coit Road, Plano, TX 75075; tel. 972/596-7930; Ms. Bobbie M Sechovec
Hilltop Haven, PO Box 39, Gunter, TX 75058; tel. 903/433-2415; Mr. Greg Losher
IHS of Dallas at Treemont, 5550 Harvest Hill Road, Dallas, TX 75230; tel. 972/661-1862; Mr. Rodney Smith
Integrated Health Services at Woodridge, 1500 Autumn Drive, Grapevine, TX 76051; tel. 817/488-8585; Dr. Robert Elkins
Integrated Health Services of Texoma, 1000 Highway 82 East, Sherman, TX 75090; tel. 903/893-9636; Mr. Michael J Flugstad
Lake Shore Village Health Care Center, 2320 Lake Shore Drive, Waco, TX 76708; tel. 817/752-1075; Mr. Kraig A Turpen
Lakewood Village Health Care Center, 5100 Randol Mill Road, Fort Worth, TX 76112; tel. 817/451-8001; Ms. Shelly Young
Lexington Place Health Care Center, 1737 North Loop West, Houston, TX 77008; tel. 713/869-5551; Ms. Gail Baschnagel
ManorCare Health Services, 3326 Burgoyne Street, Dallas, TX 75233; tel. 214/330-9291; Ms. Ann Rayner
ManorCare Health Services, 7625 Glenview Drive, Fort Worth, TX 76180; tel. 817/284-1427; Ms. Kay Severson
ManorCare Health Services, 8800 Fourwinds, San Antonio, TX 78239; tel. 210/656-7800; Ms. Tamara Myatt
ManorCare Health Services - San Antonio (Babcock), 1975 Babcock Road, San Antonio, TX 78229; tel. 210/341-8681; Mr. Paul A Ormond
ManorCare Health Services - Webster, 750 West Texas Avenue, Webster, TX 77598; tel. 281/332-3496; Ms. Robin Ricondo, Jr.
ManorCare Health Services Nursing & Rehabilitation Ctr., 7505 Bellerive, Houston, TX 77036; tel. 713-774-9611; Mr. John E Dugan
Mariner Health of Arlington, 2645 West Randol Mill Road, Arlington, TX 76012; tel. 817/277-6789; Mr. Kendal Nelson
Mariner Health of Fort Worth, 4825 Wellesley Avenue, Fort Worth, TX 76107; tel. 817/732-6608; Ms. Lynne F Jones
Mariner Health of Northwest Houston, 17600 Cali Drive, Houston, TX 77090; tel. 713/440-9000; Mr. David Stroud
Mariner Health of San Antonio, 5757 North Knoll, San Antonio, TX 78240; tel. 210/699-8535; Ms. Karen Kohlleppel
Marshall Manor Healthcare and Rehab, PO Box 1629, Marshall, TX 75670; tel. 903/935-7971; Mr. J. Walter Cook
Memorial Medical, 307 W. Cypress, San Antonio, TX 78212; tel. 210/223-5521; Ms. Janet Tennis
Retama Manor Laredo South, 1100 Galveston Street, Laredo, TX 78040; tel. 956/723-2068; Mr. Ricardo Gonzalez
Retama Manor North San Antonio, 501 Ogden, San Antonio, TX 78212; tel. 210/225-4588; Mr. Greg Moore
Retama Manor Nursing Center, 1505 South Closner, Edinburg, TX 78539; tel. 956/383-5656; Ms. Lilly E Molina
Seven Acres Jewish Senior Care Services, 6200 North Braeswood, Houston, TX 77074; tel. 713/778-5701; Mr. Malcolm P Slatko
Silver Creek Manor, 9014 Timber Path, San Antonio, TX 78250; tel. 210/523-2455; Ms. Cynthia Brown
Silver Leaves Nursing Center, 505 West Centreville Road, Garland, TX 75041; tel. 972/278-3566; Mr. Larry LaFrensen
Southfield Health Care Center, 802 Fresa Street, Pasadena, TX 77502; tel. 713/946-3360; Ms. Coral A Gooden
Southwood Care Center, 3759 Valley View, Austin, TX 78704; tel. 512/443-3436; Ms. Sharlyn Threadgall
The Clairmont - Longview, 3201 North Fourth Street, Longview, TX 75605; tel. 903/236-4291; Robert Snukal
The Village Healthcare Center, 1341 Blalock Road, Houston, TX 77055; tel. 713/468-7821; Ms. Johnnie Richardson
Victoria Nursing and Rehabilitation Center, 114 Medical Drive, Victoria, TX 77904; tel. 361/576-6128; Mr. Brent Limmer
Ware Memorial Care Center, 1300 South Harrison, Amarillo, TX 79101; tel. 806/373-0471; T.H. Holloway
Weatherford Health Care Center, 521 West 7th, Weatherford, TX 76086; tel. 817/594-8713; Ms. Lezlie McWhorter
West Oaks Geriatric Center, 3625 Greencrest Drive, Houston, TX 77082; tel. 281/558-1166; Mr. Bill Thurman

UTAH
Rocky Mountain Care - Clearfield, 1450 South 1500 East, Clearfield, UT 84015; tel. 801/728-4300; Ms. Heather M Zigliara
South Davis Community Hospital, 401 South 400 East, Bountiful, UT 84010; tel. 801/295-2361; Mr. Gordon W Bennet
Sunshine Terrace Foundation, Inc., 225 North 200 West, Logan, UT 84321-3805; tel. 801/752-0411; Ms. Sara V Sinclair
Washington Terrace Nursing Center, 400 East 5350 South, Ogden, UT 84405; tel. 801/479-9855; Ms. Kelly Ogden

VERMONT
Bennington Health and Rehabilitation Center, Blackberry Lane, Bennington, VT 05201; tel. 802/442-8525; Mr. Mark Finkelstein
Berlin Health and Rehab Center, RR 3, Box 6684, Barre, VT 05641; tel. 802/229-0308; Mr. Mark Finkelstein
Birchwood Terrace Healthcare, 43 Starr Farm Road, Burlington, VT 05401; tel. 802/863-6384; Mr. Thomas N DePoy
Burlington Health and Rehabilitation Center, 300 Pearl Street, Burlington, VT 05401; tel. 802/658-4200; Mr. Mark Finkelstein
Rowan Court Health and Rehabilitation Center, 378 Prospect Street, Barre, VT 05641; tel. 802/476-4166; Dr. Mark Finkelstein
Springfield Health and Rehab Center, 105 Chester Road, Springfield, VT 05156; tel. 802/885-5741; Mr. Mark J Finkelstein
St. Johnsbury Health and Rehab Center, Hospital Drive, Saint Johnsbury, VT 05819; tel. 802/748-8757; Mr. Mark Finkelstein
Starr Farm Nursing Center, 98 Starr Farm Road, Burlington, VT 05401; tel. 802/658-6717; Ms. Claudette Werner
Verdelle Village Extended Care Facility, Box 80 Sheldon Road, St Albans, VT 05478; tel. 802/524-6534; Mr. Paul Richards

VIRGINIA
Annaburg Manor, 9201 Maple Street, Manassas, VA 20110; tel. 703/335-8300; Ms. Ann A Finley
Appomattox Healthcare Center, Route 5, Box 800, Appomattox, VA 24522; tel. 804/352-7420; Mr. W. Heywood Fralin
Autumn Care of Norfolk, PO Box 12569, Norfolk, VA 23502; tel. 757/857-0481; Mr. Gerald P Cox
Bayside Healthcare Center, PO Box 68039, Virginia Beach, VA 23471; tel. 757/464-4058; Mr. W. Heywood Fralin
Beaufont Healthcare Center, 200 Hioaks Road, Richmond, VA 23225-4048; tel. 804/272-2918; Mr. W. Heywood Fralin
Beth Sholom Home of Eastern Virginia, 6401 Auburn Drive, Virginia Beach, VA 23464; tel. 757/420-2512; Mr. Bryan R Mesh
Beth Sholom Home of Virginia, 1600 John Rolfe Parkway, Richmond, VA 23233; tel. 804/750-2183; Mr. Mark W Finkle
Beverly Healthcare - Ridgecrest, PO Box 280, Duffield, VA 24244; tel. 540/431-2841; Ms. James O Strom
Bon Secours - Maryview Nursing Care Center, 4775 Bridge Road, Suffolk, VA 23435; tel. 757/686-0488; Ms. Eileen D Malo
Bowling Green Healthcare Center, PO Box 967, Bowling Green, VA 22427; tel. 804/633-4839; Mr. W. Heywood Fralin
Brian Center Health and Rehabilitation - Scott County, 105 Clonce Street, Weber City, VA 24290; tel. 540/386-9444; Mr. Scott Shearin
Burke Healthcare Center, 9640 Burke Lake Road, Burke, VA 22015-3022; tel. 703/425-9765; Ms. Amanda L Gannon
Camelot Hall of Lynchburg, 5615 Seminole Avenue, Lynchburg, VA 24502-2201; tel. 804/239-2657; Mr. Heywood Fralin
Camelot Health and Rehabilitation Center, 1225 South Reservoir Street, Harrisonburg, VA 22801-4499; tel. 540/433-2623; Mr. W. Heywood Fralin
Cherrydale Healthcare Center, 3710 Lee Highway, Arlington, VA 22207-3796; tel. 703/243-7640; Mr. W. Heywood Fralin
Chesapeake Healthcare Center, 688 Kingsborough Square, Chesapeake, VA 23320-4908; tel. 757/547-9111; Mr. Rick Oros
Courtland Healthcare Center, 23020 Main Street, Courtland, VA 23837-1207; tel. 757/653-0908; Mr. Heywood Fralin
Culpeper Healthcare Center, 602 Madison Road, Culpeper, VA 22701-3324; tel. 540/825-2884; Mr. W. Heywood Fralin
Elizabeth Adam Crump Manor, 1300 Mountain Road, Glen Allen, VA 23060; tel. 804/672-8725; Ms. Sandra Harless
Fairfax Nursing Center, Inc., 10701 Main Street, Fairfax, VA 22030; tel. 703/273-7705; Ms. Renee Bainum-Carlson
Franklin Healthcare Center, PO Box 555, Rocky Mount, VA 24151; tel. 540/489-3467; Mr. W. Heywood Fralin
Friendship Manor, Inc., 327 Hershberger Road, NW, Roanoke, VA 24012; tel. 540/265-2111; Mr. Monty Plymale
Goodwin House West, 3440 South Jefferson Street, Falls Church, VA 22041; tel. 703/578-7645; Mr. Marvin Ogburn
Gretna Healthcare Center, PO Box 577, Gretna, VA 24557-0577; tel. 804/656-1206; Mr. W. Heywood Fralin
Hanover Healthcare Center, 8139 Lee Davis Road, Mechanicsville, VA 23111; tel. 804/559-5030; Mr. J. Michael Williams
Health of Virginia, 2420 Pemberton Road, Richmond, VA 23233-2099; tel. 804/747-9200; Mr. Walter W Regirer
Henrico Healthcare Center, PO Box 319, Highland Springs, VA 23075-2100; tel. 804/737-0172; Mr. W. Heywood Fralin

Providers / JCAHO Accredited Freestanding Long-Term Care Care Organizations

Iliff Nursing and Rehabilitation Center, 8000 Iliff Drive, Dunn Loring, VA 22027; tel. 703/560-1000; Mr. Dick Richardson

Inova Cameron Glen Care Center, 1800 Cameron Glen Drive, Reston, VA 20190; tel. 703/834-5800; Ms. Pamela S Clark

Inova Commonwealth Care Center, 4315 Chain Bridge Road, Fairfax, VA 22030; tel. 703/934-5000; Ms. Shelly L Kobuck

Integrated Health Services of Northern Virginia, 900 Virginia Avenue, Alexandria, VA 22302; tel. 703/684-9100; Mr. David C Burke

James River Convalescent Center, 540 Aberthaw Avenue, Newport News, VA 23601; tel. 757/595-2273; Mr. Jeffrey L Mendelsohn

Jefferson Park Center Genesis ElderCare Network, P O Box 3815, Charlottesville, VA 22903; tel. 804/295-1161; Mr. Stephen Reynalds

Louisa Healthcare Center, PO Box 1310, Louisa, VA 23093; tel. 540/967-2250; Mr. W. Heywood Fralin

Lovingston Healthcare Center, PO Box 398, Lovingston, VA 22949; tel. 804/263-4823; Mr. W. Heywood Fralin

Lucy Corr Village, PO Drawer 170, Chesterfield, VA 23832; tel. 804/748-1511; Mr. Jacob W Mast, Jr.

Manor Care Skilled Nursing & Rehabilitation, 550 South Carlin Springs Road, Arlington, VA 22204; tel. 703/379-7200; Mr. Barry E Grofic

Norfolk Healthcare Center, 901 East Princess Anne Road, Norfolk, VA 23504-2732; tel. 757/626-1642; Mr. Willie E Alston

Oak Hill Center, PO Box 2565, Staunton, VA 24402-2565; tel. 540/886-2335; Mr. Richard J Shelley

Oakwood Nursing and Rehabilitation Center, 5520 Indian River Road, Virginia Beach, VA 23464; tel. 757/420-3600; Mr. Loren O King

Parham Healthcare and Rehabilitation Center, 2400 East Parham Road, Richmond, VA 23228-3100; tel. 804/264-9185; Mr. Joe Cicatko

Pheasant Ridge Nursing and Rehabilitation Center, 4355 Pheasant Ridge Road, Roanoke, VA 24014; tel. 540/725-8210; Ms. Debbie Petrine

Piney Forest Healthcare Center, 450 Piney Forest Road, Danville, VA 24540; tel. 804/799-1565; Mr. W. Heywood Fralin

Potomac Center – Genesis ElderCare Network, 1785 South Hayes Street, Arlington, VA 22202; tel. 703/920-5700; Ms. Cynthia M Martin

Pulaski Healthcare Center, 2401 Lee Highway, Pulaski, VA 24301-2329; tel. 540/980-3111; Mr. W. Heywood Fralin

Raleigh Court Healthcare Center, 1527 Grandin Road Southwest, Roanoke, VA 24015-2305; tel. 540/342-9525; Mr. Heywood Fralin

Regency Healthcare Center, 112 North Constitution Drive, Yorktown, VA 23692-2792; tel. 757/890-0675; Mr. W. Heywood Fralin

Riverside Healthcare Center, 2344 Riverside Drive, Danville, VA 24540-4212; tel. 804/791-3800; Mr. W. Heywood Fralin

Riverside Regional Convalescent Center, 1000 Old Denbigh Boulevard, Newport News, VA 23602; tel. 757/875-2000; Ms. Patricia A Iannetta

Salem Health and Rehabilitation Center, 1945 Roanoke Boulevard, Salem, VA 24153-6487; tel. 540/345-3894; Mr. W. Heywood Fralin

Shenandoah Valley Health Care Center, PO Box 711, Buena Vista, VA 24416; tel. 540/261-7444; Ms. Barbara Cathey

Stanleytown Healthcare Center, PO Box 538, Stanleytown, VA 24168; tel. 540/629-1772; Mr. W. Heywood Fralin

The Berkshire Health Care Center, 705 Clearview Drive, Vinton, VA 24179; tel. 540/982-6691; Mr. Heywood Fralin

Virginia Beach Healthcare and Rehabilitation Center, 1801 Camelot Drive, Virginia Beach, VA 23454; tel. 757/481-3500; Mr. Heywood Fralin

Virginia Veterans Care Center, 4550 Shenandoah Avenue, Northwest, Roanoke, VA 24017; tel. 540/982-2860; Thomas M Shelor

Warrenton Overlook Health and Rehabilitation Center, 360 Hospital Drive, Warrenton, VA 20186; tel. 540/349-1919; Ms. Mary M Smith

Warsaw Healthcare Center, 5373 Richmond Road, Warsaw, VA 22572; tel. 804/333-3616; Mr. Bob Fabian

Waverly Healthcare Center, PO Box 641, Waverly, VA 23890-0641; tel. 804/834-3975; Mr. W. Heywood Fralin

Williamsburg Center Genesis ElderCare, 1235 Mt. Vernon Avenue, Williamsburg, VA 23185; tel. 757/229-4121; Mr. Michael Walker

Woodbine Rehabilitation and Healthcare Center, 2729 King Street, Alexandria, VA 22302; tel. 703/836-8838; Ms. Mary Ann Sleigh

Woodmont Center, PO Box 419, Fredericksburg, VA 22404-0419; tel. 540/371-9414; Ms. Sharon Bartlett

WASHINGTON

Bessie Burton Sullivan, 1020 East Jefferson, Seattle, WA 98122; tel. 206/323-1028; Ms. Carmen Steiner

Cascade Vista Convalescent Center, Inc., 7900 Willows Road Northeast, Redmond, WA 98052; tel. 425/885-0808; Ms. Pearl K Barnes

Evergreen Vista Convalescent Center, Inc., 11800 Northeast 128th Street, Kirkland, WA 98034-7201; tel. 425/821-0404; Ms. Mary G Southwick

Mercer Island Care and Rehabilitation, 7445 Southeast 24th Street, Mercer Island, WA 98040; tel. 206/232-6600; Mr. Mark G Wimer

Meydenbauer Medical and Rehabilitation Center, 150 102nd Avenue Southeast, Bellevue, WA 98004; tel. 206/454-6166; Mr. Andrew L Turner

Sunbridge Care and Rehabilitation of Oyster Bay, 3517 11th Street, Bremerton, WA 98312; tel. 360/377-5537; Mr. Dale J Zulauf

SunRise Care & Rehabilitation for Vancouver, 5220 NE Hazel Dell Avenue, Vancouver, WA 98663; tel. 360/693-1474; Ms. Zendi Meharry

SunRise Care & Rehabilitation for Walla Walla Valley, 1200 Southeast 12th Street, College Place, WA 99324; tel. 509/529-4080; Mr. Andrew Turner

SunRise Care & Rehabilitation for Walla Walla Valley, 1200 Southeast 12th Street, College Place, WA 99324; tel. 509/529-4080; Mr. Andrew Turner

Sunrise Care and Rehabilitation for Richmond Beach, 19235 15th Avenue Northwest, Shoreline, WA 98177; tel. 206/546-2666; Mr. Andrew Turner

The Care Center at Kelsey Creek, 2210 132nd Avenue Southeast, Bellevue, WA 98005; tel. 425/957-2400; Mr. Russell Akiyama

Wedgwood Care and Rehabilitation, 9132 Ravenna Avenue Northeast, Seattle, WA 98115; tel. 206/524-6535; Ms. Nancy Ratliff

WEST VIRGINIA

Bishop Joseph H. Hodges Continuous Care Center, 600 Medical Park, Wheeling, WV 26003; tel. 304/243-3812; Mr. Gary R Gould

Brightwood Nursing and Rehabilitation Center, 840 Lee Road, Follansbee, WV 26037; tel. 304/527-1100; Ms. Kathy D Haddon

Canterbury Center, Genesis ElderCare, Route 2, Box 5, Shepherdstown, WV 25443; tel. 304/876-9422; Ms. Susan Hockensmith

Care Haven Center, Route 5, Box A167, Martinsburg, WV 25401; tel. 304/263-0933; Mr. Drew Leroy

Dawnview Center, PO Box 686, Fort Ashby, WV 26719; tel. 304/298-3602; Mr. Joseph W Mason, II

GlenWood Park, Inc. dba Glenwood Park Retirement, Village 1924 Glenwood Park Road, Princeton, WV 24740-7969; tel. 304/425-8128; Dr. Daniel W Farley

Heartland of Charleston, 3819 Chesterfield Avenue, Charleston, WV 25304; tel. 304/925-4771; Ms. Karen Lawson

Rosewood Nursing and Rehabilitation Center, 8 Rose Street, Grafton, WV 26354; tel. 304/265-0095; Ms. Rebecca Skarbek

Shenandoah Nursing and Rehabilitation Center, 219 Prospect Avenue, Charles Town, WV 25414; tel. 304/724-1101; Ms. Cheryl L Martin

Sistersville Nursing and Rehabilitation Center, 201 Wood Street, Sistersville, WV 26175; tel. 304/652-1032; Mr. Robert Dahl

SunBridge Care and Rehabilitation for Parkersburg, 1716 Gihon Road, Parkersburg, WV 26101; tel. 304/485-5511; Mr. Rodney L Hannah

SunRise Care & Rehabilitation for Putnam, 300 Seville Road, Hurricane, WV 25526; tel. 304/757-6805; Ms. Angie Booker

SunRise Pine Lodge Care and Rehabilitation, 405 Stanaford Road, Beckley, WV 25801; tel. 304/252-6317; Ms. Sherry Johnson

The Madison, 161 Bakers Ridge Road, Morgantown, WV 26505; tel. 304/285-0692; Mr. Eric T Nichols

The Willows Center, 723 Summers Street, Parkersburg, WV 26101; tel. 304/428-5573; Mr. Thomas M Kelley, Jr.

WISCONSIN

Ashland Health and Rehabilitation Center, 1319 Beaser Avenue, Ashland, WI 54806; tel. 715/682-3468; Ms. Judith A Wheeler

Bel Air Health Care Center/ Alzheimers Center, 9350 West Fond Du Lac Avenue, Milwaukee, WI 53225; tel. 414/438-4360; Ms. Jane Clemente-Elliott

Bethel Center, 8014 Bethel Road, Arpin, WI 54410; tel. 715/652-2103; Ms. Gerri Mast

Beverly Health and Rehabilitation, 6735 West Bradley Road, Milwaukee, WI 53223; tel. 414/354-3300; Ms. Lisa Thomson

Beverly Health and Rehabilitation Center/Superior, 1612 North 37th Street, Superior, WI 54880; tel. 715/392-5144; Mr. Marvin Benedict

Beverly Healthcare, Sherwood Heights, 3710 North Oakland Avenue, Shorewood, WI 53211; tel. 414/964-6200; Mr. Daniel W Langenwalter

Clement Manor Health Center, 3939 South 92nd Street, Greenfield, WI 53228; tel. 414/321-1800; Mr. Dennis Ferger

Colonial Center, 702 West Dolf Street, Colby, WI 54421; tel. 715/223-2352; Ms. Tracy Hogden

Colonial Manor Medical and Rehabilitation Center, 1010 East Wausau Avenue, Wausau, WI 54403; tel. 715/842-2028; Mrs. N. Jean Burgener

Columbus Center, 825 Western Avenue, Columbus, WI 53925; tel. 920/623-2520; Ms. Debbie Barth

Continental Manor Health and Rehabilitation Center, 502 South High Street, Randolph, WI 53956; tel. 920/326-3171; Ms. Victoria L Grant

Dorchester Health and Rehabilitation Center, 200 North 7th Avenue, Sturgeon Bay, WI 54235; tel. 920/743-6274; Mr. Chad Stroschein

Eastview Medical and Rehab Center, 729 Park Street, Antigo, WI 54409-2798; tel. 715/623-2356; Ms. Tina A Ver Hagen

Franciscan Villa, 3601 South Chicago Avenue, South Milwaukee, WI 53172; tel. 414/764-4100; Mr. Roger DeMark

Franciscan Woods, 19525 West North Avenue, Brookfield, WI 53045; tel. 414/785-1114; Ms. Mary Piette

Greendale Health and Rehabilitation Center, 3129 Michigan Avenue, Sheboygan, WI 53081; tel. 920/458-1155; Ms. Suzanne M Bruner

Heartland Health Care Center – Pewaukee, N26W23977 Watertown Road, Waukesha, WI 53188; tel. 414/523-0933; Mr. Wayne Brow

Heartland Health Care Center – Washington Manor, 3100 Washington Road, Kenosha, WI 53144; tel. 414/658-4622; Mr. Thomas O'Neal

Heritage Square Healthcare Centre, 5404 West Loomis Road, Greendale, WI 53129; tel. 414/421-0088; Mr. Dennis Mattes

Honey Creek Health and Rehabilitation Center, 2730 West Ramsey Avenue, Milwaukee, WI 53221; tel. 414/282-2600; Mr. John F Flynn

Karmenta Center, 4502 Milwaukee Street, Madison, WI 53714; tel. 608/249-2137; Ms. Cheri McCormick

ManorCare Health Services, 1335 South Oneida Street, Appleton, WI 54915; tel. 920/731-6646; Ms. Christine Wales

ManorCare Health Services, 265 South National Avenue, Fond Du Lac, WI 54935; tel. 920/922-7342; Mr. Dale Anderson

ManorCare Health Services – Green Bay, 600 South Webster Avenue, Green Bay, WI 54301; tel. 920/432-3213; D.J. Swant

Marian Catholic Center, 3333 West Highland Boulevard, Milwaukee, WI 53208; tel. 414/344-8100; Mr. Michael R Zimmerman

Marian Franciscan Center, 9632 West Appleton Avenue, Milwaukee, WI 53225; tel. 414/461-8850; Mr. James D Gresham

Northwest Health Care Center, 7800 West Fond Du Lac Avenue, Milwaukee, WI 53218-2603; tel. 414/464-3950; Mr. Mark Radmer

Outagamie County Health Center, 3400 West Brewster Street, Appleton, WI 54914-1699; tel. 920/832-5400; Mr. David A Rothmann

Parkview Manor Health and Rehabilitation Center, 2961 St. Anthony Drive, Green Bay, WI 54311; tel. 920/468-0861; Mr. Chris Orr

River Pines Center, 1800 Sherman Avenue, Stevens Point, WI 54481; tel. 715/344-1800; Ms. Sara Mahoney

Riverside Health and Rehabilitation, 101 First Street, Oconto, WI 54153; tel. 920/834-4575; Ms. Amy J Kurzynske

Shady Lane, 1235 South 24th Street, Manitowoc, WI 54220; tel. 414/682-8254; Ann Eisner

South Shore Manor, 1915 East Tripoli Avenue, Saint Francis, WI 53235; tel. 414/483-3611; Ms. Sue Blackwell

The Terrace at St. Francis, 3200 South 20th Street, Milwaukee, WI 53215; tel. 414/389-3200; Ms. Geri Wandrey

The Village at Manor Park, Inc, 3023 South 84th Street, West Allis, WI 53227–3798; tel. 414/607–4100; Mr. Reginald M Hislop, III

Western Village Health and Rehabilitation, 1640 Shawano Avenue, Green Bay, WI 54303; tel. 920/499–5177; Ms. Linda D Kessenich

Woodland Health Center, 18740 West Bluemound Road, Brookfield, WI 53045; tel. 414/782–0230; Ms. Margaret Christenson

WYOMING

Cheyenne Health Care Center, 2700 East 12th Street, Cheyenne, WY 82001; tel. 307/634–7986; Aletha Shawver

Poplar Living Center, 4305 Poplar Avenue, Casper, WY 82601; tel. 307/237–2561; Mr. Steven P Monroe

JCAHO Accredited Freestanding Mental Health Care Organizations

The accredited freestanding mental health care organizations listed have been accredited as of March, 2000 by the Joint Commission on Accreditation of Healthcare Organizations by decision of the Accreditation Committee of the Board of Commissioners.

The organizations listed here have been found to be in compliance with the Joint Commissions standards for Accreditation Manual for Mental Health, Chemical Dependency, and Mental Retardation/Development Disabilities Services.

Please refer to section A of the AHA Guide for information on hospitals with inpatient and/or outpatient services. These hospitals are identified by Facility Codes F57, F58, F59, F60, F61, F62, F63, and F64. In section A, those hospitals identified by Approval Code 1 are JCAHO accredited.

We present this list simply as a convenient directory. Inclusion or omission of any organization's name indicates neither approval nor disapproval by Health Forum LLC, an American Hospital Association company.

United States

ALABAMA
Alabama Clinical Schools, 1221 Alton Drive P.O. Box 100968, Birmingham, AL 35210; tel. 205/836–9923; Ms. Karen Downs
Behavioral Healthcare Center, 306 Paul W Bryant Drive East, Tuscaloosa, AL 35401; tel. 205/349–1033; Karima Nasrat
Bradford Health Services – Huntsville, 1600 Browns Ferry Road, Madison, AL 35758; tel. 256/461–7272; Mr. Robert S Hinds
Bradford Health Services – Warrior, PO Box 129, Warrior, AL 35180; tel. 205/647–1945; Mr. Roy M Ramsey
New Perspectives, 1000 Fairfax Park, Tuscaloosa, AL 35406; tel. 205/391–4738; Ms. Martha Hinkle
Pathway, Inc., PO Box 311206, Enterprise, AL 36331; tel. 334/894–5591; Mr. Norman G Hemp
Thomasville Mental Health Rehabilitation Center, PO Box 309, Thomasville, AL 36784; tel. 334/636–5421; Ms. Beatrice McLean

ALASKA
Akeela Treatment Services, Inc, 2805 Bering Street, Suite 4, Anchorage, AK 99503; tel. 907/561–5206; Mr. Robert P Galea
Alaska Children's Services Inc., 4600 Abbott Road, Anchorage, AK 99507–4314; tel. 907/346–2101; Mr. James E Maley
Alaska North Addictions Recovery Center, 4330 Bragaw Street, Anchorage, AK 99508; tel. 907/561–5537; Ms. Gloria O'Neill
Anchorage Charter North Counseling Center, 1650 South Bragaw, Anchorage, AK 99508; tel. 907/258–7575; Ms. Kathleen Cronen
Charter North Residential Treatment Center, 1650 South Bragaw, Anchorage, AK 99508; tel. 907/274–7313; Ms. Kathleen Cronen
Juneau Youth Services, Inc., PO Box 32839, Juneau, AK 99803; tel. 907/789–7610; Mr. Charles Bennett
Providence Adolescent Residential Treatment Program, 3400 East 20th, Anchorage, AK 99508; tel. 907/272–2148; Mr. Doug Bruce

ARIZONA
Arizona Baptist Children's Services, P O Box 39239, Phoenix, AZ 85069–9239; tel. 602/943–7760; P. David Jakes
Arizona's Children Association, PO Box 7277, Tucson, AZ 85725–7277; tel. 520/622–7611; Mr. Fred J Chaffee
Calvary Rehabilitation Center, 720 East Montebello Avenue, Phoenix, AZ 85014; tel. 602/279–1468; Mr. Jeffrey Shook
Chandler Valley Hope, PO Box 1839, Chandler, AZ 85244–1839; tel. 602/899–3335; Mr. Dennis Gilhousen
Community Behavioral Health Services, PO Box 790, Page, AZ 86040; tel. 520/645–5133; Mr. Thomas J Wright
Cottonwood de Tucson, 4110 West Sweetwater Drive, Tucson, AZ 85745; tel. 520/743–0411; Mr. Ronald B Welch
Devereux/Arizona – Richard L. Raskin Treatment Network, 11000 N. Scottsdale Road Suite 260, Scottsdale, AZ 85254; tel. 602/998–2920; Mr. Stephen A Vitali
La Paloma Family Services, Inc, PO Box 41565, Tucson, AZ 85717–1565; tel. 520/750–9667; Mr. David Bradley
META Services, Inc., 2701 N. 16th St., Suite 106, Phoenix, AZ 85006; tel. 602/650–1212; Mr. Eugene Johnson
Mingus Mountain Estate Residential Center, Inc., 10451 Palmeras Drive, Ste 105N, Sun City, AZ 85373–2052; tel. 602/780–1963; Dr. Pauline H Don Carlos
Parc Place, 5116 East Thomas Road, Phoenix, AZ 85018; tel. 602/840–4774; Mr. Gene Cavallo
PREHAB of Arizona, Inc., PO Drawer 5860, Mesa, AZ 85211–5860; tel. 602/969–4024; Mr. Michael T Hughes
PREHAB of Arizona, Inc., PO Drawer 5860, Mesa, AZ 85211–5860; tel. 602/969–4024; Mr. Michael T Hughes
Remuda Ranch Center for Anorexia and Bulimia, One East Apache Street, Wickenburg, AZ 85390; tel. 520/684–3913; Mr. Ward E Keller
Rosewood Ranch L.P., 36075 South Rincon Road, Wickenburg, AZ 85390; tel. 520/684–9594; Ms. Margaret Allen
Sierra Tucson,LLC, 39580 S. Lago del Oro Parkway, Tucson, AZ 85739; tel. 520/624–4000; Mr. Terry A Stephens
Southeastern Arizona Psychiatric Health Facility, PO Box 1296, Benson, AZ 85602; tel. 520/586–7737; Mr. Dana S Johnson
Superstition Mountain Mental Health Center, Inc., PO Box 3160, Apache Junction, AZ 85217; tel. 602/983–0065; Mr. Gary W Selvy
the EXCEL Group, 106 East First Street, Yuma, AZ 85364; tel. 520/329–8995; Mr. Michael P Puthoff
The Guidance Center, Inc., 2187 North Vickey Street, Flagstaff, AZ 86004; tel. 520/527–1899; Mr. J Michael Thompson
The Meadows, 1655 North Tegner, Wickenburg, AZ 85390; tel. 520/684–3926; Mr. James P Mellody
The New Foundation, P O Box 3828, Scottsdale, AZ 85257; tel. 602/945–3302; Mr. David S Hedgcock
Touchstone Community, Inc., 6153 West Olive Avenue Suite 1, Glendale, AZ 85302; tel. 602/930–8705; Mr. Timothy Dunst
Verde Valley Guidance Clinic, Inc., 600 South Willard Street, Cottonwood, AZ 86326; tel. 520/634–2236; Mr. Robert D Cartia
Vista Care Facility, 4120 East Ramsey Road, Hereford, AZ 85615; tel. 520/378–6466; Mr. Siamak Khadjenoury
Youth Development Institute, 1830 East Roosevelt Street, Phoenix, AZ 85006; tel. 602/254–0884; Mr. David J Cocoros

ARKANSAS
Birch Tree Communities, Inc., P.O. Box 1589, Benton, AR 72018–1589; tel. 501/315–3344; Mr. C.Tucker Steinmetz
Centers for Youth and Families, PO Box 251970, Little Rock, AR 72225–1970; tel. 501/666–8686; Doug Stadter
Community Counseling Services, Inc., PO Box 6399, Hot Springs National Park, AR 71902; tel. 501/624–7111; Dr. Donald G Martin
Delta Counseling Associates, Inc., PO Box 820, Monticello, AR 71657; tel. 870/367–9732; Mr. Patrick W Haynie
Habilitation Center, Inc., PO Box 727, Fordyce, AR 71742; tel. 870/352–8203; Mr. Barry Staggs
Ozark Counseling Services, Inc, PO Box 1776, Mountain Home, AR 72654–1776; tel. 870/425–7929; Mr. John C Greer
Ozark Guidance Center, Inc., PO Box 6430, Springdale, AR 72762–6430; tel. 501/750–2020; Dr. David L Williams
Timber Ridge Ranch NeuroRehabilitation Center, PO Box 90, Benton, AR 72015–0090; tel. 501/594–5211; Ms. Sharon Burleson
United Methodist Children's Home Inc., PO Box 4848, Little Rock, AR 72214–4848; tel. 501/661–0720; Rev. Robert A Regnier
University of Arkansas for Medical Sciences, 4301 West Markham Street, Mail Slot 554, Little Rock, AR 72205; tel. 501/686–5483; Dr. Frederick G Guggenheim
Youth Home, Inc., 20400 Colonel Glenn Road, Little Rock, AR 72210–5323; tel. 501/821–5500; Ms. Beth Cartwright

CALIFORNIA
A Touch of Care, Inc., 2231 South Carmelina Avenue, Los Angeles, CA 90064; tel. 310/473–6525; Mr. Richard B Cohen
Betty Ford Center, 39000 Bob Hope Drive, Rancho Mirage, CA 92270; tel. 760/773–4100; Mr. John T Schwarzlose
Broad Horizons, PO Box 1920, Ramona, CA 92065; tel. 760/789–7060; Ms. Celia Engelman
Cornerstone of Southern California, 13682 Yorba Street, Tustin, CA 92680; tel. 714/730–5399; Ms. Lynda Klinger
Creative Care, Inc., 18850 Devonshire Street, Northridge, CA 91324; tel. 818/363–5630; Dr. Morteza Khaleghi
Impact Drug and Alcohol Treatment Center, 1680 North Fair Oaks Avenue, Pasadena, CA 91103; tel. 818/798–0884; Mr. James M Stillwell
Kings View Center, 42675 Road 44, Reedley, CA 93654; tel. 559/638–2505; Mr. Mike Waters
Oak Grove Institute, 24275 Jefferson Avenue, Murrieta, CA 92562; tel. 909/677–5599; Dr. Thomas C Lester
R House, Inc., PO Box 2587, Santa Rosa, CA 95405; tel. 707/539–2948; Ms. Mimi G Donohue
S T E P S, 224 East Clara Street, Port Hueneme, CA 93041; tel. 805/488–6424; Mr. Charles D Morris
San Diego Center for Children, 3002 Armstrong Street, San Diego, CA 92111–5798; tel. 619/277–9550; Mr. Edwin Kofler
Sharp Vista Pacifica, 7989 Linda Vista Road, San Diego, CA 92111; tel. 858/576–1200; Dr. Daniel R Valentine
Solano Psychiatric Health Facility, PO Box 2866, Fairfield, CA 94533–0286; tel. 707/435–2130; Dr. Linda Reese
Spencer Recovery Centers, Inc., PO Box 118, Monrovia, CA 91017; tel. 949/376–3705; Mr. Christopher C Spencer
Tarzana Treatment Center, Inc., 18646 Oxnard Street, Tarzana, CA 91356; tel. 818/996–1051; Mr. Albert Senella
The Discovery Adolescent Program, 4136 Ann Arbor Road, Lakewood, CA 90712; tel. 562/425–6918; Dr. Craig M Brown
The Linden Center, 5750 Wilshire Blvd, Ste 535, Los Angeles, CA 90036; tel. 323/937–3999; Dr. Ronald E Ricker
The Sycamores, 210 S DeLacey Avenue, Ste 110, Pasadena, CA 91105–2006; tel. 626/395–7100; Mr. William P Martone
Twin Town Treatment Center, 10741 Los Alamitos Boulevard, Los Alamitos, CA 90720; tel. 562/594–8844; Mr. David Lisonbee
Vista Del Mar Child and Family Services, 3200 Motor Avenue, Los Angeles, CA 90034; tel. 310/836–1223; Mr. Gerald Zaslaw
Vista San Diego Center, 3003 Armstrong Street, San Diego, CA 92111; tel. 619/268–3343; Ms. Judith K Williams

Providers / JCAHO Accredited Freestanding Mental Health Care Organizations

Watts Health Foundation, Inc., 10300 South Compton Avenue, Los Angeles, CA 90002; tel. 323/564-4331; Dr. Clyde W Oden

COLORADO
Adolescent and Family Institute of Colorado, Inc., 10001 West 32nd Avenue, Wheat Ridge, CO 80033; tel. 303/238-1231; Dr. Eric Meyer
Colorado Boys Ranch, PO Box 681, La Junta, CO 81050; tel. 719/384-5981; Mr. Charles M Thompson
Forest Heights Lodge, PO Box 789, Evergreen, CO 80437-0789; tel. 303/674-6681; Ms. Linda Clefisch
Harmony Foundation, Inc., PO Box 1989, Estes Park, CO 80517; tel. 970/586-4491; Mr. Donald R Hays
Managed Adolescent Care, PC, 1025 Pennock, Suite 111, Fort Collins, CO 80524; tel. 970/495-8860; Mr. Ken Henschke
Parker Valley Hope, PO Box 670, Parker, CO 80134; tel. 303/841-7857; Mr. Dennis Gilhousen
Pikes Peak Mental Health Center Systems, Inc., 220 Ruskin Drive, Colorado Springs, CO 80910; tel. 719/572-6100; Mr. Charles J Vorwaller
Southern Colorado Healthcare System, Bldg 5, Room 139, 'C' Street, Fort Lyon, CO 81038; tel. 719/384-3136; Mr. Stuart C Collyer

CONNECTICUT
Capitol Region Mental Health Center, 500 Vine Street, Hartford, CT 06112; tel. 860/297-0903; Ms. Pat Rehmer
Community Mental Health Affiliates, Inc., 300 Main Street, Bristol, CT 06010; tel. 860/583-9954; Dr. Mark Muradian
Community Prevention and Addiction Services, Inc., 1491 West Main Street, Willimantic, CT 06226; tel. 860/456-3215; Ms. Leanne M Dillian
Cornerstone of Eagle Hill, Inc., 32 Alberts Hill Road, Sandy Hook, CT 06482; tel. 203/426-8085; Mr. Norman J Sokolow
Datahr Rehabilitation Institute, 135 Old State Road, Brookfield, CT 06804; tel. 203/775-4700; Mr. Thomas H Fanning
Datahr Rehabilitation Institute, 135 Old State Road, Brookfield, CT 06804; tel. 203/775-4700; Mr. Thomas H Fanning
Greater Bridgeport Community Mental Health Center, 1635 Central Avenue, Bridgeport, CT 06610; tel. 203/551-7449; Mr. James Pisciotta
Klingberg Family Centers, Inc., 370 Linwood Street, New Britain, CT 06052; tel. 860/224-9113; Ms. Rosemarie Burton
LMG Programs, Inc., 4 Elmcrest Terrace, Norwalk, CT 06850; tel. 203/325-1511; Mr. Robert Rimmer
North Central Counseling Services, Inc., 995 Day Hill Road, Windsor, CT 06095; tel. 860/253-5020; Ms. Heather M Gates
Perception Programs, Inc., PO Box 407, Willimantic, CT 06226; tel. 860/450-7122; M. Deborah Walsh
Reid Treatment Center, Inc., PO Box 1357, Avon, CT 06001-1357; tel. 203/673-6115; Mr. Mark Muradian
River Valley Services, PO Box 351, Middletown, CT 06457; tel. 860/262-5207; Mr. Howard Reid
Riverview Hospital for Children and Youth, PO Box 2797, Middletown, CT 06457; tel. 860/704-4090; Dr. Louis Ando
Rushford Center Inc., 1250 Silver Street, Middletown, CT 06457; tel. 860/346-0300; Mr. Jeffrey L Walter
Stonington Institute, 75 Swantown Hill Road, North Stonington, CT 06359; tel. 860/535-1010; Mr. Michael J Angelides
The Children's Center, Inc., 1400 Whitney Avenue, Hamden, CT 06517; tel. 203/248-2116; Mr. Anthony DelMastro
The Wellspring Foundation, Inc., 21 Arch Bridge Road, Bethlehem, CT 06751; tel. 203/266-7235; Dr. Richard E Beauvais
The Wheeler Clinic, 91 Northwest Drive, Plainville, CT 06062; tel. 860/793-3500; Dr. David Berkowitz
United Services, Inc., Post Office Box 839, Dayville, CT 06241; tel. 860/774-2020; Mr. Theodore L Ver Haagh
Vitam Center, Inc., 57 W Rocks Road, Norwalk, CT 06851-0730; tel. 203/846-2091; Dr. Leonard A Kenowitz

DELAWARE
Brandywine Counseling, Inc., 2713 Lancaster Avenue, Wilmington, DE 19805; tel. 302/656-2348; Ms. Sara T Allshouse
Connections Community Support Programs, Inc., 500 West 10th Street, Wilmington, DE 19801; tel. 302/984-3380; Ms. Catherine Devaney McKay
Delaware Guidance Services for Children and Youth, Inc., 1213 Delaware Avenue, Wilmington, DE 19806; tel. 302/652-3948; Mr. Bruce Kelsey
Open Door, Incorporated, 3301 Green Street, Claymont, DE 19703; tel. 302/798-9555; Mr. Albert Meyer
Silver Lake Treatment Consortium, 493 East Main Street, Middletown, DE 19709; tel. 302/378-5238; Dr. Thomas L Olson
SODAT – Delaware, Inc., 625 North Orange Street, Wilmington, DE 19801; tel. 302/656-4044; Mr. Thomas C Maloney
Terry Children's Psychiatric Center, 10 Central Avenue, New Castle, DE 19720; tel. 302/577-4270; Dr. Anita L Amurao

DISTRICT OF COLUMBIA
Devereux Children's Center of Washington, D.C., 3050 R Street, Northwest, Washington, DC 20007; tel. 202/282-1200; Mr. Andre Cooper
New York Avenue Presbyterian Church/McClendon Center, 1313 New York Avenue, NW, Washington, DC 20005; tel. 202/737-6191; Ms. Alice V Anderson

FLORIDA
45th Street Mental Health Center, Inc., 1041 45th Street, West Palm Beach, FL 33407; tel. 561/844-1233; Mr. Terry H Allen
Act Corporation, 1220 Willis Avenue, Daytona Beach, FL 32114; tel. 904/947-4270; Mr. J W Dreggors
Alcohol and Drug Abuse Services, 1211 Southeast Second Avenue, Fort Lauderdale, FL 33316; tel. 954/728-2704; Mr. Michael De Lucca
Alternate Family Care, Inc., 10001 W Oakland Park Blvd, Suite 302, Sunrise, FL 33351; tel. 954/746-5200; Dr. David Ferguson
Alternatives In Treatment, Inc., 7601 North Federal Highway, Suite 100B, Boca Raton, FL 33487; tel. 561/998-0866; Mr. Jacob Frydman
Apalachee Center for Human Services, Inc., PO Box 1782, Tallahassee, FL 32302; tel. 850/487-2930; Mr. Ronald P Kirkland
Bayview Center for Mental Health, Inc., 12550 Biscayne Blvd, Suite 919, North Miami, FL 33181; tel. 305/892-4646; Mr. Robert S Ward
Beachcomber Rehab, Inc., 4493 North Ocean Boulevard, Delray Beach, FL 33483; tel. 561/734-1818; Mr. James A Bryan
Behavioral Health Network of West Dade, 11924-32 SW 8th Street, Miami, FL 33184; tel. 305/227-6757; Mr. Nelson Salazar
Camelot Care Centers, Inc., 9160 Oakhurst Road Building One, Seminole, FL 33776; tel. 813/596-9960; Mr. James V Doramus
Charlotte Community Mental Health Services, Inc., 1700 Education Avenue, Punta Gorda, FL 33950; tel. 941/639-8300; Dr. Gerald N Ross
Charter Behavioral Health System of Manatee Palms, LP, 4480 51st Street, West, Bradenton, FL 34210; tel. 941/792-2222; Mr. James, Jr.
Citrus Health Network, Inc, 4175 West 20th Avenue, Hialeah, FL 33012; tel. 305/825-0300; Mr. Mario E Jardon
Coastal Recovery Centers, Inc., 3830 Bee Ridge Road, Sarasota, FL 34233; tel. 941/927-8900; Dr. Christine Cauffield
Creekside Retreat, Inc., 8889 Corporate Square Court, Jacksonville, FL 32216; tel. 904/725-7073; Dr. Joseph A Virzi
Daniel Memorial Hospital, Inc., 4203 Southpoint Blvd, Jacksonville, FL 32216; tel. 904/296-1055; Mr. James D Clark
David Lawrence Center, 6075 Golden Gate Parkway, Naples, FL 34116; tel. 941/455-1031; Mr. David C Schimmel
Devereux Florida Treatment Network, 5850 T. G. Lee Boulevard, Suite 400, Orlando, FL 32822; tel. 407/384-5950; Mr. Michael C Becker
Eckerd Alternative Treatment Program at E-How-Kee, 397 Culbreath Road, Brooksville, FL 34602; tel. 352/796-9493; Mr. Les R Smout
Fairwinds Treatment Center, 1569 S Fort Harrison Avenue, Clearwater, FL 34616; tel. 813/449-0300; Mr. Mazhar K Al-Abed
Florida Institute for Neurologic Rehabilitation, Inc, PO Box 1348, Wauchula, FL 33873-1348; tel. 800/697-5390; Mr. Anthony J Chioccarelli, Jr.
Focus Healthcare of Florida, 5960 Southwest 106th Avenue, Cooper City, FL 33328; tel. 954/680-2700; Mr. Frank Fanella
Green Cross Health Systems, Inc., 2645 Douglas Road, Suite 601, Miami, FL 33133; tel. 305/443-9990; Dr. Miguel A Nunez, Jr.
Gulf Coast Treatment Center, 1015 Mar Walt Drive, Fort Walton Beach, FL 32547; tel. 850/863-4160; Mr. Jeffrey M Kaplan
Hanley–Hazelden Center at St. Mary's, 5200 East Avenue, West Palm Beach, FL 33407; tel. 561/841-1000; Mr. Jerry Singleton
Homestead Behavioral Clinic, 447 Northeast 8th Street, Homestead, FL 33030; tel. 305/248-3488; Ms. Aidelyn Lopez
Hope Horizon Center, Inc., 7821 SW 24th Street, Suite 100, Miami, FL 33155; tel. 305/269-8550; Mr. Ramon Trabazo
Kendall Behavioral Healthcare Center, Inc., 13500 SW 88th Street, Ste 265, Miami, FL 33186; tel. 305/383-3713; Ms. Rita Martinez
La Amistad Behavioral Health Services, 1650 Park Avenue North, Maitland, FL 32751; tel. 407/647-0660; Ms. Leslie Mathes
Lakeside Alternatives, Inc., 434 West Kennedy Boulevard, Orlando, FL 32810; tel. 407/875-3700; Mr. Duane Zimmerman
Lakeview Center, Inc., 1221 West Lakeview Avenue, Pensacola, FL 32501; tel. 850/432-1222; Dr. Morris L Eaddy
Lifeskills of Boca Raton, Inc., 7301 W Palmetto Park Road, Suite 108B, Boca Raton, FL 33433; tel. 561/392-1199; Dr. Gregory Mavrides
LifeStream Behavioral Center, PO Box 491000, Leesburg, FL 34749-1000; tel. 352/360-6575; Mr. Jack H Hargrove, Jr.
Manatee Glens Corporation, PO Box 9478, Bradenton, FL 34206-9478; tel. 941/741-3111; Ms. Mary Ruiz
Marion–Citrus Mental Health Centers, Inc., P.O. Box 771929, Ocala, FL 34474-1929; tel. 352/873-6500; Mr. Russell Rasco
Mental Health Care, Inc. Main Center, 5707 North 22nd Street, Tampa, FL 33610; tel. 813/237-2244; Mr. Julian I Rice
Mental Health Resource Center, Inc., PO Box 19249, Jacksonville, FL 32245-9249; tel. 904/743-1883; Dr. Robert A Sommers
Meridian Behavioral Healthcare, Inc., PO Box 141750, Gainesville, FL 32614; tel. 352/374-5600; Dr. Douglas L Starr
Northside Mental Health Center, 12512 Bruce B. Downs Boulevard, Tampa, FL 33612-9209; tel. 813/977-8700; Ms. Marsha L Brown
Operation PAR, Inc., 6655 66th Street North, Pinellas Park, FL 33781; tel. 727/545-7564; Ms. Shirley Coletti
Pathways to Recovery, Inc., 13132 Barwick Road, Delray Beach, FL 33445; tel. 561/496-7532; Mr. Lew Hoechstetter
Peace River Center for Personal Development, Inc., 1745 Highway 17 South, Bartow, FL 33830; tel. 863/534-7020; Mr. Hubert (Bert) Lacey
Personal Enrichment through Mental Health Services, Inc., 11254 58th Street North, Pinellas Park, FL 33782; tel. 813/545-6477; Mr. Thomas C Wedekind
Renaissance Institute of Palm Beach, Inc., 7000 N Federal Hwy, 2nd Floor, Boca Raton, FL 33487; tel. 561/241-7977; Mr. Sidney Goodman
Safe Passage CMHC, 5046 Biscayne Boulevard, Miami, FL 33137; tel. 305/756-1519; Ms. Denise Ascencio
SandyPines Hospital, 11301 SE Tequesta Terrace, Tequesta, FL 33469; tel. 561/744-0211; Ms. Mary Szczepanski–Bohne'
South County Mental Health Center, Inc., 16158 South Military Trail, Delray Beach, FL 33484; tel. 561/637-1004; Mr. Joseph S Speicher
St. Francis Community Mental Health Center, Inc., 214 Southeast 13th Street, Fort Lauderdale, FL 33316; tel. 954/779-2880; Mr. John Goudie
Stewart–Marchman Center for Chemical Dependency, Inc., 3875 Tiger Bay Road, Daytona Beach, FL 32124; tel. 904/947-1300; Dr. Ernest D Cantley
Sunny Day CMHC, Inc., 4890 Northwest 7th Street, Miami, FL 33126; tel. 305/569-0707; Ms. Zoe Gonzalez
Tampa Bay Academy, 12012 Boyette Road, Riverview, FL 33569; tel. 813/677-6700; Mr. Edward C Hoefle
The Center for Alcohol and Drug Studies, Inc., 321 Northlake Blvd, Suite 214, North Palm Beach, FL 33408; tel. 561/848-1332; Mr. Donald K Mullaney
The Renfrew Center of Florida, Inc., 7700 Renfrew Lane, Coconut Creek, FL 33073; tel. 561/698-9222; Ms. Barbara Peterson
The Village South, Inc., 3180 Biscayne Boulevard, Miami, FL 33137; tel. 305/573-3784; Mr. Matthew Gissen
The Watershed, 3350 NW Boca Raton Boulevard, Suite A-28, Boca Raton, FL 33431; tel. 561/362-7116; Ms. Jackie Glass

Providers / JCAHO Accredited Freestanding Mental Health Care Organizations

The Willough at Naples, 9001 Tamiami Trail East, Naples, FL 34113; tel. 941/775-4500; Ms. Patricia Perfetto
Transitions Recovery Program, 1928 Northeast 154th Street, North Miami Beach, FL 33162; tel. 305/949-9001; Mr. Lee Barchan
Treatment Resources, Inc., 25 Northeast 167th Street, North Miami Beach, FL 33162; tel. 305/653-4944; Mr. Dale P Redlich
Turning Point of Tampa, 5439 Beaumont Center Blvd, Suite 1010, Tampa, FL 33634; tel. 813/882-3003; Ms. Robin Piper
Twelve Oaks, 2068 Healthcare Avenue, Navarre, FL 32566; tel. 850/939-1200; Ms. Candance Henderson
University Behavioral Health Center, 2500 Discovery Drive, Orlando, FL 32826; tel. 407/281-7000; Mr. David Beardsley
Wellness Resource Center, Inc., 660 Linton Boulevard, Ste 112, Delray Beach, FL 33444; tel. 561/278-8411; Ms. Michele Michael
Wynwood Community Mental Health, Inc., 3550 Biscayne Blvd, Suite 510, Miami, FL 33137; tel. 305/573-3052; Ms. Martha Porro

GEORGIA
Albany Area Community Service Board, PO Box 1988, Albany, GA 31701; tel. 912/430-4042; Dr. John C Burns, III
Albany Association for Retarded Citizens, PO Box 71026, Albany, GA 31708-1026; tel. 912/888-6852; Ms. Annette T Bowling
Behavioral Health Services of South Georgia, PO Box 3409 206 S. Patterson Street, Valdosta, GA 31604-3409; tel. 912/333-7095; Mr. W. David McCracken
Bridges Outpatient Center, Inc., 1209 Columbia Drive, Milledgeville, GA 31061; tel. 912/454-1727; Mr. James M Simmons
Brightmore Day Hospital, 115 Davis Road, Martinez, GA 30907; tel. 706/868-1735; Ms. Joy Beaird
Charter Behavioral Hlth System of Atlanta at Laurel Hgts, LL, 934 Briarcliff Road, Northeast, Atlanta, GA 30306; tel. 404/888-7860; Ms. Jewel W Norman
Cobb/Douglas Community Service Board, 361 North Marietta Parkway, Marietta, GA 30060; tel. 770/429-5000; Ms. Patricia A Redmond
Community Mental Health Center of East Central Georgia, 3421 Mike Padgett Highway, Augusta, GA 30906; tel. 706/771-4833; Mr. F. Campbell Peery
Community Service Board of Middle Georgia, 2121A Bellevue Road, Dublin, GA 31021-2998; tel. 912/272-1190; Ms. Patsy H Thomas
Decatur Seminole Service Center, 333 Airport Road, Bainbridge, GA 31717; tel. 912/246-6108; Mr. Ben H Strickland
DeKalb Community Service Board, PO Box 1648, Decatur, GA 30031; tel. 404/294-3836; Dr. R. Derril Gay
Devereux Georgia Treatment Network, PO Box 1688, Kennesaw, GA 30144-8688; tel. 770/427-0147; Ms. Elizabeth Chadwick
Fulton County Dept of Mental Health, Retardation/SA, 141 Pryor Street, SW, Ste 4035, Atlanta, GA 30303; tel. 404/730-0210; Wyeuca B Johnson
Gateway Community Service Board, 1609 Newcastle Street, Brunswick, GA 31520; tel. 912/267-0760; Ms. Susan Broome
Georgia Pines Community Service Board, PO Box 1659, Thomasville, GA 31799; tel. 912/225-4335; Mr. Robert H Jones, Jr.
Gracewood State School and Hospital, PO Box 1299, Gracewood, GA 3081211299; tel. 706/790-2030; Dr. Bruce D Callander
Green Oaks M. R. Service Center, PO Box 2677, Moultrie, GA 31776; tel. 912/891-7300; Mr. Lemuel (Zeke) J Cothern
Inner Harbour Hospitals, Ltd., 4685 Dorsett Shoals Road, Douglasville, GA 30135; tel. 770/942-2391; Mr. Ron Scroggy
LARC, Inc., 1646 East Park Avenue, Valdosta, GA 31602; tel. 912/244-8290; Mr. Lonnie Smith
McIntosh Trail MH/MR/SA Community Service Board, PO Box 1320, Griffin, GA 30224; tel. 770/358-8250; Ms. Cathy Johnson
Metro Atlanta Recovery Residences, Inc., 2801 Clearview Place, Doraville, GA 30340; tel. 770/457-1222; Mr. Douglas Brush
Mitchell-Baker Mental Retardation Service Center, 65 Industrial Boulevard, Camilla, GA 31730; tel. 912/336-7977; Mr. J Dale Goodman
Murphy - Harpst - Vashti, Inc., 740 Fletcher Street, Cedartown, GA 30125; tel. 770/748-1500; Ms. Joanne G Simmons
New Horizons Community Service Board, PO Box 5328, Columbus, GA 31906-0328; tel. 706/596-5581; Mr. Perry Alexander
Oconee Center, PO Box 1827, Milledgeville, GA 31061; tel. 912/445-4817; Mr. John W Prather
Ogeechee Behavioral Health Services, PO Box 1259, Swainsboro, GA 30401; tel. 912/289-2522; Mr. J. Frank Brantley
River Edge Behavioral Health Center, 175 Emery Highway, Macon, GA 31217; tel. 912/751-4586; Mr. Frank Fields
Schizophrenia Treatment and Rehabilitation, LLC, 208 Church Street, Decatur, GA 30030; tel. 404/377-9844; Ms. Jewel Norman
Skyland Trail, 2573 Skyland Trail, Northeast, Atlanta, GA 30319; tel. 404/248-0687; Ms. Elizabeth E Finnerty
Talbott Recovery Campus, 5448 Yorktowne Drive, Atlanta, GA 30349; tel. 770/994-0185; Mr. Benjamin H Underwood
Thomas Grady Service Center, PO Box 2507, Thomasville, GA 31799; tel. 912/225-4065; Ms. Marianne Ellis
Tidelands Community Service Board, PO Box 23407, Savannah, GA 31403-3407; tel. 912/651-2171; Mr. Malcolm D Strickler
Turning Point Hospital, PO Box 1177, Moultrie, GA 31768; tel. 912/985-4815; Mr. Ben Marion
Willingway Hospital, 311 Jones Mill Road, Statesboro, GA 30458; tel. 912/764-6236; Mr. Jimmy Mooney

IDAHO
Sun Behavioral System for Boise, 8050 Northview Street, Boise, ID 83704; tel. 208/327-0504; Mr. Gregory P Hassakis
Walker Center, 1120A Montana Street, Gooding, ID 83330; tel. 208/934-8461; Dr. Douglas Smith

ILLINOIS
Alexian Brothers Behavioral Health Resources, 901 Biesterfield Road Suite 400, Elk Grove Village, IL 60007; tel. 847/437-5500; Mr. T J Vaughan
Alexian Brothers Northwest Mental Health Center, 1606 Colonial Parkway, Inverness, IL 60067; tel. 847/952-7460; Denis Ferguson
Allendale Association, PO Box 1088, Lake Villa, IL 60046; tel. 847/356-2351; Ms. Mary Shahbazian
Alternative Behavior Treatment Centers, 27255 North Fairfield Road, Mundelein, IL 60060; tel. 847/487-9455; Ms. Robin McGinnis
Association House of Chicago, 1116 North Kedzie Ave, Chicago, IL 60651; tel. 773/772-7170; Ms. Harriet Sadauskas
Aunt Martha's Youth Service Center, Inc., 4343 Lincoln Highway, Ste 340, Matteson, IL 60443; tel. 708/747-2701; Mr. C. Gary Leofanti
Beacon Therapeutic Diagnostic and Treatment Center, 1912 West 103rd Street, Chicago, IL 60643; tel. 773/298-1243; Ms. Margaret M Morley
Ben Gordon Center, 12 Health Services Drive, De Kalb, IL 60115; tel. 815/756-4875; Mr. James W Graves
Center on Deafness, 3444 Dundee Road, Northbrook, IL 60062; tel. 847/559-0110; Mr. Robert Van Dyke
Champaign County Association for the Mentally Retarded, PO Box 92, Champaign, IL 61824; tel. 217/359-9204; Mr. Kenston Chism
Chestnut Health Systems, 1003 Martin Luther King Drive, Bloomington, IL 61701; tel. 309/827-6026; Mr. Russell J Hagen
Circle Family Care, 5002 West Madison Street, Chicago, IL 60644-4127; tel. 773/921-8100; Mr. Len Sharber
Coles County Mental Health Association, Inc., PO Box 1307, Mattoon, IL 61938; tel. 217/234-6405; Ms. Kathleen Roberts
Community Counseling Center of Northern Madison County, Inc., 2615 Edwards Street, Alton, IL 62002; tel. 618/462-4883; Ms. Debra Sloan
Community Counseling Center of the Fox Valley, Inc., 400 Mercy Lane, Aurora, IL 60506; tel. 630/897-0584; Ms. Elaine M Hegy
Community Counseling Centers of Chicago, 4740 North Clark Street, Chicago, IL 60640-4633; tel. 773/769-0205; Dr. Anthony A Kopera
Community Mental Health Center of Fulton & McDonough Countie, 229 Martin Avenue, Canton, IL 61520; tel. 309/647-1881; Ms. Debra Dix
Comprehensive Mental Health Center of St. Clair County, 3911 State Street, East Saint Louis, IL 62205; tel. 618/482-7330; Ms. Delores S Ray
Counseling Center of Lake View, 3225 North Sheffield Avenue, Chicago, IL 60657; tel. 773/549-5886; Mr. Norman J Groetzinger
DuPage County Health Dept./ Behavioral & Mental Health Ser, 111 North County Farm Road, Wheaton, IL 60187; tel. 630/682-7979; Mr. Leland Lewis
Family Service and Community Mental Health Center/McHenry, 5320 West Elm Street, Mc Henry, IL 60050; tel. 815/385-6400; Mr. Robert M Martens
Gateway Youth Care Foundation, 819 South Wabash, Suite 300, Chicago, IL 60605; tel. 312/663-1130; Mr. Michael Darcy
Grand Prairie Services, 17746 South Oak Park Avenue, Tinley Park, IL 60477; tel. 708/444-1012; Dr. Carolyn W Thompson
Heartland Human Services, PO Box 1047, Effingham, IL 62401; tel. 217/347-7179; Ms. Cheryl Compton
Heritage Behavioral Health Center, Inc., P.O. Box 710, Decatur, IL 62524-2820; tel. 217/362-6262; Mr. Grady L Wilkinson
Horizons Wellness Center, 970 South McHenry Avenue, Crystal Lake, IL 60014; tel. 815/477-8881; Ms. Linda D Simko
Human Service Center, PO Box 1346, Peoria, IL 61654-1346; tel. 309/671-8000; Mr. Michael G Kennedy
Inter Agency, Inc., 1610 West 89th Street, Chicago, IL 60620-4924; tel. 773/233-9083; Ms. Deborah Young
Interventions - Du Page Adolescent Center, 11 S 250 Route 83, Hinsdale, IL 60521; tel. 630/325-5050; Ms. Leslie Balonick
Interventions - Southwood, 5701 South Wood, Chicago, IL 60636; tel. 773/737-4600; Ms. Leslie Balonick
Interventions - Woodridge, 2221 64th Street, Woodridge, IL 60517; tel. 630/968-6477; Ms. Leslie Balonick
Interventions City Girls, 140 North Ashland Avenue, Chicago, IL 60607; tel. 312/433-7777; Ms. Leslie Balonick
Jane Addams, Inc., 1133 W Stephenson Str, Ste 401, Freeport, IL 61032; tel. 815/232-4183; Mr. Daniel E Neal
Janet Wattles Center, Inc., 526 West State Street, Rockford, IL 61101; tel. 815/968-9300; Mr. Frank H Ware
Josselyn Center for Mental Health, 405 Central Avenue, Northfield, IL 60093-3097; tel. 847/441-5600; Dr. John W Shustitzky
Lake County Health Department / Behavioral Health Services, 3012 Grand Avenue, Waukegan, IL 60085; tel. 847/360-6729; Mr. Dale W Galassie
Leyden Family Service and Mental Health Center, 10001 West Grand Avenue, Franklin Park, IL 60131; tel. 847/451-0330; Mr. Dennis P Vaccaro
McHenry County Youth Service Bureau, 101 South Jefferson Street, Woodstock, IL 60098; tel. 815/338-7360; Ms. Susan H Krause
McLean County Center for Human Services, Inc., 108 West Market Street, Bloomington, IL 61701; tel. 309/827-5351; Mr. Thomas Axley
Mental Health and Deafness Resources, Inc., 3444 Dundee Road, Northbrook, IL 60062; tel. 847/559-0110; Ms. Patricia A Scherer
North Central Behavioral Health Systems, Inc., PO Box 1488, La Salle, IL 61301; tel. 815/223-0160; Mr. Donald P Miskowiec
Perry County Counseling Center, Inc., 1016 S. Madison St. Suite A, Du Quoin, IL 62832; tel. 618/542-4357; Mr. John R Venskus
ProCare Centers, 1820 South 25th Avenue, Broadview, IL 60153; tel. 708/681-2324; Mr. J. Melvin Smith
Provena Behavioral Health, 1801 Fox Drive, Champaign, IL 61820; tel. 217/398-8080; Ms. Alexandria Lewis
RocVale Children's Home, 4450 North Rockton Avenue, Rockford, IL 61103; tel. 815/654-3050; Mr. Robert H Cook
Rosecrance on Alpine, 1505 North Alpine Road, Rockford, IL 61107; tel. 815/399-5351; Mr. Philip W Eaton
Rosecrance on Harrison, 3815 Harrison Avenue, Rockford, IL 61108; tel. 815/391-1000; Mr. Philip W Eaton
Sinnissippi Centers, Inc., 325 Illinois Route 2, Dixon, IL 61021; tel. 815/284-6611; Mr. James R Sarver
Sojourn House, Inc., 565 North Turner Avenue, Freeport, IL 61032; tel. 815/232-5121; Ms. Brenda J Bombard
Southeastern Illinois Counseling Centers, Inc., Drawer M, Olney, IL 62450; tel. 618/395-4306; Mr. Gary Robertson

Providers / JCAHO Accredited Freestanding Mental Health Care Organizations

Southern Illinois Regional Social Services, 604 East College, Suite 101, Carbondale, IL 62901; tel. 618/457–6703; Ms. Karen Frietag

Stepping Stones of Rockford, Inc., 706 North Main Street, Rockford, IL 61103; tel. 815/963–0683; Mr. Stephen Langley

Tazwood Center for Human Services, Inc., 1421 Valle Vista Boulevard, Pekin, IL 61554; tel. 309/347–5522; Mr. Robert J Moore

The Ecker Center for Mental Health, 1845 Grandstand Place, Elgin, IL 60123; tel. 847/695–0484; Mr. Daniel P Boehmer

The Kenneth W. Young Centers, 1001 Rohlwing Road, Elk Grove Village, IL 60007; tel. 847/524–8800; Mr. Mitchell Bruski

The South Suburban Council on Alcoholism and Substance Abuse, 1909 Cheker Square, East Hazel Crest, IL 60429; tel. 708/957–2854; Mr. Allen Sandusky

The Women's Treatment Center, 140 North Ashland Avenue, Chicago, IL 60607; tel. 312/850–0050; Dr. Jewell Oates

Triangle Center, 120 North 11th Street, Springfield, IL 62703–1002; tel. 217/544–9858; Mr. Stephen J Knox

White Oaks Companies of Illinois, 3400 New Leaf Lane, Peoria, IL 61614; tel. 309/692–6900; Dr. John F Gilligan

INDIANA

Adult and Child Mental Health Center, Inc., 8320 Madison Avenue, Indianapolis, IN 46227; tel. 317/882–5122; Mr. A Robert Dunbar

BehaviorCorp, 697 Pro–Med Lane, Carmel, IN 46032–5323; tel. 317/587–0500; Mr. Larry L Burch

Community Mental Health Center, Inc., 285 Bielby Road, Lawrenceburg, IN 47025; tel. 812/537–1302; Mr. Joseph D Stephens

Comprehensive Mental Health Services, Inc., 240 North Tillotson Avenue, Muncie, IN 47304; tel. 765/288–1928; Dr. Suzanne Gresham

Evansville Psychiatric Children's Center, 3300 East Morgan Avenue, Evansville, IN 47715; tel. 812/477–6436; Mr. Tom Andis

Fairbanks Hospital, Inc., 8102 Clearvista Parkway, Indianapolis, IN 46256–4698; tel. 317/849–8222; Ms. Barbara Porter-Norris

Four County Counseling Center, 1015 Michigan Avenue, Logansport, IN 46947; tel. 219/722–5151; Mr. Laurence R Ulrich

Grant–Blackford Mental Health, Inc., 505 Wabash Avenue, Marion, IN 46952; tel. 765/662–3971; Mr. Paul G Kuczora

Hamilton Center, Inc, PO Box 4323, Terre Haute, IN 47804–0323; tel. 812/231–8271; Mr. Galen Goode

LaVerna Lodge, Inc., 1950 East Greyhound Pass, Suite 18, PMB 349, Carmel, IN 46033; tel. 317/867–4330; Mr. Martin Berg

LifeSpring Mental Health Services, 207 West 13th Street, Jeffersonville, IN 47130; tel. 812/283–4491; Mr. George E Hill

Madison Center, Inc., PO Box 80, South Bend, IN 46617; tel. 219/234–0061; Mr. Jack Roberts

Oaklawn, PO Box 809, Goshen, IN 46527–0809; tel. 219/537–2635; Mr. Harold C Loewen

Park Center, Inc., 909 East State Boulevard, Fort Wayne, IN 46805; tel. 219/481–2721; Mr. Paul D Wilson

Porter–Starke Services, Inc., 601 Wall Street, Valparaiso, IN 46383; tel. 219/531–3500; Mr. Lee E Grogg

Quinco Behavioral Health Systems, PO Box 628, Columbus, IN 47202–0628; tel. 888/348–7449; Dr. Robert J Williams

R.T.C. Resource, Inc., 1404 South State, Indianapolis, IN 46203; tel. 317/783–4003; Ms. Michelle Vetter

Sharing and Caring Community Mental Health Center, Inc., 2511 East 46th Street, Ste 0–1, Indianapolis, IN 46205; tel. 317/377–5300; Ms. Debra Henderson

South Central Community Mental Health Centers, Inc., 645 South Rogers Street, Bloomington, IN 47403; tel. 812/339–1691; Dr. Dennis Morrison

Southlake Center for Mental Health, 8555 Taft Street, Merrillville, IN 46410–6199; tel. 219/769–4005; Mr. Lee Strawhun

Southwestern Indiana Mental Health Center, Inc., 415 Mulberry Street, Evansville, IN 47713–1298; tel. 812/423–7791; Mr. John K Browning

Swanson Center, 450 St. John Road, Suite 501, Michigan City, IN 46360–7350; tel. 219/879–4621; Mr. Larry D Miller

Tara Treatment Center, Inc., 6231 South US 31, Franklin, IN 46131; tel. 812/526–2611; Ms. Ann Daugherty

The Center for Mental Health, Inc., PO Box 1258, Anderson, IN 46015; tel. 765/649–8161; Mr. C. Richard DeHaven

The Children's Campus, Inc., 1411 Lincoln Way West, Mishawaka, IN 46544–1690; tel. 219/259–5666; Ms. Sylvia Sebert

The Midwest Center for Youth and Families, PO Box 669, Kouts, IN 46347; tel. 219/766–2999; Ms. Jeanne Walsh

The Otis R. Bowen Center for Human Services, Inc., PO Box 497, Warsaw, IN 46581–0497; tel. 219/267–7169; Mr. Kurt Carlson

Tri–City Comprehensive Comm Mental Health Center Inc., 3903 Indianapolis Boulevard, East Chicago, IN 46312; tel. 219/398–7050; Mr. Robert Krumwied

Universal Behavioral Services CMHC of Lake County, 8500 Broadway, Suite H, Merrillville, IN 46410; tel. 219/736–5963; Ms. Cassandra Hall

Universal Behavioral Services Community Mental Health Center, 820 Fort Wayne Avenue, Indianapolis, IN 46204; tel. 317/684–0442; Ms. Rosa L Brown

Wabash Valley Hospital, Inc., 2900 North River Road, West Lafayette, IN 47906; tel. 765/463–2555; Mr. R. Craig Lysinger

IOWA

Boys and Girls Home and Family Services, Inc., PO Box 1197, Sioux City, IA 51104; tel. 712/293–4700; Mr. Robert P Sheehan

Children and Families of Iowa, 1111 University Avenue, Des Moines, IA 50314; tel. 515/288–1981; Mr. David Stout

Christian Home Association – Children's Square U.S.A., PO Box 8–C, Council Bluffs, IA 51502–3008; tel. 712/322–3700; Ms. Carol D Wood

Four Oaks, Inc. of Iowa, Psych Medical Instit. for Children, 5400 Kirkwood Boulevard, Southwest, Cedar Rapids, IA 52404; tel. 319/364–0259; Mr. James A Ernst

Gerard, PO Box 1353, Mason City, IA 50402; tel. 515/423–3222; Ms. Rita Paxson

Gordon Recovery Centers, Inc., 800 5th Street Suite 200, Sioux City, IA 51101; tel. 712/234–2300; Mr. Kermit A Dahlen

Hillcrest Family Services, PO Box 1160, Dubuque, IA 52001; tel. 319/583–7357; Mr. Gary L Gansemer

Orchard Place – Child Guidance Center, 925 Southwest Porter Drive, Des Moines, IA 50315–0304; tel. 515/285–6781; Dr. Earl P Kelly

Tanager Place, 2309 C Street Southwest, Cedar Rapids, IA 52404–3707; tel. 319/365–9164; Mr. George Estle

KANSAS

Atchison Valley Hope, PO Box 312, Atchison, KS 66002; tel. 913/367–1618; Mr. Dennis Gilhousen

Catholic Community Services, Inc., 2220 Central Avenue, Kansas City, KS 66102–4797; tel. 913/621–5090; Mr. Mark Henke

Columbia Health Systems, Inc., 10114 West 105th Street, Suite 100, Overland Park, KS 66212; tel. 913/492–9876; Mr. Robert Reed

Jewish Family and Children Services, 5801 West 115th, Suite 103, Overland Park, KS 66211; tel. 913/327–8250; Dr. Todd Ephraim

Kaw Valley Center, Inc., 4300 Brenner Drive, Kansas City, KS 66104; tel. 913/334–0294; Mr. B. Wayne Sims

Norton Valley Hope, PO Box 510, Norton, KS 67654; tel. 785/877–5101; Mr. Dennis Gilhousen

Parkview Hospital of Topeka, 3707 Southwest 6th Avenue, Topeka, KS 66606–2085; tel. 785/295–4014; Ms. Joyce E Nuss

Parkview Passages Residential Treatment Center, 3707 Southwest 6th Avenue, Topeka, KS 66606–2085; tel. 785/295–4014; Ms. Joyce Nuss

The Saint Francis Academy, Incorporated, 509 East Elm Street, Salina, KS 67401; tel. 785/825–0541; Rev. Canon Phillip J Rapp

The Saint Francis Academy, Incorporated, Lake Placid, 509 East Elm Street, Salina, KS 67401; tel. 518–523–1718; Rev. Canon Phillip J Rapp

The Wichita Children's Home, 810 North Holyoke, Wichita, KS 67208; tel. 316/684–6581; Ms. Sarah Robinson

United Methodist Youthville, Inc., PO Box 210, Newton, KS 67114; tel. 316/283–1950; Mr. Robert D Smith

KENTUCKY

Adanta Behavioral Health Services, 259 Parkers Mill Road, Somerset, KY 42501; tel. 606/679–4782; Ms. Cathy Epperson

Bluegrass Regional Mental Health – Mental Retardation Bd, PO Box 11428, Lexington, KY 40575; tel. 606/253–1686; Mr. Joseph A Toy

Brooklawn, Inc., 2125 Goldsmith Lane, Louisville, KY 40218–1206; tel. 502/451–5177; Mr. David A Graves

Central State ICF/MR, 10510 LaGrange Road, Louisville, KY 40223; tel. 502/253–7311; Ms. T. Richelle Jones

Christian Church Homes Children's and Family Services, PO Box 45, Danville, KY 40422–0045; tel. 606/236–5507; Ms. Kathy Miles

Cumberland River Regional MH/MR Board, Inc., PO Box 568, Corbin, KY 40702; tel. 606/528–7010; Mr. Danny Jones

Kentucky Baptist Homes for Children, Inc., 10801 Shelbyville Road, Louisville, KY 40243; tel. 502/245–2101; Dr. William K Smithwick

NorthKey Community Care, PO Box 2680, Covington, KY 41012; tel. 606/578–3252; Dr. Edward G Muntel

Presbyterian Child Welfare Agency, 116 Buckhorn Lane, Buckhorn, KY 41721; tel. 606/398–7000; Mr. Charles L Baker

RiverValley Behavioral Health, PO Box 1637, Owensboro, KY 42302–1637; tel. 270/689–6500; Ms. Gayle DiCesare

Seven Counties Services, Inc., 101 W Muhammad Ali Boulevard, Louisville, KY 40202; tel. 502/589–8600; Dr. Howard F Bracco

Spectrum Care Academy, Inc., PO Box 911, Columbia, KY 42728; tel. 502/384–6444; Mr. Tony C Harvey

The Home of the Innocents, Inc, 485 East Gray Street, Louisville, KY 40202; tel. 502/561–6600; Mr. Gordon S Brown

The Kentucky United Methodist Homes for Children and Youth, PO Box 749, Versailles, KY 40383; tel. 606/873–4481; Dr. Don E Rankin

LOUISIANA

Acadiana Day Treatment, Inc., 604 Highway 3043, Opelousas, LA 70570; tel. 318/942–8088; Ms. Gwen Bertrand

Addiction Recovery Resources of New Orleans, 4836 Wabash Street, Suite 202, Metairie, LA 70001; tel. 504/837–9988; Mr. Franklin D Polk

CHARIS Community Mental Health Center, Inc., 8264 One Calais Avenue, Baton Rouge, LA 70809; tel. 504/767–8478; Ms. Carolyn Carroll

Crescent Community Care, Inc. dba Center for Better Living, 951 Gause Boulevard Suite 2, Slidell, LA 70458; tel. 504/641–0505; Eric Oleson

Hope Haven Center, 1101 Barataria Boulevard, Marrero, LA 70072; tel. 504/347–5581; Mr. Robert J Guasco

Jennings Behavioral Health, 1712 Johnson Street, Jennings, LA 70546; tel. 318/824–4300; Ms. Tehjan Martin

LA United Methodist Children and Family Services, Inc., PO Box 929, Ruston, LA 71273–0929; tel. 318/255–5020; Mr. Terrel J DeVille

New Beginnings Of Opelousas Inc., 1692 Linwood Loop, Opelousas, LA 70570; tel. 318/942–1171; Mr. Kim Signorelli

Southwest Ambulatory Behavioral Services, Inc., 112 East Hutchinson Avenue, Crowley, LA 70526; tel. 318/788–3600; Mr. Ernie P Broussard

St. Patrick's Psychiatric Hospital, PO Box 1901, Monroe, LA 71201–1901; tel. 318/327–4370; Ms. Cindy J Rogers

Vermilion Hospital for Psychiatric and Addictive Med, 2520 North University Avenue, Lafayette, LA 70507; tel. 318/234–5614; Mr. William A Ferry

MAINE

Community Health and Counseling Services, PO Box 425, Bangor, ME 04402–0425; tel. 207/947–0366; Mr. Joseph H Pickering, Jr.

KidsPeace National Ctrs for Kids in Crisis New England,Inc, PO Box 787, Ellsworth, ME 04605; tel. 207/667–0909; Mr. George W Russell, III

MARYLAND

Allegany County Health Department Addictions Program, PO Box 1745, Cumberland, MD 21501–1745; tel. 301/777–5680; Mr. Rodger D Simons

Ashley, Inc., PO Box 240, Havre de Grace, MD 21078; tel. 410/273–6600; Mr. Leonard Angus Dahl

Baltimore Behavioral Health, Inc., 200 South Arlington Avenue, Baltimore, MD 21223; tel. 410/962–7180; Ms. Sandra K Hill

Providers / JCAHO Accredited Freestanding Mental Health Care Organizations

Charter Behavioral Health Systems at Warwick Manor, 3680 Warwick Road, East New Market, MD 21631; tel. 410/943-8108; Mr. A. Jay Rimovsky
Chesapeake Youth Center, Inc., PO Box 1238, Cambridge, MD 21613; tel. 410/221-0288; Mr. David Ennis
Crossroads Centers, Inc., 2 West Madison Street, Baltimore, MD 21201; tel. 410/752-6505; Ms. Barbara Q McKenna
Edgemeade, 13400 Edgemeade Road, Upper Marlboro, MD 20772; tel. 301/888-1330; Dr. James A Filipczak
Glass Substance Abuse Program, Inc., 821 N Eutaw Street, Suite 201, Baltimore, MD 21201; tel. 410/225-9185; Mr. Herman Jones
Good Shepherd Center, 4100 Maple Avenue, Baltimore, MD 21227; tel. 410/247-2770; Sister Mary Rosaria Baxter
Hope House, PO Box 546, Crownsville, MD 21032; tel. 410/923-6700; Ms. Ruth A Hudicek
Hudson Health Services, Inc., PO Box 1096, Salisbury, MD 21802-1096; tel. 410/219-9000; Mr. Charles F Andrews
Jewish Family Services, Inc., 5750 Park Heights Avenue, Baltimore, MD 21215; tel. 410/466-9200; Mr. Steve M Solomon
Maple Shade Youth & Family Services, 23704 Ocean Gateway, Mardela Springs, MD 21837; tel. 410/742-7400; Mr. Gary Frye
Maryland Treatment Centers, Inc., PO Box E, Emmitsburg, MD 21727; tel. 301/447-2361; Ms. Mary A Roby
New Life Addiction Counseling Services, Inc., 2528 Mountain Road, Suite 204, Pasadena, MD 21122; tel. 410/255-4475; Mr. Thomas S Porter
Oakview Treatment Center, 3635 Old Court Road, Suite 203, Pikesville, MD 21208-3906; tel. 410/461-9922; Mr. Ned Rubin
Partners in Recovery, 6509 North Charles Street, Baltimore, MD 21204; tel. 410/296-9747; Mr. Robert P Kowal
Pathways, 2620 Riva Road, Annapolis, MD 21401; tel. 410/573-5400; Ms. Martha Pitzer
Quarterway Houses, Inc., PO Box 31419, Baltimore, MD 21216-6119; tel. 410/233-0684; Dr. John E Hickey
Regional Institute for Children and Adolescents, 15000 Broschart Road, Rockville, MD 20850; tel. 301/251-6800; Mr. John L Gildner
Regional Institute for Children and Adolescents, 605 South Chapel Gate Lane, Baltimore, MD 21229-3999; tel. 410/368-7800; Ms. Penny Makris
RICA – Southern Maryland, 9400 Surratts Road, Cheltenham, MD 20623; tel. 301/372-1800; Ms. Audrey B Chase
Saint Luke Institute, Inc., 8901 New Hampshire Avenue, Silver Spring, MD 20903; tel. 301/445-7970; Mr. Stephen J Rossetti
Villa Maria, 2300 Dulaney Valley Road, Timonium, MD 21093-2799; tel. 410/252-4700; Mr. Mark Greenberg
Woodbourne Center, Inc., 1301 Woodbourne Avenue, Baltimore, MD 21239; tel. 410/433-1000; Dr. John Hodge-Williams
Worcester County Health Department, PO Box 249, Snow Hill, MD 21863; tel. 410/632-1100; Ms. Deborah Goeller

MASSACHUSETTS
AdCare Hospital of Worcester, Inc., 107 Lincoln Street, Worcester, MA 01605-2499; tel. 508/799-9000; Mr. David W Hillis
Baldpate Hospital, Baldpate Road, Georgetown, MA 01833; tel. 978/352-2131; Ms. Lucille Batal
Brighton Center for Children and Families, 77 Warren Street, Building 4, Brighton, MA 02135; tel. 617/787-4884; Ms. Julie Heuberger
Brockton Multi Service Center, 165 Quincy Street, Brockton, MA 02402; tel. 508/897-2000; Mr. Daniel K Amigone
Cape Cod Alcoholism Intervention & Rehabilitation, PO Box 929, Falmouth, MA 02541; tel. 508/540-6550; Mr. Raymond V Tamasi
Cape Cod and Islands Community Mental Health Center, 259 North Street, Hyannis, MA 02601; tel. 508/775-1199; Mr. Richard W Dunnells
Center for Health and Human Services, Inc., PO Box 2097, New Bedford, MA 02745; tel. 508/995-5733; Ms. Jennifer Davis
Centerpoint, PO Box 374, Tewksbury, MA 01876; tel. 978/858-3776; Ms. Carolyn F Ingalls
Chauncy Hall Academy, PO Box 732, Westborough, MA 01581; tel. 508/898-3280; Mr. Steven R Hahn
Doctor Franklin Perkins School, 971 Main Street, Lancaster, MA 01523; tel. 978/368-6423; Dr. Charles P Conroy
Dr. John C. Corrigan Mental Health Center, 49 Hillside Street, Fall River, MA 02720; tel. 508/678-2901; Ms. Elaine M Hill
Dr. Solomon Carter Fuller Mental Health Center, 85 East Newton Street, Boston, MA 02118-2337; tel. 617/626-8860; Dr. Jean Wilkinson
Erich Lindemann Mental Health Center, 25 Staniford Street, Boston, MA 02114; tel. 617/626-8510; Ms. Carla M Saccone
Fuller Intensive Residential Treatment Program, 85 East Newton Street, 6 East, Boston, MA 02118; tel. 617/536-1227; Mr. Kenneth Davis
High Point Treatment Center, Inc., 1233 State Road, Plymouth, MA 02360-5133; tel. 508/224-7701; Mr. Daniel S Mumbauer
Intensive Treatment Unit at Hillcrest Educational Centers, PO Box 4699, Pittsfield, MA 01202-4699; tel. 413/499-7924; Mr. Gerard E Burke
Lake Grove at Maple Valley, Inc., PO Box 767, Wendell, MA 01379; tel. 978/544-6913; Mr. Roland Paulauskas
Meadowridge Behavioral Health Center, 664 Stevens Road, Swansea, MA 02777; tel. 508/676-8740; Ms. Stephanie Ward
Quincy Mental Health Center, 460 Quincy Avenue, Quincy, MA 02169; tel. 617/626-9000; Ms. Christina Browne
Spectrum Health Systems, Inc., 100 Locke Drive, Marlborough, MA 01752; tel. 508/303-6878; Mr. Charles Faris
The Grove Adolescent Treatment Center, 272 Grove Street, Northampton, MA 01060; tel. 413/586-6210; Mr. Hal Gibber
The Home for Little Wanderers Intensive Residential Treatme, 60 Hodges Avenue – Goss 3, Taunton, MA 02780; tel. 508/824-7575; Dr. Steven Feinberg
The May Institute, Inc., PO Box 899, South Harwich, MA 02661; tel. 508/432-5530; Dr. Walter P Christian
The Three Rivers Treatment Program, 26 Ridgewood Terrace, Springfield, MA 01105; tel. 413/733-4032; Mr. Carl B Cutchins
The Whitney Academy, Inc., PO Box 619, East Freetown, MA 02717; tel. 508/763-3737; Mr. George E Harmon
University of Massachusetts Medical School, TIRTP, 305 Belmont Street, 7th Flr C, Worcester, MA 01604; tel. 508/856-1455; Dr. Aaron Lazare
Wild Acre Inns, Inc., PO Box 9112, Arlington, MA 02174; tel. 781/643-0643; Dr. Bernard S Yudowitz

MICHIGAN
ACAC, Inc., 3949 Sparks Drive SE, Ste 103, Grand Rapids, MI 49546; tel. 616/957-5850; Mr. Michael R Durco
Advanced Counseling Services, P.C., 30700 Telegraph Rd. Ste 2560, Bingham Farms, MI 48025; tel. 248/203-1770; Dr. Arthur L Hughett
Antrim Kalkaska Community Mental Health, PO Box 220, Bellaire, MI 49615-0220; tel. 731/533-8619; Mr. Ross L Gibson
Auro Medical Center, 1711 South Woodward, Suite 102, Bloomfield Hills, MI 48302; tel. 248/335-1130; Ms. Sue Comer
Bay-Arenac Community Mental Health, 201 Mulholland, Bay City, MI 48708; tel. 517/895-2239; William B Cammin
Beaumont Orchard Hills Behavioral Medicine Center, 30301 Woodward Avenue, Ste 200, Royal Oak, MI 48073; tel. 248/288-9922; Dr. Hiten Patel
Berrien Mental Health Authority, P.O. Box 547, Benton Harbor, MI 49023; tel. 616/927-6065; Mr. Allen R Edlefson
Boniface Human Services, 25050 W Outer Drive, Suite 201, Lincoln Park, MI 48146; tel. 313/928-8940; Dr. Shara Johnson
Brighton Hospital, 12851 East Grand River, Brighton, MI 48116; tel. 810/227-1211; Mr. Ramon Royal
Catholic Services of Macomb, Inc., 15980 19 Mile Road, Clinton Township, MI 48038; tel. 810/416-2300; Mr. Thomas J Reed
Center For Behavior and Medicine, 2004 Hogback Road, Suite 16, Ann Arbor, MI 48105; tel. 313/677-0809; Dr. Gerard M Schmit
Center for Life Management, In, 3800 Woodward Avenue Suite 208, Detroit, MI 48201; tel. 313/831-1533; Ms. Wendie D Lee
Center of Behavioral Therapy, PC, 24453 Grand River Avenue, Detroit, MI 48219; tel. 313/592-1765; Mr. Hollis M Evans
Central Michigan Community Mental Health Services, 301 South Crapo, Suite 100, Mount Pleasant, MI 48858; tel. 517/773-6961; Mr. George Rouman
Central Therapeutic Services, Inc., 17600 W Eight Mile Road, Ste 7, Southfield, MI 48075; tel. 248/559-4340; Dr. K. G Thimotheose
Children's Home of Detroit, 900 Cook Road, Grosse Pointe Woods, MI 48236; tel. 313/886-0800; Mr. Michael R Horwitz
CHIP Counseling Center, 6777 U.S. 31 South, Charlevoix, MI 49720; tel. 231/547-6551; Mr. Scott L Hickman
City of Detroit Dept of Human Services/Drug Treatment Div, 5031 Grandy, Detroit, MI 48211; tel. 313/267-6695; Mr. William Warren
Clinton – Eaton – Ingham Community Mental Health Board, 808 Southland, Suite B, Lansing, MI 48910; tel. 517/346-8246; Mr. Robert Sheehan
Community Care Services, 26184 West Outer Drive, Lincoln Park, MI 48146; tel. 313/389-7525; Mr. William P Walsh
Community Mental Health Services of Muskegon County, 376 Apple Avenue, Muskegon, MI 49442; tel. 231/724-1111; Mr. James Borushko
Community Mental Health Services of St. Joseph County, 210 South Main Street, Three Rivers, MI 49093; tel. 616/273-5000; Ms. Kristine Kirsch
Comprehensive Psychiatric Services, PC, 28800 Orchard Lake Rd, Ste 250, Farmington Hills, MI 48334; tel. 248/932-2500; Toby Hazan
Comprehensive Services, Inc., 4630 Oakman Boulevard, Detroit, MI 48204; tel. 313/934-8400; Ms. Mary L Doss
Cruz Clinic, 17177 North Laurel Park Drive, Suite 131, Livonia, MI 48152; tel. 734/462-3210; Ms. Suzanne M Willmott
DBA Spectrum Prevention & Treatment Services, 2301 Platt Road, Ann Arbor, MI 48104; tel. 734/971-7900; Susan Custer
Delta Family Clinic, 2303 East Amelith Road, Bay City, MI 48706; tel. 517/684-9313; Mr. Gary R West
Desgranges Psychiatric Center, PC, G 8145 South Saginaw Street, Grand Blanc, MI 48439; tel. 810/694-2730; Dr. Louise Desgranges
Detroit Central City Community Mental Health, Inc., 10 Peterboro, Suite 208, Detroit, MI 48201; tel. 313/831-3160; Ms. Irva Faber-Bermudez
DOT Caring Centers, Inc., 3190 Hallmark Court, Saginaw, MI 48603-2107; tel. 517/790-3366; Mr. Christopher Zalba
Downriver Guidance Clinic, 13101 Allen Road, Southgate, MI 48195; tel. 734/287-1700; Mr. Leroy A Lott
Evergreen Counseling Centers, 6902 Chicago Road, Warren, MI 48092; tel. 810/268-4239; Mr. Donald L Warner
Fairlane Behavioral Services, 23400 Michigan Avenue, Ste P24, Dearborn, MI 48124; tel. 313/562-6730; Mr. Carlos P Ruiz
Gateway Services, 1910 Shaffer Road, Kalamazoo, MI 49001; tel. 616/382-9827; Ms. Lisa Martin
Gerontology Network, 4695 Danvers Southeast, Ste B, Grand Rapids, MI 49512; tel. 616/977-3300; Dr. Thomas A Hartwig
Growth Works Incorporated, PO Box 6115, Plymouth, MI 48170-0115; tel. 734/455-4095; Mr. Dale F Yagiela
Guest House for Women Religious, PO Box 420, Lake Orion, MI 48361; tel. 248/391-3100; Mr. Daniel Kidd
Hegira Programs, Inc., 8623 N Wayne Road, Suite 200, Westland, MI 48185; tel. 734/458-4601; Mr. Edward L Forry
Huron Valley Consultation Center, 955 W Eisenhower Circle, Ste B, Ann Arbor, MI 48103; tel. 734/662-6300; Dr. Joseph Meadows
Ionia County Community Mental Health, 5827 North Orleans Road, Orleans, MI 48865-0155; tel. 616/761-3151; Ms. Cheryl Bass
Jensen Counseling Centers, PC, 26105 Orchard Lake Rd, Ste 301, Farmington Hills, MI 48334; tel. 248/478-4411; Dr. Mary Robin Peters
Kairos Healthcare, Inc., 141 Harrow Lane, Saginaw, MI 48603; tel. 517/792-4357; Mr. Frederick E Wigen, Jr.
Lapeer County Community Mental Health Center, 1570 Suncrest Drive, Lapeer, MI 48446-1154; tel. 810/667-0500; Dr. Richard I Berman
Lapeer County Health Departmen, 1575 Suncrest Drive, Lapeer, MI 48446; tel. 810/667-0243; Mr. John D Niederhauser
Latino Family Services, Inc., 3815 West Fort Street, Detroit, MI 48216; tel. 313/841-7380; Ms. Amanda Caballero

Providers / JCAHO Accredited Freestanding Mental Health Care Organizations

London Brook Associates, PLC, 26677 West Twelve Mile Road, Suite 146, Southfield, MI 48034; tel. 248/391-0050; Ms. Debra Scheck
Macomb Child Guidance Clinic, Inc., 40600 Van Dyke, Suite 9, Sterling Heights, MI 48313; tel. 810/978-2476; Ms. Elizabeth Boyce
Meridian Professional Psychological Consultants, PC, 5031 Park Lake Road, East Lansing, MI 48823; tel. 517/332-0811; Dr. Thomas S Gunnings
Metro East Substance Abuse Treatment Corporation, PO Box 13408, Detroit, MI 48213; tel. 313/371-0055; Ms. Leslie B Carroll
Michiana Addictions and Prevention Services, 1020 Millard Street, Three Rivers, MI 49093-1658; tel. 616/279-5187; Ms. Sally Reames
Michigan Counseling Services, 1400 East 12 Mile Road, Madison Heights, MI 48071; tel. 248/547-2223; Mr. Anthony C Clemente
Nardin Park Recovery Center, Inc., PO Box 04506, Detroit, MI 48204; tel. 313/834-5930; Ms. Annie B Scott
National Council on Alcoholism / Lansing Regional Area, Inc., 3400 S Cedar Street, Suite 200, Lansing, MI 48910; tel. 517/887-0226; Ms. Nancy L Siegrist
National Council on Alcoholism and Addictions, 202 E Boulevard Drive, Ste 310, Flint, MI 48503; tel. 810/767-0350; Ms. Rebecca Jagos
National Council on Alcoholism and Drug Dependence / Vantage, 16647 Wyoming, Detroit, MI 48221; tel. 313/861-0666; Mr. Benjamin A Jones
Neighborhood Service Organization, 220 Bagley, Suite 1200, Detroit, MI 48226; tel. 313/961-4890; Ms. Angela G Kennedy
New Center Community Mental Health Services, 2051 West Grand Boulevard, Detroit, MI 48208; tel. 313/961-3200; Ms. Roberta V Sanders
New Era Alternative Treatment Center, Inc., P.O. Box 03828, Highland Park, MI 48203; tel. 313/869-6328; Dr. Joseph A Pitts
Newaygo County Mental Health Center, PO Box 867, White Cloud, MI 49349; tel. 231/689-7330; Mr. Hank W Boks
Northeast Guidance Center, 13340 East Warren, Detroit, MI 48215; tel. 313/824-8000; Ms. Cheryl C Coleman
Northeast Health Services, 3800 Woodward Avenue Suite 1002, Detroit, MI 48234-1263; tel. 313/832-6386; Mrs. Rose V Jackson
Northeast Michigan Community Mental Health Services, 400 Johnson Street, Alpena, MI 49707; tel. 517/356-2161; Mr. Charles A White
Northern Michigan Community Mental Health, One MacDonald Drive, Suite A, Petoskey, MI 49770; tel. 616/347-7890; Ms. Alexis Kaczynski
Northpointe Behavioral Healthcare Systems, 715 Pyle Drive, Kingsford, MI 49802; tel. 906/779-0542; Mr. James G Gaynor, II
Oakland Psychological Clinic, PC, PO Box 888, Bloomfield Hills, MI 48303-0888; tel. 248/594-1200; Dr. Barry H Tigay
Orchard Hills Psychiatric Center, 40000 Grand River Ave, Ste 306, Novi, MI 48375-2112; tel. 248/426-9900; Dr. Hiten C Patel
Orchards Children's Services, Inc., 30215 Southfield Road, Southfield, MI 48076; tel. 248/433-8600; Mr. Gerald L Levin
Ottawa County Community Mental Health, 12251 James Street, Suite 100, Holland, MI 49424; tel. 616/393-5600; Dr. Rudolph Lie
Parkview Company, dba Parkview Counseling Centers, 18609 West Seven Mile Road, Detroit, MI 48219; tel. 313/532-8015; Mrs. Yvette Woodruff
Perspectives of Troy, PC, 2690 Crooks Road, Suite 300, Troy, MI 48084; tel. 248/244-8644; Dr. Tim Coldiron
Psychological Consultants of Michigan, PC, 151 North Avenue, Battle Creek, MI 49017-3467; tel. 616/968-2811; Dr. Jeffrey N Andert
Quality Behavioral Health, Inc, 3455 Woodward Avenue, Ste 101, Detroit, MI 48201; tel. 313/832-5555; Mr. Naveed Syed
Redford Counseling Center, 25945 West Seven Mile Road, Redford Township, MI 48240; tel. 313/535-5560; Ms. JoAnn Sadler
Rivendell Center for Behavioral Health, 101 West Townsend Road, St. Johns, MI 48879; tel. 517/224-1177; Mr. Roger Rohall
River's Bend, P.C., 33975 Dequindre, Troy, MI 48083; tel. 248/585-3239; Mr. James L Keener
Rose Hill Center, Inc., 5130 Rose Hill Boulevard, Holly, MI 48442; tel. 248/634-5530; Mr. Daniel J Kelly
Sacred Heart Rehabilitation Center, Inc., 400 Stoddard Road P.O. Box 41038, Memphis, MI 48041; tel. 810/392-2167; Mr. John Sass, Jr.
Saginaw County Community Mental Health Authority, 500 Hancock Street, Saginaw, MI 48602; tel. 517/797-3400; Mr. Donald G Miller
Star Center, Inc., 13575 Lesure, Detroit, MI 48227; tel. 313/493-4410; Ms. Lucila S Ryder
STM Clinic – Mental Health and Substance Abuse Services, One Tuscola Street, Suite 302, Saginaw, MI 48607-1287; tel. 517/755-2532; Ms. Sara Terry–Moton
Suburban West Community Center, 11677 Beech Daly Road, Redford Twp, MI 48239; tel. 313/937-9500; Dr. William R Hart
Summit Pointe, 140 West Michigan Avenue, Battle Creek, MI 49017; tel. 616/966-1460; Mr. Ervin R Brinker
Taylor Psychological Clinic, PC, 1172 Robert T Longway Blvd, Flint, MI 48503; tel. 810/232-8466; Dr. Maxwell F Taylor, II
The Center for Human Resources, 1001 Military Street, Port Huron, MI 48060; tel. 810/985-5168; Dr. Robert E Gamble
The Kalamazoo Child Guidance Clinic, 2615 Stadium Drive, Kalamazoo, MI 49008; tel. 616/343-1651; Mr. Steven L Smith
The Montcalm Center for Behavioral Health, 611 North State Street, Stanton, MI 48888; tel. 517/831-7520; Mr. Robert L Brown
Turning Point Programs, 1931 Boston, Southeast, Grand Rapids, MI 49506; tel. 616/235-1565; Mr. Robert E Byrd
Tuscola Behavioral Health Systems, PO Box 239, Caro, MI 48723; tel. 517/673-6191; Mr. Robert E Chadwick, II
West Michigan Community Mental Health Service Programs, 920 Diana Street, Ludington, MI 49431; tel. 231/845-6294; Dr. Kim Halladay

MINNESOTA
Andrew Residence, 1215 South 9th Street, Minneapolis, MN 55404; tel. 612/333-0111; Ms. Karen Foy
Fountain Centers, 408 West Fountain Street, Albert Lea, MN 56007; tel. 507/377-6411; Dr. Ron Harmon
Guest House, PO Box 954, Rochester, MN 55903; tel. 507/288-4693; Mr. Daniel Kidd
Hazelden Recovery Services, PO Box 11, Center City, MN 55012; tel. 612/257-4010; Mr. Jerry Spicer
Omegon, Inc., 2000 Hopkins Crossroads, Minnetonka, MN 55343; tel. 612/541-4738; Ms. Barbara J Danielsen
Pride Institute, 14400 Martin Drive, Eden Prairie, MN 55344; tel. 612/934-7554; Mr. Joseph M Amico
St. Joseph's Home for Children, 1121 East 46th Street, Minneapolis, MN 55407; tel. 612/827-6241; Charles E Lawler

MISSISSIPPI
CARES Center, Inc., 402 Wesley Avenue, Jackson, MS 39202; tel. 601/360-0583; Mr. Christopher M Cherney
COPAC, Inc., 3949 Highway 43 North, Brandon, MS 39047; tel. 601/829-2500; Dr. J. Stacy Hughes
Diamond Grove Center for Children and Adolescents, PO Box 848, Louisville, MS 39339; tel. 601/779-0119; Ken O'Rourke
Male/Female Receiving Med Psych Services, PO Box 157–A, Whitfield, MS 39193; tel. 601/351-8000; Mr. James G ChastainIV
Millcreek, PO Box 1160, Magee, MS 39111; tel. 601/849-4221; Ms. Margaret F Tedford
Pine Belt Mental Healthcare Resources, PO Drawer 1030, Hattiesburg, MS 39401; tel. 601/544-4641; Mr. Jerry Mayo

MISSOURI
Boonville Valley Hope, PO Box 376, Boonville, MO 65233; tel. 660/882-6547; Mr. Dennis Gilhousen
Boys Town of Missouri, Inc., PO Box 189, St. James, MO 65559; tel. 573/265-3251; Mr. Richard C Dunn
Centrec Care, Inc., 11720 Borman Drive, Suite 103, Saint Louis, MO 63146; tel. 314/991-5388; Dr. Mohammed A Kabir
Child Advocacy Services Ctr, Inc./The Children's Place, 2 East 59th Street, Kansas City, MO 64113-2116; tel. 816/363-1898; Ms. Deborah Howland
Child Center of Our Lady, 7900 Natural Bridge Rd., St. Louis, MO 63121; tel. 314/383-0200; Mr. Edward S Koszykowski
Comprehensive Mental Health Services, Inc., 10901 Winner Road, Independence, MO 64052; tel. 816/254-3652; Mr. William H Kyles
Edgewood Children's Center, 330 North Gore Avenue, Webster Groves, MO 63119; tel. 314/968-2060; Ms. Sue S Stepleton
Epworth Children and Family Services, 110 North Elm Avenue, Saint Louis, MO 63119; tel. 314/961-5718; Mr. Kevin Drollinger
Industrial Rehabilitation Center, 429 Northeast 69 Highway, Kansas City, MO 64119; tel. 816/452-8777; Mr. Maurice L Cummings
Marillac Center, 2826 Main Street, Kansas City, MO 64118; tel. 816/508-3300; Mr. R. Michael Bowen
Piney Ridge Center, Inc., PO Box 4067, Waynesville, MO 65583; tel. 573/774-5353; Ms. Jacqueline S Howard
Provident Counseling, Inc., 2650 Olive Street, Saint Louis, MO 63103-1489; tel. 314/371-6500; Ms. Kathleen E Buescher
Research Mental Health Services, 901 NE Independence Avenue, Lees Summit, MO 64086; tel. 816/246-8000; Mr. Alan Flory

MONTANA
Intermountain Children's Home, 500 South Lamborn, Helena, MT 59601; tel. 406/442-7920; Mr. John H Wilkinson
Rocky Mountain Treatment Center, 920 Fourth Avenue North, Great Falls, MT 59401; tel. 406/727-8832; Mr. Mark Sallee
Yellowstone Boys and Girls Ranch, 1732 South 72nd Street West, Billings, MT 59106-3599; tel. 406/655-2100; Mr. Ry Sorensen

NEBRASKA
Alpha School, 1615 South 6th Street, Omaha, NE 68108; tel. 402/444-6557; Mr. Ray Christensen
Behavioral Health Specialists, Inc., 600 South 13th Street, Norfolk, NE 68701; tel. 402/370-3140; Ms. Connie Barnes
Blue Valley Mental Health Clinic, 1121 N. 10th Street, Beatrice, NE 68310; tel. 402/228-3386; Dr. Wayne R Price
Camelot Care Centers, Inc., 7501 'O' Street, Suite 104, Lincoln, NE 68510; tel. 402/484-6060; Mr. James V Doramus
Community Mental Health Center of Lancaster County, 2200 St. Mary's Avenue, Lincoln, NE 68502; tel. 402/441-7940; Mr. George Hanigan
Epworth Village, Inc., P O Box 503, York, NE 68467-0503; tel. 402/362-3353; Mr. Thomas G McBride
Father Flanagan's Boys' Home, 13603 Flanagan Boulevard, Boys Town, NE 68010; tel. 402/498-3214; Father Val J Peter, JCD,STD
Lincoln Lancaster County Child Guidance Center, 215 Centennial Mall South, Suite 312, Lincoln, NE 68508; tel. 402/475-7666; Dr. Carol Crumpacker
Mid–East Nebraska Behavioral Healthcare Services, Inc., PO Box 682, Columbus, NE 68602-0682; tel. 402/564-1426; Dr. Roberta Saunders
O'Neill Valley Hope, PO Box 918, O' Neill, NE 68763-0918; tel. 402/336-3747; Mr. Dennis Gilhousen
OMNI Behavioral Health, 4150 S 87th Street, Suite 100, Omaha, NE 68127; tel. 402/331-1598; Mr. William E Reay
Uta Halee Girls Village, 10625 Calhoun Road, Omaha, NE 68112; tel. 402/453-0803; Mr. Denis D McCarville

NEVADA
Desert Willow Treatment Center, 6171 W Charleston Boulevard, Building 17, Las Vegas, NV 89102; tel. 702/486-6100; Ms. Barbara L Qualls

NEW HAMPSHIRE
Beech Hill Hospital, LLC, PO Box 254, Dublin, NH 03444; tel. 603/563-8511; Mr. Matthew J Feehery
Community Council of Nashua, NH, Inc., 7 Prospect Street, Nashua, NH 03060-3990; tel. 603/889-6147; Dr. Zlatko M Kuftinec
Lakeview Neurorehabilitation Center, Inc., 101 Highwatch Road, Effingham, NH 03814; tel. 603/539-7451; Ms. Carolyn M Ramsay
Seacoast Mental Health Center, Inc., 1145 Sagamore Avenue, Portsmouth, NH 03801; tel. 603/431-6703; Dr. Jeffrey C Connor
The Mental Health Center of Greater Manchester, 401 Cypress Street, Manchester, NH 03103; tel. 603/668-4111; Mr. Peter Janelle

NEW JERSEY
Arthur Brisbane Child Treatment Center, PO Box 625, Farmingdale, NJ 07727; tel. 732/938-5061; Mr. Raymond Grimaldi
AtlantiCare Behavioral Health, 201 Tilton Road, Unit 13–A, Northfield, NJ 08225; tel. 609/645-7601; Mr. Donald J Parker

Providers / JCAHO Accredited Freestanding Mental Health Care Organizations

Bancroft Rehabilitation Services, PO Box 20, Haddonfield, NJ 08033; tel. 609/429-0010; Dr. George W Niemann

Bonnie Brae, PO Box 825, Liberty Corner, NJ 07938-0825; tel. 908/647-0800; Susan G Roth

Cape Counseling Services, 128 Crest Haven Road, Cape May Court House, NJ 08210; tel. 609/465-4100; Mr. Barry Keefe

Care Plus NJ, Inc., 610 Industrial Avenue, Paramus, NJ 07652; tel. 201/265-8200; Mr. Joseph A Masciandaro

Catholic Charities – Diocese of Metuchen, 319 Maple Street, Perth Amboy, NJ 08861; tel. 732/257-6677; Sister Florence Edward Kearney

Community Centers for Mental Health, Inc., 2 Park Avenue, Dumont, NJ 07628; tel. 201/385-4400; Ms. Victoria L Sidrow

Comprehensive Behavioral Healthcare, Inc., PO Box 750, Lyndhurst, NJ 07071; tel. 201/935-3322; Mr. Peter Scerbo

CPC Behavioral Healthcare, Inc, Parkway 100 3535 Route 66 Building #5, Suite D, Neptune, NJ 07753; tel. 732/643-4300; Dr. Jeanne H Wurmser

Daytop, New Jersey, Post Office Box 310, Mendham, NJ 07945; tel. 973/543-0162; Mr. Joseph Hennen

Discovery Institute for Addictive Disorders, Inc., PO Box 177, Marlboro, NJ 07746; tel. 732/946-9444; Mr. Robert C Denes

Drenk Mental Health Center, Inc., 795 Woodland Road, Suite 300, Mount Holly, NJ 08060; tel. 609/267-5656; Mr. Brian Levin

Ewing Residential Treatment Center, 1610 Stuyvesant Avenue, Trenton, NJ 08618; tel. 609/530-3350; Ms. Elizabeth A McGinnis

Family and Children's Services, 1900 Route 35 South, Oakhurst, NJ 07755; tel. 732/531-9111; Dr. Jurgen H Schwermer

Family Service of Burlington County, 770 Woodlane Road, Mount Holly, NJ 08060; tel. 609/267-5928; Ms. Mary Wells

High Focus Centers, 299 Market Street, Suite 110, Saddle Brook, NJ 07663; tel. 201/291-0055; Dr. David Nyman

Honesty House, 1272 Long Hill Road, Stirling, NJ 07980; tel. 908/647-3211; Mr. Charles H Stucky

Lighthouse at Mays Landing, PO Box 899, Mays Landing, NJ 08330; tel. 609/625-4900; Ms. Regina LaVerde

New Hope Foundation, Inc, PO Box 66, Marlboro, NJ 07746; tel. 732/946-3030; Mr. George J Mattie

NewBridge Services, Inc., PO Box 336, Pompton Plains, NJ 07444; tel. 201/839-2520; Mr. Robert L Parker

Ocean Mental Health Services, Inc., 160 Route 9, Bayville, NJ 08721; tel. 732/349-5550; Dr. Charles J Langan

Preferred Behavioral Health of New Jersey, PO Box 2036, Lakewood, NJ 08701; tel. 732/364-4590; Mr. William J Sette

Seabrook House, Inc., PO Box 5055, Seabrook, NJ 08302-0655; tel. 609/455-7575; Mr. Edward M Diehl

SERV Centers of New Jersey, Inc., 380 Scotch Road, West Trenton, NJ 08628; tel. 609/406-0100; Ms. Kathleen Enerrich

Sunrise House Foundation, PO Box 600, Lafayette, NJ 07848; tel. 973/383-6300; Dr. Philip N Horowitz

UCPC Behavioral Health Care, 117-119 Roosevelt Avenue, Plainfield, NJ 07060; tel. 908/756-6870; Ms. Marcyann E Sosnoski

UMDNJ – University Behavioral HealthCare, PO Box 1392, Piscataway, NJ 08855-1392; tel. 732/235-5900; Mr. Christopher Kosseff

Vineland Children's Residential Treatment Center, 2000 Maple Avenue, Vineland, NJ 08361-2990; tel. 856/696-6620; Mr. Theodore Allen

West Bergen Mental Healthcare, Inc., 120 Chestnut Street, Ridgewood, NJ 07450; tel. 201/444-3550; Mr. Philip E Wilson

Willowglen Academy – New Jersey, Inc., 6 Gail Court, Unit 4, Sparta, NJ 07871; tel. 973/579-3700; Mr. Leonard F Dziubla

Woodbridge Child Diagnostic and Treatment Center, 15 Paddock Street, Avenel, NJ 07001; tel. 732/499-5050; Mr. William Falvo

Youth Consultation Service, 260 Union Street, Hackensack, NJ 07601; tel. 201/343-8803; Mr. Richard Mingoia

NEW MEXICO

BHC Pinon Hills Residential Treatment Center, Inc., PO Box 428, Velarde, NM 87582; tel. 505/852-2704; Ms. Kim Whitelock

Desert Hills of New Mexico, 5310 Sequoia Northwest, Albuquerque, NM 87120; tel. 505/836-7330; Ms. Carol Bickelman

Family Opportunity Resources, 851 Magee Lane, Santa Fe, NM 87501; tel. 409/740-0442; Mr. Gordon W McKee

Four Corners Regional Adolescent Treatment Center, PO Box 220, Shiprock, NM 87420; tel. 505/368-4712; Mr. Hoskie Benally, Jr.

Namaste Child and Family Development Center, PO Box 270, Peralta, NM 87042; tel. 505/865-6176; Ms. Patricia Nugent

Sequoyah Adolescent Treatment Center, 3405 W Pan American Freeway NE, Albuquerque, NM 87107; tel. 505/344-4673; Dr. W. Henry Gardner

The Adolescent Pointe, PO Box 6, Santa Teresa, NM 88008; tel. 505/589-4054; Dr. Truett Maddox

NEW YORK

A.R.E.B.A.– Casriel, Inc., 500 West 57th Street, New York, NY 10019; tel. 212/293-3000; Mr. Steven Yohay

Arms Acres, 75 Seminary Hill Road, Carmel, NY 10512; tel. 914/225-3400; Dr. Ed Spauster

August Aichhorn R.F.T., 23 West 106th Street, New York, NY 10025; tel. 212/316-9353; Dr. Michael A Pawel

Baker Victory Services, Inc., 780 Ridge Road, Lackawanna, NY 14218; tel. 716/828-9515; Mr. James J Casion

Bronx Addiction Treatment Center, 1500 Waters Place, Building 13, Bronx, NY 10461; tel. 718/904-0026; Mr. Hermon Lockhart

Charles K. Post Addiction Treatment Center, Building 1, PPC Campus, West Brentwood, NY 11717; tel. 516/434-7209; Mr. Phillip A Dawes

Conifer Park, Inc., 79 Glenridge Road, Schenectady, NY 12302; tel. 518/399-6446; Mr. John A Duffy

Conners Residential Treatment Facility, Inc., 824 Delaware Avenue, Buffalo, NY 14209; tel. 716/884-3802; Mr. James D Lawson

Cornerstone of Medical Arts Center Hospital, 57 West 57th Street, New York, NY 10019; tel. 212/755-0200; Mr. Thomas C Puzo

Cornerstone of Rhinebeck, NY, 500 Milan Hollow Road, Rhinebeck, NY 12572; tel. 914/266-3481; Dr. Chandra Singh

Creedmoor Addiction Treatment Center, 80-45 Winchester Boulevard Building 19 – CBU 15, Queens Village, NY 11427; tel. 718/264-3743; Mr. Gerlando A Verruso

Crestwood Children's Center, 2075 Scottsville Road, Rochester, NY 14623-2098; tel. 716/436-4442; Ms. Donna M Cimino

Crossings Recovery Centers, 450 Waverly Avenue, Suite 5, Patchogue, NY 11772; tel. 516/447-0155; Dr. William Bue

Dick Van Dyke Addiction Treatment Center, 1330 County Road 132, Ovid, NY 14521; tel. 607/869-9500; Mr. Thomas Nightingale

Green Chimneys Children's Services, Caller Box 719, Brewster, NY 10509; tel. 914/279-2995; Mr. Joseph A Whalen

Hillside Children's Center, 1183 Monroe Avenue, Rochester, NY 14620; tel. 716/256-7501; Mr. Dennis M Richardson

Hope House, Inc., 517 Western Avenue, Albany, NY 12203; tel. 518/482-4673; Ms. Mary Ann DiChristopher-Finn

Hopevale, Inc., 3780 Howard Road, Hamburg, NY 14075; tel. 716/648-1964; vacant .

Jewish Board of Family and Children's Services, 120 West 57th Street, New York, NY 10019; tel. 212/582-9100; Dr. Alan B Siskind

John L. Norris Addiction Treatment Center, 1111 Elmwood Avenue, Rochester, NY 14620; tel. 716/461-0410; Mr. Thomas E Nightingale

Julia Dyckman Andrus Memorial, 1156 North Broadway, Yonkers, NY 10701; tel. 914/965-3700; Dr. Gary O Carman

Kingsboro Addiction Treatment Center, 754 Lexington Avenue, Brooklyn, NY 11221; tel. 718/453-6747; Ms. Jacqueline Cole

Manhattan Addiction Treatment Center, 600 East 125th Street, Ward's Island, New York, NY 10035; tel. 212/369-0703; Mr. Jeffrey Spitz

McPike Addiction Treatment Center, 1213 Court Street, Utica, NY 13502; tel. 315/738-4400; Mr. John F Crowley

National Expert Care Consultants, Inc., 455 West 50th Street, New York, NY 10019-6504; tel. 212/262-6000; Mr. Brian J McDowell

Parsons Child and Family Center, 60 Academy Road, Albany, NY 12208; tel. 518/426-2600; Mr. Raymond Schimmer

Passages Counseling Center, 3680 Route 112, Coram, NY 11727; tel. 516/698-9222; Mr. Arnt Monge

Psych Systems of Long Island, 1600 Stewart Avenue, Suite 202, Westbury, NY 11590; tel. 516/683-1200; Ms. Marci Zaslav

Restorative Management Corporation, 15 King Street, Middletown, NY 10940; tel. 914/342-5941; Mr. Dean Scher

Richard C. Ward Addiction Treatment Center, 117 Seward Avenue Building 92, Suite 12/16, Middletown, NY 10940; tel. 914/341-2500; Mr. Erwin G Michel

Rochester Mental Health Center, 490 East Ridge Road, Rochester, NY 14621; tel. 716/922-2500; Ms. Heide George

Russell E. Blaisdell Addiction Treatment Center, PO Box 140, Orangeburg, NY 10962; tel. 914/359-8500; Ms. Tamara Miller-Kammerer

Saint Peter's Addiction Recovery Center, Inc., 3 Mercycare Lane, Guilderland, NY 12084; tel. 518/452-6701; Ms. Karen A Giles

Salamanca Hospital District Authority, 150 Parkway Drive, Salamanca, NY 14779; tel. 716/945-1900; Dr. Kenneth L Oakley

Seafield Center, Inc., 7 Seafield Lane, Westhampton Beach, NY 11978; tel. 516/288-1122; Mr. John C Haley

South Beach Addiction Treatment Center, 777 Seaview Avenue, Building 1, Staten Island, NY 10305; tel. 718/667-4218; Mr. Gerlando A Verruso

St. Christopher-Ottilie, 101 Downing Avenue, Sea Cliff, NY 11579; tel. 516/671-1253; Mr. Robert J McMahon

St. Joseph's Rehabilitation Center, Inc., PO Box 470, Saranac Lake, NY 12983-0470; tel. 518/891-3950; Rev. Arthur M Johnson

St. Joseph's Villa of Rochester, 3300 Dewey Avenue, Rochester, NY 14616; tel. 716/865-1550; Mr. Roger C Battaglia

St. Lawrence Addiction Treatment Center, 1 Chimney Point Drive, Hamilton Hall, Ogdensburg, NY 13669; tel. 315/393-1180; Mr. Phillip Dranger

St. Mary's Children and Family Services, 525 Convent Road, Syosset, NY 11791-3864; tel. 516/921-0808; Ms. Liz Giordano

Stutzman Addiction Treatment Center, 360 Forest Avenue, Buffalo, NY 14213; tel. 716/882-4900; Mr. Steven Schwartz

The Astor Home for Children, PO Box 5005, Rhinebeck, NY 12572-5005; tel. 914/876-4081; Sr. Rose Logan

The Children's Home RTF, Inc., 638 Squirrel Hill Road, Chenango Forks, NY 13746; tel. 607/656-9004; Ms. Karen Wright

The Children's Village, Wetmore Hall, Dobbs Ferry, NY 10522; tel. 914/693-0600; Ms. Nan Dale

The Health Association – MAIN QUEST Treatment Center, 774 West Main Street, Rochester, NY 14611; tel. 716/464-8870; Ms. Susan L Costa

The House of the Good Shepherd, 1550 Champlin Avenue, Utica, NY 13502; tel. 315/733-0436; Mr. William F Holicky, Jr.

The Long Island Center for Recovery, PO Box 774, Hampton Bays, NY 11946; tel. 516/728-3100; Mr. Jack Hamilton

The Support Center, Inc., 181 Route 209, Port Jervis, NY 12771; tel. 800/724-9322; Mr. Carmine Mosca

Tully Hill Alcohol & Drug Treatment Center, PO Box 920, Tully, NY 13159-0920; tel. 315/696-6114; Ms. Cathy L Palm

Veritas Villa, Inc., PO Box 610, Kerhonkson, NY 12446-0610; tel. 914/626-3555; Mr. Lester McCandless

Villa Outpatient Center, 290 Madison Avenue, 6th Floor, New York, NY 10017; tel. 212/679-4960; Mr. Richard Partridge

Westchester Jewish Community Services, Inc., 845 North Broadway, Suite 2, White Plains, NY 10603-2427; tel. 914/761-0600; Mr. Alan Trager

NORTH CAROLINA

Alexander Children's Center, Inc., PO Box 220632, Charlotte, NC 28222-9979; tel. 704/362-8470; Mr. N.Craig Bass

Amethyst, PO Box 32861, Charlotte, NC 28232-2861; tel. 704/554-8373; Mr. Steven Johnson

CenterPoint Human Services, 725 North Highland Avenue, Winston-Salem, NC 27101; tel. 336/725-7777; Mr. Ronald W Morton

Fellowship Hall, Inc., PO Box 13890, Greensboro, NC 27415; tel. 336/621-3381; Mr. Rodney Battles

Providers / JCAHO Accredited Freestanding Mental Health Care Organizations

Grandfather Home for Children, PO Box 98, Banner Elk, NC 28604; tel. 704/898–5465; Mr. James Swinkola
Julian F. Keith Alcohol and Drug Abuse Treatment Center, 301 Tabernacle Road, Black Mountain, NC 28711; tel. 828/669–3421; Mr. William A Rafter
The Wilmington Treatment Center, 2520 Troy Drive, Wilmington, NC 28401; tel. 910/762–2727; Mr. Charles Sharp
The Wilmington Treatment Center, 2520 Troy Drive, Wilmington, NC 28401; tel. 910/762–2727; Mr. Charles Sharp
Three Springs of North Carolina, PO Box 1370, Pittsboro, NC 27312; tel. 919/542–1104; Ms. Peggy Reeder–Moore
Timber Ridge Treatment Center, 14225 Stokes Ferry Road, Gold Hill, NC 28071; tel. 704/279–1199; Mr. Thomas A R Hibbert
Unity Regional Youth Treatment Center, PO Box C–201, Cherokee, NC 28719; tel. 828/497–3958; Ms. Margaret Jenks

NORTH DAKOTA
The Dakota Boys Ranch, PO Box 5007, Minot, ND 58703; tel. 701/852–3628; Mr. Gene Kasemen

OHIO
2 North Park, Inc., 720 Pine Avenue Southeast, Warren, OH 44483; tel. 330/399–3677; Mr. Kenneth Lloyd
Akron–Urban Minority Alcoholism Drug Abuse Outreach, 665 W Market Street, Suite 2D, Akron, OH 44303; tel. 330/379–3467; Ms. Janice T Mayes
Beech Brook, 3737 Lander Road, Cleveland, OH 44124; tel. 216/831–2255; Dr. Mario Tonti
Behavioral Care Management, 5800 Monroe Street, Building A, Sylvania, OH 43560; tel. 419/885–2391; Dr. Ronald Dozoretz
Behavioral Connections of Wood County, Inc., 320 West Gypsy Lane Road, Bowling Green, OH 43402; tel. 419/352–2551; Mr. Randall J LaFond
Bellefaire Jewish Children's Bureau, 22001 Fairmount Boulevard, Shaker Heights, OH 44118; tel. 216/932–2800; Dr. Adam G Jacobs
Blick Clinic, Inc., 640 West Market Street, Akron, OH 44303; tel. 330/762–5425; Dr. Gregory L LaForme
Catholic Charities Services Corporation, 1111 Superior Avenue, Cleveland, OH 44114; tel. 216/696–6525; Mr. Thomas W Woll
Center for Chemical Addictions Treatment, 830 Ezzard Charles Drive, Cincinnati, OH 45214; tel. 513/381–6672; Ms. Sandra L Kuehn
Charles B. Mills Center, Inc., 715 South Plum Street, Marysville, OH 43040; tel. 513/644–9192; Dr. John R Lauritsen
Child Guidance Centers, 312 Locust Street, Akron, OH 44302–1878; tel. 330/762–0591; Mr. Charles M Vehlow, Jr.
Children's Aid Society, 10427 Detroit Avenue, Cleveland, OH 44102–1694; tel. 216/521–6511; Ms. Roberta King
Children's Resource Center, PO Box 738, Bowling Green, OH 43402; tel. 419/352–7588; Mr. R. Anthony Marcson
Community Drug Board, 725 East Market Street, Akron, OH 44305; tel. 330/434–4141; Mr. Theodore P Ziegler
Community Support Services, Inc., 150 Cross Street, Akron, OH 44311; tel. 330/996–9141; Mr. Arthur G Wickersham
Comprehensive Psychiatry Specialists, 955 Windham Court, Suite 2, Boardman, OH 44512; tel. 330/726–9570; Dr. Pradeep Mathur
Crisis Intervention Center of Stark County, Inc., 2421 13th Street Northwest, Canton, OH 44708; tel. 330/452–9812; Dr. Bernard S Jesiolowski
D & E Counseling Center, 142 Javit Court, Youngstown, OH 44515; tel. 330/793–2487; Mr. Gregory Cvetkovic
Family Recovery Center, PO Box 464, Lisbon, OH 44432; tel. 330/424–1468; Ms. Eloise V Traina
Focus Health Care, 5701 North High Street, Suite 8, Worthington, OH 43085; tel. 614/885–1944; Dr. Brad Lander
Glenbeigh Health Sources, PO Box 298, Rock Creek, OH 44084–0298; tel. 440/563–3400; Ms. Pat Weston-Hall
Harbor Behavioral Healthcare, 4334 Secor Road, Toledo, OH 43623–4234; tel. 419/475–4449; Mr. Dale E Shreve
Interval Brotherhood Home Inc., 3445 South Main Street, Akron, OH 44319; tel. 330644–4095; Fr. Samuel R Ciccolini
Lake Area Recovery Center, 2801 'C' Court, Ashtabula, OH 44004; tel. 440/998–0722; Ms. Kathleen Kinney
McKinley Hall, Inc., 1101 East High Street, Springfield, OH 45505; tel. 937/328–5300; Ms. Judith O Hoy
Mental Health Services for Clark County, Inc., 1345 Fountain Boulevard, Springfield, OH 45504; tel. 937/399–9500; Dr. James P Perry
Miami Valley Labor Management Healthcare Delivery Systems, 136 Heid Avenue, Dayton, OH 45404; tel. 937/208–2327; Ms. Linda VanBourgondien
Mount Carmel Behavioral Healthcare, 1808 East Broad Street, Columbus, OH 43203; tel. 614/251–8242; Dr. Marc Clemente
Neil Kennedy Recovery Clinic, 2151 Rush Boulevard, Youngstown, OH 44507; tel. 330/744–1181; Mr. Jerry V Carter
NEO Psych Consultants, 831 Southwestern Run, Suite 2, Youngstown, OH 44514; tel. 330/726–7785; Mr. Charles L Boris
New Directions, Inc., 30800 Chagrin Boulevard, Pepper Pike, OH 44124; tel. 216/591–0324; Mr. Michael E Matoney
Nova Behavioral Health, Inc., 832 McKinley Avenue Northwest, Canton, OH 44703; tel. 330/455–9407; Mr. Michael D Flora
Parkside Behavioral Healthcare, Inc., 349 Olde Ridenour Road, Columbus, OH 43230; tel. 614/471–2552; Dr. Christine N Gerber
Portage Path Behavioral Health, 340 South Broadway, Akron, OH 44308; tel. 330/376–6144; Mr. Jerome T Kraker
PsyCare, Inc., 2980 Belmont Avenue, Youngstown, OH 44505; tel. 330/759–2310; Dr. Douglas C Darnall
PsyCare, Inc., 2980 Belmont Avenue, Youngstown, OH 44505; tel. 330/759–2310; Dr. Douglas C Darnall
Quest Recovery Services, 1341 Market Avenue, North, Canton, OH 44714–2675; tel. 330/453–8252; Mr. Donald C Davies
Ravenwood Mental Health Center, 12557 Ravenwood Drive, Chardon, OH 44024; tel. 440/285–3400; Mr. David A Boyle
Rescue Mental Health Services, 3350 Collingwood Boulevard, Toledo, OH 43610; tel. 419/255–9585; Mr. Frank C Ayers
Serenity Living, Inc., PO Box 217, Vandalia, OH 45377; tel. 937/898–2788; Dr. Joseph J Trevino
Specialty Care Psychiatric Services, Inc., 2657 Niles Courtland Road, SE, Warren, OH 44484; tel. 330/652–3533; Mr. JB Mitroo
Springview Developmental Center, 3130 East Main Street, Springfield, OH 45505; tel. 937/325–9263; Mr. Dominick S Dennis
St. Joseph Children's Treatment Center, 650 St. Paul Avenue, Dayton, OH 45410; tel. 937/254–3562; Mr. Bob Pawlak
Substance Abuse Services, Inc., 1832 Adams Street, Toledo, OH 43624; tel. 419/243–7274; Mr. Carroll Parks
The Buckeye Ranch, Inc., 5665 Hoover Road, Grove City, OH 43123; tel. 614/875–2371; Mr. Richard E Rieser
The Crossroads Center, 311 Martin Luther King Drive, Cincinnati, OH 45219–3116; tel. 513/475–5300; Mrs. Jacqueline P Butler
Transitional Living, Inc. and Affiliates, 2052 Princeton Road, Hamilton, OH 45011; tel. 513/863–6383; Mr. David F Craft
Unison Behavioral Health Group, PO Box 10015, Toledo, OH 43699–0015; tel. 419/242–9577; Mr. James D Wares
Wellspring Retreat & Resource Center, PO Box 67, Albany, OH 45710; tel. 740/698–6277; Dr. Paul R Martin
Zepf Community Mental Health Center, Inc., 6605 West Central Avenue, Toledo, OH 43617; tel. 419/841–7813; Ms. Virginia Ferree

OKLAHOMA
Brookhaven Hospital, 201 South Garnett Road, Tulsa, OK 74128–1800; tel. 918/438–4257; Dr. Rolf B Gainer
Carl Albert Community Mental Health Center, PO Box 579, Mcalester, OK 74502; tel. 918/426–1000; Mr. George R Jones
Christopher Youth Center, Inc., 2741 East 7th Street, Tulsa, OK 74104; tel. 918/583–0612; Dr. Thomas E McKee
Cushing Valley Hope, PO Box 472, Cushing, OK 74023–0472; tel. 918/225–1736; Mr. Dennis Gilhousen
High Pointe, 6501 Northeast 50th Street, Oklahoma City, OK 73141; tel. 405/424–3383; Johnny Smith
Jim Taliaferro Community Mental Health Center, 602 Southwest 38th Street, Lawton, OK 73505–6999; tel. 580/248–5780; Ms. Starr Paul
Oklahoma Youth Center, 320 12th Avenue Northeast, Norman, OK 73071; tel. 405/364–9004; Mr. Paul Bouffard
Parkside, Inc., 1620 East 12th Street, Tulsa, OK 74120; tel. 918/588–8807; Mr. Paul Greever
Western State Psychiatric Center, 1222 10th, Suite 211, Woodward, OK 73801; tel. 580/571–3233; Mr. Steve Norwood
Willow Crest Hospital, 130 'A' Street Southwest, Miami, OK 74354; tel. 918/542–1836; Ms. Anne G Anthony

OREGON
BHC Pacific View RTC, 4101 Northeast Division Street, Gresham, OR 97030; tel. 503/661–0775; Mr. Michael Amador
Christie School, PO Box 368, Marylhurst, OR 97036; tel. 503/635–3416; Mr. William M Powers
Eastern Oregon Adolescent Multi–Treatment Center, Inc., 622 Airport Road, Pendleton, OR 97801; tel. 541/276–0057; Mr. Ronald E Humiston
Edgefield Children's Center, 2408 Southwest Halsey Street, Troutdale, OR 97060; tel. 503/665–0157; Mr. Jay Bloom
Kerr Youth and Family Center, 722 Northeast 162nd Avenue, Portland, OR 97230; tel. 503/255–4205; Mr. Christopher J Krenk
RiverBend Youth Center, Inc., 15544 S Clackamas River Drive, Oregon City, OR 97045; tel. 503/656–8005; Ms. Marcia L McClocklin
Ryles Center, 3339 Southeast Division Street, Portland, OR 97202; tel. 503/238–1477; Ms. Patti Williamson
Serenity Lane, Inc., 616 East Sixteenth Avenue, Eugene, OR 97401; tel. 503/687–1110; Mr. Neil H McNaughton
Southern Oregon Adolescent Study and Treatment Center, 210 Tacoma Street, Grants Pass, OR 97526; tel. 541/476–3302; Mr. Robert E Lieberman
Springbrook Northwest, Inc., 2001 Crestview Drive, Newberg, OR 97132; tel. 503/537–7000; Mr. Mark W Knudsen
Trillium Family Services, 3550 Southeast Woodward Street, Portland, OR 97202; tel. 503/234–7532; Mr. Robert L Roy
VA Domiciliary, 8495 Crater Lake Highway, White City, OR 97503; tel. 541/826–2111; Mr. George H Andries, Jr.

PENNSYLVANIA
Abraxas I, PO Box 59, Marienville, PA 16239; tel. 814/927–6615; Mr. James E Newsome
ACS Psychological Associates, Inc. – Community Services, 136 East Fayette Street, Uniontown, PA 15401; tel. 724/438–2342; Mr. Adam C Sedlock, Jr.
Adelphoi Village, Inc., 1003 Village Way, Latrobe, PA 15650; tel. 724/520–1111; Mr. John P Bukovac
American Day Treatment Centers, 468 Thomas Jones Way Suite 150, Exton, PA 19341; tel. 610/524–2680; Mr. Kerry Teel
Beacon Light Behavioral Health Systems, 800 East Main Street, Bradford, PA 16701; tel. 814/362–5250; Mr. Thomas E Urban
Bowling Green of Brandywine, Inc., 1375 Newark Road, Kennett Square, PA 19348; tel. 610/268–3588; Claire F Beckwith
Brighter Beginnings, 23062 Jericho Road, Edinboro, PA 16412; tel. 814/398–1805; Ms. Christine Brotherson
Charter Behavioral Health System at Cove Forge, New Beginnings Road, Williamsburg, PA 16693; tel. 814/832–2121; Mr. Mark Sarneso
Child Guidance Resource Centers, 600 North Olive Street, Media, PA 19063–2418; tel. 610/565–6000; Mr. Edward Maguire
Children's Aid Home Programs of Somerset County, Inc., PO Box 1195, Somerset, PA 15501; tel. 814/443–1637; Mr. Robert C Miller, Jr.
Clear Brook, Inc., 1003 Wyoming Avenue, Forty Fort, PA 18704; tel. 570/288–6692; Dr. Nicholas F Colangelo
Conewago Place, 424 Nye Road, Hummelstown, PA 17036–0406; tel. 717/533–0428; Mr. A. E Cox, Jr.
Diversified Family Services, 3679 East State Street, Hermitage, PA 16148; tel. 412/346–2123; Ms. Marilyn Klemens
Diversified Treatment Alternatives, Inc., 201 Fairfield Road, Lewisburg, PA 17837; tel. 570/523–3457; Mr. Timothy J Kelleher
Eagleville Hospital, PO Box 45, Eagleville, PA 19408–0045; tel. 610/539–6000; Ms. Kendria Kurtz
Friendship House, PO Box 3778, Scranton, PA 18505; tel. 570/342–8305; Mr. Robert H Angeloni

Providers / JCAHO Accredited Freestanding Mental Health Care Organizations

Gateway Rehabilitation Center, Moffett Run Road, Aliquippa, PA 15001; tel. 412/766-8700; Dr. Kenneth S Ramsey
Gaudenzia, Inc. - Common Ground, 2835 North Front Street, Harrisburg, PA 17110; tel. 717/238-5553; Mr. Michael B Harle
Glade Run Lutheran Services, PO Box 70, Zelienople, PA 16063-0070; tel. 724/452-4453; Dr. Charles T Lockwood
Greenbriar Treatment Center, 800 Manor Drive, Washington, PA 15301; tel. 724/225-9700; Ms. Mary G Banaszak
Greenway Center, PO Box 188, Henryville, PA 18332; tel. 800/831-6402; Mr. Wallace M Slatinsky
Hoffman Homes, Inc., PO Box 4777, Gettysburg, PA 17325-4777; tel. 717/359-7148; Mr. George Sepic
KidsPeace Corporation – National Headquarters, 5300 KidsPeace Drive, Orefield, PA 18069-9101; tel. 610/799-8005; Mr. C T O'Donnell, II
Lehigh Valley Community Mental Health Centers, Inc., PO Box 5349, Bethlehem, PA 18015-5349; tel. 610/691-4357; Ms. Melissa Chlebowski
Livengrin Foundation, Inc., 4833 Hulmeville Road, Bensalem, PA 19020-3099; tel. 215/638-5200; Mr. Richard M Pine
Malvern Institute, 940 King Road, Malvern, PA 19355; tel. 610/647-0330; Mr. Thomas J Connell
Marworth, PO Box 36, Waverly, PA 18471; tel. 717/563-1112; Mr. James J Dougherty
Milestones Community Healthcare, Inc., 614 North Easton Road, Glenside, PA 19038; tel. 215/884-5566; Dr. Paul Volosov
Mirmont Treatment Center, 100 Yearsley Mill Road, Glen Riddle Lima, PA 19063-5593; tel. 610/744-1400; Mr. Thomas F Cain
New Vitae Partial Hospitalization Program, PO Box 181, Limeport, PA 18060-0181; tel. 610/965-6231; Mr. Adam Devlin
NorthEast Treatment Centers (NET), 499 North 5th Street, Suite A, Philadelphia, PA 19123; tel. 215/451-7000; Mr. Terence McSherry
Northern Tier Children's Home Residential Services, Inc., PO Box 94, Harrison Valley, PA 16927; tel. 814/334-5226; Mr. J. Merle Herr
Penn Foundation, Inc., PO Box 32, Sellersville, PA 18960; tel. 215/453-5183; Dr. Vernon H Kratz
Presbyterian Children's Village Services, 452 South Roberts Road, Rosemont, PA 19010; tel. 610/525-5400; Mr. Loren Preheim
Renewal Centers, PO Box 107, Zionhill, PA 18981; tel. 215/536-9070; Mr. Charles Beem
Richard J. Caron Foundation, PO Box A, Wernersville, PA 19565-0501; tel. 610/678-2332; Mr. Douglas D Tieman
Roxbury, PO Box L, Shippensburg, PA 17257; tel. 717/532-4217; Mr. Joseph Barszczewski
Salisbury House of Northeast Pennsylvania, Inc., 451 Lelugh Street, Allentown, PA 18103; tel. 610/428-2698; Dr. Paul Volosov
Sarah A. Reed Children's Center, 2445 West 34th Street, Erie, PA 16506; tel. 814/838-1954; Mr. John J Kovacs
Serenity Hall, Inc., 414 West Fifth Street, Erie, PA 16507; tel. 814/459-4775; Ms. Suzanne C Mack
Silver Springs - Martin Luther School, 512 West Township Line Road, Plymouth Meeting, PA 19462-1099; tel. 610/825-4440; Ruth W Bartelt
Southern Home Services, 3200 South Broad Street, Philadelphia, PA 19145-5899; tel. 215/334-4319; Mr. Gregory W Jones
St. John Vianney Hospital, 151 Woodbine Road, Downingtown, PA 19335-3057; tel. 610/269-2600; Mr. Thomas F Dugan
Stairways, 138 East 26th Street, Erie, PA 16504; tel. 814/453-5806; Mr. William F McCarthy
The Bradley Center, Inc., 3710 Saxonburg Boulevard, Pittsburgh, PA 15238; tel. 412/767-5306; Mr. Walter Goedeke
The Bridge, 8400 Pine Road, Philadelphia, PA 19111; tel. 215/342-5000; Ms. Star Weiss
The Mitchell Clinic, 1259 S Cedar Crest Boulevard, Suite 317, Allentown, PA 18103; tel. 610/435-9257; Dr. John F Mitchell
The Renfrew Center, Inc., 475 Spring Lane, Philadelphia, PA 19128; tel. 215/482-5353; Ms. Barbara Peterson
The Terraces, PO Box 729, Ephrata, PA 17522; tel. 717/859-4100; Ms. Patricia Bixler
TODAY, Inc., PO Box 908, New Town, PA 18940; tel. 215/968-4713; Mr. John E Howell
UHS Recovery Foundation, Inc., 2001 Providence Avenue, Chester, PA 19013-5504; tel. 610/876-9000; Mr. Jimmy Patton
Westmeade Center Warwick, 940 W Valley Road–Ste. 2102, Wayne, PA 19087; tel. 215/491-9400; Mr. Thomas T Fleming
White Deer Run, Inc., Devitt Camp Road, Allenwood, PA 17810-0097; tel. 570/538-2567; Mr. Stephen T Wicke
Wordsworth Human Services, Pennsylvania Avenue and Camp Hill Road, Fort Washington, PA 19034; tel. 215/635-6600; Dr. Jerome Gibbs

RHODE ISLAND

Alternatives, 350 Duncan Drive, Providence, RI 02906; tel. 401/453-4742; Dr. Yitzhak Bakal
CODAC Treatment Centers, Inc., 1052 Park Avenue, Cranston, RI 02910; tel. 401/461-5056; Mr. Craig S Stenning
Community Counseling Center, 101 Bacon Street, Pawtucket, RI 02860; tel. 401/722-5573; Mr. Richard H LeClerc
East Bay Mental Health Center, Inc., 52 Amaral Street, East Providence, RI 02915; tel. 401/431-9875; Mr. John P Digits, Jr.
Fellowship Health Resources, Inc., 25 Blackstone Valley Place, Suite 300, Lincoln, RI 02865-1163; tel. 401/333-3980; Mr. Joseph F Dziobek
Mental Health Services of Cranston, Johnston, 1443 Hartford Avenue, Johnston, RI 02919-3236; tel. 401/553-1000; Mr. Richard H Leclerc
Newport County Community Mental Health Center, Inc., 127 Johnnycake Hill Road, Middletown, RI 02842; tel. 401/846-1213; Mr. J Clement Cicilline
Riverwood Rehabilitation Services, Inc., PO Box 897, Bristol, RI 02809; tel. 401/253-1812; Mr. Daniel Kubas-Meyer
South Shore Mental Health Center, Inc., PO Box 899, Charlestown, RI 02813; tel. 401/364-7705; Mr. Richard C Antonelli
The Providence Center for Counseling & Psychiatric Svcs, 520 Hope Street, Providence, RI 02906; tel. 401/276-4000; Mr. Charles E Maynard
Tri-Hab, Inc., 58 Hamlet Avenue, Woonsocket, RI 02895; tel. 401/765-4040; Mr. David Spencer

SOUTH CAROLINA

Lexington County Community Mental Health Center, 301 Palmetto Park Blvd, Lexington, SC 29072; tel. 803/996-1500; Dr. Louis H Muzekari
New Hope Treatment Centers, Inc., 225 Midland Parkway, Summerville, SC 29485; tel. 843/851-5010; Mr. William E Turner, III
Southbridge Center, 7901 Farrow Road, Building 1, Columbia, SC 29202-0041; tel. 803/935-0663; Mr. Michael J Cavanaugh
York Place Episcopal Church Home for Children, 234 Kings Mountain Street, York, SC 29745; tel. 803/684-8005; Mr. Steve Polak

SOUTH DAKOTA

Black Hills Children's Home, 24100 South Rockerville Road, Rapid City, SD 57701-9277; tel. 605/343-5422; Mr. David P Loving
Keystone Treatment Center, PO Box 159, Canton, SD 57013; tel. 605/987-5659; Ms. Carol Regier
Sioux Falls Children's Home, PO Box 1749, Sioux Falls, SD 57101-1749; tel. 605/334-6004; Mr. David P Loving

TENNESSEE

Academy for Academic Excellence, PO Box 3906, Clarksville, TN 37043; tel. 931/647-9831; Ms. Mercy E Yrabedra
Agency for Youth and Family Development, 5050 Poplar Avenue, Suite 525, Memphis, TN 38137; tel. 901/682-6775; Mr. Donnie Houpt
Buffalo Valley, Inc., PO Box 879, Hohenwald, TN 38462; tel. 931/796-5427; Mr. Jerry T Risner
Camelot Care Center, Inc., 102 Woodmont Blvd Suite 450, Nashville, TN 37205; tel. 615/386-6755; Mr. James V Doramus
Camelot Care Center, Inc., 667 – B Emory Valley Road, Oak Ridge, TN 37830; tel. 423/220-8927; Mr. James V Doramus
Child and Family Services of Knox County, Inc., 901 East Summit Hill Drive, Knoxville, TN 37915; tel. 423/524-7483; Mr. Charles E Gentry
Compass Intervention Center, LLC, 7900 Lowrance Road, Memphis, TN 38125; tel. 901/758-2002; Mr. Jack Bice
Cornerstone of Recovery, 1120 Topside Road, Louisville, TN 37777; tel. 423/970-7747; Mr. Dan R Caldwell
Council for Alcohol and Drug Abuse Services, Inc., PO Box 4797, Chattanooga, TN 37405; tel. 423/756-7644; Mr. James F Marcotte
Cumberland Heights, PO Box 90727, Nashville, TN 37209; tel. 615/353-1757; Mr. James B Moore
Daybreak Treatment Center, 2262 Germantown Road South, Germantown, TN 38138; tel. 901/753-4300; Ms. Tina C Mills
FHC – Cumberland Hall of Chattanooga, 7351 Standifer Gap Road, Chattanooga, TN 37421; tel. 423/499-9007; Mr. Charles A Dickens
Greene Valley Developmental Center, PO Box 910, Greeneville, TN 37744-0910; tel. 423/787-6800; Dr. Henry C Meece
Jackson Academy, LLC, 222 Church Street, Dickson, TN 37055; tel. 615/446-3900; Dr. Lindley Murray, III
Ridgeview Psychiatric Hospital and Center, Inc., 240 West Tyrone Road, Oak Ridge, TN 37830; tel. 423/482-1076; Mr. Robert J Benning
The Chad Youth Enhancement Center, 1751 Oak Plains Road, Ashland City, TN 37015; tel. 931/362-4723; Dr. Robert D Glasner
Three Springs Outdoor Therapeutic Program, PO Box 297, Centerville, TN 37033; tel. 615/729-5040; Ms. Susan Hardy
Youth Villages, 2890 Bekemeyer Drive, Arlington, TN 38002; tel. 901/252-7200; Mr. Patrick W Lawler

TEXAS

Alternatives Centre for Behavioral Health, 5001 Alabama Street, El Paso, TX 79930; tel. 915/565-4800; Ms. Carol J Anderson
Austin Child Guidance Center, 810 West 45th Street, Austin, TX 78751; tel. 512/451-2242; Dr. Donald J Zappone
Burke Center, 4101 South Medford Drive, Lufkin, TX 75901-5699; tel. 936/639-1141; Ms. Susan Rushing
Camelot Care Centers, Inc., 7400 Blanco Road, Suite 123, San Antonio, TX 78216; tel. 210/348-8801; Mr. James V Doramus
Canyon Lakes Residential Treatment Center, 2402 Canyon Lake Drive, Lubbock, TX 79415; tel. 806/762-5782; Dr. Ray H Brown
Cedar Crest Hospital & RTC, 3500 South IH-35, Belton, TX 76513; tel. 254/939-2100; Mr. Richard N Rickey
Child Study Center, 1300 West Lancaster, Fort Worth, TX 76102; tel. 817/336-8611; Dr. Joyce E Mauk
Continuum, 8455 Fannin, Suite A-1, Houston, TX 77054-4816; tel. 713/383-0888; Ms. Barbara Candley
Continuum Healthcare System, Inc., 260 N Sam Houston Parkway E, Suite 300, Houston, TX 77060; tel. 281/260-0799; Mr. Don R Johnson
DePelchin Children's Center, 100 Sandman, Houston, TX 77007; tel. 713/861-8136; Dr. Curtis C Mooney
Family Service Center, 2707 North Loop West, Ste 520, Houston, TX 77008; tel. 713/868-4466; Mr. Lloyd H Sidwell
Houston Preferred Care, Inc., 6614 Hornwood, Houston, TX 77074; tel. 713/270-8000; Mr. Darron Broadus
La Hacienda Treatment Center, PO Box 1, Hunt, TX 78024; tel. 830/238-4222; Dr. Frank J Sadlack
Life Resource, 2750 South 8th Street, Beaumont, TX 77701; tel. 409/839-1000; Dr. N. Charles Harris
Meridell Achievement Center, PO Box 87, Liberty Hill, TX 78642; tel. 512/515-6650; Ms. Patricia Mitchell
New Dimensions, 18333 Egret Bay Blvd, Ste 560, Houston, TX 77058; tel. 281/333-2284; Dr. Larry M Nahmias
New Horizons of Corpus Christi, 4455 South Padre Island Drive, Suite 50, Corpus Christi, TX 78411; tel. 361/853-9355; Ms. Jacqueline Ungerleider
New View Partial Hospitalization Centre, Inc., 4310 Dowlen Road – Suite 13, Beaumont, TX 77706; tel. 409/892-0009; Dr. D. Sue Horne
Paul Meier New Life Day Hospital and Outpatient Clinic, 2071 North Collins Boulevard, Richardson, TX 75080; tel. 972/437-4698; Ms. Jacquelyn Williams
River Oaks Day Hospital, 10600 Richmond Avenue, Houston, TX 77042; tel. 713/783-7200; Dr. Sandra E Phares
San Marcos Treatment Center, 120 Bert Brown Road, San Marcos, TX 78666; tel. 512/396-8500; Mr. Mack Wigley
Shiloh Treatment Center, Inc., 3926 Bahler Street, Manvel, TX 77578; tel. 281/489-1290; Dr. Brenda Gardner
Shoreline, Inc., PO Box 68, Taft, TX 78390; tel. 361/528-3356; Dr. Sharel Zacharias
Starlite Village Hospital, PO Box 317, Center Point, TX 78010-0317; tel. 830/634-2212; Mr. John Lacy
Summer Sky, Inc., 1100 McCart Street, Stephenville, TX 76401; tel. 254/968-2907; Mr. Al Conlan
Sundown Ranch, Inc., Route 4, Box 182, Canton, TX 75103; tel. 903/479-3933; Mr. Richard Boardman

Providers / JCAHO Accredited Freestanding Mental Health Care Organizations

The Oaks Treatment Center, Inc, 1407 West Stassney Lane, Austin, TX 78745; tel. 512/464-0400; Mr. Mack Wigley
The Patrician Movement, 222 East Mitchell Street, San Antonio, TX 78210; tel. 210/532-3126; Dr. Patrick Clancey
Upward Reach Residential Treatment Center, 1120 Cypress Station Drive, Houston, TX 77090; tel. 281/893-7200; Mr. Darrell M Koch
Waco Center for Youth, 3501 North 19th Street, Waco, TX 76708; tel. 254/745-5121; Mr. Stephen R Anfinson

UTAH
Blue Mountain Family Center / Wilderness Quest, PO Box 12, Monticello, UT 84535; tel. 435/587-2801; Mr. Larry Wells
Brightway at St. George, 115 West, 1470 South, St. George, UT 84770; tel. 435/673-0303; Ms. Sherry Shake
Center for Change, Inc., 1790 North State Street, Orem, UT 84057; tel. 801/224-8255; Dr. Michael E Berrett
Cinnamon Hills Youth Crisis Center, 770 East St. George Boulevard, St George, UT 84770; tel. 435/674-0984; Mr. Jim Downey
Copper Hills Youth Center, 5899 West Rivendell Drive, West Jordan, UT 84088; tel. 801/561-3377; Mr. David Damshen
Heritage School, 5600 N. Heritage School Drive, Provo, UT 84604; tel. 801/226-4600; Mr. Gerald H Spanos
Highland Ridge Hospital, 175 West 7200 South, Midvale, UT 84047; tel. 801/272-9851; Mr. Richard Bell
Island View Residential Treatment Center, 2650 West 2700 South, Syracuse, UT 84075; tel. 801/773-0200; Dr. Jared U Balmer
New Haven, Post Office Box 50238, Provo, UT 84605; tel. 801/794-1218; Mr. Mark McGregor
Provo Canyon School, PO Box 1441, Provo, UT 84603; tel. 801/227-2100; Mr. Jeffrey R Smith
Sorenson's Ranch School, Inc., Box 440219, Koosharem, UT 84744; tel. 435/638-7318; Mr. Shane Sorenson
Vista Adolescent Treatment Center, PO Box 69, Magna, UT 84044; tel. 801/250-9762; Mr. H. Matthew Dixon, Jr.
Youth Care of Utah, Inc., PO Box 909, Draper, UT 84020; tel. 801/572-6989; Ms. Robin P Stephens

VIRGINIA
Alice C. Tyler Village of Childhelp East, 23164 Dragoon Road, Lignum, VA 22726; tel. 540/399-1926; Mr. Edward J Murphy
DeJarnette Center, PO Box 2309, Staunton, VA 24402-2309; tel. 540/332-2100; Mr. William J Tuell
Graydon Manor, 801 Children's Center Road, SW, Leesburg, VA 20175-2598; tel. 703/777-3485; Mr. Bernard J Haberlein
Inova Comprehensive Addiction Treatment Services, 3300 Gallows Road, Falls Church, VA 22046-3300; tel. 703/698-1530; Mr. Steven E Brown
Inova Kellar Center, 10396 Democracy Lane, Fairfax, VA 22030; tel. 703/218-8500; Dr. Richard Leichtweis
Marion Correctional Treatment Center, PO Box 1027, Marion, VA 24354-1027; tel. 540/783-7154; Mr. Kenneth L Osborne
Mount Regis Center, 405 Kimball Avenue, Salem, VA 24153; tel. 540/389-4761; Ms. Gail S Basham
The Barry Robinson Center, 443 Kempsville Road, Norfolk, VA 23502; tel. 757/455-6100; Mr. Thomas D Pittman
The Life Center of Galax, PO Box 27, Galax, VA 24333; tel. 540/236-2994; Ms. Tina R Bullins
The Pines Residential Treatment Center, 825 Crawford Parkway, Portsmouth, VA 23704; tel. 757/393-0061; Ms. Debra Goldstein
Williamsburg Place, 5477 Mooretown Road, Williamsburg, VA 23188; tel. 757/565-0106; Mr. Thomas Brennan

WASHINGTON
Pearl Street Center / Comprehensive Mental Health, 815 South Pearl Street, Tacoma, WA 98465; tel. 253/396-5930; Dr. Michael K Laederich
Seattle Children's Home, 2142 Tenth Avenue West, Seattle, WA 98119; tel. 206/83-3300; Mr. R. David Cousineau
Seattle Mental Health, 1600 East Olive Street, Seattle, WA 98122; tel. 206/324-2400; Mr. David Stone
Spokane Mental Health, 107 South Division, Spokane, WA 99202; tel. 509/838-4651; Mr. David Panken
SunHealth Youth Treatment Center, 6911 226th Place Southwest, Mountlake Terrace, WA 98043; tel. 425/672-9323; Mr. David Watkins
Tamarack Center, 2901 W Ft. George Wright Drive, Spokane, WA 99204; tel. 509/326-8100; Mr. Tim Davis
The Martin Center, 2806 Douglas Avenue, Bellingham, WA 98225; tel. 360/676-2187; Ms. Gail A Estes
Valley Cities Counseling and Consultation, 2704 'I' Street Northeast, Auburn, WA 98002; tel. 206/833-7444; Ms. Marilyn La Celle

WEST VIRGINIA
Elkins Mountain School, 100 Bell Street, Elkins, WV 26241; tel. 304/637-8000; Ms. Carolyn J Yokum
Olympic Center – Preston, Inc., PO Box 158, Kingwood, WV 26537; tel. 304/329-2400; Ms. Arlene Glover
Shawnee Hills, Inc., PO Box 3698, Charleston, WV 25336-3698; tel. 304/341-0511; Ms. Martha Eades
Worthington Center, Inc., 3199 Core Road, Parkersburg, WV 26104; tel. 304/485-0082; Dr. Lance McCoy

WISCONSIN
Family Services Lakeshore, Inc, 333 Reed Avenue, Manitowoc, WI 54220; tel. 920/686-8608; Mr. Thomas Aronson
Libertas Treatment Center, 1701 Dousman Street, Green Bay, WI 54303; tel. 920/498-8600; Mr. David B Fish

WYOMING
Cathedral Home for Children, PO Box 520, Laramie, WY 82073; tel. 307/745-8997; Mr. David R Christiansen
Normative Services, Inc., PO Box 3075, Sheridan, WY 82801; tel. 307/674-6878; Ms. Julia George
St. Joseph's Children's Home, PO Box 1117, Torrington, WY 82240; tel. 307/532-4197; Mr. Robert C Mayor
Wyoming Recovery Program for Addictions, LLC, 231 South Wilson, Casper, WY 82601; tel. 307/265-3791; Ms. Carolyn Toews

U.S. Associated Areas

APO/AE
Wellness Branch, ODCSPER, USAREUR 7 Army 1 (Belgium), Hammonds Barracks, Bldg 968 Room 213 – Badenerplatz 1, APO, AE 09014; tel. 011/496-2148; Dr. G. Ed Browning

PUERTO RICO
Clinica Interdisciplinaria de Psiquiatria Avanzada, 650 Lloveras Cond Centro Plaza Suite 101, San Juan, PR 00909-2113; tel. 787/721-4020; Dr. Carlos A Caban
Instituto Psicoterapeutico de Puerto Rico, Ave Hostos 431, 433, 435, Hato Rey, PR 00919; tel. 787/753-9515; Dr. Alberto Varela

JCAHO Accredited Freestanding Substance Abuse Organizations

The accredited freestanding substance abuse programs listed have been accredited as of March, 2000 by the Joint Commission on Accreditation of Healthcare Organizations by decision of the Accreditation Committee of the Board of Commissioners.

The organizations listed here have been found to be in compliance with the Joint Commission standards for substance abuse organizations, as found in the Accreditation Manual for Mental Health, Chemical Dependency, and Mental Retardation/Developmental Disabilities Services.

Please refer to section A of the AHA Guide for information on hospitals with inpatient and/or outpatient alcohol and chemical dependency services. These hospitals are identified by Facility Codes F2 and F3. In section A, those hospitals identified by Approval Code 1 are JCAHO accredited.

We present this list simply as a convenient directory. Inclusion or omission of any organization's name indicates neither approval nor disapproval by Health Forum LLC, an American Hospital Association company.

United States

ALABAMA
Behavioral Healthcare Center, 306 Paul W Bryant Drive East, Tuscaloosa, AL 35401; tel. 205/349-1033; Karima Nasrat
Bradford Health Services – Huntsville, 1600 Browns Ferry Road, Madison, AL 35758; tel. 256/461-7272; Mr. Robert S Hinds
Bradford Health Services – Warrior, PO Box 129, Warrior, AL 35180; tel. 205/647-1945; Mr. Roy M Ramsey

ALASKA
Akeela Treatment Services, Inc, 2805 Bering Street, Suite 4, Anchorage, AK 99503; tel. 907/561-5206; Mr. Robert P Galea
Alaska North Addictions Recovery Center, 4330 Bragaw Street, Anchorage, AK 99508; tel. 907/561-5537; Ms. Gloria O'Neill
Anchorage Charter North Counseling Center, 1650 South Bragaw, Anchorage, AK 99508; tel. 907/258-7575; Ms. Kathleen Cronen

ARIZONA
Arizona's Children Association, PO Box 7277, Tucson, AZ 85725-7277; tel. 520/622-7611; Mr. Fred J Chaffee
Calvary Rehabilitation Center, 720 East Montebello Avenue, Phoenix, AZ 85014; tel. 602/279-1468; Mr. Jeffrey Shook
Chandler Valley Hope, PO Box 1839, Chandler, AZ 85244-1839; tel. 602/899-3335; Mr. Dennis Gilhousen
Cottonwood de Tucson, 4110 West Sweetwater Drive, Tucson, AZ 85745; tel. 520/743-0411; Mr. Ronald B Welch
META Services, Inc., 2701 N. 16th St., Suite 106, Phoenix, AZ 85006; tel. 602/650-1212; Mr. Eugene Johnson
Parc Place, 5116 East Thomas Road, Phoenix, AZ 85018; tel. 602/840-4774; Mr. Gene Cavallo
PREHAB of Arizona, Inc., PO Drawer 5860, Mesa, AZ 85211-5860; tel. 602/969-4024; Mr. Michael T Hughes
Rosewood Ranch L.P., 36075 South Rincon Road, Wickenburg, AZ 85390; tel. 520/684-9594; Ms. Margaret Allen
Sierra Tucson,LLC, 39580 S. Lago del Oro Parkway, Tucson, AZ 85739; tel. 520/624-4000; Mr. Terry A Stephens
Superstition Mountain Mental Health Center, Inc., PO Box 3160, Apache Junction, AZ 85217; tel. 602/983-0065; Mr. Gary W Selvy
the EXCEL Group, 106 East First Street, Yuma, AZ 85364; tel. 520/329-8995; Mr. Michael P Puthoff
The Guidance Center, Inc., 2187 North Vickey Street, Flagstaff, AZ 86004; tel. 520/527-1899; Mr. J. Michael Thompson
The Meadows, 1655 North Tegner, Wickenburg, AZ 85390; tel. 520/684-3926; Mr. James P Mellody
The New Foundation, P O Box 3828, Scottsdale, AZ 85257; tel. 602/945-3302; Mr. David S Hedgcock
Verde Valley Guidance Clinic, Inc., 600 South Willard Street, Cottonwood, AZ 86326; tel. 520/634-2236; Mr. Robert D Cartia
Vista Care Facility, 4120 East Ramsey Road, Hereford, AZ 85615; tel. 520/378-6466; Mr. Siamak Khadjenoury

ARKANSAS
Ozark Counseling Services, Inc, PO Box 1776, Mountain Home, AR 72654-1776; tel. 870/425-7929; Mr. John C Greer
Ozark Guidance Center, Inc., PO Box 6430, Springdale, AR 72762-6430; tel. 501/750-2020; Dr. David L Williams
University of Arkansas for Medical Sciences, 4301 West Markham Street, Mail Slot 554, Little Rock, AR 72205; tel. 501/686-5483; Dr. Frederick G Guggenheim

CALIFORNIA
Betty Ford Center, 39000 Bob Hope Drive, Rancho Mirage, CA 92270; tel. 760/773-4100; Mr. John T Schwarzlose
Cornerstone of Southern California, 13682 Yorba Street, Tustin, CA 92680; tel. 714/730-5399; Ms. Lynda Klinger
Impact Drug and Alcohol Treatment Center, 1680 North Fair Oaks Avenue, Pasadena, CA 91103; tel. 818/798-0884; Mr. James M Stillwell
Kings View Center, 42675 Road 44, Reedley, CA 93654; tel. 559/638-2505; Mr. Mike Waters
R House, Inc., PO Box 2587, Santa Rosa, CA 95405; tel. 707/539-2948; Ms. Mimi G Donohue
S T E P S, 224 East Clara Street, Port Hueneme, CA 93041; tel. 805/488-6424; Mr. Charles D Morris
Sharp Vista Pacifica, 7989 Linda Vista Road, San Diego, CA 92111; tel. 858/576-1200; Dr. Daniel R Valentine
Spencer Recovery Centers, Inc., PO Box 118, Monrovia, CA 91017; tel. 949/376-3705; Mr. Christopher C Spencer
Tarzana Treatment Center, Inc., 18646 Oxnard Street, Tarzana, CA 91356; tel. 818/996-1051; Mr. Albert Senella
The Discovery Adolescent Program, 4136 Ann Arbor Road, Lakewood, CA 90712; tel. 562/425-6918; Dr. Craig M Brown
Twin Town Treatment Center, 10741 Los Alamitos Boulevard, Los Alamitos, CA 90720; tel. 562/594-8844; Mr. David Lisonbee
Vista San Diego Center, 3003 Armstrong Street, San Diego, CA 92111; tel. 619/268-3343; Ms. Judith K Williams
Watts Health Foundation, Inc., 10300 South Compton Avenue, Los Angeles, CA 90002; tel. 323/564-4331; Dr. Clyde W Oden

COLORADO
Harmony Foundation, Inc., PO Box 1989, Estes Park, CO 80517; tel. 970/586-4491; Mr. Donald R Hays
Managed Adolescent Care, PC, 1025 Pennock, Suite 111, Fort Collins, CO 80524; tel. 970/495-8860; Mr. Ken Henschke
Parker Valley Hope, PO Box 670, Parker, CO 80134; tel. 303/841-7857; Mr. Dennis Gilhousen
Pikes Peak Mental Health Center Systems, Inc., 220 Ruskin Drive, Colorado Springs, CO 80910; tel. 719/572-6100; Mr. Charles J Vorwaller

CONNECTICUT
Community Mental Health Affiliates, Inc., 300 Main Street, Bristol, CT 06010; tel. 860/583-9954; Dr. Mark Muradian
Community Prevention and Addiction Services, Inc., 1491 West Main Street, Willimantic, CT 06226; tel. 860/456-3215; Ms. Leanne M Dillian
Cornerstone of Eagle Hill, Inc., 32 Alberts Hill Road, Sandy Hook, CT 06482; tel. 203/426-8085; Mr. Norman J Sokolow
Greater Bridgeport Community Mental Health Center, 1635 Central Avenue, Bridgeport, CT 06610; tel. 203/551-7449; Mr. James Pisciotta
LMG Programs, Inc., 4 Elmcrest Terrace, Norwalk, CT 06850; tel. 203/325-1511; Mr. Robert Rimmer
Perception Programs, Inc., PO Box 407, Willimantic, CT 06226; tel. 860/450-7122; M. Deborah Walsh
Reid Treatment Center, Inc., PO Box 1357, Avon, CT 06001-1357; tel. 203/673-6115; Mr. Mark Muradian
Rushford Center Inc., 1250 Silver Street, Middletown, CT 06457; tel. 860/346-0300; Mr. Jeffrey L Walter
Stonington Institute, 75 Swantown Hill Road, North Stonington, CT 06359; tel. 860/535-1010; Mr. Michael J Angelides
The Children's Center, Inc., 1400 Whitney Avenue, Hamden, CT 06517; tel. 203/248-2116; Mr. Anthony DelMastro
The Wellspring Foundation, Inc., 21 Arch Bridge Road, Bethlehem, CT 06751; tel. 203/266-7235; Dr. Richard E Beauvais
The Wheeler Clinic, 91 Northwest Drive, Plainville, CT 06062; tel. 860/793-3500; Dr. David Berkowitz
United Services, Inc., Post Office Box 839, Dayville, CT 06241; tel. 860/774-2020; Mr. Theodore L Ver Haagh
Vitam Center, Inc., 57 W Rocks Road, Norwalk, CT 06851-0730; tel. 203/846-2091; Dr. Leonard A Kenowitz

DELAWARE
Brandywine Counseling, Inc., 2713 Lancaster Avenue, Wilmington, DE 19805; tel. 302/656-2348; Ms. Sara T Allshouse
Connections Community Support Programs, Inc., 500 West 10th Street, Wilmington, DE 19801; tel. 302/984-3380; Ms. Catherine Devaney McKay
Open Door, Incorporated, 3301 Green Street, Claymont, DE 19703; tel. 302/798-9555; Mr. Albert Meyer
SODAT – Delaware, Inc., 625 North Orange Street, Wilmington, DE 19801; tel. 302/656-4044; Mr. Thomas C Maloney

FLORIDA
Act Corporation, 1220 Willis Avenue, Daytona Beach, FL 32114; tel. 904/947-4270; Mr. J W Dreggors
Alcohol and Drug Abuse Services, 1211 Southeast Second Avenue, Fort Lauderdale, FL 33316; tel. 954/728-2704; Mr. Michael De Lucca
Alternatives In Treatment, Inc., 7601 North Federal Highway, Suite 100B, Boca Raton, FL 33487; tel. 561/998-0866; Mr. Jacob Frydman
Apalachee Center for Human Services, Inc., PO Box 1782, Tallahassee, FL 32302; tel. 850/487-2930; Mr. Ronald P Kirkland
Bayview Center for Mental Health, Inc., 12550 Biscayne Blvd, Suite 919, North Miami, FL 33181; tel. 305/892-4646; Mr. Robert S Ward
Beachcomber Rehab, Inc., 4493 North Ocean Boulevard, Delray Beach, FL 33483; tel. 561/734-1818; Mr. James A Bryan
Camelot Care Centers, Inc., 9160 Oakhurst Road Building One, Seminole, FL 33776; tel. 813/596-9960; Mr. James V Doramus
Charlotte Community Mental Health Services, Inc., 1700 Education Avenue, Punta Gorda, FL 33950; tel. 941/639-8300; Dr. Gerald N Ross
Coastal Recovery Centers, Inc., 3830 Bee Ridge Road, Sarasota, FL 34233; tel. 941/927-8900; Dr. Christine Cauffield

Providers / JCAHO Accredited Freestanding Substance Abuse Organizations

Creekside Retreat, Inc., 8889 Corporate Square Court, Jacksonville, FL 32216; tel. 904/725-7073; Dr. Joseph A Virzi

David Lawrence Center, 6075 Golden Gate Parkway, Naples, FL 34116; tel. 941/455-1031; Mr. David C Schimmel

Fairwinds Treatment Center, 1569 S Fort Harrison Avenue, Clearwater, FL 34616; tel. 813/449-0300; Mr. Mazhar K Al-Abed

Focus Healthcare of Florida, 5960 Southwest 106th Avenue, Cooper City, FL 33328; tel. 954/680-2700; Mr. Frank Fanella

Hanley-Hazelden Center at St. Mary's, 5200 East Avenue, West Palm Beach, FL 33407; tel. 561/841-1000; Mr. Jerry Singleton

Lakeside Alternatives, Inc., 434 West Kennedy Boulevard, Orlando, FL 32810; tel. 407/875-3700; Mr. Duane Zimmerman

Lakeview Center, Inc., 1221 West Lakeview Avenue, Pensacola, FL 32501; tel. 850/432-1222; Dr. Morris L Eaddy

Lifeskills of Boca Raton, Inc., 7301 W Palmetto Park Road, Suite 108B, Boca Raton, FL 33433; tel. 561/392-1199; Dr. Gregory Mavrides

LifeStream Behavioral Center, PO Box 491000, Leesburg, FL 34749-1000; tel. 352/360-6575; Mr. Jack H Hargrove, Jr.

Manatee Glens Corporation, PO Box 9478, Bradenton, FL 34206-9478; tel. 941/741-3111; Ms. Mary Ruiz

Marion-Citrus Mental Health Centers, Inc., P.O. Box 771929, Ocala, FL 34474-1929; tel. 352/873-6500; Mr. Russell Rasco

Meridian Behavioral Healthcare, Inc., PO Box 141750, Gainesville, FL 32614; tel. 352/374-5600; Dr. Douglas L Starr

Operation PAR, Inc., 6655 66th Street North, Pinellas Park, FL 33781; tel. 727/545-7564; Ms. Shirley Coletti

Pathways to Recovery, Inc., 13132 Barwick Road, Delray Beach, FL 33445; tel. 561/496-7532; Mr. Lew Hoechstetter

Renaissance Institute of Palm Beach, Inc., 7000 N Federal Hwy, 2nd Floor, Boca Raton, FL 33487; tel. 561/241-7977; Mr. Sidney Goodman

South County Mental Health Center, Inc., 16158 South Military Trail, Delray Beach, FL 33484; tel. 561/637-1004; Mr. Joseph S Speicher

Stewart-Marchman Center for Chemical Dependency, Inc., 3875 Tiger Bay Road, Daytona Beach, FL 32124; tel. 904/947-1300; Dr. Ernest D Cantley

Tampa Bay Academy, 12012 Boyette Road, Riverview, FL 33569; tel. 813/677-6700; Mr. Edward C Hoefle

The Center for Alcohol and Drug Studies, Inc., 321 Northlake Blvd, Suite 214, North Palm Beach, FL 33408; tel. 561/848-1332; Mr. Donald K Mullaney

The Village South, Inc., 3180 Biscayne Boulevard, Miami, FL 33137; tel. 305/573-3784; Mr. Matthew Gissen

The Watershed, 3350 NW Boca Raton Boulevard, Suite A-28, Boca Raton, FL 33431; tel. 561/362-7116; Ms. Jackie Glass

The Willough at Naples, 9001 Tamiami Trail East, Naples, FL 34113; tel. 941/775-4500; Ms. Patricia Perfetto

Transitions Recovery Program, 1928 Northeast 154th Street, North Miami Beach, FL 33162; tel. 305/949-9001; Mr. Lee Barchan

Turning Point of Tampa, 5439 Beaumont Center Blvd, Suite 1010, Tampa, FL 33634; tel. 813/882-3003; Ms. Robin Piper

Twelve Oaks, 2068 Healthcare Avenue, Navarre, FL 32566; tel. 850/939-1200; Ms. Candance Henderson

Wellness Resource Center, Inc., 660 Linton Boulevard, Ste 112, Delray Beach, FL 33444; tel. 561/278-8411; Ms. Michele Michael

GEORGIA

Albany Area Community Service Board, PO Box 1988, Albany, GA 31701; tel. 912/430-4042; Dr. John C Burns, III

Behavioral Health Services of South Georgia, PO Box 3409 206 S. Patterson Street, Valdosta, GA 31604-3409; tel. 912/333-7095; Mr. W. David McCracken

Bridges Outpatient Center, Inc., 1209 Columbia Drive, Milledgeville, GA 31061; tel. 912/454-1727; Mr. James M Simmons

Brightmore Day Hospital, 115 Davis Road, Martinez, GA 30907; tel. 706/868-1735; Ms. Joy Beaird

Charter Behavioral Hlth System of Atlanta at Laurel Hgts, LL, 934 Briarcliff Road, Northeast, Atlanta, GA 30306; tel. 404/888-7860; Ms. Jewel W Norman

Cobb/Douglas Community Service Board, 361 North Marietta Parkway, Marietta, GA 30060; tel. 770/429-5000; Ms. Patricia A Redmond

Community Mental Health Center of East Central Georgia, 3421 Mike Padgett Highway, Augusta, GA 30906; tel. 706/771-4833; Mr. F. Campbell Peery

Community Service Board of Middle Georgia, 2121A Bellevue Road, Dublin, GA 31021-2998; tel. 912/272-1190; Ms. Patsy H Thomas

DeKalb Community Service Board, PO Box 1648, Decatur, GA 30031; tel. 404/294-3836; Dr. R. Derril Gay

Fulton County Dept of Mental Health, Mental Retardation/SA, 141 Pryor Street, SW, Ste 4035, Atlanta, GA 30303; tel. 404/730-0210; Wyeuca B Johnson

Gateway Community Service Board, 1609 Newcastle Street, Brunswick, GA 31520; tel. 912/267-0760; Ms. Susan Broome

Georgia Pines Community Service Board, PO Box 1659, Thomasville, GA 31799; tel. 912/225-4335; Mr. Robert H Jones, Jr.

McIntosh Trail MH/MR/SA Community Service Board, PO Box 1320, Griffin, GA 30224; tel. 770/358-8250; Ms. Cathy Johnson

Metro Atlanta Recovery Residences, Inc., 2801 Clearview Place, Doraville, GA 30340; tel. 770/457-1222; Mr. Douglas Brush

New Horizons Community Service Board, PO Box 5328, Columbus, GA 31906-0328; tel. 706/596-5581; Mr. Perry Alexander

Oconee Center, PO Box 1827, Milledgeville, GA 31061; tel. 912/445-4817; Mr. John W Prather

Ogeechee Behavioral Health Services, PO Box 1259, Swainsboro, GA 30401; tel. 912/289-2522; Mr. J. Frank Brantley

River Edge Behavioral Health Center, 175 Emery Highway, Macon, GA 31217; tel. 912/751-4586; Mr. Frank Fields

Talbott Recovery Campus, 5448 Yorktowne Drive, Atlanta, GA 30349; tel. 770/994-0185; Mr. Benjamin H Underwood

Tidelands Community Service Board, PO Box 23407, Savannah, GA 31403-3407; tel. 912/651-2171; Mr. Malcolm D Strickler

Turning Point Hospital, PO Box 1177, Moultrie, GA 31768; tel. 912/985-4815; Mr. Ben Marion

Willingway Hospital, 311 Jones Mill Road, Statesboro, GA 30458; tel. 912/764-6236; Mr. Jimmy Mooney

IDAHO

Sun Behavioral System for Boise, 8050 Northview Street, Boise, ID 83704; tel. 208/327-0504; Mr. Gregory P Hassakis

Walker Center, 1120A Montana Street, Gooding, ID 83330; tel. 208/934-8461; Dr. Douglas Smith

ILLINOIS

Alexian Brothers Behavioral Health Resources, 901 Biesterfield Road Suite 400, Elk Grove Village, IL 60007; tel. 847/437-5500; Mr. T J Vaughan

Association House of Chicago, 1116 North Kedzie Ave, Chicago, IL 60651; tel. 773/772-7170; Ms. Harriet Sadauskas

Aunt Martha's Youth Service Center, Inc., 4343 Lincoln Highway, Ste 340, Matteson, IL 60443; tel. 708/747-2701; Mr. C. Gary Leofanti

Ben Gordon Center, 12 Health Services Drive, De Kalb, IL 60115; tel. 815/756-4875; Mr. James W Graves

Chestnut Health Systems, 1003 Martin Luther King Drive, Bloomington, IL 61701; tel. 309/827-6026; Mr. Russell J Hagen

Community Counseling Center of Northern Madison County, Inc., 2615 Edwards Street, Alton, IL 62002; tel. 618/462-4883; Ms. Debra Sloan

Community Counseling Center of the Fox Valley, Inc., 400 Mercy Lane, Aurora, IL 60506; tel. 630/897-0584; Ms. Elaine M Hegy

Community Counseling Centers of Chicago, 4740 North Clark Street, Chicago, IL 60640-4633; tel. 773/769-0205; Dr. Anthony A Kopera

Community Mental Health Center of Fulton & McDonough Countie, 229 Martin Avenue, Canton, IL 61520; tel. 309/647-1881; Ms. Debra Dix

Comprehensive Mental Health Center of St. Clair County, 3911 State Street, East Saint Louis, IL 62205; tel. 618/482-7330; Ms. Delores S Ray

Counseling Center of Lake View, 3225 North Sheffield Avenue, Chicago, IL 60657; tel. 773/549-5886; Mr. Norman J Groetzinger

Family Service and Community Mental Health Center/McHenry, 5320 West Elm Street, Mc Henry, IL 60050; tel. 815/385-6400; Mr. Robert M Martens

Gateway Youth Care Foundation, 819 South Wabash, Suite 300, Chicago, IL 60605; tel. 312/663-1130; Mr. Michael Darcy

Heartland Human Services, PO Box 1047, Effingham, IL 62401; tel. 217/347-7179; Ms. Cheryl Compton

Heritage Behavioral Health Center, Inc., P.O. Box 710, Decatur, IL 62524-2820; tel. 217/362-6262; Mr. Grady L Wilkinson

Human Service Center, PO Box 1346, Peoria, IL 61654-1346; tel. 309/671-8000; Mr. Michael G Kennedy

Interventions – Du Page Adolescent Center, 11 S 250 Route 83, Hinsdale, IL 60521; tel. 630/325-5050; Ms. Leslie Balonick

Interventions – Southwood, 5701 South Wood, Chicago, IL 60636; tel. 773/737-4600; Ms. Leslie Balonick

Interventions – Woodridge, 2221 64th Street, Woodridge, IL 60517; tel. 630/968-6477; Ms. Leslie Balonick

Interventions City Girls, 140 North Ashland Avenue, Chicago, IL 60607; tel. 312/433-7777; Ms. Leslie Balonick

Josselyn Center for Mental Health, 405 Central Avenue, Northfield, IL 60093-3097; tel. 847/441-5600; Dr. John W Shustitzky

Lake County Health Department / Behavioral Health Services, 3012 Grand Avenue, Waukegan, IL 60085; tel. 847/360-6729; Mr. Dale W Galassie

Leyden Family Service and Mental Health Center, 10001 West Grand Avenue, Franklin Park, IL 60131; tel. 847/451-0330; Mr. Dennis P Vaccaro

McHenry County Youth Service Bureau, 101 South Jefferson Street, Woodstock, IL 60098; tel. 815/338-7360; Ms. Susan H Krause

North Central Behavioral Health Systems, Inc., PO Box 1488, La Salle, IL 61301; tel. 815/223-0160; Mr. Donald P Miskowiec

Perry County Counseling Center, Inc., 1016 S. Madison St. Suite A, Du Quoin, IL 62832; tel. 618/542-4357; Mr. John R Venskus

ProCare Centers, 1820 South 25th Avenue, Broadview, IL 60153; tel. 708/681-2324; Mr. J. Melvin Moore

Rosecrance on Alpine, 1505 North Alpine Road, Rockford, IL 61107; tel. 815/399-5351; Mr. Philip W Eaton

Rosecrance on Harrison, 3815 Harrison Avenue, Rockford, IL 61108; tel. 815/391-1000; Mr. Philip W Eaton

Sinnissippi Centers, Inc., 325 Illinois Route 2, Dixon, IL 61021; tel. 815/284-6611; Mr. James R Sarver

Sojourn House, Inc., 565 North Turner Avenue, Freeport, IL 61032; tel. 815/232-5121; Ms. Brenda J Bombard

Southeastern Illinois Counseling Centers, Inc., Drawer M, Olney, IL 62450; tel. 618/395-4306; Mr. Gary Robertson

Southern Illinois Regional Social Services, 604 East College, Suite 101, Carbondale, IL 62901; tel. 618/457-6703; Ms. Karen Frietag

Tazwood Center for Human Services, Inc., 1421 Valle Vista Boulevard, Pekin, IL 61554; tel. 309/347-5522; Mr. Robert J Moore

The South Suburban Council on Alcoholism and Substance Abuse, 1909 Cheker Square, East Hazel Crest, IL 60429; tel. 708/957-2854; Mr. Allen Sandusky

The Women's Treatment Center, 140 North Ashland Avenue, Chicago, IL 60607; tel. 312/850-0050; Dr. Jewell Oates

Triangle Center, 120 North 11th Street, Springfield, IL 62703-1002; tel. 217/544-9858; Mr. Stephen J Knox

White Oaks Companies of Illinois, 3400 New Leaf Lane, Peoria, IL 61614; tel. 309/692-6900; Dr. John F Gilligan

INDIANA

Adult and Child Mental Health Center, Inc., 8320 Madison Avenue, Indianapolis, IN 46227; tel. 317/882-5122; Mr. A Robert Dunbar

BehaviorCorp, 697 Pro-Med Lane, Carmel, IN 46032-5323; tel. 317/587-0500; Mr. Larry L Burch

Community Mental Health Center, Inc., 285 Bielby Road, Lawrenceburg, IN 47025; tel. 812/537-1302; Mr. Joseph D Stephens

Comprehensive Mental Health Services, Inc., 240 North Tillotson Avenue, Muncie, IN 47304; tel. 765/288-1928; Dr. Suzanne Gresham

Fairbanks Hospital, Inc., 8102 Clearvista Parkway, Indianapolis, IN 46256-4698; tel. 317/849-8222; Ms. Barbara Porter-Norris

Providers / JCAHO Accredited Freestanding Substance Abuse Organizations

Four County Counseling Center, 1015 Michigan Avenue, Logansport, IN 46947; tel. 219/722-5151; Mr. Laurence R Ulrich
Grant-Blackford Mental Health, Inc., 505 Wabash Avenue, Marion, IN 46952; tel. 765/662-3971; Mr. Paul G Kuczora
Hamilton Center, Inc, PO Box 4323, Terre Haute, IN 47804-0323; tel. 812/231-8271; Mr. Galen Goode
LaVerna Lodge, Inc., 1950 East Greyhound Pass, Suite 18, PMB 349, Carmel, IN 46033; tel. 317/867-4330; Mr. Martin Berg
LifeSpring Mental Health Services, 207 West 13th Street, Jeffersonville, IN 47130; tel. 812/283-4491; Mr. George E Hill
Madison Center, Inc., PO Box 80, South Bend, IN 46617; tel. 219/234-0061; Mr. Jack Roberts
Oaklawn, PO Box 809, Goshen, IN 46527-0809; tel. 219/537-2635; Mr. Harold C Loewen
Park Center, Inc., 909 East State Boulevard, Fort Wayne, IN 46805; tel. 219/481-2721; Mr. Paul D Wilson
Porter-Starke Services, Inc., 601 Wall Street, Valparaiso, IN 46383; tel. 219/531-3500; Mr. Lee E Grogg
Quinco Behavioral Health Systems, PO Box 628, Columbus, IN 47202-0628; tel. 888/348-7449; Dr. Robert J Williams
Sharing and Caring Community Mental Health Center, Inc., 2511 East 46th Street, Ste 0-1, Indianapolis, IN 46205; tel. 317/377-5300; Ms. Debra Henderson
South Central Community Mental Health Centers, Inc., 645 South Rogers Street, Bloomington, IN 47403; tel. 812/339-1691; Dr. Dennis Morrison
Southlake Center for Mental Health, 8555 Taft Street, Merrillville, IN 46410-6199; tel. 219/769-4005; Mr. Lee Strawhun
Southwestern Indiana Mental Health Center, Inc., 415 Mulberry Street, Evansville, IN 47713-1298; tel. 812/423-7791; Mr. John K Browning
Swanson Center, 450 St. John Road, Suite 501, Michigan City, IN 46360-7350; tel. 219/879-4621; Mr. Larry D Miller
Tara Treatment Center, Inc., 6231 South US 31, Franklin, IN 46131; tel. 812/526-2611; Ms. Ann Daugherty
The Center for Mental Health, Inc., PO Box 1258, Anderson, IN 46015; tel. 765/649-8161; Mr. C. Richard DeHaven
The Otis R. Bowen Center for Human Services, Inc., PO Box 497, Warsaw, IN 46581-0497; tel. 219/267-7169; Mr. Kurt Carlson
Tri-City Comprehensive Comm Mental Health Center Inc., 3903 Indianapolis Boulevard, East Chicago, IN 46312; tel. 219/398-7050; Mr. Robert Krumwied
Wabash Valley Hospital, Inc., 2900 North River Road, West Lafayette, IN 47906; tel. 765/463-2555; Mr. R. Craig Lysinger

IOWA
Children and Families of Iowa, 1111 University Avenue, Des Moines, IA 50314; tel. 515/288-1981; Mr. David Stout
Gordon Recovery Centers, Inc., 800 5th Street Suite 200, Sioux City, IA 51101; tel. 712/234-2300; Mr. Kermit A Dahlen
Hillcrest Family Services, PO Box 1160, Dubuque, IA 52001; tel. 319/583-7357; Mr. Gary L Gansemer

KANSAS
Atchison Valley Hope, PO Box 312, Atchison, KS 66002; tel. 913/367-1618; Mr. Dennis Gilhousen
Columbia Health Systems, Inc., 10114 West 105th Street, Suite 100, Overland Park, KS 66212; tel. 913/492-9876; Mr. Robert Reed
Jewish Family and Children Services, 5801 West 115th, Suite 103, Overland Park, KS 66211; tel. 913/327-8250; Dr. Todd Ephraim
Norton Valley Hope, PO Box 510, Norton, KS 67654; tel. 785/877-5101; Mr. Dennis Gilhousen

KENTUCKY
Adanta Behavioral Health Services, 259 Parkers Mill Road, Somerset, KY 42501; tel. 606/679-4782; Ms. Cathy Epperson
Bluegrass Regional Mental Health - Mental Retardation Bd, PO Box 11428, Lexington, KY 40575; tel. 606/253-1686; Mr. Joseph A Toy
Cumberland River Regional MH/MR Board, Inc., PO Box 568, Corbin, KY 40702; tel. 606/528-7010; Mr. Danny Jones
NorthKey Community Care, PO Box 2680, Covington, KY 41012; tel. 606/578-3252; Dr. Edward G Muntel

RiverValley Behavioral Health, PO Box 1637, Owensboro, KY 42302-1637; tel. 270/689-6500; Ms. Gayle DiCesare
Seven Counties Services, Inc., 101 W Muhammad Ali Boulevard, Louisville, KY 40202; tel. 502/589-8600; Dr. Howard F Bracco

LOUISIANA
Addiction Recovery Resources of New Orleans, 4836 Wabash Street, Suite 202, Metairie, LA 70001; tel. 504/837-9988; Mr. Franklin D Polk
CHARIS Community Mental Health Center, Inc., 8264 One Calais Avenue, Baton Rouge, LA 70809; tel. 504/767-8478; Ms. Carolyn Carroll
Crescent Community Care, Inc. dba Center for Better Living, 951 Gause Boulevard Suite 2, Slidell, LA 70458; tel. 504/641-0505; Eric Oleson
New Beginnings Of Opelousas Inc., 1692 Linwood Loop, Opelousas, LA 70570; tel. 318/942-1171; Mr. Kim Signorelli
Vermilion Hospital for Psychiatric and Addictive Med, 2520 North University Avenue, Lafayette, LA 70507; tel. 318/234-5614; Mr. William A Ferry

MAINE
Community Health and Counseling Services, PO Box 425, Bangor, ME 04402-0425; tel. 207/947-0366; Mr. Joseph H Pickering, Jr.

MARYLAND
Allegany County Health Department Addictions Program, PO Box 1745, Cumberland, MD 21501-1745; tel. 301/777-5680; Mr. Rodger D Simons
Ashley, Inc., PO Box 240, Havre de Grace, MD 21078; tel. 410/273-6600; Mr. Leonard Angus Dahl
Baltimore Behavioral Health, Inc, 200 South Arlington Avenue, Baltimore, MD 21223; tel. 410/962-7180; Ms. Sandra K Hill
Charter Behavioral Health Systems at Warwick Manor, 3680 Warwick Road, East New Market, MD 21631; tel. 410/943-8108; Mr. A. Jay Rimovsky
Crossroads Centers, Inc., 2 West Madison Street, Baltimore, MD 21201; tel. 410/752-6505; Ms. Barbara Q McKenna
Glass Substance Abuse Program, Inc., 821 N Eutaw Street, Suite 201, Baltimore, MD 21201; tel. 410/225-9185; Mr. Herman Jones
Hope House, PO Box 546, Crownsville, MD 21032; tel. 410/923-6700; Ms. Ruth A Hudicek
Hudson Health Services, Inc., PO Box 1096, Salisbury, MD 21802-1096; tel. 410/219-9000; Mr. Charles F Andrews
Maryland Treatment Centers, Inc., PO Box E, Emmitsburg, MD 21727; tel. 301/447-2361; Ms. Mary A Roby
New Life Addiction Counseling Services, Inc., 2528 Mountain Road, Suite 204, Pasadena, MD 21122; tel. 410/255-4475; Mr. Thomas S Porter
Oakview Treatment Center, 3635 Old Court Road, Suite 203, Pikesville, MD 21208-3906; tel. 410/461-9922; Mr. Ned Rubin
Partners in Recovery, 6509 North Charles Street, Baltimore, MD 21204; tel. 410/296-9747; Mr. Robert P Kowal
Pathways, 2620 Riva Road, Annapolis, MD 21401; tel. 410/573-5400; Ms. Martha Potter
Quarterway Houses, Inc., PO Box 31419, Baltimore, MD 21216-6119; tel. 410/233-0684; Dr. John E Hickey
Saint Luke Institute, Inc., 8901 New Hampshire Avenue, Silver Spring, MD 20903; tel. 301/445-7970; Mr. Stephen J Rossetti
Worcester County Health Department, PO Box 249, Snow Hill, MD 21863; tel. 410/632-1100; Ms. Deborah Goeller

MASSACHUSETTS
AdCare Hospital of Worcester, Inc., 107 Lincoln Street, Worcester, MA 01605-2499; tel. 508/799-9000; Mr. David W Hillis
Baldpate Hospital, Baldpate Road, Georgetown, MA 01833; tel. 978/352-2131; Ms. Lucille Batal
Cape Cod Alcoholism Intervention & Rehabilitation, PO Box 929, Falmouth, MA 02541; tel. 508/540-6550; Mr. Raymond V Tamasi
Center for Health and Human Services, Inc., PO Box 2097, New Bedford, MA 02745; tel. 508/995-5733; Ms. Jennifer Davis
High Point Treatment Center, Inc., 1233 State Road, Plymouth, MA 02360-5133; tel. 508/224-7701; Mr. Daniel S Mumbauer
Spectrum Health Systems, Inc., 100 Locke Drive, Marlborough, MA 01752; tel. 508/303-6878; Mr. Charles Faris

MICHIGAN
ACAC, Inc., 3949 Sparks Drive SE, Ste 103, Grand Rapids, MI 49546; tel. 616/957-5850; Mr. Michael R Durco
Advanced Counseling Services, P.C., 30700 Telegraph Rd. Ste 2560, Bingham Farms, MI 48025; tel. 248/203-1770; Dr. Arthur L Hughett
Antrim Kalkaska Community Mental Health, PO Box 220, Bellaire, MI 49615-0220; tel. 731/533-8619; Mr. Ross L Gibson
Auro Medical Center, 1711 South Woodward, Suite 102, Bloomfield Hills, MI 48302; tel. 248/335-1130; Ms. Sue Comer
Boniface Human Services, 25050 W Outer Drive, Suite 201, Lincoln Park, MI 48146; tel. 313/928-8940; Dr. Shara Johnson
Brighton Hospital, 12851 East Grand River, Brighton, MI 48116; tel. 810/227-1211; Mr. Ramon Royal
Catholic Services of Macomb, Inc., 15980 19 Mile Road, Clinton Township, MI 48038; tel. 810/416-2300; Mr. Thomas J Reed
Center For Behavior and Medicine, 2004 Hogback Road, Suite 16, Ann Arbor, MI 48105; tel. 313/677-0800; Dr. Gerard M Schmit
Center for Life Management, In, 3800 Woodward Avenue Suite 208, Detroit, MI 48201; tel. 313/831-1533; Ms. Wendie D Lee
Center of Behavioral Therapy, PC, 24453 Grand River Avenue, Detroit, MI 48219; tel. 313/592-1765; Mr. Hollis M Evans
Central Therapeutic Services, Inc., 17600 W Eight Mile Road, Ste 7, Southfield, MI 48075; tel. 248/559-4340; Dr. K. G Thimotheose
CHIP Counseling Center, 6777 U.S. 31 South, Charlevoix, MI 49720; tel. 231/547-6551; Mr. Scott L Hickman
City of Detroit Dept of Human Services/Drug Treatment Div, 5031 Grandy, Detroit, MI 48211; tel. 313/267-6695; Mr. William Warren
Clinton - Eaton - Ingham Community Mental Health Board, 808 Southland, Suite B, Lansing, MI 48910; tel. 517/346-8246; Mr. Robert Sheehan
Community Care Services, 26184 West Outer Drive, Lincoln Park, MI 48146; tel. 313/389-7525; Mr. William P Walsh
Comprehensive Services, Inc., 4630 Oakman Boulevard, Detroit, MI 48204; tel. 313/934-8400; Ms. Mary L Doss
DBA Spectrum Prevention & Treatment Services, 2301 Platt Road, Ann Arbor, MI 48104; tel. 734/971-7900; Susan Custer
Delta Family Clinic, 2303 East Amelith Road, Bay City, MI 48706; tel. 517/684-9313; Mr. Gary R West
Detroit Central City Community Mental Health, Inc., 10 Peterboro, Suite 208, Detroit, MI 48201; tel. 313/831-3160; Ms. Irva Faber-Bermudez
DOT Caring Centers, Inc., 3190 Hallmark Court, Saginaw, MI 48603-2107; tel. 517/790-3366; Mr. Christopher Zalba
Downriver Guidance Clinic, 13101 Allen Road, Southgate, MI 48195; tel. 734/287-1700; Mr. Leroy A Lott
Evergreen Counseling Centers, 6902 Chicago Road, Warren, MI 48092; tel. 810/268-4239; Mr. Donald L Warner
Fairlane Behavioral Services, 23400 Michigan Avenue, Ste P24, Dearborn, MI 48124; tel. 313/562-6730; Mr. Carlos P Ruiz
Gateway Services, 1910 Shaffer Road, Kalamazoo, MI 49001; tel. 616/382-9827; Ms. Lisa Martin
Growth Works Incorporated, PO Box 6115, Plymouth, MI 48170-0115; tel. 734/455-4095; Mr. Dale F Yagiela
Guest House for Women Religious, PO Box 420, Lake Orion, MI 48361; tel. 248/391-3100; Mr. Daniel Kidd
Hegira Programs, Inc., 8623 N Wayne Road, Suite 200, Westland, MI 48185; tel. 734/458-4601; Mr. Edward L Forry
Huron Valley Consultation Center, 955 W Eisenhower Circle, Ste B, Ann Arbor, MI 48103; tel. 734/662-6300; Dr. Joseph Meadows
Kairos Healthcare, Inc., 141 Harrow Lane, Saginaw, MI 48603; tel. 517/792-4357; Mr. Frederick E Wigen, Jr.
Lapeer County Community Mental Health Center, 1570 Suncrest Drive, Lapeer, MI 48446-1154; tel. 810/667-0500; Dr. Richard I Berman
Lapeer County Health Department, 1575 Suncrest Drive, Lapeer, MI 48446; tel. 810/667-0243; Mr. John D Niederhauser
Latino Family Services, Inc., 3815 West Fort Street, Detroit, MI 48216; tel. 313/841-7380; Ms. Amanda Caballero

Providers / JCAHO Accredited Freestanding Substance Abuse Organizations

London Brook Associates, PLC, 26677 West Twelve Mile Road, Suite 146, Southfield, MI 48034; tel. 248/391-0050; Ms. Debra Scheck
Meridian Professional Psychological Consultants, PC, 5031 Park Lake Road, East Lansing, MI 48823; tel. 517/332-0811; Dr. Thomas S Gunnings
Metro East Substance Abuse Treatment Corporation, PO Box 13408, Detroit, MI 48213; tel. 313/371-0055; Ms. Leslie B Carroll
Michiana Addictions and Prevention Services, 1020 Millard Street, Three Rivers, MI 49093-1658; tel. 616/279-5187; Ms. Sally Reames
Michigan Counseling Services, 1400 East 12 Mile Road, Madison Heights, MI 48071; tel. 248/547-2223; Mr. Anthony C Clemente
Nardin Park Recovery Center, Inc., PO Box 04506, Detroit, MI 48204; tel. 313/834-5930; Ms. Annie B Scott
National Council on Alcoholism / Lansing Regional Area, Inc., 3400 S Cedar Street, Suite 200, Lansing, MI 48910; tel. 517/887-0226; Ms. Nancy L Siegrist
National Council on Alcoholism and Addictions, 202 E Boulevard Drive, Ste 310, Flint, MI 48503; tel. 810/767-0350; Ms. Rebecca Jagos
National Council on Alcoholism and Drug Dependence / Vantage, 16647 Wyoming, Detroit, MI 48221; tel. 313/861-0666; Mr. Benjamin A Jones
Neighborhood Service Organization, 220 Bagley, Suite 1200, Detroit, MI 48226; tel. 313/961-4890; Ms. Angela G Kennedy
New Center Community Mental Health Services, 2051 West Grand Boulevard, Detroit, MI 48208; tel. 313/961-3200; Ms. Roberta V Sanders
New Era Alternative Treatment Center, Inc., P.O. Box 03828, Highland Park, MI 48203; tel. 313/869-6328; Dr. Joseph A Pitts
Northeast Guidance Center, 13340 East Warren, Detroit, MI 48215; tel. 313/824-8000; Ms. Cheryl C Coleman
Northeast Health Services, 3800 Woodward Avenue Suite 1002, Detroit, MI 48234-1263; tel. 313/832-6386; Mrs. Rose V Jackson
Oakland Psychological Clinic, PC, PO Box 888, Bloomfield Hills, MI 48303-0888; tel. 248/594-1200; Dr. Barry H Tigay
Orchard Hills Psychiatric Center, 40000 Grand River Ave, Ste 306, Novi, MI 48375-2112; tel. 248/426-9900; Dr. Hiten C Patel
Parkview Company, dba Parkview Counseling Centers, 18609 West Seven Mile Road, Detroit, MI 48219; tel. 313/532-8015; Mrs. Yvette Woodruff
Perspectives of Troy, PC, 2690 Crooks Road, Suite 300, Troy, MI 48084; tel. 248/244-8644; Dr. Tim Coldiron
Psychological Consultants of Michigan, PC, 151 North Avenue, Battle Creek, MI 49017-3467; tel. 616/968-2811; Dr. Jeffrey N Andert
Quality Behavioral Health, Inc, 3455 Woodward Avenue, Ste 101, Detroit, MI 48201; tel. 313/832-5555; Mr. Naveed Syed
Redford Counseling Center, 25945 West Seven Mile Road, Redford Township, MI 48240; tel. 313/535-6560; Ms. JoAnn Sadler
River's Bend, P.C., 33975 Dequindre, Troy, MI 48083; tel. 248/585-3239; Mr. James L Keener
Sacred Heart Rehabilitation Center, Inc., 400 Stoddard Road P.O. Box 41038, Memphis, MI 48041; tel. 810/392-2167; Mr. John Sass, Jr.
Star Center, Inc., 13575 Lesure, Detroit, MI 48227; tel. 313/493-4410; Ms. Lucila S Ryder
STM Clinic – Mental Health and Substance Abuse Services, One Tuscola Street, Suite 302, Saginaw, MI 48607-1287; tel. 517/755-2532; Ms. Sara Terry-Moton
Taylor Psychological Clinic, PC, 1172 Robert T Longway Blvd, Flint, MI 48503; tel. 810/232-8466; Dr. Maxwell F Taylor, II
The Center for Human Resources, 1001 Military Street, Port Huron, MI 48060; tel. 810/985-5168; Dr. Robert E Gamble
The Kalamazoo Child Guidance Clinic, 2615 Stadium Drive, Kalamazoo, MI 49008; tel. 616/343-1651; Mr. Steven L Smith
Turning Point Programs, 1931 Boston, Southeast, Grand Rapids, MI 49506; tel. 616/235-1565; Mr. Robert E Byrd
Tuscola Behavioral Health Systems, PO Box 239, Caro, MI 48723; tel. 517/673-6191; Mr. Robert E Chadwick, II

MINNESOTA
Fountain Centers, 408 West Fountain Street, Albert Lea, MN 56007; tel. 507/377-6411; Dr. Ron Harmon
Guest House, PO Box 954, Rochester, MN 55903; tel. 507/288-4693; Mr. Daniel Kidd
Hazelden Recovery Services, PO Box 11, Center City, MN 55012; tel. 612/257-4010; Mr. Jerry Spicer
Omegon, Inc., 2000 Hopkins Crossroads, Minnetonka, MN 55343; tel. 612/541-4738; Ms. Barbara J Danielsen
Pride Institute, 14400 Martin Drive, Eden Prairie, MN 55344; tel. 612/934-7554; Mr. Joseph M Amico

MISSISSIPPI
CARES Center, Inc., 402 Wesley Avenue, Jackson, MS 39202; tel. 601/360-0583; Mr. Christopher M Cherney
COPAC, Inc., 3949 Highway 43 North, Brandon, MS 39047; tel. 601/829-2500; Dr. J. Stacy Hughes
Pine Belt Mental Healthcare Resources, PO Drawer 1030, Hattiesburg, MS 39401; tel. 601/544-4641; Mr. Jerry Mayo

MISSOURI
Boonville Valley Hope, PO Box 376, Boonville, MO 65233; tel. 660/882-6547; Mr. Dennis Gilhousen
Boys Town of Missouri, Inc., PO Box 189, St. James, MO 65559; tel. 573/265-3251; Mr. Richard C Dunn
Centrec Care, Inc., 11720 Borman Drive, Suite 103, Saint Louis, MO 63146; tel. 314/991-5388; Dr. Mohammed A Kabir
Comprehensive Mental Health Services, Inc., 10901 Winner Road, Independence, MO 64052; tel. 816/254-3652; Mr. William H Kyles
Industrial Rehabilitation Center, 429 Northeast 69 Highway, Kansas City, MO 64119; tel. 816/452-8777; Mr. Maurice L Cummings
Marillac Center, 2826 Main Street, Kansas City, MO 64118; tel. 816/508-3300; Mr. R. Michael Bowen
Piney Ridge Center, Inc., PO Box 4067, Waynesville, MO 65583; tel. 573/774-5353; Ms. Jacqueline S Howard
Provident Counseling, Inc., 2650 Olive Street, Saint Louis, MO 63103-1489; tel. 314/371-6500; Ms. Kathleen E Buescher
Research Mental Health Services, 901 NE Independence Avenue, Lees Summit, MO 64086; tel. 816/246-8000; Mr. Alan Flory

MONTANA
Rocky Mountain Treatment Center, 920 Fourth Avenue North, Great Falls, MT 59401; tel. 406/727-8832; Mr. Mark Sallee

NEBRASKA
Behavioral Health Specialists, Inc., 600 South 13th Street, Norfolk, NE 68701; tel. 402/370-3140; Ms. Connie Barnes
Blue Valley Mental Health Clinic, 1121 N. 10th Street, Beatrice, NE 68310; tel. 402/228-3386; Dr. Wayne R Price
Mid-East Nebraska Behavioral Healthcare Services, Inc., PO Box 682, Columbus, NE 68602-0682; tel. 402/564-1426; Dr. Roberta Saunders
O'Neill Valley Hope, PO Box 918, O' Neill, NE 68763-0918; tel. 402/336-3747; Mr. Dennis Gilhousen

NEW HAMPSHIRE
Beech Hill Hospital, LLC, PO Box 254, Dublin, NH 03444; tel. 603/563-8511; Mr. Matthew J Feehery
Seacoast Mental Health Center, Inc., 1145 Sagamore Avenue, Portsmouth, NH 03801; tel. 603/431-6703; Dr. Jeffrey C Connor
The Mental Health Center of Greater Manchester, 401 Cypress Street, Manchester, NH 03103; tel. 603/668-4111; Mr. Peter Janelle

NEW JERSEY
AtlantiCare Behavioral Health, 201 Tilton Road, Unit 13-A, Northfield, NJ 08225; tel. 609/645-7601; Mr. Donald J Parker
Bonnie Brae, PO Box 825, Liberty Corner, NJ 07938-0825; tel. 908/647-0800; Susan G Roth
Cape Counseling Services, 128 Crest Haven Road, Cape May Court House, NJ 08210; tel. 609/465-4100; Mr. Barry Keefe
Care Plus NJ, Inc., 610 Industrial Avenue, Paramus, NJ 07652; tel. 201/265-8200; Mr. Joseph A Masciandaro
Catholic Charities – Diocese of Metuchen, 319 Maple Street, Perth Amboy, NJ 08861; tel. 732/257-6677; Sister Florence Edward Kearney
Community Centers for Mental Health, Inc., 2 Park Avenue, Dumont, NJ 07628; tel. 201/385-4400; Ms. Victoria L Sidrow
CPC Behavioral Healthcare, Inc, Parkway 100 3535 Route 66 Building #5, Suite D, Neptune, NJ 07753; tel. 732/643-4300; Dr. Jeanne H Wurmser
Daytop, New Jersey, Post Office Box 310, Mendham, NJ 07945; tel. 973/543-0162; Mr. Joseph Hennen
Discovery Institute for Addictive Disorders, Inc., PO Box 177, Marlboro, NJ 07746; tel. 732/946-9444; Mr. Robert C Denes
Family Service of Burlington County, 770 Woodlane Road, Mount Holly, NJ 08060; tel. 609/267-5928; Ms. Mary Wells
High Focus Centers, 299 Market Street, Suite 110, Saddle Brook, NJ 07663; tel. 201/291-0055; Dr. David Nyman
Honesty House, 1272 Long Hill Road, Stirling, NJ 07980; tel. 908/647-3211; Mr. Charles H Stucky
Lighthouse at Mays Landing, PO Box 899, Mays Landing, NJ 08330; tel. 609/625-4900; Ms. Regina LaVerde
New Hope Foundation, Inc, PO Box 66, Marlboro, NJ 07746; tel. 732/946-3030; Mr. George J Mattie
NewBridge Services, Inc., PO Box 336, Pompton Plains, NJ 07444; tel. 201/839-2520; Mr. Robert L Parker
Ocean Mental Health Services, Inc., 160 Route 9, Bayville, NJ 08721; tel. 732/349-5550; Dr. Charles J Langan
Preferred Behavioral Health of New Jersey, PO Box 2036, Lakewood, NJ 08701; tel. 732/364-4590; Mr. William J Sette
Seabrook House, Inc., PO Box 5055, Seabrook, NJ 08302-0655; tel. 609/455-7575; Mr. Edward M Diehl
SERV Centers of New Jersey, Inc., 380 Scotch Road, West Trenton, NJ 08628; tel. 609/406-0100; Ms. Kathleen Enerrich
Sunrise House Foundation, PO Box 600, Lafayette, NJ 07848; tel. 973/383-6300; Dr. Philip N Horowitz
UCPC Behavioral Health Care, 117-119 Roosevelt Avenue, Plainfield, NJ 07060; tel. 908/756-6870; Ms. Marcyann E Sosnoski
UMDNJ – University Behavioral HealthCare, PO Box 1392, Piscataway, NJ 08855-1392; tel. 732/235-5900; Mr. Christopher Kosseff
West Bergen Mental Healthcare, Inc., 120 Chestnut Street, Ridgewood, NJ 07450; tel. 201/444-3550; Mr. Philip E Wilson

NEW MEXICO
Desert Hills of New Mexico, 5310 Sequoia Northwest, Albuquerque, NM 87120; tel. 505/836-7330; Ms. Carol Bickelman
Family Opportunity Resources, 851 Magee Lane, Santa Fe, NM 87501; tel. 409/740-0442; Mr. Gordon W McKee
Four Corners Regional Adolescent Treatment Center, PO Box 220, Shiprock, NM 87420; tel. 505/368-4712; Mr. Hoskie Benally, Jr.

NEW YORK
A.R.E.B.A.– Casriel, Inc., 500 West 57th Street, New York, NY 10019; tel. 212/293-3000; Mr. Steven Yohay
Arms Acres, 75 Seminary Hill Road, Carmel, NY 10512; tel. 914/225-3400; Dr. Ed Spauster
Bronx Addiction Treatment Center, 1500 Waters Place, Building 13, Bronx, NY 10461; tel. 718/904-0026; Mr. Hermon Lockhart
Charles K. Post Addiction Treatment Center, Building 1, PPC Campus, West Brentwood, NY 11717; tel. 516/434-7209; Mr. Phillip A Dawes
Conifer Park, Inc., 79 Glenridge Road, Schenectady, NY 12302; tel. 518/399-6446; Mr. John A Duffy
Cornerstone of Medical Arts Center Hospital, 57 West 57th Street, New York, NY 10019; tel. 212/755-0200; Mr. Thomas C Puzo
Cornerstone of Rhinebeck, NY, 500 Milan Hollow Road, Rhinebeck, NY 12572; tel. 914/266-3481; Dr. Chandra Singh
Creedmoor Addiction Treatment Center, 80-45 Winchester Boulevard Building 19 – CBU 15, Queens Village, NY 11427; tel. 718/264-3743; Mr. Gerlando A Verruso
Crossings Recovery Centers, 450 Waverly Avenue, Suite 5, Patchogue, NY 11772; tel. 516/447-0155; Dr. William Bue
Dick Van Dyke Addiction Treatment Center, 1330 County Road 132, Ovid, NY 14521; tel. 607/869-9500; Mr. Thomas Nightingale
Hope House, Inc., 517 Western Avenue, Albany, NY 12203; tel. 518/482-4673; Ms. Mary Ann DiChristopher-Finn
Jewish Board of Family and Children's Services, 120 West 57th Street, New York, NY 10019; tel. 212/582-9100; Dr. Alan B Siskind
John L. Norris Addiction Treatment Center, 1111 Elmwood Avenue, Rochester, NY 14620; tel. 716/461-0410; Mr. Thomas E Nightingale

Providers / JCAHO Accredited Freestanding Substance Abuse Organizations

Kingsboro Addiction Treatment Center, 754 Lexington Avenue, Brooklyn, NY 11221; tel. 718/453–6747; Ms. Jacqueline Cole

Manhattan Addiction Treatment Center, 600 East 125th Street, Ward's Island, New York, NY 10035; tel. 212/369–0703; Mr. Jeffrey Spitz

McPike Addiction Treatment Center, 1213 Court Street, Utica, NY 13502; tel. 315/738–4400; Mr. John F Crowley

National Expert Care Consultants, Inc., 455 West 50th Street, New York, NY 10019–6504; tel. 212/262–6000; Mr. Brian J McDowell

Passages Counseling Center, 3680 Route 112, Coram, NY 11727; tel. 516/698–9222; Mr. Arnt Monge

Restorative Management Corporation, 15 King Street, Middletown, NY 10940; tel. 914/342–5941; Mr. Dean Scher

Richard C. Ward Addiction Treatment Center, 117 Seward Avenue Building 92, Suite 12/16, Middletown, NY 10940; tel. 914/341–2500; Mr. Erwin G Michel

Rochester Mental Health Center, 490 East Ridge Road, Rochester, NY 14621; tel. 716/922–2500; Ms. Heide George

Russell E. Blaisdell Addiction Treatment Center, PO Box 140, Orangeburg, NY 10962; tel. 914/359–8500; Ms. Tamara Miller–Kammerer

Saint Peter's Addiction Recovery Center, Inc., 3 Mercycare Lane, Guilderland, NY 12084; tel. 518/452–6701; Ms. Karen A Giles

Salamanca Hospital District Authority, 150 Parkway Drive, Salamanca, NY 14779; tel. 716/945–1900; Dr. Kenneth L Oakley

Seafield Center, Inc., 7 Seafield Lane, Westhampton Beach, NY 11978; tel. 516/288–1122; Mr. John C Haley

South Beach Addiction Treatment Center, 777 Seaview Avenue, Building 1, Staten Island, NY 10305; tel. 718/667–4218; Mr. Gerlando A Verrusc

St. Joseph's Rehabilitation Center, Inc., PO Box 470, Saranac Lake, NY 12983–0470; tel. 518/891–3950; Rev. Arthur M Johnson

St. Joseph's Villa of Rochester, 3300 Dewey Avenue, Rochester, NY 14616; tel. 716/865–1550; Mr. Roger C Battaglia

St. Lawrence Addiction Treatment Center, 1 Chimney Point Drive, Hamilton Hall, Ogdensburg, NY 13669; tel. 315/393–1180; Mr. Phillip Dranger

Stutzman Addiction Treatment Center, 360 Forest Avenue, Buffalo, NY 14213; tel. 716/882–4900; Mr. Steven Schwartz

The Astor Home for Children, PO Box 5005, Rhinebeck, NY 12572–5005; tel. 914/876–4081; Sr. Rose Logan

The Health Association – MAIN QUEST Treatment Center, 774 West Main Street, Rochester, NY 14611; tel. 716/464–8870; Ms. Susan L Costa

The Long Island Center for Recovery, PO Box 774, Hampton Bays, NY 11946; tel. 516/728–3100; Mr. Jack Hamilton

The Support Center, Inc., 181 Route 209, Port Jervis, NY 12771; tel. 800/724–9322; Mr. Carmine Mosca

Tully Hill Alcohol & Drug Treatment Center, PO Box 920, Tully, NY 13159–0920; tel. 315/696–6114; Ms. Cathy L Palm

Veritas Villa, Inc., PO Box 610, Kerhonkson, NY 12446–0610; tel. 914/626–3555; Mr. Lester McCandless

Villa Outpatient Center, 290 Madison Avenue, 6th Floor, New York, NY 10017; tel. 212/679–4960; Mr. Richard Partridge

NORTH CAROLINA

Amethyst, PO Box 32861, Charlotte, NC 28232–2861; tel. 704/554–8373; Mr. Steven Johnson

CenterPoint Human Services, 725 North Highland Avenue, Winston–Salem, NC 27101; tel. 336/725–7777; Mr. Ronald W Morton

Fellowship Hall, Inc., PO Box 13890, Greensboro, NC 27415; tel. 336/621–3381; Mr. Rodney Battles

Julian F. Keith Alcohol and Drug Abuse Treatment Center, 301 Tabernacle Road, Black Mountain, NC 28711; tel. 828/669–3421; Mr. William A Rafter

The Wilmington Treatment Center, 2520 Troy Drive, Wilmington, NC 28401; tel. 910/762–2727; Mr. Charles Sharp

Unity Regional Youth Treatment Center, PO Box C–201, Cherokee, NC 28719; tel. 828/497–3958; Ms. Margaret Jenks

NORTH DAKOTA

The Dakota Boys Ranch, PO Box 5007, Minot, ND 58703; tel. 701/852–3628; Mr. Gene Kasemen

OHIO

2 North Park, Inc., 720 Pine Avenue Southeast, Warren, OH 44483; tel. 330/399–3677; Mr. Kenneth Lloyd

Akron–Urban Minority Alcoholism Drug Abuse Outreach, 665 W Market Street, Suite 2D, Akron, OH 44303; tel. 330/379–3467; Ms. Janice T Mayes

Behavioral Care Management, 5800 Monroe Street, Building A, Sylvania, OH 43560; tel. 419/885–2391; Dr. Ronald Dozoretz

Behavioral Connections of Wood County, Inc., 320 West Gypsy Lane Road, Bowling Green, OH 43402; tel. 419/352–2551; Mr. Randall J LaFond

Bellefaire Jewish Children's Bureau, 22001 Fairmount Boulevard, Shaker Heights, OH 44118; tel. 216/932–2800; Dr. Adam G Jacobs

Catholic Charities Services Corporation, 1111 Superior Avenue, Cleveland, OH 44114; tel. 216/696–6525; Mr. Thomas W Woll

Center for Chemical Addictions Treatment, 830 Ezzard Charles Drive, Cincinnati, OH 45214; tel. 513/381–6672; Ms. Sandra L Kuehn

Charles B. Mills Center, Inc., 715 South Plum Street, Marysville, OH 43040; tel. 513/644–9192; Dr. John R Lauritsen

Community Drug Board, 725 East Market Street, Akron, OH 44305; tel. 330/434–4141; Mr. Theodore P Ziegler

Community Support Services, Inc., 150 Cross Street, Akron, OH 44311; tel. 330/996–9141; Mr. Arthur G Wickersham

Comprehensive Psychiatry Specialists, 955 Windham Court, Suite 2, Boardman, OH 44512; tel. 330/726–9570; Dr. Pradeep Mathur

Crisis Intervention Center of Stark County, Inc., 2421 13th Street Northwest, Canton, OH 44708; tel. 330/452–9812; Dr. Bernard S Jesiolowski

Family Recovery Center, PO Box 464, Lisbon, OH 44432; tel. 330/424–1468; Ms. Eloise V Traina

Focus Health Care, 5701 North High Street, Suite 8, Worthington, OH 43085; tel. 614/885–1944; Dr. Brad Lander

Glenbeigh Health Sources, PO Box 298, Rock Creek, OH 44084–0298; tel. 440/563–3400; Ms. Pat Weston–Hall

Harbor Behavioral Healthcare, 4334 Secor Road, Toledo, OH 43623–4234; tel. 419/475–4449; Mr. Dale E Shreve

Interval Brotherhood Home Inc., 3445 South Main Street, Akron, OH 44319; tel. 330/644–4095; Fr. Samuel R Ciccolini

Lake Area Recovery Center, 2801 'C' Court, Ashtabula, OH 44004; tel. 440/998–0722; Ms. Kathleen Kinney

McKinley Hall, Inc., 1101 East High Street, Springfield, OH 45505; tel. 937/328–5300; Ms. Judith O Hoy

Mental Health Services for Clark County, Inc., 1345 Fountain Boulevard, Springfield, OH 45504; tel. 937/399–9500; Dr. James P Perry

Miami Valley Labor Management Healthcare Delivery Systems, 136 Heid Avenue, Dayton, OH 45404; tel. 937/208–2327; Ms. Linda VanBourgondien

Mount Carmel Behavioral Healthcare, 1808 East Broad Street, Columbus, OH 43203; tel. 614/251–8242; Dr. Marc Clemente

Neil Kennedy Recovery Clinic, 2151 Rush Boulevard, Youngstown, OH 44507; tel. 330/744–1181; Mr. Jerry V Carter

New Directions, Inc., 30800 Chagrin Boulevard, Pepper Pike, OH 44124; tel. 216/591–0324; Mr. Michael E Matoney

Nova Behavioral Health, Inc., 832 McKinley Avenue Northwest, Canton, OH 44703; tel. 330/455–9407; Mr. Michael D Flora

Parkside Behavioral Healthcare, Inc., 349 Olde Ridenour Road, Columbus, OH 43230; tel. 614/471–2552; Dr. Christine N Gerber

PsyCare, Inc., 2980 Belmont Avenue, Youngstown, OH 44505; tel. 330/759–2310; Dr. Douglas C Darnall

Quest Recovery Services, 1341 Market Avenue, North, Canton, OH 44714–2675; tel. 330/453–8252; Mr. Donald C Davies

Ravenwood Mental Health Center, 12557 Ravenwood Drive, Chardon, OH 44024; tel. 440/285–3400; Mr. David A Boyle

Serenity Living, Inc., PO Box 771, Vandalia, OH 45377; tel. 937/898–2788; Dr. Joseph J Trevino

Specialty Care Psychiatric Services, Inc, 2657 Niles Courtland Road, SE, Warren, OH 44484; tel. 330/652–3533; Mr. JB Mitroo

Substance Abuse Services, Inc., 1832 Adams Street, Toledo, OH 43624; tel. 419/243–7274; Mr. Carroll Parks

The Buckeye Ranch, Inc., 5665 Hoover Road, Grove City, OH 43123; tel. 614/875–2371; Mr. Richard E Rieser

The Crossroads Center, 311 Martin Luther King Drive, Cincinnati, OH 45219–3116; tel. 513/475–5300; Mrs. Jacqueline P Butler

Transitional Living, Inc. and Affiliates, 2052 Princeton Road, Hamilton, OH 45011; tel. 513/863–6383; Mr. David F Craft

OKLAHOMA

Brookhaven Hospital, 201 South Garnett Road, Tulsa, OK 74128–1800; tel. 918/438–4257; Dr. Rolf B Gainer

Cushing Valley Hope, PO Box 472, Cushing, OK 74023–0472; tel. 918/225–1736; Mr. Dennis Gilhousen

Jim Taliaferro Community Mental Health Center, 602 Southwest 38th Street, Lawton, OK 73505–6999; tel. 580/248–5780; Ms. Starr Paul

Western State Psychiatric Center, 1222 10th, Suite 211, Woodward, OK 73801; tel. 580/571–3233; Mr. Steve Norwood

OREGON

BHC Pacific View RTC, 4101 Northeast Division Street, Gresham, OR 97030; tel. 503/661–0775; Mr. Michael Amador

Serenity Lane, Inc., 616 East Sixteenth Avenue, Eugene, OR 97401; tel. 503/687–1110; Mr. Neil H McNaughton

Springbrook Northwest, 2001 Crestview Drive, Newberg, OR 97132; tel. 503/537–7000; Mr. Mark W Knudsen

VA Domiciliary, 8495 Crater Lake Highway, White City, OR 97503; tel. 541/826–2111; Mr. George H Andries, Jr.

PENNSYLVANIA

Abraxas I, PO Box 59, Marienville, PA 16239; tel. 814/927–6615; Mr. James E Newsome

Adelphoi Village, Inc., 1003 Village Way, Latrobe, PA 15650; tel. 724/520–1111; Mr. John P Bukovac

Bowling Green of Brandywine, Inc., 1375 Newark Road, Kennett Square, PA 19348; tel. 610/268–3588; Claire F Beckwith

Charter Behavioral Health System at Cove Forge, New Beginnings Road, Williamsburg, PA 16693; tel. 814/832–2121; Mr. Mark Sarneso

Child Guidance Resource Centers, 600 North Olive Street, Media, PA 19063–2418; tel. 610/565–6000; Mr. Edward Maguire

Clear Brook, Inc., 1003 Wyoming Avenue, Forty Fort, PA 18704; tel. 570/288–6692; Dr. Nicholas F Colangelo

Conewago Place, 424 Nye Road, Hummelstown, PA 17036–0406; tel. 717/533–0428; Mr. A. E Cox, Jr.

Eagleville Hospital, PO Box 45, Eagleville, PA 19408–0045; tel. 610/539–6000; Ms. Kendria Kurtz

Gateway Rehabilitation Center, Moffett Run Road, Aliquippa, PA 15001; tel. 412/766–8700; Dr. Kenneth S Ramsey

Gaudenzia, Inc. – Common Ground, 2835 North Front Street, Harrisburg, PA 17110; tel. 717/238–5553; Mr. Michael B Harle

Greenbriar Treatment Center, 800 Manor Drive, Washington, PA 15301; tel. 724/225–9700; Ms. Mary G Banaszak

Greenway Center, PO Box 188, Henryville, PA 18332; tel. 800/831–6402; Mr. Wallace M Slatinsky

Livengrin Foundation, Inc., 4833 Hulmeville Road, Bensalem, PA 19020–3099; tel. 215/638–5200; Mr. Richard M Pine

Malvern Institute, 940 King Road, Malvern, PA 19355; tel. 610/647–0330; Mr. Thomas J Connell

Marworth, PO Box 36, Waverly, PA 18471; tel. 717/563–1112; Mr. James J Dougherty

Milestones Community Healthcare, Inc., 614 North Easton Road, Glenside, PA 19038; tel. 215/884–5566; Dr. Paul Volosov

Mirmont Treatment Center, 100 Yearsley Mill Road, Glen Riddle Lima, PA 19063–5593; tel. 610/744–1400; Mr. Thomas F Cain

NorthEast Treatment Centers (NET), 499 North 5th Street, Suite A, Philadelphia, PA 19123; tel. 215/451–7000; Mr. Terence McSherry

Penn Foundation, Inc., PO Box 32, Sellersville, PA 18960; tel. 215/453–5183; Dr. Vernon H Kratz

Renewal Centers, PO Box 107, Zionhill, PA 18981; tel. 215/536–9070; Mr. Charles Beem

Providers / JCAHO Accredited Freestanding Substance Abuse Organizations

Richard J. Caron Foundation, PO Box A, Wernersville, PA 19565–0501; tel. 610/678–2332; Mr. Douglas D Tieman
Roxbury, PO Box L, Shippensburg, PA 17257; tel. 717/532–4217; Mr. Joseph Barszczewski
Sarah A. Reed Children's Center, 2445 West 34th Street, Erie, PA 16506; tel. 814/838–1954; Mr. John J Kovacs
Serenity Hall, Inc., 414 West Fifth Street, Erie, PA 16507; tel. 814/459–4775; Ms. Suzanne C Mack
Stairways, 138 East 26th Street, Erie, PA 16504; tel. 814/453–5806; Mr. William F McCarthy
The Bridge, 8400 Pine Road, Philadelphia, PA 19111; tel. 215/342–5000; Ms. Star Weiss
The Terraces, PO Box 729, Ephrata, PA 17522; tel. 717/859–4100; Ms. Patricia Bixler
TODAY, Inc., PO Box 908, New Town, PA 18940; tel. 215/968–4713; Mr. John E Howell
UHS Recovery Foundation, Inc., 2001 Providence Avenue, Chester, PA 19013–5504; tel. 610/876–9000; Mr. Jimmy Patton
White Deer Run, Inc., Devitt Camp Road, Box 97, Allenwood, PA 17810–0097; tel. 570/538–2567; Mr. Stephen T Wicke

RHODE ISLAND
CODAC Treatment Centers, Inc., 1052 Park Avenue, Cranston, RI 02910; tel. 401/461–5056; Mr. Craig S Stenning
Community Counseling Center, 101 Bacon Street, Pawtucket, RI 02860; tel. 401/722–5573; Mr. Richard H LeClerc
East Bay Mental Health Center, Inc., 52 Amaral Street, East Providence, RI 02915; tel. 401/431–9875; Mr. John P Digits, Jr.
Mental Health Services of Cranston, Johnston, 1443 Hartford Avenue, Johnston, RI 02919–3236; tel. 401/553–1000; Mr. Richard H Leclerc
South Shore Mental Health Center, Inc., PO Box 899, Charlestown, RI 02813; tel. 401/364–7705; Mr. Richard C Antonelli
The Providence Center for Counseling & Psychiatric Svcs, 520 Hope Street, Providence, RI 02906; tel. 401/276–4000; Mr. Charles E Maynard
Tri–Hab, Inc., 58 Hamlet Avenue, Woonsocket, RI 02895; tel. 401/765–4040; Mr. David Spencer

SOUTH DAKOTA
Keystone Treatment Center, PO Box 159, Canton, SD 57013; tel. 605/987–5659; Ms. Carol Regier

TENNESSEE
Academy for Academic Excellence, PO Box 3906, Clarksville, TN 37043; tel. 931/647–9831; Ms. Mercy E Yrabedra
Buffalo Valley, Inc., PO Box 879, Hohenwald, TN 38462; tel. 931/796–5427; Mr. Jerry T Risner
Camelot Care Center, Inc., 102 Woodmont Blvd Suite 450, Nashville, TN 37205; tel. 615/386–6755; Mr. James V Doramus
Camelot Care Center, Inc., 667 – B Emory Valley Road, Oak Ridge, TN 37830; tel. 423/220–8927; Mr. James V Doramus
Child and Family Services of Knox County, Inc., 901 East Summit Hill Drive, Knoxville, TN 37915; tel. 423/524–7483; Mr. Charles E Gentry
Compass Intervention Center, LLC, 7900 Lowrance Road, Memphis, TN 38125; tel. 901/758–2002; Mr. Jack Bice
Cornerstone of Recovery, 1120 Topside Road, Louisville, TN 37777; tel. 423/970–7747; Mr. Dan R Caldwell
Council for Alcohol and Drug Abuse Services, Inc., PO Box 4797, Chattanooga, TN 37405; tel. 423/756–7644; Mr. James F Marcotte
Cumberland Heights, PO Box 90727, Nashville, TN 37209; tel. 615/353–1757; Mr. James B Moore
Ridgeview Psychiatric Hospital and Center, Inc., 240 West Tyrone Road, Oak Ridge, TN 37830; tel. 423/482–1076; Mr. Robert J Benning

TEXAS
Alternatives Centre for Behavioral Health, 5001 Alabama Street, El Paso, TX 79930; tel. 915/565–4800; Ms. Carol J Anderson
Burke Center, 4101 South Medford Drive, Lufkin, TX 75901–5699; tel. 936/639–1141; Ms. Susan Rushing
Cedar Crest Hospital & RTC, 3500 South IH–35, Belton, TX 76513; tel. 254/939–2100; Mr. Richard N Rickey
Continuum Healthcare System, Inc., 260 N Sam Houston Parkway E, Suite 300, Houston, TX 77060; tel. 281/260–0799; Mr. Don R Johnson
Family Service Center, 2707 North Loop West, Ste 520, Houston, TX 77008; tel. 713/868–4466; Mr. Lloyd H Sidwell
La Hacienda Treatment Center, PO Box 1, Hunt, TX 78024; tel. 830/238–4222; Dr. Frank J Sadlack
Life Resource, 2750 South 8th Street, Beaumont, TX 77701; tel. 409/839–1000; Dr. N. Charles Harris
New Dimensions, 18333 Egret Bay Blvd, Ste 560, Houston, TX 77058; tel. 281/333–2284; Dr. Larry M Nahmias
New View Partial Hospitalization Centre, Inc., 4310 Dowlen Road – Suite 13, Beaumont, TX 77706; tel. 409/892–0009; Dr. D. Sue Horne
Paul Meier New Life Day Hospital and Outpatient Clinic, 2071 North Collins Boulevard, Richardson, TX 75080; tel. 972/437–4698; Ms. Jacquelyn Williams
River Oaks Day Hospital, 10600 Richmond Avenue, Houston, TX 77042; tel. 713/783–7200; Dr. Sandra E Phares
San Marcos Treatment Center, 120 Bert Brown Road, San Marcos, TX 78666; tel. 512/396–8500; Mr. Mack Wigley
Shoreline, Inc., PO Box 68, Taft, TX 78390; tel. 361/528–3356; Dr. Sharel Zacharias
Starlite Village Hospital, PO Box 317, Center Point, TX 78010–0317; tel. 830/634–2212; Mr. John Lacy
Summer Sky, Inc., 1100 McCart Street, Stephenville, TX 76401; tel. 254/968–2907; Mr. Al Conlan
Sundown Ranch, Inc., Route 4, Box 182, Canton, TX 75103; tel. 903/479–3933; Mr. Richard Boardman
The Patrician Movement, 222 East Mitchell Street, San Antonio, TX 78210; tel. 210/532–3126; Dr. Patrick Clancey

UTAH
Blue Mountain Family Center / Wilderness Quest, PO Box 12, Monticello, UT 84535; tel. 435/587–2801; Mr. Larry Wells
Brightway at St. George, 115 West, 1470 South, St. George, UT 84770; tel. 435/673–0303; Ms. Sherry Shake
Heritage School, 5600 N. Heritage School Drive, Provo, UT 84604; tel. 801/226–4600; Mr. Gerald H Spanos
Highland Ridge Hospital, 175 West 7200 South, Midvale, UT 84047; tel. 801/272–9851; Mr. Richard Bell
Vista Adolescent Treatment Center, PO Box 69, Magna, UT 84044; tel. 801/250–9762; Mr. H. Matthew Dixon, Jr.
Youth Care of Utah, Inc., PO Box 909, Draper, UT 84020; tel. 801/572–6989; Ms. Robin P Stephens

VIRGINIA
Inova Comprehensive Addiction Treatment Services, 3300 Gallows Road, Falls Church, VA 22046–3300; tel. 703/698–1530; Mr. Steven E Brown
Inova Kellar Center, 10396 Democracy Lane, Fairfax, VA 22030; tel. 703/218–8500; Dr. Richard Leichtweis
Mount Regis Center, 405 Kimball Avenue, Salem, VA 24153; tel. 540/389–4761; Ms. Gail S Basham
The Life Center of Galax, PO Box 27, Galax, VA 24333; tel. 540/236–2994; Ms. Tina R Bullins
Williamsburg Place, 5477 Mooretown Road, Williamsburg, VA 23188; tel. 757/565–0106; Mr. Thomas Brennan

WASHINGTON
Valley Cities Counseling and Consultation, 2704 'I' Street Northeast, Auburn, WA 98002; tel. 206/833–7444; Ms. Marilyn La Celle

WEST VIRGINIA
Olympic Center – Preston, Inc., PO Box 158, Kingwood, WV 26537; tel. 304/329–2400; Ms. Arlene Glover
Shawnee Hills, Inc., PO Box 3698, Charleston, WV 25336–3698; tel. 304/341–0511; Ms. Martha Eades
Worthington Center, Inc., 3199 Core Road, Parkersburg, WV 26104; tel. 304/485–0082; Dr. Lance McCoy

WISCONSIN
Family Services Lakeshore, Inc, 333 Reed Avenue, Manitowoc, WI 54220; tel. 920/686–8608; Mr. Thomas Aronson
Libertas Treatment Center, 1701 Dousman Street, Green Bay, WI 54303; tel. 920/498–8600; Mr. David B Fish

WYOMING
Wyoming Recovery Program for Addictions, LLC, 231 South Wilson, Casper, WY 82601; tel. 307/265–3791; Ms. Carolyn Toews

U.S. Associated Areas

APO/AE
Wellness Branch, ODCSPER, USAREUR 7 Army 1 (Belgium), Hammonds Barracks, Bldg 968 Room 213 – Badenerplatz 1, APO, AE 09014; tel. 011/496–2148; Dr. G. Ed Browning
Wellness Branch, ODCSPER, USAREUR and Army 1 (Germany), Hammonds Barracks, Bldg 968 Room 213, Badenerplatz 1, APO, AE 09014; tel. 011/496–2148; Dr. G. Ed Browning

PUERTO RICO
Clinica Interdisciplinaria de Psiquiatria Avanzada, 650 Lloveras Cond Centro Plaza Suite 101, San Juan, PR 00909–2113; tel. 787/721–4020; Dr. Carlos A Caban

Abbreviations Used in the AHA Guide

AB, Army Base
ACSW, Academy of Certified Social Workers
AEC, Atomic Energy Commission
AFB, Air Force Base
AHA, American Hospital Association
AK, Alaska
AL, Alabama
AODA, Alcohol and Other Drug Abuse
APO, Army Post Office
AR, Arkansas
A.R.T., Accredited Record Technician
A.S.C., Ambulatory Surgical Center
A.T.C., Alcoholism Treatment Center
Ave., Avenue
AZ, Arizona

B.A., Bachelor of Arts
B.B.A., Bachelor of Business Administration
B.C., British Columbia
Blvd., Boulevard
B.S., Bachelor of Science
B.S.Ed., Bachelor of Science in Education
B.S.H.S., Bachelor of Science in Health Studies
B.S.N., Bachelor of Science in Nursing
B.S.W., Bachelor of Science and Social Worker
CA, California; Controller of Accounts

C.A.A.D.A.C., Certified Alcohol and Drug Abuse Counselor
CAC, Certified Alcoholism Counselor
CAE, Certified Association Executive
CAP, College of American Pathologists
CAPA, Certified Ambulatory Post Anesthesia
C.A.S., Certificate of Advanced Study
CCDC, Certified Chemical Dependency Counselor
C.D., Commander of the Order of Distinction
CDR, Commander
CDS, Chemical Dependency Specialist
CFACHE, Certified Fellow American College of Healthcare Executives
CFRE, Certified Fund Raising Executive
C.G., Certified Gastroenterology
CHC, Certified Health Consultant
C.L.D., Clinical Laboratory Director
CLU, Certified Life Underwriter, Chartered Life Underwriter
CMA, Certified Medical Assistant
C.M.H.A., Certified Mental Health Administrator
CNHA, Certified Nursing Home Administrator
CNM, Certified Nurse Midwife
CNOR, Certified Operating Room Nurse
C.N.S., Clinical Nurse Specialist
CO, Colorado; Commanding Officer
COA, Certified Ophthalmic Assistant
COMT, Commandant
C.O.M.T., Certified Ophthalmic Medical Technician
Conv., Conventions
Corp., Corporation; Corporate
C.O.T., Certified Ophthalmic Technician
CPA, Certified Public Accountant
C.P.H.Q., Certified Professional in Health Care Quality
CPM, Certified Public Manager
CRNA, Certified Registered Nurse Anesthetist
CRNH, Certified Registered Nurse Hospice
C.S.J.B., Catholic Saint John the Baptist
CSW, Certified Social Worker
CT, Connecticut
CWO, Chief Warrant Officer

D.B.A., Doctor of Business Administration

DC, District of Columbia
D.D., Doctor of Divinity
D.D.S., Doctor of Dental Surgery
DE, Delaware
Diet, Dietitian; Dietary; Dietetics
D.M.D., Doctor of Dental Medicine
D.MIN., Doctor of Ministry
D.O., Doctor of Osteopathic Medicine and Surgery, Doctor of Osteopathy
DPA, Doctorate Public Administration
D.P.M., Doctor of Podiatric Medicine
Dr., Drive
Dr.P.H., Doctor of Public Health
D.Sc., Doctor of Science
D.S.W., Doctor of Social Welfare
D.V.M., Doctor of Veterinary Medicine

E., East
Ed.D., Doctor of Education
Ed.S., Specialist in Education
ENS, Ensign
Esq., Esquire
Expwy., Expressway
ext., extension

FAAN, Fellow of the American Academy of Nursing
FACATA, Fellow of the American College of Addiction Treatment Administrators
FACHE, Fellow of the American College of Healthcare Executives
FACMGA, Fellow of the American College of Medical Group Administrators
FACP, Fellow of the American College of Physicians
FACS, Fellow of the American College of Surgeons
FAX, Facsimile
FL, Florida
FPO, Fleet Post Office
FRCPSC, Fellow of the Royal College of Physicians and Surgeons of Canada
FT, Full-time

GA, Georgia
Govt., Government; Governmental

HHS, Department of Health and Human Services
HI, Hawaii
HM, Helmsman
HMO, Health Maintenance Organization
Hon., Honorable; Honorary
H.S.A., Health System Administrator
Hts., Heights
Hwy., Highway

IA, Iowa
ID, Idaho
IL, Illinois
IN, Indiana
Inc., Incorporated

J.D., Doctor of Law
J.P., Justice of the Peace
Jr., Junior

KS, Kansas
KY, Kentucky

LA, Louisiana
LCDR, Lieutenant Commander
LCSW, Licensed Certified Social Worker
L.H.D., Doctor of Humanities

L.I.S.W., Licensed Independent Social Worker
LL.D., Doctor of Laws
L.L.P., Limited Licensed Practitioner
L.M.H.C., Licensed Master of Health Care
L.M.S.W., Licensed Master of Social Work
L.N.H.A., Licensed Nursing Home Administrator
L.P.C., Licensed Professional Counselor
LPN, Licensed Practical Nurse
L.P.N., Licensed Practical Nurse
L.S.W., Licensed Social Worker
Lt., Lieutenant
LTC, Lieutenant Colonel
Ltd., Limited
LT.GEN., Lieutenant General
LTJG, Lieutenant (junior grade)

MA, Massachusetts
M.A., Master of Arts
Maj., Major
M.B., Bachelor of Medicine
M.B.A., Masters of Business Administration
MC, Medical Corps; Marine Corps
M.C., Member of Congress
MD, Maryland
M.D., Doctor of Medicine
ME, Maine
M.Ed., Master of Education
MFCC, Marriage/Family/Child Counselor
MHA, Mental Health Association
M.H.S., Masters in Health Science; Masters in Human Service
MI, Michigan
MM, Masters of Management
MN, Minnesota
M.N., Master of Nursing
MO, Missouri
M.P.A., Master of Public Administration; Master Public Affairs
M.P.H., Master of Public Health
M.P.S., Master of Professional Studies; Master of Public Science
MS, Mississippi
M.S., Master of Science
MSC, Medical Service Corps
M.S.D., Doctor of Medical Science
MSHSA, Master of Science Health Service Administration
M.S.N., Master of Science in Nursing
M.S.P.H., Master of Science in Public Health
M.S.S.W., Master of Science in Social Work
M.S.W., Master of Social Work
MT, Montana
Mt., Mount

N., North
NC, North Carolina
N.C.A.D.C., National Certification of Alcohol and Drug Counselors
ND, North Dakota
NE, Nebraska
NH, New Hampshire
NHA, National Hearing Association; Nursing Home Administrator
NJ, New Jersey
NM, New Mexico
NPA, National Perinatal Association
NV, Nevada
NY, New York

OCN, Oncology Certified Nurse
O.D., Doctor of Optometry
O.F.M., Order Franciscan Monks, Order of Friars Minor
OH, Ohio
OK, Oklahoma
OR, Oregon
O.R., Operating Room
O.R.S., Operating Room Supervisor

OSF, Order of St. Francis

PA, Pennsylvania
P.A., Professional Association
P.C., Professional Corporation
Pharm.D., Doctor of Pharmacy
Ph.B., Bachelor of Philosophy
Ph.D., Doctor of Philosophy
PHS, Public Health Service
Pkwy., Parkway
Pl., Place
PR, Puerto Rico
PS, Professional Services
PSRO, Professional Standards Review Organization

RADM, Rear Admiral
RD, Rural Delivery
Rd., Road
R.F.D., Rural Free Delivery
RI, Rhode Island
R.M., Risk Manager
RN, Registered Nurse
RNC, Republican National Committee; Registered Nurse or Board Certified
R.Ph., Registered Pharmacist
RRA, Registered Record Administrator
R.S.M., Religious Sisters of Mercy
Rte., Route

S., South
SC, South Carolina
S.C., Surgery Center
SCAC, Senior Certified Addiction Counselor
Sc.D., Doctor of Science
Sci., Science, Scientific
SD, South Dakota
SHCC, Statewide Health Coordinating Council
Sgt., Sergeant
SNA, Surgical Nursing Assistant
SNF, Skilled Nursing Facility
Sq., Square
Sr., Senior, Sister
St., Saint, Street
Sta., Station
Ste., Saint; Suite

Tel., Telephone
Terr., Terrace
TN, Tennessee
Tpke., Turnpike
Twp., Township
TX, Texas

USA, United States Army
USAF, United States Air Force
USMC, United States Marine Corps
USN, United States Navy
USPHS, United States Public Health Service
UT, Utah

VA, Virginia
VADM, Vice Admiral
VI, Virgin Islands
Vlg., Village
VT, Vermont

W., West
WA, Washington
WI, Wisconsin
WV, West Virginia
WY, Wyoming

Index

Abbreviations Used in the AHA Guide, D1
Acknowledgements, v
AHA Offices, Officers, and Historical Data, viii
AHA Registered Hospitals, A2
Alliances, B163
    defined, B2
Ambulatory Centers and Home Care Agencies, A588
Annual Survey, A6
AOHA Listed Hospitals, A3
Approval Codes, A4
Associate Members, A588
    defined, A569
Associated University Programs in Health Administration, A583
Blue Cross–Blue Shield Plans, C30
Blue Cross Plans, A588
Canadian Hospitals, A588
Classification Codes, A5
Description of Lists, C2
Explanation of Hospital Listings, A4
Facility Codes
    alphabetically, A4
    defined, A6
    numerically, A4
Freestanding Ambulatory Surgery Centers, C71
    state government agencies, C98
Freestanding Hospices, C100
    state government agencies, C120
Headings, A5
    defined, A5
    expense, A5
    facilities, A4
    personnel, A5
    utilization data, A5
Health Care Professionals
    alphabetically, A521
Health Care Providers, C57
    defined, C2
Health Care Systems
    and their hospitals, B50
    defined, B2
    geographically, B156
    introduced, B2
    Statistics for Multihospital Health Care Systems and their Hospitals, B49
Health Maintenance Organizations, C57
    state government agencies, C69
Health Systems Agencies, C34

Healthfinder, C12
Hospital Associations, C35
Hospital Licensure Agencies, C37
Hospital Schools of Nursing, A584
Hospitals in Areas Associated with the United States, by Area, A481
Hospitals in the United States, A11
    by state, A11
Index of Health Care Professionals, A521
Index of Hospitals, A486
Other Institutional Members, A582
    defined, A582
International Organizations, C29
    defined, C2
Introduction, vi
Joint Commission on Accreditation of Healthcare Organizations
    accredited Freestanding Long–Term Care Organizations, C122
    accredited Freestanding Mental Health Care Organizations, C146
    accredited Freestanding Substance Abuse Organizations, C156
    accredited Hospitals, A11
Medical and Nursing Licensure Agencies, C39
Membership Categories, A581
National Organizations, C3
Networks and their Hospitals, B3
    defined, B2
Nonhospital Preacute and Postacute Care Facilities, A585
Nonreporting defined, A4
Other Associate Members, A588
Peer Review Organizations, C42
Provisional Hospitals, A587
Registration Requirements, A2
Shared Services Organizations, A588
State and Local Organizations and Agencies, C32
    defined, C2
State and Provincial Government Agencies, C44
State Health Planning and Development Agencies, C43
Types of Hospitals, A3
    general, A3
    psychiatric, A3
    rehabilitation and chronic disease, A3
    special, A3
U.S. Government Agencies, C31
    defined, C2
U.S. Government Hospitals Outside the United States, by Area, A485

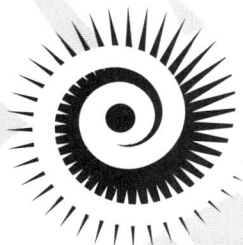
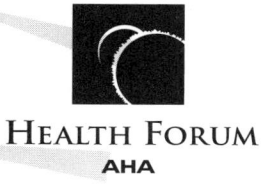

Focusing on the provider market?
Healthcare QuickDisc 2.0
can help you...

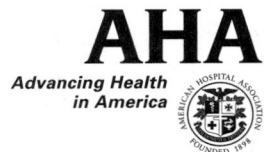

- Segment the hospital market.
- Choose your target market.
- Get comprehensive profiles to understand your target customers.
- Create strategically sound mailing and contact lists.

Healthcare QuickDisc 2.0 provides the quality of the *AHA Guide* information that you've come to expect, in a flexible database for your marketing and planning needs.

AHA
Advancing Health in America

To order or to try a **FREE DEMO,** call **(800) AHA-2626** or visit **www.ahaonlinestore.com** today.

■ Discover relationships. And understand the health care field more thoroughly than ever before.

Dig deeper.

AHA Healthcare System & Network Directory

The perfect complement to the AHA Guide. Available fall 2000.

Get to the root of system and network relationships and target these key organizations:

Hospitals
Outpatient Facilities
Extended-Care Facilities
Psychiatric Facilities
Alcohol/Drug Abuse Facilities
Rehabilitation Facilities
Community Health Centers
Home Health Agencies
Laboratory Facilities
Diagnostic Imaging Facilities

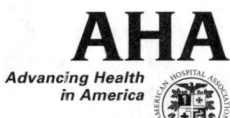

To learn more, visit **www.ahaonlinestore.com** today. And visit again over the coming weeks as the complete picture unfolds.